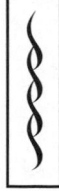 Infectious Diseases of the Fetus
and Newborn Infant

Infectious Diseases of the Fetus and Newborn Infant

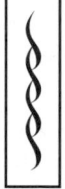

FIFTH EDITION

Jack S. Remington, M.D.

Professor of Medicine
Division of Infectious Diseases and Geographic Medicine
Stanford University School of Medicine
Stanford, California
Marcus A. Krupp Research Chair and Chairman
Department of Immunology and Infectious Diseases
Research Institute
Palo Alto Medical Foundation
Palo Alto, California

Jerome O. Klein, M.D.

Professor of Pediatrics
Boston University School of Medicine
Vice Chairman for Academic Affairs
Department of Pediatrics
Maxwell Finland Laboratory for Infectious Diseases
Boston Medical Center
Boston, Massachusetts

W.B. Saunders Company

A Harcourt Health Sciences Company

Philadelphia London New York St. Louis Sydney Toronto

W.B. SAUNDERS COMPANY
A Harcourt Health Sciences Company

The Curtis Center
Independence Square West
Philadelphia, Pennsylvania 19106

Library of Congress Cataloging-in-Publication Data

Infectious diseases of the fetus and newborn infant / [edited by] Jack S. Remington, Jerome O. Klein.—5th ed.

p.   cm.

Includes bibliographical references and index.

ISBN 0–7216–7976–5

1. Communicable diseases in newborn infants.   2. Communicable diseases in pregnancy—Complications.   3. Fetus—Diseases.   4. Neonatal infections.   I. Remington, Jack S.   II. Klein, Jerome O.
[DNLM: 1. Communicable Diseases—Infant, Newborn.   2. Fetal Diseases.   3. Infant, Newborn, Diseases.   WC 100 I42 2001]

RJ275.I54 2001   618.92'01—dc21

DNLM/DLC   99-050228

Acquisitions Editor: Judith Fletcher
Developmental Editor: Melissa Dudlick
Production Manager: Paul Nigel Harris
Supervising Copy Editor: Lee Ann Draud
Illustration Specialist: Rita Martello

Infectious Diseases of the Fetus and Newborn Infant   ISBN 0–7216–7976–5

Printed in the United States of America.

Last digit is the print number: 9   8   7   6   5   4   3   2   1

TO OUR MOST IMPORTANT PEOPLE

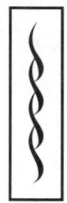

Linda and Françoise

David, Whindy, and Amanda, Lynne, Geoff, and Nathan

Andrea, Bennett, Adam, and Zachary

Alexander, Evan, and Dana

# Contributors

Charles A. Alford, Jr., M.D.
Professor Emeritus of Pediatrics, University of
Alabama School of Medicine, University of Alabama at
Birmingham, Birmingham, Alabama
Rubella

Ann M. Arvin, M.D.
Professor of Pediatrics, Stanford University School of
Medicine, Stanford, California
*Herpes Simplex Virus Infections; Other Viral Infections
of the Fetus and Newborn*

Carol J. Baker, M.D.
Professor of Pediatrics, Microbiology, and Immunology
and Head, Section of Infectious Diseases, Baylor
College of Medicine; Chair in Pediatric Infectious
Diseases, Texas Children's Hospital Foundation, Texas
Children's Hospital, Houston, Texas
Group B Streptococcal Infections

Elizabeth D. Barnett, M.D.
Assistant Professor of Pediatrics, Boston University
School of Medicine; Director, International Health
Clinic, Boston Medical Center, Maxwell Finland
Laboratory for Infectious Diseases, Boston,
Massachusetts
Bacterial Infections of the Respiratory Tract

Robert Bortolussi, M.D.
Professor of Pediatrics and Professor of Microbiology
and Immunology, Dalhousie University Faculty of
Medicine; Chief of Research, IWK-Grace Health
Centre for Children, Halifax, Nova Scotia, Canada
Listeriosis

Gail H. Cassell, Ph.D.
Professor and Chairman, Department of Microbiology,
Professor, Department of Pediatrics, University of
Alabama at Birmingham, Birmingham, Alabama; Vice
President, Infectious Diseases Drug Discovery
Research and Clinical Investigation, Eli Lilly and
Company, Indianapolis, Indiana
Mycoplasmal Infections

James D. Cherry, M.D., M.Sc.
Professor of Pediatrics, University of California, Los
Angeles, UCLA School of Medicine; Chief, Division of
Infectious Diseases, Mattel Children's Hospital at
UCLA, Los Angeles, California
Enteroviruses

Thomas G. Cleary, M.D.
Professor of Pediatrics, University of Texas Medical
School; Attending Physician, University Children's at
Hermann Hospital and M. D. Anderson Hospital and
Tumor Institute, Houston, Texas
Microorganisms Responsible for Neonatal Diarrhea

Louis Z. Cooper, M.D.
Professor of Pediatrics, Columbia University College
of Physicians and Surgeons, New York, New York
Rubella

Dennis T. Crouse, M.D.
Professor, Department of Pediatrics, Obstetrics, and
Gynecology, University of Tennessee at Memphis,
Memphis, Tennessee
Mycoplasmal Infections

Clyde S. Crumpacker, M.D.
Professor of Medicine, Harvard Medical School; Chief,
Division of Infectious Diseases, Beth Israel Deaconess
Medical Center, Boston, Massachusetts
Hepatitis

Jill K. Davies, M.D.
Instructor, Department of Obstetrics and Gynecology,
University of Colorado Health Sciences Center,
Denver, Colorado
*Obstetric Factors Associated with Infections of the Fetus
and Newborn Infant*

Georges Desmonts, M.D.
Chief (retired), Laboratoire de Sérologie Néonatale et
de Recherche sur la Toxoplasmose, Institut de
Puériculture, Paris, France
Toxoplasmosis

Morven S. Edwards, M.D.
Professor of Pediatrics, Baylor College of Medicine;
Active Staff, Texas Children's Hospital and Ben Taub
General Hospital, Houston, Texas
Group B Streptococcal Infections

Tessa Gardner, M.D.
Division of Pediatric Infectious Diseases, St. John's
Mercy Medical Center; Assistant Professor of Clinical
Pediatrics, Washington University School of Medicine,
St. Louis, Missouri
Lyme Disease

Roberto P. Garofalo, M.D.
Associate Professor of Pediatrics and Microbiology and
Immunology, University of Texas Medical Branch,
University of Texas Medical School at Galveston;
Investigator, National Institute of Environmental
Health Sciences, Center in Environmental Toxicology,
University of Texas Medical Branch Hospitals,
Galveston, Texas
Human Milk

Anne A. Gershon, M.D.
Professor of Pediatrics and Director of Pediatric
Infectious Diseases, Columbia University College of
Physicians and Surgeons, New York, New York
Chickenpox, Measles, and Mumps

Ronald S. Gibbs, M.D.
Professor and Chair, Department of Obstetrics and
Gynecology, University of Colorado Health Sciences
Center, Denver, Colorado
*Obstetric Factors Associated with Infections of the Fetus
and Newborn Infant*

Donald A. Goldmann, M.D.
Professor of Pediatrics, Harvard Medical School;
Hospital Epidemiologist and Vice Chairman for Health
Outcomes, Department of Medicine, Children's
Hospital, Boston, Massachusetts
*Infections Acquired in the Nursery: Epidemiology and
Control*

Moses Grossman, M.D.
Professor of Pediatrics (Emeritus), University of
California, San Francisco, San Francisco, California
Chlamydia

Richard L. Guerrant, M.D.
Thomas H. Hunter Professor of International
Medicine; Chief, Division of Geographic and
International Medicine; Professor of Medicine and
Attending Physician; University of Virginia Health
System, Charlottesville, Virginia
Microorganisms Responsible for Neonatal Diarrhea

Laura T. Gutman, M.D.
Director of Pediatric Sexually Transmitted Diseases
Program, Duke University Medical Center, Durham,
North Carolina
Gonococcal Infections

Jo-Ann S. Harris, M.D.
Associate Professor of Pediatrics, Boston University
School of Medicine; Director of Infection Control,
Franciscan Children's Hospital and Rehabilitation
Center, Boston, Massachusetts
*Infections Acquired in the Nursery: Epidemiology and
Control*

David Ingall, M.D.
Professor Emeritus, Departments of Pediatrics and
Obstetrics and Gynecology, Northwestern University
Medical School, Chicago; Chairman Emeritus,
Department of Pediatrics, Evanston Northwestern
Health Care, Evanston, Illinois
Syphilis

Jerome O. Klein, M.D.
Professor of Pediatrics, Boston University School of
Medicine; Vice Chairman for Academic Affairs,
Department of Pediatrics, Maxwell Finland Laboratory
for Infectious Diseases, Boston Medical Center,
Boston, Massachusetts
*Bacterial Infections of the Respiratory Tract; Bacterial
Infections of the Urinary Tract; Bacterial Sepsis and
Meningitis; Current Concepts of Infections of the Fetus
and Newborn Infant*

David B. Lewis, M.D.
Associate Professor of Pediatrics, Stanford University
School of Medicine, Stanford; Attending Physician,
Lucile Salter Packard Children's Hospital at Stanford,
Palo Alto, California
*Developmental Immunology and Role of Host Defenses in
Fetal and Neonatal Susceptibility to Infection*

Sarah S. Long, M.D.
Professor of Pediatrics, MCP Hahnemann School of
Medicine; Chief, Section of Infectious Diseases, St.
Christopher's Hospital for Children, Philadelphia,
Pennsylvania
Bacterial Infections of the Urinary Tract

Yvonne A. Maldonado, M.D.
Associate Professor of Pediatrics, Stanford University
School of Medicine, Stanford; Attending Physician,
Lucile Salter Packard Children's Hospital at Stanford
and Stanford Hospital, Palo Alto, California
*Other Viral Infections of the Fetus and Newborn;
Protozoan and Helminth Infections (Including
Pneumocystis carinii)*

S. Michael Marcy, M.D.
Clinical Professor of Pediatrics, University of Southern
California School of Medicine and University of
California, Los Angeles, UCLA School of Medicine,
Los Angeles; Staff Pediatrician, Kaiser Foundation
Hospital, Panorama City, California
*Bacterial Infections of the Bones and Joints; Focal
Bacterial Infections*

George H. McCracken, Jr., M.D.
Professor of Pediatrics, The Sarah M. and Charles E.
Seay Chair in Pediatric Infectious Diseases, University
of Texas Southwestern Medical Center; Attending
Physician, Children's Medical Center, Dallas, Texas
Clinical Pharmacology of Antibacterial Agents

Rima McLeod, M.D.
Jules and Doris Stein RPB Professor, University of
Chicago, Division of the Biological Sciences, Pritzker
School of Medicine; Attending Physician, University of
Chicago Hospitals, Michael Reese Hospital and
Medical Center, Chicago, Illinois
Toxoplasmosis

Michael J. Miller, M.D.
Professor of Pediatrics, Oregon Health Sciences
University School of Medicine, Portland, Oregon
Fungal Infections

Brigitta U. Mueller, M.D.
Assistant Professor of Pediatrics, Harvard Medical
School; Associate in Medicine, Children's Hospital,
Boston, Massachusetts
Acquired Immunodeficiency Syndrome in the Infant

Pearay L. Ogra, M.D.
Professor, Department of Pediatrics, State University
of New York at Buffalo, School of Medicine and
Biomedical Sciences, Buffalo, New York
Human Milk

Gary D. Overturf, M.D.
Professor of Pediatrics, University of New Mexico
School of Medicine; Director, Pediatric Infectious
Diseases, University of New Mexico Health Sciences
Center, Children's Hospital of New Mexico,
Albuquerque, New Mexico
*Bacterial Infections of the Bones and Joints; Focal
Bacterial Infections*

Larry K. Pickering, M.D.
Professor of Pediatrics and Microbiology/Immunology,
Eastern Virginia Medical School; Director, Center for
Pediatric Research, Children's Hospital of The King's
Daughters, Norfolk, Virginia
Microorganisms Responsible for Neonatal Diarrhea

Philip A. Pizzo, M.D.
Thomas Morgan Rotch Professor of Pediatrics,
Harvard Medical School; Physician-in-Chief and Chair,
Department of Medicine, Children's Hospital, Boston,
Massachusetts
Acquired Immunodeficiency Syndrome in the Infant

Keith R. Powell, M.D.
Professor and Chairman of Pediatrics, Northeastern
Ohio Universities College of Medicine, Rootstown;
Vice President and Dr. Noah Miller Chair,
Department of Pediatrics, Children's Hospital Medical
Center of Akron, Akron, Ohio
Laboratory Aids for Diagnosis of Neonatal Sepsis

David K. Rassin, Ph.D.
Professor, Department of Pediatrics, University of
Texas Medical Branch, University of Texas Medical
School at Galveston, Galveston, Texas
Human Milk

Jack S. Remington, M.D.
Professor of Medicine, Division of Infectious Diseases
and Geographic Medicine, Stanford University School
of Medicine, Stanford; Marcus A. Krupp Research
Chair and Chairman, Department of Immunology and
Infectious Diseases, Research Institute, Palo Alto
Medical Foundation, Palo Alto, California
*Current Concepts of Infections of the Fetus and Newborn
Infant; Toxoplasmosis*

Xavier Sáez-Llorens, M.D.
Professor of Pediatrics, University of Panama School of
Medicine; Head, Infectious Disease Service, Hospital
Del Niño, Panama City, Panama
Clinical Pharmacology of Antibacterial Agents

Joseph W. St. Geme III, M.D.
Associate Professor of Pediatrics and Molecular
Microbiology, Washington University School of
Medicine; Director of Pediatric Infectious Diseases, St.
Louis Children's Hospital, St. Louis, Missouri
Staphylococcal Infections

Pablo J. Sánchez, M.D.
Associate Professor of Pediatrics, Divisions of
Neonatal-Perinatal Medicine and Pediatric Infectious
Diseases, University of Texas Southwestern Medical
School; Attending Physician, Parkland Health and
Hospital System and Children's Medical Center of
Dallas, Dallas, Texas
Syphilis

Julius Schachter, Ph.D.
Professor of Laboratory Medicine, University of
California, San Francisco; Director, World Health
Organization Collaborating Center for Reference and
Research on Chlamydiae, San Francisco, California
Chlamydia

Walter F. Schlech III, M.D.
Professor of Medicine, Division of Infectious Diseases,
Dalhousie University Faculty of Medicine; Division of
Infectious Diseases, Queen Elizabeth II Health
Sciences Centre, Halifax, Nova Scotia, Canada
Listeriosis

Henry R. Shinefield, M.D.
Clinical Professor of Pediatrics and Dermatology,
University of California, San Francisco, School of
Medicine; Co-Director, Kaiser Permanente Vaccine
Study Center, Kaiser Permanente Medical Group, San
Francisco, California
Staphylococcal Infections

Margaret H. D. Smith, M.D.
Professor Emeritus of Pediatrics, Tulane University
School of Medicine, New Orleans, Louisiana
Tuberculosis

Sergio Stagno, M.D.
Professor and Chairman, University of Alabama School
of Medicine, University of Alabama at Birmingham;
Physician in Chief, Children's Hospital of Alabama,
Birmingham, Alabama
Cytomegalovirus

Jeffrey R. Starke, M.D.
Associate Professor of Pediatrics, Baylor College of
Medicine; Deputy Chief of Pediatrics and Director,
Children's Tuberculosis Clinic, Ben Taub General
Hospital, Houston, Texas
Tuberculosis

Barbara J. Stoll, M.D.
Professor of Pediatrics, Emory University School of
Medicine, Atlanta, Georgia
Neonatal Infections: A Global Perspective

Philippe Thulliez, M.D.
Chief, Laboratoire d'Immunoanalyses et Recherche sur la Toxoplasmose, Institut de Puériculture, Paris, France
Toxoplasmosis

Thomas J. Török, M.D.
Medical Epidemiologist Supervisor, State Branch, Division of Applied Public Health Training, Epidemiology Program Office, Centers for Disease Control and Prevention, Atlanta, Georgia
Human Parvovirus B19

Ken B. Waites, M.D.
Associate Professor, Departments of Pathology and Microbiology and Rehabilitation Medicine; Director of Clinical Microbiology, University of Alabama at Birmingham, Birmingham, Alabama
Mycoplasmal Infections

Geoffrey A. Weinberg, M.D.
Associate Professor of Pediatrics, University of Rochester School of Medicine and Dentistry; Director, Pediatric HIV Program, Children's Hospital at Strong, Strong Memorial Hospital, Rochester, New York
Laboratory Aids for Diagnosis of Neonatal Sepsis

Richard J. Whitley, M.D.
Loeb Eminent Scholar Chair in Pediatrics, Professor of Pediatrics, Microbiology and Medicine, and Director, Division of Pediatric Infectious Diseases, University of Alabama at Birmingham; Associate Director for Clinical Studies, Center for AIDS Research; Vice-Chairman, Department of Pediatrics, University of Alabama at Birmingham, Birmingham, Alabama
Herpes Simplex Virus Infections

Christopher B. Wilson, M.D.
Chair, Department of Immunology, and Professor of Immunology and Pediatrics, University of Washington School of Medicine; Attending Physician, Children's Hospital and Regional Medical Center, Seattle, Washington
Developmental Immunology and Role of Host Defenses in Fetal and Neonatal Susceptibility to Infection

Preface

Major advances in biology and medicine made during the past four decades have contributed greatly to our understanding of infections that affect the fetus and newborn. As the medical, social, and economic impact of these infections becomes more fully appreciated, the time is again appropriate for an intensive summation of existing information on this subject. Our goal for the fifth edition of this text is to provide a complete, critical, and contemporary review of this information. We have directed the book to all students of medicine interested in the care and well-being of children and hope to include among our readers medical students, practicing physicians, microbiologists, and health care workers. We believe the text to be of particular importance for obstetricians and physicians who are responsible for the pregnant woman and her developing fetus; pediatricians and family doctors who care for newborn infants; and primary care physicians, neurologists, audiologists, ophthalmologists, psychologists, and other specialists who are responsible for children who suffer the sequelae of infections acquired in utero or during the first month of life.

The scope of this book encompasses infections of the fetus and newborn, including those acquired in utero, during the delivery process, and in the early months of life. When appropriate, sequelae of these infections that affect older children and adults are included as well. Infection in the adult is described when pertinent to the developing fetus and newborn infant. Each chapter includes a review of the history, microbiology, epidemiology, pathogenesis and pathology, clinical signs and symptoms, diagnosis, prognosis, treatment, and prevention of the infection. The length of the chapters varies considerably. In some instances, this variation is related to the available fund of knowledge on the subject; in others (e.g., the chapters on toxoplasmosis, neonatal diarrhea, varicella, measles, and mumps), the length of the chapter is related to the fact that no recent comprehensive reviews of these subjects are available.

The first, second, third, and fourth editions of this text were published in 1976, 1983, 1990, and 1995, respectively. As of this writing, in the spring of 2000, it is most interesting to observe the changes that have occurred in the interval since publication of the last edition. New authors provide fresh perspectives. Major revisions of most chapters suggest the importance of new information about other infections of the fetus and newborn infant.

Each of the authors of the different chapters is a recognized authority in the field and has made significant contributions to our understanding of infections in the fetus and newborn infant. Most of these authors are individuals whose major investigative efforts on this subject have taken place during the past 20 years. Almost all were supported, in part or totally, during their training period and subsequently, by funds obtained from the National Institutes of Health or private agencies such as The National Foundation. It is clear that the major advances of this period would not have been possible without these funding mechanisms and the freedom given the investigators to pursue programs of their own choosing. Thus, the advances present in this text are also a testimony to the trustees of agencies and the legislators and other federal officials who provided unencumbered research funds in the 1960s through the 1990s.

We were Fellows at the Thorndike Memorial Laboratory (Harvard Medical Unit, Boston City Hospital) in the early 1960s. Although subsequently we worked in separate areas of investigation on the two coasts, one of us as an internist and the other as a pediatrician, we maintained close contact and, because of a mutual interest in infections of the fetus and newborn infant and their long-term effects, we joined our efforts to develop this text.

We are indebted to our teachers and associates and especially to the one individual who had a dominant influence in our training, Dr. Maxwell Finland. We deeply appreciate the example he set, his wise counsel, and his interest in and support of our investigative programs. We also wish to express our appreciation to Judith Fletcher, Melissa Dudlick, and the staff of W.B. Saunders Company for guiding this project to a successful conclusion; to Ms. Nancy Ahonen for secretarial assistance; and to Ms. Trisha Mitchell for her editorial assistance.

Jack S. Remington
Jerome O. Klein

Contents

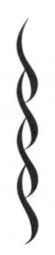

Current Concepts of Infections of the Fetus and Newborn Infant

JEROME O. KLEIN, M.D., and JACK S. REMINGTON, M.D.

Current concepts of pathogenesis, microbiology, diagnosis, and management of infections of the fetus and newborn infant are briefly reviewed in this chapter. Chapters dealing with immunology and resistance to infection, human breast milk, obstetric factors, infection control in the nursery, a global perspective of fetal and neonatal infections and clinical pharmacology of antimicrobial agents follow, as does detailed information about the various infectious diseases of importance to the fetus and newborn infant.

Since preparation of the fourth edition of this textbook in 1994, major changes have occurred in diagnosis, prevention, and management of infectious diseases of the fetus and newborn infant. Some of these changes are noted in Table 1–1 and are discussed in this and the relevant chapters.

Substantial progress has taken place to reduce the burden of infectious diseases, including reduction of the incidence of early-onset group B streptococcal disease by aggressive use of intrapartum antibiotics; reduction of vertical transmission of human immunodeficiency virus (HIV) by identification and treatment of the infected mother; extension of uses of polymerase chain reaction (PCR), permitting more rapid and specific diagnosis of microbial pathogens; increased recognition that infectious diseases cross national and regional borders; and greater access to information for physicians and parents through use of the Internet.

Setbacks in initiatives to reduce the burden of infectious diseases of the fetus and newborn infant include the explosive outbreak of HIV in developing countries and the lack of finances to provide treatment for the infected mother and her newborn infant, the intrusion of insurance plans into medical decisions in the nursery, and the increase in antibiotic resistance among pathogens responsible for nursery-acquired infections.

The expansion of use of the Internet permits access to information hitherto unavailable to physicians or parents. The physician may obtain current information about diseases and management and various guidelines for diagnosis and treatment. The interested parent who has access to the Internet may access a variety of Web sites with a vast array of information. The quality of information available to the parent is variable and in some cases may lead to danger for the patient. As an example, a case of neonatal tetanus was associated with the use of a cosmetic facial clay, Indian Healing Clay, as a dressing on an umbilical cord stump. The product had been publicized as a healing salve by midwives on an Internet site "cordcare."[1] Because much of the information on the Internet is from commercial sources and parties with varying interests and expertise, the physician should assist the interested patient in finding Web sites of value. A selected list of Web sites pertinent to infectious diseases of the fetus and newborn infant is provided in Table 1–2.

TABLE 1–1
Recent Changes in Epidemiology and Management of Infectious Diseases of the Fetus and Newborn Infant

EPIDEMIOLOGY

Increased viability of very low birth weight infants at risk for invasive infectious diseases

Increased number of multiple births (often of very low birth weight) due to successful techniques for management of infertility

Global perspective of vertically transmitted infectious diseases

Early discharge from the nursery mandated by insurance programs leading to concern for decreased time of observation for infants at risk for sepsis

DIAGNOSIS

Polymerase chain reaction for diagnosis of infection in mother, fetus, and neonate

Decreased use of fetal blood sampling and chorionic villus sampling for diagnosis of infectious diseases

PREVENTION

Peripartum antibiotics to prevent early-onset group B streptococcal infection

Antiretroviral therapy in pregnancy to prevent transmission of human immunodeficiency virus (HIV) to fetus

TREATMENT

Antiretroviral therapy in the mother to treat the HIV-infected fetus

Antitoxoplasmosis therapy in the mother to treat the infected fetus

Spread within nurseries of antibiotic-resistant bacterial pathogens

Increased use of vancomycin for multidrug-resistant gram-positive infections

Increased use of acyclovir for infants with suspected herpes simplex meningoencephalitis

The vital statistics relevant to concern for infectious disease in neonates are provided in the U.S. Department of Health and Human Services Chartbook for 1998.[2] Selected data for the United States for 1996 are listed in Table 1–3. Of importance are the racial disparities in low birth weight, prenatal care, breast-feeding, and neonatal mortality.

The number of infectious diseases in fetuses and newborn infants must be extrapolated from selected studies (see chapters for diseases). Approximately 1% of newborn infants excrete cytomegalovirus; up to 15% of infants are infected with *Chlamydia trachomatis*, and 1 to 8 infants per 1000 live births develop bacterial sepsis (a rate that will decrease with adoption of use of intrapartum prophylaxis for group B streptococcal infections). The incidence of perinatal acquired immunodeficiency syndrome (AIDS) has decreased with the use of antiretroviral therapy in pregnancy from about 25% in infants born to untreated mothers to less than 8% in those whose mothers were enrolled in therapeutic programs. Among sexually transmitted diseases, 1200 cases of congenital syphilis (30.4 per 100,000 live births) were reported in 1996 in the United States, but some communities had much higher rates. In Baltimore the rate for congenital syphilis increased from 62 to 282 per 100,000 live births from 1993 to 1996.[3] Although immunization has reduced the incidence of measles, mumps, rubella, and varicella, gaps in vaccinating children and adults has led to failure to eradicate these infections; 12 infants with laboratory-confirmed congenital rubella syndrome were reported between 1994 and 1996.[4]

Infection acquired in utero may result in resorption of the embryo, abortion, stillbirth, malformation, intrauterine growth retardation, prematurity, and the untoward sequelae of chronic postnatal infection. Infection acquired during the birth process or soon after birth may result in severe systemic disease that leads to death or persistent postnatal infection. Both in utero infection and infection acquired during the birth process may lead to late-onset disease. The infection may not be apparent at birth but may manifest with signs of disease weeks, months, or years later, as exemplified by the chorioretinitis of *Toxoplasma gondii*, the hearing loss of rubella virus, and the immunologic defects that result from HIV. The immediate as well as the long-term effects of these infections are a major problem throughout the world.

TABLE 1–2
Selected Web Sites of Value for Physicians Interested in Infectious Diseases of the Fetus and Newborn Infant

Agency for Health Care Policy and Research	http://www.ahcpr.gov
American Academy of Pediatrics	http://www.aap.org
American College of Obstetricians and Gynecologists	http://www.acog.org
Centers for Disease Control and Prevention	http://www.cdc.gov
Food and Drug Administration	http://www.fda.gov
Immunization Action Coalition	http://www.immunize.org
Information on AIDS Trials	http://www.actis.org
Morbidity and Mortality Weekly Report	http://www.cdc.gov/epo/mmwr/mmwr.html
National Center for Health Statistics	http:www.cdc.gov/nchs
Pediatric Infectious Diseases and selected bibliography*	http://www.pedid.uthscsa.edu

* Described in Jenson HB, Baltimore RS. A World Wide Web selected bibliography for pediatric infectious diseases. Clin Infect Dis 28:395–398, 1999.

TABLE 1–3
Vital Statistics Relevant to Newborn Health in the United States in 1996*

FEATURE	RACE/ETHNIC ORIGIN OF MOTHER			
	All	White	Black	Hispanic*
Number live births	3.891 m†	3.093 m	.594 m	.701 m
Birthweight				
<2500 g	7.4%	6.3%	13.0%	6.3%
<1500 g	1.37%	1.1%	3.0%	1.1%
Prenatal care				
Began 1st trimester	81.9%	84.0%	71.4%	72.2%
Began in 3rd trimester or no prenatal care	4.0%	3.3%	7.3%	6.7%
Babies breast fed	58.1%	61.2%	27.5%	67.4%
Mortality rate (<28 d)				
Per 1000 live births (1995)	4.9	4.1	9.6	4.1

* Hispanic statistics extrapolated from data for selected states.
† m = 10^6.
From Pamuk E, Makuc D, Heck K, et al. Socioeconomic Status and Health Chartbook. Health, United States, 1998. Hyattsville, Md, National Center for Health Statistics, 1998.

INFECTIONS OF THE FETUS

Pathogenesis

Pregnant women not only are exposed to the infections prevalent in the community but also are likely to reside with young children, who represent a significant additional factor in exposure to infectious disease. The vast majority of infections in the pregnant woman affect the upper respiratory and gastrointestinal tracts and either resolve spontaneously without therapy or are readily treated with antimicrobial agents. Such infections usually remain localized and have no effect on the developing fetus. However, the infecting organism may invade the bloodstream and infect the placenta and fetus.

Pregnancy induces an immunologic bias in the mother toward humoral immunity and away from cell-mediated immunity. The latter is most important against many intracellular pathogens and requires a strong Th1 response. The Th2 bias established during normal gestation may compromise successful immunity against these organisms, such as *T. gondii*. In addition, it has been proposed that a strong curative Th1 response against an organism may overcome the protective Th2 cytokines at the maternal-fetal interface and result in fetal loss.[5, 6]

Transplacental spread after maternal infection and invasion of the bloodstream is the usual route by which the fetus becomes infected. Uncommonly, the fetus may be infected by extension of infection in adjacent tissues and organs, including the peritoneum or the genitalia, or as a result of invasive methods for the diagnosis and therapy of fetal disorders, such as the use of monitors, sampling of fetal blood, and intrauterine transfusion.

The microorganisms of concern are listed in Table 1–4 and include those identified in the acronym TORCH: *T. gondii*, rubella virus, cytomegalovirus (CMV), and herpes simplex virus (HSV). A new acronym is needed to include the other well-described causes of in utero infection: syphilis, enteroviruses, varicella-zoster virus (VZV) and HIV, Lyme disease (*Borrelia burgdorferi*), and parvovirus. In selected areas, *Plasmo-dium* and *Trypanosoma cruzi* are responsible for in utero infections. TORCHES CLAP (see Table 1–4) is an inclusive acronym. THE BAC PORCH is easily remembered but relies on an idealized spelling for the word *back*. CHAST LOVER includes a truncated spelling of the word *chaste*.[7] CHEAP TORCHES has been suggested to include congenital and perinatal infections; it includes an H for hepatitis B and C and an E for everything else that is sexually transmitted (gonorrhea, *Chlamydia*, *Ureaplasma*, and papillomavirus) but ignores Lyme disease. Because there is no clear successor to TORCH, other acronyms are still welcome.[8]

Case reports indicate that other organisms are unusual causes of infections transmitted by the pregnant woman to her fetus, including *Brucella melitensis*,[9] *Coxiella burnetii* (Q fever),[10] *Babesia microti* (babesiosis),[11] human T lymphotropic virus types I and II,[12, 13] hepatitis G,[14] human herpesvirus 6,[15] and dengue.[16]

Before rupture of fetal membranes, organisms in the genital tract may invade the amniotic fluid and produce infection of the fetus. These organisms can invade the fetus through microscopic defects in the membranes, particularly in devitalized areas overlying the cervical os. It is also possible that microorganisms gain access to the fetus from descending infection via the fallopian tubes

TABLE 1–4
Suggested Acronym for the Microorganisms Responsible for Infection of the Fetus

Toxoplasma gondii	To
Rubella virus	R
Cytomegalovirus	C
Herpes simplex virus	H
Enteroviruses	E
Syphilis (*Treponema pallidum*)	S
Chickenpox (varicella-zoster virus)	C
Lyme disease (*Borrelia burgdorferi*)	L
AIDS (human immunodeficiency virus)	A
Parvovirus B19	P

in women with salpingitis or peritonitis or from direct extension of an infection in the uterus, such as myometrial abscess or cellulitis. There are few data, however, to suggest that transtubal or transmyometrial passage of microbial agents is a significant route of fetal infection.

The invasive techniques that have been developed for in utero diagnosis and therapy are potential sources of infection for the fetus. Abscesses have been observed in infants who had scalp punctures for fetal blood sampling or electrocardiographic electrodes clipped on their scalps. Osteomyelitis of the skull and streptococcal sepsis have followed a local infection at the site of a fetal monitoring electrode.[17] Intrauterine transfusion for severe erythroblastosis diagnosed in utero has also resulted in infection of the fetus: in one case, CMV infection reportedly resulted from intrauterine transfusion[18]; in another instance, contamination of donor blood with a gram-negative coccus, *Acinetobacter calcoaceticus,* led to an acute placentitis and subsequent fetal bacteremia.[19]

Fetal infection in the absence of rupture of maternal membranes usually occurs by the transplacental route after invasion of the maternal bloodstream. Microorganisms in the blood may be carried within white blood cells or attached to erythrocytes, or they may be independent of cellular elements.

RESULTS OF MICROBIAL INVASION OF THE MATERNAL BLOODSTREAM

The consequences that may follow invasion of the mother's bloodstream by microorganisms or their products (Fig. 1–1) include (1) placental infection without infection of the fetus, (2) fetal infection without infection of the placenta, (3) absence of both fetal and placental infection, and (4) infection of both placenta and fetus.

Placental Infection Without Infection of the Fetus. After reaching the intervillous spaces on the maternal side of the placenta, organisms can remain localized in the placenta without affecting the fetus. Evidence that placentitis does occur independently of fetal involvement has been demonstrated after maternal tuberculosis, syphilis, malaria, coccidioidomycosis, CMV infection, and rubella. The reasons for the lack of spread to the fetus after the placental infection has been established are unknown. Defenses of the fetus that may operate after infection of the placenta include the villous trophoblast, placental macrophages, and local production of immune factors such as antibodies and cytokines.

Fetal Infection Without Infection of the Placenta. Microorganisms may traverse the chorionic villi directly through pinocytosis, placental leaks, or diapedesis of infected maternal leukocytes and erythrocytes. Careful histologic studies, however, usually reveal areas of placentitis sufficient to serve as a source of fetal infection.

Absence of Both Fetal and Placental Infection. Invasion of the bloodstream by microorganisms is not uncommon in pregnant women, yet in most cases neither fetal nor placental infection results. Bacteremia may accompany abscesses or cellulitis, bacterial pneumonia, pyelonephritis, appendicitis, endocarditis, or other pyogenic infections; nevertheless, placental or fetal infection as a consequence of such bacteremias is rare. In most cases, the fetus is probably protected through efficient clearance of microbes by the maternal reticuloendothelial system and circulating leukocytes.

A number of bacterial diseases of the pregnant woman, including typhoid fever, pneumonia, sepsis caused by gram-negative bacteria, and urinary tract infections, may affect the developing fetus without direct microbial invasion of the placenta or fetal tissues. Simi-

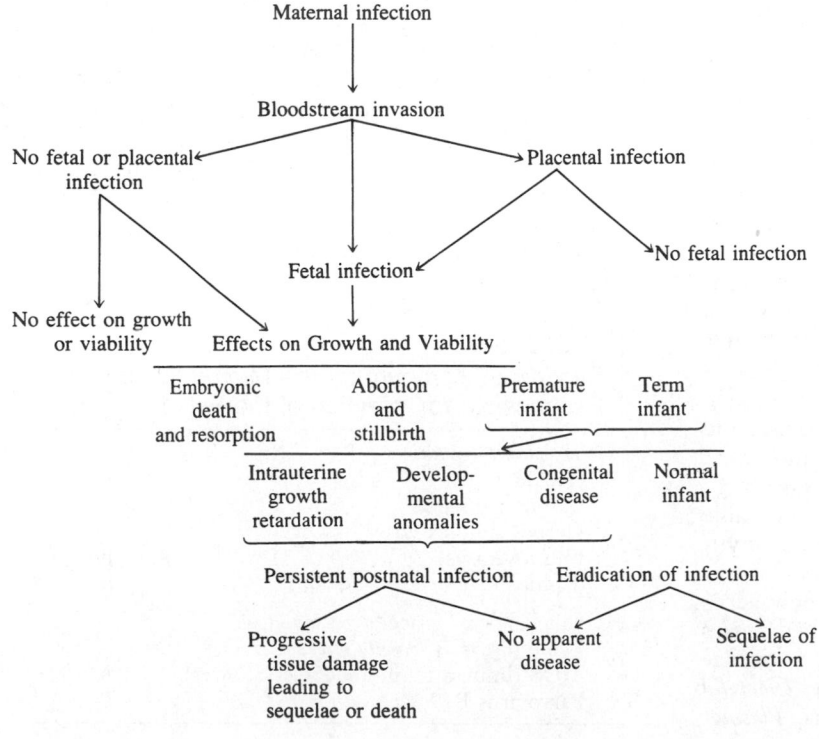

FIGURE 1–1 Pathogenesis of hematogenous transplacental infections.

larly, protozoan infection of the mother, such as malaria, and systemic viral infections, including varicella, variola, and measles, may also affect the fetus indirectly. Fever, anoxia, circulating toxins, or metabolic derangements in the mother during these infections can affect the pregnancy; abortion, stillbirth, and premature delivery are among the possible results.

The effect of microbial toxins on the developing fetus is uncertain. The fetus may be adversely affected by toxic shock in the mother due to *Staphylococcus aureus* or *Streptococcus pyogenes* infection. Botulism in pregnant women has not been associated with disease in the infant.[20, 21] A unique case of Guillain-Barré syndrome in mother and child raises questions about the possibility of a transmissible agent, toxin, or immune factor. The disease was diagnosed in the mother during the twenty-ninth week of pregnancy. While the mother was quadriplegic and on respiratory support, a healthy infant was delivered per vagina at 38 weeks' gestation. On the twelfth day of life, the infant developed flaccid paralysis of all limbs, deep tendon reflexes were absent, and cerebrospinal fluid had increased protein concentration (243 mg/dl) without white blood cells. The infant improved following administration of intravenous immunoglobulin.[22]

The association of maternal urinary tract infection with premature delivery and low birth weight is a well-studied example of a maternal infection that affects growth and development of the fetus adversely, even though there is no evidence of fetal or placental infection. Asymptomatic bacteriuria in pregnancy has been linked to an excess in the number of low-birth-weight infants.[23, 24] When the bacteriuria was eliminated by appropriate antibiotic therapy, the treated women had a lower incidence of pyelonephritis than did the untreated women, and they had the same rate of premature and low birth-weight infants as did nonbacteriuric women.[25] The basis for the premature delivery and low birth weight of infants of bacteriuric women remains obscure. Kincaid-Smith[26] suggested that all bacteriuric women face the risk of premature delivery but that the women at greatest risk are those with evidence of renal involvement as manifested by mild azotemia or minimal clinical signs of pyelonephritis. Lymphocytes from infants whose mothers had pyelonephritis caused by *Escherichia coli* proliferate in the presence of *E. coli* antigen.[27] This finding suggests that the fetal lymphocytes were exposed and sensitized to the antigen in utero.

Infection of Both Placenta and Fetus. Microbes may be disseminated from the infected placenta to the fetal bloodstream through infected emboli of necrotic chorionic tissues or through direct extension of placental infection to the fetal membranes, with secondary amniotic fluid infection and aspiration by the fetus.

RESULTS OF INFECTION OF THE EMBRYO AND FETUS

Results of infection after hematogenous transplacental spread include death and resorption of the embryo, abortion and stillbirth of the fetus, and live birth of a premature or term infant who may or may not be normal. The effects of fetal infection may appear in the live-born infant as low birth weight (resulting from intrauterine retardation of growth), developmental anomalies, congenital disease, or none of these. Infection acquired in utero may persist after birth and cause significant abnormalities in growth and development that may be apparent soon after birth or may not be recognized for months or years. The variability of the effects of fetal infection is emphasized by reports of binovular twin pregnancies that produced one severely damaged infant and another with minimal or no detectable abnormalities.[28–34]

Embryonic Death and Resorption. A variety of organisms may infect the pregnant woman in the first few weeks of gestation and produce death and resorption of the embryo. Because this usually occurs before the woman realizes she is pregnant or seeks medical attention, it is difficult to estimate the incidence of this outcome for any single infectious agent. The incidence of early pregnancy loss after implantation from all causes has been estimated to be 31%. The proportion of this loss due to infection is unknown.[35]

Abortion and Stillbirth. The earliest recognizable effects of fetal infection are seen after the sixth to eighth week of pregnancy and include abortion and stillbirth. Intrauterine death may result from overwhelming fetal infection, or the microorganisms may interfere with organogenesis to such an extent that the development of functions necessary for continued viability is interrupted. The precise mechanisms responsible for early spontaneous termination of pregnancy are unknown; in many cases, it is difficult to ascertain whether fetal death caused or resulted from the expulsion of the fetus. A number of modifying factors probably determine the ultimate outcome of intrauterine infection; these include virulence or tissue tropism of the microorganisms, stage of pregnancy, associated placental damage, and severity of the maternal illness. Primary infection is likely to have a more important effect on the fetus than recurrent infection[36]; recurrent CMV infections are less severe than primary infection, but this does not appear to be the case for recurrent infections caused by HIV, with AIDS of equivalent clinical significance in sequential pregnancies. Available studies do not distinguish between the direct effect of the microorganisms on the developing fetus and the possibility of an indirect effect attributable to illness or poor health of the mother.

Prematurity. Prematurity is defined as the birth of a viable infant before the thirty-seventh week of gestation; premature birth may result from almost any agent capable of establishing fetal infection during the last trimester of pregnancy. Those microorganisms commonly responsible for stillbirth and abortion are also implicated as significant causes of prematurity (Table 1–5).

Previous studies have demonstrated that women in premature labor whose amniotic fluid cultures for bacteria are positive have elevated levels of interleukin (IL)-6 and other proinflammatory cytokines (including tumor necrosis factor [TNF] and IL-1β) in their amniotic fluid.[37–39] Levels of IL-6 in amniotic fluid have not proved to be predictive of infection, because in many patients with elevated levels of IL-6, cultures of the

TABLE 1–5
Effects of Transplacental Fetal Infection on the Fetus and Newborn Infant

ORGANISM OR DISEASE	PREMATURITY	INTRAUTERINE GROWTH RETARDATION AND LOW BIRTH WEIGHT	DEVELOPMENTAL ANOMALIES	CONGENITAL DISEASE	PERSISTENT POSTNATAL INFECTION
Viruses					
Rubella	−	+	+	+	+
Cytomegalovirus	+	+	+	+	+
Herpes simplex	+	−	−	+	+
Varicella-zoster	−	(+)	+	+	+
Mumps	−	−	−	(+)	−
Rubeola	+	−	−	+	−
Vaccinia	−	−	−	+	−
Smallpox	+	−	−	+	−
Coxsackieviruses B	−	−	(+)	+	−
Echoviruses	−	−	−	−	−
Polioviruses	−	−	−	+	−
Influenza	−	−	−	−	−
Hepatitis B	+	−	−	+	+
Human immunodeficiency virus	(+)	(+)	(+)	+	+
Lymphocytic choriomeningitis virus	−	−	−	+	−
Parvovirus	−	−	−	+	−
Bacteria					
Treponema pallidum	+	−	−	+	+
Mycobacterium tuberculosis	+	−	−	+	+
Listeria monocytogenes	+	−	−	+	−
Campylobacter fetus	+	−	−	+	−
Salmonella typhosa	+	−	−	+	−
Borrelia burgdorferi	−	−	−	+	−
Protozoa					
Toxoplasma gondii	+	+	−	+	+
Plasmodium	(+)	+	−	+	+
Trypanosoma cruzi	+	+	−	+	−

+ = evidence for effect; − = no evidence for effect; (+) = association of effect with infection has been suggested and is under consideration.

amniotic fluid were negative.[37–39] However, premature births are invariably observed in women in premature labor whose amniotic fluid cultures are positive or who have elevated amniotic fluid levels of IL-6.[37–39] To further clarify the role of measurement of levels of IL-6 in amniotic fluid, Hitti and colleagues[39] amplified bacterial 16S rRNA encoding DNA by PCR to detect amniotic fluid infection in women in premature labor whose membranes were intact. PCR detected bacterial infection in significantly more patients whose amniotic fluid cultures were negative but had elevated IL-6 levels. Their data suggest that as many as 33% of women in premature labor whose amniotic fluid cultures are negative but in whom IL-6 amniotic fluid levels are elevated have amniotic fluid infection. The investigators concluded that the association between amniotic fluid infection and premature labor may be underestimated on the basis of amniotic fluid cultures. They further suggested that use of the broad-spectrum bacterial 16S rDNA PCR may be useful for diagnosis of infected amniotic fluid.

Intrauterine Growth Retardation and Low Birth Weight. Infection of the fetus may result in infants who are small for their gestational age. Although "small-for-date" infants appear to be associated with many maternal infections, there is sufficient evidence to establish a causal relationship only for rubella, CMV infection, and toxoplasmosis.

The organs of infants dying with congenital rubella syndrome or CMV infection contain a decreased number of morphologically normal cells.[40, 41] In contrast, the parenchymal cells of small-for-date infants who are small because of noninfectious causes such as maternal toxemia or placental abnormalities are normal in number but have a reduced amount of cytoplasm, presumably because of fetal malnutrition.[42, 43]

Developmental Anomalies and Teratogenesis. CMV, rubella virus, and VZV cause developmental anomalies in the human fetus. Coxsackieviruses B3 and B4 have been associated with congenital heart disease.[44] The pathogenetic mechanisms responsible for the fetal abnormalities produced by most infectious agents remain obscure. Histologic studies of abortuses and congenitally infected infants have suggested, however, that the ultimate mode of action of some viruses rests in their ability to cause cell death, alterations in cell growth, or chromosomal damage. Lesions resulting from the inflammatory process caused by the microorganisms must be distinguished from defects that arise from a direct effect of the organisms on the growth of cells and tissues in the developing embryo or fetus. Inflammation and tissue destruction, rather than teratogenic activity, appear to be responsible for the widespread structural abnormalities characteristic of congenital syphilis, transplacental HSV infection, and toxoplasmosis. Infants with congenital toxoplasmosis may have microcephaly, hydrocephalus, or microphthalmia, but these manifestations usually result from an intense necrotizing process containing numerous organisms and are more appropriately defined as lesions of congenital infection rather than as effects of teratogenic activity of the organism.

Some mycoplasmas[45] and viruses[46, 47] produce chromosomal damage in circulating human lymphocytes or in human cells in tissue culture. The relationship of these changes in structure to the production of congenital abnormalities in the fetus is unknown.

Congenital Disease. Clinical evidence of intrauterine infections may be present at birth, soon thereafter, or years later. The signs result from tissue damage or secondary physiologic changes caused by the invading organisms. The clinical manifestations in the newborn infant of infection acquired in utero or at delivery are given in Table 1–6. Infants with congenital rubella, toxoplasmosis, or CMV or enterovirus infections may have signs of widely disseminated infection during the neonatal period; such signs include jaundice, hepatosplenomegaly, and pneumonia, all of which reflect lesions caused by microbial invasion and proliferation rather than by defects in organogenesis. These signs of congenital infection are not detected until the neonatal period, although the pathologic processes responsible for their occurrence have been progressing for weeks or months before delivery. In some infants, the constellation of signs is sufficient to suggest the likely congenital infection (Table 1–7). In other infants, the signs are transient and self-limited and resolve as neonatal defense mechanisms control the spread of the microbial agent and tissue destruction. If damage is severe and widespread at the time of delivery, the infant is likely to die.

It is frequently difficult to determine whether the infection in the newborn infant was acquired in utero, during the delivery process, or post partum. If the onset of clinical signs and symptoms after birth is within the minimal incubation period for the disease (i.e., 3 days for enteroviruses, 10 days for varicella and rubella viruses), it is likely that the infection was acquired before delivery. The interval between exposure to malaria in the mother and congenital malaria in the infant can be prolonged; one case of congenital malaria resulting from *Plasmodium malariae* occurred in the United States in an infant born 25 years after its mother had emigrated from China.[48] Most HIV-infected children can now be diagnosed by 6 months of age using culture, the PCR method, or serologic detection of p24 antigen. About one half of HIV-infected children are virus-positive at birth. Virus-negative children who later become virus-positive may have been infected at or shortly before delivery and are in a culture-negative incubation period during the days after birth.[49]

Normal Infants. The majority of newborn infants infected in utero by rubella virus, *T. gondii*, CMV, or HIV have no signs of congenital disease. Fetal infection by a limited inoculum of organisms or with a strain of low virulence or minimal potential for teratogenicity may be responsible for this low incidence of clinical disease in infected infants. Alternatively, gestational age may be important in determining the ultimate consequences of prenatal infection. When congenital rubella and toxoplasmosis are acquired during the last trimester of pregnancy, the incidence of clinical disease in the infected infants is lower than when microbial invasion occurs during the first or second trimester.

Absence of clinically apparent disease in the newborn may be misleading. Careful observation of infected but asymptomatic children over the course of months or years often reveals defects that were not apparent at birth. The failure to recognize such defects early in life may be due to the inability to test young infants for the functions involved. Hearing defects identified years after birth may be the only manifestation of congenital rubella. Significant sensorineural deafness and other central nervous system deficiencies have afflicted children with congenital CMV infection who were considered to be normal during the neonatal period. Delayed recognition of other manifestations of in utero infection, including failure to thrive, visual defects, and minimal to severe brain dysfunction (including motor, learning, language, and behavioral disorders), may follow toxoplasmosis, rubella, and CMV infections. Infants infected with HIV are usually asymptomatic at birth and for the first few months of life. The median age for onset of signs of congenital HIV infection is approximately 3 years, but many children remain asymptomatic for more than 5 years. Failure to thrive, persistent diarrhea, recurrent suppurative infections, and diseases associated with opportunistic infections that occur weeks to months or years after birth are signs of perinatal infection related to HIV. Of particular concern is the report by Wilson and colleagues[50] that found stigmata of congenital *T. gondii* infection, including chorioretinitis and blindness, in almost all of 24 children at follow-up evaluations; the children had serologic evidence of infection but were without apparent signs of disease at birth and were largely untreated.

Because abnormalities may become obvious only as the child develops and succeeds or fails to reach appropriate physiologic or developmental milestones, it is of utmost importance to give careful and thorough follow-up examinations to infants born to women known to be infected during pregnancy.

Persistent Postnatal Infection. Microbial agents may continue to survive and replicate in tissues for months or years after in utero infection. Rubella virus and CMV have been isolated from various body fluids and tissues for long periods of time from children who were symptomatic or asymptomatic at birth. In some congenital infections, including rubella, HSV infection, cytomegalic inclusion disease, HIV infection, toxoplasmosis, syphilis, tuberculosis, and malaria, progressive tissue destruction has been demonstrated. Recurrent eye and skin infections may occur as a result of HSV infection acquired in utero or at the time of delivery. A progressive encephalitis has occurred with congenital rubella infection.[51, 52] The clinical manifestations of congenital infection in these children had been stable for many years when deterioration of motor and mental functions

TABLE 1-6
Clinical Manifestations of Neonatal Infection Acquired In Utero or at Delivery

CLINICAL SIGN	Rubella Virus	Cytomegalovirus	Toxoplasma gondii	Herpes simplex Virus	Treponema pallidum	Enteroviruses	Group B Streptococcus or Escherichia coli
Hepatosplenomegaly	+	+	+	+	+	+	+
Jaundice	+	+	+	+	+	+	+
Adenopathy	+	−	+	−	+	+	−
Pneumonitis	+	+	+	+	+	+	+
Lesions of skin or mucous membranes							
Petechiae or purpura	+	+	+	+	+	+	+
Vesicles	−	+	−	++	+	−	−
Maculopapular exanthems	−	−	+	+	++	+	−
Lesions of nervous system							
Meningoencephalitis	+	+	+	+	+	+	+
Microcephaly	−	++	+	+	−	−	−
Hydrocephalus	+	+	++	+	−	−	−
Intracranial calcifications	−	++	++	−	−	++	−
Paralysis	−	−	−	−	−	−	−
Hearing deficits	+	+	−	−	+	−	−
Lesions of heart							
Myocarditis	+	−	+	+	−	++	−
Congenital defects	++	−	−	−	−	−	−
Bone lesions	++	−	+	−	++	−	−
Eye lesions							
Glaucoma	++	−	−	−	+	−	−
Chorioretinitis or retinopathy	++	+	++	+	+	−	−
Cataracts	++	−	+	+	−	−	−
Optic atrophy	−	+	+	−	−	−	−
Microphthalmia	+	−	+	−	−	−	−
Uveitis	−	−	+	−	+	−	−
Conjunctivitis or keratoconjunctivitis	−	−	−	++	−	+	−

− = either not present or rare in infected infants; + = occurs in infants with infection; ++ = has special diagnostic significance for this infection.

TABLE 1–7
Syndromes in the Neonate Caused by
Congenital Infections

MICROORGANISM	SIGNS
Toxoplasma gondii	Hydrocephalus, diffuse intracranial calcification, chorioretinitis
Rubella virus	Cardiac defects, sensorineural hearing loss, cataracts
Cytomegalovirus	Microcephalus, periventricular calcification
Herpes simplex virus	Vesicular lesions, keratoconjunctivitis
Treponema pallidum	Bullous, macular, and eczematous skin lesions involving the palms and soles; rhinorrhea; dactylitis and other signs of osteochondritis and periostitis
Varicella-zoster virus	Limb abnormalities, cicatricial lesions
Parvovirus	Diffuse edema (in utero hydrops fetalis)
Human immunodeficiency virus (HIV)	Severe thrush, failure to thrive, recurrent bacterial infections, calcification of the basal ganglia

occurred at ages 11 to 14 years. Rubella virus was isolated from the brain biopsy specimen of a 12-year-old child. Fetal parvovirus B19 infection can persist for months after birth with persistent anemia due to suppressed medullary hematopoiesis.[53]

The mechanisms responsible for maintaining or terminating chronic fetal and postnatal infections are only partially understood. Humoral immune responses, as determined by measurement of either fetal immunoglobulin M (IgM) antibodies or specific IgG antibodies that develop in the neonatal period, appear to be intact in almost all infants (see Chapter 2). The importance of cell-mediated immunity, cytokines, complement, and other nonspecific host defense mechanisms remains to be defined; however, there is insufficient evidence at present to support a causal relation between deficiencies in any of these factors and persistent postnatal infection. It is noteworthy that all of the diseases associated with persistent postnatal infection, with the exception of rubella but including HSV and VZV infections, cytomegalic inclusion disease, HIV infection, syphilis, tuberculosis, malaria, toxoplasmosis, and hepatitis, may also produce prolonged, and in certain instances lifelong, infection when acquired later in life.

Efficiency of Transmission of Microorganisms from Mother to Fetus

The efficiency of transmission from the infected, immunocompetent mother to the fetus varies among microbial agents and may also vary with the trimester of pregnancy. In utero transmission of rubella virus and *T. gondii* occurs only as a result of primary infection, whereas in utero transmission of CMV and HIV has been described for multiple pregnancies.

The risk of congenital rubella infection in fetuses of mothers with symptomatic rubella was high in the first trimester (90% before 11 weeks' gestation), declined to a low of 25% at 23 to 26 weeks, and then rose to 67% after 31 weeks. Infection in the first 11 weeks of gestation was uniformly teratogenic, whereas no birth defects occurred in infants infected after 16 weeks.[54]

In contrast, the frequency of stillbirth and clinical and subclinical congenital *T. gondii* infection among offspring of 500 women who acquired *T. gondii* infection during pregnancy was least in the first trimester (14%), increased in the second trimester (29%), and was highest in the third trimester (59%).[55]

Congenital CMV infection may result from both primary and recurrent infections. On the basis of studies in Birmingham, Alabama, and other centers, Stagno and Whitley[56] estimate that 1 to 4% of women have primary infection during pregnancy, that 40% of these women transmit the infection to the fetus, and that 5 to 15% of the infants have signs of CMV disease. Congenital infection due to recurrent CMV infection is 0.5 to 1%, and fewer than 1% of the infected infants have clinically apparent disease.

The transmission rate of HIV infection from the untreated infected mother to the fetus is estimated to be about 25%, but the data are insufficient to identify efficiency of transmission by trimester. Infants at risk for congenital infection are those born to symptomatic women who have more advanced disease or who have low CD4$^+$ T lymphocyte counts.[57]

Diagnosis of Infection in the Pregnant Woman

CLINICAL DIAGNOSIS

Symptomatic or Clinical Infection. The major mode of diagnosis of infection in the pregnant woman and of congenital infection in the newborn infant is based on clinical signs and symptoms. Careful examination may be sufficient to suggest a diagnosis, particularly when typical signs and symptoms are accompanied by a well-documented history of exposure (see Tables 1–6 and 1–7).

Asymptomatic or Subclinical Infection. Many infectious diseases with serious consequences for the fetus are difficult or impossible to diagnose in the mother solely on clinical grounds. These asymptomatic, or subclinical, infections include the following as causes: rubella virus, CMV, *T. gondii*, HSV, and HIV. The vast majority of women infected during pregnancy with these organisms have no apparent signs of disease; only 50% of women infected with rubella virus have a rash, and although occasional cases of CMV mononucleosis are recognized, these make up a very small proportion of women who are infected during pregnancy. Similarly, the number of women with clinical manifestations of toxoplasmosis is less than 10%, and few women have systemic illness associated with primary HSV infection. The genital lesions of infections related to HSV and syphilis may go unrecognized because of their location.

Recurrent and Chronic Infection. Some organisms

may infect an individual more than once, and when such reinfections take place in a pregnant woman, the organism may affect the fetus.[36] These reinfections are generally associated with waning host immunity, but low levels of circulating antibody may be detectable. Such antibody would be expected to provide some protection against hematogenous spread and transplacental infection. Fetal disease, however, has followed reexposure of immune mothers to vaccinia,[58] variola,[59] and rubella[60] viruses.

In addition, an agent capable of persisting in the mother as a chronic asymptomatic infection could infect the fetus long after the initial infection had occurred. Reports of infection of the fetus as a result of such chronic infection of the mother have been cited in cases of malaria,[61] T. gondii infection,[62] syphilis,[63] hepatitis,[64] herpes zoster,[29] and herpes simplex.[65] Congenital CMV and HIV infections have been observed in infants from consecutive pregnancies of the same mother. In the case of T. gondii, congenital transmission from the chronically infected woman occurs almost solely when the woman is immunocompromised during gestation.

Preconceptional Infection. Acute infection immediately before conception may result in infection of the fetus, and the association may go unrecognized. Congenital rubella has occurred in the fetus in cases in which the mother was infected 3 weeks to 3 months before conception. A prolonged viremia or persistence of virus in the maternal tissues may be responsible for infection of the embryo or fetus. The same has occurred rarely in cases of maternal infection with T. gondii.[66]

ISOLATION AND IDENTIFICATION OF THE INFECTIOUS AGENT

Routine and Special Diagnostic Tests for Infection. Diagnostic tests for microorganisms or infectious diseases are part of routine obstetric care; special care is warranted for selected patients who are known or suspected to be exposed to the infectious agent or have clinical signs of the infectious disease. A list of diagnostic tests and the types of intervention that may be required if a diagnosis is made is provided in Table 1–8. The specific interventions for each disease are provided in subsequent chapters.

The most direct mode of diagnosis is isolation of the microbial agent from tissues and body fluids such as blood, cerebrospinal fluid, or urine. Isolation of the agent must be considered with knowledge of its epidemiology and natural history in the host. For example, isolation of an enterovirus from feces during the summer months may represent colonization rather than significant infection that might result in hematogenous spread to the fetus. Isolation of an enterovirus from a body

TABLE 1–8
Management of Infections in the Pregnant Woman[a]

MICROORGANISM OR DISEASE	DIAGNOSTIC TEST	First Visit	Third Trimester	At Delivery	Intervention[a]
Routine Care					
Mycobacterium tuberculosis	Purified protein derivative	+			Therapy
Gonorrhea	Culture	+	+		Therapy
Hepatitis B	Serology	+			—[b]
Chlamydia	Antigen	+	+		Therapy
Syphilis	Serology	+	+	+[c]	Therapy
Rubella	Serology	+			Postpartum vaccine
Group B Streptococcus	Culture or antigen		+	+[d]	Intrapartum therapy
Herpes simplex	Examination	+	+	+	Cesarean section
	Culture				Therapy
Special Care If Exposed or with Clinical Signs					
Human immunodeficiency virus (HIV)	Serology				Therapy
Parvovirus	Ultrasound				Intrauterine transfusion
	Serology				
Toxoplasmosis	Serology				Therapy
	Polymerase chain reaction (PCR)				
	Culture (amniotic fluid, fetal blood)				
Varicella-zoster virus	Cytology				VZIG[e]
					Therapy

[a] See appropriate chapters.
[b] Hepatitis B immune globulin for neonate.
[c] At delivery in areas with high prevalence of infection.
[d] Intrapartum culture for women with risk features.
[e] Varicella-zoster immune globulin (VZIG) following exposure of the susceptible patient.
Modified from table prepared by Riley L, Fetter S, Geller D, Boston City Hospital and Boston University School of Medicine.

fluid in which it is never present under normal circumstances or identification of a significant rise in antibody titer would be necessary to define an acute infectious process.

Tests for the presence of hepatitis B virus surface antigen (HB₅Ag) should be performed in all pregnant women. The Centers for Disease Control and Prevention has estimated that 16,500 births occur each year in the United States to women who are positive for HB₅Ag. Infants born to mothers who are positive for this antigen have up to a 90% chance of acquiring perinatal hepatitis B virus infection. If infection is identified soon after birth, use of hepatitis B immune globulin combined with hepatitis B vaccine is an effective mode of prevention of infection. For these reasons, the Advisory Committee on Immunization Practices of the U.S. Public Health Service[67] and the American Academy of Pediatrics[67a] recommend universal screening of all pregnant women for HB₅Ag.

Amniocentesis and the analysis of desquamated fetal cells have been used for the early diagnosis of chromosomal and metabolic disorders. Because the amniotic fluid contains viruses or bacteria shed from the placenta, skin, urine, or tracheal fluid of the infected fetus, studies of such fluid to recover the infecting organism or immunofluorescent staining of exfoliated cells may prove valuable in confirming suspected intrauterine infection. Isolation of CMV[68] or rubella virus[69] and demonstration of HB₅Ag[70] from amniotic fluid obtained by amniocentesis have been reported.[71]

The PCR technique has proved to be both sensitive and specific for diagnosis of many of these infections in the pregnant woman, fetus, and newborn. Thus, detection of the DNA/RNA of an organism has, in many instances, replaced the necessity for its isolation to make a definitive diagnosis. The PCR method is rapidly becoming more available to physicians in primary care practice and will markedly decrease the time to diagnosis of many of these infectious agents, as exemplified by the prenatal diagnosis of infections caused by parvovirus,[72, 73] CMV,[74–76] T. gondii,[77] and rubella[78] by PCR.[79, 80]

The sentinel publication in 1983 by Daffos and colleagues,[81] in which fetal blood sampling for prenatal diagnosis was first described, provided a method for diagnosing a variety of infections in the fetus that previously could only be diagnosed after birth. Their methods were widely adopted and have contributed significantly to our understanding of both the immune response of the fetus to a variety of pathogens, including rubella virus, varicella virus, CMV, and T. gondii,[71, 82–86] and a more objective approach to treatment of infection in the fetus before birth. Fetal blood sampling and amniocentesis are performed under ultrasound guidance. The method is not free of risk in that amniocentesis alone carries a risk of complications as high as 1%.[87, 88] Amniotic fluid may be examined for the presence of the infecting organism, its antigens, or its nucleic acid. Fetal blood can be examined for the same parameters as well as to detect antibodies formed by the fetus against the pathogen (e.g., IgA or IgM antibodies that do not normally cross the placental barrier). Fetal blood sampling is usually performed during or after the eighteenth week

of gestation. The fetus that is diagnosed as being infected with a specific pathogen or that is at high risk for infection (e.g., the fetus of a non-immune woman who acquires her infection with T. gondii or rubella virus during gestation) may be followed by ultrasound to detect abnormalities such as development of dilation of the cerebral ventricles. Although fetal blood sampling is still performed in some situations, it has largely been supplanted by PCR on amniotic fluid.

Cytologic and Histologic Diagnosis. Review of cytology and sections of tissue may provide a presumptive diagnosis of certain infections. As examples, cervicovaginal smears or cell scrapings from the base of vesicles are valuable in diagnosing VZV and HSV infections. Typical changes include multinucleated giant cells and intranuclear inclusions. Diagnosis of VZV, HSV, and CMV infection may also be accomplished by electron microscopy and direct immunofluorescence techniques as well as by immunoperoxidase staining. The urine sediment should be examined for the presence of intranuclear inclusions in epithelial cells when CMV infection is suspected. The diagnosis of acute toxoplasmosis can be made from the characteristic histologic changes in lymph nodes or by demonstration of the tachyzoite in tissue specimens obtained by biopsy of infected tissues or at autopsy.

Detailed descriptions of the changes associated with infections of the placenta are presented in a monograph by Fox.[88a] Examination of the placental parenchyma, the membranes, and the cord may provide valuable information leading to diagnosis of the infection and distinguishing the mode of transmission to the fetus (in utero or ascending infection).

Serologic Diagnosis. The serologic diagnosis of infection in the pregnant woman most often requires demonstration of a significant rise in antibody titer against the agent suspected of causing illness. Ideally, the physician should have available information about the serologic status of the woman at the onset of pregnancy to identify those who are unprotected against *Treponema pallidum*, T. gondii, and rubella virus or who are infected with hepatitis B virus or HIV. This valuable procedure has already been adopted by many obstetricians.

Difficulties in interpretation of serologic test results seldom arise when patients are seen shortly after exposure or at the onset of symptoms. However, the relatively rapid increase in antibody levels that may accompany certain infections (e.g., rubella and toxoplasmosis) may preclude the demonstration of a significant rise in titer in patients who are tested more than 7 days after the onset of the suspected illness. A diagnosis may be obtained in these circumstances through the measurement of antibodies that rise more slowly over a period of several weeks. Identification of the usefulness of demonstration of IgA and IgE antibodies (in addition to the more conventional use of tests for IgG and IgM antibodies) for the early diagnosis of infection in the pregnant woman, fetus, and newborn should serve as an impetus to commercial firms to make these methods available for use by health care providers as soon as possible. The same pertains to IgG avidity tests. For example, the latter have proven accurate in ruling out recently acquired infection with *T. gondii*. IgG avidity tests for other infections, for example, CMV, are being developed. Because, at present, these tests require special techniques and are not performed routinely by most laboratories, local or state health departments should be consulted for further information regarding their availability.

The U.S. Public Health Service[67] and the American Academy of Pediatrics[67a] recommend universal screening of all pregnant women for Hb$_s$Ag. The screening recommendation is part of a comprehensive program to reduce the burden of hepatitis B infection by immunization of high-risk children and all infants.

Use of Skin Tests. Routine skin tests for diagnosis of tuberculosis should be considered a part of prenatal care. Skin-testing antigens, including those for tuberculosis and other mycobacteria, may be administered to the mother without risk to the fetus.

UNIVERSAL SCREENING

Prenatal care includes routine screening for serologic evidence of syphilis and rubella; culture or antigen evidence of *Chlamydia* infection, group B streptococci, hepatitis B virus, and urinary tract pathogens, and skin test for tuberculosis. The demonstration that treatment of the HIV-infected mother significantly reduces the transmission of the virus to the fetus has led to recommendations for universal HIV screening for all pregnant women in the United States, but the method of implementing such a program is controversial. A Congressionally mandated study by a committee of the Institute of Medicine reported in October 1998 that HIV testing as part of routine prenatal care would more than pay for itself by reducing the cost of management of infected children.[89] Most medical authorities support programs coupling counseling education about HIV infection with serologic testing, and some states have passed legislation that mandates counseling and testing for all pregnant women.[90] Although mandatory testing for pregnant women has been suggested, most experts believe such a program would discourage women from seeking prenatal care and thereby would decrease the number of women tested.[91] At present, pregnant women diagnosed as having been infected with HIV should have CD4$^+$ counts and viral load measured at the first prenatal visit. These should be repeated at least once during the second and third trimesters and more often when needed to assess the response to treatment. Other tests, such as those for β$_2$-microglobulin and serum neopterin, are used by some physicians to assist in predicting the progression of HIV infection. Pregnant women should be examined carefully for the presence of HIV-related infections including gonorrhea, syphilis, and *Chlamydia*. Baseline antibody titers should be obtained for those opportunistic infections, such as *T. gondii*, which are observed commonly in HIV-infected women and which may be transmitted to their fetuses.

DIAGNOSIS OF FETAL INFECTION

Infants with congenital infection due to rubella virus, CMV, HSV, *T. gondii*, or *T. pallidum* may present simi-

larly with one or more of the following signs: purpura, jaundice, hepatosplenomegaly, pneumonitis, and meningoencephalitis. Some signs have specific diagnostic significance (see Tables 1–5 and 1–6).

In selected congenital infections the organism may be isolated from tissues and body fluids. Infants may excrete CMV and rubella in the urine for weeks to months after birth. *T. pallidum* may be found in the cerebrospinal fluid, in nasal secretions, and in the rash of syphilis. HIV culture or PCR is positive at birth in approximately 30 to 50% of congenitally infected infants but nearly 100% of infected infants are positive by 4 to 6 months of life.

Serologic tests are available through state or commercial laboratories for the TORCH group of microorganisms (*T. gondii*, rubella virus, CMV, and HSV) and for other congenitally acquired infections such as *T. pallidum*. To distinguish passively transferred maternal antibody from antibody derived from infection in the neonate, it is necessary to obtain two blood specimens from the infant. Because the half-life of IgG is 23 days, the first sample is obtained soon after birth, and the second sample should be obtained at least two half-lives or approximately 6 weeks after the first specimen. IgM antibodies do not cross the placenta. Measurement of IgM antibody provides evidence of current infection in the neonate, but few commercial laboratories supply reliable assays for IgM for congenital infections, as described in a Public Health Advisory from the Food and Drug Administration outlining the limitations of *Toxoplasma* IgM commercial test kits.[92]

Although most congenital infections occur as a single entity, many mothers who are HIV positive are co-infected with other infectious agents that may be transmitted to the newborn. The neonate born to an HIV-infected mother should be considered at risk for other sexually transmitted infections such as syphilis, gonorrhea, and *Chlamydia*. In addition co-infection has been documented for CMV.[93, 94]

Prevention and Management of Infection in the Pregnant Woman

PREVENTION OF INFECTION

Pregnant women should avoid contact with persons with communicable diseases, particularly if the women are known to be seronegative or have no prior history of exposure to the disease. In some cases, specific measures can be taken. The pregnant woman should avoid intercourse with her sexual partner if he has a vesicular lesion on the penis that may be due to HSV or if he is known or suspected to be infected with HIV. Pregnant women should avoid eating raw or undercooked lamb, pork, and beef because such products sometimes contain *T. gondii*. Such women should also avoid contact with cat feces or objects or materials contaminated with cat feces because these are highly infectious if they harbor *T. gondii* oocysts (see Chapter 5).

IMMUNIZATION

Routine immunization schedules for children with currently available live vaccines, including measles, poliomyelitis, mumps, and rubella, should confer protection against these infections throughout the childbearing years.

There is general agreement among public health authorities and obstetricians on the following issues as to immunization of the pregnant woman[95]:

1. Inactivated vaccines, such as those available for influenza and typhoid fever as well as tetanus and diphtheria toxoids, are not considered hazardous to the pregnant woman or her fetus and may often be of major benefit. One example is the use of tetanus toxoid in areas in which infection has significant risks for the newborn.

2. As a general rule, live vaccines should not be given to pregnant women. However, live polio virus vaccine may be considered for unprotected pregnant women if exposure is significant and unavoidable but only if inactivated vaccine is not available.

A report of IgM antibodies to yellow fever in the infant of a woman immunized during pregnancy suggests that transplacental transmission of the yellow fever vaccine virus does occur, although the incidence of congenital infection is unknown.[96]

Varicella vaccine should not be administered to pregnant women, because the possible effects on fetal development are unknown. When postpubertal females are immunized, pregnancy should be avoided for at least 1 month following immunization. Merck and Company has established a varicella vaccine pregnancy registry for women who were inadvertently immunized when pregnant (telephone: 800-986-8999).

3. Because several weeks may elapse before pregnancy is evident, there is also need for caution and selectivity in administering a live virus vaccine to any woman of childbearing age. The demonstration of prolonged virus shedding after immunization with live virus vaccine suggests that pregnancy should be avoided when possible for 2 to 3 months subsequent to the administration of any live immunizing agent.

4. The risk to the mother or fetus from immunization of members of her immediate family or other intimate contacts is uncertain. The use of attenuated measles, rubella, mumps, and varicella vaccines rarely results in dissemination of these viruses to susceptible subjects in the immediate environment, but household spread of attenuated polioviruses through contact with recently vaccinated, susceptible individuals in the family is common. Because the varicella vaccine virus may be transmitted to susceptible contacts, although at a very low rate, some experts would defer immunization of the child in the household of a susceptible pregnant woman until the third trimester or after delivery.

USE OF IMMUNE GLOBULIN

Human immune serum globulin administered after exposure to rubella, varicella, measles, or hepatitis A virus may prevent or modify clinical signs and symptoms of the disease but has not proved to be consistently effective in preventing disease, and presumably viremia, in susceptible persons. Human immune serum globulin is

therefore of undetermined value in protecting the fetus of a susceptible woman against infection with these viruses. Its use after maternal exposure to rubella virus should be limited to women to whom, in the event of documented infection during pregnancy, therapeutic abortion is unacceptable.

CHEMOTHERAPY

Almost without exception, antimicrobial agents administered systemically to the mother pass to the fetus. Management of pregnant women with acute infections amenable to therapy should be the same as that of nonpregnant patients but with attention paid to the possible effects on the fetus of the antimicrobial drug. The pregnant woman with recently acquired acute toxoplasmosis, Lyme disease, and syphilis should be treated as outlined in the specific chapters devoted to those topics. Women who are colonized with *Chlamydia trachomatis* or group B streptococci may be treated under selected circumstances and are considered in the next section. Of importance are the recent data documenting reduction of maternal-infant transmission of HIV with the administration of zidovudine.[97] Zidovudine therapy of selected HIV-infected pregnant women (those who had peripheral CD4+ T lymphocyte counts of more than 200 cells/μL and were mildly symptomatic) reduced in utero transmission by about two thirds (8.3% vs. 25.5%). The currently recommended treatment regimen is oral zidovudine to pregnant women beginning at 14 to 34 weeks' gestation and continuing throughout pregnancy, intravenous zidovudine during labor and delivery, and oral zidovudine to the newborn for the first 6 weeks of life.[98]

INFECTIONS ACQUIRED BY THE NEWBORN INFANT DURING BIRTH

Pathogenesis

The developing fetus is protected from the microbial flora of the maternal genital tract. Initial colonization of the newborn and of the placenta usually occurs after rupture of maternal membranes. If delivery is delayed after membranes rupture, the vaginal microflora may ascend and in some cases produce inflammation of fetal membranes, umbilical cord, and placenta. Fetal infection may also result from aspiration of infected amniotic fluid. Some viruses are present in the genital secretions (HSV, CMV, hepatitis B virus, or HIV) or blood (hepatitis B virus or HIV). If delivery follows shortly after rupture of the membranes, the infant may be colonized during passage through the birth canal. The variety of microorganisms that may be present in the maternal birth canal is indicated in Table 1–8 and includes gram-positive cocci (staphylococci and streptococci), gram-negative cocci (*Neisseria meningitidis* and *Neisseria gonorrhoeae*), gram-negative enteric bacilli (*E. coli*, *Proteus* sp., *Klebsiella* sp., *Pseudomonas* sp., *Salmonella*, and *Shigella*), anaerobic bacteria, viruses (CMV, HSV, rubella virus, and HIV), fungi, chlamydiae, mycoplasmas, and protozoa (*Trichomonas vaginalis* and *T. gondii*). As indicated in Table 1–8, some of these organisms are significantly associated with disease in the newborn infant, whereas others affect the neonate rarely, if at all.

The newborn is initially colonized on the skin and mucosal surfaces, including the nasopharynx, oropharynx, conjunctivae, umbilical cord, and external genitalia. In most infants, the organisms proliferate at these sites without causing illness. A few infants become infected by direct extension from the sites of colonization (e.g., sinusitis and otitis from nasopharyngeal colonization). Alternatively, invasion of the bloodstream may ensue, with subsequent dissemination of infection. The umbilical cord is a particularly common portal of entry for systemic infection because the devitalized tissues are an excellent medium for bacterial growth and because the recently thrombosed umbilical vessels provide direct access to the bloodstream. Microorganisms may also infect abrasions or skin wounds.

Infants who develop bacterial sepsis may have certain risk factors not evident in infants who do not develop significant infections. Among these factors are low birth weight, premature and prolonged rupture of maternal membranes, septic or traumatic delivery, fetal anoxia, and maternal peripartum infection. Relative immaturity of the immune system is considered to be one cause of increased risk of infection during the neonatal period. The immunology of the neonate is further discussed in Chapter 2.

Prematurity is the most important risk feature for infections acquired at birth and in the nursery. The increasing number of very low birth weight infants has increased concern for infection as a cause of morbidity and mortality. In addition, multiple births with a high incidence of low-birth-weight infants are common following various modalities for treatment of infertility. A survey of 114 infants in Cleveland with birth weights of 500 to 750 g between 1990 and 1992 identified an overall mortality of 57%. Immaturity was the predominant cause of death, but septicemia was responsible for death in 9%; septicemia occurred in 53% of survivors.[99]

The value of certain defense mechanisms is still widely debated. Vernix caseosa has no specific antibacterial properties, but retention of vernix is probably of value because it provides a protective coating to the skin. Breast milk influences the composition of the fecal flora by suppression of *E. coli* and other gram-negative enteric bacilli and encouragement of growth of lactobacilli. In addition, breast milk contains secretory IgA, lysozymes, white blood cells, and lactoferrin (an iron-binding protein that significantly inhibits the growth of *E. coli* and other microorganisms); however, the importance of these constituents for colonization and systemic infection in the neonate is uncertain (see Chapter 4).

The usual predominance of males in most series of neonates with sepsis acquired during delivery or during the newborn period has suggested a sex-linked factor in host susceptibility. In contrast to perinatal infection, the incidence of intrauterine infection is equal for males and females (see Chapter 21).

The virulence of the invading microorganism must also be considered as a factor in the pathogenesis of neonatal sepsis. As an example, certain phage types of *S. aureus* (types 80 and 81 in particular) were responsible for most disease in the staphylococcal pandemic of the 1950s. More recently, strains of *S. aureus* of phage group 2 have been responsible for the scalded skin syndrome (toxic epidermal necrolysis). Another example is evidence suggesting that the K1 capsular antigens of some strains of *E. coli* may be related to virulence.

Microbiology

The agents responsible for neonatal sepsis are those usually found in the maternal birth canal.[100, 101] Most of these organisms are considered to be saprophytic, but on occasion they may be responsible for maternal infection, including endometritis, septic abortion, and puerperal fever. The microbial flora of the adult female genital tract and its association with neonatal infection and disease are presented in Table 1–9.

Before the introduction of the sulfonamides and penicillin, gram-positive cocci, particularly group A streptococci, were responsible for most cases of neonatal sepsis. After the introduction of antimicrobial agents, gram-negative bacilli were the predominant causes of serious bacterial infections of the newborn. An increase in serious neonatal infection caused by group B streptococci has been noted in hospitals throughout the United States. Currently, group B streptococci and *E. coli* are the most important causative agents of neonatal sepsis. The bacteria responsible for neonatal sepsis are discussed in Chapter 21.

Mycoplasmas, anaerobic bacteria, and viruses (including HSV, hepatitis B virus, CMV, and HIV) that colonize the maternal genital tract are also acquired during birth.

Diagnosis

Review of the maternal record provides important clues for diagnosis of infection in the neonate. Signs of illnesses during pregnancy, exposures to sexual partners with transmissible infections, and results of cultures, serologic and skin tests, and chest radiographs should be reviewed from the record of the pregnancy. The delivery chart should be checked for peripartum events that indicate risk of sepsis in the neonate, including premature rupture of membranes, prolonged duration of rupture of membranes, evidence of fetal distress and fever or other signs of maternal infection, indications of large concentrations of pathogens in the genitalia (as reflected in urinary tract infection due to group B streptococci), and evidence of invasive bacterial infections in prior pregnancies.

The clinical diagnosis of systemic infection in the newborn may be difficult. The initial signs of infection may be subtle and nonspecific. Not only may the signs of infectious and noninfectious processes be similar, but also the signs of in utero infection may be indistinguishable from those of infections acquired during the birth process or subsequently, during the first few days of life. Respiratory distress, lethargy, poor feeding, jaundice,

TABLE 1–9

Association of Neonatal Disease with Microorganisms Present in the Maternal Birth Canal

	ASSOCIATION WITH NEONATAL DISEASE		
	Significant	Uncommon	Rare or None
Bacteria			
Lactobacillus			+
Staphylococcus epidermidis			+
Staphylococcus aureus		+	
Alpha-Hemolytic			
Streptococcus		+	
Group A *Streptococcus*	+		
Group B *Streptococcus*	+		
Group D *Streptococcus*			
Enterococcus	+		
Escherichia coli	+		
Proteus sp.		+	
Klebsiella sp.		+	
Pseudomonas sp.		+	
Salmonella sp.		+	
Shigella sp.		+	
Alkaligenes faecalis		+	
Neisseria meningitidis		+	
Neisseria gonorrhoeae	+		
Haemophilus influenzae		+	
Haemophilus parainfluenzae		+	
Haemophilus vaginalis		+	
Listeria monocytogenes	+		
Vibrio fetus		+	
Corynebacterium			+
Bacillus subtilis			+
Anaerobic Bacteria[100]			
Bacteroides		+	
Peptostreptococcus			+
Veillonella			+
Clostridium sp.		+	
Bifidobacterium			+
Eubacterium			+
Mycobacterium tuberculosis			+
Viruses			
Cytomegalovirus	+		
Herpes simplex (type 2)	+		
Rubella			+
Hepatitis B	+		
Human papillomavirus			+
Lymphocytic choriomeningitis virus			+
Human immunodeficiency virus		+	
Fungi			
Candida albicans	+		
Torulopsis glabrata			+
Coccidioides immitis		+	
Saccharomyces			+
Chlamydiaceae			
Chlamydia trachomatis	+		
Mycoplasmataceae			
Mycoplasma hominis		+	
Ureaplasma urealyticum		+	
Protozoa			
Toxoplasma gondii		+	
Trichomonas vaginalis		+	

vomiting, and diarrhea may be associated with a variety of infectious and noninfectious causes.

Some clinical manifestations, such as hepatomegaly, jaundice, pneumonitis, purpura, and meningoencephalitis, are common to many of the infections that are acquired in utero or during delivery. However, some signs are related to specific infections (see Tables 1–6 and 1–7). Many signs of congenital infection are not evident at birth: hepatitis B infection should be considered in the infant with onset of jaundice and hepatosplenomegaly between 1 and 6 months of age; CMV infection acquired at or soon after delivery is associated with an afebrile protracted pneumonitis; enterovirus infection should be considered in the infant with acute central nervous system findings and pleocytosis in the first months of life. Most infants with congenital HIV infection do not have signs of disease during the first months of life. Uncommonly, signs may be present at birth. Srugo and colleagues[102] described an infant with signs of meningoencephalitis at 6 hours of life; HIV was isolated from cerebrospinal fluid.

Focal infections, including pneumonia, otitis, soft tissue infections, urinary tract infections, septic arthritis, osteomyelitis, and peritonitis, may occur in the neonate. Bacterial meningitis is of particular concern because of the high mortality rate and the significant morbidity in survivors. Few infants have overt meningeal signs, and a high index of suspicion is required for early diagnosis.

Routine laboratory methods now available are of limited assistance in the diagnosis of systemic infections in the newborn infant. In bacterial sepsis, the total white blood cell count is variable and supports a diagnosis of bacterial sepsis only if it is high (more than 30,000 cells per mm^3) or very low (fewer than 5000 cells per mm^3). Immunoglobulin is produced by the fetus and newborn infant in response to infection. Increased levels of IgM have been measured in the serum of newborns with infections (i.e., syphilis, rubella, cytomegalic inclusion disease, toxoplasmosis, and malaria) acquired transplacentally. Increased levels of IgM also result from postnatally acquired bacterial infections. But not all infected infants have increased levels of serum IgM, and some infants who do have elevated concentrations of total IgM are apparently uninfected. Thus, identification of increased levels of total IgM in the newborn is suggestive of an infectious process acquired before or shortly after birth, but it is not specific and is of limited assistance in diagnosis and management.

Because inflammation of the placenta and umbilical cord may accompany peripartum sepsis, pathologic sections of these tissues may assist in the diagnosis of infection in the newborn. However, histologic evidence of inflammation is also noted in the absence of sepsis and therefore is not a specific sign of infection. In the immediate postnatal period, gastric aspirate, pharyngeal mucus, or fluid from the external ear canal has been used to assist in the diagnosis of bacterial infection. These materials are smeared, stained, and examined for polymorphonuclear leukocytes and bacteria. The presence of microorganisms and polymorphonuclear leukocytes indicates probable exposure to a significant infectious source and may be of diagnostic value in some infants with suspected bacterial sepsis.

Isolation of microorganisms from a significant focus, such as blood, cerebrospinal fluid, skin vesicle fluid, a suppurative lesion, or a properly obtained sample of urine, remains the most valid method of diagnosing systemic infection. Aspiration of any focus of infection in a critically ill infant (e.g., needle aspiration of middle ear fluid in an infant with otitis media or from the lung of an infant with pneumonia) should be considered to obtain the etiologic organism. Infectious agents cultured from the nose, throat, skin, umbilicus, or stool indicate colonization and may include the pathogens that are responsible for the disease but in themselves do not establish the presence of active systemic infection.

Antigen identification (latex agglutination, counterimmunoelectrophoresis for group B streptococci and *Pneumocystis carinii*, PCR for a variety of important pathogens, enzyme immunoassay for *T. gondii*) and use of electron microscopy (CMV and rotaviruses) are now available. Evidence of the microorganism should be sought in blood and other body fluids and may be of particular value if antimicrobial agents had been administered previously to mother or infant.

When appropriate, serologic studies should be performed to ascertain the presence of in utero or postnatal infection. Serologic tests are available through state or federal laboratories for the TORCH group of microorganisms and for other agents, such as *T. pallidum*. In most laboratories, these serologic tests measure IgG. To distinguish passively transferred maternal antibody from antibody derived from infection in the neonate, it is necessary to obtain two blood specimens from the infant. Because the half-life of IgG is 23 days, the first sample is obtained soon after birth, and the second sample should be obtained at least two half-lives or approximately 6 weeks after the first specimen. Measurement of IgM antibody provides evidence of current infection in the neonate, but the only assay of proven reliability at present is that for *T. gondii*.

Management

Successful management of neonatal bacterial sepsis depends on early diagnosis and prompt initiation of appropriate antimicrobial therapy and supportive measures. If the physician considers a newborn to be septic, cultures should be taken and treatment with antibiotics should be started immediately. In general, initial therapy must include coverage for gram-positive cocci, particularly group B streptococci and gram-negative enteric bacilli. A penicillin is the choice for gram-positive cocci. Choice of therapy for gram-negative infections depends on the current pattern of antibiotic susceptibility in the local hospital. Most experts prefer ampicillin and gentamicin as therapy for presumptive sepsis and ampicillin and cefotaxime for presumptive bacterial meningitis.[103] Intrapartum therapy results in concentrations of drug in the blood of the newborn infant that may suppress growth of group B streptococci in blood obtained for culture. The inability to use the culture of blood for microbiologic diagnosis has placed a substantial burden on the clinician. Although various algorithms have been prepared to guide empirical management of the neonate born to a mother who received intrapartum antimicrobial prophylaxis for prevention of early-onset group B streptococcal infection,[104] management of these infants may be categorized into three groups: (1) infants who have signs of sepsis should receive a full diagnostic evaluation and should be treated; (2) infants who are term, do not have clinical signs of sepsis, and whose mothers received two or more doses of antibiotic before delivery do not have to be evaluated or treated but should be observed for 48 hours; and (3) infants who do not have signs of sepsis but who are younger than 35 weeks' gestation and whose mothers received only one dose of antibiotic should be observed for 48 hours or more and should receive a limited evaluation, including white blood cell count and differential and culture of blood. The first two categories are readily identified, but the third often leads to concern because of the vague end points. Recent recommendations for prevention and treatment of early-onset group B streptococcal infection are discussed in Chapter 26.

The choice of antibacterial drugs should be reviewed when results of cultures and susceptibility tests become available. The duration of therapy depends on the initial response to the appropriate antibiotics but should be 7 to 10 days in most infants with sepsis, pneumonia, or minimal or absent focal infection; the minimal duration of therapy for meningitis caused by group B streptococci or gram-negative enteric bacilli is 21 days.

The clinical pharmacology of antibiotics administered to the newborn infant is unique and cannot be extrapolated from the data of absorption, excretion, and toxicity in the adult. The safety of new antimicrobial agents is a particular concern because toxic effects may not be detected until several years later (see Chapter 35).

Development of resistance of microbial pathogens to antimicrobial agents is a constant concern. Group B streptococci remain uniformly susceptible to penicillins and cephalosporins (with the exception of a few strains relatively resistant to cefoxitin), but some isolates are resistant to erythromycin and clindamycin.[105] The few doses of a penicillin administered as part of peripartum prophylactic regimen for prevention of group B streptococcal infection in the neonate would not be expected to significantly affect the genital flora, but surveillance for alteration in the flora and antibiotic susceptibility should be maintained. A case report of penicillin-resistant *Streptococcus pneumoniae* responsible for an intrauterine fetal death in the second half of pregnancy underlines concern about antibiotic resistance in infections in the pregnant woman.[106] Because the nursery is a small, closed community, development of resistance is a greater concern for iatrogenic infections than infections acquired in utero or at delivery.

Despite the use of appropriate antimicrobial agents and optimal supportive therapy, mortality from neonatal sepsis remains high. With the hope of improving survival and decreasing the severity of sequelae in survivors, investigators have turned their attention to studies of adjunctive modes of treatment that provide materials for the demonstrated deficits in the host defenses of the infected neonate. These therapies include use of granulocyte transfusion, exchange transfusion, and standard and modified hyperimmune immunoglobulins.

Antiviral therapies are now available for treatment of newborns infected with HSV (acyclovir and vidarabine), VZV (acyclovir), and HIV (zidovudine). Acyclovir and zidovudine are well tolerated in the pregnant woman.[107] Because early use of acyclovir or vidarabine for herpes simplex infections in neonates appears associated with improved outcome, physicians may choose to begin therapy for presumptive disease due to HSV and reevaluate therapy when results of cultures are known and more information is available about the clinical course.

The results of a phase II trial of safety and pharmacodynamics of ganciclovir treatment of symptomatic congenital CMV infection was reported by Whitley and colleagues.[108] Neutropenia, thrombocytopenia, and altered hepatic enzymes were noted in the majority of children. Although uncontrolled, the data suggested decreased mortality and morbidity in this group of severely affected children.

Prevention

IMMUNOPROPHYLAXIS

Immune globulins may be valuable for prevention of certain infections that occur during the neonatal period. Zoster immune globulin is effective in the prevention or the attenuation of neonatal varicella. Hepatitis B immune globulin is effective for the interruption of perinatal transmission of hepatitis B virus carrier state. Intravenous immune globulin (IGIV) reduced the number of first infections in low-birth-weight premature infants and delayed development of such infections in a recent multicenter study.[109] The results have not been corroborated by other investigators, and appropriate use of IGIV remains to be determined.

Use of a vaccine prepared from purified capsular polysaccharide of various types of group B streptococci has been investigated. In addition, cross-reactivity between type III group B streptococcus and type 14 pneumococcus (contained in the pneumococcal vaccine) has been demonstrated and may provide a mode of prevention of streptococcal infection in the neonate by use of pneumococcal vaccine in susceptible mothers (see Chapter 26).

Universal immunization of infants with hepatitis B vaccine was recommended by the American Academy of Pediatrics in April 1992.[110] Prior selective strategies of vaccination of high-risk populations and serologic screening of all pregnant women for HB$_s$Ag had little impact on control of hepatitis B infections or their sequelae, and public health authorities believe that infant immunization offers the most feasible approach to protection of all persons and eventual elimination of the disease. Infants born to HB$_s$Ag-positive women should receive hepatitis B immune globulin at or shortly after birth and should be immunized at birth.

CHEMOPROPHYLAXIS

Antimicrobial agents capable of crossing biologic membranes can achieve concentrations of drug in the fetus comparable to concentrations in other well-vascularized tissues after administration to the mother. Prevention of group B streptococcal infection in the newborn by administration of ampicillin to the mother was demonstrated by Boyer and colleagues[111] and other investigators as early as 1983 (see Chapter 30). A protocol for usage of the prophylactic regimen was presented in 1992 by the American College of Obstetrics and Gynecology[112] and the American Academy of Pediatrics.[113] These guidelines were revised in 1996 by the Centers for Disease Control and Prevention[99] and in 1997 by the American Academy of Pediatrics,[104] and additional revisions have been suggested.[114] Concentrations of drug are achieved in the fetus that are more than 30% of the concentrations in the blood of the mother[115] (see Chapter 35). Parenteral antibiotic therapy administered to the mother in labor is essentially treating the fetus earlier in the course of the intrapartum infection. If the fetus has been infected, the regimen is treatment, not prophylaxis, and for some infected fetuses the treatment administered in utero will be insufficient to prevent early-onset group B streptococcal disease.[116] Although the prophylactic regimen has decreased the incidence of early-onset group B streptococcal disease (by more than 80% in a Pittsburgh survey[117]), the regimen has had no impact on the incidence of late-onset disease.

Other modes of chemoprophylaxis administered to the neonate are the use of ophthalmic drops or ointments for prevention of gonococcal ophthalmitis and the administration of zidovudine to the infant born to the HIV-infected mother. Usage of antibacterial agents for infants with minimal or ambiguous clinical signs is therapy for presumed sepsis and should not be considered prophylaxis.

INFECTIONS OF THE NEWBORN INFANT IN THE FIRST MONTH OF LIFE

When fever or other signs of systemic infection occur in the first weeks or months of life, appropriate management requires consideration of the various sources of infection. Five types of such infection based on source can be recognized: (1) congenital infections with onset in utero; (2) infections acquired during the birth process from the maternal genital tract; (3) infections acquired in the nursery; (4) infections acquired in the household after discharge from the nursery; and (5) infection that highlights an anatomic defect, physiologic disability, or metabolic abnormality.

Pathogenesis and Microbiology

CONGENITAL INFECTIONS

Signs of congenital infection may not appear for weeks, months, or years following birth. Diagnosis and management are discussed in the disease chapters.

INFECTIONS ACQUIRED DURING DELIVERY

Although peripartum prophylaxis has reduced the incidence of early-onset group B streptococcal disease, the regimen has not altered the incidence of late-onset disease, with signs occurring after 4 to 7 days of life. The pathogenesis of late-onset group B streptococcal diseases remains obscure. Why an infant without risk features for sepsis remains well for days to weeks and without warning develops sepsis with or without meningitis remains a mystery. Even more perplexing is the occurrence of late-onset disease in infants whose mothers received intrapartum ampicillin or infants who received two or more days of therapy for suspected sepsis following delivery. It is possible the organism was acquired at the time of delivery and not eradicated from a mucosal site by the antibiotic regimen or that the infant was reinfected in the nursery by personnel or other infants or in the home by the colonized mother. Similar late-onset disease has been identified in cases of sepsis due to *E. coli* and *Listeria monocytogenes*.

NURSERY-ACQUIRED INFECTIONS

After arrival in the nursery, the newborn may become infected by various pathways involving either human carriers or contaminated materials and equipment.

Human sources in the hospital include personnel, mothers, and other infants. The methods of transmission may include the following:

1. Droplets spread from the respiratory tract of adults or other newborn infants. Outbreaks of respiratory virus infections in prolonged-stay nurseries are frequent; viruses present include influenza, respiratory syncytial, and parainfluenza viruses.[118] Methods for identification and control are provided in Chapter 34.
2. Carriage of the microorganism on the hands of hospital personnel. A study has suggested that the hands may be not only a means of transmission but also a significant reservoir of bacteria.[119]
3. Suppurative lesions. Although spread of staphylococcal and streptococcal infections to infants or mothers may be associated with asymptomatic carriers, the most serious outbreaks have been caused by a member of the medical or nursing staff with a significant lesion.
4. Human milk. CMV, HIV, HSV, human T cell lymphotropic virus type I (HTLV-I),[120] HTLV-II,[121] and HB$_s$Ag have been identified in mother's milk and may be transmitted to the neonate by this route.

CMV-infected milk from banks may be dangerous for infants without passively transferred maternal antibody.

The role of breast milk in transmission of HIV is of concern because of the importance of breast-feeding in providing nutrition and immunologic protection in the first year of life. Breast milk has been documented to be the likely source of HIV infection in the neonate in reports of mothers who were transfused with HIV-infected blood after the delivery or developed disease post partum through sexual contact.[122] These acute infections need to be differentiated from the usual event in which the mother is infected throughout pregnancy. Infection during the acute period occurs before development of antibody and may be a time when breast milk has a high titer of transmissible virus. Because of the importance of breast-feeding in the nutrition of infants in developing countries, the World Health Organization (WHO) first recommended that women in developing countries be encouraged to breast-feed even if they were known to be infected with HIV.[123] In contrast, in the United States and Western Europe, HIV-infected mothers were discouraged from breast-feeding because other forms of nutrition were available.[124] In July 1998, the United Nations changed its position and issued recommendations to discourage women infected with HIV from breast-feeding. The statement recognized that many infants were infected by the breast milk of HIV-infected mothers. The recommendation also noted that in some cultures women may become stigmatized for not breast-feeding and in some places alternatives like formula are unaffordable or unsafe. The number of congenitally infected infants in developing countries that have no resources for prevention in pregnancy has reached alarming proportions: 70% of women at a prenatal clinic in Zimbabwe and 30% of women in urban areas in six African countries were infected. The United Nations survey indicated that by the year 2000 breast-feeding would be responsible for more than one third (>200,000) of children newly infected with HIV unless some attempts were made to limit this route of transmission.[125]

Infection of breast milk by bacterial pathogens such as *S. aureus*, group B streptococci, *L. monocytogenes*,[126] and *Salmonella* sp. may result in neonatal disease. Bacteria that are components of skin flora, including *Staphylococcus epidermidis* and alpha-hemolytic *Streptococcus*, are frequently cultured from freshly expressed human milk and are unlikely to be of importance to the breast-fed infant. If these bacteria are allowed to multiply in banked breast milk, infection of the neonate is possible in theory, but no substantive data have been presented to suggest that this is an important problem.

5. Blood products. Blood used for replacement or exchange transfusion in neonates should be determined to be safe by techniques of proven efficacy, including tests for hepatitis B antigen, hepatitis C, HIV antibody, CMV antibody, and *Plasmodium* sp. in malarious areas.

Equipment has been implicated in common-source nursery outbreaks. The most common factors in transmission of infection in such instances have been contaminated solutions used in nebulization equipment, room humidifiers, and bathing solutions. Several gram-negative bacteria, including *Pseudomonas*, *Serratia marcescens*, and *Flavobacterium*, have been so troublesome that they have been termed "water bugs" because of their ability to multiply in aqueous environments at room temperature.

Catheterization of the umbilical vein and artery has been associated with sepsis, umbilical cellulitis, and abscesses. Intravenous alimentation using central venous catheters has been lifesaving for some infants but has also been associated with line sepsis.

Parenteral feeding with lipid emulsions has been associated with neonatal sepsis due to coagulase-negative staphylococci. Strains of staphylococci isolated from infected ventricular shunts or intravascular catheters produce a slime or glycocalyx that promotes adherence and growth of microcolonies on the surfaces of synthetic polymers used in the manufacture of catheters. The slime layer also protects the bacteria against the action of antibiotics and phagocytosis. The introduction of lipid emulsion through the venous catheter provides nutrients for growth of the bacteria.[127]

Hand washing remains the single most important element in the control of the spread of infectious diseases in the nursery. Hand washing should occur before and after every patient contact. Surveys of hospital employees indicate that, although the most simple of infection control techniques, hand washing is still not compulsively adhered to as a hospital rule. A study by Brown and colleagues in a Denver neonatal intensive care unit indicated that compliance with appropriate hand-washing techniques was low for both medical and nursing personnel.[128] Compliance was monitored using a direct observation technique; of 252 observed encounters of nurses, physicians, and respiratory therapists with babies, 25% of the personnel broke contact with the infant by touching self (69%) or touching another baby (4%), and 25% did not wash before patient contact. Hospitals should not accept less than complete compliance with hand washing in the nurseries.

Early discharge at 24 or 48 hours has become a common practice as hospitals and third-party payers attempt to reduce costs of health care. Study of a cohort of more than 300,000 births in Washington documented that newborns discharged home early (<30 hours after birth) were at increased risk for rehospitalization during the first month of life; the leading causes occurred within 7 days after discharge and were jaundice, dehydration, and sepsis. Of 1253 infants who were rehospitalized within the first month of life, sepsis was the cause in 55 cases (4.4%) who were discharged early contrasted with 42 (3.4%) who were discharged late.[129]

Prevention of disease in the first months of life may be accomplished by immunization of the mother with passive transfer of protective antibody to the neonate. Immunization of women in the child-bearing years or during pregnancy is of proven value in prevention of neonatal tetanus but has also been considered for prevention of invasive disease in the first months of life. Maternal immunization with polysaccharide and conjugate *Haemophilus influenzae* type b vaccines provided protective levels of antibody to the infant.[130] Immunization of the mother during pregnancy is likely to be protective for other diseases in the neonate due to encapsulated organisms including group B streptococci, pneumococci, and meningococci and has been considered for prevention of respiratory syncytial virus[131] and *Bordetella pertussis*.

HOUSEHOLD-ACQUIRED INFECTIONS

The newborn infant is susceptible to many of the infectious agents that colonize other members of the household. The physician should consider illnesses in members of the household before discharging the infant from the hospital. If an infant who is well when discharged from the nursery and whose gestation and delivery did not involve significant risk factors develops signs of an infectious disease in the latter half of the first month of life, it is probable that the infection was acquired from a household contact. A careful history of illness in family members may suggest the source of the infant's disease.

An infant may be a source of infection for members of the household. The infant with congenital rubella syndrome may shed virus for many months and is a significant source of infection for close contacts. The same is true for the infant with the vesicular lesions of herpes simplex or the syphilitic infant with rhinitis. Suppurative lesions related to *S. aureus* in an infant may introduce a virulent strain into the household that can be a source of significant disease for family members.

INFECTIONS THAT INDICATE UNDERLYING DISABILITIES

Infection may serve as the signal for identification of an underlying anatomic, metabolic, or physiologic disability. Infants with galactosemia or iron overload are susceptible to invasive gram-negative infections. Genitourinary infection early in life may serve to identify an anatomic or physiologic defect of the urinary tract. Similarly, otitis media in the first month of life may be an indication of a midline defect of the palate or of a eustachian tube dysfunction.

Infants with underlying immune defects may not have systemic infections until passively acquired maternal antibody has dissipated. Because the half-life of IgG is 23 days, such infections are likely to occur after 3 months of age.

Epidemiology

Nursery-acquired infection is frequently epidemic, and a common source may often be identified by simple epidemiologic techniques. Organisms that are frequently epidemic in nurseries include *S. aureus*, the enteric bacilli, the enteroviruses, and respiratory viruses.

The most complete documentation of nursery-acquired infection was developed during the worldwide pandemic of staphylococcal disease in the 1950s. A variety of preventive measures were attempted, including environmental manipulations, hexachlorophene bathing, and systemic antibiotics. For unknown reasons, the pandemic began to subside about 1963. These factors are further discussed in Chapter 30.

Epidemic diarrhea of the newborn infant that is associated with infection with *E. coli*, *Salmonella*, and other agents is discussed in Chapter 31. In addition, several viruses have been implicated in nursery outbreaks of gastrointestinal and respiratory diseases. They include rotaviruses, various enteroviruses (see Chapter 10), respiratory syncytial virus, parainfluenza virus, influenza virus, and adenoviruses.

Hospital personnel may acquire infection from neonates with communicable diseases. Studies of the carriage of staphylococci and streptococci usually note a significant incidence in personnel. In many cases, the infections are acquired from the infants. Studies of the shedding of rubella virus and CMV in the urine and saliva of infants with congenital infections indicate that these materials may be infectious for susceptible adults working in the nursery. Infection control is discussed in Chapter 34.

Each hospital should consider a specific program for personnel. Serologic screening of female hospital personnel for rubella antibodies should be done at the time of employment. Vaccination is advised for nonpregnant females who are seronegative and may come in contact with infectious children. All hospital employees, including those working in nurseries, should have skin tests with tuberculin annually; those who have positive test results should have periodic chest radiographs. Assignment of pregnant nurses to duties involving minimal contact with infectious patients should be considered.

Diagnosis and Management

The diagnosis and management of infection acquired by the infant in the nursery or at home are similar to those of infection acquired during delivery. The management of late-onset bacterial infections is discussed in Chapters 21, 26, 27, and 30.

References

1. U.S. Food and Drug Administration Medical Bulletin. Summer:4, 1998.
2. Pamuk E, et al. Socioeconomic Status and Health Chartbook. Health, United States. Hyattsville, Md, National Center for Health Statistics, 1998.
3. Epidemic of congenital syphilis—Baltimore, 1996–1997. MMWR Morb Mortal Wkly Rep 47:904–907, 1998.
4. Rubella and congenital rubella syndrome—United States, 1994–1997. MMWR Morb Mortal Wkly Rep 46:350–354, 1997.
5. Lea RG, Calder AA. The immunology of pregnancy. Curr Opin Infect Dis 10:171–176, 1997.
6. Raghupathy R. Th1-type immunity is incompatible with successful pregnancy (see comments). Immunol Today 18:478–482, 1997.
7. Ronel DN, Klein JO, Ware KG. New acronym needed for congenital infections. Pediatr Infect Dis J 14:921, 1995.
8. Ford-Jones EL, Kellner JD. "CHEAP TORCHES": an acronym for congenital and perinatal infections. Letter to the editor. Pediatr Infect Dis J 14:638–640, 1995.
9. Chheda S, Lopez SM, Sanderson EP. Congenital brucellosis in a premature infant. Pediatr Infect Dis J 16:81–83, 1997.
10. Stein A, Raoult D. Q fever during pregnancy: a public health problem in southern France. Clin Infect Dis 27:592–596, 1998.
11. New DL, et al. Vertically transmitted babesiosis. Letter to the editor; comment. J Pediatr 131:163–164, 1997.
12. Fujino T, et al. HTLV-I transmission from mother to fetus via placenta. Letter to the editor. Lancet 340:1157, 1992.
13. Van Dyke RB, et al. Mother-to-child transmission of human T-lymphotropic virus type II. J Pediatr 127:924–928, 1995.
14. Feucht HH, et al. Vertical transmission of hepatitis G. Letter to the editor; see comments. Lancet 347:615–616, 1996.
15. Adams O, et al. Congenital infections with human herpesvirus 6. J Infect Dis 178:544–546, 1998.

16. Chye JK, et al. Vertical transmission of dengue. Clin Infect Dis 25:1374–1377, 1997.

17. Overturf GD, Balfour G. Osteomyelitis and sepsis: severe complications of fetal monitoring. Pediatrics 55:244–247, 1975.

18. King-Lewis PA, Gardner SD. Congenital cytomegalic inclusion disease following intrauterine transfusion. BMJ 2:603–605, 1969.

19. Scott JM, Henderson A. Acute villous inflammation in the placenta following intrauterine transfusion. J Clin Pathol 25:872–875, 1972.

20. St. Clair EH, DiLiberti JH, O'Brien ML. Letter: Observations of an infant born to a mother with botulism. J Pediatr 87:658, 1975.

21. Robin L, Herman D, Redett R. Botulism in a pregnant woman. Letter to the editor. N Engl J Med 335:823–824, 1996.

22. Luijckx GJ, et al. Guillain-Barré syndrome in mother and newborn child. Lancet 349:27, 1997.

23. Savage WE, Hajj SN, Kass EH. Demographic and prognostic characteristics of bacteriuria in pregnancy. Medicine (Baltimore) 46:385–407, 1967.

24. Naeye RL. Causes of the excessive rates of perinatal mortality and prematurity in pregnancies complicated by maternal urinary-tract infections. N Engl J Med 300:819–823, 1979.

25. Norden CW, Kass EH. Bacteriuria of pregnancy—a critical appraisal. Annu Rev Med 19:431, 1969.

26. Kincaid-Smith P. Bacteriuria in pregnancy. In Kass EH (ed). Progress in Pyelonephritis. Philadelphia, FA Davis, 1965, p 11.

27. Wallach EE, Brody JI, Oski FA. Fetal immunization as a consequence of bacilluria during pregnancy. Obstet Gynecol 33:100–105, 1969.

28. Stokes JH, Beerman H, Ingraham NR Jr. Modern Clinical Syphilology: Diagnosis, Treatment, Case Study, 3rd ed. Philadelphia, WB Saunders, 1944, 1968.

29. Feldman GV. Herpes zoster neonatorum. Arch Dis Child 27:126, 1952.

30. Forrester RM, Lees VT, Watson GH. Rubella syndrome: escape of a twin. BMJ 5500:1403, 1966.

31. Shearer WT, et al. Cytomegalovirus infection in a newborn dizygous twin. J Pediatr 81:1161–1165, 1972.

32. Marsden JP, Greenfield CRM. Inherited smallpox. Arch Dis Child 9:309, 1934.

33. Miller MJ, Seaman E, Remington JS. The clinical spectrum of congenital toxoplasmosis. Problems in recognition. J Pediatr 70:714–723, 1967.

34. Ray GC, Wedgewood RJ. Neonatal listeriosis. Six case reports and a review of the literature. Pediatrics 34:378, 1964.

35. Wilcox AJ, et al. Incidence of early loss of pregnancy. N Engl J Med 319:189–194, 1988.

36. Brabin BJ. Epidemiology of infection in pregnancy. Rev Infect Dis 7:579–603, 1985.

37. Hillier SL, et al. The relationship of amniotic fluid cytokines and preterm delivery, amniotic fluid infection, histologic chorioamnionitis, and chorioamnion infection. Obstet Gynecol 81:941–948, 1993.

38. Romero R, et al. The diagnostic and prognostic value of amniotic fluid, white blood cell count, glucose, interleukin-6, and Gram stain in patients with preterm labor and intact membranes. Am J Obstet Gynecol 169:805–816, 1993.

39. Hitti J, et al. Broad-spectrum bacterial rDNA polymerase chain reaction assay for detecting amniotic fluid infection among women in premature labor. Clin Infect Dis 24:1228–1232, 1997.

40. Naeye RL. Cytomegalic inclusion disease. The fetal disorder. Am J Clin Pathol 47:738–744, 1967.

41. Naeye RL, Blanc W. Pathogenesis of congenital rubella. JAMA 194:1277–1283, 1965.

42. Naeye RL. Infants of prolonged gestation. A necropsy study. Arch Pathol 84:37–41, 1967.

43. Naeye RL, Kelly JA. Judgment of fetal age. 3. The pathologist's evaluation. Pediatr Clin North Am 13:849–862, 1966.

44. Brown GC, Karunas RS. Relationship of congenital anomalies and maternal infection with selected enteroviruses. Am J Epidemiol 95:207–217, 1972.

45. Allison AC, Paton GR. Chromosomal abnormalities in human diploid cells infected with mycoplasma and their possible relevance to the aetiology of Down's syndrome (mongolism). Lancet 2:1229–1230, 1966.

46. Nichols WW. The role of viruses in the etiology of chromosomal abnormalities. Am J Hum Genet 18:81–92, 1966.

47. Nusbacher J, Hirschhorn K, Cooper LZ. Chromosomal abnormalities in congenital rubella. N Engl J Med 276:1409–1413, 1967.

48. Congenital malaria in children of refugees—Washington, Massachusetts, Kentucky. MMWR Morb Mortal Wkly Rep 30:53–55, 1981.

49. McIntosh K. Guidelines for initial management of an infant at risk of HIV infection. Rep Pediatr Infect Dis 3:3, 1993.

50. Wilson CB, et al. Development of adverse sequelae in children born with subclinical congenital Toxoplasma infection. Pediatrics 66:767–774, 1980.

51. Townsend JJ, et al. Progressive rubella panencephalitis. Late onset after congenital rubella. N Engl J Med 292:990–993, 1975.

52. Weil ML, et al. Chronic progressive panencephalitis due to rubella virus simulating subacute sclerosing panencephalitis. N Engl J Med 292:994–998, 1975.

53. Donders GG, et al. Survival after intrauterine parvovirus B19 infection with persistence in early infancy: a two-year follow-up. Pediatr Infect Dis J 13:234–236, 1994.

54. Miller E, Cradock-Watson JE, Pollock TM. Consequences of confirmed maternal rubella at successive stages of pregnancy. Lancet 2:781–784, 1982.

55. Desmonts G, Couvreur J. Congenital toxoplasmosis: a prospective study of the offspring of 542 women who acquired toxoplasmosis during pregnancy. Pathophysiology of congenital disease. In Thalhammer O, Baumgarten K, Pollack A (eds). Perinatal Medicine, Sixth European Congress. Stuttgart, Georg Thieme, 1979, pp 51–60.

56. Stagno S, Whitley RJ. Herpesvirus infections of pregnancy. Part I: cytomegalovirus and Epstein-Barr virus infections. N Engl J Med 313:1270–1274, 1985.

57. Oxtoby MJ. Perinatally acquired HIV infection. In Pizzo PA, Wilfert CM (eds). Pediatric AIDS. Baltimore, Williams & Wilkins, 1991, p. 12.

58. Green DM, Reid SM, Rhaney K. Generalised vaccinia in the human foetus. Lancet 1:1296–1298, 1966.

59. Sharma R, Jagdev DK. Congenital smallpox. Scand J Infect Dis 3:245–247, 1971.

60. Eilard T, Strannegard O. Rubella reinfection in pregnancy followed by transmission to the fetus. J Infect Dis 129:594–596, 1974.

61. Harvey B, Remington JS, Sulzer AJ. IgM malaria antibodies in a case of congenital malaria in the United States. Lancet 1:333–335, 1969.

62. Desmonts G, Couvreur J, Thulliez P. [Congenital toxo-

plasmosis. 5 cases of mother-to-child transmission of pre-pregnancy infection]. Presse Med 19:1445–1449, 1990.

63. Nelson NA, Struve VR. Prevention of congenital syphilis by treatment of syphilis in pregnancy. JAMA 161:869, 1956.

64. Zuckerman AJ, Taylor PE. Persistence of the serum hepatitis (SH-Australia) antigen for many years. Nature 223:81–82, 1969.

65. Nahmias AJ, Alford CA, Korones SB. Infection of the newborn with herpesvirus hominis. Adv Pediatr 17:185–226, 1970.

66. Vogel N, et al. Congenital toxoplasmosis transmitted from an immunologically competent mother infected before conception. Clin Infect Dis 23:1055–1060, 1996.

67. Prevention of perinatal transmission of hepatitis B virus: prenatal screening of all pregnant women for hepatitis B surface antigen. MMWR Morb Mortal Wkly Rep 37:341–346, 351, 1988.

67a. American Academy of Pediatrics. Hepatitis B. *In* Peter G (ed). 1997 Red Book. Report of the Committee on Infectious Diseases, 24th ed. Elk Grove Village, Ill, American Academy of Pediatrics, 1997, p 256.

68. Davis LE, et al. Intrauterine diagnosis of cytomegalovirus infection: viral recovery from amniocentesis fluid. Am J Obstet Gynecol 109:1217–1219, 1971.

69. Levin MJ, et al. Diagnosis of congenital rubella in utero. N Engl J Med 290:1187–1188, 1974.

70. Papaevangelou G, et al. Hepatitis B antigen and antibody in maternal blood, cord blood, and amniotic fluid. Arch Dis Child 49:936–939, 1974.

71. Daffos F, et al. Prenatal management of 746 pregnancies at risk for congenital toxoplasmosis. N Engl J Med 318:271–275, 1988.

72. Torok TJ, et al. Prenatal diagnosis of intrauterine infection with parvovirus B19 by the polymerase chain reaction technique. Clin Infect Dis 14:149–155, 1992.

73. Wattre P, et al. A clinical and epidemiological study of human parvovirus B19 infection in fetal hydrops using PCR Southern blot hybridization and chemiluminescence detection. J Med Virol 54:140–144, 1998.

74. Lazzarotto T, et al. Prenatal diagnosis of congenital cytomegalovirus infection. J Clin Microbiol 36:3540–3544, 1998.

75. Revello MG, et al. Improved prenatal diagnosis of congenital human cytomegalovirus infection by a modified nested polymerase chain reaction. J Med Virol 56:99–103, 1998.

76. Revello MG, et al. Polymerase chain reaction for prenatal diagnosis of congenital human cytomegalovirus infection. J Med Virol 47:462–466, 1995.

77. Hohlfeld P, et al. Prenatal diagnosis of congenital toxoplasmosis with a polymerase-chain-reaction test on amniotic fluid. N Engl J Med 331:695–699, 1994.

78. Bosma TJ, et al. Use of PCR for prenatal and postnatal diagnosis of congenital rubella. J Clin Microbiol 33:2881–2887, 1995.

79. McLean LK, Chehab FF, Goldberg JD. Detection of viral deoxyribonucleic acid in the amniotic fluid of low-risk pregnancies by polymerase chain reaction. Am J Obstet Gynecol 173:1282–1286, 1995.

80. Van den Veyver IB, et al. Detection of intrauterine viral infection using the polymerase chain reaction. Mol Genet Metab 63:85–95, 1998.

81. Daffos F, Capella-Pavlovsky M, Forestier F. Fetal blood sampling via the umbilical cord using a needle guided by ultrasound. Report of 66 cases. Prenat Diagn 3:271–277, 1983.

82. Daffos F, Capella-Pavlovsky M, Forestier F. Fetal blood sampling during pregnancy with use of a needle guided by ultrasound: a study of 606 consecutive cases. Am J Obstet Gynecol 153:655–660, 1985.

83. Daffos F, et al. Prenatal diagnosis of congenital rubella. Lancet 2:1–3, 1984.

84. Grangeot-Keros L, et al. Prenatal and postnatal production of IgM and IgA antibodies to rubella virus studied by antibody capture immunoassay. J Infect Dis 158:138–143, 1988.

85. Hohlfeld P, et al. Cytomegalovirus fetal infection: prenatal diagnosis. Obstet Gynecol 78:615–618, 1991.

86. Lynch L, et al. Prenatal diagnosis of fetal cytomegalovirus infection (see comments). Am J Obstet Gynecol 165:714–718, 1991.

87. Hanson FW, et al. Ultrasonography-guided early amniocentesis in singleton pregnancies. Am J Obstet Gynecol 162:1376–1381; discussion 1381–1383, 1990.

88. Terzian E, et al. A survey of diagnostic amniocenteses in Oxford from 1974–1981. Prenat Diagn 5:401–414, 1985.

88a. Fox H. Pathology of the Placenta. Philadelphia, WB Saunders, 1978.

89. Leary WE. Medical panel urges HIV tests for all pregnant women. New York Times, national ed. New York, 1998, A24.

90. Wilfert CM. Prevention of perinatal transmission of human immunodeficiency virus: a progress report 2 years after completion of AIDS Clinical Trials Group trial 076. Clin Infect Dis 23:438–441, 1996.

91. Peckham CS, Newell ML. Controversy in mandatory HIV screening of pregnant women. Curr Opin Infect Dis 10:18–21, 1997.

92. Public Health Service. FDA Public Health Advisory: Limitations of *Toxoplasma* IgM commercial test kits. Rockville, Md, Department of Health and Human Services, U.S. Food and Drug Administration, 1997.

93. Mussi-Pinhata MM, et al. Congenital and perinatal cytomegalovirus infection in infants born to mothers infected with human immunodeficiency virus. J Pediatr 132:285–290, 1998.

94. Thomas DL, et al. Perinatal transmission of hepatitis C virus from human immunodeficiency virus type 1–infected mothers. Women and Infants Transmission Study. J Infect Dis 177:1480–1488, 1998.

95. Immunization during pregnancy. ACOG Technical Bulletin, vol. 64. Washington DC, American College of Obstetrics and Gynecology, 1982.

96. Tsai TF, et al. Congenital yellow fever virus infection after immunization in pregnancy (see comments). J Infect Dis 168:1520–1523, 1993.

97. Connor EM, et al. Reduction of maternal-infant transmission of human immunodeficiency virus type 1 with zidovudine treatment. Pediatric AIDS Clinical Trials Group Protocol 076 Study Group (see comments). N Engl J Med 331:1173–1180, 1994.

98. Public Health Service Task Force recommendations for the use of antiretroviral drugs in pregnant women infected with HIV-1 for maternal health and for reducing perinatal HIV-1 transmission in the United States. Centers for Disease Control and Prevention [published errata appear in MMWR Morb Mortal Wkly Rep 1998 Apr 17;47(14):287 and 1998 Apr 24;47(15):315]. MMWR Morb Mortal Wkly Rep 47:1–30, 1998.

99. Prevention of perinatal group B streptococcal disease: a public health perspective. Centers for Disease Control and Prevention [published erratum appears in MMWR Morb Mortal Wkly Rep 1996 Aug 9;45(31):679]. MMWR Morb Mortal Wkly Rep 45:1–24, 1996.

100. Rosebury, T. Microorganisms Indigenous to Man. New York, McGraw-Hill, 1962.
101. Gorbach SL, et al. Anaerobic microflora of the cervix in healthy women. Am J Obstet Gynecol 117:1053–1055, 1973.
102. Srugo I, et al. Meningoencephalitis in a neonate congenitally infected with human immunodeficiency virus type 1. J Pediatr 120:93–95, 1992.
103. Klass PE, Klein JO. Therapy of bacterial sepsis, meningitis and otitis media in infants and children: 1992 poll of directors of programs in pediatric infectious diseases. Pediatr Infect Dis J 11:702–705, 1992.
104. Revised guidelines for prevention of early-onset group B streptococcal (GBS) infection. American Academy of Pediatrics Committee on Infectious Diseases and Committee on Fetus and Newborn (see comments). Pediatrics 99:489–496, 1997.
105. Fernandez M, Hickman ME, Baker CJ. Antimicrobial susceptibilities of group B streptococci isolated between 1992 and 1996 from patients with bacteremia or meningitis. Antimicrob Agents Chemother 42:1517–1519, 1998.
106. Kremer JA, et al. Fatal intrauterine infection associated with penicillin-resistant Streptococcus pneumoniae. Pediatr Infect Dis J 15:467–468, 1996.
107. Sperling RS, et al. A survey of zidovudine use in pregnant women with human immunodeficiency virus infection (see comments). N Engl J Med 326:857–861, 1992.
108. Whitley RJ, et al. Ganciclovir treatment of symptomatic congenital cytomegalovirus infection: results of a phase II study. National Institute of Allergy and Infectious Diseases Collaborative Antiviral Study Group. J Infect Dis 175:1080–1086, 1997.
109. Baker CJ, et al. Intravenous immune globulin for the prevention of nosocomial infection in low-birth-weight neonates. The Multicenter Group for the Study of Immune Globulin in Neonates (see comments). N Engl J Med 327:213–219, 1992.
110. American Academy of Pediatrics Committee on Infectious Diseases: universal hepatitis B immunization [published erratum appears in Pediatrics 1992 Nov;90(5):715] (see comments). Pediatrics 89:795–800, 1992.
111. Boyer KM, et al. Selective intrapartum chemoprophylaxis of neonatal group B streptococcal early-onset disease. I. Epidemiologic rationale. J Infect Dis 148:795–801, 1983.
112. Group B streptococcal infections in pregnancy. ACOG Technical Bulletin, vol. 170. Washington, DC, American College of Obstetrics and Gynecology, 1992.
113. American Academy of Pediatrics Committee on Infectious Diseases and Committee on Fetus and Newborn: guidelines for prevention of group B streptococcal (GBS) infection by chemoprophylaxis. Pediatrics 90:775–778, 1992.
114. Gotoff SP, Boyer KM. Prevention of early-onset neonatal group B streptococcal disease. Pediatrics 99:866–869, 1997.
115. MacAulay MA, Abou-Sabe M, Charles D. Placental transfer of ampicillin. Am J Obstet Gynecol 96:943–950, 1966.
116. Yancey MK, et al. Risk factors for neonatal sepsis. Obstet Gynecol 87:188–194, 1996.
117. Brozanski BS, et al. Prevention of early-onset group B streptococcal sepsis (EOGBSS): implementation of the CDC guidelines. American Pediatric Society 108th Annual Meeting/Society for Pediatric Research 67th Annual Meeting, New Orleans, La, 1998.
118. Moisiuk SE, et al. Outbreak of parainfluenza virus type 3 in an intermediate care neonatal nursery. Pediatr Infect Dis J 17:49–53, 1998.
119. Knittle MA, Eitzman DV, Baer H. Role of hand contamination of personnel in the epidemiology of gram-negative nosocomial infections. J Pediatr 86:433–437, 1975.
120. Nagamine M, et al. DNA amplification of human T lymphotropic virus type I (HTLV-I) proviral DNA in breast milk of HTLV-I carriers. Letter to the editor. J Infect Dis 164:1024–1025, 1991.
121. Heneine W, et al. Detection of HTLV-II in breastmilk of HTLV-II infected mothers. Letter to the editor. Lancet 340:1157–1158, 1992.
122. Dunn DT, et al. Risk of human immunodeficiency virus type 1 transmission through breastfeeding (see comments). Lancet 340:585–588, 1992.
123. World Health Organization. Breast feeding/breast milk and human immunodeficiency virus (HIV). Wkly Epidemiol Rec 33:245, 1987.
124. Breastfeeding and the use of human milk. American Academy of Pediatrics. Work Group on Breastfeeding. Pediatrics 100:1035–1039, 1997.
125. Altman LK. AIDS brings a shift on breast-feeding. The New York Times, 1998, pp 1 & 6.
126. Svabic-Vlahovic M, et al. Transmission of Listeria monocytogenes from mother's milk to her baby and to puppies. Letter to the editor. Lancet 2:1201, 1988.
127. Klein JO. From harmless commensal to invasive pathogen—coagulase-negative staphylococci (editorial; comment). N Engl J Med 323:339–340, 1990.
128. Brown J, et al. High rate of hand contamination and low rate of hand washing before infant contact in a neonatal intensive care unit. Pediatr Infect Dis J 15:908–910, 1996.
129. Liu LL, et al. The safety of newborn early discharge. The Washington State experience (see comments) [published erratum appears in JAMA 1997 Dec 17;278(23):2067]. JAMA 278:293–298, 1997.
130. Englund JA, et al. Transplacental antibody transfer following maternal immunization with polysaccharide and conjugate Haemophilus influenzae type b vaccines. J Infect Dis 171:99–105, 1995.
131. Englund JA. Passive protection against respiratory syncytial virus disease in infants: the role of maternal antibody. Pediatr Infect Dis J 13:449–453, 1994.

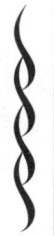

C H A P T E R   2

Developmental Immunology and Role of Host Defenses in Fetal and Neonatal Susceptibility to Infection

DAVID B. LEWIS, M.D., and CHRISTOPHER B. WILSON, M.D.

Studies of the ontogeny of the immune system in the human and in animal models provide insight into normal pathways of the development of lymphocytes and other components of the immune system, as well as the cellular and molecular basis for the susceptibility of the fetus and neonate to severe infection. This chapter focuses on the ontogeny of the cellular and humoral components of the immune system and their function in the human fetus and neonate. Antigen presentation and antigen-specific immunity, including responses to vaccines, are presented first, followed by innate mechanisms of host defense. Recent understanding of the linkage between innate immune mechanisms and those that are antigen-specific is included. The relation between deficiencies in immune function in the neonate and fetus and their increased susceptibility to bacterial, viral, and protozoan infections is examined for representative pathogens. The current and potential application of immunotherapy for these infections is briefly discussed. Finally, clues to the recognition of primary immunodeficiency during the neonatal period are presented.

The immune system is composed of hematopoietic cells, including lymphocytes, mononuclear phagocytes, dendritic cells, and granulocytes; certain nonhematopoietic cells, such as follicular dendritic cells; and humoral factors produced by cells, such as cytokines (Tables 2–1 and 2–2) and complement components. The mature hematopoietic cells of mammals are derived from pluripotent hematopoietic stem cells (HSCs). HSCs are generated sequentially during ontogeny from the para-aortic tissue (the splanchnopleure), yolk sac, fetal liver, and bone marrow. HSCs may be derived from an even more primitive precursor cell capable of also differentiating into endothelial cells.[1] In humans, the principal site of hematopoiesis is the yolk sac, starting at about the third week of embryonic development, followed by the fetal liver at 8 weeks, and, finally, the bone marrow after 5 months of gestation. HSCs are also found in the para-aortic tissue region by 5 weeks of gestation in humans.[2] Hematopoiesis by the fetal liver and bone marrow may be established by seeding of these sites with circulating HSCs derived from para-aortic tissue.[2]

T LYMPHOCYTES AND ANTIGEN PRESENTATION

Overview

T cells are lymphocytes that bear cell surface receptors for a specific antigen. Most T cells recognize antigen in the form of peptides bound to major histocompatibility complex (MHC) molecules on antigen-presenting cells (APCs). Antigen-specific T cell receptors (TCRs) are heterodimeric molecules composed of either α and β chains (αβ-TCRs) (Fig. 2–1) or γ and δ chains (γδ-TCRs). The amino-terminal portion of each of these chains is variable and is involved in antigen recognition. As discussed later, the highly variable nature of this portion of the TCR is generated, in large part, as a result of TCR gene rearrangement. In contrast, the carboxy-terminal region of each of the four TCR chains is monomorphic or constant. The TCR on the cell surface is invariably associated with the nonpolymorphic complex of CD3 proteins (see Fig. 2–1). The cytoplasmic domains of proteins of the CD3 complex include immunoreceptor tyrosine-based activation motifs (ITAMs), which serve as docking sites for intracellular tyrosine kinases that transduce activation signals to the interior of the cell after the TCR has been engaged by antigen.

Alpha-beta T cells, which bear αβ-TCRs, predominate in lymphoid organs, including the thymus, lymph nodes, and spleen, as well as in the circulation. Most αβ T cells recognize protein antigen in the form of peptide fragments bound to classical MHC. As a consequence of a rigorous selection process that occurs in the thymus, the αβ-TCR recognition of antigenic peptide–MHC complexes by mature T cells is MHC-restricted: That is, there is preferential recognition of peptides bound to self-MHC of class I or class II as opposed to non-self MHC alleles. Activation and proliferation of T cells typically occur when their TCRs recognize antigenic peptide in conjunction with other non-TCR-mediated signals provided by the APC. Activated αβ T cells, especially those that express surface CD4 (hereafter referred to as CD4 T cells), critically influence immune

TABLE 2–1
Major Human Cytokines: Their Structure, Cognate Receptors, and Receptor-Mediated Signal Transduction Pathways

CYTOKINE FAMILY	MEMBERS	STRUCTURE AND LOCUS OF EXPRESSION	COGNATE RECEPTOR FAMILY	PROXIMAL SIGNAL TRANSDUCTION PATHWAYS
IL-1	IL-1α, IL-1β, IL-18 (IL-1γ), and IL-1 receptor antagonist	β-trefoil, monomers; processed and secreted	IL-1 receptor	Receptor-associated serine threonine kinase IRAK; c-Jun N terminal kinase
Hematopoietin	IL-2 through IL-7, IL-9 through IL-15, colony-stimulating factors, oncostatin-M; interferon-α, -β, and -γ and IL-10 constitute a subfamily	Four α-helical; monomers except IL-5 and interferons (homodimers) and IL-12 (heterodimer); secreted	Hematopoietin receptors	JAK tyrosine kinases; signal transducers and activators of transcription (STAT); src and syk tyrosine kinases
Tumor necrosis factor (TNF) ligand	TNF, lymphotoxin-α and -β, CD27 ligand (L), CD30-L, CD40-L, OX40-L, and others	β-jellyroll; homotrimers; type 2 membrane proteins and secreted	TNF receptor family	TRAFS and proteins mediating apoptosis
Transforming growth factor-β (TGF-β)	TGF-β1, -β2, and -β3, bone morphogenetic proteins	Cysteine knot; processed and secreted	TGF-β receptor type 1 and 2 heterodimers (intrinsic serine-threonine kinases)	Mad and Smad proteins
Chemokines		Three-stranded β sheet; all but fractalkine are secreted	Seven membrane spanning domains	G-protein–mediated
CXC subfamily	CTAP-III, IL-8, GCP-2, GRO-α, -β, -γ, Nap-2, ENA-78, IP-10, Mig, Platelet factor 4, SDF-α, β, β-thromboglobulin		CXCR1–CXCR4	
CC subfamily	MCP-1–5, eotaxin, I309, MIP-1α, -β, -γ, -δ, MIP-3α, -3β, RANTES, TARC, I309, TECK		CCR1–CCR8	
C subfamily	Lymphotactin		XCR1	
CX3C subfamily	CX3C (fractalkine or neurotactin)		CX3CR1	

CTAP = connective tissue activating peptide; ENA-78 = epithelial cell–derived neutrophil activating peptide-78; GCP = granulocyte chemotactic protein; GRO = growth-regulated gene; IL = interleukin; IP-10 = gamma-induced protein 10 kilodaltons; MCP = monocyte chemotactic protein; MIG = monokine-induced by interferon-γ; MIP = macrophage inflammatory protein; NAP = neutrophil-activating peptide; RANTES = regulated activated normal T cells expressed secreted; SDF = stromal cell-derived factor; TARC = thymus and activation-regulated chemokine; TECK = thymus-expressed chemokine.

responses, such as B cell immunoglobulin production and memory cell generation, activation of APCs, and generation of T cells capable of cytotoxicity. This is mediated in large part by cytokines secreted by or expressed on the surface of αβ T cells. Cytokines are glycoproteins produced by cells of the immune system that act as molecular signals for cell-to-cell communication and as systemic mediators of the host's response to infection. In some respects, their function is analogous to that of neurotransmitters and hormones, respectively. In addition, activated αβ T cells, particularly those that have CD8 on their surface (hereafter referred to as CD8 T cells), carry out cell-mediated cytotoxicity and directly kill host cells that bear antigenic peptide derived from intracellular pathogens, such as viruses.

In humans, γδ T cells, which express surface γδ-TCRs, are found in only small numbers in the lymph nodes, spleen, and circulation. They are more abundant in certain mucosal tissues, such as the intestinal epithelium,[3] or specialized tissues, such as the decidua of the placenta.[4] In contrast to most αβ T cells, most γδ T cells appear to recognize nonpeptide antigens, such as host or pathogen-derived lipids, presented by specialized, nonclassic MHC molecules. Activated γδ T cells are similar to αβ T cells, in that they produce cytokines and, in some cases, kill target cells. However, because

TABLE 2–2
Immunoregulatory Effects of Selected Cytokines and Their Production by Human Neonatal Cells

CYTOKINE	PRINCIPAL CELL SOURCE	MAJOR BIOLOGIC EFFECTS	PRODUCTION BY NEONATAL VERSUS ADULT CELLS	REFERENCES
IL-1α and -β	Many cell types, Mφ are a major source	Fever, inflammatory response, cofactor in T and B cell growth	MNC: normal after LPS treatment; ? reduced in premature	823, 827, 834, 835
IL-2	T cells	T > B cell growth, increased cytotoxicity by T and NK cells, increased cytokine production and sensitivity to apoptosis by T cells	T cells: normal with most stimuli; neonatal < adult after CD3 monoclonal antibody treatment	215, 227, 230
IL-3	T cells	Growth of early hematopoietic precursors (also known as multi-CSF)	T cells: Neonatal and adult naive < adult memory MNC: neonatal < adult	227, 902, 1151
IL-4	T cells, mast cells, basophils, and eosinophils	Required for IgE synthesis, enhances B cell growth and class II MHC expression, promotes T cell growth and TH2 differentiation, mast cell growth factor, enhances endothelial VCAM-1 expression	T cells: Neonatal and adult naive < adult memory	227, 230, 232
IL-5	T cells, NK cells, mast cells, basophils, eosinophils	Eosinophil growth, differentiation, and survival	T cells: neonatal and adult naive < adult memory	227
IL-6	Mφ, fibroblasts, T cells	Hepatic acute-phase protein synthesis, fever, T and B cell growth and differentiation	T cells: Neonatal < adult naive < adult memory MNC: Term normal to slightly reduced; premature ~25% of adult Mφ: neonatal < adult after RSV infection Whole blood: neonatal = adult	838, 1152–1155
IL-7	Stromal cells of bone marrow and thymus	Essential thymocyte growth factor	Not known	
IL-8	Mφ, endothelial cells, fibroblasts, epithelial cells, T cells	Chemotaxis and activation of neutrophils	MNC: neonatal < adult or normal in different studies using LPS stimulation; preterm < term Mφ: decreased after GBS incubation Whole blood: neonatal = adult	828, 830, 838, 1156
IL-9	T cells, mast cells	T cells and mast cell growth factor	Not known	
IL-10	Mφ, T cells, B cells, NK cells, keratinocytes, and eosinophils	Inhibits cytokine production by T cells and mononuclear cell inflammatory function; promotes B cell growth and isotype switching, NK cell cytotoxicity	T cells: neonatal and adult naive < adult memory MNC: neonatal < adult (lectin or LPS) Mφ: neonatal < adult Whole blood: neonatal = adult	225, 449, 832, 838, 1157
IL-11	Marrow stromal cells, fibroblasts	Hematopoietic precursor growth, acute phase reactants by hepatocytes	Fibroblasts: neonatal > adult	1158

Table continued on following page

TABLE 2–2

Immunoregulatory Effects of Selected Cytokines and Their Production by Human Neonatal Cells *Continued*

CYTOKINE	PRINCIPAL CELL SOURCE	MAJOR BIOLOGIC EFFECTS	PRODUCTION BY NEONATAL VERSUS ADULT CELLS	REFERENCES
IL-12	Dendritic cells, Mφ	Enhances TH2 differentiation, T cell growth, T cell and NK cell cytotoxicity, induces IFN-γ secretion by T cells and NK cells; enhances B cell response to TI antigens	MNC: neonatal < adult or normal after LPS in different studies; normal in response to *Staphylococcus aureus*	607, 616, 837
IL-13	T cells, mast cells, basophils, and eosinophils	Very similar to those of IL-4, with possible exception of lacking direct T cell effects	T cell: Neonatal and adult naive < adult memory	226
IL-15	Epithelial cells, bone marrow stromal cells, activated monocytes	Enhances NK cell development, growth, survival, cytotoxicity, and cytokine production; T cell chemoattractant and growth factor	MNC: neonatal MNC < adult after LPS stimulation	597
IL-17	T cells	Enhances T cell proliferation; proinflammatory cytokine release by macrophages	Not known	
IL-18	Hepatic Kupffer cells, splenic macrophages (?), intestinal and skin epithelia	Promotes TH1 differentiation, production of IL-2 and GM-CSF by T cells, and IFN-γ by T cells, NK cells, and B cells; T cell– and NK cell–mediated cytotoxicity	Not known	
IFN-α	Mφ, lymphocytes, especially NK cells	Inhibits viral replication; increases class I MHC expression and NK cell cytotoxicity	MNC: normal in term; ? reduced in premature	834, 835, 1159
IFN-β	Fibroblasts, epithelial cells	Same as IFN-α	MNC: normal	834
IFN-γ	T cells, NK cells, eosinophils (?), IL-18–stimulated B cells	Same as IFN-α and -β and also activates Mφ, increases class II MHC and antigen presentation molecules, inhibits IgE production, and enhances B cell response to TI antigens, promotes TH1 differentiation	T cells: Neonatal and adult naive < adult memory; NK cells: normal after HSV and IL-2 stimulation; MNC: neonatal < adult after IL-12 and IL-15 treatment	215, 217, 230, 597, 615, 616, 837
Tumor necrosis factor	Mφ, T cells, NK cells	Fever and inflammatory response effects similar to those of IL-1, shock, hemorrhagic necrosis of tumors, increased VCAM-1 expression on endothelium, induces catabolic state	T cells: neonatal < adult; MNC: neonatal < adult after IL-15 or LPS treatment; Mφ: neonatal < adult after RSV infection; preterm ≤ adult after LPS treatment; Whole blood: neonatal = adult	224, 597, 827. 838, 1155, 1160

TABLE 2–2
Immunoregulatory Effects of Selected Cytokines and Their Production by Human Neonatal Cells *Continued*

CYTOKINE	PRINCIPAL CELL SOURCE	MAJOR BIOLOGIC EFFECTS	PRODUCTION BY NEONATAL VERSUS ADULT CELLS	REFERENCES
CD40 ligand	T cells, lower amounts by B cells and dendritic cells	B cell growth factor; promotes isotype switching, promotes IL-12 production by dendritic cells, activates Mφ	T cells: neonatal < adult naive = or adult memory; ? normal after CD3 monoclonal antibody activation	238–241, 245
Fas ligand	Activated T cells, NK cells, retina, testicular epithelium	Induces apoptosis of cells expressing fas, including effector B and T cells	Unknown	
Flt-3 ligand	Bone marrow stromal cells	Potent dendritic cell growth factor, and promotes growth of myeloid and lymphoid progenitor cells in conjunction with other cytokines	Unknown	
G-CSF	Mφ, fibroblasts, epithelial cells	Growth of granulocyte precursors	MNC: neonate normal or slightly < than adults Mφ: term similar and preterm < adult	228, 662, 1161
GM-CSF	Mφ, endothelial cells, T cells	Growth of granulocyte-Mφ precursors and dendritic cells; enhances granulocyte-Mφ function and B cell antibody production	T cells: neonatal < adult MNC: neonatal < adult Mφ: normal after LPS stimulation	227, 228, 1161, 1162
MIP-1α	Mφ, T cells	Mφ chemoattractant; enhances T cell activation	MNC: neonatal < adult	828
RANTES	Mφ, T cells, fibroblasts, epithelial cells	Mφ and memory cell chemoattractant; enhances T cell activation; blocks HIV co-receptor	Unknown	
TGF-β	Mφ, T cells, fibroblasts, epithelial cells, others	Inhibits Mφ activation; inhibits TH1 T cell responses	MNC: neonate < adult	828

CSF = cerebrospinal fluid; G-CSF = granulocyte colony-stimulating factor, GM-CSF = granulocyte-macrophage colony-stimulating factor; HIV = human immunodeficiency virus; IFN = interferon; IgE = immunoglobulin E; IL = interleukin; LPS = lipopolysaccharide; Mφ = mononuclear phagocyte; MIP = macrophage inflammatory protein; MNC = circulating mononuclear cell; NK = natural killer; RANTES = regulated activated normal T cells expressed secreted; RSV = respiratory syncytial virus; VCAM-1 = vascular cell adhesion molecule-1.

they appear to have immune functions that are distinct from those of most αβ T cells, they are discussed separately later.

Basic Aspects of Antigen Presentation

ANTIGEN PRESENTATION BY CLASS I MAJOR HISTOCOMPATIBILITY COMPLEX MOLECULES

MHC molecules have a special cleft for presenting antigenic peptides (Figs. 2–1 and 2–2). In class I MHC, this cleft is formed by the heavy chain.[5] There are three major types of class I heavy chains in humans, human leukocyte antigen (HLA)-A, -B, and -C, encoded by three genes clustered on chromosome 6. Class I MHC

heavy chains on the cell surface are associated with a monomorphic light chain, β2-microglobulin.[5] The association of β2-microglobulin with the heavy chain is essential for effective presentation of antigenic peptide. Peptides bound to class I MHC are preferentially recognized by the CD8 subset rather than the CD4 subset of α-β T cells. This process is due, at least in part, to an affinity of the CD8 molecule for a region of the class I heavy chain distinct from that involved in binding peptide.[6]

Most peptides bound to class I MHC molecules are derived from proteins synthesized de novo within the APC (see Fig. 2–2).[7] In the uninfected APC these are derived from normal host proteins, that is, they are self-peptides.[5, 7] After intracellular infection, for example with a virus, peptides derived from viral proteins endog-

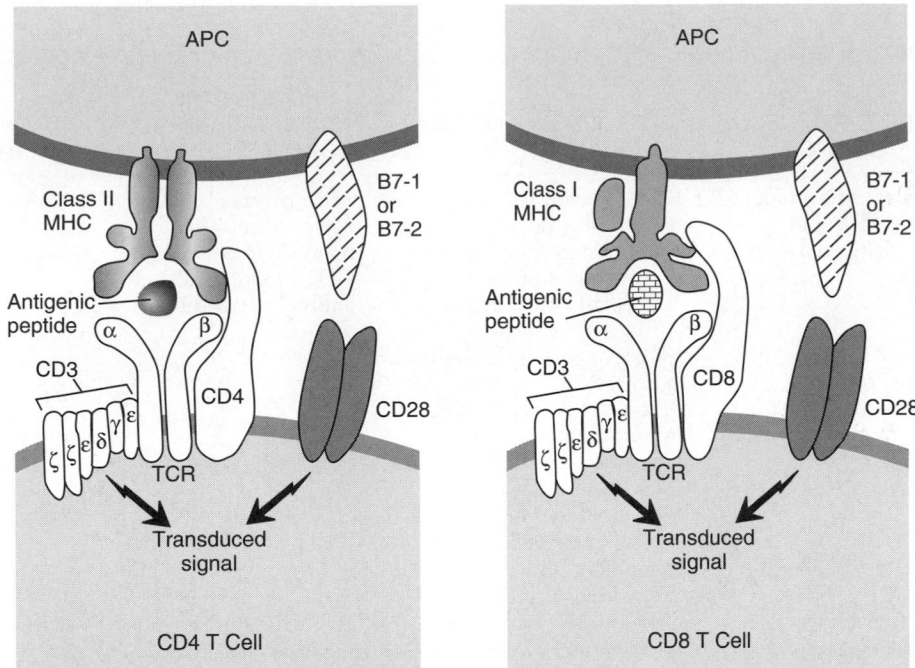

FIGURE 2–1 T cell recognition of antigen and activation. The αβ-T cell receptor (TCR) recognizes antigen from the antigen-presenting cell (APC) in the form of antigenic peptides bound to MHC molecules on the APC surface. Most CD4 T cells recognize peptides bound to class II MHC, whereas most CD8 T cells recognize peptides bound to class I MHC. This MHC restriction is the result of a thymic selection process, and is due, in part, to an intrinsic affinity of the CD4 and CD8 molecules for the class II and class I MHC molecules, respectively. Once antigen is recognized, the CD3 protein complex, which is invariably associated with the αβ-TCR, acts as docking site for tyrosine kinases that transmit activating intracellular signal. Interaction of the T cell CD28 molecule with either B7-1 or B7-2 provides an important co-stimulatory signal to the T cell, leading to complete activation, rather than functional inactivation (anergy).

enously synthesized within the cell bind to and are presented by class I MHC (see Fig. 2–2). Antigenic peptides are predominantly derived by enzymatic cleavage of proteins in the cytoplasm by a specialized organelle called the proteosome.[5] A specific peptide transporter, the transporter associated with antigen processing (TAP), then shuttles peptides formed in the cytoplasm to the endoplasmic reticulum, where peptide binding to recently synthesized class I MHC can take place.[5] Peptide binding stabilizes the association of the heavy chain with β₂-microglobulin in this compartment.

Peptides bound to class I MHC molecules in vivo are typically 8 to 10 amino acids in length.[5, 7, 8] The peptide binding groove is closed at both ends so that larger peptides cannot be accommodated. For a given MHC allele, certain positions within the peptide can only be encoded by certain amino acids for effective binding to the cleft (anchor residues). Amino acid residues at other, more variable positions point out of the cleft and are those recognized by the TCR (epitope residues). The antigen recognition process clearly imposes significant restrictions on the ability of peptides from a particular protein to be immunogenic, because the peptide must both bind to the MHC molecule and be recognized by the TCR. These constraints on peptide immunogenicity are offset by the availability of three different types of class I MHC molecules for antigen presentation, HLA-A, -B, and -C, each of which is highly polymorphic. The human HLA-A, -B, and -C heavy chain genes have

at least 86, 185, and 45 different molecularly defined alleles, respectively, with the greatest degree of polymorphism found in the region encoding the antigenic cleft.[9] MHC polymorphism ensures that at the individual and population levels the APC is able to bind and present a wide variety of peptides to T cells. It has been proposed that populations in which the MHC alleles are less polymorphic, such as Native Americans, may be generally at risk for severe infection on the basis of limitations in presenting antigenic peptides.[10]

Class I MHC and the cell components required for peptide generation, transport, and class I binding are virtually ubiquitous in the cells of vertebrates.[11] The advantage to the host is that this allows cytotoxic CD8 T cells the capacity to recognize and lyse cells infected with intracellular pathogens in most tissues. Adult neuronal cells are among the few cell types that constitutively lack class I MHC.[11] Because neurons are predominantly postmitotic cells, lack of class I MHC may help limit immune-mediated destruction of a cell type with a limited capacity to be replaced. On the other hand, recent studies indicate that class I MHCs are expressed by some populations of fetal neuronal cells, suggesting that these molecules may play a role in processes distinct from antigen presentation during early development.[12] Class I HLA-A, -B, and -C molecules are also absent from the trophoblast of the human placenta.[13] This may serve to limit the recognition of fetal-derived trophoblast cells as foreign by maternal T cells, as discussed later.

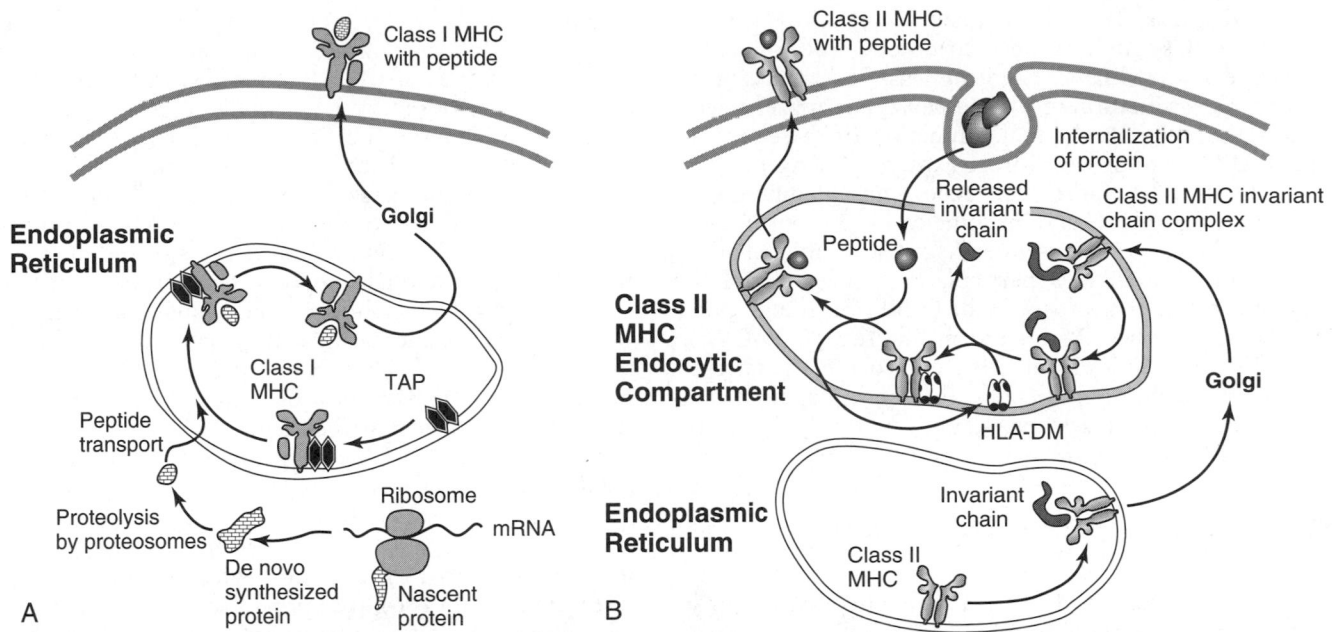

FIGURE 2–2 Intracellular pathways of antigen presentation. *A*, Foreign peptides that bind to class I MHC are derived predominantly from cytoplasmic proteins synthesized de novo within the cell. Proteins entering into the cytoplasm by macropinocytosis or after fusion of a virus with the cell membrane may also enter this pathway. Cytoplasmic proteins are degraded by proteosomes into peptides, which then enter into the endoplasmic reticulum via the TAP transporter system. Peptide binding by de novo synthesized class I MHC takes place within the endoplasmic reticulum. *B*, Foreign peptides that bind to class II MHC are mainly derived from internalization proteins that are found in the extracellular space or are components of cell membrane. The invariant chain binds to recently synthesized class II MHC and prevents peptide binding until a specialized cellular compartment for class II MHC peptide loading is reached. In this compartment, the invariant chain is proteolytically cleaved and released, and peptides derived from internalized proteins may now bind to class II MHC. The HLA-DM molecule facilitates the loading of peptide within this compartment.

An additional pathway for antigen presentation by class I MHC may operate in which extracellular proteins that are taken up as large particles (phagocytosis), as small particles (macropinocytosis), or in soluble form (micropinocytosis) are subsequently transferred from endocytic vesicles to the cytoplasm by an unknown mechanism.[14] Such a pathway may account for the ability of αβ CD8 T cells from humans infected with *Mycobacterium tuberculosis* to respond to soluble *M. tuberculosis* antigens presented by monocytes in a class I MHC–restricted manner.[15] An alternative pathway for antigen presentation by class I MHCs may also occur when dendritic cells, which are specialized for antigen presentation to T cells, take up protein from host cells that have undergone apoptosis (programmed cell death), for example, as a result of cell-mediated cytotoxicity.[16]

ANTIGEN PRESENTATION BY CLASS II MAJOR HISTOCOMPATIBILITY COMPLEX MOLECULES

In class II MHC, an α and a β chain each contribute to the formation of the cleft for antigenic peptide (see Figs. 2–1 and 2–2).[17] Class II MHC–peptide complexes on APCs are preferentially but not invariably recognized by αβ T cells of the CD4 but not the CD8 subset. This recognition is due, at least in part, to an affinity of the CD4 molecule for a domain of the class II MHC β chain distinct from the region forming part of the peptide cleft.[18] In contrast with peptides that bind to class I MHC, peptides that bind to class II MHC proteins are mostly derived from phagocytosis or endocytosis of soluble or membrane-bound proteins (see Fig. 2–2).[17] In the absence of foreign proteins, the majority of peptides bound to class II in APCs are self-peptides derived from proteins either found on the cell surface or secreted by the APC itself.[19] Newly synthesized class II MHC molecules associate in the endoplasmic reticulum with a protein called the invariant chain that impedes their binding of endogenous peptides in this compartment. This effectively separates peptides binding to class I and to class II MHC into two distinct pools.[17] The loading of exogenously derived peptides and the removal of invariant chain from class II MHC are facilitated by HLA-DM (see Fig. 2–2), a relatively nonpolymorphic heterodimeric protein that is encoded in the MHC locus.[17] This appears to occur in a specialized endocytic compartment.[17] Unlike the class I MHC cleft, the class II MHC cleft is open at both ends, allowing the binding of larger peptides than in the case of class I MHC. Most class II MHC peptides are 14 to 18 amino acids in length, although they can also be substantially longer.[8] As for class I MHC molecules, the genes that encode the α and β chains of the three major human class II MHC molecules, HLA-DR, -DP, and -DQ, are highly polymorphic, particularly in the region encoding the peptide binding cleft.[20]

The distribution of class II MHC in uninflamed tissues is more restricted than that of class I MHC,[21] as constitutive class II MHC is mainly limited to "professional" APCs, such as dendritic cells, mononuclear phagocytes, and B cells. Limiting class II MHC expression in most situations to these cell types makes teleologic sense, because the major function of these professional APCs is to process foreign antigen for recognition by CD4 T cells. Other cell types can be induced to express class II MHC and, in some cases, present antigen to CD4 T cells, as a consequence of tissue inflammation or exposure to cytokines, particularly interferon-γ (IFN-γ), but also tumor necrosis factor (TNF) or granulocyte-macrophage colony-stimulating factor (GM-CSF). These include endothelial cells, enterocytes, renal epithelial cells, thyroid epithelial cells, microglia, epidermal keratinocytes, myoblasts, eosinophils, natural killer cells, and T cells themselves.[22]

NONCLASSIC ANTIGEN-PRESENTATION MOLECULES

HLA-E, a nonclassic MHC molecule encoded on chromosome 6, is nonpolymorphic, with only two human alleles known. Like peptides bound to conventional class I MHC, peptides bound to HLA-E molecules are loaded by the TAP peptide transport system, and, like class I MHC, the HLA-E heavy chain is associated with β_2-microglobulin.[23] However, in contrast with conventional class I MHCs, HLA-E preferentially binds hydrophobic peptides derived from the amino-terminal leader sequences of most alleles of HLA-A, -B, and -C.[23] Low levels of HLA-E surface expression can be detected on most cells,[24] consistent with the nearly ubiquitous distribution of HLA-A, -B, and -C and the TAP system. As discussed in the section Natural Killer Cells, surface HLA-E interacts with CD94-NKG2-A, an inhibitory surface receptor expressed by natural killer (NK) cells.[23] This may help limit the NK cell–mediated lysis of target cells to those that have an overall reduction in the expression of classic class I MHC molecules.

HLA-G is also encoded on chromosome 6 and is expressed by human cytotrophoblasts and macrophages within the maternal uterine wall.[23] HLA-G has limited polymorphism but is otherwise quite similar to class I MHC in its association with β_2-microglobulin and its predicted structure.[25] HLA-G produced by the placenta occurs as either an integral membrane protein or a secreted protein isoform.[25] As discussed in ·the section on NK cells, a lack of conventional class I MHC may make cells highly susceptible to NK cell–mediated lysis. Because trophoblast cells lack expression of most conventional class I molecules, their surface expression of HLA-G, which is particularly high during the first trimester of pregnancy, may limit their potential lysis by maternal or fetal NK cells. This inhibition probably occurs, at least in part, by HLA-G's engaging CD94-NKG2-A, the same inhibitory receptor utilized by HLA-E.[26] The function of the soluble isoform of HLA-G remains unclear.

A group of nonclassic MHC molecules encoded by the CD1 locus on human chromosome 1 also appear to have specialized immune functions. The human CD1 locus includes four nonpolymorphic genes, CD1a

through CD1d.[27] CD1 molecules associate with β_2-microglobulin but have limited structural homology with either class I or class II MHC proteins. In humans they are mainly expressed by hematopoietic cells with APC function, including dendritic cells,[28] which are discussed in detail later. CD1b efficiently binds and appears to be involved in the presentation of highly hydrophobic lipoglycan molecules of mycobacteria, such as lipoarabinomannans, mycolic acid, and glucose monomycolate.[27, 29] Mycobacterial lipoglycans undergo processing and loading onto CD1b in an endosomal compartment that is similar or identical to that where class II MHC molecule peptide loading takes place.[27] CD1c may be involved in the presentation of lipidated bacterial polysaccharides, such as polyribosylribitol phosphate component of the capsule of *Haemophilus influenzae* type b.[30]

CD1d, the only member of the human CD1 cluster that is also expressed in the mouse, appears to be specialized for the presentation of hydrophobic nonpeptide molecules, such as the glycosylphosphatidylinositol (GPI) moiety of GPI-linked proteins.[31] Such GPI-linked proteins are found at particularly high levels on the surface of certain protozoa pathogens, such as *Plasmodium* and *Trypanosoma* species. As in the case of CD1b, the compartment for the loading of antigens onto CD1d is similar or identical to that for class II MHC peptide loading. Nonprotein antigens bound to CD1d predominantly activate a specialized subset of $\alpha\beta$ T cells that lack CD4 and CD8, rather than conventional CD4 or CD8 T cells.[27] One of these T cell subsets, NK T cells, preferentially recognizes CD1d-restricted antigens and is discussed in detail in the section Basic Aspects of T Cell Development and Function.

Two proteins encoded in the MHC locus, MHC class I–related chains A and B (MICA and MICB), have limited but clear homology with conventional class I MHC molecules. However, in contrast with conventional class I MHCs, they lack a binding site for CD8, are not associated with β_2-microglobulin, and do not appear to be involved with the presentation of peptide antigens.[32] Instead, these molecules are expressed on stressed intestinal epithelial cells, such as those experiencing heat shock, and are recognized by $\gamma\delta$ T cells that bear $V_\delta 1$-containing $\gamma\delta$-TCR. Their role in $\gamma\delta$ T cell responses is discussed in the section Gamma-Delta T Cells and Their Ontogeny.

Studies in mice indicate that other molecules with some homology to class I MHC are specialized for the presentation of peptides containing *N*-formylmethionine derived from the amino terminus of bacterial proteins.[33] Whether analogous human class I MHC–like proteins are specialized for the presentation of bacterially derived peptides remains uncertain.

DENDRITIC CELLS

Dendritic cells are often referred to as the sentinels of the immune system.[34] They are bone marrow–derived cells that express both class I and class II MHC molecules. In their resting form they are found in epithelia as well as in the interstitium of solid organs, such as heart and kidney.[35] Dendritic cells are the most efficient

APCs for activating T cells during their first encounter with antigen and for inducing B cell responses to T-dependent antigens, such as intact proteins.[34] Although the precise relationship between dendritic cells and less mature precursor cells in vivo remains poorly understood, cells with dendritic morphologic features, function, and characteristic surface expression of proteins can be derived from pluripotent stem cells of the bone marrow, monocytes or their immediate precursors, and even neutrophil precursors by incubation with various combinations of cytokines (e.g., GM-CSF and interleukin-4 [IL-4]).[34] Flt3 ligand, a cytokine produced by stromal cells within the bone marrow microenvironment, is a particularly potent inducer of dendritic cell growth and function in vivo.[36, 37] Bone marrow–derived dendritic cells enter into the circulation and preferentially migrate into epithelia and interstitial space of solid organs, where they are found at a low frequency.

Dendritic cells that initially encounter potential antigens in epithelia and the solid organs appear to be specialized for the initiation of the process of antigen presentation in that they are highly phagocytic but lack high levels of MHC surface expression. Some dendritic cells in the spleen may also serve this function. Dendritic cell phagocytosis, in contrast with that mediated by monocytes and macrophages, is not markedly enhanced by the binding of antibody, complement, or both to the target particle (opsonophagocytosis) and may occur independently of such binding.[35] Dendritic cells also express high levels of carbohydrate-specific receptors that may enhance glycoprotein uptake and entry into intracellular antigen presentation compartments.[38] They are also highly efficient at taking up extracellular fluid by macropinocytosis and micropinocytosis.[35] Finally, dendritic cells may efficiently phagocytose cells or cell fragments that have undergone apoptosis.[35, 39] Proteins that enter into dendritic cells by pinocytosis or in association with apoptotic cells can enter into both the class II pathway[39] as well as the class I MHC pathway by a TAP-dependent mechanism.[40]

Once antigens are taken up by dendritic cells in the tissues, dendritic cells move into areas of the lymph nodes and spleen, where they are more likely to encounter T cells that can specifically recognize antigen.[34] Dendritic cells undergoing this migration have a unique cytologic appearance and are known as veiled cells and increase their surface expression of class II MHC molecules.[41] This mechanism enhances the chance that they will evoke CD4 T cell antigen recognition. Dendritic cell maturation and migration can be triggered by proinflammatory stimuli, such as bacterial peptides, cell walls, DNA, or lipopolysaccharide (LPS), or host proinflammatory cytokines, such as IL-1 and TNF.[35, 42] This sequence of events has been best documented for Langerhans dendritic cells of the skin, but it is likely that a similar process occurs for dendritic cells found in the other epithelia or in solid organs.

The migration from nonlymphoid to lymphoid tissue appears to be due, at least in part, to the expression of receptors on the dendritic cell for chemokines, such as EB-11-ligand chemokine (ELC)/macrophage inflammatory protein-3β (MIP-3β), that are elaborated by peripheral lymphoid tissue.[43, 44] Chemokines constitute a large cytokine superfamily, most of which are secreted and of relatively low molecular weight. Chemokines are produced by a large number of cell types and selectively chemoattract various leukocyte populations by binding G-protein–linked receptors (see Tables 2–1 and 2–2). They can be divided into two major subfamilies, α-chemokines, most of which act as chemoattractants for neutrophils, and β-chemokines, most of which act as chemoattractants for mononuclear phagocytes and eosinophils. Both of the major subfamilies contain members that influence the migration of T cells and B cells.

Most dendritic cells found in peripheral lymphoid tissue express high levels of adhesion molecules (Table 2–3); co-stimulatory molecules, such as B7-1 and B7-2 (see Table 2–3); cytokine receptors, such as CD40; and chemokine receptors that may facilitate dendritic–T or –B cell interactions and lymphocyte activation.[34] The production of the cytokine IL-12 in response to engagement of the CD40 molecule on the dendritic cell by CD40 ligand on the T cell may be particularly important for the T cells to acquire the capacity to produce cytokines, such as IFN-γ,[45] which provide protection against infection with intracellular pathogens. Dendritic cells may also directly interact with B cells independently of T cells and regulate their production of antibody.[46]

Recent studies, most of them carried out in mice, suggest that lymphoid dendritic cells constitute a distinct cell lineage from myeloid dendritic cells.[47] Lymphoid dendritic cells appear to be derived from precursor cells that also have the capacity for differentiation into T cells, B cells, or natural killer lymphocytes rather than from mononuclear phagocyte precursors. Murine lymphoid dendritic cells have a distribution cell that is distinct from myeloid dendritic cells and appear to be generated in situ in the thymus and peripheral lymphoid organs. As discussed later, those in the thymus appear particularly important for a process of negative selection of developing thymocytes that can recognize self-antigens. It has been suggested that lymphoid dendritic cells of the peripheral lymphoid organs may serve a similar function and participate in the deletion of peripheral T cells that are autoreactive.[47] Such a negative regulatory role is suggested by rodent studies that indicate that some dendritic cells may inhibit rather than stimulate T cell responses with antigen.[48, 49] Whether peripheral lymphocyte dendritic cells in humans have a similar regulatory role is not yet clear.

Antigen Presentation in the Fetus and Neonate

By 12 weeks of gestation, the expression of class I and class II MHC molecules by a variety of fetal tissues is evident[50, 51] and all of the major "professional" APCs (macrophages, B cells, and dendritic cells) are present. Class I MHC expression by neonatal lymphocytes has been reported to be lower than that by adult cells,[52] although this difference needs confirmation and may not be functionally significant. Class II MHC molecule expression by fetal APC in tissues appears to be similar to that of the adult,[53-55] and expression by neonatal

TABLE 2–3
Pairs of Surface Molecules Involved in the Interactions Between T Cells and Antigen-Presenting Cells

T CELL SURFACE MOLECULE	T CELL DISTRIBUTION	CORRESPONDING LIGAND(S) ON APC	APC DISTRIBUTION
CD2	Most T cells, higher on memory cells, lower on adult virgin and neonatal T cells	LFA-3 (CD58), CD59	Leukocytes
CD4	Subset of αβ T cells with predominantly helper activity	Class II MHC β chain	Dendritic cells, Mφ, B cells, and others (see text)
CD5	All T cells	CD72	B cells, Mφ
CD8	Subset of αβ T cells with predominantly helper activity	Class I MHC heavy chain	Ubiquitous
LFA-1 (CD11a-CD18)	All T cells, higher on memory cells, lower on adult virgin and neonatal T cells	ICAM-1 (CD54) ICAM-2 (CD102) ICAM-3 (CD50)	Leukocytes (ICAM-3 > 1, 2) and endothelium (ICAM-1 and ICAM-2); most ICAM-1 expression requires activation
CD28	Most CD4 T cells, subset of CD8 T cells	B7-1 (CD80) B7-2 (CD86)	Dendritic cells, Mφ, activated B cells
CD45R0	High levels on memory cells, lower levels on adult virgin and neonatal T cells	CD22 (?)	B cells
VLA-4 (CD49d/CD29)	All T cells; higher on memory cells, lower on adult virgin and neonatal T cells	VCAM-1 (CD106)	Activated or inflamed endothelium (increased by TNF, IL-1, IL-4)
ICAM-1 (CD54)	All T cells; higher on memory cells, lower on adult virgin and neonatal T cells	LFA-1 (CD11a-CD18)	Leukocytes
CTLA-4 (CD152)	Activated T cells	B7-1 (CD80) B7-2 (CD86)	Dendritic cells, Mφ, activated B cells
CD40 ligand (CD154)	Activated CD4 T cells; lower on neonatal CD4 T cells	CD40	Dendritic cells, Mφ, B cells, thymic epithelial cells

ICAM-1 = intercellular adhesion molecule 1; IL = interleukin; LFA = leukocyte function antigen; Mφ = mononuclear phagocyte; TNF = tumor necrosis factor; VACAM-1 = vascular cell adhesion molecule-1; VLA = very late antigen.

monocytes and B cells is either similar to or greater than that by adult cells.[52] Fetal tissues are frequently vigorously rejected after transplantation into non–MHC-matched hosts. This indicates that the level of surface MHC expression on fetal tissue is sufficient to initiate a vigorous allogeneic response by the host in which the foreign cells are killed by cytotoxic T cells, which are predominantly of the CD8 subset. Because most allogeneic responses of T cells are directed against self-peptide–allogeneic MHC molecule complexes rather than to MHC molecules alone,[56] the vigor of rejection of fetal allografts suggests that antigen presentation by class I MHCs for the generation of cytolytic T cells is largely intact. However, these results do not exclude the possibility of more subtle deficiencies in antigen presentation in the fetus and neonate, particularly under conditions that more stringently test APC function, such as during infection with herpesviruses that inhibit peptide loading of class I MHC by multiple mechanisms.[57]

Class II MHC–mediated antigen presentation also appears to be grossly intact, because neonatal and adult monocytes are similarly effective in presenting soluble protein antigens or alloantigens to induce T prolifera-

tion,[58, 59] a response that is mainly class II MHC–dependent. However, one study[60] suggested that class II antigen presentation was reduced in infants between 6 and 12 months of age compared with older children or adults: This conclusion was mainly based on activation of responder T cells contained in the peripheral blood mononuclear cell fraction by alloantigen, with the cellular source of alloantigen consisting of blood mononuclear cells depleted of adherent cells (mostly monocytes and dendritic cells). In this system, alloantigen presentation to the responder T cells is dependent on autologous class II MHC antigen presentation by APCs contained in the responder rather than the stimulator cell population.[60] Surprisingly, this reduced T cell proliferative response to indirectly presented alloantigen was not observed for cord blood, but its adequacy during the first 6 months of life was not studied.[60] Given these findings, it will be of interest to determine whether class II MHC antigen presentation for conventional soluble antigens, rather than alloantigens, is intact during the first year of life. Interestingly, a recent report suggests that a substantial fraction of class II MHC molecules on neonatal but not adult B cells appears to be "empty," that is, without peptides in the binding groove.[61] This observation, which needs independent confirmation, raises the possibility that certain populations of neonatal APCs may be more limited than adult cells in class II MHC antigen processing, peptide loading, or both.

As discussed in detail later, antigen-specific T cell responses of the fetus and neonate, including T cell–mediated cytotoxicity and T cell–dependent antibody production, tend to be reduced or delayed compared with the responses of older individuals. Because these reduced or delayed responses could reflect limitations in the function of dendritic cells, which are critical for the initiation of the T cell response to new antigens (referred to as neoantigens), the adequacy of dendritic cell function in the fetus and neonate is of interest. Animal models support the possibility of functional immaturity in neonatal dendritic cell function, in that dendritic cell recruitment into the rat lung after infectious challenge is markedly limited during the first several weeks of life compared with that during adulthood.[62]

The adequacy of dendritic cell function in the human neonate and fetus remains unclear, particularly for those cells found in the epithelium, interstitium, or peripheral lymphoid organs. In a study using circulating dendritic cells that were isolated by a combination of cell fractionation and culture overnight in vitro, those from cord blood were substantially less effective than cells from adult peripheral blood in activating T cell proliferation from unrelated donors.[63] This decreased activity was associated with substantially reduced levels of HLA-DR molecules and intercellular adhesion molecule 1 (ICAM-1) (see Table 2–3).[63] In contrast, another group, using a protocol that did not involve overnight incubation, found that freshly isolated neonatal dendritic cells from cord blood were effective stimulators of allogeneic T cell responses in vitro.[64] Whether circulating dendritic cells in the neonate have a capacity similar to that of adult cells to produce cytokines, such as IL-12, and to express various surface molecules, such as CD40 and B7 molecules, in response to proinflammatory mediators or other maturation signals is also unclear.

Basic Aspects of T Cell Development and Function

PROTHYMOCYTES

Differentiation within the thymus is an obligatory step for most αβ T cells. Small populations of αβ T cells may develop extrathymically in bone marrow, gut epithelium, and liver.[65–68] The development of lymphocytes of the T cell, B cell, and NK cells from less committed hematopoietic cells involves a common lymphocyte progenitor.[69] This progenitor gives rise to the prothymocyte, a lymphoid cell that lacks TCR-α or TCR-β chains, expresses CD3 molecules in its cytoplasm and the CD7 protein on its surface, and has little or no expression of CD4 or CD8. CD7 is also found on mature T cells and NK cells, suggesting a close relationship between these two cell types.[70] Differentiation within the thymus is an obligatory step for most αβ T cells and begins when the prothymocyte enters the subcapsular region of the thymus from the circulation

(Fig. 2–3). Prothymocytes appear to retain the ability to differentiate into the NK lineage even after entering the thymus.[70] The human thymus does not have a population of self-replenishing stem cells, and therefore probably requires a continual input of thymocyte progenitor cells (prothymocytes) to maintain thymocytopoiesis.[71]

THYMOCYTE DEVELOPMENT AND THE GENERATION OF T CELL RECEPTOR DIVERSITY

The thymocyte microenvironment somehow triggers the rearrangement of widely dispersed gene variable (V), diversity (D), and joining (J) segments for the TCR-β and TCR-γ chain genes, and V and J segments for the TCR-α and TCR-δ chain genes, so that the segments within these genetic loci are contiguous and can be transcribed (Fig. 2–4). Rearrangement of TCR-β or TCR-γ by immature thymocytes occurs in the subcapsular region of the thymus and precedes TCR-α or TCR-δ rearrangement. Thymocytes in which rearrangement of both the TCR-β and TCR-α chain genes is productive (able to be expressed as full-length protein) express αβ-TCR protein on the cell surface and are the precursors of peripheral αβ T cells, including the CD4 and CD8 T cell subsets. Thymocytes in which rearrangement of both TCR-γ and TCR-δ is productive express surface γδ-TCR and are precursors of some peripheral γδ T cells. The events within the thymus that commit developing thymocytes to differentiate along the alpha-beta lineage versus the gamma-delta lineage remain poorly understood.[72]

Rearrangement of TCR genes and, as discussed later, immunoglobulin molecules requires a complex of DNA binding proteins and enzymes. These include recombination activating gene 1 (RAG-1) and RAG-2 proteins, a high-molecular-weight DNA-dependent protein kinase and its associated Ku70 and Ku80 proteins, and DNA ligase IV and its associated XRCC4 protein.[73] The RAG proteins are critically involved in the initiation of the recombination process by recognizing and cleaving conserved sequences flanking each V, D, and J segment. The DNA-dependent protein kinase and DNA ligase and their associated proteins are involved in the subsequent joining of DNA segments. Humans with genetic deficiency of either RAG-1 or RAG-2 have a form of severe combined immunodeficiency (SCID),[74] because T cell and B cell development depends on the surface expression of rearranged TCR and immunoglobulin genes, respectively.

The TCR-β chain gene is rearranged before the TCR-α chain gene. The unrearranged human TCR-β chain gene spans 685 kilobases of DNA on human chromosome 7 and consists of 46 potentially functional variable (V) gene segments located upstream of two constant (C) regions, each associated with one diversity (D) and six joining (J) segments (see Fig. 2–4).[75] The D segment first rearranges to a downstream J segment, with the deletion of intervening DNA. This is followed by rearrangement of a V segment to the DJ segment, resulting in a contiguous (VDJC) β-chain gene segment. If this segment lacks premature translation stop codons,

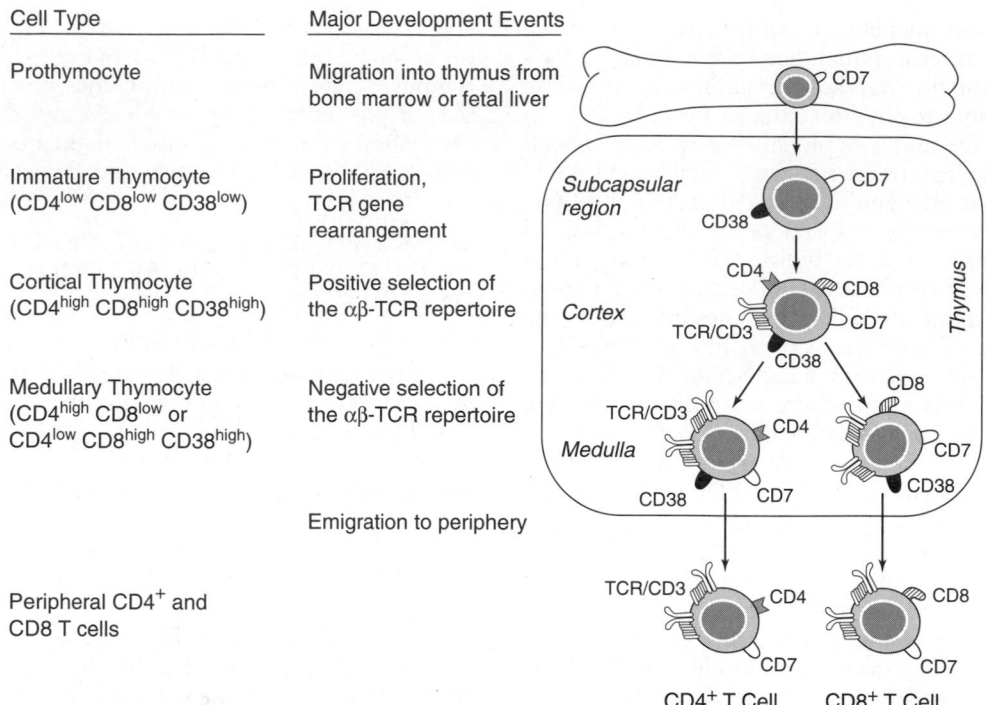

FIGURE 2–3 Putative stages of human αβ thymocyte development. Prothymocytes from the bone marrow or fetal liver, which express CD7, enter the thymus subcapsular region and give rise to progressively mature αβ-TCR thymocytes, defined by their pattern of expression of the αβ-TCR–CD3 complex, CD4, CD8, and CD38. TCR-α and TCR-β chain genes are rearranged in the subcapsular region, positive selection occurs mainly in the thymic cortex, and negative selection occurs mainly in the medulla. After these selection processes, medullary thymocytes emigrate into the circulation and colonize the peripheral lymphoid organs as CD4 and CD8 T cells with high levels of the αβ-TCR–CD3 complex and lacking CD38 surface expression. In neonates, most peripheral T cells retain surface expression of CD38.

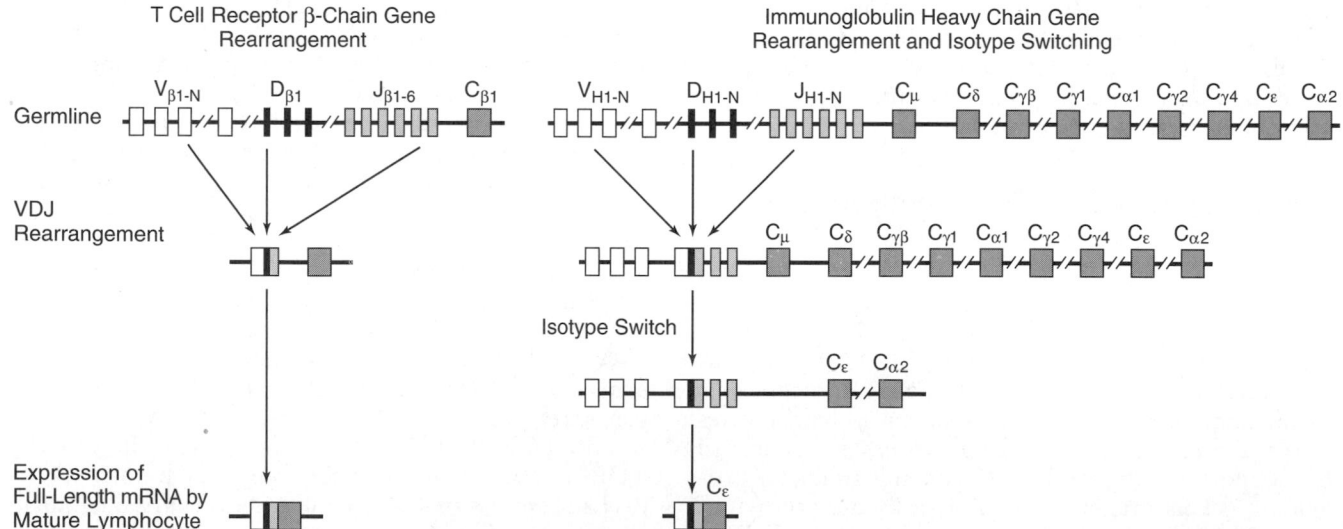

FIGURE 2–4 The T cell receptor and immunoglobulin genes are formed by rearrangement in immature lymphocytes. The TCR-β chain gene and the immunoglobulin heavy chain genes are shown as examples. A similar process is involved with rearrangement of the TCR-α, -γ, and -δ chain genes, and with the immunoglobulin light chain genes. Rearrangement involves the joining of dispersed segments of variable (V), diversity (D), and junctional (J) gene segments with the deletion of intervening DNA. This allows expression of a full-length mRNA transcript, which can be translated into a functional protein, provided that there are no premature translational stop codons. Immunoglobulin heavy chain genes undergo an additional rearrangement called isotype switching, in which the constant (C) region segment is changed without alteration of the antigen-combining host site formed by the V, D, and J segments. The isotype switch from IgM to IgE is shown.

the TCR-β chain protein may be expressed on the thymocyte surface in association with a pre–TCR-α chain protein and the CD3 signaling complex.[76] This complex instructs the thymocyte to increase its surface expression of CD4 and CD8, to start rearrangement of the TCR-α chain gene, and to stop rearrangement of the other TCR-β chain allele. This inhibition of TCR-β chain gene rearrangement results in allelic exclusion, so that more than 99% of αβ T cells express only a single type of TCR-β chain gene.[77]

Rearrangement of the TCR-α chain gene then occurs; it involves the joining of V segments directly to J segments, without intervening D segments. The human TCR-α chain gene locus is less well characterized, but is known to contain approximately 100 V segments and 50 to 100 J segments. Allelic exclusion is relatively ineffective for the TCR-α chain gene, and it is estimated that as many as one third of peripheral human αβ T cells may express two types of TCR-α chains.[78] RAG protein expression normally ceases in cortical thymocytes, limiting gene rearrangement to early thymocyte development. However, recent experiments using mice bearing an αβ-TCR encoded by a transgene suggest that peripheral T cells may also have the capacity to reexpress RAG proteins and undergo secondary TCR-β chain gene rearrangement.[79] Whether this process, known as immune receptor editing,[80] occurs in human T cells or in genetically unmanipulated mice remains to be shown.

TCR diversity is generated by the largely random use of V, (D), and J segments in assembling the TCR-α and TCR-β chain genes.[81] The CDR3 region, where the distal portion of the V segment joins the (D)J segment, appears to be a particularly important source of αβ-TCR diversity for peptide-MHC recognition.[81] In addition to this combinatorial diversity, several other mechanisms increase potential diversity at the junctions among V, D, and J. First, the recombinase is imprecise in cleaving the ends of segments for recombination so that a variable number of nucleotides are lost.[82] Second, terminal deoxytransferase (TdT), an enzyme expressed at high levels in TCR gene-rearranging thymocytes, randomly adds nucleotides (called N-nucleotides) to the ends of segments undergoing rearrangement.[82, 83] TdT addition is a particularly important mechanism for diversity generation because every three additional nucleotides encode a potential codon, potentially increasing repertoire diversity by a factor of 20. Finally, one or two nucleotides that are palindromic to the end of the gene segment (termed P nucleotides) can be added.[84] Together, these mechanisms for generating diversity can theoretically result in as many as 10^{15} types of αβ-TCR. However, actual αβ-TCR diversity is likely to be less than this theoretical maximal value, because particular V, D, and J segments may be used less frequently than would be predicted on a random basis.[85] The reasons for this deviation from random segment usage remain unclear, but it may be due to differences among segments in their accessibility to the protein complex involved in the recombination process.[85]

Thymocytes that have successfully rearranged and express αβ-TCRs have a CD4[high]CD8[high] surface phenotype (see Fig. 2–3). Cells at this stage must pass a selective process that tests the appropriateness of their TCR receptor specificity, known as positive selection. Positive selection requires that the αβ-TCR recognize self-peptides bound to MHC molecules displayed on epithelial cells of the thymic cortex. The generation of a diverse αβ-TCR repertoire appears to require that cortical epithelial cells express a diverse group of self-peptides bound to MHC.[86] The αβ-TCR interacts not only with the MHC-associated peptide but also with regions of the MHC that form the groove,[87] for which it has an intrinsic affinity.[88] This presumably applies to positive selection in the thymus as well as to the recognition of foreign antigen by peripheral αβ T cells. If the TCR has sufficient affinity for self-peptide–MHC complexes, the thymocyte receives a signal allowing its survival.[89] If this signal is absent or weak, the thymocyte dies by apoptosis as a result of activation of caspases, a family of intracellular cysteine proteases. Positive selection is also influenced by interactions between MHC molecules and the CD4 and CD8 molecules. As mentioned previously, class I MHC and class II MHC molecules have constant domains located outside their peptide binding grooves that have affinity for CD8 and CD4, respectively. As a result of these interactions, most CD4[high]CD8[low] thymocytes (and their peripheral CD4 T cell descendants) recognize peptides bound to class II MHC molecules, and most CD4[low]CD8[high] T cells (and peripheral CD8 T cells) recognize peptides bound to class I MHC molecules (see Fig. 2–3).

Positively selected CD4[high]CD8[low] and CD4[low]CD8[high] thymocytes enter the medulla, where they undergo a second selection process called negative selection, in which they are eliminated by apoptosis if their TCR has too high an affinity for peptide-MHC complexes expressed on medullary dendritic cells.[90] Negative selection helps eliminate αβ T cells with TCRs that could pose a risk of autoimmune reactions and is an important influence on the final TCR repertoire.[91] Thymic epithelial cells found in the medulla may express a diverse array of self-antigens, such as insulin and myelin basic protein, which help in this elimination.[92] In vitro studies have shown that murine thymocytes activated via the αβ-TCR–CD3 complex express the cytotoxic T lymphocyte antigen 4 (CTLA-4)(CD152) molecule and that co-engagement of this molecule may play a role in negative selection by enhancing apoptosis.[93] A ligand for CTLA-4, the B7-1 molecule (CD80), is expressed by human medullary dendritic cells, particularly during fetal development,[94] supporting the notion that CTLA-4 is involved in negative selection. As a net result of either the failure to rearrange the TCR-α or TCR-β chain genes productively, the lack of positive selection, or the occurrence of negative selection, most (~95%) thymic precursors die rather than become mature single-positive thymocytes. Positively selected thymocytes that are not eliminated by negative selection enter into the circulation as antigenically naive αβ T cells and preferentially home to the peripheral lymphoid organs (see Fig. 2–3).

Because the region forming the peptide binding groove of MHC molecules is highly polymorphic in the human population,[9, 20, 95] a result of positive selection is that T cells have a strong preference for recognizing a particular foreign peptide bound to self-MHC, rather than to the MHC of an unrelated individual. On the other hand, the fact that TCR has intrinsic affinity for MHC molecules[88] accounts for the ability of an APC bearing foreign MHC molecules to activate a substantial proportion (up to 5 to 10%) of T cells (the allogeneic response). In the allogeneic response, T cells are activated by novel antigen specificities that result from the combination of a foreign MHC with multiple self-peptides.[56] Because these self-peptide–foreign MHC specificities are not expressed in the thymus, T cells capable of recognizing them have not been eliminated by the negative selection process in the medulla.

THYMOCYTE GROWTH AND DIFFERENTIATION FACTORS

The cell-cell interactions and factors secreted within the thymic microenvironment that are essential for thymocyte development are only partly understood, but cytokines play a critical role. IL-7 is a cytokine produced by nonhematopoietic cells in the thymus that is essential for immature thymocyte proliferation. Humans lacking a functional IL-7 receptor, as a result of a genetic deficiency of either the IL-7 receptor α chain[96] or the common γ chain (γc) with which the α chain associates[97] have abortive thymocyte development and lack mature αβ T cells. A similar phenotype is observed with genetic deficiency of the JAK-3 tyrosine kinase. This kinase is associated with the cytoplasmic domain of the γc and delivers activation signals to the interior of the cell.[98] B cell development is spared in these human genetic immunodeficiencies.

THYMOCYTE POSTSELECTION MATURATION AND SURVIVAL

Alpha-beta $CD4^+CD8^-$ and $CD4^-CD8^+$ thymocytes are the most mature T cell populations in the thymus and predominate in the thymic medulla. Many of the functional differences between peripheral CD4 and CD8 T cells appear to be established during the later stages of thymic maturation, presumably as a result of differentiation induced by positive selection: $CD4^+CD8^-$ thymocytes, like peripheral $CD4^+$ T cells, are enriched in cells that can secrete certain cytokines, such as IL-2, and can provide help for B cells in producing immunoglobulin.[99] $CD4^-CD8^+$ thymocytes, like peripheral $CD8^+$ T cells, are relatively limited in their ability to produce IL-2, but, once primed by antigen, are effective in mediating cytotoxic activity.[100] $CD4^+CD8^-$ and $CD4^-CD8^+$ thymocytes enter into the circulation, where they colonize peripheral lymphoid tissue as antigenically naive CD4 and CD8 T cells, respectively. Mouse studies indicate that the long-term survival of peripheral αβ T cells, particularly the antigenically naive population, requires engagement of their αβ-TCR by self-MHC.[101] Whether this process is analogous to positive selection in the thymus in its requirements for a diverse self-peptide repertoire remains unclear.

T CELL ACTIVATION AND EFFECTOR FUNCTIONS

Activation of peripheral αβ T cells by engagement of the TCR with foreign antigenic peptide bound to MHC leads to tyrosine phosphorylation of the cytoplasmic ITAM domains of the CD3 complex.[76] The complex consists of four different proteins encoded by separate genes (CD3δ, CD3ε, CD3γ, and CD3ζ). The phosphorylated ITAMs, particularly those contained in CD3ε and CD3ζ, in turn act as docking sites for tyrosine kinases (e.g., zap-70, lck, and fyn) that propagate the activation signal. More downstream activation signal events are mediated by enzymes, such as phospholipase C, protein kinase C, calcineurin, and ras,[102] which act through adaptor molecules[103] and other intermediaries to turn on transcription of genes encoding key proteins for activation, such as cytokines, cell cycle regulators, and, in cytotoxic T cells, proteins involved in killing other cells, such as perforins. The expression of more than 100 genes is altered as a result of the activation process.[104]

T cell activation is not necessarily an all-or-none phenomenon, and alterations in the amino acids that constitute the epitope of the antigenic peptide seen by the αβ-TCR can result in partial activation of only certain responses (e.g., cytokine production but not cell proliferation) or complete block of all responses (antagonism) when the T cell is subsequently exposed to the wildtype peptide.[105] The mechanisms that underlie partial activation and antagonism remain only partly understood but may involve peptide-induced internalization of αβ-TCR, partial or altered intracellular signaling, or both.[106]

In addition to recognition of a suitable peptide-MHC complex by the TCR, αβ T cell activation often requires additional signals provided by the APCs, which are collectively referred to as co-stimulation.[107] Major sources of co-stimulation are due to interactions between the B7 molecules, B7-1 (CD80) and B7-2 (CD86) on the APC, and CD28 on the T cell,[107] and CD40 on the APC with CD40 ligand on the T cell (Fig. 2–5) (see Table 2–3).[45, 108] The CD28 molecule is constitutively expressed on most αβ T cells, whereas CD40 ligand is rapidly expressed (within a few hours) after TCR engagement by antigen.[45] CD28 signaling potently augments T cell cytokine production and the percentage of cells that enter into the cell cycle after engagement of the αβ-TCR/CD3 complex.[107] Engagement of CD40 ligand also enhances T cell proliferation and cytokine production.[109]

In addition to co-stimulation, a number of molecules on the T cell and APC surfaces may selectively bind to each other (see Table 2–3) and enhance T cell activation as a result of stabilizing the interaction between the T cell and APCs. Such adhesive interactions may be physiologically important because the affinity of the TCR for peptide-MHC complexes appears to be relatively low.[81] Some molecules may serve both in costimulatory pathways and adhesive interactions. In addition, co-stimulatory interactions may induce increased expression of surface molecules on the APC that further augment co-stimulation or adhesion.[45, 110] For example, the engagement of the CD40 molecule on the APC may increase its surface expression of B7 molecules.

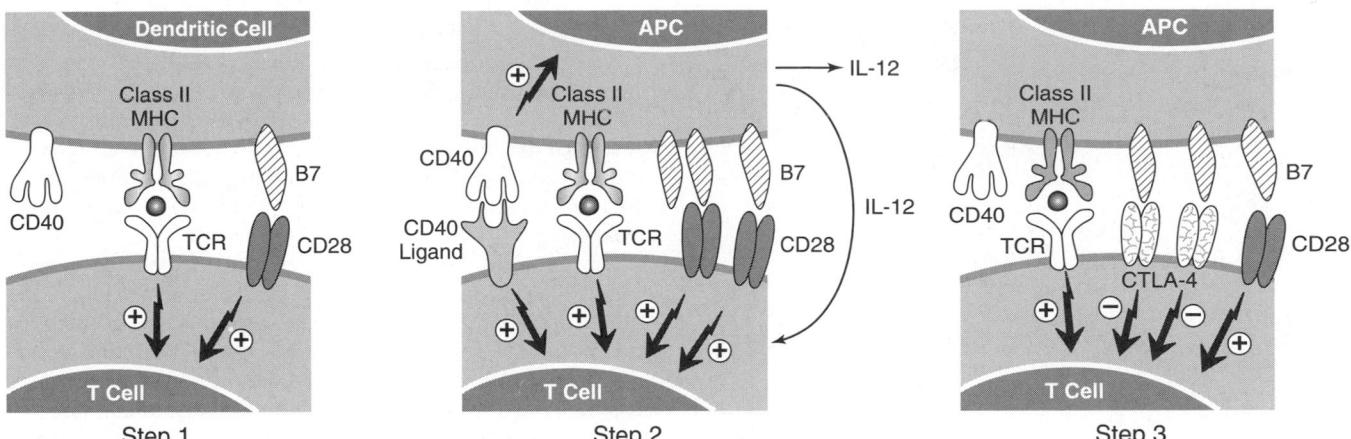

FIGURE 2–5 T cell–APC interactions early during the immune response to peptide antigens. A class II MHC–restricted response by CD4 T cells is shown as an example. Dendritic cells are probably the most important APCs for antigenically naive T cells and constitutively express B7, CD40, and class II MHC molecules on their cell surface. Engagement of the CD4 T cell by antigenic peptide bound to MHC on the dendritic cell, in conjunction with co-stimulation by B7-CD28 interactions, leads to T cell activation (step 1). The activated T cell expresses CD40 ligand on its surface, which engages CD40; this increases B7 expression on the dendritic cell, enhancing T cell co-stimulation (step 2). CD40 engagement also activates the dendritic cells to produce cytokines, such as IL-12. IL-12, in turn, promotes the differentiation of T cells into TH1-type effector cells that produce high levels of IFN-γ and low or undetectable amounts of IL-4. CTLA-4 is expressed on the T cells during the later stages of T cell activation. Engagement of CTLA-4 by B7 molecules on the APC delivers negative signals that help terminate T cell activation (step 3).

Co-stimulation appears to be particularly important if antigenic peptide-MHC is relatively limited in terms of dose or of duration (e.g., after immunization with protein). In cases of limited antigen exposure, engagement of the TCR without co-stimulation may not only fail to activate the T cell but render it anergic.[111] Anergic T cells do not subsequently respond to antigen even when normally adequate co-stimulatory signals are provided by the APC. Anergy is an attractive but controversial model for the maintenance of tolerance by mature T cells to certain antigens, particularly those that may not be expressed at sufficiently high levels in the thymus to induce negative selection.

Antigenically naive CD4 and CD8 T cells, once activated, undergo clonal expansion and differentiation into effector T cell populations (Fig. 2–6).[112] Effector T cells are lymphoblasts in the active phases of the cell cycle (i.e., not G_0) and have a greater capacity for cytokine production and cell-mediated cytotoxicity and a lower co-stimulatory requirement than antigenically naive T cells.[113] Unlike resting antigenically naive T cells, effector T cells express on their surface high-affinity IL-2 receptors, the CD69 molecule, and fas (a TNF receptor family member)[114] and have relatively low intracellular levels of bcl-2, a protein that protects against apoptosis.[115, 116] Effector T cells tend to undergo apoptosis, particularly when fas is engaged by fas ligand, a TNF ligand family cytokine, unless anti-apoptotic signals are provided by cytokines, such as IL-2 or IL-6.[115, 117] Apoptosis is important for limiting the accumulation of effector T cells once they are no longer needed for the immune response, as humans with genetic deficiencies of fas are prone to development of persistent lymphoadenopathy and hematologic autoimmune disease.[118]

ACTIVATION AND DIFFERENTIATION OF CD4 T CELLS

An important function of activated T cells, particularly those of the CD4 subset, is to produce cytokines, which amplify or regulate multiple aspects of the immune response. Most of these cytokines are secreted, although some may be predominantly expressed on the T cell surface. T cell–derived cytokines include IL-2, IL-3, IL-4, IL-5, IL-9, IL-10, IL-13; IFN-γ; GM-CSF; CD40 ligand; TNF; and fas ligand.[119] Table 2–2 summarizes the major immunomodulatory effects of T cell–derived cytokines as well as those produced by other cell types. Some key effects of cytokines in T cell proliferation, differentiation, and effector function, and in B cell, NK cell, and mononuclear phagocyte function, are discussed in detail later.

When antigenically naive CD4 αβ T cells first encounter foreign peptide-MHC complexes (the primary immune response), they produce a limited number of cytokines, including IL-2 and CD40 ligand (see Fig. 2–6).[45, 112] IL-2 is secreted and acts as an autocrine and paracrine growth factor of T cells, helping to expand a pool of antigen-specific effector cells. IL-2 increases the capacity of effector T cells to produce additional cytokines upon their reactivation by antigen,[112] including IFN-γ, IL-3, IL-4, and IL-5, and influences effector T cell differentiation so that these cells become susceptible to apoptosis. This pro-apoptotic effect appears to be important for maintaining the appropriate size of the peripheral lymphoid compartment after an immune response,[120] because humans with a genetic deficiency of high-affinity IL-2 receptor expression are prone to lymphocytic infiltration of the tissues.[121]

CD40 ligand, a member of the TNF ligand family

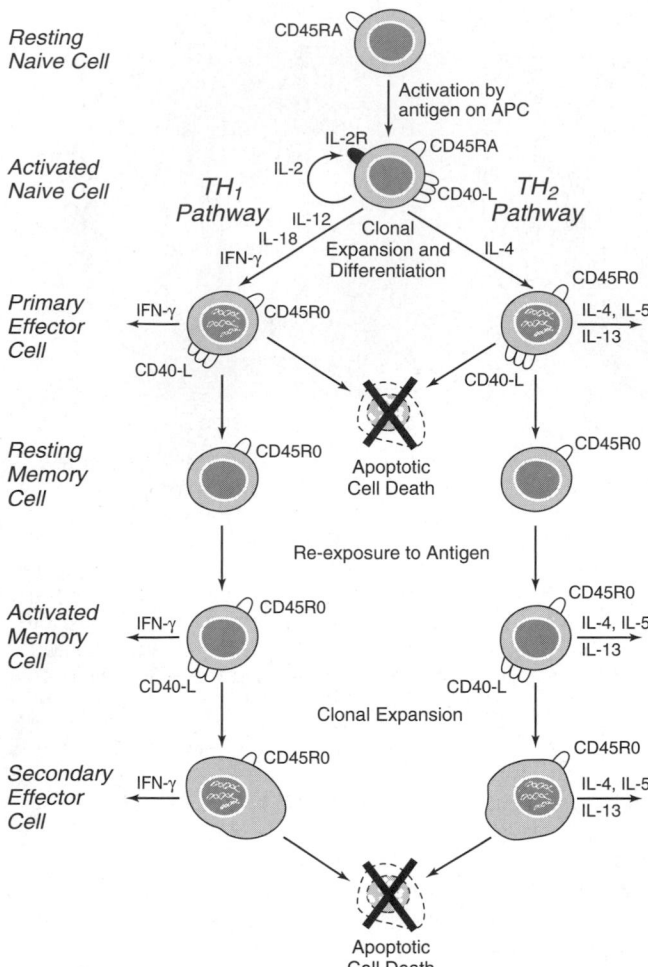

FIGURE 2–6 Differentiation of antigenically naive and memory CD4 T cells into TH1 and TH2 effector T cells by antigen exposure. Antigenically naive CD4 T cells express high levels of the CD45RA isoform of a surface protein tyrosine phosphatase. They are activated by antigen presented by APC to express CD40 ligand and IL-2 and undergo clonal expansion and differentiation, which are accompanied by expression of the CD45R0 isoform. Exposure of these expanding cells to IL-12, IL-18, and IFN-γ favors their differentiation into TH1 effector cells that secrete IFN-γ, whereas exposure to IL-4 favors their differentiation into TH2 effector cells that secrete IL-4, IL-5, and IL-13. Most effector cells die by apoptosis, but a few probably persist as memory cells that express high levels of CD45R0. Memory cells rechallenged with antigen undergo rapid clonal expansion into TH1 or TH2 secondary effector cells, most of which eventually die by apoptosis.

(see Tables 2–1 and 2–2), engages the CD40 molecule on B cells, dendritic cells, and mononuclear phagocytes.[45] CD40 engagement on the B cell surface transduces intracellular signals that promote the expression of antibody isotypes and differentiation of the B cell into a memory cell.[45] CD40 ligand is also an important activator of the microbicidal activity of mononuclear phagocytes in some infections, such as *Pneumocystis carinii* infections, and is also important in the initial priming

of antigenically naive CD4 T cells into an effector population.[122] As mentioned previously, CD40 engagement may also induce dendritic cells to produce IL-12[45] and other cytokines (see Fig. 2–5) and to express increased levels of B7 molecules. IL-12 and increased CD28 costimulation by B7 molecules, in turn, act independently to augment the production by T cells of cytokines, such as IFN-γ.[123]

Three major types of CD4 effector T cells have been identified, helper T cell 1 (TH1), TH2, and TH0. TH1 effector cells produce IFN-γ at high levels, and little or no IL-4, IL-5, and IL-13. IFN-γ is particularly important in the activation of mononuclear phagocytes for increased microbicidal activity and enhanced antigen presentation by the class I and class II MHC pathways. The TH1 cytokine profile is critical for limiting infection by nonviral intracellular pathogens,[124] such as *Toxoplasma* sp., mycobacteria, and *Listeria* sp., as discussed later. TH2 cells produce IL-4, IL-5, and IL-13 but little or no IFN-γ. This cytokine profile favors immunoglobulin production by B cells, particularly the immunoglobulin E (IgE) and IgG₄ isotypes; mast cell and basophil activation; and increased eosinophil production and survival. A TH2 pattern of cytokine production is characteristic of mucosal T cells during the immune response to helminth parasites or to allergens.[124] TH0-type responses are often seen after vaccination with protein antigens or after viral infections, such as influenza or cytomegalovirus (CMV).[125–127] Their generation in vitro seems to be favored by the presence of large amounts of IL-2 in the absence of cytokines that polarize differentiation toward either TH1 or TH2 effector cells.[128] In addition to their differing cytokine profiles, TH1 and TH2 cells also differ in their surface expression of chemokine receptors and cell adhesion molecules.[43, 129] This feature may allow TH1 and TH2 cells to localize differentially to particular tissues to mediate immune responses; for example, TH2 cells are often found in the mucosa.

TH1 effector development is favored by the exposure of CD4 T cells during the primary immune response to high levels of IL-12, IL-18, IFN-α, and IFN-γ, particularly in the absence of IL-4 (see Fig. 2–6). This process is in part due to direct effects of these cytokines on T cell differentiation, as well as ability of IL-12 and IL-18 to induce IFN-γ production by NK cells and T cells.[124, 130] The major sources of IL-12 are dendritic cells and mononuclear phagocytes,[131] whereas IL-18 is produced at high levels by Kupffer cells of the liver[130] and other mononuclear phagocyte populations. The importance of IL-12–dependent TH1 effector generation and cytokine production in human host defense is demonstrated by the increased susceptibility of patients with genetic defects in either IL-12[132] or components of the receptors for IL-12[133] or IFN-γ[134] to infection with intracellular pathogens, particularly mycobacteria and *Salmonella* sp. TH2 effector development is favored when CD4 T cells of the primary immune response encounter high amounts of IL-4, particularly in the absence of IL-12, IL-18, IFN-α, or IFN-γ (see Fig. 2–6).[135, 136] The source of this early IL-4 production remains controversial but may include conventional αβ T cells, NK T cells, mast cells, or basophils. The engagement of OX40 on the T cell by OX40 ligand, a member of the TNF ligand superfamily expressed by B cells, may also favor TH2 rather than TH1 effector development.[137] TH0 effector cell generation may be favored when IL-12, IL-18, IFN-γ, or IL-4 do not predominate at the site of the CD4 T cell primary immune response. Factors other than cytokines, such as different APCs, or the degree of signaling via the αβ-TCR–CD3 complex, also may influence the ultimate cytokine profile of effector T cells.

TERMINATION OF THE CD4 T CELL EFFECTOR RESPONSE

Effector CD4 T cell activation is limited by the interaction of B7-1 and B7-2 on the APC with CTLA-4, a molecule that is mainly expressed on the T cell surface during the later stages of cell activation. In mice genetically deficient in CTLA-4 a fatal autoimmune syndrome mediated by CD4 T cells develops, indicating the physiologic importance of this pathway in the normal control of T cell activation.[107] How CTLA-4 acts at a cellular level to terminate T cell activation is controversial, and engagement of this molecule has been variously reported to induce anergy, apoptosis, and secretion of antiproliferative cytokines, such as transforming growth factor–β(TGF-β).[138–140] The process through which CTLA-4 decreases or terminates T cell activation at the molecular level is also controversial; engagement appears to recruit the tyrosine phosphatase shp to the cytoplasmic domain of CTLA-4, resulting in T cell activation.[141] Because CTLA-4 is associated with CD3ζ, such engagement may cause shp dephosphorylation of the ITAM motifs of CD3ζ and blocking of activation.[142]

T CELL HELP FOR ANTIBODY PRODUCTION

T cells are particularly important in the regulation of B cell proliferation and enhanced immunoglobulin secretion. This help is provided both by contact-dependent mechanisms, mainly interactions between members of the TNF ligand–TNF receptor families, such as CD40 ligand–CD40, OX40 ligand–OX40, and TNF–p55 TNF receptor, and by secretion of soluble cytokines.[137, 143, 144] The contact-dependent interactions between T and B cells include both cognate (antigen-specific) recognition through the TCR of antigenic peptides associated with MHC molecules on B cells and those interactions mediated by pairs of receptor-ligand molecules. The importance of contact-dependent T cell help is clearly illustrated by the phenotype of X-linked hyper-IgM patients, who have genetic defects in the expression of the CD40 ligand.[122] The marked paucity of immunoglobulin isotypes other than IgM and the inability to generate memory B cell responses in these patients indicate that these responses critically depend on the binding of the CD40 molecule of the B cell to CD40 ligand on the T cell.[122] As discussed in the section on B cells and immunoglobulin, engagement of CD40 on the B cell in conjunction with other signals provided by cytokines, such as IL-4 or IL-10, can markedly enhance immunoglobulin production and class switching and B cell survival.[45] Other

ligand pairs, such as B7-CD28 and leukocyte function antigen-1 (LFA-1)–CD54, may promote interaction between B cells and T cells during the immune response and may enhance activation of these cells.[145, 146]

Soluble cytokines produced by activated T cells may influence the type of immunoglobulin produced by B cells. Experiments in mice in which the IL-2, IL4, IL-5, or IFN-γ genes or, in some cases, their specific receptors and associated signal transducer and activator of transcription (STAT) signaling molecules have been disrupted by gene targeting suggest that these cytokines help to regulate B cell immunoglobulin isotype expression. For example, inactivation of the IL-4 gene, components of the high-affinity IL-4 receptor, or the STAT6 protein involved in IL-4 receptor signal transduction results in a more than 90% decrease in IgE production, although the production of other antibody isotypes is largely unperturbed.[147, 148]

ACTIVATION, DIFFERENTIATION, AND HOMEOSTASIS OF CYTOTOXIC T CELLS

Cytotoxic T lymphocytes (CTLs) mediate antigen-specific, MHC-restricted cytolysis, an activity that is critical for resistance to viral infection. Alpha-beta T cells, particularly those of the CD8 subset, are typically the major source of CTLs in vivo. CD8 T cells when first activated by antigen are not effective killers but, under the influence of cytokines such as IL-2, proliferate and differentiate into an effector cell lymphoblast population that efficiently kills.[149] This differentiation includes increased expression of molecules involved in cytotoxicity, such as perforin, granzymes, and fas ligand,[150] which are discussed later, as well as an increased capacity to produce cytokines, such as IFN-γ and TNF.[150]

Recent studies have documented that viral-specific CD8 T cells undergo a dramatic expansion in vivo so that in some instances, such as Epstein-Barr virus (EBV) infection, more than 40% of circulating CD8 T cells may be reactive with a single viral peptide epitope.[151] This marked expansion again points out the importance of lymphocyte homeostatic mechanisms. Like CD4 effector T cells, most CD8 effector T cells have a relatively short life span and are probably eliminated by apoptosis after antigen clearance. The induction of apoptosis of CD8 effector T cells when compared with that of CD4 effector cells may be more dependent on engagement of the type I TNF receptor than the fas molecule.[152] CD4 T cells may directly aid in the generation of CD8 CTLs by the production of several cytokines, including IL-2 and IFN-γ. In addition, CD4 T cells may indirectly influence this process by enhancing dendritic cell function via a CD40 ligand–CD40 interaction; dendritic cells, in turn, may then help promote CD8 CTL generation by secreting cytokines and engaging co-stimulatory molecules.[153] For some viral infections, CD4 T cells may also be required for CD8 effector cells to maintain their cytotoxic function in vivo.[154] Depending on the particular viral pathogen, the generation of CD8 CTLs may be either CD4-dependent or -independent.

Some CD4 T cells, in addition to secreting cytokines

and providing help for CD8 CTL generation, mediate antigen-specific cytotoxicity directed against target cells bearing class II MHC–antigenic peptide complexes. This may be particularly important in cases of human viral infection in which class I MHC antigen presentation is substantially inhibited, such as with herpesviruses. When CD8 T cells are absent or deficient in mice, cytotoxic CD4 T cells can effectively clear certain viral infections, such as influenza, with only a slight lag compared with mice that have normal levels of CD8 T cells.

T cell–mediated cytotoxicity requires that the T cells bind to the target cell via multiple intercellular adhesion molecule interactions. CTL activation is enhanced by the interaction of CD2, LFA-1, and CD28 with their respective ligands on the target cell (see Table 2–3). After adherence, if the TCR is engaged by antigenic peptide–MHC of the target cell, a killing program is executed in which the T cell secretes proteins (perforin and granzymes) and expresses fas ligand on its surface (Fig. 2–7).[155] Perforin disrupts the target cell membrane, promoting osmotic lysis, and also allows the entry of granzyme molecules, a group of serine esterases, which induce apoptosis by cleaving intracellular substrates of the target cell.[155] Activated cytotoxic T cells also express fas ligand, which is stored in granules of specialized lysosomes.[156] CTL activation via TCR engagement results in the directed release of fas ligand to the cell surface, where interaction with fas on the target cell can occur, resulting in target cell apoptosis.[155] Finally, cytokines produced by effector T cells, such as IFN-γ and TNF,[150] may also directly inhibit intracellular viral replication in tissues, such as the liver, by a noncytotoxic mechanism; this has best been described in hepatitis B infection of hepatocytes.[157]

GENERATION OF MEMORY T CELLS AND SECONDARY EFFECTOR T CELLS

After antigenically naive T cells are activated and expanded by antigen as part of the primary immune response, a small number of these cells persist as memory T cells (see Fig. 2–6).[112, 158] The cellular and molecular interactions that are involved in the generation and maintenance of human memory T cells remain poorly understood. Some studies in mice suggest that memory CD8 T cells can differentiate directly from antigenically

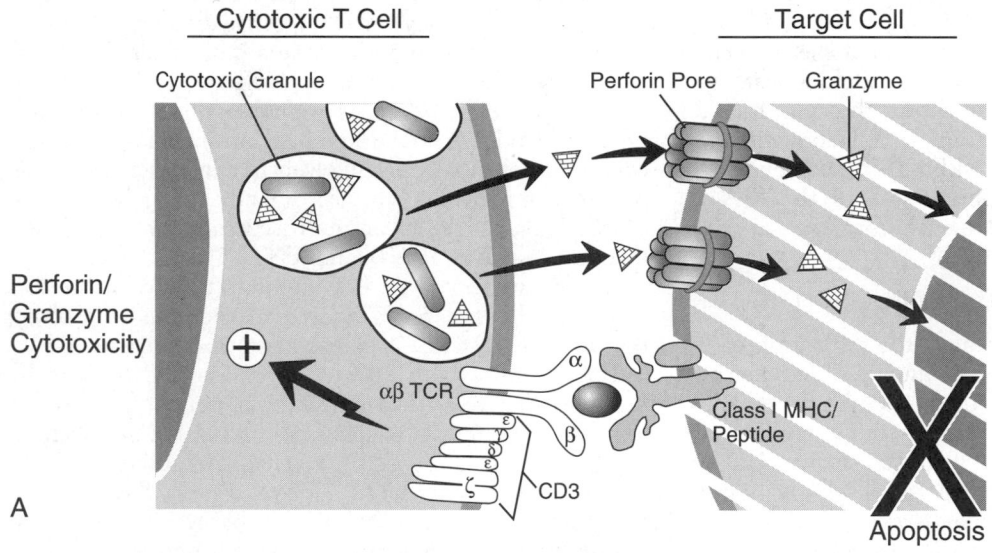

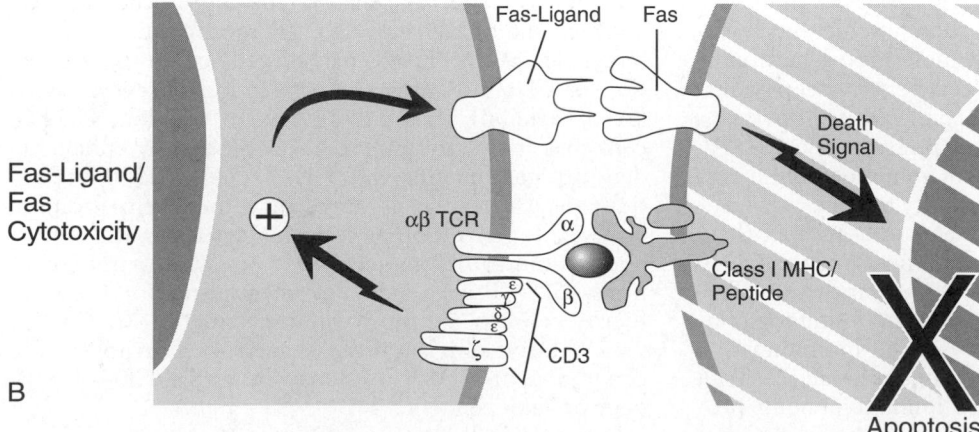

FIGURE 2–7 Two major mechanisms of antigen-specific class I MHC–restricted T cell–mediated cytotoxicity. Engagement of αβ-TCR of CD8 T cells by antigenic peptide bound to class I MHC on the target cell leads to T cell activation and target cell death. A, Cytotoxicity may occur by the extracellular release of the contents of cytotoxic granules from the T cell, including perforins and granzymes. Perforins introduce pores by which granzymes can enter into the target cell, leading to the triggering of apoptosis and cell death. B, Activation of T cells results in their surface expression of fas ligand, which engages fas on the target cell, resulting in the delivery of death signal, culminating in apoptosis.

naive CD8 T cells rather than via an effector cell intermediate, and that the CD28-B7 interaction is obligatory for effector cell generation but not for memory cell generation in vivo.[159] The CD40-CD40 ligand seems to play some role in either the generation or the function of human memory CD4 T cells, because humans genetically deficient in CD40 ligand tend to have reduced recall responses to previously administered protein vaccines.[160] It has been estimated that the expansion of human memory T cells from antigenically naive T cells is the result, on average, of 14 cell divisions.[161] Unlike effector T cells, memory T cells are not lymphoblasts and most are in a G_{0-1} phase of the cell cycle, rather than in an active phase (i.e., S or G_2/MD). Memory T cells resemble effector T cells in that they have a reduced dependence on co-stimulation and a greater capacity to produce cytokines than antigenically naive T cells.[112]

Most human memory CD4 T cells can be distinguished from antigenically naive cells by their surface expression of the CD45R0 rather than the CD45RA isoform of CD45, a protein tyrosine phosphatase (see Fig. 2–6).[162, 163] In addition, memory and effector T cells typically express higher levels of adhesion molecules, such as the VLA-4 β_1 integrin, than antigenically naive T cells.[164] About 40% of circulating adult CD4 T cells have this CD45RA^{low}CD45R0^{high} (VLA-4^{high}) memory-effector surface phenotype. Another 10 to 15% of circulating CD4 T cells have a CD45RA^{medium}CD45R0^{medium} surface phenotype and memory-effector–like function,[165] but their relationship to CD45R0^{high} T cells remains unclear. In contrast to memory-effector T cells, most antigenically naive CD4 T cells have a CD5RA^{high}CD45R0^{low} surface phenotype,[163] although some of these CD45RA^{high} T cells may be revertants from either CD45R0^{high} or CD45R0^{medium} cells.[164]

Activation and propagation of CD45RA^{high}CD45R0^{low} CD4 T cells in vitro result in their acquisition of memory-effector cell–like features, including reduced co-stimulatory requirements, a CD45RA^{low}CD45R0^{high} phenotype, an enhanced ability to produce certain cytokines (e.g., IFN-γ and IL-4), and an increased ability to provide help for B cell antibody production.[164, 166] This characteristic supports the notion that CD45RA^{high} T cells are precursors of CD45R0^{high} T cells and that this differentiation follows T cell activation. In addition, when CD4 T cells are stimulated in vitro with protein neoantigens, the CD45RA^{high}CD45R0^{low} subset but not the CD45RA^{low}CD45R0^{high} subset responds.[167] This is also consistent with the CD45RA^{low}CD45R0^{high} subset's consisting mainly of memory T cells reactive with previously encountered antigens.

Memory CD8 T cells are similar to those of the CD4 subset in expressing a CD45RA^{low}CD45R0^{high} surface phenotype and an enhanced capacity to produce multiple cytokines when compared with their antigenically naive precursors.[150] In addition, unlike memory CD4 T cells, a substantial subset of these CD45R0^{high} CD8 T cells express CD11b, CD57, and killer inhibitory receptors (KIRs).[168] KIRs bind self-HLA-A, -B, or -C alleles, thereby delivering an inhibitory signal into the cell. They are expressed at high levels on most or all human

NK lymphocytes; they are discussed in detail in the section Natural Killer Cells. The importance of KIR expression by CD8 T cells remains unclear; but it is hypothesized to regulate effector function, such as cytotoxicity, by raising the threshold for potential activation by antigenic peptide-MHC complexes.[168] Human memory CD8 T cells can also be distinguished from circulating effector CD8 T cells by surface phenotype: Most human CD8 effector cells have a CD45RA^{high}CD27$^-$CD28$^-$ surface phenotype and a high capacity to mediate cytotoxicity and to produce certain cytokines, such as TNF and IFN-γ.[150] In contrast, antigenically naive CD8 T cells have a CD45RA^{high}CD27$^+$CD28$^+$ surface phenotype and a limited ability to mediate cytotoxicity and to secrete cytokines.[150]

When memory T cells reencounter antigenic peptide–MHC complexes (recall antigen) as part of the secondary response, they are activated and undergo expansion and differentiation into a secondary effector population (see Fig. 2–6). The secondary immune response to recall antigen is typically more rapid and robust than the primary response to an antigen that has previously never been encountered. This is because of the greater frequency of antigen-specific T cells in the circulation and, presumably, lymphoid tissue,[163, 164] as well as a lower threshold for activation and enhanced function of these memory T cells and their secondary effector progeny.[112] Like effector T cells, memory T cells are more readily activated to proliferate than antigenically naive T cells with a variety of stimuli, such as anti-CD2 or anti-CD3 monoclonal antibodies,[169] a feature that may contribute to the more rapid and vigorous secondary response they mediate in vivo. Enhanced secondary responses by T cells can be observed months to decades after a single exposure to a new antigen, indicating that T cell memory overall is stable.[170] Whether most memory T cells are long-lived or are continually generated in vivo by low levels of proliferation remains controversial. Unlike antigenically naive T cells, which appear to migrate preferentially from the blood to peripheral lymphoid tissue, circulating memory T cells preferentially adhere to and migrate across the endothelium of inflamed tissues.[171]

NATURAL KILLER T CELLS

A small population of circulating $\alpha\beta$ T cells express NKR-P1A, the human homologue of the mouse NK1.1 protein, and lack expression of CD4 or CD8. These $\alpha\beta$ T cells have some surface phenotypic features (e.g., expression of NKR-P1A, CD56, and CD57) and a dependence on cytokines for their development (IL-15)[172] that are suggestive of NK cells, a non–T cell lymphocyte population that is discussed in detail later. For this reason they are frequently referred to as NK T cells or natural T cells. Like murine T cells expressing NK1.1, human NK T cells have a highly restricted repertoire of $\alpha\beta$-TCR and mainly recognize antigens presented by the nonclassic MHC molecule, CD1d, rather than by class I or class II MHC molecules. These antigens include certain lipid molecules or highly hydrophobic peptides. NK T cells also have the ability to produce high levels of IL-4 and IFN-γ and fas ligand upon primary stimulation, a capacity that is not observed with most antigenically naive αβ T cells.

The function of NK T cells remains controversial. In mice, NK T cells appear to provide help to B cells, presumably in the form of cytokines, for the production of antibodies against GPI-linked proteins.[31] These proteins are found in particularly high amounts on the surface of malarial parasites and trypanosomes, but it remains unclear whether NK T cells play an important role in host defense against these pathogens by this mechanism. There is also evidence that NK T cells may limit *Toxoplasma* infection, as discussed later. In addition to their role in host defense, NK T cells may act as negative regulators of certain T cell–mediated immune responses, such as those involved in the pathogenesis of experimental diabetes mellitus, and in graft-versus-host disease.[173] This function of NK T cells may be relevant to humans because there is evidence that a lack of NK T cells may predispose to the development of insulin-dependent diabetes mellitus.[174]

T Cell Development and Function in the Fetus and Neonate

THYMIC ONTOGENY IN THE FETUS AND NEONATE

The fetal liver between 6 to 8 weeks of gestation contains CD34+ lymphoid cells that appear to include prothymocytes, in that they can undergo differentiation into T-lineage cells in vitro under suitable conditions.[175] The fetal thymus is first colonized with prothymocytes, probably derived from the fetal liver, at approximately 8.5 weeks of gestation.[176] Shortly thereafter, thymocytes express proteins characteristic of T-lineage cells, including CD4, CD8, and the TCR-α and TCR-β chain proteins.[176] By 12 weeks of gestation, a clear architectural separation between the thymic cortex and medulla is apparent,[177] and Hassall corpuscles are evident shortly thereafter.[178] Medullary dendritic cells in the fetus but not the adult express high levels of B7-1.[94] B7-1 is a ligand of CD28,[107] a protein that is expressed by most fetal and postnatal thymocytes and mature T cells. It is also a ligand for CTLA-4 (CD152), a protein expressed by activated T cells and thymocytes.[93] It is unclear whether B7-1 plays a role in human fetal thymocyte development, although in vitro experiments described previously suggest that a B7–CTLA-4 interaction could enhance the process of negative selection.[93]

By 14 weeks of gestation the three major human thymocyte subsets defined by surface expression of the CD4 and CD8 molecules—double-negative (CD4low CD8low), double-positive (CD4highCD8high), and single-positive (CD4highCD8low or CD4lowCD8high)—are found in the subcapsular, cortical, and medullary regions, respectively, a pattern that persists in the postnatal thymus (see Fig. 2–3). The subcapsular region mainly contains large blast cells, whereas the cortex and medulla contain smaller thymocytes. By this age, the pattern of expression of a number of other proteins expressed by thymocytes, such as CD2, CD5, CD38, and the CD45 iso-

forms, matches that in the postnatal thymus. At this time, CD4 and CD8 T cells are found in the fetal liver and spleen, and CD4 T cells are detectable in primary lymph node follicles,[179] demonstrating the emigration of mature T-lineage cells from the thymus.

Thymic cellularity increases dramatically during the last trimester and continues to do so postnatally, with peak thymus size reached at about 10 years of age. When complete thymectomy is performed during the first year of life, subsequent numbers of CD4 and CD8 T cells are decreased in the circulation, indicating the importance of postnatal production of thymocytes for the peripheral T cell compartment.[180] After puberty, the thymus gradually involutes, with the gradual replacement of the cortex and medulla with fat. Single-positive thymocytes within the medulla are relatively spared during the involutionary process compared with double-positive thymocytes in the cortex.[181] However, the thymus is capable of increasing its output of antigenically naive T cells in response to severe T cell lymphopenia, for example, after intense cytoablative chemotherapy[182] or treatment with highly active antiretroviral therapy for human immunodeficiency virus (HIV) infection,[183] at least through early adulthood.

FETAL AND NEONATAL T CELL SURFACE PHENOTYPE

The percentage of T cells in the fetal or premature circulation gradually increases during the second and third trimesters of pregnancy through about 6 months of age,[184] followed by a gradual decline to adult levels during childhood.[185] The ratio of CD4 to CD8 T cells in the circulation is high (about 3.5) during fetal life and gradually declines with age.[185] The levels of expression of the αβ-TCR, CD3, CD4, CD5, CD8, and CD28 proteins on fetal and neonatal αβ T cells are similar to those of adult T cells (D Lewis, unpublished data.)[59, 109]

Unlike adult virgin T cells, virtually all peripheral fetal and neonatal T cells express the CD38 molecule.[186] CD38 is also found on most thymocytes, suggesting that peripheral T cells in the fetus and neonate may represent an immature transitional population. In contrast to circulating T cells, a significant fraction of T cells in the fetal spleen between 14 and 20 weeks of gestation are CD38−.[187] The precursor-product relationship between CD38+ and CD38− peripheral T cells in humans is unknown. In premature or term neonates who are stressed, a portion of circulating T-lineage cells are CD3low, express CD1, and co-express CD4 and CD8,[186] a phenotype characteristic of immature thymocytes of the cortex (see Fig. 2–3).[188] It is likely that stress results in the premature release of cortical thymocytes into the circulation, but the immunologic consequences of this release are unclear.

Circulating T cells in the term and preterm (22 to 30 weeks of gestation) neonate and in the second-trimester fetus predominantly express a CD45RAhighCD45R0low surface phenotype,[189, 190] which is also found on antigenically naive T cells of adults. About 30% of circulating T cells of the term neonate are CD45RAlowCD45R0low, a surface phenotype that is rare or absent in circulating adult T cells.[191] Because these CD45RA^{low}CD45R0^{low} T cells are functionally similar to neonatal CD45RA^{high}CD45R0^{low} T cells and become CD45RA^{mid}CD45R0^{low} T cells when incubated in vitro with fibroblasts,[191] they appear to be immature recent thymic emigrants. These cells may undergo extrathymic maturation to an antigenically naive (CD45RA^{high}CD45R0^{low}) T cell population over a period of days, as has been described in rodents.[192]

Most studies have found that the healthy neonate and late gestation fetus lack circulating CD45R0^{high} T cells, as is consistent with their limited exposure to foreign antigens. The surface expression of other markers, such as CD29, and, in the case of CD8 T cells, a lack of KIRs, is also consistent with predominance of an antigenically naive population in the healthy neonate.[168] A postnatal precursor-product relationship between CD45RA^{high}CD45R0^{low} and CD45RA^{low}CD45R0^{high} T cells is suggested by the fact that the proportion of $\alpha\beta$ T cells with a memory-effector phenotype, and the capacity of circulating T cells to produce cytokines, such as IFN-γ, both gradually increase, whereas the proportion of antigenically naive T cells decreases with increasing postnatal age.[185, 193] These increases in the ability to produce cytokines and expression of the CD45R0^{high} phenotype are presumably due to cumulative antigenic exposure and T cell activation, leading to the generation of memory T cells from antigenically naive T cells.

About 5% of circulating CD4 T cells in neonates, infants, and young children express high levels of CD45RA and IL-2 receptor α chains and contain CD45R0 transcripts.[194] This T cell subset may be a transitional population between antigenically naive and memory-effector T cells, although its antigen specificity has not been reported. Approximately 10 to 20% of neonatal CD45RA^{high}CD45R0^{low} T cells also lack expression of CD31, a protein found on virtually all adult CD45RA^{high}CD45R0^{low} T cells.[195] Whether this neonatal CD31$^-$ subset is functionally distinct from neonatal CD31$^+$ CD4 T cells or adult antigenically naive CD4 T cells remains to be shown. Neonatal CD8 T cells also lack a CD28$^-$CD11b$^+$ subset found in adults that may contribute to memory or effector CTL activity.[196, 197]

FETAL AND NEONATAL T CELL RECEPTOR REPERTOIRE

The usage of D and J segments in rearrangement of the TCR-β chain gene in the thymus at approximately 8 weeks' gestation is less diverse than at 11 to 13 weeks' gestation or subsequently.[198, 199] This restriction is not explained by an effect of positive or negative selection in the thymus, because it applies to D-J rearrangements, which are not expressed on the immature thymocyte cell surface.[198, 200] The CDR3 region of the TCR-β chain transcripts is reduced in length and sequence diversity in the human fetal thymus between 8 and 15 weeks of gestation, most likely as a result of decreased amounts of the TdT enzyme.[198, 199, 201] Because the CDR3 region of the TCR chains is a major determinant of antigen specificity,[81] such decreased CDR3 diversity, in conjunction with restricted usage, theoretically could limit rec-

ognition of foreign antigens by the first-trimester fetal $\alpha\beta$-TCR repertoire, particularly during the first trimester. However, any potential "holes" in the $\alpha\beta$-TCR repertoire of the human fetus from limitations in CDR3 are likely to be very subtle, particularly after the second trimester, when V segment usage is diverse. This possibility is suggested by the fact that the T cell response to immunization and viral challenge is normal in mice that are completely deficient in TdT as a result of selective gene targeting,[202] indicating that the T cell repertoire is probably not significantly limited at this age.

By the second trimester TdT activity and CDR3 length are both increased,[198, 199] and V$_{\beta}$ and V$_{\alpha}$ segment usage in the thymus and peripheral lymphoid organs is diverse.[199, 200, 203-205] The $\alpha\beta$-TCR repertoire expressed by cord blood T cells has a diversity of TCR-β usage and CDR3 length that is similar to that of antigenically naive adult T cells, indicating that the functional preimmune repertoire is fully formed by birth.[206] Repertoire analysis also suggests that there is greater oligoclonal expansion of $\alpha\beta$ T cells during the third trimester, particularly after 28 weeks' gestation, than in adulthood and that these oligoclonal expansions involve a variety of different V$_{\beta}$ segment families.[207] Whether this oligoclonal expansion is antigen driven, for example, by a response to idiotypes encoded on maternally derived immunoglobulins,[207] or is an antigen-independent process is unknown.

Positive selection of thymocytes appears to be an important influence on the $\alpha\beta$-TCR repertoire during human fetal and neonatal development. This effect can be assessed by determining whether the frequency of preimmune (antigenically naive) $\alpha\beta$ T cells, such as those predominantly found in the healthy neonate, expressing a particular V segment is skewed toward either CD4 or CD8 T cells. Such skewing suggests that these particular V segments have been positively selected primarily by class I or class II MHC molecules, respectively. Analysis of neonatal T cells has revealed that V$_{\alpha}$12.1 segments are expressed at a higher frequency by CD8 T cells, whereas V$_{\beta}$6.7, V$_{\beta}$8, and V$_{\beta}$12 segments are expressed at a higher frequency by CD4 T cells.[208-210] This skewing is also evident in the frequency with which these V segments are expressed by CD4$^+$CD8$^-$ thymocytes versus CD4$^-$CD8$^+$ thymocytes in the infant.[208] Skewing also occurs when human fetal liver is used as a source of stem cells to reconstitute human fetal thymic development in SCID mice.[205]

FETAL T CELL PROLIFERATION AND CYTOKINE RESPONSIVENESS

A substantial minority of T cells in the second trimester fetal spleen are CD45RA^{low}CD45R0^{high}, a T cell population that is absent from the spleen of young infants.[189] These fetal CD45R0^{high} T cells express high levels of the IL-2 receptor α chain and proliferate with IL-2, suggesting that they have recently been activated and are undergoing expansion.[189] In contrast with adult CD45R0^{high} T cells, these fetal spleen CD45R0^{high} T cells express low surface levels of CD2 and LFA-1 and proliferate poorly after activation with either anti-CD2 or anti-CD3 monoclonal antibodies, suggesting that they are not fully functional.[189] Their αβ-TCR repertoire is diverse, suggesting that these T cells are expanding in a non–antigen-specific manner. Such antigen-independent expansion can occur when the number of niches for T cells in the peripheral lymphoid tissue is large relative to the number of T cells (e.g., after adoptive transfer of T cells into lymphopenic recipients), and it is possible that this may be the case in the rapidly growing fetus. However, it is unknown whether these fetal spleen CD45R0[high] T cells contribute to the postnatal T cell compartment.

NEONATAL T CELL PROLIFERATION, CYTOKINE RESPONSIVENESS, AND SOLUBLE CYTOKINE PRODUCTION

Most studies have found that circulating neonatal T cells and adult T cells have similar amounts of proliferation and IL-2 production in response to mitogenic lectins, bacterial superantigens, or allogeneic cells.[60, 206, 211-215] Basal expression by neonatal T cells of the IL-2 receptor γ chain is lower than that by either adult CD45RA[high] or CD45R0[high] T cells.[216] However, activated neonatal T cells express high-affinity IL-2 receptors and proliferate in response to IL-2 as well as or better than adult T cells.[215, 217]

Interestingly, two in vitro studies suggest that neonatal T cells may be less able to differentiate into effector cells in response to neoantigen (see the section Costimulation of Neonatal T Cells and Anergy). One older study, using limiting dilution techniques and circulating mononuclear cells from CMV-nonimmune donors, found that the frequency of neonatal T cells proliferating to whole inactivated CMV antigen was significantly less than that of adult T cells.[58] Another study[218] found that neonatal mononuclear cells had decreased antigen-specific T cell proliferation and IL-2 production in response to the protein neoantigen keyhole limpet hemocyanin compared with those of adult cells. These findings, which need confirmation, contrast with findings of normal IL-2 production by neonatal T cells in response to alloantigen. As discussed later, the function of circulating dendritic cells may be reduced in the neonate,[63] and these cells are critical for activation of antigenically naive T cells by antigen, including in vitro.[219] Therefore, it is plausible that decreased dendritic function in the neonate might compromise the presentation of soluble proteins to a greater degree than alloantigens, which are presented effectively by monocytes as well as dendritic cells.[220]

In most studies, neonatal T cells and antigenically naive (CD45RA[high]) adult T cells do not proliferate as well or produce as much IL-2 as unfractionated adult T cells after activation by anti-CD2 or anti-CD3 monoclonal antibodies.[166, 221-223] The production of most other T cell–derived cytokines or expression of their cognate messenger RNAs (mRNAs) by neonatal T cells has been reported to be either slightly reduced (TNF)[224] or markedly reduced (IL-3, IL-4, IL-5, IL-6, IL-10, IL-13, IFN-γ, and GM-CSF)[225-230] compared with that of adult T cells when using polyclonal stimuli for activation.

Again, adult antigenically naive T cells are similar to neonatal T cells in their reduced capacity to produce these cytokines compared with that of adult memory-effector T cells.[231-233]

These results, taken together, suggest that in most instances the apparent cytokine deficiency of neonatal T cells can be accounted for by their antigenically naive status, rather than by developmental immaturity. In support of this idea, IFN-γ production by circulating neonatal and adult peripheral blood mononuclear cells has been reported to be similar after allogeneic stimulation,[211] although it remains to be shown that the source of this IFN-γ is T cell derived. However, some studies in which antigenically naive CD45RA[high] CD4 T cells from neonates and adults were directly compared for their response to anti-CD2 monoclonal antibody stimulation found that neonatal cells produced less IL-2 mRNA and expressed reduced amounts of high-affinity IL-2 receptors.[234, 235] These differences between neonatal and adult CD45RA[high] CD4 T cells were abrogated when phorbol ester, which induces ras and protein kinase C activation, was included in the stimulation.[234, 235] This suggests that the capacity of neonatal CD4 T cells to express these proteins is not intrinsically more limited than that of adult antigenically naive CD4 T cells, but that there may be differences in the capacity for generation of activation signals after CD2 engagement. However, the relevance of these findings to neonatal and adult T cell activation in vivo, in which the αβ-TCR–CD3 complex and multiple other surface signaling molecules in addition to CD2 are simultaneously engaged, remains unclear.

Reduced IL-4 and IFN-γ mRNA expression by polyclonally activated neonatal T cells is primarily due to reduced transcription of these cytokine genes.[230] IFN-γ genomic DNA is methylated to a greater degree in neonatal and adult CD45RA[high] T cells than in adult CD45R0[high] T cells, potentially decreasing the accessibility of this gene to transcriptional activator proteins.[236] In the case of decreased IL-3 production by neonatal T cells, reduced IL-3 mRNA stability rather than decreased gene transcription may be the major mechanism.[229] As with antigenically naive adult T cells, polyclonal activation of neonatal T cells results in their acquisition of the characteristics of effector T cells. These acquired characteristics include a CD45RA[low] CD45R0[high] surface phenotype, an enhanced ability to be activated by anti-CD2 or anti-CD3 monoclonal antibodies, and an increased capacity to produce cytokines (e.g., IL-4 and IFN-γ).[166, 213, 227, 237] Again this favors the notion that when optimal stimuli are used, neonatal T cells are not intrinsically deficient in the capacity to produce cytokines compared with antigenically naive adult T cells or, after priming in vitro, compared with adult memory T cells.

FETAL AND NEONATAL T CELL EXPRESSION OF CD40 LIGAND

The pattern of expression of CD40 ligand by fetal and neonatal T cells is distinct from that of all other T cell–derived cytokines reported to date: In one report[238] a substantial proportion of circulating fetal T cells between 19 and 31 weeks of gestation expressed CD40 ligand in vitro in response to polyclonal activation. Whether fetal T cells that can express CD40 ligand have a surface phenotype distinct from that of those lacking this capacity is not known. In contrast, T cells from later gestational age fetuses and from neonates have much more limited capacity to produce CD40 ligand.[238–241] Expression of CD40 ligand by activated neonatal CD4 T cells remains reduced for at least 10 days postnatally but appears to be almost equal to that of adult cells by 3 to 4 weeks after birth (D Lewis, unpublished data).[238] In most studies activated neonatal T cells express markedly lower amounts of CD40 ligand surface protein and mRNA than either adult CD45RA^{high} or CD45R0^{high} CD4 T cells.[238, 240, 241] Thus, decreased CD40 ligand expression may not be due to the lack of a memory-effector population in the neonatal T cell compartment but may represent a true developmental limitation in cytokine production. Interestingly, decreased CD40 ligand production by neonatal T cells has also been more recently documented in the mouse,[242] suggesting that it may be a general feature of T cells that have recently emigrated from the thymus. Consistent with this idea, human CD4$^+$CD8$^-$ thymocytes, the immediate precursors of antigenically naive CD4 T cells, also have a low capacity to express CD40 ligand.[241] As for most other T cell–derived cytokines, when neonatal T cells are activated in vitro into an effector T cell population, they acquire a markedly increased capacity to produce CD40 ligand, demonstrating that this reduction in cytokine expression is not a fixed phenotype.[238, 241]

Given the importance of CD40 ligand in multiple aspects of the immune response,[45] limitations in CD40 ligand production could contribute to decreased antigen-specific immunity mediated by TH1 effector cells and B cells in the neonate. However, all of the initial studies that reported a relative deficiency of CD40 ligand expression by neonatal T cells used stimulation by calcium ionophore and phorbol ester, a combination of pharmacologic agents that maximizes the production of most cytokines but may not accurately mimic physiologic T cell activation, at least in some respects. Preliminary studies in 1998 by Reen[243] suggested that neonatal CD4 T cells may be as responsive as adult cells to the induction of CD40 ligand by ionomycin alone but may be less responsive than adult cells to the doses of phorbol ester typically used for T cell activation. Some CD40 ligand can be expressed by neonatal T cells in response to allogeneic stimulation in vitro, a potentially more physiologic stimulus, and this CD40 ligand can induce IL-12 production by dendritic cells.[244] However, it is unclear whether such CD40 ligand production is equivalent to that by adult T cells in this context. CD40 ligand surface expression by neonatal T cells after activation by anti-CD3 monoclonal antibody has also been observed to be either similar to that of adult cells[243, 245] or substantially reduced (D Lewis, unpublished data). Given these conflicting results, it is important to assess whether expression of CD40 ligand is reduced during antigen-specific T cell activation in the neonatal period and early infancy.

CO-STIMULATION OF NEONATAL T CELLS AND ANERGY

Neonatal T cells produce IL-2 and proliferate as well as adult T cells in response to mouse APC expressing human B7-1 or B7-2 and anti-CD3 monoclonal antibody, indicating that CD28-mediated signaling is intact.[109] This is also supported by a study showing that anti-CD28 monoclonal antibody treatment of neonatal T cells also markedly augments their ability to produce IL-2 and proliferate in response to anti-CD2 monoclonal antibody stimulation.[234] However, neonatal T cells differ from adult CD45RA^{high} T cells in their tendency to become anergic rather than competent for increased cytokine secretion after priming with bacterial superantigen bound to class II MHC–transfected murine fibroblasts.[214] This tendency appears to be developmentally regulated in that CD4$^+$CD8$^-$ thymocytes, the immediate precursors of antigenically naive CD4 T cells, are also prone to anergy when treated under these conditions.[246] Superantigens activate T cells by binding to a portion of the TCR-β chain outside the peptide antigen recognition site but otherwise appear to mimic activation by peptide-MHC complexes in most respects. In addition, neonatal but not adult CD4 T cells primed by alloantigen, in the form of EBV-transformed human B cells, have also been reported to become nonresponsive to restimulation by alloantigen or by a combination of anti-CD3 and anti-CD28 monoclonal antibodies[247, 248]; preliminary studies implicate a lack of ras signaling as the basis for this reduced responsiveness.[248] These results, which need confirmation, suggest that neonatal, and presumably fetal, T cells have a greater tendency than antigenically naive adult T cells to become anergic, particularly under conditions in which co-stimulation (e.g., via B7 or CD40 on the APC) may be limiting.

NEONATAL HELPER T CELL TYPES 1 AND 2 EFFECTOR GENERATION AND PHENOTYPE

Activated neonatal T cells can also be differentiated in vitro into either TH1- or TH2-like effector cells with the addition of IL-12 and anti–IL-4 antibody or IL-4 and anti–IL-12 antibody, respectively.[195, 249–251] This indicates that neonatal T cells express functional surface receptors for IL-4 and IL-12, including the activation-induced IL-12 receptor β$_2$ subunit.[250] Interestingly, purified CD4 CD45RA^{high} T cells from neonates have been reported to proliferate substantially more in response to IL-4 than these cells from adults,[252] suggesting a mechanism by which neonatal T cells might be more prone to become TH2 effectors than antigenically naive adult T cells. More detailed studies by Delespesse and colleagues[195] also suggest that neonatal and adult CD45RA^{high} CD4 T cells may differ in their tendency to become TH2-like effector cells under certain conditions in vitro: When these cells are primed, using anti-CD3 monoclonal antibody, a fibroblast cell line expressing low amounts of the B7-1 co-stimulatory molecule, and exogenous IL-12, there is enhanced production of IL-4 by neonatal CD4 T cells compared with that by adult cells. The extent to which these in vitro priming conditions may mimic those in vivo remains to be determined.

TH1 and TH2 effectors derived from antigenically naive neonatal T cells express different patterns of chemokine receptors: TH1 effectors express CXCR3 and CCR5, whereas TH2 effectors express CCR4 and, to a lesser extent, CCR3.[43] It is likely that this differential expression may be important in targeting TH1 and TH2 cells in vivo to different microenvironments for immune responses. Whether these patterns of differential expression apply similarly to TH1 and TH2 effectors from adult antigenically naive CD4 T cells remains to be determined. It is also not known whether neonatal TH1 effector cells are similar to adult TH1 cells in their expression of a functional ligand for the P- and E-selectin adhesion molecules.[129]

FETAL AND NEONATAL T CELL–MEDIATED CYTOTOXICITY

The recent and growing use of cord blood for bone marrow transplantation, and, in particular, the finding that its use is associated with a reduced incidence of graft-versus-host disease compared with that of adult bone marrow, have led to a renewed interest in the capacity of neonatal T cells to mediate cytotoxicity and potential graft rejection. Early studies mostly used unfractionated mononuclear cells as a source of killer cells in a variety of non–antigen-specific assays, such as lectin-mediated cytotoxicity or redirected cytotoxicity using anti-CD3 monoclonal antibodies. Reduced cytotoxicity was observed with lectin-activated cord blood lymphocytes, particularly if purified T cells were used.[253–255] T cells can also be sensitized in vitro for cytotoxicity by using allogeneic (MHC other than self) stimulator cells followed by testing for cytotoxic activity against allogeneic target cells. Using this approach, most studies have found that neonatal T cells are moderately less effective than adult T cells as cytotoxic effector cells.[256–260]

Part of this apparent deficiency could reflect the absence of effector and memory T cells from the neonatal samples, because CD8 effector and memory T cells kill more efficiently than antigenically naive T cells after stimulation with lectin or anti-CD3 monoclonal antibody[261] or after allogeneic sensitization.[149, 150, 262] However, more limited studies of virus-specific T cell–mediated cytotoxicity in the neonate and infant (discussed in the section T Cell Reactivity to Specific Antigens) also suggest that the capacity for the fetus or neonate to generate a functional T cell effector population is reduced compared with that of the adult. The mechanism for reduced neonatal T cell–mediated cytotoxicity remains poorly understood. Neonatal CD8 T cells have also been reported to lack constitutive expression of perforin, whereas approximately 30% of adult CD8 T cells contain this protein.[263] Whether these differences are accounted for by the lack of memory-effector CD8 T cells in the neonate is unclear.

NEONATAL NATURAL KILLER T CELLS

T cells expressing markers for NK T cells (CD16, CD56, CD57, or $V_\alpha 24$) are undetectable in the neonate by flow cytometry; they are present by late infancy and subsequently increase in numbers with aging.[264] This suggests that NK T cells may either undergo postnatal expansion, for example, in relation to exposure of a ubiquitous antigen presented by CD1d molecules, or that their production by the thymus or at extrathymic sites occurs mainly postnatally. These possibilities are not mutually exclusive. Treatment of cord blood lymphocytes with IL-2 results in the appearance of $V_\alpha 24^+$ NK T cells.[264] Whether this reflects differentiation from an immature T cell population or expansion of a rare preexisting mature NK T cell population remains unclear. The capacity of cytokine-derived neonatal NK T cells and those directly isolated from the infant to produce cytokines or to mediate cytotoxicity has not been reported.

Gamma-Delta T Cells and Their Ontogeny

Gamma-delta T cells express a TCR heterodimer consisting of a gamma (γ) and a delta (δ) chain in association with the CD3 complex proteins. Gamma-delta T cells are rarer than $\alpha\beta$ T cells in most human tissues with a few exceptions, such as the intestinal epithelium, where they predominate.[265] Although some $\gamma\delta$ T cells can recognize conventional peptide antigens presented by MHC, this is probably not true of most.[266] For example, recognition of the herpes simplex virus (HSV)–encoded glycoprotein I (gpI) by murine $\gamma\delta$ T cells is direct and does not require antigen processing. Human $\gamma\delta$ T cells can proliferate and secrete IFN-γ after recognition of the nonpeptide antigens isopentenyl and prenyl phosphates, derived from mycobacteria.[267, 268] The putative antigen combining site of the $\gamma\delta$-TCR also shares some structural features with that of immunoglobulin molecules.[269] This is consistent with the idea that the $\gamma\delta$-TCR may be similar to immunoglobulin in recognizing three-dimensional structures, including those of nonproteins, rather than processed antigenic peptides bound to MHC molecules. Extracts from a variety of other bacteria can activate $\gamma\delta$ T cells, including some important neonatal pathogens, such as *Listeria* sp., and the $V_{\gamma}2$-$V_{\delta}2$ subset (using proposed 1995 standard nomenclature for V segments)[270] proliferates strongly in response to extracts from streptococci and plasmodia (malarial parasites).[265, 271] This in vitro activation is probably relevant in vivo because increased numbers of $\gamma\delta$ T cells are found in the skin lesions of leprosy patients and in the blood of patients with malaria.[265, 271] However, with the exception of mycobacteria, the pathogenic antigens recognized by gamma-delta T cells remain to be defined.

Like $\alpha\beta$ cytolytic T cells, activated $\gamma\delta$ T cells express high levels of perforins and serine esterases and are capable of cytotoxicity against tumor cells and other cell targets. Gamma-delta T cells can also secrete a variety of cytokines in vitro, including TNF, IFN-γ, and IL-4,[265, 271] as well as lymphotactin and other chemokines, which may help recruit inflammatory cells to the tissues.[272] Experiments with mice genetically deficient in $\gamma\delta$ T cells or in which these cells are depleted by antibody treatment suggest that these cells are critical for mucosal immunity. Mice lacking $\gamma\delta$ cells have markedly decreased numbers of intestinal plasma cells for IgA and decreased production of IgA when immunized orally with a foreign protein and adjuvant[273]; whether this mechanism is due to direct effects of $\gamma\delta$ T cells on the function of intestinal epithelial cells or B cells, or on the generation of $\alpha\beta$ TH2-like effector cells that may provide help to B cells in the mucosa remains unclear. In other contexts, such as mucosal allergic disease, $\gamma\delta$ T cells may produce cytokines, such as IL-4, which are required for allergic sensitization and generation of $\alpha\beta$ TH2 effector cells.[274] Gamma-delta T cells may also contribute to defense of the host against intracellular pathogens, including HSV, *Listeria* sp., and *M. tuberculosis*, particularly if $\alpha\beta$ T cell function is compromised.[275-277]

More recent studies indicate that human $\gamma\delta$ T cells with TCR-bearing $V_\delta 1$ segments can recognize and be activated by the class I MHC–like MICA and MICB molecules, which are induced on heat-shock-stressed epithelial cells[278] and, presumably, stressed or infected epithelium in vivo. This suggests a role of $\gamma\delta$ T cells in regulating host epithelial function under stressful conditions, such as infection. Consistent with this idea, resident $\gamma\delta$ T cells of the murine skin can produce epithelium-specific growth factors, which may help maintain epithelial integrity during stress.[279]

In the thymus and peripheral blood of most individuals only about 2 to 5% of T-lineage cells express $\gamma\delta$-TCR.[3] Unlike most $\alpha\beta$ T cells, whose development requires an intact thymus, a significant portion of $\gamma\delta$ T cells can develop by a thymic-independent pathway, and normal numbers of $\gamma\delta$ T cells are found in cases of complete thymic aplasia.[3] This effect may be explained, at least in part, by the differentiation of $\gamma\delta$ T cells directly from primitive lymphohematopoietic precursor cells found in clusters in the lamina propria of the small intestine, as has been demonstrated in the mouse.[280] In contrast with $\alpha\beta$-TCR, the γ- and δ-TCR chain genes show no evidence of allelic exclusion.[281] The human γ- and δ-TCR chain genes undergo a programmed rearrangement of dispersed segments analogous to that of the β- and α-TCR genes. However, most $\gamma\delta$ T cells lack surface expression of either the CD4 or the CD8 β chain, suggesting that they may not undergo the same process of positive selection that is obligatory for $\alpha\beta$ T cells.[282] It is also unclear whether $\gamma\delta$ T cells undergo negative selection.[266]

Rearrangement of the human γ- and δ-TCR genes begins shortly after colonization of the thymus with lymphoid cells during fetal gestation, and TCR-δ protein is detectable by 9.5 weeks of gestation.[176] Whether differentiation of $\gamma\delta$ T cells occurs by a pathway that is largely or completely independent of that for $\alpha\beta$ thymocytes remains unclear.[72, 283] Gamma-delta T cells constitute about 10% of the circulating T cell compartment at 16 weeks, a percentage that gradually declines to less than 3% at term.[190, 284]

Although there is potential for the formation of a highly diverse $\gamma\delta$-TCR repertoire, peripheral $\gamma\delta$ T cells use only a small number of V segments, which vary with age and with tissue location. These can be divided into two major groups—$V_\gamma 2$-$V_\delta 2$ cells and $V_\delta 1$ cells, in which a $V_\delta 1$-bearing TCR δ chain predominantly pairs with a TCR-γ chain using a V_γ segment other than $V_\gamma 1$. Most $\gamma\delta$ thymocytes in the first trimester of fetal life express $V_\delta 2$ segments. This is followed by $\gamma\delta$ thymocytes that express $V_\delta 1$ and that predominate at least through infancy in the thymus. Most circulating fetal and neonatal $\gamma\delta$ T cells are also $V_\delta 1$, with only about 10% bearing $V_\delta 2$,[264] and these $V_\delta 1$ cells are the predominant $\gamma\delta$ T cell population of the small intestinal epithelium after birth. In contrast with the fetal thymus and fetal and neonatal circulation during early gestation, $V_\delta 2$ T cells predominate in the fetal liver and spleen early during the second trimester[285, 286] and appear before $\gamma\delta$ thymocytes,[176, 287] suggesting that they are produced extrathymically by the fetal liver. By 6 months after birth, $\gamma\delta$ T cells bearing $V_\gamma 2$-$V_\delta 2$ segments become predominant in the circulation and remain so during adulthood,[288] most likely as a result of their preferential expansion in response to ubiquitous antigen(s).

Although neonatal $\gamma\delta$ T cells proliferate in vitro in response to mycobacterial lipid antigens,[289] they express lower levels of serine esterases than adult $\gamma\delta$ T cells, suggesting they may be less effective as cytotoxic cells.[290] Gamma-delta T cell clones derived from cord blood also have a markedly reduced capacity to mediate cytotoxicity against tumor cell extracts compared with that of $\gamma\delta$ T cell clones derived from adult peripheral blood.[284] Because these neonatal clones also have lower CD45R0 surface expression than adult clones, their reduced activity may reflect their relative antigenic naivete compared with that of most adult $\gamma\delta$ T cells. However, in contrast with neonatal $\alpha\beta$ T cells, activation and propagation of these cells in culture do not appear to enhance their function relative to that of the adult $\gamma\delta$ T cell population. The function of fetal liver $\gamma\delta$ T cells remains unclear. A single report suggests that they are enriched in cytotoxic reactivity against noninherited maternal class I MHC[287] and could help prevent the engraftment of maternal T cells into the fetus.

Practical Aspects of T Cell Function in the Neonate

DELAYED CUTANEOUS HYPERSENSITIVITY AND GRAFT REJECTION

Skin test reactivity to cell-free antigens assesses a form of delayed-type hypersensitivity (DTH) that requires the function of antigen-specific CD4 T cells. Skin test reactivity to common antigens such as *Candida* sp., streptokinase-streptodornase, and tetanus toxoid is usually not detectable in neonates.[291-293] This reflects primarily a lack of antigen-specific sensitization because in vitro reactivity of these antigens is also absent. However, when leukocytes, and presumably antigen-specific CD4 T cells, from sensitized adults are adoptively transferred to neonates, children, or adults, only neonates fail to respond to antigen-specific skin tests.[294] As discussed later, this indicates that the neonate may be deficient in other components of the immune system required for DTH, such as monocyte chemotaxis. Such deficiencies may account, in least in part, for diminished skin reactivity by the neonate compared with that of the adult after specific sensitization or after intradermal injection with T cell mitogens.[295, 296] Diminished skin reactivity after sensitization appears to persist postnatally up to 1 year of age.[297]

Nevertheless, neonates, including those who are premature, are capable of rejecting foreign grafts.[298] Results of experiments using human SCID mouse chimeras also suggest that second trimester human fetal T cells are capable of becoming cytotoxic effector T cells in responding to foreign antigens and in rejecting solid tissue allografts.[299] Transplantation of fetal blood from one unaffected fraternal twin to another with β-thalassemia did not result in marrow engraftment, despite a sharing of similar MHC haplotypes, and instead produced a detectable postnatal recipient cytotoxic T cell response against donor leukocytes.[300] A T cell response to alloantigens can also be detected in newborns after in utero irradiated red blood cell transfusions from unrelated donors, and these neonates also have a significantly greater percentage of CD45R0[high] T cells than healthy controls.[301, 302] These observations support the notion that fetal T cells have the capacity to mediate allogeneic responses, including graft rejection, in vivo, although it is unclear whether these responses are equivalent to those that would occur postnatally after transplantation or transfusion.

Another indication of the capacity of neonatal T cells to mediate allogeneic responses is that blood transfusions rarely induce graft-versus-host disease in the term neonate. However, rare cases of persistence of donor lymphocytes and of graft-versus-host disease have developed subsequent to intrauterine transfusion in the last trimester as well as in transfused premature neonates,[303–306] but the precise age-related risk for this complication is not known. Because the infusion of fresh leukocytes into the neonate has been shown to induce a state of partial tolerance to skin grafts,[298] the induction of tolerance for transfused lymphocytes might occur by a similar mechanism, predisposing the fetus or neonate to graft-versus-host disease. Together, these observations suggest a partial immaturity in T cell and inflammatory mechanisms required for DTH and for graft rejection.

T CELL REACTIVITY TO SPECIFIC ANTIGENS

Specific antigen reactivity can theoretically develop in the fetus by exposure to antigens transferred from the mother, by transfer of specific cellular immunity derived from maternal lymphocytes, or by infection of the fetus itself.[307] Several independent studies suggest that fetal T cells can become primed to environmental or dietary protein allergens as a result of maternal exposure and transfer to the fetus.[308–311] Interestingly, in one study, protein allergen–specific T cell proliferation detected at birth appeared to be more common when allergen exposure occurred in the first or second trimester rather than the third trimester of gestation.[311] Whether this reflects decreased maternal-to-fetal transport of antigen during late pregnancy or is an intrinsic difference between the capacity of early- and late-gestation fetal T cells to be primed remains unclear. Whether allergen priming of fetal T cells is a risk factor for the postnatal development of atopic disease also remains controversial.

In contrast with that of protein allergens, antigen-specific fetal T cell priming to vaccines has not been documented, for example, after maternal vaccination during the last trimester of pregnancy with tetanus toxoid or influenza A or influenza B.[312] This suggests that fetal sensitization to foreign proteins may be relatively inefficient, particularly when exposure is temporally limited. Whether this reflects relatively inefficient maternal-fetal transfer of protein antigens, intrinsic limitations of the fetus for antigen presentation and T cell priming, or both is unclear. Even if it is assumed that the capacity of fetal T cells to be primed by foreign antigens is similar to that of antigenically naive adult T cells, the immune response to maternally derived foreign proteins by fetal T cells would be expected to be poor compared with the maternal response, because foreign antigen may enter into the fetal circulation without accompanying activation of the innate response required for efficient T cell activation (discussed later).

Cord blood lymphocyte proliferation or cytokine production in response to in vitro incubation with specific microbial antigens, particularly those used in tests of cellular immunity, has also been described. In studies in which in vitro reactivity of lymphocytes was studied between birth and the first week of life, specific reactivity to tuberculin purified protein derivative (PPD),[313, 314] *Mycobacterium leprae*,[315] measles,[316] and rubella[317] was observed. However, infants with reactive lymphocytes usually constituted less than 20% of those born to mothers without evidence of active infection, and the data were interpreted as evidence for the transfer of maternal cellular immunity.[317, 318] Responses are usually small and may, at least in some instances, represent laboratory artifacts rather than true sensitization. In vitro reactivity of neonatal T cells to various whole preparations of gram-negative bacteria or *Staphylococcus aureus* has been reported to demonstrate variable frequency.[319–321] The interpretation of these studies is confounded by the ability of some of these stimuli to act as mitogens or superantigens rather than as MHC-restricted peptide antigens. For example, T cells, including those from the neonate, are effectively activated by superantigen toxins produced by *S. aureus* and other bacteria.[206, 213] Bacterial superantigens activate T cells primarily on the basis of the expression by the T cell of particular TCR V_β segments rather than the ability of the TCR to recognize specific antigenic peptide–MHC complexes. Mycobacterial products, such as PPD or *M. leprae* extracts, can activate many γδ T cells in the absence of specific prior sensitization with mycobacteria. These responses may be mediated, at least in part, by the presentation of lipoglycan antigens bound to CD1. Although maternal-to-fetal and fetal-to-maternal transfer of a low percentage of leukocytes does occur, the frequency of maternal leukocytes in the fetus is very low (usually less than 0.1%)[322] and is unlikely to result in detectable antigen-specific cellular immunity. Thus, reports of neonatal T cell responses as a result of transfer of maternal immunity should remain suspect unless the T cell population that mediates the response is identified and its antigen specificity and MHC restriction are demonstrated. With the possible exception of some environmental protein allergens, specific cellular immunity is probably rare in the neonate in the absence of fetal infection.

Pathogen-specific T cell proliferative responses and cytokine (IL-2 and IFN-γ) responses of infants and children who have been congenitally infected (e.g., with syphilis, CMV, varicella-zoster virus [VZV], or *Toxoplasma gondii*) are often absent or are markedly lower than in those with postnatally acquired infection.[323–328] This is particularly evident when these infections occur in the first or second trimester. For severe infections occurring during the first trimester, a direct deleterious effect on T cell development is a possible mechanism. However, T cells from infants and children with congenital toxoplasmosis retain the ability to respond to alloantigen, mitogen, and, in at least one case, tetanus toxoid.[325] This suggests that these reduced pathogen-specific responses may be more often due to mechanisms that result in antigen-specific unresponsiveness (such as antigen-specific anergy, deletion, or ignorance [the failure of the T cell to be initially activated by antigen]).[329] As discussed, it is unlikely that a decreased TCR repertoire limits these immune responses, particularly in cases that occur from the second trimester onward. Decreased responses may also not apply to all congenital pathogens: In one study, most 10-year-old children who were congenitally infected with mumps had delayed-type hypersensitivity reactions to mumps antigen, indicating the persistence of functional mumps-specific memory-effector T cells.[330]

Postnatal infection of neonates with HSV results in antigen-specific proliferation and cytokine (IL-2 and IFN-γ) production by CD4 T cells. However, these responses are delayed in their appearance compared with that of adults with primary HSV infection.[331, 332] Infants between 6 and 12 months of age also have moderately lower IL-2 production in response to tetanus toxoid than older children and adults.[60] Taken together, these findings suggest that either antigen-specific memory CD4 T cell generation or function is decreased during early infancy, particularly soon after infection or immunization. Whether this reflects limitations in antigen processing; in T cell activation and co-stimulation, proliferation, and differentiation; or in all of these processes remains unclear.

There have been few studies of antigen-specific cytotoxic T cell responses in the fetus or neonate. In one case of congenital HIV-1 infection, the expansion of HIV-specific cytotoxic T cells was detected at birth. This indicates that the ability of the fetal T cells to be activated by viral antigen and undergo expansion is at least partially intact.[333] As discussed in the section on viral host defense mechanisms, studies of cytotoxic responses to HIV in perinatally infected infants suggest that the cytotoxic response may be reduced and delayed in appearance compared with that in adults with recent infection.[334] It is possible that these decreased responses may be due to a greater suppressive effect on immune function of HIV-1 in the young infant than in the adult rather than to intrinsic immunologic immaturity. How-

ever, studies of viral-specific cytotoxicity in infants with acute respiratory syncytial virus (RSV) infection also suggest that RSV-specific cytotoxicity is more pronounced and frequent in cells from infants 6 to 24 months of age than in cells from 0- to 5-month-old infants,[335] suggesting that the neonate may have a reduced capacity to generate antiviral CTL populations. However, this study did not determine the nature of the effector cells mediating the cytotoxicity.

Congenital infection with viruses or *T. gondii* during the second and third trimesters may result in the appearance of CD45R0^{high} T cells in the circulation and an inversion in the ratio of CD4 to CD8 T cells.[336–338] This suggests that fetal CD8 T cells can be activated and expanded in vivo in response to serious infection. These alterations may also be present in the circulation at birth as well as through early infancy,[339, 340] although their sensitivity and specificity for diagnosing congenital infection remain unclear. It is also uncertain whether these memory-effector–like T cells are functionally competent.

Summary

Overall, T cell function in the fetus and neonate is impaired compared with that in adults. Diminished functions include T cell–mediated cytotoxicity, T cell participation in delayed-type hypersensitivity, and, as discussed in more detail later, T cell help for B cell differentiation. Selective decreases in production of cytokines, such as CD40 ligand, by T cells may contribute to all of these deficits. Limitations in the available repertoire of αβ T cell receptors are unlikely to limit immune responses by the fetus from mid-gestation onward, although it is possible they could do so earlier during development. After neonatal infection, the acquisition of detectable T cell–dependent antigen-specific responses is delayed, and this likely applies to fetal infection. The basis for this delay remains to be defined, but preliminary in vitro results raise the possibility that limitations in dendritic cell function, activation and differentiation of antigenically naive T cells into memory and effector T cells, or both may be contributory. Although there is no compelling evidence that the mother transfers T cell–specific immunity to the fetus, it is likely that T cell sensitization to environmental allergens can occur during fetal life.

B CELLS AND IMMUNOGLOBULIN

Basic Aspects of B Cells and Immunoglobulin Production

OVERVIEW

Mature B cells are lymphocytes that are identifiable by their surface expression of immunoglobulin. Immunoglobulin, which is synonymous with antibody, is a heterodimeric protein consisting of two identical heavy chains and two identical light chains linked by disulfide bonds (Fig. 2–8).[341] Like the TCR, the amino terminal portion of the antibody chains is highly variable as a

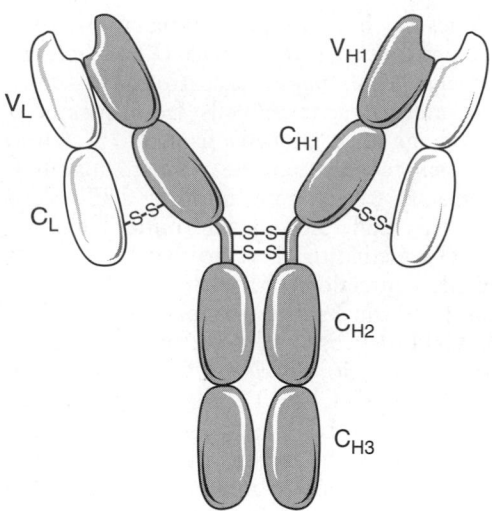

FIGURE 2–8 Structure of an immunoglobulin molecule: two heavy chains (dark shading) and two light chains (unshaded) linked by disulfide bonds. The antigen-combining site is formed by amino-terminal region of the heavy and light chains contained in the V_H and V_L domains of the heavy and light chains, respectively. For IgG, IgD, and IgA, the constant region C_{H3} domain of the heavy chain determines isotype or subclass specificity, which determines the ability of the immunoglobulin to fix complement, bind to Fc receptors, and be actively transported from the mother to the fetus during gestation. Not shown, IgM and IgE are structurally similar except that they contain an additional C_{H4} domain conferring these properties, and they lack a hinge region.

consequence of the assembly of V, D, and J gene segments (heavy chain) or V and J segments (light chain) to a monomorphic or C region. However, antibody molecules are distinct from the αβ-TCR in that they typically recognize antigens found on intact proteins or other molecules, such as complex carbohydrates. Thus, the B cell recognition of antigen is typically highly sensitive to its three-dimensional structure.

B cells are activated to proliferate and differentiate into antibody-secreting cells after surface immunoglobulin (sIg) binds antigen. The sIg molecule is invariably associated with the nonpolymorphic membrane proteins, Ig-α (CD79a) and Ig-β (CD79b), which, in conjunction with sIg, constitute the B cell receptor (BCR).[341] Ig-α and Ig-β, which are structural and functional homologues of the CD3 complex proteins, are expressed as disulfide-linked heterodimers and contain ITAM motifs in their cytoplasmic tails. As in T cells, these ITAMs act as docking sites for signaling molecules, such as the lyn and syk tyrosine kinases.

For B cells to be activated effectively and to produce antibody against protein antigens requires help from T cells in most cases. This help is in the form of soluble cytokines, such as IL-4, and of cell surface–associated signals, such as the cytokine CD40 ligand, which is transiently expressed on the T cell surface. The engagement of CD40, which is constitutively expressed by the B cell, is also instrumental in inducing B cells to undergo immunoglobulin isotype switching, for example, from

IgM to IgE (see Fig. 2–4). This is a process in which a portion of the C region of the immunoglobulin heavy chain gene is replaced with another isotype-specific segment but the antigen-combining site is preserved. In cases in which the antigen has multiple and identical surface determinants (e.g., complex polysaccharides or certain viral proteins with repetitive motifs) and multiple surface immunoglobulins are cross linked, antigen binding alone may be sufficient to induce B cell activation without cognate (direct cell-cell interaction) help from T cells. In this case, other signals derived from non–T cells, such as cytokines, or microorganisms, such as bacterial lipoproteins, may enhance antibody responses.

As for T cells, B cells receive additional regulatory signals from the engagement of surface molecules other than the BCR that act as either co-stimulatory or inhibitory molecules. Of the co-stimulatory molecules, a complex consisting of CD19, CD21, and CD81 is best defined. CD21, also known as complement receptor 2, binds fragments of the C3 complement component, C3dg or C3d. CD19 and CD81 transmit intracellular activation signals after complement binding to CD21.[342] Gene disruption experiments indicate that both CD19 and CD21 expression by B cells is essential for production of antibody to protein antigens,[343] whereas the lack of CD19 or CD21 has little or no effect on the production of antibodies to polysaccharide antigens, at least in mice.

The activation of B cells by BCR engagement and co-stimulation is counterbalanced by a number of surface molecules on the B cell that transmit inhibitory intracellular signals. For example, B cell activation is suppressed when a surface receptor for the crystallizable fragment (Fc) portion of IgG, FcγRIIB, is engaged concurrently with the BCR by antigen-IgG complexes. This serves as a negative feedback mechanism to limit antibody production; for example, gene knockout mice lacking FcγRIIB have substantially increased levels of circulating antibody after immunization.[344] Activated B cells, like T cells, also express CTLA-4,[345] but whether CTLA-4 inhibits B cell activation and proliferation in a manner analogous to that of its suppressive effects on T cell activation remains to be shown.

In addition to their secretion of antibodies, mature B cells express class II MHC and may also participate in antigen processing and presentation to CD4 T cells. Memory B cells are probably more effective than antigenically naive B cells, because they constitutively express higher surface levels of B7 molecules that provide co-stimulatory signals to T cells. The preferential source of protein for antigenic peptides is probably sIg–protein complexes internalized from the cell surface. The internalized proteins are degraded to peptides that can then be presented back on the cell surface bound to class II MHC molecules. Because the sIg-antigen interaction is of high affinity, B cell antigen presentation theoretically permits T cells to be activated at relatively low concentrations of antigen. However, depending on the particular antigen, the presentation of protein antigen by resting (antigenically naive) B cells can result in effective T cell activation or, in other instances, T cell apoptosis or antigen-specific tolerance.[346] In general, antigenically naive T cells are more likely to become anergic than to be activated when antigen is presented by antigenically naive B cells, whereas this is not the case for memory T cells. The relative importance of B cells versus other APCs, such as dendritic cells, for presenting protein antigens to CD4 T cells in vivo remains controversial.

IMMUNOGLOBULIN STRUCTURE AND THE GENETIC BASIS FOR IMMUNOGLOBULIN DIVERSITY

The amino-terminal region of each pair of heavy and light chains is variable; together these form the antigen-binding fragment (Fab) portion of immunoglobulin, which contains the antigen binding site (see Fig. 2–8). The variable region of each chain can be subdivided into three hypervariable complementarity-determining regions (CDRs), CDR1, CDR2, and CDR3, and four intervening, less-variable framework regions. The three-dimensional folding of the antibody molecules results in the approximation of the three CDR regions into a contiguous antigen-recognition site, with CDR3 located at the center and the CDR1 and CDR2 regions forming the outer border of the site.[347] The carboxy-terminal portion of the heavy and light chain genes is monomorphic or C and consists of three constant heavy (CH) domains and one constant light (CL) domain, respectively (see Fig. 2–8). The heavy chains also have a hinge region at which the two halves are joined by disulfide bonds. The heavy chain C region is the Fc portion of immunoglobulin and contains sites that determine complement fixation, placental transport, and binding to leukocyte Fc receptors. The portion of the heavy chain C region encoded by the last exon of heavy chain gene defines antibody isotype or isotype subclass, of which there are nine in humans, IgM, IgD, IgG_1, IgG_2, IgG_3, IgG_4, IgA_1, IgA_2, and IgE. There are two types of light chains, kappa and lambda, each containing a distinct type of constant region.

The heavy chain and kappa and lambda light chains are synthesized independently from genes located on human chromosomes 14, 2, and 22, respectively. Analogous to the β chain of the TCR, the heavy immunoglobulin chain is encoded by variable (V), diversity (D), joining (J), and constant (C) regions. Approximately 44 functional V segments and 20 different D segments are dispersed over 1100 kb of DNA upstream of the J-C region[348, 349]; 39 of the 44 V segments are expressed.[348] There are 6 different J segments located near the C region. Antibody gene rearrangement is required to bring the V, D, and J-C regions into proximity so that the gene can be expressed (see Fig. 2–4). The same recombinase enzyme complex required for TCR gene rearrangement, including the RAG-1 and RAG-2 proteins, mediates this process. The assembly of the light chain genes from multiple potential segments is similar, except that D segments are not used. The human kappa light chain gene locus consists of at least 32 potentially functional V segments and 5 J segments, and a single C segment.[350] The human lambda light chain gene locus encodes at least 40 potentially functional V segments

and 4 functional J segments, each associated with its own C segment.[351] The CDR1 and CDR2 regions of the antigen-combining site are entirely encoded by the V segments. The CDR3 is encoded at the junction of the V, D, and J segments.

Similar to that of the TCR genes, antibody diversity is generated by (1) the juxtaposition of various combinations of V, D, and J segments and (2) the imprecision in the joining process itself: Nucleotides at junctions may be removed by exonucleolytic activity or, alternatively, added by the TdT enzyme or as P nucleotides. Finally, in the case of the heavy chain gene, D-D joining can occur and D segments can also rearrange by inversion or deletion.[352] Together these mechanisms permit a theoretical immunoglobulin repertoire of more than 10^{12} specificities to be generated from fewer than 10^3 somatic gene segments. However, for reasons that are not clear, immunoglobulin heavy chain V segment usage by immature pre-B cells and antigenically naive B cells appears to be dominated by relatively few segments.[353, 354] Thus, actual immunoglobulin diversity is less than would be predicted if segment usage were completely random. As in the case of the TCR genes, the CDR3 region appears to be the most important source of diversity.[81]

The rearrangement process maximizes the generation of diversity at the expense of precision. Consequently the majority of pre-B cells fail to produce a functional immunoglobulin molecule, do not mature, and subsequently die. The inefficiency of generating productive rearrangements for both heavy and light chains is offset by the high rate of proliferation of immature pro- and pre-B cells. Still further diversification is possible later in B cell differentiation by processes known as somatic mutation and receptor editing, which are described later.

B CELL MATURATION AND PREIMMUNE SELECTION

The pro-B cell is the most immature cell type that is known to be committed to differentiate along the B lineage. Human pro-B cells have a $CD34^{high}$ $CD19^{low}$ surface phenotype. They also express the RAG and TdT proteins, although the immunoglobulin heavy chain gene remains in its unrearranged, germline configuration.[355] Immunoglobulin heavy chain gene rearrangement occurs at the next stage, the pre-B cell, which lacks surface CD34 and expresses high amounts of CD19. Pro-B cells and pre-B cells are found only in the bone marrow of the adult. In the fetus, these cells are found in the liver and omentum and in smaller numbers in the lung and kidney.[356]

In immature pre-B cells, the heavy chain gene usually, but not invariably, rearranges first, initially with a joining of a D segment to a J segment.[357] Rearrangement results in the excision of intervening DNA so that the heavy chain gene segments can be transcribed as a single unit. If the DJ segment is productively rearranged, its transcripts are translated into DJ heavy chain protein. If a nonproductive DJ rearrangement occurs, a second attempt at productive DJ rearrangement is made by the heavy chain gene on the other chromosome 14. DJ heavy chain gene rearrangement and protein expression are followed by the joining of a V segment to the DJ segment. Productive VDJ rearrangement results in the expression of full-length heavy chain protein in the cytoplasm. In humans, the first easily recognized pre-B cells are those that contain cytoplasmic IgM heavy chains but no light chains or sIg.

The late pre-B cell stage occurs when the heavy chain protein associates on the cell surface with VpreB and a λ5/14.1 segment, two proteins that together form a functional surrogate light chain.[341, 358] The heavy chain and surrogate light chain proteins are associated with Ig-α/Ig-β heterodimers, forming the pre–B cell receptor (pre-BCR). The pre-BCR is essential for proliferation and development of human B cells, for blocking of rearrangement of the other heavy chain gene allele (allelic exclusion), and for promotion of light chain rearrangement.[341] In some pre-B cells productive light chain rearrangements can occur in the absence of productive heavy chain rearrangements, at least in the fetal bone marrow, suggesting that heavy chain gene rearrangement is not obligatory for light chain rearrangement.[357]

After the expression of the pre-BCR, a similar process of gene rearrangement subsequently occurs to assemble light chain genes from V and J segments. Allelic exclusion also usually acts at the light chain level so that only a single type of light chain is produced. Kappa light chain gene rearrangement usually occurs first, and if neither kappa chain gene rearrangement is productive, this apparently permits lambda chain gene rearrangement to proceed. Approximately 60% of human immunoglobulin molecules utilize kappa light chains, and the remainder use lambda light chains.[351] If rearrangement and expression of a complete kappa or lambda light chain subsequently occur, a functional immunoglobulin molecule is assembled and expressed as sIg. The end result of allelic exclusion is that a B cell usually synthesizes only a single immunoglobulin protein, although each cell has the genetic information to produce two heavy chains and four light chains. Compared with that of the heavy chain, allelic exclusion of immunoglobulin light chains is relatively "leaky" such that 0.2 to 0.5% of circulating B cells express both a kappa and a lambda light chain in their surface IgM.[359]

The initial expression of sIg by B-lineage cells is in the form of both the IgM and IgD isotypes. This is the result of alternative RNA splicing of the exons of the heavy chain gene that encode isotype specificity. B cells, like T cells, also appear to undergo negative and positive selection processes in the bone marrow prior to their entry into the periphery and their activation by foreign antigens. Evidence for positive and negative selection of B cells in human adults comes from an analysis of the B cell immunoglobulin repertoire.[360] Positive selection of immature B cells in the bone marrow requires an intact BCR complex and presumably involves some interaction of the BCR with self-molecules.[341, 361–363] In the absence of positive selection, B cells fail to enter into the recirculating pool in which antigenically naive B cells transit among the circulation, spleen, lymph nodes, Peyer's patches, and tonsils. Antigenically naive B cells that survive this selection process leave the bone marrow and colonize the T cell–rich areas of peripheral lymphoid organs.[364]

Extensive murine experiments utilizing B cells expressing self-reactive transgenic sIg have shown that negative selection can either eliminate (clonal deletion) or inactivate (clonal anergy) potential autoreactive antigenically naive B cells.[365] In some cases negative selection may occur after the entry of B cells into the peripheral lymphoid organs.[366] CD4 T cells can also potentially rescue autoreactive B cells from negative selection[367] and, hence, may play an important role in autoantibody-mediated diseases.

B CELL ACTIVATION, CLONAL EXPANSION, AND IMMUNE SELECTION

Mature antigenically naive B cells that survive positive and negative selection are IgM^{high}IgD^{high} [368] and recirculate between the peripheral lymphoid organs via the circulation and lymph. The encounter of these B cells with antigen recognized by the sIg triggers their activation and proliferation under appropriate conditions. In T cell–dependent activation of B cells, it appears that antigenically naive CD4 T cells are first activated by dendritic cells independently of B cells in the periarteriolar lymphoid sheath region of the spleen and the paracortical region of the lymph nodes.[369] These activated T cells express surface CD40 ligand and OX40, a member of the TNF receptor family. Some activated T cells leave the lymphoid organ to become effector or memory T cells; others move to the outer border of the T cell zone to contact antigen-activated B cells at the edge of the follicular zone (also known as the mantle region).[369] Interactions between B cells and dendritic cells that occur independently of T cells may also enhance B cell activation.[46] During the initial immune response, most antigenically naive B cells are derived from clones expressing antibody-variable regions with relatively low affinity for antigen. As in the case of the TCR, activation via the BCR is also not necessarily an all-or-none phenomenon. For example, high-affinity binding to IgM of the BCR may allow B cell proliferation to occur in the absence of any T cell help, whereas lower-affinity binding may only result in proliferation in the presence of additional T cell–derived signals.[370]

The interaction of CD40 ligand and OX40 on the T cell with CD40 and OX40 ligand on the B cell appears to enhance B cell activation further.[371] In addition, OX40 engagement of the T cell promotes its differentiation into an IL-4–producing effector cell and the expression of the CXCR5 α-chemokine receptor, also known as blr-1; blr-1 appears to mediate the entry of small numbers of B cells and T cells into B cell follicles, where an α-chemokine ligand for this receptor is expressed.[137] Antigen-specific B cells proliferate strongly within the B cell follicle, leading to the formation of germinal centers.[372] The more avidly the B cell binds antigen, the stronger is the stimulus to proliferate. The source of antigen for triggering the extensive B cell proliferation of the germinal center is probably provided by follicular dendritic cells. Follicular dendritic cells are nonhematopoietically derived and have the unusual capacity to bind antigen-antibody complexes for long periods on their cell surface.[373]

Immunoglobulin variants are generated among germinal center B cells by the process of somatic hypermutation, in which immunoglobulin genes accumulate apparently random point mutations within existing V, D, and J segments. These variants undergo a selection process favoring B cells that bear immunoglobulin with high affinity for antigen. Such high-affinity immunoglobulin provides high levels of BCR signaling, favoring germinal center B cell survival rather than a default pathway of apoptosis.[374] The identity of the proteins the somatic mutator comprises remains obscure, although one component appears to be certain general DNA mismatch repair enzymes.[375] It also remains unclear how the effects of the mutator are focused on the variable region of immunoglobulin and its immediate flanking sequences. The peak of somatic mutation is approximately 10 to 12 days after immunization with a protein antigen.[376]

In cases in which the affinity of the germinal center B cell surface immunoglobulin for antigen and, as a consequence, BCR signaling is relatively weak, T cell–derived signals, such as CD40 ligand and soluble cytokines, may result in the reinduction of the RAG recombinase machinery and receptor editing.[377] Receptor editing may occur via secondary V-to-J light chain gene rearrangements or replacement of V heavy chain gene segments with previously unrearranged upstream V segments in mature B cells.[80] Strong signaling via the BCR inhibits RAG complex expression, terminating further rearrangement and ensuring that high-affinity surface immunoglobulins are prevented from undergoing further editing.[377] There is evidence for light chain receptor editing in human germinal centers,[378] but the importance of this process to shaping the final immunoglobulin repertoire in humans remains unclear.

Germinal center B cells that receive appropriate survival signals leave the germinal center to persist as memory B cells. The engagement of CD40 on germinal center B cells by CD40 ligand on T cells is absolutely required for memory B cell generation but is apparently not involved in initial germinal center B cell proliferation.[379] Experiments in mice also suggest that memory B cell generation requires the binding by CD21 on B cells of C3 complement components, apparently derived from the classic complement pathway.[343] Memory B cells enter the recirculating lymphocyte pool, where they preferentially colonize the skin and mucosa, sites that are likely to have direct contact with antigen,[159] as well as the marginal zone of the spleen and its equivalent at other sites of peripheral lymphoid tissue. The marginal zone region is a major draining site for antigens found in the bloodstream, and such a localization may permit memory B cells to respond rapidly to antigen reexposure. Spleen marginal zone memory B cells can be distinguished from antigenically naive B cells by their high levels of surface expression of CD148, a protein-tyrosine phosphatase, and CD27, a member of the TNF receptor family.[380] CD27 expression also appears to be a reliable marker for circulating memory B cells.[381] Once a memory B cell is generated, further somatic mutation of its immunoglobulin genes apparently does not occur.[382]

Memory B cells can persist in a nonmitotic state in lymphoid organs for at least 6 months.[383]

GENERATION OF PLASMA CELLS AND THE MOLECULAR BASIS FOR IMMUNOGLOBULIN SECRETION

Some activated B cells migrate to extrafollicular regions of the lymph node or spleen, where they become short-lived plasma cells that mainly produce IgM, an outcome that may be favored by the production of IL-12 by dendritic cells.[384] Differentiation of these plasma cells does not appear to require CD40 ligand–CD40 interaction, accounting for relatively normal IgM responses in patients with genetic deficiency of CD40 ligand.[122] In the absence of CD40 engagement, germinal center B cells that have survived the selection process probably differentiate by a default pathway to become long-lived plasma cells,[159] which can persist in the spleen and bone marrow for at least a year.[385] This plasma cell differentiation pathway may also be favored by engagement of the CD27 molecule on the B cell.[386] In mice, long-lived plasma cells are distinguishable from short-lived plasma cells by their lack of class II MHC expression.[385] Plasma cells are concentrated in peripheral lymphoid tissue, liver, and bone marrow, as well as in lymphoid tissue of the gastrointestinal and respiratory tracts.

The membrane-bound form of immunoglobulin is slightly longer than the secreted form and contains a carboxy-terminal region that anchors the molecule in the cell membrane. The secretory form of immunoglobulin lacks this membrane-anchoring segment as a result of a change in splicing of the heavy chain mRNA. Maturation of B cells into plasma cells is associated with a marked increase in their capacity to secrete immunoglobulin and with loss of surface Ig expression. Plasma cells rather than mature B cells account for most of the secreted antibody during both primary and secondary immune responses.

SWITCHING OF IMMUNOGLOBULIN ISOTYPE AND CLASS

Human B cells produce five isotypes of antibody, IgM, IgD, IgG, IgA, and IgE. The IgG and IgA isotypes can be, respectively, divided into the IgA_1 and IgA_2, and the IgG_1, IgG_2, IgG_3, and IgG_4 subclasses. During their process of differentiation into plasma cells, B cells are able to change from IgM to other antibody isotypes without changing antigen specificity (see Fig. 2–4). With the exception of IgD expression, this usually involves isotype recombination, the genetic replacement of the IgM-specific portion of the constant region ($C\mu$) of the heavy chain with a new isotype-specific gene segment. The intervening DNA is excised as a large circle. Isotype recombination is mediated by switch regions that are positioned immediately upstream of each of the isotype-specific C regions with the exception of IgD. However, the precise identity and mechanism of the "switch recombinase" remain enigmatic. Successive multiple isotype switching by a single B cell can also occur, for example, IgM to IgA to IgG to IgE.[387]

The CD40–CD40 ligand interaction is critical for most isotype switching. Mutations in the CD40 ligand that prevent its expression or efficient binding to CD40, or defects in CD40 signaling, result in the hyperimmunoglobulin M syndrome, an immunodeficiency in which B cell antibody production is largely limited to the IgM isotype.[122] Secreted cytokines derived from T cells or other cell types play an important role in promoting or inhibiting switching to a specific isotype. For example, IL-4 or IL-13 is absolutely required for isotype switching to IgE, a process that can be inhibited by the presence of IFN-γ.[388] Cytokine-induced switching to a particular isotype segment strongly correlates with the cytokine-inducing transcription that is initiated immediately upstream of this region. In some instances, hormones may also play a role in isotype switching. For example, vasoactive intestinal peptide in conjunction with CD40 engagement can induce human B cells to produce high levels of IgA$_1$ and IgA$_2$.[389]

Isotype switching typically occurs after somatic hypermutation within the germinal center, when B cells encounter antigen-specific CD4 T cells that produce CD40 ligand and various cytokines.[159, 390] Switch recombination after primary immunization is evident in peripheral lymphoid tissue 4 days after immunization with protein antigen and peaks between 10 and 18 days.[391] Switch recombination is also triggered during memory B cell responses, is detectable within 24 hours of secondary immunization, and peaks between 3 and 4 days.[391] Most memory B cells or plasma cells switch to another isotype by gene rearrangement, and somatic mutations are most common in antibodies other than IgM. However, some adult B cells express surface IgM but not IgD or other isotypes, and these cells appear to consist of memory B cells that have not undergone isotype switching.[392] Thus, isotype switching is not obligatory for somatic hypermutation or for memory cell generation.

REGULATION OF B CELL PROLIFERATION AND DIFFERENTIATION

B cell activation and differentiation are subject to regulation at multiple steps by cell-cell contact and soluble factors as well as intracellular signaling molecules and transcription factors. Such regulation may be specific for particular stages of B cell development. For example, btk, a tyrosine kinase expressed by B-lineage cells, appears to play a role in cell activation after engagement of the pre-BCR or BCR complexes. Functional mutations in btk result in the syndrome of X-linked agammaglobulinemia, in which B cell development is arrested at a pre–B cell stage.[393] In contrast, the engagement of CD40 by CD40 ligand is not required for B cell development but is essential for the generation of memory B cells from mature antigenically naive B cells.[122] IL-6, in addition to its role in inducing complement proteins within germinal centers, may serve as an autocrine factor for the proliferation of plasma cells. As previously discussed, most cytokines secreted by T cells, such as IL-2, IL-4, and IFN-γ, are not essential for B cell development but are important regulators of expression of B cell isotype.

SPLENIC FUNCTION AND IMMUNOGLOBULIN PRODUCTION

The human spleen has distinct anatomic sites that may play specialized roles in antibody responses and has an important role in the production of antibody against repetitive carbohydrate antigens, such as the capsular polysaccharides of pathogenic bacteria, such as *Streptococcus pneumoniae*, *Neisseria meningitidis*, and *H. influenzae*. Antigens and lymphocytes enter the spleen through vascular sinusoids located in the red pulp that are in proximity to the marginal zone area. The white pulp area contains periarteriolar sheaths of lymphocytes, mainly T cells, as well as periarteriolar follicles, which are mainly B cells. These, in turn, are surrounded by a microanatomic site known as the marginal zone that contains loose clusters of B cells, macrophages, and some CD4 T cells.[394] The precise pathways of lymphocyte and dendritic cell migration in the human spleen, particularly during immune responses, remain unknown.

Immunization with polysaccharide antigens before splenectomy maintains the capacity of the immune system to respond to these antigens subsequently.[395] This suggests that the activation of splenic B cells recognizing polysaccharide antigens may result in their migration and persistence in other lymphoid organs, such as the subepithelial region of the tonsil.[396] The appearance of splenic marginal zone postnatally as well 1 to 2 years after bone marrow transplantation correlates with an ability to produce antibodies in response to immunization with polysaccharide vaccines. Marginal zone B cells are predominantly IgM^{high}IgD^{low} and CD21^{high} [397] and include antigenically naive B cells that appear to be important for responses to polysaccharide antigens,[398, 399] as well as memory B cells that have not undergone isotype switching. Marginal zone B cells are more easily stimulated by T cell–independent stimuli, such as LPS, than are follicular B cells.[400]

B-1 AND B-2 CELLS

B cells that express CD5 and that have low levels of surface expression of CD45RA appear to represent a distinct B cell subset that has been termed B-1. The B-1 subset can be further divided into B-1a cells, in which CD5 is expressed on the cell surface, and B-1b cells, in which CD5 expression is limited to the RNA level.[401] B cells that lack CD5 mRNA or protein expression and that are CD45RA^{high} compose the B-2 lineage; they include most of the peripheral B cells in the adult. B-1 and B-2 cells appear to be subject to different positive and negative influences of the preimmune (i.e., before exposure to foreign antigen) immunoglobulin repertoire.[402, 403] B-1 cells have a tendency to produce antibodies that are mainly of the IgM isotype and that are polyreactive; that is, individual antibodies are typically of low affinity but are able to react with multiple unrelated antigens. These include self-antigens, such as DNA, and foreign antigens, such as viral proteins or bacterial-derived products, such as phosphorylcholine. In contrast, B-2 cells typically produce high-affinity antibodies that are usually monoreactive, bind only a single antigen or highly related antigens,[404] and are often of isotypes other than IgM.[405, 406] In the adult, somatic hypermutation of immunoglobulin molecules is common for both B-1 and B-2 cells. This suggests that both cell types are subject to an antigen-driven selection process after activation[403, 407] and that activated B-1 cells tend to become memory cells that have not undergone isotype switching. Whether B-1 cells are derived from a separate lineage or, as recent evidence suggests, are induced to differentiate from a common precursor that is shared with B-2 cells[408] remains controversial. As discussed later, B-1 cells predominate during early fetal development. These cells have been proposed to play a role in regulation and development of the immune system in early ontogeny, perhaps in the induction of tolerance to self-antigens, or in host defense, by provision of polyreactive IgM antibodies that are pathogen-reactive.

Ontogeny of B Cells and Immunoglobulins

B CELL DEVELOPMENT AND ISOTYPE EXPRESSION

Pre-B cells are first detected in human fetal liver and omentum by 8 weeks of gestation and in fetal bone marrow by 13 weeks of gestation.[409, 410] Between 18 and 22 weeks of gestation pro- or pre-B cells can also be detected in substantial numbers in the liver, lung, and kidney,[356] whether these cells represent B cell lymphopoiesis in situ or are derived from other sites remains to be determined. By mid-gestation, bone marrow is the predominant site of pre–B cell development.[411] After 30 weeks of gestation, B cell lymphopoiesis occurs solely in bone marrow for the remainder of life.[356]

B cells expressing surface IgM are present by 10 weeks of gestation.[409] Unlike surface IgM-positive adult B cells found in the peripheral lymphoid organs, most of which also express surface IgD, fetal B cells at this stage have been reported to express IgM without IgD.[409, 412] Such IgM$^+$IgD$^-$ B cells appear to constitute a transitory stage between pre-B cells and mature IgM$^+$IgD$^+$ B cells, and it is at this stage that the CD21 surface molecule is expressed. Experiments in mice have shown that exposure of IgM$^+$IgD$^-$ B cells to antigens, including those found in the adult bone marrow, results in clonal anergy rather than activation.[413] It is hypothesized that the susceptibility of IgM$^+$IgD$^-$ cells to clonal anergy throughout life helps to maintain B cell tolerance to soluble self-antigens present at high concentrations. This raises the possibility that antigen exposure in utero may tend to induce specific B cell tolerance rather than an antibody response. This may account for the observation that early congenital infection sometimes results in pathogen-specific defects in immunoglobulin production. In some cases, such as congenital mumps, these defects may occur despite normal T cell responses, such as delayed-type hypersensitivity,[330] suggesting a direct inhibitory effect on antigen-specific B cell function.

Between 8 and 11 weeks of gestation, transcripts for IgA and IgG can be detected in the liver,[414] followed shortly by the appearance of B cells bearing sIg of the IgA, IgG, and IgD isotypes. By 16 weeks of gestation, fetal bone marrow B cells expressing sIg of all heavy chain isotypes are detectable.[415] The source of stimulation for isotype switching during fetal development remains unclear because in the adult it is typically seen in response to B cell activation by foreign protein antigens. The frequency of B cells in tissues then rapidly increases so that by 22 weeks of gestation the proportion of B cells in the spleen, blood, and bone marrow is similar to that in the adult.[409, 412] In contrast to adult B cells, which bear IgM plus IgD or IgG or IgA alone, neonatal B cells have been reported to express IgG or IgA with IgM plus IgD.[409] This result, which was based on fluorescent microscopy using polyclonal antisera, has not yet been confirmed by multiparameter flow cytometry. In a flow cytometric study in which nonspecific binding was carefully excluded, neonatal B cells expressing surface IgG or IgA were below the limit of detectability by the assay (that is, less than 1% of circulating B cells).[416] True germinal centers in the spleen and lymph nodes are absent during fetal life but appear in the first months after birth, presumably as a result of postnatal antigenic stimulation.[372]

In adults, CD10 surface expression ceases at the antigenically naive B cell stage. In contrast, most fetal bone marrow and spleen B cells express CD10.[417, 418] Although this raises the possibility that CD10$^+$ B cells might constitute an immature transitional population, these cells appear to be functionally mature on the basis of their ability to undergo isotype switching, as discussed later. Another distinct feature of fetal and neonatal B cells is their high frequency of CD5, indicating they belong to the B-1a subset.[418] More than 40% of B cells in the fetal spleen, omentum, and circulation at midgestation are CD5$^+$,[405, 406, 419] but lesser numbers are found in the fetal liver and bone marrow.[419] The preponderance of CD5$^+$ B cells noted in the fetus is also observed in the neonatal circulation[185] and gradually declines with postnatal age.[405, 420, 421] Like adult B-1a cells, those of the fetus and newborn have a greater tendency to express IgM antibodies that are polyreactive, including reactivity with self-antigens, such as DNA, than do B-2 cells.[404–406, 422] Although CD5$^+$ B cells have been proposed to play a role in regulation of the immune system in early ontogeny, perhaps in the induction of tolerance to self-antigens, they lack most surface markers characteristic of previously activated B cells.[405]

B-1 cells are also likely to be the major source of the low amounts of circulating "natural" IgM present at birth, which is largely produced in the absence of stimulation by foreign antigens. Murine studies that defined a role for such natural IgM are of interest: Mice in which secretory IgM but not surface IgM was eliminated by selective gene targeting had decreased primary responses to T cell–dependent antigens.[423] These mice also have an increased susceptibility to acute peritonitis caused by endogenous bacteria, which is apparently due, in part, to the lack of natural IgM antibodies with reactivity against phosphatidylcholine.[424] Although natural IgM may have low affinity, it is, nevertheless, effective in activating complement, and this may allow antigenically naive B cells to be more efficiently activated as a result of receiving a BCR signal in conjunction with co-stimulation via complement receptor 2 (CD21). Interestingly, natural IgM does not appear to play a role in enhancing the response to polysaccharide antigens, at least in mice.[423–425]

THE IMMUNOGLOBULIN REPERTOIRE IN THE FETUS AND NEONATE

The primary or preimmune immunoglobulin repertoire consists of all antibodies that the individual potentially can express prior to the first encounter with antigen. It is determined by the number of different B cell clones with distinct antigen specificity. The preimmune immunoglobulin repertoire is more limited during the initial stages of B cell development in the fetus than in the adult. In the early to mid-gestation human fetus, the set of V segments used to generate the heavy chain gene is smaller than in the adult.[426, 427] The V segments that are expressed are scattered throughout the heavy chain gene locus.[428] There are also clear differences in the usage of particular heavy chain D and J segments between the first and second trimesters and term.[352] These developmental differences in segment usage appear to be genetically determined rather than to result from environmental influences, such as stimulation by endogenous antigens, because they apply to early immature B cell precursors that do not express a pre-BCR complex.

The length of the heavy chain's CDR3, which is formed at the junction of the V segment with the D and J segments, is shorter in the fetus at mid-gestation than at birth[429] or in adulthood, including in pre-B cells.[430] As in the case of fetal thymocytes and T cells, this characteristic is due, at least in part, to decreased TdT, which is responsible for N additions. Up to 25% of heavy chain fetal CDR3 regions lack N additions, and in the remaining, the size of the N additions is smaller than in neonatal or adult CDR3 regions. The CDR3 region is the most hypervariable portion of immunoglobulins, and a short CDR3 region significantly reduces the diversity of the fetal immunoglobulin repertoire.[431] Moreover, because the CDR3 region is at the center of the antigen-binding pocket of antibodies,[347] such reduced diversity could limit the efficiency of the antibody response. A complete lack of N-terminal additions would be predicted to produce antibodies with combining sites that are relatively flat and potentially inefficient at combining with antigen.[352] However, the importance of shortened CDR3 regions, by themselves, in limiting antibody responses is doubtful, because gene knockout mice lacking TdT produce normal antibody responses after immunization or infection.[202] Although it remains theoretically possible that a combination of a relative lack of TdT and limitations in V and D usage could compromise the ability of the fetal B cells to recognize the full range of possible foreign antigens, particularly prior to mid-gestation, such a "hole in the repertoire" has not yet been documented.

The B cell repertoire increases during gestation,[432] and by birth it is substantially more diverse in the use of heavy chain V segments and length of the CDR3 region for IgM and IgA, but not IgG transcripts.[433]

Modest limitations in V segment repertoire may persist through the neonatal period, because some heavy chain V segments expressed by the adult repertoire are not found in the neonate.[431, 434] On the other hand, certain other V segments, such as VH3, are present at a greater frequency in the preimmune Ig repertoire of the neonate than in older individuals.[435] It is hypothesized that this increased representation of VH3 segments, which confers on antibody molecules an ability to bind protein A of S. aureus, may help provide intrinsic protection against bacterial pathogens during the perinatal period. Although most neonatal and fetal immunoglobulin heavy chain gene variable regions appear not to have undergone somatic mutation,[429, 434] these studies examined heavy chain transcripts for IgM, an isotype in which somatic mutation is uncommon in the adult, except in IgM$^+$IgD$^-$ memory cells.[436, 437] In contrast, somatic mutations are detectable in rare neonatal B cells expressing IgG or IgA transcripts.[433] Among neonatal B cells that bear somatic mutations, the mutational frequency per length of DNA is similar to that of adult B cells. Together, these observations indicate that somatic hypermutation occurs normally by birth in the B cell compartment.

NEONATAL B CELL SURFACE PHENOTYPE

Neonatal B cells, including the CD5$^-$ subset consisting of B-1b and B-2 cells, have increased surface levels of IgM compared with adult B cells; these differences persist until at least several years of age.[438] In a study by Macardle and co-workers[438] surface expression of CD19, CD21, CD22, and CD81 was similar in neonatal and adult B cells, including the CD5$^+$ and CD5$^-$ subsets, although another group reported that CD21 expression by neonatal B cells was reduced.[439] Surface expression of the FcγRII receptor (CD32) is reduced on neonatal B cells,[438] raising the possibility that they might be less subject to the inhibitory effect of antigen-antibody complexes, although this remains to be shown.

Circulating neonatal CD5$^-$ B cells have been reported to have reduced expression of a number of adhesion molecules compared with adult CD5$^-$ B cells, including CD11a, CD44, CD54 (ICAM-1), and CD62-L (L-selectin).[440] A similar reduction is found in the CD5$^-$ B cells of adult patients during the first 3 months that follow either autologous or heterologous bone marrow transplantation but resolves by approximately 14 months post-transplantation.[440] The postnatal age by which adult levels of expression of these adhesion molecules by B cells is typically achieved and the contribution of this reduced expression to defects in humoral immunity are unknown. Circulating neonatal B cells have also been reported to have lower surface levels of class II MHC than adult splenic B cells and, in contrast with adult cells, an inability to increase their intracellular calcium concentration after engagement of class II MHC by monoclonal antibodies.[441] It is unclear whether this also applies to neonatal and adult B cells that are more closely matched on the basis of their cell source and surface phenotype. Moreover, because neonatal B cells proliferate as well as or better than adult splenic B cells after class II engagement,[441] these alterations in signaling appear unlikely to compromise neonatal B cell function.

Cerutti and colleagues[442] reported that circulating neonatal B cells, of which approximately 90% were of the B-1a subset, expressed substantially more B7-1 (CD80), CD27, and CD28 than adult spleen B cells, in which more than 95% of the cells were of the B-2 subset. Whether this unusual surface phenotype for neonatal B-1a cells also applies to the adult B-1a subset was not determined. It is also unclear what role CD28 on B cells plays in the immune response in vivo. However, the presence of B7-1 as well as CD27, which is a reliable marker for memory B cells in the adult, raises the possibility that at least some circulating neonatal B-1a cells have undergone some form of activation in vivo.

FETAL AND NEONATAL T CELL–DEPENDENT IMMUNOGLOBULIN PRODUCTION AND ISOTYPE SWITCHING

Most early in vitro studies of immunoglobulin production by neonatal B cells utilized pokeweed mitogen, a polyclonal activator of both T and B cells. In this system, immunoglobulin production in cultures of neonatal lymphocytes was low compared with that of adults, and cell mixing experiments suggested that neonatal T cells acted as suppressors of immunoglobulin production by either adult or neonatal B cells. Further fractionation of the T cell populations in this assay suggested that in the absence of memory-effector T cells, antigenically naive (CD45RA^{high}CD45R0^{low}) CD4 T cells of either the neonate or the adult acted as suppressors of antibody production.[166] Priming of neonatal or adult antigenically naive CD4 T cells in vitro resulted in their acquisition of a CD45RA^{low}CD45R0^{high} phenotype and, concurrently, an ability to enhance rather than suppress pokeweed mitogen–induced immunoglobulin production.[166] However, the relevance of this nonspecific activation system to in vivo B cell immune responses mediated by the neonate remains unclear, in part because of our limited understanding of the cellular and molecular nature of suppression by T cells in vivo.

When B cells are activated by exogenous cytokines (e.g., IL-4, IL-10, or cytokine-containing supernatants from activated T cells) and a cellular source of CD40 ligand (e.g., CD40 ligand–expressing fibroblasts), neonatal B cell production of IgM, IgG$_1$, IgG$_2$, IgG$_3$, IgG$_4$, and IgE in most studies is similar to that of adult antigenically naive B cells.[241, 388, 443] The capacity for isotype switching appears to be established at the pre–B cell stage, including during human fetal ontogeny: Isotype switching and IgE and IgG$_4$ production have been observed using fetal B cells and pre-B cells from as early as 12 weeks of gestation.[418, 444–446] IgA$_1$ and IgA$_2$ are also produced in similar amounts by fetal antigenically naive B cells and adult B cells in response to stimulation with anti-CD40 antibody and the hormone vasoactive intestinal peptide,[389] and fetal pre-B cells are also competent for IgA production under these conditions.[389] Experiments in which human B and T cells either develop in or are adoptively transferred into SCID mice also suggest that fetal or neonatal B cells are capable of

isotype switching and immunoglobulin production when appropriate T cell–derived signals are present.[299, 447, 448]

However, other studies suggest that isotype switching and antibody production by fetal and neonatal B cells may be more limited compared with that of antigenically naive (IgD$^+$) adult B cells. One study found that IgM, IgG, and IgE production by fetal B cells was substantially lower at mid-gestation than that by neonatal or adult B cells, indicating that these cells are intrinsically less responsive to the engagement of CD40, cytokine receptors, or both.[238] Neonatal B cells have also been shown to produce substantially less IgA than adult antigenically naive B cells in response to anti-CD3 monoclonal antibody–stimulated adult T cells from a third-party donor (which provides a source of cell-surface CD40 ligand) and exogenous cytokines, such as IL-10.[449] Thus, it is possible that there may be limitations in B cell isotype switching and antibody production in the fetus and neonate that reflect intrinsic limitations of B cell function, particularly under conditions in which T cell help may be limited.

When neonatal T cells are activated for only hours and then fixed, they provide substantially less help for B cell immunoglobulin production and isotype switching by antigenically naive B cells than do similarly activated and fixed adult T cells.[241] The major source of help provided by such fixed T cells is likely to be mediated by CD40 ligand. Taken together with the studies of in vitro isotype switching and antibody production described, these results suggest that a reduced production of T cell–derived cytokines, particularly CD40 ligand, may limit fetal and neonatal B cell immune responses. It is also plausible that limitations in neonatal dendritic cell function may limit B cell responses, by both a direct mechanism[46] and an indirect mechanism involving T cells.

IgM and IgG synthesis has first been detected as early as 12 weeks in fetal organ cultures.[450] Immunoglobulin-secreting plasma cells are detectable by the fifteenth week of gestation, and those secreting IgG and IgA are first observed at the twentieth and thirtieth weeks, respectively.[451] In general, neonatal B cells can differentiate into IgM-secreting plasma cells as efficiently as adult cells and, as discussed, can undergo isotype switching effectively when their CD40 molecule is engaged. One study has found that T cell–dependent immunoglobulin production by neonatal CD5$^+$ and CD5$^-$ B cells is more readily inhibited by agents that raise intracellular cyclic adenosine monophosphate (cAMP), such as prostaglandin E$_2$ than is that by adult B cells.[452] It is unclear whether adult memory B cells are resistant to these inhibitory effects mediated by cAMP.

DEVELOPMENT OF B CELL CAPACITY TO RESPOND TO T CELL–DEPENDENT AND T CELL–INDEPENDENT ANTIGENS

The ability to respond to specific antigens develops chronologically in a manner distinctive for whether the antigen response occurs independently of cognate T cell help or requires it (Table 2–4). As indicated largely by work in the mouse, antigens can be divided into antigens

TABLE 2–4
Hierarchy of Antibody Responsiveness to Different Antigens

SPECIES	TYPE OF ANTIGEN	EXAMPLES OF ANTIGEN	AGE AT ONSET OF ANTIBODY RESPONSE
Mouse	T cell–dependent	TNP-KLH	Birth
	T cell–independent type I	TNP-*Brucella abortus*	Birth
	T cell–independent type II	TNP-Ficoll	Delayed (2–3 wk of age)
Human	T cell–dependent	Tetanus toxoid, HBSAg, *Haemophilus influenzae* conjugate vaccine, bacteriophage φ × 174	Birth
	T cell–independent type I	TNP-*B. abortus*	Birth
	T cell–independent type II	Bacterial capsular polysaccharides (*H. influenzae* type b, *Neisseria meningitidis, Streptococcus pneumoniae*, GBS)	Delayed (6–24 mo of age)

TNP = trinitrophenol; KLH = keyhole limpet hemocyanin; HB$_s$Ag = hepatitis B surface antigen, GBS = group B streptococcus.

that are dependent on a functional thymus and cognate help (direct cell-cell interactions) provided by mature αβ T cells (T-dependent antigens) and those that are independent of such T cell help, the T-independent antigens. The T-independent (TI) antigens can be further divided into type 1 or type 2, on the basis of their dependence on cytokines produced by T cells or other cell types. Most proteins are T-dependent antigens, which absolutely require cognate T cell–B cell interaction for production of antibodies other than small amounts of IgM. The antibody response to T-dependent antigens is characterized by the generation of memory B cells with somatically mutated immunoglobulin and the potential for a wide range of isotype switching. TI type 1 antigens are those that bind to B cells and directly activate them in vitro to produce antibody in the absence of T cells or exogenous cytokines. In the human, these include fixed *Brucella abortus*. TI type 2 antigens are mostly polysaccharides composed of multiple identical subunits, as well as certain proteins that contain multiple determinants with similar antigenic specificity. TI type 2 antigen responses are enhanced in vitro or in vivo by a variety of cytokines, including IL-6, IL-12, IFN-γ, and GM-CSF.[453–456] These may be provided by NK cells, T cells, or macrophages.[455] In addition, TI type 2 responses are also enhanced by bacterially derived LPS, lipoproteins, porin proteins, or DNA.[455, 457] In contrast with that to T-dependent antigens, the human antibody response to TI type 2 antigens is characterized by the lack of B cell memory or somatic hypermutation and is largely restricted to the IgM and IgG$_2$ isotype.[439]

The capacity of the neonate to respond to T-dependent antigens is established at birth (see Table 2–4), and is, in most instances, only modestly reduced compared with the response of the adult. The mechanism for this modest reduction is unclear and could reflect limitations in antigen presentation to CD4 T cells by dendritic cells, CD4 T cell activation and expansion into an effector population, CD4–B cell interactions, dendritic cell–B cell interactions, or intrinsic B cell function, possibilities that are not mutually exclusive. Most studies of the neonatal immune response to T-dependent vaccine antigens have also not evaluated antibody affinity, a reflection of somatic mutation, or isotype expression.

Given the recent finding of substantially reduced production of CD40 ligand by neonatal T cells,[238–241] it is of interest to determine whether production of this cytokine by vaccine antigen–specific T cells is also reduced in the neonate and the very young infant, and whether this correlates with reduced memory B cell development and decreased isotype switching and somatic hypermutation.

Antibody production by human neonatal B cells to a TI type 1 antigen in vitro (*B. abortus*) is also only modestly reduced,[458] indicating that the neonate can effectively respond to this type of antigen (see Table 2–4). This modest reduction appears to reflect a decreased ability of antigen-activated B cells to proliferate rather than a decreased precursor frequency of antigen-specific clones.[458] Human B cells (from both adults and neonates) are nonresponsive to high doses of LPS alone, a TI type 1 stimulus that is effective for murine B cells. However, low doses of LPS are capable of augmenting the response of human B cells to certain TI type 2–like stimuli,[455] suggesting that these cells express functional LPS receptors and signaling pathways.

In humans and mice, the response to TI type 2 antigens is the last to appear chronologically (see Table 2–4). This accounts for the poor antibody response of neonates to polysaccharide vaccine and to infection with encapsulated bacteria such as group B streptococci,[459–461] and for the poor response of children to vaccination with the unconjugated capsular polysaccharides of *H. influenzae* type b, meningococci, and most strains of pneumococci, until approximately 2 to 3 years of age. Whether decreased responses to TI type 2 antigens during early childhood reflect an intrinsic B cell immaturity; decreased function of non-B cells, such as APCs; or both remains unclear. Rijkers and colleagues[439] have reported that CD21 surface expression on neonatal B cells is lower than on adult B cells,[462, 463] and that the acquisition of competence to respond to bacterial polysaccharides at approximately 2 to 3 years of age correlates with the appearance of B cells expressing CD21 in the spleen's marginal zone region.[464] As described, CD21 is expressed in association with CD19, the type 2 complement receptor, and appears mainly to transduce B cell activating signals when CD19 is engaged by C3 complement components, so it is plausible that reductions in this protein could limit B cell activation. Incubation of human spleen tissue with pneumococcal polysaccharides with complement-containing serum results in preferential binding of the polysaccharide and C3 complement components, presumably as a complex, to CD21+ B cells of this area of the spleen.[465] In vitro studies using human spleen tissue suggest that TI type 2 antigens activate complement and bind the C3 component, then localize to marginal zone splenic B cells expressing type 2 complement receptors.[439] This localization would presumably induce polysaccharide-reactive B cells to proliferate in vivo.

Although a limitation in CD21-dependent signaling is an attractive mechanism to explain limitations in the TI type 2 response, decreased expression of CD21 by neonatal B cells has not been independently confirmed by others.[438] Moreover, animal experiments argue that decreased CD21 signaling is not a plausible explanation for the relatively intact antibody responses to T cell–dependent protein antigens and the severely decreased responses to polysaccharide antigens of the human neonate: Immunization of mice genetically deficient in the type 2 complement receptor or CD21 indicates that this complex is essential for T cell–dependent antigens, but has only a modest effect on the response to polysaccharide antigens.[342, 343] Therefore, this suggests either that other mechanisms besides decreased CD21 surface expression may play a role in decreased polysaccharide responses during the first 2 to 3 years after birth or that these mouse experiments do not accurately model the requirements for human antibody response to TI type 2 antigens.

Snapper and colleagues have used dextran-conjugated anti-Ig monoclonal antibodies as a means of multivalent engagement of B cells to mimic the events in TI type 2 antibody responses in vitro. Murine B cells treated in this manner proliferate but do not produce antibodies unless additional stimuli, such as NK cells, cytokines, or bacterial-derived products, are provided. Human neonatal B cells respond to this stimulus as well as do adult B cells, suggesting that the lack of the TI type 2 response in the neonate may not be due to an intrinsic limitation in B cell function.[466] However, dextran-conjugated anti-Ig monoclonal antibodies can potentially activate any B cell regardless of its particular sIg specificity, and it remains possible that the B cell population that is reactive with polysaccharides or other TI type 2 antigens in vivo, and that appears to localize preferentially to the marginal zone of the spleen and peripheral lymphoid organs, may be functionally distinct from most B cells in the circulation.

SPECIFIC ANTIBODY RESPONSES BY THE FETUS TO MATERNAL IMMUNIZATION AND CONGENITAL INFECTION

Early studies by Silverstein and colleagues examining the antibody response of fetal sheep and rhesus monkeys to immunization with foreign proteins were conceptually important in establishing two major features of the ontogeny of B cell immune competence for T cell–

dependent antigens in large mammals. First, immune competence for T cell–dependent antigens is established relatively early during fetal ontogeny: Primary immunization of fetal rhesus monkeys between 103 and 127 days of gestation (of a total of 160 days) with sheep red blood cells (SRBCs), a T cell–dependent antigen, results in the expansion of SRBC-reactive B cells in the spleen; reimmunization 3 weeks later results in a more rapid response and includes SRBC-reactive B cells utilizing IgG.[467] In the case of fetal sheep, the antibody response to bacteriophage φX174 occurs as early as 40 days postconception,[468] and, again, isotype switching is evident during the fetal response. Together, this suggests that B cell responses to protein antigens, including isotype switching and probably memory cell generation, are functional during fetal life. Second, the development of this competence occurs in a predictable, stepwise fashion for particular antigens. For example, in fetal sheep, the antibody response to keyhole limpet hemocyanin and lymphocytic choriomeningitis virus is first detectable at about 80 and 120 days post conception, respectively.[468] The immunologic basis for this sequential immune competence for antibody responses remains unclear. These differences in the responsiveness to particular antigens are very unlikely to be explained by limitations in the repertoires of sIg or αβ-TCR, because it is likely that a diverse repertoire of these antigen receptors is established early in ontogeny in the sheep, similarly to what has been observed in the human. There is also no clear correlation between the physical or chemical characteristics of particular antigens and their immunogenicity during ontogeny. For example, bacteriophage φX174 and bacteriophage T-4 are both particulate antigens and would be expected to enter into antigen processing pathways similarly. However, during fetal gestation in the sheep, bacteriophage T-4 only becomes immunogenic 60 days after φX174.

Antibody responses by the human fetus may follow maternal immunization with tetanus toxoid during the third trimester but not earlier, as shown by the presence of tetanus-specific IgM antibodies at birth.[469, 470] Those infants with tetanus-specific antibodies at birth also were shown to have enhanced secondary antibody responses after tetanus toxoid immunization, indicating priming rather than tolerance.[470] Although this suggests that fetal memory B cell generation and antigen-specific T cell priming can occur in utero in response to vaccination with T-dependent antigens, another group was unable to demonstrate either neonatal tetanus toxoid–specific IgM antibody or T cell proliferation after maternal tetanus toxoid vaccination in the third trimester.[312] These antigen-specific neonatal responses were also not observed after maternal immunization with inactivated trivalent influenza vaccine.[312] It is not known whether fetal antibody responses occur after vaccination with polysaccharide-protein conjugate vaccines, many of which have been proposed for use during pregnancy to ensure that protective levels of antibody are present at birth.

Specific antibody production has been documented at birth in response to a variety of intrauterine infections, including with rubella virus, CMV, HSV, VZV, and *T. gondii*, and is often the basis for the diagnosis of congenital infection. However, not all fetuses mount a detectable antibody response to intrauterine infection even at term: Specific IgM antibody was absent in 34% of infants with congenital rubella,[471] 19 to 33% of infants with congenital *T. gondii* infection,[472, 473] and 11% of infants with congenital CMV infection.[474] In cases in which congenital infection is severe and occurs during the first or second trimester, specific immunoglobulin production may not occur until late childhood.[326] This unresponsiveness may reflect, at least in part, a lack of T cell help, because antigen-specific T cell responses are also frequently reduced in parallel with B cell responses, as discussed previously.

Interestingly, congenital infection with *T. gondii* frequently results in detectable circulating IgE and IgA anti-*Toxoplasma* protein antibodies at birth or during early infancy.[475] Similarly, filarial- and schistosome-specific IgE is detectable in the majority of newborns after maternal filariasis or schistosomiasis.[476] This indicates that T cell–dependent isotype switching and immunoglobulin production can occur during fetal life, at least for certain pathogens, and that in some infections, such as with *T. gondii*, specific non-IgM isotype antibodies may be more sensitive than specific IgM antibodies for the diagnosis of infection. Nevertheless, it is important to note that IgA- and IgE-specific antibodies for the diagnosis of established congenital toxoplasmosis may still be less sensitive using fetal blood obtained between 20 and 30 weeks of gestation than after birth.[477–479] These results suggest that production of such antigen-specific antibodies by the fetus may also be delayed in appearance relative to that by adults.

SPECIFIC ANTIBODY RESPONSES BY THE TERM NEONATE TO IMMUNIZATION WITH PROTEIN ANTIGENS

Immunization of neonates elicits a protective response to most protein antigens, including tetanus and diphtheria toxoids,[480] oral poliovirus vaccine,[481] *Salmonella* sp. flagellar antigen,[459, 460] bacteriophage φX174,[482] and hepatitis B surface antigen (HB$_s$Ag) vaccine.[483] However, the magnitude of the response to certain vaccines may be less in the neonate than in older children or adults. This has been observed with the primary response to recombinant HB$_s$Ag vaccine given to healthy term neonates lacking maternally derived HB$_s$Ag antibody, in comparison with children and adults who have never been infected or previously vaccinated.[483, 484] The ultimate HB$_s$Ag-specific antibody levels that are achieved with secondary and tertiary immunization when immunization is begun in the neonatal period are similar to those of older children, indicating that neonatal immunization with this particular protein antigen does not result in tolerance.[483] If immunization is delayed until infants are at least 1 month of age, the antibody response to primary HB$_s$Ag vaccination is increased and nearly equivalent to that of older children, suggesting that the developmental limitations responsible for reduced antibody responses are quite transient.[483, 485] Similarly, 2-week-old infants immunized with a single dose of diphtheria or tetanus toxoid had delayed production of

specific antibody compared with that of older infants; by 2 months of age, the response was similar to that of 6-month-old infants,[486] suggesting rapid postnatal maturation of T-dependent responses. The switch from IgM to IgG production may also be delayed after neonatal vaccination as, for example, with *Salmonella* sp. H vaccine,[460] although not with others, such as bacteriophage φX174.[482]

Interestingly, in contrast with most other vaccines, whole cell pertussis vaccine given to neonates may produce a poor initial antibody response to certain vaccine protein antigens, and subsequent antibody response to certain pertussis antigens, such as lymphocyte-promoting toxin, may be less than that of children immunized at 1 month of age or older.[487–489] This suggests the induction of partial tolerance by early immunization. Whole cell pertussis vaccine immunization of premature infants (28 to 36 weeks' gestation) at 2 months of age elicited a response similar to that of 2-month-olds born at term.[481] This suggests that the tolerogenic period for vaccination with pertussis proteins rapidly wanes during the postnatal period and is relatively independent of gestational age. This tolerogenic effect is apparently highly antigen-dependent, because no inhibitory effect was observed on antibody titer between 2 and 6 months of age after primary administration of diphtheria or tetanus toxin at 4 days of age rather than at 2 months[480] or after primary immunization of neonates with HB$_s$Ag vaccine within 48 hours of birth rather than at 1 month of age or older.[483] Oral polio vaccine given to neonates also enhanced rather than inhibited the response to subsequent oral immunization during infancy, suggesting that tolerance does not necessarily occur for antigens that are delivered via a mucosal route.[490]

Interestingly, there may be more persistent limitations in the antibody response to certain protein antigens postnatally. For example, the antibody response to a dose of measles vaccine administered at 6 months of age is significantly less than to that given at 9 or 12 months of age, even when the inhibitory effect of maternal antibody is controlled for.[491] This difference does not appear to be due to the lack of generation of a measles-specific T cell population, because measles virus–specific T cell proliferation was similar in the three groups,[491] but limitations in T cell help, such as CD40 ligand production, or in intrinsic B cell function remain possible.

SPECIFIC ANTIBODY RESPONSES BY THE TERM NEONATE TO IMMUNIZATION WITH POLYSACCHARIDE ANTIGENS AND POLYSACCHARIDE-PROTEIN CONJUGATES

In contrast with protein antigens, many polysaccharide antigens elicit no response or a severely blunted response, as demonstrated by the inability of many neonates to produce a detectable antibody to *H. influenzae* type b polyribosylphosphate (PRP) unconjugated vaccine or to group B streptococcus type–specific capsular antigens after infection. In humans the response to some polysaccharide antigens can be demonstrated by 6 months of age, but the response to vaccination with

H. influenzae polysaccharides, *N. meningitidis* type C, or many of the pneumococcal polysaccharides included in the 23 valent vaccine remains poor until approximately 18 to 24 months.[492] As discussed, the basis for the inability of infants to respond to polysaccharides and other TI type 2 antigens is not clearly understood but does not appear to be a lack of the appropriate antibody repertoire, at least for *H. influenzae*.[493]

Conjugation of the *H. influenzae* bacterial capsular polysaccharide covalently to protein carriers renders it immunogenic in infants as young as 2 months of age. This results in a subsequent enhanced antibody response to unconjugated vaccine at 12 months of age. Because this is an age when responses to the unconjugated vaccine are usually poor, this finding indicates that the conjugate vaccine induces polysaccharide-specific B cell memory.[494] Similarly, the administration of a single dose of *H. influenzae* type b polysaccharide–tetanus toxoid conjugate to term neonates as early as a few days after birth may enhance the antibody response to unconjugated *H. influenzae* type b polysaccharide vaccine at 4 months of age.[495] This also suggests that polysaccharide antigen–specific B cells can be primed to some degree by conjugate vaccine administered shortly after birth. However, the enhanced response is relatively weak and is not seen when neonates are primed with tetanus toxoid followed by immunization with conjugate vaccine at 2 months of age.[496] Coupling of the *H. influenzae* type b polysaccharide to protein carriers appears to convert it from TI type 2 antigen to a T cell–dependent antigen, with increased antibody avidity compared with that of unconjugated vaccine.[497] This is presumably the result of the T-dependent memory B cell generation, which favors affinity maturation after somatic hypermutation. The likely early interactions between T cells and B cells in response to such carbohydrate-protein conjugate vaccines are summarized in Figure 2–9. In the case of *H. influenzae* type b polysaccharide, conjugation to tetanus

toxoid or diphtheria protein does not change the repertoire of the antibodies produced in response to the conjugate as compared with that to the free polysaccharide.[493, 494] This suggests that the conjugation to these proteins does not alter the initial repertoire of B cells that interacts with the polysaccharide moiety. The response to conjugate vaccines in the neonate and young infant is also consistent with their ability to respond to other T cell–dependent antigens, such as proteins. Vaccines in which capsular polysaccharides of *S. pneumoniae* (types 4, 6B, 9V, 14, 18C, 19F, and 23F)[498-500] and *N. meningitidis* (types A and C)[501] have been conjugated with proteins are also immunogenic in infants as young as 2 months of age. It is likely but unproven that these newer conjugate vaccines are also able to prime term neonates for enhanced antibody production at least to some degree.

SPECIFIC ANTIBODY RESPONSES BY THE PRETERM NEONATE TO IMMUNIZATION

Preterm neonates of 24 weeks of gestation or older produce antibody in response to protein antigens such as diphtheria toxoid alone, diphtheria-pertussis-tetanus vaccine, and oral and inactivated poliovirus vaccines, as well as do term neonates or infants, when these are administered at the usual intervals of 2, 4, and 6 months of postnatal age.[481, 502–504] The antibody response of premature infants to multiple doses of HB$_s$Ag vaccine, initially administered at birth, is clearly reduced compared with that of term infants.[505] These titers are substantially increased if immunization of premature infants is delayed until 5 weeks of age and appear to reflect the importance of postnatal age to the response rather than the achievement of a particular body weight.[506] However, the antibody levels achieved after three doses of *H. influenzae* type b capsular polysaccharide–tetanus conju-

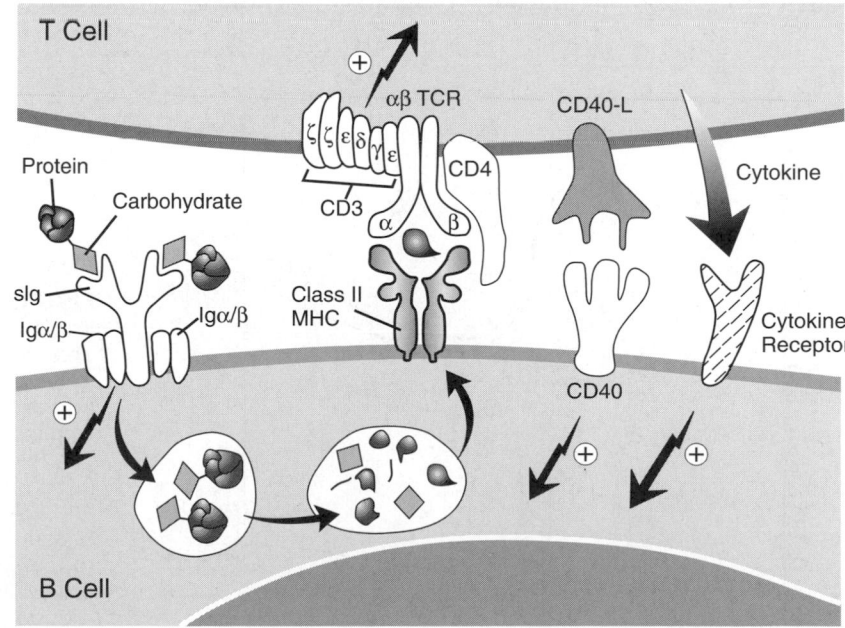

FIGURE 2–9 Interactions between B cells and T cells in the response to conjugate vaccines consisting of carbohydrate (e.g., bacterial capsular polysaccharide) covalently linked to protein carrier. The carbohydrate moiety of the conjugate is bound by surface immunoglobulin (sIg) on B cells, resulting in the internalization of the conjugate. Peptides derived from the protein moiety of the conjugate are presented by class II MHC on the B cell, resulting in the activation of the T cell and expression of CD40 ligand. Engagement of CD40 on the B cell by CD40 ligand, in conjunction with cytokines secreted by the T cell, results in carbohydrate-specific B cell proliferation, immunoglobulin isotype switching, and secretion of antibody, as well as memory B cell generation.

gate vaccine are significantly lower in premature than in term infants when vaccination is begun at 2 months of postnatal age,[507] particularly in those who have chronic lung disease.[508] As discussed later, treatment with glucocorticoids can have adverse effects on specific antibody responses, and it is uncertain to what extent such decreased responses in infants with chronic lung disease are due to glucocorticoid therapy versus other factors. As in term infants, the ability to respond to polysaccharide antigens remains diminished during the first 2 years of life.

MATERNALLY DERIVED IMMUNOGLOBULIN G ANTIBODY

IgG is the predominant immunoglobulin isotype at all ages.[509] Human IgG is composed of four different subclasses (IgG$_1$, IgG$_2$, IgG$_3$, and IgG$_4$) and is the only isotype that crosses the placenta. All subclasses, with the exception of IgG$_4$, can activate the classic complement pathway. In adults, IgG$_1$ is the predominant subclass (70%), whereas IgG$_2$, IgG$_3$, and IgG$_4$ are approximately 20%, 7%, and 3% of the total, respectively.[510]

The mechanism by which IgG is transferred to the fetus is only partially understood but clearly depends on the recognition of maternal IgG via its Fc domain. Although maternally derived placental syncytiotrophoblasts express surface type III Fc receptors for IgG, which are particularly abundant over the area in direct contact with the maternal circulation,[511] it is unclear whether these or other surface Fc receptors are important for internalizing maternal IgG to be transported to the fetus.[512] Such uptake might potentially occur by pinocytosis.[513] Once IgG is internalized by the trophoblast, the next step in transport probably involves FcRn, an intracellular IgG receptor that is an unusual β2-microglobulin–associated nonpolymorphic member of the class I MHC family.[513–515] FcRn lacks a functional peptide binding groove and, instead, utilizes a different region of the molecule for binding IgG via its Fc do-

main. IgG that is bound to FcRn receptor is presumed to undergo transcytosis across the syncytiotrophoblast, followed by its release into the interstitium in the vicinity of endothelial cells surrounding fetal villus vessels.[514] The way that IgG is internalized and transported across the endothelium of fetal villus vessels remains unclear, as these cells express only low or undetectable amounts of FcRn.[513, 515] In addition to the syncytiotrophoblast, FcRn is widely expressed by nonplacental tissues, where it is likely to bind IgG taken up by pinocytosis and recycle it to the circulation. This recycling system appears to account for the relatively long half-life of IgG compared with that of other plasma proteins.

Maternal IgG and FcRn expression can be detected in placental syncytiotrophoblasts during the first trimester,[515] but transport does not occur because circulating fetal concentrations of IgG remain below 100 mg/dl until about 17 weeks. The maternally derived placental cytotrophoblast, which is found between the syncytiotrophoblast and the fetal endothelium during the first trimester, may act as an additional barrier of IgG transport; the cytotrophoblast layer becomes discontinuous as the villus surface area expands during the second trimester.[515] After 17 weeks of gestation, circulating IgG levels in the fetus rise steadily, reaching half of the term serum concentration by about 30 weeks and equaling that of the mother by about 33 weeks.[516, 517] In some instances fetal IgG concentrations may exceed those of the mother by twofold.[518] The mechanism through which greater circulating levels of IgG are achieved in the fetus than in the mother is unknown, but it is hypothesized that IgG may undergo concentration within the syncytiotrophoblast before its release into the fetal interstitial space.[512]

Because the fetus synthesizes little IgG, the concentration in utero reflects almost solely maternally derived antibody (Fig. 2–10).[519] Accordingly, prematurity is reflected in proportionately lower neonatal IgG concentrations. There is a relatively low ratio of the IgG$_2$ concentration in cord blood from term infants compared

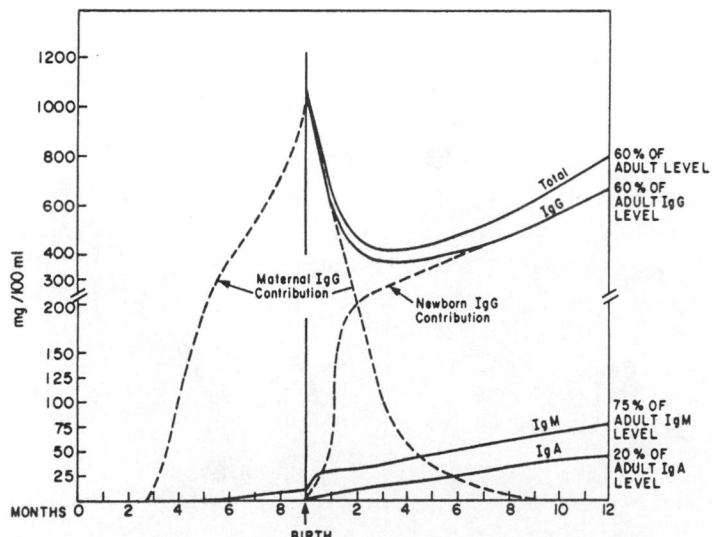

FIGURE 2–10 Immunoglobulin (IgG, IgM and IgA) levels in the fetus and infant in the first year of life. The IgG of the fetus and newborn infant is solely of maternal origin. The maternal IgG disappears by the age of 9 months, by which time endogenous synthesis of IgG by the infant is well established. The IgM and IgA of the neonate are entirely endogenously synthesized because maternal IgM and IgA do not cross the placenta. (From Saxon A, Stiehm ER. The B-lymphocyte system. *In* Stiehm ER [ed]. Immunologic Disorders in Infants and Children, 3rd ed. Philadelphia, WB Saunders, 1989, pp 40–67, with permission.)

TABLE 2–5
Levels of Immunoglobulins in Sera of Normal Subjects, by Age[a]

AGE	IgG		IgM		IgA		TOTAL IMMUNOGLOBULINS	
	mg/dl	Percentage of Adult Level	mg/dl	Percentage of Adult Level	mg/dl	Percentage of Adult Level	mg/dl	Percentage of Adult Level
Newborn	1031 ± 200[b]	89 ± 17	11 ± 5	11 ± 5	2 ± 3	1 ± 2	1044 ± 201	67 ± 13
1–3 mo	430 ± 119	37 ± 10	30 ± 11	30 ± 11	21 ± 13	11 ± 7	481 ± 127	31 ± 9
4–6 mo	427 ± 186	37 ± 16	43 ± 17	43 ± 17	28 ± 18	14 ± 9	498 ± 204	32 ± 13
7–12 mo	661 ± 219	58 ± 19	54 ± 23	55 ± 23	37 ± 18	19 ± 9	752 ± 242	48 ± 15
13–24 mo	762 ± 209	66 ± 18	58 ± 23	59 ± 23	50 ± 24	25 ± 12	870 ± 258	56 ± 16
25–36 mo	892 ± 183	77 ± 16	61 ± 19	62 ± 19	71 ± 37	36 ± 19	1024 ± 205	65 ± 14
3–5 yr	929 ± 228	80 ± 20	56 ± 18	57 ± 18	93 ± 27	47 ± 14	1078 ± 245	69 ± 17
6–8 yr	923 ± 256	80 ± 22	65 ± 25	66 ± 25	124 ± 45	62 ± 23	1112 ± 293	71 ± 20
9–11 yr	1124 ± 235	97 ± 20	79 ± 33	80 ± 33	131 ± 60	66 ± 30	1334 ± 254	85 ± 17
12–16 yr	946 ± 124	82 ± 11	59 ± 20	60 ± 20	148 ± 63	74 ± 32	1153 ± 169	74 ± 12
Adult	1158 ± 305	100 ± 26	99 ± 27	100 ± 27	200 ± 61	100 ± 31	1457 ± 353	100 ± 24

[a]The values were derived from measurements made for 296 normal children and 30 adults. Levels were determined by the radial diffusion technique, using specific rabbit antisera to human immunoglobulins.

[b]One standard deviation.

Adapted with permission from Stiehm ER, Fudenberg HH. Serum levels of immune globulins in health and disease: a survey. Pediatrics 37:715, 1966.

with that of maternal blood (approximately 30%), whereas this ratio is usually close to 100% for other subclasses.[520] This potentially may reflect the relatively low affinity of the type III Fc receptor for IgG_2. IgM, IgA, IgD, and IgE do not cross the placenta. There is also no evidence for transamniotic transfer of IgG to the fetus.[512]

By approximately 2 months of life, the amount of circulating IgG synthesized by the infant equals the amount derived from transplacental transfer; by 10 to 12 months of age the IgG is nearly all derived from synthesis by the infant. As a consequence of the fall in passively derived IgG and increased synthesis of IgG, values reach a nadir of ~400 mg/dl in term infants at 3 to 4 months of age and rise thereafter (Table 2–5) (see Fig. 2–10). The premature infant has proportionately lower IgG concentration at birth and values reach a lower nadir: At 3 months of age values of 82 and 104 mg/dl are observed in infants born at 25 to 28 and 29 to 32 weeks of gestation, respectively. Although passively transferred maternal antibody plays an important role in protection, it confounds the use of antibody tests that measure IgG or total antibody for the diagnosis of infection in the fetus, neonate, and infant.

PLACENTAL TRANSFER OF SPECIFIC ANTIBODIES

The fetus receives IgG antibodies against antigens to which the mother has been exposed by means of infection or vaccination (Table 2–6). For example, in mothers immunized with H. influenzae type b capsular PRP polysaccharide antigen at 34 to 36 weeks of gestation, anti-PRP antibody is effectively transferred to the fetus. This transfer results in protective circulating antibody levels for approximately the first 4 months of life. However, the mother may be protected by antibody against infection, whereas the fetus is not. For example, the mother

may have levels of specific antibody that are too low to be protective to the neonate. She, but not the neonate, can have a rapid recall antibody response with infectious challenge. In addition, if protective antibodies are not of the IgG isotype, as is the case of IgM antibodies directed against gram-negative bacterial pathogens, such as Escherichia coli and Salmonella sp.[459, 460] the fetus does not receive them. Finally, premature neonates may not receive amounts of IgG sufficient for protection, because most maternal IgG is transferred to the fetus after 34 weeks of gestation.[521]

Maternally derived antibody may also inhibit active production by the fetus or neonate of antibodies of the same specificity. The degree to which antibody inhibits the neonatal antibody response varies with the antigen, dose, and adjuvants used in the vaccine and with antibody titer. A marked inhibition of the response to measles and rubella vaccine, but not to mumps vaccine,[522] has been the reason for delaying these immunizations until at least 12 months of age. A potential mechanism for this inhibitory effect is that the optimal antibody response to these live attenuated vaccines may require viral replication in the recipient, which may be blocked by maternally derived neutralizing antibodies Maternal antibodies have also been shown to inhibit modestly the response of the neonate to immunization with "dead," that is, nonreplicating, vaccines or antigens, such as whole cellular pertussis vaccine,[488] diphtheria toxoid,[523] Salmonella sp. flagellar antigen,[460] and inactivated poliovirus vaccine.[524] In the case of these nonreplicating antigens, one possible inhibitory mechanism is that maternal IgG may form antigen-antibody complexes with the immunogen and block B cell activation via simultaneous engagement of the FcγRII receptor by the IgG component of the complex and the sIg by immunogen. These antigen-antibody complexes may also cause more rapid clearance of vaccine antigen, resulting in decreased immunogenicity. However, in the case of neonatal HB_sAg

TABLE 2–6
Neonatal Passive Immunity: Placental Passage of Maternal Antibodies

GOOD PASSIVE TRANSFER (IgG)	POOR PASSIVE TRANSFER	NO PASSIVE TRANSFER[a]
Tetanus antitoxin	*B. pertussis* Ab	*Salmonella* somatic (O) Ab
Diphtheria antitoxin	*Shigella flexneri* Ab	*Escherichia coli* H and O Ab
Bordetella pertussis agglutinin	*Streptococcus* Mg Ab	Heterophile Ab
Antistreptolysin Ab[b]		Wassermann Ab
Antistaphylolysin Ab		Natural (anti-A, anti-B)
Poliomyelitis Ab		isoagglutinins
Measles, mumps, rubella Ab		Rh saline (complete) agglutinins
Herpes simplex Ab		Reaginic Ab (IgE)
Haemophilus influenzae Ab (see text)		
Group B streptococcal Ab		
Salmonella flagellar (H) Ab		
Rh incomplete (Coombs') Ab		
Immune (anti-A, anti-B) isoagglutinins		
VDRL Ab		
Long-acting thyroid stimulator		
Antinuclear Ab (ANA)		

[a]Mostly IgM.
[b]Ab = antibodies.
Adapted from Miller ME, Stiehm ER. Immunology and resistance to infection. *In* Remington JS, Klein JO. Infectious Diseases of the Fetus and Newborn Infant, 2nd ed. Philadelphia, WB Saunders, 1983, with permission.

immunization, neither maternal antibody nor hepatitis B hyperimmune globulin administration appears to have a substantial inhibitory effect on the immune response. Thus, if B cell inhibition by FcγRII engagement occurs after vaccination of infants with high titers of preexisting passively obtained antibody, it does not appear to apply to all antigens.

Immunoglobulin Synthesis by the Fetus and Neonate

IMMUNOGLOBULIN M AND IMMUNOGLOBULIN G

IgM is the only isotype besides IgG that binds and activates complement, with only a single IgM required for such activation. IgM increases from a mean of 6 mg/dl in premature neonates at less than 28 weeks of gestation to 11 mg/dl, approximately 8% of maternal levels, at term.[525, 526] This IgM is likely to be preimmune (not the result of the responses of B cells to foreign antigens) and may be enriched for polyreactive antibodies produced by B-1 cells. Experiments in mice suggest that such natural IgM may fix complement and allow antigenically naive B cells to be more efficiently activated via complement receptor 2 (CD21) co-stimulation.[423, 425] However, at least some of this IgM in the human neonate may be monomeric and, therefore, nonfunctional, as opposed to its usual pentameric functional form.[527, 528] Postnatally, IgM concentrations rise rapidly for the first month and then more gradually thereafter, presumably in response to antigenic stimulation (see Fig. 2–10). By 1 year of age, values are approximately 60% of those in adults. The postnatal rise is similar in premature and term infants.[527] Elevated (more than 20 mg/dl) IgM

concentrations in cord blood suggest possible intrauterine infections,[529] but many infants with congenital infections have normal IgM concentrations in cord blood.[474]

Passively derived maternal IgG is the source of virtually all the IgG subclasses detected in the normal fetus and neonate, and levels of these subclasses fall rapidly after birth. IgG concentrations synthesized by the neonate and those derived from the mother are approximately equal when the neonate reaches 2 months of age. IgG in the plasma has a half-life of about 21 days, and by 10 to 12 months of postnatal age, virtually all maternally derived IgG has been catabolized. As discussed, maternal IgG may inhibit certain postnatal antibody responses by binding to FcγRII receptors and by rapidly clearing potential antigens. However, the slow onset of IgG synthesis in the neonate appears predominantly to reflect an intrinsic limitation of the neonate rather than these factors or other theoretical mechanisms, for example, by idiotypic networking by maternal antibody, because a similar pattern was observed in a neonate born to a mother with agammaglobulinemia.[530] By 1 year, the total IgG concentration is approximately 60% of that of adults. IgG_1 and IgG_3 subclasses reach adult concentrations by 8 years, whereas IgG_2 and IgG_4 do so by 10 and 12 years of age, respectively.[531] The slow rise in IgG_2 concentrations parallels the poor antibody response to bacterial polysaccharide antigens (e.g., *H. influenzae* PRP), antibodies to which after natural infection are predominantly IgG_2.[532] Interestingly, the order in which the adult levels of isotype expression are achieved after birth closely parallels the order of the heavy chain gene segments that encode these isotypes. This raises the possibility that there may be postnatal developmental regulation of isotype switching mediated, in part, at the level of the heavy chain gene locus; for example, the chromatin configuration of this region may be developmentally regulated.

IMMUNOGLOBULIN A

IgA is found in significant concentrations in both serum and secretions and is the isotype produced in greatest amount per day in humans. IgA exists as both a monomer and a dimer containing a covalently linked J chain. The J chain is not absolutely required for IgA dimerization but may play an important role in facilitating IgA secretion into the bile.[533] There are two subclasses of IgA: IgA$_1$, which makes up 90% of that found in serum, and IgA$_2$, which makes up 60% of that found in secretions. This indicates preferential localization of IgA$_2$-secreting plasma cells adjacent to mucosal surfaces, which may be significant because IgA$_1$ but not IgA$_2$ is susceptible to specific bacterial proteases. IgA does not cross the placenta and serum concentrations in cord blood are usually 0.1 to 5.0 mg/dl, approximately 0.5% of the levels in maternal serum.[526] Concentrations are similar in term and premature–neonates,[525] and both IgA$_1$ and IgA$_2$ are present. At birth, the frequencies of IgA$_1$- versus IgA$_2$-bearing B cells are equivalent. Subsequently there is a preferential expansion of IgA$_1$-bearing cells, presumably as a result of postnatal exposure to environmental antigens.[534] Concentrations in serum increase to 20% of those in adults by 1 year of age and rise progressively through adolescence. Increased cord blood IgA concentrations are observed in some infants with congenital infection.[529] Elevated IgA concentration is common in infants infected by vertical transmission with HIV. IgA has a relatively short half-life in plasma of approximately 5 days.

IMMUNOGLOBULIN D

IgD in serum from cord blood is detectable by sensitive techniques in term and premature infants.[525, 535] Mean serum levels at term are approximately 0.05 mg/dl[526] and increase during the first year of life. Circulating IgD has no clear functional role. The immune responses of mice in which IgD expression has been eliminated by gene targeting appear to be normal. On the other hand, surface IgD can perform the function of surface IgM in B cell function in mice. Together, these results suggest that the functions of IgM and IgD are largely redundant.

IMMUNOGLOBULIN E

Although the synthesis of IgE by the fetus is detectable as early as 11 weeks, levels in cord blood at term are typically low, with a mean of approximately 0.5% of those of maternal levels.[526] These small levels of IgE are likely to be mainly fetally derived and are higher in samples at 40 to 42 weeks' gestation than those at 37 to 39 weeks' gestation.[526] The rate of postnatal increase varies, being greater in those infants predisposed to allergic disease and having greater environmental exposure to allergens.[536, 537]

Summary

The neonate is in part passively protected by placental transfer of maternal IgG antibody in the latter part of pregnancy. Immunoglobulin concentrations similar to or higher than maternal concentrations are achieved after 34 weeks of gestation. However, the ability of the neonate to produce antibodies in response to polysaccharides, including bacterial capsular polysaccharides, limits resistance to bacterial pathogens to which the mother has little or no IgG antibody. The basis for this immaturity remains unclear; it may reflect an intrinsic limitation in B cell function, a deficiency in the anatomic microenvironment required for these cells to be activated and differentiated into plasma cells, or both. In contrast, the neonatal response to most protein antigens is relatively intact for IgM production and is only limited for IgG responses to certain vaccines. Nevertheless, there are clear differences between neonates and older infants in the magnitude of their response to many protein neoantigens, indicating an immunologic limitation that rapidly resolves after birth. The limited antibody response of premature neonates to immunization with protein antigens during the first month of life but not subsequently is also consistent with the idea that chronologic (i.e., postnatal) age is a more important determinant of T cell–dependent antibody responses than gestational age. Limitations in isotype expression by B cells after immunization with T cell–dependent antigens appear to reflect a combination of limitations in help provided by T cells and possibly reduced CD40 ligand production, as well as an intrinsic limitation of the B cell. These intrinsic limitations may be most pronounced in the fetus.

NATURAL KILLER CELLS

Basic Aspects of Natural Killer Cells and Their Function

OVERVIEW

NK cells are large granular lymphocytes with cytotoxic function. They do not rearrange either the TCR or immunoglobulin genes and as a consequence lack surface expression of TCR/CD3 and sIg. Virtually all circulating human NK cells in the adult express p46, a 46-kDa protein that appears to be NK cell–specific.[538] Most of these cells also express the CD2, CD16, CD56, and NKR-P1A (CD161) molecules,[539, 540] which are not unique to the NK cell lineage and are also found on T cells or other cell types. Approximately 50% of adult NK cells express CD57.[539] p46 and NKR-P1A appear to activate NK cells when they are engaged by unknown ligands on target cells. CD16 is a component of the FcγRIIIB receptor, which is activated by binding IgG coated on target cells. CD2, CD56, and CD57 are primarily involved in NK cell adhesion to either target cells or endothelium. All NK cells also express cytoplasmic CD3ζ and FcεR1γ, which are involved in the intracellular propagation of activation signals, and most or all probably express DAP-12, a CD3-like homologue with similar function. NK cells are probably mainly produced in the bone marrow and, as discussed later, appear to be derived from a common T and NK cell precursor cell.

NK cells are functionally defined by their ability to lyse virally infected or tumor target cells in a non–MHC-restricted manner that does not require prior sensitization.[541] NK cells recognize the absence of self–class I MHC expression (natural cytotoxicity), in contrast with cytotoxic T cells, which are triggered to lyse targets after the recognition of foreign antigenic peptides bound to self-MHC (MHC-restricted cytotoxicity) or of self-peptides bound to foreign MHC (allogeneic cytotoxicity). This property also endows NK cells with the capacity to reject bone-marrow grafts from individuals lacking recipient MHC alleles even if they do not express foreign MHC alleles. This phenomenon is known as hybrid resistance and may be important immunologically in the rejection of nonautologous bone marrow grafts.[542] NK cells also have the ability to kill target cells that are coated with IgG antibodies, a process known as antibody-dependent cellular cytotoxicity (ADCC). ADCC requires the recognition of the target cell IgG by the NK cell FcγRIIIB receptor.[543] Viral infection of host cells, particularly by those of the herpesvirus group, including HSV, CMV, and VZV, and by some adenoviruses leads to decreased surface expression of class I MHC molecules. For example, CMV encodes proteins that inhibit class I MHC surface expression by causing nascent class I MHC in the endoplasmic reticulum to be translocated to the cytoplasm to undergo rapid degradation.[57] Such decreased expression of class I MHC may limit the ability of CD8 T cells to lyse virally infected cells. This limitation is likely to be particularly important during early infection, when CD8 T cells with appropriate antigen specificity are present at a low frequency. In contrast, decreased class I MHC expression may facilitate recognition and lysis by NK cells. The importance of NK cells in the initial control of human herpesvirus infections is suggested by the observation that individuals with selective deficiency of NK cells are prone to severe infection with HSV, CMV, and VZV (D Lewis, unpublished data).[544]

NATURAL KILLER CELL DEVELOPMENT

The bone marrow is assumed to be the major site for postnatal NK cell production. CD34$^+$ cells lacking markers for mature cell lineages (lin$^-$) and expressing CD7 or CD38 are found in the adult bone marrow and the neonatal or adult circulation and appear to be enriched for NK cell progenitors.[70, 545] In vitro treatment of these putative progenitor cells with cytokines, stromal cells, or both results in the appearance of CD56$^+$ cells with NK cell functional characteristics, such as natural cytotoxicity.[546, 547] Cells with these or similar characteristics in the thymus can also differentiate into thymocytes or lymphoid dendritic cells, depending on the culture conditions employed, suggesting the existence of a common T–NK-lymphoid dendritic cell progenitor.[548, 549] A close relationship of NK cells to T lymphocytes is also suggested by the transient cytoplasmic expression of the CD3ε and CD3δ components by unactivated human fetal liver NK cells.[539, 550] The precise developmental sequence of NK cell maturation in the bone marrow remains poorly understood. In vitro studies suggest a NK-lineage cell developmental sequence in which NKR-P1A expression is acquired early, followed by the appearance of CD56, CD16, the capacity for natural cytotoxicity and cytokine production, and, finally, CD2 surface expression.[545, 549, 551] The finding of a small population of CD3$^-$ CD7$^+$ CD16$^-$ CD56$^-$ NKR-P1A$^+$ lymphocytes in the neonatal and adult circulation suggests that this cell type is a normal intermediate stage in NK cell development.[551]

IL-15 is particularly important for directing uncommitted lymphocyte precursors to differentiate into the NK cell lineage[552] and for promoting the survival of mature NK cells.[553] This is supported by studies in mice that have shown that IL-15 and an intact high-affinity IL-15 receptor, which consists of the IL-15 receptor α chain, the IL-2 receptor β chain, and the γc chain, are essential for NK cell development.[554, 555] NK cells as well as T cells are absent in patients with X-linked SCID, in which there is a genetic deficiency of γc chain. The γc chain is utilized by the receptors for IL-7, IL-15, and several other cytokines. Both IL-7 and IL-15 and their cognate receptors are expressed at sites of lymphoid development in the bone marrow and thymus. The absence of IL-15–mediated signaling is most likely to account for the absence of NK cells in γc deficiency in humans, rather than a lack of IL-7, because patients with deficiency of the IL-7 receptor α chain lack T cells but have normal numbers of NK cells.[96]

NATURAL KILLER CELL INHIBITORY RECEPTORS

NK cell cytotoxicity appears to be regulated by a complex array of inhibitory and activating receptor-ligand interactions with target cells (Fig. 2–11). NK cells are inhibited by recognition of class I MHCs or segments derived from them that are expressed on nontransformed, uninfected cells. Binding of the NK cell to class I MHC molecules is presumed to provide a net inhibitory signal that predominates over activating signals. Infection of the host target cell may downregulate inhibitory ligands, such as class I MHCs, and upregulate other molecules promoting NK cell–mediated cytotoxicity, such as LFA-3. How these multiple signals are integrated biologically to regulate cytotoxicity remains unclear.[541] There are two major families of class I MHC receptors, the KIRs and the CD94-containing C-type lectins.[541, 556] The major inhibitory receptor of the CD94 family consists of a heterodimer of CD94 and NKG2-A, each of which is encoded by a single nonpolymorphic gene.

KIRs vary in size, depending on whether they contain two (KIR2D) or three (KIR3D) extracellular immunoglobulin-like domains. The cytoplasmic domain of KIRs includes an immunoreceptor tyrosine-based inhibitory motif (ITIM). This ITIM segment is tyrosine phosphorylated after KIR engagement and recruits protein tyrosine phosphatases that inhibit NK cell activation and

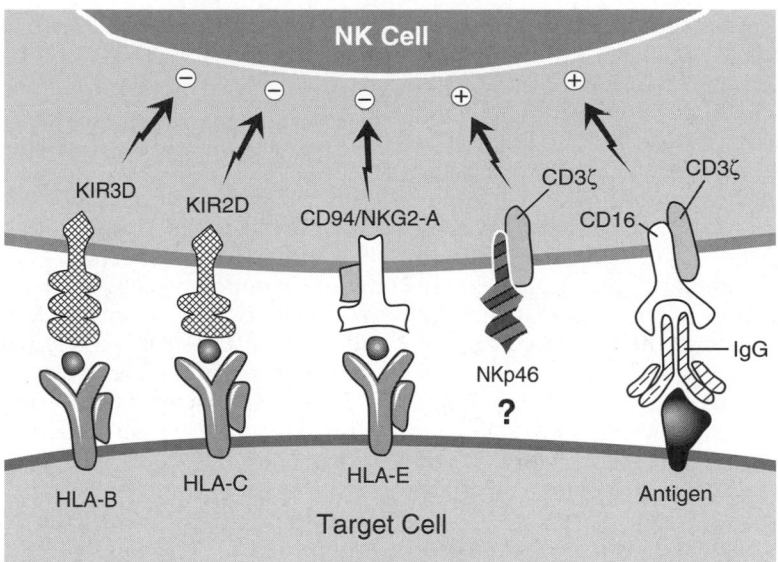

FIGURE 2–11 Positive and negative regulation of NK cell cytotoxicity by receptor-ligand interactions. NK cell cytotoxicity is inhibited by engagement of killer inhibitory receptors (KIRs) by class I MHC molecules, such as HLA-B and HLA-C. In addition, NK cells are inhibited when CD94-NKG2 complex, a member of the C-type lectin family, on the NK cell is engaged by HLA-E. HLA-E binds hydrophobic leader peptides derived from HLA-A, -B, and -C molecules and requires these for its surface expression. Thus, HLA-E surface expression on a potential target cell indicates its overall production of conventional class I MHC molecules. These inhibitory influences on NK cell cytotoxicity are overcome if viral infection of the target cell results in decreased class I MHC and HLA-E levels. NK cell cytotoxicity is positively regulated by the engagement of NKp46 as well as CD16, an Fc receptor for IgG. These positive receptors are complexed with CD3ζ, which acts as a docking site for tyrosine kinases that mediate intracellular activation signals.

cytotoxicity.[557] There are at least four KIR genes that encode inhibitory ITIM-containing receptors, all of which have multiple alleles.[558, 559] The expression of particular KIRs by individuals is heterogeneous and appears to be genetically regulated but not by MHC-encoded loci.[560] Human KIRs that recognize alleles of HLA-A, -B, and -C molecules have been identified.[541, 561] Particular KIRs often recognize closely related class I MHC alleles but are typically uninfluenced by the nature of the peptide bound to these molecules.[168] The HLA allele-binding specificity is known for only a small fraction of the more than 30 KIR family members that have been identified in the human.[168] No KIRs have been identified as yet for binding HLA-A alleles other than HLA-A3,[561, 562] or for binding certain HLA-B alleles, such as HLA-Bw6.[556]

These potential limitations in KIR recognition of self–class I MHC alleles, which could theoretically lead to NK cell autoreactivity, may be overcome by CD94-NKG2-A. Consistent with this idea, an analysis of multiple NK cell clones from normal human donors found that fewer NK cells that lacked all KIR expression invariably expressed CD94-NKG2-A.[558] Although the external domains of the proteins constituting CD94-NKG2-A are both C-type lectins and are structurally distinct from KIRs, the NKG2-A protein is similar to KIRs in having a cytoplasmic ITIM that mediates NK cell inhibition. In contrast to KIRs, CD94-NKG2-A recognizes HLA-E,[24] which preferentially binds nine amino acid hydrophobic peptides derived from the leader sequences of HLA-A, -B, and -C molecules.[23] Because HLA-E requires these leader sequences for its intracellular assembly, stability, and transport,[24] the amount of HLA-E on the cell surface is an indication of the overall levels of conventional class I MHC molecules that are expressed by the potential target cell.[541]

NATURAL KILLER CELL ADHESION, ACTIVATING RECEPTORS, AND CYTOTOXICITY

Most resting NK cells are found in the circulation and spleen. The small population of circulating NK cells that are CD16− or low and CD56+ NK cells may be a subpopulation specialized in the surveillance of solid organs, including the maternal decidua.[563] As for cytotoxic T cells, target cell recognition can be divided into a binding phase and an effector phase of either NK cell triggering or inactivation. A number of NK cell–target cell interactions may be utilized for binding, including interactions between CD2 and CD58, CD27 and CD70, CD11a-CD18 or CD11b-CD18 and ICAM-2, and CD44 and mucosal addressin cell adhesion molecule-1 (MadCAM-1).[564] Certain of these interactions may play a role in both binding and triggering. The critical activating receptors for natural cytotoxicity remain poorly defined but may include NKp46, which is associated with CD3ζ,[565] and NKp44, which associates with DAP-12.[566] Like CD3ζ, DAP-12 contains ITAMs and promotes NK cell activation via intracellular tyrosine kinases, such as zap-70 and syk.[541] NKR-P1A may also be an activating receptor because its crosslinking by monoclonal antibodies results in NK cell–mediated cytotoxicity. The ligands on target cells that engage NKp44, NKp46, and NKR-P1A are not known.

Certain members of the class I MHC KIR and CD94 receptor families are also candidates to contribute to NK cell activation. These activating KIRs are also referred to as killer activating receptors (KARs). KARs retain the characteristic extracellular immunoglobulin-like domains of KIRs but lack ITIMs and instead associate with DAP-12. Similarly, the NKG2-C component of the CD94-NKG2-C heterodimeric receptor lacks an ITIM and activates NK cells by its association with DAP-12.[541, 567, 568] The KARs and the CD94-containing C-type lectin receptors have ligand specificity identical or very similar to that of their respective inhibitory forms. At present, it is unclear how NK cells integrate the effects of inhibitory and activating forms of the KIR family or C-type lectin receptors to regulate natural cytotoxicity appropriately.

As for T cells, NK cell–mediated cytotoxicity involves the release of perforins and granzymes from preformed cytotoxic granules. NK cell–mediated cytotoxicity may also be mediated by fas ligand[569] or TNF-related apoptosis-inducing ligand (TRAIL)[570] expressed on the activated NK cell surface. Fas ligand–mediated cytotoxicity appears to occur mainly after treatment of NK cells with stimulatory cytokines, such as IL-2,[571] or during ADCC[572] rather than during natural cytotoxicity. Most mouse studies suggest that fas ligand–mediated cytotoxicity in NK cells is of minor or no importance compared with that of perforin-granzyme–dependent cytotoxicity in the control of viral infections.[573] In contrast with murine NK cells, which have been reported to express CD28 after activation by cytokines or in vivo infection[574] and to respond to B7 co-stimulatory molecules with increased IFN-γ production,[575] human NK cells do not appear to express CD28 or CTLA-4 and do not respond positively to B7 engagement, regardless of their activation state.[576]

ANTIBODY-DEPENDENT CELLULAR CYTOTOXICITY

In addition to natural cytotoxicity, NK cell–mediated ADCC is triggered when IgG bound to target cells engages the FcγRIIIA receptor on the NK cell.[543] The FcγRIIIA receptor, which is also found on macrophages and a small subset of T cells, consists of the CD16 molecule, which binds IgG via its Fc domain, and its associated homo- or heterotrimers of CD3ζ, or the FcεRIγ chain,[543] CD3ζ and FcεRIγ both contain ITAMs that contribute to NK cell activation after CD16 engagement. Because of the relative ease with which ADCC can be triggered experimentally, substantially more is known of the events in activation and effector function than of natural cytotoxicity. As in the case of T cell activation, FcγRIIIA engagement appears sequentially to activate tyrosine kinases of the src and syk families, followed by downstream signals, including increased concentrations of intracellular calcium and activated ras proteins.[543] In contrast to natural cytotoxicity, in which perforin-granzyme–dependent mechanisms appear to be predominant, ADCC appears to utilize both

perforin-granzyme– and fas ligand–dependent cytotoxic mechanisms.[572]

NATURAL KILLER CELL CYTOKINE RESPONSIVENESS AND DEPENDENCE

NK cell proliferation and cytotoxicity are enhanced in vitro by cytokines produced by T cells (IL-2, IFN-γ), APCs (IL-1, IL-10, IL-12, IL-18, and IFN-α), and nonhematopoietic cells, such as bone marrow mesenchymal cells (IL-15, stem cell factor, and flt3 ligand) and fibroblasts (IFN-β).[577, 578] Certain β-chemokines, such as macrophage inflammatory protein-1α (MIP-1α), MIP-1β, and monocyte chemotactic protein-1 (MCP-1), may also enhance NK cell function. IL-15, which appears critical for the development of NK cells in the bone marrow, also promotes the survival of mature NK cells[553] and, like IL-12, increases the expression of perforin and granzymes.[579] The positive effect of IL-15 on NK cell differentiation and mature NK cell lytic function can be blocked by IL-4, which decreases expression of a component of the IL-15 receptor.[579, 580] NK cell cytotoxicity in vivo is modestly decreased in mice genetically deficient in IFN-γ,[581] IL-12,[582] or IL-18[583] and is markedly depressed in combined IL-12 and IL-18 deficiency. This suggests that IL-12 and IL-18 largely act in a nonredundant fashion to help maintain NK cell cytotoxicity in vivo, and this maintenance is mediated, at least in part, by the induction of IFN-γ by these cytokines.

When NK cells are primed by cytokine exposure or are triggered in vitro for ADCC, they also become prone to apoptosis in the absence of exogenous cytokine exposure. Apoptosis of primed NK cells can occur in vitro after engagement of their surface CD2, CD16, or CD94 molecules.[584] Analogous to that in effector T cell populations, this tendency for NK effector cells to undergo apoptosis may help limit total NK cell numbers and prevent abnormal lymphoproliferation. The extent to which NK cell apoptosis occurs in vivo, particularly after natural cytotoxicity, is unknown.

NATURAL KILLER CELL CYTOKINE PRODUCTION

NK cells are also important producers of IFN-γ and TNF in the early phase of the immune response to viruses, and these cytokines may promote the development of CD4 T cells into TH1 effector cells. NK cell–mediated IFN-γ production may be induced by the ligation of surface β₁ integrins on the NK cell surface,[585] as well as by the cytokines IL-1, IL-12, and IL-18,[586] which are produced by dendritic cells and mononuclear phagocytes. The combination of IL-12 and IL-15 potently induces NK cells to produce the β-chemokine MIP-1α,[587] which may help chemoattract other types of mononuclear cells to sites of infection where NK cell–mediated lysis takes place. NK cells from HIV-infected individuals are also able to produce a variety of β-chemokines, including MIP-1α, MIP-1β, and regulated upon activation normal T cell expressed secreted (RANTES) chemokine in response to treatment with IL-2 alone; these chemokines may help prevent HIV

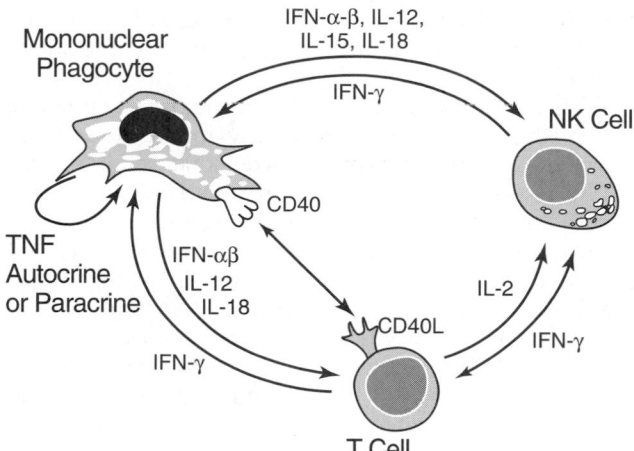

FIGURE 2–12 Cytokines link innate and antigen-specific immune mechanisms against intracellular pathogens. Activation of T cells by APCs, such as mononuclear phagocytes, results in the expression of CD40 ligand and the secretion cytokines, such as IL-2 and IFN-γ. Mononuclear phagocytes are activated by IFN-γ and the engagement of CD40 with increased microbicidal activity. Mononuclear phagocytes produce TNF, which enhances their microbicidal activity in a paracrine or autocrine manner. Mononuclear phagocytes also secrete the cytokines IFN-α/β, IL-12, IL-15, and, in the case of Kupffer cells, IL-18. These cytokines promote TH1 effector cell differentiation and also promote NK cell activation. NK cell activation is further augmented by IL-2. Activated NK cells in turn secrete IFN-γ, which further enhances mononuclear phagocyte activation and TH1 effector cell differentiation.

infection of T cells and mononuclear phagocytes by acting as antagonists of the HIV co-receptor.[588] NK cells can also be triggered to produce a similar array of cytokines during ADCC in vitro, but the role of such ADCC-derived cytokines in regulating immune responses in vivo remains poorly defined.

Some of the cytokine-dependent mechanisms by which NK cells, T cells, and APCs may influence each other's function, such as in response to infection with viruses and other intracellular pathogens, are summarized in Figure 2–12. In addition, studies in mice indicate that cytokines produced by NK cells, such as IFN-γ, may also allow the B cells to respond to TI-type antigens, such as polysaccharides and certain protein antigens with repetitive B cell epitopes.[589] Human NK cells have also been shown to produce IL-5, a cytokine that promotes eosinophil production, function, and survival.[590] The importance of IL-5 production by NK cells in immunologic situations in which IL-5 and other TH2 cytokines play a role, such as helminth infection or allergic disease, remains to be shown.

NATURAL KILLER CELLS OF THE MATERNAL DECIDUA AND THEIR REGULATION BY HUMAN LEUKOCYTE ANTIGEN G

The maternal decidua contains a prominent population of NK cells. Recent studies suggest that these cells are important for successful pregnancy, in that genetically manipulated mice lacking maternal NK cells have marked fetal loss, placental insufficiency, and vascular abnormalities at the fetal-maternal interface.[591] It is unclear what beneficial function maternal NK cells provide in this context, although these cells have the potential when triggered to produce multiple cytokines typical of circulating NK cells. Human trophoblasts and, possibly, maternal placental macrophages express HLA-G, a β2-microglobulin–associated molecule with limited polymorphism that is structurally quite similar to conventional class I MHC molecules. Because placental trophoblasts lack expression of conventional class I MHC molecules, and HLA-G expression is particularly high during the first trimester of pregnancy, it has been hypothesized that HLA-G may engage inhibitory receptors on maternal NK cells of the decidua or circulation in order to prevent maternal NK cell–mediated fetal rejection. HLA-G–mediated inhibition of NK cell cytotoxicity may involve engagement of CD94-NKG2-A,[592] certain KIRs,[593] and LIR1,[594] an inhibitory member of the leukocyte inhibitory receptor (LIR) family. The immunologic role of particular LIRs, which are also expressed by B cells, mononuclear phagocytes, and dendritic cells, is unknown.

Natural Killer Cell Development and Function in the Fetus and Neonate

FETAL AND NEONATAL NATURAL KILLER CELL DEVELOPMENT AND SURFACE PHENOTYPE

The development of human NK cells precedes that of αβ T cells during ontogeny, demonstrating their thymic independence. Cells with an NK cell–like surface phenotype predominate in the fetal liver mononuclear cell compartment and are detected as early as 6 weeks of gestation. They become increasingly abundant during the second trimester.[539] CD34+ lin− cells of the second trimester fetal liver, particularly those that are CD38+, give rise to NK-like cells rather than T-lineage cells after culture in vitro with cytokines.[595] This suggests that the fetal liver is a site of development of NK cells but not of extrathymic T cells. In the mouse fetal thymus, NK cells occur before αβ thymocytes,[596] and it is likely that a similar sequence of events applies to humans.

Neonatal mononuclear cells have been reported to produce less IL-15 than adult cells after LPS stimulation.[597] IL-15 is considered likely to be essential for human NK cell development, on the basis of a number of mouse studies,[554, 555] and it is unclear whether production of this cytokine at the major sites of NK cell development, such as the fetal bone marrow and fetal liver, is decreased. A biologically significant decrease in IL-15 production appears unlikely because NK cells are present in greatest numbers in the circulation during the second trimester of fetal development,[598] and their number in the neonatal circulation is typically equal to or higher than that in adults.[539, 599]

In contrast with adult NK cells, a substantial proportion of fetal liver NK cells express in their cytoplasm CD3ε and CD3δ components and lack CD16 surface expression[539]: Virtually all fetal and neonatal NK cells lack expression of CD57. The fraction of fetal and neonatal NK cells that express CD2 or CD56 is also reduced by about 50% compared with that in the adult.[539, 540, 600] Incubation of CD2[−] NK cells with IL-2 results in the gradual appearance of CD2 on the cell surface,[540] suggesting that CD2[−] NK cells may give rise to those expressing CD2; however, it remains to be shown that this cell precursor–product relationship occurs during human NK cell maturation in vivo. Fetal NK cells, unlike those of the adult, have also been reported to express CD28,[601] but it is unclear whether these cells functionally respond to engagement by B7 molecules, the ligands of CD28.

FETAL AND NEONATAL NATURAL KILLER CELL FUNCTION

NK cells from the fetus or premature infant have reduced cytotoxic function compared with those of the term neonate.[539, 602] Decreased cytotoxic activity by neonatal NK cells compared with that by adult cells is also consistently observed with HSV-infected target cells and with some tumor cell lines, but not with all.[539, 603, 604] In contrast, neonatal and adult NK cells have equivalent cytotoxic activity against HIV-1–infected cells.[602, 605] Although the mechanisms underlying these pathogen-related differences in natural cytotoxicity by neonatal versus adult NK cells remain unclear, these findings, taken together, suggest that there is a developmentally regulated limitation in NK cell–mediated cytotoxicity. Reduced cytolytic activity parallels the reduced numbers of CD56[+] NK cells in the neonate, consistent with their usually poor cytolytic activity.[600] When only CD56[+] neonatal NK cells are studied, their cytolytic activity is similar to that of adult NK cells.[539, 606] ADCC mediated by circulating neonatal mononuclear cells is approximately 50% of that by adult mononuclear cells, including against HIV-infected targets.[602]

Like adult NK cells, IL-2, IL-12, and IFN-α, -β, and -γ can rapidly (within hours) augment the cytolytic activity of neonatal NK cells.[607] Consistent with the findings for IL-2 and IFN-γ, neonatal NK cells have surface levels of receptors for IL-2 and IFN-γ that are similar to those of adult NK cells or higher.[608] Circulating neonatal NK cells also acquire substantially greater natural cytotoxic activity when they are incubated overnight to several days with IL-2, IL-12, IL-15, or combinations of these to generate lymphokine-activated killer (LAK) cells.[52, 600, 602, 604, 609–612] Neonatal LAK cells in many studies have cytotoxic activity equivalent to that of adult LAK cells, suggesting that neonatal NK cells have a normal capacity to be primed by exogenous cytokines. The generation of neonatal LAK cells from NK cells also increases their surface expression of CD56[612, 613] as a result of differentiation of CD56[−] NK cells into CD56[+] LAK cells, rather than expansion from the preexisting neonatal CD56[+] NK population.[612] Although this suggests that the neonatal CD56[−] NK cell population might be a phenotypically and functionally immature NK cell subset that gives rise to a more mature CD56[+] population, whether this precursor-

product relationship between CD56[−] and CD56[+] cells occurs during NK cell development in vivo remains to be shown.

The mechanisms responsible for decreased spontaneous NK cell–mediated cytotoxicity in the neonate remain unclear. It has been reported that soluble class I MHC is present at a 10-fold greater concentration in cord blood serum than in adult serum, and it is hypothesized that this could contribute to decreased NK cell–mediated cytotoxicity in the neonate, perhaps by engaging KIRs.[604] However, because the use of physiologic levels of soluble class I MHC found in cord blood has only a modest inhibitory effect on NK cell–mediated cytotoxicity in vitro,[604] this is unlikely to be a major mechanism for reduced neonatal NK cell cytotoxicity. Cell-mediated suppression has also been proposed, although this has not been directly shown in mixing experiments.[614] Decreased natural cytotoxicity by neonatal NK cells does not appear to be due to decreased binding to target cells[604] or to decreased levels of intracellular perforin or granzyme B compared with those of adult cells.[612] Treatment of neonatal NK cells, including the CD56[−] subset, with ionomycin and phorbol myristate acetae (PMA) results in a substantial enhancement of natural cytotoxicity, achieving levels similar to that of adult NK cells.[612] This increased natural cytotoxicity is blocked by inhibitors of granule exocytosis, indicating the involvement of perforin-granzyme cytotoxic mechanisms. This suggests that decreased release of cytotoxic granules could account for decreased NK cell–mediated cytotoxicity in the neonate. The role of fas ligand or TRAIL in neonatal NK cell–mediated cytotoxicity is unknown.

Neonatal NK cells have been reported to produce IFN-γ as effectively as adult NK cells in response to exogenous IL-2 and HSV.[615] Conflicting results have been obtained as to whether IL-12–induced production of IFN-γ by neonatal mononuclear cells (most likely mediated by NK cells) is reduced compared with that of adult cells,[607, 616] and further studies using purified NK cell populations may help resolve this issue. Whether the production of other cytokines by neonatal NK cells, particularly with stimuli other than HSV, is reduced compared with that of adult NK cells remains to be determined.

NATURAL KILLER CELLS IN CONGENITAL INFECTION

Congenital viral or *T. gondii* infection during the second trimester may result in a substantial increase in the number of circulating NK cells,[598] suggesting that fetal NK cells can respond to infections, at least to some degree. In such cases, persistent increases in NK cells can continue until birth and may be accompanied by decreased NK cell expression of CD45RA and increased expression of CD45R0.[340] This CD45RA[low]CD45R0[high] surface phenotype suggests that these cells have been activated in vivo, because similar alterations occur when NK cells are incubated in vitro with either IL-2 or tumor cell targets.[616, 617] Whether congenital infection results in enhanced natural cytotoxicity by fetal or neonatal NK cells remains to be determined.

Summary

Although NK cells appear early during gestation and are present in normal numbers by mid- to late gestation, approximately 50% of these cells at birth are CD56⁻. Although this surface phenotype may be a marker for NK cell immaturity, the precursor-product relationship between CD56⁻ and CD56⁺ cells during adult NK cell development remains unclear. These CD56⁻ cells have decreased natural cytotoxicity, including against virus-infected target cells, compared with that of cells from adults, which are uniformly CD56⁺. The precise mechanism for this remains unclear. Neonatal NK cell cytotoxicity can be augmented to levels that are similar to those of adult cells by incubation with exogenous cytokines, suggesting a potential immunotherapeutic strategy of increasing cytotoxicity in vivo.

PHAGOCYTES

Origin and Differentiation of Phagocytes

Phagocytes are derived from a common precursor myeloid stem cell, which is often referred to as the colony-forming unit–granulocyte-monocyte (CFU-GM) (Fig. 2–13). The formation of myeloid stem cells from pluripotent HSCs and further differentiation of the myeloid

precursor into mature granulocytes and monocytes are governed (1) by stromal cells present in the bone marrow environment and the cell-cell contacts between these cells and the hematopoietic progenitors and (2) by soluble colony-stimulating factors and other cytokines produced by these and other cells (see Table 2–2).[618-620] Factors that act primarily on early hematopoietic stem cells include stem cell factor (also known as steel factor or *c-kit* ligand) and Flt-3 ligand. The response to these factors is enhanced by granulocyte colony-stimulating factor (G-CSF) and thrombopoietin, hematopoietic growth factors originally identified by their ability to enhance the production of neutrophils and platelets, respectively, and by IL-1, IL-3, and IL-6. Other factors act later and are more specific for given myeloid lineages: GM-CSF acts to increase the production of neutrophils, eosinophils, and monocytes; G-CSF acts to increase neutrophil production; M-CSF acts to increase monocyte production; and IL-5 enhances eosinophil production.

The precise role of these mediators in normal steady-state hematopoiesis is becoming more clear, primarily as a result of studies in mice with targeted disruptions of the relevant genes. Genetic defects in the production of biologically active stem cell factor or its receptor *c kit* lead to mast cell deficiency and severe anemia, with less severe defects in granulocytopoiesis and in formation of megakaryocytes,[621] whereas deficiency of Flt-3 has no overt effect except on B cell progenitors. Deficiency for both Flt-3 ligand and c-kit has a more severe phenotype than for either alone, indicating partial redundancy in their function. Deficient production of M-CSF is associ-

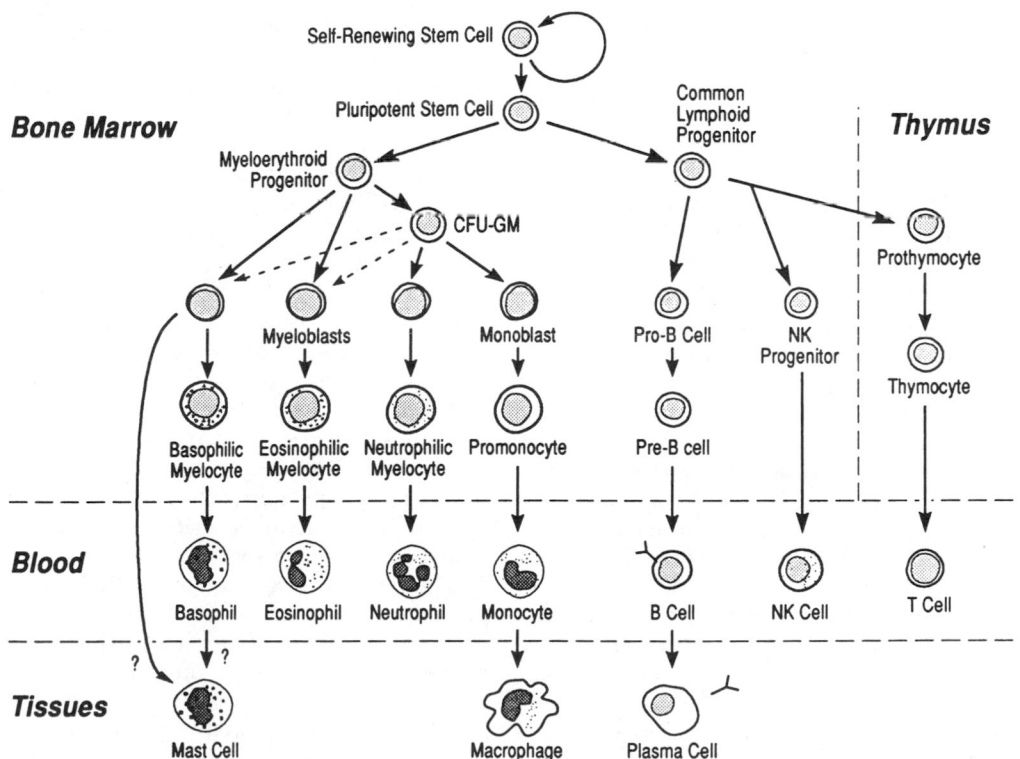

FIGURE 2–13 Myeloid and lymphoid differentiation and tissue compartments in which they occur. CFU-GM = colony-forming unit–granulocyte-monocyte.

ated with some diminution in macrophage numbers and a marked deficiency in maturation of osteoclasts (presumably from monocyte precursors), which results in a form of osteopetrosis.[622] Mice with a targeted disruption of G-CSF or its receptor and humans with mutations in the G-CSF receptor are neutropenic (though they do not completely lack neutrophils) and have fewer multilineage hematopoietic progenitor cells.[620] In contrast, in mice GM-CSF deficiency causes pulmonary alveolar proteinosis but does not affect the numbers of neutrophils, monocytes, or eosinophils, whereas IL-5 deficiency results in an inability to increase the numbers of eosinophils in response to parasites or allergens. Thus, hematopoietic growth factors appear to play complex and, in some cases, partially overlapping roles in normal steady-state production of myeloid cells.

In response to an infectious or inflammatory stimulus, the production of the CSFs is increased. Under these conditions, concentrations sufficient to enhance growth and differentiation of myeloid cells are produced and are believed to play an important role in the enhanced marrow production and release of granulocytes and monocytes that are observed. Similarly, when given exogenously, these factors enhance production of the indicated cell lineages.[623, 624]

Neutrophilic Polymorphonuclear Leukocytes

ORIGIN AND DERIVATION OF NEUTROPHILS IN THE MATURE HOST

Polymorphonuclear leukocytes or granulocytes are derived from CFU-GM. Neutrophilic granulocytes are the principal cells of interest in relation to defense against common neonatal pyogenic pathogens. This section specifically addresses these cells. The first identifiable committed granulocyte precursor is the myeloblast, which sequentially matures into myelocytes, metamyelocytes, bands, and mature neutrophilic granulocytes or polymorphonuclear leukocytes. Myelocytes and more mature neutrophilic granulocytes cannot replicate and constitute the postmitotic neutrophilic storage pool.[625] Mature neutrophils enter the circulation, where they remain for 8 to 10 hours and are distributed equally and dynamically between circulating cells and those adherent to the vascular endothelium.[625] After leaving the circulation, neutrophils do not normally recirculate. After about 24 hours in tissues, they die.

The postmitotic neutrophil storage pool is an important reserve because these cells can be rapidly released into the circulation in response to inflammation. Furthermore, increased production of stem cells in response to inflammation requires approximately 5 to 7 days before it can contribute to increased neutrophil output. Accelerated maturation or replication from nonstem cells in the mitotic compartment may enhance this somewhat. Nevertheless, the storage pool size is a critical determinant of the host's capacity to increase neutrophil output in response to infection.

As indicated, the control of granulocyte production and release is regulated by colony-stimulating or hematopoietic growth factors. Neutrophil production is specifically favored by G-CSF but is also facilitated by the more broadly acting IL-3 and GM-CSF. These factors enhance the proliferation of neutrophil precursors by driving progenitor cells to enter the cell cycle and, in the case of G-CSF, biasing progenitors capable of differentiating into granulocytes or monocytes into the neutrophil differentiation pathway. Granulocyte production also appears to be under potential negative regulation by prostaglandins and iron-containing proteins such as lactoferrin.[619, 625, 626] These negative regulators are produced by granulocytes and monocytes, suggesting that mature cells may self-regulate production. Release of neutrophils from the marrow may be enhanced in part by cytokines, including IL-1 and TNF, in response to infection or inflammation.[618]

MIGRATION TO SITES OF INFECTION

After release from the bone marrow into the blood, neutrophils circulate until they are called upon to enter the tissues at sites of infection or injury. Neutrophils adhere selectively to endothelium in inflamed tissues but not in normal tissues. The adhesion and subsequent migration of neutrophils through blood vessels and into the tissues are governed by cell adhesins expressed on the neutrophil and on the vascular endothelium and by specific chemotactic factors.

Adhesion

The adhesion molecules that are known to play a central role in neutrophil adherence are derived from one of three families of cell surface glycoproteins: the selectins, the integrins, and certain members of the immunoglobulin gene superfamily.[627–629]

The selectins are named by the cell types in which they are primarily expressed: L-selectin by leukocytes, E-selectin by endothelial cells, and P-selectin by platelets and endothelial cells. Selectins are named for their ability to bind to specific types of carbohydrates that are selectively expressed on different tissues; binding is mediated through a lectin-like domain found in all family members. L-selectin is constitutively expressed on leukocytes and appears to bind to tissue- or inflammation-specific carbohydrate-containing ligands on endothelial cells. E-selectin and P-selectin are expressed only on activated, not resting, endothelial cells or platelets. E- and P-selectin bind to sialylated glycoproteins on the surface of leukocytes, including PSGL-1. L-selectin binds to glycoproteins (including CD34 and MadCAM-1) and to glycolipids that are expressed on vascular endothelial cells in specific tissues.

The integrins are a large family of heterodimeric proteins composed of an α and a β chain. Integrins expressing a β_2 (CD18) chain, which associates on the plasma membrane with one of four α (CD11) chains, are found only on leukocytes. β_2 integrins play a critical role in neutrophil function, because unlike other types of leukocytes, neutrophils do not express other integrins in substantial amounts. The β_2 integrins (also known as leukocyte integrins) are constitutively expressed on neutrophils, but both their abundance and their avidity for their endothelial ligands are increased after activation of neutrophils—for example, in response to chemotactic factors. LFA-1 (CD11a-CD18) and Mac-1 (CD11b-CD18) appear to play the predominant role in leukocyte–endothelial cell interactions, whereas CD11c-CD18 plays a lesser role and CD11d-CD18 participates in leukocyte-leukocyte interactions. The endothelial ligands for LFA-1 are members of the immunoglobulin-like family and include ICAM-1 and ICAM-2. Both are constitutively expressed on endothelium, but ICAM-1 expression is increased markedly by exposure to inflammatory mediators, including IL-1, TNF, and LPS.

These adhesion molecules and chemotactic factors act in a coordinated fashion to allow neutrophil recruitment into tissues in response to infection or injury. In response to injury or inflammatory cytokines, P-selectin is transferred from endothelial or platelet stores to the surface of the endothelium of capillaries or postcapillary venules within minutes. This mechanism allows neutrophils in the blood to adhere in a low-avidity fashion, which results in rolling of these cells along the vessel walls. This step is transient and reversible unless a second, high-avidity interaction is triggered. If, at the time of the low-avidity binding, neutrophils also encounter chemotactic factors (discussed later) released from the tissues or from the endothelium itself, they rapidly upregulate the avidity of the LFA-1 and Mac-1 integrins and translocate additional LFA-1 and Mac-1 from specific granules to the neutrophil cell surface. This process enhances binding to ICAM-1 and ICAM-2 on endothelial cells. The high-avidity interaction of these integrins with ICAMs, in the presence of a gradient of chemotactic factors from the tissue to the blood vessel, appears to trigger the migration of neutrophils across the endothelium and into the tissues. Over a matter of several hours, the intensity of this response can be further upregulated by the de novo expression of E-selectin and increased expression of ICAM-1 on endothelium in response to mediators (e.g., platelet activating factor [PAF], TNF) produced at the site of infection or injury. The profound importance of integrin- and selectin-mediated leukocyte adhesion processes in the normal inflammatory response is illustrated by the genetic leukocyte adhesion deficiency syndromes.[628] Deficiency of the common β_2 integrin results in the absence on the plasma membrane of all β_2 integrins. This results in inability of leukocytes to exit the bloodstream and reach sites of infection and injury in the tissues. These patients are profoundly susceptible to infections with pathogenic and nonpathogenic bacteria, have poor tissue healing, and commonly die in the first years of life. Such patients not uncommonly present in early infancy with delayed separation of the umbilical cord, omphalitis, and severe pyogenic infection. A related syndrome—leukocyte adhesion deficiency syndrome type II—is due to a defect in synthesis of the carbohydrate selectin ligands. This results in a similar defect in neutrophil function and predisposition to infection but is also associated with more general problems related to defects in proper glycosylation of proteins. Studies of mice deficient in specific selectins indicate that P-selectin and E-selectin play partially redundant roles, and that L-selectin acts in concert with either of these two selectins and their ligands to facilitate neutrophil recruitment to sites of inflammation.

CHEMOTAXIS

Chemotaxis is important for focusing the delivery of leukocytes to the site of infection or injury. Random movement of leukocytes, even if accelerated by stimuli, would be inefficient. Sensing of chemotactic gradients is achieved through cell surface receptors for specific chemotactic factors. A number of receptors for specific chemotactic factors have been molecularly cloned and are related by their common structure. This is consistent with their interaction with heterotrimeric G proteins, which serve to transduce the signal from these receptors. Chemotactic agents may be derived directly from bacterial components, such as formyl-leucyl-phenylalanine (FMLP); from activated complement, such as C5a; and from host cell lipids, such as leukotriene B_4 (LTB$_4$) and PAF. These chemotactic agents are produced within minutes, because they are derived from preexisting microbial or host components.[630, 631] In addition, a large family of chemotactic cytokines (chemokines) are synthesized by macrophages and other cells within hours[632] (see Table 2–2). Chemokines may be displayed on the luminal side of the vascular endothelium through binding to proteoglycans and appear to play an important role in the maintenance and evolution of the inflammatory response.

The receptors for chemotactic agents are located on the cell surface, and additional stores are present in cytoplasmic granules. On exposure to low concentrations of chemotactic agents, the cells express additional receptors on the plasma membrane[633]; some of these are of higher affinity and increase the ability of the cell to sense the chemotactic agent. The cells also sense the spatial gradient of chemotactic agents; a difference of as little as 0.1% can be detected.[633, 634] The cells then orient so that they are flattened at the end toward the highest concentration (the lamellipodium) and have a thin tail (the uropod) at the opposite end. This polarization of the cell requires an intact cytoskeleton network and a fluid cell membrane. The polarized cell contains increased numbers of receptors for chemotactic agents and for IgG at the flattened lamellipodium.[633–635] Chemotactic agents engaged to receptors on the neutrophil lamellipodium trigger a local and selective release of granules, which contain a pool of the β_2 integrins, including Mac-1. Adhesion to the endothelium is thereby augmented at this point of contact, and translocation between endothelial cells is facilitated. Neutrophils may then attach to and ultimately pass through the basement membrane to reach the tissues. Platelet-endothelial cell adhesion molecule-1 (PECAM-1, CD31), which is expressed on both neutrophils and endothelial cells, and components of the extracellular matrix (e.g., fibronectin and laminin) contribute at this stage.[627, 629] Release of digestive enzymes from lysosomes may also facilitate movement of neutrophils through the endothelium and tissues. Neutrophils must undergo considerable deformation to allow diapedesis through the endothelium. Migration through the tissues is also likely to be facilitated by the reversible adhesion and deadhesion between ligands on the neutrophil surface, including the integrins, with components of the extracellular matrix, such as fibronectin and collagen.

PHAGOCYTOSIS AND KILLING

Phagocytosis by neutrophils occurs in two phases: recognition and ingestion. The recognition phase usually involves binding of opsonized bacteria to specific receptors on the cell surface. Opsonin-independent surface phagocytosis may also occur but is less efficient, particularly for encapsulated organisms. Opsonization, a process whereby immunoglobulin, complement, certain other host-derived proteins, or all three are bound to the surface of the organism, is discussed later in this chapter. Neutrophils contain specific receptors for the Fc portion of the IgG molecule (Fcγ receptors) and receptors for two different forms of the activated third component of complement.[636, 637] C3b is bound by CR1 and C3bi by CR3 and CR4; CR3 and CR4, respectively, are the CD11b-CD18 and CD11c-CD18 integrins described previously.[627, 635] Opsonized bacteria bind and cross link Fcγ and C3b-C3bi receptors, and this transmits a signal for ingestion and, in the case of Fcγ receptors, for the activation of the cell's microbicidal mechanisms. Signal transduction from these receptors is not fully elucidated but appears to involve a series of intracellular events, including activation of tyrosine kinases, increased intracellular Ca^{2+} concentration, activation of serine-threonine protein kinases including protein kinase C, activation of phospholipase A_2, and activation of small guanosine triphosphate (GTP)-binding proteins.[638–640]

Once ingested, microbes are exposed to a variety of potent microbicidal products. Oxygen-dependent microbicidal mechanisms are of central importance, as illustrated by the severe compromise in defenses against a wide range of pyogenic pathogens (with the exception of catalase-negative bacteria) observed in children with a genetic defect in this system.[641] This disorder—chronic granulomatous disease—results from a defect in one of four intracellular proteins that together form the phagocyte oxidase. This oxidase consists of two plasma membrane–associated and two cytosolic components. In response to activation of the cell—for example, during receptor-mediated phagocytosis—these four components are assembled in the plasma membrane into an enzymatic complex that transfers an electron to oxygen. This forms superoxide anion, which has weak microbicidal activity and is a precursor for more toxic compounds, including hydrogen peroxide and hydroxyl radicals. The assembly of the oxidase in the plasma membrane allows these products to be secreted into the nascent or fully formed phagocytic vacuole, where their activity can be focused on the microbe. The activity of hydrogen peroxide can also be augmented by myeloperoxidase, a protein stored in neutrophil granules, which are discharged into the phagocytic vacuole.

In addition to myeloperoxidase, the neutrophil contains other granule proteins with potent microbicidal activity. These mediate oxygen-independent killing. Many of these are relatively small, cationic proteins with direct microbicidal activity, including the defensins, cathepsin G, and a protein that binds selectively to gram-negative lipopolysaccharide—bactericidal permeability-increasing (BPI) protein.[642, 643]

PRODUCTION OF INFLAMMATORY MEDIATORS BY NEUTROPHILS

Neutrophils produce leukotrienes, primarily LTB$_4$, PAF, and certain cytokines that facilitate the inflammatory response. These include IL-1,[644] TNF,[645] and members of the chemokine family, such as IL-8.[631] Thus, in addition to playing a direct role in microbicidal killing, neutrophils may modulate the inflammatory response.

Neutrophils in the Fetus and Neonate

NEUTROPHIL PRODUCTION AND RELEASE

Neutrophil precursors are first detected in the yolk sac and then in the liver, spleen, and bone marrow, appearing somewhat later than macrophage precursors.[646, 647] Mature neutrophils are first detected by 14 to 16 weeks of gestation. The numbers of circulating neutrophil precursors (CFU-GMs) are 10- to 20-fold higher in the fetus and neonate than in the adult, and neonatal bone marrow also contains an abundance of neutrophil precursors.[646, 648–650] However, the rate of proliferation of circulating neutrophil precursors in both human and rat neonates appears to be near maximal,[648–650] suggesting that the capacity to increase the numbers of CFU-GMs in response to infection may be limited. In contrast to the numbers of CFU-GMs, in the midgestation human fetus the numbers of postmitotic neutrophils in the fetal liver and bone marrow are markedly lower than in term newborns and adults.[651] Further, at this stage of gestation neutrophils constitute less than 10% of circulating leukocytes, rising to values of 50 to 60% at term.

Within hours of birth, the numbers of circulating neutrophils increase sharply in term and preterm neonates.[652] One study of healthy term neonates reported absolute neutrophil counts at 4 hours of 9.5 to 21.5 $\times$ 10^3/mm^3 (10th to 90th percentile) and an immature-to-mature neutrophil ratio of 0.05 to 0.27.[653] The number of neutrophils normally peaks shortly thereafter, whereas the fraction of neutrophils that are immature (bands and less mature forms) remains constant at about 15% (Fig. 2–14). Values may be influenced by a number of factors. Most important is the response to sepsis. Septic infants may have normal or increased neutrophil counts. However, sepsis and other perinatal complications, including maternal hypertension, periventricular hemorrhage, and severe asphyxia, can cause neutropenia, and severe or fatal sepsis often is associated with persistent neutropenia, particularly in preterm neonates.[654, 655] Neutropenia may be associated with increased margination of circulating neutrophils, which occurs early in response to infection.[625] However, neutropenia that is sustained often reflects depletion of the neonate's, particularly the

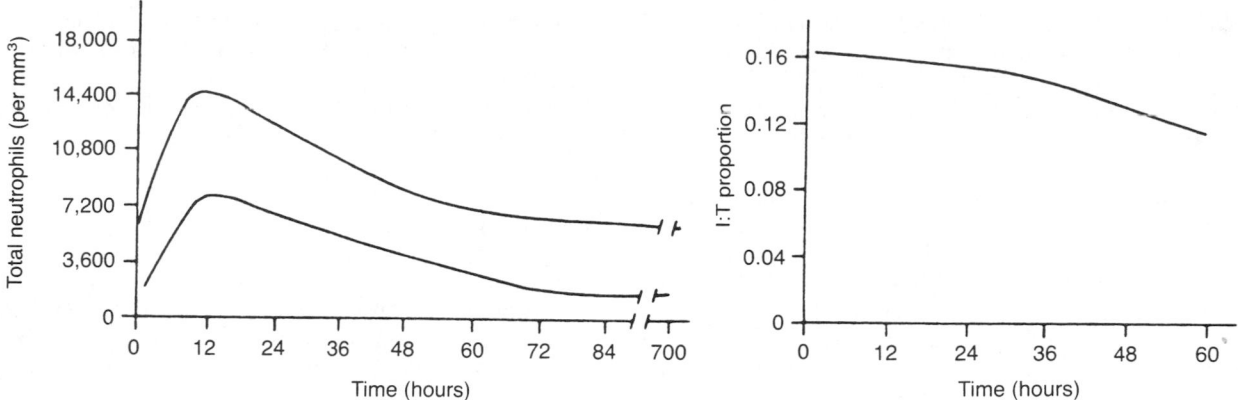

FIGURE 2–14 Change in total number of neutrophils and in ratio of immature to total neutrophils in the neonate. (From Manroe BL, Weinberg AG, Rosenfeld CR, et al. The neonatal blood count in health and disease. I. Reference values for neutrophilic cells. J Pediatr 95:89–98, 1979, with permission.)

premature neonate's, limited postmitotic neutrophil storage pool. Consistently with this, septic neutropenic neonates in whom the neutrophil storage pool is depleted are more likely to die than are those with normal neutrophil storage pools.[655] Leukemoid reactions are also observed at a frequency of ~1% in term neonates in the absence of infection or other definable cause. They appear to reflect increased marrow production of neutrophils, and are not consistently associated with increased G-CSF concentrations.[656]

As discussed earlier, CSFs, particularly G-CSF, are important for neutrophil production, survival, and optimal function. Mononuclear cells and monocytes from mid-gestation fetuses and premature neonates generally produce less G-CSF and GM-CSF after stimulation in vitro than do similar cell populations from adults, whereas cells from term neonates produce amounts that are similar to or modestly less than those of adults (see Table 2–2). In contrast with these findings, circulating G-CSF levels in healthy individuals are highest in the first hours after birth, and levels in premature neonates are generally higher than in term neonates.[657–660] Levels rapidly decline in the neonatal period and subsequently decline more slowly with aging. One study reported a direct correlation between circulating levels of G-CSF and the blood absolute neutrophil count, although this has not been confirmed by others.[658] Plasma G-CSF levels tend to be elevated in infected mature and premature neonates,[657] although some studies have found considerable overlap with the levels of those who are uninfected.[661] In one report G-CSF levels in neutropenic neonates without sepsis were not elevated above normal, whereas, in contrast, levels in neutropenic adults undergoing chemotherapy were markedly increased.[662] Although the cause of neutropenia in these neonates was not described, these observations raise the possibility that deficient G-CSF production might be a contributory factor to neutropenia in some neonates.

Overall, the available data suggest that the most critical deficiency in phagocyte defenses in the fetus and neonate, particularly the premature neonate, is their limited ability to accelerate neutrophil production in response to infection. This appears to result in large part from a limited neutrophil storage pool, and perhaps a more limited ability to increase neutrophil production in response to infection. This is not clearly due to a deficiency in the production of G-CSF in vivo, though this may be a factor in some cases. As discussed in the section Adjunct Therapy of Pyogenic Infections—Colony-Stimulating Factors, trials of G-CSF or GM-CSF have recently been undertaken to determine whether this form of intervention can ameliorate these deficits.

MIGRATION TO SITES OF INFECTION

In addition to defects in neutrophil production in response to infection, a substantial body of evidence suggests that the ability of neonatal neutrophils to migrate from the blood into sites of infection and inflammation may be reduced or delayed.[663, 664] In human neonates, the early inflammatory response in the skin often contains a larger number of eosinophils than in adults, and the transition from a neutrophilic to a mononuclear cell–dominated response is delayed.[665] Similarly, the influx of neutrophils into the peritoneal cavity in response to FMLP, group B streptococci, or E. coli[666] or into implanted polyvinyl sponges[655] was markedly reduced in neonatal rats compared with that in adult rats; this occurred in spite of greater release of marrow neutrophil stores in neonates than in adults. This diminished delivery of neutrophils may result in part from defects in adhesion and chemotaxis.

Adhesion of neonatal neutrophils under resting conditions is normal or at most modestly impaired, whereas adhesion of activated cells is deficient.[667, 668] Adhesion of neonatal neutrophils to activated endothelium under conditions of flow similar to those found in capillaries or postcapillary venules is variable but on average only 40 to 45% of that observed with adult neutrophils.[669, 670] This appears to reflect, at least in part, a deficiency in the abundance of L-selectin and ability to shed this protein from the surface of neonatal neutrophils, and decreased binding of these cells to P-selectin.[669–672] Many studies[669, 670, 673, 674] find that resting neonatal and adult neutrophils have similar amounts of the β_2 integrins Mac-1 (CD11b-CD18) and LFA-1 (CD11a-CD18) on their plasma membrane. However, neutrophils from term and, in particular, preterm neonates have a reduced ability to upregulate expression of these integrins after exposure to chemotactic agents, which is due in part to reduced intracellular stores of these molecules in their granules. This is associated with a parallel decrease in adhesion to activated endothelium or purified ICAM-1.[675] However, two studies have concluded that expression of Mac-1 and LFA-1 is not reduced on resting or stimulated neonatal neutrophils, and that diminished expression observed in other studies may be an artifact of the methods used to purify neutrophils.[672, 676] Nonetheless, the preponderance of data suggests that a deficit in adhesion underlies in part the diminished ability of neonatal neutrophils to migrate through endothelium into tissues.[669, 675]

In nearly all studies in which neutrophil migration has been compared in vitro, chemotaxis of neonatal neutrophils was less than that of adult neutrophils (Table 2–7).[663, 667, 677–679] When compared directly, chemotaxis of neonatal peripheral blood neutrophils seems to be more impaired than that of cord blood neutrophils.[678] Some studies have found that chemotaxis remains less than that of adult cells at least until 1 to 2 years of age,[678, 679] whereas others have suggested more rapid maturation.[680] The response of neonatal neutrophils is reduced to a variety of chemotactic factors, including FMLP, LTB$_4$, PAF, and IL-8.[681–683] Neutrophil chemotaxis in premature infants is at least as impaired as that of term neonates.[680, 684, 685] Most[667, 686, 687] but not all studies[688] have found that the number and affinity of receptors for FMLP are similar in adult and neonatal neutrophils, whereas receptors for C5a may be reduced.[689] Thus, decreased chemotaxis is probably due, in large part, to an event downstream of binding of the chemotaxin to its specific receptor, such as the increases in intracellular

calcium and inositol phospholipid generation, and the change in cell membrane potential within the neutrophil.[687, 690] An additional factor may be the reduced deformability of neonatal neutrophils, particularly immature granulocytes, which may limit their ability to enter the tissues after binding to the vascular endothelium.[668] This defect appears to reflect a diminished capacity of neonatal neutrophils to reorganize their cytoskeleton in response to stimulation, rather than altered amounts of tubulin or actin.[663, 677, 691] Because chemotaxis by neonatal neutrophils is relatively more impaired at low than at high concentrations of chemotactic factors,[692] decreased generation of chemotactic factors in neonatal serum[678, 692] may compound the intrinsic deficits of neonatal neutrophils (as discussed previously). However, the generation of other chemotactic agents, such as LTB$_4$, by neonatal neutrophils appears to be normal.[693] Finally, not all changes in response to chemotactic factors are abnormal in neonatal neutrophils: Upregulation of the type 1 complement receptor (CR1) is normal or at most slightly impaired.[694, 695]

PHAGOCYTOSIS AND KILLING OF BACTERIA BY NEONATAL NEUTROPHILS

Under optimal in vitro conditions, neutrophils from healthy human term and preterm neonates bind and ingest gram-positive and gram-negative bacteria as well as or slightly less efficiently than do cells from adults.[684, 696, 697] Levels of opsonins, including IgG, and of complement are reduced in serum from neonates, in particular in serum from preterm neonates. Consistent with this, phagocytosis of bacteria by neutrophils from preterm but not term neonates is reduced compared with that of cells from adults when assayed in whole blood.[698–700] This deficiency appears primarily to be due to differences in plasma components rather than differences between neutrophils.[700] This is the case even though neutrophils from preterm neonates have reduced numbers

TABLE 2–7
Chemotaxis of Neonatal Granulocytes

CELL SOURCE	ASSAY	STIMULUS[a]	PERCENTAGE OF ADULT RESPONSE	COMMENT	REFERENCE
Cord blood	3-μm filter (Nucleopore)	EAS	79	Normal random motility	678
Peripheral blood	Agarose	ZAS	27	Low until 2 yr of age	679
Cord blood	3-μm filter (Nucleopore)	EAS	125	Still low at 6 mo of age; normal chemokinesis	677
Peripheral blood			53		
Cord blood	Agarose	ZAS	$\geq$30	More severe with lower concentrations of ZAS	692
Peripheral blood	5-μm cellulose filter, whole blood	ZAS	79	Ill neonates = 62%	1163
Cord blood	Cellulose filter, 3, 5, or 8 μm	Casein	37–60	Normal random motility, normal chemokinesis	1164
Cord blood	Agarose	EAS	60–80	Normal random motility	1165
	3-μm cellulose		<15		
Peripheral blood	5-μm cellulose filter	ZAS	88		1166
Peripheral blood	Cellulose filter	ZAS	~50	Equal to adult by 2 wk	1167
Cord blood	Agarose	FMLP	70	Low until 1 yr of age	683

[a]EAS = endotoxin-activated serum; ZAS = zymosan-activated serum; FMLP = formylated bacterial peptide.

of receptors for IgG and complement, that is, FcγRIII (CD16) and C3bi (CD11b-CD18), compared with neutrophils from term neonates and adults.[676, 694, 698, 701] When concentrations of opsonins are even more limiting,[702] neutrophils from term neonates ingest bacteria less efficiently than those from adults. The basis for this is unknown, because FcγRII, FcγRIII, CR1, and CR3 expression is similar.[699] Decreased upregulation of the C3bi receptor, which is the β_2 integrin Mac-1, by neonatal neutrophils in response to chemotactic factor or LPS priming may play a role.[694, 695, 703, 704]

Killing of ingested gram-positive and gram-negative bacteria and *Candida* organisms by neutrophils from healthy neonates has been normal in most studies.[696, 705, 706] However, variable and usually mildly decreased bactericidal activity has been noted against *Pseudomonas aeruginosa*,[707] *S. aureus*,[708] and certain strains of group B streptococci[709, 710] but not others.[709, 711] Deficits in killing by neonatal neutrophils were found to be more apparent at high ratios of bacteria to neutrophils.[712] Sick or stressed neonates (most of whom were preterm with sepsis, respiratory impairment, hyperbilirubinemia, premature rupture of membranes, or hypoglycemia) also have clearer differences in microbicidal activity[713, 714] in spite of normal[714] or only variably decreased[713] phagocytosis. However, it should be noted that neutrophils from adults with similar illnesses may also have diminished microbicidal activity.[713] It remains to be determined whether neonatal neutrophils are more severely compromised by illness than those of comparable adults.

Studies to elucidate the mechanisms for differences in microbicidal activity of human neonatal neutrophils have focused on the generation of toxic oxygen metabolites. In most studies, generation of superoxide anion by human neonatal[711, 715] and fetal[716] neutrophils is similar to that by adult cells. Similarly, neutrophils from term and preterm neonates generate hydrogen peroxide at least as efficiently as cells from adults.[700] In contrast, production of the toxic hydroxyl radical, and chemiluminescence (an index of oxygen radical production) may be decreased.[715, 717, 718] Efficient killing of a strain of group B streptococcus type Ic (in contrast with most non–group B streptococci) by polymorphonuclear neutrophils required generation of oxygen metabolites,[710] and group B streptococci are highly susceptible to killing by hydroxyl radical but relatively resistant to the action of superoxide anion and hydrogen peroxide.[719] Thus, if generation of hydroxyl radical by neutrophils from some neonates is deficient, it may contribute to a defect in microbicidal activity.

Oxygen-independent microbicidal mechanisms of neonatal neutrophils remain poorly characterized. Their ability to release the lysosomal enzymes lysozyme and β glucuronidase appears to be intact.[720] However, their content of specific granules[703, 721] and the release of specific granule contents (e.g., lactoferrin) on activation appear to be reduced. Because a diminished content of microbicidal defensins has been observed in individuals with inherited specific granule deficiency,[722] it is possible that neonatal neutrophils may have reduced amounts of defensins.

EFFECTS OF IMMUNOMODULATORS

After systemic treatment with G-CSF and GM-CSF, expression of CR3 (CD11b-CD18) on neonatal neutrophil increases.[723] Studies performed in vitro indicate that IFN-γ and GM-CSF enhance the chemotactic response of neonatal neutrophils.[724–726] However, GM-CSF inhibits chemotaxis at higher concentrations, which are associated with enhancement of oxygen radical production.[725, 726] The methylxanthine pentoxifylline exhibits a biphasic enhancement of chemotaxis by neonatal neutrophils.[663] None of these agents causes full normalization of chemotaxis compared with that by adult cells. Of potential concern, indomethacin, which is used clinically to facilitate ductal closure in premature neonates, impairs chemotaxis of cells from term and preterm neonates.[685] Clinical trials of immunomodulators are discussed in the Adjunct Therapy of Pyogenic Infections sections.

Eosinophilic Granulocytes

In adults and older children, eosinophils represent a small percentage of the circulating granulocytes. Their numbers are increased in allergic states, parasitic (particularly metazoan) infections, and in certain autoimmune or malignant disease states. In the fetus and neonate, eosinophils commonly represent a sizable fraction of the total number of circulating granulocytes. At 18 to 30 weeks of gestation, total granulocytes represent only about 10% of total circulating leukocytes, whereas eosinophils constitute 10 to 20% of total granulocytes.[727] Similarly, in premature neonates the numbers of eosinophils are increased relative to those of term neonates, often reaching values of 1500 to 3000 cells per mm³ and representing up to one third of total granulocytes in the first month of life.[728, 729] The postnatal increase of eosinophils lags behind that of neutrophils, peaking at the third to fourth week of postnatal life. There is a relative increase in the abundance of eosinophils in inflammatory exudates in neonates, paralleling their greater numbers in the circulation.[670] In addition to prematurity, certain conditions have been associated with a relatively greater degree of eosinophilia; these include Rh disease, total parenteral nutrition, and transfusions.[728] In contrast with conditions such as allergic and parasitic diseases, neonatal eosinophilia is not associated with increased amounts of circulating IgE.[729] The basis or the significance of the eosinophilic tendency of the neonate is not known. Certain of the functional deficits observed in neonatal neutrophils, such as the diminished expression of adhesion molecules important in leukocyte migration into tissues, have been observed in neonatal eosinophils.[670]

Mononuclear Phagocytes

ORIGIN AND DIFFERENTIATION IN THE ADULT

Mononuclear phagocytes are the most phylogenetically primitive cells of the innate immune system, functioning to phagocytose microbes and debris. In vertebrates they have additional functions, including presentation of antigen to T cells, secretion of inflammatory mediators, and cell-mediated cytotoxicity. Mononuclear phagocytes are derived from bone marrow precursors (monoblasts and promonocytes) and include the blood monocytes and tissue macrophages. Under steady-state conditions, monocytes are released from the marrow within 24 hours and circulate in the blood for 1 to 3 days before moving to the tissues.[730] Once they have left the blood, monocytes do not recirculate but differentiate into macrophages, which are present in all tissues. Monocytes lose granule myeloperoxidase as they differentiate into tissue macrophages.[731] Other changes vary with the local tissue conditions. For example, monocytes and peritoneal macrophages rely primarily on anaerobic glycolysis, whereas alveolar (lung) macrophages utilize aerobic cytochrome oxidation as well.[732] The function of macrophages is readily modulated by cytokines, and macrophages can fuse to form multinucleated giant cells.[730] The estimated life span of macrophages in the tissues is 4 to 12 weeks, and they are capable of limited replication in situ.[732, 733]

MIGRATION TO THE SITES OF INFECTION: ADHERENCE, CHEMOTAXIS, AND DELAYED HYPERSENSITIVITY REACTIONS

Like neutrophils, mononuclear phagocytes express the adhesion molecules L-selectin and β_2 integrin. These cells, unlike neutrophils, also express robust amounts of the $\alpha_4\beta_1$ integrin very late antigen–4 (VLA-4).[734, 735] Thus, in addition to allowing adherence to the ligands recognized by the adhesion molecules expressed on neutrophils, monocytes are able to adhere to endothelium expressing vascular cell adhesion molecule-1 (VCAM-1), the ligand for VLA-4. VCAM-1 is a member of the immunoglobulin gene superfamily, which is expressed only on endothelial cells that have been activated by exposure to cytokines or bacterial products such as LPS. Like that of the β_2 integrins, the avidity of the β_1 integrins for VCAM-1 is upregulated when monocytes are activated, enhancing adhesion and presumably transendothelial migration.[735] VLA-4 allows monocytes to enter tissues in states in which there is little or no neutrophilic inflammation, such as delayed hypersensitivity. The expression of VLA-4 may also account for the capacity of monocytes but not neutrophils to enter tissues in patients with the type I leukocyte adhesion deficiency syndrome (discussed previously).

Many of the factors that are chemotactic for neutrophils also induce monocyte chemotaxis. These include bacterial products such as FMLP and host products such as PAF. However, those chemokines (see Table 2–2) that are chemotactic for neutrophils are not generally chemotactic for monocytes, and vice versa. For example, the α-chemokine IL-8 is chemotactic for neutrophils but not for monocytes, whereas MCP-1, a β-chemokine, selectively activates and attracts monocytes.[632] The normal inflammatory response induced by a transient irritant (e.g., dermal abrasion) is characterized by an initial infiltration of neutrophils that is followed within 6 to 12 hours by a response consisting predominantly of mononuclear phagocytes.[730] The orchestration of this sequential influx of leukocytes appears to be governed by the temporal order in which specific chemokines and endothelial adhesins are expressed and by the slower migration rate of monocytes versus neutrophils.

Delayed cutaneous hypersensitivity responses are characterized by an influx of mononuclear phagocytes and lymphocytes. This response reaches maximum at 24 to 72 hours after antigen infiltration. Experimental evidence in mice and humans undergoing delayed hypersensitivity reactions suggests that this process is governed, at least in part, by cytokines. These include IL-1 and TNF, which are produced by Langerhans cells (epidermal dendritic cells) and by epithelial cells, and IL-2 and IFN-γ, which are produced by T cells infiltrating the subcutaneous tissues.[736, 737] The expression of these cytokines and the induction by IFN-γ of class II MHC antigen reach their maximum before the peak influx of cells and induration, consistent with a role in causation.

ANTIMICROBIAL PROPERTIES OF MONOCYTES AND MACROPHAGES

Although neutrophils ingest and kill pyogenic bacteria more efficiently, resident macrophages are the initial line of phagocyte defense in the tissues against microbial invasion. When the microbial insult is modest, these cells may be sufficient to clear the microbes fully. If not, mononuclear phagocytes, through production of LTB$_4$, PAF, and chemokines, assist in the recruitment of circulating neutrophils and monocytes. Monocytes and macrophages express each of the three Fcγ receptors for IgG[640, 738]; Fcα receptors for IgA[739]; CR1 and CR3 receptors for C3b and C3bi, respectively[637, 740]; CD14 and Toll receptors for LPS[740–743]; and receptors that allow them nonspecifically to recognize unencapsulated bacteria, yeast, certain viruses, and effete cells, such as mannose/fucose, CD14, and scavenger receptors.[744–747] Mononuclear phagocytes are capable of nonspecific phagocytosis, but this process is greatly facilitated by coating of the microbe or particle with immunoglobulin, complement, or both (i.e., opsonization, discussed later). Phagocytosis of particles and subsequent microbicidal mechanisms of mononuclear phagocytes parallel those of neutrophils in most respects. Mononuclear phagocytes generate reactive oxygen metabolites, but in lesser amounts than do neutrophils. Circulating monocytes but not tissue macrophages contain myeloperoxidase, which facilitates the microbicidal activity of hydrogen peroxide. The expression of microbicidal granule proteins differs somewhat in mononuclear phagocytes versus neutrophils; for example, human mononuclear phagocytes have not been shown to contain defensins.[748] Several unique mechanisms of antimicrobial activity are expressed primarily by activated macrophages.

In contrast with that of neutrophils, the microbicidal activity of resident tissue macrophages is relatively modest. This may be important in allowing macrophages to remove small numbers of microbes and tissue debris without excessively damaging tissues through release of microbicidal materials, which also may be toxic to host cells. Macrophage microbicidal and proinflammatory functions are enhanced in a process commonly referred to as macrophage activation.[664, 749, 750] Macrophages are primed for increased function through engagement of CD40 on the macrophage plasma membrane by CD40 ligand expressed on antigen-stimulated T cells and by exposure to cytokines secreted by antigen-stimulated T cells or NK cells, including IFN-γ and, to a more limited extent, TNF or GM-CSF. Macrophages that have been primed through these mechanisms have augmented responses (e.g., greater proinflammatory cytokine production and antimicrobial activity) and are fully activated in response to microbes and microbial products (e.g., LPS, lipoteichoic acid, bacterial DNA), activated complement components, or immune complexes. Cytokines produced by activated macrophages, including TNF, GM-CSF, IL-12, and IL-15, can further amplify their activation through autocrine or paracrine mechanisms, as described in more detail later. Their increased antimicrobial activity reflects increased expression of FcγRI,[751, 752] enhanced phagocytic activity, and increased production of reactive oxygen metabolites in response to phagocytic or other stimuli. Other antimicrobial mechanisms induced by activation of these cells include the catabolism of tryptophan, scavenging of iron, and production of nitric oxide and its metabolites by the inducible nitric oxide synthase (iNOS). The latter is a major mechanism by which activated murine macrophages inhibit or kill a variety of intracellular pathogens. Expression of iNOS by human macrophages is less consistently observed and less robust than that by murine macrophages, and the role of nitric oxide in the antimicrobial activity of human macrophages is uncertain.[753]

Activated macrophages play a critical role in defense against infection with bacteria and parasites that replicate within host cells, which are commonly referred to as intracellular pathogens. Support for this notion comes from studies in humans and mice with genetic deficiencies in proteins that participate in macrophage activation. Humans with IFN-γ receptor, IL-12, or IL-12 receptor deficiency suffer unduly from infections with *Mycobacteria* species.[132, 754, 755] They may also be at increased risk for infections with other intracellular bacteria, including *Listeria monocytogenes* and *Salmonella* sp. Similarly, mice deficient in these cytokines or their receptors are much more susceptible to these infections and to infections with other intracellular pathogens, including *T. gondii*. Deficiency of TNF or its receptors also impairs defenses to certain of these pathogens, including *L. monocytogenes* and mycobacteria.[756] Patients with the X-linked hyper-IgM syndrome,[122] which is due to a deficiency in CD40 ligand expression, have defects in antibody production that result from the importance of CD40 ligand in T cell–mediated help for B cell responses. In addition, these patients are predisposed to disease due to *P. carinii* and *Cryptosporidium parvum* and may also be at greater risk for disease due to mycobacteria and *Cryptococcus neoformans*. Mice with CD40 ligand deficiency are also at greater risk for infection with *P. carinii*, but unlike those with IFN-γ, IL-12, or TNF deficiency, are not more susceptible to infection with *L. monocytogenes*.[749] This suggests that secreted cytokine- and CD40 ligand–mediated macrophage activation may play, at least in part, distinct roles in host defense.

REGULATION OF THE IMMUNE AND INFLAMMATORY RESPONSES BY CYTOKINES PRODUCED BY MONONUCLEAR PHAGOCYTES

Monocytes and macrophages play important roles in regulation of the afferent and efferent phases of the immune response. As noted, mononuclear phagocytes and dendritic cells that arise from the mononuclear phagocyte cell lineage are important APCs, which express class II MHC antigens and process and present antigens efficiently to T cells. The production of cytokines facilitates this process and modulates the efferent immune and inflammatory responses (see Table 2–2). Most cytokines produced by mononuclear phagocytes have potent and diverse effects.[750, 757] Whether macrophages or other cells (e.g., endothelial cells) are the major source of these cytokines varies, depending on the inciting stimulus for their production and the tissue.

Cytokines produced by mononuclear phagocytes contribute to the systemic response to infection, including the induction of fever and the acute phase response, and play important local roles in the regulation of inflammation. IL-1, TNF, IL-6, and type 1 interferons (α/β) induce fever.[758–761] This effect is mediated at least in part by stimulating vascular endothelial cells in the hypothalamic area to produce prostaglandin E_2 (PGE$_2$), accounting for the antipyretic effect of drugs that inhibit prostaglandin synthesis. PGE$_2$ acts in turn on cells within the anterior hypothalamus to cause fever. Fever may have a beneficial role in host resistance to infection both by inhibiting the growth of certain microorganisms directly and by enhancing certain host immune responses.[762, 763] TNF, IL-1, and IL-6 act on the liver to induce the acute phase response, which is associated with decreased albumin synthesis and increased synthesis of complement components C3 and factor B, haptoglobin, fibrinogen, C-reactive protein, and other proteins. G-, GM-, and M-CSFs enhance the production of their respective target cell populations, increasing the numbers of phagocytes available. At the sites of infection or injury, TNF and IL-1 increase the adhesive properties of endothelial cells, in part as a result of increased synthesis and expression of cell adhesion molecules on endothelial cells, such as ICAM-1 and VCAM-1; increase endothelial cell procoagulant activity; and enhance neutrophil adhesiveness by upregulating β$_2$ integrin expression.[758, 764–767] α-Chemokines enhance the avidity of neutrophil integrin binding to ligands on the endothelium and direct these cells to migrate into the inflammatory-infectious focus; β-chemokines play a similar role in attracting mononuclear phagocytes and lymphocytes.[632, 768] Mononuclear phagocytes produce these chemokines directly, and do so indirectly through the production of TNF and IL-1, which in turn trigger their own production by other cells (e.g., endothelial cells). These and additional effects contribute to edema, redness, and leukocyte infiltration, which characterize inflammation.

The production of cytokines by mononuclear phagocytes is normally restricted temporally and anatomically to cells in contact with microbial products, antigen-stimulated T cells, or other agonists (discussed previously) found at sites of infection or secondary lymphoid organs draining these sites. Nonetheless, TNF and IL-1, along with IFN-γ produced by NK cells and T cells, contribute to the clinical sepsis syndrome. When produced in excess, these cytokines, along with other mediators, can induce septic shock and disseminated intravascular coagulation, underscoring the importance of closely regulated and anatomically restricted production of proinflammatory cytokines.[769–771] This is achieved in part by a combination of positive and negative feedback regulation. For example, TNF and IL-1 directly induce production of IL-1, TNF, IL-6, and G-, M-, and GM-CSFs by mononuclear phagocytes and other cells such as endothelial cells. Conversely, macrophages produce cytokines that attenuate the production of proinflammatory and TH1-type cytokines by macrophages and lymphocytes. These anti-inflammatory cytokines include IL-10,[772] TGF-β,[773] and the IL-1 receptor antagonist (IL-1ra).[764] IL-6 attenuates proinflammatory cytokine production (e.g., TNF) but also has proinflammatory effects. IL-6, IL-10, and IL-1ra are expressed a few hours later than TNF and IL-1, after stimulation of macrophages, and inhibit production of TNF and IL-1.[644, 774–777] The production of these anti-inflammatory cytokines is also enhanced by exposure of macrophages to cytokines produced by TH2 T cells, including IL-4, IL-10, IL-13, and TGF-β. In contrast, cytokines produced by TH1 T cells, particularly IFN-γ, attenuate the production of IL-10.[761]

Mononuclear phagocytes are also important sources of IFN-α/β, IL-12, IL-15, and IL-18, which enhance NK cell lytic function and production of IFN-γ.[555, 583, 778–780] These cytokines also collectively facilitate the development of antigen-specific TH1 and CD8 T cells, which play a critical role in control of infection with intracellular bacterial, protozoan, and viral pathogens and inhibit the development of TH2 T cells.[750, 781] IFN-α/β inhibits viral replication in host cells, as do IFN-γ and TNF. IFN-γ enhances the capacity of macrophages to produce IL-12 and TNF and inhibits IL-10 production,[750, 761, 781] thereby amplifying its own production and TH1 T cell responses.

Mononuclear phagocytes also secrete a number of noncytokine products that are potentially important in host defense mechanisms. These include a variety of complement components, fibronectin, and lysozyme.[782] Lysozyme, an enzyme active against the cells of gram-positive bacteria, is constitutively secreted in large quantities. Complement and fibronectin are discussed later.

Mononuclear Phagocytes in the Fetus and Neonate

Macrophages are detectable as early as 4 weeks of fetal life in the yolk sac, soon thereafter in the liver, and then in the bone marrow.[783] The capacity of the fetus and the neonate to produce monocytes, as indicated by development of macrophage colonies when fetal liver or bone marrow or blood of neonates is grown in culture, appears to be equal to or greater than that of adults.[784] The number of monocytes per volume of blood in neonates is also equal to or greater than that in adults.[646, 785]

The numbers of tissue macrophages in human neonates are less well characterized. The lung contains few macrophages until shortly before term in rabbits, rats, and monkeys,[786, 787] and limited data suggest that this is true in humans.[788] Postnatally, this number increases rapidly to adult levels by 24 to 48 hours in healthy monkeys but not in those with hyaline membrane disease, perhaps because of the absence of stimuli, such as surfactant, to attract monocytes to the lungs.[786] An indirect measure of splenic (and perhaps hepatic) macrophage number is the efficiency with which these cells, acting as part of the reticuloendothelial system, remove damaged erythrocytes from the blood. The blood of infants younger than 36 weeks of gestation has increased numbers of such erythrocytes, a condition that suggests decreased splenic macrophage function or mass compared with that of term infants and adults.[789]

MIGRATION TO SITES OF INFECTION AND DELAYED HYPERSENSITIVITY

The influx of monocytes into sites of inflammation and cellular immune reactions are delayed and attenuated in neonates compared with those in adults. After dermal abrasion, polymorphonuclear leukocytes infiltrate initially, but by 6 to 12 hours mononuclear leukocytes are the predominant cells in adults.[730] However, in term and preterm neonates, the influx of monocytes is delayed and remains below that of adults even after 24 hours (Table 2–8).[790, 791] The delayed and diminished influx of neonatal mononuclear phagocytes observed in vivo could result from a decreased capacity of neonatal monocytes to migrate to sites of inflammation or decreased generation of factors attracting these cells.

Results from studies of neonatal monocyte chemotaxis have varied. Most studies used cord blood mononuclear cells and a micropore assay, although chemotactic stimuli varied; all studies except that by Weston and associates[792] concluded that neonatal and adult monocytes had normal chemotaxis. However, in the two studies in which peripheral blood rather than cord blood was the

TABLE 2–8
Delayed Monocyte Response in Rebuck Skin Windows in Human Neonates and Adults

POPULATION	% MONOCYTES			
	2 hr	4 hr	6 hr	24 hr
Premature[a]	4	13	18	30
Term < 24 hr[a]	4	9	13	20
Term 24–108 hr[a]	2	7	11	19
Adult[b]	5	21	38	76

[a]Data from Bullock JD, Robertson AF, Bodenbender JB, et al. Inflammatory responses in the neonate re-examined. Pediatrics 44:58–61, 1969; with permission.
[b]Data from van Furth R, Raeburn JA, van Zwet TL. Characteristics of human mononuclear phagocytes. Blood 54:485–500, 1979; with permission.

source of cells,[677, 679] chemotaxis of neonatal cells was less than that of adult cells and remained less until 6 to 10 years of age.[679] The basis for reduced chemotaxis is uncertain and has not been addressed in detail. Data regarding adhesion molecules on monocytes from neonates are limited to two reports on the expression of the β_2 integrins. One study reported increased amounts of the β_2 integrin Mac-1 (CD11b-CD18) on resting and activated neonatal monocytes,[676] whereas the other found expression to be modestly lower.[793]

Monocyte chemotaxis, like that of polymorphonuclear leukocytes, is induced by activated complement components, bacterial factors, LTB_4, and certain chemokines (see Table 2–2). As described later, the production of LTB_4 and of some chemokines by neonatal monocytes may be reduced. Delayed cutaneous hypersensitivity, which depends on an influx of monocytes and lymphocytes into the site, is diminished in neonates[294, 298, 794] even when in vitro tests indicate sensitivity. This suggests that a decreased influx of cells in vivo may contribute to the diminished skin test response.

ACTIVITY OF MONOCYTES AND MACROPHAGES AGAINST PYOGENIC PATHOGENS

Monocytes from human neonates ingest and kill *S. aureus*, *E. coli*, and group B streptococci as well as do monocytes from adults,[709, 792, 795–797] although the rate at which they ingest unopsonized latex particles is lower.[664, 798] The production of microbicidal oxygen metabolites by neonatal and adult monocytes is similar.[796, 799] The ability of neonatal monocyte-derived macrophages (monocytes cultured in vitro) to phagocytose bacteria or other particles through receptors for mannose-fucose, IgG, complement, and opsonin-independent pathways appears not to differ from that of similarly prepared cells from adults. Neonatal monocytes have comparable oxygen radical generation and microbicidal activity against staphylococci.[800, 801]

There are few studies of the microbicidal activity of tissue macrophages from neonates because such cells are difficult to obtain. Because tissue macrophages are derived from monocytes, it might be assumed that these functions of neonatal tissue macrophages would also be mature. However, local tissue conditions in neonates may differ from those in adults and may be reflected by differences in macrophage function. Studies with alveolar macrophages are illustrative.

One study compared macrophages obtained from aspirated bronchial fluid of neonates with alveolar macrophages obtained by bronchoalveolar lavage from adults. A qualitative difference in killing of *Candida* sp. was observed. Cells from neonates killed the yeast form less well, but total killing was normal because surviving yeast cells then formed intracellular pseudohyphae, which cells from neonates killed normally[802]; concern must be raised that the cell preparations were not truly equivalent. However, parallel studies with alveolar macrophages obtained from monkeys, rabbits, and rats present a relatively consistent picture: There is a marked paucity in numbers of alveolar macrophages at birth, particularly in preterm neonates; when alveolar macrophages are challenged with a wide variety of bacteria in vivo, the rate at which they ingest the bacteria in neonatal animals is diminished, particularly in premature neonates[803–806]; phagocytosis in vitro is diminished in most but not all studies[805, 806]; and the microbicidal activity of macrophages is impaired to a modest degree.[709, 786, 787, 802, 807] This correlates with diminished generation of microbicidal oxygen metabolites[808, 809] and a lower content of microbicidal defensins in alveolar macrophages of neonatal rabbits.[810] In one study of rabbits, decreased killing of *Candida albicans* could be induced by exposure of adult alveolar macrophages to crude surfactant-containing material from the alveoli of neonates.[811] The authors concluded that the excess surfactant present in the alveoli at 1 day of age, which exceeded the amounts in adults severalfold, was ingested by neonatal alveolar macrophages and induced the defects in their function. Nonetheless, the extent to which these results can be extrapolated to human neonates is uncertain.

ACTIVITY OF MONOCYTES AND MACROPHAGES AGAINST INTRACELLULAR PATHOGENS

Certain neonatal pathogens, including all viruses and some nonviral pathogens, require replication or are capable of replicating within cells. Control of infection with these intracellular pathogens is mediated by factors that limit viral entry into cells, inhibit their replication, induce their killing within cells, or destroy infected cells.

Neonatal monocytes ingest and kill *Toxoplasma*[787, 812] and *Listeria* organisms (C Wilson, unpublished data). Further, both cultured blood monocytes and placental macrophages from human neonates are activated by IFN-γ as efficiently as are adult cells to kill or restrict the growth of these neonatal pathogens. In contrast, IFN-γ treatment did not activate monocyte-derived macrophages from human neonates to kill *C. albicans* and to generate superoxide anion as effectively as it did cells from adults.[813] Macrophages derived from the lungs of a small number of sick neonates post mortem allowed the intracellular replication of HSV, which was not observed with cells from adults.[814] However, two other studies that used neonatal monocytes, monocyte-derived macrophages, and fetal macrophages from the placenta found no difference in permissiveness for the replication of this virus.[815, 816] Whether results in the former study were due to the tissue from which the macrophages were obtained or the compromised status of the infants studied is not known. In general, neonatal macrophages do not appear to be more permissive for the replication of HSV. Monocytes and macrophages also restrict viral replication by inhibiting it in other cells[817] or by lysing virus-infected cells in the absence or in the presence of antibody.[818] Monocytes from neonates may be slightly less cytotoxic than those from adults in the absence of antibody,[819] but they are as active in the presence of antibody.[819, 820] Exogenous IFN-γ induces resistance to *Listeria* sp. infection in neonatal rats and to HSV infection in neonatal mice. This suggests that in these species the antimicrobial activity of host macrophages (and other host cells mediating resistance to these microbes) can be enhanced sufficiently to be protective, given the provision of this cytokine.[821–823] This also implies that the deficit in production of IFN-γ and certain other cytokines (e.g., TNF) that facilitate resistance to these microbes may be an important factor in the neonate's increased susceptibility (discussed later).

CYTOKINE AND INFLAMMATORY MEDIATOR PRODUCTION BY MONONUCLEAR PHAGOCYTES FROM THE FETUS AND NEONATE

CD14 is a ligand-binding receptor for lipopolysaccharide and other bacterial products that triggers monocyte cytokine production. Neonatal and adult monocytes express comparable amounts of CD14.[824] The relative abundance of Toll proteins, which are the signal transducing receptors for LPS,[741, 825, 826] on adult and neonatal cells is not known. A deficiency in neonatal cord blood of an as yet uncharacterized plasma protein that facilitates the response of monocytes to lipopolysaccharide has been reported.[824]

In response to stimulation with various agonists (e.g., LPS, IL-1), monocytes from term neonates produce mediators that enhance neutrophil and monocyte production (i.e., G-, GM-, and M-CSF) or contribute to acute inflammatory and acute-phase responses (i.e., IL-1, TNF, IL-6, IL-8, LTB$_4$) in amounts varying from ~25 to 75% of the amounts produced by adult cells (summarized in Table 2–2); however, in some studies, production of G-CSF, IL-1, and IL-6 has been similar to that in adult cells.[22, 228, 616, 662, 824, 827–831] Monocytes from preterm neonates produce less TNF, G-CSF, and IL-8 than those from term neonates and adults. Production of TNF by monocyte-derived and tissue (placental) macrophages from term neonates is reduced to a greater extent than that by blood monocytes and appears to be upregulated less by IFN-γ than in cells from adults.[827] Deficient production of IFN-γ by neonatal T cells may further compound the deficit in TNF-α production in humans (see earlier discussion). This is similar to results in neonatal rats challenged with lipopolysaccharide or *L. monocytogenes*,[822, 823] in which decreased production of IFN-γ by NK cells and T cells may be a contributing factor to the decreased production of TNF and diminished resistance to *Listeria* sp.[822] Although these findings suggest that neonatal monocytes have a modest deficiency in the production of proinflammatory cytokines, this appears to be balanced by similar reductions in the production of cytokines that dampen inflammation, including IL-10 and TGF-β.[225, 828, 832] However, one report suggests that alveolar macrophages from preterm neonates with hyaline membrane disease produce less IL-10 in vivo than those from term neonates,[833] although other differences in the patient populations may account for this finding.

The production by monocytes of cytokines that enhance defenses against intracellular pathogens appears to be reduced to a modest extent. Production of IFN-α/β by neonatal mononuclear cells and monocytes appears to be relatively normal in response to a variety of inducers including HSV and other viruses,[834, 835] although one study suggested that production in response to HSV may be diminished.[836] One group reported that the production of IL-12 and IL-15 by blood mononuclear cells (and presumably monocytes) from term neonates after stimulation with lipopolysaccharide was approximately 25% of that by cells from adults,[597, 616] whereas others found that neonatal and adult blood mononuclear cells stimulated with *S. aureus* or with meningococcal outer membrane proteins produce similar amounts of IL-12.[597, 616, 837] There are no reports regarding IL-18 production by cells from neonates. Production of the β-chemokine MIP-1α by cord blood mononuclear cells stimulated with mitogen was reported to be ~20 to 25% of that by adult cells,[828] whereas bioassays that measured total production of cytokines that are chemotactic for monocytes found similar responses by neonatal and adult cell preparations.[795, 796]

Collectively, these results suggest a variable diminution in the production of cytokines by monocytes from neonates. However, one group has found that when whole blood was used for the assays and cells were stimulated with LPS, TNF, IL-6, IL-8, and IL-10 production by cells from term neonates and adults was similar.[838] These results are likely to reflect monocyte cytokine production, though indirect effects mediated in part through cytokines produced by NK cells and T cells are possible.

Antigen presentation is discussed above in the section Antigen Presentation in the Fetus and Neonate.

Summary

The most clearly defined deficits in neonatal phagocytic defenses are the diminished neutrophil storage pool and diminished ability of the neonatal neutrophil to adhere to endothelium and migrate to sites of infection. Deficiencies in phagocytosis and killing appear to be less significant but may be exacerbated by a limitation in opsonins or high local bacterial density.

Blood monocytes from human neonates are normal in number and are generally as competent as those from adults in phagocytic and microbicidal activity. However, the diminished chemotactic activity of neonatal monocytes may reduce their delivery to sites of infection. The few data available on the function of tissue macrophages from neonates parallel data from certain animal species that suggest that phagocytosis and microbicidal activity by macrophages in the tissues may not be fully competent. The capacity of mononuclear phagocytes to produce both pro- and anti-inflammatory cytokines may be modestly reduced in term neonates and further reduced in premature neonates; this modest deficiency in cytokine production may be further compromised by the deficiency in production of IFN-γ by neonatal T cells and NK cells, and perhaps the ability of neonatal mononuclear phagocytes to respond fully to IFN-γ.

HUMORAL MEDIATORS OF INFLAMMATION AND OPSONIZATION

In response to infection and inflammation, a wide range of mediators are produced or activated.[839–841] Certain factors are derived from components normally present in plasma, including the complement system, mannan-binding lectin, fibronectin, the kinin system, and the coagulation system. Others, such as products of arachidonic acid metabolism (the prostaglandins, PAF, and leukotrienes), endorphins, amines (including histamine, catecholamines, and serotonin), and lysosomal enzymes, are produced and released from leukocytes, endothelial cells, neuronal cells, and other cell types. The balance in the production of these substances and their interactions may be critical determinants of outcome.

Studies with experimental animals suggest direct involvement of certain of these mediators in the unfavorable response of the neonate to infection.[842–845] Certain of these studies and limited studies with human adults[839, 840] and neonates[845] suggest that therapy directed toward modulating production of the mediators may be beneficial. However, for the most part, results are not yet sufficient to provide a clear understanding of the relative role of most mediators or to warrant recommendation of specific therapy.

Complement

The complement system is composed of serum proteins that, under specific conditions, interact in an orderly and sequential cascade. Interaction occurs along one of two pathways—the classic or the alternative—that converge on a final common pathway. Detailed reviews of the complement system are available[637, 846]; they are summarized in Figure 2–15.

CLASSIC PATHWAY

When antibodies that are capable of fixing complement to their Fc portion (IgM, IgG_1, IgG_2, and IgG_3 in hu-

mans) complex with microbial (or other) antigens, they bind C1. C1 is actually composed of three different proteins—C1q, C1r, and C1s—that are sequentially bound. Bound C1 then acts enzymatically on C4 and C2, components of which (C2a, C4b) are bound to the antigen. These then act on C3 to form C3b, which remains bound to the antigen, and C3a, which is released. Mannan-binding lectin can also activate the complement cascade via the classic pathway, although two proteases specific for mannan-binding lectin–induced activation are used instead of C1r and C1s to initiate cleavage of C4 and C2. C-reactive protein, a host-derived acute-phase protein[847] that binds to carbohydrate found in certain bacteria, particularly *S. pneumoniae*, also may substitute for antibody in the activation of the classic pathway. Bound C3b, C4b, and C2a together act on C5 to release C5a. The larger C5b fragment on the particle binds the terminal C6789 components, which form a complex. This complex forms pores in cell membranes and thereby causes cytolysis.

ALTERNATIVE PATHWAY

The alternative pathway is phylogenetically older. Although it is facilitated by the $F(ab')_2$ portion of antibody, antibody is not required for its activation. The continuous, but inefficient interaction of factor B with factor D and C3 in the fluid phase generates low levels of C3b and Bb continuously. If C3b and Bb bind to a microorganism, they form a more efficient system, which binds and acts on additional C3 to yield bound C3b. This interaction is facilitated by factor P (properdin) and inhibited by alternative pathway factors H and I.

Bacteria vary in their capacity to activate the alternative pathway, which is determined by their ability to bind C3b and to protect the complex of C3b and Bb

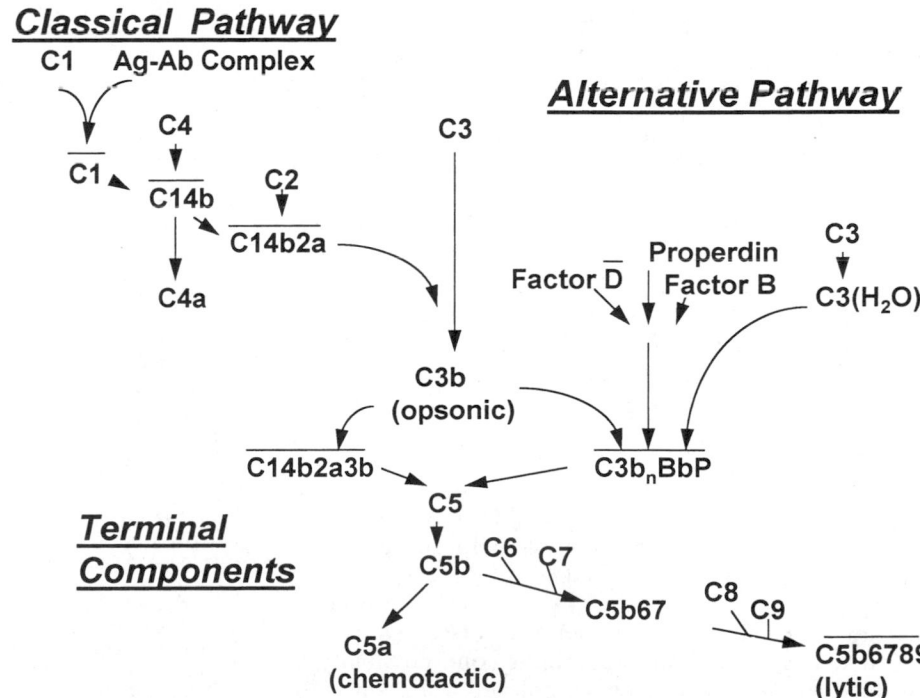

FIGURE 2–15 Complement activation. The classical and alternative pathways intersect at C3. This is followed by activation of the terminal components, which generate the membrane attack complex (C5b6789). Enzymatically active proteases, which serve to cleave and activate subsequent components, are shown with an overbar.

from the inhibitory effects of factors H and I. Sialic acid, a component of many bacterial polysaccharide capsules, including those of group B streptococci and *E. coli* K1, favors factor H binding. Thus, many virulent pathogens are protected from the alternative pathway by their capsules, although this protection may vary from strain to strain. Antibody is needed for efficient opsonization of such organisms.

It should also be apparent that the classic pathway, by creating particle-bound C3b, can activate the alternative pathway. Thus, the alternative pathway can act as an autocatalytic amplification mechanism. This may be particularly important in the presence of small amounts of antibody.

BIOLOGIC CONSEQUENCES OF COMPLEMENT ACTIVATION

Binding of specific complement components on the microbial surface facilitates microbial killing or removal. C3b binds to CR1 receptors. C3b is also cleaved to C3bi, which binds to the CR3 receptor (Mac-1, Cd11b-CD18) and CR4 receptor (CD11c-CD18). These receptors are found on neutrophils, macrophages, and certain other cell types. Along with IgG antibody, which binds to Fcγ receptors on these phagocytes, C3b and C3bi promote the ingestion of the organism. This is an important mechanism by which most bacteria and fungi are cleared.

C3b is also a key component of the C5a convertase, which leads to the cleavage of C5, release of C5a into the fluid phase, and binding of C5b on the microbial surface. C5b acts to assemble the membrane attack complex, which consists of C5b and the terminal C6–C9 complement components. Once assembled, this complex may lyse the cell to which it is bound. This mechanism appears to be the principal defense mechanism mediating systemic resistance to meningococci and gonococci; however, all gram-positive organisms and many gram-negative organisms are resistant to complement lysis. Thus, it may play a limited role in defense against neonatal bacterial pathogens. Virus-infected cells and certain parasites, including *Toxoplasma* sp., may also be lysed in this manner, but the role of such mechanisms in resistance to these infections is probably limited.

C5a, and to a more limited degree C3a, complement cleavage products that are released into the fluid phase, cause vasodilatation and increase vascular permeability. C5a is also a potent chemotactic factor for neutrophils, monocytes, and eosinophils. It stimulates these cells to degranulate, adhere to endothelium, and release leukotrienes, which themselves are potent mediators of inflammation.

In addition to these roles for complement in innate immunity, complement facilitates B cell responses to T cell–dependent antigens. Mice that are genetically deficient in C3, C4, or the complement receptors for C3b and C3d have diminished antibody responses to immunization with protein antigens.[343] The precise mechanism for this is uncertain. As discussed in the section B Cells and Immunoglobulin, one possibility is that C3d bound to antigen complexed with antibody (produced as part of the initial B cell response) amplifies the antibody response by simultaneous engagement of the C3d receptor (CD21) along with the B cell antigen receptor.

COMPLEMENT BIOSYNTHESIS

The hepatocyte appears to be the principal cell type that synthesizes complement components.[450, 848] However, macrophages synthesize complement proteins except those in the terminal membrane attack complex. Other cell types, including fibroblasts, may produce certain complement proteins.

COMPLEMENT IN THE FETUS AND NEONATE

Little, if any, maternal complement is transferred to the fetus. Fetal synthesis of complement components can be detected in tissues as early as 6 to 14 weeks of gestation, depending on the specific complement component and tissue examined.[450, 849]

Table 2–9 summarizes published reports on complement hemolytic activity of the classic pathway (CH_{50}) or alternative pathway (AP_{50}) and individual complement components in neonates. It should be emphasized that there is substantial variability among individuals and that many term neonates have values of individual complement components or of CH_{50} or AP_{50} within the adult

TABLE 2–9
Summary of Published Complement Levels in Neonates[a]

COMPLEMENT COMPONENT	MEAN % OF ADULT LEVELS	
	Term Neonate	Preterm Neonate
CH_{50}	56–90 (5)[b]	45–71 (4)
AP_{50}	49–65 (4)	40–55 (3)
C1q	61–90 (4)	27–58 (3)
C4	60–100 (5)	42–91 (4)
C2	76–100 (3)	67–96 (2)
C3	60–100 (5)	39–78 (4)
C5	73–75 (2)	67 (1)
C6	47–56 (2)	36 (1)
C7	67–92 (2)	72 (1)
C8	20–36 (2)	29 (1)
C9	<20–52 (3)	<20–41 (2)
B	35–64 (4)	36–50 (4)
P	33–71 (6)	16–65 (3)
H	61 (1)	—
C3bi	55 (1)	—

[a]Number of studies.
[b]Data are derived from the review of Johnston RB, Stroud RM. Complement and host defense against infection. J Pediatr 90:169–179, 1977; from Notarangelo LD, Chirico G, Chiara A, et al. Activity of classical and alternative pathways of complement in preterm and small-for-gestational-age infants. Pediatr Res 18:281–285, 1984; from Davis CA, Vallota EH, Forristal J. Serum complement levels in infancy: age-related changes. Pediatr Res 13:1043–1046, 1979; from Lassiter HA, Watson SW, Seifring ML, Tanner JE. Complement factor 9 deficiency in serum of human neonates. J Infect Dis 166:53–57, 1992; from Wolach B, Dolfin T, Regev R, et al. The development of the complement system after 28 weeks' gestation. Acta Paediatr 86:523–527, 1997; Zilow G, Bruessau J, Hauck W, Zilow EP. Quantitation of complement component C9 deficiency in term and preterm neonates. Clin Exp Immunol 97:52–59, 1994, with permission.

range. As indicated by the data (see Table 2–9), alternative pathway activity (AP_{50}) and alternative pathway components (B, P) are more consistently decreased than classic pathway (CH_{50}) activity and components. A marked deficiency in the terminal complement component C9, which is important for lytic activity against serum-sensitive gram-negative microbes, correlates with poor killing of these organisms by serum from neonates. C9 deficiency of cord blood serum appears to be quantitatively more important in the inefficient killing of *E. coli* K1 than does a deficiency in specific IgG.[850] In addition to this quantitative deficiency, a qualitative difference in the function of C3, which is deposited on microbes but not efficiently cross linked, could contribute to decreased opsonic activity.[851] Preterm infants have a clearer and more consistent decrease in both classic and alternative pathway activity.[852] Mature but small-for-gestational-age infants have CH_{50} and AP_{50} values similar to those for healthy term infants.[853] The concentration of most complement proteins increases postnatally and approaches adult mean values by 6 to 18 months of age.[854]

Fibronectin

Fibronectin, a ubiquitous glycoprotein that plays a key role in cell adhesion and spreading, is important in adherence of neutrophils and monocytes necessary for migration from the blood to the tissues.[855] Fibronectin also has opsonic properties; it appears to enhance binding of certain bacteria, including staphylococci and group B streptococci, to phagocytes.[856–859] This action is inefficient relative to that of antibody or complement, but it may facilitate binding of organisms opsonized with suboptimal amounts of antibody and complement.[856, 858, 860] It may also have a direct phagocytosis-enhancing effect on monocytes and stimulated neutrophils.[861] Fragments of fibronectin also have chemotactic activity for monocytes[862] and fibroblasts and may be important in chronic inflammation and tissue repair.[863] There are two major forms of fibronectin. Most plasma fibronectin is produced by the liver, whereas cellular or tissue fibronectin is produced by multiple cell types, including fibroblasts and endothelial cells.[864, 865]

Plasma fibronectin concentrations are diminished in neonates, particularly premature neonates.[863, 866, 867] Values are further reduced in septic neonates and those with birth asphyxia or respiratory distress syndrome[863, 867]; this also occurs in septic adults. Plasma fibronectin concentrations approach the lower limit of adult norms by 1 year of age.[868]

C-Reactive Protein

As noted earlier, C-reactive protein may act as an opsonin; it appears not to cross the placenta. The capacity of term and preterm neonates to produce this protein, as indicated by serum concentrations, appears to be similar to that of adults.[869] Serum concentrations are frequently higher in healthy neonates than in healthy adults.

Mannan-Binding Lectin, Lipopolysaccharide-Binding Protein, and Surfactant Apoproteins

With rare exception, glycoproteins containing terminal mannose sugars are not found on extracellular proteins in mammals, since they are modified in the endoplasmic reticulum before transport through the Golgi complex. In contrast, terminal mannose, fucose, glucose, and *N*-acetyl glucosamine are found on the surfaces of gram-positive and gram-negative bacteria, mycobacteria, yeast, and certain viruses and parasites.[870] As noted, tissue macrophages contain mannose-fucose receptors, which bind high-mannose–containing carbohydrate polymers, mediate phagocytosis, and trigger the microbicidal processes of these cells. In contrast, neutrophils and blood monocytes lack these mannose-fucose receptors. However, the liver produces a homologous secreted protein, mannan-binding lectin (also referred to as mannose-binding protein), which binds to and opsonizes these microbes for subsequent ingestion by neutrophils and monocytes.[870] Mannan-binding lectin is a member of a family of structurally homologous proteins known as collectins.[870] Mannan-binding lectin is a calcium-dependent lectin that circulates as an 18-mer composed of 3 to 6 identical homotrimeric structural units. It is homologous to C1q and can bind to C1q receptors on mononuclear phagocytes, facilitating phagocytosis of microbes to which it is bound. This protein also enhances activation of complement on the surface of such organisms and is an acute-phase protein, so that its concentration in blood increases in inflammation. Engagement of mannan-binding lectin is impeded by capsular polysaccharides of most virulent gram-negative pathogens. Approximately 5 to 7% of the general population is deficient in mannose-binding lectin, as a result of a polymorphism in codon 54.[871, 872] Although some individuals with this deficiency may experience increased numbers of infections, most do not, suggesting that mannan-binding lectin plays an auxiliary rather than a critical role in host defense. The concentration of mannan-binding lectin in the blood of term neonates is similar to that in adults, but values in preterm neonates are approximately 50% lower.[871, 872] However, there is no evidence to date that the reduced amounts of this protein in preterm neonates contribute to their greater risk of infection.[871]

Surfactant apoproteins A and D are also members of the collectin family. They are synthesized by the type 2 alveolar epithelial cells and Clara cells in the lung epithelium, and by certain other cell types outside the lung.[870, 873] Like mannan-binding lectin, surfactant apoprotein A binds to mannose-glucose polymers found on the surface of gram-positive and gram-negative bacteria, mycobacteria, and yeast. Mice rendered deficient in surfactant apoprotein A are much more susceptible to pulmonary infection with the group B streptococcus and *P. aeruginosa*,[874, 875] and perhaps other microbes. The role of surfactant apoprotein D is uncertain at present. These results raise the possibility that surfactant deficiency may be one factor in the greater risk of the preterm neonate for pulmonary infections.

The LPS-binding protein is also produced by the liver

constitutively and as an acute-phase protein. It facilitates binding of LPS to the high-affinity CD14 receptor, which is expressed by mononuclear phagocytes and to a lesser extent by neutrophils,[740] and presumably thereafter to the Toll proteins.[741, 826] LPS-binding protein and CD14 together lower by orders of magnitude the concentration of LPS needed to prime or activate macrophages and promote binding of gram-negative bacteria by these cells. At present there are no published data regarding the content of LPS-binding protein in the blood of neonates. However, a deficiency in neonatal cord blood of an as yet uncharacterized plasma protein that facilitates the response of monocytes to lipopolysaccharide has been reported.[824]

Opsonic Activity

Opsonic activity of serum measures the ability of serum to enhance the phagocytosis (or phagocytosis and killing) of a particular organism or particle. Some organisms are effective activators of the alternative pathway, whereas others require antibody to activate complement. Thus, depending on the organism or particle tested, opsonic activity reflects specific antibody, mannose-binding lectin, classic or alternative complement pathway activity, or combinations of these.

Not surprisingly, the efficiency with which neonatal sera opsonize organisms is quite variable. For example, although opsonization of S. aureus was normal in neonatal sera in all studies,[702, 706, 876] opsonization of group B streptococci,[706, 877] S. pneumoniae,[876] E. coli,[706, 878] and other gram-negative rods[706, 878] was decreased against certain strains and in some studies but not in others.

Certain studies have examined the basis for decreased opsonization in more detail. Mills and colleagues[879] used a strain of E. coli opsonized efficiently by the alternative pathway. Phagocytosis of this strain when opsonized with neonatal sera was approximately 40% as efficient as when opsonized with adult sera. In contrast, neonatal and adult sera opsonized two strains that required the classic pathway equally well.[879] Similarly, Marodi and co-workers[880] found decreased opsonization by neonatal compared with adult sera of a strain of E. coli that required the alternative pathway but normal opsonization of a strain of S. aureus and of group B streptococci that required the classic pathway. This effect was most apparent at lower serum concentrations. This finding, also noted by others with different organisms,[881] is compatible with the moderate reduction in alternative pathway components described and does not appear to reflect a failure of alternative pathway activation in neonatal sera.[882] Edwards and colleagues[877] and Eads and colleagues[883] have also examined a less common mechanism of opsonization. They used a strain of type Ia group B streptococcus that is opsonized by the classic pathway in the absence of antibody; 8 of 20 neonates had markedly decreased opsonization, which correlated with low values of CH_{50} and complement components in these sera. Together, these studies indicate that a relative immaturity of complement-dependent, antibody-independent opsonization exists in the neonate. This is accentuated in sera from premature neonates and

may be further impaired by the depletion of complement components in some neonates with sepsis.[461]

Chemotactic Factor Generation

Complement activation also generates fluid phase components with chemotactic activity for neutrophils and monocytes, most of which are derived from C5a.[884] Miller[885] found that sera from term neonates generated less chemotactic activity than did adult sera. Because this effect also occurred with antigen-antibody complexes, a complement rather than an antibody deficiency was suggested as the cause. Pahwa and co-workers[678] had similar results. Anderson and associates[884] found that sera from healthy term neonates incubated with type III group B streptococci generated less chemotactic activity than did adult sera even when exogenous IgG was added in amounts similar to those in adult sera. Because each of these studies used sera from term neonates, it is probable that differences would be more striking in sera of preterm neonates,[884] but this remains to be determined. Despite a reduction in the abundance of complement proteins, preterm and term neonates do generate substantial amounts of activated complement products in response to infection in vivo.[886] Lower chemotactic activity of activated neonatal sera may also reflect greater generation of a chemotactic factor inactivator.[887]

Summary

Compared with adults, neonates have moderately diminished alternative complement pathway activity, slightly diminished classic complement pathway activity, and decreased activity of the terminal complement components with the exception of C7. Fibronectin and mannan-binding lectin concentrations are also slightly lower. This effect correlates with diminished ability of neonatal sera to opsonize certain organisms in the absence of antibody or when antibody or serum concentrations are limiting. Generation of complement-derived chemotactic activity is also moderately diminished. These differences are greater in preterm than in term neonates. Preterm neonates may also have compromised lung defenses as a result of reduced abundance of surfactant apoprotein A. Along with the differences in phagocyte function, these factors may contribute to a delayed inflammatory response and impaired bacterial clearance in neonates.

CONDITIONS AFFECTING NEONATAL IMMUNITY

Small-for-Gestational-Age Neonates

The effects of prematurity on immune function are multiple and are described in the relevant sections. Intrauterine growth retardation appears to have a greater effect on T cell function than on other aspects of the immune system.[888] These infants have a smaller thymus,[889] decreased numbers of T cells,[890–892] and diminished delayed hypersensitivity skin test reactions.[891, 892]

Proliferation of lymphocytes in response to mitogens in vitro was diminished in intrauterine growth–retarded infants from India[891, 892] but not in those from Italy or Canada.[893] This may reflect more severe malnutrition or other militating factors in the Indian children. The greater impairment of skin test reactivity than of in vitro reactivity is consistent with the diminished inflammatory response of neonates. It could reflect impairment of migration of leukocytes into inflammatory sites. Abnormal chemotaxis has been observed in malnourished 2-month-old infants[894] but has not been studied in intrauterine growth–retarded neonates. These abnormalities of cellular immunity are present for at least the first year of life.[891, 893] In contrast with these results, the activity of NK cells from neonates with intrauterine growth retardation is greater than that of healthy neonates but still less than that of adults.[892]

Immunoglobulin levels are more variable in intrauterine growth–retarded infants; variability may in part reflect difficulties in determining whether certain infants are growth-retarded, preterm, or both. IgM values have been normal or increased in some growth-retarded infants compared with those in healthy term infants.[892, 894, 895] IgA levels have been normal,[892, 896] and total IgG concentration was normal in studies by Evans and Smith[895] and Bhaskaram and co-workers[892] but low in studies by Yeung and Hobbs[896] and Catty and colleagues.[897] Catty and associates noted that levels of IgG_1 and to a lesser extent of IgG_2 were decreased compared with those of healthy infants.

Glucocorticoids and Other Immunosuppressants

Glucocorticoids have potent effects on inflammation and on the innate and adaptive immune responses.[898-901] At doses produced in response to the stress of infection or injury, or when used in therapeutic amounts, they inhibit inflammation by reducing the production of prostaglandins, leukotrienes, PAF, and proinflammatory cytokines, including TNF and IL-1. Conversely, glucocorticoids either do not inhibit or enhance the production of the anti-inflammatory cytokines IL-10 and TGF-β. Adhesion and migration of leukocytes to sites of infection or injury are also reduced. T cell proliferation and the production of cytokines characteristic of a TH1 response, such as IL-2 and IFN-γ, are inhibited, as are antigen presentation and production of IL-12. Conversely, the production of TH2 cytokines is less impaired. Physiologically these actions of glucocorticoids serve to impede host injury through an excessive immune and inflammatory response. In addition, under basal conditions glucocorticoids appear to contribute to the normal homeostasis of the immune system.

When proliferation and IL-2 and IL-3 production by blood mononuclear cells in response to T cell mitogens are assessed in vitro, cells from term and preterm neonates and infants younger than 9 months of age appear to be more sensitive to the inhibitory effects of therapeutic concentrations of glucocorticoids than cells from adults.[902, 903] Although neonatal but not adult T cells are almost solely naive and enriched in recent thymic emigrants, and such T cells are more sensitive to glucocorticoids than are memory T cells, this difference is probably not the only reason for the difference in sensitivity to glucocorticoids. One possibility is that this is an adaptive change in response to the lower concentrations of circulating hydrocortisone in neonates.[903]

Glucocorticoids are used therapeutically to reduce inflammation or impede an undesired immune response. The not surprising consequence of this is that daily or more frequent administration of these agents in therapeutic amounts predisposes adults to infection in proportion to the dose and duration of therapy. The concentrations of dexamethasone achieved in neonates treated for bronchopulmonary dysplasia ($\sim 0.5 \times 10^{-8}$ M) are sufficient partially to impede proliferation and cytokine production by cells tested in vitro.[902-904] Preterm neonates who experience bronchopulmonary dysplasia and continue to receive corticosteroid therapy beyond the neonatal period have had persistent hypogammaglobulinemia throughout infancy, reduced production of antibody in response to vaccines (i.e., tetanus and diphtheria toxoids), diminished T cell responses to mitogens, and increased risk of respiratory and gastrointestinal tract infection.[905] Correlation among corticosteroid dose, persistently low IgG concentrations, and rate of infections has been noted. This has prompted some to treat these infants with intravenous immune globulin (IGIV). However, these analyses have been retrospective and the use of IGIV has not been studied in a controlled manner, so it is not certain to what extent corticosteroids, rather than (or in addition to) factors leading to prolonged corticosteroid use, contributed to the impairment in immunity. Prolonged glucocorticoid use in older children with severe asthma has been associated with hypogammaglobulinemia, but with specific antibody production intact.[906] This suggests that infants born prematurely (and with chronic lung disease) may be more sensitive to the effects of corticosteroids. In contrast, children who were treated with two doses of hydrocortisone on the first day of life and then evaluated at 5 years of age had normal lymphocyte counts, immunoglobulin and complement levels, and antibody response to immunization. However, they did have a slightly lower (53 versus 69%) percentage of T cells than controls.[907] In general, the results suggest that prolonged daily glucocorticoid treatment in infants with underlying lung disease, at least in those born prematurely, may be associated with an increased risk of infection and substantive immune impairment, whereas short courses are not.

Brief antenatal administration of corticosteroids for the prevention of respiratory distress syndrome does not appear to affect neonatal lymphocyte count, lymphocyte response to mitogens,[908] or capacity to produce immunoglobulin.[909] Neonatal neutrophilia has been observed after maternal corticosteroid treatment.[910] Maternal betamethasone slightly decreased phagocytosis of *Candida* organisms by neonatal neutrophils.[911] However, neither maternal betamethasone nor postnatal dexamethasone substantially impaired chemotaxis by neutrophils from preterm neonates; however, the number of infants studied was small.[912]

One child born to a mother who had had a renal transplant and received azathioprine and prednisone during pregnancy was found to have a unique primary immunodeficiency associated with a defect in T cell signal transduction; however, there is no direct evidence that the defect was due to the treatment.[913] Evidence against such a relationship is provided by other studies, which suggest that minimal or no long-term immunologic effects are derived by infants born to mothers treated with cyclosporine, azathioprine, and prednisone to suppress transplant rejection during pregnancy.[914] However, four children (8 to 10 years of age when evaluated) born to mothers receiving only azathioprine during pregnancy had smaller numbers of naive T cells, perhaps reflecting decreased thymic output. Larger studies are needed to determine the degree to which immune function of children born to mothers receiving nonsteroidal immunosuppressants is impaired in the neonatal period and at later stages of life.

Hyperbilirubinemia

Infants with hyperbilirubinemia of diverse causes have impairment of several immune functions compared with healthy neonates.[915] Decreased neutrophil microbicidal activity, lymphocyte proliferation to phytohemagglutinin,[916] and antibody response to subsequent immunization with diphtheria, pertussis, and tetanus but not to naturally encountered E. coli antigens[917] have been noted. However, whether these findings were a direct effect of bilirubin or related to factors leading to hyperbilirubinemia has not been determined. Bilirubin inhibits complement function in vitro; that effect may account for decreased complement-dependent serum bactericidal activity in neonates with hyperbilirubinemia. Bilirubin was found to inhibit lymphocyte proliferation in a study by Rola-Pleszcynski and colleagues.[918] Additional studies with humans and experimental animals suggest that bilirubin may impair T cell function.[919] However, a direct effect of hyperbilirubinemia on infection-related morbidity rate has not been shown.

Effects of Maternal Drug Abuse

The fetal alcohol syndrome has been associated with a decreased percentage of T cells, diminished T cell responses to mitogens, and reduced hypersensitivity responses when compared with responses of healthy or intrauterine growth–retarded controls.[920] This may persist until the child is 10 years of age and has been suggested to contribute to an increased risk of subsequent infections. Animal models support the notion that fetal alcohol exposure leads to impaired T cell function.[921] In contrast, neonates born to mothers who smoked had normal or increased T cell mitogen and immunoglobulin levels, neutrophil mobility, and T cell numbers compared with those of neonates of nonsmokers.[922]

Maternal intravenous drug abuse (~50% heroin and 50% cocaine or amphetamines) was associated with a diminished absolute lymphocyte count, percentage of CD4$^+$ cells (presumably mostly T cells), and prolifera-

tion to phytohemagglutinin by blood mononuclear cells at the time of birth in one study of 17 infants.[923] However, two European multicenter studies with much larger patient bases found no association between maternal drug abuse and lymphocyte or CD4 numbers in populations at risk for HIV infection.[924, 925] In utero cocaine exposure may cause a modest reduction in proliferative responses, but the effect is small in magnitude, transient, and of doubtful biologic significance.[926]

Intravenous Lipid Emulsions

Administration of intravenous lipid emulsions to premature or ill neonates is associated with an increased risk of colonization and infection with *Pityrosporon orbiculare*. Data suggest that this relates directly to the ability of high concentrations of lipid to support the growth of this fungus. Although some studies suggest that lipid emulsions may impair certain immune functions, others do not.[927–933] In some of the studies the effects observed may be an artifact[930] or may represent effects of concentrations higher than those observed in vivo.

HOST DEFENSE AGAINST SPECIFIC CLASSES OF NEONATAL PATHOGENS

In general terms, there are four major classes of neonatal pathogens as defined by the immune mechanisms mediating protection: pyogenic bacteria, fungi, viruses, and nonviral intracellular pathogens. This section describes the interaction of the previously discussed immune mechanisms believed to be important in resistance to prototypical pathogens representative of pyogenic bacteria, viruses, and nonviral intracellular pathogens. Developmental differences in immune mechanisms that predispose the neonate to infection are discussed, as are potential avenues for immunologic intervention. Additional detail regarding the virulence determinants of specific microbes and certain aspects of host defense is provided in the chapters on the specific organisms. Host defense mechanisms for the response to fungal pathogens and their adequacy in the human neonate have been reviewed.[829]

Pyogenic Bacteria—Group B Streptococci

OVERVIEW OF HOST DEFENSE MECHANISMS

In most cases, infection of the neonate with group B streptococci (GBS) likely involves adherence to and subsequent invasion through the respiratory mucosa. Initial colonization is influenced by the organism's ability to adhere to epithelial cells, through an as yet uncharacterized receptor(s). Physical disruption of mucosa may not be required for GBS invasion, as GBS can enter into the cytoplasm of cultured respiratory epithelial cells via an actin microfilament–dependent process.[934] Specific secretory IgA antibody and fibronectin may decrease bacterial adherence to the mucosa.[935, 936] β defensins are potent antimicrobial peptides expressed by epithelial cells of the tongue and airways of humans and other mammals.[722, 937, 938] Defensins may attenuate the growth or invasion of GBS in these sites, though this effect remains to be tested directly.

Phagocytes and opsonins are the critical elements of defense against invasive GBS infection. Antibody and complement are required to opsonize bacteria for phagocytosis and do not kill GBS in the absence of phagocytes, in contrast to certain normally avirulent strains of E. coli and other gram-negative bacteria that are lysed by antibody and complement alone; such strains are usually incapable of causing invasive infections but may do so in neonates.[850] GBS and strains of E. coli that cause serious neonatal infections possess type-specific capsular polysaccharide, which generally prevents direct activation of the alternative complement pathway at their surface, thus protecting them from opsonization for phagocytosis and from bacteriolysis.[461, 939]

Optimal opsonization of type III GBS, the strain best studied, requires both type-specific IgM or IgG antibody and complement.[461] This likely reflects the fact that type III capsule confers resistance of GBS to opsonophagocytic killing by the alternative complement pathway: Among type III GBS strains there is an inverse correlation between the degree of encapsulation and the deposition of C3b on the bacteria by the alternative pathway,[940] although some studies have not found an effect of capsule on complement deposition.[941] This latter result notwithstanding, deposition of C3b and C3bi on the bacteria is enhanced by the presence of type-specific anticapsular antibody for all types of GBS (Ia, Ib/c, II [with or without c protein], and III).[942] Consistent with these findings, susceptibility to infection with type III GBS strain is essentially limited to infants lacking type-specific antibody (see Chapter 26), and complement contributes to protection against type III GBS in animal models.[943] IgG-coated and, in the lung, surfactant apoprotein A–coated bacteria are bound and ingested by phagocytes,[874] and phagocytosis is augmented by C3b and C3bi. IgM-coated bacteria are not bound or ingested in the absence of C3b or C3bi, but neutrophils and activated macrophages can phagocytose IgM- and C3b-coated bacteria via the C3b receptors.[944] Fibronectin facilitates binding and ingestion of GBS by phagocytes but only in the presence of antibody and complement[856, 858, 860]; the phagocyte respiratory burst and cytoskeletal reorganization that follow GBS ingestion are also enhanced in this context.[945] In conjunction with monoclonal anti-GBS antibodies of the IgG, IgM, and, surprisingly, the IgA isotypes, fibronectin protects neonatal rats from GBS infection.[856]

Opsonized bacteria in small numbers may be effectively cleared by macrophages, which are the resident tissue phagocytes.[805, 946] If the bacteria are not cleared, circulating phagocytes, primarily neutrophils, are recruited to the site by chemotactic factors, including the complement fragment C5a and products released by local macrophages, such as leukotrienes, chemokines (e.g., IL-8), and bacterially derived components, such as N-formyl-methyl peptides.[947–949] Circulating monocytes incubated with GBS opsonized with type-specific antibody and complement release LTB_4 and IL-8, both of which contribute to the chemoattraction of neutrophils.[830] Many strains of GBS contain an enzyme, C5a-ase, that degrades C5a and may thereby impede the recruitment of phagocytes to sites of infection.[950] However, the importance of C5a-ase in GBS virulence has not been established.

The neutrophil response requires that the bone marrow produce and release sufficient numbers into the circulation. Receptors on neutrophils bind chemotactic factors, thereby enhancing the avidity and abundance of β_2 integrins, allowing these cells to bind firmly to the vascular endothelium.[629] Neutrophils migrate through the vascular endothelium to the site of infection, where they bind and ingest bacteria opsonized with IgG and C3b or C3bi.[663, 664] Adhesion of neutrophils to the endothelium is enhanced by TNF and IL-1 produced by monocytes and macrophages in response to microbial products. The ingested bacteria are exposed to a variety of potentially microbicidal products (discussed earlier). Although streptococci generate hydrogen peroxide, it appears that neutrophils must generate oxygen metabolites to kill these bacteria efficiently. Non–oxygen-dependent microbicidal factors, including acid and cationic proteins, may also contribute to killing of bacteria by neutrophils. IL-12 facilitates IFN-γ production, and both enhance the resistance of neonatal rats to GBS infection.[951, 952] The mechanism by which IFN-γ enhances resistance is not known, but it may be due in part to enhanced phagocyte microbicidal activity. Whether IFN-γ contributes to protection in humans is not known.

In cases in which GBS is not cleared from the circulation, it may elicit a host response leading to septic shock. Septic shock is the most frequent cause of death due to systemic GBS infection in neonates. In gram-negative bacteria, such as E. coli, endotoxin-mediated production of proinflammatory cytokines, such as TNF, IL-1, and IL-6, by mononuclear phagocytes appears to play a critical role in the pathogenesis of septic shock. The importance of TNF in the pathogenesis of GBS is suggested by the finding of TNF in the circulation of type III GBS–infected human neonates,[953] and in neonatal piglets and rats.[954, 955] Both encapsulated and unencapsulated type III GBS can induce TNF production by human monocytes in vitro,[953] and exogenous fibronectin synergizes with GBS in this induction.[956] Like other gram-positive bacteria, GBS lacks endotoxin, but lipoteichoic acid and polysaccharides from GBS stimulate the release of TNF, IL-1, and IL-6 by blood monocytes.[957] Exotoxins produced by GBS may also induce mononuclear phagocytes to produce TNF and other proinflammatory cytokines.[958] Neutralization of TNF with antiserum significantly enhances survival in animal models,[955] even when begun 12 hours after GBS inoculation.[959] Similarly, administration of IL-10, which inhibits production of TNF and other proinflammatory cytokines, enhances survival.[960]

NEONATAL DEFENSES

Of the host factors that determine risk, the absence of passively derived maternal antibody appears to be the most critical, because, with rare exceptions,[961] neonatal GBS infection occurs only in infants who lack specific antibody.[962-964] Before 32 weeks' gestation, fetal IgG concentrations are less than 50% of maternal values; at term, they are usually somewhat greater than those of the mother.[896] Despite this, most studies have demonstrated that the amount of GBS type III–specific antibody in cord sera is slightly less than that in maternal sera.[961, 965] In infants born before 34 weeks' gestation the specific antibody titer is often markedly reduced compared with that of the maternal antibody titer.[966] Therefore, preterm neonates younger than 34 weeks of gestation may lack antibody even when maternal sera contain protective amounts of IgG antibody. Even when infected, most neonates do not make detectable type-specific antibody during the first month after infection; a few transiently synthesize IgM but not IgG antibody.[962] Type III–specific IgM antibodies are found by 3 months of age in most normal neonates as well as in those who have been infected with type III GBS.[967, 968] However, it is not clear that these antibodies require the exposure of normal infants to type III GBS; they could result, at least in part, from a cross reactive immune response to another source of antigens to which the infant is exposed postnatally. Although lack of type-specific antibody is an important risk factor, disease develops in less than 10% of infants who lack specific antibody and who are born to mothers colonized with GBS type III.[969] Among neonates lacking type-specific antibody, the risk for development of GBS disease appears to be greater in those born to mothers with high-density genital tract colonization or GBS amnionitis and also may vary with the virulence of the strain. As noted, antibody is required for opsonization of organisms that do not spontaneously activate complement; these include most strains of type III GBS and many strains of types I and II GBS. It is not surprising that the efficiency with which neonatal sera opsonize GBS (and other bacteria) is variable.[706, 878] This reflects variability in the amounts of passively derived type-specific antibody and variability in alternative[879] and, to a lesser extent, classic[877] complement pathway activity. For example, Marodi and co-workers[880] found that in the presence of type-specific antibody, neonatal sera activated complement and opsonized GBS as well as sera from adults, indicating normal opsonization via the classic complement pathway. This finding has been substantiated by other investigators using different test organisms[881] and is compatible with the greater reduction in neonates of alternative pathway as compared with classic pathway complement components.[854, 970] Nonetheless, classic pathway–dependent opsonization may be impaired in neonates under some conditions. For example, the classic pathway mediates antibody-independent opsonization of certain strains of type Ia GBS, perhaps acting through a mannan-binding lectin-dependent mechanism (a hypothesis that has not been tested directly), and this activity is reduced in many neonates.[877, 883] Complement-mediated opsonization may be further impaired by the depletion of complement components in some neonates with sepsis.

Besides these factors, overall deficits in mucosal defenses and the number and function of phagocytes con-

tribute to the neonate's, and in particular the premature neonate's, susceptibility to colonization and to invasive infection. Greater adherence of pathogenic type III group B streptococci to mucosal epithelial cells of neonates, particularly ill neonates, may facilitate colonization.[971, 972] The mechanism for this difference has not been determined. The lack of secretory IgA and decreased fibronectin in the secretions of neonates also may contribute to susceptibility. The paucity of alveolar macrophages in the lungs of term and particularly preterm neonates at the time of birth and the diminished rates of phagocytosis and killing of bacteria by these cells may allow greater microbial replication by those bacteria entering through the respiratory tract, as GBS may. Because surfactant apoprotein A is an important lung opsonin for GBS, the reduced amounts of this protein in the lungs of preterm neonates with hyaline membrane disease may predispose them to infection. Limited generation of chemotactic factors may be a factor in a delayed recruitment of neutrophils along with the well-established deficit in the ability of neonatal polymorphonuclear neutrophils to respond appropriately to chemotactic stimuli in vitro, as indicated by consistently observed abnormalities in adherence, aggregation, deformability, and migration. Once at the site of infection, neutrophils may kill bacteria less efficiently because of limited amounts of opsonins, because the local bacterial density has reached high levels as a result of a delayed influx of neutrophils, or because the microbicidal activity of neutrophils from certain neonates is decreased. Rapidly progressive infection may then deplete the limited marrow neutrophil reserve to compound the problem.

OVERVIEW OF IMMUNOLOGIC INTERVENTIONS FOR NEONATAL GROUP B STREPTOCOCCAL SEPSIS

As summarized in the preceding section, the principal host defense deficits in the neonate that predispose to infections with GBS and other pyogenic pathogens appear to be a deficiency of opsonins, particularly protective antibodies, and a limited capacity to increase neutrophil production and mobilize neutrophils to sites of infection. Attempts have been made to address both of these deficits through immunologic interventions. However, evidence supporting the routine use of any form of immunologic augmentation for prevention or as an adjunct to antimicrobial therapy for infections in the neonate is currently lacking.

PREVENTION

Selective intrapartum chemoprophylaxis with penicillin or ampicillin has proved useful in reducing the rate of early onset disease due to GBS by preventing colonization of at-risk neonates. However, both the screening-based (preferred) and risk-factor–based approaches are imperfect, and the administration of intrapartum antibiotics within 4 hours of delivery cannot prevent all neonatal disease. A more appealing strategy would be to ensure that mothers have adequate amounts of IgG anti-

GBS antibodies to protect their infants passively. Initial results of immunization of pregnant women with purified GBS type III polysaccharide were encouraging but limited by a relatively low response rate of 60%. The development of GBS polysaccharide-protein conjugate vaccines may surmount this problem. Initial results of phase 1 and 2 clinical studies using these candidate vaccines in healthy nonpregnant women showed improved immunogenicity compared with that of the earlier vaccines,[973] and further studies are in progress.

Five prospective studies have evaluated the use of IGIV to prevent nosocomial or late-onset pyogenic infections in premature neonates, a group at increased risk of infection.[974, 975] Only one study has shown a reduction in the frequency of infections,[976] and no study has shown a reduction in mortality rate or duration of hospitalization.[974, 976–980] Thus, the preponderance of the evidence suggests that IGIV administered to low-birth-weight infants in an attempt to prevent subsequent nosocomial infection is not effective. Whether modifications in patient selection or in the nature of the IGIV preparation would improve efficacy is not known. Nonetheless, on the basis of the currently available data, routine administration of IGIV to low-birth-weight infants in an attempt to prevent subsequent late-onset or nosocomial infection is not justified.

The recombinant colony-stimulating factors G-CSF and GM-CSF augment granulocyte production and function in neonatal animals and provide some protection against challenge with pyogenic bacteria including GBS. Administration of recombinant G-CSF and GM-CSF to nonseptic, non-neutropenic human neonates has been well tolerated and resulted in increased levels of circulating neutrophils and augmentation of the neutrophil storage pool.[723] Two studies have shown that G-CSF administration to neutropenic low-birth-weight infants born to mothers with pre-eclampsia rapidly increases the circulating neutrophil counts,[981] presumably as a result of increased release of postmitotic neutrophils from the bone marrow storage pool.[982] In a preliminary report one group found that prophylactic administration of recombinant G-CSF to neutropenic low-birth-weight infants born to mothers with pre-eclampsia led to a reduction in proven bacterial infections in these patients.[983] In contrast, another study found that prophylactic administration of recombinant GM-CSF to very-low-birth-weight (less than 1000 g) neonates during the first 28 days of life, although well tolerated, was not associated with a reduction in nosocomial infections.[723] Additional studies will be required before either prophylactic G- or GM-CSF therapy can be generally recommended. In contrast with its beneficial effect on pre-eclampsia-associated neonatal neutropenia, G-CSF has not been useful in neonates with alloimmune neutropenia.[984]

ADJUNCT THERAPY OF PYOGENIC INFECTIONS—PASSIVE ANTIBODY

In some early studies, IGIV appeared to be efficacious in animal models of GBS and E. coli K1 infection. However, because very high doses of IGIV were found to impede resistance to GBS in some animal models of infection, perhaps through the blockade of mononuclear phagocyte Fc receptors, trials of IGIV as adjunct therapy in neonatal sepsis have been cautiously pursued.[975] Nevertheless, three pilot studies in humans, each of which evaluated a different population of patients and each of which used a different preparation of IGIV or, in one study, a preparation of mixed immune globulins, concluded that mortality rate was reduced. However, because of the small numbers of neonates studied, lack of controls, or absence of a prospective design, these studies do not provide sufficient information to form a firm conclusion regarding efficacy.[974, 985] There was no evidence of toxicity of the IGIV in these or in two more recent prospective, controlled studies.[980, 986] In one of these studies, improvement in neutrophil counts, perhaps reflecting improved mobilization of storage pools, and opsonic capacity was observed in IGIV-treated but not albumin placebo–treated neonates with clinical or proven sepsis[986]; there were no deaths in either group. In the study by Weisman and co-workers,[980] which also assessed prophylactic efficacy (described previously), all premature neonates were randomly assigned to receive IGIV selected for high titers of antibody to GBS or albumin placebo within 12 hours of birth. Although no efficacy in prevention of late-onset infection was found, IGIV may have been beneficial among the 31 patients with early-onset sepsis, which was most commonly due to GBS. Among these 31, 5 of 16 placebo recipients died within the first 7 days of life, in contrast with none of 14 IGIV-treated neonates, a statistically significant difference. However, 2 late deaths occurred in the IGIV group, so that survival at 8 weeks of age did not differ in the two groups, although the trend still favored the IGIV group. The treatment arm of the study was terminated early, because the monitoring group concluded that the prophylactic arm of the trial did not show efficacy of IGIV. Another study performed in Saudi Arabia suggested benefit from therapeutic administration of an IgM-containing immunoglobulin preparation not available in the United States, but this study did not include a randomized control group.[987] At the present time data are insufficient to recommend the use of IGIV for adjunct therapy of neonatal sepsis. Further study of this approach, and of the long-term effects of neonatal IGIV therapy on subsequent production of antibody in infants, is warranted.

An alternative to the use of IVIG may be the use of hyperimmune GBS immunoglobulin and monoclonal antibody preparations. Hyperimmune GBS IGIV administered before infectious challenge significantly reduced the mortality rate of newborn rhesus monkeys infected with GBS by the intragastric route; however, the control group in this experiment received neither conventional IGIV nor antibiotic therapy.[988] Although preliminary studies with GBS IGIV suggested that it is well tolerated by neonates with suspected neonatal sepsis,[988] there have been no published reports of its efficacy in a controlled trial. Murine monoclonal antibodies to GBS provide protection in animal models[989–991] and have been considered for human therapy. Potential advantages of this approach include the uniformity of the preparation and the prevention of nonspecific immunosuppressant effects that results from the administration of large doses of IGIV. However, because antibodies have developed in response to other murine monoclonal antibody preparations, such as OKT3, human or humanized monoclonal antibodies against GBS have been developed. In the case of a human monoclonal antibody directed against the GBS group carbohydrate, differences in efficacy of antibodies with identical antigen-binding domains have been observed in which the Fc (constant region) domain was either IgM or IgG$_1$; the IgM isotype of this GBS monoclonal antibody appears to be more effective than the IgG isotype in opsonophagocytosis assays and in protection of neonatal rats from GBS infectious challenge with several capsular serotypes, presumably because of its higher valency. On the basis of studies in neonatal macaques, this antibody also appears to be safe.[992–994] Clinical trials with such preparations have yet to be undertaken.

ADJUNCT THERAPY OF PYOGENIC INFECTIONS—NEUTROPHIL TRANSFUSIONS

Neutrophil transfusions enhance survival rate in certain animal models of neonatal sepsis, but the clinical efficacy of neutrophil transfusion in septic human neonates is uncertain. Three of five controlled studies have shown statistically significant improvement in survival rate of neonates receiving granulocyte transfusions compared with those not receiving this therapy.[995–1001] However, small sample size and variable entry criteria for treated patients and controls, methods of neutrophil preparation, numbers of neutrophils per transfusion, numbers of transfusions, and bacterial pathogens causing disease preclude a meaningful meta-analysis of these studies.[995] Though neutrophil storage pool depletion has been used as a selection criterion for neonates for whom transfusion may be beneficial, the difficulty in ascertainment of neutrophil storage pool size in clinical practice and the failure of this parameter to predict outcome in some studies make this measure an imperfect one in clinical practice. The utility of neutrophil transfusions is further compromised by the difficulty in obtaining neutrophils in a timely fashion and the potential complications of transfusions, including the risk of infection. In the absence of additional clinical data, neutrophil transfusions cannot be recommended as routine therapy for neonates with suspected or proven overwhelming sepsis.

ADJUNCT THERAPY OF PYOGENIC INFECTIONS—COLONY-STIMULATING FACTORS

Another approach to augmenting neutrophil numbers, function, or both is the administration of recombinant G-CSF or GM-CSF. Both of these CSFs have shown benefit as adjunct therapy for established pyogenic infections in experimental animals.[723] In initial studies, administration of G-CSF to human neonates ranging from 26 to 40 weeks of gestation with presumed early-onset sepsis significantly increased the numbers of circulating neutrophils, bone marrow neutrophil storage pool size,

and neutrophil expression of CR3 receptors (CD11b-CD18) without short- or long-term adverse effects.[1002–1004] Further, several anecdotal reports and one case-control study[1005] suggested that G-CSF might be beneficial in cases of bacterial sepsis in premature neonates with neutropenia. However, the first randomized, placebo-controlled, double-blinded trial of recombinant G-CSF in neutropenic neonates with clinical signs of early-onset sepsis not only did not demonstrate an increase in circulating neutrophils in the neonates receiving G-CSF, but also found no difference in severity of illness, morbidity rate, or mortality rate between the two groups.[1006] Additional randomized, controlled trials of recombinant G-CSF are required to evaluate this strategy fully, but the use of G- or GM-CSF in septic neonates cannot be recommended at present.

Viruses

The neonate experiences more severe or rapidly progressive infection with certain viruses, most notably those due to HSV, CMV, and HIV, and enteroviruses. Because viruses replicate intracellularly, it is not surprising that mechanisms that act to control or block infection within cells, spread of virus from cell to cell, or both are critical for effective host defense. With the exception of the enteroviruses, the most important components of the immune response are cellular. This discussion focuses on defenses operative against HSV-1 and HSV-2 (referred to collectively as HSV), mentioning, where relevant, information on CMV, another herpesvirus family member.

The antiviral immune response can generally be divided into an early non–antigen-specific phase (in HSV infection, the first 5 to 7 days) and a later antigen-specific phase.[757, 1007] In the early phase, infection may either be contained by innate defenses or disseminate widely, whereas in the later phase, antigen-specific immunity acts to eliminate active infection. This late-phase response results either in the eradication of virus or the cessation of viral replication and establishment of latency. Of the viruses mentioned, eradication is achieved in most individuals only in the case of enterovirus infection. In the others, the antigen-specific immune system, and particularly T cells, appears to play an important role in the maintenance of viral latency, as indicated by the frequency of recurrent and severe infections with HSV and CMV in patients with congenital or acquired immune deficiency. In the case of HSV infection, the tempo of the disease is initially acute, so that the early containment phase of the response may be relatively more important than it is in the less rapidly progressive infection with CMV. In either case, the tempo with which antigen-specific T cell–mediated immunity develops is an important determinant of the outcome. An untimely delay in the development of an effective T cell response in the neonate compared with the adult appears to be a major factor in the ability of HSV and CMV to produce severe or fatal disease in this age group.

INNATE IMMUNITY

The importance of mononuclear phagocytes in protection against HSV is suggested by the increased severity of infection in mice treated with agents that deplete these cells, such as silica or antimacrophage sera.[1008] Mononuclear phagocytes are an important source of cytokines during the early phase of infection with murine CMV.[1009, 1010] Macrophages, NK cells, and IFN-α/β appear to be the key components of innate defense to HSV. Mononuclear phagocytes, when activated, become capable of mediating several distinct antiviral activities. Viral replication within adjacent nonphagocytic cells is suppressed by an IFN-α/β independent mechanism.[1011] Mononuclear phagocytes have also been shown to lyse virally infected cell directly, at least in vitro,[1012] but the importance of this process to the control of infection in vivo has yet to be established. Infected macrophages and dendritic cells produce multiple cytokines, including IFN-α/β, IL-1, TNF, chemokines, and perhaps IL-12; whether HSV induces production of IL-15, a cytokine that enhances NK and T cell function, is not known.[1013, 1014] Most IFN-α is produced by dendritic cells and mononuclear phagocytes,[1015] whereas IFN-β is produced by fibroblasts and other epithelial cell types; substantial amounts of these IFNs are found in the tissues of HSV-infected animals and humans.[1016, 1017]

Studies in which the biologic activity of cytokines is inhibited in vivo by antibody treatment, in which cytokines are administered therapeutically, or in which both occur suggest that IFN-α/β and IL-12 limit the early phase of infection with HSV and murine CMV[1009, 1018] and that TNF may also contribute to this antiviral effect, at least in mice lacking T and NK cells.[1009] As discussed later, these three cytokines have important effects on NK cell–mediated antiviral immunity and also appear to have antiviral effects that are independent of NK cells.[1009] IFN-α/β and TNF may act in part by directly inducing an antiviral state in cells.[1019] TNF also increases class II MHC expression on mononuclear phagocytes via an autocrine or paracrine mechanism and helps recruit these cells to sites of viral infection.[1020] Each of these cytokines can enhance NK cell cytotoxicity in vitro. However, in mice infected with murine CMV, endogenously produced IFN-α/β rather than IL-12 or TNF accounts for most enhanced NK cell–mediated cytotoxicity and proliferation[1009]; in contrast, the production of IFN-γ by NK cells in vivo during the early phase of infection requires IL-12 and is enhanced by TNF but not by IFN-α/β. Chemokines secreted by mononuclear phagocytes and dendritic cells are likely to play an important role in the recruitment of NK cells and subsequently T cells to sites of infection. HSV-1 infection of mice induces the expression of a number of β-chemokines in the cornea and trigeminal ganglia.[1021, 1022] However, human CMV encodes a protein that sequesters β-chemokines, which may impede the immune response to this infection.[1023] The overall importance and role of particular chemokines in the host response to HSV and other herpesviruses remain to be defined.

NK cells appear critical for the initial control of herpesvirus infections in humans. Patients lacking NK cells have severe primary herpesvirus infections, including with HSV, CMV, and VZV; although the initial disease is severe, these patients are able eventually to clear these viruses, presumably by T cell–mediated immunity (D Lewis, unpublished data).[544] It is interesting that these patients do not appear to be markedly susceptible to viruses other than herpesvirus. Murine models of HSV and CMV infection also support the importance of NK cells in the early control of infection.[1024–1026] As discussed in the section Natural Killer Cells, the control of viral infection by NK cells may be mediated by (1) direct lysis of virally infected cells, (2) lysis of virally infected cells via ADCC, and (3) production of proinflammatory cytokines that increase intrinsic antiviral resistance (e.g., IFN-α/β) and promote the development of effective antigen-specific T cell immunity (e.g., IFN-γ). IFN-α/β and IFN-γ may facilitate the subsequent development of an effective CD8 T cell response to these infections, through the enhancement of MHC class I and TAP expression (discussed later). However, HSV, CMV, and other human herpesviruses express proteins (discussed later) that block MHC class I or TAP expression and function.[57] However, NK cells can lyse HSV- and CMV-infected cells with reduced class I MHC expression, which would not be recognized and lysed by CD8 T cells. As discussed in the Natural Killer Cells section, engagement of MHC class I by receptors on the NK cell surface normally provides an inhibitory signal blocking NK cell activation. Thus, reduced or absent MHC class I on the cell surface allows NK cells to be activated to produce cytokines and to lyse infected target cells. Notably, human CMV encodes a protein that acts as a surrogate class I MHC to impede NK cell–mediated lysis, which may impede recognition of infected cells by NK cells.[57] The inhibitory effects of HSV and CMV on class I MHC expression can be overcome to a substantial extent by IFN-α.[57] IFN-γ produced by NK cells also increases class II MHC expression on mononuclear phagocytes and dendritic cells,[1020] an effect that facilitates antigen presentation to CD4 T cells. IFN-γ produced by NK cells during the initiation of the antigen-specific immune response may also favor the development of T cells with an enriched capacity to secrete TH1-type cytokines (IL-2, IFN-γ, and lymphotoxin-α),[1027] which help to limit viral infection. However, human CMV may counter the actions of IFN-γ by inhibiting signal transduction through its receptor[1028]; but the extent to which this impedes the effects of IFN-γ in vivo is not known. Nonetheless, NK cells may contribute to both the innate and antigen-specific phases of host defense against herpesvirus infections and do so by multiple mechanisms.

ANTIGEN-SPECIFIC IMMUNITY

Antigen-specific T cell and B cell responses are first detected 5 to 7 days after the onset of HSV infection in adult humans, and the peak response is achieved approximately 3 weeks after primary infection with HSV.[331, 1029, 1030] In most individuals, antigen-specific immunity does not eradicate infection but does terminate active viral replication and the acute infection. T cells play the critical role in resolution of active HSV infection and maintenance of viral latency.[1030–1032] The importance of T cells in the control of HSV and other herpesvirus infections is indicated by the increased susceptibility of hosts with quantitative (late HIV infection) or qualitative defects in T cells, antigen presentation (Wiskott-Aldrich syndrome), or both. Both CD4 and CD8 T cells appear to contribute to clearance of HSV after acute infection in mice, acting in part through the production of IFN-γ, whereas B cells are not able to provide protection in the absence of T cells.[1030–1038] The relative importance of CD4 and CD8 T cells and the mechanisms by which they contribute to the control of HSV infection in humans are uncertain.

Two gene products of HSV block presentation of viral proteins by class I MHC: the viral host shutoff protein, which is present in the viral particle, and the immediate-early protein ICP47, which is expressed early after infection of the host cell and binds to human TAP. The ICP47-TAP interaction blocks loading of peptides on class I MHC and transport of class I MHC to the cell surface.[1039–1042] The net effect of these proteins is to mask the recognition of HSV-infected cells by CD8 T cells. The importance of these immune evasion strategies in the pathogenicity of HSV and CMV has not yet been formally tested in vivo. Notably, NK cells and HSV antigen–specific CD4 T cells are detected earlier than antigen-specific CD8 T cells in lesions of adult humans with recurrent HSV-2 disease.[1043] This has led to the proposal that IFN-γ produced by infiltrating NK and CD4 T cells overrides the inhibitory effects of ICP47 on class I MHC expression,[1041, 1044] thereby allowing the subsequent eradication of virus by CD8 T cells, which increase in lesions around the time of viral clearance.[1031, 1043] This possibility is supported by the finding that in patients with acquired immunodeficiency syndrome (AIDS), a lower frequency of circulating HSV antigen–specific CD8 CTL precursors is associated with more frequent and severe recurrences of genital disease.[1045] These correlative data suggest that CD8 T cells may play an important role in the clearance of HSV in humans, at least from recurrent mucocutaneous lesions. However, the validity of this hypothesis and its applicability to acute infection have not been formally tested. The ability to address this question through the use of murine models of HSV infection is partly compromised by the fact that HSV ICP47 inhibits murine TAP poorly[1039, 1042]; that limitation may explain the greater ease with which anti-HSV CD8 CTLs have been detected in mice compared with humans.[1031, 1032, 1043, 1046–1048] Even so, studies in the mouse suggest that CD4 T cells may play the most critical role in protection,[1034] although CD8 T cells contribute, particularly in the nervous system.[1033, 1049–1051] The inhibitory effects of ICP47 on MHC class I–mediated antigen presentation are almost certainly greater in the human nervous system than in that of the mouse. Thus, either CD8 T cells are likely to contribute less to protection in humans than in mice or IFN-γ produced by NK cells and CD4 T cells is likely to play a critical role in overriding the effects of the viral host shutoff protein and ICP47 on class I MHC expression and antigen presentation to CD8 T cells.

CMV also contains proteins that block class I MHC expression.[57] Thus, the finding that the therapeutic administration of donor-derived anti-CMV CD8 CTL provides considerable protection of bone marrow transplant recipients against disease due to CMV supports the notion that CD8 CTL plays a role in host defense against herpesviruses despite viral-mediated inhibition of class I MHC expression.

CD4 T cells appear to play a key role in protection from HSV. The following are likely to be important mechanisms, reflecting the central and diverse roles of CD4 T cells in mediating and regulating antigen-specific immunity: (1) CD4 T cells may directly inhibit viral replication through the production of IFN-γ, TNF, and CD40 ligand, each of which has antiviral activity against HSV,[1033, 1052] as discussed previously. (2) CD4 T cells appear to be required for the generation and survival of anti-HSV effector CD8 CTL in mice.[1038, 1053, 1054] This effect may be mediated in part by the ability of CD4 T cells to prime dendritic cells (and perhaps other antigen-presenting cells) through CD40 ligand.[1055, 1056] Consistent with this, CD4 T cells are not required for the development of CD8 CTL if primed dendritic cells are used as the source of APCs.[1053] The need for CD4 T cell help suggests that HSV does not efficiently prime dendritic cells. Perhaps consistent with this, HSV infection of dendritic cells from adult humans stimulates them to secrete IFN-α and IL-1, but not to secrete IL-12 or express increased amounts of CD80 or CD86.[1013] Production of IL-2 by CD4 T cells may also contribute to the expansion and differentiation of CTL. Finally, as discussed, IFN-γ produced by CD4 T cells may play a central role in overriding HSV ICP47–mediated class I MHC inhibition.[1031, 1041] (3) CD4 T cells may lyse cells expressing viral peptides bound to class II MHC.[1057] Such cytotoxic CD4 T cells have been frequently isolated from humans after infection with HSV and appear to constitute about 30% of the cytotoxic T cells in murine HSV infection.[1043, 1058] Human CD4 cytotoxic cells can recognize peptides derived from viral glycoproteins found in the HSV lipid envelope,[1032, 1059, 1060] and it is likely that these viral glycoproteins enter into the class II antigen-processing endocytic pathway by first fusing with the host cell membrane. Although class II MHC is normally expressed only by APCs, such as B cells, mononuclear phagocytes, and dendritic cells, a wide variety of cell types can express class II MHC and, in most cases, present antigen, after exposure to IFN-γ as well as to GM-CSF or TNF (see the section Basic Aspects of Antigen Presentation). Whether CD4 CTL is essential in the control of HSV infection or primarily plays an immunoregulatory role in this disease remains to be determined.[1032, 1045] In any case, because IFN-γ may play a critical role in inducing or enhancing class I and class II MHC expression by cells infected by HSV and CMV, it is likely to play an important role in human host defenses against these viruses that may not be fully apparent from studies in mice.

Gamma-delta T cells, particularly those bearing $V_\gamma 2$-$V_\delta 2$ T cell receptors, obtained from HSV seropositive donors can lyse HSV-infected cells in a non–MHC–restricted manner.[284] The ligands on the target cells that activate these T cells via their TCR remain to be defined but do not appear to be restricted by class I or class II MHC molecules. Murine experiments suggest that γδ

T cells may also contribute to defense of the host against HSV, particularly if αβ T cell function is compromised.[275] Whether this process also applies to humans is unknown.

Antibody does not appear to play an essential role in the control of most viral infection, including that by herpesviruses, because patients with X-linked agammaglobulinemia, who lack mature B cells and antibody production, are not generally susceptible to these pathogens. A notable exception are enteroviral infections, in which agammaglobulinemic or hypogammaglobulinemic patients may experience paralytic poliomyelitis or severe chronic encephalitis with enteric cytopathic human orphan viruses (echoviruses) or coxsackieviruses.[393] Nevertheless, antibody may serve an auxiliary role in host defense against herpesvirus infection, particularly when cellular components of the response are deficient, as in the human neonate.

The production of most antiviral antibodies by B cells is T cell dependent, although, as discussed, some viral antigens, particularly those encoding repeated epitopes, may act as T-independent type 2 antigens.[589] Such T-independent type 2 antibody responses have not yet been documented for human HSV infection. If antibody is passively acquired, as in the case of maternal-to-fetal transfer, humoral immunity may exist independently of T cell immunity. Although enveloped viruses can be lysed by antibody and complement in vitro, this is unlikely to be an important mechanism in vivo because of the high concentrations of antibody required. Under relatively physiologic conditions, IgG and complement components can coat the surfaces of many viruses, including HSV, and effectively neutralize their infectivity, possibly by preventing their attachment or fusion with cell membranes.[1061] However, the importance of complement in viral host defense is uncertain because serious viral infection is not a feature of patients with severe inherited complement deficiency or of animals made acutely hypocomplementemic.[1062, 1063] A potentially more effective system for the elimination of virus-infected cells by specific antibody is ADCC. NK cells are probably the most efficient effector cells for ADCC,[757] though neutrophils may contribute. The specificity of cytotoxicity is due to the specific recognition by antibody of viral antigens present on the infected cell surface. In vitro ADCC requires low concentrations of antibody and occurs rapidly (within hours), making it less likely that the virus will have had sufficient time to produce infectious particles. ADCC mediated by all types of effectors is upregulated by IFN-γ.[757, 1064–1066] Although in vitro ADCC activity correlates, in some cases, with protection against serious viral infections in humans and in animal models,[1067, 1068] it remains uncertain to what extent this is due to occurrence of ADCC in vivo.

Because most antibody production by B cells in response to viral antigens is T cell dependent, it is often difficult to assess independently the actual in vivo role of T and B cell immunity in viral host defense in humans. In cases of severe and relatively selective primary T cell immunodeficiency, a predilection for severe infection with herpesviruses is seen with some disorders (nucleoside phosphorylase deficiency) but not others (thymic hypoplasia in DiGeorge's syndrome).[829, 1069] This may reflect, in part, the degree to which T cell function is reduced in these disorders. Nude mice, which have markedly depressed T cell function from birth, are also predisposed to severe HSV infection and die during its later phases when antigen-specific immunity usually develops.[1070] Adoptive transfer of T cells in these mice is protective and also results in some endogenous antibody production, whereas passive antibody administration is not ultimately protective but does appear to limit viral spread.[1070] We have found that B cell–deficient mice are substantially more susceptible to acute HSV infection than normal controls (C Wilson, unpublished data), supporting a role for antibody in protection. Antibody is not essential for the resolution of primary murine CMV infection but does limit the dissemination of virus during reactivation from latency.[1071] These observations suggest that B cell immunity does contribute to the control of HSV and other herpesviruses.

NEONATAL DEFENSES

Characteristically, HSV infection in neonates spreads rapidly to produce either disseminated or central nervous system disease. Deficiencies in the function of neonatal NK cells and, possibly, macrophages are probably important contributors to poor early control of infection by the innate immune response. Also, unlike in adults, in neonates critical antigen-specific T cell responses to the virus appear to develop too slowly to prevent the virus from producing irreparable tissue injury or death.

Deficits in the early nonspecific phase of viral resistance have been reported in neonatal humans and animals, consistent with the functional differences between neonatal and adult macrophages and NK cells described. Although the production of IFN-α/β by blood monocytes from term neonates in response to HSV and other viruses appears to be similar to that by cells from adults, production by cells from preterm neonates may be reduced. As discussed in the section Natural Killer Cells, the cytotoxic activity of blood mononuclear cells, monocytes, and purified NK cells from neonates is generally impaired against a variety of targets, including those infected with HSV.[757] Such deficits have been apparent in assays measuring natural cytotoxicity and ADCC, including with HSV- and CMV-infected target cells. In addition, IFN-α/β enhances NK cell lytic activity by adult cells more than that by neonatal cells. Nevertheless, ADCC may still provide some measure of protection because the presence of passively acquired maternal ADCC antibody is associated with less severe disease in infected neonates.[757] As discussed, exposure of neonatal blood mononuclear cells to IL-2, IL-12, and IL-15 enhances their NK cell cytolytic activity to values equivalent to those of similarly treated cells from adults and induces IFN-γ production (probably reflecting NK cell production) at values ranging from ~25 to 100% of that of adult cells.[597, 607, 615, 616, 837] However, the in vitro production of certain of these cytokines that enhance NK cell function is decreased in neonates. Whether such cytokines are produced in amounts sufficient to mediate these effects on NK cells in neonates with HSV infection is not known. Collectively these results suggest that diminished cytolytic activity, and perhaps IFN-γ production, by neonatal NK cells may contribute to less efficient containment of HSV.

Consistent with these observations and the apparent role of NK cells in resistance to infection with herpes group viruses, Kohl has demonstrated in a murine model that the age-related maturation of NK cell function parallels the development of resistance to HSV.[757, 821] Neonatal mice, which, like human neonates, are more susceptible to HSV, can be protected by adoptive transfer of human blood mononuclear cells from adults but not from neonates. Addition of IL-2 augments protection mediated by cells from adults but not cells from neonates, and protection is dependent on IFN-γ production by the transferred cells. The failure of human neonatal cells to transfer resistance in this model also can be corrected by the addition of IFN-γ, a cytokine produced poorly by neonatal T cells (see Table 2–2). This suggests that lack of IFN-γ production may be one important difference between adult and neonatal cells. Whether deficits in NK cell IFN-γ production and cytotoxicity may contribute to the failure of neonatal mononuclear cells to confer protection in this model is uncertain.

HSV-specific T cell–mediated immune responses are commonly diminished, delayed, or both in their development in human neonates compared with those in adults with primary HSV infection. As noted, under most conditions neonatal T cells express less TNF (~25 to 50% of adult cells) and much less IFN-γ and CD40 ligand (~10 to 20% of adult T cells) than adult T cells. These reduced functions of neonatal T cells reflect in part their naive status: When restimulated as early as 5 to 7 days after initial stimulation in vitro, neonatal T cells develop into effector T cells that produce these and other cytokines and that are cytotoxic for allogeneic target cells, with activities comparable to those of similarly treated adult T cells. If neonatal T cells proliferated and acquired these functions with similar efficiency in response to HSV in vivo, it is unlikely that the basal differences in function could account for the neonate's greater susceptibility. However, development of detectable antigen-specific T cell responses in neonates with HSV infection is much slower (3 to 6 weeks) than in adults (~1 week) with primary HSV infection.[331, 332] Once antigen-specific T cells develop in neonates (as indicated by HSV-induced T cell proliferation), their capacity to produce IFN-γ in response to HSV antigens is equal to that of T cells from adults, consistent with the notion that the deficit in production of IFN-γ by neonatal T cells largely reflects the lack of antigen-specific memory-effector T cells.[331] Other reports indicate that antigen-specific T cell responses are commonly slow to develop in neonates infected perinatally or in utero with CMV.[1072] Whether there is a similar delay in the development of cytotoxic T cells is uncertain, though limited data in infants with perinatal HIV infection suggest that this may be the case.

The basis for the delayed development of antigen-specific T cells in neonates is not known. It may reflect in part a lower frequency of precursors able to respond to HSV and other antigens.[1073] As discussed earlier in the section Co-stimulation of Neonatal T Cells and Anergy, it may also reflect the tendency of neonatal T cells to become anergic, unless antigen is presented by primed-mature dendritic cells expressing co-stimulatory molecules and cytokines,[244, 247, 248] and reduced dendritic cell–APC function in neonates and young infants.[60, 63] Dendritic cells derived from immature precursors in neonatal or adult blood can be primed for efficient antigen presentation by engagement of their CD40 molecule by CD40 ligand expressed by activated T cells, or by their exposure to microbial products or inflammatory cytokines induced by these products. Thus, it is possible that both the lack of prior exposure to microbes, which occurs in a cumulative manner after birth, as well as the paucity of effector T cells expressing CD40 ligand account in part for diminished dendritic cell function and the slow rate at which antigen-specific T cells develop. This delay in the acquisition of antigen-specific T cells and cytokine production may be an important factor in the neonate's greater susceptibility to infections with HSV and other pathogens against which such defenses play an important role. It is unknown whether this is accompanied by a similar delay or deficit in T cell–mediated, antigen-specific cytotoxicity. The data on antiviral cytotoxicity of neonatal cells to virus-infected targets are limited[335] and lack clear evidence for antigen-specific MHC-restricted T cell–mediated cytotoxicity, with the exception of studies in infants and children with acquired perinatal HIV infection. In such children HIV-1–specific CTL responses were usually not detectable during the first few months of life.[333, 1074] When evaluated beyond infancy, CTL directed to HIV envelope proteins was commonly detected, whereas CTL directed against *gag* or *pol* proteins rarely was.[333] These results suggest that there may be a delay in the development of CTL compared to that in adults, and that the nature of the target antigens recognized by neonatal CTL may be more limited. It remains to be determined whether neonates have similar deficits in development of CTL directed to other viruses, such as HSV. In addition, no studies have examined cytolytic activity mediated by neonatal CD4 T cells, although CD4 T cell–mediated viral clearance is likely to play an important role in the resolution of HSV infection in humans.

In addition to the neonate's own immune response, antibody-mediated protection can be passively provided from the mother. The risk of transmission of HSV from mother to infant in cases of primary or initial maternal infection is much higher (~35%) than in cases of recurrent maternal infection. This may reflect, in part, lesser amounts of virus in the maternal genital tract in recurrent infection but also appears to correlate with presence of HSV type-specific antibody, particularly to glycoprotein G.[1075] Kohl and colleagues[1076] have also shown that of HSV-infected infants, those with greater concentrations of ADCC antibody had less severe disease. It is important to note that healthy adults and older children with primary HSV infection, who by definition lack antibody to HSV, do not experience severe disease, as do neonates with primary infection. This indicates that the deficits intrinsic to the neonate are the important factors predisposing the neonate to infection. Nevertheless, passively acquired antibody may play a role in decreasing transmission or ameliorating disease severity.

HSV infection is severe in term infants infected at the time of parturition, as well as in the uncommon infants who acquire it in utero. In contrast, congenital infection with CMV produces considerably greater damage when primary maternal infection, and thereby fetal infection, occurs in the first half of gestation.[1077] When infection is acquired after mid-gestation, severe sequelae are uncommon, although some sequelae, particularly sensorineural hearing loss, may result. Similarly, congenital rubella virus infection produces sequelae essentially only when maternal infection occurs in the first 16 weeks of gestation. Infections that occur in the first 10 weeks of gestation do so at a time when the fetus has few detectable T or B cells, and if infection begins before the sixth week of gestation, NK cells also are absent. Furthermore, the numbers and repertoire for antigen recognition of T cells, B cells, and antibody-secreting plasma cells are low in the first half of gestation. Thus, it is plausible, but unproven, that the extraordinary susceptibility to infection with these agents in the first half of gestation may reflect, at least in part, quantitative deficits in these cells of the immune system. The less severe sequelae that are due to congenital CMV when infection develops after mid-gestation may result from the functional deficiencies in the fetal and neonatal immune system described, as proposed for HSV infection.

Enterovirus infections are severe and may be fatal when acquired in the perinatal period. The absence of protective neutralizing antibody appears to be the major factor predisposing to enterovirus infection.[1078, 1079] It is likely that T cell–mediated immune responses also play a role in defense with these agents.

ADJUNCT THERAPY OF HERPESVIRUS INFECTIONS

The studies cited raise the possibility that neonates could be passively protected by administration of antibody to HSV, particularly antibody that would facilitate ADCC. Human monoclonal antibodies, murine monoclonal antibodies that have been humanized, and specific hyperimmunoglobulin could potentially be employed for this purpose. The phage display technique has recently been used to select human monoclonal antibodies with an ability to neutralize effectively either HSV-1 or HSV-2 at a relatively low concentration in vitro,[1080] but it remains to be seen whether these or related antibodies will be efficacious in limiting the extent of primary HSV infection in humans. The unique capacity of IFN-γ to endow human neonatal blood mononuclear cells with the ability to protect neonatal mice from infection suggests that exogenous IFN-γ may also be a potentially useful means to enhance the human neonate's resistance to HSV. However, in the experimental models described by Kohl[757] passive immunotherapy must be given before or at the time of infection. This raises the concern that such therapy, if administered once infection is established, may be less effective, at least in controlling viral-induced tissue damage. In addition, recent unanticipated

fatal toxicity and mortality due to administration of IL-12 to adult cancer patients[1081] indicate that there is reason to be cautious in using exogenous cytokine therapy in the seriously ill neonate. It should also be noted that there is as yet no direct evidence that the initial innate immune response of the neonate to HSV infection is deficient in terms of cytokine production (e.g., for IL-12, TNF, and IFN-γ) derived from cells other than T cells. Facilitating the more rapid development of antigen-specific CD4 and CD8 T cells with appropriate effector function might be a more physiologically appropriate approach, allowing these cells and the cytokines they produce to localize properly to the sites of infection. Further elucidation of the cellular and molecular mechanisms that underlie the lag in the development of antigen-specific immunity in the neonate in response to HSV may help in devising therapies to overcome these limitations in host defenses.

An HSV vaccine consisting of recombinant glycoprotein D and B HSV-2 antigens induced antibody neutralization titers and T cell proliferative responses that were equal to or greater than those with naturally acquired HSV-2 infection.[1078, 1082] It is likely that this vaccine also induced substantial titers of IgG antibodies that mediate ADCC. Such vaccines might be useful to increase the titer of antibodies in young women who are either HSV-1 and/or HSV-2 seronegative and, therefore, are at risk to acquire primary or first episode HSV infection during pregnancy. However, initial trials with this vaccine did not provide sufficient protection to adults, and it is unlikely to be marketed for clinical use. Further efforts to develop a vaccine that will prevent disease in adults and in neonates are indicated.

Nonviral Intracellular Pathogens

OVERVIEW OF HOST DEFENSE MECHANISMS

In addition to viruses, certain nonviral intracellular pathogens can replicate within cells and cause severe fetal or neonatal infection. These include *Salmonella* sp., *L. monocytogenes*, and *M. tuberculosis*, which are facultative intracellular pathogens, and *T. gondii* (hereafter referred to as *Toxoplasma*) and *Chlamydia trachomatis*, which are obligate intracellular pathogens. Unlike pyogenic bacteria, for which phagocytosis usually results in death, phagocytosis for these pathogens is a means of entering into an intracellular haven. Each of these pathogens readily infects tissue macrophages of the reticuloendothelial system. In addition, *Toxoplasma* can infect virtually any mammalian cell type, and this has important consequences for the pathogenesis of toxoplasmosis. This discussion of host defense mechanisms focuses primarily on *Toxoplasma*. Relevant information from studies of *Listeria* sp. and the protozoan *Leishmania*, an extensively studied obligate intracellular pathogen in rodents, is included.

During acute toxoplasmosis in humans, the replicating form, the tachyzoite, is found both extracellularly and intracellularly. A 30-kDa tachyzoite surface protein, P30, appears to be involved in the initial attachment of *Toxoplasma* to host cells.[1083] Antibodies are frequently made against this protein after infection and are the basis for serodiagnosis.[1083, 1084] Intracellular *Toxoplasma* organisms are found principally in specialized parasitophorous vacuoles that are derived from the host cell membrane. These vacuoles, although resistant to fusion with lysosomes, allow the free exchange of nutrients with the host cell cytoplasm, facilitating parasite replication.[1085] Cellular invasion by tachyzoites occurs without generating a respiratory burst in human macrophages[1086] or activating microbicidal nitric oxide production in murine macrophages.[1087] In response to adverse intracellular conditions that slow its replication,[1088] the tachyzoite is somehow induced to convert into a less metabolically active form, the bradyzoite. Bradyzoites can persist in many tissues for years or decades in the form of cysts. As discussed later, limiting chronic *Toxoplasma* organism infection to this quiescent state depends on antigen-specific cellular immunity; acquired T cell immunodeficiency, such as pharmacologic immunosuppression or HIV infection, may allow bradyzoites to reconvert to tachyzoites that resume invasive infection.

Murine studies suggest that the control of acute infection by *Toxoplasma* and other nonviral intracellular pathogens, such as *Listeria* and *Leishmania* sp., involves an initial innate response involving dendritic cells, NK cells, and mononuclear phagocytes, followed by an antigen-specific response in which T cell immunity is critical.[1089, 1090] Alpha-beta T cells are particularly important for the chronic maintenance of *Toxoplasma* organisms in a quiescent state within infected host cells.[1089] The distinctiveness of the early innate response compared with the later antigen-specific response in mice is demonstrated by the observation that genetic susceptibility of common laboratory strains to acute *Toxoplasma* infection does not correlate with the susceptibility to chronic infection.[1091]

The following is a model for how cytokines link the activity of innate and antigen-specific immune mechanisms (see Fig. 2–12) in acute toxoplasmosis and during infection with other nonviral intracellular pathogens. This model is largely based on studies in mice utilizing spontaneously occurring or genetically manipulated immunodeficient strains, antibody treatment, or both to deplete particular cell types or to neutralize cytokine and cytokine receptors: *Toxoplasma* tachyzoites, or products they secrete, induce dendritic cells or mononuclear phagocytes to produce cytokines, such as IL-1, IL-12, TNF,[1092, 1093] and, possibly, IL-15.[1094] These cytokines in conjunction with *Toxoplasma* organism–derived products induce NK cells to produce IFN-γ.[1092, 1095] NK cell–derived IFN-γ, in turn, increases toxoplasmacidal activity within mononuclear phagocytes, helping limit the initial extent of infection.[1096] IFN-γ, IL-12, and TNF produced by innate (i.e., NK cells, dendritic cells, and monocytes) rather than antigen-specific mechanisms (i.e., T cells) appear essential for the initial control of acute infection.[1089, 1092, 1097] IFN-γ in conjunction with IL-12 also favors the differentiation of antigen-specific T cells into a TH1-type effector population that is able to secrete IFN-γ at high levels.[1089] This provides a T cell–derived source of IFN-γ that contains the parasite during the late phase of acute infection and also helps

limit the spread of infection in tissues should *Toxoplasma* cysts reactivate into tachyzoites.

In normal mice, the production and effects of proinflammatory cytokines are counterbalanced by IL-10, an anti-inflammatory cytokine produced by mononuclear phagocytes and T cells. This counterregulation is biologically important because mice that are genetically deficient in IL-10 and acutely infected with *Toxoplasma* have increased expression of IL-12, TNF, and IFN-γ and die, probably as a result of inflammatory liver necrosis.[1098] Some cytokines may mediate both positive and negative roles in the immune response to *Toxoplasma* organisms. For example, IL-4 production occurs relatively late in primary murine toxoplasmosis and, in this context, may enhance, rather than inhibit, the differentiation of protective IFN-γ–producing TH1 effector cells.[1099] This effect contrasts with *Leishmania* infection of certain mouse strains, in which IL-4 production occurs very early and potently inhibits TH1 effector cell generation.[124] On the other hand, IL-4 produced during the chronic phase of murine infection appears to inhibit the host's ability to control *Toxoplasma* cyst replication within the central nervous system.[1100] These observations emphasize the importance of the temporal sequence of cytokine expression for appropriate immunoregulation.

INNATE IMMUNITY: NATURAL KILLER CELLS, MONONUCLEAR PHAGOCYTES, AND DENDRITIC CELLS

Most murine studies are supportive of a role for NK cells in linking the initial innate response and the development of persistent antigen-specific immunity to *Toxoplasma*: NK cell depletion or neutralization of NK cell–derived IFN-γ prevents the development of a protective immune response after vaccination with attenuated *Toxoplasma* in mice that have CD4 T cells but are genetically deficient in αβ CD8 T cells and NK T cells.[1101] However, this pathway may be less important in the fully immunocompetent host, because experiments with wild-type mice depleted of NK cells have yielded conflicting results as to whether NK cells are important for the control of early primary *Toxoplasma* infection.[1102, 1103] Interestingly, *Toxoplasma* infection of SCID mice, which lack T and B cells, results in the appearance of NK cells that express CD28. These NK cells respond to B7 engagement with enhanced IFN-γ secretion.[575] However, there is no evidence as yet that this is relevant to human infection, because CD28 expression by human NK cells is not detectable after in vitro activation with exogenous cytokines.[576] The role of NK cell–mediated cytolysis in the control of *Toxoplasma* infection in vivo is also unclear, although IL-2–treated NK cells are capable of lysing *Toxoplasma* organism–infected cells in vitro.

As mentioned, cytokines produced by nonlymphoid cells during the early phase of toxoplasmosis may play a critical role in the early control of infection by multiple mechanisms, including induction of IFN-γ production by NK cells and NK T cells, enhancement of TH1 effector cell generation, and activation of mononuclear phagocyte microbicidal activity in an autocrine or paracrine fashion. Although mononuclear phagocytes are a potent source of cytokines, such as IL-12, when incubated in vitro with *Toxoplasma* organisms or their products, dendritic cells, particularly those in the spleen, are also a major source of early IL-12 production in vivo.[1090, 1104] This suggests that mononuclear phagocytes may act downstream of dendritic cells in the innate phase of the immune response to infection.

The critical role of macrophages in resistance to intracellular nonviral pathogens was first demonstrated in animal studies of *Listeria* organisms in which depletion of macrophages increased susceptibility.[1105] In the first days of infection, the rate at which monocytes are recruited to the site of infection and the microbicidal activity of these cells correlate with the control of *Toxoplasma* in animals.[1106] As discussed in the section Mononuclear Phagocytes, monocyte entry into infected tissues appears to require the coordinated interaction of selectins, integrins (particularly those of the β_1 group), and β-chemokine receptors on the monocyte with counter-ligands on the endothelium and extracellular matrix. Transcripts for the β-chemokine MIP-1α are present in the central nervous system of SCID mice with *Toxoplasma* encephalitis, suggesting that this β-chemokine serves as a mononuclear phagocyte chemoattractant in vivo.[1107] Infection of human monocytes by *Toxoplasma* tachyzoites also results in the induction of B7-1 (CD80) and increased expression of B7-2 (CD86).[1108] The increased expression of these co-stimulatory molecules may enhance proliferation and IFN-γ production by T cells early in *Toxoplasma* infection[1109] and may assist in the generation of TH1 effector cells from antigenically naive T cells.[1109] In general there is greater microbicidal activity of human monocytes than macrophages against *Toxoplasma*.[1110, 1111] In vitro studies with mononuclear phagocytes or microglial cells, which are mononuclear phagocyte–derived cells of the central nervous system, demonstrate that both oxidative and nonoxidative mechanisms are involved in limiting intracellular *Toxoplasma* replication. The ability of human monocytes to kill *Toxoplasma* organisms in the absence of exogenous cytokines depends mainly on oxidative mechanisms,[1110] whereas human macrophages, including those from lung alveoli and peritoneum, kill *Toxoplasma* by a nonoxidative mechanism.[1112, 1113] Microbicidal activity against and phagocytosis of *Toxoplasma* by monocyte-derived human macrophages are substantially reduced when these cells are infected in vitro with HIV-1. This effect appears to be due to the induction of PGE_2 by HIV-1, a mechanism that could contribute to the reactivation of *Toxoplasma* observed in HIV-1–infected patients.[1114]

Cytokines are critical regulators of mononuclear phagocyte activity during infection with intracellular nonviral pathogens. IFN-γ produced by activated T cells or NK cells is the most important activator of macrophages for toxoplasmacidal activity.[1089, 1115] In vitro studies have demonstrated that macrophages first primed by treatment with IFN-γ can be triggered for toxoplasmacidal activity by incubation with TNF; treatment with IFN-γ alone is ineffective.[1116] IFN-γ is able to induce toxoplasmacidal activity in monocytes or monocyte-derived macrophages from patients with chronic granulo-

matous disease, confirming the existence of cytokine-dependent, nonoxidative mechanisms for the intracellular killing.[1110] One such mechanism is the induction of the enzyme indoleamine 2,3,-dioxygenase, which catalyzes the first step in tryptophan degradation and deprives replicating *Toxoplasma* organisms of this essential nutrient.[1117] Whether this mechanism is important in limiting *Toxoplasma* in vivo remains to be shown.

Experiments with gene knockout mice lacking iNOS indicate that this enzyme is required for the control of persistent *Toxoplasma* infection.[1118] Pharmacologic blockade of iNOS activity results in exacerbation of chronic infection.[1119] As discussed in the section Mononuclear Phagocytes, iNOS is a nitric oxide–producing enzyme expressed mainly by mononuclear phagocytes. In murine toxoplasmosis, the induction of iNOS appears dependent on the production of IFN-γ and TNF, both of which can directly activate mononuclear phagocytes for increased iNOS expression.[1097, 1120] The mechanism by which iNOS mediates an antitoxoplasmal effect in vivo remains unclear. In most cytokine-activated human mononuclear phagocyte populations, iNOS activity has been low or undetectable except in certain contexts, such as alveolar macrophages from tuberculosis patients, and the importance of iNOS in limiting *Toxoplasma* or other intracellular pathogens in humans remains unclear.[753]

ANTIGEN-SPECIFIC IMMUNITY: $\alpha\beta$ AND $\gamma\delta$ T CELLS AND B CELLS

The importance of T lymphocytes in protection of humans from *Toxoplasma* infection is suggested by the marked increase in the incidence of severe infection in HIV-1–infected patients who have quantitative and qualitative CD4 T cell deficiency. This critical role for T lymphocytes in controlling toxoplasmosis is supported by the marked susceptibility of rodents with genetic T cell immunodeficiencies (e.g., nude or SCID rodents) and by the ability of splenocytes or T cells from immune animals to transfer resistance adoptively to susceptible recipients.[1089, 1105, 1121] The importance of CD4 and CD8 T cells in protection depends on the phase of infection. In acute infection, CD8 T cells appear to be more protective than CD4 T cells, although both subsets afford some protection to unvaccinated rodents.[1122] CD4 and CD8 T cells are both necessary in order to limit the extent of central nervous system (CNS) infection in the brain,[1123] and CD4 T cells are required for the development of long-term protective immunity.[1124] In contrast, once protective immunity has developed, CD4 or CD8 T cells can independently limit acute reactivation of chronic *Toxoplasma* infection; this requires the secretion of IFN-γ.[1125]

Studies with perforin knockout mice suggest that the perforin-granzyme cytotoxicity mechanism is more important in the control of chronic toxoplasmosis, particularly in the brain, than in acute infection.[1126] Such cytotoxicity is more likely to be mediated by T cells rather than NK cells, although this remains to be shown. *Toxoplasma* infection of potential target cells may also broadly inhibit the induction of apoptosis, including by granzymes or fas ligand,[408] thus limiting the efficacy of cell-mediated cytotoxic mechanisms. Human CD4 and CD8 T cells can lyse *Toxoplasma*-infected cells,[1127] and, in the case of CD4 T cells, this cytotoxicity has been demonstrated to be self–class II MHC–restricted.[1128, 1129] However, it is unclear that lysis results in the intracellular death of *Toxoplasma*, and, if not, whether any released viable tachyzoites are cleared by mononuclear cell phagocytosis, direct lysis by antibody and complement, or both. If such released tachyzoites were able to infect new cellular targets, such cytotoxicity might be detrimental to the host.

The production of cytokines by TH1 effector and memory cells, such as IFN-γ, is critical for the control of acute toxoplasmosis, as well as prevention of the reactivation of chronic infection.[1089, 1115] In most immune responses, IFN-γ production by T cells is mediated mainly by effector cell populations that have previously undergone clonal expansion from antigenically naive precursor cells. However, a novel pathway for inducing IFN-γ production by antigenically naive CD45RA^high CD45R0^low αβ T cells has been identified. Cells with this phenotype obtained from donors seronegative for *Toxoplasma* organisms, including neonates, produce IFN-γ and proliferate in response to autologous monocytes infected with *Toxoplasma* tachyzoites.[1109] This response is dependent on the upregulation of the B7 molecules on infected monocytes and appears to utilize class II MHC antigen presentation.[1109] This response does not have the restricted V_β repertoire characteristic of responses to a superantigen, but whether an antigenic peptide or nonprotein antigen is involved remains unclear. It will be of interest to determine whether a *Toxoplasma*-specific response by antigenically naive αβ CD4 T cells can be documented in vivo during either human or murine toxoplasmosis.

Gamma-delta T cells, mainly those encoding V_γ2-V_δ2 T cell receptors, are increased in the circulation of children with postnatally acquired primary toxoplasmosis.[1130, 1131] These cells are predominantly of a CD45RA^low CD45R0^high surface phenotype, suggesting that they have been activated in vivo.[1131] This expansion appears to be a direct effect of *Toxoplasma* organisms on this cell population because V_γ2-V_δ2–bearing T cells, when incubated with peripheral blood mononuclear cells that have internalized killed parasites, are activated to secrete cytokines (IL-2, IFN-γ, and TNF) and to proliferate.[1132] Interestingly, lysis of *Toxoplasma*-infected cells by these V_γ2-V_δ2 T cells occurs in an MHC-unrestricted manner and does not require previous infection of the donor by *Toxoplasma*.[1132]

The role of γδ T cells in host defense against *Toxoplasma* remains controversial. Mice depleted of γδ T cells by monoclonal antibody treatment and administered a large dose of *Toxoplasma* bradyzoites die more rapidly than untreated mice[1133]; untreated mice have increases in the number of γδ T cells in the spleen and peritoneum in response to *Toxoplasma* infection. Gamma-delta T cells also undergo expansion in mice lacking αβ T cells, and the transfer of these cells into mice lacking CD4 and CD8 T cells, NK T cells, and NK cells affords protection.[1134] These γδ cells produce IFN-γ and lyse autologous *Toxoplasma*-infected macro-

phages.[1134] It is unclear whether γδ T cells improve the outcome of infection in these systems by the secretion of cytokines, cell-mediated cytotoxicity, or other mechanisms. In contrast to these studies, Sayles and colleagues,[1135] using a lower inoculum of bradyzoites, found no evidence either for the in vivo expansion of γδ T cells in wild-type mice or for any deleterious effects of γδ T cell depletion.

In contrast with *Listeria* organisms, in which immunoglobulin appears to play no role in the host resistance to infection,[1136] immunoglobulin probably contributes some protection against protozoa, including *Toxoplasma*, at least in experimental animals. Mice that cannot mount an antibody response are slightly more susceptible to late death from *Toxoplasma* organisms than are normal mice, and antiserum from convalescent animals has only a slight protective effect.[1137] Antibody and complement lyse extracellular *Toxoplasma*, and this is the basis of Sabin-Feldman dye assay for anti–*Toxoplasma* antibodies. Antibody-coated *Toxoplasma* organisms are also killed by resting mouse and human macrophages, probably via Fc-receptor–mediated entry into an intracellular vacuole that, unlike the parasitophorous vacuole, fuses with lysosomes.[1138] Antibody alone provides minimal protection in adult and newborn mice, but antibody enhances protection by activated macrophages,[1139] perhaps via Fc-receptor–mediated mechanisms. However, T cell–deficient mice are much more susceptible than are antibody-deficient animals and are not protected by antibody. The fact that *Toxoplasma* encephalitis in adult AIDS patients typically develops as a recrudescence of a chronic latent infection despite the presence of preexisting antibodies to *Toxoplasma* organisms[1140] underscores the importance of T cells rather than B cells in the control of chronic infection with this pathogen.

FETAL AND NEONATAL DEFENSES

The initial immune response of the human fetus to *Toxoplasma* is largely unknown. However, on the basis of animal studies with *Toxoplasma* and other nonviral intracellular pathogens, it is likely that limitations in responses by mononuclear phagocytes, NK cells, and T cells may all contribute to fetal susceptibility. Limitations in cytokine production, particularly for IFN-γ, TNF, and IL-12, would be expected to be particularly deleterious. Studies in neonatal rodents, which are highly susceptible to infection with *L. monocytogenes*, support the idea that reduced cytokine production or responsiveness may limit neonatal immunity. In neonatal mice and rats administration of recombinant IFN-γ before or at the time of infection protects from acute infection and allows the development of protective immunity.[822, 823, 1141] In adult animals, TNF, or agents that induce TNF, enhance resistance, whereas this effect is not observed in the neonates. Co-administration of suboptimal doses of IFN-γ and TNF protects neonatal rats. Acquisition of resistance to infection correlates with acquisition of adult competence for TNF production[822]; this also is likely to correlate with competence for IFN-γ production, but this correlation has not been reported. During fetal *Toxoplasma* infection, the ability of NK cells to produce IFN-γ and TNF and for mononuclear phagocytes to produce TNF and other proinflammatory cytokines is unknown.

Infection with *Toxoplasma*, like that for many congenital viral pathogens, such as CMV, is much more likely to produce severe untoward infection when the mother acquires primary infection early in pregnancy. As discussed, the most severely damaged infants are likely to have acquired infection during the first trimester, when their numbers of T cells and their $\alpha\beta$-TCR repertoire for antigen recognition are limited compared with those of the fetus in the latter half of gestation. However, $\alpha\beta$-TCR repertoire limitations are unlikely to be an important mechanism in most cases of fetal toxoplasmosis, because severe sequelae may occur in infants infected during mid- to late gestation, and in most infants infected at any time during gestation sequelae ultimately develop. Similarly, *Listeria* infection occurring in infants in the latter part of gestation is usually severe. This suggests that mechanisms acting to contain *Toxoplasma* and *Listeria* infection are still immature in late gestation and at term relative to those of older individuals.

As noted, antigenically naive CD45RA[high]CD45R0[low] CD4 T cells from donors who have not been infected with toxoplasmosis can proliferate in response to autologous *Toxoplasma*-infected mononuclear cells.[1109] However, CD4 T cells from neonates proliferate less well than antigenically naive CD4 T cells from adults. The relationship between this novel in vitro response, which requires high concentrations of infected cells or antigen, and the development of *Toxoplasma*-specific effector memory T cells in vivo, particularly in the fetus, remains to be defined. In contrast, *Toxoplasma*-specific recall CD4 T cell responses, which are evident in response to low concentrations of soluble antigen, are often delayed in their appearance in congenital toxoplasmosis and may not be detectable until weeks or months after birth. When memory T cells first appear they may also have a reduced capacity to proliferate and to produce IL-2 or IFN-γ compared with that of memory T cells from adults with postnatal *Toxoplasma* infection.[325] A similar impairment, lag, or both in development of recall antigen–specific CD4 T cell responses has also been observed in infants with congenital infection due to syphilis, CMV, VZV, and rubella,[323-328] and, as previously discussed, in neonates infected postnatally with HSV.[331, 332] Whether this initial poor response, lag in its appearance, or both are due to (1) failure initially to activate or to expand antigenically naive T cells (immunologic ignorance); (2) deletion of antigen-specific T cells; or (3) the tendency of cells undergoing expansion to differentiate into anergic cells that are unable to respond to restimulation, as has been observed with in vitro priming of neonatal T cells with alloantigen[248] or superantigen,[214] or all of these mechanisms remains unknown. Regardless of the precise mechanism, these findings suggest that infection occurring at a time of greater immunologic immaturity, such as in the fetus, may lead to a state of complete or partial antigen-specific nonresponsiveness.

At least some neonates and young infants with congenital *Toxoplasma* infection demonstrate increased expansion of $V_\gamma 2$-$V_\delta 2$–bearing T cells, most of which express a CD45RA[low]CD45R0[high] surface phenotype, indicating prior activation in vivo.[339] An analysis of a very limited number of patients has found that the $\gamma\delta$ T cell population in the congenitally infected neonate has a poor proliferative response to stimulation by peripheral blood mononuclear cells infected with viable or irradiated *Toxoplasma* organisms.[339] However, other functions, such as the secretion of cytokines by these cells, were not assessed, and rigorous age-matched controls were not employed. These results, which need to be confirmed, raise the possibility of an anergic state in human $\gamma\delta$ T cells in certain contexts, such as congenital infection.

Although cell-mediated immunity against *Toxoplasma* organisms appears to be compromised in the human neonate, an antibody response against the P30 *Toxoplasma* antigen is frequently detectable in the fetus and neonate after congenital infection and is useful for serodiagnosis. Anti-P30 IgA antibodies are found in most neonates after congenital infection, whereas anti-P30 IgM antibodies are found in few of these individuals.[1084, 1142] *Toxoplasma*-specific IgE antibodies are also frequently present within the first 2 months of life in congenitally infected infants.[1143] Anti-P30 IgA and IgE antibodies are not unique to the fetus and neonate but are also common in older individuals with postnatally acquired toxoplasmosis. Together these results suggest that isotype switching of antibodies from IgM to the IgA and IgE isotypes can occur in utero, particularly in the face of continuing antigenic stimulation. Because IL-4 or IL-13 produced by CD4 T cells is likely to be required for the production of protein antigen–specific IgE antibodies,[1144] these results also suggest that the CD4 T cell response to *Toxoplasma* organisms in the fetus may include the production of these cytokines.

IMPLICATIONS FOR IMMUNOLOGIC INTERVENTION

The findings in human neonates in concert with the results of studies in rodents suggest that correction of the deficits in NK function, cytokine production, and the T cell response could facilitate treatment of infections with nonviral intracellular pathogens, such as *Toxoplasma*. However, several limitations are apparent. For example, treatment of neonatal rats with IFN-γ or -α after establishment of infection with *Listeria* sp. is not effective, whereas concomitant therapy or pretreatment is effective.[1145] This is perhaps not surprising given the evidence that IFN-γ is important only in the early phase of this infection. In the case of congenital infection with *Toxoplasma*, therapy would need to be initiated and maintained in utero, when maternal infection is often asymptomatic, and there is no obvious way by which this could be safely targeted to the fetus. In fact, there are data in mouse models that increased production of IFN-γ during maternal infection may contribute to fetal loss as a result of maternal rejection of the fetus as a foreign allograft.[1146] After birth it may be possible to provide exogenous IFN-γ (or perhaps TNF, IL-12, or IL-15), but the same caveats noted for treatment in cases of viral infection would apply. If studies in other patient populations (e.g., those with HIV infection) provide evidence that IFN-γ, TNF, IL-12, or IL-15 alone or in some combination can contribute to resolution of established disease with *Toxoplasma* in conjunction with antimicrobial therapy, its use in neonates might be considered. Alternatively, approaches that seek to modify the deficit in development of antigen-specific effector T cells may prove to be more effective.

A live attenuated *Toxoplasma* vaccine has been developed for veterinary use.[1147] However, live *Toxoplasma* vaccines in humans that result in latent infection are not desirable, because they pose the risk of reactivation and dissemination in the immunocompromised individual. Immunization with recombinant *Toxoplasma* proteins would prevent this problem, and two proteins, the P30 surface antigen and a 58-kDa cytoplasmic protein, appear to have potential as vaccine antigens, on the basis of studies in rodents.[1148] In rodents, the co-administration of certain cytokines, such as IL-15, may enhance the development of CD8 T cell responses to soluble *Toxoplasma* antigen,[1094] suggesting the potential utility of this cytokine as part of a vaccination strategy. Human vaccine trials with recombinant *Toxoplasma* proteins have not been reported.

IMMUNOPROPHYLAXIS IN THE NEONATE

Passive Immunization

There is currently no established use for IGIV in the immunoprophylaxis or adjunctive treatment of infection in the neonate. Intramuscular immune globulin (0.02 ml/kg) is indicated for prophylaxis of exposure to hepatitis A, as soon as possible after exposure.[1149] Immune globulin (0.25 ml/kg) may also be given to prevent or modify measles in neonates when the mother has active infection. Specific human hyperimmune globulin preparations are indicated in some situations.[1149] Hyperimmune hepatitis B immune globulin (HBIG) is indicated in conjunction with hepatitis B vaccine in infants born to mothers who are hepatitis B surface antigen positive. HBIG is given at a dose of 0.5 ml at a site different from that used for vaccine administration. Both HBIG and hepatitis B vaccine should be given as soon as possible, preferably within 12 hours after birth.[1149] Infants with neonatal tetanus or at risk for it may be given tetanus immune globulin. Precise dosages for treatment in this age group are not established; older individuals are generally treated with 3000 to 5000 U, whereas dosages of 500 U may be effective for the neonate.[1149] Varicella-zoster immune globulin (VZIG) is available from local distribution centers and is indicated (125 units, 1.25 ml) for the prophylaxis of infection in those cases in which clinical maternal chickenpox develops between 5 days before and 48 hours after the time of delivery.[1149] Infants born to mothers who have hypogammaglobulinemia may benefit from prophylactic administration of immune globulin in cases in which mothers have not received adequate immune globulin replacement therapy near term and IgG levels in the neonate are documented to be low or are likely to be so.

Active Immunization

The rationale for and against immunization in the neonatal period is described more fully in the section B Cells and Immunoglobulin and the section T Cell Reactivity to Specific Antigens. The only vaccines commonly administered to neonates are bacille Calmette-Guérin and hepatitis B, both of which are immunogenic in neonates. Hepatitis B vaccination may also be started at 2 months of age unless the neonate may have been exposed to the virus during delivery, in which case vaccination and treatment with HBIG within 12 hours of birth are indicated.[1149] Most other vaccines for T cell–dependent antigens, such as whole or acellular pertussis, *H. influenzae* type b polysaccharide protein conjugate, diphtheria, and oral or inactivated poliovirus vaccine, are begun at approximately 2 months of age.[1149] Although immunization at birth is attractive from a public health point of view, vaccine responses to some T cell–dependent antigens may be low or even suppressed compared with responses when vaccination is delayed until 2 months of age. Premature or small-for-gestational-age infants may also be immunized with these vaccines at this age.

Recognition of Primary Immunodeficiency in the Neonate

Recognition of primary immunodeficiency in the neonate is often possible. Several syndromes have characteristic clinical findings that permit early diagnosis—for example, the thrombocytopenia with low mean platelet volume of Wiskott-Aldrich syndrome; the hypocalcemia, facies, and congenital heart disease of DiGeorge's syndrome; and the skeletal dwarfing in cartilage-hair hypoplasia. Others may present with laboratory abnormalities in the neonatal period that are suggestive of the diagnosis, such as marked elevations of IgE level in some patients with hyperimmunoglobulin E syndrome, and hypereosinophilia seen in patients with Omenn's syndrome, a form of SCID due to partial RAG deficiency. Patients with leukocyte adhesion defect (LAD) due to CD18 deficiency may have omphalitis and late (after 3 weeks of age) separation of the umbilical cord; because the predictive value of late cord separation for LAD is relatively low, it may be useful to check the complete blood count in such a situation; those with LAD have a persistent leukocytosis even when they are uninfected. Patients with SCID may present with severe or recalcitrant mucocutaneous candidiasis, protracted diarrhea, *P. carinii* pneumonia, severe eczema, or all those symptoms, often associated with lymphopenia. A family history of immunodeficiency or early unexplained death is suggestive. HIV infection, particularly congenitally acquired, is always considered in the differential diagnosis of neonates who appear to have SCID. Chronic granulomatous disease may present in the neonatal period and should be considered in a term neonate who experiences severe bacterial infection with oxidase-positive bacteria or with fungi and who does not have risk factors for these. In general, unusually severe, recalcitrant, or recurrent infections—that is, those related to organisms of low virulence, especially if they occur in infants without predisposing factors (such as extreme prematurity, multiple courses of empirical antibiotic therapy, multiple catheters, or other aspects of prolonged intensive care)—should prompt consideration of primary immunodeficiency.

Normal term neonates lack delayed-type hypersensitivity responses to antigens, have IgG values similar to those of their mother, and have little or no circulating IgM and IgA. Thus, these common screening tests for immunodeficiency in older children are of little value in the neonate. Useful tests include (1) chest radiograph for thymus size; (2) a total lymphocyte count, which is helpful when low (fewer than 1500 lymphocytes per mm³), although a normal count does not exclude immunodeficiency; (3) enumeration of T, B, and NK cell numbers by flow cytometry; (4) lymphocyte proliferative responses to mitogens, superantigens, anti-CD3, and anti-CD28 monoclonal antibodies, or allogeneic cells; (5) effector cell responses, including cytotoxicity and lymphokine release; (6) staining for CD11a, CD11b, and CD18 and, in the appropriate setting, neutrophil function tests; (7) tests to screen for defects in the neutrophil oxidative burst, the cause of chronic granulomatous disease, which include an analysis of neutrophil hydrogen peroxide generation by flow cytometry and the nitroblue tetrazolium (NBT) test. More detailed discussion of the evaluation of neonates for primary immunodeficiency is available.[1150] Early aggressive antimicrobial therapy, appropriate isolation, and early specific treatment of the immunologic disorder (e.g., IGIV for B immunodeficiency) are indicated whenever possible.

References

1. Sharkis S, Kanz L, Brugger W, et al. The fascinating life of hematopoietic stem cells. Nat Med 4:1118–1119, 1998.
2. Tavian M, Coulombel L, Luton D, et al. Aorta-associated CD34⁺ hematopoietic cells in the early human embryo. Blood 87:67–72, 1996.
3. Borst J, Vroom TM, Bos JD, et al. Tissue distribution and repertoire selection of human gamma delta T cells: comparison with the murine system. Curr Top Microbiol Immunol 173:41–46, 1991.
4. Mincheva NL, Kling M, Hammarstrom S, et al. Gamma delta T cells of human early pregnancy decidua: evidence for local proliferation, phenotypic heterogeneity, and extrathymic differentiation. J Immunol 159:3266–3277, 1997.
5. York IA, Rock KL. Antigen processing and presentation by the class I major histocompatibility complex. Annu Rev Immunol 14:369–396, 1996.
6. Salter RD, Benjamin RJ, Wesley PK, et al. A binding site for the T-cell co-receptor CD8 on the alpha 3 domain of HLA-A2. Nature 345:41–46, 1990.
7. Pamer E, Cresswell P. Mechanisms of MHC class I–restricted antigen processing. Annu Rev Immunol 16:323–358, 1998.
8. Wilson IA, Bjorkman PJ. Unusual MHC-like molecules: CD1, Fc receptor, the hemochromatosis gene product, and viral homologs. Curr Opin Immunol 10:67–73, 1998.
9. Mason PM, Parham P. HLA class I region sequences, 1998. Tissue Antigens 51:417–466, 1998.
10. Black FL. Why did they die? Science 258:1739–1740, 1992.
11. Daar AS, Fuggle SV, Fabre JW, et al. The detailed distribution of HLA-A, B, C antigens in normal human organs. Transplantation 38:287–292, 1984.
12. Corriveau RA, Huh GS, Shatz CJ. Regulation of class I MHC gene expression in the developing and mature CNS by neural activity. Neuron 21:505–520, 1998.
13. Lata JA, Tuan RS, Shepley KJ, et al. Localization of major histocompatibility complex class I and II mRNA in human first-trimester chorionic villi by in situ hybridization. J Exp Med 175:1027–1032, 1992.
14. Jondal M, Schirmbeck R, Reimann J. MHC class I–restricted CTL responses to exogenous antigens. Immunity 5:295–302, 1996.
15. Canaday D, Ziebold C, Noss E, et al. Activation of human CD8⁺ alpha/beta-TCR⁺ cells by the *Mycobacterium tuberculosis* via an alternate class I MHC antigen-processing pathway. J Immunol 162:372–379, 1999.
16. Kurts C, Miller JF, Subramaniam RM, et al. Major histocompatibility complex class I–restricted cross-presentation is biased towards high dose antigens and those released during cellular destruction. J Exp Med 188:409–414, 1998.
17. Busch R, Mellins ED. Developing and shedding inhibitions: how MHC class II molecules reach maturity. Curr Opin Immunol 8:51–58, 1996.
18. Konig R, Huang LY, Germain RN. MHC class II interaction with CD4 mediated by a region analogous to the MHC class I binding site for CD8. Nature 356:796–798, 1992.
19. Chicz RM, Urban RG, Lane WS, et al. Predominant naturally processed peptides bound to HLA-DR1 are derived from MHC-related molecules and are heterogeneous in size. Nature 358:764–768, 1992.
20. Marsh S. HLA class II region sequences, 1998. Tissue Antigens 51:467–507, 1998.
21. Daar AS, Fuggle SV, Fabre JW, et al. The detailed distribution of MHC class II antigens in normal human organs. Transplantation 38:293–298, 1984.
22. Lewis DB. Host defense mechanisms against bacteria, fungi, viruses, and non-viral intracellular pathogens. *In* Polin R, Fox W (eds). Neonatal and Fetal Medicine. Philadelphia, WB Saunders, 1998, pp 1869–1919.
23. O'Callaghan CA, Bell JI. Structure and function of the human MHC class Ib molecules HLA-E, HLA-F and HLA-G. Immunol Rev 163:129–138, 1998.
24. Braud VM, Allan DS, Wilson D, et al. TAP- and tapasin-dependent HLA-E surface expression correlates with the binding of an MHC class I leader peptide. Curr Biol 8:1–10, 1998.
25. McMaster M, Zhou Y, Shorter S, et al. HLA-G isoforms produced by placental cytotrophoblasts and found in amniotic fluid are due to unusual glycosylation. J Immunol 160:5922–5928, 1998.
26. Rouas-Freiss N, Gonecalves RM, Menier C, et al. Direct evidence to support the role of HLA-G in protecting the fetus from maternal uterine natural killer cytolysis. Proc Natl Acad Sci USA 94:11520–11525, 1997.
27. Porcelli SA, Segelke BW, Sugita M, et al. The CD1 family of lipid antigen-presenting molecules. Immunol Today 19:362–368, 1998.
28. Melian A, Beckman EM, Porcelli SA, et al. Antigen presentation by CD1 and MHC-encoded class I–like molecules. Curr Opin Immunol 8:82–88, 1996.

29. Ernst WA, Maher J, Cho S, et al. Molecular interaction of CD1b with lipoglycan antigens. Immunity 8:331–340, 1998.

30. Fairhurst RM, Wang CX, Sieling PA, et al. CD1-restricted T cells and resistance to polysaccharide-encapsulated bacteria. Immunol Today 19:257–259, 1998.

31. Schofield L, McConville MJ, Hansen D, et al. CD1d-restricted immunoglobulin G formation to GPI-anchored antigens mediated by NK T cells. Science 283:225–229, 1999.

32. Steinle A, Groh V, Spies T. Diversification, expression, and gamma delta T cell recognition of evolutionarily distant members of the MIC family of major histocompatibility complex class I–related molecules. Proc Natl Acad Sci USA 95:12510–12515, 1998.

33. Lindahl KF, Byers DE, Dabhi VM, et al. H2-M3, a full-service class Ib histocompatibility antigen. Annu Rev Immunol 15:851–879, 1997.

34. Hart DN. Dendritic cells: unique leukocyte populations which control the primary immune response. Blood 90:3245–3287, 1997.

35. Austyn JM. New insights into the mobilization and phagocytic activity of dendritic cells. J Exp Med 183:1287–1292, 1996.

36. Pulendran B, Lingappa J, Kennedy MK, et al. Developmental pathways of dendritic cells in vivo: distinct function, phenotype, and localization of dendritic cell subsets in flt3 ligand–treated mice. J Immunol 159:2222–2231, 1997.

37. Pulendran B, Smith J, Jenkins M, et al. Prevention of peripheral tolerance by a dendritic cell growth factor: flt3 ligand as an adjuvant. J Exp Med 188:2075–2082, 1998.

38. Jiang W, Swiggard WJ, Heufler C, et al. The receptor DEC-205 expressed by dendritic cells and thymic epithelial cells is involved in antigen processing. Nature 375:151–155, 1995.

39. Inaba K, Turley S, Yamaide F, et al. Efficient presentation of phagocytosed cellular fragments on major histocompatibility complex class II products of dendritic cells. J Exp Med 188:2163–2173, 1998.

40. Albert ML, Sauter B, Bhardwaj N. Dendritic cells acquire antigen from apoptotic cells and induce class I–restricted CTLs. Nature 392:86–89, 1998.

41. Pierre P, Turley SJ, Gatti E, et al. Developmental regulation of MHC class II transport in mouse dendritic cells. Nature 388:787–792, 1997.

42. Sparwasser T, Koch ES, Vabulas RM, et al. Bacterial DNA and immunostimulatory CpG oligonucleotides trigger maturation and activation of murine dendritic cells. Eur J Immunol 28:2045–2054, 1998.

43. Sallusto F, Schaerli P, Loetscher P, et al. Rapid and coordinated switch in chemokine receptor expression during dendritic cell maturation. Eur J Immunol 28:2760–2769, 1998.

44. Sozzani S, Allavena P, D'Amico G, et al. Differential regulation of chemokine receptors during dendritic cell maturation: a model for their trafficking properties. J. Immunol 161:1083–1086, 1998.

45. van Kooten C, Banchereau J. CD40-CD40 ligand: a multifunctional receptor-ligand pair. Adv Immunol 61:1–77, 1996.

46. Wykes M, Pombo A, Jenkins C, et al. Dendritic cells interact directly with naive B lymphocytes to transfer antigen and initiate class switching in a primary T-dependent response. J Immunol 161:1313–1319, 1998.

47. de St. Groth B-F. The evolution of self-tolerance: a new cell arises to meet the challenge of self-reactivity. Immunol Today 19:448–454, 1998.

48. Kronin V, Winkel K, Suss G, et al. A subclass of dendritic cells regulates the response of naive CD8 T cells by limiting their IL-2 production. J Immunol 157:3819–3827, 1996.

49. Finkelman FD, Lees A, Birnbaum R, et al. Dendritic cells can present antigen in vivo in a tolerogenic or immunogenic fashion. J Immunol 157:1406–1414, 1996.

50. Hofman FM, Danilovs JA, Taylor CR. HLA-DR (Ia)–positive dendritic-like cells in human fetal nonlymphoid tissues. Transplantation 37:590–594, 1984.

51. Oliver AM, Thomson AW, Sewell HF, et al. Major histocompatibility complex (MHC) class II antigen (HLA-DR, DQ, and DP) expression in human fetal endocrine organs and gut. Scand J Immunol 27:731–737, 1988.

52. Keever CA, Abu HM, Graf W, et al. Characterization of the alloreactivity and anti-leukemia reactivity of cord blood mononuclear cells. Bone Marrow Transplant 15:407–419, 1995.

53. Foster CA, Holbrook KA. Ontogeny of Langerhans cells in human embryonic and fetal skin: cell densities and phenotypic expression relative to epidermal growth. Am J Anat 184:157–164, 1989.

54. Edwards JA, Jones DB, Evans PR, et al. Differential expression of HLA class II antigens on human fetal and adult lymphocytes and macrophages. Immunology 55:489–500, 1985.

55. Harvey J, Jones DB, Wright DH. Differential expression of MHC- and macrophage-associated antigens in human fetal and postnatal small intestine. Immunology 69:409–415, 1990.

56. Sherman L. The molecular basis of allorecognition. Annu Rev Immunol 11:385–402, 1993.

57. Ploegh HL. Viral strategies of immune evasion. Science 280:248–253, 1998.

58. Chilmonczyk BA, Levin MJ, McDuffy R, et al. Characterization of the human newborn response to herpesvirus antigen. J Immunol 134:4184–4188, 1985.

59. Roncarolo MG, Bigler M, Ciuti E, et al. Immune responses by cord blood cells. Blood Cells 20:573–585, 1994.

60. Clerici M, DePalma L, Roilides E, et al. Analysis of T helper and antigen-presenting cell functions in cord blood and peripheral blood leukocytes from healthy children of different ages. J Clin Invest 91:2829–2836, 1993.

61. Garban F, Ericson M, Roucard C, et al. Detection of empty HLA class II molecules on cord blood B cells. Blood 87:3970–3976, 1996.

62. Nelson DJ, Holt PG. Defective regional immunity in the respiratory tract of neonates is attributable to hyporesponsiveness of local dendritic cells to activation signals. J Immunol 155:3517–3524, 1995.

63. Hunt DW, Huppertz HI, Jiang HJ, et al. Studies of human cord blood dendritic cells: evidence for functional immaturity. Blood 84:4333–4343, 1994.

64. Sorg S. Dendritic cell function in the neonate. Vaccine 100:1–10, 1998.

65. Dejbakhsh JS, Jerabek L, Weissman IL, et al. Extrathymic maturation of alpha beta T cells from hematopoietic stem cells. J Immunol 155:3338–3344, 1995.

66. Ohteki T, Wilson A, Verbeek S, et al. Selectively impaired development of intestinal T cell receptor gamma delta$^+$ cells and liver CD4$^+$ NK1$^+$ T cell receptor alpha/beta$^+$ cells in T cell factor-1–deficient mice. Eur J Immunol 26:351–355, 1996.

67. Ohteki T, Okuyama R, Seki S, et al. Age-dependent increase of extrathymic T cells in the liver and their appearance in the periphery of older mice. J Immunol 149:1562–1570, 1992.

68. Lefrancois L, Puddington L. The role of the thymus in intestinal intraepithelial T-cell development. Ann NY Acad Sci 778:36–46, 1996.

69. Kondo M, Weissman IL, Akashi K. Identification of clonogenic common lymphoid progenitors in mouse bone marrow. Cell 91:661–672, 1997.

70. Blom B, Res PC, Spits H. T cell precursors in man and mice. Crit Rev Immunol 18:371–388, 1998.

71. Donskoy E, Goldschneider I. Thymocytopoiesis is maintained by blood-borne precursors throughout postnatal life: a study in parabiotic mice. J Immunol 148:1604–1612, 1992.

72. Robey E, Fowlkes BJ. The alpha beta versus gamma delta T-cell lineage choice. Curr Opin Immunol 10:181–187, 1998.

73. Gao Y, Sun Y, Frank K, et al. A critical role for DNA end-joining proteins in both lymphogenesis and neurogenesis. Cell 95:891–902, 1998.

74. Schwarz K, Notarangelo L, Spanopoulou E, et al. Recombination defects. In Ochs HD, Edvard Smith CIE, Puck JM (eds). Primary Immunodeficiency Diseases: A Molecular and Genetic Approach. New York, Oxford University Press, 1999, pp 155–166.

75. Rowen L, Koop BF, Hood L. The complete 685-kilobase DNA sequence of the human beta T cell receptor locus. Science 272:1755–1762, 1996.

76. Malissen B, Malissen M. Functions of TCR and pre-TCR subunits: lessons from gene ablation. Curr Opin Immunol 8:383–393, 1996.

77. Padovan E, Giachino C, Cella M, et al. Normal T lymphocytes can express two different T cell receptor beta chains: implications for the mechanism of allelic exclusion. J Exp Med 181:1587–1591, 1995.

78. Padovan E, Casorati G, Dellabona P, et al. Expression of two T cell receptor alpha chains: dual receptor T cells. Science 262:422–424, 1993.

79. McMahan C, Fink P. RAG re-expression and DNA recombination at T cell receptor loci in peripheral CD4+ T cells. Immunity 9:637–647, 1998.

80. Nussenzweig M. Immune receptor editing: revise and select. Cell 95:875–878, 1998.

81. Davis MM, Lyons DS, Altman JD, et al. T cell receptor biochemistry, repertoire selection and general features of TCR and Ig structure. Ciba Found Symp 204:94–100, 1997.

82. Siu G, Kronenberg M, Strauss E, et al. The structure, rearrangement and expression of D beta gene segments of the murine T-cell antigen receptor. Nature 311:344–350, 1984.

83. Komori T, Okada A, Stewart V, et al. Lack of N regions in antigen receptor variable region genes of TdT-deficient lymphocytes. Science 261:1171–1175, 1993.

84. Lewis SM. P nucleotides, hairpin DNA and V(D)J joining: making the connection. Semin Immunol 6:131–141, 1994.

85. Jores R, Meo T. Few V gene segments dominate the T cell receptor beta-chain repertoire of the human thymus. J Immunol 151:6110–6122, 1993.

86. Barton G, Rudensky A. Requirement for diverse, low-abundance peptides in positive selection of T cells. Science 283:67–70, 1999.

87. Garcia KC, Teyton L. T-cell receptor peptide-MHC interactions: biological lessons from structural studies. Curr Opin Biotechnol 9:338–343, 1998.

88. Zerrahn J, Held W, Raulet DH. The MHC reactivity of the T cell repertoire prior to positive and negative selection. Cell 88:627–636, 1997.

89. Alam SM, Travers PJ, Wung JL, et al. T-cell-receptor affinity and thymocyte positive selection [see comments]. Nature 381:616–620, 1996.

90. Laufer TM, DeKoning J, Markowitz JS, et al. Unopposed positive selection and autoreactivity in mice expressing class II MHC only on thymic cortex. Nature 383:81–85, 1996.

91. van Meerwijk JP, Marguerat S, Lees RK, et al. Quantitative impact of thymic clonal deletion on the T cell repertoire. J Exp Med 185:377–383, 1997.

92. Farr AG, Rudensky A. Medullary thymic epithelium: a mosaic of epithelial "self"? J Exp Med 188:1–4, 1998.

93. Cilio CM, Daws MR, Malashicheva A, et al. Cytotoxic T lymphocyte antigen 4 is induced in the thymus upon in vivo activation and its blockade prevents anti-CD3–mediated depletion of thymocytes. J Exp Med 188:1239–1246, 1998.

94. Vandenberghe P, Delabie J, de Boer M, et al. In situ expression of B7/BB1 on antigen-presenting cells and activated B cells: an immunohistochemical study. Int Immunol 5:317–321, 1993.

95. Bodmer J. World distribution of HLA alleles and implications for disease. Ciba Found Symp 197:233–253, 1996.

96. Puel A, Ziegler SF, Buckley RH, et al. Defective IL7R expression in T(-)B(+)NK(+) severe combined immunodeficiency. Nat Genet 20:394–397, 1998.

97. Puck JM, Pepper AE, Henthorn PS, et al. Mutation analysis of IL2RG in human X-linked severe combined immunodeficiency. Blood 89:1968–1977, 1997.

98. Candotti F, Oakes SA, Johnston JA, et al. Structural and functional basis for JAK3-deficient severe combined immunodeficiency. Blood 90:3996–4003, 1997.

99. Ceredig R, Dialynas DP, Fitch FW, et al. Precursors of T cell growth factor producing cells in the thymus: ontogeny, frequency, and quantitative recovery in a subpopulation of phenotypically mature thymocytes defined by monoclonal antibody GK-1.5. J Exp Med 158:1654–1671, 1983.

100. Ceredig R, Glasebrook AL, MacDonald HR. Phenotypic and functional properties of murine thymocytes. I. Precursors of cytolytic T lymphocytes and interleukin 2–producing cells are all contained within a subpopulation of "mature" thymocytes as analyzed by monoclonal antibodies and flow microfluorometry. J Exp Med 155:358–379, 1982.

101. Tanchot C, Rosado MM, Agenes F, et al. Lymphocyte homeostasis. Semin Immunol 9:331–337, 1997.

102. Crabtree GR, Clipstone NA. Signal transmission between the plasma membrane and nucleus of T lymphocytes. Annu Rev Biochem 63:1045–1083, 1994.

103. Rudd CE. Adaptors and molecular scaffolds in immune cell signaling. Cell 96:5–8, 1999.

104. Ullman K, Northrop J, Verewij C, et al. Transmission of signals from the T lymphocyte antigen receptor to the genes responsible for cell proliferation and immune function: the missing link. Annu Rev Immunol 8:421–452, 1990.

105. Jameson SC, Bevan MJ. T cell receptor antagonists and partial agonists. Immunity 2:1–11, 1995.

106. Kersh E, Shaw A, Allen P. Fidelity of T cell activation through multistep T cell receptor phosphorylation. Science 281:572–575, 1998.

107. Chambers CA, Allison JP. Co-stimulation in T cell responses. Curr Opin Immunol 9:396–404, 1997.

108. Grewal IS, Flavell RA. The CD40 ligand: at the center of the immune universe? Immunol Res 16:59–70, 1997.
109. Cayabyab M, Phillips JH, Lanier LL. CD40 preferentially costimulates activation of CD4+ T lymphocytes. J Immunol 152:1523–1531, 1994.
110. Clark EA, Berberich I, Klaus SJ, et al. Accessory molecules that influence signaling through B lymphocyte antigen receptors. Adv Exp Med Biol 365:35–43, 1994.
111. Schwartz RH. Models of T cell anergy: is there a common molecular mechanism? J Exp Med 184:1–8, 1996.
112. Swain SL, Croft M, Dubey C, et al. From naive to memory T cells. Immunol Rev 150:143–167, 1996.
113. Dubey C, Croft M, Swain SL. Naive and effector CD4 T cells differ in their requirements for T cell receptor versus costimulatory signals. J Immunol 157:3280–3289, 1996.
114. Miyawaki T, Uehara T, Nibu R, et al. Differential expression of apoptosis-related Fas antigen on lymphocyte subpopulations in human peripheral blood. J Immunol 149:3753–3758, 1992.
115. Akbar AN, Borthwick N, Salmon M, et al. The significance of low bcl-2 expression by C-D45R0 T cells in normal individuals and patients with acute viral infections: the role of apoptosis in T cell memory. J Exp Med 178:427–438, 1993.
116. Salmon M, Pilling D, Borthwick NJ, et al. The progressive differentiation of primed T cells is associated with an increasing susceptibility to apoptosis. Eur J Immunol 24:892–899, 1994.
117. Uehara T, Miyawaki T, Ohta K, et al. Apoptotic cell death of primed CD45R0+ T lymphocytes in Epstein-Barr virus–induced infectious mononucleosis. Blood 80:452–458, 1992.
118. Puck JM, Sneller MC. ALPS: an autoimmune human lymphoproliferative syndrome associated with abnormal lymphocyte apoptosis. Semin Immunol 9:77–84, 1997.
119. Liles WC, Van Voorhis WC. Review: nomenclature and biologic significance of cytokines involved in inflammation and the host immune response. J Infect Dis 172:1573–1580, 1995.
120. Lenardo MJ. Fas and the art of lymphocyte maintenance. J Exp Med 183:721–724, 1996.
121. Sharfe N, Dadi HK, Shahar M, et al. Human immune disorder arising from mutation of the alpha chain of the interleukin-2 receptor. Proc Natl Acad Sci U S A 94:3168–3171, 1997.
122. Ramesh N, Geha RS, Notarangelo LD. CD40 ligand and the hyper-IgM syndrome. In Ochs HD, Edvard Smith CIE, and Puck JM (eds). Primary Immunodeficiency Diseases: A Molecular and Genetic Approach. New York, Oxford University Press, 1999, pp 233–249.
123. McDyer JF, Goletz TJ, Thomas E, et al. CD40 ligand/CD40 stimulation regulates the production of IFN-gamma from human peripheral blood mononuclear cells in an IL-12– and/or CD28–dependent manner. J Immunol 160:1701–1707, 1998.
124. Fearon DT, Locksley RM. The instructive role of innate immunity in the acquired immune response. Science 272:50–53, 1996.
125. Carding SR, Allan W, McMickle A, et al. Activation of cytokine genes in T cells during primary and secondary murine influenza pneumonia. J Exp Med 177:475–482, 1993.
126. Waldrop SL, Davis KA, Maino VC, et al. Normal human CD4+ memory T cells display broad heterogeneity in their activation threshold for cytokine synthesis. J Immunol 161:5284–5295, 1998.
127. Toellner KM, Luther SA, Sze DM, et al. T helper 1 (Th1) and Th2 characteristics start to develop during T cell priming and are associated with an immediate ability to induce immunoglobulin class switching. J Exp Med 187:1193–1204, 1998.
128. Rogers PR, Huston G, Swain SL. High antigen density and IL-2 are required for generation of CD4 effectors secreting Th1 rather than Th0 cytokines. J Immunol 161:3844–3852, 1998.
129. Austrup F, Vestweber D, Borges E, et al. P- and E-selectin mediate recruitment of T-helper-1 but not T-helper-2 cells into inflamed tissues. Nature 385:81–83, 1997.
130. Okamura H, Kashiwamura S, Tsutsui H, et al. Regulation of interferon-gamma production by IL-12 and IL-18. Curr Opin Immunol 10:259–264, 1998.
131. Heufler C, Koch F, Stanzl U, et al. Interleukin-12 is produced by dendritic cells and mediates T helper 1 development as well as interferon-gamma production by T helper 1 cells. Eur J Immunol 26:659–668, 1996.
132. Altare F, Lammas D, Revy P, et al. Inherited interleukin 12 deficiency in a child with Bacille Calmette-Guérin and Salmonella enteritidis disseminated infection. J Clin Invest 102:2035–2040, 1998.
133. de Jong R, Altare F, Haagen IA, et al. Severe mycobacterial and Salmonella infections in interleukin-12 receptor–deficient patients. Science 280:1435–1438, 1998.
134. Newport MJ, Huxley CM, Huston S, et al. A mutation in the interferon-gamma–receptor gene and susceptibility to mycobacterial infection. N Engl J Med 335:1941–1949, 1996.
135. Parronchi P, Mohapatra S, Sampognaro S, et al. Effects of interferon-alpha on cytokine profile, T cell receptor repertoire and peptide reactivity of human allergen-specific T cells. Eur J Immunol 26:697–703, 1996.
136. Murphy KM. T lymphocyte differentiation in the periphery. Curr Opin Immunol 10:226–232, 1998.
137. Flynn S, Toellner KM, Raykundalia C, et al. CD4 T cell cytokine differentiation: the B cell activation molecule, OX40 ligand, instructs CD4 T cells to express interleukin 4 and upregulates expression of the chemokine receptor, Blr-1. J Exp Med 188:297–304, 1998.
138. Scheipers P, Reiser H. Fas-independent death of activated CD4(+) T lymphocytes induced by CTLA-4 crosslinking. Proc Natl Acad Sci USA 95:10083–10088, 1998.
139. Chen W, Jin W, Wahl S. Engagement of cytotoxic T lymphocyte–associated antigen 4 (CTLA-4) induces transforming growth factor beta (TGF-beta) production by murine CD4(+) T cells. J Exp Med 188:1849–1857, 1998.
140. Perez VL, Van Parijs L, Biuckians A, et al. Induction of peripheral T cell tolerance in vivo requires CTLA-4 engagement. Immunity 6:411–417, 1997.
141. Marengere LE, Waterhouse P, Duncan GS, et al. Regulation of T cell receptor signaling by tyrosine phosphatase SYP association with CTLA-4. Science 272:1170–1173, 1996.
142. Lee K, Chuang E, Khattri M, et al. Molecular basis of T cell inactivation by CTLA-4. Science 282:2263–2266, 1998.
143. Macchia D, Almerigogna F, Parronchi P, et al. Membrane tumor necrosis factor–alpha is involved in the polyclonal B-cell activation induced by HIV-infected human T cells. Nature 363:464–466, 1993.
144. Lipsky PE, Attrep JF, Grammer AC, et al. Analysis of CD40-CD40 ligand interactions in the regulation of human B cell function. Ann N Y Acad Sci 815:372–383, 1997.

145. Ochs HD, Nonoyama S, Farrington ML, et al. The role of adhesion molecules in the regulation of antibody responses. Semin Hematol 30:72–79, 1993.
146. Lane P. Molecular mechanisms involved in T-B interactions. Chem Immunol 67:1–13, 1997.
147. Kuhn R, Rajewsky K, Muller W. Generation and analysis of interleukin-4 deficient mice. Science 254:707–710, 1991.
148. Takeda K, Tanaka T, Shi W, et al. Essential role of Stat6 in IL-4 signaling. Nature 380:627–630, 1996.
149. Mescher MF. Molecular interactions in the activation of effector and precursor cytotoxic T lymphocytes. Immunol Rev 14:177–210, 1995.
150. Hamann D, Baars PA, Rep MH, et al. Phenotypic and functional separation of memory and effector human CD8+ T cells. J Exp Med 186:1407–1418, 1997.
151. Callan MFC, Tan L, Annels N, et al. Direct visualization of antigen-specific CD8+ T cells during the primary immune response to Epstein-Barr virus in vivo. J Exp Med 187:1395–1402, 1998.
152. Zheng L, Fisher G, Miller RE, et al. Induction of apoptosis in mature T cells by tumor necrosis factor. Nature 377:348–351, 1995.
153. Lanzavecchia A. Immunology. Licence to kill. Nature 393:413–414, 1998.
154. Kalams S, Walker B. The critical need for CD4 help in maintaining effective cytotoxic T lymphocyte responses. J Exp Med 188:2199–2204, 1998.
155. Shresta S, Pham CT, Thomas DA, et al. How do cytotoxic lymphocytes kill their targets? Curr Opin Immunol 10:581–587, 1998.
156. Bossi G, Griffiths G. Degranulation plays an essential part in regulating cell surface expression of fas ligand in T cells and natural killer cells. Nat Med 5:90–96, 1999.
157. Guidotti LG, Ishikawa T, Hobbs MV, et al. Intracellular inactivation of the hepatitis B virus by cytotoxic T lymphocytes. Immunity 4:25–36, 1996.
158. Doherty PC. Cytotoxic T cell effector and memory function in viral immunity. Curr Top Microbiol Immunol 206:1–14, 1996.
159. Liu YJ. Tracing antigen-driven B cell development in humans. Chem Immunol 67:14–26, 1997.
160. Ameratunga R, Lederman HM, Sullivan KE, et al. Defective antigen-induced lymphocyte proliferation in the X-linked hyper-IgM syndrome. J Pediatr 131:147–150, 1997.
161. Weng NP, Levine BL, June CH, et al. Human naive and memory T lymphocytes differ in telomeric length and replicative potential. Proc Natl Acad Sci USA 92:11091–11094, 1995.
162. Rabin RL, Roederer M, Maldonado Y, et al. Altered representation of naive and memory CD8 T cell subsets in HIV-infected children. J Clin Invest 95:2054–2060, 1995.
163. Young JL, Ramage JM, Gaston JS, et al. In vitro responses of human CD45R0brightRA- and CD45R0-RAbright T cell subsets and their relationship to memory and naive T cells. Eur J Immunol 27:2383–2390, 1997.
164. Sanders ME, Makgoba MW, Sharrow SO, et al. Human memory T lymphocytes express increased levels of three cell adhesion molecules (LFA-3, CD2, and LFA-1) and three other molecules (UCHL1, CDw29, and Pgp-1) and have enhanced IFN-gamma production. J Immunol 140:1401–1407, 1988.
165. Hamann D, Baars PA, Hooibrink B, et al. Heterogeneity of the human CD4+ T-cell population: two distinct CD4+ T-cell subsets characterized by coexpression of CD45RA and CD45R0 isoforms. Blood 88:3513–3521, 1996.
166. Clement LT. Isoforms of the CD45 common leukocyte antigen family: markers for human T-cell differentiation. J Clin Immunol 12:1–10, 1992.
167. Plebanski M, Saunders M, Burtles SS, et al. Primary and secondary human in vitro T-cell responses to soluble antigens are mediated by subsets bearing different CD45 isoforms. Immunology 75:86–91, 1992.
168. D'Andrea A, Lanier LL. Killer cell inhibitory receptor expression by T cells. Curr Top Microbiol Immunol 230:25–39, 1998.
169. Sanders ME, Makgoba MW, June CH, et al. Enhanced responsiveness of human memory T cells to CD2 and CD3 receptor-mediated activation. Eur J Immunol 19:803–808, 1989.
170. Ahmed R, Gray D. Immunological memory and protective immunity: understanding their relation. Science 272:54–60, 1996.
171. Pitzalis C, Kingsley GH, Covelli M, et al. Selective migration of the human helper-inducer memory T cell subset: confirmation by in vivo cellular kinetic studies. Eur J Immunol 21:369–376, 1991.
172. Ohteki T, Ho S, Suzuki H, et al. Role for IL-15/IL-15 receptor beta-chain in natural killer 1.1+ T cell receptor-alpha/beta+ cell development. J Immunol 159:5931–5935, 1997.
173. Zeng D, Lewis D, Dejbaksh-Jones S, et al. Bone marrow NK1.1- and NK1.1+ T cells reciprocally regulate lethal graft-versus-host-disease. J Exp Med 189:1073–1082, 1999.
174. Wilson SB, Kent SC, Patton KT, et al. Extreme Th1 bias of invariant Valpha24JalphaQ T cells in type 1 diabetes. Nature 391:177–181, 1998.
175. Poggi A, Demarest JF, Costa P, et al. Expression of a wide T cell receptor V beta repertoire in human T lymphocytes derived in vitro from embryonic liver cell precursors. Eur J Immunol 24:2258–2261, 1994.
176. Haynes BF, Heinly CS. Early human T cell development: analysis of the human thymus at the time of initial entry of hematopoietic stem cells into the fetal thymic microenvironment. J Exp Med 181:1445–1458, 1995.
177. Horst E, Meijer CJ, Duijvestijn AM, et al. The ontogeny of human lymphocyte recirculation: high endothelial cell antigen (HECA-452) and CD44 homing receptor expression in the development of the immune system. Eur J Immunol 20:1483–1489, 1990.
178. Gilhus NE, Matre R, Tonder O. Hassall's corpuscles in the thymus of fetuses, infants and children: immunological and histochemical aspects. Thymus 7:123–135, 1985.
179. Asano S, Akaike Y, Muramatsu T, et al. Immunohistologic detection of the primary follicle (PF) in human fetal and newborn lymph node anlages. Pathol Res Pract 189:921–927, 1993.
180. Ramos SB, Garcia AB, Viana SR, et al. Phenotypic and functional evaluation of natural killer cells in thymectomized children. Clin Immunol Immunopathol 81:277–281, 1996.
181. Baroni CD, Valtieri M, Stoppacciaro A, et al. The human thymus in ageing: histologic involution paralleled by increased mitogen response and by enrichment of OKT3+ lymphocytes. Immunology 50:519–528, 1983.
182. Mackall CL, Fleisher TA, Brown MR, et al. Age, thymopoiesis, and CD4+ T-lymphocyte regeneration after intensive chemotherapy. N Engl J Med 332:143–149, 1995.

183. Douek D, McFarland R, Keiser P, et al. Changes in thymic function with age and during the treatment of HIV infection. Nature 396:690–695, 1998.

184. Settmacher U, Volk HD, Jahn S, et al. Characterization of human lymphocytes separated from fetal liver and spleen at different stages of ontogeny. Immunobiology 182:256–265, 1991.

185. Hannet I, Erkeller YF, Lydyard P, et al. Developmental and maturational changes in human blood lymphocyte subpopulations. Immunol Today 13:215, 218, 1992.

186. Wilson M, Rosen FS, Schlossman SF, et al. Ontogeny of human T and B lymphocytes during stressed and normal gestation: phenotypic analysis of umbilical cord lymphocytes from term and preterm infants. Clin Immunol Immunopathol 37:1–12, 1985.

187. Asma GE, Van den Bergh RL, Vossen JM. Use of monoclonal antibodies in a study of the development of T lymphocytes in the human fetus. Clin Exp Immunol 53:429–436, 1983.

188. Lanier LL, Allison JP, Phillips JH. Correlation of cell surface antigen expression on human thymocytes by multi-color flow cytometric analysis: implications for differentiation. J Immunol 137:2501–2507, 1986.

189. Byrne JA, Stankovic AK, Cooper MD. A novel subpopulation of primed T cells in the human fetus. J Immunol 152:3098–3106, 1994.

190. Peakman M, Buggins AG, Nicolaides KH, et al. Analysis of lymphocyte phenotypes in cord blood from early gestation fetuses. Clin Exp Immunol 90:345–350, 1992.

191. Bofill M, Akbar AN, Salmon M, et al. Immature CD45RA(low)R0(low) T cells in the human cord blood. I. Antecedents of CD45RA+ unprimed T cells. J Immunol 152:5613–5623, 1994.

192. Yang CP, Bell EB. Functional maturation of recent thymic emigrants in the periphery: development of alloreactivity correlates with the cyclic expression of CD45RC isoforms. Eur J Immunol 22:2261–2269, 1992.

193. Frenkel L, Bryson YJ. Ontogeny of phytohemagglutinin-induced gamma interferon by leukocytes of healthy infants and children: evidence for decreased production in infants younger than 2 months of age. J Pediatr 111:97–100, 1987.

194. Kanegane H, Miyawaki T, Kato K, et al. A novel subpopulation of CD45RA+ CD4+ T cells expressing IL-2 receptor alpha-chain (CD25) and having a functionally transitional nature into memory cells. Int Immunol 3:1349–1356, 1991.

195. Delespesse G, Yang LP, Ohshima Y, et al. Maturation of human neonatal CD4+ and CD8+ T lymphocytes into Th1/Th2 effectors. Vaccine 16:1415–1419, 1998.

196. Azuma M, Cayabyab M, Phillips JH, et al. Requirements for CD28-dependent T cell–mediated cytotoxicity. J Immunol 150:2091–2101, 1993.

197. Azuma M, Phillips JH, Lanier LL. CD28-T lymphocytes. Antigenic and functional properties. J Immunol 150:1147–1159, 1993.

198. George JFJ, Schroeder HWJ. Developmental regulation of D beta reading frame and junctional diversity in T cell receptor–beta transcripts from human thymus. J Immunol 148:1230–1239, 1992.

199. Raaphorst FM, van Bergen J, van den Bergh RL, et al. Usage of TCRαV and TCRβV gene families in human fetal and adult TCR rearrangements. Immunogenetics 39:343–350, 1994.

200. Raaphorst FM, Kaijzel EL, Van Tol MJ, et al. Nonrandom employment of V beta 6 and J beta gene elements and conserved amino acid usage profiles in CDR3 regions of human fetal and adult TCR beta chain rearrangements. Int Immunol 6:1–9, 1994.

201. Bonati A, Zanelli P, Ferrari S, et al. T-cell receptor beta-chain gene rearrangement and expression during human thymic ontogenesis. Blood 79:1472–1483, 1992.

202. Gilfillan S, Bachmann M, Trembleau S, et al. Efficient immune responses in mice lacking N-region diversity. Eur J Immunol 25:3115–3122, 1995.

203. Doherty PJ, Roifman CM, Pan SH, et al. Expression of the human T cell receptor V beta repertoire. Mol Immunol 28:607–612, 1991.

204. Paganelli R, Cherchi M, Scala E, et al. Activated and "memory" phenotype of circulating T lymphocytes in intrauterine life. Cell Immunol 155:486–492, 1994.

205. Vandekerckhove BA, Baccala R, Jones D, et al. Thymic selection of the human T cell receptor V beta repertoire in SCID-hu mice. J Exp Med 176:1619–1624, 1992.

206. Garderet L, Dulphy N, Douay C, et al. The umbilical cord blood alpha/beta T-cell repertoire: characteristics of a polyclonal and naive but completely formed repertoire. Blood 91:340–346, 1998.

207. Schelonka RL, Raaphorst FM, Infante D, et al. T cell receptor repertoire diversity and clonal expansion in human neonates. Pediatr Res 43:396–402, 1998.

208. Grunewald J, Shankar N, Wigzell H, et al. An analysis of alpha/beta TCR V gene expression in the human thymus. Int Immunol 3:699–702, 1991.

209. DerSimonian H, Band H, Brenner MB. Increased frequency of T cell receptor V alpha 12.1 expression on CD8+ T cells: evidence that V alpha participates in shaping the peripheral T cell repertoire. J Exp Med 174:639–648, 1991.

210. Cossarizza A, Kahan M, Ortolani C, et al. Preferential expression of V beta 6.7 domain on human peripheral CD4+ T cells: implication for positive selection of T cells in man. Eur J Immunol 21:1571–1574, 1991.

211. Trivedi HN, HayGlass KT, Gangur V, et al. Analysis of neonatal T cell and antigen presenting cell functions. Hum Immunol 57:69–79, 1997.

212. Caux C, Massacrier C, Vanbervliet B, et al. Interleukin 10 inhibits T cell alloreaction induced by human dendritic cells. Int Immunol 6:1177–1185, 1994.

213. Hayward A, Cosyns M. Proliferative and cytokine responses by human newborn T cells stimulated with staphylococcal enterotoxin B. Pediatr Res 35:293–298, 1994.

214. Takahashi N, Imanishi K, Nishida H, et al. Evidence for immunologic immaturity of cord blood T cells: cord blood T cells are susceptible to tolerance induction to in vitro stimulation with a superantigen. J Immunol 155:5213–5219, 1995.

215. Wilson CB, Westall J, Johnston L, et al. Decreased production of interferon-gamma by human neonatal cells. Intrinsic and regulatory deficiencies. J Clin Invest 77:860–867, 1986.

216. Saito S, Morii T, Umekage H, et al. Expression of the interleukin-2 receptor gamma chain on cord blood mononuclear cells. Blood 87:3344–3350, 1996.

217. Lewis DB, Larsen A, Wilson CB. Reduced interferon-gamma mRNA levels in human neonates: evidence for an intrinsic T cell deficiency independent of other genes involved in T cell activation. J Exp Med 163:1018–1023, 1986.

218. Hassan J, Reen DJ. Reduced primary antigen-specific T-cell precursor frequencies in neonates is associated with deficient interleukin-2 production. Immunology 87:604–608, 1996.

219. Mehta DA, Markowicz S, Engleman EG. Generation

of antigen-specific CD4$^+$ T cell lines from naive precursors. Eur J Immunol 25:1206–1211, 1995.

220. Crow MK, Kunkel HG. Human dendritic cells: major stimulators of the autologous and allogeneic mixed leucocyte reactions. Clin Exp Immunol 49:338–346, 1982.

221. Gerli R, Bertotto A, Crupi S, et al. Activation of cord T lymphocytes. I. Evidence for a defective T cell mitogenesis induced through the CD2 molecule. J Immunol 142:2583–2589, 1989.

222. Splawski JB, Jelinek DF, Lipsky PE. Delineation of the functional capacity of human neonatal lymphocytes. J Clin Invest 87:545–553, 1991.

223. Splawski JB, Lipsky PE. Cytokine regulation of immunoglobulin secretion by neonatal lymphocytes. J Clin Invest 88:967–977, 1991.

224. English BK, Burchett SK, English JD, et al. Production of lymphotoxin and tumor necrosis factor by human neonatal mononuclear cells. Pediatr Res 24:717–722, 1988.

225. Chheda S, Palkowetz KH, Garofalo R, et al. Decreased interleukin-10 production by neonatal monocytes and T cells: relationship to decreased production and expression of tumor necrosis factor–alpha and its receptors. Pediatr Res 40:475–483, 1996.

226. Dolganov G, Bort S, Lovett M, et al. Coexpression of the interleukin-13 and interleukin-4 genes correlates with their physical linkage in the cytokine gene cluster on human chromosome 5q23-31. Blood 87:3316–3326, 1996.

227. Ehlers S, Smith KA. Differentiation of T cell lymphokine gene expression: the in vitro acquisition of T cell memory. J Exp Med 173:25–36, 1991.

228. English BK, Hammond WP, Lewis DB, et al. Decreased granulocyte-macrophage colony-stimulating factor production by human neonatal blood mononuclear cells and T cells. Pediatr Res 31:211–216, 1992.

229. Lee SM, Knoppel E, van de Ven C, et al. Transcriptional rates of granulocyte-macrophage colony-stimulating factor, granulocyte colony-stimulating factor, interleukin-3, and macrophage colony-stimulating factor genes in activated cord versus adult mononuclear cells: alteration in cytokine expression may be secondary to post-transcriptional instability. Pediatr Res 34:560–564, 1993.

230. Lewis DB, Yu CC, Meyer J, et al. Cellular and molecular mechanisms for reduced interleukin 4 and interferon-gamma production by neonatal T cells. J Clin Invest 87:194–202, 1991.

231. Jung T, Wijdenes J, Neumann C, et al. Interleukin-13 is produced by activated human CD45RA$^+$ and CD45R0$^+$ T cells: modulation by interleukin-4 and interleukin-12. Eur J Immunol 26:571–577, 1996.

232. Lewis DB, Prickett KS, Larsen A, et al. Restricted production of interleukin 4 by activated human T cells. Proc Natl Acad Sci USA 85:9743–9747, 1988.

233. Salmon M, Kitas GD, Bacon PA. Production of lymphokine mRNA by CD45R$^+$ and CD45R$^-$ helper T cells from human peripheral blood and by human CD4$^+$ T cell clones. J Immunol 143:907–912, 1989.

234. Hassan J, O'Neill S, O'Neill LA, et al. Signaling via CD28 of human naive neonatal T lymphocytes. Clin Exp Immunol 102:192–198, 1995.

235. Hassan J, Reen DJ. Cord blood CD4$^+$ CD45RA$^+$ T cells achieve a lower magnitude of activation when compared with their adult counterparts. Immunology 90:397–401, 1997.

236. Melvin AJ, McGurn ME, Bort SJ, et al. Hypomethylation of the interferon-gamma gene correlates with its

237. Pirenne H, Aujard Y, Eljaafari A, et al. Comparison of T cell functional changes during childhood with the ontogeny of CDw29 and CD45RA expression on CD4$^+$ T cells Pediatr Res 32:81–86, 1992.

238. Durandy A, De-Saint-Basile G, Lisowska GB, et al. Undetectable CD40 ligand expression on T cells and low B cell responses to CD40 binding agonists in human newborns. J Immunol 154:1560–1568, 1995.

239. Brugnoni D, Airo P, Graf D, et al. Ineffective expression of CD40 ligand on cord blood T cells may contribute to poor immunoglobulin production in the newborn. Eur J Immunol 24:1919–1924, 1994.

240. Fuleihan R, Ahern D, Geha RS. Decreased expression of the ligand for CD40 in newborn lymphocytes. Eur J Immunol 24:1925–1928, 1994.

241. Nonoyama S, Penix LA, Edwards CP, et al. Diminished expression of CD40 ligand by activated neonatal T cells. J Clin Invest 95:66–75, 1995.

242. Flamand V, Donckier V, Demoor FX, et al. CD40 ligation prevents neonatal induction of transplantation tolerance. J Immunol 160:4666–4669, 1998.

243. Reen DJ. Activation and functional capacity of human neonatal CD4 T cells. Vaccine 16:1401–1408, 1998.

244. Ohshima Y, Delespesse G. T cell–derived IL-4 and dendritic cell–derived IL-12 regulate the lymphokine-producing phenotype of alloantigen-primed naive human CD4 T cells. J Immunol 158:629–636, 1997.

245. Splawski JB, Nishioka J, Nishioka Y, et al. CD40 ligand is expressed and functional on activated neonatal T cells. J Immunol 156:119–127, 1996.

246. Imanishi K, Seo K, Kato H, et al. Post-thymic maturation of migrating human thymic single-positive T cells: thymic CD1a$^-$ CD4$^+$ T cells are more susceptible to anergy induction by toxic shock syndrome toxin-1 than cord blood CD4$^+$ T cells. J Immunol 160:112–119, 1998.

247. Risdon G, Gaddy J, Horie M, et al. Alloantigen priming induces a state of unresponsiveness in human umbilical cord blood T cells. Proc Natl Acad Sci USA 92:2413–2417, 1995.

248. Porcu P, Gaddy J, Broxmeyer HE. Alloantigen-induced unresponsiveness in cord blood T lymphocytes is associated with defective activation of Ras. Proc Natl Acad Sci USA 95:4538–4543, 1998.

249. Demeure CE, Wu CY, Shu U, et al. In vitro maturation of human neonatal CD4 T lymphocytes II: cytokines present at priming modulate the development of lymphokine production. J Immunol 152:4775–4782, 1994.

250. Rogge L, Barberis ML, Biffi M, et al. Selective expression of an interleukin-12 receptor component by human T helper 1 cells. J Exp Med 185:825–831, 1997.

251. Sornasse T, Larenas PV, Davis KA, et al. Differentiation and stability of T helper 1 and 2 cells derived from naive human neonatal CD4$^+$ T cells, analyzed at the single-cell level. J Exp Med 184:473–483, 1996.

252. Early E, Reen D. Antigen-independent responsiveness to interleukin-4 demonstrates differential regulation of newborn human T cells. Eur J Immunol 26:2885–2889, 1996.

253. Campbell AC, Waller C, Wood J, et al. Lymphocyte subpopulations in the blood of newborn infants. Clin Exp Immunol 18:469–482, 1974.

254. Andersson U, Bird AG, Britton BS, et al. Humoral and cellular immunity in humans studied at the cell level from birth to two years of age. Immunol Rev 57:1–38, 1981.

255. Lubens RG, Gard SE, Soderberg-Warner M, et al. Lectin-dependent T-lymphocyte and natural killer cytotoxic deficiencies in human newborns. Cell Immunol 74:40–53, 1982.

256. Rayfield LS, Brent L, Rodeck CH. Development of cell-mediated lympholysis in human foetal blood lymphocytes. Clin Exp Immunol 42:561–570, 1980.

257. Granberg C, Hirvonen T. Cell-mediated lympholysis by fetal and neonatal lymphocytes in sheep and man. Cell Immunol 51:13–22, 1980.

258. Harris DT, LoCascio J, and Besencon FJ. Analysis of the alloreactive capacity of human umbilical cord blood: implications for graft-versus-host disease. Bone Marrow Transplant 14:545–553, 1994.

259. Risdon G, Gaddy J, Broxmeyer HE. Allogeneic responses of human umbilical cord blood. Blood Cells 20:566–570, 1994.

260. Risdon G, Gaddy J, Stehman FB, et al. Proliferative and cytotoxic responses of human cord blood T lymphocytes following allogeneic stimulation. Cell Immunol 154:14–24, 1994.

261. de Jong R, Brouwer M, Miedema F, et al. Human CD8$^+$ T lymphocytes can be divided into CD45RA$^+$ and CD45R0$^+$ cells with different requirements for activation and differentiation. J Immunol 146:2088–2094, 1991.

262. Akbar AN, Salmon M, Ivory K, et al. Human CD4$^+$CD45R0$^+$ and CD4$^+$CD45RA$^+$ T cells synergize in response to alloantigens. Eur J Immunol 21:2517–2522, 1991.

263. Berthou C, Legros MS, Souli'e A, et al. Cord blood T lymphocytes lack constitutive perforin expression in contrast to adult peripheral blood T lymphocytes. Blood 85:1540–1546, 1995.

264. Musha N, Yoshida Y, Sugahara S, et al. Expansion of CD56$^+$ NK T and gamma delta T cells from cord blood of human neonates. Clin Exp Immunol 113:220–228, 1998.

265. Kaufmann SH. Gamma/delta and other unconventional T lymphocytes: what do they see and what do they do? Proc Natl Acad Sci USA 93:2272–2279, 1996.

266. Chien YH, Jores R, Crowley MP. Recognition by gamma/delta T cells. Annu Rev Immunol 14:511–532, 1996.

267. Tanaka Y, Morita CT, Nieves E, et al. Natural and synthetic non-peptide antigens recognized by human gamma delta T cells. Nature 375:155–158, 1995.

268. Garcia VE, Sieling PA, Gong J, et al. Single-cell cytokine analysis of gamma delta T cell responses to non-peptide mycobacterial antigens. J Immunol 159:1328–1335, 1997.

269. Li H, Lebedeva MI, Llera AS, et al. Structure of the Vdelta domain of a human gamma/delta T-cell antigen receptor. Nature 391:502–506, 1998.

270. Arden B, Clark SP, Kabelitz D, et al. Human T-cell receptor variable gene segment families. Immunogenetics 42:455–500, 1995.

271. Kabelitz D. Function and specificity of human gamma/delta-positive T cells. Crit Rev Immunol 11:281–303, 1992.

272. Boismenu R, Feng L, Xia YY, et al. Chemokine expression by intraepithelial gamma delta T cells: implications for the recruitment of inflammatory cells to damaged epithelia. J Immunol 157:985–992, 1996.

273. Fujihashi K, McGhee JR, Kweon MN, et al. Gamma/delta T cell–deficient mice have impaired mucosal immunoglobulin A responses. J Exp Med 183:1929–1935, 1996.

274. Zuany AC, Ruffi'e C, Hail'e S, et al. Requirement for gamma/delta T cells in allergic airway inflammation. Science 280:1265–1267, 1998.

275. Sciammas R, Kodukula P, Tang Q, et al. T cell receptor–gamma/delta cells protect mice from herpes simplex virus type 1–induced lethal encephalitis. J Exp Med 185:1969–1975, 1997.

276. Ladel CH, Blum C, Dreher A, et al. Protective role of gamma/delta T cells and alpha/beta T cells in tuberculosis. Eur J Immunol 25:2877–2881, 1995.

277. Ladel CH, Blum C, Kaufmann SH. Control of natural killer cell–mediated innate resistance against the intracellular pathogen Listeria monocytogenes by gamma/delta T lymphocytes. Infect Immun 64:1744–1749, 1996.

278. Groh V, Steinle A, Bauer S, et al. Recognition of stress-induced MHC molecules by intestinal epithelial gamma/delta T cells. Science 279:1737–1740, 1998.

279. Boismenu R, Havran WL. Modulation of epithelial cell growth by intraepithelial gamma delta T cells. Science 266:1253–1255, 1994.

280. Saito H, Kanamori Y, Takemori T, et al. Generation of intestinal T cells from progenitors residing in gut cryptopatches. Science 280:275–278, 1998.

281. Sleckman BP, Khor B, Monroe R, et al. Assembly of productive T cell receptor delta variable region genes exhibits allelic inclusion. J Exp Med 188:1465–1471, 1998.

282. Bigby M, Markowitz JS, Bleicher PA, et al. Most gamma delta T cells develop normally in the absence of MHC class II molecules. J Immunol 151:4465–4475, 1993.

283. Burtrum DB, Kim S, Dudley EC, et al. TCR gene recombination and alpha beta–gamma delta lineage divergence: productive TCR-beta rearrangement is neither exclusive nor preclusive of gamma delta cell development. J Immunol 157:4293–4296, 1996.

284. Bukowski JF, Morita CT, Brenner MB. Recognition and destruction of virus-infected cells by human gamma delta CTL. J Immunol 153:5133–5140, 1994.

285. Erbach GT, Semple JP, Osathanondh R, et al. Phenotypic characteristics of lymphoid populations of middle gestation human fetal liver, spleen and thymus. J Reprod Immunol 25:81–88, 1993.

286. Wucherpfennig KW, Liao YJ, Prendergast M, et al. Human fetal liver gamma/delta T cells predominantly use unusual rearrangements of the T cell receptor delta and gamma loci expressed on both CD4$^+$ CD8$^-$ and CD4$^-$ CD8$^-$ gamma/delta T cells. J Exp Med 177:425–432, 1993.

287. Miyagawa Y, Matsuoka T, Baba A, et al. Fetal liver T cell receptor gamma/delta$^+$ T cells as cytotoxic T lymphocytes specific for maternal alloantigens. J Exp Med 176:1–7, 1992.

288. Parker CM, Groh V, Band H, et al. Evidence for extrathymic changes in the T cell receptor gamma/delta repertoire. J Exp Med 171:1597–1612, 1990.

289. Tsuyuguchi I, Kawasumi H, Ueta C, et al. Increase of T-cell receptor gamma/delta–bearing T cells in cord blood of newborn babies obtained by in vitro stimulation with mycobacterial cord factor. Infect Immun 59:3053–3059, 1991.

290. Smith MD, Worman C, Yuksel F, et al. T gamma delta–cell subsets in cord and adult blood. Scand J Immunol 32:491–495, 1990.

291. Steele RW, Suttle DE, LeMaster PC, et al. Screening for cell-mediated immunity in children. Am J Dis Child 130:1218–1221, 1976.

292. Munoz AI, Limbert D. Skin reactivity to Candida and streptokinase-streptodomase antigens in normal pediat-

ric subjects: influence of age and acute illness. J Pediatr 91:565–568, 1977.

293. Franz ML, Carella JA, Galant SP. Cutaneous delayed hypersensitivity in a healthy pediatric population: diagnostic value of diphtheria-tetanus toxoids. J Pediatr 88:975–977, 1976.

294. Warwick W, Good RA, Smith RT. Failure of passive transfer of delayed hypersensitivity in the newborn human infant. J Lab Clin Med 56:139–147, 1960.

295. Uhr J, Cancis J, Neumann CG. Delayed-type hypersensitivity in premature neonatal humans. Nature 187:1130–1131, 1960.

296. Bonforte RJ, Topilsky M, Siltzbach LE, et al. Phytohemagglutinin skin test: a possible in vivo measure of cell-mediated immunity. J Pediatr 81:775–780, 1972.

297. Kniker WT, Lesourd BM, McBryde JL, et al. Cell-mediated immunity assessed by Multitest CMI skin testing in infants and preschool children. Am J Dis Child 139:840–845, 1985.

298. Fowler R, Schubert WK, West CD. Acquired partial tolerance to homologous skin grafts in the human infant at birth. Ann NY Acad Sci 87:403–428, 1960.

299. Rouleau M, Namikawa R, Antonenko S, et al. Antigen-specific cytotoxic T cells mediate human fetal pancreas allograft rejection in SCID-hu mice. J Immunol 157:5710–5720, 1996.

300. Orlandi F, Giambona A, Messana F, et al. Evidence of induced non-tolerance in HLA-identical twins with hemoglobinopathy after in utero fetal transplantation. Bone Marrow Transplant 18:637–639, 1996.

301. Vietor HE, Bolk J, Vreugdenhil GR, et al. Alterations in cord blood leukocyte subsets of patients with severe hemolytic disease after intrauterine transfusion therapy. J Pediatr 130:718–724, 1997.

302. Vietor HE, Hawes GE, van den Oever C, et al. Intrauterine transfusions affect fetal T-cell immunity. Blood 90:2492–2501, 1997.

303. Naiman JL, Punnett HH, Lischner HW, et al. Possible graft-versus-host reaction after intrauterine transfusion for Rh erythroblastosis fetalis. N Engl J Med 281:697–701, 1969.

304. Parkman R, Mosier D, Umansky I, et al. Graft-versus-host disease after intrauterine and exchange transfusions for hemolytic disease of the newborn. N Engl J Med, 290:359–363, 1974.

305. Berger RS, Dixon SL, Fulminant transfusion-associated graft-versus-host disease in a premature infant. J Am Acad Dermatol 20:945–950, 1989.

306. Flidel O, Barak Y, Lifschitz-Mercer B, et al. Graft versus host disease in extremely low birth weight neonate. Pediatrics 89:689–690, 1992.

307. Field EJ, Caspary EA. Is maternal lymphocyte sensitization passed to the child? Lancet 2:337–342, 1971.

308. Szepfalusi Z, Nentwich I, Gerstmayr M, et al. Prenatal allergen contact with milk proteins. Clin Exp Allergy 27:28–35, 1997.

309. Prescott S, Macaubas C, Yabuhara A, et al. Developing patterns of T cell memory to environmental allergens during the first two years of life. Int Arch Allergy Immunol 113:75–79, 1997.

310. Prescott S, Macaubas C, Holt B, et al. Transplacental priming of the human immune system to environmental allergens: universal skewing of initial T cell responses toward the Th2 cytokine profile. J Immunol 160:4730–4737, 1998.

311. Van Duren Schmidt K, Pichler J, Ebner C, et al. Prenatal contact with inhalant allergens. Pediatr Res 41:128–131, 1997.

312. Englund JA, Mbawuike IN, Hammill H, et al. Maternal immunization with influenza or tetanus toxoid vaccine for passive antibody protection in young infants. J Infect Dis 168:647–656, 1993.

313. Schlesinger JJ, Covelli HD. Evidence for transmission of lymphocyte responses to tuberculin by breast-feeding. Lancet 2:529–532, 1977.

314. Shiratsuchi H, Tsuyuguchi I. Tuberculin purified protein derivative–reactive T cells in cord blood lymphocytes. Infect Immun 33:651–657, 1981.

315. Barnetson RS, Bjune G, Duncan ME. Evidence for a soluble lymphocyte factor in the transplacental transmission of T-lymphocyte responses to Mycobacterium leprae. Nature 260:150–151, 1976.

316. Gallagher MR, Welliver R, Yamanaka T, et al. Cell-mediated immune responsiveness to measles: its occurrence as a result of naturally acquired or vaccine-induced infection and in infants of immune mothers. Am J Dis Child 135:48–51, 1981.

317. Thong YH, Hurtado RC, Rola-Pleszczynski M, et al. Transplacental transmission of cell-mediated immunity. Lancet 1:1286–1287, 1974.

318. Leikin S, Oppenheim JJ. Differences in transformation of adult and newborn lymphocytes stimulated by antigen, antibody, and antigen-antibody complexes. Cell Immunol 1:468–475, 1970.

319. Brody JI, Oski FA, Wallach EE. Neonatal lymphocyte reactivity as an indicator of intrauterine bacterial contact. Lancet 1:1396–1398, 1968.

320. Ivanyi L, Lehner T. Interdependence of in vitro responsiveness of cord and maternal blood lymphocytes to antigens from oral bacteria. Clin Exp Immunol 30:252–258, 1977.

321. Rubin HR, Sorensen RU, Polmar SH. Lymphocyte responses of human neonates to bacterial antigens. Cell Immunol 57:307–315, 1981.

322. Lo Y, Lo E, Watson N, et al. Two-way traffic between mother and fetus: biologic and clinical implications. Blood 88:4390–4395, 1996.

323. Buimovici-Klein E, Cooper LZ. Cell-mediated immune response in rubella infections. Rev Infect Dis 7(Suppl 1):S123–S128, 1985.

324. Friedmann PS. Cell-mediated immunological reactivity in neonates and infants with congenital syphilis. Clin Exp Immunol 30:271–276, 1977.

325. McLeod R, Mack DG, Boyer K, et al. Phenotypes and functions of lymphocytes in congenital toxoplasmosis. J Lab Clin Med 116:623–635, 1990.

326. Paryani SG, Arvin AM. Intrauterine infection with varicella-zoster virus after maternal varicella. N Engl J Med 314:1542–1546, 1986.

327. Pass RF, Stagno S, Britt WJ, et al. Specific cell-mediated immunity and the natural history of congenital infection with cytomegalovirus. J Infect Dis 148:953–961, 1983.

328. Starr SE, Tolpin MD, Friedman HM, et al. Impaired cellular immunity to cytomegalovirus in congenitally infected children and their mothers. J Infect Dis 140:500–505, 1979.

329. Wood KJ. New concepts in tolerance. Clin Transplant 10:1–9, 1996.

330. Aase JM, Noren GR, Reddy DV, et al. Mumps-virus infection in pregnant women and the immunologic response of their offspring. N Engl J Med 286:1379–1382, 1972.

331. Burchett SK, Corey L, Mohan KM, et al. Diminished interferon-gamma and lymphocyte proliferation in neo-

natal and postpartum primary herpes simplex virus infection. J Infect Dis 165:813–818, 1992.

332. Sullender WM, Miller JL, Yasukawa LL, et al. Humoral and cell-mediated immunity in neonates with herpes simplex virus infection. J Infect Dis 155:28–37, 1987.

333. Luzuriaga K, Holmes D, Hereema A, et al. HIV-1–specific cytotoxic T lymphocyte responses in the first year of life. J Immunol 154:433–443, 1995.

334. Pikora CA, Sullivan JL, Panicali D, et al. Early HIV-1 envelope-specific cytotoxic T lymphocyte responses in vertically infected infants. J Exp Med 185:1153–1161, 1997.

335. Chiba Y, Higashidate Y, Suga K, et al. Development of cell-mediated cytotoxic immunity to respiratory syncytial virus in human infants following naturally acquired infection. J Med Virol 28:133–139, 1989.

336. Bruning T, Daiminger A, Enders G. Diagnostic value of CD45R0 expression on circulating T lymphocytes of fetuses and newborn infants with pre-, peri- or early post-natal infections. Clin Exp Immunol 107:306–311, 1997.

337. Hohlfeld P, Forestier F, Marion S, et al. *Toxoplasma gondii* infection during pregnancy: T lymphocyte subpopulations in mothers and fetuses. Pediatr Infect Dis J 9:878–881, 1990.

338. Thilaganathan B, Carroll SG, Plachouras N, et al. Fetal immunological and haematological changes in intrauterine infection. Br J Obstet Gynaecol 101:418–421, 1994.

339. Hara T, Ohashi S, Yamashita Y, et al. Human V delta 2+ gamma/delta T-cell tolerance to foreign antigens of *Toxoplasma gondii*. Proc Natl Acad Sci USA 93:5136–5140, 1996.

340. Michie C, Harvey D. Can expression of CD45R0, a T cell surface molecule, be used to detect congenital infection? Lancet 343:1259–1260, 1994.

341. Rajewsky K. Clonal selection and learning in the antibody system. Nature 381:751–758, 1996.

342. Tedder TF, Inaoki M, Sato S. The CD19-CD21 complex regulates signal transduction thresholds governing humoral immunity and autoimmunity. Immunity 6:107–118, 1997.

343. Carroll MC. The role of complement and complement receptors in induction and regulation of immunity. Ann Rev Immunol 16:545–568, 1998.

344. Takai T, Ono M, Hikida M, et al. Augmented humoral and anaphylactic responses in Fc gamma RII–deficient mice. Nature 379:346–349, 1996.

345. Hintzen RO, Lens SM, Lammers K, et al. Engagement of CD27 with its ligand CD70 provides a second signal for T cell activation. J Immunol 154:2612–2623, 1995.

346. Yuschenkoff VN, Sethna MP, Freeman GJ, et al. Coexpression of B7-1 and antigen blocks tolerance induction to antigen presented by resting B cells. J Immunol 157:1987–1995, 1996.

347. Padlan EA. Anatomy of the antibody molecule. Mol Immunol 31:169–217, 1994.

348. Matsuda F, Ishii K, Bourvagnet P, et al. The complete nucleotide sequence of the human immunoglobulin heavy chain variable region locus. J Exp Med 188:2151–2162, 1998.

349. Tomlinson IM, Cook GP, Walter G, et al. A complete map of the human immunoglobulin V_H locus. Ann NY Acad Sci 764:43–46, 1995.

350. Klein R, Zachau HG. Expression and hypermutation of human immunoglobulin kappa genes. Ann NY Acad Sci 764:74–83, 1995.

351. Blomberg BB, Glozak MA, Donohoe ME. Regulation of human lambda light chain gene expression. Ann NY Acad Sci 764:84–98, 1995.

352. Schroeder HWJ, Ippolito GC, Shiokawa S. Regulation of the antibody repertoire through control of HCDR3 diversity. Vaccine 16:1383–1390, 1998.

353. Stewart AK, Huang C, Stollar BD, et al. High-frequency representation of a single VH gene in the expressed human B cell repertoire. J Exp Med 177:1227, 1993.

354. Kraj P, Rao SP, Glas AM, et al. The human heavy chain Ig V region gene repertoire is biased at all stages of B cell ontogeny, including early pre-B cells. J Immunol 158:5824–5832, 1997.

355. Bertrand FE, Billips LG, Burrows PD, et al. Ig D H gene segment transcription and rearrangement before surface expression of the pan–B-cell marker CD19 in normal human bone marrow. Blood 90:736–744, 1997.

356. Nunez C, Nishimoto N, Gartland GL, et al. B cells are generated throughout life in humans. J Immunol 156:866–872, 1996.

357. Kubagawa H, Cooper MD, Carroll AJ, et al. Light-chain gene expression before heavy-chain gene rearrangement in pre-B cells transformed by Epstein-Barr virus. Proc Natl Acad Sci USA 86:2356–2360, 1989.

358. Minegishi Y, Coustan-Smith E, Wang YH, et al. Mutations in the human lambda5/14.1 gene result in B cell deficiency and agammaglobulinemia. J Exp Med 187:71–77, 1998.

359. Giachino Padovan E, Lanzavecchia A. Kappa+lambda+ dual receptor B cells are present in the human peripheral repertoire. J Exp Med 181:1245–1250, 1995.

360. Brezinschek HP, Brezinschek RI, Lipsky PE. Analysis of the heavy chain repertoire of human peripheral B cells using single-cell polymerase chain reaction. J Immunol 155:190–202, 1995.

361. Torres RM, Flaswinkel H, Reth M, et al. Aberrant B cell development and immune response in mice with a compromised BCR complex. Science 272:1804–1808, 1996.

362. Lam KP, Kuhn R, Rajewsky K. In vivo ablation of surface immunoglobulin on mature B cells by inducible gene targeting results in rapid cell death. Cell 90:1073–1083, 1997.

363. Rosado MM, Freitas AA. The role of the B cell receptor V region in peripheral B cell survival. Eur J Immunol 28:2685–2693, 1998.

364. MacLennan IC. B-cell receptor regulation of peripheral B cells. Curr Opin Immunol 10:220–225, 1998.

365. Goodnow CC. Balancing immunity and tolerance: deleting and tuning lymphocyte repertoires. Proc Natl Acad Sci USA 93:2264–2271, 1996.

366. Healy JI, Goodnow CC. Positive versus negative signaling by lymphocyte antigen receptors. Annu Rev Immunol 16:645–670, 1998.

367. Fulcher DA, Lyons AB, Korn SL, et al. The fate of self-reactive B cells depends primarily on the degree of antigen receptor engagement and availability of T cell help. J Exp Med 183:2313–2328, 1996.

368. Klein U, Kuppers R, Rajewsky K. Human IgM+IgD+ B cells, the major B cell subset in the peripheral blood, express V kappa genes with no or little somatic mutation throughout life. Eur J Immunol 23:3272–3277, 1993.

369. Garside P, Ingulli E, Merica RR, et al. Visualization of specific B and T lymphocyte interactions in the lymph node. Science 281:96–99, 1998.

370. Kouskoff V, Famiglietti S, Lacaud G, et al. Antigens varying in affinity for the B cell receptor induce differ-

ential B lymphocyte responses. J Exp Med 188:1453–1464, 1998.

371. Tarlinton D. Germinal centers: getting there is half the fun. Curr Biol 8:R753–R756, 1998.

372. Zheng B, Kelsoe G, Han S. Somatic diversification of antibody responses. J Clin Immunol 16:1–11, 1996.

373. Tew JG, Wu J, Qin D, et al. Follicular dendritic cells and presentation of antigen and costimulatory signals to B cells. Immunol Rev 15:39–52, 1997.

374. Smith KG, Weiss U, Rajewsky K, et al. Bcl-2 increases memory B cell recruitment but does not perturb selection in germinal centers. Immunity 1:803–813, 1994.

375. Cascalho M, Wong J, Steinberg C, et al. Mismatch repair co-opted by hypermutation. Science 279:1207–1210, 1998.

376. Jacob J, Kelsoe G, Rajewsky K, et al. Intraclonal generation of antibody mutants in germinal centres. Nature 354:389–392, 1991.

377. Meffre E, Papavasiliou F, Cohen P, et al. Antigen receptor engagement turns off the V(D)J recombination machinery in human tonsil B cells. J Exp Med 188:765–772, 1998.

378. deWildt R, Hoet R, van Venrooij WJ, et al. Analysis of heavy and light chain pairings indicates that receptor editing shapes the human antibody repertoire. J Mol Biol 285:895–901, 1999.

379. Gray D, Dullforce P, Jainandunsing S. Memory B cell development but not germinal center formation is impaired by in vivo blockade of CD40-CD40 ligand interaction. J Exp Med 180:141–155, 1994.

380. Tangye SG, Liu YJ, Aversa G, et al. Identification of functional human splenic memory B cells by expression of CD148 and CD27. J Exp Med 188:1691–1703, 1998.

381. Klein U, Rajewsky K, Kuppers R. Human immunoglobulin (Ig)M+IgD+ peripheral blood B cells expressing the CD27 cell surface antigen carry somatically mutated variable region genes: CD27 as a general marker for somatically mutated (memory) B cells. J Exp Med 188:1679–1689, 1998.

382. McHeyzer-William MG, Nossal GJ, Lalor PA. Molecular characterization of single memory B cells. Nature 350:502–505, 1991.

383. Schittek B, Rajewsky K. Maintenance of B-cell memory by long-lived cells generated from proliferating precursors. Nature 346:749–751, 1990.

384. Dubois B, Massacrier C, Vanbervliet B, et al. Critical role of IL-12 in dendritic cell–induced differentiation of naive B lymphocytes. J Immunol 161:2223–2231, 1998.

385. Slifka MK, Ahmed R. Long-lived plasma cells: a mechanism for maintaining persistent antibody production. Curr Opin Immunol 10:252–258, 1998.

386. Nagumo H, Agematsu K, Shinozaki K, et al. CD27/CD70 interaction augments IgE secretion by promoting the differentiation of memory B cells into plasma cell. J Immunol 161:6496–6502, 1998.

387. Zhang K, Mills FC, Saxon A. Switch circles from IL-4–directed epsilon class switching from human B lymphocytes: evidence for direct, sequential, and multiple step sequential switch from mu to epsilon Ig heavy chain gene. J Immunol 152:3427–3435, 1994.

388. Banchereau J, Briere F, Liu YJ, et al. Molecular control of B lymphocyte growth and differentiation. Stem Cells (Dayt) 12:278–288, 1994.

389. Kimata H, Fujimoto M. Induction of IgA1 and IgA2 production in immature human fetal B cells and pre-B cells by vasoactive intestinal peptide. Blood 85:2098–2104, 1995.

390. Butch AW, Chung GH, Hoffmann JW, et al. Cytokine

391. Toellner KM, Gulbranson JA, Taylor DR, et al. Immunoglobulin switch transcript production in vivo related to the site and time of antigen-specific B cell activation. J Exp Med 183:2303–2312, 1996.

392. Klein U, Kuppers R, Rajewsky K. Evidence for a large compartment of IgM-expressing memory B cells in humans. Blood 89:1288–1298, 1997.

393. Ochs HD, Smith CI. X-linked agammaglobulinemia: a clinical and molecular analysis. Medicine (Baltimore) 75:287–299, 1996.

394. Timens W, Poppema S. Lymphocyte compartments in human spleen: an immunohistologic study in normal spleens and uninvolved spleens in Hodgkin's disease. Am J Pathol 120:443–454, 1985.

395. Amlot PL, Hayes AE. Impaired human antibody response to the thymus-independent antigen, DNP-Ficoll, after splenectomy: implications for post-splenectomy infections. Lancet 1:1008–1011, 1985.

396. Dono M, Zupo S, Grossi CE, et al. Subepithelial B cells of the human tonsil. Chem Immunol 67:58–69, 1997.

397. Timens W, Boes A, Rozeboom-Uiterwijk T, et al. Immaturity of the human splenic marginal zone in infancy: possible contribution to the deficient infant immune response. J Immunol 143:3200–3206, 1989.

398. Spencer J, Perry ME, Dunn-Walters DK. Human marginal-zone B cells. Immunol Today 19:421–426, 1998.

399. Dunn-Walters DK, Isaacson PG, Spencer J. Analysis of mutations in immunoglobulin heavy chain variable region genes of microdissected marginal zone (MGZ) B cells suggests that the MGZ of human spleen is a reservoir of memory B cells. J Exp Med 182:559–566, 1995.

400. Oliver AM, Martin F, Gartland GL, et al. Marginal zone B cells exhibit unique activation, proliferative and immunoglobulin secretory responses. Eur J Immunol 27:2366–2374, 1997.

401. Kasaian MT, Ikematsu H, Casali P. Identification and analysis of a novel human surface CD5–B lymphocyte subset producing natural antibodies. J Immunol 148:2690–2702, 1992.

402. Brezinschek HP, Foster SJ, Brezinschek R, et al. Analysis of the human VH gene repertoire: differential effects of selection and somatic hypermutation on human peripheral CD5(+)/IgM+ and CD5(-)/IgM+ B cells. J Clin Invest 99:2488–2501, 1997.

403. Dorner T, Brezinschek HP, Foster SJ, et al. Comparable impact of mutational and selective influences in shaping the expressed repertoire of peripheral IgM+/CD5– and IgM+/CD5+ B cells. Eur J Immunol 28:657–668, 1998.

404. Chen ZJ, Wheeler CJ, Shi W, et al. Polyreactive antigen-binding B cells are the predominant cell type in the newborn B cell repertoire. Eur J Immunol 28:989–994, 1998.

405. Bhat NM, Kantor AB, Bieber MM, et al. The ontogeny and functional characteristics of human B-1 CD5+ B cells. Int Immunol 4:243–252, 1992.

406. Kipps TJ, Robbins BA, Carson DA. Uniform high frequency expression of autoantibody-associated crossreactive idiotypes in the primary B cell follicles of human fetal spleen. J Exp Med 171:189–196, 1990.

407. Schettino EW, Chai SK, Kasaian MT, et al. VHDJH gene sequences and antigen reactivity of monoclonal antibodies produced by human B-1 cells: evidence for somatic selection. J Immunol 158:2477–2489, 1997.

408. Clarke SH, Arnold LW. B-1 cell development: evidence for an uncommitted immunoglobulin (Ig)M+ B cell

expression by germinal center cells. J Immunol 150:39–47, 1993.

precursor in b-1 cell differentiation. J Exp Med 187:1325–1334, 1998.

409. Gathings WE, Lawton AR, Cooper MD. Immunofluorescent studies of the development of pre-B cells, B lymphocytes and immunoglobulin isotype diversity in humans. Eur J Immunol 7:804–810, 1977.

410. Solvason N, Chen X, Shu F, et al. The fetal omentum in mice and humans: a site enriched for precursors of CD5 B cells early in development. Ann NY Acad Sci 651:10–20, 1992.

411. Nishimoto N, Kubagawa H, Ohno T, et al. Normal pre-B cells express a receptor complex of mu heavy chains and surrogate light-chain proteins. Proc Natl Acad Sci USA 88:6284–6288, 1991.

412. Gupta S, Pahwa R, O'Reilly R, et al. Ontogeny of lymphocyte subpopulations in human fetal liver. Proc Natl Acad Sci USA 73:919–922, 1976.

413. Metcalf ES, Klinman NR. In vitro tolerance induction of neonatal murine B cells. J Exp Med 143:1327–1340, 1976.

414. Baskin B, Islam KB, Smith CI. Characterization of the CDR3 region of rearranged alpha heavy chain genes in human fetal liver. Clin Exp Immunol 112:44–47, 1998.

415. Dosch HM, Lam P, Hui MF, et al. Concerted generation of Ig isotype diversity in human fetal bone marrow. J Immunol 143:2464–2469, 1989.

416. Wedgwood JF, Weinberger BI, Hatam L, et al. Umbilical cord blood lacks circulating B lymphocytes expressing surface IgG or IgA. Clin Immunol Immunopathol 84:276–282, 1997.

417. LeBien TW, Wormann B, Villablanca JG, et al. Multiparameter flow cytometric analysis of human fetal bone marrow B cells. Leukemia 4:354–358, 1990.

418. Punnonen J, Aversa GG, Vandekerckhove B, et al. Induction of isotype switching and Ig production by $CD5^+$ and $CD10^+$ human fetal B cells. J Immunol 148:3398–3404, 1992.

419. Antin JH, Emerson SG, Martin P, et al. Leu-1$^+$ ($CD5^+$) B cells: a major lymphoid subpopulation in human fetal spleen: phenotypic and functional studies. J Immunol 136:505–510, 1986.

420. Griffiths CS, Patterson JA, Berger CL, et al. Characterization of immature T cell subpopulations in neonatal blood. Blood 64:296–300, 1984.

421. Small TN, Keever C, Collins N, et al. Characterization of B cells in severe combined immunodeficiency disease. Hum Immunol 25:181–193, 1989.

422. Lydyard PM, Quartey PR, Broker B, et al. The antibody repertoire of early human B cells. I. High frequency of autoreactivity and polyreactivity. Scand J Immunol 31:33–43, 1990.

423. Ehrenstein MR, O'Keefe TL, Davies SL, et al. Targeted gene disruption reveals a role for natural secretory IgM in the maturation of the primary immune response. Proc Natl Acad Sci USA 95:10089–10093, 1998.

424. Boes M, Prodeus A, Schmidt T, et al. A critical role of natural immunoglobulin M in immediate defense against systemic bacterial infection. J Exp Med 188:2381–2386, 1998.

425. Boes M, Esau C, Fischer MB, et al. Enhanced B-1 cell development, but impaired IgG antibody responses in mice deficient in secreted IgM. J Immunol 160:4776–4787, 1998.

426. Schroeder HJ, Hillson JL, Perlmutter RM. Early restriction of the human antibody repertoire. Science 238:791–793, 1987.

427. Cuisinier AM, Guigou V, Boubli L, et al. Preferential expression of VH5 and VH6 immunoglobulin genes in early human B-cell ontogeny. Scand J Immunol 30:493–497, 1989.

428. Schutte ME, Ebeling SB, Akkermans-Koolhaas KE, et al. Deletion mapping of Ig V_H gene segments expressed in human CD5 B cell lines: JH proximity is not the sole determinant of the restricted fetal V_H gene repertoire. J Immunol 149:3953–3960, 1992.

429. Raaphorst FM, Timmers E, Kenter MJ, et al. Restricted utilization of germ-line VH3 genes and short diverse third complementarity-determining regions (CDR3s) in human fetal B lymphocyte immunoglobulin heavy chain rearrangements. Eur J Immunol 22:247–251, 1992.

430. Raaphorst FM, Raman CS, Tami J, et al. Human Ig heavy chain CDR3 regions in adult bone marrow pre-B cells display an adult phenotype of diversity: evidence for structural selection of D_H amino acid sequences. Int Immunol 9:1503–1515, 1997.

431. Sanz I. Multiple mechanisms participate in the generation of diversity of human H chain CDR3 regions. J Immunol 147:1720–1729, 1991.

432. Cuisinier AM, Fumoux F, Moinier D, et al. Rapid expansion of human immunoglobulin repertoire V_H, V kappa, V lambda expressed in early fetal bone marrow. New Biol 2:689–699, 1990.

433. Mortari F, Wang JY, Schroeder HJ. Human cord blood antibody repertoire: mixed population of V_H gene segments and CDR3 distribution in the expressed C alpha and C gamma repertoires. J Immunol 150:1348–1357, 1993.

434. Mortari F, Newton JA, Wang JY, et al. The human cord blood antibody repertoire: frequent usage of the VH7 gene family. Eur J Immunol 22:241–245, 1992.

435. Silverman GJ, Sasano M, Wormsley SB. Age-associated changes in binding of human B lymphocytes to a VH3-restricted unconventional bacterial antigen. J Immunol 151:5840–5855, 1993.

436. van Ess J, Meyling FH, Logtenberg T. High frequency of somatically mutated IgM molecules in the human adult blood B cell repertoire. Eur J Immunol 22:2761–2764, 1992.

437. Nicholson IC, Brisco MJ, Zola H. Memory B lymphocytes in human tonsil do not express surface IgD. J Immunol 154:1105–1113, 1995.

438. Macardle PJ, Weedon H, Fusco M, et al. The antigen receptor complex on cord B lymphocytes. Immunology 90:376–382, 1997.

439. Rijkers GT, Sanders EA, Breukels MA, et al. Infant B cell responses to polysaccharide determinants. Vaccine 16:1396–1400, 1998.

440. Parra C, Rold'an E, Brieva JA. Deficient expression of adhesion molecules by human CD5$^-$ B lymphocytes both after bone marrow transplantation and during normal ontogeny. Blood 88:1733–1740, 1996.

441. Garban F, Truman JP, Lord J, et al. Signal transduction via human leucocyte antigen class II molecules distinguishes between cord blood, normal, and malignant adult B lymphocytes. Exp Hematol 26:874–884, 1998.

442. Cerutti A, Trentin L, Zambello R, et al. The CD5/CD72 receptor system is coexpressed with several functionally relevant counterstructures on human B cells and delivers a critical signaling activity. J Immunol 157:1854–1862, 1996.

443. Servet DC, Bridon JM, Djossou O, et al. Delayed IgG2 humoral response in infants is not due to intrinsic T or B cell defects. Int Immunol 8:1495–1502, 1996.

444. Punnonen J, Aversa G, de Vries JE. Human pre-B cells differentiate into Ig-secreting plasma cells in the pres-

ence of interleukin-4 and activated CD4$^+$ T cells or their membranes. Blood 82:2781–2789, 1993.

445. Punnonen J, Cocks BG, de Vries JE. IL-4 induces germ-line IgE heavy chain gene transcription in human fetal pre-B cells: evidence for differential expression of functional IL-4 and IL-13 receptors during B cell ontogeny. J Immunol 155:4248–4254, 1995.

446. Punnonen J, de Vries JE. IL-13 induces proliferation, Ig isotype switching, and Ig synthesis by immature human fetal B cells. J Immunol 152:1094–1102, 1994.

447. Ueno Y, Ichihara T, Hasui M, et al. T-cell–dependent production of IgG by human cord blood B cells in reconstituted SCID mice. Scand J Immunol 35:415–419, 1992.

448. Vandekerckhove BA, Jones D, Punnonen J, et al. Human Ig production and isotype switching in severe combined immunodeficient–human mice. J Immunol 151:128–137, 1993.

449. Splawski J, Yamamoto K, Lipsky P. Deficient interleukin-10 production by neonatal T cells does not explain their ineffectiveness at promoting neonatal B cell differentiation. Eur J Immunol 28:4248–4256, 1998.

450. Gitlin D, Biasucci A. Development of gamma G, gamma A, gamma M, beta IC–beta IA, Ca 1 esterase inhibitor, ceruloplasmin, transferrin, hemopexin, haptoglobin, fibrinogen, plasminogen, alpha 1–antitrypsin, orosomucoid, beta-lipoprotein, alpha 2 macroglobulin, and prealbumin in the human conceptus. J Clin Invest 48:1433–1446, 1969.

451. Gathings WE, Kubagawa H, Cooper MD. A distinctive pattern of B cell immaturity in perinatal humans. Immunol Rev 5:107–126, 1981.

452. Splawski JB, Lipsky PE. Prostaglandin E2 inhibits T cell–dependent Ig secretion by neonatal but not adult lymphocytes. J Immunol 152:5259–5267, 1994.

453. Ambrosino DM, Delancy NR, Shamberger RC. Human polysaccharide-specific B cells are responsive to pokeweed mitogen and IL-6. J Immunol 144:1221–1226, 1990.

454. Peeters CC, Tenbergen-Meekes AM, Heijnen CJ, et al. Interferon-gamma and interleukin-6 augment the human in vitro antibody response to the Haemophilus influenzae type b polysaccharide. J Infect Dis 165 (Suppl 1):S161–S162, 1992.

455. Snapper CM, Mond JJ. A model for induction of T cell–independent humoral immunity in response to polysaccharide antigens. J Immunol 157:2229–2233, 1996.

456. Buchanan RM, Arulanandam BP, Metzger DW. IL-12 enhances antibody responses to T-independent polysaccharide vaccines in the absence of T and NK cells. J Immunol 161:5525–5533, 1998.

457. Snapper CM, Rosas FR, Jin L, et al. Bacterial lipoproteins may substitute for cytokines in the humoral immune response to T cell–independent type II antigens. J Immunol 155:5582–5589, 1995.

458. Golding B, Muchmore AV, Blaese RM. Newborn and Wiskott-Aldrich patient B cells can be activated by TNP–Brucella abortus: evidence that TNP–Brucella abortus behaves as a T-independent type 1 antigen in humans. J Immunol 133:2966–2971, 1984.

459. Fink C, Miller WE, Dorward B, et al. The formation of macroglobulin antibodies. II. Studies on neonatal infants and older children. J Clin Invest 41:1422–1428, 1962.

460. Smith R, Eitzman DV, Catlin ME, et al. The development of the immune response. Pediatrics 33:163–183, 1964.

461. Baker CJ, Edwards MS. Group B streptococcal infections. In Remington JS, Klein JO (eds). Infectious Diseases of the Fetus and Newborn Infant, 4th ed. Philadelphia, WB Saunders, 1995, pp 980–1054.

462. Griffioen AW, Toebes EA, Zegers BJ, et al. Role of CR2 in the human adult and neonatal in vitro antibody response to type 4 pneumococcal polysaccharide. Cell Immunol 143:11–22, 1992.

463. Griffioen AW, Franklin SW, Zegers BJ, et al. Expression and functional characteristics of the complement receptor type 2 on adult and neonatal B lymphocytes. Clin Immunol Immunopathol 69:1–8, 1993.

464. Timens W, Rozeboom T, Poppema S. Fetal and neonatal development of human spleen: an immunohistological study. Immunology 60:603–609, 1987.

465. Peset-Llopis MJ, Harms G, Hardonk MJ, et al. Human immune response to pneumococcal polysaccharides: complement-mediated localization preferentially on CD21-positive splenic marginal zone B cells and follicular dendritic cells. J Allergy Clin Immunol 97:1015–1024, 1996.

466. Halista SM, Johnson-Robbins LA, El-Mohandes A-E, et al. Characterization of early activation events in cord blood B cells after stimulation with T cell–independent activators. Pediatr Res 43:496–503, 1998.

467. Silverstein AM, Prendergast RA, Parshall CJJ. Cellular kinetics of the antibody response by the fetal rhesus monkey. J Immunol 104:269–271, 1970.

468. Silverstein A. Ontogeny of the immune response: a perspective. In Cooper MD, Dayton DH (eds). Development of Host Defenses. New York, Raven Press, 1977, pp 1–10.

469. Vanderbeeken Y, Sarfati M, Bose R, et al. In utero immunization of the fetus to tetanus by maternal vaccination during pregnancy. Am J Reprod Immunol Microbiol 8:39–42, 1985.

470. Gill TJ, Repetti CF, Metlay LA, et al. Transplacental immunization of the human fetus to tetanus by immunization of the mother. J Clin Invest 72:987–996, 1983.

471. Enders G, Serologic test combinations for safe detection of rubella infections. Rev Infect Dis 7 (Suppl 1):S113–S122, 1985.

472. Naot Y, Desmonts G, Remington JS. IgM enzyme-linked immunosorbent assay test for the diagnosis of congenital Toxoplasma infection. J Pediatr 98:32–36, 1981.

473. Chumpitazi BF, Boussaid A, Pelloux H, et al. Diagnosis of congenital toxoplasmosis by immunoblotting and relationship with other methods. J Clin Microbiol 33:1479–1485, 1995.

474. Griffiths PD, Stagno S, Pass RF, et al. Congenital cytomegalovirus infection: diagnostic and prognostic significance of the detection of specific immunoglobulin M antibodies in cord serum. Pediatrics 69:544–549, 1982.

475. Pinon JM, Toubas D, Marx C, et al. Detection of specific immunoglobulin E in patients with toxoplasmosis. J Clin Microbiol 28:1739–1743, 1990.

476. King CL, Malhotra I, Mungai P, et al. B cell sensitization to helminthic infection develops in utero in humans. J Immunol 160:3578–3584, 1998.

477. Decoster A, Darcy F, Caron A, et al. Anti-P30 IgA antibodies as prenatal markers of congenital toxoplasma infection. Clin Exp Immunol 87:310–315, 1992.

478. Stepick-Biek P, Thulliez P, Araujo FG, et al. IgA antibodies for diagnosis of acute congenital and acquired toxoplasmosis. J Infec Dis 162:270–273, 1990.

479. Desmonts G, Daffos F, Forestier F, et al. Prenatal diag-

nosis of congenital toxoplasmosis. Lancet 1:500–504, 1985.

480. Dengrove J, Lee EJ, Heiner DC, et al. IgG and IgG subclass specific antibody responses to diphtheria and tetanus toxoids in newborns and infants given DTP immunization. Pediatr Res 20:735–739, 1986.

481. Smolen P, Bland R, Heiligenstein E, et al. Antibody response to oral polio vaccine in premature infants. J Pediatr 103:917–919, 1983.

482. Uhr J, Dancis J, Franklin E, et al. The antibody response to bacteriophage in newborn premature infants. J Clin Invest 41:1509–1513, 1962.

483. West DJ. Clinical experience with hepatitis B vaccines. Am J Infect Control 17:172–180, 1989.

484. Lee SS, Lo YC, Young BW, et al. A reduced dose approach to hepatitis B vaccination for low-risk newborns and preschool children. Vaccine 13:373–376, 1995.

485. Greenberg DP. Pediatric experience with recombinant hepatitis B vaccines and relevant safety and immunogenicity studies. Pediatr Infect Dis J 12:438–445, 1993.

486. Dancis J, Osborn JJ, Junz HW. Studies of the immunology of the newborn infant. Pediatrics 1953:151–156, 1953.

487. Provenzano R, Wetterlow HL, Sullivan CL. Immunization and antibody response in the newborn infant. N Engl J Med 273:959–965, 1965.

488. Baraff LJ, Leake RD, Burstyn DG, et al. Immunologic response to early and routine DTP immunization in infants. Pediatrics 73:37–42, 1984.

489. Peterson J. Immunization in the young infant: response to combined vaccines: I-IV. Am J Dis Child 81:484–491, 1951.

490. Schoub BD, Johnson S, McAnerney J, et al. Monovalent neonatal polio immunization—a strategy for the developing world. J Infect Dis 157:836–839, 1988.

491. Gans HA, Arvin AM, Galinus J, et al. Deficiency of the humoral immune response to measles vaccine in infants immunized at age 6 months. JAMA 80:527–532, 1998.

492. Smith DH, Peter G, Ingram DL, et al. Responses of children immunized with the capsular polysaccharide of *Haemophilus influenzae*, type b. Pediatrics 52:637–644, 1973.

493. Adderson EE, Shackelford PG, Quinn A, et al. Restricted Ig H chain V gene usage in the human antibody response to *Haemophilus influenzae* type b capsular polysaccharide. J Immunol 147:1667–1674, 1991.

494. Granoff DM, Holmes SJ, Osterholm MT, et al. Induction of immunologic memory in infants primed with *Haemophilus influenzae* type b conjugate vaccines. J Infect Dis 168:663–671, 1993.

495. Eskola J, Keayhty H. Early immunization with conjugate vaccines. Vaccine 16:1433–1438, 1998.

496. Lieberman JM, Greenberg DP, Wong VK, et al. Effect of neonatal immunization with diphtheria and tetanus toxoids on antibody responses to *Haemophilus influenzae* type b conjugate vaccines. J Pediatr 126:198–205, 1995.

497. Schlesinger Y, Granoff DM. Avidity and bactericidal activity of antibody elicited by different *Haemophilus influenzae* type b conjugate vaccines: The Vaccine Study Group. JAMA 267:1489–1494, 1992.

498. Siber G. Pneumococcal disease: prospects for a new generation of vaccines. Science 265:1385–1387, 1994.

499. Anderson EL, Kennedy DJ, Geldmacher KM, et al. Immunogenicity of heptavalent pneumococcal conjugate vaccine in infants. J Pediatr 128:649–653, 1996.

500. Daum RS, Hogerman D, Rennels MB, et al. Infant immunization with pneumococcal CRM197 vaccines: effect of saccharide size on immunogenicity and interactions with simultaneously administered vaccines. J Infect Dis 176:445–455, 1997.

501. Fairley CK, Begg N, Borrow R, et al. Conjugate meningococcal serogroup A and C vaccine: reactogenicity and immunogenicity in United Kingdom infants. J Infect Dis 174:1360–1363, 1996.

502. Bernbaum JC, Daft A, Anolik R, et al. Response of preterm infants to diphtheria-tetanus-pertussis immunizations. J Pediatr 107:184–188, 1985.

503. Koblin BA, Townsend TR, Muanoz A, et al. Response of preterm infants to diphtheria-tetanus-pertussis vaccine. Pediatr Infect Dis J 7:704–711, 1988.

504. Adenyi-Jones SC, Faden H, Ferdon MB, et al. Systemic and local immune responses to enhanced-potency inactivated poliovirus vaccine in premature and term infants. J Pediatr 120:686–689, 1992.

505. Lau YL, Tam AY, Ng KW, et al. Response of preterm infants to hepatitis B vaccine. J Pediatr 121:962–965, 1992.

506. Kim SC, Chung EK, Hodinka RL, et al. Immunogenicity of hepatitis B vaccine in preterm infants. Pediatrics 99:534–536, 1997.

507. Greenberg DP, Vadheim CM, Partridge S, et al. Immunogenicity of *Haemophilus influenzae* type b tetanus toxoid conjugate vaccine in young infants: The Kaiser-UCLA Vaccine Study Group. J Infect Dis 170:76–81, 1994.

508. Washburn LK, O'Shea TM, Gillis DC, et al. Response to *Haemophilus influenzae* type b conjugate vaccine in chronically ill premature infants. J Pediatr 123:791–794, 1993.

509. Stiehm ER, Fudenberg HH. Serum levels of immune globulins in health and disease: a survey. Pediatrics 37:715–727, 1966.

510. Lee SI, Heiner DC, Wara D. Development of serum IgG subclass levels in children. Monogr Allergy 19:108–121, 1986.

511. Kameda T, Koyama M, Matsuzaki N, et al. Localization of three subtypes of Fc gamma receptors in human placenta by immunohistochemical analysis. Placenta 12:15–26, 1991.

512. Landor M. Maternal-fetal transfer of immunoglobulins. Ann Allergy Asthma Immunol 74:279–283, 1995.

513. Leach JL, Sedmak DD, Osborne JM, et al. Isolation from human placenta of the IgG transporter, FcRn, and localization to the syncytiotrophoblast: implications for maternal-fetal antibody transport. J Immunol 157:3317–3322, 1996.

514. Story CM, Mikulska JE, Simister NE. A major histocompatibility complex class I–like Fc receptor cloned from human placenta: possible role in transfer of immunoglobulin G from mother to fetus. J Exp Med 180:2377–2381, 1994.

515. Simister NE, Story CM, Chen HL, et al. An IgG-transporting Fc receptor expressed in the syncytiotrophoblast of human placenta. Eur J Immunol 26:1527–1531, 1996.

516. Gusdon JPJ. Fetal and maternal immunoglobulin levels during pregnancy. Am J Obstet Gynecol 103:895–900, 1969.

517. Kohler PF, Farr RS. Elevation of cord over maternal IgG immunoglobulin: evidence for an active placental IgG transport. Nature 210:1070–1071, 1966.

518. Pitcher-Wilmott RW, Hindocha P, Wood CB. The placental transfer of IgG subclasses in human pregnancy. Clin Exp Immunol 41:303–308, 1980.

519. Martensson L, Fudenberg HH. Gm genes and gamma

G–globulin synthesis in the human fetus. J Immunol 94:514–520, 1965.

520. Hay FC, Hull MG, Torrigiani G. The transfer of human IgG subclasses from mother to foetus. Clin Exp Immunol 9:355–358, 1971.

521. Morell A, Sidiropoulos D, Herrmann U, et al. IgG subclasses and antibodies to group B streptococci, pneumococci, and tetanus toxoid in preterm neonates after intravenous infusion of immunoglobulin to the mothers. Pediatr Res 20:933–936, 1986.

522. Sato H, Albrecht P, Reynolds DW, et al. Transfer of measles, mumps, and rubella antibodies from mother to infant: its effect on measles, mumps, and rubella immunization. Am J Dis Child 133:1240–1243, 1979.

523. Vahlquist B. Response of infants to diphtheria immunization. Lancet 1:16–18, 1949.

524. Perkins F, Yetto R, Gaisford W. Response of infants to a third dose of poliomyelitis vaccine given 10 to 12 months after primary immunization. Br Med J 1:680–682, 1959.

525. Cederqvist LL, Ewool LC, Litwin SD. The effect of fetal age, birth weight, and sex on cord blood immunoglobulin values. Am J Obstet Gynecol 131:520–525, 1978.

526. Avrech OM, Samra Z, Lazarovich Z, et al. Efficacy of the placental barrier for immunoglobulins: correlations between maternal, paternal and fetal immunoglobulin levels. Int Arch Allergy Immunol 103:160–165, 1994.

527. Allansmith M, McClellan BH, Butterworth M, et al. The development of immunoglobulin levels in man. J Pediatr 72:276–290, 1968.

528. Perchalski JE, Clem LW, Small PJ. 7S Gamma–M immunoglobulins in normal human cord serum. Am J Med Sci 256:107–111, 1968.

529. Alford CJ, Stagno S, Reynolds DW. Diagnosis of chronic perinatal infections. Am J Dis Child 129:455–463, 1975.

530. Kobayashi RH, Hyman CJ, Stiehm ER. Immunologic maturation in an infant born to a mother with agammaglobulinemia. Am J Dis Child 134:942–944, 1980.

531. Ochs IID, Wedgwood RJ. IgG subclass deficiencies. Annu Rev Med 38:325–340, 1987.

532. Granoff DM, Shackelford PG, Pandey JP, et al. Antibody responses to Haemophilus influenzae type b polysaccharide vaccine in relation to Km(1) and G2m(23) immunoglobulin allotypes. J Infect Dis 154:257–264, 1986.

533. Hendrickson BA, Conner DA, Ladd DJ, et al. Altered hepatic transport of immunoglobulin A in mice lacking the J chain. J Exp Med 182:1905–1911, 1995.

534. Conley ME, Kearney JF, Lawton AR, et al. Differentiation of human B cells expressing the IgA subclasses as demonstrated by monoclonal hybridoma antibodies. J Immunol 125:2311–2316, 1980.

535. Josephs SH, Buckley RH. Serum IgD concentrations in normal infants, children, and adults and in patients with elevated IgE. J Pediatr 96:417–420, 1980.

536. Young M, Geha RS. Ontogeny and control of human IgE synthesis. Clin Immunol Allergy 5:339–349, 1985.

537. Bazaral M, Orgel HA, Hamburger RN. IgE levels in normal infants and mothers and an inheritance hypothesis. J Immunol 107:794–801, 1971.

538. Sivori S, Vitale M, Morelli L, et al. p46, A novel natural killer cell–specific surface molecule that mediates cell activation. J Exp Med 186:1129–1136, 1997.

539. Phillips JH, Hori T, Nagler A, et al. Ontogeny of human natural killer (NK) cells: fetal NK cells mediate cytolytic function and express cytoplasmic CD3 epsilon, delta proteins. J Exp Med 175:1055–1066, 1992.

540. Nakazawa T, Agematsu K, Yabuhara A. Later development of Fas ligand–mediated cytotoxicity as compared with granule-mediated cytotoxicity during the maturation of natural killer cells. Immunology 92:180–187, 1997.

541. Lanier LL. NK cell receptors. Annu Rev Immunol 16:359–393, 1998.

542. George T, Yu YY, Liu J, et al. Allorecognition by murine natural killer cells: lysis of T-lymphoblasts and rejection of bone-marrow grafts. Immunol Rev 15:29–40, 1997.

543. Perussia B. Fc receptors on natural killer cells. Curr Top Microbiol Immunol 230:63–88, 1998.

544. Biron CA, Byron KS, Sullivan JL. Severe herpesvirus infections in an adolescent without natural killer cells. N Engl J Med 320:1731–1735, 1989.

545. Miller JS, Alley KA, McGlave P. Differentiation of natural killer (NK) cells from human primitive marrow progenitors in a stroma-based long-term culture system: identification of a CD34^{++} NK progenitor. Blood 83:2594–2601, 1994.

546. Carayol G, Robin C, Bourhis JH, et al. NK cells differentiated from bone marrow, cord blood and peripheral blood stem cells exhibit similar phenotype and functions. Eur J Immunol 28:1991–2002, 1998.

547. Mrozek E, Anderson P, Caligiuri MA. Role of interleukin-15 in the development of human CD56^{+} natural killer cells from CD34^{+} hematopoietic progenitor cells. Blood 87:2632–2640, 1996.

548. Marquez C, Trigueros C, Franco JM, et al. Identification of a common developmental pathway for thymic natural killer cells and dendritic cells. Blood 91:2760–2771, 1998.

549. Poggi A, Costa P, Morelli L, et al. Expression of human NKRP1A by CD34^{+} immature thymocytes: NKRP1A-mediated regulation of proliferation and cytolytic activity. Eur J Immunol 26:1266–1272, 1996.

550. Hori T, Phillips JH, Duncan B, et al. Human fetal liver–derived CD7^{+}CD2^{low}CD3^{-}CD56^{-} clones that express CD3 gamma, delta, and epsilon and proliferate in response to interleukin-2 (IL-2), IL-3, IL-4, or IL-7: implications for the relationship between T and natural killer cells. Blood 80:1270–1278, 1992.

551. Bennett IM, Zatsepina O, Zamai L, et al. Definition of a natural killer NKR-P1A^{+}/CD56^{-}/CD16^{-} functionally immature human NK cell subset that differentiates in vitro in the presence of interleukin 12. J Exp Med 184:1845–1856, 1996.

552. Mingari MC, Vitale C, Cantoni C, et al. Interleukin-15–induced maturation of human natural killer cells from early thymic precursors: selective expression of CD94/NKG2-A as the only HLA class I–specific inhibitory receptor. Eur J Immunol 27:1374–1380, 1997.

553. Carson WE, Fehniger TA, Haldar S, et al. A potential role for interleukin-15 in the regulation of human natural killer cell survival. J Clin Invest 99:937–943, 1997.

554. Ogasawara K, Hida S, Azimi N, et al. Requirement for IRF-1 in the microenvironment supporting development of natural killer cells. Nature 391:700–703, 1998.

555. Lodolce JP, Boone DL, Chai S, et al. IL-15 receptor maintains lymphoid homeostasis by supporting lymphocyte homing and proliferation. Immunity 9:669–676, 1998.

556. Moretta A, Sivori S, Ponte M, et al. Stimulatory receptors in NK and T cells. Curr Top Microbiol Immunol 230:15–23, 1998.

557. Oxenius A, Campbell KA, Maliszewski CR, et al. CD40-CD40 ligand interactions are critical in T-B cooperation but not for other anti-viral CD4+ T cell functions. J Exp Med 183:2209–2218, 1996.

558. Valiante NM, Uhrberg M, Shilling HG, et al. Functionally and structurally distinct NK cell receptor repertoires in the peripheral blood of two human donors. Immunity 7:739–751, 1997.

559. Uhrberg M, Valiante NM, Shum BP, et al. Human diversity in killer cell inhibitory receptor genes. Immunity 7:753–763, 1997.

560. Gumperz JE, Valiante NM, Parham P, et al. Heterogeneous phenotypes of expression of the NKB1 natural killer cell class I receptor among individuals of different human histocompatibility leukocyte antigen types appear genetically regulated, but not linked to major histocompatibility complex haplotype. J Exp Med 183:1817–1827, 1996.

561. Pende D, Biassoni R, Cantoni C, et al. The natural killer cell receptor specific for HLA-A allotypes: a novel member of the p58/p70 family of inhibitory receptors that is characterized by three immunoglobulin-like domains and is expressed as a 140-kD disulphide-linked dimer. J Exp Med 184:505–518, 1996.

562. Dohring C, Scheidegger D, Samaridis J, et al. A human killer inhibitory receptor specific for HLA-A1,2. J Immunol 156:3098–3101, 1996.

563. Moller MJ, Kammerer R, von Kleist S. A distinct distribution of natural killer cell subgroups in human tissues and blood. Int J Cancer 78:533–538, 1998.

564. Helander TS, Timonen T. Adhesion in NK cell function. Curr Top Microbiol Immunol 230:89–99, 1998.

565. Pessino A, Sivori S, Bottino C, et al. Molecular cloning of NKp46: a novel member of the immunoglobulin superfamily involved in triggering of natural cytotoxicity. J Exp Med 188:953–960, 1998.

566. Vitale M, Bottino C, Sivori S, et al. NKp44, a novel triggering surface molecule specifically expressed by activated natural killer cells, is involved in non–major histocompatibility complex–restricted tumor cell lysis. J Exp Med 187:2065–2072, 1998.

567. Cantoni C, Biassoni R, Pende D, et al. The activating form of CD94 receptor complex: CD94 covalently associates with the Kp39 protein that represents the product of the NKG2-C gene. Eur J Immunol 28:327–338, 1998.

568. Lanier LL, Corliss B, Wu J, et al. Association of DAP12 with activating CD94/NKG2C NK cell receptors. Immunity 8:693–701, 1998.

569. Oshimi Y, Oda S, Honda Y, et al. Involvement of Fas ligand and Fas-mediated pathway in the cytotoxicity of human natural killer cells. J Immunol 157:2909–2915, 1996.

570. Zamai L, Ahmad M, Bennett I, et al. Natural killer (NK) cell–mediated cytotoxicity: differential use of TRAIL and Fas ligand by immature and mature primary human NK cells. J Exp Med 188:2375–2380, 1998.

571. Medvedev AE, Johnsen AC, Haux J, et al. Regulation of Fas and Fas-ligand expression in NK cells by cytokines and the involvement of Fas-ligand in NK/LAK cell–mediated cytotoxicity. Cytokine 9:394–404, 1997.

572. Eischen CM, Schilling JD, Lynch DH, et al. Fc receptor–induced expression of Fas ligand on activated NK cells facilitates cell–mediated cytotoxicity and subsequent autocrine NK cell apoptosis. J Immunol 156:2693–2699, 1996.

573. Van-den-Broek MF, Kagi D, Hengartner H. Effector pathways of natural killer cells. Curr Top Microbiol Immunol 230:123–131, 1998.

574. Chambers BJ, Wilson JL, Salcedo M, et al. Triggering of natural killer cell mediated cytotoxicity by costimulatory molecules. Curr Top Microbiol Immunol 230:53–61, 1998.

575. Hunter CA, Ellis NL, Gabriel KE, et al. The role of the CD28/B7 interaction in the regulation of NK cell responses during infection with Toxoplasma gondii. J Immunol 158:2285–2293, 1997.

576. Lang S, Vujanovic NL, Wollenberg B, et al. Absence of B7.1-CD28/CTLA-4–mediated co-stimulation in human NK cells. Eur J Immunol 28:780–786, 1998.

577. Tomura M, Zhou XY, Maruo S, et al. A critical role for IL-18 in the proliferation and activation of NK1.1+ CD3− cells. J Immunol 160:4738–4746, 1998.

578. Shaw SG, Maung AA, Steptoe RJ, et al. Expansion of functional NK cells in multiple tissue compartments of mice treated with Flt3-ligand: implications for anti-cancer and anti-viral therapy. J Immunol 161:2817–2824, 1998.

579. Salvucci O, Mami-Chouaib F, Moreau JL, et al. Differential regulation of interleukin-12– and interleukin-15–induced natural killer cell activation by interleukin-4. Eur J Immunol 26:2736–2741, 1996.

580. Aiba Y, Hirayama F, Ogawa M. Clonal proliferation and cytokine requirement of murine progenitors for natural killer cells. Blood 89:4005–4012, 1997.

581. Dalton DK, Pitts-Meek S, Keshav S, et al. Multiple defects of immune cell function in mice with disrupted interferon-gamma genes. Science 259:1739–1742, 1993.

582. Magram J, Sfarra J, Connaughton S, et al. IL-12-deficient mice are defective but not devoid of type 1 cytokine responses. Ann NY Acad Sci 795:60–70, 1996.

583. Takeda K, Tsutsui H, Yoshimoto T, et al. Defective NK cell activity and Th1 response in IL-18–deficient mice. Immunity 8:383–390, 1998.

584. Ida H, Anderson P. Activation-induced NK cell death triggered by CD2 stimulation. Eur J Immunol 28:1292–1300, 1998.

585. Mainiero F, Gismondi A, Soriani A, et al. Integrin-mediated ras–extracellular regulated kinase (ERK) signaling regulates interferon gamma production in human natural killer cells. J Exp Med 188:1267–1275, 1998.

586. Hunter CA, Chizzonite R, Remington JS. IL-1 beta is required for IL-12 to induce production of IFN-gamma by NK cells: a role for IL-1 beta in the T cell–independent mechanism of resistance against intracellular pathogens. J Immunol 155:4347–4354, 1995.

587. Bluman EM, Bartynski KJ, Avalos BR, et al. Human natural killer cells produce abundant macrophage inflammatory protein–1 alpha in response to monocyte-derived cytokines. J Clin Invest 97:2722–2727, 1996.

588. Oliva A, Kinter AL, Vaccarezza M, et al. Natural killer cells from human immunodeficiency virus (HIV)–infected individuals are an important source of CC-chemokines and suppress HIV-1 entry and replication in vitro. J Clin Invest 102:223–231, 1998.

589. Tay CH, Szomolanyi-Tsuda E, Welsh RM. Control of infections by NK cells. Curr Top Microbiol Immunol 230:193–220, 1998.

590. Warren HS, Kinnear BF, Phillips JH, et al. Production of IL-5 by human NK cells and regulation of IL-5 secretion by IL-4, IL-10, and IL-12. J Immunol 154:5144–5152, 1995.

591. Guimond MJ, Wang B, Croy BA. Engraftment of bone marrow from severe combined immunodeficient (SCID) mice reverses the reproductive deficits in natural killer

cell–deficient tg epsilon 26 mice. J Exp Med 187:217–223, 1998.

592. Lopez-Botet M, Carretero M, Bellon T, et al. The CD94/NKG2 C-type lectin receptor complex. Curr Top Microbiol Immunol 230:41–52, 1998.

593. Munz C, Holmes N, King A, et al. Human histocompatibility leukocyte antigen (HLA)–G molecules inhibit NKAT3 expressing natural killer cells. J Exp Med 185:385–391, 1997.

594. Colonna M, Navarro F, Bell'on T, et al. A common inhibitory receptor for major histocompatibility complex class I molecules on human lymphoid and myelomonocytic cells. J Exp Med 186:1809–1818, 1997.

595. Jaleco AC, Blom B, Res P, et al. Fetal liver contains committed NK progenitors, but is not a site for development of CD34$^+$ cells into T cells. J Immunol 159:694–702, 1997.

596. Carlyle JR, Michie AM, Cho SK, et al. Natural killer cell development and function precede alpha beta T cell differentiation in mouse fetal thymic ontogeny. J Immunol 160:744–753, 1998.

597. Qian JX, Lee SM, Suen Y, et al. Decreased interleukin-15 from activated cord versus adult peripheral blood mononuclear cells and the effect of interleukin-15 in upregulating antitumor immune activity and cytokine production in cord blood. Blood 90:3106–3117, 1997.

598. Thilaganathan B, Abbas A, Nicolaides KH. Fetal blood natural killer cells in human pregnancy. Fetal Diagn Ther 8:149–153, 1993.

599. Moretta L, Ciccone E, Moretta A, et al. Allorecognition by NK cells: nonself or no self? Immunol Today 13:300–306, 1992.

600. Gaddy J, Risdon G, Broxmeyer HE. Cord blood natural killer cells are functionally and phenotypically immature but readily respond to interleukin-2 and interleukin-12. J Interferon Cytokine Res 15:527–536, 1995.

601. Azuma M, Cayabyab M, Buck D, et al. Involvement of CD28 in MHC-unrestricted cytotoxicity mediated by a human natural killer leukemia cell line. J Immunol 149:1115–1123, 1992.

602. Merrill JD, Sigaroudinia M, Kohl S. Characterization of natural killer and antibody-dependent cellular cytotoxicity of preterm infants against human immunodeficiency virus–infected cells. Pediatr Res 40:498–503, 1996.

603. Cicuttini FM, Martin M, Petrie HT, et al. A novel population of natural killer progenitor cells isolated from human umbilical cord blood. J Immunol 151:29–37, 1993.

604. Webb BJ, Bochan MR, Montel A, et al. The lack of NK cytotoxicity associated with fresh HUCB may be due to the presence of soluble HLA in the serum. Cell Immunol 159:246–261, 1994.

605. Jenkins M, Mills J, Kohl S. Natural killer cytotoxicity and antibody-dependent cellular cytotoxicity of human immunodeficiency virus–infected cells by leukocytes from human neonates and adults. Pediatr Res 33:469–474, 1993.

606. Sancho L, de la Hera A, Casas J, et al. Two different maturational stages of natural killer lymphocytes in human newborn infants. J Pediatr 119:446–454, 1991.

607. Lau AS, Sigaroudinia M, Yeung MC, et al. Interleukin-12 induces interferon-γ expression and natural killer cytotoxicity in cord blood mononuclear cells. Pediatr Res 39:150–155, 1996.

608. Han P, Hodge G, Story C, et al. Phenotypic analysis of functional T-lymphocyte subtypes and natural killer cells in human cord blood: relevance to umbilical cord blood transplantation. Br J Haematol 89:733–740, 1995.

609. Harris DT. In vitro and in vivo assessment of the graft-versus-leukemia activity of cord blood. Bone Marrow Transplant 15:17–23, 1995.

610. Umemoto M, Azuma E, Hirayama M, et al. Two cytotoxic pathways of natural killer cells in human cord blood: implications in cord blood transplantation. Br J Haematol 98:1037–1040, 1997.

611. Condiotti R, Nagler A. Effect of interleukin-12 on antitumor activity of human umbilical cord blood and bone marrow cytotoxic cells. Exp Hematol 26:571–579, 1998.

612. Gaddy J, Broxmeyer HE. Cord blood CD16$^+$56$^-$ cells with low lytic activity are possible precursors of mature natural killer cells. Cell Immunol 180:132–142, 1997.

613. Malygin AM, Timonen T. Non–major histocompatibility complex–restricted killer cells in human cord blood: generation and cytotoxic activity in recombinant interleukin-2–supplemented cultures. Immunology 79:506–508, 1993.

614. Dominguez E, Madrigal JA, Layrisse Z, et al. Fetal natural killer cell function is suppressed. Immunology 94:109–114, 1998.

615. Hayward AR, Herberger M, Saunders D. Herpes simplex virus–stimulated interferon-γ production by newborn mononuclear cells. Pediatr Res 20:398–401, 1986.

616. Lee SM, Suen Y, Chang L, et al. Decreased interleukin-12 (IL-12) from activated cord versus adult peripheral blood mononuclear cells and upregulation of interferon-gamma, natural killer, and lymphokine-activated killer activity by IL-12 in cord blood mononuclear cells. Blood 88:945–954, 1996.

617. Braakman E, Sturm E, Vijverberg K, et al. Expression of CD45 isoforms by fresh and activated human gamma delta T lymphocytes and natural killer cells. Int Immunol 3:691–697, 1991.

618. Furman WL, Crist WM. Biology and clinical applications of hemopoietins in pediatric practice. Pediatrics 90:716–728, 1992.

619. Metcalf D. Control of granulocytes and macrophages: molecular, cellular, and clinical aspects. Science 254:529–533, 1991.

620. Metcalf D. The molecular control of hematopoiesis: progress and problems with gene manipulation. Stem Cells (Dayt) 16:314–321, 1998.

621. Zsebo KM, Williams DA, Geissler EN, et al. Stem cell factor is encoded at the Sl locus of the mouse and is the ligand for the c-kit tyrosine kinase receptor. Cell 63:213–224, 1990.

622. Wiktor-Jedrzejczak W, Bartocci A, Ferrante AJ, et al. Total absence of colony-stimulating factor 1 in the macrophage-deficient osteopetrotic op/op mouse. Proc Natl Acad Sci USA 87:4828–4832, 1990.

623. Lieschke GJ, Burgess AW. Granulocyte colony-stimulating factor and granulocyte-macrophage colony-stimulating factor 2. N Engl J Med 327:99–106, 1992.

624. Mueller BU, Pizzo PA. Cytokines and biological response modifiers in the treatment of infection. Cancer Treat Res 96:201–222, 1998.

625. Walker RI, Willemze R. Neutrophil kinetics and the regulation of granulopoiesis. Rev Infect Dis 2:282–292, 1980.

626. Engle WA, Schreiner RL, Baehner RL. Neonatal white blood cell disorders. Semin Perinatol 7:184–200, 1983.

627. Dunon D, Piali L, Imhof BA. To stick or not to stick: the new leukocyte homing paradigm. Curr Opin Cell Biol 8:714–723, 1996.

628. Etzioni A, Harlan JM. Cell adhesion and leukocyte

adhesion defects. *In* Ochs HD, Edvard Smith CIE, Puck JM (eds). Primary Immunodeficiency Diseases: A Molecular and Genetic Approach. New York, Oxford University Press, 1999, pp 375–388.

629. Springer TA. Traffic signals on endothelium for lymphocyte recirculation and leukocyte emigration. Annu Rev Phys 57:827–872, 1995.

630. Harvath L. Neutrophil chemotactic factors. EXS 59:35–52, 1991.

631. Miller MD, Krangel MS. Biology and biochemistry of the chemokines: a family of chemotactic and inflammatory cytokines. Crit Rev Immunol 12:17–46, 1992.

632. Luster AD. Chemokines—chemotactic cytokines that mediate inflammation. N Engl J Med 338:436–445, 1998.

633. Snyderman R, Pike MC. Chemoattractant receptors on phagocytic cells. Annu Rev Immunol 2:257–281, 1984.

634. Snyderman R, Goetzl EJ. Molecular and cellular mechanisms of leukocyte chemotaxis. Science 213:830–837, 1981.

635. Springer TA. Adhesion receptors of the immune system. Nature 346:425–434, 1990.

636. Ravetch JV, Clynes RA. Divergent roles for Fc receptors and complement in vivo. Annu Rev Immunol 16:421–432, 1998.

637. Colten HR, Rosen FS. Complement deficiencies. Annu Rev Immunol 10:809–834, 1992.

638. Allen LA, Aderem A. Mechanisms of phagocytosis. Curr Opin Immunol 8:36–40, 1996.

639. Caron E, Hall A. Identification of two distinct mechanisms of phagocytosis controlled by different Rho GTPases. Science 282:1717–1721, 1998.

640. Ravetch JV. Fc receptors: rubor redux. Cell 78:553–560, 1994.

641. Smith RM, Curnutte JT. Molecular basis of chronic granulomatous disease. Blood 77:673–686, 1991.

642. Spitznagel JK. Antibiotic proteins of human neutrophils. J Clin Invest 86:1381–1386, 1990.

643. Martin E, Ganz T, Lehrer RI. Defensins and other endogenous peptide antibiotics of vertebrates. J Leukoc Biol 58:128–136, 1995.

644. Dinarello CA. Interleukin-1 and interleukin-1 antagonism. Blood 77:1627–1652, 1991.

645. Vassalli P. The pathophysiology of tumor necrosis factors. Annu Rev Immunol 10:411–452, 1992.

646. Christensen RD. Hematopoiesis in the fetus and neonate. Pediatr Res 26:531–535, 1989.

647. Playfair J, Wolfendale M, Kay H. The leucocytes of peripheral blood in the human foetus. Br J Haematol 9:336–344, 1963.

648. Shapiro L, Bassen F. Sternal marrow changes during the first week of life: correlation with peripheral blood findings. Am J Med Sci 292:341–354, 1941.

649. Christensen RD, Rothstein G. Pre- and postnatal development of granulocytic stem cells in the rat. Pediatr Res 18:599–602, 1984.

650. Ohls RK, Li Y, Abdel-Mageed A, et al. Neutrophil pool sizes and granulocyte colony-stimulating factor production in human mid-trimester fetuses. Pediatr Res 37:806–811, 1995.

651. Laver J, Duncan E, Abboud M, et al. High levels of granulocyte and granulocyte-macrophage colony-stimulating factors in cord blood of normal full-term neonates. J Pediatr 116:627–632, 1990.

652. Manroe BL, Weinberg AG, Rosenfeld CR, et al. The neonatal blood count in health and disease. I. Reference values for neutrophilic cells. J Pediatr 95:89–98, 1979.

653. Schelonka RL, Yoder BA, des Jardins SE, et al. Periph-

654. Squire E, Favara B, Todd J. Diagnosis of neonatal bacterial infection: hematologic and pathologic findings in fatal and nonfatal cases. Pediatrics 64:60–64, 1979.

655. Christensen RD, Rothstein G. Exhaustion of mature marrow neutrophils in neonates with sepsis. J Pediatr 96:316–318, 1980.

656. Calhoun DA, Kirk JF, Christensen RD. Incidence, significance, and kinetic mechanism responsible for leukemoid reactions in patients in the neonatal intensive care unit: a prospective evaluation. J Pediatr 129:403–409, 1996.

657. Gessler P, Kirchmann N, Kientsch-Engel R, et al. Serum concentrations of granulocyte colony-stimulating factor in healthy term and preterm neonates and in those with various diseases including bacterial infections. Blood 82:3177–3182, 1993.

658. Ishiguro A, Inoue K, Nakahata T, et al. Reference intervals for serum granulocyte colony-stimulating factor levels in children. J Pediatr 128:208–212, 1996.

659. Shimada M, Minato M, Takada M, et al. Plasma concentration of granulocyte colony-stimulating factor in neonates. Acta Paediatr 85:351–355, 1996.

660. Wilimas JA, Wall JE, Fairclough DL, et al. A longitudinal study of granulocyte colony-stimulating factor levels and neutrophil counts in newborn infants. J Pediatr Hematol Oncol 17:176–179, 1995.

661. Kennon C, Overturf G, Bessman S, et al. Granulocyte colony-stimulating factor as a marker for bacterial infection in neonates. J Pediatr 128:765–769, 1996.

662. Schibler KR, Liechty KW, White WL, et al. Production of granulocyte colony-stimulating factor in vitro by monocytes from preterm and term neonates. Blood 82:2478–2484, 1993.

663. Hill HR. Biochemical, structural, and functional abnormalities of polymorphonuclear leukocytes in the neonate. Pediatr Res 22:375–382, 1987.

664. Johnston RB, Jr. Function and cell biology of neutrophils and mononuclear phagocytes in the newborn infant. Vaccine 16:1363–1368, 1998.

665. Weisman LE, Stoll BJ, Kueser TJ, et al. Intravenous immune globulin therapy for early-onset sepsis in premature neonates. J Pediatr 121:434–443, 1992.

666. Schuit KE, Homisch L. Inefficient in vivo neutrophil migration in neonatal rats. J Leukoc Biol 35:583–586, 1984.

667. Anderson DC, Hughes BJ, Smith CW. Abnormal mobility of neonatal polymorphonuclear leukocytes: relationship to impaired redistribution of surface adhesion sites by chemotactic factor or colchicine. J Clin Invest 68:863–874, 1981.

668. Anderson DC, Hughes BJ, Wible LJ, et al. Impaired motility of neonatal PMN leukocytes: relationship to abnormalities of cell orientation and assembly of microtubules in chemotactic gradients. J Leukoc Biol 36:1–15, 1984.

669. Anderson DC, Abbassi O, Kishimoto TK, et al. Diminished lectin-, epidermal growth factor–, complement binding domain–cell adhesion molecule–1 on neonatal neutrophils underlies their impaired CD18-independent adhesion to endothelial cells in vitro. J Immunol 146:3372–3379, 1991.

670. Smith JB, Kunjummen RD, Kishimoto TK, et al. Expression and regulation of L-selectin on eosinophils from human adults and neonates. Pediatr Res 32:465–471, 1992.

671. Koenig JM, Simon J, Anderson DC, et al. Diminished

soluble and total cellular L-selectin in cord blood is associated with its impaired shedding from activated neutrophils. Pediatr Res 39:616–621, 1996.

672. Rebuck N, Gibson A, Finn A. Neutrophil adhesion molecules in term and premature infants: normal or enhanced leucocyte integrins but defective L-selectin expression and shedding. Clin Exp Immunol 101:183–189, 1995.

673. Abughali N, Berger M, Tosi MF. Deficient total cell content of CR3 (CD11b) in neonatal neutrophils. Blood 83:1086–1092, 1994.

674. McEvoy LT, Zakem-Cloud H, Tosi MF. Total cell content of CR3 (CD11b/CD18) and LFA-1 (CD11a/CD18) in neonatal neutrophils: relationship to gestational age. Blood 87:3929–3933, 1996.

675. Anderson DC, Rothlein R, Marlin SD, et al. Impaired transendothelial migration by neonatal neutrophils: abnormalities of Mac-1 CD11b/CD18-dependent adherence reactions. Blood 76:2613–2621, 1990.

676. Adinolfi M, Cheetham M, Lee T, et al. Ontogeny of human complement receptors CR1 and CR3: expression of these molecules on monocytes and neutrophils from maternal, newborn and fetal samples. Eur J Immunol 18:565–569, 1988.

677. Raghunathan R, Miller ME, Everett S, et al. Phagocyte chemotaxis in the perinatal period. J Clin Immunol 2:242–245, 1982.

678. Pahwa SG, Pahwa R, Grimes E, et al. Cellular and humoral components of monocyte and neutrophil chemotaxis in cord blood. Pediatr Res 11:677–680, 1977.

679. Klein RB, Fischer TJ, Gard SE, et al. Decreased mononuclear and polymorphonuclear chemotaxis in human newborns, infants, and young children. Pediatrics 60:467–472, 1977.

680. Carr R, Huizinga TW, Kleijer M, et al. Changes in plasma FcRIII demonstrate increasing receptor production. Pediatr Res 32:505–508, 1992.

681. Dos SC, Davidson D. Neutrophil chemotaxis to leukotriene B4 in vitro is decreased for the human neonate. Pediatr Res 33:242–246, 1993.

682. Tan ND, Davidson D. Comparative differences and combined effects of interleukin-8, leukotriene B4, and platelet-activating factor on neutrophil chemotaxis of the newborn. Pediatr Res 38:11–16, 1995.

683. Yasui K, Masuda M, Tsuno T, et al. An increase in polymorphonuclear leucocyte chemotaxis accompanied by a change in the membrane fluidity with age during childhood. Clin Exp Immunol 81:156–159, 1990.

684. Bektas S, Goetze B, Speer CP. Decreased adherence, chemotaxis and phagocytic activities of neutrophils from preterm neonates. Acta Paediatr Scand 79:1031–1038, 1990.

685. Kamran S, Usmani SS, Wapnir RA, et al. In vitro effect of indomethacin on polymorphonuclear leukocyte function in preterm infants. Pediatr Res 33:32–35, 1993.

686. Strauss RG, Snyder EL. Chemotactic peptide binding by intact neutrophils from human neonates. Pediatr Res 18:63–66, 1984.

687. Sacchi F, Hill HR. Defective membrane potential changes in neutrophils from human neonates. J Exp Med 160:1247–1252, 1984.

688. Nunoi H, Endo F, Chikazawa S, et al. Chemotactic receptor of cord blood granulocytes to the synthesized chemotactic peptide N-formyl-methionyl-leucyl-phenylalanine. Pediatr Res 17:57–60, 1983.

689. Nybo M, Sorensen O, Leslie R, et al. Reduced expression of C5a receptors on neutrophils from cord blood. Arch Dis Child 78:129–132, 1998.

690. Santoro P, Agosti V, Viggiano D, et al. Impaired D-myo-inositol 1,4,5-triphosphate generation from cord blood polymorphonuclear leukocytes. Pediatr Res 38:564–567, 1995.

691. Merry C, Puri P, Reen DJ. Defective neutrophil actin polymerisation and chemotaxis in stressed newborns. J Pediatr Surg 31:481–485, 1996.

692. Boner A, Zeligs BJ, Bellanti JA. Chemotactic responses of various differentiational stages of neutrophils from human cord and adult blood. Infect Immun 35:921–928, 1982.

693. Kikawa Y, Shigematsu Y, Sudo M. Leukotriene B4 biosynthesis in polymorphonuclear leukocytes from blood of umbilical cord, infants, children, and adults. Pediatr Res 20:402–406, 1986.

694. Bruce MC, Baley JE, Medvik KA, et al. Impaired surface membrane expression of C3bi but not C3b receptors on neonatal neutrophils. Pediatr Res 21:306–311, 1987.

695. Smith JB, Campbell DE, Ludomirsky A, et al. Expression of the complement receptors CR1 and CR3 and the type III Fc gamma receptor on neutrophils from newborn infants and from fetuses with Rh disease. Pediatr Res 28:120–126, 1990.

696. McCracken GJ, Eichenwald HF. Leukocyte function and the development of opsonic and complement activity in the neonate. Am J Dis Child 121:120–126, 1971.

697. Harris MC, Stroobant J, Cody CS, et al. Phagocytosis of group B streptococcus by neutrophils from newborn infants. Pediatr Res 17:358–361, 1983.

698. Falconer AE, Carr R, Edwards SW. Impaired neutrophil phagocytosis in preterm neonates: lack of correlation with expression of immunoglobulin or complement receptors. Biol Neonate 68:264–269, 1995.

699. Falconer AE, Carr R, Edwards SW. Neutrophils from preterm neonates and adults show similar cell surface receptor expression: analysis using a whole blood assay. Biol Neonate 67:26–33, 1995.

700. Fujiwara T, Kobayashi T, Takaya J, et al. Plasma effects on phagocytic activity and hydrogen peroxide production by polymorphonuclear leukocytes in neonates. Clin Immunol Immunopathol 85:67–72, 1997.

701. Payne NR, Fleit HB. Extremely low birth weight infants have lower Fc gamma RIII (CD16) plasma levels and their PMNs produce less Fc gamma RIII compared to adults. Biol Neonate 69:235–242, 1996.

702. Miller ME. Phagocyte function in the neonate: selected aspects. Pediatrics 64:709–712, 1979.

703. Jones DH, Schmalstieg FC, Dempsey K, et al. Subcellular distribution and mobilization of MAC-1 CD11b/CD18 in neonatal neutrophils. Blood 75:488–498, 1990.

704. Qing G, Rajaraman K, Bortolussi R. Diminished priming of neonatal polymorphonuclear leukocytes by lipopolysaccharide is associated with reduced CD14 expression. Infect Immun 63:248–252, 1995.

705. Park BH, Holmes B, Good RA. Metabolic activities in leukocytes of newborn infants. J Pediatr 76:237–241, 1970.

706. Dossett JH, Williams RC, Jr, Quie PG. Studies on interaction of bacteria, serum factors and polymorphonuclear leukocytes in mothers and newborns. Pediatrics 44:49–57, 1969.

707. Cocchi P, Marianelli L. Phagocytosis and intracellular killing of Pseudomonas aeruginosa in premature infants. Helv Paediatr Acta 22:110–118, 1967.

708. Coen R, Grush O, Kauder E. Studies of bactericidal activity and metabolism of the leukocyte in full-term neonates. J Pediatr 75:400–406, 1969.

709. Becker ID, Robinson OM, Bazaan TS, et al. Bactericidal capacity of newborn phagocytes against group B beta-hemolytic streptococci. Infect Immun 34:535–539, 1981.

710. Stroobant J, Harris MC, Cody CS, et al. Diminished bactericidal capacity for group B *Streptococcus* in neutrophils from "stressed" and healthy neonates. Pediatr Res 18:634–637, 1984.

711. Shigeoka AO, Charette RP, Wyman ML, et al. Defective oxidative metabolic responses of neutrophils from stressed neonates. J Pediatr 98:392–398, 1981.

712. Mills EL, Thompson T, Bjeorkstaen B, et al. The chemiluminescence response and bactericidal activity of polymorphonuclear neutrophils from newborns and their mothers. Pediatrics 63:429–434, 1979.

713. Wright WJ, Ank BJ, Herbert J, et al. Decreased bactericidal activity of leukocytes of stressed newborn infants. Pediatrics 56:579–584, 1975.

714. Shigeoka AO, Santos JI, Hill HR. Functional analysis of neutrophil granulocytes from healthy, infected, and stressed neonates. J Pediatr 95:454–460, 1979.

715. Ambruso DR, Altenburger KM, Johnston RJ. Defective oxidative metabolism in newborn neutrophils: discrepancy between superoxide anion and hydroxyl radical generation. Pediatrics 64:722–725, 1979.

716. Newburger PE. Superoxide generation by human fetal granulocytes. Pediatr Res 16:373–376, 1982.

717. Strauss RG, Rosenberger TG, Wallace PD. Neutrophil chemiluminescence during the first month of life. Acta Haematol 63:326–329, 1980.

718. Van-Epps DE, Goodwin JS, Murphy S. Age-dependent variations in polymorphonuclear leukocyte chemiluminescence. Infect Immun 22:57–61, 1978.

719. Wilson CB, Weaver WM. Comparative susceptibility of group B streptococci and *Staphylococcus aureus* to killing by oxygen metabolites. J Infect Dis 152:323–329, 1985.

720. Yasui K, Masuda M, Matsuoka T, et al. Abnormal membrane fluidity as a cause of impaired functional dynamics of chemoattractant receptors on neonatal polymorphonuclear leukocytes: lack of modulation of the receptors by a membrane fluidizer. Pediatr Res 24:442–446, 1988.

721. Ambruso DR, Bentwood B, Henson PM, et al. Oxidative metabolism of cord blood neutrophils: relationship to content and degranulation of cytoplasmic granules. Pediatr Res 18:1148–1153, 1984.

722. Ganz T, Lehrer RI. Defensins. Curr Opin Immunol 6:584–589, 1994.

723. Cairo MS, Agosti J, Ellis R, et al. A randomized double-blind, placebo-controlled trial of prophylactic recombinant human granulocyte-macrophage colony-stimulating factor to reduce nosocomial infections in very low birth weight neonates. J Pediatr 134:64–70, 1999.

724. Hill HR, Augustine NH, Jaffe HS. Human recombinant interferon gamma enhances neonatal polymorphonuclear leukocyte activation and movement, and increases free intracellular calcium. J Exp Med 173:767–770, 1991.

725. Frenck RJ, Buescher ES, Vadhan-Raj S. The effects of recombinant human granulocyte-macrophage colony stimulating factor on in vitro cord blood granulocyte function. Pediatr Res 26:43–48, 1989.

726. Cairo MS, van de Ven C, Toy C, et al. Recombinant human granulocyte-macrophage colony-stimulating factor primes neonatal granulocytes for enhanced oxidative metabolism and chemotaxis. Pediatr Res 26:395–399, 1989.

727. Forestier F, Daffos F, Galactaeros F, et al. Hematologi-cal values of 163 normal fetuses between 18 and 30 weeks of gestation. Pediatr Res 20:342–346, 1986.

728. Bhat AM, Scanlon JW. The pattern of eosinophilia in premature infants: a prospective study in premature infants using the absolute eosinophil count. J Pediatr 98:612–616, 1981.

729. Rothberg AD, Cohn RJ, Argent AC, et al. Eosinophilia in premature neonates: phase 2 of a biphasic granulopoietic response. S Afr Med J 64:539–541, 1983.

730. van Furth R, Raeburn JA, van Zwet TL. Characteristics of human mononuclear phagocytes. Blood 54:485–500, 1979.

731. Nichols BA, Bainton DF, Farquhar MG. Differentiation of monocytes: origin, nature, and fate of their azurophil granules. J Cell Biol 50:498–515, 1971.

732. Hocking WG, Golde DW. The pulmonary-alveolar macrophage (first of two parts). N Engl J Med 301:580–587, 1979.

733. Bitterman PB, Saltzman LE, Adelberg S, et al. Alveolar macrophage replication: one mechanism for the expansion of the mononuclear phagocyte population in the chronically inflamed lung. J Clin Invest 74:460–469, 1984.

734. Butcher EC. Leukocyte–endothelial cell recognition: three or more steps to specificity and diversity. Cell 67:1033–1036, 1991.

735. Hemler ME. VLA proteins in the integrin family: structures, functions, and their role on leukocytes. Annu Rev Immunol 8:365–400, 1990.

736. Enk AH, Katz SI. Early molecular events in the induction phase of contact sensitivity. Proc Natl Acad Sci USA 89:1398–1402, 1992.

737. Tsicopoulos A, Hamid Q, Varney V, et al. Preferential messenger RNA expression of Th1-type cells IFN-gamma$^+$, IL-2$^+$ in classical delayed-type tuberculin hypersensitivity reactions in human skin. J Immunol 148:2058–2061, 1992.

738. Daeron M. Fc receptor biology. Annu Rev Immunol 15:203–234, 1997.

739. Maliszewski CR, March CJ, Schoenborn MA, et al. Expression cloning of a human Fc receptor for IgA. J Exp Med 172:1665–1672, 1990.

740. Wright SD. Multiple receptors for endotoxin. Curr Opin Immunol 3:83–90, 1991.

741. Poltorak A, He X, Smirnova I, et al. Defective LPS signaling in C3H/HeJ and C57BL/10ScCr mice: mutations in *Tlr4* gene. Science 282:2085–2088, 1998.

742. Pugin J, Heumann ID, Tomasz A, et al. CD14 is a pattern recognition receptor. Immunity 1:509–516, 1994.

743. Kirschning CJ, Wesche H, Merrill-Ayres T, et al. Human toll-like receptor confers responsiveness to bacterial lipopolysaccharide. J Exp Med 188:2091–2097, 1998.

744. Ezekowitz RA, Sastry K, Bailly P, et al. Molecular characterization of the human macrophage mannose receptor: demonstration of multiple carbohydrate recognition-like domains and phagocytosis of yeasts in Cos-1 cells. J Exp Med 172:1785–1794, 1990.

745. Devitt A, Moffatt OD, Raykundalia C, et al. Human CD14 mediates recognition and phagocytosis of apoptotic cells. Nature 392:505–509, 1998.

746. Franc NC, Dimarcq JL, Lagueux M, et al. Croquemort, a novel *Drosophila* hemocyte/macrophage receptor that recognizes apoptotic cells. Immunity 4:431–443, 1996.

747. Haworth R, Platt N, Keshav S, et al. The macrophage scavenger receptor type A is expressed by activated mac-

rophages and protects the host against lethal endotoxic shock. J Exp Med 186:1431–1439, 1997.

748. Lehrer RI, Ganz T, Selsted ME. Defensins: endogenous antibiotic peptides of animal cells. Cell 64:229–230, 1991.

749. Grewal IS, Flavell RA. CD40 and CD154 in cell-mediated immunity. Annu Rev Immunol 16:111–135, 1998.

750. Locksley RM, Wilson CB. Cell mediated immunity and its role in host defense. In Mandell GL, Bennett JE, Dolin R (eds). Principles and Practice of Infectious Diseases, 4th ed. New York, Churchill Livingstone, 1995, pp 102–149.

751. van de Winkel JG, Anderson CL. Biology of human immunoglobulin G Fc receptors. J Leukoc Biol 49:511–524, 1991.

752. Clarkson SB, Ory PA. CD16: developmentally regulated IgG Fc receptors on cultured human monocytes. J Exp Med 167:408–420, 1988.

753. Nathan C. Inducible nitric oxide synthase: what difference does it make? J Clin Invest 100:2417–2423, 1997.

754. Altare F, Durandy A, Lammas D, et al. Impairment of mycobacterial immunity in human interleukin-12 receptor deficiency. Science 280:1432–1435, 1998.

755. Altare F, Jouanguy E, Lamhamedi S, et al. Mendelian susceptibility to mycobacterial infection in man. Curr Opin Immunol 10:413–417, 1998.

756. Flynn JL, Goldstein MM, Chan J, et al. Tumor necrosis factor–alpha is required in the protective immune response against Mycobacterium tuberculosis in mice. Immunity 2:561–572, 1995.

757. Kohl S. The neonatal human's immune response to herpes simplex virus infection: a critical review. Pediatr Infect Dis J 8:67–74, 1989.

758. Beutler B. Endotoxin, tumor necrosis factor, and related mediators: new approaches to shock. New Horiz 1:3–12, 1993.

759. Bluethmann H, Rothe J, Schultze N, et al. Establishment of the role of IL-6 and TNF receptor 1 using gene knockout mice. J Leukoc Biol 56:565–570, 1994.

760. Chai Z, Gatti S, Toniatti C, et al. Interleukin (IL)–6 gene expression in the central nervous system is necessary for fever response to lipopolysaccharide or IL-1 beta: a study on IL-6–deficient mice. J Exp Med 183:311–316, 1996.

761. Chomarat P, Rissoan MC, Banchereau J, et al. Interferon-γ inhibits interleukin 10 production by monocytes. J Exp Med 177:523–527, 1993.

762. Dinarello CA, Cannon JG, Wolff SM. New concepts on the pathogenesis of fever. Rev Infect Dis 10:168–189, 1988.

763. Mackowiak PA. Direct effects of hyperthermia on pathogenic microorganisms: teleologic implications with regard to fever. Rev Infect Dis 3:508–520, 1981.

764. Dinarello CA. The biological properties of interleukin-1. Eur Cytokine Netw 5:517–531, 1994.

765. Shanley TP, Warner RL, Ward PA. The role of cytokines and adhesion molecules in the development of inflammatory injury. Mol Med Today 1:40–45, 1995.

766. Smart SJ, Casale TB. Pulmonary epithelial cells facilitate TNF-alpha–induced neutrophil chemotaxis: a role for cytokine networking. J Immunol 152:4087–4094, 1994.

767. Ward PA. Recruitment of inflammatory cells into lung: roles of cytokines, adhesion molecules, and complement. J Lab Clin Med 129:400–404, 1997.

768. Strieter RM, Standiford TJ, Huffnagle GB, et al. The good, the bad, and the ugly: the role of chemokines in models of human disease. J Immunol 156:3583–3586, 1996.

769. Calandra T, Baumgartner JD, Grau GE, et al. Prognostic values of tumor necrosis factor/cachectin, interleukin-1, interferon-alpha, and interferon-gamma in the serum of patients with septic shock. Swiss-Dutch J5 Immunoglobulin Study Group. J Infect Dis 161:982–987, 1990.

770. Car BD, Eng VM, Schnyder B, et al. Interferon gamma receptor deficient mice are resistant to endotoxic shock. J Exp Med 179:1437–1444, 1994.

771. Casey LC, Balk RA, Bone RC. Plasma cytokine and endotoxin levels correlate with survival in patients with the sepsis syndrome. Ann Intern Med 119:771–778, 1993.

772. Mosmann TR. Properties and functions of interleukin-10. Adv Immunol 56:1–26, 1994.

773. Letterio JJ, Roberts AB. Regulation of immune responses by TGF-beta. Annu Rev Immunol 16:137–161, 1998.

774. Howard M, O'Garra A. Biological properties of interleukin 10. Immunol Today 13:198–200, 1992.

775. Aderka D, Le JM, Vilacek J. IL-6 inhibits lipopolysaccharide-induced tumor necrosis factor production in cultured human monocytes, U937 cells, and in mice. J Immunol 143:3517–3523, 1989.

776. Fiorentino DF, Zlotnik A, Mosmann TR, et al. IL-10 inhibits cytokine production by activated macrophages. J Immunol 147:3815–3822, 1991.

777. Gerard C, Bruyns C, Marchant A, et al. Interleukin 10 reduces the release of tumor necrosis factor and prevents lethality in experimental endotoxemia. J Exp Med 177:547–550, 1993.

778. Boehm U, Klamp T, Groot M, et al. Cellular responses to interferon-gamma. Annu Rev Immunol 15:749–795, 1997.

779. Gately MK, Renzetti LM, Magram J, et al. The interleukin-12/interleukin-12–receptor system: role in normal and pathologic immune responses. Annu Rev Immunol 16:495–521, 1998.

780. He YW, Malek TR. The structure and function of gamma c–dependent cytokines and receptors: regulation of T lymphocyte development and homeostasis. Crit Rev Immunol 18:503–524, 1998.

781. Pearce EJ, Reiner SL. Induction of Th2 responses in infectious diseases. Curr Opin Immunol 7:497–504, 1995.

782. Nathan CF. Secretory products of macrophages. J Clin Invest 79:319–326, 1987.

783. Kelemen E, Jaanossa M. Macrophages are the first differentiated blood cells formed in human embryonic liver. Exp Hematol 8:996–1000, 1980.

784. Ueno Y, Koizumi S, Yamagami M, et al. Characterization of hemopoietic stem cells in cord blood. Exp Hematol 9:716–722, 1981.

785. Weinberg AG, Rosenfeld CR, Manroe BL, et al. Neonatal blood cell count in health and disease. II. Values for lymphocytes, monocytes, and eosinophils. J Pediatr 106:462–466, 1985.

786. Jacobs RF, Wilson CB, Smith AL, et al. Age-dependent effects of aminobutyryl muramyl dipeptide on alveolar macrophage function in infant and adult Macaca monkeys. Am Rev Respir Dis 128:862–867, 1983.

787. Wilson C. Lung antimicrobial defenses in the newborn. Semin Respir Med 6:149–154, 1984.

788. Alenghat E, Esterly JR. Alveolar macrophages in perinatal infants. Pediatrics 74:221–223, 1984.

789. Freedman RM, Johnston D, Mahoney M, et al. Devel-

opment of splenic reticuloendothelial function in neonates. J Pediatr 96:466–468, 1980.

790. Bullock JD, Robertson AF, Bodenbender JG, et al. Inflammatory response in the neonate re-examined. Pediatrics 44:58–61, 1969.

791. Sheldon W, Caldwell J. The mononuclear cell phase of inflammation in the newborn. Bull Johns Hopkins Hosp 112:258–269, 1963.

792. Weston WL, Carson BS, Barkin RM, et al. Monocyte-macrophage function in the newborn. Am J Dis Child 131:1241–1242, 1977.

793. Marwitz PA, Van Arkel-Vigna E, Rijkers GT, et al. Expression and modulation of cell surface determinants on human adult and neonatal monocytes. Clin Exp Immunol 72:260–266, 1988.

794. Smith S, Jacobs RF, Wilson CB. The immunobiology of childhood tuberculosis: a window on the ontogeny of cellular immunity. J Pediatr 131:16–26, 1997.

795. Kretschmer RR, Stewardson P, Paperniak CK, et al. Chemotactic and bactericidal capacities of human newborn monocytes. J Immunol 117:1303–1307, 1976.

796. Hawes CS, Kemp AS, Jones WR. In vitro parameters of cell-mediated immunity in the human neonate. Clin Immunol Immunopathol 17:530–536, 1980.

797. Orlowski JP, Sieger L, Anthony BF. Bactericidal capacity of monocytes of newborn infants. J Pediatr 89:797–801, 1976.

798. Schuit KE, Powell DA. Phagocytic dysfunction in monocytes of normal newborn infants. Pediatrics 65:501–504, 1980.

799. Speer CP, Ambruso DR, Grimsley J, et al. Oxidative metabolism in cord blood monocytes and monocyte-derived macrophages. Infect Immun 50:919–921, 1985.

800. Conly ME, Speert DP. Human neonatal monocyte-derived macrophages and neutrophils exhibit normal nonopsonic and opsonic receptor-mediated phagocytosis and superoxide anion production. Biol Neonate 60:361–366, 1991.

801. Speer CP, Gahr M, Wieland M, et al. Phagocytosis-associated functions in neonatal monocyte-derived macrophages. Pediatr Res 24:213–216, 1988.

802. D'Ambola JB, Sherman MP, Tashkin DP, et al. Human and rabbit newborn lung macrophages have reduced anti-*Candida* activity. Pediatr Res 24:285–290, 1988.

803. Coonrod JD, Jarrells MC, Bridges RB. Impaired pulmonary clearance of pneumococci in neonatal rats. Pediatr Res 22:736–742, 1987.

804. Martin TR, Rubens CE, Wilson CB. Lung antibacterial defense mechanisms in infant and adult rats: implications for the pathogenesis of group B streptococcal infections in the neonatal lung. J Infect Dis 157:91–100, 1988.

805. Martin TR, Ruzinski JT, Rubens CE, et al. The effect of type-specific polysaccharide capsule on the clearance of group B streptococci from the lungs of infant and adult rats. J Infect Dis 165:306–314, 1992.

806. Sherman MP, Johnson JT, Rothlein R, et al. Role of pulmonary phagocytes in host defense against group B streptococci in preterm versus term rabbit lung. J Infect Dis 166:818–826, 1992.

807. Kurland G, Cheung AT, Miller ME, et al. The ontogeny of pulmonary defenses: alveolar macrophage function in neonatal and juvenile rhesus monkeys. Pediatr Res 23:293–297, 1988.

808. Bellanti JA, Nerurkar LS, Zeligs BJ. Host defenses in the fetus and neonate: studies of the alveolar macrophage during maturation. Pediatrics 64:726–739, 1979.

809. Sherman MP, Lehrer RI. Oxidative metabolism of neonatal and adult rabbit lung macrophages stimulated with opsonized group B streptococci. Infect Immun 47:26–30, 1985.

810. Ganz T, Sherman MP, Selsted ME, et al. Newborn rabbit alveolar macrophages are deficient in two microbicidal cationic peptides, MCP-1 and MCP-2. Am Rev Respir Dis 132:901–904, 1985.

811. Zeligs BJ, Nerurkar LS, Bellanti JA. Chemotactic and candidacidal responses of rabbit alveolar macrophages during postnatal development and the modulating roles of surfactant in these responses. Infect Immun 44:379–385, 1984.

812. Berman JD, Johnson WJ. Monocyte function in human neonates. Infect Immun 19:898–902, 1978.

813. Marodi L, Káposzta R, Campbell DE, et al. Candidacidal mechanisms in the human neonate: impaired IFN-gamma activation of macrophages in newborn infants. J Immunol 153:5643–5649, 1994.

814. Trofatter KJ, Daniels CA, Williams RJ, et al. Growth of type 2 herpes simplex virus in newborn and adult mononuclear leukocytes. Intervirology 11:117–123, 1979.

815. Mintz L, Drew WL, Hoo R, et al. Age-dependent resistance of human alveolar macrophages to herpes simplex virus. Infect Immun 28:417–420, 1980.

816. Plaeger-Marshall S, Ank BJ, Altenburger KM, et al. Replication of herpes simplex virus in blood monocytes and placental macrophages from human neonates. Pediatr Res 26:135–139, 1989.

817. Morahan PS, Morse SS, McGeorge MG. Macrophage extrinsic antiviral activity during herpes simplex virus infection. J Gen Virol 46:291–300, 1980.

818. Kohl S. Herpes simplex virus immunology: problems, progress, and promises. J Infect Dist 152:435–440, 1985.

819. Kohl S, Frazier JJ, Greenberg SB, et al. Interferon induction of natural killer cytotoxicity in human neonates. J Pediatr 98:379–384, 1981.

820. Milgrom H, Shore SL. Assessment of monocyte function in the normal newborn infant by antibody-dependent cellular cytotoxicity. J Pediatr 91:612–614, 1977.

821. Kohl S. Protection against murine neonatal herpes simplex virus infection by lymphokine-treated human leukocytes. J Immunol 144:307–312, 1990.

822. Bortolussi R, Rajaraman K, Serushago B. Role of tumor necrosis factor–alpha and interferon-gamma in newborn host defense against *Listeria monocytogenes* infection. Pediatr Res 32:460–464, 1992.

823. Bortolussi R, Issekutzj T, Burbridge S, et al. Neonatal host defense mechanisms against *Listeria monocytogenes* infection: the role of lipopolysaccharides and interferons. Pediatr Res 25:311–315, 1989.

824. Cohen L, Haziot A, Shen DR, et al. CD14-independent responses to LPS require a serum factor that is absent from neonates. J Immunol 155:5337–5342, 1995.

825. Medzhitov R, Preston-Hurlburt P, Janeway CA Jr. A human homologue of the *Drosophila* Toll protein signals activation of adaptive immunity. Nature 388:394–397, 1997.

826. Yang RY, Mark MR, Gray A, et al. Toll-like receptor–2 mediates lipopolysaccharide-induced cellular signalling. Nature 395:284–288, 1998.

827. Burchett SK, Weaver WM, Westall JA, et al. Regulation of tumor necrosis factor/cachectin and interleukin-1 secretion in human mononuclear phagocytes. J Immunol 140:3473–3481, 1988.

828. Chang M, Suen Y, Lee SM, et al. Transforming growth factor–beta 1, macrophage inflammatory protein–1

alpha, and interleukin-8 gene expression is lower in stimulated human neonatal compared with adult mononuclear cells. Blood 84:118–124, 1994.

829. Lewis DB. Host defense mechanisms against bacteria, fungi, viruses, and nonviral intracelluar pathogens. *In* Polin RA, Fox WW (eds). Neonatal and Fetal Medicine. Philadelphia, WB Saunders, 1998, pp 1869–1919.

830. Rowen JL, Smith CW, Edwards MS. Group B streptococci elicit leukotriene B4 and interleukin-8 from human monocytes: neonates exhibit a diminished response. J Infect Dis 172:420–426, 1995.

831. Sautois B, Fillet G, Beguin Y. Comparative cytokine production by in vitro stimulated mononucleated cells from cord blood and adult blood. Exp Hematol 25:103–108, 1997.

832. Kotiranta-Ainamo A, Rautonen J, Rautonen N. Interleukin-10 production by cord blood mononuclear cells. Pediatr Res 41:110–113, 1997.

833. Jones CA, Cayabyab RG, Kwong KY, et al. Undetectable interleukin (IL)-10 and persistent IL-8 expression early in hyaline membrane disease: a possible developmental basis for the predisposition to chronic lung inflammation in preterm newborns. Pediatr Res 39:966–975, 1996.

834. Ray CG. The ontogeny of interferon production by human leukocytes. J Pediatr 76:94–98, 1970.

835. Kohl S, and Harmon MW. Human neonatal leukocyte interferon production and natural killer cytotoxicity in response to herpes simplex virus. J Interferon Res 3:461–463, 1983.

836. Cederblad B, Riesenfeld T, Alm GV. Deficient herpes simplex virus–induced interferon-alpha production by blood leukocytes of preterm and term newborn infants. Pediatr Res 27:7–10, 1990.

837. Scott ME, Kubin M, Kohl S. High level interleukin-12 production, but diminished interferon-gamma production, by cord blood mononuclear cells. Pediatr Res 41:547–553, 1997.

838. Seghaye MC, Heyl W, Grabitz RG, et al. The production of pro- and anti-inflammatory cytokines in neonates assessed by stimulated whole cord blood culture and by plasma levels at birth. Biol Neonate 73:220–227, 1998.

839. Glauser MP, Zanetti G, Baumgartner JD, et al. Septic shock: pathogenesis. Lancet 338:732–736, 1991.

840. Pollack M, Ohl C. Endotoxin-based molecular strategies for the prevention and treatment of gram-negative sepsis and septic shock. Curr Top Microbiol Immunol 216:275–297, 1996.

841. van Zee KJ, DeForge LE, Fischer E, et al. IL-8 in septic shock, endotoxemia, and after IL-1 administration. J Immunol 146:3478–3482, 1991.

842. O'Brien WF, Golden SM, Bibro MC, et al. Short-term responses in neonatal lambs after infusion of group B streptococcal extract. Obstet Gynecol 65:802–806, 1985.

843. Peevy KJ, Chartrand SA, Wiseman HJ, et al. Myocardial dysfunction in group B streptococcal shock. Pediatr Res 19:511–513, 1985.

844. Hemming VG, O'Brien WF, Fischer GW, et al. Studies of short-term pulmonary and peripheral vascular responses induced in oophorectomized sheep by the infusion of a group B streptococcal extract. Pediatr Res 18:266–269, 1984.

845. Gibson RL, Truog WE, Henderson WJ, et al. Group B streptococcal sepsis in piglets: effect of combined pentoxifylline and indomethacin pretreatment. Pediatr Res 31:222–227, 1992.

846. Frank MM. The complement system in host defense and inflammation. Rev Infect Dis 1:483–501, 1979.

847. Gewurz H. Biology of C-reactive protein and the acute phase response. Hosp Pract (Hospital Edition) 17:67–81, 1982.

848. Colten HR. Molecular basis of complement deficiency syndromes. Lab Invest 52:468–474, 1985.

849. Kohler PF. Maturation of the human complement system. I. Onset time and sites of fetal Clq, C4, C3, and C5 synthesis. J Clin Invest 52:671–677, 1973.

850. Lassiter HA, Watson SW, Seifring ML, Tanner JE. Complement factor 9 deficiency in serum of human neonates. J Infect Dis 166:53–57, 1992.

851. Zach TL, Hostetter MK. Biochemical abnormalities of the third component of complement in neonates. Pediatr Res 26:116–120, 1989.

852. Johnston RB, Jr, Altenburger KM, Atkinson AW, Jr, et al. Complement in the newborn infant. Pediatrics 64:781–786, 1979.

853. Notarangelo LD, Chirico G, Chiara A, et al. Activity of classical and alternative pathways of complement in preterm and small for gestational age infants. Pediatr Res 18:281–285, 1984.

854. Davis CA, Vallota EH, Forristal J. Serum complement levels in infancy: age related changes. Pediatr Res 13:1043–1046, 1979.

855. Marino JA, Pensky J, Culp LA, et al. Fibronectin mediates chemotactic factor–stimulated neutrophil substrate adhesion. J Lab Clin Med 105:725–730, 1985.

856. Hill HR, Shigeoka AO, Augustine NH, et al. Fibronectin enhances the opsonic and protective activity of monoclonal and polyclonal antibody against group B streptococci. J Exp Med 159:1618–1628, 1984.

857. Proctor RA, Mosher DF, and Olbrantz PJ. Fibronectin binding to *Staphylococcus aureus*. J Biol Chem 257:14788–14794, 1982.

858. Jacobs RF, Kiel DP, Sanders ML, et al. Phagocytosis of type III group B streptococci by neonatal monocytes: enhancement by fibronectin and gammaglobulin. J Infect Dis 152:695–700, 1985.

859. Yang KD, Bohnsack JF, Hawley MM, et al. Effect of fibronectin on IgA-mediated uptake of type III group B streptococci by phagocytes. J Infect Dis 161:236–241, 1990.

860. Jacobs RF, Kiel DP, Sanders ML, et al. Neonatal macrophage phagocytosis of group B streptococci III: enhancement by fibronectin and gammaglobulin. J Infect Dis 152:695–700, 1985.

861. Pommier CG, O'Shea J, Chused T, et al. Studies on the fibronectin receptors of human peripheral blood leukocytes: morphologic and functional characterization. J Exp Med 159:137–151, 1984.

862. Norris DA, Clark RA, Swigart LM, et al. Fibronectin fragments are chemotactic for human peripheral blood monocytes. J Immunol 129:1612–1618, 1982.

863. Gerdes JS, Yoder MC, Douglas SD, et al. Decreased plasma fibronectin in neonatal sepsis. Pediatrics 72:877–881, 1983.

864. Matsuura H, Hakomori S. The oncofetal domain of fibronectin defined by monoclonal antibody FDC-6: its presence in fibronectins from fetal and tumor tissues and its absence in those from normal adult tissues and plasma. Proc Natl Acad Sci USA 82:6517–6521, 1985.

865. Peters JH, Ginsberg MH, Bohl BP, et al. Intravascular release of intact cellular fibronectin during oxidant-induced injury of the in vitro perfused rabbit lung. J Clin Invest 78:1596–1603, 1986.

866. Barnard DR, Arthur MM. Fibronectin cold insoluble globulin in the neonate. J Pediatr 102:453–455, 1983.

867. Yoder MC, Douglas SD, Gerdes J, et al. Plasma fibronectin in healthy newborn infants: respiratory distress syndrome and perinatal asphyxia. J Pediatr 102:777–780, 1983.

868. McCafferty MH, Lepow M, Saba TM, et al. Normal fibronectin levels as a function of age in the pediatric population. Pediatr Res 17:482–485, 1983.

869. Ainbender E, Cabatu EE, Guzman DM, et al. Serum C-reactive protein and problems of newborn infants. J Pediatr 101:438–440, 1982.

870. Epstein J, Eichbaum Q, Sheriff S, et al. The collectins in innate immunity. Curr Opin Immunol 8:29–35, 1996.

871. Lau YL, Chan SY, Turner MW, et al. Mannose-binding protein in preterm infants: developmental profile and clinical significance. Clin Exp Immunol 102:649–654, 1995.

872. Super M, Thiel S, Lu J, et al. Association of low levels of mannan-binding protein with a common defect of opsonisation. Lancet 2:1236–1239, 1989.

873. Lu J. Collectins: collectors of microorganisms for the innate immune system. Bioessays 19:509–518, 1997.

874. LeVine AM, Bruno MD, Huelsman KM, et al. Surfactant protein A–deficient mice are susceptible to group B streptococcal infection. J Immunol 158:4336–4340, 1997.

875. LeVine AM, Kurak KE, Bruno MD, et al. Surfactant protein-A–deficient mice are susceptible to Pseudomonas aeruginosa infection. Am J Respir Cell Mol Biol 19:700–708, 1998.

876. Geelen SP, Fleer A, Bezemer AC, et al. Deficiencies in opsonic defense to pneumococci in the human newborn despite adequate levels of complement and specific IgG antibodies. Pediatr Res 27:514–518, 1990.

877. Edwards MS, Buffone GJ, Fuselier PA. Deficient classical complement pathway activity in newborn sera. Pediatr Res 17:685–688, 1983.

878. Winkelstein JA, Kurlandsky LE, Swift AJ, et al. Defensive activation of the third component of complement in the sera of newborn infants. Pediatr Res 13:1093–1096, 1979.

879. Mills EL, Bjorkste'n B, Quie PG. Deficient alternative complement pathway activity in newborn sera. Pediatr Res 13:1341–1344, 1979.

880. Marodi L, Leijh PC, Braat A, et al. Opsonic activity of cord blood sera against various species of microorganism. Pediatr Res 19:433–436, 1985.

881. Kobayashi Y, Usui T. Opsonic activity of cord serum—an evaluation based on determination of oxygen consumption by leukocytes. Pediatr Res 16:243–246, 1982.

882. Adamkin D, Stitzel A, Urmson J, et al. Activity of the alternative pathway of complement in the newborn infant. J Pediatr 93:604–608, 1978.

883. Eads ME, Levy NJ, Kasper DL, et al. Antibody-independent activation of C1 by type Ia group B streptococci. J Infect Dis 146:665–672, 1982.

884. Anderson DC, Hughes BJ, Edwards MS, et al. Impaired chemotaxigenesis by type III group B streptococci in neonatal sera: relationship to diminished concentration of specific anticapsular antibody and abnormalities of serum complement. Pediatr Res 17:496–502, 1983.

885. Miller ME. Chemotactic function in the human neonate: humoral and cellular aspects. Pediatr Res 5:496–502, 1971.

886. Zilow EP, Hauck W, Linderkamp O, et al. Alternative pathway activation of the complement system in preterm infants with early onset infection. Pediatr Res 41:334–339, 1997.

887. Tannous R, Spitzer RE, Clarke WR, et al. Decreased chemotactic activity in activated newborn plasma. J Lab Clin Med 99:331–341, 1982.

888. Chandra RK. Interactions between early nutrition and the immune system. Ciba Found Symp 156:77–89, 1991.

889. Naeye R, Diener M, Harcke H, et al. Relation of poverty and race to birth weight and organ and cell structure in the newborn. Pediatr Res 5:17–22, 1971.

890. Ferguson AC, Lawlor GJ, Neuman CG, et al. Decreased rosette-forming lymphocytes in malnutrition and intrauterine growth retardation. J Pediatr 85:717–723, 1974.

891. Chandra RK. Fetal malnutrition and postnatal immunocompetence. Am J Dis Child 129:450–454, 1975.

892. Bhaskaram C, Raghuramulu N, Reddy V. Cell-mediated immunity and immunoglobulin levels in light-for-date infants. Acta Paediatr Scand 66:617–619, 1977.

893. Ferguson AC. Prolonged impairment of cellular immunity in children with intrauterine growth retardation. J Pediatr 93:52–56, 1978.

894. Anderson DC, Krishna GS, Hughes BJ, et al. Impaired polymorphonuclear leukocyte motility in malnourished infants: relationship to functional abnormalities of cell adherence. J Lab Clin Med 101:881–895, 1983.

895. Evans D, Smith J. Response of the young infant to active immunization. Br Med Bull 19:225–229, 1963.

896. Yeung CY, Hobbs JR. Serum gamma globulin levels in normal premature, postmature, and "small-for-dates" newborn babies. Lancet 1:1167–1170, 1968.

897. Catty D, Seger R, Drew R, et al. IgG-subclass concentrations in cord sera from premature, full term and small-for-dates babies. Eur J Pediatr 125:89–96, 1977.

898. Chrousos GP. The hypothalamic-pituitary-adrenal axis and immune-mediated inflammation. N Engl J Med 332:1351–1362, 1995.

899. Sternberg EM. Neural-immune interactions in health and disease. J Clin Invest 100:2641–2647, 1997.

900. Stuck AE, Minder CE, Frey FJ. Risk of infectious complications in patients taking glucocorticosteroids. Rev Infect Dis 11:954–963, 1989.

901. Wilckens T, De Rijk R. Glucocorticoids and immune function: unknown dimensions and new frontiers. Immunol Today 18:418–424, 1997.

902. Bessler H, Straussberg R, Gurary N, et al. Effect of dexamethasone on IL-2 and IL-3 production by mononuclear cells in neonates and adults. Arch Dis Child Fetal Neonatal Ed 75:F197–F201, 1996.

903. Kavelaars A, Cats B, Visser GH, et al. Ontogeny of the responses of human peripheral blood T cells to glucocorticoids. Brain Behavior Immun 10:288–297, 1996.

904. Schwarze J, Bartmann P. Influence of dexamethasone on lymphocyte proliferation in whole blood cultures of neonates. Biol Neonate 65:295–301, 1994.

905. Wheeler W, Kurachek S, McNamara J, et al. Consequences of hypogammaglobulinemia and steroid therapy in severe bronchopulmonary dysplasia. Pediatr Pulmonol 22:96–100, 1996.

906. Lack G, Ochs HD, Gelfand EW. Humoral immunity in steroid-dependent children with asthma and hypogammaglobulinemia. J Pediatr 129:898–903, 1996.

907. Gunn T, Reece ER, Metrakos K, et al. Depressed T cells following neonatal steroid treatment. Pediatrics 67:61–67, 1981.

908. Ryhanen P, Kauppila A, Koivisto M. Unaltered neonatal

cell-mediated immunity after prenatal dexamethasone treatment. Obstet Gynecol 56:182–185, 1980.

909. Gleicher N, Siegel I, Cederqvist LL. Do glucocorticosteroids affect the fetal immune system? Am J Reprod Immunol 1:184–185, 1981.

910. Otero L, Conlon C, Reynolds P, et al. Neonatal leukocytosis associated with prenatal administration of dexamethasone. Pediatrics 68:778–780, 1981.

911. Lazzarin A, Capsoni F, Moroni M, et al. Leucocyte function after antenatal betamethasone given to prevent respiratory distress. Lancet 2:1354–1355, 1977.

912. Eisenfeld L, Rosenkrantz TS, Block C, et al. Effect of corticosteroids on the maturation of neutrophil motility in very low birthweight neonates. Am J Perinatol 11:163–166, 1994.

913. Chatila T, Wong R, Young M, et al. An immunodeficiency characterized by defective signal transduction in T lymphocytes. N Engl J Med 320:696–702, 1989.

914. Pilarski LM, Yacyshyn BR, Lazarovits AI. Analysis of peripheral blood lymphocyte populations and immune function from children exposed to cyclosporine or to azathioprine in utero. Transplantation 57:133–144, 1994.

915. Miler I, Sima P, Vetvicka V, et al. The potential immunosuppressive effect of bilirubin. Allerg Immunol (Paris) 34:177–184, 1988.

916. Rubaltelli FF, Piovesan AL, Semenzato G, et al. Immune competence assessment in hyperbilirubinemic newborns before and after phototherapy. Helv Paediatr Acta 32:129–133, 1977.

917. Nejedlaa Z. The development of immunological factors in infants with hyperbilirubinemia. Pediatrics 45:102–104, 1970.

918. Rola-Plezczynski M, Hensen SA, Vincent MM, et al. Inhibitory effects of bilirubin on cellular immune responses in man. J Pediatr 86:690–696, 1975.

919. Sevjcar J, Miler I, Pekarek J. Effects of bilirubin on an in vitro correlate of cell-mediated immunity—the migration inhibition test. J Clin Lab Immunol 3:145–149, 1984.

920. Johnson S, Knight R, Marmer DJ, et al. Immune deficiency in fetal alcohol syndrome. Pediatr Res 15:908–911, 1981.

921. Chiappelli F, Taylor AN. The fetal alcohol syndrome and fetal alcohol effects on immune competence. Alcohol Alcohol 30:259–262, 1995.

922. Paganelli R, Ramadas D, Layward L, et al. Maternal smoking and cord blood immunity function. Clin Exp Immunol 36:256–259, 1979.

923. Culver KW, Ammann AJ, Partridge JC, et al. Lymphocyte abnormalities in infants born to drug-abusing mothers. J Pediatr 111:230–235, 1987.

924. European Collaborative Study. Risk factors for mother-to-child transmission of HIV-1. Lancet 339:1007–1012, 1992.

925. de Martino M, Tovo PA, Galli L, et al. Prognostic significance of immunologic changes in 675 infants perinatally exposed to human immunodeficiency virus: The Italian Register for Human Immunodeficiency Virus Infection in Children. J Pediatr 119:702–709, 1991.

926. Karlix JL, Behnke M, Davis-Eyler F, et al. Cocaine suppresses fetal immune system. Pediatr Res 44:43–46, 1998.

927. Fischer GW, Hunter KW, Wilson SR, et al. Diminished bacterial defences with Intralipid. Lancet 2:819–820, 1980.

928. Nugent KM. Intralipid effects on reticuloendothelial function. J Leukoc Biol 36:123–132, 1984.

929. Nordenstrom J, Jarstrand C, Wiernik A. Decreased chemotactic and random migration of leukocytes during Intralipid infusion. Am J Clin Nutr 32:2416–2422, 1979.

930. English D, Roloff JS, Lukens JN, et al. Intravenous lipid emulsions and human neutrophil function. J Pediatr 99:913–916, 1981.

931. Usmani SS, Harper RG, Sia CG, et al. In vitro effect of Intralipid on polymorphonuclear leukocyte function in the neonate. J Pediatr 109:710–712, 1986.

932. Ladisch S, Poplack DG, Blaese RM. Inhibition of human lymphoproliferation by intravenous lipid emulsion. Clin Immunol Immunopathol 25:196–202, 1982.

933. Loo LS, Tang JP, Kohl S. Inhibition of cellular cytotoxicity of leukocytes for herpes simplex virus–infected cells in vitro and in vivo by Intralipid. J Infect Dis 146:64–70, 1982.

934. Rubens CE, Smith S, Hulse M, et al. Respiratory epithelial cell invasion by group B streptococci. Infect Immun 60:5157–5163, 1992.

935. VandeWater L, Destree AT, Hynes RO. Fibronectin binds to some bacteria but does not promote their uptake by phagocytic cells. Science 220:201–204, 1983.

936. Walker WA. Host defense mechanisms in the gastrointestinal tract. Pediatrics 57:901–916, 1976.

937. Schnapp D, Harris A. Antibacterial peptides in bronchoalveolar lavage fluid. Am J Respir Cell Mol Biol 19:352–356, 1998.

938. Bals R, Wang X, Wu Z, et al. Human beta-defensin 2 is a salt-sensitive peptide antibiotic expressed in human lung. J Clin Invest 102:874–880, 1998.

939. Pluschke G, Achtman M. Degree of antibody-independent activation of the classical complement pathway by K1 Escherichia coli differs with O antigen type and correlates with virulence of meningitis in newborns. Infect Immun 43:684–692, 1984.

940. Marques MB, Kasper DL, Pangburn MK, et al. Prevention of C3 deposition by capsular polysaccharide is a virulence mechanism of type III group B streptococci. Infect Immun 60:3986–3993, 1992.

941. Campbell JR, Baker CJ, Edwards MS. Deposition and degradation of C3 on type III group B streptococci. Infect Immun 59:1978–1983, 1991.

942. Campbell JR, Baker CJ, Edwards MS. Influence of serotype of group B streptococci on C3 degradation. Infect Immun 60:4558–4562, 1992.

943. Wessels MR, Butko P, Ma M, et al. Studies of group B streptococcal infection in mice deficient in complement component C3 or C4 demonstrate an essential role for complement in both innate and acquired immunity. Proc Natl Acad Sci USA 92:11490–11494, 1995.

944. Janeway CA, Travers P. The humoral immune response. In Immunobiology: The Immune System in Health and Disease. London, Current Biology, and New York, Garland Publishing, 1997, pp 8.1–8.54.

945. Yang KD, Augustine NH, Shaio MF, et al. Effects of fibronectin on actin organization and respiratory burst activity in neutrophils, monocytes, and macrophages. J Cell Physiol 158:347–353, 1994.

946. Martin TR, Ruzinski JT, Wilson CB, et al. Effects of endotoxin in the lungs of neonatal rats: age-dependent impairment of the inflammatory response. J Infect Dis 171:134–144, 1995.

947. Harada A, Sekido N, Akahoshi T, et al. Essential involvement of interleukin-8 (IL-8) in acute inflammation. J Leukoc Biol 56:559–564, 1994.

948. Strieter R, Kunkel S. Acute lung injury: the role of

cytokines in the elicitation of neutrophils. J Invest Med 42:640–651, 1994.

949. Wilkinson PC. Leukocyte locomotion and chemotaxis: effects of bacteria and viruses. Rev Infect Dis 2:293–318, 1980.

950. Bohnsack JF, Zhou XN, Gustin JN, et al. Bacterial evasion of the antibody response: human IgG antibodies neutralize soluble but not bacteria-associated group B streptococcal C5a-ase. J Infect Dis 165:315–321, 1992.

951. Cusumano V, Mancuso G, Genovese F, et al. Role of gamma interferon in a neonatal mouse model of group B streptococcal disease. Infect Immun 64:2941–2944, 1996.

952. Mancuso G, Cusumano V, Genovese F, et al. Role of interleukin 12 in experimental neonatal sepsis caused by group B streptococci. Infect Immun 65:3731–3735, 1997.

953. Williams PA, Bohnsack JF, Augustine NH, et al. Production of tumor necrosis factor by human cells in vitro and in vivo, induced by group B streptococci. J Pediatr 123:292–300, 1993.

954. Gibson RL, Redding GJ, Henderson WR, et al. Group B streptococcus induces tumor necrosis factor in neonatal piglets: effect of the tumor necrosis factor inhibitor pentoxifylline on hemodynamics and gas exchange. Am Rev Respir Dis 143:598–604, 1991.

955. Teti G, Mancuso G, Tomasello F. Cytokine appearance and effects of anti-tumor necrosis factor alpha antibodies in a neonatal rat model of group B streptococcal infection. Infect Immun 61:227–235, 1993.

956. Peat EB, Augustine NH, Drummond WK, et al. Effects of fibronectin and group B streptococci on tumour necrosis factor–α production by human culture-derived macrophages. Immunology 84:440–445, 1995.

957. von Hunolstein C, Totolian A, Alfarone G, et al. Soluble antigens from group B streptococci induce cytokine production in human blood cultures. Infect Immun 65:4017–4021, 1997.

958. Schlievert PM, Gocke JE, Deringer JR. Group B streptococcal toxic shock–like syndrome: report of a case and purification of an associated pyrogenic toxin. Clin Infect Dis 17:26–31, 1993.

959. Givner LB, Gray L, O'Shea TM. Antibodies to tumor necrosis factor–alpha: use as adjunctive therapy in established group B streptococcal disease in newborn rats. Pediatr Res 38:551–554, 1995.

960. Cusumano V, Genovese F, Mancuso G, et al. Interleukin-10 protects neonatal mice from lethal group B streptococcal infection. Infect Immun 64:2850–2852, 1996.

961. Hemming VG, Hall RT, Rhodes PG, et al. Assessment of group B streptococcal opsonins in human and rabbit serum by neutrophil chemiluminescence. J Clin Invest 58:1379–1387, 1976.

962. Baker CJ, Edwards MS, Kasper DL. Role of antibody to native type III polysaccharide of group B Streptococcus in infant infection. Pediatrics 68:544–549, 1981.

963. Gotoff SP, Papierniak CK, Klegerman ME, et al. Quantitation of IgG antibody to the type-specific polysaccharide of group B streptococcus type 1b in pregnant women and infected infants. J Pediatr 105:628–630, 1984.

964. Klegerman ME, Boyer KM, Papierniak CK, et al. Estimation of the protective level of human IgG antibody to the type-specific polysaccharide of group B Streptococcus type Ia. J Infect Dis 148:648–655, 1983.

965. Edwards MS, Fuselier PA, Rench MA, et al. Class specificity of naturally acquired and vaccine-induced anti-

body to type III group B streptococcal capsular polysaccharide: determination with a radioimmunoprecipitin assay. Infect Immun 44:257–261, 1984.

966. Christensen KK, Christensen P, Duc G, et al. Correlation between serum antibody levels against group B streptococci and gestational age in newborns. Eur J Pediatr 142:86–88, 1984.

967. Boyer KM, Klegerman ME, Gotoff SP. Development of IgM antibody to group B Streptococcus type III in human infants. J Infect Dis 165:1049–1055, 1992.

968. Edwards MS, Hall MA, Rench MA, et al. Patterns of immune response among survivors of group B streptococcal meningitis. J Infect Dis 161:65–70, 1990.

969. Anthony BF, Concepcion NF, Wass CA, et al. Immunoglobulin G and M composition of naturally occurring antibody to type III group B streptococci. Infect Immun 46:98–104, 1984.

970. Wolach B, Dolfin T, Regev R, et al. The development of the complement system after 28 weeks' gestation. Acta Paediatr 86:523–527, 1997.

971. Broughton RA, Baker CJ. Role of adherence in the pathogenesis of neonatal group B streptococcal infection. Infect Immun 39:837–843, 1983.

972. Nealon TJ, Mattingly SJ. Role of cellular lipoteichoic acids in mediating adherence of serotype III strains of group B streptococci to human embryonic, fetal, and adult epithelial cells. Infect Immun 43:523–530, 1984.

973. Kasper DL, Paoletti LC, Wessels MR, et al. Immune response to type III group B streptococcal polysaccharide–tetanus toxoid conjugate vaccine. J Clin Invest 98:2308–2314, 1996.

974. Hill HR. Intravenous immunoglobulin use in the neonate: role in prophylaxis and therapy of infection. Pediatr Infect Dis J 12:549–558, 1993.

975. Schreiber JR, Berger M. Intravenous immune globulin therapy for sepsis in premature neonates. J Pediatr 121:401–404, 1992.

976. Baker CJ, Melish ME, Hall RT, et al. Intravenous immune globulin for the prevention of nosocomial infection in low-birth-weight neonates: The Multicenter Group for the Study of Immune Globulin in Neonates. N Engl J Med 327:213–219, 1992.

977. Fanaroff AA, Korones SB, Wright LL, et al. A controlled trial of intravenous immune globulin to reduce nosocomial infections in very-low-birth-weight infants: National Institute of Child Health and Human Development Neonatal Research Network. N Engl J Med 330:1107–1113, 1994.

978. Kinney J, Mundorf L, Gleason C, et al. Efficacy and pharmacokinetics of intravenous immune globulin administration to high-risk neonates. Am J Dis Child 145:1233–1238, 1991.

979. Magny JF, Bremard OC, Brault D, et al. Intravenous immunoglobulin therapy for prevention of infection in high-risk premature infants: report of a multicenter, double-blind study. Pediatrics 88:437–443, 1991.

980. Weisman LE, Stoll BJ, Kueser TJ, et al. Intravenous immune globulin prophylaxis of late-onset sepsis in premature neonates. J Pediatr 125:922–930, 1994.

981. Makhlouf RA, Doron MW, Bose CL, et al. Administration of granulocyte colony-stimulating factor to neutropenic low birth weight infants of mothers with preeclampsia. J Pediatr 126:454–456, 1995.

982. La Gamma EF, Alpan O, Kocherlakota P. Effect of granulocyte colony-stimulating factor on preeclampsia-associated neonatal neutropenia. J Pediatr 126:457–459, 1995.

983. Kocherlakota P, La Gamma EF. Preliminary report:

rhG-CSF may reduce the incidence of neonatal sepsis in prolonged preeclampsia-associated neutropenia. Pediatrics 102:1107–1111, 1998.

984. Bedu A, Baumann C, Rohrlich P, et al. Failure of granulocyte colony-stimulating factor in alloimmune neonatal neutropenia. J Pediatr 127:508–509, 1995.

985. Friedman CA, Wender DF, Temple DM, et al. Intravenous gamma globulin as adjunct therapy for severe group B streptococcal disease in the newborn. Am J Perinatol 7:1–4, 1990.

986. Christensen RD, Brown MS, Hall DC, et al. Effect on neutrophil kinetics and serum opsonic capacity of intravenous administration of immune globulin to neonates with clinical signs of early-onset sepsis. J Pediatr 118:606–614, 1991.

987. Haque KN, Remo C, Bahakim H. Comparison of two types of intravenous immunoglobulins in the treatment of neonatal sepsis. Clin Exp Immunol 101:328–333, 1995.

988. Fischer GW, Weisman LE, Hemming VG. Directed immune globulin for the prevention or treatment of neonatal group B streptococcal infections: a review. Clin Immunol Immunopathol 62:92–97, 1992.

989. Hill HR, Kelsey DK, Gonzales LA, et al. Monoclonal antibodies in the therapy of experimental neonatal group B streptococcal disease. Clin Immunol Immunopathol 62:87–91, 1992.

990. Ricci ML, von Hunolstein C, Gomez MJ, et al. Protective activity of a murine monoclonal antibody against acute and chronic experimental infection with type IV group B streptococcus. J Med Microbiol 44:475–481, 1996.

991. Shigeoka AO. Murine type-specific monoclonal antibodies in experimental group B streptococcal infection: interaction with complement components and phagocytes. Semin Perinatol 14:30–39, 1990.

992. Raff HV, Bradley C, Brady W, et al. Comparison of functional activities between IgG1 and IgM class-switched human monoclonal antibodies reactive with group B streptococci or *Escherichia coli* K1. J Infect Dis 163:346–354, 1991.

993. Raff HV, Shuford W, Wolff E, et al. Pharmacokinetic and pharmacodynamic analysis of a human immunoglobulin M monoclonal antibody in neonatal *Macaca fascicularis*. Pediatr Res 29:310–314, 1991.

994. Raff HV. Bacterial carbohydrates in neonatal sepsis: targets for immunotherapy. Springer Semin Immunopathol 15:173–181, 1993.

995. Sweetman RW, Cairo MS. Blood component and immunotherapy in neonatal sepsis. Transfus Med Rev 9:251–259, 1995.

996. Baley JE, Stork EK, Warkentin PI, et al. Buffy coat transfusions in neutropenic neonates with presumed sepsis: a prospective, randomized trial. Pediatrics 80:712–720, 1987.

997. Cairo MS, Worcester C, Rucker R, et al. Role of circulating complement and polymorphonuclear leukocyte transfusion in treatment and outcome in critically ill neonates with sepsis. J Pediatr 110:935–941, 1987.

998. Cairo MS, Worcester CC, Rucker RW, et al. Randomized trial of granulocyte transfusions versus intravenous immune globulin therapy for neonatal neutropenia and sepsis. J Pediatr 120:281–285, 1992.

999. Christensen RD, Rothstein G, Anstall HB, et al. Granulocyte transfusions in neonates with bacterial infection, neutropenia, and depletion of mature marrow neutrophils. Pediatrics 70:1–6, 1982.

1000. Laurenti F, Ferro R, Isacchi G, et al. Polymorphonuclear leukocyte transfusion for the treatment of sepsis in the newborn infant. J Pediatr 98:118–123, 1981.

1001. Wheeler JG, Chauvenet AR, Johnson CA, et al. Buffy coat transfusions in neonates with sepsis and neutrophil storage pool depletion. Pediatrics 79:422–425, 1987.

1002. Drossou-Agakidou V, Kanakoudi-Tsakalidou F, Sarafidis K, et al. Administration of recombinant human granulocyte-colony stimulating factor to septic neonates induces neutrophilia and enhances the neutrophil respiratory burst and beta2 integrin expression: results of a randomized controlled trial. Eur J Pediatr 157:583–588, 1998.

1003. Gillan ER, Christensen RD, Suen Y, et al. A randomized, placebo-controlled trial of recombinant human granulocytes colony stimulating factor administration in newborn infants with presumed sepsis: significant induction of peripheral and bone marrow neutrophilia. Blood 84:1427–1433, 1994.

1004. Rosenthal J, Healey T, Ellis R, et al. A two-year follow-up of neonates with presumed sepsis treated with recombinant human granulocyte colony-stimulating factor during the first week of life. J Pediatr 128:135–137, 1996.

1005. Kocherlakota P, La Gamma EF. Human granulocyte colony-stimulating factor may improve outcome attributable to neonatal sepsis complicated by neutropenia. Pediatrics 100:E6, 1997.

1006. Schibler KR, Osborne KA, Leung LY, et al. A randomized placebo-controlled trial of granulocyte colony-stimulating factor administration to newborn infants with neutropenia and clinical signs of early-onset sepsis. Pediatrics 102:6–13, 1998.

1007. Zinkernagel RM. Immunology taught by viruses. Science 271:173–178, 1996.

1008. Zisman B, Hirsch MS, Allison AC. Selective effects of anti-macrophage serum, silica and anti-lymphocyte serum on pathogenesis of herpes virus infection of young adult mice. J Immunol 104:1155–1159, 1970.

1009. Orange JS, Biron CA. Characterization of early IL-12, IFN-alpha/beta, and TNF effects on antiviral state and NK cell responses during murine cytomegalovirus infection. J Immunol 156:4746–4756, 1996.

1010. Wang B, Biron C, She J, et al. A block in both early T lymphocyte and natural killer cell development in transgenic mice with high-copy numbers of the human CD3ε gene. Proc Natl Acad Sci USA 91:9402–9406, 1994.

1011. Morse SS, Morahan PS. Activated macrophages mediate interferon-independent inhibition of herpes simplex virus. Cell Immunol 58:72–84, 1981.

1012. Stanwick TL, Campbell DE, Nahmias AJ. Cytotoxic properties of human monocyte-macrophages for human fibroblasts infected in herpes simplex virus: interferon production and augmentation. Cell Immunol 70:132–147, 1982.

1013. Ghanekar S, Zheng L, Logar A, et al. Cytokine expression by human peripheral blood dendritic cells stimulated in vitro with HIV-1 and herpes simplex virus. J Immunol 157:4028–4036, 1996.

1014. Kanangat S, Thomas J, Gangappa S, et al. Herpes simplex virus type–1–mediated up-regulation of IL-12 (p40) mRNA expression. J Immunol 156:1110–1116, 1996.

1015. Stanwick TL, Campbell DE, Nahmias AJ. Cells infected with herpes simplex virus induce human monocyte-macrophages to produce interferon. Immunobiology 158:207–212, 1981.

1016. Lebon P, Ponsot G, Aicardi J. Early intrathecal synthesis of interferon in herpes encephalitis. Biomedicine 31:267–271, 1979.

1017. Zawatzky R, Engler H, Kirchner H. Experimental infection of inbred mice with herpes simplex virus. III. Comparison between newborn and adult C57BL/6 mice. J Gen Virol 60:25–29, 1982.

1018. Carr JA, Rogerson J, Mulqueen MJ, et al. Interleukin-12 exhibits potent antiviral activity in experimental herpesvirus infections. J Virol 71:7799–7803, 1997.

1019. Wong GH, Goeddel DV. Tumour necrosis factors alpha and beta inhibit virus replication and synergize with interferons. Nature 323:819–822, 1986.

1020. Heise MT, Virgin HW. The T-cell–dependent role of gamma interferon and tumor necrosis factor alpha in macrophage activation during murine cytomegalovirus and herpes simplex virus infections. J Virol 69:904–909, 1995.

1021. Rosler A, Pohl M, Braune HJ, et al. Time course of chemokines in the cerebrospinal fluid and serum during herpes simplex type 1 encephalitis. J Neurol Sci 157:82–89, 1998.

1022. Tumpey TM, Cheng H, Yan XT, et al. Chemokine synthesis in the HSV-1–infected cornea and its suppression by interleukin-10. J Leukoc Biol 63:486–492, 1998.

1023. Bodaghi B, Jones TR, Zipeto D, et al. Chemokine sequestration by viral chemoreceptors as a novel vital escape strategy: withdrawal of chemokines from the environment of cytomegalovirus-infected cells. J Exp Med 188:855–866, 1998.

1024. Habu S, Akamatsu K, Tamaoki N, et al. In vivo significance of NK cell on resistance against virus (HSV-1) infections in mice. J Immunol 133:2743–2747, 1984.

1025. Rager-Zisman B, Quan PC, Rosner M, et al. Role of NK cells in protection of mice against herpes simplex virus–1 infection. J Immunol 138:884–888, 1987.

1026. Tay CH, Welsh RM, Brutkiewicz RR. NK cell response to viral infections in β2-microglobulin–deficient mice. J Immunol 154:780–789, 1995.

1027. O'Garra A. Cytokines induce the development of functionally heterogeneous T helper cell subsets. Immunity 8:275–283, 1998.

1028. Miller DM, Rahill BM, Boss JM, et al. Human cytomegalovirus inhibits major histocompatibility complex class II expression by disruption of the Jak/Stat pathway. J Exp Med 187:675–683, 1998.

1029. Lafferty WE, Brewer LA, Corey L. Alteration of lymphocyte transformation response to herpes simplex virus infection by acyclovir therapy. Antimicrob Agents Chemother 26:887–891, 1984.

1030. Whitley RJ. Herpes simplex virus. In Fields BN, Knipe DM, Howley PM (eds). Fields Virology, 3rd ed. Philadelphia, Lippincott-Raven, 1996, pp 2297–2342.

1031. Posavad CM, Koelle DM, Corey L. Tipping the scales of herpes simplex virus reactivation: the important responses are local. Nat Med 4:381–382, 1998.

1032. Schmid DS, Rouse BT. The role of T cell immunity in control of herpes simplex virus. Curr Top Microbiol Immunol 179:57–74, 1992.

1033. Holterman A-X, Rogers K, Edelmann K, et al. An important role for MHC class–restricted T cells, and limited role for interferon-γ, in protection of mice against lethal herpes simplex virus infection. J Virol 73:2058–2063, 1999.

1034. Manickan E, Rouse BT. Roles of different T-cell subsets in control of herpes simplex virus infection determined by using T-cell–deficient mouse-models. J Virol 69:8178–8179, 1995.

1035. Manickasingham SP, Hill TJ, Williams NA. Modulation of Langerhans cell phenotype, migration and maturation by agents known to cause herpes simplex virus reactivation in a mouse model. Clin Exp Immunol 106:304–311, 1996.

1036. Milligan GN, Bernstein DI. Analysis of herpes simplex virus–specific T cells in the murine female genital tract following infection with herpes simplex virus type 2. Virology 212:481–489, 1995.

1037. Milligan GN, Bernstein DI. Interferon-gamma enhances resolution of herpes simplex virus type 2 infection of the murine genital tract. Virology 229:259–268, 1997.

1038. Smith PM, Wolcott RM, Chervenak R, et al. Control of acute cutaneous herpes simplex virus infection: T cell–mediated viral clearance is dependent upon interferon-gamma. Virology 202:76–88, 1994.

1039. Ahn K, Meyer TH, Uebel S, et al. Molecular mechanism and species specificity of TAP inhibition by herpes simplex virus ICP47. EMBO J 15:3247–3255, 1996.

1040. Hill A, Jugovic P, York I, et al. Herpes simplex virus turns off the TAP to evade host immunity. Nature 375:411–415, 1995.

1041. Tigges MA, Leng S, Johnson DC, et al. Human herpes simplex virus (HSV)–specific CD8+ CTL clones recognize HSV-2–infected fibroblasts after treatment with IFN-gamma or when virion host shutoff functions are disabled. J Immunol 156:3901–3910, 1996.

1042. Tomazin R, van Schoot NE, Goldsmith K, et al. Herpes simplex virus type 2 ICP47 inhibits human TAP but not mouse TAP. J Virol 72:2560–2563, 1998.

1043. Koelle DM, Posavad CM, Barnum GR, et al. Clearance of HSV-2 from recurrent genital lesions correlates with infiltration of HSV-specific cytotoxic T lymphocytes. J Clin Invest 101:1500–1508, 1998.

1044. Mikloska Z, Kesson AM, Penfold MET, et al. Herpes simplex virus protein targets for CD4 and CD8 lymphocyte cytotoxicity in cultured epidermal keratinocytes treated with interferon-gamma. J Infect Dis 173:7–17, 1996.

1045. Posavad CM, Koelle DM, Shaughnessy MF, et al. Severe genital herpes infections in HIV-infected individuals with impaired herpes simplex virus–specific CD8+ cytotoxic T lymphocyte responses. Proc Natl Acad Sci USA 94:10289–10294, 1997.

1046. Bonneau RH, Salvucci LA, Johnson DC, et al. Epitope specificity of H-2Kb–restricted, HSV-1–, and HSV-2–cross-reactive cytotoxic T lymphocyte clones. Virology 195:62–70, 1993.

1047. Cose SC, Kelly JM, Carbone FR. Characterization of a diverse primary herpes simplex virus type 1 gb-specific cytotoxic T-cell response showing a preferential Vbeta bias. J Virol 69:5849–5852, 1995.

1048. Simmons A, Tscharke DC. Anti-CD8 impairs clearance of herpes simplex virus from the nervous system: implications for the fate of virally infected neurons. J Exp Med 175:1337–1344, 1992.

1049. Gold R, Toyka KV, Hartung HP. Synergistic effect of IFN-gamma and TNF-alpha on expression of immune molecules and antigen presentation by Schwann cells. Cell Immunol 165:65–70, 1995.

1050. Goldsmith K, Chen W, Johnson DC, et al. Infected cell protein (ICP)47 enhances herpes simplex virus neurovirulence by blocking the CD8+ T cell response. J Exp Med 187:341–348, 1998.

1051. Simmons A, Tscharke D, Speck P. The role of immune mechanisms in control of herpes simplex virus infection of the peripheral nervous system. Curr Top Microbiol Immunol 179:31–56, 1992.

1052. Ruby J, Bluethmann H, Aguet M, et al. CD40 ligand has potent antiviral activity. Nat Med 1:437–441, 1995.

1053. Mercadal CM, Martin S, Rouse BT. Apparent requirement for CD4+ T cells in primary anti–herpes simplex virus cytotoxic T-lymphocyte induction can be overcome by optimal antigen presentation. Viral Immunol 4:177–186, 1991.

1054. Stohlman SA, Bergmann CC, Lin MT, et al. CTL effector function within the central nervous system requires CD4+ T cells. J Immunol 160:2896–2904, 1998.

1055. Bennett SRM, Carbone FR, Karamalis F, et al. Help for the cytotoxic T-cell responses is mediated by CD40 signalling. Nature 393:478–480, 1998.

1056. Ridge JP, Di Rosa F, Matzinger P. A conditioned dendritic cell can be a temporal bridge between a CD4+ T-helper and a T-killer cell. Nature 393:474–478, 1998.

1057. Borysiewicz LK, Sissons JG. Cytotoxic T cells and human herpes virus infections. Curr Top Microbiol Immunol 189:123–150, 1994.

1058. Koelle DM, Abbo H, Peck A, et al. Direct recovery of herpes simplex virus (HSV)–specific T lymphocyte clones from recurrent genital HSV-2 lesions. J Infect Dis 169:956–961, 1994.

1059. Schmid DS, Mawle AC. T cell responses to herpes simplex viruses in humans. Rev Infect Dis 13 (Suppl 11):S946–S949, 1991.

1060. Yasukawa M, Zarling JM. Human cytotoxic T cell clones directed against herpes simplex virus–infected cells. III. Analysis of vital glycoproteins recognized by CTL clones by using recombinant herpes simplex viruses. J Immunol 134:2679–2682, 1985.

1061. Gollins SW, Porterfield JS. A new mechanism for the neutralization of enveloped viruses by antiviral antibody. Nature 321:244–246, 1986.

1062. Berger M, Frank MM. The serum complement system. In Stiehm ER (ed). Immunologic Disorders in Infants and Children, 5th ed. Philadelphia, WB Saunders, 1996, pp 133–158.

1063. McKendall RR. IgG-mediated viral clearance in experimental infection with herpes simplex virus type 1: role for neutralization and Fc-dependent functions but not C′ cytolysis and C5 chemotaxis. J Infect Dis 151:464–470, 1985.

1064. Kohl S, Starr SE, Oleske JM, et al. Human monocyte-macrophage–mediated antibody-dependent cytotoxicity to herpes simplex virus–infected cells. J Immunol 118:729–735, 1977.

1065. Petroni KC, Shen L, Guyre PM. Modulation of human polymorphonuclear leukocyte IgG Fc receptors and Fc receptor–mediated functions by IFN-γ and glucocorticoids. J Immunol 140:3467–3472, 1988.

1066. Trinchieri G, Perussia B. Immune interferon: a pleiotropic lymphokine with multiple effects. Immunol Today 6:130–136, 1985.

1067. Kohl S, Loo LS, Greenberg SB. Protection of newborn mice from a lethal herpes simplex virus infection by human interferon, antibody, and leukocytes. J Immunol 128:1107–1111, 1982.

1068. Kohl S, Stewart-West M, Prober CG, et al. Serologic determinants of neonatal herpes simplex virus (HSV) infection. Pediatr Res 23:373A, 1988.

1069. Nahmias AJ, Coleman RM. The significance of herpes simplex virus infections in humans. In Rouse BT, Lopez C (eds). Immunobiology of Herpes Simplex Virus Infection. Boca Raton, Fla, CRC Press, 1984, pp 1–8.

1070. Nagafuchi S, Oda H, Mori R, et al. Mechanism of acquired resistance to herpes simplex virus infection as studied in nude mice. J Gen Virol 44:715–723, 1979.

1071. Jonjic S, Pavic I, Polic B, et al. Antibodies are not essential for the resolution of primary cytomegalovirus infection but limit dissemination of recurrent virus. J Exp Med 179:1713–1717, 1994.

1072. Stagno S. Cytomegalovirus. In Remington JS, Klein JO (eds). Infectious Diseases of the Fetus and Newborn Infant, 4th ed. Philadelphia, WB Saunders, 1995, pp 312–353.

1073. Hayward AR, Herberger MJ, Groothuis J, et al. Specific immunity after congenital or neonatal infection with cytomegalovirus or herpes simplex virus. J Immunol 133:2469–2473, 1984.

1074. Buseyne F, Blanche S, Schmitt D, et al. Detection of HIV-specific cell-mediated cytotoxicity in the peripheral blood from infected children. J Immunol 150:3569–3581, 1993.

1075. Ashley RL, Dalessio J, Burchett S, et al. Herpes simplex virus-2 (HSV-2) type-specific antibody correlates of protection in infants exposed to HSV-2 at birth. J Clin Invest 90:511–514, 1992.

1076. Kohl S, West MS, Prober CG, et al. Neonatal antibody-dependent cellular cytotoxic antibody levels are associated with the clinical presentation of neonatal herpes simplex virus infection. J Infect Dis 160:770–776, 1989.

1077. Stagno S, Pass RF, Cloud G, et al. Primary cytomegalovirus infection in pregnancy: incidence, transmission to fetus, and clinical outcome. JAMA 256:1904–1908, 1986.

1078. Hammond GW, Lukes H, Wells B, et al. Maternal and neonatal neutralizing antibody titers to selected enteroviruses. Pediatr Infect Dis J 4:32–35, 1985.

1079. Modlin JF, Polk BF, Horton P, et al. Perinatal echovirus infection: risk of transmission during a community outbreak. N Engl J Med 305:368–371, 1981.

1080. Burioni R, Williamson RA, Sanna PP, et al. Recombinant human Fab to glycoprotein D neutralizes infectivity and prevents cell-to-cell transmission of herpes simplex viruses 1 and 2 in vitro. Proc Natl Acad Sci USA 91:355–359, 1994.

1081. Cohen J. IL-12 deaths: explanation and a puzzle. Science 270:908, 1995.

1082. Straus SE, Corey L, Burke RL, et al. Placebo-controlled trial of vaccination with recombinant glycoprotein D of herpes simplex virus type 2 for immunotherapy of genital herpes. Lancet 343:1460–1463, 1994.

1083. Mineo JR, McLeod R, Mack D, et al. Antibodies to Toxoplasma gondii major surface protein SAG-1, P30 inhibit infection of host cells and are produced in murine intestine after peroral infection. J Immunol 150:3951–3964, 1993.

1084. Decoster A. Detection of IgA anti-P30 SAG1 antibodies in acquired and congenital toxoplasmosis. Curr Top Microbiol Immunol 219:199–207, 1996.

1085. Schwab JC, Beckers CJ, Joiner KA. The parasitophorous vacuole membrane surrounding intracellular Toxoplasma gondii functions as a molecular sieve. Proc Natl Acad Sci USA 91:509–513, 1994.

1086. Wilson CB, Tsai V, Remington JS. Failure to trigger the oxidative metabolic burst by normal macrophages: possible mechanism for survival of intracellular pathogens. J Exp Med 151:328–346, 1980.

1087. Adams LB, Hibbs JBJ, Taintor RR, et al. Microbiostatic effect of murine-activated macrophages for Toxoplasma gondii: role for synthesis of inorganic nitrogen oxides from L-arginine. J Immunol 144:2725–2729, 1990.

1088. Bohne W, Heesemann J, Gross U. Reduced replication of Toxoplasma gondii is necessary for induction of bradyzoite-specific antigens: a possible role for nitric oxide in triggering stage conversion. Infect Immun 62:1761–1767, 1994.

1089. Alexander J, Hunter CA. Immunoregulation during toxoplasmosis. Chem Immunol 70:81–102, 1998.

1090. Johnson LL, Sayles PC. Interleukin-12, dendritic cells, and the initiation of host-protective mechanisms against *Toxoplasma gondii*. J Exp Med 186:1799–1802, 1997.

1091. Suzuki Y, Orellana MA, Wong SY, et al. Susceptibility to chronic infection with *Toxoplasma gondii* does not correlate with susceptibility to acute infection in mice. Infect Immun 61:2284–2288, 1993.

1092. Gazzinelli RT, Amichay D, Scharton-Kersten T, et al. Role of macrophage-derived cytokines in the induction and regulation of cell-mediated immunity to *Toxoplasma gondii*. Curr Top Microbiol Immunol 219:127–139, 1996.

1093. Pelloux H, Ambroise-Thomas P. Cytokine production by human cells after *Toxoplasma gondii* infection. Curr Top Microbiol Immunol 219:155–163, 1996.

1094. Khan IA, Kasper LH. IL-15 augments CD8+ T cell–mediated immunity against *Toxoplasma gondii* infection in mice. J Immunol 157:2103–2108, 1996.

1095. Denkers EY, Scharton KT, Barbieri S, et el. A role for CD4+ NK1.1+ T lymphocytes as major histocompatibility complex class II independent helper cells in the generation of CD8+ effector function against intracellular infection. J Exp Med 184:131–139, 1996.

1096. Hunter CA, Subauste CS, Van Cleave VH, et al. Production of gamma interferon by natural killer cells from *Toxoplasma gondii*–infected SCID mice: regulation by interleukin-10, interleukin-12, and tumor necrosis factor alpha. Infect Immun 62:2818–2824, 1994.

1097. Deckert SM, Bluethmann H, Rang A, et al. Crucial role of TNF receptor type 1 (p55), but not of TNF receptor type 2 (p75), in murine toxoplasmosis. J Immunol 160:3427–3436, 1998.

1098. Gazzinelli RT, Wysocka M, Hieny S, et al. In the absence of endogenous IL-10, mice acutely infected with *Toxoplasma gondii* succumb to a lethal immune response dependent on CD4+ T cells and accompanied by overproduction of IL-12, IFN-gamma and TNF-alpha. J Immunol 157:798–805, 1996.

1099. Suzuki Y, Yang Q, Yang S, et al. IL-4 is protective against development of toxoplasmic encephalitis. J Immunol 157:2564–2569, 1996.

1100. Roberts CW, Ferguson DJ, Jebbari H, et al. Different roles for interleukin-4 during the course of *Toxoplasma gondii* infection. Infect Immun 64:897–904, 1996.

1101. Denkers EY, Gazzinelli RT, Martin D, et al. Emergence of NK1.1+ cells as effectors of IFN-gamma–dependent immunity to *Toxoplasma gondii* in MHC class I–deficient mice. J Exp Med 178:1465–1472, 1993.

1102. Johnson LL, VanderVegt FP, Havell EA. Gamma interferon–dependent temporary resistance to acute *Toxoplasma gondii* infection independent of CD4+ or CD8+ lymphocytes. Infect Immun 61:5174–5180, 1993.

1103. Shirahata T, Yamashita T, Ohta C, et al. CD8+ T lymphocytes are the major cell population involved in the early gamma interferon response and resistance to acute primary *Toxoplasma gondii* infection in mice. Microbiol Immunol 38:789–796, 1994.

1104. Sousa CR, Hieny S, Scharton-Kersten T, et al. In vivo microbial stimulation induces rapid CD40 ligand–independent production of interleukin 12 by dendritic cells and their redistribution to T cell areas. J Exp Med 186:1819–1829, 1997.

1105. Hahn H, Kaufmann SH. The role of cell-mediated immunity in bacterial infections. Rev Infect Dis 3:1221–1250, 1981.

1106. McLeod R, Estes RG, Mack DG, et al. Immune response of mice to ingested *Toxoplasma gondii*: a model of *Toxoplasma* infection acquired by ingestion. J Infect Dis 149:234–244, 1984.

1107. Hunter CA, Abrams JS, Beaman MH, et al. Cytokine mRNA in the central nervous system of SCID mice infected with *Toxoplasma gondii*: importance of T-cell–independent regulation of resistance to *T. gondii*. Infect Immun 61:4038–4044, 1993.

1108. Subauste CS, de-Waal-Malefyt R, Fuh F. Role of CD80 (B7.1) and CD86 (B7.2) in the immune response to an intracellular pathogen. J Immunol 160:1831–1840, 1998.

1109. Subauste CS, Fuh F, de-Waal-Malefyt R, et al. Alpha beta T cell response to *Toxoplasma gondii* in previously unexposed individuals. J Immunol 160:3403–3411, 1998.

1110. Murray HW, Rubin BY, Carriero SM, et al. Human mononuclear phagocyte antiprotozoal mechanisms: oxygen-dependent vs oxygen-independent activity against intracellular *Toxoplasma gondii*. J Immunol 134:1982–1988, 1985.

1111. Wilson CB, Remington JS. Activity of human blood leukocytes against *Toxoplasma gondii*. J Infect Dis 140:890–895, 1979.

1112. Catterall JR, Sharma SD, Remington JS. Oxygen-independent killing by alveolar macrophages. J Exp Med 163:1113–1131, 1986.

1113. Catterall JR, Black CM, Leventhal JP, et al. Nonoxidative microbicidal activity in normal human alveolar and peritoneal macrophages. Infect Immun 55:1635–1640, 1987.

1114. Biggs BA, Hewish M, Kent S, et al. HIV-1 infection of human macrophages impairs phagocytosis and killing of *Toxoplasma gondii*. J Immunol 154:6132–6139, 1995.

1115. Suzuki Y, Orellana MA, Schreiber RD, et al. Interferon-gamma: the major mediator of resistance against *Toxoplasma gondii*. Science 240:516–518, 1988.

1116. Sibley LD, Adams LB, Fukutomi Y, et al. Tumor necrosis factor-alpha triggers antitoxoplasmal activity of IFN-gamma–primed macrophages. J Immunol 147:2340–2345, 1991.

1117. Thomas SM, Garrity LF, Brandt CR, et al. IFN-gamma–mediated antimicrobial response: indoleamine 2,3-dioxygenase-deficient mutant host cells no longer inhibit intracellular *Chlamydia* spp. or *Toxoplasma* growth. J Immunol 150:5529–5534, 1993.

1118. Scharton KTM, Yap G, Magram J, et al. Inducible nitric oxide is essential for host control of persistent but not acute infection with the intracellular pathogen *Toxoplasma gondii*. J Exp Med 185:1261–1273, 1997.

1119. Hayashi S, Chan CC, Gazzinelli R, et al. Contribution of nitric oxide to the host parasite equilibrium in toxoplasmosis. J Immunol 156:1476–1481, 1996.

1120. Gazzinelli RT, Eltoum I, Wynn TA, et al. Acute cerebral toxoplasmosis is induced by in vivo neutralization of TNF-alpha and correlates with the down-regulated expression of inducible nitric oxide synthase and other markers of macrophage activation. J Immunol 151:3672–3681, 1993.

1121. Frenkel JK. Adoptive immunity to intracellular infection. J Immunol 98:1309–1319, 1967.

1122. Suzuki Y, Remington JS. Dual regulation of resistance against *Toxoplasma gondii* infection by Lyt-2+ and Lyt-

1+, L3T4+ T cells in mice. J Immunol 140:3943–3946, 1988.

1123. Brown CR, McLeod R. Class I MHC genes and CD8+ T cells determine cyst number in *Toxoplasma gondii* infection. J Immunol 145:3438–3441, 1990.

1124. Araujo FG. Depletion of L3T4+ CD4+ T lymphocytes prevents development of resistance to *Toxoplasma gondii* in mice. Infect Immun 59:1614–1619, 1991.

1125. Gazzinelli R, Xu Y, Hieny S, et al. Simultaneous depletion of CD4+ and CD8+ T lymphocytes is required to reactivate chronic infection with *Toxoplasma gondii*. J Immunol 149:175–180, 1992.

1126. Denkers EY, Yap G, Scharton-Kersten T, et al. Perforin-mediated cytolysis plays a limited role in host resistance to *Toxoplasma gondii*. J Immunol 159:1903–1908, 1997.

1127. Montoya JG, Lowe KE, Clayberger C, et al. Human CD4+ and CD8+ T lymphocytes are both cytotoxic to *Toxoplasma gondii*–infected cells. Infect Immun 64:176–181, 1996.

1128. Curiel TJ, Krug EC, Purner MB, et al. Cloned human CD4+ cytotoxic T lymphocytes specific for *Toxoplasma gondii* lyse tachyzoite-infected target cells. J Immunol 151:2024–2031, 1993.

1129. Prigione I, Facchetti P, Ghiotto F, et al. *Toxoplasma gondii*–specific CD4+ T cell clones from healthy, latently infected humans display a Th0 profile of cytokine secretion. Eur J Immunol 25:1298–1305, 1995.

1130. Scalise F, Gerli R, Castellucci G, et al. Lymphocytes bearing the gamma delta T-cell receptor in acute toxoplasmosis. Immunology 76:668–670, 1992.

1131. De-Paoli P, Basaglia G, Gennari D, et al. Phenotypic profile and functional characteristics of human gamma delta T cells during acute toxoplasmosis. J Clin Microbiol 30:729–731, 1992.

1132. Subauste CS, Chung JY, Do D, et al. Preferential activation and expansion of human peripheral blood gamma delta T cells in response to *Toxoplasma gondii* in vitro and their cytokine production and cytotoxic activity against *T. gondii*–infected cells. J Clin Invest 96:610–619, 1995.

1133. Hisaeda H, Nagasawa H, Maeda K, et al. Gamma delta T cells play an important role in hsp65 expression and in acquiring protective immune responses against infection with *Toxoplasma gondii*. J Immunol 155:244–251, 1995.

1134. Kasper LH, Matsuura T, Fonseka S, et al. Induction of gamma/delta T cells during acute murine infection with *Toxoplasma gondii*. J Immunol 157:5521–5527, 1996.

1135. Sayles PC, Rakhmilevich AL, Johnson LL. Gamma delta T cells and acute primary *Toxoplasma gondii* infection in mice. J Infect Dis 171:249–252, 1995.

1136. Mackaness G. The immunological basis of acquired cellular immunity. J Exp Med 120:104–120, 1964.

1137. Frenkel JK, Taylor DW. Toxoplasmosis in immunoglobulin M–suppressed mice. Infect Immun 38:360–367, 1982.

1138. Joiner KA, Fuhrman SA, Miettinen HM, et al. *Toxoplasma gondii*: fusion competence of parasitophorous vacuoles in Fc receptor–transfected fibroblasts. Science 249:641–646, 1990.

1139. Eisenhauer P, Mack DG, McLeod R. Prevention of peroral and congenital acquisition of *Toxoplasma gondii* by antibody and activated macrophages. Infect Immun 56:83–87, 1988.

1140. Luft BJ, Brooks RG, Conley FK, et al. Toxoplasmic

encephalitis in patients with acquired immune deficiency syndrome. JAMA 252:913–917, 1984.

1141. Chen Y, Nakane A, Minagawa T. Recombinant murine gamma interferon induces enhanced resistance to *Listeria monocytogenes* infection in neonatal mice. Infect Immun 57:2345–2349, 1989.

1142. Huskinson J, Thulliez P, Remington JS. Toxoplasma antigens recognized by human immunoglobulin A antibodies. J Clin Microbiol 28:2632–2636, 1990.

1143. Wong SY, Hajdu MP, Ramirez R, et al. Role of specific immunoglobulin E in diagnosis of acute toxoplasma infection and toxoplasmosis. J Clin Microbiol 31:2952–2959, 1993.

1144. de Vries JE, Zurawski G. Immunoregulatory properties of IL-13: its potential role in atopic disease. Int Arch Allergy Immunol 106:175–179, 1995.

1145. Bortolussi R, Burbridge S, Durnford P, et al. Neonatal *Listeria monocytogenes* infection is refractory to interferon. Pediatr Res 29:400–402, 1991.

1146. Krishnan L, Guilbert LJ, Wegmann TG, et al. T helper 1 response against *Leishmania major* in pregnant C57BL/6 mice increases implantation failure and fetal resorptions: correlation with increased IFN-gamma and TNF and reduced IL-10 production by placental cells. J Immunol 156:653–662, 1996.

1147. Buxton D, Innes EA. A commercial vaccine for ovine toxoplasmosis. Parasitology 110(Suppl):S11–S16, 1995.

1148. Darcy F, Maes P, Gras-Masse H, et al. Protection of mice and nude rats against toxoplasmosis by a multiple antigenic peptide construction derived from *Toxoplasma gondii* P30 antigen. J Immunol 149:3636–3641, 1992.

1149. Peter G (ed). 1997 Red Book: Report of the Committee on Infectious Diseases, 24th ed. Elk Grove, Ill, American Academy of Pediatrics, 1997.

1150. Stiehm ER (ed). Immunologic Disorders in Infants and Children, 5th ed. Philadelphia, WB Saunders, 1996.

1151. Cairo MS, Suen Y, Knoppel E, et al. Decreased G-CSF and IL-3 production and gene expression from mononuclear cells of newborn infants. Pediatr Res 31:574–578, 1992.

1152. Yachie A, Takano N, Ohta K, et al. Defective production of interleukin-6 in very small premature infants in response to bacterial pathogens. Infect Immun 60:749–753, 1992.

1153. Liechty KW, Koenig JM, Mitchell MD, et al. Production of interleukin-6 by fetal and maternal cells in vivo during intraamniotic infection and in vitro after stimulation with interleukin-1. Pediatr Res 29:1–4, 1991.

1154. Schibler KR, Liechty KW, White WL, et al. Defective production of interleukin-6 by monocytes: a possible mechanism underlying several host defense deficiencies of neonates. Pediatr Res 31:18–21, 1992.

1155. Matsuda K, Tsutsumi H, Sone S, et al. Characteristics of IL-6 and TNF-alpha production by respiratory syncytial virus–infected macrophages in the neonate. J Med Virol 48:199–203, 1996.

1156. Taniguchi T, Matsuzaki N, Shimoya K, et al. Fetal mononuclear cells show a comparable capacity with maternal mononuclear cells to produce IL-8 in response to lipopolysaccharide in chorioamnionitis. J Reprod Immunol 23:1–12, 1993.

1157. Mehrotra PT, Donnelly RP, Wong S, et al. Production of IL-10 by human natural killer cells stimulated with IL-2 and/or IL-12. J Immunol 160:2637–2644, 1998.

1158. Suen Y, Chang M, Lee SM, et al. Regulation of interleukin-11 protein and mRNA expression in neonatal and adult fibroblasts and endothelial cells. Blood 84:4125–4134, 1994.

1159. Handzel ZT, Levin S, Dolphin Z, et al. Immune competence of newborn lymphocytes. Pediatrics 65:491–496, 1980.

1160. Weatherstone KB, Rich EA. Tumor necrosis factor/cachectin and interleukin-1 secretion by cord blood monocytes from premature and term neonates. Pediatr Res 25:342–346, 1989.

1161. Cairo MS, Suen Y, Knoppel E, et al. Decreased stimulated GM-CSF production and GM-CSF gene expression but normal numbers of GM-CSF receptors in human term newborns compared with adults. Pediatr Res 30:362–367, 1991.

1162. Buzby JS, Lee SM, Van Winkle P, et al. Increased granulocyte-macrophage colony-stimulating factor mRNA instability in cord versus adult mononuclear cells is translation-dependent and associated with increased levels of A + U–rich element binding factor. Blood 88:2889–2897, 1996.

1163. Krause PJ, Maderazo EG, Scroggs M. Abnormalities of neutrophil adherence in newborns. Pediatrics 69:184–187, 1982.

1164. Fontan G, Lorente F, Garcia R, et al. In vitro human neutrophil movement in umbilical cord blood. Clin Immunol Immunopathol 20:224–230, 1981.

1165. Tono-Oka T, Nakayama M, Uehara H, et al. Characteristics of impaired chemotactic function in cord blood leukocytes. Pediatr Res 13:148–151, 1979.

1166. Usmani S, Schlessel J, Sia C, et al. Polymorphonuclear leukocyte function in the preterm neonate. Pediatrics 87:675–679, 1991.

1167. Eisenfeld L, Krause P, Herson V, et al. Longitudinal study of neutrophil adherence and motility. J Pediatr 117:926–929, 1990.

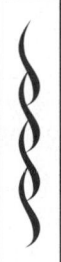

Neonatal Infections:
A Global Perspective

BARBARA J. STOLL, M.D.

One of the greatest challenges to global public health is to eliminate the gaps in health care resources, in access to preventive and curative services, and in health outcomes between rich and poor countries. Although infant mortality has declined by more than 50% since 1955,[1] neonatal mortality has changed little in some of the world's poorest countries. Worldwide, neonatal mortality accounts for a substantial proportion of mortality in both infants and children younger than 5 years.[2, 3] The World Health Organization (WHO) estimates that approximately 5 million neonates die each year and that 98% of these deaths occur in developing countries.[4] Causes of neonatal mortality, especially in developing countries, are difficult to ascertain, partly because many of these deaths occur at home, unattended by medical personnel, and partly because critically ill neonates often present with nondiagnostic signs and symptoms of disease. Infectious diseases, birth asphyxia, and prematurity are thought to be the major causes of neonatal death worldwide.[5]

Although access to sophisticated technology is limited in developing countries, neonatal mortality related to infection could be substantially reduced by simple, known interventions before and during pregnancy, labor, and delivery; in the immediate postpartum period; and in the early days of life. This chapter is an expansion and update of an earlier article on the global impact of neonatal infection.[6] The global burden of infectious diseases in the newborn, the proportion of neonatal mortality attributed to infection, specific infections of relevance to developing countries, and strategies to reduce both the incidence of neonatal infection and morbidity and mortality in those who do become infected are presented.

THE MAGNITUDE OF THE PROBLEM

Infection as a Cause of Neonatal Death: Hospital- and Community-Based Studies

In developing countries, where most births and neonatal deaths occur at home and are not attended by doctors or other trained health care workers, information on cause of death is often incomplete. Accurate data on causes of death are useful for many reasons. It is important for providers of primary care, for investigators as they design interventions for prevention and treatment, for local and national health administrators, and for decision makers who implement and evaluate health care programs.

To evaluate the impact of infection as a cause of neonatal death, hospital- and community-based studies from developing countries (in Africa, Asia, the Indian Subcontinent, the Pacific, the Middle East, and the Americas) that report neonatal mortality rates and present data on infection as a cause of death were reviewed. Neonatal deaths are defined as deaths among liveborn infants during the first 28 days of life, and the neonatal mortality rate (NMR) is reported per 1000 livebirths.[4] Early neonatal deaths are those that occur in the first week of life, and late neonatal deaths are those that occur between 8 and 28 days of life. Infections associated with neonatal death in these studies included bacterial sepsis and meningitis, respiratory infection, neonatal tetanus, omphalitis, and diarrhea.

Twenty-seven hospital-based studies published from 1980 onward were reviewed.[7–33] Epidemiologic studies varied in size, ranging from approximately 1000 to more than 100,000 livebirths and approximately 50 to 800 neonatal deaths. Data on infection as a cause of early neonatal death were presented in 16 of 27 studies; infection was associated with 7 to 54% of early neonatal deaths in these studies. Five studies reported data on infection as a cause of late neonatal death: 30 to 73% of these late deaths were associated with infection. Seventeen of the 27 studies presented data on infection as a cause of neonatal deaths overall (birth–28 days). In these studies, infection was associated with 4 to 56% of all neonatal deaths.

Twenty-nine community-based studies were reviewed.[16, 34–64] Total population in each study ranged from several thousand to 60 million people, numbers of births in each study ranged from under 1000 to more than 1 million, and numbers of neonatal deaths ranged from 7 to approximately 7000. Twelve of the 29 studies presented data on infection as a cause of early neonatal death: 0 to 43% of early neonatal deaths were associated with infection. Six community studies reported numbers of infections responsible for late neonatal deaths: 44 to 100% of late neonatal deaths were associated with infection. Twenty-four of the 29 studies presented data on infection as a cause of all neonatal deaths. Infection

was associated with 8 to 84% of all deaths in these studies.

It is well known that neonatal deaths in developing countries are under-reported and that infection as a cause of death is underestimated because of imprecision in diagnosis. Remarkably few published studies worldwide present detailed surveillance data on numbers of births and neonatal deaths and on probable causes of death. Although hospital-based studies are important for accurately determining causes of morbidity and mortality, they do not always reflect what is happening in the community. Carefully conducted community studies are needed. Furthermore, in many parts of the developing world, neonatal deaths are underestimated, owing to inadequate vital registration—especially of home births. If a child dies before the birth has been reported, there is a good chance that neither the birth nor the death will be recorded. If we estimate that 30 to 40% of neonatal deaths are associated with infections and use WHO's 1996 estimate of 4,984,000 neonatal deaths per year in the less developed regions of the world,[4] we estimate that infection is responsible for between 1.5 and 2 million neonatal deaths per year—or between 4000 and 5000 deaths per day in the less developed countries of the world.

Incidence of Neonatal Sepsis and Meningitis and Associated Mortality

Hospital-based studies from developing countries were reviewed to determine the incidence of neonatal sepsis and meningitis, the case:fatality rates (CFRs) associated with these infections, and the spectrum of bacterial pathogens in different regions of the world. Cases reported occurred among infants born in hospital, as well as those referred from home or other health facilities. Forty-nine studies[9, 65–112] from developing countries, published between 1980 and 1998, were reviewed to evaluate neonatal sepsis and meningitis in different geographic regions. Thirty-eight of these studies are primarily reports of neonatal sepsis, and 14 studies present data on bacterial meningitis. The vast majority of studies do not distinguish between maternally acquired, community-acquired, or nosocomial infections. Table 3–1 summarizes data by region.

In all regions, sepsis was responsible for a substantial burden of disease, with high CFRs reported in the vast majority of studies. Overall, incidence of neonatal sepsis ranged from 2 to 21 per 1000 livebirths (average 6/1000 livebirths) with CFRs of 1 to 69%. Of note, only two studies reported CFRs under 10%, whereas the majority of studies reported sepsis CFRs above 30%. There were fewer studies on neonatal meningitis from which to present incidence and CFRs by region. The incidence of neonatal meningitis ranged from 0.33 to 2.8 per 1000 livebirths (average 1/1000 livebirths) and CFRs ranged from 13 to 59% in these reports. Using these hospital-based rates and recent United Nations estimates of approximately 126,377,000 births per year in the less developed countries of the world,[113] we estimate that approximately 750,000 cases of neonatal sepsis and 126,000 cases of neonatal meningitis occur in developing

TABLE 3–1

Incidence and Case:Fatality Rates (CFRs) for Sepsis and Meningitis from Hospital-Based Studies in Developing Countries

REGION	INCIDENCE OF SEPSIS	CFR (%)	INCIDENCE OF MENINGITIS	CFR (%)
India/Pakistan/SE Asia/Pacific	2.4–16/1000 LB	2–69	—	45
Sub-Saharan Africa	6–21/1000 LB	27–56	0.7–1.9/1000	18–59
Middle East/N. Africa	1.8–12/1000 LB	13–45	0.33–1.5/1000	16–32
Americas/Caribbean	2, 9/1000 LB	1–31	0.4, 2.8/1000	13, 35

LB = livebirths.
Adapted from Stoll BJ. The global impact of neonatal infection. Clin Perinatol 24:1–21, 1997, with permission.

countries each year. Because the vast majority of neonates in developing countries are born at home and because many lack access to medical care if they become ill, these numbers are undoubtedly a gross underestimate of the true numbers of these infections. The high CFRs for both sepsis and meningitis (compared with those in developed countries) suggest that early detection and improved management of infected neonates would reduce mortality.

Bacterial Pathogens Associated with Infections in Different Geographic Regions

Historical reviews from developed countries have demonstrated that the predominant organisms responsible for neonatal infections change over time.[114, 115] Prospective microbiologic surveillance is therefore important to guide empirical therapy, to identify new agents of importance to neonates, to recognize epidemics, and to monitor changes over time. Moreover, the organisms associated with neonatal infection are different in different geographic areas, reinforcing the need for local microbiologic surveillance. In areas where blood cultures of sick neonates cannot be performed, knowledge of the bacterial flora of the maternal genital tract may serve as a surrogate marker for organisms causing early-onset neonatal sepsis, meningitis, and pneumonia. The vast majority of studies on the causes of neonatal sepsis and meningitis are hospital reviews that include data on infants born in hospital as well as those transferred from home or other facilities. Fifty-eight studies were reviewed to determine the spectrum of bacterial pathogens responsible for neonatal sepsis and meningitis in developing countries and to compare these pathogens with the organisms prevalent in the developed world.* In most of these studies, it is difficult to determine whether infections were of maternal origin or hospital or community acquired. Also, the infants' ages at the time of infection are not always specified. The studies vary in the detail with which culture methods are presented. It is therefore difficult to judge the quality and reliability of the microbiologic data presented.

Forty-seven studies present data on bacterial sepsis.† The spectrum of organisms presented in these studies does indeed differ from what is known from developed countries. Although the group B *Streptococcus* (GBS) continues to be the most important bacterial pathogen associated with early-onset neonatal sepsis in many developed countries,[114, 115, 131] studies from developing countries present a different picture (Table 3–2). The most striking finding from the 20 studies from India, Pakistan, Asia, and the Pacific is the low rate of GBS sepsis.‡ Half of these studies, summarizing data from approximately 1000 patients with positive blood cultures, report no isolates of GBS, and the other studies report 63 cases among 4167 infected neonates (1.5%). Gram-negative organisms were isolated significantly more frequently than gram-positive organisms, with *Klebsiella* being the most frequently isolated pathogen in

---

*See references 9, 65–76, 78–100, 102, 103, 106, 108–111, and 116–130.
†See references 9, 67, 69, 70, 72, 74, 78–83, 85–88, 90–100, 102, 103, 106, 108–110, 116–119, and 121–130.
‡See references 69, 70, 72, 80, 83, 85, 87, 94, 96, 97, 99, 100, 102, 117, 118, and 126–130.

TABLE 3–2

Organisms Associated with Sepsis and Meningitis in Developing Countries

REGION	ORGANISMS ASSOCIATED WITH SEPSIS		ORGANISMS ASSOCIATED WITH MENINGITIS	
	% Gram-Negative	% GBS	% Gram-Negative	% GBS
India/Pakistan/SE Asia/Pacific	21–85	0–5	22–100	0–15
Sub-Saharan Africa	16–68	0–30	22–77	0–61
Middle East/N. Africa	25–98	0–24	20–87	0–70
Americas/Caribbean	31–71	2–37	33, 63	3, 56

GBS = Group B *Streptococcus*.
Adapted from Stoll BJ. The global impact of neonatal infection. Clin Perinatol 24:1–21, 1997, with permission.

half of the studies. Eleven studies present data from sub-Saharan Africa.* Again, GBS was uncommon, isolated in only 8% of the 1324 patients with bacteremia. However, in two studies, group B streptococci were the most common agents found.[9, 78] In half of the studies, *Staphylococcus aureus* was the most frequently isolated agent. Overall, there was an almost equal distribution of gram-negative and gram-positive infections. Among 10 of 11 studies from the Middle East or North Africa,† GBS infection was also uncommon (44/1119, 4%), with only one study reporting group B streptococci in a substantial number of infected neonates (25/106, 24%).[81] Gram-negative organisms were somewhat more likely to be associated with sepsis in these studies. The five studies from the Americas[86, 106, 121, 124, 125] present a varying range of gram-negative and gram-positive pathogens. The two largest of these studies, from Mexico[124] and Panama,[86] identified only 18/804 (2%) infants with GBS, whereas a study from the French West Indies reported 40/107 (37%) septic neonates infected with GBS.[106]

Nineteen studies are summarized that present data on bacterial meningitis in developing countries (see Table 3–2).‡ Among 721 culture-confirmed cases, 470 (65%) were caused by gram-negative pathogens. Group B streptococci were uncommon in the majority of studies.

World Health Organization Young Infant Study

A multicenter project to determine the bacterial etiology and clinical signs of serious infections in infants younger than 90 days was sponsored by WHO in four developing countries—Ethiopia, The Gambia, Papua New Guinea, and the Philippines.[103, 129, 130, 132–136] This is the largest prospective study of early infant infections in developing countries. At the four sites, 2453 sick young infants had blood cultures performed and 507 had lumbar punctures. Seven percent (167/2453) of all blood cultures were positive: 10% in The Gambia, 9% in Ethiopia, 5% in Papua New Guinea, and 4% in the Philippines. Eight percent (40/507) of all cerebrospinal fluid cultures were positive. As might have been predicted, clinical symptoms were not helpful in distinguishing infections caused by different pathogens. Overall, 30% of infants with positive blood cultures died. Serious infection was most common in the first week of life, with the majority of deaths occurring in infants younger than 1 week of age.

There were 1673 infants evaluated in the first 4 weeks of life. Among these patients, 5% had positive blood cultures; 57% had gram-positive organisms, and 43% had gram-negative organisms. The most frequently isolated organisms were *S. aureus* (23%), *Streptococcus pyogenes* (20%), *Escherichia coli* (18%), and *Streptococcus pneumoniae* (10%). The virtual absence of GBS in this large study in four countries is striking (only 2/84 positive blood cultures). Nineteen patients had neonatal meningitis (11 had bacteremia as well)—63% of these were due

to gram-negative organisms and 37% to gram-positive organisms. The most frequent isolates were *S. pneumoniae* (5/19, 26%) and *E. coli* (4/19, 21%). Only one neonate had GBS meningitis. Of interest, *S. pneumoniae* was the most frequent organism isolated in the second and third months of life, accounting for 30% (25/83) of all positive blood cultures and 55% (12/22) of all positive cerebrospinal fluid cultures. An important conclusion of this study is that the pneumococcus must be considered in any case of serious infection in a young infant in a developing country, particularly if signs of meningitis are present.

Group B Streptococcal Infections

It is unclear why neonates in some developing countries are rarely infected with GBS. The most important risk factor for invasive GBS disease in the neonate is exposure to the organism via the mother's genital tract. Other known risk factors include young maternal age, preterm birth, prolonged rupture of the membranes, maternal chorioamnionitis, exposure to a high inoculum of a virulent GBS strain, and a low maternal serum concentration of antibody to the capsular polysaccharide of the colonizing GBS strain.[137] In the United States, differences in GBS colonization rates have been identified among women of different ethnic groups that appear to correlate with infection in newborns. In an attempt to understand the low rates of invasive GBS disease reported among neonates in many developing countries, Stoll and Schuchat[138] reviewed 34 studies that evaluated GBS colonization rates in women. These studies reported culture results from 7730 women, with an overall colonization rate of 12.7%. Studies that used culture methods that were judged to be appropriate found significantly higher colonization rates than those that used inadequate methods (675 of 3801 women [17.8%] vs. 308 of 3929 [7.8%]). When analyses were restricted to studies with adequate methods, the prevalence of colonization by region was Middle East/North Africa, 22%; Asia/Pacific, 19%; sub-Saharan Africa, 19%; India/Pakistan, 12%; and Americas, 14%.

The distribution of GBS serotypes varied among studies. GBS serotype III, the most frequently identified invasive serotype in the West, was identified in all studies reviewed and was the most frequently identified serotype in one half of the studies. Serotype V, which has only recently been recognized as a cause of invasive disease in developed countries,[139] was identified in studies from Peru[140] and The Gambia.[141] Monitoring serotype distribution is important as candidate GBS vaccines are considered for areas with high rates of disease.

With estimated colonization rates among women in developing countries as high as 18%, one would expect higher rates of invasive neonatal disease than have been reported. Low rates of invasive GBS disease in some developing countries may be explained by less virulent strains, by genetic differences in susceptibility to disease, by as yet unidentified beneficial cultural practices, or by high concentrations of transplacentally acquired protective antibody in serum (i.e., mother colonized but has

---

*See references 9, 67, 78, 88, 92, 93, 98, 103, 116, 122, and 123.
†See references 74, 79, 81, 82, 90, 91, 95, 108–110, 119.
‡See references 65, 66, 68, 71, 73, 75, 76, 81, 84, 86, 89, 103, 109–112, 120, 126, and 129.

protective concentrations of type-specific GBS antibody).

Hospital-based surveillance in developing countries may be insensitive at detecting sepsis in very young infants. In developing countries, where most deliveries occur at home, infants with early-onset sepsis often get sick and die at home or are taken to local health care facilities where a diagnosis of possible sepsis may be missed or where blood cultures cannot be performed. In this setting there may be underdiagnosis of early-onset pathogens, including GBS. In the WHO Young Infant Study,[132] 1673 infants were evaluated in the first month of life and only 2 had cultures positive for GBS. The absence of GBS in this study cannot be explained by the evaluation of insufficient numbers of sick neonates (360/1673 were infants younger than 1 week of age).

Increasing evidence suggests that heavy colonization with GBS increases the risk of delivering a preterm low-birth-weight (LBW) infant.[142] Population differences in the prevalence of heavy GBS colonization have been reported in the United States, where African Americans have a significantly higher risk of heavy colonization. If heavy colonization is more prevalent among women in developing countries and results in an increase in preterm LBW infants, GBS-related morbidity may appear as illness and death related to prematurity. By contrast, heavy colonization could increase maternal type-specific GBS antibody concentrations, resulting in lower risk of neonatal disease. Further studies in developing countries are needed to explore these important issues.

Antibiotic Therapy

These studies of bacterial etiology have implications for presumptive antibiotic therapy of bacterial infection in neonates. Currently, the drugs most frequently used to treat suspected severe neonatal infections, in both developed and developing countries, are a combination of penicillin or ampicillin and an aminoglycoside (usually gentamicin).[143] Antibiotic therapy must be tailored to the specific microbiologic needs of a particular geographic region, especially if blood cultures are not performed and cannot be used to guide therapy. The problem of antibiotic resistance is now recognized to be a global problem. There are limited data, however, on the extent of antibiotic resistance in organisms responsible for severe bacterial infections (sepsis, meningitis, pneumonia) among neonates in developing countries.[143a] The possibility of resistance must be considered in infants who deteriorate despite recommended antibiotic therapy. Moreover, in developing countries, drug supply, availability, quality, and cost are issues that must be addressed.

ACUTE RESPIRATORY INFECTIONS

The WHO estimates that almost 800,000 deaths due to acute respiratory infections (ARIs) occur in neonates in developing countries each year.[5, 144] Among young infants, most of these deaths are due to pneumonia, bronchiolitis, or laryngotracheitis. Pneumonia in neonates,

like neonatal sepsis, is of both early and late onset (i.e., acquired during birth from organisms that colonize or infect the maternal genital tract or acquired later from organisms in the hospital, home, or community). Although there are only few studies of the bacteriology of neonatal pneumonia, they suggest that organisms causing disease are similar to those that cause neonatal sepsis.[145, 146]

In a review of the magnitude of ARI mortality in developing countries, Garenne and co-workers[144] estimated that 21% of all ARI deaths in children younger than age 5 years occur in the neonatal period (1254/6041 ARI deaths in 12 countries). In a carefully conducted community study, Bang and associates[147] determined that 66% of ARI deaths in the first year of life occurred in the neonatal period.

It is difficult to determine the incidence of neonatal ARI in developing countries because many sick neonates are never referred for medical care. In a large community study of ARI in Bangladeshi children, the highest incidence of ARI was in children younger than 5 months old.[148] In the Bang and associates study,[147] there were 64 cases of pneumonia among 3100 children (21/1000), but this underestimates the true incidence because it was known that many neonates were never brought for care. In a study of LBW infants in India,[149] in which infants were visited weekly and mothers queried about disease, there were 61 episodes of moderate to severe ARI among 211 LBW infants and 125 episodes among 448 normal weight infants. Although 33% episodes occurred in LBW infants, 79% deaths occurred in this weight group.

Tuberculosis

Tuberculosis (TB) remains a major global public health threat and has become the biggest killer of young women worldwide, with an estimated 1 million deaths annually among women of childbearing age (15–44 years). The vast majority of TB infections and deaths occur in developing countries. TB during pregnancy may increase the risk of miscarriage, prematurity, and LBW.[153, 154] Adverse perinatal outcomes are increased in mothers who have late diagnosis or incomplete or irregular therapy.[154] Ideally, diagnosis and treatment of women with TB should occur before pregnancy. The lung remains the most common site of infection. However, the prevalence of extrapulmonary TB is increasing. A recent study from India reviewed the outcome of 33 pregnancies complicated by extrapulmonary TB.[154a] Extrapulmonary TB confined to the lymph nodes had no adverse effect on maternal or fetal outcome. However, disease at other sites (skeleton, intestines, kidney, meninges, endometrium) was associated with increased maternal disability and reduced fetal growth. Although congenital TB is rare, the fetus may become infected by hematogenous spread in a woman with placentitis, by swallowing or aspirating infected amniotic fluid, or by direct contact with an infected cervix at the time of delivery.[153] The most common route of infection of the neonate is through airborne transmission of *Mycobacterium tuberculosis* from an infected untreated mother to her infant. Infected newborns are at particularly high risk of developing severe disease.[153]

The resurgence of TB and the increased risk of TB among those who are infected with the human immunodeficiency virus (HIV) is well known. In one report from South Africa,[155] 11 neonates with culture-confirmed perinatal TB were described. Six infants were categorized as having congenital TB; and in five, postnatal transmission could not be excluded. Six mothers were HIV positive and three of their infants were also HIV infected. The predominant clinical features were intrauterine growth retardation (7/11), progressive pneumonia (9/11), fever (9/11), and hepatomegaly (7/11). One infant died. Pregnant women who are co-infected with HIV may be at increased risk for placental or genital TB, resulting in an increased risk of transmission to the fetus.[155, 156] In areas of the world where both TB and HIV are endemic, there must be a high index of suspicion for both diseases in the mother and neonate.

HOME-BASED NEONATAL CARE

Several studies have evaluated community-based care to identify sick neonates in a timely fashion and to treat them in their own homes. Datta and colleagues[149] implemented a program of ARI control at the primary health care level and demonstrated that improved detection and treatment could reduce mortality among LBW infants (less than 2500 g). Interventions involved training primary health care workers and treating moderate-severe ARI with oral penicillin (125 mg twice a day for 5 days) using a "decision and action" classification. They compared numbers of episodes of ARI and CFRs among LBW infants in intervention and control villages. ARI-specific mortality was 30 per 1000 live births in the intervention area versus 71 per 1000 live births in the control area (6/199 versus 15/211, respectively). In a similar study of the feasibility of managing neonatal pneumonia in the community, Bang and colleagues[147] also demonstrated reduction in ARI mortality with a primary health care program. Community interventions used by this group included extensive health education of possible caregivers (traditional birth attendants, paramedics, and village health workers) and specific case management—continued breast-feeding and oral co-trimoxazole syrup for 7 days. Community-based management of pneumonia had a significant impact in reducing pneumonia-associated mortality. In the intervention area, the neonatal mortality rate from all causes was 64 per 1000 children and the pneumonia-specific mortality rate was 17 per 1000 versus 84 per 1000 and 29 per 1000, respectively, in control villages, representing a 24% reduction in mortality overall and a 40% reduction in pneumonia-specific mortality in the intervention villages. The CFR for neonatal pneumonia in the Bang study was 15% (10/65 died) in the intervention area. This CFR is lower than what has been reported from hospital-based studies in India (22–56%),[145, 150, 151] suggesting that cases managed in the community were diagnosed and treated earlier than hospitalized cases.

Both of these intervention studies identified cultural barriers to care, including noncompliance with referral and medication use. Bhandari and associates[152] studied 2007 infants (aged 0–2 months) at two urban slum clinics in Delhi, India. Because of severe illness, hospital admission was advised for 273 (14%) of these infants, including 104 patients with ARI. Only 24% of families of sick infants and 20% of those with ARI complied with recommendations for admission. The other infants were treated as outpatients and at home (with no deaths in the ARI group). These data suggest that improved community or domiciliary management of sick newborns may be the only way to improve outcome in some settings.

In a recent study, Bang and colleagues[149a] implemented a comprehensive program of home-based neonatal care in a remote rural area of India. Trained female village health care workers identified pregnant women, visited them in their homes during the pregnancy, attended the delivery (with traditional birth attendants), observed the neonate at birth and resuscitated the infant if necessary (using a simple resuscitation device), and visited the mother and baby in the home on days 1, 3, 5, 7, 14, 21, and 28 and any other time if called by the family. These health care workers were specifically trained to encourage mothers to breast-feed in the first hour after birth, to maintain a normal body temperature in the newborn by keeping the home warm and using clothing appropriately, and to identify severe illnesses including clinical sepsis, pneumonia, or meningitis. Criteria used to diagnose presumed sepsis, pneumonia, or meningitis included a baby who cried well at birth who then developed a weak or abnormal cry; a baby who sucked well initially but stopped sucking; a baby who became drowsy or unconscious; a skin temperature above 99° F or below 95° F; pus on the skin or umbilicus; diarrhea, persistent vomiting, or abdominal distention; grunting or severe retractions; and a respiratory rate of 60 or more per minute in a quiet baby. If an infant was diagnosed to have presumed sepsis, pneumonia, or meningitis, the parents were advised to take the infant to hospital. If parents were unwilling to take the child to hospital, home-based care was offered. This care included antibiotics (intramuscular gentamicin [15 mg bid × 10 days for preterm newborns or those with birth weights under 2500 g and 7.5 mg bid × 7 days for term newborns or those with birth weights above 2500 g] and oral co-trimoxazole [sulphamethoxazole 200 mg and trimethoprim 40 mg/5 ml] 1.25 ml bid for 7 days), support to maintain a normal temperature and to promote breast-feeding, and very close follow-up with home visits twice a day for 7 to 10 days. Investigators compared health outcomes in 39 intervention and 47 control villages that had similar population characteristics and baseline mortality rates (1993–1995). Specific home-based neonatal care was studied in the intervention villages in 1995–1998. The vast majority of births in the intervention villages occurred at home (95%), and 43% of the neonates were low birth weight (under 2500 g). Very few neonates in the intervention villages were hospitalized for a severe illness (under 1% during study period). In this study, the CFR for severe neonatal illness

TABLE 3–3

Projected Cumulative Total of HIV-Infected Women and Their Children by Geographic Area in the Year 2000[a]

AREA	HIV+ WOMEN	HIV+ INFANTS	PEDIATRIC AIDS	ORPHANS <5 YEARS	ORPHANS <15 YEARS
North America & Western Europe	320,000 (2)	25,000 (1)	20,000 (1)	35,000 (2)	120,000 (1)
Southeast Asia	5,000,000 (32)	440,000 (14)	300,000 (14)	270,000 (17)	870,000 (13)
Latin America & Caribbean	1,400,000 (9)	230,000 (7)	170,000 (7)	180,000 (11)	640,000 (10)
Sub-Saharan Africa	8,800,000 (57)	2,500,000 (78)	1,700,000 (78)	1,100,000 (70)	5,200,000 (76)
Total	15,520,000 (100)	3,195,000 (100)	2,190,000 (100)	1,585,000 (100)	6,830,000 (100)

[a]The numbers of perinatally infected infants (HIV+ infants) were adjusted for competing causes of perinatal mortality; numbers of pediatric AIDS and maternal AIDS orphans were adjusted for competing causes of child (younger than 5) mortality; numbers < 10,000 were rounded off to the nearest 1000; numbers > 10,000 and < 100,000 were rounded off to the nearest 5000; numbers > 100,000 were rounded off to the nearest 10,000; numbers in brackets denote percentage of the column total.

From Chin J. The growing impact of the HIV/AIDS pandemic on children born to HIV-infected women. Clin Perinatol 21:1–14, 1994, with permission.

declined from 16.6% before the intervention to 2.8% after the intervention ($p < 0.05$). Moreover, early neonatal mortality, overall neonatal mortality, and infant mortality rates all declined significantly in the intervention villages (50% reduction, 62% reduction, and 46% reduction, respectively). Of interest, mortality was reduced at all birth weights (under 1500 g, 1500–1999 g, 2000–2499 g, and ≥ 2500 g). This comprehensive home-based system for neonatal care was accepted by families and was successful in reducing mortality. It must be replicated in other areas of the world, where referral to hospital for the sick neonate may not currently be acceptable to families or even possible.

HUMAN IMMUNODEFICIENCY VIRUS INFECTION

The Joint United Nations Programme on HIV/AIDS (UNAIDS) and the WHO estimate that by the year 2000 more than 40 million people worldwide will be infected with HIV and that approximately 16,000 new infections occur each day. Most HIV infections occur in the developing world; more than 90% of those infected live in sub-Saharan Africa, Asia, Latin America, or the Caribbean. Worldwide, more than 40% of cases occur in women and more than 500,000 children are infected with HIV each year, mostly by maternal-to-infant transmission either in utero, intrapartum, or through breast-feeding.[157]

Because HIV increases deaths among young adults—both male and female—the acquired immunodeficiency syndrome (AIDS) epidemic has resulted in a generation of AIDS orphans. It is projected that by 2000 more than 1.5 million children younger than 5 years will have been orphaned by AIDS, the vast majority in sub-Saharan Africa.[2] It is well known that maternal mortality increases neonatal and infant deaths, independent of HIV status. Global estimates for the numbers of HIV-infected women, perinatally infected infants, children with AIDS, and maternal AIDS orphans projected to the year 2000 are presented in Table 3–3 and Figure 3–1.[158]

Transmission

There is a clear gap between developed and developing countries in mother-to-child transmission of HIV.[157, 159] Whereas transmission rates as low as 4 to 11% have been reported for Europe and North America in the post-zidovudine (azidothymidine [AZT]) era,[160–165] rates in developing countries range from 21 to 48%.[166–172] These differences are primarily due to differences in access to antiretroviral drugs (to reduce transmission) and to differences in breast-feeding practices.[157, 159] Other factors that may influence transmission rates in developing countries include co-infection with other sexually transmitted diseases (STDs)[173]; poor nutritional status of the mother[174]; micronutrient deficiencies, particularly vitamin A deficiency[175]; maternal anemia[168, 171]; specific obstetric factors, including abruption, premature or prolonged rupture of the membranes, chorioamnionitis, and mode of delivery[161, 167, 168, 171, 176–181b]; virulence of the infecting HIV strain; and advanced maternal disease.[159, 167, 168, 180, 182]

Breast-Feeding and Human Immunodeficiency Virus

HIV is present in breast milk, and postnatal transmission by means of breast-feeding is an important mode of transmission in developing countries.[182–188] A review of published studies evaluated transmission risk among mothers who were infected prenatally and postnatally.[183] Based on five studies in which the mother had been infected prenatally (as is most often the case), the additional risk of HIV transmission with breast-feeding (above the in-utero and delivery risks) was estimated to be 14% (95% CI 7–22%). By contrast, when the mother

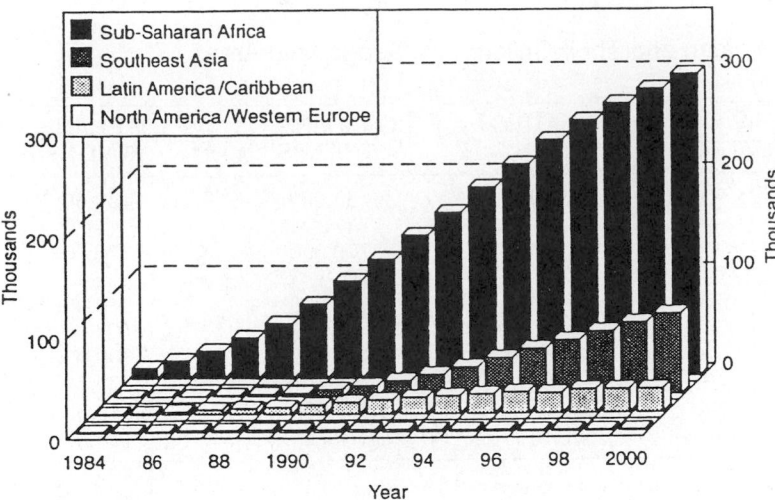

FIGURE 3–1 Estimated and projected number of infants infected with human immunodeficiency virus (HIV) born annually to HIV-infected mothers. (From Chin J. The growing impact of the HIV/AIDS pandemic on children born to HIV-infected women. Clin Perinatol 21:1–14, 1994.)

developed her primary infection after birth, transmission risk increased substantially—estimated from four studies to be 29% (95% CI 16–42%). Worldwide, it is estimated that between one third and one half of all HIV-infected infants acquire infection postnatally from breast-feeding.[188]

The risk of postnatal transmission increases as duration of breast-feeding increases.[172, 187, 189, 190] Therefore, prolonged breast-feeding may be an important risk factor for transmission. A recent study from South Africa[190a] compared HIV-transmission rates in exclusively breast-fed, mixed-fed, and never breast-fed (formula-fed) infants to assess whether the pattern of breast feeding has an impact on early mother-to-infant transmission of HIV. Of 547 infants followed prospectively, 156 never breast-fed, 103 were exclusively breast-fed, and 288 received breast milk and other foods in the first 3 months of life. Transmission rates by day 1, which reflect in-utero transmission, did not differ among groups (~6%). Excluding those who were HIV positive on day 1, the proportion of infants infected at 3 months of age did not differ in those who never received breast milk (13.2%) versus those who were exclusively breast-fed (8.3%). However, the infection rate was significantly higher in the group of infants who were not exclusively breast-fed (19.9%, $p = 0.01$). This preliminary study, if confirmed, suggests that exclusive breast-feeding and early weaning might reduce postnatal HIV transmission. Further studies are needed to better define risk factors for HIV transmission via breast-feeding and interventions to reduce risk. Although mainly speculative, other factors that might influence the infectivity of breast milk and breast-feeding include the concentration of cell-free or cell-associated HIV in breast milk; viral strain; the presence or absence of HIV-specific antibodies, particularly secretory IgA or IgM, or cytotoxic T cells in breast milk, lactoferrin, lysozymes, and other factors with specific antiviral activity; and the presence of mastitis with or without overt nipple cracks and bleeding.[186, 191, 191a] Furthermore, infant susceptibility to infection through breast-feeding might be affected by stomach pH, oral ulceration, gastroenteritis, prematurity or low birth weight, nutritional status, and the presence of mucosal (salivary, gastrointestinal) or serum anti-HIV antibodies or cytotoxic T lymphocytes.[186, 191]

Although breast-feeding by HIV-positive mothers is discouraged in Europe and North America, where safe and affordable alternatives to breast milk are available, the issue of breast-feeding and HIV is much more complicated in developing countries, where breast-feeding has proven benefits and where artificial feeding has known risks. Benefits of breast-feeding include decreased risk of diarrhea and other infectious diseases, improved nutritional status, and decreased infant mortality (see later section on breast-feeding).

In 1998, UNAIDS, WHO, and UNICEF issued a joint policy statement on HIV and infant feeding to help decision makers in different countries develop their own policies regarding feeding practices in the context of HIV.[188] The statement addresses several issues: the human rights perspective, preventing HIV infection in women, the health of mothers and children, and elements for establishing a policy on HIV and infant feeding. As a general principle, the document supports breast-feeding. Furthermore, the statement encourages access to voluntary and confidential HIV testing for both women and men of reproductive age, as well as education regarding the implications of their HIV status for the health and welfare of their children. Because mothers may wish to keep their HIV status confidential, the statement acknowledges that women must be empowered to make decisions regarding infant feeding and supported to carry out their decision. "This should include efforts to promote a hygienic environment, essentially clean water and sanitation, that will minimize health risks when a breast milk substitute is used. When children born to women living with HIV can be ensured uninterrupted access to nutritionally adequate breast milk substitutes that are safely prepared and fed to them, they are at less risk of illness and death if they are not breast-fed. However, when these conditions are not fulfilled, in particular in an environment where infectious diseases and malnutrition are the primary causes of death during infancy, artificial feeding substantially increases children's risk of illness and death."[188]

Several issues are implicit in this document. Breast-feeding has been actively promoted for many years to improve child survival. Discouraging breast-feeding is contrary to these policies and may be socially unacceptable in certain settings as well as unsafe. The risks of breast-feeding in the context of maternal HIV infection must be explained in a clear, supportive, and nonjudgmental manner. Moreover, universal access to voluntary HIV testing, although a clear human right, has broad social as well as financial implications.[192] Women may feel coerced into being tested, rather than it being a truly voluntary decision. There is a stigma to being infected with HIV, which in some settings may lead to spousal rejection or abuse, loss of friends and family support networks, and loss of jobs or livelihood. Programs to reduce breast-feeding or limit its duration among HIV-infected women (and therefore decrease transmission to their infants) must not reduce breast-feeding among women who are uninfected as well and must ensure that safe and affordable (maybe even free) breast milk substitutes are readily available. Although scientists have attempted, through mathematical modeling, to define levels of HIV seroprevalence and non–HIV-related child mortality at which breast-feeding might be either discouraged or promoted, there are no simple solutions to this very complicated issue.[193, 194] A possible decline in breast-feeding in developing countries could have grave consequences.

Prevention of Human Immunodeficiency Virus Infection in Developing Countries

Primary prevention of HIV infection among women of childbearing age is the most successful but most difficult way to prevent the infection of infants. Improving the social status of women, education of both men and women, ensuring access to information about HIV and HIV prevention, promotion of safer sex through condom use, social marketing of condoms, and treatment of other STDs that increase the risk of HIV transmission are potential strategies that have been successful at reducing infection.[188]

Prevention of Transmission of Human Immunodeficiency Virus from Infected Mother to Infant

With approximately 550,000 infants infected perinatally each year worldwide, prevention strategies are urgently needed. In 1994, a clinical trial performed in the United States and France (Pediatric AIDS Clinical Trials Group [ACTG] Protocol 076)[160] demonstrated that zidovudine (AZT, 100 mg, five times per day) administered orally to HIV-infected pregnant women with no prior treatment with antiretroviral drugs during pregnancy, beginning at 14 to 34 weeks' gestation and continuing throughout pregnancy, intravenously during labor (2 mg/kg over 1 hour followed by 1 mg/kg per hour until

delivery), and orally to the newborn for the first 6 weeks of life (2 mg/kg every 6 hours) reduced perinatal transmission by 67.5% from 25.5% (95% CI 18.4–32.5%) to 8.3% (95% CI 3.9–12.8%). The regimen was recommended as standard care in the United States and quickly became common practice.[195] However, because of feasibility and high costs ($800 per pregnancy), this regimen is unavailable to the vast majority of HIV-infected pregnant women in developing countries. For example, a country such as Côte d'Ivoire, with a high prevalence of HIV and high fertility rates, would have to spend the majority of its drug budget just to treat all HIV-infected pregnant women using this regimen, which obviously is impossible. Moreover, in many developing countries women receive limited or no prenatal care; intravenous dosing may be unsafe, impractical, or impossible; and women either give birth at home or come to a hospital or clinic only when they are already in labor. Thus, newer, simpler, less expensive, methods to reduce mother-to-infant transmission of HIV are needed for the majority of women and children in the world.

A number of modified AZT trials have been completed, are in progress, or are being planned. These trials are evaluating a shorter prenatal course, oral rather than intravenous dosing in labor, a shorter newborn course, or no AZT to the neonate. In a joint U.S. Centers for Disease Control and Prevention and Thai Ministry of Public Health trial, 397 asymptomatic Thai women were randomized to receive either placebo or AZT in the last month of pregnancy (300 mg tablets orally twice daily from 36 weeks until labor, one tablet at the onset of labor, and one tablet every 3 hours until delivery). Infants did not receive AZT and were not breast-fed (infant formula was provided free for 18 months). Transmission was reduced 50% from 18.9% (95% CI 13.2 to 24.2%) in the placebo group to 9.4% (95% CI 5.2 to 13.5%) in the AZT group.[196] The cost of treatment was about $50 per woman. The Thai trial, although highly effective, did not address the issue of whether short-course AZT would be effective in a more symptomatic population and one in which breast-feeding is the norm. In Côte d'Ivoire, as in the rest of Africa, most HIV-infected women are counseled to breast-feed their infants because of high infant mortality without breast-feeding, the cost of infant formula, and the stigma associated with alternative feeding regimens. A trial using the Thai treatment regimen was performed in Côte d'Ivoire among a cohort of pregnant women who breast-fed their infants from birth.[197] The trial was stopped in February 1988 when results of the Thai trial became available. In the Côte d'Ivoire trial, transmission was reduced from 21.7% in the placebo group (n = 140) to 12.2% in the treatment group (n = 140) at 1 month (44% reduction) and from 24.9% to 15.7% at 3 months (37% reduction). To further investigate the efficacy of this regimen in breast-feeding women, the results of similar studies performed in Burkina Faso and Côte d'Ivoire were combined.[198] At 6 months of age, the probability of HIV infection was 18.0% in the AZT group (n = 192) versus 27.5% in the placebo group (n = 197), a 38% reduction of early vertical transmission of HIV, despite breast-feeding.

UNAIDS is sponsoring the PETRA (PErinatal TRAnsmission) study designed in conjunction with African scientists and ongoing at five sites in South Africa, Tanzania, and Uganda.[199] The study is evaluating the efficacy of three different antiviral regimens using two drugs (AZT and lamivudine [3TC]) versus placebo in HIV-infected pregnant women in populations in which breast-feeding is the norm. Preliminary results suggest that the two-drug regimen begun at the time of delivery and continued in both mother and baby for 1 week following delivery reduces transmission from 17% (no drugs) to 10% at 6 weeks of age (38% decline). When drugs are started at 36 weeks' gestation, transmission is further reduced to 8% (53% decline). When drugs were given only during the intrapartum period, there was no reduction in transmission. Infants in this trial will be followed to 18 months of age.[199a]

Nevirapine is a non-nucleoside reverse-transcriptase inhibitor that has potent antiviral activity, is rapidly absorbed orally, and passes quickly through the placenta. The safety and efficacy of short-course nevirapine compared with AZT given to women during labor and to neonates in the first week of life were compared in the HIVNET 012 trial conducted in Uganda.[199b] Six-hundred-twenty-six HIV-infected women (313 in each group) were randomly assigned to single-dose nevirapine (200 mg orally at onset of labor and 2 mg/kg to their babies within 72 hours of birth) or AZT (600 mg orally at onset of labor and 300 mg every 3 hours until delivery; and 4 mg/kg orally twice a day to babies for 7 days after birth). Almost all infants were breast-fed from birth (98.8%), and 95.6% were still breast-feeding at 14 to 16 weeks. The HIV transmission rates in the nevirapine and AZT groups were 8.2% versus 10.4% at birth ($p =$ NS), 11.9% versus 21.3% at 6 to 8 weeks ($p = 0.0027$), and 13.1% versus 25.1% at 14 to 16 weeks of age ($p = 0.0006$). When nevirapine and AZT were both started at the onset of labor, nevirapine reduced HIV transmission by almost 50% in a breast-feeding population. Of note, the 25.1% transmission rate in the AZT group was higher than reported in the AZT trials from Côte d'Ivoire,[197, 198] but drug was started at 36 weeks (not at the onset of labor) in those studies. Although nevirapine appeared to be safe, long-term follow-up of infants is needed. Single-dose nevirapine administered to mother and infant is the cheapest antiviral regimen studied to date (~$4 per mother-infant pair) and represents a deliverable, cost-effective regimen for the prevention of mother-to-child transmission of HIV in sub-Saharan Africa.[199c] If the HIVNET 012 results are confirmed in other developing country settings, implementation of single-dose nevirapine programs could have a major public health impact.

In 1998, the WHO published recommendations on the safe and effective use of short course AZT for the prevention of mother-to-child transmission of HIV.[200] The Thai regimen is recommended for use in settings in which practical and budgetary considerations preclude use of the ACTG 076 regimen (i.e., most of the developing world) and in which there is an adequate infrastructure for short-course therapy. As the results of newer trials using different drug regimens become available, the specific recommendations may change. However, the recommendations note that antiretroviral therapy requires the identification of HIV-infected women early enough in pregnancy to allow them access to therapy; and, therefore, a system for voluntary, confidential HIV counseling and testing must be in place. Furthermore, women must understand the implications of HIV, the drug intervention, and the possibility that even with antiviral therapy they might transmit infection to their infants. Interventions to reduce mother-to-child transmission of HIV, especially the administration of antiretroviral drugs and the avoidance of breast-feeding, make it difficult for HIV-positive women to keep their infection status private. If women fear stigmatization, discrimination, and even violence if they are identified as HIV-infected, they will be unable or reluctant to take advantage of strategies to reduce transmission to their infants. Providing voluntary counseling and testing, antiviral drugs, and alternatives to breast-feeding to reduce maternal-to-child HIV transmission has potential wider benefits for society, including improvement in the quality of health care services for mothers and children, and opportunities to address primary prevention of HIV; care for HIV-infected men, women, and children; support for HIV orphans; and discriminatory societal attitudes.[200a]

In a joint initiative, UNICEF, WHO, and UNAIDS are working together to reduce mother-to-infant transmission by initiating a pilot program in selected low-income countries, including Botswana, Burkina Faso, Cambodia, Côte d'Ivoire, Honduras, Rwanda, Tanzania, Thailand, Uganda, Zambia, and Zimbabwe.[201] The initiative will support 30,000 HIV-infected women and will provide the following: early access to adequate antenatal care; voluntary and confidential counseling and HIV testing for women and their partners; AZT during pregnancy and delivery for HIV-positive women (provided at lower cost by Glaxo Wellcome); improved care during labor and delivery; counseling for HIV-positive women explaining a range of choices for infant feeding; and support for HIV-positive women who choose not to breast-feed. UNICEF will work with governments and infant formula companies to identify ways of providing safe and affordable alternatives to breast milk. At the same time, UNICEF, WHO, and UNAIDS continue to promote breast-feeding as the best feeding method for mothers who are HIV negative or who do not know their HIV status.

Alternatives to antiretroviral drugs are also being studied in developing countries. These include giving pregnant women or their newborns, or both, an intravenous dose of anti-HIV immunoglobulin (passive immunization) to prevent HIV transmission (much like the use of hepatitis B immunoglobulin [HBIG] to prevent perinatal transmission of hepatitis B); use of vaginal microbicides in labor and delivery to reduce the amount of HIV the neonate comes in contact with during delivery; vitamin A supplementation to reduce transmission in areas with high prevalence of vitamin A deficiency; and supplementation with other micronutrients (folate,

TABLE 3–4
Percentage of Infant Deaths Due to AIDS:
Projections for the Year 2010

COUNTRY	U.S. BUREAU OF THE CENSUS[a]	U.N. POPULATION DIVISIONS[b]
Botswana	61	35
Zimbabwe	58	27
Kenya	41	12
Zambia	40	17
Rwanda	31	6
Uganda	31	10
Malawi	30	9
Tanzania	29	6
Burkina Faso	27	6
Côte d'Ivoire	26	8
Central African Rep.	23	6
Lesotho	20	5
Burundi	18	3
Cameroon	18	3
Congo	16	11
Brazil	13	0
Congo, Democratic Rep.	10	3
Haiti	7	7
Thailand	5	7

[a]Data from U.S. Bureau of the Census. The Demographic Impacts of HIV/AIDS: perspectives from the World Population Profile, 1996.

[b]Data from U.N. Population Division, World Population Prospects: the 1996 Revision, 1997.

Modified from The Progress of Nations. New York, UNICEF, 1997, with permission.

iron, multivitamins).[202, 203] The effect of breast-feeding on any new intervention needs to be evaluated as well.

Human Immunodeficiency Virus and Child Survival

Although there have been tremendous gains in child survival over the past 25 years with reductions worldwide in deaths due to diarrhea, pneumonia, and vaccine-preventable diseases, the AIDS epidemic threatens to undermine this dramatic trend (Table 3–4).[204, 205] In parts of the developing world, AIDS has already had a negative impact on child survival; in sub-Saharan Africa, AIDS has become a leading cause of death among infants and children. In Harare, Zimbabwe, for example, infant mortality doubled between 1990 and 1996 from 30 to 60 per 1000 livebirths, and deaths among children aged 1 to 5 years (the years when most childhood AIDS deaths occur in developing countries) increased from 8 to 20 per 1000 livebirths.[157] Obviously, methods to reduce mother-to-child transmission of HIV are desperately needed in developing countries.

NEONATAL TETANUS

More is known about neonatal tetanus than about any other newborn infection occurring in developing countries. There is a vast published literature on neonatal tetanus. Neonatal tetanus has traditionally been an un-

der-reported "silent" illness. Because it attacks newborns in the poorest countries of the world in the first few days of life while they are still confined to home, because of a high and rapid CFR, and because of poor access to medical care, the disease may be unrecognized.[206, 207] Retrospective community surveys of neonatal tetanus have been conducted since the late 1970s to determine burden of disease and mortality rates.[208, 209] The surveillance case definition of neonatal tetanus is relatively straightforward—that is, the ability of a newborn to suck at birth and for the first few days of life, followed by inability to suck starting between 3 and 10 days of age, spasms, stiffness, convulsions, and death. Using this definition and the verbal autopsy technique, country surveys have estimated the magnitude of the problem worldwide. As of 1989, 42 countries conducted more than 75 neonatal tetanus surveys[210] and, by 1995, 93% of developing countries were reporting data on neonatal tetanus.[207] In 1998, the WHO estimated that approximately 400,000 cases of neonatal tetanus occur annually in the developing world. The vast majority of cases occur in a limited number of countries.[207] With a CFR (untreated) of 85% in developing countries,[211] approximately 340,000 deaths per year are still caused by neonatal tetanus. In some of the least developed countries, neonatal tetanus is still a major cause of neonatal death.[206] Between 1990 and 1997, five countries with large populations and high birth rates made significant progress in reducing neonatal tetanus deaths. Deaths declined by 82% in China (75,700 to 13,700), by 69% in Indonesia (22,800 to 7,100), by 46% in Bangladesh (38,000 to 20,700), by 24% in India (77,700 to 59,100), and by 18% in Pakistan (36,300 to 29,700).[212]

Neonatal tetanus is a completely preventable disease. It can be prevented by immunizing mothers before or during pregnancy and/or by ensuring a clean delivery, clean cutting of the umbilical cord, and proper care of the cord in the days after birth. Clean delivery practices have additional benefits—prevention of other neonatal and maternal infections, in addition to tetanus. Maternal immunization—ideally immunization of girls before they reach reproductive age—has the added benefit of preventing maternal tetanus–related mortality, a complication of both induced abortion and childbirth in unimmunized women.[212a] The global elimination of tetanus by the year 2000 was among the goals agreed on by almost all of the world's governments after the 1990 World Summit for Children.[213] Although not yet achieved, this goal can be met, but it will require increased political and financial commitment.

OMPHALITIS

In developed countries, aseptic delivery techniques and cord care have decreased the occurrence of umbilical infection or omphalitis. Furthermore, prompt diagnosis and antimicrobial therapy have decreased morbidity and mortality if omphalitis develops. However, omphalitis continues to be a problem in developing countries, where hygienic cord care practices are not universal.[214] The necrotic tissue of the umbilical cord is an excellent medium for bacterial growth. The umbilical stump is rapidly colonized by bacteria from the maternal genital tract and from the environment. This colonized necrotic tissue, in close proximity to umbilical vessels, provides microbial pathogens with direct access to the bloodstream. It is not surprising that umbilical infection is common in the developing country setting with the triad of home births, unsterile cutting of the cord, and unhygienic cord care after birth. Omphalitis may remain a localized infection or may spread to the abdominal wall, the peritoneum, the umbilical or portal vessels, or the liver. Infants who present with abdominal wall cellulitis or necrotizing fasciitis have a high incidence of associated bacteremia (often polymicrobial) and a high mortality rate.[214–216]

There are only a limited number of recent studies on umbilical infection from developing countries.[39, 59, 129, 217–220] Overall, incidence of omphalitis in these studies ranged from 2 to 54 per 1000 livebirths, with the CFR ranging from 0 to 15%. Guvenc and associates[219] identified 88 newborns with omphalitis at a university hospital in eastern Turkey over a 2-year period. These included 54 patients with only local symptoms and 34 with systemic symptoms. The overall CFR was 15%, but all deaths occurred among patients with systemic signs, with a CFR of 38% in this group. Gram-positive organisms were isolated from 68% of umbilical cultures, gram-negative organisms were isolated from 60%, and multiple organisms were cultured in 28% of patients. Airede[217] studied 33 Nigerian neonates with omphalitis. The incidence of omphalitis was 2 per 1000 livebirths, and the prevalence was 16 per 1000 admissions to hospital. There were no deaths in this series. Aerobic bacteria were isolated from 70%, and anaerobic bacteria were isolated from 30%. Sixty percent of the aerobic isolates were gram-positive organisms, and polymicrobial isolates were common. Three studies from India were identified that present data on omphalitis or umbilical sepsis. Singhal and associates[59] reported that 28 of 920 livebirths developed umbilical sepsis (30/1000) and two of these infants died (CFR 7%). Four percent of all neonatal deaths in this study were attributed to umbilical sepsis. Bhardwaj and Hasan[39] reported that 11 of 204 livebirths (54/1000) developed umbilical sepsis; there were no deaths in this group. Faridi and colleagues[218] studied 182 Indian neonates with omphalitis, including 104 hospital-born and 78 home-delivered infants. The incidence of omphalitis in the hospital-born group was 24/1000 livebirths. Overall, gram-negative organisms were isolated more frequently than gram-positive organisms (57% versus 43%), but *S. aureus* was the single most frequent isolate (28%). In one report from Turkey, 85 neonates with bacteriologically proven omphalitis were evaluated.[220] *S. aureus* and *E. coli* were the most frequent organisms isolated. Overall CFR was 13% with no difference between term and preterm infants. In a study from Papua New Guinea, 116 young infants with signs suggestive of omphalitis had umbilical cultures performed. The most frequently isolated organisms were group A beta-hemolytic *Streptococcus* (44%), *S. aureus* (39%), *Klebsiella* (17%), *E. coli* (17%), and *Proteus mirabilis* (16%).[129] In infants with both omphalitis and bacter-

emia, the same organism may be cultured from both umbilicus and blood. In the Papua New Guinea study cited earlier, newborns with sepsis and omphalitis had *S. aureus*, group A beta-hemolytic streptococci, and *Klebsiella pneumoniae* each isolated from both sites.

The method of caring for the umbilical cord after birth affects both bacterial colonization and time to cord separation.[221, 222] It is generally agreed that application of antimicrobial agents to the umbilical cord reduces bacterial colonization. The effect of such agents on reducing infection is less clear.[222] During a study of pregnancy in a rural area of Papua New Guinea, Garner and colleagues[223] detected a high prevalence of neonatal fever and umbilical infection, which were associated with the subsequent development of neonatal sepsis. They designed an intervention program for umbilical cord care that included maternal health education and umbilical care packs containing acriflavine spirit and new razor blades. Neonatal sepsis was significantly less frequent in the intervention group (1/67 versus 8/64, $p = 0.02$). This study documented the importance of umbilical infection in the etiology of neonatal sepsis in a rural developing country setting and demonstrated that a simple cord care intervention could reduce infectious morbidity.

DIARRHEA

It is generally agreed that diarrheal episodes are more common in infants older than 6 months than in those who are younger.[224, 225] It is thought that the high prevalence of breast-feeding in the first month of life, the fact that most of the world's children are born at home rather than in hospital, and the relative segregation of infants for a period of time after birth are factors that protect the newborn from diarrhea. Mortality from diarrhea is thought to be greatest in the first year of life.

Numerous studies have investigated the epidemiology of diarrhea in hospital and community settings and the role of breast milk and breast-feeding in protection against disease.[226–231a] Clemens and colleagues followed a cohort of 198 breast-fed Egyptian neonates for the first 6 months of life.[231a] Neonates who had breast-feeding initiated within the first 3 days of life, when breast milk contains colostrum (early group, n = 151), had a 26% lower rate of diarrhea during the first 6 months of life than infants who started breast-feeding later (late group, n = 47; early versus late: 6.4 episodes versus 9.0 episodes per child year, $p < 0.05$). Huilan and associates[226] studied the agents associated with diarrhea in children from birth to 35 months of age from five hospitals in China, India, Mexico, Myanmar, and Pakistan. A total of 3640 cases of diarrhea were studied, 28% of which occurred in infants younger than 6 months of age. Data on the detection of rotavirus, enterotoxigenic *E. coli* and *Campylobacter* were provided by age. Five percent of isolates of these agents (17/323) were from neonates (birth–29 days). Black and colleagues[228] performed community studies of diarrheal epidemiology and etiology in a periurban community in Peru. The incidence of diarrhea was 9.8 episodes per child in the first year of life and did not differ significantly by month of age (0.64–1.0 episode per child-month) with infants having diarrhea from birth. Mahmud and colleagues[229] prospectively followed a cohort of 1476 Pakistani newborns from four different communities. Eighteen percent of infants evaluated in the first month of life (180/1028) had diarrhea.

Although most infants in developing countries are born at home, those born in hospital are at risk for nosocomial diarrheal infections. Aye and co-workers[231] studied diarrheal morbidity in neonates born at the largest maternity hospital in Rangoon, Myanmar. Diarrhea was a significant problem, with rates of 7 per 1000 livebirths for infants born vaginally and 50 per 1000 for infants delivered by cesarean section. These differences were attributed to the following: infants born by cesarean section remain hospitalized longer, are handled more by staff and less by their own mothers, and are less likely to be fully breast-fed.

Rotavirus is one of the most important causes of diarrhea among infants and children worldwide, occurring most commonly in infants aged 3 months to 2 years. In developing countries, an estimated 800,000 children die of rotavirus diarrhea each year and infections occur earlier in infancy.[232, 233] There are few reports of rotavirus in newborns.[234] It appears that in most cases neonatal infection is asymptomatic and that neonatal infection may protect against severe diarrhea in subsequent infections.[235, 236] Neonates are generally infected with unusual rotavirus strains that may be less virulent and may serve as natural immunogens.[237] The rate of infection among neonates may be more common than previously thought. Cicirello and associates[237] screened 169 newborns at six hospitals in Delhi, India, and found a rotavirus prevalence of 26%. Prevalence increased directly with length of hospital stay. The high prevalence of neonatal infections in Delhi (and perhaps in other developing country settings) could lead to priming of the immune system and have implications for vaccine efficacy.

Several of the community-based studies reviewed earlier present data on diarrhea as a cause of neonatal death.[40, 43, 46, 48, 50–53, 59, 60] In these studies, diarrhea was responsible for 1 to 12% of all neonatal deaths. In 9 of the 10 studies, 70 of 2673 neonatal deaths (3%) were attributed to diarrhea. Whereas diarrhea is more common in infants after 6 months of age, it is clearly a problem, with both morbidity and mortality, for neonates in developing countries. The WHO estimates that there are 4,984,000 neonatal deaths per year in the less developed regions of the world.[4] If 3% of all neonatal deaths are due to diarrhea, we estimate that approximately 150,000 neonatal deaths per year are associated with diarrhea.

OPHTHALMIA NEONATORUM

Ophthalmia neonatorum, defined as purulent conjunctivitis in the first 28 days of life, remains a common problem in many developing countries. Data on incidence and bacteriologic spectrum from specific countries are limited. Although a wide array of agents are cultured from infants with ophthalmia neonatorum (*S. aureus*, coagulase-negative *Staphylococcus*, *S. pneumoniae*, *S. pyogenes*, *Streptococcus viridans*, *Pseudomonas aeruginosa*, *K. pneumoniae*, and *E. coli*[238–241]), *Neisseria gonorrhoeae* (gonococcus), and *Chlamydia trachomatis* are the most important etiologic agents from a global perspective.[136, 241–246] The pathogenesis of infection is similar for these two agents—that is, infection is acquired from an infected mother during passage through the birth canal or via an ascending route. The etiologic agent cannot be distinguished by clinical examination: both produce a purulent conjunctivitis. However, gonococcal ophthalmia may appear earlier and is more severe than chlamydial conjunctivitis. Untreated gonococcal conjunctivitis may lead to corneal scarring and blindness, whereas the risk of severe ocular damage is low with chlamydial infection. Without ocular prophylaxis, ophthalmia neonatorum will develop in 30 to 42% of infants born to mothers with untreated *N. gonorrhoeae* infection,[242, 243, 245] and in approximately 30% of infants exposed to *Chlamydia*.[243]

The risk of infection in the neonate is directly related to the prevalence of maternal infection and the frequency of ocular prophylaxis. Infants born in areas of the world with high rates of STDs are at greatest risk. Although data from developing countries are limited,[247–249] the WHO has estimated that there are approximately 32 million new cases of gonococcal conjunctivitis and 46 million new cases of chlamydial infection among women in the world annually. The vast majority of cases occur in developing countries; areas with the highest numbers of new cases are South and Southeast Asia, sub-Saharan Africa, Latin America, and the Caribbean.[250]

Strategies to prevent or ameliorate ocular morbidity related to ophthalmia neonatorum include (1) primary prevention of STDs; (2) antenatal screening for and treatment of STDs (particularly gonorrhea and *Chlamydia*); (3) eye prophylaxis at birth; and (4) early diagnosis and treatment of ophthalmia neonatorum.[245] For developing countries, eye prophylaxis soon after birth is the most cost-effective and feasible strategy. Eye prophylaxis is used primarily to prevent gonococcal ophthalmia. Primary prevention of STDs in developing countries is limited, although promotion of condom use has been successful in reducing STDs in some countries.[251, 252] Screening women at prenatal and STD clinics and treatment based on a syndromic approach (i.e., treat for possible infections in all women with vaginal discharge without laboratory confirmation) is cost effective and promising but may lead to overtreatment of uninfected women and missed cases. Because primary infection with both *N. gonorrhoeae* and *Chlamydia* is usually asymptomatic, pregnant women need to be specifically screened for STDs to ensure early diagnosis and treatment of the mother before delivery of her neonate.

Eye prophylaxis consists of cleaning the eyelids and instilling an antimicrobial agent into the eyes as soon after birth as possible. The agent should be placed directly into the conjunctival sac (using clean hands), and the eyes should not be flushed after instillation. Infants born both vaginally and by cesarean section should receive prophylaxis. Although no agent is 100% effective at preventing disease, the use of 1% silver nitrate solution (introduced by Credé in 1881)[253] dramatically reduced the incidence of ophthalmia neonatorum. This inexpensive agent is still widely used in many parts of the world and is the most successful prophylactic antimicrobial agent in history. The major problems with silver nitrate are that it may cause chemical conjunctivitis in up to 50% of infants and that it has limited antimicrobial activity against *Chlamydia*.[244, 254, 255] In developing countries in which heat and improper storage may be a problem, evaporation and concentration are particular concerns. Although 1% tetracycline and 0.5% erythromycin ointments are commonly used in developed countries, and are as effective as silver nitrate for the prevention of gonococcal conjunctivitis, these agents are more expensive and unavailable in many parts of the world. Moreover, silver nitrate appears to be a better prophylactic agent in areas where penicillinase-producing *N. gonorrhoeae* (PPNG) is a problem.[256]

The ideal prophylactic agent for developing countries would have a broad antimicrobial spectrum and also be available and affordable. Povidone-iodine is an inexpensive, nontoxic topical agent that is potentially widely available in developing countries. Preliminary studies suggest that it may be useful in preventing ophthalmia neonatorum. A prospective masked controlled trial of ocular prophylaxis using 2.5% povidone-iodine solution, 1% silver nitrate solution, or 0.5% erythromycin ointment was conducted in Kenya.[257] Of 3117 neonates randomized to study drug, 13.1% in the povidone-iodine group versus 15.2% of those who received erythromycin and 17.5% in the silver nitrate group developed infectious conjunctivitis ($p < 0.01$). The high rates of infection in this group, despite ocular prophylaxis are striking. Whereas there was no significant difference among agents in prevention of gonococcal ophthalmia ($\leq 1\%$ for each agent), povidone-iodine was more effective than either other agent in preventing chlamydial conjunctivitis (5.5% versus 7.4% versus 10.5%—povidone-iodine versus erythromycin versus silver nitrate; $p < 0.01$). Although the antimicrobial spectrum of povidone-iodine is wider than that of other topical agents[258] and antibacterial resistance has not been demonstrated,[259] published data on the efficacy of povidone-iodine against PPNG are not yet available. Of note, 2.5% povidone-iodine might also be useful as an antimicrobial agent for cord care—of relevance to preventing omphalitis (see earlier). Further studies of the safety and efficacy of this agent are particularly important for its use in developing countries.

The efficacy of topical therapy in the prevention of chlamydial conjunctivitis is unclear. Moreover, topical prophylaxis does not prevent nasopharyngeal colonization and subsequent pneumonia.[254] Therefore, it is recommended that neonates born to mothers with untreated chlamydial infection be treated with oral erythromycin for 14 days to prevent or eradicate nasopharyngeal colonization and reduce the risk of pneumonia.[256] Unfortunately, this recommendation is impractical for many developing country settings.

The frequency of ocular prophylaxis in developing countries is unknown. Given high rates of STD among pregnant women in many developing countries, eye prophylaxis is an important blindness prevention strategy that must become part of routine neonatal care for infants born in clinics or hospitals.[242] For infants born at home, a single dose of antimicrobial agent for ocular prophylaxis should be added to traditional birth attendant or home delivery kits. The strategy of ocular prophylaxis is more cost effective than early diagnosis and appropriate treatment. Furthermore, in areas of the world in which access to medical care is limited and effective drugs are scarce or unavailable, it may be the only viable strategy.

No prevention strategy is 100% effective. Even with prophylaxis, 5 to 10% of infants will develop ophthalmia. All infants with ophthalmia must be treated—even if they received prophylaxis at birth. A single dose of either ceftriaxone (125 mg or 50 mg/kg intramuscularly) or cefotaxime (100 mg/kg intramuscularly) is effective therapy for gonococcal ophthalmia caused by both PPNG and non-PPNG strains.[256, 260, 261] Gentamicin and kanamycin have also been shown to be effective therapy and may be more readily available in some settings. Rarely, gonococcal infection acquired at birth may become disseminated, resulting in arthritis, septicemia, and even meningitis. Neonates with disseminated gonococcal disease require systemic therapy with ceftriaxone (25–50 mg/kg IV or IM once daily) or cefotaxime (50–100 mg/kg twice daily) for 7 days (arthritis, sepsis) or 10 to 14 days (meningitis). If a lumbar puncture cannot be performed (and meningitis cannot be ruled out) in an infant with evidence of dissemination, the longer period of therapy should be chosen.[256] Infants with proven or presumed chlamydial conjunctivitis should receive a 2-week course of oral erythromycin (50 mg/kg per day in four divided doses). After the immediate neonatal period, oral sulfonamides may be used, if erythromycin is unavailable or not tolerated by the infant.[256] Human milk has been used as a traditional remedy for ophthalmia neonatorum in some developing countries. An interesting study from Nigeria demonstrated that colostrum (but not mature milk) resulted in in-vitro inhibition of growth of *S. aureus* and a variety of coliform organisms.[262] Although an unorthodox therapy, use of colostrum deserves further study—especially for rural areas with limited access to health care facilities.

MALARIA

From a global perspective, malaria is one of the most important infectious diseases. More than 40% of the world's population live in areas with malaria risk. The WHO estimates that 300 to 500 million cases occur annually with 1.5 to 3 million deaths. More than half of all malaria deaths occur in children younger than 5.[263] The disease is mainly confined to poorer tropical areas of Africa, Asia, and Latin America. Countries in sub-Saharan Africa account for more than 90% of malaria cases. Each year approximately 24 million African women become pregnant in malaria-endemic areas and are at risk for malaria during pregnancy.[264] Four species of the malaria parasite infect humans: *Plasmodium falciparum, P. vivax, P. ovale, and P. malariae. P. falciparum* is responsible for the severest form of disease and is the predominant parasite in tropical Africa, Southeast Asia, the Amazon area, and Oceania. Groups at greatest risk are young nonimmune children, pregnant women (especially primigravidas), and nonimmune adults.

Malaria in Pregnancy

Preexisting levels of immunity determine susceptibility to infection and severity of disease.[264–267] In areas of high endemicity, where there are high levels of protective immunity, the effects of malaria on the mother and fetus are less severe than in areas where malaria transmission is low or unstable (i.e., sporadic, periodic). It is unclear why pregnant women (even with preexisting immunity) are at increased risk for malaria. Severe maternal complications (cerebral malaria, pulmonary edema, renal failure) occur most commonly in women with little or no immunity and are most frequent with infections due to *P. falciparum*. Severe malaria may result in pregnancy-related maternal mortality.

Malaria parasitemia is more common, and the parasite burden is higher in pregnant than in nonpregnant women.[265, 266] This increase in both prevalence and density of parasitemia is highest in primiparous women and decreases with increasing parity.[266] The parasite burden is highest in the second trimester and decreases with increasing gestation. The most important effects of malaria on pregnant women are severe anemia[265, 267–269] and placental infection.[264–267, 270, 271] A recent study highlighted the importance of *P. vivax* infection (as well as the much more studied *P. falciparum*) as a cause of pregnancy-related morbidity, including anemia.[271a] The prevalence of anemia can be as high as 78%, and anemia is more common and more severe in primigravidas.[271]

Perinatal Outcome

Perinatal outcome is directly related to placental malaria. Malaria is associated with an increase in spontaneous abortions and stillbirths,[267] particularly in areas where malaria is acquired by nonimmune women. Reported rates of fetal loss range from 9 to 50%.[266] The uteroplacental vascular space is thought to be a relatively protected site for parasite sequestration and replication.[270, 272] Placental malaria is characterized by the presence of parasites and leukocytes in the intervillous space, pigment within macrophages, proliferation of cytotrophoblasts, and thickening of the trophoblastic basement membrane.[271] Placental infection may alter the function of the placenta, reducing oxygen and nutrient transport and resulting in intrauterine growth retardation, and/or may allow the passage of infected red blood cells to the fetus, resulting in congenital infection. In primigravidas living in endemic areas, placental malaria occurs in 16 to 63% of women, whereas in multigravidas, the prevalence is much lower, 12 to 33%.[265, 266] The most profound effect of placental malaria is the reduction of birth weight.[267, 273, 274] Both *P. falciparum* and *P. vivax* infection during pregnancy are associated with a reduction in birthweight.[271a] Steketee and associates[273] have estimated that in highly endemic settings, placental malaria may account for approximately 13% of LBW secondary to intrauterine growth retardation. In Africa, malaria is thought to be an important contributor to the almost 3.5 million LBW infants born annually.[275] Importantly, malaria is one of the few preventable causes of LBW. Because LBW is a major determinant of neonatal and infant mortality in developing countries, malaria may indirectly increase mortality by increasing LBW. An important benefit of malaria prevention programs will be a reduction of LBW and LBW-associated infant mortality.[276]

Congenital Malaria

Transplacental infection of the fetus may also occur. It is relatively rare in populations with prior immunity (0.1%–1.5%)[265] but more common in nonimmune mothers. It is thought that the low rate of fetal infection in the face of a high incidence of placental infection is due in part to protection from transplacental maternal antibodies.[277, 278]

The clinical characteristics of neonates with congenital malaria (i.e., malaria parasitemia on peripheral blood smear) include fever, respiratory distress, pallor, anemia, hepatomegaly, jaundice, and diarrhea. There is a high mortality rate with congenital infection.[279] The global burden of disease related to congenital malaria is unknown.

Antimalarial Drugs in Pregnancy

Chloroquine is the safest, cheapest, most widely available antimalarial drug. It has been the drug of choice for the prevention and treatment of malaria in pregnancy.[280] However, in all areas where *P. falciparum* is prevalent, the parasite is at least partially resistant to chloroquine (Table 3–5).[263] There are a limited number of safe and effective antimalarials available for use in pregnancy. Antimalarial drug resistance, especially to chloroquine, makes policy decisions and recommendations for prophylaxis and treatment increasingly difficult.

Effect of Malaria Chemoprophylaxis on Mother and Newborn

A systematic review of randomized controlled trials of maternal chemoprophylaxis was conducted by Garner and Brabin.[281] Chemoprophylaxis with chloroquine, proguanil, and/or mefloquine is associated with reduced maternal disease, including anemia and placental infection. Placental malaria is reduced by chemoprophylaxis, even when chloroquine is used in areas with chloroquine-resistant malaria.[282] The review also demonstrated a positive effect of chemoprophylaxis on birth weight. No single study was large enough to evaluate the effect of chemoprophylaxis on perinatal mortality.

Other Malaria Control Measures

Although the benefits of antimalarial chemoprophylaxis have been established, poor compliance[283] and increasing

TABLE 3–5
Countries Reporting Chloroquine-Resistant Malaria

Sub-Saharan Africa

Angola	Liberia
Benin	Madagascar
Botswana	Malawi
Burkina Faso	Mali
Burundi	Mauritania
Cameroon	Mozambique
C. African Rep.	Namibia
Chad	Niger
Congo	Nigeria
Congo, Dem. Rep.	Rwanda
Côte d'Ivoire	Senegal
Eritrea	Sierra Leone
Ethiopia	Somalia
Gabon	South Africa
The Gambia	Tanzania
Ghana	Togo
Guinea	Uganda
Guinea-Bissau	Zambia
Kenya	Zimbabwe

Middle East and North Africa

Iran	Sudan
Oman	Yemen

Central Asia

Afghanistan

East/South Asia and Pacific

Bangladesh	Nepal
Cambodia[a]	Pakistan
China	Papua New Guinea
India	Philippines
Indonesia	Sri Lanka
Lao Rep.	Thailand[a]
Malaysia	Viet Nam
Myanmar[a]	

Americas

Bolivia	Panama
Brazil[a]	Paraguay
Colombia	Peru
Ecuador	Venezuela

[a]*P. falciparum* has widespread resistance to more than one drug.
Data from World Health Organization. International Travel and Health–Vaccination Requirements and Health Advice. Geneva, World Health Organization, 1997.
Produced from The Progress of Nations. New York, UNICEF, 1997, with permission.

drug resistance have led to trials of alternative prevention strategies. Use of insecticide-treated bed nets has been successful in reducing childhood morbidity and mortality in malaria-endemic areas.[284–286] However, the effects of bed nets on malaria in pregnancy are less promising. A study from the Thai-Myanmar border found a significant reduction in maternal anemia, with only a marginal effect on peripheral parasitemia[287]; a study from The Gambia found a reduction in severe anemia in the dry season and fewer preterm deliveries in the rainy season,[288] but studies from Ghana[289] and Kenya[290] showed no significant impact of impregnated bed nets on malaria-associated morbidity in pregnant women, including anemia and LBW. Given the number of pregnant women living in malarious areas, other control strategies are needed for this high-risk group.

SUMMARY OF THE GLOBAL BURDEN OF INFECTIOUS DISEASES AMONG NEWBORNS

Table 3–6 summarizes our estimates of the global burden for the most important neonatal infections. These estimates are based on the review of studies presented earlier and selected WHO and United Nations documents.[4, 5, 113, 207] In summary, of the estimated 126,377,000 children born in developing countries each year, more than 20% (or almost 30 million children) develop a neonatal infection and more than 1,500,000 infants die of infection in the neonatal period each year.

DIRECT AND INDIRECT CAUSES OF NEONATAL DEATH RELATED TO INFECTION

The immediate or direct medical causes of neonatal death related to infection include sepsis, meningitis, omphalitis, neonatal tetanus, pneumonia, TB, diarrhea, malaria, and HIV/AIDS. There are, however, a vast array of indirect causes for many of the infectious deaths in developing countries (Table 3–7). These contributory factors have social as well as medical roots. Sociocultural factors include poverty (not just of individuals, but of governments as well), illiteracy, low social status of women, lack of political power (for women and children) and lack of will in those who have power, gender discrimination (for both mother and neonate), harmful traditional or cultural practices, poor hygiene, lack of clean water and sanitation, the cultural belief that a sick newborn is doomed to die and is, moreover, replaceable, the family's inability to recognize danger signs in the newborn, inadequate access to high-quality medical care either because it is unavailable or because of the lack of transport for emergency care or the lack of supplies or appropriate drugs, and maternal death.[2, 3, 291, 292] Medical factors that may also contribute to an infectious neonatal death include poor maternal health, untreated maternal infections (including STDs, urinary tract infection, and chorioamnionitis), failure to fully immunize the mother against tetanus, inappropriate management of labor and delivery, unsanitary cutting and care of the umbilical cord, failure to promote early and exclusive breast-feeding, and prematurity and/or LBW.[2, 3, 5, 293, 294] To promote change, families must know enough to identify illness and must want and be able to seek care. Health care workers (of all levels) must know what to do and must have the resources to support needed therapy. Moreover, better maternal care—both preventive and curative—is preventive medicine for the newborn.

With the scientific knowledge currently available, it is possible to address the medical causes of infectious death and to make a significant impact on mortality. It is far

TABLE 3–6
Estimated Global Burden of Disease—Major Neonatal Infections

INFECTION	ESTIMATED NO. CASES	ESTIMATED CASE-FATALITY RATE (%)	ESTIMATED NO. DEATHS
Neonatal sepsis	750,000	40	300,000
Neonatal meningitis	126,000	40	50,400
Neonatal tetanus	400,000	85	340,000
Acute respiratory infection	2,650,000	30	800,000
Diarrhea	25,000,000	0.6	150,000
Human immunodeficiency virus	550,000	?[a]	?[a]
Total	29,476,000		1,640,400

[a]Data unavailable: Most HIV-related deaths occur after the neonatal period.
Adapted from Stoll BJ. The global impact of neonatal infection. Clin Perinatol 24:1–21, 1997, with permission.

harder to address and solve the sociocultural factors that, in some settings, make a medical approach to preventing and treating these diseases impossible. Coordinated activities are needed to bring about change that is sustainable by countries on their own, over the long haul. This will involve a multidisciplinary approach—bringing together people with different interests, from different backgrounds, different agencies, different government ministries—to seek solutions to problems and to implement change at the local level. Finally, it will involve the global acknowledgment that this is the right thing to do (i.e., a moral imperative) and, therefore, the long-term commitment of substantial funding to help provide needed services to poor countries. The challenge for the next decade is to link science and medicine with social solutions through a global commitment to long-term, long-lasting change so that improvements in both maternal and newborn health can be achieved and sustained.

STRATEGIES TO REDUCE INFECTION IN THE NEONATE AND TO REDUCE INFECTION-ASSOCIATED MORTALITY

Strategies to prevent or reduce neonatal infections and to reduce morbidity and mortality in those newborns

TABLE 3–7
Direct and Indirect Causes of Neonatal Death Related to Infections in Less Developed Countries

DIRECT CAUSES OF DEATH	INDIRECT CAUSES OF DEATH
Medical	**Sociocultural**
Sepsis	Poverty
Meningitis	Illiteracy
Omphalitis with sepsis	Low social status of women
Tetanus	Lack of political power
Pneumonia	Gender discrimination (for mother and newborn)
Tuberculosis	Harmful traditional practices
Diarrhea	Poor hygiene
Malaria	Lack of clean water and sanitation
HIV/AIDS	Cultural belief that a sick newborn is doomed to die
	Inability to recognize danger signs in sick newborn
	Poor care-seeking behavior
	Inadequate access to high quality medical care
	Lack of transport for emergency care
	Lack of appropriate drugs
	Maternal death
	Medical
	Poor maternal health
	Untreated maternal infections including sexually transmitted diseases, urinary tract infection, chorioamnionitis
	Failure to fully immunize mother against tetanus
	Inappropriate management of labor and delivery
	Unsanitary cutting and care of the umbilical cord
	Failure to promote early and exclusive breast feeding (HIV dilemma noted)
	Prematurity/low birth weight

Adapted from Stoll BJ. The global impact of neonatal infection. Clin Perinatol 24:1–21, 1997, with permission.

who develop infection involve putting into practice what is known and inventing creative ways to make these interventions workable in a developing country context. Use of simple, cost-effective technologies that are potentially available at the village or district hospital level could have a major impact in reducing morbidity and mortality related to neonatal infection. Moreover, public health, medical, and social interventions all have a role to play in reducing the global burden of neonatal infection. Several potential interventions are reviewed here (Table 3–8).

Maternal Immunization to Prevent Neonatal Disease

There is growing interest in the possibility of using maternal immunization to protect neonates and very young infants from infection through passively acquired transplacental or breast milk antibodies, or both.[295] Immunization of pregnant women with tetanus toxoid has dramatically reduced cases of neonatal tetanus and is the classic example of maternal immunization and subsequent passive immunization to protect the newborn. Because most IgG antibody is transported across the placenta in the last 4 to 6 weeks of pregnancy, maternal immunization to prevent neonatal disease through transplacental antibodies is most promising for term newborns who will have adequate antibody levels at birth. By contrast, this strategy will be less successful for preterm infants because of insufficient passage of maternal antibodies. Boosting breast milk antibodies by immunizing the mother is a potential strategy for reducing infection in both term and preterm infants. Vaccines being currently developed or field tested to reduce or prevent neonatal infection by passive immunization include vaccines against GBS, *S. pneumoniae*, and *Haemophilus influenzae*.[296–301]

Because most neonatal GBS disease—especially that which is most severe—occurs in the first hours of life, maternal immunization to provide passive protection to the neonate is a potentially important strategy. A problem with GBS vaccines has been poor immunogenicity. Recent studies have focused on the immunogenicity of polysaccharide-protein conjugate vaccines and suggest that conjugate vaccines may be highly effective in pregnant women.[297] Multivalent vaccines, which could provide protection against multiple GBS serotypes, are particularly promising.

Pneumococcal polysaccharide vaccines have been administered safely to pregnant women.[298, 299] One study from Bangladesh reported that pneumococcal vaccination during pregnancy increased type-specific IgG serum antibody in both mother and infant.[298] Cord blood levels of antibody were about half those of the mother, with IgG1 subclass antibodies preferentially transferred to the infant. The estimated antibody half-life in the infant was 35 days. Immunization increased breast milk antibody as well. If passive immunization does not interfere with active immunization of young infants, vaccination of pregnant women could be used to prevent pneumococcal disease in early infancy. The recent finding from the WHO young infant study that *S. pneumoniae* is an

TABLE 3–8

Interventions to Reduce Neonatal Infections or to Reduce Infection-Associated Mortality in Developing Countries

Antenatal Care
Tetanus immunization
Maternal immunization with new vaccines in the future (e.g., group B streptococci, *Haemophilus influenzae* type b, pneumococcus)
Primary prevention of sexually transmitted diseases, including HIV, through maternal education and safer sex using condoms
Diagnosis and treatment of sexually transmitted diseases, urinary tract infection, malaria, tuberculosis, other infections
Plan clean and safe delivery

Intrapartum/Delivery Care
Prevent prolonged labor
Optimal management of complications, including fever, premature rupture of membranes, puerperal sepsis
Clean delivery
Clean cutting of cord/optimal cord care

Breast-feeding
Promote early and exclusive breast-feeding (HIV dilemma noted)

Gender Issues
Promote gender equality
Encourage education of girls

Interventions to Decrease Low Birth Weight and/or Prematurity
Delay childbearing in young adolescents
Promote maternal education
Improve maternal nutrition: caloric supplementation before and during pregnancy
Reduce tobacco use
Diagnose and treat sexually transmitted diseases
Malaria prophylaxis and treatment
Limit maternal work load during pregnancy
Maternal support to decrease stress/anxiety

Community-Based Interventions
Train birth attendants to identify problems in the newborn, treat simple problems, refer newborns with serious illness
Promote and support breastfeeding (HIV dilemma noted)
Maternal education regarding personal and domestic hygiene, newborn care, childhood immunization
Home-based diagnosis and treatment of newborn infections

Early Identification and Improved Treatment of Neonates with Infection
Integrated approach to the sick young infant (WHO/UNICEF)
Improve newborn care at all levels: home, village, health center, district hospital, referral hospital

Neonatal Immunization
Bacillus Calmette-Guérin, hepatitis B, other new vaccines (e.g., rotavirus)

Adapted from Stoll BJ. The global impact of neonatal infection. Clin Perinatol 24:1–21, 1997, with permission.

important cause of sepsis and meningitis in young infants[132] supports the continued investigation of maternal immunization with pneumococcal vaccines as a prevention strategy for developing countries.

In developed countries, invasive disease resulting from

H. influenzae type b (HIB) has been almost completely eliminated by the use of HIB conjugate vaccines.[302] However, in many parts of the world, HIB remains an important cause of life-threatening infections in infancy, particularly pneumonia and meningitis. Although HIB infection is rare in the neonatal period, approximately 40% of HIB disease in developing countries occurs in infants younger than 6 months.[303, 304] Both neonatal and maternal immunization strategies are being explored to target populations in which HIB infections occur in young infants.[295, 300, 301] A study from The Gambia[300] showed that maternal immunization with HIB polysaccharide-tetanus protein conjugate vaccine increased both maternal and neonatal antibody concentrations. At 2 months of age, 60% of infants of vaccinated mothers had antibody concentrations considered to be protective.

Further studies of the safety, efficacy, and effectiveness of immunizing pregnant women with specific vaccines are needed. They must address issues of safety to the mother, fetus, and young infant. Furthermore, they must assess protection against specific diseases (e.g., sepsis, pneumonia, meningitis) as well as protection against all causes of neonatal and infant mortality. The subsequent response of the infant to active immunization must also be evaluated, to ensure that passive immunization does not interfere with the infant's ability to mount an immune response. Therefore, in developing countries, studies must be carried out in settings where it is possible to maintain surveillance throughout infancy.

Neonatal Immunization

The bacillus Calmette-Guérin (BCG) vaccine, developed early in this century, is a live attenuated strain of *Mycobacterium bovis*. The WHO promotes the use of BCG in newborns to prevent TB, and this vaccine is widely used in developing countries in which TB is a common and potentially lethal disease. Although approximately 3 billion doses have been given, the efficacy of this vaccine is still debated. Vaccine efficacy in many prospective trials and case-control studies of vaccine use at all ages ranges from possibly harmful to 90% protective.[305] One meta-analysis of BCG studies in newborns and infants concluded that the vaccine was effective and reduced infection in children by more than 50%.[306] BCG reduced the risk of pulmonary TB, TB meningitis, disseminated TB, and death from TB. Factors that may explain the variability of responses to BCG vaccination in different studies/populations include use of a wide variety of vaccine preparations, regional differences in environmental flora that may alter vaccine response, and population differences.[295] The safety of BCG in immunocompromised patients (e.g., those with HIV) is unclear.

Hepatitis B vaccination of newborns has proved that neonatal immunization can prevent neonatal infections and their sequelae.[307] Studies from both developed and developing countries have shown that hepatitis B vaccine administered in the immediate newborn period can significantly reduce the rate of neonatal infection and the development of a chronic HB_sAg carrier state.[308] The efficacy of vaccine alone (without HBIG) has allowed developing countries that cannot screen pregnant women and do not have HBIG to make a major impact in reducing the infection of newborns. Recently, the WHO recommended that all countries add hepatitis B vaccine to their routine childhood immunization programs.[309] In addition, studies of neonatal immunization with polio vaccine, HIB conjugate vaccines, and pneumococcal conjugate vaccines suggest some protection with neonatal vaccination that might reduce but not eliminate disease.[295]

Rotavirus diarrhea is a major killer of young infants in developing countries, causing approximately 800,000 childhood deaths per year. The development of a live oral quadrivalent rhesus rotavirus vaccine, which has been shown to be highly effective in young infants, particularly at preventing severe disease, is exciting and potentially very important.[310] Additional studies in developing countries are needed before rotavirus vaccines can be added to routine childhood vaccination programs. The quadrivalent rhesus rotavirus vaccine, highly effective in preventing severe disease in Venezuelan children,[311] has never been tested in African or Asian children. Factors that might influence efficacy in developing countries include younger age of infection, potentially larger viral inoculum, presence of different or unusual strains of rotavirus, and poorer nutritional status.[232] Unlike children in developed countries, in developing countries children experience most severe episodes of rotavirus diarrhea in the first year of life. Vaccines will need to be delivered early—perhaps at birth. Further studies on the safety and efficacy of rotavirus vaccine in neonates are needed.[237, 310]

With the global problem of increasing antibiotic resistance, maternal and neonatal immunization have become even more important strategies to pursue. In developing countries, issues of vaccine cost, availability, and efficacy in the field are particularly pressing and are major barriers to the use of vaccines that are known to be safe and effective in developed countries. Efforts to reduce vaccine cost by studying lower doses of vaccine and use of single-dose vials for multiple-dose use are promising.[312] Ultimately, the reduction of vaccine cost is in the hands of vaccine manufacturers.

Role of Antenatal Care in the Prevention of Neonatal Infection

The care and general well-being of the mother is inextricably linked to the health of her newborn. Antenatal care can play an important role in the prevention or reduction of neonatal infections.[313] Both preventive and curative interventions directed toward the mother can have beneficial effects on the fetus or newborn or both. Tetanus immunization of the pregnant woman is an essential component of any developing country antenatal care program and, as discussed earlier, will prevent neonatal tetanus.[294, 314] The diagnosis and treatment of STDs—especially syphilis, gonorrhea, and chlamydia—can have a significant impact on neonatal morbidity and mortality.[247, 248, 293, 315] In areas of the world in which syphilis is endemic, congenital syphilis may be a major cause of neonatal morbidity and mortality.[315] Antenatal treatment of gonorrhea and chlamydia can prevent neonatal infection with these agents—ophthalmia neonatorum (for gonorrhea and chlamydia), disseminated gonorrhea, and neonatal respiratory disease (for chlamydia).[247, 248, 293] Moreover, STDs and maternal urinary tract infection increase the mother's risk of puerperal sepsis with its associated increased risk of neonatal sepsis. In malaria-endemic areas, treatment of maternal malaria can have an impact on newborn health, particularly through a reduction in the incidence of LBW.[293, 316]

Antenatal care is also an important setting for maternal education regarding danger signs during pregnancy, labor, and delivery—especially maternal fever, prolonged or premature rupture of the membranes, and prolonged labor—and danger signs to watch for in the newborn. Moreover, it is the time and place for the mother to plan where and by whom she will be delivered and to stress the importance of a clean delivery.

Role of Intrapartum and Delivery Care in the Prevention of Neonatal Infection

It is universally recognized that poor aseptic techniques during labor and delivery, including unclean hands, unclean instruments, and unhygienic cutting of the umbilical cord are major risk factors for both maternal and neonatal infections.[313] It is essential to promote safe and hygienic practices at every level of the health care system where women deliver (i.e., home, health center, district or referral hospital). Proper management of labor and delivery can have a significant impact on the prevention of neonatal infection. It is important to emphasize the need for clean hands, clean perineum, clean delivery surface, clean instruments, clean cord care, use of an appropriate clean delivery kit, avoidance of harmful traditional practices, prevention of unnecessary vaginal examinations, prevention of prolonged labor, and optimal management of pregnancy complications including prolonged rupture of the membranes, maternal fever, and chorioamnionitis/puerperal sepsis.[5]

If the mother does develop a puerperal infection, the newborn requires special attention and should be treated for presumed sepsis.[313] Prolonged rupture of the membranes, maternal fever during labor, and chorioamnionitis are particular risk factors for early-onset neonatal sepsis and pneumonia in both developed and developing countries.[317–319] Ideally, high-risk infants who are born at home should be referred to the nearest health care facility for observation and antibiotic therapy. In practice this may be either impossible or unacceptable to the family, and ways to deliver care to the mother and newborn in the home must be developed and evaluated. The traditional birth attendant or other health care worker who attends the birth has a critical role to play in the early health of the newborn.

Breast-Feeding

The promotion of early and exclusive breast-feeding is one of the most important interventions for the maintenance of newborn health and the promotion of optimal growth and development.[5] Breast-feeding is especially important in developing countries, where safe alternatives to breast milk are often unavailable or too expensive. Moreover, poor hygiene and a lack of clean water and clean feeding utensils make artificial formula an important vehicle for the transmission of infection. Breast milk has many unique anti-infective factors, including secretory immunoglobulin A antibodies, lysozyme, and lactoferrin. In addition, breast milk is rich in receptor analogues for certain epithelial structures that microorganisms need for attachment to host tissues, an initial step in infection.[320] Many studies have shown that breast-feeding reduces the risk of infectious diseases, including neonatal sepsis, diarrhea, and possibly respiratory tract infection.[119, 227, 321–325] Moreover, there is evidence that breast-feeding protects against infection-related neonatal and infant mortality.[326–329] The HIV epidemic has raised questions about the safety of breast-feeding in areas in which there is a high prevalence of HIV infection among lactating women.[182–188, 191, 330, 331] HIV may be transmitted through breast-feeding. A major question for any setting is whether the benefits of breast-feeding outweigh the risk of postnatal transmission of HIV via breast milk.[331] For many areas of the world, where infectious diseases, especially diarrheal diseases, are a primary cause of infant death, breast-feeding, even when the mother is HIV infected, remains the safest mode of infant feeding. Countries with high and low reported rates of exclusive breast-feeding are listed in Table 3–9.[263]

Maternal Education and Socioeconomic Status

Maternal education, literacy, and overall socioeconomic status are powerful influences on the health of both

TABLE 3–9
Breast-Feeding Rates in Developing Countries[a]

EXCLUSIVE BREAST-FEEDING RATES OF 10% OR LESS		EXCLUSIVE BREAST-FEEDING RATES OF 50% OR MORE	
Country	%	Country	%
Niger	1	Rwanda	90
Nigeria	2	Burundi	89
Angola	3	Ethiopia	74
Côte d'Ivoire	3	Tanzania	73
Haiti	3	Uganda	70
Central African Rep.	4	Egypt	68
Thailand	4	Eritrea	65
Cameroon	7	China	64
Paraguay	7	Mauritania	60
Maldives	8	Bangladesh	54
Senegal	9	Turkmenistan	54
Dominican Rep.	10	Bolivia	53
Togo	10	Iran	53
Trinidad/Tobago	10	India	51
		Guatemala	50

[a]Data refer to infants younger than 4 months of age.
From DHS MICS and other nationwide surveys, 1987–1996.
Reproduced from The Progress of Nations. New York, UNICEF, 1997, with permission.

mother and newborn.[332–335] Education of girls must be promoted and expanded so that women of reproductive age know enough to seek preventive services, understand the implications of danger signs during labor and delivery and in their newborns, and know that they must obtain referral care for obstetric or newborn complications, or both. Improvements in education and socioeconomic status are obviously linked. They may affect child health by allowing the mother a greater voice in the family with greater decision-making power, making her better informed about domestic hygiene, disease prevention, or disease recognition, or enhancing her ability to seek medical attention outside the home and to comply with medical advice.

Low Birth Weight and Prematurity

Infants who have birth weights of 2500 g or less are a major public health problem. Worldwide approximately 90% of LBW infants are born in developing countries.[336] LBW is caused by impaired fetal growth, by shortened gestation, or by a combination of both. In developing countries, LBW is more frequently caused by intrauterine growth retardation than by prematurity.[275, 336] There are data to suggest that both preterm and LBW infants are at increased risk for infection and infection-related mortality.[131, 337, 338] Therefore, strategies to reduce LBW and prematurity could have a measurable impact on neonatal infection. Potential interventions to improve intrauterine growth or to lengthen gestation, or both, include delayed childbearing in adolescents, improved maternal education, caloric supplementation before and during pregnancy, general improvements in nutrition, malaria prophylaxis or treatment, treatment of STDs and other maternal infections, efforts to reduce tobacco use, improved water and sanitation, limitation of maternal work during pregnancy, and general improvement in socioeconomic conditions.[275]

Community-Based Interventions

In parts of the world in which the majority of births occur at home, primary health care at the village level will need to put added emphasis on care of the newborn. The birth attendant is responsible for observation of the newborn at and after birth and deciding that the newborn is healthy and ready to be "discharged" to the care of the mother. It is important to link postpartum care of the mother with surveillance and care of the newborn. The postpartum visit should be used to detect and treat the sick newborn as well as to evaluate the mother. Birth attendants need to be trained to identify problems in the newborn, to treat simple problems (e.g., skin infections), and to refer those that are potentially life-threatening (e.g., suspected sepsis). Moreover, they should provide all new mothers with breast-feeding support and give advice regarding personal hygiene/cleanliness and other prevention strategies such as immunization. Improvement in domestic hygiene should be encouraged, including sanitary disposal of wastes, use of clean water, and hand washing—so that the newborn enters a clean home and is less likely to encounter pathogenic organisms. In some settings, families will refuse to take even a sick newborn to hospital and care will need to be brought into the village or home. Community interventions need to be designed and modified to meet the needs of mothers and newborns in different settings in different countries and need further evaluation.

Early Identification and Improved Treatment of Neonates with Infection

If untreated, infections in newborns can rapidly become severe and life threatening. Therefore, early identification and treatment of the infected newborn is essential. It is important to treat localized infections (e.g., skin, umbilical, or ear infections) before they become systemic. Mothers, birth attendants, and other health care workers and family members must be educated so that they can identify danger signs in the newborn and understand that prompt and appropriate therapy may make the difference between life and death. An integrated approach to the sick child, including sick young infants, has been developed by the WHO and UNICEF.[339] This strategy promotes prompt recognition of disease, appropriate therapy using standardized case management, referral of serious cases, and prevention through improved nutrition (breast-feeding of the neonate) and immunization. This approach stresses diagnosis using simple clinical signs that can be taught to health care workers at all levels. The health care worker assesses the child by questioning the mother and examining the child, classifies the illness as serious or not, and determines if the infant needs urgent treatment and referral, specific treatment and advice, or only simple advice and home management. Breast-feeding is stressed, and follow-up instructions are given. All young infants are checked for specific danger signs that equate with need for emergency care and urgent referral. Because the signs of serious bacterial infection in the newborn cannot easily be distinguished, every young infant with danger signs is treated for a possible bacterial infection. All newborns with suspected severe infection receive antibiotics as soon as possible and are then referred to hospital. In situations where referral is impossible or unacceptable to the family, community-based interventions must be designed, implemented, and evaluated.

CONCLUSION

The 1996 World Health Report[3] highlights the global importance of infectious diseases, especially among young children, and stresses the impact of new or emerging diseases. Neonatal infections are old diseases. Furthermore, each infection-related death should be considered a potentially preventable death. What is needed is a new recognition that they are important causes of morbidity and mortality and that simple interventions are available that can make a significant impact on reducing both the incidence of infection and death related to infection in developing countries.

References

1. World Health Report 1998. Geneva, World Health Organization, 1998.
2. The State of the World's Children. UNICEF. New York, Oxford University Press, 1995.
3. World Health Report 1996: fighting disease, fostering development. Geneva, World Health Organization, 1996.
4. World Health Organization. Perinatal mortality: A listing of available information. Geneva, World Health Organization, 1996.
5. Mother-Baby Package: Implementing safe motherhood in countries. WHO/FHE/MSM/94. 11.
6. Stoll BJ. The global impact of neonatal infection. Clin Perinatol 24:1–21, 1997.
7. Adeyokunnu AA, Taiwo O, Antia AU. Childhood mortality among 22,255 consecutive admissions in the University College Hospital, Ibadan. Niger J Paediatr 7:7–15, 1980.
8. Agarwal VK, Gupta SC, Chowdhary SR, et al. Some observations on perinatal mortality. Indian Pediatr 19:233–238, 1982.
9. Aiken CGA. The causes of perinatal mortality in Bulawayo, Zimbabwe. Cent Afr J Med 38:263–281, 1992.
10. Baja-Panlilio H, Cabigas-Resurreccion J, Matanguihan AT, et al. Perinatal morbidity and mortality in the Philippines. Asia-Oceania J Obstet Gynaecol 12:331–339, 1986.
11. Boo NY, Nasri NM, Cheong SK, et al. A 2-year study of neonatal mortality in a large Malaysian Hospital. Singapore Med J 32:142–147, 1991.
12. Chaturvedi P, Potdar S. Change in neonatal care pattern and neonatal mortality in a rural medical college. Indian Pediatr 25:171–178, 1988.
13. Dawodu AH, Umran KA, Faraidy AA. Neonatal vital statistics: a 5-year review in Saudi Arabia. Ann Trop Paediatr 8:187–192, 1988.
14. Dommisse J. The causes of perinatal deaths in the Greater Cape Town area: a 12-month survey. S Afr Med J 80:270–275, 1991.
15. Dutta D, Bhattacharya MK, Bhattacharya SK, et al. Influence of admission weight on neonatal mortality amongst hospitalised neonates in Calcutta. J Indian Med Assoc 90:308–309, 1992.
16. Geetha T, Chenoy R, Stevens D, et al. A multicentre study of perinatal mortality in Nepal. Paediatr Perinat Epidemiol 9:74–89, 1995.
17. Gupta PK, Gupta AP. Perinatal mortality. Indian Pediatr 22:201–205, 1985.
18. Horpaopan S, Ratrisawasdi V, Vichitpahanakarn P, et al. Perinatal mortality at Children's and Rajvithi Hospitals in 1983–1987. J Med Assoc Thai 72:376–381, 1989.
19. Hotrakitya S, Tejavej A, Siripoonya P. Early neonatal mortality and causes of death in Ramathibodi Hospital: 1981–1990. J Med Assoc Thai 76:119–129, 1993.
20. Kazimoto TPK. Review of perinatal mortality at Muhimbili maternity block. J Gynecol East Cent Afr 1:105–108, 1982.
21. Maouris P. Reducing perinatal mortality in Vila Central Hospital, Vanuatu. PNG Med J 37:178–180, 1994.
22. Njokanma OF, Olanrewaju DM. A study of neonatal deaths at the Ogun State University Teaching Hospital, Sagamu, Nigeria. J Trop Med Hyg 98:155–160, 1995.
23. Njokanma OF, Sule-Odu AO, Akesode FA. Perinatal mortality at the Ogun State University Teaching Hospital, Sagamu, Nigeria. J Trop Pediatr 40:78–81, 1994.
24. Okolo AA, Omene JA. Trends in neonatal mortality in Benin City, Nigeria. Int J Gynaecol Obstet 23:191–195, 1985.
25. Oyedeji GA, Olamijulo SK, Joiner KT. Experience at Wesley: 1,391 consecutive admissions into the neonatal unit (Hurford Ward). J Trop Pediatr 29:206–212, 1983.
26. Panja S, Bhattacharyya I, Das Gupta M. Low birth weight infants—study of mortality. Indian Pediatr 21:201–205, 1984.
27. Pengsa K, Taksaphan S. Perinatal mortality at Srinagarind Hospital. J Med Assoc Thai 70:667–672, 1987.
28. Sangamnerkar M, Sutaria UD, Shrotri AN. Pattern of neonatal mortality in a government teaching institute. Asia-Oceania J Obstet Gynaecol 14:219–225, 1988.
29. Santhanakrishnan BR, Gopal S, Jayam S. Perinatal mortality in a referral teaching hospital in Madras city. Indian J Pediatr 53:359–363, 1986.
30. Singh M. Hospital-based data on perinatal and neonatal mortality in India. Indian Pediatr 23:579–584, 1986.
31. Singh M, Deorari AK, Khajuria RC, et al. Perinatal and neonatal mortality in a hospital. Indian J Med Res 94:1–5, 1991.
32. Siripoonya P, Tejavej A, Boonpasat Y. Early neonatal mortality at Ramathibodi Hospital: 1969–1978. J Med Assoc Thai 64:546–549, 1981.
33. Vince JD. Neonatal care in perspective: results of neonatal care at Port Moresby. Papua New Guinea Med J 30:127–134, 1987.
34. Bang AT, Bang RA, Sontakke PG, & the SEARCH team. Management of childhood pneumonia by traditional birth attendants. Bull World Health Organ 72:897–905, 1994.
35. Barros FC, Victora CG, Vaughan JP, et al. Perinatal mortality in southern Brazil: a population-based study of 7392 births. Bull World Health Organ 65:95–104, 1987.
36. Bartlett AV, Paz de Bocaletti ME. Intrapartum and neonatal mortality in a traditional indigenous community in rural Guatemala. Acta Paediatr Scand 80:288–296, 1991.
37. Bartlett AV, Paz de Bocaletti ME, Bocaletti MA. Neonatal and early postneonatal morbidity and mortality in a rural Guatemalan community: the importance of infectious diseases and their management. Pediatr Infect Dis J. 10:752–757, 1991.
38. Ben-Li L, Dao-zhong Z, Hong-qi T, et al. Perinatal mortality rate in 11 Jiangsu cities. Chin Med J 98:157–160, 1985.
39. Bhardwaj N, Hasan SB. High perinatal and neonatal mortality in rural India. J R Soc Health 113:60–63, 1993.
40. Bhatia S. Patterns and causes of neonatal and postneonatal mortality in rural Bangladesh. Stud Fam Plann 20:136–146, 1989.
41. Bourne DE, Rip MR, Woods DL. Characteristics of infant mortality in the RSA 1929–1983: II. Causes of death among white and coloured infants. S Afr Med J 73:230–232, 1988.
42. Choudhary SR, Jayaswal ON. Infant and early childhood mortality in urban slums under ICDS scheme—a prospective study. Indian Pediatr 26:544–549, 1989.
43. De Francisco A, Hall AJ, Armstrong Schellenberg JRM, et al. The pattern of infant and childhood mortality in Upper River Division, The Gambia. Ann Trop Paediatr 13:345–352, 1993.
44. Fauveau V, Wojtyniak B, Mostafa G, et al. Perinatal mortality in Matlab, Bangladesh: a community-based study. Int J Epidemiol 19:606–612, 1990.
45. Fonseka P, Wijewardene K, Harendra de Silva DG, et al. Neonatal and post-neonatal mortality in the Galle district. Ceylon Med J 39:82–85, 1994.

46. Garg SK, Mishra VN, Singh JV, et al. Neonatal mortality in Meerut district. Indian J Med Sci 47:222–225, 1993.

47. Greenwood AM, Greenwood BM, Bradley AK, et al. A prospective survey of the outcome of pregnancy in a rural area of The Gambia. Bull World Health Organ 65:635–643, 1987.

48. Islam MS, Rahaman MM, Aziz KMS, et al. Infant mortality in rural Bangladesh: an analysis of causes during neonatal and postneonatal periods. J Trop Pediatr 28:294–298, 1982.

49. Jalil F, Lindblad BS, Hanson LA, et al. Early child health in Lahore, Pakistan: IX. Perinatal events. Acta Paediatr 390(Suppl):95–107, 1993.

50. Kandeh BS. Causes of infant and early childhood deaths in Sierra Leone. Soc Sci Med 23:297–303, 1986.

51. Khan SR, Jalil F, Zaman S, et al. Early child health in Lahore, Pakistan: X. Mortality. Acta Paediatr 390(Suppl):109–177, 1993.

52. Knobel RH, Yang WS, Ho MS. Urban-rural and regional differences in infant mortality in Taiwan. Soc Sci Med 39:815–822, 1994.

53. Kumar V, Datta N, Saini SS. Infant mortality in a rural community development block in Haryana. Indian J Pediatr 49:795–802, 1982.

54. Moir JS, Garner PA, Heywood PF, et al. Mortality in a rural area of Madang Province, Papua New Guinea. Ann Trop Med Parasitol 83:305–319, 1989.

55. Rahman S, Nessa F. Neonatal mortality patterns in rural Bangladesh. J Trop Pediatr 35:199–202, 1989.

56. Rip MR, Bourne DE, Woods DL. Characteristics of infant mortality in the RSA 1929–1983: I. Components of the white and coloured infant mortality rate. S Afr Med J 73:227–229, 1988.

57. Shah U, Pratinidhi AK, Bhatlawande PV. Perinatal mortality in rural India: intervention through primary health care: II. Neonatal mortality. J Epidemiol Commun Health 38:138–142, 1984.

58. Singhal PK, Mathur GP, Mathur S, et al. Perinatal mortality: in ICDS urban slum area. Indian Pediatr 23:339–343, 1986.

59. Singhal PK, Mathur GP, Mathur S, et al. Neonatal morbidity and mortality in ICDS urban slums. Indian Pediatr 27:485–488, 1990.

60. Sivagnanasundram C, Sivarajah N, Wijayaratnam A. Infant deaths in a health unit area of Northern Sri Lanka. J Trop Med Hyg 88:401–406, 1985.

61. Taha TE, Gray RH, Abdelwahab MM. Determinants of neonatal mortality in central Sudan. Ann Trop Paediatr 13:359–364, 1993.

62. Thora S, Awadhiya S, Chansoriya M, et al. Perinatal and infant mortality in urban slums under I.C.D.S. scheme. Indian Pediatr 23:595–598, 1986.

63. Urrutia JJ, Sosa R, Kennell JH, et al. Prevalence of maternal and neonatal infections in a developing country: possible low-cost preventive measures. In Perinatal Infections, vol 77. Amsterdam, Ciba Foundation Symposium, 1980, pp 171–186.

64. Woodruff AW, Adamson EA, El-Suni A, et al. Infants in Juba, Southern Sudan: the first six months of life. Lancet 2:262–264, 1983.

65. Adhikari M, Coovadia YM, Singh D. A 4-year study of neonatal meningitis: clinical and microbiological findings. J Trop Pediatr 41:81–85, 1995.

66. Airede AI. Neonatal bacterial meningitis in the middle belt of Nigeria. Dev Med Child Neurol 35:424–430, 1993.

67. Airede AK. Neonatal septicaemia in an African city of high altitude. J Trop Pediatr 38:189–191, 1992.

68. Ali Z. Neonatal meningitis: a 3-year retrospective study at the Mount Hope Women's Hospital, Trinidad, West Indies. J Trop Pediatr 41:109–111, 1995.

69. Bhutta ZA, Naqvi SH, Muzaffar T, et al. Neonatal sepsis in Pakistan: presentation and pathogens. Acta Paediatr Scand 80:596–601, 1991.

70. Boo NY, Chor CY. Six year trend of neonatal septicaemia in a large Malaysian maternity hospital. J Paediatr Child Health 30:23–27, 1994.

71. Chotpitayasunondh T. Bacterial meningitis in children: etiology and clinical features, an 11-year review of 618 cases. Southeast Asian J Trop Med Public Health 25:107–115, 1994.

72. Chugh K, Aggarwal BB, Kaul VK, et al. Bacteriological profile of neonatal septicemia. Indian J Pediatr 55:961–965, 1988.

73. Coovadia YM, Mayosi B, Adhikari M, et al. Hospital-acquired neonatal bacterial meningitis: the impacts of cefotaxime usage on mortality and of amikacin usage on incidence. Ann Trop Paediatr 9:233–239, 1989.

74. Daoud AS, Abuekteish F, Obeidat A, et al. The changing face of neonatal septicaemia. Ann Trop Paediatr 15:93–96, 1995.

75. Dawodu AH, Ashiru JO. The changing pattern of causative bacterial organisms in neonatal meningitis. Niger J Paediatr 10:1–5, 1983.

76. Elzouki AY, Vesikari T. First international conference on infections in children in Arab countries. Pediatr Infect Dis J 4:527–531, 1985.

77. Gupta PK, Murali MV, Faridi MM, et al. Clinical profile of Klebsiella septicemia in neonates. Indian J Pediatr 60:565–572, 1993.

78. Haffejee IE, Bhana RH, Coovadia YM, et al. Neonatal group B streptococcal infections in Indian (Asian) babies in South Africa. J Infect 22:225–231, 1991.

79. Haque KN, Chagia AH, Shaheed MM. Half a decade of neonatal sepsis, Riyadh, Saudi Arabia. J Trop Pediatr 36:20–23, 1990.

80. Khatua SP, Das AK, Chatterjee BD, et al. Neonatal septicemia. Indian J Pediatr 53:509–514, 1986.

81. Koutouby A, Habibullah J. Neonatal sepsis in Dubai, United Arab Emirates. J Trop Pediatr 41:177–180, 1995.

82. Kuruvilla AC. Neonatal septicaemia in Kuwait. J Kwt Med Assoc 14:225–231, 1980.

83. Lim NL, Wong YH, Boo NY, et al. Bacteraemic infections in a neonatal intensive care unit—a nine-month survey. Med J Malaysia 50:59–63, 1995.

84. Longe AC, Omene JA, Okolo AA. Neonatal meningitis in Nigerian infants. Acta Paediatr Scand 73:477–481, 1984.

85. Mondal GP, Raghavan M, Vishnu BB, et al. Neonatal septicaemia among inborn and outborn babies in a referral hospital. Indian J Pediatr 58:529–533, 1991.

86. Moreno MT, Vargas S, Poveda R, et al. Neonatal sepsis and meningitis in a developing Latin American country. Pediatr Infect Dis J 13:516–520, 1994.

87. Namdeo UK, Singh HP, Rajput VJ, et al. Bacteriological profile of neonatal septicemia. Indian Pediatr 24:53–56, 1987.

88. Nathoo KJ, Mason PR, Chimbira THK, and the Puerperal Sepsis Study Group. Neonatal septicaemia in Harare Hospital: aetiology and risk factors. Cent Afr J Med 36:150–156, 1990.

89. Nathoo KJ, Pazvakavamba I, Chidede OS, et al. Neonatal meningitis in Harare, Zimbabwe: a 2-year review. Ann Trop Paediatr 11:11–15, 1991.

90. Ohlsson A, Bailey T, Takieddine F. Changing etiology

and outcome of neonatal septicemia in Riyadh, Saudi Arabia. Acta Paediatr Scand 75:540–544, 1986.

91. Ohlsson A, Serenius F. Neonatal septicemia in Riyadh, Saudi Arabia. Acta Paediatr Scand 70:825–829, 1981.

92. Okolo AA, Omene JA. Changing pattern of neonatal septicaemia in an African city. Ann Trop Paediatr 5:123–126, 1985.

93. Owa JA, Olusanya O. Neonatal bacteraemia in Wesley Guild Hospital, Ilesha, Nigeria. Ann Trop Paediatr 8:80–84, 1988.

94. Prasertsom W, Ratrisawadi V, Thanasophon Y, et al. Early versus late onset neonatal septicemia at Children's Hospital. J Med Assoc Thai 73:106–109, 1990.

95. Rajab A, DeLouvois J. Survey of infection in babies at the Khoula Hospital, Oman. Ann Trop Paediatr 10:39–43, 1990.

96. Sharma PP, Halder D, Dutta AK, et al. Bacteriological profile of neonatal septicemia. Indian Pediatr 24:1011–1017, 1987.

97. Sinha N, Deb A, Mukherjee AK. Septicemia in neonates and early infancy. Indian J Pediatr 53:249–256, 1986.

98. Tafari N, Ljungh-Wadstrom A. Consequences of amniotic fluid infection: early neonatal septicaemia. In Perinatal Infections, vol 77. Amsterdam, Ciba Foundation Symposium, 1980, pp 55–67.

99. Yardi D, Gaikwad S, Deodhar L. Incidence, mortality and bacteriological profile of septicemia in pediatric patients. Indian J Pediatr 51:173–176, 1984.

100. Saxena S, Anand NK, Saini L, et al. Bacterial infections among home delivered neonates: clinical picture and bacteriological profile. Indian Pediatr 17:17–24, 1980.

101. Wong NACS, Hunt LP, Marlow N. Risk factors for developing neonatal septicaemia at a Malaysian Hospital. J Trop Pediatr 43:54–58, 1997.

102. Bhutta ZA, Yusuf K. Neonatal sepsis in Karachi: factors determining outcome and mortality. J Trop Pediatr 43:65–70, 1997.

103. Muhe L, Tilahun M, Lulseged S, et al. Etiology of pneumonia, sepsis, and meningitis in young infants below 3 months of age in Ethiopia. Pediatr Infect Dis J Suppl 18:S56–S61, 1999.

104. Ghiorghis B. Neonatal sepsis in Addis Ababa, Ethiopia: a review of 151 bacteremic neonates. Ethiopian Med J 35:169–176, 1997.

105. Kago I, Wouafo Ndayo M, Tchokoteu PF, et al. Neonatal septicemia and meningitis caused by gram-negative bacilli in Yaonde: clinical, bacteriological and prognostic aspects. Bull Soc Pathol Exot 84:573–581, 1991.

106. Robillard PY, Nabeth P, Hulsey TC, et al. Neonatal bacterial septicemia in a tropical area: four-year experience in Guadeloupe (French West Indies). Acta Paediatr 82:687–689, 1993.

107. Rodriguez CJ, Fraga JM, Garcia Riestra C, et al. Neonatal sepsis: epidemiologic indicators and relation to birth weight and length of hospitalization time. Anal Español Pediatr 48:401–408, 1998.

108. Dawodu A, Al Umran K, Twum-Danso K. A case control study of neonatal sepsis: experience from Saudi Arabia. J Trop Pediatr 43:84–88, 1997.

109. Greenberg D, Shinwell ES, Yagupsky P. A prospective study of neonatal sepsis and meningitis in Southern Israel. Pediatr Infect Dis J 16:768–773, 1997.

110. Leibovitz E, Flidel-Rimon O, Juster-Reicher A, et al. Sepsis at a neonatal intensive care unit: a four-year retrospective study (1989–1992). Isr J Med Sci 33:734–738, 1997.

111. Daoud AS, Al-Sheyyab M, Abu-Ekteish F, et al. Neonatal meningitis in Northern Jordan. J Trop Pediatr 42:267–270, 1996.

112. Campagne G, Djibo S, Schuchat A, et al. Epidemiology of bacterial meningitis in Niamey, Niger, 1981–1996. Bull World Health Organ 77:499–508, 1999.

113. World Population Prospects: the 1994 revision. New York, United Nations Publications (ST/ESA/SER.A/145), 1995.

114. Bennett R, Eriksson M, Melen B, et al. Changes in the incidence and spectrum of neonatal septicemia during a fifteen-year period. Acta Paediatr Scand 74:687–690, 1985.

115. Gladstone IM, Ehrenkranz RA, Edberg SC, et al. A ten-year review of neonatal sepsis and comparison with the previous fifty-year experience. Pediatr Infect Dis J 9:819–825, 1990.

116. Antia-Obong OE, Utsalo SJ. Bacterial agents in neonatal septicaemia in Calabar, Nigeria: review of 100 cases. Trop Doct 21:169–170, 1991.

117. Bhatia BD, Chugh SP, Narang P, et al. Bacterial flora in mothers and babies with reference to causative agent in neonatal septicemia. Indian Pediatr 26:455–459, 1989.

118. Chaturvedi P, Agrawal M, Narang P. Analysis of blood-culture isolates from neonates of a rural hospital. Indian Pediatr 26:460–465, 1989.

119. El Rifai MR. A study of 214 neonates with infection in the Maternity and Children's Hospital of Riyadh, Saudi Arabia. Ann Trop Paediatr 2:119–122, 1982.

120. Liebowitz LD, Koornhof HJ, Barrett M, et al. Bacterial meningitis in Johannesburg—1980–1982. S Afr Med J 66:677–679, 1984.

121. MacFarlane DE. Neonatal group B streptococcal septicaemia in a developing country. Acta Paediatr Scand 76:470–473, 1987.

122. Musoke RN, Malenga GJ. Bacterial infections in neonates at the Kenyatta Hospital nursery. A prospective study. East Afr Med J 61:909–916, 1984.

123. Nathoo KJ, Mason PR, Gwanzure L, et al. Severe Klebsiella infection as a cause of mortality in neonates in Harare, Zimbabwe: evidence from postmortem blood cultures. Pediatr Infect Dis J 12:840–844, 1993.

124. Solorzano-Santos F, Diaz-Ramos RD, Arredondo-Garcia JL. Diseases caused by group B Streptococcus in Mexico. Letter. Pediatr Infect Dis J 9:66, 1990.

125. St. John MA, Lewis DB, Archer E. Current problems of neonatal septicaemia in Barbados. West Indian Med J 35(Suppl):16, 1986.

126. Rao PS, Baliga M, Shivananda PG. Bacteriology of neonatal septicaemia in a rural referral hospital in South India. J Trop Pediatr 39:230–233, 1993.

127. Monga K, Fernandez A, Deodhar L. Changing bacteriological patterns in neonatal septicaemia. Indian J Pediatr 53:505–508, 1986.

128. Pruekprasert P, Chongsuvivatwong V, Patamasucon P. Factors influencing case-fatality rate of septicemic children. Southeast Asian J Trop Med Public Health 25:678–683, 1994.

129. Lehmann D, Michael A, Omena M, et al. The bacterial and viral etiology of severe infection in children aged less than three months in the highlands of Papua New Guinea. Pediatr Infect Dis J Suppl 18:S42–S49, 1999.

130. Gatchalian SR, Quiambao BP, Morelos AMR, et al. Bacterial and viral aetiology of serious infections in very young Filipino infants. Pediatr Infect Dis J Suppl 18:S50–S55, 1999.

131. Stoll BJ, Gordon T, Korones SB, et al. Early-onset sepsis in very low birthweight neonates: a report from the

NICHD Neonatal Research Network. J Pediatr 129:72–80, 1996.

132. WHO Young Infants Study Group. The bacterial etiology of serious infections in young infants in developing countries—results of a multicenter study. Pediatr Infect Dis J Suppl 18:S17–S22, 1999.

133. Mulholland EK, Ogunlesi OO, Adegbola RA, et al. Etiology of serious infections in young Gambian infants. Pediatr Infect Dis J 18(10 Suppl):S35–41, 1999.

134. WHO Young Infants Study Group. Clinical prediction of serious bacterial infections in young infants in developing countries. Pediatr Infect Dis J Suppl 18:S23–S31, 1999.

135. Lehmann D, Sanders RC, Marjen B, et al. High rates of *Chlamydia trachomatis* infections in young Papua New Guinean infants. Pediatr Infect Dis J Suppl 18:S62–S69, 1999.

136. WHO Young Infants Study Group. Conclusions from the WHO multicenter study of serious infections in young infants. Pediatr Infect Dis J Suppl 18:S32–S34, 1999.

137. Baker CJ. Group B streptococcal infections. Clin Perinatol 24:59–70, 1997.

138. Stoll BJ, Schuchat A. Maternal carriage of group B streptococci in developing countries. Pediatr Infect Dis J 17:499–503, 1998.

139. Blumberg HM, Stephens DS, Modansky M, et al. Invasive group B streptococcal disease: the emergence of serotype V. J Infect Dis 173:365–373, 1996.

140. Collins TS, Calderon M, Gilman RH, et al. Group B streptococcal colonization in a developing country: its association with sexually transmitted disease and socioeconomic factors. Am J Trop Med 59:633–636, 1998.

141. Suara RO, Adegbola RA, Baker CJ, et al. Carriage of group B streptococci in pregnant Gambian mothers and their infants. J Infect Dis 70:1316–1319, 1994.

142. Regan JA, Klebanoff MA, Nugent RP, et al, for the VIP Study Group. Colonization with group B streptococci in pregnancy and adverse outcome. Am J Obstet Gynecol 174:1354–1360, 1996.

143. Klein JO, Marcy SM. Bacterial sepsis and meningitis. *In* Remington JS, Klein JO (eds): Infectious Diseases of the Fetus and Newborn Infant, 5th ed. Philadelphia, WB Saunders, 2000.

143a. Duke T, Michael A. Increase in sepsis due to multiresistant enteric gram-negative bacilli in Papua New Guinea. Lancet 353:2210–2211, 1999.

144. Garenne M, Ronsmans C, Campbell H. The magnitude of mortality from acute respiratory infections in children under 5 years in developing countries. World Health Stat Q 45:180–191, 1992.

145. Misra S, Bhakoo ON, Ayyagiri A, et al. Clinical and bacteriological profile of neonatal pneumonia. Indian J Med Res 93:366–370, 1991.

146. Patwari AK, Bisht S, Srinjvasari A, et al. Aetiology of pneumonia in hospitalized children. J Trop Pediatr 42:15–19, 1996.

147. Bang AT, Bang RA, Morankar VP, et al. Pneumonia in neonates: can it be managed in the community? Arch Dis Child 68:550–556, 1993.

148. Zaman K, Baqui AH, Yunas M, et al. Acute respiration infections in children: a community-based longitudinal study in rural Bangladesh. J Trop Pediatr 43:133–137, 1997.

149. Datta N, Kumar V, Kumar L, et al. Application of case management to the control of acute respiratory infections in low-birth-weight infants: a feasibility study. Bull World Health Organ 65:77–82, 1987.

149a. Bang AT, Bang RA, Baitule SB, et al. Effect of home-based neonatal care and management of sepsis to reduce neonatal mortality: field trial in rural India. Lancet 354:1955–1961, 1999.

150. Thomas S, Verma IC, Singh M, et al. Spectrum of respiratory distress syndrome in the newborn in North India: a prospective study. Indian J Pediatr 48:61–65, 1981.

151. Misra PK. Respiratory distress in newborn: a prospective study. Indian Pediatr 24:77–80, 1987.

152. Bhandari N, Bahl R, Bhatnagar V, et al. Treating sick young infants in urban slum setting. Letter. Lancet 347:1774–1775, 1996.

153. Starke JR. Tuberculosis: an old disease but a new threat to the mother, fetus, and neonate. Clin Perinatol 24:107–127, 1997.

154. Jana N, Vasishta K, Jindal SK, et al. Perinatal outcome in pregnancies complicated by pulmonary tuberculosis. Int J Gynecol Obstet 44:119–124, 1994.

154a. Jana N, Vasishta K, Saha SC, et al. Obstetrical outcomes among women with extrapulmonary tuberculosis. N Engl J Med 341:645–649, 1999.

155. Adhikari M, Pillay T, Pillay D. Tuberculosis in the newborn: an emerging disease. Pediatr Infect Dis J 16:1108–1112, 1997.

156. Cantwell MF, Shehab ZM, Costello AM, et al. Brief report: congenital tuberculosis. N Engl J Med 330:1051–1054, 1994.

157. World Health Organization. Global HIV/AIDS and STD Surveillance Report, June 1998.

158. Chin J. The growing impact of the HIV/AIDS pandemic on children born to HIV-infected women. Clin Perinatol 21:1–14, 1994.

159. Bulterys M, Lepage P. Mother-to-child transmission of HIV. Curr Opin Pediatr 10:143–150, 1998.

160. Connor EM, Sperling RS, Gelber R, et al. Reduction of maternal-infant transmission of human immunodeficiency virus type 1 with zidovudine treatment. N Engl J Med 331:1173–1180, 1994.

161. Boyer PJ, Dillon M, Navaie M, et al. Factors predictive of maternal-fetal transmission of HIV-1: preliminary analysis of zidovudine given during pregnancy and/or delivery. JAMA 271:1925–1930, 1994.

162. Cooper ER, Nugent RP, Diaz C, et al. After AIDS clinical trial 076: the changing pattern of zidovudine use during pregnancy, and the subsequent reduction in the vertical transmission of human immunodeficiency virus in a cohort of infected women and their infants. Women and Infants Transmission Study Group. J Infect Dis 174:1207–1211, 1996.

163. Mayaux MJ, Teglas JP, Mandelbrot L, et al. Acceptability and impact of zidovudine for prevention of mother-to-child human immunodeficiency virus-1 transmission in France. J Pediatr 131:857–862, 1997.

164. Simonds RJ, Steketee R, Nesheim S, et al. Impact of zidovudine use on risk and risk factors for perinatal transmission of HIV. Perinatal AIDS Collaborative Transmission Studies. AIDS 12:301–308, 1998.

165. Henderson SL, Lindsay MK, Higgins J, et al. Perinatal zidovudine to prevent mother to infant HIV transmission: impact of a ten-year program of routine voluntary prenatal HIV counseling and testing in an inner-city hospital. Submitted for publication.

166. Hira SK, Kamanga J, Bhat GJ, et al. Perinatal transmission of HIV-1 in Zambia. BMJ 299:1250–1252, 1989.

167. Ryder RW, Nsa W, Hassig SE, et al. Perinatal transmission of the human immunodeficiency virus type 1 to infants of seropositive women in Zaire. N Engl J Med 320:1637–1642, 1989.

168. St. Louis ME, Kamenga M, Brown C, et al. Risk for perinatal HIV-1 transmission according to maternal im-

munologic, virologic, and placental factors. JAMA 269:2853–2859, 1993.

169. Srison D, Thisyakorn U, Paupunwatana S, et al. Perinatal HIV infections in Thailand. Southeast Asian J Trop Med Public Health 26:659–663, 1995.

170. The Working Group on Mother-to-Child Transmission of HIV. Rates of mother-to-child transmission of HIV-1 in Africa, America, and Europe: results from 13 perinatal studies. J Acquir Immune Defic Syndr Hum Retrovirol 8:506–510, 1995.

171. Bobat R, Coovadia H, Coutsoudis A, et al. Determinants of mother-to-child transmission of human immunodeficiency virus type 1 infection in a cohort from Durban, South Africa. Pediatr Infect Dis J 15:604–610, 1996.

172. Datta P, Embree JE, Kreiss JK, et al. Mother-to-child transmission of human immunodeficiency virus type 1: report from the Nairobi study. J Infect Dis 170:1134–1140, 1994.

173. Mandelbrot L, Mayaux MJ, Bongain A, et al. Obstetrics: obstetric factors and mother-to-child transmission of human immunodeficiency virus type 1: the French perinatal cohorts. Am J Obstet Gynecol 175:661–667, 1996.

174. Landers DV. Nutrition and immune function: II. Maternal factors influencing transmission. J Nutr 126:2637s–2640s, 1996.

175. Semba RD. Overview of the potential role of vitamin A in mother-to-child transmission of HIV-1. Acta Paediatr Suppl 421:107–112, 1997.

176. Dunn DT, Newell ML, Mayaux MJ, et al. Mode of delivery and vertical transmission of HIV-1: a review of prospective studies. J Acquir Immune Defic Syndr 7:1064–1066, 1994.

177. Minkoff H, Burns DN, Landesman S, et al. Obstetrics: the relationship of the duration of ruptured membranes to vertical transmission of human immunodeficiency virus. Am J Obstet Gynecol 173:585–589, 1995.

178. Mofenson LM. A critical review of studies evaluating the relationship of mode of delivery to perinatal transmission of human immunodeficiency virus. Pediatr Infect Dis J 14:169–177, 1995.

179. Landesman SH, Kalish LA, Burns DN, et al. Obstetrical factors and the transmission of human immunodeficiency virus type 1 from mother to child. N Engl J Med 334:1617–1623, 1996.

180. Newell ML, Dunn DT, Peckham CS, et al. Vertical transmission of HIV-1: maternal immune status and obstetric factors. The European Collaborative Study. AIDS 10:1675–1681, 1996.

181. Newell ML, Dunn DT, Peckham CS, et al for the European Collaborative Study. Caesarean section and risk of vertical transmission of HIV-1 infection. Lancet 343:1464–1467, 1994.

181a. The European Mode of Delivery Collaboration. Elective caesarean-section versus vaginal delivery in prevention of vertical HIV-1 transmission: a randomised clinical trial. Lancet 353:1035–1039, 1999.

181b. The International Perinatal HIV Group. The mode of delivery and the risk of vertical transmission of human immunodeficiency virus type 1—a meta-analysis of 15 prospective cohort studies. N Engl J Med 340:977–987, 1999.

182. Tess BH, Rodrigues LC, Newell ML, et al. Breastfeeding, genetic, obstetric and other risk factors associated with mother-to-child transmission of HIV-1 in Sao Paulo State, Brazil. AIDS 12:513–520, 1998.

183. Dunn DT, Newell ML, Ades AE, et al. Risk of human immunodeficiency virus type 1 transmission through breastfeeding. Lancet 340:585–588, 1992.

184. Bertolli J, St. Louis ME, Simonds RJ, et al. Estimating the timing of mother-to-child transmission of human immunodeficiency virus in a breastfeeding population in Kinshasa, Zaire. J Infect Dis 174:722–726, 1996.

185. Ekpini ER, Wiktor SZ, Satten GA, et al. Late postnatal mother-to-child transmission of HIV-1 in Abidjan, Côte d'Ivoire. Lancet 349:1054–1059, 1997.

186. Kreiss J. Breastfeeding and vertical transmission of HIV-1. Acta Paediatr Suppl 421:113–117, 1997.

187. Bobat R, Moodley D, Coutsoudis A, et al. Breastfeeding by HIV-1 infected women and outcome in their infants: a cohort study from Durban, South Africa. AIDS 11:1627–1633, 1997.

188. World Health Organization/UNAIDS. HIV and infant feeding: A policy statement developed collaboratively by UNAIDS, WHO, and UNICEF, 1998, pp 20–21.

189. de Martino M, Pier-Angelo T, Tozzi AE, et al. HIV-1 transmission through breast-milk: appraisal of risk according to duration of feeding. AIDS 6:991–997, 1992.

190. Leroy V, Newell ML, Dabis F, et al. International multicentre pooled analysis of late postnatal mother-to-child transmission of HIV-1 infection. Lancet 352:597–600, 1998.

190a. Coutsoudis A, Pillay K, Spooner E, et al. Influence of infant-feeding patterns on early mother-to-child transmission of HIV-1 in Durban, South Africa: a prospective cohort study. Lancet 354:471–476, 1999.

191. Van de Perre P. Postnatal transmission of human immunodeficiency virus type 1: the breastfeeding dilemma. Am J Obstet Gynecol 173:483–487, 1995.

191a. Semba RD, Kumwenda N, Hoover DR, et al. Human immunodeficiency virus load in breast milk, mastitis, and mother-to-child transmission of human immunodeficiency virus type 1. J Infect Dis 180:93–98, 1999.

192. Abdool-Karim Q, Abdool-Karim SS, Coovadia HM, et al. Informed consent for HIV testing in a South African hospital: is it truly informed and truly voluntary? Am J Public Health 88:637–640, 1998.

193. Del Fante P, Jenniskens F, Lush L, et al. HIV, breastfeeding and under-5 mortality: modelling the impact of policy decisions for or against breastfeeding. J Trop Med Hyg 96:203–211, 1993.

194. Kuhn L, Stein Z. Infant survival, HIV infection, and feeding alternatives in less-developed countries. Am J Public Health 87:926–931, 1997.

195. Centers for Disease Control and Prevention. Public Health Service Task Force recommendations for the use of antiretroviral drugs in pregnant women infected with HIV-1 for maternal health and for reducing perinatal HIV-1 transmission in the United States. MMWR Morb Mortal Wkly Rep 47(rr-2):1–30, 1998.

196. Centers for Disease Control and Prevention. Administration of zidovudine during late pregnancy and delivery to prevent perinatal HIV transmission—Thailand, 1996–1998. MMWR Morb Mortal Wkly Rep 47(8):151–154, 1998.

197. UNAIDS. Perinatal TRAnsmission Study (PETRA). A clinical trial for the prevention of mother-to-child transmission of HIV. Press release, July 1996.

198. Mansergh G, Haddix AC, Steketee RW, et al. Cost-effectiveness of short-course zidovudine to prevent perinatal HIV type 1 infection in a sub-Saharan African developing country setting. JAMA 276:139–145, 1996.

199. Marseille E, Kahn JG, Saba J. Cost-effectiveness of antiviral drug therapy to reduce mother-to-child HIV transmission in sub-Saharan Africa. AIDS 12:939–948, 1998.

199a. Saba J for the PETRA Trial Management Committee. A multicentre, randomized, double-blind, placebo-controlled clinical trial to evaluate efficacy, tolerance, and effectiveness of three drug regimens using zidovudine + lamivudine for the prevention of mother-to-child transmission of HIV-1. Presented at the Global Strategies for Prevention of Mother-to-Child Transmission Conference held in Montreal, Canada, September 1–4, 1999.

199b. Guay LA, Musoke P, Fleming T, et al. Intrapartum and neonatal single-dose nevirapine compared with zidovudine for prevention of mother-to-child transmission of HIV-1 in Kampala, Uganda: HIVNET 012 randomised trial. Lancet 354:795–802, 1999.

199c. Marseille E, Kahn JG, Mmiro F, et al. Cost effectiveness of single-dose nevirapine regimen for mothers and babies to decrease vertical HIV-1 transmission in sub-Saharan Africa. Lancet 354:803–809, 1999.

200. World Health Organization. Recommendations on the safe and effective use of short-course ZDV for prevention of mother-to-child transmission of HIV. Wkly Epidemiol Rec 73:313–320, 1998.

200a. UNAIDS. Prevention of HIV transmission from mother to child: strategic options, 1999.

201. World Health Organization. New initiative to reduce HIV transmission from mother-to-child in low-income countries. WHO/UNAIDS press release, June 1998.

202. Fowler MG, Rogers MF. Overview of perinatal HIV infection. J Nutr 126:2602s–2607s, 1996.

203. Cohen J. Bringing AZT to poor countries. Science 269:624–626, 1995.

204. Valleroy LA, Harris JR, Way PO. The impact of HIV-1 infection on child survival in the developing world. AIDS 4:667–672, 1990.

205. Bennett JV, Rogers MF. Child survival and perinatal infections with human immunodeficiency virus. Am J Dis Child 145:1242–1247, 1991.

206. Whitman C, Beigharbi L, Gasse F, et al. Progress towards the global elimination of neonatal tetanus. World Health Stat Q 45:248–256, 1992.

207. World Health Organization. Eliminating neonatal tetanus: how near, how far? WHO/EPI/GEN/96.01. Geneva, World Health Organization, 1996.

208. Galazka A, Gasse F, Henderson RH. Neonatal tetanus and the global expanded programme on immunization. In Kessel E, Awan AK (eds). Maternal and Child Care in Developing Countries: Assessment, Promotion, Implementation. Proceedings of the Third International Congress for Maternal and Neonatal Health. Thun, Ott, 1989.

209. Galazka A, Stroh G. Neonatal Tetanus: guidelines on the community-based survey on neonatal tetanus mortality. WHO/EPI/GEN/86/8. Geneva, World Health Organization, 1995.

210. Gasse F. Neonatal tetanus elimination initiative: Progress report and recommendation. EPI/MCHINNT/GEN/90.1. Geneva, World Health Organization, 1990.

211. Stroh G, Aye KU, Thaung U, et al. Measurement of mortality from neonatal tetanus in Burma. Bull World Health Organ 65:309–316, 1987.

212. The Progress of Nations 1998. New York, UNICEF, 1998.

212a. Rochat R, Akhter HH. Tetanus and pregnancy-related mortality in Bangladesh. Lancet 354:565, 1999.

213. The State of the World's Children 1996. UNICEF. New York, Oxford University Press, 1996.

214. Cushing AH. Omphalitis: a review. Pediatr Infect Dis J 4:282–285, 1985.

215. Samuel M, Freeman NV, Vaishnav A, et al. Necrotizing fasciitis: a serious complication of omphalitis in neonates. J Pediatr Surg 29:1414–1416, 1994.

216. Sawin RS, Schaller RT, Tapper D, et al. Early recognition of neonatal abdominal wall necrotizing fasciitis. Am J Surg 167:481–484, 1994.

217. Airede AI. Pathogens in neonatal omphalitis. J Trop Pediatr 38:129–131, 1992.

218. Faridi MM, Rattan A, Ahmad SH. Omphalitis neonatorum. J Indian Med Assoc 91:283–285, 1993.

219. Guvenc H, Guvenc M, Yenioglu H, et al. Neonatal omphalitis is still common in eastern Turkey. Scand J Infect Dis 23:613–616, 1991.

220. Guvenc H, Aygun AD, Yasar F, et al. Omphalitis in term and preterm appropriate for gestational age and small for gestational age infants. J Trop Pediatr 43:368–372, 1997.

221. Baley JE, Fanaroff AA. Neonatal infections: I. Infection related to nursery care practices. In Sinclair JC, Bracken MB (eds). Effective Care of the Newborn Infant. New York, Oxford University Press, 1992, pp 454–476.

222. Rush J, Chalmers I, Enkin M. Care of the new mother and baby. In Chalmers I, Enkin M, Keirse MJNC (eds). Effective Care in Pregnancy and Childbirth, vol 2. New York, Oxford University Press, 1989, pp 1333–1346.

223. Garner P, Lai D, Baea M, et al. Avoiding neonatal death: an intervention study of umbilical cord care. J Trop Pediatr 40:24–28, 1994.

224. Bern C, Martines J, de Zoysa I, et al. The magnitude of the global problem of diarrhoeal disease: a ten-year update. Bull World Health Organ 70:705–714, 1992.

225. Snyder JD, Merson MH. The magnitude of the global problem of acute diarrhoeal disease: a review of active surveillance data. Bull World Health Organ 60:605–613, 1982.

226. Huilan S, Zhen LG, Mathan MM, et al. Etiology of acute diarrhoea among children in developing countries: a multicentre study in five countries. Bull World Health Organ 89:s49–s55, 1991.

227. de Zoysa I, Rea M, Martines J. Why promote breastfeeding in diarrhoeal disease control programmes? Health Pol Plan 6:371–379, 1991.

228. Black RE, Lopez de Romana G, Brown KH, et al. Incidence and etiology of infantile diarrhea and major routes of transmission in Huascar, Peru. Am J Epidemiol 129:785–799, 1989.

229. Mahmud A, Jalil F, Karlberg J, et al. Early child health in Lahore, Pakistan: VII. Diarrhoea. Acta Paediatr Suppl 390:79–85, 1993.

230. Stoll BJ, Glass RI, Huq MI, et al. Surveillance of patients attending a diarrhoeal disease hospital in Bangladesh. BMJ 285:1185–1188, 1982.

231. Aye DT, Sack DA, Wachsmuth IK, et al. Neonatal diarrhea at a maternity hospital in Rangoon. Am J Public Health 81:480–481, 1991.

231a. Clemens J, Elyazeed RA, Rao M, et al. Early initiation of breastfeeding and the risk of infant diarrhea in rural Egypt. Pediatrics 104:e3, 1999.

232. Parashar UD, Bresee JS, Gentsch JR, et al. Rotavirus. Emerg Infect Dis 4:1–10, 1998.

233. Espinoza F, Paniagua M, Hallander H, et al. Rotavirus infections in young Nicaraguan children. Pediatr Infect Dis J 16:564–571, 1997.

234. Haffejee IE. The epidemiology of rotavirus infections: a global perspective. J Pediatr Gastroenterol Nutr 20:275–286, 1995.

235. Bishop RF, Barnes GL, Cipriani E, et al. Clinical immunity after neonatal rotavirus infection: a prospective longitudinal study in young children. N Engl J Med 309:72–76, 1983.

236. Bhan MK, Lew JF, Sazawal S, et al. Protection conferred by neonatal rotavirus infection against subsequent diarrhea. J Infect Dis 168:282–287, 1993.

237. Cicirello HG, Das BK, Gupta A, et al. High prevalence of rotavirus infection among neonates born at hospitals in Delhi, India: predisposition of newborns for infection with unusual rotavirus. Pediatr Infect Dis J 13:720–724, 1994.

238. Nsanze H, Dawodu A, Usmani A, et al. Ophthalmia neonatorum in the United Arab Emirates. Ann Trop Paediatr 16:27–32, 1996.

239. Verma M, Chhatwal J, Varughese PV. Neonatal conjunctivitis: a profile. Indian Pediatr 31:1357–1361, 1994.

240. Pandey KK, Bhat BV, Kanungo R, et al. Clinico-bacteriological study of neonatal conjunctivitis. Indian J Pediatr 57:527–531, 1990.

241. Sergiwa A, Pratt BC, Eren E, et al. Ophthalmia neonatorum in Bangkok: the significance of Chlamydia trachomatis. Ann Trop Paediatr 13:233–236, 1993.

242. Galega FP, Heymann DL, Nasah BT. Gonococcal ophthalmia neonatorum: the case for prophylaxis in tropical Africa. Bull World Health Organ 62:95–98, 1984.

243. Laga M, Plummer FA, Nzanze H, et al. Epidemiology of ophthalmia neonatorum in Kenya. Lancet 2:1145–1148, 1986.

244. Laga M, Plummer FA, Piot P, et al. Prophylaxis of gonococcal and chlamydial ophthalmia neonatorum: a comparison of silver nitrate and tetracycline. N Engl J Med 318:653–657, 1988.

245. Laga M, Meheus A, Piot P. Epidemiology and control of gonococcal ophthalmia neonatorum. Bull World Health Organ 67:471–478, 1989.

246. Fransen L, Nsanze H, Klauss V, et al. Ophthalmia neonatorum in Nairobi, Kenya. The roles of Neisseria gonorrhoeae and Chlamydia trachomatis. J Infect Dis 153:862–869, 1986.

247. Wasserheit JN. The significance and scope of reproductive tract infections among Third World women. Int J Gynecol Obstet Suppl 3:145–168, 1989.

248. De Schryver A, Meheus A. Epidemiology of sexually transmitted diseases: the global picture. Bull World Health Organ 68:639–654, 1990.

249. Bergstrom S. Genital infections and reproductive health: infertility and morbidity of mother and child in developing countries. Scand J Infect Dis Suppl 69:99–105, 1990.

250. Gerbase AC, Rowley JT, Mertens TE. Global epidemiology of sexually transmitted diseases. Lancet 351(Suppl):2–4, 1998.

251. Hanenberg RS, Rojanapithayakorn W, Kunasol P, et al. Impact of Thailand's HIV-control programme as indicated by the decline of sexually transmitted diseases. Lancet 344:243–246, 1994.

252. Nelson KE, Celentano DD, Eiumtrakol S, et al. Changes in sexual behavior and decline in HIV infection among young men in Thailand. N Engl J Med 335:297–303, 1996.

253. Credé KSF. Die Verhütung der Augenentzündung der Neugeborenen. Arch Gynekol 17:50–53, 1881.

254. Hammerschlag MR, Cummings C, Roblin PM, et al. Efficacy of neonatal ocular prophylaxis for the prevention of chlamydial and gonococcal conjunctivitis. N Engl J Med 320:769–772, 1989.

255. Zanoni D, Isenberg SJ, Apt L. A comparison of silver nitrate with erythromycin for prophylaxis against ophthalmia neonatorum. Clin Pediatr 31:295–298, 1992.

256. American Academy of Pediatrics. 1997 Red Book: Report of the Committee on Infectious Diseases, 24th ed. Chicago, American Academy of Pediatrics, 1997.

257. Isenberg SJ, Apt L, Wood M. A controlled trial of povidone-iodine as prophylaxis against ophthalmia neonatorum. N Engl J Med 332:562–566, 1995.

258. Benevento WJ, Murray P, Reed CA, et al. The sensitivity of Neisseria gonorrhoeae, Chlamydia trachomatis, and herpes simplex type II to disinfection with povidone-iodine. Am J Ophthalmol 109:329–333, 1990.

259. Hounag ET, Gilmore OJA, Reid C, et al. Absence of bacterial resistance to povidone iodine. J Clin Pathol 29:752–755, 1976.

260. Lapage P, Bogaerts J, Kestelyn P, et al. Single-dose cefotaxime intramuscularly cures gonococcal ophthalmia neonatorum. Br J Ophthalmol 72:518–520, 1988.

261. Haase DA, Nash RA, Nsanze H, et al. Single-dose ceftriaxone therapy of gonococcal ophthalmia neonatorum. Sex Transm Dis 13:53–55, 1986.

262. Ibhanesebhor SE, Otobo ES. In vitro activity of human milk against the causative organisms of ophthalmia neonatorum in Benin City, Nigeria. J Trop Pediatr 42:327–329, 1996.

263. The Progress of the Nations 1997. New York, UNICEF, 1997.

264. Steketee RW, Wirima JJ, Slutsker L, et al. The problem of malaria and malaria control in pregnancy in sub-Saharan Africa. Am J Trop Med Hyg 55:2–7, 1996.

265. Brabin BJ. An analysis of malaria in pregnancy in Africa. Bull World Health Organ 61:1005–1016, 1983.

266. McGregor IA. Epidemiology, malaria, and pregnancy. Am J Trop Med Hyg 33:517–525, 1984.

267. Nosten F, ter Kuile F, Maelankirri L, et al. Malaria during pregnancy in an area of unstable endemicity. Trans R Soc Trop Med Hyg 85:424–429, 1991.

268. Gilles HM, Lawson JB, Sibelas M, et al. Malaria, anaemia and pregnancy. Ann Trop Med Parasitol 63:245–263, 1969.

269. Egwunyenga OA, Ajayi JA, Duhlinska-Popova DD. Malaria in pregnancy in Nigerians: seasonality and relationship to splenomegaly and anaemia. Indian J Malariol 34:17–24, 1997.

270. McGregor IA, Wilson ME, Billewicz WZ. Malaria infection of the placenta in The Gambia, West Africa; its incidence and relationship to stillbirth, birthweight and placental weight. Trans R Soc Trop Med Hyg 77:232–244, 1983.

271. Matteelli A, Caligaris S, Castelli F, et al. The placenta and malaria. Ann Trop Med Parasitol 91:803–810, 1997.

271a. Nosten F, McGready R, Simpson A, et al. Effects of Plasmodium vivax malaria in pregnancy. Lancet 354:546–549, 1999.

272. Galbraith RM, Fox H, Hsi B, et al. The human materna-foetal relationship in malaria: II. Histological, ultrastructural and immunopathological studies of the placenta. Trans R Soc Trop Med Hyg 74:61–72, 1980.

273. Steketee RW, Wirima JJ, Hightower AW, et al. The effect of malaria and malaria prevention in pregnancy on offspring birthweight, prematurity, and intrauterine growth retardation in rural Malawi. Am J Trop Med Hyg 55:33–41, 1996.

274. Bouvier P, Breslow N, Doumbo O, et al. Seasonality, malaria, and impact of prophylaxis in a West African village: II. Effect on birthweight. Am J Trop Med Hyg 56:384–389, 1997.

275. Kramer MS. Determinants of low birth weight: methodological assessment and metaanalysis. Bull World Health Organ 65:663–737, 1987.

276. Greenwood AM, Armstrong JRM, Byass P, et al. Malaria chemoprophylaxis, birth weight and child survival. Trans R Soc Trop Med Hyg 86:483–485, 1992.

277. Nguyen-Dinh P, Steketee RW, Greenberg AE, et al.

Rapid spontaneous post-partum clearance of *Plasmodium falciparum* parasitemia in African women. Lancet 2:751–752, 1988.

278. Chizzolini C, Trottein R, Bernard FX, et al. Isotypic analysis, antigen specificity, and inhibitory function of maternally transmitted *Plasmodium falciparum*–specific antibodies in Gabonese newborns. Am J Trop Med Hyg 45:57–64, 1991.

279. Ibhanesebhor SE. Clinical characteristics of neonatal malaria. J Trop Pediatr 41:330–333, 1995.

280. Wolfe MS, Cordero JF. Safety of chloroquine in chemosuppression of malaria during pregnancy. BMJ 290:1466–1467, 1985.

281. Garner P, Brabin B. A review of randomized controlled trials of routine antimalarial drug prophylaxis during pregnancy in endemic malarious areas. Bull World Health Organ 72:89–99, 1994.

282. Cot M, Roisin A, Barro D, et al. Effect of chloroquine chemoprophylaxis during pregnancy on birthweight: results of a randomized trial. Am J Trop Med Hyg 46:21–27, 1992.

283. Heyman DL, Steketee RW, Wirima JJ, et al. Antenatal chloroquine prophylaxis in Malawi: chloroquine resistance, compliance, protective efficacy and cost. Trans R Soc Trop Med Hyg 84:496–498, 1990.

284. Alonso PL, Lindsay SW, Armstrong JRM, et al. The effect of insecticide-treated bed nets on mortality of Gambian children. Lancet 337:1499–1502, 1991.

285. Nevill CG, Some ES, Mung'ala VO, et al. Insecticide-treated bednets reduce mortality and severe morbidity from malaria among children on the Kenyan Coast. Trop Med Intern Health 1:139–146, 1996.

286. Binka FN, Kubaaje A, Adjuik M, et al. Impact of permethrin-impregnated bednets on child mortality in Kassena-Nankana district, Ghana: a randomized controlled trial. Trop Med Intern Health 1:147–154, 1996.

287. Dolan G, ter-Kuile FO, Jacovtot V, et al. Bednets for the prevention of malaria and anaemia in pregnancy. Trans R Soc Trop Med Hyg 87:620–626, 1993.

288. D'Alessandro U, Langerock P, Bennett S, et al. The impact of a national impregnated bednet programme on the outcome of pregnancy in primigravidae in The Gambia. Trans R Soc Trop Med Hyg 90:487–492, 1996.

289. Browne ENL. Insecticide treated nets for malaria control in pregnancy in rural Ghana. 18th African Health Sciences Congress, Cape Town, South Africa.

290. Shulman CE, Dorman EK, Talisuna AO, et al. A community randomized controlled trial of insecticide-treated bednets for the prevention of malaria and anaemia among primigravid women on the Kenyan coast. Trop Med Intern Health 3:197–204, 1998.

291. The World's Women 1995: Trends and Statistics. Social Statistics and Indicators. New York, United Nations Publication, 1995.

292. Tomasevski K: Women and Human Rights. Atlantic Highlands, NJ, Zed Books, 1993.

293. Maternal and Perinatal Infections: a practical guide: report of a WHO consultation WHO/MCH/91.10. Geneva, World Health Organization, 1991.

294. Maternal care for the reduction of perinatal and neonatal mortality. Geneva, World Health Organization, 1986.

295. Fischer GW, Ottolini MG, Mond JJ. Prospects for vaccines during pregnancy and in the newborn period. Clin Perinatol 24:231–249, 1997.

296. Baker C, Rench M, Edwards M, et al. Immunization of pregnant women with a polysaccharide vaccine of group B streptococcus. N Engl J Med 319:1180–1185, 1988.

297. Baker CJ. Vaccine prevention of group B streptococcal disease. Pediatr Ann 22:711–714, 1993.

298. Shahid NS, Steinhoff MC, Hoque SS, et al. Serum, breast milk, and infant antibody after maternal immunisation with pneumococcal vaccine. Lancet 346:1252–1257, 1995.

299. O'Dempsey TJD, McArdle T, Ceesay SJ, et al. Immunization with a pneumococcal capsular polysaccharide vaccine during pregnancy. Vaccine 14:963–970, 1996.

300. Mulholland K, Suara RO, Siber G, et al. Maternal immunization with *Haemophilus influenzae* type b polysaccharide-tetanus protein conjugate vaccine in The Gambia. JAMA 275:1182–1188, 1996.

301. Englund JA, Glezen WP, Thompson C, et al. *Haemophilus influenzae* type b-specific antibody in infants after maternal immunization. Pediatr Infect Dis J 16:1122–1130, 1997.

302. Bisgard KM, Kao A, Leake J, et al. *Haemophilus influenzae* invasive disease in the United States, 1994–1995: near disappearance of a vaccine-preventable childhood disease. Emerg Infect Dis 4:229–237, 1998.

303. Bijlmer HA. Epidemiology of *Haemophilus influenzae* invasive disease in developing countries and intervention strategies. *In* Ellis RW, Granoff DM (eds). Development and uses of *Haemophilus* b conjugate vaccines. New York, Marcel Dekker, 1994, pp 247–264.

304. Funkhouser A, Steinhoff MD, Ward J. *Haemophilus influenzae* disease and immunization in developing countries. Rev Infect Dis 13(Suppl 6):S542–S554, 1991.

305. Smith PG. Case-control studies of the efficacy of BCG against tuberculosis. *In* International Union Against Tuberculosis (ed). Proceedings of the XXVIth IUAT World Conference on Tuberculosis and Respiratory Diseases, Singapore. Japan, Professional Postgraduate Services International, 1987, pp 73–79.

306. Colditz GA, Berkey CS, Mosteller F, et al. The efficacy of bacillus Calmette-Guérin vaccination of newborns and infants in the prevention of tuberculosis: meta-analyses of the published literature. Pediatrics 96:29–35, 1995.

307. Delage G, Remy-Prince S, Montplaisir S. Combined active-passive immunization against the hepatitis B virus: five-year follow-up of children born to hepatitis B surface antigen-positive mothers. Pediatr Infect Dis J 12:126–130, 1993.

308. Andre FE, Zuckerman AJ. Review: Protective efficacy of hepatitis B vaccines in neonates. J Med Virol 44:144–151, 1994.

309. World Health Organization. Expanded programme on immunization: Global advisory group. Wkly Epidemiol Rec 3:11–16, 1992.

310. Glass RI, Bresee JS, Parashar U, et al. Rotavirus vaccines at the threshold. Nature Med 3:1324–1325, 1997.

311. Perez-Schael I, Guntinas MJ, Perez M, et al. Efficacy of the rhesus rotavirus-based quadrivalent vaccine in infants and young children in Venezuela. N Engl J Med 337:1181–1187, 1997.

312. Lagos R, Valenzuela MT, Levine OS, et al. Economisation of vaccination against *Haemophilus influenzae* type b: a randomised trial of immunogenicity of fractional-dose and two-dose regimens. Lancet 351:1472–1476, 1998.

313. World Health Organization. The prevention and management of puerperal infections. Geneva, World Health Organization, 1992.

314. World Health Organization. The global elimination of neonatal tetanus: progress to date. Bull World Health Organ 72:155–164, 1994.

315. McDermott J, Steketee R, Larsen S, et al. Syphilis-asso-

ciated perinatal and infant mortality in rural Malawi. Bull World Health Organ 71:773–780, 1993.

316. Kuate DB. Epidemiology and control of infant and early childhood malaria: a competing risks analysis. Int J Epidemiol 24:204–217, 1995.

317. Airede AI. Prolonged rupture of membranes and neonatal outcome in a developing country. Ann Trop Paediatr 12:283–288, 1992.

318. Asindi AA, Omene JA. Prolonged rupture of membrane and neonatal morbidity. East Afr Med J 57:707–711, 1980.

319. Raghavan M, Mondal GP, Vishnu BB, et al. Perinatal risk factors in neonatal infections. Indian J Pediatr 59:335–340, 1992.

320. Hanson LA, Hahn-Zoric M, Berndes M, et al. Breast feeding: overview and breast milk immunology. Acta Paediatr Jpn 36:557–561, 1994.

321. Ashraf RN, Jalil F, Zaman S, et al. Breast feeding and protection against neonatal sepsis in a high risk population. Arch Dis Child 66:488–490, 1991.

322. Brown KH, Black RE, Lopez de Romana G, et al. Infant-feeding practices and their relationship with diarrheal and other diseases in Huascar (Lima), Peru. Pediatrics 83:31–40, 1989.

323. Feachem G, Koblinsky MA. Interventions for the control of diarrhoeal diseases among young children: promotion of breast-feeding. Bull World Health Organ 62:271–291, 1984.

324. Glezen WP. Epidemiological perspective of breastfeeding and acute respiratory illnesses in infants. *In* Mestecky J (ed): Immunology of Milk and the Neonate. New York, Plenum Press, 1991, pp 235–240.

325. Narayanan I, Murthy NS, Prakash K, et al. Randomised controlled trial of effect of raw and holder pasteurised human milk and of formula supplements on incidence of neonatal infection. Lancet 2:1111–1113, 1984.

326. Habicht JP, DaVanzo J, Butz XVP. Does breastfeeding really save lives, or are apparent benefits due to biases? Am J Epidemiol 123:279–290, 1986.

327. Srivastava SP, Sharma VK, Jha SP. Mortality patterns in breast versus artificially fed term babies in early infancy: a longitudinal study. Indian Pediatr 31:1393–1396, 1994.

328. Victora CG, Smith PG, Vaughan JP, et al. Infant feeding and deaths due to diarrhea: a case-control study. Am J Epidemiol 129:1032–1041, 1989.

329. Victora CG, Vaughan JP, Lombardi C, et al. Evidence for protection by breast-feeding against infant deaths from infectious diseases in Brazil. Lancet 11:319–322, 1987.

330. Cutting WAM. Breast-feeding and HIV—a balance of risks. J Trop Pediatr 40:6–11, 1994.

331. Kennedy KI, Fortney JA, Bonhomme MG, et al. Do the benefits of breastfeeding outweigh the risk of postnatal transmission of HIV via breastmilk? Trop Doct 20:25–29, 1990.

332. Bicego GT, Boerma JT. Maternal education and child survival: a comparative study of survey data from 17 countries. Soc Sci Med 36:1207–1227, 1993.

333. Victora CG, Huttly SRA, Barros FC, et al. Maternal education in relation to early and late child health outcomes: findings from a Brazilian cohort study. Soc Sci Med 34:899–905, 1992.

334. World Development Report 1993: Investing in health. New York, Oxford University Press, 1993.

335. van Ginneken JK, Lob-Levyt J, Gove S. Potential interventions for preventing pneumonia among young children in developing countries: promoting maternal education. Trop Med Intern Health 1:283–294, 1996.

336. Villar J, Belizan JM. The relative contribution of prematurity and fetal growth retardation to low birth weight in developing and developed societies. Am J Obstet Gynecol 143:793–798, 1982.

337. Victora CG, Barros FC, Vaughan JP, et al. Birthweight and infant mortality: a longitudinal study of 5914 Brazilian children. Int J Epidemiol 16:239–245, 1987.

338. Victora CG, Smith PG, Vaughan JP, et al. Influence of birth weight on mortality from infectious diseases: a case-control study. Pediatrics 81:807–811, 1988.

339. World Health Organization. Integrated management of the sick child. Bull World Health Organ 73:735–740, 1995.

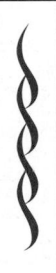

C H A P T E R 4

Human Milk

DAVID K. RASSIN, Ph.D., ROBERTO P. GAROFALO, M.D., and PEARAY L. OGRA, M.D.

In the intervening years since the last edition of this chapter (1995), considerable new evidence has been reported regarding the importance of human milk for the healthy term infant. This new information provides further documentation of protection by human milk against infectious diseases in the infant, the role of breast-feeding in cognitive development, the importance of nutrients such as long chain polyunsaturated fatty acids (especially docosahexaenoic acid [DHA]) and nucleotides, and the growing catalog of bioactive compounds, such as cytokines found in human milk. In addition, there is improved understanding of the potential role of breast-feeding in the transmission of infectious agents such as human immunodeficiency virus (HIV). These findings, added to what was already known about the benefits of human milk, stimulated the American Academy of Pediatrics to strengthen its recommendations about breast-feeding. These recommendations now urge mothers to breast-feed for the full first year of the life of the infant and urge both pediatricians and obstetricians to take a much more active role in the promotion and support of breast-feeding.[1]

Mother's milk delivered naturally via breast-feeding has been the sole source of infant feeding in human and other mammalian species for millions of years. Since humanity learned to domesticate cattle (about 10,000 years ago), nonhuman mammalian milk has also been used to supplement or replace maternal breast-feeding in the human infant. The development and widespread use of commercially prepared infant formula products have been phenomena of the twentieth century and notably of the past 50 years.

On a related historical note, the immune responses on intestinal and respiratory mucosal surfaces to local infections have been intensely studied over the past few decades. These investigations have led to the development of concepts of relative compartmentalization of immunity on mucosal surfaces of gastrointestinal, respiratory, and genitourinary tracts and identification of mucosa-associated lymphoid tissue and local mechanisms of defense that are distinct from the internal (systemic) immune system. With the increasing awareness that the human neonate is initially limited in its capacity to respond efficiently to infectious or environmental antigens on mucosal surfaces, especially in the gut, a rapidly expanding area of investigation on the development of immune competence in the fetus and neonate has evolved.

The intent of this chapter is to examine some of the major aspects of the physiologic, nutritional, immunologic, and anti-infective components and the products of lactation. The available evidence about the contribution of human milk to the development of immunologic integrity in the infant and its influence on the outcome of infectious and other host-antigen interactions in the neonate is discussed in some detail.

TABLE 4–1
Possible Endocrine Factors Involved in Growth of Human Female Mammary Glands

CLINICAL STATE	GROWTH CHARACTERISTICS	MATURATIONAL HORMONES
Prenatal	Rudimentary	None
Infancy	Rudimentary	None
Puberty	Growth and budding of milk ducts	Growth hormone, prolactin-estrogen, adrenocortical steroids, prolactin (high doses)
Pregnancy	Growth of acinar lobules and alveoli	Estrogen, progesterone, prolactin, growth hormone, adrenocortical steroids
Parturition	Alveolar growth	Prolactin, adrenocortical steroids
Lactational growth of tissue	None	None
Secretory products	Casein, alpha-lactalbumin	Prolactin, insulin, adrenocortical steroids

PHYSIOLOGY OF LACTATION

Anatomic Development

The rudimentary mammary tissue undergoes several developmental changes during morphogenesis and lactogenesis: In the 4-mm human embryo, the breast tissue appears as a tiny mammary band on the chest wall[2, 3]; by the 7-mm embryonic stage, the mammary band develops into the mammary line, along which eventually develops the true mammary anlage; by the 12-mm stage, a primitive epithelial nodule develops; by the 30-mm stage, the primitive mammary bud appears. These initial phases of development take place in both sexes (Table 4–1). However, further development in the male appears to be limited by androgenic or other male-associated substances.[4, 5] Castration in male rat embryos early in gestation leads to female breast development, whereas ovariectomy of the female does not alter the course of development of the mammary anlage. Toward the end of pregnancy, initial phases of fetal mammary differentiation seem to occur under the influence of placental and transplacentally acquired maternal hormones, with the transient development of the excretory and lactiferous ductular systems. Such growth, differentiation, and secretory activities are transient and regress soon after birth.[5, 6]

At the larche, and later on at menarche, true mammary growth and development begin in association with rapidly increasing levels of estrogens, progesterone, growth hormone, insulin, adrenocorticosteroids, and prolactin.[6, 7] Estrogens appear to be important for the growth and development of the ductular system and progestins for lobuloalveolar development (see Table 4–1). Final differentiation of the breast associated with growth and proliferation of the acinar lobes and alveoli continues to be influenced by the levels of estrogen and progesterone. Other peptide hormones, such as prolactin, insulin, and placental chorionic somatomammotropin, appear to be far more important for the subsequent induction and maintenance of lactation (see Table 4–1).

There are data suggesting that prolactin secretion from the pituitary gland is under neural control and that the increasing innervation of the breast observed throughout pregnancy is regulated by estrogens.[7] Intense neural input in virgin and parturient, but not in currently pregnant mammals has been shown to result in lactation. For example, lactation in goats can be induced by milking. Adoptive breast-feeding is also well documented in primitive human societies. Sudden and permanent cessation of suckling can result in the termination of milk secretion and involution of the breast to prepregnant state as the concentrations of prolactin decline. Estrogen and progesterone may also amplify the direct effects of prolactin or induce additional receptors for this peptide hormone on appropriate target tissues in the breast.

DEVELOPMENTAL ANATOMY OF THE MAMMARY GLAND AND ENDOCRINE CONTROL

Breast tissue is responsive to hormones, even as a rudimentary structure, as illustrated by the secretion of "witch's milk" by both male and female newborns in response to exposure to maternal secretion of placental lactogen, estrogens, and progesterone.[3] The secretion of this early milk ceases after exposure to maternal hormones has waned. Sexual differentiation, marked by puberty, is the next major stage in mammary development. As pointed out earlier, androgens inhibit the development of mammary tissue in the male, whereas the development of mammary tissue in the female is dependent on estrogen, progesterone, and pituitary hormones.[8] The postpubertal mammary gland undergoes cyclical changes in response to the release of hormones that takes place during the menstrual cycle. The last stage of development occurs during menopause, when the decline in estrogen secretion results in some atrophy of mammary tissue.

During the menstrual cycle, the mammary gland responds to the sequential release of estrogen and progesterone with a hyperplasia of the ductal system that continues through the secretory phase and declines with the onset of menstruation. Prolactin increases mildly during the follicular stage of the menstrual cycle but remains constant during the secretory phase.[9] Prolactin secretion appears to be held in readiness for the induction and maintenance of lactation.

Initiation and Maintenance of Lactation. Pregnancy is marked by profound hormonal changes reflecting major secretory contributions from the placenta, the hypothalamus, and the pituitary gland, with contributions from a number of other endocrine glands (e.g., the pancreas, thyroid, and parathyroid). Increased estrogen and progesterone levels during pregnancy stimulate secretion of prolactin from the pituitary, whereas placental lactogen appears to inhibit the release of a prolactin-inhibiting factor from the hypothalamus. Prolactin, lactogen, estrogen, and progesterone all aid in preparing the mammary gland for lactation. Initially in gestation there is an increased growth of ductule and alveolobular tissue in response to estrogen and progesterone. In the beginning of the second trimester, secretory material begins to appear in the luminal cells. By the middle of the second trimester, mammary development has proceeded sufficiently to permit lactation to occur should parturition take place.

Once the infant is delivered, a regulatory factor (the placenta) is lost and a new regulatory factor (the maternal-infant interaction or neuroendocrine regulation) is gained for control of lactation. Loss of placental hormone secretion results in an endocrine hypothalamic stimulation of prolactin release from the anterior pituitary gland as well as neural stimulation of oxytocin from the posterior pituitary. The stimulation of the nipple by suckling activates a neural pathway that results in release of both prolactin and oxytocin. Prolactin is responsible for stimulating milk production, whereas oxytocin stimulates milk ejection (the combination is known as the let-down reflex). Oxytocin also stimulates uterine contractions, which the mother may feel while she is breast-feeding; this response helps to restore the uterus to prepregnancy tone.

Milk production and ejection are thus dependent on the complex interaction of stimulation by the infant, neural reflex of the hypothalamus to such stimulation, release of hormones from the anterior and posterior pituitary, and response of the mammary gland to these hormones to complete the cycle.

Milk Secretion. Milk is produced as the result of synthetic mechanisms within the mammary gland as well as the transport of components from blood. Milk-specific proteins are synthesized in the mammary secretory cells, packaged in secretory vesicles, and exocytosed into the alveolar lumen. Lactose is secreted into the milk in a similar manner, whereas many monovalent ions, such as sodium, potassium, and chloride, are dependent on active transport systems based on sodium, potassium adenosine triphosphatases (Na^+,K^+-ATPases). In some situations, the mammary epithelium, which may behave as a "mammary barrier" between interstitial fluid derived from blood and the milk because of the lack of space between these cells, may "leak," permitting direct diffusion of components into the milk. This barrier results in the formation of different pools or compartments of milk components within the mammary gland and is responsible for maintaining gradients of these components from the blood to the milk.

Lipid droplets can be observed within the secretory cells of the mammary gland and are surrounded by a milk fat globule membrane. These fat droplets appear to fuse with the apical membrane of the secretory cells and then to be either exocytosed or "pinched off" into the milk.[8] Some whole cells are also found in milk, including leukocytes, macrophages, lymphocytes, and broken or shed mammary epithelial cells. The process by which these cells enter the milk is unclear.

As the structure of the mammary gland is compartmentalized, so is that of the milk. The gross composition of milk consists of cytoplasm encased by cellular membranes in milk fat globule membranes (a fat compartment made up of fat droplets), a soluble compartment containing water-soluble constituents, a casein-micelle compartment containing acid-precipitable proteins with calcium and lactose, and a cellular compartment. The relative amounts of these components change during the course of lactation, generally with less fat and more protein in early lactation than in late lactation. Thus, the infant consumes a dynamic complex solution that has physical properties permitting unique separation of different functional constituents from one another, presumably in forms that best support growth and development.

Lactation Performance. Successful lactation performance depends on continued effective contributions from the neural, endocrine, and maternal-infant interactions that were initiated at the time of delivery. The part of this complex behavior most liable to inhibition is the mother-child interaction. An early attachment of the infant to the breast is mandatory to begin stimulation of the neural pathways essential to maintaining prolactin and oxytocin release.

A healthy newborn infant placed between its mother's breasts will locate the mother's nipple and begin to suck spontaneously within the first hour of birth.[10] This rapid attachment to the mother may reflect olfactory stimuli from the breast received by the infant at birth.[11] Frequent feedings are necessary for the mother to maintain an appropriate level of milk production for the infant's proper growth and development. Programs to support lactation performance must emphasize proper maternal-infant bonding, relaxation of the mother, support for the mother, technical assistance to initiate breast-feeding properly and to cope with problems, and reduction of environmental hindrances. These latter may include lack of rooming-in in the hospital, use of extra formula feeds, and lack of convenient day care for working mothers.

Lactation ceases when suckling stops; therefore, in effect, any behavior that reduces the amount of suckling by the infant initiates weaning or the end of lactation. Introduction of water in bottles or of one or two bottles of formula a day may begin the weaning process regardless of the time post parturition but can be most damaging to the process when the mother-infant dyad is first establishing lactation.

Secretory Products of Lactation

NUTRITIONAL COMPONENTS OF HUMAN COLOSTRUM AND MILK

Colostrum and milk contain a rich diversity of nutrients, including electrolytes, vitamins, minerals, and trace metals; nitrogenous products; enzymes; and immunologically specific cellular and soluble products. The distribution and relative content of various nutritional

TABLE 4–2
Distribution of Secretory Products in Human Colostrum and Milk[a]

Water 86–87.5%; Total Solids 11.5 g

Nutritional Components
Lactose 6.9–7.2 g
Fat 3.0–4.4 g
Protein 0.9–1.03 g
Alpha-lactalbumin 150–170 mg
Beta-lactoglobulin trace
Serum albumin 50 mg

Electrolytes, Minerals, Trace Metals
Sodium 15–17.5 mg
Potassium 51–55 mg
Calcium 32–43 mg
Phosphorus 14–15 mg
Chloride 38–40 mg
Magnesium 3 mg
Iron 0.03 mg
Zinc 0.17 mg
Copper 15–105 μg
Iodine 4.5 μg
Manganese 1.5–2.4 μg
Fluoride 5–25 μg
Selenium 1.8–3.2 μg
Boron 8–10 μg

Nitrogen Products Total 0.15–2 g
Whey protein nitrogen 75–78 mg
Casein protein nitrogen 38–41 mg
Nonprotein nitrogen 25% of total nitrogen
Urea 0.027 g
Creatinine 0.021 g
Glucosamine 0.112 g

Vitamins
C 4.5–5.5 mg
Thiamine (B_1) 12–15 μg
Niacin 183.7 μg
B_6 11–14 μg
B_{12} <0.05 μg
Biotin 0.6–0.9 μg
Folic acid 4.1–5.2 μg
Choline 8–9 mg
Inositol 40–46 mg
Pantothenic acid 200–240 μg
A (retinol) 54–56 μg
D <0.42 IU
E 0.56 μg
K 1.5 μg

[a]Estimates based on amount per deciliter.

substances found in human milk are presented in Table 4–2. The chemical composition often exhibits considerable variation among individuals and in the same individual at different times of lactation,[12] as well as between samples obtained from mothers of low-birth-weight infants and full-term infants.[13, 14] Mature milk contains the following average amounts of major chemical constituents per deciliter: total solids, 11.3 g; fat, 3.0 g; protein, 0.9 g; whey protein nitrogen, 760 mg; casein nitrogen, 410 mg; alpha-lactalbumin, 150 mg; serum albumin, 50 mg; lactose, 7.2 g; lactoferrin, 150 mg; and

lysozyme, 50 mg. Human milk contains relatively low amounts of vitamins D and E (see Table 4–2) and contains little or no beta-lactoglobulin (the major whey protein in bovine milk). The fat globule membrane appears to have a high content of oleic acid, linoleic acid, phosphatidylpeptides, and inositol.[15] In addition, a binding ligand, which promotes absorption of zinc, has been identified in human milk.[16, 17] Temporal studies have indicated that concentrations of many chemical components, especially nitrogen, calcium, and sodium, decrease significantly as the duration of lactation increases.[18, 19] However, several components have been found to change in concentration as a function of water content because their total daily output appears to be remarkably constant, at least during the first 8 weeks of lactation.[20, 21]

Milk production progresses through three distinct phases, characterized by the secretion of colostrum, transitional (early) milk, and mature milk. Colostrum defines lactational products detected just before and for the first 3 to 4 days of lactation. It consists of yellowish, thick fluid, with a mean energy value of over 66 kilocalories (kcal)/dl, and contains high concentrations of immunoglobulin, protein, fat, fat-soluble vitamins, and ash. Transitional milk is usually observed between the fifth and fourteenth days of lactation, and mature milk is found thereafter. The concentrations of many nutritional components decline as milk production progresses to synthesis of mature milk. The content of fat-soluble vitamins and proteins decreases as the water content of milk increases. However, levels of lactose, fat, water-soluble vitamins, and total caloric content have been shown to increase as lactation matures.[22, 23]

As the result of several manufacturing errors, the nutrient composition of infant formulas has been legislated,[24] resulting in the paradoxical situation that human milk may not always meet the recommended standards for some nutrients, whereas infant formulas may exceed the recommendation. Human milk nutrient composition varies with time of lactation (colostrum versus early milk versus mature milk) and, to some extent, maternal nutritional status. The appropriate amounts of each nutrient must be considered within these constraints.

Minerals. The mineral content of human milk is low relative to that of infant formulas and very low compared to that of cow's milk, from which most formulas are prepared, so that, although it is sufficient to support growth and development, it also represents a fairly low solute load to the developing kidney. The levels of major minerals tend to decline during lactation, with the exception of that of magnesium, but with considerable variability among individuals.[25] Sodium, potassium, chloride, calcium, zinc, and phosphorus all appear to be more bioavailable in human milk than in infant formulas, reflecting their lower concentrations in human milk. Iron is readily bioavailable to the infant from human milk but may have to be supplemented later in lactation.[26, 27] Preterm infants fed human milk may need supplements of calcium and sodium.[28]

Vitamins. Human milk contains sufficient vitamins to maintain infant growth and development, with the caveat that water-soluble vitamins are particularly dependent on maternal intake of these nutrients.[29] The preterm infant may require supplements of vitamins D, E, and K when fed human milk.[30, 31] The low content of vitamin D in human milk has been related to the induction of rickets in a few breast-fed infants, as discussed later.[32] Vitamin D deficiency may be a particular problem in breast-fed infants who are not exposed to at least 30 minutes of sunshine a week.[33]

Carbohydrates and Energy. Lactose is the primary sugar found in human milk and is usually the carbohydrate chosen for the preparation of commercial formulas. Lactose supplies approximately half the energy (of a total 67 kcal/dl) taken in by the infant from human milk. Lactose (a disaccharide of glucose and galactose) may also be important to the neonate as a carrier of galactose, which may be more readily incorporated into gangliosides in the central nervous system than galactose derived from glucose in the neonate.[34] Also, glycogen may be synthesized more efficiently from galactose than glucose in the neonate because of the relatively low activity of glucokinase in early development.[35] Human milk also contains other sugars, including glucose and galactose and more than one hundred different oligosaccharides.[36] These oligosaccharides may have protective functions for the infant, especially with respect to their ability to bind to gastrointestinal pathogens.[37]

Lipids. Fats provide almost half the calories in human milk, primarily in the form of triacylglycerols (triglycerides).[38] These lipids are supplied in the form of fat globules enclosed in plasma membranes derived from the mammary epithelial cells.[39] The essential fatty acid, linoleic acid, supplies about 10% of the calories derived from the lipid fraction. The triacylglycerols serve as precursors for prostaglandins, steroids, and phospholipids and as carriers for fat-soluble vitamins. The lipid profiles of human milk differ dramatically from those of commercial formulas, and, despite considerable adaptation of such formulas, human milk lipids are absorbed more efficiently by the infant.

Cholesterol, an important lipid constituent of human milk (12 mg/dl), is usually found in only trace amounts in commercial formulas. It has been suggested that cholesterol may be an essential nutrient for the neonate.[40] A lack of cholesterol in early development may result in turning on of cholesterol synthetic mechanisms that are difficult to turn off later in life, influencing induction of hypercholesterolemia.[41] Some studies suggest that breast-feeding the neonate is associated with lowered adult serum cholesterol level and reduced deaths from ischemic heart disease.[42]

Recently there has been increased interest in the role that long-chain polyunsaturated fatty acids (LC-PUFAs) may play in human milk—especially DHA and arachidonic acid (AA). These LC-PUFAs are not found in unsupplemented infant formulas but are present in human milk. They are structural components of brain and retinal membranes and, thus, may be important for both cognitive and visual development. In addition, they may have a role in preventing atopy.[43] Numerous studies have found that infants fed formula without DHA or AA have reduced red blood cell amounts of these fatty acids[44, 45]; however, findings of visual and cognitive functional studies in term infants have been inconsistent.[46, 47] These studies have been complicated by the finding of slower growth in some preterm infants fed LC-PUFA–supplemented formulas.[48] The inconsistent findings in supplemented formula-fed babies may reflect the difficulty in determining the optional ratios of DHA to AA, and their precursors linoleic and linolenic acids, that must be fed. Thus, these lipids appear to be best delivered from human milk.

Protein and Nonprotein Nitrogen. The exact protein content of mature human milk is variable but falls close to 1.0 g/dl, in contrast to that of infant formulas, which usually contain 1.5 g/dl; the milk from mothers who deliver preterm infants may have slightly more protein.[49] The nutritionally available protein may be even less than 1.0 g/dl—as low as 0.8 g/dl—as a result of the proportion of proteins that is utilized for non-nutritional purposes. In addition, human milk contains a considerably greater percentage of nonprotein nitrogen (25% of the total nitrogen) when compared with formulas (5% of the total nitrogen).[50]

Human milk protein is primarily whey-predominant (acid soluble protein), whereas formulas prepared from bovine milk classically reflect the 18% whey:82% casein protein composition of that animal. The whey:casein protein ratio may change during lactation, from 90% whey (early milk) to 60% (mature milk) to 50% (late milk).[51] Formulas for preterm infants have been reconstituted from bovine milk to provide 60% whey:40% casein proteins; all the major formulas for term infants in the United States are now bovine whey protein–predominant preparations in an attempt to make them closer to human milk in composition. These protein quality differences are reflected by differences in the plasma and urine amino acid responses of infants fed human milk or formulas that are casein protein–predominant or whey protein–predominant.[52–54] However, in general, term infants do not respond with the dramatic differences of preterm infants when fed formulas with different protein quality.[55–58]

The nonprotein nitrogen component of human milk contains a variety of compounds that may be of importance to the development of the neonate: polyamines, nucleotides, creatinine, urea, free amino acids, carnitine, and taurine.[59] The significance of the presence of these components is not always clear, but when they are not fed, as in the case of infant formulas that contain little taurine[52] or of soy formulas that contain little carnitine,[60] apparent deficiencies that may influence the development of the infant occur. Taurine is important for bile salt conjugation as well as for support of appropriate development of the brain and retina,[40] whereas carnitine appears to be important for appropriate fatty acid metabolism.[61]

Nucleotides, in particular, appear to bridge the gap between the nutritional and immunologic roles of human milk components. Human milk contains a majority of these compounds in the form of polymeric nucleotides or nucleic acids,[62, 63] whereas formulas contain nucleotides (when they are supplemented) only in the monomeric forms (Table 4–3). Nucleotides appear to enhance intestinal development, promote iron absorption, and modify lipid metabolism in their nutritional

TABLE 4–3
Nucleotides in Human Milk and Supplemented Formula

	HUMAN MILK[a]	HUMAN MILK[b] (%)	FORMULA[a]
Nucleic acid	48	42	4
Nucleotides	36	52	81
Nucleotides	8	7	15
Total (μmol/liter)	402	163	141

[a]See reference 62.
[b]See reference 63.

role.[64] On the other hand, these compounds perform an immunologic function by promoting killer cell cytotoxicity and interleukin-2 production by stimulated mononuclear cells from infants either breast-fed or fed nucleotide supplemented formulas.[65] Nucleotide supplementation has also been reported to reduce the number of episodes of infant diarrhea in a group of lower-socioeconomic-class infants in Chile, in a manner analogous to the protection afforded by human milk.[66] In 1998 it was reported that nucleotide supplemented formulas promote the immune response of infants to *Haemophilus influenzae* type b polysaccharide immunization at 7 months of age, and a similar response was observed for diphtheria immunization.[67] Infants fed human milk for more than 6 months had a similar response and also had an enhanced titer response to oral polio vaccine; this latter response was not observed in the nucleotide formula supplemented group.[67] Thus, nucleotides are emerging as both nutritional and immunologic components of human milk.

Nutritional Proteins. As noted, the nutritional proteins in human milk are classified as either whey (acid-soluble) or casein (acid-precipitable). Within these two classes of proteins, several specific proteins are responsible for supporting the nutritional needs of the infant.

Human casein is primarily made up of beta- and kappa-casein, although it is not clear what the actual distribution of these two proteins is.[68] In contrast, bovine milk contains alpha$_{s1}$- and alpha$_{s2}$-casein (neither of which is found in human milk) in addition to beta- and kappa-casein.[69] These two human milk casein proteins appear to make up approximately 30% of the protein found in human milk, in contrast to the earlier calculation of 40% (the amount commonly used to prepare reconstituted, so-called humanized formulas from bovine milk, which normally contains 82% casein proteins).

The whey protein fraction contains all the proposed functional proteins in human milk (immunoglobulins, lysozyme, lactoferrin, enzymes, cytokines, peptide hormones) in addition to the major nutritional protein alpha-lactalbumin. The whey proteins make up approximately 70% of human milk proteins, in contrast to 18% in bovine milk. Whereas alpha-lactalbumin is the major whey protein in human milk, beta-lactoglobulin is the major whey protein in bovine milk (and is not found in

human milk).[50] A consistent fraction of human milk whey protein is made up of serum albumin. Its source remains unclear; there is some evidence that it may be synthesized in the mammary gland.[70] However, most of the serum albumin is probably synthesized outside the mammary gland.

Thus, milk proteins are characterized by their site of synthesis as well as being species-specific. Therefore, proteins such as alpha-lactalbumin and beta-lactoglobulin are species- and organ-specific, whereas proteins such as serum albumin are species-, but not organ-specific.[71] The net result of these differences in proteins utilized for nutrition by the neonate is that different amounts of amino acids are ingested by the neonate, depending on the source of milk, and even reconstitution of the whey and casein classes of proteins from one species into a ratio similar to that of another does not result in an identical amino acid intake. These differences are reflected in plasma amino acid profiles of infants fed commercial milks versus human milk regardless of the ratios of reconstitution.[54]

Bioactive Proteins and Peptides. Whereas a major proportion of human milk protein is composed of the nutritional proteins just described, a significant proportion of these proteins subserves a variety of functions, either other than or in addition to the nutritional support of the neonate. These proteins include carrier proteins, enzymes, hormones, growth factors, immunoglobulins, and cytokines (the latter two are discussed in the following section). It has not always been established that these proteins are still functional once they have been ingested by the neonate, but it is clear that human milk supplies a mixture that is potentially far more complex than just nutritional substrate.

Carrier Proteins. A number of nutrients are supplied to the neonate bound to proteins found in human milk. This binding may play an important role in making these nutrients bioavailable. Lactoferrin is an iron-binding protein (a property that may also play a role in its bacteriostatic action) that is apparently absorbed intact by the infant.[72] Lactoferrin may be important in the improved absorption of iron by the infant from human milk compared with that from cow's milk preparations, which contain little lactoferrin.[26] Lactoferrin may also bind other minerals, including zinc and manganese, although the preferred mineral form appears to be the ferric ion.

A number of other proteins appear to be important as carriers of vitamins and hormones. Folate-binding, vitamin B_{12}–binding, and vitamin D–binding proteins have all been identified in human milk. These proteins appear to have some resistance to proteolysis, especially when they are saturated with the appropriate vitamin ligand.[73] Serum albumin acts as a carrier of a number of ligands, whereas alpha-lactalbumin acts as a carrier for calcium. Finally, proteins that bind thyroid hormone and corticosteroids have been reported to be present in human milk,[74, 75] although serum albumin may in part fulfill this function.

Enzymes. The activity of more than 30 enzymes has been detected in human milk.[76] Most of these enzymes appear to originate from the blood, with a few originating from secretory epithelial cells of the mammary gland. Little is known about the role of these enzymes, other than lysozyme and the lipases, in human milk. The enzymes found in human milk range from adenosine triphosphatases (ATPases) to antioxidant enzymes, such as catalase, to phosphatases and glycolytic enzymes. Although these enzymes have important roles in normal body metabolism, it is not clear how many of them either function in the milk itself or survive ingestion by the infant to function in the neonate.

Lysozyme appears to have a part in the antibacterial function of human milk, whereas the lipases have a more nutrient-related role in modulating fat metabolism for the neonate. Two lipases have been identified in human milk, a lipoprotein lipase and a bile salt–stimulated lipase.[77] Lipoprotein lipase appears to be involved in determining the pattern of lipids found in human milk by regulating uptake into milk at the level of the mammary gland. Human milk bile salt–stimulated lipase is an acid-stable protein that compensates for the low activity of lipases secreted into the digestive tract during early development.[78] Thus, these two enzymes regulate both the amount and the pattern of lipid that appears in milk as well as the extremely efficient absorption of lipid by the infant. Human milk lipid is absorbed much more readily than lipid from commercial milk formulas despite the many adaptations that have been made to improve absorption, illustrating the effective mechanisms supported by the lipases.

Hormones and Growth Factors. Both peptide and steroid hormones, as well as growth factors, have been identified in trace amounts in human milk, although, as with most of the enzymes, it is not clear to what degree they function in the neonates to whom they have been supplied. As discussed previously, binding proteins for corticosteroids and thyroxine have been identified in milk and, by extrapolation from other milk components, may play a role in making these bioactive compounds more readily available to the infant.

Among the hormones identified in human milk are insulin, oxytocin, calcitonin, and prolactin. Most of these hormones appear to be absorbed by the infant, but their role in in vivo function remains unclear.[79] Breast-fed infants appear to have a different endocrine response than formula-fed infants, presumably reflecting the intake of hormones from human milk.[80] However, the advantages or disadvantages to the infant of these responses are unknown.

Human milk also contains a rich mixture of growth factors, including epidermal growth factor and nerve growth factor.[81] In addition, a variety of gastrointestinal peptides have been identified in human milk. Presumably the supply of these various factors to the infant via the milk compensates for their possible deficiency in the infant during early development.

The composition of human milk provides a complex and complete nutritional substrate to the neonate. Human milk supplies not only individual nutrients but also enzymes involved in metabolism, carriers to improve absorption, and hormones that may regulate metabolic rates. Commercial formulas have not yet been developed to the point that they can provide an analogous complete nutritional system.

RESISTANCE TO INFECTION

Component Mechanisms of Defense: Origin and Distribution

Fresh human milk contains a wealth of components that provide specific, as well as nonspecific, defenses against infectious agents and environmental macromolecules (Table 4–4). These include cells, such as T and B lymphocytes, polymorphonuclear leukocytes (PMNs), and macrophages; soluble products, especially immunoglobulins; secretory immunoglobulin A (sIgA); immunomodulatory cytokines and cytokine receptors; components of the complement system; several carrier proteins; enzymes; and a number of endocrine hormones or hormone-like substances. Additional soluble factors that are active against streptococci, staphylococci, and tumor viruses have also been identified.[22] Other soluble milk factors with potential implications in host defense include the bifidus factor, which promotes growth of bifidobacteria, and an epidermal growth factor, which promotes growth of mucosal epithelium and maturation of intestinal brush border. The developmental characteristics of sIgA have been studied more extensively than those of other components.[82–84]

On the basis of available information, it is clear that the majority of IgA-producing cells observed in milk have their origin in the precursor immunocompetent cells in the gut-associated lymphoid tissues (GALTs) and bronchus-associated lymphoid tissues (BALTs). Exposure of IgA precursor B lymphocytes in the GALT or BALT to microbial and dietary antigens in the mucosal lumen is an important prerequisite for their initial activation and proliferation. Such antigen-sensitized cells are eventually transported via the systemic circulation to other mucosal surfaces, including the mammary glands, and, as plasma cells, initiate the synthesis of immunoglobulin against specific antigens previously experienced in the mucosa of the respiratory or alimentary tract.[82, 83] It has been proposed that T cells observed in the milk may also be derived from GALT and BALT in a manner similar to that of IgA-producing cells. Little or no information is available regarding the site of origin of other cellular or soluble immunologic components normally present in human milk. Specific antibody and cellular immune reactivity against many respiratory and enteric bacterial and viral pathogens and ingested food proteins is also present in human breast milk (Table 4–5).

SOLUBLE PRODUCTS

Immunoglobulin A. As observed in other peripheral mucosal sites, the major class of immunoglobulin in human colostrum and milk is the 11S sIgA. Other isotypes, namely, 7S IgA, IgG, IgM, IgD, and IgE, are also present. The IgA exists as a dimer of two 7S IgA molecules linked together by a polypeptide chain, the J-chain, and is associated with a nonimmunoglobulin protein

TABLE 4–4

Immunologically and Pharmacologically Active Components and Hormones Observed in Human Colostrum and Milk

SOLUBLE	CELLULAR	HORMONES AND HORMONE-LIKE SUBSTANCES
Immunologically Specific	**Immunologically Specific**	Epidermal growth factors
Immunoglobulin sIgA (11S), 7S IgA, IgG, IgM, IgE, IgD, secretory component	T lymphocytes	Prostaglandins
	B lymphocytes	Relaxin
T Cell Products	**Accessory Cells**	Neurotensin
Histocompatibility Antigens	Neutrophils	Somatostatin
Nonspecific Factors	Macrophages	Bombesin
Complement	Epithelial cells	Gonadotropins
Chemotactic factors		Ovarian steroids
Properdin		Thyroid-releasing hormone
Interferon		Thyroid-stimulating hormone
Alpha-fetoprotein		Thyroxine and triiodothyronine
Bifidus factor		Adrenocorticotropin
Antistaphylococcal factor(s)		Corticosteroids
Antiadherence substances		Prolactin
Epidermal growth factor		Erythropoietin
Folate uptake enhancer		Insulin
Antiviral factor(s)		
Migration inhibition factor		
Carrier Proteins		
Lactoferrin		
Transferrin		
B_{12}-binding protein		
Corticoid-binding protein		
Enzymes		
Lysozyme		
Lipoprotein lipase		
Leukocyte enzymes		

referred to as the secretory component. The sIgA protein constitutes about 75% of the total nitrogen content of human milk. The IgA dimers produced by plasma cells at the basal surface of the mammary epithelium are transported to specialized columnar epithelial cells, where they acquire the secretory component before their discharge into the alveolar spaces.[83, 84]

Sequential quantitation of class-specific immunoglobulin in human colostrum and milk has demonstrated that the highest levels of sIgA and IgM are present

TABLE 4–5

Specific Antibody or Cell-Mediated Immunologic Reactivity in Human Colostrum and Milk

BACTERIA	VIRUSES	OTHER
Escherichia coli (O + K antigens and enterotoxin)	Rotavirus	*Candida albicans*
Salmonella	Rubella	*Giardia* sp.
Shigella sp.	Poliovirus types 1, 2, 3	*Entamoeba histolytica*
Vibrio cholerae	Echoviruses	Food proteins
Bacteroides fragilis	Coxsackieviruses A and B	
Streptococcus pneumoniae	Respiratory syncytial virus[a]	
Bordetella pertussis	Cytomegalovirus[a]	
Clostridium tetani and *C. difficile*	Influenza A virus	
Corynebacterium diphtheriae	Herpes simplex virus type 1	
Streptococcus mutans	Arboviruses	
Haemophilus influenzae type B	Semliki Forest	
Mycobacterium tuberculosis[a]	Ross River	
Poliovirus types 1, 2, 3	Japanese B	
Echoviruses	Dengue	
	Human immunodeficiency virus (HIV)	

[a]Evidence of reactivity for both antibody and cellular immunity.

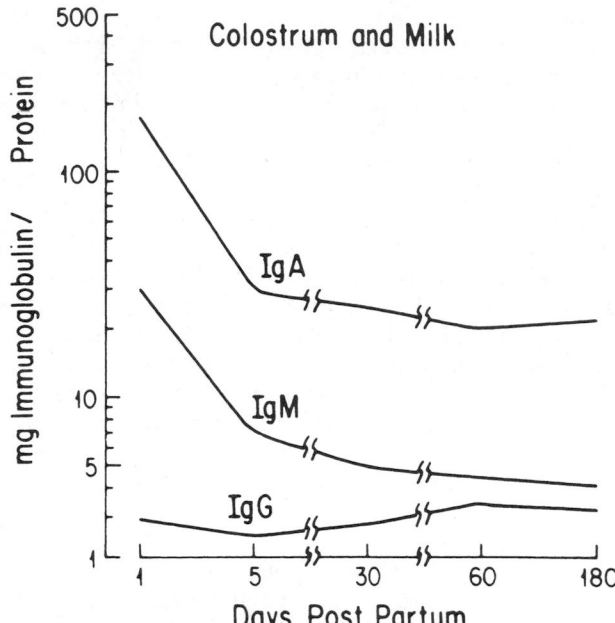

FIGURE 4–1. Comparison of the mean levels of IgG, IgA, and IgM in colostrum and milk at different intervals after the onset of lactation in mothers who were breast-feeding. (Modified from Ogra SS, Ogra PL. Immunologic aspects of human colostrum and milk. II. Characteristics of lymphocyte reactivity and distribution of E-rosette forming cells at different times after the onset of lactation. J Pediatr 92:550–555, 1978.)

during the first few days of lactation (Fig. 4–1). Levels of IgA are 4- to 5-fold higher than those of IgM, 20- to 30-fold higher than those of IgG, and 5- to 6-fold higher than those of serum IgA.[84] As lactation progresses, IgA declines to levels that range from 20 to 27 mg/g protein and IgM levels decline from 3.5 to 4.1 mg/g protein. IgG levels do not show any significant change during early and late lactation and are usually maintained in the range of 1.4 to 4.9 mg/g protein (see Fig. 4–1). Although a dramatic and rapid decline in milk IgA and IgM occurs during the first week of life, this is more than balanced by an increase in the volume of milk produced as the process of lactation becomes established (see Fig. 4–1).

IgA antibodies found in milk possess specificity for infectious agents endemic to or pathogenic for the intestinal and respiratory tracts (see Table 4–4). These may be present in the milk in the absence of specific circulating IgA. In a study in which pregnant women were given oral feedings of *Escherichia coli* 083, development of IgA antibody in human milk was evident in the absence of detectable serum antibody–specific responses.[85] Other investigators have observed similar responses in animal models using intrabronchial immunization with *Streptococcus pneumoniae*. These and other studies[86–89] have strongly supported the concept of a bronchomammary, as well as an enteromammary, axis of immunologic reactivity in the breast.

Despite the elegance of studies that have defined the mechanisms of IgA cell traffic from GALT and BALT to the mammary glands, it is clear that the actual number of B cells or IgA plasma cells in the mammary glands is sparse. At the same time, colostrum and milk may contain large amounts of IgA (as much as 11 g in colostrum and as much as 1 to 3 g per day in later milk), as shown in Table 4–6. The reasons underlying the apparent disparity between the content of immunoglobulin-producing cells and concentrations of immunoglobulin are not known. It may be related to the unique hormonal environment of the mammary glands. The hormones that have been consistently observed in human milk are listed in Table 4–4.

The effect of pregnancy- and lactation-related hormones on regulation of immunologic reactivity present in the resting and lactating breast has been examined.[90] In a study on immunoglobulin production in the nonlactating human breast, several interesting findings were noted.[91] Few mononuclear cells were present in the nulliparous and parous nonlactating breast, although IgA-containing cells predominated. Synthesis of IgA appeared to be slightly increased in the parous subjects. IgA was found in the mammary tissues during the proliferative stage of the menstrual cycle in the nulliparous subjects and during the luteal phase in the parous subjects. The number of IgA-producing cells in the nonlactating breast was observed to increase with parity. These findings suggest that the immunologic makeup of the nonlactating, as well as the lactating, breast may be

---

TABLE 4–6

Level of Immunoglobulins in Colostrum and Milk and Estimates of Delivery of Lactational Immunoglobulins to the Breast-Feeding Neonate[a]

Day Post Partum	PERCENTAGE OF TOTAL PROTEINS REPRESENTED BY IMMUNOGLOBULIN			OUTPUT OF IMMUNOGLOBULIN, MG/24 HR		
	IgG	IgM	IgA	IgG	IgM	IgA
1	7	3	80	80	120	11,000
3	10	45	45	50	40	2000
7	1–2	4	20	25	10	1000
7–28	1–2	2	10–15	10	10	1000
<50	1–2	0.5–1	10–15	10	10	1000

[a]Estimates based on the available data for total immunoglobulin and daily protein synthesis (see references 6, 83, 84).

significantly influenced by the hormonal milieu. In another study of virgin mice given exogenously administered hormones,[92] an extended exposure to estrogen, progesterone, and prolactin was necessary for maximal increments in IgA-producing plasma cells in the breast. Similarly, castrated males exposed to these hormones became moderately receptive to mammary gland homing of cells specific for IgA synthesis. As would be expected, testosterone eliminated female breast receptivity to these cells. These studies suggest the existence of a hormonally determined homing mechanism in the mammary gland for class-specific, immunoglobulin-producing cells.

More recent studies have proposed another possible influence of lactational hormones on immunocompetent cells. In limited observations, combinations of prolactin with estrogen and progesterone (in concentrations observed normally at the beginning of parturition) appeared to have an amplifying effect on the synthesis and secretion of IgA from peripheral blood lymphocytes.[93] This observation raises the possibility that the high levels of sIgA observed in colostrum and milk may be the result of selective, hormonally mediated proliferation of antigen-sensitized IgA cells in the peripheral blood and its rapid clearance and bioconcentration in the mammary secretions. The immunoglobulin could acquire secretory component during its passage through the mammary epithelium and eventually appear in the colostrum or milk as mature sIgA. Although the appearance of sIga antibody in milk characteristically follows antigenic exposure in the GALT or BALT, the precise nature of the IgA content in milk appears to be determined by a variety of other factors operating in the mucosal lymphoid tissue. These include the regulatory T cell network in the GALT and possibly in the BALT,[94] the nature of antigens (soluble proteins versus particulate microbial agents),[95] and the route of primary versus secondary antigenic exposure.[96]

It has been estimated that the breast-fed infant may consistently receive an amount of about 1 g IgA each day. Approximately 1/100 of this amount each day is IgM and IgG.[97, 98] The estimates of lactational immunoglobulin delivered to the breast-fed infant at different periods of lactation are presented in Table 4–6. Most ingested IgA is eliminated in the feces, although up to 10% may be absorbed from the intestine into the circulation within the first 18 to 24 hours after birth. Approximately 70 to 75% of ingested milk IgA survives passage through the gut and is excreted in the feces.[99] Feces of breast-fed infants contain functional antibodies present in the ingested milk.[100] Other studies also support the finding of prolonged survival of milk IgA in the gastrointestinal tract. Infants fed human milk have demonstrated the presence of all immunoglobulin classes in the feces. Fecal IgA content was three- to fourfold higher than that of IgM after human milk feeding. Comparative studies on survival of human milk IgA and bovine IgG in the neonatal intestinal tract have suggested that the fecal content of IgA may be 14- to 20-fold higher after human milk feeding than that of bovine IgG after feeding of bovine immune globulin.[101]

Direct information about the role of milk IgA in antimicrobial defense is available in several studies. sIgA interferes with bacterial adherence to cell surfaces.[102] Colostrum and milk can inhibit the activity of E. coli and Vibrio cholerae enterotoxins in experimental settings.[103] The antitoxic activity of human milk appears to correlate well with its IgA content but not with its IgM and IgG content. Precoating of V. cholerae with specific sIgA protects infant mice from disease.[104] Similar results have been obtained by using specific purified milk sIgA in preventing E. coli– and Shigella dysenteriae–induced disease in rabbits.[105] Less definite, but suggestive, is a study conducted with human milk feeding relative to the intestinal implantation of orally administered live poliovirus vaccine.[106] This study found that breast-feeding may reduce the degree of seroconversion for poliovirus antibody in the vaccinated infants. Because antipolio IgA is present in human milk and colostrum, the authors concluded that specific IgA may bind poliovirus and influence viral replication in the intestinal mucosa. Extensive experience with oral polio immunization worldwide, however, has not associated breast-feeding with live vaccine failures. Other studies have clearly shown that the magnitude of poliovirus replication in the intestine is determined by the presence and level of preexisting sIgA antibody. With high levels of intestinal IgA antibody, little or no replication of vaccine virus was observed in the gut. With lower levels, varying degrees of viral replication could be demonstrated.[107]

Indirect evidence, obtained from a more clinical perspective, suggests a protective role for milk against a variety of mucosal infections. Breast-feeding has been strongly implicated in supporting gastrointestinal homeostasis in the neonate and in establishing normal gut flora. Observations have shown the absence of diarrheal disease in breast-fed infants, even in the face of contamination of the fed milk with E. coli and Shigella species.[108] A preventive and therapeutic role for breast-feeding has also been suggested in nursery outbreaks with enteropathogenic strains of E. coli[109] and diarrhea associated with rotavirus.[110] Breast-feeding plays an inhibitory role in the appearance of E. coli 083 agglutinins found in the feces of colonized infants. A decrease in the incidence of neonatal sepsis, specifically that associated with gram-negative bacilli and E. coli K1 serotypes, has also been linked to breast-feeding.[111, 112] Milk IgA, possibly by limiting ingestion of foreign antigens by the neonate, or by binding of foreign proteins with specific antibodies to prevent absorption, or by both processes, may decrease the incidence of atopic-allergic diseases.[113–115] The frequency of IgE skin test–positive results in individuals has been described as being lower among breast-fed infants, possibly because of decreased exposure to cow's milk proteins or presence of maternal blocking antibodies.[116] Indirect epidemiologic data suggest that breast-feeding is protective against certain respiratory bacterial and viral infections.[117, 118] Whereas the epidemiologic studies strongly support a protective role of breast-feeding, it is not possible in these studies to dissect the relative contribution of sIgA from that of other soluble or cellular components present in colostrum and milk.

IgG and IgM. Normal neonates exhibit characteristic paucity or lack of IgA during the first 7 to 10 days after birth. At this time, the presence of IgM and IgG in milk may be important to compensate for immunologic functions not present in the mucosal sites. For example, both IgG and IgM participate in complement fixation and specific bactericidal activity, functions not associated with IgA. Studies carried out after oral feeding of immune serum globulin (mostly IgG) have suggested that IgG may survive in the gastrointestinal tract of low-birth-weight infants.[119] Thus, other immunoglobulin isotypes in milk may also be able to serve as effective substitutes for IgA in the neonates of IgA-deficient mothers in prevention of infection with enteric or respiratory pathogens.

IgE and IgD. Studies on the distribution and role of IgE or IgD in colostrum and milk are few. Normal cord blood contains little or no IgE or IgD. The highest IgE concentrations observed in normal neonates are usually less than 5 ng/ml. Investigations have failed to demonstrate local synthesis of IgE in the breast.[120–122] Although IgE may be detected in up to 40% of colostrum and milk samples, the concentrations are extremely low, and many samples of colostrum and milk contain no IgE activity when paired samples of serum contain high IgE levels. On the other hand, IgD has been detected in most colostrum and milk samples. It has been suggested that subjects with high serum IgD levels are more likely to have high IgD concentrations in the milk. The possibility of some local production of both IgE and IgD cannot be ruled out.[122]

CELLULAR ELEMENTS

Human colostrum and milk contain lymphocytes, monocytes-macrophages, neutrophils, and epithelial cells.[123] Early colostrum contains the highest concentration of cells, approximately 1 to 3 $\times$ 10^6 cells per ml. By the end of the first week of lactation, cell concentration is of the order of 10^5 cells per ml. Total cell numbers delivered to the newborn throughout lactation may, however, remain constant when adjustments are made for the increase in volume of milk produced.[124] The two major cell populations in human milk are difficult to distinguish by common staining methods because of the large number of intracytoplasmic inclusions, neutrophils, and macrophages. More accurate estimates by flow cytometry analysis suggest that the relative frequencies of neutrophils, macrophages, and lymphocytes in early milk samples are approximately 80%, 15%, and 4%, respectively.[125, 126] The remaining cells are present in smaller amounts, especially in the absence of active suckling, engorgement, or local breast infection.

Macrophages. Histochemically, the milk macrophage differs from the blood monocyte in having decreased peroxidase staining and increased lysosomes and significant amounts of immunoglobulin, especially IgA, in the cytoplasm.[127–129] The intracellular immunoglobulin in macrophages represents up to 10% of milk IgA.[130] Kinetic studies on the release of IgA by human milk macrophages suggest that immunoglobulin release by macrophages, unlike that by other phagocytic cells, is a time-dependent phenomenon and is not significantly influenced by the use of secretagogues or stimulants,

such as phorbol myristate acetate.[130] However, active phagocytosis is associated with significant increase in release of IgA.[131] In other studies, milk macrophages have been found to be efficient in release of superoxide anions after in vitro stimulation with phorbol myristate acetate.[132, 133] Milk macrophages have the capacity to be primed by appropriate stimulation for greater release of superoxide anions.[133] It has been shown that milk macrophages obtained from preterm-delivered lactating mothers have a significantly higher phagocytic index than the macrophages in term milk. However, the bactericidal activity appears to be similar in pre- and full-term milk macrophages.[132] In neutrophils, milk macrophages appear to be activated, as demonstrated by the increased expression of CD11b and decreased expression of L-selectin.[125]

The precise functions of macrophages in colostrum or milk have not been explored fully. These cells have been suggested as potential transport vehicles for IgA.[128, 129] Milk macrophages possess phagocytic activity against *Staphylococcus aureus*, *E. coli*, and *Candida albicans*, with possible cytocidal activity against the first two organisms.[134] Milk macrophages participate in antibody-dependent, cell-mediated cytotoxicity of herpes simplex virus type 1–infected cells.[135] Infection of milk macrophages by respiratory syncytial virus results in the production of the proinflammatory cytokines interleukin-1β (IL-1β), IL-6, and tumor necrosis factor–alpha (TNF-α).[136] They are also involved in a variety of other biosynthetic and excretory activities, including production of lactoferrin, lysozyme,[137] components of complement,[138] properdin factor B, epithelial growth factor(s), T lymphocyte suppressive factor(s), and IgA B cell helper factor(s).[82] There is also a suggestion that milk macrophages may be important in regulation of T cell function.[139, 140]

Lymphocytes. Milk contains a small number of lymphocytes, 80% of which are T cells and 4 to 6% of which are B cells.[126] The small number of B cells reflects the sessile nature of these cells, which enter the lamina propria of the mammary gland to transform into plasma cells. Although several investigators have been unable to show in vitro antibody synthesis by milk lymphocytes, studies performed with colostral B cells transformed by Epstein-Barr virus have shown production of IgG, as well as J-chain–containing IgM and IgA.[141] A small population of CD16$^+$ natural killer cells can be also identified in most milk samples but cannot be accurately quantitated.[126] In functional studies, however, colostral cells exhibit natural killer cytotoxicity, which is enhanced by interferon and interleukin-2. Colostral cells also elicit antibody- and lectin-dependent cellular cytotoxic responses. However, the natural killer, as well as the antibody- and lectin-dependent, responses in colostral cells have been observed to be significantly lower than those of autologous peripheral blood cells. Reduced cellular cytotoxicity of colostral cells has also been observed against virus-infected targets and certain bacteria. In fact, with several specific virus-infected targets, colostrum and milk cells conspicuously lack cellular cytotoxicity when compared with autologous peripheral blood cells. There is also an apparent exclusion of cytolytic T

TABLE 4–7

Lymphocyte Subpopulations in Human Milk and Autologous Blood[a]

LYMPHOCYTE SUBPOPULATIONS	HUMAN MILK	BLOOD
CD3[+b]	83 ± 11	75 ± 7
CD3[+] CD4[+b]	36 ± 13	44 ± 6
CD3[+] CD8[+b]	43 ± 12	27 ± 4
CD4[+]/CD8[+c]	0.88 ± 0.35	1.70 ± 0.45
CD19[+b]	6 ± 4	14 ± 5

[a]Expressed as mean ± standard deviation (SD).
[b]Expressed as percentage of total lymphocytes.
[c]Ratio of CD3[+]/CD4[+] to CD3[+]/CD8[+] lymphocytes.

Adapted from Wirt DP, Adkins LT, Palkowetz KH, et al. Activated-memory T lymphocytes in human milk. Cytometry 13:282–290, 1992. Copyright © 1992. Reprinted by permission of John Wiley & Sons, Inc.

cells in the milk for certain human leukocyte antigen (HLA) phenotypes.[142, 143]

The majority of T lymphocytes in colostrum and milk are mature CD3[+] cells. Both CD4[+] (helper) and CD8[+] (cytotoxic and suppressor) populations are present in human milk, with a proportion of CD8[+] T cells higher than that found in human blood T cells (Table 4–7). The CD4[+]/CD8[+] ratio in milk is significantly lower than that observed in peripheral blood and is not due to an increase of CD8[+] cells in the peripheral blood of women during the postpartum period. Colostral and milk T lymphocytes manifest in vitro proliferative responses on stimulation with a number of mitogens and antigens. Several studies have shown a selectivity in lymphocyte stimulation responses in colostral and milk lymphocytes to various antigens when compared with peripheral blood lymphocyte responses.[124, 144] Antigens such as rubella virus stimulate T lymphocytes in secretory sites and milk as well as in systemic sites.[124] In contrast, E. coli K1 antigen, whose exposure is limited to mucosal sites, produces stimulation of lymphoproliferative responses only in milk lymphocytes. These studies support the concept of select T cell populations in the mammary gland. In addition to antigen selectivity, there is a general hyporesponsiveness to mitogenic stimulation of milk lymphocytes relative to peripheral blood lymphocytes.[124, 140] The decreased reactivity of milk lymphocytes to phytohemagglutinin (PHA) may be partly the result of a relative deficiency of certain populations of T cells in milk. Macrophage–T cell interactions have also been postulated as being responsible for this relative hyporesponsiveness,[84] although it is not known whether the effects are the result of decreased helper or increased suppressor function. Recent studies have shown that milk lymphocytes exhibit reduced responses to allogenic cells but display good ability to stimulate alloreactivity.[142] Treatment of milk lymphocytes with monoclonal antibodies cytotoxic for T lymphocytes or with anti–HLA class II antigen-specific monoclonal antibodies has resulted in a substantial reduction in in vitro proliferative responses to bacterial antigens. It appears that, in general, the T cell proliferative responses to PHA and tetanus toxoid in breast-fed infants are significantly higher than those in bottle-fed infants, possibly secondary to the presence of maternally derived cell growth factors and other lymphokines present in human milk.[140, 145]

Virtually all CD4[+] and CD8[+] T cells in milk bear the CD45 isoform CD45RO that is associated with immunologic memory.[126, 146] In addition, the proportion of T cells that display other phenotypic markers of activation, including CD25 (IL-2R) and HLA-DR, is much greater than that in blood.[126, 147] Consistent with their memory phenotype, T cells in human milk produce interferon γ.[146] Furthermore, a significantly greater number of CD4[+] T cells in colostrum express the CD40 ligand (CD40-L) compared with autologous or heterologous blood T cells.[148] Cognate interaction between the CD40-L on T cells and CD40 on B cells is a necessary step for antibody production in vivo and is congenitally deficient in the newborn. However, the function of these memory T cells in the recipient human infant is currently unknown. Mucous membrane sites in the upper alimentary–respiratory tract of the recipient infant would seem to be potential sites for human milk leukocytes to enter. It is of considerable interest that very small numbers of memory T cells are detected in blood in infancy.[149] Thus, it may be possible that maternal memory T cells in milk compensate for the developmental delay in their production in the infant. In this regard, the proportion of T lymphocytes bearing the T cell receptor-γδ (TCR-γδ) is approximately twofold greater in colostrum than in blood.[150, 151] Human TCR-γδ[+] cells populate organized lymphoid tissues and represent half of the intraepithelial lymphocytes in the gut.[152] Thus, the intestinal epithelia may have a selective affinity for TCR-γδ[+] cells and provide a favorable environment for maternal T cells in milk to be transferred to the breast-fed infants. There is evidence from experimental animal studies that milk lymphocytes enter tissues of the neonate,[153–156] but this has not been demonstrated in humans. In addition, the possible transfer of histocompatibility antigens and T cells to the neonate through breast-feeding has been examined by determining the fate of skin grafts in suckling rats fed by allogenic mothers.[157] Such foster feeding of milk may result not only in increased allogenic graft survival but also in development of "runting" syndrome, possibly as a result of a graft-versus-host–like reaction in the breast-fed animal. Effects of the transfer may be related to dosage of ingested allogenic cells, in that increasing cell numbers transferred may prolong skin graft survival but may also increase the likelihood of a graft-versus-host reaction. It is important to note that the suckling rat gut has a higher degree of permeability to whole proteins than does the human intestine. Furthermore, clinical experience in immunodeficient neonates has never supported the development of graft-versus-host–like disease in the breast-fed human infant. In humans, possible transfer of maternal T cell reactivity to tuberculin protein from the mother to the neonate has been observed via the process of breast-feeding.[99, 158, 159] The implications of these observations are that maternal cellular products or soluble mediators of cellular reactivity may be transferred passively to the neonate via the process of breast-feeding. Admittedly, however, the occurrence of such phenomena in humans has not been studied carefully. Thus, it must be emphasized that at this time there is no evidence to suggest any T cell–mediated immunologic risks associated with breast-feeding in humans. On the other hand, it is still unknown whether milk T cells, either TCR-$\alpha\beta^+$ or -$\gamma\beta^+$, play a role in the transfer of adoptive immunoprotection to the recipient infant.

Neutrophils. Milk contains large numbers of neutrophils. Although the absolute counts collected from actively nursing mothers exhibit considerable variability between different samples, highest numbers are generally observed during the first 3 to 4 days of lactation. The numbers of neutrophils decrease significantly after 3 to 4 weeks of lactation, and only rare neutrophils are observed in samples collected after 60 to 80 days post partum. Leukocytes in human milk appear to be metabolically activated. Indeed, although the neutrophils are phagocytic and produce toxic oxygen radicals, they do not respond well to chemoattractants by increasing their adherence, polarity, or directed migration in in vitro systems.[160] This diminished response was found to be due to prior activation in that the neutrophils in milk displayed a phenotypic pattern that is typical of activated neutrophils. The expression of CD11b, the alpha chain subunit of Mac-1, was increased, and the expression of L-selectin was decreased.[125]

Epithelial Cells. On the basis of their anatomic distribution, epithelial cells in the human mammary gland can be classified into two main types: myoepithelial and luminal. However, these cells appear to be more heterogeneous on histologic and physicochemical testing.[142, 161, 162] They include secretory cells, which contain abundant rough endoplasmic reticulum; lipid droplets; and Golgi apparatus. The secretory cells appear to produce casein micelle. The squamous epithelial cells are usually seen in the regions of the cutaneous junction of the nipples, especially near the galactophores. The ductal or luminal cells, which exist in clusters, have many short microvilli, tight junctions, and remnants of desmosomes.[161, 162] Studies with the use of monoclonal antibodies have shown that, in rodents, there may be as many as 10 different types of epithelial cells in the adult mammary glands. These cell types probably represent various stages of differentiation of mammary gland epithelium. These include, in the mammary end buds, the distinct cell types of the tip and the main compartment peripheral cell types I and II; and in alveoli, as well as in the ducts of the mammary glands, the luminal cell types I and II and myoepithelial cells.[161] It is, however, not known whether similar epithelial cell differentiation occurs in the human mammary gland.

In human milk, relatively few epithelial cells are observed in the early phases of lactation. Most epithelial cells appear after 2 to 3 weeks and are seen in appreciable numbers, even as long as 180 to 200 days after the onset of lactation. With the possible exception of the synthesis of secretory component and casein and possibly other products, with which secretory epithelial cells have been associated in the stroma of the mammary gland, the role of epithelial cells in the milk remains to be defined.

The information reviewed thus far provides strong evidence for the existence of a number of dynamic cellular reactions in the mammary gland, colostrum, and milk. Unfortunately, the specific functional role, collectively or individually, for the epithelial cells, monocytes, neutrophils, or lymphocytes in the mammary gland or the milk remains to be defined. In view of the high degree of selectivity and the differences in the quantitative and functional distribution of cellular elements, it is suggested that the mammary gland, like mucosal surfaces, may function somewhat partitioned from the cellular elements in peripheral blood, similarly to other peripheral sites (such as the genital tract) of the common mucosal system. It is, however, not known whether the characteristic proportions of macrophages, T lymphocytes, other cytotoxic cells, or epithelial cells are designed for any specific functions locally in the mammary gland in the lactating mother or in epithelium or lumen of the intestinal or respiratory mucosa of the breast-feeding infant, or both. The observations on the transfer of delayed hypersensitivity reactions in human neonates and of graft-versus-host reactivity in the rat raise the possibility that milk cells may function as important vehicles in transfer of maternal immunity to neonates. However, the potential beneficial and harmful roles of such cell-mediated transfer via the mucosal routes need to be investigated further. The paucity of natural killer and other cytotoxic cells in the colostrum may have a role for the breast-feeding neonate, especially in influencing the antigen processing and uptake of replicating microorganisms and their immune response at systemic or mucosal levels or both. Although colostral cells await further elucidation of their function in the mammary glands and the suckling neonate, it is likely that their presence in the milk represents a highly selective phenomenon and not a mere contamination with peripheral blood cells.

OTHER POSSIBLE DEFENSE FACTORS

Human colostrum and milk contain all components of the complement system. Active production of C3 has been reported in vitro in breast milk cell cultures.[163, 164] Interferon,[165] migration-inhibition factor,[158] and alpha-fetoprotein[148] are also present in human milk, although their roles have not been fully elucidated at this time (see Table 4–4).

Iron-binding proteins present in colostrum and milk, such as lactoferrin,[166] have bacteriostatic activity in vitro against *E. coli*, *S. aureus*, and *C. albicans*.[137] There is evidence of enhanced bactericidal activity of lactoferrin in association with IgA. Lysozyme and bifidus factor (a collection of glycosamides that promote growth of *Lactobacillus* and bifidobacterial species, whose growth in turn inhibits growth of enteric gram-negative aerobic bacilli) may function as ancillary inhibitors of gut and skin pathogens. Antistaphylococcal factors appear to be active against experimental staphylococcal infections and may be important for local mammary gland protection.[166, 167] Of particular interest is the demonstration of certain oligosaccharides that prevent attachment of *S. pneumoniae* to human epithelial cells[168] and of high-molecular-weight substances that inhibit virulence of enterotoxins of Enterobacteriaceae (see Table 4–4).

Nonimmunoglobulin antiviral factors have been demonstrated in lipid and aqueous phases of human milk. These include activity against influenza A and B viruses, herpes simplex virus, Semliki Forest virus, Japanese B encephalitis virus, rubella virus, rhinovirus, and rotavirus (see Table 4–4). The milk-associated antiviral factors have been shown to have inhibitory functions only in vitro. Their in vivo role in neonatal and maternal infections remains to be elucidated. Recent studies have also demonstrated the presence of other substances in human milk that promote growth and maturation of intestinal epithelial tissue[169] and uptake of folate by the intestinal cells.[170]

Several recent studies have generated interest in the potential role of nonantibody proteins, bile salt lipases, whey proteins, and trace metals present in human milk on the course of enteric infections.[171–174] Several species of gram-positive and gram-negative bacteria can frequently be killed by incubation with human milk whey but not commercial infant formula.[171] The mechanisms responsible for such antibacterial activity are not known. The synergistic interaction among IgA, lactoferrin, and iron has been suggested to play a role in such defense.[171–172]

Concentrations of free fatty acid and possibly monoglycerides seem to increase during storage of milk because of spontaneous lipolysis generated by lipoprotein lipase.[175, 176] Antibody-independent antiparasitic effect of stored, but not fresh, human milk against Giardia lamblia or Entamoeba histolytica has been attributed to such free fatty acids.[177] In additional studies in vitro, bile salt–stimulated lipase, the major lipase in human milk, has been found to cause hydrolysis of milk triglycerides. It remains to be seen whether free fatty acids induce significant in vivo protection in the intestine against intestinal parasites. On the other hand, bile salts themselves may stimulate the growth of G. lamblia.[173]

Nonantibody proteins, several carrier proteins, and cellular enzyme proteins are present in milk in high concentrations. Concentrations of lysozyme range from 30 to 50 mg/100 ml in early colostrum to 5 to 10 mg/100 ml in late milk. The susceptibility of an organism to lysozyme depends on the availability of the peptidoglycan substrate. In certain situations in which the peptidoglycan may be blocked by lipoproteins, the organisms are relatively resistant to lysozymes.[173, 174]

Direct-Acting Antimicrobial Agents

General Features. The defense agents in human milk, although biochemically diverse, share certain features: (1) They are usually common to mucosal sites, and (2) they are adapted to resist digestion in the gastrointestinal tract of the recipient infant. (3) They protect by noninflammatory mechanisms. (4) They act synergistically with each other or with factors produced by the infant. (5) Most components of the immune system in human milk are produced throughout lactation and during gradual weaning, but (6) there is often an inverse relationship between the production of these factors in

the mammary gland and their production by the infant during the same time frames of lactation and postnatal development. Indeed, as lactation proceeds, the concentration of many factors in human milk declines. Concomitantly, the mucosal production of these factors rises in the developing infant. It is unclear whether the inverse relationship between these processes is due to feedback mechanisms or whether the processes are independent.

Oligosaccharides and Glycoconjugates. The oligosaccharides and glycoconjugates include monosialogangliosides that are receptor analognes for heat-labile toxins produced by V. cholerae and E. coli[178]; fucose-containing oligosaccharides that inhibit the hemagglutinin activity of the classical strain of V. cholerae[179]; fucosylated oligosaccharides that protect against heat-stable enterotoxin of E. coli[180]; mannose-containing high-molecular-weight glycoproteins that block the binding of the eltor strain of V. cholerae[178]; and glycoproteins and glycolipids that interfere with the binding of colonization factor (CFA/II) fimbriae on enterotoxigenic E. coli.[181] The inhibition of toxin binding is associated with acidic glycolipids containing sialic acid (gangliosides). Although the quantities of total gangliosides in human and bovine milk are similar, the relative frequencies of each type of ganglioside in milk from these two species are distinct. More than 50 types of monosialylated oligosaccharides have been identified in human milk, and new types are still being recognized.[182] Monosialoganglioside 3 constitutes about 74% of total gangliosides in human milk, but it is much lower in bovine milk.[183, 184] Also, the level of the enterotoxin receptor ganglioside G_{M1} is 10-fold greater in human than in bovine milk.[184] This may be of clinical importance because G_{M1} inhibits enterotoxins of E. coli and V. cholerae.[185]

It is also of interest that intact human milk fat globules, as well as the mucin from the membranes of these structures, inhibit the binding of S-fimbriated E. coli to human buccal epithelial cells.[186]

Oligosaccharides in human milk also interfere with the attachment of H. influenzae and S. pneumoniae.[187] In this regard, N-acetylglucosamine (G1cNAc) (1–3) Gal-disaccharide subunits block the attachment of S. pneumoniae to respiratory epithelium. Moreover, there is recent evidence that human milk interferes with the binding of HIV envelope antigen gp120 to CD4 molecules on T cells.[188]

Some data from animal models suggest that the oligosaccharides and glycoconjugates in human milk protect in vivo,[189–191] but there are few clinical data that pertain to the question.[192]

In addition to the direct antimicrobial effects of the carbohydrates in human milk, nitrogen-containing oligosaccharides in human milk are growth promoters for Lactobacillus bifidus var. Pennsylvania,[193] glycoproteins, and glycopeptides.[194, 195] The bifidus growth promoter activity associated with caseins may reside in the oligosaccharide moiety of those complex molecules.[196] It appears that these factors are responsible to a great extent for the predominance of Lactobacillus sp. in the bacterial flora of the large intestine of the breast-fed infant. These bacteria produce large amounts of acetic acid, which aids in suppressing the multiplication of enteropathogens. It has also been reported that *Lactobacillus* sp. strain GG aids in the recovery from acute rotavirus infections[197] and may enhance the formation of circulating cells that produce specific antibodies of the IgG, IgA, and IgM isotypes as well as serum levels of those antibodies.[198]

Generation of Antiviral, Antiparasitic Lipids from Substrata in Human Milk. Human milk supplies defense agents from fat as it is partially digested in the recipient's alimentary tract. Fatty acids and monoglycerides produced from milk fats by bile salt–stimulated lipase or lipoprotein lipase in human milk,[199] lingual/gastric lipase from the recipient from birth,[200] or pancreatic lipase after a few weeks of age is able to disrupt enveloped viruses.[201–205] These antiviral lipids may aid in preventing coronavirus infections of the intestinal tract[206] and may also defend against intestinal parasites such as *G. lamblia* and *E. histolytica*.[207, 208]

Proteins. The principal proteins in human milk that have direct antimicrobial properties follow.

Lactoferrin. Lactoferrin, the dominant whey protein in human milk, is a single-chain glycoprotein with two globular lobes, both of which display a site that binds ferric iron.[209] More than 90% of the lactoferrin in human milk is in the form of apolactoferrin (i.e., does not contain ferric iron),[210] which competes with siderophilic bacteria and fungi for ferric iron[211–215] and thus disrupts the proliferation of these microbial pathogens. The epithelial growth–promoting activities of lactoferrin in human milk may also aid in the defense of the recipient infant.[216] The mean concentration of lactoferrin in human colostrum is between 5 and 6 mg/ml.[217] As the volume of milk production increases, the concentration falls to about 1 mg/ml at 2 to 3 months of lactation.[218, 219]

Because of its resistance to proteolysis,[220–222] the excretion of lactoferrin in stool is higher in human milk–fed than cow's milk–fed infants.[72, 223–225] The mean intake of milk lactoferrin per day in healthy, breast-fed, full-term infants is about 260 mg/kg at 1 month of lactation and 125 mg/kg by 4 months.[223] The quantity of lactoferrin excreted in the stools of low-birth-weight infants fed human milk is approximately 185 times that in stools of infants fed a cow's milk formula.[226] That estimate, however, may be too high because of the presence of immunoreactive fragments of lactoferrin in the stools of human milk–fed infants.[227]

In addition, there is a significant increment in the urinary excretion of intact and fragmented lactoferrin as a result of human milk feedings.[227–229] Recent stable isotope studies suggest that the increments in urinary lactoferrin and its fragments are principally from ingested human milk lactoferrin.[230]

Lysozyme. Relatively high concentrations of lysozyme single-chain protein are present in human milk.[218, 219, 231–235] This 15-kilodalton agent lyses susceptible bacteria by hydrolyzing β-1,4 linkages between *N*-acetylmuramic acid and 2-acetylamino-2-deoxy-D-glucose residues in cell walls.[236] Lysozyme is relatively resistant to digestion by trypsin or denaturation due to acid. The mean concentration of lysozyme is about 70 μ/ml in colostrum,[218] about 20 μg/ml at 1 month of lactation, and 250 μ/ml by 6 months.[219] The approximate mean daily intake of

milk lysozyme in healthy, full-term, completely breast-fed infants is 3 to 4 mg/kg at 1 month of lactation and 6 mg/kg by 4 months.[223]

Few studies have been conducted concerning the fate of human milk lysozyme ingested by the infant. The amount of lysozyme excreted in the stools of low-birth-weight infants fed human milk is about eight times that found in the stools of infants fed a cow's milk formula,[226] but the urinary excretion of this protein does not increase as a result of human milk feedings.

Fibronectin. Fibronectin, a high-molecular-weight protein that facilitates the uptake of many types of particulates by mononuclear phagocytic cells, is present in human milk (mean concentration in colostrum, 13.4 mg/liter).[237] The in vivo effects and fate of this broad-spectrum opsonin in human milk are not known.

Complement Components. The components of the classical and alternative pathways of complement are present in human milk, but the concentrations of these components, except C3, are exceptionally low.[163, 164]

Anti-inflammatory Agents

Although a direct anti-inflammatory effect of human milk has not been demonstrated in vivo, a number of clinical observations suggest that breast-feeding protects the recipient infant from injury to the intestinal or respiratory mucosa.[238, 239] This protection may be due in part to the more rapid elimination or neutralization of microbial pathogens in the lumen of the gastrointestinal tract by specific or broad-spectrum defense agents from human milk, but other features of human milk suggest that this is not the sole explanation. Phlogistic agents and the systems that give rise to them are poorly represented in human milk.[240] In contrast, human milk contains a host of anti-inflammatory agents,[241] including a heterogeneous group of growth factors with cytoprotective and trophic activity for the mucosal epithelium, antioxidants, antiproteases, cytokines and cytokine receptors and antagonists, and other bioactive agents that inhibit inflammatory mediators or block the selected activation of leukocytes. Like the antimicrobial factors, some of these factors are well adapted to operate in the hostile environment of the recipient's alimentary tract.

Growth factors in human milk include epidermal growth factor[169, 242] and the transforming growth factors (TGFs)–α[243] and –β,[244] lactoferrin,[216] mammary gland–derived growth factor,[245] and polyamines.[246, 247] These and a host of hormones,[248] including cortisol,[249] may affect the growth and maturation of epithelial barriers, limit the penetration of pathogenic microorganisms and free antigens, and prevent allergic sensitization. Corticosterone, a glucocorticoid that is present in high concentrations in rat milk, speeds gut closure in the neonatal rat.[250] Although macromolecular absorption does not appear to be as marked in the human neonate,[251–253] the function of the mucosal barrier system in early infancy is important to host defense, and this system may be affected by factors in human milk. In this regard, the maturation of the intestinal tract as measured by mucosal mass, DNA, and protein content of the small intestinal tract appears to be influenced by milk, particularly early milk, secretions.[254]

Antioxidant activity in colostrum has been shown to be associated with an ascorbate compound and uric acid.[255] In addition, two other antioxidants present in human milk, alpha-tocopherol[256, 257] and beta-carotene,[257] are absorbed into the circulation by the recipient gastrointestinal mucosa. Serum vitamin E concentrations rise in breast-fed infants, from a mean of 0.3 mg/ml at birth to approximately 0.9 mg/ml on the fourth day of life.[256]

The pleiotropic cytokine IL-10, a potent suppresser of macrophage, T cell, and natural killer (NK) cell function, has been demonstrated at very high concentrations in samples of human milk collected during the first 80 hours of lactation.[258] IL-10 is present not only in the aqueous phase of the milk, but also in the lipid layer. Its bioactive properties were confirmed by the finding that human milk samples inhibited blood lymphocyte proliferation and that this property was greatly reduced by the treatment with anti–IL-10 antibody. Interestingly, mice with a targeted disruption in the IL-10 gene, when raised under conventional housing conditions, spontaneously develop a generalized enterocolitis that becomes apparent at the age of 4 to 8 weeks (time of weaning).[259] These observations suggest that IL-10 in human milk may play a critical role in the homeostasis of the immature intestinal barrier by regulating aberrant immune responses to foreign antigens. Soluble receptors and cytokine receptor antagonists are also potent anti-inflammatory agents. Human colostrum and mature milk have been shown to contain biologically active levels of IL-1 receptor antagonist (IL-1Ra) and soluble TNF-α receptors I and II (sTNF-αRI and -RII).[260] The in vivo relevance of these observations has also been confirmed in a chemically induced colitis model of rats. Animals with colitis fed human milk had significantly lower neutrophilic inflammation than animals fed either chow or infant formula.[261] Similar "protective" effects were seen in rats with colitis fed an infant formula supplemented with IL-1Ra,[261] suggesting that this anti-inflammatory agent present in milk may contribute to the broad protection against different injuries provided by human milk feeding. The presence in human milk of platelet-activating factor acetylhydrolase (PAF-AH), the enzyme that catalyzes the degradation and inactivation of PAF, is intriguing.[262] Indeed, elevated serum concentrations of PAF have been found in rat and human neonates with necrotizing enterocolitis, whereas the concentrations of PAF-AH were found to be significantly lower than in control unaffected neonates.[263, 264] It is also of interest that serum concentrations of PAF-AH are below those of adults at birth and then gradually rise.[265] The enzyme is actively transferred from the mucosal to the serosal fluid in intestine of neonatal rats, particularly in the earliest postnatal period.[266] Other anti-inflammatory factors present in human milk include an IgE-binding factor, related antigenically to the Fc,RII (the lower-affinity receptor for IgE), that suppresses the in vitro synthesis of human IgE,[267] and the glycophosphoinositol-containing molecule protectin (CD59) that inhibits insertion of the complement membrane-attack complex to cell targets.[268] The in vivo fate and effects of these anti-inflammatory factors in human milk are still poorly understood.

Modulators of the Immune System

Several seemingly unrelated types of observations suggest that breast-feeding modulates the development of the immune system of the recipient infant:

1. Both prospective and retrospective epidemiologic studies have shown that breast-fed infants are at less risk for development of certain chronic immunologically mediated disorders later in childhood, including allergic diseases,[269] Crohn's disease,[270] ulcerative colitis,[271] insulin-dependent diabetes mellitus,[272] and some lymphomas.[273]

2. Humoral and cellular immune responses to specific antigens (i.e., vaccines) given during the first year of life appear to develop differently in breast-fed and formula-fed infants. Several studies have reported increased serum antibody titers to *H. influenzae* type b polysaccharide,[274] oral polio virus,[275] tetanus,[276] and diphtheria toxoid[277] immunizations in breast-fed infants. In regard to cell-mediated immunity, breast-fed infants given bacille Calmette-Guérin (BCG) vaccine either at birth or later show a significantly higher lymphocyte transformation response to purified protein derivative (PPD) than those who were never breast-fed.[277] Moreover, maternal renal allografts survive better in individuals who were breast-fed rather than non-breast-fed.[278–280] In this respect, the in vitro allogeneic responses between the blood lymphocytes of mothers (stimulating cells) and their infants (responding cells), as measured by an analysis of the cytotoxic T lymphocyte (CTL) precursor frequencies directed against HLA alloantigens (CTL allorepertoire), are low in breast-fed infants.[281]

3. Increased levels of certain immune factors in breast-fed infants, levels that could not be explained simply by passive transfer of those substances, also suggest an immunomodulatory activity of human milk. Breast-fed infants produce higher blood levels of interferon in response to respiratory syncytial virus infection.[282] It was also found that the increments in blood levels of fibronectin that were achieved by breast-feeding could not be due to the amounts of that protein in human milk.[237] In addition, it was found that human milk feeding led to a more rapid development in the appearance of sIgA in external secretions,[226, 228, 229, 276, 283] some of which, such as urine, are far removed anatomically from the route of ingestion.[228, 229]

These and other observations suggest that the ability of human milk to modulate the development of the infant's own mucosal and systemic immune systems may be associated with immunoregulatory factors present in colostrum and in more mature milk. Several different types of immunomodulatory agents can be identified in human milk.[241] Among the numerous substances with proven or potential ability to modulate the infant immune response are prolactin,[284] alpha-tocopherol,[256] lactoferrin,[285] nucleotides,[67] anti-idiotypic sIgA,[286] and cytokines.[287] It is evident that many of these factors in milk have other primary biologic functions, as in the case of hormones or growth factors, and that their potential as immune regulatory agents overlaps with their antimicrobial or anti-inflammatory properties.[241]

Cytokines in Human Milk

In the 1990s, several cytokines that mediate the effector phases of natural and specific immunity were discovered in human milk. Human milk displays a number of cytokine-like biologic activities, including the stimulation of growth, differentiation of immunoglobulin production by B cells,[288-290] enhancement of thymocyte proliferation,[291] inhibition of IL-2 production by T cells,[292] and suppression of IgE production.[267] IL-1β[293] and TNF-α[294] were the first two cytokines quantified in human milk. In colostrum, TNF-α is mainly present in molecular weight fractions between 80 and 195 kDa, probably bound to its soluble receptors.[260] Milk TNF-α is secreted both by milk macrophages[294, 295] and by the mammary epithelium.[296] IL-6 was first demonstrated in human milk by a specific bioassay.[297] In those studies, anti–IL-6 neutralizing antibodies inhibited IgA production by colostrum mononuclear cells, suggesting that IL-6 may be involved in the production of IgA in the mammary gland. The presence of IL-6 in milk has been also demonstrated by immunoassays.[294, 296, 298, 299] In like manner, IL-6 is localized in high molecular fractions of human milk.[298] The association of IL-6 with its own receptor has not been studied in milk, although the expression of IL-6 receptor by the mammary epithelium[296] and in secreted form in the milk[260] may explain the high molecular weight of this cytokine in human milk. The expression of IL-6 messenger ribonucleic acid (mRNA) and protein in milk cells and in the mammary gland epithelium suggests that both milk mononuclear cells and the mammary gland are likely major sources of this cytokine.[295, 296, 300] The presence of interferon γ (IFN-γ) in human milk has also been reported,[151, 296, 299] although some investigators have found significant levels of IFN-γ only in milk samples obtained from mothers who had delivered by cesarean section (MF Böttcher et al, personal communication).[299] The significance of this observation is not clear at the present moment. IFN-γ bioactivity as well as its association with specific subsets of milk T cells also remains to be determined.[151] (The presence and possible function of IL-10 in human milk are discussed in the section Anti-inflammatory Agents.)

Chemokines are a novel class of small cytokines with discrete target-cell selectivity that are able to recruit and activate different populations of leukocytes.[301] Two major subfamilies, the CXC and the CC chemokines, are defined by the splicing of the conserved cysteine residues, which are either separated by one amino acid (CXC chemokines) or adjacent amino acids (CC chemokines). IL-8 and growth related peptide–α (GRO-α) belong to the CXC family and are mainly chemotactic factors for neutrophils. On the other hand, CC chemokines, which include monocyte chemotactic protein–1 (MCP-1), macrophage inflammatory protein–1α (MIP-1α), and regulated upon activation, normal T cell expressed and secreted (RANTES), are chemotactic fac-

TABLE 4–8
Cytokines, Chemokines, and Colony-Stimulating Factors in Human Milk

CYTOKINES	CHEMOKINES	COLONY-STIMULATING FACTORS
IL-1β	IL-8	G-CSF
IL-6	GRO-α	M-CSF
IL-10	MCP-1	GM-CSF
IL-16[a]		
IFN-γ	RANTES	
TNF-α	Eotaxin[a]	

[a]MF Böttcher et al, personal communication.
Adapted from Garofalo RP, Goldman AS. Cytokines, chemokines, and colony stimulating factors in human milk: the 1997 update. Biol Neonate 74:134–142, 1998, with permission.

tors for monocytes, basophils and eosinophils, and T lymphocytes.[302] The presence of both CXC and CC chemokines has been described in human milk (Table 4–8). IL-8 concentration was first determined in a small group of milk samples by Basolo and colleagues[296] and soon after by Palkowetz and associates.[303] Both groups have identified the expression and secretion of IL-8 by mammary epithelial cells, although milk cells appear also to produce this chemokine.[295, 300] Another member of the CXC chemokine found in human milk is GRO-α, along with the two CC chemokines MCP-1 and RANTES.[300] Expression of MCP-1 and to a lesser extent RANTES mRNA was confirmed in studies of milk cells.[300] Recently, high levels of the CC chemokine eotaxin, a potent and specific chemotactic factor for eosinophils and helper T cell subtype 2 (T_H2) have also been demonstrated in human milk (MF Böttcher et al, personal communication).

Colony-stimulating factors, highly specified protein factors that regulate cell proliferation and differentiation in the process of hematopoiesis, have been discovered very recently in human milk. Although colony-stimulating activity was demonstrated in milk in 1983,[304] granulocyte colony-stimulating factor (G-CSF), macrophage colony-stimulating factor (M-CSF), and granulocyte-macrophage colony-stimulating factor (GM-CSF) were not specifically identified and measured in human milk until the 1990s.[151, 305-307] The concentrations of M-CSF in particular appear to be 10- to 100-fold higher than those in serum and to be produced by epithelial cells of the ducts and alveoli of the mammary gland under the regulatory activity of female sex hormones.[306]

Although it is tempting to speculate that cytokines present in milk may be able to interact with mucosal tissues in the respiratory and alimentary tracts of the recipient infant, the functional expression of specific receptors for cytokines on epithelial or lymphoid cells in the airway and gastrointestinal mucosa has not been fully explored.[241] A receptor-independent mechanism of cytokine uptake by the gastrointestinal mucosa during the neonatal period has not been demonstrated to date.

Milk and Altered Pregnancy

Several investigators have examined the effects of prematurity, early weaning, galactorrhea, and maternal malnutrition on the process of lactation. The immunologic aspects of these studies have focused largely on evaluation of the total content of sIgA and specific antibody activity. As described previously, the mammary secretions of nonlactating breast contain sIgA, although the amount appears to be much lower than in the lactating breast.[308] Mammary secretions of patients with galactorrhea appear to contain sIgA in concentrations similar to those of normal postpartum colostrum.[309] Although malnutrition has been associated with reduced secretory antibody response in other external secretions, maternal malnutrition does not seem to affect the total sIgA concentration or antimicrobial-specific antibody activity in the milk.[310]

The nutritional, as well as immunologic, composition of milk from mothers of prematurely delivered neonates appears to be significantly different from that of the milk of mothers delivering at term.[14, 219, 311, 312] Comparative studies conducted during the first 12 weeks of lactation suggest that the mean concentrations of lactoferrin and lysozyme are higher in preterm than in term milk. sIgA is the predominant immunoglobulin in preterm as well as term milk, although the sIgA concentration appears to be significantly higher in preterm milk collected during the first 8 to 12 weeks of lactation. sIgA antibody activity against certain organisms (E. coli somatic antigen) in the preterm milk was observed to be somewhat lower than, or at best similar to, the levels found in term milk. In addition, the number of lymphocytes and macrophages in milk appears to be lower at 2 weeks but significantly higher at 12 weeks in the milk from mothers with preterm (34 to 38 weeks' gestation) infants than in those with full-term milk.[311] The authors of these investigations have proposed that some of the observed changes may reflect the lower volume of milk produced by mothers delivering preterm infants. The possibility remains that changes in the immunologic profile of preterm milk may be a consequence of inadequate stimulation by the preterm infant, alterations in the maternal hormonal milieu, or other factors underlying premature delivery itself.

BENEFITS AND RISKS OF HUMAN MILK

Benefits

GASTROINTESTINAL HOMEOSTASIS AND PREVENTION OF DIARRHEA

Development of mucosal integrity in the gut appears to depend on maturation of the mucosal tissue itself and the establishment of a normal gut flora. The former represents an anatomic and enzymatic blockage to invasion of microorganisms and antigens and the latter an inhibition to colonization by pathogenic bacteria. Although permeability of the neonatal gut to immunoglobulin is rather short-lived or incompletely developed, unprotected or damaged neonatal gut is permeable to a host of other proteins and macromolecules for several weeks or longer. Large milk protein peptides and bovine serum albumin have been shown to enter the circulation and produce a circulating antibody response. The inflamed or ischemic gut is even more porous to both antigens and pathogens. A variety of proven and presumed mechanisms for the role of both IgA and the normal flora have been proposed to compensate for these temporary inadequacies. Evidence for gut-trophic substances in humans is still preliminary. There is ample epidemiologic evidence of a positive effect of breast-feeding in establishing the normal gut flora. Most compelling are the observations in rural Guatemala of gross contamination of milk by potentially pathogenic, aerobic, gram-negative bacilli, including E. coli and Shigella sp., with an absence both of diarrheal illness and of significant quantities of these species in the feces of infants during the period of lactation. In addition, the presence of diverse serotypes of aerobic, gram-negative bacilli in the oropharynx and gastrointestinal tract of the neonates may serve as a source of antigen to boost the presensitized mammary glands, leading to a further modulation of specific bacterial growth in the mucosa.[313] The precise role of antibody that blocks adherence of these pathogens to the gut and the effects of other factors, such as lactoperoxidase, lactoferrin, lysozyme, and Bifidobacterium bifidum, in those situations are undetermined.

Extensive epidemiologic literature on the "prophylactic value" of breast-feeding in the prevention or amelioration of diarrheal disease is available in several reviews.[22, 82, 314, 315] Ample experimental animal data on the value of specific colostral antibody in preventing diarrheal illness are available on colostral deprivation. These include colibacteriosis associated with E. coli K88 in swine; rotaviral gastroenteritis in cattle, swine, and sheep; and diarrheal illness associated with transmissible gastroenteritis of swine.[316] In humans, cholera is rare in infancy, especially in endemic areas where the prevalence of breast-feeding is high. The experience with an outbreak of cholera in the Persian Gulf lends support to the possibility that the absence of breast-feeding is an important variable in increasing the risk of cholera in infancy.

There have been a few claims that nursery outbreaks of diarrhea associated with enteropathogenic strains of E. coli can be interrupted by use of breast milk. Conflicting data exist regarding prevention of human rotaviral disease. Evaluation of nursery outbreaks of rotavirus has suggested that the incidence both of infection and of illness was lower in breast-fed infants, but the incidence of symptoms in formula-fed infants was also very low. Studies carried out in Japan have noted a fivefold decrease in incidence of rotaviral infection among breast-fed infants younger than 6 months of age. It must be emphasized that most rotavirus infections in neonates are asymptomatic, regardless of breast- or bottle-feeding.[317–321] Careful clinical observations by Bishop and co-workers[322] in Australia first questioned the positive effects of breast-feeding in rotavirus infection. More recent case-control studies of enteric viral infections in breast-fed infants have suggested that breast-feeding may protect infants from hospitalization rather than from infection itself.[323, 324] Longitudinal follow-up of a large cohort of infants during a community outbreak of rotavirus has shown that attack rates of rotavirus were similar in breast-fed and bottle-fed infants. However, the frequency of clinical disease with diarrhea appeared to be significantly lower in breast-fed infants. Interestingly, the protection observed in these patients was more a reflection of altered microbial flora from breast-feeding than of specific immunologic protection against rotavirus. Thus, it appears that breast-feeding provides significant protection against diarrheal disease, although the mechanism of such protection remains to be defined.[323, 324]

NECROTIZING ENTEROCOLITIS

Necrotizing enterocolitis (NEC) is a complex illness of the stressed premature infant, often associated with hypoxia, gut mucosal ischemia, and necrolysis and death.[325, 326] Clinical manifestations have, on a few occasions, been associated with bacteremia and invasion by gram-negative bacilli, particularly *Klebsiella pneumoniae*, into the intestinal submucosa. Clinical manifestations include abdominal distention, gastric retention, and bloody diarrhea. Classic radiographic findings include air in the bowel wall (pneumatosis intestinalis), air in the portal system, and free infradiaphragmatic air (signifying perforation). Treatment involves decompression, systemic antibiotics, and, often, surgery.[327-329]

A number of studies have suggested a beneficial role of breast milk in preventing or modifying the development of NEC in high-risk human infants. Some pediatric centers have claimed virtual absence of NEC in breast-fed infants. However, there have also been many reports of the failure of milk feeding to prevent human NEC. In fact, there have been outbreaks of NEC related to *Klebsiella* and *Salmonella* spp. secondary to banked human milk feedings.[127, 330, 331] In an asphyxiated neonatal rat model of NEC, the entire syndrome could be prevented with feeding of maternal milk. The crucial factor in the milk appeared to be the cells, probably the macrophages.[127] It is also possible that antibody and nonspecific factors play a role, as does establishment of a gut flora. Prophylactic oral administration of immunoglobulin has been found to have a profound influence on the outcome of NEC in well-controlled studies.[331] Penetration of the gut by pathogens and antigens is increased with ischemic damage, and noncellular elements of milk may aid in blockage of this transit.[332] The role of enteric anaerobic organisms has been seriously considered in the pathogenesis of NEC. Cytolytic toxins of *Clostridium difficile* and other clostridial species have been demonstrated in infants with NEC, often significantly more frequently than in normal infants.[333-336] Clearly, NEC is a complex disease entity whose pathogenesis and cause remain to be defined. Although breast-feeding may be protective, a number of other factors are clearly related to the mechanism of mucosal injury and the pathogenesis of this syndrome.

NEONATAL SEPSIS

It has been suggested that the incidence of bacteremia among premature infants fed breast milk is significantly lower than that among those receiving formula feeding or no feeding.[337-339] It has been shown that a high percentage of neonatal bacteremias and meningitis caused by gram-negative bacilli are associated with the *E. coli* K1 serotype. Both antibody and compartmentalized cellular reactivity to this serotype have been demonstrated in human colostrum. High colostral antibody titers are associated most often with the colonization by the organism in the maternal gut. Other studies have, however, failed to demonstrate clear evidence of protection against systemic infection in breast-fed infants.[340-342]

PREVENTION OF ATOPY AND ASTHMA

One of the most challenging developments in human milk research has been the demonstration in breast-fed infants of a reduced incidence of diseases with auto- or dysregulated immunity, long after the termination of breast-feeding.[269-273] Since the first report in 1936,[343] numerous studies have appeared concerning the effect of infant feeding on the development of atopic disease and asthma. Although beneficial results of breast-feeding as prophylaxis against atopy have been observed in most of the studies, other findings have reported beneficial effects only in infants with a genetically determined risk for atopic disease. Finally, no beneficial effects at all or even an increased risk has been suggested in some breast-fed infants. Kramer, in an extensive meta-analysis of 50 studies published before 1986 that focused on infant feeding and atopic disease, has attempted to shed some light on the controversy.[344] Seven of the 13 studies on asthma included in this analysis claimed a protective effect of breast-feeding, whereas 6 claimed no protection. However, several serious methodologic drawbacks have been noted in this analysis. In a number of the studies analyzed, early infant feeding history was obtained months or years after the feeding period, ascertainment of the infant feeding history was obtained by interviewers who were aware of the disease outcome, or insufficient duration and exclusivity of breast-feeding were documented; all were confounding variables that considered inappropriate "exposure standards." Nonblind ascertainment of disease outcome was found to be the most common violation of the "outcome standards." Failure to control for confounding variables was a common violation in "statistical analysis standards" identified in several studies. Indeed, the effect of infant feeding on subsequent asthma may be confounded by other variables that are associated both with infant feeding and with unique investigational conditions. Factors that seem to have the greatest potential for confounding effects include the family history of atopic disease, socioeconomic status, and parental cigarette smoking. Only 1 of 13 studies on asthma included in the meta-analysis adequately controlled for these confounding factors. Moreover, 3 of the studies that did not demonstrate a protective effect of breast-feeding on asthma were afflicted by inadequate statistical power. The effect of infant feeding on the severity of outcome and on the age at onset of the disease was virtually ignored in most of the studies.[344]

Although this extensive meta-analysis may suggest

some uncertainty about the prophylactic benefit of breast-feeding, two recent studies strongly support a positive effect of breast-feeding on the development of atopic disease and asthma. In the first study,[269] a prospective, long-term follow-up from infancy until 17 years of age, the group of subjects with short (less than 1 month) or no breast-feeding had a significantly higher prevalence of atopy, which increased to a demonstrable difference at 17 years of age, when compared with the subject groups with intermediate (1 to 6 months) or prolonged (longer than 6 months) breast-feeding. The differences in the prevalence of atopy persisted when the groups were divided according to positive or negative atopic heredity. Furthermore, the atopy manifestations between the infant feeding groups did not remain constant with age. In particular, respiratory allergy, including asthma, increased greatly in prevalence up to 17 years of age, with a prevalence as high as 64% in the group with short or no breast-feeding.[269] In the second study, a prospective, longitudinal study of the prevalence and risk factors for acute and chronic respiratory illness in childhood, the authors investigated the relationship of infant feeding to recurrent wheezing at age 6 years and the association with lower respiratory tract illnesses associated with wheezing early in life.[345] Children who were never breast-fed had significantly higher rates of recurrent wheezing at 6 years of age. Increasing duration of breast-feeding beyond 1 month was not associated with significantly lower rates of a recurrent wheeze. The effect of breast-feeding was apparent for children both with and without wheezing lower respiratory tract illnesses in the first 6 months of life. However, in contrast to the findings of the first study, the effect of breast-feeding was significant only among nonatopic children.[345]

The exact mechanisms by which breast-feeding seems to confer long-lasting protection against allergic sensitization are poorly understood. It is likely, however, that multiple synergistic mechanisms may be responsible for this effect, including (1) maturation of the recipient gastrointestinal and airway mucosa, promoted by growth factors present in human milk[242–244]; (2) inhibition of antigen absorption by milk secretory IgA[346]; (3) reduced incidence of mucosal infections and consequent sensitization to bystander antigens[347]; (4) changes in the microbial flora of the intestine of breast-fed infants[325]; and (5) direct immunomodulatory activity of human milk components on the recipient infant.[241] A number of earlier and current studies have greatly contributed to the understanding of macromolecular transport across the immature gut and its consequences in terms of the generation of circulating antibody or immune complexes, the processes that are blocked predominantly by sIgA, the glycocalyx, and the intestinal enzymes. These mucosal immunologic events have been the basis for the concept of immune exclusion. However, immune exclusion is not absolute, because uptake of some antigens across the gut may be enhanced rather than blocked by interaction with antibody at the mucosal surface. Beginning with the observations of IgA-deficient patients, it has become clear that the absence of the IgA barrier in the gut is associated with both an increased incidence of circulating antibodies directed against many food antigens and an increased occurrence of atopic-allergic diseases.[346] Other studies have noted complement activation in serum after feeding of bovine milk to children with cow's milk allergy. The neonate is somewhat analogous to the IgA-deficient patient,[348] and increased transintestinal uptake of food antigen with consequent circulating antibody formation in the premature infant has been reported.[349] Other studies have suggested that early breast-feeding, even of short duration, is associated with a decreased serum antibody response to cow's milk proteins.[253] Prolonged breast-feeding may not only partially exclude foreign antigens through immune exclusion, but also, by the nature of being the sole food source, prevent their ingestion.[350] It must, however, be emphasized that intact bovine milk proteins and other food antigens and antibodies have been observed in samples of colostrum and milk.[6]

OTHER BENEFITS

As described previously, there is epidemiologic evidence to suggest that bacterial and viral respiratory infections are less frequent and less severe among breast-fed infants in a variety of cultures and socioeconomic settings. Antibodies and immunologic reactivity directed against herpes simplex virus, respiratory syncytial virus, and other infectious agents[86, 95, 118, 351, 352] have been quantitated in colostrum and milk. Adoptive experiments in suckling ferrets have shown that protection of the young against respiratory syncytial virus can be transferred via colostrum containing specific antibody. However, the neonatal ferret gut is quite permeable to macromolecules and permits passage of large quantities of virus-specific IgG. In the absence of either documented antibody or cellular transfer in the human neonate across the mucosa, any mechanisms of protection against respiratory syncytial virus and other respiratory pathogens remain obscure.

There are no data in humans on passive protection in other mucosal surfaces, such as the eye, ear, or genitourinary tract. Some epidemiologic evidence is available to suggest that recurrence of otitis media with effusion is strongly associated with early bottle-feeding and that breast-feeding may confer protection against otitis media with effusion for the first 3 years of life.[353] Foster feeding–acquired antibody to herpes simplex virus has been found to result in significant protection against reinfection challenge in experimental animal studies.[351]

A number of other benefits have been associated with breast-feeding, including natural contraception during active nursing[354] and protection against sudden infant death syndrome,[355] diabetes,[356] obesity,[357] and high cholesterol level and ischemic heart disease later in life.[42] Of particular recent interest has been the association of breast-feeding with higher intellectual performance in older children. Several studies have now demonstrated enhanced cognitive outcome in breast-fed children, although controversy exists regarding the mechanisms by which such improved performance may occur.[358–360] There may even be health benefits to the mother in breast-feeding, reflected in a reduced incidence of breast cancer in mothers who have lactated.[361]

Potential Risks

NONINFECTIOUS RISKS

There are several potentially harmful effects associated with breast-feeding. Some provocative data suggest that nonautologous human milk may, under certain conditions, be nutritionally inadequate for the premature infant.[22, 23] The concentration of anti–Rhesus factor (anti-Rh) antibodies in milk appears to be too low to pose any threat to the incompatible neonate. Variable concentrations of medicinal products and their metabolites are excreted in colostrum and milk (Table 4–9). Environmental contaminants, such as dichlorodiphenyl trichloroethane (DDT), polychlorinated biphenyls, and mercury, have been demonstrated in high concentrations in human milk.[22, 362]

The failure to initiate lactation properly during early breast-feeding may present a risk of dehydration to the infant as insufficient fluids may be ingested. Inappropriate introduction of bottles and pacifiers may also interfere with proper induction of lactation. Later in lactation, introduction of bottles may induce premature weaning as the result of a reduction in the milk supply.

Although human milk is the optimal form of nutrition for most healthy term infants, there are some circumstances in which breast-feeding is contraindicated and some in which continued breast-feeding should be conducted with caution to protect the infant. Infants with inherited metabolic diseases may be best nourished by treatment with alternative forms of nutrition. In particular, neonates with diagnosed galactosemia need to have galactose removed from their diet; in other words, they need to be switched to a milk containing lactose-free (a glucose-galactose disaccharide) carbohydrate. Infants diagnosed with phenylketonuria may receive some human milk to support their requirement for phenylalanine but may often be better managed by use of specially prepared commercial milks.

Hyperbilirubinemia associated with breast-feeding, so-called breast milk jaundice, has been an area of some controversy. The mechanism responsible for this form of jaundice is unknown but has been suggested to reflect inhibitors of glucuronidation, deficiency of related enzymes, excessive lipid breakdown, and insufficient milk intake.[363, 364] Recent recommendations suggest that a more laissez-faire approach to this problem is appropriate.[365] Increasing milk volume by increasing feeds may be the most appropriate approach to breast milk jaundice; however, severe cases may necessitate phototherapy. Increased intake of fluids in breast-feeding infants appears to be effective in many cases.[366]

Several instances of specific nutrient deficiencies in breast-fed infants have been described, specifically related to lack of vitamin K, vitamin D, vitamin B_{12}, folic

TABLE 4–9
Drugs in Maternal Circulation Known to Pose Potential Health Problems for the Breast-Feeding Infant

DRUGS		ENVIRONMENTAL CONTAMINANTS
Anticoagulants	Autonomic drugs	DDT
Ethyl biscoumacetate	Atropine	Polybromated biphenyls (PBBs)
Phenindione	Laxatives	Polychlorinated biphenyls (PCBs)
Anticonvulsants	Anthraquinone derivatives	Heptachlor
Mysoline	(Dialose Plus, Dorbane,	Mirex
Phenobarbital	Doxidan, Peri-Colace)	Lead
Phenytoin	Aloe	Radioisotopes
(diphenylhydantoin)	Calomel	Caffeine
Carbamazepine	Cascara	Food proteins
Antidepressants	Narcotics	Nicotine
Lithium	Heroin	Cadmium
Antihypertensives	Methadone	Alcohol
Reserpine	Oral contraceptives	
Antimetabolites	Pain killers	
Cyclophosphamide	Propoxyphene (Darvon)	
Methotrexate	Sedatives	
Antimicrobials	Barbiturates	
Chloramphenicol	Bromides	
(Chloromycetin)	Chloral hydrate	
Metronidazole (Flagyl)	Diazepam (Valium)	
Nalidixic acid	Steroids	
Nitrofurantoin[a]	Prednisone	
Sulfonamides[a]	Prednisolone	
Antithyroid drugs	Miscellaneous	
Iodide	Dihydrotachysterol (DHT)	
Thiouracil	Ergot alkaloids	
Radioactive iodine	Gold thioglucose	

[a]This drug causes problems mainly in infants suffering from the inherited deficiency of glucose-6-phosphate dehydrogenase.

Adapted from Packard VS. Human milk and infant formula. *In* Stewart GE (ed). Food and Science Technology Series. New York, Academic Press, 1982, p 118, with permission.

TABLE 4–10
Spectrum of Infectious Agents[a] Recovered in Human Milk and Their Possible Role in Infections in the Neonate

Agent in Milk	EFFECT ON BREAST-FED NEONATE[b]		
	Seroconversion	Replication of Agent with Illness	Replication of Agent Without Illness
Rubella virus	+ + (25–30)	0	+ + (56)
Cytomegalovirus	+	±	+ + (58)
Hepatitis B virus	–	?	+ +
Herpes simplex virus	–	+	–
Human immunodeficiency virus (HIV)	+	±	+ +
Tumor viruses	–	–	+
HTLV-1	+	±	+
HTLV-2	+	±	+
Coxiella burnetii	–	–	–
Streptococcus sp.	–	±	+
Staphylococcus sp.	–	±	+
Enterotoxin	–	–	–
Mycobacterium sp.	–	–	–
Salmonella sp.	–	–	+ +
Escherichia coli	–	–	+

[a]All agents listed can be rendered noninfectious by heat inactivation at 62.5° C.
[b]+ to + + = modest to strong evidence; ± = presumptive evidence; ? = inconclusive data; – = not known; 0 = absent; ( ) = percentage of subjects reported.

acid, vitamin C, and carnitine. In each of these instances, several case reports have appeared warning against deficiencies that have resulted in clinical consequences to the neonate. For example, a few breast-fed infants with hemorrhagic disease who have been reported have been successfully treated with vitamin K.[367] These infants did not receive vitamin K at birth. Mothers who practice unusual dietary habits, such as strict vegetarianism, may have reduced levels of vitamin B_{12} and folic acid in their milk, and deficient breast-fed infants of such mothers have been reported.[368, 369] Cases of rickets in breast-fed infants have been reported, particularly during winter among infants not exposed to the sun.[32, 370] Deficiency of carnitine, a nutrient responsible for modulating fat absorption, has also been reported to result in clinical symptoms in breast-fed infants in mothers ingesting unusual diets.[61, 371]

These various clinical expressions of nutrient deficiency in milk are of concern, but they should also be put in the context of nutrient deficiencies observed in formula-fed infants. Clearly, millions of infants in developing countries are at severe risk of malnutrition when they are formula-fed because of the economic stress of supplying sufficient formula. Even in developed countries, large numbers of nutrient deficiencies and associated clinical symptoms have occurred as a result of accidents in the manufacture of formulas.[372] The most notable of these accidents have taught us the effects of early vitamin B_6 deficiency, folic acid deficiency, and chloride deficiency. Formula feeding has also been associated with an increased incidence of diabetes.[373]

Thus, some situations arise in which breast-feeding must be carefully considered as an appropriate feeding for the infant. However, commercial formulas also represent risks. The infant is best served by observant pediatricians and mothers who promptly respond to any clinical signs in the neonate.

INFECTIOUS RISKS

The presence of microbial contamination in both directly fed and banked milk is of serious concern. Contaminated milk has been implicated in neonatal infection with *S. aureus*, group B hemolytic streptococcus, mycobacteria, and, possibly, *Salmonella* sp. (Table 4–10).

Viral contaminants of milk include rubella, herpes simplex virus, hepatitis B virus, cytomegalovirus, HIV-1, human T-lymphotropic virus (HTLV), and, possibly, HTLV-2 (see Table 4–10). For most viruses, although transmission has been documented as evidenced by seroconversion, no serious illness in the neonate secondary to breast-feeding has been reported.[22, 314] One report of possible severe neonatal herpes simplex virus infection associated with the virus in milk may just as easily have been caused by an infant-to–mammary gland rather than a mammary gland–to-infant route of inoculation.[374] Both the RNA-dependent DNA polymerase and structural proteins of C-type tumor viruses, possibly related to mouse mammary tumor and Mason-Pfizer viruses, have been identified in human breast tissues and products of lactation.[82] There has been speculation on the risks of breast-feeding of female infants in families with a strong history of carcinoma of the breast. However, there is no epidemiologic evidence to support such a notion. Breast-feeding may, in fact, be a protective factor relative to maternal risk of such neoplastic disease.[375] Therefore, given reasonable maternal hygiene and in the absence of intense chemical contamination, there are generally few proven or well-defined contraindications to natural breast-feeding.

Breast-Feeding and Human Immunodeficiency Virus Infection. Recently, serious concern has been voiced regarding the potential risk of the transmission of HIV from infected mothers to their suckling neonates via the process of breast-feeding. The possibility of postnatal transmission of this virus from mother to child has been considered in a large number of infants breast-fed in the United States and in other parts of the world. In some of these infants, breast-feeding has been implicated as one of the major risk factors for acquisition of HIV infection. Since 1985, more than 25 infants with possible development of HIV infection via the process of breast-feeding have been reported.[376] In virtually all cases, maternal seroconversion for HIV antibody probably occurred after delivery of the infant. More than 50% of these mothers acquired the infection via heterosexual transmission, and about 30% via blood transfusion. One subject was judged to be an intravenous drug user. Although acquisition of HIV infection prior to delivery cannot be ruled out with certainty, the likely route of transmission in these infants has been presumed to be via breast-feeding. The most convincing observations are based on several maternal-infant pairs in whom maternal seroconversion to HIV antibody occurred 4 months or longer after delivery.[377]

A number of studies have demonstrated HIV in milk.[378–382] These include isolation of HIV from milk supernatants collected from symptom-free subjects and from cellular fractions of maternal milk, recovery of HIV virions in the histiocytes and cell-free extracts of milk by electron microscopy, and detection of viral DNA by polymerase chain reaction in 25 of 38 (73%) milk samples from HIV-seropositive women. However, limited epidemiologic studies carried out to date have failed to demonstrate the magnitude of risk of HIV infection in breast-fed infants. Cohort studies[383] in different populations have suggested increased, reduced, or similar transmission rates to the infants of breast-feeding and non–breast-feeding (bottle-feeding) mothers (Table 4–11). Thus, it appears that although precise epidemiologic data are still lacking, the majority of breast-fed infants born to HIV-seropositive mothers remain uninfected despite the presence of HIV DNA in the milk in a high proportion of such mothers. Nevertheless, the risk of acquisition of HIV infection via breast-feeding must not be ignored. On the basis of meta-analysis of available data it has been estimated that the additional

risk of HIV infection through breast-feeding is 7 to 22%.[384] Some studies have suggested that breast-feeding contributes up to a 50% increase in the overall vertical transmissions of HIV infection.[385]

Despite the potential risk of HIV infection perceived in HIV-infected breast-feeding mothers, consideration of cessation of breast-feeding must be balanced against other beneficial effects outlined in this chapter. In a 1990 study, breast-fed HIV-infected children progressed to acquired immunodeficiency syndrome (AIDS) at a slower rate than bottle-fed subjects.[386]

Most HIV-infected children in whom breast-feeding has been implicated in the transmission of infection reside in developing countries, where the use of bottle-feeding and other alternatives to breast-feeding is associated with a significantly increased rate of malnutrition and death. In such situations, the benefits of breast-feeding may exceed the potential added risk of HIV transmission. As a result, the World Health Organization has recommended continued breast-feeding regardless of HIV status in most developing countries, especially where safe and effective alternatives to breast-feeding are not available.[386] However, 1998 recommendations were more discouraging regarding HIV positive mothers' breast-feeding their infants in developing countries.[387] On the other hand, in industrialized nations such as the United States, and those of Australia, Russia, Japan, Western Europe, HIV-seropositive women have been more strongly advised not to breast-feed.

MOTHER'S OWN MILK: MILK BANKING

On the basis of the information reviewed in the preceding sections of this chapter, it is apparent that human colostrum and milk are richly endowed with a wide variety of cellular and soluble components that participate in many nutritional, immunologic, and anti-infective processes of specific benefit to the neonate. The function of the products of lactation and maternal breast-feeding best characterized to date is nutritional support and, possibly, compensation for the transient mucosal immune deficiency against infectious and dietary macromolecules in the autologous infant.

In general, it is quite safe for the mother to collect and feed or to breast-feed her own neonate. However, increasing concerns regarding contamination of human milk by infectious agents have resulted in the limited utility of either milk banks or wet nursing. Because of the transfer of infectious agents from maternal blood to milk (see Table 4–10), it is recommended by several national advisory committees that patients who have known transmissible infectious viral diseases, such as hepatitis B, rubella, cytomegalovirus, and HIV, or bacterial diseases, such as active tuberculosis, should not breast-feed.[388] Although it is appropriate to exercise caution in such situations, little or no evidence is available to suggest that breast-feeding of infants by their biologic mothers is associated with increased infection in the neonate, even when the infectious agents identified here are in question. Acute mastitis has been observed in up

---

TABLE 4–11

Comparisons of HIV-I Transmission Rates in Infants Born to HIV-Infected Mothers Relative to Breast- and Bottle-Feeding

| | PERCENTAGE OF INFECTED INFANTS | |
Country of Study Population	Breast-Fed (N = 353)	Bottle-Fed (N = 108)
Haiti	25	0
USA	0	29
USA	28	33
Congo	52	0
Zaire	18	25

Adapted from Ruff AJ, Halsey NA, Coberly J. Breast-feeding and maternal-infant transmission of human immunodeficiency virus type 1. J Pediatr 121:325–329, 1992, with permission.

to 3% of lactating women. *S. aureus* is the causative organism of infection in about 50% of such patients. Such mothers may represent another group who should not nurse during active infection. Other clinical situations in which withholding breast-feeding, because of high metabolite content in the milk, is appropriate include presence of galactosemia (galactose from lactose), phenylketonuria (phenylalanine), or other amino acid disorders in the infant.

As shown in Tables 4–9 and 4–10, many drugs, infectious agents, and environmental agents can be transferred to the infant via maternal milk. Rather than stopping breast-feeding, a nursing mother should avoid use of any drugs, unless it is absolutely essential. Many organohalides and fat-soluble environmental products, such as DDT and polychlorinated biphenyls, may be present in higher concentrations in human milk.[22] Although not much is known about their risk to the infant, it is generally agreed that, unless the degree of exposure in mothers is extremely high, the benefits of breast-feeding outweigh the possible risks associated with environmental contaminants. Caffeine, alcohol, and nicotine are other potential hazards to the infant (see Table 4–9). It is advisable to reduce the intake of tobacco, caffeine-bearing products, and alcoholic beverages during lactation and nursing.

CURRENT TRENDS IN BREAST-FEEDING

Both international[389] and national[1, 390, 391] organizations have endorsed breast-feeding as the optimal feeding for the healthy term infant. In general, the percentage of mothers initiating breast-feeding in developing countries is 80% or higher and often 90% or more.[392] However, the health and economic consequences to the proportion of bottle-fed infants in these countries are severe. In the United States, at one point in the early 1970s, the rate of breast-feeding initiation was as low as 25%. This low point was followed by an increase to a high of 61.9% in 1982. After 1982 a slow decline was observed (to 52.2% in 1989), after which a modest increase to 59.7% in 1995 took place.[393]

The pattern of breast-feeding initiation is accompanied by concomitant changes in maintenance of breast-feeding to 6 months, from 24% (1984) to 18% (1989) to 21.6% (1995).[393, 394] These changes took place despite goals set by the U.S. Surgeon General for 75% of infants to be breast-feeding in the first week of life and 35% at 6 months.[395] These goals were re-established for the year 2000, but the current trend indicates that it is unlikely that they will be met.[396]

Within the United States, a variety of demographic patterns appear to be associated with breast-feeding behavior. Older mothers, mothers with a college education, and higher-income mothers are all more likely to breast-feed. In contrast, black and Hispanic mothers, mothers who are Women, Infants, and Children (WIC) participants, and mothers who live in the southern sections of the United States are much less likely to breast-feed. The low rate of breast-feeding by mothers enrolled in WIC is of particular concern, as that agency has a specific policy to encourage breast-feeding. However, many states now depend on formula company rebates in order to fund part of their WIC programs, creating something of a conflict of interest. The disturbing part of the demographic pattern of breast-feeding in the United States is that the infants of lower socioeconomic mothers, who would accrue the greatest health and economic benefits from breast-feeding, are those least likely to be breast-fed.

Although demographic studies indicate who is breast-feeding, they do not explain the behavioral differences among groups of mothers. One of the more complete models designed to explain breast-feeding behavior includes components that address maternal attitudes and family, societal, cultural, and environmental variables.[397] Individual studies have shown that the maternal decision-making process is closely related to the social support and influence that come from the family members surrounding the mother.[398] The husband, in particular, appears to be a strong positive influence, whereas the mother's mother may be a negative influence on the breast-feeding decision. Social support appears to be different among ethnic groups, as are maternal attitudes; such differences may provide one explanation for differences in breast-feeding behavior among ethnic groups.[399, 400]

SUMMARY AND CONCLUSIONS

Human colostrum and milk contain a wide variety of cellular and soluble components that participate in many biologic functions in the mother and neonate. Passively transferred components can be targeted to enhance protection in the neonate against a variety of mucosal insults. Animal investigation and field application have demonstrated that through planned maternal immunization, generally by local gut priming and parenteral boosting, high sIgA titers directed against most enteric and respiratory pathogens can be consistently induced in milk.

Investigations in humans have primarily focused on IgA and gut mucosa. The immediate practical aim of such investigations should be to extend to intestinal and respiratory mucosal surfaces in the neonate the benefits of passively transferred, anti-infective milk factors directed against major pathogens of infancy, such as viral and bacterial pathogens in the gut; respiratory syncytial virus and *Chlamydia trachomatis* in the respiratory tract; and some intestinal parasitic infestations.

An evaluation of the soluble factors in the products of lactation, which may contribute to the growth and development of the gut and, perhaps, of other organ systems, has just begun. This promises to become an exciting field of inquiry distinct from the immune function of the breast.

The intrinsic suppressive qualities both of the products of lactation and of the neonate itself may have a profound regulatory role in the eventual expression of mucosal immunity and development of the systemic immune response. Such modulation of immunologic reactivity may be necessary to prevent the immunologically virgin infant from overreacting to the heavy exposure to antigens to which it is forced to react for the first time immediately after birth. The idea of preventive elimination of infectious agents and the possible role of immune exclusion of dietary antigens and other macromolecules in the modulation of atopic disease are consistent with such a concept.

Although there has been much investigation of the interaction of colostrum and milk with bacterial and viral pathogens, as well as with macromolecules, the relationship of the products of lactation to other major classes of luminal pathogens, namely, the intestinal protozoa and metazoa, is just beginning to be explored. Investigation of the possible role of immunocompetent cells, basophils, and IgE in defense against these pathogens is also under way. There is some evidence to suggest a role for passively acquired neutralizing IgA antibody in the antiparasitic defenses of young animals. Because parasitic disease is of major consequence in much of the world, more investigation on the possible contribution of breast-feeding to resistance against parasitic and perhaps inflammatory bowel disease in the infant is of particular interest. Fortunately, parasitic diseases are relatively uncommon in the neonatal period.

The contribution of the cells in milk to the well-being of the neonate remains obscure, and not all breast milk cells have been fully characterized as to class and function. Additional studies need to be directed toward an in-depth examination of the nature of macrophage-lymphocyte interaction, immune cell–epithelial cell interaction, and neurohormonal control of immune responsiveness in the mammary glands and other mucosal surfaces.

Clearly, breast-feeding under natural conditions by the infant's own mother remains the best approach to foster the use of human milk. The continued use of stored milk from natural mother or milk banks or the continuous nasogastric feeding of milk must be re-examined relative to its many potential and several documented risks to the neonates. It would be advisable to limit the use of nasogastric feeding to intermittent periods and discontinue the use of foster milk feeding until such specimens can be adequately tested and standardized for the benefit versus risk factors. It would also seem that the risks associated with the feeding of unpasteurized human milk outweigh the potential benefits related to the milk components (mostly cellular elements) lost by pasteurization. Under most circumstances, breast-feeding the healthy term infant promotes optimal growth, health, and development.

References

1. American Academy of Pediatrics, Workgroup on Breast-Feeding. Breast-feeding and the use of human milk. Pediatrics 100:1035–1039, 1997.
2. Kratochwil K. Experimental analysis of the prenatal development of the mammary gland. *In* Kretchmer N, Rossi E, Sereni F (eds). Milk and Lactation, Modern Problems in Paediatrics, vol. 15. Basel, S. Karger, 1975, pp 1–15.
3. Vorherr H. The Breast: Morphology, Physiology and Lactation. New York, Academic Press, 1974.
4. Goldman AS, Shapiro B, Neumann F. Role of testosterone and its metabolites in the differentiation of the mammary gland in rats. Endocrinology 99:1490–1495, 1976.
5. Kleinberg DL, Niemann W, Flamm E. Primate mammary development: effects of hypophysectomy, prolactin inhibition, and growth hormone administration. J Clin Invest 75:1943–1950, 1985.
6. Ogra SS, Ogra PL. Components of immunologic reactivity in human colostrum and milk. *In* Ogra PL, Dayton D. (eds). Immunology of Breast Milk. New York, Raven Press, 1979, pp 185–195.
7. Pasteels JL. Control of mammary growth and lactation by the anterior pituitary: an attempt to correlate classic experiments on animals with recent clinical findings. *In* Kretchmer N, Rossi E, Sereni F (eds). Milk and Lactation: Modern Problems in Paediatrics, vol. 15. Basel, S. Karger, 1975, pp 80–95.
8. Mepham TB. Physiology of Lactation. Milton Keynes, England, Open University Press, 1987.
9. Frantz AG. Prolactin. N Eng J Med 298:201–207, 1978.
10. Widström AM, Ransjo-Arvisson AB, Christensson K, et al. Gastric suction in healthy newborn infants. Acta Paediatr Scand 76:566–572, 1987.
11. Varendi H, Porter RH, Winberg J. Does the newborn baby find the nipple by smell. Lancet 344:989–990, 1994.
12. Lönnerdal B, Forsum E, Hambraeus L. The protein content of human milk. I. A transversal study of Swedish normal mothers. Nutr Rep Int 13:125–134, 1976.
13. Schanler RJ, Oh W. Composition of breast milk obtained from mothers of premature infants as compared to breast milk obtained from donors. J Pediatr 96:679–681, 1980.
14. Sann L, Bienvenu F, Lahet C. Comparison of the composition of breast milk from mothers of term and preterm infants. Acta Paediatr Scand 70:115–116, 1981.
15. Mata L. Breast-feeding: main promoter of infant health. Am J Clin Nutr 31:2058–2065, 1978.
16. Hurley LS, Lonnerdal B, Stanislowski AG. Zinc citrate, human milk and acrodermatitis enteropathica. Lancet 1:677–678, 1979.
17. Eckhert CD, Sloan MV, Duncan JR. Zinc binding: a difference between human and bovine milk. Science 195:789–790, 1977.
18. Fomon SJ. Infant Nutrition, 2nd ed. Philadelphia, WB Saunders, 1974.
19. Woodruff CW. The science of infant nutrition and the art of infant feeding. JAMA 240:657–661, 1978.
20. Moran R, Vaughn R, Orth DN, et al. Epidermal growth factor concentrations and daily production in breast milk during seven weeks post delivery in mothers of premature infants. Pediatr Res 16:171A, 1982.
21. Moran R, Bonum P, Vaughn R, et al. The concentration and daily output of trace elements, vitamins and carnitine in breast milk from mothers of premature infants for seven postnatal weeks. Pediatr Res 16:172A, 1982.
22. Ogra PL, Greene HL. Human milk and breast-feeding: an update on the state of the art. Pediatr Res 16:266–271, 1982.
23. Greene HL, Courtney ME. Breast-feeding and infant nutrition. *In* Ogra PL (ed). Neonatal Infections: Nutritional and Immunologic Interactions. Orlando, Fla, Grune & Stratton, 1984, pp 265–284.
24. Code of Federal Regulations, Title 21, Pat 107.100. Washington, DC, U.S. Government Printing Office, 1992, p 84.
25. Anderson RR. Variations in major minerals of human

milk during the first 5 months of lactation. Nutr Res 12:701–711, 1992.

26. Saarinen UM, Siimes MA, Dallman PR. Iron absorption in infants: high bioavailability of breast milk iron as indicated by extrinsic tag method of iron absorption and by the concentration of serum ferritin. J Pediatr 91:36–39, 1977.

27. McMillan JA, Oski FA, Louire G, et al. Iron absorption from human milk, simulated human milk, and proprietary formulas. Pediatrics 60:896–900, 1977.

28. Fomon S, Ziegler E, Vasquez H. Human milk and the small premature infant. Am J Dis Child 131:463–467, 1977.

29. Gopalan C, Belavady B. Nutrition and lactation. Fed Proc 20(Suppl 7):177–184, 1961.

30. Gorten MK, Cross ER. Iron metabolism in premature infants. II. Prevention of iron deficiency. J Pediatr 64:509–520, 1964.

31. Committee on Nutrition, American Academy of Pediatrics. Nutritional needs of low-birth-weight infants. Pediatrics 60:519–530, 1977.

32. O'Connor P. Vitamin D-deficiency rickets in two breast-fed infants who were not receiving vitamin D supplementation. Clin Pediatr 16:361–363, 1977.

33. Specker BL, Valonis B, Hertzberg V, et al. Sunshine exposure and serum 25-hydroxyvitamin D concentrations in exclusively breast-fed infants. J Pediatr 107:372–376, 1985.

34. Moser HW, Karnovsky ML. Studies on the biosynthesis of glycolipids and other lipids of the brain. J Biol Chem 234:1990–1997, 1959.

35. Kliegman RM, Miettinen EL, Morton S. Potential role of galactokinase in neonatal carbohydrate assimilation. Science 220:302–304, 1983.

36. Newburg DS, Neubauer SH. Carbohydrate in milks: analysis, quantities and significance. *In* Jensen RG (ed). Handbook of Milk Composition, San Diego, Academic Press, 1995, pp 273–349.

37. Newburg DS. Do the binding properties of oligosaccharides in milk protect human infants from gastrointestinal bacteria? J Nutr 127:980S–984S, 1997.

38. Department of Health and Social Security. The composition of mature human milk. Report 12. London, Her Majesty's Stationery Office, 1977.

39. Jensen RG, Ferris AM, and Lammi-Keefe CJ. Lipids in human milk and infant formulas. Annu Rev Nutr 12:417–441, 1992.

40. Rassin DK, Räihä NCR, Gaull GE. Protein and taurine nutrition in infants. *In* Lebenthal E (ed). Textbook of Gastroenterology and Nutrition in Infancy. New York, Raven Press, 1981, pp 391–401.

41. Reiser R, Sidelman Z. Control of serum cholesterol homeostasis by cholesterol in the milk of the suckling rat. J Nutr 102:1009–1016, 1972.

42. Fall CHD, Barker DJP, Osmond C, et al. Relation of infant feeding to adult serum cholesterol concentration and death from ischaemic heart disease BMJ 304:801–805, 1992.

43. Galli E, Picardo M, Chini L, et al. Analysis of polyunsaturated fatty acids in newborn seRA: a screening tool for atopic disease. Br J Dermatol 130:752–756, 1994.

44. Innis SM, Auestad N, Siegman JS. Blood lipid docosahexaenoic acid in term gestation infants fed formulas with high docosahexaenoic acid, low eicosapentaenoic acid fish oil. Lipids 31:617–625, 1996.

45. Carlson SE, Ford AJ, Werkman SH, et al. Visual acuity and fatty acid status of term infants fed human milk and formulas with and without docosahexaenoate and arachidonate from egg yolk lecithin. Pediatr Res 39:882–888, 1996.

46. Auestad N, Montalto MB, Hall RT, et al. Visual acuity, erythrocyte fatty acid composition and growth in term infants fed formulas with long chain polyunsaturated fatty acids for one year. Pediatr Res 41:1–10, 1997.

47. Birch EE, Hoffman DR, Usuy R, et al. Visual acuity and the eosentiality of docosahexaenoic acid and acndridonic acid in the diet of term infants. Pediatr Res 44:201–209, 1998.

48. Carlson SE, Werkman SH, Tolley EA. Effect of long-chain n-3 fatty acid supplementation on visual acuity and growth of preterm infants with and without bronchopulmonary dysplasia. Am J Clin Nutr 63:687–689, 1996.

49. Gross SJ, Geller J, Tomarelli RM. Composition of breast milk from mothers of preterm infants. Pediatrics 68:490–493, 1981.

50. Hambraeus L. Proprietary milk versus human breast milk in infant feeding: a critical appraisal from the nutritional point of view. Pediatr Clin North Am 24:17–36, 1977.

51. Kunz C, Lönnerdal B. Re-evaluation of the whey protein/casein ratio of human milk. Acta Paediatr 81:107–112, 1992.

52. Järvenpää A-L, Räihä NCR, Rassin DK, et al. Milk protein quantity and quality in the term infant. II. Effects on acidic and neutral amino acids. Pediatrics 70:221–230, 1982.

53. Janas LM, Picciano MF, Hatch TF. Indices of protein metabolism in term infants fed human milk, whey-predominant formula, or cow's milk formula. Pediatrics 75:775–784, 1985.

54. Picone TA, Benson JD, Moro G, et al. Growth, serum biochemistries, and amino acids of term infants fed formulas with amino acid and protein concentrations similar to human milk. J Pediatr Gastroenterol Nutr 9:351–360, 1989.

55. Gaull GE, Rassin DK, Räihä NCR, et al. Milk protein quantity and quality in low-birth-weight infants. III. Effects on sulfur-containing amino acids in plasma and urine. J Pediatr 90:348–355, 1977.

56. Rassin DK, Gaull GE, Heinonen K, et al. Milk protein quantity and quality in low-birth-weight infants. II. Effects on selected essential and nonessential amino acids in plasma and urine. Pediatrics 59:407–422, 1977.

57. Rassin DK, Gaull GE, Räihä NCR, et al. Milk protein quantity and quality in low-birth-weight infants. IV. Effects on tyrosine and phenylalanine in plasma and urine. J Pediatr 90:356–360, 1977.

58. Räihä NCR, Heinonen K, Rassin DK, et al. Milk protein quantity and quality in low-birth-weight infants. I. Metabolic responses and effects on growth. Pediatrics 57:659–674 1976.

59. Gaull GE, Jensen RG, Rassin DK, et al. Human milk as food. Adv Perinatal Med 2:47–120, 1982.

60. Novak M, Wieser PB, Buch M, et al. Acetyl-carnitine and free carnitine in body fluids before and after birth. Pediatr Res 13:10–15, 1979.

61. Schmidt-Sommerfeld E, Novak M, Penn D, et al. Carnitine and development of newborn adipose tissue. Pediatr Res 12:660–664, 1978.

62. Thorell L, Sj'berg L-B, Hernell O. Nucleotides in human milk: sources and metabolism by the newborn infant. Pediatr Res 40:845–852, 1996.

63. Leach JL, Baxter JH, Molitor BE, et al. Total potentially available nucleotides of human milk by stage of lactation. Am J Clin Nutr 61:1224–1230, 1995.

64. Uauy R. Dietary nucleotides and requirements in early life. *In* Lebenthal E (ed). Textbook of Gastroenterology

and Nutrition in Infancy. New York, Raven Press, 1989, pp 265–280.

65. Carver JD, Pimentel B, Cox WI, et al. Dietary nucleotide effects upon immune function in infants. Pediatrics 88:359–363, 1991.

66. Brunser O, Espinosa J, Araya M, et al. Effect of dietary nucleotide supplementation on diarrhoeal disease in infants. Acta Paediatr 83:188–191, 1994.

67. Pickering L, Granoff DM, Erickson JR, et al. Modulation of the immune system by human milk and infant formula containing nucleotides. Pediatrics 101:242–249, 1998.

68. Lönnerdal B, Forsum E. Casein content of human milk. Am J Clin Nutr 41:113–120, 1985.

69. Kunz C, Lönnerdal B. Casein micelles and casein subunits in human milk. *In* Atkinson SA, Lönnerdal B (eds). Protein and Non-Protein Nitrogen in Human Milk. Boca Raton, Fla, CRC Press, 1989, pp 9–27.

70. Phillippy BO, McCarthy RD. Multi-origins of milk serum albumin in the lactating goat. Biochim Biophys Acta 584:298–303, 1979.

71. Jenness R. Biosynthesis and composition of milk. J Invest Dermatol 63:109–118, 1974.

72. Spik G, Brunet B, Mazunier-Dehaine C, et al. Characterization and properties of the human and bovine lactoferrins extracted from the faeces of newborn infants. Acta Paediatr Scand 71:979–985, 1982.

73. Trugo NMF, Newport MJ. Vitamin B_{12} absorption in the neonatal piglet. II. Resistance of the vitamin B_{12}-binding protein in cow's milk to proteolysis in vivo. Br J Nutr 54:257–267, 1985.

74. Oberkotter LV, Tenore A, Pasquariello PS, et al. Tyroxine-binding proteins in human breast milk similar to serum thyroxine-binding globulin. J Clin Endocrinol Metab 57:1133–1139, 1983.

75. Payne DW, Peng LH, Pearlman WH. Corticosteroid-binding proteins in human colostrum and milk and rat milk. J Biol Chem 251:5272–5279, 1976.

76. Blanc B. Biochemical aspects of human milk-comparison with bovine milk. World Rev Nutr Diet 36:1–89, 1981.

77. Olivecrona T, Hernell O. Human milk lipases and their possible role in fat digestion. Pädiät Pädo 11:600–604, 1976.

78. Hamosh M. Linguinal and breast milk lipases. Adv Pediatr 29:33–67, 1982.

79. Koldovsky O, Thornburg W. Peptide hormones and hormone-like substances in milk. *In* Atkinson SA, Lönnerdal B (eds). Protein and Non-Protein Nitrogen in Human Milk. Boca Raton, Fla, CRC Press, 1989, pp 53–65.

80. Lucas A, Blackburn AM, Green AA, et al. Breast vs bottle: endocrine responses are different with formula feeding. Lancet 1:1267–1269, 1980.

81. Koldovsky O, Štrbák V. Hormones and growth factors in human milk. *In* Jensen RG (ed). Handbook of Human Milk Composition. San Diego, Academic Press, 1995, pp 428–436.

82. Ogra PL, Losonsky GA. Defense factors in products of lactation. *In* Ogra PL (ed). Neonatal Infections: Nutritional and Immunologic Interactions. Orlando, Fla, Grune & Stratton, 1984, pp 67–68.

83. Losonsky GA, Ogra PL. Mucosal immune system. *In* Ogra PL (ed). Neonatal Infections: Nutritional and Immunologic Interactions. Orlando, Fla, Grune & Stratton, 1984, pp 51–65.

84. Ogra SS, Ogra PL. Immunologic aspects of human colostrum and milk. I. Distribution characteristics and concentrations of immunoglobulins at different times after the onset of lactation. J Pediatr 92:546–549, 1978.

85. Goldblum RM, Ahlatedt S, Carlson B, et al. Antibody forming cells in human colostrum after oral immunization. Nature 257:797–799, 1975.

86. Fishaut JM, Murphy D, Neifert M, et al. The bronchomammary axis in the immune response to respiratory syncytial virus. J Pediatr 99:186–191, 1981.

87. Orskov F, Sorenson KB. *Escherichia coli* serogroups in breast-fed and bottle-fed infants. Acta Pathol Microbiol Scand Sect B, Microbiol 83:25–30, 1975.

88. van Genderen J. Diphtheria-antitoxin in Kolostrum und Muttermilch bei Menschen. Z Immunutaetsforsch Allerg Klin Immunol 83:54–59, 1934.

89. Montgomery PC, Rosner BR, Cohn J, et al. The secretory antibody response: anti-DNP antibodies induced by dinitrophenylated type III pneumococcus. Immunol Commun 3:143–156, 1974.

90. Lamm M, Weisz-Carrington P, Roux ME, et al. Mode of induction of an IgA response in the breast and other secretory sites by oral antigen. *In* Ogra PL, Dayton D (eds). Immunology of Breast Milk. New York, Raven Press, 1979, pp 105–114.

91. Drife J, McClelland DB, Pryde A, et al. Immunoglobulin synthesis in the "resting" breast. BMJ 2:503–506, 1976.

92. Weisz-Carrington P, Roux ME, McWilliams M, et al. Hormonal induction of the secretory immune system in the mammary gland. Proc Natl Acad Sci U S A 75:2928–2932, 1978.

93. Cumella JC, Ogra PL. Pregnancy associated hormonal milieu and bronchomammary cell traffic. *In* Hamosh M, Goldman AS (eds). Human Lactation 2. New York, Plenum Publishing, 1986, pp 507–524.

94. Strober, W, Elson CO, Graeff A, et al. Class specific T cell regulation of mucosal immune responses. *In* Strober W, et al (eds). Recent Advances in Mucosal Immunity. New York, Raven Press, 1982, pp. 121–130.

95. Peri BA, Theodore CM, Losonsky GA, et al. Antibody content of rabbit milk and serum following inhalation or ingestion of respiratory syncytial virus and bovine serum albumin. Clin Exp Immunol 48:91–101, 1982.

96. Losonsky GA, Fiskaut JM, Strussenberg JG, et al. Effect of immunization against rubella on lactation products. I. Development and characterization of specific immunologic reactivity in breast milk. J Infect Dis 145:654–660, 1982.

97. McClelland DBL, McGrath J, Samson, RR. Antimicrobial factors in human milk: studies of concentration and transfer to the infant during the early stages of lactation. Acta Paediatr Scand Suppl 271:1–20, 1978.

98. Pitt J. The milk mononuclear phagocyte. Pediatrics 64:745–749, 1979.

99. Ogra SS, Weintraub D, Ogra PL. Immunologic aspects of human colostrum and milk. III. Fate and absorption of cellular and soluble components in the gastrointestinal tract of the newborn. J Immunol 119:245–248, 1977.

100. Kenny JF, Boesman MI, Michaels RH. Bacterial and viral copro-antibodies in breast-fed infants. Pediatrics 39:201–213, 1967.

101. Haneberg B. Immunoglobulins in feces from infants fed human or bovine milk. Scand J Immunol 3:191–197, 1974.

102. McClelland DBL, Samson RR, Parkin DM, et al. Bacterial agglutination studies with secretory IgA prepared from human gastrointestinal secretions and colostrum. Gut 13:450–458, 1972.

103. Stoliar OA, Pelley RP, Kaniecki-Green E, et al. Secretory IgA against enterotoxins in breast milk. Lancet 1:1258–1261, 1976.

104. Steele EJ, Chicumpa W, Rowley D. Isolation and biological properties of three classes of rabbit antibody in *Vibrio cholerae*. J Infect Dis 130:93–103, 1974.

105. Cantey JR. Prevention of bacterial infections of mucosal surfaces of immune secretory IgA. Adv Exp Med Biol 107:461–470, 1978.

106. Plotkin SA, Katz M, Brown RE, et al. Oral poliovirus vaccination in newborn African infants: the inhibitory effect of breast-feeding. Am J Dis Child 111:27–30, 1966.

107. Ogra PL, Karzon DT. The role of immunoglobulins in the mechanism of mucosal immunity to virus infection. Pediatr Clin North Am 17:385–390, 1970.

108. Mata LJ, Wyatt RG. The uniqueness of human milk: host resistance to infection. Am J Clin Nutr 24:976–986, 1971.

109. Svirsky-Gross S. Pathogenic strains of coli (0;111) among prematures and the cause of human milk in controlling the outbreak of diarrhea. Ann Pediatr (Paris) 190:109–115, 1958.

110. Yolken RH, Wyatt RG, Mata L, et al. Secretory antibody directed against rotavirus in human milk-measurement by means of an ELISA. J Pediatr 93:916–921, 1978.

111. Glode MP, Sutton A, Robbins JB, et al. Neonatal meningitis due to *Escherichia coli* K1. J Infect Dis 136 (Suppl):S93–S97, 1977.

112. Ellestad-Sayed J, Coodin FJ, Dilling LA, et al. Breast-feeding protects against infection in Indian infants. Can Med Assoc J 120:295–298, 1979.

113. Chandra RK. Prospective studies on the effect of breast-feeding on incidence of infection and allergy. Acta Paediatr Scand 68:691–694, 1979.

114. Eastham EJ Walker, WA. Adverse effects of milk formula ingestion on the gastrointestinal tract: an update. Gastroenterology 76:365–374, 1979.

115. Soothill JF. Immunodeficiency, allergy and infant feeding. *In* Hambraeus L, Hanson LA, McFarlane H (eds). Food and Immunology: Proceedings of a Symposium Co-sponsored by the Swedish Medical Research Council. Stockholm, Almqvist & Wiksell, 1977, pp 88–91.

116. Stevenson DD, Orgal HA, Hamburger RN. Development of IgE in newborn human infants. J Allergy Clin Immunol 48:61–72, 1971.

117. Downham MAPS, Scott R, Sims DG, et al. Breast-feeding protects against respiratory syncytial virus infections. BMJ 2:274–276, 1976.

118. Scott R, de Landazuri MO, Gardner PS, et al. Human antibody dependent cell-mediated cytotoxicity against target cells infected with respiratory syncytial virus. Clin Exp Immunol 28:19–26, 1977.

119. Blum P, Phelps DL, Ank BJ, et al. Survival of oral human immune serum globulin in the gastrointestinal tract of low birth weight infants. Pediatr Res 15:1256–1260, 1981.

120. Bahna SL, Keller MA, Heiner DC. IgE and IgD in human colostrum and plasma. Pediatr Res 16:604–607, 1982.

121. Keller MA, Heiner, DC, Kidd RM, et al. Local production of IgG4 in human colostrum. J Immunol 130:1654–1657, 1983.

122. Keller MA, Heiner DC, Myers, AS, et al. IgD in human colostrum. Pediatr Res 19:122–126, 1985.

123. Smith CW, Goldman AS: The cells of human colostrum. I. In vitro studies of morphology and functions. Pediatr Res 2:103–109, 1968.

124. Ogra SS, Ogra PL. Immunologic aspects of human colostrum and milk. II. Characteristics of lymphocyte reactivity and distribution of E-rosette forming cells at different times after the onset of lactation. J Pediatr 92:550–555, 1978.

125. Keeney SE, Schmalstieg FC, Palkowetz KH, et al. Activated neutrophils and neutrophil activators in human milk: Increased expression of CD116 and decreased expression of L-selectin. J Leukocyte Biol 54(2):97–104, 1993.

126. Wirt DP, Adkins LT, Palkowetz KH, et al. Activated-memory T lymphocytes in human milk. Cytometry 13:282–290, 1992.

127. Pitt J, Barlow B, Heird, WC. Protection against experimental necrotizing enterocolitis by maternal milk. I. Role of milk leucocytes. Pediatr Res 11:906–909, 1977.

128. Pittard WB, and Bill K. Immunoregulation by breast milk cells. Cell Immunol 42:437–441, 1979.

129. Pittard WB, III, Polmar SH, and Fanaroff AA. The breast milk macrophage: potential vehicle for immunoglobulin transport. J Reticuloendothel Soc 22:597–603, 1977.

130. Clemente J, Leyva-Cobian F, Hernandez M, et al. Intracellular immunoglobulins in human milk macrophages: ultrastructural localization and factors affecting the kinetics of immunoglobulin release. Int Arch Allergy Appl Immunol 80:291–299, 1986.

131. Weaver EA, Goldblum RM, Davis CP, et al. Enhanced immunoglobulin A release from human colostral cells during phagocytosis. Infect Immun 34:498–502, 1981.

132. Schlesinger L, Munoz C, Arevalo M, et al. Functional capacity of colostral leukocytes from women delivering prematurely. J Pediatr Gastroenterol Nutr 8:89–94, 1989.

133. Cummings NP, Neifert MR, Pabst MJ, et al. Oxidative metabolic response and microbicidal activity of human milk macrophages: effect of lipopolysaccharide and muramyl dipeptide. Infect Immun 49:435–439, 1985.

134. Robinson JE, Harvey BA, and Sothill JF. Phagocytosis and killing of bacteria and yeast by human milk after opsonization in aqueous phase of milk. BMJ 1:1443–1445, 1978.

135. Kohl S, Malloy MM, Pickering LK, et al. Human colostral antibody dependent cellular cytotoxicity against herpes simplex virus infected cells mediated by colostral cells. J Clin Lab Immunol 1:221–224, 1978.

136. Sone S, Tsutsumi H, Takeuchi R, et al. Enhanced cytokine production by milk macrophages following infection with respiratory syncytial virus. J Leukoc Biol 61:630–636, 1997.

137. Kirkpatrick CH, Green I, Rich RR, et al. Inhibition of growth of *Candida albicans* by iron-unsaturated lactoferrin: relation to host defense mechanisms in chronic mucocutaneous candidiasis. J Infect Dis 124:539–544, 1971.

138. Murillo GJ, Goldman AS. The cells of human colostrum. II. Synthesis of IgA and B-1C. Pediatr Res 4:71–75, 1970.

139. Diaz-Uanen E, Williams RC, Jr. T and B lymphocytes in human colostrum. Clin Immunol Immunopathol 3:248–255, 1974.

140. Oksenberg JR, Persity E, Brautbar C. Cellular immunity in human milk. Am J Reprod Immunol Microbiol 8:125–129, 1985.

141. Hanson LA, Ahlstedt S, Andersson B., et al. Protective factors in milk and development of the immune system. J Pediatr 75:172–175, 1985.

142. Ogra PL, Ogra SS. Cellular aspects of immunologic reactivity in human milk. *In* Hanson LA (ed). Biology of Human Milk. Nestlé Nutrition Workshop Series, vol. 15. New York, Raven Press, 1988, pp 171–184.

143. Nair MP, Schwartz SA, Slade HB, et al. Comparison of the cellular cytotoxic activities of colostral lymphocytes

and maternal peripheral blood lymphocytes. J Reprod Immunol 7:199–213, 1985.

144. Parmely MJ, Beer AE, Billingham RE. In vitro studies on the T-lymphocyte population of human milk. J Exp Med 144:358–370, 1976.

145. Shinmoto H, Kawakami H, Dosako S, et al. IgA specific helper factor in human colostrum Clin. Exp Immunol 66:223–230, 1986.

146. Bertotto A, Gerli R, Fabietti G, et al. Human breast milk T lymphocytes display the phenotype and functional characteristics of memory T cells. Eur J Immunol 20:1877–1880, 1990.

147. Gibson CE, Eglinton BA, Penttila IA, et al. Phenotype and activation of milk-derived and peripheral blood lymphocytes from normal and coeliac subjects. Immunol Cell Biol 69:387–391, 1991.

148. Bertotto A, Castellucci G, Pradicioni M, et al. CD40 ligand expression on the surface of colostral T cells. Arch Dis Child 74:F135–136, 1996.

149. Hayward AR, Lee J, Beverley PCL. Ontogeny of expression of UCHL1 antigen on TcR-1⁺ (CD4/8) and TcR⁺ T cells. Eur J Immunol 19:771–773, 1989.

150. Bertotto A, Castellucci G, Fabietti G, et al. Lymphocytes bearing the T cell receptor γδ in human breast milk. Arch Dis Child 65:1274–1275, 1990.

151. Eglinton BA, Roberton DM, Cummins AG: Phenotype of T cells, their soluble receptor levels, and cytokine profile of human breast milk. Immunol Cell Biol 72:306–313, 1994.

152. Trejdosiewicz LK. Intestinal intraepithelial lymphocytes and lymphoepithelial interactions in the human gastrointestinal mucosa. Immunol Lett 32:13–19, 1992.

153. Head JR, Beer AE, Billingham RE. Significance of the cellular component of the maternal immunologic endowment in milk. Transplant Proc 9:1465–1471, 1977.

154. Jain L, Vidyasagar D, Xanthou M, et al. In vivo distribution of human milk leucocytes after ingestion by newborn baboons. Arch Dis Child 64:930–933, 1989.

155. Schnorr KL, Pearson LD. Intestinal absorption of maternal leukocytes by newborn lambs. J Reprod Immunol 6:329–337, 1984.

156. Weiler IJ, Hickler W, Spenger R. Demonstration that milk cells invade the neonatal mouse. Am J Reprod Immunol 4:95–98, 1983.

157. Beer AE, Billingham RE, Head J. The immunologic significance of the mammary gland. J Invest Dermatol 63:65–74, 1974.

158. Mohr JA, Leu R, Mabry W. Colostral leukocytes. J Surg Oncol 2:163–167, 1970.

159. Schlesinger JJ, Covelli HD. Evidence for transmission of lymphocyte response to tuberculin by breast-feeding. Lancet 2:529–532, 1977.

160. Thorpe LW, Rudloff HE, Powell LC, et al. Decreased response of human milk leukocytes to chemoattractant peptides. Pediatr Res 20:373–377, 1986.

161. Dulbecco R, Unger M, Armstrong B, et al. Epithelial cell types and their evolution in the rat mammary gland determined by immunological markers. Proc Natl Acad Sci U S A 80:1033–1037, 1983.

162. Allen R, Dulbecco R, Syka P, et al. Developmental regulation of cytokeratins in cells of the rat mammary gland studies with monoclonal antibodies. Proc Natl Acad Sci U S A 81:1203–1207, 1984.

163. Ballow M, Fang F, Good RA, et al. Developmental aspects of complement components in the newborn. Clin Exp Immunol 18:257–266, 1974.

164. Nakajima S, Baba AS, and Tamura N. Complement system in human colostrum. Int Arch Allergy Appl Immunol 54:428–433, 1977.

165. Tomasi TB, Jr. New areas arising from studies of secretory immunity. Adv Exp Med Biol 107:1–8, 1978.

166. Gyorgy P. A hitherto unrecognized biochemical difference between human milk and cow's milk. Pediatrics 11:98–108, 1953.

167. György P, Dhanamitta S, Steers E. Protective effects of human milk in experimental staphylococcus infection. Science 137:338–340, 1962.

168. Hanson LA, Ahlstedt S, Anderson B, et al. Mucosal immunity. Ann NY Acad Sci 409:1–21, 1983.

169. Carpenter G. Epidermal growth factor is a major growth-promoting agent in human milk. Science 210:198–199, 1980.

170. Colman N, Hettiarachchy N, Herbert V. Detection of a milk factor that facilitates folate uptake by intestinal cells. Science 211:1427–1429, 1981.

171. Dolan SA, Boesman-Finkelstein M, Finkelstein RA. Antimicrobial activity of human milk against pediatric pathogens. J Infect Dis 154:722–725, 1986.

172. Boesman-Finkelstein M, Finkelstein RA. Antimicrobial effects of human milk: inhibitory activity on enteric pathogens. FEMS Microbiol 27:167–174, 1985.

173. Farthing MJG, Keusch GT, Carey MC. Effects of bile and bile salts on growth and membrane lipid uptake by Giardia lamblia. J Clin Invest 76:1727–1732, 1985.

174. Reiter B. Role of nonantibody proteins in milk in the protection of the newborn. In Williams AF, Baum JD (eds). Human Milk Banking. New York, Nestlé Nutrition, Raven Press, 1984, pp 29–53.

175. Hernell O, Bläckberg L, Olivecrona T. Human milk lipases. In Lebenthal E. (ed). Gastroenterology and Nutrition in Infancy. New York, Raven Press, 1981, pp 347–354.

176. Hernell O, Bläckberg L. Lipase and esterase activities in human milk. In Jensen RG, Neville MC. (eds). Human Lactation: Milk Components and Methodologies. New York, Plenum Publishing, 1985, pp 267–276.

177. Hernell O, Blackberg L. Antiparasitic factors in human milk. In Hanson LA (ed). Biology of Human Milk. Nestlé Nutrition Workshop Series, vol. 15. New York, Raven Press, 1988, pp 159–170.

178. Holmgren J, Svennerholm AM, Ahren C. Nonimmunoglobulin fraction of human milk inhibits bacterial adhesion (hemagglutination) and enterotoxin binding of Escherichia coli and Vibrio cholera. Infect Immun 33:136–141, 1981.

179. Holmgren J, Svennerholm AM, Lindblad M. Receptor-like glycocompounds in human milk that inhibit classical and El Tor Vibrio cholerae cell adhererence (hemagglutination). Infect Immun 39:147–154, 1983.

180. Newburg DS, Pickering LK, McCluer RH, et al. Fucosylated oligosaccharides of human milk protect suckling mice from heat-stable enterotoxin of Escherichia coli. J Infect Dis 162:1075–1080, 1990.

181. Holmgren J, Svennerholm A-M, Lindblad M, et al. Inhibition of bacterial adhesion and toxin binding by glycoconjugate and oligosaccharide receptor analogues in human milk. In Goldman AS, Atkinson SA, and Hanson LNA (eds). Human Lactation 3: The Effects of Human Milk on the Recipient Infant. New York and London, Plenum Press, 1987, pp 251–259.

182. Grönberg G, Lipniunas P, Lundgren T, et al. Structural analysis of five new monosialyated oligosaccharides from human milk. Arch Biochem Biophys 296:597–610, 1992.

183. Laegreid A, Kolsto Otnaess, AB, and Bryn K. Purification of human milk gangliosides by silica gel chromatog-

raphy and analysis of trifluoroacetate derivatives by gas chromatography. J Chromatogr 377:59–67, 1986.

184. Laegreid A, Kolsto Otnaess AB, Fuglesang J. Human and bovine milk: comparison of ganglioside composition and enterotoxin-inhibitory activity. Pediatr Res 20:416–421, 1986.

185. Laegreid A, Kolsto Otnaess AB. Trace amounts of ganglioside GM1 in human milk inhibit enterotoxins from *Vibrio cholerae* and *Escherichia coli*. Life Sci 40:55–62, 1987.

186. Schroten H, Hanisch FG, Plogmann R, et al. Inhibition of adhesion of S-fimbriated *Escherichia coli* to buccal epithelial cells by human milk fat globule membrane components: a novel aspect of the protective function of mucins in the nonimmunoglobulin fraction. Infect Immun 60:2893–2899, 1992.

187. Andersson B, Porras O, Hanson LA, et al. Inhibition of attachment of *Streptococcus pneumoniae* and *Haemophilus influenzae* by human milk and receptor oligosaccharides. J Infect Dis 153:232–237, 1986.

188. Newburg DS, Viscidi RP, Ruff A, et al. A human milk factor inhibits binding of human immunodeficiency virus to the CD4 receptor. Pediatr Res 31:22–28, 1992.

189. Otnaess AB, Svennerholm AM. Non-immunoglobulin fraction in human milk protects rabbit against enterotoxin-induced intestinal fluid secretion. Infect Immun 35:738–740, 1982.

190. Ashkenazi S, Newburg DS, Cleary TG. The effect of human milk on the adherence of enterohemorrhagic *E. coli* to rabbit intestinal cells. *In* Mesteky J, Blair C, Ogra PL (eds). Immunology of Milk and the Neonate. New York, Plenum Press, 1991, pp 173–177.

191. Cleary TG, Chambers JP, and Pickering LK, Protection of suckling mice from the heat-stable enterotoxin of *Escherichia coli* by human milk. J Infect Dis 148:1114–1119, 1983.

192. Glass RL, Svenneholm AM, Stoll BJ, et al. Protection against cholera in breast-fed children by antibodies in breast milk. N Engl J Med 308:1389–1392, 1983.

193. György P, Jeanloz RW, Nicolai H, et al. Undialyzable growth factors for *Lactobacillus bifidus var. Pennsylvanicus*: protective effect of sialic acid bound to glycoprotein and oligosaccharides against bacterial degradation. Eur J Biochem 43:29–33, 1974.

194. Bezkorovainy A, Grohlich D, Nichols JH. Isolation of a glycopeptide fraction with *Lactobacillus bifidus* subspecies *Pennsylvanicus* growth-promoting activity from whole human milk casein. Am J Clin Nutr 32:1428–1432, 1979.

195. Nichols JH, Bezkorovainy A, and Paque R. Isolation and characterization of several glycoproteins from human colostrum whey. Biochim Biophys Acta 412:99–108, 1975.

196. Bezkorovainy A, Topouzian N. *Bifidobacterium bifidus* var. *Pennsylvanicus* growth promoting activity of human milk casein and its derivates. Int J Biochem 13:585–590, 1981.

197. Isolauri E, Juntanen M, Rautanen T, et al. A human Lactobacillus strain (Lactobacillus GG) promotes recovery from acute diarrhea in children. Pediatrics 88:90–97, 1991.

198. Kaila M, Isolauir E, Elina S, et al. Enhancement of the circulating antibody secreting cell response in human diarrhea by a human Lactobacillus strain. Pediatr Res 32:141–144, 1992.

199. Hamosh M. Enzymes in human milk: their role in nutrient digestion, gastrointestinal function, and nutrient delivery to the newborn infant. *In* Lebenthal E (ed). Textbook of Gastroenterology and Nutrition in Infancy, 2nd ed. New York, Raven Press, pp 121–134.

200. Institute of Medicine (U.S.) Subcommittee on Nutrition During Lactation, et al. Nutrition During Lactation: Summary, Conclusions and Recommendations. Washington, DC, National Academy Press, 1991.

201. Issacs CE, Thormar H, Pessolano T. Membrane-disruptive effect of human milk: inactivation of enveloped viruses. J Infect Dis 154:966–971, 1986.

202. Stock CC, and Francis T, Jr. The inactivation of the virus of epidemic influenza by soaps. J Exp Med 71:661–681, 1940.

203. Thormar H, Isaacs CE, Brown HR, et al. Inactivation of enveloped viruses and killing of cells by fatty acids and monoglycerides. Antimicrobiol Agents Chemother 31:27–31, 1987.

204. Welsh JK, Arsenakis M, Coelen RJ, et al. Effect of antiviral lipids, heat, and freezing on the activity of viruses in human milk. J Infect Dis 140:322–328, 1979.

205. Welsh JK, May JT. Anti-infective properties of breast milk. J Pediatr 94:1–9, 1979.

206. Resta S, Luby JP, Rosenfeld CR, et al. Isolation and propagation of a human enteric coronavirus. Science 229:978–981, 1985.

207. Gillin FD, Reiner DS, Wang C-S. Human milk kills parasitic protozoa. Science 221:1290–1292, 1983.

208. Gillin FD, Reiner, DS, Gault MJ. Cholate-dependent killing of *Giardia lamblia* by human milk. Infect Immun 47:619–622, 1985.

209. Anderson BF, Baker HM, Dodson EJ, et al. Structure of human lactoferrin at 3.1-resolution. Proc Natl Acad Sci U S A 84:1769–1773, 1987.

210. Fransson G-B, Lonnerdal B. Iron in human milk. J Pediatr 96:380–384, 1980.

211. Arnold RR, Cole MF, McGhee JR. A bactericidal effect for human milk lactoferrin. Science 197:263–265, 1977.

212. Bullen JJ, Rogers HJ, Leigh L. Iron-binding proteins in milk and resistance of *Escherichia coli* infection in infants. BMJ 1:69–75, 1972.

213. Spik G, Cheron A, Montreuil J, et al. Bacteriostasis of a milk-sensitive strain of *Escherichia coli* by immunoglobulins and iron-binding proteins in association. Immunology 35:663–671, 1978.

214. Stephens S, Dolby JM, Montreuil J, et al. Differences in inhibition of the growth of commensal and enteropathogenic strains of *Escherichia coli* by lactoferrin and secretory immunoglobulin A isolated from human milk. Immunology 41:597–603, 1980.

215. Stuart J, Norrel S, Harrington JP. Kinetic effect of human lactoferrin on the growth of *Escherichia coli*. Int J Biochem 16:1043–1047, 1984.

216. Nichols BL, McKee KS, Henry JF, et al. Human lactoferrin stimulates thymidine incorporation into DNA of rat crypt cells. Pediatr Res 21:563–567, 1987.

217. Goldblum RM, Garza CA, Johnson GA, et al. Human milk banking. II. Relative stability of immunologic factors in stored colostrum. Acta Paediatr Scand 71:143–144, 1981.

218. Goldblum RM, Garza CA, Johnson CA, et al. Human milk banking I. Effects of container upon immunologic factors in mature milk. Nutr Res 1:449–459, 1981.

219. Goldman AS, Garza CA, Johnson CA, et al. Immunologic factors in human milk during the first year of lactation. J Pediatr 100:563–567, 1982.

220. Brines RD, Brock JH. The effect of trypsin and chymotrypsin on the *in vitro* antimicrobial and iron-binding properties of lactoferrin in human milk and bovine colostrum. Biochim Biophys Acta 759:229–235, 1983.

221. Samson RR, Mirtle C, McClelland DBL. The effect of digestive enzymes on the binding and bacteriostatic

properties of lactoferrin and vitamin B$_{12}$ binder in human milk. Acta Paediatr Scand 69:517–523, 1980.

222. Spik G, Montreuil J. Études comparatives de la structure de la tranferrine de la lactotransferrine humaines. Fingerprinting des hydrolytes protéasiques des deux glycoproteides. CR Seances Soc Biol Paris 160:94–98, 1996.

223. Butte NF, Goldblum RM, Fehl LM, et al. Daily ingestion of immunologic components in human milk during the first four months of life. Acta Paediatr Scand 73:296–301, 1984.

224. Davidson LA, Lonnerdal B. Lactoferrin and secretory IgA in the feces of exclusively breast-fed infants. Am J Clin Nutr 41:852A, 1985.

225. Davidson LA, Lonnerdal B. The persistence of human milk proteins in the breast-fed infant. Acta Paediatr Scand 76:733–740, 1987.

226. Schanler RJ, Goldblum RM, Garza C, et al. Enhanced fecal excretion of selected immune factors in very low birth weight infants fed fortified human milk. Pediatr Res 20:711–715, 1986.

227. Goldman AS, Garza C, Schanler RJ, et al. Molecular forms of lactoferrin in stool and urine from infants fed human milk. Pediatr Res 27:252–255, 1990.

228. Goldblum RM, Schanler RJ, Garza C, et al. Human milk feeding enhances the urinary excretion of immunologic factors in birth weight infants. Pediatr Res 25:184–188, 1989.

229. Prentice A. Breast-feeding increases concentrations of IgA in infants' urine. Arch Dis Child 62:792–795, 1987.

230. Hutchens TW, Henry JF, Yip T-T, et al. Origin of intact lactoferrin and its DNA-binding fragments found in the urine of human milk-fed preterm infants: evaluation of stable isotopic enrichment. Pediatr Res 29:243–250, 1991.

231. Chandan RC, Shahani KM, Holly RG. Lysozyme content of human milk. Nature (London) 204:76, 1964.

232. Jolles J, Jolles P. Human tear and human milk lysozymes. Biochemistry 6:411–417, 1967.

233. Goldman AS, Garza C, Johnson CA, et al. Immunologic components in human milk during weaning. Acta Paediatr Scand 72:133–134, 1983.

234. Goldman AS, Goldblum RM, Garza C. Immunologic components in human milk during the second year of lactation. Acta Paediatr Scand 72:461–462, 1983.

235. Peitersen B, Bohn L, Anderson H. Quantitative determination of immunoglobulins, lysozyme, and certain electrolytes during a 24-hour period, and in milk from the individual mammary gland. Acta Paediatr Scand 64:709–717, 1975.

236. Chipman DM, Sharon N. Mechanism of lysozyme action. Science 165:454–465, 1969.

237. Friss HE, Rubin LG, Carsons S, et al. Plasma fibronectin concentrations in breast-fed and formula fed neonates. Arch Dis Child 63:528–532, 1988.

238. Cunningham AS, Jelliffe DB, Jelliffe EFP. Breast-feeding and health in the 1980s: a global epidemiologic review. J Pediatr 118:659–666, 1991.

239. Glass RI, Stoll BJ. The protective effect of human milk against diarrhea. Acta Paediatr Scand 351:131–136, 1989.

240. Goldman AS, Thorpe LW, Goldblum RM, et al. Anti-inflammatory properties of human milk. Acta Paediatr Scand 75:689–695, 1986.

241. Garofalo RP, Goldman AS. Expression of functional immunomodulatory and anti-inflammatory factors in human milk. Clin Perinatol 26:361–377, 1999.

242. Klagsbrun M. Human milk stimulates DNA synthesis and cellular proliferation in cultured fibroblasts. Proc Natl Acad Sci U S A 75:5057–5061, 1978.

243. Okada M, Ohmura E, Kamiya Y, et al. Transforming growth factor (TGF)-α in human milk. Life Sci 48:1151–1156, 1991.

244. Saito S, Yoshida M, Ichijo M, et al. Transforming growth factor-beta (TGF-β) in human milk. Clin Exp Immunol 94:220–224, 1993.

245. Kidwell WR, Bano M, Burdette K, et al. Human lactation. Mammary derived growth factors in human milk. In Jensen RG, Neville MC (eds). Human Lactation: Milk Components and Methodologies. New York and London, Plenum Press, 1985, pp 209–219.

246. Sanguansermsri J, György P, Zilliken F. Polyamines in human and cow's milk. Am J Clin Nutr 27:859–865, 1974.

247. Romain N, Dandrifosse G, Leusette C, et al. Polyamine concentration in rat milk and food, human milk, and infant formulas. Pediatr Res 32:58–63, 1992.

248. Koldovsky O, Bedrick A, Pollack P, et al. Hormones in milk: their presence and possible physiological significance. In Goldman AS, Atkinson SA, Hanson LA (eds). Human Lactation 3: The Effects of Human Milk on the Recipient Infant. New York and London, Plenum Press, 1987, p 183–193.

249. Kulski JK, Hartmann PE. Milk insulin, GH and TSH: relationship to changes in milk lactose, glucose and protein during lactogenesis in women. Endocrinol Exp 17:317–326, 1983.

250. Teichberg S, Wapnir RA, Moyse J, et al. Development of the neonatal rat small intestinal barrier to nonspecific macromolecular absorption. II. Role of dietary corticosterone. Pediatr Res 32:50–57, 1992.

251. Weaver LT, Walker WA. Uptake of macromolecules in the neonate. In Lebenthal E (ed). Human Gastrointestinal Development. New York, Raven Press, pp 731–748.

252. Axelsson I, Jakobsson I, Lindberg T, et al. Macromolecular absorption in preterm and term infants. Acta Paediatr Scand 78:532–537, 1989.

253. Eastham EJ, Lichauco T, Grady ML, et al. Antigenicity of infant formulas: role of immature intestine on protein permeability. J Pediatr 93:561–564, 1978.

254. Widdowson EM, Colombo VE, Artavanis CA. Changes in the organs of pigs in response to feeding for the first 24 h after birth. II. The digestive tract. Biol Neonate 28:272–281, 1976.

255. Buescher ES, McIlheran SM. Colostral antioxidants: separation and characterization of two activities in human colostrum. J Pediatr Gastroenterol Nutr 14:47–56, 1992.

256. Chappell JE, Francis T, Clandinin MT. Vitamin A and E content of human milk at early stages of lactation. Early Hum Dev 11:157–167, 1985.

257. Ostrea EM, Jr, Balun JE, Winkler R, et al. Influence of breast-feeding on the restoration of the low serum concentration of vitamin E and -carotene in the newborn infant. Am J Obstet Gynecol 154:1014–1017, 1986.

258. Garofalo R, Chheda S, Mei F, et al. Interleukin-10 in human milk. Pediatr Res 37:444–449, 1995.

259. Kühn R, Löhler J, Rennick D, et al. Interleukin-10-deficient mice develop chronic enterocolitis. Cell 25:263–274, 1993.

260. Buescher ES, Malinowska I. Soluble receptors and cytokine antagonists in human milk. Pediatr Res 40:839–844, 1996.

261. Grazioso C, Werner A, Alling D, et al. Anti-inflammatory effects of human milk on chemically induced colitis in rats. Pediatr Res 42:639–643, 1997.

262. Furukawa M, Narahara H, Johnston JM. The presence of platelet-activating factor acetylhydrolase activity milk. J Lipid Res 34:1603–1609, 1993.

263. Caplan MS, Kelly A, Hsueh W. Endotoxin and hypoxia-induced intestinal necrosis in rats: the role of platelet activating factor. Pediatr Res 31:428–434, 1992.

264. Caplan MS, Sun X-M, Hsueh W, et al. The role of platelet activating factor and tumor necrosis factor-alpha in neonatal necrotizing enterocolitis. J Pediatr 116:960–964, 1990.

265. Caplan MM, Hsueh W, Kelly A, et al. Serum PAF acetyl-hydrolase increases during neonatal maturation. Prostaglandins 39:705–714, 1990.

266. Furukawa M, Frenkel RA, Johnston JM. Absorption of platelet-activating factor acetylhydrolase by rat intestine. Am J Physiol 266:G935–G939, 1994.

267. Sarfati M, Vanderbeeken Y, Rubio-Trujillo M, et al. Presence of IgE suppressor factors in human colostrum. Eur J Immunol 16:1005–1008, 1986.

268. Bjørge L, Jensen TS, Kristoffersen EK, et al. Identification of the complementary regulatory protein CD59 in human colostrum and milk. Am J Reprod Immunol 35:43–50, 1996.

269. Saarinen UM, Kajosaari M. Breast-feeding as prophylaxis against atopic disease: prospective follow-up study until 17 years old. Lancet 346:1065–1069, 1995.

270. Koletzko S, Sherman P, Corey M, et al. Role of infant feeding practices in development of Crohn's disease in childhood. BMJ 298:1617–1618, 1989.

271. Koletzko S, Griffiths A, Corey M, et al. Infant feeding practices and ulcerative colitis in childhood. BMJ 302:1580–1581, 1991.

272. Mayer EJ, Hamman RF, Gay EC, et al. Reduced risk of IDDM among breast-fed children. Diabetes 37:1625–1632, 1988.

273. Davis MK, Savitz DA, Grauford B. Infant feeding in childhood cancer. Lancet 2:365–368, 1988.

274. Pabst HF, Spady DW. Effect of breast-feeding on antibody response to conjugate vaccines. Lancet 336:269–270, 1990.

275. Hahn-Zoric M, Fulconis F, Minoli I, et al. Antibody responses to parenteral and oral vaccines are impaired by conventional and low protein formula as compared to breast-feeding. Acta Paediatr Scand 79:1137–1142, 1990.

276. Stephens S, Kennedy CR, Lakhani PK, et al. *In-vivo* immune responses of breast- and bottle-fed infants to tetanus toxoid antigen and to normal gut flora. Acta Paediatr Scand 73:426–432, 1984.

277. Pabst HF, Grace M, Godel J, et al. Effect of breast-feeding on immune response to BCG vaccination. Lancet 1:295–297, 1989.

278. Campbell DA, Jr, Lorber MI, Sweeton JC, et al. Maternal donor-related transplants: influence of breast-feeding on reactivity to the allograft. Transplant Proc 15:906–909, 1983.

279. Campbell DA Jr, Lorber MI, Sweeton JC, et al. Breast-feeding and maternal-donor renal allografts. Transplantation 37:340–344, 1984.

280. Kois WE, Campbell DA, Jr., Lorber MI, et al. Influence of breast-feeding on subsequent reactivity to a related renal allograft. J Surg Res 37:89–93, 1984.

281. Zhang L, an Bru S, van Road JJ, et al. Influence of breast-feeding on the cytotoxic T cell allorepertoire in man. Transplantation 52:914–916, 1991.

282. Chiba Y, Minagawa T, Miko K, et al. Effect of breast-feeding on responses of systemic interferon and virus-specific lymphocyte transformation in infants with respiratory syncytial virus infection. J Med Virol 21:7–14, 1987.

283. Stephens S. Development of secretory immunity in breast-fed and bottle fed infants. Arch Dis Child 61:263–269, 1986.

284. Gala RR. Prolactin and growth hormone in the regulation of the immune system. Proc Soc Exp Biol Med 198:513–527, 1991.

285. Nuijens JH, van Berkel PH, Schanbacher FL. Structure and biological action of lactoferrin. J Mammary Gland Biol Neoplasia 1:285–295, 1996.

286. Hahn-Zoric M, Carlsson B, Jeansson S, et al. Anti-idiotypic antibodies to polio virus in commercial immunoglobulin preparations, human serum, and milk. Pediatr Res 33:475–480, 1993.

287. Garofalo RP, Goldman AS. Cytokines, chemokines, and colony-stimulating factors in human milk: the 1997 update. Biol Neonate 74:134–142, 1998.

288. Pittard BK, III. Differentiation of cord blood lymphocytes into IgA-producing cells in response to breast milk stimulatory factor. Clin Immunol Immunopathol 13:430–434, 1979.

289. Juto P. Human milk stimulates B cell function. Arch Dis Child 60:610–613, 1985.

290. Julius MH, Janusz M, Lisowski J. A colostral protein that induces the growth and differentiation of resting B lymphocytes. J Immunol 140:1366–1371, 1988.

291. Soder O. Isolation of interleukin-1 from human milk. Int Arch Allergy Appl Immunol 83:19–23, 1987.

292. Hooton JW, Pabst HF, Spady DW, et al. Human colostrum contains an activity that inhibits the production of IL-2. Clin Exp Immunol 86:520–524, 1991.

293. Munoz C, Endres S, van der Meer J, et al. Interleukin-1 beta in human colostrum. Res Immunol 141:501–513, 1990.

294. Rudloff HE, Schmalstieg FC, Mushtaha AA, et al. Tumor necrosis factor-α in human milk. Pediatr Res 31:29–33, 1992.

295. SkansJn-Saphir U, Linfors A, Andersson U. Cytokine production in mononuclear cells of human milk studied at the single-cell level. Pediatr Res 34:213–216, 1993.

296. Basolo F, Conaldi PG, Fiore L, et al. Normal breast epithelial cells produce interleukins-6 and 8 together with tumor-necrosis factor: defective IL-6 expression in mammary carcinoma. Int J Cancer 55:926–930, 1993.

297. Saito S, Manuyama M, Kato Y, et al. Detection of IL-6 in human milk and its involvement in IgA production. J Reprod Immunol 20:267–276, 1991.

298. Rudloff HE, Schmalstieg FC, Palkowetz KH, et al. Interleukin-6 in human milk. J Reprod Immunol 23:13–20, 1993.

299. Bocci V, von Bremen K, Corradeschi F, et al. Presence of interferon-α and interleukin-6 in colostrum of normal women. Lymphokine Cytok Res 12:21–24, 1993.

300. Srivastava MD, Srivastava, A, Brouhard B, et al. Cytokines in human milk. Res Commun Mol Pathol Pharmacol 93:263–287, 1996.

301. Oppenheim JJ, Zachariae COC, Mukaida N, et al. Properties of the novel proinflammatory supergene "intercrine" cytokine family. Annu Rev Immunol 9:617–648, 1991.

302. Baggiolini M, Dewald B, Moser B. Interleukin-8 and related chemotactic cytokines - CXC and CC chemokines. Adv Immunol 55:97–179, 1994.

303. Palkowetz KH, Royer CL, Garofalo R, et al. Production of interleukin-6 and interleukin-8 by human mammary gland epithelial cells. J Reprod Immunol 26:57–64, 1994.

304. Sinha SK, Yunis AA. Isolation of colony stimulating factor from milk. Biochem Biophys Res Commun 114:797–803, 1983.

305. Gilmore WS, McKelvey-Martin, VJ, Rutherford S, et

al. Human milk contains granulocyte-colony stimulating factor (G-CSF). Eur J Clin Nutr 48:222–224, 1994.

306. Hara T, Irie K, Saito S, et al. Identification of macrophage colony-stimulating factor in human milk and mammary epithelial cells. Pediatr Res 37:437–443, 1995.

307. Gasparoni A, Chirico G, De Amici M, et al. Granulocyte-macrophage colony stimulating factor in human milk. Eur J Pediatr 156:69, 1996.

308. Yap PL, Miller WR, Humeniuk V, et al. Milk protein concentrations in the mammary secretions of non-lactating women. J Reprod Immunol 3:49–58, 1981.

309. Yap PL, Pryde EA, McClelland DB. Milk protein concentrations in galactorrhoeic mammary secretions. J Reprod Immunol 1:347–357, 1980.

310. Carlsson BS, Ahlstedt S, Hanson LA, et al. *Escherichia coli*–O antibody content in milk from healthy Swedish mothers from a very low socioeconomic group of a developing country. Acta Paediatr Scand 65:417–423, 1976.

311. Goldman AS, Garza C, Nichols B, et al. Effects of prematurity on the immunologic system in human milk. J Pediatr 101:901–905, 1982.

312. Gross SJ, Buckley RH, Wakel SS, et al. Elevated IgA concentrations in milk produced by mothers delivered of preterm infants. J Pediatr 99:389–393, 1981.

313. Lodinova R, Jouya V. Antibody production by the mammary gland in mothers after oral colonization of their infants with a nonpathogenic strain *E. coli* O83. Acta Paediatr Scand 66:705–708, 1977.

314. May JT. Antimicrobial properties and microbial contaminants of breast milk-an update. Aust Paediatr J 20:265–269, 1984.

315. The breast-fed infant: a model for performance. Report of the 91st Ross Conference on Pediatric Research. Columbus, Ohio, Ross Laboratories, 1986.

316. Sandine W, Muralidh KS, Elliker PR, et al. Lactic acid bacteria in food and health: a review with special references to enteropathogenic *Escherichia coli* as well as certain enteric diseases and their treatment with antibiotics and lactobacilli. J Milk Food Technol 35:691–702, 1972.

317. Bishop RF, Cameron DJ, Barnes GL, et al. The aetiology of diarrhea in newborn infants. Ciba Found Symp 42:223–236, 1976.

318. Cameron DJ, Bishop RF, Veenstra AA, et al. Noncultivable viruses and neonatal diarrhea: fifteen-month survey in a newborn special care nursery. J Clin Microbiol 8:93–98, 1978.

319. Cameron DJ, Bishop RF, Veenstra AA, et al. Pattern of shedding of two noncultivable viruses in stools of newborn babies. J Med Virol 2:7–13, 1978.

320. Chrystei IL, Totterdell BM, Bonatvala JE. Asymptomatic endemic rotavirus infections in the newborn. Lancet 1:1176–1178, 1978.

321. Murphy AM, Albrey MB, Crewe EB. Rotavirus infections of neonates. Lancet 2:1149–1150, 1977.

322. Bishop RF, Cameron DJ, Veenstra AA, et al. Diarrhea and rotavirus infection associated with differing regimens for postnatal care of newborn babies. J Clin Microbiol 9:525–529, 1979.

323. Duffy LC, Riepenhoff-Talty M, Byers TE, et al. Modulation of rotavirus enteritis during breast-feeding. Am J Dis Child 140:1164–1168, 1986.

324. Duffy LC, Byers TE, Riepenhoff-Taltz M, et al. The effects of infant feeding on rotavirus-induced gastroenteritis: a prospective study. Am J Public Health 76:259–263, 1986.

325. Frantz ID, III, L'Heureux P, Engel RR, et al. Necrotizing enterocolitis. J Pediatr 86:259–263, 1975.

326. Bell MJ, Feigen RD, Ternberg JL. Changes in the incidence of necrotizing enterocolitis associated with variation of the gastrointestinal microflora in neonates. Am J Surg 138:629–631, 1979.

327. Book LS, Overall JC, Herbst JJ, et al. Clustering of necrotizing enterocolitis: interruption by infection-control measures. N Engl J Med 297:984–986, 1977.

328. Bunton GL, Durbin GM, McIntosh M, et al. Necrotizing enterocolitis. Arch Dis Child 52:772–777, 1977.

329. Kliegman RM, Pittard WB, Fanaroff AA. Necrotizing enterocolitis in neonates fed human milk. J Pediatr 95:450–453, 1979.

330. Moriartey RR, Finer NN, Cox SF, et al. Necrotizing enterocolitis and human milk. J Pediatr 94:295–296 1979.

331. Eibl MM, Wolf HM, Furnkranz H, et al. Prophylaxis of necrotizing enterocolitis by oral IgA-IgG: review of a clinical study in low birth weight infants and discussion of the pathogenic role of infection. J Clin Immunol 10:72S–775, 1990.

332. Pitt J. Necrotizing enterocolitis: a model for infection-immunity interaction. *In* Ogra PL (ed). Neonatal Infections: Nutritional and Immunologic Interactions. Orlando, Fla, Grune & Stratton, 1984, pp 173–184.

333. Donta ST, Myers MG. *Clostridium difficile* toxin in asymptomatic neonates. J Pediatr 100:431–434, 1982.

334. Howard FM, Flynn DM, Bradley JM, et al. Outbreak of necrotizing enterocolitis caused by *Clostridium butyricum*. Lancet 2:1099–1102, 1977.

335. Zeissler J, Rossfeld-Sternberg L. Enteritis necroticans due to *Clostridium welchii* type F. BMJ 1:267–269, 1949.

336. Pederson PV, Hansen FH, Halveg AB, et al. Necrotizing enterocolitis of the newborn-is it gas gangrene of the bowel? Lancet 2:715–716, 1976.

337. Weinberg RJ, Tipton G, Klish WJ, et al. Effect of breast-feeding on morbidity in rotavirus gastroenteritis. Pediatrics 74:250–253, 1984.

338. Research Subcommittee of the South-East England Faculty. The influence of breast-feeding on the incidence of infectious illness during the first year of life. Practitioner 209:356–362, 1972.

339. Fallot ME, Boyd JL, Oski FA. Breast-feeding reduces incidence of hospital admissions for infection in infants. Pediatrics 65:1121–1124, 1980.

340. Elger MS, Rausen AR, Silverio J. Breast vs. bottle feeding. Clin Pediatr 23:492–495, 1984.

341. Habicht J-P, DaVanzo J, Butz WP. Does breast-feeding really save lives, or are apparent benefits due to biases? Am J Epidemiol 123:279–290, 1986.

342. Bauchner H, Leventhal JM, Shapiro ED. Studies of breast-feeding and infections. How good is the evidence? JAMA 256:887–892, 1986.

343. Grulee CG, Sanford HN. The influence of breast and artificial feeding on infantile eczema. J Pediatr 9:223–225, 1936.

344. Kramer MS. Does breast-feeding help protect against atopic disease? Biology, methodology, and a golden jubilee of controversy. J Pediatr 112:181–190, 1988.

345. Wright AL, Holberg CJ, Taussig LM, et al. Relationship of infant feeding to recurrent wheezing at age 6 years. Arch Pediatr Adolesc Med 149:758–763, 1995.

346. Hanson LA, Ahlstedt S, Carlsson B, et al. Secretory IgA antibodies against cow's milk proteins in human milk and their possible effect in mixed feeding. Int Arch Allergy Appl Immunol 54:457–462, 1977.

347. Uhnoo IS, Freihort J, Riepenhoff-Talty M, et al. Effect of rotavirus infection and malnutrition on uptake of dietary antigen in the intestine. Pediatr Res 27:153–160, 1990.

348. Brandtzaeg P. The secretory immune system of lactating

human mammary glands compared with other exocrine organs. Ann N Y Acad Sci 409:353–382, 1983.

349. Rieger CHL, Rothberg RM. Development of the capacity to produce specific antibody to an ingested food antigen in the premature infant. J Pediatr 87:515–518, 1975.

350. Businco L, Marchetti F, Pellegrini G, et al. Prevention of atopic disease in "at risk newborns" by prolonged breast-feeding. Ann Allergy 51:296–299, 1983.

351. Kohl S, Loo LS. The relative role of transplacental and milk immune transfer in protection against lethal neonatal herpes simplex virus infection in mice. J Infect Dis 149:38–42, 1984.

352. Laegreid A, Kolsto Otnuess AB, Orstorik I, et al. Neutralizing activity in human milk fractions against respiratory syncytial virus. Acta Paediatr Scand 75:696–701, 1986.

353. Saarinen, UM. Prolonged breast-feeding as prophylaxis for recurrent otitis media. Acta Paediatr Scand 71:567–571, 1982.

354. Short RV. Breast-feeding. Sci Am 250:35–41, 1984.

355. Gunther M. The neonate's immunity gap, breast-feeding and cot death. Lancet 1:441–442, 1975.

356. Pettitt DJ, Forman MR, Hanson RL, et al. Breast-feeding and incidence of non-insulin-dependent diabetes mellitus in Pima Indians. Lancet 350:166–168, 1997.

357. Kramer MS. Do breast-feeding and delayed introduction of solid foods protect against subsequent obesity? J Pediatr 98:883–887, 1981.

358. Rodgers B. Feeding in infancy and later ability and attainment: a longitudinal study. Dev Med Child Neurol 20:421–426, 1978.

359. Rogan WJ, Gladen BC. Breast-feeding and cognitive development. Early Hum Dev 31:181–193, 1993.

360. Horwood LJ, Fergusson DM. Breast-feeding and later cognitive and academic outcomes. Pediatrics 101:99, 1998.

361. Katsouyani K, Lipworth L, Trichopoulou A, et al. A case-control study of lactation and cancer of breast. Br J Cancer 73:814–818, 1996.

362. Packard VS. Human Milk and Infant Formula. New York, Academic Press, 1982, p 118–119.

363. Lawrence RA. Breast-Feeding: A Guide for the Medical Profession, 2nd ed. St. Louis, CV Mosby, 1985.

364. Arias IM, Gartner LM. Production of unconjugated hyperbilirubinemia in full-term new-born infants following administration of pregnane-3, 20-diol. Nature 203:1292–1293, 1966.

365. Newman TB, Maisels ML. Evaluation and treatment of jaundice in the term newborn: a kinder, gentler approach. Pediatrics 89:809–818, 1992.

366. Gartner L. Management of jaundice in the well baby. Pediatrics 89:826–827, 1992.

367. O'Connor ME, Livingston DS, Hannah J, et al. Vitamin K deficiency and breast-feeding. Am J Dis Child 137:601–602, 1983.

368. Zmora E, Gorodescher R, Bar-Ziv J. Multiple nutritional deficiencies in infants from a strict vegetarian commune. Am J Dis Child 133:141–144, 1979.

369. Nau SB, Stickler, GB, Hawort JC. Serum 25-hydroxyvitamin D in infantile rickets. Pediatrics 57:221–225, 1976.

370. Higinbotham MC, Sweetman L, Nyhan WL. A syndrome of methylmalonic aciduria, homocystinuria, megaloblastic anemia and neurologic abnormalities in a vitamin B_{12}-deficient breast-fed infant of a strict vegetarian. N Engl J Med 299:317–323, 1978.

371. Kanaka C, Schütz B, Zuppinger KA. Risks of alternative nutrition in infancy: a case report of severe iodine and carnitine deficiency. Eur J Pediatr 151:786–788, 1992.

372. Anderson SA, Chinn HI, Fisher KD. A background paper on infant formulas. Bethesda, Md, Life Sciences Research Office, FASEB, 1980.

373. Saukkonen T, Virtanen SM, Karppinen M, et al. Childhood Diabetes in Finland Study Group: Significance of cow's milk protein antibodies as risk factor for childhood IDDM: interactions with dietary cow's milk intake and HLA-DQB1 genotype. Diabetologia 41:72–78, 1998.

374. Dunkle LM, Schmidt RR, Connor DM. Neonatal herpes simplex infection possibly acquired via maternal breast milk. Pediatrics 63:250–251, 1979.

375. Vorherr H. Hormonal and biochemical changes of pituitary and breast during pregnancy. Semin Perinatol 3:193–198, 1979.

376. Ziegler JB, Cooper DA, Johnson RO, et al. Postnatal transmission of AIDS-associated retrovirus from mother to infant. Lancet 1:896–898, 1985.

377. Van de Perre P, Simonon A, Msellati P, et al. Postnatal transmission of the human immunodeficiency virus type 1 from mother to infant: a prospective cohort study in Kigali, Rwanda. N Engl J Med 325:593–598, 1991.

378. Thiry L, Sprecher-Goldberger S, Joncksheer T, et al. Isolation of AIDS virus from cell-free breast milk of three healthy virus carriers. Letter. Lancet 2:891–892, 1985.

379. Vogt MW, Witt DJ, Craven DE, et al. Isolation of HTLV-III/LAV from cervical secretions of women at risk of AIDS. Letter. Lancet 1:525–527, 1986.

380. Bucens M, Armstrong J, Stuckey M. Virologic and electron microscopic evidence for postnatal HIV transmission via breast milk. Fourth International Conference on AIDS, Stockholm, 1988, abstract.

381. Pezzella M, Caprilli F, Cordiali Fei P, et al. The presence of HIV-1 genome in human colostrum from asymptomatic seropositive mothers, vol. 6. International Conference on AIDS, 1990, p 165.

382. Ruff A, Coberly J, Farzadegan H, et al. Detection of HIV-1 by PCR in breast milk, vol. 7. International Conference on AIDS, 1991, p 300.

383. Ruff AJ, Halsey NA, Coberly J. Breast-feeding and maternal-infant transmission of human immunodeficiency virus type 1. J Pediatr 121:325–329, 1992.

384. Newell M-L, Gray G, Bryson YJ. Prevention of mother-to-child transmission of HIV-1 infection. AIDS 11 (Suppl A):S165–S172, 1997.

385. European Collaborative Study. Caesarian section and risk of vesticle transmission of HIV-1 infection. Lancet 343:1464–1467, 1994.

386. Tozzi A, Pezzotti P, Greco D. Does breast-feeding delay progression to AIDS in HIV-infected children? AIDS 4:1293–1294, 1990.

387. Gottlieb S. UN amends policy on breast-feeding. BMJ 317:297, 1998.

388. American College of Obstetricians and Gynecologists Committee statement: Breast-feeding. Washington, DC, 1985.

389. ESPGAN Committee on Nutrition. Guidelines on infant nutrition. I. Recommendations for the composition of an adapted formula. Acta Paediatr Scand 262 (Suppl):1–20, 1977.

390. Nutrition Committee of the Canadian Pediatric Society and the Committee on Nutrition of the American Academy of Pediatrics. Breast-feeding: a commentary in celebration of the International Year of the Child, 1979. Pediatrics 62:591–601, 1978.

391. Ambulatory Pediatric Association. The World Health Organization code of marketing of breastmilk substitutes. Pediatrics 68:432–434, 1981.

392. Kent MM. Breast-Feeding in the Developing World: Current Patterns and Implications for Future Trends. Washington, DC, Population Reference Bureau, 1981.

393. Ryan AS. The resurgence of breast-feeding in the United States. Pediatrics 99:1–5, 1997.

394. Ryan AS, Rush D, Krieger FW, et al. Recent declines in breast-feeding in the United States, 1984 through 1989. Pediatrics 88:719–727, 1988.

395. Report of the Surgeon General's Workshop on Breast-feeding and Human Lactation. Washington, DC, U.S. Department of Health and Human Services, Public Health Service, 1984.

396. Healthy People 2000: National Health Promotion and Disease Prevention Objectives. Washington, DC, U.S. Department of Health and Human Services, Public Health Service, 1990, pp 379–380.

397. Bentovim A. Shame and other anxieties associated with breast-feeding: a systems theory and psychodynamic approach. Ciba Found Symp 45:159–178, 1976.

398. Baranowski T, Bee DE, Rassin DK, et al. Social support, social influence, ethnicity and the breast-feeding decision. Soc Sci Med 17:1599–1611, 1983.

399. Baranowski T, Rassin DK, Richardson CJ, et al. Attitudes toward breast-feeding. J Dev Behav Pediatr 7:367–372, 1986.

400. Baranowski T, Rassin DK, Richardson CJ, et al. Expectancies of infant-feeding methods among mothers in three ethnic groups. Psychol Health 5:59–75, 1990.

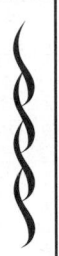

C H A P T E R 5

Toxoplasmosis

JACK S. REMINGTON, M.D., RIMA McLEOD, M.D., PHILIPPE THULLIEZ, M.D., and GEORGES DESMONTS, M.D.

Among the most tragic infectious diseases of humans are those that pass from the pregnant woman to her unborn child. *Toxoplasma gondii* is a protozoan parasite that can cause devastating disease in the fetus and newborn yet remain unrecognized in women who acquire the infection during gestation. In addition, in most countries, congenital infection and congenital toxoplasmosis in the newborn go undiagnosed, thereby predisposing to the occurrence of untoward sequelae of the infection, including decreased vision or blindness, decreased hearing or deafness, and mental and psychomotor retardation. The cost estimates for special care of children with congenital toxoplasmosis born each year is in the hundreds of millions of dollars.

An early estimate of the lifetime cost for special services for the infected children born each year was $221.9 million.[1] In 1990, Roberts and Frenkel estimated preventable medical costs to be $369 million as a low estimate of the number of congenital cases born each year and many hundreds of millions as a high estimate.[2] Only relatively recently have most physicians, veterinarians, research scientists, and economists recognized the important position of *T. gondii* among the significant pathogens of humans and animals. The organism is ubiquitous in nature and is the cause of a variety of illnesses that were previously thought to be due to other agents or to be of unknown cause. Toxoplasmic encephalitis has now proved to be a significant cause of morbidity and mortality in immunodeficient patients, including infants, children, and adults with acquired immunodeficiency syndrome (AIDS). Toxoplasmosis in domestic animals is of economic importance in countries such as England and New Zealand, where it causes abortion in sheep, and in Japan, where it has caused abortion in swine. It has been estimated that as many as 4100 of the 4.1 million infants born annually in recent years in the

United States have the congenital infection. The majority of infected infants do not have clinical signs at birth but have sequelae of the congenital infection recognized or developing later in life. In this text, the term *congenital toxoplasmosis* refers to cases in which signs of disease related to congenital infection are present.

The history of *T. gondii* began in 1908, when Nicolle and Manceaux observed a parasite in mononuclear cells of the spleen and liver of a North African rodent, the gondi (*Ctenodactylus gondi*); this organism so closely resembled *Leishmania* that they tentatively named it *Leishmania gondi*.[3] The next year they decided, on the basis of morphologic criteria, that it was not a *Leishmania* organism and proposed the name *Toxoplasma* (from the Greek *toxon*, "arc") *gondii*.[4] It might just as well have been called *Toxoplasma cuniculi*, for at the same time, and independently, Splendore found it in a rabbit that had died with paralysis in Brazil.[5] The organism soon attracted attention as a cause of disease in animals, and, in 1923, Janku, an ophthalmologist in Prague, described the first recognized case in humans.[6] He found parasitic cysts in the retina of an 11-month-old child with congenital hydrocephalus and microphthalmia with coloboma in the macular region. The parasite noted by Janku was later (1928) recognized by Levaditi to be *T. gondii*, and he suggested a possible connection between congenital hydrocephalus and toxoplasmosis.[7]

However, it was not until 1937 that toxoplasmosis as a disease entity in humans really had an impact on medicine. In that year, Wolf and Cowen in the United States reported a fatal case of infantile granulomatous encephalitis that they believed to be caused by an encephalitozoon.[8] Sabin and Olitski, who had previously encountered *T. gondii* in guinea pigs,[9] were able to make the correct diagnosis. Wolf and associates later recognized and reclassified the cases described by Torres in 1926 and by Richter in 1936 as earlier reports of congenital cases.[10–12] Wolf and Cowen and collaborators then performed numerous studies and established *T. gondii* as a cause of prenatally transmitted human disease.[13, 14] (Case 4 in reference 12 is of special interest because it established beyond question that the infantile form of the infection was prenatal in origin.)

The discovery of *T. gondii* as a cause of disease acquired later in life has been credited to Pinkerton and Weinman. In 1940, they described a generalized fatal illness in a young man that was caused by this organism.[15] In 1941, Pinkerton and Henderson provided a clinical description of two fatal cases of an acute febrile exanthematous disease in adults,[16] and in the same year Sabin described cases of toxoplasmic encephalitis in children.[17]

In 1948, Sabin and Feldman originated a serologic test, the dye test, that allowed numerous investigators to study epidemiologic and clinical aspects of toxoplasmosis, to demonstrate that *T. gondii* is the cause of a highly prevalent and widespread (most often asymptomatic) infection in humans, and to define the spectrum of disease in humans.[18] It was not until 1969, some 60 years after the discovery of the parasite, that *T. gondii* was found to be a coccidian and the definitive host was found to be the cat.

THE ORGANISM

T. gondii is a coccidian and exists in three forms outside the cat intestine: an oocyst in which sporozoites are formed[19, 20]; a proliferative form, formerly referred to as a *trophozoite* and more recently as an *endozoite* or *tachyzoite*; and a tissue cyst, which has an intracystic form termed a *cystozoite* or *bradyzoite*. (Because a single nomenclature has not been agreed on, the terms for each form are used as synonyms in this chapter.) For a more thorough discussion of the organism itself, including its cell biology, molecular biology, genetics, antigenic structure, and immunobiology, the reader is referred to recent reviews on these subjects.[21–30]

Oocyst

The enteroepithelial cycle occurs in the intestines of members of the cat family (see section on Transmission) and results in oocyst formation (Figs. 5–1*F* and 5–2). Schizogony and gametogony appear to take place throughout the small intestine but especially in the tips of the villi in the ileum. In cats, the prepatent period from the ingestion of cysts to oocyst production varies from 3 to 10 days after ingestion of tissue *T. gondii*, 19 to 48 days after ingestion of tachyzoites,[31] and 21 to 40 days after ingestion of oocysts.[32]

Gametocytes appear throughout the small intestine from 3 to 15 days after infection. Fertilization is effected by a mature microgamete emerging from an epithelial cell into the lumen of the gut and then swimming to and penetrating a mature macrogamete, which most likely resides in the epithelium, to form a zygote. After zygote and oocyst formation, no further development occurs within the gut of the cat.

Oocysts pass out with the feces; peak oocyst production occurs between days 5 and 8. Oocysts are shed in the feces for periods that vary from 7 to 20 days. As many as 10 million oocysts may be shed in the feces in a single day.

The zygote divides into two sporoblasts. Each sporoblast develops a wall, the sporocyst, within which two further divisions take place to produce four sporozoites within each sporocyst and eight altogether within the oocyst. The fully sporulated oocyst is infective when ingested, giving rise to the extraintestinal forms. Within the cat, it can also give rise to the enteroepithelial cycle.

Oocysts are spherical at first, but after sporulation they become more oval, measuring 11 to 14 μm × 9 to 11 μm (mean, 12.5 × 11 μm). The two sporocysts are approximately 8.5 × 6 μm, and the sporozoites are about 8 × 2 μm. Depending on the temperature and availability of oxygen, sporulation occurs in 1 to 21 days.[33, 34] Sporulation takes place in 2 to 3 days at 24° C, 5 to 8 days at 15° C, and 14 to 21 days at 11° C.[35] Oocysts do not sporulate below 4° C or above 37° C.[33]

Tachyzoite (Endozoite)

Tachyzoites are crescentic or oval, with one end attenuated (pointed) and the other end rounded (see Fig. 5–1*A* and *B*); they are 2 to 4 μm wide and 4 to 8 μm long. The organisms stain well with either Wright or Giemsa

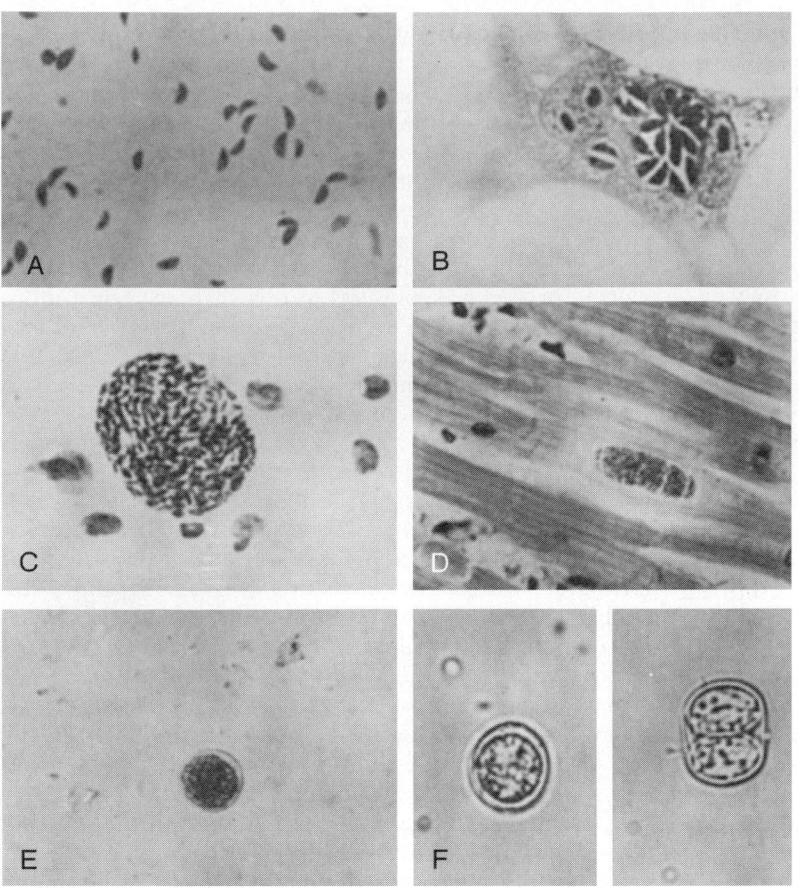

FIGURE 5–1 The three forms of *Toxoplasma*. *A*, Tachyzoite from peritoneal fluid of a 3-day infected mouse. *B*, Tachyzoite in cytoplasm of chick embryo fibroblast. *C*, Cyst in brain stained with periodic acid–Schiff. *D*, Cyst in myocardium of fatal human case. *E*, Microisolated cyst from brain in mouse. *F*, Unsporulated (left) and sporulated (right) oocysts. (From Remington JS. Toxoplasmosis. *In* Brennemann's Practice of Pediatrics, vol. 2. New York, Harper & Row, 1970, with permission.)

stain. This form of the organism is employed in serologic tests (e.g., Sabin-Feldman dye test, fluorescent antibody methods, and agglutination test). Locomotion is by gliding or by body flexion.[36, 37]

The tachyzoite form requires an intracellular habitat to survive and multiply. It cannot survive desiccation, freezing and thawing, or the digestive juices of the human stomach.[38] This form of the parasite is destroyed within a few minutes in gastric juice but can survive in tryptic digestive fluid for at least 3 hours but not as long as 6 hours. The organism is propagated in the laboratory in the peritoneum of mice,[39] in tissue cultures of mammalian cells,[40] and in embryonated hens' eggs.[39] Variations in strain virulence correlate positively with invasiveness and with the rate of multiplication of this form in tissue culture.[41]

Norrby and Lycke and colleagues[42–44] extracted a factor from *T. gondii* tachyzoites that enhances their ability to penetrate mammalian cells. The penetration-enhancing factor has the characteristics of an enzyme and appears to modify the host cell membrane. A parasite serine protease is critical for invasion.[45] The organism is able to enter both phagocytic and nonphagocytic cells by direct penetration as well as by being phagocytosed.[46–49]

The tachyzoites occur within vacuoles in their host cells (see Fig. 5–1*B*), and there is a definite space and an intravacuolar network between the parasite and the vacuole wall.[50–52] Mitochondria are often concentrated in the host cell at the edge of the vacuole. Reproduction in the tissues is by endodyogeny.[53] This is a process of internal budding in which two daughter cells are formed

within the parent cell and are released with disruption of the parent cell. When additional nuclear divisions occur before the daughter organisms are completely separated, rosettes are formed; repeated endodyogeny results in cyst formation.

The tachyzoite form is seen in the acute stage of the infection, during which it invades every kind of mammalian cell (see section on Pathology). After host cell invasion, the organisms multiply within their vacuoles approximately every 4 to 6 hours and form rosettes. The cytoplasm becomes so filled with tachyzoites that ultimately the cell is disrupted, releasing organisms that then invade contiguous cells[54–56] or are phagocytosed.[57] Colonies of pseudocysts containing tachyzoites produced by endodyogeny may persist within host cells for prolonged periods without forming a true cyst. The duration of this type of infection in vivo is not known.

Recently, biochemical, genetic, and chemotherapeutic evidence for the presence of enzymes of the shikimate pathway in Apicomplexan parasites including *T. gondii* has been reported; this pathway, previously demonstrated in plastids of plants, may prove to be a valuable target for development of new anti–*T. gondii* drugs. The impetus for this study was the knowledge that *T. gondii* as well as all other Apicomplexan parasites has a plastid-like organelle, most likely of plant origin.[58–61]

Cyst

The tissue cyst (see Fig. 5–1*C* and *D*) is formed within the host cell and may vary in size from cysts that contain

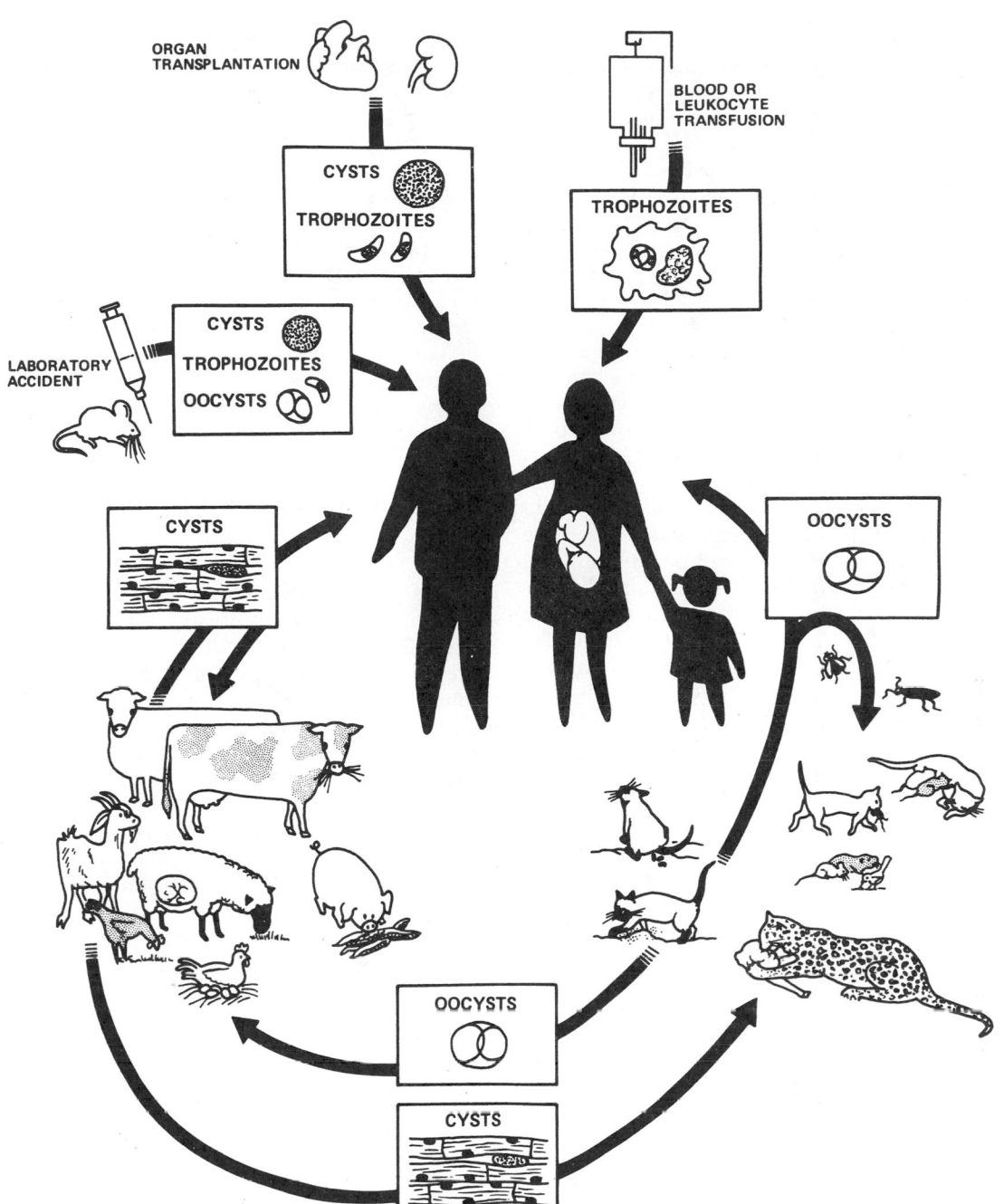

FIGURE 5–2 The life cycle of *Toxoplasma gondii*. The cat appears to be the definitive host. (From Remington JS, McLeod R. Toxoplasmosis. *In* Braude AI [ed]. International Textbook of Medicine, vol. II, Medical Microbiology and Infectious Disease. Philadelphia, WB Saunders, 1981, p 1818.)

only a few organisms to large cysts, 200 μm in size, that contain approximately 3000 organisms.[62] This form of *T. gondii* stains well with periodic acid–Schiff (PAS) stain, which causes it to stand out from the background tissue. The cyst wall is argyrophilic and weakly positive for PAS. The bradyzoites are rich in amylopectin granules, whereas tachyzoites have few of them and more lipid.[63, 64] Such cysts are demonstrable as early as the first week of infection in animals[65] and probably persist as viable parasites throughout the life of the host.[31] Although they may exist in virtually every organ, the brain and skeletal

and heart muscles (see Fig. 5–1*C* and *D*) appear to be the most common sites of latent infection.[66] Cysts are spherical in the brain and conform to the shape of muscle fibers in heart and skeletal muscles (see Fig. 5–1*D*). Because of this persistence in tissues, the demonstration of cysts in histologic sections does not necessarily mean that the infection was recently acquired. The cyst wall is disrupted by peptic or tryptic digestion, and the liberated parasites remain viable for at least 2 hours in pepsin–hydrochloric acid and for as long as 6 hours in trypsin,[38] thereby allowing them to survive the normal digestive period in the stomach and even longer in the duodenum. In the presence of tissue, the liberated organisms remain viable for 3 hours in peptic digestive fluid and for at least 6 hours in tryptic digestive fluid. Freezing and thawing, heating above 66° C and desiccation destroy this tissue cyst form; however, the organisms can survive as long as 2 months at 4° C.[38] Tissue cysts are rendered nonviable when internal temperatures have reached 66° C or −12° C.[67] Until more data are available, it appears that freezing at −20° C for 18 to 24 hours, followed by thawing, should be considered ample means for cyst destruction.[38, 68, 69]

Like the tachyzoite, the cyst develops within a host cell vacuole. However, whereas the mass of tachyzoites ruptures the cell, the cyst may attain a relatively enormous size while still within the host cell. In one report it was suggested that tissue cysts in the brain are preferentially located within neurons and are retained within viable host cells irrespective of size or age. This would explain the long-term survival of latent infection because the intracellular location could provide the minimal metabolic requirements of the resting stage (bradyzoite).[70] It is not clear whether cysts are formed by tachyzoites that differ from those that rupture out of the host cell or whether cyst formation results mainly from extraneous factors.[71, 72] Development of immunity has been suggested as a factor in cyst formation, but the presence of cysts in the brains of neonates 7 to 8 days old[73] and the formation of cysts in tissue culture systems devoid of antibody and complement[73–75] do not support the theory that immunity is the sole mechanism involved. Nevertheless, immunity is of prime importance in regard to the presence of the different forms of the parasite during the extraintestinal cycle in the infected host. During the acute, initial state of the infection, parasites are present mainly as tachyzoites, which are responsible for parasitemia and systemic infection. When the host has developed an immune response, the infection usually reaches a latent or chronic* stage, during which cysts are present in many tissues, and, in the immunocompetent host, parasitemia and systemic infection with tachyzoites have subsided. These schematic definitions of the stages of the infection are important to the later discussion on congenital transmission. These two stages were defined by Frenkel and Friedlander in 1952[76] as the first and third stages of *T. gondii* infection. They also described a second, subacute stage as a hypothesis to explain the pathogenesis of lesions observed in congenital toxoplasmosis. It seems likely that there is also an intermediate stage of uncertain duration in cases with subclinical infection during which both encysted parasites and low-grade systemic infection with tachyzoites are present in the immune host. Whether "dormant" tachyzoites are present during chronic infection in addition to tissue cysts is not known.

TRANSMISSION

Congenital transmission of *T. gondii* from an infected mother to her fetus was the first form of transmission

---

*The term *chronic infection* is used synonymously with the term *latent infection*, both implying the persistence of *T. gondii* in multiple tissues of the body months or years after initial infection.

to be recognized.[13] The investigators raised two hypotheses in an attempt to explain congenital transmission. They considered that transmission might occur as a consequence of the acute, initial stage of the infection in a pregnant woman or as a consequence of a recrudescence (either local or systemic with recurrent parasitemia) of a chronic (latent) maternal infection during pregnancy.

Experimental studies of congenital infections in different animal species were helpful for understanding this form of transmission, but definitive data were not obtained until prospective studies were performed in humans in nations such as Austria, where screening for the diagnosis of *T. gondii* infection among pregnant women is routinely performed, and France, where screening is compulsory.

Congenital Transmission

EXPERIMENTAL STUDIES

Laboratory Animals. Experiments performed to study congenital transmission during the acute stage of the infection in mice and rats revealed that only rarely are all of the offspring infected.[77–81] However, others found that transmission varied with time during gestation; infection of outbred mice on the eleventh day[82] of gestation consistently resulted in infection of almost all offspring. However, the rate of transmission depends on a number of variables, including time during gestation the animal is infected, the site of infection, and the strain of the parasite and of the mice or rats.

In studies with acutely infected pregnant rats, Hellbrügge noted that parasitemia persisted for 18 days, corresponding to the length of gestation (21 days).[79] *T. gondii* did not infect the fetuses until the sixteenth day; hence, despite the duration of parasitemia, transmission to the fetus occurred only in the last third of pregnancy. The organisms could be found in the placentas earlier but not in the fetuses. By the seventeenth to eighteenth day, all placentas and all fetuses were infected.

Congenital transmission of *T. gondii* from chronically infected animals to their offspring has been reported in rats,[83–88] guinea pigs,[89] rabbits,[90] and mice.[84, 91] The strain of the parasite appears to be important in determining whether transmission occurs. Some young animals born to chronically infected mothers develop to maturity without signs of toxoplasmosis, and infected females in those litters have, in turn, given birth to infected progeny.[84, 91]

In a study of persistent parasitemia in mice used for transmission studies, 50% of the mice with chronic infection (with a strain of *T. gondii* that was frequently transmitted to the offspring) showed parasitemia.[92, 93] A similar percentage of such mice produced *T. gondii*–infected offspring. Mice chronically infected with another strain of *T. gondii* and rats with chronic infection produced far fewer infected fetuses, and such animals did not have demonstrable parasitemia. During the course of the chronic infection in rats, Hellbrügge was able to produce a 100% rate of infection in the fetuses, but this depended on the size of the original inoculum.[79] Thus, in rodents, congenital transmission can occur during both acute and chronic maternal infections. These experimental results suggest a close relationship between maternal parasitemia and transmission to the fetus. They also highlight the importance of the placental barrier in delaying fetal infection. *T. gondii* is found earlier in the placenta than in the fetus.

Domestic Animals. Congenital infection with *T. gondii* has been observed during both natural and experimental infections in most domestic animal species, including cats, dogs, pigs, goats, and sheep.[94-101] Congenital infection is frequent in sheep and goats, is less frequent in pigs, and has not been documented in cattle. Toxoplasmosis occurs as an epizootic in pregnant ewes and causes early embryonic death, mummification of the fetus, abortion, stillbirth, or birth of weakened lambs with congenital infection. Embryonic death and stillbirth may result from fetal infection but occur most often from the focal necrotic lesions present in the placental cotyledons. In sheep as well, the placenta is invaded first and the fetus only some days later. In a series of studies on experimental congenital transmission of ovine toxoplasmosis, Jacobs and Hartley found that transmission occurred only in ewes infected during pregnancy, not before pregnancy.[102] If seronegative ewes were infected at 30 days of gestation, early death or mummification of congenitally infected fetuses frequently followed. In ewes infected at 90 days of pregnancy, congenital transmission occurred frequently, but only a small proportion of these ewes aborted. In many cases they gave birth to live lambs, of which about 20% died. In studies of ewes with naturally acquired infection and antibodies before experimental challenge, Hartley noted substantial immunity, but he also observed congenital transmission and some abortions among these ewes.[103] Beverley and colleagues reported similar results.[104] These investigators found that experimental infection of ewes before mating generally prevented abortion related to *T. gondii* infection acquired in midpregnancy.[104] In a trial with a killed vaccine, only ewes developing relatively high antibody titers manifested any protection against fetal death after challenge.[105] The protection was only partial in that the pregnancy was often normal, but the fetus and placenta were both infected. In a trial with live, attenuated parasite vaccine, protection of sheep was manifested as increased live births of healthy lambs.[106]

STUDIES IN HUMANS

The excellent correlation between isolation of *T. gondii* from placental tissue and infection of the neonate, along with results obtained at autopsy of neonates with congenital toxoplasmosis suggesting that the infection is acquired by the fetus in utero through the bloodstream, has led to the concept that infection of the placenta is an obligatory step between maternal and fetal infection. A likely scenario is that organisms reach the placenta during parasitemia in the mother. They then invade and multiply within cells of the placenta, and eventually some gain access to the fetal circulation.

Maternal Parasitemia

Acute Infection. From pathology studies of patients with toxoplasmosis as well as from experiments in animals, it can be concluded that parasitemia occurs during the acute, initial stage of both subclinical and symptomatic infections. In an attempt to define the magnitude and duration of the parasitemia during subclinical infection, inoculation of mice was performed with clots of blood taken from women with recent subclinical infections (G Desmonts, unpublished data); these were the first seropositive blood samples obtained from pregnant women who were previously seronegative and who had been tested repeatedly during pregnancy. Approximately 50 patients were examined, and none proved positive. Because this method has proved to be valuable for isolation of *T. gondii* from patients with congenital toxoplasmosis (Table 5-1) and from newborns with subclinical infections, the absence of demonstrable organisms in these women suggests that parasitemia during the acute stage of acquired subclinical infection is no longer present, at least by the method employed, once serum antibodies are detectable. Attempts at isolation of *T. gondii* from blood of more than 30 patients with toxoplasmic lymphadenopathy was unsuccessful (JS Remington, unpublished data).

If it is accepted that transmission of *T. gondii* from a mother to her fetus reflects that parasitemia occurred in the mother, there is evidence that parasitemia occurs at an early stage of the mother's infection before the appearance of serum antibodies[107] and clinical signs (if signs occur). We have observed this in several cases of acquired toxoplasmosis in pregnant women in whom lymphadenopathy appeared during the first month after they had been delivered of newborns with congenital *T. gondii* infection. Precise data are not available on the timing of events that occur after initial infection in humans. The delay between initial infection and occurrence of parasitemia is not known. This includes the duration of parasitemia during the initial stage of the infection and the actual time between the initial infection and the earliest appearance of demonstrable specific antibodies.

Chronic Infection (Persistent or Recurrent Parasitemia). A systematic search for persistent parasitemia

---

TABLE 5-1

Parasitemia in Clinical Forms of Congenital Toxoplasmosis[a]

CLINICAL FORM	NO. OF INFANTS	NO. WITH PARASITEMIA (%)
Generalized	21	15 (71)
Neurologic or ocular	29	5 (17)
Subclinical	19	10 (52)
Total	69	30 (43)

[a]Infants were studied during the first 2 months of life, but no infants had detectable parasitemia after 4 weeks of age.

Adapted from Desmonts G, Couvreur J. Toxoplasmosis: epidemiologic and serologic aspects of perinatal infection. *In* Krugman S, Gershon AA (eds). Infections of the Fetus and the Newborn Infant. Progress in Clinical and Biological Research, vol 3. New York, Alan R. Liss, 1975, pp 115–132, with permission.

in humans, especially during pregnancy (as has been performed in animals), has not been reported. However, one case report bearing on this subject is pertinent here. Persistent parasitemia was evident in a clinically asymptomatic, otherwise healthy, 19-year-old primigravid woman during 14 months after the delivery of her congenitally infected infant who died during delivery.[108] This parasitemia persisted despite treatment with pyrimethamine and sulfadiazine. During the period of parasitemia, the patient again became pregnant; the result of this second pregnancy was a healthy baby with no evidence of congenital toxoplasmosis. This case of persistent parasitemia is unique in our experience.

Huldt (G Huldt, personal communication to JS Remington, 1987) isolated *T. gondii* from the blood of an elderly but otherwise healthy woman 1 year after clinical lymphadenopathy; in another case, a woman 60 years of age with a suspected lymphoma had detectable parasitemia on several occasions during a period of 2 years.

Similar to what has been observed in normal laboratory animals, parasitemia may be observed during chronic infection in the immunodeficient patient despite the presence of neutralizing antibodies in the serum.[109]

Recurrent parasitemia may be associated with an increase in the IgG *T. gondii* antibody titer. An example is given in Table 5–2 in which data from one of the AIDS cases reported by Derouin and colleagues are shown.[110] This case demonstrates that, in the presence of a low antibody titer, recurrent parasitemia may induce an anamnestic response with an increase in IgG titer but with no evidence of stimulation of formation of IgM antibody. Thus, the possibility of recurrent parasitemia should be considered when a significant increase in IgG antibody titer occurs in a patient known to have had a low stable preexisting titer.[111] Although uncommon, such increases are sometimes observed even in immunologically competent patients, suggesting that a low-grade systemic infection with possible recurrence of parasitemia can persist for several months as long as cell-mediated immunity is not fully established.

Demonstration of *Toxoplasma gondii* in Placentas

Histologic Demonstration. *T. gondii* organisms have been demonstrated histologically in human placentas in cases described by Garcia,[112] Glasser and Delta,[113] Beckett and Flynn,[114] and Neghme and associates.[115] (See also section on Pathology.)

In 1967, Sarrut reported histologic findings in the placentas of eight patients with congenital toxoplasmosis, with microscopic demonstration of the organism in four of them.[116] She noted a correlation between the clinical pattern of neonatal disease and the presence of histologically demonstrable parasites. Both cysts and tachyzoites were numerous and easily demonstrated in three patients with severe systemic fetal disease, whereas parasites were microscopically demonstrable in only one of five patients (see also section on Pathology) with milder disease. Parasites were not noted in cases in which clinical signs of the infection were delayed until weeks after birth. On the contrary, injection of placental tissue into mice proved positive in patients with congenital toxoplasmosis as well as in those with subclinical infection.[117]

Isolation Studies

Toxoplasma gondii in Placentas During Acute Infection. From the original studies performed in France in the 1960s it was concluded that *T. gondii* could frequently be isolated from the placenta when acute infection occurred during pregnancy but rarely, if ever, when it occurred before conception.[118] This was true even for women with high antibody titers at the beginning of pregnancy, which suggested that infection might have been acquired shortly before conception. Similar results were obtained by Aspöck and colleagues.[119] These authors examined 2451 women who had decided on termination of their pregnancy. Of these women, 1139 (46%) were seropositive and 77 (3%) had a *T. gondii* indirect fluorescent antibody test titer of 1:256 or higher. The researchers injected the products of conception of 51 of these 77 women into mice. None of the results was positive. Because they had used the whole product of conception after induced abortion, this negative result suggests that this conclusion—that placental infection is seldom if ever present at the time of delivery of women with high antibody titers at the beginning of pregnancy—might also be true for decidua, embryos, and placental tissues obtained early in pregnancy from such women.

When infection is acquired during pregnancy, the

TABLE 5–2

Serologic Results Associated with Recurrent Parasitemia in a Patient with Acquired Immunodeficiency Syndrome (AIDS)

DATE OF SAMPLE IN 1985	IMMUNOFLUORESCENT ANTIBODY TEST[a] (IU/ml)	IgG AGGLUTINATION TEST[b] (IU/ml)	IgM ISAGA[a]
March 5	40	25	0
May 3	40	25	0
May 20	40	25	0
September 25[c]	400	1600	0
November 19	400	800	0

[a]Performed at St. Louis Hospital (F. Derouin). ISAGA = immunosorbent agglutination assay.
[b]Performed at Institute of Puericulture (G. Desmonts).
[c]Parasitemia was demonstrated in this sample, drawn during an episode of fever, without clinical evidence of neurologic involvement.

TABLE 5–3

Attempts to Isolate *Toxoplasma*[a] from the Placenta at Time of Delivery of Women Who Acquired *Toxoplasma* Infection During Pregnancy

MATERNAL TREATMENT DURING PREGNANCY	INFECTION ACQUIRED DURING FIRST TRIMESTER		INFECTION ACQUIRED DURING SECOND TRIMESTER		INFECTION ACQUIRED DURING THIRD TRIMESTER		TOTAL	
	No. Examined	No. Positive (%)	No. Examined	No. Positive (%)	No. Examined	No. Positive (%)	No. Examined	No. Positive (%)
None	16	4 (25)	13	7 (54)	23	15 (65)	52	26 (50)
Spiramycin	89	7 (8)	144	28 (19)	36	16 (44)	269	51 (19)
Total	105	11 (10)	157	35 (22)	59	31 (53)	321	77 (24)

[a]By mouse inoculation.

Adapted from Desmonts G, Couvreur J. Congenital toxoplasmosis: a prospective study of the offspring of 542 women who acquired toxoplasmosis during pregnancy: pathophysiology of congenital disease. *In* Thalhammer O, Baumgarten K, Pollak A (eds). Perinatal Medicine, Sixth European Congress, Vienna. Stuttgart, Georg Thieme, 1979, pp 51–60, with permission.

frequency of isolation of *T. gondii* from placentas obtained at the time of delivery is dependent on when seroconversion occurred during pregnancy. Table 5–3 shows the results obtained in 321 such cases. The frequency of positive isolation depended on the trimester of pregnancy in which maternal infection was acquired: the later it was acquired, the more frequently were parasites isolated. The frequency of isolation also depended on whether the women were treated. Organisms were isolated less often if spiramycin was administered before delivery. These data were collected in the 1960s and 1970s during surveys carried out by Desmonts and Couvreur[120] and were feasibility studies of measures for prevention of congenital toxoplasmosis. The measures became compulsory in France in 1978. For many years (in the laboratory of one of us [GD]), placental tissue of women considered to be at risk of giving birth to a child with congenital *T. gondii* infection was routinely injected into mice for attempts at isolation of the parasite. (The number of placental inoculations performed in the Laboratoire de Sérologie Néonatale et de Recherche sur la Toxoplasmose, Institut de Puériculture de Paris, averaged 800 per year.) The results support the conclusions of the initial surveys: *T. gondii* organisms were frequently present in the placenta on delivery when the acute infection occurred during pregnancy; the later the infection was acquired, the more frequently the placenta was involved. When infection occurred during the last few weeks of pregnancy, placental infection was demonstrable in more than 80% of cases.

There was a virtually perfect correlation between neonatal and placental infection (see section on Diagnosis) when the mother was not treated during gestation or when she was treated for too brief a period or with an inadequate dose of spiramycin (less than 3 g).[121] Among 85 pregnancies ending in delivery of a child with congenital *T. gondii* infection, isolation of *T. gondii* from placental tissue was successful in 76 of 85 (89%) cases. If the fact that only a relatively small portion of the placenta was digested for the inoculation into mice is taken into account, the high proportion of positive results supports the concept that placental infection is an obligatory occurrence between maternal and fetal

infection. It also demonstrates that if the mother is not treated or if she is treated insufficiently, placental infection persists until delivery. However, placental infection may not be demonstrable by mouse inoculation on delivery of a child with congenital *Toxoplasma* infection when the mother was treated during pregnancy. In the series of cases reported by Couvreur and colleagues,[121] the proportion of placentas from which *T. gondii* was isolated was 89 of 118 (75%) if the mothers had been treated for more than 15 days with 3 g per day of spiramycin. It was 10 of 20 (50%) if pyrimethamine plus sulfonamides were added to treatment during the last months of pregnancy.

Toxoplasma gondii in Placentas During Chronic Infection. A study was performed by Remington and colleagues in Palo Alto, California, to determine whether *T. gondii* can be isolated from placentas of women with stable dye test titers (unpublished observations*). Of the 499 placentas obtained consecutively, 112 (22%) were from women with positive dye test results. The digestion procedure (see section on Isolation Procedures) was performed on 101 of these placentas. *T. gondii* organisms were not isolated from any of them. Thus, in the population studied, chronic (latent) infection with *T. gondii* does not appear to involve the placenta significantly. In contrast, *T. gondii* has been isolated with relative ease from the adult human brain,[66] skeletal muscle,[66] and uterus.[122]

Another study in which an attempt was made to isolate the organism from placental tissue is that of Ruiz and associates in Costa Rica.[123] Much smaller amounts of tissue were injected into mice, but isolation was successful in 1 of 100 placentas. The dye test titer in the mother from whose placenta the organism was isolated was 1:1024. Adequate clinical and serologic data for the offspring were not provided. The researchers stated that no *T. gondii* organisms were found in the placental tissue by microscopic examination. This is not surprising when one considers the findings of Sarrut.[116] The high dye test titer in this case might have been due to an infection acquired during pregnancy. Ruoss and Bourne failed to

---

*This study was performed in collaboration with Dr. Beverly Koops.

isolate *T. gondii* from 677 placentas of mothers who were delivered of viable infants and who had low *T. gondii* antibody titers.[124] It can be concluded from these studies that placental infection is extremely rare in pregnant women with chronic *T. gondii* infection.

Fetal *Toxoplasma gondii* Infection and Congenital Toxoplasmosis

Acute Infection in the Mother. Direct data that demonstrate the frequency with which *T. gondii* is transmitted to the fetus during the period of acute infection in the mother come from prospective studies such as those performed by Desmonts and Couvreur,[118] Kräubig,[125] Kimball and colleagues,[126] and Stray-Pedersen.[127] Fetal infection, the consequence of placental infection, depends on the time during gestation when maternal infection was acquired. Table 5–4 (contains the same group of cases as in Table 5–3, but the number of cases in both tables is not the same because placentas were available in only 321 of the 542 pregnancies) shows data collected in the 1960s and 1970s by Couvreur and Desmonts. In Table 5–4, children are classified into five groups: no congenital infection, subclinical congenital infection, mild congenital toxoplasmosis, severe congenital toxoplasmosis, and stillbirth or children who died shortly after birth. Children were considered to be free of congenital infection if they had no clinical manifestations suggesting congenital toxoplasmosis and if their *T. gondii* serology became negative after disappearance of passively transmitted maternal antibodies. Congenitally infected infants were classified as subclinical if no clinical signs of disease related to toxoplasmosis occurred during infancy. Clinical disease was considered to be mild if the infant was apparently normal and developed normally on follow-up. An example would be a child with no

mental retardation or neurologic disorder on later examination but with isolated retinal scars discovered during a prospective eye examination (or, in one case, isolated intracranial calcifications on radiographic examination) performed because the child was at risk of having congenital *T. gondii* infection, having been born to a mother who acquired the infection during gestation. Cases were considered to be severe if both chorioretinitis and intracranial calcifications were present or if mental retardation or neurologic disorders were present. From the results shown in Table 5–4, the subclinical form is by far the most frequent presentation of congenital *T. gondii* infection. Severe cases with survival of the fetus are scarce. In 500 pregnancies, it was possible to ascertain the trimester during which *T. gondii* infection had been acquired (Table 5–5). *T. gondii* infection occurred in the fetus or was present in the newborn in 14%, 29%, and 59% of cases of maternal infection acquired during the first, second, and third trimesters, respectively. The proportion of cases of congenital toxoplasmosis was higher in the first- and second-trimester groups than in the third-trimester group. This was especially true for severe congenital toxoplasmosis (including cases with stillbirths, perinatal deaths, or severe neonatal disease). No case of severe toxoplasmosis was observed among the 76 offspring of mothers who had acquired *T. gondii* infection during their third trimester.

Experience acquired since 1978[128–131] has confirmed these earlier findings: transmission of the parasite to the fetus was dependent on the time of acquisition of maternal infection during pregnancy. The proportion of cases that resulted in congenital *T. gondii* infection was very low if maternal infection was acquired during the first few weeks after conception. The later maternal infection was acquired, the more frequent the transmission to the fetus. The frequency of congenital infection was 80% or higher if maternal infection was acquired during the last few weeks before delivery and if it was not treated. Table 5–6 shows the frequency of transmission observed in a group of 930 women with acute *Toxoplasma* infection acquired during pregnancy who were referred to the Institut de Puériculture de Paris for prenatal diagnosis. The incidence of transmission rose from 1.2% when maternal infection occurred around the time of conception to 75% when it occurred close to term. These data were updated by Hohlfeld and co-workers,[132] whose report includes the 2632 pregnant women for whom a prenatal diagnosis was performed between 1983 and 1992 (Table 5–7). The observed incidence of transmission rose from 0% when maternal infection was acquired before week 2 of pregnancy to 67% when it was acquired between weeks 31 and 34. The incidence of transmission remained very low, less than 2%, when maternal infection was acquired during the first 10 weeks of gestation. It rose sharply when maternal infection was acquired from week 15 to week 34. To appropriately interpret the data provided by Hohlfeld and co-workers, a number of points deserve discussion. Their patients were referred to the Institut de Puériculture for prenatal diagnosis. Thus, cases with fetal death in utero before the time of amniocentesis were not included. The consequence is that the incidence of congenital infection when maternal

TABLE 5–4

Outcome of 542 Pregnancies in Which Maternal *Toxoplasma* Infection Was Acquired During Gestation: Incidence of Congenital Toxoplasmosis and Effect of Treatment with Spiramycin of Mother During Pregnancy

OUTCOME IN OFFSPRING	NO TREATMENT No. (%)	TREATMENT No. (%)
No congenital *Toxoplasma* infection	60 (39)	297 (77)
Congenital toxoplasmosis		
Subclinical	64 (41)	65 (17)
Mild	14 (9)	13 (3)
Severe	7 (5)	10 (2)
Stillbirth or perinatal death[a]	9 (6)	3 (1)
Total	154 (100)	388 (100)

[a]See text.

Adapted from Desmonts G, Couvreur J. Congenital toxoplasmosis: a prospective study of the offspring of 542 women who acquired toxoplasmosis during pregnancy: pathophysiology of congenital disease. *In* Thalhammer O, Baumgarten K, Pollak A (eds). Perinatal Medicine, Sixth European Congress, Vienna. Stuttgart, Georg Thieme, 1979, pp 51–60, with permission.

TABLE 5-5
Frequency of Stillbirth, Clinical Congenital Toxoplasmosis, and Subclinical Infection Among Offspring of 500 Women Who Acquired *Toxoplasma* Infection During Pregnancy[a]

OUTCOME IN OFFSPRING	INFECTION ACQUIRED DURING FIRST TRIMESTER No. (%)	INFECTION ACQUIRED DURING SECOND TRIMESTER No. (%)	INFECTION ACQUIRED DURING THIRD TRIMESTER No. (%)
No congenital *Toxoplasma* infection	109 (86)	173 (71)	52 (41)
Congenital toxoplasmosis			
Subclinical	3 (2)	49 (20)	68 (53)
Mild	1 (1)	13 (5)	8 (6)
Severe	7 (6)	6 (2)	0 (0)
Stillbirth or perinatal death[b]	6 (5)	5 (2)	0 (0)
Total	126 (100)	246 (100)	128 (100)

[a]Forty-two pregnancies are not included from Table 5-3 because it was not possible to ascertain the trimester during which infection occurred in the mother.
[b]See text.
Adapted from Desmonts G, Couvreur J. Congenital toxoplasmosis: a prospective study of the offspring of 542 women who acquired toxoplasmosis during pregnancy: pathophysiology of congenital disease. *In* Thalhammer O, Baumgarten K, Pollak A (eds). Perinatal Medicine, Sixth European Congress, Vienna. Stuttgart, Georg Thieme, 1979, pp 51-60, with permission.

infection occurred during the first few weeks of pregnancy is slightly underestimated. For example, when Daffos and colleagues reported the first 746 cases from this same series, they[130] estimated the incidence of transmission to be 0.6% among 159 women with "periconceptional infection" and 3.7% among 487 women whose infection was acquired between weeks 6 and 16 of gestation. The observed incidences were 1.8% and 4.7%, respectively, if those fetuses who died in utero because of congenital toxoplasmosis before the time of blood sampling were included in the report. Another consequence of the recruitment of the cases reported by Hohlfeld and co-workers is that the number of cases with acquired maternal infection after week 26 of gestation is small, because maternal infection acquired late during pregnancy was not discovered early enough to allow for performance of a prenatal diagnosis. The incidence of congenital infection was reported to be 194 of 2632 (7.4%). If, however, one excludes 100 cases of maternal infection acquired before week 2, and 351

whose gestational age at the time of maternal infection was unknown, the distribution of patients would be as follows: maternal infection acquired at gestational age 3 to 14 weeks—1398 cases; 15 to 26 weeks—745 cases; and 27 to 34 weeks—38 cases. Most of the cases studied by Hohlfeld and co-workers occurred in women who acquired infection early in pregnancy. If cases of maternal acquired infection had been equally distributed through each of the weeks of gestation, from week 3 to week 34, the adjusted mean transmission rate would have been 19.5%. The transmission rate observed by Jenum and associates in Norway[133] was 11 of 47 (23%). A higher transmission rate, 65 of 190 (34%), was observed in a series of 190 consecutive cases of maternal

TABLE 5-6
Fetal *Toxoplasma* Infection as a Function of Duration of Pregnancy[a]

TIME OF MATERNAL INFECTION	NO. OF WOMEN	% INFECTED
Periconception	182	1.2
6-16 wk	503	4.5
17-20 wk	116	17.3
21-35 wk	88	28.9
Close to term	41	75

[a]Women were treated during gestation as soon as feasible after diagnosis of the acute acquired infection was established or strongly suspected. If prenatal diagnosis was made in the fetus, treatment was with pyrimethamine-sulfadiazine; otherwise it was spiramycin.
Adapted from Forestier F. Fetal diseases, prenatal diagnosis and practical measures. Presse Med 20:1448-1454, 1991, with permission.

TABLE 5-7
Incidence of Congenital *Toxoplasma gondii* Infection by Gestational Age at Time of Maternal Infection[a]

WEEK OF GESTATION	INFECTED FETUSES/ TOTAL NO. FETUSES	INCIDENCE (%)
0-2	0/100	0
3-6	6/384	1.6
7-10	9/503	1.8
11-14	37/511	7.2
15-18	49/392	13
19-22	44/237	19
23-26	30/116	26
27-30	7/32	22
31-34	4/6	67
Unknown	8/351	
Total	194/2632	7.4

[a]Maternal infection was treated with spiramycin in a dose of 9 million IU (3 g) daily.
Adapted from Hohlfeld P, et al. Prenatal diagnosis of congenital toxoplasmosis with polymerase-chain-reaction test on amniotic fluid. N Engl J Med 331:695-699, 1994.

acute *Toxoplasma* infection, each of whose sera were examined in a single laboratory in Paris (P Thulliez, personal communication to G Desmonts, 1999). These cases were more equally distributed in regard to gestational ages at time of infection. The incidences of congenital infection in this series of 190 women were as follows: 4 to 16 weeks—5 of 44 (11%); 17 to 28 weeks—15 of 71 (21%); and 29 to 40 weeks—45 of 75 (60%). In another series, reported by Dunn and associates,[131] the mean rate of transmission was 29% in 603 cases studied in Lyon between 1987 and 1995. *A critical point to remember, when reviewing the data obtained in the European countries where screening for* Toxoplasma *infection during pregnancy is routinely performed, is that most patients are treated during pregnancy. This likely reduces the incidence of transmission of the parasite.*

The frequency of congenital toxoplasmosis (i.e., of fetal lesions or of clinical manifestations in the infant with congenital infection) is also highly dependent on the time of acquisition of maternal infection during pregnancy. The earlier maternal infection was acquired, the higher the prevalence of fetal or neonatal disease among infants with congenital *T. gondii* infection.

A number of observations suggest that *T. gondii* may be present in the placenta but is transmitted to the previously uninfected fetus only after a delay. This delay has been termed the *prenatal incubation period* by Thalhammer.[134, 135] Placental infection is a potential source of infection of the infant even long after maternal parasitemia has subsided. This has been documented in studies in which, after induced abortions, samples of fetal tissues and placentas were injected into mice in an attempt to isolate *T. gondii*. Table 5–8 shows the results obtained in 177 such cases in which no attempt at prenatal diagnosis of fetal infection had been made. Isolation attempts were successful from placentas in 10 cases (6%). In 8 of the 10 cases, placental and fetal tissues were injected separately and *T. gondii* organisms were isolated solely from the placentas and not from the fetus

in 4 of those 8 cases. The fetuses were not infected at the time the pregnancies were terminated. In one of these cases, pregnancy was terminated at week 21 in a woman who had acquired her infection shortly before the fourth week of gestation. This case demonstrates that delay between maternal and fetal infection may be longer than 16 weeks. In other cases, the delay may be much shorter. Among 22 pregnancies terminated because congenital *T. gondii* infection had been demonstrated in the fetus by prenatal diagnosis (see section on Prenatal Diagnosis of Fetal *Toxoplasma gondii* Infection; data not included in Table 5–8), there was evidence that the time that elapsed between maternal and fetal infection was less than 8 weeks in 2 cases, less than 6 weeks in 2 cases, and less than 4 weeks in 1 case. The case histories also suggested that the later during gestation maternal infection occurred, the shorter was the delay between maternal and fetal *T. gondii* infection (Table 5–9). The data of Daffos demonstrate that it is almost always first- and second-trimester infections that are associated with substantial brain necrosis and hydrocephalus.[130]

The severity of the disease depends on the age of the fetus at the time of transmission. This is determined both by the time during pregnancy when maternal infection occurs and by the duration of the delay between maternal infection and transmission to the fetus (prenatal incubation period). The earlier the fetus is infected, the more severe is the disease in the newborn. The likelihood that transmission will occur early in fetal life is greater when the mother acquires her infection during the first or second trimester of pregnancy.

Results of examination of fetuses after induced abortion agree with these conclusions. Among the 177 cases in which pregnancies were terminated without any prior attempt at prenatal diagnosis (see Table 5–8), inoculation tests of fetal tissues were positive in 4 cases. In each of these 4, macroscopic lesions were evident on gross examination of the aborted fetus at autopsy. The same was true for 22 fetuses of women in whom the decision to terminate the pregnancy was made after fetal infection was demonstrated by isolation of *T. gondii* from amniotic fluid or from cord blood samples obtained in an attempt at prenatal diagnosis.[130] Each of these 22 had multiple necrotic foci in the brain; this was true even for women who previously had normal ultrasound examination results before their pregnancy was terminated. Congenital infection in these infants would not have been subclinical if the pregnancies had been allowed to continue to term.

Transmission during the third trimester almost always results in either subclinical infection or mild congenital toxoplasmosis. There are exceptions, however. Two cases have been observed in which maternal infection was acquired after 30 weeks of gestation and the offspring had severe systemic disease (G Desmonts, unpublished observations) and died in the newborn period.

By collecting data from pregnancies that resulted in delivery of severely damaged infants, it was possible to define more precisely the weeks of pregnancy during which infection produces the greatest risk of delivery of a child with severe congenital toxoplasmosis. The period

---

TABLE 5–8

Isolation of *Toxoplasma* from Placental and Fetal Tissue After Termination of Pregnancy in 177 Women Who Acquired Their Infection Just Before or During Gestation

Maternal infection category I[a]	
No. of cases	115
No. of positive isolations	10 (9%)[b]
Maternal infection category II[a]	
No. of cases	62
No. of positive isolations	0

[a]Category I: *Toxoplasma* infection was proved to have been acquired during pregnancy; category II: *Toxoplasma* infection was noted to have been recently acquired; it occurred either before or soon after conception as judged by serologic test results obtained at the time of first examination, when patients were in their fourth to eighth weeks of gestation. No attempt at prenatal diagnosis was made in any of the cases.

[b]*Toxoplasma* was isolated in two cases from mixed placental and fetal tissues after curettage, in four cases from both placenta and fetal tissues injected separately, and in four cases solely from the placenta.

Adapted from Desmonts G, Forestier F, Thulliez P, et al. Prenatal diagnosis of congenital toxoplasmosis. Lancet 1:500–504, 1985, with permission.

TABLE 5–9
Frequency of Findings in the Fetus Correlated with Gestational Age When Infection Was Acquired

FETAL GESTATIONAL AGE (WEEKS) WHEN INFECTED	FREQUENCY OF ULTRASOUND EVIDENCE[a] OF INFECTION	FREQUENCY (%) OF CEREBRAL VENTRICULAR DILATION
<16	31 (60%) of 52	48
17–23	16 (25%) of 63	12
>24	1 (3%) of 33	0

[a]Ascites, pericarditis, necrotic foci in brain.
Data from Daffos F, et al. Letter to the editor. Lancet 344:541, 1994.

of highest risk was weeks 10 to 24.[128] Although the incidence of transmission to the fetus is highest during weeks 26 to 40, it results in milder infection in the newborn. Weeks 1 to 10 were a low-risk period because transmission to the fetus was infrequent. Although infrequent, cases have been observed in which infection was acquired before week 7 or even shortly before conception, which resulted in delivery of severely damaged infants. The attempt at prenatal diagnosis by Daffos and associates[130] in 159 cases of periconceptional maternal infection (i.e., infections that, as judged by serologic test results, had been acquired at the time of conception or within a few weeks after conception) revealed fetal infection in only 1.8% of cases (see earlier). Thus, in these circumstances, transmission of parasites is infrequent.

A question that is frequently asked when toxoplasmic lymphadenopathy is diagnosed in women of childbearing age or when serologic test results in a sample of serum drawn for routine testing very early in pregnancy suggest recently acquired *T. gondii* infection is How long before pregnancy is acquisition of *T. gondii* infection to be considered a risk for transmission of the parasite to the fetus in a future pregnancy? The answer is that if toxoplasmic lymphadenopathy was already present at the time of conception, and/or if two samples of serum, the first drawn before the eighth week of gestation and the second 3 weeks later, are examined in parallel and have identical IgG titers, the initial stage of the infection most likely occurred before conception. In these conditions, the risk for congenital *T. gondii* infection is extremely low. Unfortunately, accumulated data do not allow for a more definitive answer. Cases that demonstrate that the exception does occur have been reported. Of special interest are cases in which the diagnosis of toxoplasmic lymphadenopathy was well established before pregnancy occurred, because they provide reliable information in regard to the timing of events (clinical signs in the mother, beginning of pregnancy, and the development of signs, if any, in the infant). A summary of the history of the first reported case[128, 136] appeared in the third and fourth editions of this book.[137, 138] Another case was reported by Marty and co-workers in 1991,[139] and a third was reported by Vogel and associates in 1996.[140] The time elapsed between the occurrence of lymphadenopathy and conception was 2 months, 3 months, and 2 months, respectively. The patient reported by Marty and co-workers received spiramycin for 6 weeks at the time of lymphadenopathy;

however, she was not treated during pregnancy. Neither the first (studied by Desmonts)[138] nor the third (Vogel) mothers received any treatment. In the three cases, no specific sign of congenital toxoplasmosis was present in the newborn (except possibly for the case reported by Marty and co-workers in whom slight splenomegaly was noted in the neonate). Strabismus occurred at 3 months of age in the first case. None of the infants was treated before the diagnosis of congenital toxoplasmosis infection was established. This occurred in two infants when obstructive hydrocephalus developed, at the ages of 4 months and 9 months, respectively. In the case described by Marty and co-workers, infection was still subclinical when the diagnosis was made at age 8 months because of an increase in the antibody load (see section on Diagnosis).

The clinical patterns and the delayed antibody response observed in the infants are highly suggestive that transmission of the parasite to the fetuses occurred after maternal IgG had reached a significant level in the fetal blood (i.e., after 17 to 20 weeks of gestation), and probably later in the patient (described by Marty and co-workers) whose infection remained subclinical, despite absence of treatment before the eighth month of life.

These three cases demonstrate that infection in the 3 months before conception does not always confer effective immunity against congenital transmission. However, transmission rarely occurs in these conditions. In our personal experience,[128] there has been no other example of congenital infection among several hundred cases in which toxoplasmic lymphadenopathy had occurred before pregnancy. Advice given (G Desmonts) was that patients should be treated with spiramycin if lymphadenopathy had occurred during the 6 months preceding pregnancy. This possibly reduced the incidence of congenital infection among the offspring of these patients.

That fetal infection is rare when maternal acquisition of *T. gondii* infection has occurred even a short time before pregnancy is in agreement with the observation first made by Feldman and Miller,[141] and amply confirmed since, that congenital infection does not occur in siblings (except twins) of a child with congenital toxoplasmosis. Several exceptions have occurred. One was the report by Garcia of what appears to be congenital *T. gondii* infection in two successive siblings.[112] The first infant, born by cesarean section for fetal distress at the seventh month of gestation, died at 24 hours with multiple organ involvement with *T. gondii*. About 5 months after delivery of this infant, the mother again became pregnant. This pregnancy ended in spontaneous abortion of a macerated fetus at about the sixth month of gestation. Microscopic examination revealed *T. gondii* infection of both infants and their respective placentas. Although the proof rests solely on histologic examination, the data presented in these cases appear incontrovertible.

Two cases of transmission to the fetuses of women with subclinical infection acquired before pregnancy have also been published in France. Both were well established because sera drawn before conception were available for comparison with the mandatory sample taken at the beginning of pregnancy.[142, 143] In both cases sera were negative for *T. gondii* antibodies 7 months before pregnancy and found positive with a high, but not rising, titer of IgG antibodies at 3 and 4 weeks of gestation, respectively. Thus, infection had occurred about 1 to 2 months before conception in both cases. In both, prenatal diagnosis proved positive and severe fetal lesions were demonstrated after termination of the pregnancies. Therefore, it is well established that the acute subclinical infection in a pregnant woman can result in fetal infection and congenital toxoplasmosis, even when acquired by the mother before conception.

Serologic tests for screening acute *T. gondii* infection during pregnancy are usually performed at the eighth to twelfth weeks of gestation. If the results suggest a recently acquired infection, it is often difficult, even with the help of a second sampling of serum 3 weeks later, to decide whether infection occurred before or after the time of conception (see section on Diagnosis). These cases can be classified as "periconceptional," and in our practice (G Desmonts)[129, 136] these women were cared for as if they had been infected during gestation (spiramycin treatment and prenatal diagnosis). The transmission rate observed after "periconceptional" infection was 3 of 161 (1.8%).[130]

It is apparent that the transmission rate of the parasite from a woman to her fetus after the acute infection rises from virtually zero when *T. gondii* infection was acquired several months (the exact number is unclear) before pregnancy to about 2% (or slightly less) when acquired at about the time of conception. An important point is that the transmission rate remains low for several weeks, approximately 10, after the beginning of pregnancy. After the tenth week of gestation there is a shift from this low transmission rate toward a steeply increasing incidence of congenital infection in relation to the gestational age. This shift is observed in the 11 to 14 weeks' gestational age group in the series reported by Hohlfeld and co-workers[132] and after the thirteenth week in the series reported by Dunn and associates.[131] Several hypotheses might explain this shift from a low toward a steeply rising risk of transmission. One relies on a truism: Congenital toxoplasmosis is a fetopathy, resulting from a placental infection. Thus, a placenta and a fetus are necessary for observing the disease. Hence, congenital *T. gondii* infection, when resulting from an infection acquired by the mother before the formation of the placenta, is the consequence of a recurrent parasitemia. The incidence of transmission in this situation depends on the frequency of recurrent parasitemia in a woman

whose cell-mediated immunity has not yet fully developed (see section on Pathogenesis). When maternal infection is acquired later during pregnancy, the parasite can reach the placenta during the initial parasitemia, which occurs in the mother before the development of any immune response. This is more effective for the colonization of the placenta by the parasite. However, the later the infection occurs in the fetus, the less severe the disease, because immunologic maturation has had time to develop.

A summary of the just-presented data is shown in Figure 5–3, in which percentages of risk are given, to suggest a range in magnitude and not necessarily exact data. It should also be noted that the data used in this figure were obtained from women almost all of whom were treated with spiramycin during pregnancy. Hence, the outcome in the fetuses would have been more severe, both for transmission rates and for severity of infection, if only results from untreated pregnancies had been used.

Chronic Maternal *Toxoplasma gondii* Infection. Data obtained in prospective studies have established that chronic (or latent) maternal infection, per se, is not a risk for congenital infection.[141] Also, as a rule, evidence of previous chronic (latent) infection signifies that the future mother is not at risk of giving birth to a child with congenital *T. gondii* infection. These observations are the basis for the preventive measures that have been adopted by and have proved effective in countries such as Austria and France.[144–146] Immunity associated with chronic (latent) infection is only relative in laboratory animals (see section on Pathogenesis) and in sheep.[103, 104] Four cases have been published that suggest that this statement might be true for humans as well.[136, 147–149] Each was observed in France. This is not surprising because such cases can only be observed in countries where screening for *Toxoplasma* infection during pregnancy is systematic. A summary of the histories of the four cases follows: The women were known from previous pregnancies to have low and stable titers of IgG antibodies characteristic of past infection and immunity. The same low titer of IgG was present at the beginning of their new pregnancy. Thus, they were considered as being immune and that their fetus was not at risk. Treatment was therefore not given during gestation. Congenital *T. gondii* infection was demonstrated in each of their offspring. A subclinical infection was noted at 12 months of age in one case (the history of which was published in the third and fourth editions of the present chapter[137, 138]); spontaneous abortion at 12 weeks of gestation with demonstration of parasite in fetal tissues in another case[147]; congenital toxoplasmosis (chorioretinitis) diagnosed at birth[148] in the third case; and at 9 months of age in the fourth case.[149] In each of the four cases, a serologic relapse occurred during pregnancy, as evidenced by a significant increase in IgG antibodies that reached high titers in each woman. In three of the women, samples of sera drawn during pregnancy were available for retrospective examination. Of interest is that in these three cases, IgA antibodies were present at the beginning of the serologic relapse. An IgM response was noted in only one woman. Serologic relapse had

Weeks of Gestation When Maternal Infection Occurred	Transmission Rate* (Incidence of Congenital Infection)	Prevalence* of Congenital Toxoplasmosis (Mild or Severe) Among Fetuses or Infants with Congenital Infection	Risk for the Mother of Giving Birth to a Child with Severe Congenital Infection

6 months (?) before pregnancy
 	
Conception
	Virtually 0
	                   ↓
	                   2%
		≥80%	Low risk
			
			(low transmission rate)

10th week		High prevalence ≥80% ≥80%	
24th week	3% ↓ Increasing to	≥80% ↓ 20%	Highest risk
30th week			Low risk (congenital infection is frequent but mainly mild)
Delivery	≥80%	Low prevalence ↓ 6%	

*Percentages are given as a range according to what has been observed among women, most of whom were treated with spiramycin during pregnancy.

FIGURE 5–3 Transmission rate and prevalence of congenital *Toxoplasma* infection or congenital toxoplasmosis among offspring of women with acute *Toxoplasma* infection in relation to gestational age at time of maternal infection.

occurred between weeks 8 and 11 of gestation in the case ending in abortion and after weeks 10, 16, and 19, respectively, in the other three cases.

Even if some cases have gone unpublished (Dr. Jacques Couvreur has data on two more cases, personal communication to G Desmonts, 1999), the examples of offspring with congenital *T. gondii* infection born to mothers who, at the beginning of pregnancy, had serologic test results that established the presence of a chronic (latent) infection are exceptional. When this does occur, immunologic dysfunction must be suspected as having been the cause. The first case we observed (in the third and fourth editions of the present chapter[137, 138]) was that of a woman who had a low CD4/CD8 ratio associated with Hodgkin's disease from which she had recovered 2 years before becoming pregnant. She also previously had a splenectomy. No immunologic dysfunction was demonstrated in the other three women. Reinfection with oocysts of another *T. gondii* strain was suggested as an explanation for the cases observed by both Fortier and Gavinet and their co-workers.[147, 149] Each woman had contact with kittens at the beginning or during the twentieth week of gestation, respectively.

Transmission of *T. gondii* from mother to fetus has

been observed in immunodeficient women owing to reactivation of the chronic infection, primarily in patients with AIDS (see section on Congenital *Toxoplasma gondii* Infection and Acquired Immunodeficiency Syndrome). However, it has occurred as a consequence of other immunocompromised states that appear to have resulted in an active but subclinical infection in the chronically infected pregnant woman. One case was reported in this chapter in the third and fourth editions of this book.[137, 138, 150] Two additional cases were published in 1990,[136] and a fourth in 1995 by d'Ercole and colleagues.[151] The immunologic dysfunction was associated with lupus erythematosus in three of the four patients and with pancytopenia in one. This last patient, as well as one of those with lupus also previously had a splenectomy. Each of the four patients was treated with corticosteroids during gestation. Three[136] were not treated for their *T. gondii* infection. The serologic evidence for (chronic) active infection was the unusually high IgG titers that had been present since childhood in two of the cases (titers of greater than 4000 IU for more than 5 and 10 years, respectively). One of these women gave birth to an infant with severe congenital toxoplasmosis that resulted in the death of the child at the age of 3 months.

Congenital toxoplasmosis was diagnosed in the other case when chorioretinitis occurred at 4 months of age. In one of the four mothers, the IgG titer rose from a relatively low titer at the beginning of pregnancy to 800 IU and she developed a weakly positive IgM test titer. One of her twin infants, a boy, died when 9 days old due to toxoplasmic encephalomyelitis. His twin sister had subclinical congenital *T. gondii* infection.

The case published by d'Ercole and colleagues[151] is of special interest because the woman was known to have both lupus erythematosus and high *T. gondii* IgG antibody titers together with a strongly positive IgA test titer before becoming pregnant. For this reason she was monitored with *T. gondii* serologies for two consecutive pregnancies. During both pregnancies serologic signs of activity of *T. gondii* infection were observed to recur. She had an increase in IgG titers and an IgM test that became temporarily positive. Despite treatment with spiramycin, prenatal diagnosis revealed that the infection was transmitted to the fetuses in both of these pregnancies. During the first pregnancy, the fetus died in utero at a gestational age of 23 weeks. In the second pregnancy, the mother received pyrimethamine and sulfonamide after polymerase chain reaction (PCR) was observed to be positive on amniotic fluid at a gestational age of 23 weeks. This pregnancy ended in a delivery of a child who was considered to have *T. gondii* infection based on the presence of IgA serum antibodies in the newborn. The infant was treated and at 1 year of age had no signs of congenital toxoplasmosis or *T. gondii* antibodies.

The cases just described conclusively demonstrate that the presence of a chronic, yet active *T. gondii* infection in an immunocompromised pregnant woman results in a significant risk of congenital infection for the fetus and newborn. In addition to women with AIDS, this is especially true for women who must receive long-term treatment with corticosteroids during gestation.

In the past, chronic *Toxoplasma* infection in the mother was considered to be responsible for repeated abortions, stillbirths, or perinatal fetal mortality. In an attempt to determine whether *T. gondii* is indeed a contributing cause of stillbirth and perinatal infant mortality in women with chronic (latent) infection, Remington and colleagues performed a study in El Salvador, where the incidence of the infection in the childbearing age group was approximately 65% and there was a very high incidence of perinatal infant mortality.[152, 153] In the Maternity Hospital in San Salvador, a dye test was performed on serum obtained from 103 mothers on the day of the death of their newborn infants or, in the case of death in utero, at the time of delivery. The dye test was repeated 1 month later to determine if the titers were stable, and a skin test was performed at the same time. A high percentage of the mothers had dye test titers of 1:1000 or higher,[153] a marked contrast to the test results in the pregnant population in the United States. Sixty-five percent of the 103 women in this study had a positive dye test result. One hundred ten infants were examined. The diagnostic categories were as follows: cranial deformities, 5; premature births, 45; stillbirths, 40; and miscellaneous, 70. Fifty-eight of the mothers

had had previous abortions; 26 had had one abortion, 12 had had two or more abortions, and more than 7 had given birth to dead infants. At least 20 g of each infant's brain and a similar amount of liver were injected into 10 to 20 mice. *T. gondii* was not isolated from any of the infants, which suggested that in this population *T. gondii* was not an important cause of perinatal fetal mortality. Ferraris and Avitto, in Rome, obtained similar results for their population.[154]

Several prospective surveys have been performed to determine whether chronic *T. gondii* infection is a cause of abortion. In a study in Palo Alto, California, and its immediate surroundings, tissue specimens were obtained from abortions in 272 women. (For the initial portion of this study, see the work of Remington and co-workers.[155]) Twenty-nine percent (79) of these women had positive dye test titers. Of these 79 women, at least 18 had had one abortion and at least 8 had had two or more abortions. *T. gondii* was isolated from two specimens obtained from two chronically infected women— one specimen came from decidual tissue obtained at curettage after spontaneous abortion and the other from the aborted fetus and decidual tissues. Chronic *T. gondii* infection in the first case was evident from the stable dye and hemagglutination test titers, at levels lower than those usually associated with acute *T. gondii* infection, and a positive skin test. Subsequent attempts to isolate the organism from endometrial tissue and from menstrual blood were unsuccessful. The second case was that of a 27-year-old white woman whose first two pregnancies (in 1960 and 1962) had resulted in the births of normal offspring. In February 1963, she aborted at approximately 5 weeks of gestation. A dye test performed at that time showed a titer of 1:512, and an attempt to isolate *T. gondii* from the abortion tissues was unsuccessful. She aborted again in March 1964, and her serum again showed a titer of 1:512. *T. gondii* was isolated from the aborted fetus and decidual tissues. The presence in this case of identical dye test titers in serum samples collected 1 year apart is proof of chronic infection with *T. gondii* and appears to establish the fact that *T. gondii* can be associated with abortion during the chronic stage of infection in women in the United States. A similar case, in which *T. gondii* was isolated from products of abortion, has been described by Meylan in Switzerland.[156]

Ruoss and Bourne, in England, failed to isolate *T. gondii* from products of conception in 104 cases of abortion (25 occurred in patients with low titers of *T. gondii* antibodies).[124] Janssen and colleagues attempted to isolate *T. gondii* from 218 samples of maternal or fetal tissue obtained from 172 cases of abortion and from 10 cases of curettage of nonpregnant women who had had abortions.[157] Of these women, 70% had positive dye test titers and 29% showed positive results in the complement fixation (CF) test. Janssen and colleagues were successful in isolating *T. gondii* from only one case—from curettage material taken after a second abortion in a woman who had a proven chronic (latent) infection. An attempt to isolate the parasite from products of a previous abortion in this woman 5 months earlier had been unsuccessful; at that time, her dye test titer was 1:256 and her CF test titer was 1:5. A third abortion occurred 7 months later and was thoroughly studied; however, attempts to isolate the parasite from placenta, fetus, and tissue obtained at curettage were all unsuccessful. Like Remington and co-workers,[108, 158] Janssen and colleagues concluded that they could not state unequivocally that *T. gondii* was responsible for the abortion in their cases. They believed that isolation of *T. gondii* from abortion tissues of women with latent infection is possible, but only in rare cases.

Kimball and colleagues from the United States studied a population of 5033 pregnant women in New York City and found no evidence to suggest an association of *T. gondii* infection with habitual abortions.[159] In contrast, their evidence suggesting an association between chronic *T. gondii* infection and sporadic abortion was substantial. This association was particularly significant in white patients, especially in those with positive CF tests. Whether these sporadic abortions are related to recurrent parasitemia or to persistence of encysted *T. gondii* in uterine tissue[122] is not known.

The significance of *T. gondii* infection as a cause of abortion has been a subject of considerable conjecture among workers in this field throughout the world. A detailed review of this subject has been presented in the first two editions of this book[160, 161]; it is omitted from the present edition because no new data are available.

Transmission by Ingestion

Whether the mode of transmission consists of infective oocysts or meat that contains cysts, it appears that the natural route of transmission usually proceeds from animals (and contaminated soil) to humans by way of ingestion.

MEAT

Because the results of feeding tissues from chronically infected mice or rats to other mice were much more successful than the results of similar feedings of tissues from acutely infected animals,[38, 39, 93, 162, 163] it was hypothesized that the cyst form, found in the chronic infection, was better able to withstand the digestive process. Microscopically, the cyst wall was seen to be destroyed immediately on contact with pepsin hydrochloride; however, the liberated parasites were infective for mice as long as after 2 hours of exposure to peptic digestive fluid but not after 3 hours.[38] When trypsin was used, liberated parasites were infective for up to 6 hours of digestion, the longest period tested.[38]

These data, combined with those on the seroepidemiology of *T. gondii* infection in domestic animals used for human consumption, led a number of workers to suggest that meat may serve as a source of human *T. gondii* infection.[38]

In 1956, Weinman and Chandler published a classic article suggesting a meat-to-human route to explain the spread of *T. gondii*.[164] Their investigations stemmed from a study in which they noted that humans are more likely to have antibody titers to *T. gondii* if they eat undercooked pork. This observation led Jacobs and co-

workers to explore the occurrence of *T. gondii* cysts in the edible flesh of meat animals. Samples of mutton, pork, and beef from abattoirs in Baltimore were digested in artificial gastric juice; infection was demonstrated in 12 (24%) of 50 samples of pork, 8 (9.3%) of 86 samples of mutton, and only 1 (1.7%) of 60 samples of beef.[38] (The single isolation from beef was questionable, according to the authors.) Similar results have been found in samples of meat from butcher shops in Palo Alto, California, and from other areas of the world.[157–180] Dubey and colleagues have reported on the distribution of *T. gondii* tissue cysts in commercial cuts of pork.[181] In a genotypic analysis of 43 isolates of *T. gondii* from pigs in Iowa, 87% were type II. Type III genotype was identified in only 16.3% of the isolates. These prevalences are similar to the frequencies with which they occur in cases of the disease in humans. Type I strains were not identified, although these strains have previously been shown to account for 10 to 25% of cases of toxoplasmosis in humans.[182] Isolation of *T. gondii* from beef was reported by Catár and colleagues in Bratislava, Czechoslovakia.[176] The cyst form was found in 8 (9.4%) of 85 cattle. *T. gondii* has not been isolated from cattle slaughtered in the United States.[73, 173, 183] It should be recognized, however, that only relatively small specimens have been evaluated. Other workers have shown that persons who handle raw meat, even without consuming it, have a higher prevalence of antibodies to *T. gondii*. A listing of isolation of *T. gondii* from muscle of domestic animals from around the world is presented in Table 5–10.[184–201]

In 1965, Desmonts and colleagues in Paris published what appears to be definitive evidence in favor of the meat-to-human hypothesis.[202] They found that children in a French hospital developed antibodies to *T. gondii* at a rate five times that in the general population. Because it was the custom in this hospital to serve undercooked meat (mainly beef or horsemeat) as a therapeutic measure, these workers reasoned that this fact explained the higher incidence of infection among this hospitalized population. To test this hypothesis, they added undercooked mutton to the diet and observed that the yearly rate of acquisition of antibody to *T. gondii* doubled. Some of the children developed clinical signs of infection, mainly lymphadenopathy. Severe illness was not observed in any of them. Four years later, Kean and colleagues in New York reported a miniepidemic of toxoplasmosis in five medical students.[203] Epidemiologic evidence strongly implicated the ingestion of undercooked hamburgers, which the authors recognized might have been contaminated with mutton or pork, as the source of infection in these cases.[204, 205]

There have been a number of isolated cases and recent miniepidemics of acute acquired *T. gondii* infection, which resulted in at least one case of congenital toxoplasmosis, associated with consumption of undercooked venison or preparation of venison (R. McLeod, personal observation), another that resulted in significant illness in adults who ingested undercooked lamb (J. Remington, unpublished data),[206] one in which undercooked kangaroo meat resulted in acute infection in 12 adults and a case of congenital toxoplasmosis,[207] and another linked

TABLE 5–10

Isolation of *Toxoplasma gondii* from Muscle of Domestic Animals

SPECIES	COUNTRY	PROPORTION POSITIVE FOR *T. GONDII* (%)	REFERENCE NO.
Sheep	Australia	8/32 (25)	a
	New Zealand	3/5 (60)	184
	United States	8/86 (9.3)	185
	Germany	6/50 (12)	186
	Denmark	7/31 (23)	187
	Norway	69/174 (39.6)	188
	Iran	5/66 (7.5)	189
	Japan	3/26 (11.5)	190
Cattle	Czechoslovakia	8/85 (9.4)	191
	New Zealand	0/80 (0)	184
	United States	1/60[b] (1.7)	185
	United States	0/350[c]	183
	Germany	0/500	192
	Germany	0/74	186
	Germany	0/1260	193
	Denmark	0/30	187
Swine	Czechoslovakia	14 (432) (3.2)	194
	United States	12/50 (24)	185
	United States	170/1000 (17)	195
	Germany	54/500 (10.8)	196
	Italy	18/60 (30)	197
	Denmark	10/29 (35)	187
	Norway	20/63 (31.7)	198
	Japan	3/61 (5)	199
	Japan	25/130 (19)	200
	Japan	4/190 (2.1)	201

[a]Munday, unpublished data.

[b]Result was considered to be equivocal, suggesting that there were actually no isolates.

[c]Tissues fed to cats; the rest were inoculated into mice.

Adapted from Munday BL. The epidemiology of toxoplasmosis with particular reference to the Tasmanian environment. Thesis, University of Melbourne, Melbourne, Australia, 1971, 95 pp.

to undercooked pork.[208] In regard to venison, a high prevalence of *T. gondii* antibodies has been reported in white-tailed deer in the United States.[209, 210]

The prevalence rates in various countries indicate that the habits and customs of various populations in regard to the handling and preparation of meat products are an important factor in the spread of toxoplasmosis.[211–214]

OOCYST

Although ingestion of undercooked meat (especially mutton or pork) explained one mode of transmission, such a hypothesis did not explain how herbivorous animals and vegetarian humans became infected. In humans, the prevalence of *T. gondii* antibodies was the same among vegetarian populations (e.g., Hindus) as among meat-eating populations in the same geographic area (e.g., Christians and Muslims in India).[215, 216] A possible explanation was forthcoming when Hutchison and associates,[217] as well as several others working independently,[218, 219] described a new form of the parasite, the oocyst.

Oocyst formation has been found to occur only in members of the cat family (e.g., domestic cat, bobcat, mountain lion). Cats may excrete up to 10 million oocysts in a single day, and excretion may continue for 2

weeks. Immunity to the intestinal stages in cats is apparently not absolute, because renewed oocyst production may occur when a cat becomes reinfected[220] or infected with the related coccidian, *Isospora*. Once shed, the oocyst sporulates in 1 to 5 days and becomes infectious; it may remain so for more than 1 year under appropriate conditions (e.g., in warm, moist soil).[221, 222] This form of the parasite may be inactivated by freezing, heating to a temperature of 45° C to 55° C, drying, or treating with formalin, ammonia, or tincture of iodine. (For further information on the biology of the oocyst, the reader is referred to the works of Frenkel and Dubey.[19, 223]) Its buoyancy allows it to float to the top layers of soil after rain, a location more conducive to transmission than the deeper soil where cats usually bury their feces. Transport of the oocyst from the site of deposit may occur by a number of vectors. Coprophagous invertebrates such as cockroaches and flies may mechanically carry oocysts to food.[224–226] Earthworms may also play a role by carrying oocysts to the soil surface.[34, 227, 228]

A number of attempts have been made to demonstrate oocysts in the feces of cats in their natural surroundings. Whereas Dubey was unable to demonstrate oocysts of *T. gondii* in the feces of 510 domiciled seropositive and seronegative cats in Kansas City,[229] Wallace detected them in the feces of 12 (0.7%) of 1604 stray or unwanted cats on the island of Oahu, Hawaii.[230] In his studies in the South Pacific, Wallace had previously noted that *T. gondii* antibodies were far more common in humans, rats, and pigs on Pacific atolls on which cats were present than on atolls without cats.[231–233] Munday made similar epidemiologic observations for sheep on the Tasmanian islands.[234] In a study performed in Germany, Janitschke and Kühn found oocysts in the feces of approximately 1% of privately owned cats[235] or cats from animal care facilities[236]; Werner and Walton found a similar ratio in the house cats of U.S. Armed Forces families in the Kanto Plain (Tokyo) area of Japan.[237] These low prevalence rates markedly contrast to results of a series of epidemiologic studies in Costa Rica. Ruiz and Frenkel noted that 23% of 237 cats were excreting oocysts. Of interest is the fact that 64% of the excreters were kittens.[220] A report from Beirut, Lebanon, described the incidence of "*T. gondii*–like oocysts" in the feces of 9.9% of 313 cats.[238] In a similar study from Brno, Czechoslovakia, oocysts of *T. gondii* were demonstrated in feces of 1.9% of 620 cats.[239] The prevalence of *T. gondii* oocysts in the feces of naturally infected cats in which their presence was proved by mouse inoculation is shown in Table 5–11.

The relative importance of the oocyst versus undercooked or raw meat in transmission of *T. gondii* to humans remains to be defined. Whereas meat appears to be of primary importance in most areas of the United States, as shown by Etheredge and Frenkel,[240] this is not true for other geographic areas. Epidemics of toxoplasmosis associated with presumptive exposure to infected cats support the importance of this mode of transmission.[241–244]

TABLE 5–11
Prevalence of *Toxoplasma* Oocysts in Feces of Naturally Infected Cats

COUNTRY	NO. EXAMINED	NO. POSITIVE	% POSITIVE
Australia	74	1	1.3
Brazil	185	1	0.5
Costa Rica	237	55	23.2
Czechoslovakia	91	4	4.4
	161	3	1.9
Germany			
Berlin	502	5	0.9
Hannover	308	4	1.3
Munich	694	4	0.5
Hungary	200	2	1.0
Italy	250	1	0.4
Japan	90	1	1.1
	446	4	0.8
Netherlands	567	2	0.4
Nigeria	200	14	7.0
Spain	104	1	0.9
United Kingdom	100	2	2.0
United States	510	0	0.0
	1604	12	0.7
	1000	7	0.7

Adapted from Dubey JP. Toxoplasmosis in cats. Feline Pract 16:12–26, 1986, with permission.

MILK

T. gondii has been transmitted successfully through milk directly to suckling young in experimental mouse models.[78, 84] The organism has also been found in the milk during acute experimental infection in cats, dogs, goats,[245] guinea pigs, rabbits, and sheep[246] (see Fig. 5–2). It has been isolated from the colostrum of a cow and from the milk of naturally infected asymptomatic pigs.[97, 247]

Langer reported isolation of *T. gondii* from the milk of 3 of 18 women.[165] Remarkably, in two of the three women, the dye tests and CF tests were negative. This is the first such report of isolation from human milk. However, interpretation of Langer's results is complicated by the fact that pollen grains contaminated his preparations, which were being examined microscopically for the presence of cysts, and he was unable to decide retrospectively which of his preparations showed pollen grains or *T. gondii* cysts.[169] Transmission during breast-feeding in humans has not been demonstrated. It is conceivable that such might be the case if a mother were to acquire her infection during the last weeks of pregnancy. In these circumstances, the risk of transplacental transmission is so high (approaching 100%) that the possible additional risk of breast-feeding would be insignificant.[248]

It is conceivable that unpasteurized milk (goat milk has been especially implicated) could be a vehicle for transmission of *T. gondii*,[249–251] but the process of pasteurization would kill all forms of the organism.

CHICKEN AND EGGS

Latent infection was found in chickens obtained from a poultry processing plant by Jacobs and Melton[252] (see Fig. 5–2). Because chicken is usually well cooked before eating, it is unlikely that it plays a significant role in transmission. These investigators also were able to isolate *T. gondii* from 1 of 327 eggs laid by 16 chickens with experimentally induced chronic infections. The epidemiologic significance of this finding may be assessed in relation to the number of raw eggs consumed by different population groups. The report by Pande and co-workers of isolation from chicken eggs[253] was fraudulently illustrated,[254] and thus their data are open to question.

Other Means of Transmission

BLOOD TRANSFUSION

Neto and associates recovered *T. gondii* from blood donated by an asymptomatic person for transfusion.[255] *T. gondii* was shown to survive in whole citrated blood stored at 4° C for up to 50 days.[184, 256, 257] Kimball and co-workers inferred that the risk of transmission of *T. gondii* through blood to children who had received numerous transfusions was not great because the prevalence of positive serologic tests for *T. gondii* antibodies in these children was no different from that in children in the normal population.[185] However, the majority of their patients had received transfusions of packed red blood cells; if *T. gondii* remains viable in leukocytes,[186] transfusion of whole blood may be a mode of transmission of the parasite. Because prolonged parasitemia has been observed during latent toxoplasmosis in experimental animals[92] and in humans with asymptomatic acquired toxoplasmosis,[108, 187] blood transfusions must be considered a potential vehicle for transmission of the infection.

Siegal and colleagues described four patients with acute leukemia who developed overt toxoplasmosis after receipt of leukocytes from donors with chronic myelogenous leukemia.[258] Three of the four patients died. Retrospective serologic analyses suggested that the transfused donor white cells were the source of the parasite. If a pregnant woman is to be transfused with whole blood, it would seem advisable to choose as a donor an individual without antibodies to *T. gondii* whenever possible. Patients with chronic myelogenous leukemia and high titers of antibody to *T. gondii* should not be used as blood or blood cell donors.[192, 197]

LABORATORY-ACQUIRED INFECTIONS (INCLUDING INFECTIONS ACQUIRED AT AUTOPSY)

A number of cases of toxoplasmosis have been acquired by laboratory personnel who handle infected animals or contaminated needles and glassware.[199, 200, 259–261] We are aware of numerous cases of laboratory-acquired infection with *T. gondii* that have occurred in recent years. At the Palo Alto Medical Foundation laboratory and Stanford University there have been more than a dozen such instances. Some were in pregnant women (JS Remington, unpublished data). Certainly, this experience indicates that pregnancy is a contraindication to working with *T. gondii* for women who have no demonstrable *T. gondii* antibodies.

One instance has been reported of toxoplasmosis acquired during performance of an autopsy.[262]

ARTHROPODS

The data derived from studies of multiple potential insect vectors are negative and inconclusive.[19] Flies and cockroaches may serve as carriers of oocysts[224, 225, 245] (see Fig. 5–2).

MISCELLANEOUS

Free organisms have been identified within the alveoli of infants with congenital toxoplasmosis (see section on Lungs under Pathology) and have been isolated from saliva[263] and sputum.[264] *T. gondii* has been reported to survive for 4 to 6 days in saliva, tears, and milk.[265] The demonstrated presence of organisms in the glomeruli and tubules of the kidneys and in the mucosa of the bladder and intestine suggests that contamination by urine and feces might be a source of infection in persons caring for such infants. Transmission from such sources has never been proved. *T. gondii* has been transmitted by organ transplantation, most often through organs from a seropositive donor transplanted into a seronegative recipient.[266–268]

EPIDEMIOLOGY

General Considerations

Toxoplasmosis is a zoonosis; the definitive host is the cat, and all other hosts are incidental. The organism occurs in nature in herbivorous, omnivorous, and carnivorous animals, including all orders of mammals, some birds, and probably some reptiles, although in reptiles this suggestion rests solely on interpretation of histologic preparations.[269] In regard to *T. gondii* in cold-blooded hosts, data suggest that natural infection might occur under suitable environmental conditions.[270, 271]

The organism is ubiquitous in nature and is one of the most common infections of humans throughout the world. (For a review of *T. gondii* infection in domestic animals, the reader is referred to Dubey and Beattie.[94]) In humans, the prevalence of positive serologic test titers increases with age, indicating past exposure, and there is no significant difference in prevalence between men and women in reports from the United States.

There are considerable geographic differences in prevalence rates. Differences in the epidemiology of the infection in various geographic locales and between population groups within the same locale may be explained by differences in exposure to the two main sources of the infection, the tissue cyst (in flesh of animals) and the oocyst (in soil contaminated by cat feces). The high prevalence of infection in France has been attributed to a preference for consumption of undercooked meat.[202] A similarly high prevalence in Central America has been related to the frequency of stray cats in a climate favoring survival of oocysts and to the type of dwelling.[220, 221] Examples of factors affecting the frequency of the infection are shown in Table 5–12. Of special note are reports of outbreaks of *T. gondii* infections among family members.[272–276]

In 1993, The European Network on Congenital Toxoplasmosis, which includes approximately 50 institutions in Europe with investigators interested in different aspects of congenital toxoplasmosis, was organized and has been funded by the Biomedicine Research Program of the Commission of the European Union. The Network is overseen by Dr. Eskild Petersen of Copenhagen and Dr. Ruth Gilbert of London. Its initial focus has been on diagnosis, including quality control, education and prevention, and identification of risk factors for infection during gestation. In 1995, the European Multicenter Study on Congenital Toxoplasmosis (EMSCOT) was organized to gain further knowledge of the epidemiology and natural history of congenital toxoplasmosis and to perform prospective, controlled trials of new treatments and treatment regimens (written communication from Dr. Eskild Petersen to JS Remington, 1998).

Among studies designed to identify the risk factors for *T. gondii* infection during pregnancy, results from France, Italy, Norway, and Yugoslavia were reported.[212,

TABLE 5–12
Factors Affecting the Incidence of *Toxoplasma* Infection Among Different Populations

FACTOR	CONSIDERATIONS
Cat population (mainly feral and stray cats)	If present, the size of the population of cats within the locale inhabited by the specific human population in question.
Climatic conditions	Certain temperatures and humidity levels favor maturation and survival of oocysts in soil. Very cold and hot, dry climates are adverse conditions.
Method of farming of food animals	Access of cats to food of these animals varies according to whether the animals are in the fields, in pens, or in stables.
Hygienic habits in regard to food for human consumption	Whether food is exposed to coprophagous insects (flies and cockroaches) and whether meat has been previously frozen influence the incidence.
Cultural habits in regard to cooking of food	Principally, meat is important—the size of portions and whether served raw, rare, or well-cooked.
Hygienic conditions and occupational situations favoring acquisition of infection from contaminated soil	

[214, 277, 278] Three of these studies reported a comparison between pregnant women who had recently seroconverted or who had evidence of recently acquired infection with seronegative matched controls. The study from Yugoslavia compared seronegative with seropositive individuals who had past infection. The conclusions of these four studies, for example, that ingestion of raw or undercooked meat, use of kitchen knives that have not been sufficiently washed, and ingestion of unwashed raw vegetables or fruits are factors associated with an increased risk, are not unexpected. Consumption of meat that had been frozen was associated with a lower risk. Surprisingly, in Naples, Italy, Buffolano and colleagues[214] observed an increased risk associated with consumption of cured pork; this might be related to the fact that in southern Italy cured pork usually contains only 1% salt to fresh weight, is stored at less than 12° C, and may be eaten within 10 days of slaughter. A pet cat at home was not associated with an increased risk in any of these studies, but cleaning the cat litter box was a significant risk factor among women in the study from Norway.[212] Health education was associated with a lower risk when written and found in a book or magazine.[277] This improved efficacy of written information was observed in the past in Saint Antoine Hospital in Paris (Table 5–13); the yearly seroconversion rate decreased from 37 per 1000 to 11 per 1000 when explanatory drawings were given to every seronegative pregnant woman.

Prevalence of *Toxoplasma gondii* Antibodies in Women of Childbearing Age

Knowledge of the prevalence of antibodies in women in the childbearing age group is important because of its relevance to the strategic approach for prevention of congenital toxoplasmosis. When evaluating results obtained in any serologic survey, the factors noted earlier under General Considerations must be examined, in addition to two potential causes of differences that may not be real: the serologic method used (and its accuracy) for collection of the data and the dates of collection of the sera.

Data from studies of pregnant women in New York City, London, and Paris are shown in Table 5–14. These data were obtained in surveys performed during the

TABLE 5–13
Effect of Attempts at Health Education on Incidence Rate of *Toxoplasma* Infection in Selected Populations of Pregnant Women in the Paris Area

HOSPITAL[a]	PERIOD	SEROCONVERSION[b]	YEARLY SEROCONVERSION RATE (PER 1000)
Pinard and Baudelocque[c]	Pre-1960	11/356	60
Centres Medico-Sociaux CPCAM[d]	1961–1970	73/2496	64
Hospital X[e]	1973–1975	18/710	59
Saint Antoine[f]	1973	7/463	37
	1974	3/658	11
Longjumeau[g]	1974–1981	20/1938	22

[a]Patients from several obstetric departments. Sera were examined in one laboratory (G. Desmonts) with the same level of sensitivity of the serologic methods.
[b]Number of seroconversions observed/number of seronegative women screened in the dye test and/or agglutination test.
[c]Serum samples, taken during pregnancy, were examined only after delivery.
[d]No information was given as to how to avoid becoming infected. The mode of transmission of *Toxoplasma* was not known at that time.
[e]Little or no information was given as to how to avoid becoming infected.
[f]There was an intensive attempt at health education of seronegative women as to how to avoid becoming infected. In 1973, only verbal instructions were given. In 1974, patients were given drawings illustrating the cycle and transmission of the parasite, with explanations in the language of the patient.
[g]Only verbal instructions were given.
Modified from Roux C, Desmonts G, Mulliez N, et al. Toxoplasmose et grossesse: bilan de deux ans de prophylaxie de la toxoplasmose congénitale à la maternité de l'hôpital Saint-Antoine (1973–1974). J Gynecol Obstet Biol Reprod 5:249–264, 1976, with permission.

TABLE 5–14
Prevalence of *Toxoplasma* Dye Test Antibodies in Three Populations of Pregnant Women

AGE GROUP (YR)	% POSITIVE			
	New York	London	Paris	
			French	Others[a]
15–19	16	15	80	56
20–24	27	27	81	53
25–29	33	33	86	78
30–34	40	34	95	77
≥35	50	36	96	80
Total	32	22	87	70

[a]Spaniards, North African Muslims, and Portuguese.
Adapted from Desmonts G, Couvreur J. Toxoplasmosis in pregnancy and its transmission to the fetus. Bull NY Acad Med 50:146–159, 1974, with permission.

years 1960 to 1970 and were largely from results of the dye test. They are shown here for comparison with more recent data.

Data on the prevalence of antibodies in pregnant women or women in the childbearing age group for the United States and for other areas of the world are shown in Tables 5–15[211, 279–353] and 5–16. There has been a remarkable decrease in the prevalence rate among pregnant women in Palo Alto, California, from 27% in 1964 and 24% in 1974 to 10% in 1987 and 1998.

In regard to the variability in prevalence of infection among populations within a given geographic area are the observations of Ades and associates.[354] They studied the prevalence of maternal antibody in an anonymous neonatal serosurvey in London in 1991. Among women born in the United Kingdom, the seroprevalence was estimated to be 12.7% in inner London, 7.5% in suburban London, and 5.5% in nonmetropolitan areas. The prevalence in those from India was 7.6%; Africa, 15% to 41%; Pakistan and Bangladesh, 21%; Ireland, 31%; and the Caribbean, 33%. Thus, much of the variation between districts might be explained by ethnic group or country of birth composition. Recent data from France are available from a national survey performed in 1995 for the Direction Générale de la Santé.[355] The seroprevalence was 54.3%, with considerable geographic differences. Lower prevalences were noted in the northeast of the country (30 to 40%) than in the southwest or northwest (55 to 65%). Differences were also noted depending on the country of origin: France, 55%; other European countries, 46%; North Africa, 51%; and South Saharan Africa, 40%. A high prevalence (64%) was observed among women practicing, or whose husband practiced, a learned profession. In the Paris area, the seroprevalence had decreased from more than 80% in the 1960s to 72% in the 1970s. It was still higher than 65% in 1995. In Liege, Belgium, Thoumsin[356] reported that the seroprevalence decreased from 70% between 1966 and 1975 to 62% between 1976 and 1981 and to 47% between 1982 and 1987. In Norway, Jenum and colleagues[331] reported a prevalence of 10.9%, ranging from 13% in the southeastern part of the country and in Oslo to 6.7% in the north. These findings observed from 1992 to 1994 are similar to those reported in the mid-1970s.

Cultural habits regarding food are probably the major cause of the differences in frequency of *T. gondii* infection from one country to another, from one region to another in the same country, and from one ethnic group to another in the same region. The data just described all reveal a decrease in the prevalence rate of *T. gondii* antibodies in the United States and in Europe during the past three decades. This decrease is more striking in countries that had a high prevalence than in those in which it was low. Because meat is probably the main vector of infection in most developed countries, it seems logical to relate this decrease to a less frequent presence of *T. gondii* in meat, which likely results from improved methods in the way the animals are raised and in the processing of meat.[357, 358]

Incidence of Acquired Infection During Pregnancy

ESTIMATES FROM PREVALENCE RATES: MATHEMATICAL EPIDEMIOLOGIC MODELS

Once seroconversion occurs, IgG antibodies essentially persist for the life of the individual. Thus, the prevalence of antibodies increases with increasing age and the proportion of uninfected individuals decreases. If the hypothesis is accepted that the risk of acquiring *T. gondii* infection from the environment is the same at any age of life, and if this yearly seroconversion rate is known, the prevalence of antibodies in relation to age, and the proportion of negative individuals in this population at a given age can be computed easily. Consider as an example a population of infants of 1 year of age who are not infected and thus are seronegative: if they are exposed to a risk of acquiring *T. gondii* infection equal to 10% per year, that is, to a yearly seroconversion rate of 10%, the probability of these infants still being free of infection (seronegative) will be 0.9 at 2 years of age, 0.81 at 3 years of age, 0.729 at 4 years of age, and so on. At age 20, the prevalence of antibodies will be 86.5% and the proportion of seronegative individuals will be 13.5%. The curves shown in Figure 5–4 depict the theoretical antibody prevalence rates, in relation to age, for a fixed yearly seroconversion rate ranging from 0.1 to 20% (representative of possible rates in various locations). The frequency of acquisition of *T. gondii* infection at a given age (the incidence of *T. gondii* infection at that age) is dependent on both the proportion of the population that is seronegative at that age and on the rate of seroconversion. In the example just given, in a population exposed to a 10% yearly seroconversion rate from the age of 1 year, the incidence of acquired infection between 20 and 21 years of age will be 10% of 13.5%, that is, 13.5 per 1000. The balance between the prevalence of immunity due to past infection and the risk of acquiring infection can result in apparently paradoxical findings when one examines the incidence of infection in the young adult. For example, if a population has been exposed from the age of 1 year to a yearly seroconversion rate of 5%, the prevalence of antibodies

TABLE 5–15

Published Figures on the Prevalence of *Toxoplasma* Antibodies Among Pregnant Women in the Childbearing Age Group from Various Geographic Locales

LOCALE	REFERENCE NO.	% POSITIVE	LOCALE	REFERENCE NO.	% POSITIVE
Central African Republic	279	81	Guatemala	316	≈45
Gabon, Africa	280	60	Szeged, Hungary	317	69
Senegal, Africa	281	4.2	Delhi, India	318	≈2
Tanzania, Africa	282	48.5	Jakarta, Indonesia	319	14
Togo, Tropical Africa	283	≈50	Central Italy	320	49
Tunis, Africa	284	46.5	Hyogo Prefecture, Japan	321	6
Zambia, Africa	285	23	Kuwait	322	58
Buenos Aires, Argentina	286	58.9	Islamic Republic of Mauritania	323	≈22
Buenos Aires Province, Argentina	287	53.4	Casablanca, Morocco	324	51
Melbourne, Australia	288	4	Nepal	325	54.8
Western Australia	289	35	Tilburg, The Netherlands	326	≈40
Vienna, Austria	290	36.7	Papua New Guinea	327	18
Bangladesh	291	38.5	Benue River Basin Area, Nigeria	328	43.7
Brussels, Belgium	292	56	Ibadan, Nigeria	329	78
Belgium	293	46	Niger Delta, Nigeria	330	≈60
Cotonou, Republic of Benin	294	53.6	Norway	331	10.9
Yadunde, Cameroon	295	77	Panama City, Panama	332	≈63
Santiago, Chile	296	59	Zakopane, Poland	333	36
Chengdu, China	297	39	Lisbon, Portugal	334	64
Lanzhou, China	298	7.3	Santo Domingo	335	47
Taiwan, China	299	9	Riyadh, Saudi Arabia	336	30
Quindio, Colombia	300	60	Western Scotland	337	13
Pointe-Noire, Congo	301	43	Central Scotland and Midland England	338	15
Copenhagen, Denmark	302	28.7	Ljubljana, Slovenia	339	37
Denmark	303	27	Barcelona, Spain	340	50
Egypt (rural area)	304	43	Malmo, Sweden	341	40
Eastern England	305	7.7	Basel, Switzerland	342	53
Ethiopia	211	>75	Geneva, Switzerland	343	42
Southern Finland	306	20	Switzerland	344	46.9
Strasbourg, France	307	36	Dar Es Salaam, Tanzania	345	35
Franceville (Gabon)	308	71.2	Chiang Mai, Thailand	346	3
La Guadeloupe, French West Indies	309	≈60	Bangkok, Thailand	347	13
Lower Saxony, Germany	310	46	Bangkok, Thailand	348	14
Berlin, Germany	311	54	Turkey	349	65
Greifswald, Germany (Northeast)	312	68	United Arab Emirates	350	22.9
Würzberg, Germany	313	41.6	Timok Region, Eastern Yugoslavia	351	46
Germany	314	36	Slovenia, Yugoslavia	352, 353	≈50
Patras, Greece	315	52			

TABLE 5–16
Prevalence of *Toxoplasma* Antibodies Among Pregnant Women and Nonpregnant Women in Childbearing Age Group, from Various Geographic Locales in the United States

LOCALE	% POSITIVE
Palo Alto, California	10[a]
Birmingham, Alabama	30[b]
Chicago, Illinois	12[c]
Massachusetts	14[d]
Denver, Colorado	3.3[e]
Los Angeles, California	30[f]
Houston, Texas	12[g]
New Hampshire	13[h]

[a]J. S. Remington, unpublished data, 1998.
[b]From Hunter, 1983.[368]
[c]Personal communication from Dr. Rima McLeod, 1987.
[d]Personal communication from Dr. Roger Eaton, 1998.
[e]Personal communication from Dr. Douglas Hershey, 1986.
[f]Personal communication from Dr. Andrea Kovacs, 1993.
[g]Personal communication from Dr. Fred Bakht, 1993.
[h]Personal communication from Dr. Roger Eaton, 1998.

will be 62% at age 20 and the incidence of infection between age 20 and 21 will be 18.9 per 1000. Thus, owing to the higher number of seronegatives, a lower constant risk of infection, 5% instead of 10% per year, results in a higher frequency of infection acquired by the young adult.

Taking into account the number of pregnancies by age group, and the age distribution of pregnant women in France, Papoz and co-workers[359] set up a mathematical epidemiologic model to determine the expected frequency of acquired infection in France. This model was applied to a survey of the prevalence of *T. gondii* antibodies that they performed during 1982 and 1983; 7605 women from ages 14 to 44 years were tested. The prevalence of antibodies rose from 52% before the age of 20 to 83% after the age of 40 years and averaged 63.5%. The yearly seroconversion rate, calculated for each of the 1-year age groups ranged from 2.7 to 5.1%; the average rate was 3.69%. The authors calculated that in the absence of intervention during pregnancy, the incidence of infection during pregnancy should be 10.6 per 1000 pregnancies. This is close to the highest possible rate during pregnancy in those epidemiologic conditions. These estimations of the frequency of acquired toxoplasmosis during pregnancy calculated from the increase in prevalence of antibodies with increasing age are based on the hypothesis that the risk of infection has been constant over time. However, as discussed earlier, there is evidence that the prevalence of antibodies among pregnant women has decreased over the past decades in France as well as in other countries. This suggests a decrease in the risk of acquiring infection and, thus, in seroconversion rates. Larsen and Lebech[360] published a modified mathematical epidemiologic model for prediction of the frequency of *T. gondii* infection during pregnancy in situations of changing infection rates. They concluded that in countries in transition from high to low infection rates, it is likely that the

influence of decreasing immunity of the population will at least temporarily more than outweigh the influence of the falling infection rates, resulting in a higher number of infected pregnant women. This important conclusion is used in the following discussion.

ESTIMATES FROM PROSPECTIVE STUDIES OF ACQUIRED INFECTION DURING PREGNANCY AND CONSEQUENCES OF HEALTH EDUCATION

During the early 1950s, congenital toxoplasmosis was recognized as a frequent cause of severe neonatal disease in France,[117, 361] and the feasibility of screening pregnant women for acquired infection during pregnancy was investigated. During the first survey performed in Paris at Pinard and Baudelocque hospitals, sera obtained from pregnant women at first prenatal visit (i.e., at the end of the second month of gestation) were stored frozen. After delivery, these sera were examined in parallel with cord sera. Of the 2228 pregnancies examined, 1872 women had a positive dye test at the beginning of pregnancy, a prevalence of 84%; 356 (16%) were seronegative at first prenatal examination. Seroconversion from a negative to a positive dye test was observed in 11 women, an incidence of 11 of 356 (3%) among *seronegative* women. Because the mean time elapsed between the first prenatal examination and delivery was 6 months, the yearly seroconversion rate was estimated to be 60 per 1000. If we refer to the entire group of 2228 pregnant women, both seronegative and seropositive, the incidence of seroconversion was 11 of 2228 (0.49%). Because these women were observed for a period of 6 months and because the duration of pregnancy is 9 months, this corresponds to an incidence rate of 7.3 per 1000 pregnancies. (These

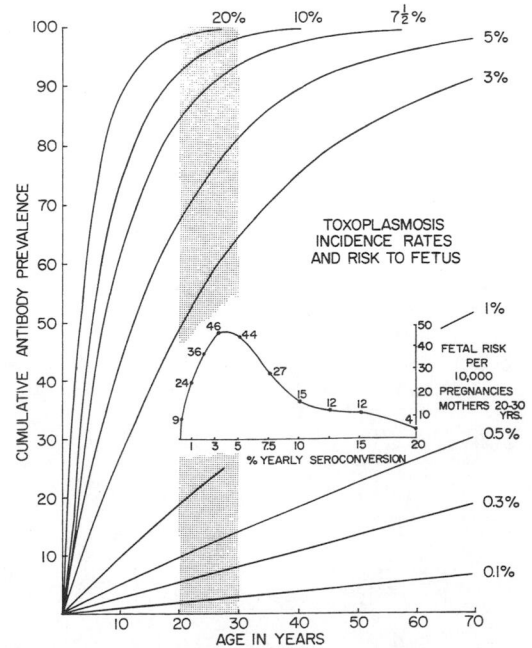

FIGURE 5–4 Incidence rates in mother and risk to fetus. (From Frenkel JK. BioScience 23:343–352. Copyright 1973 by the American Institute of Biological Science.)

different means of expressing the frequency of *T. gondii* infection during pregnancy frequently result in misunderstandings when comparing data reported by different investigators.)

The high prevalence of antibodies in the female population of childbearing age in the Paris area suggested that a simple program for screening *T. gondii* infection during pregnancy was possible. From 1961 to 1970, women in their second month of gestation who attended the Centres Prénataux of the Caisse d'Assurance Maladie were examined for *T. gondii* antibodies. Those with a negative dye test result were examined again at month 7 and again at the time of delivery. This was designed to identify and treat women who seroconverted and to allow for examination of their newborns specifically for the presence of *T. gondii* infection at birth. In the 2493 seronegative women who were repeatedly tested during pregnancy, 73 seroconversions were observed. Because the mean time elapsed between the first and last serum sampling was 5½ months, the yearly seroconversion rate was 64 per 1000. During the years of the study, the prevalence of dye test antibodies was observed to be decreasing among the study population of women: The prevalence was 83.5% in 1961 and 72% in 1970 (Seror and Hazemann, personal communication to G Desmonts). Thus, according to the mathematical epidemiologic model set up by Larsen and Lebech,[360] the incidence rate of *T. gondii* infection acquired during pregnancy was probably rising.

Serologic screening for *T. gondii* infection during pregnancy became a common practice in France and in several European countries during those years. It should also be noted that the life cycle of the parasite was elucidated in the years 1970 to 1971, so that it became possible to instruct women about the mode of transmission of *T. gondii* and how they could avoid becoming infected. Whereas this health education was carefully attempted in some obstetric centers, there was no attempt at education in others. Table 5–13 shows the yearly conversion rates observed before 1970 and those observed after 1970 in three obstetric centers. Each of the departments for which results are shown is situated in the Paris area. The sera were all tested in a single laboratory (G Desmonts). In one department (Hospital X), little or no information was provided as to how seronegative women might avoid infection. The observed seroconversion rate was 59 per 1000, a rate that was essentially identical to the values observed before 1970 (60 or 64 per 1000). The seroconversion rate was significantly lower when health education was attempted, especially when explanatory drawings were provided to seronegative women. Thoumsin and colleagues reported a summary of 22 years of screening for *T. gondii* infection during pregnancy in Liege, Belgium.[356] From 1966 to 1987, 20,901 pregnant women attending the Department of Obstetric of the C.H.R. of Liege were screened. The numbers of seroconversions observed were 129 (6.4%) among 2027 seronegative women from 1966 to 1975 and 74 (2.8%) among 2601 from 1976 to 1981. After 1981, prophylactic counseling was provided by a specially trained nurse to all seronegative pregnant women. From 1982 to 1987, the number

of seroconversions observed was 48 of 3859 (1.2%). The authors do not state the mean time during which their patients were examined for possible seroconversion. If it was approximately 6 months, these data would suggest that the yearly seroconversion rate was greater than 120 per 1000 before 1975, 56 per 1000 from 1976 to 1981, and 24 per 1000 from 1982 to 1987. These values demonstrate a decrease in the risk of infection quite similar to that shown in Table 5–13.

Since 1978, it is obligatory under French law to test pregnant women for *T. gondii* infection acquired during gestation. The common practice is to perform a test for *T. gondii* antibodies at the first prenatal visit (usually week 10 to 15). The result is reported to the patient and, if negative, the laboratory that performed the test must send a letter to the woman describing hygienic measures she can practice to avoid infection with *T. gondii*. Serologic testing of seronegative women is repeated monthly until delivery to identify those who seroconvert. If the test performed at the first prenatal visit is suggestive of a recently acquired infection, either from the high titer of antibody or from the presence of IgM antibodies, or both, a second sample of serum is obtained to determine whether the infection was acquired during the first few weeks of pregnancy or earlier. One consequence of this procedure is that the surveillance for acquired *T. gondii* infection now encompasses the entire pregnancy, including the first 10 weeks and not solely the last 30 weeks of gestation, as was the case during the first surveys performed in France (discussed earlier).

Jeannel and associates[362] reported the results of a survey performed in the Paris area between 1981 and 1983. The prevalence rate of *T. gondii* antibodies was estimated to be 67.3%. Among 2216 pregnant women at risk, the rate of seroconversion was 1.6% per 9 months of pregnancy, which corresponds to a yearly seroconversion rate equal to 21 per 1000. A national inquiry regarding the present status of *T. gondii* infection during pregnancy in France was set up by the "Réseau National de la Santé Publique" in 1995.[355] The medical data of each of the 13,459 women whose delivery occurred in France during the first week of February 1995 were analyzed. The overall prevalence of *T. gondii* antibodies was 54.3%. *T. gondii* infection was acquired during pregnancy by 89 women, an incidence of 6.6 per 1000 pregnancies. If the incidence was reported in only those women who were seronegative at the beginning of pregnancy, the percentage was 1.48%. This corresponds approximately to a yearly seroconversion rate of 19 per 1000, essentially the same as it was 20 years ago among patients who received health education (see Table 5–13) and the same as the rate observed by Jeannel and associates between 1981 and 1983. The incidence among primiparous women was twice that of multiparous women. This suggests that women who knew they were seronegative because they had been repeatedly tested for infection with *T. gondii* during a previous pregnancy tried to avoid acquiring this infection when they again became pregnant.

Jenum and co-workers[133] reported the results of a screening program that was conducted in Norway from

1992 to 1994. The prevalence of *T. gondii* infection in Norway is very low when compared with France, where it is still high. All 35,940 women examined received an information folder that contained health care advice with specific precautions to be taken to prevent *T. gondii* infection. The first sample of serum was collected at approximately the tenth gestational week and examined for *T. gondii* antibodies. Retesting was requested for seronegative women at about weeks 22 and 38 of gestation. Tests for evidence of acute infection were also performed on the serum sample obtained during the tenth week to identify infections that had occurred during the first 10 weeks of pregnancy. Hence, the model of the survey was planned to encompass the first 38 weeks of gestation. The average time during which women remained under observation for the study was, in fact, 34 weeks. The prevalence of antibodies due to infection acquired before pregnancy was 10.9%. Among 32,033 seronegative women, 47 (0.147%) fulfilled the criteria for acquired infection during pregnancy. The seroconversion rate calculated for 40 weeks of pregnancy was 0.173%. This percentage corresponds to a yearly seroconversion rate of 2.3 per 1000. Jenum and co-workers observed a higher number of seroconversions during the first trimester of pregnancy (0.287% per 40 weeks, which is a yearly seroconversion rate equal to 3.8 per 1000) than during the second and third trimesters. They suggest that this might be related to the health education advice given at the first prenatal visit.

The differences in the frequency of *T. gondii* infection from one country to another can be illustrated by the differences in the incidence rates as well as by the differences in the prevalence rates. As an example, the yearly seroconversion rates calculated from the data from Norway[133] are nearly eight times lower than those calculated from the data obtained in 1995 in France[355] and the antibody prevalence rate at the age of pregnancy is five times lower in Norway than it is in France. In the Paris area the yearly seroconversion rate observed during pregnancy was approximately 60 per 1000 during the late 1950s and early 1960s, and it was about 19 per 1000 in 1995. But this lower seroconversion rate was observed as early as 1974 when instruction became available to pregnant women as to how they could avoid becoming infected (see Table 5–13).[363] As judged by the results of recent studies,[355, 362] there has been no significant decrease in seroconversion rates between 1974 and 1995. The decrease from approximately 60 per 1000 to approximately 20 per 1000 occurred during the early 1970s. If we consider the incidence rates, that is, the frequency of seroconversions in the total population of pregnant women (seropositive as well as seronegative), there is no significant difference between the incidence rates observed in the late 1950s and in 1995; the incidence rate during the first prospective study performed in Paris before 1960 was 7.3 per 1000 pregnancies. The incidence reported by Ancelle and colleagues[355] in 1996 was 6.6 (± 1.4) per 1000 pregnancies. However, in this epidemiologic situation, that is, in a country in transition from a very high to a lower infection rate, the influence of decreasing immunity in the population should have outweighed the influence of the falling infection rate,

resulting in a higher number of women who acquired the infection during gestation (despite the decreasing risk of acquiring the infection in the general population).[360] This was not observed, and the reason most likely is that health care education of pregnant women reduced the risk of acquiring *T. gondii* infection during pregnancy.

The seroconversion rates observed during these recent surveys from France and from Norway can be used to calculate an expected prevalence rate according to the methods discussed earlier.[360, 364, 365] This calculated "expected" prevalence rate is lower than the observed prevalence rates in both surveys. This suggests that the risk of becoming infected with *T. gondii* is lower among pregnant women than in nonpregnant women, perhaps also the result of health care education provided at the first prenatal visit. Thus, the timing of providing pregnant women the appropriate information on prevention of infection with *T. gondii* at the first prenatal visit probably skews results of prospective studies of acquired *T. gondii* infection during pregnancy by selectively reducing the frequency of infection acquired during the second half of pregnancy.

Prevalence of Congenital *Toxoplasma gondii* Infection

INDIRECT ESTIMATES FROM INCIDENCE RATES OF MATERNAL *TOXOPLASMA GONDII* INFECTION

The prevalence of congenital *T. gondii* infection can be estimated from the incidence rate of *T. gondii* infection acquired during pregnancy by multiplying the figure for the number of mothers who acquire infection during pregnancy by the transmission rate of the parasite to the fetus. For example, according to Frenkel (see Fig. 5–4), if the yearly seroconversion rate in a population is 30 per 1000, the rate of neonatal *T. gondii* infection will be 4.6 per 1000 births. From the epidemiologic model derived from a survey performed in France in 1982–1983, Papoz and colleagues[359] calculated that the risk of neonatal *T. gondii* infection was 6.4 per 1000 births.

A recent study of the age-specific prevalence of *T. gondii* antibodies in the United States used data and sera from the third National Health and Nutrition Examination and Survey (NHANES III, 1989–94, N = 17,658). The investigators modeled the incidence of acute infection in pregnant women using the declining prevalence from the study in military recruits and the age-specific prevalence from the NHANES III study. They estimate that the incidence among seronegative women is 0.27% during pregnancy in the United States. With a birth cohort of 4 million and assuming an overall transmission rate of 33% there should be approximately 3500 children born with congenital toxoplasmosis each year in the United States. This rate should vary by region and may be declining if the trend demonstrated in the military recruit study is continuing (J McAuley, written communication to JS Remington, 1998). Unfortunately, at present, we do not have objective data on the prevalence of congenital *T. gondii* infection or congenital toxoplasmosis for the United States. Because screening of pregnant women in the United States is not systematic, our ability to accurately assess the incidence of *T. gondii* infection among pregnant women in different populations and of congenital *T. gondii* infection is limited. Data from one city or single population within that city may not accurately reflect the true prevalence or incidence of infection either in that city or elsewhere. Although the prevalence of the infection has decreased in some areas of the United States during the past 20 years, this is not necessarily the case in subpopulations even in those same areas.

DIRECT ESTIMATES FROM STUDIES AT BIRTH OR DURING INFANCY

Estimates from Clinical Information or from Findings at Autopsy. These data are mainly from older studies.[123, 124] They underestimated the actual prevalence because congenital infection uncommonly results in stillbirth or neonatal death and frequently is not diagnosed during infancy because of subclinical infection in the infant and delayed occurrence of signs of infection.[366, 367]

Estimates from Serologic Screening of Neonates or Infants. One of the first studies that relied on determination of total IgM levels in cord blood, followed by serologic testing of infants who had elevated levels, was performed at the University of Alabama.[368] As stressed by the investigators, such studies result in an underestimate of the true incidence of the infection and the disease because infants with congenital infection may not have an increase in total IgM in their cord blood or demonstrable IgM *T. gondii* antibodies. This survey revealed what has proved to be an historical trend toward a decrease in prevalence of congenital *T. gondii* infection in Alabama; the observed rate was 2 per 1000 during the first year of the study and 0.6 per 1000 during the last year. Although different methods were used in a later study by this same group, the observed rate was approximately 0.1 per 1000 births.[368]

The Commonwealth of Massachusetts began screening newborn sera in January 1986 to determine the incidence of congenital *T. gondii* infection. Blood specimens are collected on filter paper and utilized to test for IgM antibodies by the sensitive IgM enzyme-linked immunosorbent assay (ELISA). From 1986 to 1998, 99 infants were detected who had IgM *T. gondii* antibodies, an incidence of approximately 1 in 10,000 births (R Eaton, personal communication to JS Remington, 1998). Although a careful follow-up was not performed for all seronegative infants, it is known that the diagnosis was missed in at least six infants in whom IgM antibodies were not detected but who were referred by local physicians. In one of these later children, *T. gondii* was isolated from cerebrospinal fluid (CSF); the infection was suspected on clinical grounds in this child, who was born prematurely with hydrocephalus, cerebral calcifications, and bilateral chorioretinitis. Thus, their incidence figure is lower than the actual incidence despite the sensitivity of the method used to detect IgM antibodies of *T. gondii*.[369] Nevertheless, if as many as 50% of cases were

missed (which is unlikely) with the methodology used by the New England Regional Screening Program, an incidence of 1 per 10,000 births is strikingly different from the incidence of 1.3 per 1000 reported by Kimball and co-workers in 1971 from a prospective screening study of pregnant women in New York City.[126] With the discovery of the importance of detecting IgA and IgE antibodies (see section on Diagnosis) in the newborn, serologic studies of newborns such as those being performed in Massachusetts should detect a higher percentage of infected infants. The Danish Congenital Toxoplasmosis Study Group has published results of their feasibility study of neonatal screening for *T. gondii* infection in the absence of prenatal treatment.[370] The focus of their study was different from that of the Massachusetts group in that they sought to determine the prevalence of the infection among live neonates and the maternofetal transmission rate in untreated, infected mothers. Secondarily they assessed the feasibility and acceptability of neonatal screening using *T. gondii* IgM antibody testing on samples from PKU cards. They reported a surprisingly low transmission rate of 19.4. The researchers concluded that a neonatal screening program based on detection of IgM *T. gondii* antibodies alone identifies between 70% and 80% of cases of congenital toxoplasmosis. Although this detection rate is certainly preferable to no screening, the possible occurrence of significant numbers of false-negative reactions is disturbing. Yet Lebech and his colleagues stated that their IgM method with PKU cards could be used in large-scale newborn screening for congenital *T. gondii* infection. Before this can be widely accepted, it is hoped that improved technology will be developed to reduce the numbers of infected infants who will go undetected using presently available methods.[371] The group in Massachusetts uses a special IgM method that is designed to be highly sensitive, thereby attempting to lessen the likelihood of false-negative results. No data are provided in the publication of the Danish group on the sensitivity or specificity, or of the Boston Group on the sensitivity, of their IgM antibody method in newborns. (Denmark began screening of all newborns rather than pregnant women beginning in 1999 [E Petersen, personal communication to JS Remington].[370, 372])

But even if underestimated, the present data (at least from Alabama and Massachusetts) strongly suggest that the prevalence of congenital infection has significantly decreased during the recent two decades in the United States. This decrease in the prevalence rate of congenital *T. gondii* infection parallels the historic decrease in antibody prevalence rate observed in the adult. This would be expected from the epidemiologic models discussed earlier; in a population in which the seroprevalence rate was rather low (well below 50% in the adult as it is in the United States), a decrease in the risk of acquiring infection immediately results in a decrease in the incidence rate of acquired infection in women in the childbearing age group.

An attempt to define the prevalence of congenital *T. gondii* infection in infants in the Paris area was made in a cooperative study with the Centre de Bilans de Santé de la Caisse Primaire d'Assurance Maladie de Paris.[373]

An opportunity arose to perform serologic tests because infants at 10 months of age underwent a general health examination. From 1970 to 1980, 26,402 infants were examined. *T. gondii* antibodies were present in the serum of 295 (1.1%), and all had high titers in the dye test. Among their mothers, 51 had high dye test titers, suggesting that the infection present in the infant was congenital in origin. Two-hundred-ten mothers either had a negative or a low dye test titer, suggesting that their infection had been acquired long before the recent pregnancy. In their infants, congenital infection was considered as excluded or unlikely; their infection was postnatally acquired. In 34 cases, it was not possible to decide between congenital or postnatally acquired infection. Thus, the incidence of acquired infection during the first 10 months of life was between 7.9 and 9.2 per 1000. The prevalence of congenital infection was between 1.9 and 3.2 per 1000. None of the infants had severe toxoplasmosis. The fact that congenital infection was asymptomatic would be expected because this cohort was recruited by taking the opportunity of a general health examination of 10-month-old infants. However, on yearly follow-up of these children, chorioretinitis was present or was discovered in 12 of 54 (22%). This prevalence rate of congenital infection of approximately 2 per 1000, observed between 1970 and 1980, is three times lower than the risk (6.4 per 1000) calculated by Papoz and associates[359] from their epidemiologic model and the antibody prevalence survey among pregnant women that they performed in 1982 and 1983. During this decade (1970–1980), screening for *T. gondii* infection during pregnancy was becoming a common practice in France and information on how to avoid acquiring the infection was provided to seronegative women. We believe that health education might have been responsible for this difference between the expected risk calculated by Papoz and associates and the lower prevalence rate that was observed.

Effects of Systematic Screening of Pregnant Women at Risk on the Prevalence of Congenital *Toxoplasma gondii* Infection and of Congenital Toxoplasmosis

The purpose of the first attempts at systematic serologic screening was to identify pregnant women at risk to try to prevent congenital toxoplasmosis or, if present, to allow for early instigation of treatment. Once the life cycle of the parasite was elucidated, primary preventive measures were possible through education of seronegative women (see section on Prevention, Table 5–57). This is now currently done in several European countries and has proved moderately effective, as judged by the data discussed earlier; acquired *T. gondii* infection during pregnancy is apparently three times less frequent in France than it would be were no information provided to seronegative pregnant women in regard to the sources of infection and how they may reduce their risk of acquiring the infection. This estimation is very close to the conclusions of Foulon and colleagues,[292] who

calculated that in Brussels, Belgium, primary preventive measures reduced the seroconversion rates during pregnancy by 63%. Better results would be expected. One critical point is the time at which this education is provided. In most cases, it is during the first prenatal visit, at about the tenth week of pregnancy. This timing does not reduce the number of infections acquired during the first 10 weeks of gestation or the number of seroconversions that occur within 2 weeks after the first prenatal visit because women whose seroconversion occurs at this time were probably in the initial stage of the infection (during which parasitemia occurs before antibodies become detectable in the serum) at the time they received the instruction. Thus, the results of such an education program can only be a reduction in the number of infections that occur later during pregnancy. Because late acquired infections are those for which the rate of congenital transmission is the highest (primarily resulting in subclinical cases) it is understandable that in addition to a lower number of infections acquired during gestation, health education, if provided at first prenatal visit at about the tenth week of pregnancy, should result in a lower rate of transmission than observed in the previous surveys performed before the means by which *T. gondii* is horizontally transmitted to humans was known. In addition, the proportion of infected fetuses with the more severe form of congenital toxoplasmosis might be higher unless treatment during gestation is effective in the infected fetus.

Screening for *T. gondii* infection during pregnancy is now a common practice in several European countries. After surveys performed in Austria in the 1950s and 1960s a national program was introduced in 1975 that required serologic examination of every pregnant woman for *T. gondii* infection. In cases with suspect primary infection acquired during pregnancy, the woman is immediately treated. From 1975 through 1998 no cases of congenital toxoplasmosis have been registered in women who had been tested and (in instances of recent infection) treated in accordance with the regulations. Moreover, no recommendations for induced abortion had to be given, and no serious side-effects of chemotherapy were observed. The incidence of congenital *T. gondii* infection in Austria is now 1 to 2 cases per 10,000 newborns compared with 20 to 35 per 10,000 that would be expected without the screening and its consequences[374, 375] (H Aspöck, personal communication to JS Remington, 1998).

In France, congenital toxoplasmosis was the most frequent fetopathy in the years 1950 to 1960. For example, in the years 1950 to 1960, several cases of congenital toxoplasmosis were diagnosed each year among approximately 1000 premature infants admitted annually to the Hôpital de l'Institut de Puériculture de Paris. In 1957, for instance, 7 cases were diagnosed among 1085 newborns. However, in the same hospital, only two cases have been observed between 1980 and 1990. Within 40 years the pediatrician was witness to a dramatic change in the presenting signs of the disease (J Couvreur, written communication to JS Remington, 1998). In the past, patients were referred to the specialized toxoplasmosis clinic in Paris because they had clinical symptoms or often severe signs that suggested congenital toxoplasmosis. For instance, in a group of 147 neonates or infants with congenital *T. gondii* infection studied between 1949 and 1960, 62.5% had signs of central nervous system (CNS) involvement (with hydrocephalus in two thirds of them) and 32.5% had retinochoroiditis, without clinical evidence of CNS involvement. Despite their being asymptomatic, most patients now attend the specialized clinic because they are suspected of, or diagnosed as having, congenital *T. gondii* infection. Congenital *T. gondii* infection is subclinical and remains subclinical in the majority of them. For example, congenital infection remained subclinical in 166 of 234 (71%) infants observed between 1984 and 1992. In this group, 60 of 234 (26%) had a retinal scar but no CNS involvement; CNS involvement with or without hydrocephalus was present in 8 of 234 (3%) of these infants. At present, severe neurologic or ocular involvement, or both, is observed only in the following circumstances: patients referred from foreign countries where screening is not performed during pregnancy (e.g., Morocco, Algeria, United Kingdom), mothers who for any reason were not screened during pregnancy, those who were immunodeficient, and those who were erroneously considered as immune. With the exception of these circumstances, which may be considered abnormal (see sections on Transmission During Chronic Infection and Toxoplasmosis and AIDS), prenatal screening for maternal *T. gondii* infection during pregnancy has proved effective as a preventive measure for congenital toxoplasmosis in France.

PATHOGENESIS

Factors Operative During Initial Infection

VIRULENCE OF *TOXOPLASMA GONDII*

An isoenzyme analysis of *T. gondii* isolates demonstrated that certain patterns correlated with virulence of tachyzoites for mice.[376] Similar results have been obtained by restriction fragment length polymorphism (RFLP) analysis.[377] Population genetic analysis revealed three predominant lineages designated strain types I, II, and III.[378, 379] The majority of human cases of toxoplasmosis (both postnatally acquired and congenital) are due to type II[379, 380]; 10 to 25% are due to type I. It is likely that virulence, as well as inoculum size and the genetic background of the infected individual, influences transmission and severity of congenital toxoplasmosis.

ROLE OF CELLS AND ANTIBODY

After local invasion (usually in the intestines), the organisms invade cells directly or are phagocytosed.[46] They multiply intracellularly, causing host cell disruption, and then invade contiguous cells. Whereas human monocytes and neutrophils kill the vast majority of ingested *T. gondii*, tachyzoites survive within macrophages derived in vitro from peripheral blood monocytes.[381–383] Data have shown that human peritoneal and alveolar macrophages kill *T. gondii*.[384] However, cytotoxic T lymphocyte–mediated lysis of *T. gondii*–infected target cells did not lead to death of the intracellular parasites and indicated that intracellular *T. gondii* remains alive after lysis of host cells by cytolytic T cells.[385, 386] The presence of persistent parasitemia observed in humans[108] and animals[92, 387] can best be explained by the existence of intracellular parasites in the circulation.

T. gondii organisms invade every organ and tissue of the human host except non-nucleated red blood cells, although there is evidence that this may occur as well.[388] Termination of continued tissue destruction by *T. gondii* depends both on the development of cell-mediated immunity and on antibodies. Continued destruction may occur in those sites where ready access to circulating antibody is impeded (e.g., CNS and eye). Despite the ability of antibody in the presence of complement to kill extracellular *T. gondii* effectively in vitro, the intracellular habitat of this protozoon in vivo protects it from the effects of circulating antibody.[18]

Cyst formation can be demonstrated as early as the eighth day of experimental infection.[65] Cysts persist in multiple organs and tissues after immunity is acquired, probably for the life of the host.

The barrier to passive diffusion of antibodies into brain and eye has been given as an explanation of the continued proliferation of the parasite in these sites at the same time that it is disappearing from extraneural sites.[389] This barrier has also been employed as an explanation of what has been interpreted as a greater latent infection of the CNS than of extraneural tissues. However, cysts may persist and may be abundant in tissues where antibody is not opposed by such a barrier (e.g., cardiac and skeletal muscle).[66]

The ability of the pregnant woman to control multiplication and spread of *T. gondii* depends not only on specific antibody synthesis but also on the time of appearance of cell-mediated immunity. In addition to the immunosuppression associated with pregnancy itself, cell-mediated immunity, at least as measured by antigen-specific lymphocyte transformation, may not be demonstrable for weeks or even months after acute infection with *T. gondii* in humans.[390, 391] Although the importance of cellular immunity in the control of the initial acute infection in humans has not been defined, it is likely, from what we know of the immunology of toxoplasmosis on animal models[29, 30] and studies with human immune cells,[392–395] that cell-mediated immunity plays a major role. The helper T cell 2 (Th2) bias (toward humoral immunity and away from cellular immunity) established during normal gestation may compromise successful immunity against *T. gondii*, which requires a strong Th1 response. In addition, it has been proposed that a strong Th1 response against *T. gondii* may overcome the protective Th2 cytokines at the maternal-fetal interface and result in fetal loss.[396, 397] For a discussion of the immunoregulation of *T. gondii* infection and toxoplasmosis, the reader is referred to references 28 through 30 and 398.

AGE

Evidence for the supposition that maturity is an important factor in host resistance to *T. gondii* comes not only from experiments that have revealed remarkable resistance to *T. gondii* in adult rats[399] and chickens[400] when compared with newborns of those species but from the situation in humans as well. The infection in the mother frequently goes unrecognized, whereas the newborn may be severely damaged, even when infection of the fetus occurs after the fifth month of gestation (when maternal antibody first becomes available to the fetus and immunoglobulin and complement synthesis[401, 402] can occur). Deckert-Schlüter and co-workers have established a model of congenital *T. gondii* encephalitis in mice following prenatal infection with the parasite.[403] Disease in the newborn mice during the first 2 weeks of life exhibited the key histopathologic features of human congenital toxoplasmic encephalitis, including foci of necrosis, intracerebral calcifications, and ventriculitis. Importantly, the findings differed significantly from the histopathology found in adult mice with toxoplasmic encephalitis. The immune response in the prenatally infected mice was predominantly mediated by the innate immune system with preferential recruitment of macrophages and granulocytes to the brain.

GENDER

That the lymphadenopathic form of toxoplasmosis is more commonly observed in females has been recognized for many years.[404] In studies in laboratory animals, Kittas and colleagues demonstrated that female mice are more susceptible than male mice to death after *T. gondii* infection and that gonadectomized male and female mice treated with estrogens had increased mortality.[405, 406] Results of Alexander and his group[29] conclusively demonstrated that sex differences in susceptibility to *T. gondii* operate at the level of the innate immune response (as measured by interleukin-12 and interferon gamma [IFN-γ] production). Female mice were observed to suffer more severe pathology and mortality than their male counterparts; production of the cytokines at high levels was significantly earlier in the male mice.

ROLE OF HLA CLASS II GENES

The frequency of the HLA class II gene DQ3 was found to be increased in infants with congenital toxoplasmosis and hydrocephalus relative to the frequency of this gene in the U.S. population or in infants with congenital toxoplasmosis without hydrocephalus.[407] Of interest is that this unique frequency of DQ3 was also noted to be a susceptibility marker in AIDS patients who developed toxoplasmic encephalitis.[408] HLA class II DQ genes function in transgenic mice to protect against brain parasite burden. DQ1 protects better than DQ3. This observation is consonant with the observation that the DQ3 gene is more frequent in infants with congenital toxoplasmosis with hydrocephalus than in those without hydrocephalus, and than in the U.S. population.[407] Interestingly, AIDS patients with toxoplasmic encephalitis also have greater than predicted DQ3 gene frequency.[408]

REINFECTION

Although survival from the acute stages of the initial *T. gondii* infection usually results in resistance to reinfec-

tion, the immunity associated with the chronic (latent) infection is only relative. Immunity to *T. gondii* in mice protects against but does not necessarily prevent reinfection.[409–413] Mice immunized with one strain of *T. gondii* and subsequently challenged with another strain have both strains encysted in their tissues. This undoubtedly occurs in humans also, but its significance is unknown (see Transmission section).

Factors Operative During Latent Infection

CYST RUPTURE

Factors that influence tachyzoite and bradyzoite interconversion are critical to understanding the pathogenesis of recrudescent infection.

Whether cyst rupture occurs in vivo is unclear, but histologic evidence suggesting that it does has been reported.[414, 415] Indirect evidence in favor of cyst rupture in the normal host is suggested by the frequent development of new retinal lesions contiguous to the border of older scars and is reported in the studies of Lainson[65] and van der Waaij.[416] In the brains of chronically infected mice, it is not unusual to find large and small cysts close together, suggesting the possibility that cyst rupture or "leakage" of bradyzoites has caused the satellite cysts. It is not clear whether the satellite cysts are the result of cyst rupture or whether they simply developed at the same time as the larger cysts in the same area.

Huldt has demonstrated fluorescence around *T. gondii* cysts by using the immunofluorescent antibody (IFA) method.[417] Her results suggest that antigen may "leak" from cysts. That this antigen does not excite an inflammatory response is suggested by the lack of any cellular reaction around almost all cysts observed in histologic sections of chronically infected animals. Under certain circumstances, leakage may excite an inflammatory response in which previously committed lymphocytes participate, perhaps releasing a cytokine that disrupts the cyst wall. Release of enzymes from intact or degenerating neutrophils or macrophages might also result in destruction of the cyst wall with liberation of parasites.

Organisms that are intracellular or located within cysts are apparently protected from the action of antibody and perhaps also from cell-mediated immunity, although changes in the host cell membrane that may occur at the time of infection might predispose the infected cell to disruption by lymphokine-activated killer cells[392] or lymphocytes.[30, 418, 419] Cyst rupture would lead to release of viable organisms that, if released into areas deficient in antibody (e.g., brain and retina), could result in significant tissue damage. In addition, a hypersensitivity reaction probably results from release of organisms and cyst fluid, thereby resulting in further tissue destruction.

PERSISTENCE OF "ACTIVE" INFECTION

Frenkel has suggested that cyst rupture is responsible for underlying persistent immunity and antibody and that the encysted form of the organism causes localized or generalized relapse.[19] Another possibility is that organisms that have resided intracellularly as terminal colonies or pseudocysts for months or years are released after cell destruction from other causes. Such intracellular persistence of the tachyzoite form of the parasite in humans and animals appears probable. Indirect evidence for this comes from experimental observations in a number of mammalian species. Persistent parasitemia has been demonstrated not only in laboratory animals[92, 387, 420] but also in humans.[108, 258, 421] In addition, there appears to be a constant antigenic stimulus to account for the persistence of T. gondii antibodies, which may remain at high titers for years after the acute infection and at lower titers for the life of the infected host. Antigen-specific lymphocyte proliferation has been demonstrated in persons who had acquired the infection as long as 19 years previously.[390] Another observation pointing to the persistence of active infection during chronicity is that, despite having high levels of neutralizing antibody titers, hypergammaglobulinemia,[422, 423] and resistance to challenge with an ordinarily lethal dose of T. gondii, laboratory rats and mice chronically infected with T. gondii can transmit the organism to their offspring transplacentally[84, 91] (see section on Transmission).

"IMMUNOLOGIC TOLERANCE"

Results of studies in laboratory animals suggest that maternal IgG antibody may inhibit antibody formation to T. gondii in the fetus.[424] The studies revealed that significant suppression of the antibody response to living tachyzoites of T. gondii occurs when passive antibody is present even in very low concentrations and that passive administration of IgG T. gondii antibody to newborn rabbits infected with T. gondii may significantly delay IgM T. gondii antibody formation.[425]

Although previous reports on the in vitro response of human T cells to T. gondii did not demonstrate proliferation of T cells from seronegative individuals,[426, 427] McLeod and co-workers described blastogenic response of lymphocytes from uninfected individuals to relatively high concentrations of T. gondii antigens.[428] Subauste and colleagues[394] also have clearly demonstrated in vitro reactivity to T. gondii of presumably unprimed CD4+ αβ T cells from T. gondii–seronegative adults and newborns. In addition, they demonstrated that αβ T cells produce IFN-γ in response to T. gondii, an effector function that may be critical to the early immune response to the parasite. This rapid and remarkable αβ T cell response in previously unexposed individuals, the explanation for which remains to be defined, may play an important role in the early events of the immune response to T. gondii.

The observation that T. gondii induces expansion of the particular V region, Vδ2, of the γδ T cell response in acquired infection[429, 430] led Hara and associates to examine Vδ2+ γδ T cell tolerance in infants with congenital T. gondii infection.[430a] Important in this regard is the observation by Subauste and colleagues[393] that γδ T cells produce IFN-γ, a major mediator of resistance against T. gondii.[431] Hara and associates noted that Vδ2+ γδ T cells were anergic with or without clonal expansion during the newborn period in two infants with the congenital infection. Clonal expansion of Vδ2 was not observed to be associated with T cell response downregulation and no deletion of Vδ2+ γδ T cells was observed. At 1 month of age T cell anergy was noted, and T. gondii–specific anergy was noted at 5 months of age. Cord blood of infants with congenital toxoplasmosis has been reported to have increased numbers of CD45RO+ T cells.[432] In the study by Hara and associates, most of the CD45RO+ T cells were γδ T cells and these T cell levels were not always elevated, especially in an infant with severe disease in the newborn period.[430a] In their study, despite persistent αβ T cell unresponsiveness, γδ T cells became reactive to live T. gondii–infected cells and produced IFN-γ after two infants with congenital toxoplasmosis reached 1 year of age. The investigators postulated that because treatment of congenital toxoplasmosis is usually discontinued after 1 year without evidence of clinical relapse, the reversal of peripheral tolerance of γδ T cells may contribute to the spread of T. gondii after 1 year of age in congenitally infected infants in whom toxoplasmosis is severe and in whom T cell unresponsiveness to T. gondii (lysate antigen) persists.

McLeod and co-workers demonstrated absence of lymphocyte response to T. gondii antigens in some infants (usually those with the most severe manifestations) with congenital toxoplasmosis.[433] For almost all infants, response to T. gondii antigens was present by 1 year of age, when medications had been discontinued. Their lymphocyte response was often of lesser magnitude than that of their mothers or other infected adults. The mechanism or mechanisms of this absence of response and its restoration by 1 year of age remain to be determined.

Other aspects of immunologic tolerance are discussed in the section on Special Problems Concerning Pathogenesis in the Eye and in the section on Diagnosis.

IMMUNODEPRESSION

The immunodepression observed in mice infected with T. gondii is further evidence of the persistence of active infection and the persistent immunologic effect of the organism. Strickland and co-workers[434] and Hibbs and associates[435] have noted that mice infected with T. gondii have significantly depressed levels of hemagglutinins and hemolysins after immunization with sheep red blood cells. Huldt and co-workers found that neonatal infection in the mouse affects both the anatomy and the function of the thymus.[436] Additional studies by Hibbs and associates revealed an impaired responsiveness to tetanus toxoid and remarkable prolongation of allograft rejection time in T. gondii–infected animals.[437] Pregnant mice have a remarkably decreased resistance to T. gondii infection.[438] Whether similar immunodepression occurs in humans in the acute congenital or acquired infection remains to be determined. As mentioned earlier, failure of lymphocyte recognition of T. gondii antigens and significant functional and quantitative alterations in T lymphocyte subpopulations have been reported in the acute acquired infections in humans,[390, 391, 439–441] but the mechanisms underlying these effects have not been identified.

SPECIAL PROBLEMS CONCERNING PATHOGENESIS IN THE EYE

The plethora of data and the controversy that exists about immunity and hypersensitivity as they pertain to toxoplasmic chorioretinitis related to congenital toxoplasmosis preclude complete coverage of the subject here. The reader is referred to reviews of the subject by O'Connor and colleagues[442–445] and to related work in the mouse model of congenital ocular toxoplasmosis.[446–452] Whereas Frenkel fostered the theory that toxoplasmic chorioretinitis in older children and adults is a hypersensitivity phenomenon,[453] O'Connor and colleagues concluded that both the acute and the recurrent forms of necrotizing chorioretinitis are due to multiplication of T. gondii tachyzoites in the retina and that release of antigen into the retina of previously sensitized individuals does not result in recurrence of the inflammatory response. T. gondii antigen and antibody have been detected in ocular fluids in experimental ocular toxoplasmosis.[454] The rapid improvement in inflammation that occurs with antimicrobial treatment in infants, children, and adults with congenital toxoplasmosis[455] suggests that parasite replication and the resulting destruction of retinal tissue causes the eye disease. Support for the role of the parasite per se also comes from studies in which the PCR was positive on samples of vitreous of adults with the acute acquired infection.[456–459]

There are no available data in humans that clarify whether in young children the pathogenesis of eye disease related to T. gondii is the same as or different from that in adults. It is difficult to extrapolate data directly from animal models to humans. The immunologic parameters that may or may not operate in each situation are a major factor in determining the severity and outcome of eye infection and disease.

Recurrent parasitemia may provide at least one clue to the means whereby toxoplasmic chorioretinitis occurs without concurrent systemic infection. Uveitis usually develops in individuals with relatively low and stable antibody levels. Because spontaneous parasitemia can occur during the chronic (latent) infection in humans, wandering cells containing T. gondii could distribute these organisms into tissues with very low antibody levels, thereby allowing for invasion of susceptible cells. In contrast, the contiguity of old and new lesions[455] and the presence of parasites in areas of retina without lesions[460] in eyes of congenitally infected fetuses also suggest that pathogenesis of new lesions may be due to cyst rupture.

A substantial degree of antibody-induced tolerance to T. gondii has been demonstrated in experimental animals,[424, 425, 461] and it is probable that this also occurs in humans—but to what degree is unknown. It may be that maternal antibody–induced tolerance in the newborn contributes to continued multiplication of T. gondii, resulting in numerous cysts in the retina and other tissues. When, in later life, cysts or pseudocysts are for some reason recognized and destroyed or simply rupture with release of parasites that invade and destroy new host cells, perhaps when the cytokine milieu is altered due to stress or other factors, so that the immune response is less effective, clinically apparent chorioretinitis occurs. The occurrence of cyst destruction in other tissues (e.g., skeletal muscle) would not usually lead to clinical illness. A small inflammatory focus in a large muscle mass would hardly be noticed, whereas its occurrence in the retina could cause impaired vision, especially if macular in location.

Although the peak incidence of chorioretinitis related to congenital T. gondii infection usually occurs between the ages of 15 and 20 years, it may not occur until late in adult life. Crawford described a patient in whom the first eye symptoms occurred at the age of 61 years.[462] For the next 9 years, the inflammatory activity in the posterior segment of one eye continued relentlessly, causing pain and ultimately blindness. The severity of the pain necessitated enucleation. Masses of cysts were found in the retina. In such cases, it is impossible to determine whether the primary infection was congenital or acquired. In approximately 10% of 240 cases of probable ocular toxoplasmosis studied by Hogan and associates, the onset of eye disease occurred after the age of 50 years.[463] A prolonged recurrent course involving only one eye is not unusual. For example, Jacobs and co-workers isolated T. gondii from the eye of a man who had had unilateral chorioretinitis for 8.5 years, which illustrates the ability of the parasite (and reactions to it) to persist in tissues for years.[464] In a similar case, Hogan and associates made a retrospective diagnosis of congenital toxoplasmosis from a history of neonatal pneumonia and chorioretinitis in a patient at age 1.5 years and of cerebral calcifications at the age of 14 years.[465] The patient experienced recurrent attacks of chorioretinitis, which resulted in a loss of vision by age 12 and, finally, in enucleation of the left eye at age 20; T. gondii was isolated from the enucleated eye.

Recent reports of significant numbers of cases of toxoplasmic chorioretinitis that occurred during the acute acquired infection in adults highlight the difficulties in assigning all the cases of toxoplasmic chorioretinitis occurring later in life to the congenital infection.[466, 467]

The unique predilection of T. gondii for maculae, brain periaqueductal and periventricular areas, and basal ganglia in congenital toxoplasmosis remains unexplained. In the mouse model of Deckert-Schlüter and associates,[403] it is of interest that congenitally infected mice have similar periventricular lesions, unlike adult mice. It remains to be determined whether this is due to immaturity of the fetal immune system, unique interaction of T. gondii antigens with the fetal immune system, development of the fetal brain at the time infection is initiated, or some combination of these.

PATHOLOGY

In reviewing the literature about the pathology of congenital toxoplasmosis, it is immediately apparent that the genesis of the natural infection in the fetus is entirely comparable to that observed in experimental toxoplasmosis in animals. The position of necrotic foci and lesions in general suggests that the organisms reach the brain and all other organs through the bloodstream. Noteworthy is the remarkable variability in distribution of lesions and parasites among the different reported cases[468–471] (Table 5–17). Age at the time of autopsy is a major modifying factor, but others include the virulence of the strain of *T. gondii*, the number of organisms actually transmitted from the mother to the fetus, the time during pregnancy when the infection occurred, the developmental maturity of the infant's immune system, and the number of organs and tissues carefully examined. After the appearance of early reports of cases of congenital toxoplasmosis, there was a prevailing impression that the infection manifested itself in infants mainly as an encephalomyelitis and that visceral lesions were uncommon and insignificant. This view reflected the observation of a marked degree of damage to the CNS without a comparable degree of extraneural involvement in these infants. In some cases, however, extraneural lesions are severe and may even predominate.[12, 471, 472] Thus, at autopsy in some cases only the CNS and eyes may be involved, whereas in others there is wide dissemination of lesions and parasites. Between these two extremes are wide variations in the degree of organ and tissue involvement, but the CNS is never spared. The clinical importance of lesions in the CNS and eye is magnified by the lack of ability of these tissues to regenerate when compared with the remarkable regenerative capacity of other tissues in the body. Active regeneration of extraneural tissues may be observed even in the most acute stages of infection in the infant.[473] Thus, in extraneural organs, residual lesions may be so slight and insignificant that they are easily overlooked. In the CNS and eye, on the other hand, the inability of nerve cells to regenerate leads to more severe permanent damage.[473]

The presence of *T. gondii* in the cells lining alveoli and in the endothelium of pulmonary vessels led Callahan and co-workers to suggest that aspiration of infected amniotic fluid may be a route of entry of the organism into the fetus.[468] That infection by this route may occur cannot be disputed. The diffuse character of the lung changes differs from the more focal lesions found in other organs and tissues. Zuelzer pointed out that this difference may be due to the position of the lungs in the route of circulation; because all parasites in the blood pass through the alveolar capillaries, the lungs are exposed to more parasites than any other single organ.[473]

Placenta

The first description of *T. gondii* in placental tissues was by Neghme and co-workers.[115] Subsequently, a number of similar observations have been made.[114, 116, 474–477] Evidence for the likelihood of the hematogenous route of spread of *T. gondii* to the placenta is supplied by the fact that groups of tachyzoites can be found widely dispersed in the chorionic plate, decidua, and amnion and organisms have been observed in the placental villi and umbilical cord without associated significant lesions (Fig. 5–5).[113–115, 478–480] The first description of the histopathologic features of a *T. gondii*–infected placenta of a woman with AIDS was by Piche and colleagues in 1997.[481] The woman had a spontaneous abortion associated with fever and *T. gondii* pneumonia.

In five cases studied by Benirschke and Driscoll, the most consistent findings in the placentas were chronic inflammatory reactions in the decidua capsularis and focal reactions in the villi.[476] The lesions appeared to be more severe in infants who died soon after birth. Villous lesions develop at random throughout the placenta. These include single or multiple neighboring villi with low-grade chronic inflammation, activation of Hofbauer cells, necrobiosis of component cells, and proliferative fibrosis. Although villous lesions are frequently observed in placental toxoplasmosis, histologic examination of these foci does not reveal parasites; they occur in free villi and in villi attached to the decidua. Lymphocytes and other mononuclear cells, rarely plasma cells, make up the intravillous and perivillous infiltrates. The decidual infiltrate consists primarily of lymphocytes. Inflammation of the umbilical cord is uncommon. When fetal hydrops is present, the placenta is also hydropic.

The organism is seen mainly in the tissue cyst form and may be present in the connective tissues of the amnionic and chorionic membranes and Wharton's jelly and in the decidua. Benirschke and Driscoll observed one specimen from which the parasite was isolated in which contiguous decidua capsularis, chorion, and amnion contained organisms.[476] In a retrospective histologic examination of 13 placentas of newborns with serologic test results suggestive of congenital *T. gondii* infection, Garcia and associates observed organisms that had the morphology of *T. gondii* tachyzoites in 4 cases.[482] Of interest is that in 10 of their cases, on gross examination, the placenta was found to be abnormal and suggested the diagnosis of prolonged fetal distress, hematogenous infection, or both.

In some cases, the diagnosis was made initially from examination of the placenta.[113, 483] Altshuler made a premortem diagnosis by noting cysts in connective tissue beneath the amnion in a very hydropic placenta.[483] The fetal villi showed hydrops, an abundance of Hofbauer cells, and vascular proliferation. Numerous erythroblasts were present within the vessels of the terminal villi.

Elliott described lesions in a placenta of a macerated fetus (third-month spontaneous abortion).[475] The placenta showed nodular accumulations of histiocytes beneath the syncytial layer. In villi that had pronounced histiocytic infiltrates, the syncytial layer was raised away from the villous stroma and the infiltrate had spilled into the intervillous space. Disruption of the syncytium was associated with coagulation necrosis of the villous stroma and fibrinous exudate. Both encysted and free forms of *T. gondii* were present in the areas of histiocytic inflammation, in the zones of coagulation necrosis, and in the villi without either necrotizing inflammation or syncytial loss. The location of the organisms varied, but they seemed to be concentrated at the interface between the stroma and the trophoblast. This aggregation of histiocytes and organisms at the stroma–trophoblast interface suggested to Elliott that this is a favored site of growth for the parasite.

TABLE 5-17

Organ Involvement in 21 Cases of Congenital Toxoplasmosis

ORGAN/SYSTEM	M 11–16 MO	F 2 DAYS	F 120 DAYS	F 26 DAYS	F 42 DAYS	F 30 DAYS	M 31 DAYS	F 63 DAYS	M STILLBORN	F 3.5 DAYS
Central nervous system	—ᵃ	Cᵇ	BᶜC	Aᵈ	BC	ABC	BC	ABC	ABC	ABC
Eyes	AB	C	—	—	—	ABC	BC	ABC	ABC	AB
Heart	—	—	—	AB	—	AB	—	—	AB	AB
Lungs	—	—	—	A	0ᵉ	0	—	—	0	B
Spleen	—	0	—	B	—	B?	—	—	0	0
Liver	—	0	—	0	—	0	—	—	0	0
Pancreas	—	—	—	0	—	0	—	—	0	
Adrenal gland	—	0	—	A	—	0	—	—	AB	AB
Kidney	—	—	—	0	—	0	0	—	0	0
Testes	—			—					0	
Ovary		—	—	—	—	0	—	—		ABC
Uterus		—	—	—	—	0	—	—		—
Bladder		—	—	—	—	—	0	—		—
Gastrointestinal organs	0	—	—	—	—	0	—	—	—	A
Thyroid	—	0	—	—	—	0	—	—	—	—
Thymus	—	—	—	—	—	0	—	—	—	—
Pituitary	—	—	—	—	—	0	—	—	—	A
Striated muscle	—	C	—	—	—	0	—	—	AB	A
Skin, subcutaneous tissue	—	C	—	—	—	0	—	—	—	A
Umbilicus	—	—	—	0	—	0	—	—	0	AC
Blood vessels	—	0	—	—	—	0	—	—	0	—
Lymph nodes	—	—	—	—	—	—	—	—	—	—
Diaphragm	—	—	—	0	—	—	—	—	—	—
Bone marrow	—	—	—	—	—	0	—	—	—	0

ᵃNot described.
ᵇC = typical inflammatory picture—parasites.
ᶜB = typical inflammatory picture—no parasites.
ᵈA = parasites found—no inflammatory infiltrate.
ᵉ0 = examined—no lesions of toxoplasmosis.
M = male; F = female.
Adapted from Rodney MB, Mitchell H, Redner B, et al. Infantile toxoplasmosis: report of a case with autopsy. Pediatrics 5:649–663, 1950, with permission.

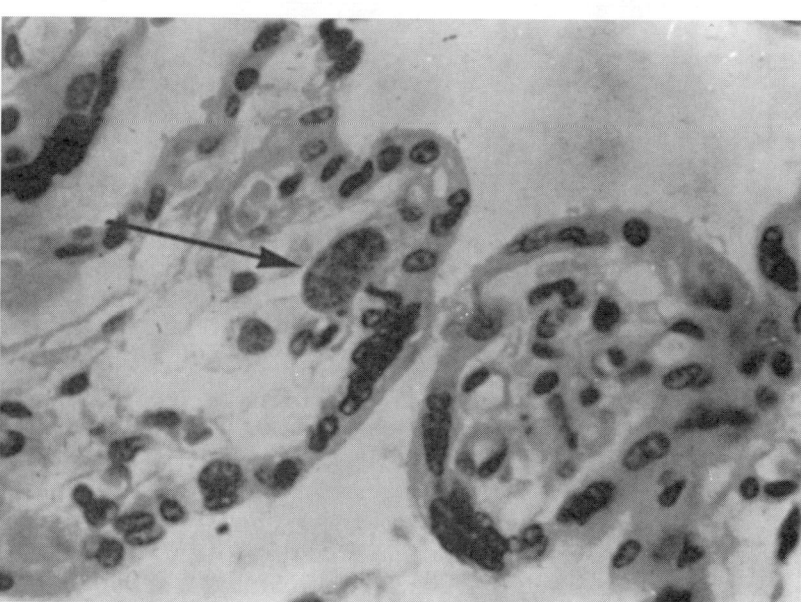

FIGURE 5–5 *Toxoplasma* cyst in the placenta of an infected fetus (arrow).

Central Nervous System

In infants who die in the newborn period, the severity of the cellular reaction in the leptomeninges of both brain and spinal cord reflects the amount of damage done to underlying tissue. The pia-arachnoid overlying destructive cortical or spinal cord lesions shows congestion of the vessels and infiltration of large numbers of lymphocytes, plasma cells, macrophages, and eosinophils. This type of change is particularly noticeable around small arterioles, venules, and capillaries. There may be complete obliteration of the gyri and sulci; the line of demarcation between the pia-arachnoid and brain substance is obscured. Parasites are frequently found within intimal cells of the arterioles, venules, and capillaries.[468]

In the cerebral hemispheres, brain stem, and cerebellum there are extensive diffuse and focal alterations of the parenchymal architecture[76, 468, 473, 484, 485] (Figs. 5–6D and 5–7D). The most characteristic change is the extensive necrosis of the brain parenchyma because of vascular involvement by lesions. The lesions are most intense in the cortex and basal ganglia and at times in the periventricular areas; they are marked by the formation of glial nodules,[76] which Wolf and co-workers referred to as characteristic miliary granulomas.[485] Necrosis may progress to actual formation of cysts, which have a homogeneous eosinophilic material at the center of the cyst cavity. At the periphery of these cystic areas, focal calcification of necrotic individual nerve cells may be evident. Calcification within zones of necrosis may be extensive, forming broad bands of calcific material involving most of the cortical layers, or it may be scattered diffusely throughout the foci of necrosis. The calcium salts are deposited in coarse granules or in finely divided particles, which give the appearance of "calcium dust." Many cells become completely calcified, whereas others contain only a few particles of finely divided calcium. Some pathologists have suggested that the *T. gondii* organisms themselves become encrusted with calcium salts.[11, 473] (Cells containing fine particles of calcium are also observed in cytomegalovirus infection of the fetus or newborn and may be misdiagnosed as evidence of *T. gondii*.) The extent of calcification appears to depend on the severity of the reaction and the duration of the infection.[468] *T. gondii* tachyzoites and cysts are seen in and adjacent to the necrotic foci, near or in the glial nodules, in perivascular regions, and in cerebral tissue uninvolved by inflammatory change (see Figs. 5–6D and 5–7D).[484]

Hervas and colleagues described an infant who developed progressive drowsiness, a weak cry, and grunting in the newborn period.[486] Computed tomography (CT) revealed cerebral calcifications, multiple ring-enhanced lesions mimicking a brain abscess, and moderate ventricular enlargement. At autopsy, *T. gondii* organisms were seen in the ventricular CSF. There was widespread necrosis and granulomatous lesions with mononuclear infiltrates.

The degree of change in the spinal cord is extremely variable. It may consist of local infiltration of lymphocytes and plasma cells, or, on the other hand, there may be almost complete disruption of the normal architecture, caused by the transformation of the gray and white matter into a mass of necrotic granulation tissue. *T. gondii* cysts, which can be identified in the white matter, are usually unassociated with inflammatory reaction.

Periaqueductal and periventricular vasculitis with necrosis is a lesion that occurs only in toxoplasmosis.[76] The large areas of necrosis have been attributed to vascular thrombosis. The necrotic brain tissue autolyzes and is gradually sloughed into the ventricles. The protein content of such ventricular fluid may be in the range of grams per deciliter and has been shown to contain significant amounts of *T. gondii* antigens.[487] If the cerebral aqueduct of Sylvius becomes obstructed by the ependymitis, the lateral and third ventricles begin to resemble an abscess cavity containing accumulations of *T. gondii* and inflammatory cells.[488] Hydrocephalus develops in such children, and the necrotic brain tissue may

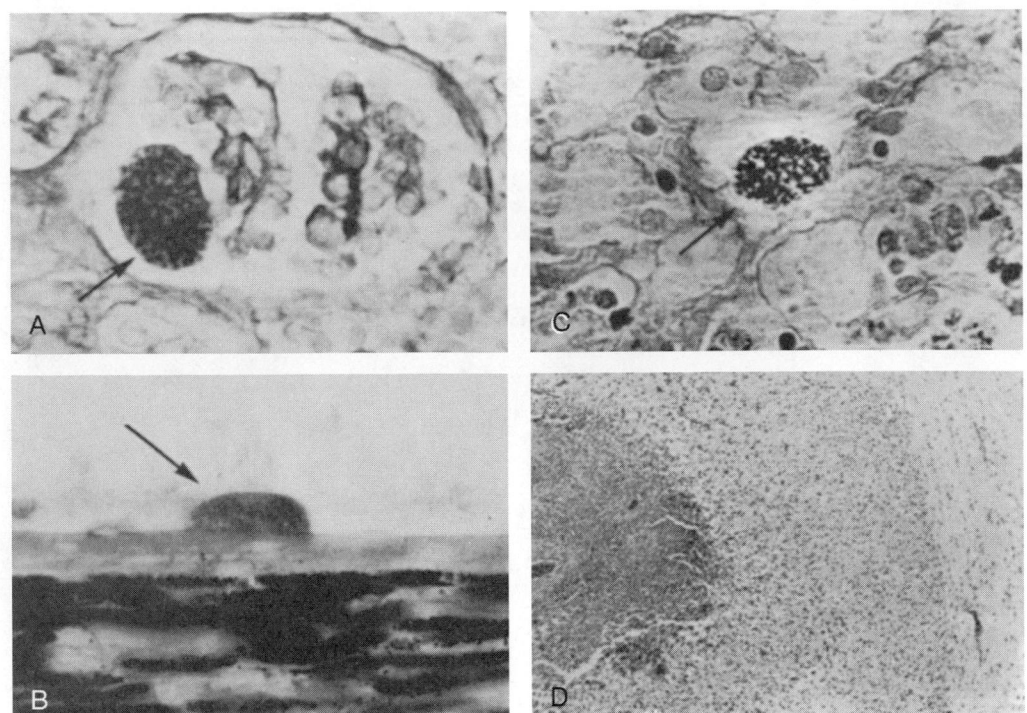

FIGURE 5–6 *A,* Large cyst (arrow) in glomerular space. *B, Toxoplasma* cyst (arrow) in the retina. Note incomplete pigmentation of the choroid. *C, Toxoplasma* cyst (arrow) in the fetal cortex of the adrenal gland. *D,* Section of brain showing abscess to the left, normal brain on right, and area of gliosis between. Encysted parasites were abundant at the periphery of these areas. (From Miller MJ, Seaman E, Remington JS. The clinical spectrum of congenital toxoplasmosis: problems in recognition. J Pediatr 70:714–723, 1967, with permission.)

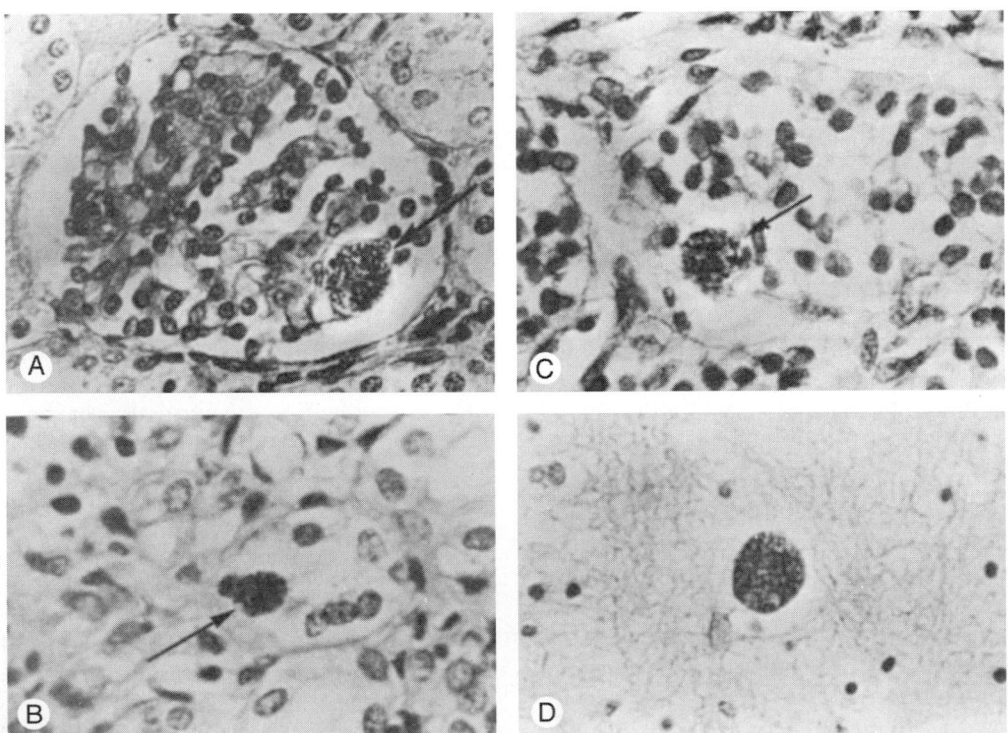

FIGURE 5–7 *A, Toxoplasma* cyst (arrow) within a glomerulus. Similar cysts were identified in endothelial cells of the glomeruli as well as free in the glomerular spaces. *B,* Encysted parasites (arrow) in a renal tubule cell. Other cysts were present within lumina of several tubules. *C, Toxoplasma* cyst (arrow) in immature testicular tissue. *D, Toxoplasma* cyst in cerebral cortex. Note lack of inflammatory response. (From Miller MJ, Seaman E, Remington JS. The clinical spectrum of congenital toxoplasmosis: problems in recognition. J Pediatr 70:714–723, 1967, with permission.)

calcify and become visible on radiographs. The fourth ventricle may show ulcers and ependymal nodules but is free from periventricular vasculitis and necrosis, apparently as a consequence of adequate drainage of its fluid through the foramina of Luschka and Magendie. The CSF that communicates with the fourth ventricle often contains several hundred milligrams per deciliter of protein and fewer inflammatory cells than the lateral ventricle.[488] Frequently, there is inflammation and necrosis involving the hypothalamus surrounding the third ventricle. Wolf and co-workers suggested that such lesions in the floor of the third ventricle probably cause the temperature lability so often observed in infants with congenital toxoplasmosis.[485, 489] Destruction of brain tissue—especially intense periventricular necrosis—rather than obstruction of ventricular passages appears to account for the development of hydrocephalus in some cases.[473, 485]

Eye

The histopathologic features of the ocular lesions depend on their stage of development at the time of the examination; a number of studies describing lesions in the earliest recognized cases have been published[12, 16, 490–495] and have been reviewed by Hogan in his classic thesis.[495] The description that follows is based on Hogan's summary of his and other cases.

The primary and principal lesions are found in the retina and choroid; secondary changes, such as iridocyclitis and cataracts,[491] that occur in other portions of the eye are considered to be complications of the chorioretinitis. Intraocular inflammation may cause microphthalmia owing to arrest in development of the eye, or a secondary atrophy may result in shrinkage of the globe. The frequently reported failure of regression of the fetal pupillary vessels may indicate that an arrest in development occurred.

The inflammation commences in the retina (see Fig. 5–6B), and copious exudation into the vitreous produces a marked haze. Secondary involvement of the choroid causes marked elevation; small satellite foci are common. After healing, the lesions are atrophic and pale, with a variable amount of pigmentation at the margins.

The organisms first lodge in the capillaries of the inner layers of the retina, invade the endothelium, and extend into adjacent tissues. An intense focal inflammatory reaction results, with edema and infiltration of polymorphonuclear leukocytes, lymphocytes, plasma cells, mononuclear cells, and, in some cases, eosinophils. The reaction results in disruption and disorganization of the retinal layers. Cells are dislocated from the nuclear layers into the adjacent fiber layers. The external limiting membrane may be ruptured, displacing retinal cells into the subretinal space. The inner limiting membrane may also be interrupted, and cells from the inner nuclear layers are then displaced into the adjacent vitreous. Glial tissue, vascular connective tissue, and inflammatory exudate also extend through the interruptions in the inner and outer limiting membranes. In the zones of most acute inflammation, all retinal supporting and neural tissues are completely destroyed. The pigmentary epithelium shows extensive destruction. The retina may detach.[460]

In the healing process, proliferation of the pigment bordering the inflammatory foci occurs. Large lesions cause considerable necrosis and destruction, resulting in marked central atrophy of the retina and choroid. Disorganization of retinal cells has occurred.[460]

Inflammation in the choroid is most acute beneath the retinal foci and is rather well demarcated. Bruch's membrane is frequently destroyed, and there is proliferation of connective tissue into the subretinal space. Retina and choroid thereby become fixed to each other by a scar. The choroidal vessels are usually engorged and show perivascular infiltration of lymphocytes, plasma cells, mononuclear cells, and eosinophils. Lymphocytes predominate, and there are both CD4 and CD8 lymphocytes.[445, 460]

Organisms are present in the retinal lesions and, in general, are most numerous where the lesions are most severe (see Fig. 5–6B). Occasional parasites without an accompanying reaction are observed in relatively normal portions of the retina near the margins of inflammatory foci. The organisms may occur singly or in clusters, free or intracellularly, or as cysts (see Fig. 5–1C and D). They are rarely seen in the choroid. They have also been found in the tissues of the optic papilla and in optic nerve association with inflammatory cells in congenital cases.[460, 470]

Serofibrinous exudate and inflammatory cells extend into the vitreous through dehiscences in the inner limiting membrane of the retina. The exudate may be accompanied by masses of budding capillaries, and the vitreous becomes infiltrated with granulation tissue.

The optic disk may show papillitis sometimes associated with optic neuritis[460] and sometimes secondary to inflammation in the adjacent retina or a papilledema caused by the hydrocephalus. Leptomeningeal inflammation may be present around the optic nerve.

Ear

The presence of the parasite in the mastoid and inner ear and the accompanying inflammatory and pathologic changes have been considered to be causes of deafness in congenital toxoplasmosis.[468, 496] Also, brain stem involvement affecting auditory nuclei can lead to inability to process auditory input.

Lungs

The alveolar septa may be widened, edematous, and infiltrated with mononuclear cells, occasional plasma cells, and rare eosinophils. The walls of small blood vessels may be infiltrated with lymphocytes and mononuclear cells, and parasites may be found in endothelial cells.[468] In many cases, there is some degree of bronchopneumonia, often caused by suprainfection with other agents. T. gondii has been identified in the epithelial cells lining alveoli and within the endothelium of small blood vessels in such patients, and, in some, the pneumonic process was considered to be a prominent part of the general disease.[468] Single organisms have been found free in alveoli in the cases described by Zuelzer[473] and Paige and co-workers.[12] Interestingly, their pathologic findings are identical to those described for adults in whom the lungs were particularly involved.[16] For a review of this subject in congenital and acquired cases, see references 497 and 498.

Heart

T. gondii is almost always found in the heart in the form of cysts in myocardial fibers and is accompanied by the presence of pathologic changes in the heart muscle. There is a focal infiltration with lymphocytes, plasma cells, mononuclear cells, and occasional eosinophils. These foci usually do not contain organisms. In the focal areas of infiltration, the myocardial cells may undergo hyaline necrosis and fragmentation. Parasites are found in myocardial fibers in large aggregates and in cysts without any accompanying inflammatory reaction (see Fig. 5–1D). Single parasites may often be present in areas of beginning necrosis and peripherally in larger areas of necrosis.[468, 473, 484] Extensive calcification of the heart, involving primarily the right ventricle and intraventricular septum, was observed in a 3-hour-old infant and was attributed to congenital toxoplasmosis.[499] Of interest in this regard is the consistent finding of marked calcification in hearts of mice experimentally infected with less virulent strains. As is the case with other tissues, the organisms can invade the myocardial fibers without destroying them or producing inflammatory reactions in the surrounding tissue. Myocarditis is probably produced by the rupture of parasitized cells, which liberates the organisms, which in turn cause an inflammatory reaction in the surrounding tissue.[468] Involvement of the heart in a congenitally infected infant has been described. The infant had AIDS and died of *Pneumocystis carinii* pneumonia and toxoplasmosis. Autopsy was limited to cardiac biopsy and revealed marked autolytic changes without evidence of inflammatory reaction or fibrosis. *T. gondii* organisms were identified in the muscle fibers.[500]

Spleen

Marked engorgement of the splenic pulp may be noted, along with erythropoiesis. In general, no significant pathologic changes that could be attributed to direct destruction by the parasite have been noted in the spleen. In some cases, an eosinophilic leukocytic infiltration has been described.[76, 473] Organisms are rarely seen in the spleen.

Liver, Ascites

In most cases, parasites are not identified in the liver, and neither necrosis nor inflammatory cell infiltrations are present. In some instances, areas of marked hepatocellular degenerative changes do occur but without associated cellular infiltration.[76, 471, 473] The periportal spaces may be infiltrated with mononuclear cells, neutrophils, and eosinophils. Enlargement of the liver is frequently pronounced and is accompanied by erythropoiesis, as

occurs also in the spleen. In a few cases, hepatic cirrhosis has been observed as a sequel to congenital toxoplasmosis.[501] Caldera and co-workers have described calcification in the liver seen both radiologically and at autopsy.[502]

Congenital toxoplasmosis was diagnosed by exfoliative cytology of ascitic fluid in a 7-week-old infant delivered at 38 weeks' gestation. The infant developed hepatomegaly and anemia shortly after birth and liver failure and ascites during the first week of life. Because an extensive workup failed to reveal a cause, a paracentesis was performed that revealed tachyzoites both in Wright-stained smear preparations and in electron microscopy sections. This case is reminiscent of an adult AIDS patient in whom the diagnosis of toxoplasmosis was first established on examination of Wright-Giemsa–stained smears of ascitic fluid obtained because of suspect bacterial peritonitis.[503]

Kidney

Numerous foci of hematopoiesis may be seen in the kidney. Focal glomerulitis has often been observed; in such cases, the majority of glomeruli remain intact.[468, 473] In fully developed lesions, glomerular tufts undergo massive necrosis and there may be necrosis of adjacent tubules. In the earlier stages of the glomerular lesion, some capillary loops are still intact; in others, necroses of the basement membrane and epithelium are observed and the lumina are occluded by fibrin thrombi. In some of these partly preserved glomeruli, single parasites have been found in cells of the exudate within the capsular space or embedded in the necrotic remains of the capillary loop.[473] *T. gondii* cysts have been found in glomeruli and renal tubules of kidneys in which there were no other associated lesions[504, 505] (see Figs. 5–6A and 5–7A and B). In severely affected kidneys, focal areas of necrosis are also found in the collecting tubules in the medulla. The inflammatory infiltrations are predominantly mononuclear, although in some cases there are also numerous eosinophils scattered throughout. In 1966, Fediushina and Sherstennikova reported the pathologic findings in the kidneys of nine cases of congenital toxoplasmosis.[506] In three of these cases, there were distinct changes in the glomeruli, and, from their description, many of the changes appear to resemble those observed in glomerulonephritis from other causes, including streptococcal infection.

In 1972, Wickbom and Winberg reported a case of a 10-week-old boy with congenital toxoplasmosis who developed severe nephritis with the nephrotic syndrome.[507] Inasmuch as Huldt had previously demonstrated antigen-antibody complexes in glomeruli of mice infected with an avirulent strain of *T. gondii*,[417] there was experimental evidence to support these authors' hypothesis that their case represented immune complex nephritis induced by *T. gondii*; no renal biopsy was made to support this suggestion. In 1974, a case of what appears to have been acute acquired toxoplasmosis was reported in a 10-year-old girl; light microscopy showed interstitial nephritis without glomerular lesions. Eleven months after treatment with pyrimethamine, sulfisomidine, and spiramycin, a second renal biopsy revealed slight granular segmental deposits of IgM and β_1C in the glomeruli. No immune deposits were found in the glomeruli of a renal biopsy specimen taken 4 months after treatment.[508]

In that same year, Shahin and associates reported a case of nephrotic syndrome in a 4-month-old infant with congenital toxoplasmosis.[509] Granular and pseudolinear glomerular deposits of IgM, fibrinogen, and *T. gondii* antigen and antibody were demonstrated in the glomeruli of the initial biopsy of renal tissue. After about 7 months of treatment, a second renal biopsy showed no evidence of the *T. gondii* antigen-antibody complexes previously noted, but IgM, fibrinogen, and the fourth component of complement (C4) were present. IgG and C3 were not demonstrable in the glomeruli in either biopsy specimen. Light microscopy of the first renal biopsy revealed glomeruli with a diffuse mild increase in mesangial cells and matrix. One glomerulus contained a segmented area of sclerosis that adhered to Bowman's capsule. There were rare foci of tubular atrophy and associated interstitial fibrosis, occasional hyaline casts, focal tubular and interstitial calcification, and prominent tubular hyaline droplets. The second renal biopsy, obtained after treatment with prednisone for 7 months and pyrimethamine and sulfadiazine for 3 weeks, revealed glomeruli with varying degrees of damage, ranging from total hyalinization to partial collapse and segmental sclerosis. The tubulointerstitial changes were not significantly different from those observed in the first biopsy specimen. The results of electron microscopy were also reported. Couvreur and associates have reported two cases of nephrotic syndrome associated with congenital toxoplasmosis.[510] Outcome was fatal in one, and *T. gondii* cysts were demonstrated in glomeruli.

Adrenals, Pituitary, Pancreas, and Thyroid

Parasites and numerous foci of necrosis have been identified in the adrenal cortex (see Fig. 5–6C). Similar areas of necrosis have been found in the pancreas.[12, 468, 472, 473] Parasites, usually without associated inflammation, have been found in the pituitary.[468, 472] Large clusters of organisms, without accompanying inflammation or necrosis, have been found in the acini of the thyroid gland.[12]

Testes and Ovaries

There is frequently an acute interstitial inflammation with focal areas of necrosis.[12, 76, 468, 472, 473] Necrosis of the seminiferous tubules with preservation of adjacent units is common, with infiltration with plasma cells, lymphocytes, mononuclear cells, and eosinophils. Parasites are often observed in the spermatogonia of intact tubules (see Fig. 5–7C). Focal hematopoiesis has been observed in the interstitium of these organs.

Skeletal Muscle

Involvement varies from parasitized fibers without pathologic changes to focal areas of infiltration or widespread myositis with necrosis. The organisms in parasitized fibers are found beneath the sarcolemmal sheaths. Hundreds of organisms may be present in a single long tubular space in a fiber, and *T. gondii* cysts are frequently seen in muscle fibers. The affected fibers are swollen and lose their striations, but as a rule no inflammatory reactions are noted. In contrast, focal areas of inflammation and necrosis may be present in areas where only a few parasites or none can be identified. The cellular infiltrate consists mainly of mononuclear cells, but lymphocytes, plasma cells, and eosinophils are also present. In rare instances, one finds focal inflammatory lesions adjacent to heavily parasitized but unbroken muscle fibers.[473] Noteworthy is the description of severe involvement of the extraocular muscles in the case described by Rodney and co-workers.[484]

Thymus

Sarrut observed a hypoplastic thymus in an infant who died of congenital toxoplasmosis at the age of 1 month (personal communication to G Desmonts, 1980). The disease was not diagnosed before autopsy. *T. gondii* organisms were isolated from the brain and heart. The histologic picture in this case was quite different from that described in experimental infection in newborn mice[436] in that, in the former, hypoplasia involved both lymphocytes and Hassall's corpuscles.

Skin

Torres found *T. gondii* tachyzoites without formation of lesions in the subcutaneous tissue of one infant.[511] In case 5 reported by Paige and associates, there were *T. gondii* organisms in the subcutaneous tissue, again with no associated inflammatory lesion or necrosis.[12] No rash was noted in the infant.

Bone

Milgram described osseous changes in a fatal case of congenital toxoplasmosis.[472] The infant died on day 17, and at autopsy widespread active infection was discovered. The parasite was found in almost all tissues of the body. Large numbers of inflammatory cells were found in the bone marrow, and there was deficient osteogenesis and remodeling in the primary spongiosa. Intracellular aggregates of *T. gondii* were present in macrophages in the bone marrow.

Immunoglobulin Abnormalities

Subtle abnormalities have been noted in the development of immunoglobulins in infants with subclinical congenital toxoplasmosis.[512] In several infants, retarded development of IgA for the first 3 years of life and excessive development of IgG and IgM were noted. The latter abnormality is also seen in congenital rubella, cytomegalic inclusion disease, and syphilis. In the *T. gondii*–infected children, the degree of increase in IgG and IgM appeared to be directly related to the severity of the infection.

Macroglobulinemia in infants with congenital infections was apparently first described in infants with congenital syphilis.[513–515] The first such report involving a case of congenital toxoplasmosis appeared in 1959 in a newborn with hydrocephalus who died at approximately 2 months of age.[516] A serum protein abnormality was suspected when blood taken for routine laboratory work became clotted in the syringe in the absence of cryoglobulins in the blood.

Oxelius described monoclonal (M) immunoglobulins in the serum and CSF of three newborns with severe clinical signs of congenital toxoplasmosis.[517] The M components belonged to the IgG class and included both κ and λ types. Because the M proteins were found in the sera of newborns but not in the sera of their mothers, Oxelius concluded that the M immunoglobulins were either selectively transferred or synthesized by the newborn. There appeared to be either local production or a selective local accumulation of the M immunoglobulins in the CSF. The M components disappeared, and the IgM level in serum and CSF decreased after therapy. Dye test antibodies were localized to the site of the M components in the electrophoretic patterns of both serum and CSF. Rheumatoid factors were also found in the serum and CSF of newborns with congenital toxoplasmosis, but, interestingly, they were not present in the sera of their mothers. These findings are especially interesting because long-standing bacterial and parasitic infections are usually associated with hypergammaglobulinemia of the diffuse polyclonal type. Oxelius was unable to absorb the dye test activity from the gamma globulin exhibiting the M components. She did not describe the nature of the antigen she employed but acknowledged that the amount of antigen used may have been inadequate. It has been shown that intact *T. gondii* organisms can effectively absorb dye test antibodies.[423] It is of interest that the M components have also been described in congenital syphilis.[518]

Reports by Van Camp and associates[519] and Griscelli and colleagues[520, 521] suggest that the observation by Oxelius may not be uncommon. Griscelli and colleagues performed a survey of 27 newborns and older infants who had the severe form of congenital toxoplasmosis. In 11 of the infants, M-IgG components were noted. These authors concluded that these components were synthesized by the fetus because they could be detected up to the seventy-fifth postpartum day and were absent in maternal serum. They were unable to define any anti–*T. gondii* antibody in isolated M-IgG. Four of the clonal M components in their 11 cases could be assigned to the κ light chain and five to the λ type. In the other two cases, it was not possible to assign the M component to either light chain type. Separation of the serum into IgM and IgG fractions by gel filtration confirmed that the M component was IgG. They noted that, whereas early treatment induced a shift of IgG concentration toward physiologic ranges, the levels of IgA and IgD remained elevated in most infants with congenital toxoplasmosis. Absorption of the hypergammaglobulinemic sera with antigens of *T. gondii* resulted in almost complete loss of the dye test antibodies but did not affect the presence of the M component or significantly reduce the immunoglobulin levels. Similar results have been

reported in *T. gondii*–infected mice; hypergammaglobulinemia and a condition that appeared to be a monoclonal spike was observed.[423] The underlying mechanism or the cause of the appearance of M components in infants with congenital toxoplasmosis is unknown.

Toxoplasma gondii–Cytomegalovirus Infection

A number of reports of this dual infection have appeared.[522–526] In systematically searching for cytomegalovirus infection among nine autopsies in cases of congenital toxoplasmosis, Vinh and co-workers found these two diseases coexisting in two instances.[522] Sotelo-Avila and associates described a case of coexisting congenital toxoplasmosis and cytomegalovirus infection in a microcephalic infant who died at the age of 15 days.[523] Microscopically, there were numerous areas of calcification and necrosis and large cells with the characteristic nuclear inclusions of cytomegalovirus. Aggregates of *T. gondii* were found in the cytoplasm of many of the cytomegalic inclusion cells in the CNS, lungs, retina, kidneys, and liver. Maszkiewicz and colleagues described a case of cytomegalic inclusion disease and toxoplasmosis in a premature infant.[524]

CLINICAL MANIFESTATIONS

Infection in the Pregnant Woman

Because acute acquired *T. gondii* infection in the pregnant woman usually is unrecognized, the infection in such cases has been said to be asymptomatic. A diagnosis of asymptomatic infection is based largely on retrospective questioning of mothers who gave birth to infected infants and requires prospective clinical studies for documentation. Even if signs and symptoms are more frequently associated with the acute infection, they are often so slight as to escape the memory of the vast majority of women.

The most commonly recognized clinical manifestations of acquired toxoplasmosis are lymphadenopathy and fatigue without fever.[259, 527–532] The groups of nodes most commonly involved are the cervical, suboccipital, supraclavicular, axillary, and inguinal. The adenopathy may be localized (e.g., most commonly a single posterior cervical node is enlarged), or it may involve multiple areas, including retroperitoneal and mesenteric nodes.[533] Palpable nodes are usually discrete, vary in firmness, and may or may not be tender; there is no tendency toward suppuration. The lymphadenopathy may occasionally have a febrile course accompanied by malaise, headache, fatigue, sore throat, and myalgia—features that closely simulate those of infectious mononucleosis. The spleen[534] and liver[535] may also be involved.[241, 536–539] Atypical lymphocytes indistinguishable from those seen in infectious mononucleosis may be present in smears of peripheral blood. In some patients, lymphadenopathy may persist for as long as 1 year and malaise may also be persistent, although this is more difficult to relate directly to the infection.[529] An exanthem may be present—it has been described in a pregnant patient.[470] An association of *T. gondii* infection and the clinical syndromes of polymyositis and dermatomyositis has been reported.[540–546] Chorioretinitis rarely occurs in the acute acquired infection, but such cases have been documented.[547–551]

Infection in the Infant

GENERAL CONSIDERATIONS

A diagnosis of congenital *T. gondii* infection is usually considered in infants who show signs of hydrocephalus, chorioretinitis, and intracranial calcifications. These signs, often described as the classic triad,[552] were present in the first proven case of congenital toxoplasmosis described by Wolf and colleagues in 1939.[11] However, since this original observation was made, they, as well as others, have seen and described congenitally infected infants who presented with a variety of clinical signs; the clinical spectrum may vary from normal appearance at birth to a picture of erythroblastosis, hydrops fetalis, the classic triad of toxoplasmosis, or a variety of other manifestations.[552, 553] Thus, such wide variation in clinical signs precludes a diagnosis according to strict adherence to a set of specific clinical criteria. Such adherence may lead to misdiagnoses, especially in cases of congenital toxoplasmosis in which the signs mimic those of other disease states. Until the variability in the clinical picture of congenital *T. gondii* infection is appreciated by pediatricians and until the diagnosis is considered more often in infants with mild nonspecific illness, the blindness, mental retardation, and even death related to *T. gondii* will continue to go unrecognized.

Congenital *T. gondii* infection may occur in one of four forms: (1) a neonatal disease; (2) a disease (severe or mild) occurring in the first months of life; (3) sequelae or relapse of a previously undiagnosed infection during infancy, childhood, or adolescence; (4) a subclinical infection. When clinically recognized in the neonate, the infection is usually severe. Symptoms and signs of generalized infection may be prominent, and signs referable to the CNS are always present. The neurologic signs are frequently more extensive than might be suspected at first.

In other neonates, neurologic signs (e.g., convulsions, bulging fontanelle, nystagmus, abnormal increase in circumference of the skull) are the major indications of the diagnosis. Such manifestations are not always associated with gross cerebral damage; instead, they may be related to an active encephalitis not yet associated with irreversible cerebral necrosis or to obstruction of the cerebral aqueduct of Sylvius caused by edema or inflammatory cells, or both, rather than to permanent obstruction. In these latter infants who are treated, signs and symptoms may disappear and development may be normal thereafter.

Mild cases in the neonate are usually not recognized. Identification of the disease has been possible in prospective studies, however, when infants born to mothers known to have acquired *T. gondii* infection during pregnancy are examined. The most frequent signs include isolated chorioretinal scars. Such cases prove that the infection was active during fetal life without causing detectable systemic damage.

Most children with congenital *T. gondii* infection are said to have been normal at birth, as signs or symptoms become manifest weeks, months, or years later. Obviously, in many cases this is not delayed onset of disease but late recognition of disease. Nevertheless, it has been possible to verify delayed onset of disease weeks or months or years after birth in neonates who had no abnormalities that could be related to toxoplasmosis.[113, 118, 361, 512] Disease with delayed onset may be severe and occurs most often in premature infants in whom severe CNS and eye lesions appear during the first 3 months after birth. In the full-term infant, delayed onset of disease occurs mainly during the first 2 months of life. Clinical signs may be related to generalized infection (e.g., hepatosplenomegaly, delayed onset of icterus, lymphadenopathy); CNS involvement (e.g., encephalitis or hydrocephalus), which may occur after a more protracted period; or eye lesions, which may occur months or years after birth in infants and children whose fundi are checked repeatedly.

Sequelae are most often ocular (e.g., chorioretinitis occurring at school age or adolescence), but in some cases they are neurologic—for instance, convulsions may lead to the discovery of cerebral calcifications or retinal scars. Ocular lesions may recur during childhood, adolescence, or adulthood. In some instances, neurologic relapses (e.g., late obstruction of the aqueduct) have been observed.

Congenital *T. gondii* infection in the newborn in the series from France, as well as in a study performed in the United States,[361, 554] was most frequently a subclinical or inapparent infection, not, as had previously been thought, an obvious and fulminant one. In those infants who were clinically normal at birth, the infection was diagnosed by demonstration of persistent serologic test titers. Such asymptomatic infants may suffer no untoward sequelae of the infection, or they may develop chorioretinitis, strabismus, blindness, hydrocephaly or microcephaly, psychomotor and mental retardation, epilepsy, or deafness months or even years later.[555–557] Such patients—asymptomatic at birth but developing untoward sequelae later—were noted by Callahan and coworkers in the early 1940s (their cases 3 and 4).[468] Frequently, neurologic signs or hydrocephalus appears between the third and twelfth months.[558] In patients with encephalitic lesions, CNS abnormalities that produce clinical signs rarely develop after the first year[559] (see section on Follow-up).

At present, there are no parameters with which to predict the outcome of the infection in a newborn with asymptomatic *T. gondii* infection. However, there are hundreds of reports attesting to the crippling effects of the infection when severe disease is apparent at birth.

Clinically Apparent Disease. One of the most complete studies was that of Eichenwald, who in 1947 initiated a study to discover the clinical forms of congenital toxoplasmosis and to determine the natural history of the infection and its effect on the infant.[552] The cases were referred by a group of cooperating hospitals in a systematic and prearranged manner. Sera were obtained from three groups of infants and their mothers. The first two groups consisted of 5492 infants examined because they had either undiagnosed CNS disease in the first year of life (neurologic disease group) or undiagnosed non-neurologic diseases during the first 2 months of life (generalized disease group). The third group consisted of 5761 normal infants. The incidences of serologically proven cases in the three groups was 4.9%, 1.3%, and 0.07%, respectively. Of the 11,253 infants studied, 156 had serologically proven congenital toxoplasmosis; 69% were in the neurologic disease group, and 28% were in the generalized disease group. The signs and symptoms in the infants in these two groups are shown in Table 5–18. Approximately one third showed signs and symptoms of an acute infectious process, with splenomegaly, hepatomegaly, jaundice, anemia, chorioretinitis, and abnormal CSF as the most common findings. The so-called classic triad of toxoplasmosis was demonstrated in only a small proportion of the patients. The

TABLE 5–18
Signs and Symptoms Occurring Before Diagnosis or During the Course of Acute Congenital Toxoplasmosis

SIGNS AND SYMPTOMS	FREQUENCY OF OCCURRENCE (%) IN INFANTS WITH	
	Neurologic Disease[a] (108 Cases)	Generalized Disease[b] (44 Cases)
Chorioretinitis	94	66
Abnormal spinal fluid	55	84
Anemia	51	77
Convulsions	50	18
Intracranial calcification	50	4
Jaundice	29	80
Hydrocephalus	28	0
Fever	25	77
Splenomegaly	21	90
Lymphadenopathy	17	68
Hepatomegaly	17	77
Vomiting	16	48
Microcephaly	13	0
Diarrhea	6	25
Cataracts	5	0
Eosinophilia	4	18
Abnormal bleeding	3	18
Hypothermia	2	20
Glaucoma	2	0
Optic atrophy	2	0
Microphthalmia	2	0
Rash	1	25
Pneumonitis	0	41

[a]Infants with otherwise undiagnosed central nervous system diseases in the first year of life.
[b]Infants with otherwise undiagnosed non-neurologic diseases during the first 2 months of life.
Adapted from Eichenwald HF. A study of congenital toxoplasmosis. In Siim JC (ed). Human Toxoplasmosis. Copenhagen, Munksgaard, 1960, pp 41–49, with permission. Study performed in 1947.

fact that 98% of the infants had clinical evidence of infection can be explained by the manner in which the case material was collected for the study. Despite the fact that Eichenwald clearly defined this, his data for years have been misinterpreted to show that all infants with congenital T. gondii infection have signs and symptoms of infection, as set forth in Table 5–18. Most of the patients were followed from birth to 5 or more years of age. The overall mortality rate was 12% (no significant differences in mortality rate existed between the clinical groups), and approximately 85% of the survivors were mentally retarded. Almost 75% developed convulsions, spasticity, and palsies, and about 50% had severely impaired vision (Table 5–19). It is noteworthy that deafness, usually attributed to congenital viral infections (e.g., cytomegalovirus and rubella), also occurs as a sequel to congenital T. gondii infection. The signs and symptoms in this series of patients differ in many respects from those recorded in reports published earlier, owing undoubtedly to the fact that the cases studied by Eichenwald were drawn from a relatively unselected group rather than from a limited survey based on infants tested solely because they showed most of the so-called classic signs of congenital toxoplasmosis.

Subclinical Infection. Studies of subclinical infection have been performed in an attempt to determine the following: how often congenital T. gondii infection is subclinical; whether it is really subclinical or whether, in fact, initial signs have gone unrecognized; and what the prognosis is of subclinical infection. For information on prognosis, see the section on Follow-up.

Alford and colleagues performed a series of studies to determine the medical significance of the subclinical form of congenital T. gondii infection.[512] Their serologic screening program (see section on Diagnosis) was performed in a moderately low socioeconomic urban population in the southern United States, and 10 infants with congenital T. gondii infection were detected of 7500 newborns screened (1 proven case per 750 deliveries over a study period of 2.5 years). The findings in the 10 newborns are shown in Table 5–20. Only 1 infant had signs that suggested T. gondii infection (hepatosplenomegaly, chorioretinitis, cerebral calcification). Thus, 9 of the infected infants would have escaped detection were it not for the laboratory screening program. The investigators pointed out that there were, nevertheless, significant abnormalities in this group of newborns with so-called subclinical infection. Half were premature, and the average birth weight of the infected infants, 2664 g, was 349 g less than that of control infants (3013 g). Although there were no signs or symptoms referable to the nervous system in the 9 infants, abnormalities in the CSF were noted in each of the 8 infants in whom this examination was performed. CSF lymphocytosis (10 to 110 cells per μl) and elevated protein levels (150 to 1000 mg/dl) persisted for 2 weeks to 4 months or more (average: at least 3 months for the group), even in infants treated in the first 4 weeks after birth. The findings in a severe case and a mild case are depicted graphically in Figures 5–8 and 5–9, respectively. The infant whose data are shown in Figure 5–8 was premature but had no sign of infection during the neonatal period. The elevated

TABLE 5–19
Major Sequelae of Congenital Toxoplasmosis Among 105 Patients Followed 4 Years or More

CONDITION	NO. (%) WITH NEUROLOGIC DISEASE[a] (70 PATIENTS)	NO. (%) WITH GENERALIZED DISEASE[b] (31 PATIENTS)	NO. (%) WITH SUBCLINICAL DISEASE (4 PATIENTS)
Mental retardation	69 (89)	25 (81)	2 (50)
Convulsions	58 (83)	24 (77)	2 (50)
Spasticity and palsies	53 (76)	18 (58)	0
Severely impaired vision	48 (69)	13 (42)	0
Hydrocephalus or microcephaly	31 (44)	2 (6)	0
Deafness	12 (17)	3 (10)	0
Normal	6 (9)	5 (16)	2 (50)

[a]Infants with otherwise undiagnosed central nervous system diseases in the first year of life.
[b]Infants with otherwise undiagnosed non-neurologic diseases during the first 2 months of life.
Adapted from Eichenwald HF. A study of congenital toxoplasmosis. *In* Siim JC (ed). Human Toxoplasmosis. Copenhagen, Munksgaard, 1960, pp 41–49, with permission. Study performed in 1947.

level of CSF protein suggested severe CNS involvement from birth onward. At 2.5 months of age, retarded growth of the head, generalized intracranial calcification, chorioretinitis, and hepatosplenomegaly first became evident; these signs became worse despite treatment with pyrimethamine and sulfadiazine, which was, however, instituted late in the course of the infection. At the age of 4 years, this child had a developmental level of 2 years.

Figure 5–9 shows a representative example of the eight patients with milder diseases, in six of whom CSF abnormalities were present. Persistent lymphocytosis was detected in all, and elevations of CSF protein levels were distinctly lower (150 to 285 mg/dl) in this group

than in the two infants who proved to have severe disease.

Follow-up evaluation in infants who were asymptomatic at birth is discussed under Follow-up. The data indicate that nearly all children born with subclinical congenital *T. gondii* infection develop adverse sequelae.

How often is congenital infection subclinical? The only prospective data are from studies performed in France, where serologic examination of pregnant women for *T. gondii* infection is obligatory. Couvreur and colleagues reported a series of 210 infants referred to them because acute acquired infection with *T. gondii* was diagnosed in the mothers before delivery.[560] The series includes all cases of congenital infection prospectively diagnosed from 1972 to 1981. Infants referred because of the presence of clinical signs but who were born of mothers in whom the diagnosis of acute acquired infection had not been previously made during pregnancy

TABLE 5–20
Data in 10 Newborns with Congenital *Toxoplasma* Infection Identified by the Presence of IgM *Toxoplasma* Antibodies

FINDING	NO. OF INFANTS
Maternal illness ("flu")	2
Diagnosis suspected (neonate)	1
Gestational prematurity[a]	5
Intrauterine growth retardation[b]	2
Hepatosplenomegaly	1
Jaundice	1
Thrombocytopenia	1
Anemia	1
Chorioretinitis	2
Abnormal head size	0
Hydrocephalus	1
Microcephaly	0
Abnormal spinal fluid	8[c]
Abnormal neurologic examination	1
Serum IgM elevated	9
Serum IgM *Toxoplasma* antibody	10

[a]<37 weeks of gestation.
[b]Lower tenth percentile (Grunewald).
[c]Only eight were examined.
Adapted from Alford CA Jr, Stagno S, Reynolds DW. Congenital toxoplasmosis: clinical, laboratory, and therapeutic considerations, with special reference to subclinical disease. Bull N Y Acad Med 50:160–181, 1974, with permission.

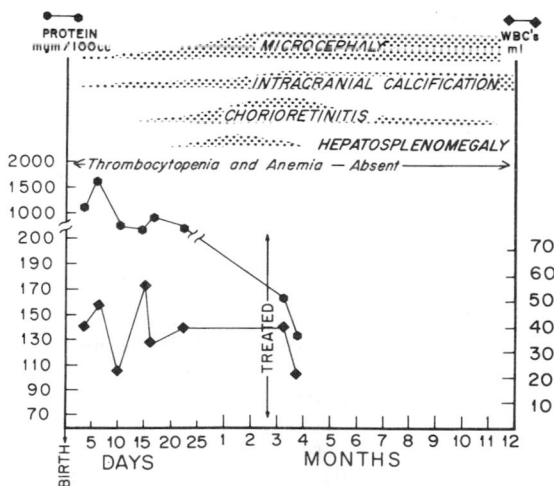

FIGURE 5–8 Severe form of congenital toxoplasmosis. Spinal fluid and clinical findings. (From Alford CA, Foft JW, Blankenship WJ, et al. Subclinical central nervous system disease of neonates: a prospective study of infants born with increased levels of IgM. J Pediatr 75:1167–1178, 1969, with permission.)

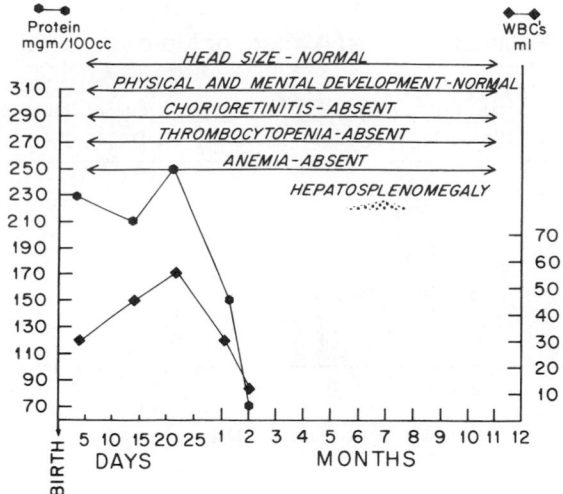

FIGURE 5–9 Mild form of congenital toxoplasmosis. Spinal fluid and clinical findings. (From Alford CA, Foft JW, Blankenship WJ, et al. Subclinical central nervous system disease of neonates: a prospective study of infants born with increased levels of IgM. J Pediatr 75:1167–1178, 1969, with permission.)

were not included (because diagnosis in these cases was retrospective). Among these 210 infants, 2 died during the first year of life; the cause of death in 1 was systemic congenital toxoplasmosis and in the other was probably not related to *T. gondii* infection. Twenty-one infants

(10%) had severe congenital toxoplasmosis with CNS involvement. Eye lesions were present in most cases, and systemic disease was present in some. Seventy-one cases (34%) were mild, with a normal clinical examination except for the presence of peripheral retinal scarring or isolated intracranial calcifications in an asymptomatic child.

One hundred sixteen infants (55%) had subclinical infections both at initial examination and at a subsequent examination at 12 months of age. The frequency of the signs observed is shown in Table 5–21. As pointed out by the investigators, these figures for the respective frequency of severe, mild, or subclinical cases are biased. Several biases probably decreased the relative frequency of severe congenital infection. The most severe cases with neonatal death were not referred to the investigators, nor probably were those in which congenital toxoplasmosis was so evidently severe that therapy did not appear worthwhile. In addition, abortion is often performed when acquired infection is diagnosed sufficiently early during pregnancy. This likely decreased the number of infected infants born alive despite early transmission of the parasites, which would probably have resulted in delivery of severely damaged infants (see section on Transmission). Also, when diagnosis in the mother is made before delivery, treatment with spiramycin has resulted in fewer severely infected offspring and might have decreased the severity of infection in the fetus.[561] In the studies of Couvreur and colleagues,[560] the numbers of severe cases were 16 (14%) among 116 infants

---

TABLE 5–21

Prospective Study of Infants Born to Women Who Acquired *Toxoplasma* Infection During Pregnancy: Signs and Symptoms in 210 Infants with Proven Congenital Infection

FINDING	NO. EXAMINED	NO. POSITIVE (%)
Prematurity	210	
Birth weight < 2500 g		8 (3.8)
Birth weight 2500–3000 g		5 (7.1)
Dysmaturity (intrauterine growth retardation)		13 (6.2)
Postmaturity	108	9 (8.3)
Icterus	201	20 (10)
Hepatosplenomegaly	210	9 (4.2)
Thrombocytopenic purpura	210	3 (1.4)
Abnormal blood count (anemia, eosinophilia)	102	9 (4.4)
Microcephaly	210	11 (5.2)
Hydrocephalus	210	8 (3.8)
Hypotonia	210	2 (5.7)
Convulsions	210	8 (3.8)
Psychomotor retardation	210	11 (5.2)
Intracranial calcifications on radiography	210	24 (11.4)
Abnormal ultrasound examination	49	5 (10)
Abnormal computed tomography scan of brain	13	11 (84)
Abnormal electroencephalographic result	191	16 (8.3)
Abnormal cerebrospinal fluid	163	56 (34.2)
Microphthalmia	210	6 (2.8)
Strabismus	210	11 (5.2)
Chorioretinitis	210	
Unilateral		34 (16.1)
Bilateral		12 (5.7)

Data are adapted from Couvreur J, Desmonts G, Tournier G, et al. [A homogeneous series of 210 cases of congenital toxoplasmosis in 0 to 11-month-old infants detected prospectively.] Ann Pediatr (Paris) (in French) 31:815–819, 1984.

born of untreated mothers and 3 (4%) in the 79 cases in which the mothers were known to have been treated.

This study also allows for an estimation of the proportion of cases in which infection is really subclinical and of those in which initial signs have in fact not been recognized. Among 116 cases in which infection was considered to be subclinical by the referring physicians, 39 (33%) were discovered to have one or several signs of congenital toxoplasmosis; the most frequent sign was an abnormal CSF.

In a newborn serologic screening program in Massachusetts, more thorough evaluations of the apparently asymptomatic newborns revealed 20% with eye disease and 20% with neurologic findings.[562]

PREMATURITY

Prematurity and low Apgar scores are common among newborns with congenital *T. gondii* infection who have clinically apparent disease at birth.[141, 512, 556, 563, 564] In larger series, prematurity has been reported in 25 to more than 50% of the infants. When Lelong and coworkers searched for cases of congenital toxoplasmosis on a single ward of premature infants, they found 7 (0.6%) among 1085 infants.[361]

TWINS

In 1965, Glasser and Delta reviewed reports of congenital toxoplasmosis in twins that had appeared in the literature up to that year.[113] Later, Couvreur and colleagues reviewed this subject and added 14 of their own previously unpublished cases to the literature. Through 1980, we are aware of 35 cases of congenital toxoplasmosis in twins: 11 in monozygotic twins,[113, 473, 505, 565–571] 13 in dizygotic twins,[93, 505, 565, 572–576] and 11 whose type is undetermined.[565, 571, 577–580] In 1986, Sibalic and associates reported a series of 21 pairs of twins with congenital toxoplasmosis in 38 of the infants.[581] *T. gondii* was isolated from four infants. In the remainder, the diagnosis was made by serology alone. The data are difficult to evaluate because the serologic test results were not presented individually for each infant. Wiswell and coworkers reported congenital toxoplasmosis in triplets.[582] *T. gondii* was demonstrated in the CSF of each infant; no mention was made as to whether the infants were polyzygotic. Each of the three infants had severe disease. In 1991, Couvreur and colleagues added six additional cases.[583] The diagnosis of infection was made in two cases by prenatal sampling of blood from each of the fetuses.

The diagnosis of congenital toxoplasmosis would likely be missed in an asymptomatic twin were it not for specific lesions in the other twin, which lead the physician to consider this diagnosis in both twins in the set.[505, 565] Thus, variable clinical patterns have been noted in pairs of twins, and in some sets one twin died and a subclinical infection existed in the other.[505, 553, 573] It is doubtful that the diagnosis of congenital toxoplasmosis would have been suspected in the surviving twins without benefit of the results of autopsy in their respective twins.[505]

A distinct difference in clinical patterns has been observed between monozygotic and dizygotic twins. In nine pairs of monozygotic twins, the clinical pattern in each twin of a pair most often appears to be similar.[113] For example, chorioretinitis was found in each twin in seven pairs. In addition, with one exception,[473] the lesions were either bilateral or unilateral in each twin of each pair considered. Each twin in four sets had hydrocephalus, in four sets cerebral calcification, in four sets convulsions, and in one set mental and motor retardation. In only two sets, in which each infant had hyperbilirubinemia, was there a marked variation from this similarity in clinical pattern in single sets. In each of these sets, one twin died and the other survived.[473, 505, 565] Among the monozygotic twins, there was a remarkable predominance of males (eight of nine pairs), a phenomenon as yet unexplained.

In dizygotic twins, on the other hand, discrepancies in clinical findings within single sets are frequent and marked. In 11 sets of dizygotic twins,[505, 565, 572–575] chorioretinitis was present in 13 of the 22 twins but was observed in both twins of a set in only two instances,[565, 573, 574] and even in these the lesions were not identical. Such discrepancies were also true for virtually all other clinical features in these twins. In many cases, one of the twins had a subclinical infection whereas, in the other, it was severe.[505, 565, 584] In two sets of twins, one bichorial and biamniotic and the other monochorial and biamniotic, one infant in each set completely escaped infection.[565]

CENTRAL NERVOUS SYSTEM

Other clinical manifestations of CNS destruction are described in the sections on Mental Retardation, Down Syndrome, and Radiologic Studies.

Although in infants with clinically manifested disease, the clinical signs of congenital toxoplasmosis may vary considerably, widespread destruction of the CNS usually gives rise to the first clinical indications of disease. Among the most common manifestations are internal obstructive hydrocephalus,[585] which is often present at birth or appears shortly thereafter and is usually progressive; seizures, which may range from muscular twitching and spasticity to major motor seizures; stiff neck with retraction of the head and, in some cases, opisthotonos; and spinal or bulbar involvement manifested by paralysis of the extremities, difficulty in swallowing, and respiratory distress. Thus, the spectrum of neurologic manifestations is protean and may vary from a massive acute encephalopathy to a subtle neurologic syndrome. That the infection can involve the spinal cord is highlighted by a case in a 4-week-old girl who presented with macrocephaly and paralysis of both legs. CT revealed hydrocephalus, and magnetic resonance imaging revealed numerous lesions in the cerebral parenchyma and spinal cord.[586] Eighty-four cases (6.5%) of toxoplasmosis were found among 1282 children younger than the age of 1 year who had signs of neurologic disease without obvious reasons.[559] (A similar figure, 4.9%, was reported by Eichenwald.[552]) The proportion of cases of congenital *T. gondii* infection was strikingly greater in infants with retinal lesions associated with CNS involvement (62 [23%] of 266 cases examined) than in those who had CNS lesions but no ocular lesions (22 [2.2%] of 1016 cases examined).

It is important to recognize that hydrocephalus due to aqueductal obstruction may be the sole clinical manifestation associated with congenital *T. gondii* infection. Occasionally, the hydrocephalus may be stable but in most cases it requires a neurosurgical shunt procedure.[587] In a significant number of infants, the prognosis is good, especially after a shunt procedure; the intelligence quotient may be within the normal range. The performance of CT in the months after shunt placement is useful in determining long-term prognosis—which is good if the results of the CT are normal, even in some cases with clinically apparent encephalitis. The prognosis is less promising when there is little expansion of the cortical mantle in the months after ventriculoperitoneal shunt placement. Follow-up CT after shunt placement is also important to exclude subdural collections associated with bleeding from small vessels associated with reduction of pressure when the obstructive hydrocephalus is corrected. Kaiser has presented a follow-up study of 10 children with hydrocephalus resulting from congenital toxoplasmosis.[588] Hydrocephalus was present at birth in only 3 of the 10 patients and was noted for the first time as late as 11 and 15 months in 2 patients. All children had progressive hydrocephalus, which required placement of a shunt. In the U.S. (Chicago) National Collaborative Treatment Trial, hydrocephalus was present in 45 children. It usually was detected clinically at birth, occasionally prenatally, and after 2 weeks of age in 16 infants. Occasionally, hydrocephalus developed after birth. All children with substantial hydrocephalus in which there was evidence of aqueductal obstruction and increased intracranial pressure had placement of ventriculoperitoneal shunts.

From 1949 to 1960, Couvreur and Desmonts observed 300 cases of congenital toxoplasmosis.[559] These patients were found by clinical selection. Ocular disorders, particularly chorioretinitis (76%), and neurologic disturbances (51%) were present in most cases. Twenty-six percent had abnormalities in cranial volume and 32% had intracranial calcifications.

Toxoplasmosis in children with abnormal cranial volume is uncommon without associated ocular lesions. Of 261 children younger than the age of 2 years with hydrocephalus, 16 (6%) had congenital *T. gondii* infection; and of 178 children of the same age group with microcephaly, only 3 (1.7%) had congenital *T. gondii* infection. (See also the next section, Microcephaly.)

An interesting case of what appears to have been congenital *T. gondii* infection that manifested as a brain tumor at approximately 1 year of age was reported by Tognetti and associates.[589]

For information on the special problem of congenital toxoplasmosis in infants infected with human immunodeficiency virus (HIV) the reader is referred to the section on Congenital *Toxoplasma gondii* Infection and Acquired Immunodeficiency Syndrome.

MICROCEPHALY

Baron and co-workers examined the role of *T. gondii* in microcephaly and mental retardation.[590] Normal, nor-mocephalic children served as controls, and adequate numbers of microcephalic children ranging in age from 5 months to 5 years were tested in the dye test. Their data did not reveal significant evidence of an association of *T. gondii* infection and microcephaly. Similar results were obtained by Thalhammer[578, 591] and Remington.[592] However, it should be remembered that many microcephalic infants have died before 5 years of age. Microcephaly in this infection usually reflects severe brain damage, but patients with microcephaly have also developed normally or near-normally.

INSTABILITY OF REGULATION OF BODY TEMPERATURE

As mentioned in the section Central Nervous System, under Pathology, hypothermia may be present and may persist for weeks.[12, 76, 468, 593] Wide fluctuations in temperature, from hypothermia to hyperthermia, have been reported.[473]

EYE

Chorioretinitis

Because toxoplasmosis is one of the most common causes of chorioretinitis in the United States and much of the rest of the world, it is important to note that most workers consider toxoplasmic chorioretinitis in older children and adults to be the result of a congenital infection rather than a manifestation of acquired toxoplasmosis. From data derived from extensive surveys of cases of uveitis, Perkins concluded that only about 1.5% of patients with toxoplasmic lymphadenopathy have chorioretinitis related to the acquired infection.[594] As he pointed out, population surveys have always shown that the incidence of infection with *T. gondii* increases with age; if toxoplasmic chorioretinitis results from chronic acquired infection, the number of cases should also rise with increasing age. However, in contrast to nontoxoplasmic uveitis, the incidence of which increases with age to reach its maximum in the fourth decade, toxoplasmic chorioretinitis occurs most frequently in the second and third decade of life and is rare after age 50.[595] In addition, if the ocular lesions resulted from acquired infection, it would be expected that the patients would have higher levels of circulating antibodies than asymptomatic persons among the normal population. Actually, high dye test titers are exceptional in toxoplasmic uveitis and, even when found, are not necessarily evidence of acquired infection, because some patients with congenital infection have dye test titers of 100 IU or greater in adult life. There is a report of what seems to be a reappearance of IgM, IgA, and IgE antibodies in some patients diagnosed as having an exacerbation of chorioretinitis due to congenital toxoplasmosis,[596] whereas others have not found this to occur.[455] Studies have revealed that postnatally acquired toxoplasmic chorioretinitis occurs more frequently than previously appreciated; however, its actual incidence is not known.[466, 467, 597]

Attesting to the potential severity of the outcome of congenital ocular toxoplasmosis are results of studies such as those of Fair.[598, 599] In a survey of almost 1000 children in state schools for the blind in the southern United States, Fair concluded that 51 (5%) of the students owed their visual disability to bilateral congenital central chorioretinitis, and, of these, a diagnosis of congenital toxoplasmosis was certain or very probable in 40 (4%).[600] All showed the nystagmus and squint that always call for further examination. Kazdan and co-workers stated that the most common cause of posterior uveitis in children 15 years of age and younger at the Hospital for Sick Children in Toronto was congenital toxoplasmosis.[601]

Congenital bilateral toxoplasmic macular scars, optic atrophy, and congenital cataracts were the major causes (43.5%) of low vision in a retrospective review of a population of 395 consecutive children younger than 14 years of age who were attended by the Low Vision Service of the State University of Campinas in São Paulo, Brazil, from 1982 to 1992.[602] Previous studies have revealed similar results.[603, 604] Fortunately, use of low magnification (telescopic prescriptions) significantly improved vision in these children and, in 63%, provided both social and personal benefits.[602]

To assess the extent of ocular and systemic involvement in adolescent and adult patients with severe congenital toxoplasmosis, Meenken and co-workers[605] from the Netherlands reviewed clinical data, available since birth, in 15 patients whose severe toxoplasmosis was confirmed during the first year of life. The patients were residents of an institute for mentally and visually handicapped children and adults. Nine of them had been treated postnatally for 2 to 10 months. Mean follow-up was 27 years. Although the diagnosis was made more than 25 years earlier when more reliable serologic methods were not available, the serodiagnosis seems clear in 13 of the 15. Each of the 15 patients also had the combination of psychomotor retardation, epilepsy, and focal necrotizing retinitis diagnosed as being due to congenital toxoplasmosis. Intracerebral calcifications were present in 12 cases, and in 10 cases, obstructive hydrocephalus had been diagnosed in the first months of life; all were treated and all required repeated shunting procedures. In addition to chorioretinitis, the most common abnormal ocular features were optic nerve atrophy (83%), visual acuity of less than 0.1 (85%), strabismus (76%), and microphthalmos (53%). One half exhibited iridic abnormalities, and approximately 40% developed a cataract. The majority with iris atrophy were in children aged 5 to 10 years. Of the 8 patients (16 eyes) with iridic atrophy, 12 (75%) had atrophic changes in the eyeball. In only one case was the chorioretinitis unilateral; it was bilateral in 97% of the cases. In the majority of cases, severe visual impairment was associated with optic nerve atrophy. The documented recurrence rate was low (9%) when compared with the recurrence rate in patients who suffer solely from ocular involvement.[606] Some factors that appeared to account for this low documentation of recurrences were difficulties in examination including the presence of cataract, extreme microphthalmos, band keratopathy, and lack of patient cooperation. The endocrinologic involvement in these patients is described in the section on Endocrine Organs.

The risk of development of chorioretinitis in congenital cases appears to increase with increasing age during the early years of life. For example, in one case, unilateral (followed by bilateral) chorioretinitis developed between days 90 and 115 in an untreated premature infant in whom ophthalmoscopic examination was performed every 10 days.[607] In contrast, between 1981 and 1999 in 93 treated children in the U.S. (Chicago) National Collaborative Treatment Trial there has been no progression or development of new lesions during the first year of life while infants were being treated but there are a small number of children with later recurrence.[455] Recurrences were documented in a subset of the children in the U.S. (Chicago) National Collaborative Treatment Trial who were treated during their first year of life. All these children were examined by a single observer at specified intervals. The examinations are when they reach 1, 3.5, 5, 7.5, 10, and 15 years of age. The median age for the treated children is approximately 5 years old. The presence of new eye lesions was noted. The children in this cohort who have developed eye lesions are listed in Table 5–22, as well as various aspects of their clinical findings.

Another group of children were referred to the U.S. (Chicago) National Collaborative Treatment Trial. This latter group of children were called historical "untreated" patients because they had not received treatment during their first year of life. They were usually referred because quiescent retinal disease was noted (see Table 5–22).

Among 47 patients with subclinical congenital toxoplasmosis at birth, the overall incidence of retinal lesions was 30%[608] (Table 5–23). It was less in the first 4 years of life (approximately 23%) than after 5 years of age (40 to 50%). Thus, localized ocular phenomena frequently develop as a late manifestation.[1, 554, 557, 609] De Roever-Bonnet and colleagues[557] postulated that late development of eye lesions may be caused by second infections rather than by relapses, although there have been no supporting data for this hypothesis.

The occurrence of consecutive cases of ocular toxoplasmosis has been reported in siblings.[235, 610] Data are not adequate to prove that these cases were not due to postnatally acquired infection.

Lappalainen and her colleagues observed typical retinal scars of congenital toxoplasmosis in three infants who were seronegative by the age of 1 year. They were born to mothers who had seroconverted during the first trimester.[611] By the age of 5 years, one of these children had seroconverted. Seronegativity in congenital ocular disease had also been observed by Koppe and co-workers in two children who had become seronegative by the ages of 9 and 14 years.[366] Gross and co-workers[612] reported a congenitally infected child in whom attempts at diagnosis had failed with relatively insensitive serologic techniques (the CF test) but succeeded with immunoblot and PCR; one wonders if IgG antibody would indeed have been demonstrable had serology been performed with more sensitive and specific serologic methods (e.g., the Sabin-Feldman dye test). This raises the question as to how frequently negative *T. gondii* serology (and thus a missed diagnosis) actually occurs in children with clinical

TABLE 5–22
New or Recrudescent Retinal Lesions in Treated and Historical Patients That Occurred After 1 Year of Age

GROUP	PATIENT NUMBER	AGE (YR) NOTED[a]	PREVIOUS EYE LESION	ACTIVE	LOCATION	VISUAL ACUITY BEFORE; AFTER	SEROLOGY DURING RELAPSE
Treated	7	6[A], 10[A]	No, Yes	Yes	Perimacular, peripheral[b]	20/20; 20/20[c]	Not acute, N/A
	9	5[A]	No	No	Posterior pole	Nl; 20/50	N/A
	12	3[A], 10[A]	No, Yes	Yes	Peripheral, peripapillary[b]	20/20; 20/30	Not acute
	13	7[B]	Yes	Yes[d]	Perimacular[b]	6/400; 20/200	Not acute
	15	3[A]	Yes	No	Peripheral[b]	20/30; 20/30	N/A
	19	5[C], 8[C]	Yes	Yes[d]	Peripheral[b]	20/20; 20/20	Not acute
	21	4[A]	Yes	No	Perimacular[b]	Abnl; 1/30	N/A
Historical (untreated)	20	3[A]	Yes	Yes[d]	Peripheral	1/30; 20/400	Not acute
	25	10[A]	Yes	No	Peripheral	20/400; 18/200	Not acute
	27	7[A]	Yes	No	Perimacular	3/30; 5/30	N/A
	42	10[A]	Yes	Yes[d]	Perimacular[b]	20/30; 20/30	Not acute
	46	24[A]	Yes	Yes[d]	Perimacular[b]	20/60; 20/60	Not acute
	62	11[C], 13[C], 15[B]	Yes	Yes[d]	Perimacular, peripheral	20/20; 20/15	N/A
	82	16[A]	Yes	Yes[d]	Peripapillary	20/400; 20/400	Not acute
	89	12[B]	Yes	Yes[d]	Perimacular	20/100; N/A	Not acute

These data are from the U.S. (Chicago) National Collaborative Treatment Trial; patient numbers are those used in all prior publications. Recurrences were documented in a subset of the children in the U.S. (Chicago) National Collaborative Treatment Trial who were treated during their first year of life. All these children were examined in Chicago by a single observer at specified intervals. The examinations are when they reach 1, 3.5, 5, 7.5, 10, and 15 years of age. The median age for the treated children is approximately 5 years old. The presence of new eye lesions was noted. Historical patients were not treated in the first year of life and were referred after that time. There were 18 historical patients and 76 treated patients.

[a]Recurrence documented at visit in Chicago (A), recurrence documented by history (B), photographs reviewed in Chicago, and recurrence documented by history only (C).
[b]Satellites of earlier lesion.
[c]Quantitative visual acuity measured using Snellen chart or Allen cards.
[d]Symptoms present during active disease.
N/A = not available; Nl = normal; Abnl = abnormal.
From Mets MB, et al. Eye manifestations of congenital toxoplasmosis. Am J Ophthalmol 122:309–324, 1996.

TABLE 5–23
Results of Funduscopic Examination in 47 Patients with Congenital Toxoplasmosis Who Were Asymptomatic at Birth[a]

AGE[b]	NO. OF PATIENTS WITH NORMAL FUNDI	NO. OF PATIENTS WITH CHORIORETINITIS	ESTIMATED INCIDENCE OF OCULAR LESIONS (%)
0–11 mo	8	3	27
1–4 yr	17	5	23
5–9 yr	6	4	40
>10 yr	2	2	50

[a]Children were selected who had congenital toxoplasmosis, either clinical or subclinical, with normal fundi at birth.

[b]Age = the age at the time of the last normal funduscopic examination or the first examination showing chorioretinitis, if chorioretinitis developed.

Adapted from Desmonts G. Some remarks on the immunopathology of toxoplasmic uveitis. In Böke W, Luntz MH (eds). Modern Problems in Ophthalmology. Ocular Immune Responses, vol 16. Basel, S. Karger, 1976.

features considered diagnostic of congenital toxoplasmic retinochoroiditis. In such cases, sera should be tested by multiple methods in a reference laboratory.

Features of External Clinical Examination

Microphthalmia, small cornea, posterior cortical cataract, anisometropia, strabismus, and nystagmus may be present. Leukocoria has been reported.[455, 613] Nystagmus may result either from poor fixation related to the chorioretinitis or from involvement of the CNS. A history of "dancing eyes" should always raise the possibility of a bilateral congenital central chorioretinitis—the typical ocular lesion of congenital toxoplasmosis. Convergent or divergent strabismus may be caused by direct involvement of the extraocular muscles or may result from involvement of the brain.

The iris and ciliary body may be affected by foci of inflammation with formation of synechiae. As a result, dilatation of the pupils with mydriatics may be difficult.

Features of Funduscopic Examination

The characteristic lesion of ocular toxoplasmosis is a focal necrotizing retinitis (Fig. 5–10), which is most often bilateral.[614] Such lesions in the acute or subacute stage of inflammation appear as yellowish white, cotton-like patches in the fundus. They may be solitary lesions that are about the same size as the optic disk or a little larger. More often, however, they appear in small clusters, among which lesions of various ages can be discerned. The more acute lesions are soft and cotton-like, with indistinct borders; the older lesions are whitish gray, sharply outlined, and spotted by accumulations of choroidal pigment. The inflammatory exudate that is cast off from the surface of the acute lesions is often so dense that clear visualization of the fundus is impossible. In such cases, the most that can be discerned is a whitish mass against the pale orange background of the fundus. The posterior hyaloid membrane is often detached, and

precipitates of inflammatory cells—the equivalents of keratic precipitates in the anterior segment of the eye—are seen on the posterior face of the vitreous.

Retinal edema, that affects especially the macular and peripapillary areas, is commonly observed in the subacute phase of inflammation. Edema of the macula is almost always present when acute inflammatory foci in the retina are situated above the macula. In older children, this edema is the principal cause of blurred vision when other causes, such as a central retinal lesion, involvement of the optic nerve, or extensive clouding of the vitreous, can be excluded. Macular edema is usually temporary, although cystic changes in the fovea sometimes occur as a result of long-standing edema. In this instance, central visual acuity may be permanently impaired despite the absence of central lesions or involvement of the optic nerve.

The optic nerve may be affected either primarily, resulting from destruction of the macula and other portions of the retina, or secondarily, resulting from papilledema. Manschot and Daamen and others have described T. gondii in the optic nerve itself,[470] or optic nerve inflammation.[460]

What at first appears to be primary involvement of the optic nerve head, with papilledema and exudation of cells into the overlying vitreous, often turns out to be a juxtapapillary lesion. A retinal lesion contiguous to the head of the optic nerve can produce swelling and inflammation in the nerve, but when the acute lesion subsides it becomes clear that the optic nerve itself has been spared and that a narrow rim of normal tissue separates the lesion from the nerve head.

Segmental atrophy of the optic nerve, characterized by pallor and loss of substance, especially of the temporal portion of the nerve head, often occurs in the wake of a macular lesion. In these cases, the prognosis is, of course, for limited vision.

Although the majority of lesions described in the older

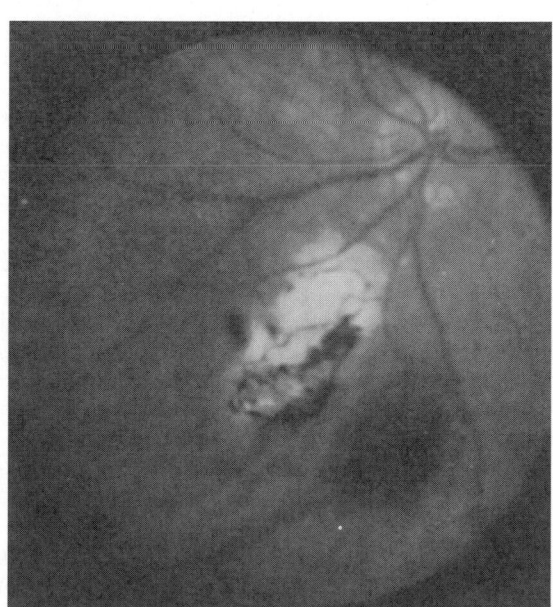

FIGURE 5–10 Chorioretinitis in congenital toxoplasmosis.

literature are at or near the posterior pole of the retina, peripheral lesions have been described. In one series of more than 100 children with congenital toxoplasmosis,[455] there were more peripheral lesions. However, considering the relative size of the macula and peripheral retina, macular lesions were predominant. These have roughly the same morphology as the more central lesions, but they tend to be less significant as a cause of visual loss unless they are accompanied by massive contractures of the overlying vitreous and subsequent retinal detachment.

The anterior uvea is often the site of intense inflammation characterized by redness of the external eye, cells and protein in the anterior chamber, large keratic precipitates, posterior synechiae, nodules on the iris, and, occasionally, neovascular formations on the surface of the iris. This reaction may be accompanied by high rises of intraocular pressure and by cataracts.

Isolated iritis should not be taken as an indication of toxoplasmosis. To be considered as a manifestation of toxoplasmosis, iritis should be preceded or at least accompanied by a posterior lesion. The same can be said of scleritis, which may be observed external to a focus of toxoplasmic chorioretinitis; it has no significance by itself as a sign of toxoplasmosis.

Ophthalmoscopic features of the intraocular lesions of congenital toxoplasmosis in infants are those listed in Table 5–26 (see later) and have been reported[491] to include (1) unilateral or bilateral involvement of the macular region; (2) bilateral occurrence of other lesions; (3) involvement of the periphery in one or more quadrants of the retina and choroid; (4) punched-out appearance of large and small lesions in the late phase; (5) occurrence of massive chorioretinal degeneration; (6) extensive connective tissue proliferation and heavy pigmentation, as contrasted to the dissociation of these changes in other chorioretinal lesions; (7) presence of an essentially normal retina and vasculature surrounding the lesions in all stages of the infection; (8) occurrence of associated congenital defects in the eyes; (9) rapid development of sequential optic nerve atrophy; and (10) frequent clarity of the media in the presence of severe chorioretinitis.

Hogan and co-workers tabulated the data from 22 cases of chorioretinitis in infants 6 months of age or younger with congenital toxoplasmosis (in 81%, the lesions were bilateral) from the literature published through 1949.[463] A precise determination of prevalence cannot be gleaned from these reports because for many of the infants the data were incomplete—for example, in some, no description of the fundus was provided, but other features such as microphthalmia were described. Of those infants for whom sufficient information was available, there were 7 with only healed retinal lesions, 5 with only acute lesions, and 4 with both acute and healed lesions. Macular involvement was seen in 5, and peripheral retinal involvement in 10; diffuse retinal involvement was present in 3. Twelve had microphthalmia, 5 had optic nerve atrophy, 3 had papilledema, 8 had strabismus, 7 had nystagmus, 10 had anterior segment involvement, and 2 had cataracts; in 10, parasites were noted in the retina at autopsy.

Franceschetti and Bamatter reviewed the signs in 243 cases of congenital ocular toxoplasmosis and found the following percentages: bilateral involvement in 66%, unilateral involvement in 34%, microphthalmia in 23%, optic atrophy in 27%, nystagmus in 23%, strabismus in 28%, cataract in 8%, iritis and posterior synechiae in 8%, persistence of pupillary membrane in 4%, and vitreous changes in 11%.[615]

The findings of Mets and colleagues[455] in the children in the United States (U.S. [Chicago] National Collaborative Treatment Trial) are shown in Table 5–24.

Differential Diagnosis of Eye Lesions

Congenital Anomalies. The healed foci of toxoplasmic chorioretinitis may resemble a colobomatous defect[6] (Fig. 5–11). The associated ocular, systemic, and serologic changes make toxoplasmosis the most likely diagnosis. Abnormal retinal morphology has been described in one fetal eye[460] and similar findings have been described in a variety of animal models of the congenital infection. Chromosome analysis was not available for the fetus, however.

Other Inflammatory Lesions. The differential diagnosis of eye lesions includes many of the inflammatory lesions described in Chapters 6, 7, 8, and 12. Lymphochoriomeningitis virus can also cause similar lesions.

TABLE 5–24
Ophthalmologic Manifestations of Congenital Toxoplasmosis in Children in U.S. (Chicago) National Collaborative Treatment Trial[a]

	NUMBER WITH FINDING (%)		
	Treated Patients n = 76	Historical Patients n = 18	Total n = 94
Strabismus	26 (34)	5 (28)	31 (33)
Nystagmus	20 (26)	5 (28)	25 (27)
Microphthalmia	10 (13)	2 (11)	12 (13)
Phthisis	4 (5)	0 (0)	4 (4)
Microcornea	15 (20)	3 (17)	18 (19)
Cataract	7 (9)	2 (11)	9 (10)
Vitritis (active)	3 (4)[b]	2 (11)	5 (5)
Retinitis (active)	6 (8)	4 (22)	10 (11)
Chorioretinal scars	56 (74)	18 (100)	74 (79)
Macular	39/72 (54)[c]	13/17 (76)	52/89 (58)
Juxtapapillary	37/72 (51)	9/17 (53)	46/89 (52)
Peripheral	43/72 (58)	14/17 (82)	57/89 (64)
Retinal detachment	7 (9)	2 (11)	9 (10)
Optic atrophy	14 (18)	5 (28)	19 (20)

[a]Children were either treated with pyrimethamine and sulfadiazine during their first year of life (treated patients) or referred after their first year of life when they had not been treated (historical patients). In general, historical patients were referred because they had eye disease. Current mean ages of the children in these groups are in Table 5–53.

[b]Two additional patients, not included in this table, were receiving treatment, and retinochoroiditis had resolved but vitreous cells and veils persisted at time of examination.

[c]Numerator represents number with finding. Denominator represents n, unless otherwise specified. Number in parentheses is percentage. Patients with bilateral retinal detachment in whom the location of scars was not possible were excluded from the denominator.

From Mets MB, et al. Eye manifestations of congenital toxoplasmosis. Am J Ophthalmol 122:309–324, 1996.

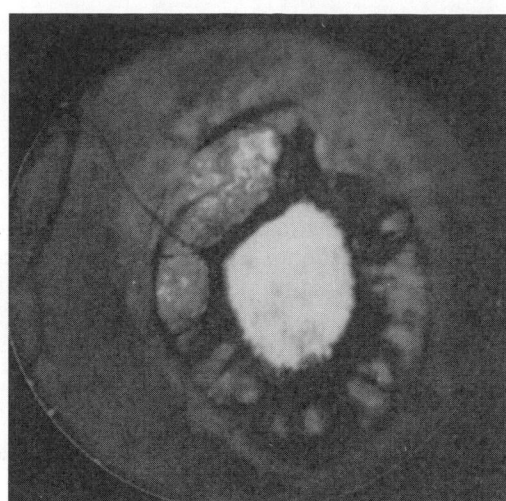

FIGURE 5–11 Macular pseudocoloboma of the retina in congenital toxoplasmosis.

Birth Injury. Intraocular hemorrhage may be unrecognized and may cause retinal damage with gliosis and fibrosis. The lesion is usually unilateral, associated cerebral damage is absent, and there is no serologic evidence to support a diagnosis of toxoplasmosis. Retinopathy of prematurity may occur in conjunction with toxoplasmic chorioretinitis.

Circulatory Disturbances. Congenital aneurysms and telangiectasia of retinal vessels may result in extensive retinal fibrosis, with pigmentation and detachment. The disease is usually unilateral and is not associated with cerebral involvement or other changes.

Neoplasms. Retinoblastoma rarely may cause the picture described for ocular toxoplasmosis. It is most often unilateral and is unassociated with visceral or cerebral damage unless an advanced stage has been reached. Pseudoglioma may be difficult to distinguish from a healed chorioretinitis but is usually single and unilateral. Gliomas may be bilateral, progressing from a small nodule to a large polypoid mass protruding into the vitreous.

MENTAL RETARDATION

Numerous studies have attempted to establish a causative relationship between mental retardation and congenital toxoplasmosis. A prospective study on this subject is that of Alford and colleagues.[512, 616] When these workers noted that changes in CSF protein concentration and cell count were common in newborns with subclinical congenital toxoplasmosis, they set out to determine the significance of these changes in relation to later mental development. They compared the intellectual and social development of eight children, aged 2 to 4 years, who were identified at birth as having subclinical congenital toxoplasmosis, with those of eight matched controls. Their results revealed that there may be varying degrees of intellectual impairment in children who are asymptomatic at birth, reflecting the fact that brain damage does occur with subclinical congenital toxoplasmosis. The investigators concluded that although sub-

clinical congenital toxoplasmosis does not necessarily cause overt mental retardation, it may be associated with some degree of intellectual impairment. Further studies along these lines have corroborated these findings (see Follow-up section), but until a much larger number of infants are examined over a longer time, these data can be considered only tentative.

The total contribution of congenital toxoplasmosis, including the less severe and clinically inapparent forms at birth, to mental retardation is uncertain. One of the earliest studies from Europe was that of Thalhammer in Vienna, who classified congenital toxoplasmosis into three broad categories: (1) generalized, with hepatomegaly, jaundice, myocarditis, pneumonitis, and similar effects; (2) cerebral, accompanied by at least one of the two characteristic signs, namely, chorioretinitis and intracerebral calcification; and (3) cerebral, accompanied by damage but without these signs.[578] Thalhammer concluded that the first type was rare, the second not common enough to be a problem, and the third a common condition creating serious medical and social problems. He studied 1332 children with congenital cerebral damage that could not be accounted for by postnatal encephalitic illness. The results of this study are summarized in Table 5–25. In children with cerebral defects of all types, the prevalence of *T. gondii* infection was about 17% higher than in normal children. Although the frequency of *T. gondii* infection in this series was not measurably greater in children with microcephaly, hydrocephalus, and cerebral palsy than it was in normal children, it was much greater in those with epilepsy and mental retardation. Thalhammer concluded from these statistics that in about 20% of the cases of mental retardation the most important cerebral defects were due to congenital toxoplasmosis. Others have similarly concluded from their data that congenital toxoplasmosis is or may be an important cause of mental retardation.[592, 617, 620]

Through a series of computations from the data of others, Hume concluded that toxoplasmosis is the cause of at least 4% of the group composed of the "mentally retarded and [those with] cerebral dysfunction."[621] Inter-

TABLE 5–25

Frequency of *Toxoplasma* Infections in 1332 Children (Ages 1–14 Years) with Congenital Cerebral Defects Compared with 600 Normal Children

TYPE OF DEFECT	NO. TESTED	NO. POSITIVE[a] (%)
Microcephaly	57	2 (3.5)
Hydrocephalus	191	17 (8.9)
Cerebral palsy	55	5 (9.1)
Epilepsy	344	73 (21.2)
Mental retardation	685	167 (24.4)
Cerebral defects (all types)	1332	264 (19.8)
None (normal)	600	20 (3.3)

[a]Dye test titers of 1 : 4 or higher were considered to be positive.
Adapted from Thalhammer O. Congenital toxoplasmosis. Lancet 1:23–24, 1962, with permission.

pretation of many of these studies, as well as those by workers who found little or no significant difference between mentally retarded and control populations,[559, 590, 622-630] is complicated by the high prevalence of acquired toxoplasmosis in control subjects, which may mask the possible role of congenital toxoplasmosis in mental retardation (as well as other sequelae of encephalopathy such as convulsions). For example, if the proportion of cases of mental retardation is small and the prevalence of *T. gondii* antibody titers in the control population is high, it is not possible with presently available diagnostic techniques to distinguish those cases in which *T. gondii* is the cause of mental retardation. Another cause of the variations in reported results is the choice of controls. In many studies, subjects were not properly matched, and the differences or lack of differences found was due solely to differences in populations from which the patients were chosen.[624]

Only through large-scale prospective studies of infection with *T. gondii* acquired during the course of pregnancy, compiled by means of long-term observations of the infants, will accurate figures be obtained on the contribution of congenital *T. gondii* infection to mental deficiency (as well as epilepsy, blindness, and other disorders).

DOWN SYNDROME

Although numerous investigators have interpreted their data as evidence of an association between toxoplasmosis in the mother and Down syndrome in the offspring,[631-636] such an association has never been proved satisfactorily.[636] In a study of 71 such children, Thalhammer found a higher than normal prevalence of *T. gondii* antibodies.[591] He attributed the higher prevalence to their mental deficiency and suggested that their institutional environment probably favored a higher rate of acquired infection; the prevalence of *T. gondii* antibodies was no different from that of normal controls in the age group birth to 5 years and rose to levels higher than those demonstrated in controls only in the older age groups. Until adequate data to the contrary are furnished, the association between Down syndrome and toxoplasmosis in a newborn must be considered coincidental. Frenkel[637] points out that, in view of the chromosomal aberrations in Down syndrome, it would be necessary to demonstrate that toxoplasmosis is related to the nonhereditary or nondisjunction form of Down syndrome; if this is true, one would have to postulate an influence of *T. gondii* on the ovum, which thus far has not been demonstrated.[631] Much of the literature on this subject, as well as that on the relationship of toxoplasmosis to other entities in the newborn, is purely speculative.

ENDOCRINE ORGANS

The endocrine disorders that have been associated with congenital toxoplasmosis are nonspecific, because they reflect the severity of the infection in those areas of the brain that are related to endocrine function. Two cases in which congenital toxoplasmosis and congenital myxedema occurred simultaneously have been reported.[638, 639] Because each of these conditions is relatively uncommon, their concurrent appearance suggests more than mere coincidence. *T. gondii* has been demonstrated in histologic sections of the pituitary and thyroid glands of infants dying of toxoplasmosis, and it may be that such involvement contributed to or resulted in myxedema in these patients. Silver and Dixon described persistent hypernatremia in an infant who had evidence of vasopressin-sensitive diabetes insipidus without polyuria or polydipsia.[593] This was associated with a marked eosinophilia in blood and bone marrow. A similar case was described by Margit and Istvan.[640] Diabetes insipidus has occurred in the perinatal period or developed later in childhood.[489, 641] This is most likely secondary to pituitary-hypothalamic *T. gondii* infection. It has occurred in infants and children with severe brain damage and hydrocephalus as well as in children who have only intracerebral calcifications.[489, 642, 643]

Bruhl and colleagues reported sexual precocity in association with congenital toxoplasmosis in a male infant who, at the age of 2 years, showed rapid growth of the external genitalia and appearance of pubic hair, along with generalized convulsions, microcephaly, severe mental retardation, bilateral microphthalmia, and blindness (deafness was suspected, because the child did not respond to noises).[644] After 9 years of hospitalization, he died at the age of 13.5 years. The early onset of growth of the penis and testes and the development of pubic hair, as well as testicular biopsy and hormone assays, established the diagnosis of true precocity in this case. A cause-and-effect relationship between toxoplasmosis and precocious puberty could not be proved, but the presence of two rare disorders in the same patient suggested such a relationship. Also, a variety of lesions involving the hypothalamus has been associated with precocious puberty, and the third ventricle was dilated and the hypothalamus was distorted in this patient. The anterior pituitary appeared normal at autopsy—a prerequisite to development of precocious puberty in patients with lesions in or near the hypothalamus. Partial anterior hypopituitarism was observed in the infant reported by Coppola and co-workers.[645] Massa and associates described three cases with growth hormone deficiency, two of whom were gonadotropin deficient and one of whom had precocious puberty in addition to central diabetes insipidus.[641]

In the study performed by Meenken and associates[605] (described previously under the section on Chorioretinitis), overt endocrinologic disease was diagnosed in 5 of 15 patients with severe congenital toxoplasmosis, all of whom had serious eye disease due to the infection. Panhypopituitarism was observed in 2, gonadal failure with dwarfism in 1, precocious puberty with dwarfism and thyroid deficiency in 1, and diabetes mellitus and thyroid deficiency in 1. The investigators found that the major manifestations of the endocrine disease in these patients occurred at the mean age of 12 years (range, 9–16 years) and was associated with obstructive hydrocephalus and dilated third ventricle in each case.

NEPHROTIC SYNDROME

In infants with congenital toxoplasmosis, generalized edema and ascites may reflect the presence of the nephrotic syndrome.[507, 508, 510, 646] Protein and casts have been reported in the urine in these cases, as have hypoproteinemia, hypoalbuminemia, and hypercholesterolemia. In one case, there was a marked decrease in the serum IgG level, but IgM and IgA levels were normal.[508] (Hypogammaglobulinemia has been reported to be associated with congenital toxoplasmosis in the absence of nephrosis.[647])

RADIOLOGIC STUDIES

Brain

Hydrocephalus is characteristically due to periaqueductal involvement. Obstruction of the aqueduct of Sylvius leads to enlargement of the third and lateral ventricles (Fig. 5–12A). Obstruction of the foramen of Monro can lead to unilateral hydrocephalus (Fig. 5–12B and Fig. 5–13).[489] Dramatic resolution and brain cortical expansion and growth can occur in conjunction with ventriculoperitoneal shunt placement and antimicrobial therapy

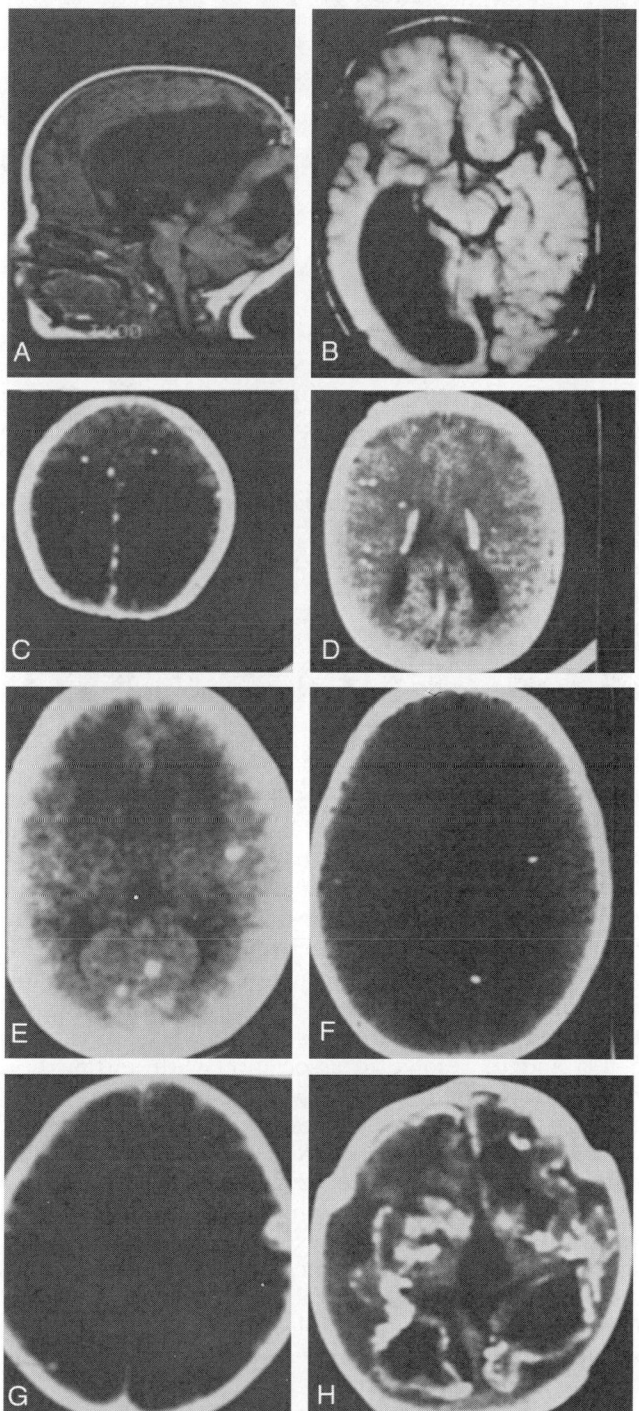

FIGURE 5–12 Neuroradiographic findings in congenital toxoplasmosis. The remarkable clinical improvements in the treated children and their brain radiographs in C to F are particularly noteworthy. A, MRI of the brain demonstrating obstruction of the aqueduct of Sylvius and consequent dilation of the third and lateral ventricles. B, MRI of the brain demonstrating unilateral hydrocephalus. C and D, Brain CT scans in the early newborn period (C) and of the same child at 1 year of age (D) following shunt placement and antimicrobial therapy. This child is developmentally and neurologically normal at 1 year of age. E and F, Brain CT scans of another child in the early newborn period (E) and of this same child at 1 year of age (F) following antimicrobial therapy. The resolution or diminution of calcifications is noteworthy and has occurred in a substantial number (but not all) of treated children in the Chicago study. This child is also developmentally and neurologically normal. G, Brain CT scan that demonstrates a ring-enhancing lesion and calcifications. H, Brain CT scan showing extremely extensive intracerebral calcifications and hydrocephalus. (These figures were reproduced from McAuley J, Roizen N, Patel D, et al. Early and longitudinal evaluations of treated infants and children and untreated historical patients with congenital toxoplasmosis: the Chicago Collaborative Treatment Trial. Clin Infect Dis 18:38–72, 1994; Patel D, Vogel N, Roizen N, et al. Neuroradiologic findings in 65 patients with congenital toxoplasmosis. In progress; McLeod R, Wisner J, Boyer K. Toxoplasmosis. In Krugman S, Katz S, Wilfert C, et al [eds]. Infectious Diseases of Children, 8th ed. St. Louis, CV Mosby, 1992, pp 518–550, with permission.)

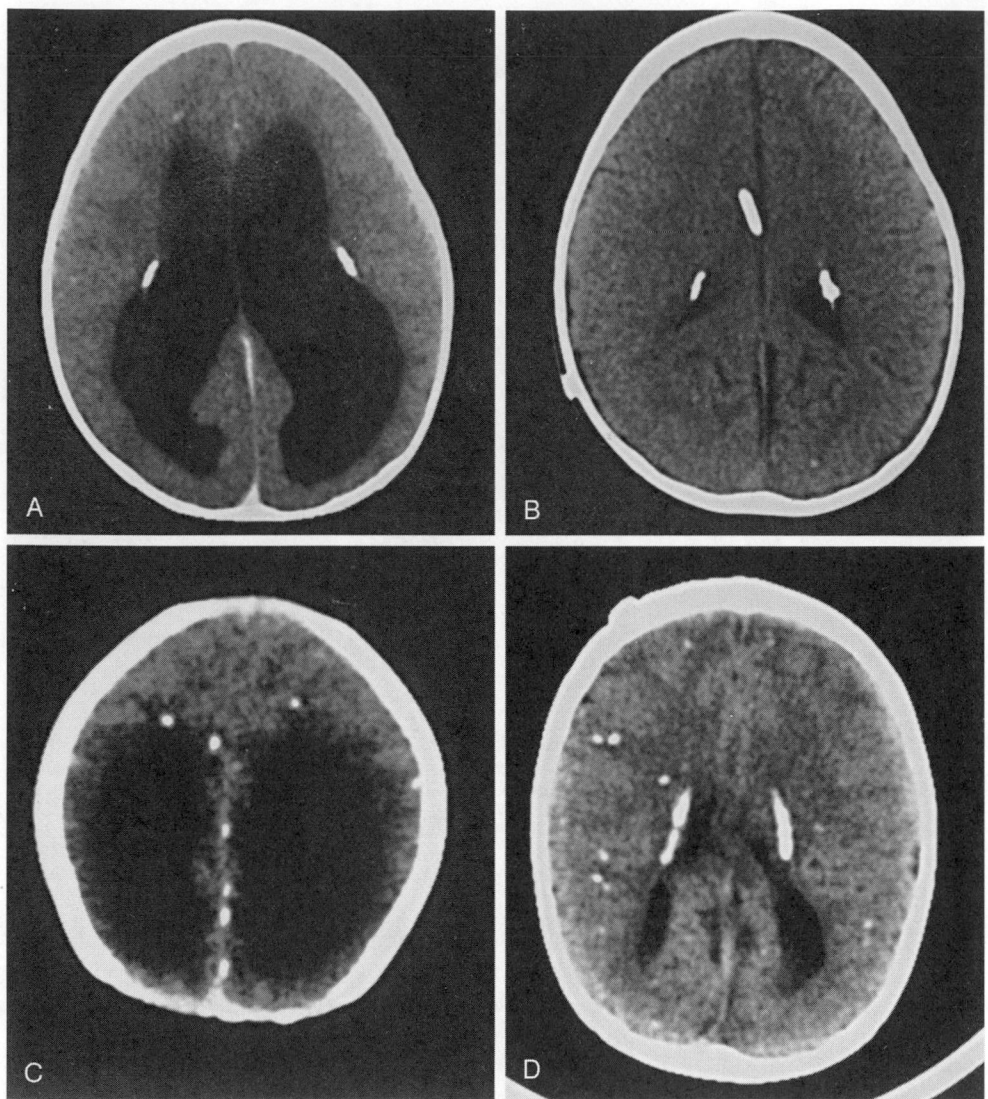

FIGURE 5–13 Cranial CT scans of two infants (one represented in *A* and *B*, the other in *C* and *D*) before (*A* and *C*) and after (*B* and *D*) placement of ventriculoperitoneal shunts. Both infants have developed normally. CT scans and the subsequent normal development of these children indicate that it is not possible to predict ultimate cognitive outcome from the initial appearance of the CT scan. (From Boyer KM, McLeod RL. *Toxoplasma gondii* [toxoplasmosis]. *In* Long SS, Prober CG, Pickering LK [eds]. Principles and Practice of Pediatric Infectious Diseases. New York, Churchill Livingstone, 1997, pp 1421–1448.)

(see Figs. 5–12*C* and *D* and 5–13) Calcifications may be single or multiple (see Figs. 5–12*E* to *H* and 5–14 and, surprisingly, in some cases have resolved with antimicrobial therapy during the first year of life (see Figs. 5–12*E* and *F* and 5–14).[648] Contrast-enhancing lesions have been detected, indicating active encephalitis (see Fig. 5–12*G*).[489] Massive hydrocephalus, as documented by ultrasound, has been noted to develop in fetuses and newborns within a period as brief as 1 week (see Fig. 5–14) and to resolve in association with antimicrobial treatment in one fetus (Fig. 5–15).[649]

Radiologic signs in newborns exposed to primary *T. gondii* infection in utero were described by Virkola and colleagues.[650] There were 42 mothers (37 delivered of live born infants and 5 who had spontaneous abortions) with follow up. The findings on brain ultrasonography associated with infection included calcifications, cysts, and candlestick sign; and those on abdominal ultrasonography were enlarged spleen and ascites. In some instances, these findings were associated with abnormalities in the newborn period.

Puri and co-workers described a 2-week-old infant with hydrocephalus.[651] A brain scan with ^{99m}Tc-pertechnetate showed an area of increased uptake in the left temporoparietal region. A four-vessel angiogram showed large ventricles with a mass lesion in the left hemisphere pushing midline structures to the right. An electroencephalogram was abnormal, with sharp θ activity in the left parietotemporal area. A bubble ventriculogram showed obstruction of the left foramen of Monro. Because of the rapid deterioration of the patient's condition, a craniotomy was performed; it revealed a large granular infiltrating tumor in the left temporal region. *T. gondii* organisms were seen in great profusion in the operative specimen of brain. A similar cerebral mass lesion was described by Hervei and Simon in a case of congenital toxoplasmosis[652] and by Bobowski and Reed in a case of acquired toxoplasmosis.[653] Hervas and colleagues reported a newborn with congenital toxoplasmosis whose cranial CT scan with contrast medium enhancement demonstrated calcifications and multiple ring-enhanced lesions not dissimilar to those seen in adult patients with AIDS with multiple brain abscesses related to *T. gondii*.[486] McAuley and co-workers[489] also

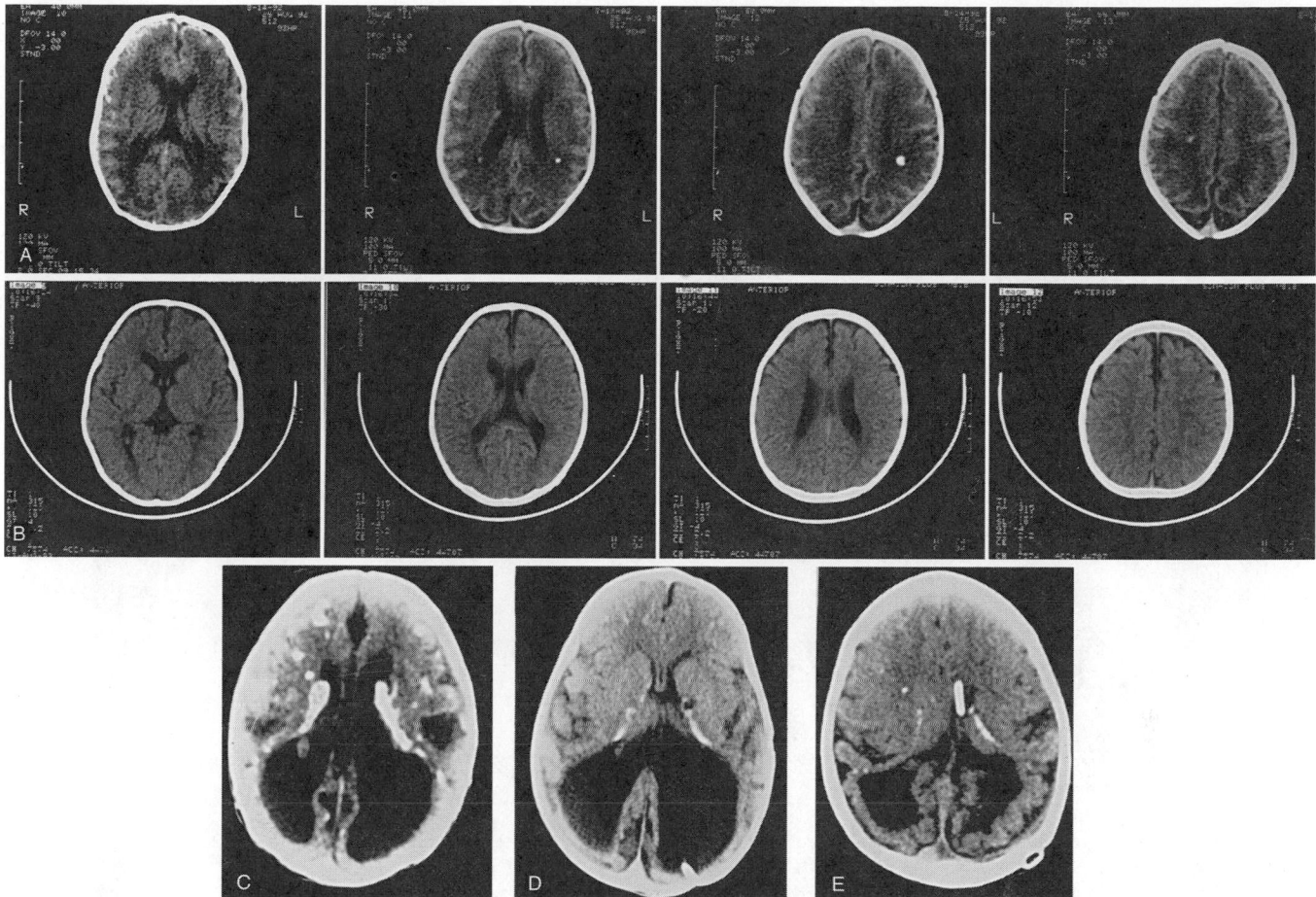

FIGURE 5–14 Additional examples of cranial CT scans that demonstrate resolution of calcifications in treated children. *A* and *B*, CT scans in a treated infant obtained at birth, August 1992 *(A)* and August 1993 *(B)*. *C–E*, Diminution and/or resolution of large areas of calcification are seen in these representative cranial CT scans from another treated infant. Cranial CT scans in this treated infant obtained *(C)* at birth, February 1987, *(D)* at follow-up, May 1988, and *(E)* July 1991.

Illustration continued on following page

described enhancement around a lesion that resolved with antimicrobial treatment.

CT, which allows for neuroanatomic localization of intracranial calcifications, delineation of ventricular size, and recognition of cortical atrophy, has proved to be valuable in evaluation of congenital toxoplasmosis.[654–657] Diebler and associates published results of CT in 32 cases of congenital toxoplasmosis.[655] They reported a clear relationship between the lesions observed on these scans, neurologic signs, and date of maternal infection. The destructive lesions were porencephalic cysts that when multiple may constitute multicystic encephalomalacia or even hydranencephaly. Dense and large calcifications were seen in the basal ganglia of seven cases, with or without periventricular calcifications. Hydrocephalus was always secondary to aqueductal stenosis. In one case, ocular calcification was noted. In a retrospective study of cases in which pachygyria-like changes were observed on CT or magnetic resonance imaging, a single case of congenital toxoplasmosis was noted.[658] Ultrasonography has also been suggested as useful for diagnosis of congenital toxoplasmosis. CT of the brain detects calcifications not seen with ultrasonography of the brain.[659, 660]

Intracranial Calcification

With rare exceptions,[502] the deposits of calcium noticed in congenital toxoplasmosis have been limited to the intracranial structures. The deposits are scattered throughout the brain and in some studies have been reported to have no characteristic distribution. In other studies, many children were observed to have prominent basal ganglia and periventricular califications.[648, 661–665] Masherpa and Valentino described two types of calcifications: (1) multiple, dense round deposits 1 to 3 mm in diameter scattered in the white matter and, more frequently, in the periventricular areas of the occipitoparietal and temporal regions; and (2) curvilinear streaks in the basal ganglia, mostly in the head of the caudate nucleus.[663] Some workers consider that evidence of both nodular calcifications and linear calcifications is pathognomonic of toxoplasmosis (Figs. 5–16 and 5–17).

Although in cytomegalic inclusion disease the calcifications are chiefly located subependymally and are bilaterally symmetrical, mostly in the walls of the dilated ventricles,[664, 665] these locations are also found in congenital toxoplasmosis. The largest series of cases of cerebral calcification related to congenital toxoplasmosis are

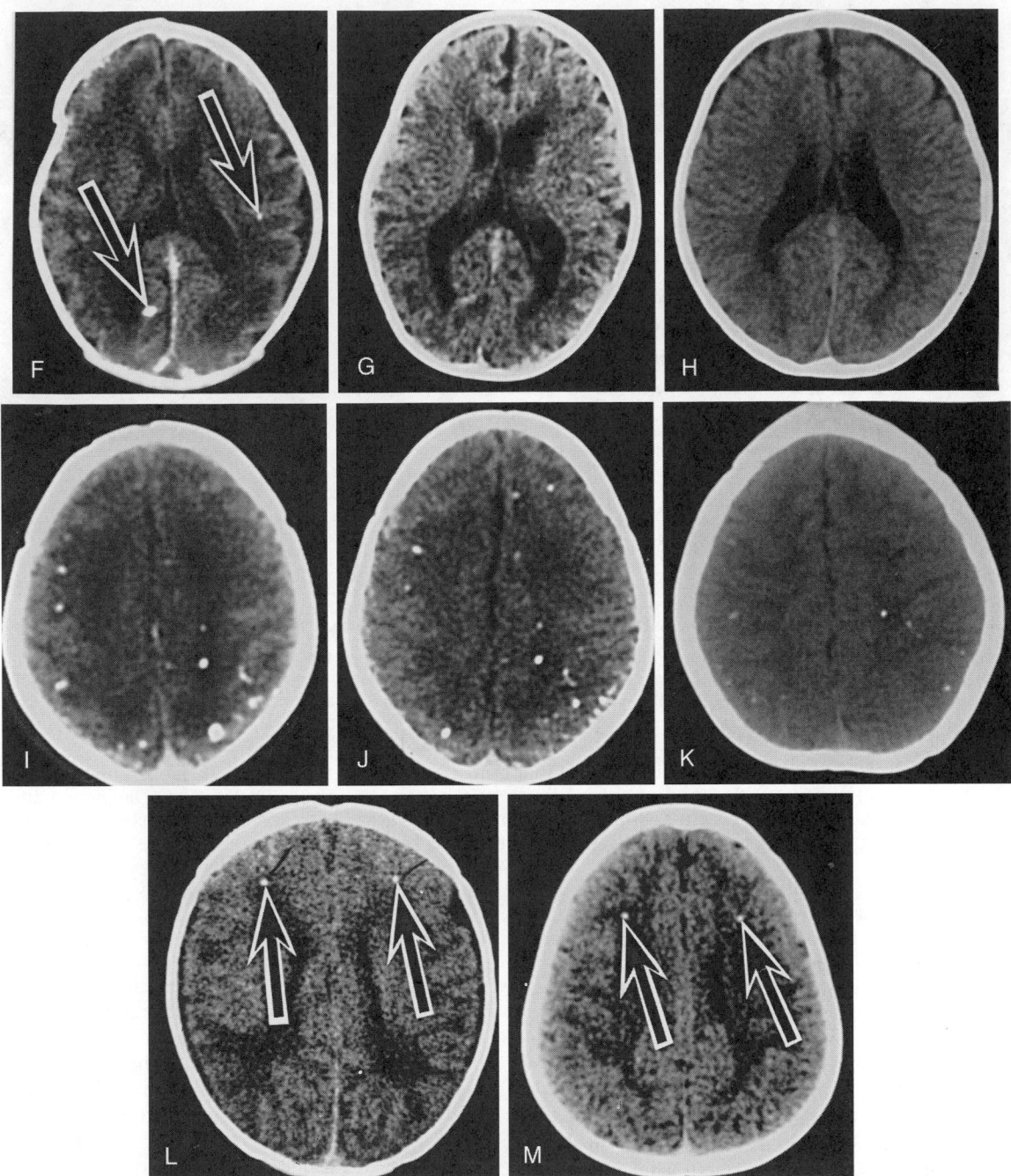

FIGURE 5–14 *Continued F–H,* Cranial CT scans of the dizygotic twin of patient in Figure 5–4 (*A* and *B*). Newborn scan obtained *(F)* August 1992. The calcifications (arrows) were seen to have resolved on follow-up scans obtained *(G)* November 1992 and *(H)* August 1993. *Note:* patient in Figure 5–4 (*A* and *B*) was randomized to receive initial higher dose therapy (6 months of 1 mg/kg/day of pyrimethamine) and patient in Figure 5–4 *(F–H)* was randomized to receive initial lower dose therapy (2 months of 1 mg/kg/day of pyrimethamine). Both infants completed 1 year of treatment with pyrimethamine 1 mg/kg each Monday, Wednesday, and Friday and sulfadiazine. Calcifications were seen to have resolved completely in cranial CT scans of both twins. *I–K,* Cranial CT scans obtained for another infant in the newborn period *(I),* January 1993, *(J)* at follow-up, February 1993, and *(K)* January 1994 demonstrate diminution and/or resolution of calcifications. This child has developed normally. *L* and *M,* Cranial CT scans obtained in the newborn period *(L),* May 1991, and *(M)* August 1992 in a different, noncompliant child who was treated in our study for only 1 month. Arrows mark calcifications that remained the same size. (From Patel DV, et al. Resolution of intracranial calcifications in infants with treated congenital toxoplasmosis. Radiology 199:433–440, 1996, with minor modifications and permission.)

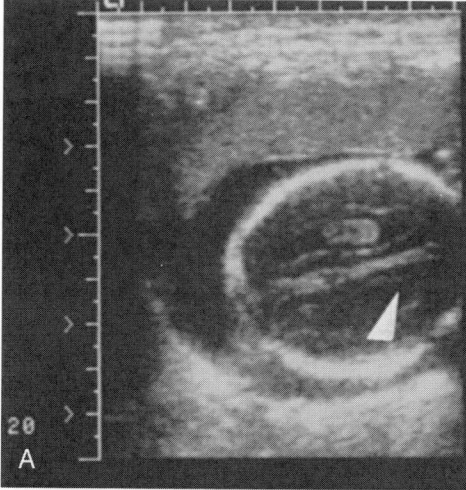

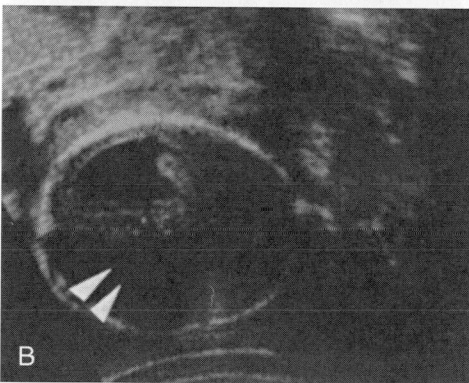

FIGURE 5–15 Rapid development of massive hydrocephalus in a fetus between 20 *(A)* and 21 *(B)* weeks of gestation. Single arrowhead indicates cerebral ventricles in *A* and double arrowheads indicate massively dilated ventricles in *B.*

studied at approximately 1 year of age; in these children, a diagnosis of congenital toxoplasmosis had been made through a systematic survey. The increase in size and number of calcific lesions during a period of months or years in some cases suggests that the process of healing (and perhaps also of destruction) may occur long after the onset of the infection. Calcifications can diminish in size or resolve with treatment.[648]

Osseous Changes

In 1974, Milgram described the radiographic signs present in an infant who died 17 days after birth with a severe clinical form of congenital toxoplasmosis.[472] Roentgenograms of several ribs and vertebrae and one femur revealed bands of metaphyseal lucency and irregularity of the line of provisional calcification at the epiphyseal plates. Periosteal reaction was not present. (Syphilis may also cause this same finding.)

Liver

Although it has been stated that calcifications do not occur outside the CNS in infants with congenital toxoplasmosis, Caldera and colleagues described cases of three infants with calcifications in the liver.[502] The calcifications were evident both radiologically and in the liver at autopsy.

Kove and co-workers described the pattern of serum transaminase activity in a newborn with cytomegalic

those of Dyke and colleagues[666] and of Müssbichler.[667] The latter reviewed material from 32 clinically well-documented cases. Approximately one third of the patients were 3 months of age or less, and 80% were younger than 2 years of age. Müssbichler's findings—some original and others confirming the findings of others—revealed that calcifications in the caudate nucleus, choroid plexuses, meninges, and subependyma are characteristic in toxoplasmosis, although some of these locations have also been described in cytomegalic inclusion disease. Because calcifications were present in multiple areas of the brain in the cases he reviewed, he concluded that calcifications found in the choroid plexuses alone should not be regarded as evidence of toxoplasmosis. Müssbichler found calcifications in the meninges that had not previously been described and attributed his ability to locate them to the use of appropriate projections that delineated them clearly. For these untreated children calcifications in the meninges and caudate nucleus were signs of a poor prognosis; they were found only in the youngest children, who died early. Conversely, disseminated nodular calcifications do not necessarily suggest a poor prognosis and have been discovered fortuitously in "normal" infants who were

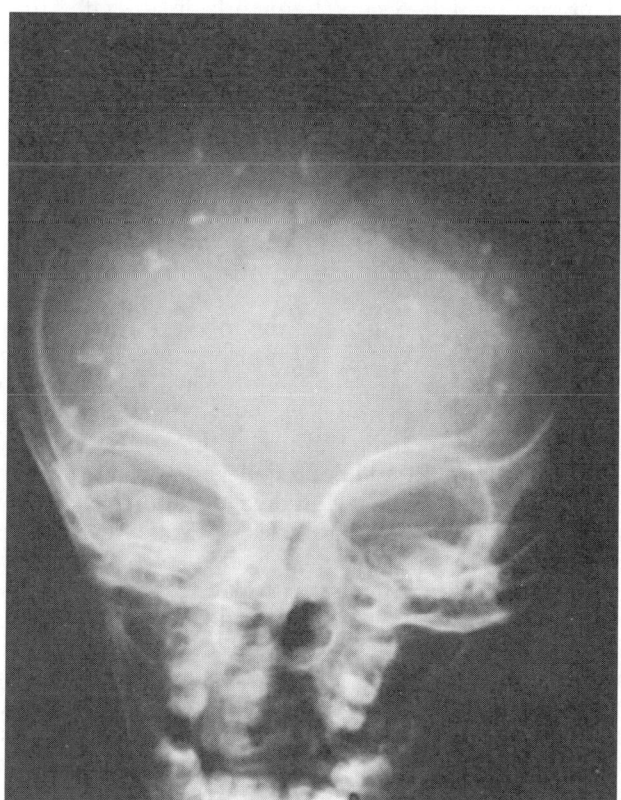

FIGURE 5–16 Cerebral calcifications in congenital toxoplasmosis in a 10-month-old infant; the infection was subclinical. (Courtesy of J Couvreur, Paris.)

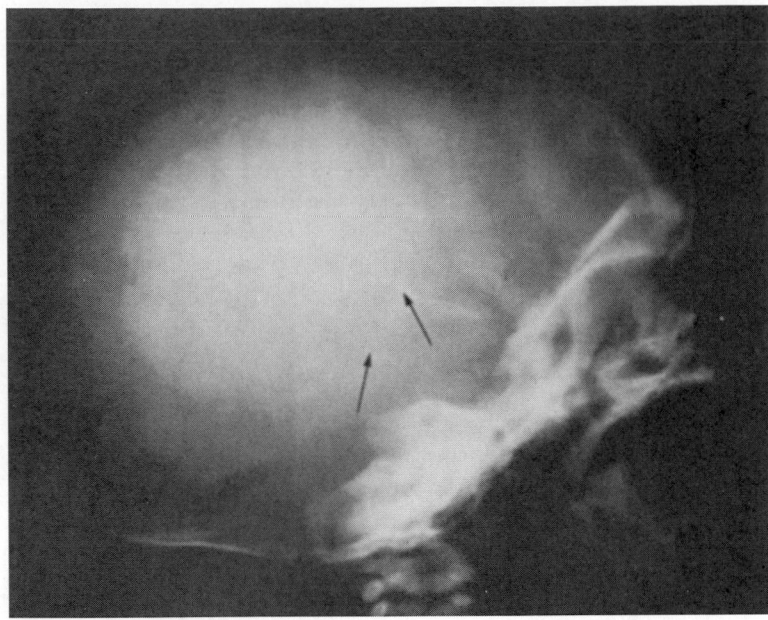

FIGURE 5–17 Cerebral calcifications in congenital toxoplasmosis in a neonate with calcifications lining the ventricles (arrows). (Courtesy of J Couvreur, Paris.)

inclusion disease and in another with congenital toxoplasmosis.[668] Both developed jaundice. The patterns were unique and unlike those observed in infants with other causes of neonatal jaundice. The investigators pointed out that more studies are necessary to determine if serial measurements of serum transaminase will actually be a useful tool in the diagnosis of congenital toxoplasmosis and cytomegalic inclusion disease.

Jaundice, which occurs frequently, may reflect liver damage or hemolysis, or both. Among 225 infants with neonatal icterus studied by Couvreur and Desmonts, 5 (2.2%) were found to have congenital toxoplasmosis.[559] The conjugated hyperbilirubinemia and jaundice seen in untreated infants with congenital toxoplasmosis may persist for months.[485] In treated infants, hyperbilirubinemia and jaundice usually resolve in a few weeks.

Skin

Like almost all other signs of the infection, those referable to the skin are varied and nonspecific.[669, 670] Thrombocytopenia may be associated with petechiae, ecchymoses, or even gross hemorrhages into the skin. Zuelzer described a fine punctate rash over the entire body of a 3-day-old infant.[473] Miller and colleagues noted albinism in one of the infants they studied but did not consider this to be caused by toxoplasmosis.[505] Wolf and associates noted a diffuse maculopapular rash in two infants with jaundice, beginning on the sixth day in one and on the ninth day in the other.[485] Reiss and Verron described a premature infant with a lenticular, deep blue-red, sharply defined macular rash over the entire body, including the palms and soles.[671] Diffuse blue papules were noted in the patient described by Justus.[672] Korovitsky and co-workers, in a discussion of skin lesions in toxoplasmosis, mentioned an exfoliative dermatitis in cases of congenital toxoplasmosis,[673] but, according to Justus, a cause-and-effect relationship between these two conditions was not shown in the infant he described.[672] In

1968, Justus reported complete calcification of the skin, except for the palms and soles, in a premature infant who died 10 minutes after birth.[674] The mother had experienced tetany during delivery and required supplemental calcium thereafter. Thus, the calcifications may not have been due solely, or even in part, to congenital toxoplasmosis in the infant but rather to a metabolic defect in calcium metabolism in the mother.

MALFORMATIONS

The possibility that *T. gondii* can cause fetal malformations has been the subject of much conjecture. Thalhammer, commenting on the accumulated data on this subject, stated that he did not believe that *T. gondii* causes malformations.[591] He found 4 instances of malformations among 326 cases of congenital toxoplasmosis (1.2%), and this was less than the average incidence of malformations in his geographic area. Of 144 children with malformations, only 2 had *T. gondii* antibodies.

In contrast, workers in Germany,[125, 169, 477, 675, 676] Greece,[677] the former Czechoslovakia,[635, 678] and the former Soviet Union[679] interpret their data as proof that *T. gondii* causes fetal malformations. Most of these studies were performed in an uncontrolled and uncritical manner. For example, in the United States, Erdélyi suggested that some cases of palatal cleft malformations may be due to congenital toxoplasmosis[680]; a similar conclusion was reached by Jírovec and co-workers in Prague.[635] The evidence in the former consisted of dye test data and in the latter of skin test data drawn from investigations of mothers of children with cleft palate and harelip defects; the prevalence of positive tests in mothers of such children was found to be higher than that in controls from the general population. Carefully chosen controls should be a necessary feature of all such studies; results obtained from the general population are not applicable or valid.

Although involvement of the placenta by infection

early in pregnancy may cause damage without direct infection of the developing embryo, the available data are insufficient either to support or to reject the hypothesis that *T. gondii* can cause fetal malformations. This problem is easily approached with existing epidemiologic methods and awaits careful controlled study.

OTHER SIGNS AND SYMPTOMS

Erythroblastosis and Hydrops Fetalis. Congenital toxoplasmosis may be confused with erythroblastosis related to isosensitization.[479, 631, 681–686] The peripheral blood picture and clinical course may be identical to those observed in other forms of erythroblastosis. This is exemplified by cases such as those reported by Callahan and colleagues[468] and by Beckett and Flynn.[114] A negative Coombs' test result is helpful in distinguishing erythroblastosis caused by congenital infection from that caused by blood group factor sensitization.

Cardiovascular Signs. Severe toxoplasmic myocarditis may be manifested clinically as edema.[468]

Gastrointestinal Signs. In some cases, the first sign of the disease appears to be vomiting or diarrhea.[468] Feeding problems are also common.

Respiratory Difficulty. Respiratory difficulty,[12, 468] often with cyanosis, may be due to an interstitial toxoplasmic pneumonitis, to viral or bacterial suprainfection, or to CNS lesions affecting the respiratory control centers of the brain.

Deafness. From the follow-up studies of Eichenwald[552] and others,[687] ample clinical and histologic[76, 468, 496, 565, 688] data are available to show that congenital infection with *T. gondii* can lead to deafness. The well-documented cases of profound hearing loss have been almost totally confined to infants with severe clinical disease, but in the series of children with subclinical infection at birth reported by Wilson and associates,[687] there were 17% with significant hearing loss. In some instances, serologic and skin test surveys among deaf patients have suggested a cause-and-effect relationship,[689] whereas in others no such relationship has been found.[690] An association between epilepsy, cerebral palsy, and nerve deafness and presence of antibodies to *T. gondii* in sera of Israeli children was noted (relative risk 2.5, $p = 0.03$; nerve deafness relative risk 7.1, $p = 0.01$).[691] Such studies are frequently open to criticism, owing to the choice of controls. Thus, there are no satisfactory data to support the contention that congenital toxoplasmosis may be a frequent cause of deafness.[692] In the U.S. (Chicago) National Collaborative Treatment Trial, hearing loss has not been noted in treated children[693] (Table 5–26). One child with brain stem lesions involving the auditory nucleus has auditory perceptual difficulties.

Ascites. Vanhaesebrouck and co-workers reported a case of a preterm congenitally infected infant with isolated transudative ascites caused by *T. gondii*.[694] Neonatal[695] and fetal[132, 696, 697] ascites due to congenital toxoplasmosis have been reported.

FOLLOW-UP

Adequate follow-up studies (see also the previous section Eye) to gain information on the natural course of con-

genital toxoplasmosis are lacking in most series of reported cases. In the vast majority, the original diagnosis was made in a retrospective manner, in most cases because of the presence of clinical signs of the infection. Most accumulated data, therefore, are from infants and older children with the most atypical form of congenital toxoplasmosis, that is, clinically apparent disease, in the newborn period. It is in those infants who are actually in the majority—those who were asymptomatic at birth—that there is the greatest need for follow-up studies, such as those performed by Alford and colleagues[512, 616] described previously. (See also Hedenström and colleagues.[698, 699]) Follow-up in the infants who were asymptomatic at birth in the Paris study is difficult to interpret, because most were treated in the newborn period. However, in some, recognition of the first clinical finding (usually chorioretinitis) was delayed until several weeks or months after birth, thereby illustrating an often reported observation in congenital toxoplasmosis—a child who appears normal for some months before overt disease is recognized.[113, 554, 587, 700]

Follow-up studies of those patients reported by Eichenwald have already been mentioned. Two patients reported by Wolf and co-workers in 1942[485] were still alive in 1959 and were being cared for in mental institutions.[701] One of them, first seen at the age of 3 years and 9 months, was about 22 years old at the time of the second report. She was mentally and physically retarded, oblivious to her environment, drooled constantly, was resistant to care and feeding, and was losing weight. She continued to have petit mal and grand mal seizures. Old chorioretinal scars were still present. The second patient was 2 years old when the diagnosis was made and about 18 years of age at the time of the last report. His IQ was only 40. He was said to have a pleasant personality and could engage in some project activities. Vision was 20/100 in one eye and 20/70 in the other.

Feldman and Miller analyzed 187 patients with congenital toxoplasmosis: among 176 of these patients, 119 were 4 years old or younger, 38 were 5 to 9 years old, and 19 were 10 to 19 years old.[141] Thirty-six had been delivered prematurely; 20% of the premature infants and 7% of those born at term died. Residual damage varied in degree, but most of the patients exhibited chorioretinitis, mental retardation, and abnormalities of head size. In this series, reported frequencies were intracerebral calcification in 59%, psychomotor retardation in 45%, seizures in 39%, chorioretinitis in 94%, microphthalmia in 36%, hydrocephalus in 22%, and microcephaly in 21%.[553]

Puissan and co-workers observed the late onset of convulsions in an 8-year-old girl with congenital toxoplasmosis.[702] Interesting in this case was the demonstration of what appears to have been local production of *T. gondii* antibody in the CSF when the convulsions began.

In the first report of the prospective study by Koppe and colleagues, follow-up data were obtained for 7 years for 12 congenitally infected children.[556] Four children had clinical signs (ocular only), and 1 was clinically normal but *T. gondii* had been isolated from the placenta and CSF; these 5 were treated with pyrimethamine and sulfadiazine. No signs of cerebral damage or intracranial

TABLE 5–26
Definitions of Hearing Impairment and Outcome in Reported Studies of Hearing in Cases of Congenital Toxoplasmosis

DEGREE OF HEARING IMPAIRMENT	DEFINITIONS			RESULTS		
	U.S. (Chicago) National Collaborative Treatment Trial		Wilson et al	Eichenwald	U.S. (Chicago) National Collaborative Treatment Trial	Wilson et al	Eichenwald
	ABR (dB/HL)	**Audiogram (dB/HL)**					
Normal	≤20	0–20	<25 dB[a]	Not available	104	14	Not available
Mild	>20–40	25–40	25–50 dB	Not available	0	3	Not available
Moderate	>40–60	>40	51–80 dB	Not available	0	2	Not available
Severe	>60	>70–90	Not found	Not available	0	0	Not available
Profound		>90	Not found	"Deaf"	0	0	15
TOTAL					104	19	105

dB = decibels; HL = hearing level.
[a]Defined as "hearing reception threshold" by Wilson and McLeod.[555]
Adapted from McGee T, et al. Absence of sensorineural hearing loss in treated infants and children with congenital toxoplasmosis. Otolaryngol Head Neck Surg 106:75–80, 1992, with minor modifications and permission.

calcifications developed in any of the children, and all were said to be "mentally normal" at the age of 7 years.[556] Their development was judged by their performance in school, which was stated to be normal. In fact, in a later report, two thirds of these children had developed chorioretinitis,[557] and, because they were still younger than 15 years of age when last reported, they remained at risk for the development of additional sequelae. (See the Amsterdam Study section later for the final report.)

CONGENITAL *TOXOPLASMA GONDII* INFECTION AND ACQUIRED IMMUNODEFICIENCY SYNDROME

Congenital transmission of *T. gondii* from pregnant women co-infected with *T. gondii* and HIV has been recognized as a unique problem[703–710] but fortunately a relatively uncommon one.[711–717] Unfortunately, we have insufficient data on what the CD4+ T lymphocyte counts were in these dually infected women during their pregnancies because transmission of *T. gondii* from these chronically infected women would be most likely to occur in the setting of severe immunosuppression. This would assist in determining the importance of this and other parameters of immunosuppression that place their fetuses at risk for congenital *T. gondii* infection. Data available at present reveal that these mothers have chronic *T. gondii* infection and do not have demonstrable IgM *T. gondii* antibodies. Noteworthy are the observations that most of these dually infected newborns do not have clinical signs of either infection at birth even though each of the cases thus far examined has revealed dual infection of the infant with the parasite and HIV. Many of these infants go on to develop severe signs of disseminated infection within the first weeks or months of life.

Mitchell and colleagues described four young infants, two of whom were siblings, who were dually infected with HIV-1 and *T. gondii*.[703] Their mothers were similarly co-infected. The mother of the first infant had toxoplasmic encephalitis diagnosed at delivery. The other mothers had no clinical evidence of toxoplasmosis but did have *T. gondii* antibodies. The investigators concluded that the mother was the source of the infection in each of the infants. Of interest is that in three of the seven cases (three cases were diagnosed after the initial publication) documented at the University of Miami, the diagnosis was not suspected before the patient's death and was made only at autopsy (C Mitchell, personal communication to JS Remington, 1993). Three of the four cases from the original publication are briefly presented here as examples of the problem.

CASE HISTORY: INFANTS 2 AND 3

The mother of the siblings with congenital *T. gondii* infection had given birth to five children, four of whom were infected with HIV-1. The siblings with toxoplasmosis were the third and fifth born. The mother developed AIDS 1 month after the birth of this fifth child but never developed clinical or tomographic

evidence of toxoplasmic encephalitis. She died 8 months later of tuberculosis and bacterial sepsis. An autopsy was not performed. One sibling, born at term and appropriate for gestational age, was discharged from the hospital at 3 days of age in good condition, only to return at 3 months of age with complications of AIDS. He remained hospitalized until he died at age 6 months. At autopsy, he was found to have disseminated cytomegalovirus infection involving most visceral organs and all lobes of the lung, *T. gondii* pneumonitis, and diffuse CNS toxoplasmosis. The other sibling was a full-term female appropriate for gestational age. She had an unremarkable neonatal course. When seen at 5 weeks of age, she was in septic shock and emaciated and had severe oral thrush. She died within 1 hour after admission to the hospital. Blood cultures were positive for *Propionibacterium*; autopsy revealed disseminated candidiasis involving the lungs and esophagus and diffuse intracerebral toxoplasmosis. ■

CASE HISTORY: INFANT 4

This infant was an appropriate-for-gestational-age, full-term female recognized at birth to be at risk for congenital toxoplasmosis and HIV-1 infection because her mother was known to be seropositive for *T. gondii* and had previously been delivered of a child who died of AIDS. Results of examination at birth were normal, but the infant was treated expectantly for toxoplasmosis with pyrimethamine and sulfadiazine because of the presence of IgM *T. gondii* antibodies in her serum. After an extended course of therapy complicated by hepatitis of unclear etiology, she died; permission for autopsy was denied. This child's mother died of AIDS 3 years later, never having developed clinical toxoplasmosis. ■

Marty and co-workers[718] reported a 22-week pregnant, HIV-infected woman who was observed to have reactivation of her *T. gondii* serologic test titer (from an IgG dye test titer of 5 IU/ml in 1992 to 400 IU one year later). She had a CD4+ cell count of 90 per mm³. An ultrasound revealed fetal hydrocephaly, and a therapeutic abortion was performed. The external morphology of the fetus was normal, but autopsy revealed multiple abscesses in the brain and liver, and *T. gondii* was isolated from amniotic fluid, placenta, liver, spleen, heart, and brain.

Pathology

There is a relative paucity of information on the pathology in the CNS in fetuses or newborns co-infected with *T. gondii* and HIV-1. In three of the cases reported by Mitchell and co-workers, there was histologic evidence of meningitis, as evidenced by chronic leptomeningeal inflammatory cell infiltrates.[703] *T. gondii* cysts as well as microglial nodules that suggested an immune response against the parasite were seen in the brains of two of the cases. Examination of numerous slides from the brain of one infant, who had been treated for toxoplasmosis, revealed only a single *T. gondii* cyst and no microglial nodules. The brain revealed chronic inflammation and widespread foci of necrosis surrounded by macrophages, lymphocytes, and plasma cells. Gliosis was also present. Immunoperoxidase staining demonstrated *T. gondii* in the CNS of this infant.

There are insufficient data to estimate how frequently the diagnosis of congenital *T. gondii* infection in these dually infected infants might be suggested by serologic examination. IgM and IgG *T. gondii* antibodies have been demonstrable in some of these infants[705] (C Mitchell and A Kovacs, personal communication to JS Remington, 1993).

Treatment

Treatment of the Newborn. There are insufficient data on the outcome of treatment of congenital *T. gondii* infection in these newborns. The diagnosis of co-infection with HIV is usually made late and often a month or more after birth. Thus, at least at present, whether to use drugs directed against HIV in combination with anti-*T. gondii* therapy in the early newborn period does not appear to be a major consideration. This is important because toxicity to the bone marrow may be considerably increased when, for example, zidovudine, pyrimethamine, and sulfadiazine are used together. When the diagnosis in the newborn is suspected or proved, we recommend that the pyrimethamine-sulfadiazine combination be used. Because relapse uniformly occurs in the adult if maintenance treatment is not given, such treatment is administered for the duration of the patient's life. Such relapse is to be expected in infants, but the duration of maintenance therapy in these infants remains to be defined especially in view of recent data in adults on highly active antiviral treatment (protease inhibitors). Discontinuation of prophylaxis against *P. carinii* pneumonia did not result in a significant number of cases of toxoplasmosis in those AIDS patients at risk.[719] Until such information is available, it seems prudent to maintain the infants on their primary therapy (pyrimethamine-sulfadiazine). We recommend consultation with experts in regard to dosage and dosing regimens for this purpose. A number of the drugs being used or studied at present for maintenance therapy in adults have not been used or studied in newborns or young infants, although some of them will, it is hoped, prove useful for this purpose.

Treatment and Primary Prophylaxis in the Human Immunodeficiency Virus– and *Toxoplasma gondii*–Infected Pregnant Woman. Treatment with pyrimethamine-sulfadiazine (and leukovorin) should be started in patients with active toxoplasmosis.[720] Clindamycin may be used as an alternative to sulfadiazine in the combination.[721] Use of pyrimethamine in the first trimester is usually contraindicated, as discussed earlier. The decision whether to use this drug should be made in consultation with experts.

Until there is more complete information on the special factors that predispose to congenital transmission of *T. gondii* in these women, we recommend that primary prophylaxis be used in those with CD4+ T cell counts of fewer than 200 cells per mm³. The combination trimethoprim-sulfamethoxazole is commonly used in these patients to prevent *P. carinii* pneumonia and has been reported to be effective in prevention of toxoplasmic encephalitis in AIDS patients who can tolerate the drug combination.[722] This and other drug regimens for *T. gondii* primary prophylaxis are common practice in nonpregnant HIV-infected adults who also have chronic *T. gondii* infection.[722] More complete treatment of this subject is beyond the scope of this chapter. For a commentary on this issue in general, the reader is referred to reference 722. It should be noted, however, that there are no data in regard to whether pyrimethamine-sulfadiazine and pyrimethamine-clindamycin combinations are of comparable efficacy in preventing transmission of *T. gondii* to the fetus.

Of interest in regard to the transmission from mother to her fetus are two cases of CNS toxoplasmosis in HIV-infected pregnant women who gave birth to infants who were not infected with *T. gondii*.[723, 724]

DIAGNOSIS

The diagnosis of acute infection with *T. gondii* may be established by isolation of the organism from blood or body fluids, demonstration of the presence of cysts in the placenta or tissues of a fetus or newborn, demonstration of the presence of antigen or organisms or both in sections or preparations of tissues and body fluids, demonstration of antigenemia and antigen in serum and body fluids, specific nucleic acid sequences (e.g., PCR), or serologic tests.

Diagnostic Methods

LABORATORY EXAMINATION

Cerebrospinal Fluid (see also the sections on Serologic Diagnosis in the Newborn and Serology and Polymerase Chain Reaction on Cerebrospinal Fluid and Polymerase Chain Reaction on Urine). Approximately four decades ago, Callahan and colleagues, in reviewing the CSF changes in 108 patients with congenital toxoplasmosis, stated, "Examination of the CSF affords the most constant significant laboratory examination for the presence of infantile toxoplasmosis."[468] Although the patients studied by these investigators had the most severe form of the disease, this statement is pertinent even today. Despite the fact that CSF changes in infants with congenital toxoplasmosis are not specific for toxoplasmosis, the demonstration of these changes should lead the physician to consider a diagnosis of toxoplasmosis even in subclinical cases. The findings of xanthochromia and mononuclear pleocytosis in cases of congenital toxoplasmosis are also common in many other generalized infections of the newborn. Almost unique to infants with neonatal toxoplasmosis, however, is the very high protein content of the ventricular fluid. Although in some infants the protein level is just slightly above normal, in others it can be measured in grams per deciliter rather than in milligrams per deciliter.[76, 512, 725]

Alford and associates considered that, in most infants with congenital toxoplasmosis who appear clinically normal at birth, there is a "silent" CNS involvement as reflected by persistent CSF pleocytosis and the elevated protein content[512] (see also Central Nervous System in Pathology and Clinical Manifestations sections). Increases in protein levels and pleocytosis were not as common in a prospective study performed in France (G Desmonts, unpublished data). The difference is probably due to the difference in method of selection of cases. In the study by Alford and associates, only those infants in whom an elevated serum IgM was present at birth were screened for *T. gondii* antibody, and the development of the infection in these infants by the time of birth may have differed significantly from that in the French studies, in which infants were examined because of suspicion of maternal toxoplasmosis acquired during pregnancy. In the French study, the infants, who were infected very close to the time of labor or during labor may not have had elevated serum IgM levels at birth and therefore would have been missed in the studies in which IgM screening alone was the criterion for case selection.

Persistence of IgM antibodies to *T. gondii* in the CSF has been observed in some infected infants and may suggest continued active infection. Such persistence of IgM antibodies in the CSF has also been reported in congenital rubella.[726]

Specific IgG antibody formation in the CNS has been demonstrated in infants with congenital toxoplasmosis.[727] Two hundred forty-two examinations were performed in 206 congenitally infected infants as part of the routine workup for CSF. Only three cases (1.8%) had demonstrable local IgG antibody formation in the CNS. *T. gondii* has been detected by PCR in CSF of newborns with congenital toxoplasmosis (see Polymerase Chain Reaction section). Woods and Englund[728] described a newborn with severe congenital toxoplasmosis who presented with signs of brain destruction and whose CSF was hazy and xanthochromic, with 302 white blood cells per mm^3 and 106 red blood cells per mm^3. The differential count revealed 1% neutrophils, 8% mononuclear cells, and 91% eosinophils. The CSF glucose level was 23 mg/dl, and the CSF protein level was 158 mg/dl. At the same time, her peripheral blood showed 16% eosinophils (absolute count 432 eosinophils per mm^3). Although peripheral blood eosinophilia is common in newborns with congenital toxoplasmosis, as are eosinophilic infiltrations of the pia-arachnoid overlying destructive cortical lesions, eosinophilia has not previously been reported in the CSF of such newborns. A newborn whose congenital toxoplasmosis caused hydrocephalus and cerebral atrophy and quadriparesis due to spinal cord atrophy had peripheral blood eosinophilia (40%) and markedly abnormal CSF (13% of 98 white blood cells) (W Barson, personal communication to R McLeod, 1999).

Blood and Blood-Forming Elements. Leukocytosis or leukopenia may be present, and, early in the course of the infection, lymphocytosis and monocytosis are usually found.[12, 468, 593] Marked polymorphonuclear leukocytosis frequently reflects suprainfection with bacteria.

Thrombocytopenia is common in infants who have clinical signs of the infection as well as in subclinical cases[483, 505, 698, 729]; petechiae or ecchymoses may be the earliest clue to this congenital infection.[468, 473, 479, 483, 698] Eosinophilia in the newborn period has been frequently observed and may exceed 30% of the differential white blood cell count.[12, 76, 468, 565, 593, 730–732]

HISTOLOGIC DIAGNOSIS

Demonstration of tachyzoites in tissues (e.g., brain biopsy, bone marrow aspirate) or body fluids (ventricular fluid or CSF,[469, 486, 733–736] aqueous humor,[737] sputum[264]) establishes the diagnosis of acute toxoplasmosis. Unfortunately, it is frequently difficult to visualize the tachyzoite form in tissues or impression smears stained by ordinary methods. For this reason, the fluorescent antibody technique has been suggested for this purpose.[127, 738–742] Because of its greater sensitivity and specificity, the peroxidase-antiperoxidase technique has largely supplanted the fluorescent antibody method.[743] Both methods are applicable to unfixed or formalin-fixed paraffin-embedded tissue sections. The pitfalls in interpretation of these methods have been discussed by Frenkel and Piekarski.[744] In the retina, because the retinal pigment epithelium is brown or black, a method that stains the parasites red, rather than brown, has proved useful for detection of the parasites.[460] Histologic demonstration of the cyst form establishes that the patient has toxoplasmosis but does not warrant the conclusion that the infection is acute unless there is associated inflammation and necrosis. On the other hand, because cysts may form early in infection, their demonstration does not exclude the possibility that the infection is still in the acute stages.[745]

In the case of acute acquired toxoplasmosis in the pregnant patient, lymphadenopathy may reflect a variety of infectious agents.[532] Distinctive histologic changes in toxoplasmic lymphadenitis enable a pathologist to make a presumptive diagnosis of acute acquired toxoplasmosis.[746] These histologic changes represent the characteristic reaction of the host to the infection, but the organisms themselves are only rarely demonstrable. The histologic signs of infection in other tissues range from areas of no inflammation around cysts to acute necrotizing lesions associated with tachyzoites. The latter are seen almost solely in immunocompromised individuals. None of these changes confirms the diagnosis of toxoplasmosis unless the organism can be demonstrated.

ISOLATION PROCEDURES

General Considerations

Isolation of the parasite from an infant provides unequivocal proof of infection, but, unfortunately, such isolation usually takes too long to permit an early diagnosis. *T. gondii* is readily isolated from tissue obtained at autopsy (e.g., brain, skeletal muscle, or heart muscle); the organism may also be isolated from biopsy material from the neonate (e.g., skeletal muscle). In our experience, isolates from congenitally infected infants are most often avirulent for mice, and a period of 4 to 6 weeks is usually required for definitive demonstration of the parasite when this method is used. In cases in which the organism is virulent for mice, the parasite can often be demonstrated in the peritoneal fluid after 5 to 10 days. *T. gondii* has been isolated from body fluids (e.g., ventricular fluid or CSF,[485, 733, 734, 747–753] subretinal fluid,[754] aqueous humor,[755] or amniotic fluid[751, 756, 757]) of infants and adults. Isolation from tissues (e.g., skeletal muscle, lung, brain, or eye) obtained by biopsy or at autopsy from older children and adults may only reflect the presence of tissue cysts and thus is not definitive proof of active acute infection. One possible exception is the isolation of *T. gondii* from lymph nodes in older children and adults; such evidence probably indicates relatively recently acquired infection, because cysts are rarely found in lymph nodes. Attempts at isolation are usually performed by injection of suspect material into laboratory mice but may also be accomplished by inoculation into tissue culture preparations (see later).[469, 752, 758, 759] One can observe plaque formation and both extracellular and intracellular parasites in unstained or stained preparations. Abbas found cell cultures less sensitive than mouse inoculation for isolation of the parasite.[760] Thus, if cell cultures are used in attempts at primary isolation, it is advisable also to use mouse inoculation when feasible. Tissue culture isolation is quite rapid (usually 1 week or less) and should be used when early isolation is critical for the management of the patient. Because physicians frequently request that isolation procedures be performed, the following are offered as guidelines for the laboratory.

Specimens should be injected into animals and cell cultures as soon as possible after collection to prevent death of the parasite. Formalin kills the parasite, and freezing may result in death of both tachyzoite and cyst forms. If storage of specimens is necessary, refrigeration at 4° C is preferred. This maintains the encysted form in tissues, if kept moist, for up to 2 months and prevents death of the tachyzoite for several days. The parasite survives in blood for a week or longer (see Transmission section). For antibody determination, serum may be removed from clotted cord blood or blood obtained later in the newborn period; the clot should be stored at 4° C until the results of the serologic tests are known. If the serologic tests are not diagnostic and the reason for suspecting congenital toxoplasmosis remains, the blood clot should be injected into mice (or tissue culture) in the same way as any other tissue specimen. Body fluids and heparinized blood can be injected directly, but we prefer to remove the plasma from the formed elements of blood and amniotic fluid to eliminate the possibility of introducing the majority of *T. gondii* antibodies into the recipient animals. Passively transferred human antibody may interfere with infection of the mice, and thus with isolation of the organisms, as well as produce false-positive serologic tests in the inoculated animals for 6 weeks or longer.[108] Because the organisms are most likely to reside within white blood cells in patients with parasitemia, the buffy coat layer may be suspended in a small volume of sterile saline and inoculated into mice by the intraperitoneal or subcutaneous route or onto tissue culture.

Biopsy specimens and blood clots may be triturated with a mortar and pestle or tissue homogenizer in a small amount of normal saline before animal or tissue culture inoculation. After trituration, we generally add enough sterile saline so that the suspension can be drawn into a syringe. If connective tissue prevents aspiration through the needle, the suspension can be filtered through several layers of sterile gauze. Depending on the size of the mice, 0.5 to 2 ml is injected intraperitoneally, subcutaneously, or both. For isolation attempts from superficial enlarged lymph nodes, material can be obtained by needle aspiration of the node.

To isolate *T. gondii* from large amounts of tissue (e.g., placenta), we use trypsin digestion (0.25% trypsin in buffered saline, pH 7.2).[118] The trypsin method makes it possible to isolate both tachyzoite and cyst forms. The former are killed more rapidly by pepsin–hydrochloric acid (HCl).[38] The tissue is first minced with scissors and passed through a meat grinder or ground in a blender; it is then placed in a volume of trypsin solution (10 to 20 ml trypsin solution per gram of tissue) and incubated with constant agitation for 1.5 to 2 hours at 37° C. (If there is gross contamination of the tissue, antibiotics may be added both to the digestion fluid and to the tissue digest before injection.) The suspension is passed through several layers of gauze to remove large particles and then is centrifuged. After the sediment has been washed three or four times in saline to remove trypsin, the digested material is resuspended in saline, and 0.5 to 1 ml is injected both intraperitoneally and subcutaneously into mice. If peptic digestion is desired, the solution is prepared by dissolving 4 g pepsin (Difco 1:10,000), 7.5 g sodium chloride, and 10.5 ml concentrated HCl in water to a volume of 1500 ml.

Mouse Inoculation

In most countries, it is not necessary to perform serologic testing in laboratory mice to determine if they are infected before they are used in isolation attempts. In areas of the world where normal laboratory mice have been found to be infected, serologic testing of individual mice must be performed before such use. Five to 10 days after intraperitoneal injection, the peritoneal fluid should be examined either fresh or in stained smears (Wright or Giemsa stain) for the presence of intracellular and extracellular tachyzoites (see Fig. 5–1*A*). Demonstration of the organism is proof of the infection. Mice that die before 6 weeks have elapsed are examined for the presence of the organism in their peritoneal fluid; stained impression smears of liver and spleen can also be examined. If no organisms are found, suspensions of liver, spleen, and brain may be injected into fresh mice. Surviving mice are bled from the tail vein or orbital sinus for serologic testing after 6 weeks but may be bled from the tail vein more often (e.g., at 2-week intervals). (The dye test, agglutination test, IFA test, or ELISA can be used for this purpose.) We prefer to use the agglutination test as a screening method for this purpose because only a single drop of blood from the tail vein can be tested using microtiter plate wells. If antibodies are present, proof of infection must be obtained by demonstration of the parasite. This can be accomplished most easily by examining Giemsa-stained smears of fresh brain for demonstration of cysts (see Fig. 5–1E). Examination of wet preparations of brain tissue may be hazardous if done by inexperienced workers; pine pollen has been confused with *T. gondii* cysts and has led to the erroneous diagnosis of the infection. Examination is easier under phase microscopy. If cysts are not seen, injection into fresh mice of a suspension of brain, liver, and spleen should be performed to determine the presence of the parasite.

Tissue Culture

Isolation by tissue culture has routinely been used by Derouin and colleagues with a high degree of success.[757] They use coverslip cultures of human embryonic fibroblasts (MRC5, bioMérieux, France) in wells of 24-well plates (Nunc, Denmark).[759] The sediment of approximately 10 ml of amniotic fluid is resuspended in 8 ml of minimum essential medium (MEM) supplemented with 10% fetal calf serum, penicillin (5 IU/ml) and streptomycin (50 mg/ml). One milliliter of the suspension is inoculated into each of six cell culture wells and incubated for 72 to 96 hours at 37° C. Thereafter, they are washed with phosphate-buffered saline and fixed with cold acetone. Indirect immunofluorescence is then performed on the coverslip cultures, using rabbit anti–*T. gondii* IgG as the first antibody and fluorescein-labeled rabbit anti-IgG as the second antibody. After the coverslips are mounted onto slides, they are examined for the presence of *T. gondii* by fluorescence microscopy. Parasite division is readily observed in the cells as is pseudocyst formation; if cells are heavily infected, foci of extracellular parasites may be present. Some workers stain the coverslips with Wright-Giemsa stain or use the immunoperoxidase method to demonstrate *T. gondii* in the cultures. However, these methods are less sensitive than immunofluorescence for detection of low numbers of parasitized cells.

Special Considerations

Placenta. If congenital toxoplasmosis is suspected in a newborn, either because acute toxoplasmosis was diagnosed during pregnancy in the mother or because clinical signs raise suspicion of this diagnosis in the neonate, approximately 100 g of placenta should be kept without fixative and stored at 4 °C until it can be injected into mice. Digestion with trypsin is preferable. This procedure yielded positive results in 25% of placentas obtained from 123 mothers who acquired toxoplasmosis during pregnancy, and in each of these positive cases it was associated with a congenitally infected neonate.[747] Conversely, cases in which infants were proved to be infected, despite the inability to isolate *T. gondii* from their placentas, are rare unless mothers have been treated during pregnancy.[121, 761] Injection of placental tissue into mice is a very useful tool for the diagnosis of congenital toxoplasmosis.

Blood. *T. gondii* may be isolated from cord or peripheral blood of the newborn,[733] and such isolation should

be attempted whenever possible, because serologic diagnosis may be uncertain during the first weeks or months of life. In a study of 69 infants with congenital toxoplasmosis, Desmonts and Couvreur isolated *T. gondii* from peripheral blood in 30 (43%) of them[762] (see Table 5–1). The high incidence (52%) of parasitemia in infants with subclinical infection is noteworthy, as is the overall frequency of parasitemia in congenital cases.

Relatively few positive results were obtained in infants with only neurologic or ocular signs of the disease. This might be related to the fact that these infants are usually not examined during the first days of life, unlike those with generalized disease or those in whom the possibility of disease is suspected because of prospective studies in their mothers. Seventy-one percent of the positive results were obtained from samples of blood taken during the first week of life. The percentage decreased to 33% when blood for isolation purposes was obtained during the following 3 weeks, and there were no positive results in infants older than 1 month of age.[762]

Saliva. Levi and co-workers have reported the isolation of *T. gondii* from saliva of 12 of 20 patients, mostly with the lymphadenopathic form of the disease.[264] This report is interesting but requires confirmation. Whether the parasite can be isolated (or demonstrated by PCR) from sputum or saliva in the newborn period remains to be determined, but the presence of the organism in the alveoli of the lung suggests that attempts at isolation from such material might prove successful.

Post Mortem. *T. gondii* is most easily isolated from brain and skeletal muscle specimens of infants who die months or years after birth, although it has also been isolated from virtually every organ and tissue of infants with congenital toxoplasmosis. Here again, digestion with either pepsin or trypsin is preferred, because it allows for sampling of sufficiently large amounts of tissue. If necessary, brain specimens passed several times through a syringe and No. 20 needle can be injected into mice directly without prior digestion. It is noteworthy that isolation of *T. gondii* from the placenta is common in cases in which fetal death has occurred in utero. Although the organisms are regularly isolated from infected fetuses after induced abortion, they usually cannot be isolated from infected macerated fetuses that have remained in utero for an extended period of time after the fetus has died.

TESTS OF CELL-MEDIATED IMMUNITY

Toxoplasmin Skin Test. At present, the skin test is not used in diagnosis of congenital infection, and no systematic study has been performed to define its potential usefulness for this purpose. It is discussed here for the sake of completeness.

Infection with *T. gondii* results in the development of cell-mediated immunity against the parasite. This may be demonstrated with the toxoplasmin skin test,[763] which elicits delayed hypersensitivity. The large-scale use of the skin test, especially in population surveys, has yielded excellent agreement between the results of this test for delayed hypersensitivity and the presence or absence of antibody.[268, 763–767] False-positive skin test results are rare.[768] Delayed skin hypersensitivity to *T. gondii* antigens in cases of acquired infection appears not to develop until months or years after the initial infection.[122, 269, 769–771] For this reason, the skin test appears to be most useful in the diagnosis of chronic (latent) infection; when positive, the possibility that the patient had a very recently acquired infection seems remote.

Antigen-Specific Lymphocyte Transformation. Lymphocyte transformation to *T. gondii* antigens has been shown to be a specific indicator of prior *T. gondii* infection in adults.[390, 391, 439, 772] This technique has been found useful in establishing the diagnosis of congenital *T. gondii* infection in some infants.[687, 773, 774] Whereas depressed lymphocyte responsiveness to antigens of the infecting organisms has been reported in infants with congenital cytomegalovirus infection,[775, 776] congenital rubella,[777, 778] and congenital syphilis,[779] specific cell-mediated immunity appears to develop for most infants with congenital *T. gondii* infection by 1 year of age, although the magnitude of the response is often less than that of their mothers.[687, 780] In one series,[687] lymphocyte proliferation to *T. gondii* antigen was both a sensitive (84%) and a specific (100%) indicator of congenital *T. gondii* infection; the sensitivity was similar in asymptomatic (82%) and in symptomatic (88%) infants.[687] Wilson and co-workers concluded that as a diagnostic tool this method compared favorably with isolation of *T. gondii* and was superior in sensitivity to the IgM IFA test. In the study by Wilson and co-workers, the majority of patients were not symptomatic or had mild infection and tests of lymphocyte transformation were performed only once; it is possible that even greater sensitivity would be achieved with repeated testing (as was done in the IgM IFA test). Such repeated testing was done in the cases reported by McLeod and colleagues[774] and Yano and associates.[781] The patients described by McLeod and colleagues[433] had more severe involvement, and a substantial proportion of them did not have lymphocyte blastogenic responses to *T. gondii* antigens in the first month of life.

For the present, lymphocyte transformation to *T. gondii* antigens can be regarded as strong evidence of the congenital infection in both symptomatic and asymptomatic children. Additional diagnostic information provided by tests of lymphocyte proliferation may allow more careful selection of children to be treated. An infant with a positive lymphocyte-transformation test would be a candidate for treatment and should also have sequential serologic tests to confirm the diagnosis. A potentially infected infant whose lymphocytes do not respond to *T. gondii* antigens should have serologic and, if feasible, lymphocyte-proliferation tests periodically.

POLYMERASE CHAIN REACTION

In 1990, Grover and colleagues described the usefulness of PCR for rapid prenatal diagnosis of congenital *T. gondii* infection.[782] In a prospective study of 43 documented cases of acute maternal *T. gondii* infection acquired during gestation, PCR correctly identified the presence of *T. gondii* in all five samples of amniotic fluid from 4 proven cases of congenital infection and in 3 of 5 positive cases from a nonprospective group. Detection of IgM antibodies in fetal blood and inoculation of amniotic fluid into tissue cultures identified the infection in two and four of the nine infants with PCR-positive samples, respectively. Mouse inoculation of blood and amniotic fluid detected seven and six of the nine infants with PCR-positive samples, respectively. There were no false-positive results by any of the methods. PCR has subsequently been used successfully on samples of ascitic fluid, amniotic fluid, CSF, blood, urine, and tissues, including placenta and brain of infants with congenital toxoplasmosis.[132, 612, 783–795] False-negative results have been reported, but the data are often[796] difficult to evaluate because there are multiple reasons for such an occurrence, including mishandling of the sample before it is received by the laboratory and use of a single-copy target gene that limits the sensitivity and thus is not able to detect the *T. gondii* DNA in the sample.

Perhaps the greatest advancement in prenatal diagnosis of *T. gondii* infection in the fetus has been the use of PCR on amniotic fluid without having to resort to a percutaneous umbilical blood sample.[132] PCR testing will likely replace many of the methods described in this section for diagnosis of the infection in the newborn.

DEMONSTRATION OF ANTIGEN IN SERUM AND BODY FLUIDS

The ELISA has been used to demonstrate *T. gondii* antigenemia in humans and animals with the acute infection,[797–803] and antigen has been demonstrated in CSF and amniotic fluid of newborns with congenital toxoplasmosis.[804] *T. gondii* antigens have also been demonstrated in urine of a congenitally infected infant by the ELISA.[805] Dot immunobinding has also been used for this purpose.[806] The studies by Araujo and associates[797, 804] were performed in a population of individuals in whom the infection was carefully defined. The ELISA detected antigenemia in 15 (65.2%) of 23 serum samples from 22 adults with recently acquired acute toxoplasmosis. Antigenemia was not detected in sera from 28 normal (seronegative for antibodies to *T. gondii*) individuals or from 55 individuals chronically infected with *T. gondii*. These investigators[804] have also used mouse monoclonal antibodies to detect antigenemia.

DEMONSTRATION OF ANTIBODIES IN SERUM AND BODY FLUIDS

The most widely used serologic tests for the diagnosis of *T. gondii* infection and toxoplasmosis are the Sabin-Feldman dye test,[18] the indirect hemagglutination (IHA) test,[807] the IFA test,[808] the agglutination test,[809] the ELISA,[369, 810–812] and the immunosorbent agglutination assay (ISAGA).[813–815] Certain serologic methods are of little help in diagnosing congenital toxoplasmosis. This is especially true for some CF or IHA tests.[816] These may be weakly positive or even negative in a newborn with congenital toxoplasmosis as well as in the infant's mother. The diagnosis of acute acquired toxoplasmosis may be established by the demonstration of rising sero-

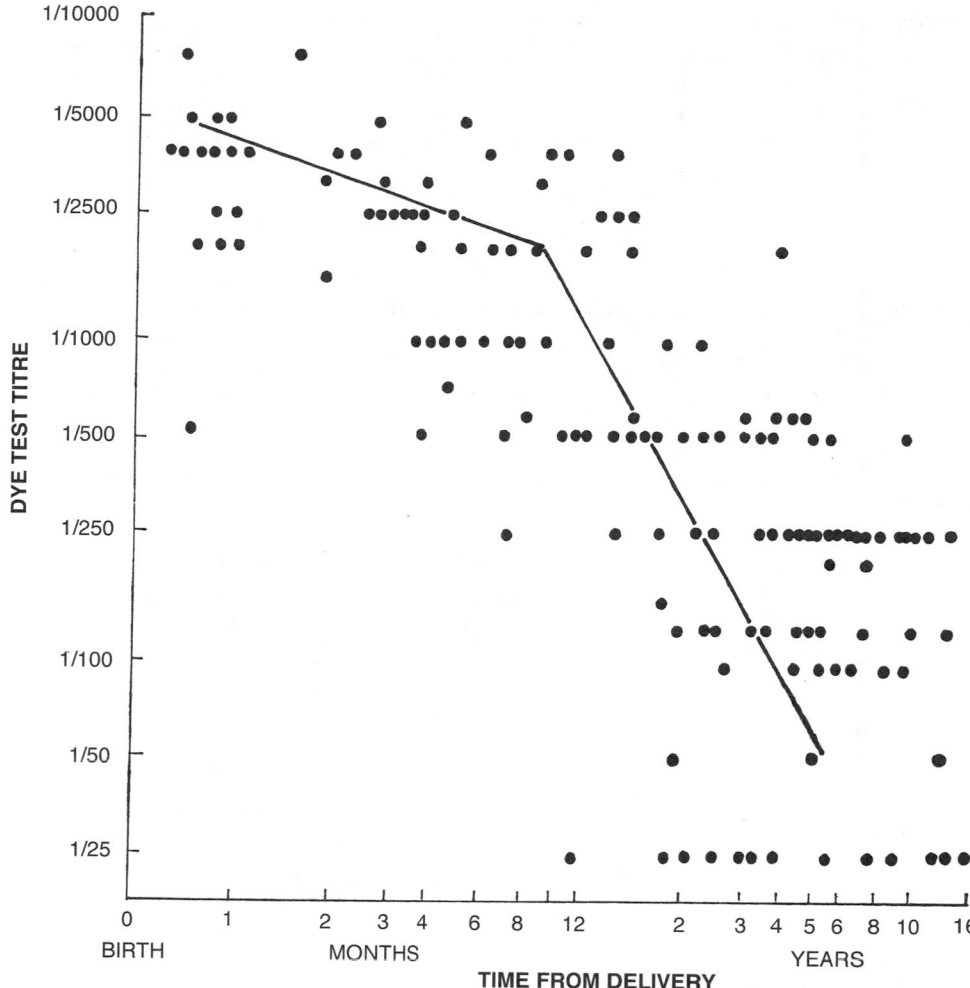

FIGURE 5–18 Dye test titers in 117 mothers of children with congenital toxoplasmosis in relation to time since delivery. (From Couvreur J, Desmonts G. Congenital and maternal toxoplasmosis. A review of 300 congenital cases. Dev Med Child Neurol 4:519–530, 1962, with permission.)

logic test titers.[259] However, a stable high titer may have been reached by the time the patient is first seen by a physician. Because high titers (e.g., 300 to 1000 IU) may persist for many years after acute infection[817] (Figs. 5–18 and 5–19) and are present in the general population, one cannot conclude from a single high serologic test titer in any one method that a clinical illness is definitely due to toxoplasmosis.

Sabin-Feldman Dye Test. The Sabin-Feldman dye test is based on the observation that when living organisms (e.g., from the peritoneal exudate of mice) are incubated with normal serum, they become swollen and stain deeply blue when methylene blue is added to the suspension.[18] Parasites exposed to antibody-containing serum, under the same conditions, appear thin and distorted and are not stained when the dye is added. This is due to lysis of the organisms.[818] The membrane is disrupted because of activation of the complement system.[819] The titer reported is that dilution of serum at which half of the organisms are not killed (stained) and the other half are killed (unstained). (The stain is not required. Differentiation of lysed from nonlysed organisms may be readily accomplished under phase microscopy.) The World Health Organization has recommended that titers in most serologic tests be expressed in international units (IU) per milliliter of serum, com-

pared with an international standard reference serum, which is available on request from the World Health Organization.[820]*

Indirect Hemagglutination Test. In the IHA test, red blood cells tagged with *T. gondii* antigen agglutinate when serum that contains antibodies to *T. gondii* is added.[807] Titers in the IHA test may lag several weeks or more behind those in the dye test,[821–823] attain levels as high as or higher than titers in the dye test, and tend to remain elevated at higher levels even longer.[824, 825] The IHA test has frequently been negative in cases of congenital toxoplasmosis with high dye test titers and is therefore *not recommended* for the diagnosis of congenital toxoplasmosis (Table 5–27). In addition, because a rise in titer in the IHA test may not be demonstrable for months, it is not satisfactory as a screening method in pregnant women with *T. gondii*.[821, 824–829] Because of these problems and the variations in titers obtained in different laboratories, the IHA test cannot at present supplant the dye test, IFA test, or ELISA for demonstration of IgG antibodies. It is, however, an additional test that may be useful in serologic surveys.

*World Health Organization, National Institute of Biological Standards and Control (NIBSC), P.O. Box 1193, Potters Bar, Hertfordshire EN6 3QG, United Kingdom. Telephone (+44)-1707-646399; Fax (+44)-1707-646977.

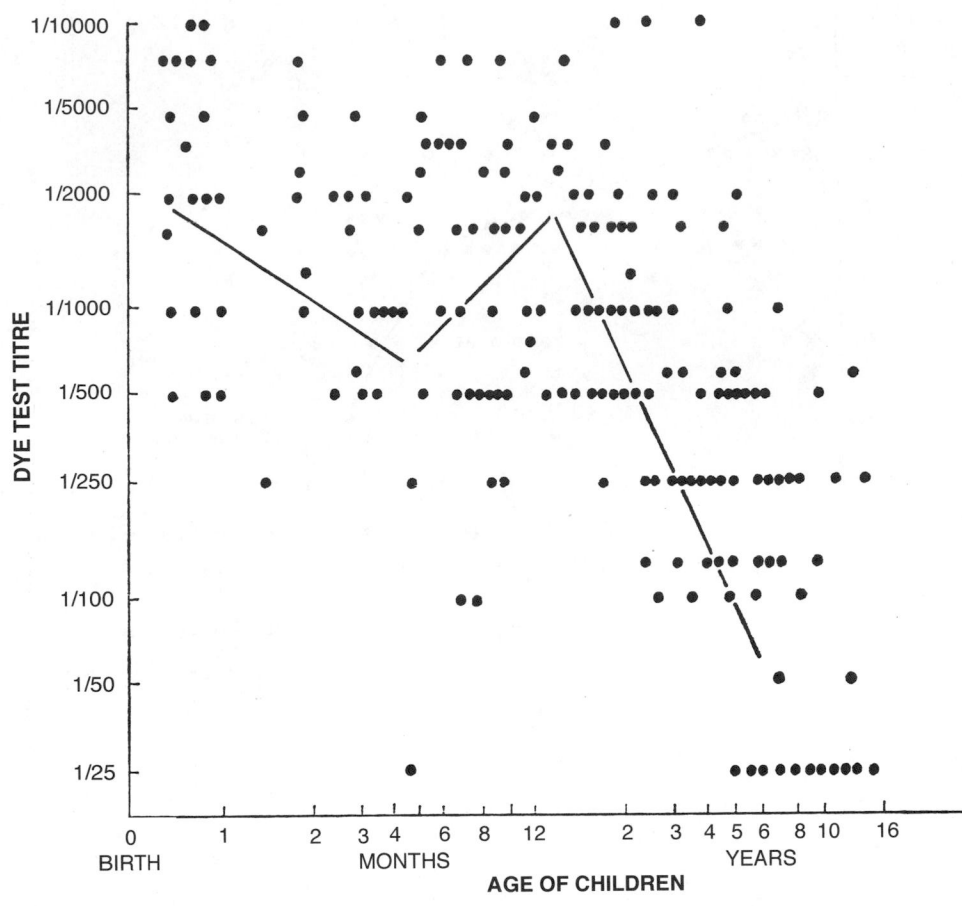

FIGURE 5–19 Dye test titers in 119 children with congenital toxoplasmosis in relation to age. (From Couvreur J, Desmonts G. Congenital and maternal toxoplasmosis. A review of 300 congenital cases. Dev Med Child Neurol 4:519–530, 1962, with permission.)

Complement Fixation Test. Complement-fixing antibodies have been studied mainly in acquired toxoplasmosis. They appear later than those demonstrable by the dye test. Because of this difference, the special usefulness of the CF test was the demonstration of rising titers when dye test or IFA test titers are already high and stable.[821, 830] A negative CF test result that becomes positive or increasing CF test titers, together with stable high dye test titers, indicate active infection. The CF test result may become negative within a few years after acquisition of infection[821, 830] or, in some instances, may remain positive for as long as 10 years.[553] The antigen preparations employed in the CF test have not been standardized. The test is not available to most physicians in the United States.

Agglutination Test. The agglutination test[828, 831] is available commercially in Europe and has been evaluated by a number of investigators.[832–837] The test employs whole parasites that have been preserved in formalin. The method is very sensitive to IgM antibodies. Nonspecific agglutination (apparently related to "naturally" occurring IgM *T. gondii* agglutinins) has been observed

TABLE 5–27
Results of the Dye Test and IHA Test in Twins with Congenital Toxoplasmosis[a]

AGE (MO)	FIRST TWIN (MALE)[b]		SECOND TWIN (FEMALE)[c]	
	Dye Test Titer	IHA Test Titer[d]	Dye Test Titer	IHA Test Titer[d]
1	4000	Negative	250	Negative
2	4000	Negative	125	Negative
4½	2000	64	80	Negative
8	4000	4096	1000	256
11	4000	1024	500	1024

[a]Titers are expressed as the reciprocal of the serum dilution.
[b]Clinical congenital toxoplasmosis with encephalitis and chorioretinitis.
[c]Subclinical infection.
[d]Sera were examined in parallel; negative indicates < 16.
Adapted from Desmonts G. Congenital toxoplasmosis: problems in early diagnosis. *In* Hentsch D (ed). Toxoplasmosis. Bern, Hans Huber, 1971, pp 137–149, with permission.

in individuals devoid of antibody in the dye test and conventional IFA test.[838] These natural IgM antibodies do not cross the placenta but are detected at low titers as early as the second month of life. However, they do not develop in infants with maternal IgG antibody to *T. gondii* as long as IgG antibody is present. False-positive results because of these natural antibodies may be avoided.[839] When they are, this test is excellent for wide-scale screening of pregnant women because it is accurate, simple to perform, and inexpensive.[1, 839] A method that employs latex-tagged particles may also be available commercially.[840–842] A chemical alteration of the outer membrane of the parasite led to the development of a unique differential agglutination method (HS/AC test) that is very useful for helping to differentiate between acute and chronic infections in the pregnant patient.[814, 831, 843, 844]

Differential Agglutination Test. The differential agglutination test compares titers obtained with formalin-fixed tachyzoites (HS antigen) with those obtained with acetone- or methanol-fixed tachyzoites (AC antigen).[306, 814, 831] The AC antigen preparation contains stage-specific antigens that are recognized by IgG antibodies early during infection; these antibodies have different specificities than those found later in the infection.[845] Guidelines for interpretation of results for this test are shown in Figure 5–20. In a study of patients with recently acquired infection, Dannemann and co-workers reported that use of this method in the appropriate clinical setting is useful for diagnosis of the acute infection using a single serum sample from the patient.[814] In practice, to assist with a clinical decision, it is important to take into regard the results of other serologic tests along with those found in the HS/AC test. It is our practice to use the HS/AC test only in adults, and only in those who have IgG and IgM antibodies to *T. gondii* and in whom there is a question as to whether the infection was recently acquired. In adults, it appears to be more valuable than does demonstration of the presence of IgA antibodies, which, during the acute infection, may simply parallel the presence of IgM antibody. In the study by Dannemann and co-workers in which a single serum specimen was tested in each patient, the HS/AC test correctly identified all the pregnant and almost all (31 of 33) of the nonpregnant patients with recently acquired toxoplasmic lymphadenopathy or asymptomatic infections. Each of the seven women in their study who seroconverted during gestation had an acute pattern in the HS/AC test within 0 to 8 weeks after seroconversion in the dye test. Thirteen percent of 15 individuals who had been infected for at least 2 years had an acute pattern, but the wide range in duration of time from original infection (2 to 14 years) did not allow for an estimate of when the pattern in the HS/AC test changed from an acute to a nonacute pattern.

Conventional Indirect Fluorescent Antibody Test. In this test, slide preparations of killed *T. gondii* are incubated with serial dilutions of the patient's serum. If a specific reaction between the antigenic sites on the organisms and the patient's antibody occurs, it can be detected by a fluorescein-tagged antiserum prepared against serum immune globulins. A positive reaction is detected by the bright yellow-green fluorescence of the organisms when examined by fluorescence microscopy. In general, qualitative agreement with the dye test and IFA test has been excellent.[808] Despite the claims of many workers, reliable and reproducible quantitative titers are frequently difficult to obtain. To permit valid comparisons of results from different laboratories that express their titers as the last positive serum dilution, it should be noted that, depending on the laboratory, the dye test may vary in sensitivity between 0.1 and 0.5 IU/ml for the 50% end point. Thus, a positive serum with a titer of 1000 IU/ml could be reported as 1:2000 or 1:10,000 in the dye test. The range is even greater with the IFA test.

Although most workers consider the IFA test to equal the dye test in specificity, false-positive results occur with some sera that contain antinuclear antibodies.[846] For this reason, in patients with connective tissue disorders (e.g., systemic lupus erythematosus), a dye test or ELISA can be performed to document a positive IFA test.

To avoid misinterpretation of the polar staining of organisms that is due to naturally occurring IgM antibodies,[847, 848] the fluorescein-tagged conjugate should be only anti-IgG.[849]

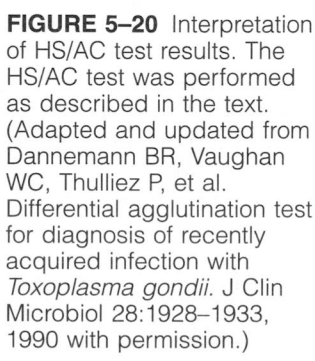
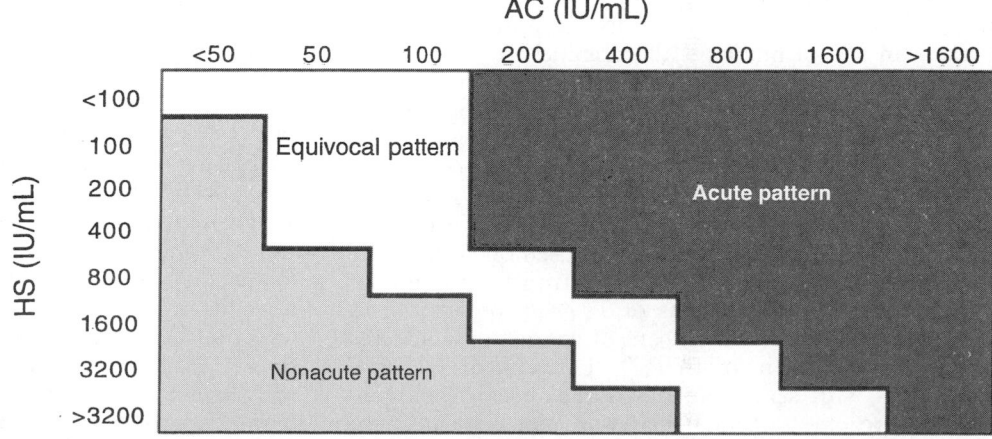

FIGURE 5–20 Interpretation of HS/AC test results. The HS/AC test was performed as described in the text. (Adapted and updated from Dannemann BR, Vaughan WC, Thulliez P, et al. Differential agglutination test for diagnosis of recently acquired infection with *Toxoplasma gondii*. J Clin Microbiol 28:1928–1933, 1990 with permission.)

Conventional Enzyme-Linked Immunosorbent Assay. The ELISA technology has largely replaced other methodologies in the routine clinical laboratory. It has been used successfully to demonstrate IgG, IgM, IgA, and IgE[850, 851] antibodies in the pregnant woman, fetus, and newborn.[811, 852, 853] Most workers have employed an enzyme-conjugated antibody directed against human IgG[854–856] or against total immunoglobulins.[857–861] Titers in the IgG ELISA correlated well with titers in the dye, IHA, IFA, and CF tests in some studies[860] but not in others.[861, 862] Commercial kits are widely available for detection of IgG or IgM antibodies. However, their reliability for detection of IgM antibodies varies considerably and false-positive results have been a serious problem.[863, 864]

Capture Enzyme-Linked Immunosorbent Assay. The capture ELISA is routinely employed by many laboratories for demonstration of IgM[369, 836, 865] and IgA[852, 853, 862] *T. gondii* antibodies in the fetus, newborn, and pregnant patient. In appropriately standardized methods (commercial kits), the IgA ELISA is more sensitive than the IgM ELISA or IgM ISAGA for diagnosis of the infection in the fetus and newborn. IgA antibodies may persist for 8 months or longer in congenitally infected infants.[811, 853] Demonstration of IgA *T. gondii* antibodies in an adult with the early acute acquired infection is comparable to demonstration of IgM antibody, although IgA antibody may appear somewhat later than IgM antibody. In the adult, IgA *T. gondii* antibodies usually disappear earlier than do IgM antibodies, but, as with the latter, they may remain positive for a year or longer. Very high titers in either ELISA appear to correlate with more recent onset of the infection. Many cases in adults have been observed in which the IgM ELISA and HS/AC (see earlier) tests were positive and the IgA ELISA was negative. We and others have only rarely found the IgA test to be useful for diagnosis of the acute infection in the pregnant woman.[866]

Enzyme-Linked Immunofiltration Assay (ELIFA). This method makes use of a micropore membrane[867] and permits simultaneous study of antibody specificity by immunoprecipitation and characterization of antibody isotypes by immunofiltration with enzyme-labeled antibodies. This method has detected as high as 85% of cases of congenital infection in the first few days of life. This test is not available to physicians in the United States. By this method, IgE may be found at birth in the CSF or serum of the newborn. IgA antibodies were present in 5% of infants with congenital infection after the fifth month of age and were never found in the CSF. In Pinon and colleagues' study,[868] the combination of their ELIFA with the IgA and IgM ISAGA provided a positive diagnosis in 90% of the infants within 1 month of birth and in 94% by the end of the first 3 months of life. The method is excellent for diagnosis of congenital infection in the newborn and can be used on cord serum.

Protein Blot. The protein-blotting technique has been used to detect antigens of *T. gondii* recognized by IgG and IgM antibodies in sera of congenitally infected newborns and their mothers.[869] Patterns of IgG and IgM blots with sera from newborns revealed antigen-antibody reactions (bands) that were not present in the respective blots obtained with sera from their mothers.

These results confirm and extend the results of Pinon and Gruson.[870] The method has proved to be of value for difficult to diagnose cases of congenital *T. gondii* infection in the newborn.

IgG Avidity. Testing for the avidity of antibodies against *T. gondii* stems from the knowledge that after primary antigenic stimulation, antibody-binding avidity (affinity) for an antigen is initially low but increases thereafter. IgG antibodies that are present owing to prior antigenic stimulus are most often of high avidity; this pertains to the secondary antibody response as well. (For a review, the reader is referred to reference 871.) The most widely used method is one that employs the hydrogen-bond disrupting agent urea, which preferentially dissociates complexes formed by low-affinity antibodies. An avidity "index" may be determined as the percentage of antibodies that resist elution by 6M urea (e.g., in an ELISA plate). The method has been used by numerous investigators in an attempt to differentiate between recently acquired infection and infection acquired in the more distant past.[872–876] Commercial kits are available in Europe.[877] At present, despite the many publications using the ELISA format, there is no consensus on a standard procedure. Thus, each investigator has had to define what constitutes a low, high, or equivocal avidity result. What is generally agreed on is that a low avidity cannot be interpreted to mean that the patient has had a recently acquired infection because low avidity antibodies may persist for more than 5 months, depending on the method used. However, a high avidity result in the first trimester virtually rules out a recently acquired infection. Unfortunately, for all methods thus far reported, the equivocal range is broad, and a result in this range requires additional testing in a reference laboratory. For diagnosis in the pregnant woman, the avidity method is most useful when used early during gestation, because a high avidity result late in gestation does not rule out an infection acquired in the first trimester or earlier. With the method used in their laboratory, Lappalainen and colleagues[878] reported that the predictive value of a high avidity test result for excluding infection in the prior 5 months was 100%. In the Palo Alto laboratory, a high avidity result obtained by an ELISA method during the first 12 weeks of gestation essentially excludes an infection acquired within the prior 3 months. Jenum and associates[879] concluded from their results that acquisition of *T. gondii* infection in early pregnancy can be excluded on the basis of results in a single serum sample collected in the first trimester. By confirming latent infection on the basis of a high IgG avidity result early during gestation, the need to collect a second serum sample would be eliminated. It is important to appreciate that antibiotic treatment (e.g., spiramycin) may affect the kinetics of IgG avidity maturation[880] and thereby prolong the duration of detectable low-avidity antibodies. The avidity test in its present form is an excellent adjunctive method for ruling out infection acquired during the first 3 months of gestation.[878, 881–883] Agreement between the HS/AC method and the avidity ELISA was 97% in sera obtained in the first 12 weeks of gestation (JS Remington, unpublished data).

DEMONSTRATION OF SPECIFIC IGM ANTIBODIES

Because of the widespread use of IgM antibody tests for diagnosis of the infection during pregnancy and in the fetus and neonate, further discussion of these tests seems warranted.

IgM Fluorescent Antibody Test. The IFA test has been adapted for the demonstration of IgM antibodies to *T. gondii*, and the method has been successfully used to establish acute congenital and acquired infections.[512, 826, 828, 884–890] The use of IgM antibody for diagnosis of congenital infection stems from the discovery in 1963 by Eichenwald and Shinefield[891] that the fetus is able to produce IgM-specific antibody. Critical to this method is the choice of an antiserum that is specific for IgM, as discussed previously.[532, 892] Serious and misleading errors related to the use of antisera that have specificity not only for IgM but also for IgG have been reported in the literature.

Failure to demonstrate IgM antibodies in the IgM IFA test in sera from some patients with the acute acquired infection has been shown to be due to an inhibitory effect of high titers of IgG antibodies to *T. gondii* in these sera.[893, 894] This may be avoided by removal of the IgG before testing in the IgM IFA test. Commercial kits are available for this purpose.

The presence of IgM antibodies in cord serum or in serum obtained from the neonate is evidence of specific antibody synthesis by the infected fetus in utero. Maternal IgM antibodies do not normally pass the placental barrier as do maternal IgG antibodies. The IgM IFA test was the first designed to make an early diagnosis of congenital toxoplasmosis by distinguishing between passively transferred maternal antibodies and the response of the fetus and neonate to infection.[884] The test has also been successfully used to detect active acute acquired toxoplasmosis.[259, 746, 821, 895, 896] After acute acquired infection, the IgM IFA test titer may rise rapidly (and at times earlier than titers in the dye test or conventional IFA test) to high titers.[821] The titer usually declines and may disappear within several months; in some patients, however, the IgM IFA test has remained positive at a low titer for several years. IgM antibodies to *T. gondii* may not be demonstrable in immunodeficient patients with acute toxoplasmosis and in patients with isolated active ocular toxoplasmosis. Only 25 to 50% of congenitally infected infants have *T. gondii*–specific IgM antibodies demonstrable by IgM IFA tests.[369, 687, 892] With two qualifications, demonstration of IgM antibodies to *T. gondii* in the serum of a newborn should be considered as diagnostic of congenital toxoplasmosis. First, if cord serum is tested, or if the serum is obtained in the early newborn period in an infant during whose delivery a placental "leak" occurred, which enabled maternal blood to mix with that of the infant, a false-positive result could occur in any serologic test for IgM, IgA, or IgE antibodies. This can be checked by performing the test on the mother's serum. If the mother's serum is negative for IgM antibodies and the infant's serum is positive, the infant is infected. If both mother and infant are positive, the infant should be tested again several days later; a

marked fall in the IgM IFA test titer will have occurred if the IgM was maternally acquired, because the half-life of IgM is only approximately 5 days.[897, 898] If the IgM IFA test titer in the infant remains high or is rising, it is diagnostic of infection.

The second qualification is the presence of rheumatoid factor. False-positive IgM IFA test results may occur in sera that contain rheumatoid factor.[899] Rheumatoid factor may be present not only in adults but in infected newborns as well,[517, 900] purportedly as a result of an IgM immune response of the fetus in utero to passively transferred maternal IgG. After treatment of sera containing rheumatoid factor with heat-aggregated IgG, false-positive IgM IFA test titers become negative. In contrast, titers in cases of acute congenital or acquired toxoplasmosis are unaffected by this treatment. Thus, treatment with heat-aggregated IgG or other commercially available adsorbent can be used to differentiate false-positive IgM IFA test titers related to rheumatoid factor from those related to specific IgM antibody to *T. gondii*. The incidence of rheumatoid factor in sera of infants with congenital toxoplasmosis is unknown. All infants who respond positively to the IgM IFA test should be tested for rheumatoid factor as well.

IgM Enzyme-Linked Immunosorbent Assay. The double-sandwich IgM ELISA for detection of IgM antibodies to *T. gondii* was developed by Naot and Remington and colleagues.[369, 810, 865] It is presently the most widely used method for demonstration of IgM antibodies to *T. gondii* in adults, the fetus, and newborns. In contrast to the conventional method in which the wells of microtiter plates are coated with antigen, the wells are coated with specific antibody to IgM. The double-sandwich IgM ELISA is more sensitive than the IgM IFA test for diagnosis of the recently acquired infection, and serum samples that are negative in the dye test but that contain either antinuclear antibodies or rheumatoid factor and thus cause false-positive results in the IgM IFA test are negative in the double-sandwich IgM ELISA. This latter observation is attributed to the fact that serum IgM fractions are separated from IgG fractions during the initial step in the double-sandwich IgM ELISA procedure.

The double-sandwich IgM ELISA is also useful for diagnosis of congenital *T. gondii* infection.[369] The double-sandwich IgM ELISA was positive in 43 (72.7%) of 55 serum samples from newborns with proven congenital *T. gondii* infection, whereas the IgM IFA test was positive in only 14 (25.4%) of these samples. Of the sera obtained from the infected newborns during the first 30 days of life, 81.2% were positive in the double-sandwich IgM ELISA, whereas only 25% were positive in the IgM IFA test. The double-sandwich IgM ELISA avoids false-positive results related to rheumatoid factor and false-negative results related to competition from high levels of maternal IgG antibody that occur in the IgM IFA test. A number of modifications of the method have been described.[562, 901–907] The double-sandwich IgM ELISA is superior to the IgM IFA test for diagnosis both of acute acquired and congenital *T. gondii* infections.

Immunosorbent Agglutination Assay for Demonstration of IgM, IgA, and IgE Antibodies. The

ISAGA[813, 815, 863, 908–910] is widely used by investigators because it combines the advantages of both the direct agglutination test and the double-sandwich (capture) ELISA in its specificity and sensitivity for demonstration of IgM, IgA, and IgE[815] antibodies to *T. gondii*. The ISAGA does not require use of an enzyme conjugate; it is as simple to perform as the direct agglutination test and is read in the same manner as that test. It avoids false-positive results related to the presence of rheumatoid factor and/or antinuclear antibodies in serum samples. A commercial kit for IgM antibodies is available (bioMérieux, Lyon, France).

The ISAGA is more sensitive and more specific than the IgM IFA and IgM ELISA[911, 912] and has been used effectively for diagnosis of congenital infection.[913] Specific IgA antibodies in the ISAGA test indicated congenital toxoplasmosis in three infants in the absence of associated IgM antibodies.[914] The ISAGA method has also been used by Pinon and co-workers for detection of IgA antibodies.[868, 912] These investigators found such antibodies in serum and CSF of seven cases of congenital toxoplasmosis in the neonatal period.

Because of its high sensitivity, the ISAGA detects IgM antibodies earlier after the acute acquired infection (e.g., 1 to 2 weeks) than do other tests for IgM antibody. This sensitivity also results in the longest duration of detection of IgM antibody after infection. The method has been standardized by the recognition of this greater sensitivity to provide greater diagnostic power during early infections in adults.[911] Pinon and co-workers[815] and Wong and associates[850] have found the IgE ISAGA to be useful for diagnosis of acute acquired infection in the pregnant woman and in the congenitally infected newborn. Its advantage is related to its early rise along with IgM and IgA antibodies and its much earlier disappearance. In the study by Pinon and co-workers, IgE antibodies in the adult persisted for less than 4 months. At present, this test is only available in a few specialty laboratories. As is true for appropriate interpretation of all other serologic tests for diagnosis of the acute infection, it should be used only in combination with other serologic methods.[844, 910]

Enzyme-Linked Immunofiltration Assay. Please see earlier section for discussion of this method.[867]

Guidelines for Evaluation of the Newborn After Diagnosis of Congenital Toxoplasmosis Is Suspected

Guidelines for evaluation of the newborn of a mother who acquired her infection during gestation to include or exclude the diagnosis of congenital *T. gondii* infection are shown in Table 5–28.

Serologic Diagnosis of Acquired *Toxoplasma gondii* Infection in the Pregnant Woman

The presence of a positive titer (except for the rare false-positive results mentioned earlier) in any of the

---

TABLE 5–28

Guidelines for Evaluation of Newborn of Mother Who Acquired Her Infection During Gestation to Determine Whether Infant Has Congenital *Toxoplasma* Infection and to Assess Degree of Involvement

History and physical examination
Pediatric neurologic evaluation
Pediatric ophthalmologist examination of retinae
Complete blood cell count with differential, platelet count
Liver function tests (bilirubin, GGTP)
Urinalysis, serum creatinine
Serum quantitative immunoglobulins
Serum Sabin-Feldman dye test (IgG), IgM ISAGA, IgA ELISA, IgE ISAGA/ELISA[a] (with maternal serum, perform same tests as for infant except substitute IgM ELISA for the IgM ISAGA and also obtain AC/HS[a])
Cerebrospinal fluid cell count, protein, glucose, and *T. gondii*–specific IgG and IgM antibodies as well as quantitative IgG to calculate antibody load
Subinoculate into mice or tissue culture 1 ml peripheral blood buffy coat or clot and digest of 100 g placenta (see Diagnosis section for method of digestion). Consider PCR of buffy coat from approximately 1 ml blood, cell pellet from approximately 1 ml cerebrospinal fluid, and cell pellet from 10–20 ml amniotic fluid (see Diagnosis section)
Brain computed tomography scan with and without contrast medium enhancement
Auditory brain-stem response to 20 dB

GGTP = gamma-glutamyltranspeptidase; PCR = polymerase chain reaction.
[a]When performed in combination in our laboratories, these tests have demonstrated a high degree of specificity and sensitivity in establishing the diagnosis of acute infection in the pregnant woman and congenital infection in the fetus and newborn.

---

serologic tests discussed earlier establishes the diagnosis of *T. gondii* infection. Because titers in each of these tests may remain elevated for years, a single high titer does not indicate whether the infection is acute or chronic, nor does it necessarily mean that the clinical findings are due to toxoplasmosis. Before a diagnosis of acute *T. gondii* infection or toxoplasmosis can be made by means of serologic tests, it is necessary to demonstrate a rising titer in serial specimens (either conversion from a negative to a positive titer or a rise from a low to a higher titer).[259, 915] Because the diagnosis is frequently considered relatively late in the course of the patient's illness, serologic test titers (e.g., dye test, IFA test, or ELISA) may have already reached their peak at the time the first serum is obtained for testing. The IgM IFA test, IgM ELISA, IgM ISAGA, and tests for IgA and IgE antibodies and IgG avidity appear to be of considerable help in these circumstances.[259, 532, 810, 813, 863, 896, 910] The most important fact for the clinician is that any patient with a positive IgG titer and a positive IgM IFA or IgM ELISA titer must be presumed to have recently acquired infection with *T. gondii* and be tested further in a reference laboratory.[863, 916] Most mothers of children with congenital toxoplasmosis are unable to recall being ill during pregnancy. Some (10 to 20%) notice enlarged lymph nodes, mostly in the posterior cervical area, a sign that suggests acquired infection. These enlarged nodes are sometimes still present at delivery. Clinical signs of infection in the pregnant woman are not necessarily associated with an increased predilection for transmission, as shown by the reports of cases in which, although the parasite was present in a lymph node biopsy performed as part of the diagnostic evaluation of lymphadenopathy, the offspring were uninfected.[527, 917, 918] Examples of similar cases of lymphadenopathy (with demonstration of the parasite in the nodes) in which congenital transmission did occur are those of Siim,[919] Beckett and Flynn,[114] Macer,[631] and Couvreur.[920]

Because the majority (> 80%) of cases of acquired T. gondii infection are subclinical, the diagnosis relies mainly on the results of serologic tests. To interpret serologic test results in the pregnant woman, it is important to understand how antibodies of different immunoglobulin classes and different specificities for antigenic determinants develop after the infection is acquired and which antibodies are detected in the different serologic methods used for diagnosis of this infection. In addition, the physician should have knowledge of the relationship of the time of acquisition of the infection to the onset of parasitemia (which results in infection of the placenta) and also to the onset of clinical manifestations (when present). The answers to many of these questions are unknown or only partly understood. What follows in this section is information and guidelines for interpretation of test results, as adopted from our personal experiences and supplemented by pertinent data from the literature. We have attempted whenever possible to distinguish between hypothesis and established fact.

The antigenic structure of T. gondii is complex; both cytoplasmic antigens, which are liberated when the organisms are lysed, and membrane antigens are involved in the immune response.[921–927] We know that certain antigens cross react, because normal human sera contain IgM antibodies that bind to these antigens.[928–930] It seems reasonable to suggest that antibodies formed in response to these different antigens differ both in their specificity and in their class and subclass of immunoglobulins.[931] These variations account for the fact that different antibodies may or may not be detected, depending on the serologic method employed.

In Table 5–29, we have attempted to describe the evolution of the IgM, IgG, IgA, and IgE antibody responses as they relate to interpretation of serologic test results in the diagnosis of T. gondii infection in the pregnant woman.[811] An example of their usefulness is shown in Table 5–30. The usefulness of the IgG avidity method is shown in Table 5–31. Agreement between the avidity test and the HS/AC test is 97% in the Palo Alto laboratory.

ANTIBODY RESPONSE IN RELATION TO THE SEROLOGIC METHOD USED

The methods for demonstration of specific IgM antibodies have been discussed earlier. They are valuable as long as it is possible to ascertain that a positive result is not due to the presence of "natural" IgM antibodies,[932] rheumatoid factor, or antinuclear antibodies. For this reason, methods that rely on differences in titers after

sera have been treated with 2-mercaptoethanol (e.g., the IHA and agglutination tests) are not satisfactory. Specific IgM antibodies may not be detectable within a few weeks after their first demonstration or may persist for years. In studies of women who seroconverted during gestation, IgA antibodies as measured by ELISA appeared at approximately the same time as did IgM antibodies.[853] Similar results have been observed with the IgE ISAGA.[815, 933] Antibody titers in the IgE ISAGA decrease more rapidly than do IgA antibodies. In the study by Pinon and co-workers,[815] they persisted for less than 4 months in 23 patients tested serially. In the study by Wong and associates, the IgE ISAGA results were similar to those reported by Pinon and co-workers whereas IgE antibodies measured by ELISA persisted significantly longer in some seroconverters.[850]

Titers in the dye test, the agglutination test, and the IHA test (when these latter two tests are performed with 2-mercaptoethanol) depend on the concentration of IgG antibodies; this is true also for the conventional IFA test when performed with a conjugate specific for IgG. Nevertheless, depending on which test is used, differences in the rise and fall of IgG antibody titers are noted; titers in the dye test rise more rapidly, whereas those measured in the agglutination and IHA tests in the presence of 2-mercaptoethanol rise slowly.

A summary of the IgG antibody responses to T. gondii infection, as measured by different serologic methods, is given in Table 5–32. For a discussion of the IgG avidity method, see earlier under IgG Avidity in the section on Demonstration of Antibodies in Serum and Body Fluids.

A special comment regarding the agglutination test is made here because of its commercial availability and increasing usefulness for screening and diagnosis of the acute infection in pregnant women. With the whole-cell agglutination test, agreement with the dye test was virtually 100% except in some patients tested within a few days after they became infected, when only IgM antibodies were present.[831] With these serum samples, the dye test was at times positive while the agglutination test was still negative. In contrast, the agglutination test may be positive at times when the dye test is negative in chronically infected persons. This is due to the greater sensitivity of the agglutination test for detection of low titers of IgG antibodies. Because it takes more than 2 months (2 to 6 months) for IgG antibodies detected with the whole-cell agglutination test to reach a steady high titer, the existence of a steady high titer signifies that the infection was acquired more than 2 months earlier. As a consequence, if the first sample of serum has been obtained during the first 2 months of pregnancy, a stable agglutination test titer demonstrates that the infection occurred before the time of conception and that there is little risk of a congenitally infected infant.[831]

It is exceedingly difficult to establish guidelines for interpretation of serologic methods that measure both IgM and IgG antibodies. For example, in examining paired sera that were stated to have high stable titers in the conventional IFA test (performed with a conjugate against total immunoglobulins), we have frequently observed a definite rise in titer between the samples when a method specific for IgG antibody was used (e.g., the

TABLE 5–29
General Considerations of IgM, IgG, IgA, and IgE Antibody Responses to Postnatally Acquired Infection with *Toxoplasma*

ANTIBODIES	UNINFECTED INDIVIDUAL	RECENT (ACUTE) INFECTION	CHRONIC (LATENT) INFECTION
IgM			
Directed toward antigens that cross-react	Present	Present	Present
Directed toward specific *Toxoplasma* antigens	Absent	Present in almost all cases. Period that IgM antibodies are present may vary from a few weeks to many months. Ability to detect these antibodies depends on serologic technique used.	Most often absent, but IgM antibodies may persist for years in some patients (about 5%). In such cases, titers are almost always low, but in some cases they remain high. Persistence of IgM antibodies is generally associated with low or medium titers of IgG antibodies.
IgG			
Directed toward antigens that cross-react	Absent	Absent (?)	Absent (?)
Directed toward specific *Toxoplasma* antigens	Absent (<2 IU/ml)[a]	Present. Rise from a low titer (2 IU/ml) to a high titer (300–6000 IU/ml). In a few asymptomatic patients, titers remain low (100–200 IU/ml). Duration of rise varies with patient and with serologic test used. Depending on serologic techniques, it may take from 2 to 6 mo for the IgG antibody titer to reach its peak.	Present. Stable or slowly decreasing titers (to a titer of 2–200 IU/ml). High titers (>300 IU/ml) persist for years in some patients (about 5%). A significant rise in titer is sometimes observed after a normal decrease in titer has occurred.
IgA			
Directed toward antigens that cross-react	Absent	Absent (?)	Absent (?)
Directed toward specific *Toxoplasma* antigens	Absent	Present in almost all cases. Period that IgA antibodies are present may vary from several months to 1 year or more. The most common disappear by 7 months.	Most often absent
IgE			
Directed toward antigens that cross-react	Absent	Absent (?)	Absent (?)
Directed toward specific *Toxoplasma* antigens	Absent	Present	Absent

[a]Titers are expressed in international units (IU) to minimize technical differences that might occur among different laboratories.

dye test or the agglutination test performed with 2-mercaptoethanol). Although both samples had the same titer in the conventional IFA test, the titer in the first sample was the sum of the anti-IgM and anti-IgG antibody activities of the conjugate whereas the titer in the second sample reflected only the anti-IgG antibody activity of the conjugate.

Establishing guidelines for the IHA and CF tests is made difficult by the fact that different antigen preparations cause markedly different results; some preparations detect IgM antibodies, some detect IgG antibodies, and others detect both. Thus, the evolution of the antibody response may differ not only when different tests are used but also when the same test is used in different laboratories. This problem has been paramount in the confusion surrounding the subject of the practical approach to diagnosing acute infection.

In a systematic screening program (data of G Des-monts and P Thulliez, Paris, France) in which follow-up sera from pregnant women are examined monthly, IgM antibodies are usually the first to appear, but low titers of IgG antibodies, as measured in the dye test, also appear early. Sera in which only IgM antibodies are detectable are uncommon. A rise in IgM antibody titer is infrequently observed, suggesting that the IgM antibody titer rise is steep and that this rise does not last longer than 1 or 2 weeks before reaching its peak. In contrast, the rise in IgG antibody titer is initially slow. The titer, as measured in the dye test, usually remains relatively low (2 to 100 IU/ml or 1:10 to 1:100) for 3 to 6 weeks. This fact is critical for proper interpretation of serologic test results when serum samples obtained 2 to 3 weeks apart are tested in parallel, especially if the dye test is performed with fourfold dilutions of the sera, which would require an eightfold (two-tube) rise in titer to be considered significant. When testing such sera in paral-

TABLE 5–30
Serologic Test Results in Women Who Seroconverted During Pregnancy

PATIENT	DATE	DYE TEST (IgG) (IU/ml)	IgM ELISA[a]	IgM ISAGA[a]	IgA ELISA[a]	AC/HS[b]	IgE ELISA[c]	IgE ISAGA[a]
1	12/29/89	<2	0.4	0	0.6	NA	−	0
	02/23/90	200	5.0	12	1.8	A	+	6
	03/30/90	400	2.1	12	1.0	A	+	3
	04/30/90	800	1.3	12	0.8	A	+	3
	05/28/90	800	0.6	8	1.0	A	−	3
	06/26/90	800	1.1	6	1.0	A	+	3
2	02/17/89	<2	0.7	0	0.2	NA	−	0
	04/20/89	<2	0.2	0	0.0	NA	−	0
	05/18/89	160	6.4	12	2.8	NA	+	4
	08/23/89	200	2.7	12	0.8	A	±	0
3	03/09/82	Negative	0.0	QNS	QNS	QNS	−	6
	03/24/82	16	8.3	12	2.6	NA	+	9
	08/10/82	1000	4.9	12	2.6	A	+	6
	09/13/82	500	4.8	12	2.5	A	+	6
	12/07/82	200	4.1	12	1.0	A	+	3
	08/24/83	64	2.2	11	0.6	(A)	±	0

[a]Positive results (in an adult): IgM ELISA = ≥ 1.7; IgM ISAGA = >3; IgA ELISA = 1.4; IgE ISAGA = 4 (3 is considered borderline).
[b]AC/HS results: A = acute; NA = not acute; (A) = borderline acute.
[c]IgE ELISA: − = negative; + = positive; ± = equivocal (see reference 850).
QNS = quantity not sufficient.
Adapted from Wong SY, Hajdu M-P, Ramirez P, et al. Role of specific immunoglobulin E in diagnosis of acute *Toxoplasma* infection and toxoplasmosis. J Clin Microb 31:2952–2959, 1993, with permission.

lel, it is imperative to use twofold dilutions so that a fourfold (two-tube) rise can be detected. In our experience, this rise is difficult to detect in the IgG IFA test. After the initial 3 to 6 weeks, the rise in IgG antibody titer becomes steeper; high titers (> 400 IU/ml or 1:1000) are usually reached within an additional 3 weeks. Thereafter, the rise in titer is slower but may still be detectable over an additional 3 to 6 weeks if careful quantitative methodology is used (here again, this rise will be missed if fourfold dilutions of sera are used). Thus, although the rise in IgG antibody titer as detected in the dye test differs from one case to another, it lasts for more than 2 months and sometimes as long as 3 months. The rise in IgG antibody titer, as detected in the agglutination test (in the presence of 2-mercaptoethanol), may parallel exactly the pattern described for the dye test or the titer may rise more slowly; the peak may not occur earlier than 6 months after infection. As mentioned earlier, by 6 months, titers in the IgM IFA test are no longer demonstrable in most cases. Titers in the capture IgM ELISA and in the IgM ISAGA, however, usually remain positive for this period; and in women who acquire the infection during pregnancy, the titers in these latter two tests are almost always positive at the time of parturition (the level of the titer depends on the duration of infection before delivery).

Although definitive data are not available, when specific treatment for *T. gondii* infection is administered early during the initial antibody response (when the IgG antibody titer is still low), it appears that the antibody response may be slowed and the titer (e.g., in the dye test, conventional IFA test, or ELISA) may remain relatively low as long as treatment is continued. A late (delayed) rise is often observed after cessation of treatment.

TABLE 5–31
Usefulness of a High Avidity Test Result in Women with a Positive IgM Test Titer in the First 12 Weeks of Gestation

PATIENT NO.	WEEKS OF GESTATION	DYE TEST TITER IU/ml	IgM ELISA[a]	PERCENT AVIDITY[b]	AVIDITY INTERPRETATION
1	10	51	4.7	44.4	High
2	9	51	2.3	41.6	High
3	11	102	2.6	31.2	High
4	8	102	5.8	33.8	High
5	12	410	2.9	47.3	High

[a]Negative 0.0–1.6, equivocal 1.7–1.9, positive ≥2.0.
[b]Low <15, borderline 15–30, high >30.

TABLE 5–32
IgG Antibody Responses to *Toxoplasma* Infection as Measured by Different Serologic Methods[a]

SEROLOGIC METHOD	UNINFECTED INDIVIDUAL	RECENT (ACUTE) INFECTION	CHRONIC (LATENT) INFECTION
Dye test	Negative (<1:4)	Rising from a negative or low titer (1:4) to a high titer (1:256 to 1:128,000).	Stable or slowly decreasing titer. Titers are usually low (1:4 to 1:256) but may remain high (≥1:1024) for years.
Agglutination test (after treatment of sera with 2-mercaptoethanol)	Negative (<1:4)	Rising slowly from a negative or low titer (1:4) to a high titer (1:512). If a high-sensitivity antigen is used, the titer may reach 1:128,000.	Stable or slowly decreasing titer. Titers are usually higher than in the dye test if a high-sensitivity antigen is used. Striking differences between dye test and agglutination test titers are observed in some patients.
IHA test (after treatment of sera with 2-mercaptoethanol)	Negative (<1:16)	Rising very slowly from a negative or low titer (1:16) to a high titer (1:1024). It may take 6 mo before a high titer is reached; in some patients, high titers are never observed.	Stable or slowly decreasing high or low titer.
Conventional IFA test (conjugated antiserum to IgG)	Negative (<1:20)	Rise in titer is parallel to rise in dye test titer, but decrease in titer might be slower than that in dye test.	

[a]Similar data for the IgG ELISA have not been published.

PRACTICAL GUIDELINES FOR DIAGNOSIS OF INFECTION IN THE PREGNANT WOMAN

Three examples are discussed: (1) A woman pregnant for a few weeks has had a serologic test for *T. gondii* infection performed on a routine basis by her physician or at her request; (2) a woman pregnant for a few months is suspected of having acute toxoplasmosis; and (3) a woman has just delivered, and congenital toxoplasmosis is suspected in the infant. In almost all cases in the United States, the diagnosis in these situations must be considered on two pieces of data: the results of a test for IgG antibodies (e.g., dye test, ELISA, IFA) and the results of a test for IgM antibody (e.g., IgM IFA, IgM ISAGA, or IgM ELISA). At the time of writing, commercial kits for IgA continue to vary in their reliability and are not available for IgE. The accuracy of some ELISA kits being sold at present is unsatisfactory, and proper interpretation of the results of titers obtained for many of these kits has not been defined clearly. A number of studies attest to the false-positive and false-negative results obtained with certain kits that employ IFA or ELISA technology.[133, 863, 864, 916, 934, 935]

1. *Pregnant for a few weeks.* If no antibody is demonstrable, the patient has not been infected and must be considered at risk of infection. A positive IgG test titer and a negative test result for IgM antibodies or high avidity antibody test can be interpreted as reflecting infection that occurred months or years before the pregnancy. Essentially, there is no risk of the patient giving birth to a congenitally infected child (unless she is immunosuppressed) regardless of the level of antibody titer. No matter how high the titer is, it should not be considered prognostically meaningful.

If IgM antibodies are present, the IgG test should be performed in parallel with a second sample taken 3 weeks after the first. If no rise in IgG antibody test titer occurs, the infection was acquired before pregnancy and there is almost no risk to the fetus. If a rise in IgG antibody test titer is observed, the infection was probably acquired less than 2 months previously, perhaps around the time of conception. In this situation, the risk of giving birth to an infected child is very low (see Table 5–8).

2. *Pregnant a few months with suspected acute infection.* The diagnosis depends on three criteria: (1) the presence of lymphadenopathy in areas compatible with the diagnosis of acute acquired toxoplasmosis,[529, 532, 739, 746, 936, 937] (2) a high IgG test titer (≥ 300 IU/ml), and (3) IgM antibody. If two of the three criteria are present, for purposes of management, the diagnosis of acute acquired toxoplasmosis should be considered likely. If, however, the IgG test titer is less than 300 IU/ml, a significant rise in titer should be demonstrable in a second serum sample obtained 2 to 3 weeks later. Confirmatory testing should be requested.

3. *Woman recently delivered of an infant in whom congenital toxoplasmosis is suspected.* The diagnosis of the acute acquired infection in these mothers is rarely difficult. As a rule, diagnosis of recent infection in a mother delivered of a child with suspected congenital toxoplasmosis relies on the IgG test titer and the results of tests for IgM antibodies. Paradoxically, examination of maternal sera is frequently more useful for diagnosing subclinical or atypical congenital toxoplasmosis in a neonate than is examination of the child's serum. If IgM antibody is detected in the mother and no prior serologic test results are available, her newborn should be examined clinically and serologically to rule out congenital infection.

Because IgM antibodies as measured by ELISA or

ISAGA may persist for many months or even years, their greatest value is in determining that a pregnant woman examined early in gestation has not recently been infected. A negative result virtually rules out recently acquired infection unless sera are tested late in gestation (in which case IgM antibodies may no longer be detectable) or so early after the acute infection that an antibody response has not yet occurred (in which case, the acute infection would be identified in a screening program in which follow-up serology is performed in seronegative pregnant women). A positive IgM test result is more difficult to evaluate unless a significant rise in IgG or IgM titer can be demonstrated when sera are run in parallel or when other tests (e.g., tests for IgA and IgE antibody and the AC/HS test) suggest recent infection. A very high IgM, IgA, or IgE titer is more likely to reflect recent infection, although such high titers may persist for months. Such positive sera should be tested with additional methods, such as the HS/AC or avidity test. In most cases, this will require use of, and consultation with, a reference laboratory. In the Palo Alto laboratory, a "chronic" pattern in the HS/AC test agrees virtually 100% with a "chronic" titer in the ELISA avidity test.

In the unusual situation in which a pregnant woman has a positive IgM antibody titer and a persistently negative IgG titer, a false-positive IgM result must be considered, and, where feasible, all such patients should have IgG antibodies measured by a different method.[938, 939] Examples of the serologic response in women who seroconverted during pregnancy are shown in Table 5–29. These sera were from women who were treated with spiramycin as soon as seroconversion was observed. This treatment may have partially curbed their antibody response.

Pinon and colleagues in France fortuitously diagnosed two cases of congenital toxoplasmosis in newborns whose mothers did not have detectable T. gondii antibodies at the time of birth. These cases prompted the investigators to perform a study over an 18-month period to determine by postnatal serologic follow up whether they could detect women who were infected but whose serology was negative at the time of delivery. They detected four cases of perinatal maternal infection, and two of them resulted in infected offspring. In view of these results, and to prevent missing maternal infection at the end of pregnancy, they suggest that serologic testing of seronegative women should continue such that the last blood sample is obtained at approximately 30 days *after* they have given birth.[107]

Prenatal Diagnosis of Fetal *Toxoplasma gondii* Infection

Although PCR on amniotic fluid is now the method of choice, cordocentesis[940–942] may still be used when PCR is unavailable or in the rare instances when the PCR is negative and the ultrasonographic findings suggest fetal infection. For this reason, results using this method are described here along with those obtained with PCR.

CORDOCENTESIS

When a diagnosis of acquired toxoplasmosis is established in a pregnant woman, either based on clinical manifestations or as a result of systematic serologic screening performed during pregnancy, it is possible to demonstrate either the presence or the absence of congenital T. gondii infection or congenital toxoplasmosis, or both, in the *fetus, before delivery.*[129, 130, 758, 943, 944] The method was initially described by Desmonts and colleagues,[129] and the overall results obtained by this same group were reported by Daffos and co-workers.[130] These investigators reported a prospective study of 746 documented cases of maternal T. gondii infection in which prenatal diagnosis was attempted with follow-up of the live-born infants for at least 3 months. Pathologic and parasitologic examinations of aborted fetuses were performed. The complication rate related to the procedure in general was 0.3 fetal losses per 1000. A volume of 1 to 3 ml of pure fetal blood was usually obtained at the first attempt. In 3% of cases, a second attempt was necessary; this was performed 1 hour later or 1 week later, depending on the reason for the failure in the initial attempt (F Daffos, personal communication to JS Remington, 1993). In only 4 of 1356 pregnancies were they unable to obtain pure fetal blood.[130]

Definitive diagnosis of fetal infection relied on isolation (by mouse inoculation) of the parasite from fetal blood or amniotic fluid usually obtained at 20 to 26 weeks of gestation and on serologic examination of serum of the fetus for evidence of synthesis of IgM T. gondii antibodies. Nonspecific tests included ultrasound scans; white blood cell, platelet, and eosinophil counts; and measurement of total IgM, γ-glutamyltransferase, and lactate dehydrogenase. An ultrasound examination was performed every 2 weeks from the time of fetal blood sampling to the end of pregnancy, with special focus on the size of the lateral cerebral ventricles (Fig. 5–21A and B), the thickness of the placenta, and the presence of ascites, hepatomegaly, or cerebral calcification.

To allow for a comprehensive analysis of the indications for and results of these diagnostic procedures, the 746 pregnant women were divided into three groups. Group 1 included 159 women in whom a recently acquired acute infection was discovered when the first serologic screening test was performed at the beginning of pregnancy. Serologic or clinical data suggested that they had acquired the infection either shortly before conception or, at the latest, before week 6 of gestation. Group 2 included 487 women whose infection was acquired between weeks 6 and 16 of gestation. Tests for possible seroconversion are as a rule performed monthly in seronegative women in France, a practice that facilitates determination of the time at which infection was acquired. In these groups, cases were referred for prenatal diagnosis but were not included in the study if the fetus was dead in utero because of congenital toxoplasmosis before the time of blood sampling. The incidences of congenital infection were 0.6% and 3.7%, respectively. Group 3 was composed of 100 women who acquired the infection between weeks 17 and 25; fetal

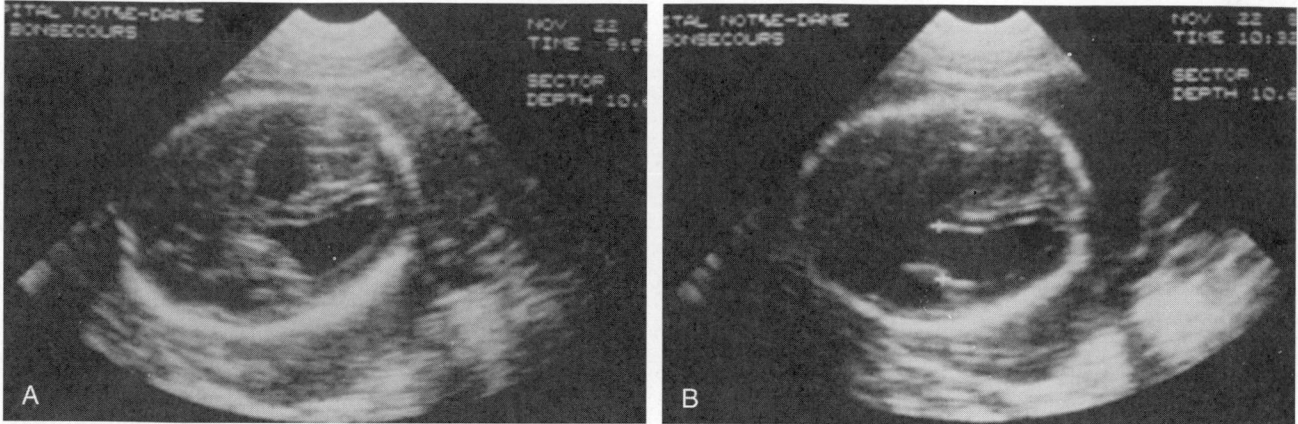

FIGURE 5–21 *A* and *B,* Ultrasound study of fetus with hydrocephalus resulting from toxoplasmosis. (Courtesy of F Daffos, Paris.)

blood and amniotic fluid were sampled between weeks 24 and 29. In this group, the incidence of congenital infection was 20%.

The presence of *T. gondii* infection in the fetus was demonstrated at prenatal examination in 39 of these 746 pregnancies. Infection was parasitologically proved by isolation of *T. gondii* from fetal blood or amniotic fluid, or both, in 34 of the 39 cases. *T. gondii*–specific IgM antibodies were detected in fetal blood in only 9 cases, despite the high sensitivity of the method used (ISAGA). None of the samples taken before week 24 was positive. Signs of congenital toxoplasmosis were recognized at ultrasound examination in 9 of the 39 cases; these were principally unilateral or bilateral ventricular dilations demonstrated by an increase in the ventricle:hemisphere ratio. In 10 additional cases, the ultrasound examination result was normal at the time of fetal blood sampling (24 weeks) but ventricular dilation appeared during the following weeks and was present at the time of termination of the pregnancy. Ascites were observed twice as an early but transitory sign. Intrahepatic calcifications were found in one case, and intracranial calcifications were noted in two cases.

One or more laboratory measurements of fetal blood proved to be abnormal in most cases. The most frequent signs were an increase in the total IgM level (22 of the 37 samples examined) and an increase in γ-glutamyl-transferase level (28 of the 33 samples examined). It is evident from these results that none of the examinations performed proved to be 100% reliable for demonstration of congenital toxoplasmosis in the fetus. However, when the results of the various tests were grouped together, they had a remarkably high predictive value and a high degree of specificity.

POLYMERASE CHAIN REACTION

In 1994, Hohlfeld and co-workers from Paris[132] published a follow-up to their cordocentesis study reported in 1988.[130] Prenatal diagnosis, which included amniocentesis, ultrasonography, and fetal blood sampling, was performed in 2632 women who had acquired *T. gondii* infection during gestation. One hundred ninety-four cases of congenital toxoplasmosis were identified, and 178 of them were diagnosed by conventional methods of prenatal diagnosis. There were no false-positive results. The overall sensitivity was 92%, the specificity was 100%, and the negative predictive value was 99%. The sensitivity of the IgM antibody test was 28%; of mouse inoculation with fetal blood, 72%; of mouse inoculation with amniotic fluid, 64%; and of tissue culture of amniotic fluid, 64%. The overall rate of spontaneous fetal loss was 1.3%. PCR was performed on the amniotic fluid in 339 consecutive women, and the results were compared with those obtained by the conventional methods. By conventional testing, congenital infection was demonstrated in 34 fetuses, and in each the PCR test was also positive. In three additional fetuses, only the PCR was positive, and in each the diagnosis of congenital infection was confirmed on follow-up (autopsy findings in two and serology in one). There was one false-negative result with the PCR and no false-positive results. The investigators concluded that the PCR is a more reliable, safer, simpler, and less expensive method than the conventional methods they had been using and that it can be used from the eighteenth week of gestation until term. They also concluded that fetal blood sampling is no longer necessary and that amniocentesis together with the PCR test and inoculation of mice (tissue culture is less sensitive) is preferred (Table 5–33). The authors did not have data on the efficacy of testing amniotic fluid before 18 weeks' gestation. They stated that prenatal diagnosis should not be attempted until at least 4 weeks after the acute infection in the mother.

AMNIOCENTESIS: POLYMERASE CHAIN REACTION IN AMNIOTIC FLUID

In 1998, Forestier (a member of the original Daffos group) and his colleagues published additional data from 1867 consecutive new cases of prenatal diagnosis using the PCR on amniotic fluid as the sole diagnostic method. The overall risk of fetal infection was 7.6%, when compared with the 7.4% they had observed in their previous study, which included both PCR and fetal

TABLE 5–33

Diagnostic Value of the Polymerase Chain Reaction Compared with Conventional Methods of Prenatal Diagnosis of Congenital *Toxoplasma gondii* Infection in 339 Pregnancies

VARIABLE	PCR[a]	CONVENTIONAL METHODS[a, b]
Sensitivity	37/38 (97.4; 86.1–99.9)	34/38 (89.5; 72.2–97.0)[c]
Specificity	301/301 (100; 98.8–100)	301/301 (100; 98.8–100)
Positive predictive value	37/37 (100; 90.5–100)	34/34 (100; 89.7–100)
Negative predictive value	301/302 (99.7; 98.7–100)	301/305 (98.7; 97.4–99.9)

[a]Positive tests/all tests (%; 95% confidence interval).
[b]Tissue culture of amniotic fluid, inoculation of mice with fetal blood and amniotic fluid, and determination of specific IgM in fetal blood.
[c]The sensitivity of conventional methods in the study overall was somewhat higher (92%; 95% confidence interval, 88 to 96%).

Adapted from Hohlfeld P, et al. Prenatal diagnosis of congenital toxoplasmosis with polymerase-chain-reaction test on amniotic fluid. N Engl J Med 331:695–699, 1994.

blood sampling.[132] As previously observed, the incidence of congenital infection increased with gestational age at the time of maternal infection, but the investigators did not have sufficient data to accurately assess the risk beyond the thirty-second week of gestation. Their results clearly demonstrate the value of PCR on amniotic fluid owing to its reliability, relative safety, and speed with which results can be obtained. The inclusion in the PCR methodology of specific decontamination with uracil DNA glycosylase to prevent carry-over contamination was emphasized by the authors.

In 1998, Jenum and associates published the Norwegian experience with a nested PCR on amniotic fluid collected from 67 women diagnosed as having acquired the infection during gestation.[794] They also used mouse inoculation on each of the samples. They commented on the greater sensitivity of the PCR because mouse inoculation results were affected by treatment of the mothers. Whereas Hohlfeld and co-workers[132] found a specificity of 100%, Jenum and associates observed a specificity of only 94% despite careful technical steps to avoid contamination of their samples. Their positive predictive value was 67%, with 10 true positives among 15 positive results. Three of 8 infants with congenital toxoplasmosis diagnosed after birth had a negative PCR and mouse inoculation on prenatal examination. Thus, in their study, a positive PCR result did not confirm infection in the fetus. For this reason, the researchers stated that positive results also require serologic follow-up for confirmation of the diagnosis. Prenatal diagnosis using PCR performed on amniotic fluid from each twin in a dizygotic pregnancy was recently reported by Tjalma and colleagues.[945]

Because a physician must make decisions regarding management of a pregnancy after results of amniocentesis are obtained, it is of utmost importance that the PCR be specific insofar as there are no false-positive results. For example, the recent report of the use of a nested PCR[794] did not appear to yield results that fit this requirement, and thus that nested PCR cannot be considered as an improvement over conventional methods for prenatal diagnosis.

One shortcoming of the study reported by Hohlfeld and co-workers[132] is that the sensitivity and negative predictive value of the PCR on amniotic fluid were compared with those of conventional methods but not with the status of the infection in the live-born infants. The enthusiasm that has been generated for the reliability of the PCR should be tempered by the fact that, because of the delay that can occur between the time of maternal infection and transmission of the parasite to the fetus (transmission may occur after the date of the amniocentesis), all congenital infections are not and cannot be identified by prenatal diagnosis. One case that suggests such a delay is reported in the publication by Hohlfeld and co-workers.[132] Before PCR was used for prenatal diagnosis, it was well recognized that not all cases of congenital *T. gondii* infection could be detected prenatally. Of 89 congenital infections, Hohlfeld and co-workers[946] reported 9 cases (10%) with a negative prenatal diagnosis. In other published series, the rate of congenital infections with no prenatally identified abnormal findings varied from 3% in the study by Pratlong and co-workers[947] to 8% in that by Berrebi and associates.[948] Actually, the number of infections that were not detected by the prenatal diagnostic procedures was underestimated in each of these studies because a significant number of the offspring were lost to follow-up, 50 (24%) of 211,[947] or data were not provided by the investigators.[132] Before the use of PCR, it was not possible to define whether these discrepancies were due to a lack of sensitivity of the diagnostic procedures or to the fact that transmission of the parasite occurred after the amniocentesis or cordocentesis was performed. The higher sensitivity of PCR when compared with conventional methods explains why congenital infection had been missed in the past when the less-sensitive conventional methods were used. Preliminary data from a prospective study (P Thulliez and colleagues, study in progress) in which follow-up of infants is being performed reveal that approximately 15% of congenitally infected infants are not detected by the prenatal diagnostic procedure despite use of PCR. This is likely due to a delay in transmission of the parasite to the fetus. Thus, a negative prenatal diagnosis does not rule out the possibility of the congenital infection and consequently emphasizes the necessity to continue clinical and serologic follow-up of infants born to women who acquired the infection during pregnancy.

IGA ANTIBODIES

The value of demonstration of IgA *T. gondii* antibodies in the fetus is now well recognized,[853, 868, 947, 949, 950] and testing for these antibodies for this purpose should be routine in reference laboratories.

INTERFERON

Interferon has been demonstrated in blood of fetuses infected with *T. gondii*, suggesting that the fetus is able to synthesize this cytokine as early as 26 weeks of gestation.[951] Its demonstration appears helpful when used with other nonspecific tests for diagnosing *T. gondii* infection in the fetus. Interferon serum levels that were significantly higher than in controls were also demonstrated in sera of pregnant women during seroconversion for *T. gondii* antibodies.[951]

T CELL SUBSETS

T cell subsets were evaluated in a group of uninfected and infected fetuses.[952] Significant differences from controls were noted in that the infected fetuses were characterized by a smaller percentage of CD3 and CD4 T cells and a decrease in absolute number of CD4 cells and lower CD4:CD8 ratio. The mothers in this study were receiving treatment, and the possible results of this treatment on T cells could not be excluded. In addition, because the number of infected fetuses was small, it was not possible to compare the values obtained according to gestational age as was done in the control, uninfected fetuses.

In another study, Lecolier and co-workers studied T lymphocyte subpopulations in normal and in six *T. gondii*–infected fetuses.[949] They noted a significant increase of CD8[+] T cells in two cases investigated soon after maternal infection (3 and 6 weeks, respectively) and a significant decrease of CD4[+] T cells in the four other cases that were investigated later (7 to 13 weeks after maternal infection). These observations suggest that alterations in T lymphocyte subsets in the infected fetus are similar to those that occur in the acute acquired infection in adults.[422] In another study by Foulon and associates, these results were not confirmed.[758] Thus, further study is necessary to evaluate whether study of T cell subsets will be useful as an adjunctive test for prenatal diagnosis.

COMPLEMENT

It appears that the C4 component of complement is significantly increased in fetuses congenitally infected with *T. gondii*. Gestational age is important in interpretation of results, but the demonstration of elevated levels of C4 in a fetus may be a useful nonspecific adjunctive test for prenatal diagnosis.[953]

Serologic Diagnosis in the Newborn

Because of the pleomorphism of congenital toxoplasmosis, because the infection is most often subclinical in the newborn, and because the infection may be mimicked by other infections and diseases of the neonate, the diagnosis of congenital *T. gondii* infection is far more complicated than is diagnosis of the acquired infection.

The serologic diagnosis of congenital *T. gondii* infection in the newborn is particularly difficult because of the prevalence of antibodies to *T. gondii* in the normal childbearing population in the United States and in much of the rest of the world (see Table 5–14). Thus, a high antibody titer in a newborn may merely reflect past or recent infection in the mother (maternal IgG antibody having passed transplacentally to her fetus).

The fact that infection in the fetus may stimulate production of sufficient IgM to result in abnormally high levels of this immunoglobulin in the newborn has been shown in a variety of congenital infections by Stiehm and associates[897] and by Alford and co-workers.[954, 955] Thus, quantification of IgM in cord serum may be a valuable screening device for detecting infection in the newborn. At present, the consensus of those working on immunologic responses to perinatal infection is that enough "false-negative" results occur to suggest that quantification of IgM in the newborn may not be universally applicable for diagnosing infection.[956–958] Such false-negative results are not infrequent in premature infants with proven rubella.[956] For a nonspecific test to be beneficial as a screen, it seems that a slight excess in sensitivity resulting in overdiagnosis (false-positive results) can be accepted but that lack of sensitivity in known cases, resulting in underdiagnosis (false-negative results), cannot be accepted.

As mentioned previously, demonstration of IgM, IgA, or IgE antibodies to *T. gondii* in cord serum or serum of the newborn is diagnostic of congenital *T. gondii* infection if contamination with maternal blood has not occurred. When an appropriate fluorescein-tagged antiserum to IgM has been employed, we have not had any false-positive results except for the qualifications mentioned earlier under the description of the IgM IFA method. Because high levels of maternal IgG antibodies to *T. gondii* may compete for antigenic sites on the surface of the organisms[894] with the relatively low IgM antibody levels usually found in the fetus or neonate, weak reactions and low IgM antibody titers (1:2) indicate infection in the newborn. However, even allowing for these weakly positive reactions, detectable specific IgM antibody is absent in the sera of most neonates with congenital toxoplasmosis (approximately 75%) when the IgM IFA test is used.[687] This false-negative result rate was only approximately 20% if the double-sandwich IgM ELISA method was used.[369] Because of the high incidence of false-negative results in the IgM IFA test, we recommend that the capture IgM ELISA or ISAGA method be used instead. It is noteworthy that the proportion of infants showing IgM antibody is the same whether illness is clinically manifest or subclinical. IgA antibodies have been demonstrated in approximately 90% of newborns with the congenital infection,[853, 959] which further attests to the great value of testing for these antibodies (Table 5–34). A number of investigators have reported greater sensitivity of IgA antibody determination for diagnosis in infected children than for IgM.[812, 852, 853, 960, 961] As stated by Foudrinier and co-workers, specificity of IgA detected at birth must be confirmed, because equivocal and positive IgA test results were found in newborns during the first days of

TABLE 5–34

Serologic Test Results for IgM and IgA Antibodies at Birth and During the Newborn Period in Sera of 23 Congenitally Infected and 49 Uninfected Offspring of Mothers Infected During Gestation[a]

TRIMESTER MOTHER ACQUIRED INFECTION (TIME TEST PERFORMED)	IgM− IgA−	IgM+ IgA+	IgM+ IgA−	IgM− IgA+
Uninfected (at birth)	47	0	1	1
Infected (at birth)				
1st trimester	1	1	0	2
2nd trimester	1	0	0	5
3rd trimester	2	8	1	0
Infected (follow-up 1 wk to 3 mo)	3	11	0	9

[a]All mothers were treated with spiramycin during gestation from time seroconversion was noted.

Adapted from Decoster A, Slizwicz B, Simon J, et al. Platelia-toxo IgA, a new kit for early diagnosis of congenital toxoplasmosis by detection of anti-P30 immunoglobulin A antibodies. J Clin Microbiol 29:2291–2295, 1991, with permission.

life whereas subsequent sera became negative within less than 10 days.[961] They concluded that in a neonate born to a mother with IgA or IgM *T. gondii* antibodies, a positive IgA or IgM test result must be interpreted with caution and be confirmed after approximately 10 days of life unless the diagnosis is established before this time. Additional data are needed to clarify whether all newborns with a positive IgA or IgM antibody titer at approximately 10 days of age are indeed infected, especially in those cases in which the maternal IgA or IgM antibody titers were very high. Determination of levels of β-human chorionic gonadotropin and total IgA may prove of value as adjunctive tests. However, we have never observed a false-positive result after the first day of life when the ISAGA was used for detection of IgM antibodies. The value of demonstration of IgE antibodies is also clear. In one of our laboratories (JS Remington), 19 (90%) of 21 infants (ages birth to 5 weeks) with congenital toxoplasmosis and signs of CNS involvement tested positive for IgE antibodies (92% by ELISA and 62% by ISAGA)[850]; of the 10 tested in the first week of life, 9 had IgM antibody and all 7 of those tested for IgA antibodies were positive. Seven of the 21 were first tested in the second week of life; 6 had IgM antibodies, and all 5 of those tested for IgA were positive. Of the 4 first tested at 3 to 5 weeks of life, 3 had both IgM and IgA antibody; 1 infant had neither.[850] In ongoing studies by Pinon and colleagues, 52 cases of congenital *T. gondii* infection (5 symptomatic and 47 "asymptomatic" cases) were studied; at birth or during the first month of life, none of the symptomatic and 13 (25%) of the "asymptomatic" infants were positive by IgE ISAGA. Thirty-five (67%) of the 52 infants were positive for IgA antibody by ISAGA.[962]

The results from the laboratory of J. S. Remington using the IgE ELISA in infants with neurologic sequelae are encouraging.[850] The apparent differences from the

results of Pinon and colleagues are likely due to differences in methodology for detection of IgE antibodies and the excellent antenatal screening program in France, which enables early diagnosis and treatment of women who acquire the acute infection during gestation. Such treatment may blunt the serologic response in the fetus and newborn.

If the infant is infected in utero at a time when it is immunologically competent to produce IgM antibodies but before the passage of maternal IgG *T. gondii* antibodies across the placenta has occurred, there is no reason to suspect competition for recognition of antigenic sites on the parasite. Data derived from studies of infants with very high IgM titers in the early newborn period support this hypothesis. Table 5–35 displays clinical and serologic data representing such an instance in a mother and her infant. The mother had a high but not rising dye test titer since the ninth week of pregnancy and a negative IgM IFA test titer. The same results were obtained during the thirteenth week. This suggests that infection occurred at about the time of conception or a few weeks earlier. She was not treated and gave birth to a severely infected infant with generalized toxoplasmosis who died 8 days after delivery. This newborn had an unusually high IgM test titer. If, however, high titers of maternal antibody are present in the fetus before the organism reaches the fetus—as a consequence of delay by the placental barrier discussed earlier—it is possible that IgG antibody might compete (and "cover") for recognition sites[894] on the parasite or may by other means (e.g., feedback mechanism) suppress fetal IgM antibody synthesis. (This might also explain the paradoxical occurrence of an elevated IgM level in the serum of an infected infant in the presence of a negative IgM test titer.) That this may occur has been shown in an experimental animal model.[425] Thus, a negative IgM test titer in a newborn does not rule out the possibility of congenital infection.

In our experience, IgM antibody titers usually decrease rapidly after the infant's own IgG antibodies have reached a high titer; at 1 year of age, IgM antibodies are usually not demonstrable or are present in very low titer.

In the absence of demonstration of the parasite, IgM or IgA antibodies to *T. gondii*, follow-up testing of infants with suspected toxoplasmosis is the only means of making a serologic diagnosis of subclinical toxoplasmosis. For proper interpretation of test titers in infants who are past the immediate newborn period, the physician must understand how passively transmitted maternal IgG decreases in the uninfected infant. Because the literature is replete with misinformation on the interpretation of *T. gondii* serology in older infants, this important subject is dealt with here. In Figure 5–22, curve 1 shows the total serum IgG values in milligrams per deciliter in the newborn and infant to the age of 1 year. The values in the newborn at birth are frequently somewhat higher than they are in the mother and subsequently decrease. Minimal values (e.g., 300 to 400 mg/dl) are observed at about the third or fourth month, after which time the level increases with increasing production of IgG by the infant. Maternally transmitted antibodies (curve 2)

TABLE 5–35

Data in a Mother Who Acquired *Toxoplasma gondii* Infection at About the Time of Conception or a Few Weeks Earlier Who Had a Negative IgM Test Titer and Whose Infant Had a High IgM Test Titer

SUBJECT	STAGE OF PREGNANCY OR AGE	CLINICAL MANIFESTATIONS	TITER		*T. GONDII* ISOLATED
			Dye Test[a] (IU/ml)	IgM Test[b]	
Mother	9 wk	None	2000	Negative	
	13 wk	None	2000	Negative	
	8 mo	Delivery			
	1 mo after delivery	None	2000	Negative	Blood negative
Infant	4 days	Hydrocephalus, microphthalmia, convulsions, abnormal cerebrospinal fluid	1000	Positive	Blood positive
	8 days	Death			Brain positive

[a]Dye test titers are approximately 8000 in the mother and 4000 in the infant if expressed as reciprocal of serum dilution.

[b]Titers are expressed as the reciprocal of the serum dilution.

Adapted from Desmonts G, Couvreur J. Toxoplasmosis in pregnancy and its transmission to the fetus. Bull NY Acad Med 50:146–159, 1974, with permission. The mother was not treated.

progressively disappear, because they are not synthesized by the infant. Their half-life is approximately 30 days, that is, they decrease by approximately one half per month (Fig. 5–23).

Figure 5–24 shows actual data from an uninfected infant plotted against the background of the theoretical decay curve for IgG maternal antibody (approximately one half the value every 30 days). Thus, a titer of 1000 IU/ml at birth should drop to 1 IU/ml in 300 days. The infant whose titers are shown here had titers of 400 IU/ml at birth, 60 IU/ml at 75 days, and 3 IU/ml at 212 days. These are exactly the expected values. Figure 5–23

shows results obtained in 430 paired sera from 93 uninfected infants with passively transmitted maternal antibodies plotted against their theoretical values. Ninety-three percent of the actual titers are less than one twofold dilution different from the expected values. These data preclude acceptance of such statements as "all infants with a positive titer at 4 to 6 months have congenital toxoplasmosis." The same rate of decrease applies to both high and low titers. It takes approxi-

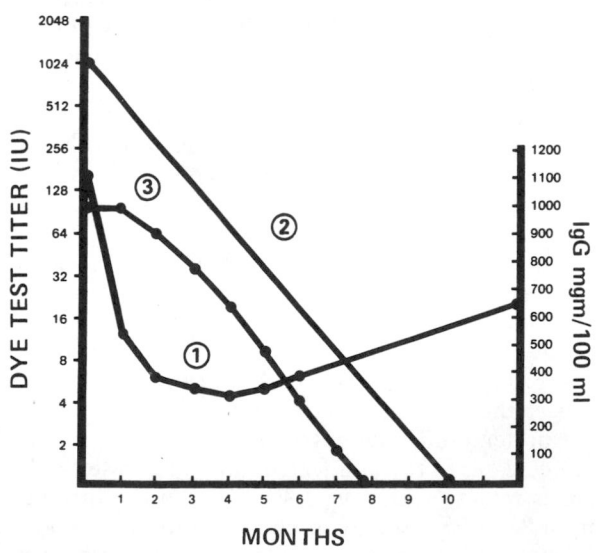

FIGURE 5–22 IgG and *Toxoplasma* antibodies: uninfected child. Curve 1, mg of IgG/dl; curve 2, IU of *Toxoplasma* antibody per ml; curve 3, IU of *Toxoplasma* antibody per mg of IgG. (From Desmonts G, Couvreur J. Toxoplasmosis: epidemiologic and serologic aspects of perinatal infection. *In* Krugman S, Gershon AA [eds]. Infections of the Fetus and the Newborn Infant. Progress in Clinical and Biological Research, vol. 3. New York, Alan R Liss, 1975, pp 115–132, with permission.)

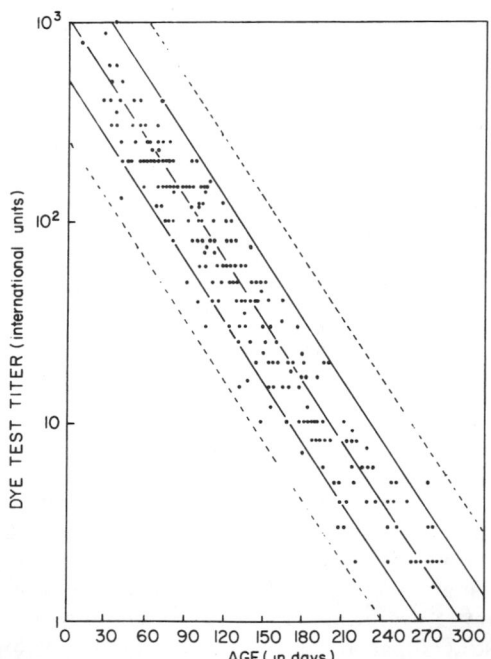

FIGURE 5–23 Decrease in maternally transmitted *Toxoplasma* antibodies (dye test) in uninfected infants. The two parallel lines indicate one half and twice the titer, plus or minus one twofold dilution. The result in one serum sample of each pair is on the theoretical line and is not represented by a dot. The result in the other serum sample of each pair is represented by a dot.

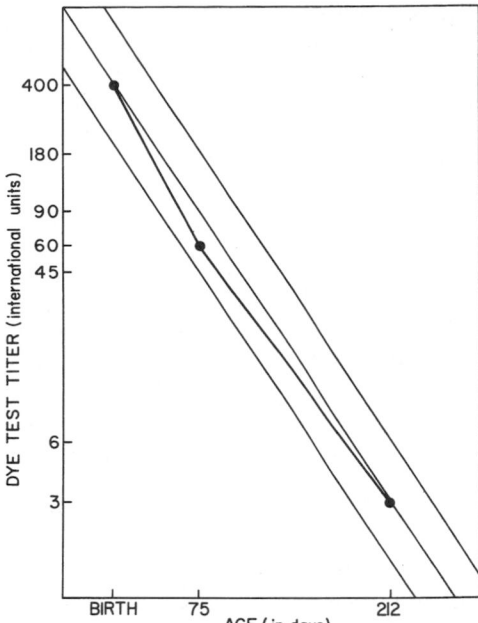

FIGURE 5–24 Evolution of maternally transmitted antibody (dye test) in an uninfected infant from birth to the age of 212 days.

mately the same amount of time for a decrease from 1000 to 250 IU/ml, a seemingly very significant variation, as for a decrease from 4 to 1 IU/ml, a titer difference that most investigators would consider negligible (i.e., no significant difference).

For a better estimate of this decrease in passively transmitted maternal antibodies, it is useful to compare the antibody titer to the level of IgG and to compute the specific *antibody load*, that is, the ratio of specific antibodies (number of IU/ml) to total IgG. This is represented diagrammatically in Figure 5–22 by curve 3 and in Table 5–35. In Figure 5–22, as late as the fourth to sixth week of life, there is usually no change in the antibody load; the IgG is still mainly maternal in origin. Although the titer of antibodies decreases, the total IgG decreases in a similar manner. As a result, the ratio remains constant. During the second and third months, the amount of IgG synthesized by the infant increases. Because this newly synthesized IgG does not contain antibodies to *T. gondii*, the antibody load decreases and will continue to decrease as IgG synthesis in the child progresses.

The production of antibody in infants with congenital toxoplasmosis varies considerably from one case to another and is also affected by treatment. Cases in which antibody production during fetal life can be demonstrated by antibody load are scarce. Early and delayed antibody production can, however, be demonstrated by the antibody load method. An example of early production is shown in Figure 5–25. During the first month of life, the titer in the infant decreases in proportion to the decrease in total IgG (curve 4). At 1 month of age, the situation is similar to that in an uninfected infant: the antibody titer and the total amount of IgG have dimin-

ished in the same proportions, and the antibody load is constant. However, during the second and third months, the antibody titer in the infected infant does not decrease at the rate expected and the antibody load remains the same or may increase. This finding demonstrates that the IgG being synthesized by the infant contains at least as many specific antibodies to *T. gondii* as does the maternal IgG, and this becomes obvious between the fourth and sixth months, when a definite increase in antibody titer and in antibody load occurs. In some cases, the rise in titer is not demonstrable until even later (Fig. 5–26).

The pattern observed in infants with a delayed onset of antibody response is shown in Figure 5–27. In this situation, the antibody titer remains parallel to the expected titer of passively transferred maternal antibodies. The antibody load decreases, proving that the infant has begun to synthesize IgG, which apparently does not contain significant amounts of antibodies to *T. gondii*. This situation may persist for several months before the onset of specific antibody production is demonstrable.

Another pattern of antibody development is that observed in infants born of mothers who acquire their infection very near to the time of delivery. Such infants have been found in prospective studies.[118, 120] Serologic test titers may be negative in the cord blood or show very low titers, especially during the first weeks of life. In such cases, the diagnosis would usually be missed— and, in fact, because of the low titer in the infant, probably never suspected.

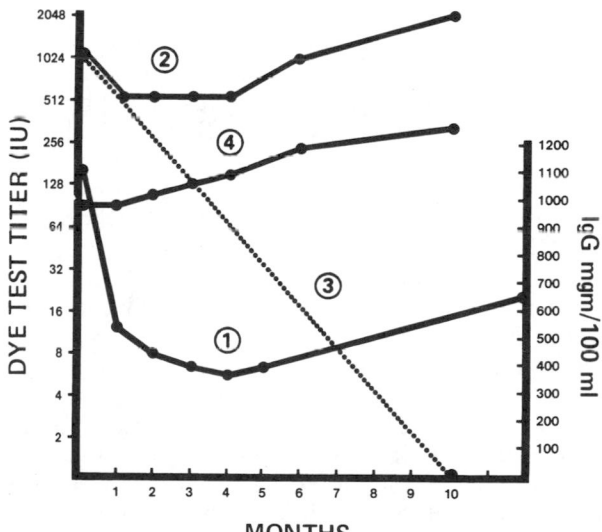

FIGURE 5–25 Antibodies in congenital toxoplasmosis (cases with early synthesis of antibodies). Curve 1, mg of IgG/dl; curve 2, IU of *Toxoplasma* antibody per ml; curve 3, expected titer if antibodies were maternal in origin; curve 4, IU of *Toxoplasma* antibody per mg of IgG. (From Desmonts G, Couvreur J. Toxoplasmosis: epidemiologic and serologic aspects of perinatal infection. *In* Krugman S, Gershon AA [eds]. Infections of the Fetus and the Newborn Infant. Progress in Clinical and Biological Research, vol. 3. New York, Alan R Liss, 1975, pp 115–132, with permission.)

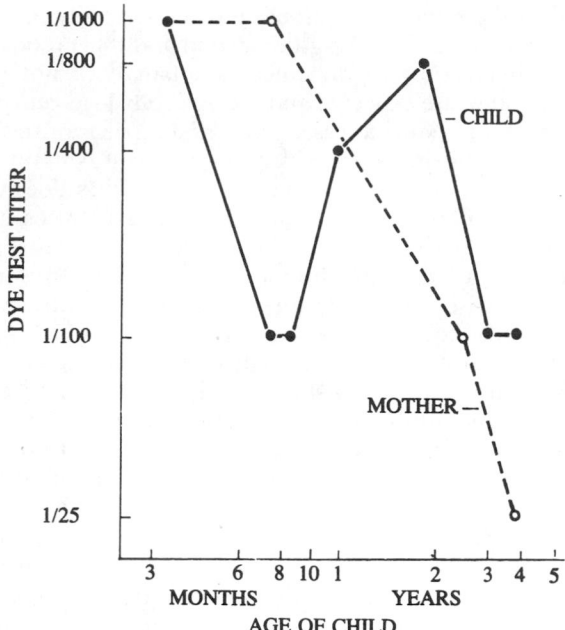

FIGURE 5–26 Example of antibody development (dye test) in a child with congenital toxoplasmosis in relation to time since birth. (From Couvreur J, Desmonts G. Congenital and maternal toxoplasmosis. A review of 300 congenital cases. Dev Med Child Neurol 4:519–530, 1962, with permission.)

SEROLOGY AND POLYMERASE CHAIN REACTION ON CEREBROSPINAL FLUID AND POLYMERASE CHAIN REACTION ON URINE

High titers of *T. gondii* antibodies are often observed in CSF of newborns with congenital toxoplasmosis. This does not prove that antigenic stimulus or antibody formation has occurred within the CNS, because the antibody load in the CSF of these neonates, as a rule, is equal to that in their serum. High titers of *T. gondii* antibodies can be observed in the CSF of newborns with other CNS diseases (e.g., congenital diseases due to syphilis[963] or cytomegalovirus), even when they are not infected with *T. gondii*. Because of passively transferred maternal *T. gondii* antibodies,[959] and when the protein concentration is very high in the CSF, the IgG concentration may reach the sensitivity level of the serologic test used. Thus, demonstration of high titers of IgG antibodies in the CSF in newborns is not useful diagnostically. Demonstration of IgM antibodies in the CSF, especially in the absence of IgM antibodies in the serum, supports the diagnosis of *T. gondii* infection in the CNS. In contrast to this situation in the newborn, serologic testing of CSF and determination of antibody load are sometimes diagnostic during infancy or childhood in patients with CNS toxoplasmosis. The diagnosis is also established if *T. gondii* antigens are demonstrable in the CSF. The method of choice for detection of the parasite in CSF is PCR. It is both highly sensitive and specific for this purpose.[642, 788, 964] Fuentes and colleagues[788] detected the parasite by PCR in blood and CSF of three of four newborns suspected of being congenitally in-

fected with *T. gondii* and by PCR in the urine of each of the four newborns. The investigators cautioned that because only urine from symptomatic newborns was examined, it will be necessary to assess the utility of PCR in urine from asymptomatic infants as well.

EFFECT OF TREATMENT

T. gondii–specific IgM is rarely present in serum of an infant at birth who has been treated with pyrimethamine and sulfadiazine in utero from the seventeenth week of gestation until birth.[946] Data on the effects of treatment on production of IgM, IgA, and IgE antibodies are insufficient for comment.[512, 762, 868] Adequate data, however, are available on the effects of treatment on the dye test (IgG antibody) and antibody load method. These are described here. Alterations in antibody response vary among different cases and appear to depend in large part on the stage of synthesis of antibody in the child when treatment is begun.

If the infant does not begin producing antibody before treatment is started or if synthesis is at a low level, treatment apparently curbs the low-grade synthesis and prevents antibody formation. (This is not surprising because treatment kills the tachyzoite form and thereby halts the production of antigen.)

Data on the IgM antibody response and on the development of IgG antibody by the fetus and infant presented in this section support the hypothesis discussed

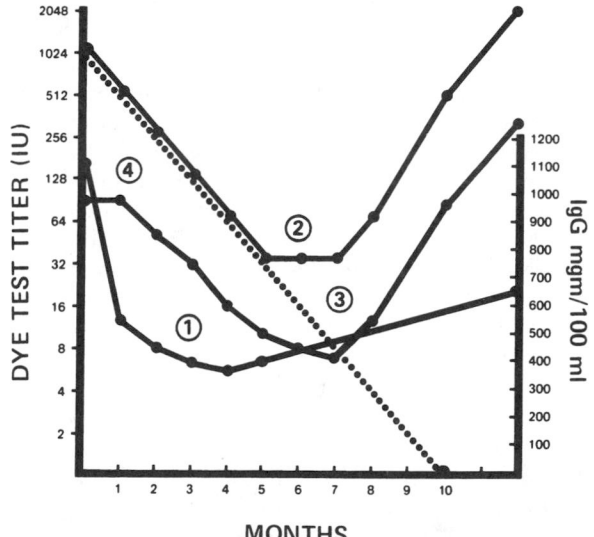

MONTHS

FIGURE 5–27 Antibodies in congenital toxoplasmosis (cases with delayed synthesis of antibodies). (Synthesis is usually not delayed more than 3 or 4 months if the child receives no treatment. It may be delayed up to the sixth or ninth month, if treated.) Curve 1, mg of IgG/dl; curve 2, IU of *Toxoplasma* antibody per ml; curve 3, expected titer if antibodies were maternal in origin; curve 4, IU of *Toxoplasma* antibody per mg of IgG. (From Desmonts G, Couvreur J. Toxoplasmosis: epidemiologic and serologic aspects of perinatal infection. *In* Krugman S, Gershon AA [eds]. Infections of the Fetus and the Newborn Infant. Progress in Clinical and Biological Research, vol. 3. New York, Alan R Liss, 1975, pp 115–132, with permission.)

TABLE 5–36

Correlation of Age of Infant and Presence of Demonstrable Parasitemia

AGE	NO. OF INFANTS	NO. WITH PARASITEMIA (%)
Cord–1st wk	28	20 (71)
2nd wk	15	5 (33)
3rd–4th wk	15	5 (33)
2nd mo	11	9 (0)

Adapted from Desmonts G, Couvreur J. Toxoplasmosis: epidemiologic and serologic aspects of perinatal infection. *In* Krugman S, Gershon AA (eds). Infections of the Fetus and the Newborn Infant. Progress in Clinical and Biological Research, vol 3. New York, Alan R. Liss, 1975, pp 115–132, with permission.

earlier (see Transmission section) that some infants are not infected during intrauterine life but are infected during labor, from the infected placenta. The data reveal that some newborns and fetuses are able to recognize *T. gondii* antigens and actively synthesize IgM and IgG antibodies. Once established, this synthesis of IgG and IgM antibodies does not appear to be affected by treatment. Other infants do not produce *T. gondii* antibodies until maternally transmitted antibody decreases to a low titer or until specific treatment is discontinued, thereby allowing renewed proliferation of the organism. Thus, in infants in whom a marked decrease in antibodies has occurred after birth—only to increase again when the infant is 3 or 4 months of age—it seems plausible to suggest that the infection occurred not during fetal life but during labor. The delay in antibody synthesis could be related solely to the late infection; this is substantiated by the fact that parasitemia is frequently demonstrable in cord blood or in the blood of the neonate during the first days of life (Table 5–36). But even if infection occurred during parturition, this explanation alone is insufficient to explain certain other observations. Antibodies develop readily during the first weeks of life in infants infected shortly before delivery as long as they received little or no maternal IgG antibody, whereas synthesis of antibody is often poor or completely lacking in infants whose early lesions prove that they were definitely infected during fetal life. Inhibition of fetal recognition of *T. gondii* antigen appears to offer the most satisfactory explanation for the delay in antibody synthesis observed in most infected infants. Maternal IgG is the most likely effector of this inhibitory effect. This is not solely of academic interest, because such inhibition of antibody synthesis, whether by maternal IgG or by specific treatment, has important implications for the diagnosis of congenital toxoplasmosis. If treatment is begun early in these infants and is continued for some months, the diagnosis cannot be established serologically before the sixth to twelfth month of life.

Serologic Rebound After Treatment. Serologic rebound (Table 5–37) occurs commonly when pyrimethamine and sulfadiazine are discontinued.[489, 965, 966] In the study by Villena and associates, rebound occurred in 90% of the infants, mainly 2 to 6 months after treatment was discontinued.[967] This serologic rebound indicates that although these antimicrobial agents eliminate active disease, probably through their effect on tachyzoites, not all organisms are eliminated in spite of 1 year of therapy. A small number of infants with very mild disease or minimal manifestations of infection, or both, have not had such serologic rebound. In almost all children, serologic rebound has been asymptomatic without changes on ophthalmoscopic examination. One infant with serologic rebound and symptoms had fever, failure to thrive, and new seizures in association with this serologic rebound. His illness resolved with resumption of 2 weeks of pyrimethamine and sulfadiazine therapy and did not recur when these medications were discontinued. Thus, it appears to be uncommon for an infant to develop symptomatic disease at the time serologic rebound occurs. Nonetheless, it seems prudent to closely observe infants (especially with an ophthalmologic examination), particularly during the months after therapy is discontinued. At present, no serologic markers have reliably been associated with recurrences of chorioretinitis in congenitally infected children. It was reported that the IgM level was often elevated with recurrences,[596] but this has not been found to be the case in the patients in the U.S. (Chicago) National Collaborative Treatment Trial[433] (see Table 5–22).

TABLE 5–37

Examples of Serologic Rebound in a Child Who Developed Symptoms (Patient 2) and in One Who Did Not (Patient 1)[a]

PATIENT	AGE SERUM OBTAINED (MO)	DYE TEST	IgM ISAGA	IgM ELISA	IgA ELISA	IgE ISAGA	IgE ELISA
1	1	1:4096	9	Negative	Negative	Negative	Positive
	5[b]	1:128	Negative	Negative	Negative	Negative	Negative
	12[c]	1:2048	12	7.8	Negative	Negative	Positive
2	1.5	1:8000	QNS	6.3	11.4	QNS	QNS
	15[b]	1:128	Negative	Negative	Negative	Negative	Negative
	17[c]	1:8000	12	Negative	3.5	12	Positive

[a]Serologic tests were performed in the laboratory of Dr. Jack S. Remington.
[b]Sample obtained while still taking pyrimethamine and sulfadiazine.
[c]Sample obtained after pyrimethamine and sulfadiazine were stopped.
QNS = quantity not sufficient.

DIFFERENTIAL DIAGNOSIS

The diseases to be considered in the differential diagnosis of toxoplasmosis are essentially the same as those described in Chapter 7 and should also include congenital lymphocytic choriomeningitis virus syndrome.[968]

THERAPY

General Comments

We recommend specific therapy in every case of congenital toxoplasmosis or congenital *T. gondii* infection in infants younger than 1 year of age. There are insufficient data to evaluate properly treatment in the asymptomatic infected infant. However, most investigators, including ourselves, consider that treatment of such infants should be undertaken in the hope of preventing the remarkably high incidence of late untoward sequelae.[1]

Evaluation of the efficacy of treatment of congenital *T. gondii* infection is made difficult because of the high morbidity (both early and late) and mortality rates associated with this congenital infection; most workers are understandably reluctant to perform studies that would entail withholding specific therapy. Evaluation of treatment is difficult because of variations in severity and outcome of the infection and the disease. The parasite is probably never completely eliminated by specific therapy, and cure of disease (in contrast to infection) in humans apparently depends on the strain of parasite involved, the organs infected, and the time during the course of infection when treatment is initiated. The agents that can be recommended for specific therapy at present are beneficial against the tachyzoite form, but none has been shown to effectively eradicate the encysted form, especially from the CNS and eye.

NEURORADIOLOGIC FOLLOW-UP AFTER SHUNT PLACEMENT

Because it has not been possible to determine with certainty at the time of presentation what the response to shunt placement and antimicrobial therapy will be, a therapeutic approach expectant for good outcome is recommended for most infants with congenital toxoplasmosis. It is often difficult to predict whether such therapy will result in brain cortical growth and expansion. A follow-up CT scan in the perioperative period after shunt placement to assess adequacy of drainage and whether subdural collections have occurred is advisable and may be useful prognostically.

Specific Therapy

PYRIMETHAMINE PLUS SULFONAMIDES

Pyrimethamine, a substituted phenylpyrimidine antimalarial drug (Daraprim), brings about not only survival but also a radical cure of animals given experimental *T. gondii* infection. The persistence of this medicine in the blood was recognized many years ago in patients who received antimalarial prophylaxis with 25-mg weekly doses. The plasma half-life in adults is approximately 100 hours.[969–972] Pyrimethamine pharmacokinetics in newborns and those younger than 1.5 years of age have been reported (Fig. 5–28).[973] Pyrimethamine serum half-life in infants is approximately 60 hours. Pyrimethamine dosages of 1 mg/kg per day yield serum pyrimethamine levels of approximately 1000 to 2000 ng/ml 4 hours after a dose. Dosages of 1 mg/kg each Monday, Wednesday, and Friday yield serum levels of approximately 500 ng/ml 4 hours after a dose. Serum levels at intervals after these two dosages are shown in Figure 5–25. CSF levels are 10 to 20% of concomitant serum levels. Phenobarbital induces hepatic enzymes that degrade pyrimethamine, and phenobarbital therapy resulted in lower serum levels and shortened the half-life of pyrimethamine. Pyrimethamine and sulfadiazine therapy has been associated with resolution of signs of active congenital toxoplasmosis, usually within the first weeks after initiation of therapy.[973] Favorable outcomes for newborns with substantial disease (e.g., microcephaly, multiple cerebral calcifications, hydrocephalus, meningoencephalitis, thrombocytopenia, hepatosplenomegaly, active chorioretinitis) have occurred in conjunction with therapy during their first year of life, which resulted in pyrimethamine levels 4 hours after a dose that ranged from 300 to 2000 ng/ml.[973] Seizures have been reported in association with pyrimethamine serum levels of approximately 5000 ng/ml (R Hoff, personal communication to R McLeod, 1986).

Pyrimethamine and sulfadiazine act synergistically against *T. gondii* with a combined activity eight times that which would be expected if their effects were merely additive.[974–976] Consequently, the simultaneous use of both drugs is indicated in all cases. Comparative tests have shown that sulfapyrazine, sulfamethazine, and sulfamerazine are about as effective as sulfadiazine.[977, 978] All the other sulfonamides tested (sulfathiazole, sulfapyridine, sulfadimidine, sulfisoxazole) are much less effective and are not recommended. It would appear logical to use multiple sulfonamides for the treatment of toxoplasmosis to achieve an additive effect with less toxicity. The usual dosage of sulfadiazine is 100 mg/kg of body weight every 24 hours in two to four equal doses by mouth in addition to pyrimethamine. Administration of pyrimethamine, sulfadiazine, and leucovorin to infants can be difficult because pediatric suspensions are not commercially available. The method shown in Figure 5–29[489] was developed to facilitate administration of these medications to infants in the U.S. (Chicago) National Collaborative Treatment Trial. It is suggested that treatment of infants in the United States be done in conjunction with the U.S. (Chicago) National Collaborative Treatment Trial* to facilitate obtaining knowledge concerning optimal medication dosages and outcome of treatment of the congenital infection and disease. The U.S. (Chicago) National Collaborative Treatment Trial treatment regimen is summarized in Table 5–38 and Figure 5–29 and Table 5–39. An alternative method,

---

*National Institutes of Health–supported National (Chicago) Collaborative Treatment Trial, telephone number 773-834-4152.

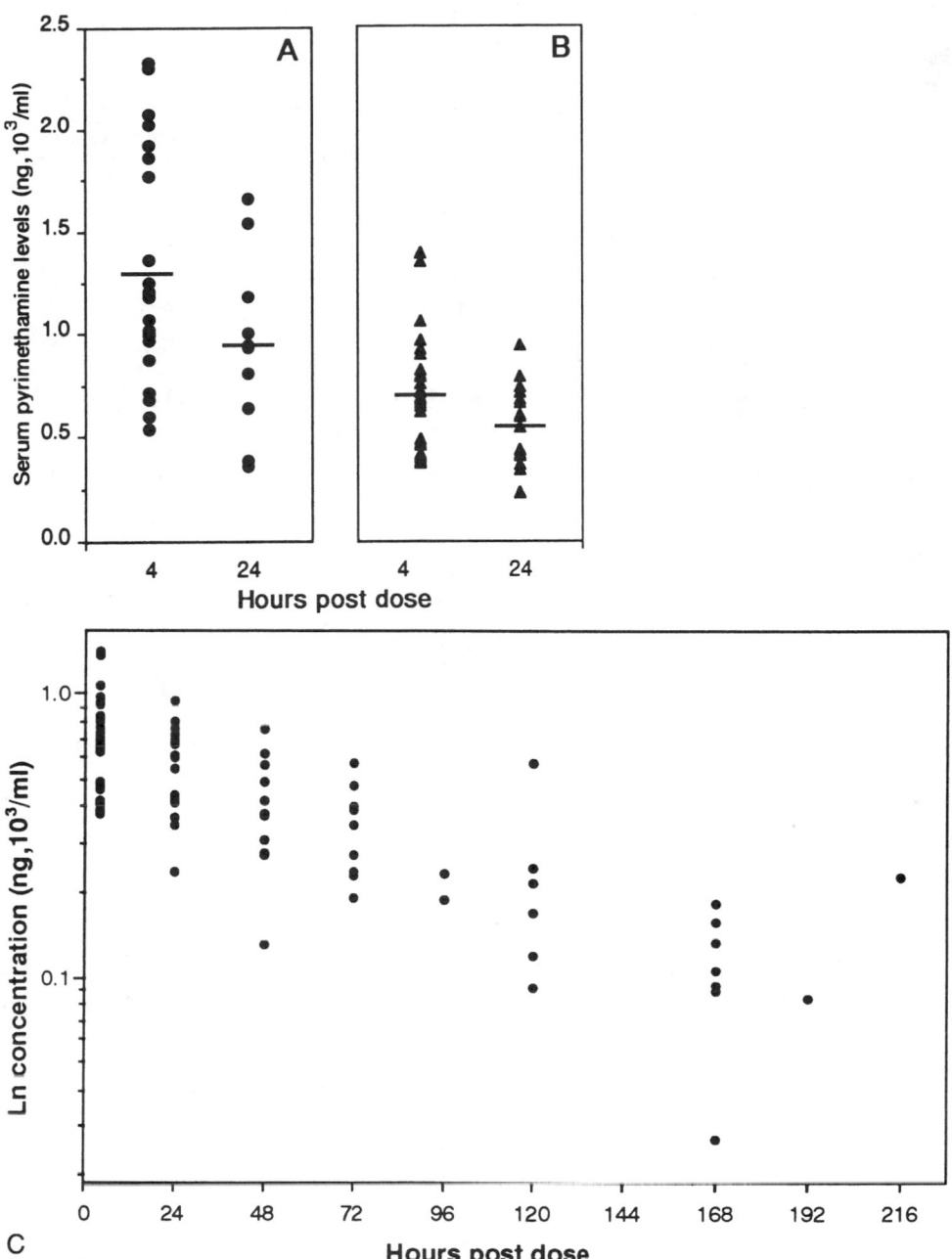

FIGURE 5–28 Serum pyrimethamine levels obtained in infants with congenital *Toxoplasma* infection. *A,* Pyrimethamine serum levels (4 and 24 hours after a dose) of children given 1 mg of pyrimethamine per kg daily. *B,* Pyrimethamine serum levels (4 and 24 hours after a dose) of children given 1 mg of pyrimethamine per kg on Monday, Wednesday, and Friday of each week. Values for children taking phenobarbital are not included. *C,* Pyrimethamine levels in sera of the entire population of infants taking 1 mg of pyrimethamine per kg on Monday, Wednesday, and Friday of each week. Values for children taking phenobarbital are not included. (Adapted from McLeod R, Mack D, Foss R, et al. Levels of pyrimethamine in sera and cerebrospinal and ventricular fluids from infants treated for congenital toxoplasmosis. Antimicrob Agents Chemother 36:1040–1048, 1992, with permission.)

which incorporates pyrimethamine, sulfadiazine, and spiramycin, formerly was used extensively for treatment of infants in France. Treatment of the fetus in utero, by treatment of the mother with pyrimethamine, sulfadiazine, and leucovorin (see Outcome of Treatment of the Fetus in Utero section and Figure 5–30), has been followed by treatment during the first year of life.

Dorangeon and co-workers studied the transplacental passage of the combination pyrimethamine-sulfadoxine (Fansidar) by measuring drug levels in mother and neonate at time of delivery.[979] They noted that the levels of pyrimethamine in the newborn were 50 to 100% and those of sulfadoxine essentially 100% of the maternal levels, depending on when the drug was last administered to the mother. The authors recognized the limitations of their study; they did not evaluate levels in the

WEIGH BABY <u>EACH</u> WEEK.
INCREASE MEDICATIONS ACCORDINGLY.

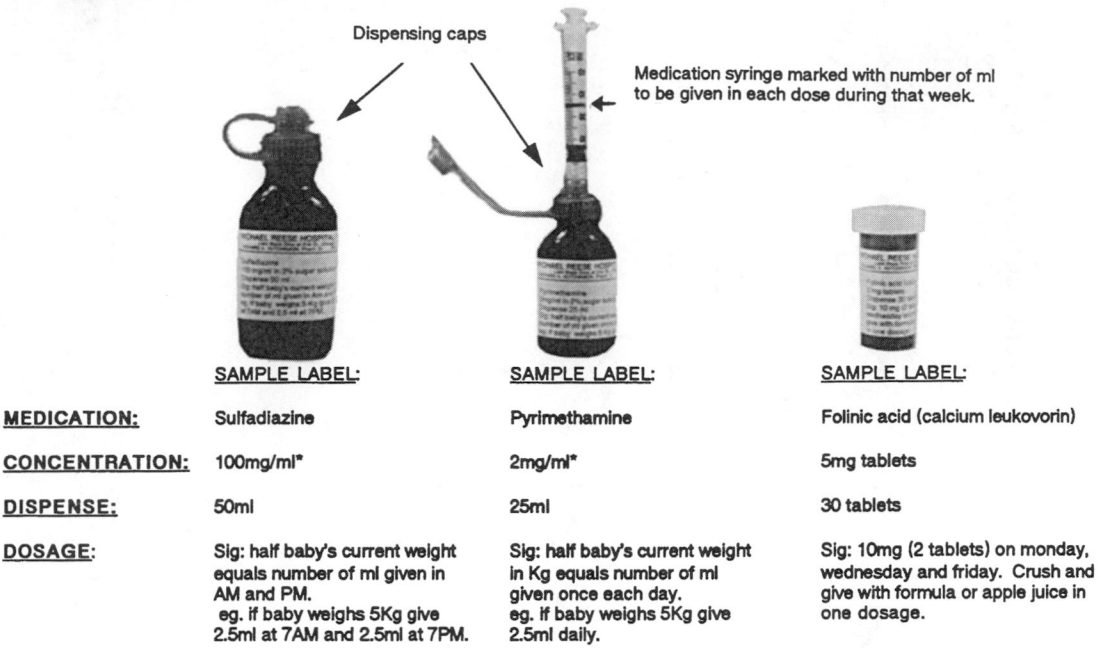

MEDICATION:	Sulfadiazine	Pyrimethamine	Folinic acid (calcium leukovorin)
CONCENTRATION:	100mg/ml*	2mg/ml*	5mg tablets
DISPENSE:	50ml	25ml	30 tablets
DOSAGE:	Sig: half baby's current weight equals number of ml given in AM and PM. eg. if baby weighs 5Kg give 2.5ml at 7AM and 2.5ml at 7PM.	Sig: half baby's current weight in Kg equals number of ml given once each day. eg. If baby weighs 5Kg give 2.5ml daily.	Sig: 10mg (2 tablets) on monday, wednesday and friday. Crush and give with formula or apple juice in one dosage.

*Suspended in 2% sugar solution. Suspension at usual concentration must be made up each week. Store refrigerated.

FIGURE 5–29 Preparation of pyrimethamine, sulfadiazine, and leucovorin in treatment of congenital toxoplasmosis. (Adapted from McAuley J, Roizen N, Patel D, et al. Early and longitudinal evaluations of treated infants and children and untreated historical patients with congenital toxoplasmosis: the Chicago Collaborative Treatment Trial. Clin Infect Dis 18:38–72, 1994. University of Chicago, publisher.)

fetus at different times during gestation, when adequate drug levels are so critical.

Villena and colleagues, in France, have reported an extensive experience with pyrimethamine-sulfadoxine treatment of congenital toxoplasmosis and in the mother when prenatal diagnosis was positive.[143, 967] Although in the United States at present, pyrimethamine-sulfadoxine is not recommended for use in pregnant women, newborns, or children with *T. gondii* infection, this drug combination is increasingly being used in Europe. For this reason, the studies by Trenque and colleagues in Reims, France, are summarized here.[980] To evaluate the fetal/maternal concentration (F/M) ratio of the drugs, these investigators studied placental transfer of pyrimethamine and sulfadoxine at the end of gestation in 10 women who had seroconverted during pregnancy and had been taking the drug combination by mouth twice monthly along with folinic acid. Blood samples were collected at delivery from the mother and from the umbilical vein. The F/M ratios for pyrimethamine and sulfadoxine ranged from 0.43 to 1.03 (mean ± SD = 0.66 ± 0.22) and from 0.65 to 1.16 (mean ± SD = 0.97 ± 0.14), respectively. The patients had steady-state drug concentrations at the time of study. Concentrations of pyrimethamine in the fetus ranged from 50 to 100% (mean 66%) of simultaneous serum concentrations in the mothers. Their results agree with those obtained in monkeys by Schoondermark-van de Ven and co-workers.[981] Trenque and colleagues concluded that the effec-

tive concentrations of both drugs at 14 days after the last dose justifies twice-monthly dosing of the drug combination in cases of documented fetal infection.

It was reported[143, 967, 982] that preliminary follow-up studies suggest that such treatment with Fansidar (1.25 mg/kg pyrimethamine each 14 or each 10 days after treatment of the fetus in utero by treatment of the mother) may lead to a lower incidence of subsequent ocular disease with less sequelae than described for untreated children in the earlier literature.[552, 983] There does not appear to be randomization, statistical analysis, or long-term follow-up in these studies, and whether there was consistency in the evaluations was not specified.

Issues of dosing, pharmacokinetics, serum and tissue levels, efficacy, toxicity, and safety are relevant to considerations concerning use of Fansidar to treat congenital toxoplasmosis. Sulfadoxine was found to be less active than sulfadiazine when sulfonamides were tested in vitro either alone or in conjunction with pyrimethamine against a standard laboratory strain, the type I, RH strain of *T. gondii*. Concentrations of pyrimethamine alone or in conjunction with sulfadiazine that were needed to inhibit *T. gondii* were greater than 25 ng/ml.[973, 984] Although the clinical relevance of these in vitro tests is not known, it seems that brain and retinal tissue trough levels (i.e., minimum levels) should exceed this minimum amount, unless both other data correlating outcomes with lower tissue levels using a variety of

TABLE 5–38

Guidelines for Treatment of *Toxoplasma gondii* Infection in the Pregnant Woman and Congenital *Toxoplasma* Infection in the Fetus, Infant, and Older Child

MANIFESTATION OF INFECTION	MEDICATION	DOSAGE	DURATION OF THERAPY
In pregnant women with acute toxoplasmosis			
First 21 weeks of gestation or until term if fetus not infected	Spiramycin[a]	1 g every 8 hr without food	A = until fetal infection documented or excluded at 21 wk; if documented, in alternate months with pyrimethamine, leucovorin, and sulfadiazine[b]
If fetal infection confirmed after 18th week of gestation	Pyrimethamine *plus*	Loading dose: 100 mg per day in two divided doses for 2 days then 50 mg per day	As in A[b]
	Sulfadiazine *plus*	Loading dose: 75 mg/kg per day in two divided doses (maximum 4 g per day) for 2 days, then 100 mg/kg per day in two divided doses (maximum 4 g per day)	As in A[b]
	Leucovorin (folinic acid)	10–20 mg daily[c]	During and for 1 wk after pyrimethamine therapy
Congenital *Toxoplasma* infection in the infant[d]	Pyrimethamine[d] *plus*	Loading dose: 2 mg/kg per day for 2 days, then 1 mg/kg per day for 2 or 6 mo,[e] then this dose every Monday, Wednesday, Friday[d]	1 yr[f]
	Sulfadiazine[d] *plus*	100 mg/kg per day in two divided doses	1 yr[f]
	Leucovorin[d]	10 mg three times weekly[c]	During and for 1 wk after pyrimethamine therapy
	Corticosteroids[g] (prednisone) have been used when cerebrospinal fluid protein is ≥ 1 g/dl and when active chorioretinitis threatens vision	B = 1 mg/kg per day in two divided doses	C = Until resolution of elevated (≥ 1 g/dl) cerebrospinal fluid protein level or active chorioretinitis that threatens vision
Active chorioretinitis in older children	Pyrimethamine *plus*	Loading dose: 2 mg/kg per day (maximum 50 mg) for 2 days, then maintenance, 1 mg/kg per day (maximum 25 mg)	D = Usually 1–2 wk beyond the time that signs and symptoms have resolved
	Sulfadiazine *plus*	Loading dose: 75 mg/kg, then maintenance, 50 mg/kg every 12 hr	As in D
	Leucovorin	10–20 mg three times weekly[c]	During and for 1 wk after pyrimethamine therapy
	Corticosteroids[g]	As in B	As in C

[a]Available only on request from the U.S. Food and Drug Administration, telephone number 301-443-5680.

[b]The only studies are those of Daffos et al. However, because Daffos and colleagues found pyrimethamine-sulfadiazine therapy to be superior to spiramycin for treatment of the fetus, continuous therapy with pyrimethamine, sulfadiazine, and leucovorin should be considered in the third trimester. This regimen has been used extensively in France and appears to be safe and feasible. Alternatively, in the United States, daily administration of pyrimethamine (50 mg per day) and sulfadiazine (1 g each 6 hr) plus leucovorin (10 mg) administered every other day to the mother has been used in the treatment of a limited number of fetuses in utero. This treatment was begun after the eighteenth week of gestation and continued until birth of the infant. Subsequent treatment of the infant is the same as that described under treatment of congenital infection. This appears to have been feasible and safe treatment for a small number of patients. When the diagnosis of infection in the fetus is established earlier, we suggest that sulfadiazine be used alone until approximately 20 weeks of gestation, at which time pyrimethamine should be added to the regimen.

[c]Adjusted for megaloblastic anemia, granulocytopenia, or thrombocytopenia; blood cell counts, including platelets, should be monitored as described in text.

[d]Optimal dosage, feasibility, and toxicity currently being evaluated or planned in ongoing Chicago-based National Collaborative Treatment Trial, telephone number 773-834-4152.

[e]These two regimens are currently being compared in a randomized manner in the National Collaborative Treatment Trial. Data are not yet available to determine which, if either, is superior. Both regimens appear to be feasible and relatively safe.

[f]The duration of therapy is unknown for infants and children, especially those with AIDS. See discussion in the Congenital *Toxoplasma* Infection and AIDS section.

[g]Corticosteroids should be used only in conjunction with pyrimethamine, sulfadiazine, and leucovorin treatment and should be continued until signs of inflammation (high cerebrospinal fluid protein > 1 g/dl) or active chorioretinitis that threatens vision have subsided—dosage can then be tapered and discontinued; use only with pyrimethamine, sulfadiazine, and leucovorin.

Adapted from information appearing in *The New England Journal of Medicine*, Daffos F, Forestier F, Capella-Pavlovsky M, et al. Prenatal management of 746 pregnancies at risk for congenital toxoplasmosis. N Engl J Med 31:271–275, 1988.

TABLE 5–39
Oral Suspension Formulations for Pyrimethamine and Sulfadiazine in the United States

Pyrimethamine, 2 mg/ml suspension[a]

1. Crush four 25-mg pyrimethamine tablets in a mortar to a fine powder.
2. Add 10 ml of syrup vehicle.[c]
3. Transfer mixture to an amber bottle.
4. Rinse mortar with 10 ml of sterile water and transfer.
5. Add enough of the serum vehicle to q.s. to 50 ml final volume.
6. Shake very well until this is a fine suspension.
7. Label and give a 7-day expiration.
8. Store refrigerated.

Sulfadiazine, 100 mg/ml suspension[b]

1. Crush ten 500-mg sulfadiazine tablets in a mortar to a fine powder.
2. Add enough sterile water to make a smooth paste.
3. Slowly triturate the syrup vehicle[c] close to the final volume of 50 ml.
4. Transfer the suspension to a larger amber bottle.
5. Add sufficient syrup vehicle to q.s. to 50 ml final volume.
6. Shake well.
7. Label and give a 7-day expiration.
8. Store refrigerated.

---

[a]Pyrimethamine: 25-mg tablets (Daraprim, Glaxo Wellcome Inc.) NDC #0173-0201-55.

[b]Sulfadiazine: 500-mg tablets (Eon Labs Manufacturing, Inc.) NDC #00185-0757-01.

[c]Syrup vehicle: suggest 2% sugar suspension for pyrimethamine. If the infant is not lactose intolerant, 2% sugar suspension can be 2 g lactose per 100 ml distilled water. Suggest simple syrup or alternatively cherry syrup for sulfadiazine suspension.

strains of *T. gondii* and clinical trials were to demonstrate that lower levels are beneficial. The observation that CSF levels of pyrimethamine were 10 to 25% of serum pyrimethamine levels in infants with congenital toxoplasmosis therefore is relevant.[973] The serum levels of pyrimethamine following 1.25 mg Fansidar administered every 14 days to infants were approximately 350 ng/ml peak and 25 ng/ml trough.[979] Thus, CSF, brain, and retinal levels may not exceed 25 ng/ml for much of the time that this dosage regimen is administered with twice-monthly dosing. Consequently, potential therapeutic brain and retinal levels may not be achieved for substantial periods of time with twice-monthly dosing.

Administration of Fansidar each 2 weeks is a more convenient regimen than daily administration of pyrimethamine and sulfadiazine. There was no reported hematologic toxicity when this regimen was administered,[967] as contrasted to relatively frequent, but easily reversible, neutropenia (requiring frequent hematologic monitoring) in children treated with 1 mg/kg pyrimethamine daily or three times each week.[489, 973] Serious and life-threatening toxicity has been reported with use of Fansidar in other clinical settings, and this finding has led to reluctance to recommend its use when other medicines, especially sulfonamides with shorter half-lives, are equally or potentially more effective.[984] There have been no such serious side effects reported in the studies of congenital toxoplasmosis treated with Fansidar, but although the incidence of lethal hepatotoxicity[985] is estimated to be quite low, the numbers of women and children treated to date are not sufficient to exclude the possibility that it may occur.[982, 986, 987]

Both pyrimethamine and the sulfonamides are potentially toxic. Because most physicians are familiar with untoward reactions to sulfonamides (e.g., crystalluria, hematuria and hypersensitivity, marrow suppression), only the toxic effects of pyrimethamine are considered here.

Toxic Effects of Pyrimethamine

Pyrimethamine inhibits dihydrofolate reductase, which is important in the synthesis of folic acid, thus producing

---

Diagnosis mother:	Systematic serologic screening, before conception and intrapartum
Treatment of mother:	If acute serology, spiramycin reduces transmission Untreated 94 (60%) of 154 vs. treated 91 (23%) of 388*
Treatment of fetus:	pyrimethamine, sulfadiazine, or termination N = 54 livebirths; 34 terminations†
Diagnosis fetus:	Ultrasounds; amniocentesis, PCR at ≥ 18 weeks' gestation Sensitivity 37 (97%) of 38: specificity 301 of 301‡
Outcome:	All 54 normal development; initial report was 19% subtle findings: 7 (13%) intracranial calcifications, 3 (6%) chorioretinal scars§; follow-up of 18 children (median age 4.5 yr; range, 1–11 yr): 39% retinal scars, most scars were peripheral‖

*From Desmonts and Couvreur.[120]
†From Daffos, et al.[130]
‡From Hohlfeld, et al.[132]
§From Hohlfeld, et al.[946]
‖From Brézin, et al.[1087]

FIGURE 5–30 Paris approach to prenatal prevention, diagnosis, and treatment. (Adapted from Roberts F, McLeod R, Boyer K. Toxoplasmosis. *In* Katz S, Gershon A, Hotez P [eds]. Krugman's Infectious Diseases of Children, 10th ed. St. Louis, CV Mosby, pp 538–570, with minor modifications and permission.)

reversible and usually gradual depression of the bone marrow.[988, 989] Reversible neutropenia is the most frequent toxicity, although platelet depression and anemia may occur as well. Other, less serious side effects are gastrointestinal distress, headaches, and a bad taste in the mouth. Accidental overdosing in infants has resulted in vomiting, tremors, convulsions, and bone marrow depression.[990] All patients treated with pyrimethamine should have a peripheral blood cell and platelet count twice each week. Folinic acid (in the form of leucovorin calcium) has been used to protect the bone marrow from toxic effects of pyrimethamine.[200, 991] We usually administer 5 to 20 mg leucovorin calcium each Monday, Wednesday, and Friday or even daily in infants or young children. We usually employ 10 to 20 mg per day orally in older children and adults. Data suggesting that oral leucovorin calcium can be used to reverse the toxic effects of pyrimethamine have been presented. Nixon and Bertino clearly demonstrated that leucovorin calcium in tablet form was well absorbed (in adult subjects), thereby expanding the serum pool of reduced folates.[992] Under fasting conditions, the quantitative absorption of the orally administered preparation was close to 90%. The parenteral form (Calcium Leucovorin Injection, Lederle Laboratories) may be ingested with equal effectiveness (CJ Masur, Lederle Laboratories, written communication to JS Remington, 1975). These substances, in contrast to folic acid, do not appear to inhibit the action of pyrimethamine on the proliferative form of *T. gondii*, because of an active transport mechanism for folinic acid,[993] and thus may be used in conjunction with the latter drug to allay toxicity.

Garin and colleagues have used Fansidar in a small number of infants and consider this agent to be well tolerated, with a much simpler treatment regimen.[994–996] The potential for serious toxicity of medication with so long a half-life as that of sulfadoxine has led others to avoid this regimen. Whether its potential for toxicity is as great in infants as in adults is not known, although it has recently been administered safely to large numbers of French and Italian infants. Until further information becomes available on this point, we do not recommend routine use of Fansidar.

Teratogenic Effects of Pyrimethamine

In experiments with pyrimethamine, Thiersch reported an effect on rat fetuses ranging from stunting to death, depending on the amount of pyrimethamine administered to the mothers during pregnancy.[997] The effect on the fetuses could be moderated, with a higher yield of live litters but also of stunted and malformed animals, when the mother was given leucovorin calcium at the time of drug administration. The malformations resulted from enormous doses (e.g., 12 mg/kg compared with the usual dose in humans of 0.5 to 1 mg/kg) and were similar to those obtained with closely related folic acid analogues: general stunting of growth, general hydrops, cranial bone defects, incomplete cranial and brain development, rachischisis, internal hydrocephalus, ventral hernias, situs inversus, and combinations of all of these. An even more severe teratogenic effect was reported

in the studies of Anderson and Morse, who similarly employed doses far higher than could ever be employed in humans.[998] Similar studies in rats are those of Dyban and associates.[999, 1000] In another study in rats, Krahe used doses more comparable to those employed in humans and noted fetal resorption but no teratogenic effects after large doses of pyrimethamine.[1001] In 1971, Sullivan and Takacs pointed out the lack of comparative data about the teratogenic effects of pyrimethamine in different mammalian species[1002]—a lack that adds to the difficulty in estimating the extent of teratogenic risk in humans. Their results in rats and hamsters emphasize the shortcomings of attempts to determine a safe clinical dose on the basis of tests limited to a single species of test animal. The drug was less teratogenic in golden hamsters than in Wistar rats. About 70% of rat fetuses were dead or malformed (the malformations included brachygnathia, cleft palate, oligodactyly, and phocomelia) as a result of administration of single oral doses of 5 mg (approximately 20 mg/kg) to pregnant females. Less than 10% of hamster fetuses died or were malformed after similar doses that on a milligram per kilogram basis were eight to nine times greater than those given to rats. Repeated doses nearer to those used in humans were also teratogenic in rats but not in hamsters. These investigators also demonstrated that folinic acid can significantly reduce the incidence of dead and malformed fetuses when administered during pyrimethamine treatment.

Puchta and Simandlová, using doses of 2, 5, and 10 mg/kg in rats, could demonstrate no malformations in rat fetuses.[1003] Their results are in marked contrast to those of most other workers, and the differences remain to be explained.

In all of these studies, pyrimethamine was administered during the period of early organogenesis, which is the period of maximum susceptibility to damage by teratogenic agents.

SPIRAMYCIN

Spiramycin, a macrolide antibiotic that is available to physicians in the United States only by request to the U.S. Food and Drug Administration, has an antibacterial spectrum comparable to that of erythromycin and is active against *T. gondii*, as demonstrated in animal experiments.[1004, 1005] In vitro studies have also been reported.[1006] The actual concentration necessary to inhibit growth of or kill the organism is unknown. It has been described as having exceptional persistence in the tissues[1007, 1008] when compared with erythromycin, oleandomycin, or carbomycin. Such high tissue levels may account for the observations that spiramycin is much more active in vivo against susceptible bacteria than is erythromycin, despite higher serum levels attained with comparable doses of erythromycin and greater sensitivity of the bacteria to erythromycin in vitro.[1009] A review of this antimicrobial agent has been published.[1010]

Spiramycin is supplied as a syrup and in capsules. The usual dose in adults is 1 g three times a day daily in three divided doses. Garin and co-workers studied the concentration in humans in maternal serum, cord serum, and placenta.[1011] On a daily regimen of 2 g by mouth, the average levels were 1.19 µg/ml (range, 0.50 to 2.0 µg/ml), 0.63 µg/ml (range, 0.20 to 1.8 µg/ml), and 2.75 µg/ml (range, 0.70 to 5.0 µg/ml), respectively. On a dosage schedule of 3 g daily, the results were 1.69 µg/ml (range, 1 to 4 µg/ml), 0.78 µg/ml (range, 0.75 to 2.0 µg/ml), and 6.2 µg/ml (range, 3.25 to 10 µg/ml), respectively. (These serum levels in the mother are similar to those obtained by Hudson and colleagues at 2 and 4 hours after a given dose in persons receiving 1 g every 6 hours.[1012]) Thus, a total dose of 3 g daily resulted in levels in the placenta that were twice as high as those attained with a total dose of 2 g daily. (This is one reason for the recommendation of 3 g administered as a 1-g thrice-daily dose during gestation.) In both regimens, the concentration in cord serum was approximately one half and the placental levels approximately three to five times greater than the level in the corresponding maternal serum. The investigators stated that the levels achieved in the placenta are ample for treatment of T. gondii in that organ, but whether the levels in cord serum are sufficient for treatment of the fetus in utero remains to be verified. Forestier and associates published another study of spiramycin concentrations in the mother and fetus (fetal blood sampling).[1013]

There are individual variations in spiramycin pharmacokinetics. Fetomaternal concentrations were studied in 20 cases of maternal infection acquired between the third and the tenth weeks of pregnancy and treated with a daily dose of 3 g. The maternal plasma concentration of spiramycin was 0.682 ± 0.132 mg/liter in the first month of treatment; 0.618 ± 0.102 mg/liter during the twentieth to the twenty-fourth weeks of pregnancy; and 1.015 ± 0.22 mg/liter in the sixth month. The mean fetal concentration was 0.290 mg/liter during the twentieth to the twenty-fourth weeks of pregnancy (i.e., 47% of maternal values), with a lack of correlation between mothers and fetuses. At birth, the placental concentration (2.3 µg/ml) was four times the average blood concentration in mothers (0.47 mg/liter) and six and one-half times the cord blood values (0.34 mg/liter). There was a good correlation between maternal blood and placental values and a fair correlation between cord blood and placental values. These facts suggest that monitoring of spiramycin treatment by measuring maternal spiramycin blood concentrations might be useful in determining effective individual dosage.[121]

Unfortunately, as with pyrimethamine plus sulfonamides, there is very little definitive information on the efficacy of spiramycin in congenital toxoplasmosis in the newborn. In a study of 12 cases (mainly of severe clinical disease) by Martin and co-workers in which spiramycin was employed, the data are impossible to interpret, because tetracyclines, pyrimethamine, sulfonamides, and corticosteroids were frequently used as well in the same infants.[1014]

In a carefully designed study, Beverley and colleagues treated congenitally infected mice from the age of 4 to 8 weeks with spiramycin or with a combination of sulfadimidine and pyrimethamine.[1015] The levels of spiramycin in the heart, liver, kidney, and spleen were approximately 50 to 140 times greater than the serum levels after 4 weeks of treatment. Both treatment regimens were effective in preventing the histopathologic changes noted in congenitally infected but untreated mice. Regardless of the form of treatment, a smaller number of cysts were found in the brains of treated mice than in those of untreated mice (probably because treatment prevented the development of new cysts rather than destroying cysts formed before instigation of therapy). The authors suggested that because spiramycin was as effective as the potentially toxic combination of pyrimethamine and sulfadimidine, it will be found to be preferable to the combination agent in treatment of congenital toxoplasmosis.

Because the optimal dose and route of administration of spiramycin in infants and adults have never been established for toxoplasmosis, the study by Back and co-workers on the pharmacology of parenteral spiramycin as an antineoplastic agent is pertinent.[1016] Twelve patients with various types of far-advanced neoplastic diseases were treated intravenously with daily doses ranging from 5 to 160 mg/kg. Doses above 35 mg/kg produced local vasospasm, a feeling of coolness, strange taste, vertigo, dizziness, flushing of the face, tearing of the eyes, nausea, vomiting, diarrhea, and anorexia. No hematologic toxicity, electrocardiographic changes, or impairment of liver or kidney function was noticed. However, QT interval prolongation and life-threatening arrhythmias (cardiac arrest) have been reported in two neonates being treated with spiramycin (300,000 IU/kg per day by mouth).[1017] The infants recovered completely after immediate cardiopulmonary resuscitation maneuvers.

At present the only indication for which we use spiramycin is in the actively infected mother to attempt to reduce transmission to her fetus.[1018] It should be noted that spiramycin failed to prevent neurotoxoplasmosis in immunosuppressed patients.[1019] Spiramycin may reduce the severity of infection in a fetus because it delays transmission to a later time in gestation when transmission is associated with less severe manifestations of infection. There are no data that conclusively demonstrate efficacy of spiramycin in treatment of the infected fetus.

OTHER DRUGS

At present, there are no clinical data available to allow for recommendation of any of the drugs described next for treatment of the immunocompetent pregnant patient, fetus, or newborn.

Trimethoprim plus Sulfamethoxazole. Despite reports of successful treatment of murine toxoplasmosis with a combination of trimethoprim and sulfamethoxazole (TMP-SMZ),[1020, 1021] trimethoprim alone has been found to have less effect against T. gondii both in vitro and in vivo.[1022–1025] The combination of this drug with sulfamethoxazole is synergistic in vitro[1021] but is significantly less active in vitro and in vivo than the combination of pyrimethamine and sulfonamide. Previously, there have been a number of reports on the use of the combination in human toxoplasmosis but whether the effect of the combination was solely due to the sulfonamide component was unclear.[1026–1028] A recent, randomized trial of TMP-SMZ versus pyrimethamine-sulfadiazine in toxoplasmic encephalitis in AIDS patients by Torre and colleagues[1029] revealed that TMP-SMZ was a valuable alternative to pyrimethamine-sulfadiazine for that purpose. However, we do not recommend its use for treatment of the infected fetus or newborn in the absence of carefully designed trials that reveal efficacy of TMP-SMZ in congenital toxoplasmosis.

Clindamycin. This antibiotic has been shown to be effective in treatment of murine toxoplasmosis[1030, 1031] and ocular infection in rabbits.[1032] However, studies are needed before it can be recommended for routine treatment of congenitally infected infants or pregnant women. When used in combination with pyrimethamine in AIDS patients with toxoplasmic encephalitis, results have been comparable to treatment with pyrimethamine-sulfadiazine.[1033, 1034]

Tetracyclines. Both doxycycline[1035] and minocycline[1036, 1037] have efficacy in murine toxoplasmosis. Their mechanism of action on *T. gondii* is unknown. Doxycycline was used successfully in two AIDS patients with toxoplasmic encephalitis when it was administered at 300 mg per day intravenously in three divided doses.[1038] When doxycycline was used orally at doses of 100 mg twice a day in six patients intolerant to pyrimethamine-sulfadiazine, five patients had associated neurologic and radiologic recurrences while receiving the drug.[1039] Further study of the tetracyclines in the treatment of toxoplasmosis in adults is likely to involve their use in combination with other antimicrobial agents. There are no data on their use in the newborn or young children with toxoplasmosis, nor are they recommended for this purpose.

Rifampin. Rifampin in high doses was not effective against *T. gondii* in a murine model.[1040]

Macrolides. Three new macrolides—roxithromycin,[1041, 1042] clarithromycin,[1043] and azithromycin[1044]—have been shown to have activity against *T. gondii* in vivo in a mouse model. Stray-Pederson studied levels of azithromycin in placental tissue, amniotic fluid, and maternal and cord blood.[1045] Levels in maternal serum ranged from 0.017 to 0.073 mg/ml (mean, 0.028 mg/ml). Whole blood levels were higher (mean, 0.313 mg/ml). Mean levels in amniotic fluid and cord blood were 0.040 and 0.027 mg/ml, respectively. Placental levels were higher (mean, 2.067 mg/ml). It should be understood, however, that azithromycin is concentrated in tissues and intracellularly; and thus it is levels at these sites that are likely more important than serum or blood levels.

When used in combination with pyrimethamine, both clarithromycin and azithromycin have been successful in treating toxoplasmic encephalitis in adult patients with AIDS.[1046]

The related compounds, the ketolides, are also active both in utero and in vivo in the mouse model of toxoplasmosis.[1047]

Atovaquone. Atovaquone has been reported to have potent in vitro activity against both tachyzoite and cyst forms.[1048, 1049] It reduced mortality in murine toxoplasmosis significantly and had remarkable, although differing, activity against strains of *T. gondii*.[1049] Atovaquone has been used in AIDS patients with toxoplasmic encephalitis with encouraging results.[1050–1052] Unfortunately, relapse occurred in approximately 50% of patients in whom atovaquone was used for acute therapy and continued alone as maintenance therapy.[1050, 1052] Seventeen (26%) of 65 patients treated with atovaquone as a single agent for maintenance therapy of toxoplasmic encephalitis experienced a relapse.[1053] The combination of pyrimethamine and atovaquone may prove more useful.[1050] Serum levels of atovaquone in patients with toxoplasmic encephalitis were not predictive of clinical response or failure.[1051] Bioavailability of the drug is improved when medication is ingested with food. The reliability of absorption of this drug continues to be a problem. Survival time was significantly better among those patients with higher steady-state plasma concentrations of the drug.[1052] Although a new formulation of atovaquone is reported to achieve higher plasma concentrations, prospective trials are needed to compare the efficacy of this drug with that obtained in standard drug regimens. This drug should never be used alone for the treatment of the acute infection, but rather it should be used in combination with drugs such as pyrimethamine. The adverse events observed in these studies included hepatic enzyme abnormalities (50%), rash (25%), nausea (21%), and diarrhea (19%).[1051] Between 3% and 10% of patients treated with atovaquone were reported to discontinue the drug because of rash, hepatic enzyme abnormalities, nausea, or vomiting.[1050, 1051, 1053] Leukopenia associated with the combination of pyrimethamine and atovaquone has responded to folinic acid (leucovorin) and granulocyte colony-stimulating factor therapy.[1050]

Fluoroquinolones. A number of fluoroquinolones have been tested against *T. gondii* in vitro and in vivo in a mouse model of the acute infection. Among those tested, only trovafloxacin had excellent activity both in vitro and in vivo. Its activity was enhanced when used in combination with pyrimethamine, sulfadiazine, clarithromycin, or atovaquone.[1054, 1055]

Duration of Therapy

The optimal duration of therapy in congenitally infected infants is not known. Infants treated with the combination of pyrimethamine and sulfadiazine for relatively brief periods have subsequently developed untoward sequelae of the disease.[555, 1056] We, as well as other investigators (including our colleague Dr. J Couvreur in Paris), recommend that therapy be continued for 1 year as outlined in Table 5–39). We recommend using the combination of pyrimethamine and sulfonamide for the entire 1-year period.

In some areas of Europe, treatment is continued for the first 2 years of life. We have not noted active disease or progression of signs or symptoms when treatment is discontinued when children are 1 year old. For the special issue of treatment of the HIV- and *T. gondii*–infected newborn of an HIV-infected mother, see the Congenital *Toxoplasma gondii* Infection and Acquired Immunodeficiency Syndrome section.

Treatment of the Fetus In Utero

With the advent of prenatal diagnosis (see earlier discussion), attempts are being made to treat the infected fetus of mothers who have decided to carry their pregnancy to term by treatment of the mother with pyrimethamine and sulfadiazine. Couvreur, in close cooperation with Daffos and colleagues, has made certain observations that should prove helpful.[1018] Their data suggest that spiramycin, although effective in reducing the frequency of transmission of the organism from mother to fetus, does not alter significantly the pathology of the infection in the fetus. For this reason, after the seventeenth week of gestation, they treat with pyrimethamine-sulfadiazine for the duration of pregnancy when fetal infection has been proved or is highly probable. (In a commentary, Jeannel and colleagues raise the question of whether spiramycin was of value in the pregnancies studied by Daffos and colleagues.[1057]) During this treatment period, the mother is carefully monitored for development of hematologic toxicity. If significant toxicity appears despite treatment with folinic acid, the drug combination is discontinued until the hematologic abnormalities are corrected and the drug regimen is then restarted. Pyrimethamine (in combination with sulfonamides) appears to be the most efficacious treatment for infection in the fetus and newborn. Whether it has untoward toxic effects on the fetus, even after organogenesis has occurred, is unknown. Thus, its use cannot be recommended as routine in every woman who acquires the acute infection during pregnancy. Because of this, we consider it important to employ prenatal diagnosis in every case of acquired *T. gondii* infection during pregnancy, even late in gestation, if there is no ethical or technical reason for not performing the procedure. Demonstration of fetal infection will allow for this treatment regimen to be chosen. If, however, extenuating circumstances preclude prenatal diagnosis in a mother whose infection was proved to have occurred during the second or third trimester, the same course of treatment as that used for cases in which the diagnosis has been established in the fetus may be considered because infection acquired during the second trimester is associated with the highest risk for fetal disease and in the third trimester with the highest rate of transmission to the fetus.

The original report by Daffos and colleagues in 1988 was the first to highlight the importance of attempting to treat the infected fetus to improve clinical outcome.[130] In 24 of the 39 positive cases, pregnancy was terminated at the request of the mother. Toxoplasmic encephalitis was noted in each of these 24 fetuses, including those in whom the ultrasound examination was normal when the pregnancy was terminated. In every case, extensive necrotic foci were present, which suggested that sequelae might have been severe were the pregnancy not terminated. These findings also strongly suggest that early transmission (before week 24) usually results in severe congenital toxoplasmosis and not in subclinical infection (see also Table 5–9).

In 15 of the 39 positive cases, the mother decided to continue her pregnancy. In these women, maternal infection was acquired between weeks 17 and 25; in these cases, fetal ultrasound examination results were normal. Treatment with sulfonamides and pyrimethamine was prescribed as soon as the diagnosis of fetal infection was established; this treatment was begun between 8 and 17 weeks after acquisition of the infection by the mother. After delivery, the presence of congenital *T. gondii* infection was demonstrated in the 15 newborns (the infant whose serology test turned totally negative became positive again a few weeks after treatment was discontinued; the infection was only suppressed, not eradicated). The 15 infants were asymptomatic despite the presence of cerebral calcifications in 4. Fundi were normal, as was the CSF examination. Children were treated after birth, and all remained asymptomatic without neurologic signs or mental retardation. Ocular fundi remained normal in 13 children; retinal lesions were noted in 2 (one at 4 months of age, the other at 18 months of age; the duration of follow-up was 3 to 30 months). Thus, despite rather early (before week 26) transmission of parasites from mother to fetus, infection remained either subclinical or mild in those fetuses whose mothers received pyrimethamine and sulfonamide treatment during pregnancy. Positive findings at prenatal diagnosis should be considered an indication for this therapeutic regimen, which would not usually be considered because of its potential toxicity to both fetus and mother. It should be understood that for ethical reasons, controlled trials (treated and untreated patients) have not been performed and likely will never be performed if an untreated group is required. Thus, one is left with studies in which historical data are used for comparison. Comparative trials will be performed in the future as newer therapies are developed.

SUBSEQUENT STUDIES

Couvreur and colleagues studied the outcome in 52 cases of congenital *T. gondii* infection diagnosed by prenatal examination in mothers who were then treated with the pyrimethamine, sulfadiazine, and spiramycin regimen described by Daffos and colleagues.[130, 946] Results in these infants were compared with those obtained in 51 infants with congenital toxoplasmosis whose mothers had received only spiramycin. Treatment of the infants after birth was the same in both groups. Although these two groups were not strictly comparable, certain information that is valuable can be gleaned as long as the quantitative data are not emphasized but, rather, the qualitative direction of the results is focused on. Remarkable were the lesser number of isolates from the placentas, the lower IgG antibody titers at birth and at 6 months of age, the lower prevalence of positive IgM antibody tests, and the higher number of subclinical infections in the offspring of mothers who received the pyrimethamine-sulfadiazine regimen. These data further support those discussed earlier that treatment of the fetus is possible and that such treatment may result in a more favorable outcome if pyrimethamine-sulfadiazine is in the regimen[1018] (Table 5–40).

Boulot and colleagues[1058] described two infants born of mothers who had had positive prenatal diagnoses and who were subsequently treated with pyrimethamine plus

TABLE 5–40

Outcome of In Utero Treatment of Congenitally Infected Fetuses with Spiramycin or Spiramycin Followed by Pyrimethamine and Sulfadiazine

IN UTERO TREATMENT	NO. OF PATIENTS	DATES OF STUDY	DATES OF MATERNAL INFECTION[a]	DURATION OF FOLLOW-UP	NO. OF ISOLATES FROM PLACENTA	IMMUNE LOAD OF IgG		IgM PREVALENCE	NO. (%) OF SUBCLINICAL INFECTIONS
						At Birth	At 6 Mo		
Spiramycin	51	1972–82	22.8 (10–35)	46.7 mo (2 mo–11 yr)	23/30 (77%)	139	137	18/26 (69%)	17/51 (33%)
Spiramycin + pyrimethamine + sulfadiazine	52	1983–9	22.6 (10–30)	76 wk (11–46 wk)	16/38[b] (42%)	86	70	8/46 (17%)[c]	30/52 (57%)

[a]Weeks of gestation.
[b]$p < 0.01$.
[c]$p < 0.001$.
Adapted from Couvreur J, et al. In utero treatment of toxoplasmic fetopathy with the combination pyrimethamine-sulfadiazine. Fetal Diagn Ther 8:45–50, 1993.

sulfadiazine alternated with spiramycin as described by Daffos and co-workers. Despite prolonged treatment of the mothers, the offspring of these two pregnancies had congenital toxoplasmosis; *T. gondii* was isolated from the placentas. Although the success of treatment of the fetus will depend on a number of variables discussed earlier, these results serve as a note of caution in regard to the information given to parents about the effectiveness of such prenatal treatment.

In 1989, Hohlfeld and co-workers[946] updated information published earlier by their same group.[130] Because these are the first such available data, and although only relatively short-term follow-up is provided, a reasonably comprehensive presentation of their data seems justified. They reported 89 fetal infections in 86 pregnancies (39 of these infected fetuses were included in the original report by Daffos and co-workers as discussed earlier). All of the women were treated with spiramycin, 3 g daily, throughout their pregnancy from the time maternal infection was proved or strongly suspected on the basis of serologic studies until fetal infection was documented or considered to be highly likely. Spiramycin treatment was instigated a mean of 36 ± 27 days after the estimated onset of infection. On prenatal examination, 80 had had positive specific test results and the remaining 9 had evidence of congenital *T. gondii* infection at birth. When fetal infection was confirmed, 34 terminations were performed at the request of the parents. The mean interval between infection and beginning of therapy for continued pregnancies was remarkably and significantly shorter than for terminated pregnancies. The terminations were considered if severe lesions (marked hydrocephaly) were present on ultrasonography at the time of prenatal diagnosis or when maternal infection had occurred very early in pregnancy. The main reason for termination was demonstration of cerebral lesions on ultrasonograms. Of interest is that the evolution of hydrocephalus was remarkably rapid in some of their cases, with ventricular dilation being observed to develop within 10 days. (Ventricular dilation is an indirect sign of the presence of lesions due to *T. gondii*.) For most of the 52 pregnancies allowed to continue, treatment with pyrimethamine and sulfadiazine for 3 weeks alternating with spiramycin for 3 weeks was instigated along with folinic acid. In 47 of 54 cases, postnatal treatment consisted of courses of pyrimethamine and sulfadiazine alternating with spiramycin except in 3 infants, in whom only spiramycin was used. The mean period of follow-up was 19 months (range, 1 to 48 months).

Subclinical infection was defined as complete absence of symptoms. The benign form included isolated subclinical signs, including intracerebral calcifications, normal neurologic status, and chorioretinal scars without visual impairment. This form was mainly found in older infants observed during the follow-up period and in younger infants when retinal scars were peripheral and did not involve the macular region (P Hohlfeld, personal communication to JS Remington, 1993). The severe form included hydrocephaly, microcephaly, bilateral chorioretinitis with impaired vision, and abnormal immunologic findings.

The overall risk of fetal infection was 7%, and this risk varied with time of maternal infection, as shown in Table 5–7. A more complete breakdown by week of gestation was published by the same group in 1994 (see Table 5–8).[132] At prenatal diagnosis, the nonspecific signs were not predictive of the severity of the fetal lesions; they were not found to differ significantly when subsequently terminated pregnancies were compared with those pregnancies that were allowed to continue. Fifty-five infants were born of the 52 pregnancies that were allowed to continue; no intrauterine growth retardation was noted. The findings are shown in Table 5–41. Each of the seven infants with cerebral calcifications had normal ophthalmologic and neurologic examinations (benign form).

Attempts at isolation of the parasite from the placenta were positive in 23 cases, negative in 20, and inconclusive in 3; isolation was not attempted in 9 cases. Cord blood was positive for IgM antibodies in 8 cases, negative in 46 cases, and not performed in 1 case.

Follow-up was for 6 months to 4 years in 54 of the infants. The overall subclinical infection rate was 76%. The outcomes are shown in Table 5–42, where they are compared with historical controls from a study performed from 1972 to 1981.[1059]

The additional information provided by this publication further supports and extends the indirect evidence these authors published earlier,[130] that such treatment of the fetus reduces the number of biologic signs at birth and can reduce the likelihood of severe damage in the newborn. Thus, prenatal management as discussed by Hohlfeld and co-workers and previously by Daffos and co-workers appears to have resulted in an increase in the proportion of subclinical infections in first- and second-trimester infections as well as in a reduction of severe congenital toxoplasmosis and a shift from benign forms to subclinical infections. In the earlier study, a large percentage of the cases had been third-trimester infections, which are known to have a better prognosis. Hohlfeld and colleagues recognized that their superior results, at least in part, may have been due to accurate

TABLE 5–41
Findings at Birth in 55 Live Infants Born of 52 Pregnancies in Which Prenatal Diagnosis Was Positive

OBSERVATIONS	NO.[a]	%
Subclinical infection	44/54	81
Multiple intracranial calcifications	5/54	9
Single intracranial calcification	2/54	4
Chorioretinitis scar	3/54	6
Abnormal lumbar puncture	1/54	2
Positive findings on inoculation of placenta	23/46	50
Positive cord blood IgM antibody	8/53	15

[a]Denominator = number of birth findings; numerator = total number of infants examined for findings.

Adapted from Hohlfeld P, Daffos F, Thulliez P, et al. Fetal toxoplasmosis: outcome of pregnancy and infant follow-up after in utero treatment. J Pediatr 115:767, 1989, with permission.

TABLE 5–42

Comparison with Historical Controls (1972–1981) of the Outcome of Live-Born Infants Diagnosed with Congenital *Toxoplasma* Infection in a Study of Prenatal Diagnosis (1982–1988) in Which the Mothers Were Treated with a Regimen of Pyrimethamine-Sulfadiazine Alternated with Spiramycin

	TRIMESTER										
	First				Second				Third		
OUTCOME	1972–1981 (No.)	(%)	1982–1988 (No.)	(%)	1972–1981 (No.)	(%)	1982–1988 (No.)	(%)	1972–1981 (No.)	(%)	1982–1988 (No.)a
Subclinical	1	10	6	67	23	37	33	77	74	68	2
Benign	5	50	2	22	28	45	10	23	31	29	0
Severe	4	40	1	11	11	18	0	0	3	3	0
Total	10		9		62		43		108		2

aSee text.

Adapted from Hohlfeld P, Daffos F, Thulliez P, et al. Fetal toxoplasmosis: outcome of pregnancy and infant follow-up after in utero treatment. J Pediatr 115:767, 1989, with permission.

diagnosis and selective termination in the few cases of severely affected fetuses (2.7% of all referred cases in their experience) as well as to the effect of spiramycin on prevention of congenital transmission and the apparent reduction in the severity of fetal infection associated with the regimen of pyrimethamine-sulfadiazine. In Hohlfeld and co-workers' series, only 4% were third-trimester infections because, in the first years of their experience, prenatal diagnosis was not performed for late infections during gestation. Now that more rapid methods are available for diagnosis the authors consider that the third trimester can also be considered for prenatal diagnosis and treatment.

OUTCOME OF TREATMENT OF THE FETUS IN UTERO

Outcome was not uniformly favorable[943] when the algorithm of Daffos and co-workers[130] and Hohlfeld and co-workers[946] for patient care was applied. As mentioned earlier, part of the favorable outcome of Hohlfeld and co-workers can be attributed to termination of pregnancies in which the fetus had severe involvement (e.g., hydrocephalus). Nonetheless, the individual outcomes reported are better than would have been expected for first-trimester and early second-trimester infections. Almost all the infected children from pregnancies managed according to this algorithm have had normal development, and those who have had clinical signs do not appear to have manifestations that will significantly impair normal function.[946] Thus, at present, the approach of Daffos and Hohlfeld and their co-workers[130, 946] appears to provide the best possible outcome.

There were 148 fetal infections in 2030 cases of maternal infection. The only predictive feature for fetal infection was fetal gestational age when infected: If this was less than 16 weeks, there were 31 of 52 (60%) with ultrasonographic evidence of infection. This included ascites, pericarditis, or necrotic foci; 48% had cerebral ventricular dilation. If pregnancy was terminated, they found large areas of necrosis in the fetal brain; in those who terminated their pregnancies at 17 to 23 weeks'

gestation, there were 16 of 63 (25%) infected fetuses who had signs on ultrasonographic examination; 12% had ventricular dilation. If termination was later than 24 weeks, 1 of 33 fetuses had signs on ultrasonographic evaluation. Hydrocephalus was not observed. Thus, they offer termination at less than 16 weeks' gestation (see Table 5–9).

In the Paris studies, when mothers were found to be infected well before 16 weeks' gestation (i.e., in the first weeks of gestation) and the fetus was found to be infected by amniocentesis at 17 to 18 weeks' gestation, many of the pregnancies were terminated and almost uniformly the fetus was found to have brain necrosis and 48% had cerebral ventricular dilation[130] (see Table 5–9). In contrast, Wallon and co-workers[1060] do not terminate pregnancies of women who are acutely infected after 13 weeks' gestation and who are treated, unless fetal brain ultrasonographic evaluations are markedly abnormal. This was because most infected children in their series were not severely impaired. In their experience with 116 congenitally infected children, there were only 2 children (2%) with some visual impairment due to macular lesions and these children had no neurologic or mental deficits. There were 31 (27%) with cerebral calcifications or retinal lesions, but they were neurologically and developmentally normal and without severe impairment of their vision.

Mirlesse and associates[1061] described the outcome of 2684 maternal infections. There were 133 fetuses without cerebral dilation diagnosed and treated prenatally, and 104 infants without ventricular dilation were followed for a prolonged period postnatally. These patients were treated prenatally and postnatally. Several different types of important information are included in this report. The first is the overall outcome of treatment for children detected and treated in this manner. Specifically, there were 201 fetal infections (7.4%) in these 2684 mothers and 60 (39.8%) pregnancies were terminated. Termination was usual for infections before the sixteenth week of gestation or when there was hydrocephalus. There were 140 (70%) of 201 pregnancies with 141 live-born children. One hundred four children were observed for a mean of 31 months. Two children died of malignant hyperthermia, 1 child had seizures, 1 child had a psychiatric disorder, and 12 had new eye lesions that developed between 6 months and 2 years of age. Sixteen (12%) of 133 children had eye lesions when they were born (Table 5–43).

Prenatally, fetal ultrasounds were performed fortnightly and head ultrasonographic evaluations and sometimes brain CT also were performed in the newborn period for some of the infants. The prenatal ultrasonographic evaluation was performed through the endovaginal route with a 7-MHZ probe when there was a cephalic presentation of the fetus.

These investigators describe important correlations with a finding of heterogeneous granular brain parenchyma in some of the congenitally infected infants. These findings predominated in the periventricular re-

gion but were found throughout the parenchyma. These areas ranged in size from a few millimeters to more than 1 cm. When they were calcified, they sometimes generated a shadow. The authors emphasize that it was important to distinguish these hyperechogenic areas (HEAs) from cross-sectional vascular images by opening a color Doppler window (see Table 5–43).

In 133 children, HEAs were present in 37 (26%) and HEAs were identified antenatally in 17 (46%) of 37. HEAs were never seen before 29 to 30 weeks' gestation. Ultrasound examinations underestimated lesions identified in CT at birth in 6 cases.

An important finding was that there were more fetuses with HEAs if there was a longer interval between diagnosis of material and fetal infection (see Table 5–43). This implies that with frequent maternal serologic monitoring and prompt initiation of treatment, there will be

TABLE 5–43
Significant Correlations of Brain Hyperechogenic Areas in Fetal and Newborn Ultrasounds with Other Clinical Aspects of Congenital Toxoplasmosis

	CEREBRAL HYPERECHOGENICITY[a]	NO CEREBRAL HYPERECHOGENICITY	TOTAL OR [SIGNIFICANCE OF DIFFERENCE]
Interval between diagnosis of maternal and fetal infection	8.5 Weeks	6.5 Weeks	[$p = 0.03$]
Interval between maternal infection and beginning pyrimethamine and sulfadiazine	9.5 Weeks	8.5 Weeks	[$p = 0.06$]
Ocular lesions	9/37 (24%)[b]	7/96 (7%)	16/133 (12%) [$p < 0.008$]
New eye lesions	7/37 (18%)	5/67 (7%)	12/104 (12%) [$p < 0.058$]

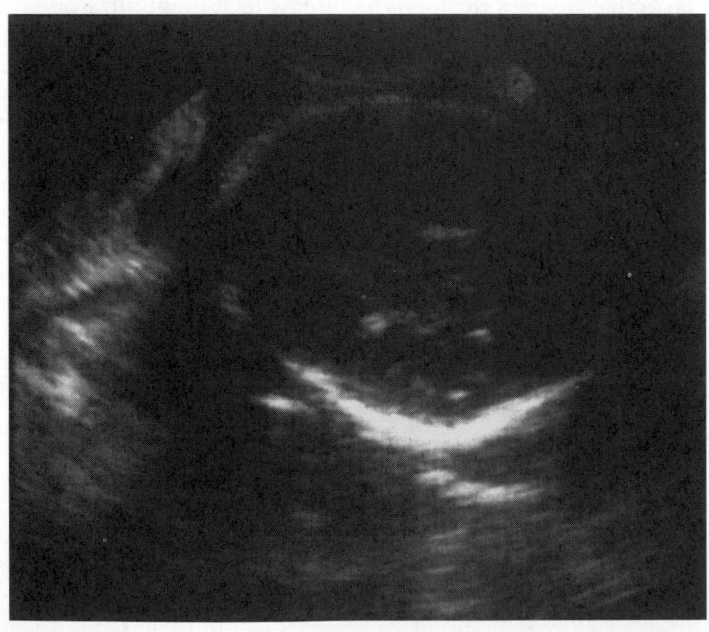

[a]See ultrasound for hyperechogenicity.

[b]Number with finding/number in group (%). Maximum duration of follow-up was until 2 years old. *Note:* delays in diagnosis and treatment were associated with cerebral hyperechogenicity on brain ultrasound and such hyperechogenicity was associated with more ocular lesions and development of new eye lesions.

From Mirlesse V, et al. Long-term follow-up of fetuses and newborn with congenital toxoplasmosis diagnosed and treated prenatally. In preparation.

fewer neurologic lesions and less ophthalmologic disease.

Another important implication of these investigators' findings is that HEA and its correlation with more frequent ophthalmologic disease demonstrates homogeneity of neurosensory involvement. In the U.S. (Chicago) National Collaborative Treatment Trial, this finding of frequent concordance of neurologic and ophthalmologic involvement also was noted. HEA predicts ophthalmologic findings, but they are not always present. Developmental outcome in these treated children, whether HEAs were present or not, was normal (see Table 5–43).

Sequelae of Congenital Toxoplasmosis in Untreated Children

STANFORD-ALABAMA STUDY

Results of a collaborative study performed in the United States suggest that a very significant number of children born with subclinical congenital T. gondii infection develop adverse sequelae.[555]

In this study,[555] the children were divided into two groups on the basis of differences in the reason for which serologic studies for toxoplasmosis were initially performed. Group I consisted of 13 children: of these, 8 cases were detected as a result of routine screening of cord serum for IgM T. gondii antibodies[512] and as a result of testing for IgG and IgM antibodies to T. gondii. These tests were performed either because acute T. gondii infection was diagnosed during pregnancy or at term in the mother or because the children were screened for nonspecific findings in the newborn period. Although each of these 13 children was carefully evaluated, none had signs of neurologic, ophthalmologic, or severe generalized disease at birth or at the time of diagnosis of congenital T. gondii infection; they would not have been detected if screening tests for antibodies to T. gondii had not been performed. (Data regarding earlier clinical and laboratory evaluations of eight of the children from Alabama had been reported previously.[512, 1056, 1062]) Group II consisted of 11 children in whom neither their parents nor their physicians detected signs of congenital infection during the newborn period. The diagnosis was entertained only after they presented with ophthalmologic or neurologic signs suggestive of congenital T. gondii infection. Because these children were preselected as a result of having developed complications of their initially subclinical infection and because it is possible that a more detailed evaluation during the newborn period might have detected abnormalities in some of them, they were analyzed separately from the children in group I. The characteristics of both groups are shown in Table 5–44.

Of the 24 children, 11 (5 in group I and 6 in group II) were never treated (Table 5–45). Four children (1 in group I and 3 in group II) were treated only after they developed adverse sequelae or for less than 2 weeks or both; for purposes of analysis, these children were referred to as untreated. Nine children (7 in group I and 2 in group II) were treated for at least 3 weeks before 1 year of age and before the development of neurologic

TABLE 5–44

Characteristics of Children Born with Subclinical Congenital *Toxoplasma* Infection: Results of Stanford University and University of Alabama Study

CHARACTERISTIC	GROUP I[a] (N = 13)	GROUP II[a] (N = 11)
Sex		
Male	4	9
Female	9	2
Race		
White	8	10
Black	5	0
Hispanic	0	1
Mean socioeconomic class[b]	4.08 ± 1.04	3.27 ± 1.19
Birth weight percentile		
<10	5	3
>10, <50	5	8
>50	3	0
Mean gestational age (wk)	37	38
Range	27.5–42.0	33.0–43.0
Mean age at diagnosis (wk)	2	34
Range	0.0–26.0	17.0–52.0
Mean age at most recent examination (yr)	8.26	8.68
Range	3.50–11.17	1.25–17.25
Treatment history for *Toxoplasma* infection[c]		
Never treated	5	6
Treated after sequelae developed and/or for < 2 wk	1	3
Treated	7	2

[a]Group I = children for whom serologic tests were performed either because *Toxoplasma* infection was diagnosed in the mother during pregnancy or at term or because the children were screened for nonspecific findings in the newborn period. Group II = children in whom no signs of congenital infection were found during the newborn period. Diagnosis was first entertained after these children presented with signs suggestive of congenital *Toxoplasma* infection.

[b]Hollingshead's classification, mean ± SD (Hollingshead AB. Social Class and Mental Illness: A Community Study. New York, John Wiley, 1958).

[c]See text for definition and details of treatment.

Adapted from Wilson CB, Remington JS, Stagno S, et al. Development of adverse sequelae in children born with subclinical congenital *Toxoplasma* infection. Pediatrics 66:767–774, 1980, with permission.

or intellectual deficits. Treatment in all cases consisted of pyrimethamine and sulfadiazine or pyrimethamine and trisulfapyrimidines.

All children were evaluated at least once. The methods of evaluation are indicated in Table 5–45. A detailed history was taken, and a physical and neurologic examination was performed for each child. Birth weight percentiles, based on the appropriate gender and presence or absence of twin births, were used.[1063]

The results of the study revealed that 22 (92%) of the 24 children ultimately developed untoward sequelae of their congenital infection. The two children who had not developed sequelae were in group I; they were 8 and 10 years of age at the time of last examination.

Ophthalmologic Outcome. In group I, 11 (85%) of 13 children developed sequelae, and chorioretinitis was the initial manifestation of disease in all 11 (Table 5–46). The age at onset of eye disease ranged from 1 month to

TABLE 5–45

Methods of Evaluation of Children Born with Subclinical Congenital *Toxoplasma* Infection: Results of Stanford University and University of Alabama Study

METHOD	GROUP I[a] (N = 13)	GROUP II[a] (N = 11)
History; physical and neurologic examination	13	11
Urinalysis	13	11
Complete blood cell count	13	11
Detailed ophthalmologic examination	13	10
Skull roentgenograms	10	6
Pneumoencephalograms or angiograms	0	2
Intelligence testing		
University of Alabama		
Revised 1974 Wechsler Intelligence Scale for Children	5	1
McCarthy Scales of Children's Abilities	2	1
Stanford-Binet Intelligence Scale (1972 Standards)	1	0
Not performed	0	2
Stanford University		
Stanford-Binet Intelligence Scale (1972 Standards)	5	6
Cattell Infant Intelligence Scale	0	1
Audiometry	13	11

[a]Group I = children for whom serologic tests were performed either because *Toxoplasma* infection was diagnosed in the mother during pregnancy or at term or because the children were screened for nonspecific findings in the newborn period. Group II = children in whom no signs of congenital infection were found during the newborn period. Diagnosis was first entertained after these children presented with signs suggestive of congenital *Toxoplasma* infection.

Adapted from Wilson CB, Remington JS, Stagno S, et al. Development of adverse sequelae in children born with subclinical congenital *Toxoplasma* infection. Pediatrics 66:767–774, 1980, with permission.

9.3 years of age, with a mean of 3.7 years of age. At their most recent examination, 3 children had unilateral functional blindness and the remaining 8 had chorioretinitis without loss of visual function. Subsequent to the initial episode of chorioretinitis, 3 of these 11 children had one or more additional episodes of active chorioretinitis at ages ranging from 1 to 8.7 years of age; 1 of the 3 children developed unilateral chorioretinitis at 1 year of age, experienced four additional episodes of active chorioretinitis in that eye, and also developed chorioretinitis in the previously uninvolved eye at 5 years of age. Although temporarily decreased visual function was associated with the recurrent episodes of active chorioretinitis in some of these children, no permanent, additional loss of visual function has resulted.

In group II, eight children initially presented with abnormal eye findings (see Table 5–46). The age at onset of eye disease ranged from 3 months to 1 year of age, with a mean of 0.4 year of age. The two other children in group II in whom ophthalmologic examinations were performed had chorioretinitis at the time they presented with neurologic abnormalities. At their most recent examination, five children had bilateral functional blindness, three had unilateral functional blindness, one had moderate unilateral visual loss, and one had chorioretinitis without loss of visual function. Subsequent to the initial episode of chorioretinitis, two of these children had recurrences of active chorioretinitis, at 2.3 to 3.5 years of age. One child in group II did not have an adequate ophthalmologic evaluation at the time of last follow-up and is not included in the results of ophthalmologic outcome.

Neurologic Outcome. Neurologic sequelae (Table 5–47) developed less frequently than did chorioretinitis

and were always associated with eye pathology. Five (38.5%) of 13 children in group I suffered neurologic sequelae. Major neurologic sequelae developed in 1 (8%) and minor neurologic sequelae developed in 4 (31%) children in group I. In the child with major neurologic sequelae, severe psychomotor retardation and microcephaly became evident 19 months after the onset of chorioretinitis and 22 months after the diagnosis of congenital infection was made. This child subsequently developed a seizure disorder at 5 years of age. Two of the 4 children with minor neurologic sequelae in group I had delayed psychomotor development during the first 6 months of life, but their subsequent psychomotor development and neurologic status were normal when they were last examined at 3.7 and 8.7 years of age. The other two children in group I had minor cerebellar signs when most recently evaluated at 3.5 and 6.6 years of age.

Eight (73%) of 11 children in group II suffered neurologic sequelae (see Table 5–47). Of the children in group II, major neurologic sequelae developed in 3, minor followed by major neurologic sequelae developed in 2, and minor neurologic sequelae developed in 3. Two of these 5 children with major neurologic sequelae initially presented with eye abnormalities at 3 and 4 months of age; 1 subsequently developed a seizure disorder at 3 years of age, and the other was first noted to be microcephalic at 2 years of age. The other 3 children with major neurologic sequelae in group II included 1 child who presented with hydrocephalus at 8.5 months of age and subsequently developed a seizure disorder and severe psychomotor retardation; 1 child who first exhibited transiently delayed psychomotor development between 6 and 12 months of age and subsequently developed severe psychomotor retardation; and 1 child who pre-

TABLE 5–46
Ophthalmologic Outcome in Children Born with Subclinical Congenital *Toxoplasma* Infection: Results of Stanford University and University of Alabama Study

OPHTHALMOLOGIC FINDING	GROUP I[a] (N = 13)	GROUP II[a] (N = 10)[b]
No sequelae (7.6, 10)[c]	2	0
Chorioretinitis		
Bilateral		
Bilateral blindness[d]	0	5
Unilateral blindness	3	3
Moderate unilateral visual loss	0	1[e]
Minimal or no visual loss	5	1
Unilateral		
Minimal or no visual loss	3	0
Mean age at onset (yr)	3.67	0.42
Range	0.08–9.33	0.25–1.00
Recurrences of active chorioretinitis	3	2

[a]Group I = children for whom serologic tests were performed either because *Toxoplasma* infection was diagnosed in the mother during pregnancy or at term or because the children were screened for nonspecific findings in the newborn period. Group II = children in whom no signs of congenital infection were found during the newborn period. Diagnosis was first entertained after these children presented with signs suggestive of congenital *Toxoplasma* infection.

[b]One of the 11 children in group II was excluded because an adequate follow-up ophthalmologic examination was not performed.

[c]Age (yr) at most recent examination.

[d]Blindness = vision not correctable to > 20/200.

[e]Macular involvement but vision correctable to 20/40.

Adapted from Wilson CB, Remington JS, Stagno S, et al. Development of adverse sequelae in children born with subclinical congenital *Toxoplasma* infection. Pediatrics 66:767–774, 1980, with permission.

sented with seizures at 4 months of age and subsequently developed a seizure disorder associated with minor cerebellar dysfunction. Two additional children in group II had minor cerebellar dysfunction only, and 1 child had minor cerebellar dysfunction after showing transiently delayed psychomotor development in the first year of life.

Of the 16 children from both groups I and II for whom skull roentgenograms during infancy were available, 5 (mean age, 5.2 months) had intracranial calcifications and 11 (mean age, 4.8 months) did not. One of these children had normal skull roentgenograms in the first month of life, but calcifications were noted on repeat roentgenograms at 3 months of age. Intracranial calcifications were noted on initial roentgenograms taken between 3 and 10 months of age in the remaining 4 children. All 5 children with intracranial calcifications and 4 of the 11 children without intracranial calcifications developed major or minor neurologic sequelae (p = 0.03). In this group of 9 children, the neurologic sequelae that developed were classified as major sequelae in 4 children (3 with intracranial calcifications and 1 without intracranial calcifications). Thus, of the 16 children, major neurologic sequelae developed in 3 of 5 children with intracranial calcifications and 1 of 11 children without intracranial calcifications (p = 0.06). No correlation was found between neurologic outcome and birth weight, race, or age at most recent examination.

Eight children in group I had CSF examinations performed during the newborn period. In 7 of them, abnormalities were detected; such abnormalities did not correlate with the development of any type of sequelae.

Intelligence Testing. Intelligence testing was performed in 22 of the 24 children by the methods that are indicated in Table 5–45. The results of intelligence testing are presented in Table 5–48. IQ scores correlated directly with upper socioeconomic class (r = 0.37, p < 0.05). In addition, the 16 white children had a higher mean IQ (89.6 ± 26.3) than did the 6 nonwhite children (81.2 ± 15), but this difference was not statistically significant. Two of the children in group I (1 white, 1 African American) had moderately severe retardation (IQ scores of 36 and 62, respectively), as did 2 of the children (both white) in group II (IQ scores of 43 and 53). There was a tendency for IQ scores to decrease on later testing among the 7 children (6 in group I and 1 in group II) who were tested more than once. The mean IQ score of these children fell from 96.9 to 74 over an average of 5.5 years, with all but 1 child showing a decrease on repeat testing.

There was no significant correlation between IQ scores and the finding of abnormal CSF in the newborn period, intracranial calcifications on skull roentgenograms, age at time of testing, or birth weight below the tenth percentile. There was, in fact, a trend toward

TABLE 5–47
Neurologic Outcome in Children Born with Subclinical Congenital *Toxoplasma* Infection: Results of Stanford University and University of Alabama Study

NEUROLOGIC FINDING	GROUP I[a] (N = 13)	GROUP II[a] (N = 11)
No sequelae	8	3
Major sequelae[b]		
Hydrocephalus	0	1[c]
Microcephaly	1[d]	1
Seizures	1	3[e]
Severe psychomotor retardation	1	2[f]
Minor sequelae		
Mild cerebellar dysfunction	2	4
Transiently delayed psychomotor development	2	2

[a]Group I = children for whom serologic tests were performed either because *Toxoplasma* infection was diagnosed in the mother during pregnancy or at term or because the children were screened for nonspecific findings in the newborn period. Group II = children in whom no signs of congenital infection were found during the newborn period. Diagnosis was first suspected when they presented with signs suggestive of congenital *Toxoplasma* infection.

[b]Microcephaly was diagnosed when the head circumference was below the third percentile; hydrocephalus was diagnosed on the basis of pneumoencephalography.

[c]The same child had a seizure disorder and severe psychomotor retardation and was included in the figures under those categories in group II.

[d]The same child had a seizure disorder and severe psychomotor retardation and was included in the figures under those categories in group I.

[e]One of these three children had mild cerebellar dysfunction and was included in the figures under that category in group II.

[f]One of these two children first exhibited transiently delayed psychomotor development and was included in the figures under that category in group II.

Adapted from Wilson CB, Remington JS, Stagno S, et al. Development of adverse sequelae in children born with subclinical congenital *Toxoplasma* infection. Pediatrics 66:767–774, 1980, with permission.

TABLE 5–48
Intelligence Testing in Children Born with Subclinical Congenital *Toxoplasma* Infection: Results of Stanford University and University of Alabama Study

AGE AND INTELLIGENCE TEST FINDING	GROUP I[a] (N = 13)	GROUP II[a] (N = 9)[b]
Mean age at most recent testing (yr)	7.40	10.20
Range	2.75–10.00	2.50–17.25
IQ[c]	88.6 ± 23.4[d]	85.3 ± 25.6[e]

[a]Group I = children for whom serologic tests were performed either because *Toxoplasma* infection was diagnosed in the mother during pregnancy or at term or because the children were screened for nonspecific findings in the newborn period. Group II = children in whom no signs of congenital infection were found during the newborn period. Diagnosis was first suspected when they presented with signs suggestive of congenital *Toxoplasma* infection.

[b]Two of 11 children in group II were excluded because they did not have intelligence formally evaluated.

[c]Mean ± SD.

[d]Evaluation was performed with the Stanford-Binet Intelligence Scale, 6 children; Revised 1974 Wechsler Intelligence Scale for Children, 5 children; and McCarthy Scales of Children's Abilities, 2 children.

[e]Evaluation was performed with the Stanford-Binet Intelligence Scale, 6 children; Revised 1974 Wechsler Intelligence Scale for Children, 1 child; McCarthy Scales of Children's Abilities, 1 child; and Cattell Infant Intelligence Scale, 1 child.

Adapted from Wilson CB, Remington JS, Stagno S, et al. Development of adverse sequelae in children born with subclinical congenital *Toxoplasma* infection. Pediatrics 66:767–774, 1980, with permission.

higher IQ scores (mean, 96.9) in children with birth weight below the tenth percentile. These results of intelligence testing must be interpreted with caution. The range of IQ scores was wide, testing was performed by different individuals, and different tests were employed. The low mean socioeconomic class of the children also may have accounted for the low mean IQ scores that were observed. It is likely, however, that the results for the 2 children in group I and the 2 children in group II who had moderately severe retardation would not have been substantially different under other circumstances. It is particularly disturbing to note the downward trend in IQ scores for those children who were evaluated more than once. Although the finding is not statistically significant, all 6 children in group I had lower IQ scores when tested an average of 5.5 years after initial intelligence testing was performed. The mean age of the total study population was lower than that of the children who had repeat IQ testing, all of whom were older than 9 years of age when last tested. Thus, the true extent of intellectual impairment in the study population may be greater than the investigators observed.

Other Abnormalities. Several other abnormalities noted in the children are shown in Table 5–49. The incidence of sensorineural hearing loss in the study population also appeared to be excessive. In an earlier study on certain of these children,[1056] the incidence of mild sensorineural hearing loss in 41 normal control children (mean age, 3.8 years) was 5%; no children with more severe sensorineural hearing loss were observed. In this study,[555] the incidence of sensorineural hearing loss in children tested in group I was 30% and that in group II

was 22%. One child in each group had moderate unilateral hearing loss.

Effect of Treatment. One of the 2 children in group I who had not developed sequelae at the time of the study was treated (this child's mother also was treated during the last trimester of pregnancy), and the other was never treated. Of the 22 children in groups I and II who presented with chorioretinitis in the absence of neurologic disease, major neurologic sequelae developed in 5 of 13 untreated children but none of 9 treated children ($p = 0.05$). Because abnormal skull roentgenograms correlated with development of neurologic sequelae, the researchers examined the results of skull roentgenograms in treated and untreated children. Skull roentgenograms were available from 8 of the 13 untreated and 5 of the 9 treated children. Whereas no treated child had abnormal skull roentgenograms (each had roentgenograms obtained before and 1 had roentgenograms obtained after treatment), 4 of the untreated children had intracranial calcifications ($p = 0.01$). No factors other than abnormal skull roentgenograms differed significantly between treated and untreated children. The mean IQ score (97 ± 22) of those children treated for 3 weeks or more at or before 1 year of age was higher than the mean IQ score (93 ± 22) of those who received no treatment or the mean IQ score (82.5 ± 29.7) of those who were treated for a shorter duration or at a later age (usually after obvious sequelae were evident); these differences were not significant ($p > 0.1$).

Special Considerations. Because this study was not controlled and was only in part prospective, certain limitations must be considered in interpreting the data. Children in group II were detected because they developed sequelae that were sufficiently significant to attract medical attention. Thus, it would be inappropriate to

TABLE 5–49
Other Abnormalities in Children Born with Subclinical Congenital *Toxoplasma* Infection: Results of Stanford University and University of Alabama Study

ABNORMALITY	GROUP I[a]	GROUP II[a]
Sensorineural hearing loss		
Moderate unilateral	1/10[b]	1/9[b]
Mild unilateral	1/10	0/9
Mild bilateral	1/10	1/9
Precocious puberty	2/13[c]	0/11
Premature thelarche	0/13	1/11[d]
Miscellaneous[e]	3/13	1/11

[a]Group I = children for whom serologic tests were performed either because *Toxoplasma* infection was diagnosed in the mother during pregnancy or at term or because the children were screened for nonspecific findings in the newborn period. Group II = children in whom no signs of congenital infection were found during the newborn period. Diagnosis was first suspected when they presented with signs suggestive of congenital *Toxoplasma* infection.

[b]Number with abnormality/number evaluated.

[c]Onset at 6 and 8 years of age.

[d]Onset at 2 years of age.

[e]Includes one genu recurvatum, one clubfoot, one low-set umbilicus, and one slow weight gain.

Adapted from Wilson CB, Remington JS, Stagno S, et al. Development of adverse sequelae in children born with subclinical congenital *Toxoplasma* infection. Pediatrics 66:767–774, 1980, with permission.

use data from this group to determine the frequency with which children born with subclinical infection develop sequelae. Nevertheless, data from group II do provide information regarding the potential seriousness of ocular disease in children born with subclinical congenital *T. gondii* infection and regarding the risk of subsequent neurologic sequelae in children who have previously developed chorioretinitis. There are no data from this study or from other studies that indicate that a significant bias toward more severe disease was introduced by the different screening methods employed in group I. It is likely, therefore, that the data from group I provide a reasonable estimate both of the seriousness and of the frequency of complications in children with initially subclinical congenital *T. gondii* infection. Because of the small sample size and the lack of a matched control group, these data must, however, be considered estimates. In addition, because more than half of the children in this study were younger than the age of 9 years, it should be appreciated that additional sequelae may have developed among them. This study and the early Eichenwald studies are profound descriptions of the tragedy of untreated or inadequately treated children.

PARIS STUDIES

Of 108 infants with congenital *T. gondii* infection who were diagnosed and followed prospectively by Couvreur and colleagues[560] and discussed by Szusterkac,[1064] 27 had chorioretinitis. In 26 of them, the lesions were present at the time of the first ophthalmoscopic examination after birth. In only 1 infant was the eye examination result normal at birth with subsequent development of chorioretinitis. In 3 other infants, a retinal lesion was noted at the time of first examination, and a new lesion was discovered on follow-up. It is noteworthy that only 16 of the 108 infants were examined after the age of 2 years and only 3 were examined after the age of 5 years. Only 6 of these 19 children had chorioretinitis on initial examination. Of interest is the observation that there was a striking difference between the children who were treated and those not treated during the first year of life. Among the treated children, no lesions were discovered after the age of 2 years, whereas 8% of the untreated children developed chorioretinitis between 10 months and 4 years of age. It is possible to assume from the experience of Koppe and colleagues[556, 557] and Wilson

and co-workers[555] that careful follow-up in these 108 children would reveal additional cases of chorioretinitis and additional lesions in the 27 children who already had eye disease. Follow-up in the series is important because all of these children were identified prospectively and were treated for approximately 1 year either from birth or from the time that the diagnosis was established in the first months of life.

Additional data in children in whom congenital *T. gondii* infection was not recognized in the newborn period have been published by Briatte.[1065] These data were obtained in collaboration with Couvreur, Hazemann, and Desmonts in Paris. Hazemann established a program at a number of medical centers in the Paris area in which any infant could be examined free of charge at the request of the mother. The infant was first examined at the age of 10 months. Among the blood tests performed in this program was the dye test to detect cases of previously undiagnosed congenital *T. gondii* infection. Forty-eight infants with subclinical congenital *T. gondii* infection were detected among the 20,513 infants examined from 1971 through 1979. (The data were corrected for those cases in which the infection was most likely acquired postnatally.) Infants with clinical toxoplasmosis were probably not examined in this program because these infants would already be under medical care and thus their mothers would not likely request their participation in this medical screening program. For the same reason, it is likely that the vast majority of infants screened had few or no problems during infancy.

The frequency of probable congenital *T. gondii* infection in the entire study population averaged 2.33 per 1000 (range, 0.38 to 5.2 per 1000 per study year). The frequency of chorioretinitis in the 48 infants is shown in Table 5–50. Of these 48 children (who were, of course, not treated for their *T. gondii* infection during their first 10 months of life), 18% developed chorioretinitis by the age of 4 years. Eight developed chorioretinitis after the age of 10 months and before the age of 4 years. This latter finding differs considerably from that reported by Szusterkac[1064] in infants who were treated in the early weeks or months of life (see earlier discussion). Cerebral calcifications were present in 3 of the 48 previously unrecognized and untreated infants.[1065]

INTERPRETATION OF STANFORD-ALABAMA AND PARIS STUDIES

For proper interpretation of the data presented for the Stanford-Alabama study[555] and the study reported by

TABLE 5–50
Frequency of Chorioretinitis in Infants with Subclinical Congenital *Toxoplasma* Infection First Discovered in a Systematic Serologic Screening Program

AGE WHEN FUNDUS WAS EXAMINED	NO. OF CHILDREN	CHORIORETINITIS PREVIOUSLY RECOGNIZED	NEW CASES OF CHORIORETINITIS DISCOVERED	TOTAL NO. OF CHILDREN WITH CHORIORETINITIS IN THIS AGE GROUP (%)
10 mo	48	0	5	5 (10)
Examined again at 2 yr	31	5	3	8 (16)
Examined again at 4 yr	28	8	1	9 (18)

Data are adapted from patients studied by Drs. J. Couvreur, J. J. Hazemann, and G. Desmonts. Cases are discussed by Briatte.[1065]

Briatte,[1065] it is important to understand how the data might be biased because of the method of case selection. The method used in the studies in Alabama for detection of subclinical congenital infection (detection of an increase in cord serum IgM) might have selected for the most "severe" (heavily infected) cases among subclinically infected newborns. In the studies performed by the Stanford group, some of the patients were selected because manifestations of the infection occurred during infancy. Thus, in both of these studies, the method of selection might have predisposed to an increased frequency of more severe cases in the Stanford-Alabama study. In contrast, in the study reported by Briatte, it is probable that the most "benign" cases were selected among subclinically infected newborns because these investigators studied infants who had few or no medical problems during the first 10 months of life. Despite this bias toward "mild" infection, 18% of the infants that the Paris group observed had ocular lesions by the age of 4 years.

AMSTERDAM STUDY

As mentioned earlier, in 1964 a prospective study was started in Amsterdam to determine the frequency of congenital toxoplasmosis.[556] Of 1821 pregnancies screened, 249 infants were followed—21 because of seroconversion in the dye test; 42 because of a high baseline dye test titer; 183 because of a slight rise in dye test titer; and 3 because their mothers had toxoplasmosis shortly before gestation. At birth, 4 infants had chorioretinitis and parasites were isolated from placenta and CSF of 1 other infant. Each of these 5 children was treated. Seven children who were asymptomatic and whose dye test titer did not revert to negative were not treated. Ten other questionably infected children who had no symptoms but whose dye test titer became negative 18 months after birth were also not treated. These 22 children were followed annually for 5 years by physical examinations and dye and CF tests. No new abnormalities were detected except in 1 patient with chorioretinitis, who required surgery to correct a squint at the age of 2 years.[556] The 12 congenitally infected children continued to be examined yearly until the age of 20 years. The authors' original optimistic view was revised in their 1986 publication.[366] One of the 5 treated children and 1 of the symptom-free children had new scars in their eyes at the age of 6 years. Additional new scars or acute lesions were observed in both treated and untreated children. In 3 children, scars appeared at ages 11, 12, and 13 years. One patient had a new scar in his right eye when examined for the first time at age 17, and another had no severe eye abnormalities until the age of 18 years, when an acute lesion appeared in the right macula that led to blindness in that eye. Another patient had a new acute lesion in her right eye at the age of 12 years and again in both eyes at the age of 13 years. Thus, after a total of 20 years of follow-up, of 11 congenitally infected children, 9 had scars in one or both eyes. Four of these children had vision severely impaired in one eye, and 3 were blind in one eye. Among the 10 questionably infected children, 1 had a scar in the right macula at 5 years of age that led to severe visual impairment. Another, whose mother had toxoplasmosis during gestation, remained persistently seropositive. He had not developed any scars in his eyes. The other 8 children remained seronegative for 5 to 19 years, and some acquired toxoplasmosis during this time. When compared for school performance, the 11 congenitally infected children did not differ from controls in their school performance. None of the 11 was mentally retarded.

From the results of this prospective study, it is apparent that 9 (82%) of 11 children after 20 years of follow-up had significant sequelae of toxoplasmosis and that 5 of these 11 had severely impaired vision. Although the report by Wilson and associates described earlier demonstrated a similar percentage of untoward sequelae by the age of 10 years, theirs was not a prospective study.[555]

In regard to the above described results the prospective clinical study reported by Sever and associates and performed in children born of mothers whose sera were sampled during pregnancy between 1959 and 1966,[1066] the investigators suggested that maternal *T. gondii* infection may be associated with greater damage to women and children than had previously been recognized. Of special interest is the increased rate of deafness, microcephaly, and low IQ values at an examination of the children at 7 years of age. This suggests that late sequelae of congenital *T. gondii* infection are not limited to eye disease but occur also in the CNS.

U.S. (CHICAGO) NATIONAL COLLABORATIVE TREATMENT TRIAL STUDY

A national, collaborative, prospective study is being carried out by a group based in Chicago. This study group is evaluating long-term outcome for infants treated with pyrimethamine (comparing two doses), in combination with leucovorin and sulfadiazine (100 mg/kg per day in two divided doses). Medications are begun when a child is younger than 2.5 months of age according to the method shown in Figure 5–29 and continued for 12 months. Therapy is monitored by parents with a nurse case manager and the primary physician, and compliance is also documented with serum pyrimethamine levels. Children who have not been treated during the first year of life and are referred to the study group when they are older than 1 year are also followed. Patients are evaluated comprehensively by the study group near the time of birth and at 1, 3.5, 5, 7.5, 10, and 15 years of age.

The following parameters are evaluated: history; physical examination; audiologic, ophthalmologic, neurologic, and cognitive function and development; and a number of laboratory tests, including tests of hematologic status and serologic and lymphocyte response to *T. gondii* antigens, and neuroradiologic studies. As of March 1999, 104 treated children have been evaluated. They range in age from .07 to 17.1 years (mean age, 6.8 years). Twenty-eight untreated historical controls have been followed. They range in age from 5.6 to 33.6 years (mean age, 14.1 years) (Table 5–51).

Preliminary results of this study indicate that early outcomes for many, but not all, congenitally infected

TABLE 5–51

Ages (Years) of Patients in U.S. (Chicago) National Collaborative Treatment Trial[a]

	ALL PATIENTS			PATIENTS ≥5 YEARS OLD		
	Mean ± s.d.	Range	N	Mean ± s.d.	Range	N
Historical patients[a]	13.9 ± 8.9	5.4–33.4	28	15.3 ± 8.9	5.4–33.4	28
Treatment A: feasibility	11.7 ± 1.1	10.0–14.3	13	11.7 ± 1.1	10.0–14.3	13
Randomized	5.7 ± 1.9	1.9–8.8	38	6.7 ± 1.2	5.0–8.8	26
Treatment C: feasibility	3.5 ± 4.6	0.5–15	7	12.7 ± 3.2	10.5–15.0	2
Randomized	5.4 ± 2.0	0.9–10.0	28	6.7 ± 1.4	5.1–10.0	16

[a]Historical patients were untreated patients diagnosed after 1 year of age. Treated children received 2 months (Treatment A) or 6 months (Treatment C) of daily pyrimethamine and sulfadiazine, followed by pyrimethamine on Monday, Wednesday, and Friday and continued daily sulfadiazine for the remainder of the year of therapy.

children treated in this decade, in this manner, appear to be substantially better than outcomes reported in earlier decades for children who were untreated or treated for 1 month or less (Tables 5–26, 5–52, and 5–53). Specifically, the early results from this study indicate that such therapy has been feasible for 104 children. The only substantial toxicity was transient neutropenia, which has responded to increased dosages of leucovorin or withholding of pyrimethamine. This appeared to occur primarily during the prodrome of concomitant viral infections. Dental caries occurred in one of the first children studied (Table 5–54). Thereafter, parents were cautioned to clean teeth of older infants because medications were administered in sugar suspensions. Pediatricians were cautioned to avoid using a second sulfonamide to treat concomitant infections such as otitis media, because more prolonged neutropenia occurred in one child in conjunction with such therapy.

Pharmacokinetics of pyrimethamine were characterized in the initial feasibility phase of the study, and serum levels associated with the two-dosage regimens of pyrimethamine were noted (see Pyrimethamine plus Sulfonamides section) (Fig. 5–31).

All signs of active infection (e.g., thrombocytopenia, hepatitis, rash, meningitis, hypoglycorrhachia, active chorioretinitis, and vitritis) resolved within weeks of initiation of therapy.[973] Chorioretinitis did not progress or relapse during therapy.

Audiologic outcome was significantly better than that reported in the earlier literature[693] (see Table 5–26). There has been no sensorineural hearing loss in the 104 treated children in contrast to a 14% incidence of "deafness"[552] or 26% incidence of "hearing loss"[555] in earlier studies. Contrasts of outcomes in this and earlier studies are summarized in Table 5–26 (see also the next section, Comparison of Outcomes).

Retinal disease became quiescent with therapy within weeks and did not recrudesce during therapy.[973] New lesions (primarily those "satelliting" preexisting lesions) occurred in older children (see Table 5–37). The oldest treated child was 17 years of age in 1999. Lesions have also occurred in previously normal-appearing retinae. These were noted first at study evaluations at 3.5, 5, or 7.5 years of age and had not been present at the preceding evaluation. Evaluations were near birth and at 1, 3.5, 5, and 7.5 years of age. To date, no loss in visual acuity

has occurred when prompt treatment of active recurrent chorioretinitis was initiated. Comparison of early outcome with 2 versus 6 months of 1 mg/kg per day of pyrimethamine followed by this dosage administered on Monday, Wednesday, and Friday, both administered with sulfadiazine and leucovorin are shown in Table 5–53. At present, there are no statistically significant differences. Thus, treatment during the first year of life with pyrimethamine and sulfonamides, unfortunately, did not prevent recrudescent chorioretinitis uniformly. Determination of whether it reduces the incidence of recurrent or new chorioretinitis compared with the almost uniform occurrence of this complication in untreated children diagnosed in earlier decades requires longer follow-up of more children. It is especially important to try to determine whether treatment prevents subsequent chorioretinitis when no retinal lesions are present at birth.

Visual acuity that is adequate for all usual activities and reading has been noted to occur in some children with large macular scars. Nonetheless, impairment of vision has been one of the two most prominent sequelae (Table 5–55). Visual impairment has presented a challenge in the care of children of school age; that is, special attention is needed to optimize their ability to read, and participation in learning activities is needed so that their visual impairments do not impair cognitive development. Retinal scars have been central, peripheral, unilateral, and bilateral and have resulted in partial and complete retinal detachment. Loss of sight at presentation (e.g., due to retinal detachment) has usually been associated with the most profound neurologic impairment. Visual outcomes to date are contrasted with those of earlier studies in the Comparison of Outcomes section. Neurologic and cognitive function of most of these treated children has been significantly better than reported in earlier decades.[489, 1067–1069] This is summarized in Table 5–56.

In an earlier report,[552] more than 80% of children who had substantial generalized and neurologic involvement at birth and who were not treated or were treated for 1 month had IQ scores below 70 at 4 years of age. In that report, initial involvement in the perinatal period appears to have been less severe or similar in severity to that of children in the U.S. (Chicago) National Collaborative Treatment Trial. In contrast to the outcome in

TABLE 5-52
Comparison of Ophthalmologic, Developmental, and Audiologic Outcomes with Postnatal Treatment

AUTHOR(S), YEAR OF PUBLICATION [REFERENCE]	NO. STUDIED	TREATMENT	MEAN AGE IN YEARS WHEN DATA TABULATED (RANGE)	PERCENT WITH FINDING OR IMPAIRMENT					
				Ophthalmologic			Neurologic		Audiologic
				Lesions[a]	Vision[b]	New[c]	Cognitive	Motor or Seizures	
Eichenwald, 1959 [17]	104	0 or 1 mo P, S	4 (minimum)	NA	0, 42, 67[d]	NA	50, 81, 89[d]	0, 58, 76[d]	0, 10, 17[d]
Wilson et al, 1980 [18]	23	0 or 1 mo P, S	8.5 (1–17)	93	47	22	55 (20 severe)	20	22, 30[e]
Koppe et al, 1986 [19]	12	0 or 1 mo P, S	20 (NA)	80	NA	NA	0	0	NA
Labadie and Hazemann, 1984 [20]	17	0	1 (NA)	28	NA	NA	NA	NA	NA
Couvreur et al, 1984 [21]	172	1 yr P, S, Sp	NA (2–11)	NA	NA	8	NA	NA	NA
Hohlfeld 1989 [15]	43	Prenatal, 1 yr P, S, Sp	NA (0.5–4)	12	NA	NA	0	0	NA
Villena, 1998 [23]	47	F, Sp	NA [born 1980–89]	—	—	15/45 (33)[f]	—	—	—
	19	1 yr F	NA [born 1990–96]	—	—	2/18 (11)	—	—	—
	12	2 yr F	NA [born 1990–97]	—	—	1/11 (9)	—	—	—
Peyron, 1996 [24]	121	F'	12 (5–22)	—	—	37/121 (31)	—	—	—
Chicago study (historical patients)	7	0	5.6 (2–10)	100	86	29	25	25	14
Chicago study (treated patients)	37[g]	Most for 1 yr P, S	3.4 (0.3–10)	81	81	8	0, 24[h]	0, 24	0

[a]Lesions = any chorioretinal lesions.
[b]Vision = vision impaired.
[c]New = new lesions.
[d]Subclinical, generalized, neurologic.
[e]Subclinical, generalized, neurologic.
[f]Number with finding/number in group (%).
[g]These data are for the first 37 children studied before May 1991.
F = Fansidar (pyrimethamine 1.25 mg/kg each 14 days); F' = Fansidar (in utero and postnatally pyrimethamine 6 mg/5 kg each 10 days; small numbers also treated in utero); NA = not available; P = pyrimethamine; S = sulfonamides; Sp = spiramycin.
Adapted from McAuley J, et al. Early and longitudinal evaluations of treated infants and children and untreated historical patients with congenital toxoplasmosis: the Chicago Collaborative Treatment Trial. Clin Infect Dis 18:38–72, 1994.

TABLE 5–53
Early Outcomes for Children ≥5 Years Old in the U.S. (Chicago) National Collaborative Treatment Trial

A	% in Literature 5 yr, 10 yr[c]	Historical Patients[d]	MILD[a] Treatment A[b] Feasibility	Randomized	Treatment C[b] Feasibility	Randomized
Vision <20/20	25, 50	11/14 (79)[e]	0/4	0/3	0/0	0/0
New retinal lesions	25, 85	5/9 (56)	0/4	1/3	0/0	0/0
Motor abnormality	10, 10	0/14 (0)	0/4	0/3	0/0	0/0
IQ < 70	0–50, 0–50	0/13 (0)	0/4	0/3	0/0	0/0
ΔIQ ≥ 15	50, 50	0/5 (0)	0/4	1/3	0/0	0/0
Hearing loss	30, 30	0/14 (0)	0/4	0/3	0/0	0/0

B	% in Literature 5 yr, 10 yr[f]	Historical Patients	SEVERE[a] Treatment A Feasibility	Randomized	Treatment C Feasibility	Randomized
Vision <20/20	70, 70	10/10 (100)	7/9 (78)	8/9 (89)	1/2	6/9 (67)
New retinal lesions	50, 90	4/9 (44)	3/9 (33)	1/8 (13)	2/2	0/9 (0)
Motor abnormality	60, 60	1/10 (10)	3/9 (33)	2/9 (22)	0/2	1/9 (11)
IQ < 70	90, >90	1/10 (10)	4/9 (44)	4/9 (44)	0/2	2/9 (22)
ΔIQ ≥ 15	95, 95	0/8 (0)	0/9 (0)	2/9 (22)	0/2	1/9 (11)
Hearing loss	30, 30	0/10 (0)	0/9 (0)	0/9 (0)	0/2	0/9 (0)

Note: Percentages not shown when ≤ 4 patients per group.

[a]Clinical disease considered "Mild" if infant is apparently normal and develops normally on follow-up (e.g., but has isolated nonmacular retinal scars or < 3 intracranial calcifications on CT. Clinical disease considered "Severe" if neurologic signs or symptoms present, symptomatic chorioretinitis that threatened vision, ≥3 intracranial calcifications on CT.

[b]Treated children received 2 months (Treatment A) or 6 months (Treatment C) of daily pyrimethamine and sulfadiazine, followed by pyrimethamine on Monday, Wednesday, and Friday and continued daily sulfadiazine for the remainder of the year of therapy. Feasibility patients were treated in the early phase of the study before randomized study.

[c]Data from Wilson et al.[555]

[d]Historical patients were untreated patients diagnosed after 1 year of age.

[e]Number with abnormality/number in group (% affected). No differences between treatment regimens achieved statistical significance ($p > 0.05$ using Fisher Exact test).

[f]Data from Eichenwald.[552]

this earlier series, only 24% of the children treated in the decade 1982–1992 in the U.S. (Chicago) National Collaborative Treatment Trial had substantial cognitive impairments. The remaining 76% of the treated children in the U.S. (Chicago) National Collaborative Treatment Trial who presented with substantial generalized or neurologic manifestations of infection or both in the perinatal period are developing normally and are likely to be capable of self-care. The same trends have been present in children tested through 1999. The rela-

tive contribution of shunt placement, antimicrobial therapy, and adjunctive supportive care to this improved outcome cannot be determined with certainty. The observation that almost all children without hydrocephalus in the U.S. (Chicago) National Collaborative Treatment Trial have at least average cognitive function contrasts dramatically with the 81% incidence rate of mental retardation at 4 years of age in children presenting with generalized disease in Eichenwald's series who were untreated or treated for 1 month.[552] This suggests that

TABLE 5–54
Episodes of Reversible Neutropenia Requiring Temporary Withholding of Medications for the U.S. National Collaborative Study[a]

	NO. OF EPISODES MEDICATION WITHHELD (MEAN ± S.D. [RANGE])	NUMBER WHO STOPPED MEDICATION/NO. IN GROUP WHO HAVE COMPLETED 1 YEAR OF THERAPY (%)	NO. OF CHILDREN WHO STOPPED MEDICATIONS TEMPORARILY/NO. IN GROUP (%) Feasibility	Randomized	DISCONTINUED MEDICATIONS DUE TO NEUTROPENIA ≥ 4 TIMES
Treatment A	1.8 ± 1.1 [1–4]	11/32 (34)	6/14 (43)	11/34 (32)	4
Treatment C	3.8 ± 3.1 [1–11]	17/48 (35)	1/4 (25)	10/28 (36)	5

[a]Children received 2 mo (Treatment A) or 6 mo (Treatment C) of daily pyrimethamine and sulfadiazine, followed by pyrimethamine on Monday, Wednesday, and Friday and continued daily sulfadiazine for the remainder of the year of therapy. Feasibility patients were treated in the early phase of the study before randomized study. Toxicity for Treatments A and C was measured as episodes of reversible neutropenia requiring temporary withholding of medications.

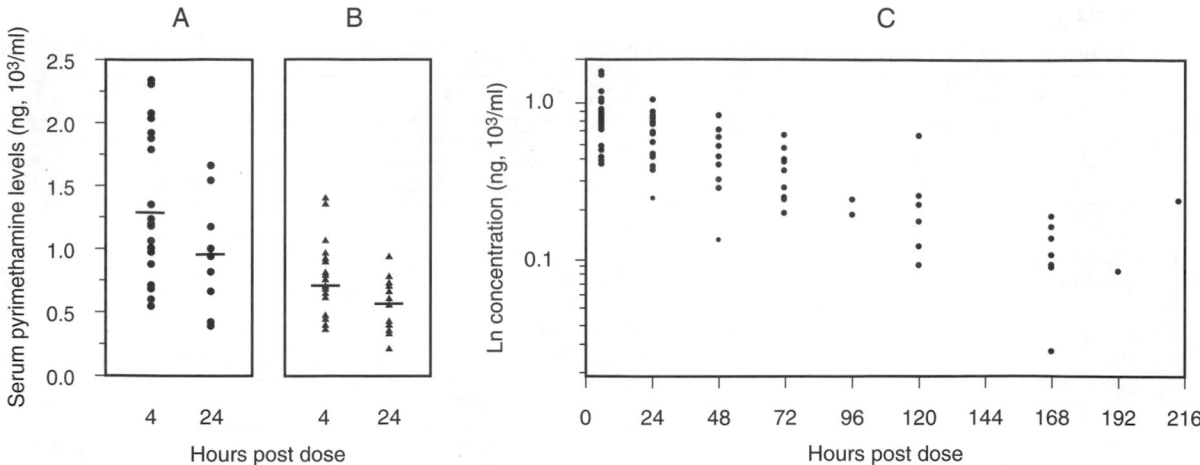

FIGURE 5–31 Pyrimethamine pharmacokinetics. *A*, Pyrimethamine serum levels (4 and 24 hours post dose) of children given 1 mg of pyrimethamine per kg daily. *B*, Pyrimethamine serum levels (4 and 24 hours post dose) of children given 1 mg of pyrimethamine per kg on Monday, Wednesday, and Friday of each week. Values for children taking phenobarbital are not included. *C*, Pyrimethamine serum levels of the entire study population of infants taking 1 mg of pyrimethamine per kg on Monday, Wednesday, and Friday of each week. Values for children taking phenobarbital are not included. (From McLeod R, Mack D, Foss R, et al: Levels of pyrimethamine in sera and cerebrospinal and ventricular fluids from infants treated for congenital toxoplasmosis. Antimicrob Agents Chemother 36:1040–1948, 1992.)

antimicrobial therapy may contribute significantly to the more favorable outcome. There has not been deterioration of cognitive function over time in these treated children, although visual impairment clearly has affected school performance and ability to acquire information and skills for some children.[1067] This contrasts with earlier reports of diminished cognitive function over time for untreated children or those treated for less than 1 month who had subclinical disease in the perinatal period (described by Wilson and associates[555]). Avoiding the negative effects of visual impairment on learning will be important for children in the U.S. (Chicago) National Collaborative Treatment Trial. In spite of the remarkably good cognitive outcome for many of these children, the impact of the infection on their cognitive function is reflected in the fact that their IQ scores are often 15 points less than those of their nearest-age siblings ($p < 0.05$).[1067]

It has been possible to discontinue antiepileptic medications for four infants who have had seizures (presumably due to active encephalitis) in the perinatal period without recurrence of seizures. Before September 1991 (see Table 5–56), four children had developed new onset of seizures after the perinatal period. Hypsarrhythmia occurred in two children. One of these latter children responded dramatically and promptly to adrenocorticotropic hormone injections (pyrimethamine and sulfadiazine were administered concomitantly), and one responded to clonazepam treatment.

In many instances, a number of considerations may make it reasonable to withhold antiepileptic therapy after a short course of such medications. These considerations include the potential adverse interactions of each antiepileptic medication with the antimicrobial agents needed to treat *T. gondii* infection.[973] If antimicrobial therapy results in resolution of active encephalitis, which was the seizure focus, antiepileptic medications would

no longer be needed. In the U.S. (Chicago) National Collaborative Treatment Trial, the lack of recurrence of seizures when antiepileptic medications were discontinued[1067–1069] supports this approach.

The remarkable reduction in size or disappearance of calcifications, as well as the dramatic improvement in brain CT scans (see Figs. 5–10*C* to *F* and 5–14), occurred in association with antimicrobial therapy in this study.[489, 973, 1067]

Factors in the newborn period that were often associated with poorer prognosis included apnea and bradycardia, hypoxia, hypotension, delays in shunt placement and/or initiation of therapy, blindness, retinal detachment, CSF protein greater than 1 g/dl, diabetes insipidus in the perinatal period, hypsarrhythmia, and markedly diminished size of brain cortical mantle that did not increase after shunt placement.[1067] However, favorable outcomes have also been noted when some of these findings were present.[1067–1069]

Comparison of Outcomes. Comparison of outcomes with no treatment, 1 month of treatment, 1 year of pyrimethamine plus sulfonamides in alternate months with spiramycin, and 1 year of pyrimethamine plus sulfadiazine is shown in Table 5–52. Early treatment in the U.S. (Chicago) National Collaborative Treatment Trial appears to have resulted in more favorable outcome than was reported to occur for untreated infants or infants who were treated for only 1 month.

Treatment of Relapsing Chorioretinitis. The factors that lead to relapse of chorioretinitis are not known. It is of interest that this has been reported to occur most often during adolescence. An antimicrobial agent that eliminates encysted organisms in the eye is needed, because it is clear that treatment with presently available antimicrobial agents does not uniformly prevent or eliminate relapsing chorioretinitis.[489, 1070] Longer follow-up of large numbers of treated infants (especially those who

TABLE 5–55

Quantitative Visual Acuity in U.S. (Chicago) National Collaborative Treatment Trial in Patients with Macular Lesions (m) in at Least One Eye

GROUP	PATIENT NO.	RIGHT EYE	LEFT EYE
Treated[a]	7	20/20	20/20 (m)
	13	6/400 (m)	20/50 (m)[b]
	15	4/30 (m)	20/30 (m)
	19	20/200[c]	20/20 (m)
	21	1/30 (m)	1/30 (m)
	26	3/30 (m)	1/30 (m)
	28	20/30 (m)	15/30 (m)
	30	1/30 (m)	12/30[d]
	36	20/30	8/30 (m)
Historical[a]	20	20/400 (m)	20/25
	25	20/400 (m)	20/30
	27	5/30 (m)	1/30[e]
	31	20/25	3/200 (m)
	38	20/400 (m)	20/25[e]
	41	20/30	20/200 (m)
	42	20/70 (m)	20/30 (m)
	46	20/200 (m)	20/60 (m)
	47	3/30 (m)	3/30[e]
	82	20/400 (m)	20/15
	89	20/100 (m)	20/25

[a]Treated: n = 39 (30 too young or with cognitive limitations that made it not possible for the child to cooperate with quantitative vision). Historical: n = 13 (2 too young for quantitative vision).
[b]Rectangle indicates surprisingly good vision in spite of foveal lesion.
[c]Strabismus, microphthalmia, and amblyopia present.
[d]Poor cooperation, patient 4 years old.
[e]Peripheral lesion with dragging of the macula.
From Mets MB, et al. Eye manifestations of congenital toxoplasmosis. Am J Ophthalmol 122:309–324, 1996.

acquired their infection in the third trimester and have no retinal involvement at birth) is needed to determine whether treatment reduces this sequela. After treatment during the first year of life, because they are at risk for relapse, congenitally infected infants and young children should have ophthalmoscopy at 3- to 4-month intervals until they can reliably report visual symptoms. Studies are ongoing to determine whether continued frequent follow-up ophthalmologic evaluations and earlier treatment can prevent the devastating consequences of recurrent chorioretinitis. Careful evaluation, including retinal examination, should be performed whenever there are ocular symptoms that may be due to active chorioretinitis.

In infants and in the limited number of older children followed to date in the U.S. (Chicago) National Collaborative Treatment Trial, active chorioretinitis appeared to resolve within 1 to 2 weeks of beginning treatment with pyrimethamine and sulfonamides as described in Table 5–22. With recurrence of lesions after the first year of life, antimicrobial treatment has been continued 1 to 2 weeks beyond resolution of signs and symptoms. It is standard practice to administer prednisone (1 mg/kg daily in two divided doses) in conjunction with pyrimethamine and sulfonamides if there is inflammation threatening the macula, optic disk, or optic nerve. The efficacy of this practice is unknown. Some investigators have recommended clindamycin or tetracycline therapy.[1071] There are no convincing data that make it possible to determine whether inclusion of these medications would be beneficial.

Because transmission occurs frequently when acute infection is acquired in the later part of the third trimester, it is reasonable to treat the fetus by treating the recently infected mother with pyrimethamine and sulfadiazine. A diagnostic procedure for the fetus (see Prenatal Diagnosis of Fetal *Toxoplasma gondii* Infection section) should be performed before starting this therapy, because such treatment may obscure the diagnosis at birth. When this happens, it significantly complicates decision making concerning treatment of the infant during the first year of life if there is no accurate diagnostic information.

PREVENTION

Seronegative pregnant women and immunodeficient patients are two populations in which avoidance of infection by *T. gondii* is most important. We consider that the data on morbidity, incidence, and cost of congenital toxoplasmosis warrant a major attempt to define and initiate means whereby congenital toxoplasmosis can be prevented.[1072] Several methods for the prevention of congenital toxoplasmosis have been proposed. Attention to the specific hygienic measures outlined in Table 5–57 is the only method available for the *primary* prevention of congenital toxoplasmosis.[364] It is the responsibility of all physicians caring for pregnant women and women attempting to conceive (women at risk) to inform them of these preventive measures so that they will not place their fetus at risk. Lack of a systematic screening program in the United States leaves education as the principal means of preventing this tragic disease. The impact of these measures on the incidence of acquired toxoplasmosis in a given population has been discussed earlier in the section on Epidemiology. A substantial effort to educate women at risk and the physicians who care for them is clearly an important aspect of any program for prevention and should be undertaken.[1073–1075] A cost-benefit analysis of preventive measures for the United States is beyond the scope of this chapter. For a discussion of this matter, the reader is referred to the article by Roberts and Frenkel.[2]

In addition to primary preventive measures, it is necessary to identify those women who acquire the infection during pregnancy (so that treatment during gestation, or abortion, can be considered). A mechanism for identification of these women must also be a part of any program for prevention of congenital toxoplasmosis. Because approximately 90% of women infected during pregnancy have no clinical illness and because there are no pathognomonic clinical signs of the infection in the adult, diagnosis in the pregnant woman must be made by serologic methods. This makes prospective testing desirable.

Food

The tissue cyst can be rendered noninfective by heating meat thoroughly to 66° C (150° F) or by having it

TABLE 5–56
Comparison of Neurologic and Developmental Outcomes in the Chicago, Wilson et al, and Eichenwald Studies

OUTCOME	CHICAGO (1991) Subclinical (N = 3)	Generalized/ Neurologic (N = 34)	WILSON ET AL (1980) Subclinical I (N = 13)	Subclinical II (N = 11)	EICHENWALD (1959) Subclinical (N = 4)	Generalized (N = 31)	Neurologic (N = 70)
Seizures requiring therapy after first months	0 (0)[a]	4 (12)	1 (8)	3 (27)	2 (50)	24 (77)	58 (82)
Motor/tone permanent impairment	0 (0)	8 (24)	3 (23)	2 (18)	0 (0)	18 (58)	53 (76)
IQ < 70	0 (0)	8 (24)	2 (15)	2 (18)	2 (50)	25 (81)	62 (89)
Sequentially lower IQ score	0/2 (0)	3[b]/13 (0)	6/6 (100)	0/1 (0)	NA	NA	NA

[a]Number affected/number tested if different from N (%).
[b]Three children had a >15-point diminution and 2 children had a >15-point increase in IQ score. The differences over time for the entire group were not statistically significant (p > .05).
NA = not available.
Data from references 484, 552, 555, 987, 1067, and 1069.

smoked or cured. Curing may not eliminate the organism.[69] Freezing meat is a less reliable method of killing the cyst[69]; freezing meat at −20° C for 24 hours may be sufficient to destroy the tissue cyst,[38] but not all freezers available in the United States can maintain this temperature even when new. To minimize the chance of infection resulting from handling raw meat, the hands should be thoroughly washed with soap and water after contact with the meat, and the mucous membranes of the mouth

TABLE 5–57
Methods for Prevention of Congenital Toxoplasmosis

Prevention of Infection in Pregnant Women
Women should take these precautions:
1. Cook meat to well done, smoke it, or cure it in brine.
2. Avoid touching mucous membranes of mouth and eyes while handling raw meat. Wash hands thoroughly after handling raw meat.
3. Wash kitchen surfaces that come into contact with raw meat.
4. Wash fruits and vegetables before consumption.
5. Prevent access of flies, cockroaches, and so on to fruits and vegetables.
6. Avoid contact with materials that are potentially contaminated with cat feces (e.g., cat litter boxes) or wear gloves when handling such materials or when gardening.
7. Disinfect cat litter box for 5 minutes with nearly boiling water.

Prevention of Infection in Fetuses
1. Identify women at risk by serologic testing.
2. Treat during pregnancy, which results in an approximate 60% reduction in infected infants. Perform therapeutic abortion, which prevents birth of infected infant; used only for women who acquired infection in first or second trimester (<50% of cases).

Adapted from Wilson CB, Remington JS. What can be done to prevent congenital toxoplasmosis? Am J Obstet Gynecol 138:357–363, 1980, with permission.

and eyes should not be touched with potentially contaminated hands while meat is handled. Eggs should not be eaten raw. Vegetables and fruits should be washed before they are eaten.

Oocysts and Cats

To avoid infection by oocysts, several measures can be suggested. Cat feces may be disposed of daily by burning or flushing down the toilet, and the empty litter pan may be made free of viable oocysts by pouring nearly boiling water into it (an exposure time of 5 minutes is sufficient).[1076] Strong ammonia (7%) also kills oocysts, but contact for at least 3 hours is necessary. Drying, disposing as part of ordinary garbage, surface burial, freezing, or using chlorine bleach, dilute ammonia, quaternary ammonium compounds, or any general disinfectant cannot be relied on.[1077] Women who are seronegative during pregnancy and immunodeficient persons should avoid contact with cat feces altogether. When handling litter boxes or when working in sand or soil that may have been contaminated by cat feces, disposable gloves should be worn. Because sandboxes are often used by cats as litter boxes, covers should be placed over them when not in use and the hands should be washed after exposure to the sand. Flies, cockroaches, and probably other coprophagic animals serve as transport hosts for *T. gondii* and should be controlled and their access to food prevented.[19] Fruits and vegetables may have oocysts on their surfaces and should be washed before ingestion. Because the cat is the only animal known to produce the oocyst form, efforts should be directed toward preventing infection in cats. Feeding them dried, canned, or cooked food rather than allowing them to depend on hunting (e.g., for birds and mice) as their source of food reduces the likelihood of their becoming infected. Frozen raw meat should also be avoided, because freezing may not always eliminate *T. gondii*.[1077]

Although it has been recommended that pet cats

should be banished for the duration of pregnancy,[1078, 1079] this is hardly feasible under most circumstances. Repeated requests for serologic testing of cats are being received by veterinarians in the United States, and, in many instances, serologic test results are misinterpreted in respect to the danger of transmission. Patients are being misguided, unnecessary anxiety is being produced, and cats are being sacrificed without good reason. The fact is that cats with antibodies are safer pets than cats without antibodies because the presence of antibodies offers some degree of immunity to reinfection and thereby prevents or markedly decreases repetition of oocyst discharge.[19] Antibody determinations are not practical for the determination of infectivity of cats because the infectious oocysts are usually discharged before cats have developed antibodies[223, 237]; routine serologic testing for this purpose should be discouraged.

Veterinarians and their lay staff caring for cats are probably at increased risk, and special precautionary measures must be exercised to protect pregnant personnel. Large numbers of cats are handled annually by animal practitioners and their staffs, and as much as 1% of these cats may excrete oocysts. Feces from caged cats should be collected (preferably on a disposable tray or material) and discarded daily (preferably incinerated) before sporulation occurs. Care must be taken when handling feces for worm counts and similar procedures; samples should be examined within 24 hours of collection, and care must be exercised to avoid contamination of hands, centrifuges, benches, and microscopes. Gloves should be worn at all times by those handling cat feces.[1078, 1080]

Serologic Screening

The cost effectiveness of screening women during pregnancy depends on a variety of factors, including the cost of tests and how frequently they are employed compared with the cost to society of caring for the diseased children who would be born in the absence of screening.[1, 313, 317, 374, 1081–1084] Wilson and Remington[1] and McCabe and Remington[1075] have proposed that a screening program should be considered in the United States. This would include the performance of a serologic test equal in sensitivity, specificity, and reproducibility to the Sabin-Feldman dye test in all pregnant women. It is crucial that initial testing be performed as early as possible, but at least by 10 to 12 weeks' gestation. (Ideally, testing of all women just before pregnancy would identify those at risk.)

Presentation and discussion of the pros and cons of a systematic screening program for the United States is beyond the scope of this chapter. Each of the authors is in favor of a screening program for the United States similar to that being used at present in France (see Fig. 5–30). However, we recognize that constraints of present-day health care systems may not permit such screening on a monthly basis or, in some instances, screening of pregnant women per se. Cost-benefit analyses are especially relevant to mandated, state-supported screening programs. However, it seems to us that almost all parents, given the choice, would select a simple, not very costly, and direct measure that could prevent cognitive and ocular damage to their child as part of their health care coverage.

Introduction of prenatal screening and, in particular, use of PCR testing on amniotic fluid at 18 weeks of gestation has altered the approach to screening of women who are not tested on a monthly basis as is done in France. Wilson and Remington[1] and others previously suggested that such women be screened for seroconversion with the first serum being obtained as early as possible in the first trimester and again in the second and third trimesters. This would allow for detection of those women whose fetuses are at greatest risk of being infected and would allow for appropriate management decisions to be made in regard to the newborn. With the introduction of treatment of the fetus through administration of specific therapy to the pregnant woman, it has become even more important to establish the diagnosis in the fetus at the earliest possible time; PCR on amniotic fluid provides for this. Therefore, women must be informed of the importance of their being seen by a physician as early as possible in pregnancy so as to allow for early serologic testing. The second serum sample should be drawn at a time in the second trimester such that, if it reveals recently acquired infection, it will allow for PCR on the amniotic fluid at 17 to 18 weeks' gestation. If that second serum does not reveal recently acquired infection, a third serum sample can be drawn in the early third trimester. If seroconversion is observed at that time, we recommend PCR on amniotic fluid; if the PCR reveals infection in the fetus, the mother should receive pyrimethamine-sulfadiazine in an attempt to treat the fetus. A final serum sample is obtained at the time of parturition to detect those mothers who acquired their infection very late in gestation but whose fetuses are at greatest risk of infection. Luyasu and associates[1085] reported seven cases of subclinical congenital *T. gondii* infection born of mothers who acquired their infection between 2 and 4 weeks before delivery. They emphasized that because children born to mothers who become infected close to term are at greatest risk of the congenital infection and must be treated to attempt to prevent untoward sequelae of the infection, it is important to screen seronegative pregnant women until the time of delivery.

A woman whose serum is positive on initial testing would ideally have a test for IgM antibodies and an avidity test performed on the same serum. If the avidity test results reveal chronic infection in the first trimester (e.g., high avidity antibody), acute infection during the first trimester is essentially excluded. For further decisions regarding patient management and desirability of confirmatory testing if the IgM test is positive and the avidity test result is low or equivocal, the reader is referred to the discussion in the section on Diagnosis. In patients with a positive IgG test titer and a negative test for IgM antibodies in the first trimester and no clinical signs of acute toxoplasmosis, no further testing would be performed, because in the United States the probability of these women being acutely infected is low (probably < 0.2%).

Some of the possible negative effects of reducing the

frequency of screening as described earlier, as contrasted to the approach in France of screening every month, are as follows: Screening early in and throughout pregnancy provides the opportunity to reduce transmission to the fetus.[132, 1018, 1086] The data of Mirlessi and colleagues (see Table 5–43)[1061] indicate that a shorter time interval between diagnosis and treatment yields a better outcome for the newborn and that eye and neurologic involvement are directly correlated. The data of Brézin and associates indicate that there is less, and also less severe, later retinal disease for the patients treated according to the method used by the group in Paris.[1087] Furthermore, in the third trimester, transmission rates are high and 40% of infants detected in neonatal screening programs (most infected late in gestation) already have evidence of retinal or CNS involvement or both.[128, 562, 946, 1088, 1089] Prompt detection of infection permits prompt treatment of infection that can cause irreversible destruction of ocular and CNS tissue in utero. Postnatal treatment leads to rapid resolution of signs of active infection.[489] Early outcomes for such treated children are considerably better than those for children who were untreated or treated for only 1 month.[455, 489, 1067] Nonetheless, retinal scars and neurologic damage in utero may be irreversible.[455, 1090] Although postnatal treatment improves outcome, some treated children do not have significant improvement; and even for those that function normally, the in utero infection is not without late consequences because cognitive outcomes for treated children are in some instances less favorable than for their uninfected siblings.[1067]

Whereas the data from France that describe better outcomes were derived from an algorithm of screening pregnant women each month,[132] it should be noted that there are no outcomes data for a method with less frequent screening described earlier. Based on the data of Mirlesse and associates,[1061] it is likely that delays in treatment will lead to worse outcomes (see Table 5–43).

In late 1998 we examined the trimester of gestation of 211 consecutive women whose sera were submitted for testing to the Palo Alto laboratory: 36% of the samples were drawn in the first, 46% in the second, and 17% in the third trimester. Despite the fact that some of these sera were submitted for confirmatory testing, more than 60% were received too late in pregnancy to allow for evaluation of an avidity test result (for discussion of avidity testing, see the section on Diagnosis). This experience again emphasizes the need for an organized systematic screening program. For recent discussions of the aspects (pros and cons) of systematic serologic screening the reader is referred to references 1084, and 1091 through 1093.

At present in the United States, T. gondii serology is performed haphazardly by laboratories of varying quality for physicians who may understand little of the disease or the tests; and, unfortunately, in many cases inappropriate decisions are made on the basis of unreliable information.[863, 864] For these reasons, our present lack of systematic screening—in a setting of sporadic screening that is inadequately supervised—may result in more harm than good. We and the U.S. Food and Drug Administration recommend that any serologic test re-sults that suggest that infection was acquired during pregnancy be confirmed and interpreted by a reference laboratory before decisions regarding treatment, prenatal diagnosis, or therapeutic abortion are made.[863, 916] In late 1998, the Centers for Disease Control and Prevention (CDC) in Atlanta, Georgia, convened a committee of international experts to consider a number of topics in regard to T. gondii, primarily transmission and prevention of the infection. The major focus was on prevention of the congenital infection and infection in the pregnant woman. In early 1999, a working group was appointed to help evaluate whether a serologic screening program in pregnant women, newborns, or both is justified in the United States and, if so, how this might best be accomplished.

Treatment of the Pregnant Woman

For the special instance of the pregnant woman with HIV infection, see the Congenital *Toxoplasma gondii* Infection and Acquired Immunodeficiency Syndrome section.

ACUTE INFECTION

Antimicrobial Therapy

Treatment during pregnancy has been employed in an attempt to decrease both the incidence and the severity of congenital infection. This treatment is administered to a pregnant woman with a recently acquired (acute) infection in the hope that such treatment will prevent spread of infection to the fetus. The rationale for such treatment is based on the observation that there is a significant lag period between the onset of maternal infection and infection of the fetus. In the first such study, performed in Germany, Kräubig used a combination of sulfonamides and pyrimethamine.[125, 1094] Because of its potential teratogenic effects, pyrimethamine was not administered during the first 12 to 14 weeks of gestation. Kräubig noted a definite reduction in incidence of congenitally infected infants born to treated (5%) versus untreated (16.6%) mothers—a 70% reduction (prevention). Kräubig considered these data an indication that treatment is necessary if a diagnosis of acute acquired toxoplasmosis is made during pregnancy. Thalhammer, who closely collaborated in these studies with Kräubig, agreed with this statement because it appears that all congenital toxoplasmosis might be prevented by such an approach.[1095, 1096] In 1982, Hengst from Berlin reported similar results in a prospective study.[1097]

In a separate and independent study performed in France, daily oral doses of 2 to 3 g of spiramycin in four divided doses were administered for 3 weeks to women who acquired toxoplasmosis during pregnancy. Such courses of treatment were arbitrarily repeated at 2-week intervals up to the time of delivery. Only women who completed at least one such course were considered to be treated. Cases of congenital T. gondii infection were significantly more frequent among 154 untreated women (58%) than among 388 treated women (23%). Clinically apparent disease in the newborns, however, was just as frequent among children born with congenital *T. gondii* infection from both groups of women (28 and 27% of infected offspring).[120] This suggests that spiramycin treatment of the pregnant woman might have reduced by 60% the frequency of transmission of *T. gondii* to the offspring but did not apparently modify the pattern of infection in the infected fetus. However, although the difference between treated and untreated groups is highly significant, the untreated pregnant women in this study do not represent a good control group for several reasons. Most women diagnosed in their first trimester were treated, whereas the proportion of untreated women is rather low among women who acquired *T. gondii* infection during the last months of pregnancy. Thus, more infections occurred earlier among the treated than among the untreated women, a fact that of itself might have led to fewer congenital infections and to a higher proportion of clinical disease among infected infants, if untreated. Nevertheless, congenital infections were less frequent among the treated group in each trimester of pregnancy. Consequently, one could assume that the decrease in fetal infections reflects not only bias in the selection of cases but treatment as well.

Variability in the clinical aspects of congenital infection also must be considered. Table 5–58 shows the comparison between treated and untreated pregnant women. There was no difference in the proportion of mild and subclinical cases. In contrast, the number of stillbirths decreased and the proportion of children born alive with severe disease increased slightly in the treated group. The numbers are too small to be significant, but the reason that such results could occur because of treatment during fetal life is that treatment, although undertaken too late to prevent severe damage, might sometimes have prevented fetal death.

A prospective study that compares the efficacy of spiramycin versus pyrimethamine plus sulfonamide for prevention of congenital transmission has not been performed. There are, however, data that, when compared with recently obtained but historical controls, suggest the importance of the pyrimethamine plus sulfonamide regimen. Each of the studies involved an attempt to isolate the organism from placentas. In one such study of 32 women, each of whose fetuses was diagnosed as being infected by isolation of the parasite from amniotic fluid or blood between weeks 24 and 30 of gestation (update of data presented in reference 121), infection in the mothers was documented to have occurred between the tenth and twenty-ninth weeks of gestation. The mothers were treated with 3 g of spiramycin daily as soon as the diagnosis of their acute acquired infection was made. Pyrimethamine plus sulfonamide was given during the last 2 months of gestation. Because of the potential hazard for mother or fetus, use of the combination of pyrimethamine plus sulfonamide is restricted by Couvreur and colleagues to the last 2 months of gestation and to a high-risk group in which fetal infection has been documented during pregnancy. *T. gondii* was isolated from 47% of the placentas (examined after delivery) from these 32 cases. In marked contrast, *T. gondii* was isolated from 71.5% of placentas of 21 infants born to mothers treated with spiramycin alone and, using historical controls, from 89% of placentas of 85 infants born to mothers who were insufficiently treated with spiramycin (treatment for less than 2 weeks or with a dose of 2 g daily, which is considered by the investigators to be too low) or who were not treated. In Austria, Aspöck and colleagues routinely use spiramycin before the sixteenth week of gestation and pyrimethamine plus sulfonamide after the fifteenth week of gestation. In their prospective study, this treatment regimen was highly successful.[290]

Although critical appraisal of these studies does not permit a definite conclusion about the efficacy of treatment during pregnancy in the prevention of congenital toxoplasmosis, the data strongly suggest that treatment is effective. In addition, because spiramycin may also delay transmission of the parasite to the fetus, it should have the added benefit of reducing the severity of the disease in the fetus and newborn due to the increased maturity of the maternal immune response and of the fetus at the time infection occurs. Critically designed studies are needed to clarify this question. However, until such data become available—and noting the prevention rate of congenital infection of 60 to 70% achieved in the two studies quoted earlier—it would appear prudent to advise treatment in women who acquire the infection during pregnancy. *The optimal dose of spiramycin is 3 g per day.* Toxicity has not proved to be a problem with spiramycin in such cases. This drug is at present available in the United States only by request to the U.S. Food and Drug Administration. It is hoped that it will be made more widely available in the near future. Pyrimethamine plus sulfadiazine can be employed in the second and third trimester of pregnancy with the precautionary measures mentioned earlier in the Therapy section (see also Treatment of the Fetus In Utero section). Whether sequelae in prenatally treated

TABLE 5–58

Effect of Spiramycin Treatment on Relative Frequency of Stillbirth and on Different Aspects of Congenital Toxoplasmosis

	NO. (%) OF OFFSPRING WITH OUTCOME FOR	
OUTCOME IN OFFSPRING	Mothers Not Treated During Pregnancy	Mothers Treated During Pregnancy
Congenital toxoplasmosis		
Subclinical	64 (68)	65 (72)
Mild	14 (15)	13 (14)
Severe	7 (7)	10 (11)
Stillbirth or perinatal death[a]	9 (10)	3 (3)
Total	94 (100)	91 (100)

[a]See text.

Adapted from Desmonts G, Couvreur J. Congenital toxoplasmosis: a prospective study of the offspring of 542 women who acquired toxoplasmosis during pregnancy: pathophysiology of congenital disease. *In* Thalhammer O, Baumgarten K, Pollak A (eds). Perinatal Medicine, Sixth European Congress, Vienna. Stuttgart, Georg Thieme, 1979, pp 51–60, with permission.

but infected children are as frequent or as serious as those in untreated children is a question that can be answered only by long-term observation.

Termination of Pregnancy

The decision whether to treat with antimicrobial agents or to perform an abortion in a woman suspected of acquiring *T. gondii* infection during pregnancy should ultimately be made by the patient in conjunction with her physician after careful consideration of the potential results of both modalities of intervention. Therapeutic abortion may be considered in women who are known to have acquired acute *T. gondii* infection early during gestation or in whom the likelihood of their having acquired acute infection early during gestation is very high. Only approximately 22% of women who acquire primary *T. gondii* infection during the first 22 to 24 weeks of gestation transmit the infection to their offspring. Even if all women who acquire the infection during the first two trimesters were to elect abortion, less than one half of all cases of congenital toxoplasmosis would be prevented because more than 50% of infected offspring result from maternal infection acquired in the last trimester. Prenatal examination has for the first time allowed for an objective decision by the pregnant woman in regard to abortion and whether her aborted fetus would indeed be congenitally infected. Such a decision was previously based on a statistical estimation of the risk to the fetus. Since the last edition of this book, considerable controversy has arisen in regard to whether and under what circumstances abortion might be considered. The controversy appears to have stemmed from the publication by Berrebi and associates in *The Lancet* in 1994,[941] who conclude that only ultrasonographic evidence of hydrocephalus indicates a poor outcome and for this reason they no longer use the gestational age-related statistics that Daffos and colleagues propose[130] to counsel affected couples.[948] Berrebi and associates studied 163 mothers who acquired infection with *T. gondii* before 28 weeks of gestation. All were treated with spiramycin and 23 also received pyrimethamine and sulfadiazine. Each had cordocentesis and regular ultrasound examinations. Their 162 live-born infants were followed for 15 to 71 months. Three fetuses died in utero, and 27 of 162 live-born infants had congenital toxoplasmosis: 10 had clinical signs of the infection, 5 with isolated or multiple intracranial calcifications, 7 with peripheral chorioretinitis, and 2 with moderate ventricular dilation. Because each of the 27 was free of symptoms and had normal neurologic development at 15 to 71 months of age the investigators concluded that acute fetal infection identified in first- and second-trimester pregnancies need not be an indication for interruption of the pregnancy if fetal ultrasonographic evaluation results are normal (no evidence of fetal death or hydrocephalus) and treatment of the fetus is instigated.

In a letter to the editor of *The Lancet* commenting on the results of Berrebi and associates, Wallon and co-workers[1060] were also conservative in their conclusions. From the results of their studies, they recommend that termination should not be performed unless fetal ultra-sonographic examination reveals morphologic abnormalities. In contrast, in a simultaneously published letter to the editor of *The Lancet*, Daffos and colleagues[1098] concurred that too many pregnancies are terminated because congenital toxoplasmosis is diagnosed prenatally but were far less optimistic than Berrebi and associates about the outcome for the fetus infected early in gestation. Daffos and colleagues stated that in a study of 148 fetal infections diagnosed by prenatal examination, "the best (and perhaps the only) factor with predictive value for the severity of the fetal infection is gestational age at the time of maternal infection." In their study, they noted that if the infection occurred before 16 weeks of gestation, 31 (60%) of 52 fetuses had ultrasonographic evidence of infection, including ascites, pericarditis, or necrotic foci in their brains, and 48% had cerebral ventricular dilation. If infection had occurred between 17 and 23 weeks, 16 (25%) of 63 fetuses had ultrasonographic signs and only 12% had ventricular dilation. In those cases of infection after 24 weeks, only 1 (.03%) of 33 fetuses had ultrasonographic signs and none had hydrocephalus. Thus, the approach that Daffos and his colleagues had recommended 6 years earlier[130] appeared to still be valid. These workers accept parental requests for termination in those cases in which infection occurs before 16 weeks because of the severe prognosis in such fetuses. In such instances, they have always found large areas of brain necrosis at necropsy even when there was no evidence of ventricular dilation on ultrasound evaluation. They conclude that such dilation of the ventricles would have developed in many of these cases if the pregnancies had been allowed to continue even if treatment with pyrimethamine and sulfadiazine was used. It is hoped that in the near future this issue will be resolved by a collaborative effort to review all pertinent data by interested investigators and, if necessary, to design studies, the results of which will lead to a consensus and guidelines for providing the patient with objective information during counseling about termination of pregnancy.

Despite the fact that IgM tests do not differentiate between the acute and chronic infection accurately, their results strongly influence pregnant women as to whether they choose to terminate their pregnancy. In the United States such decisions are often made on the basis of results of *T. gondii* serology on a single serum specimen in which the IgM antibody test is positive and confirmatory testing is not done. We previously estimated that approximately 20% of women who are told that they have a positive IgM antibody test will request therapeutic abortion.[1099] In that study, approximately 60% of the IgM tests reported as positive by commercial laboratories were negative in the IgM test in the Palo Alto reference laboratory. They were also negative for evidence of recently acquired infection as determined by results in the *T. gondii* serologic profile. Thus, at a minimum, 12 of every 20 fetuses who were not infected were aborted. In a more recent study, Liesenfeld and associates[1099] from the same laboratory determined the accuracy of *T. gondii* serologic test results obtained in commercial laboratories and the role of confirmatory testing in preventing unnecessary abortion. These investigators demonstrated clearly that confirmatory testing, along with a discussion of the results with the patient's physician by an expert on toxoplasmosis in pregnancy, can remarkably (> 50%) and significantly decrease the number of abortions in women with positive IgM *T. gondii* antibody test results.

Every physician who recommends or performs an abortion must be knowledgeable about the subject so that an intelligent decision can be made. Because abortions are performed as late as 22 to 24 weeks' gestation in the United States, one has time to obtain an initial serologic specimen early in gestation and a follow-up specimen later in gestation to define those women at risk of transmitting *T. gondii* to their offspring (see Serologic Screening section). Guidelines for the interpretation of serologic tests obtained during pregnancy have been given previously in the Diagnosis section. If tests for IgM antibodies to *T. gondii* are unavailable to assist in establishing the diagnosis of acute infection, it should be understood that the risk of congenital toxoplasmosis is almost zero in a patient whose serum shows a high titer in the dye test or IFA test in the second month of pregnancy. A high titer at that time indicates an infection that occurred at least 2 months before (and perhaps much earlier) in all but rare exceptions in which the serologic test titer rises steeply for several weeks. On the contrary, women who will later deliver a congenitally infected infant, when examined during the second or third month of pregnancy, either have no antibody (not yet infected) or may have a low titer (associated with IgM antibody) as a result of an infection acquired during the past few days or weeks. A careful follow-up examination and confirmatory testing in a reference laboratory along with amniocentesis for PCR and mouse inoculation may reveal infection in the fetus in time to allow for consideration of termination of the pregnancy in these cases. Treatment of the infected mother to attempt to prevent transmission of the infection to the fetus appears more worthy of consideration in such circumstances.

CHRONIC (LATENT) INFECTION

The controversial subjects of congenital transmission, repeated abortion, and perinatal fetal mortality during chronic (latent) infection have already been discussed. In an attempt to prevent infection and reduce fetal wastage, a series of women who had had previous abortions, premature births, or similar misfortunes were treated with pyrimethamine by Cech and Jírovec of Prague.[678] A marked reduction in perinatal fetal mortality rate was observed in these treated women. The investigators interpreted their results as showing a remarkable effect of pyrimethamine on the outcome of pregnancy in the skin test–positive women. Their results appear to be very favorable, but, because the study was uncontrolled, these results must be interpreted with caution. Studies along the same line are those of Eckerling and associates in Israel[1100] and others.[167, 1101, 1102] Results reported by Sharf and co-workers in Israel[1103] suggested an etiologic relationship between latent maternal toxoplasmosis and spontaneous abortions, premature deliveries, and stillbirths. A number of such women were treated with pyrimethamine and triple sulfonamides before their next pregnancy and with sulfonamides alone during pregnancy. The researchers interpreted their results as evidence that such treatment significantly increased the chance of a successful outcome of the pregnancy. Unfortunately, their controls were poorly defined and appear inadequate for statistical analysis.

Kimball and colleagues stated that, despite the association of antibodies to *T. gondii* with sporadic abortion noted by them, there is no evidence that therapy to prevent abortion should be administered routinely to pregnant women with antibodies to *T. gondii*—even those with high titers.[159] In their series, there was a significantly greater incidence of abortions in patients with CF test titers of 1:8 or higher than in those with titers 1:4 or lower ($p < 0.01$). But they believed it unwarranted to recommend therapy to a group of pregnant women of whom only 10% could be expected to abort without therapy. Whether therapy for toxoplasmosis in patients with CF test titers of 1:8 or higher who are threatening to abort would be beneficial is unknown.

The question must now be raised whether there is sufficient evidence to warrant the routine prophylactic use of a drug with toxic and teratogenic potential against *T. gondii* in pregnant women who have positive serologic titers and a history of chronic abortion. Until the controversy is resolved by further evidence justifying

TABLE 5–59
Some Pertinent Resources and Phone Numbers/Internet Sites

Reference laboratory for serology, isolation, and PCR (U.S.)	650-853-4828
Reference laboratory for serology, isolation, and PCR (France)	33-1-40-44-39-41
FDA for IND number to obtain spiramycin for treatment of a pregnant woman (U.S.)	301-827-2335
FDA Public Health Advisory	301-594-3060
Spiramycin (Rhone Poulenc) for treatment of a pregnant woman (U.S.)	610-454-8469
Congenital Toxoplasmosis Study Group (U.S.)	773-834-4152
Education Pamphlet/The March of Dimes (U.S.)	312-435-4007 or
Educational pamphlet: "Congenital Toxoplasmosis: The Hidden Threat"	1-800-323-9100
Educational pamphlet: "Toxoplasmosis," NIH publication No. 83-308	301-496-5717
	www.niaid.nih.gov
Information concerning AIDS and congenital toxoplasmosis (U.S.)	305-243-6522
Information for European families: The Toxoplasmosis Trust (U.K.)	44-171-713-0663
Educational information on the Internet	http://www.lit.edu/≈toxo/pamphlet

the risk of therapy, the only conclusion that can be made is that pyrimethamine must not be used in such cases.[158, 1104] There are continued reports of use of such treatment.[1105]

RESOURCES

A summary of useful resources and means to contact them is presented in Table 5–59.

ACKNOWLEDGMENTS

We are sincerely grateful to Drs. Jacques Couvreur, Fernand Daffos, J. P. Dubey, José Montoya, and Oliver Liesenfeld for their advice and help in the preparation of this chapter.

We thank Drs. V. Mirlesse and F. Daffos for providing their soon-to-be published data for inclusion in this chapter. We appreciate Trisha Mitchell's tireless and enthusiastic administrative help in preparation of this chapter and also the assistance of Vicki Aitchison and Ellen Holfels.

This work was supported by grants AI 04717, AI 302230, AI 27530, and AI 16945 from the National Institutes of Health.

References

1. Wilson CB, Remington JS. What can be done to prevent congenital toxoplasmosis? Am J Obstet Gynecol 138:357–363, 1980.
2. Roberts T, Frenkel JK. Estimating income losses and other preventable costs caused by congenital toxoplasmosis in people in the United States. J Am Vet Med Assoc 196:249–256, 1990.
3. Nicolle C, Manceaux L. Sur une infection à corps de Leishman (ou organismes voisins) du gondi. C R Hebdomadaire Séances Acad Sci 146:207–209, 1908.
4. Nicolle C, Manceaux L. Sur un protozoaire nouveau de Gondi, *Toxoplasma*. Arch Inst Pasteur (Tunis) 2:97–103, 1909.
5. Splendore A. A new protozoan parasite in rabbits. *In* Kean BH, Mott KKE, Russell AJ (eds). Tropical Medicine and Parasitology: Classical Investigations. Ithaca, NY, Cornell University Press, 1908, pp 272–274.
6. Janku, J. Pathogenesa a pathologicka anatomie tak nazvaneho vrozeneho kolobomu zlute skvrny v oku normalne velikem a mikrophthalmickem s nalezem parazitu v sitnici. Cas Lek Ces 62:1021–1027, 1054–1059, 1081–1085, 1111–1115, 1138–1144, 1923.
7. Levaditi C. Au sujet de certaines protozooses héréditaires humaines à localization oculaires et nerveuses. C R Soc Biol (Paris) 98:297–299, 1928.
8. Wolf A, Cowen D. Granulomatous encephalomyelitis due to an encephalitozoon (encephalitozoic encephalomyelitis): a new protozoan disease of man. Bull Neurol Inst NY 6:306–371, 1937.
9. Sabin AB, Olitsky PK. *Toxoplasma* and obligate intracellular parasitism. Science 85:336–338, 1937.
10. Wolf A, Cowen D. Granulomatous encephalomyelitis due to a protozoan (*Toxoplasma* or Encephalitozoon): II. Identification of a case from the literature. Bull Neurol Inst NY 7:266–283, 1938.
11. Wolf A, Cowen D, Paige BH. Toxoplasmic encephalomyelitis: III. A new case of granulomatous encephalomyelitis due to a protozoon. Am J Pathol 15:657–694, 1939.
12. Paige BH, Cowen D, Wolf A. Toxoplasmic encephalomyelitis: V. Further observations of infantile toxoplasmosis: intrauterine inception of the disease; visceral manifestations. Am J Dis Child 63:474–514, 1942.
13. Wolf A, Cowen D. Human toxoplasmosis: occurrence in infants as an encephalomyelitis verification by transmission to animals. *In* Kean BH, Mott KKE, Russell AJ (eds). Tropical Medicine and Parasitology: Classical Investigations. Ithaca, NY, Cornell University Press, 1939, pp 282–284.
14. Wolf A. Cowen C, Paige BH. Toxoplasmic encephalomyelitis. Trans Am Neurol Assoc 65:76–79, 1939.
15. Pinkerton H, Weinman D. *Toxoplasma* infection in man. Acta Pathol 30:374–392, 1940.
16. Pinkerton H, Henderson RG. Adult toxoplasmosis. JAMA 116:807–814, 1941.
17. Sabin AB. Toxoplasmic encephalitis in children. JAMA 116:801–807, 1941.
18. Sabin AB, Feldman HA. Dyes as microchemical indicators of a new immunity phenomenon affecting a protozoan parasite (*Toxoplasma*). Science 108:660–663, 1948.
19. Frenkel JK. Toxoplasmosis: parasite life cycle pathology and immunology. *In* Hammond DM, Long PL (eds): The Coccidia. Baltimore, University Park Press, 1973, pp 343–410.
20. Levine N. Sarcocystis, *Toxoplasma*, and related protozoa. *In* Protozoan Parasites of Domestic Animals and of Man, 2nd ed. Minneapolis, Burgess, 1973, pp 288–316.
21. Beaman M, Remington J. Cytokines and resistance against *Toxoplasma gondii*: evidence from in vivo and in vitro studies. *In* Sonnenfeld G, et al (eds). Cytokines and Resistance to Nonviral Pathogenic Infections. New York, Biomedical Press, 1992, pp 111–119.
22. McLeod R, Mack D, Brown C. *Toxoplasma gondii*—new advances in cellular and molecular biology. Exp Parasitol 72:109–121, 1991.
23. Wong SY, Remington JS. Biology of *Toxoplasma gondii*. *In* Broder S, Merigan TC, Bolognesi D (eds). Textbook of AIDS Medicine. Baltimore, Williams & Wilkins, 1994, pp 223–258.
24. Cesbron M-F, Dubremetz J-F, Sher A. The immunobiology of toxoplasmosis. Res Immunol 144:7–8, 1993.
25. Dubey JP, Lindsay DS, Speer CA. Structures of *Toxoplasma gondii* tachyzoites, bradyzoites, and sporozoites and biology and development of tissue cysts. Clin Microbiol Rev 11:267–299, 1998.
26. Mercier C, Cesbron-Delauw MF, Sibley LD. The amphipathic alpha helices of the *Toxoplasma* protein GRA2 mediate post-secretory membrane association. J Cell Sci 111:2171–2180, 1998.
27. Sibley LD, Howe DK. Genetic basis of pathogenicity in toxoplasmosis. *In* Gross U (ed). Current Topics in Microbiology and Immunity: *Toxoplasma gondii*. New York, Springer, 1996, pp 3–15.
28. Hunter CA, Subauste CS, Remington JS. The role of cytokines in toxoplasmosis. Biotherapy 7:237–247, 1994.
29. Alexander J, Hunter CA. Immunoregulation during toxoplasmosis. Chem Immunol 70:81–102, 1998.
30. Denkers EY, Gazzinelli RT. Regulation and function of T-cell–mediated immunity during *Toxoplasma gondii* infection. Clin Microbiol Rev 11:569–588, 1998.
31. Dubey JP, Frenkel JK. Feline toxoplasmosis from acutely infected mice and the development of *Toxoplasma* cysts. J Protozool 23:537–546, 1976.

32. Freyre A, et al. Oocyst-induced *Toxoplasma gondii* infections in cats. J Parasitol 75:750–755, 1989.

33. Dubey JP, Miller NL, Frenkel JK. Characterization of the new fecal form of *Toxoplasma gondii*. J Parasitol 56:447–456, 1970.

34. Dubey JP, Miller NL, Frenkel JK. The *Toxoplasma gondii* oocyst from cat feces. J Exp Med 132:636–662, 1970.

35. Frenkel JK, Dubey JP, Miller NL. *Toxoplasma gondii* in cats: fecal stages identified as coccidian oocysts. Science 167:893–896, 1970.

36. Manwell RD, Drobeck HP. The behavior of *Toxoplasma* with notes on its taxonomic status. J Parasitol 39:577–584, 1953.

37. Sibley LD, Hakansson S, Carruthers VB. Gliding motility: an efficient mechanism for cell penetration. Curr Biol 8:R12–R14, 1998.

38. Jacobs L, Remington JS, Melton ML. The resistance of the encysted form of *Toxoplasma gondii*. J Parasitol 46:11–21, 1960.

39. Jacobs L. The biology of *Toxoplasma*. Am J Trop Med Hyg 2:365–389, 1953.

40. Cook MK, Jacobs L. Cultivation of *Toxoplasma gondii* in tissue cultures of various derivations. J Parasitol 44:172–182, 1958.

41. Kaufman HE, et al. Strain differences of *Toxoplasma gondii*. J Parasitol 45:189–190, 1959.

42. Norrby R, Lycke E. Factors enhancing the host-cell penetration of *Toxoplasma gondii*. J Bacteriol 93:53–58, 1967.

43. Lycke E, Norrby R, Remington JS. Penetration-enhancing factor extracted from *Toxoplasma gondii* which increases its virulence for mice. J Bacteriol 96:785–788, 1968.

44. Lycke E, Carlberg K, Norrby R. Interactions between *Toxoplasma gondii* and its host cells: function of the penetration-enhancing factor of *Toxoplasma*. Infect Immun 11:853–861, 1975.

45. Conseil V, Soete M, Dubremetz JF. Serine protease inhibitors block invasion of host cells by *Toxoplasma gondii*. Antimicrob Agents Chemother 43:1358–1361, 1999.

46. Jones TC, Hirsch JG. The interaction between *Toxoplasma gondii* and mammalian cells: II. The absence of lysosomal fusion with phagocytic vacuoles containing living parasites. J Exp Med 136:1173–1194, 1972.

47. Klainer AS, Krahenbuhl JL, Remington JS. Scanning electron microscopy of *Toxoplasma gondii*. J Gen Microbiol 75:111–118, 1973.

48. Zaman V, Colley FC. Ultrastructural study of penetration of macrophages by *Toxoplasma gondii*. Trans R Soc Trop Med Hyg 66:781–784, 1972.

49. Nguyen BT, Stadtsbaeder S. [Modes of entry of *Toxoplasma gondii* trophozoites into normal mouse peritoneal macrophage and HeLa cell monolayers: a phase-contrast microcinematographic study.] Z Parasitenkd (in French) 60:135–146, 1979.

50. Gustafson PV, Agar HD, Cramer DI. An electron microscope study of *Toxoplasma*. Am J Trop Med Hyg 3:1008–1021, 1954.

51. Sibley LD, et al. *Toxoplasma* modifies macrophage phagosomes by secretion of a vesicular network rich in surface proteins. J Cell Biol 103:867–874, 1986.

52. Sibley LD, Weidner E, Krahenbuhl JL. Characterization of membrane vesicles secreted by intracellular *Toxoplasma gondii*. Thirty-fourth Annual Meeting of the American Society of Tropical Medicine and Hygiene, Miami, 1985.

53. Goldman M, Carver RK, Sulzer AJ. Similar internal morphology of *Toxoplasma gondii* and *Besnoitia jellisoni* stained with silver protein. J Parasitol 43:490–491, 1957.

54. Bommer W, Hofling KH, Heunert HH. Multiplication of *Toxoplasma gondii* in cell cultures. Dtsch Med Wochenschr 94:1–14, 1969.

55. Lund E. Lycke E, Sourander P. A cinematographic study of *Toxoplasma gondii* in cell cultures. Br J Exp Pathol 42:357–362, 1961.

56. Hirai K, Hirato K, Yanagwa R. A cinematographic study of the penetration of cultured cells by *Toxoplasma gondii*. Jpn J Vet Res 14:83–90, 1996.

57. Jones TC, Yeh S, Hirsch JG. The interaction between *Toxoplasma gondii* and mammalian cells: I. Mechanism of entry and intracellular fate of the parasite. J Exp Med 136:1157–1172, 1972.

58. Roberts F, et al. Evidence for the shikimate pathway in apicomplexan parasites. Nature 393:801–805, 1998.

59. Kohler S, et al. A plastid of probable green algal origin in apicomplexan parasites. Science 275:1485–1489, 1997.

60. Fichera ME, Roos DS. A plastid organelle as a drug target in apicomplexan parasites. Nature 290:407–409, 1997.

61. Wilson RJ, et al. Complete gene map of the plastid-like DNA of the malaria parasite *Plasmodium falciparum*. J Mol Biol 261:155–172, 1996.

62. Remington JS, in discussion, Laison R. Observations on the nature and transmission of *Toxoplasma* in the light of its wide host and geographical range. Surv Ophthalmol 6:721–758, 1961.

63. Van der Zypen E, Piekarski G. Licht- und elektgronen-mikroskopische Betgrachtungen über absterbende Toxoplasmen unter natürlichen Lebensbedingungen. Zentralbl Bakteriol 203:232–245, 1967.

64. Speer CA, Clark S, Dubey JP. Ultrastructure of the oocysts, sporocysts, and sporozoites of *Toxoplasma gondii*. J Parasitol 84:505–512, 1998.

65. Lainson R. Observations on the development and nature of pseudocysts and cysts of *Toxoplasma gondii*. Trans R Soc Trop Med Hyg 52:396–407, 1958.

66. Remington JS, Cavanaugh EN. Isolation of the encysted form of *Toxoplasma gondii* from human skeletal muscle and brain. N Engl J Med 273:1308–1310, 1965.

67. Kotula AW, et al. Effect of freezing on infectivity of *Toxoplasma gondii* tissue cysts in pork. J Food Protect 54:687–690, 1991.

68. Dubey JP. Effect of freezing on the infectivity of *Toxoplasma* cysts to cats. J Am Vet Med Assoc 165:534–536, 1974.

69. Work K. Resistance of *Toxoplasma gondii* encysted in pork. Acta Pathol Microbiol Scand 73:85–92, 1968.

70. Ferguson DJ, Hutchison WM. The host-parasite relationship of *Toxoplasma gondii* in the brains of chronically infected mice. Virchows Arch [A] 411:39–43, 1987.

71. Bohne W, Hessemann J, Gross U. Reduced replication of *Toxoplasma gondii* is necessary for induction of bradyzoite-specific antigens: a possible role for nitric oxide in triggering stage conversion. Infect Immun 62:1761–1767, 1994.

72. Soete M, Camus D, Dubremetz J. Experimental induction of bradyzoite-specific antigen expression and cyst formation by the RH strain of *Toxoplasma gondii* in vitro. Exp Parasitol 78:361–370, 1994.

73. Jacobs L. New knowledge of *Toxoplasma* and toxoplasmosis. Adv Parasitol 11:631–669, 1973.

74. Hogan MJ, et al. Morphology and culture of toxoplasma. Arch Ophthalmol 64:655–667, 1960.

75. Linday DS, Dubey JP, Blagburn BL. Examination of

tissue cyst formation by *Toxoplasma gondii* in cell cultures using bradyzoites, tachyzoites, and sporozoites. J Parasitol 77:126–132, 1991.

76. Frenkel JK, Friedlander S. Toxoplasmosis: pathology of neonatal disease. *In* Public Health Service publication No. 141. Washington, D. C., U. S. Government Printing Office, 1952, p 108.

77. Cowen D, Wolf A. Experimental congenital toxoplasmosis: II. Transmission of toxoplasmosis to the placenta and fetus following vaginal infection in the pregnant mouse. J Exp Med 92:403–416, 1950.

78. Eichenwald H. Experimental toxoplasmosis: I. Transmission of the infection in utero and through the milk of lactating female mice. Am J Dis Child 76:307–315, 1948.

79. Hellbrügge T. [Fetal infection in the course of the acute and chronic phase in latent rat toxoplasmosis.] Arch Gynakol (in German) 186:384–388, 1955.

80. Dubey JP, Shen SK. Rat model of congenital toxoplasmosis. Infect Immun 59:3301–3302, 1991.

81. Zenner L, et al. Rat model of congenital toxoplasmosis: rate of transmission of three *Toxoplasma gondii* strains to fetuses and protective effect of a chronic infection. Infect Immun 61:360–363, 1993.

82. McLeod R, et al. Subcutaneous and intestinal vaccination with tachyzoites of *Toxoplasma gondii* and acquisition of immunity to peroral and congenital *Toxoplasma* challenge. J Immunol 140:1632–1637, 1988.

83. Dubey JP, et al. Toxoplasmosis in rats (*Rattus norvegicus*): congenital transmission to first and second generation offspring and isolation of *Toxoplasma gondii* from seronegative rats. Parasitology 115:9–14, 1997.

84. Remington JS, Jacobs L, Melton ML. Congenital transmission of toxoplasmosis from mother animals with acute and chronic infections. J Infect Dis 108:163–173, 1961.

85. Hellbrügge T, Dahme E. Experimentelle Toxoplasmose: Bemergungen zur Arbeit von Schultz und Bauer über Placentarbefunde bei Ratten. Klin Wochenschr 31:789–791, 1953.

86. Wildführ G. Tierexperimentelle Untersuchungen bveim vor der Gravidatät infizierten Muttertier. *In* Forschung Untersuchungen Ergebnisse. Leipzig, Universität Klinisches Institut, 1954, p 161.

87. Thiermann E. Transmission congénita del *Toxoplasma gondii* enratas con infection leve. Biologica (Chile) 23:59–67, 1957.

88. Wildführ G. Experimental animal studies to study the diaplacental transmission of toxoplasmen in a mother animal infected before pregnancy. Z Immun Exp Ther 111:110–120, 1954.

89. Huldt G. Experimental toxoplasmosis: transplacental transmission in guinea pigs. Acta Pathol Microbiol Scand 49:176–188, 1960.

90. Janitschke K, Jorren H. [Studies on the significance of intrauterine infection for the prevalence of *Toxoplasma* in domestic rabbits.] (in German) Z Tropenmed Parasitol 21:246–251, 1970.

91. Beverley JKA. Congenital transmission of toxoplasmosis through successive generations of mice. Nature 183:1348–1349, 1959.

92. Remington JS, Melton ML, Jacobs L. Induced and spontaneous recurrent parasitemia in chronic infections with avirulent strains of *Toxoplasma gondii*. J Immunol 87:578–581, 1961.

93. Remington JS. Experiments on the transmission of toxoplasmosis. Surv Ophthalmol 6:856–876, 1961.

94. Dubey JP, Beattie CP. Toxoplasmosis of Animals and Man. Boca Raton, Fla, CRC Press, 1988.

95. Work K, Eriksen L, Fennestad KL. Experimental toxoplasmosis in pregnant sows: I. Clinical, parasitological and serological observations. Acta Pathol Microbiol Scand [B] 78:129–139, 1970.

96. Møller T, et al. Experimental toxoplasmosis in pregnant sows. Acta Pathol Microbiol Scand [A] 78:241–255, 1970.

97. Sanger VL, Cole CR. Toxoplasmosis: VI. Isolation of *Toxoplasma* from milk, placentas, and newborn pigs of asymptomatic carrier sows. 16:536–539, 1955.

98. Hartley WJ, Moyle G. Observations on an outbreak of ovine congenital toxoplasmosis. Aust Vet J 44:105–107, 1968.

99. Watson WA, Beverley JKA. Epizootics of toxoplasmosis causing ovine abortion. Vet Rec 88:120–124, 1971.

100. Munday BL. The epidemiology of toxoplasmosis with particular reference to the Tasmanian environment. University of Melbourne, 1971, pp 1–95.

101. Munday BL, Mason RW. Toxoplasmosis as a cause of perinatal death in goats. Aust Vet J 55:485–487, 1979.

102. Jacobs L, Hartley WJ. Ovine toxoplasmosis: studies on parasitaemia, tissue infection, and congenital transmission in ewes infected by various routes. Br Vet J 120:347–364, 1964.

103. Hartley WJ. Experimental transmission of toxoplasmosis in ewes showing high and low dye test titres. NZ Vet J 12:6–8, 1964.

104. Beverley JKA, Watson WA, Centre VI. Prevention of experimental and of naturally occurring ovine abortion due to toxoplasmosis. Vet Rec 88:39–41, 1970.

105. Beverley JK, et al. Trial of a killed vaccine in the prevention of ovine abortion due to toxoplasmosis. Br Vet J 127:529–535, 1971.

106. Vermeulen AN, Bos HJ. Vaccination of sheep with Toxovax: field trial data from UK, France and the Netherlands. Fourth International Biennial Toxoplasma Conference. Drymen, Scotland, 1996.

107. Marx-Chemla C, et al. Should immunologic monitoring of toxoplasmosis seronegative pregnant women stop at delivery? Presse Med 19:367–368, 1990.

108. Miller MJ, Aronson WJ, Remington JS. Late parasitemia in asymptomatic acquired toxoplasmosis. Ann Intern Med 71:139–145, 1969.

109. Derouin F, et al. Abstract: Detection of *Toxoplasma* parasitemia in immunocompromised patients. IXth International Congress of Infectious and Parasitic Diseases, Munich, July 20–26, 1986.

110. Vittecoq D, et al. *Toxoplasma* parasitemia associated to serological reactivation of chronic toxoplasmosis in an immunocomprised (sic) patient. IXth International Congress of Infectious and Parasitic Diseases, Munich, July 20–26, 1986.

111. Luft BJ, et al. Primary and reactivated *Toxoplasma* infection in patients with cardiac transplants: clinical spectrum and problems in diagnosis in a defined population. Ann Intern Med 99:27–31, 1983.

112. Garcia AG. Congenital toxoplasmosis in two successive sibs. Arch Dis Child 43:705–710, 1968.

113. Glasser L, Delta BG. Congenital toxoplasmosis with placental infection in monozygotic twins. Pediatrics 35:276–283, 1965.

114. Beckett RS, Flynn FJ Jr. Toxoplasmosis: report of two new cases, with a classification and a demonstration of the organisms in the human placenta. N Engl J Med 249:345–350, 1953.

115. Neghme A, Thiermann E, Pino F. Toxoplasmosis humana en Chile. Bol Infect Parasitol Chile 7:6–8, 1952.
116. Sarrut S. [Histological study of the placenta in congenital toxoplasmosis.] Ann Pediatr (Paris) (in French) 14:2429–2435, 1967 (English summary, p 2434).
117. Desmonts G, Couvreur J. [The clinical expression of infection in the newborn: III. Congenital toxoplasmosis.] (in French) 21st Congress Pediatres de Langue Française 3:453–488, 1967.
118. Desmonts G, Couvreur J. Toxoplasmosis in pregnancy and its transmission to the fetus. Bull N Y Acad Med 50:146–159, 1974.
119. Aspöck H, et al. Attempts for detection of *Toxoplasma gondii* in human embryos of mothers with preconceptional Toxoplasma infections. Mitt Österr Ges Tropenmed Parasitol 5:93–97, 1983.
120. Desmonts G, Couvreur J. Congenital toxoplasmosis: a prospective study of the offspring of 542 women who acquired toxoplasmosis during pregnancy: pathophysiology of congenital disease. *In* Thalhammer O, Pollak A, Baumgarten K (eds). Perinatal Medicine, 6th European Congress, Vienna. Stuttgart, Georg Thieme, 1979, pp 51–60.
121. Couvreur J, Desmonts G, Thulliez P. Prophylaxis of congenital toxoplasmosis: effects of spiramycin on placental infection. J Antimicrob Chemother 22(Suppl. B):193–200, 1988.
122. Remington JS, Melton ML, Jacobs L. Chronic *Toxoplasma* infection in the uterus. J Lab Clin Med 56:879–883, 1960.
123. Ruiz A, Flores M, Kotcher E. The prevalence of *Toxoplasma* antibodies in Costa Rican postpartum women and their neonates. Am J Obstet Gynecol 95:817–819, 1966.
124. Ruoss CF, Bourne GL. Toxoplasmosis in pregnancy. J Obstet Gynaecol Br Commonw 79:1115–1118, 1972.
125. Kräubig H. [Preventive method of treatment of congenital toxoplasmosis.] *In* Kirchhoff H, Kräubig H (eds). Toxoplasmose: Praktische Fragen und Ergebnisse. Stuttgart, Georg Thieme, 1966, pp 104–122.
126. Kimball AC, Kean BH, Fuchs F. Congenital toxoplasmosis: a prospective study of 4,048 obstetric patients. Am J Obstet Gynecol 111:211–218, 1971.
127. Stray-Pedersen B. A prospective study of acquired toxoplasmosis among 8,043 pregnant women in the Oslo area. Am J Obstet Gynecol 136:399–406, 1980.
128. Desmonts G. Acquired toxoplasmosis in pregnant women: evaluation of the frequency of transmission of *Toxoplasma* and of congenital toxoplasmosis. Lyon Med 248:115–123, 1982.
129. Desmonts G, et al. Prenatal diagnosis of congenital toxoplasmosis. Lancet 1:500–504, 1985.
130. Daffos F, et al. Prenatal management of 746 pregnancies at risk for congenital toxoplasmosis. N Engl J Med 318:271–275, 1988.
131. Dunn D, et al. Mother-to-child transmission of toxoplasmosis: risk estimates for clinical counselling. Lancet 353:1829–1833, 1999.
132. Hohlfeld P, et al. Prenatal diagnosis of congenital toxoplasmosis with polymerase-chain-reaction test on amniotic fluid. N Engl J Med 331:695–699, 1994.
133. Jenum PA, et al. Incidence of *Toxoplasma gondii* infection in 35,940 pregnant women in Norway and pregnancy outcome for infected women. J Clin Microbiol 36:2900–2906, 1998.
134. Thalhammer O, Fetale und angeborene Cytomegalie: zur Bedeutung die präntalen Inkubationszeit. Monatsschr Kinderheilkd 116:209–211, 1968.
135. Thalhammer O. Prenatal incubation period. *In* Thalhammer O (ed). Prenatal Infections, Stuttgart, Georg Thieme Verlag, 1971, pp 70–71.
136. Desmonts G, Couvreur J, Thulliez P. [Congenital toxoplasmosis: five cases with mother-to-child transmission of pre-pregnancy infection.] Presse Med (in French) 19:1445–1449, 1990.
137. Remington JS, Klein JO. Infectious Diseases of the Fetus and Newborn Infant, 3rd ed. Philadelphia, WB Saunders, 1983.
138. Remington JS, Klein JO. Infectious Diseases of the Fetus and Newborn Infant, 4th ed. Philadelphia, WB Saunders, 1995.
139. Marty P, et al. Toxoplasmose congénitale et toxoplasmose ganglionnaire maternelie préconceptionnelle. Presse Med 20:387, 1991.
140. Vogel N, et al. Congenital toxoplasmosis transmitted from an immunologically competent mother infected before conception. Clin Infect Dis 23:1055–1060, 1996.
141. Feldman HA, Miller LT. Congenital human toxoplasmosis. Ann NY Acad Sci 64:180–184, 1956.
142. Pons J, et al. Congenital toxoplasmosis: mother-to-fetus transmission of pre-pregnancy infection. Presse Med 24:179–182, 1995.
143. Villena I, Quereux C, Pinon JM. Congenital toxoplasmosis: value of prenatal treatment with pyrimethamine-sulfadoxine combination. Prenat Diagn 18:754–756, 1998.
144. Aspöck H, Flamm H, Picher O. Toxoplasmosis surveillance during pregnancy—10 years of experience in Austria (English summary). Mitt Österr Ges Tropenmed Parasitol 8:105–113, 1986.
145. Flamm H, Aspöck H. [Toxoplasmosis surveillance during pregnancy in Austria—results and problems.] Padiatr Grenzgeb (in German) 20:27–34, 1981.
146. Desmonts G. Prevention de la toxoplasmose: remarques sur l'experience poursuivie en France. *In* Marois M (ed). Prevention of Physical and Mental Congenital Defects, Part B: Epidemiology, Early Detection and Therapy, and Environmental Factors. New York, Alan R. Liss, 1985, pp 313–316.
147. Fortier B, et al. Spontaneous abortion and reinfection by *Toxoplasma gondii* [letter to the editor]. Lancet 338:444, 1991.
148. Hennequin C, et al. Congenital toxoplasmosis acquired from an immune woman. Pediatr Infect Dis 16:75–76, 1997.
149. Gavinet MF, et al. Congenital toxoplasmosis due to maternal reinfection during pregnancy. J Clin Microbiol 35:1276–1277, 1997.
150. Wechsler B, et al. [Toxoplasmosis and disseminated lupus erythematosus: four case reports and a review of the literature.] Ann Med Interne (Paris) (in French) 137:324–330, 1986.
151. D'Ercole C, et al. Recurrent congenital toxoplasmosis in a woman with lupus erythematosus. Prenat Diagn 15:1171–1175, 1995.
152. Remington JS. Congenital transmission of *Toxoplasma* during chronic infection of the mother. First International Congress of Parasitology, Rome (abstract). Oxford, London, Pergamon Press, 1994, pp 184–186.
153. Remington JS, et al. Studies on toxoplasmosis in El Salvador: prevalence and incidence of toxoplasmosis as measured by the Sabin-Feldman dye test. Trans R Soc Trop Med Hyg 64:252–267, 1970.
154. Ferraris G, Avitto P. [Biological research on toxoplasmosis: attempts of isolation of the parasite in fetal and adnexal tissues.] Minerva Ginecol 17:781–783, 1965.

155. Remington JS, Newell JW, Cavanaugh E. Spontaneous abortion and chronic toxoplasmosis: report of a case, with isolation of the parasite. Obstet Gynecol 24:25–31, 1964.

156. Meylan J. Toxoplasmosis as a cause of repeated abortion. *In* Hentsch D (ed). Toxoplasmosis. Bern, Stuttgart, Vienna, Hans Huber, 1971, pp 151–158.

157. Janssen P, Piekarski G, Korte W. [Problem of abortions because of latent *Toxoplasma* infection in women.] Klin Wochenschr (in German) 48:25–30, 1970.

158. Remington JS. *Toxoplasma* and chronic abortion [Editorial]. Obstet Gynecol 24:155–157, 1964.

159. Kimball AC, Kean BH, Fuchs F. The role of toxoplasmosis in abortion. Am J Obstet Gynecol 111:219–226, 1971.

160. Remington JS, Desmonts G. Toxoplasmosis. *In* Remington JS, Klein JO (eds). Infectious Diseases of the Fetus and Newborn Infant. Philadelphia, WB Saunders, 1983, pp 143–263.

161. Remington JS, Desmonts G. Toxoplasmosis. *In* Remington JS, Klein JO (eds). Infectious Diseases of the Fetus and Newborn Infant. Philadelphia, WB Saunders, 1976, pp 191–332.

162. Wildführ G. Experimentelle Versuche zur Resistenz der Toxoplasmen. Z Hyg Infekt 143:134–139, 1956.

163. Kass E. Undersokelser over *Toxoplasma* og toxoplasmose. In Inaugural Dissertation, Oslo, 1954.

164. Weinman D, Chandler AH. Toxoplasmosis in man and swine—an investigation of the possible relationship. JAMA 161:229–232, 1956.

165. Langer H. Repeated congenital infection with *Toxoplasma gondii*. Obstet Gynecol 21:318–329, 1963.

166. Langer H. [Intrauterine *Toxoplasma* infection.] (in German) Stuttgart, Georg Thieme, 55, 1963.

167. Langer H. [Toxoplasma infection during pregnancy.] Zentralbl Gynakol (in German) 86:745–750, 1964.

168. Langer H. Toxoplasmose und gestation. 202:79–91, 1965.

169. Langer H. [The significance of a latent *Toxoplasma* infection during gestation.] In Kirchhoff H, Kräubig H (eds). Toxoplasmose. Praktische Fragen und Ergebnisse. Stuttgart, Georg Thieme, 1966, pp 123–138.

170. Langer H. [On prenatal toxoplasma infection.] Landarzt (in German) 43:1300–1305, 1967.

171. Remington JS. Toxoplasmosis and congenital infection. Intrauterine Infect 4:47–56, 1968.

172. Jacobs L, Moyle G, Ris RR. The prevalence of toxoplasmosis in New Zealand sheep and cattle. Am J Vet Res 24:673–675, 1963.

173. Jacobs L, Remington JS, Melton ML. A survey of meat samples from swine, cattle, and sheep for the presence of encysted *Toxoplasma*. J Parasitol 46:23–28, 1960.

174. Janitschke K, Weiland G, Rommell MQ. Untersuchungen über den Befall von Schlactälbvern und -schafen mit *Toxoplasma gondii*. Fleischwirtschaft 47:135–136, 1967.

175. Work K. Isolation of *Toxoplasma gondii* from the flesh of sheep, swine and cattle. Acta Pathol Microbiol Scand 71:296–306, 1967.

176. Catár G, Bergendi L, Holkova R. Isolation of *Toxoplasma gondii* from swine and cattle. J Parasitol 55:952–955, 1969.

177. Boch J, Janitschke K, Rommel M. Untersuchungen über das Vorkommen von Toxoplasma-Infektionen bei Schlachtrindern. Wien Tierarztl Monatsschr 52:1029–1036, 1965.

178. Lalla F, Bechelli G, Sampieri L. Osservazioni sierologiche e parassitologiche sulla diffusione della toxoplasmosi nei maiali dell'area de Siena. Clin Vet Milano 90:439–454, 1967.

179. Komiya Y, Kobayashi A, Koyama T. Human toxoplasmosis, particularly on the possible source of its infection in Japan: a review. Jpn J Med Sci Biol 14:157–172, 1961.

180. Fujita J. Parasitic disease of livestock in Japan. Off Int Epizoot Bull 69:203–213, 1968.

181. Dubey JP, et al. Distribution of *Toxoplasma gondii* tissue cysts in commercial cuts of pork. J Am Vet Med Assoc 188:1035–1037, 1986.

182. Mondragon R, et al. Genotypic analysis of *Toxoplasma gondii* isolates from pigs. J Parasitol 84:639–641, 1998.

183. Dubey JP, Streitel RH. Prevalence of *Toxoplasma* infection in cattle slaughtered at an Ohio abattoir. J Am Vet Med Assoc 169:1197–1199, 1976.

184. Raisanen S. Toxoplasmosis transmitted by blood transfusions. Transfusion 18:329–332, 1978.

185. Kimball AC, Kean BH, Kellner A. The risk of transmitting toxoplasmosis by blood transfusion. Transfusion 5:447–451, 1965.

186. Matsubayashi H, Akao S. Immuno-electron microscopic studies on *Toxoplasma gondii*. Am J Trop Med Hyg 15:486–491, 1966.

187. Shevkunova EA, Rokhina LA, Nugumanova MF. [A case of chronic acquired toxoplasmosis with positive agents detectable in the blood.] Med Parazitol (Mosk) (in Russian) 44:235–238, 1975.

188. Waldeland H. Toxoplasmosis in sheep: *Toxoplasma gondii* in muscular tissue, with particular reference to dye test titres and haemoglobin type. Acta Vet Scand 17:403–411, 1976.

189. Ghorbani M, et al. Animal toxoplasmosis in Iran. J Trop Med Hyg 86:73–76, 1983.

190. Maitani T. [Serological investigation of toxoplasmosis in human and various animals, and isolation of *Toxoplasma gondii*.] Niigata Med J (in Japanese) 84:325, 1970.

191. Siegel SE, et al. Transmission of toxoplasmosis by leukocyte transfusion. Blood 37:388–394, 1971.

192. Beauvais B, et al. [Toxoplasmosis and transfusion.] Ann Parasitol Hum Comp (in French) 51:625–635, 1976.

193. Rommel M, et al. [Investigations into the epizootiology of infections with cystforming coccidia (Toxoplasmidae, Sarcocystidae) in cats, cattle and free-living rodents.] DTW Dtsch Tierarztl Wochenschr (in German) 89:57–62, 1982.

194. Prosek F, Hejlícek K. V'yskyt protilátek proti toxoplazmóze u jatecnych vírat ze socialistického sektoru. Veterinarstvi 30:405, 1980.

195. Dubey J, Thulliez P, Powell E. *Toxoplasma gondii* in Iowa sows: comparison of antibody titers to isolation of *T. gondii* by bioassays in mice and cats. J Parasitol 81:48–53, 1995.

196. Boch J, Rommel M, Janitschke K. Beiträge zur toxoplasmose des Schweines: I. Ergebnisse künstlicher *Toxoplasma*-infektionnen bei schweinen. Berl Munch Tierarztl Wochenschr 77:161, 1964.

197. Beauvais B, et al. [Toxoplasmosis and chronic myeloid leukemia.] Nouv Rev Fr Hematol (in French) 16:169–184, 1976.

198. Hellesnes I, Mohn SF, Melhuus B. *Toxoplasma gondii* in swine in south-eastern Norway. Acta Vet Scand 19:574–587, 1978.

199. Kayhoe DE, et al. Acquired toxoplasmosis: observations on two parasitologically proved cases treated with pyrimethamine and triple sulfonamides. N Engl J Med 257:1247–1254, 1957.

200. Frenkel JK, Weber RW, Lunde MN. Acute toxoplasmosis. Effective treatment with pyrimethamine, sulfadia-

zine, leucovorin, calcium, and yeast. JAMA 173:1471–1476, 1960.

201. Hagiwara T, Katsube Y. Detection of *Toxoplasma* infection in pork by Sabin-Feldman's dye test with meat extract. Nippon Juigaku Zasshi 43:763–765, 1981.

202. Desmonts G, et al. Étude epidemiologique sur la toxoplasmose: l'influence de la cuisson des viandes de boucherie sur la frequence de l'infection humaine. Revue Française d'Études Cliniques et Biologiques 10:952–958, 1965.

203. Kean BH, Kimball AC, Christenson WN. An epidemic of acute toxoplasmosis. JAMA 208:1002–1004, 1969.

204. Schantz PM, Juaranek DD, Schultz MG. Trichinosis in the United States, 1975: increase in cases attributed to numerous common-source outbreaks. J Infect Dis 136:712–715, 1977.

205. Dubey JP. Toxoplasmosis. J Am Vet Med Assoc 189:166–170, 1986.

206. Passos JN, Bonametti AM, Passos EM. Surto de toxoplasmose aguda transmitida atraves da ingestao de carne de gado ovino. Congresso da Sociedade de Medicina Tropical, Salvador, Resumos, 1994, p 30.

207. Robson MB, et al. A probable foodborne outbreak of toxoplasmosis. Commun Dis Intell 19:517–522, 1995.

208. Choi WY, et al. Foodborne outbreaks of human toxoplasmosis. J Infect Dis 175:1280–1282, 1997.

209. Vanek JA, et al. Prevalence of *Toxoplasma gondii* antibodies in hunter-killed white-tailed deer (*Odocoileus virginianus*) in four regions of Minnesota. J Parasitol 82:41–44, 1996.

210. Humphreys JG, Stewart RL, Dubey JP. Prevalence of *Toxoplasma gondii* antibodies in sera of hunter-killed white-tailed deer in Pennsylvania. Am J Vet Res 56:172–173, 1995.

211. Guebre-Xabier M, et al. Sero-epidemiological survey of *Toxoplasma gondii* infection in Ethiopia. Ethiop Med J 31:201–208, 1993.

212. Kapperud G, et al. Risk factors for *Toxoplasma gondii* infection in pregnancy. Am J Epidemiol 144:405–412, 1996.

213. Raz R, et al. Seroprevalence of antibodies against *Toxoplasma gondii* among two rural populations in Northern Israel. Isr J Med Sci 29:636–639, 1993.

214. Buffolano W, et al. Risk factors for recent *Toxoplasma* infection in pregnant women in Naples. Epidemiol Infect 116:347–351, 1996.

215. Rawal BD. Toxoplasmosis: a dye-test survey on sera from vegetarians and meat eaters in Bombay. Trans R Soc Trop Med Hyg 53:61–63, 1959.

216. Jacobs L. The interrelation of toxoplasmosis in swine, cattle, dogs and man. Public Health Rep 72:872–882, 1957.

217. Hutchison WM, Dunachie JF, Work K. The fecal transmission of *Toxoplasma gondii* (brief report). Acta Pathol Microbiol Scand 74:462–464, 1968.

218. Sheffield HG, Melton ML. *Toxoplasma gondii*: transmission through feces in absence of *Toxocara cati* eggs. Science 164:431–432, 1969.

219. Frenkel JK, Dubey JP, Miller NL. *Toxoplasma gondii*: fecal forms separated from eggs of the nematode *Toxocara cati*. Science 164:432–433, 1969.

220. Ruiz A, Frenkel JK. *Toxoplasma gondii* in Costa Rican cats. Am J Trop Med Hyg 29:1150–1160, 1980.

221. Frenkel JK, Ruiz A, Chinchilla M. Soil survival of *Toxoplasma* oocysts in Kansas and Costa Rica. Am J Trop Med Hyg 24:439–443, 1975.

222. Coutinho SG, Lobo R, Dutra G. Isolation of *Toxoplasma* from the soil during an outbreak of toxoplasmosis in a rural area in Brazil. J Parasitol 68:866–868, 1982.

223. Dubey JP, Frenkel JK. Cyst-induced toxoplasmosis in cats. J Protozool 19:155–177, 1972.

224. Wallace GD. Experimental transmission of *Toxoplasma gondii* by filth-flies. Am J Trop Med Hyg 20:411–413, 1971.

225. Wallace GD. Experimental transmission of *Toxoplasma gondii* by cockroaches. J Infect Dis 126:545–547, 1972.

226. Smith DD, Frenkel JK. Cockroaches as vectors of *Sarcocystis muris* and of other coccidia in the laboratory. J Parasitol 64:315–319, 1978.

227. Markus MB. Earthworms and coccidian oocysts. Ann Trop Med Parasitol 68:247–248, 1974.

228. Ruiz A, Frenkel JK. Intermediate and transport hosts of *Toxoplasma gondii* in Costa Rica. Am J Trop Med Hyg 29:1161–1166, 1981.

229. Dubey JP. Feline toxoplasmosis and coccidiosis: a survey of domiciled and stray cats. J Am Vet Med Assoc 162:873–877, 1973.

230. Wallace GD. Isolation of *Toxoplasma gondii* from the feces of naturally infected cats. J Infect Dis 124:227–228, 1971.

231. Wallace GD, Marshall L, Marshall M. Cats, rats, and toxoplasmosis on a small Pacific island. Am J Epidemiol 95:475–482, 1972.

232. Wallace GD. Serologic and epidemiologic observations on toxoplasmosis on three Pacific atolls. Am J Epidemiol 90:103–111, 1969.

233. Wallace GD. The role of the cat in the natural history of *Toxoplasma gondii*. Am J Trop Med Hyg 22:313–322, 1973.

234. Munday BL. Serological evidence of *Toxoplasma* infection in isolated groups of sheep. Res Vet Sci 13:100–102, 1972.

235. Stern GA, Romano PE. Congenital ocular toxoplasmosis: possible occurrence in siblings. Arch Ophthalmol 96:615–617, 1978.

236. Janitschke K, Kühn D. *Toxoplasma*-Oozysten im Kot naturlich infizierter Katzen. Berl Munch Tierarztl Wochenschr 3:46–47, 1972.

237. Werner JK, Walton BC. Prevalence of naturally occurring *Toxoplasma gondii* infections in cats from U.S. military installations in Japan. J Parasitol 58:1148–1150, 1972.

238. Deeb BJ, Sufan MM, DiGiacomo RF. *Toxoplasma gondii* infection of cats in Beirut, Lebanon. J Trop Med Hyg 88:301–306, 1985.

239. Svobodova V, Svoboda M. The occurrence of the oocysts of *Toxoplasma gondii* in the feces of cats. Vet Med (Praha) 31:621–628, 1986.

240. Etheredge GD, Frenkel JK. Human *Toxoplasma* infection in Kuna and Embera children in the Bayano and San Blas, Eastern Panama. Am J Trop Med Hyg 53:448–457, 1995.

241. Teutsch SM, et al. Epidemic toxoplasmosis associated with infected cats. N Engl J Med 300:695–699, 1979.

242. Stagno S, et al. An outbreak of toxoplasmosis linked to cats. Pediatrics 65:706–712, 1980.

243. Benenson MW, et al. Oocyst-transmitted toxoplasmosis associated with ingestion of contaminated water. N Engl J Med 307:666–669, 1982.

244. Bowie WR, et al. Outbreak of toxoplasmosis associated with municipal drinking water. Lancet 350:173–177, 1997.

245. Mayer H. Investigaciones sobre toxoplasmosis. Bol Sanit Panam 58:485–497, 1965.

246. Rommel M, Breuning J. [Research into the occurrence

of *Toxoplasma gondii* in the milk of some animals and the possibility of lactogenous infection.] Berl Munch Tierarztl Wochenschr (in German) 80:365–369, 1967.

247. Sanger VL, Chamberlain DM, Chamberlain KW. Toxoplasmosis: V. Isolation of *Toxoplasma* from cattle. J Am Vet Med Assoc 123:87–91, 1953.

248. Bonametti AM, Passos JN (Correspondence). Probable transmission of acute toxoplasmosis through breast feeding. J Trop Pediatr 43:16, 1997.

249. Riemann HP, et al. Toxoplasmosis in an infant fed unpasteurized goat milk. J Pediatr 87:573–576, 1975.

250. Chiari C, Neves DP. [Human toxoplasmosis acquired by ingestion of goat's milk.] Mem Inst Oswaldo Cruz (in Spanish) 79:337–340, 1984.

251. Sacks JJ, Roberto RR, Brooks NF. Toxoplasmosis infection associated with raw goat's milk. JAMA 248:1728–1732, 1982.

252. Jacobs L, Melton ML. Toxoplasmosis in chickens. J Parasitol 52:1158–1162, 1966.

253. Pande PG, Shukla RR, Sekariah PC. *Toxoplasma* from the eggs of domestic fowl *(Gallus gallus)*. Science 133:648, 1961.

254. DuShane G, et al. An unfortunate event. Science 134:945–946, 1961.

255. Neto VA, Cotrim JX, Laus WC. Nota scircumflex obre o encontro de *Toxoplasma gondii* en sangue destinado a transfusao. Rev Inst Med Trop São Paulo 5:68–69, 1963.

256. Talice RV, et al. Researches on toxoplasmosis in Uruguay: survival of *Toxoplasma gondii* in human blood "in vitro." An Fac Med Montevideo 42:143–147, 1957.

257. Vasina SG, Dunaeva ZV. [The survival of *Toxoplasma* outside the host organism.] J Med Parazitol (Mosk) (in Russian) 29:451–454, 1960.

258. Siegal SE, Lunde MN, Gelderman AH. Transmission of toxoplasmosis by leukocyte transfusion. Blood 37:388–394, 1971.

259. Remington JS, Gentry LO. Acquired toxoplasmosis: infection versus disease. Ann NY Acad Sci 174:1006–1017, 1970.

260. Miller NL, Frenkel JK, Dubey JP. Oral infections with *Toxoplasma* cysts and oocysts in felines, other mammals, and in birds. J Parasitol 58:928–937, 1972.

261. Markvart K, Rehnova M, Ostrovska A. Laboratory epidemic of toxoplasmosis. J Hyg Epidemiol Microbiol Immunol 22:477–484, 1978.

262. Neu HC. Toxoplasmosis in childhood. Lancet 1:813–814, 1954.

263. Cathie IAG. Toxoplasmosis in childhood. Lancet 266:813–814, 1954.

264. Levi GC, et al. [Presence of *Toxoplasma gondii* in the saliva of patients with toxoplasmosis. Eventual importance of such verification concerning the transmission of the disease (preliminary report).] Rev Inst Med Trop São Paulo (in Portuguese) 10:54–58, 1968.

265. Saari M, Raisanen S. Transmission of acute *Toxoplasma* infection: the survival of trophozoites in human tears, saliva, and urine and in cow's milk. Acta Ophthalmol (Copenh) 52:847–852, 1974.

266. Brooks RG, Remington JS. Transplant-related infections. *In* Bennett JV, Brachman PS (eds). Hospital Infections. Boston, Little, Brown, 1986, pp 581–618.

267. Israelski DM, Remington JS. Toxoplasmosis in the non-AIDS immunocompromised host. *In* Remington JS, Swartz M (eds). Current Clinical Topics in Infectious Diseases. London, Blackwell Scientific, 1993, pp 322–356.

268. Mayes J, et al. Transmission of *Toxoplasma gondii* infec-

tion by liver transplantation. Clin Infect Dis 21:511–515, 1995.

269. Jacobs L. Propagation, morphology and biology of *Toxoplasma*. Ann NY Acad Sci 64:154–179, 1956.

270. Stone WB, Manwell RB. Toxoplasmosis in cold-blooded hosts. J Protozool 16:99–102, 1969.

271. Levine ND, Nye RR. *Toxoplasma ranae* sp. m. from the leopard frog *Rana linnaeus*. J Parasitol 23:488–490, 1976.

272. Luft BJ, Remington JS. Acute *Toxoplasma* infection among family members of patients with acute lymphadenopathic toxoplasmosis. Arch Intern Med 144:53–56, 1984.

273. Coutinho SG, et al. Concomitant cases of acquired toxoplasmosis in children of a single family: evidence of reinfection. J Infect Dis 146:30–33, 1982.

274. Coutinho SG, et al. Outbreak of human toxoplasmosis in a rural area: a three year serologic follow-up study. Mem Inst Oswaldo Cruz 77:29–36, 1982.

275. Humphreys H, Hillary IB, Kiernan T. Toxoplasmosis: a family outbreak. Ir Med J 79:191, 1986.

276. Shenep JL, et al. An outbreak of toxoplasmosis on an Illinois farm. Pediatr Infect Dis 3:518–522, 1984.

277. Baril L, Ancelle T, Thulliez P, et al. Facteurs de risque de la toxoplasmose chez les femmes enceintes en 1995 (France). Bulletin Épidémiologique Hebdomadaire, 16, 1996.

278. Bobic B, et al. Risk factors for *Toxoplasma* infection in a reproductive age female population in the area of Belgrade, Yugoslavia [In Process Citation]. Eur J Epidemiol 14:605–610, 1998.

279. Dumas N, Meunier DM, Seguela JP. [Toxoplasmosis in the Central African Republic: first survey.] Bull Soc Pathol Exot Filiales (in French) 78:221–225, 1985.

280. Billiault X, et al. [Toxoplasmosis in pregnant women in Haut Ogooue Province (Gabon).] Bull Soc Pathol Exot Filiales (in French) 80:74–83, 1987.

281. Vercruysse J, Deschampheleire IL, Van De Velden L. Contribution à l'étude de la toxoplasmose humaine à Pikine (Sénégal). Med Afr Noire 31:619–620, 1984.

282. Gill HS, Mtimavalye LA. Prevalence of *Toxoplasma* antibodies in pregnant African women in Tanzania. Afr J Med Sci 11:167–170, 1982.

283. Dumas N, et al. [Toxoplasmosis in the African tropical zone. Preliminary prevalence studies.] Bull Soc Pathol Exot Filiales (in French) 78:795–800, 1985.

284. Kennou MF. [Epidemiology of toxoplasmosis in pregnant Tunisian women.] Epidemiologie de la toxoplasmose chez les femmes enceintes tunisiennes. Arch Inst Pasteur Tunis 59:205–211, 1982.

285. Rudolph C. [Seroepidemiologic study of the incidence of *Toxoplasma* infections in black African females in Zambia.] Off Gesundheitsw (in German) 49:41–43, 1987.

286. Fuente MC, Bovone NS, Cabral GE. Profilaxis de la toxoplasmosis prenatal. Medicina 57:155–160, 1997.

287. Rickard E, et al. Toxoplasmosis antibody prevalence in pregnancy in Buenos Aires Province, Argentina. *In* 9th European Congress of Clinical Microbiology and Infectious Diseases. Berlin, The European Society of Clinical Microbiology and Infectious Diseases, 1999.

288. Sfameni SF, Skurrie IJ, Gilbert GL. Antenatal screening for congenital infection with rubella, cytomegalovirus and *Toxoplasma*. Aust NZ J Obstet Gynaecol 26:257–260, 1986.

289. Walpole IR, Hodgen N, Bower C. Congenital toxoplasmosis: a large survey in Western Australia. Med J Aust 154:720–724, 1991.

290. Aspöck H, Pollak A. Prevention of prenatal toxoplasmosis by serological screening of pregnant women in Austria. Scand J Infect Dis Suppl 84:32–38, 1992.

291. Ashrafunnessa, et al. Seroprevalence of *Toxoplasma* antibodies among the antenatal population in Bangladesh. J Obstet Gynaecol Res 24:115–119, 1998.

292. Foulon W, Naessens A, Derde M. Evaluation of the possibilities for preventing congenital toxoplasmosis. Am J Perinatol 11:57–62, 1994.

293. Luvasu V, et al. Screening of pregnant women for antibodies against toxoplasma and CMV with the IMX analyzer in Belgium. Sixth European Congress of Clinical and Microbiological Infectious Disease, Seville, Spain, 1993.

294. Rodier MH, et al. Seroprevalences of *Toxoplasma*, malaria, rubella, cytomegalovirus, HIV, and treponemal infections among pregnant woman in Cotonou, Republic of Benin. Acta Trop 59:271–277, 1995.

295. Martin P, Andela A. Sexual and other infections of foetal interest during pregnancy in Yadunde, Cameroon [abstract]. VIII International Conference on AIDS, Amsterdam, The Netherlands, 1992.

296. Vial P, et al. Serologic screening for cytomegalovirus, rubella virus, herpes simplex virus, hepatitis B virus, and *Toxoplasma gondii* in two urban populations of pregnant women in Chile. Bull Pan Am Health Org 20:53–61, 1986.

297. Rong-guo S, Zheng-le L, De-cheng W. The prevalence of *Toxoplasma* infection among pregnant women and their newborn infants in Chengdu. Chung Hua Liu Hsing Ping Hsueh Tsa Chih 16:98–100, 1995.

298. Zhang W, Zhao R, Qiu H. [Toxoplasmosis infection in pregnant women in Lanzhou.] Chung Hua Fu Chan Ko Tsa Chih (in Chinese) 32:208–210, 1997.

299. Yu JC. [A seroepidemiological study on *Toxoplasma gondii* infection among pregnant women and neonates in Taiwan.] Taiwan I Hsueh Hui Tsa Chih (in Chinese) 84:286–295, 1985.

300. Gomez-Marin JE, Montoya-de-Londondo MT, Castano-Osorio JC. A maternal screening program for congenital toxoplasmosis in Quindio, Columbia and application of mathematical models to estimate incidences using age-stratified data. Am J Trop Med Hyg 57:180–186, 1997.

301. Candolfi E, Berg M, Kien T. Approche de la prévalence de la toxoplasmose a pointe-noire au Congo. Bull Soc Pathol Exot 86:358–362, 1993.

302. Lebech M, et al. Neonatal screening for congenital toxoplasmosis based on material seroconversion during pregnancy. Unpublished, 1996.

303. Lebech M, Petersen E. Neonatal screening for congenital toxoplasmosis in Denmark: presentation of the design of a prospective study. Scand J Infect Dis 84(Suppl):75–79, 1992.

304. El-Nawawy A, et al. Maternal and neonatal prevalence of *Toxoplasma* and cytomegalovirus (CMV) antibodies and hepatitis-B antigens in an Egyptian rural area. J Trop Pediatr 42:154–157, 1996.

305. Allain JP, Palmer CR, Pearson G. Epidemiological study of latent and recent infection by *Toxoplasma gondii* in pregnant women from a regional population in the U.K. J Infect 36:189–196, 1998.

306. Lappalainen M, et al. Incidence of primary *Toxoplasma* infections during pregnancy in Southern Finland: a prospective cohort study. Scand J Infect Dis 24:97–104, 1992.

307. Candolfi E, Wittersheim P, Kien T. Prevalence de la Toxoplasmose humaine à Strasbourg en 1992 (unpublished).

308. Nabias R, et al. [Serological investigation of toxoplasmosis in patients of the M.I.P. center of Franceville (Gabon).] Bull Soc Pathol Exot (in French) 91:318–320, 1998.

309. Barbier D, Ancelle T, Martin-Bouyer G. Seroepidemiological survey of toxoplasmosis in La Guadeloupe, French West Indies. Am J Trop Med Hyg 32:935–942, 1983.

310. Sander J, Niehaus C. [Incidence of primary toxoplasmosis infection in pregnant women.] Dtsch Med Wochenschr (in German) 108:455–457, 1983 (English summary, p 455).

311. Janitschke K, Busch W, Kellershofen C. [Direct agglutination as a tool for *Toxoplasma* control in pregnancy care.] Immun Infekt (in German) 16:189–191, 1988.

312. Krausse T, et al. Toxoplasmoscreening in der schwangershaft—ein pilotprogramm im Nordosten Deutschlands. Geburtshilfe Frauenheilkd 53:613–618, 1993.

313. Roos T, et al. Systematic serologic screening for toxoplasmosis in pregnancy. Obstet Gynecol 81:243–250, 1993.

314. Friese K, et al. Incidence of congenital infections. Geburtshilfe Frauenheilkd 51:890–896, 1991.

315. Decavalas G, et al. Prevalence of *Toxoplasma gondii* antibodies in gravidas and recently aborted women and study of risk factors. Eur J Epidemiol 6:223–226, 1990.

316. Sinibaldi J, De Ramirez I. Incidence of congenital toxoplasmosis in live Guatemalan newborns. Eur J Epidemiol 8:516–520, 1992.

317. Szenasi Z, et al. Prevention of congenital toxoplasmosis in Szeged, Hungary. Int J Epidemiol 26:428–435, 1997.

318. Mittal V, Bhatia R, Sehgal S. Prevalence of *Toxoplasma* antibodies among women with BOH and general population in Delhi. J Commun Dis 22:223–226, 1991.

319. Gandahusada S. Study on the prevalence of toxoplasmosis in Indonesia. Southeast Asian J Trop Med Public Health Suppl 1:93–98, 1991.

320. Ricci N, et al. [Epidemiology of toxoplasmosis: occurrence and risk of congenital toxoplasmosis in the province of Isernia.] Nuovi Ann Ig Microbiol (in Italian) 35:13–21, 1984.

321. Konishi E, et al. Prevalence of antibody to *Toxoplasma gondii* among pregnant women and umbilical cords in Hyogo Prefecture, Japan. Jpn J Parasitol 36:198–200, 1987.

322. Al-Nakib W, et al. Seroepidemiology of viral and toxoplasmal infections during pregnancy among Arab women of child-bearing age in Kuwait. Int J Epidemiol 12:220–223, 1983.

323. Monjour L, et al. An epidemiological survey of toxoplasmosis in Mauritania. Trop Geogr Med 35:21–25, 1983.

324. Guessous-Idrissi N, et al. [Toxoplasmosis and rubella in Moroccan women: results of a serological survey.] Pathol Biol (Paris) (in French) 32:761–765, 1984.

325. Rai SK, et al. Immuno-serological study of human toxoplasmosis in Nepal. *In* Third Congress Asia Pacific Societies of Pathologists and Eleventh National Convention Bangladesh Society of Pathologists, Bangladesh, 1993.

326. van der Veen J, Polak MF. Prevalence of *Toxoplasma* antibodies according to age with comments on the risk of prenatal infection. J Hyg (Lond) 85:165–174, 1980.

327. Klufio C, et al. The prevalence of *Toxoplasma* antibodies in pregnant patients attending the Port Moresby Gen-

eral Hospital antenatal clinic: a seroepidemiological survey. Papua New Guinea Med J 36:4–9, 1993.

328. Olusi T, Grob U, Ajayi J. High incidence of toxoplasmosis during pregnancy in Nigeria. Scand J Infect Dis 28:645–646, 1996.

329. Onadeko MO, Joynson DHM, Payne RA. The prevalence of *Toxoplasma* infection among pregnant women in Ibadan, Nigeria. J Trop Med Hyg 95:143–145, 1992.

330. Arene FO. The prevalence of toxoplasmosis among inhabitants of the Niger Delta. Fol Parasitol (Praha) 33:311–314, 1986.

331. Jenum PA, et al. Prevalence of *Toxoplasma gondii*–specific immunoglobulin G antibodies among pregnant women in Norway. Epidemiol Infect 120:87–92, 1998.

332. Sousa OE, Saenz RE, Frenkel JK. Toxoplasmosis in Panama: a 10-year study. Am J Trop Med Hyg 38:315–322, 1988.

333. Ziobrowski S. [Occurrence of positive toxoplasmosis reactions in mothers and newborn infants.] Klin Oczna (in Polish) 86:209–211, 1984.

334. Antunes F. Toxoplasmose, estudo la epidemiologia e da infeccao congenita na regiao de Lisboa. Fotocomposicao e Impressao: Santelmo, Portugal, Coop de Arted Graficas, C.R.L. Lisboa, Julho 1984.

335. Matos Aybar O, Mendoza HR. Prevalence of congenital toxoplasmosis in Santo Domingo. Arch Dominican Pediatr 18:137–144, 1982.

336. Al-Meshari AA, et al. Screening for toxoplasmosis in pregnancy. Int J Gynecol Obstet 29:39–45, 1982.

337. Williams KA, et al. Congenital toxoplasmosis: a prospective survey in the West of Scotland. J Infect 3:219–229, 1981.

338. Jackson MH, Hutchison WM, Siim JC. A seroepidemiological survey of toxoplasmosis in Scotland and England. Ann Trop Med Parasitol 81:359–365, 1987.

339. Logar J. Novak-Antolic Z, Zore A. Serological screening for toxoplasmosis in pregnancy in Slovenia. Scand J Infect Dis 27:163–164, 1995.

340. Sierra M, Lite J, Matas E. Significance of IgM antibodies to *Toxoplasma gondii* in pregnancy [abstract]. Fourth European Congress of Clinical Microbiology, Nice, France, 1989.

341. Ahlfors K, et al. Incidence of toxoplasmosis in pregnant women in the City of Malmo, Sweden. Scand J Infect Dis 21:315–321, 1989.

342. Sturchler D, Berger R, Just M. [Congenital toxoplasmosis in Switzerland: seroprevalence, risk factors and recommendations for prevention.] Schweiz Med Wochenschr (in German) 117:161–167, 1987.

343. Bornand JE, Piguet JD. Infestation toxoplasmique: prévalence, risque d'infection congénitale et évolution à Genéve de 1973 à 1987. Schweiz Med Wochenschr 121:21–29, 1991.

344. Zuber PLF, et al. *Toxoplasma* infection among pregnant women in Switzerland: a cross-sectional evaluation of regional and age-specific lifetime average annual incidence. Am J Epidemiol 141:659–666, 1995.

345. Doehring E, et al. *Toxoplasma gondii* antibodies in pregnant women and their newborns in Dar es Salaam, Tanzania. Am J Trop Med Hyg 52:546–548, 1995.

346. Morakote N, et al. Prevalence of *Toxoplasma* antibodies in Chiang Mai population. Southeast Asian J Trop Med Public Health 15:80–85, 1984.

347. Chintana T, et al. *Toxoplasma gondii* antibody in pregnant women with and without HIV infection. Southeast Asian J Trop Med Public Health 29:383–386, 1998.

348. Taechowisan T, et al. Immune status in congenital infections by TORCH agents in pregnant Thais. Asian Pac J Allergy Immunol 15:93–97, 1997.

349. Dilmen U, et al. Antenatal screening for toxoplasmosis [Letter to the editor]. Lancet 336:818–819, 1990.

350. Dar FK, et al. Gestational and neonatal toxoplasmosis: regional seroprevalence in the United Arab Emirates. Eur J Epidemiol 13:567–571, 1997.

351. Stojanovic D. [The effect of toxoplasmosis on occurrence of spontaneous abortions and anomalies in neonates in the Timok region.] Vojnosanit Pregl (in Serbo-Croatian [Cyrillic]) 55:151–159, 1998.

352. Logar J, et al. Incidence of congenital toxoplasmosis in the Republic of Slovenia. Scand J Infect Dis 24:105–108, 1992.

353. Logar J. Toxoplasmosis in Slovenia, one of the socialist republics of Yugoslavia [abstract]. Abstracts of the 5th International Congress of Parasitology, Toronto, August 7–14, 1982, p 540.

354. Ades A, et al. Maternal prevalence of *Toxoplasma* antibody based on anonymous neonatal serosurvey: a geographical analysis. Epidemiol Infect 110:127–133, 1993.

355. Ancelle T, et al. La toxoplasmose chez la femme enceinte en France en 1995. Bull Epidemiol Hebdomadaire Direction Generale Santé 51:227–228, 1996.

356. Thoumsin H, Senterre J, Lambotte R. Twenty-two years screening for toxoplasmosis in pregnancy: Liege, Belgium. Scand J Infect Dis 84(Suppl):82–83, 1992.

357. Dubey JP, et al. Sources and reservoirs of *Toxoplasma gondii* infection on 47 swine farms in Illinois. J Parasitol 81:723–729, 1995.

358. Edelhofer R, Aspöck H. Modes and sources of infections with *Toxoplasma gondii* in view of the screening of pregnant women in Austria. Mitt Osterr Ges Tropenmed Parasitol 18:59–70, 1996.

359. Papoz L, et al. A simple model relevant to toxoplasmosis applied to epidemiologic results in France. Arch Pathol Lab Med 110:42–46, 1986.

360. Larsen SO, Lebech M. Models for prediction of the frequency of toxoplasmosis in pregnancy in situations changing infection rates. Int J Epidemiol 23:1309–1314, 1994.

361. Lelong M, et al. [Thoughts on 7 cases of congenital toxoplasmosis: different clinical aspects of this infirmity.] Arch Fr Pediatr (in French) 15:433–448, 1959.

362. Jeannel D, et al. Epidemiology of toxoplasmosis among pregnant women in the Paris area. Int J Epidemiol 17:595–602, 1988.

363. Bronstein R. Toxoplasmose et grossesse. Concours Med 104:4177–4186, 1982.

364. Frenkel JK. *Toxoplasma* in and around us. Bio Sci 23:343–352, 1973.

365. Papoz L, et al. A simple model relevant to toxoplasmosis applied to epidemiologic results in France. Am J Epidemiol 123:154–161, 1986.

366. Koppe JG, Loewer-Sieger DH, De Roever-Bonnet H. Results of 20-year follow-up of congenital toxoplasmosis. Am J Ophthalmol 101:248–249, 1986.

367. Koppe JG, Kloosterman GJ. Congenital toxoplasmosis: long-term follow-up. Padiatr Padol 17:171–179, 1982.

368. Hunter K, et al. Prenatal screening of pregnant women for infections caused by cytomegalovirus, Epstein-Barr virus, herpesvirus, rubella, and *Toxoplasma gondii*. Am J Obstet Gynecol 145:269–273, 1983.

369. Naot Y, Desmonts G, Remington JS. IgM enzyme-linked immunosorbent assay test for the diagnosis of congenital *Toxoplasma* infection. J Pediatr 98:32–36, 1981.

370. Lebech M, et al. Feasibility of neonatal screening for

Toxoplasma infection in the absence of prenatal treatment. Danish Congenital Toxoplasmosis Study Group. Lancet 353:1834–1837, 1999.

371. Lynfield R, Hsu HW, Guerina NG. Screening methods for congenital *Toxoplasma* and risk of disease. Lancet 353:1899–1900, 1990.

372. Lebech M, Petersen E, Angeborene D. Toxoplasmose-Studiengruppe, Neonatal screening for congenital toxoplasmosis in Denmark based on maternal seroconversion during pregnancy. Mitt Osterr Ges Tropenmed Parasitol 18:33–40, 1996.

373. Labadie MD, Hazemann JJ. [Contribution of health check-ups in children to the detection and epidemiologic study of congenital toxoplasmosis.] Ann Pediatr (Paris) (in French) 31:823–828, 1984.

374. Aspöck H, Pollak A. Prevention of prenatal toxoplasmosis by serological screening of pregnant women in Austria. Scand J Infect Dis Suppl 84:32–37, 1992.

375. Aspöck H. Österreichs Betrag zur Toxoplasmose-Forschung und 20 Jahre Toxoplasmose-Überwachung der Schwangeren in Österreich. Mitt Österr Ges Tropenmed Parasitol 18:59–70, 1996.

376. Darde ML, Bouteille B, Pestre-Alexandre M. Isoenzymic characterization of seven strains of *Toxoplasma gondii* by isoelectrofocusing in polyacrylamide gels. Am J Trop Med Hyg 39:551–558, 1988.

377. Sibley LD, Boothroyd JC. Virulent strains of *Toxoplasma gondii* comprise a single clonal lineage. Nature 359:82–85, 1992.

378. Darde ML, Bouteille B, Pestre-Alexandre M. Isoenzyme analysis of 35 *Toxoplasma gondii* isolates and the biological and epidemiological implications. J Parasitol 78:786–794, 1992.

379. Howe DK, Sibley DL. *Toxoplasma gondii* comprises three clonal lineages: correlation of parasite genotype with human disease. J Infect Dis 172:1561–1566, 1995.

380. Howe DK, et al. Determination of genotypes of *Toxoplasma gondii* strains isolated from patients with toxoplasmosis. J Clin Microbiol 35:1411–1414, 1997.

381. Wilson CB, Remington JS. Activity of human blood leukocytes against *Toxoplasma gondii*. J Infect Dis 140:890–895, 1979.

382. Wilson CB, Tsai V, Remington JS. Failure to trigger the oxidative metabolic burst by normal macrophages: possible mechanism for survival of intracellular pathogens. J Exp Med 151:328–346, 1980.

383. McLeod R, et al. Effects of human peripheral blood monocytes, monocyte-derived macrophages, and spleen mononuclear phagocytes on *Toxoplasma gondii*. Cell Immunol 54:330–350, 1980.

384. Catterall JR, et al. Nonoxidative microbicidal activity in normal human alveolar and peritoneal macrophages. Infect Immun 55:1635–1640, 1987.

385. Brown C, Estes R, McLeod R. Fate of an intracellular parasite during lysis of its host cell by cytotoxic T cells. 1995 (unpublished).

386. Yamashita K, et al. Cytotoxic T-lymphocyte–mediated lysis of *Toxoplasma gondii*–infected target cells does not lead to death of intracellular parasites [In Process Citation]. Infect Immun 66:4651–4655, 1998.

387. Huldt G. Experimental toxoplasmosis: parasitemia in guinea pigs. Acta Pathol Microbiol Scand 58:457–470, 1963.

388. Jadin JM, Creemers J. [Ultrastructure and biology of *Toxoplasma*: III. Observations on intraerythrocytic *Toxoplasma* in a mammal.] Acta Trop (in French) 25:267–270, 1968.

389. Frenkel JK. Pathogenesis of toxoplasmosis with a consideration of cyst rupture in *Besnoitia* infection. Surv Ophthalmol 6:799–825, 1961.

390. Krahenbuhl JL, Gaines JD, Remington JS. Lymphocyte transformation in human toxoplasmosis. J Infect Dis 125:283–288, 1972.

391. Anderson SEJ, Krahenbuhl JL, Remington JS. Longitudinal studies of lymphocyte response to *Toxoplasma* antigen in humans infected with *T. gondii*. J Clin Lab Immunol 2:293–297, 1979.

392. Subauste CS, Dawson L, Remington JS. Human lymphokine-activated killer cells are cytotoxic against cells infected with *Toxoplasma gondii*. J Exp Med 176:1511–1519, 1992.

393. Subauste CS, et al. Preferential activation and expansion of human peripheral blood T cells in response to *Toxoplasma gondii* in vitro and their cytokine production and cytotoxic activity against *T. gondii*–infected cells. J Clin Invest 96:610–619, 1995.

394. Subauste CS, et al. T cell response to *Toxoplasma gondii* in previously unexposed individuals. J Immunol 160:3403–3411, 1998.

395. Purner MB, Berens RL, Nash PB, et al. CD4-mediated and CD8-mediated cytotoxic and proliferative immune responses to *Toxoplasma gondii* in seropositive humans. Infect Immun 64:4330–4338, 1996.

396. Lea RG, Calder AA. The immunology of pregnancy. Curr Opin Infect Dis 10:171–176, 1997.

397. Raghupathy R. Th1-type immunity is incompatible with successful pregnancy [see comments]. Immunol Today 18:478–482, 1997.

398. Hunter CA, Remington JS. Immunopathogenesis of toxoplasmic encephalitis. J Infect Dis 170:1057–1067, 1994.

399. Lewis WP, Markell EP. Acquisition of immunity to toxoplasmosis by the newborn rat. Exp Parasitol 7:463–467, 1958.

400. Harboe A, Erichsen S. Toxoplasmosis in chickens: III. Attempts to provoke a systemic disease in chickens by infection with a chicken strain and a human strain of toxoplasma. APMIS 35:495–502, 1954.

401. Kohler PF. Maturation of the human complement system: I. Onset time and site of fetal C1q, C4, C3, and C5 synthesis. J Clin Invest 52:671–677, 1973.

402. Johnston RB Jr, et al. Complement in the newborn infant. Pediatrics 64(Suppl):781–786, 1979.

403. Deckert-Schlüter M, Schlüter D, Theisen F, et al. Activation of the innate immune system in murine congenital *Toxoplasma* encephalitis. J Neuroimmunol 53:47–51, 1994.

404. Beverley JK, et al. Age-sex distribution of various diseases with particular reference to toxoplasmic lymphadenopathy. J Hyg (Lond) 76:215–228, 1976.

405. Kittas C, Henry L. Effect of sex hormones on the response of mice to infection with *Toxoplasma gondii*. Br J Exp Pathol 61:590–600, 1980.

406. Kittas S, et al. A histological and immunohistochemical study of the changes induced in the brains of white mice by infection with *Toxoplasma gondii*. Br J Exp Pathol 65:67–74, 1984.

407. Mack D, et al. Role of murine and human MHC class II genes in pathogenesis of and protection against toxoplasmosis. Fourth International Biennial Toxoplasma Conference, Drymen, Scotland, 1996.

408. Suzuki Y, et al. Evidence for genetic regulation of susceptibility to toxoplasmic encephalitis in AIDS patients. J Infect Dis 173:265–268, 1996.

409. Werner H, Egger I. [Protective effect of *Toxoplasma*

antibody against re-infection.] Trop Med Parasitol (in German) 24:174–180, 1973.

410. Rodhain J. Formation de pseudokystes au cours d'essais d'immunité croisée entre souches différentes de toxoplasmes. C R Soc Biol (Paris) 144:719–722, 1950.

411. Dubey JP, Frenkel JK. Experimental *Toxoplasma* infection in mice with strains producing oocysts. J Parasitol 59:505–512, 1973.

412. de Roever-Bonnet H. Mice and golden hamsters infected with an avirulent and virulent *Toxoplasma* strain. Trop Geogr Med 15:45–60, 1963.

413. Nakayama I. Persistence of the virulent RH strain of *Toxoplasma gondii* in the brains of immune mice. Keio J Med 13:7–12, 1964.

414. Remington JS, in discussion, Zimmerman LE. Ocular pathology of toxoplasmosis. Surv Ophthalmol 6:832–856, 1961.

415. Werner H, Pichl H. [Comparative investigations on cyst-forming *Toxoplasma* strains: II. Development of cysts and formation of humoral antibodies.] Zentralbl Bakteriol (in German) 210:402–416, 1969.

416. van der Waaij D. Formation, growth and multiplication of *Toxoplasma gondii* cysts in mouse brains. Trop Geogr Med 11:345–370, 1959.

417. Huldt G. Studies on experimental toxoplasmosis. Ann NY Acad Sci 177:146–155, 1971.

418. Yano A, et al. Antigen presentation by *Toxoplasma gondii*–infected cells to CD4+ proliferative T cells and CD8+ cytotoxic cells. J Parasitol 75:411–416, 1989.

419. Purner MB, Berens RL, Nash PB, et al. CD4-mediated and CD8-mediated cytotoxic and proliferative immune responses to *Toxoplasma gondii* in seropositive humans. Infect Immun 64:4330–4338, 1996.

420. Ito S, et al. Demonstration by microscopy of parasitemia in animals experimentally infected with *Toxoplasma gondii*. Natl Inst Anim Health Q (Tokyo) 6:8–23, 1966.

421. Beverley JKA. A rational approach to the treatment of toxoplasmic uveitis. Trans Ophthalmol Soc 78:109–121, 1958.

422. Remington JS, Hackman R. Changes in serum proteins of rats infected with *Toxoplasma gondii*. J Parasitol 51:865–870, 1965.

423. Remington JS, Hackman R. Changes in mouse serum proteins during acute and chronic infection with an intracellular parasite (*Toxoplasma gondii*). J Immunol 95:1023–1033, 1966.

424. Araujo FG, Remington JS. Immune response to intracellular parasites: suppression by antibody. Proc Soc Exp Biol Med 139:254–258, 1972.

425. Araujo FG, Remington JS. IgG antibody suppression of the IgM antibody response to *Toxoplasma gondii* in newborn rabbits. J Immunol 115:335–338, 1975.

426. Canessa A, et al. An in vitro model for *Toxoplasma* infection in man: interaction between CD4+ monoclonal T cells and macrophages results in killing of trophozoites. J Immunol 140:3580–3588, 1988.

427. Saavedra R, Herion P. Human T-cell clones against *Toxoplasma gondii*: production of interferon-, interleukin-2, and strain cross-reactivity. Parasitol Res 77:379–385, 1991.

428. McLeod R, et al. Secretory IgA, antibody to SAG1, H-2 Class I–restricted CD8+ T-lymphocytes and the Int-1 locus in protection against *Toxoplasma gondii*. In Smith J (ed). Toxoplasmosis. Series H: Cell Biology. New York, Springer-Verlag, 1993, pp 131–151.

429. de Paoli P, et al. Phenotypic profile and functional characteristics of human gamma and delta T cells during acute toxoplasmosis. J Clin Microbiol 30:729–731, 1992.

430. Scalise F, et al. Lymphocytes bearing the T-cell receptor in acute toxoplasmosis. Immunology 76:668–670, 1992.

430a. Hara T, Ohashi S, Yamashita Y, et al. Human Vδ2+ γδ T-cell tolerance to foreign antigens of *Toxoplasma gondii*. Proc Natl Acad Sci U S A 93:5136–5140, 1996.

431. Suzuki Y, et al. Interferon-γ: the major mediator of resistance against *Toxoplasma gondii*. Science 240:516–518, 1988.

432. Michie C, Harvey D. Can expression of CD45RO, a T-cell surface molecule, be used to detect congenital infection? Lancet 343:1259–1260, 1994.

433. McLeod R, et al. Phenotypes and functions of lymphocytes in congenital toxoplasmosis. J Lab Clin Med 116:623–635, 1990.

434. Strickland GT, Petitt LE, Voller A. Immunodepression in mice infected with *Toxoplasma gondii*. Am J Trop Med Hyg 22:452–455, 1973.

435. Hibbs JB Jr, Remington JS, Stewart CC. Modulation of immunity and host resistance by micro-organisms. Pharmacol Ther 8:37–69, 1980.

436. Huldt G, Gard S, Olovson SG. Effect of *Toxoplasma gondii* on the thymus. Nature 244:301–303, 1973.

437. Hibbs JB, Lambert LH, Remington JS. Activated macrophage-mediated nonspecific tumor resistance [abstract]. J Reticul Soc 13:368, 1973.

438. Luft BJ, Remington JS. Effect of pregnancy on resistance to *Listeria monocytogenes* and *Toxoplasma gondii* infections in mice. Infect Immun 38:1164–1171, 1982.

439. Tremonti L, Walton BC. Blast transformation and migration-inhibition in toxoplasmosis and leishmaniasis. Am J Trop Med Hyg 19:49–56, 1970.

440. Luft BJ, et al. Functional and quantitative alterations in T lymphocyte subpopulations in acute toxoplasmosis. J Infect Dis 150:761–767, 1984.

441. De Waele M, et al. Activated T-cells with suppressor/cytotoxic phenotype in acute *Toxoplasma gondii* infection. Clin Exp Immunol 62:256–261, 1985.

442. O'Connor GR. The influence of hypersensitivity on the pathogenesis of ocular toxoplasmosis. Trans Am Ophthalmol Soc 68:501–547, 1970.

443. Dutton GN. The causes of tissue damage in toxoplasmic retinochoroiditis. Trans Ophthalmol Soc UK 105:404–412, 1986.

444. O'Connor GR. Ocular toxoplasmosis. Trans New Orleans Acad Ophthalmol 108–121, 1983.

445. Holland GN, et al. Toxoplasmosis. *In* Pepose JS, Holland GN, Wilhelmus KR (eds). Ocular Infection and Immunity. St. Louis, Mosby–Year Book, 1996, pp 1183–1223.

446. Roberts F, McLeod R. Pathogenesis of toxoplasmic retinochoroiditis. Parasitol Today 15:51–57, 1999.

447. Hay J, et al. Congenital toxoplasmic retinochoroiditis in a mouse model. Ann Trop Med Parasitol 78:109–116, 1984.

448. Hay J, et al. Congenital neuro-ophthalmic toxoplasmosis in the mouse. Ann Trop Med Parasitol 81:25–28, 1987.

449. Hutchison WM, et al. A study of cataract in murine congenital toxoplasmosis. Ann Trop Med Parasitol 76:53–70, 1982.

450. Hay J, Dutton GN, Ralston J. Congenital toxoplasmic retinochoroiditis in the mouse—the use of the peroxidase anti-peroxidase method to demonstrate *Toxoplasma* antigen. Trans R Soc Trop Med Hyg 79:106–109, 1985.

451. Dutton GN, et al. Clinicopathological features of a

congenital murine model of ocular toxoplasmosis. Graefes Arch Clin Exp Ophthalmol 224:256–264, 1986.

452. Graham DI, et al. Encephalitis in mice with congenital ocular toxoplasmosis. J Pathol 142:265–277, 1984.

453. Frenkel JK. Pathogenesis of toxoplasmosis and of infections with organisms resembling *Toxoplasma*. Ann NY Acad Sci 64:215–251, 1956.

454. Rollins DF, et al. Detection of toxoplasmal antigen and antibody in ocular fluids in experimental ocular toxoplasmosis. Arch Ophthalmol 101:455–457, 1983.

455. Mets MB, et al. Eye manifestations of congenital toxoplasmosis. Am J Ophthalmol 122:309–324, 1996.

456. Montoya JG, et al. Use of the polymerase chain reaction for diagnosis of ocular toxoplasmosis. Ophthalmology 106:1554–1563, 1999.

457. Chan C-C, et al. Diagnosis of ocular toxoplasmosis by the use of immunocytology and the polymerase chain reaction. Am J Ophthalmol 117:803–805, 1994.

458. Manners R, et al. Use of the polymerase chain reaction in the diagnosis of acquired ocular toxoplasmosis in an immunocompetent adult. Br J Ophthalmol 78:583–584, 1994.

459. Norose K, Tokushima T, Yano A. Quantitative polymerase chain reaction in diagnosing ocular toxoplasmosis. Am J Ophthalmol 121:441–442, 1996.

460. Roberts F, Mets M, Ferguson D, et al. The histopathological features of ocular toxoplasmosis in the fetus and infant. Presented by F. Roberts. Fifth International Toxoplasma Conference, Marshall, Calif, May 1–6, 1999.

461. Araujo FG, Remington JS. Induction of tolerance to an intracellular protozoan *(Toxoplasma gondii)* by passively administered antibody. J Immunol 113:1424–1428, 1974.

462. Crawford JB. *Toxoplasma* retinochoroiditis. Arch Ophthalmol 76:829–832, 1966.

463. Hogan MJ, Kimura SJ, O'Connor R. Ocular toxoplasmosis. Clin Sci 72:592–600, 1964.

464. Jacobs L, Fair MJR, Bickerton MJH. Adult ocular toxoplasmosis: a preliminary report of a parasitologically proved case. Arch Ophthalmol 51:287, 1954.

465. Hogan MJ, Zweigart PA, Lewis AB. Recovery of *Toxoplasma* from a human eye. Arch Ophthalmol 60:548–554, 1958.

466. Montoya JG, Remington JS. Toxoplasmic chorioretinitis in the setting of acute acquired toxoplasmosis. Clin Infect Dis 23:277–282, 1996.

467. Couvreur J, Thulliez P. [Acquired toxoplasmosis with ocular or neurologic involvement.] Presse Med (in French) 25:438–442, 1996.

468. Callahan WP Jr, Russell WO, Smith M. Human toxoplasmosis. Medicine 25:343–397, 1946.

469. Hayes K, et al. Cell culture isolation of *Toxoplasma gondii* from an infant with unusual ocular features. Med J Aust 1:1297–1299, 1973.

470. Manschot WA, Daamen CB. Connatal ocular toxoplasmosis. Arch Ophthalmol 74:48–54, 1965.

471. Pratt-Thomas HR, Cannon WM. Systemic infantile toxoplasmosis. Am J Pathol 22:779–795, 1946.

472. Milgram JW. Osseous changes in congenital toxoplasmosis. Arch Pathol 97:150–151, 1974.

473. Zuelzer WW. Infantile toxoplasmosis, with a report of three cases, including two in which the patients were identical twins. Arch Pathol 38:1–19, 1944.

474. Mellgren J, Alm L, Kjessler A. The isolation of *Toxoplasma* from the human placenta and uterus. Separatum Acta Pathologica 30:59–67, 1952.

475. Elliott WG. Placental toxoplasmosis: a report of a case. Am J Clin Pathol 53:413–417, 1970.

476. Benirschke K, Driscoll SG. The Pathology of the Human Placenta. New York, Springer-Verlag, 1967, p 512.

477. Werner H, Schmidtke L, Thomascheck G. [*Toxoplasma* infection and pregnancy: histologic demonstration of the intrauterine route of infection.] Klin Wochenschr (in German) 41:96–101, 1963.

478. Driscoll SG. Fetal infections in man. *In* Benirschke K (ed). Comparative Aspects of Reproductive Failure. New York, Springer-Verlag, 1996, pp 270–295.

479. Farber S, Craig JM. Clinical Pathological Conference (Children's Medical Center, Boston, Mass). J Pediatr 49:752–764, 1956.

480. Cardoso RA, et al. Congenital toxoplasmosis. *In* Siim JC (ed): Human Toxoplasmosis. Copenhagen, Munksgaard, 1960, pp 20–33.

481. Piche M, Battaglione V, Monticelli I, et al. [Placenta toxoplasmosis in the course of AIDS. Immunohistochemical and ultrastructural study of a case.] Ann Pathol (in French) 17:337–339, 1997.

482. Garcia AG, et al. Placental morphology of newborns at risk for congenital toxoplasmosis. J Trop Pediatr 29:95–103, 1983.

483. Altshuler G. Toxoplasmosis as a cause of hydranencephaly. Am J Dis Child 125:251–252, 1973.

484. Rodney MB, et al. Infantile toxoplasmosis: report of a case with autopsy. Pediatrics 5:649–663, 1950.

485. Wolf A, Cowen D, Paige BH. Toxoplasmic encephalomyelitis: VI. Clinical diagnosis of infantile or congenital toxoplasmosis: survival beyond infancy. Am J Pathol 48:689–739, 1942.

486. Hervas JA, et al. Central nervous system congenital toxoplasmosis mimicking brain abscesses. Pediatr Infect Dis J 6:491–492, 1987.

487. Frenkel JK. Pathology and pathogenesis of congenital toxoplasmosis. Bull NY Acad Med 50:182–191, 1974.

488. Frenkel JK. Toxoplasmosis: mechanisms of infection, laboratory diagnosis and management. Curr Top Pathol 54:27–75, 1971.

489. McAuley J, Roizen N, Patel D, et al. Early and longitudinal evaluations of treated infants and children and untreated historical patients with congenital toxoplasmosis: the Chicago Collaborative Treatment Trial. Clin Infect Dis 18:38–72, 1994.

490. Heath P, Zuelzer WW. Toxoplasmosis (report of eye findings in infant twins). Trans Am Ophthalmol Soc 42:119–131, 1944.

491. Koch FL, et al. Toxoplasmic encephalomyelitis: VII. Significance of ocular lesions in the diagnosis of infantile or congenital toxoplasmosis. Arch Ophthalmol 29:1–25, 1943.

492. Bamatter F. La choriorétinite toxoplasmique. Ophthalmologica 114:340–358, 1947.

493. Binkhorst CD. Toxoplasmosis: report of four cases, with demonstration of parasites in one case. Ophthalmologica 115:65–67, 1948.

494. Hogan MJ. Toxoplasmic chorioretinitis. Trans Pac Coast Otoophthalmol Soc 28:83–102, 1947.

495. Hogan MJ. Ocular Toxoplasmosis. New York, Columbia University Press, 1951, p 86.

496. Kelemen G. Toxoplasmosis and congenital deafness. Arch Ophthalmol 68:547–561, 1958.

497. Couvreur J. [The lungs in toxoplasmosis.] Rev Mal Respir (in French) 3:525–532, 1975.

498. Pomeroy C, Filice GA. Pulmonary toxoplasmosis: a review. Clin Infect Dis 14:863–870, 1992.

499. Garcia AG, Torres AC, Pegado CS. Congenital toxo-

plasmic myocarditis: case report of an unusual presentation. Ann Trop Paediatr 5:227–230, 1985.

500. Medlock MD, Tilleli JT, Pearl GS. Congenital cardiac toxoplasmosis in a newborn with acquired immunodeficiency syndrome. Pediatr Infect Dis J 9:129–132, 1990.

501. Lelong M, Lepage F, Alison F, et al. Toxoplasmose du nouveau-né avec ictére et cirrhose du foie. Arch Fr Pediatr 10:530–536, 1953.

502. Caldera R, Sarrut S, Rossier A. [Hepatic calcifications in the course of congenital toxoplasmosis.] Arch Fr Pediatr (in French) 19:1087–1093, 1962.

503. Israelski DM, et al. *Toxoplasma* peritonitis in a patient with acquired immunodeficiency syndrome. Arch Intern Med 148:1655–1657, 1988.

504. Kean BH, Grocott RG. Sarcosporidiosis or toxoplasmosis in man and guinea pig. Am J Pathol 21:467–483, 1945.

505. Miller MJ, Seaman E, Remington JS. The clinical spectrum of congenital toxoplasmosis: problems in recognition. J Pediatr 70:714–723, 1967.

506. Fediushina NA, Sherstennikova GE. [Damage of the kidneys in congenital toxoplasmosis.] Vrach Delo (in Russian) 4:121–122, 1966.

507. Wickbom B, Winberg J. Coincidence of congenital toxoplasmosis and acute nephritis with nephrotic syndrome. Acta Paediatr Scand 61:470–472, 1972.

508. Guignard JP, Torrado A. Interstitial nephritis and toxoplasmosis in a 10-year-old child. J Pediatr 85:381–382, 1974.

509. Shahin B, Papadopoulou ZL, Jenis EH. Congenital nephrotic syndrome associated with congenital toxoplasmosis. J Pediatr 85:366–370, 1974.

510. Couvreur J, et al. [The kidney and toxoplasmosis.] Ann Pediatr (in French) 31:847–852, 1984.

511. Torres CM. Affinité de l'encephalitozoon chagasi agent étiologique d'une méningoencephalomyélitis congénitale avec myocardite et myosite chez l'homme. C R Soc Biol 86:1797–1799, 1927.

512. Alford CA Jr, Stagno S, Reynolds DW. Congenital toxoplasmosis: clinical, laboratory, and therapeutic considerations, with special reference to subclinical disease. Bull N Y Acad Med 50:160–181, 1974.

513. Willi H, Koller F, Raaflaub J. Symptomatische makroglobulinamie bei lues congenita; beitrag zur frage der "fibrinasthenie" faconi. Acta Haematol 11:316–320, 1954.

514. Koch F, Schlagetter K, Schultze HE, et al. Symptomatische makroglobulinamie bei les connata. Z Kinderheilkd 78:283–300, 1956.

515. Oehme J. Symptomatische makroglobulinamie bei lues connata. Klin Wochenschr 36:369–382, 1958.

516. Koch F, Schultze HE, Schwick G. [Symptomatic Makroglobulinamie in congenital toxoplasmosis.] Z Kinderheilkd (in German) 82:44–49, 1959.

517. Oxelius VA. Monoclonal immunoglobulins in congenital toxoplasmosis. Clin Exp Immunol 11:367–380, 1972.

518. Aiuti F, Ungari S, Turbessi G, et al. Immunologic aspects of congenital syphilis. Helv Paediatr Acta 21:66–71, 1966.

519. Van Camp B, Reynaert P, Van Beers D. Congenital toxoplasmosis associated with transient monoclonal IgGl-lambda gammopathy. Rev Infect Dis 4:173–178, 1982.

520. Griscelli C, et al. Congenital toxoplasmosis: fetal synthesis of oligoclonal immunoglobulin G in intrauterine infection. J Pediatr 83:20–26, 1973.

521. Arnaud JP, et al. [Hematological and immunological

522. Vinh LT, et al. Association of congenital toxoplasmosis and cytomegaly in infants: study of two anatomo-clinical cases. Arch Fr Pediatr 27:511–521, 1970.

523. Sotelo-Avila C, et al. Coexistent congenital cytomegalovirus and toxoplasmosis in a newborn infant. J Tenn Med Assoc 67:588–592, 1974.

524. Maszkiewicz W, Wojnar A, Sujakowa A, Ostrowska-Ryng W. [Coexistence of cytomegalic inclusion disease, toxoplasmosis and in a premature infant.] Pediatr Pol (in Polish) 57:821–826, 1982.

525. De Zegher F, et al. Concomitant cytomegalovirus infection and congenital toxoplasmosis in a newborn. Eur J Pediatr 147:424–425, 1988.

526. Demian SD, Donnelly WJ, Monif GR. Coexistent congenital cytomegalovirus and toxoplasmosis in a stillborn. Am J Dis Child 125:420–421, 1973.

527. Stanton MF, Pinkerton H. Benign acquired toxoplasmosis with subsequent pregnancy. Am J Clin Pathol 23:1199–1207, 1953.

528. Remington JS, et al. Toxoplasmosis and infectious mononucleosis. Arch Intern Med 110:744–753, 1962.

529. Siim JC. Clinical and diagnostic aspects of human acquired toxoplasmosis. Human Toxoplasmosis 53–79, 1960.

530. Tenhunen A. Glandular Toxoplasmosis: Occurrence of the Disease in Finland. Helsinki, Finland, Department of Pathology, University of Helsinki, 1964, pp 9–72.

531. Beverley JKA, Beattie CP. Glandular toxoplasmosis: a survey of 30 cases. Lancet 2:379–384, 1958.

532. Remington JS. Toxoplasmosis in the adult. Bull NY Acad Med 50:211–227, 1974.

533. Joseph R, et al. Abdominal lymphadenopathy as first localization of acquired toxoplasmosis. Human Toxoplasmosis 120–123, 1960.

534. Jones TC, Kean BH, Kimball AC. Acquired toxoplasmosis. NY State J Med 69:2237–2242, 1969.

535. Vischer TL, Bernheim C, Engelbrecht E. Two cases of hepatitis due to *Toxoplasma gondii*. Lancet 2:919–921, 1967.

536. Masur H, Jones TC. Hepatitis in acquired toxoplasmosis [Letter to the editor]. N Engl J Med 301:613, 1979.

537. Frenkel JK, Remington JS. Hepatitis in toxoplasmosis [Letter to the editor with reply]. N Engl J Med 302:178–179, 1980.

538. Weitberg AB, et al. Acute granulomatous hepatitis in the course of acquired toxoplasmosis. N Engl J Med 300:1093–1096, 1979.

539. Vethanyagam A, Bryceson ADM. Acquired toxoplasmosis presenting as hepatitis. Trans R Soc Trop Med Hyg 70:524–525, 1976.

540. Greenlee JE, et al. Adult toxoplasmosis presenting as polymyositis and cerebellar ataxia. Ann Intern Med 82:367–371, 1975.

541. Samuels BS, Rietschel RL. Polymyositis and toxoplasmosis. JAMA 235:60–61, 1976.

542. Phillips PE, Kassan SS, Kagen LJ. Increased *Toxoplasma* antibodies in idiopathic inflammatory muscle disease: a case-controlled study. Arthritis Rheum 22:209–214, 1979.

543. Kagen LJ, Kimball AC, Christian CL. Serologic evidence of toxoplasmosis among patients with polymyositis. Am J Med 56:186–191, 1974.

544. Pollock JL. Toxoplasmosis appearing to be dermatomyositis. Arch Dermatol 115:736–737, 1979.

545. Pointud P, et al. [Positive toxoplasmic serology in poly-

myositis.] Ann Med Interne (Paris) (in French) 127:881–885, 1976.

546. Topi GC, et al. Dermatomyositis-like syndrome due to *Toxoplasma*. Br J Dermatol 101:589–591, 1979.

547. Gump DW, Holden RA. Acquired chorioretinitis due to toxoplasmosis. Ann Intern Med 90:58–60, 1979.

548. Masur H, et al. Outbreak of toxoplasmosis in a family and documentation of acquired retinochoroiditis. Am J Med 64:396–402, 1978.

549. Michelson JB, et al. Retinitis secondary to acquired systemic toxoplasmosis with isolation of the parasite. Am J Ophthalmol 86:548–552, 1978.

550. Saari M, et al. Acquired toxoplasmic chorioretinitis. Arch Ophthalmol 94:1485–1488, 1976.

551. Wising PJ. Lymphadenopathy and chorioretinitis in acute adult toxoplasmosis. Nord Med 47:563–565, 1952.

552. Eichenwald HF. A study of congenital toxoplasmosis, with particular emphasis on clinical manifestations, sequelae and therapy. *In* Siim JC (ed). Human Toxoplasmosis. Copenhagen, Munksgaard, 1960, p 41.

553. Feldman HA. Toxoplasmosis. Pediatrics 22:559–574, 1958.

554. Alford C, et al. Subclinical central nervous system disease of neonates: a prospective study of infants born with increased levels of IgM. J Pediatr 75:1167–1178, 1969.

555. Wilson CB, Remington JS, Stagno S, Reynolds DW. Development of adverse sequelae in children born with subclinical congenital *Toxoplasma* infection. Pediatrics 66:767–774, 1980.

556. Koppe JG, et al. Toxoplasmosis and pregnancy, with a long-term follow-up of the children. Eur J Obstet Gynecol Reprod Biol 4:101–110, 1974.

557. De Roever-Bonnet H, Koppe JG, Loewer-Sieger DH. Follow-up of children with congenital *Toxoplasma* infection and children who become serologically negative after 1 year of age, all born in 1964–1965. *In* Thalhammer O, Baumgarten K, Pollak A (eds). Perinatal Medicine, Sixth European Congress. Stuttgart, Georg Thieme, 1969, pp 61–75.

558. Rossier A, Blancher G, Designolle L, et al. Toxoplasmose congénitale à manifestation retardée: effet du traitement. Sem Hop 37:1266–1268, 1961.

559. Couvreur J, Desmonts G. Congenital and maternal toxoplasmosis: a review of 300 congenital cases. Dev Med Child Neurol 4:519–530, 1962.

560. Couvreur J, et al. [A homogeneous series of 210 cases of congenital toxoplasmosis in 0 to 11-month-old infants detected prospectively.] Ann Pediatr (Paris) (in French) 31:815–819, 1984.

561. Foulon W, et al. Treatment of toxoplasmosis during pregnancy: a multicenter study of impact on fetal transmission and children's sequelae at age 1 year. Am J Obstet Gynecol 180:410–415, 1999.

562. Guerina N, et al. Neonatal serologic screening and early treatment for congenital *Toxoplasma gondii* infection. N Engl J Med 330:1858–1863, 1994.

563. Sever JL. Perinatal infections affecting the developing fetus and newborn. *In* Eichenwald HF (ed). The Prevention of Mental Retardation Through Control of Infectious Diseases. Public Health Service Publication No. 1692. Washington, DC, U.S. Government Printing Office, 1968, pp 37–68.

564. Paul J. Früngeburt und Toxoplasmose. Munich, Urban & Schwarzenberg, 1962.

565. Couvreur J, Desmonts G, Girre JY. Congenital toxoplasmosis in twins: a series of 14 pairs of twins: absence of infection in one twin in two pairs. J Pediatr 89:235–240, 1976.

566. Abbott KH, Camp JD. Extensive symmetrical cerebral calcification and chorioretinitis in identical twins (toxoplasmosis?): clinical report of cases. Bull Los Angeles Neurol Soc 12:38–47, 1947.

567. Fendel H. Eine toxoplasmotische Zwillingsgeburt. Virchows Arch Pathol Anat 327:293–303, 1955.

568. François J. La toxoplasmose et ses manifestations oculaires. Paris, Masson, 1963, p 614.

569. Granström KO, Magnusson JH. Convergent strabismus, macular foci and toxoplasmosis in monozygotic twins. Br J Ophthalmol 34:105–107, 1950.

570. Hoppeler H, Sadoun R. Encéphalophatie chronique chez deux jumeaux: role éventuel de la toxoplasmose. Arch Fr Pediatr 12:212–214, 1955.

571. Murphy WF, Flannery JL. Congenital toxoplasmosis occurring in identical twins. Am J Dis Child 84:223–226, 1952.

572. Binkhorst CD. Toxoplasmosis: A Clinical, Serological Study with Special Reference to Eye Manifestations. Leiden, HE Stenfert, 1948, p 163.

573. Farquhar HG. Congenital toxoplasmosis: report of two cases in twins. Lancet 259:562–564, 1950.

574. Rieger H. Toxoplasmosis congenital und Zwillingsschwangerschaft. Klin Monatsbl Augenheilkd 134:862–871, 1959.

575. Yukins RE, Winter FC. Ocular disease in congenital toxoplasmosis in nonidentical twins. Am J Ophthalmol 62:44–46, 1966.

576. Statz A, Wenzel D, Heimann G. [Clinical course of congenital toxoplasmosis in dizygotic twins.] Klin Padiatr (in German) 190:599–602, 1978.

577. Benjamin B, Brickman HF, Neaga A. A congenital toxoplasmosis in twins. Can Med Assoc J 80:639–643, 1958.

578. Thalhammer O. Congenital toxoplasmosis. Lancet 1:23–24, 1962.

579. Beverley JK. A discussion on toxoplasmosis: congenital *Toxoplasma* infections. Proc R Soc Med 53:111–113, 1960.

580. Juurikkala A. Posterior uveitis and toxoplasmosis. Acta Ophthalmol 39:367–369, 1961.

581. Sibalic D, Djurkovic DO, Nikolic R. Congenital toxoplasmosis in premature twins. Folia Parasitol (Praha) 33:7–13, 1986.

582. Wiswell TE, et al. Congenital toxoplasmosis in triplets. J Pediatr 105:59–61, 1984.

583. Couvreur J, Thulliez P, Daffos F, et al. Six cases of toxoplasmosis in twins. Ann Pediatr 38:63–68, 1991.

584. Tolentino P, Bucalossi A. Due casi de encefalomielite infantile di natura toxoplasmica. Policlin Infant 16:265–284, 1948.

585. Martinovic J, et al. Frequency of toxoplasmosis in the appearance of congenital hydrocephalus. J Neurosurg 56:830–834, 1982.

586. Wende-Fischer R, et al. Toxoplasmosis. Monatsschr Kinderheilkd 141:789–791, 1993.

587. Ribierre M, Couvreur J, Canetti J. Les hydrocéphalies par sténose de l'aqueduc de Sylvius dans la toxoplasmose congenitale. Arch Fr Pediatr 27:501–510, 1970.

588. Kaiser G. Hydrocephalus following toxoplasmosis. Z Kinderchir 40(Suppl 1):10–11, 1985.

589. Tognetti F, Galassi E, Gaist G. Neurological toxoplasmosis presenting as a brain tumor: case report. J Neurosurg 56:716–721, 1982.

590. Baron J, et al. The incidence of cytomegalovirus, herpes simplex, rubella, and *Toxoplasma* antibodies in microce-

phalic, mentally retarded, and normocephalic children. Pediatrics 44:932–939, 1969.

591. Thalhammer O. Die angeborene Toxoplasmose. *In* Kirchhoff H, Kräubig H (eds): Toxoplasmose: Praktische Fragen und Ergebnisse. Stuttgart, Georg Thieme, 1966, pp 151–173.

592. Remington JS, cited by Frenkel JK. Some data on the incidence of human toxoplasmosis as a cause of mental retardation. *In* Eichenwald HF (ed). The Prevention of Mental Retardation Through Control of Infectious Diseases. Public Health Service Publication No. 1692. Washington, DC, U.S. Government Printing Office, 1968, pp 89–97.

593. Silver HK, Dixon MS. Congenital toxoplasmosis: report of case with cataract, "atypical" vasopressin-sensitive diabetes insipidus, and marked eosinophilia. Am J Dis Child 88:84–91, 1954.

594. Perkins ES. Ocular toxoplasmosis. Br J Ophthalmol 57:1–17, 1973.

595. Desmonts G. Toxoplasmose oculaire: étude épidemiologique (bilan de 2030 examené d'humeur agueuse). Arch Ophthalmol (Paris) 33:87–102, 1973.

596. Sibalic D, Djurkovic-Djakovic O, Bobic B. Onset of ocular complications in congenital toxoplasmosis associated with immunoglobulin M antibodies to *Toxoplasma gondii*. Eur J Clin Microbiol Infect Dis 9:671–674, 1990.

597. Burnett AJ, et al. Multiple cases of acquired toxoplasmosis retinitis presenting in an outbreak. Ophthalmology 105:1032–1037, 1998.

598. Fair JR. Congenital toxoplasmosis: III. Ocular signs of the disease in state schools for the blind. Am J Ophthalmol 48:165–172, 1959.

599. Fair JR. Congenital toxoplasmosis—diagnostic importance of chorioretinitis. JAMA 168:250–253, 1958.

600. Fair JR. Congenital toxoplasmosis: V. Ocular aspects of the disease. J Med Assoc Ga 48:604–607, 1959.

601. Kazdan JJ, McCulloch JC, Crawford JS. Uveitis in children. Can Med Assoc J 96:385–391, 1967.

602. de Carvalho KM, et al. Characteristics of a pediatric low-vision population. J Pediatr Ophthalmol Strabismus 35:162–165, 1998.

603. Kara-José N, et al. Estudos retrospectivos dos primeiros 140 caves atendidos na Clinica de Visao Subnormal do Hospital das Clinicas da UNICAMP. Arq Bras Oftalmol 51:65–69, 1988.

604. Buchignani BPC, Silva MRBM. Levantamento das causes e resultados. Arq Bras Oftalmol 50:49–54, 1991.

605. Meenken C, et al. Long-term ocular and neurological involvement in severe congenital toxoplasmosis. Br J Ophthalmol 79:581–584, 1995.

606. Rothova A. Ocular involvement in toxoplasmosis. Br J Ophthalmol 77:371–377, 1993.

607. Hogan MJ, et al. Early and delayed ocular manifestations of congenital toxoplasmosis. Trans Am Ophthalmol Soc 55:275–296, 1957.

608. Parissi G. Essai d'évaluation du risque de poussée évolutive secondaire de choriorétinite dans la toxoplasmose congénitale. Paris, Thése Paris-Saint-Antoine, 1973.

609. De Vroede M, et al. Congenital toxoplasmosis: late appearance of retinal lesions after treatment. Acta Paediatr Scand 68:761–762, 1979.

610. Lou P, Kazdan J, Basu PK. Ocular toxoplasmosis in three consecutive siblings. Arch Ophthalmol 96:613–614, 1978.

611. Lappalainen M, et al. Outcome of children after maternal primary *Toxoplasma* infection during pregnancy with emphasis on avidity of specific IgG. Pediatr Infect Dis J 14:354–361, 1995.

612. Gross U, et al. Possible reasons for failure of conventional tests for diagnosis of fatal congenital toxoplasmosis: report of a case diagnosed by PCR and immunoblot. Infection 20:149–152, 1992.

613. Pettapiece MC, Hiles DA, Johnson BL. Massive congenital ocular toxoplasmosis. J Pediatr Ophthalmol 13:259–265, 1976.

614. O'Connor GR. Manifestations and management of ocular toxoplasmosis. Bull NY Acad Med 50:192–210, 1974.

615. Franceschetti A, Bamatter F. Toxoplasmose oculaire: diagnostique, clinique, anatomique et histoparasitologique des affections toxoplasmiques. Acta I Congr Latinus Ophthalmol 1:315–437, 1953.

616. Saxon SA, et al. Intellectual deficits in children born with subclinical congenital toxoplasmosis: a preliminary report. J Pediatr 82:792–797, 1973.

617. Berengo A, et al. [Serological research on diffusion of toxoplasmosis: study of 1720 patients hospitalized in a psychiatric hospital.] Minerva Med (in Italian) 57:2292–2305, 1966.

618. Kvirikadze VV, Yourkova IA. On the role of congenital toxoplasmosis in the origin of oligophrenia and of its certain other forms of mental ailments. Zh Nevropatol Psikhiatr 61:1059–1062, 1961.

619. Kozar Z, et al. Toxoplasmosis as a cause of mental deficiency. Neurol Neurochir Pol 4:383–396, 1954.

620. Caiaffa W, et al. Toxoplasmosis and mental retardation—report of a case-control study. Mem Inst Oswaldo Cruz 88:253–261, 1993.

621. Hume OS. Toxoplasmosis and pregnancy. Am J Obstet Gynecol 114:703–715, 1972.

622. Fleck DG. Epidemiology of toxoplasmosis. J Hyg 61:61–65, 1963.

623. Burkinshaw J, Kirman BH, Sorsby A. Toxoplasmosis in relation to mental deficiency. BMJ 1:702–704, 1953.

624. Mackie MJ, Fiscus AG, Pallister P. A study to determine causal relationships of toxoplasmosis to mental retardation. Am J Epidemiol 94:215–221, 1971.

625. Stern H, et al. Microbial causes of mental retardation: the role of prenatal infections with cytomegalovirus, rubella virus, and *Toxoplasma*. Lancet 2:443–448, 1969.

626. Fisher OD. *Toxoplasma* infection in English children: a survey with toxoplasmin intradermal antigen. Lancet 2:904–906, 1951.

627. Cook I, Derrick EH. The incidence of *Toxoplasma* antibodies in mental hospital patients. Aust Ann Med 10:137–141, 1961.

628. Fair JR. Congenital toxoplasmosis: IV. Case finding using the skin test and ophthalmoscope in state schools for mentally retarded children. Am J Ophthalmol 48:813–819, 1959.

629. Labzoffsky NA, et al. A survey of toxoplasmosis among mentally retarded children. Can Med Assoc J 92:1026–1028, 1965.

630. Hoejenbos E, Stronk MG. In quest of toxoplasmosis as a cause of mental deficiency. Psychiatr Neurol Neurochir 69:33–41, 1966.

631. Macer G. Toxoplasmosis in obstetrics, its possible relation to mongolism. Am J Obstet Gynecol 87:66–70, 1963.

632. Thiers H, Romagny G. Mongolisme chez une enfant atteinte de toxoplasmose: discussion du rapport étiologique. Lyon Med 185:145–151, 1951.

633. Kleine HO. Toxoplasmose als ursache von mongolismus. Z Geburtschilfe Gynaekol 147:13–27, 1956.

634. Hostomská L, et al. Mongolismus und latente toxoplasmose der mutter. Endokrinologie 34:296–304, 1957.

635. Jírovec O, et al. [Studies with the toxoplasmin test: I. Communication.] Zeutralbl Bakteriol (in German) 169:129–159, 1957.

636. Kleif AD, Kerner GI. [On the role of toxoplasmosis in the genesis of Down's syndrome.] Zh Nevropatol Psikhiatr (in Russian) 67:1462–1466, 1967.

637. Frenkel JK. Toxoplasmosis. In Benirschke K (ed). Comparative Aspects of Reproductive Failure. New York, Springer-Verlag, 1966, pp 296–322.

638. Andersen H. Toxoplasmosis in a child with congenital myxoedema. Acta Paediatr 44:98–99, 1955.

639. Aagaard K, Melchior J. The simultaneous occurrence of congenital toxoplasmosis and congenital myxoedema. Acta Paediatr 48:164–168, 1959.

640. Margit T, Istvan ER. Congenital toxoplasmosis causing diabetes insipidus. Orv Hetil 124:827–829, 1983.

641. Massa G, et al. Hypothalamo-pituitary dysfunction in congenital toxoplasmosis. Eur J Pediatr 148:742–744, 1989.

642. Yamakawa R, et al. Congenital toxoplasmosis complicated by central diabetes insipidus in an infant with Down syndrome. Brain Dev 18:75–77, 1996.

643. Oygür N, et al. Central diabetes insipidus in a patient with congenital toxoplasmosis. Am J Perinatol 15:191–192, 1998.

644. Bruhl HH, Bahn RC, Hayles AB. Sexual precocity associated with congenital toxoplasmosis. 33:682–686, 1958.

645. Coppola A, et al. [Partial anterior hypopituitarism caused by toxoplasmosis congenita: description of a clinical case.] Minerva Med (in Italian) 78:403–410, 1987.

646. Roussel B, et al. [Congenital nephrotic syndrome associated with congenital toxoplasmosis.] Arch Fr Pediatr (in French) 44:795–797, 1987.

647. Farkas-Bargeton E. Personal communication cited by Rabinowicz T. Acquired cerebral toxoplasmosis in the adult. In Hentsch D (ed). Toxoplasmosis. Bern, Hans Huber, 1971, pp 197–219.

648. Patel DV, et al. Resolution of intracranial calcifications in infants with treated congenital toxoplasmosis. Radiology 199:433–440, 1996.

649. Friedman S, et al. Congenital toxoplasmosis: prenatal diagnosis, treatment and postnatal outcome. Prenat Diagn 19:330–333, 1999.

650. Virkola K, et al. Radiological signs in newborns exposed to primary Toxoplasma infection in utero. Pediatr Radiol 27:133–138, 1997.

651. Puri S, Spencer RP, Gordon ME. Positive brain scan in toxoplasmosis. J Nucl Med 15:641–642, 1974.

652. Hervei S, Simon K. [Congenital toxoplasmosis mimicking a cerebral tumor. Special aspects in serodiagnostics of connatal toxoplasmosis.] Monatsschr Kinderheilkd (in German) 127:43–47, 1979.

653. Bobowski SJ, Reed WG. Toxoplasmosis in an adult, presenting as a space-occupying cerebral lesion. Arch Pathol Lab Med 65:460–464, 1958.

654. Collins AT, et al. Computed tomography in the evaluation of congenital cerebral toxoplasmosis. J Comput Assist Tomogr 4:326–329, 1980.

655. Diebler C, Dusser A, Dulac O. Congenital toxoplasmosis: clinical and neuroradiological evaluation of the cerebral lesions. Neuroradiology 27:125–130, 1985.

656. Dunn D, Weisberg LA. Serial changes in a patient with congenital CNS toxoplasmosis as observed with CT. Comput Radiol 8:133–139, 1984.

657. Grant EG, et al. Intracranial calcification in the infant and neonate: evaluation by sonography and CT. Radiology 157:63–68, 1985.

658. Titelbaum DS, Hayward JC, Zimmerman RA. Pachygyric-like changes: topographic appearance at MR imaging and CT and correlation with neurologic status. Radiology 173:663–667, 1989.

659. Neuenschwander S, Cordier MD, Couvreur J. [Congenital toxoplasmosis: contribution of transfontanelle echotomography and computed tomography.] Ann Pediatr (Paris) (in French) 31:837–839, 1984.

660. Calabet A, et al. [Congenital toxoplasmosis and transfontanelle brain echography: apropos of 8 cases observed in newborn infants and infants.] J Radiol (in French) 65:367–373, 1984.

661. Brodeur AE. Radiologic Diagnosis in Infants and Children. St. Louis, CV Mosby, 1965, p 503.

662. Lindgren E. Röntgenologie: einschliesslich Kontrastmethoden. In Olivecrona H, Tönnis W (eds). Handbuch der Neurochirurgie, Band II. Berlin, Springer–Verlag, 1954, p 296.

663. Masherpa F, Valentino V. Intracranial Calcifications. Springfield, Ill, Charles C Thomas, 1959.

664. Potter KH. Pathology of the Fetus and Infant. Chicago, Year Book, 1961.

665. Traveras JM, Wood EH. Diagnostic Neuroradiology. Baltimore, Williams & Wilkins, 1964, p 960.

666. Dyke CG, et al. Toxoplasmic encephalomyelitis: VIII. Significance of roentgenographic findings in the diagnosis of infantile or congenital toxoplasmosis. AJR Am J Roentgenol 47:830–844, 1942.

667. Müssbichler H. Radiologic study of intracranial calcifications in congenital toxoplasmosis. Acta Radiol [Diagn] (Stockh) 7:369–379, 1968.

668. Kove S, et al. Pattern of serum transaminase activity in neonatal jaundice due to cytomegalic inclusion disease and toxoplasmosis with hepatic involvement. J Pediatr 63:660–662, 1963.

669. Freudenberg E. Akute infantile Toxoplasmosis-Enzephalitis. Schweiz Med Wochenschr 77:680–682, 1947.

670. Hellbrügge T. Über Toxoplasmose. Dtsch Med Wochenschr 74:385–389, 1949.

671. Reiss HJ, Verron T. Beiträge zur Toxoplasmose. Dtsch Gesundheitsw 6:646–653, 1951.

672. Justus J. Cutaneous manifestations of toxoplasmosis. Curr Probl Dermatol 4:24–47, 1972.

673. Korovitsky LK, et al. [Skin lesions in toxoplasmosis.] Vestn Dermatol Venerol (in Russian) 38:28–32, 1962.

674. Justus J. [Congenital toxoplasmosis with dermatitis calcificans toxoplasmatica and tetany of the mother during delivery.] Dtsch Med Wochenschr (in German) 93:349–353, 1968.

675. Schmidtke L. [On toxoplasmosis, with special reference to care in pregnancy.] Monatsschrift für Gesundheitsverwaltung und Sozialhygiene (in German) 23:587–591, 1961.

676. Mohr W. Toxoplasmose. In Handbuch für Innere Medizin. Berlin, Springer-Verlag, 1952, pp 730–770.

677. Georgakopoulos PA. Etiologic relationship between toxoplasmosis and anencephaly. Int Surg 59:419–420, 1974.

678. Cech JA, Jírovec O. The importance of latent maternal infection with Toxoplasma in obstetrics. Prog Obstet Gynecol 11:41–90, 1961.

679. Korovickij LK, et al. Toksoplazmoz. Kiev, Gosmedizdat Kkr SSR, 1962, p 188.

680. Erdélyi R. The influence of toxoplasmosis on the incidence of congenital facial malformations: preliminary report. Plast Reconstr Surg 20:306–310, 1957.

681. Bain A, et al. Congenital toxoplasmosis simulating

haemolytic disease of the newborn. Br J Obstet Gynaecol 63:826–832, 1956.

682. Hall EG, et al. Congenital toxoplasmosis in newborn. Arch Dis Child 28:117–124, 1953.

683. Schubert W. Fruchttod und Hydrops universalis durch Toxoplasmose. Virchows Arch 330:518–524, 1957.

684. Siliaeva NF. A case of congenital toxoplasmic meningoencephalitis complicated by an edematous form of symptomatic erythroblastosis. Arkh Patol 27:67–70, 1965.

685. Nelson LG, Hodgman JE. Congenital toxoplasmosis with hemolytic anemia. Calif Med 105:454–457, 1966.

686. Roper HP. A treatable cause of hydrops fetalis. J R Soc Med 79:109–110, 1986.

687. Wilson CB, et al. Lymphocyte transformation in the diagnosis of congenital Toxoplasma infection. N Engl J Med 302:785–788, 1980.

688. Koch F, Schorn J, Ule G. Über Toxoplasmose. Dtsch Z Nervenheilkd 166:315–348, 1951.

689. Tós-Luty S, Chrzastek-Spruch H, Uminski J. [Studies on the frequency of a positive toxoplasmosis reaction in mentally deficient, deaf and normally developed children.] Wiad Parazytol (in Polish) 10:374–376, 1964.

690. Ristow W. [On the problem of the etiological importance of toxoplasmosis in hearing disorders, especially in deaf-mutism.] Z Laryngol Rhinol Otol (in German) 45:251–264 (English summary, 261), 1966.

691. Potasman I, et al. Congenital toxoplasmosis: a significant cause of neurological morbidity in Israel? Clin Infect Dis 20:259–262, 1995.

692. Wright I. Congenital toxoplasmosis and deafness: an investigation. Pract Otorhinolaryngol (Basel) 33:377–387, 1971.

693. McGee T, et al. Absence of sensorineural hearing loss in treated infants and children with congenital toxoplasmosis. Otolaryngol Head Neck Surg 106:75–80, 1992.

694. Vanhaesebrouck P, et al. Congenital toxoplasmosis presenting as massive neonatal ascites. Helv Paediatr Acta 43:97–101, 1988.

695. Griscom NT, et al. Diagnostic aspects of neonatal ascites: report of 27 cases. AJR Am J Roentgenol 128:961–969, 1977.

696. Blaakaer J. Ultrasonic diagnosis of fetal ascites and toxoplasmosis. Acta Obstet Gynecol Scand 65:653–654, 1986.

697. Daffos F. Technical aspects of prenatal samplings and fetal transfusion. Curr Stud Hematol Blood Transfus 55:127–129, 1988.

698. Hedenström G. Toxoplasmosis in children: a study of 83 Swedish cases. Acta Paediatr 50:304–312, 1961.

699. Hedenström G. The variability of the course of congenital toxoplasmosis on some relatively mild cases. In Siim JC (ed). Human Toxoplasmosis. Copenhagen, Munksgaard, 1960, pp 34–40.

700. Couvreur J, Desmonts G. Les poussées évolutives tardives de la toxoplasmose congénitale. Cah Coll Med Hop Paris 5:752–758, 1964.

701. Wolf A, Cowen D. Perinatal infections of the central nervous system. J Neuropathol Exp Neurol 18:191–243, 1959.

702. Puissan C, Desmonts G, Mozziconacci P. Evolutivité neurologique tardive d'une toxoplasmose congénitale démontrée par l'étude du L.C.R. Ann Pediatr (Paris) 18:224–227, 1971.

703. Mitchell CD, et al. Congenital toxoplasmosis occurring in infants perinatally infected with human immunodeficiency virus 1. Pediatr Infect Dis J 9:512–518, 1990.

704. Cohen-Addad NE, et al. Congenital acquired immuno-deficiency syndrome and congenital toxoplasmosis: pathologic support for a chronology of events. J Perinatol 8:328–331, 1988.

705. Velin P, et al. [Double contamination materno-foetale par le VIH 1 et le toxoplasme] [Letter to the editor]. Presse Med 20:960, 1991.

706. O'Donohoe JM, Brueton MJ, Holliman RE. Concurrent congenital human immunodeficiency virus infection and toxoplasmosis. Pediatr Infect Dis J 10:627–628, 1991.

707. Taccone A, et al. An unusual CT presentation of congenital cerebral toxoplasmosis in an 8-month-old boy with AIDS. Pediatr Radiol 22:68–69, 1992.

708. Tovo PA, et al. Prognostic factors and survival in children with perinatal HIV-1 infection. Lancet 339:1249–1253, 1992.

709. Miller MJ, Remington JS. Toxoplasmosis in infants and children with HIV infection or AIDS. In Pizzo PA, Wilfert CM (eds). Pediatric AIDS: The Challenge of HIV Infection in Infants, Children, and Adolescents. Baltimore, Williams & Wilkins, 1990, pp 299–307.

710. Castelli G, et al. Toxoplasma gondii infection in AIDS children in Italy. IXth International Conference on AIDS. Berlin, IVth STD World Congress, 1993.

711. Minkoff H, et al. Vertical transmission of Toxoplasma by human immunodeficiency virus–infected women. Am J Obstet Gynecol 176:555–559, 1997.

712. European Collaborative. Low incidence of congenital toxoplasmosis in children born to women infected with human immunodeficiency virus. Eur J Obstet Gynecol Reprod Biol 68:93–96, 1996.

713. Shanks GD, Redfield RR, Fischer GW. Toxoplasma encephalitis in an infant with acquired immunodeficiency syndrome. Pediatr Infect Dis J 6:70–71, 1987.

714. Bernstein LJ, et al. Defective humoral immunity in pediatric acquired immune deficiency syndrome. J Pediatr 107:352–357, 1985.

715. Scott GB, et al. Mothers of infants with the acquired immunodeficiency syndrome: evidence for both symptomatic and asymptomatic carriers. JAMA 253:363–366, 1985.

716. Desmonts G. Central nervous system toxoplasmosis [Letter to the editor]. Pediatr Infect Dis J 6:872–873, 1987.

717. O'Riordan SE, Farkas AG. Maternal death due to cerebral toxoplasmosis. Br J Obstet Gynaecol 105:565–566, 1998.

718. Marty P, et al. Prenatal diagnosis of severe fetal toxoplasmosis as a result of toxoplasmic reactivation in an HIV-1 seropositive woman. Prenat Diagn 14:414–415, 1994.

719. Furrer H, et al. Discontinuation of primary prophylaxis against Pneumocystis carinii pneumonia in HIV-1–infected adults treated with combination antiretroviral therapy. Swiss HIV Cohort Study [see comments]. N Engl J Med 340:1301–1306, 1999.

720. Luft BJ, Remington JS. Toxoplasmic encephalitis in AIDS (AIDS commentary). Clin Infect Dis 15:211–222, 1992.

721. Beaman M, Luft B, Remington J. Prophylaxis for toxoplasmosis in AIDS. Ann Intern Med 117:163–164, 1992.

722. Liesenfeld O, Wong SY, Remington JS. Toxoplasmosis in the setting of AIDS. In Bartlett JD, Merigan TC, Bolognesi D (eds). Textbook of AIDS Medicine. Baltimore, Williams & Wilkins, 1999, pp 225–259.

723. Hedriana H, et al. Normal fetal outcome in a pregnancy with central nervous system toxoplasmosis and human

immunodeficiency virus infection. J Reprod Med 38:747–750, 1993.

724. Vanhems P, Irion O, Hirschel B. Toxoplasmic encephalitis during pregnancy. AIDS 7:142–143, 1992.

725. Wallon M, et al. Value of cerebrospinal fluid cytochemical examination for the diagnosis of congenital toxoplasmosis at birth in France. Pediatr Infect Dis J 17:705–710, 1998.

726. Vesikari T, Meurman OH, Mäki R. Persistent rubella-specific IgM-antibody in the cerebrospinal fluid of a child with congenital rubella. Arch Dis Child 55:46–48, 1980.

727. Couvreur J, et al. [Increased local production of specific G immunoglobulins in the cerebrospinal fluid in congenital toxoplasmosis.] Ann Pediatr (Paris) (in French) 31:829–835, 1984.

728. Woods CR, Englund J. Congenital toxoplasmosis presenting with eosinophilic meningitis. Pediatr Infect Dis J 12:347–348, 1993.

729. Hohlfeld P, et al. Fetal thrombocytopenia: a retrospective survey of 5,194 fetal blood samplings. Blood 84:1851–1856, 1994.

730. Riley ID, Arneil GC. Toxoplasmosis complicated by chickenpox and smallpox. Lancet 2:564–565, 1950.

731. Magnusson JH, Wahlgren F. Human toxoplasmosis: an account of twelve cases in Sweden. Acta Pathol Microbiol Scand 25:215–236, 1948.

732. Schwarz GA, Rose EK, Fry WE. Toxoplasmic encephalomyelitis (clinical report of 6 cases). Pediatrics 1:478–494, 1948.

733. Verlinde JD, Makstenieks O. Repeated isolation of Toxoplasma from the cerebrospinal fluid and from the blood, and the antibody response in four cases of congenital toxoplasmosis. Antonie Van Leeuwenhoek 16:366–372, 1950.

734. Dorta AF, et al. [Congenital toxoplasmosis. (second case parasitologically proved during life, in Venezuela).] Arch Venez Puericult Pediatr (in Spanish) 27:332–339, 1964.

735. Embil JA, et al. Visualization of Toxoplasma gondii in the cerebrospinal fluid of a child with a malignant astrocytoma. Can Med Assoc J 133:213–214, 1985.

736. Coffey JJ. Congenital toxoplasmosis 38 years ago [Letter to the editor]. Pediatr Infect Dis J 4:214, 1985.

737. Habegger H. Toxoplasmose humaine; mise en évidence des parasites dan les milieux intra-oculaires; humeur aquese, exudat rétrorétinien. Arch Ophthalmol (Paris) 14:470–488, 1954.

738. Hoffbauer H, et al. [Demonstration of Toxoplasma in the menstrual blood using the immunofluorescence technic.] Munch Med Wochenschr (in German) 111:969–976, 1969.

739. Terragna A. Toxoplasmic lymphadenitis. In Hentsch D (ed). Toxoplasmosis. Bern, Hans Huber, 1971, pp 159–178.

740. Tsunematsu Y, Shioiri K, Kusano N. Three cases of lymphadenopathia toxoplasmotica—with special reference to the application of fluorescent antibody technique for detection of Toxoplasma in tissue. Jpn J Exp Med 34:217–230, 1964.

741. Shioiri-Nakano K, Aoyama Y, Tsuenmatsu Y. The application of fluorescent-antibody technique to the diagnosis of glandular toxoplasmosis. Rev Med 8:429–436, 1971.

742. Khodr G, Matossian R. Hydrops fetalis and congenital toxoplasmosis: value of direct immunofluorescence test. Obstet Gynecol 51(Suppl 1):74S–77S, 1978.

743. Conley FK, Jenkins KA, Remington JS. Toxoplasma gondii infection of the central nervous system: use of the peroxidase-antiperoxidase method to demonstrate Toxoplasma in formalin fixed, paraffin embedded tissue sections. Hum Pathol 12:690–698, 1981.

744. Frenkel JK, Piekarski G. The demonstration of Toxoplasma and other organisms by immunofluorescence: a pitfall [Editorial]. J Infect Dis 138:265–266, 1978.

745. Kass EH, et al. Toxoplasmosis in the human adult. Arch Intern Med 89:759–782, 1952.

746. Dorfman RF, Remington JS. Value of lymph-node biopsy in the diagnosis of acute acquired toxoplasmosis. N Engl J Med 289:878–881, 1973.

747. Desmonts G, Couvreur J. [Isolation of the parasite in congenital toxoplasmosis: its practical and theoretical importance.] Arch Fr Pediatr (in French) 31:157–166, 1974.

748. Deutsch AR, Horsley ME. Congenital toxoplasmosis. Am J Ophthalmol 43:444–448, 1957.

749. Ariztía A, et al. Toxoplasmose connatal activa en un rec ién nacido con demonstracion del parasito in vivo: primer caso en Chile. Rev Chil Pediatr 25:501–510, 1954.

750. De Roever-Bonnet H. Congenital toxoplasmosis. Trop Geogr Med 13:27–41, 1961.

751. Schmidtke L. [Demonstration of Toxoplasma in amniotic fluid: preliminary report.] Dtsch Med Wochenschr (in German) 82:1342, 1957.

752. Chang CH, et al. Isolation of Toxoplasma gondii in tissue culture. J Pediatr 81:790–791, 1972.

753. Dos Santos Neto JG. Toxoplasmosis: a historical review, direct diagnostic microscopy, and report of a case. Am J Clin Pathol 63:909–915, 1975.

754. Matsubayashi H, et al. A case of ocular toxoplasmosis in an adult, the infection being confirmed by the isolation of the parasite from subretinal fluid. Keio J Med 10:209–224, 1961.

755. Frezzotti R, et al. A case of congenital toxoplasmosis with active chorioretinitis: parasitological and histopathological findings. Ophthalmologica 169:321–325, 1974.

756. Teutsch SM, et al. Toxoplasma gondii isolated from amniotic fluid. Obstet Gynecol 55(Suppl 3):2S–4S, 1980.

757. Derouin F, et al. Early prenatal diagnosis of congenital toxoplasmosis using amniotic fluid samples and tissue culture. Eur J Clin Microbiol Infect Dis 7:423–425, 1988.

758. Foulon W, et al. Detection of congenital toxoplasmosis by chronic villus sampling and early amniocentesis. Am J Obstet Gynecol 163:1511–1513, 1990.

759. Derouin F, Mazeron MC, Garin YJ. Comparative study of tissue culture and mouse inoculation methods for demonstration of Toxoplasma gondii. J Clin Microbiol 25:1597–1600, 1987.

760. Abbas AM. Comparative study of methods used for the isolation of Toxoplasma gondii. Bull World Health Organ 36:344–346, 1967.

761. Philippe F, et al. [Why monitor infants born to mothers who had a seroconversion for toxoplasmosis during pregnancy? Reality and risk of subclinical congenital toxoplasmosis in children: review of 30,768 births.] Ann Pediatr (Paris) (in French) 35:5–10, 1988.

762. Desmonts G, Couvreur J. Toxoplasmosis: epidemiologic and serologic aspects of perinatal infection. In Krugman S, Gershon AA (eds). Infections of the Fetus and the Newborn Infant. Progress in Clinical and Biological Research, vol 3. New York, Alan R. Liss, 1975, pp 115–132.

763. Frenkel JK. Dermal hypersensitivity to Toxoplasma antigens (toxoplasmins). Proc Soc Exp Biol Med 68:634–639, 1948.

764. Frenkel JK. Uveitis and toxoplasmin sensitivity. Am J Ophthalmol 32:127–135, 1949.

765. Beverley JKA, Beattie CP, Roseman C. Human *Toxoplasma* infection. J Hyg 52:37–46, 1954.

766. Jacobs L, et al. A comparison of the toxoplasmin skin tests, the Sabin-Feldman dye tests, and the complement fixation tests for toxoplasmosis in various forms of uveitis. Bull Johns Hopkins Hosp 99:1–15, 1956.

767. Frenkel JK, Jacobs L. Ocular toxoplasmosis: pathogenesis, diagnosis and treatment. Arch Ophthalmol 59:260–279, 1958.

768. Kaufman HE. Uveitis accompanied by a positive *Toxoplasma* dye test. Arch Ophthalmol 63:767–773, 1960.

769. Remington JS, et al. *Toxoplasma* antibodies among college students. N Engl J Med 269:1394–1398, 1963.

770. Frenkel JK. Pathogenesis, diagnosis and treatment of human toxoplasmosis. JAMA 140:369–377, 1949.

771. Jacobs L. Toxoplasmosis. N Z Med J 2–9, 1962.

772. Maddison SE, et al. Lymphocyte proliferative responsiveness in 31 patients after an outbreak of toxoplasmosis. Am J Trop Med Hyg 28:955–961, 1979.

773. Stray-Pedersen B. Infants potentially at risk for congenital toxoplasmosis: a prospective study. Am J Dis Child 134:638–642, 1980.

774. McLeod R, Beem MO, Estes RG. Lymphocyte anergy specific to *Toxoplasma gondii* antigens in a baby with congenital toxoplasmosis. J Clin Lab Immunol 17:149–153, 1985.

775. Gehrz RC, et al. Specific cell-mediated immune defect in active cytomegalovirus infection of young children and their mothers. Lancet 2:844–847, 1977.

776. Reynolds DW, Dean PH. Cell mediated immunity in mothers and their offspring with cytomegalovirus (CMV) infection. Pediatr Res 12:498, 1978.

777. Alford CA Jr. Rubella. *In* Remington JS, Klein JO (eds). Infectious Diseases of the Fetus and Newborn Infant. Philadelphia, WB Saunders, 1976, pp 71–106.

778. Fuccillo DA, et al. Impaired cellular immunity to rubella virus in congenital rubella. Infect Immun 9:81–84, 1974.

779. Friedmann PS. Cell-mediated immunological reactivity in neonates and infants with congenital syphilis. Clin Exp Immunol 30:271–276, 1977.

780. McLeod R, et al. In preparation.

781. Yano A, et al. Immune response to *Toxoplasma gondii*: I. *Toxoplasma*-specific proliferation response of peripheral blood lymphocytes from patients with toxoplasmosis. Microbiol Immunol 27:455–463, 1983.

782. Grover CM, et al. Rapid prenatal diagnosis of congenital *Toxoplasma* infection by using polymerase chain reaction and amniotic fluid. J Clin Microbiol 28:2297–2301, 1990.

783. van de Ven E, et al. Identification of *Toxoplasma gondii* infections by BI gene amplification. J Clin Microbiol 19:2120–2124, 1991.

784. Cazenave J, et al. Contribution of a new PCR assay to the prenatal diagnosis of congenital toxoplasmosis. Prenat Diagn 12:119–127, 1992.

785. Gross U, et al. Improved sensitivity of the polymerase chain reaction for detection of *Toxoplasma gondii* in biological and human clinical specimens. Eur J Clin Microbiol 11:33–39, 1992.

786. Dupouy-Camet J, et al. Comparative value of polymerase chain reaction and conventional biological tests. Ann Biol Clin 50:315–319, 1992.

787. Bergstrom T, et al. Congenital *Toxoplasma gondii* infection diagnosed by PCR amplification of peripheral mononuclear blood cells from a child and mother. Scand J Infect Dis 30:202–204, 1998.

788. Fuentes I, et al. Urine sample used for congenital toxoplasmosis diagnosis by PCR. J Clin Microbiol 34:2368–2371, 1996.

789. Knerer B, et al. Detection of *Toxoplasma gondii* with polymerase chain reaction for the diagnosis of congenital toxoplasmosis. Wien Klin Wochenschr 107:137–140, 1995.

790. Liesenfeld O, et al. Use of the polymerase chain reaction on amniotic fluid for prenatal diagnosis of congenital infection with *Toxoplasma gondii*. *In* 97th General Meeting of the ASM, Miami, May 4–8, 1997.

791. Pelloux H, et al. A new set of primers for the detection of *Toxoplasma gondii* in amniotic fluid using polymerase chain reaction. FEMS Microbiol Lett 138:11–15, 1996.

792. Paugam A, et al. Seroconversion toxoplasmique pendant la grossesse. Presse Med 11:1235, 1993.

793. Fricker-Hidalgo H, et al. Detection of *Toxoplasma gondii* in 94 placentae from infected women by polymerase chain reaction, in vivo, and in vitro cultures. Placenta 19:545–549, 1998.

794. Jenum PA, et al. Diagnosis of congenital *Toxoplasma gondii* infection by polymerase chain reaction (PCR) on amniotic fluid samples: the Norwegian experience. Apmis 106:680–686, 1998.

795. Gratzl R, et al. Follow-up of infants with congenital toxoplasmosis detected by polymerase chain reaction analysis of amniotic fluid. Eur J Clin Microbiol Infect Dis 17:853–858, 1998.

796. Pelloux H, et al. A second European collaborative study on polymerase chain reaction for *Toxoplasma gondii*, involving 15 teams. FEMS Microbiol Lett 165:231–237, 1998.

797. Araujo FG, Remington JS. Antigenemia in recently acquired acute toxoplasmosis. J Infect Dis 141:144–150, 1980.

798. van Knapen F, Panggabean SO. Detection of circulating antigen during acute infections with *Toxoplasma gondii* by enzyme-linked immunosorbent assay. J Clin Microbiol 6:545–547, 1977.

799. Lindenschmidt EG. Enzyme-linked immunosorbent assay for detection of soluble *Toxoplasma gondii* antigen in acute-phase toxoplasmosis. Eur J Clin Microbiol 4:488–492, 1985.

800. Asai T, et al. Detection of nucleoside triphosphate hydrolase as a circulating antigen in sera of mice infected with *Toxoplasma gondii*. Infect Immun 55:1332–1335, 1987.

801. Turunen HJ. Detection of soluble antigens of *Toxoplasma gondii* by a four-layer modification of an enzyme immunoassay. J Clin Microbiol 17:768–773, 1983.

802. Hassl A, Picher O, Aspöck H. Studies on the significance of detection of circulation antigen (cag) for the diagnosis of a primary infection with *T. gondii* during pregnancy. Mitt Osterr Ges Tropenmed Parasitol 9:91–94, 1987.

803. Hafid J, et al. Detection of circulating antigens of *Toxoplasma gondii* in human infection. Am J Trop Med Hyg 52:336–339, 1995.

804. Araujo FG, Handman E, Remington JS. Use of monoclonal antibodies to detect antigens of *Toxoplasma gondii* in serum and other body fluids. Infect Immun 30:12–16, 1980.

805. Huskinson J, Stepick-Biek P, Remington JS. Detection of antigens in urine during acute toxoplasmosis. J Clin Microbiol 27:1099–1101, 1989.

806. Brooks RG, Sharma SD, Remington JS. Detection of

Toxoplasma gondii antigens by a dot-immunobinding technique. J Clin Microbiol 21:113–116, 1985.

807. Jacobs L, Lunde M. A hemagglutination test for toxoplasmosis. J Parasitol 43:308–314, 1957.

808. Walton BC, Benchoff BM, Brooks WH. Comparison of the indirect fluorescent antibody test and methylene blue dye test for detection of antibodies to *Toxoplasma gondii*. Am J Trop Med Hyg 15:149–152, 1966.

809. Sérologie de l'Infection Toxoplasmique en Particulier à Son Début: Méthodes et Interprétation des Résultats. Lyon, Fondation Mérieux, 1975.

810. Naot Y, Remington JS. An enzyme-linked immunosorbent assay for detection of IgM antibodies to *Toxoplasma gondii*: use for diagnosis of acute acquired toxoplasmosis. J Infect Dis 142:757–766, 1980.

811. Bessieres MH, et al. IgA antibody response during acquired and congenital toxoplasmosis. J Clin Pathol 45:605–608, 1992.

812. Decoster A, et al. IgA antibodies against P30 as markers of congenital and acute toxoplasmosis. Lancet 2:1104–1106, 1988.

813. Desmonts G, Naot Y, Remington JS. Immunoglobulin M–immunosorbent agglutination assay for diagnosis of infectious diseases: diagnosis of acute congenital and acquired *Toxoplasma* infections. J Clin Microbiol 14:486–491, 1981.

814. Dannemann BR, et al. Differential agglutination test for diagnosis of recently acquired infection with *Toxoplasma gondii*. J Clin Microbiol 28:1928–1933, 1990.

815. Pinon JM, et al. Detection of specific immunoglobulin E in patients with toxoplasmosis. J Clin Microbiol 28:1739–1743, 1990.

816. Fleck CG. The antigens of *Toxoplasma gondii*. *In* Proceedings of the First International Congress of Parasitology. Oxford, Pergamon Press, 1966.

817. Feldman HA, Miller LT. Serological study of toxoplasmosis prevalence. Am J Hyg 64:320–335, 1956.

818. Lelong M, Desmonts G. Sur la nature de phénomene de Sabin et Feldman. C R Soc Biol 146:207–209, 1952.

819. Feldman HA. To establish a fact: Maxwell Finland lecture. J Infect Dis 141:525–529, 1980.

820. WHO Expert Committee on Biological Standardization. World Health Organ Tech Rep Ser 1:1–100, 1968.

821. Welch PC, et al. Serologic diagnosis of acute lymphadenopathic toxoplasmosis. J Infect Dis 142:256–264, 1980.

822. BenRachid MS, Ferraro G, Desmonts G. Data on HA tests in newborns. Arch Inst Pasteur Tunis 44:391–400, 1967.

823. Desmonts G. Congenital toxoplasmosis: problems in early diagnosis. *In* Hentsch D (ed). Toxoplasmosis. Bern, Hans Huber, 1971, pp 137–149.

824. Camargo ME, Leser PG. Diagnostic information from serological tests in human toxoplasmosis: II. Evolutive study of antibodies and serological patterns in acquired toxoplasmosis, as detected by hemagglutination, complement fixation, IgG- and IgM-immunofluorescence tests. Rev Inst Med Trop São Paulo 18:227–238, 1976.

825. Camargo ME, Leser PG, Leser WS. Diagnostic information from serological tests in human toxoplasmosis: I. A comparative study of hemagglutination, complement fixation, IgG- and IgM-immunofluorescence tests in 3,752 serum samples. Rev Inst Med Trop São Paulo 18:215–226, 1976.

826. Karim KA, Ludlam GB. The relationship and significance of antibody titres as determined by various serological methods in glandular and ocular toxoplasmosis. J Clin Pathol 28:42–49, 1975.

827. Ambroise-Thomas P, Simon J, Bayard M. Indirect hemagglutination using whole mixed antigen for checking toxoplasmosis immunity and for serodiagnosis of human toxoplasmosis, compared with immunofluorescence. Biomedicine 29:245–248, 1978.

828. Camargo ME, et al. Serology in early diagnosis of congenital toxoplasmosis. Rev Inst Med Trop São Paulo 20:152–160, 1978.

829. Balfour AH, Bridges JB, Harford JP. An evaluation of the ToxHA test for the detection of antibodies to *Toxoplasma gondii* in human serum. J Clin Pathol 33:644–647, 1980.

830. Kean BH, Kimball AC. The complement-fixation test in the diagnosis of congenital toxoplasmosis. Am J Dis Child 131:21–28, 1977.

831. Thulliez P, et al. A new agglutination test for the diagnosis of acute and chronic *Toxoplasma* infection. Pathol Biol 34:173–177, 1986.

832. Niel G, Gentilini M. Immunofluorescence quantitative, test de Remington et agglutination directe: confrontation et apport de leur pratique simultanée dans le diagnostic sérologique de la toxoplasmose. *In* Sérologie de l'Infection Toxoplasmique en Particulier à Son Début: Méthodes et Interprétation des Résultats. Lyon, Fondation Mérieux, 1975.

833. Couzineau P. La réaction d'agglutination dans le diagnostic sérologique de la toxoplasmose. *In* Sérologie de l'Infection Toxoplasmique en Particulier à Son Début: Méthodes et Interprétation des Résultats. Lyon, Fondation Mérieux, 1975.

834. Baufine-Ducrocq H. Les anticrops naturels dans de serodiagnostic de la toxoplasmose par agglutination directe. *In* Sérologie de l'Infection Toxoplasmique en Particulier à Son Début: Méthodes et Interprétation des Résultats. Lyon, Fondation Mérieux, 1975.

835. Garin JP, et al. Immunofluorescence et agglutination dans le diagnostic serologique de la toxoplasmose valeur comparative de la recherche des IgM et du test au 2-mercapto-éthanol. *In* Sérologie de l'Infection Toxoplasmique en Particulier à Son Début: Méthodes et Interprétation des Résultats. Lyon, Fondation Mérieux, 1975.

836. Laugier M. Notre experience du depistage de la toxoplasmose congenitale dans la region Marseillaise (méthodes-interprétation des résultats). *In* Sérologie de l'Infection Toxoplasmique en Particulier a Son Début: Méthodes et Interprétation des Résultats. Lyon, Fondation Mérieux, 1975

837. Desmonts G, Thulliez P. The *Toxoplasma* agglutination antigen as a tool for routine screening and diagnosis of *Toxoplasma* infection in the mother and infant. Dev Biol Stand 62:31–35, 1985.

838. Desmonts G, et al. [Natural antibodies against Toxoplasma.] Nouv Presse Med 3:1547–1549, 1974.

839. Desmonts G, Remington JS. Direct agglutination test for diagnosis of *Toxoplasma* infection: method for increasing sensitivity and specificity. J Clin Microbiol 11:562–568, 1980.

840. Payne RA, Francis JM, Kwantes W. Comparison of a latex agglutination test with other serological tests for the measurement of antibodies to *Toxoplasma gondii*. J Clin Pathol 37:1293–1297, 1984.

841. Nagington J, Martin AL, Balfour AH. Technical method: a rapid method for the detection of antibodies to *Toxoplasma gondii* using a modification of the Toxoreagent latex test. J Clin Pathol 36:361–362, 1983.

842. Wilson M, Ware DA, Walls KW. Evaluation of commercial serology kits for toxoplasmosis. *In* Joint Meet-

ing of the Royal and American Societies of Tropical Medicine and Hygiene, the 33rd annual meeting of the American Society of Tropical Medicine and Hygiene. Baltimore, 1984.

843. Wong S, Remington JS. Toxoplasmosis in Pregnancy. Clin Infect Dis 18:853–862, 1994.

844. Liesenfeld O, et al. Study of Abbott toxo IMx system for detection of immunoglobulin G and immunoglobulin M Toxoplasma antibodies: value of confirmatory testing for diagnosis of acute toxoplasmosis. J Clin Microbiol 34:2526–2530, 1996.

845. Suzuki Y, et al. Antigen(s) responsible for immunoglobulin G responses specific for the acute stage of Toxoplasma infection in humans. J Clin Microbiol 26:901–905, 1988.

846. Araujo FG, et al. False-positive anti-Toxoplasma fluorescent-antibody tests in patients with antinuclear antibodies. Appl Microbiol 22:270–275, 1971.

847. Hobbs KM, Sole E, Bettelheim KA. Investigation into the immunoglobulin class responsible for the polar staining of Toxoplasma gondii in the fluorescent antibody test. Zentralbl Bakteriol [Orig A] 239:409–413, 1977.

848. Sulzer AJ, Wilson M, Hall EC. Toxoplasma gondii: polar staining in fluorescent antibody test. Exp Parasitol 29:197–200, 1971.

849. De Meuter F, De Decker H. [Indirect fluorescent antibody test in toxoplasmosis: advantage of the use of fluorescent anti-IgG conjugate.] Zentralbl Bakteriol Mikrobiol Hyg [A] 233:421–430, 1975.

850. Wong SY, et al. The role of specific immunoglobulin E in diagnosis of acute Toxoplasma infection and toxoplasmosis. J Clin Microbiol 31:2952–2959, 1993.

851. Pinon JM, et al. Evaluation of risk and diagnostic value of quantitative assays for anti-Toxoplasma gondii immunoglobulin A (IgA), IgE, and IgM and analytical study of specific IgG in immunodeficient patients. J Clin Microbiol 33:878–884, 1995.

852. Decoster A, et al. Platelia-toxo IgA, a new kit for early diagnosis of congenital toxoplasmosis by detection of anti-P30 immunoglobulin A antibodies. J Clin Microbiol 29:2291–2295, 1991.

853. Stepick-Biek P, et al. IgA antibodies for diagnosis of acute congenital and acquired toxoplasmosis. J Infect Dis 162:270–273, 1990.

854. Balsari A, et al. ELISA for Toxoplasma antibody detection: a comparison with other serodiagnostic tests. J Clin Pathol 33:640–643, 1980.

855. van Loon A, van der Veen J. Enzyme-linked immunosorbent assay for quantitation of toxoplasma antibodies in human sera. J Clin Pathol 33:635–639, 1980.

856. Ruitenberg EJ, van Knapen F. The enzyme-linked immunosorbent assay and its application to parasitic infections. J Infect Dis 136(Suppl):S267–S273, 1977.

857. Carlier Y, et al. Evaluation of the enzyme-linked immunosorbent assay (ELISA) and other serological tests for the diagnosis of toxoplasmosis. Bull World Health Organ 58:99–105, 1980.

858. Denmark JR, Chessum BS. Standardization of enzyme-linked immunosorbent assay (ELISA) and the detection of Toxoplasma antibody. Med Lab Sci 35:227–232, 1978.

859. Capron A, et al. Application of immunoenzyme methods in diagnosis of human parasitic diseases. Ann NY Acad Sci 254:331, 1975.

860. Walls KW, Bullock SL, English DK. Use of the enzyme-linked immunosorbent assay (ELISA) and its microadaptation for the serodiagnosis of toxoplasmosis. J Clin Microbiol 5:273–277, 1977.

861. Voller A, et al. A microplate enzyme-immunoassay for Toxoplasma antibody. J Clin Pathol 29:150–153, 1976.

862. Milatovic D, Braveny I. Enzyme-linked immunosorbent assay for the serodiagnosis of toxoplasmosis. J Clin Pathol 33:841–844, 1980.

863. Liesenfeld O, et al. False-positive results in immunoglobulin M (IgM) Toxoplasma antibody tests and importance of confirmatory testing: the Platelia toxo IgM test. J Clin Microbiol 35:174–178, 1997.

864. Wilson M, et al. Evaluation of six commercial kits for detection of human immunoglobulin M antibodies to Toxoplasma gondii. J Clin Microbiol 35:3112–3115, 1997.

865. Siegel JP, Remington JS. Comparison of methods for quantitating antigen-specific immunoglobulin M antibody with a reverse enzyme-linked immunosorbent assay. J Clin Microbiol 18:63–70, 1983.

866. Gorgievski-Hrisoho M, Germann D, Matter L. Diagnostic implications of kinetics of immunoglobulin M and A antibody responses to Toxoplasma gondii. J Clin Microbiol 34:1506–1511, 1996.

867. Pinon JM, Thoannes H, Gruson N. An enzyme-linked immuno-filtration assay used to compare infant and maternal antibody profiles in toxoplasmosis. J Immunol Methods 77:15–23, 1985.

868. Pinon JM, et al. Early neonatal diagnosis of congenital toxoplasmosis: value of comparative enzyme-linked immunofiltration assay, immunological profiles and anti-Toxoplasma gondii immunoglobulin M (IgM) or IgA immunocapture and implications for postnatal therapeutic strategies. J Clin Microbiol 34:579–583, 1996.

869. Remington JS, Araujo FG, Desmonts G. Recognition of different Toxoplasma antigens by IgM and IgG antibodies in mothers and their congenitally infected newborns. J Infect Dis 152:1020–1024, 1985.

870. Pinon JM, Gruson N. Interest of ELISA specific and compared immunological profiles in the early diagnosis of congenital toxoplasmosis. Lyon Med 248:27–30, 1982.

871. Hedman K, et al. Avidity of IgG in serodiagnosis of infectious diseases. Rev Med Microbiol 4:123–129, 1993.

872. Cozon G, et al. IgG Avidity for Diagnosis of Chronic T. gondii Infection in Pregnant Women. In 8th ECCMID. Lausanne, Switzerland, May 25–28, 1997.

873. Rossi CL. A simple, rapid enzyme-linked immunosorbent assay for evaluating immunoglobulin G antibody avidity in toxoplasmosis. Diagn Microbiol Infect Dis 30:25–30, 1998.

874. Ashburn D, et al. Do IgA, IgE, and IgG avidity tests have any value in the diagnosis of Toxoplasma infection in pregnancy? J Clin Pathol 51:312–315, 1998.

875. Ambroise-Thomas P, et al. Standardization by the Vidas system of an avidity test for toxoplasmosis diagnosis in pregnant women. In 38th Interscience Conference on Antimicrobial Agents and Chemotherapy. San Diego, Calif, ASM, 1998.

876. Cozon GJ, et al. Estimation of the avidity of immunoglobulin G for routine diagnosis of chronic Toxoplasma gondii infection in pregnant women. Eur J Clin Microbiol Infect Dis 17:32–36, 1998.

877. Pelloux H, et al. Determination of anti-Toxoplasma gondii immunoglobulin G avidity: adaptation to the Vidas system (bioMérieux). Diagn Microbiol Infect Dis 32:69–73, 1998.

878. Lappalainen M, et al. Toxoplasmosis acquired during pregnancy: improved serodiagnosis based on avidity of IgG. J Infect Dis 167:691–697, 1993.

879. Jenum PA, Stray-Pedersen B, Gundersen A-G. Im-

proved diagnosis of primary *Toxoplasma gondii* infection in early pregnancy by determination of anti-*Toxoplasma* immunoglobulin G activity. J Clin Microbiol 35:1972–1977, 1997.

880. Sensini A, et al. IgG avidity in the serodiagnosis of acute *Toxoplasma gondii* infection: a multicenter study. Clin Microbiol Infect 2:25–29, 1996.

881. Hedman K, et al. Recent primary *Toxoplasma* infection indicated by a low avidity of specific IgG. J Infect Dis 159:736–739, 1989.

882. Camargo ME, et al. Avidity of specific IgG antibody as a marker of recent and old *Toxoplasma gondii* infections. Rev Inst Med Trop São Paulo 33:213–218, 1991.

883. Joynson DHM, Payne RA, Rawal BK. Potential role of IgG avidity for diagnosing toxoplasmosis. J Clin Pathol 43:1032–1033, 1990.

884. Remington JS, Miller MJ, Brownlee I. IgM antibodies in acute toxoplasmosis: I. Diagnostic significance in congenital cases and a method for their rapid demonstration. Pediatrics 41:1082–1091, 1968.

885. Remington JS, Miller MJ, Brownlee I. IgM antibodies in acute toxoplasmosis: II. Prevalence and significance in acquired cases. J Lab Clin Med 71:855–866, 1968.

886. Remington JS. The present status of the IgM fluorescent antibody technique in the diagnosis of congenital toxoplasmosis. J Pediatr 75:1116–1124, 1969.

887. Lunde MN. Laboratory methods in the diagnosis of toxoplasmosis. Health Lab Sci 10:319–328, 1973.

888. Stagno S, Thiermann E. [Value of indirect immunofluorescence test in the serological diagnosis of acute toxoplasmosis.] Bol Chil Parasitol (in Spanish) 25:9–15, 1970.

889. Aparicio GJ, Cour BI. [Application of immunofluorescence to the study of immunoglobulin fractions in the diagnosis of acquired and congenital toxoplasmosis. Clinical value.] Rev Clin Esp (in Spanish) 125:37–42, 1972.

890. Dropsy G, Carquin J, Croix JC. [Technics of demonstration of IgM type antibodies in congenital infections.] Ann Biol Clin (Paris) (in French) 29:67–73, 1971.

891. Eichenwald HF, Shinefield HR. Antibody production by the human fetus. J Pediatr 63:870, 1963.

892. Remington JS, Desmonts G. Congenital toxoplasmosis: variability in the IgM-fluorescent antibody response and some pitfalls in diagnosis. J Pediatr 83:27–30, 1973.

893. Pyndiah N, et al. Simplified chromatographic separation of immunoglobulin M from G and its application to *Toxoplasma* indirect immunofluorescence. J Clin Microbiol 9:170–174, 1979.

894. Filice GA, Yeager AS, Remington JS. Diagnostic significance of immunoglobulin M antibodies to *Toxoplasma gondii* detected after separation of immunoglobulin M from immunoglobulin G antibodies. J Clin Microbiol 12:336–342, 1980.

895. Lunde MN, et al. Serologic diagnosis of active toxoplasmosis complicating malignant diseases: usefulness of IgM antibodies and gel diffusion. Cancer 25:637–643, 1970.

896. Desmonts G, et al. [Early diagnosis of acute toxoplasmosis: critical study of Remington's test.] Nouv Presse Med (in French) 1:339–342, 1972.

897. Stiehm ER, Amman AJ, Cherry JD. Elevated cord macroglobulins in the diagnosis of intrauterine infections. N Engl J Med 275:971–977, 1966.

898. Barth WF, et al. Metabolism of human gamma macroglobulins. J Clin Invest 43:1036–1048, 1964.

899. Hyde B, Barnett EV, Remington JS. Method for differentiation of nonspecific from specific *Toxoplasma* IgM fluorescent antibodies in patients with rheumatoid factor. Proc Soc Exp Biol Med 148:1184–1188, 1975.

900. Reimer CB, et al. The specificity of fetal IgM: antibody or anti-antibody? Ann N Y Acad Sci 254:77–93, 1975.

901. Filice G, et al. Detection of IgM–anti-*Toxoplasma* antibodies in acute acquired and congenital toxoplasmosis. Boll Ist Sieroter Milan 76:271–273, 1984.

902. Pouletty P, et al. An anti-human immunoglobulin M monoclonal antibody for detection of antibodies to *Toxoplasma gondii*. Eur J Clin Microbiol 3:510–515, 1984.

903. Santoro F, et al. Serodiagnosis of *Toxoplasma* infection using a purified parasite protein (P30). Clin Exp Immunol 62:262–269, 1985.

904. Pouletty P, et al. An anti-human chain monoclonal antibody: use for detection of IgM antibodies to *Toxoplasma gondii* by reverse immunosorbent assay. J Immunol Methods 76:289–298, 1985.

905. Cesbron JY, et al. [A new ELISA method for the diagnosis of toxoplasmosis: assay of serum IgM by immunocapture with an anti–*Toxoplasma gondii* monoclonal antibody.] Presse Med (in French) 19:737–740, 1986.

906. Lindenschmidt EG. Demonstration of immunoglobulin M class antibodies to *Toxoplasma gondii* antigenic component p3500 by enzyme-linked antigen immunosorbent assay. J Clin Microbiol 24:1045–1049, 1986.

907. Herbrink P, et al. Interlaboratory evaluation of indirect enzyme-linked immunosorbent assay, antibody capture enzyme-linked immunosorbent assay, and immunoblotting for detection of immunoglobulin M antibodies to *Toxoplasma gondii*. J Clin Microbiol 25:100–105, 1987.

908. Filice G, et al. IgM-IFA, IgM-ELISA, DS-IgM-ELISA, IgM-ISAGA, performed on whole serum and IgM fractions, for detection of IgM anti-*Toxoplasma* antibodies during pregnancy. Boll Ist Sieroter Milan 65:131–137, 1986.

909. Saathoff M, Seitz HM. [Detection of *Toxoplasma*-specific IgM antibodies—comparison with the ISAGA (immunosorbent agglutination assay) and immunofluorescence results.] Z Geburtshilfe Perinatol (in German) 189:73–78, 1985.

910. Montoya JG, Remington JS. Studies on the serodiagnosis of toxoplasmic lymphadenitis. Clin Infect Dis 20:781–790, 1995.

911. Thulliez P, et al. Evaluation de trois reactifs de detection par immunocapture des IgM specifiques de la toxoplasmose. Ref Fr des Lab, Fev 1988, No. 169; 25–31.

912. Pinon JM, et al. Detection of IgA specific for toxoplasmosis in serum and cerebrospinal fluid using a nonenzymatic IgA-capture assay. Diagn Immunol 4:223–227, 1986.

913. Plantaz D, et al. [Value of the immunosorbent agglutination assay (ISAGA) in the early diagnosis of congenital toxoplasmosis.] Pediatrie (in French) 42:387–391, 1987.

914. Le Fichoux Y, Marty P, Chan H. [Contribution of specific serum IgA assay to the diagnosis of toxoplasmosis.]. Ann Pediatr (Paris) (in French) 34:375–379, 1987.

915. Krogstad DJ, Juranek DD, Walls KW. Toxoplasmosis: with comments on risk of infection from cats. Ann Intern Med 77:773–778, 1972.

916. Service PH. FDA Public Health Advisory: Limitations of *Toxoplasma* IgM Commercial Test Kits. Rockville, Md, Department of Health and Human Services, Food and Drug Administration, 1997, p 3.

917. Gard S, Magnusson JH. A glandular form of toxoplasmosis in connection with pregnancy. Acta Med Scand 141:59–64, 1951.

918. Jeckeln E. Lymph node toxoplasmosis. Frankfurter Zeitschr Pathol 70:513–522, 1960.
919. Siim JC. Toxoplasmosis acquisita lymphonodosa: clinical and pathological aspects. Ann N Y Acad Sci 64:185–206, 1956.
920. Couvreur J. Prospective study of acquired toxoplasmosis in pregnant women with a special reference to the outcome of the fetus. *In* Hentsch D (ed). Toxoplasmosis. Bern, Hans Huber, 1971, pp 119–136.
921. Handman E, Remington JS. Serological and immunochemical characterization of monoclonal antibodies to *Toxoplasma gondii*. Immunology 40:579–588, 1980.
922. Handman E, Remington JS. Antibody responses to *Toxoplasma* antigens in mice infected with strains of different virulence. Infect Immun 29:215–220, 1980.
923. Li S, et al. Serodiagnosis of recently acquired *T. gondii* infection with a recombinant antigen. J Clin Microbiol 38:in press, 2000.
924. Johnson AM, Roberts H, Tenter AM. Evaluation of a recombinant antigen ELISA for the diagnosis of acute toxoplasmosis and comparison with traditional antigen ELISAs. J Med Microbiol 37:404–409, 1992.
925. Martin V, et al. Detection of human *Toxoplasma*-specific immunoglobulins A, M, and G with recombinant *Toxoplasma gondii* ROP2 protein. Clin Diagn Lab Immunol 5:627–631, 1988.
926. Redlich A, Muller WA. Serodiagnosis of acute toxoplasmosis using a recombinant form of the dense granule antigen GRA6 in an enzyme-linked immunosorbent assay. Parasitol Res 84:700–706, 1998.
927. Tenter AM, Johnson AM. Recognition of recombinant *Toxoplasma gondii* antigens by human sera in an ELISA. Parasitol Res 77:197–203, 1991.
928. Sharma SD, et al. Western blot analysis of the antigens of *Toxoplasma gondii* recognized by human IgM and IgG antibodies. J Immunol 131:977–983, 1983.
929. Erlich HA, et al. Identification of an antigen-specific immunoglobulin M antibody associated with acute *Toxoplasma* infection. Infect Immun 41:683–690, 1983.
930. Potasman I, et al. *Toxoplasma gondii* antigens recognized by sequential samples of serum obtained from congenitally infected infants. J Clin Microbiol 25:1926–1931, 1987.
931. Huskinson J, et al. *Toxoplasma* antigens recognized by immunoglobulin G subclasses during acute and chronic Infection. J Clin Microbiol 27:2031–2038, 1989.
932. Potasman I, Araujo FG, Remington JS. *Toxoplasma* antigens recognized by naturally occurring human antibodies. J Clin Microbiol 24:1050–1054, 1986.
933. Gross U, Keksel O, Dardé ML. The value of detecting immunoglobulin E (IgE) antibodies for the serological diagnosis of *Toxoplasma gondii* infection. Clin Diagn Lab Immunol 4:247–251, 1997.
934. Petithory JC, et al. Performance of European laboratories testing serum samples for *Toxoplasma gondii*. Eur J Clin Microbiol Infect Dis 15:45–49, 1996.
935. Hofgartner WT, Plorde JJ, Fritsche TR. Detection of IgG and IgM antibodies to *Toxoplasma gondii*: evaluation of 4 newer commercial immunoassays. ASM 97th General Meeting, Miami, Fla, 1997.
936. Jones TC, Kean BH, Kimball AC. Toxoplasmic lymphadenitis. JAMA 192:87–91, 1965.
937. Lelong M, et al. [Acquired toxoplasmosis (study of 227 cases).] Arch Fr Pediatr (in French) 17:1–51, 1960.
938. Gussetti N, D'Elia R. Natural immunoglobulin M antibodies against *Toxoplasma gondii* during pregnancy. Am J Obstet Gynecol 51:1359–1360, 1990.
939. Konishi E. A pregnant woman with a high level of naturally occurring immunoglobulin M antibodies to *Toxoplasma gondii*. Am J Obstet Gynecol 157:832–833, 1987.
940. Hezard N, et al. Prenatal diagnosis of congenital toxoplasmosis in 261 pregnancies. Prenat Diagn 17:1047–1054, 1997.
941. Berrebi A, et al. Termination of pregnancy for maternal toxoplasmosis. Lancet 344:36–39, 1994.
942. Pratlong F, et al. Fetal diagnosis of toxoplasmosis in 190 women infected during pregnancy. Prenat Diagn 14:191–198, 1994.
943. Boulet P, et al. Pure fetal blood samples obtained by cordocentesis: technical aspects of 322 cases. Prenat Diagn 10:93–100, 1990.
944. Legras B, et al. Blood chemistry of human fetuses in the second and third trimesters. Prenat Diagn 10:801–807, 1990.
945. Tjalma W, et al. Discordant prenatal diagnosis of congenital toxoplasmosis in a dizygotic pregnancy. Eur J Obstet Gynecol Reprod Biol 79:107–108, 1998.
946. Hohlfeld P, et al. Fetal toxoplasmosis: outcome of pregnancy and infant follow-up after in utero treatment. J Pediatr 115:765–769, 1989.
947. Pratlong F, et al. Antenatal diagnosis of congenital toxoplasmosis: evaluation of the biological parameters in a cohort of 286 patients. Br J Obstet Gynaecol 103:552–557, 1996.
948. Berrebi A, Kobuch W. Toxoplasmosis in pregnancy. Lancet 344:950, 1994.
949. Lecolier B, et al. T-cell subpopulations of fetuses infected by *Toxoplasma gondii*. Eur J Clin Microbiol Infect Dis 8:572–573, 1989.
950. Decoster A, et al. Anti-P30 IgA antibodies as prenatal markers of congenital *Toxoplasma* infection. Clin Exp Immunol 87:310–315, 1992.
951. Raymond J, et al. Presence of gamma interferon in human acute and congenital toxoplasmosis. J Clin Microbiol 28:1434–1437, 1990.
952. Hohlfeld P, et al. *Toxoplasma gondii* infection during pregnancy: T lymphocyte subpopulations in mothers and fetuses. Pediatr Infect Dis J 9:878–881, 1990.
953. Cohen-Khallas Y, et al. La fraction C4 du complément: un nouveau marqueur indirect pour le diagnostic anténatal de la toxoplasmose. Presse Med 23:908, 1992.
954. Alford CA, et al. A correlative immunologic, microbiologic and clinical approach to the diagnosis of acute and chronic infections in newborn infants. N Engl J Med 277:437–449, 1967.
955. Alford CA. Immunoglobulin determinations in the diagnosis of fetal infection. Pediatr Clin North Am 18:99–113, 1971.
956. McCracken GH Jr, et al. Evaluation of a radial diffusion plate method for determining serum immunoglobulin levels in normal and congenitally infected infants. J Pediatr 75:1204–1210, 1969.
957. Korones SB, et al. Neonatal IgM response to acute infection. J Pediatr 75:1261–1270, 1969.
958. Miller MJ, Sunshine PJ, Remington JS. Quantitation of cord serum IgM and IgA as a screening procedure to detect congenital infection: results in 5,006 infants. J Pediatr 75:1287–1291, 1969.
959. Thorley JD, et al. Passive transfer of antibodies of maternal origin from blood to cerebrospinal fluid in infants. Lancet 1:651–653, 1975.
960. Patel B, et al. Immunoglobulin—a detection and the investigation of clinical toxoplasmosis. J Med Microbiol 38:286–292, 1993.
961. Foudrinier F, et al. Value of specific immunoglobulin A

detection by two immunocapture assays in the diagnosis of toxoplasmosis. Eur J Clin Microbiol Infect Dis 14:585–590, 1995.

962. Villena I., et al. Detection of specific IgE during maternal, fetal and congenital toxoplasmosis. J Clin Microbiol 37:3487–3490, 1999.

963. McCracken GH Jr, Kaplan JM. Penicillin treatment for congenital syphilis: a critical reappraisal. JAMA 228:855–858, 1974.

964. Parmley SF, Goebel FD, Remington JS. Detection of *Toxoplasma gondii* DNA in cerebrospinal fluid from AIDS patients by polymerase chain reaction. J Clin Microbiol 30:3000–3002, 1992.

965. Fortier B, et al. [Study of developing clinical outbreak and serological rebounds in children with congenital toxoplasmosis and follow-up during the first 2 years of life.] Arch Pediatr (in French) 4:940–946, 1997.

966. Kahi S, et al. Circulating *Toxoplasma gondii*–specific antibody-secreting cells in patients with congenital toxoplasmosis. Clin Immunol Immunopathol 89:23–27, 1998.

967. Villena I, et al. Pyrimethamine-sulfadoxine treatment of congenital toxoplasmosis: follow-up of 78 cases between 1980 and 1997. Reims Toxoplasmosis Group. Scand J Infect Dis 30:295–300, 1998.

968. Wright R, et al. Congenital lymphocytic choriomeningitis virus syndrome: a disease that mimics congenital toxoplasmosis or cytomegalovirus infections. Pediatrics 100:E91–E100, 1997.

969. Smith CC, Ihrig J. Persistent excretion of pyrimethamine following oral administration. Am J Trop Med Hyg 8:60–62, 1959.

970. Stickney DR, et al. Pharmacokinetics of pyrimethamine (PRM) and 2,4-diamino-5-(3′,4′-dichlorophenyl)-6-methylpyrimidine (DMP) relevant to meningeal leukemia. Proc Am Assoc Cancer Res 14:52, 1973.

971. Weidekamm E, et al. Plasma concentrations of pyrimethamine and sulfadoxine and evaluation of pharmacokinetic data by computerized curve fitting. Bull World Health Organ 60:115–122, 1982.

972. Ahmad RA, Rogers HJ. Pharmacokinetics and protein binding: interactions of dapsone and pyrimethamine. Br J Clin Pharmacol 10:519–524, 1980.

973. McLeod R, et al. Levels of pyrimethamine in sera and cerebrospinal and ventricular fluids from infants treated for congenital toxoplasmosis. Antimicrob Agents Chemother 36:1040–1048, 1992.

974. Eyles DE, Coleman N. Synergistic effect of sulfadiazine and daraprim against experimental toxoplasmosis in the mouse. Antibiot Chemother 3:483–490, 1953.

975. Eyles DE, Coleman N. An evaluation of the curative effects of pyrimethamine and sulfadiazine, alone and in combination, on experimental mouse toxoplasmosis. Antibiot Chemother 5:529–539, 1955.

976. Sheffield HG, Melton ML. Effect of pyrimethamine and sulfadiazine on the fine structure and multiplication of *Toxoplasma gondii* in cell cultures. J Parasitol 61:704–712, 1972.

977. Eyles DE, Coleman N. The relative activity of the common sulfonamides against toxoplasmosis in the mouse. Am J Trop Med Hyg 2:54–63, 1953.

978. Eyles DE, Coleman N. The effect of sulfadimetine, sulfisoxazole, and sulfapyrazine against mouse toxoplasmosis. Antibiot Chemother 5:525–528, 1955.

979. Dorangeon PH, et al. Passage transplacentaire de l'association pyriméthamine-sulfadoxine lors du traitement anténatal de lat toxoplasmose congénitale. Presse Med 19:2036, 1990.

980. Trenque T, et al. Human maternofoetal distribution of pyrimethamine-sulphadoxine [Letter to the editor]. Br J Clin Pharmacol 45:179–180, 1998.

981. Schoondermark-van de Ven E, et al. Study of treatment of congenital *Toxoplasma gondii* infection in rhesus monkeys with pyrimethamine and sulfadiazine. Antimicrob Agents Chemo 39:137–144, 1995.

982. Peyron F, Wallon M, Bernardoux C. Long-term follow-up of patients with congenital ocular toxoplasmosis. N Engl J Med 334:993–994, 1996.

983. Wilson CB. Treatment of congenital toxoplasmosis during pregnancy. J Pediatr 116:1003–1005, 1990.

984. Mack DG, McLeod R. New micromethod to study the effect of antimicrobial agents on *Toxoplasma gondii*: comparison of sulfadoxine and sulfadiazine individually and in combination with pyrimethamine and study of clindamycin, metronidazole, and cyclosporin A. Antimicrob Agents Chemother 26:26–30, 1984.

985. Zitelli BJ, et al. Fatal hepatic necrosis due to pyrimethamine-sulfadoxine (Fansidar). Ann Intern Med 106:393–395, 1987.

986. Matsui D. Prevention, diagnosis, and treatment of fetal toxoplasmosis. Clin Perinatol 21:675–689, 1994.

987. McLeod R. Treatment of congenital toxoplasmosis. Plenary Symposium: Advances in Therapy of Protozoal Infections. ICAAC, Orlando, Florida, 1994.

988. Ryan RW, et al. Diagnosis and treatment of toxoplasmic uveitis. Trans Am Acad Ophthalmol Otolaryngol 58:867–884, 1954.

989. Perkins ES, Smith CH, Schofield PB. Treatment of uveitis with pyrimethamine (Daraprim). Br J Ophthalmol 40:577–586, 1956.

990. Elmalem J, et al. [Severe complications arising from the prescription of pyrimethamine for infants being treated for toxoplasmosis.] Therapie (in French) 40:357–359, 1989.

991. Frenkel JK, Hitchings GH. Relative reversal by vitamins (*p*-aminobenzoic, folic and folinic acids) of the effects of sulfadiazine and pyrimethamine on *Toxoplasma*, mouse and man. Antibiot Chemother 7:630–638, 1957.

992. Nixon PF, Bertino JR. Effective absorption and utilization of oral formyltetrahydrofolate in man. N Engl J Med 286:175–179, 1972.

993. Allegra CJ, et al. Potent in vitro and in vivo anti-*Toxoplasma* activity of the lipid-soluble antifolate trimetrexate. J Clin Invest 79:478–482, 1987.

994. Maisonneuve H, et al. [Toxoplasmose congenitale. Tolerance de l'association sulfadoxine-pyrimethamine. Vingt-quatre observations.] Presse Med (in French) 13:859–862, 1984.

995. Garin JP, et al. [Effect of pyrimethamine sulfadoxine (Fansidar) on an avirulent cystogenic strain of *Toxoplasma gondii* (Prugniaud strain) in white mice.] Bull Soc Pathol Exot Filiales (in French) 78:821–824, 1985.

996. Garin JP, Paillard B. [Experimental toxoplasmosis in mice: comparative activity of clindamycin, midecamycin, josamycin, spiramycin, pyrimethamine-sulfadoxine, and trimethoprim-sulfamethoxazole.] Ann Pediatr (Paris) (in French) 31:841–845, 1984.

997. Thiersch JB. Effect of certain 2,4-diaminopyrimidine antagonists of folic acid on pregnancy and rat fetus. Proc Soc Exp Biol Med 87:571–577, 1954.

998. Anderson SI, Morse LM. The influence of solvent on the teratogenic effect of folic acid antagonist in the rat. Exp Mol Pathol 5:134–145, 1966.

999. Dyban AP, Akimova IM. Characteristic features of the action of chloridine on various stages of embryonic

development (experimental investigation). Akush Ginekol (Rus) 41:21–38, 1965.

1000. Dyban AP, Akimova IM, Svetlova VA. Effects of 2,4-diamino-5-chlorphenyl-6-ethylpyrimidine on embryonic development of rats. Dokl Akad Nauk (Moskova) 163:1514–1517, 1965.

1001. Krahe M. [Investigations on the teratogen effect of medicine for the treatment of toxoplasmosis during pregnancy.] Arch Gynakol (in German) 202:104–109, 1965.

1002. Sullivan GE, Takacs E. Comparative teratogenicity of pyrimethamine in rats and hamsters. Teratology 4:205–210, 1971.

1003. Puchta V, Simandlová E. Zur frage der fruchtschadigung durch pyrimethamin (Daraprim) [On the question of fetus injury due to pyrimethamine (Daraprim)]. In Kirchhoff H, Langer H (eds). Toxoplasmose. Stuttgart, Georg Thieme, 1971, p 19.

1004. Garin J-P, Eyles DE. [Spiramycin therapy of experimental toxoplasmosis in mice.] Presse Med (in French) 66:957–958, 1958.

1005. Mas Bakal P. [Deferred spiramycin treatment of acute toxoplasmosis in white mice.] Ned Tijdschr Geneeskd (in German) 109:1014–1017, 1965.

1006. Niel G, Videau D. Activité de la spiramycione in vitro sur Toxoplasma gondii. Réunion Inter Discipl Chimioth Antiinfect, Paris 121:8, 1981.

1007. MacFarlane JA, et al. Spiramycin in the prevention of postoperative staphylococcal infection. Lancet 1:1–4, 1968.

1008. Benazet F, Dubost M. Apparent paradox of antimicrobial activity of psiramycin. Antibiot Ann 211–220, 1958–1959.

1009. Sutherland R. Spiramycin: a reappraisal of its antibacterial activity. Br J Pharmacol 19:99–110, 1962.

1010. Kernbaum S. [Spiramycin; therapeutic value in humans.] Sem Hop Paris (in French) 58:289–297, 1982.

1011. Garin JP, et al. Bases theoriques de la prevention par la spiramycine de la toxoplasmose congenitale chez la femme enceinte. Presse Med 76:2266, 1968.

1012. Hudson DG, Yoshihara GM, Kirby WM. Spiramycin: clinical and laboratory studies. Arch Intern Med 97:57–61, 1956.

1013. Forestier F, et al. Suivi therapeutique foetomaternel de la spiramycine en cours de grossesse. Arch Fr Pediatr 44:539–544, 1987.

1014. Martin C, et al. [The course of congenital toxoplasmosis: critical study of 12 treated cases.] Ann Pediatr (Paris) (in French) 16:117–128, 1969.

1015. Beverley JKA, et al. Prevention of pathological changes in experimental congenital toxoplasma infections. Lyon Medical 230:491–498, 1973.

1016. Back N, et al. Clinical and experimental pharmacology of parenteral spiramycin. Clin Pharmacol Ther 3:305–313, 1962.

1017. Stramba-Badiale M, et al. QT interval prolongation and risk of life-threatening arrhythmias during toxoplasmosis prophylaxis with spiramycin in neonates. Am Heart J 133:108–111, 1997.

1018. Couvreur J, et al. In utero treatment of toxoplasmic fetopathy with the combination pyrimethamine-sulfadiazine. Fetal Diagn Ther 8:45–50, 1993.

1019. Leport C, et al. Failure of spiramycin to prevent neurotoxoplasmosis in immunosuppressed patients [Letter to the editor]. Med Clin North Am 70:677–692, 1986.

1020. Stadtsbaeder S, Calvin-Preval MC. [The trimethoprim-sulfamethoxazole association in experimental toxoplasmosis in mice.] Acta Clin Belg (in French) 28:34–39, 1973.

1021. Grossman PL, Remington JS. The effect of trimethoprim and sulfamethoxazole on Toxoplasma gondii in vitro and in vivo. Am J Trop Med Hyg 28:445–455, 1979.

1022. Feldman HA. Effects of trimethoprim and sulfisoxazole alone and in combination on murine toxoplasmosis. Addendum by JS Remington. J Infect Dis 128(Suppl): S774–S776, 1973.

1023. Remington JS. Addendum to Feldman HA. Effects of trimethoprim and sulfisoxazole alone and in combination on murine toxoplasmosis. J Infect Dis 128 (Suppl):S774–S776, 1973.

1024. Sander J, Midtvedt T. The effect of trimethoprim on acute experimental toxoplasmosis in mice. Acta Pathol Microbiol Scand [B] 78:664–668, 1970.

1025. Brus R, et al. Antitoxoplasmic activity of sulfonamides with various radicals in experimental toxoplasmosis in mice. Z Tropenmed Parasitol 22:98–103, 1971.

1026. Norrby R, et al. Treatment of toxoplasmosis with trimethoprim-sulphamethoxazole. Scand J Infect Dis 7:72–75, 1975.

1027. Domart A, Robineau M, Carbon C. [Acquired toxoplasmosis: a new chemotherapy: the sulfamethoxazole-trimethoprim combination.] Nouv Presse Med (in French) 2:321–322, 1973.

1028. Mössner G. Klinische ergebnisse mit dem kombinationspraparat sulfamethoxazole + trimethoprim. Progress in Antimicrobial and Anticancer Chemotherapy. Baltimore, University Park Press, 1970, pp 966–970.

1029. Torre D, et al. Randomized trial of trimethoprim-sulfamethoxazole versus pyrimethamine-sulfadiazine for therapy of toxoplasmic encephalitis in patients with AIDS. Italian Collaborative Study Group. Antimicrob Agents Chemother 42:1346–1349, 1998.

1030. Araujo FG, Remington JS. Effect of clindamycin on acute and chronic toxoplasmosis in mice. Antimicrob Agents Chemother 5:647–651, 1974.

1031. McMaster PR, et al. The effect of two chlorinated lincomycin analogues against acute toxoplasmosis in mice. Am J Trop Med Hyg 22:14–17, 1973.

1032. Tabbara KF, Nozik RA, O'Connor GR. Clindamycin effects on experimental ocular toxoplasmosis in the rabbit. Arch Ophthalmol 92:244–247, 1974.

1033. Dannemann BR, Israelski DM, Remington JS. Treatment of toxoplasmic encephalitis with intravenous clindamycin. Arch Intern Med 148:2477–2482, 1988.

1034. Dannemann BR, et al. Treatment of toxoplasmic encephalitis in patients with AIDS: a randomized trial comparing pyrimethamine plus clindamycin to pyrimethamine plus sulfadiazine. Ann Intern Med 1992. 116:33–43, 1992.

1035. Chang HR, Comte R, Pechere JC. In vitro and in vivo effects of doxycycline on Toxoplasma gondii. Antimicrob Agents Chemother 34:775–780, 1990.

1036. Tabbara KF, Sakuragi S, O'Connor GR. Minocycline in the chemotherapy of murine toxoplasmosis. Parasitology 84:297–302, 1982.

1037. Chang HR, et al. Activity of minocycline against Toxoplasma gondii infection in mice. J Antimicrob Chemother 27:639–645, 1991.

1038. Pope-Pegram L, et al. treatment of presumed central nervous system toxoplasmosis with doxycycline [abstract]. Program and Abstracts of VII International Conference on AIDS. Florence, Italy, 1991.

1039. Turett G, et al. Failure of doxycycline in the treatment of cerebral toxoplasmosis [abstract]. Sixth International Conference on AIDS. San Francisco, 1990.

1040. Remington JS, Yagura T, Robinson WS. The effect of rifampin on *Toxoplasma gondii*. Proc Soc Exp Biol Med 135:167–172, 1970.

1041. Chan J, Luft BJ. Activity of roxithromycin (RU 28965), a macrolide, against *Toxoplasma gondii* infection in mice. Antimicrob Agents Chemother 30:323–324, 1986.

1042. Luft BJ. In vivo and in vitro activity of roxithromycin against *Toxoplasma gondii* in mice. Eur J Clin Microbiol 6:479–481, 1987.

1043. Araujo FG, et al. Activity of clarithromycin alone or in combination with other drugs for treatment of murine toxoplasmosis. Antimicrob Agents Chemother 36:2454–2457, 1992.

1044. Araujo FG, Guptill DR, Remington JS. Azithromycin, a macrolide antibiotic with potent activity against *Toxoplasma gondii*. Antimicrob Agents Chemother 32:755–757, 1988.

1045. Stray-Pederson B. Azithromycin levels in placental tissue, amniotic fluid and blood. 36th Interscience Conference on Antimicrobial Agents and Chemotherapy, 1996.

1046. Liesenfeld O, Wong SY, Remington JS. Toxoplasmosis in the Setting of AIDS. *In* Bartlett JG, Merigan TC, Bolognesi D (eds): Textbook of AIDS Medicine. Baltimore, Williams & Wilkins, 1999.

1047. Araujo FG, et al. Use of ketolides in combination with other drugs to treat experimental toxoplasmosis. J Antimicrob Chemother 42:665–667, 1998.

1048. Huskinson-Mark J, Araujo FG, Remington JS. Evaluation of the effect of drugs on the cyst form of *Toxoplasma gondii*. J Infect Dis 164:170–177, 1991.

1049. Araujo FG, Huskinson J, Remington JS. Remarkable in vitro and in vivo activities of the hydroxynaphthoquinone 566C80 against tachyzoites and tissue cysts of *Toxoplasma gondii*. Antimicrob Agents Chemother 35:293–299, 1991.

1050. Kovacs JA. Efficacy of atovaquone in treatment of toxoplasmosis in patients with AIDS. Lancet 340:637–638, 1992.

1051. Clumeck N, et al. Abstract Atovaquone (1.4 hydroxynaphthoquinone, 566C80) in the treatment of acute cerebral toxoplasmosis (CT) in AIDS patients (P). 32nd Interscience Conference on Antimicrobial Agents and Chemotherapy. Anaheim, Calif, 1992.

1052. Torres RA, et al. Atovaquone for salvage treatment and suppression of toxoplasmic encephalitis in patients with AIDS. Atovaquone/Toxoplasmic Encephalitis Study Group. Clin Infect Dis 24:422–429, 1997.

1053. Katlama C, et al. Atovaquone as long-term suppressive therapy for toxoplasmic encephalitis in patients with AIDS and multiple drug intolerance. AIDS 10:1107–1112, 1996.

1054. Khan AA, et al. Trovafloxacin is active against *Toxoplasma gondii*. Antimicrob Agents Chemother 40:1855–1859, 1996.

1055. Khan AA, et al. Activity of trovafloxacin in combination with other drugs for treatment of acute murine toxoplasmosis. Antimicrob Agents Chemother 41:893–897, 1997.

1056. Stagno S, et al. Auditory and visual defects resulting from symptomatic and subclinical congenital cytomegaloviral and toxoplasma infections. Pediatrics 59:669–678, 1977.

1057. Jeannel D, et al. What is known about the prevention of congenital toxoplasmosis? Lancet 336:359–361, 1990.

1058. Boulot P, Pratlong F, Sarda P, et al. [Limitations of the prenatal treatment of congenital toxoplasmosis with the sulfadiazine-pyrimethamine combination.] Presse Med (in French) 12:570, 1990.

1059. Couvreur J, et al. Étude d'une serie homogene de 210 cas de toxoplasmose congenitale chez des nourrissons ages de 0 a 11 mois et depistes de facon prospective. Sem Hop Paris 61:3015–3019, 1985.

1060. Wallon M, et al. Letter to the editor. Lancet 344:541, 1994.

1061. Mirlesse V, et al. Long-term follow-up of fetuses and newborn with congenital toxoplasmosis diagnosed and treated prenatally. In preparation, 2000.

1062. Alford CA Jr, Reynolds DW, Stagno S. Current concepts of chronic perinatal infections. *In* Gluck L (ed). Modern Perinatal Medicine. Chicago, Year Book, 1975, pp 285–306.

1063. Cunningham GC, Hawes WE, Madore C. Intrauterine Growth and Neonatal Risk in California. Sacramento, State of California Department of Health, 1976.

1064. Szusterkac M. A propos de 124 cas de toxoplasmose congénitale: aspects cliniques et paracliniques en fonction des circonstances du diagnostic retrospectif ou prospectif; resultats du traitement. Paris, Faculté de Médécine Saint-Antoine, 1980.

1065. Briatte C. Étude de 55 cas de toxoplasmose congenitale dépistes lors de bilans de santé systematiques après l'age de 10 mois. Centre de Bilans de Santé de la Securité Sociale de la Region Parisienne. Paris, Faculté de Médécine Saint-Antoine, 1980.

1066. Sever JL, et al. Toxoplasmosis: maternal and pediatric findings in 23,000 pregnancies. Pediatrics 82:181–192, 1988.

1067. Roizen N, et al. Developmental and neurologic function in treated congenital toxoplasmosis [abstract no. 2101]. Pediatr Res 31:353A, 1992.

1068. McLeod R, et al. Treatment of congenital toxoplasmosis [abstract]. 17th International Congress of Chemotherapy. Berlin, Futuramed, 1991.

1069. Swisher CN, et al. Congenital toxoplasmosis. Semin Pediatr Neurol 1:4–25, 1994.

1070. Mets MG, Mack DG, Boyer K. Congenital ocular toxoplasmosis. *In* Mets MB, Group TTS (eds): Ophthalmologic Findings in Congenital Toxoplasmosis [abstract No. 2009–16]. Invest Ophthalmol Vis Sci 1094, 1992.

1071. Engstrom REJ, et al. Current practices in the management of ocular toxoplasmosis. Am J Ophthalmol 111:601–610, 1991.

1072. Desmonts G. Prevention de la toxoplasmose: remarques sur l'experience poursuivie en France. *In* Marois M (ed). Prevention of Physical and Mental Congenital Defects, Part B: Epidemiology, Early Detection and Therapy, and Environmental Factors. New York, Alan R. Liss, 1985, pp 313–316.

1073. Frenkel JK. Congenital toxoplasmosis: prevention or palliation? Am J Obstet Gynecol 141:359–361, 1981.

1074. Henderson JB, et al. The evaluation of new services: possibilities for preventing congenital toxoplasmosis. Int J Epidemiol 13:65–72, 1984.

1075. McCabe R, Remington JS. Toxoplasmosis: the time has come [Editorial]. N Engl J Med 318:313–315, 1988.

1076. Frenkel JK. Breaking the transmission chain of Toxoplasma: a program for the prevention of human toxoplasmosis. Bull NY Acad Med 50:228–235, 1974.

1077. Frenkel JK. Toxoplasmosis in cats and man. Feline Practice, pp 28–41, 1975.

1078. Hartley WJ, Munday BL. Felidae in the dissemination of toxoplasmosis to man and other animals. Aust Vet J 50:224–228, 1974.

1079. Hutchison WM. *Toxoplasma gondii* and its development in domestic felines. Victorian Vet Proc, pp 17–21, 1973–1974.

1080. Frenkel JK, Dubey JP. Rodents as vectors for feline coccidia, *Isospora felis* and *Isospora rivolta*. J Infect Dis 125:69–72, 1972.

1081. Hassl A. Efficiency analysis of toxoplasmosis screening in pregnancy: comment (correspondence). Scand J Infect Dis 28:211–212, 1996.

1082. Lappalainen M, et al. Cost-benefit analysis of screening for toxoplasmosis during pregnancy. Scand J Infect Dis 27:265–272, 1995.

1083. Lappalainen M, et al. Screening of toxoplasmosis during pregnancy. Isr J Med Sci 30:362–363, 1994.

1084. Bader TJ, Macones GA, Asch DA. Prenatal screening for toxoplasmosis. Obstet Gynecol 90:457–464, 1997.

1085. Luyasu V, et al. [Congenital toxoplasmosis and seroconversion at the end of pregnancy: clinical observations.] Acta Clin Belg (in French) 52:381–387, 1997.

1086. Couvreur J. [In utero treatment of congenital toxoplasmosis with a pyrimethamine-sulfadiazine combination.] Presse Med (in French) 20:1137, 1991.

1087. Brézin AP, et al. Ophthalmic outcome after pre- and post-natal treatment of congenital toxoplasmosis. ARVO, 1998.

1088. Desmonts G, Jones TC. Congenital toxoplasmosis. N Engl J Med 291:365–366, 1974.

1089. Desmonts G, Couvreur J. [Congenital toxoplasmosis: prospective study of the outcome of pregnancy in 542 women with toxoplasmosis acquired during pregnancy.] Ann Pediatr (Paris) (in French) 31:805–809, 1984.

1090. Roberts F, et al. Histopathological features of ocular toxoplasmosis in the fetus and infant. Arch Ophthalmol. Submitted 2000.

1091. Holliman RE. Congenital toxoplasmosis: prevention, screening and treatment. J Hosp Infect 30(Suppl):179–190, 1995.

1092. Ledger WJ. Preventative care in obstetrics—toxoplasmosis, cytomegalovirus, and hepatitis B. J Matern Fetal Med 5:100–105, 1996.

1093. Mittendorf R, et al. Is routine antenatal toxoplasmosis screening justified in the United States? Statistical considerations in the application of medical screening tests [in process citation]. Clin Obstet Gynecol 42:163–173, 1999.

1094. Kräubig H. Erste praktische erfahrungen mit der prophylaze der konnatalen toxoplasmose. Med Klin 58:1361–1364, 1963.

1095. Thalhammer O. Congenital toxoplasmosis in Vienna. Summering (sic) findings and opinions. *In* Specia L (ed). Colloque sur la Toxoplasmose de la Femme Enceinte et la Prevention de la Toxoplasmose Congenitale. Lyon, Medical, 1969, pp 109–129.

1096. Thalhammer O. [Prevention of congenital toxoplasmosis.] Neuropediatrie (in French) 4:233–237, 1973.

1097. Hengst VP. [Effectiveness of general testing for *Toxoplasma gondii* infection in pregnancy.] Zentralbl Gynakol (in German) 104:949–956, 1982.

1098. Daffos F, et al. Letter to the editor. Lancet 344:541, 1994.

1099. Liesenfeld O, et al. Confirmatory serological testing results in remarkable decrease in unnecessary abortion among pregnant women in the United States with positive toxoplasma serology. 35th Annual Meeting of the Infectious Diseases Society of America. San Francisco, 1997.

1100. Eckerling B, Neri A, Eylan E. Toxoplasmosis: a cause of infertility. Fertil Steril 19:883–891, 1968.

1101. Vlaev S. Opyt profilaktiki vrozdennogo toksoplazmoza. Vop Okrany Materin Dets 10:78–82, 1965.

1102. Isbruch F. [Contributions to the problem of toxoplasmosis: I. Should we, at the present state of knowledge, treat pregnant women with positive toxoplasmosis titers, with daraprim and supronal?] Zentralbl Gynakol (in German) 82:1522–1544, 1960.

1103. Sharf M, Eibschitz I, Eylan E. Latent toxoplasmosis and pregnancy. Obstet Gynecol 42:349–354, 1973.

1104. Feldman HA. Congenital toxoplasmosis [Letter to the editor]. N Engl J Med 26:1212, 1963.

1105. Cengir SD, Ortac F, Soylemex F. Treatment and results of chronic toxoplasmosis. Gynecol Obstet Invest 33:105–108, 1992.

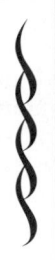

C H A P T E R   6

Rubella

LOUIS Z. COOPER, M.D., and CHARLES A. ALFORD, JR., M.D.

The impact of rubella virus infection and the progress made toward controlling congenital rubella infection have been well chronicled.[1-9] Rubella was first recognized as a clinical entity by German researchers in the mid-eighteenth century, who called it Rötheln. However, they considered it to be a modified form of measles or scarlet fever.[1] Manton first described it as a separate disease in the English literature in 1815.[10] In 1866, Veale gave it a "short and euphonious" name, rubella.[11] The disease was considered mild and self-limited. It became a focus of major interest in 1941, only after Gregg, an Australian ophthalmologist, associated intrauterine acquisition of infection with production of cataracts and heart disease.[12] Although his findings were initially doubted, numerous reports of infants with congenital defects after maternal rubella soon appeared in the literature.[1] Subsequent investigations showed that the major defects associated with congenital rubella infection include congenital heart disease, cataracts, and deafness. Mental retardation and many defects, involving almost every organ, have also been noted.[2-4, 7, 13, 14] Before the availability of specific viral diagnostic studies, the frequency of fetal damage after maternal infection in the first trimester was estimated to be in excess of 20%, a figure now known to be much too low.

Recognition of the teratogenic potential of rubella infection led to increased efforts to isolate the etiologic agent. The viral etiology of rubella was suggested by experimental infections in humans and monkeys as early as 1938 but was not confirmed until reports of the isolation of the viral agent in cell cultures were made independently in 1962 by Weller and Neva at Harvard University School of Public Health and by Parkman, Buescher, and Artenstein at Walter Reed Army Institute for Research.[15-20] This accomplishment paved the way for the development of serologic tests and a vaccine.[2-4, 21-23] Efforts to develop a vaccine were hastened by the tragic events associated with a worldwide rubella pandemic from 1962 through 1964, which, in the United States, resulted in approximately 12.5 million cases of clinically acquired rubella, 11,000 fetal deaths, and 20,000 infants born with defects collectively referred to as the congenital rubella syndrome; 2100 infants with congenital rubella syndrome died in the neonatal period.[24] The estimated cost to the U.S. economy was approximately $2 billion.

In 1969, three strains of live, attenuated rubella vaccine were licensed in various countries: HPV-77 (high-passage virus, 77 times), grown in duck embryo for five passages (DE-5) or dog kidney for 12 passages (DK-12); Cendehill, grown in primary rabbit cells; and RA 27/3 (rubella abortus, twenty-seventh specimen, third explant), grown in human diploid fibroblast culture.[25–27] Although these and other strains of vaccine are now used globally, the RA 27/3 vaccine has been used exclusively in the United States since 1979.[2–4, 7, 28]

In addition to providing the impetus for vaccine research and development, the rubella pandemic also provided the scientific community with a unique opportunity to gain new knowledge about the nature of both intrauterine and extrauterine infections and the immunity stimulated by both. The quest for more knowledge using the tools of molecular biology has continued since vaccine licensure and serves as a tribute to Gregg's historic contribution to our understanding of intrauterine infection.

Much current interest has focused on the epidemiology of rubella and congenital rubella syndrome in countries with immunization programs, the desirability of introducing vaccine in countries without a program, and the optimal strategy to control congenital rubella (universal immunization versus selective immunization of females).[3, 5–7, 29–34] Vaccination of all children, as well as susceptible adolescents and young adults, particularly females, has had such a dramatic impact on the occurrence of rubella and congenital rubella in the United States that efforts are now in progress to eliminate congenital rubella syndrome from the United States.[5, 24, 30, 35] Given the magnitude of international travel, this goal will remain elusive until similar goals are adopted by other countries, particularly in Latin America, and vaccine use is increased in certain communities that in the past have been resistant to immunization efforts.[35]

Duration and quality of vaccine-induced immunity[5, 8, 36–55] and adverse events associated with immunization, particularly arthritis and the risk of the vaccine to the fetus,[5, 8, 56–63] have been of concern, but the vaccine continues to confer long-lasting immunity while placing the vaccinated person at minimal risk of adverse events.

Rubella research on the characteristics of the virus, its effect on the developing fetus, the host's immune response, and diagnostic methodology has yielded new information about the structural proteins of the virus as well as the difference in the immune response to these proteins after congenital and acquired infections.[64–84] Differences in antibody profile may be useful in diagnosing congenital infection retrospectively and may provide further information on the pathogenesis of congenital infection.[82, 83, 85] Techniques that detect rubella-specific antibodies within minutes have been developed by using latex agglutination and passive hemagglutination.[86–92]

Studies to examine the subclass distribution of IgG immunoglobulin and the kinetics of rubella-specific immunoglobulins (including IgA, IgD, and IgE) after acquired rubella, congenital infection, and vaccination may eventually lead to the development of additional diagnostic tools.[93–97]

Improved laboratory methods have further defined the risk of fetal infection and congenital damage in all stages of pregnancy.[98–105] It now appears that the risk of fetal infection after first-trimester maternal infection and subsequent congenital anomalies after fetal infection may be higher than previously noted (81% and 85%, respectively, in one study).[100] There is also evidence that the fetus is at risk of infection throughout pregnancy, even near term, although the occurrence of defects after infection beyond 16 to 18 weeks of gestation appears to be small. Use of more sensitive laboratory assays has also shown that subclinical reinfection after previous natural infection, as after vaccination, may be accompanied by an IgM response, making differentiation between subclinical reinfection and asymptomatic primary infection at times difficult.[39, 49, 51, 53] Although reinfection usually poses no threat to the fetus, rare instances of congenital infection after maternal reinfection have been reported.[39, 40, 43, 45, 49–51, 53, 106–111]

Finally, follow-up of patients with congenital rubella has provided new information about the pathogenesis, immune status, interplay between congenital infection, and human leukocyte antigen (HLA) haplotypes and long-term outcome associated with congenital infection.[112–129] These studies continue to document that congenital infection is persistent, that virtually every organ may be affected, and that autoimmunity and immune complex formation are probably involved in many of the disease processes, particularly in the delayed and persistent clinical manifestations. They also confirm earlier studies, noting an increased risk of diabetes mellitus and other endocrinopathies in patients with congenital rubella syndrome compared with the general population.

THE VIRUS

Morphology and Physical and Chemical Composition

Rubella virus is a generally spherical particle, 50 to 70 nm in diameter, with a dense central nucleoid measuring 30 nm in diameter. The central nucleoid is surrounded by a 10-nm-thick, single-layered envelope acquired during budding of the virus into cytoplasmic vesicles or through the plasma membrane.[130–135] Surface projections or spikes with knobbed ends that are 5 to 6 nm in length have been reported. The specific gravity of the complete viral particle is 1.184 ± 0.004 g/ml, corresponding to a sedimentation constant of 360 ± 50 Svedberg units.[130]

The wild virus contains infectious RNA (molecular weight 3 to 4 × 10^6) within its core.[115] The rubella virus envelope contains lipids that differ quantitatively from those of the plasma membrane and are essential for infectivity.[145, 146] Rubella virus is heat labile and has a half-life of 1 hour at 57° C.[147] However, in the presence of protein (e.g., 2% serum albumin), infectivity is maintained for a week or more at 4° C and indefinitely at −60° C. Storage at freezer temperatures of −10° C to −20° C should be avoided because infectivity is rapidly lost.[147, 148] Rubella virus can also be stabilized against heat inactivation by the addition of magnesium sulfate to virus suspensions.[149] Thus, specimens to be examined virologically should be transported to distant laboratories packed in ice rather than frozen, with the addition of stabilizer if possible. Infectivity is also rapidly lost at pH levels below 6.8 or above 8.1, and in the presence of ultraviolet light, lipid-active solvents, or other chemicals such as formalin, ethylene oxide, and β-propiolactone.[147, 150–152] Infectivity of rubella in cell culture is inhibited by amantadine, but the drug appears to have no therapeutic effect.[153–156]

Several laboratories have described the structural proteins of rubella virus and determined the nucleotide sequence of the genes coding for these proteins.[64, 79, 130, 157–160] Originally, three structural proteins were identified and designated as VP-1, VP-2, and VP-3.[157] These three major structural proteins now are designated E1, E2, and C, with relative molecular weights of 58,000, 42,000 to 47,000, and 33,000, respectively.[65–67] E1 and E2 are envelope glycoproteins and make up the characteristic spikelike projections that are located on the viral membrane. Structural protein C, which is not glycosylated, is associated with the infectious 40S genomic RNA to form the nucleocapsid.[69] The E2 glycopeptide has been shown on polyacrylamide gels to be heterogeneous with two bands, which are designated E2a (relative molecular weight of 42,000) and E2b (relative molecular weight of 47,000).[65]

Monoclonal antibody studies have begun to delineate the functional activities of these structural proteins. E1 appears to be the viral hemagglutinin and binds hemagglutination-inhibiting, as well as hemolysis-inhibiting, antibody; E2 does not appear to be involved in hemagglutination.[64, 66, 68, 70–73] Monoclonal antibodies specific for both E1 and E2 have neutralizing activity.[64, 68, 74, 83, 84] Studies also indicate that there are multiple epitopes on the structural proteins that are involved in hemagglutination inhibition (HI) and neutralizing activities.[73, 76] Molecular analyses of rubella viruses isolated during the period 1961 and 1997 from specimens obtained in North America, Europe, and Asia have documented the remarkable antigenic stability of the E1 envelope glycoprotein.[78] E1 amino acid sequences have differed by no more than 3%, indicating no major antigenic variation over the 36-year period that spanned the major worldwide pandemic of 1962 to 1964 and the 30 years since introduction of rubella vaccine. However, two genotypes were evident: genotype I isolated before 1970 grouped into a single diffuse clade, indicating intercontinental circulation, whereas most of the post-1975 viruses segregated into geographic clades from each continent, indicating evolution in response to vaccination programs. The availability of molecular analysis and the minor variations in amino acid sequences have provided an additional tool for monitoring the sources of infection in areas where indigenous rubella has been greatly reduced by high levels of immunization. As discussed in more detail later, the complexity of the antigenic nature of the rubella virion affects the ability of the host to respond to the full complement of antigens, as well as the various antibody assays required to detect all the corresponding antibody responses (see the later section on Natural History).

Classification

Rubella has been classified as a member of the togavirus family (from the Latin word *toga*, meaning "cloak"), genus rubivirus.[161, 162] No serologic relationship exists between rubella and other known viruses. Minor biologic differences identified in different passaged strains of rubella virus are not reflected in antigenic differences, as assessed by comparing protein composition or serologic reactions.[130, 160, 163, 164] Thus, differences in the immune response after immunization with the various vaccines now in use are not caused by inherent differences in the viral strain but rather by modification of the viruses during their attenuation in cell culture.[28] The reported variation in the virulence of rubella epidemics does not appear to be explained by the molecular analyses noted earlier, but they may be due to differences in population susceptibility and under-reporting of cases of congenital rubella.[165–172]

Antigen and Serologic Testing

Purified rubella virus has a number of antigenic components associated with both the viral envelope and the ribonucleoprotein core.[152, 158] These antigens and the ability of specific antiserum to neutralize virus form the basis for the wide variety of serologic methods available to measure humoral immunity after natural and vaccine-induced infection.

The ability of antibodies to inhibit agglutination of erythrocytes by the surface hemagglutinin (HA antigen) forms the basis for the HI test, which at one time was the most popular rubella serologic test. The HA antigen was originally prepared from BHK tissue culture fluids and then from alkaline extracts of infected BHK-21 cells.[23, 173] This antigen can agglutinate a variety of red blood cells, including newborn chick, adult goose, pigeon, and human group O erythrocytes.[174] Rubella hemagglutinin is unique in its dependency on calcium ions to attach to red blood cell receptors.[174, 175] After extraction from infected cells, rubella hemagglutinin is stable for months at −20° C, several weeks at 4° C, and overnight at 37° C but is destroyed within minutes after heating to 56° C.[173, 175] The HA antigen can be protected from ether inactivation by pretreatment with Tween 80. Cells and serum both contain heat-stable β-lipoproteins that can inhibit rubella hemagglutination and give rise to false-positive results.[23, 152] Although it has been reported that nonspecific inhibitors do not interfere in the HI test if the HA antigen and erythrocytes are mixed before addition of serum, the recommended method is to pretreat the sera to remove these inhibitors.[152, 176] Earlier test procedures used kaolin adsorption for removal of these nonspecific inhibitors; however, a number of faster and more specific methods are now used, such as treatment with heparin-MnCl$_2$ or dextran sulfate-CaCl.[177, 178]

Cell-associated complement fixation antigen was first derived from infected rabbit kidney (RK-13) and African green monkey kidney cell cultures and later prepared from alkaline extracts of infected BHK-21 cells.[22, 179] There are two complement fixation antigens—one similar in size and weight to both the hemagglutinin and infectious virus, and the other smaller and "soluble."[180-182] The antibody response as measured by the soluble antigen is slower than that of the larger antigen, which parallels the HI response. In contrast to the HA antigen, complement fixation antigens do not lose their antigenicity after ether treatment.[179, 181]

A variety of precipitin antigens have been serologically demonstrated; two of these, the theta and iota antigens, are associated with the viral envelope and core, respectively.[183-185] The antibody response to these two antigens is of interest. Antibodies to the theta antigen rise promptly and persist. Antibodies to the iota antigen are detectable later and for a shorter time.[186] The RA 27/3 vaccine appears to be unique among vaccine strains in its ability to elicit a response to the iota antigen, thus making its immune response more like natural infection. The significance of this observation remains unclear.[187]

Rubella virus antigen-antibody complexes (involving both the envelope and the core antigens) cause aggregation of platelets.[188, 189] However, the main platelet aggregation activity appears to reside with the viral envelope.

Antibody directed against the rubella virus can also be measured by virus neutralization in tissue culture.[2-4, 21, 190-192] Whereas the presence of neutralizing antibodies correlates best with protective immunity, neutralization assays are time consuming, expensive, and relatively difficult to perform. Thus, laboratories have traditionally performed the complement fixation and HI tests. Because the complement fixation test is insensitive for screening purposes and cannot detect an early rise in antibody in acute acquired infection, the HI test has been the most widely used assay.[2-4, 152, 186, 190, 193, 194] However, over the past decade a number of more rapid, easily performed, reliable, and sensitive tests have replaced the HI test in popularity.[86, 194, 195] These include passive (or indirect) hemagglutination; single radial hemolysis (also known as hemolysis in gel), which is used widely abroad; radioimmunoassay; immunofluorescence; and enzyme immunoassay tests, also referred to as enzyme-linked immunosorbent assays.[190, 193-224] Rapid latex agglutination and passive hemagglutination assays can provide results in minutes for both screening and diagnostic purposes.[86-92] The large number of assays now available and their greater sensitivity compared with the HI test have led to some confusion about the level of antibody that should be considered indicative of immunity (see Update on Vaccine Characteristics section).[42, 52, 55, 194, 222] The HI test still, however, remains the reference test against which other assays are compared.

Immunoglobulin class-specific antibody can be measured in most of the serologic systems.[152, 201-205, 208, 210, 219-222, 225-233] This most frequently involves detection of IgM in either whole or fractionated sera. A number of techniques are used to fractionate and then test the serum. An important consideration in any IgM assay is the possibility of false-positive results because of the presence of rheumatoid factor. Solid-phase IgM capture assays, however, appear to be unaffected by rheumatoid factor.[97, 205, 220, 231]

Growth in Cell Culture

Rubella replicates in a wide variety of cell culture systems, primary cell strains and cell lines.[148, 152, 234] The time required for virus recovery varies markedly, depending in part on the culture system being employed.

As a generalization, rubella growing in primary cell cultures (human, simian, bovine, rabbit, canine, or duck) produces interference to superinfection by a wide variety of viruses (especially enteroviruses, but also myxoviruses, papovaviruses, arboviruses, and, to some extent, herpesviruses) but no cytopathic effect.[19, 20, 147] In contrast, a cytopathic effect of widely varying natures results from infection of continuous cell lines (hamster, rabbit, simian, and human). Generally, primary cells, especially African green monkey kidney, have proved superior for isolation of virus from human material by the interference technique. However, the continuous RK-13 and Vero (vervet kidney) cell lines are also used because cytopathic effect is produced and there is no problem with adventitious simian agents.[148] Continuous cell lines, such as BHK-21 and Vero, are best suited for antigen production because of the higher levels of virus produced.

All cell lines support chronic infection with serial propagation, but some are limited by the occurrence of cytopathic effect. These cells grow slowly and can be subcultivated fewer times than when not infected.[148] The mechanisms of rubella-induced interference and persistent infection in cell cultures are not completely understood. Although interferon production has been described after rubella infection of cell cultures, interference appears to be an intrinsic phenomenon.[148, 152, 235-237] As with other viruses, generation of defective interfering particles can be found in tissue culture.[238] However, these particles are thought to be nonessential for persistence.

Rubella virus can be plaqued in RK-13, BHK-21, SIRC (rabbit cornea), and Vero cells.[152] Plaquing forms the basis of neutralization assays, and differences in plaquing characteristics can be used as markers to distinguish among strains.[21, 152, 164, 190-192]

Pathogenicity for Animals

Rubella virus grows in primates and in various small laboratory animals. However, in no animal has the acquired or congenital disease been completely reproduced.

Vervet and, particularly, rhesus monkeys are susceptible to infection by the intranasal, intravenous, or intramuscular routes.[239-241] Although no rash develops, there is nasopharyngeal excretion of viruses in all of the inoculated monkeys and demonstrable viremia in 50%. Attempts to produce transplacental infection in pregnant monkeys have been partially successful. Rubella virus has been recovered from the amnion and the placenta, but the embryo itself has not been shown to be consistently infected.[242, 243]

The ferret is by far the most useful of the small laboratory animals in rubella studies. Ferret kits are highly sensitive to subcutaneous and, particularly, intracerebral inoculations. Virus has been recovered from the heart, liver, spleen, lung, brain, eye, blood, and urine for a month or longer after inoculation, and both neutralizing and complement fixation antibodies have developed.[244] Ferret kits inoculated at birth develop corneal clouding. Virus appears in fetal ferrets after inoculation of pregnant animals.[245]

Rabbits, hamsters, guinea pigs, rats, and suckling mice have all been infected with rubella virus, but none has proved to be a consistent and reliable animal model system for study of rubella infection.[165, 166, 246–249] Studies indicating that Japanese strains of rubella virus were less teratogenic to offspring of infected rabbits than U.S. strains have not been confirmed.[165, 166] These experiments were conducted to examine further the hypothesis referred to earlier that there is a difference in the virulence among rubella virus strains circulating in Japan and other parts of the world.[163, 165–169, 171]

EPIDEMIOLOGY

Humans are the only known host for rubella virus. Continuous cycling in humans is the only apparent means for the virus to be maintained in nature. Because rubella is predominantly a self-limited infection seen in late winter and spring, questions have arisen as to how the virus persists throughout the remainder of the year. Person-to-person transmission probably occurs at very low levels in the general population throughout summer and winter and probably at much higher levels in closed populations of susceptible individuals.[250–270] Congenitally infected infants can shed virus from multiple sites and can serve as reservoirs of virus during periods of low transmission.[156, 271–276] This is of particular concern in the hospital setting.[156, 268] Efficiency of transmission may also vary among individuals, with some being better "spreaders" than others. This phenomenon may contribute to continued circulation of the virus.[277]

Rubella is worldwide in distribution.[278–284] The virus circulates almost continually, at least in continental populations. In the northern hemisphere's continental temperate zones, rubella is consistently more prevalent in the spring, with peak attack rates in March, April, and May; infection is much less prevalent during the remainder of the year, increasing or decreasing during the 2 months before or after the peak period.[281, 283] Before widespread rubella immunization, in most of the world, sizable epidemics occurred every 6 to 9 years, with major ones at intervals ranging from 10 to 30 years. Epidemics usually built up and receded gradually over a 3- to 4-year interval, peaking at the midpoint.[9, 278, 281, 283] The apparent increased infectivity and virulence of rubella as exemplified in the major epidemics have been the subject of considerable speculation and interest in recent years. One popular thesis, referred to previously, is the un-

proven emergence of a more virulent strain of virus at widely separated intervals.[163, 165–169, 171] However, convincing evidence for the existence of biologically different strains of rubella of clinical significance has yet to be presented. At least, molecular analysis of the E1 envelope glycoprotein does not support the hypothesis of an epidemic versus endemic strain difference.[78] The apparent severity of the epidemic appears to be related to the number of susceptible adults, especially pregnant women, in any given population at the outset of an epidemic.[170, 172, 283, 285] Host factors, such as the differences in the ability to transmit rubella, as well as still unknown factors, may also be involved.[277, 285]

Attack rates in open populations have not been defined precisely for a number of reasons. First, because rubella is such a mild disease, it is under-reported, even in areas where reporting has been mandatory for years. Mandatory reporting did not begin in the United States until 1966 (Fig. 6–1A).[281, 286] In addition, the high and variable rate of inapparent infection poses a major problem when attempting to interpret the recorded data, which are based usually on clinical findings.[254, 287–292]

In childhood, the most common time of infection, 50% or more of serologically confirmed infections result in inapparent illness. The ratio may rise as high as 6:1 or 7:1 in adults, perhaps as a result of silent reinfection in naturally immune individuals who have lost detectable antibody.[254, 290] The frequent occurrence of infections that clinically mimic rubella makes it even more difficult to determine attack rates in open populations.[293] Finally, attack rates are undoubtedly dependent on the number of susceptible individuals, which varies widely in different locations.

Serologic assessments of rubella attack rates have been performed in closed populations, such as military recruits, isolated island groups with small populations, boarding home residents, and household members.[254–256, 277, 289, 291, 292, 294–299] In such situations, individual exposure to the virus is more intense than that encountered in open populations. Under these circumstances, 90 to 100% of both children and adults who are susceptible may become infected. Attack rates in susceptible persons on college and university campuses and in other community settings range from 50 to 90%.[9, 285] Like primary infection, reinfection is also likely to be increased as exposure becomes more intense.[254, 290, 297, 298]

In most of the world, including the United States before the introduction of mass immunization of children in 1969, rubella was typically a childhood disease that was most prevalent in the 5- to 14-year-old age group.[2, 3, 7, 279–286] It was rare in infants younger than 1 year of age. As noted in Figure 6–2A, the incidence increased slowly for the first 4 years, rose steeply between 5 and 14 years, peaked around 20 to 24 years, and then leveled off. In developed countries, the incidence of infection did not reach 100% before ages 35 to 40; 5 to 20% of women of childbearing age remain susceptible to infection.

In isolated or island populations, such as in Trinidad, some areas of Japan, Panama, rural Peru, and Hawaii, a relatively high rate of susceptibility is found in young adults (see Fig. 6–2B).[279, 280, 282, 283, 296] From 26 to 70%

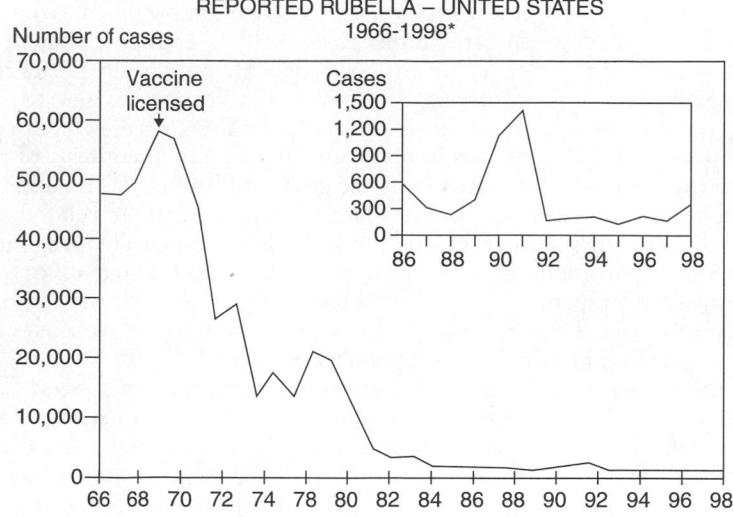

REPORTED RUBELLA – UNITED STATES
1966-1998*

A   *1998 provisional total

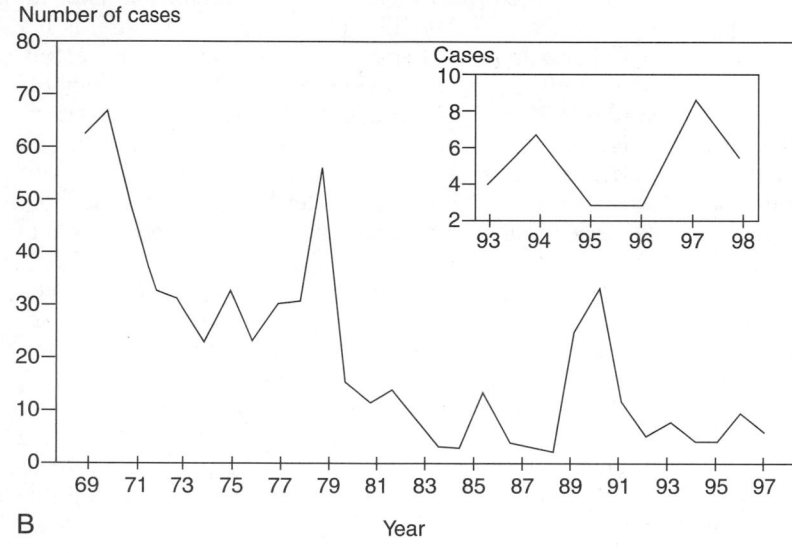

REPORTED CONGENITAL RUBELLA SYNDROME – UNITED STATES
1969-1998

B   Year

FIGURE 6–1 *A,* Incidence rates of reported rubella—United States, 1966–1998. (Data from Centers for Disease Control and Prevention, 1999.) *B,* Incidence rates of reported congenital rubella—United States, 1969–1998. (Data from Centers for Disease Control and Prevention, 1999.)

of women of childbearing age remain susceptible. This situation exists even though rubella is endemic. There is ample opportunity for multiple introductions of virus from the outside. Low population density, tropical climate, low concentration of effective spreaders, and genetic factors have all been invoked to explain these low attack rates, but none can adequately account for this peculiar epidemiologic phenomenon by itself.[277, 282, 283, 285]

As depicted in Figure 6–2C, in other areas, particularly South America, infection begins earlier in life and peak incidence occurs before puberty.[282] However, infection rates in most South American countries reach a plateau at approximately the same level as that seen in Europe and North America, leaving 10% or more of young women who are susceptible, based on serologic tests. Chile appears to be an exception, with almost all persons being infected before puberty.[282]

Initial mass vaccination of children, followed by routine vaccination of 1-year-old children, as well as vaccination of susceptible adolescents and adults, has been extremely successful in controlling rubella and congenital rubella syndrome in the United States.[5, 24, 30, 35, 252, 286] The characteristic 6- to 9-year epidemic cycle has been interrupted, and the reported incidence of rubella has ranged from approximately 200 to 400 cases annually during the period 1992 through 1998. For comparison, there were approximately 58,000 cases reported in 1969, the year of vaccine licensure in the United States (see Fig. 6–1A). Age-specific declines in the occurrence of rubella have been greatest in children, who, because they were the major reservoir of the virus, have been the primary target of the U.S. immunization program. However, the risk of rubella has now decreased by 99% in all age groups after efforts to increase vaccination

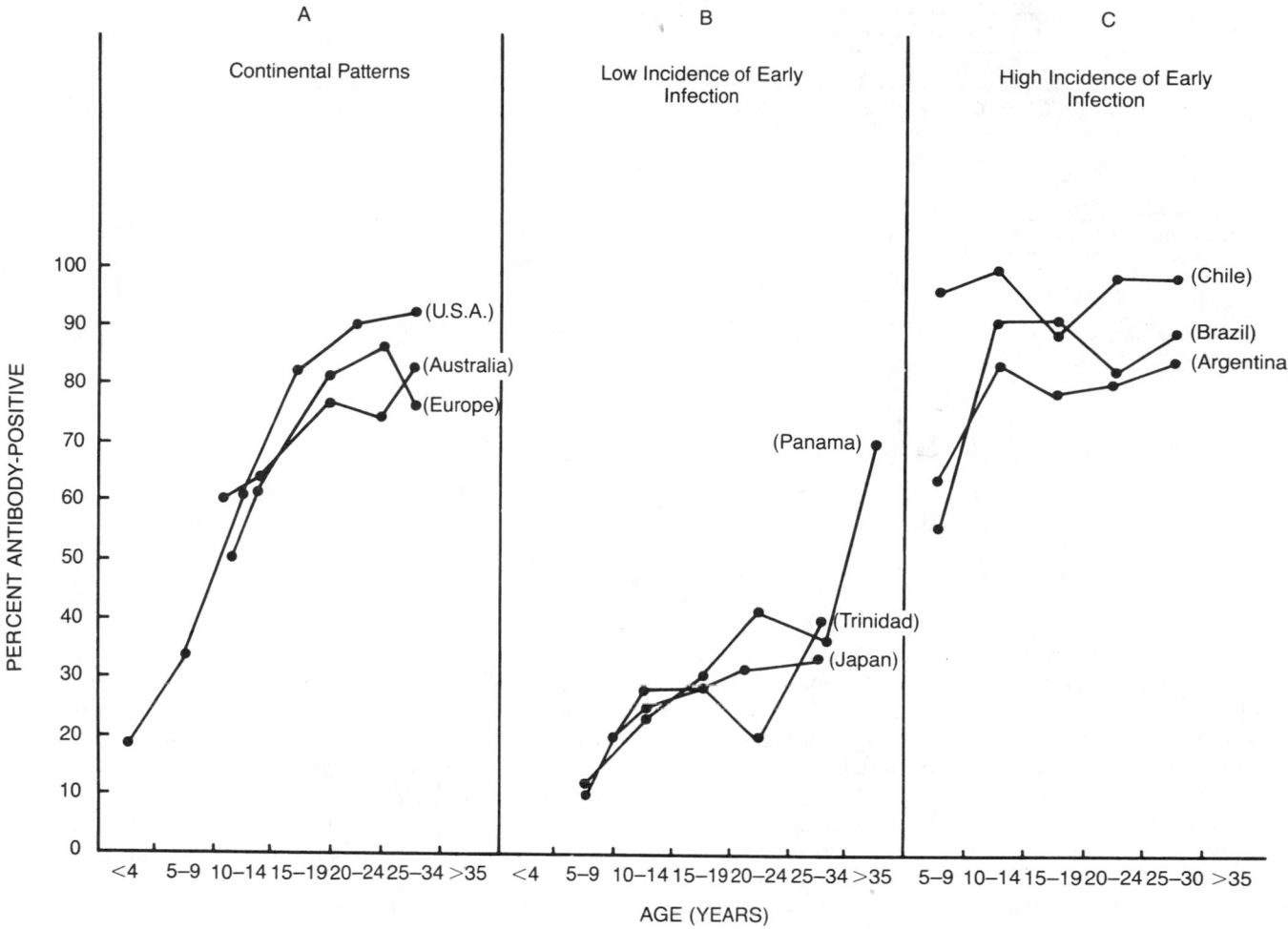

FIGURE 6–2 *A* to *C,* Seroepidemiology of rubella in different populations throughout the world, by age (see text). (Data from references 259, 261–263.)

levels in older, susceptible persons, especially childbearing-aged females (see also Prevention of Congenital Rubella section).[250, 251] Nonetheless, serologic surveys continue to document 10 to 20% susceptibility in this population because of less-than-optimal immunization coverage rates.[258, 286, 300–306] Adolescents and young adults now account for the majority of reported cases, with more cases reported among those older than age 15 years than in children. Outbreaks are still reported in colleges, hospitals, cruise ships, and other settings in which persons live or work in proximity.[260–262, 265–270] Outbreaks no longer occur among military recruits because they receive rubella vaccine as soon as they arrive for basic training.[257] Whereas the reported incidence of cases of congenital rubella syndrome has also decreased dramatically, the number of cases of rubella and congenital rubella reported in the United States increased in 1989 to 1991, documenting that the potential for cases will continue as long as children and women of childbearing age remain underimmunized.[35] The outbreak of rubella and congenital rubella among the Amish in Pennsylvania in 1991 and 1992 was a tragic reminder that there are still pockets of susceptible individuals in the United States.[264]

TRANSMISSION IN UTERO

During the period of viremia in clinical or inapparent primary rubella in pregnancy, virus infects the placenta, and, subsequently, infects the fetus (Fig. 6–3).[2, 6, 278, 293, 307–313] Intrauterine transmission of virus associated with maternal reinfection is extremely rare. It is presumed that this difference is a reflection that viremia is either absent or greatly reduced because of immunity induced by the primary infection (natural or vaccine-induced).* Maternal infection may result in (1) no infection of the conceptus, (2) resorption of the embryo (seen only with infections occurring in the earliest stages of gestation), (3) spontaneous abortion, (4) stillbirth, (5) infection of the placenta without fetal involvement, or (6) infection of both the placenta and fetus.[6] Infected infants can have obvious multiple organ system involvement or, as is frequently observed, no immediately evident disease.[6, 13, 102, 323–330] However, after long-term follow-up, many of these seemingly unaffected infants have evidence of hearing loss or central nervous system or other defects.†

---

*See references 5, 6, 39, 40, 43, 45, 49–51, 53, 106, 111, and 314–322.
†See references 6, 13, 14, 102, 126, 127, 323, 324, and 326–329.

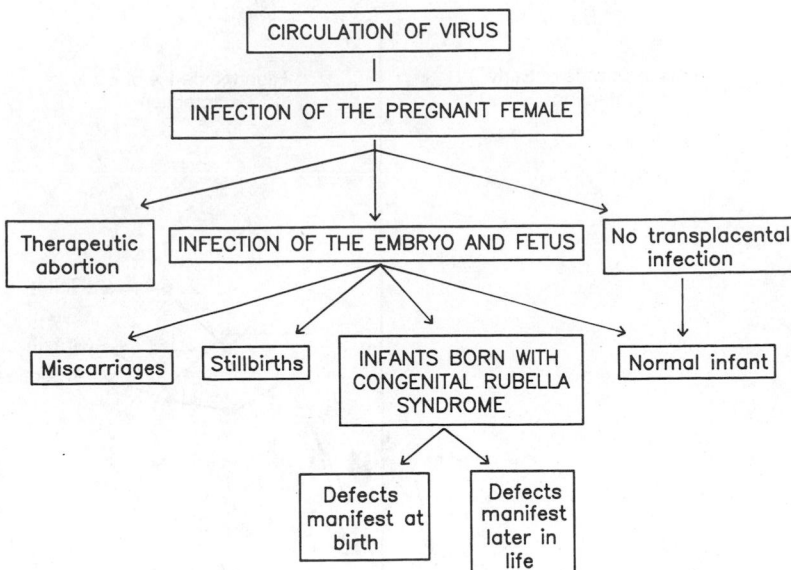

FIGURE 6–3 Schematic of events after rubella infection of the susceptible pregnant female.

Gestational age at the time of maternal infection is the most important determinant of intrauterine transmission and fetal damage.[2–4, 6, 278, 293, 310] The risk of fetal infection and congenital anomalies decreases with increasing gestational age. Fetal damage is rare much beyond the first trimester of pregnancy.

Availability of more sensitive antibody assays has, however, led to refinement of our understanding of the risk of fetal infection and subsequent congenital defects throughout all stages of pregnancy.[98, 105] Although the risk of defects does decrease with increasing gestational age, fetal infection can occur at any time during pregnancy. Data on the risk of fetal infection when maternal rubella occurs before conception are inconsistent.[1, 12, 103, 105, 331–334] If some risk exists, the risk is small.

Risk of Fetal Infection

Early attempts to define the risk of fetal infection relied on isolation of virus from products of conception.[307–313] Between 40% and 90% of products of conception obtained from women with clinical rubella during the first trimester were found to be infected. The higher rates were observed in serologically confirmed cases of maternal rubella and when improved isolation techniques were employed.[312, 313] Attempts were made to refine the risk estimates by evaluating placental and fetal tissue separately. In some of these studies, equal rates of persistent placental and fetal infection were observed, ranging from 80 to 90%.[312, 313] In others, persistent placental infection was found to be twice as frequent as fetal infection—50 to 70% versus 20 to 30%.[307, 310] However, high rates of fetal infection accompanied placental infection when specimens obtained during the first 8 weeks of gestation were examined. For example, of 14 cases in which virus was cultured from placental tissue, six of seven fetuses were culture positive when maternal rubella occurred during the first 8 weeks of pregnancy. In contrast, only one of seven fetal specimens was positive

when infection occurred between 9 and 14 weeks of gestation.[307] In another similar study, fetal infection rates decreased sharply after the eighth week of gestation, whereas placental infection rates decreased but less rapidly.[310] Thus, after the eighth week, placental infection occurred in 36% (8/22) and fetal infection occurred in 10% (2/20) of cases. Although fetal infection was not documented beyond the tenth week of gestation, placental infections were noted up to the sixteenth week.

Further data on the risk of fetal infection have been obtained from studies using sensitive laboratory tests to detect congenital infection in children born to mothers with serologically confirmed rubella.[98, 105] Because congenital rubella is often subclinical in infants and young children, use of such tests is necessary to assess accurately the risk of congenital infection.[6, 98–103, 324, 326–329] In recent investigations in which this approach was used, with detection of rubella-specific IgM antibody in sera to document congenital infection, the discrepancy between rates of placental and fetal infection noted in viral isolation studies is less apparent. Furthermore, these studies have provided new information on the events after maternal infection in the second and third trimester.

In a study involving a total of 273 children (269 of whom had IgM antibody assessment), Miller and colleagues reported that fetal infection after serologically documented symptomatic maternal rubella in the first trimester was, as expected, quite high: 81% (13/16), with rates of 90% and 67% for those exposed before 11 weeks and at 11 to 12 weeks, respectively (Table 6–1).[100] Of greater interest is that the infection rate was 39% (70/178) after exposure in the second trimester (decreasing steadily from 67% at 13 to 14 weeks to 25% at 23 to 26 weeks) but rose to 53% (34/64) with third-trimester infection (with infection rates of 35%, 60%, and 100% during the last 3 months of pregnancy, respectively).

In another investigation of fetal infection after first-trimester maternal rubella infection, based on IgM de-

TABLE 6–1
Risk of Serologically Confirmed Congenital Rubella Infection and Associated Defects in Children Exposed to Symptomatic Maternal Rubella Infection, by Weeks of Gestation

WEEKS OF GESTATION	INFECTION		DEFECTS[a]		OVERALL RISK OF DEFECTS (%)[b]
	No. Tested	Rate (%)	No. Followed	Rate (%)	
<11	10	90 (9)[c]	9	100	90
11–12	6	67 (4)	4	50	33
13–14	18	67 (12)	12	17	11
15–16	36	47 (17)	14	50	24
17–18	33	39 (13)	10		
19–22	59	34 (20)			
23–26	32	25 (8)			
27–30	31	35 (11)	53		
31–36	25	60 (15)			
>36	8	100 (8)			
Total	258[d]	45 (117)	102	20	

[a]Defects in seropositive patients only.
[b]Overall risk of defects = rate of infection × rate of defects.
[c]Numbers in parentheses are number of children infected.
[d]None of 11 infants whose mothers had subclinical rubella were infected.
Adapted from Miller E, Cradock-Watson JE, Pollock TM. Consequences of confirmed maternal rubella at successive stages of pregnancy. Lancet 2:781, 1982, with permission.

termination, Cradock-Watson and associates noted that 32% of 166 children were infected after second-trimester exposure and a comparable proportion were infected after infection in the third trimester (24% of 100).[98] The rate of infection increased during the latter stages of gestation after initially decreasing to a low of 12% by the twenty-eighth week and was 58% (11/19) when maternal infection occurred near term. Even higher rates were observed if persistence of IgG antibody was used as the criterion for congenital infection. The true fetal infection rate probably lies between the rates calculated by using the IgM and persistent IgG data.

In both of these studies, the fetal infection rate declined between 12 and 28 weeks, suggesting that the placenta may prevent transfer of virus, but not completely.[98] Although some of the infections recorded during the last weeks of pregnancy could have been perinatally or postnatally acquired (e.g., by means of exposure to virus in the birth canal or from breast milk), the available evidence indicates that the placental barrier to infection may be relatively ineffective during the last month, perhaps to the same degree as that seen during the first trimester, and that the fetus is susceptible to infection throughout pregnancy, albeit to varying degrees.[335–337]

Risk of Congenital Defects

Estimates of the risk of congenital anomalies in live-born children after fetal infection have been affected by a number of factors. Early retrospective and hospital-based studies led to overestimates of the risk of congenital defects after first-trimester infection (up to 90%).[6, 102, 285] The risk of abnormalities as determined by prospective studies relying on a clinical diagnosis of maternal rubella varied considerably (10 to 54% overall, with a 10 to 20% risk for major defects recognizable at up to

3 years of age) and tended to underestimate the risk because serologic evaluation of infants was not performed.[102, 331, 338–342] The proportion of pregnancies electively terminated can affect observed malformation rates. The fact that fetal infection can occur during all stages of pregnancy also influences assessments of the risk of congenital defects.

Because most infants born with congenital rubella who were exposed after the twelfth week of gestation do not have grossly apparent defects, long-term follow-up is necessary to detect subtle, late-appearing abnormalities, such as deafness and mental impairment.* This is especially true for infants infected beyond the sixteenth to twentieth week of gestation, who at present appear to be at little, if any, risk of congenital anomalies.[98, 104] Studies by Peckham and associates demonstrate that estimates of the risk of defects are affected by the serologic status and age at evaluation of the child.[102, 328] The overall incidence of defects in 218 children studied at about 2 years of age was 23%; it was 52% after maternal infection before 8 weeks of gestation, 36% at 9 to 12 weeks, and 10% at 13 to 20 weeks. No defects were observed when maternal infection occurred after 20 weeks. When considering only seropositive children, the overall risk of defects increased to 38%, with increased risks of 75%, 52%, and 18%, respectively, for the three gestational periods just cited. At follow-up at 6 to 8 years of age, the overall risk of abnormalities in infected children who were seropositive at 2 years of age increased from 38 to 59%; the risk after first-trimester infection increased from 58 to 82%.

Miller and co-workers observed higher rates of defects in infected children observed for only 2 years (see Table 6–1).[100] Defects were noted in 9 of 9 seropositive children exposed during the first 11 weeks, 2 of 4 exposed

---

*See references 6, 13, 14, 102, 126, 127, 323, 324, and 326–329.

at 11 to 12 weeks, 2 of 12 exposed at 13 to 14 weeks, and 7 of 14 exposed at 15 to 16 weeks. Congenital heart disease and deafness were observed after infection before the eleventh week; deafness was the sole defect noted after infection at 11 to 16 weeks. No defects were observed in 63 children infected after 16 weeks. However, some children infected in the third trimester had growth retardation.

Although the number of subjects is small, this study indicates that the risk of damage in seropositive infants is 85% if fetal infection occurs in the first trimester and 35% after infection during weeks 13 to 16. These rates of defects are higher than previously reported, but they may be an accurate reflection of intrauterine events because all maternal cases were serologically confirmed and sensitive antibody assays were used to detect congenital infection. It is possible that with further follow-up, higher rates of defects will be observed.

These rates pertain to offspring known to be infected and are useful in evaluating the risk of defects given fetal infection. For counseling purposes, it is essential to know the risk of congenital defects after confirmed maternal infection. This can be derived by multiplying the rates of defects in infected fetuses by the rates of fetal infection. Based on the reported experience of Miller and colleagues, the risks are 90% for maternal infection before the eleventh week, 33% for infection during weeks 11 to 12, 11% for weeks 13 to 14, and 24% for weeks 15 to 16 (see Table 6–1). The risk after maternal infection in the first trimester is 69%.

NATURAL HISTORY

Postnatal Infection

VIROLOGIC FINDINGS

The pertinent virologic findings of postnatal infection are depicted in Figure 6–4. The portal of entry for rubella virus is believed to be the upper respiratory tract. Virus then spreads through the lymphatics, or by a transient viremia, to regional lymph nodes, where replication first occurs. Between the seventh and ninth day after exposure, virus is released into the blood and may seed multiple tissues, including the placenta. By the

ninth to eleventh day, viral excretion begins from the nasopharynx, as well as from the kidneys, cervix, gastrointestinal tract, and various other sites.[9, 272, 288, 295, 335-337, 343]

The viremia peaks at 10 to 17 days, just before rash onset, which usually occurs 16 to 18 days after exposure. Virus disappears from the serum in the next few days, as antibody becomes detectable.[272, 288, 295, 343] However, infection may persist in peripheral blood lymphocytes and monocytes for 1 to 4 weeks.[57, 62, 344, 345] Virus is excreted in high titers from nasopharyngeal secretions. Nasopharyngeal shedding may be detected rarely for up to 3 to 5 weeks. Although virus can usually be cultured from the nasopharynx from 7 days before to 14 days after rash onset, the highest risk of virus transmission is believed to be from 5 days before to 6 days after appearance of rash. Viral shedding from other sites is not as consistent, intense, or prolonged.[288, 343] Rubella virus has been cultured from skin at sites where rash was both present and absent.[346, 347]

HUMORAL IMMUNE RESPONSE

In challenge studies conducted in the early 1960s, Green and co-workers demonstrated that neutralizing antibody was first detected in serum 14 to 18 days after exposure (usually 2 to 3 days after rash onset), peaked within a month, and persisted for the duration of the follow-up period of 6 to 12 months.[288] The HI test soon became the standard method for detecting rubella antibodies after acute postnatal rubella infection because of its reliability and ease compared with the neutralization test. A number of other methods for measuring rubella antibody responses have supplanted the HI test in popularity (see The Virus section).[86, 194, 195] The kinetics of the immune response to acute infection detected by these various serologic assays, which have been exhaustively compared with the HI technique, is depicted in Figure 6–5.*

In general, there are three distinct patterns of antibody kinetics. Antibodies of the IgG class measured by HI, latex agglutination, neutralization, immunofluorescence, single radial hemolysis (or hemolysis in gel) (not shown in Fig. 6–5), radioimmunoassay, and enzyme-

---

*See references 86–90, 186, 190–200, 202, 209–219, 221, and 224.

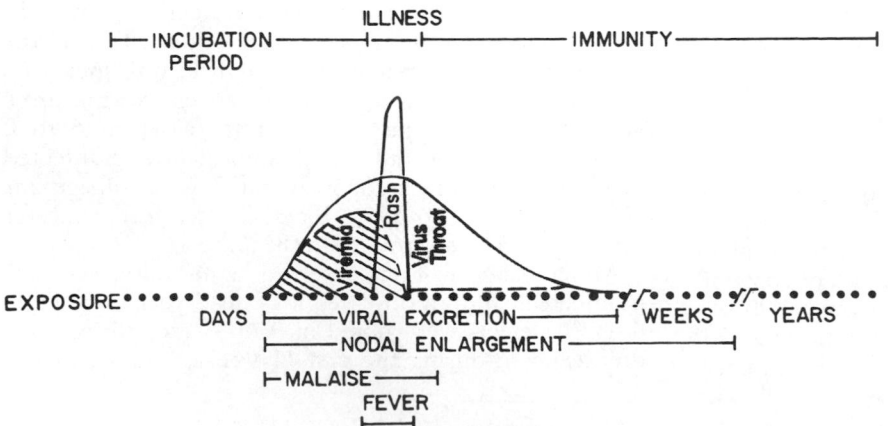

FIGURE 6–4 Relation of viral excretion and clinical findings in postnatally acquired rubella. (From Alford CA. Chronic congenital and perinatal infections. In Avery GB [ed]. Neonatology. Philadelphia, JB Lippincott, 1987, with permission.)

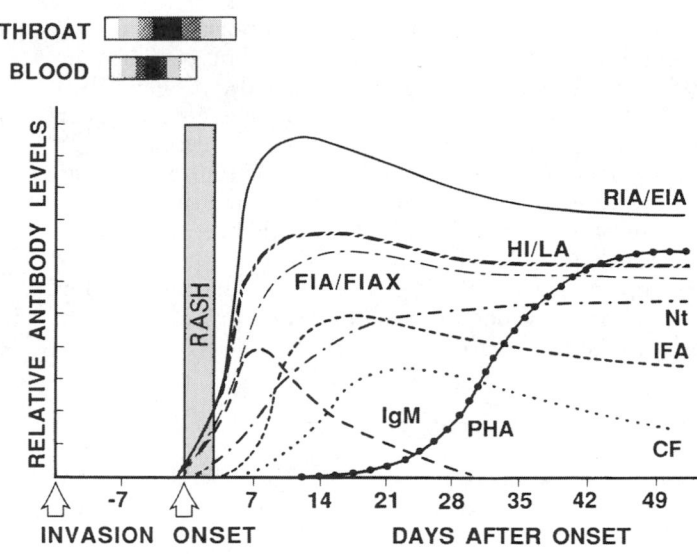

FIGURE 6–5 Schematic of the immune response in acute rubella infection. CF = complement fixation; EIA = enzyme immunoassay; FIA/FIAX and IFA = immunofluorescence; HI = hemagglutination inhibition; IgM = immunoglobulin M; LA = latex agglutination; Nt = neutralization; PHA = passive agglutination; RIA = radioimmunoassay. (Adapted from Herrmann KL. Rubella virus. *In* Lennette EH, Schmidt NJ. [eds]. Diagnostic Procedures for Viral, Rickettsial and Chlamydial Infections. Washington, DC, American Public Health Association, 1979, p 725; and Herrmann KL. Available rubella serologic tests. Rev Infect Dis 7 [Suppl 1]: S108, 1985, University of Chicago, publisher. With permission.)

linked immunoassay theta precipitation (not shown) follow the first pattern. Such antibodies usually become detectable 5 to 15 days after rash onset, although they may appear earlier and may even be present 1 or 2 days before the rash appears. The antibody titers rapidly increase to reach peak values at 15 to 30 days and then gradually decline over a period of years to a constant titer that varies from person to person. In some patients with low levels of residual antibody, a second exposure to rubella virus may lead to low-grade reinfection of the pharynx. A booster antibody response can then be detected with any of the assays. This rapidly terminates the new infection, which is most often subclinical, and little, if any, viremia occurs.[36, 42, 45, 48, 52, 54, 254, 298, 322]

A second pattern of immune response to rubella infection is noted when IgG antibodies are measured by passive hemagglutination. The peak titer of these antibodies is similar to that measured by HI, but the passive hemagglutination antibodies are relatively delayed in appearance and rise only slowly to their maximal titers. They first become detectable 15 to 50 days after the onset of the rash and often take 200 days to reach peak titers. The antibodies probably persist for life. Booster responses may be seen with reinfections.

Studies indicate that the predominant IgG subclass detected by all these various assays is probably IgG1.[93, 95] Failure to detect IgG3 may be indicative of reinfection.[96]

A third distinct pattern of antibody production is represented in Figure 6–5 by the IgM antibody class immune response. Rubella-specific IgM antibody can be measured by HI, immunofluorescence, radioimmunoassay, or enzyme immunoassay.* IgM antibodies are most consistently detectable 5 to 10 days after the onset of the rash, rise rapidly to peak values at around 20 days, and then decline so rapidly that they usually disappear by 50 to 70 days. In a few patients, however, low levels may persist for up to 1 year.[348–350] The booster IgG antibody response to reinfection noted earlier does not usually involve the IgM class of antibody, so that the

presence of high-titer IgM antibodies indicates recent primary infection with rubella. However, more sensitive techniques, such as radioimmunoassay or enzyme immunoassay, may occasionally detect low levels of specific IgM antibodies in some patients with reinfections, which may cause some difficulty in differentiating subclinical reinfection, which is almost always of no consequence, from acute primary subclinical infection.[39, 49, 51, 53] Determination of avidity of rubella-specific IgG may help resolve this problem.[351–353] Primary infection appears to be associated with low-avidity IgG, and reinfection seems to be associated with high-avidity IgG.

The kinetics of the immune response to rubella infection detected by other serologic assays is not as distinct as the three patterns just described, and marked variability between patients has been noted. Complement fixation antibodies or iota precipitins (not shown in Fig. 6–5) are not present in the first 10 days after the rash and rise slowly to peak at 30 to 90 days.[186] These antibodies persist for several years in one third of patients and may reappear during reinfections. Iota precipitins do not persist for more than a few months and do not usually reappear with reinfections.

Antibodies of the IgA class appear within 10 days but may either disappear within a further 20 days or persist for several years.[94, 97, 201, 226] IgD and IgE antibodies appear rapidly (6 to 9 days) after infection, remain high for at least 2 months, and then decline slightly at 6 months.[94] IgE antibodies reach an early peak similar to that seen for IgM and IgA. In contrast, the IgD response is somewhat delayed, like that of IgG.

The antibody response after infection is generally considered to confer complete and permanent immunity. As noted earlier, clinical reinfection is rare, and reinfections in general pose little risk to the fetus because placental exposure to the virus is minimal.[36, 39, 42, 45, 48, 49, 51–54, 322] Some of the rare instances of fetal infection after maternal reinfection may be due to an incomplete immune response to the various antigenic domains on each of the virus' structural proteins (see The Virus section).[72–74, 106, 110, 314, 319–321] For example, three cases

*See references 97, 152, 201–205, 208, 210, 219, 220, and 225–233.

after natural infection have been reported involving women who had positive HI results but who had no detectable levels of neutralizing antibody.[314, 319, 321] Obviously, the sensitivity of the neutralizing assay itself is an important determinant in interpreting these results.[106, 191] This phenomenon might also account for the four reported cases of congenital infection that followed reinfection of women who had presumably been immunized previously.[40, 43, 50, 111] It is also worth noting that some of the reported instances of maternal reinfection probably, and in at least one case definitely, represent cases of primary acute infection.[5, 6, 108, 316–318]

CELLULAR IMMUNE RESPONSE

Cellular immunity to rubella virus has been measured by lymphocyte transformation response, secretion of interferon, secretion of macrophage migration inhibitory factor, induction of delayed hypersensitivity to skin testing, and release of lymphokines by cultured lymphocytes.[354–365] Peripheral blood lymphocytes from seropositive individuals respond better in each of these tests than do lymphocytes from uninfected persons, suggesting that these assays measure parameters of the cellular immune response to rubella virus. The results from other studies in which chromium-51 microcytotoxicity assays have been used are difficult to interpret because syngeneic cell lines have not been used to control for HLA-restricted responses.[355, 358]

In the first weeks after natural rubella infection, some degree of transient lymphocyte suppression may occur.[359, 361] Generally, cell-mediated immune responses precede the appearance of humoral immunity by 1 week, reach a peak value at the same time as the antibody response, and subsequently persist for many years, probably for life.[324] Acute infection may suppress skin reactivity to tuberculin testing for approximately 30 days.[366]

LOCAL IMMUNE RESPONSE

The local antibody response at the portal of entry in the nasopharynx is essentially IgA in character; low levels of short-lived IgG antibody are rarely detectable in nasopharyngeal secretions. The nasopharyngeal IgA antibody persists at detectable levels for at least 1 year after infection. Its persistence apparently minimizes the tendency for reinfection after natural rubella infection. The lack of local IgA nasopharyngeal response after parenteral administration of live rubella vaccines (less so with the RA 27/3 strain than with other strains) probably plays a key role in the increased incidence of subclinical reinfection after vaccination.[36, 38, 42, 48, 52, 54, 367–370] Local antibody levels tend to be higher in individuals resistant to challenge with live virus, but no specific titer of antibody has been associated with complete protection.

A cell-mediated immune response in tonsillar cells has been detected by lymphocyte transformation and secretion of migration inhibitory factor after both natural rubella and intranasal challenge with live RA 27/3 vaccine.[371] In guinea pigs, the response first becomes detectable 1 to 2 weeks after intranasal vaccination, peaks at 4 weeks, and then disappears at around 6 weeks.[372]

Congenital Infection

VIROLOGIC FINDINGS

An important feature that distinguishes congenital infection from postnatal infection is that the former is chronic.[2, 13, 278, 303, 310, 373, 374] During the period of maternal viremia, the placenta may become infected and in turn transmit virus to the fetus (see Transmission in Utero section).[2, 6, 278, 293, 307–313] Although virus may persist for months in the placenta, recovery of virus from the placenta at birth is infrequent.[375] In contrast, once the fetus is infected, the virus persists typically throughout gestation and for months postnatally. It can infect many fetal organs or only a few.[310] In infected infants, virus can be recovered from multiple sites (pharyngeal secretions, urine, conjunctival fluid, feces) and is detectable in cerebrospinal fluid, bone marrow, and circulating white blood cells.* Pharyngeal shedding of virus is more common, prolonged, and intense during the early months after delivery (Fig. 6–6). By 1 year of age, only 2 to 20% of infants shed virus.[271–273] In rare instances, shedding may continue beyond the age of 2 years.[274–276] Virus can be isolated from the eye and cerebrospinal fluid, particularly when disease is evident in the corresponding organs, and can persist for over a year in the eye and central nervous system.[377–380] Virus has been isolated from the brain of a 12-year-old boy with later-appearing subacute panencephalitis occurring after congenital rubella infection.[381, 382]

HUMORAL IMMUNE RESPONSE

It is clear that placental infection does not prevent passive transfer of maternal antibody and that the infected fetus can mount an immune response.[278, 307–313, 383–385] Although the development and function of the other components of the immune response of the fetus may be important, critical factors that allow fetal infection to occur in the presence of antibody may be the timing when antibody is present in the fetal circulation, the quality of the antibody that the fetus produces, or both.

Although placental transfer of antibody occurs in spite of persistent infection, levels of antibody in fetal blood during the first half of gestation are only 5 to 10% of those in maternal serum.[385–389] As the placental transfer mechanisms mature by mid gestation (16 to 20 weeks), increasing levels of maternal IgG antibody are transferred to the fetus (Fig. 6–7).[388]

The development of the fetal humoral immune system also appears to be too late to limit the effects of the virus. Cells with membrane-bound immunoglobulins of all three major classes—IgM, IgG, and IgA—appear in the fetus as early as 9 to 11 weeks of gestation.[389] However, circulating fetal antibody levels remain low until mid-gestation, despite the presence of high titers of virus and the development of antigen receptors on the cell

---

*See references 2, 13, 156, 271–276, 278, 307, 308, 310, 312, and 373–377.

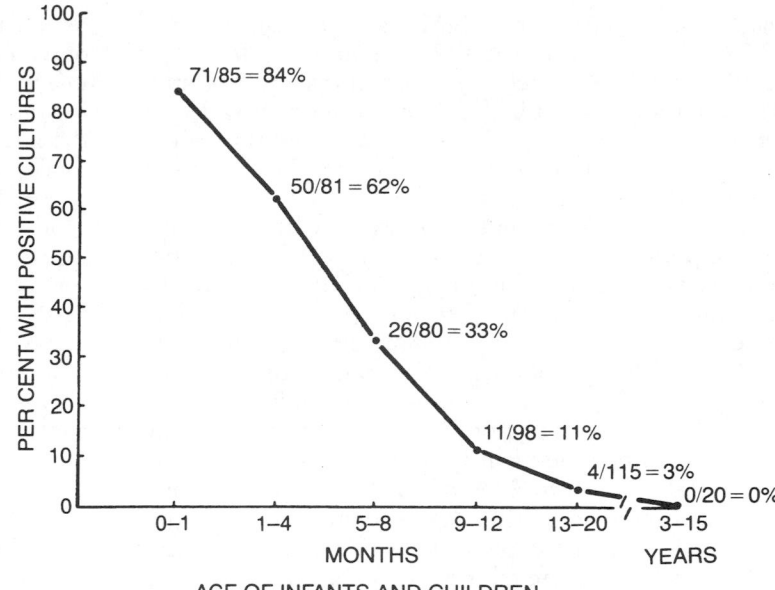

FIGURE 6–6 Rate of virus excretion in infants and children with congenital rubella infection, by age. (From Cooper LZ, Krugman S. Clinical manifestations of postnatal and congenital rubella. Arch Ophthalmol 77:434, 1967. Copyright 1967, American Medical Association.)

surface (see Fig. 6–7). At this time, levels of fetal antibody increase, with IgM antibody predominating.[385, 390-394] Fetal IgA, IgD, and IgG are also made, but in lesser amounts.[94, 391, 394] As in the case with other chronic intrauterine infections, congenital rubella infection may lead to an increase in total IgM antibody levels.[383, 385, 386, 394] Total IgA levels are also occasionally raised, but IgG levels seldom exceed those of uninfected infants.[383, 385, 394, 395]

At the time of delivery of infected infants, levels of IgG rubella antibodies in cord sera are equal to or greater than those in maternal sera, even if the infant is born prematurely.[385] IgG is the dominant antibody present at delivery in rubella-infected infants and is mainly maternal in origin. In contrast, the IgM levels are lower but are totally fetus derived.

In the first 3 to 5 months after birth, the levels of maternally derived IgG decrease as maternal antibody is catabolized (see Fig. 6–7).[385] In contrast, IgM antibodies increase in titer and can predominate. Later, as viral excretion wanes and disappears, the IgM antibody levels diminish and IgG becomes the dominant and persistent antibody type. Cradock-Watson and colleagues noted that total IgM was elevated in nearly all sera obtained from infected infants during the first 3 months of life and in one half of sera from infected infants 3 to 6 months old.[394] Rubella-specific IgM has been shown to persist consistently for 6 months, frequently for a year, and rarely longer when assayed by sensitive serologic procedures, such as radioimmunoassay and immunofluorescence.[207, 394] For example, Cradock-Watson and col-

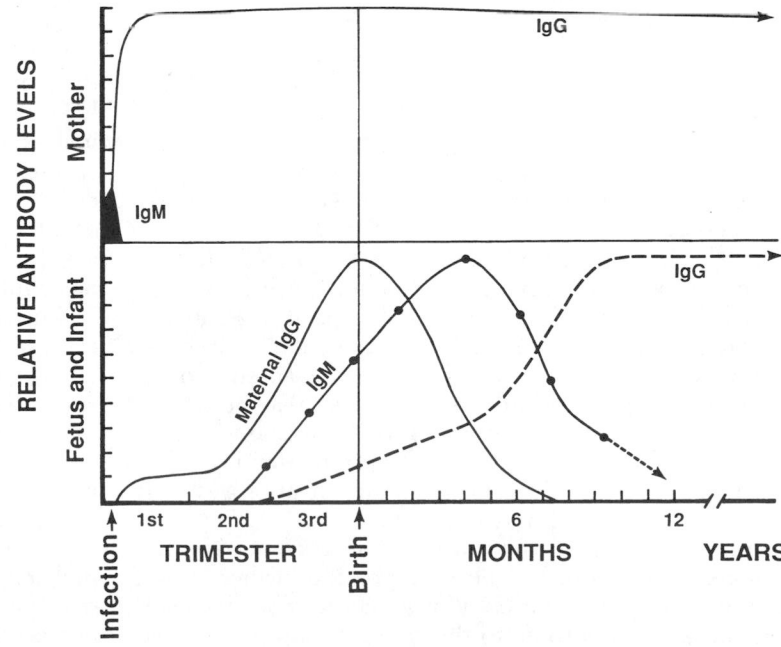

FIGURE 6–7 Schematic of the immune response in the mother, fetus, and infant after maternal and fetal rubella infections in the first trimester of pregnancy. (Adapted from Alford CA. Immunology of rubella. In Friedman H, Prier JE [eds]. Rubella. Springfield, Ill, Charles C Thomas, 1972.)

leagues also reported that IgM was detectable in 48 of 50 (96%) sera during the first 6 months of life and in 11 of 38 (29%) sera between 6.5 months and 2 years.[394] The total level of antibody, as measured by a variety of serologic tests, remains virtually unchanged throughout the first year of life, in spite of the fluctuations in immunoglobulin composition.[385, 394]

High levels of IgG antibody are usually maintained for a number of years after detectable virus excretion ends, suggesting that there may be continued antigenic stimulation. During the first few years of life, some patients have a relative hypergammaglobulinemia, particularly of the IgM and IgG classes of antibody, which results from the increased antigenic stimulus accompanying the chronic infection.[394, 396] With increasing time, however, antibody levels may decrease and even become undetectable in 10 to 20% of patients.[328, 397–399] Cooper and co-workers noted that the geometric mean HI titer decreased by a factor of 16 by 5 years of age in 223 children with congenital rubella syndrome.[399] No HI antibodies were detected in 8 of 29 five-year-old children. In contrast, in a study from Japan, only 3% of 381 children with congenital infection observed for more than 17 years had undetectable HI titers.[400] There was an initial rapid decline from a geometric mean titer of 1:416 ($2^{8.7}$) to 1:84 ($2^{6.4}$) over the first 2 years of follow-up. After this, there was a modest continuing decline; the final geometric mean titer was 1:42 ($2^{5.4}$).

Cooper and co-workers have also reported that congenitally infected children who have lost detectable rubella-specific antibody do not develop a boost in antibody titer after rubella vaccination.[399] This may reflect some sort of immunologic tolerance that follows intrauterine exposure to rubella virus. None of the children with congenital rubella in Japan had evidence of significant boosts in antibody or a history of clinical disease when exposed during recent outbreaks of rubella.[400, 401]

Hypogammaglobulinemia, with low levels of all three major classes of immunoglobulins, has been reported in a few instances of congenital rubella.[128, 156, 402, 403] Usually only IgA is affected. There may also be instances when IgG levels are low whereas levels of IgM are two or three times the upper limit of normal for adults. These IgG and IgM abnormalities may occur with or without IgA abnormalities.[402] Over time, immunoglobulin development may become normal. This can occur despite continued viral excretion but is more likely if viral titers are decreasing.[274]

In addition to defects in the immune globulin levels, defects in specific antibody production have been observed. One such defect is a complete lack of antibody response to any antigen, including the rubella virus itself. Response only to the virus, in the absence of a response to most other antigens, has also been reported.[274] This state of immunologic unresponsiveness resolves in many patients. Antibody production becomes normal as the patient's general condition improves and as immune globulin levels normalize.

Immunoprecipitation studies of sera from patients with congenital rubella syndrome provide further information on defective antibody production. They indicate that the antibody profile to the three structural proteins of the rubella virus is qualitatively different from that observed in sera from persons with postnatally acquired infection (see The Virus section).[82, 83, 85] Little or no antibody to the core structural protein (C) is found, and the absolute and relative amounts of antibody to structural proteins E1 and E2 appear to vary with age.[82, 83] These findings further suggest that the immune response of the infected fetus may be incomplete and may explain why detectable antibodies are not present in some sera.[85, 328, 397–400] If a serum contains relatively little antibody to structural protein E1 (the hemagglutinin), assays that detect antibody to the whole virion will be more likely to be positive than those that detect antibody only to E1 (e.g., the HI assay). It is not yet clear if these abnormal antibody patterns persist for life.

CELLULAR IMMUNE RESPONSE

Like the cells responsible for the humoral immune response (B cells), the cells involved in cellular immunity (T cells, macrophages) develop some of their functions early in gestation.[404–406] However, little is known about their response in utero because appropriate specimens have not been obtainable for study. Therefore, the cellular immune response of the infected fetus has been inferred from studies of infected infants and children. Available evidence indicates that some infants with congenital rubella have impaired cellular immune responses.

Retarded development of the thymus and lymphocyte depletion have both been reported, but these abnormalities may result from the stress of infection rather than the virus itself.[407] Abnormal delayed hypersensitivity skin reactions to a number of antigens (e.g., diphtheria toxoid, *Candida*, dinitrofluorobenzene) have also been reported.[274, 408] This defect has been associated with abnormalities in the humoral system and resolves as antibody production returns to normal.

Results of studies of in vitro lymphocyte blastogenesis in congenitally infected infants and children have been confusing. Early studies demonstrated a poor response to phytohemagglutinin, vaccinia, and diphtheria toxoid.[408–411] However, because rubella virus could depress the lymphocyte blastogenic response and the virus could be isolated from lymphocytes of chronically infected infants, the abnormality may be a result of viral infection of the circulating blood cells rather than an inherent defect in cell-mediated immunity.[409–412] This diminished cellular response may normalize over time because elevated lymphocyte responses have been detected in some older infected children.[408, 413]

Buimovici-Klein and colleagues showed that lymphocytes from older children and adolescents with congenital rubella had no or very poor lymphocyte proliferative responses to rubella virus antigens, as well as markedly reduced interferon and migration-inhibition factor production.[365, 414] These studies indicated that these defects were greater in children exposed early in gestation than those exposed later, with the greatest degree of abnormality in those whose mothers had been infected during the first 8 weeks of pregnancy. They also pointed out that these defects could persist long after viral excretion had ceased. It remains unclear if these cellular immune defects are responsible for viral persistence or are yet another manifestation of intrauterine infection.[414]

A number of other investigators have confirmed that patients with congenital rubella have defects in cell-mediated immunity.[115, 128, 129] Verder and colleagues noted a decreased proportion of suppressor/cytotoxic (T8) cells in an infant with congenital rubella.[129] Rabinowe and co-workers documented persistent T cell abnormalities in patients with congenital infection who were 9 to 21 years of age.[128] Compared with normal subjects, the congenitally infected patients had depressed ratios of T4 cells (helper/inducer) to T8 cells (from a decreased proportion of T4 and an increased percentage of T8 cells). Such findings persist for only 1 month after acute postnatal rubella infection.[415]

Lymphocytes of infected children were unable to kill rubella-infected cells in a cytotoxicity assay.[416] These results were questioned because syngeneic target cells were not used, and these responses are known to be HLA restricted. However, similar results have been found by Verder and associates, who observed abnormal killer and natural killer cell activities.[129]

INTERFERON RESPONSE

It has long been suggested that the fetus has a deficient interferon response to viral infections, including rubella, but this evidence has been derived from indirect studies with in vitro cell systems or animal models.[168, 169, 312, 417, 418] Technical difficulties have hampered direct studies of humans. However, interferon that appeared to be specifically stimulated by the presence of rubella virus in rubella-infected human embryos has been demonstrated.[419] The interferon was found as early as 7 weeks' gestation and as long as 12 weeks after symptoms ceased in the mothers. Direct study of fetal blood and amniotic fluid has also shown that the fetus can produce interferon in response to the virus.[420]

Children with congenital infection do have the capacity to make interferon on challenge. For example, Desmyter and co-workers reported that interferon could not be detected from the serum or urine of nine such children 11 to 18 months of age who were excreting virus.[421] However, after vaccination with live measles vaccine (Edmonston B or Schwarz strains), all the children seroconverted and produced detectable levels of interferon.

PATHOGENESIS

Postnatal Infection

The events leading to acute postnatal infection are relatively well known and have been detailed in the section on natural history. Available information indicates that both viral replication and postinfection immune phenomena are involved in the clinical manifestations of the illness.

Viremia may lead to seeding of multiple organs, but few are clinically affected.[6] Speculation that the rash may be an immune phenomenon caused by circulating immune complexes has not been documented. In fact,

few persons with uncomplicated illness have immune complexes containing rubella virus, and virus has been isolated from uninvolved, as well as involved, skin.[118, 123, 346, 347] Virus has been isolated from lymph nodes and conjunctiva, accounting for the lymph node enlargement and conjunctivitis observed in many patients.[343, 422] Virus has been isolated from synovial fluid, but immune mechanisms may play a role in some cases of arthralgia and arthritis, particularly if symptoms are persistent.[118, 423–426] Encephalitis is probably a manifestation of the immune response, but direct viral invasion may be involved, particularly in the rare case of progressive panencephalitis that has been reported to follow postnatal infection.[116, 427–429]

It has been suggested that pregnant women are at increased risk of serious complications because of the impaired immune response associated with pregnancy, but there are few data to support this claim.[430, 431] There has also been interest, especially in Japan, in the influence of HLA type and other genetic factors on the incidence and severity of postnatal infection.[113, 114, 117, 119, 122, 432] To date, no consistent pattern has been reported.

Congenital Infection

The outcome of maternal rubella infection follows a logical sequence of events, beginning with maternal infection, followed by viremia, placental seeding, and dissemination of infection to the fetus (see Transmission in Utero and Natural History sections).[2, 6, 278, 293, 307–313] The fetus, in turn, may escape infection entirely, succumb in utero, be born with multiple obvious defects, or appear to be normal at birth only to develop abnormalities later in life (see Fig. 6–3).[6, 13, 102, 272, 323–330] The variability in outcome is highlighted by the observation that one identical twin may be infected and the other spared.[6, 433, 434]

The most important determinant of fetal outcome is gestational age at the time of infection.[2, 3, 6, 98, 105, 278, 293, 307, 310] The disease is more severe and has a greater tendency to involve multiple organs when acquired during the first 8 weeks of gestation. However, the factors that govern the influence of gestation are unknown. It is possible that immature cells are more easily infected and support the growth of virus better than older, more differentiated cells. It is also possible that the placenta becomes increasingly resistant to infection (or at least more able to limit infection) as it rapidly matures during the first trimester. A third possibility is that maturing fetal defense mechanisms become capable of confining and clearing the infection. This last explanation is probably important after 18 or 20 weeks of gestation but seems unlikely in the latter half of the first trimester, when attenuation of fetal infection begins. It is likely that a combination of these and other factors are responsible for the decrease in virulence of fetal infection with increasing gestational age.

The hallmark of fetal infection is its chronicity, with the tendency for virus to persist throughout fetal life and after birth.* The fact that virus can be isolated long after birth also raises the possibility of reactivation, at

---

*See references 2, 13, 156, 271–276, 278, 293, 307–313, and 372–382.

least in brain tissue.[381, 382] It is not clear why the virus has these properties, because the fetus is not truly immunologically tolerant and appears to be able to produce interferon.[207, 278, 324, 384, 385, 394, 417–421] In any case, chronic and/or reactivated infection can lead to ongoing pathologic processes.*

The causes of cellular and tissue damage from congenital rubella infection are poorly defined.[417, 418] Only a variable, small number of cells are infected (1 per 1000 to 1 per 250,000).[313] In tissue culture, infection with rubella virus has diverse effects, ranging from no obvious effect to cell destruction (see The Virus section); this is also likely to be the case in vivo,[152] but, in fact, cytolysis is relatively rare (see Pathology section).[2, 3, 6, 9, 435–439] Furthermore, inflammation is minimal and consists mainly of infiltration of small lymphocytes. Both polymorphonuclear leukocytes and plasma cells are lacking, particularly in comparison with other viral infections of the human fetus, in which inflammation and general necrosis are quite extensive. In contrast, vascular insufficiency appears to be more important than cell destruction or secondary inflammatory damage in the genesis of congenital defects.[2, 3, 6, 9, 435–439] This suggestion is supported by the observation that rubella virus has low destructive potential for cells growing in vitro, including those of human origin. A number of investigators have maintained multiple types of rubella-infected human fetal cells in culture for years without loss of viability or evidence of cytopathic effect (see also CA Alford Jr, unpublished data).[440–442]

Other defects have been reported in chronically infected cells that might help explain the mechanism of congenital defects. These include chromosomal breaks, reduced cellular multiplication time, and increased production of a protein inhibitor that causes mitotic arrest of certain cell types.[373, 440, 443–448]

A report by Bowden and associates indicates that rubella virus may interfere with mitosis by having an adverse effect on actin microfilaments.[449] Yoneda and coworkers have observed that rubella virus may alter cell receptors to specific growth factors.[450] All of these abnormalities, if occurring in vivo, could result in decreased cell multiplication because of slow growth rates and limited doubling potential during the period of embryogenesis, when cell division and turnover are normally very rapid. Naeye and Blanc found histopathologic evidence for mitotic arrest and reduced cell numbers in infants who died of congenital rubella syndrome.[451] These observations have been offered to explain the increased incidence of intrauterine growth retardation seen in infants with congenital rubella, but this explanation probably represents an oversimplification of the actual mechanisms involved.

Immunologic responses also have been proposed as causes of cellular damage. Although cellular immune defects may be a result of chronic infection, it is possible that these defects actually contribute to ongoing tissue damage.[365, 414, 452] Excessive serum immunoglobulin development, persistent antibody production in the face of viral replication for prolonged periods, and production of rheumatoid factor, all indicative of overstimulation of the immune system, may also have a role in the pathogenesis of congenital rubella syndrome.[453, 454] The presence of immune complexes and autoantibodies and the influence of certain HLA types may contribute to the delayed expression of some signs of congenital rubella, such as pneumonitis, diabetes mellitus, thyroid dysfunction, and progressive rubella panencephalitis (see Clinical Manifestations section).* Some of these immunologic events may be directly involved in tissue damage (e.g., immune complexes and autoantibodies), whereas others may allow the virus to persist or reactivate.

PATHOLOGY

Postnatal Infection

Little is known about the pathology of postnatally acquired rubella because patients seldom die of this mild disease. As noted by Cherry, the histologic findings of tissues that have been examined (lymph nodes and autopsy specimens from patients dying with encephalitis) are unremarkable.[9] Changes in lymphoreticular tissue have been limited to mild edema, nonspecific follicular hyperplasia, and some loss of normal follicular morphology. Examination of brain tissue has revealed diffuse swelling, nonspecific degeneration, and little meningeal and perivascular infiltrate.

Congenital Infection

In contrast to the situation with postnatal rubella, much is known about the pathology of congenital rubella infection.[2, 3, 6, 9, 435–439, 455] In general, small foci of infected cells are seen in apparently normal tissue. Cellular necrosis and secondary inflammation are seldom very marked, although a generalized vasculitis predominates (see Pathogenesis section).

The pathologic findings of the placenta include hypoplasia, inflammatory foci in chorionic villi, granulomatous changes, mild edema, focal hyalinization, and necrosis.[435, 436, 455, 456] There is usually extensive damage to the endothelium of the capillaries and smaller blood vessels of the chorion. The vessel lesions consist mainly of endothelial necrosis, with fragmentation of intraluminal blood cells. Töndury and Smith have postulated that emboli of infected endothelial cells originating from the chorion may seed target organs in the fetus.[435] These emboli may also contribute to organ damage by obstructing the fetal blood supply. Petechiae and the presence of hemosiderin-laden phagocytes in surrounding tissue are evidence of functional vascular damage.[436]

Although not nearly as common as vascular lesions, specific cytolysis, presumably caused by direct viral effect on the cell, is also present in the placenta. This is characterized by cytoplasmic eosinophilia, nuclear pyknosis or karyorrhexis, and cellular necrosis. Specific cellular inclusion bodies, both nuclear and cytoplasmic,

---

*See references 6, 13, 14, 102, 126, 127, 323, 324, and 326–329.

*See references 13, 14, 112, 115, 116, 118, 120, 121, 124–129, 381, and 382.

are rare but have been observed.[456] Whereas placentitis would be expected to be present in all affected placentas, regardless of when fetal infection occurred, Garcia and colleagues have noted that placental lesions appeared to be more intense when infection occurred in the last trimester of pregnancy.[456] This finding is consistent with the observation that the placenta is not a barrier to fetal infection in the latter stages of pregnancy.[98, 104, 326, 328]

Autopsies show that virtually every organ may be involved, with hypoplasia being a common finding. The necrotizing angiopathy of small blood vessels seen in the placenta is the most characteristic lesion in fetal organs. Cytolysis with tissue necrosis and accompanying inflammatory changes are also far less common but have been found in the myocardium, brain, spinal cord, skeletal muscle, viscera, and epithelial cells of the developing lens, inner ear (organ of Corti), and teeth.

The overall pathologic process of congenital rubella, in keeping with its chronic nature, is progressive. Both healing and new lesions can be found in specimens obtained in the later stages of gestation.[435, 436] The pathologic changes vary among embryos in quantity and in organ distribution, and the location and nature of organ lesions depend somewhat on the gestational age at the time of infection.[435] The pathologic findings parallel the enormous variability of the clinical disease seen in infected newborns.

CLINICAL MANIFESTATIONS

Postnatal Infection

Rubella is usually a mild disease with few complications. Clinical illness may be more severe in adults.[6, 9, 285, 288, 343, 457] The relationship between viral and clinical events is depicted in Figure 6–4. Measles, varicella, and some enteroviruses acquired close to delivery may be associated with serious illness in the newborn, probably because of fetal exposure to transplacental viremia in the absence of protective levels of maternal antibody (see appropriate chapters). One case report suggests that the same may be true in rubella. Sheinis and associates reported the death of a neonate with rash onset at 12 days of age; the mother developed rash on the day of delivery.[458] This single observation needs to be confirmed. There are no conclusive data to indicate that infection in the immunocompromised host is associated with an increased risk of complications.

The first symptoms of rubella occur after an incubation period of 16 to 18 days, with a range of 14 to 21 days. In the child, rash is often the first sign detected. In adolescents and adults, however, the eruption is commonly preceded by a 1- to 5-day prodromal period characterized by low-grade fever, headache, malaise, anorexia, mild conjunctivitis, coryza, sore throat, cough, and lymphadenopathy, usually involving suboccipital, postauricular, and cervical nodes.

The constitutional symptoms often subside rapidly with the appearance of the rash. The rash can last from 1 to 5 days or more and in adults can be pruritic. Infection without a rash is quite common. The ratio of subclinical to clinical infections has varied from 1:9 to 7:1.[254, 290] Subclinical infection can lead to fetal infection, although it is not clear whether the risk is as great as that associated with clinically apparent infection.[2, 3, 6, 100, 103, 328, 334]

Arthralgia and frank arthritis with recrudescence of low-grade fever and other constitutional symptoms may appear after the rash fades. Joint involvement typically lasts 5 to 10 days but may be more persistent. The frequency of these symptoms is variable, but it is more common in adults, particularly women.[9] In some studies of adult patients, the frequency has been as high as 70%.[459] Thrombocytopenia (occurring at a rate of approximately 1 per 3000 cases) and acute postinfection encephalitis (occurring at a rate of 1 per 5000 to 1 per 6000 cases) are rare complications that usually occur 2 to 4 days after rash onset.[9] Rare complications associated with postnatal rubella include myocarditis, Guillain-Barré syndrome, relapsing encephalitis, optic neuritis, and bone marrow aplasia.[9, 460–464] Two cases of a progressive panencephalitis, similar to measles-associated subacute sclerosing panencephalitis, have been reported.[427, 428] As noted next, this central nervous system disturbance is more likely to occur in patients with congenital rubella syndrome, although still infrequently.[382, 465, 466] Testalgia has also been reported in patients with rubella, but this may have been a coincidental finding.[467, 468]

Congenital Infection

Gregg's original report in 1941 defined the rubella syndrome as a constellation of defects, usually involving some combination of congenital heart, eye, and hearing abnormalities, with or without mental retardation and microcephaly.[12] After the extensive studies in the mid 1960s, in which virologic and serologic methods of assessment were used, the pathologic potential associated with intrauterine rubella had to be greatly expanded.[2, 3] In fact, the recognition of various new defects associated with congenital rubella infection led to speculation that they had not existed before the 1962 to 1964 pandemic. However, a review of the abnormalities in infants born during previous nonepidemic periods indicated that they were, in fact, not new but simply had not been appreciated previously because of the small number of affected infants studied.[469]

As previously discussed, it was found that the virus can infect one or virtually all fetal organs and, once established, can persist for long periods (see Transmission in Utero, Natural History, Pathogenesis and Pathology sections).* Congenital rubella, a chronic infection, may kill the fetus in utero, causing miscarriage or stillbirth. At the other extreme, the infection may have no apparent effect clinically detectable at the delivery of normal-appearing infants. Alternatively, severe multiple birth defects may be obvious in the newborn period. The wide spectrum of disease is summarized later in Tables 6–3 and 6–4 (see also references 6 and 9).

Silent infections in the infant are much more common

---

*See references 6, 13, 14, 102, 126, 127, 156, 271–276, 278, 293, 307–313, 323–330, and 373–382.

than symptomatic ones. Schiff and colleagues examined prospectively 4005 infants born after the 1964 rubella epidemic.[327] Based on virologic and serologic techniques to detect infection in the newborns, the overall rate of congenital rubella was in excess of 2% compared with only approximately 0.1% in endemic years.[327, 334] Sixty-eight percent of the infected newborns had subclinical infection during the neonatal period. Among those who were followed, 71% developed manifestations of infection at various times in the first 5 years of life. Many important rubella defects can be undetectable or overlooked in the early months of life. Furthermore, existing manifestations of infection can progress and new manifestations may appear throughout life.[6, 13, 14, 102, 126, 127, 323-330] Later in the chapter Table 6–3 lists congenital rubella syndrome abnormalities that usually are not detected until the second year of life or later. The silent and progressive nature of congenital rubella infection has important implications for accurate, timely diagnosis and appropriate management, both short term and long term.

It is useful to group the clinical features of congenital rubella into three categories: (1) transient manifestations in newborns and infants; (2) permanent manifestations, which may be present at birth or become apparent during the first year of life; and (3) developmental and late-onset manifestations, which usually appear and progress during childhood, adolescence, and early adult life.[13, 434, 470] These groupings obviously overlap.

TRANSIENT MANIFESTATIONS

Transient manifestations appear to reflect ongoing heavy viral infection, perhaps abetted by the newborn's emerging, often abnormal immune function.[6, 115, 129] Examples of these manifestations include hepatosplenomegaly, hepatitis, jaundice, thrombocytopenia with petechiae and purpura, discrete bluish-red ("blueberry muffin") lesions of dermal erythropoiesis, hemolytic anemia, chronic rash, adenopathy, meningoencephalitis (in some cases), large anterior fontanelle, interstitial pneumonia, myositis, myocarditis, diarrhea, cloudy cornea, and disturbances in bone growth that appear as striated radiolucencies in the long bones. Infants with these transient findings usually have evidence of intrauterine growth retardation (≥50%) and may continue to fail to thrive during infancy.[272] These transient abnormalities were referred to as the *expanded rubella syndrome* when widely reported after the pandemic of 1962 to 1964. In fact, careful review of the early observations during the 1940s and 1950s revealed that these were not new manifestations of congenital rubella.

These conditions usually are self-limiting and clear spontaneously over days or weeks.[2] These lesions are important from a diagnostic and prognostic standpoint. They may be associated with other, more severe defects. This applies especially to thrombocytopenia and bone lesions.[13, 470] The mortality rate was approximately 35% in one group of infants who presented with neonatal thrombocytopenia. Extreme prematurity, gross cardiac lesions or myocarditis with early heart failure, rapidly progressive hepatitis, extensive meningoencephalitis, and fulminant interstitial pneumonitis contributed to the mortality during infancy.[434]

PERMANENT MANIFESTATIONS

Permanent manifestations include heart and other blood vessel defects, eye lesions, central nervous system abnormalities, deafness, and a variety of other congenital anomalies. These structural defects result from defective organogenesis (e.g., some cardiac, eye, and other organ defects), as well as from tissue destruction and scarring (e.g., hearing loss, brain damage, cataracts, chorioretinopathy, and vascular stenosis). Relatively few defects result from gross anatomic abnormalities. It is not certain that all of the malformations given in Table 6–2 are actually associated with congenital rubella.[13, 308, 374, 447, 469-497] Because many of them occur in the absence of intrauterine rubella infection, their presence in affected infants may be coincidental.[9]

Congenital heart disease is present in more than one half of children infected during the first 2 months of gestation. The most common lesions, in descending order, are patent ductus arteriosus, pulmonary artery stenosis, and pulmonary valvular stenosis. Aortic valvular stenosis and tetralogy of Fallot have also been recorded. A patent ductus arteriosus occurs alone in approximately one third of cases; otherwise, it is frequently found in association with pulmonary artery or valvular stenosis.[13, 470, 482] Stenosis of other vessels plays an important role in the spectrum of congenital rubella syndrome.[438, 491, 492] These lesions may be related to coronary, cerebral, renal, and peripheral vascular disease seen in adults.[126, 521]

A "salt and pepper" retinopathy due to disturbed growth of the pigmentary layer of the retina is the most common of all ocular findings.[6, 13, 434, 470] Cataracts, often accompanied by microphthalmia, occur in approximately one third of all cases of congenital rubella. Bilateral cataracts are found in one half of affected children. Primary glaucoma is relatively uncommon; it does not affect a cataractous eye. Cataracts and infantile glaucoma may not be present or detectable at birth but usually become apparent during the early weeks of life. Other ocular abnormalities occur later in life (see Developmental and Late-Onset Manifestations).

Children with congenital rubella syndrome exhibit a number of central nervous system abnormalities that follow widespread insult to the brain. Microcephaly can be a feature of this syndrome. Mental retardation and motor retardation are common and are directly related to the acute meningoencephalitis that is present in 10 to 20% of affected children at birth.[9] Behavioral and psychiatric disorders have been noted in many patients.[13, 434] Of particular interest is autism, which has been reported to occur with a frequency of approximately 6%.[434] Chronic encephalitis has been reported in young children.[6] However, a late-onset progressive panencephalitis may occur in the second decade of life.[382, 465, 466] This is discussed later with other developmental manifestations.

The incidence of deafness has been underestimated because many cases had been missed in infancy and early childhood. However, based on follow-up studies,

TABLE 6–2
Clinical Findings and Their Estimated Frequency of Occurrence in Young Symptomatic Infants with Congenitally Acquired Rubella

CLINICAL FINDINGS	FREQUENCY[a]	REFERENCES
Adenopathies	+ +	470, 471
Anemia	+	471, 472
Bone		
Micrognathia	+	469
Extremities	+	469
Bony radiolucencies	+ +	470, 473–476
Brain		
Encephalitis (active)	+ +	477, 478
Microcephaly	+	308, 478, 479
Brain calcification	Rare	478, 480, 481
Bulging fontanelle	+	374, 470
Cardiovascular system		
Pulmonary arterial hypoplasia	+ +	482
Patent ductus arteriosus	+ +	482
Coarctation of aortic isthmus	+	482
Interventricular septal defect	Rare	
Interauricular septal defect	Rare	
Others	Rare	13
Chromosomal abnormalities	?	447
Dermal erythropoiesis (blueberry muffin syndrome)	+	483, 484
Dermatoglyphic abnormalities	+	485, 486
Ear		
Hearing defects (severe)	+ + +	470
Peripheral	+ + +	470
Central	+	
Eye	+ +	470, 487–489
Retinopathy	+ + +	13
Cataracts	+ +	308, 374, 469–471, 477, 487, 490
Cloudy cornea	Rare	470
Glaucoma	Rare	471, 477, 487
Microphthalmos	+	470, 487
Genitourinary tract	+	470, 491–493
Undescended testicle	+	470, 494
Polycystic kidney[b]	Rare	492
Bilobed kidney with reduplicated ureter[b]	Rare	492
Hypospadias	Rare	14, 493
Unilateral agenesis[b]	Rare	492
Renal artery stenosis with hypertension[b]	Rare	493
Hydroureter and hydronephrosis[b]	Rare	478
Growth retardation		
Intrauterine	+ + +	308, 374, 469–471, 477, 490
Extrauterine	+ +	308, 494
Hepatitis	Rare	469, 470, 477, 495
Hepatosplenomegaly	+ + +	308, 374, 469–471, 477, 490
Immunologic dyscrasias	Rare	496
Interstitial pneumonitis (acute, subacute, chronic)	+ +	121, 470, 477, 497
Jaundice (regurgitative)	+	477, 490
Leukopenia	+	472
Myocardial necrosis	Rare	477, 478, 488, 495
Neurologic deficit	+ +	13, 479
Prematurity	+	308, 374, 469–471, 477, 490, 495
Thrombocytopenia with/without purpura	+ +	308, 374, 469–471, 477, 490

Table continued on following page

TABLE 6–2
Clinical Findings and Their Estimated Frequency of Occurrence in Young Symptomatic Infants with Congenitally Acquired Rubella *Continued*

CLINICAL FINDINGS	FREQUENCY[a]	REFERENCES
Others[b]	Rare	
Esophageal atresia		308
Tracheoesophageal fistula		490
Anencephaly		490
Encephalocele		469, 490
Meningomyelocele		479
Cleft palate		308, 490
Inguinal hernia		
Asplenia		
Nephritis (vascular)		478
Clubfoot		490
High palate		494
Talipes equinovarus		494
Depressed sternum		494
Pes cavus		494
Clinodactyly		494
Brachydactyly		494
Syndactyly		494
Elfin facies		494

[a]Frequency of occurrence is classified as follows: +, less than 20%; + +, 20 to 50%; + + +, 50 to 75%.
[b]Rarely associated with rubella syndrome (whether caused by infection unknown). Incidence seemingly increased in infants with congenital rubella.

deafness is now known to be the most common manifestation of congenital rubella, occurring in 80% or more of those infected.* In contrast to other serious defects, hearing impairment often is the only significant consequence of congenital rubella. Defects dependent on organogenesis (i.e., cataracts and some heart lesions) are uncommon after infection beyond the eighth week of gestation. However, the organ of Corti is vulnerable to the effects of the virus up to the first 16 weeks and perhaps up to the first 18 to 20 weeks. The deafness, ranging from mild to profound and from unilateral or bilateral, is usually peripheral (sensorineural) and is more commonly bilateral. Central auditory impairment and language delay may lead to a misdiagnosis of mental retardation.[13, 498–502]

DEVELOPMENTAL AND LATE-ONSET MANIFESTATIONS

Developmental and late-onset manifestations have been reviewed by Sever and Shaver and their colleagues.[126, 127] They include endocrinopathies, deafness, ocular damage, vascular effects, and progression of central nervous system disease (Table 6–3).† A number of mechanisms may be responsible for the continuing disease process that leads to these abnormalities: persistent viral infection, viral reactivation, vascular insufficiency, and immunologic insult. The last may be mediated by circulating immune complexes and autoantibodies. Abnormalities in cellular immunity and genetic factors have also been studied.

Insulin-dependent diabetes mellitus is the most frequent of all these manifestations, occurring in approximately 20% of patients by adulthood.[13, 112, 120, 125–127, 505] This reported prevalence is 100 to 200 times that observed for the general population. Studies of HLA type indicate that congenital rubella syndrome patients with diabetes have the same frequencies of selected HLA haplotypes as diabetic patients without the syndrome (e.g., increased HLA DR3 and decreased HLA DR2). The presence of pancreatic islet cell and cytotoxic surface antibodies in children with congenital rubella syndrome does not appear to be related to any specific HLA type. Thus, it has been postulated that congenital infection increases the penetrance of a preexisting susceptibility to diabetes in these patients.[125] Rabinowe and associates have also reported an elevation in the number of Ia-positive ("activated") T cells in patients with congenital rubella syndrome.[128] They suggested that this T cell abnormality may be related, in these patients, to the increased incidence of diabetes mellitus and other diseases associated with autoantibodies.

Thyroid dysfunction has been reported in about 5% of patients and manifests as hyperthyroidism, hypothyroidism, and thyroiditis.[112, 124, 506–511] Autoimmune mechanisms appear to be responsible for these abnormalities. For example, Clarke and colleagues reported that 23% of 201 deaf teenagers with congenital infection had autoantibodies to the microsomal and/or globulin fractions of the thyroid and that 20% of those with autoantibodies had thyroid gland dysfunction.[124] Coexistence of diabetes and thyroid dysfunction has been reported, but the significance of the association is unknown.[112, 128]

Two cases of growth hormone deficiency have been reported.[512] The defect appears to be hypothalamic in origin. However, among eight growth-retarded older

*See references 6, 9, 13, 14, 102, 126, 127, 323, 324, and 326–329.
†See references 13, 14, 112, 120, 125, 126, 128, 323, 328, 382, 434, 466, 467, 479, 492, 498–512, and 515–521.

TABLE 6–3
Abnormalities of Congenital Rubella Usually Not Detected Until Second Year or Later

DEFECTS	REFERENCES
Hearing	
Peripheral	13, 323, 328, 498–501
Central	
Language	13, 492, 501, 502
Developmental	
Motor	13, 503, 504
Intellectual	13, 479, 503
Behavioral	13, 503
Psychiatric	13, 503
Autism	13, 434
Endocrine	
Diabetes	13, 112, 120, 125, 126, 128, 505
Precocious puberty	13, 14
Hypothyroidism	506–510
Thyroiditis	507–509
Hyperthyroidism	112, 511
Growth hormone deficiency	512–514
Addison's disease	14
Visual	
Glaucoma (later onset)	515
Subretinal neovascularization	516, 517
Keratic precipitates	515
Keratoconus	518
Corneal hydrops	518
Lens absorption	519
Dental	494, 520
Progressive panencephalitis	382, 466, 467
Educational difficulties	13
Hypertension	521

children with congenital rubella syndrome, Oberfield found no evidence of functional abnormality in the hypothalamic-pituitary axis and normal or elevated levels of somatomedin C.[513] Growth patterns in a group of 105 late adolescents revealed three patterns: (1) growth consistently below the fifth percentile; (2) growth in the normal range, but early cessation of growth, usually with final height below the fifth percentile; and (3) normal growth. The magnitude of the cognitive deficits was closely correlated with growth failure.[514] Ziring has commented on a case with Addison's disease.[14] Precocious puberty has also been noted.[13, 14]

The delayed diagnosis of preexisting deafness has already been referred to. However, the hearing deficit can increase over time, and sudden onset of sensorineural deafness may occur after years of normal auditory acuity.[338, 503, 522] As noted by Sever and co-workers, the latter has been observed in a child 10 years of age.[126]

A number of late-onset ocular defects can occur. Glaucoma has been reported in patients between 3 and 22 years of age who did not previously have the congenital or infantile variety of glaucoma associated with congenital rubella syndrome.[515] Other reported manifestations are keratic precipitates, keratoconus, corneal hydrops, and spontaneous lens absorption.[518, 519]

The retinopathy of congenital rubella, which was previously believed to be completely benign, has more recently been associated with the delayed occurrence of visual difficulties caused by subretinal neovascularization.[516, 517, 523] Another delayed manifestation associated with vascular changes is hypertension resulting from renal artery and aortic stenosis.[521]

Mental retardation, autism, and other behavioral problems may be delayed in appearance and can be progressive.[13, 434] However, the most interesting and serious delayed central nervous system manifestation is the occurrence of a progressive and fatal panencephalitis resembling subacute sclerosing panencephalitis that presents during the second decade of life. The first cases were reported by Weil and Townsend and their co-workers.[382, 465] At the time of their review, Waxham and Wolinsky noted that 10 cases of progressive rubella panencephalitis had been reported in patients with congenital rubella syndrome.[466] As noted previously, 2 cases have been reported after postnatally acquired rubella.[427, 428] Patients with this condition present with increasing loss of mental function, seizures, and ataxia. These symptoms continue to progress until the patient is in a vegetative state and ultimately dies. Rubella virus has been recovered from the brain of one congenitally infected patient.[381, 382] Elevated serum and cerebrospinal fluid antibodies and increased amounts of cerebrospinal fluid protein and gamma globulin have been detected. Virus has also been isolated from lymphocytes, and rubella-specific immune complexes have been identified.[116, 524] Although rare, this syndrome focuses attention on the ability of the virus to persist and perhaps become reactivated after years of latency.

LONG-TERM PROGNOSIS

Fifty survivors of the congenital rubella epidemic of 1939 to 1943 in Australia were seen at age 25, and their status was reviewed again in 1991.[571] Seven subjects had died in the interval—three with malignancies, three with cardiovascular disease, and one with the acquired immunodeficiency syndrome. Among the 1991 survivors, 5 were diabetic, all 40 examined were deaf, 23 had eye defects, and 16 had cardiovascular defects. In spite of these conditions, the group was characterized by remarkably good social adjustment. Most (29) were married, and they had 51 children—only 1 with a congenital defect (deafness presumed to be hereditary from his deaf father, who did not have congenital rubella). Most were of normal stature, although 6 (of the 40) were less than the third percentile for height. This group of survivors is quite different from the approximately 300 survivors followed in New York since the rubella epidemic of 1963 to 1965.[572] Among these survivors, in their late twenties, approximately one third were leading relatively normal lives in the community, one third live with their parents and may have "noncompetitive" employment, and one third require care in facilities with round-the-clock (24-hour) care. Neither the Australian nor the New York group is a representative sample of all survivors of maternal rubella infection, but these groups do offer insight on long-term prognosis. The differences in outcome between the Australian group (survivors of Norman

Gregg's original patients) and the New York group probably reflect both the different methods by which the groups were collected and the significant differences in the medical technology of the 1940s compared with the 1960s.

LABORATORY DIAGNOSIS

Timely, accurate diagnosis of acute primary rubella infection in the pregnant woman and congenital rubella infection in the infant is imperative if appropriate management is to be undertaken (see Management Issues section). The diagnosis must be confirmed either serologically or virologically because clinical diagnosis of both postnatal and congenital rubella is unreliable. In any suspected exposure of a pregnant woman, every effort should be made to confirm rubella infection so that accurate counseling can be offered about the risks to the fetus. Laboratory proof of congenital infection facilitates proper treatment, follow-up, and long-term management.

Maternal Infection

Because of inapparent infection, the variable clinical manifestations of rubella, and the mimicking of rubella by other viral exanthems, laboratory diagnosis is essential in managing potential rubella infection during pregnancy (see Natural History and Clinical Manifestations sections).[152, 194, 221, 222, 301] Although virus can be cultured from the nose and throat, isolation techniques are impractical. Thus, laboratory confirmation is realistically limited to serologic testing (see The Virus section). Acute primary infection can usually be documented by demonstrating a significant rise in antibody level between acute and convalescent sera or the presence of rubella-specific IgM antibody. Appropriate timing of specimen collection with regard to rash onset (or exposure in the case of subclinical infection) is critical for accurate interpretation of results (see Fig. 6–5). Diagnosis is greatly facilitated if the immune status is known before disease onset or exposure.[253] Women with laboratory evidence of immunity are not at risk. From a practical point of view, women with a history of vaccination on or after the first birthday should also be considered immune.[250, 251] However, because seroconversion is not 100% (see Prevention of Congenital Rubella section), serologic testing may be indicated on an individual basis in vaccinated women who have a known exposure or a rash and illness consistent with rubella to rule out acute primary infection.

Traditionally, a fourfold or greater rise in antibody titer (e.g., HI, complement fixation, or latex agglutination) has been considered a significant rise in antibody. However, with the advent of enzyme immunoassay the diagnosis may be based on significant changes in optical density expressed as an "index" rather than a titer. The acute-phase specimen should be taken as soon as possible after onset of the rash, ideally within 7 days. If a positive titer is obtained for a specimen taken on the day of rash onset or 1 to 2 days later, the risk of acute infection is low but cannot be excluded. The convalescent-phase serum sample should be taken 10 to 14 days later. If the first serum sample is from more than 7 days after rash onset, some assays, such as HI, may not be able to detect a significant antibody rise because titers may have already peaked. In this situation, measurement of antibodies that appear later in the course of infection may be useful. A significant rise in complement fixation titer or, for example, a high HI, latex agglutination, or enzyme immunoassay titer and little or no antibody, as measured by passive hemagglutination, is very suggestive of recent infection (see Fig. 6–5).

When multiple serum samples are obtained in the course of the diagnostic workup, all should be tested simultaneously in the same laboratory to avoid misinterpretation of laboratory-related variations in titer. Although a single high titer is consistent with recent infection, its presence is not specific enough to conclude that recent infection has, in fact, occurred.[253]

Detection of rubella-specific IgM (RIgM) is a very useful method for confirming acute, recent infection. Although RIgM testing is very useful, a number of factors can affect test results. Results must be interpreted with careful attention to the timing of the specimens. Samples taken within the first several days after onset of rash may have low or even undetectable levels of RIgM, but a specimen taken 7 to 14 days later will invariably show higher titers of antibody. The levels of RIgM may decline promptly thereafter (see Fig. 6–5). It should be remembered that many of the various methods previously described for detecting IgM have some limitations (see The Virus section). IgM antibody testing may involve pretreatment of the serum by a variety of techniques to separate IgM from IgG, such as column chromatography, sucrose gradient centrifugation, or adsorption of IgG with staphylococcal protein A. The serum IgM fraction can then be assayed by HI, immunofluorescence, radioimmunoassay, or enzyme immunoassay.[152, 201–205, 208, 210, 219–222, 225–233] A false-positive result may occur if the serum was pretreated with protein A because about 5% of IgG is not removed. The radioimmunoassay and enzyme immunoassay techniques can directly detect specific IgM antibodies in unfractionated sera, but false-positive results may be produced by the presence of rheumatoid factor.[152, 202, 204] A solid-phase, immunosorbent (i.e., capture) technique, however, appears to be unaffected by rheumatoid factor.[97, 205, 220, 231] A final note of caution is necessary. Whereas high or moderate titers provide very good evidence of recent infection, low rubella-specific IgM titers detected by sensitive assays must be interpreted cautiously. As noted earlier, low titers have been shown to persist for many months in a few patients after natural infection and can be detected in some immune patients with subclinical reinfection.[39, 49, 51, 53, 348–350]

Diagnosis of subclinical infection is relatively straightforward if the woman is known to be susceptible, the exposure is recognized, and a serum sample is obtained approximately 28 days after exposure. The diagnosis is more difficult if the immune status of the woman is unknown. However, it can be facilitated if the acute-phase serum specimen is obtained as soon as possible after a recognized exposure that did not occur more than 5 weeks previously.[253] The convalescent serum sample, if necessary, should then be obtained approximately 3 weeks later. If the first specimen lacks detectable antibody, continued close clinical and serologic follow-up is necessary. If the first specimen has detectable antibody and was obtained within a week to 10 days of exposure, there is no risk of infection and further evaluation is unnecessary. On the other hand, a positive titer in a specimen obtained after this period indicates a need for further serologic investigation. If test results of paired serum specimens are inconclusive, RIgM testing may be helpful, but a negative test result may be difficult to interpret. Passive hemagglutination testing may also be employed.

More significant diagnostic difficulties arise when women of unknown immune status are exposed at an unknown time, were exposed more than 5 weeks previously, or had rash onset more than 3 weeks previously.[253] In these situations, expert consultation may be necessary if positive titers are present. Unfortunately, conclusive information about the timing of past infection and risk to the fetus is often not available, even when a combination of antibody assays is used. These situations can be minimized if prenatal rubella testing is carried out routinely. Furthermore, laboratories performing prenatal screening should store these specimens until delivery in case retesting is necessary.[250, 525]

Congenital Infection

A presumptive diagnosis of congenital rubella infection should be entertained in any infant born to a mother who had documented or suspected rubella infection at any time during pregnancy (see Transmission in Utero section).[98, 104] The diagnosis should also be considered in any infant with evidence of intrauterine growth retardation and other stigmata consistent with congenital infection, regardless of maternal history (see Clinical Manifestations section). Although such findings are sensitive for clinically apparent disease, they are nonspecific because many of them can be associated with other intrauterine infections, such as cytomegalovirus infection, syphilis, and toxoplasmosis (see appropriate chapters). In addition, many affected infants are asymptomatic. Thus, as with maternal rubella, congenital infection must be confirmed by laboratory tests.

In contrast to maternal rubella, attempting to isolate rubella virus in tissue culture is a valuable tool for diagnosing congenital rubella in newborns. The virus is most readily isolated from the posterior pharynx and less consistently so from the conjunctivae, cerebrospinal fluid, or urine.* Virus isolation should be attempted as soon as congenital rubella is suspected clinically because viral excretion wanes during infancy (see Fig. 6–6). In older children in whom virus shedding has ceased from other sites, virus may still be isolated from cataractous lens

tissue.[380] In children with encephalitis, virus may persist in the cerebrospinal fluid for several years.[353–355, 357, 358, 479]

There are two approaches for serologic diagnosis. First, cord serum can be assayed for the presence of rubella-specific IgM antibody.[383, 385, 386, 394] Detectable IgM antibody is a reliable indicator of congenital infection because IgM is fetally derived. However, false-positive results may occur because of rheumatoid factor or incomplete removal of IgG (largely maternal), depending on the techniques used. In addition, a minority of newborns with stigmata of congenital rubella may not have detectable levels of RIgM in sera taken during the first days of life and some infections may go undiagnosed if infection occurred late in pregnancy because it is theoretically possible that there was inadequate time for the fetus to produce detectable levels of specific IgM antibodies by the time of delivery.[13, 98, 104]

A second approach is to monitor IgG levels in the infant over time to see if they persist. Maternally derived antibodies have a half-life of approximately 30 days.[383, 385, 386] As measured by the HI test, they usually decline at a rate of one twofold dilution per month and would be expected to disappear by 6 to 12 months of age (see Fig. 6–7). Persistence of IgG antibody at this age, especially in high titer, is presumptive evidence of intrauterine infection with rubella virus. Sera should be drawn at 3 and 5 to 6 months of age, with a repeat specimen at 12 months of age if necessary. As noted earlier, all serum samples should be tested in parallel.

Important limitations of this method are the delay in diagnosis and the fact that rubella infections occurring after birth may be mistaken for congenital infections.[98, 526] The latter is usually more of a problem when attempting to diagnose congenital infection retrospectively in patients beyond infancy, especially if the incidence of rubella in childhood is high or vaccine has already been administered. A third limitation is that some infants and children with congenital rubella syndrome (particularly older children) may lack antibody as measured by HI.[328, 397–399] If the diagnosis is still suspected, and HI, IgM, and culture results are negative, retesting with an assay that detects antibody to all components of the virion, such as some enzyme immunoassays, is advised.[85] Some cases with undetectable HI antibody may be from an incomplete immune response to all the structural proteins of the virus, including the hemagglutinin (see The Virus section).[82, 83] Other diagnostic methods, such as measurement of cellular immunity and response to vaccine (i.e., a failure to boost antibody titer), may also be helpful in this situation, but, all too frequently, a definitive retrospective diagnosis cannot be made.[365, 414, 527, 528] Cerebrospinal fluid may also be examined for the presence of rubella-specific IgM.[529] Finally, as in the case for acquired infection, determination of avidity of IgG may be useful.[351, 353, 530]

The availability of sensitive and specific tests for prenatal diagnosis of fetal infection after suspected or documented maternal rubella can greatly facilitate counseling. Although positive diagnoses were reported from examination of amniotic fluid, fetal blood, and chorionic villus sampling for virus isolation, rubella-specific IgM and antigens, interferon, and RNA,[97, 420, 531–537] the low

---

*See references 2, 13, 156, 271–276, 278, 307, 308, 310, 312, 376, and 377.

sensitivity of these assays added little to the counseling process. More recently, reverse transcription-nested polymerase chain reaction has been reported to offer a far more reliable and rapid tool and thus, where available, a valuable aid to counseling.[538–540] Timing of the specimen collection related to the timing of maternal infection may influence sensitivity, which reached 100% for amniotic fluid, eight of eight specimens in one study, and 83% for chorionic villus sampling, five of six specimens in another study. Repeat testing may increase the yield of positive specimens.[531, 540]

MANAGEMENT ISSUES

The major management issues associated with postnatal infection arise when a pregnant woman is at risk of acquiring infection. Confirming the diagnosis, counseling about the risks of infection of and damage to the fetus, and discussing courses of action, including the use of immune globulin and consideration of termination of pregnancy, require a thorough understanding of the natural history and consequences of rubella in pregnancy. In the case of congenital infection, the emphasis is on diagnosis and acute and long-term management. Isolation may be important to reduce spread of infection.

Use of Immune Globulin

The role of passive immunization with immune globulin after exposure to rubella is controversial.[2, 6, 9, 288, 294, 325, 328, 541–544] Brody and co-workers reported that large doses of immune globulin may have some efficacy,[542] but, in general, it proved to be more useful when given prophylactically than when administered after exposure. This is not surprising because extensive viral replication is demonstrable a week or more before symptoms appear, with initial replication probably beginning even earlier. In addition, the amount of antirubella antibody in commercial immune globulin preparations is variable and unpredictable; specific hyperimmune globulin preparations are not available.[544, 545] Theoretically, the role of circulating antibodies in rubella is mainly to limit the viremia and possibly to prevent replication at the portal of entry; antibody is less valuable once infection has begun. Indeed, fetal infection occurred when immune globulin was administered to the mother in what appeared to be adequate amounts soon after exposure. Another disadvantage of immune globulin is that it may eliminate or reduce clinical findings without affecting viral replication. Thus, clinical clues of maternal infection would be masked without adequate protection of the fetus, resulting in a false sense of security.

It is currently recommended that use of immune globulin be confined to those women known to have been exposed to rubella who do not wish to interrupt their pregnancy under any circumstances.[250, 251] In this situation, large doses (20 ml in adults) should be administered. The patient should be advised, however, that protection from fetal infection cannot be guaranteed.

Termination of Pregnancy

A discussion of the complex issues involved in the decision about termination of pregnancy for maternal rubella is beyond the scope of this chapter. Needless to say, the decision must be carefully weighed by the physician and the prospective parents. The physician must have a thorough understanding of the known facts about the pathogenesis and diagnosis of congenital rubella and the risks to the fetus depending on the timing of maternal infection. Where available, analysis of amniotic fluid, fetal blood, or chorionic villus sampling by reverse transcription-nested polymerase chain reaction may assist in antenatal diagnosis of infection.[538–540] Expert consultation is desirable to ensure that the most current information is used in the decision-making process.

Clinical Management

Acute rubella infection usually requires little clinical management. However, the patient with congenital infection may require medical, surgical, educational, and rehabilitative management. Many lesions are not apparent at birth because they either have not yet appeared or cannot be detected. In keeping with its chronicity, congenital rubella must be managed as a dynamic rather than a static disease state. A continuing effort on the part of the physician must be made to define initially the extent of the problem and to detect evidence of progressive disease or emergence of new problems over time. Because of the broad range of problems, a multidisciplinary team approach to care is essential.

Complete pediatric, neurologic, cardiac, ophthalmologic, and audiologic examinations should be complemented by complete blood cell count, by radiologic bone surveys, and often by evaluation of cerebrospinal fluid for all newborns in whom the diagnosis is suspected, whether the infant is symptomatic or not. Some defects, such as interstitial pneumonitis, can be slowly progressive and apparently cause their major functional difficulties months after birth. Infected infants require close scrutiny during the first 6 months of life. Serial assessment for immunologic dyscrasias is necessary during this period because the humoral defects may be masked by the presence of maternal immunoglobulin.

Hearing defects and psychomotor difficulties are by far the most important problems because of their high incidence. Both of these often occur in infants who are initially asymptomatic. The new techniques for detection of hearing impairment in newborns and the increasingly state-by-state, mandated universal newborn hearing screening testing requirements have been initiated too recently to determine their utility in detection of unsuspected congenital rubella. It is clear that delay in diagnosis and therapeutic intervention has profound impact on language development and skills acquisition and can magnify psychosocial adjustment problems within the entire family constellation.

Because many children with congenital rubella are multihandicapped, early, interdisciplinary treatment is warranted. Appropriate hearing aids; visual aids, including contact lenses; speech, language, occupational, and physical therapy; and special educational programs are frequently required for such children. Serial psychologic and perceptual testing may be very helpful for ongoing management, particularly when performed by individuals experienced in assessing multihandicapped, sensorially deprived children. Repeated testing is important because, in many cases, the problems appear to be progressive and require continuing assessment of the therapeutic approach.

In the United States, most infants suspected of congenital rubella will be eligible for early intervention and habilitation services authorized by the Federal Individuals with Disabilities Education Act of 1997. These programs offer such services to affected children beginning in infancy, a critical time for children who may be hearing impaired. The impact of universal newborn hearing screening programs as another tool for early detection of congenital rubella remains to be seen.

Chemotherapy

Because postnatal rubella is usually mild, there has been little need to pursue chemotherapeutic regimens, and the literature on this subject is sparse. Interferon has been used to treat chronic arthritis, and Isoprinosine has been administered to a patient with postnatally acquired progressive rubella panencephalitis.[428, 524, 546] Chance temporal association between interferon administration and reported improvement in joint symptoms cannot be differentiated from potential therapeutic benefits of the interferon. In the trial of Isoprinosine, no improvement was observed.

The number of reports regarding treatment of infants with congenital rubella is also somewhat limited. The course of congenital infection does not appear to be altered by any currently available chemotherapeutic agent. Because amantadine reduces the replication of rubella virus in vitro, it has theoretical possibilities as a chemotherapeutic agent.[153–155] Its use, however, has been confined to a 5-month-old infant with congenital infection.[156] Neither virus excretion nor clinical status was affected. Interferon has also been administered to a few infants with congenital rubella syndrome. Arvin and associates reported that nasopharyngeal excretion in three infants (3 to 5 months of age) persisted throughout interferon administration but at reduced titers compared with baseline.[547] There was, however, no clinical effect. Larsson and co-workers administered interferon to a 14-month-old child and reported regression of a cutaneous eruption resulting from vasculitis and disappearance of viremia.[548] However, viruria and other signs of viral persistence (e.g., rubella-specific IgM in the cerebrospinal fluid) were unaffected. It is also not certain if the improvement in the rash was from the interferon or was coincidental. A 10-month-old infant treated by Verder and co-workers may have benefited from interferon, but it is noteworthy that improvement was also noted after exchange transfusions that preceded the interferon treatment.[129] Finally, Isoprinosine has been administered to some patients with progressive rubella panencephalitis.[524, 549] As for postnatally acquired disease, the results in this case have been disappointing.

Isolation

Patients with rubella are considered infectious from the fifth day before to the seventh day after the onset of the rash and should be placed in contact isolation.[550] Exposed rubella-susceptible patients confined to hospital should be placed in contact isolation from the seventh through the twenty-first day after exposure and tested appropriately to rule out asymptomatic infection.[551] Infectious patients with congenital rubella should also be in contact isolation.[550] Isolation precautions should be instituted as soon as either rubella or congenital rubella is suspected. Only persons known to be immune (i.e., those with serologic evidence of immunity or documentation of vaccination on or after the first birthday) should care for infectious or potentially infectious patients.[250, 251]

Children with congenital rubella syndrome should be considered infectious for the first year of life unless repeated pharyngeal and urine culture results are negative.[251, 550] Culture results are unlikely to become negative until 3 to 6 months of age (see Fig. 6–6). From a practical point of view, children older than 1 year of age are unlikely to be a significant source of infection. In the home situation, susceptible pregnant visitors should be informed of the potential risk of exposure.

PREVENTION OF CONGENITAL RUBELLA

Rubella Vaccine and Immunization Strategies

Active immunization is the only practical means to prevent congenital rubella because passive immunization provides unreliable, transient protection (see Management Issues section). However, there has been considerable debate about the best way to utilize the vaccine.[3, 5–7, 29, 34, 552] Because rubella vaccination is not aimed primarily at protecting the individual, but, rather, the unborn fetus, two basic strategies have been proposed: universal childhood immunization and selective vaccination of susceptible girls and women of childbearing age. The former approach is designed to interrupt transmission of virus by vaccinating the reservoir of infection, reduce the overall risk of infection in the general population, and provide indirect protection of unvaccinated, postpubertal women. The latter approach directly protects those at risk of being infected when pregnant, limits overall vaccine use, and allows virus to circulate and boost vaccine-induced immunity in the population. Experience gained over the past 30 years indicates that integration of both is necessary to achieve maximum control in the shortest possible time.[5, 29, 32, 34]

At the time of licensure in 1969, available information indicated that the live, attenuated rubella vaccines were safe, noncommunicable and highly effective (see introductory section).[3, 4, 25–27] Although information on the duration of vaccine-induced immunity was limited, public health policy makers in the United States believed that vaccination of all children would provide protection into the childbearing years. The duration and quality of the immunity would obviously have to be monitored continually. Because vaccine virus could cross the placenta and infect the fetus, cautious recommendations for vaccination of susceptible women of childbearing age were also proposed.[553-555] Specifically, vaccine was to be administered in this population only after susceptibility had been documented by serologic testing. Vaccinated women were also advised to avoid conception for 2 months after vaccination. After Fleet and colleagues isolated virus from the fetus of a woman who had conceived 7 weeks before vaccination, this time interval was increased to 3 months as an extra precaution.[250, 251, 556]

In England and other areas of the world, mass vaccination was considered undesirable because of concerns about the duration of vaccine-induced immunity.[5-7, 31, 102] Rather, vaccine was targeted for all schoolgirls 11 to 14 years of age and postpubertal females known to be seronegative. As with the U.S. program, pregnancy was to be avoided for up to 3 months after immunization. The goal was to immunize at least 90% of the women immediately at risk and simultaneously provide a higher level of immunity throughout the childbearing-age group. It was recognized that this approach would take many years to have a significant effect on the incidence of congenital infection.

As noted previously, the U.S. strategy prevented epidemic disease but initially had little effect on the occurrence of infection in young adults, particularly women of childbearing age (see Epidemiology section).[5, 24, 30, 35, 252, 286] Although vaccine was recommended for susceptible women, concerns about the effect of the vaccine on the fetus led to low immunization coverage in this population. There was no evidence that infection was occurring in individuals who had been vaccinated years earlier (see Update on Vaccine Characteristics section). Thus, childhood vaccination decreased the overall risk of infection, but virus could still circulate in the community, especially wherever unvaccinated adolescents and adults congregated.[254-262, 265-270] Although congenital rubella syndrome could eventually be eliminated as vaccinated cohorts of children entered the childbearing years, this process would take many years, and potentially preventable cases of congenital infection would continue to occur.[262] Accordingly, specific recommendations to increase vaccination levels in older individuals, particularly women of childbearing age, were made (see Vaccine Recommendations section).[250, 251]

Selective vaccination programs have not been successful because of the inability to immunize a sufficient proportion of the female population.[7, 32, 33] With this immunization approach, large-scale epidemics continue to occur, and the incidence of congenital rubella has not declined significantly since the introduction of vaccines. Because of these problems, Great Britain, in 1988, implemented a program of measles-mumps-rubella (MMR) vaccination for all children in the second year of life; began a mass measles-rubella vaccine program for 5- to 16-year olds in 1994; and added a preschool MMR booster in 1996 (personal communication from P Tookey, National Congenital Rubella Surveillance Program, June 1999).[32, 34]

Update on Vaccine Characteristics

Approximately 200 million doses of vaccine have been administered in the United States since rubella vaccines were licensed in 1969. The RA 27/3 strain of vaccine was licensed for use in the United States in 1979 and is now the only vaccine available. Although it has been used intranasally, it is licensed only for subcutaneous administration. The RA 27/3 vaccine elicits an immune response that more closely resembles that following natural infection than either the Cendehill or HPV-77 strains of vaccines.[187, 369, 370, 557] However, there are no data to indicate the need for revaccination of persons who had not previously received the RA 27/3 vaccine. Although comparative data are not available, at least one study has shown that the RA 27/3 vaccine induces antibody formation to the three major rubella virus structural proteins.[80]

Appropriate administration of vaccine induces an antibody response in 95% or more of persons 12 months of age or older who were vaccinated. Vaccine efficacy and challenge studies indicate that more than 90 to 95% of vaccinated persons are protected against clinical illness or asymptomatic viremia. Whereas vaccine-induced titers are lower than those after natural infection and are more likely to increase after reexposure, protection after a single dose of vaccine is, for the most part, solid and lasts for at least 18 years, if not for life.*

Detectable HI antibodies persist in almost all vaccinated subjects who initially seroconvert.[37, 41, 44, 46, 52, 55] Furthermore, long-term studies of vaccinated persons who initially seroconverted and then lost detectable HI antibodies indicate that the vast majority of these individuals are also immune because they either have detectable antibodies as measured by other more sensitive assays or have a booster immune response (i.e., absence of IgM antibody and a rapid rise and decline in IgG antibody) after revaccination.[41, 47, 559] Viremia and reinfection have been documented in some vaccinated persons, as well as in some naturally immune individuals, who had very low titers of antibody.[36, 38, 42, 48, 54] It is not known how often this phenomenon occurs or places the fetus at risk, but the incidence of both events is believed to be low.[8] As noted earlier, there are rare case reports of congenital infection after reinfection of mothers who had either been previously infected or vaccinated (see The Virus and Natural History sections).[40, 43, 50, 106, 111, 314, 319-321]

The lack of an international standard level of antibody considered to be protective frequently complicates the interpretation of serologic data when antibodies are detected only by tests more sensitive than the HI test. Cutoff levels ranging from 5 to 15 IU have been used.[52, 55, 194, 222, 559, 562] Currently available information indicates that any appropriately measured level of detectable antibody should be considered presumptive evidence of past infection and immunity.[250, 251] This applies to both naturally acquired and vaccine-induced immunity.

Rubella vaccine is remarkably safe. Rash, low-grade

---

*See references 36–38, 41, 42, 44, 46–48, 52, 54, 55, 254, 298, and 558–561.

fever, and lymphadenopathy are occasionally observed. The polyneuropathies, myositis, and vasculitis associated with the HPV-77 strain of vaccine have not been reported after administration of the RA 27/3 strain.[9, 563]

On the other hand, vaccine-related arthralgia and arthritis remain a concern, particularly for susceptible adult women.[5, 8, 57, 59, 60, 62] Although arthralgia has been reported in up to 3% of susceptible children, arthritis has been reported rarely in these vaccinated subjects. In contrast, joint pain occurs in up to 40% of susceptible vaccinated females, with arthritis-like signs and symptoms reported in 10 to 20%.[5, 62] Persistent and recurring joint complaints have been reported, but most studies indicate that they occur infrequently. The high frequency (5%) of persistent joint symptoms reported by one group of investigators has not yet been confirmed.[8, 62] However, this rate is still far less than that (30%) after natural infection, as reported by the same group of researchers.[62] Permanent disability and joint destruction have also been reported, but only rarely.[59, 62]

The vast majority of published data indicate that these and other adverse events associated with rubella vaccine occur only in susceptible vaccinated persons.[5, 8] There is no conclusive evidence that there is an increased risk of reactions in persons who are already immune at the time of vaccination.[8, 62, 118] Vaccination programs of adults have not led to significant rates of absenteeism or disruption in everyday, work-related activities.[8, 265, 267–270]

Although some vaccinated persons intermittently shed virus in low titers from the pharynx 7 to 28 days after vaccination, there is no evidence that vaccine virus is spread to susceptible contacts.[5, 557] Vaccine virus can, however, be recovered from breast milk and may be transmitted to the breast-fed neonate.[59, 336, 564, 565] The vaccine virus may elicit an immune response in some exposed neonates. At present, there is no evidence of a significant alteration in the immune response or increased risk of reactions after vaccination at a later date.[60, 62] Although a mild clinical infection from transmitted vaccine virus has been reported, infection with wild-type virus may actually have occurred.[566]

The fetotropic and teratogenic potential of rubella vaccine virus has greatly influenced vaccination practices, not only in the United States but also worldwide. With the increased emphasis on vaccinating susceptible, postpubertal females in the United States, especially recent immigrants, the need to have accurate information on the risks of the vaccine virus on the fetus became even more important.

From 1971 through 1988, the Centers for Disease Control followed to term prospectively 321 pregnant women known to be susceptible to rubella by serologic testing who were vaccinated in the period from 3 months before to 3 months after conception (Table 6–4).[63, 250] Approximately one third received vaccine during the highest risk period for viremia and fetal defects (1 week before to 4 weeks after conception).[56, 63] Ninety-four received HPV-77 or Cendehill vaccines, 1 received a vaccine of unknown strain, and 226 received RA 27/3 vaccine. None of the 229 offspring (three mothers who received RA 27/3 vaccine were delivered of twins) had malformations consistent with congenital rubella infection.

Although the observed risk of congenital defects is zero, the maximal estimated theoretical risk of serious malformations attributable to any rubella vaccine, based on the 95% confidence limits of the binomial distribution, is 1.2%. If only the infants exposed to the RA 27/3 vaccine are considered, the maximal theoretical risk is 1.7%. The overall maximal theoretical risk remains far less than that for congenital rubella syndrome after maternal infection with wild virus during the first trimester of pregnancy (up to 70%) and is no greater than the 2 to 3% rate of major birth defects in the absence of exposure to rubella vaccine.[63, 100]

Four children were born with various congenital malformations consistent with congenital rubella whose mothers were later found to have received rubella vaccine within 3 months of conception.[5, 365] Clinical, epidemiologic, and laboratory data indicate that all the mothers had natural rubella infection.

These favorable data are consistent with the experience reported with Cendehill and RA 27/3 vaccines in the Federal Republic of Germany and the United Kingdom.[58, 61] None of 98 infants in the Federal Republic of Germany and none of 21 infants in Great Britain whose mothers were known to be susceptible when vaccinated was born with congenital anomalies consistent with congenital rubella syndrome.

Although the vaccines have not been shown to be teratogenic, the data continue to document the ability of the vaccine viruses to cross the placenta and infect the fetus.[63] The reported isolation rate from the products of conception is 20% (17/85) for the HPV-77 and Cendehill strains and 3% (1/35) for the RA 27/3 strain. Subclinical infection has also been documented to occur in approximately 2% of infants exposed to any strain of vaccine virus. No abnormalities in growth and development attributable to the vaccine have been noted in the small number of infected children followed.

Vaccination Recommendations

The control of rubella and congenital rubella in the United States has been predicated on universal immunization of children, with a single dose of vaccine given after the first birthday, and selective immunization of postpubertal and susceptible postpartum women. This approach remains the basis for current recommendations of the Immunization Practices Advisory Committee (ACIP) of the Public Health Service and the American Academy of Pediatrics (AAP).[250, 251] However, it is clear that success, in part, has come from the recommended use of rubella vaccine as a component of the combined MMR vaccine, which in the United States is given routinely at 15 months of age. As concerns arose about measles in adolescents and adults, attributed to both the existence of a cohort of young adults representing the 2 to 10% failure rate for a single dose of measles vaccine and the theoretical possibility of waning immunity after successful immunization in early childhood, in 1989, the expert committees just mentioned added a second dose to the measles immunization schedule. The specific rec-

TABLE 6–4
Maximal Theoretical Risks of Congenital Rubella Syndrome (CRS) After Rubella Vaccination, by Vaccine Strain, United States, 1971 to 1988[a]

VACCINE STRAIN	SUSCEPTIBLE VACCINATED SUBJECTS	NORMAL LIVE BIRTHS	RISK OF CRS	
			Observed	Theoretical
RA 27/3	226	229[b]	0	0–1.8
Cendehill or HPV-77	94	94		0–3.8
Unknown	1	1	0	
Total	321	324	0	0–1.2

[a]No women entered in the register after 1980 were vaccinated with Cendehill or HPV-77 vaccine.
[b]Includes three twin births.

ommendation was that the second dose be given just before school entry or in the prepubertal period and that the vaccine be given as the MMR vaccine.[250, 251]

These new recommendations for rubella immunization in childhood do not eliminate the need for continued selective immunization of susceptible women of childbearing age. In fact, 38% of the reported cases of congenital rubella in the United States during the past decade have represented second or subsequent pregnancies and could have been prevented by appropriate screening and postpartum or postabortion rubella immunization. These events go under the heading of "missed opportunities." Ideally, adults would be screened for susceptibility to rubella before being immunized. In many settings, including some where there is relatively higher risk that women may be susceptible, antibody screening is not practical. In such settings, when women have neither histories of immunization nor of serologic tests showing immunity, the current recommendation is to (1) ask women if they are pregnant and exclude those who are or may be, (2) explain the theoretical risks related to pregnancy, and (3) immunize those who understand and accept the responsibility to avoid pregnancy for 3 months after immunization. This approach may be used in family planning clinics and in freestanding abortion centers and during routine medical and gynecologic visits.

Missed opportunities should not be confused with bona fide contraindications for rubella immunization. These include the following:

1. Severe febrile illness
2. Altered immunity from congenital immunodeficiency; from acquired diseases such as leukemia, lymphoma, and generalized malignancy; and from therapy with radiation, corticosteroids, alkylating drugs, and antimetabolites
3. History of an anaphylactic reaction to neomycin (the vaccine does not contain penicillin)
4. Pregnancy, albeit because of theoretical concerns

Because vaccine virus is not transmitted through the nasopharynx, the presence of a susceptible pregnant woman in a household is not a contraindication for vaccination of other household members. As previously noted, vaccine virus is present in the milk and can infect the neonate, but breast-feeding also is not a contraindi-

cation to vaccination. Although vaccination is usually deferred for 8 to 12 weeks after receipt of immune globulin, receipt of anti-Rho (D) immune globulin (human) or blood products does not generally interfere with seroconversion and is not a contraindication to postpartum vaccination.[567–570] However, in this situation, 6- to 8-week postvaccination serologic testing should be performed to ensure that seroconversion has taken place.[569] This is the only situation in which postvaccination testing is recommended as routine.

Outbreak Control

Although outbreak control is an after-the-fact method of prevention, rapid, aggressive responses to outbreaks are necessary to limit the spread of infection and can serve as a catalyst to increase immunization levels. Although there is no conclusive evidence that vaccination after exposure prevents rubella, there are also no data to suggest that vaccinating an individual incubating rubella is harmful. Thus, vaccination programs initiated in the midst of an outbreak serve to protect persons not adequately exposed in the current outbreak from future exposures.

Although laboratory confirmation of cases is important, control measures—including isolation of suspected cases or susceptible exposed persons, vaccination or exclusion of susceptible persons, and confirmation of the immune status of exposed pregnant women—should be implemented as soon as a suspected case has been identified (see Management Issues section). Ideally, mandatory exclusion and vaccination of susceptible individuals should be practiced to ensure high rates of vaccination in the shortest possible time frame, particularly in the medical setting. Vaccination during an outbreak has not been associated with significant absenteeism in the workplace.[8, 265, 267–270] However, vaccination before the occurrence of an outbreak is preferable because vaccination causes far less disruption of routine work activities and schedules than rubella infection.

Surveillance

Surveillance of rubella and congenital rubella is necessary for rubella prevention because the information can be used to evaluate the progress of the immunization program, to identify high-risk groups that would benefit from specific interventions, and to monitor the safety, efficacy, and durability of the vaccine. Surveillance can also draw attention to small numbers of cases before they develop into sizable outbreaks. Because rubella and congenital rubella are reportable diseases, all suspected cases should be reported to local health officials.

Prospects for the Future

In theory, full implementation of the two-dose MMR vaccine recommendation should eliminate congenital rubella from the United States. However, until that schedule is expanded to Latin America, the major source of rubella importation to the United States, the magnitude of intra-American travel will remain a barrier to achieving the goal now met for polio.[573] The sporadic nature of the cases will likely add to delay in diagnosis. The need for maintaining high levels of immunization, ongoing surveillance, and prompt outbreak control measures remains critical for ultimate eradication of rubella. Given the efficacy of MMR vaccine, full commitment to immunization in the Western Hemisphere can make these diseases matters of historic interest only during the coming decade and can be a model for ultimate worldwide efforts.[574]

References

1. Wesselhoff C. Rubella (German measles). N Engl J Med 236:943, 1947.
2. Krugman S (ed). Rubella symposium. Am J Dis Child 110:345, 1965.
3. Krugman S (ed). Proceedings of the International Conference on Rubella Immunization. Am J Dis Child 118:2, 1969.
4. Regamy RH, deBarbieri A, Hennessen W, et al (eds). International Symposium on Rubella Vaccines. Symp Ser Immunobiol Stand 11:1, 1969.
5. Preblud SR, Serdula MK, Frank JA Jr, et al. Rubella vaccination in the United States: a ten-year review. Epidemiol Rev 2:171, 1980.
6. Hanshaw JB, Dudgeon JA, Marshall WC (eds). Viral Diseases of the Fetus and Newborn, 2nd ed. Philadelphia, WB Saunders, 1985, p 13.
7. Krugman S (ed). International Symposium on Prevention of Congenital Rubella Infection. Rev Infect Dis 7(Suppl 1):S1, 1985.
8. Preblud SR. Some current issues relating to rubella vaccine. JAMA 254:253, 1985.
9. Cherry JD. Rubella. In Feigin RD, Cherry JD (eds). Textbook of Pediatric Infectious Diseases, 3rd ed. Philadelphia, WB Saunders, 1992, p 1792.
10. Manton WG. Some accounts of rash liable to be mistaken for scarlitina. Med Trans R Coll Physicians (London) 5:149, 1815.
11. Veale H. History of epidemic Rötheln, with observations on its pathology. Edinburgh Med J 12:404, 1896.
12. Gregg NM. Congenital cataract following German measles in the mother. Trans Ophthalmol Soc Aust 3:35, 1941.
13. Cooper LZ. Congenital rubella in the United States. In Krugman S, Gershon AA (eds). Infections of the Fetus and the Newborn Infant. New York, Alan R. Liss, 1975, p 1.
14. Ziring PR. Congenital rubella: the teenage years. Pediatr Ann 6:762, 1977.
15. Hiro Y, Tasaka S. Die Röteln sind eine Viruskrankheit. Monatsschr Kinderheilkd 76:328, 1938.
16. Habel K. Transmission of rubella to Macaca mulatta monkeys. Public Health Rep 57:1126, 1942.
17. Anderson SB. Experimental rubella in human volunteers. J Immunol 62:29, 1949.
18. Krugman S, Ward R, Jacobs KG, et al. Studies on rubella immunization: I. Demonstration of rubella without rash. JAMA 151:285, 1953.
19. Weller TH, Neva FA. Propagation in tissue culture of cytopathic agents from patients with rubella-like illness. Proc Soc Exp Biol Med 111:215, 1962.
20. Parkman PD, Buescher EL, Artenstein MS. Recovery of rubella virus from army recruits. Proc Soc Exp Biol Med 111:225, 1962.
21. Parkman PD, Mundon FK, McCown JM, et al. Studies of rubella: II. Neutralization of the virus. J Immunol 93:608, 1964.
22. Sever JL, Huebner RJ, Castellano GA, et al. Rubella complement fixation test. Science 148:385, 1965.
23. Stewart GL, Parkman PD, Hopps HE, et al. Rubella-virus hemagglutination-inhibition test. N Engl J Med 276:554, 1967.
24. Orenstein WA, Bart KJ, Hinman AR, et al. The opportunity and obligation to eliminate measles from the United States. JAMA 251:1988, 1984.
25. Meyer HM Jr, Parkman PD, Panos TC. Attenuated rubella virus: II. Production of an experimental live-virus vaccine and clinical trial. N Engl J Med 275:575, 1966.
26. Prinzie A, Huygelen C, Gold J, et al. Experimental live attenuated rubella virus vaccine: clinical evaluation of Cendehill strain. Am J Dis Child 118:172, 1969.
27. Plotkin JA, Farquhar JD, Katz M. Attenuation of RA 27/3 rubella virus in WI-38 human diploid cells. Am J Dis Child 118:178, 1969.
28. Perkins FT. Licensed vaccines. Rev Infect Dis 7(Suppl 1):S73, 1985.
29. Hinman AR, Bart KJ, Orenstein WA, et al. Rational strategy for rubella vaccination. Lancet 1:39, 1983.
30. Bart KJ, Orenstein WA, Preblud SR, et al. Universal immunization to interrupt rubella. Rev Infect Dis 7(Suppl 1):S177, 1985.
31. Dudgeon JA. Selective immunization: protection of the individual. Rev Infect Dis 7(Suppl 1):S185, 1985.
32. Walker D, Carter H, Jones IJ. Measles, mumps, and rubella: the need for a change in immunisation policy. BMJ 292:1501, 1986.
33. Best JM, Welch JM, Baker DA, et al. Maternal rubella at St. Thomas' Hospital in 1978 and 1986: support for augmenting the rubella vaccination programme. Lancet 2:88, 1987.
34. Badenoch J. Big bang for vaccination: eliminating measles, mumps, and rubella. BMJ 297:750, 1988.
35. Centers for Disease Control. Increase in rubella and congenital rubella in the United States, 1988–1990. MMWR Morb Mortal Wkly Rep 40:93, 1991.
36. Harcourt GC, Best JM, Banatvala JE. Rubella-specific serum and nasopharyngeal antibodies in volunteers with naturally acquired and vaccine-induced immunity after intranasal challenge. J Infect Dis 142:145, 1980.
37. Weibel RE, Buynak EB, McLean AA, et al. Persistence of antibody in human subjects 7 to 10 years following administration of combined live attenuated measles, mumps, and rubella virus vaccines (40967). Proc Soc Exp Biol Med 165:260, 1980.
38. Balfour HH, Groth KE, Edelman C, et al. Rubella virae-

mia and antibody responses after rubella vaccination and reimmunisation. Lancet 1:1078, 1981.

39. Cradock-Watson JE, Ridehalgh MKS, Anderson MJ, et al. Outcome of asymptomatic infection with rubella virus during pregnancy. J Hyg (London) 87:147, 1981.

40. Bott LM, Eizenberg DH. Congenital rubella after successful vaccination. Med J Aust 1:514, 1982.

41. Herrmann KL, Halstead SB, Wiebenga NH. Rubella antibody persistence after immunization. JAMA 247:193, 1982.

42. O'Shea S, Best JM, Banatvala JE. Viremia, virus excretion, and antibody responses after challenge in volunteers with low levels of antibody to rubella virus. J Infect Dis 148:639, 1983.

43. Enders G, Calm A, Schaub J. Rubella embryopathy after previous maternal rubella vaccination. Infection 12:96, 1984.

44. Hillary IB, Griffith AH. Persistence of rubella antibodies 15 years after subcutaneous administration of Wistar 27/3 strain live attenuated rubella virus vaccine. Vaccine 2:274, 1984.

45. Morgan-Capner R, Hodgson J, Sellwood J, et al. Clinically apparent rubella reinfection. J Infect 9:97, 1984.

46. O'Shea S, Best JM, Banatvala JE, et al. Persistence of rubella antibody 8–18 years after vaccination. BMJ 288:1043, 1984.

47. Serdula MK, Halstead SB, Wiebenga NH, et al. Serological response to rubella revaccination. JAMA 251:1974, 1984.

48. Banatvala JE, Best JM, O'Shea S, et al. Persistence of rubella antibodies after vaccination: detection after experimental challenge. Rev Infect Dis 7(Suppl 1):S86, 1985.

49. Cradock-Watson JE, Ridehalgh MKS, Anderson MJ, et al. Rubella reinfection and the fetus. Lancet 1:1039, 1985.

50. Forsgren M, Soren L. Subclinical rubella reinfection in vaccinated women with rubella-specific IgM response during pregnancy and transmission of virus to the fetus. Scand J Infect Dis 17:337, 1985.

51. Grangeot-Keros L, Nicolas JC, Bricout F, et al. Rubella reinfection and the fetus. N Engl J Med 313:1547, 1985.

52. Horstmann DM, Schluederberg A, Emmons JE, et al. Persistence of vaccine-induced immune responses to rubella: comparison with natural infection. Rev Infect Dis 7(Suppl 1):S80, 1985.

53. Morgan-Capner P, Hodgson J, Hambling MH, et al. Detection of rubella-specific IgM in subclinical rubella reinfection in pregnancy. Lancet 1:244, 1985.

54. Schiff GM, Young BC, Stefanovic GM, et al. Challenge with rubella virus after loss of detectable vaccine-induced antibody. Rev Infect Dis 7(Suppl 1):S157, 1985.

55. Chu SY, Bernier RH, Stewart JA, et al. Rubella antibody persistence after immunization: sixteen-year follow-up in the Hawaiian Islands. JAMA 259:3133, 1988.

56. Bart SW, Stetler HC, Preblud SR, et al. Fetal risk associated with rubella vaccine: an update. Rev Infect Dis 7(Suppl 1):S95, 1985.

57. Chantler JK, Tingle AJ, Perry RE. Persistent rubella virus infection associated with chronic arthritis in children. N Engl J Med 313:1117, 1985.

58. Enders G. Rubella antibody titers in vaccinated and non-vaccinated women and results of vaccination during pregnancy. Rev Infect Dis 7(Suppl 1):S103, 1985.

59. Tingle AJ, Chantler JK, Pot KH, et al. Postpartum rubella immunization: association with development of prolonged arthritis, neurological sequelae, and chronic rubella viremia. J Infect Dis 152:606, 1985.

60. Preblud PR, Orenstein WA, Lopez C, et al. Postpartum rubella immunization. Letter to the editor. J Infect Dis 154:367, 1986.

61. Sheppard S, Smithells RW, Dickenson A, et al. Rubella vaccination and pregnancy: preliminary report of a national survey. BMJ 292:727, 1986.

62. Tingle AJ. Postpartum rubella immunization (reply). J Infect Dis 154:368, 1986.

63. Centers for Disease Control. Rubella vaccination during pregnancy—United States, 1971–1988. MMWR Morb Mortal Wkly Rep 38:290, 1989.

64. Ho-Terry L, Cohen A. Degradation of rubella virus envelope components. Arch Virol 65:1, 1980.

65. Oker-Blom C, Kalkkinen N, Kaariainen L, et al. Rubella virus contains one capsid protein and three envelope glycoproteins, E1, E2a, and E2b. J Virol 46:964, 1983.

66. Waxham MN, Wolinsky JS. Immunochemical identification of rubella virus hemagglutinin. Virology 126:194, 1983.

67. Bowden DS, Westway EG. Rubella virus: structural and non-structural proteins. J Gen Virol 65:933, 1984.

68. Ho-Terry L, Cohen A, Tedder RS. Immunologic characterisation of rubella virion polypeptides. J Med Microbiol 17:105, 1984.

69. Oker-Blom C, Ulmanen I, Kaariainen L, et al. Rubella virus 40S genome RNA specifies a 24S subgenomic mRNA that codes for a precursor to structural proteins. J Virol 49:403, 1984.

70. Dorsett PH, Miller DC, Green KY, et al. Structure and function of the rubella virus proteins. Rev Infect Dis 7(Suppl 1):S150, 1985.

71. Pettersson RF, Oker-Blom C, Kalkkinen N, et al. Molecular and antigenic characteristics and synthesis of rubella virus structural proteins. Rev Infect Dis 7(Suppl 1):S140, 1985.

72. Waxham MN, Wolinsky JS. A model of the structural organization of rubella virions. Rev Infect Dis 7(Suppl 1):S133, 1985.

73. Waxham MN, Wolinsky JS. Detailed immunologic analysis of the structural polypeptides of rubella virus using monoclonal antibodies. Virology 143:153, 1985.

74. Green KY, Dorsett PH. Rubella virus antigens: localization of epitopes involved in hemagglutination and neutralization by using monoclonal antibodies. J Virol 57:893, 1986.

75. Vidgren G, Takkinen K, Kalkkinen N, et al. Nucleotide sequence of the genes coding for the membrane glycoproteins E1 and E2 of rubella virus. J Gen Virol 68:2347, 1987.

76. Terry GM, Ho-Terry L, Londesborough P, et al. Localization of the rubella E1 epitopes. Arch Virol 98:189, 1988.

77. Clarke DM, Loo TW, McDonald H, et al. Expression of rubella virus cDNA coding for the structural proteins. Gene 65:23, 1988.

78. Frey TK, Marr LD. Sequence of the region coding for virion proteins C and E2 and the carboxy terminus of the nonstructural proteins of rubella virus: comparison with alphaviruses. Gene 62:85, 1988.

79. Takkinen K, Vidgren G, Ekstrand J, et al. Nucleotide sequence of the rubella virus capsid protein gene reveals an unusually high G/C content. J Gen Virol 69:603, 1988.

80. Cusi MG, Rossolini GM, Cellesi C, et al. Antibody response to wild rubella virus structural proteins following immunization with RA 27/3 live attenuated vaccine. Arch Virol 101:25, 1988.

81. Frey TK, Abernathy ES, Bosma TJ, et al. Molecular

analysis of rubella virus epidemiology across three continents, North America, Europe and Asia, 1961–1997. J Infect Dis 178:642–60, 1998.

82. Katow S, Sugiura A. Antibody response to the individual rubella virus proteins in congenital and other rubella virus infections. J Clin Microbiol 21:449, 1985.

83. de Mazancourt A, Waxman MN, Nicholas JC, et al. Antibody response to the rubella virus structural proteins in infants with the congenital rubella syndrome. J Med Virol 19:111, 1986.

84. Chaye H, Chong P, Tripet B, et al. Localization of the virus neutralizing and hemagglutinin epitopes of E1 glycoprotein of rubella virus. Virology 189(2):483, 1992.

85. Hancock EJ, Pot K, Puterman ML, et al. Lack of association between titers of HAI antibody and whole-virus ELISA values for patients with congenital rubella syndrome. J Infect Dis 154:1031, 1986.

86. Castellano GA, Madden DL, Hazzard GT, et al. Evaluation of commercially available diagnostic kits for rubella. J Infect Dis 143:578, 1981.

87. Storch GA, Myers N. Latex-agglutination test for rubella antibody: validity of positive results assessed by response to immunization and comparison with other tests. J Infect Dis 149:459, 1984.

88. Safford JW, Abbott GG, Diemier CM. Evaluation of a rapid passive hemagglutination assay for anti-rubella antibody: comparison to hemagglutination inhibition and a vaccine challenge study. J Med Virol 17:229, 1985.

89. Skendzel LP, Edson DC. Latex agglutination test for rubella antibodies: report based on data from the College of American Pathologists surveys, 1983 to 1985. J Clin Microbiol 24:333, 1986.

90. Vaananen P, Haiva VM, Koskela P, et al. Comparison of a simple latex agglutination test with hemolysis-in-gel, hemagglutination inhibition, and radioimmunoassay for detection of rubella virus antibodies. J Clin Microbiol 21:973, 1985.

91. Chernesky MA, DeLong DJ, Mahony JB, et al. Differences in antibody responses with rapid agglutination tests for the detection of rubella antibodies. J Clin Microbiol 23:772, 1986.

92. Pruneda RC, Dover JC. A comparison of two passive agglutination procedures with enzyme-linked immunosorbent assay for rubella antibody status. Am J Clin Pathol 86:768, 1986.

93. Linde GA. Subclass distribution of rubella virus-specific immunoglobulin G. J Clin Microbiol 21:117, 1985.

94. Salonen E-M, Hovi T, Meurman O, et al. Kinetics of specific IgA, IgD, IgE, IgG, and IgM antibody responses in rubella. J Med Virol 16:1, 1985.

95. Stokes A, Mims A, Grahame R. Subclass distribution of IgG and IgA responses to rubella virus in man. J Med Microbiol 21:283, 1986.

96. Thomas HIJ, Morgan-Capner P. Specific IgG subclass antibody in rubella virus infections. Epidemiol Infect 100:443, 1988.

97. Grangeot-Keros L, Pillot J, Daffos F, et al. Prenatal and postnatal production of IgM and IgA antibodies to rubella virus studied by antibody capture immunoassay. J Infect Dis 158:138, 1988.

98. Cradock-Watson JE, Ridehalgh MKS, Anderson MJ, et al. Fetal infection resulting from maternal rubella after the first trimester of pregnancy. J Hyg (London) 85:381, 1980.

99. Vejtorp M, Mansa B. Rubella IgM antibodies in sera from infants born after maternal rubella later than the twelfth week of pregnancy. Scand J Infect Dis 12:1, 1980.

100. Miller E, Cradock-Watson JE, Pollock TM. Consequences of confirmed maternal rubella at successive stages of pregnancy. Lancet 2:781, 1982.

101. Grillner L, Forsgren M, Barr B, et al. Outcome of rubella during pregnancy with special reference to the 17th-24th weeks of gestation. Scand J Infect Dis 15:321, 1983.

102. Peckham C. Congenital rubella in the United Kingdom before 1970: the prevaccine era. Rev Infect Dis 7(Suppl 1):S11, 1985.

103. Bitsch M. Rubella in pregnant Danish women 1975–1984. Dan Med Bull 34:46, 1987.

104. Munro ND, Shephard S, Smithells RW, et al. Temporal relations between maternal rubella and congenital defects. Lancet 2:201, 1987.

105. Enders G, Miller E, Nickerl-Pacher U, et al. Outcome of confirmed periconceptional maternal rubella. Lancet 1:1445, 1988.

106. Best JM, Harcourt GC, Banatvala JE, et al. Congenital rubella affecting an infant whose mother had rubella antibodies before conception. BMJ 282:1235, 1981.

107. Partridge JW, Flewett TH, Whitehead JEM. Congenital rubella affecting an infant whose mother had rubella antibodies before conception. BMJ 282:187, 1981.

108. Levine JB, Berkowitz CD, St. Geme JW. Rubella virus reinfection during pregnancy leading to late-onset congenital rubella syndrome. J Pediatr 100:589, 1982.

109. Sibille G, Sarda P, Jalaguier J, et al. Rubéole de réinfection et syndrome polymalformatif congénital. J Genet IIum 34:305, 1986.

110. Hornstein L, Levy U, Fogel A. Clinical rubella with virus transmission to the fetus in a pregnant woman considered to be immune. Letter to the editor. N Engl J Med 319:1415, 1988.

111. Saule H, Enders G, Zeller J, et al. Congenital rubella infection after previous immunity of the mother. Eur J Pediatr 147:195, 1988.

112. Floret D, Rosenberg D, Hage GN, et al. Hyperthyroidism, diabetes mellitus and the congenital rubella syndrome. Acta Paediatr Scand 69:259, 1980.

113. Hansen HE, Larsen SO, Leerhoy J. Lack of correlation between the incidence of rubella antibody and the distribution of HLA antigens in a Danish population. Tissue Antigens 15:325, 1980.

114. Kato S, Kimura M, Takakura I, et al. HLA-linked genetic control in natural rubella infection. Tissue Antigens 15:86, 1980.

115. Tardieu M, Grospierre B, Durandy A, et al. Circulating immune complexes containing rubella antigens in late-onset rubella syndrome. J Pediatr 97:370, 1980.

116. Coyle PK, Wolinsky JS. Characterization of immune complexes in progressive rubella panencephalitis. Ann Neurol 9:557, 1981.

117. Ishii K, Nakazono N, Sawada H, et al. Host factors and susceptibility to rubella virus infection: the association of HLA antigens. J Med Virol 7:287, 1981.

118. Coyle PK, Wolinsky JS, Buimovici-Klein E, et al. Rubella-specific immune complexes after congenital infection and vaccination. Infect Immun 36:498, 1982.

119. Kato S, Muranaka S, Takakura I, et al. HLA-DR antigens and the rubella-specific immune response in man. Tissue Antigens 19:140, 1982.

120. Rubinstein P, Walker ME, Fedun B, et al. The HLA system in congenital rubella patients with and without diabetes. Diabetes 31:1088, 1982.

121. Boner A, Wilmott RW, Dinwiddie R, et al. Desquamative interstitial pneumonia and antigen-antibody complexes in two infants with congenital rubella. Pediatrics 72:835, 1983.

122. Ilonen J, Antila A-C, Lehtinen M, et al. HLA antigens

in rubella seronegative young adults. Tissue Antigens 22:379, 1983.

123. Ziola B, Lund G, Meurman O, et al. Circulating immune complexes in patients with acute measles and rubella virus infections. Infect Immun 41:578, 1983.

124. Clarke WL, Shaver KA, Bright GM, et al. Autoimmunity in congenital rubella syndrome. J Pediatr 104:370, 1984.

125. Ginsberg-Fellner F, Witt ME, Fedun B, et al. Diabetes mellitus and autoimmunity in patients with congenital rubella syndrome. Rev Infect Dis 7(Suppl 1):S170, 1985.

126. Sever JL, South MA, Shaver KA. Delayed manifestations of congenital rubella. Rev Infect Dis 7(Suppl 1):S164, 1985.

127. Shaver KA, Boughman JA, Nance WE. Congenital rubella syndrome and diabetes: a review of epidemiologic, genetic, and immunologic factors. Am Ann Deaf 130:526, 1985.

128. Rabinowe SL, George KL, Loughlin R, et al. Congenital rubella: monoclonal antibody-defined T cell abnormalities in young adults. Am J Med 81:779, 1986.

129. Verder H, Dickmeiss E, Haahr S, et al. Late-onset rubella syndrome: coexistence of immune complex disease and defective cytotoxic effector cell function. Clin Exp Immunol 63:367, 1986.

130. Bardeletti G, Kessler N, Aymard-Henry M. Morphology, biochemical analysis and neuraminidase activity of rubella virus. Arch Virol 49:175, 1975.

131. Best JM, Banatvala JE, Almeida JD, et al. Morphological characteristics of rubella virus. Lancet 2:237, 1967.

132. Murphy FA, Halonen PE, Harrison AK. Electron microscopy of the development of rubella virus in BHK-21 cells. J Virol 2:1223, 1968.

133. Oshiro LS, Schmidt NJ, Lennette EH. Electron microscopic studies of rubella virus. J Gen Virol 5:205, 1969.

134. Bardeletti G, Tektoff J, Gautheron D. Rubella virus maturation and production in two host cell systems. Intervirology 11:97, 1979.

135. Holmes IH, Wark MC, Warburton MF. Is rubella an arbovirus? II. Ultrastructural morphology and development. Virology 37:15, 1969.

136. Maes R, Vaheri A, Sedwick D, et al. Synthesis of virus and macromolecules by rubella-infected cells. Nature 210:384, 1966.

137. Nakhasi HL, Zheng D, Hewlett IK, et al. Rubella virus replication: effect of interferons and actinomycin D. Virus Res 10:1, 1988.

138. Sato M, Yamada T, Yamamoto K, et al. Evidence for hybrid formation between rubella virus and a latent virus of BHK21/WI-2 cells. Virology 69:691, 1976.

139. Sato M, Tanaka H, Yamada T, et al. Persistent infection of BHK21/WI-2 cells with rubella virus and characterization of rubella variants. Arch Virol 54:333, 1977.

140. Sato M, Urade M, Maeda N, et al. Isolation and characterization of a new rubella variant with DNA polymerase activity. Arch Virol 56:89, 1978.

141. Sato M, Maeda N, Urade M, et al. Persistent infection of primary human cell cultures with rubella variant carrying DNA polymerase activity. Arch Virol 56:181, 1978.

142. Sato M, Maeda N, Shirasuna K, et al. Presence of DNA in rubella variant with DNA polymerase activity. Arch Virol 61:251, 1979.

143. Mifune K, Matsuo S. Some properties of temperature-sensitive mutant of rubella virus defective in the induction of interference to Newcastle disease virus. Virology 63:278, 1975.

144. Norval M. Mechanism of persistence of rubella virus in LLC-MK2 cells. J Gen Virol 43:289, 1979.

145. Bardeletti G, Gautheron DC. Phospholipid and choles-terol composition of rubella virus and its host cell BHK21 grown in suspension cultures. Arch Virol 52:19, 1978.

146. Voiland A, Bardeletti G. Fatty acid composition of rubella virus and BHK21/13S infected cells. Arch Virol 64:319, 1980.

147. Parkman PD, Buescher EL, Artenstein MS, et al. Studies of rubella. I. Properties of the virus. J Immunol 93:595, 1964.

148. McCarthy K, Taylor-Robinson CH. Rubella. Br Med Bull 23:185, 1967.

149. Wallis C, Melnick JL, Rapp F. Different effects of MgCl₂ and MgSO₄ on the thermostability of viruses. Virology 26:694, 1965.

150. Chagnon A, Laflamme P. Effect of acidity on rubella virus. Can J Microbiol 10:501, 1964.

151. Fabiyi A, Sever JL, Ratner N, et al. Rubella virus. Growth characteristics and stability of infectious virus and complement-fixing antigen. Proc Soc Exp Biol Med 122:392, 1966.

152. Herrmann KL. Rubella virus. In Lennette EH, Schmidt NJ (eds). Diagnostic Procedures for Viral, Rickettsial and Chlamydial Infections. Washington, DC, American Public Health Association, 1979, p 725.

153. Cochran KW, Maassab HF. Inhibition of rubella virus by 1-adamantanamine hydrochloride. Fed Proc 23:387, 1964.

154. Plotkin SA. Inhibition of rubella virus by amantadine. Arch Gesamte Virusforsch 16:438, 1965.

155. Oxford JS, Schild GC. In vitro inhibition of rubella virus by 1-adamantanamine hydrochloride. Arch Gesamte Virusforsch 17:313, 1965.

156. Plotkin SA, Klaus RM, Whitely JA. Hypogammaglobulinemia in an infant with congenital rubella syndrome: failure of 1-adamantanamine to stop virus excretion. J Pediatr 69:1085, 1966.

157. Vaheri A, Hovi T. Structural proteins and subunits of rubella virus. J Virol 9:10, 1972.

158. Vesikari T. Immune response in rubella infection. Scand J Infect Dis (Suppl 4):1, 1972.

159. Liebhaber H, Gross PA. The structural proteins of rubella virus. Virology 47:684, 1972.

160. Chantler JK. Rubella virus: intracellular polypeptide synthesis. Virology 98:275, 1979.

161. Fenner F. The classification and nomenclature of viruses. Intervirology 6:1, 1975–1976.

162. Melnick JL. Taxonomy of viruses. Prog Med Virol 22:211, 1976.

163. Best JM, Banatvala JE. Studies on rubella virus strain variation by kinetic hemagglutination-inhibition tests. J Gen Virol 9:215, 1970.

164. Fogel A, Plotkin SA. Markers of rubella virus strains in RK13 culture. J Virol 3:157, 1969.

165. Kono R. Antigenic structures of American and Japanese rubella virus strains and experimental vertical transmission of rubella virus in rabbits. Symp Ser Immunobiol Stand 11:195, 1969.

166. Kono R, Hayakawa Y, Hibi M, et al. Experimental vertical transmission of rubella virus in rabbits. Lancet 1:343, 1969.

167. Banatvala JE, Best JM. Cross-serological testing of rubella virus strains. Lancet 1:695, 1969.

168. Potter JE, Banatvala JE, Best JM. Interferon studies with Japanese and U.S. rubella virus. BMJ 1:197, 1973.

169. Banatvala JE, Potter JE, Webster MJ. Foetal interferon responses induced by rubella virus. Ciba Found New Ser 10:77, 1973.

170. Ueda K, Nishida Y, Oshima K, et al. An explanation for

the high incidence of congenital rubella syndrome in Ryukyu. Am J Epidemiol 107:344, 1978.

171. Kono R, Hirayama M, Sugishita C, et al. Epidemiology of rubella and congenital rubella infection in Japan. Rev Infect Dis 7(Suppl 1):S56, 1985.

172. Ueda K, Tokugawa K, Nishida Y, et al. Incidence of congenital rubella syndrome in Japan (1965–1985): a nationwide survey of the number of deaf children with history of maternal rubella attending special schools for the deaf in Japan. Am J Epidemiol 124:807, 1986.

173. Halonen PE, Ryan JM, Stewart JA. Rubella hemagglutinin prepared with alkaline extraction of virus grown in suspension culture of BHK-21 cells. Proc Soc Exp Biol Med 125:162, 1967.

174. Schmidt NJ, Dennis J, Lennette EH. Rubella virus hemagglutination with a wide variety of erythrocyte species. Appl Microbiol 22:469, 1971.

175. Furukawa T, Plotkin SA, Sedwick WD, et al. Studies on hemagglutination by rubella virus. Proc Soc Exp Biol Med 126:745, 1967.

176. Haukenes G. Simplified rubella haemagglutination inhibition test not requiring removal of nonspecific inhibitors. Lancet 2:196, 1979.

177. Liebhaber H. Measurement of rubella antibody by hemagglutination inhibition: I. Variables affecting rubella hemagglutination. J Immunol 104:818, 1970.

178. Liebhaber H. Measurement of rubella antibody by hemagglutination inhibition: II. Characteristics of an improved test employing a new method for the removal of non-immunoglobulin HA inhibitors from serum. J Immunol 104:826, 1970.

179. Schmidt NJ, Lennette EH. Rubella complement-fixing antigens derived from the fluid and cellular phases of infected BHK-21 cells: extraction of cell-associated antigen with alkaline buffers. J Immunol 97:815, 1966.

180. Schmidt NJ, Lennette EH, Gee PS. Demonstration of rubella complement-fixing antigens of two distinct particle sizes by gel filtration on Sephadex G-200. Proc Soc Exp Biol Med 123:758, 1966.

181. Schmidt NJ, Lennette EH. Antigens of rubella virus. Am J Dis Child 118:89, 1969.

182. Ho-Terry L, Londesborough P, Cohen A. Analysis of rubella virus complement-fixing antigens by polyacrylamide gel electrophoresis. Arch Virol 87:219, 1986.

183. Schmidt NJ, Styk B. Immunodiffusion reactions with rubella antigens. J Immunol 101:210, 1968.

184. Salmi AA. Gel precipitation reactions between alkaline extracted rubella antigens and human sera. Acta Pathol Microbiol Scand 76:271, 1969.

185. LeBouvier GL. Precipitinogens of rubella virus infected cells. Proc Soc Exp Biol Med 130:51, 1969.

186. Cappel R, Schluederberg A, Horstmann DM. Large-scale production of rubella precipitinogens and their use in the diagnostic laboratory. J Clin Microbiol 1:201, 1975.

187. LeBouvier GL, Plotkin SA. Precipitin responses to rubella vaccine RA27/3. J Infect Dis 123:220, 1971.

188. Vaheri A, Vesikari T. Small size rubella virus antigens and soluble immune complexes, analysis by the platelet aggregation technique. Arch Gesamte Virusforsch 35:10, 1971.

189. Penttinen K, Myllyla G. Interaction of human blood platelets, viruses, and antibodies: I. Platelet aggregation test with microequipment. Ann Med Exp Biol Fenn 46:188, 1968.

190. Lennette EH, Schmidt NJ. Neutralization, fluorescent antibody and complement fixation tests for rubella. In Friedman H, Prier JE (eds). Rubella. Springfield, Ill, Charles C Thomas, 1973, p 18.

191. Schluederberg A, Horstmann DM, Andiman WA, et al. Neutralizing and hemagglutination-inhibition antibodies to rubella virus as indicators of protective immunity in vaccinees and naturally immune individuals. J Infect Dis 138:877, 1978.

192. Sato H, Albrecht P, Krugman S, et al. Sensitive neutralization test for rubella antibody. J Clin Microbiol 9:259, 1979.

193. Meurman OH. Antibody responses in patients with rubella infection determined by passive hemagglutination, hemagglutination inhibition, complement fixation, and solid-phase radioimmunoassay tests. Infect Immun 19:369, 1978.

194. Herrmann KL. Available rubella serologic tests. Rev Infect Dis 7(Suppl 1):S108, 1985.

195. Skendzel LP, Wilcox KR, Edson DC. Evaluation of assays for the detection of antibodies to rubella: A report based on data from the College of American Pathologists surveys of 1982. Am J Clin Pathol 80(Suppl):594, 1983.

196. Hauknes G. Experience with an indirect (passive) hemagglutination test for the demonstration of rubella virus antibody. Acta Pathol Microbiol Scand 88:85, 1980.

197. Kilgore JM. Further evaluation of a rubella passive hemagglutination test. J Med Virol 5:131, 1980.

198. Inouye S, Satoh K, Tajima T. Single-serum diagnosis of rubella by combined use of the hemagglutination inhibition and passive hemagglutination tests. J Clin Microbiol 23:388, 1986.

199. Harnett GB, Palmer CA, Mackay-Scollay EM. Single-radial-hemolysis test for the assay of rubella antibody in antenatal, vaccinated, and rubella virus-infected patients. J Infect Dis 140:937, 1979.

200. Nommensen FE. Accuracy of single radial hemolysis test for rubella immunity when internal reference standards are used to estimate antibody levels. J Clin Microbiol 25:22, 1987.

201. Halonen P, Meurman O, Matikainen M-T, et al. IgA antibody response in acute rubella determined by solid-phase radioimmunoassay. J Hyg (London) 83:69, 1979.

202. Kangro HO, Pattison JR, Heath RB. The detection of rubella-specific IgM antibodies by radioimmunoassay. Br J Exp Pathol 59:577, 1978.

203. Meurman OH, Viljanen MK, Granfors K. Solid-phase radioimmunoassay of rubella virus immunoglobulin M antibodies: comparison with sucrose density gradient centrifugation test. J Clin Microbiol 5:257, 1977.

204. Meurman OH, Ziola BR. IgM-class rheumatoid factor interference in the solid-phase radioimmunoassay of rubella-specific IgM antibodies. J Clin Pathol 31:483, 1978.

205. Mortimer PP, Tedder RS, Hambling MH, et al. Antibody capture radioimmunoassay for anti-rubella IgM. J Hyg (London) 86:139, 1981.

206. Brown GC, Maassab HF, Veronelli JA, et al. Rubella antibodies in human serum: detection by the indirect fluorescent-antibody technic. Science 145:943, 1964.

207. Cradock-Watson JE, Ridehalgh MKS, Pattison JR, et al. Comparison of immunofluorescence and radioimmunoassay for detecting IgM antibody in infants with the congenital rubella syndrome. J Hyg (London) 83:413, 1979.

208. Leinikki PO, Shekarchi I, Dorsett P, et al. Determination of virus-specific IgM antibodies by using ELISA: elimination of false-positive results with protein A-Sepharose absorption and subsequent IgM antibody assay. J Lab Clin Med 92:849, 1978.

209. Vejtorp M. Enzyme-linked immunosorbent assay for de-

termination of rubella IgG antibodies. Acta Pathol Microbiol Scand 86:387, 1978.

210. Vejtorp M, Fanoe E, Leerhoy J. Diagnosis of postnatal rubella by the enzyme-linked immunosorbent assay for rubella IgM and IgG antibodies. Acta Pathol Microbiol Scand 87:155, 1979.

211. Bidwell D, Chantler SM, Morgan-Capner P, et al. Further investigation of the specificity and sensitivity of ELISA for rubella antibody screening. J Clin Pathol 33:200, 1980.

212. Skendzel LP, Edson DC. Evaluation of enzyme immunosorbent rubella assays. Arch Pathol Lab Med 109:391, 1985.

213. Morgan-Capner P, Pullen HJM, Pattison JR, et al. A comparison of three tests for rubella antibody screening. J Clin Pathol 32:542, 1979.

214. Champsaur H, Dussaix E, Tournier P. Hemagglutination inhibition, single radial hemolysis, and ELISA tests for the detection of IgG and IgM to rubella virus. J Med Virol 5:273, 1980.

215. Deibel R, D'Areangelis D, Ducharme CP, et al. Assay of rubella antibody by passive hemagglutination and by a modified indirect immunofluorescence test. Infection 8(Suppl 3):S255, 1980.

216. Zartarian MV, Friedly G, Peterson EM, et al. Detection of rubella antibodies by hemagglutination inhibition, indirect fluorescent-antibody test, and enzyme-linked immunosorbent assay. J Clin Microbiol 14:640, 1981.

217. Weissfeld AS, Gehle WD, Sonnenworth AC. Comparison of several test systems used for the determination of rubella immune status. J Clin Microbiol 16:82, 1982.

218. Truant AL, Barksdale BL, Huber TW, et al. Comparison of an enzyme-linked immunosorbent assay with indirect hemagglutination inhibition for determination of rubella virus antibody: evaluation of immune status with commercial reagents in a clinical laboratory. J Clin Microbiol 17:106, 1983.

219. Field PR, Gong CM. Diagnosis of postnatally acquired rubella by use of three enzyme-linked immunosorbent assays for specific immunoglobulins G and M and single radial hemolysis for specific immunoglobulin G. J Clin Microbiol 20:951, 1984.

220. Cubie H, Edmond E. Comparison of five different methods of rubella IgM antibody testing. J Clin Pathol 38:203, 1985.

221. Enders G. Serologic test combinations for safe detection of rubella infections. Rev Infect Dis 7(Suppl 1):S113, 1985.

222. Forsgren M. Standardization of techniques and reagents for the study of rubella antibody. Rev Infect Dis 7(Suppl 1):S129, 1985.

223. Grillner L, Forsgren M, Nordenfelt E. Comparison between a commercial ELISA, Rubazyme, and hemolysis-in-gel test for determination of rubella antibodies. J Virol Methods 10:111, 1985.

224. Chernesky MA, Smaill F, Mahony JB, et al. Combined testing for antibodies to rubella non-structural and envelope proteins sentinels infections in two outbreaks. Diagn Microbiol Infect Dis 8:173, 1987.

225. Ankerst J, Christensen P, Kjellen L, et al. A routine diagnostic test for IgA and IgM antibodies to rubella virus: absorption of IgG with Staphylococcus aureus. J Infect Dis 130:268, 1974.

226. Pattison JR, Mace JE. Elution patterns of rubella IgM, IgA, and IgG antibodies from a dextran and an agarose gel. J Clin Pathol 28:670, 1975.

227. Pattison JR, Mace JE, Dane DS. The detection and

228. Pattison JR, Mace JE. The detection of specific IgM antibodies following infection with rubella virus. J Clin Pathol 28:377, 1975.

229. Pattison JR, Jackson CM, Hiscock JA, et al. Comparison of methods for detecting specific IgM antibody in infants with congenital rubella. J Med Microbiol 11:411, 1978.

230. Caul EO, Hobbs SJ, Roberts PC, et al. Evaluation of a simplified sucrose gradient method for the detection of rubella-specific IgM in routine diagnostic practice. J Med Virol 2:153, 1978.

231. Krech U, Wilhelm JA. A solid-phase immunosorbent technique for the rapid detection of rubella IgM by haemagglutination inhibition. J Gen Virol 44:281, 1979.

232. Morgan-Capner P, Davies E, Pattison JR. Rubella-specific IgM detection using Sephacryl S-300 gel filtration. J Clin Pathol 33:1072, 1980.

233. Kobayashi N, Suzuki M, Nakagawa T, et al. Separation of hemagglutination-inhibiting immunoglobulin M antibody to rubella virus in human serum by high-performance liquid chromatography. J Clin Microbiol 23:1143, 1986.

234. Cunningham AL, Fraser JRE. Persistent rubella virus infection of human synovial cells cultured in vitro. J Infect Dis 151:638, 1985.

235. Parkman PD, Meyer HM, Kirschstein RL, et al. Attenuated rubella virus: I. Development and laboratory characterization. N Engl J Med 275:569, 1966.

236. Desmyter J, DeSomer P, Rawls WE, et al. The mechanism of rubella virus interference. Symp Ser Immunobiol Stand 11:139, 1969.

237. Kleiman MB, Carver DH. Failure of the RA 27/3 strain of rubella virus to induce intrinsic interference. J Gen Virol 36:335, 1977.

238. Frey TK, Hemphill ML. Generation of defective-interfering particles by rubella virus in Vero cells. Virology 164:22, 1988.

239. Sigurdardottir B, Givan KF, Rozee KR, et al. Association of virus with cases of rubella studied in Toronto: propagation of the agent and transmission to monkeys. Can Med Assoc J 88:128, 1963.

240. Heggie AD, Robbins FC. Rubella in naval recruits: a virologic study. N Engl J Med 271:231, 1964.

241. Parkman PD, Phillips PE, Kirschstein RL, et al. Experimental rubella virus infection in the rhesus monkey. J Immunol 95:743, 1965.

242. Parkman PD, Phillips PE, Meyer HM. Experimental rubella virus infection in pregnant monkeys. Am J Dis Child 110:390, 1965.

243. Sever JL, Meier GW, Windle WF, et al. Experimental rubella in pregnant rhesus monkeys. J Infect Dis 116:21, 1966.

244. Fabiyi A, Gitnick GL, Sever JL. Chronic rubella virus infection in the ferret (Mustela putorius fero) puppy. Proc Soc Exp Biol Med 125:766, 1967.

245. Barbosa L, Warren J. Studies on the detection of rubella virus and its immunogenicity for animals and man. Semiannual contract progress report to the National Institute for Neurological Diseases and Blindness, September 1, 1966 to March 1, 1967.

246. Belcourt RJ, Wong FC, Walcroft MJ. Growth of rubella virus in rabbit foetal tissues and cell cultures. Can J Public Health 56:253, 1965.

247. Oxford JS. The growth of rubella virus in small laboratory animals. J Immunol 98:697, 1967.

248. Cotlier E, Fox J, Bohigian G, et al. Pathogenic effects

of rubella virus on embryos and newborn rats. Nature 217:38, 1968.

249. Carver DH, Seto DSY, Marcus PI, et al. Rubella virus replication in the brains of suckling mice. J Virol 1:1089, 1967.

250. Centers for Disease Control. Recommendation of the Immunization Practices Advisory Committee (ACIP). Rubella prevention. MMWR Morb Mortal Wkly Rep 39(RR-15):1, 1990.

251. Committee on Infectious Diseases. Rubella. *In* Peter G (ed). Report of the Committee on Infectious Diseases, 22nd ed. Elk Grove Village, Ill, American Academy of Pediatrics, 1991, p 410.

252. Bart KJ, Orenstein WA, Preblud SR, et al. Elimination of rubella and congenital rubella from the United States. Pediatr Infect Dis 4:14, 1985.

253. Mann JM, Preblud SR, Hoffman RE, et al. Assessing risks of rubella infection during pregnancy: a standardized approach. JAMA 245:1647, 1981.

254. Horstmann DM, Liebhaber H, LeBouvier GL, et al. Rubella: reinfection of vaccinated and naturally immune persons exposed in an epidemic. N Engl J Med 283:771, 1970.

255. Lehane DE, Newberg NR, Beam WE Jr. Evaluation of rubella herd immunity during an epidemic. JAMA 213:2236, 1970.

256. Pollard RB, Edwards EA. Epidemic survey of rubella in a military recruit population. Am J Epidemiol 101:435, 1975.

257. Crawford GE, Gremellion DH. Epidemic measles and rubella in Air Force recruits: impact of immunization. J Infect Dis 144:403, 1981.

258. Blouse LE, Lathrop GD, Dupuy HJ, et al. Rubella screening and vaccination program for US Air Force trainees: an analysis of findings. Am J Public Health 72:280, 1982.

259. Chretien JH, Esswein JG, McGarvey MA, et al. Rubella: pattern of outbreak in a university. South Med J 69:1042, 1976.

260. Centers for Disease Control. Rubella in colleges—United States, 1983–1984. MMWR Morb Mortal Wkly Rep 34:228, 1985.

261. Centers for Disease Control. Rubella outbreaks in prisons—New York City, West Virginia, California. MMWR Morb Mortal Wkly Rep 34:615, 1985.

262. Centers for Disease Control. Rubella and congenital rubella syndrome—New York City. MMWR Morb Mortal Wkly Rep 35:770, 779, 1986.

263. Centers for Disease Control. Increase in rubella and congenital rubella syndrome in the United States. MMWR Morb Mortal Wkly Rep 40:93, 1991.

264. Centers for Disease Control. Congenital rubella syndrome among the Amish—Pennsylvania, 1991–1992. MMWR Morb Mortal Wkly Rep 41:468, 1992.

265. Goodman AK, Friedman SM, Beatrice ST, et al. Rubella in the workplace: the need for employee immunization. Am J Public Health 77:725, 1987.

266. McLaughlin MC, Gold LH. The New York rubella incident: a case for changing hospital policy regarding rubella testing and immunization. Am J Public Health 79:287, 1979.

267. Polk BF, White JA, DeGirolami PC, et al. An outbreak of rubella among hospital personnel. N Engl J Med 303:541, 1980.

268. Greaves WL, Orenstein WA, Stetler HC, et al. Prevention of rubella transmission in medical facilities. JAMA 248:861, 1982.

269. Strassburg MA, Stephenson TG, Habel LA, et al. Rubella in hospital employees. Infect Control 5:123, 1984.

270. Storch GA, Gruber C, Benz B, et al. A rubella outbreak among dental students: description of the outbreak and analysis of control measures. Infect Control 6:150, 1985.

271. Sever JL, Monif G. Limited persistence of virus in congenital rubella. Am J Dis Child 110:452, 1965.

272. Cooper LZ, Krugman S. Clinical manifestations of postnatal and congenital rubella. Arch Ophthalmol 77:434, 1967.

273. Rawls WE, Philips CA, Melnick JL, et al. Persistent virus infection in congenital rubella. Arch Ophthalmol 77:430, 1967.

274. Michaels RH. Immunologic aspects of congenital rubella. Pediatrics 43:339, 1969.

275. Menser MA, Forrest JM, Slinn RF, et al. Rubella viruria in a 29-year-old woman with congenital rubella. Lancet 2:797, 1971.

276. Shewman DA, Cherry JD, Kirby SE. Shedding of rubella virus in a 4½-year-old boy with congenital rubella. Pediatr Infect Dis 1:342, 1982.

277. Hattis RP, Halstead SB, Herrmann KL, et al. Rubella in an immunized island population. JAMA 223:1019, 1973.

278. Weller TH, Alford CA Jr, Neva FA. Changing epidemiologic concepts of rubella, with particular reference to unique characteristics of the congenital infection. Yale J Biol Med 37:455, 1965.

279. Rawls WE, Melnick JL, Bradstreet CMP, et al. WHO collaborative study on the seroepidemiology of rubella. Bull World Health Organ 37:79, 1967.

280. Cockburn WC. World aspects of the epidemiology of rubella. Am J Dis Child 118:112, 1969.

281. Witte JJ, Karchmer AW, Case G, et al. Epidemiology of rubella. Am J Dis Child 118:107, 1969.

282. Dowdle WR, Ferreira W, Gomes LFD, et al. WHO collaborative study on the seroepidemiology of rubella in Caribbean and Middle and South American populations in 1968. Bull World Health Organ 42:419, 1970.

283. Horstmann DM. Rubella: the challenge of its control. J Infect Dis 123:640, 1971.

284. Assad R, Ljungars-Esteves K. Rubella—world impact. Rev Infect Dis 7(Suppl 1):S29, 1985.

285. Horstmann DM. Rubella. *In* Evans AS (ed). Viral Infections of Humans: Epidemiology and Control, 2nd ed. New York, Plenum Publishing, 1985, p 519.

286. Centers for Disease Control. Rubella Surveillance, January 1976–December 1978, issued May 1980. U.S. Department of Health and Human Services Publication No. (CDC)80-8023.

287. Buescher EL. Behavior of rubella virus in adult populations. Arch Gesamte Virusforsch 16:470, 1965.

288. Green RH, Balsame MR, Giles JP, et al. Studies of the natural history and prevention of rubella. Am J Dis Child 110:348, 1965.

289. Horstmann DM, Riordan JT, Ohtawara M, et al. A natural epidemic of rubella in a closed population. Arch Gesamte Virusforsch 16:483, 1965.

290. Brody JA. The infectiousness of rubella and the possibility of reinfection. Am J Public Health 56:1082, 1966.

291. Bisno AL, Spence LP, Stewart JA, et al. Rubella in Trinidad: seroepidemiologic studies of an institutional outbreak. Am J Epidemiol 89:74, 1969.

292. Gale JL, Detels R, Kim KSW, et al. The epidemiology of rubella on Taiwan: III. Family studies in cities of high and low attack rates. Int J Epidemiol 1:261, 1972.

293. Neva FA, Alford CA Jr, Weller TH. Emerging perspective of rubella. Bacteriol Rev 28:444, 1964.

294. Brody JA, Sever JL, McAlister R, et al. Rubella epidemic

on St. Paul Island in the Pribilofs, 1963. I. Epidemiologic, clinical, and serologic findings. JAMA 191:619, 1965.

295. Sever JL, Brody JA, Schiff GM, et al. Rubella epidemic on St. Paul Island in the Pribilofs, 1963: II. Clinical and laboratory findings for the intensive study population. JAMA 191:624, 1965.

296. Halstead SB, Diwan AR, Oda AI. Susceptibility to rubella among adolescents and adults in Hawaii. JAMA 210:1881, 1969.

297. Wilkins J, Leedom JM, Portnoy B, et al. Reinfection with rubella virus despite live vaccine-induced immunity. Am J Dis Child 118:275, 1969.

298. Chang TW, DesRosiers S, Weinstein, L. Clinical and serologic studies of an outbreak of rubella in a vaccinated population. N Engl J Med 283:246, 1970.

299. Gross PA, Portnoy B, Mathies AW, et al. A rubella outbreak among adolescent boys. Am J Dis Child 119:326, 1970.

300. Shlian DM. Screening and immunization of rubella-susceptible women: experience in a large, prepaid medical group. JAMA 240:662, 1978.

301. Preblud SR, Gross F, Halsey NA, et al. Assessment of susceptibility to measles and rubella. JAMA 247:1134, 1982.

302. Miller KA. Rubella susceptibility in an adolescent female population. Mayo Clin Proc 59:31, 1984.

303. Allen S. Rubella susceptibility in young adults. J Fam Pract 21:271, 1985.

304. Cohen ZB, Rice LI, Felice ME. Rubella seronegativity in a low socioeconomic adolescent female population. Clin Pediatr (Phila) 24:387, 1985.

305. Dorfman SF, Bowers CH Jr. Rubella susceptibility among prenatal and family planning clinic populations. Mt Sinai J Med 52:248, 1985.

306. Serdula MK, Marks JS, Ibara CM, et al. Premarital rubella screening program: from identification to vaccination of susceptible women in the state of Hawaii. Public Health Rep 101:329, 1986.

307. Alford CA, Neva FA, Weller TH. Virologic and serologic studies on human products of conception after maternal rubella. N Engl J Med 271:1275, 1964.

308. Horstmann DJ, Banatvala JE, Riordan JT, et al. Maternal rubella and the rubella syndrome in infants. Am J Dis Child 110:408, 1965.

309. Monif GRG, Sever JL, Schiff GM, et al. Isolation of rubella virus from products of conception. Am J Obstet Gynecol 91:1143, 1965.

310. Alford CA Jr. Congenital rubella: a review of the virologic and serologic phenomena occurring after maternal rubella in the first trimester. South Med J 59:745, 1966.

311. Heggie AD. Intrauterine infection in maternal rubella. J Pediatr 71:777, 1967.

312. Rawls WE, Desmyter J, Melnick JL. Serologic diagnosis and fetal involvement in maternal rubella. JAMA 203:627, 1968.

313. Thompson KM, Tobin JO. Isolation of rubella virus from abortion material. BMJ 2:264, 1970.

314. Strannegard O, Holm SE, Hermodsson S, et al. Case of apparent reinfection with rubella. Lancet 1:240, 1970.

315. Boué A, Nicholas A, Montagnon, B. Reinfection with rubella in pregnant women. Lancet 2:1251, 1971.

316. Haukenes G, Haram KO. Clinical rubella after reinfection. N Engl J Med 287:1204, 1972.

317. Northrop RL, Gardner WM, Geittman WF. Rubella reinfection during early pregnancy. Obstet Gynecol 39:524, 1972.

318. Northrop RI, Gardner WM, Geittmann WF. Low-level immunity to rubella. N Engl J Med 287:615, 1972.

319. Eilard T, Strannegard O. Rubella reinfection in pregnancy followed by transmission to the fetus. J Infect Dis 129:594, 1974.

320. Snijder JAM, Schroder, FP, Hoekstra, J. H. Importance of IgM determination in cord blood in cases of suspected rubella infection. BMJ 1:23, 1977.

321. Forsgren M, Carlstrom G, Strangert K. Congenital rubella after maternal reinfection. Scand J Infect Dis 11:81, 1979.

322. Fogel A, Handsher R, Barnea B. Subclinical rubella in pregnancy—occurrence and outcome. Isr J Med Sci 21:133, 1985.

323. Sheridan MD. Final report of a prospective study of children whose mothers had rubella in early pregnancy. BMJ 2:536, 1964.

324. Butler NR, Dudgeon JA, Hayes K, et al. Persistence of rubella antibody with and without embryopathy: a follow-up study of children exposed to maternal rubella. BMJ 2:1027, 1965.

325. Phillips GA, Melnick JL, Yow MD, et al. Persistence of virus in infants with congenital rubella and in normal infants with a history of maternal rubella. JAMA 193:1027, 1965.

326. Hardy JB, McCracken GH Jr, Gilkeson MR, et al. Adverse fetal outcome following maternal rubella after the first trimester of pregnancy. JAMA 207:2414, 1969.

327. Schiff GM, Sutherland J, Light I. Congenital rubella. In Thalhammer O (ed). Prenatal Infections. International Symposium of Vienna, September 2–3, 1970. Stuttgart, Georg Thieme Verlag, 1971, p 31.

328. Peckham GS. Clinical and laboratory study of children exposed in utero to maternal rubella. Arch Dis Child 47:571, 1972.

329. Menser MA, Forrest JM. Rubella—high incidence of defects in children considered normal at birth. Med J Aust 1:123, 1974.

330. Dudgeon JA. Infective causes of human malformations. Br Med Bull 32:77, 1976.

331. Lundstrom R. Rubella during pregnancy: A follow-up study of children born after an epidemic of rubella in Sweden, 1951, with additional investigations on prophylaxis and treatment of maternal rubella. Acta Paediatr 51(Suppl 133):1, 1962.

332. Whitehouse WL. Rubella before conception as a cause of foetal abnormality. Lancet 1:139, 1963.

333. Monif GRG, Hardy JB, Sever JL. Studies in congenital rubella, Baltimore 1964–65: I. Epidemiologic and virologic. Bull Johns Hopkins Hosp 118:85, 1966.

334. Sever JL, Hardy JB, Nelson KB, et al. Rubella in the Collaborative Perinatal Research Study: II. Clinical and laboratory findings in children through 3 years of age. Am J Dis Child 118:123, 1969.

335. Seppala M, Vaheri A. Natural rubella infection of the female genital tract. Lancet 1:46, 1974.

336. Buimovici-Klein E, Hite RL, Byrne T, et al. Isolation of rubella virus in milk after postpartum immunization. J Pediatr 91:939, 1977.

337. Klein EB, Bryne T, Cooper LZ. Neonatal rubella in a breast-fed infant after postpartum maternal infection. J Pediatr 97:774, 1980.

338. Manson MM, Logan WPD, Loy RM. Rubella and other virus infections during pregnancy. In Reports on Public Health and Medical Subjects, No. 101. London, Her Majesty's Stationery Office, 1960.

339. Siegel M, Greenberg M. Fetal death, malformation and

prematurity after maternal rubella: results of prospective study, 1949–1958. N Engl J Med 262:389, 1960.

340. Liggins GC, Phillips LI. Rubella embryopathy: an interim report on a New Zealand epidemic. BMJ 1:711, 1963.

341. Pitt D, Keir EH. Results of rubella in pregnancy: III. Med J Aust 2:737, 1965.

342. Sallomi SJ. Rubella in pregnancy: a review of prospective studies from the literature. Obstet Gynecol 27:252, 1966.

343. Heggie AD, Robbins FC. Natural rubella acquired after birth: clinical features and complications. Am J Dis Child 118:12, 1969.

344. Chantler JK, Tingle AJ. Isolation of rubella virus from human lymphocytes after acute infection. J Infect Dis 145:673, 1982.

345. O'Shea S, Mutton D, Best JM. In vivo expression of rubella antigens on human leucocytes: detection by flow cytometry. J Med Virol 25:297, 1988.

346. Heggie AD. Pathogenesis of the rubella exanthem: isolation of rubella virus from the skin. N Engl J Med 285:664, 1971.

347. Heggie AD. Pathogenesis of the rubella exanthem: distribution of rubella virus in the skin during rubella with and without rash. J Infect Dis 137:74, 1978.

348. Al-Nakib W, Best JM, Banatvala JE. Rubella-specific serum and nasopharyngeal immunoglobulin responses following naturally acquired and vaccine-induced infection: prolonged persistence of virus-specific IgM. Lancet 1:182, 1975.

349. Pattison JR, Dane DS, Mace JE. The persistence of specific IgM after natural infection with rubella virus. Lancet 1:185, 1975.

350. Meurman OH. Persistence of immunoglobulin G and immunoglobulin M antibodies after postnatal rubella infection determined by solid-phase radioimmunoassay. J Clin Microbiol 7:34, 1978.

351. Rousseau S, Hedman K. Rubella infection and reinfection distinguished by avidity of IgG. Letter to the editor. Lancet 1:1108, 1988.

352. Hedman K, Seppälä I. Recent rubella virus infection indicated by a low avidity of specific IgG. J Clin Immunol 8:214, 1988.

353. Morgan-Capner P, Thomas HIJ. Serological distinction between primary rubella and reinfection. Letter to the editor. Lancet 1:1397, 1988.

354. Smith KA, Chess L, Mardiney MR Jr. The relationship between rubella hemagglutination inhibition antibody (HIA) and rubella induced in vitro lymphocyte tritiated thymidine incorporation. Cell Immunol 8:321, 1973.

355. Steele RW, Hensen SA, Vincent MM, et al. A ^{52}Cr microassay technique for cell-mediated immunity to viruses. J Immunol 110:1502, 1973.

356. Honeyman MC, Forrest JM, Dorman DC. Cell-mediated immune response following natural rubella and rubella vaccination. Clin Exp Immunol 17:665, 1974.

357. McMorrow L, Vesikari T, Wolman SR, et al. Suppression of the response of lymphocytes to phytohemagglutinin in rubella. J Infect Dis 130:464, 1974.

358. Steele RW, Hensen SA, Vincent MM, et al. Development of specific cellular and humoral immune responses in children immunized with liver rubella virus vaccine. J Infect Dis 130:449, 1974.

359. Kanra GY, Vesikari T. Cytotoxic activity against rubella-infected cells in the supernatants of human lymphocyte cultures stimulated by rubella virus. Clin Exp Immunol 19:17, 1975.

360. Vesikari T, Kanra GY, Buimovici-Klein E, et al. Cell-mediated immunity in rubella assayed by cytotoxicity of

supernatants from rubella virus-stimulated human lymphocyte cultures. Clin Exp Immunol 19:33, 1975.

361. Ganguly R, Cusumano CL, Waldman RH. Suppression of cell-mediated immunity after infection with attenuated rubella virus. Infect Immun 13:464, 1976.

362. Buimovici-Klein E, Weiss KE, Cooper LZ. Interferon production in lymphocyte cultures after rubella infection in humans. J Infect Dis 135:380, 1977.

363. Rossier E, Phipps PH, Polley JR, et al. Absence of cell-mediated immunity to rubella virus 5 years after rubella vaccination. Can Med Assoc J 116:481, 1977.

364. Rossier E, Phipps PH, Weber JM, et al. Persistence of humoral and cell-mediated immunity to rubella virus in cloistered nuns and in schoolteachers. J Infect Dis 144:137, 1981.

365. Buimovici-Klein E, Cooper LZ. Cell-mediated immune response to rubella infections. Rev Infect Dis 7(Suppl 1):S123, 1985.

366. Mori T, Shiozawa K. Suppression of tuberculin hypersensitivity caused by rubella infection. Am Rev Respir Dis 131:886, 1985.

367. Ogra PL, Kerr-Grant D, Umana G, et al. Antibody response in serum and nasopharynx after naturally acquired and vaccine-induced infection with rubella virus. N Engl J Med 285:1333, 1971.

368. Al-Nakib W, Best JM, Banatvala JE. Detection of rubella-specific serum IgG and IgA and nasopharyngeal IgA responses using a radioactive single radial immunodiffusion technique. Clin Exp Immunol 22:293, 1975.

369. Plotkin SA, Farquhar JD. Immunity to rubella: comparison between naturally and artificially induced resistance. Postgrad Med J 48(Suppl):47, 1972.

370. Plotkin SA, Farquhar JD, Ogra PL. Immunologic properties of RA 27/3 rubella virus vaccine: a comparison with strains presently licensed in the United States. JAMA 225:585, 1973.

371. Morag A, Beutner KR, Morag B, et al. Development and characteristics of in vitro correlates of cellular immunity to rubella virus in the systemic and mucosal sites in guinea pigs. J Immunol 113:1703, 1974.

372. Morag A, Morag B, Bernstein JM, et al. In vitro correlates of cell-mediated immunity in human tonsils after natural or induced rubella virus infection. J Infect Dis 131:409, 1975.

373. Selzer G. Virus isolation, inclusion bodies, and chromosomes in a rubella-infected human embryo. Lancet 2:336, 1963.

374. Rudolph AJ, Yow MD, Phillips A, et al. Transplacental rubella infection in newly born infants. JAMA 191:843, 1965.

375. Catalano LW Jr, Fuccillo DA, Traub RG, et al. Isolation of rubella virus from placentas and throat cultures of infants: a prospective study after the 1964–65 epidemic. Obstet Gynecol 38:6, 1971.

376. Schiff GM, Dine MS. Transmission of rubella from newborns: a controlled study among young adult women and report of an unusual case. Am J Dis Child 110:447, 1965.

377. Plotkin SA, Cochran W, Lindquist JM, et al. Congenital rubella syndrome in late infancy. JAMA 200:435, 1967.

378. Monif GRG, Sever JL. Chronic infection of the central nervous system with rubella virus. Neurology 16:111, 1966.

379. Desmond MM, Wilson GS, Melnick JL, et al. Congenital rubella encephalitis. J Pediatr 71:311, 1967.

380. Menser MA, Harley JD, Herzberg R, et al. Persistence of virus in lens for three years after prenatal rubella. Lancet 2:387, 1967.

381. Cremer NE, Oshiro LS, Weil ML, et al. Isolation of

rubella virus from brain in chronic progressive panencephalitis. J Gen Virol 29:143, 1975.

382. Weil ML, Itabashi HH, Cremer NE, et al. Chronic progressive panencephalitis due to rubella virus simulating subacute sclerosing panencephalitis. N Engl J Med 292:994, 1975.

383. Alford CA Jr. Immunoglobulin determinations in the diagnosis of fetal infection. Pediatr Clin North Am 18:99, 1971.

384. Weller TH, Alford CA, Neva FA. Retrospective diagnosis by serologic means of congenitally acquired rubella infections. N Engl J Med 270:1039, 1964.

385. Alford CA Jr. Studies on antibody in congenital rubella infections: I. Physicochemical and immunologic investigations of rubella-neutralizing antibody. Am J Dis Child 110:455, 1965.

386. Alford CA Jr, Blankenship WJ, Straumfjord JV, et al. The diagnostic significance of IgM-globulin elevations in newborn infants with chronic intrauterine infections. In Bergsma D (ed). Birth Defects—Original Articles Series, vol 4, no 5. New York, National Foundation–March of Dimes, 1968.

387. Gitlin D. The differentiation and maturation of specific immune mechanisms. Acta Paediatr Scand Suppl 172:60, 1967.

388. Gitlin D, Biasucci A. Development of gamma G, gamma A, beta IC-beta IA, CI esterase inhibitor, ceruloplasmin, transferrin, hemopexin, haptoglobin, fibrinogen, plasminogen, alpha 1-antitrypsin, orosomucoid, beta-lipoprotein, alpha 2-macroglobulin, and prealbumin in the human conceptus. J Clin Invest 48:1433, 1969.

389. Lawton AR, Self KS, Royal SA, et al. Ontogeny of lymphocytes in the human fetus. Clin Immunol Immunopathol 1:104, 1972.

390. Bellanti JA, Artenstein MS, Olson LC, et al. Congenital rubella: clinicopathologic, virologic, and immunologic studies. Am J Dis Child 110:464, 1965.

391. Baublis JV, Brown GC. Specific response of the immunoglobulins to rubella infection. Proc Soc Exp Biol Med 128:206, 1968.

392. Cohen SM, Ducharme CP, Carpenter CA, et al. Rubella antibody in IgG and IgM immunoglobulins detected by immunofluorescence. J Lab Clin Med 72:760, 1968.

393. Vesikari T, Vaheri A, Pettay O, et al. Congenital rubella: immune response of the neonate and diagnosis by demonstration of specific IgM antibodies. J Pediatr 75:658, 1969.

394. Cradock-Watson JE, Ridehalgh MKS, Chantler S. Specific immunoglobulins in infants with the congenital rubella syndrome. J Hyg (London) 76:109, 1976.

395. McCracken GH Jr, Hardy JB, Chen TC, et al. Serum immunoglobulin levels in newborn infants: II. Survey of cord and follow-up sera from 123 infants with congenital rubella. J Pediatr 74:383, 1969.

396. Alford CA Jr. Fetal antibody in the diagnosis of chronic intra-uterine infections. In Thalhammer O (ed). Prenatal Infections. International Symposium of Vienna, September 2–3, 1970. Stuttgart, Georg Thieme, 1971, p 53.

397. Kenrick KG, Slinn RF, Dorman DC, et al. Immunoglobulins and rubella-virus antibodies in adults with congenital rubella. Lancet 1:548, 1968.

398. Hardy JB, Sever JL, Gilkeson MR. Declining antibody titers in children with congenital rubella. J Pediatr 75:213, 1969.

399. Cooper LZ, Florman AL, Ziring PR, et al. Loss of rubella hemagglutination-inhibition antibody in congenital rubella. Am J Dis Child 122:397, 1971.

400. Ueda K, Tokugawa K, Fukushige J, et al. Hemagglutination inhibition antibodies in congenital rubella: a 17-year follow-up in the Ryukyu Islands. Am J Dis Child 141:211, 1987.

401. Ueda K, Tokugawa K, Fukushige J, et al. Continuing problem in congenital rubella syndrome in southern Japan: its outbreak in Fukuoka and the surrounding areas after the 1965–1969 and 1975–1977 rubella epidemics. Fukuoka Acta Med 77:309, 1986.

402. Soothill JF, Hayes K, Dudgeon JA. The immunoglobulins in congenital rubella. Lancet 1:1385, 1966.

403. Hancock MP, Huntley CC, Sever JL. Congenital rubella syndrome with immunoglobulin disorder. J Pediatr 72:636, 1968.

404. Hayward AR, Ezer G. Development of lymphocyte populations in the human foetal thymus and spleen. Clin Exp Immunol 17:169, 1974.

405. Cooper MD, Dayton DH. In Cooper MD, Dayton DH (eds). Development of Host Defenses. New York, Raven Press, 1977.

406. Miller ME. In Miller ME (ed). Host Defenses in the Human Neonate. Monographs in Neonatology. New York, Grune & Stratton, 1978.

407. Berry CL, Thompson EN. Clinicopathological study of thymic dysplasia. Arch Dis Child 43:579, 1968.

408. White LR, Leikin S, Villavicencio O, et al. Immune competence in congenital rubella: lymphocyte transformation, delayed hypersensitivity and response to vaccination. J Pediatr 73:229, 1968.

409. Montgomery JR, South MA, Rawls WE, et al. Viral inhibition of lymphocyte response to phytohemagglutinin. Science 157:1068, 1967.

410. Olson GB, South MA, Good RA. Phytohemagglutinin unresponsiveness of lymphocytes from babies with congenital rubella. Nature 214:695, 1967.

411. Olson GB, Dent PB, Rawls WE, et al. Abnormalities of in vitro lymphocyte responses during rubella virus infections. J Exp Med 128:47, 1968.

412. Simmons JJ, Fitzgerald MG. Rubella virus and human lymphocytes in culture. Lancet 2:937, 1968.

413. Marshall WC, Cope WA, Soothill JF, et al. In vitro lymphocyte response in some immunity deficiency diseases and in intrauterine virus infections. Proc R Soc Med 63:351, 1970.

414. Buimovici-Klein E, Lang PB, Ziring PR, et al. Impaired cell-mediated immune response in patients with congenital rubella: correlation with gestational age at time of infection. Pediatrics 64:620, 1979.

415. Hyyp iä T, Eskola J, Laine M, et al. B-cell function in vitro during rubella infection. Infect Immun 43:589, 1984.

416. Fuccillo DA, Steele RW, Hensen SA, et al. Impaired cellular immunity to rubella virus in congenital rubella. Infect Immun 9:81, 1974.

417. Mims CA. Pathogenesis of viral infections in the fetus. Prog Med Virol 10:194, 1968.

418. Rawls WE. Congenital rubella: the significance of virus persistence. Prog Med Virol 10:238, 1968.

419. Alford CA Jr. Production of interferon-like substance by the rubella-infected human conceptus. Program and Abstracts, American Pediatric Society and Society of Pediatric Research Meeting, Atlantic City, April 29–May 2, 1970, p 203.

420. Lebon P, Daffos F, Checoury A, et al. Presence of an acid-labile alpha-interferon in sera from fetuses and children with congenital rubella. J Clin Microbiol 21:755, 1985.

421. Desmyter J, Rawls WE, Melnick JL, et al. Interferon in

congenital rubella: response to live attenuated measles vaccine. J Immunol 99:771, 1967.

422. McCarthy K, Taylor-Robinson CH, Pillinger SE. Isolation of rubella virus from cases in Britain. Lancet 2:593, 1963.

423. Hildebrandt HM, Maassab HF. Rubella synovitis in a 1-year-old patient. N Engl J Med 274:1428, 1966.

424. Yanez JE, Thompson GR, Middelsen WM, et al. Rubella arthritis. Ann Intern Med 64:772, 1966.

425. McCormick JN, Duthie JJR, Gerber H, et al. Rheumatoid polyarthritis after rubella. Ann Rheum Dis 37:266, 1978.

426. Graham R, Armstrong R, Simmons NA, et al. Isolation of rubella virus from synovial fluid in five cases of seronegative arthritis. Lancet 2:649, 1981.

427. Lebon P, Lyon G. Noncongenital rubella encephalitis. Lancet 2:468, 1974.

428. Wolinsky JS, Berg BO, Maitland CJ. Progressive rubella panencephalitis. Arch Neurol 33:722, 1976.

429. Squadrini F, Taparelli F, De Rienzo B, et al. Rubella virus isolation from cerebrospinal fluid in postnatal rubella encephalitis. BMJ 2:1329, 1977.

430. Thong YH, Steele RW, Vincent MM, et al. Impaired in vitro cell-mediated immunity to rubella virus during pregnancy. N Engl J Med 289:604, 1973.

431. Weinberg ED. Pregnancy-associated depression of cell-mediated immunity. Rev Infect Dis 6:814, 1984.

432. Honeyman MC, Dorman DC, Menser MA, et al. HL-A antigens in congenital rubella and the role of antigens 1 and 8 in the epidemiology of natural rubella. Tissue Antigens 5:12, 1975.

433. Forrester RM, Lees VT, Watson GH. Rubella syndrome: escape of a twin. BMJ 1:1403, 1966.

434. Cooper LZ. The history and medical consequences of rubella. Rev Infect Dis 7(Suppl 1):S1, 1985.

435. Töndury G, Smith DW. Fetal rubella pathology. J Pediatr 68:867, 1966.

436. Driscoll SG. Histopathology of gestational rubella. Am J Dis Child 118:49, 1969.

437. Dudgeon JA. Teratogenic effect of rubella virus. Proc R Soc Med 63:1254, 1970.

438. Menser MA, Reye RDK. The pathology of congenital rubella: a review written by request. Pathology 6:215, 1974.

439. Esterly JR, Oppenheimer EH. Intrauterine rubella infection. In Rosenberg HS, Bolande RP (eds). Perspectives in Pediatric Pathology, vol. 1. Chicago, Year Book Medical Publishers, 1973, p 313.

440. Boué A, Boué JG. Effects of rubella virus infection on the division of human cells. Am J Dis Child 118:45, 1969.

441. Smith JL, Early EM, London WT, et al. Persistent rubella virus production in embryonic rabbit chondrocyte cell cultures (37465). Proc Soc Exp Biol Med 143:1037, 1973.

442. Heggie AD. Growth inhibition of human embryonic and fetal rat bones in organ culture by rubella virus. Teratology 15:47, 1977.

443. Rawls WE, Melnick JL, Rosenberg HA, et al. Spontaneous virus carrier cultures and postmortem isolation of virus from infants with congenital rubella. Proc Soc Exp Biol Med 120:623, 1965.

444. Boué A, Plotkin SA, Boué JG. Action du virus de la rubéole sur différents systèmes de cultures de cellules embryonnaires humaines. Arch Gesamte Virusforsch 16:443, 1965.

445. Plotkin SA, Boué A, Boué JG. The in vitro growth of rubella virus in human embryo cells. Am J Epidemiol 81:71, 1965.

446. Chang TH, Moorhead PS, Boué JG, et al. Chromosome studies of human cells infected in utero and in vitro with rubella virus. Proc Soc Exp Biol Med 122:236, 1966.

447. Nusbacher J, Hirschhorn K, Cooper LZ. Chromosomal studies on congenital rubella. N Engl J Med 276:1409, 1967.

448. Plotkin SA, Vaheri A. Human fibroblasts infected with rubella virus produce a growth inhibitor. Science 156:659, 1967.

449. Bowden DS, Pedersen JS, Toh BH, et al. Distribution by immunofluorescence of viral products and actin-containing cytoskeleton filaments in rubella virus-infected cells. Arch Virol 92:211, 1987.

450. Yoneda T, Urade M, Sakuda M, et al. Altered growth, differentiation, and responsiveness to epidermal growth factor of human embryonic mesenchymal cells of palate by persistent rubella virus infection. J Clin Invest 77:1613, 1986.

451. Naeye RL, Blanc W. Pathogenesis of congenital rubella. JAMA 194:1277, 1965.

452. Dent PB, Olson GB, Good RA, et al. Rubella-virus/leukocyte interaction and its role in the pathogenesis of the congenital rubella syndrome. Lancet 1:291, 1968.

453. Reimer CB, Black CM, Phillips DJ, et al. The specificity of fetal IgM: antibody or anti-antibody? Ann NY Acad Sci 254:77, 1975.

454. Robertson PW, Kertesz V, Cloonan MJ. Elimination of false-positive cytomegalovirus immunoglobulin M-fluorescent-antibody reactions with immunoglobulin M serum fractions. J Clin Microbiol 6:174, 1977.

455. Altshuler G. Placentitis with a new light on an old TORCH. Obstet Gynecol Ann 6:197, 1977.

456. Garcia AGP, Marques RLS, Lobato YY, et al. Placental pathology in congenital rubella. Placenta 6:281, 1985.

457. Krugman S, Katz SL, Gershon AA, et al (eds). Rubella. In Infectious Diseases of Children, 8th ed. St. Louis, CV Mosby, 1985, p 307.

458. Sheinis M, Sarov I, Maor E, et al. Severe neonatal rubella following maternal infection. Pediatr Infect Dis 4:202, 1985.

459. Judelsohn RG, Wyll SA. Rubella in Bermuda: termination of an epidemic by mass vaccination. JAMA 223:401, 1973.

460. Fujimoto T, Katoh C, Hayakawa H, et al. Two cases of rubella infection with cardiac involvement. Jpn Heart J 20:227, 1979.

461. Saeed AA, Lange LS. Guillain-Barré syndrome after rubella. Postgrad Med J 54:333, 1978.

462. Callaghan N, Feely M, Walsh B. Relapsing neurological disorder associated with rubella virus infection in two sisters. J Neurol Neurosurg Psychiatry 40:1117, 1977.

463. Connolly JH, Hutchinson WM, Allen IV, et al. Carotid artery thrombosis, encephalitis, myelitis and optic neuritis associated with rubella virus infections. Brain 98:583, 1975.

464. Choutet P, Binet CH, Goudeau A, et al. Bone-marrow aplasia and primary rubella infection. Lancet 2:966, 1979.

465. Townsend JJ, Baringer JR, Wolinsky JS, et al. Progressive rubella panencephalitis: late onset after congenital rubella. N Engl J Med 292:990, 1975.

466. Waxham MN, Wolinsky JS. Rubella virus and its effect on the nervous system. Neurol Clin 2:267, 1984.

467. Schlossberg D, Topolosky MR. Military rubella. JAMA 238:1273, 1974.

468. Preblud SR, Dobbs HI, Sedmak GV, et al. Testalgia associated with rubella infection. South Med J 73:594, 1980.

469. White LR, Sever JL, Alepa FP. Maternal and congenital

rubella before 1964: frequency, clinical features, and search for isoimmune phenomena. Pediatrics 74:198, 1969.

470. Cooper LZ. Rubella: a preventable cause of birth defects. *In* Bergsma D (ed). Birth Defects—Original Article Series, vol. 4, no. 23. New York, National Foundation–March of Dimes, 1968.

471. Cooper LZ, Green RH, Krugman S, et al. Neonatal thrombocytopenic purpura and other manifestations of rubella contracted in utero. Am J Dis Child 110:416, 1965.

472. Zinkham WH, Medearis DN, Osborn JE. Blood and bone marrow findings in congenital rubella. J Pediatr 71:512, 1967.

473. Rudolph AJ, Singleton EB, Rosenberg HS, et al. Osseous manifestations of the congenital rubella syndrome. Am J Dis Child 110:428, 1965.

474. Rabinowitz JG, Wolf BS, Greenberg EI, et al. Osseous changes in rubella embryopathy. Radiology 85:494, 1965.

475. Wall WL, Altman DH, Gair DR, et al. Roentgenological findings in congenital rubella. Clin Pediatr 4:704, 1965.

476. Reed GB Jr. Rubella bone lesions. J Pediatr 74:208, 1969.

477. Korones SB, Ainger LE, Monif GRG, et al. Congenital rubella syndrome: study of 22 infants. Am J Dis Child 110:434, 1965.

478. Rorke LB, Spiro AJ. Cerebral lesions in congenital rubella syndrome. J Pediatr 70:243, 1967.

479. Streissguth AP, Vanderveer BB, Shepard TH. Mental development of children with congenital rubella syndrome: a preliminary report. Am J Obstet Gynecol 108:391, 1970.

480. Rowen M, Singer MI, Moran ET. Intracranial calcification in the congenital rubella syndrome. Am J Roentgenol 115:86, 1972.

481. Peters ER, Davis RL. Congenital rubella syndrome: cerebral mineralizations and subperiosteal new bone formation as expressions of this disorder. Clin Pediatr (Phila) 5:743, 1966.

482. Hastreiter AR, Joorabchi B, Pujatti G, et al. Cardiovascular lesions associated with congenital rubella. J Pediatr 71:59, 1967.

483. Klein HZ, Markarian M. Dermal erythropoiesis in congenital rubella: description of an infected newborn who had purpura associated with marked extramedullary erythropoieses in the skin and elsewhere. Clin Pediatr (Phila) 8:604, 1969.

484. Brough AJ, Jones D, Page RH, et al. Dermal erythropoieses in neonatal infants. Pediatrics 40:627, 1967.

485. Achs R, Harper KG, Siegal M. Unusual dermatoglyphic findings associated with the rubella embryopathy. N Engl J Med 274:148, 1966.

486. Purvis-Smith SG, Howard PR, Menser MA. Dermatoglyphic defects and rubella teratogenesis. JAMA 209:1865, 1969.

487. Murphy AM, Reid RR, Pollard I, et al. Rubella cataracts: further clinical and virologic observations. Am J Ophthalmol 64:1109, 1967.

488. Collis WJ, Cohen DN. Rubella retinopathy: a progressive disorder. Arch Ophthalmol 84:33, 1970.

489. Kresky B, Nauheim JS. Rubella retinitis. Am J Dis Child 113:305, 1967.

490. Schiff GM, Sutherland JM, Light IJ, et al. Studies on congenital rubella. Am J Dis Child 110:441, 1965.

491. Menser MA, Dorman DC, Reye RDK, et al. Renal artery stenosis in the rubella syndrome. Lancet 1:790, 1966.

492. Menser MA, Robertson SEJ, Dorman DC, et al. Renal lesions in congenital rubella. Pediatrics 40:901, 1967.

493. Kaplan GW, McLaughlin AP III. Urogenital anomalies and congenital rubella syndrome. Urology 2:148, 1973.

494. Forrest JM, Menser MA. Congenital rubella in schoolchildren and adolescents. Arch Dis Child 45:63, 1970.

495. Korones SB, Ainger LE, Monif GR, et al. Congenital rubella syndrome: new clinical aspects with recovery of virus from affected infants. J Pediatr 67:166, 1965.

496. South MA, Alford CA Jr. The immunology of chronic intrauterine infections. *In* Stiehm ER, Fulginiti VA (eds). Immunologic Disorders in Infants and Children. Philadelphia, WB Saunders, 1973, p 565.

497. Phelan P, Campbell P. Pulmonary complications of rubella embryopathy. J Pediatr 75:202, 1969.

498. Karmody GS. Subclinical maternal rubella and congenital deafness. N Engl J Med 278:809, 1968.

499. Ames MD, Plotkin SA, Winchester RA, et al. Central auditory imperception: a significant factor in congenital rubella deafness. JAMA 213:419, 1970.

500. Peckham CS, Martin JAM, Marshall WC, et al. Congenital rubella deafness: a preventable disease. Lancet 1:258, 1979.

501. Rossi M, Ferlito A, Polidoro F. Maternal rubella and hearing impairment in children. J Laryngol Otol 94:281, 1980.

502. Weinberger MM, Maslund MW, Asbed R, et al. Congenital rubella presenting as retarded language development. Am J Dis Child 120:125, 1970.

503. Desmond MM, Fisher ES, Vorderman AL, et al. The longitudinal course of congenital rubella encephalitis in nonretarded children. J Pediatr 93:584, 1978.

504. Zausmer E. Congenital rubella: pathogenesis of motor deficits. Pediatrics 47:16, 1971.

505. Menser MA, Forrest JM, Bransby RD. Rubella infection and diabetes mellitus. Lancet 1:57, 1978.

506. Hanid TK. Hypothyroidism in congenital rubella. Lancet 2:854, 1976.

507. Nieberg PI, Gardner LI. Thyroiditis and congenital rubella syndrome. J Pediatr 89:156, 1976.

508. Perez Comas A. Congenital rubella and acquired hypothyroidism secondary to Hashimoto thyroiditis. J Pediatr 88:1065, 1976.

509. Ziring PR, Gallo G, Finegold M, et al. Chronic lymphocytic thyroiditis: identification of rubella virus antigen in the thyroid of a child with congenital rubella. J Pediatr 90:419, 1977.

510. AvRuskin TW, Brakin M, Juan C. Congenital rubella and myxedema. Pediatrics 69:495, 1982.

511. Ziring PR, Fedun BA, Cooper LZ. Thyrotoxicosis in congenital rubella. J Pediatr 87:1002, 1975.

512. Preece MA, Kearney PJ, Marshall WC. Growth hormone deficiency in congenital rubella. Lancet 2:842, 1977.

513. Oberfield SE, Cassulo AM, Chiriboga-Klein S, et al. Growth hormone dynamics in congenital rubella syndrome. Brain Dysfunction 1:303, 1988.

514. Chiriboga-Klein S, Oberfield SE, Cassulo AM, et al. Growth in congenital rubella syndrome and correlation with clinical manifestations. J Pediatr 115:251, 1989.

515. Boger WP III. Late ocular complications in congenital rubella syndrome. Ophthalmology 87:1244, 1980.

516. Deutman AF, Grizzard WS. Rubella retinopathy and subretinal neovascularization. Am J Ophthalmol 85:82, 1978.

517. Frank KE, Purnell EW. Subretinal neovascularization following rubella retinopathy. Am J Ophthalmol 86:462, 1978.

518. Boger WP III, Petersen RA, Robb RM. Keratoconus and acute hydrops in mentally retarded patients with

congenital rubella syndrome. Am J Ophthalmol 91:231, 1981.

519. Boger WP III, Petersen RA, Robb RM. Spontaneous absorption of the lens in the congenital rubella syndrome. Arch Ophthalmol 99:433, 1981.

520. Gullikson JS. Tooth morphology in rubella syndrome children. J Dent Child 42:479, 1979.

521. Fortuin NJ, Morrow AG, Roberts WC. Late vascular manifestations of the rubella syndrome: a roentgenographic-pathologic study. Am J Med 51:134, 1971.

522. Anderson H, Barr B, Wedenberg E. Genetic disposition—a prerequisite for maternal rubella deafness. Arch Otolaryngol 91:141, 1970.

523. Orth DH, Fishman GA, Segall M, et al. Rubella maculopathy. BMJ 64:201, 1980.

524. Wolinsky JS, Dau PC, Buimovici-Klein E, et al. Progressive rubella panencephalitis: immunovirological studies and results of isoprinosine therapy. Clin Exp Immunol 35:397, 1979.

525. Preblud SR, Kushubar R, Friedman HM. Rubella hemagglutination inhibition titers. JAMA 247:1181, 1982.

526. Munro ND, Wild HJ, Sheppard S, et al. Fall and rise of immunity to rubella. BMJ 294:481, 1987.

527. Hoskins CS, Pyman C, Wilkins B. The nerve deaf child—intrauterine rubella or not? Arch Dis Child 58:327, 1983.

528. Iurio JL, Hosking CS, Pyman C. Retrospective diagnosis of congenital rubella. BMJ 289:1566, 1984.

529. Vesikari T, Meurman OH, Maki R. Persistent rubella-specific IgM-antibody in the cerebrospinal fluid of a child with congenital rubella. Arch Dis Child 55:46, 1980.

530. Fitzgerald MG, Pullen GR, Hosking CS. Low affinity antibody to rubella antigen in patients after rubella infection in utero. Pediatrics 81:812, 1988.

531. Alestig K, Bartsch FK, Nilsson L-A, et al. Studies of amniotic fluid in women infected with rubella. J Infect Dis 129:79, 1974.

532. Levine MJ, Oxman MN, Moore MG, et al. Diagnosis of congenital rubella in utero. N Engl J Med 290:1187, 1974.

533. Cederqvist LL, Zervoudakis IA, Ewool LC, et al. Prenatal diagnosis of congenital rubella. BMJ 276:615, 1977.

534. Daffos F, Forestier F, Grangeot-Keros L, et al. Prenatal diagnosis of congenital rubella. Lancet 2:1, 1984.

535. Terry GM, Ho-Terry L, Warren RC, et al. First trimester prenatal diagnosis of congenital rubella: a laboratory investigation. BMJ 292:930, 1986.

536. Enders G, Jonatha W. Prenatal diagnosis of intrauterine rubella. Infection 15:162, 1987.

537. Ho-Terry L, Terry GM, Londesborough P, et al. Diagnosis of fetal rubella infection by nucleic acid hybridization. J Med Virol 24:175, 1988.

538. Bosma TJ, Corbett SO, Banatvala JE, Best JM. PCR for detection of rubella virus RNA in clinical samples. J Clin Microbiol 33:1075–1079, 1995.

539. Tanemura M, Suzumori K, Yagami Y, Katow S. Diagnosis of fetal rubella infection with reverse transcription and nested polymerase chain reaction: a study of 34 cases diagnosed in fetuses. Am J Obstet Gynecol 174:578–582, 1996.

540. Revello MG, Baldanti F, Sarasini A, et al. Prenatal diagnosis of rubella virus infection by direct detection and semiquantitation of viral RNA in clinical samples by reverse transcription-PCR. J Clin Microbiol 35:708–713, 1997.

541. McDonald JC. Gamma-globulin for prevention of rubella in pregnancy. BMJ 2:416, 1963.

542. Brody JA, Sever JL, Schiff GM. Prevention of rubella by gamma globulin during an epidemic in Barrow, Alaska, in 1964. N Engl J Med 272:127, 1965.

543. McCallin PF, Fuccillo DA, Ley AC, et al. Gammaglobulin as prophylaxis against rubella-induced congenital anomalies. Obstet Gynecol 39:185, 1972.

544. Urquhart GED, Crawford RJ, Wallace J. Trial of high-titre human rubella immunoglobulin. BMJ 2:1331, 1978.

545. Schiff GM, Sever JL, Huebner RJ. Rubella virus: neutralizing antibody in commercial gamma globulin. Science 142:58, 1963.

546. Armstrong RD, Sinclair A, O'Keefe G, et al. Interferon treatment of chronic rubella associated arthritis. Clin Exp Rheumatol 3:93, 1985.

547. Arvin AM, Schmidt NJ, Cantell K, et al. Alpha interferon administration to infants with congenital rubella. Antimicrob Agents Chemother 21:259, 1982.

548. Larsson A, Forsgren M, Hardaf-Segerstad S, et al. Administration of interferon to an infant with congenital rubella syndrome involving persistent viremia and cutaneous vasculitis. Acta Paediatr Scand 65:105, 1976.

549. Jan JE, Tingle AJ, Donald G, et al. Progressive rubella panencephalitis: clinical course and response to "Isoprinosine." Dev Med Child Neurol 21:648, 1979.

550. Garner JS, Simmons BP. CDC guidelines for isolation precautions in hospitals. Infect Control 4:245, 1983.

551. Williams WW. CDC guidelines for infection control in hospital personnel. Infect Control 4:326, 1983.

552. Schoenbaum SC, Hyde JN, Bartoshesky L, et al. Benefit-cost analysis of rubella vaccination policy. N Engl J Med 294:306, 1976.

553. Furukawa T, Miyata T, Kondo K, et al. Clinical trials of RA 27/3 (Wistar) rubella vaccine in Japan. Am J Dis Child 118:262, 1969.

554. Vaheri A, Vesikari T, Oker-Blom N, et al. Transmission of attenuated rubella vaccines to the human fetus: a preliminary report. Am J Dis Child 118:243, 1969.

555. Recommendations of the Public Health Service Advisory Committee on Immunization Practices. Rubella vaccine. Am J Dis Child 118:397, 1969.

556. Fleet WF Jr, Benz EW Jr, Karzon DT, et al. Fetal consequences of maternal rubella immunization. JAMA 227:621, 1974.

557. Plotkin SA. Rubella vaccine. In Plotkin SA, Mortimer EA Jr (eds). Vaccines. Philadelphia, WB Saunders, 1988, p 235.

558. Brunell PA, Weigle K, Murphy MD. Antibody response following measles-mumps-rubella vaccine under conditions of customary use. JAMA 250:1409, 1983.

559. Mortimer PP, Edwards JMB, Porter AD, et al. Are many women immunized against rubella unnecessarily? J Hyg (London) 87:131, 1981.

560. Greaves WL, Orenstein WA, Hinman AR, et al. Clinical efficacy of rubella vaccine. Pediatr Infect Dis 2:284, 1982.

561. Balfour HH Jr, Amren DP. Rubella, measles and mumps antibodies following vaccination of children. Am J Dis Child 132:573, 1978.

562. Orenstein WA, Herrmann KL, Holmgreen P, et al. Prevalence of rubella antibodies in Massachusetts schoolchildren. Am J Epidemiol 124:290, 1986.

563. Rutledge SL, Snead OC III. Neurologic complications of immunizations. J Pediatr 109:917, 1986.

564. Losonsky GA, Fishaut JM, Strussenberg J, et al. Effect of immunization against rubella on lactation products: I. Development and characterization of specific immunologic reactivity in breast milk. J Infect Dis 145:654, 1982.

565. Losonsky GA, Fishaut JM, Strussenberg J, et al. Effect of immunization against rubella on lactation products: II. Maternal-neonatal interactions. J Infect Dis 145:661, 1982.

566. Landes RD, Bass JW, Millunchick EW, et al. Neonatal rubella following maternal immunization. J Pediatr 97:465, 1980.

567. Centers for Disease Control. Immunization practices in colleges—United States. MMWR Morb Mortal Wkly Rep 36:209, 1987.

568. Edgar WM, Hambling MH. Rubella vaccination and anti-D immunoglobulin administration in the puerperium. Br J Obstet Gynaecol 84:754, 1977.

569. Watt RW, McGucken RB. Failure of rubella immunization after blood transfusion: birth of congenitally infected infant. BMJ 281:977, 1980.

570. Black NA, Parsons A, Kurtz JB, et al. Post-pubertal rubella immunisation: a controlled trial of two vaccines. Lancet 2:990, 1983.

571. McIntosh ED, Menser MA. A fifty-year follow-up of congenital rubella. Lancet 340:414, 1992.

572. Noticeboard. Congenital rubella—50 years on. Lancet 337:668, 1991.

573. Schluter WW, Reef SE, Redd C, et al. Changing epidemiology of congenital rubella syndrome in the United States. J Infect Dis 178:636–641, 1998.

574. Plotkin SA, Katz M, Cordero JF. The eradication of rubella. JAMA 281:561–562, 1999.

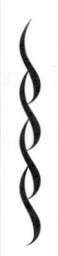

C H A P T E R 7

Cytomegalovirus

SERGIO STAGNO, M.D.

Cytomegaloviruses (CMV) comprise a group of agents in the herpesvirus family known for their ubiquitous distribution in humans and in numerous other mammals. In vivo and in vitro infections with CMV are highly species specific and result in a characteristic cytopathology of greatly enlarged (cytomegalic) cells containing intranuclear and cytoplasmic inclusions.[1] The strikingly large, inclusion-bearing cells with a typical owl's eye appearance were first reported by Ribbert in 1881 from the kidneys of a stillborn infant with congenital syphilis.[2] Subsequently, Jesionek and Kiolemenoglou reported similar findings for another stillborn infant with congenital syphilis.[3] In 1907, Lowenstein described inclusions in 4 of 30 parotid glands obtained from children from 2 months to 2 years of age.[4] Subsequently, Goodpasture and Talbot noted the similarity of these cells to the inclusion-bearing cells (giant cells) found in cutaneous lesions caused by varicella virus, and they postulated that cytomegaly was the result of a similar agent.[5] The observation of a similar cytopathic effect after infection with herpes simplex led Lipschutz and then others to suggest that these characteristic cellular changes were a specific reaction of the host to infection with a virus.[6] The observation by Cole and Kuttner that inclusion-

bearing salivary glands from older guinea pigs were infectious for younger animals after being passed through a Berkefeld N filter in a highly species-specific manner led to the denomination of these agents as *salivary gland viruses*.[7] The cellular changes observed in tissue sections from patients with a fatal infection led to the use of the term *cytomegalic inclusion disease* (CID) years before the causative agent was identified.

In 1954, Smith succeeded in propagating murine CMV in explant cultures of mouse embryonic fibroblasts.[8] Utilization of similar techniques led to the independent isolation of human CMV shortly thereafter by Smith,[9] Rowe and co-workers,[10] and Weller and associates.[11] Smith isolated the agent from two infants with CID. Rowe and associates isolated three strains of CMV from adenoidal tissue of children undergoing adenoidectomy. The term *AD169* to designate a common laboratory-adapted strain of CMV comes from these studies. Weller and associates isolated the virus from the urine and liver of living infants with generalized CID. The term *cytomegalovirus* was proposed in 1960 by Weller and colleagues to replace the names CID and salivary gland virus, which were misleading because the virus usually involved other organs and because the name salivary gland virus had been used to designate unrelated agents obtained from bats.[12]

The propagation of CMV in vitro led to the rapid development of serologic methods such as neutralization and complement fixation. Using such antibody assays and viral isolation, several investigators quickly established that human CMV was a significant pathogen in humans. This ancient virus, like other members of the herpesvirus family, infects almost all humans at some time during their lives.[13, 14] Evidence of infection has been found in all populations tested. The age at acquisition of infection differs in various geographic groups and socioeconomic settings, which results in major differences in prevalence among groups. The natural history of human CMV infection is very complex. After a primary infection, viral excretion, occasionally from several sites, persists for weeks, months, or even years before the virus becomes latent. Episodes of recurrent infection with renewed viral shedding are common, even years after the primary infection. These episodes of recurrent infection are most often due to reactivation of latent viruses, but reinfections with an antigenically diverse strain of CMV are also possible. In immunocompetent hosts, CMV infections are generally subclinical. However, when infection occurs during pregnancy without consequences for the mother, it can have serious repercussions for the fetus. Even though most immunocompromised hosts tolerate CMV infections relatively well, in some instances, such as acquired immunodeficiency syndrome (AIDS) and bone marrow transplants, CMV can cause disease of diverse severity and the infection can be life threatening. As a result of a long-standing and close host-parasite relationship, many—probably thousands—genetically different strains of CMV have evolved and circulate in the general population.[15]

THE VIRUS

Morphology

Electron microscopic studies have shown that CMV is morphologically similar to the other human herpesviruses. It is, however, the largest member of the family, with a diameter of approximately 200 nm.[16, 17] The virus consists of a 64-nm core enclosed by a 110-nm icosahedral capsid composed of 162 capsomeres, each of which is a hollow hexagon in cross-section. The capsid is surrounded by a poorly defined amorphous tegument, which is itself surrounded by a loosely applied lipid-containing envelope.[16, 17] The envelope is most likely acquired during the budding process through the nuclear membrane into a cytoplasmic vacuole, which contains the protein components of the envelope. The mature virions exit the cells by a process similar to reverse pinocytosis. When CMV is propagated in vitro, several morphologically defective forms of CMV can be found within the cytoplasm of infected cells as well as in the extracellular medium. The best-known form is the so-called dense body, which is often present in 1000-fold excess of infectious virions.[18] Dense bodies contain nearly all the protein components of the virion, with

the exception of viral nucleic acids.[19] The second most abundant and well-studied form has been termed *noninfectious enveloped particles*, which consist of an empty capsid surrounded by a lipid envelope.[19]

Genome

The genome of CMV consists of a linear double-stranded DNA molecule of approximately 240 kilobases in size (150×10^6 daltons).[20–23] The genome of CMV is similar to that of herpes simplex virus in that it has long and short unique sequences, both of which are bounded by homologous repetitive sequences. Each long and short sequence can be arranged in one of two directions so that four DNA isomeres are produced by cells in culture (Fig. 7–1). The GC content of human CMV is high (58%) and, together with its genomic structure, has placed CMV into the beta-herpesvirus subgroup.[24] The massive CMV genome, which is approximately 50% larger than the genome of herpes simplex, encodes for at least 35 unique virion proteins and an undefined number of nonstructural proteins.[18, 25–27] At least five electrophoretically distinct capsid proteins ranging in size from 155,000 to 11,000 daltons have been identified within mature virions.[28] Many of the CMV capsid proteins appear to share structural, functional, and even antigenic similarities with capsid proteins from other human herpesviruses.[29, 29a] All (five) capsid proteins are immunogenic, as shown by specific antibody responses in convalescent sera. Outside the capsid but beneath the envelope is the tegument or matrix. Within this region are five of the most abundant and immunogenic proteins encoded by CMV. They induce both rapid and durable antibody responses. Their molecular masses range from 28,000 to 220,000 daltons.[30–32] The tegument region also contains proteins that probably contribute to early gene expression after delivery of incoming viral genomes to the cell nucleus, and in the late stages of infection tegument proteins probably play a critical role in virion morphogenesis.[33] The lipid-containing envelope is composed of virion glycoproteins and host-derived membrane lipids. Although the CMV genome has been shown to contain over 50 open reading frames that could encode glycoproteins, only 6 or 7 have thus far been identified and characterized.[33] The envelope of CMV is thought to play an essential role in the initial steps of virus–host cell interactions, and host immune responses against virion components are thought to be important in protective immunity.[33] The most abundant and most immunogenic glycoprotein of the envelope is glycoprotein B (gB).[34–36]

Replicative Cycle

The replication of CMV is very similar to the pattern described for herpes simplex virus, but the replicative cycle is much slower.[37] In contrast to herpes simplex virus, CMV does not shut off host cell protein synthesis until late in the replication cycle. In fact, CMV initially increases host cell protein, suggesting that it may depend on several key host cell enzymes for replication and assembly. After attachment, possibly through specific

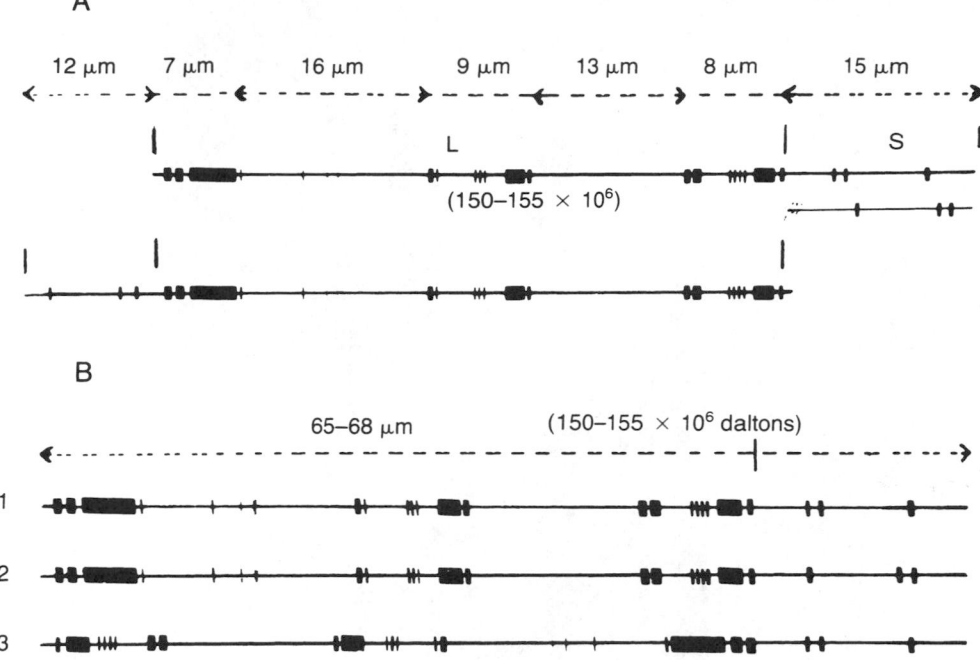

FIGURE 7–1 Molecular arrangement of human CMV DNA. Dark bars represent denatured regions. *A,* Summary of observed features and length obtained from study of partial denaturation of viral DNA. *B,* Four possible orientations of CMV DNA. L = long segment; S = short segment.

cell surface molecules such as proteoglycan heparan sulfate,[38, 39] higher affinity interactions occur through virus-specific receptors. Attachment and cell membrane fusion and penetration are mediated by viral envelope glycoproteins, and antibodies directed against these proteins can neutralize infectious virus.[40, 41] The virus penetrates the cell membrane and is enclosed within a cytoplasmic vacuole. The virus then uncoats, and the nucleocapsids proceed rapidly to the nucleus by a pathway that may involve the cellular cytoskeleton.[42] Shortly thereafter, restricted expression of virus-specified RNA immediate-early or alpha gene transcripts can be found in the absence of de novo protein synthesis or viral DNA replication.[43–46] This phase has been called the "immediate-early" period. The expression of these proteins is essential for the expression of the next set of viral genes, the early or beta genes, which represent the second major class of RNA transcripts. These genes are transcribed from throughout the genome and encode for a variety of proteins, including viral DNA polymerase and other enzymes necessary for replication of viral DNA. In contrast to the immediate-early phase, the "early" phase of gene expression lasts longer, extending well past the first 24 hours of infection and into the late phase of transcription. Some structural proteins, most notably components of the tegument, are also synthesized at this early time. This class of genes includes replicative enzymes such as the viral polymerases.[33]

The "late" period of CMV replication can be defined as the time after viral DNA replication; it occurs from 36 to 48 hours after viral infection. This period coincides with the production of structural proteins of the virion and with the release of infectious virions.

The synthesis of the CMV genome proceeds along an orderly cascade in which each phase controls the progression into the next period. Metabolic inhibitors (cyclohexamide, phosphonoacetic acid, or cytarabine) can be employed to modify this cascade.[47–49] For instance, if cells are infected with CMV in the presence of an inhibitor of protein synthesis, the net effect is a high concentration of messenger RNA. To prevent the progression from immediate-early to early protein synthesis, one can incorporate inhibitors of transcription into the medium. Finally, to inhibit the progression from early to late protein synthesis, inhibitors of DNA synthesis can be added to cultures. Virus assembly begins in the nucleus of the infected cells with the formation of the capsid structure.[50] Newly replicated DNA is packaged in the capsid, and tegument components are added before exiting the nucleus. Final envelopment occurs in the cytoplasm. Mature virions are released by the lysis of infected cells or by reverse endocytosis.[33]

Growth in Tissue Culture

Although human CMV infection in vivo involves primarily epithelial cells, the only cells that are fully permissive for CMV replication in the laboratory are human fibroblasts.[1] Permissive infection is routinely obtained only in terminally differentiated cells. CMV can be recovered from epithelial cells, peripheral blood mononuclear cells, cells from the central nervous system, and endothelial cells.[51, 52] Common sources of fibroblasts include embryonic skin, muscle, lung, and foreskin. The characteristic cytopathic changes induced by CMV in tissue culture appear more slowly than the

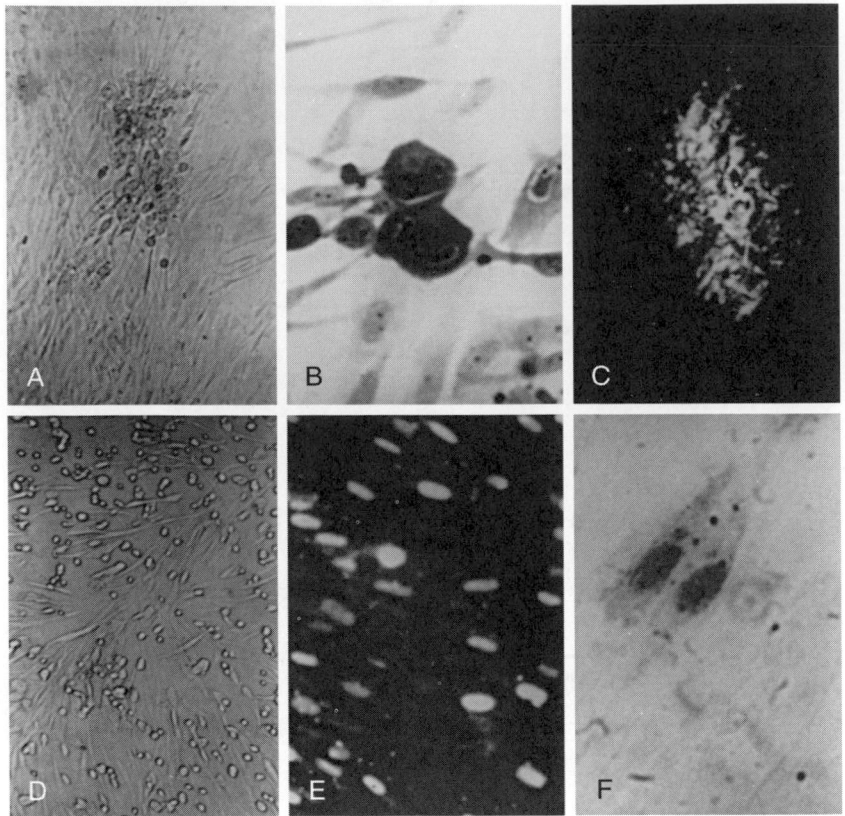

FIGURE 7–2 *A,* Focal cytopathic effect of clinical isolate of CMV in human foreskin fibroblasts (unstained preparation). *B,* Cytopathic effect of clinical isolate of CMV in human foreskin fibroblasts. Note prominent intranuclear inclusion, nuclear halo, and eosinophilic cytoplasmic inclusion. (H & E × 500.) *C,* Focal cytopathic effect detected by anticomplement immunofluorescence. *D,* Generalized cytopathic effect 24 hours after inoculation of a clinical isolate of CMV with a high multiplicity of infection. The specimen is urine from an infant with congenital CMV infection. *E,* CMV-specific early antigens detected by monoclonal antibodies, 24 hours after inoculation of a clinical specimen with a high multiplicity of infection. Similar staining can be obtained with fluorescein-labeled monoclonal antibodies to CMV early antigens. *F,* Detection of CMV-specific early antigens by enzyme-linked immunosorbent assay.

changes induced by other viruses, such as herpes simplex.

Depending on the amount of CMV present in the preparations, a characteristic cytopathic effect may develop within hours or weeks after inoculation.[53] In unstained specimens, early cytopathic changes consist of small, round or elongated foci of enlarged refractile cells (Fig. 7–2*A*). Because infectious CMV is mainly cell associated, infection usually spreads from cell to cell, and the foci gradually enlarge. When the amount of infectious virus contained in the inoculum is large, generalized cell rounding may appear within 24 hours (see Fig. 7–2*D*). A similar phenomenon can be observed with laboratory-adapted strains of CMV inoculated at high multiplicity of input. The phenomenon is believed to be related to the synthesis of immediate-early and early protein. Of great diagnostic significance, these early antigens can be detected with CMV-specific monoclonal antibodies within 24 hours of inoculation of clinical specimens (see Fig. 7–2*E* and *F*).

The adaptation of clinical isolates in the laboratory leads to higher yields of both intracellular and extracellular virus, and as a result the progression of cytopathology is markedly enhanced.

In infected monolayers fixed with Bouin's solution and stained with hematoxylin and eosin, cell enlargement or rounding (or both) is visualized within 6 hours after infection. By 24 hours, the nucleus is eccentrically placed with prominent nuclei (see Fig. 7–2*B*). An eosinophilic paranuclear inclusion develops, and cell enlargement is more apparent. Between 48 and 72 hours after infection, an irregular skeinlike basophilic nuclear inclu-

sion appears. The cytoplasm stains more basophilic, and the eosinophilic paranuclear inclusion is more prominent. Multinucleated cells can be seen, with inclusion-bearing nuclei arranged concentrically around the large eosinophilic inclusion.

Antigenic Structure

A number of studies have shown that all known strains of CMV are genetically homologous but that none appear to be genetically identical unless they were obtained from epidemiologically related cases.[54, 55]

Early serologic studies used relatively crude sources of antigen. In recent years it has been possible, by using more refined immunologic techniques, to assess the humoral immune response of the host to individual CMV-encoded proteins. For instance, antibodies against all five components of the capsid have been demonstrated.[34, 56–58] In fact, tegument proteins pp 150 and pp 65 are the most immunogenic proteins within the virion.[59–62] The most likely reason for the consistency of these observations is that this particular protein is by far the most abundant virus-encoded protein, accounting for more than 50% of the mass of the virus.[63] Other proteins, including nonstructural proteins 49 and 72, are readily detectable.[57, 58, 64] Antibodies reactive with these proteins are unlikely to be protective in vivo, because these structures do not exist on either the surface of infected cells or infectious viruses and thus are not accessible to antiviral antibodies.[33, 62]

In contrast, antibodies against the major components of the virion envelope, gB and gH, neutralize virus infectivity and appear to provide some protection in vivo.[33, 65-67] A correlation exists between clinical presentation/outcome and the presence of virus-neutralizing antibodies in both normal individuals and immunocompromised hosts.[68, 69] The most immunogenic component of the envelope is gB. Anti-gB antibodies represent the bulk of neutralizing antibodies generated in vivo.[66-68] The next most immunogenic component of the envelope is gH. This protein appears to be less immunogenic than gB, although it does induce a neutralizing response in vivo and is also expressed on the surface of the infected cells. Other virus-encoded proteins also induce strong antibody responses, but most of these do not appear to provide protective immunity in the host.[33] These antibody responses are important in serodiagnosis of CMV. Tegument proteins pp 65 and pp 150 have high degrees of specificity and sensitivity for detecting IgG antibodies.[70] In addition, pp 50 may be useful in serologic assays for the detection of CMV-specific IgM antibodies.[71] Cross-reactive antibodies against homologous proteins of other herpesviruses have been described.[72]

Studies in allograft recipients have repeatedly shown that deficits in T lymphocyte responses are associated with more severe CMV infections in the post-transplant period.[33, 73, 74] The absence of CMV-specific major histocompatibility complex (MHC) restricted CD8+ cytotoxic T lymphocytes is also correlated with severe disease in bone marrow allograft recipients.[73] On the other hand, the passive transfer of CMV-specific cytotoxic T lymphocytes to patients in the post-transplant period improves patient outcome.[75] Two tegument proteins, pp 65 and pp 150, are dominant targets of CMV-specific T lymphocyte responses.[76] In addition, proliferative responses of CD4 lymphocytes after stimulation with recombinant pp 65 and pp 150 have been reported.[33, 77]

EPIDEMIOLOGY

Overall

Human CMV is highly species specific, and humans are believed to be its only reservoir.[1] CMV infection is endemic and without seasonal variation.[14] Seroepidemiologic surveys have found CMV infection in every human population that has been tested.[13, 14] The prevalence of antibody to CMV increases with age, but, according to geographic and ethnic and socioeconomic backgrounds, the patterns of acquisition of infection vary widely among populations (Fig. 7-3).[15] In general, the prevalence of CMV infection is higher in developing countries and among the lower socioeconomic strata of the more developed nations. These differences are particularly striking during childhood. For instance, in Africa and the South Pacific, the rate of seropositivity was 95 to 100% among preschool children studied, whereas surveys in Great Britain and in certain populations in the United States have generally found that less than 20% of children of similar ages are seropositive.

The level of immunity among women of childbearing age, which is an important factor in determining the incidence and significance of congenital and perinatal CMV infections, also varies widely among different populations. Several reports indicate that seropositivity rates in young women in the United States and Western Europe range from less than 50 to 85%.[13, 78] In contrast, in the Ivory Coast,[79] Japan,[80] and Chile,[81] the rate of seropositivity is greater than 90% by the end of the second decade of life. More important, from the point of view of congenital infection, prospective studies of pregnant women in the United States indicate that the rate of CMV acquisition for childbearing-aged women of middle to higher socioeconomic background is approximately 2% per year, whereas it is 6% per year among women of lower socioeconomic background.[82]

The modes of transmission from person to person are incompletely understood. The following features of CMV infection make it difficult to study the modes of acquisition.[78] In the majority of individuals, CMV infections are subclinical, including those acquired in utero and during the perinatal period. Infected persons continue to expose other susceptible people. Virus excretion persists for years after congenital, perinatal, and early postnatal infections. Prolonged viral shedding is

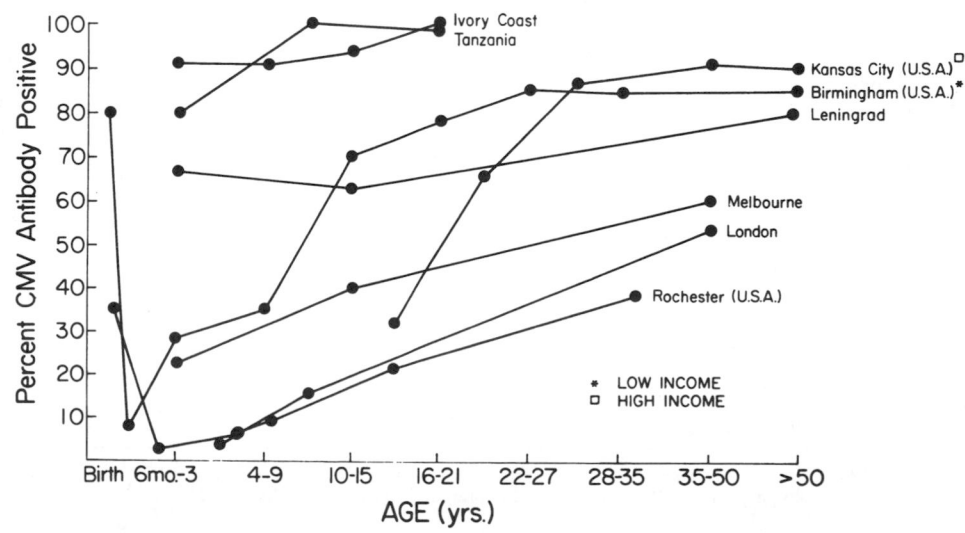

FIGURE 7-3 Age-related prevalence of antibody to CMV in various populations. (From Alford CA, et al. Epidemiology of cytomegalovirus. *In* Nahmias AJ, Dowdle WR, Schinazi RE [eds]. The Human Herpesviruses. New York, Elsevier/North-Holland, 1981, p 161, with permission.)

also a feature of primary infection in older children and adults. Because recurrent infections are fairly common, intermittent excretion of virus can be anticipated in a significant proportion of seropositive adults.

It is clear that a large reservoir of CMV exists in the population at all times. Transmission occurs by direct or indirect person-to-person contact. Sources of virus include urine, oropharyngeal secretions, cervical and vaginal secretions, semen, milk, tears, blood products, and organ allografts.[83-87]

CMV is not very contagious because the spread of infection appears to require close or intimate contact with infected secretions. As indicated, the prevalence of CMV infection and the risk of seroconversion are higher for populations of low socioeconomic status, presumably a reflection of factors that account for increased exposure to CMV such as crowding, sexual practices, and increased exposure to infants and toddlers. Sexual contact contributes to the spread of CMV. Higher rates of seropositivity have been observed among males and females with multiple sex partners and histories of sexually transmitted diseases.[88-91]

Certain child-rearing practices influence the spread of CMV among children. Because seropositive women often excrete CMV in milk, the incidence of perinatal CMV infection is high where breast-feeding is a common practice. As shown in Table 7–1, in countries where the vast majority of women of childbearing age have already been infected with CMV and the practice of breast-feeding is almost universal, the rates of infection of infants ranged from 28 to 100% at an average of 1 year of age.[86] These observations indicate that as breast-feeding regains popularity in the United States, the incidence of perinatal transmission of CMV will increase, thus creating an even larger pool of infected children.[92, 93]

In 1971, Weller suggested that the high rate of seropositivity among Swedish children was probably due to the frequent use of day-care centers.[1] Swedish children had a rate of infection that was three to four times higher than that observed in London or in Rochester, New York. As shown in Table 7–2, high rates of CMV infection among children attending day-care centers were later confirmed in Sweden and have been reported in several studies in the United States.[94-98] The studies, which included a control group of children, confirmed that the rate of CMV infection was substantially higher among those in day care than in those who stayed at home.[94, 95] In the study of Pass and co-workers, in a group of 70 children of middle- to upper-income background whose ages ranged from 3 to 65 months, the rate of CMV excretion in urine and saliva was 51%.[94] The lowest rate of excretion (9%) occurred in infants younger than 1 year of age, and the highest rate (88%) was among toddlers in their second year of life. Infants younger than 12 months of age in group day care who excrete CMV are more likely to have acquired CMV congenitally or perinatally from maternal cervical secretions or breast milk. Twelve children whose mothers were seronegative excreted CMV, which indicated that their infection was not perinatally acquired. The findings of Pass and co-workers have been subsequently confirmed by other investigators. There is now compelling evidence that the high rate of CMV infection among children in group day care is caused by horizontal transmission from child to child. The route of transmission that appears most likely is the transfer of virus that occurs through saliva on hands and toys.[99, 100] No data have indicated CMV transmission through respiratory droplets.

The strongest evidence supporting child-to-child transmission was obtained by analysis of the restriction

TABLE 7–1
Breast-Feeding Patterns and Prevalence of CMV Infections in Young Children of Various Nations

| NATION | BREAST-FEEDING RATE | | % SEROPOSITIVE | |
	Ever	At 3 mo	Mothers	Children (Age)
Solomon Islands	100	97	100	100 (5 mo to 4 yr)
India				
Vellore	96	64	98	80 (1yr)
Pondicherry			97	67 (1–5 yr)
Barbados	96	?	77	62 (1–5 yr)
Guatemala	95	?	98	47 (6 mo to 1 yr)
Chile	89	?	92	42 (1–2 yr)
Japan				
Sapporo	?	56	67	42 (6 mo to 2 yr)
Sendai			85	38 (1 yr)
Finland (Helsinki)	95	50	55	28 (1 yr)
United States				
Houston, Texas	46	?	48	15 (1 yr)
Birmingham, Alabama	8	?	85	8 (1 yr)
France (Paris)	85	?	56	10 (10 mo)
Canada (Nova Scotia)	49	26	34	12 (6 mo to 1 yr)
United Kingdom (Manchester)	51	13	59	12 (3–11 mo)

Modified from Pass RF. Transmission of viruses through human milk. *In* Howell RR, Morris FH Jr, Pickering K (eds). Role of Human Milk in Infant Nutrition and Health. Courtesy of Charles C Thomas, Publisher, Springfield, Illinois, 1986, pp 205–224.

TABLE 7–2
Prevalence of CMV Excretion Among Children in Day-Care Centers

INVESTIGATOR	YEAR	LOCATION	% INFECTED (NO.)
Stangert	1976	Stockholm	35 (7/20)
Strom	1979	Stockholm	72 (13/18)
Pass	1982	Birmingham, Alabama	51 (36/70)
Adler	1985	Richmond, Virginia	24 (16/66)
Hutto	1985	Birmingham, Alabama	41 (77/188)
MMWR	1985	Birmingham, Alabama	29 (66/231)
Jones	1985	San Francisco, California	22 (31/140)
Murph	1986	Iowa City, Iowa	22 (9/41)
Adler	1987	Richmond, Virginia	53 (55/104)

Data from Adler SP. Cytomegalovirus transmission among children in daycare, their mothers and caretakers. Pediatr Infect Dis J 7:279–285, 1988.

enzyme digestion patterns of CMV DNA of the isolates obtained from infected children attending day care. Adler examined the restriction endonuclease patterns of isolates obtained from 16 children at a single day-care center.[97] Four children older than 28 months who shared a common room were shedding a common strain. A second strain was shed by seven children younger than 28 months who had little contact with the older group but who played with one another daily. Only five of the infected children were shedding unique strains. In a subsequent study, Adler identified by endonuclease analysis 14 different strains of CMV among 104 children in a single day-care center who were monitored at 4-month intervals for over 26 months.[101] Three of these 14 strains infected 44 children, all of whom were younger than 3 years of age. Of 75 initially seronegative children, 34 acquired day-care–associated strains, whereas 4 were infected with unique isolates. The findings of Adler, which have been confirmed by others, demonstrate that CMV is very efficiently transmitted from child to child in the day-care setting and that it is not unusual to find excretion rates as high as 20 to 40% in young toddlers.[96, 102] In many instances, these rates of infection are substantially higher than the seroprevalence rates for the parents of the children and young adults in the cities where the studies were done.[93]

These observations in day-care centers indicate that as children become mobile and engage in close interpersonal contact, CMV can be expected to spread rapidly among them.[93] With the changes in child-rearing practices now occurring in the United States and the resurgence of breast-feeding, significant changes in the epidemiology of CMV can be expected within the next decades.[93]

An important issue is whether children excreting CMV can become a source of infection for serosusceptible child-care personnel and parents, particularly women of childbearing age. Transmission of CMV from an infant to his or her mother and from an infant to a pregnant aunt with subsequent transmission to her infant has been confirmed by restriction endonuclease mapping of CMV DNA.[103, 104] Seroepidemiologic studies suggest that parents often acquire CMV from their children who became infected outside the family. For instance, Yeager reported that 7 of 15 (47%) seronegative mothers of premature infants who acquired CMV in a nursery seroconverted within 1 year.[105] Dworsky and colleagues reported that the rate of seroconversion for women with at least one child living at home was 5.5%, significantly higher than the 2.3% rate for women from the same clinic who were pregnant for the first time or the rates for susceptible nursery nurses and for physicians in training.[106] Taber and associates monitored the acquisition of CMV in 68 Houston families observed for a mean of 3.5 years per family.[107] The study showed a significant association between seroconversion among children and seroconversion among susceptible parents. Taber and associates found that in 10 of the 18 families in which the index case was known, CMV infection in a child preceded seroconversion in the parents. Adler and Pass and co-workers have presented more compelling evidence linking the acquisition of CMV by children in day care with subsequent infection in their mothers and caregivers.[101–103, 108–110] Pass and co-workers did a longitudinal serologic follow-up study of seronegative parents whose children attended a day-care center and of seronegative parents whose children did not attend day care.[108] The groups were followed for a mean of 17 and 21 months, respectively. The study revealed that 14 of 67 seronegative parents with children in day-care centers acquired CMV, compared with none of 31 serosusceptible parents whose children did not attend day care. More significant, all 14 parents of the day-care group who seroconverted had a child who was shedding CMV in saliva or urine. In fact, seroconversion occurred in 14 to 48 parents of children who shed CMV, compared with none of 21 whose children did not excrete CMV. The highest risk of seroconversion (45%) was for parents with a child shedding CMV who was 18 months of age or younger at enrollment. In 2 of the 14 cases, DNA analysis indicated the child as the source of CMV infection. In a subsequent study, this group of investigators also demonstrated by means of restriction enzyme analysis that infections acquired by a mother from a child can be transmitted to her fetus.[102] In a very similar study, Adler observed that of 18 seronegative mothers whose children shed CMV strains associated with day care, 6 seroconverted and excreted CMV strains identical to the strains shed by their children.[101] On average, these mothers acquired the infection within 4.2 months

TABLE 7–3
Rate of Congenital CMV Infection in Relation to Rate of Maternal Immunity in Various Locales

LOCATION AND DATE	NO. OF INFANTS	% CONGENITAL CMV INFECTION	% MATERNAL SEROPOSITIVITY
Manchester, England, 1978	6051	0.24	25
Aarhus-Viborg, Denmark, 1979	3060	0.4	52
Hamilton, Canada, 1980	15,212	0.42	44
Halifax, Canada, 1975	542	0.55	37
Birmingham, Alabama (upper SES), 1981	2698	0.6	80
Houston, Texas (upper SES), 1980	461	0.6	50
London, England, 1973	720	0.69	58
Houston, Texas (low SES), 1980	493	1.2	83
Abidjan, Ivory Coast, 1978	2032	1.38	100
Sendai, Japan, 1970	132	1.4	83
Santiago, Chile, 1976	118	1.7	98
Helsinki, Finland, 1977	200	2.0	85
Birmingham, Alabama (low SES), 1980	1412	2.2	85

SES = socioeconomic status.
From Stagno S, et al. Maternal cytomegalovirus infection and perinatal transmission. Clin Obstet Gynecol 25:564, 1982, with permission.

(range, 3 to 7 months) after their children became infected.

In assessing the risk to caretakers working with young children in day-care centers, Adler has reported an annual seroconversion rate of 11% among 202 seronegative women employed at 33 day-care centers in Richmond, Virginia.[110] This rate was significantly higher than the 2% annual rate occurring among a group of 229 female hospital employees matched for age, race, and marital status. The restriction endonuclease DNA patterns of 17 of 31 isolates of CMV obtained from day-care workers were compared with the DNAs of isolates shed by the children cared for by these women. Nine of the 17 isolates were identical to the DNAs of isolates shed by one or more children. These observations provide compelling evidence that serosusceptible women who work with children in day care have an occupational risk of acquiring CMV.

From the data generated from these studies, it is reasonable to expect that approximately 50% of susceptible children between the ages of 1 and 3 years who attend group day care will acquire CMV from their playmates and become an important potential source of infection for susceptible parents and caregivers.[93] Of particular concern is the risk to seronegative mothers who have children in group day care and who become pregnant.[93]

Fomites may also play some role in transmission because CMV has been shown to retain infectivity for hours on plastic surfaces and has been isolated from randomly selected toys and surfaces in a day-care center.[99, 100]

Maternal Infection and Vertical Transmission

Because maternal CMV infection is the origin of congenital infections and of most perinatal infections, it is important to review the relevant issues that pertain to vertical transmission. As used here, vertical transmission implies transmission from mother to infant.

CONGENITAL INFECTION

Congenital infection is assumed to be the result of transplacental transmission. In the United States, congenital CMV infection occurs in between 0.2 and 2.2% (average, 1%) of all newborns. However, as shown in Table 7–3, the incidence of congenital infection is quite variable among different populations. The natural history of CMV during pregnancy is particularly complex and has not been fully explained. Infections such as rubella and toxoplasmosis cannot serve as models. With these infections, in utero transmission occurs only as a result of a primary infection acquired during pregnancy, whereas the in utero transmission of CMV can occur as a consequence of both primary and recurrent infections.[80, 111] Far from being a rare event, congenital infection resulting from recurrent CMV infection has been shown to be common, especially in highly immune populations. The initial clue was provided by three independent reports of congenital CMV infections that occurred in consecutive pregnancies.[112–114] In all three instances, the first infant was severely affected or died and the second born in each case was subclinically infected. More convincing evidence came from a prospective study of women known to be seroimmune before conception.[111] As shown in Table 7–4, the rate of congenital CMV infection was 1.9% among 541 infants born to these seropositive women. Clearly, the 10 congenitally infected infants were not infected as a result of primary maternal CMV infection because all mothers were known to have been infected with CMV from one to several years before the onset of pregnancy. Shortly after our studies were published, Schopfer and associates found that in an Ivory Coast population in which virtually all inhabitants are infected in childhood, the prevalence of congenital CMV infection was 1.4%.[80]

This remarkable phenomenon of intrauterine trans-

TABLE 7–4

Incidence of Congenital CMV Infection in a Low-Income Population

PARAMETER	TOTAL	NO. INFECTED (%)
Incidence in general infant population	1412	31 (2.2)
Incidence with recurrent maternal infection		
Previously seropositive	457	8 (1.8)
Prior CMV excretion	58	1 (1.7)
Prior intrauterine transmission	26	1 (3.8)
Total	541	10 (1.9)

From Stagno S, et al. Maternal cytomegalovirus infection and perinatal transmission. Clin Obstet Gynecol 25:567, 1982, with permission.

mission that occurs in the presence of substantial humoral immunity has been attributed to reactivation of endogenous virus. Of particular significance is our observation that the viruses isolated from each of three pairs of congenitally infected siblings were identical when examined by restriction endonuclease analysis.[115] In two of these three pairs, the first-born infant was severely affected, whereas the second-born sibling was subclinically infected, which suggested that virulence of infection was not related to strain and that maternal immunity in some way attenuated the fetal infection.

This unique characteristic of intrauterine transmission in immune women accounts for the direct relationship

between the incidence of congenital CMV infection and the rate of seropositivity shown in Table 7–3. At present, it is impossible to define by either virologic or serologic markers which patient may undergo a reactivation of CMV, nor is it possible to define the time of intrauterine transmission with such reactivation during pregnancy. The sites from which CMV reactivates to produce congenital infection are not known and are likely inaccessible to sampling during pregnancy. Figure 7–4 summarizes our estimates of the maternal risk of acquiring both primary and recurrent CMV infections during pregnancy and the risk of intrauterine transmission with the consequences to the offspring in women both of low-income and of high-income backgrounds in the United States.

Although CMV excretion is a relatively common event during and after pregnancy, studies have demonstrated that the simple isolation of virus during pregnancy is a poor indicator of the risk of intrauterine infection.

Virus can be shed at variable rates from single or multiple sites after primary or recurrent infections in females whether pregnant or not. Sites of excretion include the genital tract, cervix, urinary tract, pharynx, and breast. Table 7–5 summarizes the results of one study of the prevalence of viral shedding according to site and pregnant status in women of low socioeconomic background.[115] In pregnant women, virus was excreted most commonly from the cervix (8.6%) and, in decreasing order, from the urinary tract (3.9%) and the throat (1.8%). From women shedding at other sites, 37 speci-

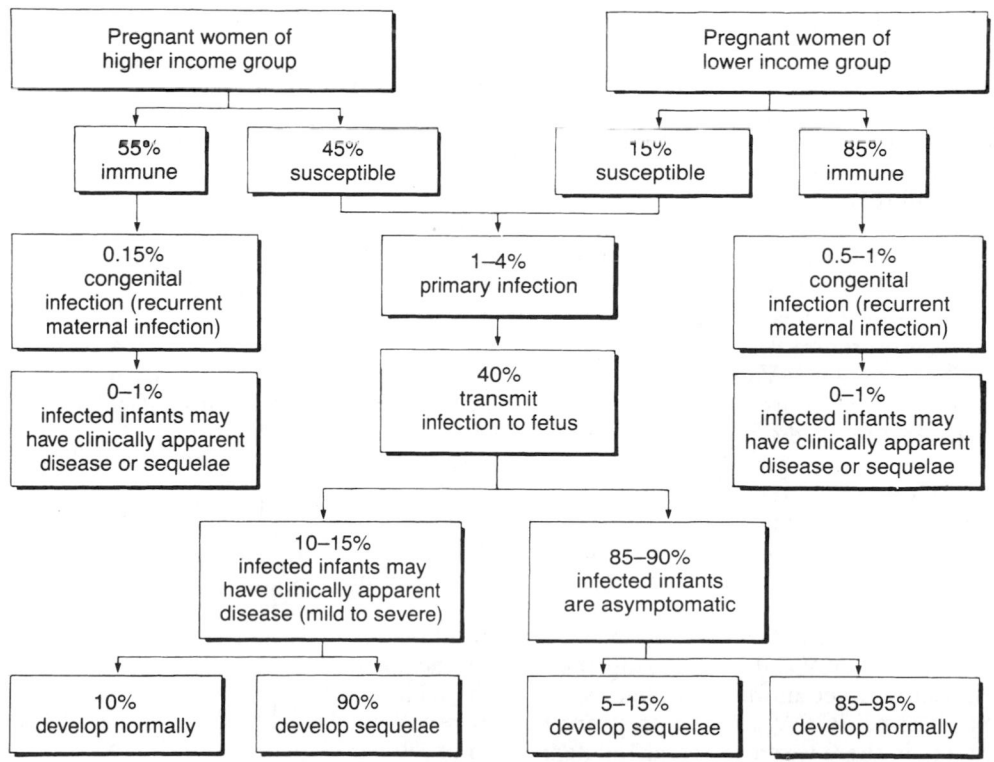

FIGURE 7–4 Characteristics of CMV infection in pregnancy. (From Stagno S, Whitley RJ. Herpesvirus infection of pregnancy. N Engl J Med 313:1270–1274, 1985.)

TABLE 7–5

Rate of CMV Excretion by Site in Pregnant and Nonpregnant Women of Low Socioeconomic Background in Birmingham, Alabama

SITE	PREGNANT WOMEN, NO. POSITIVE/TOTAL (%)	NONPREGNANT WOMEN, NO. POSITIVE/ TOTAL (%)
Cervix	134/1552 (8.6)	43/398 (10.8)
Urine	27/684 (3.9)	6/230 (2.6)
Throat	10/562 (1.8)	
Amniotic fluid[a]	0/37 (0)	
Buffy coat[a]	2/108 (1.8)	
Milk[b]	51/353 (14.4)	

[a]Specimens collected from women excreting CMV in other sites.
[b]Immediate post partum.
From Stagno S, et al. Maternal cytomegalovirus infection and perinatal transmission. Clin Obstet Gynecol 25:570, 1982, with permission.

mens of amniotic fluid and 108 buffy-coat specimens of heparinized blood were examined. CMV was isolated twice from buffy coats but not from amniotic fluid. In the immediate postpartum period, viral shedding into breast milk occurred in 14.4% of the patients. The rates of cervical and urinary tract shedding in nonpregnant women are comparable to those found in pregnant cohorts of similar demographic and socioeconomic characteristics. In general, rates of cervical shedding range from 5.2% for nonpregnant women drawn from private practice or family planning clinics to 24.5% among women attending a sexually transmitted disease clinic.[88–91]

Pregnancy per se has no discernible effect on the overall prevalence of viral shedding. However, gestational age has a significant influence on the rate of CMV excretion. The prevalence of excretion is lower (2.6%) in the first trimester than near term (7.6%).[115] This phenomenon was initially interpreted as an indication that pregnancy enhances productive CMV infection in the genital tract. It was assumed that the lower rate seen during the first trimester was similar to the frequency in the nonpregnant state. However, in controlled studies the prevalence of genital tract infection in nonpregnant women was comparable to that found in pregnant women near term, and the majority of pregnant women who shed virus near term were seropositive before the onset of excretion.[116]

The rates of CMV excretion in the genital and urinary tracts of women are inversely related to age after puberty. In one study, the rate of genital CMV excretion fell from 15% in girls between 11 and 14 years of age to undetectable levels in women age 31 years and older.[117] From a peak of 8% in the younger group, urinary excretion fell to zero in women age 26 years and older. No CMV excretion occurred from either site in postmenopausal women.

The transient depression of cellular immune responses to CMV antigens during the second and third trimesters is yet another peculiar aspect of the relationship between CMV and the pregnant human host.[118] In this study there was no generalized depression of cellular

immunity because numbers of T lymphocytes, T cell proliferative responses to other mitogens, and serum antibody titers remained unchanged. None of these mothers shed virus during the period of depressed cellular immune response, nor did they transmit the infection to their infants. It has been shown that antibody responses to glycoprotein B are significantly higher at the time of delivery in women with primary CMV infection who transmitted the infection in utero compared with those who did not, suggesting that the amount of antiviral antibody is not reflective of protection from transmission.[119] However, analysis of the qualitative antibody response revealed lower neutralizing antibody titers in transmitters, suggesting an association between neutralizing activity and intrauterine transmission. In this study, a significant correlation was found between neutralizing titers and antibody avidity, indicating that antibody avidity maturation is critical for production of high levels of neutralizing antibodies during primary CMV infection.[119] In a separate study, higher levels of transplacentally acquired maternal antibodies against glycoprotein B and neutralizing antibodies were observed in infants with symptomatic infection at birth and who went on to develop sequelae.[120]

PERINATAL INFECTION

In contrast to the poor correlation that exists between CMV excretion during pregnancy and congenital infection, there is a good correlation between maternal shedding in the genital tract and milk and perinatal acquisition. As shown in Table 7–6, in one study[86] the two most efficient sources of transmission in the perinatal period were infected breast milk, which resulted in a 63% rate of perinatal infection, and the infected genital tract, particularly in late gestation, which was associated with transmission in 26 and 57% of the cases (natal

TABLE 7–6

Association Between Maternal Excretion of CMV from Various Sites and Subsequent Infection of the Infant

ONLY SITE OF MATERNAL EXCRETION	NO. OF INFANTS INFECTED/NO. EXPOSED (%)
Breast milk	
Breast-fed infant	19/30 (63)
Bottle-fed infant	0/9 (0)
Cervix	
Third trimester and post partum	8/14 (57)
Third trimester	18/68 (26)
First and second trimester	1/8 (12)
Urine[a]	0/11 (0)
Saliva[b]	0/15 (0)
Nonexcreting women	
Bottle-fed infant	0/125 (0)
Breast-fed infant	0/11 (9)

[a]Late third trimester.
[b]Excretion 1 day post partum.
From Stagno S, et al. Breast milk and the risk of cytomegalovirus infection. N Engl J Med 302:1073, 1980.

infection). Viral shedding from the pharynx and urinary tract of the mother late in gestation and during the first months post partum has not been associated with perinatal transmission.

As shown in Table 7–1, there is considerable variability in perinatal transmission of CMV throughout the world.[121] The age of the mother and her prior experience with CMV, which in turn influence the frequency of viral excretion into the genital tract and breast milk, are certainly important factors. Younger seropositive women who breast-feed are at a greater risk for transmitting virus in early infancy, especially in lower socioeconomic groups.[93] It is remarkable that in Japan, Guatemala, Finland, and India, where the rates of CMV excretion within the first year of life are extremely high (39 to 56%), the practice of breast-feeding is almost universal and the majority of women of childbearing age are seroimmune for CMV.

Sexual Transmission

In general, in developing areas of the world, 90 to 100% of the population is infected during childhood, even as early as 5 years of age. Sexual transmission in these populations plays a minor role as a source of primary CMV infection, but its importance in reinfection is unclear. In developed countries, the infection is acquired at a lower rate, and in some population groups there is a burst in the prevalence of infection after puberty.

Several lines of evidence indicate that sexual transmission of CMV is at least partly responsible for this increase in seroprevalence. CMV is frequently recovered from semen and cervical secretions.[84, 85, 89] Increased seroprevalence of CMV and excretion of virus have been found in women attending sexually transmitted disease clinics and in young male homosexuals.[88–91, 122] Chretien and co-workers reported a cluster of cases with CMV mononucleosis that occurred in sex partners but not in persons who shared living quarters but did not engage in sexual contact.[122] Handsfield and colleagues showed that, in two pairs of sex partners with CMV infections attending a sexually transmitted disease clinic, strains of virus were identical by restriction endonuclease analyses of DNA.[123] Evidence has also been provided for sexual transmission in less promiscuous populations.[90, 91] Among the many variables investigated, a significant correlation was found among seropositivity to CMV, greater numbers of lifetime sexual partners, and past or present infection with *Chlamydia trachomatis*.

Nosocomial Transmission

Nosocomial CMV infection is an important hazard of blood transfusion and organ transplantation. In compromised hosts such as small premature newborns and bone marrow transplant recipients, transfusion-acquired CMV infection has been associated with serious morbidity and even fatal infection. The association between the acquisition of CMV infection and blood transfusion was first suggested in 1960 by Kreel and co-workers, who described a syndrome characterized by fever and leukocytosis occurring 3 to 8 weeks after open heart surgery.[124] The reports that followed soon after expanded the syndrome to include fever, atypical lymphocytosis, splenomegaly, rash, and lymphadenopathy.[125–129] The term *postperfusion mononucleosis* was then proposed. Prospective studies incriminated blood transfusion as the major risk factor and demonstrated that although the clinical syndrome occurred in approximately 3% of the patients undergoing transfusion, inapparent acquisition of CMV infection ranged from 9 to 58% as determined by seroconversion, a fourfold rise in complement-fixing antibody titers, and/or viral excretion occurring between 3 and 12 weeks after surgery. It has been estimated that the percentage of blood donors capable of transmitting CMV ranges from 2.5 to 12%. In a study of seronegative children receiving blood for cardiac surgery, the risk of acquiring CMV was calculated to be 2.7% per unit of blood.[126] There is a significant correlation between the risk of acquisition of CMV by patients labeled seronegative and the number of units of blood (total volume) transfused. In one study, the incidence of primary infection increased from 7% among patients receiving 1 unit of blood to 21% among those receiving more than 15 units.[127] For seronegative marrow transplant patients who receive standard blood products, the risk of CMV infection is between 28 and 57%.[130] Under conditions found in blood banks, CMV inoculated in whole blood persisted for 28 days and in freshly frozen plasma for 97 days.

The observation that two newborns who received large volumes of fresh blood subsequently developed symptomatic CMV infections led McCracken and associates to suggest an association between blood transfusion and clinically apparent postnatal CMV infection.[131] Subsequent reports indicated an association between postnatal CMV infection and exchange transfusions.[132] With exchange transfusions, the probability that a seropositive infant receiving seropositive blood becomes infected is 20%, whereas for a seronegative infant receiving seropositive blood the probability is 50%.[132] This remarkably high incidence after exchange transfusions is most likely because infants who receive the transfusions usually receive large volumes (150 to 200 ml/kg) of fresh whole blood from a single donor. Intrauterine transfusions were implicated by King-Lewis and Gardner as the source of CMV in two pregnant women who subsequently seroconverted and whose infants developed viruria between 2 and 8 weeks of postnatal life.[133] Pass and associates reported that the risk of CMV infections in newborns was significantly greater for infants (13 of 37) receiving blood from donors with complement fixation titers to CMV greater than 1:8 than for those (2 of 28) receiving blood from donors with titers of less than 1:8.[134]

Two prospective studies have proved that seropositive blood is the source of acquired CMV in neonates undergoing multiple transfusions. In the study to Yeager, 10 of 74 infants of seronegative mothers who were exposed to one or more seropositive blood donors acquired CMV.[135] The risk of infection increased to 24% for patients who received more than 50 ml of packed red blood cells from at least one seropositive donor.[135, 136] The use of only seronegative blood completely eliminated the acquisition of CMV by seronegative infants.[136] A subsequent study by Adler and associates confirmed these findings and proved further that significant risk factors for transmission of CMV and subsequent disease included transfusions from multiple seropositive donors, lack of passively acquired maternal antibody to CMV, and low birth weight (<1250 g).[137, 138]

Transplantation of a kidney from a seropositive donor into a seronegative recipient results in primary CMV in around 80% of transplant patients.[139-143] The clinical manifestations of the infection vary widely, depending principally on immunosuppressive regimens. Most investigators have found that CMV infection has an adverse effect on the survival of the allograft. CMV is also a major cause of morbidity and mortality in bone marrow recipients.[144-146] Interstitial pneumonitis is the most significant manifestation of the infection; its mortality approaches 100% in some series. Factors that adversely affect the incidence and severity of CMV infections are the degree of immunosuppression, hematologic malignancies (as opposed to aplastic anemia), and acquisition of CMV infection after the transplant.

From 70 to 100% of recipients of heart transplants excrete CMV.[147, 148] In fact, in one series, all patients who had antibody to CMV before transplantation excreted CMV after surgery. Primary CMV infection occurs in a high proportion (60%) of patients who are seronegative before surgery. Severe disease is more likely to be associated with primary than with reactivated infection.[149, 150] but primary infection is not associated with an increased risk of rejection of the transplant.[150] The incidence of CMV infection is higher among seronegative patients who receive grafts from seropositive donors than among seronegative recipients of hearts from seronegative donors.[147]

There is evidence from restriction endonuclease analysis of CMV isolates obtained from a nursery population that nosocomial transmission is possible in this setting, which suggests that workers' hands or contaminated fomites might be involved.[103, 104] CMV has been recovered from objects used in the care of an infected newborn and from surfaces in a day-care center, with recovery of virus for up to 8 hours.[99, 100, 151] The very low rate of CMV infection in newborn infants of seronegative mothers who are not exposed to other important sources such as banked human milk or seropositive blood products indicates that transmission of CMV via fomites or workers' hands is very rare.

Transmission to Hospital Workers

Because hospital workers are often women of childbearing age, there has been concern about occupational risk through contact with patients shedding CMV. As illustrated in Table 7–7, the majority of the studies carried out during the last decade indicates that the risk is not significantly different from the general population.[152] The studies showing differences in the rate of seroconversion between health care workers and controls did not show that the risks were statistically significant.[153, 154]

The risk for hospital personnel is a function of the prevalence of CMV excretion among patients, the prevalence of seronegativity in health care workers, and the degree of their exposure to infected patients. In general, among hospitalized infants and children, viruria occurs in approximately 1% of newborns and 5 to 10% of older

---

☐ **TABLE 7–7**
Rates of Primary CMV Infection Among Health Care Workers and Others

STUDY (REFERENCE NO.)	GROUP	NO. IN GROUP	SEROCONVERSIONS (%/YR)
Yeager 1975 (158)	Nonnurses	27	0
	Neonatal nurses	34	4.1
	Pediatric nurses	31	7.7
Dworsky et al 1983 (106)	Medical students	89	0.6
	Pediatric residents	25	2.7
	Neonatal nurses	61	3.3
Friedman et al 1984ᵃ (159)	"High risk": pediatric intensive care unit, blood IV team	57	12.3
	"Low risk": pediatric ward nurses, noncontact	151	3.3
Brady et al 1985 (162)	Pediatric residents	122	3.8
Adler et al 1986 (163)	Pediatric nurses	31	4.4
	Neonatal nurses	40	1.8
Demmler et al 1986 (164)	Pediatric nurses	43	0
	Pediatric "therapists"	76	0
Balfour and Balfour 1986 (160)	Transplant/dialysis nurses	117	1.04
	Neonatal intensive care unit nurses	96	2.28
	Nursing students	139	2.25
	Blood donors	167	1.57
Stagno et al 1986	Middle-income pregnant women	4692	2.5
	Low-income pregnant women	507	6.8

ᵃOnly study in a children's hospital reporting a statistically significant difference in relation to occupational contact.
Modified from Pass RF, Stagno S. Cytomegalovirus. *In* Donowitz LG (ed). Hospital Acquired Infection in the Pediatric Patient. © 1988. The Williams & Wilkins Co., Baltimore.

infants and toddlers. As discussed earlier, the rate of viral excretion in infants depends on the rates of natal and perinatal transmission from mother to infant, breast-feeding practices, and blood transfusion policies. In toddlers and older children, the rate of CMV excretion depends on factors such as crowding, socioeconomic status, child-rearing practices (e.g., breast-feeding), and attendance at day-care centers. On the other hand, age, race, and, to some extent, gender influence the prevalence of seronegative hospital personnel.

Working with hospitalized children inevitably leads to contact with a child shedding CMV; however, it is important that workers who develop a primary infection not assume that their occupational exposure or contact with a specific patient is the source of infection. Two case reports illustrate this point well. Yow and co-workers[155] and Wilfert and associates[156] described health care workers who acquired CMV while pregnant and after attending a patient known to be excreting CMV. In each of these reports, restriction endonuclease analysis of DNA from CMV isolates indicated that the source of CMV for the worker and her aborted fetus was not the patient under suspicion. Adler and associates used restriction enzyme methods to study CMV strains from 34 newborns and a nurse who seroconverted; all 35 strains were different, which supported the conclusion that nosocomial spread of CMV to workers or among newborns was not occurring in their nursery.[157]

PATHOGENESIS

Routes of Transmission

Many women acquire or reactivate CMV infection during pregnancy, but only a minority transmit the virus to their fetuses to cause acute and/or long-term morbidity in a small number of offspring. Generalized CID of the newborn is almost always the result of primary maternal infection.[82, 157a–166] Even so, clinically apparent infection occurs in less than 15% of the infected newborns. Damage after recurrent maternal infection is clearly uncommon. Only a handful of symptomatic infants are known to have been born to mothers who were seropositive before pregnancy.[157a, 158, 162–170] Several of these patients were immunosuppressed or experienced a primary infection close to the time of conception.

Although not clearly established, intrauterine infection is assumed to result from maternal viremia, with subsequent placental infection and hematogenous dissemination to the fetus. Because maternal CMV infection is generally asymptomatic, it has been difficult to study the sequence of events that lead to intrauterine infection. Still undefined is whether cell-free virus or leukocyte-associated virus is required for the spread from the mother to the fetus through the placenta. Maternal antibody response against CMV-encoded proteins is greater in women with primary infection who transmit virus in utero than those who do not, suggesting that women who infect their fetuses have a higher level of virus replication.[119] Because intrauterine transmission occurs in only 30 to 40% of pregnant

women with primary CMV, a mechanism that is not understood but is generally referred to as placental barrier must operate to prevent fetal infection. Placental infection has been detected both with and without fetal infection. CMV can be transmitted in utero with equal facility throughout gestation, but preliminary evidence suggests that the fetal infection is more virulent when acquired in the first half of gestation.[171]

Congenital infection frequently results from recurrent infection in immune women. It is unclear how the virus evades the immune system under these circumstances. CMV could become latent and reactivate at sites that are less accessible to virologic examination, such as the endometrium and myometrium, spread to the fetus, and cause congenital CMV infection despite maternal immunity.

Pathogenic Mechanisms

Once intrauterine infection has occurred, the incidence of harmful effects is higher than at any other time in life, perhaps with the exception of severely immunocompromised patients.

Why some infants are severely affected and others remain free of symptoms is not clear. It is possible that because of the low-grade virulence of CMV infection in general, some late-appearing abnormalities may be delayed manifestations of damage that occurred in utero. The mechanism of cell and organ damage is thought to arise from productive viral replication leading to cell lysis. Longitudinal studies of infants with congenital and perinatal infections have demonstrated that excretion of CMV into urine and saliva persists for years, as illustrated in Figure 7–5.[171a] Infants with symptomatic congenital CMV infection excrete larger amounts of virus in the first few months of life than do those with asymptomatic infection. In congenitally infected infants, viremia may be demonstrated for several months and viruria for 6 years in approximately 50% of cases. It is likely that chronic viral replication also occurs at other sites that are less accessible to virologic examination. The importance of the host immune response is clear. Failure of the immune response to stop viral replication and eliminate the infection can result in ongoing cell death. It is common to find that organ dysfunction is out of proportion to the level of viral replication.[33]

CMV is difficult to neutralize completely, even in the presence of high titers of antibody, and isolated virion-antibody complexes can remain infectious. CMV can bind to host beta-microglobulin and is thus protected from neutralization by antibody. Beta-microglobulin, which has high affinity for CMV and is found in most body fluids, provides protection from immune attack.[172] Like herpes simplex, CMV induces the production of a glycoprotein that is expressed on the surface of the infected cells and acts as an Fc receptor. By nonspecifically binding the Fc portion of IgG, this receptor could provide a protective coat against the host immune responses.[172]

Another possible factor is vasculitis, which may occur in utero or after birth. Infants with serious congenital CMV who die soon after birth usually have disseminated

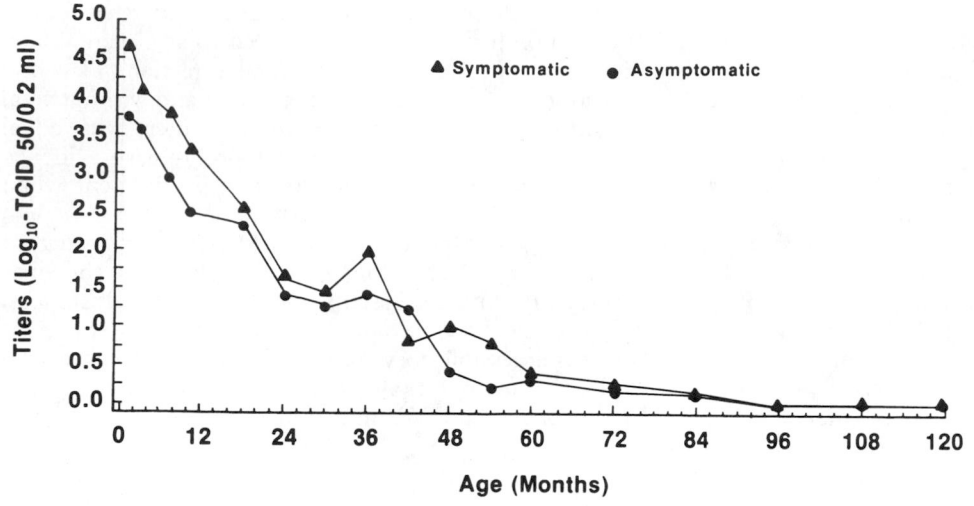

FIGURE 7–5 Quantitative assessment of CMV excretion in subjects with congenital symptomatic (▲) and congenital asymptomatic (●) infections.

intravascular coagulopathy. Vascular endothelium is a target of viral infection, and loss of blood supply due to viral replication or secondary host inflammatory response could result in additional damage to the involved organ.[33] Some reports have suggested that CMV may induce cytokine responses that could enhance the localization of inflammatory cells to areas of blood vessels in which CMV is actively replicating.[33, 173, 174] Vascular involvement with CMV could account for the widespread disease seen in some organs such as the CNS. Focal involvement may be the result of specific tropism of CMV for certain cells. For example, hearing loss, a relatively common complication of congenital CMV infection, may be the result of tropism for cells located within the cochlea and eight cranial nerves.[175]

Injury mediated by immunologic factors has also been studied. Persistence of CMV replication in the presence of an immune response is characteristic of CMV infection and may contribute to the capacity of this virus to cause disease.[33, 176] Studies have described mechanisms by which CMV can evade host-derived immunity (Table 7–8).[33] An interesting observation is that a CMV-induced glycoprotein can prevent MHC transport to the cell surface and thereby impair MHC-restricted immune recognition of CMV-infected cells, thus sheltering them

from virus-specific cytotoxic T lymphocytes.[177] Decreased expression of virus envelope glycoproteins has also been shown to result in escape of virus from the neutralizing antibodies.[178] The variable expression of CMV phenotype resulted in viruses that were resistant to neutralization but were still infectious.[33] How these various immune-mediated mechanisms operate in congenital and perinatally acquired infections remains to be elucidated. It is interesting that maternal immune response protects only 40% of exposed infants from becoming infected.[85] The ensuing infection, although chronic, remains subclinical in the vast majority of infants, which indicates that the passive transfer of maternal antibody is more protective for virulence than for transmission. Studies show that transfusion-acquired infection is more virulent in seronegative than in seropositive infants irrespective of underlying diseases or gestational age. Another indirect mechanism of cellular injury is the possible destruction of cells carrying latent or low-grade persistent infection by a cellular immune reaction.

Congenitally and perinatally infected infants have also been noted to have impaired specific cell-mediated immunity, as assessed by the lymphocyte transformation response to CMV antigen.[179–181] This test measures only the recognition, not the effector function, of T lympho-

TABLE 7–8

Persistence of CMV: Proposed Mechanisms of Immune Evasion

VIRAL FUNCTION	PROPOSED MECHANISM OF IMMUNE EVASION	REFERENCE
Genetic variation between different strains	Evasion of neutralizing antibody response	Urban et al (1992)
	Absence of major histocompatibility complex–determined lymphocyte response	Curtsinger et al (1994)
Variability in envelope protein expression	Neutralizing antibody resistance	Li et al (1995)
Loss of major histocompatibility complex:viral peptide transport	Evasion of cytotoxic T lymphocyte recognition of infected cells	Gilbert et al (1993); Wiertz et al (1996)
Restricted gene expression	Lack of recognition of virus-infected cells by immune system of major histocompatibility complex	Schnolke et al (1995)
Cell-associated dissemination	Virus spread sheltered from systematic immunity	

From Britt WJ. Cytomegalovirus: overview of the virus and its pathogenic mechanisms. Baillieres Clin Infect Dis 3:307–325, 1996.

cytes and does not require, as other techniques do, the use of syngeneic target cells. Another defect consistently observed is the inability of the lymphocytes of these infants to induce interferon production in vitro when challenged with CMV antigens. The impairments are not a reflection of a generalized disturbance because it is restricted to a blastogenic response to CMV and is highly virus specific. CMV-infected patients who have antibodies to herpes simplex virus, for example, have a normal blastogenic response to this virus.[180] Infants with impaired lymphocyte transformation responses have normal reactions to both killed and live vaccines. The impairment has no relation to the clinical presentation and outcome, but it is more intense and long lasting in patients with a symptomatic CMV infection. As patients grow older, the impairment disappears, together with viral replication.

Nature of Maternal Infection

The nature of the maternal infection is a major pathogenetic factor for congenital CMV infection. Primary infections are more likely to be transmitted to the fetus and are likely to cause more fetal injury than recurrent infections.[159] With primary CMV infection, as in other infections during pregnancy, there appears to be some innate barrier against vertical transmission.[82, 157, 161, 182–185] Intrauterine transmission after primary infection occurs in 30 to 40% of cases. How the placenta contains the infection is poorly defined. There have been a few reports of isolated placental involvement in the absence of fetal infection. Current information suggests that gestational age has no apparent influence on the risk of transmission of CMV in utero.[82, 160, 161, 182] However, with regard to the role of gestational age on the expression of disease in the fetus and offspring, it has been suggested that infection at an earlier gestational age produces the worst outcome.[82, 161, 171]

Congenital infection may also result from recurrences of infection.[79, 111–114] The term *recurrence* is used here to represent either reactivation of infection or reinfection with the same or a different strain of CMV during pregnancy. Evidence indicates that despite the inability of maternal immunity to prevent transmission of this virus to the fetus, congenital infections that result from recurrent infections are less likely to affect the offspring than those resulting from primary infections.[159] The risk of congenital CMV infection resulting from a recurrence of infection during pregnancy ranges from a high of 1.5% for a U.S. population of low socioeconomic background to 0.19% for women of middle or upper socioeconomic background from the United States,[82] Great Britain,[182] or Sweden.[157]

In recurrent infection, it is likely that preexisting immunity inhibits the occurrence of viremia at least to some extent. It is conceivable that cellular immunity is more important than humoral immunity; however, maternal IgG antibodies are transmitted to the fetus, but their precise role has not been elucidated. Several cases of symptomatic congenital infection have been reported after therapeutic immune suppression, in women with lupus or AIDS, and even in women with intact immune systems.[157a, 158, 163, 165, 167–170]

Perinatal Infection

Naturally acquired perinatal CMV infections result from exposure to infected maternal genital secretions at birth or to breast milk during the first months of postnatal life.[85, 86] The presence of CMV at these two sites may be the result of either primary or recurrent maternal infection. Iatrogenic CMV infections are acquired predominantly from transfusions of blood or blood products and breast milk from CMV-infected donors. Exposure to CMV in the maternal genital tract has resulted in a 30 to 50% rate of perinatal infection. The transmission from mother to infant through breast milk occurs in 30 to 70% if nursing lasts for more than 1 month.[121] After ingestion of the virus, CMV infection is presumably established at a mucosal surface (buccal, pharyngeal, or esophageal mucosa) or in the salivary glands, for which CMV is known to have a special tropism. Occasionally, perinatal CMV infection and, rarely, congenital CMV infections are associated with pneumonitis. Although yet unproved, it is conceivable that CMV replicates in respiratory mucosa after aspiration of infected secretions or breast milk.

Transmission of CMV by blood transfusion is more likely to occur when large quantities of blood are transfused. The failure to isolate CMV from the blood or blood elements of healthy seropositive blood donors suggests that the virus exists in a latent state, presumably within leukocytes. It has been suggested that CMV becomes reactivated after transfusion, when infected cells encounter the allogeneic stimulus. CMV genomes are activated when transfused to a recipient, particularly if immunologically immature or deficient. Chou and colleagues reported that if the recipient is HLA matched with the donor, activation is more likely to occur, presumably because of better survival of infected cells.[186]

Persistent Viral Excretion

Congenitally and perinatally acquired CMV infections are characterized by chronic viral excretion.[171a] Virus is consistently shed into the urine for up to 6 years or longer and into saliva for 2 to 4 years. Not only does excretion persist much longer in these patients than in infected older children and adults, the quantity of virus excreted is also much greater. Even asymptomatic congenitally or perinatally infected infants excrete quantities of virus that usually exceed those detectable in seriously ill immunocompromised older patients. As illustrated in Figure 7–5, the highest quantities of virus are excreted during the first 6 months of life. Infants with symptomatic congenital CMV infection excrete significantly larger amounts than those with asymptomatic congenitally or perinatally acquired infections.

PATHOLOGY

Early reports of histopathologic changes associated with CMV infections relied on a demonstration of classic changes characterized by cytomegaly and nuclear and cytoplasmic inclusions.[53, 187] The distinctive features include large cells 20 to 35 mm in diameter with a large nucleus containing round, oval, or reniform inclusions. These large inclusions are separated from the nuclear membrane by a clear zone, which gives the inclusion the so-called owl's eye appearance. The inclusions within the nucleus show DNA positivity by histochemical staining, whereas the cytoplasmic inclusions contain carbohydrates, as evidenced by periodic acid–Schiff positivity. The cytoplasmic inclusions vary from minute dots to distinct rounded bodies 3 to 4 mm in diameter. The cytoplasmic inclusions are usually aggregated opposite to the eccentrically placed inclusion-bearing nucleus. Unfortunately, the classic CMV inclusion-bearing cell may be only scattered throughout involved tissue and missed by routine sectioning. This finding has been confirmed when more refined techniques such as in situ DNA hybridization and immunofluorescence using CMV-specific monoclonal antibodies have been used to define the extent of infection with CMV in immunocompromised patients.

Commonly Involved Organ Systems

Disseminated disease can occur in the infected fetus and congenitally infected infant. CMV can cause a multisystem disease in which almost all major organ systems are involved. The interested reader is referred to a comprehensive review of this subject.[187]

Central Nervous System. Involvement of the central nervous system is perhaps the most important consequence of fetal infection with CMV. Most descriptions of the pathology of central nervous system infection are relevant only to infants with severe CID, which is occasionally fatal.[188–190] The infection can be described grossly as focal encephalitis and periependymitis. The encephalitis can involve cells of both the gray and white matter, as well as cells within the choroid plexus. Inclusion-bearing cells have been identified in neurons, glia, ependyma, choroid plexus, meninges, and vascular endothelium, and in cells lying free in the ventricles. Rarely, inclusion-bearing cells have been identified in the cerebrospinal fluid.[191] Resolution of acute encephalitis leads to gliosis and calcification. Previous descriptions have emphasized the paraventricular location of calcifications; however, these lesions can be located anywhere in the brain.[192, 193] CMV has been isolated on a few occasions from cerebrospinal fluid.[194]

Viral inclusion-bearing cells and viral antigen-containing cells can also be found within structures of the inner ear, including the organ of Corti, and in epithelial cells of striae vascularis of the cochleae.[175, 195–197] Finally, involvement of the eye, including chorioretinitis, optic neuritis, cataract formation, colobomas, and microphthalmos, has been demonstrated.[190, 195] The histopathologic changes associated with retinitis begin as an acute vasculitis that spreads into the choroid through the vascular basement membrane. CMV has been isolated from fluid of the anterior chamber of the eye.[198]

Liver. Involvement of the liver is common in congenital CMV infections. Clinical evidence of hepatitis as manifested by hepatomegaly, elevated levels of serum transaminases, and direct hyperbilirubinemia is frequently seen in infants with symptomatic congenital infections. Pathologic descriptions of hepatic involvement include mild cholangitis with CMV infections of bile duct cells, intralobular cholestasis, and obstructive cholestasis secondary to extramedullary hematopoiesis.[189] Liver calcification has been detected radiologically in infants with congenital infections.[199, 200] Clinical and laboratory evidence of liver disease eventually subsides in surviving infants.

Hematopoietic System. Hematologic abnormalities, including thrombocytopenia, anemia, and extramedullary hematopoieses, are common in symptomatically infected infants, but these abnormalities almost invariably resolve within the first year of life. The exact mechanism accounting for these disturbances is not certain, although congestive splenomegaly resulting in platelet and red blood cell trapping certainly must play some part in the overall process. Major splenomegaly is not uncommon, and congestion, extramedullary hematopoiesis, and diminished size of lymphoid follicles can be seen histologically.

In congenital CMV infections, thrombocytopenia may persist for several months, even years, with or without petechiae. At least in animal models, direct infection of megakaryocytes has been found and postulated as a possible mechanism.[201] Anemia is another feature of symptomatic congenital CMV infection. The presence of indirect hyperbilirubinemia, extramedullary hematopoiesis, and erythroblastemia indicates active hemolysis, but mechanisms for these effects have not been elucidated.

Kidneys. Macroscopically, the kidneys show no alterations. Microscopically, inclusion-bearing cells are commonly seen, especially in the cells lining the distal convoluted tubules and collecting ducts.[202, 203] Affected cells may desquamate into the lumina of the tubules and appear in the urine sediment. Inclusions can be found occasionally in Bowman's capsules and proximal tubules. Mononuclear cell infiltration may be present in the peritubular zones of the kidney.

Endocrine Glands. Secretory cells of endocrine glands commonly contain typical CMV inclusions. In the pancreas, both the endocrine and the exocrine cells are affected.[187] Some reports describe intralobular or periductal mononuclear infiltration, suggesting focal pancreatitis. To date, there is no indication of an association between congenital CMV infection and diabetes mellitus. CMV inclusion-bearing cells have been documented in follicular cells of the thyroid, the adrenal cortex, and the anterior pituitary.

Gastrointestinal Tract. The salivary glands are commonly involved in both congenital and perinatal CMV infections. However, there are no reliable figures on the frequency of involvement because the examination of the salivary glands is not always part of autopsies.[203] CMV inclusions have also been described in the mucosal surfaces of the esophagus, stomach, and intestine and in the vessels of ulcerative intestinal lesions.[204]

Lungs. Pulmonary CMV lesions are similar in the newborn and the adult. Microscopically, the majority of the inclusion-bearing cells are alveolar cells that lay free in terminal air spaces. In general, there is little inflammatory reaction; however, in the more severe cases, focal interstitial infiltration by lymphocytes and plasma cells can be found.

Placenta. Abnormalities are present in the placentas of a majority of patients with symptomatic CMV infection and are infrequent with subclinical infections.[205] Placentas are not remarkable in size or macroscopic appearance. The most specific feature histologically is the presence of inclusion-bearing cells, which may be found in endothelial cells, in cells attached to the capillary walls, or in Hofbauer's or stromal cells.[205, 206] Other lesions include focal necrosis, which in early gestation shows sparse infiltration by lymphocytes, macrophages, and a few plasma cells. The early lesions present as foci of necrosis of the stroma and occasionally of the vessels of the villi. The focus of necrosis is later invaded by inflammatory cells, histiocytes, and fibroblasts. At later gestational ages, these focal lesions become densely cellular, with plasma cells predominating over lymphocytes. Deposition of intracellular and extracellular hemosiderin can be found in stem and terminal villi and is presumably the result of fetal hemorrhage during the necrotizing phase or of maternal intervillous thrombosis. Calcification within villi or on basement membranes has also been described as a late manifestation of placental CMV infection.

CLINICAL MANIFESTATIONS

Congenital Infection

Approximately 10% of the estimated 44,000 infants (1% of all live births) born annually with congenital CMV infection in the United States have signs and symptoms at birth that would lead one to suspect a congenital infection. Only half of these symptomatic infants have typical generalized CID, characterized mainly by the clinical manifestations given in Table 7–9.[207, 208] Another 5% of these infants present with milder or atypical involvement, and 90% are born with subclinical but chronic infection. Because early studies emphasized symptomatic infections, congenital CMV was considered a rare and often fatal disease. In the early reports, many patients were referred to the investigators because of developmental problems; this may have automatically highlighted a group of patients at a higher risk for persistent abnormalities and neurologic damage. The use of more sensitive and specific methods of diagnosis, particularly viral isolation, has allowed prospective longitudinal study of newborns with symptomatic and asymptomatic congenital CMV infections. This has resulted in a better understanding of the infection and its clinical spectrum.

SYMPTOMATIC INFECTION

Acute Manifestations

Clinically apparent infections or CID is characterized by involvement of multiple organs, in particular the reticuloendothelial and central nervous system, with or

TABLE 7–9

Clinical and Laboratory Findings in 106 Infants with Symptomatic Congenital CMV Infection in the Newborn Period

ABNORMALITY	POSITIVE/TOTAL EXAMINED (%)
Prematurity (<38 wk)	36/106 (34)
Small for gestational age	53/106 (50)
Petechiae	80/106 (76)
Jaundice	69/103 (67)
Hepatosplenomegaly	63/105 (60)
Purpura	14/105 (13)
Neurologic findings	
One or more of the following:	72/106 (68)
Microcephaly	54/102 (53)
Lethargy/hypotonia	28/104 (27)
Poor suck	20/103 (19)
Seizures	7/105 (7)
Elevated alanine aminotransferase (>80 U/liter)	46/58 (83)
Thrombocytopenia	
<100 × 10³/mm³	62/81 (77)
<50 × 10³/mm³	43/81 (53)
Conjugated hyperbilirubinemia	
Direct serum bilirubin >4 mg/dl	47/68 (69)
Hemolysis	37/72 (51)
Increased cerebrospinal fluid protein (>120 mg/dl)ᵃ	24/52 (46)

ᵃDeterminations in the first week of life.

From Boppana S, Pass RF, Britt WS, et al. Symptomatic congenital cytomegalovirus infection: neonatal morbidity and mortality. Pediatr Infect Dis J 11:93–99, 1992, with permission.

without ocular and auditory damage. Weller and Hanshaw defined the abnormalities found most frequently in infants with symptomatic congenital infection as hepatomegaly, splenomegaly, microcephaly, jaundice, and petechiae.[207] As shown in Table 7–9, petechiae, hepatosplenomegaly, and jaundice are the most frequently noted presenting signs. In addition, the magnitude of the prenatal insult is noted by the occurrence of microcephaly with or without cerebral calcification, intrauterine growth retardation, and prematurity.[82, 160, 161, 208–210] Inguinal hernia in males and chorioretinitis with or without optic atrophy are less common. Clinical findings occasionally include hydrocephalus, hemolytic anemia, and pneumonitis. Among the most severely affected infants, mortality may be as high as 30%.[171a] Most deaths occur in the neonatal period and are usually due to multiorgan disease with severe hepatic dysfunction, bleeding, disseminated intravascular coagulation, and secondary bacterial infections. When death occurs after the first month but during the first year, it is usually due to progressive liver disease with severe failure to thrive. Death after the first year is usually restricted to the severely neurologically handicapped children and is due to malnutrition, aspiration pneumonia, and overwhelming infections.

Hepatomegaly. This sign, along with splenomegaly, is probably the most common abnormality found in the newborn period in infants born with a symptomatic congenital CMV infection.[211] The liver edge is smooth and nontender and usually measures 4 to 7 cm below the right costal margin. Liver function tests are often abnormal but usually not markedly so. The persistence of hepatomegaly is variable. In some infants, liver enlargement disappears by the age of 2 months. In others, significant enlargement persists throughout the first year of life. However, massive hepatomegaly extending beyond the first 12 months of life is uncharacteristic of CID.

Splenomegaly. Enlargement of the spleen exists to a greater or lesser degree in all the common human congenital infections and is especially frequent in congenital CMV infections.[208, 211] It may be the only abnormality present at birth. In some instances, splenomegaly and a petechial rash coexist as the only manifestations of the disease. Occasionally, the enlargement is such that the spleen may be felt 10 to 15 cm below the costal margin. Splenomegaly usually persists longer than does hepatomegaly.

Jaundice. Jaundice is a common manifestation of congenital CID. The pattern of hyperbilirubinemia may take several forms, ranging from high levels on the first day to undetectable jaundice on the first day with gradual elevation of the bilirubin level to clinically apparent jaundice. The level of jaundice in the early weeks of life may fluctuate considerably.[211] In some instances, jaundice is a transient phenomenon, beginning on the first day and disappearing by the end of the first week. More often, however, jaundice tends to persist beyond the time of physiologic jaundice. Transient jaundice may occasionally occur in early infancy with pronounced elevation of bilirubin levels during the third month. Bilirubin levels are high in both the direct and the indirect components. Characteristically, the direct component increases after the first few days of life and may constitute as much as 50% of the total bilirubin level. It is rare for the indirect bilirubin component to rise high enough to require an exchange transfusion, but this has been reported.

Petechiae and Purpura. There is evidence that CMV has a direct effect on the megakaryocytes of the bone marrow that results in a depression of the platelets and a localized or generalized petechial rash.[201, 211] In some patients, the rash is purpuric (Fig. 7–6), not unlike that observed in the expanded rubella syndrome. Unlike the latter infection, however, pinpoint petechiae are a more common manifestation. These petechiae are rarely present at birth but often appear within a few hours thereafter; they may be transient, disappearing within 48 hours. The petechiae may be the only clinical manifestation of CMV infection. More often, however, enlargement of the liver and spleen is associated. The petechiae may persist for weeks after birth. Crying, coughing, the application of a tourniquet, a lumbar puncture, or restraints of any kind may result in the appearance of petechiae even months after birth. Platelet counts in the first week of life range from less than 10,000 to 125,000, with a majority in the 20,000 to 60,000 range. Some infants with petechial rashes do not have associated thrombocytopenia.

Microcephaly. Microcephaly, usually defined as a

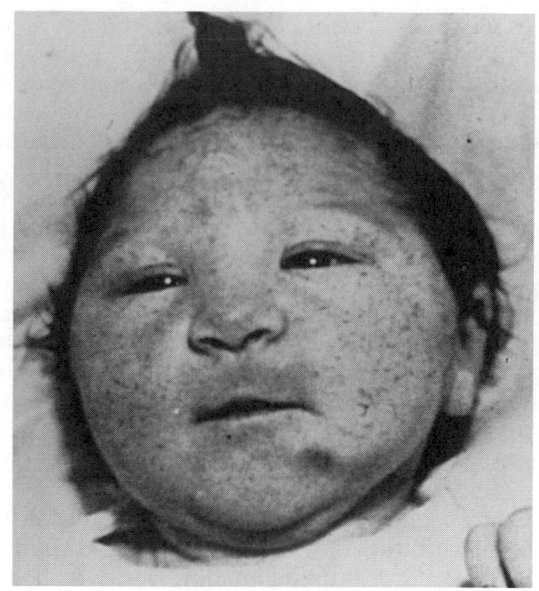

FIGURE 7–6 Symptomatic congenital CMV infection manifested by microcephaly and petechiae.

head circumference of less than the fifth percentile, was found to be present in 14 of 17 patients with CID studied by Medearis in 1964.[212] As tissue culture methods became more widely used and clinical awareness of the infection increased, microcephaly became a less prominent symptom in subsequent series that included mainly infants born with less severe disease. In a more recent examination of 106 surviving patients who were born with symptomatic CMV infection, 53% were microcephalic.[208] Not all infants with microcephaly continue to have head circumferences of less than the third percentile. This is especially true if the head measurement is close to the fifth percentile in an infant of low birth weight.[211] If intracranial calcifications are present, the growth of the brain is invariably impaired. Microcephaly is occasionally followed by obstruction of the fourth ventricle and subsequent hydrocephalus. The presence of calcification is an indication that the infant will have at least moderate and probably severe mental retardation.

Ocular Defects. The principal abnormality related to the eye in CMV infection is chorioretinitis, with strabismus and optic atrophy.[208, 208a, 211] Microphthalmos, cataracts, retinal necrosis and calcification, blindness, anterior chamber and optic disk malformations, and pupillary membrane vestige have also been described in association with generalized congenital CID. In spite of this, the presence of abnormalities such as microphthalmos and cataracts is strong presumptive evidence that the disease process is not caused by CMV. Chorioretinitis occurs in approximately 14% of infants born with symptomatic congenital infection.[208, 208a] Although chorioretinitis occurs less frequently in symptomatic congenital CMV than in congenital toxoplasmosis, lesions caused by CMV and *Toxoplasma* cannot be differentiated on the basis of location or appearance.[195, 208a] Both *Toxoplasma gondii* and CMV can induce central retinal lesions. Occasionally, the appearance of strabismus with subsequent referral to an ophthalmologist is the means by which chorioretinitis is detected. Any infant with suspected CMV infection or strabismus in early life should be examined carefully for retinal lesions. Chorioretinitis caused by CMV differs from that caused by *Toxoplasma* in that postnatal progression is uncommon.[208a]

Fetal Growth Retardation. Intrauterine growth retardation, occasionally severe, was reported in 50% of 106 patients with symptomatic congenital CMV infection, whereas prematurity occurred in 34% (see Table 7–9).[208] Infants with asymptomatic congenital infection in general show no intrauterine growth retardation or prematurity, and CMV cannot be considered an important cause of either condition.

Pneumonitis. Pneumonitis, a common clinical manifestation of CMV infection after bone marrow and renal transplants in adults, is not usually a part of the clinical presentation of congenital CMV infection in newborns. In my experience, diffuse interstitial pneumonitis occurs in less than 1% of congenitally infected infants, even when the most severely affected cases are considered. As is discussed in greater detail later, CMV-associated pneumonitis is more likely to develop in infants with perinatally acquired CMV infections.[213]

Dental Defects. Congenital CMV infection is also associated with a distinct defect of enamel, which thus far seems to affect mainly primary dentition.[214] This defect is more severe in children with the symptomatic form of the infection than in those born with asymptomatic infections (Fig. 7–7). Clinically, this defect appears on all or nearly all of the teeth and is characterized by generalized yellowish discoloration. The enamel is opaque and moderately soft and tends to chip away from dentin. Affected teeth tend to wear down rapidly and may be the basis for the rampant dental caries frequently seen in these children. In our longitudinal studies, this defect of enamel was documented in 27% of 92 children

born with symptomatic congenital CMV infection and in 4% of 267 who were born with the subclinical form and who were observed for at least 2 years. These patients usually require extensive orthodontic therapy. It is evident that these defects do not involve permanent teeth to the same degree.

Deafness. Sensorineural deafness probably is the most common handicap caused by congenital CMV infection. Medearis was the first investigator to call attention to the presence of deafness in symptomatic congenitally infected infants.[212] Subsequent reports confirmed this association and provided evidence that CMV can also cause sensorineural hearing loss in children with subclinical congenital infection.[131, 195, 215–223] In fact, CMV is now considered one of the most important causes of deafness in childhood. CMV can replicate in many structures of the inner ear, as noted by typical CMV-induced cytopathology in Reissner's membrane, stria vascularis, and semicircular canals or by CMV-specific immunofluorescence in the organ of Corti and neurones of the eighth nerve.[175, 195–197] The distribution of viral antigens is far more extensive than viral cellular cytolysis. The presence of an inflammatory response suggests the possibility that immune damage in the inner ear may also be a contributing factor. However, the inner ear may be spared of CMV, as was shown in one infant who died with fulminant congenital infection.[195]

In general, the frequency and severity of the hearing impairment are worse in patients with symptomatic infection (Table 7–10).[208] Because hearing is not commonly assessed within the first month of life, it is difficult to say how many congenitally infected infants, whether symptomatic or not, are born with hearing impairments. This handicap, however, becomes a very significant problem in infancy and early childhood. Of 100 surviving patients with symptomatic CMV infection, 58 (58%) suffer from some degree of hearing impairment.

Congenital Anomalies. There are reports suggesting an association between CMV and congenital anomalies involving various organs.[211] Most of the studies are retrospective or in the form of single case reports. To date, with the exception of inguinal hernias occurring in males, anomalies of the first branchial arch and a defect of tooth enamel that becomes apparent when teeth erupt, there is little evidence that CMV can be considered a teratogen.[214] Anatomic defects and abnormalities such as microcephaly, spastic quadriplegia, generalized hypotonia, microphthalmos, and others do occur in connection with congenital CMV infection, but they are not an indication of a teratogenic effect of this virus.

Long-Term Outcome

The likelihood of survival with normal intellect and hearing after symptomatic congenital CMV infection is small.[131, 207, 208, 212, 217, 218, 224, 225]

As shown in Table 7–10, in our prospective studies, one or more handicaps have occurred in nearly 90% of the patients with symptomatic congenital infection who survived.[208] Psychomotor retardation, usually combined with neurologic complications and microcephaly, oc-

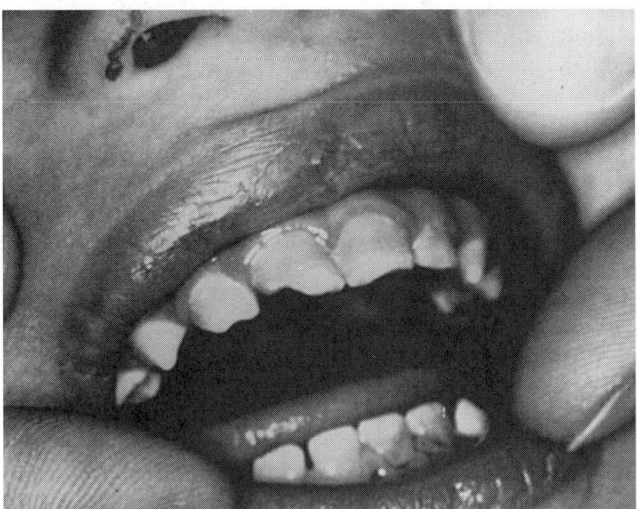

FIGURE 7–7 CMV-affected teeth. This patient had a clinically severe congenital CMV infection. Note fractured borders and opaque and hypocalcified enamel.

◻ **TABLE 7–10**
Sequelae in Children After Congenital CMV Infection

SEQUELAE	% SYMPTOMATIC (NO.)	% ASYMPTOMATIC (NO.)
Sensorineural hearing loss	58 (58/100)	7.4 (22/299)
Bilateral hearing loss	37 (37/100)	2.7 (8/299)
Speech threshold moderate to profound (60 to 90 dB)[a]	27 (27/100)	1.7 (5/299)
Chorioretinitis	20.4 (19/93)	2.5 (7/281)
IQ <70	55 (33/60)	3.7 (6/159)
Microcephaly, seizures or paresis/paralysis	51.9 (54/104)	2.7 (9/330)
Microcephaly	37.5 (39/104)	1.8 (6/330)
Seizures	23.1 (24/104)	0.9 (3/330)
Paresis/paralysis	12.5 (13/104)	0 (0/330)
Death[b]	5.8 (6/104)	0.3 (1/330)

[a]For the ear with better hearing.
[b]After newborn period.
Adapted from Pass RF, Fowler KB, Boppana S. Progress in cytomegalovirus research. *In* Landini MP (ed). Proceedings of the Third International Cytomegalovirus Workshop. Bologna, Italy, June 1991. London, Excerpta Medica, 1991, pp 3–10.

curred in nearly 70% of the patients. Sensorineural hearing loss was seen in 58%. The hearing loss is bilateral in 37% of patients with hearing loss and is progressive in 80%. Chorioretinitis or optic atrophy occurred in 20% of cases. Williamson and associates reported a longitudinal study of 17 patients with symptomatic congenital CMV.[217] In addition to the abnormalities described by previous investigators, they found that 14 children had expressive language delays. In 11, this could be related to hearing loss or cognitive deficits, but 3 other children had delayed expressive language skills that could not be directly attributed to auditory or mental impairment because these patients had normal or disproportionately high language comprehensive skills. Also, learning disabilities and visual motor dysfunction were exhibited by four school-age children with normal intelligence and hearing loss. Subsequently, Conboy and co-workers reported a longitudinal study of 32 surviving children with symptomatic congenital CMV infection with ages ranging from 19 months to 17 years.[219] The study was designed to better define prognosis and to identify clinical predictors of intelligence and developmental outcome. Sequelae in this group of children included hearing loss (in 60%, with 31% being bilateral), retinochoroiditis (16%), microcephaly (34%), neurologic deficits (47%), and mental retardation (41%; IQ < 70). Simple correlations showed that microcephaly at birth, development of neurologic problems during the first year of life, ocular lesions (chorioretinitis), and microcephaly that became apparent after birth were significantly associated with a low IQ and developmental quotient. Multiple regression analysis of 13 variables showed that age, ocular lesions, and neurologic sequelae were significantly associated with poor intellectual prognosis. The best predictor of adverse neurodevelopmental outcome is the presence of cranial computed tomographic (CT) abnormalities detected within the first month of life.[219a] In infants with symptomatic congenital CMV infection, abnormal CT findings, particularly intracerebral calcifications, are common (70%). Nearly 90% of children with abnormal newborn CT scans develop at least one sequela compared with 29% among those with a normal study.[219a] In this particular study, which included 56 children with symptomatic congenital CMV, only 1 child with a normal CT scan had an IQ of less than 70, in contrast to 59% of those with imaging abnormalities. Newborn CT abnormalities were also associated with an abnormal hearing screen at birth and hearing loss on follow-up. Of interest, none of the neonatal neurologic findings was predictive of an abnormal CT.[219a] Overall, it can be anticipated that between 90 and 95% of infants with symptomatic congenital infections who survive will develop mild to severe handicaps.

ASYMPTOMATIC INFECTION

As indicated in the previous section, nearly 90% of infants with congenital CMV infections have no early clinical manifestations, and their long-term outcome is much better. Nevertheless, there is now solid evidence derived from controlled prospective studies that at least 10% of these infants, and perhaps as many as 15%, are at risk of developing a multitude of developmental abnormalities, such as sensorineural hearing loss, microcephaly, motor defects (e.g., spastic diplegia or quadriplegia), mental retardation, chorioretinitis, dental defects, and others. These abnormalities usually become apparent within the first 2 years of life.[195, 215, 216, 220, 221, 226, 227] Table 7–10 shows results based on our prospective longitudinal study of 330 patients with asymptomatic congenital infection who were followed by using serial clinical, psychometric, audiometric, and visual assessments.[208] Follow-up studies of patients with inapparent congenital CMV infection have also been done by Kumar and colleagues,[220] Saigal and associates,[216] Melish and Hanshaw,[215] Pearl and co-workers,[222] Williamson and colleagues,[226] Preece and associates,[185] Ahlfors and co-workers,[157] Conboy and colleagues,[223] Ivarsson and associates,[227] Harris and co-workers,[228] and Fowler and colleagues.[229] In general, their findings resemble the results of our study presented in Table 7–10. The majority of the patients in these various studies and their controls were from a low socioeconomic background. Consequently, we should be careful not to extrapolate these findings to the population at large, at least until more extensive studies are carried out in other groups. An important late-appearing abnormality in children born with subclinical congenital CMV is sensorineural hearing loss.

In one study, Fowler and associates evaluated 307 children with documented asymptomatic congenital CMV infection and compared their audiometric assessments with 76 uninfected siblings of children with asymptomatic congenital CMV infection and 201 children whose neonatal screen for this infection showed negative results.[229] Sensorineural hearing loss occurred only in children with congenital CMV infection. Among them, 22 (7.2%) had hearing loss. In 11 of the 22 children (50%), the hearing loss was bilateral. Among the children with hearing loss, further deterioration of hearing occurred in 50% with a medial age at first progression of 18 months (range: 2 to 70 months). Delayed onset of sensorineural hearing loss occurred in 18% of the children with the medial age of detection at 27 months (range: 25 to 62 months). Also, fluctuating hearing loss was documented in 22.7% of the children with hearing loss. These results are very similar to those obtained by Williamson and co-workers in Houston.[226] From an audiologic viewpoint, late-onset hearing loss and, to a lesser extent, progression and fluctuation of sensorineural hearing loss indicate that hearing tests done within the first days or even during the first year of life do not rule out the possibility of hearing impairments in the future. Consequently, children at risk, whether symptomatic or not, should have careful, serial audiometric examinations.

Congenital CMV infection is a significant cause of sensorineural hearing loss in young children as demonstrated by cohort studies.[228–230] A study in Sweden of more than 10,000 newborns screened for both hearing loss and congenital CMV infection found that this congenital infection was the leading cause of sensorineural hearing loss accounting for 40% of the cases with hearing loss.[228] In our group, Hicks and co-workers[230] found 14 cases of congenital CMV infection with sensorineural hearing loss in 12,371 neonates screened for CMV, a rate of approximately 1.1 per 1,000 live births. The rate was 0.6 per 1,000 when only cases with bilateral loss of 50 dB or greater were considered. These results suggest that CMV infection accounts for at least one third of sensorineural hearing loss in young children.[230]

Prospective studies of children with subclinical congenital CMV infections have also revealed a wide but significant spectrum of neurologic complications.[226] It has been estimated that within the first 2 years of life, 2 to 7% of the infants in this group develop microcephaly with various degrees of mental retardation and neuromuscular defects. How often milder forms of brain damage, such as learning or behavioral difficulties, will occur as these patients grow older is presently unknown. Studies of the intellectual development of children with asymptomatic congenital CMV infections have shown conflicting results. One study evaluated 18 prospectively followed, normal-hearing, school-aged children with asymptomatic congenital CMV infections and 18 controls matched for age, gender, race, school grade, and socioeconomic status.[223] Children were tested by the Wechsler Intelligence Scale for Children—Revised, the Kaufman Assessment Battery for Children, and the Wide Range Achievement Test. Multivariate analysis revealed no difference between the groups on intelligence scores, achievement scores, or incidence of learning disabilities. The mean scores for infected and control infants were similar to national norms. The conclusion of this study is that infants with an asymptomatic congenital CMV infection and normal hearing are not at increased risk of developing mental impairments.

Children with asymptomatic congenital CMV infections have a low risk of chorioretinitis. The current estimate is that it occurs in 2% of these children and, like the hearing loss, may not be present at birth.

In summary, these observations underscore the need for longitudinal follow-up of patients with congenital CMV infection regardless of the initial clinical presentation. Careful assessments of perceptual functions (hearing, visual acuity), psychomotor development, and learning abilities must be made to recognize the full impact of CMV. With early identification of a problem, corrective measures can be instituted to reduce psychosocial and learning problems.

EFFECT OF TYPE OF MATERNAL INFECTION ON SYMPTOMS AND LONG-TERM OUTCOME

Studies have clearly demonstrated that preexisting maternal immunity does not prevent CMV from reactivating during pregnancy and cannot reliably prevent transmission in utero.[79, 111–114, 159, 165–170, 231] However, despite this imperfection, congenital infections resulting from a recurrence of CMV infection during pregnancy are less likely to be clinically apparent than those resulting from a primary maternal infection (Table 7–11).[159]

In recent years, we have extended our observation to include 141 children with congenital CMV infection born after primary maternal infection and 55 children infected in utero as a result of a recurrence of infection. It is important to note that these patients were born at only two hospitals and were screened as part of prospective studies of CMV infections during pregnancy. Their mothers represented women of low as well as mid to high socioeconomic backgrounds. Careful clinical assessments at birth have shown that 7 of 55 infants in the recurrent group had mild symptoms at birth (small for gestational age, hepatosplenomegaly, and petechiae each occurred in 3 of the 7 infants). All these patients were born to women in the low socioeconomic group. Long-term follow-up of these children shows that the risk of sequelae is significantly lower for infants born after recurrent infection (see Table 7–11).[159] Because of the small number of cases in which it has been possible to correlate the type of maternal infection with outcome, we cannot exclude the possibility that severe fetal infection may occasionally result from recurrent maternal infection. Indeed, there have been a handful of reports of affected infants being born to mothers who were seropositive before pregnancy.[157, 158, 164, 167, 168]

TABLE 7–11
Sequelae in Children with Congenital CMV Infection According to Type of Maternal Infection

SEQUELAE	TYPE OF MATERNAL INFECTION		
	% Primary (No.)	% Recurrent (No.)	p Value
Sensorineural hearing loss	15 (18/120)	5.4 (3/56)	0.05
Bilateral hearing loss	8.3 (10/120)	0 (0/56)	0.02
Speech threshold >60 dB[a]	7.5 (9/120)	0 (0/56)	0.03
IQ <70	13.2 (9/68)	0 (0/32)	0.03
Chorioretinitis[b]	6.3 (7/112)	1.9 (1/54)	0.20
Other neurologic sequelae[c]	6.4 (8/125)	1.6 (1/64)	0.13
Microcephaly	4.8 (6/125)	1.6 (1/64)	0.25
Seizures	4.8 (6/125)	0 (0/64)	0.08
Paresis or paralysis	0.8 (1/125)	0 (0/64)	0.66
Death[d]	2.4 (3/125)	0 (0/64)	0.29
Any sequelae	24.8 (31/125)	7.8 (5/64)	0.003

[a]For the ear with better hearing.
[b]Three of the seven children with chorioretinitis (43%) in the primary-infection group had visual impairment.
[c]Four of the eight children (50%) had more than one abnormality.
[d]After the newborn period.
From Fowler K, Stagno S, Pass RF, et al. The outcome of congenital cytomegalovirus infection in relation to maternal antibody status. N Engl J Med 326:663–667, 1992.

PUBLIC HEALTH SIGNIFICANCE

The public health impact of congenital CMV infection in the United States is significant, as shown in Table 7–12. With an average incidence of 1% and a birth rate of 4 million per annum, approximately 40,000 infants are born each year with congenital CMV infections. Of these, as many as 2800 present with signs and symptoms of infection (CID). About 336 of them can be expected to die within the first year, and nearly 2160 of the survivors develop handicaps. Another 5580 or so among the subclinically infected develop significant hearing and mental deficits. In addition to the personal and family suffering associated with these conditions, the cost to society for caring for all these children must amount to millions of dollars annually.

Perinatal Infection

As discussed in previous sections, perinatal infections can be acquired from exposure to virus in the maternal

TABLE 7–12
Public Health Impact of Congenital CMV Infection in the United States

PARAMETER	ESTIMATED FIGURE
No. of live births per year	4,000,000
Rate of congenital CMV infection (average)	1%
No. of infected infants	40,000
No. of infants symptomatic at birth (5–7%)	2800
No. with fatal disease (±12%)	336
No. with sequelae (90% of survivors)	2160
No. of infants asymptomatic at birth (93–95%)	37,200
No. with late sequelae (15%)	5580
Total no. with sequelae or fatal outcome	8076

genital tract at delivery, from breast milk, or through multiple blood transfusions.[80, 85, 86, 135, 138] To establish the diagnosis of perinatal CMV infection, one must first exclude congenital infection by showing an absence of viral excretion during the first 2 weeks of life. The incubation period of perinatal CMV infection ranges between 4 and 12 weeks. Although the quantity of virus excreted by infants with perinatal infection is less than that seen with intrauterine acquisition, the infection is also chronic, with viral excretion persisting for years.[171a]

The vast majority of infants with naturally acquired perinatal infections remain asymptomatic. Most of these infections result from reactivation of maternal virus, and therefore infants are born with variable levels of maternal antibody. Asymptomatic perinatal CMV infection in full-term and otherwise healthy infants does not appear to have an adverse effect on growth, perceptual functions, or motor or psychosocial development. CMV has been incriminated as a cause of pneumonitis in infants younger than 4 months of age.[86, 213, 232] In a study undertaken to define the possible association of CMV and other respiratory pathogens with pneumonitis in young infants, CMV was isolated in 21 of 104 patients (21%) enrolled.[213] Only 3% of 97 hospitalized controls were infected. CMV-associated pneumonitis occurs throughout the year in contrast to the common respiratory virus infections, which occur most often in winter and early spring.

CMV-associated pneumonitis is clinically and radiographically indistinguishable from other types of afebrile pneumonia caused by agents such as C. trachomatis and respiratory syncytial virus. Clinically, patients with CMV-associated pneumonitis have an afebrile course with tachypnea, apnea, cough (sometimes paroxysmal), coryza, nasal congestion, intercostal retractions, and roentgenographic evidence of diffuse lower airway obstruction (air trapping, thickened bronchial walls with prominent pulmonary markings and varying degrees of atelectasis). Expiratory wheezing is unusual. Laboratory findings include elevated levels of one or more serum immunoglobulins (especially IgM, in 66% of patients), leukocytosis of more than 12,000 white blood cells per mm³ (59%), and absolute eosinophilia. The median time of hospitalization is 17 days. Some infants require oxygen therapy and ventilatory assistance. Long-term follow-up of patients with pneumonitis associated with CMV and other respiratory pathogens provides evidence that significant mortality and morbidity do occur irrespective of the etiologic agent.[233]

In premature and ill full-term infants, Yeager and colleagues found that naturally acquired CMV infection may pose a greater risk.[234] They found that premature infants weighing less than 1500 g at birth who acquired CMV from a maternal source often developed hepatosplenomegaly, neutropenia, lymphocytosis, and thrombocytopenia, coinciding with the onset of virus excretion. Frequently, infected patients required longer treatment with oxygen than uninfected patients. In a later study, Paryani and co-workers from the same group reported a prospective study of 55 premature infants including controls and suggested that there may be a propensity for an increased incidence of neuromuscular impairments, particularly in premature infants with the onset of CMV excretion during the first 2 months of life.[235] However, sensorineural hearing loss, chorioretinitis, and microcephaly occurred with similar frequency in both groups. More recently, similar findings were reported by Vochem and colleagues.[235a]

Transfusion-acquired perinatal CMV infection can cause significant morbidity and mortality, particularly in premature infants with a birth weight of less than 1500 g born to CMV-seronegative mothers.[132, 135, 138] The syndrome of post-transfusion CMV infection in premature newborns was characterized by Ballard and co-workers.[236] They isolated CMV from 16 of 51 preterm infants of a mean birth weight of 1000 g and found that 14 of the 16 virus-positive infants had a constellation of symptoms that resembled CID. This recognizable, self-limited syndrome consisted of deterioration of respiratory function, hepatosplenomegaly, unusual gray pallor with disturbing septic appearance, both an atypical and an absolute lymphocytosis, thrombocytopenia, and hemolytic anemia. The syndrome was more severe in low-birth-weight infants and occurred 4 to 12 weeks after the transfusion, when the infants were progressing satisfactorily. Although the course of the disease was generally self-limited (lasting from 2 to 3 weeks), death occurred in 20% of the ill infants. Subsequent work by Yeager and associates[136] and Adler[137] confirmed these observations. The risk of infection is greater with an increasing number of units of blood transfused. Yeager and associates demonstrated that the risk of infection is related to the serologic status of the donor and that these infections could be prevented by transfusing seronegative newborns with blood from seronegative donors.

DIAGNOSIS

Detection of Virus

The diagnosis of congenital CMV infection should be entertained in any newborn with signs of congenital infection or if there is a history of maternal seroconversion or a mononucleosis-like illness during pregnancy. The best test is virus isolation in tissue cultures or demonstration of CMV genetic material by polymerase chain reaction (PCR), which is generally accomplished with urine and/or saliva.[53, 237–241] With both techniques, it is possible to confirm the diagnosis from blood, cerebrospinal fluid, and biopsy material. Of particular interest is the possibility of diagnosis by PCR on blood stored on filter paper.[240] To confirm a congenital CMV infection, isolation must be attempted in the first 2 weeks of life because viral excretion after that time may represent an infection acquired at birth (natal) by exposure to infected birth canal or one acquired in the neonatal period by exposure to breast milk or blood products. Although isolation of CMV during the first 2 weeks of life proves a congenital CMV infection, it does not necessarily confirm an etiologic relationship with an existing disease. Urine and saliva are the preferred specimens for culture because they contain larger amounts of virus. The viability of CMV is surprisingly good when specimens are properly stored. For instance, when positive urine specimens (without preservatives) are stored at 4° C for 7 days, the rate of isolation drops to only 93%; it drops to only 50% after 1 month of storage.[242] However, storage and transport at ambient temperature or freezing should never be used because infectivity is rapidly and significantly reduced.

Specimens must be inoculated into monolayers of human fibroblasts and incubated at 37° C. Viral cytopathic effect is detected with light microscopy (see Fig. 7–2A). Initially, this effect consists of small, round or elongated foci of enlarged, refractile cells. Often the affected cells have brownish refractile granules. The spread of infection in the monolayer is quite slow, involving adjacent cells first. Foci then gradually enlarge, often with central degeneration. Satellite foci usually form, but generally the initial infection progresses to involve the entire monolayer unless the inoculum is quite large. When the inoculum contains large quantities of CMV, generalized cell rounding may appear within 24 hours (see Fig. 7–2D). The CMV cytopathic effect is confirmed by hematoxylin-eosin staining or by immunofluorescence with monoclonal or polyclonal antibodies (see Fig. 7–2B and C).

Since 1980, methods for rapid viral diagnosis became available. Several modifications of the standard tissue culture method combined with immunologic detection of immediate-early CMV-induced antigens have maintained high specificity and sensitivity yet allowed the confirmation of diagnosis within 24 hours of inoculation of the clinical specimen.[162, 242–246]

Typically, this test includes the use of monoclonal antibodies to CMV-specific early antigens with low-speed centrifugation of the clinical specimens onto the monolayer of fibroblasts growing on coverslips inside shell vials.[243–245] When this method was evaluated with clinical specimens (blood; urine; bronchoscopy lavage; lung, liver, and kidney biopsy samples; sputum; and others), obtained primarily from immunosuppressed patients, the sensitivity approached 80% and the specificity ranged from 80 to 100%. Subsequently, another adaptation of this rapid immunofluorescent assay used 96-well microtiter plates and a monoclonal antibody that is reactive with the major immediate-early human CMV protein polypeptide 72.[246] This rapid assay detected all but 1 of 19 specimens identified by standard virus isolation method from 1676 newborn urine specimens, achieving a sensitivity of 94.5% and a specificity of 100%. This test retained high sensitivity and specificity when saliva instead of urine was tested.[238] To date, this microtiter plate method using either saliva or urine samples is the most rapid, simple to perform, and inexpensive alternative to the standard virus isolation method. It is perfectly suitable for mass screening, and there is no drop in sensitivity for specimens at 4° C for up to 3 days. Our study also showed that the sensitivity of the microtiter plate method declined rapidly for specimens from older infants and children with congenital CMV infection and from virus-infected children attending day-care centers. Thus, it is not recommended for either screening or diagnosing CMV infections in older infants and children.

Rapid diagnosis of CMV can also be accomplished by DNA hybridization.[247–251] However, the methodology is cumbersome, owing to the need to concentrate virus at high speed centrifugation and the need to extract DNA and hybridize it with a DNA probe labeled with phosphorus-32. The sensitivity and specificity of this method is good when the specimens contain 10^3 or more tissue culture infective doses per milliliter.

Detection of viral nucleic acid by PCR amplification DNA has proven extremely sensitive for the detection of CMV genetic material in a variety of clinical samples, including urine, cerebrospinal fluid, blood, plasma, saliva, and biopsy material.[237, 239–241, 252, 253] Using primers directed at both major immediate-early protein and late antigen genes, Demmler found 41 urine specimens positive by PCR from a total of 44 specimens positive by tissue culture. No positive PCR results were found in 27 urine specimens that were negative by tissue culture.[237] Warren and co-workers used the PCR technique to detect CMV in saliva from children who were between the ages of 1 month and 14 years and who had either congenital or perinatal CMV infection and compared the results with a standard tissue culture method and microtiter plate detection of early antigen with tissue culture results as a reference.[238] The sensitivity of PCR was 89.2%, and the specificity was 95.8%. Reproducibility was excellent. If primer selection and amplification conditions are carefully chosen, PCR can give results comparable to standard tissue culture test. Some advantages include the minute amount of specimen and the fact that infectious virus is not required, allowing for retrospective diagnosis of CMV infection if the appropriate specimens are available.[240] Nelson and colleagues showed that PCR detection of CMV-DNA in serum is a sensitive, specific, and rapid method for diagnosis of infants with symptomatic congenital CMV infection.[254] The PCR detected CMV DNA in the serum of 18 infants with symptomatic infection, 1 of 2 with asymptomatic infection, and 0 of 32 controls.

An assay to detect CMV antigenemia by means of monoclonal antibodies to pp 65 in polymorphonuclear leukocytes has shown good sensitivity when compared to conventional methods (serology, culture) for the diagnosis of CMV disease in immunocompromised adult subjects.[255–258] More recently, this assay has proven to be sensitive for the diagnosis of primary CMV infection in normal adults with Epstein-Barr virus–negative mononucleosis syndrome and in women with primary CMV infections during pregnancy.[259, 260] There is no evidence that the CMV antigenemia assay is applicable to the diagnosis of congenital CMV infection.

Detection of Immune Response

With congenital CMV infection, antibody production begins in utero and is continued probably during the life span of the host. Antibodies are also produced for prolonged periods after postnatally acquired infections.

Detection of IgG Antibodies. Serologic tests that measure IgG antibody are readily available and are easier to perform than are most virologic methods. However, their correct interpretation is complicated by the presence of antibodies (IgG class) that are normally transmitted from the mother to the fetus.[176] Of course, a negative antibody titer in cord and maternal sera is sufficient evidence to exclude the diagnosis of congenital CMV infection. In uninfected infants born to seropositive mothers, IgG antibodies serially decrease with a half-life of approximately 1 month and finally disappear between 4 and 9 months of age. In contrast, in infected infants, IgG antibody levels persist for long periods at comparable or sometimes higher levels than in their mothers. CMV infections are commonly acquired during the neonatal period mostly from maternal sources (milk, genital secretions) and blood or blood products. When neonatal infections are transmitted from the mother, the distinction from congenital involvement is not possible by routine serologic means. In both situations, IgG antibody titers tend to remain stable for many months. Of course, a neonatal infection in the face of a negative maternal IgG antibody titer should point to transmission from other sources, for example, blood transfusion or nosocomial.

Many serologic assays have been described and evaluated for the detection of CMV IgG antibodies. Among these, complement fixation, enzyme-linked immunosorbent assay (ELISA), anticomplement immunofluorescence, radioimmunoassay, and indirect hemagglutination are perfectly adequate.[56]

Detection of IgM Antibodies. Infected fetuses usually produce specific IgM antibodies. IgM antibodies are not transferred by the placenta, and thus their presence in cord or neonatal blood represents a fetal antibody response. There are a number of different means to test for IgM antibodies, but before deciding on the use of any particular test it is important to know its specificity, sensitivity, and reproducibility. None has thus far reached a level of specificity and sensitivity to match the virologic assays described in the previous section.

The solid-phase radioimmunoassay RIA described by Griffiths and Kangro is among the best, with a reported sensitivity of 89% and a specificity of 100% for diagnosis of congenital CMV infections.[261] With the IgM ELISA, the specificity was nearly 95% with a sensitivity of approximately 70% when evaluating congenitally infected infants.[262] The IgM capture ELISA and radioimmunoassay have not fared much better when testing for congenital CMV infection. Recent modifications of the IgM tests yet to be appropriately tested in newborns include an ELISA test that uses purified recombinant CMV polypeptides shown to be highly immunogenic as the antigens for the assay.[263] Another version with proven greater sensitivity in blood donors, pregnant women, and transplant recipients with active CMV infection is a Western blot test for IgM antibodies against viral structural polypeptides pp 150 and pp 52.[264] Until IgM antibody tests are better perfected for general use, clinicians should not rely solely on one of these assays to diagnose congenital CMV infection. Continued research in this area may provide a simple and generally available method for rapid, definitive diagnosis of congenital infections in both ill and asymptomatic neonates.

Prenatal Diagnosis

The prenatal diagnosis of congenital CMV infection is possible by isolation of virus and PCR on amniotic fluid.[265, 273] While a positive result confirms the infection, the predictive value of a negative culture is not known, particularly during the first 20 weeks of gestation. After a primary maternal infection, it may take from weeks to months for transplacental transmission to occur. In several reports, the cases were referred for study for suspected maternal infection and the presence of fetal abnormalities, raising the possibility of selection bias. In addition, in almost all cases amniotic fluid was obtained after the twenty-first week of gestation. Recent publications have shown that PCR detection of CMV in amniotic fluid has a sensitivity of 80 to 100% in antenatal diagnosis after 21 weeks of gestation. The study of Donner and co-workers, tested 36 amniotic fluid specimens collected between 14 and 20 weeks of gestation from women with primary CMV infection and found the test to be 45% sensitive and 100% specific.[274] To counsel pregnant women, it is important to know that the majority of children with congenital CMV infection escape central nervous system sequelae. The presence or absence of ultrasonographic evidence of fetal abnormalities should be taken into consideration before deciding on whether to terminate pregnancy.

The value of other diagnostic methods such as IgM-specific antibodies or elevation of gamma-glutamyl transpeptidase in amniotic fluid and fetal blood is not known.

Diagnosis of Perinatally Acquired Infections

For perinatally acquired infections, viral culture or CMV-DNA detection by PCR from urine and saliva are the preferred diagnostic methods, but CMV excretion does not begin until 3 to 12 weeks after exposure.[85, 176] For diagnostic specificity, it is imperative to have a negative result from urine or saliva specimens collected within the first 2 weeks of life.[238] In early infancy, anti-

body assays have the same limitations described earlier for infants with congenital CMV infection. The desire to differentiate between congenital and perinatal CMV infections stems from the fact that their risks for acute morbidity and for long-term sequelae are very different.

DIFFERENTIAL DIAGNOSIS

During the newborn period, the constellation of hepatosplenomegaly, petechiae, and direct hyperbilirubinemia with or without pneumonitis, microcephaly, and ocular and neurologic abnormalities that characterize CID is common to several disease entities, including other congenital infections such as congenital rubella syndrome, toxoplasmosis, syphilis, neonatal herpes simplex virus infections, and, less likely, hepatitis B and varicella virus infections.[211] The differential diagnosis of symptomatic congenital CMV infection also includes bacterial sepsis and noninfectious disorders such as hemolytic diseases related to Rh or ABO incompatibilities or red blood cell defects; metabolic disorders such as galactosemia and tyrosinemia; immune thrombocytopenia; reticuloendotheliosis; congenital leukemia; and others. The list of diseases that must be considered in the differential diagnosis becomes obviously broader as the clinical manifestations diminish in severity.

It is known that infections may coexist in the same patient. Consequently, the laboratory workup for differential diagnosis must be thorough.

Congenital Rubella Syndrome

Congenital rubella has been virtually eliminated in the United States after the successful immunization program adopted years ago. Although symptomatic congenital rubella and CMV infections share many signs and symptoms, central cataracts, congenital heart defects, raised purpuric rather than petechial rash, salt-and-pepper lesions as opposed to chorioretinitis, and the absence of cerebral calcifications are more likely to occur with congenital rubella syndrome than with CID.[211, 223]

Congenital Toxoplasmosis

Almost all the manifestations observed in CID have been described for symptomatic congenital toxoplasmosis. Some differences are worthy of note.[211] For instance, the calcifications of toxoplasmosis are generally scattered throughout the cerebral cortex, whereas the calcifications of CID tend to occur in the periventricular areas. The rash associated with toxoplasmosis is usually maculopapular but is not petechial or purpuric. Chorioretinitis in the two diseases cannot be differentiated on the basis of appearance or distribution. However, it is more likely that chorioretinitis related to CMV is associated with other major clinical manifestations, such as microcephaly. Not uncommonly, the chorioretinitis of toxoplasmosis is an isolated finding.

Congenital Syphilis

The most consistent signs of early congenital syphilis are osteochondritis and epiphysitis on the roentgenogram of the long bones.[211] These occur in approximately 90% of infected patients and are more likely to appear in patients who become symptomatic in the first week of life. Rhinitis, sometimes associated with laryngitis, is another common manifestation of congenital syphilis; it is often followed by a dark red maculopapular, spotted rash. Lesions of the skin and mucous membranes are also seen. Hepatosplenomegaly occurs but is less common in early syphilis than in CID. Calcifications of the brain are not characteristic of congenital syphilis. However, choroiditis may be seen.

Neonatal Herpes Simplex Virus Infections

Congenital herpes simplex virus infections are less common than neonatal herpes simplex virus infections, yet they are more likely to pose a diagnostic dilemma because they may resemble CID. Microcephaly, intracranial calcifications, chorioretinitis with and without optic atrophy and hepatosplenomegaly are common clinical manifestations of intrauterine herpes simplex virus infections. The presence of skin vesicles or scarring present at birth is valuable for the differential diagnosis. The more common form of herpes simplex virus infection, neonatal infection, is acquired during parturition and does not usually present as an acute disease until 5 to 21 days of age. Unlike the situation in typical CID, the infant is well during most of the first week of life. When illness does occur, it may be accompanied by seizures, encephalitis, respiratory distress, bleeding disorders, and vesicular lesions that tend to cluster. The presence of skin and mucous membranous lesions is valuable for the differential diagnosis of CID.

TREATMENT

Chemotherapy

A small number of systemically administered antiviral agents have been used in therapeutic trials of serious, life-threatening or sight-threatening CMV disease.[275] Currently, two antiviral agents, ganciclovir and foscarnet, are licensed for this purpose in immunocompromised patients. Foscarnet inhibits viral replication by inhibiting viral DNA polymerase, and ganciclovir acts as a chain terminator during elongation of the newly synthesized viral DNA.[276, 277]

Presently, a randomized controlled multicenter clinical trial evaluating the use of ganciclovir in the treatment of infants with symptomatic congenital CMV infection is in progress. The results of the Phase II study with 47 infants receiving either 8 or 12 mg/kg of ganciclovir intravenously in divided doses at 12-hour intervals for 6 weeks have been reported.[278] The study included serial clinical, pharmacokinetics, virologic, audiometric, and ophthalmologic evaluations. Ganciclovir administration was discontinued in 8 patients because of neutropenia (6), worsening liver function tests (1), and bacterial infection (1). One patient died on day 9 secondary to translocation of the great vessels, and 3 other infants died of presumed overwhelming CMV infection on days 43 (necrotizing enterocolitis), 55 (CMV pneumonia), and 90 (multiple congenital infections, including human immunodeficiency virus, syphilis, and CMV infection). The most common adverse effects included neutropenia (16 patients), absolute neutropenia (2 patients), increases in aspartate aminotransferase (6 patients), and increase in direct hyperbilirubinemia (3 patients). During treatment, quantitative excretion of CMV in the urine decreased. However, after cessation of therapy, viruria returned to pretreatment levels. Clinically, the most significant observation was hearing improvement of stabilization in 5 of 30 infants (16%) at 6 months of follow-up or later, suggesting efficacy.[278] Very similar results were obtained in a smaller trial by Nigro and co-workers in 1994.[279] There are no reports on the therapeutic efficacy of combined therapy (foscarnet-ganciclovir) in the treatment of symptomatic congenital CMV infection. Confounding factors for the interpretation of therapeutic efficacy are the wide spectrum of disease resulting from symptomatic congenital CMV infection, the unpredictable natural course of the disease, and the fact that many patients incur irreversible damage before birth.

Passive Immunization

Hyperimmune plasma and globulin have been used with some success as prophylaxis for primary CMV infections in immunosuppressed transplant patients. A meta-analysis of randomized, controlled trials of immunoglobulin as prophylaxis for CMV disease in adult transplant recipients found a significant beneficial effect.[280] Studies are under way to determine if humanized monoclonal antibody such as the one that binds to gH of CMV is more efficacious for the prevention or treatment in patients at high risk for CMV infection.[281] It is unlikely that passive immunoprophylaxis will ever work for treatment of congenital infections because the cases are identified weeks and months after infection occurred in utero. However, it might be a means of preventing primary CMV infection and disease associated with transfusion-acquired infections in premature infants. No controlled studies are available.

Vaccines

Two live attenuated vaccines have been developed and have undergone efficacy trials in both CMV immune and susceptible normal individuals and renal transplant recipients.[282–285] The attenuated Towne strain of CMV was evaluated for efficacy in renal allograft recipients.[286–288] It proved immunogenic and reduced both the severity and the incidence of CMV-associated disease in seronegative patients who received a renal allograft from a seropositive donor. So far, there is no evidence that vaccine virus reactivates in these patients. In a challenge study using a low passage of a clinical isolate (Toledo) and vaccinated and control volunteers, the Towne vaccine protected against infection but only with low doses of challenge virus. At higher doses, infection and in some cases illness occurred.[289] As summarized by Britt, there is substantial evidence that a CMV vaccine will benefit populations at risk, including the serious consequences of congenital infection.[285] In a small study of 22 young women immunized with the AD169 attenuated strain who were followed for 8 years, antibody and lymphocyte antigenic response induced by the vaccine disappeared in 50% of the cases.[284] In women immunized at different intervals before pregnancy, congenital infection was not detected. In a more recent study of vaccine efficacy in normal adult women at higher-than-normal risk of acquiring CMV, the Towne strain did not provide protection against naturally acquired infection.[290] The vaccine was used at a low dose and potency and produced neutralizing antibody titers against CMV that were 10- to 20-fold lower than those produced in wild type infections.[290] Although vaccines have not been shown to reactivate, the possibility that reactivations might occur during pregnancy with transmission to the fetus raises concern about their use, even in vaccine trials. A candidate vaccine should be capable of preventing primary infection without inducing latent infection with the risk of reactivation. An attractive approach is the development of a subunit vaccine that contains antigenic targets of the host immune response.[66, 285, 291, 292] Table 7–13 summarizes the antigenic targets of immune responses to CMV that are potential targets. One of the best candidates is glycoprotein gB. This is the dominant target of antienvelope antibody response, in particular virus-neutralizing response.[285] Existing data suggest that protective immune responses, both humoral and cellular, can be generated with a limited number of CMV-encoded proteins.[285] The gene of gB has been identified, allowing for the production of this viral surface antigen in vaccinia virus and adenovirus recombinant vaccine vector system.[291, 292] Several biotechnology companies have initiated the production and testing of subunit vaccines, and preliminary reports of phase I

trials in normal human volunteers indicate that a gB subunit vaccine is capable of inducing cellular and neutralizing antibody responses. We must now await further studies on the immunogenicity and protective efficacy of these subunit vaccines.

PREVENTION

In general, CMV is not very contagious and its horizontal transmission requires close direct contact with infected material, namely, secretions that contain the virus and, less likely, fomites.[94–108, 115, 139] With the exception of a few small studies that were designed to prevent infection through blood and blood products and grafted organs, no broad-based strategies for preventing the transmission of this virus have been tested.[136, 138, 139, 293] Although there are still no effective means of preventing congenital CMV infections or most perinatally acquired CMV infections, a few common sense recommendations can be made.

Pregnant Women

An average of 2% of susceptible pregnant women acquire CMV infection during pregnancy in the United States; the majority has no symptoms, and only 40% of the episodes result in fetal infection (see Fig. 7–4).[294] Because there is no effective drug therapy and the risk of fetal morbidity is low, several investigators have concluded that routine serologic screening of pregnant women for primary CMV infections during pregnancy is of limited value.[182, 295] However, reliable and inexpensive serologic tests are now available so that women of childbearing age can be informed of their immune status.[296] Those who are seronegative should be able to make informed decisions about the risks of CMV. Primary CMV infection should be suspected in pregnant women with symptoms compatible with a heterophil-negative, mononucleosis-like syndrome. At present, there are no reliable means to determine whether intrauterine transmission has occurred after symptomatic or subclinical primary infection in early gestation or to assess the relatively small number of fetuses at risk of disease. The usefulness of amniotic fluid PCR and viral culture is good after 20 weeks of gestation. Thus, there is still limited information to serve as a basis for recommendations regarding termination of pregnancy after a primary CMV infection acquired in early gestation. Similarly, there is no information regarding how long conception should be delayed after primary infection. Viral excretion is not a good indicator because virus is shed into saliva for weeks or months after infection and into urine and the cervix for months or years.

The data on which to base recommendations for prevention of congenital CMV infection after recurrent maternal infection are even more inadequate. Preexisting immunity does not prevent the virus from reactivating, nor does it effectively control the occasional spread to the fetus.[159] However, preexisting maternal immunity affords significant protection to the fetus. At present, there are no techniques for identifying women

---

TABLE 7–13

Antigenic Targets of Immune Responses to Human Cytomegalovirus That Are Potential Components of a Subunit Vaccine[a]

PROTEIN	ORF	IMMUNE RESPONSE
Glycoproteins		
gB	UL55	Dominant target of antienvelope antibody response; principal target of virus-neutralizing response
gH	UL75	Induces potent virus-neutralizing antibodies
Phosphoproteins		
pp 65	UL62	Dominant target of virus-specific CTLs
pp 150	UL32	Dominant target of virus-specific CTLs
Nonstructural protein		
pp 72[b]		Target of virus-specific CTLs

[a]ORF, open reading frame, CTLs, cytotoxic T lymphocytes.
[b]Spliced message containing multiple CTL epitopes within first four exons.
From Britt WJ. Vaccines against human cytomegalovirus: time to test. Trends Microbiol 4:34–38, 1996.

with reactivation of CMV that results in intrauterine transmission. Because the risk of transmission is very low (see Fig. 7–4) and the risk of fetal disease even lower, women known to be seropositive before conception do not need to be virologically or serologically tested, nor do they need to be unduly worried about the very low risk of transmitting the virus to the fetus.

The principal sources of CMV infection among women of childbearing age are exposure to children excreting CMV and sexual contacts. Recommendations for prevention of sexual transmission of CMV are beyond the scope of this review. Suffice it to say that they are similar to those advocated for the prevention of other, more common sexually transmitted infections. As for the risk from exposure to children, at greater risk are susceptible pregnant mothers of CMV-infected children who attend day-care centers.[94, 95, 101–105, 108–110] Hand washing and simple hygienic measures that are routine for hospital care can be recommended, but it is unrealistic to expect all mothers to comply.

Because CMV has been found to be endemic in the day-care setting and is found everywhere in hospitals, questions often arise about the occupational risks to pregnant personnel in these facilities. Although hospital workers do not appear to be at increased risk for CMV infection,[106, 152, 154, 157] personnel who work in day-care centers certainly are.[94, 95, 99–102] In the hospital, routine procedures for hand washing and infection control should make nonparenteral acquisition of CMV infections less likely than in the community. Although the majority of patients who shed CMV are asymptomatic and go unrecognized, when caring for known CMV-excreting patients, these routine measures should be combined with a special recommendation that pregnant caretakers be especially careful in handling such patients.[297] In the day-care setting, where hygiene is difficult at best, these preventive measures may be more difficult to implement. Although there is still debate about the need for routine serologic screening of female personnel and day-care workers, I believe that it should be recommended for potentially childbearing women whose occupation exposes them to CMV. Knowing their immune status can be helpful in counseling pregnant women at risk. Those found to be seropositive can be strongly reassured. Those found to be serosusceptible should be provided with information and reassured that common sense measures such as hand washing and avoiding contact with secretions should prevent acquisition of infection.[297] Attempts to identify all congenitally CMV-infected children and children excreting this virus in the workplace so that seronegative workers and parents can avoid contact with them may become feasible in the near future with assays such as PCR.

Nosocomial Infection

Hospitalized patients who receive blood products and organ transplants are at risk for nosocomial CMV infection. Because the role of organ transplants in transmission of CMV is insignificant in the newborn period, it is not discussed here. Transfusion of blood products, on the other hand, can be an important source of perinatal CMV infections. The use of blood products from seronegative donors prevents the transmission of CMV and the subsequent risk of disease.[130, 136–138] However, this method is not practical in areas where the majority of the donor population is seropositive. Clearly, the availability of seronegative donors as well as the additional cost involved in serologic screening and processing the blood must be evaluated by regional blood banks.

The use of deglycerolized, frozen red blood cells and the use of filters to remove leukocytes are also effective means of eliminating post-transfusion CMV infection in adult dialysis patients and in newborns, even low-birth-weight infants.[130, 293, 298] Both methods result in a significant disruption and depletion of leukocytes.

Many hospitals are using one of these three approaches to prevent transfusion-acquired perinatal CMV infections.[299] It is up to the local hospital and blood bank to determine whether transfusion-associated CMV disease is a problem and which method to choose. However, many nurseries have adopted the policy that all transfusions of blood or blood products should be with seronegative blood, irrespective of the infant's birth weight and maternal immune status.

The absence of CMV infection in premature infants born to seronegative mothers and who receive only seronegative blood products suggests that spread of CMV from hands of personnel or from fomites must be rare.[297] Until more information is available, the only logical recommendation is hand washing and routine infection control measures.

Rarely is perinatal infection through breast milk a cause for concern, at least for full-term newborns who receive their mother's milk. Premature infants, who generally do not receive sufficient quantities of specific transplacental antibodies, supposedly are at higher risk for morbidity. We must also be cautious with expressed banked milk and wet nurses because CMV-infected milk might inadvertently be given to infants born to seronegative women. Storage of naturally infected breast milk at $-20°$ C (freezer temperature) significantly reduces but does not eliminate infectivity.[300]

References

1. Weller TH. The cytomegaloviruses: ubiquitous agents with protean clinical manifestations. N Engl J Med 285:203–214, 1971.
2. Ribbert H. Uber protozoenartigen Zellen in der Nire-eines syphilitischen Neugeboren und in der Parotis von Kindren. Zentralbl Allg Pathol 15:945–948, 1904.
3. Jesionek A, Kiolemenoglou B. Über einen Befund von protozoenartigen Gebilden in den Organen eines heredi-tarleustiochen Fotus Muench Med Wochenschr 51:1905–1907, 1904.
4. Lowenstein C. Über protozoenartigen Gebilden in den Organen von Dindern. Zentralbl Allg Pathol 18:513–518, 1907.
5. Goodpasture E, Talbot FB. Concerning the nature of "protozoan-like" cells in certain lesions of infancy. Am J Dis Child 21:415–425, 1921.
6. Lipschutz B. Untersuchungen uber die Aetiologic der Krankheiten d. herpes genitalis, usw. Arch Derm Syph 136:428–482, 1921.

7. Cole R, Kuttner AG. Filterable virus present in the salivary glands of guinea pigs. J Exp Med 44:855–873, 1926.

8. Smith MG. Propagation of salivary gland virus of the mouse in tissue culture. Proc Soc Exp Biol Med 86:435–440, 1954.

9. Smith MG. Propagation in tissue cultures of a cytopathogenic virus from human salivary gland virus (SGV) disease. Proc Soc Exp Biol Med 92:424–430, 1956.

10. Rowe WP, Hartley JW, Waterman S, et al. Cytopathogenic agent resembling salivary gland virus recovered from tissue cultures of human adenoids. Proc Soc Exp Biol Med 92:418–424, 1956.

11. Weller TH, Macauley JC, Craig JM, et al. Isolation of intranuclear inclusion-producing agents from infants with illnesses resembling cytomegalic inclusion disease. Proc Soc Exp Biol Med 94:4–12, 1957.

12. Weller TH, Hanshaw JB, Scott DE. Serologic differentiation of viruses responsible for cytomegalic inclusion disease. Virology 12:130–132, 1960.

13. Krech U, Jung M, Jung F. Cytomegalovirus Infections of Man. Basel, S Karger, 1971, p 28.

14. Gold E, Nankervis GA. Cytomegalovirus. In Evans AS (ed). Viral Infections of Humans: Epidemiology and Control. New York, Elsevier, 1976, pp 143–161.

15. Alford CA, Stagno S, Pass RF, et al. Epidemiology of cytomegalovirus. In Nahmias A, Dowdle W, Schinazi R (eds). The Human Herpesviruses: An Interdisciplinary Perspective. New York, Elsevier, 1981, pp 159–171.

16. Smith JD, DeHarven E. Herpes simplex virus and human cytomegalovirus replication in WI-38 cells: I. Sequence of viral replication. J Virol 12:919–930, 1978.

17. Wright HT, Goodheart CR, Lielausis A. Human cytomegalovirus morphology by negative staining. Virology 23:419–424, 1964.

18. Sarov I, Abady I. The morphogenesis of human cytomegalovirus: isolation and polypeptide characterization of cytomegalovirus and dense bodies. Virology 66:464–473, 1975.

19. Irmiere A, Gibson W. Isolation and characterization of a noninfectious virion-like particle released from cells infected with human strains of cytomegalovirus. Virology 130:118–133, 1983.

20. Geelen JL, Walig C, Wertheim P, van der Noordaa J. Human cytomegalovirus DNA. I. Molecular weight and infectivity. J Virol 26:813–816, 1978.

21. Huang ES, Chen ST, Pagano JS. Human cytomegalovirus. I. Purification and characterization of viral DNA. J Virol 12:1473–1481, 1973.

22. Sarov I, Friedman A. Electron microscopy of human cytomegalovirus DNA. Arch Virol 50:343–347, 1976.

23. Lakeman A, Osborn JE. Size and infectivity of DNA from human and murine cytomegalovirus. J Virol 30:414–416, 1979.

24. Roizman B, Carmichael LE, Deinhardt F. Herpesviridae: definition, provisional nomenclature and taxonomy. Intervirology 16:201–217, 1981.

25. Fiala M, Honess RW, Heiner DC, et al. Cytomegalovirus proteins: I. Polypeptides of virus and dense bodies. J Virol 19:243–254, 1976.

26. Kim KS, Spaienza VJ, Carp RI, et al. Analysis of structural polypeptides of purified human cytomegalovirus. J Virol 20:604–611, 1976.

27. Stinski MF. Human cytomegalovirus: glycoproteins associated with virions and dense bodies. J Virol 19:594–609, 1976.

28. Irmiere A, Gibson W. Isolation of human cytomegalovirus intranuclear capsids, characterization of their protein constituents, and demonstration that the B-capsid assembly protein is also abundant in noninfectious enveloped particles. J Virol 56:277–283, 1985.

29. Chee M, Rudolf S, Plachter B, et al. Identification of the major capsid protein gene of human CMV. J Virol 63:1345–1353, 1989.

29a. Mocarski ES. Cytomegaloviruses and their replication. In Fields BN, Knipe DM, Howley PM, et al (eds). Fields Virology, 3rd ed. Philadelphia, Lippincott–Raven, 1996, pp 2447–2492.

30. Jahn G, Kouzarides T, March M. Map position and nucleotide sequence of the gene for the large structural phosphoprotein of human cytomegalovirus. J Virol 61:1358–1367, 1987.

31. Meyer H, Bankier A, Lankini MP, et al. Identification and procaryotic expression of the gene coding for the highly immunogenic 28-kilodalton structural phosphoprotein (pp 28) of human cytomegalovirus. J Virol 62:2243–2250, 1988.

32. Ruger B, Klages S, Walla B. Primary structure and transcription of the genes coding for the two vision phosphoproteins pp 65 and pp 71 of human cytomegalovirus. J Virol 61:446–453, 1987.

33. Britt WJ. Cytomegalovirus: overview of the virus and its pathogenic mechanisms. Baillieres Clin Infect Dis 3:307–325, 1996.

34. Britt WJ. Neutralizing antibodies detect a disulfide-linked glycoprotein complex within the envelope of human cytomegalovirus. Virology 135:369–378, 1984.

35. Rasmussen L, Mullehax R, Nelson R, et al. Viral polypeptides detected by complement-dependent neutralizing murine monoclonal antibody to human cytomegalovirus. J Virol 55:274–280, 1985.

36. Gretch DR, Kari B, Rasmussen L, et al. Identification and characterization of three distinct families of glycoprotein complexes present in the envelopes of human cytomegalovirus. J Virol 62:875–888, 1988.

37. Honess RW, Roizman B. Regulation of herpesvirus macromolecular synthesis: I. Cascade regulation of the synthesis of three groups of viral proteins. J Virol 14:8–19, 1974.

38. Kari B, Gehrz R. A human glycoprotein complex designated gC-II is a major heparin-binding component of the envelope. J Virol 66:1761–1764, 1992.

39. Compton T, Nowlin DM, Cooper NR. Initiation of human cytomegalovirus infection requires initial interaction with heparan sulfate. Virology 193:834–841, 1993.

40. Rasmussen L. Immune response to human cytomegalovirus infection. Curr Top Microbiol Immunol 154:222–254, 1990.

41. Keay S, Baldwin B. Anti-idiotype antibodies that mimic gp 86 of human cytomegalovirus inhibit viral fusion but not attachment. J Virol 65:5124–5128, 1991.

42. Whittaker G, Bui M, Helenius A. The role of nuclear import and export in influenza virus infection. Trends Cell Biol 6:67–71, 1996.

43. Stinski MF, Thomsen DR, Stenberg RM, et al. Organization and expression of the immediate early genes of human cytomegalovirus. J Virol 46:1–14, 1983.

44. Stinski MF, Malone CL, Hermiston TW, Liu B. Regulation of human cytomegalovirus transcription. In Wagner EK (ed). Herpesvirus Transcription and its Control. Boca Raton, CRC Press, 1991, pp 245–260.

45. DeMarchi JM. Human cytomegalovirus DNA: restriction enzyme cleavage maps and map location for immediate early, early, and late RNA. Virology 114:23–38, 1981.

46. Gibson W. Immediate-early proteins of human cytomeg-

alovirus strains AD169, Davis and Towne differ in electrophoretic mobility. Virology 112:350–354, 1981.

47. Kemble GW, McCormick AL, Pereira L, et al. A cytomegalovirus protein with properties of herpes simplex virus ICP8: partial purification of the polypeptide and map position of the gene. J Virol 61:3143–3151, 1987.

48. Geballe AP, Leach FS, Mocarski ES. Regulation of cytomegalovirus late gene expression: genes are controlled by post-transcriptional events. J Virol 57:864–874, 1986.

49. The TH, Klein G, Langehuysen M. Antibody reactions to virus specific early antigens (EA) in patients with cytomegalovirus infection. Clin Exp Immunol 16:1–12, 1974.

50. Gibson W, McNally LM, Welch AR, et al. Cytomegalovirus maturational proteinase: site-directed mutagenesis used to probe enzymatic and substrata domains. In Michelson S, Plotkin SA (eds). Multidisciplinary Approach to Understanding Cytomegalovirus Disease. Amsterdam, Elsevier, 1993, pp 21–25.

51. Gonezol E, Andrews PW, Plotkin SA. Cytomegalovirus replicate in differentiated but not in undifferentiated human embryonal carcinoma cells. Science 224:159–161, 1984.

52. Fish KN, Depto AS, Moses AV, et al. Growth kinetics of human cytomegalovirus are altered in monocyte-derived macrophages. J Virol 69:3737–3743, 1995.

53. Reynolds DW, Stagno S, Alford CA. Laboratory diagnosis of cytomegalovirus infections. In Lennette EH, Schmidt NJ (eds). Diagnostic Procedures for Viral, Rickettsial and Chlamydial Infections, 5th ed. Washington, D.C., American Public Health Association, 1979, pp 399–439.

54. Huang ES, Huang SM, Tegtmeier GE, et al. Cytomegalovirus: genetic variation of viral genomes. Ann NY Acad Sci 354:332–346, 1980.

55. Huang ES, Alford CA, Reynolds DW, et al. Molecular epidemiology of cytomegalovirus infection in women and their infants. N Engl J Med 303:958–962, 1980.

56. Pereira L, Hoffman M, Cremer N. Electrophoretic analysis of polypeptides immune precipitated from cytomegalovirus-infected cell extracts by human sera. Infect Immun 36:933–942, 1982.

57. Nowak B, Sullivan C, Sirnow P, et al. Characterization of monoclonal antibodies and polyclonal immune sera directed against human cytomegalovirus virion proteins. Virology 132:325–338, 1984.

58. Landini MP, Re MC, Mirolo B, et al. Human immune response to cytomegalovirus structural polypeptides studied by immunoblotting. J Med Virol 17:303–311, 1985.

59. Jahn G, Scholl BC, Traupe B, et al. The two major structural phosphoproteins (pp 65 and pp 150) of human cytomegalovirus and their antigenic properties. J Gen Virol 68:1327–1337, 1987.

60. Landini MP, Rossier E, Schmitz H. Antibodies to human cytomegalovirus structural peptides during primary infection. J Virol Methods 22:309–317, 1988.

61. Pereira L, Holfman M, Cremer N. Electrophoretic analysis of polypeptides immune precipitated from cytomegalovirus-infected cell extracts by human sera. Infect Immun 36:933–942, 1982.

62. Britt WJ, Vagler L. Structural and immunological characterization of the intracellular forms of an abundant 68,000 MW human cytomegalovirus protein. J Gen Virol 68:1897–1907, 1987.

63. Gibson W, Irmiere A. Selection of particles and proteins for use as human cytomegalovirus subunit vaccines. In Plotkin SA, Michelson S, Pagano JS, et al (eds). CMV:

Pathogenesis and Prevention of Human Infection, vol 20. New York, Alan R. Liss, 1984, pp 305–324.

64. Hayes K, Alford CA, Britt WJ. Antibody response to virus-encoded proteins after cytomegalovirus mononucleosis. J Infect Dis 156:615–621, 1987.

65. Britt WJ. Recent advances in the identification of significant human cytomegalovirus-encoded proteins. Transplant Proc 23:64–69, 1991.

66. Britt WJ, Vugler L, Butfiloski EJ, et al. Cell surface expression of human cytomegalovirus (HCMV) gp 55-116 (gB): use of HCMV-vaccinia recombinant virus infected cells in analysis of the human neutralizing antibody response. J Virol 64:1079–1085, 1990.

67. Marshall GS, Rabalais GP, Stout GG, et al. Antibodies to recombinant-derived glycoprotein B after natural human cytomegalovirus infection correlate with neutralizing activity. J Infect Dis 165:381–384, 1992.

68. Rasmussen L, Morris S, Wolitz R, et al. Deficiency in antibody response to human cytomegalovirus glycoprotein gH in human immunodeficiency virus infected patients at risk for cytomegalovirus retinitis. J Infect Dis 170:673–677, 1994.

69. Boppana SB, Polis MA, Kramer AA, et al. Virus specific antibody responses to human cytomegalovirus in human immunodeficiency virus type 1–infected individuals with HCMV retinitis. J Infect Dis 171:182–185, 1995.

70. Landini MP. New approaches and perspectives in cytomegalovirus diagnosis. Prog Med Virol 40:157–177, 1993.

71. Landini MP, Lezzarotto T, Maine GT, et al. Recombinant mono- and poly-antigens to detect cytomegalovirus specific IgM in human sera by enzyme immunoassay. J Clin Microbiol 33:2535–2542, 1995.

72. Loh LC, Britt WJ, Raggo C, Laferte S. Sequence analysis and expression of the murine cytomegalovirus UL44 gene product. Virology 200:413–427, 1994.

73. Reusser P, Riddell SR, Meyers JD, Greenberg PD. Cytotoxic T-lymphocyte response to cytomegalovirus after human allogeneic bone marrow transplantation: pattern of recovery and correlation with cytomegalovirus infection and disease. Blood 78:1373–1380, 1991.

74. Ljungman P, Aschan J, Azinge JN, et al. Cytomegalovirus viremia and specific T-helper cell responses as predictors of disease after allogeneic marrow transplantation. Br J Haematol 83:118–124, 1993.

75. Walter EA, Greenberg PD, Gilbert MJ, et al. Reconstitution of cellular immunity against cytomegalovirus in recipients of allogeneic bone marrow by transfer of T-cell clones from the donor. N Engl J Med 333:1038–1044, 1995.

76. Gavin MA, Gilbert MJ, Riddell SR, et al. Alkali hydrolysis of recombinant proteins allows for the rapid identification of class I MHC-restricted CTL epitopes. J Immunol 151:3971–3980, 1993.

77. Beninga J, Kopff B, March M. Comparative analysis of fourteen individual human cytomegalovirus proteins for helper T-cell response. J Gen Virol 76:153–160, 1995.

78. Gole E, Nankervis GA. Cytomegalovirus. In Evans AS (ed). Viral Infections of Humans: Epidemiology and Control. New York, Plenum, 1982, pp 167–186.

79. Schopfer K, Lauber E, Krech U. Congenital cytomegalovirus infection in newborn infants of mothers infected before pregnancy. Arch Dis Child 53:536–539, 1978.

80. Numazaki Y, Yano N, Morizuka T, et al. Primary infection with human cytomegalovirus: virus isolation from healthy infants and pregnant women. Am J Epidemiol 91:410–417, 1970.

81. Vial P, Torres J, Stagno S, et al. Serological screening

for cytomegalovirus, rubella virus, herpes simplex virus, hepatitis B virus and *Toxoplasma gondii* in two populations of pregnant women in Chile. Bol Sanit Panam 99:528–538, 1985.

82. Stagno S, Pass RF, Cloud G, et al. Primary cytomegalovirus infection in pregnancy: incidence, transmission to fetus and clinical outcome. JAMA 256:1904–1908, 1986.

83. Hayes K, Danks DM, Gibas H, et al. Cytomegalovirus in human milk. N Engl J Med 287:177–178, 1972.

84. Lang DJ, Krummer JF. Cytomegalovirus in semen: observations in selected populations. J Infect Dis 132:472–473, 1975.

85. Reynolds DW, Stagno S, Hosty TS, et al. Maternal cytomegalovirus excretion and perinatal infection. N Engl J Med 289:1–5, 1973.

86. Stagno S, Reynolds DW, Pass RF, et al. Breast milk and the risk of cytomegalovirus infection. N Engl J Med 302:1073–1076, 1980.

87. Bowden RA. Cytomegalovirus infection in transplant patients: methods of prevention of primary cytomegalovirus. Transplant Proc 23:136–138, 1991.

88. Jordan MC, Rousseau WE, Noble GR, et al. Association of cervical cytomegaloviruses with venereal disease. N Engl J Med 288:932–934, 1973.

89. Coonrod D, Collier AC, Ashley R, et al. Association between cytomegalovirus seroconversion and upper genital tract infection among women attending a sexually transmitted disease clinic: a prospective study. J Infect Dis 177:1188–1193, 1998.

90. Drew WL, Mintz L, Miner RC, et al. Prevalence of cytomegalovirus infection in homosexual men. J Infect Dis 143:188–192, 1981.

91. Chandler SJ, Holmes KK, Wentworth BB, et al. The epidemiology of cytomegaloviral infection in women attending a sexually transmitted disease clinic. J Infect Dis 152:597–605, 1985.

92. Vochem M, Hamprecht K, Jahn G, Speer CP. Transmission of cytomegalovirus to preterm infants through breast milk. Pediatr Infect Dis J 17:53–58, 1998.

93. Stagno S, Cloud GA. Working parents: the impact of day care and breast feeding on cytomegalovirus infection in offspring. Proc Natl Acad Sci USA 91:2384–2389, 1994.

94. Pass RF, August AM, Dworsky M, et al. Cytomegalovirus infection in a day care center. N Engl J Med 307:477–479, 1982.

95. Adler SP, Wilson MS, Lawrence LT. Cytomegalovirus transmission among children attending a day care center. Pediatr Res 19:285A, 1985.

96. Murph JR, Bale JF, Perlman S, et al. The prevalence of cytomegalovirus infection in a midwest day care center. Pediatr Res 19:205A, 1985.

97. Adler SP. The molecular epidemiology of cytomegalovirus transmission among children attending a day care center. J Infect Dis 152:760–768, 1985.

98. Hutto C, Ricks R, Garvie M, et al. Epidemiology of cytomegalovirus infections in young children: day care vs. home care. Pediatr Infect Dis 4:149–152, 1985.

99. Hutto C, Little A, Ricks R, et al. Isolation of cytomegalovirus from toys and hands in a day care center. J Infect Dis 154:527–530, 1986.

100. Faix RG. Survival of cytomegalovirus on environmental surfaces. J Pediatr 106:649–652, 1985.

101. Adler SP. Molecular epidemiology of cytomegalovirus: viral transmission among children attending a day care center, their parents, and caretakers. J Pediatr 112:366–372, 1988.

102. Pass RF, Little EA, Stagno S, et al. Young children as a

probable source of maternal and congenital cytomegalovirus infection. N Engl J Med 316:1366–1370, 1987.

103. Dworsky ME, Lakeman AD, Stagno S. Cytomegalovirus transmission within a family. Pediatr Infect Dis 3:236–238, 1984.

104. Spector SA, Spector DH. Molecular epidemiology of cytomegalovirus infection in premature twin infants and their mother. Pediatr Infect Dis 1:405–409, 1982.

105. Yeager AS. Transmission of cytomegalovirus to mothers by infected infants: another reason to prevent transfusion-acquired infections. Pediatr Infect Dis 2:295–297, 1983.

106. Dworsky ME, Welch K, Cassady G, et al. Occupational risk for primary cytomegalovirus infection. N Engl J Med 309:950–953, 1983.

107. Taber LH, Frank AL, Yow MD, et al. Acquisition of cytomegaloviral infections in families with young children: a serological study. J Infect Dis 151:948, 1985.

108. Pass RF, Hutto SC, Ricks R, et al. Increased rate of cytomegalovirus infection among parents of children attending day care centers. N Engl J Med 314:1414–1418, 1986.

109. Adler SP. Molecular epidemiology of cytomegalovirus: evidence for viral transmission to parents from children infected at a day care center. Pediatr Infect Dis 5:315–318, 1986.

110. Adler SP. Cytomegalovirus and child day care: evidence for an increased infection rate among day-care workers. N Engl J Med 321:1290–1300, 1989.

111. Stagno S, Reynolds DW, Huang ES, et al. Congenital cytomegalovirus infection: occurrence in an immune population. N Engl J Med 296:1254–1258, 1977.

112. Embil JA, Ozere RJ, Haldane EV. Congenital cytomegalovirus infection in two siblings from consecutive pregnancies. J Pediatr 77:417–421, 1970.

113. Stagno S, Reynolds DW, Lakeman AD, et al. Congenital cytomegalovirus infection (C-CMV): consecutive occurrence with similar antigenic viruses. Abstract. Pediatr Res 7:141, 1973.

114. Krech U, Konjajev Z, Jung M. Congenital cytomegalovirus infection in siblings from consecutive pregnancies. Helv Paediatr Acta 26:355–362, 1971.

115. Stagno S, Pass RF, Dworsky ME, et al. Maternal cytomegalovirus infection and perinatal transmission. Clin Obstet Gynecol 25:563–576, 1982.

116. Stagno S, Reynolds DW, Tsiantos A, et al. Cervical cytomegalovirus excretion in pregnant and nonpregnant women: suppression in early gestation. J Infect Dis 131:522–527, 1975.

117. Knox GE, Pass RF, Reynolds DW, et al. Comparative prevalence of subclinical cytomegalovirus and herpes simplex virus infections in the genital and urinary tracts of low income, urban women. J Infect Dis 140:419–422, 1979.

118. Gehrz RC, Christianson WR, Linner KM, et al. Cytomegalovirus-specific humoral and cellular immune response in human pregnancy. J Infect Dis 143:391–395, 1981.

119. Boppana SB, Britt WJ. Antiviral antibody responses and intrauterine transmission after primary maternal cytomegalovirus infection. J Infect Dis 171:1115–1121, 1995.

120. Boppana SB, Miller J, Britt WJ. Transplacentally acquired antiviral antibodies and outcome in congenital human cytomegalovirus infection. Viral Immunol 9:211–218, 1996.

121. Pass RF. Transmission of viruses through human milk. *In* Howell RR, Morris FH Jr, Pickering K. (eds). Role of

Human Milk in Infant Nutrition and Health. Springfield, Ill, Charles C Thomas, 1986, pp 205–224.

122. Chretien JH, McGinnis CG, Muller A. Venereal causes of cytomegalovirus mononucleosis. JAMA 238:1644–1645, 1977.

123. Handsfield HH, Chandler SH, Caine VA, et al. Cytomegalovirus infection in sex partners: evidence for sexual transmission. J Infect Dis 151:344–348, 1985.

124. Kreel I, Zaroff LI, Canter JW, et al. A syndrome following total body perfusion. Surg Gynecol Obstet 111:317–321, 1960.

125. Seaman AJ, Starr A. Febrile postcardiotomy lymphocytic splenomegaly: a new entity. Ann Surg 156:956–960, 1962.

126. Armstrong JA, Tarr GC, Youngblood LA, et al. Cytomegalovirus infection in children undergoing open-heart surgery. Yale J Biol Med 49:83–91, 1976.

127. Prince AM, Szmuness W, Millian SJ, et al. A serologic study of cytomegalovirus infections associated with blood transfusions. N Engl J Med 284:1125–1131, 1971.

128. Stevens DP, Barker LF, Ketcham AS, et al. Asymptomatic cytomegalovirus infection following blood transfusion in tumor surgery. JAMA 211:1341–1344, 1970.

129. Kaariainen L, Klemola E, Paloheimo J. Rise of cytomegalovirus antibodies in an infectious mononucleosis-like syndrome after transfusion. BMJ 1:1270–1272, 1966.

130. Bowden RA, Slichter SJ, Sayers M, et al. A comparison of filtered leukocyte-reduced and cytomegalovirus (CMV) seronegative blood products for the prevention of transfusion-associated CMV infection after bone marrow transplant. Blood 86:3598–3603, 1995.

131. McCracken GJ, Shinefield HR, Cobb K, et al. Congenital cytomegalic inclusion disease: a longitudinal study of 20 patients. Am J Dis Child 117:522–539, 1969.

132. Kumar A, Nankervis GA, Cooper AR, et al. Acquisition of cytomegalovirus infection in infants following exchange transfusion: a prospective study. Transfusion 20:327–331, 1980.

133. King-Lewis PA, Gardner SD. Congenital cytomegalic inclusion diseases following intrauterine transfusion. BMJ 2:603–605, 1969.

134. Pass MA, Johnson JD, Schulman IA, et al. Evaluation of a walking donor blood transfusion program in an intensive care nursery. J Pediatr 89:646–651, 1976.

135. Yeager AS. Transfusion-acquired cytomegalovirus infection in newborn infants. Am J Dis Child 128:478–483, 1974.

136. Yeager AS, Grumet FC, Hafleigh EB, et al. Prevention of transfusion-acquired cytomegalovirus infection in newborn infants. J Pediatr 98:281–287, 1981.

137. Adler SP. Transfusion-associated cytomegalovirus infections. Rev Infect Dis 5:977–993, 1983.

138. Adler SP, Chandrika T, Lawrence L, et al. Cytomegalovirus infections in neonates due to blood transfusions. Pediatr Infect Dis 2:114–118, 1983.

139. Onorato IM, Morens DM, Martone WJ, et al. Epidemiology of cytomegalovirus infections: recommendations for prevention and control. Rev Infect Dis 7:479–497, 1985.

140. May AG, Betts RF, Freeman RB, et al. An analysis of cytomegalovirus infection and HLA antigen matching on the outcome of renal transplantation. Ann Surg 187:110–117, 1978.

141. Niaudet P, Raguin G, Lefevre JJ, et al. Serological status of cytomegalovirus and outcome of renal transplantation. Kidney Int 23:S50–S53, 1983.

142. Tourkantonis A, Lazaridis A. Interaction between cytomegalovirus infection and renal transplant rejection. Kidney Int 23:S46–S49, 1983.

143. Pass RF, Long WK, Whitley RJ, et al. Productive infection with cytomegalovirus and herpes simplex virus in renal transplant recipients: role of source of kidney. J Infect Dis 137:556–563, 1978.

144. Neiman PE, Reeves W, Ray G, et al. A prospective analysis of interstitial pneumonia and opportunistic viral infection among recipients of allogeneic bone marrow grafts. J Infect Dis 136:754–767, 1977.

145. Winston DJ, Gale RP, Meyer DV, et al. Infectious complications of human bone marrow transplantation. Medicine 58:1–31, 1979.

146. Meyers JD, Flournoy N, Thomas ED. Nonbacterial pneumonia after allogeneic marrow transplantation: a review of ten years' experience. Rev Infect Dis 4:1119–1132, 1982.

147. Preiksaitis JK, Rosno S, Grumet C, et al. Infections due to herpesviruses in cardiac transplant recipients: role of the donor heart and immunosuppressive therapy. J Infect Dis 147:974–981, 1983.

148. Dummer JS, Hardy A, Poorsattar A, et al. Early infections in the kidney, heart and liver transplant recipients on cyclosporine. Transplantation 36:259–267, 1983.

149. Pollard RB, Rand KH, Arvin AM, et al. Cell-mediated immunity to cytomegalovirus infection in normal subjects and cardiac transplant patients. J Infect Dis 137:541–549, 1978.

150. Pollard RB, Arvin AM, Gamberg P, et al. Specific cell-mediated immunity and infections with herpesviruses in cardiac transplant recipients. Am J Med 73:679–687, 1982.

151. Pass RF, Hutto SC, Reynolds DW, et al. Increased frequency of cytomegalovirus in children in group day care. Pediatrics 74:121–126, 1984.

152. Pass RF, Stagno S. Ctyomegalovirus. In Donowitz LG (ed). Hospital Acquired Infection in the Pediatric Patient. Baltimore, Williams & Wilkins, 1988.

153. Yeager AS. Longitudinal, serological study of cytomegalovirus infections in nurses and in personnel without patient contact. J Clin Microbiol 2:448–452, 1975.

154. Friedman HM, Lewis MR, Nemerofsky DM, et al. Acquisition of cytomegalovirus infection among female employees at a pediatric hospital. Pediatr Infect Dis 3:233–235, 1984.

155. Yow MD, Lakeman AD, Stagno S, et al. Use of restriction enzymes to investigate the source of a primary CMV infection in a pediatric nurse. Pediatrics 70:713–716, 1982.

156. Wilfert CV, Huang ES, Stagno S. Restriction endonuclease analysis of cytomegalovirus DNA as an epidemiological tool. Pediatrics 70:717–721, 1982.

157. Adler SP, Baggett J, Wilson M, et al. Molecular epidemiology of cytomegalovirus in a nursery: lack of evidence for nosocomial transmission. J Pediatr 108:117–123, 1986.

157a. Ahlfors K, Ivarsson SA, Harris S, et al. Congenital cytomegalovirus infection and disease in Sweden and the relative importance of primary and secondary maternal infections. Scand J Infect Dis 16:129–137, 1984.

158. Rutter D, Griffiths P, Trompeter RS. Cytomegalic inclusion disease after recurrent maternal infection. Lancet 2:1182, 1985.

159. Fowler KB, Stagno S, Pass RF, et al. The outcome of congenital cytomegalovirus infection in relation to maternal antibody status. N Engl J Med 326:663–667, 1992.

160. Yow MD, Williamson DW, Leeds LJ, et al. Epidemiologic characteristics of cytomegalovirus infection in

mothers and their infants. Am J Obstet Gynecol 158:1189–1195, 1988.

161. Demmler GJ. Summary of a workshop on surveillance for congenital cytomegalovirus disease. Rev Infect Dis 13:315–319, 1991.

162. Griffiths PD. Cytomegalovirus. In Zuckerman AJ, Banatvala JE, Pattison JR (eds). Principles and Practice of Clinical Virology. New York, John Wiley 1987, pp 75–109.

163. Jones MM, Lidsky MD, Brewer EJ, et al. Congenital cytomegalovirus infection and maternal systemic lupus erythematosus: a case report. Arthritis Rheum 29:1402–1404, 1986.

164. Preece PM, Pearl KN, Peckham CS. Congenital cytomegalovirus infection. Arch Dis Child 59:1120–1126, 1984.

165. Evans TJ, McCollum JPK, Valdimarssan H. Congenital cytomegalovirus infection after maternal renal transplantation. Lancet 1:1359–1360, 1975.

166. Hayes K, Symington G, Mackay IR. Maternal immunosuppression and cytomegalovirus infection of the fetus. Aust NZ J Med 9:430–433, 1979.

167. Portalini M, Cermelli S, Sabbatini AMT, et al. A fatal case of congenital cytomegalic inclusion disease following recurrent maternal infection. Microbiologica 18:427–428, 1995.

168. Morris DJ, Sims D, Chiswick M, et al. Symptomatic congenital cytomegalovirus infection after maternal recurrent infection. Pediatr Infect Dis J 13:61–64, 1994.

169. Laifer SA, Ehrlich GD, Haff DS, et al. Congenital cytomegalovirus infection in offspring of liver transplant recipient. Clin Infect Dis 20:52–55, 1995.

170. Muss-Pinhata MM, Yamamoto AY, Figueiredo LTM, et al. Congenital and perinatal cytomegalovirus infection in infants born to mothers infected with human immunodeficiency virus. J Pediatr 132:285–290, 1998.

171. Pass RF, Fowler KB, Stagno S, et al. Gestational age at time of maternal infection and outcome of congenital cytomegalovirus infection. Pediatr Res 35:191A, 1994.

171a. Stagno S, Pass RF, Dworsky ME, et al. Congenital and perinatal cytomegaloviral infections. Semin Perinatol 7:31–42, 1983.

172. Griffiths PD, Grundy JE. Molecular biology and immunology of cytomegalovirus. Biochem J 241:313–324, 1987.

173. Grundy JE, Pahal GS, Akbar AN. Increased adherence of CD2 peripheral blood lymphocytes to CMV-infected fibroblasts is blocked by anti-LFA-3 antibody. Immunology 78:413–420, 1993.

174. Sedmak DD, Knight DA, Vook NC, Waldman JW. Divergent patterns of ELAM-1, ICAM-1 and VCAM-1 expression on CMV-infected endothelial cells. Transplantation 58:1379–1385, 1994.

175. Keithley EM, Woolf NK, Harris JP. Development of morphological and physiological changes in the cochlea induced by cytomegalovirus. Laryngoscope 99:409–414, 1989.

176. Stagno S, Reynolds DW, Tsiantos A, et al. Comparative serial virologic and serologic studies of symptomatic and subclinical congenitally and natally acquired cytomegalovirus infections. J Infect Dis 132:568–577, 1975.

177. Wiertz EJHJ, Jones TR, Sun L, et al. The human cytomegalovirus US11 gene product dislocates MHC class I heavy chains from the endoplasmic reticulum to the cytosol. Cell 84:769–779, 1996.

178. Li L, Coelingh KL, Britt WJ. Human cytomegalovirus neutralizing antibody resistant phenotype is associated with reduced expression of glycoprotein H. J Virol 69:6047–6053, 1995.

179. Pass RF, Stagno S, Britt WJ, et al. Specific cell mediated immunity and the natural history of congenital infection with cytomegalovirus. J Infect Dis 148:953–961, 1983.

180. Pass RF, Dworsky ME, Whitley RJ, et al. Specific lymphocyte blastogenic responses in children with cytomegalovirus and herpes simplex virus infections acquired early in infancy. Infect Immun 34:166–170, 1981.

181. Starr SE, Tolpin MD, Friedman HM, et al. Impaired cellular immunity to cytomegalovirus in congenitally infected children and their mothers. J Infect Dis 140:500–505, 1979.

182. Griffiths PD, Baboonian C. A prospective study of primary cytomegalovirus infection during pregnancy: final report. Br J Obstet Gynaecol 91:307–315, 1984.

183. Granstrom ML. Perinatal cytomegalovirus in man. Thesis. University of Helsinki, Helsinki, Finland, 1979.

184. Monif GRG, Egan EA, Held B, et al. The correlation of maternal cytomegalovirus infection during varying stages in gestation with neonatal involvement. J Pediatr 80:17–20, 1972.

185. Preece PM, Pearl KN, Peckham CS. Congenital cytomegalovirus infection. Arch Dis Child 59:1120–1126, 1984.

186. Chou S, Kim DY, Norman DJ. Transmission of cytomegalovirus by pretransplant leukocyte transfusions in renal transplant candidates. J Infect Dis 155:565–567, 1987.

187. Becroft DMO. Prenatal cytomegalovirus infection: epidemiology, pathology and pathogenesis. In Rosenberg HS, Bernstein J (eds). Perspectives in Pediatric Pathology, vol 6. New York, Masson Publishing USA, 1981, pp 203–241.

188. Wolf A, Cowen D. Perinatal infections of the central nervous system. J Neuropathol Exp Neurol 18:191–243, 1959.

189. Naeye RL. Cytomegalic inclusion disease, the fetal disorder. Am J Clin Pathol 47:738–744, 1967.

190. Hanshaw JB. Developmental abnormalities associated with congenital cytomegalovirus infection. Adv Teratol 4:64, 1970.

191. Arey JB. Cytomegalic inclusion disease in infancy. Am J Dis Child 88:525–526, 1954.

192. Mercer RD, Luse S, Guyton DH. Clinical diagnosis of generalized cytomegalic inclusion disease. Pediatrics 11:502–514, 1953.

193. Sackett GL, Ford MM. Cytomegalic inclusion disease with calcification outlining the cerebral ventricles. AJR Am J Roentgenol 76:512, 1956.

194. Jamison RM, Hathorn AW. Isolation of cytomegalovirus from cerebrospinal fluid of a congenitally infected infant. Am J Dis Child 132:63–64, 1978.

195. Stagno S, Reynolds DW, Amos CS, et al. Auditory and visual defects resulting from symptomatic and subclinical congenital cytomegaloviral and Toxoplasma infections. Pediatrics 59:669–678, 1977.

196. Myers EN, Stool S. Cytomegalic inclusion disease of the inner ear. Laryngoscope 78:1904–1915, 1968.

197. Davis GL. Cytomegalovirus in the inner ear. Case report and electron microscopic study. Ann Otol Rhinol Laryngol 78:1179–1188, 1969.

198. Guyton TB, Ehrlich F, Blanc WA, et al. New observations in generalized cytomegalic inclusion disease of the newborn: reports of a case with chorioretinitis. N Engl J Med 257:803–807, 1957.

199. Ansari BM, Davis DB, Jones MR. Calcification in liver

associated with congenital cytomegalic inclusion disease. J Pediatr 90:661–663, 1977.

200. Alix D, Castel Y, Gouedard H. Hepatic calcification in congenital cytomegalic inclusion disease. J Pediatr 92:856, 1978.

201. Osborn JE, Shahidi NT. Thrombocytopenia in murine cytomegalovirus infection. J Lab Clin Med 81:53–63, 1973.

202. Fetterman GH, Sherman FE, Fabrizio NS, et al. Generalized cytomegalic inclusion disease of the newborn: localization of inclusions in the kidney. Arch Pathol 86:86–94, 1968.

203. Donnellan WL, Chantra-Umporn S, Kidd JM. The cytomegalic inclusion cell: an electron microscopic study. Arch Pathol 82:336–348, 1966.

204. Reyes C, Pereira S, Warden MJ, Sills J. Cytomegalovirus enteritis in a premature infant. J Pediatr Sur 32:1545–1547, 1997.

205. Blanc WA. Pathology of the placenta and cord in some viral infections. In Hanshaw JB, Dudgeon JA (eds). Viral Diseases of the Fetus and Newborn. Philadelphia, WB Saunders, 1978, pp 237–258.

206. Benirschke K, Mendoza GR, Bazeley PL. Placental and fetal manifestations of cytomegalovirus infection. Virchows Arch B 16:121, 1974.

207. Weller TH, Hanshaw JB. Virologic and clinical observations on cytomegalic inclusion disease. N Engl J Med 266:1233–1244, 1962.

208. Boppana SB, Pass RF, Britt WJ, et al. Symptomatic congenital cytomegalovirus infection: neonatal morbidity and mortality. Pediatr Infect Dis J 11:93–99, 1992.

208a. Anderson KS, Amos CS, Boppana S, Pass RF. Ocular abnormalities in congenital cytomegalovirus infection. J Am Optom Assoc 67:273–278, 1996.

209. Istes AS, Demmler GJ, Dobbins JG, et al. Surveillance for congenital cytomegalovirus disease: a report from the National Congenital Cytomegalovirus Disease Registry. Clin Infect Dis 20:665–670, 1995.

210. Demmler GJ. Congenital cytomegalovirus infection. Semin Pediatr Neurol 1:36–42, 1994.

211. Hanshaw JB, Dudgeon JA (eds). Viral Diseases of the Fetus and Newborn. Philadelphia, WB Saunders, 1978.

212. Medearis TN. Observations concerning human cytomegalovirus infection and disease. Bull Johns Hopkins Hosp 114:181–211, 1964.

213. Stagno S, Brasfield DM, Brown MC, et al. Infant pneumonitis associated with cytomegalovirus, chlamydia, pneumocystis and ureaplasma—a prospective study. Pediatrics 68:322–329, 1981.

214. Stagno S, Pass RF, Thomas JP, et al. Defects of tooth structure in congenital cytomegalovirus infection. Pediatrics 69:646–648, 1982.

215. Melish ME, Hanshaw JB. Congenital cytomegalovirus infection: developmental progress of infants detected by routine screening. Am J Dis Child 126:190–194, 1973.

216. Saigal S, Luynk O, Larke B, et al. The outcome in children with congenital cytomegalovirus infection: a longitudinal follow-up study. Am J Dis Child 136:896–901, 1982.

217. Williamson WD, Desmond MM, LaFevers N, et al. Symptomatic congenital cytomegalovirus: disorders of language, learning and hearing. Am J Dis Child 136:902–905, 1982.

218. Berenberg W, Nankervis G. Long-term follow-up of cytomegalic inclusion disease of infancy. Pediatrics 37:403, 1970.

219. Conboy TJ, Pass RF, Stagno S, et al. Early clinical manifestations and intellectual outcome in children with symptomatic congenital cytomegalovirus infection. J Pediatr 111:343–348, 1987.

219a. Boppana SB, Fowler KB, Vaid Y, et al. Neuroradiographic findings in the newborn period and long-term outcome in children with symptomatic congenital CMV infection. Pediatrics 99:409–414, 1997.

220. Kumar ML, Nankervis GA, Gold E. Inapparent congenital cytomegalovirus infection: a follow-up study. N Engl J Med 288:1370–1377, 1973.

221. Reynolds DW, Stagno S, Stubbs KG, et al. Inapparent congenital cytomegalovirus infection with elevated cord IgM levels: causal relationship with auditory and mental deficiency. N Engl J Med 290:291–296, 1974.

222. Pearl KN, Preece PM, Ades A, et al. Neurodevelopmental assessment after congenital cytomegalovirus infection. Arch Dis Child 61:232–236, 1986.

223. Conboy TJ, Pass RF, Stagno S, et al. Intellectual development in school aged children with asymptomatic congenital cytomegalovirus infection. Pediatrics 77:801–806, 1986.

224. Pass RF, Stagno S, Myers GJ, et al. Outcome of symptomatic congenital cytomegalovirus infection: results of long-term longitudinal follow-up. Pediatrics 66:758–762, 1980.

225. Ramsey MEB, Miller E, Peckham CS. Outcome of confirmed symptomatic congenital cytomegalovirus infection. Arch Dis Child 66:1068–1069, 1991.

226. Williamson WD, Percy AK, Yow MD, et al. Asymptomatic congenital cytomegalovirus infection. Audiologic, neuroradiologic and neurodevelopmental abnormalities during the first year. Am J Dis Child 144:1365–1368, 1990.

227. Ivarsson SA, Lernmark B, Svanberg L. Ten-year clinical, developmental and intellectual follow up of children with congenital cytomegalovirus infection without neurologic symptoms at one year of age. Pediatrics 99:800–803, 1997.

228. Harris S, Ahlfors K, Ivarsson S, et al. Congenital cytomegalovirus infection and sensorineural hearing loss. Ear Hear 5:352–355, 1984.

229. Fowler KB, McCollister FP, Dahle AJ, et al. Progressive and fluctuating sensorineural hearing loss in children with asymptomatic congenital cytomegalovirus infection. J Pediatr 130:624–630, 1997.

230. Hicks T, Fowler K, Richardson M, et al. Congenital cytomegalovirus infection and neonatal auditory screening. J Pediatr 123:779–782, 1993.

231. Stagno S, Pass RF, Dworsky ME, et al. Congenital cytomegalovirus infection: the relative importance of primary and recurrent maternal infection. N Engl J Med 306:945–949, 1982.

232. Whitley RJ, Brasfield D, Reynolds DW, et al. Protracted pneumonitis in young infants associated with perinatally acquired cytomegaloviral infection. J Pediatr 89:11–16, 1976.

233. Brasfield DM, Stagno S, Whitley RJ, et al. Infant pneumonitis associated with cytomegalovirus, chlamydia, pneumocystis and ureaplasma: follow-up. Pediatrics 79:76–83, 1987.

234. Yeager AS, Palumbo PE, Malachowski N, et al. Sequelae of maternally derived cytomegalovirus infections in premature infants. Pediatrics 102:918–922, 1983.

235. Paryani SG, Yeager AS, Hosford-Dunn H, et al. Sequelae of acquired cytomegalovirus infection in premature and sick term infants. J Pediatr 107:451–456, 1985.

235a. Vochem M, Hamprecht K, Jahn G, Speer CP. Transmission of cytomegalovirus to preterm infants through breast milk. Pediatr Infect Dis J 17:53–58, 1998.

236. Ballard RB, Drew WL, Hufnagle KG, et al. Acquired cytomegalovirus infection in preterm infants. Am J Dis Child 133:482–485, 1979.

237. Demmler GJ, Buffone GJ, Schimbor CM, et al. Detection of cytomegalovirus in urine from newborns by using polymerase chain reaction DNA amplification. J Infect Dis 158:1177–1184, 1988.

238. Warren WP, Balcarek K, Smith RJ, et al. Comparison of rapid methods of detection of cytomegalovirus in saliva with virus isolation in tissue culture. J Clin Microbiol 30:786–789, 1992.

239. Nelson CT, Istas AS, Wilkerson MK, et al. PCR detection of cytomegalovirus DNA in serum as a diagnostic test for congenital cytomegalovirus infection. J Clin Microbiol 33:3317–3318, 1995.

240. Johansson PJH, Jonsson M, Ahlfors K, et al. Retrospective diagnosis of congenital cytomegalovirus infection performed by polymerase chain reaction in blood stored on filter paper. Scand J Infect Dis 29:465–468, 1997.

241. Dzierzahowska D, Augustynowicz E, Gzyl A, et al. Application of polymerase chain reaction (PCR) for the detection of DNA-HCMV in cerebrospinal fluid of neonates and infants with cytomegalovirus infection. Neurol Neurochir Pol 31:447–462, 1997.

242. Stagno S, Pass RF, Reynolds DW, et al. Comparative study of diagnostic procedures for congenital cytomegalovirus infection. Pediatrics 65:251–257, 1980.

243. Shuster EA, Beneke JS, Tegtmeier GE, et al. Monoclonal antibody for rapid laboratory detection of cytomegalovirus infections: characterization and diagnostic application. Mayo Clin Proc 60:577, 1985.

244. Alpert G, Mazeron MC, Colimon R, et al. Rapid detection of human cytomegalovirus in the urine of humans. J Infect Dis 152:631–633, 1985.

245. Stirk PR, Griffiths PD. Use of monoclonal antibodies for the diagnosis of cytomegalovirus infection by the detection of early antigen fluorescent foci (DEAFF) in cell culture. J Med Virol 21:329–337, 1987.

246. Boppana SB, Smith RJ, Stagno S, et al. Evaluation of a microtiter plate fluorescent-antibody assay for rapid detection of human cytomegalovirus infection. J Clin Microbiol 30:721–723, 1992.

247. Chou S, Merigan TC. Rapid detection and quantitation of human cytomegalovirus in urine through DNA hybridization. N Engl J Med 308:921–925, 1983.

248. Spector SA, Rua JA, Spector DH, et al. Detection of human cytomegalovirus in clinical specimens by DNA-DNA hybridization. J Infect Dis 150:121–126, 1984.

249. Schuster V, Matz B, Wiegand H, et al. Detection of human cytomegalovirus in urine by DNA-DNA and RNA-DNA hybridization. J Infect Dis 154:309–314, 1986.

250. Virtanen M, Syvanen A, Oram J, et al. Cytomegalovirus in urine: detection of viral DNA by sandwich hybridization. J Clin Microbiol 20:1083–1088, 1984.

251. Lurain NS, Thompson SK, Farrand SK. Rapid detection of cytomegalovirus in clinical specimens by using biotinylated DNA probes and analysis of cross-reactivity with herpes simplex virus. J Clin Microbiol 24:724–730, 1986.

252. Spector SA, Merrill R, Wolf D, et al. Detection of human cytomegalovirus in plasma of AIDS patients during acute visceral disease by DNA amplification. J Clin Microbiol 30:2359–2365, 1992.

253. Cotte L, Drouet E, Bissuel F, et al. Diagnostic value of amplification of human cytomegalovirus DNA from gastrointestinal biopsies from human immunodeficiency virus-infected patients. J Clin Microbiol 31:2066–2069, 1993.

254. Nelson CT, Istas AS, Wilkerson MK, Demmler GJ. PCR detection of CMV DNA in serum as a diagnostic test for congenital CMV infection. J Clin Microbiol 33:3317–3318, 1995.

255. Erice A, Holm MA, Gill PC, et al. Cytomegalovirus (CMV) antigenemia assay is more sensitive than shell viral cultures for rapid detection of CMV in polymorphonuclear blood leukocytes. J Clin Microbiol 30:2822–2825, 1992.

256. Mazzulli T, Rubin RH, Ferraro MJ, et al. Cytomegalovirus antigenemia: clinical correlations in transplant recipients and in persons with AIDS. J Clin Microbiol 31:2824–2827, 1993.

257. Dodt KK, Jacobsen PH, Hofmann B, et al. Development of cytomegalovirus (CMV) disease may be predicted in HIV-infected patients by CMV polymerase chain reaction and the antigenemia test. AIDS 11:F21–28, 1997.

258. Wetherill PE, Landry ML, Alcabes P, Friedland G. Use of a quantitative cytomegalovirus (CMV) antigenemia test in evaluating HIV+ patients with and without CMV diease. J Acquir Immune Defic Syndr Hum Retrovirol 12:33–37, 1996.

259. Lesprit P, Scieux C, Lemann M, et al. Use of the cytomegalovirus (CMV) antigenemia assay for the rapid diagnosis of primary CMV infection in hospitalized adults. Clin Infect Dis 26:646–650, 1998.

260. Revello MG, Zavattoni M, Sarasini A, et al. Human cytomegalovirus in blood of immunocompetent persons during primary infection: prognostic implications for pregnancy. J Infect Dis 177:1170–1175, 1998.

261. Griffiths PD, Kangro HO. A user's guide to the indirect solid-phase radioimmunoassay for the detection of cytomegalovirus specific IgM antibodies. J Virol Methods 8:271–282, 1984.

262. Stagno S, Tinker MK, Elrod C, et al. Immunoglobulin M antibodies detected by enzyme-linked immunosorbent assay and radioimmunoassay in the diagnosis of cytomegalovirus infections in pregnant women and newborn infants. J Clin Microbiol 21:930–935, 1985.

263. Vornhagen R, Hinderer W, Sonneborn HH, et al. IgM-specific serodiagnosis of acute human cytomegalovirus infection using recombinant autologous fusion proteins. J Virol Methods 60:73–80, 1996.

264. Lazzarotto T, Maine GT, DalMonte P, et al. A novel Western Blot test containing both viral and recombinant proteins for anticytomegalovirus immunoglobulin M detection. J Clin Microbiol 35:393–397, 1997.

265. French MLV, Thompson JR, White A. Cytomegalovirus viremia with transmission from mother to fetus. Ann Intern Med 86:748–749, 1977.

266. Huikeshoven FJM, Wallenburg HCS, Jahoda MGJ. Diagnosis of severe fetal cytomegalovirus infection from amniotic fluid in the third trimester of pregnancy. Am J Obstet Gynecol 142:1053–1054, 1982.

267. Yambao TJ, Clark D, Weiner L, Aubry RH. Isolation of cytomegalovirus from the amniotic fluid during the third trimester. Am J Obstet Gynecol 141:937–938, 1981.

268. Grose C, Weiner CP. Prenatal diagnosis of congenital cytomegalovirus infection: two decades later. Am J Obstet Gynecol 163:447–450, 1990.

269. Lamy ME, Mulongo KN, Gadisseux JF, et al. Prenatal diagnosis of fetal cytomegalovirus infection. Am J Obstet Gynecol 166:91–94, 1992.

270. Grose C, Meehan T, Weiner CP. Prenatal diagnosis of congenital cytomegalovirus infection by virus isolation after amniocentesis. Pediatr Infect Dis J 11:605–608, 1992.

271. Pass RF. Commentary: is there a role for prenatal diag-

nosis of congenital cytomegalovirus infection? Pediatr Infect Dis J 11:608–609, 1992.

272. Lynch L, Daffos F, Emanuel D, et al. Prenatal diagnosis of fetal cytomegalovirus infection. Am J Obstet Gynecol 166:91–94, 1992.

273. Ruellan EG, Barjot P, Carupet M, et al. Evaluation of virological procedures to detect fetal human cytomegalovirus infection: avidity of IgG antibodies, virus detection in amniotic fluid and maternal serum. J Med Virol 50:9–15, 1996.

274. Donner C, Liesnard C, Brancart F, Rodesch F. Accuracy of amniotic fluid testing before 21 weeks of gestation in prenatal diagnosis of congenital cytomegalovirus infection. Prenat Diagn 14:1055–1059, 1994.

275. Collaborative DHPG Treatment Study Group. Treatment of serious cytomegalovirus infections with 9-(1,3-dihydroxy-2-propoxymethyl) guanine in patients with AIDS and other immunodeficiencies. N Engl J Med 314:801–805, 1986.

276. Chrisp P, Clissold SP. Foscarnet: a review of its antiviral activity, pharmacokinetic properties and therapeutic use in immunocompromised patients with cytomegalovirus retinitis. Drugs 41:104–129, 1991.

277. Faulds D, Heel RC. Ganciclovir: a review of its antiviral activity, pharmacokinetic properties and therapeutic efficacy in cytomegalovirus infections. Drugs 39:597–638, 1990.

278. Whitley RJ, Cloud G, Gruber W, et al. Ganciclovir treatment of symptomatic congenital cytomegalovirus infection: results of a Phase II study. J Infect Dis 175:1080–1086, 1997.

279. Nigro G, Scholz H, Bartmann U. Ganciclovir therapy for symptomatic congenital cytomegalovirus infection in infants: a two-regimen experience. J Pediatr 124:318–322, 1994.

280. Glowacki LS, Smaill FM. Meta-analysis of immune globulin prophylaxis in transplant recipients for the prevention of symptomatic cytomegalovirus disease. Transplant Proc 25:1408–1410, 1993.

281. Hamilton AA, Manuel DM, Grundy JE, et al. A humanized antibody against human cytomegalovirus (CMV) gp UL 75 (gH) for prophylaxis or treatment of CMV infections. J Infect Dis 176:59–68, 1997.

282. Elek SD, Stern H. Development of a vaccine against mental retardation caused by cytomegalovirus infection in utero. Lancet 1:1–5, 1974.

283. Plotkin SA, Furukawa T, Zygraich N, et al. Candidate cytomegalovirus strain for human vaccination. Infect Immun 12:521–527, 1975.

284. Stern H. Live cytomegalovirus vaccination of healthy volunteers: eight-year follow-up studies. In Plotkin SA, Michelson S, Pagano JS, et al (eds). CMV: Pathogenesis and Prevention of Human Infection. Birth Defects: Original Article Series, vol 20. New York, Alan R. Liss, 1984, pp 263–269.

285. Britt WJ. Vaccines against human cytomegalovirus: time to test. Trends Microbiol 4:34–38, 1996.

286. Plotkin SA, Starr SE, Friedman HM, et al. Effect of Towne live virus vaccine on cytomegalovirus disease after renal transplant. Ann Intern Med 114:525–531, 1991.

287. Balfour HH, Jr, Welo PK, Sachs GW. Cytomegalovirus vaccine trial in 400 renal transplant candidates. Transplant Proc 17:81–83, 1985.

288. Plotkin SA, Farquhar J, Hornberger E. Clinical trials of immunization with the Towne 125 strain of human cytomegalovirus. J Infect Dis 134:470–475, 1976.

289. Plotkin SA, Starr SE, Friedman HM, et al. Protective effects of Towne cytomegalovirus vaccine against low-passage cytomegalovirus administered as a challenge. J Infect Dis 159:860–865, 1989.

290. Adler SP, Hempfling SH, Starr SE, et al. Safety and immunogenicity of the Towne strain cytomegalovirus vaccine. Pediatr Infect Dis J 17:200–206, 1998.

291. Cranage MP, Kouzarides T, Bankier AT, et al. Identification of human cytomegalovirus glycoprotein B gene and induction of neutralizing antibodies via its expression in recombinant vaccinia virus. EMBO J 5:3057–3063, 1986.

292. Marshall GS, Ricciardi RP, Rando RF, et al. An adenovirus recombinant that expresses the human cytomegalovirus major envelope glycoprotein and induces neutralizing antibodies. J Infect Dis 162:1177–1181, 1990.

293. Brady MT, Milam JD, Anderson DC, et al. Use of deglycerolized red blood cells to prevent posttransfusion infection with cytomegalovirus in neonates. J Infect Dis 150:334–399, 1984.

294. Stagno S, Whitley RJ. Herpesvirus infection of pregnancy. N Engl J Med 313:1270–1274, 1327–1329, 1985.

295. Peckham CS, Chin KS, Coleman JC, et al. Cytomegalovirus infection in pregnancy: preliminary findings from a prospective study. Lancet 1:1352–1355, 1983.

296. Yow MD. Congenital cytomegalovirus disease: a NOW problem. J Infect Dis 159:163–167, 1989.

297. Pass RF, Stagno S. Cytomegalovirus. In Donowitz L (ed). Hospital Acquired Infection in the Pediatric Patient. Baltimore, Williams & Wilkins, 1988.

298. Gilbert GL, Hayes K, Hudson IL, et al. Prevention of transfusion-acquired cytomegalovirus infection in infants by blood filtration to remove leukocytes. Lancet 1:1228–1231, 1989.

299. Holland PV, Schmitt PJ. Standards for Blood Banks and Transfusion Services, 12th ed. Arlington, Va, Committee on Standards, American Association of Blood Banks, 1987, pp 30–31.

300. Dworsky ME, Stagno S, Pass RF, et al. Persistence of cytomegalovirus in human milk after storage. J Pediatr 101:440–443, 1982.

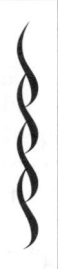

Herpes Simplex Virus Infections

ANN M. ARVIN, M.D., and RICHARD J. WHITLEY, M.D.

Herpes simplex virus (HSV) infections were recognized by the ancient Greeks. The word *herpes*, meaning "to creep or crawl," was used to describe skin lesions. Herodotus associated mouth ulcers and lip vesicles with fever[1] and called this event "herpes febrilis." Genital herpetic infections were first described by Astruc, a physician to French royalty.[2] The transmissibility of these viruses was established unequivocally by passage of virus from lip and genital lesions of humans to either the cornea or the scarified skin of the rabbit.[3] During the early twentieth century, diseases associated with HSV infections became more clearly defined by numerous clinical and pathologic case reports.

Neonatal herpes simplex infection was identified as a distinct disease 60 years ago. The first written descriptions of neonatal HSV infections were attributed to Hass, who described the histopathologic findings of a fatal case, and to Batignani, who described a newborn with herpes simplex keratitis.[4, 5] During the subsequent decades our understanding of neonatal HSV infections was based on histopathologic descriptions of the disease, which indicated a broad spectrum of organ involvement in infants.

An important scientific breakthrough occurred in the mid 1960s when Nahmias and Dowdle demonstrated two antigenic types of HSV.[6] The development of viral typing methods provided the tools required to clarify the epidemiology of these infections. HSV infections "above the belt," primarily of the lip and oropharynx, were found in most cases to be caused by HSV type 1. Those infections "below the belt," particularly genital infections, were usually caused by HSV type 2. The finding that both genital herpes infections and neonatal HSV infections were most often caused by HSV type 2 suggested a cause-and-effect relationship between these two disease entities. This causal relationship was strengthened by detection of the virus in the maternal genital tract at the time of delivery, which indicated that acquisition of the virus by the infant occurs by contact with infected genital secretions during birth.

During the past 20 years, our knowledge of the epidemiology, natural history and pathogenesis of neonatal HSV infections has been enhanced greatly. The development of antiviral therapy represents a significant advance in the management of infected children, providing the opportunity to decrease mortality and reduce the morbidity associated with these infections. Neonatal HSV infection should be more amenable to prevention and treatment than many other pathogens because it is acquired most often at birth rather than during gestation. As our understanding of the epidemiology of HSV infections has improved, postnatal acquisition of HSV type 1 has been documented from nonmaternal sources, and more cases due to HSV type 1 infections of the maternal genital tract have been identified. New perspectives on the changing presentations of neonatal HSV infection, the obstacles to diagnosis, and the value of antiviral therapy are topics addressed in this chapter.

HERPES SIMPLEX VIRUS

Structure

The biologic, molecular, antigenic, and epidemiologic characteristics of HSV types 1 and 2 have been the subject of numerous publications. Recent reviews highlight the importance of these organisms as models for viral replication and as pathogens in human infection.[7, 8]

Herpes simplex viruses are members of a family of large DNA viruses that contain centrally located, linear, double-stranded DNA. Other members of the herpesvirus family include cytomegalovirus, varicella-zoster virus, Epstein-Barr virus, and human herpesviruses 6, 7, and 8.[7, 8] As a family, these viruses are virtually indistinguishable from each other by electron microscopy. The viral DNA is packaged inside a protein structure, the capsid, which confers icosahedral symmetry to the virus. The capsid consists of 162 capsomers and is surrounded by a tightly adherent membrane known as the tegument. An envelope consisting of glycoproteins, lipids, and polyamines loosely surrounds the capsid and tegument. The glycoproteins mediate attachment of the virus to cells.

Our current understanding of HSV indicates that the genome consists of about 150,000 base pairs.[7] The DNA encodes more than 85 polypeptides. The genome consists of two components, L and S, each of which contains unique sequences that can invert, which leads to four isomers. The ability to exist as one of four isomers is a unique property of HSV. Viral DNA extracted from virions or infected cells, then, consists of four equal populations differing solely with respect to the relative orientation of these two unique components.

The DNAs of HSV types 1 and 2 are colinear, with respect to the order of genes encoding viral proteins. The percent homology of base pairs that constitute each gene varies from high to lesser degrees of conservation. Of note, there is considerable overlap in the cross-reactivity between HSV type 1 and type 2 glycoproteins, although unique regions of these gene products exist for each virus.[9, 10] The two viral types can be distinguished by using restriction enzyme analysis of viral DNA, which allows precise epidemiologic investigations of virus transmission. Whether viruses of the one type are closely related can also be determined to establish the probable source of infection.

Replication

Replication of HSV is characterized by the expression of three gene classes: alpha, beta, and gamma. These genes are expressed temporally and in a cascade sequence.[7] Two observations are of relevance as they relate to gene expression of herpes simplex viruses. First, although herpesvirus genes carry transcriptional and translational signals similar to those of other DNA viruses that infect higher eukaryotic cells, the messenger RNAs arising from the vast majority of genes are not spliced. Second, the information density is lower than that encoded in the genes of smaller viruses. This relatively low density of genetic information is important in that it permits insertion and deletion of genes in the HSV genome without significant alteration of the genomic architecture. This point is particularly relevant because it provides an opportunity for the use of genetically engineered herpesviruses as either vaccines or vectors for antigen delivery.[11]

Alpha genes are expressed at immediate early times after infection and are responsible for the initiation of replication. These genes are transcribed in infected cells in the absence of viral protein synthesis. The beta gene products, or "early" genes, include those enzymes necessary for viral replication, such as herpes simplex thymidine kinase, as well as the regulatory proteins. These genes require functional alpha gene products for expression. The onset of expression of beta genes coincides with a decline in the rate of expression of alpha genes and an irreversible shutoff of host cellular macromolecular protein synthesis.[7] Structural proteins are usually of the gamma, or "late," gene class. The gamma genes are heterogeneous and are differentiated from beta genes solely by their requirement for viral DNA synthesis for maximal expression. Most glycoproteins are expressed as late genes. In addition to its regulatory and structural genes, the virus encodes genes that allow initial evasion of the host response, notably the downregulation of major histocompatibility complex class I molecules mediated by the ICP47 protein.[12]

Replication of viral DNA occurs in the nucleus of the cell. Assembly of the virus begins in the nucleus with acquisition of the envelope as the capsid buds through the inner lamella of the nuclear membrane. Virus is transported through the cytoskeleton to the plasma membrane, where lysis of the cell results in the release of progeny virions.

HSV specifies at least 10, and probably several more, glycoproteins. The glycoproteins have been designated as B, C, D, E, G, H, I, K, L, and M.[9] Glycoprotein D (gD) is required for infectivity and is the most potent inducer of neutralizing antibodies; glycoprotein B (gB) is required for infectivity and also induces neutralizing antibodies; glycoprotein C (gC) binds to the C3b component of complement; and glycoprotein E (gE) binds to the Fc portion of IgG. The amino acid sequences of the glycoprotein G (gG) produced by HSV types 1 and 2 are sufficiently different to elicit antibody responses that are specific for each virus type. The fact that the antibody response to the two G molecules exhibits minimal cross-reactivity has provided the basis for serologic methods that can be used to detect recent or past HSV type 2 infection in individuals who have also been infected with HSV type 1.[13–16]

The close virologic relationship between HSV types 1 and 2 has clinical relevance because it interferes with the serologic diagnosis of these infections. Standard serologic assays available to clinicians in practice do not distinguish between individuals who have had past infection with HSV type 1 only, past infection with HSV type 2 only, or dual infection.[15] Although laboratory reports often indicate antibody titers to each virus, the methods used by almost all commercial laboratories do not eliminate the detection of cross-reactive antibodies. The antigenic relatedness of the two viruses interferes with identifying women with HSV type 2 infection unless accurate type-specific serologic tests are used, because many women of childbearing age have been infected with HSV type 1 during childhood.

Latency and Reactivation

All of the herpesviruses have a characteristic ability to establish latency, by mechanisms that are as yet unidentified; to persist in this latent state for various intervals of time; and to reactivate, causing virus excretion at mucosal or other sites. After infection, the viral DNA persists in the host for the entire lifetime of the individual.

The biologic phenomenon of latency has been recognized and described since the beginning of this century, particularly the association of HSV latency with neurons. In 1905, Cushing noted that patients treated for trigeminal neuralgia by sectioning a branch of the trigeminal nerve developed herpetic lesions along the innervated areas of the sectioned branch.[17] This specific association of HSV with the trigeminal ganglion was suggested by Goodpasture.[18] More recent observations have demonstrated that microvascular surgery of the trigeminal nerve tract to alleviate pain associated with tic douloureux resulted in recurrent lesions in more than 90% of seropositive individuals.[19, 20]

Accumulated experience in animal models and from clinical observations suggests that inoculation of virus at the portal of entry, usually oral or genital mucosal tissue, results in infection of sensory nerve endings, and the virus is transported to the dorsal root ganglia. Replication at the site of inoculation enhances access of the virus to ganglia but is usually not associated with any signs of mucocutaneous disease. Only a fraction of new infections with HSV type 1 and type 2 are associated with clinically recognizable disease. When reactivation is triggered, either at oral or genital sites, the virus is transported back down axons to mucocutaneous sites. Replication, along with shedding of infectious virus, occurs at these sites. Recognizing that excretion of infectious virus during reactivation is not usually associated with clinical signs of recurrent herpes lesions is essential for understanding the transmission of HSV to newborns. Clinically silent reactivations are much more common than are recurrent lesions. Reactivation, with or without symptoms, appears in the presence of both humoral and cell-mediated immunity. Reactivation is spontaneous, although symptomatic recurrences have been associated with physical or emotional stress, exposure to ultraviolet light, tissue damage, and suppression of the immune system. Persistence of viral DNA has been documented in neuronal tissue of both animal models and humans.[7, 8, 21-23]

Animal model studies indicate that the transport of virus to the ganglia is by retrograde axonal flow.[24] After transport, virus replicates for several days in sensory ganglia that innervate the sites of inoculation. Once latency is established in sensory ganglia, antiviral drugs cannot eradicate latent virus from the infected cells. Since the latent virus does not multiply, it is not susceptible to drugs, like acyclovir, that affect viral DNA synthesis. Understanding of the mechanisms by which HSV establishes a latent state and persists in this form remains limited and is a subject of intense research interest.

EPIDEMIOLOGY

Nature of Infection

Although many routes of infection have been suggested, transmission of HSV most often occurs as a consequence of intimate, person-to-person contact. Virus must come in contact with mucosal surfaces or abraded skin for infection to be initiated. Infection with HSV type 1, generally limited to the oropharynx, can be transmitted by respiratory droplets or through direct contact of a susceptible individual with infected secretions. Acquisition often occurs during childhood.

Primary HSV type 1 infection in the young child is usually asymptomatic, but clinical illness is associated with HSV gingivostomatitis. Primary infection in young adults has been associated with only pharyngitis or with a mononucleosis-like syndrome. Seroprevalence studies have demonstrated that acquisition of HSV type 1 infection, like that of other herpesvirus infections, is related to socioeconomic factors. Antibodies, indicative of past infection, are found early in life among individuals of lower socioeconomic groups, which is presumed to be the consequence of crowded living conditions that provide a greater opportunity for direct contact with infected individuals. As many as 75 to 90% of individuals from lower socioeconomic populations develop antibodies to HSV type 1 by the end of the first decade of life.[8, 25-27] In comparison, in middle and upper middle socioeconomic groups, only 30 to 40% of individuals are seropositive by the middle of the second decade of life.[8] A change in seroprevalence rates of HSV type 1 has been recognized in the past few decades that reflects a delay in acquisition of infection until later in life. The increase in the reported number of cases of genital herpes caused by HSV type 2 may be related to a lower prevalence of prior HSV type 1 infection in young adults. These individuals would not have the partial protection against HSV type 2 infection that is probably conferred by cross-reactive HSV type 1 immunity.

Because infections with HSV type 2 are usually acquired through sexual contact, antibodies to this virus are rarely found until the age at onset of sexual activity.[26] There is a progressive increase in infection rates with HSV type 2 in all populations that begins in adolescence. Until recently, the precise seroprevalence of antibodies to HSV type 2 had been difficult to determine because of cross-reactivity with HSV type 1 antigens. During the late 1980s, seroepidemiologic studies performed using type-specific antigen for HSV type 2 (glycoprotein G-2) identified antibodies to this virus in 25 to 35% of middle-class women in several geographic areas of the United States.[14, 15, 28-30] Based on national health surveys, the seroprevalence of HSV type 2 in the United States from 1988 to 1994 was 21.9% in individuals 12 years of age or older.[30] Among those with serologic evidence of infection, fewer than 10% had a history of genital herpes symptoms. This seroprevalence represented a 30% increase compared with data collected from 1976 to 1980.

The molecular epidemiology of HSV infections can be determined by restriction enzyme analysis of viral DNA obtained from infected individuals. Viruses have identical profiles when they are from the same host or are epidemiologically related.[31] In a few circumstances, however, it has been demonstrated that superinfection or exogenous reinfection with a new strain of HSV is possible. Such occurrences are uncommon in the nonimmunocompromised host with recurrent genital HSV infection.[31-33] Differences in the restriction endonuclease patterns of viral DNAs, indicating exogenous infections, are more common in immunocompromised individuals who are exposed to different herpes simplex viruses, such as patients with acquired immunodeficiency syndrome.

Maternal Infection

Genital HSV infection in the pregnant woman is common. Using assays to detect type-specific antibodies to HSV type 2, seroepidemiologic investigations have demonstrated that approximately one in five pregnant women has had HSV type 2 infection.[29, 34-38] Given the capacity of HSV to establish latency, the presence of antibodies is a marker of persistent infection of the host with the virus. The incidence of infection in women of upper socioeconomic class was 30% or higher in three large studies.[36, 38, 39] Unfortunately, these recent investigations have demonstrated that the majority of women with serologic evidence of HSV type 2 infection have no history of symptomatic primary or recurrent disease. New HSV type 2 infections also appear to be acquired during pregnancy with a frequency that is comparable to seroconversion rates among nonpregnant women, and these infections usually occur without clinical signs or symptoms.[35-39]

An evaluation of pregnant women and their partners has demonstrated that women can remain susceptible to HSV type 2 despite prolonged sexual contact with a partner who has known genital herpes.[37] One in 10 women in this study were found to be at unsuspected risk of acquiring HSV type 2 infection during pregnancy as a result of contact with a partner whose HSV type 2 infection was asymptomatic.

Most maternal infections are clinically silent during gestation. However, infection during gestation may manifest in several clinical syndromes. A particularly perplexing, but fortunately uncommon, problem encountered with HSV infections during pregnancy is that of widely disseminated disease. As first reported by Flewett and associates in 1969 and by others subsequently, infection has been documented to involve multiple visceral sites, in addition to cutaneous ones.[40-42] In a limited number of cases, dissemination after primary oropharyngeal or genital infection has led to such severe manifestations of disease as necrotizing hepatitis with or without thrombocytopenia, leukopenia, disseminated intravascular coagulopathy, and encephalitis. Although only a few patients have suffered from disseminated infection, the mortality among these pregnant women is reported to be higher than 50%. Fetal deaths were described in more than 50% of cases, although mortality did not necessarily correlate with the death of the mother. Surviving fetuses were delivered by cesarean section, either during the acute illness or at term, and none had evidence of neonatal HSV infection.

Earlier studies described an association of maternal primary infection before 20 weeks of gestation with spontaneous abortion in some women.[43] Although the original incidence of spontaneous abortion after a symptomatic primary infection during gestation was thought to be as high as 25%, this estimate was not substantiated by prospective studies and was erroneous because of the small number of women studied. More precise data obtained from a prospective analysis of susceptible women demonstrated that 2% or more acquired infection but acquisition of infection was not associated with a risk of spontaneous abortion.[44] An earlier report that suggested a risk of fetal growth impairment after maternal primary infection was superseded by this study, showing no measurable effect.[38] Infection that develops later in gestation was not associated with the premature termination of pregnancy.

Localized genital infection, whether it is associated with lesions or remains asymptomatic, is the most common form of HSV infection during pregnancy. Overall, prospective investigations using cytologic and virologic screening indicate that genital herpes occurred with a frequency of about 1% in women tested at any time during gestation.[36, 44] Most of these infections were classified as recurrent when HSV type 2–specific serologic evaluation was done concurrently. Transmission of infection to the infant is most frequently related to the actual shedding of virus at the time of delivery. Because HSV infection of the infant is usually the consequence of contact with infected maternal genital secretions at the time of delivery, the incidence of viral excretion at this time point has been of particular interest. The actual incidence of viral excretion at delivery has been reported to be 0.01 to 0.39% for all women, regardless of past history of genital herpes.[36, 39]

Several prospective studies have evaluated the frequency and nature of viral shedding in pregnant women with a known history of genital herpes. These women represent a subset of the population of women with HSV type 2 infection because they had characteristic genital lesions from which virus was isolated. In a predominantly white, middle-class population, symptomatic recurrent infection occurred during pregnancy in 84% of pregnant women with a history of symptomatic disease.[45] Viral shedding from the cervix occurred in only 0.56% of symptomatic infections and 0.66% of asymptomatic infections. These data are similar to those obtained for other populations.[28] The incidence of cervical shedding in asymptomatic pregnant women has been reported to vary from 0.2 to 7.4%, depending on the numbers of cultures that were obtained between symptomatic episodes. Overall, these data indicate that the frequency of cervical shedding is low, which may reduce the risk of transmission of virus to the infant when the infection is recurrent. The frequency of shedding does not appear to vary by trimester during gestation. No increased incidence of premature onset of labor was apparent in these prospective studies of women with reactivation of HSV type 2 infection.

The most important fact about maternal transmission is that most infants who develop neonatal disease are born to women who are completely asymptomatic for genital HSV infections during the pregnancy as well as at the time of delivery. These women usually have neither a past history of genital herpes nor a sexual partner reporting a genital vesicular rash and account for 60 to 80% of all women whose infants become infected.[46-48]

Among women being delivered of children who developed neonatal HSV infection, only 27% had either a history of or evidence of recurrent lesions indicative of HSV infection during the current pregnancy.[47] Furthermore, only half of these women reported genital HSV infection in their sexual partners.

Factors Influencing Transmission of Infection to the Fetus

The development of serologic assays that distinguish antibodies to HSV type 1 from those elicited by HSV type 2 infection has allowed an accurate analysis of risks related to perinatal transmission of HSV.[13–16] The category of maternal genital infection at the time of delivery influences the frequency of neonatal acquisition of infection. Maternal infections are classified as due to HSV type 1 or type 2 and as newly acquired or recurrent. These categories of maternal infection status are based on laboratory criteria and are independent of clinical signs. Women with recurrent infections are those who have preexisting antibodies to the virus type that is isolated from the genital tract, which is usually HSV type 2, even though the majority have no history of symptomatic genital herpes. Infections that are newly acquired, which have been referred to as "first episode" infections, are further categorized as "primary" or "first episode, nonprimary" based on type-specific serologic testing. Again, this differentiation is made whether or not clinical signs are present. "Primary" infections are those in which the mother is experiencing a new infection with HSV type 1 or type 2 and has not already been infected with the other virus type. These mothers are seronegative for any HSV antibodies (HSV-1 negative/HSV-2 negative) at the onset of infection. "Nonprimary" infections are those in which the mother has a new infection with one virus type, usually HSV type 2, but has antibodies to the other virus type, usually HSV type 1, because of an infection that was acquired previously. As transmission has been studied using type-specific serologic methods, it has become obvious that attempts to distinguish primary and recurrent disease by clinical criteria are not reliable. Serologic classification is an important advance because many "new" genital herpes infections in pregnancy represent the first symptomatic episode of infection acquired at some time in the past. In one study designed to evaluate acyclovir therapy, pregnant women who were thought to have recent acquisition of HSV type 2, based on symptoms, had all been infected previously. These women were experiencing genital symptoms, caused by the reactivation of latent virus, for the first time.[49]

A hierarchy of risk of transmission has emerged using laboratory tools to classify maternal infection. Infants born to mothers who have true primary infections at the time of delivery are at highest risk, with transmission rates of 50% or higher.[44, 48] Those born to mothers with new infections that are not primary but are acquired in the presence of preexisting immunity due to infection with the other virus type appear to be at lower risk; transmission rates are estimated at around 30%. The lowest risk of neonatal acquisition occurs when the mother has active infection caused by shedding of virus acquired before the pregnancy or at stages of gestation before the onset of labor. The attack rate for neonatal herpes among these infants is considered to be less than 2%. This estimate is reliable because it is based on the cumulative experience from large prospective studies of pregnant women, in which viral shedding was evaluated at delivery regardless of the mother's history of genital herpes or contact with a partner with suspected or documented genital herpes.

The reasons for the higher risk of transmission to the infant when the mother has a new infection can be attributed to differences in the quantity and duration of viral shedding in the mother and in the transfer of passive antibodies from the mother to the infant before delivery. Primary infection is associated with larger quantities of virus replicating in the genital tract ($> 10^6$ viral particles per 0.2 ml of inoculum) and a period of viral excretion that may persist for an average of 3 weeks.[50] Many women with new infections have no symptoms but shed virus in high titers. In some mothers, these infections cause signs of systemic illness, including fever, malaise, and myalgias. In a small percentage of cases, significant complications, such as urinary retention and aseptic meningitis, can occur. In contrast, virus is shed for an average of only 2 to 5 days and at lower concentrations (10^2 to 10^3 viral particles per 0.2 ml of inoculum) in women with symptomatic recurrent genital infections. Asymptomatic reactivation is also associated with short periods of viral replication, often less than 24 to 48 hours. To reemphasize, one of the most important observations about HSV infections that has emerged from the evaluation of pregnant women is that new HSV type 1 and type 2 infections often occur without any of the manifestations that were originally described as the classic findings in primary and recurrent genital herpes.

In parallel with the classification of maternal infection, the mother's antibody status to HSV at delivery appears to be an additional factor that influences the likelihood of transmission, and probably the clinical course of neonatal herpes. Transplacental maternal neutralizing antibodies appear to have a protective, or at least an ameliorative, effect on acquisition of infection for infants inadvertently exposed to virus.[51] Maternal primary infection late in gestation may not result in significant passage of maternal antibodies across the placenta to the fetus. Based on available evidence, the highest risk of transmission is from mothers with newly acquired genital herpes observed when the infant is born before the transfer of passive antibodies to HSV type 1 or 2, when the infant is exposed at delivery or within the first few days of life.[44, 47, 52]

The duration of ruptured membranes has also been described as an indicator of risk for acquisition of neonatal infection. Observations of a small cohort of women with symptomatic genital herpes indicated that prolonged rupture of membranes (> 6 hours) increased the risk of acquisition of virus, perhaps as a consequence of ascending infection from the cervix.[43] It is recommended that women with active genital lesions at the time of onset of labor be delivered by cesarean section.[53] The benefit of cesarean section beyond 6 hours of ruptured membranes has not been evaluated. Although some protection may be expected, infection of the newborn has occurred in spite of delivery by cesarean section.[46, 54]

Certain forms of medical intervention during labor and delivery may increase the risk of neonatal herpes if the mother has active shedding of the virus, although in most instances viral shedding is not suspected clinically. For example, fetal scalp monitors can be a site of viral entry through skin.[55, 56] The benefits and risks of these devices should be considered in women with a history of recurrent genital HSV infections. Because most women with genital infections caused by HSV are asymptomatic during labor and have no history of genital herpes, it is usually not possible to make this assessment.

Incidence of Newborn Infection

Although centers caring for infants with neonatal HSV infections have observed fluctuations in disease incidence, the estimated rate of occurrence is 1 in 2000 to 1 in 5000 deliveries per year.[8] A progressive increase in the number of cases of neonatal HSV infection to a rate of approximately 1 in 1500 deliveries was noted in King County, Washington, during the period from 1966 to 1983, when adult infection rates were also increasing.[57] Overall, the United States, with approximately 4.0 million deliveries a year, has an estimated 11 to 33 cases of neonatal infection per 100,000 live births. This estimate has been confirmed by a review of comprehensive hospital discharge data recorded in California for the years 1985, 1990, and 1995. The diagnosis of HSV infection in infants 6 weeks of age or younger was made in 11.7, 11.3, and 11.4 infants per 100,000 live births in each of these years.[58]

Neonatal HSV infection occurs far less frequently than might be expected given the high prevalence of genital HSV infections in women of childbearing age in the United States. Some countries do not report a significant number of cases of neonatal HSV infection in spite of a similar high prevalence of antibodies to HSV type 2 in women. In the United Kingdom, genital herpetic infection is relatively common, but very few cases of neonatal HSV infection are recognized. Although serologic studies in central Africa indicate that women have a high frequency of antibodies to HSV type 2, the first case of neonatal herpes was reported less than 25 years ago.[8] Although under-reporting of cases may explain some differences between countries, there may be unidentified factors that account for these differences. The interpretation of incidence data must also include the potential for postnatal acquisition of HSV infection. Not all cases of neonatal herpes are the consequence of intrapartum contact with infected maternal genital secretions, which alters the overall estimate of delivery-associated infections.

Times of Transmission of Infection

HSV infection of the newborn can be acquired in utero, intrapartum, or postnatally. The mother is the most common source of infection for the first two of these routes of transmission of infection. With regard to postnatal acquisition of HSV infection, the mother can be a source of infection from a genital or nongenital site, or other contacts or environmental sources of virus can lead to infection of the child. A maternal source should be suspected when maternal herpetic lesions are discovered shortly after the birth of the child or when the infant's illness is caused by HSV type 2. Although intrapartum transmission accounts for 85 to 90% of cases, in utero and postnatal infection must be recognized for public health and prognostic purposes.

Recognizing that some infants acquire infection in utero, this mode of transmission is extremely rare.[56–63] Although it was originally presumed that in utero acquisition of infection resulted in either a totally normal infant or premature termination of gestation,[43] it has now become apparent that intrauterine acquisition of infection can lead to the clinical signs of congenital infection. By using stringent diagnostic criteria, more than 30 infants with symptomatic congenital disease have been described in the literature to date. These criteria include identification of infected infants with lesions present at birth, virologic confirmation of infection and the exclusion of other infectious agents whose pathogenesis mimics the clinical findings of herpes simplex infections, such as congenital cytomegalovirus infection, rubella, syphilis, or toxoplasmosis. Virologic diagnosis is a necessary criterion because no standard method for detection of IgM antibodies is available and infected infants often fail to produce IgM antibodies detectable by research methods.[52, 64]

The manifestations of disease in this group of children range from simply the presence of skin vesicles at the time of delivery to the most severe neurologic abnormalities.[46, 59] In utero infection can occur as a consequence of either transplacental or ascending infection. Examination of the placenta in the cases of neonatal herpes thought to be the consequence of in utero transmission has helped to clarify this route of transmission. The placenta can show evidence of necrosis and inclusions in the trophoblasts, which suggests a transplacental route of infection.[65] This situation can result in an infant who has hydranencephaly at the time of birth, or it may be associated with spontaneous abortion and intrauterine HSV viremia. Virus has been isolated from the products of conception under such circumstances. Histopathologic evidence of chorioamnionitis suggests ascending infection as an alternative route for in utero infection.[63] Risk factors associated with intrauterine transmission are not known. Both primary and recurrent maternal infections can result in infection of the fetus in utero. The second, and most common, route of infection is intrapartum contact of the fetus with infected maternal genital secretions. Intrapartum transmission is favored by delivery of the infant to a mother with newly acquired infection.

Postnatal acquisition is the third route of transmission. Postnatal transmission of HSV type 1 has been suggested as an increasing risk. Recent data from the National Institute of Allergy and Infectious Disease (NIAID) Collaborative Antiviral Study Group indicated that the frequency of infants with neonatal HSV type 1 infections was now nearly 30%.[46] HSV type 1 has been associated with genital lesions. However, HSV type 1 infections appear to account for only 5 to 15% of all genital HSV infections, creating greater concern about postnatal acquisition of infection from nonmaternal sources.

Relatives and hospital personnel with orolabial herpes may be a reservoir of virus for infection of the newborn. The documentation of postnatal transmission of HSV type 1 has focused attention on such sources of virus.[66–70] Postpartum transmission from mother to child has been reported as a consequence of nursing on an infected breast.[71] Transmission from fathers and grandparents has also been documented.[69] When the infant's mother has not had HSV infection, the infant may be inoculated with the virus from a nonmaternal contact in the absence of any possible protection from maternally derived passive antibodies.

Because of the prevalence of HSV type 1 infections in the general population, many individuals have intermittent episodes of asymptomatic excretion of the virus from the oropharynx and therefore can provide a source of infection for the newborn. The occurrence of herpes labialis, commonly referred to as fever blisters or cold sores, has ranged from 16 to 46% in various groups of adults.[72] Population studies conducted in two hospitals indicated that 15 to 34% of hospital personnel had a past history of nongenital herpetic lesions.[72, 73] In both hospitals surveyed, at least 1 in 100 individuals documented a recurrent cold sore each week. As is true of genital herpes, many individuals have HSV type 1 infection with no clinical symptoms at the time of acquisition or during episodes of reactivation and shedding of infectious virus in oropharyngeal secretions. Prospective virologic monitoring of hospital staff increased the frequency with which infection was detected by twofold; however, no cases of neonatal HSV infection were documented in these nurseries.

The risk of nosocomial infection in the hospital environment is of concern. The demonstration of identity by restriction endonuclease analysis of virus recovered from an index case and a nursery contact leaves little doubt as to the possibility of spread of virus in a high-risk nursery population.[67, 68] The possible vectors for nosocomial transmission have not been defined. Whether personnel with herpes labialis should avoid working in the nursery while lesions are active remains a matter of debate. No cases of transmission of HSV from personnel to infants have been documented. Vigorous hand-washing procedures and continuing education of personnel in newborn nurseries can be expected to contribute to the low frequency of HSV transmission in this environment. A herpetic whitlow in a health care provider should preclude direct patient contact, regardless of the nursing unit. Because more infants are born to seronegative women now, our nursery practice is to exclude personnel with active herpes labialis from direct patient care activities until the lesion is crusted.

Because most mothers have antibodies to HSV and these antibodies are transferred to their infants, exposures to the virus in the newborn period may not often result in neonatal disease. However, if the mother was seronegative, nosocomial exposure may pose a more significant risk to the infant.

IMMUNOLOGIC RESPONSE

The host response of the newborn to HSV is impaired compared with that of older children and adults.[52, 64, 74–78] At present, there is no evidence for differences in virulence of particular HSV strains. The severity of the manifestations of HSV type 1 and 2 infections in the newborn, as described in the section on Neonatal Infection, can be attributed to immunologic factors. The relevant issues are protection of the fetus by transplacental antibodies, the innate immune response of the exposed infant, and the acquisition of adaptive immunity by the infected newborn.

Passive antibodies to HSV influence the acquisition of infection, as well as its severity and clinical signs.[38, 48, 52, 64] Transplacentally acquired antibodies from the mother are not totally protective against newborn infection but transplacentally acquired neutralizing antibodies correlate with a lower attack rate in exposed newborns.[48, 51, 52] Whereas the absence of any detectable antibodies has been associated with dissemination, the presence of antibodies at the time that clinical signs appear does not predict the subsequent outcome.[46, 64] The most important example of the failure of passive antibodies to alter progression is the occurrence of encephalitis in untreated infants whose initial symptoms were limited to cutaneous lesions. Most infected newborns eventually produce IgM antibodies, but the interval to detection is prolonged, requiring at least 2 to 4 weeks.[52] This method cannot be used for diagnostic purposes to determine the need for antiviral therapy. These antibodies increase rapidly during the first 2 to 3 months, and they may be detectable for as long as 1 year after infection. The quantity of neutralizing antibodies and antibodies that mediate antibody-dependent cellular cytotoxicity in infants with disseminated infection is lower than that in those with more limited disease.[52, 74] Humoral antibody responses to specific viral proteins, especially glycoproteins, have been evaluated by assays for antibodies to gG and immunoblot.[13, 64] Immunoblot studies indicate that the severity of infection correlates directly with the number of antibody bands to defined polypeptides. Children with a more limited infection, such as infection of the skin, eye, and/or mouth, have fewer antibody bands compared with those children with disseminated disease. A vigorous antibody response to the ICP4 alpha gene product, which is responsible for initiating viral replication, has been correlated with poor long-term neurologic outcome, suggesting that these antibodies reflect the extent of viral replication. A regression analysis that compared neurologic impairment with the quantity of antibodies to ICP4 identified the child at risk for severe neurologic impairment.[64]

Adaptive cellular immunity is a critical component of the host response to primary herpetic infections. Newborns with HSV infections have a delayed T lymphocyte proliferative response compared with older individuals.[52, 76, 77] Most infants have no detectable T lymphocyte responses to HSV when evaluated 2 to 4 weeks after the onset of clinical symptoms.[52] The delayed T lymphocyte response to viral antigens in infants whose initial disease is localized to the skin, eye, or mouth may be an important determinant of the frequent progression to more severe disease in infants.[52, 77] Lack of cell-mediated immunity is likely to permit viremia and dissemination in infants, which is otherwise controlled by the host response in older children and adults with new HSV infections.

Infected newborns have decreased interferon-α and interferon-γ production in response to HSV antigen when compared with adults with primary HSV infection.[77] The importance of interferon-α may be related to its effect on the induction of innate immune mechanisms, such as natural killer cell responses.[78] Other mechanisms of the innate immune system of the newborn that may be deficient in controlling HSV include other nonspecific cytokine responses and complement-mediated effects. T lymphocytes from infected infants have decreased interferon-γ production during the first month of life. This defect can be predicted to limit the clonal expansion of helper and cytotoxic T lymphocytes specific for herpesviral antigens, allowing more extensive and prolonged viral replication and failure to establish latency.

Antibody-dependent cell-mediated cytotoxicity has been demonstrated to be an important component of adaptive immunity to viral infection.[74] Antibodies and lymphocytes, monocytes, macrophages, or polymorphonuclear leukocytes, as well as antibodies and complement, lyse HSV-infected cells in vitro.[79] However, newborns appear to have fewer effector lymphocytes than older individuals. The immaturity of neonatal monocytes and macrophage function against HSV infection has been demonstrated in vitro and in animal models.[80, 81]

NEONATAL INFECTION

After direct exposure, replication of HSV is presumed to occur at the portal of entry, which is probably the mucous membranes of the mouth or eye, or at sites where the skin has been damaged. Factors that determine whether the infection causes symptoms at the site of inoculation or disseminates to other organs are poorly understood. Sites of replication during the incubation period have not been defined, but the virus evades the host response during this early stage, probably by mechanisms such as blocking cell-mediated immune recognition of viral peptides by preventing major histocompatibility complex class I molecules from reaching the surface of infected cells. Intraneuronal transmission of viral particles may provide a privileged site that is inaccessible to circulating humoral and cell-mediated defense mechanisms, facilitating the pathogenesis of encephalitis. Transplacental maternal antibodies may be less effective under such circumstances. Disseminated infection appears to be the consequence of viremia, and

extensive cell-to-cell spread could explain primary HSV pneumonia after aspiration of infected secretions.

Once the virus has adsorbed to cell membranes and penetration has occurred, viral replication proceeds, leading to release of progeny virus and cell death. The synthesis of cellular DNA and protein ceases as large quantities of HSV are produced. Cell death in critical organs of the newborn, such as the brain, results in devastating consequences, as reflected by the long-term morbidity of herpes encephalitis. Cellular swelling, hemorrhagic necrosis, development of intranuclear inclusions, and cytolysis all result from the replicative process. Small, punctuate, yellow-to-gray areas of focal necrosis are the most prominent gross lesion in infected organs. When infected tissue is examined by microscopy, there is extensive evidence of hemorrhagic necrosis, clumping of nuclear chromatin, dissolution of the nucleolus, cell fusion with formation of multinucleate giant cells, and, ultimately, a lymphocytic inflammatory response.[82] Lymphocytic perivascular cuffing is particularly prominent in organs that exhibit extensive hemorrhagic necrosis, especially in the central nervous system (CNS).[83] Irreversible organ damage results from ischemia as well as direct viral destruction of cells.

Clinical Presentation

Pediatricians must be prepared to consider the diagnosis of neonatal herpes in infants who have clinical signs consistent with the disease regardless of the maternal history of genital herpes. This circumstance results from the fact that only about 30% of mothers whose infants develop neonatal herpes have had symptomatic genital herpes or sexual contact with a partner who has recognized HSV infection either during or before the pregnancy.

The clinical presentation of infants with neonatal HSV infection depends on the initial site and extent of viral replication. In contrast to human cytomegalovirus, neonatal infections caused by HSV types 1 and 2 are almost invariably symptomatic. Case reports of asymptomatic infection in the newborn exist, but they are most uncommon, and long-term follow-up of these children to document absence of subtle disease or sequelae was not described.

Classification of newborns with HSV infection is mandatory for prognostic and therapeutic considerations.[84] Historically, infants with neonatal HSV infection were classified as having localized or disseminated disease, with the former group being subdivided into those with skin, eye, or mouth disease versus those with CNS infection. However, this classification system understates the significant differences in outcome within each category.[85] In a revised classification scheme, infants who are infected intrapartum or postnatally can be divided into three groups: those with (1) disease localized to the skin, eye, or mouth; (2) encephalitis, with or without skin, eye, and/or mouth involvement; and (3) disseminated infection that involves multiple organs, including those in the CNS, lung, liver, adrenals, skin, eye, and/or mouth. A few infants with intrauterine infection constitute a fourth category. Knowledge about the patterns of

TABLE 8–1
Demographic and Clinical Characteristics of Infants Enrolled in NIAID Collaborative Antiviral Study

	DISEASE CLASSIFICATION		
	Disseminated	Central Nervous System	Skin/Eye/Mouth
No. of infants	93 (32)[a]	95 (33)	102 (35)
No. male/no. female	54/39	50/46	51/51
Race			
No. white/no. other	60/33	73/23	76/26
No. premature (<36 wk)	33 (35)	20 (21)	24 (24)
Gestational age (wk)	36.5 ± 0.4	37.9 ± 0.4	37.8 ± 0.3
Enrollment age (wk)	11.6 ± 0.7	17.4 ± 0.8	12.1 ± 1.1
Maternal age (yr)	21.7 ± 0.5	23.1 ± 0.5	22.8 ± 0.5
Clinical findings (no.)			
Skin lesions	72 (77)	60 (63)	86 (84)
Brain involvement	69 (74)	96 (100)	0 (0)
Pneumonia	46 (49)	4 (4)	3 (3)
Mortality at 1 yr[b]	56 (60)	13 (14)	0 (0)
Neurologic impairment of survivors (no. affected/total no.)			
Total	15/34[b] (44)	45/81[c] (56)	10/93[c] (11)
Adenine arabinoside	13/26[c] (50)	25/51[c] (49)	3/34[c] (9)
Acyclovir	1/6[c] (17)	18/27[c] (67)	4/51[c] (8)
Placebo	1/2[c] (50)	2/3[c] (67)	3/8[c] (38)

[a]Numbers in parentheses are percentages.
[b]Regardless of therapy.
[c]Denominators vary according to number with follow-up available.

clinical disease caused by HSV types 1 and 2 in the newborn is based on prospectively acquired data obtained through the NIAID Collaborative Antiviral Study Group. These analyses have employed uniform case record forms from one study interval to the next. The presentation and outcome of infection, including the effect of antiviral therapy on prognosis, varies significantly according to the clinical categories.[86] Table 8–1 summarizes disease classification of 291 infants with neonatal herpesvirus infections of the NIAID Collaborative Antiviral Study Group.

INTRAUTERINE INFECTION

Intrauterine infection is very rare. The frequency of occurrence of these manifestations has been estimated to be approximately 3 for every 100 infected infants.[62] When it occurs, severe disease can follow acquisition of infection at virtually any time in gestation. In the most severely afflicted group of infants, it is apparent at birth and is characterized by a triad of findings, including skin vesicles or skin scarring, eye damage, and the far more severe manifestations of microcephaly or hydranencephaly. CNS damage is caused by intrauterine encephalitis. These infants do not have evidence of embryopathy. Often, chorioretinitis in combination with other eye findings, such as keratoconjunctivitis, is a component of the clinical presentation. Serial ultrasound examination of the mothers of infants infected in utero has demonstrated the presence of hydranencephaly, but these cases are seldom diagnosed before delivery. Chorioretinitis alone should alert the pediatrician to the possibility of this diagnosis, although it is a common sign for other congenital infections. A few infants have been described who have signs of HSV infection at birth, following prolonged rupture of membranes. The infants may have no other findings of invasive multiorgan involvement—specifically, no chorioretinitis, encephalitis, or evidence of other diseased organs—and can be expected to respond to antiviral therapy. Antiviral therapy is not effective for infants who are born with hydranencephaly.

DISSEMINATED INFECTION

Infants whose initial diagnosis is disseminated herpes have the worst prognosis for mortality and morbidity. Many of these infants are born to mothers who are experiencing a new HSV type 1 or type 2 infection and may lack any passively acquired antibodies against the infecting virus type.[13, 48, 87] Infants with disseminated infection have signs of illness within the first week of life, although the diagnosis may be delayed until the second week. The onset of illness may be as short as 24 hours after birth, but most infants appear well at delivery. The short incubation period of disseminated herpes reflects an acute viremia, which allows transport of the virus to all organs, with the principal organs involved being the liver, causing fulminant hepatitis in some cases, and adrenals.[84, 88, 89] There is evidence that viremia is associated with infection of circulating mononuclear cells in these infants.[89–91] Infection can affect multiple organs, including the CNS, larynx, trachea, lungs, esophagus, stomach, lower gastrointestinal tract, spleen, kidneys, pancreas, and heart. Initial signs and symptoms are irritability, seizures, respiratory distress, jaundice, bleeding diathesis, and shock. The characteristic vesicular exanthem is usually not present when the symptoms begin. Untreated infants may develop cutaneous lesions secondary to viremia. However, more than 20% of children with disseminated infection do not develop skin vesicles during the course of their illness.[46, 89] Disseminated infections caused by HSV types 1 and 2 are indistinguishable by clinical criteria.

The diagnosis of disseminated neonatal herpes is exceedingly difficult because the clinical signs are often vague and nonspecific, mimicking those of neonatal enteroviral disease or bacterial sepsis. The diagnosis of disseminated herpes should be pursued by obtaining specimens of oropharyngeal and respiratory secretions and a rectal swab to be tested by viral culture and by polymerase chain reaction (PCR) testing, if a qualified reference laboratory is available. Enzyme immunoassay methods may detect viral antigens, permitting a presumptive diagnosis that should be confirmed by viral culture. Of note, the direct immunofluorescence methods that are useful for rapid diagnosis of HSV-infected cells in skin lesion specimens must not be used to test secretions. The virus can also be detected in the peripheral blood of some infants, but confirmation of viremia is not necessary for clinical management.

Evaluation of the extent of dissemination is imperative to provide appropriate supportive interventions early in the clinical course. Infants should be assessed for hypoxemia, acidosis, hyponatremia, abnormal hepatic enzyme levels (aspartate aminotransferase and γ-glutamyltransferase), direct hyperbilirubinemia, neutropenia, thrombocytopenia, and bleeding diathesis, among others. Chest roentgenography should be done, and depending on signs and whether the infant is stable enough, abdominal radiography, electroencephalography, and computed tomography of the head should be used to further determine the extent of disease. The radiographic picture of HSV lung disease is characterized by a diffuse, interstitial pattern, which progresses to a hemorrhagic pneumonitis. Not infrequently, pneumatosis intestinalis can be detected when gastrointestinal disease is present. Meningocephalitis appears to be a common component of disseminated infection, occurring in 60 to 75% of children. Usual examinations of cerebrospinal fluid (CSF) and viral culture and PCR, if available, should be done, along with noninvasive neurodiagnostic tests, to assess the extent of brain disease.

Mortality of disseminated herpes in the absence of therapy exceeds 80%, and many survivors are impaired. The most common causes of death in infants with disseminated disease are intravascular coagulopathy or HSV pneumonitis. There is some evidence that the neurologic outcome is better for infants with disseminated HSV type 1 involving the CNS than for those who are infected with HSV type 2.[86, 92, 93]

ENCEPHALITIS

Nearly one third of all infants with neonatal HSV infection have encephalitis only as the initial manifestation of disease.[86, 94] These infants have clinical manifestations that are distinct from those who have CNS infection

associated with disseminated herpes. The pathogenesis of these two forms of brain infection is probably different. The virus is likely to reach brain parenchyma by a hematogenous route in infants with disseminated infection, resulting in multiple areas of cortical hemorrhagic necrosis. In contrast, neonates who present with only encephalitis likely develop brain disease as a consequence of retrograde axonal transport of the virus to the CNS. The evidence for this hypothesis is twofold. First, newborns with disseminated disease have documented viremia. Second, infants with encephalitis are more likely to have received transplacental neutralizing antibodies from their mothers, which may allow only intraneuronal transmission of virus to the brain.

Infants with localized herpes encephalitis as their initial manifestation of infection usually develop signs more than a week after birth, typically presenting in the second or third week, and sometimes as late as 4 to 6 weeks of age. Clinical manifestations of encephalitis include seizures (both focal and generalized), lethargy, irritability, tremors, poor feeding, temperature instability, bulging fontanelle, and pyramidal tract signs. Similar signs are observed when disseminated herpes is associated with encephalitis. As in disseminated herpes, many infants with encephalitis do not have skin vesicles when signs of illness begin. In some infants, there is a history or residual signs of mucocutaneous lesions of the skin or eye that were not recognized as herpetic. If untreated, infants with encephalitis may develop skin vesicles later in the disease course.[94] Anticipated findings on CSF examination include pleocytosis, moderately low glucose concentrations, and proteinosis. A few infants with CNS infection, proved by brain biopsy done immediately after the onset of seizures, have no abnormalities of their CSF, but most infants have some pleocytosis and mild reduction of glucose. The hemorrhagic nature of the encephalitis may result in apparent "bloody tap." Although initial protein concentrations may be normal or only slightly elevated, infants with localized brain disease usually demonstrate progressive increases in protein, up to more than 1000 mg/dl. The importance of CSF examinations in all infants is underscored by the finding that even subtle abnormalities have been associated with significant developmental sequelae.[84] Electroencephalography and computed tomography can be very useful in defining the presence of CNS abnormalities and should be done before discharge of all infants with this diagnosis.[95] These abnormalities may also be detected by ultrasound.[96]

Localized CNS disease is fatal in approximately 50% of infants who are not treated and is usually related to involvement of the brain stem. With rare exceptions, survivors are left with neurologic impairment.[84] The long-term prognosis is poor. As many as 50% of surviving children have some degree of psychomotor retardation, often in association with microcephaly, hydranencephaly, porencephalic cysts, spasticity, blindness, chorioretinitis, or learning disabilities (Fig. 8–1). There is some evidence that progressive neurologic damage occurs after neonatal herpes encephalitis, although many infants have obvious severe sequelae within a few weeks after onset of herpes encephalitis.[97, 98]

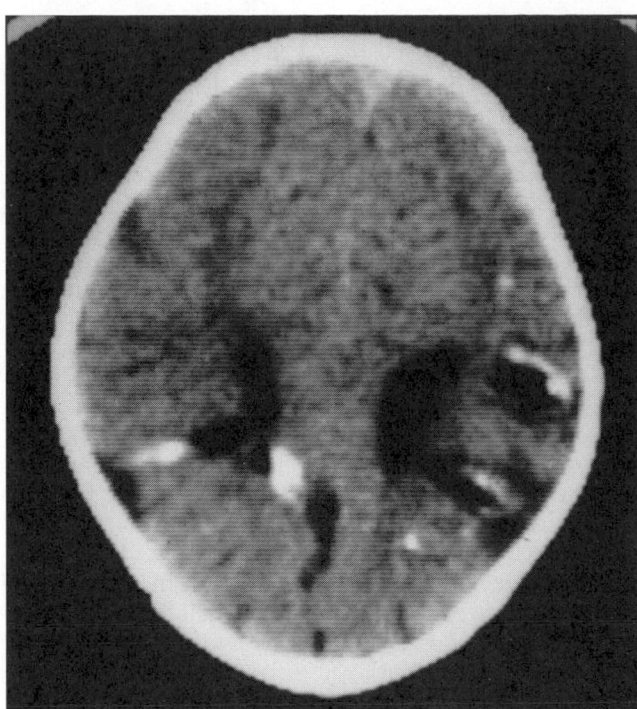

FIGURE 8–1 Herpes simplex encephalitis: Computed tomography scan of an infant with herpes simplex virus type 2 infection with severe sequelae.

Several points warrant reiteration. Clinical manifestations of disease in children with encephalitis alone are virtually identical to those findings that occur with brain infection in disseminated cases in spite of the presumed differences in pathogenesis. For infants with encephalitis, only two thirds, or approximately 60%, develop evidence of a vesicular rash characteristic of HSV infection. Thus, a newborn with pleocytosis and proteinosis of the CSF but without a rash can easily be misdiagnosed as having another viral or bacterial infection unless HSV infection is carefully considered.

SKIN, EYE, AND/OR MOUTH INFECTION

Infection localized to the skin, eye, and/or mouth appears benign at the onset, but it is associated with a high risk of progression to serious disease (Fig. 8–2). When infection is localized to the skin, the presence of discrete vesicles remains the hallmark of disease. Vesicles occur in 90% of children with skin, eye, and/or mouth infection. The skin vesicles usually erupt from an erythematous base and are usually 1 to 2 mm in diameter. The formation of new lesions adjacent to the original vesicles is typical, creating a cluster that may coalesce into larger, irregular vesicles. In some cases, the lesions can progress to large bullae more than 1 cm in diameter. Clusters of vesicles may appear initially on the presenting part of the body, presumed to occur because of prolonged contact with infected secretions during birth. Nevertheless, the first herpetic lesions in infants with localized cutaneous disease have been described on the trunk, extremities, and other sites. Children with disease localized to the skin, eye, and/or mouth generally have symptoms within the first 7 to 10 days of life.

Whereas discrete vesicles are usually encountered, crops and clusters of vesicles are described, particularly before antiviral treatment was available or when the cause of the first lesions is not recognized. In these cases, the rash can progress to involve other cutaneous sites, presumably by viremia and hematogenous spread. Scattered vesicles that resemble varicella are observed. Although progression is expected without treatment, a few infants have had infection of the skin limited to one or two vesicles, with no further evidence of cutaneous disease. These infants may be identified after the newborn period and should have a careful evaluation because many are likely to have had neurologic disease that was not detected. A zosteriform eruption is another manifestation of herpetic skin disease reported in infants.[99]

Infections affecting the eye may manifest as keratoconjunctivitis. Ocular infection may be the only involvement in the newborn. When localized eye infection is observed in infants who also have microphthalmos and retinal dysplasia, intrauterine acquisition should be suspected and a thorough neurologic evaluation should be done. Before antiviral therapy was available, persistent ocular disease resulted in chorioretinitis, caused by either HSV type 1 or type 2.[100] Keratoconjunctivitis can progress to chorioretinitis, cataracts, and retinal detachment despite therapy. Cataracts have been detected as a long-term consequence in infants with perinatally acquired HSV infections.

Localized infection of the oropharynx, involving the mouth or tongue, occurs, but newborns do not develop the classic herpetic gingivostomatitis caused by primary HSV type 1 infection in older children. Overall, approximately 10% of patients have evidence of HSV infection of the oropharynx by viral culture. Unfortunately, many of these children did not undergo a thorough oral examination to determine whether the detection of infectious virus in oropharyngeal secretions was associated with lesions.

Long-term neurologic impairment has been encountered in children whose disease appeared to be localized

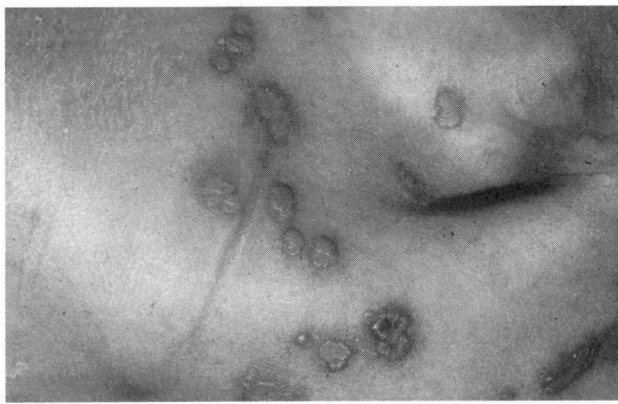

FIGURE 8–2 Cutaneous herpes simplex virus infection. Initial vesicular lesion in a premature infant with herpes simplex type 2 infection.

to the skin, eye, and/or mouth during the newborn period.[46, 84, 93, 98] The significant findings include spastic quadriplegia, microcephaly, and blindness. Important questions regarding the pathogenesis of delayed-onset neurologic debility are raised by these clinical observations. Despite normal clinical examinations in these children, neurologic impairment became apparent between 6 months and 1 year of life. At this stage of the disease, the clinical presentation may be similar to that associated with congenitally acquired toxoplasmosis or syphilis.

Newborns who have skin lesions invariably suffer from recurrences for months or years. Continued recurrences are common, particularly when the infecting virus in HSV type 2, whether or not antiviral therapy was administered. Historically, although death was not associated with disease localized to the skin, eye, or mouth, approximately 30% of these children eventually developed some evidence of neurologic impairment.[46]

SUBCLINICAL INFECTION

A few cases of apparent subclinical infection with HSV, proved by culture isolation of virus in the absence of symptoms, have been described. [101] Nevertheless, it has been difficult to document such cases in the course of prospective evaluations of several thousand infants from many centers around the United States. Conversely, infants who were exposed to active maternal infection at the time of delivery and who did not develop symptoms have been followed for the first year of life and do not have immunologic evidence of subclinical infection.[48] HSV type 1 or type 2 may be recovered from the infant's oropharyngeal secretions transiently, without representing true infection. Nevertheless, because of the propensity of the newborn to develop severe or life-threatening disease, laboratory evidence of neonatal HSV infection requires careful follow-up for clinical signs and the administration of antiviral therapy.

DIAGNOSIS

Clinical Evaluation

The clinical diagnosis of neonatal HSV infection is difficult because the appearance of skin vesicles cannot be relied on as an initial component of disease presentation. Enteroviral sepsis is a major differential diagnostic possibility in infants with signs suggesting neonatal herpes. Bacterial infections of newborns can mimic neonatal HSV infection. In addition, some infants infected by HSV have been described who had concomitant bacterial infections, including group B *Streptococcus*, *Staphylococcus aureus*, *Listeria monocytogenes*, and gram-negative bacteria. Many other disorders of the newborn can be indistinguishable from neonatal HSV infections, including acute respiratory distress syndrome, intraventricular hemorrhage, necrotizing enterocolitis, and various ocular or cutaneous diseases.

When vesicles are present, alternative causes of exanthems should be excluded. Other diagnoses include enteroviral infection, varicella-zoster virus infection, and syphilis. Laboratory methods are available to differentiate these causes of cutaneous lesions in the newborn. Such cutaneous disorders as erythema toxicum, neonatal melanosis, acrodermatitis enteropathica, or incontinentia pigmenti often confuse physicians who suspect neonatal HSV infections. Herpes lesions can be distinguished rapidly from those caused by these diseases using direct immunofluorescent stain of lesion scrapings or other methods for rapid detection of viral proteins and confirmed by viral culture.

HSV encephalitis is the most difficult clinical diagnosis to make, particularly because many children with CNS infection do not have a vesicular rash at the time of clinical presentation. Infection of the CNS should be suspected in the child who has evidence of acute neurologic deterioration, often associated with the onset of seizures and in the absence of intraventricular hemorrhage and metabolic causes. PCR to detect the viral DNA in CSF has become an important diagnostic method, largely replacing the need for diagnosis by brain biopsy.[102] Infants with localized encephalitis usually have serial increases in CSF cell counts and protein concentrations, negative bacterial cultures of the CSF, and negative antigen studies for bacteria. As noted previously, noninvasive neurodiagnostic studies can be used to attempt to define the sites of involvement.

Laboratory Assessment

The appropriate use of laboratory methods is essential if a timely diagnosis of HSV infection, allowing for effective antiviral treatment, is to be achieved.[103] Virus isolation remains the definitive diagnostic method. If skin lesions are present, a swab of skin vesicles, done vigorously enough to obtain cells from the base of the lesion, should be made and transferred in appropriate virus transport media to a diagnostic virology laboratory. Rapid diagnosis should be attempted by preparing material from lesion scrapings for direct immunofluorescence testing to detect the presence of virus-infected cells or for testing by enzyme immunoassays for viral proteins. Because of the possibility of false-positive results using immunofluorescence or other antigen detection methods, specimens should also be obtained for confirmation by viral isolation. Direct immunofluorescence staining for virus-infected cells is not reliable unless the specimen is obtained from a lesion. Cells from oropharyngeal swabs or from CSF should not be tested with this method.

Clinical specimens should be transported to the diagnostic virology laboratory without being frozen, and their processing should be expedited to permit the rapid confirmation of the clinical diagnosis. In addition to skin vesicles, other materials or sites from which virus may be isolated include the CSF, stool, urine, throat, nasopharynx, and conjunctivae. The isolation of virus from swabs of superficial sites, such as the nasopharynx, may represent transient presence of the virus in secretions, when the culture is obtained within the first 24 hours after birth and particularly when the specimen is taken immediately after birth. Typing of an HSV isolate may be done by one of several techniques. Because the outcome of antiviral treatment may be related to the virus type, typing is of prognostic as well as epidemiologic importance.[84] Viral cultures of the CSF may be positive in infants with disseminated HSV infections but are usually negative in those who have localized encephalitis.

The PCR provides a promising new tool for rapid viral diagnosis of HSV infections that can be designed to differentiate virus type simultaneously.[102–106] At present, these methods are sensitive and highly specific in research laboratories, but no commercial assay is available and contamination leading to false-positive results is difficult to control. PCR has been used for the retrospective analysis of materials collected from 34 infants enrolled in antiviral studies, demonstrating that detection of the viral DNA in CSF by PCR may allow a rapid presumptive diagnosis of HSV encephalitis in the newborn. [104] HSV was detected by PCR assay of CSF in 71% of infants before antiviral therapy was initiated. At least one specimen was positive in 76% of infants, and all samples that were positive by viral culture were also positive by PCR. Of note, PCR tests of CSF were positive in 7 of 29 infants (24%) whose clinical disease was limited to mucocutaneous lesions. Five of the 6 infants who were evaluated at 1 year of age were developmentally normal. The significance of this observation for disease classification and prognosis remains to be determined in prospective studies. Other studies of PCR for the diagnosis of HSV infections indicate sensitivities of 75% and 100% in small cohorts of infants.[105, 106] Until more information about the clinical correlates with disease and the reliability of results obtained in clinical rather than research laboratories has been determined, it is important to use standard diagnostic methods for the evaluation of infants with possible neonatal herpes.

Every effort should be made to confirm HSV infection by viral isolation. Cytologic examination of cells from the infant's lesions should not be used to diagnose HSV infection, now that reliable specific methods are available. Cytologic methods, such as Papanicolaou, Giemsa, or Tzanck staining, have a sensitivity of only 60 to 70%; therefore, a negative result must not be interpreted as excluding the diagnosis of HSV infection and a positive result should not be the sole diagnostic determinant for HSV infection in the newborn. Intranuclear inclusions and multinucleated giant cells may be indicative, but not diagnostic, of HSV infection.

In contrast to some other neonatal infections, serologic diagnosis of HSV infection has little clinical value. The interpretation of serologic assays is complicated by the fact that transplacentally acquired maternal IgG cannot be differentiated from endogenously produced antibodies, making it difficult to assess the neonate's antibody status during acute infection. Because commonly available serologic assays do not distinguish between antibodies to HSV types 1 and 2, maternal antibodies to type 1 will prevent the detection of a response to type 2 in the infected infant. Serial antibody testing may be useful for retrospective diagnosis if a mother without a prior history of HSV infection has a primary infection late in gestation and transfers little or no antibody to the fetus. In any case, therapeutic decisions cannot await a diagnostic approach based on comparing acute and convalescent antibody titers. IgM production is delayed or does not occur in infected infants because of inherent immunodeficiencies in the response to systemic viral infections in the newborn, and commercially available assays for IgM antibodies to HSV have limited reliability.

The results of specific laboratory tests for HSV should be used in conjunction with clinical findings and general laboratory tests, such as platelet counts, CSF analysis, and liver function tests, to establish a disease classification.

TREATMENT

The cumulative experience of the past two decades demonstrates that perinatally acquired HSV infections are amenable to treatment with antiviral agents. Acyclovir has emerged as the drug of choice.[86] Because most infants acquire infection at the time of delivery or shortly thereafter, antiviral therapy has the potential to decrease mortality and improve long-term outcome. As is the case with other perinatally acquired infections, the benefits that antiviral therapy can provide are influenced substantially by diagnosis early after the onset of clinical illness. The likelihood of disease progression in infants who acquire HSV infections is an established fact. Without treatment, 70% of those presenting with disease localized to the skin, eye, and/or mouth develop involvement of the CNS or disseminated infection. Treatment initiated after disease progression is not optimal because many of these children either die or are left with significant neurologic impairment. Regardless of the apparently minor clinical findings in some cases, the possibility of HSV infection in the newborn requires aggressive diagnostic evaluation, and likely or proved infection mandates the immediate initiation of acyclovir therapy, which must be given intravenously.

Antiviral Drugs

Historically, four nucleoside analogues have been used to treat neonatal herpes: idoxuridine, cytarabine, vidarabine, and acyclovir. Of these compounds, the first three are nonspecific inhibitors of both cellular and viral replication, and the last, acyclovir, is selectively activated by HSV thymidine kinase. Acyclovir acts as a competitive inhibitor of HSV DNA polymerase and terminates DNA chain elongation.[107] Idoxuridine and cytarabine have no value as systemic therapy for any viral infection because of toxicity and equivocal efficacy. Vidarabine was the first drug demonstrated to be efficacious; it decreased mortality and improved morbidity in neonatal HSV infections. [93] A comparison of vidarabine with acyclovir suggests that these compounds have a similar level of activity for this disease, but vidarabine is no longer available for clinical use.[98] Acyclovir is safe for use in newborns and is familiar to pediatricians from its other clinical uses.

In the first successes in treatment of neonatal HSV reported by the NIAID Collaborative Antiviral Study Group in 1984, the use of vidarabine in infants with

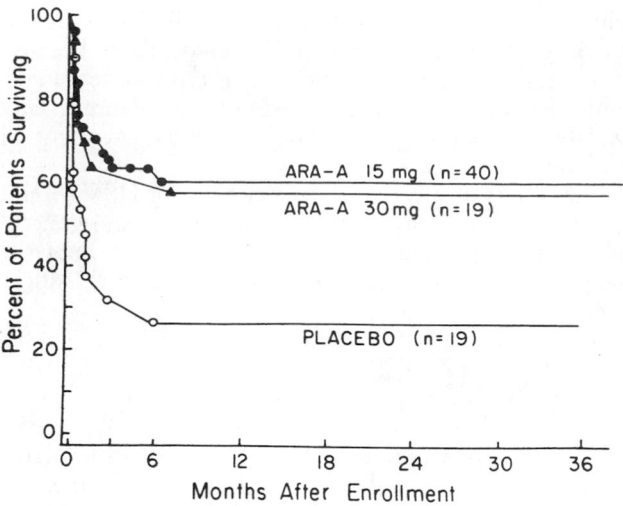

FIGURE 8–3 Survival of babies with neonatal herpes simplex virus infections—encephalitis and disseminated infections—according to therapeutic regimen. Ara-A-vidarabine. (From Whitley RJ, Nahmias J, Soong SJ, et al. Reproduced by permission of Pediatrics, vol. 73, page 778, copyright 1984.)

disseminated or localized CNS disease was associated with a decline in mortality rate from 75 to 40% (Fig. 8–3).[93] Infants received vidarabine, 15 or 30 mg/kg per day, or placebo, for 10 to 14 days. When outcome was examined according to each of the three disease classifications, as shown in Figure 8–4, the best therapeutic result was achieved in infants with either skin, eye, and/or mouth infection or encephalitis. Mortality was decreased from nearly 90% in infants with disseminated infection to approximately 70% in those with therapy. For infants with encephalitis, mortality was decreased from 50 to 15% with vidarabine treatment.

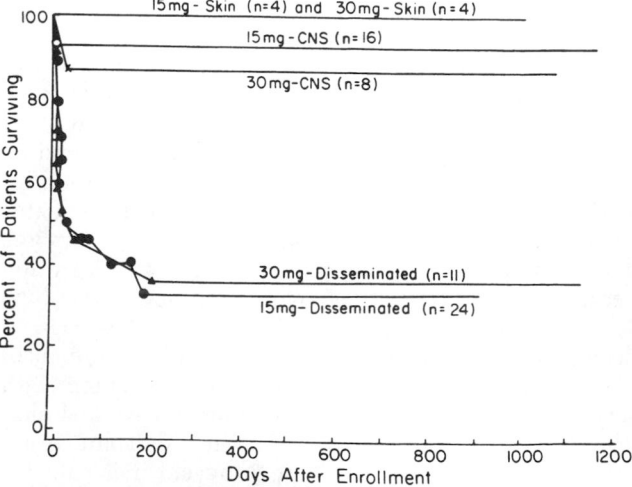

FIGURE 8–4 Survival of babies with neonatal herpes simplex virus infection according to disease classification and vidarabine dosages. (From Whitley RJ, Nahmias J, Soong S J, et al. Reproduced by permission of Pediatrics, vol. 73, page 778, copyright 1984.)

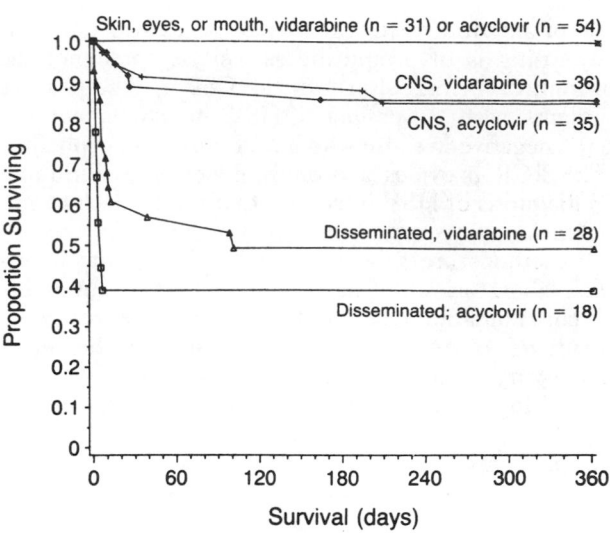

FIGURE 8–5 Survival of babies with neonatal herpes simplex virus (HSV) infection, according to treatment and the extent of disease. The infection was classified as confined to the skin, eyes, or mouth; affecting the central nervous system (CNS); or producing disseminated disease. After adjustment for the extent of disease with use of a stratified analysis, the overall comparison of vidarabine with acyclovir was not statistically significant ($p = 0.27$) by a log-rank test. No comparison of treatments within disease categories was statistically significant. (From Whitley R, Arvin A, Prober C, et al. A controlled trial comparing vidarabine with acyclovir in neonatal herpes simplex virus infection. Reprinted by permission of The New England Journal of Medicine, 324:444, 1991. © 1991, Massachusetts Medical Society. All rights reserved.)

Approximately 30% of children with either encephalitis or disseminated infection were reported as functioning normally at 1 year of life. Although there were no deaths among infants with skin, eye, and/or mouth infection, severe neurologic impairment was observed later in 30% of placebo recipients and 10% of treated infants.[93, 108] No enhanced therapeutic benefit for mortality or morbidity was noted with the higher dosage of vidarabine. For those infants receiving vidarabine at doses of 15 or 30 mg/kg per day, progression occurred in approximately 20 and 5 per cent of infected children, respectively.

Acyclovir has been established as efficacious for the treatment of primary genital herpes simplex infection when administered by intravenous, oral, and topical routes.[109, 110] Furthermore, the oral and intravenous administration of acyclovir to the immunocompromised host decreases both the frequency of reactivation after immunosuppression and the duration of disease.[111] Acyclovir has been established to be superior to vidarabine for the treatment of HSV encephalitis in older children and adults.[112] Because this compound is a selective inhibitor of viral replication, it has a low frequency of side effects.

After pharmacokinetic and tolerance evaluations of acyclovir were done in infants,[113, 114] the NIAID Collaborative Antiviral Study Group compared vidarabine and acyclovir for the treatment of neonatal HSV infection in a randomized trial.[98] The dose of vidarabine was 30 mg/kg per day, and acyclovir was given at a dose of 10 mg/kg every 8 hours. The duration of therapy was 10 days. No difference in either mortality or morbidity was observed for infected infants treated with either of these two drugs. The mortality for infants with disseminated infection 1 year after therapy for acyclovir and vidarabine was 55% and 40%, respectively ($p = 0.123$); for encephalitis, it was 10% for both treatment groups; and for disease localized to the skin, eye, and/or mouth, no infant died (Fig. 8–5). There were no differences in either adverse effects or laboratory evidence of toxicity. The overall morbidity for all treatment groups showed no statistically significant difference between vidarabine and acyclovir recipients (Table 8–2). Of the infants enrolled, more than 40% had disease localized to the skin, eye, and/or mouth. This percentage represents a threefold increase in infants with skin, eye, and/or mouth involvement from previous studies and historical data ($p < 0.001$). The number of infants with encephalitis remained constant at about 30%, and the number of those with disseminated disease decreased to 20%. The overall mortality was 19%, and morbidity for this cohort of infants was significantly reduced from previous studies (Fig. 8–6). Among infants with skin, eye, and/or mouth disease, those with HSV type 1 infections were all normal developmentally at 1 year compared with 86% of those with HSV type 2 infections. Infants who were alert or lethargic when treatment was initiated had a survival rate of 91%, compared with 54% for those who were semicomatose or comatose; similar differences in survival rates related to neurologic status were observed in infants with disseminated infection. Prematurity, pneumonitis, and disseminated intravascular coagulopathy were poor prognostic signs.

The overall change in the clinical spectrum of neonatal HSV infection and improved outcome probably reflected earlier diagnosis and institution of antiviral ther-

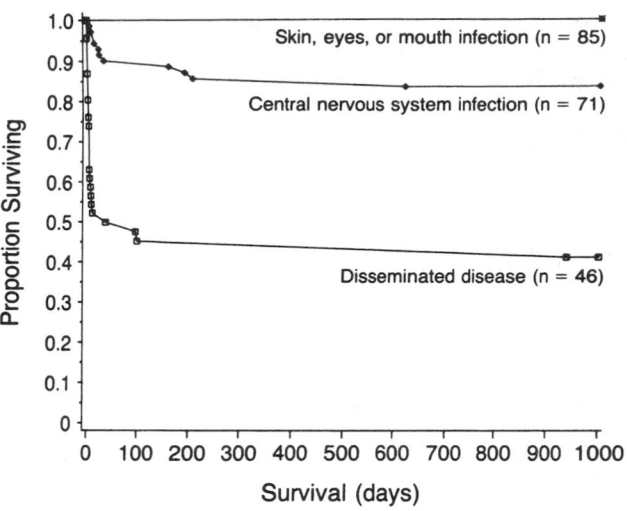

FIGURE 8–6 Survival of babies with neonatal herpes simplex virus infection, according to the extent of disease ($p < 0.001$ for all comparisons). (From Whitley R, Arvin A, Prober C, et al. Predictors of morbidity and mortality in neonates with herpes simplex infections. Reprinted by permission of The New England Journal of Medicine, 324:450, 1991. © 1991, Massachusetts Medical Society. All rights reserved.)

apy, thereby preventing progression of disease from skin, eye, and/or mouth to more severe disease. Therapy was begun an average of 3 days earlier for this group of infants. However, the mean duration of disease for all participants, regardless of disease classification, was 4 to 5 days, indicating that therapy might have been instituted even sooner. These observations suggested that further advances in therapeutic outcome might be achieved by earlier intervention.

Although the efficacy of antiviral therapy for neonatal herpes is proved, mortality remains high and many infants who survive disseminated or CNS disease have

TABLE 8–2
Assessment of Morbidity After 12 Months in Infants with Neonatal Herpes Simplex Virus Infection Treated with Vidarabine or Acyclovir

EXTENT OF DISEASE	NO. WITH MORBIDITY AFTER 12 MO					NO. ALIVE AFTER 12 MO. MORBIDITY UNKNOWN	NO. DEAD WITHIN 12 MO	TOTAL
	Normal	Mild	Moderate	Severe	Subtotal			
Skin, eye, or mouth infection								
Vidarabine	22	1	1	1	25	6	0	31
Acyclovir	45	0	1	0	46	8	0	54
Central nervous system infection								
Vidarabine	13	1	5	11	30	1	5	36
Acyclovir	8	5	6	9	28	2	5	35
Disseminated disease								
Vidarabine	7	1	0	4	12	2	14	28
Acyclovir	3	1	0	1	5	2	11	18
Total	98	9	13	26	146	21	35	202

From Whitley R, Arvin A, Prober C, et al. A controlled trial comparing vidarabine with acyclovir in neonatal herpes simplex virus infection. Reprinted by permission of The New England Journal of Medicine 324:444, 1991. © 1991. Massachusetts Medical Society. All rights reserved.

serious sequelae. This circumstance dictated the need to evaluate high doses of acyclovir and longer treatment regimens. Infants were enrolled in a Collaborative Antiviral Study Group assessment of acyclovir given at an intermediate dose (45 mg/kg per day) or high dose (60 mg/kg per day).[115] Based on initial analyses, mortality and morbidity in infants with disseminated or CNS disease were lower in infants given high-dose acyclovir than observed in earlier studies. The current recommendation for acyclovir treatment of neonatal HSV infections is 30 mg/kg per day in three doses, based on its demonstrated efficacy, with the usual duration of therapy being 14 to 21 days. These recent observations may result in a change to the use of 20 mg/kg per dose three times a day for 21 days.

The use of oral acyclovir is contraindicated for the treatment of acute HSV infections in newborns. Its limited oral bioavailability results in plasma and CSF concentrations of drug that are inadequate for therapeutic effects on viral replication. The high risk of progression from localized mucocutaneous infections requires the administration of intravenous acyclovir to these infants, regardless of how well they may appear at the time of diagnosis. In addition to intravenous therapy, infants with ocular involvement caused by HSV should receive one of the topical ophthalmic agents approved for this indication. Topical acyclovir is not necessary for treatment of mucocutaneous lesions caused by HSV because parenteral drug reaches these sites.

Acyclovir treatment should be based on a laboratory diagnosis of neonatal herpes. Rapid methods, including direct antigen detection and PCR, should be used to facilitate early laboratory confirmation of suspected cases. Acyclovir prophylaxis is not recommended. However, presumptive treatment may be a reasonable option when circumstances prevent rapid laboratory diagnosis and the clinical manifestations are those described for mucocutaneous herpes, disseminated disease, or HSV encephalitis. In all cases, specimens should be obtained for laboratory testing to guide the decision to continue treatment. During the course of therapy, careful monitoring is important to assess the therapeutic response. Even in the absence of clinical evidence of encephalitis, evaluation of the CNS should be done for prognostic purposes. Serial evaluations of certain hepatic (increased levels of aspartate and alanine aminotransferases) and bone marrow (decreased numbers of platelets) parameters may indicate changes caused by the viral infection or by drug toxicity.

Intravenous acyclovir has been tolerated well by infants given each of the doses evaluated in the prospective studies done by the Collaborative Antiviral Study Group, including 60 mg/kg per day.[115] Adequate hydration is necessary to minimize the risk of nephrotoxicity, and dosage adjustments are necessary if renal clearance is impaired. As for all drugs, the possibility of acute toxicity should be considered in any child receiving parenteral antiviral therapy and should be assessed by serially evaluating bone marrow, renal, and hepatic functions. The potential for long-term harm from these drugs remains to be defined.

Acyclovir resistance has been reported in an infant who had acute HSV infection of the larynx in the newborn period; in this case, the initial isolate was not inhibited by acyclovir, although the source of this infection could not be explained.[116] Isolates of HSV recovered from infants who received intravenous acyclovir for cutaneous disease in the newborn period and had subsequent recurrent cutaneous lesions remained sensitive to acyclovir.[117] The emergence of viral resistance to acyclovir, which usually results from the selection of thymidine kinase-negative mutants, has been described in patients requiring prolonged or repeated treatment with this drug. One infant who was given long-term oral acyclovir for suppression of recurrences during the first 6 months of life had a resistant HSV isolated from a lesion after therapy was discontinued, but subsequent isolates were susceptible.[118] Antiviral resistance does not explain the failure of infants with the disseminated or encephalitic form of the disease to respond well to antiviral therapy. Clinical deterioration, despite appropriate therapy and supportive care, can be attributed to virus-induced destruction of cells comprising infected organs, such as liver or brain, or irreversible changes, such as disseminated intravascular coagulopathy.

The observation of an association between late sequelae and frequent recurrences of skin lesions in infants who were treated for localized HSV type 2 infections during the newborn period has raised questions about the potential benefit of suppressive therapy with oral acyclovir. The Collaborative Antiviral Study Group has undertaken an assessment of the safety and efficacy of suppression as an adjunct, following the recommended treatment of mucocutaneous disease with intravenous acyclovir.[118] Infants were given 300 mg/m^2 per dose twice or three times a day, for 6 months. Of 16 infants given the thrice-daily regimen, 13 (81%) had no recurrences of lesions while receiving therapy compared with 54% of infants from earlier studies who received intravenous acyclovir only. Forty-six percent of the 26 infants developed neutropenia. In 1 infant, suppressive therapy was associated with a transient recurrence of infection due to an acyclovir resistant isolate of HSV type 2; subsequent recurrences were due to susceptible isolates. Whether this effect on cutaneous recurrences, which was limited to periods of active oral suppressive therapy, has any effect on late neurologic sequelae is not known. Oral acyclovir prophylaxis is not recommended for routine use, pending a larger trial of efficacy against this endpoint.

Other Issues in Acute Management

Isolation of the newborn with HSV infection is important to decrease the potential for nosocomial transmission. Many infants with this infection have life-threatening problems, including disseminated intravascular coagulation, shock, and respiratory failure, and require supportive care that is available only at tertiary medical centers.

At the present time, there is no indication that administration of immune globulin or hyperimmune globulin is of value for treatment of neonatal HSV infection. Although a series of studies have suggested that the quantity of transplacental neutralizing antibodies affects the attack rate among exposed infants and may influence the initial disease manifestations, the presence of antibodies may or may not influence the subsequent course of infection.[46, 48, 51, 52, 74] The administration of standard preparations of intravenous immune globulin does not enhance the titers of functional antibodies against HSV in low birth weight infants.[119] The evaluation of virus-specific monoclonal antibodies in combination with antiviral therapy may be feasible as new technologies for deriving human or humanized antibody preparations are developed.[120]

No other forms of adjunctive therapy are useful for treating neonatal HSV infections. Various experimental modalities, including bacille Calmette-Guérin, interferon, immune modulators, and immunization, have been attempted, but none has produced demonstrable effects.

Long-Term Management of Infected Infants

With the advent of antiviral therapy, an increasing number of newborns who suffered from HSV infection are surviving and require careful, long-term follow-up. The most common complications of neonatal HSV infection include neurologic and ocular sequelae that may be detected only on long-term follow-up. Therefore, it is necessary that these children receive serial long-term evaluation from qualified pediatric specialists in these areas, which should include neurodevelopmental, ophthalmologic, and hearing assessments.

Recurrent skin vesicles are present in many children, including those who did not have obvious mucocutaneous disease during the acute phase of the clinical illness. These skin vesicles provide a potential source for transmission of infection to other children or adults who have direct contact with these infants. The increasing use of day care for children, including those surviving neonatal HSV infections, stimulates many questions from day-care providers about these children. Certainly, there is some risk that children with recurrent HSV skin lesions will transmit the virus to other children in this environment. The most reasonable recommendation in this situation appears to be simply to cover the lesions to prevent direct contact. It is much more likely that HSV type 1 will be present in the day-care environment in the form of asymptomatic infection or gingivostomatitis. In both cases, virus is present in the mouth and pharynx, so that the frequent exchange of saliva and other respiratory droplets that occurs among children in this setting makes this route of transmission more likely. Education of day-care workers and the general public about herpesvirus infections, their implications, and the frequency with which they occur in the population as a whole could do much to calm fears and correct common misconceptions.

Parents of children with neonatal HSV infection often have significant feelings of guilt. Parents often require interventive support from psychologists, psychiatrists, or counselors. The family physician or pediatrician can provide a supportive role of great value to the family in this situation. Most parents, and many physicians, are not aware of the high prevalence of HSV type 2 infection in the United States and are not informed about the life-long persistence and subclinical nature of these infections. Concern about the risk of fetal and neonatal infection during subsequent pregnancies is often a major issue that can be addressed effectively based on the low risks, as proved from large prospective studies.

PREVENTION

In spite of the progress that has been made in antiviral treatment of neonatal HSV infection, the ideal approach is to prevent the exposure of infants to active maternal infection at the time of delivery. Unfortunately, the fact that genital infections caused by HSV are often clinically silent, both when they are acquired and when the virus reactivates, has been proved unequivocally. The high prevalence of HSV type 2 infections in the population in the United States, means that women are at risk of acquiring new genital infections during pregnancy and that at least one in five will have been infected before pregnancy. The problem of asymptomatic genital herpes infection means that the transmission of herpes simplex from mothers to infants cannot be eliminated even with the best obstetric management. It is now apparent that it is futile to obtain sequential genital cultures during the last weeks of gestation in women with a history of genital herpes in an effort to identify those who will have asymptomatic infection at the onset of labor.[45] These cultures do not predict the infant's risk of exposure at delivery because of the usual brief duration of asymptomatic shedding and the time required for the culture to become positive. Because of the attention of the lay press to the devastating outcome of neonatal herpes, many women who know that they have genital herpes experience severe anxiety about the potential risks to the fetus and newborn. As a consequence, these women may have an unnecessarily high frequency of cesarean deliveries. In fact, the risk of neonatal HSV infection in the newborn is approximately equivalent for women who have no prior history of genital herpes or a partner with known infection (Table 8–3).

Management of Pregnant Women with Known Genital Herpes

Women who have a history of recurrent genital herpes, whether or not recurrences are diagnosed during the pregnancy, should be reassured that the risk of fetal or neonatal infection is very low. Intrauterine infections due to herpes simplex are extremely rare, with an estimated overall risk of 1 in 200,000 pregnancies.[59] Information about the risk of exposure to asymptomatic reactivation at delivery derived from six large-scale prospective studies is now sufficient to conclude that the incidence of asymptomatic reactivation in these women is about 2% and that the attack rate for their exposed infants is approximately 3% or less; therefore, the risk of neonatal infection under these circumstances is less than 1 in 2000 deliveries. Because laboratory methods

TABLE 8–3

Projected Risk of Transmission of HSV-2 from Mothers to Infants at Delivery in a Cohort of 100,000 Pregnant Women

25% PAST HSV-2 INFECTION	75% SUSCEPTIBLE TO HSV-2
25,000 women	75,000 women
1.5% reactivation at delivery	0.02% seroconversion/wk
375 women with reactivation	30 women with infection <2 wk before delivery
<5% risk of transmission to infant	~50% risk of transmission
19 infected infants	15 infected infants

Reproduced with permission from Arvin AM. The epidemiology of perinatal herpes simplex infections. *In* Stanberry L (ed). Genital and Neonatal Herpes. New York, John Wiley & Sons, 1996, pp 179–192. Copyright John Wiley & Sons Limited.

cannot be used to detect asymptomatic infection in a timely manner, the current approach to management is to perform a careful vaginal examination at presentation and to elect cesarean delivery if the mother has signs or symptoms of recurrent genital herpes at the onset of labor. Given the low probability of neonatal infection, it is appropriate to deliver infants of women who have a history of recurrent genital herpes but who have no active clinical disease at delivery by the vaginal route.[53] An analysis of the occurrence of HSV infections in infants in California showed no change from 1985 to 1995, despite a documented decrease in deliveries by cesarean section and an increase in the proportion of women with a known past diagnosis of genital herpes whose infants were delivered vaginally.[58]

A culture for HSV obtained at the time of delivery may be useful in establishing whether the virus was present at delivery to facilitate the recognition of neonatal infection if it should occur. However, the value of this approach has not been established. Alternative diagnostic approaches, such as those based on PCR to detect virus, are being developed to expedite identification of women at risk for being delivered of infected infants.[121, 122]

Suppressive therapy of genital herpes in women with a known history of recurrent infection remains a question for clinical investigation because of risk-benefit considerations. It has already been established from the trials of suppressive therapy with acyclovir in individuals with frequently recurrent genital herpes that reactivation of virus can occur in spite of the administration of 200 mg of acyclovir three times daily.[123, 124] It is not unreasonable to think that such an event could occur in women who are given such therapy for recurrent infection during the last 4 weeks of gestation. The pharmacokinetics and metabolism of acyclovir in the human fetus are not known. The possibility of fetal nephrotoxicity related to acyclovir is a potential risk that must be considered. Whether acyclovir treatment of mothers with primary genital herpes late in gestation will reduce the neonatal risk of these infections is also a research issue. However, signs of disseminated herpes in the mother warrant the administration of intravenous acyclovir.

Management of Infants of Mothers with Genital Herpes

Infants of mothers with histories of genital herpes delivered either vaginally or by cesarean section, and whose mothers have no evidence of active genital herpetic infection, are at low risk for acquiring neonatal HSV infection. These infants need no special evaluation during the newborn period.

Infants delivered vaginally to mothers with an active genital herpes infection or who have genital cultures done at delivery that are positive for HSV should be isolated from other infants for the duration of their hospitalization up to 4 weeks of age. Parents and primary care physicians should be notified about the exposure of the infant so that the infant can be observed for the occurrence of nonspecific signs consistent with possible neonatal herpes. The parents and responsible family members should be educated about the low risk of transmission to relieve anxiety and to ensure prompt return for care in the unlikely event that signs of infection appear. Information regarding infection should include a description of the risks associated with transmission of infection to the newborn, the common signs and symptoms of neonatal herpes, the necessity for careful monitoring for the onset of illness as long as 4 weeks after birth, and the planned approach to treatment if symptoms occur.

It may be useful to obtain cultures from the exposed infant between 24 and 48 hours after delivery and at intervals during the first 4 weeks of life. Sites from which virus may be recovered include eye, oropharynx, nasopharynx, and skin lesions that are suspected to be herpetic. Several protocols have been suggested for the surveillance of exposed infants using viral cultures; the utility of this approach has not been proved by prospective studies, and it should be considered an optional addition to clinical observation. A reasonable protocol consists of performing weekly cultures of specimens from the eyes, nose, mouth, and skin for 4 to 6 weeks.[53] If cultures from any site are positive, a thorough diagnostic evaluation should be done, including obtaining additional specimens for viral culture from the site that was reported to be positive, the oropharynx, and the CSF; and treatment with vidarabine or acyclovir should be initiated. Cultures of the urine and buffy coat may also be considered to identify additional sites of viral infection.

At present, there are no data to support the administration of acyclovir to exposed infants who have no signs of infection. Parameters for duration of such prophylaxis cannot be defined. The experience from other clinical settings is that the virus is only suppressed for the period that the drug is given and is not eradicated. Careful clinical follow-up of these infants, with immediate institution of antiviral therapy should symptoms occur, is an appropriate approach to this problem.

An issue of frequent concern is whether the mother with an active genital HSV infection at delivery should be isolated from her child after delivery. Women with recurrent orolabial herpes simplex infection, as well as cutaneous herpes simplex infections at other sites (breast lesions), are at similar risk for transmission of virus to their newborn. Because transmission occurs by direct contact with the virus, appropriate precautions by the mother, including careful hand washing before touching the infant, should prevent any need to separate the mother and child. In some cases it is possible to have the exposed infant "room in" with the mother as a means of isolating the child from other newborns. Similarly, breast-feeding is contraindicated only if the mother has vesicular lesions involving the breast.

CONCLUSION

Neonatal HSV infection remains a life-threatening disease in the newborn. With an increasing prevalence of genital herpes and the recognition that many of these infections are completely asymptomatic in the mother, pediatricians, neonatologists, obstetricians, and family practitioners must continue to maintain a high index of suspicion in infants whose symptoms may be compatible with HSV infections. Early identification leads to prompt treatment. It is hoped that during this decade, the development of safe and efficacious vaccines, as well as a better understanding of factors associated with transmission of virus from mother to infant, will allow prevention of neonatal HSV infection.[125, 126]

ACKNOWLEDGMENTS

The data bases on clinical presentations, diagnosis, and antiviral therapy of neonatal herpes have been generated through the efforts of the Collaborative Antiviral Study Group for more than 20 years, with support from the National Institute of Allergy and Infectious Diseases. This work was initiated when the increased incidence of these infections was observed in the late 1970s through the leadership of Drs. C. A. Alford and A. J. Nahmias.

References

1. Mettler C. History of Medicine. Philadelphia, Blakiston, 1947, p 356.
2. Astruc J. De Morbis Venereis Libri Sex. Paris, G. Cavelier, 1736, p 361.
3. Gruter W. Das Herpesvirus, seine atiologische und klinische Bedeutung. Münch Med Wochenschr 71:1058, 1924.
4. Hass M. Hepatoadrenal necrosis with intranuclear inclusion bodies: report of a case. Am J Pathol 11:127, 1935.
5. Batignani A. Conjunctivite da virus erpetico in neonato. Boll Ocul 13:1217, 1934.
6. Nahmias A, Dowdle WR. Antigenic and biological differences in herpesvirus hominis. Prog Med Virol 10:110–159, 1968.
7. Roizman B. Herpes simplex viruses and their replication. *In* Roizman B, Knipe D, Howley P (eds). Fields Virology. Philadelphia, Lippincott-Raven, 1995, p 2231.
8. Whitley RJ. Herpes simplex viruses. *In* Roizman B, Knipe D, Howley P (eds). Fields Virology. Philadelphia, Lippincott-Raven, 1995, p 2296.
9. Spear PG. Glycoproteins of herpes simplex virus. *In* Bentz J (ed). Viral Fusion Mechanisms. Boca Raton, Fla, CRC Press, 1993, p. 201.
10. Roizman B, Norrild B, Chan C, et al. Identification of a herpes simplex virus 2 glycoprotein lacking a known type 1 counterpart. Virology 133:242, 1984.
11. Roizman B, Jenkins FJ. Genetic engineering of novel genomes of large DNA viruses. Science 229:1208, 1985.
12. Jugovic P, Hill AM, Tomazin R, et al. Inhibition of major histocompatibility complex type 1 antigen presentation in pig and primate cells by herpes simplex virus type 1 and 2 ICP47. J Virol 72:5076–5084, 1998.
13. Sullender WM, Yasukawa LL, Schwartz M, et al. Type-specific antibodies to herpes simplex virus type 2 (HSV-2) glycoprotein G in pregnant women, infants exposed to maternal HSV-2 infections at delivery, and infants with neonatal herpes. J Infect Dis 157:164, 1988.
14. Coleman RM, Pereira L, Bailey PD, et al. Determination of herpes simplex virus type-specific antibodies by enzyme-linked immunosorbent assay. J Clin Microbiol 18:287–291, 1983.
15. Ashley R, Cent A, Maggs V, et al. Inability of enzyme immunoassays to discriminate between infections with herpes simplex virus types 1 or 2. Ann Intern Med 115:520, 1991.
16. Ashley RL, Wu L, Pickering JW, et al. Premarket evaluation of a commercial glycoprotein-G based enzyme immunoassay for herpes simplex virus type-specific antibodies. J Clin Microbiol 36:845, 1998.
17. Cushing H. Surgical aspects of major neuralgia of trigeminal nerve: report of 20 cases of operation upon the gasserian ganglion with anatomic and physiologic notes on the consequence of its removal. JAMA 44:1002, 1905.
18. Goodpasture EW. Herpetic infections with special reference to involvement of the nervous system. Medicine 8:223, 1929.
19. Carton CA, Kilbourne ED. Activation of latent herpes simplex by trigeminal sensory-root section. N Engl J Med 246:172, 1952.
20. Pazin GJ, Armstrong JA, Lam MT, et al. Prevention of reactivation of herpes simplex virus infection by human leukocyte interferon after operation on the trigeminal root. N Engl J Med 301:225, 1979.
21. Stevens JG, Cook ML. Latent herpes simplex virus in spinal ganglia of mice. Science 173:843, 1971.
22. Rock DL, Fraser NW. Detection of HSV-1 genome in central nervous system of latently infected mice. Nature 302:523, 1983.
23. Baringer JR. Recovery of herpes simplex virus from human trigeminal ganglions. N Engl J Med 291:828, 1974.
24. Hill TJ. Herpes simplex virus latency. *In* Roizman B (ed). The Herpesviruses, vol 3. New York, Plenum Publishing, 1985, p 175.
25. Wentworth BB, Alexander ER. Seroepidemiology of infections due to members of the herpesvirus group. Am J Epidemiol 94:496, 1971.
26. Arvin AM. The epidemiology of perinatal herpes simplex infections. *In* Stanberry L (ed). Genital and Neonatal Herpes. New York, John Wiley & Sons, 1996, pp 179–192.

27. Nahmias AJ, Josey WE, Naib ZM, et al. Antibodies to *Herpesvirus hominis* types 1 and 2 in humans. Am J Epidemiol 91:539, 1970.

28. Wald A, Zeh J, Selke S, et al. Virologic characteristics of subclinical and symptomatic genital herpes infections. N Engl J Med 326:770, 1995.

29. Frenkel LM, Garratty E, Shen JP, et al. Clinical reactivation of herpes simplex virus type 2 in seropositive pregnant women with no history of genital herpes. Ann Intern Med 118:414, 1993.

30. Fleming DT, McQuillan GM, Johnson RE, et al. Herpes simplex virus type 2 in the United States, 1976 to 1994. N Engl J Med 337:1105–1111, 1997.

31. Buchman T, Roizman B, Nahmias AJ. Demonstration of exogenous genital reinfection with herpes simplex virus type 2 by restriction endonuclease fingerprinting of viral DNA. J Infect Dis 140:195, 1979.

32. Schmidt OW, Fife KH, Corey L. Reinfection is an uncommon occurrence in patients with symptomatic recurrent genital herpes. J Infect Dis 149:645, 1984.

33. Lakeman AD, Nahmias AJ, Whitley RJ. Analysis of DNA from recurrent genital herpes simplex virus isolates by restriction endonuclease digestion. Sex Transm Dis 13:61, 1986.

34. Boucher FD, Yasukawa LL, Bronzan RN, et al. A prospective evaluation of primary genital herpes simplex virus type 2 infections acquired during pregnancy. Pediatr Infect Dis 9:499, 1990.

35. Brown ZA, Vontver LA, Benedetti J, et al. Genital herpes in pregnancy: risk factors associated with recurrences and asymptomatic viral shedding. Am J Obstet Gynecol 153:24, 1985.

36. Prober CG, Hensleigh PA, Boucher FD, et al. Use of routine viral cultures at delivery to identify neonates exposed to herpes simplex virus. N Engl J Med 318:887, 1988.

37. Kulhanjian JA, Soroush V, Au DS, et al. Identification of women at unsuspected risk of primary infection with herpes simplex virus type 2 during pregnancy. N Engl J Med 326:916, 1992.

38. Brown Z, Vontver L, Bendetti J, et al. Effects on infants of first episode of genital herpes during pregnancy. N Engl J Med 317:1246, 1987.

39. Brown ZA, Benedetti J, Ashley R, et al. Neonatal herpes simplex virus infection in relation to asymptomatic maternal infection at the time of labor. N Engl J Med 324:1247, 1991.

40. Flewett TH, Parker RGF, Philip WM. Acute hepatitis due to herpes simplex virus in an adult. J Clin Pathol 22:60, 1969.

41. Young EJ, Killam AP, Greene JF Jr. Disseminated herpesvirus infection. Association with primary genital herpes in pregnancy. JAMA 235:2731, 1976.

42. Hensleigh PA, Glover DB, Cannon M. Systemic herpesvirus hominis in pregnancy. J Reprod Med 22:171, 1979.

43. Nahmias AJ, Josey WE, Naib ZM, et al. Perinatal risk associated with maternal genital herpes simplex virus infection. Am J Obstet Gynecol 110:825, 1971.

44. Brown ZA, Selke S, Zeh J, et al. The acquisition of herpes simplex virus during pregnancy. N Engl J Med 337:509, 1997.

45. Arvin AM, Hensleigh PA, Prober CG, et al. Failure of antepartum maternal cultures to predict the infant's risk of exposure to herpes simplex virus at delivery. N Engl J Med 315:796, 1986.

46. Whitley RJ, Corey L, Arvin A, et al. Changing presentation of neonatal herpes simplex virus infection. J Infect Dis 158:109, 1988.

47. Prober CG, Arvin AM. Genital herpes and the pregnant woman. *In* Remington JS, Swartz M (eds). Current Clinical Topics in Infectious Diseases, vol 10. Boston, Blackwell Scientific, 1989, p 1.

48. Prober CG, Sullender WM, Yasukawa LL, et al. Low risk of herpes simplex virus infections in neonates exposed to the virus at the time of vaginal delivery to mothers with recurrent genital herpes simplex virus infections. N Engl J Med 316:240, 1987.

49. Hensleigh PA, Andrews WW, Brown Z, et al. Genital herpes during pregnancy: inability to distinguish primary and recurrent infections clinically. Obstet Gynecol 89:891, 1997.

50. Corey L, Adams HG, Brown ZA, et al. Genital herpes simplex virus infections: clinical manifestations, course and complications. Ann Intern Med 98:958, 1983.

51. Yeager AS, Arvin AM, Urbani LJ, et al. Relationship of antibody to outcome in neonatal herpes simplex virus infections. Infect Immun 29:532, 1980.

52. Sullender WM, Miller JL, Yasukowa LL, et al. Humoral and cell-mediated immunity in neonates with herpes simplex virus infection. J Infect Dis 155:28, 1987.

53. Prober CG, Corey L, Brown ZA, et al. The management of pregnancies complicated by genital infections with herpes simplex virus. Clin Infect Dis 15:1031, 1992.

54. Stone KM, Brooks CA, Guinan ME, et al. National surveillance for neonatal herpes simplex virus infection. Sex Transm Dis 16:152, 1989.

55. Parvey LS, Chien LT. Neonatal herpes simplex virus infection introduced by fetal monitor scalp electrode. Pediatrics 65:1150, 1980.

56. Kaye EM, Dooling EC. Neonatal herpes simplex meningoencephalitis associated with fetal monitor scalp electrodes. Neurology 31:1045, 1981.

57. Sullivan-Bolyai J, Hull HF, Wilson C, et al. Neonatal herpes simplex virus infection in King County, Washington: increasing incidence and epidemiologic correlates. JAMA 250:3059, 1983.

58. Gutierrez KM, Halpern MF, Maldonado Y, Arvin AM. The epidemiology of neonatal herpes simplex virus (HSV) infections in California from 1985 to 1995. J Infect Dis 180:199–202, 1999.

59. Hutto C, Arvin A, Jacobs R, et al. Intrauterine herpes simplex virus infections. J Pediatr 110:97, 1987.

60. Florman AL, Gershon AA, Blackett PR, et al. Intrauterine infection with herpes simplex virus: resultant congenital malformations. JAMA 225:129, 1973.

61. South MA, Tompkins WA, Morris CR, et al. Congenital malformation of the central nervous system associated with genital type (type 2) herpesvirus. J Pediatr 75:8, 1969.

62. Baldwin S, Whitley RJ. Intrauterine HSV infection. Teratology 39:1, 1989.

63. Arvin AM. Fetal and neonatal infections. *In* Nathanson N, Murphy F (eds). Viral Pathogenesis. Philadelphia, Lippincott-Raven, 1996, pp 801–814.

64. Kahlon J, Whitley RJ. Antibody response of the newborn after herpes simplex virus infection. J Infect Dis 158:925, 1988.

65. Garcia AG. Maternal herpes-simplex infection causing abortion. Histopathologic study of the placenta. Hospital (Rio de Janeiro) 78:1266, 1970.

66. Light IJ. Postnatal acquisition of herpes simplex virus by the newborn infant: a review of the literature. Pediatrics 63:480, 1979.

67. Linnemann CC, Light IJ, Buchman TG, et al. Transmission of herpes simplex virus type 1 in a nursery for the

newborn: identification of viral isolates by DNA "fingerprinting." Lancet 1:964, 1978.

68. Hammerberg O, Watts J, Chernesky M, et al. An outbreak of herpes simplex virus type 1 in an intensive care nursery. Pediatr Infect Dis 2:290, 1983.

69. Yeager AS, Ashley RL, Corey L. Transmission of herpes simplex virus from the father to neonate. J Pediatr 103:905, 1983.

70. Douglas JM, Schmidt O, Corey L. Acquisition of neonatal HSV-1 infection from a paternal source contact. J Pediatr 103:908, 1983.

71. Sullivan-Bolyai JZ, Fife KH, Jacobs RF, et al. Disseminated neonatal herpes simplex virus type 1 from a maternal breast lesion. Pediatrics 71:455, 1983.

72. Hatherley LI, Hayes K, Jack I. Herpesvirus in an obstetric hospital. Asymptomatic virus excretion in staff members. Med J Aust 2:273, 1980.

73. Hatherley LI, Hayes K, Jack I. Herpes virus in an obstetric hospital: III. Prevalence of antibodies in patients and staff. Med J Aust 2:325, 1980.

74. Kohl S, West MS, Prober CG, et al. Neonatal antibody-dependent cellular cytotoxic antibody levels are associated with the clinical presentation of neonatal herpes simplex virus infection. J Infect Dis 160:770, 1989.

75. Dworsky ME, Whitley RJ, et al. Specific lymphocyte blastogenic responses in children with cytomegalovirus and herpes simplex virus infections acquired early in infancy. Infect Immun 34:166, 1981.

76. Chilmonczyk BA, Levin MJ, McDuffy R, et al. Characterization of the human newborn response to herpesvirus antigen. J Immunol 134:4184, 1985.

77. Burchett SK, Westall J, Mohan K, et al. Ontogeny of neonatal mononuclear cell transformation and interferon gamma production after herpes simplex virus stimulation. Clin Res 34:129, 1986.

78. Kohl S, Harmon MW. Human neonatal leukocyte interferon production and natural killer cytotoxicity in response to herpes simplex virus. J Interferon Res 3:461, 1983.

79. Kohl S. Neonatal herpes simplex virus infection. Clin Perinatol 24:129, 1997.

80. Mintz H, Drew WL, Hoo R, et al. Age dependent resistance of human alveolar macrophages to herpes simplex virus. Infect Immun 28:417, 1980.

81. Hirsch MS, Zisman B, Allison AC. Macrophages and age-dependent resistance to herpes simplex virus in mice. J Immunol 104:1160, 1970.

82. Singer DB. Pathology of neonatal herpes simplex virus infection. Perspect Pediatr Pathol 6:243, 1981.

83. Smith MC, Lennette EH, Reames HR. Isolation of the virus of herpes simplex and the demonstration of intranuclear inclusions in a case of acute encephalitis. Am J Pathol 17:538, 1971.

84. Whitley R, Arvin A, Prober C, et al. Predictors of morbidity and mortality in neonates with herpes simplex infections. N Engl J Med 324:450, 1991.

85. Nahmias A, Alford C, Korones S. Infection of the newborn with herpesvirus hominis. Adv Pediatr 17:185, 1970.

86. Whitley RJ, Kimberlin D. Treatment of viral infections during pregnancy and the neonatal period. Clin Perinatol 24:267–283, 1997.

87. Malm G, Berg U, Forsgren M. Neonatal herpes simplex: clinical findings and outcome in relation to type of maternal infection. Acta Paediatr 84:256, 1995.

88. Greenes DS, Rowitch D, Thorne G, et al. Neonatal herpes simplex virus infection presenting as fulminant liver failure. Pediatr Infect Dis J 14:242, 1995.

89. Arvin AM, Yeager AS, Bruhn FW, et al. Neonatal herpes simplex infection in the absence of mucocutaneous lesions. J Pediatr 100:715, 1982.

90. Gressens P, Langston C, Martin JR. In situ PCR localization of herpes simplex virus DNA sequences in disseminated neonatal herpes encephalitis. J Neuropathol Exp Neurol 53:469, 1994.

91. Golden SE. Neonatal herpes simplex viremia. Pediatr Infect Dis J 7:425, 1987.

92. Corey L, Stone EF, Whitley RJ, Mohan K. Difference between herpes simplex virus type I and type 2 neonatal encephalitis in neurological outcome. Lancet 1:1–4, 1988.

93. Whitley RJ, Nahmias J, Soong SJ, et al. Vidarabine therapy of neonatal herpes simplex virus infection. Pediatrics 66:495, 1980.

94. Yeager AS, Arvin AM. Reason for the absence of a history of recurrent genital infections in mothers of neonates infected with herpes simplex virus. Pediatrics 73:188, 1984.

95. Mizrahi EM, Tharp BR. A unique electroencephalogram pattern in neonatal herpes simplex virus encephalitis. Neurology 31:164, 1981.

96. O'Reilly MAR, O'Reilly PMR, de Bruyn R. Neonatal herpes simplex type 2 encephalitis: its appearances on ultrasound and CT. Pediatr Radiol 25:68, 1995.

97. Gutman LT, Wilfert CM, Eppes S. Herpes simplex virus encephalitis in children: analysis of cerebrospinal fluid and progressive neurodevelopmental deterioration. J Infect Dis 154:415, 1986.

98. Whitley R, Arvin A, Prober C, et al. A controlled trial comparing vidarabine with acyclovir in neonatal herpes simplex virus infection. N Engl J Med 324:444, 1991.

99. Musci SI, Fine EM, Togo Y. Zoster-like disease in the newborn due to herpes simplex virus. N Engl J Med 284:24, 1971.

100. Nahmias A, Hagler W. Ocular manifestations of herpes simplex in the newborn. Int Ophthalmol Clin 12:191, 1972.

101. Cherry JD, Soriano F, Jahn CL. Search for perinatal viral infection: a prospective, clinical virology and serologic study. Am J Dis Child 116:245, 1968.

102. Whitley RJ, Lakeman FD. Herpes simplex virus infections of the central nervous system: therapeutic and diagnostic considerations. Clin Infect Dis 20:414, 1995.

103. Arvin AM, Prober CG. Herpes simplex viruses. In Murphy P (ed). Manual of Clinical Microbiology, 7th ed. Washington, D.C., American Society for Microbiology, 1998.

104. Kimberlin DW, Lakeman FD, Arvin AM, et al. Application of the polymerase chain reaction to the diagnosis and management of neonatal herpes simplex virus disease. National Institute of Allergy and Infectious Diseases Collaborative Antiviral Study Group. J Infect Dis 174:1162–1167, 1996.

105. Troendle-Atksin J, Demmler GJ, Buffone GJ. Rapid diagnosis of herpes simplex virus encephalitis by using the polymerase chain reaction. J Pediatr 123:376, 1993.

106. Kimura H, Futamura M, Kito H, et al. Detection of viral DNA in neonatal herpes simplex virus infections: frequent and prolonged presence in serum and cerebrospinal fluid. J Infect Dis 164:289, 1991.

107. Elion, GB, Furman PA, Fyfe JA, et al. Selectivity of action of an antiherpetic agent 9-(2-hydroxyethoxymethyl) guanine. Proc Natl Acad Sci U S A 74:5716, 1977.

108. Whitley RJ, Yeager A, Kartus P, et al. Neonatal herpes simplex virus infection: follow-up evaluation of vidarabine therapy. Pediatrics 72:778, 1983.

109. Corey L, Benedetti J, Critchlow C, et al. Treatment of primary first-episode genital herpes simplex virus infections with acyclovir: results of topical, intravenous and oral therapy. J Antimicrob Chemother 12:79, 1983.

110. Bryson YJ, Dillon M, Lovett M, et al. Treatment of first episodes of genital herpes simplex virus infection with oral acyclovir: a randomized double-blind controlled trial in normal subjects. N Engl J Med 308:916, 1983.

111. Saral R, Burns WH, Laskin OL, et al. Acyclovir prophylaxis of herpes-simplex-virus infections. N Engl J Med 305:63, 1981.

112. Whitley RJ, Alford CA, Hirsch MS, et al. Vidarabine versus acyclovir therapy of herpes simplex encephalitis. N Engl J Med 314:144, 1986.

113. Yeager AS. Use of acyclovir in premature and term neonates. Am J Med 73:205, 1982.

114. Hintz M, Connor JD, Spector SA, et al. Neonatal acyclovir pharmacokinetics in patients with herpesvirus infections. Am J Med 73:210, 1982.

115. Kimberlin DW, Jacobs RF, Powell DA, et al. The safety and efficacy of high dose acyclovir in neonatal herpes simplex virus infections. Abstract. Society for Pediatric Research, San Francisco, 1999.

116. Nyquist A-C, Rotbart HA, Cotton M, et al. Acyclovir-resistant neonatal herpes simplex virus infection of the larynx. J Pediatr 124:967, 1994.

117. Rabalais GP, Nusinoff-Lehrman S, Arvin AM, Levin MJ. Antiviral susceptiblities of herpes simplex virus isolates from infants with recurrent mucocutaneous lesions after neonatal infection. Pediatr Infect Dis J 8:221, 1991.

118. Kimberlin D, Powell D, Gruber W, et al. Administration of oral acyclovir suppressive therapy after neonatal herpes simplex virus disease limited to the skin, eyes and mouth: results of a Phase I/II trial. Pediatr Infect Dis J 15:247, 1996.

119. Kohl S, Loo LS, Rench MS, et al. Effect of intravenously administered immune globulin on functional antibody to herpes simplex virus in low birth weight neonates. J Pediatrics 115:135, 1989.

120. Whitley RJ. Neonatal herpes simplex virus infections: is there a role for immunoglobulin in disease prevention and therapy? Pediatr Infect Dis J, 13:432, 1994.

121. Hardy DA, Arvin AM, Yasukawa LL, et al. Use of polymerase chain reaction for successful identification of asymptomatic genital infection with herpes simplex virus in pregnant women at delivery. J Infect Dis 162:1031, 1990.

122. Cone RW, Hobson AC, Brown Z, et al. Frequent detection of genital herpes simplex virus DNA by polymerase chain reaction among pregnant women. JAMA 272:792–796, 1994.

123. Douglas JM, Critchlow C, Benedetti J, et al. A double-blind study of oral acyclovir for suppression of recurrences of genital herpes simplex virus infection. N Engl J Med 310:1551, 1984.

124. Straus SE, Takiff HE, Seidlin M, et al. Suppression of frequently recurring genital herpes: a placebo-controlled double-blind trial of oral acyclovir. N Engl J Med 310:1545, 1984.

125. Arvin AM. Genital herpesvirus infections: Rationale for a vaccine strategy. In Hitchcock PJ, MacKay HT, Wasserheit JN, Binder R (eds). Sexually Transmitted Diseases and Adverse Outcomes of Pregnancy. Washington, D.C., American Society for Microbiology, 1999.

126. Arvin AM, Prober CG. Herpes simplex virus type 2, a persistent problem. N Engl J Med 337:1158–1159, 1997.

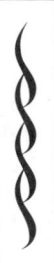

C H A P T E R   9

Acquired Immunodeficiency Syndrome in the Infant

BRIGITTA U. MUELLER, M.D., and PHILIP A. PIZZO, M.D.

The first descriptions of the acquired immunodeficiency syndrome (AIDS) in infants and children were published more than a decade ago.[1–4] As of December 1998, more than 8000 AIDS cases in children younger than the age of 13 years have been registered by the Centers for Disease Control and Prevention (CDC) in the United States.[5, 6] However, this represents only a fraction of the nearly 1.1 million children living with human immunodeficiency virus type 1 (HIV-1) infection worldwide and of the 2.7 million children who have already died of the disease. Although HIV infection in children has been acquired in the past by the transfusion of contaminated blood or coagulation products, this route has been virtually completely eliminated in the United States. AIDS cases in infants are the result of vertical transmission (i.e., from an infected mother to her child).[5, 6] During childhood, sexual abuse has been associated with the acquisition of HIV infection by some children; and both the use of contaminated needles and unprotected sexual intercourse account for the vast majority of infections in teenagers.

In this chapter the experience with HIV infection in children is reviewed with the focus on the infection in the neonate and infant. We now have a sound knowledge of the clinical presentation of HIV infection in infants and children and have made major progress in preventing vertical transmission in industrialized countries. However, there is an urgent need for the development of simpler and inexpensive interventions, as well as the need to even better understand the time point at which transmission occurs and the role of potentially protective factors. Such knowledge will impact on future recommendations for the treatment of pregnant women, on the management of very young children, and on the use of preventive measures, including immunization and other supportive care modalities, before the onset of disease manifestations.

EPIDEMIOLOGY

HIV infection is a pandemic with cases reported to the World Health Organization (WHO) from virtually every country. Through June 1998 an estimated 30.6 million people were infected, almost half of them (12.1 million) women and 1.1 million children younger than the age of 15 years (UNAIDS report on the Global HIV/AIDS Epidemic). The epidemic continues unabated in Africa and is expanding rapidly in Southeast Asia, India, and Latin America.[7–10] It has been estimated that in 1997 alone, 5.2 million adults and 590,000 children were newly infected with HIV-1 (approximately 1600 new cases per day), and 2.3 million adults and 460,000 children younger than the age of 15 years have died of HIV-related complications. If the current trend continues, 60 to 70 million people will have been infected by the year 2000.

In contrast, in the United States, HIV-infected children younger than the age of 13 years account for only 1% of all AIDS cases.[5] However, in developing nations, children comprise more than 10% of the people living with HIV/AIDS, and 23% (2.7 million) of AIDS-related deaths have been in children younger than 15 years. Furthermore, UNAIDS estimates that 8.2 million children have been orphaned by the AIDS epidemic.

As of December 1998, of the 8461 cases of AIDS in children younger than the age of 13 years that have been reported to the CDC in the United States, about half have already died of their disease.[5] Minority groups are disproportionally affected with 58% of cases occurring in black, non-Hispanic children (who account for only 14% of the U.S. pediatric population), and 23% in Hispanics (17% of U.S. pediatric population), compared with 18% in white, non-Hispanic children (64% of pediatric U.S. population).

Almost 80% of the children with AIDS are younger than the age of 5 years, reflecting the predominant mode of transmission from mother to child, which accounts currently for 91% of HIV infections in children.[5] About 28% of the women in the United States have acquired HIV infection through intravenous drug use, but a growing number (currently 54%) has been infected through sexual contact.[5] The increasing number of infected women of childbearing age will continued to greatly influence the number of infected children in the United States and worldwide.

TRANSMISSION

Current data suggest that the majority of children are infected during the immediate peripartum period. In the United States the transmission rate without intervention is estimated to be 25 to 30%, in Europe, it is lower (13 to 20%), whereas a rate of 40% has been observed in Africa.[11, 12] These differences in transmission rates are difficult to explain. Maternal disease status, especially a CD4 count less than 200 cells/mm^3 or a high viral load, is directly correlated with the risk for vertical transmission.[11, 13]

In 1994, the results of the AIDS Clinical Trials Group protocol 076 (PACTG 076) employing zidovudine during pregnancy were published, resulting in new guidelines issued by the CDC.[14–16] This trial, which resulted in a 67% reduction in perinatal transmission, is now the gold standard to which future strategies for the prevention of perinatal transmission are being compared.

Intrauterine Transmission

The female glandular epithelium can contain HIV between the columnar and squamous cells of the cervix, whereas swabs from the vagina yield fewer virus particles.[17, 18] Sperm cells do not express CD4 receptors and are therefore unlikely to be directly infected with HIV, but the virus can be detected in seminal white cells and plasma.[18]

Virus has been detected in some aborted fetuses of 8 to 20 weeks' gestational age and in amniotic fluid.[19–22] Maternal decidual leukocytes, villous macrophages

(Hofbauer cells), and endothelial cells stain positive for gp41 antigen and HIV nucleic acids.[23] The placenta can be infected through the CD4$^+$ trophoblasts or through the occasional occurrence of a chorioamnionitis.[24, 25] Notably, there is not a clear predictive value of the identification of HIV in the placenta and the infection of the fetus or newborn.[26] Moreover, there are important technical limitations to studies of fetal or placenta tissues, particularly due to the difficulty of excluding contamination with maternal blood.

A number of factors that might correlate with a heightened risk for transmission have been assessed, including the maternal viral burden, specific viral phenotypes or genotypes, the disease stage of the mother, her immune response to HIV infection, placental disruption by coexistence of other infections, and fetal susceptibility (which may be influenced by genetic factors).[11, 13, 27–32] In the absence of prophylactic zidovudine treatment, HIV-positive mothers have a potentially higher risk for transmission if they have positive p24 antigenemia, a CD4 count less than 400 cells/mm^3, and a high HIV RNA level.[13, 32, 33] A high rate of transmission was reported with advanced clinical stage of disease, with 100% transmission among 10 patients with CDC class IV (symptomatic) disease, versus 13% in 56 patients with CDC class II (asymptomatic) or CDC class III (i.e., lymphadenopathy as only symptom) disease.[34]

Intrapartum Infection

The bimodal course of disease in HIV-infected children and the fact that at the time of birth virus can only be recovered from less than 25% of the infants who are subsequently shown to be infected suggest that a large proportion of perinatal infections occur late during pregnancy or during delivery.[35] An infant is considered to have been infected in utero if the HIV-1 genome can be detected by polymerase chain reaction (PCR) or be cultured from blood within 48 hours of birth. In contrast, a child is considered to have intrapartum infection if diagnostic assays such as culture, PCR, and serum p24 antigen are negative in blood samples obtained during the first week of life, but became positive during the period from day 7 to day 90, and the infant had not been breast-fed.[36]

In a study by the French Collaborative Study Group, timing of transmission was estimated with a mathematical model.[37] Data for the 95 infected infants (those seropositive at 18 months and those who died of HIV disease before this age and who were exclusively bottle-fed), were used in the model, which indicated that one third of the infants were infected in utero, less than 2 months before delivery (ninety-fifth percentile). In the remaining 65% of cases (95% confidence interval [CI], 22–92%), the date of infection was estimated as the day of birth. Viral markers became positive after an estimated median time period of 10 days (95% CI, 6–14%), and the ninety-fifth percentile was estimated at 56 days.[37]

Discordance of infection has been described not only among the progeny of different pregnancies but even more intriguingly among twins.[38–41] In a large multinational study, data were collected on 100 sets of twins and one set of triplets born to HIV-seropositive mothers.[40] HIV-1 infection was more common in first-born than in second-born twins ($p = 0.004$), with 50% of first-born twins delivered vaginally and 38% of first-born twins delivered by cesarean section being infected, compared with 19% of second-born twins delivered by either route. Thus, passage through, or close proximity to, the birth canal appears to be an important factor, and prophylactic measures such as cleansing the birth canal before delivery might reduce the risk of intrapartum infection.[42] One study, performed in Africa, compared the HIV transmission rate of infants born to 3327 women whose infants were delivered in a conventional way with that of 3637 infants of women who were treated with manual cleansing of the birth canal with a cotton pad soaked in 0.25% chlorhexidine on admission for labor and every 4 hours until delivery.[43] Although the intervention had no significant impact on HIV transmission rates (27% in 505 intervention women compared with 28% in 477 control women), cleansing the birth canal with chlorhexidine reduced the hospitalization rates for early neonatal and maternal postpartum infectious problems.[44]

Cesarean section, although likely to reduce the risk of transmission to a certain degree (in one study from 32% to 18%, $p = 0.11$), does not prevent it altogether.[28, 40] However, it has been demonstrated that prolonged rupture of membranes over 4 hours increases the risk of transmission considerably, regardless of the mode of delivery.[45]

Postpartum Infection

Breast-feeding has been implicated as a postnatal route of maternal-infant transmission of HIV disease.[46, 47] HIV-1 has been demonstrated by culture or PCR in up to 73% of breast milk specimens from HIV-1 seropositive women.[18, 49] The prevalence of cell-free HIV-1 appears to be higher in mature milk (47%) than in colostrum (27%, $p = 0.1$).[50] Guay and colleagues collected expressed breast milk specimens from 201 HIV-1–seropositive and 86 HIV-1–seronegative Ugandan women approximately 6 weeks after delivery. Forty-seven of the 201 HIV-1–infected women had HIV-1–infected children, 143 had children who seroreverted, and 11 had children of indeterminate status. Breast milk supernatants were available for p24 antigen testing from 188 of the HIV-1–infected women and breast milk cell pellets were available and contained amplifiable DNA in 125 of them (20 transmitters, 104 nontransmitters, 1 indeterminate). HIV-1 DNA was detected by PCR in 72% (75/104) of nontransmitters and 80% (16/20) of the transmitters.[51] Other studies have also shown that the majority of breast-fed infants appear to remain uninfected.[48, 52] A study of breast-fed infants born to HIV-infected mothers was performed in Kinshasa, Democratic Republic of Congo (formerly Zaire).[53] Among 69 HIV-infected children (26% of the cohort), 23% (95% CI, 14–35%) were estimated to have had intrauterine, 65% (CI, 53–76%) intrapartum/early postpartum, and 12% (CI, 5–22%) late postpartum transmission. The authors estimated the risks for intrauterine, intrapartum/ early postpartum, and late postpartum infection, respectively, to be 6% (16/261; CI, 4–10%), 18% (45/245; CI, 14–24%), and 4% (8/189, CI, 2–8%).[53]

Comparing the risk of transmission of HIV-1 by breast-feeding and subsequent associated mortality with the mortality resulting from bottle feeding with potentially contaminated water has been reviewed, but is yielding controversial results. One study demonstrated that the benefits of breast-feeding over bottle-feeding can substantially outweigh the risk of HIV transmission unless the prevalence of HIV infection is high or the difference in mortality of breast-fed and bottle infants is very low[54]; however, another study did not support this conclusion.[55] The WHO continues to encourage breast-feeding in countries where good oral food substitutes and safe water supplies for reconstituting dried milk products are not readily available (Policy Statement developed by UNAIDS, UNICEF, and WHO, 1998). The American Academy of Pediatrics (AAP) has issued the following policy statement (abbreviated form)[56]:

- The AAP recommends documented, routine HIV education and routine testing with consent of all women seeking prenatal care so that each woman will know her HIV status and the methods available both to prevent the acquisition and transmission of HIV and to determine whether it is appropriate to breast feed.
- *Women who are known to be HIV-infected must be counseled not to breast feed or provide their milk for the nutrition of their own or other infants.* In general, women who are known to be HIV seronegative should be encouraged to breast feed. However, women who are HIV seronegative but at particularly high risk of seroconversion (injection drug users and sexual partners of known HIV-positive persons or active drug users) should be provided education about HIV infection with an individualized recommendation concerning the appropriateness of breast-feeding.

Several large studies have shown a lack of transmission of HIV infection to household contacts through casual interactions.[57–60] In fact, the American Academy of Pediatrics does not place any special restrictions on daycare or school attendance of HIV-infected children but recommends observance of universal precaution measures for all handling of blood and body fluids, regardless of the infection status of the child.[61, 62] The same guidelines apply to the handling of *all* newborns during or after birth. Gloves should be worn when handling body fluids, including amniotic fluid, and only bulb or wall suction devices should be used to avoid exposure of medical personnel.[63]

MOLECULAR BIOLOGY

HIV-1 is an enveloped virus of 80 to 120 nm with a cylindrical, electrodense core. HIV-1 and its close relative HIV-2 are members of the Lentiviridae of retroviruses and have a complex genomic structure.[64, 65] Like all retroviruses HIV-1 contains the genes for *gag*, which encodes the core nucleocapsid polypeptides (gp24, p17, p9), *env* for the surface-coat proteins of the virus (gp120 and gp41), as well as *pol*, which codes for the viral reverse transcriptase and other enzymatic activities (i.e., integrase and protease). In addition there are at least six regulatory genes present (*vif, vpr, vpx, tat, rev, vpu,* and *nef*).[66] The retroviral core also contains two copies of the viral single-stranded RNA associated with enzymes such as the reverse transcriptase, Rnase H, integrase, and protease.[65]

The life cycle of HIV-1 is characterized by several distinct stages.[67] The first step in the entry process of HIV into a cell is the interaction of the virion envelope glycoproteins (gp120 and gp41) with both the CD4 molecule as well as a chemokine receptor.[68–74] Human cord blood mononuclear cells are preferentially infected by macrophage-tropic (M-tropic) strains of HIV-1 using the CC chemokine receptor CCR5.[72, 74, 75] T cell tropic strains replicate in $CD4^+$ T cells and macrophages. They use the chemokine receptor CXCR4, a member of the CXC chemokine family.[68, 71, 72, 74]

The HIV virions enter the cell and are rapidly uncoated. The viral reverse transcriptase transforms the single-stranded viral RNA into linear double-stranded DNA, whereas the less specific ribonuclease H degrades and removes the RNA template.[76] This viral DNA is circularized and transferred to the nucleus, where it is inserted by the viral integrase at random sites as a provirus.[77, 78] It is also a common feature of all retroviruses to accumulate large amounts of unintegrated viral DNA that are fully competent templates for HIV-1 core and envelope antigen production.[79] The inactive provirus in the form of HIV-1 DNA has been found in 0.1 to 13.5% of peripheral blood mononuclear cells, compared with viral mRNA, which is found in 0.002 to 0.25% of these cells.[80–82] The latent provirus is activated by host cell responses to antigens, mitogens, cytokines such as tumor necrosis factor, and different gene products of other viruses.[82–85]

HIV gene expression follows by using host cell RNA polymerase II among other factors, forming a ribonucleoprotein core containing *gag* and *pol* gene products. The 53-kDa precursor of the *gag* protein is cleaved by the HIV-1–derived protease into the p24, p17, p9, and p7 proteins.[86–88] The assembly of new virions consists of the formation of the critical viral enzymes, including reverse transcriptase, integrase, ribonuclease, and a protease, and the aggregation into a ribonucleoprotein core.[64, 65] This core then moves to the cell surface and buds as mature virions through the plasma membrane.

Perinatal HIV infection is characterized by plasma RNA levels that rapidly reach very high levels.[89–91] In a study of 106 HIV-infected infants the median plasma HIV RNA value at 1 month of age was 318,000 copies/ml, and it was not uncommon to see viral levels that exceeded 10^6 copies/ml. In the absence of antiretroviral therapy the levels decrease only gradually over the first 24 to 36 months.[92] As in adults, higher viral loads correlate with a more rapid disease progression.[89, 93–95] This provides a strong argument for early and aggressive intervention with antiretroviral therapy (see later).

A controversial issue is the proposed clearance of HIV infection in some perinatally infected infants.[96–100] It was postulated that rarely children could have a positive culture of peripheral blood mononuclear cells for HIV-1 and positivity of plasma by PCR assay, but later become negative both by culture and PCR, as well as remain seronegative without ever having received antiretroviral therapy. However, a recent analysis of 42 cases of suspected "transient infection" among 1562 exposed seroreverting infants and one mother did not document a phylogenetic linkage between the infant's and the mother's virus in 17 cases, did not detect any HIV-1 *env* sequences in 20 cases, or demonstrated that the specimens were mistakenly attributed to the child (6 cases).[101]

IMMUNE PATHOGENESIS

Infection with HIV results in profound deficiencies in cell-mediated and humoral immunity, secondary to both quantitative and qualitative defects, leading to a progressive dysfunction of the immune system with depletion of $CD4^+$ T cells. Flow cytometric analysis of lymphocyte subpopulations in healthy children has revealed age-related changes in the number of the different subgroups.[102–104] Comparison of lymphocytes subsets in HIV-infected versus noninfected children younger than 2 years demonstrated no difference for absolute CD8 counts but clearly decreased levels of CD4 cells.[105] In the absence of early antiretroviral therapy, an abnormal CD4 count (less than the 10th percentile for uninfected children) was found in 83% and an abnormally low absolute CD4 count was observed in 67% of the infected children. As in adults, the relative risks of death or disease progression are inversely related to the CD4 cell count, which in turn is closely related to the viral load.[91, 106] A rapid increase in HIV RNA levels correlates with early disease progression and loss of CD4 cells in vertically infected infants.[106]

Other immune abnormalities include decreased lymphocyte proliferation in response to an antigen, polyclonal B cell activation resulting in hypergammaglobulinemia, and altered function of monocytes and neutrophils.[107–110] In the European Collaborative Study, hypergammaglobulinemia (IgG, IgM, and IgA) identified 77% of infected children at the age of 6 months with 97% specificity.[111] In a group of 47 HIV-infected children (17 asymptomatic and 30 symptomatic), Roilides and co-workers found an abnormality of at least one IgG subclass in 83%, including some patients who had IgG2, IgG4, or combined IgG2–IgG4 deficiencies.[107] Of note, there was no clear correlation of the incidence of bacterial infections with specific subclass deficiencies. A virus-specific cytotoxic T lymphocyte response can be demonstrated at a very early age, even in the fetus, and becomes more pronounced with longer duration of infection.[112, 113]

DIAGNOSIS

Diagnosis of HIV infection as part of routine prenatal care of pregnant women is very important, because preventive therapies are now widely available (at least in industrialized countries). The CDC recommends voluntary HIV testing for all pregnant women and strongly encourages antiretroviral therapy for HIV-positive pregnant women (see later).[16, 114]

Prenatal diagnosis in the fetus is difficult because of the risk for bleeding and contamination of the sample with maternal blood or the possibility for accidental iatrogenic infection of the fetus. Amniotic fluid has been found to be positive for p24 antigen and HIV reverse transcriptase.[19, 22] Chorionic villus sampling or percutaneous umbilical blood sampling are associated with a higher risk for the fetus, and noninvasive techniques such as fetal ultrasonography or the clinical assessment of the mother give unspecific and not very predictive information.

The diagnosis of HIV infection in an infant born to a seropositive mother used to pose a problem because of the passive transfer of maternal antibodies. However, measurement of viral RNA or DNA copy numbers as well as culture technique have become standardized and are now widely available in industrialized countries.[115] The PCR assay should not be performed on cord blood, because there is a possibility of contamination with maternal blood. However, any positive test should be repeated for confirmation. It is assumed that children who have a positive HIV PCR result within the first 48 hours after birth were infected in utero, whereas those who are infected during the intrapartum period might become positive 2 to 6 weeks after birth. In a study using dried blood spot specimens, a technique yielding equivalent results to fresh blood specimens, only 19% (5/26) of infected children had detectable HIV DNA compared with a sensitivity of 96% (25/26) at 1 month of age.[116]

In adults and in children older than 18 months, serologic tests for specific antibodies are still important tools to establish the diagnosis of HIV infection, especially if PCR assays or culture methods are not available. HIV-specific antibody is usually detectable within 4 to 24 weeks after initial infection.[117] These antibodies are directed against the envelope proteins gp160, gp120, and gp41, the core proteins p24, p55, and p18, and the enzyme bands p31 and p65/51. The response to the envelope proteins usually persists throughout life, but the antibodies to core (gag) proteins may become lost in more symptomatic patients, and severely hypogammaglobulinemic children will not produce detectable antibodies.[118] Most commercially available enzyme immunoassay tests measure IgG antibodies to HIV. Virtually all children born to seropositive mothers will therefore be positive for HIV antibodies at birth, even though only a minority are actually infected. The uninfected children will lose these passively transferred antibodies between 6 and 12 months of age (75%), but persistence of maternal antibodies has been documented in 2% up to 18 months of age.[111, 119] Tests for IgM antibodies have been problematic, probably owing to interaction with abundant IgG and the short duration of IgM production.[120] The 1994 revised CDC guidelines for the diagnosis of HIV infection in infants and children are shown in Table 9–1.

Clinical and nonspecific laboratory parameters may also suggest HIV infection. The newborn HIV-infected child is usually asymptomatic but can become seriously

TABLE 9–1
Centers for Disease Control and Prevention Definition of Human Immunodeficiency Virus Infection in Children Younger Than 13 Years of Age

HIV INFECTED

A. A child <18 mo of age who is known to be HIV seropositive or born to an HIV-infected mother
and
Has positive results on two separate determinations (excluding cord blood) from one or more of the following HIV detection tests:
- HIV culture
- HIV polymerase chain reaction
- HIV antigen (p24)
or
Meets criteria for AIDS diagnosis based on the 1987 AIDS surveillance case definition

B. A child >18 mo of age born to an HIV-infected mother or any child infected by blood, blood products, or other known modes of infection who:
- Is HIV antibody positive by repeatedly reactive EIA and confirmatory test (e.g., Western blot or immunofluorescence assay)
or
- Meets any of the criteria in A

PERINATALLY EXPOSED (PREFIX E)

A child who does not meet the criteria above and who:
- Is HIV seropositive by EIA and confirmatory test and is <18 mo of age
or
- Has unknown antibody status but was born to a mother known to be HIV infected

SEROREVERTER (SR)

A child who is born to an HIV-infected mother and who:
- Has been documented as HIV-antibody negative (i.e., two or more negative EIA tests performed at 6–18 mo of age or one negative EIA after 18 mo of age)
or
- Has had no laboratory evidence of infection
and
- Has not had an AIDS-defining condition

EIA = enzyme immunoassay.
Adapted from 1994 Revised classification system for human immunodeficiency virus infection in children less than 13 years of age. MMWR Morb Mortal Wkly Rep 43:1–10, 1994.

ill within the first weeks to months of life. Table 9–2 provides a diagram outlining the initial evaluation and the necessary follow-up tests for an asymptomatic child born to an HIV-positive mother, as recommended by the AAP.[63] Opportunistic infections, hepatosplenomegaly, and lymphadenopathy are indicators for infection in the antibody-positive child younger than age 18 months. Hypergammaglobulinemia is a nonspecific but early finding of HIV infection, and CD4 counts must be interpreted within the bounds of the age-dependent normal range.[102–104, 121] Of course, diagnosis is established if an AIDS-defining disease, as listed in Table 9–3, occurs. In developing countries with limited diagnostic resources the diagnosis often has to be based on clinical symptoms, and a modified provisional definition for pediatric cases of AIDS has been issued by the WHO.[122]

TABLE 9–2

Evaluation Schedule for Asymptomatic Infants Born to Human Immunodeficiency Virus–Seropositive Mothers

TEST	Birth	2 wk	4 wk	6 wk	2 mo	3 mo	4 mo	5 mo	6 mo
History,[a] physical examination (including weight, height, head circumference)	+	+	+	+[b]	+	+	+	+	+
Developmental testing	(+)		+		+	+	+	+	+
Complete blood cell test and platelets	+		+	+	+	+	+		+
Serum chemistry (blood urea nitrogen, creatinine, liver function tests)	+			+		+	+		+
Serum immunoglobulins							+		+
Lymphocyte subsets[c]			+			+			+
HIV peripheral blood culture and/or polymerase chain reaction[d]	+		+				+		+
Urine for cytomegalovirus	+				+				
Chest radiograph, computed tomography or magnetic resonance imaging of head[e]									(+)
Electrocardiogram or echocardiogram[e]									(+)

[a]The frequency of "common" pediatric problems, such as diaper rash, mucocutaneous *Candida* infection, diarrhea, otitis, and so on should be carefully monitored.

[b]Zidovudine to prevent perinatal transmission is discontinued at 6 wk of age; however, strongly consider initiation of other antiretroviral therapy in child who is proven to be infected. Initiate prophylaxis for *Pneumocystis carinii* pneumonia (PCP).

[c]T cell profile should be repeated at 6 mo if infection status is unclear at 6 mo.

[d]Repeat PCR or viral culture immediately if positive to confirm infection. If the initial test is negative, repeat test at 4 wk to 2 mo (earlier if clinical or laboratory parameters suggest infection).

[e]Optional in the absence of clinical symptoms.

CLINICAL MANIFESTATIONS AND PATHOLOGY

HIV infection in infants and children has a different presentation from adults, and the CDC classifies HIV infection in children younger than the age of 13 years based on clinical and immunologic parameters (see Table 9–3). Of note, children found to be HIV infected are reported to the CDC only at the time of diagnosis, and tables that list the incidence of certain marker diseases (Table 9–4) are necessarily incomplete because a child may show other symptoms after the initial registration. Growth delay is an early and frequent finding of untreated perinatal HIV infection, and the linear growth is most severely affected in children with high viral loads.[123] Children are more likely than adults to have serious bacterial infections, and lymphocytic interstitial pneumonitis is almost entirely restricted to the pediatric age group. However, toxoplasmosis, cryptococcal infection, and the occurrence of cancer, especially Kaposi's sarcoma, are less common in HIV infection of childhood.

The initial symptoms may be subtle and sometimes difficult to distinguish from manifestations caused by drug use during pregnancy, from problems associated with prematurity, or congenital infections other than HIV. Premature birth has been reported in 19% with no difference between children born to drug-using mothers and children of mothers who were infected through other routes.[111, 124] However, children of drug-addicted mothers had significantly lower birth weights and smaller head circumferences.

Common clinical features seen during the course of HIV infection are lymphadenopathy, fevers, malaise, loss of energy, hepatosplenomegaly, respiratory tract infections, as well as recurrent and chronic otitis and sinusitis. Also commonly encountered are failure to thrive, sometimes associated with chronic diarrhea, failure to grow, the presence and persistence of mucocutaneous candidiasis, and many nonspecific cutaneous manifestations.

Infectious Complications

Infections in the HIV-infected newborn or infant can be serious or life threatening. The difficulty in treating these infectious episodes, their chronicity, and their tendency to recur distinguish them from the "normal" infections of early infancy. It is therefore helpful to document each episode and to evaluate their course, as well as the frequency of their recurrence.

BACTERIAL INFECTIONS

Recurrent serious bacterial infections such as meningitis, sepsis, and pneumonia are so typical of HIV infection in children that they were included in the revised CDC definition of 1987.[125, 126] In a study of 42 vertically infected children, a mean of 1.8 febrile visits per child-

TABLE 9–3

1994 Centers for Disease Control and Prevention Revised Classification System for Human Immunodeficiency Virus (HIV) Infection in Children Younger Than 13 Years of Age

Using this system children are classified according to three parameters: infection status, clinical status, and immunologic status. The categories are mutually exclusive. Once classified in a more severe category, a child is *not* reclassified in a less severe category even if the clinical or immunologic status improves.[a]

Pediatric HIV Virus Classification

IMMUNE CATEGORIES	CLINICAL CATEGORIES			
	(N) No Symptoms	(A) Mild Symptoms	(B)[b] Moderate Symptoms	(C)[b] Severe Symptoms
(1) No Suppression	N1	A1	B1	C1
(2) Moderate Suppression	N2	A2	B2	C2
(3) Severe Suppression	N3	A3	B3	C3

Immunologic Categories Based on Age-Specific CD4$^+$ T Lymphocyte Counts and Percent of Total Lymphocytes

The immunologic category classification is based on age-specific CD4$^+$ T lymphocyte count or percent of total lymphocytes and is designed to determine severity of immunosuppression attributable to HIV for age. If either CD4 count or percent results in classification into a different category, the child should be classified into the more severe category. A value should be confirmed before reclassification of the child into a more severe category. Regardless of subsequent CD4 determinations, children should not be reclassified into a less severe category.

IMMUNOLOGIC CATEGORY	AGE GROUPS		
	0–11 mo	1–5 yr	>6 yr
(1) No Suppression	>1500 cells/µL (>25%)	>1000 cells/µL (>25%)	>500 cells/µL (>25%)
(2) Moderate Suppression	750–1499 cells/µL (15–24%)	500–999 cells/µL (15–24%)	200–499 cells/µL (15–24%)
(3) Severe Suppression	<750 cells/µL (<15%)	<500 cells/µL (<15%)	<200 cells/µL (<15%)

Clinical Categories for Children with HIV Infection

Category N: Not Symptomatic

Children who have no signs or symptoms considered to be the result of HIV infection or who have only one of the conditions listed in Category A

Category A: Mildly Symptomatic

Children with two or more of the conditions listed below but none of the conditions listed in Categories B and C
- Lymphadenopathy (>0.5 cm at more than two sites; bilateral = one site)
- Hepatomegaly
- Splenomegaly
- Dermatitis
- Parotitis
- Recurrent or persistent respiratory infection, sinusitis, or otitis media

Category B: Moderately Symptomatic

Children who have symptomatic conditions other than those listed for Category A or C that are attributed to HIV infection. Examples of conditions in clinical Category B included but are not limited to:
- Anemia (<8 g/dl), neutropenia (<1000/mm³), or thrombocytopenia (<100,000/mm³) persisting >30 d
- Bacterial meningitis, pneumonia, or sepsis (single episode)
- Candidiasis, oropharyngeal thrush, persisting for >2 mo in children >6 mo of age
- Cardiomyopathy
- Cytomegalovirus infection, with onset before 1 mo of age
- Diarrhea, recurrent or chronic
- Hepatitis
- Herpes simplex virus stomatitis, recurrent (more than two episodes within 1 yr)
- HSV bronchitis, pneumonitis, or esophagitis with onset before 1 mo of age
- Herpes zoster (shingles) involving at least two distinct episodes or more than one dermatome
- Leiomyosarcoma
- Lymphoid interstitial pneumonia or pulmonary lymphoid hyperplasia complex
- Nephropathy
- Nocardiosis
- Persistent fever (lasting >1 mo)
- Toxoplasmosis, onset before 1 mo of age
- Varicella, disseminated (complicated chickenpox)

Table continued on following page

> **TABLE 9–3**
>
> 1994 Centers for Disease Control and Prevention Revised Classification System for Human Immunodeficiency Virus (HIV) Infection in Children Younger Than 13 Years of Age *Continued*

Clinical Categories for Children with HIV Infection *Continued*

Category C: Severely Symptomatic

Children who have any condition listed in the 1987 surveillance case definition for AIDS, with the exception of lymphoid interstitial pneumonia

- Serious bacterial infections, multiple or recurrent (i.e., any combination of at least two culture-confirmed infections within a 2-yr period, of the following types: septicemia, pneumonia, meningitis, bone or joint infection, or abscess of an internal body organ or body cavity, excluding otitis media, superficial skin or mucosal abscesses, and indwelling catheter-related infections)
- Candidiasis, esophageal or pulmonary (bronchi, trachea, lungs)
- Coccidioidomycosis, disseminated (at site other than or in addition to lungs or cervical or hilar nodes)
- Cryptosporidiosis or isosporidiosis with diarrhea persisting >1 mo
- Cytomegalovirus disease with onset of symptoms at age >1 mo (other than liver, spleen, or lymph nodes)
- Encephalopathy (at least one of the following progressive findings present for at least 2 mo in the absence of a concurrent illness other than HIV infection that could explain the findings): (a) failure to attain or loss of developmental milestones or loss of intellectual ability, verified by standard developmental scale or neuropsychological tests; (b) impaired brain growth or acquired microcephaly demonstrated by head circumference measurements or brain atrophy demonstrated by computed tomography or magnetic resonance imaging (serial imaging is required for children <2 yr of age); (c) acquired symmetrical motor deficit manifested by two or more of the following: paresis, pathologic reflexes, ataxia, or gait disturbance
- Herpes simplex virus infection causing a mucocutaneous ulcer that persists for >1 mo or bronchitis, pneumonitis, or esophagitis for any duration affecting a child >1 mo of age
- Histoplasmosis, disseminated (other than or in addition to lungs or cervical lymph nodes)
- Kaposi's sarcoma
- Lymphoma, primary, in brain
- Lymphoma, small, noncleaved cell (Burkitt's), or immunoblastic or large cell lymphoma of B cell or unknown immunologic phenotype
- *Mycobacterium tuberculosis*, disseminated or extrapulmonary
- Mycobacterium, other species or unidentified species, disseminated (other than or in addition to lungs, skin, or cervical or hilar lymph nodes)
- *Mycobacterium avium-intracellulare* complex or *Mycobacterium kansasii*, disseminated (other than or in addition to lungs, skin, or cervical or hilar lymph nodes)
- *Pneumocystis carinii* pneumonia
- Progressive multifocal leukoencephalopathy
- *Salmonella* (nontyphoid) septicemia, recurrent
- Toxoplasmosis of the brain with onset >1 mo of age
- Wasting syndrome in the absence of a concurrent illness other than HIV infection that could explain the following findings: (a) persistent weight loss >10% of baseline *or* (b) downward crossing of at least two of the following percentile lines on the weight-for-age chart (e.g., 95th, 75th, 50th, 25th, 5th) in a child >1 yr of age *or* (c) <5th percentile on weight-for-height chart on two consecutive measurements >30 d apart *plus* (a) chronic diarrhea (i.e., at least two loose stools per day for >30 d) *or* (b) documented fever (for >30 d, intermittent or constant)

[a]Children whose HIV infection status is not confirmed are classified by using the grid with a letter E (for vertically exposed) placed before the appropriate classification code (e.g., EN2).

[b]Both category C and lymphoid interstitial pneumonitis in category B are reportable to state and local health departments as acquired immune deficiency syndrome.
From Centers for Disease Control and Prevention. Recommendations of the U.S. Public Health Service Task Force on the use of zidovudine to reduce perinatal transmission of human immunodeficiency virus. MMWR Morb Mortal Wkly Rep 43:1–20, 1994.

year of observation was noted.[127] Eleven of the 27 positive blood cultures grew *Streptococcus pneumoniae*, and 16 grew organisms that were considered central venous line related (coagulase-negative *Staphylococcus*, gram-negative enterics, *Staphylococcus aureus*, *Pseudomonas aeruginosa*, *Candida* species). This increased incidence of pneumococcal infections has been confirmed by other studies as well.[128, 129]

Infections in the HIV-infected newborn have the same pattern as seen commonly in the neonatal period. A syndrome of very late onset group B streptococcal disease (at the age of 3.5 to 5 months of life) has been described in HIV-infected children.[130] Other currently rare infections such as congenital syphilis or neonatal gonococcal disease may become more frequent in the future as the incidence rises in pregnant women.[131–133]

Congenital syphilis may be missed if serologic tests are not performed on both the mother and her child at the time of delivery and repeated later if indicated.

Mycobacterial infections have assumed an increasingly important role in the pathology of the HIV-infected infant and child. Although the number of HIV-infected children with *Mycobacterium tuberculosis* infection is still small, organisms resistant to multiple antituberculosis drugs cultured from adults and children pose a threat not only to other immunocompromised patients but also to health care providers.[134–138] An important issue for the neonatologist is the question whether the mother is infected with *M. tuberculosis* and can potentially transmit the disease to her child. The diagnosis of *M. tuberculosis* infection is complicated in the HIV-infected patient because of the frequent anergy leading to a negative Man-

TABLE 9–4

Acquired Immunodeficiency Syndrome Indicator Diseases Diagnosed in 8086 Children Younger Than Age 13 Years Reported to the Centers for Disease Control and Prevention Through 1997

DISEASE	NO. OF CHILDREN DIAGNOSED	% OF TOTAL[a]
Pneumocystis carinii pneumonia	2700	33
Lymphocytic interstitial pneumonitis	1942	24
Recurrent bacterial infections	1619	20
Wasting syndrome	1419	18
Encephalopathy	1322	16
Candida esophagitis	1266	16
Cytomegalovirus disease	658	8
Mycobacterium avium infection	639	8
Severe herpes simplex infection	370	5
Pulmonary candidiasis	307	4
Cryptosporidiosis	291	4
Cancer	162	2

[a]The sum of percentages is greater than 100 because some patients have more than one disease.

From Centers for Disease Control and Prevention (CDC). U.S. HIV and AIDS cases reported through December 1997. HIV/AIDS Surveillance report: year-end edition. MMWR Morb Mortal Wkly Rep 9:1–44, 1997.

toux test even in the presence of infection. To diagnose anergy, a control (e.g., for mumps, *Candida*, or tetanus) should always be placed simultaneously with the Mantoux test.[137, 139] Treatment of *M. tuberculosis* infection in children is complicated by the lack of pediatric formulations but usually includes isoniazid, rifampin, and, during the first 2 months, pyrazinamide.[140]

Infection with *Mycobacterium avium-intracellulare* complex occurs in nearly 20% of HIV-infected children with advanced disease and presents as nonspecific symptoms such as night sweats, weight loss, and low-grade fevers.[141, 142] Treatment usually consists of three or more drugs (e.g., clarithromycin, ethambutol, rifampin and/or amikacin, ciprofloxacin, clofazimine) but commonly provides only temporary symptomatic relief and not an eradication of the infection. Prophylaxis with clarithromycin or azithromycin should be initiated in infants younger than 1 year of age with a CD4 count less than 750 cells/mm^3, in children 1 to 2 years of age with a CD4 count less than 500 cells/mm^3, and in children 2 to 6 years of age with a CD4 count less than 75 cells/mm^3. In children older than 6 years, the adult threshold of 50 cells/mm^3 can be used.[143]

VIRAL INFECTIONS

Viral infections are important causes for morbidity and mortality in HIV-infected children. Primary varicella can be unusually severe and can recur as zoster, often presenting with very few, atypical lesions. The virus may become resistant to standard treatment with acyclovir.[144–146] Cytomegalovirus infection can result in esophagitis, hepatitis, enterocolitis, or retinitis.[147–150] Cytomegalovirus can become resistant to the treatment with ganciclovir, necessitating the use of foscarnet or even combination regimens.[151, 152]

Other commonly encountered viruses in the HIV-infected infant and child are hepatitis A, B, and C, often associated with a more fulminant or chronic aggressive

course than in the non–HIV-infected patient.[153–155] Hepatitis C infection is more common in children born to HIV-infected mothers (23% vs. 12% in infants born to HIV-negative mothers).[155]

Infection with the measles virus is associated with a high mortality in HIV-infected children and often presents without the typical rash and can result in a fatal giant cell pneumonia.[156–159] Infection with respiratory syncytial virus or adenovirus, alone or in combination, can also result in rapid and sometimes fatal respiratory compromise, as well as in chronic or persistent viral shedding or infection.[160–162]

An interesting observation is the occurrence of a polyclonal lymphoproliferative syndrome, often associated with evidence of primary or reactivated Epstein-Barr virus infection. These patients develop impressive lymphadenopathy and sometimes concurrent lymphocytic interstitial pneumonitis or parotitis.[163] The distinction between a self-limited benign hyperproliferation and the development of a monoclonal lymphoid malignancy is crucial for treatment and prognosis.

FUNGAL AND PROTOZOAL INFECTIONS

Oral candidiasis is common even in healthy, non–HIV-infected newborns and infants. However, infection beyond infancy, involvement of pharynx and esophagus, and persistence despite treatment with antifungal agents are more typical for the immunocompromised child. Disseminated candidiasis is, however, uncommon in the absence of predisposing factors such as central venous catheters or total parenteral nutrition.[164]

Infection with *Cryptococcus neoformans*, although common in adults with HIV infection, is less common in children.[165, 166] Colonization with *Aspergillus* species and invasive disease has been described in adult patients with HIV infection, and we have observed at least one infant with perinatally acquired HIV infection and associated myelodysplastic syndrome who developed fatal pulmonary aspergillosis.[167–169] The incidence of other fungal infections varies with the prevalence of the organism in the specific geographic area. Of note, disseminated histoplasmosis as the AIDS-defining illness has been described in a few infants.[170–172]

Only a few years ago, *Pneumocystis carinii* pneumonia (PCP) was the AIDS indicator disease in almost 40% of the pediatric cases reported to the CDC.[173] However, this has changed dramatically since the introduction of the new guidelines for PCP prophylaxis in HIV-exposed infants and HIV-infected children and in 1997 accounted for only 25% of the AIDS cases.[5, 174] The peak incidence of PCP in infancy occurs during the first 3 to 6 months of life, often as the first symptom of HIV infection. Presumably, this represents primary infection in these infants. At least one case of maternal-fetal transmission of PCP has also been documented.[175]

Most children with PCP present with an acute illness, hypoxemia, and without a "typical" radiographic picture.[176, 177] The diagnosis is usually made by obtaining an induced sputum (which can be done by experienced therapists even in very young children) or by performing a bronchoalveolar lavage, and only rarely is an open lung biopsy necessary.[178, 179] Treatment options are high dose intravenous trimethoprim/sulfamethoxazole or pentamidine as first-line drugs.[180] Early adjunctive treatment with corticosteroids has been shown to be beneficial in adults and children with moderate to severe PCP and is commonly recommended for patients with an initial arterial oxygen pressure of less than 70 mm Hg or an arterial-alveolar gradient of more than 35 mm Hg.[181–184]

Unfortunately, PCP has been associated with a mortality of 39 to 65% in infants, in spite of improved diagnosis and treatment.[185, 186] In 1991 the CDC issued guidelines for PCP prophylaxis in children, taking into account the age-dependent levels of normal CD4 cell numbers.[187] However, these recommendations were only applicable if a child was known to be HIV infected. A survey published in 1995 revealed basically no change between 1988 and 1992 in the incidence of PCP among infants born to HIV-infected mothers.[188] Two thirds of these infants had never received PCP prophylaxis, and 59% of those children were recognized as having been exposed to HIV infection within 30 days or less of PCP diagnosis. Furthermore, among the infants known to be HIV infected who had a CD4 count performed within 1 month of PCP diagnosis, 18% had a CD4 count over 1500 cells/mm³, the recommended threshold for initiation of PCP prophylaxis.[188] At the same time it was shown that primary prophylaxis during the first year of life was highly effective in the prevention of PCP.[189] These pivotal studies led to revised guidelines in 1995.[174] The major new recommendation was that all infants born to HIV-infected women should be started on PCP prophylaxis at 4 to 6 weeks of age, regardless of their CD4 counts. More details are presented in Table 9–5.

The recommended prophylactic regimen is trimethoprim/sulfamethoxazole (TMP/SMX) with 150 mg TMP/m² per day and 750 mg/m² per day of SMX given orally in divided doses twice a day during 3 consecutive days per week. Alternative regimens, if TMP/SMX is not tolerated, are dapsone orally (2 mg/kg per day) or aerosolized pentamidine. However, breakthrough infections can occur with every regimen and appear to be most frequent with intravenous pentamidine and least common with TMP/SMX.[190, 191]

It is of interest that encephalitis caused by *Toxoplasma gondii* is common in adults with HIV infection but only rarely noted in children.[92] However, several case reports of *T. gondii* encephalitis in infants between 5 weeks and 18 months of age have been published. Some of these infants probably acquired toxoplasmosis infection in utero.[193, 194] Toxoplasmosis remains an important differential diagnosis in the patient with an intracerebral mass.

Protozoal infections of the gastrointestinal tract often represent difficult diagnostic and therapeutic problems and can be associated with an intractable diarrhea. Infec-

---

TABLE 9–5

Recommendations for *Pneumocystis carinii* Pneumonia (PCP) Prophylaxis and CD4 Monitoring in HIV-Exposed Infants and HIV-Infected Children

AGE/HIV-INFECTION STATUS	PCP PROPHYLAXIS	CD4+ MONITORING
Birth to 4–6 wk, HIV exposed or infected	No prophylaxis (because PCP is rare and due to concerns regarding kernicterus with TMP/SMX)	1 mo
4–6 wk to 4 mo, HIV exposed	Prophylaxis	3 mo
4–12 mo	Prophylaxis	6, 9, 12 mo
• HIV infected or indeterminate	No prophylaxis	None
• HIV infection reasonably excluded[a]		
1–5 yr, HIV infected	Prophylaxis if • CD4+ count is <500 cells/mm³ or • CD4+ percentage is <15%	Every 3–4 mo (more frequently if indicated)
Older than 6 yr, HIV infected	Prophylaxis if • CD4+ count <200 cells/mm³ or • CD4+ percentage is <15%	Every 3–4 yr

[a]Two or more negative HIV diagnostic tests (i.e., HIV culture or polymerase chain reaction), both performed at ≥ 1 mo of age and one of which was performed at ≥ 4 mo of age, or ≥ 2 negative HIV IgG antibody tests performed at ≥ 6 mo of age among children without clinical evidence of HIV disease.

HIV = human immunodeficiency virus; TMP/SMX = trimethoprim/sulfamethoxazole.

From Centers from Disease Control and Prevention. 1995 Revised guidelines for prophylaxis against *Pneumocystis carinii* pneumonia for children infected with or perinatally exposed to human immunodeficiency virus. MMWR Morb Mortal Wkly Rep 44:1–12, 1995.

tion with cryptosporidia has a prevalence of 3.0 to 3.6% among children with diarrhea.[195] HIV-infected children are at risk for prolonged diarrheal disease with often severe wasting.

Malignancies

Several case reports of malignancies associated with HIV infection in infants and children have been published; however, cancer is the AIDS-defining illness in only 2% of children, compared with 14% of the adults.[5, 196] The most common cancer in HIV-infected children is non-Hodgkin's lymphoma, either as a systemic disease or as a primary central nervous system tumor.[197–199] Kaposi's sarcoma has been described in a few children, including a 6-day-old infant, but remains relatively uncommon.[200–202] Interestingly, an increased incidence of leiomyomas and leiomyosarcomas, a soft tissue tumor associated with Epstein-Barr virus infection in immunocompromised patients, is also increasingly common.[200, 203, 204]

Encephalopathy

Encephalopathy, often with early onset, was a frequent and typical manifestation of HIV infection in children, before the introduction of antiretroviral therapy. Symptoms of encephalopathy in the newborn or young infant initially include delayed head control or delayed acquisition of a social smile and variable degrees of truncal hypotonia.[205–207] Subsequently, impairment of cognitive, behavioral, and motor functions becomes apparent. Typical findings included a loss of, or failure to attain, normal developmental milestones, weakness, intellectual deficits, or neurologic symptoms such as ataxia and pyramidal tract signs including spasticity or rigidity.[208] Seizures are rare but have been described, and, recently, cerebrovascular disease resulting in strokes or the formation of giant aneurysms at the base of the brain has been reported.[209, 210] The course can be static, wherein the child attains milestones, albeit at a slower rate than

normal for age, or the development can reach a plateau and then the child ceases to acquire new milestones. The most severe form is manifested by a subacute-progressive course in which the child loses previously acquired capabilities.[211, 212] The older child will have impaired expressive language function whereas receptive language appears to be slightly less affected.[213, 214] Physical examination can reveal hypotonia or spasticity, and microcephaly may be present. Radiologic examination can suggest cerebral atrophy, calcifications in the basal ganglia and periventricular frontal white matter, and decreased attenuation in the white matter (Fig. 9–1).[215–219]

HIV-1 can be found in brain monocytes, macrophages, and microglia; and limited expression of the regulatory gene *nef*, but not of structural gene products, has been demonstrated in astrocytes.[220–223] Analysis of cerebrospinal fluid revealed HIV RNA in 90% of samples, and more than 10,000 copies/ml were associated with severe neurodevelopmental delay.[224, 225] It is likely that immune-mediated mechanisms or the secretion of toxic cytokines by infected cells contributes to the pathogenesis of central nervous system disease in AIDS patients.[226] The level of quinolonic acid, a neurotoxin that has been implicated in the development of HIV-related encephalopathy, is elevated in children with symptomatic central nervous system disease and decreased during treatment with zidovudine.[227, 228]

Postmortem examination shows variable degrees of white matter abnormalities, calcific deposits in the wall of blood vessels of the basal ganglia and the frontal white matter, and subacute encephalitis. At least one report described an HIV-related meningoencephalitis in a newborn, supporting the assumption of an intrauterine infection.[229] Spinal cord disease, manifested by vacuolar myelopathy, has been described in children but is less common than in adults.[230]

Dramatic improvements in the degree of encephalopathy have been achieved by treating the children with zidovudine, especially when given as a continuous intra-

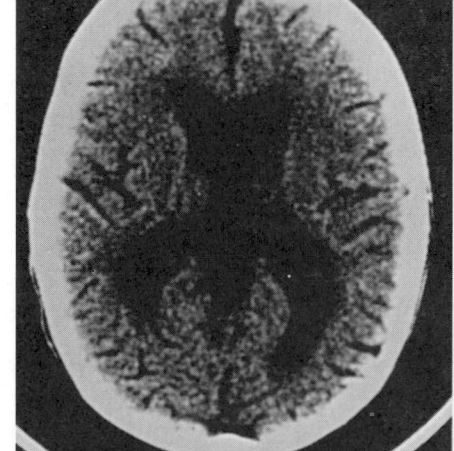
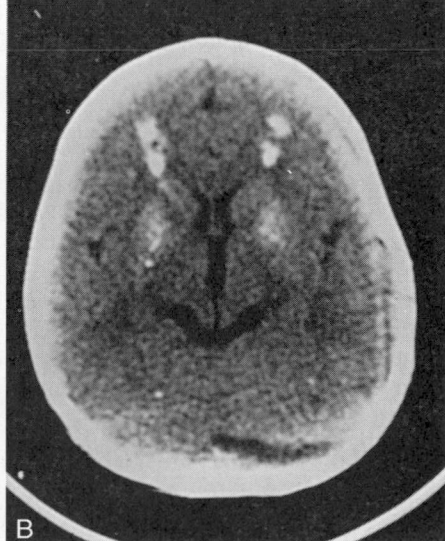

FIGURE 9–1 Computed tomographic scans of the brains of two infants with HIV-associated encephalopathy. *A,* Cerebral atrophy with enlarged ventricles and widened sulci. *B,* Calcifications in basal ganglia and frontal white matter.

venous infusion (see later).[231] Therapy with corticosteroids has also been shown to be beneficial in some patients.[232]

Ophthalmologic Pathology

The ophthalmologic complications associated with HIV infection can be particularly devastating. HIV-1 can infect the retina and presents as cotton-wool spots on examination but rarely leads to impaired vision.[233, 234] However, several other pathogens, some of them acquired in utero, can affect the eye and impact visual acuity. Fortunately, the incidence of blindness remains low in pediatric AIDS, but the infections caused by herpesviruses, and especially cytomegaloviral retinitis, can be difficult to control and require intensive intravenous treatment.[147, 149, 150] A few children have been described with congenital toxoplasmosis and associated chorioretinitis, and one of the extrapulmonary manifestations of *Pneumocystis carinii* infection is involvement of the retina.[235-237] Early recognition and aggressive intervention are crucial to prevent progression of visual impairment, and routine ophthalmologic examinations should be part of the care of all HIV-infected children.

Interstitial Lung Disease

Lymphocytic interstitial pneumonitis, or pulmonary lymphoid hyperplasia, is seen almost exclusively in the pediatric patient with HIV infection and is currently still included into the CDC definition of AIDS-defining diseases for children younger than 13 years of age (see Table 9–3). The incidence of lymphocytic interstitial pneumonitis is difficult to assess but may affect as many as 50% of the HIV-infected children.[238] Clinically there is a wide spectrum in the severity of this disease: a child may be asymptomatic with only radiologic changes, or he or she can become severely compromised with exercise intolerance or even with oxygen dependency and the need for high-dose corticosteroid therapy. Children with lymphocytic interstitial pneumonitis are at higher risk to develop frequent bacterial and viral infections.[239]

A diffuse, interstitial, often reticulonodular infiltrative process is typically observed on radiologic examination sometimes associated with hilar or mediastinal lymphadenopathy (Fig. 9–2).[238] On biopsy, peribronchiolar lymphoid aggregates or a diffuse lymphoid infiltration of the alveolar septa and peribronchiolar areas is seen.[163] Treatment of lymphocytic interstitial pneumonitis is only indicated in the symptomatic child with hypoxia and consists of oral therapy with corticosteroids, to suppress the lymphocytic proliferation.[238] Of note, lymphocytic interstitial pneumonitis has been associated in some studies with a better prognosis than other HIV-related manifestations such as encephalopathy or PCP, with a median survival of 72 months after diagnosis compared with 1 and 11 months, respectively.[240]

Cardiovascular Complications

Cardiovascular abnormalities are seen in over 50% of HIV-infected adults and have also been described in

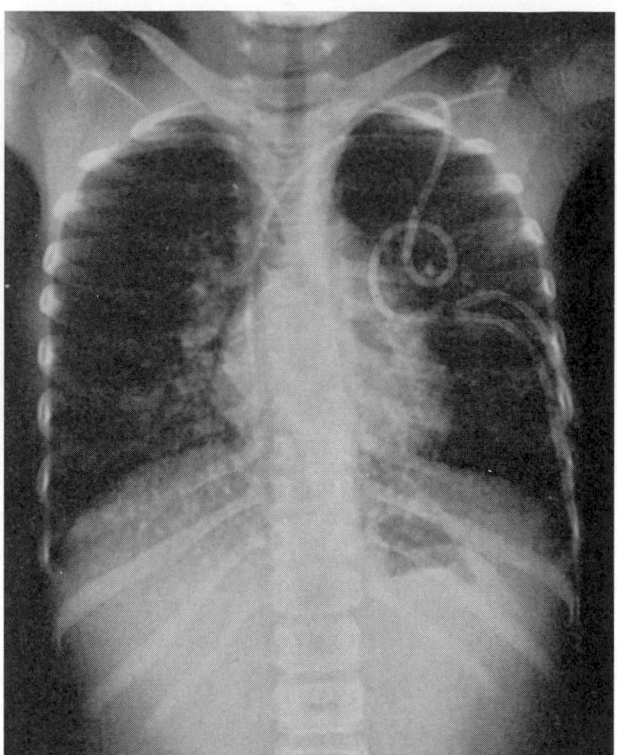

FIGURE 9–2 Chest radiograph of an 8-year-old girl with severe lymphocytic interstitial pneumonitis who is oxygen and steroid dependent.

children.[241, 242] A progressive left ventricular dilatation and an increase in ventricular afterload was demonstrated in a group of 51 children with symptomatic HIV disease but a normal initial echocardiogram.[242] Clinical manifestations include hepatosplenomegaly, tachypnea, and tachycardia, often with an S3 gallop, or another arrhythmia. Postmortem examination is remarkable for biventricular dilatation with grossly unremarkable valves and coronary arteries and, less frequently, a pericardial effusion. Interestingly, cardiomyopathy is more commonly found in children with HIV-related encephalopathy (30%) than in those without this manifestation (2%).[207]

Microscopically, a hypertrophy of the myocardium with only rare foci of inflammatory lymphocytic infiltrates is usually present.[243, 244] HIV RNA can be demonstrated in only a small number of cells, probably representing macrophages, monocytes, or endothelial cells, but the distribution does not correlate with the structural damage.[245, 246]

Another poorly understood phenomenon is the formation of aneurysms of the cerebral and coronary arteries in association with HIV infection.[210, 247, 248] We have observed a child who developed large cerebral aneurysms, leading to hypothalamic dysfunction and neurologic impairment.[249]

Pathology of the Gastrointestinal Tract

Dysfunction of the digestive tract is a frequent problem in children with AIDS. In an Italian study of 200 HIV-infected children, Galli and colleagues observed a higher incidence of hepatitis and diarrhea with onset during the first year of life (occurring in 20 to 50% of cases) than at any later time point.[250] Commonly encountered pathogens, which may cause severe diarrhea, are *Cryptosporidium*, *M. avium-intracellulare* complex, *Microsporidium*, as well as *Salmonella* and *Shigella*.[251] HIV nucleid acids have also been found in the feces of children with persistent diarrheal disease.[252] However, many HIV-infected children have a gastrointestinal dysfunction due to disaccharide intolerance, and their clinical status can be improved with a careful attention to dietary intake.[252]

Progressive weight loss, anorexia, and sometimes pathogen-negative diarrhea characterize the wasting syndrome often seen in association with HIV disease.[253–256] The etiology is not clear but probably represents a combination of a metabolic imbalance with hypermetabolism, disturbed nitrogen balance, and increased cytokine levels. No specific treatment is available, but individual patients may benefit from appetite stimulants, dietary supplements, or parenteral nutrition.[257]

Liver dysfunction secondary to an infection, including that from cytomegalovirus, Epstein-Barr virus, the hepatitis viruses, *M. avium-intracellulare* complex, or HIV-1, is a common feature and can evolve into a chronic hepatitis or cholangitis.[258, 259] *Candida albicans* and the herpesviruses are often the cause not only of infections of the oral cavity but also of esophagitis. Of note, esophagitis in the HIV-infected child does not necessarily present as the typical symptoms or dysphagia but may be the cause of poor appetite and weight loss. Pancreatitis is a rare complication of HIV infection in children and may occur as the result of opportunistic infections such as cytomegalovirus or as a side effect or therapeutic agents.[260, 261]

Nephropathy

Renal disease in children with HIV infection presents most often as focal glomerulosclerosis or mesangial hyperplasia. In one study, 12 of 155 children between the ages of 7 months and 8 years were found to have proteinuria, and 5 of them developed severe renal failure within a year of diagnosis.[262, 263] This nephrotic syndrome is often resistant to the treatment with corticosteroids, but cyclosporins may induce a remission.[264] In addition, IgA nephritis has been observed in a few HIV-infected children and adults, clinically presenting as recurrent gross hematuria.[265, 266] However, an infection with CMV or treatment with the protease inhibitor indinavir can also cause hematuria.[150, 267, 268]

Pathology of Endocrine Organs

Failure to thrive or grow is commonly seen in children with HIV infection. In a study of 35 HIV-positive hemophiliacs, a decrease of more than 15 percentile points in height or weight for age was a predictive marker for children who become symptomatic for AIDS.[269–271] Whereas a few patients may have some dysregulation of thyroid function or a lack of growth hormone, often there is no definable endocrine cause recognizable.[272, 273]

The exception is the child with adrenal insufficiency, which may be caused by CMV infection of the adrenal gland.[274] We have observed one child with severe salt craving who required therapy with fluorocortisol. In a study of 167 HIV-infected children, Hirschfeld and associates found low levels of free thyroxine in 18% and increased thyrotropin or thyroid binding globulin levels in 30% of children.[275]

Involvement of Lymphoid Organs and Thymus

Thymic abnormalities have been found in 3 of 37 fetuses aborted between 20 to 27 weeks of gestation.[276] This may represent the initial injury to the lymphoid system. In children with AIDS the thymus can show precocious involution, with marked depletion of lymphocytes and loss of corticomedullary differentiation, or a thymitis, characterized by the presence of lymphoid follicles with germinal centers or a diffuse lymphomononuclear infiltration.[277] An interesting phenomenon is the occurrence of multilocular thymic cysts, often detected as an incidental finding.[277] Lymphadenopathy is common among infected children and adults, and lymphoid organs function as reservoirs for HIV-1.[278–281]

Hematologic Problems

Anemia is the most common hematologic disorder observed in HIV-infected children with the incidence depending on the severity of HIV disease, the age group, and the use of antiretroviral therapy.[282–284] In a retrospective study of 75 HIV-infected children, 19.7% had anemia at age 6 months, 32.9% at 9 months of age, and 37.3% at 12 months of age.[285] Bone marrow aspirate or biopsy specimens may show lymphoid aggregates, some degree of dysplasia, or an ineffective erythropoiesis.[286] Pure red cell aplasia secondary to acute or persistent B19 parvovirus infection has been described in some HIV-infected children and adults and should be considered when the red blood cell production rate is less than expected for the degree of anemia.[287–289]

A white blood cell count of less than 3000 cells/mm³ has been observed in 26 to 38% of untreated pediatric patients, and neutropenia, defined as an absolute neutrophil count of less than 1500 cells/mm³, has been found in 43%.[282–284] This can be due to HIV infection, the infection with opportunistic pathogens such as *M. avium-intracellulare* complex or cytomegalovirus, or as the result of the therapy with a myelotoxic drug, including zidovudine.

In the patient population at the National Cancer Institute we found a platelet count of less than 50,000 cells/mm³ in 19% of the children; thrombocytopenia has also been described in HIV-infected infants.[290–292] Treatment options are similar to those of noninfected children and include intravenous gammaglobulins, corticosteroids, and WinRho. However, an improvement is often best achieved by optimizing the antiretroviral therapy and decreasing the circulating viral load.

Deficiency of the vitamin K–dependent factors II, VII, IX, and X is common in HIV-infected children and can result in a coagulopathy that is relatively easy to correct. Also commonly seen are autoimmune phenomena, such as lupus anticoagulants and antiphospholipid or anticardiolipid antibodies.[293-295] Disseminated intravascular coagulopathy has been described as a complication of fulminant infectious conditions, but there are no data to indicate that this complication occurs more frequently in HIV-infected individuals.

Skin

Mucocutaneous disease is very common in pediatric HIV infection but presents often in an unusual or atypical form.[296, 297] The most common lesions with an infectious etiology are oral thrush and diaper rash (C. albicans), chickenpox (acute or chronic), and recurrent shingles (Varicella zoster virus), as well as molluscum contagiosum.[298] Bacterial infections or a highly contagious form of scabies have also been reported with some frequency. Severe seborrheic dermatitis or an unspecific intensely pruritic eczematous dermatitis can pose difficult and frustrating clinical problems, necessitating prolonged therapy. Because of the atypical presentations and wide variety of possible causes it is often prudent to culture lesions (for bacteria or for Varicella zoster virus), or even to perform a scraping or biopsy. Drug eruptions appear to be more common in HIV-infected patients and can develop into a toxic epidermal necrolysis.[296] However, most drug rashes resolve after stopping the causative agent.

MORBIDITY, MORTALITY, AND PROGNOSIS

Thanks to more effective treatment of HIV infection and associated complications, as well as improved guidelines for the prophylaxis of opportunistic infections, a major decrease in morbidity and mortality of HIV infection in children and adults has occurred during the last few years. However, infants who are not known to be HIV infected or do not have access to early intervention are still at high risk for early and severe morbidity and continue to have a high mortality rate.[299-301]

Although the course of HIV infection in children is in general more accelerated than in adults, distinct subgroups are noticeable. Perinatally acquired HIV infection follows a bimodal course, with about one third of the children becoming symptomatic within the first 2 years of life and the remainder in the next several years. Only a minority of patients remains relatively asymptomatic until the age of 8 years or older. In a study of HIV-seropositive and HIV-seronegative women and their newborns in Nairobi, Kenya, no statistically significant difference was found between the groups regarding occurrence of congenital malformations, stillbirths, Apgar score, or gestational age. However, the mean birth weight of singleton neonates of HIV-positive mothers was significantly lower than that of controls.[302] Although not as pronounced, there was also a difference between the height and weight of birth of HIV-infected infants born in the United States compared with uninfected infants.[303] Of note, these studies of natural history of perinatal HIV infection were performed before the routine use of antiretroviral therapy in pregnant women and their infants.

In a European study of 392 HIV-infected children, Blanche and colleagues found that 20% of children died or developed an AIDS-defining symptom (CDC category C; see Table 9–3) within the first year of life and 4.7% per year thereafter, reaching a cumulative incidence of 36% by 6 years of age.[299] Two thirds of the children alive at 6 years of age had only minor symptoms, and one third had well preserved CD4 counts (<25%) despite prior clinical manifestations. Children with HIV infection acquired through a transfusion during the neonatal period tend to have a prolonged asymptomatic period as well.[304]

Both clinical and laboratory factors have been evaluated in regard to their prognostic value. Children born to mothers with low CD4 counts and high viral load tend to progress more rapidly to category C disease or death, emphasizing the importance of diagnosis and adequate treatment of HIV-infected pregnant women.[33, 114, 305] Early manifestation of clinical symptoms in the infant, especially opportunistic infections, encephalopathy, or hepatosplenomegaly, has repeatedly been associated with a poor prognosis.[285, 306, 307]

A high virus copy number in the blood has been shown to be a strong predictor for progression of HIV disease.[91, 308-310] Infants with very high HIV RNA copy numbers shortly after birth are presumed to have been infected in utero and tend to have early onset of symptoms.[309] Dickover and associates, when calculating HIV-infected infants followed for up to 8 years, found that a 1-log higher HIV-1 RNA copy number at birth increased the relative hazard of developing CDC class A or B symptoms by 40% ($p = 0.004$), to develop AIDS by 60% ($p = 0.01$), and the risk of death by 80% ($p = 0.023$). The peak HIV-1 RNA copy number during the period of primary viremia was also predictive of progression to AIDS (relative hazard 9.9; 95% CI, 1.8–54.1%; $p = .008$) and death (relative hazard, 6.9; 95% CI, 1.1–43.8%; $p = .04$).[309]

PREVENTION

An important goal in the care for HIV-infected people is the prevention of further infections, and especially the transmission from mother to infant. Many countries have initiated large educational programs to halt the spread of the epidemic in the heterosexual community. However, the prevalence of HIV infection is so high in certain populations, especially in developing countries, that a change in behavior will only result in a very slow decrease in the number of new infections. Identifying pregnant women who are HIV infected is essential, not only for the potential initiation of therapy but also for the coordination of optimal prenatal care.

The birth order and delivery route appear to play a role in the infection rate. In the absence of zidovudine treatment, HIV infection occurred in 35% of first-born twins and 15% of second-born twins who were delivered vaginally, compared with 16% first-born and 8% second-born twins delivered by cesarean section.[41] The European Collaborative Study of 1254 HIV-infected mothers and their children estimated that cesarean section resulted in a 50% reduction of the transmission rate.[311] However, there is a potential bias in the indication for cesarean section. Obstetricians may be less likely to perform a surgical procedure in a mother with advanced HIV infection; emergency cesarean section is more common in the case of larger infants (who are less likely to be infected), and monitoring during vaginal deliveries might itself increase the risk for transmission, especially if fetal scalp electrodes are being used.[42] Randomized clinical studies are ongoing in Europe and will be published soon. However, it has been shown that prolonged rupture of membranes (>4 hours before delivery) increases the risk for perinatal transmission and should therefore be avoided.[45]

The success of the AIDS Clinical Trials Group 076 (PACTG 076) protocol has had a major impact on the prevention of perinatal transmission of HIV-1 and has resulted in new guidelines issued by the CDC.[14, 15, 114] In that landmark study pregnant HIV-infected women received oral zidovudine, starting at 14 to 34 weeks of gestation, and intravenous zidovudine during labor and delivery, while the infants were treated with 6 weeks of oral zidovudine post partum (Table 9–6). This resulted in a 67% reduction in the perinatal transmission rate, from 25% to 8.3% ($p = 0.00006$).[15] It has also been demonstrated that a high maternal plasma concentration of HIV-1 is a risk factor for transmission to the infant.[13] The identification of HIV-infected pregnant women and

their prompt treatment has already led to a marked decrease in the number of newly HIV-infected children in industrialized countries.

However, this treatment regimen is not feasible for developing countries, where by the year 2000 about 6 million pregnant women will be infected with HIV-1.[312] Discussions regarding the ethics of clinical trials in developing countries, especially trials involving a placebo group, admittedly one of the fastest ways to detect a significant decrease in transmission rate, are ongoing.[313] An attempt to decrease the transmission rate by "cleansing" the birth canal has unfortunately so far not been successful.[43, 44] Preliminary results from a study performed in Thailand as collaboration between the Thailand Ministry of Health and the CDC have become available. This trial enrolled non–breast-feeding women who were treated with zidovudine (300 mg twice daily) beginning at week 36 of gestation. During labor and delivery the oral dose of zidovudine was increased to 300 mg every 3 hours; the newborns were not treated. The estimated efficacy of this therapy was 51% (decrease from 18.6% transmission rate in placebo group to 9.2% in treated group). Although this transmission rate is somewhat higher than the one reported with the PACTG 076 regimen, it indicates that a two-part regimen without the intravenous and postnatal component (a more feasible alternative for developing countries) merits further investigation.

Passive immunization of the fetus in combination with antiretroviral therapy is another approach that has been studied (ACTG 185). A highly purified human immune globulin prepared from asymptomatic HIV-seropositive persons has been evaluated for safety and toxicity in several small Phase I studies. HIV immune globulin (HIVIG) appeared to be safe and well tolerated.[314, 315] Immunoglobulins of the IgG class are readily transported through the placenta, and a passive immunization of the mother may protect the fetus, a model that has been extensively used in the prevention of neonatal hepatitis B infection. With further knowledge about the exact timing of perinatal HIV infection, additional strategies for intervention can be developed.

TREATMENT

Supportive Care and General Management

Optimizing prenatal care, including nutrition, avoidance of drugs and other harmful substances, as well as recognition and treatment of concurrent infections, is crucial to prevent the premature delivery of children with low birth weight. The general care of the newborn and infant is not different for children born to seropositive mothers, but special attention should be given to the documentation of developmental milestones, frequency and course of infections, and nutritional status.

The AAP recommends routine immunizations with some modifications for all seropositive children, whether they are actually infected or not.[63] Similar to other newborns, children born to HIV-infected mothers

---

TABLE 9–6
Pediatric AIDS Clinical Trials Group 076 Regimen

TIME OF ZIDOVUDINE ADMINISTRATION	REGIMEN
Antepartum	100 mg zidovudine five times daily, initiated at 14–34 wk of gestation and continued throughout pregnancy
Intrapartum	During labor, intravenous administration of zidovudine in a 1-hr initial dose of 2 mg/kg, followed by continuous infusion of 1 mg/kg per hr until delivery
Postpartum	Oral zidovudine to the newborn (zidovudine syrup at 2 mg/kg per dose every 6 hr) for the first 6 wk of life, beginning at 8–12 hr after birth. If an infant cannot tolerate oral zidovudine, it can be given intravenously at a dosage of 1.5 mg/kg every 6 hr

From Centers for Disease Control and Prevention. Public Health Service task force recommendations for the use of antiretroviral drugs in pregnant women infected with HIV-1 for maternal health and for reducing perinatal HIV-1 transmission in the United States. MMWR Morb Mortal Wkly Rep 47:1–31, 1998.

should receive hepatitis B vaccinations; but if the mother is HbsAg positive, the child should also receive HBIG within 12 hours to birth. The current recommendation is that live virus vaccine (oral poliovirus) or live bacterial vaccines (bacille Calmette-Guérin) should not be given to patients with HIV infection. The exception is MMR, because the risk for measles in immunocompromised children is much higher than the risk associated with the vaccination, although only children with mild to moderate immunosuppression should have the MMR vaccine.[157] However, varicella-zoster immunization is contraindicated in HIV-infected children and adults. A currently recommended prophylaxis in HIV-infected infants is the administration of intravenous immunoglobulin (IVIG) or specific hyperimmune globulin within 72 to 96 hours after the exposure to varicella-zoster virus or measles.[143, 316] Children older than 2 years of age with HIV infection should be administered the 23-valent polysaccharide pneumococcal vaccine, and revaccination should be offered after 3 to 5 years in children younger than 10 years of age and after 5 years in older children.[143] However, it is important to remember that prior immunization does not give complete protection from further infection, as has been described for pertussis occurring in previously immunized children.[317]

The monthly administration of IVIG has been studied in asymptomatic and symptomatic children with HIV infection. IGIV has been shown to prevent serious bacterial infections in patients with congenital immunodeficiencies. However, in a group of children who did not receive any antiretroviral treatment, only children with a CD4 count of 200 cells/mm³ or more appeared to benefit from monthly IGIV administration.[318] A study evaluating children receiving antiretroviral therapy did not find a statistically significant difference between children who received IGIV and children treated with placebo (albumin), as long as they were also receiving PCP prophylaxis with TMP/SMX. The current recommendation is to use prophylactic IGIV (400 mg/kg per dose every 28 days) in HIV-infected children with hypogammaglobulinemia, poor functional antibody developmental (i.e., lack of antibody response after immunizations), or significant recurrent infections despite therapy with appropriate antibiotics.[143]

Prophylactic measurements for the prevention of PCP have been discussed previously. Prophylaxis for *M. tuberculosis* exposure follows the guidelines used in immunocompetent children, but all children born to HIV-infected mothers should have a purified protein derivative test placed at or before 9 to 12 months of age and should be retested every 2 to 3 years.[143] Prophylaxis with clarithromycin or azithromycin for *M. avium-intracellulare* complex infection should be offered to children aged younger than 12 months of age if their CD4 count is less than 750 cells/μl, children aged 1 to 2 years with CD4 counts less than 500 cells/μl, children aged 2 to 6 years with CD4 counts less than 75 μl, and children older than 6 years if the CD4 count is less than 50 cells/μl.[143]

The evaluation and therapy of an infectious complication in the HIV-infected child mandates a high level of suspicion for unusual presentations, an aggressive approach for the establishment of the diagnosis, and often the use of intravenous antibiotics, at least during the initial days. Chronic and recurrent infections can compromise the nutritional status of the child but also influence the neurodevelopmental performance state. However, these symptoms are also typical for progressive HIV infection and should be monitored carefully.

Antiretroviral Therapy

As our knowledge about the dynamics of viral replication and its implication in regard to disease progression and prognosis have evolved, it has become clear that early and aggressive therapy offers the potential benefit of a prolonged asymptomatic time period. Panels of experts recently developed guidelines for the use of antiretroviral agents in children, adolescents, and adults, including pregnant women, with HIV infection.[114, 319, 320] The indications for the initiation of antiretroviral therapy include clinical, immunologic, and virologic parameters (Table 9–7).

Monotherapy is no longer considered appropriate treatment for the HIV-infected child or adult. The only exception is the use of zidovudine monotherapy in infants of indeterminant HIV status during the first 6 weeks of life as part of the regimen to prevent perinatal transmission. As soon as a child has been proven to be infected, therapy should be changed to a combination of agents.[320] Based on results from trials in adults, a three-drug combination is currently recommended and provides the best opportunity to preserve immune function and to prevent disease progression. This therapy should include a highly active protease inhibitor plus two dideoxynucleoside reverse transcriptase inhibitors as the initial therapeutic regimen.[320] The protease inhibitors currently recommended are nelfinavir and ritonavir (indinavir is not yet approved for children and is only available in capsule form). The combinations of dideoxynucleosides include zidovudine/didanosine or zidovudine/lamivudine and (supported by fewer data) stavudine/didanosine or stavudine/lamivudine and zidovudine/

TABLE 9–7
Initiation of Therapy

INFANTS <12 MO
- All HIV-infected infants <12 mo of age, regardless of clinical, immunologic, or virologic status, should be treated

CHILDREN >12 MO SHOULD BE TREATED IF THEY
- Are classified as clinical CDC category A, B, C (see Table 9–3) or develop frequent clinical symptoms *or*
- Have a CD4 count that classifies them into immunologic CDC category 2 or 3 (see Table 9–3) *or*
- Have rapidly declining CD4 counts (absolute or percentage) to values approaching Category 2 (moderate immune suppression) or
- Have a high (>10,000–20,000 copies/ml in the child >30 mo and definitively if >100,000 copies/ml in younger children) or a substantially increasing HIV RNA copy number (more than fivefold in children <2 yr and more than threefold in children >2 yr)

zalcitabine. Alternative regimens include the non-nucleoside reverse transcriptase inhibitors nevirapine or efavirenz (approved for children) or delavirdine in combination with dideoxynucleosides, with or without protease inhibitors. However, it is important to remember that there are currently no data available about the long-term tolerance and efficacy of any of these combinations in children. Furthermore, although ritonavir and nelfinavir are licensed for children older than 2 years of age, none of the protease inhibitors is currently approved for children younger than 2 years of age. Certain combinations are not recommended because of overlapping toxicities, including zalcitabine/didanosine or zalcitabine/stavudine or zalcitabine/lamivudine. The combination of stavudine and zidovudine is not recommended because of their antagonism.

The most commonly used antiretroviral agents in newborns and infants, the reverse transcriptase inhibitors zidovudine, didanosine, lamivudine, and nevirapine and the protease inhibitors nelfinavir and ritonavir, are briefly reviewed. For more extensive reviews it is recommended to consult specific textbooks or the current recommendations from the CDC.[320, 321] Because the standards of care are still evolving, collaboration between the child's primary health care provider and an HIV treatment center is strongly suggested. Whenever possible, children should be enrolled in clinical trials: access and information can be obtained by calling 1-800-TRIALS-A (AIDS Clinical Trials Group, ACTG), or 301-402-0696 (HIV & AIDS Malignancy Branch, National Cancer Institute).

ZIDOVUDINE

Only limited data are available regarding the appropriate dosing of antiretroviral drugs in the neonate. Zidovudine does cross the placenta and can be measured in amniotic fluid, cord blood, and fetal organs.[322, 323] The total body clearance and terminal half-life of zidovudine is similar in nonpregnant women and in women during the third trimester of pregnancy, and the half-life in the neonate is about tenfold longer than in the mother.[324, 325] Elimination of the drug and its main metabolite is markedly prolonged during the first 24 to 36 hours of life, with a mean serum half-life after maternal ingestion of 14.4 ± 7.5 hours.[322, 326–328] The total-body clearance of zidovudine increases rapidly within the first few weeks of life from 10.9 ml/minute per kilogram in infants 14 days old or younger to 19.0 ml/minute per kilogram in older infants ($p < 0.0001$).[329, 330] Oral bioavailability decreases from 89% in the younger group to 61% in infants older than 14 days of age.

Some studies have demonstrated that zidovudine is incorporated into the DNA of newborn mice and monkeys, as well as into the nuclear DNA of cord blood samples drawn from children whose mothers were being treated with zidovudine.[331, 332] Studies of the offsprings of mice who had been treated with zidovudine during the last trimester of pregnancy revealed an increased risk to develop liver and lung tumors as well as tumors of the reproductive organs. However, a similar study performed by Burroughs Wellcome, the manufacturer

of zidovudine, was not able to support these findings. A panel convened by the National Institutes of Health, although acknowledging the validity of the findings, also recognized that the benefit of preventing transmission of HIV disease in the vast majority of children currently outweighs the potential concerns of carcinogenicity.

Common side effects of zidovudine include bone marrow suppression, myopathy, and liver toxicity.[329, 333, 334]

The currently recommended dosage of zidovudine (in combination with other antiretroviral agents, see earlier[320]) is:

- Premature babies (under study): 1.5 mg/kg per dose orally every 12 hours from birth to 2 weeks of age; then increase to 2 mg/kg per dose every 8 hours
- Neonatal dosage: 2 mg/kg per dose every 6 hours orally or 1.5 mg/kg every 6 hours intravenously
- Pediatric dosage: 160 mg/m² per dose every 8 hours orally (range 90–180 mg/m² every 6 to 8 hours); intermittent intravenous dosing at 120 mg/m² every 6 hours or continuous intravenous dosing at 20 mg/m² per hour.

DIDANOSINE

Didanosine has also a plasma half-life of about an hour but, in contrast to zidovudine, a lower oral absorption rate (19 ± 17%) further characterized by high interpatient variability and a low penetration rate into cerebrospinal fluid.[335] Some of the variation in bioavailability could be because didanosine is acid labile and has to be taken with an antacid. It is conceivable that the amount of antacid necessary to neutralize gastric acidity varies between patients. Pharmacokinetic data for neonates or young infants are limited because of these problems but data from the macaque animal model indicate limited transplacental transport.[336–338]

Side effects of didanosine include pancreatitis, retinal depigmentation, and increased liver enzymes.[261, 339–341]

The currently recommended dosage of didanosine (in combination with other antiretroviral agents, see earlier[320]) is:

- Premature babies: no data available
- Neonatal dosage (infants younger than 90 days old): 50 mg/m² per dose every 12 hours orally
- Pediatric dosage: 90 mg/m² per dose every 12 hours orally (dosage range from 90 to 150 mg/m² per dose every 8 to 12 hours)

LAMIVUDINE

Lamivudine has been approved for the use in combination with zidovudine. Lamivudine at doses between 0.5 to 20 mg/kg per day given to children in two daily doses was well tolerated.[342, 343] Side effects included hyperactivity (2%), increase in liver function to more than 10 times normal (3%), neutropenia (3%), and reversible pancreatitis (8%). Lamivudine was rapidly absorbed after oral administration and 66 ± 25% of the oral dose was absorbed.

The currently recommended dosage of lamivudine

(in combination with other antiretroviral agents, see earlier[320]) is:

- Premature babies: no data available
- Neonatal dosage (infants younger than 30 days old): 2 mg/kg per dose twice daily orally
- Pediatric dosage: 4 mg/kg per dose twice daily

NEVIRAPINE

Nevirapine is also a reverse transcriptase inhibitor but, unlike zidovudine, didanosine, and lamivudine, does not belong to the dideoxynucleoside family of drugs.[344] Nevirapine therapy results in a rapid and marked decrease in HIV-1 RNA concentrations in plasma, which makes it a promising agent for the prevention of vertical transmission.[345] However, a drawback of nevirapine is that resistance develops rapidly during monotherapy due to several possible mutations.[346] Nevirapine was well tolerated in a pediatric trial including 21 children.[347] At doses of more than 240 mg/m² per day, 5 of 10 children experienced a prolonged reduction in p24 antigenemia. Eight infants born to seven HIV-infected mothers were studied, after the mothers received 200 mg of nevirapine during labor. The infants were treated with 2-mg/kg oral doses of nevirapine at a mean of 56.6 hours after birth.[348] No side effects were observed in mothers or children; and with a dose of nevirapine during labor and another 48 to 72 hours after birth, nevirapine levels of more than 100 ng/ml (10 times the IC_{50}) were achieved throughout the first week of life.

The currently recommended dosage of nevirapine (in combination with other antiretroviral agents, see earlier[320]) is:

- Premature babies: no data available
- Neonatal dosage (currently being studied): 5 mg/kg per dose once daily for 14 days, followed by 120 mg/m² every 12 hours for 14 days, followed by 200 mg/m² per dose every 12 hours
- Pediatric dosage: 120 to 200 mg/m² per dose every 12 hours. *Note:* Therapy should be initiated at 120 mg/m² per dose once daily for 14 days to decrease the risk of cutaneous reactions.

NELFINAVIR

Nelfinavir, a protease inhibitor approved for the use in children and adults with HIV infection, was studied in an as yet unpublished open-label, uncontrolled clinical trial of 38 children aged 2 to 13 years.[349] Nelfinavir should be taken with food to optimize absorption of the drug. The most common adverse event is diarrhea of mild to moderate intensity. Nelfinavir, as all the protease inhibitors, is metabolized by the hepatic cytochrome P450 enzyme system, which can lead to drug interactions with a variety of commonly used medications.[350]

The currently recommended dosage of nelfinavir (in combination with other antiretroviral agents, see earlier[320]) is:

- Premature babies: no data available
- Neonatal dosage: no data available, the dose currently being studied is 10 mg/kg per dose three times daily orally
- Pediatric dosage (limited data): 20 to 30 mg/kg per dose three times daily

RITONAVIR

Ritonavir, another protease inhibitor approved for use in children, is extensively metabolized by the P450 enzyme system, and drug interactions are very common.[350] In a phase I/II study performed by the National Cancer Institute, HIV-infected children between 6 months and 18 years of age were eligible to enroll at four different dose levels of ritonavir oral solution (250, 300, 350, and 400 mg/m² given every 12 hours.)[351] Ritonavir was administered alone for the first 12 weeks and then in combination with zidovudine and/or didanosine. Dose-related nausea, diarrhea, and abdominal pain were the most common toxicities. CD4 cell counts increased by a median of 79 cells/mm³ after 4 weeks of monotherapy and were maintained throughout the study. Plasma HIV RNA levels decreased by 1 to 2 $\log_{10}$ copies/ml within 4 to 8 weeks of ritonavir monotherapy, and this level was sustained in patients enrolled at the highest dose level of 400 mg/m² for the 24-week period.

The currently recommended dosage of ritonavir (in combination with other antiretroviral agents, see earlier[320]) is:

- Premature babies: no data available
- Neonatal dosage: no data available, currently being studied
- Pediatric dosage (limited data): 400 mg/m² (range 350–400 mg/m²) every 12 hours orally. To minimize nausea/vomiting, initiate therapy at 250 mg/m² every 12 hours and increase stepwise over 5 days to full dose.

FUTURE GOALS

The past few years have brought major advances in the understanding, prevention, and treatment of HIV disease. The application of the PACTG 076 protocol has led to a marked decrease in the perinatal transmission rate of HIV infection in industrialized countries. The increased understanding of the interactions between viral load and immunologic status and their implications for prognosis have prompted earlier and more aggressive antiretroviral therapy. The advent of the protease inhibitors and the accelerated approval of antiretroviral drugs for both children and adults have broadened the therapeutic armamentarium. However, many problems remain.

The most urgent need continues to be the prevention of further spread of HIV infection, not only among adults but also from a mother to her unborn child. Almost two decades after the description of the clinical syndrome of AIDS, we are still dealing with an ever-growing pandemic, affecting not only certain minorities, but both sexes and all age groups and social levels, but targeting mainly the developing countries with already limited resources. The staggering demands put on public health systems and their financial resources could easily create tensions regarding the distribution of available funds. Before the widespread use of combination therapy and protease inhibitors, it has been estimated that the lifetime cost of hospital-based care for children with HIV infection is $408,307.[352] Assuming that hospital-based care represents 83% of the total charges, the mean overall lifetime cost would be about $500,000. The cost of current antiretroviral therapy is even higher and life expectancy longer, although this is partially offset by fewer hospitalizations. It has become very clear that major efforts are needed to make prevention and therapy for HIV infection feasible and affordable for developing nations, because they have the highest numbers of infected people with the fewest financial and organizational resources.

New and different antiretroviral agents are needed, because of toxicities, emergence of resistance, and in order to provide more effective or even permanent inhibition of viral replication. We need to know the pharmacokinetic properties of drugs when given to the pregnant mother, the neonate, or the very young infant. Progress has been made in the early recognition and prophylaxis of opportunistic infections. However, as patients with HIV infection survive longer, problems with resistant organisms, multiple drug allergies, altered organ function, as well as long-term side effects of medications emerge and complicate adequate therapy.

Advocacy for children and pregnant women, ensuring equal access to new drugs but also providing sound data regarding dosing and potential toxicities, continues to be important. The U.S. Food and Drug Administration now allows the approval of drugs for use in children based on efficacy data gathered in adults, if the disease in children and adults is reasonably similar and if the pharmaceutical companies provide dosing (pharmacokinetic) and safety (toxicity) data from controlled trials performed in an adequate number of children. The treatment and care of HIV-infected children and adults has become increasingly complex, and close collaboration with physicians and centers specialized in their care is highly recommended.

References

1. Centers for Disease Control. Unexplained immunodeficiency and opportunistic infections in infants—New York, New Jersey, California. MMWR 31:665–667, 1982.
2. Ammann AJ, Cowan MJ, Wara DW, et al. Acquired immunodeficiency in an infant: possible transmission by means of blood products. Lancet 1:956–958, 1983.
3. Oleske J, Minnefor A, Cooper R, et al. Immune deficiency syndrome in children. JAMA 249:2345–2349, 1983.
4. Rubinstein A, Sicklick M, Gupta A, et al. Acquired immunodeficiency with reversed T4/T8 ratios in infants born to promiscuous and drug-addicted mothers. JAMA 249:2350–2356, 1983.
5. Centers for Disease Control and Prevention. U.S. HIV and AIDS cases reported through December 1997. HIV/AIDS Surveillance report: year-end edition. MMWR Morb Mortal Wkly Rep 9:1–44, 1997.

6. Centers for Disease Control and Prevention. Update: Trends in AIDS incidence, deaths and prevalence—United States, 1996. MMWR Morb Mortal Wkly Rep 46:165–173, 1997.
7. Coleman RL, Wilkinson D. Increasing HIV prevalence in a rural district of South Africa from 1992 through 1995. J Acquir Immune Defic Syndr Hum Retrovirol 16:50–53, 1997.
8. Laga M, De Cock KM, Kaleeba N, et al. HIV/AIDS in Africa: the second decade and beyond. AIDS 11:S1–S3, 1997.
9. Foster G. Today's children—challenges to child health promotion in countries with severe AIDS epidemics. AIDS Care 10(Suppl 1):S17–S23, 1998.
10. Balter M. United Nations: global program struggles to stem the flood of new cases. Science 280:1863–1864, 1998.
11. The European Collaborative Study. Vertical transmission of HIV-1: maternal immune status and obstetric factors. AIDS 10:1675–1681, 1996.
12. The Working Group on Mother-To-Child Transmission of HIV. Rates of mother-to-child transmission of HIV-1 in Africa, America, and Europe: results from 13 perinatal studies. J Acquir Immune Defic Syndr Hum Retrovirol 8:506–510, 1995.
13. Sperling RS, Shapiro DE, Coombs RW, et al. Maternal viral load, zidovudine treatment, and the risk of transmission of human immunodeficiency virus type 1 from mother to infant. Pediatric AIDS Clinical Trials Group Protocol 076 Study Group. N Engl J Med 335:1621–1629, 1996.
14. Connor EM, Sperling RS, Gelber R, et al. Reduction of maternal-infant transmission of immunodeficiency virus type 1 with zidovudine treatment. N Engl J Med 331:1173–1180, 1994.
15. Connor EM, Mofenson LK. Zidovudine for the reduction of perinatal human immunodeficiency virus transmission: Pediatric AIDS Clinical Trials Group protocol 076—results and treatment recommendations. Pediatr Infect Dis J 14:536–541, 1995.
16. Centers for Disease Control and Prevention. Recommendations of the U.S. Public Health Service Task Force on the use of zidovudine to reduce perinatal transmission of human immunodeficiency virus. MMWR Morb Mortal Wkly Rep 43:1–20, 1994.
17. Nuovo GJ, Forde A, MacConnell P, Fahrenwald R. In situ detection of PCR-amplified HIV-1 nucleic acids and tumor necrosis factor cDNA in cervical tissues. Am J Pathol 143:40–48, 1993.
18. Royce RA, Sena A, Cates W, Cohen MS. Sexual transmission of HIV. N Engl J Med 336:1072–1078, 1997.
19. Sprecher S, Soumenkoff G, Puissant F, Degueldre M. Vertical transmission of HIV in 15-week fetus. Lancet 2:288, 1986.
20. Jovaisas E, Koch MA, Schäfer A, et al. LAV/HTLV-III in 20-week fetus. Lancet 2:1129, 1985.
21. Mano H, Chermann J-C. Fetal human immunodeficiency virus type 1 infection of different organs in the second trimester. AIDS Res Hum Retroviruses 7:83–88, 1991.
22. Mundy DC, Schinazi RF, Gerber AR, et al. Human immunodeficiency virus isolated from amniotic fluid. Lancet 2:459–460, 1987.
23. Lewis SH, Reynolds-Kohler C, Fox HE, Nelson JA. HIV-1 in trophoblastic and villous Hofbauer cells, and haematological precursors in eight-week fetuses. Lancet 335:565–568, 1990.
24. Amirhessami-Aghili N, Spector SA. Human immunode-

ficiency virus type 1 infection of human placenta: Potential route for fetal infection. J Virol 65:2231–2236, 1991.

25. Zachar V, Thomas RA, Jones T, Goustin AS. Vertical transmission of HIV: detection of proviral DNA in placental trophoblasts. AIDS 8:129–130, 1994.

26. Mattern CFT, Murray K, Jensen A, Farzadegan H, Pang J, Modlin JF. Localization of human immunodeficiency virus core antigen in term human placentas. Pediatrics 89:207–209, 1992.

27. St. Louis ME, Kamenga M, Brown C, et al. Risk for perinatal HIV-1 transmission according to maternal immunologic, virologic, and placental factors. JAMA 269:2853–2859, 1993.

28. Thomas PA, Weedon J, Krasinski K, et al. Maternal predictors of perinatal human immunodeficiency virus transmission. Pediatr Infect Dis J 13:489–495, 1994.

29. Borkowsky W, Krasinski K, Cao Y, et al. Correlation of perinatal transmission of human immunodeficiency virus type 1 with maternal viremia and lymphocyte phenotypes. J Pediatr 125:345–351, 1994.

30. Fang G, Burger H, Grimson R, et al. Maternal plasma human immunodeficiency virus type 1 RNA level: A determinant and projected threshold for mother-to-child transmission. Proc Natl Acad Sci U S A 92:12100–12104, 1995.

31. Mayaux MJ, Blanche S, Rouzioux C, et al. Maternal factors associated with perinatal HIV-1 transmission: the French Cohort Study: 7 years of follow-up observation. J Acquir Immune Defic Syndr Hum Retrovirol 8:188–194, 1995.

32. Cao Y, Krogstad P, Korber BT, et al. Maternal HIV-1 viral load and vertical transmission of infection: the Ariel Project for the prevention of HIV transmission from mother to infant. Nature Med 3:549–552, 1997.

33. Lambert G, Thea DM, Pliner V, et al. Effect of maternal CD4+ cell count, acquired immunodeficiency syndrome, and viral load on disease progression in infants with perinatally acquired human immunodeficiency virus type 1 infection. J Pediatr 130:890–897, 1997.

34. D'Arminio Monforte A, Ravizza M, Muggiasca ML, et al. HIV-infected pregnant women: possible predictors of vertical transmission. Presented before the 7th International Conference on AIDS, Florence, Italy, 1991.

35. Peckham C, Gibb D. Mother-to-child transmission of the human immunodeficiency virus. N Engl J Med 333:298–302, 1995.

36. Bryson YJ, Luzuriaga K, Sullivan JL, Wara DW. Proposed definition for in utero versus intrapartum transmission of HIV-1. N Engl J Med 327:1246–1247, 1992.

37. Rouzioux C, Costagliola D, Burgard M, et al. Estimated timing of mother-to-child human immunodeficiency virus type 1 (HIV-1) transmission by use of a Markov model. The HIV Infection in Newborns French Collaborative Study Group. Am J Epidemiol 142:1330–1337, 1995.

38. Nesheim SR, Shaffer N, Vink P, et al. Lack of increased risk for perinatal human immunodeficiency virus transmission to subsequent children born to infected women. Pediatr Infect Dis J 15:886–890, 1996.

39. Young KY, Nelson RP. Discordant human immunodeficiency virus infection in dizygotic twins detected by polymerase chain reaction. Pediatr Infect Dis J 9:454–456, 1990.

40. Goedert JJ, Duliege AM, Amos CI, et al. High risk of HIV-1 infection for first-born twins. Lancet 338:1471–1475, 1991.

41. Duliege A-M, Amos CI, Felton S, et al. Birth order, delivery route, and concordance in the transmission of

human immunodeficiency virus type 1 from mothers to twins. J Pediatr 126:625–632, 1995.

42. Mofenson LM. A critical review of studies evaluating the relationship of mode of delivery to perinatal transmission of human immunodeficiency virus. Pediatr Infect Dis J 14:169–177, 1995.

43. Biggar RJ, Miotti PG, Taha TE, et al. Perinatal intervention trial in Africa: effect of a birth canal cleansing intervention to prevent HIV transmission. Lancet 347:1647–1650, 1996.

44. Taha TE, Biggar RJ, Broadhead RL, et al. Effect of cleansing the birth canal with antiseptic solution on maternal and newborn morbidity and mortality in Malawi: clinical trial. BMJ 315:216–219, 1997.

45. Landesman SH, Kalish LA, Burns DN, et al. Obstetrical factors and the transmission of human immunodeficiency virus type 1 from mother to child. N Engl J Med 334:1617–1623, 1996.

46. Van De Perre P, Simonon A, Msellati P, et al. Postnatal transmission of human immunodeficiency virus type 1 from mother to infant. N Engl J Med 325:593–598, 1991.

47. Van de Perre P, Simonon A, Hitimana D-G, et al. Infective and anti-infective properties of breast milk from HIV-1 infected women. Lancet 341:914–918, 1993.

48. Ruff AJ, Halsey NA, Coberly J, Boulos R. Breast-feeding and maternal-infant transmission of human immunodeficiency virus type 1. J Pediatr 121:325–329, 1992.

49. Thiry L, Sprecher-Goldberger S, Jonckheer T, et al. Isolation of AIDS virus from cell-free breast milk of three healthy virus carriers. Lancet 2:891–892, 1985.

50. Lewis P, Nduati R, Kreiss JK, et al. Cell-free human immunodeficiency virus type 1 in breast milk. J Infect Dis 177:34–39, 1998.

51. Guay LA, Hom DL, Mmiro F, et al. Detection of human immunodeficiency virus type 1 (HIV-1) DNA and p24 antigen in breast milk of HIV-1–infected Ugandan women and vertical transmission. Pediatrics 98:438–444, 1996.

52. de Martino M, Tovo P-A, Tozzi AE, et al. HIV-1 transmission through breast milk: appraisal of risk according to duration of feeding. AIDS 6:991–997, 1992.

53. Bertolli J, St. Louis ME, Simonds RJ, et al. Estimating the timing of mother-to-child transmission of human immunodeficiency virus in a breast-feeding population in Kinshasa, Zaire. J Infect Dis 174:722–726, 1996.

54. Lederman SA. Estimating infant mortality from human immunodeficiency virus and other causes in breast-feeding and bottle-feeding populations. Pediatrics 89:290–296, 1992.

55. Bobat R, Moodley D, Coutsoudis A, Coovadia H. Breastfeeding by HIV-1–infected women and outcome in their infants: a cohort study from Durban, South Africa. AIDS 11:1627–1633, 1997.

56. American Academy of Pediatrics Committee on Pediatric AIDS. Human milk, breastfeeding, and transmission of human immunodeficiency virus in the United States. Pediatrics 96:977–979, 1995.

57. Friedland GH, Saltzman BR, Rogers MF, et al. Lack of transmission of HTLV-III/LAV infection to household contacts of patients with AIDS or AIDS-related complex with oral candidiasis. N Engl J Med 314:334–339, 1986.

58. Mann JM, Quinn TC, Francis H, et al. Prevalence of HTLV-III/LAV in household contacts of patients with confirmed AIDS and controls in Kinshasa, Zaire. JAMA 256:721–724, 1986.

59. Centers for Disease Control and Prevention. Human immunodeficiency virus transmission in household

settings—United States. MMWR Morb Mortal Wkly Rep 43:347–356, 1994.

60. Lobato MN, Oxtoby MJ, Augustyniak L, et al. Infection control practices in the home: a survey of households of HIV-infected persons with hemophilia. Infect Control Hosp Epidemiol 17:721–725, 1996.

61. American Academy of Pediatrics Task Force of Pediatric AIDS. Education of children with human immunodeficiency virus infection. Pediatrics 88:645–648, 1991.

62. Committee on Infectious Diseases. Health guidelines for the attendance in day-care and foster care settings of children infected with human immunodeficiency virus. Pediatrics 79:466–470, 1987.

63. American Academy of Pediatrics. Evaluation and medical treatment of the HIV-exposed infant. Pediatrics 99:909–917, 1997.

64. Zeichner SL. The molecular biology of HIV: insights into pathogenesis and targets for therapy. Clin Perinatol 21:39–73, 1994.

65. Pavlakis GN. The molecular biology of human immunodeficiency virus type 1. In DeVita VT Jr, Hellman S, Rosenberg SA (eds): AIDS: Biology, Diagnosis, Treatment and Prevention. Philadelphia, Lippincott–Raven, 1997, pp 45–74.

66. Cullen BR. HIV-1 auxiliary proteins: making connections in a dying cell. Cell 93:685–692, 1998.

67. Fauci AS, Pantaleo G, Stanley S, Weissman D. Immunopathogenic mechanisms of HIV infection. Ann Intern Med 124:654–663, 1996.

68. Feng Y, Broder CC, Kennedy PE, Berger EA. HIV-1 entry cofactor: Functional cDNA cloning of a seven-transmembrane G protein-coupled receptor. Science 272:872–877, 1996.

69. Cocchi F, DeVico AL, Garzino-Demo A, et al. The V3 domain of the HIV-1 gp120 envelope glycoprotein is critical for chemokine-mediated blockade of infection. Nature Med 2:1244–1247, 1996.

70. Kinter AL, Ostrowski M, Goletti D, et al. HIV replication in CD4+ T cells of HIV-infected individuals is regulated by a balance between viral suppressive effects of endogenous β-chemokines and the viral inductive effects of other endogenous cytokines. Proc Natl Acad Sci U S A 93:14076–14081, 1996.

71. Lapham CK, Ouyang J, Chandrasekhar B, et al. Evidence for cell-surface association between fusin and the CD4-gp120 complex in human cell lines. Science 274:602–605, 1996.

72. Wu L, Gerard NP, Wyatt R, et al. CD4-induced interaction of primary HIV-1 gp120 glycoproteins with the chemokine receptor CCR-5. Nature 384:179–183, 1996.

73. Rollins BJ. Chemokines. Blood 90:909–928, 1997.

74. Cairns JS, D'Souza MP. Chemokines and HIV-1 second receptors: the therapeutic connection. Nat Med 4:563–568, 1998.

75. Reinhardt PP, Reinhardt B, Lathey JL, Spector SA. Human cord blood mononuclear cells are preferentially infected by non–syncytium-inducing, macrophage-tropic human immunodeficiency virus type 1 isolates. J Clin Microbiol 33:292–297, 1995.

76. Panganiban AT. Retroviral reverse transcription and DNA integration. Virology 1:187–194, 1990.

77. Bushman FD, Fujiwara T, Craigie R. Retroviral DNA integration directed by HIV integration protein in vitro. Science 249:1555–1558, 1990.

78. Brown PO, Bowerman B, Varmus HE, Bishop JM. Retroviral integration: structure of the initial covalent product and its precursor, and a role for the viral IN protein. Proc Natl Acad Sci U S A 86:2525–2529, 1989.

79. Stevenson M, Haggerty S, Lamonica CA, et al. Integration is not necessary for expression of human immunodeficiency virus type 1 protein products. J Virol 64:2421–2425, 1990.

80. Bagasra O, Hauptman SP, Lischner HW, et al. Detection of human immunodeficiency virus type 1 provirus in mononuclear cells by in situ polymerase chain reaction. N Engl J Med 326:1385–1391, 1992.

81. Chevret S, Kirstetter M, Mariotti M, et al. Provirus copy number to predict disease progression in asymptomatic human immunodeficiency virus type 1 infection. J Infect Dis 169:882–885, 1994.

82. Ho DD. Dynamics of HIV-1 replication in vivo. J Clin Invest 99:2565–2567, 1997.

83. Ho DD, Neumann AU, Perelson AS, et al. Rapid turnover of plasma virions and CD4 lymphocytes in HIV-1 infection. Nature 373:123–126, 1995.

84. Perelson AS, Neumann AU, Markowitz M, et al. HIV-1 dynamics in vivo: clearance rate, infected cell life-span, and viral generation time. Science 271:1582–1586, 1996.

85. Perelson AS, Essunger P, Cao Y, et al. Decay characteristics of HIV-1-infected compartments during combination therapy. Nature 387:188–191, 1997.

86. Kohl NE, Emini EA, Schleif WA, et al. Active human immunodeficiency virus protease is required for viral infectivity. Proc Natl Acad Sci U S A 85:4686–4690, 1988.

87. Swanstrom R, Kaplan AH, Manchester M. The aspartic proteinase of HIV-1. Semin Virol 1:175–186, 1990.

88. Perno C-F, Bergamini A, Pesce CD, et al. Inhibition of the protease of human immunodeficiency virus blocks replication and infectivity of the virus in chronically infected macrophages. J Infect Dis 168:1148–1156, 1993.

89. Shearer WT, Quinn TC, LaRussa P, et al. Viral load and disease progression in infants infected with human immunodeficiency virus type 1. N Engl J Med 336:1337–1342, 1997.

90. Palumbo PE, Kwok S, Wesley Y, et al. Viral measurement by polymerase chain reaction–based assays in human immunodeficiency virus–infected infants. J Pediatr 126:592–595, 1995.

91. Mofenson LM, Korelitz J, Meyer WA 3rd, et al. The relationship between serum human immunodeficiency virus type 1 (HIV-1) RNA level, CD4 lymphocyte percent, and long-term mortality risk in HIV-1-infected children. National Institute of Child Health and Human Development Intravenous Immunoglobulin Clinical Trial Study Group. J Infect Dis 175:1029–1038, 1997.

92. McIntosh K, Shevitz A, Zaknun D, et al. Age- and time-related changes in extracellular viral load in children vertically infected by human immunodeficiency virus. Pediatr Infect Dis J 15:1087–1091, 1996.

93. Balotta C, Colombo MC, Colucci G, et al. Plasma viremia and virus phenotype are correlates of disease progression in vertically human immunodeficiency virus type 1–infected children. Pediatr Infect Dis J 16:205–211, 1997.

94. Mellors JW, Kingsley LA, Rinaldo CR, et al. Quantitation of HIV-1 RNA in plasma predicts outcome after seroconversion. Ann Intern Med 122:573–579, 1995.

95. Mellors JW, Rinaldo CR, Gupta P, et al. Prognosis of HIV-1 infection predicted by the quantity of virus in plasma. Science 272:1167–1170, 1996.

96. Bryson YJ, Pang S, Wei LS, et al. Clearance of HIV infection in a perinatally infected infant. N Engl J Med 332:833–838, 1995.

97. Bryson YJ. HIV clearance in infants—a continuing saga. AIDS 9:1373–1375, 1995.

98. Roques PA, Gras G, Parnet-Mathieu F, et al. Clearance

of HIV infection in 12 perinatally infected children: clinical, virological and immunological data. AIDS 9:F19–F26, 1995.

99. Lepage P, Van de Perre P, Simonon A, et al. Transient seroreversion in children born to human immunodeficiency virus 1–infected mothers. Pediatr Infect Dis J 11:892–894, 1992.

100. Bakshi SS, Tetali S, Abrams EJ, et al. Repeatedly positive human immunodeficiency virus type 1 DNA polymerase chain reaction in human immunodeficiency virus–exposed seroreverting infants. Pediatr Infect Dis J 14:658–662, 1995.

101. Frenkel LM, Mullins JI, Learn GH, et al. Genetic evaluation of suspected cases of transient HIV-1 infection of infants. Science 280:1073–1077, 1998.

102. Erkeller-Yuksel FM, Deneys V, Hannet I, et al. Age-related changes in human blood lymphocyte subpopulations. J Pediatr 120:216–222, 1992.

103. The European Collaborative Study. Age-related standards for T lymphocyte subsets based on uninfected children born to human immunodeficiency virus 1–infected mothers. Pediatr Infect Dis J 11:1018–1026, 1992.

104. Comans-Bitter WM, de Groot R, van den Beemd R, et al. Immunophenotyping of blood lymphocytes in childhood. Reference values for lymphocyte subpopulations. J Pediatr 130:388–393, 1997.

105. McKinney RE, Wilfert CM. Lymphocyte subsets in children younger than 2 years old: Normal values in a population at risk for human immunodeficiency virus infection and diagnostic and prognostic application to infected children. Pediatr Infect Dis J 11:639–644, 1992.

106. Dickover RE, Dillon M, Gillette SG, et al. Rapid increases in load of human immunodeficiency virus correlate with early disease progression and loss of CD4 cells in vertically infected infants. J Infect Dis 170:1279–1284, 1994.

107. Roilides E, Black C, Reimer C, et al. Serum immunoglobulin G subclasses in children infected with human immunodeficiency virus type 1. Pediatr Infect Dis J 10:134–139, 1991.

108. Luzuriaga K, Koup RA, Pikora CA, et al. Deficient human immunodeficiency virus type 1–specific cytotoxic T cell responses in vertically infected children. J Pediatr 119:230–236, 1991.

109. Monforte ADA, Novati R, Galli M, et al. T-cell subsets and serum immunoglobulin levels in infants born to HIV-seropositive mothers: a longitudinal evaluation. AIDS 4:1141–1144, 1990.

110. Borkowsky W, Rigaud M, Krasinski K, et al. Cell-mediated and humoral immune responses in children infected with human immunodeficiency virus during the first four years of life. J Pediatr 120:371–375, 1992.

111. European Collaborative Study. Children born to women with HIV-1 infection: natural history and risk of transmission. Lancet 337:253–260, 1991.

112. Luzuriaga K, Holmes D, Hereema A, et al. HIV-1–specific cytotoxic T lymphocyte responses in the first year of life. J Immunol 154:433–443, 1995.

113. Pikora CA, Sullivan JL, Panicali D, Luzuriaga K. Early HIV-1 envelope-specific cytotoxic T lymphocyte responses in vertically infected children. J Exp Med 185:1153–1161, 1997.

114. Centers for Disease Control and Prevention. Public Health Service task force recommendations for the use of antiretroviral drugs in pregnant women infected with HIV-1 for maternal health and for reducing perinatal

115. Kline MW, Lewis DE, Hollinger FB, et al. A comparative study of human immunodeficiency virus culture, polymerase chain reaction and anti-human immunodeficiency virus immunoglobulin A antibody detection in the diagnosis during early infancy of vertically acquired human immunodeficiency virus infection. Pediatr Infect Dis J 13:90–94, 1994.

116. Comeau AM, Pitt J, Hillyer GV, et al. Early detection of human immunodeficiency virus on dried blood spot specimens: sensitivity across serial specimens. J Pediatr 129:111–118, 1996.

117. Horsburgh CR, Ou CY, Jason J, et al. Duration of human immunodeficiency virus infection before detection of antibody. Lancet 2:637–640, 1989.

118. Rogers MF, Ou C-Y, Kilbourne B, Schochetman G. Advances and problems in the diagnosis of human immunodeficiency virus infection in infants. Pediatr Infect Dis J 10:523–531, 1991.

119. Chantry CJ, Cooper ER, Pelton SI, et al. Seroreversion in human immunodeficiency virus–exposed but uninfected infants. Pediatr Infect Dis J 14:382–387, 1995.

120. Tudor-Williams G. Early diagnosis of vertically acquired HIV-1 infection. AIDS 5:103–105, 1991.

121. Yanase Y, Tango T, Okumura K, et al. Lymphocyte subsets identified by monoclonal antibodies in healthy children. Pediatr Res 20:1147–1151, 1986.

122. Quinn TC, Ruff A, Halsey N. Pediatric acquired immunodeficiency syndrome: special considerations for developing nations. Pediatr Infect Dis J 1992; 11:558–568, 1992.

123. Pollack H, Glasberg H, Lee E, et al. Impaired early growth of infants perinatally infected with human immunodeficiency virus: correlation with viral load. J Pediatr 130:915–922, 1997.

124. Blanche S, Tardieu M, Duliege A-M, et al. Longitudinal study of 94 symptomatic infants with perinatally acquired human immunodeficiency virus infection. Am J Dis Child 144:1210–1215, 1990.

125. Centers for Disease Control. Revision of the CDC surveillance case definition for acquired immunodeficiency syndrome. MMWR Morb Mortal Wkly Rep 36 (suppl 1s):1S–15S, 1987.

126. Andiman WA, Mezger J, Shapiro E. Invasive bacterial infections in children born to women infected with human immunodeficiency virus type 1. J Pediatr 124:846–852, 1994.

127. Lichenstein R, King JC, Farley JJ, et al. Bacteremia in febrile human immunodeficiency virus–infected children presenting to ambulatory care settings. Pediatr Infect Dis J 17:381–385, 1998.

128. Janoff EN, Breiman RE, Daley CL, Hopewell PC. Pneumococcal disease during HIV infection: epidemiology, clinical, and immunologic perspectives. Ann Intern Med 117:314–324, 1992.

129. Farley JJ, King JC, Nair P, et al. Invasive pneumococcal disease among infected and uninfected children of mothers with human immunodeficiency virus infection. J Pediatr 124:853–858, 1994.

130. Di John D, Krasinski K, Lawrence R, et al. Very late onset of group B streptococcal disease in infants infected with the human immunodeficiency virus. Pediatr Infect Dis J 9:925–928, 1990.

131. Dorfman DH, Glaser JH. Congenital syphilis presenting in infants after the newborn period. N Engl J Med 323:1299–1302, 1990.

132. Dumois JA. Potential problems with the diagnosis and

treatment of syphilis in HIV-infected pregnant women. Pediatr AIDS HIV Infect Fetus Adolesc 3:22–24, 1992.

133. McIntosh K. Congenital syphilis—breaking through the safety net. N Engl J Med 323:1339–1341, 1990.

134. Centers for Disease Control. Screening for tuberculosis and tuberculous infection in high-risk populations and the use of preventive therapy for tuberculous infections in the United States. MMWR Morb Mortal Wkly Rep 39:1–12, 1990.

135. Khoury YF, Mastrucci MT, Hutto C, et al. *Mycobacterium tuberculosis* in children with human immunodeficiency virus type 1 infection. Pediatr Infect Dis J 11:950–955, 1992.

136. Gutman LT, Moye J, Zimmer B, Tian C. Tuberculosis in human immunodeficiency virus–exposed or –infected United States children. Pediatr Infect Dis J 13:963–968, 1994.

137. Committee on Infectious Diseases. Screening for tuberculosis in infants and children. Pediatrics 93:131–134, 1994.

138. Adhikari M, Pillay T, Pillay DG. Tuberculosis in the newborn: an emerging disease. Pediatr Infect Dis J 16:1108–1112, 1997.

139. Committee on Infectious Diseases. Update on tuberculosis skin testing of children. Pediatrics 97:282–284, 1996.

140. Starke JR, Correa AG. Management of mycobacterial infection and disease in children. Pediatr Infect Dis J 14:455–470, 1995.

141. Lewis LL, Butler KM, Husson RN, et al. Defining the population of human immunodeficiency virus–infected children at risk for *Mycobacterium avium-intracellulare* infection. J Pediatr 121:677–683, 1992.

142. Rutstein RM, Cobb P, McGowan KL, et al. *Mycobacterium avium intracellulare* complex infection in HIV-infected children. AIDS 7:507–512, 1993.

143. USPHS/IDSA Prevention of Opportunistic Infections Working Group. USPHS/IDSA guidelines for the prevention of opportunistic infections in persons infected with human immunodeficiency virus. MMWR Morb Mortal Wkly Rep 46:1–46, 1997.

144. Jura E, Chadwick EG, Josephs SH, et al. Varicella-zoster virus infections in children infected with human immunodeficiency virus. Pediatr Infect Dis J 8:586–590, 1989.

145. Silliman CC, Tedder D, Ogle JW, et al. Unsuspected varicella-zoster virus encephalitis in a child with acquired immunodeficiency syndrome. J Pediatr 123:418–422, 1993.

146. Lyall EG, Ogilvie MM, Smith NM, Burns S. Acyclovir resistant varicella zoster and HIV infection. Arch Dis Child 70:133–135, 1994.

147. Chandwani S, Kaul A, Bebenroth D, et al. Cytomegalovirus infection in human immunodeficiency virus type 1–infected children. Pediatr Infect Dis J 15:310–314, 1996.

148. Nigro G, Krysztofiak A, Castelli Gattinara G, et al. Rapid progression of HIV disease in children with cytomegalovirus DNAemia. AIDS 10:1127–1133, 1996.

149. Doyle M, Atkins JT, Rivera-Matos IR. Congenital cytomegalovirus infection in infants infected with human immunodeficiency virus type 1. Pediatr Infect Dis J 15:1102–1106, 1996.

150. Kitchen BJ, Engler HD, Gill VJ, et al. Cytomegalovirus infection in children with human immunodeficiency virus infection. Pediatr Infect Dis J 16:358–363, 1997.

151. Zaknun D, Zangerle R, Kapelari K, et al. Concurrent ganciclovir and foscarnet treatment for cytomegalovirus encephalitis and retinitis in an infant with acquired immunodeficiency syndrome: case report and review. Pediatr Infect Dis J 16:807–811, 1997.

152. Walton RC, Whitcup SM, Mueller BU, et al. Combined intravenous ganciclovir and foscarnet for children with recurrent cytomegalovirus retinitis. Ophthalmology 102:1865–1870, 1995.

153. Bodsworth NJ, Cooper DA, Donovan B. The influence of human immunodeficiency virus type 1 infection on the development of the hepatitis B virus carrier state. J Infect Dis 163:1138–1140, 1991.

154. Eyster ME, Diamondstone LS, Lien J-M, et al. Natural history of hepatitis C virus infection in multitransfused hemophiliacs: effect of co-infection with human immunodeficiency virus. J Acquir Immune Defic 6:602–610, 1993.

155. Paccagnini S, Principi N, Massironi E, et al. Perinatal transmission and manifestation of hepatitis C virus infection in a high risk population. Pediatr Infect Dis J 14:195–199, 1995.

156. Kaplan LJ, Daum RS, Smaron M, McCarthy CA. Severe measles in immunocompromised patients. JAMA 267:1237–1241, 1992.

157. Palumbo P, Hoyt L, Demasio K, et al. Population-based study of measles and measles immunization in human immunodeficiency virus–infected children. Pediatr Infect Dis J 11:1008–1014, 1992.

158. Nadel S, McGann K, Hodinka RL, et al. Measles giant cell pneumonia in a child with human immunodeficiency virus infection. Pediatr Infect Dis J 10:542–544, 1991.

159. Krasinski K, Borkowsky W. Measles and measles immunity in children infected with human immunodeficiency virus. JAMA 261:2512–2516, 1989.

160. Chandwani S, Borkowsky W, Krasinski K, et al. Respiratory syncytial virus infection in human immunodeficiency virus–infected children. J Pediatr 117:251–254, 1990.

161. Ellaurie M, Schutzbank TE, Rakusan TA, Lipson SM. Spectrum of adenovirus infection in pediatric HIV infection. Pediatr AIDS HIV Infect 4:211–214, 1993.

162. King JC, Burke AR, Clemens JD, et al. Respiratory syncytial virus illnesses in human immunodeficiency virus- and noninfected children. Pediatr Infect Dis J 1993; 12:733–739, 1993.

163. Joshi VV. Systemic lymphoproliferative lesions in children with AIDS. Pediatric AIDS & HIV Infection: From Fetus to Adolescent 1:44–48, 1990.

164. Gonzales CE, Venson D, Lee S, et al. Risk factors for fungemia in children infected with human immunodeficiency virus: a case control study. Clin Infect Dis 23:515–521, 1996.

165. Leggiadro RJ, Kline MW, Hughes WT. Extrapulmonary cryptococcosis in children with acquired immunodeficiency syndrome. Pediatr Infect Dis J 10:658–662, 1991.

166. Gonzales GE, Shetty D, Lewis LL, et al. Cryptococcosis in human immunodeficiency virus–infected children. Pediatr Infect Dis J 15:796–800, 1996.

167. Minamoto GY, Barlam TF, Vander Els NJ. Invasive aspergillosis in patients with AIDS. Clin Infect Dis 14:66–74, 1992.

168. Denning DW, Follansbee SE, Scolaro M, et al. Pulmonary aspergillosis in the acquired immunodeficiency syndrome. N Engl J Med 324:654–662, 1991.

169. Shetty D, Giri N, Gonzales CE, et al. Invasive aspergillosis in human immunodeficiency virus–infected children. Pediatr Infect Dis 16:216–221, 1997.

170. Sarosi GA, Johnson PC. Disseminated histoplasmosis in patients infected with human immunodeficiency virus. Clin Infect Dis 14 (suppl 1):S60–S67, 1992.

171. Pappas PG, Pottage JC, Powderly WG, et al. Blastomycosis in patients with the acquired immunodeficiency syndrome. Ann Intern Med 116:847–853, 1992.

172. Byers M, Feldman S, Edwards J. Disseminated histoplasmosis as the acquired immunodeficiency syndrome–defining illness in an infant. Pediatr Infect Dis J 11:127–128, 1992.

173. Simonds RJ, Oxtoby MJ, Caldwell B, et al. *Pneumocystis carinii* pneumonia among US children with perinatally acquired HIV infection. JAMA 270:470–473, 1993.

174. Centers for Disease Control and Prevention. 1995 Revised guidelines for prophylaxis against *Pneumocystis carinii* pneumonia for children infected with or perinatally exposed to human immunodeficiency virus. MMWR Morb Mortal Wkly Rep 44:1–12, 1995.

175. Mortier E, Pouchot J, Bossi P, Molinié V. Maternal-fetal transmission of *Pneumocystis carinii* in human immunodeficiency virus infection. N Engl J Med 332:825–826, 1995.

176. Bye MR, Bernstein LJ, Glaser J, Kleid D. *Pneumocystis carinii* pneumonia in young children with AIDS. Pediatr Pulmonol 9:251–253, 1990.

177. Connor E, Bagarazzi M, McSherry G, et al. Clinical and laboratory correlates of *Pneumocystis carinii* pneumonia in children infected with HIV. JAMA 265:1693–1697, 1991.

178. Gosey LL, Howard RM, Witebsky FG, et al. Advantages of a modified toluidine blue O stain and bronchoalveolar lavage for the diagnosis of *Pneumocystis carinii* pneumonia. J Clin Microbiol 22:803–807, 1985.

179. Ognibene FP, Gill VJ, Pizzo PA, et al. Induced sputum to diagnose *Pneumocystis carinii* pneumonia in immunosuppressed pediatric patients. J Pediatr 115:430–433, 1989.

180. Sattler FR, Cowan R, Nielsen DM, Ruskin J. Trimethoprim-sulfamethoxazole compared with pentamidine for treatment of *Pneumocystis carinii* pneumonia in the acquired immunodeficiency syndrome: a prospective, noncrossover study. Ann Intern Med 109:280–287, 1988.

181. Gagnon S, Boota AM, Fischl MA, et al. Corticosteroids as adjunctive therapy for severe *Pneumocystis carinii* pneumonia in the acquired immunodeficiency syndrome. N Engl J Med 323:1444–1450, 1990.

182. Bozzette SA, Sattler FR, Chiu J, et al. A controlled trial of early adjunctive treatment with corticosteroids for *Pneumocystis carinii* pneumonia in the acquired immunodeficiency syndrome. N Engl J Med 1323:1451–1457, 1990.

183. The National Institutes of Health–University of California Expert Panel for Corticosteroids as Adjunctive Therapy for Pneumocystis Pneumonia. Consensus statement on the use of corticosteroids as adjunctive therapy for *Pneumocystis* pneumonia in the acquired immunodeficiency syndrome. N Engl J Med 323:1500–1504, 1990.

184. McLaughlin GE, Virdee SS, Schleien CL, et al. Effect of corticosteroids on survival of children with acquired immunodeficiency syndrome and *Pneumocystis carinii*–related respiratory failure. J Pediatr 126:821–824, 1995.

185. Bernstein LJ, Bye MR, Rubinstein A. Prognostic factors and life expectancy in children with acquired immunodeficiency syndrome and *Pneumocystis carinii* pneumonia. Am J Dis Child 143:775–778, 1989.

186. Kovacs A, Frederick T, Church J, et al. CD4 T-lymphocyte counts and *Pneumocystis carinii* pneumonia in pediatric HIV infection. JAMA 265:1698–1703, 1991.

187. Centers for Disease Control. Guidelines for prophylaxis against *Pneumocystis carinii* pneumonia for children infected with human immunodeficiency virus. MMWR Morb Mortal Wkly Rep 40:1–13, 1991.

188. Simonds RJ, Lindegren ML, Thomas P, et al. Prophylaxis against *Pneumocystis carinii* pneumonia among children with perinatally acquired human immunodeficiency

189. Thea DM, Lambert G, Weedon J, et al. Benefit of primary prophylaxis before 18 months of age in reducing the incidence of *Pneumocystis carinii* pneumonia and early death in a cohort of 112 human immunodeficiency virus–infected infants. Pediatrics 97:59–64, 1996.

190. Mueller BU, Butler KM, Husson RN, Pizzo PA. *Pneumocystis carinii* pneumonia despite prophylaxis in children with human immunodeficiency virus infection. J Pediatr 119:992–994, 1991.

191. Nachman SA, Mueller BU, Mirochnik M, Pizzo PA. High failure rate of dapsone and pentamidine as *Pneumocystis carinii* pneumonia prophylaxis in human immunodeficiency virus–infected children. Pediatr Infect Dis J 13:1004–1006, 1994.

192. Mitchell CD. Toxoplasmosis. *In* Pizzo PA, Wilfert CM (eds): Pediatric AIDS: The Challenge of HIV Infection in Infants, Children, and Adolescents. Baltimore, Williams & Wilkins, 1994, pp 419–431.

193. Mitchell CD, Erlich SS, Mastrucci MT, et al. Congenital toxoplasmosis occurring in infants infected with human immunodeficiency virus I. Pediatr Infect Dis J 9:512–518, 1990.

194. Medlock MD, Tilleli JT, Pearl GS. Congenital cardiac toxoplasmosis in a newborn with acquired immunodeficiency syndrome. Pediatr Infect Dis J 9:129–132, 1990.

195. Cordell RL, Addiss DG. Cryptosporidiosis in child care settings: a review of the literature and recommendations for prevention and control. Pediatr Infect Dis J 13:310–317, 1994.

196. Mueller BU. Cancers in human immunodeficiency virus–infected children. J Natl Cancer Inst Monogr 23:31–35, 1998.

197. Siskin GP, Haller JO, Miller S, Sundaram R. AIDS-related lymphoma: Radiologic features in pediatric patients. Radiology 196:63–66, 1995.

198. Nadal D, Caduff R, Frey E, et al. Non-Hodgkin's lymphoma in four children infected with the human immunodeficiency virus. Cancer 73:224–230, 1994.

199. Granovsky MO, Mueller BU, Nicholson HS, et al. HIV-associated tumors in children: a case series from the Children's Cancer Group and National Cancer Institute, Tenth Annual Meeting of the American Society of Pediatric Hematology/Oncology, San Francisco, CA, September 10–20, 1997.

200. Connor E, Boccon-Gibod L, Joshi V, et al. Cutaneous acquired immunodeficiency syndrome–associated Kaposi's sarcoma in pediatric patients. Arch Dermatol 126:791–793, 1990.

201. Buck BE, Scott GB, Valdes-Dapena M, Parks WP. Kaposi sarcoma in two infants with acquired immune deficiency syndrome. J Pediatr 103:911–913, 1983.

202. Gutierrez-Ortega P, Hierro-Orozco S, Sanchez-Cisneros R, Montana LF. Kaposi's sarcoma in a 6-day-old infant with human immunodeficiency virus. Arch Dermatol 125:432–433, 1989.

203. McClain KL, Leach CT, Jenson HB, et al. Association of Epstein-Barr virus with leiomyosarcomas in young people with AIDS. N Engl J Med 332:12–18, 1995.

204. Jenson HB, Leach CT, McClain KL, et al. Benign and malignant smooth muscle tumors containing Epstein-Barr virus in children with AIDS. J Acquir Immune Defic Syndr Hum Retrovirol 14:A49, 1997.

205. Lobato MN, Caldwell MB, Ng P, Oxtoby MJ, Pediatric Spectrum of Disease Clinical Consortium. Encephalopathy in children with perinatally acquired human immu-

nodeficiency virus infection. J Pediatr 126:710–715, 1995.

206. Diaz C, Hanson C, Cooper ER, et al. Disease progression in a cohort of infants with vertically acquired HIV infection observed from birth: the Women and Infants Transmission Study (WITS). J Acquir Immune Defic Syndr Hum Retrovirol 18:221–228, 1998.

207. Cooper ER, Hanson C, Diaz C, et al. Encephalopathy and progression of human immunodeficiency virus disease in a cohort of children with perinatally acquired human immunodeficiency virus infection. Women and Infants Transmission Study Group. J Pediatr 132:808–812, 1998.

208. The European Collaborative Study. Neurologic signs in young children with human immunodeficiency virus infection. Pediatr Infect Dis J 9:402–406, 1990.

209. Park YD, Belman AL, Kim T-S, et al. Stroke in pediatric acquired immunodeficiency syndrome. Ann Neurol 28:303–311, 1990.

210. Lang C, Jacobi G, Kreuz W, et al. Rapid development of giant aneurysm at the base of the brain in an 8-year-old boy with perinatal HIV infection. Acta Histochem Suppl 42:S83–S90, 1992.

211. Belman AL, Diamond G, Dickson D, et al. Pediatric acquired immunodeficiency syndrome: neurologic symptoms. Am J Dis Child 142:29–35, 1988.

212. Epstein LG, Sharer LR, Goudsmit J. Neurological and neuropathological features of human immunodeficiency virus infection in children. Ann Neurol 23(suppl):S19–S23, 1988.

213. Gay GL, Armstrong FD, Cohen D, et al. The effects of HIV on cognitive and motor development in children born to HIV-seropositive women with no reported drug use: birth to 24 months. Pediatrics 96:1078–1082, 1995.

214. Wolters PL, Brouwers P, Moss HA, Pizzo PA. Differential receptive and expressive language functioning of children with symptomatic HIV disease and relation to CT scan brain abnormalities. Pediatrics 95:112–119, 1995.

215. Brouwers P, Belman A, Epstein L. Central nervous system involvement: manifestations, evaluation, and pathogenesis. In Pizzo PA, Wilfert CA (eds): Pediatric AIDS. The Challenge of HIV Infection in Infants, Children, and Adolescents. Baltimore, Williams & Wilkins, 1994, pp 433–455.

216. Brouwers P, DeCarli C, Civitello L, et al. Correlation between computed tomographic brain scan abnormalities and neuropsychological function in children with symptomatic human immunodeficiency virus disease. Arch Neurol 52:39–44, 1995.

217. Brouwers P, DeCarli C, Tudor-Williams G, et al. Interrelations among patterns of change in neurocognitive, CT brain imaging and CD4 measures associated with antiretroviral therapy in children with symptomatic HIV infection. Adv Neuroimmunol 4:223–231, 1994.

218. DeCarli C, Civitello LA, Brouwers P, Pizzo PA. The prevalence of computed tomographic abnormalities of the cerebrum in 100 consecutive children symptomatic with the human immunodeficiency virus. Ann Neurol 34:198–205, 1993.

219. DeCarli C, Fugate L, Falloon J, et al. Brain growth and cognitive improvement in children with human immunodeficiency virus–induced encephalopathy after 6 months of continuous infusion zidovudine therapy. J Acquir Immune Defic Syndr 4:585–592, 1991.

220. Sharer LR, Saito Y, Epstein LG, Blumberg BM. Detection of HIV-1 DNA in pediatric AIDS brain tissue by two-step ISPCR. Adv Neuroimmunol 4:283–285, 1994.

221. Sharer LR. Neuropathological aspects of HIV-1 infection in children. In Gendelman HE, Lipton SA, Epstein L, Swindells S (eds): The Neurology of AIDS. New York, Chapman & Hall, 1998, pp 408–418.

222. Saito Y, Sharer LR, Epstein LG, et al. Overexpression of nef as a marker for restricted HIV-1 infection of astrocytes in postmortem pediatric central nervous tissues. Neurology 44:474–481, 1994.

223. Baba TW, Liska V, Ruprecht RM. HIV-1/SIV infection of the fetal and neonatal nervous system. In Gendelman HE, Lipton SA, Epstein L, Swindells S (eds): The Neurology of AIDS. New York, Chapman & Hall, 1998, pp 443–456.

224. Pratt RD, Nichols S, McKinney N, et al. Virologic markers of human immunodeficiency virus type 1 in cerebrospinal fluid of infected children. J Infect Dis 174:288–293, 1996.

225. Sei S, Stewart SK, Farley M, et al. Evaluation of HIV-1 RNA levels in cerebrospinal fluid and viral resistance to zidovudine in children with HIV encephalopathy. J Infect Dis 174:1200–1206, 1996.

226. Gelbard HA. HIV-1-induced neurotoxicity in the developing central nervous system. In Gendelman HE, Lipton SA, Epstein L, Swindells S (eds): The Neurology of AIDS. New York, Chapman & Hall, 1998, pp 419–424.

227. Brouwers P, Heyes MP, Moss HA, et al. Quinolinic acid in the cerebrospinal fluid of children with symptomatic human immunodeficiency virus type 1 disease: relationships to clinical status and therapeutic response. J Infect Dis 168:1380–1386, 1993.

228. Sei S, Saito K, Stewart SK, et al. Increased human immunodeficiency virus (HIV) type 1 DNA content and quinolinic acid concentration in brain tissues from patients with HIV encephalopathy. J Infect Dis 172:638–647, 1995.

229. Srugo I, Wittek AE, Israele V, Brunell PA. Meningoencephalitis in a neonate congenitally infected with human immunodeficiency virus type 1. J Pediatr 120:93–95, 1992.

230. Sharer LR, Dowling PC, Michaels J, et al. Spinal cord disease in children with HIV-1 infection: a combined molecular biological and neuropathological study. Neuropathol Appl Neurobiol 16:317–331, 1990.

231. Brouwers P, Moss H, Wolters P, et al. Effect of continuous-infusion zidovudine therapy on neuropsychologic functioning in children with symptomatic human immunodeficiency virus infection. J Pediatr 117:980–985, 1990.

232. Stiehm ER, Bryson YJ, Frenkel LM, et al. Prednisone improves human immunodeficiency virus encephalopathy in children. Pediatr Infect Dis J 11:49–50, 1992.

233. Cunningham ET, Margolis TP. Ocular manifestations of HIV infection. N Engl J Med 339:236–244, 1998.

234. de Smet MD, Nussenblatt RB. Ocular manifestations of HIV in pediatric populations. In Pizzo PA, Wilfert CM (eds): Pediatric AIDS: The Challenge of HIV Infection in Infants, Children, and Adolescents. Baltimore, Williams & Wilkins, 1994, pp 457–466.

235. Bottoni F, Gonnella P, Autelitano A, Orzalesi N. Diffuse necrotizing retinochoroiditis in a child with AIDS and toxoplasmic encephalitis. Graefes Arch Clin Exp Ophthalmol 228:36–39, 1990.

236. Lopez JS, deSmet MD, Masur H, et al. Orally administered 566C80 for treatment of ocular toxoplasmosis in a patient with the acquired immunodeficiency syndrome. Am J Ophthalmol 113:331–333, 1992.

237. Telzak EE, Cote RJ, Gold JWM, et al. Extrapulmonary Pneumocystis carinii infections. Rev Infect Dis 12:380–386, 1990.

238. Connor EM, Andiman WA. Lymphoid interstitial pneumonitis. *In* Pizzo PA, Wilfert CM (eds): Pediatric AIDS: The Challenge of HIV Infection in Infants, Children, and Adolescents. Baltimore, Williams & Wilkins, 1994, pp 467–482.

239. Sharland M, Gibb DM, Holland F. Respiratory morbidity from lymphocytic interstitial pneumonitis (LIP) in vertically acquired HIV infection. Arch Dis Child 76:334–336, 1997.

240. Scott GB, Hutto C, Makuch RW, et al. Survival in children with perinatally acquired human immunodeficiency virus type 1 infection. N Engl J Med 321:1791–1796, 1989.

241. Luginbuhl LM, Orav EJ, McIntosh K, Lipshultz SE. Cardiac morbidity and related mortality in children with HIV infection. JAMA 269:2869–2875, 1993.

242. Lipshultz SE, Orav EJ, Sanders SP, et al. Cardiac structure and function in children with human immunodeficiency virus infection treated with zidovudine. N Engl J Med 327:1260–1265, 1992.

243. Lipshultz SE, Fox CH, Perez-Atayde AR, et al. Identification of human immunodeficiency virus-1 RNA and DNA in the heart of a child with cardiovascular abnormalities and congenital acquired immune deficiency syndrome. Am J Cardiol 66:246–250, 1990.

244. Joshi VV, Gadol C, Connor E, et al. Dilated cardiomyopathy in children with acquired immunodeficiency syndrome: a pathologic study of five cases. Hum Pathol 19:69–73, 1988.

245. Lewis W. AIDS: cardiac findings from 115 autopsies. Prog Cardiovasc Dis 32:207–215, 1989.

246. Grody WW, Cheng L, Lewis W. Infection of the heart by the human immunodeficiency virus. Am J Cardiol 66:203–206, 1990.

247. Joshi VV, Pawel B, Connor E, et al. Arteriopathy in children with acquired immune deficiency syndrome. Pediatr Pathol 7:261–275, 1987.

248. Kure K, Park YD, Kim T-S, et al. Immunohistochemical localization of an HIV epitope in cerebral aneurysmal arteriopathy in pediatric acquired immunodeficiency syndrome (AIDS). Pediatr Pathol 9:655–667, 1989.

249. Husson RN, Saini R, Lewis LL, et al. Cerebral artery aneurysms in children infected with human immunodeficiency virus. J Pediatr 121:927–930, 1992.

250. Galli L, de Martino M, Tovo P-A, et al. Onset of clinical signs in children with HIV-1 perinatal infection. AIDS 9:455–461, 1995.

251. Pickering LK. Infections of the gastrointestinal tract. *In* Pizzo PA, Wilfert CM (eds): Pediatric AIDS: The Challenge of HIV Infection in Infants, Children, and Adolescents. Baltimore, Williams & Wilkins, 1994, pp 377–404.

252. Yolken RH, Li S, Perman J, Viscidi R. Persistent diarrhea and fecal shedding of retroviral nucleic acids in children infected with human immunodeficiency virus. J Infect Dis 164:61–66, 1991.

253. Grunfeld C, Feingold KR. Metabolic disturbances and wasting in the acquired immunodeficiency syndrome. N Engl J Med 327:329–337, 1992.

254. Lewis JD, Winter HS. Intestinal and hepatobiliary diseases in HIV-infected children. Gastroenterol Clin North Am 24:119–132, 1995.

255. Kotloff KL, Johnson JP, Nair P, et al. Diarrheal morbidity during the first 2 years of life among HIV-infected infants. JAMA 271:448–452, 1994.

256. Thea DM, St. Louis ME, Atido U, et al. A prospective study of diarrhea and HIV-1 infection among 429 Zairian infants. N Engl J Med 329:1696–1702, 1993.

257. Miller TL. Nutritional assessment and its clinical application in children infected with the human immunodeficiency virus. J Pediatr 129:633–636, 1996.

258. Leggiadro RJ, Lewis D, Whitington GL, et al. Chronic hepatitis associated with perinatal HIV infection. AIDS Reader March/April:57–61, 1992.

259. Persaud D, Bangaru B, Greco A, et al. Cholestatic hepatitis in children infected with the human immunodeficiency virus. Pediatr Infect Dis J 12:492–498, 1993.

260. Miller TL, Winter HS, Luginbuhl LM, et al. Pancreatitis in pediatric human immunodeficiency virus infection. J Pediatr 120:223–227, 1992.

261. Butler KM, Venzon D, Henry N, et al. Pancreatitis in human immunodeficiency virus–infected children receiving dideoxyinosine. Pediatrics 91:747–751, 1993.

262. Strauss J, Abitol C, Zilleruelo G, et al. Renal disease in children with the acquired immunodeficiency syndrome. N Engl J Med 321:625–630, 1989.

263. Strauss J, Zilleruelo G, Abitbol C, et al. Human immunodeficiency virus nephropathy. Pediatr Nephrol 7:220–225, 1993.

264. Ingulli E, Tejani A, Fikrig S, et al. Nephrotic syndrome associated with acquired immunodeficiency syndrome in children. J Pediatr 119:710–716, 1991.

265. Schoeneman MJ, Ghali V, Lieberman K, Reisman L. IgA nephritis in a child with human immunodeficiency virus: a unique form of human immunodeficiency virus–associated nephropathy? Pediatr Nephrol 6:46–49, 1992.

266. Kimmel PL, Phillips TM, Ferreira-Centeno A, et al. Brief report: Idiotypic IgA nephropathy in patients with human immunodeficiency virus infection. N Engl J Med 327:702–706, 1992.

267. Mueller BU, Sleasman J, Nelson RP Jr, et al. A phase I/II study of the protease inhibitor indinavir in children with HIV infection. Pediatrics 102:101–109, 1998.

268. Bruce RG, Munch LC, Hoven AD, et al. Urolithiasis associated with the protease inhibitor indinavir. Urology 50:513–518, 1997.

269. Gertner JM, Kaufman FR, Donfield SM, et al. Delayed somatic growth and pubertal development in human immunodeficiency virus–infected hemophiliac boys: Hemophilia Growth and Development Study. J Pediatr 124:896–902, 1994.

270. Fisher GD, Rinaldo CR, Gbadero D, et al. Seroprevalence of HIV-1 and HIV-2 infection among children diagnosed with protein-calorie malnutrition in Nigeria. Epidemiol Infect 110:373–378, 1993.

271. Brettler DB, Forsberg A, Bolivar E, et al. Growth failure as a prognostic indicator for progression to acquired immunodeficiency syndrome in children with hemophilia. J Pediatr 117:584–588, 1990.

272. Laue L, Pizzo PA, Butler K, Cutler GB. Growth and neuroendocrine dysfunction in children with acquired immunodeficiency syndrome. J Pediatr 117:541–545, 1990.

273. Schwartz LJ, St. Louis Y, Wu R, et al. Endocrine function in children with human immunodeficiency virus infection. Am J Dis Child 145:330–333, 1991.

274. Grinspoon SK, Bilezikian JP. HIV disease and the endocrine system. N Engl J Med 327:1360–1365, 1992.

275. Hirschfeld S, Laue L, Cutler GB Jr, Pizzo PA. Thyroid abnormalities in children infected with human immunodeficiency virus. J Pediatr 128:70–74, 1996.

276. Papiernik M, Brossard Y, Mulliez N, et al. Thymic abnormalities in fetuses aborted from human immunodeficiency virus type 1 seropositive women. Pediatrics 89:297–301, 1992.

277. Joshi VV, Oleske JM, Saad S, et al. Thymus biopsy in

children with acquired immunodeficiency syndrome. Arch Pathol Med 110:837–842, 1986.

278. Sei S, Kleiner DE, Kopp JB, et al. Quantitative analysis of viral burden in tissues from adults and children with symptomatic human immunodeficiency virus type 1 infection assessed by polymerase chain reaction. J Infect Dis 170:325–333, 1994.

279. Pantaleo G, Cohen OJ, Schacker T, et al. Evolutionary pattern of human immunodeficiency virus (HIV) replication and distribution in lymph nodes following primary infection: implications for antiviral therapy. Nature Med 4:341–345, 1998.

280. Pantaleo G, Fauci AS. HIV-1 infection in the lymphoid organs: a model of disease development. J NIH Res 5:68–72, 1993.

281. Mueller BU, Sei S, Anderson B, et al. Comparison of virus burden in blood and sequential lymph node biopsy specimens from children infected with human immunodeficiency virus. J Pediatr 129:410–418, 1996.

282. Scott GB, Buck BE, Leterman JG, et al. Acquired immunodeficiency syndrome in infants. N Engl J Med 310:76–81, 1984.

283. Ellaurie M, Burns ER, Rubinstein A. Hematologic manifestations in pediatric HIV infection: severe anemia as a prognostic factor. Am J Pediatr Hematol Oncol 12:449–453, 1990.

284. Mueller BU. Hematological problems and their management in children with HIV infection. In Pizzo PA, Wilfert CM (eds): Pediatric AIDS: The Challenge of HIV Infection in Infants, Children, and Adolescents. Baltimore, Williams & Wilkins, 1994, pp 591–602.

285. Forsyth BW, Andiman WA, O'Connor T. Development of a prognosis-based clinical staging system for infants infected with human immunodeficiency virus. J Pediatr 129:648–655, 1996.

286. Mueller BU, Tannenbaum S, Pizzo PA. Bone marrow aspirates and biopsies in children with human immunodeficiency virus infection. J Pediatr Hematol Oncol 18:266–271, 1996.

287. Parmentier L, Boucary D, Salmon D. Pure red cell aplasia in an HIV-infected patient. AIDS 6:234–235, 1992.

288. Nigro G, Castelli Gattinara G, Mattia S, et al. Parvovirus-B19–related pancytopenia in children with HIV infection. Lancet 340:115, 1992.

289. Abkowitz JL, Brown KE, Wood RW, et al. Clinical relevance of parvovirus B19 as a cause of anemia in patients with human immunodeficiency virus infection. J Infect Dis 176:269–273, 1997.

290. Holodniy M, Margolis D, Carroll R, et al. Quantitative relationship between platelet count and plasma virion HIV RNA. AIDS 10:232–233, 1996.

291. Ballem PJ, Belzberg A, Devine DV, et al. Kinetic studies of the mechanism of thrombocytopenia in patients with human immunodeficiency virus infection. N Engl J Med 327:1779–1789, 1992.

292. Rigaud M, Leibovitz E, Sin Quee C, et al. Thrombocytopenia in children infected with human immunodeficiency virus: long-term follow-up and therapeutic considerations. J Acquir Immune Defic Syndr 5:450–455, 1992.

293. Abuaf N, Laperche S, Rajoely B, et al. Autoantibodies to phospholipids and the coagulation proteins in AIDS. Thromb Haemost 77:856–861, 1997.

294. Sorice M, Griggi T, Arcieri P, et al. Protein S and HIV infection: the role of anticardiolipin and anti–protein S antibodies. Thromb Res 73:165–175, 1994.

295. Rodriguez-Mahou M, Lopez-Longo J, Lapointe N, et al. Autoimmune phenomena in children with human immu-nodeficiency virus infection and acquired immunodeficiency syndrome. Acta Paediatr Suppl 400:31–34, 1994.

296. Coopman SA, Johnson RA, Platt R, Stern RS. Cutaneous disease and drug reactions in HIV infection. N Engl J Med 328:1670–1674, 1993.

297. Prose NS. Skin problems. In Pizzo PA, Wilfert CM (eds): Pediatric AIDS: The Challenge of HIV Infection in Infants, Children, and Adolescents. Baltimore, Williams & Wilkins, 1994, pp 535–546.

298. von Seidlein L, Gillette SG, Bryson Y, et al. Frequent recurrence and persistence of varicella-zoster virus infections in children infected with human immunodeficiency virus type 1. J Pediatr 128:52–57, 1996.

299. Blanche S, Newell ML, Mayaux MJ, et al. Morbidity and mortality in European children vertically infected by HIV-1. The French Pediatric HIV Infection Study Group and European Collaborative Study. J Acquir Immune Defic Syndr Hum Retrovirol 14:442–450, 1997.

300. Palella FJ, Delaney KM, Moorman AC, et al. Declining morbidity and mortality among patients with advanced human immunodeficiency virus infection. N Engl J Med 338:853–860, 1998.

301. Jean SS, Reed GW, Verdier R-I, et al. Clinical manifestations of human immunodeficiency virus infection in Haitian children. Pediatr Infect Dis J 16:600–606, 1997.

302. Braddick MR, Kreiss JK, Embree JE, et al. Impact of maternal HIV infection on obstetrical and early neonatal outcome. AIDS 4:1001–1005, 1990.

303. Moye J Jr, Rich KC, Kalish LA, et al. Natural history of somatic growth in infants born to women infected by human immunodeficiency virus. Women and Infants Transmission Study Group. J Pediatr 128:58–69, 1996.

304. Frederick T, Mascola L, Eller A, et al. Progression of human immunodeficiency virus disease among infants and children infected perinatally with human immunodeficiency virus or through neonatal blood transfusion. Pedia Infect Dis J 13:1091–1097, 1994.

305. Blanche S, Mayaux M-J, Rouzioux C, et al. Relation of the course of HIV infection in children to the severity of the disease in their mothers at delivery. N Engl J Med 330:308–312, 1994.

306. Blanche S, Rouzioux C, Guihard Moscato M-L, et al. A prospective study of infants born to women seropositive for human immunodeficiency virus type 1. N Engl J Med 320:1643–1648, 1989.

307. Mayaux M-J, Burgard M, Teglas J-P, et al. Neonatal characteristics in rapidly progressive perinatally acquired HIV-1 disease. JAMA 275:606–610, 1996.

308. Zaknun D, Orav J, Kornegay J, et al. Correlation of ribonucleic acid polymerase chain reaction, acid dissociated p24 antigen, and neopterin with progression of disease. J Pediatr 130:898–905, 1997.

309. Dickover RE, Dillon M, Leung KM, et al. Early prognostic indicators in primary perinatal human immunodeficiency virus type 1 infection: importance of viral RNA and the timing of transmission on long-term outcome. J Infect Dis 178:375–387, 1998.

310. Abrams EJ, Weedon J, Steketee RW, et al. Association of human immunodeficiency virus (HIV) load early in life with disease progression among HIV-infected infants. New York City Perinatal HIV Transmission Collaborative Study Group. J Infect Dis 178:101–108, 1998.

311. The European Collaborative Study. Caesarean section and risk of vertical transmission of HIV-1 infection. Lancet 343:1464–1467, 1994.

312. Scarlatti G. Paediatric HIV infection. Lancet 348:863–868, 1996.

313. Lurie P, Wolfe SM. Unethical trials of interventions to

reduce perinatal transmission of the human immunodeficiency virus in developing countries. N Engl J Med 337:853–856, 1997.

314. Mofenson LM, Burns DN. Passive immunization to prevent mother-infant transmission of human immunodeficiency virus: current issues and future directions. Pediatr Infect Dis J 10:456–462, 1991.

315. Lambert JS, Mofenson LM, Fletcher CV, et al. Safety and pharmacokinetics of hyperimmune anti-human immunodeficiency virus (HIV) immunoglobulin administered to HIV-infected pregnant women and their newborns. Pediatric AIDS Clinical Trials Group Protocol 185 Pharmacokinetic Study Group. J Infect Dis 175:283–291, 1997.

316. American Academy of Pediatrics Committee on Infectious Diseases. Recommended timing of routine measles immunization for children who have recently received immune globulin preparations. Pediatrics 93:682–685, 1994.

317. Adamson PC, Wu TC, Meade BD, et al. Pertussis in a previously immunized child with human immunodeficiency virus infection. J Pediatr 115:598–592, 1989.

318. The National Institute of Child Health and Human Development Intravenous Immunoglobulin Study Group. Intravenous immune globulin for the prevention of bacterial infections in children with symptomatic human immunodeficiency virus infection. N Engl J Med 325:73–80, 1991.

319. Centers for Disease Control and Prevention. Report of the NIH Panel to Define Principles of Therapy of HIV Infection and Guidelines for the Use of Antiretroviral Agents in HIV-Infected Adults and Adolescents. MMWR Morb Mortal Wkly Rep 47:1–83, 1998.

320. Centers for Disease Control and Prevention. Guidelines for the use of antiretroviral agents in pediatric HIV infection. MMWR Morb Mortal Wkly Rep 47:1–44, 1998.

321. Working Group on Antiretroviral Therapy and Medical Management of Infants, Children, and Adolescents with HIV Infection. Antiretroviral therapy and medical management of pediatric HIV infection. Pediatrics 102:1005–1085, 1998.

322. Lyman WD, Tanaka KE, Kress Y, et al. Zidovudine concentrations in human fetal tissue: implications for perinatal AIDS. Lancet 335:1280–1281, 1990.

323. Garland M, Szeto HH, Daniel SS, et al. Placental transfer and fetal metabolism of zidovudine in the baboon. Pediatr Res 44:47–53, 1998.

324. Sperling RS, Roboz J, Dische R, et al. Zidovudine pharmacokinetics during pregnancy. Am J Perinatol 9:247–249, 1992.

325. O'Sullivan MJ, Boyer PJJ, Scott GB, et al. The pharmacokinetics and safety of zidovudine in the third trimester of pregnancy for women infected with human immunodeficiency virus and their infants: Phase I Acquired Immunodeficiency Syndrome Clinical Trials Group study (protocol 082). Am J Obstet Gynecol 168:1510–1516, 1993.

326. Watts DH, Brown ZA, Tartaglione T, et al. Pharmacokinetic disposition of zidovudine during pregnancy. J Infect Dis 163:226–232, 1991.

327. Lopez-Anaya A, Unadkat JD, Schumann LA, Smith AL. Pharmacokinetics of zidovudine (azidothymidine): I. Transplacental transfer. J Acquir Immune Defic Syndr 3:959–964, 1990.

328. Lopez-Anaya A, Unadkat JD, Schumann LA, Smith AL. Pharmacokinetics of zidovudine (azidothymidine): II. Development of metabolic and renal clearance pathways

in the neonate. J Acquir Immune Defic Syndr 3:1052–1058, 1990.

329. Boucher FD, Au DS, Martin DM, et al. Pharmacokinetics and safety of azidothymidine (AZT) in infants less than three months old, exposed at birth to HIV. Clin Res 37:190A, 1989.

330. Boucher FD, Modlin JF, Weller S, et al. Phase I evaluation of zidovudine administered to infants exposed at birth to the human immunodeficiency virus. J Pediatr 122:137–144, 1993.

331. Olivero OA, Anderson LM, Diwan BA, et al. Transplacental effects of 3'-azido-2',3'-dideoxythymidine (AZT): tumorigenicity in mice and genotoxicity in mice and monkeys. J Natl Cancer Inst 89:1602–1608, 1997.

332. Olivero OA, Anderson LM, Diwan BA, et al. AZT is a genotoxic transplacental carcinogen in animal models. J Acquir Immune Defic Syndr Hum Retrovirol 14:A29, 1997.

333. Dalakas MC, Illa I, Pezeshkpour GH, et al. Mitochondrial myopathy caused by long-term zidovudine therapy. N Engl J Med 322:1098–1105, 1990.

334. Brady MT, McGrath N, Brouwers P, et al. Randomized study of the tolerance and efficacy of high- versus low-dose zidovudine in human immunodeficiency virus–infected children with mild to moderate symptoms (AIDS Clinical Trial Group 128). J Infect Dis 173:1097–1106, 1996.

335. Balis FM, Pizzo PA, Butler KM, et al. Clinical pharmacology of 2',3'-dideoxyinosine in human immunodeficiency virus–infected children. J Infec Dis 165:99–104, 1992.

336. Pons JC, Boubon MC, Taburet AM, et al. Fetoplacental passage of 2',3'-dideoxyinosine. Lancet 337:732, 1991.

337. Pereira CM, Nosbisch C, Winter HR, et al. Transplacental pharmacokinetics of dideoxyinosine in pigtailed macaques. Antimicrob Agents Chemother 38:781–786, 1994.

338. Pereira CM, Nosbisch C, Unadkat JD. Pharmacokinetics of dideoxyinosine in neonatal pigtailed macaques. Antimicrob Agents Chemother 38:787–789, 1994.

339. Lai KR, Gang DL, Zawacki JK, Cooley TP. Fulminant hepatic failure associated with 2',3'-dideoxyinosine (ddI). Ann Intern Med 115:283–284, 1991.

340. Whitcup SM, Butler KM, Caruso R, et al. Retinal toxicity in human immunodeficiency virus–infected children treated with 2',3'-dideoxyinosine. Am J Ophthalmol 113:1–7, 1992.

341. Whitcup S, Butler K, Pizzo P, Nussenblatt R. Retinal lesions in children treated with dideoxyinosine. N Engl J Med 326:1226–1227, 1992.

342. Lewis LL, Venzon D, Church J, et al. Lamivudine in children with human immunodeficiency virus infection: A phase I/II study. J Infect Dis 174:16–25, 1996.

343. Mueller BU, Lewis LL, Yuen GJ, et al. Serum and cerebrospinal fluid pharmacokinetics of intravenous and oral lamivudine in human immunodeficiency virus–infected children. Antimicrob Agents Chemother 42:3187–3192, 1998.

344. Grob PM, Wu JC, Cohen KA, et al. Nonnucleoside inhibitors of HIV-1 reverse transcriptase: nevirapine as a prototype drug. AIDS Res Hum Retrovir 8:145–152, 1992.

345. Grob PM, Cao Y, Muchmore E, et al. Prophylaxis against HIV-1 infection in chimpanzees by nevirapine, a nonnucleoside inhibitor of reverse transcriptase. Nature Med 3:665–670, 1997.

346. Richman DD, Havlir D, Corbeil J, et al. Nevirapine

resistance mutations of human immunodeficiency virus type 1 selected during therapy. J Virol 68:1660–1666, 1994.

347. Luzuriaga K, Bryson Y, McSherry G, et al. Pharmacokinetics, safety, and activity of nevirapine in human immunodeficiency virus type 1–infected children. J Infect Dis 174:713–721, 1996.

348. Mirochnik M, Sullivan J, Gagnier P, et al. Safety and pharmacokinetics (PK) of nevirapine in neonates born to HIV-1 infected women. Presented before the 4th Conference on Retroviruses and Opportunistic Infections, Washington, DC, 1997.

349. Krogstad P, Kerr B, Anderson R, et al. Phase I study of the HIV protease inhibitor nelfinavir mesylate (NFV) in HIV+ children. Presented before the 4th Conference on Retroviruses and Opportunistic Infections, Washington, DC, 1997.

350. Flexner C. HIV-protease inhibitors. N Engl J Med 338:1281–1292, 1998.

351. Mueller BU, Nelson RP Jr, Sleasman J, et al. A phase I/II study of the protease inhibitor ritonavir in children with human immunodeficiency virus infection. Pediatrics 101:335–343, 1998.

352. Havens PL, Cuene BE, Holtgrave DR. Lifetime cost of care for children with human immunodeficiency virus infection. Pediatr Infect Dis J 16:607–610, 1997.

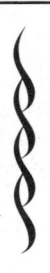

C H A P T E R   1 0

Enteroviruses

JAMES D. CHERRY, M.D., M.Sc.

Enteroviruses—coxsackieviruses, echoviruses, enteroviruses, and polioviruses—are responsible for significant and frequent human illnesses, with protean clinical manifestations.[1-12] Enteroviruses are one genus of the Picornaviridae.[13-15] They were first categorized together and named in 1957 by a committee sponsored by the National Foundation for Infantile Paralysis[16]; the human alimentary tract was believed to be the natural habitat of these agents. They are grouped together because of similarities in physical and biochemical properties, as well as shared features in their epidemiology and pathogenesis and the many disease syndromes that they cause.

Congenital and neonatal infections have been linked with many different enteroviruses, and representatives of all four major enterovirus groups—coxsackievirus, echovirus, enterovirus, and poliovirus—have been associated with disease in the neonate.[1-12, 17-29]

Poliomyelitis, the first enteroviral disease to be recognized and the most important one, has had a long history.[30] The earliest record is an Egyptian stele of the eighteenth dynasty (1580–1350 BC), which shows a young priest with a withered, shortened leg, the characteristic deformity of paralytic poliomyelitis.[31, 32] Underwood, a London pediatrician, published the first medical description in 1789 in his *Treatise on Diseases of Children*.[33] During the nineteenth century, many reports appeared in Europe and the United States describing small clusters of cases of "infantile paralysis." The authors were greatly puzzled as to the nature of the affliction; not until the 1860s and 1870s was the spinal cord firmly established as the seat of the pathologic process. The contagious nature of poliomyelitis was not appreciated until the latter part of the nineteenth century. Medin, a Swedish pediatrician, was the first to describe the epidemic nature of poliomyelitis (1890), and his pupil Wickman worked out the basic principles of the epidemiology.[34]

The virus was first isolated in monkeys by Landsteiner and Popper in 1908.[35] The availability of a laboratory animal assay system opened up many avenues of research that, in the ensuing 40 years, led to the demonstration that an unrecognized intestinal infection was common and that paralytic disease was a relatively uncommon event.

Coxsackieviruses and echoviruses have had a shorter history. Epidemic pleurodynia was clinically described in 1735 by Hannaeus more than 200 years before the coxsackieviral etiology of this disease was discovered.[36] In 1948, Dalldorf and Sickles first reported the isolation of a coxsackievirus by using suckling mouse inoculation.[37]

In 1949, Enders and associates[38] reported the growth of poliovirus type 2 in tissue culture, and their techniques paved the way for the recovery of a large number of other cytopathic viruses. Most of these "new" viruses failed to produce illness in laboratory animals. Because the relationships of many of these newly recovered agents to human disease were unknown, they were called orphan viruses.[4] Later, several agents were grouped together and called enteric cytopathogenic human orphan viruses, or echoviruses.

The three-dimensional structure of poliovirus at 2.9 Å resolution by x-ray crystallographic methods was described in 1985.[39] This event yielded important information related to the structure and function of enteroviruses and may be useful in the future for the development of both vaccines and antiviral agents.

The most notable advance during the past 15 years has been the dramatic reduction in worldwide poliomyelitis due to immunization with oral polio vaccines (OPV).[40-43] The last case of confirmed paralytic polio in the Western Hemisphere occurred in 1991,[43] and the World Health Assembly established the goal of global polio eradication by the year 2000.[44]

Aside from the polio immunization successes, there have been few major advances, new concepts, or new modes of treatment for enteroviral diseases. However, the use of nucleic acid detection systems for enteroviral diagnosis has progressed over the past 10 years such that rapid diagnosis of meningitis and other enteroviral illnesses is now possible.[45-62] In addition, there has been recent progress in the development of specific antienteroviral drugs.[63, 64]

THE VIRUSES

Morphology and Classification[11, 13, 15, 65-72]

The enteroviruses are single-stranded RNA viruses belonging to the Picornaviridae (*pico*, "small"). They are grouped together because they share certain physical and biochemical properties. In electron micrographs, the viruses are seen as 24- to 30-nm particles consisting of naked protein capsids constituting 70 to 75% of the particles and a dense central core (nucleoid) of RNA. The virion has icosahedral symmetry owing to the regular organization of identical protein subunits. The subunits are arranged in axes of fivefold, threefold, and twofold symmetry within the protein shell of the virus. The capsid of enteroviruses is made up of rather indistinct capsomeres, the exact number of which has been variously reported as 32, 42, or 60.

All enteroviruses contain polypeptide chains (structural proteins; protomers): VP1, VP2, VP3, and VP4. These coat proteins protect the RNA genomes from nucleases, are important determinants of host range and tropism, determine antigenicity, and deliver the RNA genome into the cytoplasm of new host cells.

The genome of enteroviruses is a single-stranded, positive-strand RNA molecule.[68] It contains a 5' noncoding region (5' NCR), which is followed by a single long open reading frame, a short 3' NCR and a poly (A) tail. The four capsid proteins (VP1–VP4) and seven nonstructural proteins (2A, 2B, 2C, 3A, 3B, 3C, and 3D) result from a cleaved long polyprotein that was translated from genomic RNA.

Viral components and complete virions are formed in the cytoplasm of infected cells. If the rate of virus assembly is rapid and many particles are formed in one area, crystallization may occur.

The classification of human enteroviruses is shown in Table 10–1. The enteroviral subgroups were originally differentiated from each other by their different effects

TABLE 10–1
Human Enteroviruses: Animal and Tissue Culture Spectrum[a]

VIRUS	ANTIGENIC TYPES[b]	CYTOPATHIC EFFECT (CPE)		ILLNESS AND PATHOLOGY	
		Monkey Kidney Culture	Human Tissue Culture	Suckling Mouse	Monkey
Polioviruses	1–3	+	+	–	+
Coxsackieviruses A	1–24[c]	–	–	+	–
Coxsackieviruses B	1–6	+	+	+	–
Echoviruses	1–34[d]	+	±	–	–

[a]Many enteroviral strains have been isolated that do not conform to these categories.
[b]New types, beginning with type 68, are now assigned enterovirus type numbers instead of coxsackievirus or echovirus numbers. Types 68 through 71 have been identified.
[c]Type 23 was found to be the same as echovirus 9.
[d]Echovirus 10 was reclassified as a reovirus; echovirus 26 was reclassified as a rhinovirus.

in tissue cultures and in animals. Although these differentiating factors are still useful, many strains have now been isolated that do not conform to such rigid specificities. For example, several coxsackievirus A strains grow and have a cytopathic effect (CPE) in monkey kidney tissue cultures, and some echovirus strains cause paralysis in mice. Newly characterized enteroviruses are now assigned enterovirus type numbers instead of coxsackievirus or echovirus numbers. Prototype enteroviral strains Fermon, Toluca-1, J670/71, and BrCr have been assigned enteroviral numbers 68 through 71, respectively. Definitive identification of enteroviral types is made by neutralization with type-specific antiserum.

Complete or partial genetic sequence data are now available from several enteroviruses.[68–72] In general, sequence comparisons partially support the classic subgrouping of enteroviruses as noted in Table 10–1. However, in many instances genetic relationships do not correlate with these subdivisions.[68] At the present time the analysis of different genomic regions of sequenced human enteroviruses reveals two clusters in the 5′ NCR and four clusters in the coding region and in the 3′ NCR. Therefore, all human enteroviruses with complete or partial sequence data from the coding region fall into four clusters: poliovirus-like (C-cluster); enterovirus 70-like (D-cluster); coxsackievirus B-like (B-cluster); and coxsackievirus A-like (A-cluster). The C-cluster includes coxsackieviruses A1, A11, A13, A15, A17 through A22, A24 and polioviruses 1 through 3. The D-cluster contains enteroviruses 68 and 70. The B-cluster contains coxsackieviruses A9, B1, B3 through B5, enterovirus 69, and echoviruses 1, 4, 6, 7, 11, 12, 27, and 30. The A cluster contains coxsackieviruses A2, A3, A5, A7, A8, A10, A12, A14, A16, and enterovirus 71.

Characteristics and Host Systems[11, 13, 15, 32, 66, 67]

Enteroviruses are relatively stable viruses in that they retain activity for several days at room temperature and can be stored indefinitely at ordinary freezer temperatures ($-20°$ C). They are rapidly inactivated by heat ($>56°$ C), formaldehyde, chlorination, and ultraviolet light but are resistant to 70% alcohol, 5% Lysol, quaternary ammonium compounds, ether, deoxycholate, and detergents that are effective against lipid-containing viruses.

Enteroviral strains grow rapidly when adapted to susceptible host systems and cause cytopathology in 3 to 7 days. The typical tissue culture CPE is shown in Figure 10–1; characteristic pathologic findings in mice are shown in Figures 10–2 and 10–3. Final titers of virus recovered in the laboratory vary markedly among different viral strains and the host systems employed; usually concentrations of 10^3 to 10^7 infectious doses per 0.1 ml of tissue culture fluid or tissue homogenate are obtained. Unadapted viral strains frequently require long periods of incubation in both tissue cultures or suckling mice before visible evidence of growth is observed. Blind passage is occasionally necessary for cytopathology to become apparent.

Although many different primary and secondary tissue culture systems support the growth of various enteroviruses, it is generally accepted that primary rhesus monkey kidney cultures have the most inclusive spectrum. Other simian kidney tissue cultures, although less commonly used, also have the same broad spectrum.[73] Tissue cultures of human origin have a more limited spectrum, but several echovirus types have had more consistent primary isolation in human embryonic lung fibroblastic cell strains than in monkey kidney cultures.[74–76]

Most coxsackievirus A types do not grow and produce a CPE in simian kidney tissue cultures. However, most coxsackievirus A types (except A1, A19, and A22) replicate in the RD cell line derived from a human rhabdomyosarcoma.[77] A satisfactory system for the primary recovery of enteroviruses from clinical specimens would include primary rhesus, cynomolgus, or African green monkey kidney tissue cultures; a diploid, human embryonic lung fibroblast cell strain; the RD cell line; and the intraperitoneal and intracerebral inoculation of suckling mice younger than 24 hours old. Optimally, blind passage should be carried out in the tissue culture systems.

Serologic Characteristics[11, 13, 15, 32, 66]

Although there are some minor cross-reactions between several enteroviral types, there are no common group structural protein antigens of diagnostic importance. Intratypic strain differences are common, and some strains (prime strains) are poorly neutralized by antisera to prototype viruses. These prime strains induce antibody

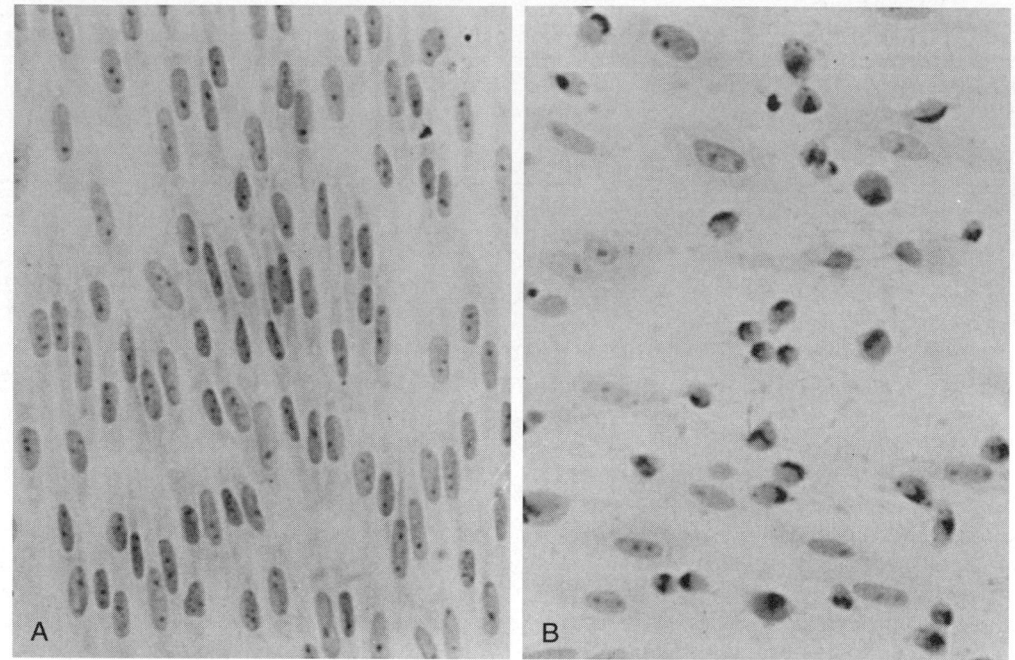

FIGURE 10–1 Fetal rhesus monkey kidney tissue culture (HL-8). *A*, Uninoculated tissue culture. *B*, Echovirus 11 cytopathic effect.

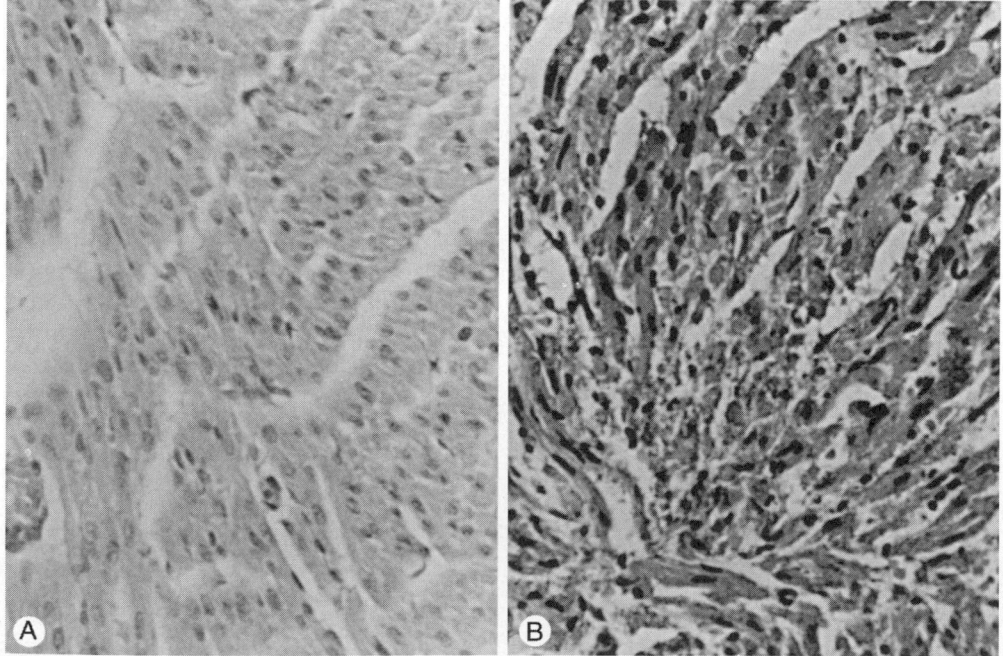

FIGURE 10–2 Suckling mouse myocardium. *A*, Normal suckling mouse myocardium. *B*, Myocardium of suckling mouse infected with coxsackievirus B1.

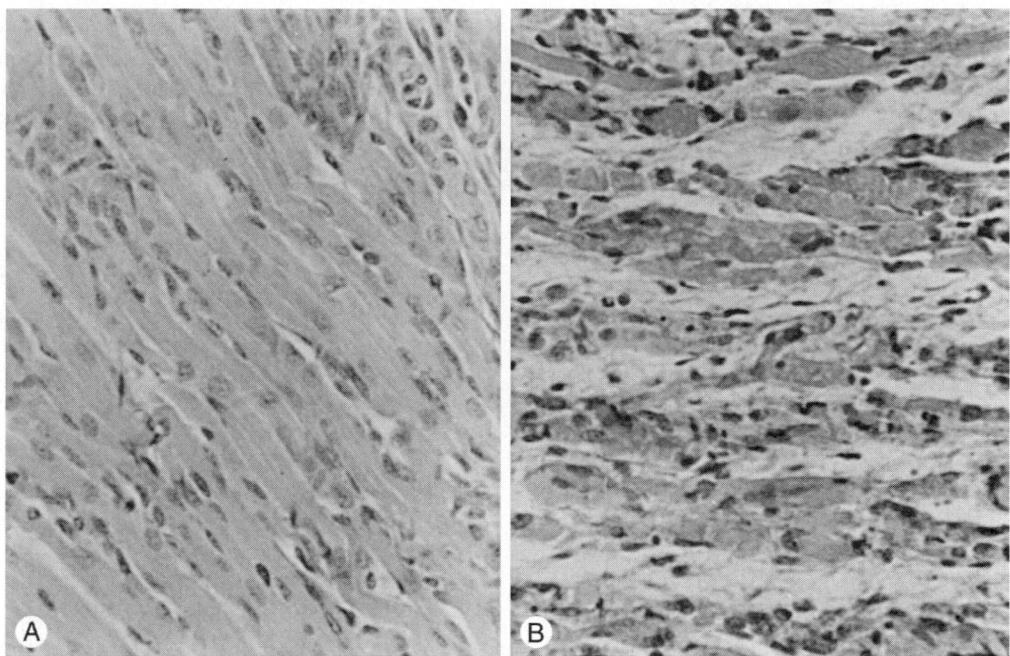

FIGURE 10–3 Suckling mouse skeletal muscle. *A,* Normal suckling mouse skeletal muscle. *B,* Skeletal muscle of a mouse infected with coxsackievirus A16.

in animals that does, however, neutralize the specific prototype viruses.

The identification of enteroviral types by neutralization in suckling mice or tissue cultures with antiserum pools is relatively well defined. Neutralization is induced by the epitopes on structural proteins VP1, VP2, and VP3; in particular, several epitopes are clustered on VP1. Prime strains do cause diagnostic difficulties because they are frequently not neutralized by the reference antisera. This is a particular problem with echoviruses 4, 9, and 11 and enterovirus 71. If suspected, this problem can be overcome by employing antisera in less dilute concentrations or using antisera prepared against several different strains of problem viruses.

EPIDEMIOLOGY AND TRANSMISSION

General

Spread of enteroviruses is from person to person by fecal-oral and possibly oral-oral (respiratory) routes.[1-11, 78] Swimming and wading pools may serve as a means of spread of enteroviruses during the summer.[79] Oral-oral transmission by way of the contaminated hands of health care personnel and transmission by fomites have been documented on a chronic care pediatric ward.[80] Enteroviruses have been recovered from trapped flies, and this carriage probably contributes to the spread of human infections, particularly in lower socioeconomic populations that have poor sanitary facilities.[81-83]

Children are the main susceptible cohort; they are immunologically susceptible, and their unhygienic habits facilitate spread. Spread is from child to child (via feces to skin to mouth) and then within family groups. Recov-

ery of enteroviruses is inversely related to age; the prevalence of specific antibodies is directly related to age. The incidence of infections and the prevalence of antibodies do not differ between boys and girls.

Transplacental Transmission

POLIOVIRUSES

Poliovirus infections in pregnancy can result in abortion, stillbirth, neonatal disease, or no evidence of fetal involvement.[84] Gresser and associates have shown that the human amniotic membrane in organ culture can be infected, resulting in a persistent low-grade infection.[85] It has been observed on many occasions that maternal poliomyelitis occurring late in pregnancy has resulted in transplacental transmission of the virus to the fetus in utero.[86-107] The evidence that transplacental passage of virus occurs in early pregnancy is meager. Schaeffer and colleagues were able to recover virus from both the placenta and the fetus after a spontaneous abortion in a 24-year-old woman with poliomyelitis.[89]

Although attenuated poliovirus vaccines have been given to pregnant women, there has never been a search for the transplacental passage of vaccine virus.[108-110] Viremia occurs after oral administration of polio vaccine, so this virus is probably also passed transplacentally to the fetus on occasion.[111-118]

COXSACKIEVIRUSES

Several investigators have studied coxsackievirus infections in pregnant animals and the transplacental passage of virus to the fetus. Dalldorf and Gifford studied two strains of coxsackievirus B1 and one of coxsackievirus A8 in gravid mice.[119] In only one instance (coxsackievirus

B1) were they able to recover virus from a fetus. They thought that this result was inconclusive because they were unable to recover virus in five other instances. Berger and Roulet noted muscle lesions in the young of gravid mice infected with both coxsackieviruses A1 and B1.[120] Selzer studied several viruses in gravid mice; coxsackievirus A9 was found in the placentas of two mice but in no fetuses, and coxsackievirus A18 was not recovered from either fetuses or placentas.[121] In contrast, both coxsackieviruses B3 and B4 were found by Selzer to pass the placental barrier. Soike also noted that in the last week of pregnancy coxsackievirus B3 reached fetal mice transplacentally.[122] Modlin and Crumpacker noted that infection in late gestational mice was more severe than that occurring in early pregnancy and that transplacental infection of the fetus occurred transiently during the maternal infection.[123] Flamm noted that coxsackievirus A9, when injected intravenously in rabbits, reached the blastocyst early in pregnancy and the amniotic fluid later in pregnancy.[124] He also demonstrated congenital infection in mice with coxsackievirus A1.[125]

Palmer and co-workers studied the gestational outcome in pregnant mice inoculated intravenously with Theiler's murine encephalomyelitis virus, a murine enterovirus.[126] In early gestational infections they found a high rate of both placental and fetal abnormalities. The rates of fetal abnormalities and placental infection were greater than the rate of fetal viral infection, suggesting that the adverse effects of the viral infections were both direct and indirect. Gestational infection could result in virus passage to the fetus and fetal damage or in placental compromise with indirect fetal damage.

In another study using the same murine model with Theiler's murine encephalomyelitis virus, Abzug found that maternal factors (compromised uteroplacental blood flow, concomitant infection, and advanced age) could increase the risk of transplacental fetal infection.[127]

In humans, the transplacental passage of coxsackieviruses at term has been noted on several occasions. Benirschke studied the placentas in three cases of congenital coxsackievirus B disease and could find no histologic evidence of infection.[128] In 1956, Kibrick and Benirschke reported the first case of intrauterine infection with coxsackievirus B3.[129] In this instance, the infant was delivered by cesarean section and had clinical evidence of infection several hours after birth. Brightman and colleagues recovered coxsackievirus B5 from the placenta and rectum of a premature infant.[130] No histologic abnormalities of the placenta were noted. Other evidence of intrauterine infection has been presented for coxsackieviruses A4 and B2 through B6.[131–138]

Evidence for intrauterine infection during the first and second trimesters of pregnancy with coxsackieviruses is less clear. Burch and co-workers presented immunofluorescent studies of two fetuses of 5 months' gestational age and one fetus of 6 months' gestational age; the 6-month-old fetus had evidence of coxsackievirus B4 myocarditis, one 5-month-old fetus showed signs of coxsackievirus B3 infection and the other 5-month-old fetus showed evidence of coxsackievirus B2, B3, and B4 infections.[139] Basso and associates recovered coxsackievirus B2 from the placenta, liver, and brain of a fetus after a spontaneous abortion at 3 months of gestation.[134] Plager and co-workers noted no evidence of intrauterine viral transmission with coxsackievirus B5 infections during the first and second trimesters of pregnancy.[140]

ECHOVIRUSES

Less is known about transplacental passage of echoviruses than about that of coxsackieviruses and polioviruses. Echovirus infections are regular occurrences in all populations, so it is apparent that women in all stages of pregnancy are frequently infected and that viremia is commonly seen in these infections.[141] In particular, epidemic disease related to echovirus 9 has been studied both epidemiologically and serologically.[142–144] In these studies, a search for teratogenesis has been made but no definitive virologic investigations have been carried out; asymptomatic transplacental infection may well have occurred.

Cherry and colleagues cultured samples from 590 newborns during a period of enteroviral prevalence without isolating an echovirus.[132] Antepartum serologic study of a group of 55 mothers in this study showed that 5 (9%) were actively infected with echovirus 17 during the 6-week period before delivery. In two other large nursery studies, there was no suggestion of intrauterine echovirus infections.[145, 146]

Berkovich and Smithwick[147] noted a newborn without clinical illness who had specific IgM echovirus 22 antibody in the cord blood, suggesting intrauterine infection with this virus. Hughes and colleagues reported a newborn with echovirus 14 infection who had a markedly elevated IgM (190 mg/dl) on the sixth day of life.[148] It seems likely that this infant was also infected in utero. Echoviruses 7, 9, 11, 19, 27, and 33 have also been noted in transplacentally acquired infections.[134, 149–156]

Ascending Infection and Contact Infection During Birth

There is no definitive evidence for either ascending infection or contact infection with enteroviruses during birth. In prospective studies of genital herpes simplex and cytomegaloviral infections, there have been no enteroviral isolations.[157, 158] These results suggest that ascending infections with enteroviruses, if they occur at all, are extremely rare. However, Reyes and associates recovered coxsackievirus B5 from the cervix of four third-trimester pregnant women.[159] Three of the four positive cultures were obtained 3 weeks or more before delivery. In the fourth case, the cervical culture was obtained the day before delivery and the child was delivered by cesarean section. All of the infants were healthy, but, unfortunately, culture for virus was obtained only from the infant delivered by cesarean section; this culture was negative. In an earlier study, Reyes and colleagues reported a child who died from a disseminated echovirus 11 infection.[153] The illness had its onset on the third day of life, and the virus was recovered from the mother's cervix at that time.

Enteroviral infection during the birth process would seem quite probable. The fecal carriage rate of enteroviruses in asymptomatic adult patients varies between 0 and 6% or higher in different population groups.[160-162] Cherry and associates noted that in 2 of 55 (4%) mothers, enteroviruses were present in the feces shortly after delivery.[132] Katz, in a discussion of a child with neonatal coxsackievirus B4 infection, suggested that the infant might have inhaled maternally excreted organisms during birth.[163] The fact that this child had pneumonia would tend to support this contention. Certainly, infections occurring 2 to 7 days after birth could have been acquired during passage through the birth canal.

Neonatal Infection

Neonatal infections and illnesses from enteroviruses are relatively common. Transmission of enteroviruses to newborns is similar to that for populations of older people. The main factor in spread of virus is human-to-human contact.

During the summer and fall of 1981 in Rochester, New York, 666 neonates were cultured for enteroviruses within 24 hours of birth and then weekly for 1 month.[164] The incidence of acquisition of nonpolio enteroviral infections during this period was 12.8%. Two risk factors were identified: lower socioeconomic status and lack of breast-feeding.

POLIOVIRUSES

Clinical poliomyelitis is rare in neonates, but the infection rate before the vaccine era was never determined. It is probable that the rarity of neonatal poliomyelitis was not related to lack of viral transmission but to the protection from disease offered by transplacentally transmitted specific polioviral antibodies. From experience gained in vaccine studies, it is apparent that infants with passively acquired antibody can be regularly infected.[165-177]

Bates, in 1955, reviewed the literature of poliomyelitis in infants younger than 1 month of age.[101] He noted six infants who apparently were not infected by their mothers and who had had other likely contacts. A neighbor was the contact in one case, siblings in two cases, nursery nurses in two cases, and an uncle in the sixth case. In the majority of the other infants, the mother had had poliomyelitis shortly before the child was born and probably was the contact. The mode of transmission—intrauterine, during birth, or postnatal contact—is not known.

More recently, Bergeisen and colleagues reported a case of paralytic poliomyelitis from a type 3 vaccine viral strain.[178] They suggested that the source of this virus may have been the child of the neonate's baby sitter, who was vaccinated about 2 weeks before the onset of the illness.

COXSACKIEVIRUSES

Several epidemics with coxsackieviruses B in newborn nurseries have been studied. Brightman and co-workers observed an epidemic of coxsackievirus B5 in a premature nursery.[130] Their data suggested that the virus was introduced into this nursery by an infant with a clinically inapparent infection who had been infected in utero. Secondary infections occurred in 12 infants and two nurses. The timing of the secondary cases suggested that three generations of infection had occurred and that the nurses had been infected during the second generation. The authors suggested that the infection had spread from infant to infant and from infant to nurse.

Javett and colleagues noted an acute epidemic of myocarditis associated with coxsackievirus B3 infection in a Johannesburg maternity home.[179] Unfortunately, no epidemiologic investigation or search for asymptomatic infected infants was performed. However, in analyzing the dates of the onset of the illnesses, it would appear that single infections occurred for five generations and then five children became ill within a 3-day period.

Kipps and colleagues carried out epidemiologic investigations in two coxsackievirus B3 nursery epidemics.[180] In the first epidemic, the initial infection was probably transmitted from a mother to her child; this infant was then the source of five secondary cases in newborns and one illness in a nurse. Infants with four of the five secondary cases were located on one side of the nursery, but only one cot was close to the cot of the index patient, and this cot did not adjoin the cots of the three other infants with contact cases. In the second outbreak, an infant who also was infected by his mother probably introduced the virus into the nursery. Infants with the three secondary cases were geographically far removed from the one with the primary case.

There have been many other instances of isolated nursery infections and small outbreaks with coxsackieviruses, and it seems that the most consistent source of original nursery infection is transmission from a mother to her child,[179-219] but introduction of virus into the nursery by personnel also occurs.[219, 220]

ECHOVIRUSES

Although many outbreaks of echovirus infections have been observed in newborn nurseries, information on viral transmission is incomplete.[29, 221-251] Cramblett and co-workers reported an outbreak of echovirus 11 disease in four infants in an intensive care nursery.[221] All infants were in enclosed incubators, and three patients became ill within 24 hours; the fourth child became ill 4 days later. Echovirus 11 was recovered from two members of the nursery staff. These data suggest that transmission from personnel to infants occurred because of inadequate washing of hands. In another outbreak in an intensive care unit, the initial patient was transferred to the nursery because of severe echovirus 11 disease.[236] After transfer, infection occurred in the senior house officer and a psychologist in the unit. It is inferred by the investigators that spread by respiratory droplets to nine other infants occurred from these infected personnel.

In a maternity unit outbreak of echovirus 11 involving six secondary cases, which was studied by Mertens and associates,[243] it was noted that infection spread through close contact between the infected newborns and the nurses. In a more recently reported nosocomial echovirus 11 outbreak, it was found that infants present in an intermediate care unit for more than 2 days were more likely to become infected than those who were there for less than 2 days. Illness was also associated with gavage feeding, mouth care, and being a twin.[244]

Modlin reviewed reports of 16 nursery outbreaks involving 206 ill infants.[246] In only 4 of the 16 outbreaks was the source noted, and in all 4 the primary case was an infant who acquired infection vertically from its mother. After introduction of an infected newborn into a nursery, spread to other infants by personnel is common.[248-251] Risk factors for nursery transmission as noted by Rabkin and co-workers were "lower gestational age or birth weight; antibiotic or transfusion therapy; nasogastric intubation or feeding; proximity in the nursery to the index patient; and care by the same nurse during the same shift as the index patient."[248]

Wilson and associates reported an intensive care nursery epidemic in which respiratory syncytial virus and echovirus 7 infections occurred concurrently.[250] This epidemic persisted from January to June 1984 in spite of an aggressive isolation cohorting program. A major factor in persistence was asymptomatic infections with both viruses.

Jack and colleagues observed the endemic occurrence of asymptomatic infection with echovirus 22 in a nursery during an 8-month period.[222] A total of 44 infants were infected during this time, and nursery infection occurred when there was no known activity of echovirus 22 in the community at large. The investigators believed that the endemic viral infection was spread by fecal contamination of hands of nursery personnel.

Interestingly, Nakao and colleagues[232] and Berkovich and Pangan[223] also noted echovirus 22 infections in nurseries. Like Jack and colleagues, they observed that the infections seemed to be endemic to the nurseries rather than related to community epidemics.

Host Range

It is the general opinion that humans are the only natural hosts of enteroviruses.[78] However, enteroviruses have been recovered in nature from sewage,[82] flies,[81-83] swine,[252, 253] dogs,[254, 255] a calf,[256] a budgerigar,[257] a fox,[258] mussels,[259] and oysters.[260] In addition, serologic evidence of infection with enteroviruses similar to human strains has been noted in chimpanzees,[261] cattle,[262] rabbits,[263] a fox,[264] a chipmunk,[265] and a marmot.[237] It is probable that infection of these animals was the result of their direct contact with an infected human or infected human excreta. As stated previously, although enteroviruses do not multiply in flies, they would appear to be a possible significant vector in situations of poor sanitation and heavy human infection. The contamination of shellfish is also intriguing[259, 260, 264-269] because, in addition to their possible role in human infection, they offer a source of enteroviral storage during cold weather. Contaminated foods are another possible source of human infection.[269]

Geographic Distribution and Season

Enteroviruses have a worldwide distribution.[1, 11, 78, 270, 271] Neutralizing antibodies for specific viral types have been noted in serologic surveys throughout the world, and most strains have been recovered in worldwide isolation studies. In any one area there are frequent fluctuations in predominant types. Epidemics probably depend on new susceptible persons in the population rather than on reinfections; they may be localized and sporadic and may vary in etiology from place to place in the same year. Pandemic waves of infection also occur.

In temperate climates, enteroviral infections occur primarily in the summer and fall, but, in the tropics, they are prevalent year round.[11, 78, 272] A basic concept in understanding their epidemiology concerns the far greater frequency of unrecognized infection in comparison with that of clinical disease. This is illustrated by poliomyelitis, which remained an epidemiologic mystery until it was appreciated that unrecognized infections were the main source of contagion. Serologic surveys were instrumental in elucidating the problem: in populations living in conditions of poor sanitation and hygiene, epidemics do not occur; but wide dissemination of polioviruses has been confirmed by demonstrating the presence of specific antibodies to all three types in nearly 100% of children by age 5 years.

Epidemics of poliomyelitis first began to appear in Europe and the United States during the latter part of the nineteenth century; they continued with increasing frequency in the economically advanced countries until the introduction of effective vaccines in the 1950s and 1960s.[30, 31, 273, 274] The evolution from endemic to epidemic follows a characteristic pattern, beginning with collections of a few cases, then endemic rates that are higher than usual, followed by severe epidemics with high attack rates.

The age group attacked in endemic areas and in early epidemics is the youngest one—more than 90% of paralytic cases begin in children younger than age 5 years. Once a pattern of epidemicity begins, it is irreversible unless preventive vaccination is carried out. Because epidemics recur over a period of years, there is a shift in age incidence such that relatively fewer cases are in the youngest children; the peak often occurs in the 5- to 14-year-old group, and an increasing proportion is in young adults. These changes are correlated with socioeconomic factors and improved standards of hygiene; when children are protected from immunizing infections in the first few years of life, the pool of susceptible persons builds up, and introduction of a virulent strain often is followed by an epidemic. Extensive use of vaccines in the past four decades has resulted in elimination of paralytic poliomyelitis from large geographic areas, but the disease remains endemic in various parts of the world, and outbreaks of true infantile paralysis continue to occur, particularly in developing countries where economic and other problems have delayed effective immunization programs.[29, 275] Although seasonal periodicity is distinct in temperate climates, some viral activity does take place during the winter.[276] Infection and acquisition of postinfection immunity occur with greater intensity and at earlier ages among crowded, economically deprived populations with less efficient sanitation facilities.

Recently, molecular techniques have allowed the study of genotypes of specific viral types in populations over time.[277-280] For example, Mulders and colleagues studied the molecular epidemiology of wild poliovirus type 1 in Europe, the Middle East, and the Indian subcontinent.[280] They found four major genotypes circulating. Two genotypes were found predominantly in Eastern Europe, a third genotype was circulating mainly in Egypt, and the fourth genotype was widely dispersed. All four genotypes were found in Pakistan.

The epidemiologic behavior of coxsackieviruses and echoviruses parallels that of polioviruses: unrecognized infections far outnumber those with distinctive symptoms. The agents are disseminated widely throughout the world, and outbreaks related to one or another type of virus occur regularly. These outbreaks tend to be localized, with different agents being prevalent in different years. In the late 1950s, however, echovirus 9 had a far wider circulation, sweeping through a large part of the world and infecting not only children but also young adults. This behavior has been repeated occasionally with other enteroviruses; after a long absence, a particular agent returns and circulates among the susceptible persons of different ages who have been born since the last epidemic occurred. Other agents remain endemic in a given area, surfacing as sporadic cases and occasionally as small outbreaks. Multiple types are frequently active at the same time, although one agent commonly predominates in a given locality.

There are no available data on the incidence of symptomatic congenital and neonatal enteroviral infections. From the frequency of reports in the literature, it would appear that severe neonatal disease caused by enteroviruses decreased slightly during the late 1960s and early 1970s and then became more common again. Shown in Table 10–2 are the five most prevalent nonpolio enterovirus isolations per year in the United States from 1961 through 1996. The majority of patients from whom viruses were isolated had neurologic illnesses. It is possible that other enteroviruses were also prevalent but without clinical disease severe enough to cause physicians to submit specimens for study. In addition, probably many coxsackievirus A infections, even in the epidemic situation, went undiagnosed because the suckling mouse inoculation assay is frequently not performed. Although 65 nonpolio enteroviral types are identified, it is of interest that in the 36 years covered in Table 10–2, only 20 different virus types are noted. Echovirus type 9 was most common, with echoviruses 4, 6, and 11 and coxsackieviruses B2 and B4 the next most common. Since 1990, echovirus type 30 has been the most common circulating viral type.

An analysis of Centers for Disease Control and Prevention nonpolio enterovirus data for 14 years found that early isolates in a particular year were predictive of isolates for the remainder of that year[281]: the six most common isolates during March, April, and May were predictive of 59% of the total isolates during July through December of the same year.

Although use of live polioviral vaccine has eliminated epidemic poliomyelitis in the United States, it is hard to determine what the effect of polio vaccine viruses has been on enteroviral ecology. In 1970, polioviruses accounted for only 6% of the total enteroviral isolations from patients with neurologic illnesses.[282] Although the figures are not directly comparable, more than one third of the enteroviral isolations in 1962 from similar patients were polioviruses.[283] However, Horstmann and associates studied specimens from sewage and asymptomatic children during the vaccine era and noted that the number of yearly polioviral isolations (presumably vaccine strains) was greater than the number of nonpolioviral enteroviruses.[284] The prevalence of vaccine viruses did not seem to affect the seasonal epidemiology of other enteroviruses.

PATHOGENESIS

Events During Pathogenesis

Congenital infections with enteroviruses result from transplacental passage of virus to fetus. The method of transport from mother to fetus is poorly understood. It is apparent that maternal viremia during enteroviral infections is common. Because virus has been recovered from the placenta on several occasions, it is probable that active infection of the placenta also occurs. Benirschke could find no histologic evidence of placental disease in three cases of established transplacentally acquired coxsackievirus B infections.[128] On the other hand, Batcup and associates noted diffuse perivillous fibrin deposition with villous necrosis and inflammatory cell infiltration of the placenta in a woman who 2 weeks earlier at 33 weeks of gestation had coxsackievirus A9 meningitis.[285] The woman was delivered of a macerated stillborn infant. At birth, virus was recovered from the placenta but not from the stillborn infant.

It is assumed that infection in the fetus results from hematogenous dissemination initiated in the involved placenta. It is also possible that some in utero infection results from the ingestion of virus contained in amniotic fluid; in this situation, primary fetal infection would involve the pharynx and lower alimentary tract.

The portal of entry of infection during both the birth process and the neonatal period is similar to that for older children and adults.

Figure 10–4 shows a schematic diagram of the events of pathogenesis. After initial acquisition of virus by the oral or respiratory route, implantation occurs in the pharynx and the lower alimentary tract. Within 1 day, the infection extends to the regional lymph nodes. On about the third day, minor viremia occurs, resulting in involvement of many secondary infection sites. In congenital infections, infection is initiated during the minor viremia phase. Multiplication of virus in secondary sites coincides with the onset of clinical symptoms. Illness can vary from minor infections to fatal ones. Major viremia occurs during the period of multiplication of virus in the secondary infection sites; this period usually lasts from the third to the seventh days of infection. In many echovirus and coxsackievirus infections, central nervous system involvement apparently occurs at the same time as other secondary organ involvement. This occasionally appears to happen with polioviral infections also; however, more commonly, the central ner-

TABLE 10–2
Predominant Types of Nonpolio Enteroviral Isolations in the United States, 1961–1996[a]

FIVE MOST COMMON VIRAL TYPES PER YEAR

Year	First	Second	Third	Fourth	Fifth
1961	Coxsackievirus B5	Coxsackievirus B2	Coxsackievirus B4	Echovirus 11	Echovirus 9
1962	Coxsackievirus B3	Echovirus 9	Coxsackievirus B2	Echovirus 4	Coxsackievirus B5
1963	Coxsackievirus B1	Coxsackievirus A9	Echovirus 9	Echovirus 4	Coxsackievirus B4
1964	Coxsackievirus B4	Coxsackievirus B2	Coxsackievirus A9	Echovirus 4	Echovirus 6, Coxsackievirus B1
1965	Echovirus 9	Echovirus 6	Coxsackievirus B2	Coxsackievirus B5	Coxsackievirus B4
1966	Echovirus 9	Coxsackievirus B2	Echovirus 6	Coxsackievirus B5	Coxsackievirus A9, A16
1967	Coxsackievirus B5	Echovirus 9	Coxsackievirus A9	Echovirus 6	Coxsackievirus B2
1968	Echovirus 9	Echovirus 30	Coxsackievirus A16	Coxsackievirus B3	Coxsackievirus B4
1969	Echovirus 30	Echovirus 9	Echovirus 18	Echovirus 6	Coxsackievirus B4
1970	Echovirus 3	Echovirus 9	Echovirus 6	Echovirus 4	Coxsackievirus B4
1971	Echovirus 4	Echovirus 9	Echovirus 6	Coxsackievirus B4	Coxsackievirus B2
1972	Coxsackievirus B5	Echovirus 4	Echovirus 6	Echovirus 9	Coxsackievirus B3
1973	Coxsackievirus A9	Echovirus 9	Echovirus 6	Coxsackievirus B2	Coxsackievirus B5, echovirus 5
1974	Echovirus 11	Echovirus 4	Echovirus 6	Echovirus 9	Echovirus 18
1975	Echovirus 9	Echovirus 4	Echovirus 6	Coxsackievirus A9	Coxsackievirus B4
1976	Coxsackievirus B2	Echovirus 4	Coxsackievirus B4	Coxsackievirus A9	Coxsackievirus B3, echovirus 6
1977	Echovirus 6	Coxsackievirus B1	Coxsackievirus B3	Echovirus 9	Coxsackievirus A9
1978	Echovirus 9	Echovirus 4	Coxsackievirus A9	Echovirus 30	Coxsackievirus B4
1979	Echovirus 11	Echovirus 7	Echovirus 30	Coxsackievirus B2	Coxsackievirus B4
1980	Echovirus 11	Coxsackievirus B3	Echovirus 30	Coxsackievirus B2	Coxsackievirus A9
1981	Echovirus 30	Echovirus 9	Echovirus 11	Echovirus 3	Coxsackievirus A9, echovirus 5
1982	Echovirus 11	Echovirus 30	Echovirus 5	Echovirus 9	Coxsackievirus B5
1983	Coxsackievirus B5	Echovirus 30	Echovirus 20	Echovirus 11	Echovirus 24
1984	Echovirus 9	Echovirus 11	Coxsackievirus B5	Echovirus 30	Coxsackievirus B2, A9
1985	Echovirus 11	Echovirus 21	Echovirus 6, 7[b]		Coxsackievirus B2
1986	Echovirus 11	Echovirus 4	Echovirus 7	Echovirus 18	Coxsackievirus B5
1987	Echovirus 6	Echovirus 18	Echovirus 11	Coxsackievirus A9	Coxsackievirus B2
1988	Echovirus 11	Echovirus 9	Coxsackievirus B4	Coxsackievirus B2	Echovirus 6
1989	Coxsackievirus B5	Echovirus 9	Echovirus 11	Coxsackievirus B2	Echovirus 6
1990	Echovirus 30	Echovirus 6	Coxsackievirus B2	Coxsackievirus A9	Echovirus 11
1991	Echovirus 30	Echovirus 11	Coxsackievirus B1	Coxsackievirus B2	Echovirus 7
1992	Echovirus 11	Echovirus 30	Echovirus 9	Coxsackievirus B1	Coxsackievirus A9
1993	Echovirus 30	Coxsackievirus B5	Coxsackievirus A9	Coxsackievirus B1	Echovirus 7
1994	Coxsackievirus B2	Coxsackievirus B3	Echovirus E6	Echovirus 30	Coxsackievirus A9
1995	Echovirus 9	Echovirus 11	Coxsackievirus A9	Coxsackievirus B2	Echovirus 30
1996	Coxsackievirus B5	Echovirus 17	Echovirus 6	Coxsackievirus A9	Coxsackievirus B4

[a]The majority of patients from whom viruses were isolated had neurologic illnesses.
[b]Third and fourth place tie.
From Cherry JD. Enteroviruses: coxsackieviruses, echoviruses, and polioviruses. *In* Feigin RD, Cherry JD (eds). Textbook of Pediatric Infectious Diseases, 4th ed. Philadelphia, WB Saunders, 1998, p 1792; and Centers for Disease Control and Prevention. Nonpolio enterovirus surveillance—United States, 1993–1996. MMWR Morb Mortal Wkly Rep 46:748, 1997, with permission.

vous system symptoms of poliomyelitis are delayed, suggesting that seeding occurred later in association with the major viremia.

Cessation of viremia correlates with the appearance of serum antibody. The viral concentration in secondary infection sites begins to diminish on about the seventh day. However, infection continues in the lower intestinal tract for prolonged periods.

Factors That Affect Pathogenesis

The pathogenesis and pathology of enterovirus infections depend on the virulence, tropism, and inoculum concentration of virus, as well as on many specific host factors. It is obvious that enteroviruses have marked differences in both tropism and virulence. Although some generalizations can be made in regard to tropism, there are marked differences even among strains of specific viral types.

It is generally believed that enterovirus infections of the fetus and neonate are more severe than similar infections in older individuals. This is undoubtedly true in coxsackievirus B infections and probably also true in coxsackievirus A, echovirus, and poliovirus infections. Although the reasons for this increased severity are largely unknown, several aspects of neonatal immune

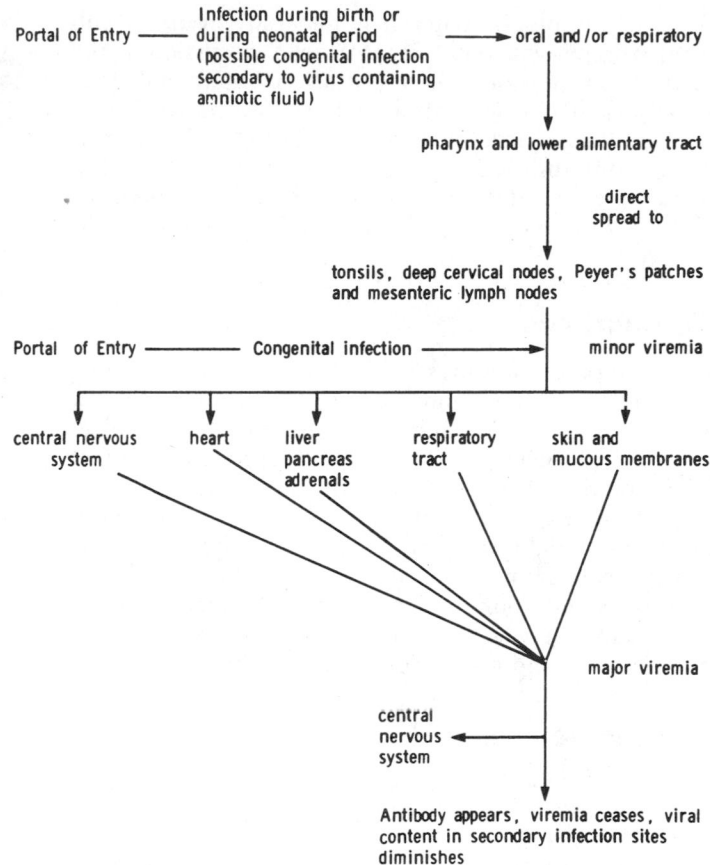

FIGURE 10–4 The pathogenesis of congenital and neonatal enteroviral infections.

mechanisms have been studied. In addition, the similarity of coxsackievirus B infections in suckling mice to those in human neonates has made available a useful animal model system. Heineberg and co-workers compared coxsackievirus B1 infections in 24-hour-old suckling mice with similar infections in older mice.[286] They noted that adult mice produced interferon in all infected tissues, whereas in suckling mice only small amounts of interferon were noted in the liver. They thought that the difference in outcome of coxsackievirus B1 infections in suckling and older mice could be explained by the inability of the cells of the immature animal to elaborate interferon.

Others have thought that the increased susceptibility of suckling mice to severe coxsackievirus infections is related to the transplacentally acquired, increased concentrations of adrenocortical hormones.[287, 288] Kunin suggested that the difference in age-specific susceptibility might be explained at the cellular level.[289] He showed that a variety of tissues of newborn mice bound coxsackievirus B3, whereas tissues of adult mice were virtually inactive in this regard.[289, 290] It is suggested that the progressive loss of receptor-containing cells or of receptor sites on persisting cells with increasing age may be the mechanism that accounts for infections of lesser severity in older animals. Teisner and Haahr[291] have suggested that the increased susceptibility of suckling mice to severe and fatal coxsackievirus infections may be from physiologic hypothermia and poikilothermia during the first week of life.

In the past, it has been assumed that specific pathology in various organs and tissues in enteroviral infections was due to the direct cytopathic effect and tropism of a particular virus. In more recent years a large number of studies using murine myocarditis model systems have suggested that host immune responses contribute to the pathology.[292–302] These studies suggest that T cell–mediated processes and virus-induced autoimmunity cause both acute and chronic myocardial damage. However, studies by McManus and associates suggest that the primary viral cytopathic effect is responsible for myocardial cell damage and that various T cell responses are a response to the damage and not the cause of the damage.[303]

Cellular Effect of Enteroviruses

Enteroviruses are usually cytolytic; infection of susceptible cells results in cell death and release of infectious virus.[13, 14] Clinical symptoms are related to the extent and location of cell death.

PATHOLOGY

General

Because there is great variation in the clinical signs of congenital and neonatal enterovirus infections, it is apparent that there are also wide variations in pathology.

Because pathologic material is generally available only from patients with fatal illnesses, the discussion in this section considers only the more severe enteroviral manifestations. It is worth emphasizing, however, that these fatal infections account for only a small portion of all congenital and neonatal enterovirus infections. The pathologic findings in infants with milder infections, such as nonspecific febrile illness, have not been described.

Polioviruses

The pathologic findings in fatal neonatal poliomyelitis are similar to those noted in disease of older children and adults.[18, 93, 99, 100, 102] The major findings have involved the central nervous system, specifically the anterior horns of the spinal cord and the motor nuclei of the cranial nerves. The involvement is usually irregular in distribution and symmetry. Microscopically, the anterior horn cells show neuronal destruction, gliosis, and perivascular small round cell infiltration. Myocarditis has also been observed,[93] characterized by focal necrosis of muscle fibers and varying degrees of cellular infiltration.

Coxsackieviruses A

Records of neonatal illnesses associated with coxsackieviruses A are rare.[304–306] Gold and co-workers, in a study of sudden unexpected death in infants, recovered coxsackievirus A4 from the brains of three children.[305] In none of these patients were histologic abnormalities noted in the brains or spinal cords. Baker and Phillips reported the death of twins in association with coxsackievirus A3 intrauterine infections; the first twin was stillborn, and the second twin died at 2 days of age with viral pneumonia.[306]

Coxsackieviruses B

Of the enteroviruses, coxsackieviruses B have most frequently been associated with severe and catastrophic neonatal disease. The most common findings in these cases have been myocarditis or meningoencephalitis, or both. Involvement of the adrenals, pancreas, liver, and lungs has also been noted.

HEART[129, 138, 179, 181, 190]

Grossly, the heart is usually enlarged, with dilatation of the chambers and flabby musculature. Microscopically, the pericardium frequently contains some inflammatory cells; and thickening, edema, and focal infiltrations of inflammatory cells may be found in the endocardium. The myocardium (Fig. 10–5) is congested and contains infiltrations of inflammatory cells (lymphocytes, mononuclear cells, reticulum cells, histiocytes, plasma cells, and polymorphonuclear and eosinophil leukocytes). The involvement of the myocardium is often patchy and focal but occasionally is diffuse. The muscle shows loss of striation as well as edema and eosinophilic degeneration. Frequently, muscle necrosis without extensive cellular infiltration is present.

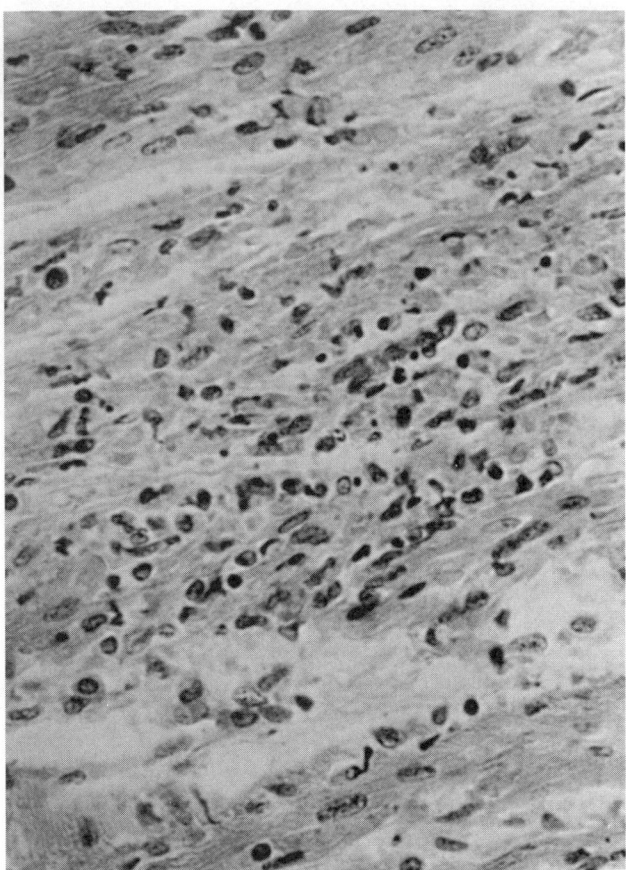

FIGURE 10–5 Coxsackievirus B4 myocarditis in a 9-day-old infant. Note myocardial necrosis and mononuclear cellular infiltration.

BRAIN AND SPINAL CORD[129, 138, 163, 181, 187, 190, 307]

The meninges are congested, edematous, and occasionally mildly infiltrated with inflammatory cells. Lesions in the brain and spinal cord are focal rather than diffuse but frequently involve many different areas. The lesions consist of areas of eosinophilic degeneration of cortical cells, clusters of mononuclear and glial cells (Fig. 10–6), and perivascular cuffing. Occasionally, areas of liquefaction necrosis unassociated with inflammation are noted.

OTHER ORGANS[129, 163, 181, 187, 308, 309]

In the lungs, there are frequently areas of mild focal pneumonitis with peribronchiolar mononuclear cellular infiltrations. Massive pulmonary hemorrhage has been observed. The liver is frequently engorged and occasionally contains isolated foci of liver cell necrosis and mononuclear cell infiltrations. In the pancreas, infiltration of mononuclear cells, lymphocytes, and plasma cells has been observed and occasional focal degeneration of the islet cells occurs. Congestion has been observed in the adrenal glands, with mild to severe cortical necrosis; inflammatory cells are present.

Echoviruses

Although frequently responsible for neonatal illnesses, echoviruses until relatively recently were rarely associ-

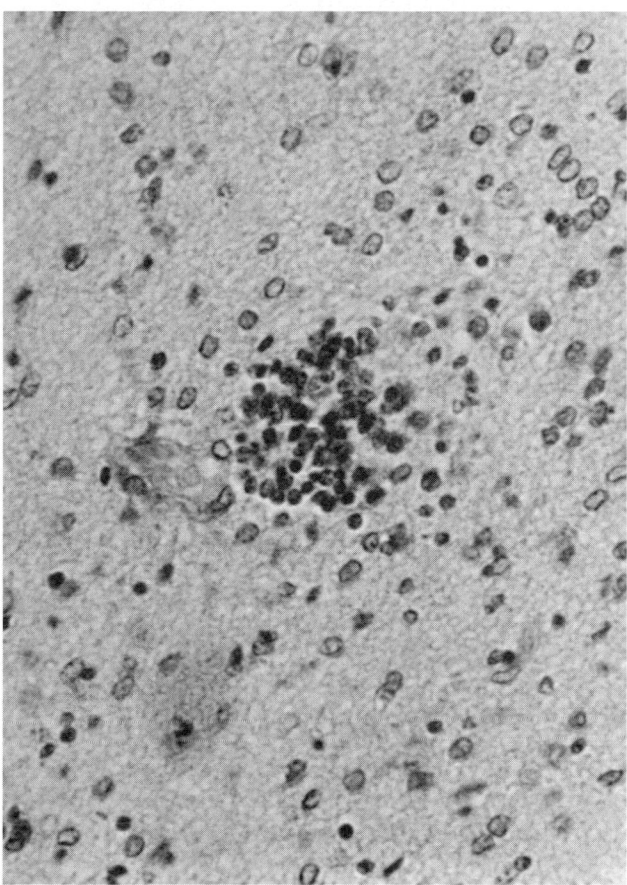

FIGURE 10–6 Coxsackievirus B4 encephalitis in a 9-day-old infant. Note focal infiltrate of mononuclear and glial cells.

ated with fatal infections. During the past 25 years, there have been many reports of fatal illnesses in newborns from echovirus type 11.[29, 151, 154, 243, 310–314] In virtually all cases, the major pathologic finding was massive hepatic necrosis; other findings included hemorrhagic necrosis of the adrenal glands, hemorrhage in other organs, myocardial necrosis, and acute tubular necrosis of the kidneys. Extensive myositis of the strap muscles of the neck was noted in one case.[314] Massive hepatic necrosis has also been noted in infections with echoviruses 3, 6, 7, 9, 14, 19, 20, and 21.[148, 149, 240, 310, 315–318] Wreghitt and associates noted a neonate with a fatal echovirus 7 infection.[319] This infant was found to have massive disseminated intravascular coagulation, with bleeding in the adrenal glands, renal medulla, liver, and cerebellum.

At autopsy, one infant with echovirus 6 infection was noted to have cloudy and thickened leptomeninges, liver necrosis, adrenal and renal hemorrhage, and mild interstitial pneumonitis.[310] One infant with echovirus 9 infection was noted to have an enlarged and congested liver with marked central necrosis,[315] and another with this virus had interstitial pneumonitis without liver involvement.[150] Three infants with echovirus 11 infections were noted to have renal and adrenal hemorrhage and small vessel thrombi in the renal medulla and in both the medulla and the inner cortex of the adrenal glands.[236] In

these patients, the livers were normal. Two infants, one with echovirus 6 and the other with echovirus 31 infection, had only extensive pneumonias.[242, 320]

CLINICAL MANIFESTATIONS

Abortion

POLIOVIRUSES

Poliomyelitis is associated with an increased incidence of abortion. Horn noted 43 abortions in 325 pregnancies complicated by maternal poliomyelitis.[84] Abortion was directly related to the severity of the maternal illness, including the degree of fever during the acute phase of illness. However, abortion also occurred in association with mild nonparalytic poliomyelitis. Schaeffer and colleagues studied the placenta and abortus 12 days after the onset of illness in the mother.[89] Poliovirus type 1 was isolated from both the placenta and the fetal tissues.

Several other investigators have reported an increased incidence of abortions with maternal poliomyelitis.[321–325] Siegel and Greenberg noted that fetal death occurred in 14 of 30 (46.7%) instances of maternal poliomyelitis during the first trimester.[103] Kaye and colleagues reviewed the literature in 1953 and noted 19 abortions in 101 cases of poliomyelitis in pregnancy.[325] In a small study in Evanston Hospital, the abortion rate in maternal poliomyelitis was little different from the expected rate.[322] In a study of 310 pregnant women who received trivalent oral polioviral vaccine, there was no increase in abortions above the expected rate.[109] In a more recent study in Finland that involved about 9000 pregnant women immunized with OPV, there was no evidence of an increase in still births.[326]

COXSACKIEVIRUSES

Although in the late 1950s and early 1960s there were extensive outbreaks of illness due to coxsackievirus A16, there was no evidence of adverse outcomes of pregnancy relating to this virus. Infections with other coxsackieviruses rarely involve large segments of the population so that population rate studies have not been performed.

Frisk and Diderholm found that 33% of women with abortions had IgM antibody to coxsackieviruses B whereas only 8% of controls had similar antibody.[327] In a second larger study the same research group confirmed their original findings.[328]

ECHOVIRUSES

There is no available evidence suggesting that echovirus infections during pregnancy are a cause of spontaneous abortion. Landsman and associates studied 2631 pregnancies during an epidemic of echovirus 9 and could find no difference in antibody to echovirus 9 in mothers who aborted and in those who delivered term infants.[144] A similar study in Finland revealed no increase in the abortion rate in mothers infected in early pregnancy with echovirus 9.[142]

Congenital Malformations

POLIOVIRUSES

The congenital malformation rate as determined in the Collaborative Perinatal Research Study of 45,000 pregnancies was 4.1%.[329] Although isolated instances of congenital malformation and maternal poliomyelitis have been noted, there is little statistical evidence that indicates that polioviruses are teratogens. In their review of the literature, Kaye and colleagues noted six anomalies in 101 infants born to mothers with poliomyelitis during pregnancy.[325] In the reviews of Horn,[84] Bates,[101] and Siegel and Greenberg,[103] no evidence of maternal poliovirus infection–induced anomalies was noted.

The possibility of congenital anomalies associated with attenuated polioviral vaccine has also been studied.[108, 109, 326, 330–332] Pearson and co-workers studied the fetal malformation rate in a community in which a large vaccine field trial had been carried out; although it is probable that pregnant women became infected with vaccine virus by secondary spread, there was no community increase in fetal malformations.[108] Prem and associates studied the infants of 69 women who received attenuated vaccine before the 20th week of gestation and found that none had anomalies.[109] In contrast, it was noted in Blackburn, England, that the rate of congenital defects increased coincident with mass vaccination with trivalent poliomyelitis vaccine.[330] However, there is no evidence of cause and effect related to this observation. Connelly and colleagues commented on a child with a unique renal disease acquired in utero.[331] The child's mother had received oral polio vaccine during the second month of pregnancy.

In February 1985, a mass vaccination program with live oral poliovirus vaccine was carried out in Finland.[332] Although pregnant women received vaccine, there was no evidence that vaccine virus had a harmful effect on developing fetuses.

COXSACKIEVIRUSES

In a large prospective study, Brown[333–335] and colleagues (Evans[336, 337] and Karunas[338]) made a serologic search for selected maternal enteroviral infections in association with congenital malformations. In this study, serum samples from 22,935 women had been collected.[338] From this group, serum samples from 630 mothers of infants with anomalies and from 1164 mothers of children without defects were carefully studied. Specifically, serologic evidence of infection during the first trimester and last 6 months of pregnancy with coxsackieviruses B1 through B5 and A9 and with echoviruses 6 and 9 was sought. In this study, infants were examined for 113 specific abnormalities; these anomalies were grouped into 12 categories for analysis. The authors demonstrated a positive correlation between maternal infection and infant anomaly with coxsackieviruses B2 through B4 and A9. The overall anomaly rate associated with first-trimester infections with coxsackievirus B4 was significantly higher than that in controls. Maternal coxsackievirus B2 infection throughout pregnancy, coxsackievirus B4 infections during the first trimester of pregnancy, and infection with at least one of the five coxsackieviruses B during pregnancy were all associated with urogenital anomalies when compared with controls. Coxsackievirus A9 infection was associated with digestive anomalies, and coxsackieviruses B3 and B4 were associated with cardiovascular defects. When coxsackieviruses B were analyzed as a group (B1 to B5), there was an overall association with congenital heart disease; the likelihood of cardiovascular anomalies was increased when maternal infection with two or more coxsackieviruses B occurred. In this study, the mothers had been instructed to keep illness "diary" sheets. There was no correlation between reported maternal clinical illnesses and serologic evidence of infection with the selected enteroviruses. This suggests that many infections that may have been causally related to the anomalies were asymptomatic. A disturbing finding in this study was the lack of seasonal occurrence of the births of children with specific defects. Because enteroviral transmission is most common in the summer and fall, it might be expected, if coxsackieviruses were a major cause of malformation, that the birth rate of children with malformations would be greatest in the spring and summer.

In the Collaborative Research Project, Elizan and co-workers were unable to find any relationships between maternal infections with coxsackieviruses B and congenital central nervous system malformations.[339] There are scattered case reports in the literature that describe congenital anomalies in association with maternal coxsackievirus infections. Makower and colleagues noted a child with congenital malformations who was born at 32 weeks of gestation and from whom a coxsackievirus A4 strain was recovered from the meconium.[131] The child's mother had been well throughout pregnancy, except for a febrile illness during the first month. The relationship of the viral infection to the congenital malformations or to the prematurity is uncertain.

Gauntt and associates studied the ventricular fluids from 28 newborn infants with severe congenital anatomic defects of the central nervous system.[340] In four infants (two with hydranencephaly, one with an occipital meningocele, and one with aqueductal stenosis), neutralizing antibody to one or more coxsackievirus B types was found in the fluid. In one case, IgM-neutralizing antibody to coxsackievirus B6 was found. The authors concluded that their data suggested the possibility of an association between congenital infections with coxsackieviruses B and severe central nervous system defects.

ECHOVIRUSES

In the large prospective study of Brown and Karunas, the possible association of maternal infections with echoviruses 6 and 9 and congenital malformations was examined.[338] Maternal infection with these selected echoviruses apparently was not associated with any anomaly. In three other studies,[142–144] no association between maternal echovirus 9 infection and congenital malformation was noted.

Prematurity and Stillbirth

POLIOVIRUSES

In the study by Horn of 325 pregnancies, 9 infants died in utero.[84] In each instance, the mother was critically ill with poliomyelitis. Horn also noted that 45 infants weighed less than 6 lb, and 17 of these had a birth weight of less than 5 lb. These low-birth-weight infants were born predominantly to mothers who had had poliomyelitis early in pregnancy. A similar finding was reported by Aycock.[87, 341] In New York City, Siegel and Greenberg also noted an increase in prematurity after maternal poliomyelitis infection.[103] This was specifically related to maternal paralytic poliomyelitis. There has been no observation of stillbirth or prematurity in relation to vaccine administration.[326]

COXSACKIEVIRUSES

Bates reported a fetus of 8 months' gestational age who was stillborn and had calcific pancarditis and hydrops fetalis at autopsy.[135] Fluorescent antibody study revealed coxsackievirus B3 antigen in the myocardium. Burch and colleagues noted three stillborn infants who had fluorescent antibody evidence of coxsackievirus B myocarditis, one each with coxsackieviruses B2, B3, and B4.[139] They also noted a premature boy who had histologic and immunofluorescent evidence of cardiac infection with coxsackieviruses B2 through B4; he lived only 24 hours. A macerated stillborn girl was delivered 2 weeks after the occurrence of aseptic meningitis caused by coxsackievirus A9 in a 27-year-old woman.[285] Virus was recovered from the placenta but not from the infant. Coxsackievirus B6 has been recovered from the brain, liver, and placenta of a stillborn infant.[134]

ECHOVIRUSES

Freedman reported the occurrence of a full-term, fresh stillbirth in a woman infected with echovirus 11.[342] Because the infant had no pathologic or virologic evidence of infection, he attributed the event to a secondary consequence of maternal infection from fever and dehydration rather than primary transplacental infection. Echovirus 27 has been associated with intrauterine death on two occasions.[134, 155]

In an extensive study of neonatal enteroviral infections in Milwaukee in 1979, Piraino and associates noted that 12 of 19 stillbirths occurred from July through October in coincidence with a major outbreak of enterovirus disease.[154] Echovirus 11 was the major agent isolated during this period.

Neonatal Infection

NONPOLIO ENTEROVIRUSES (ILLNESSES BY CLINICAL CLASSIFICATION) (Table 10–3)

Inapparent Infection

Although it is probable that inapparent infections in neonates occasionally occur with many different enteroviruses, there is little documentation of this assumption. Cherry and co-workers studied 590 normal newborns during a 6-month period and noted only one infection without clinical signs of illness.[132] This was a child infected in utero or immediately thereafter with coxsackievirus B2. The mother had an upper respiratory illness

10 days before delivery. In a similar but more comprehensive study, Jenista and associates failed to isolate any enteroviruses from cultures from 666 newborns on the first postpartum day.[164] However, during weekly cultures during the month after birth, 75 enteroviruses were isolated. Symptomatic enteroviral disease was noted in 21% (16 of 75).

During a survey of perinatal virus infections, 44 infants were found to be infected with echovirus 22 during a study period from May to December 1966.[222] The virus prevalence and the incidence of new infections during this period were fairly uniform. No illness was attributed to echovirus 22 infection, and the virus disappeared from the nursery in mid-December 1966. Inapparent infections with echovirus 22 have been noted on two other occasions.[223, 232] Infections without evidence of illness have also been noted with coxsackieviruses A9, B1, B4, and B5 and with echoviruses 3, 5, 9, 11, 13, 14, 20, 30, and 31[9, 145, 146, 164, 196, 226, 236, 242, 343–346]

Mild, Nonspecific Febrile Illness

In a review of 338 enteroviral infections in early infancy, 9% were classified as nonspecific febrile illnesses.[343] Illness may be sporadic in nature or part of an outbreak with a specific viral type. In the latter situation, clinical manifestations vary depending on the viral type; some infants have aseptic meningitis and other signs and symptoms and some only nonspecific fever. Coxsackievirus B5 and echovirus types 5, 11, and 33 have been those found most commonly in nonspecific fevers; other agents that have been noted include coxsackieviruses A9, A16, and B1 through B4 and echoviruses 4, 7, 9, and 17.*

Mild, nonspecific febrile illness occurs most commonly in full-term infants after uneventful pregnancies and deliveries without complications. Illness can occur at any time during the first month of life. In cases in which the onset occurs after 7 days of age, a careful history frequently reveals a trivial illness in a family member. The onset of illness is characterized by mild irritability and fever. The temperature is usually in the 38° C to 39° C range, but higher recordings are occasionally noted. Poor feeding is frequently observed. One or two episodes of vomiting or diarrhea, or both, may occur in some infants. The usual duration of illness is 2 to 4 days.

Routine laboratory study is not helpful, but cerebrospinal fluid (CSF) examination may reveal an increased protein concentration and leukocyte count indicative of aseptic meningitis.

Although, by definition, illness in the present category is mild, it is important to point out that the degree of viral infection may be extensive. When looked for, virus may be isolated from the blood, urine, and spinal fluid of infants with mild illnesses.[197, 344]

Sepsis-like Illness

The major diagnostic problem in neonatal enteroviral infections is the differentiation of bacterial from viral

---

*See references 28, 132, 154, 182, 193, 197, 215, 216, 224, 226–228, 235–237, 344, and 347–349.

TABLE 10–3
Major Manifestations of Neonatal Nonpolio Enteroviral Infections

SPECIFIC INVOLVEMENT	COMMON	RARE
Inapparent infection	Echo 22	Cox A9, B1, B2, B4, B5
		Echo 3, 5, 9, 11, 13, 14, 20, 30, 31
Mild nonspecific febrile illness	Cox B5	Cox B1, B2, B3, B4, A9, A16
	Echo 5, 11, 33	Echo 4, 7, 9, 17
Sepsis-like illness	Cox B2, B3, B4, B5	Cox B1, A9
	Echo 5, 11, 15	Echo 2, 3, 4, 6, 9, 14, 19, 21, 22
Respiratory illness (general)	Echo 11, 22	Cox B1, B4, B5, A9
		Echo 9, 17
Herpangina		Cox A5
Coryza		Cox A9
		Echo 11, 17, 19, 22
Pharyngitis		Cox B4
		Echo 11, 17, 18
Laryngotracheitis or bronchitis		Cox B1, B4
		Echo 11
Pneumonia		Cox B4, A9
		Echo 6, 9, 11, 17, 22, 31
Cloud baby		Echo 20
Gastrointestinal		
Vomiting or diarrhea	Echo 5, 17, 18	Cox B1, B2, B5
		Echo 4, 6, 8, 9, 11, 16, 19, 21, 22
		Entero 71
Hepatitis	Echo 11, 19	Cox B1, B3, B4, A9
		Echo 6, 7, 9, 14, 20, 21
Pancreatitis		Cox B3, B4, B5
Necrotizing enterocolitis		Cox B2, B3
Cardiovascular		
Myocarditis and pericarditis	Cox B1, B2, B3, B4	Cox B5, A9
		Echo 11, 19
Skin	Cox B5	Cox B1
	Echo 5, 17, 22	Echo 4, 7, 9, 11, 18
Neurologic		
Aseptic meningitis	Cox B2, B3, B4, B5	Cox B1, A9, A14
	Echo 3, 9, 11, 17	Echo 1, 5, 14, 21, 30
		Entero 71
Encephalitis	Cox B1, B2, B3, B4	Cox B5
		Echo 6, 9, 23
Paralysis		Cox B2
Sudden infant death		Cox B1, B3, B4, A4, A5, A8
		Echo 22

Cox = coxsackievirus; echo = echovirus; entero = enterovirus.
Modified from Cherry JD. Enteroviruses: coxsackieviruses, echoviruses and polioviruses. *In* Feigin RD, Cherry JD (eds). Textbook of Pediatric Infections Diseases, 4th ed. Philadelphia, WB Saunders, 198, p 1817, with permission.

disease. Even in the infant with mild nonspecific fever, bacterial disease must be strongly considered. The sepsis-like illness described here is always alarming. Illness is characterized by fever, poor feeding, abdominal distention, irritability, rash, lethargy, and hypotonia.[308, 350–352] Other findings include diarrhea, vomiting, seizures, shock, disseminated intravascular coagulation, thrombocytopenia, hepatomegaly, jaundice, and apnea. The onset of illness is introduced by irritability, poor feeding, and fever, followed within 24 hours by other manifestations. In a group of 27 neonates, Lake and associates observed that 54% had temperatures of 39° C or more.[271] The duration of fever varies from 1 to 8 days, most commonly 3 to 4 days. Barre and colleagues reported a 3-day-old boy with an enterovirus-associated hemophago-

cytic syndrome.[353] This neonate presented with a typical sepsis-like picture with fever, hepatosplenomegaly, coagulopathy, thrombocytopenia, and anemia. This child recovered and had no hemophagocytic relapses.

Sepsis-like illness is common. Morens noted its occurrence in one fifth of 338 enteroviral infections in infants.[343] In an attempt to differentiate bacterial from viral disease, Lake and co-workers studied 27 infants with enteroviral infections.[308] White blood cell counts were not helpful because the total count, the number of neutrophils, and the number of band form neutrophils were elevated in the majority of instances. Of most importance were historical data. The majority of mothers had evidence of a recent, febrile, viral-like illness. In addition, other factors often associated with bacterial sepsis, such as prolonged rupture of membranes, prematurity, and low Apgar scores, were unusual in the enteroviral infection group.

Sepsis-like illness has been noted most often with coxsackieviruses B2 through B5 and echovirus types 5, 11, and 16; other viruses noted include coxsackieviruses A9 and B1 and echoviruses 2 through 4, 6, 9, 14, 19, 21, and 22.*

Since the early 1980s, echovirus 11 has been associated most frequently with fatal septic events, with hepatic necrosis, and disseminated intravascular coagulation.[29, 152–154, 243, 311–314, 319]

Respiratory Illness

Respiratory complaints are generally overshadowed by other manifestations of neonatal enteroviral disease. Only 7% of 338 enteroviral infections in early infancy were classified as respiratory illness.[343] Except for echoviruses 11 and 22, respiratory illness associated with enteroviruses has been sporadic.[223, 225]

Hercík and co-workers reported an epidemic of respiratory illness in 22 newborns associated with echovirus 11 infection.[225] All of these infants had rhinitis and pharyngitis, 50% had laryngitis, and 32% had interstitial pneumonitis. Berkovich and Pangan studied respiratory illnesses in premature infants and reported 64 with illness, 18 of whom had virologic or serologic evidence of echovirus 22 infection.[223] In addition, many had high but constant levels of serum antibody to echovirus 22. Some of these latter infants were probably also infected with echovirus 22. The children with proven echovirus 22 infections could not be clinically differentiated from those without evidence of echovirus 22 infection. Ninety percent of the infants had coryza, and 39% had radiographic evidence of pneumonia.

Herpangina. Chawareewong and associates noted several infants with herpangina and coxsackievirus A5 infection.[360] A vesicular lesion on an erythematous base, on a tonsillar pillar, in a 6-day-old infant with coxsackievirus B2 meningitis, has also been reported.[361] Two 1-month-old infants were noted in an outbreak of herpangina due to coxsackievirus B3 in a welfare home in Japan.[362]

Coryza. The following agents have been noted in association with coryza: coxsackievirus A9 and echoviruses 11, 17, 19, and 22.[147, 225, 229, 232, 363]

Pharyngitis. Pharyngitis is uncommon in neonatal enteroviral infections. In more than 50 infants with enteroviral infections, studied by Linnemann and colleagues[348] and Lake and associates,[308] the occurrence of pharyngitis was not noted. Suzuki and co-workers observed pharyngitis in 3 of 42 neonates with echovirus 11 infections.[364] In contrast, in the same study, 67% of children 1 month to 4 years of age had pharyngitis. Pharyngitis has been associated with coxsackievirus B4 and echoviruses 11, 17, and 18.[193, 225, 229, 364, 365]

Laryngotracheobronchitis or Bronchitis. The following enteroviruses have been noted in laryngotracheobronchitis or bronchitis: coxsackieviruses B1 and B4 and

echovirus 11.[225, 366] Specific clinical descriptions of laryngotracheobronchitis or bronchitis associated with enteroviral infections are scanty. Hercík and co-workers observed laryngitis in 11 and croup in 4 of 22 neonates during an echovirus 11 outbreak.[225] All of the affected infants had upper respiratory tract findings, vomiting, and lethargy as well. Many were also cyanotic and had hepatosplenomegaly.

Pneumonia. Pneumonia as the main manifestation of neonatal enteroviral infection is rare. Morens noted only seven instances of pneumonia in 338 neonatal enteroviral infections.[343] Outbreaks of pneumonia in neonates have been reported with echoviruses 11 and 22.[223, 225] Pneumonia resulting from other enteroviruses is a sporadic event. The following nonpolio enteroviruses have been associated with neonatal pneumonia: coxsackieviruses A9 and B4 and echoviruses 9, 17, and 31.

During a nursery echovirus 11 outbreak, 7 of 22 neonates had pneumonia.[225] These infants all had signs of upper respiratory infection and general signs of sepsis-like illness as well. In infants with pneumonia associated with an echovirus 22 nursery epidemic, coryza, cough, and dyspnea were early signs.[223] The illnesses tended to be protracted, with radiographic changes persisting for 10 to 100 days.

"Cloud Baby." Eichenwald and associates recovered echovirus 20 from four full-term infants younger than 8 days of age.[234] Although these infants apparently were well, it was found that they were extensively colonized with staphylococci and that they disseminated these organisms into the air around them. Because of this ability to disseminate staphylococci, they were called cloud babies. The authors believed that these cloud babies contributed to the epidemic spread of staphylococci in the nursery. Because active staphylococcal dissemination occurred only during the time that echovirus 20 could be recovered from the nasopharynx, it was theorized that viral-bacterial synergistic activity was present.

Gastrointestinal Manifestations

Significant gastrointestinal illness occurs in about 7% of enteroviral infections of infancy.[343]

Vomiting or Diarrhea. Vomiting and diarrhea are common but usually just part of the overall illness complex and not the major manifestations. In 1958, Eichenwald and associates described epidemic diarrhea associated with echovirus 18 infections.[230] In a nursery unit of premature infants, 12 of 21 were mildly ill. Neither temperature elevation nor hypothermia occurred. Six infants were lethargic and listless, and two developed moderate abdominal distention. The diarrhea lasted from 1 to 5 days; there were five or six watery, greenish stools per day, occasionally expelled explosively. In two infants, a small amount of blood was noted in the stools but no mucus or pus cells. Five other infants in another nursery had similar diarrheal illness. Echovirus 18 was recovered from all ill infants.

In 22 infants with epidemic respiratory disease caused by echovirus 11, all had vomiting as a manifestation of the illness.[225] Linnemann and colleagues noted vomiting in 36% and diarrhea in 7% of neonates with echoviral

---

*See references 27–29, 149, 150, 152–154, 200, 220, 221, 229, 233, 236, 237, 243, 308, 311–313, 315, 316, 319, 348, 350, and 354–359.

infections.[348] In another study, Lake and associates found diarrhea in 81% and vomiting in 33% of neonates with nonpolio enteroviral infections.[308]

Vomiting and diarrhea in neonates have been noted in association with coxsackieviruses B1, B2, and B5; echoviruses 4 through 6, 8, 9, 11, 16 through 19, 21, and 22; and enterovirus 71.*

Hepatitis. Morens noted that 2% of neonates with clinically severe enteroviral disease had hepatitis.[343] Lake and colleagues[308] observed that hepatomegaly was present in 37% of neonates with enteroviral infections, and hepatosplenomegaly was observed by Hercík and associates[225] in 12 of 22 newborns with echovirus 11 respiratory illnesses.

Severe hepatitis, frequently with hepatic necrosis, has been noted with echoviruses 6, 7, 9, 11, 14, 19, 20, and 21.[148, 149, 249, 310, 311, 315, 318, 370] In 1980, Modlin reported four fatal echovirus 11 illnesses in premature infants.[240] All had hepatitis, disseminated intravascular coagulation, and thrombocytopenia as well as apnea, lethargy, poor feeding, and jaundice. Since 1980, there have been many reports of sepsis-like illness with fatal hepatitis related to echovirus 11.[29, 152, 154, 243, 312, 314, 316]

Philip and Larson reported three catastrophic neonatal echovirus 19 infections that resulted in hepatic necrosis and massive terminal hemorrhage.[149] One infant, infected in utero, was symptomatic at birth. The Apgar score was 3, and multiple petechiae were observed. Generalized ecchymoses and apneic episodes occurred, and the infant died at 3½ hours of age. Thrombocytopenia was noted, and echovirus 19 was isolated from the brain, liver, spleen, and lymph nodes. The other two infants who died of echovirus 19 infection were twins. They were normal during the first 3 days of life but then became mildly cyanotic and lethargic. Shortly thereafter, apneic episodes occurred and jaundice and petechiae developed. Both twins became oliguric, and they died on the eighth and ninth days of life with severe, terminal gastrointestinal bleeding. Both twins were thrombocytopenic, and virus was recovered from systemic sites in both.

Coxsackieviruses B1 and B4 and other B types have also been associated with neonatal hepatitis.[12, 28, 189, 202, 358, 359]

Pancreatitis. Pancreatitis was noted in three of four newborns with coxsackievirus B5 meningitis[186] and in coxsackievirus B3 and B4 infections at autopsy.[183] In other fatal coxsackievirus B infections, pancreatic involvement has been noted, but clinical manifestations have rarely been observed.

Necrotizing Enterocolitis. Lake and associates noted three infants with necrotizing enterocolitis.[308] Coxsackievirus B3 was recovered from two of these infants and coxsackievirus B2 from the third.

Cardiovascular Manifestations†

In contrast with enteroviral cardiac disease in children and adults, in which pericarditis is common, neonatal

---

TABLE 10–4
Findings in Neonatal Coxsackievirus B Myocarditis

FINDING	FREQUENCY (%)
Feeding difficulty	84
Listlessness	81
Cardiac signs	81
Respiratory distress	75
Cyanosis	72
Fever	70
Pharyngitis	64
Hepatosplenomegaly	53
Biphasic course	35
Central nervous system signs	27
Hemorrhage	13
Jaundice	13
Diarrhea	8

Modified from Kibrick S. Viral infections of the fetus and newborn. Perspect Virol 2:140, 1961, with permission.

disease virtually always involves the heart muscle. Most cases of neonatal myocarditis are related to coxsackievirus B infections, and nursery outbreaks have occurred on several occasions. In 1961, Kibrick[19] reviewed the clinical findings in 45 cases of neonatal myocarditis; his findings are summarized in Table 10–4. It is of interest that many of the early experiences, particularly in South Africa, involved catastrophic nursery epidemics. Except for the observation in 1972 of five newborns with echovirus 11 infections and myocarditis, there have been no recent nursery epidemics.[373]

The illness as described by Kibrick[19] was most commonly abrupt in onset, with listlessness, anorexia, and fever. A biphasic pattern was noted in about a third of the patients. Progression was rapid, and signs of circulatory failure appeared in a 2-day period. If death did not occur, recovery was occasionally rapid but usually occurred gradually during an extended period. Most patients had cardiac findings, such as tachycardia, cardiomegaly, electrocardiographic changes, and transitory systolic murmurs. Many patients showed signs of respiratory distress and cyanosis. About one third of the infants had signs suggesting neurologic involvement. Of the 45 patients analyzed by Kibrick, only 12 survived.

In the echovirus 11 nursery outbreak reported by Drew, 5 of 10 infants had tachycardia out of proportion to their fevers.[375] Three of these infants had electrocardiograms, and supraventricular tachycardia was noted in all and ST segment depression was observed in two of the records. Supraventricular tachycardia has also been seen in coxsackievirus B infections.[196] Echovirus 19 has also been noted in association with myocarditis.[363]

In recent years, neonatal myocarditis related to enteroviruses has been less common than it was three decades ago. Morens[343] in his review noted only two instances among 248 severe neonatal enteroviral illnesses.

Exanthem

Exanthem as a manifestation of neonatal enteroviral infection has been noted with coxsackieviruses B1 and B5 and echoviruses 4, 5, 7, 9, 11, 16 through 18, 21, and 22.* In most instances, rash is just a minor manifestation of moderate to severe neonatal disease. In 27 infants studied by Lake and colleagues, 41% had exanthem.[308] Similarly, Linnemann and co-workers noted exanthem in 4 of 14 neonates with echoviral infections.[348]

Cutaneous manifestations usually have their onset between the third and fifth day of illness. The rash is usually macular or maculopapular. Petechial lesions are occasionally noted. Surprisingly, vesicular lesions have not been described, nor has any rash illness in neonates been associated with coxsackievirus A16. Hall and associates reported two neonates with echovirus 16 infections in which the illnesses were roseola-like.[350] The patients had fevers for 2 and 3 days, defervescence, and then the appearance of maculopapular rashes.

Neurologic Manifestations

Meningitis and Meningoencephalitis.† As noted in Table 10–3, meningitis and meningoencephalitis have been associated with coxsackieviruses B1 through B5 and many echoviruses as well. In most instances, the differentiation of meningitis from meningoencephalitis is difficult in neonates. Meningoencephalitis is common in infants with sepsis-like illness, and autopsy studies reveal many infants with disseminated viral disease (heart, liver, adrenals) in addition to central nervous system involvement. In the review of Morens,[343] 50% of the neonates with enteroviral infections had encephalitis or meningitis.

The initial clinical findings in neonatal meningitis or meningoencephalitis are similar to those in nonspecific febrile illness or sepsis-like illness. Most often the child is quite normal and then is noted to be febrile, anorectic, and lethargic. Jaundice is frequently noted in newborns, and vomiting occurs in neonates of all ages. Less common findings include apnea, tremulousness, and general increased tonicity. Seizures occasionally occur.

CSF examination reveals considerable variation in protein, glucose, and cellular values. In seven newborns with meningitis related to coxsackievirus B5 studied by Swender and associates, the mean CSF protein value was 244 mg/dl and the highest value was 480 mg/dl.[220] The mean CSF glucose value was 57 mg/dl, and one of the seven had a pronounced hypoglycorrhachia (a value of 12 mg/dl). The mean CSF leukocyte count in the seven infants was 1069 cells per mm³, with 67% polymorphonuclear cells. The highest cell count was 4526 cells per mm³, with 85% polymorphonuclear cells. In another study involving 28 children younger than 2 months of age in which coxsackievirus B5 was the implicated pathogen, 36% of the infants had CSF leukocyte counts of 500 cells per mm³ or more.[356] In this same study, only 13% of the infants had CSF protein values of 120 mg/dl or more; 12% of the infants had glucose values of less than 40 mg/dl.

In summary, it must be stressed that the CSF findings in neonatal nonpolio enteroviral infections are frequently similar to those in bacterial disease. In particular, the most consistent finding in bacterial disease, hypoglycorrhachia, is noted in about 10% of newborns with enteroviral meningitis.[220, 308, 347, 356, 377]

Paralysis. Johnson and associates reported a 1-month-old boy with a right facial paralysis and loss of abdominal reflexes.[378] The facial paralysis persisted through convalescence; the reflexes returned to normal within 2 weeks. The boy was infected with coxsackievirus B2.

Sudden Infant Death

Balduzzi and Greendyke recovered a coxsackievirus A5 from the stool of a 1-month-old child with sudden infant death.[304] In a similar investigation of sudden infant death, Gold and co-workers recovered coxsackievirus A4 from the brains of three infants.[305] Coxsackievirus A8 was also recovered from the stool of a child in whom anorexia was noted on the day before death. Coxsackievirus B3 was recovered at autopsy from an infant who died suddenly on the eighth day of life.[304] Morens and associates[6] noted sudden infant death eight times in association with enteroviral infection; echovirus 22 was found on two occasions. In five instances of cot death in one study, echovirus 11 was isolated from the lungs in two cases, from the myocardium in one case, and from the nose or feces in the other two cases.[311]

In a more recent study, Grangeot-Keros and co-workers looked for evidence of enteroviral infections using polymerase chain reaction (PCR) and an IgM immunoassay in infants with sudden unexplained deaths.[395] They divided their infant death population into two groups: one group had clinical, biologic, or histologic signs of viral infection, and the other group had no indicators of an antecedent infection. Fifty-four percent of those infants with evidence of a preceding infection had PCR evidence of an enterovirus in samples from the respiratory tract and/or lung, whereas none of those without evidence of a prior infection had similar positive PCR findings. Their IgM antibody studies supported their PCR findings.

MANIFESTATIONS OF POLIOVIRUSES

General

Polioviral infection in children classically results in a spectrum of clinical illness. As noted by Paul[396] and accepted by others, 90 to 95% of infections are inapparent, 4 to 8% are abortive, and 1 to 2% are frank cases of poliomyelitis. Whether neonatal polioviral infection is acquired in utero, during birth, or after birth, it would appear that the more severe manifestations of clinical illness are similar to those of older children. However, the available reports in the literature suggest that the frequencies of occurrence of inapparent, abortive, and frank cases are quite different from those in older children. Most reports describe severely affected infants. Asymptomatic infection does occur, however.[87, 88]

*See references 27, 28, 138, 147, 150, 154, 184, 198, 210, 221, 224, 226, 229, 348, 350–352, 358, 363, 373, and 376.

†See references 27–29, 139, 146, 154, 198, 214, 220, 221, 224, 228, 233, 243, 245, 307, 313, 345, 351, 352, 356, 361, 367, 369, 373, and 376–394.

TABLE 10–5
Clinical Findings in 58 Cases of Neonatal Poliomyelitis

FINDING	NO. OF CASES WITH PARTICULAR FINDING PER NO. OF CASES EVALUATED	%
Time of onset after birth		
≤5 days	13/55	24
6–14 days	25/55	45
≥15 days	17/55	31
Possible source (symptomatic illness) of infection		
Mother	22/42	52
Other contact	6/42	14
Unknown	14/42	34
Acute illness		
Fever	17/29	59
Anorexia or dysphagia	16/24	67
Listlessness	24/33	73
Irritability	3/33	9
Diarrhea	2/11	18
Paralysis	43/44	98
Outcome		
Death	21/44	48
Residual paralysis	12/44	27
Recovery without paralysis	11/44	25

Adapted from Bates T. Poliomyelitis in pregnancy, fetus, and newborn. Am J Dis Child 90:189, 1955. Copyright 1955, American Medical Association.

In the excellent review by Bates[101] in 1955, 58 cases of poliomyelitis in infants younger than 1 month of age were described. Although complete data were not available on many of the cases, 51 had paralysis or died from their disease or both. Of the total number of infants for whom there were clinical data, only one had nonparalytic disease. Because follow-up observation was recorded for only a short time in many infants, the evaluation of residual paralysis, either its presence or its absence, may not be reliable. Pertinent clinical data from the study by Bates are presented in Table 10–5. From these data, it is apparent that over half of the cases were secondary to maternal disease. Because others have noted congenital infection without symptomatic maternal infection, it is probable that infection in the mother was the source for an even greater percentage of the neonatal illnesses. The incubation period of neonatal poliomyelitis has not been determined, and it is therefore difficult to know how many of the infants were infected in utero. Probably, most illnesses that occurred within the first 5 days of life were of congenital origin.

The majority of the neonates had symptoms of fever, anorexia or dysphagia, and listlessness. Almost half the infants noted in this review died, and of those surviving, 48% had residual paralysis.

Inapparent Infection

Shelokov and Habel followed a virologically proven infected newborn without signs of illness.[88] The infant was normal at 1 year of age. Wingate and co-workers studied an infant delivered by cesarean section from a woman with poliomyelitis who died 1 hour after delivery.[98] The infant was treated with gamma globulin intramuscularly at 21 hours of age. He remained asymptomatic; poliovirus 1 was recovered from a stool specimen on the fifth day of life.

Infection Acquired In Utero

Elliott and colleagues described an infant girl in whom "complete flaccidity" was noted at birth.[102] This child's mother had had mild paralytic poliomyelitis, the onset of minor illness occurring 19 days before the infant's birth. Fetal movements had ceased 6 days before delivery, suggesting that paralysis had occurred at this time. On examination, the infant was severely atonic; when supported under the back, she was passively opisthotonic. Respiratory efforts were abortive and confined to accessory muscles; laryngoscopy revealed complete flaccidity in the larynx.

Johnson and Stimson[95] reported a case in which the mother's probable abortive infection occurred 6 weeks before the birth of the infant. The newborn was initially thought to be normal but apparently had no medical examination until the fourth day of life. At this time, the physician noted a right hemiplegia. On the following day, a more complete examination revealed a lateral bulging of the right abdomen accompanied by crying and the maintenance of the lower extremities in a frog-leg position. Adduction and flexion at the hips were weak, and the knee and ankle jerks were absent. Laboratory studies were unremarkable except for the examination of the CSF, which revealed 20 lymphocytes per mm^3 and a protein concentration of 169 mg/dl. During a 6-month period, this child's paralysis gradually improved and resulted in only residual weakness of the left lower extremity.

A paresis of the left arm was noted in another child with apparent transplacentally acquired poliomyelitis shortly after birth.[105] At 2 days of age, the infant was quadriplegic, but patellar reflexes were present and there were no respiratory or swallowing difficulties. This child had pneumonia at 3 weeks of age, but, aside from this, general neurologic improvement occurred. Examination at 8 weeks of age revealed bilateral atrophy of the shoulder girdle muscles. The CSF in this case revealed 63 leukocytes per mm^3, 29% of them polymorphonuclear cells, and a protein value of 128 mg/dl.

All three of the infants just discussed were apparently infected in utero several days before birth. Their symptoms were exclusively neurologic; fever, irritability, and vomiting did not occur.

Postnatally Acquired Infection

In contrast to infections acquired in utero, those acquired postnatally are more typical of classic poliomyelitis. Shelokov and Weinstein described a child who was asymptomatic at birth.[90] Onset of minor symptoms in the mother occurred 3 weeks, and major symptoms 1 day, before delivery. On the sixth day of life, the infant became suddenly ill with watery diarrhea. He looked grayish and pale. On the following day, he was irritable, lethargic, and limp and had a temperature of 38° C. Mild opisthotonus and weakness of both lower extremities developed. He was responsive to sound, light, and touch. The CSF had an elevated protein level and an increased number of leukocytes. His condition worsened during a total period of 3 days, and then gradual improvement began. At 1 year of age, he had severe residual paralysis of the right leg and moderate weakness in the left leg.

Baskin and associates described two infants with neonatal poliomyelitis.[93] The first child, whose mother had severe poliomyelitis at the time of delivery, was well for 3 days and then developed a temperature of 38.3° C. On the fifth day of life, the boy became listless and cyanotic. CSF examination revealed a protein level of 300 mg/dl and 108 leukocytes per mm³. His condition worsened, and extreme flaccidity, irregular respiration, and progressive cyanosis developed; he died on the seventh day of life. The second infant was a boy who was well until he was 8 days old, but he then became listless and developed a temperature of 38.3° C. During the next 5 days, a flaccid quadriplegia developed as well as irregular, rapid, and shallow respirations and the inability to swallow. The child died on the 14th day of life. His mother had developed acute poliomyelitis 6 days before the onset of his symptoms.

Abramson and colleagues reported four children with neonatal poliomyelitis, two of whom died.[99] In three of the children, the illnesses were typical of acute poliomyelitis seen in older children; they were similar to the cases of Baskin and associates[93] noted previously. The other child died at 13 days of age with generalized paralysis. The onset of his illness was difficult to define, and he was never febrile. Swarts and Kercher also described a child whose illness had an insidious onset.[100] At 10 days of age, the child gradually became lethargic and anorectic and regurgitated formula through his nose. On the following day, flaccid quadriplegia developed.

Winsser and associates[106] and Bates[101] also described infants with acute poliomyelitis with clinical illnesses similar to those that occur in older individuals.

Vaccine Viral Infections

Administration of oral polio vaccines to newborns has been carried out in numerous studies.[109, 165–177] Vaccine viral infection occurs in newborns with all three types of poliovirus, although the rate of infection is less than that for immunized older children. This rate is governed by the dose of virus, transplacentally acquired maternal antibody, and antibody acquired from colostrum and breast milk. Although clinical illness has on rare occasions resulted from attenuated polioviral infections in older children and adults, there is at the present time only one specific report of paralytic poliomyelitis in a newborn associated with infection with a vaccine viral strain.[178] In this case the possible source for the infection was the recently vaccinated child of the baby sitter. In a review of 118 cases of vaccine-associated paralytic poliomyelitis in the United States between 1980 and 1992 the age of patients ranged from 1 month to 69 years, but details relating to neonates were not presented.[397]

MANIFESTATIONS OF SPECIFIC NONPOLIO ENTEROVIRUSES

Coxsackieviruses

Coxsackievirus A. There have been few reports of neonatal coxsackievirus A infections. Baker and Phillips reported a small-for-gestational-age infant with pneumonia and a sepsis-like illness with disseminated intravascular coagulation.[306] This newborn died on the second day of life, and on culture the CSF grew coxsackievirus A3. Balduzzi and Greendyke[304] recovered a coxsackievirus A5 from the stool of a 1-month-old child with sudden infant death. In a similar investigation of sudden infant death, Gold and co-workers recovered coxsackievirus A4 from the brains of three infants.[305] Coxsackievirus A8 was also recovered from the stool of a child in whom anorexia was noted on the day before death. Berkovich and Kibrick reported a 3-day-old neonate with nonspecific febrile illness (temperature 38.3° C) who was infected with coxsackievirus A9.[228] Coxsackievirus A9 was also recovered from an 11-day-old infant with rhinitis, lethargy, anorexia, and fever.[229] This illness lasted 3 days. Jack and associates[222] described a 3-day-old newborn with fever, cyanosis, and respiratory distress who died on the seventh day of life; an autopsy revealed bronchopneumonia. Coxsackievirus A9 was isolated from the feces on the fourth and sixth days of life.

Lake and associates[308] noted two neonates with coxsackievirus A9 infections, but no clinical details were presented. Jenista and co-workers recovered coxsackievirus A9 strains from seven nonhospitalized neonates who were thought to be well.[164] In the Netherlands, a neonate with coxsackievirus A9 illness had pericarditis, meningitis, pneumonitis, and hepatitis; he recovered completely.[311] Krajden and Middleton[27] noted a neonate with a sepsis-like illness who died. Coxsackievirus A9 was recovered from the liver and lung. Morens also reported a death associated with this same virus type.[343] Forty-eight of 598 neonates admitted to a regular nursery in Bangkok, Thailand, in the spring of 1977 had herpangina.[359] Coxsackievirus A5 was isolated from nine specimens from the afflicted infants, and a serum antibody titer rise was noted in 10 instances. Helin and colleagues noted 16 newborns with aseptic meningitis from coxsackievirus A14.[382] During a 2½-year follow-up period, they all developed normally and no sequelae were noted. Coxsackievirus A16 was recovered from one newborn with nonspecific illness; his mother had had hand-foot-and-mouth syndrome 4 days previously.[216]

Coxsackievirus B1. Coxsackievirus B1 has only occasionally been recovered from newborns (Table 10–6). Eckert and co-workers recovered a coxsackievirus B1 strain from the stool of a 1-month-old boy with bronchitis.[366] Jahn and Cherry noted a 4-day-old infant who became febrile and lethargic.[197] This illness persisted for 5 days without other signs or symptoms. An examination of the CSF showed a slight increase in leukocytes with a majority of mononuclear cells. Coxsackievirus B1 was recovered from the throat, stool, urine, and serum.

TABLE 10–6
Clinical and Pathologic Findings in Coxsackievirus B Infection of Newborns

FINDING	REFERENCE NUMBERS FOR COXSACKIEVIRUS				
	B1	B2	B3	B4	B5
Febrile exanthem	210, 358				138, 184, 198, 376
Nonspecific febrile illness		133	215	182, 193	349
Sepsis-like illness	28, 201, 219, 358, 359	28	27, 219	152, 306	28
Paralysis	359	378			
Diarrhea		368			
Sudden infant death	395		304, 395	395	
Pneumothorax					222
Aseptic meningitis, meningoencephalitis, encephalomyelitis	197, 200, 202	139, 185, 195, 208, 306, 307, 347, 361, 391, 392	27, 28, 129, 136, 187, 198, 209	28, 184, 189, 190, 198, 213, 307	27, 130, 138, 139, 186, 188, 196, 217, 218, 220, 345, 356, 374, 381, 390
Myocarditis	200, 202–204, 219, 358, 359	28, 139, 185, 195, 196, 205–206, 306, 347, 389	27, 28, 129, 179, 180, 187, 194, 215, 219, 309	27, 139, 154, 182, 184, 189, 190, 192, 199, 213, 306, 372, 389	27, 138, 188, 345, 381
Hepatitis	202, 219, 358, 360		219	189, 199	
Pancreatitis				183	186
Adrenal cortical necrosis			187		
Bronchitis			366		

Wright and colleagues reported an infant fatality associated with coxsackievirus B1 infection.[202] This premature boy was well until 4 days of age, when he had two episodes of cyanosis and apnea. After this he became anorexic and listless and lost the Moro reflex. On the ninth day of life, he had shallow respirations, hepatomegaly, jaundice, petechiae, and thrombocytopenia. He was edematous and lethargic, and he had a temperature of 34.5° C, a pulse rate of 130 and a respiratory rate of 20. He became weaker, unresponsive, and apneic and died. Positive laboratory findings included the following values: platelets, less than 10,000 per mm³, CSF protein, 283 mg/dl; serum bilirubin, 20.5 mg/dl; and serum aspartate aminotransferase, 100 units. Autopsy revealed hepatic necrosis, meningoencephalitis, and myocarditis. Coxsackievirus B1 was recovered from the throat, urine, liver, lung, kidney, and brain.

Twin boys with a sepsis-like illness with hepatitis and disseminated intravascular coagulation have been reported.[28] The first twin died on the 16th day of life, and the second twin survived. Three other newborns with fatal sepsis-like illnesses with hepatitis have been described.[358, 359]

Isacsohn described four severe neonatal illnesses due to coxsackievirus B1; three of the four neonates died.[219] Of the three fatalities one was from myocarditis and the other two were from multi-organ dysfunction. The surviving infant had hepatitis, congestive heart failure, thrombocytopenia, and residual neurologic damage.

McLean and colleagues described a male newborn who had a temperature of 39° C, vomiting, and diarrhea on the fourth day of life.[200] When 6 days of age, he appeared gray and mottled and developed shallow respi-

rations. He died on the seventh day of life after increased respiratory distress (90 breaths per minute), hepatomegaly, generalized edema, and cardiac enlargement. Coxsackievirus B1 was recovered from the heart and brain.

Gear studied an extensive epidemic of Bornholm disease related to coxsackievirus B1 in Johannesburg in the summer of 1960–1961.[203] After the first coxsackievirus B1 isolations, the medical officers of the area were on the alert for nursery infections and the prevention of nursery epidemics. In spite of careful isolation procedures, Gear reported that infection "was introduced into all the large maternity homes in Johannesburg." About 20 cases of neonatal myocarditis were noted, as were three deaths. The isolation procedures apparently prevented secondary nursery cases.

Volakova and Jandasek reported epidemic myocarditis related to coxsackievirus B1.[204] Cherry and Jahn noted a child with a mild febrile exanthematous illness, which had its onset within 10 minutes of birth.[210]

Coxsackievirus B2. The reported instances of coxsackievirus B2 infections in neonates are recorded in Table 10–6. In most instances, the infants had myocarditis or neurologic manifestations. Eleven of 12 of the infants with myocarditis died. The one child with myocarditis who survived was re-examined at 2 years of age and found to be normal.[205] This child's mother became ill with sore throat, coryza, and malaise on the day after delivery. At 3 days of age, the child became febrile (temperature 38.9° C) and had periods of apnea and cardiac irregularities. The cry was "pained." The electrocardiogram showed a left-sided heart pattern in the V leads and T wave abnormalities. The child's symptoms lasted less than 48 hours. Coxsackievirus B2 was isolated from the nose, urine, throat, and CSF, as well as from the mother's stool. Interestingly, the mother breast-fed the infant (while she wore a mask) during her illness. A later specimen of breast milk was cultured for virus without successful recovery of an agent.

Puschak reported a child who became febrile (temperature 39.5° C) at 8 hours of age.[133] During the next 9 days, the infant's temperature fluctuated between 36.7° C and 38.9° C. The patient had no other symptoms. Serologic evidence of coxsackievirus B2 infection was noted.

Johnson and associates described a 1-month-old infant with aseptic meningitis who developed a persistent right facial paralysis.[378] In the study of undifferentiated diarrheal syndromes, Ramos-Alvarez observed a child with coxsackievirus B2 infection.[368] Eilard and associates reported a nursery outbreak in which 12 infants were infected.[347] All had aseptic meningitis, and, in addition, two had myocarditis. One of the latter infants died on the 13th day of life. One child with thrombocytopenia and respiratory failure died.[308]

Coxsackievirus B3. Neonatal infections with coxsackievirus B3 are recorded in Table 10–6. Most reported cases have been severe illnesses with myocarditis or meningoencephalitis, or both. One case involved sudden infant death,[304] in which coxsackievirus B3 was recovered from a pool of organs from an infant who died on the eighth day of life.

Tuuteri and co-workers studied a nursery outbreak of coxsackievirus B3 infection.[215] Seven children had mild disease characterized by anorexia, listlessness, and fever, and two infants had fatal myocarditis. Of the 55 reported neonatal infections with coxsackievirus B3, 29 deaths have been noted, the majority of them associated with myocarditis and sepsis-like illness. Three infants had febrile illnesses with meningitis and have been reported to have suffered no residual effects; long-term follow-up is not available, however.[136, 198]

Isacsohn and colleagues reported two neonates with multi-organ dysfunction who survived.[219]

Chesney and associates studied a 3-week-old girl with meningoencephalitis.[377] This child was noted to have hypoglycorrhachia; the CSF glucose value on the sixth day of illness was 23 mg/dl, with a corresponding blood glucose level of 78 mg/dl. In another review, two infants who died had thrombocytopenia and respiratory failure; a clinical picture suggestive of necrotizing enterocolitis was also observed.[308]

During a 5-year period in Toronto, Krajden and Middleton noted 24 neonates with enteroviral infections who were admitted to the Hospital for Sick Children.[27] There were 9 children infected with coxsackievirus B3; 2 infants had meningitis, 3 had myocarditis, and 4 had a sepsis-like illness. Of this group, 1 infant with meningitis, 1 with myocarditis, and all with sepsis-like illness died. All the neonates with sepsis-like illness had clinical evidence of multiple organ involvement; they had respiratory distress, hepatomegaly, hemorrhagic manifestations, and congestive heart failure. Two neonates with herpangina and coxsackievirus B3 infections were noted in an outbreak involving 25 infants.[362]

Coxsackievirus B4. In Table 10–6, a review of coxsackievirus B4 neonatal infections is presented. The majority were severe and frequently fatal illnesses with neurologic and cardiac involvement. An infant with less severe disease was described by Sieber and associates.[193] This child was well until 6 days of age, when he developed pharyngitis, diarrhea, and gradually increasing lethargy. This was followed by fever for 36 hours. No other signs or symptoms were noted, and the child was well by 11 days of age. He had virologic and serologic evidence of coxsackievirus B4 infection.

Winsser and Altieri noted an infant who suddenly became cyanotic and convulsed and died at 2 days of age.[183] At autopsy, the only findings were bronchopneumonia, congestive splenomegaly, and chronic, interstitial pancreatitis. Coxsackievirus B4 was isolated from the spleen.

Barson and associates reported the survival of an infant with myocarditis.[372] In this child, cardiac calcification was noted on radiographs at 4 weeks of age and the electrocardiogram revealed a left bundle branch block. The conduction defect was still present at 7 months of age, but the myocardial calcification had resolved.

Coxsackievirus B5. The spectrum of neonatal infection with coxsackievirus B5 is greater than that with the other coxsackieviruses B. A summary of reports is given in Table 10–6. Meningitis and encephalitis are common neonatal manifestations of coxsackievirus B5 infection.* Nursery epidemics have been observed. Rantakallio and associates[217] noted 17 infants in one nursery with aseptic meningitis. None of the infants were severely ill. All had fever, with a temperature range from 38° C to 40° C. Eleven of the 17 neonates were boys. Signs included irritability, nuchal rigidity, increased tone, anorexia, opisthotonus, whimpering, loose stools, and diminution of alertness. In another nursery outbreak, Farmer and Patten found 28 infected infants.[345] Of the group of 28, 15 had aseptic meningitis, 4 had diarrhea, and 9 had no signs of illness. Six years later, the 15 children who had had meningitis were studied. Thirteen were found to be physically normal and to have normal intelligence. Two children had intelligence levels below the mean for the group and were noted to have residual spasticity. At the time of the initial illness, these two infants and one additional child had been noted to be twitching, irritable, or jittery.

Swender and associates studied seven cases of aseptic meningitis in an intensive care nursery during a 6-week period during the summer of 1972.[220] Two of the infants had apnea. One of the infants had a CSF glucose level of 12 mg/dl. During a community outbreak of coxsackievirus B5 infections, Marier and colleagues studied 32 infants with aseptic meningitis.[356] In this group, 36% had CSF leukocyte counts of 500 cells per mm³ or more and in 19% the percentage of neutrophils was 50 or more. In 12% of the patients, the CSF glucose level was less than 40 mg/dl. Thirty-eight percent of the infants had blood leukocyte counts of 15,000 cells per mm³ or more.

Of particular interest is the observation of exanthem

---

*See references 27, 130, 138, 139, 186, 188, 217, 218, 220, 345, 356, and 381.

in four reports. Cherry and co-workers noted a 3-week-old boy with fever, a maculopapular rash, and enlarged cervical and postauricular lymph nodes.[376] Examination of the CSF revealed 141 leukocytes per mm³, of which 84% were lymphocytes, and a protein value of 100 mg/dl. An electrocardiogram was normal. In this child, the rash appeared before the fever. Coxsackievirus B5 was isolated from the pharynx and the CSF. Nogen and Lepow noted an infant with a similar illness.[198] This child had a nonspecific erythematous papular rash on the face and scalp. One week later, he became febrile and irritable. The CSF contained 440 white blood cells per mm³, 96% of them mononuclear. Virus was isolated from the feces, throat, and CSF.

Artenstein and associates reported a 23-day-old girl with a fever and an erythematous macular rash that spread from the scalp to the entire body, except the palms and soles, and lasted 4 days.[184] Coxsackievirus B5 was recovered from the stool, but no evidence of serum antibody to this virus was found. McLean and co-workers also noted a child with a rash.[138] In this child, a papular rash on the trunk and limbs was present at birth. On the fourth day of life, the rash had disappeared, but the patient then developed a temperature of 39.4° C. Irritability, twitching, and fullness of the anterior fontanelle were observed, and CSF examination showed meningitis. During an 8-day period, the child had repeated vomiting and diarrhea. On the 11th day of life, hyperpnea and tachycardia were noted, as well as an enlarging liver. The child died on the 13th day of life. Autopsy revealed extensive encephalitis and focal myocardial necrosis. Virus was recovered from the brain, heart, lungs, and liver.

It would appear that neonatal infection with coxsackievirus B5 is less likely to be fatal than infection with the other coxsackieviruses B. Only 6 of 36 infants noted in Table 10–6 died. In contrast to coxsackieviruses B2, B3, and B4, coxsackievirus B5 appears to be more neurotropic than cardiotropic.

Echoviruses

Echovirus 1. Dömök and Molnár described aseptic meningitis related to echovirus 1.[214]

Echovirus 2. Krajden and Middleton noted three infants with echovirus 2 infections.[27] Two of the neonates had meningitis and recovered. The third child, who died, had a sepsis-like illness. Virus was isolated from the CSF, lung, liver, and urine. One other neonate with echovirus 2 infection has been observed, but no details are available.[308]

Echovirus 3. In the summer of 1970, Haynes and co-workers studied an epidemic of infection caused by echovirus 3.[379] Three infected neonates were observed, all of whom had meningitis. One child, a full-term girl, developed tonic seizures and an inability to suck on the third day of life. The serum bilirubin level was 28 mg/dl. Shortly thereafter, the child became cyanotic, flaccid, and apneic and developed a bulging anterior fontanelle; she was in shock. She received assisted ventilation with a respirator for 3 days. At 1 month of age, severe neurologic damage with developing hydrocephalus was obvi-

ous. Echovirus 3 was recovered from the CSF, and the CSF protein level was 880 mg/dl on the sixth day of life.

The other two infants in this study apparently had uncomplicated aseptic meningitis. The CSF findings in one child revealed 1826 white blood cells per mm³, 91% of them polymorphonuclear cells; the other child had 320 cells per mm³, 98% of which were polymorphonuclear cells.

A 4-day-old infant from whom echovirus 3 was recovered from the CSF has been reported.[27] This child had less than 3 white blood cells per mm³ in the CSF. Other neonates with echovirus 3 infection have been observed, but no details are available.[164, 308]

Echovirus 4. Linnemann and associates studied 11 infants with echovirus 4 infections.[348] All infants had fevers, and most were irritable. Four infants had a fine maculopapular rash, which was located on the face or abdomen or both. In two children, the extremities were also involved. Other neonates with echovirus 4 infections have been noted, but details of illness are not available.[164, 308]

Echovirus 5. There have been five reports of neonatal illnesses associated with echovirus 5 infections.[308, 344, 390] In one nursery epidemic, six infants were involved.[227] All infants had fever (38.3° C to 39.7° C), which lasted from 4 to 8 days. Two neonates had tachycardia that was disproportionately rapid when compared with the degree of fever, but in neither was there evidence of myocarditis. Four infants had splenomegaly and enlarged lymph nodes; these findings persisted for several weeks.

In 1966 (July to October), an epidemic of echovirus 5 infection involved 23% of the infants in the maternity unit at the Royal Air Force Hospital in Chargi, Singapore.[226] Fifty-six infants were symptomatically infected, and 10 were asymptomatically infected. Those who were ill were 2 to 12 days of age at the onset of disease. All 56 symptomatic infants had fever; 87 per cent of them had a temperature of 38.3° C or greater. The mean duration of fever was 3.5 days, with a range of 2 to 7 days. Twenty infants had a faint erythematous macular rash that was most prominent on the limbs and buttocks but also occurred on the trunk and face. The rash, which began 24 to 36 hours after the beginning of fever, lasted 48 hours. Diarrhea was noted in 17 infants, 4 of whom passed blood and mucus. Vomiting was observed in about half the neonates. All infants apparently recovered completely.

A newborn girl has been described who had a nonspecific biphasic febrile illness.[302] Echovirus 5 was recovered from the CSF, but the cell count, protein level and glucose value were normal.

In another study, a 9-day-old infant with aseptic meningitis was noted.[390] During an epidemiologic investigation in Rochester, New York, 13 of 75 enteroviral isolates were echovirus 5.[164] Six of the infants were asymptomatic; no clinical details of the other seven patients were presented.

Echovirus 6. Sanders and Cramblett reported a boy who was well until 9 days of age, when he developed a fever (38° C), severe diarrhea, and dehydration.[229] His white blood cell count was 27,900 cells per mm³, and virologic and serologic evidence of echovirus 6 infection was found. Treatment consisted of intravenous hydration, to which there was a good response. Krous and colleagues noted an infant who died on the ninth day of life with a sepsis-like illness.[310] The child had meningitis, disseminated intravascular coagulation, hepatic necrosis, and adrenal and renal hemorrhage. Echovirus type 6 has been found in association with neonatal illness on two other occasions, but no clinical details are available.[308, 348]

Echovirus 7. Piraino and colleagues reported three infants with echovirus 7 infections.[154] All three had fever, one had respiratory distress and exanthem, and one had irritability and loose stools. Two neonates with fatal sepsis-like illnesses with massive disseminated intravascular coagulation have been reported.[249, 319]

Echovirus 8. In a search for etiologic associations in infantile diarrhea, Ramos-Alvarez[368] noted one neonate from whom echovirus 8 was recovered from the stool; the antibody titer to this virus rose fourfold.

Echovirus 9. Echovirus 9 is the most prevalent of all the enteroviruses (see Table 10–2). From 1955 to 1958, epidemic waves of infection spread throughout the world.[398] Since that time, echovirus 9 has been a common cause of human illness. In spite of its prevalence and its frequent association with epidemic disease, descriptions of neonatal illness are infrequent. Unlike experiences with several other enteroviruses, newborn nursery epidemics caused by echovirus 9 have not often been described. Neonatal echovirus 9 experiences are recorded in Table 10–7. Moscovici and Maisel noted an asymptomatic infant with echovirus 9 infection.[145] When echovirus 9 was prevalent in Erie County, New York, during the summer of 1971, seven neonatal cases were observed.[367] Four children had aseptic meningitis, but only moderate elevations of CSF protein values and white blood cells were observed. One child, a 15-day-old infant, had radiologic evidence of bronchopneumonia, and two infants had gastroenteritis. Rawls and coworkers described an infant who was well until the seventh day of life, when progressive lethargy, anorexia, and irritability developed.[315] The child became moribund and jaundice, scattered petechiae, and hypothermia were observed. The pulse rate was 90, the respiratory rate was 40 breaths per minute, and the liver was enlarged. The infant died 3 days after the onset of symp-

toms. Echovirus 9 was recovered from the lung, brain, and CSF. Cho and colleagues[354] described a similar severe neonatal illness in a child from whom echovirus 9 was recovered from the CSF. This child was hypothermic and hypotonic on the third day of life. He had bilateral pneumonia and leukopenia. After a stormy course, which included an exchange transfusion for suspected sepsis and mechanical ventilation for apnea, he eventually recovered.

A child who became febrile (temperature 38.3° C), irritable, and anorectic on the sixth day of life was described by Jahn and Cherry.[197] This child became asymptomatic within 2 days; echovirus 9 was recovered from the throat, feces, serum, and CSF. Eichenwald and Kostevalov noted two children with mild irritability, fever, and diarrhea and a third child with diarrhea and convulsions in whom laboratory findings showed aseptic meningitis.[146] Haynes and colleagues studied a large outbreak of meningoencephalitis caused by echovirus 9 and described nine children who were 2 weeks to 2 months of age.[380] Cheeseman and associates[150] noted a neonate with fatal interstitial pneumonia, and Krajden and Middleton[27] reported a 4-day-old infant from whom echovirus 9 was recovered from the CSF. This child had less than 3 white blood cells per mm³ in the CSF.

Echovirus 11. Neonatal illness associated with echovirus 11 infection has been interesting and varied. Reported cases are listed in Table 10–8. Eleven of the reports involved nursery outbreaks, and in five reports the neonatal cases were part of a larger community epidemic. Miller and associates studied an epidemic of aseptic meningitis and other acute febrile illnesses in New Haven, Connecticut, in the summer of 1965.[224] This epidemic was unique in that half of the patients with meningitis from whom virus was isolated were younger than 6 months old. The echovirus 11 in this epidemic was a prime strain. Three neonatal illnesses were reported. One of the patients, a 1-month-old infant, was initially irritable and feverish and had diarrhea. Chest radiographs revealed bilateral pneumonitis. A generalized discrete maculopapular rash, which lasted 24 hours, was noted on the third day of illness. Fever persisted for 6 days. A 12-day-old girl had fever lasting 1 day (temperature 39.4°C), without other findings. Echovirus 11 was recovered from her throat. Another 1-month-old infant had aseptic meningitis.

Sanders and Cramblett noted two infants with diarrhea.[229] Both infants were acutely ill; one was jaundiced and irritable and had feeding difficulty. In another study, diarrhea was present in two infants with echovirus 11 infections.[228] One infant had a temperature of 39.3° C and a "stuffy nose," and the other had a temperature of 39.8° C and aseptic meningitis. Cramblett and co-workers observed an outbreak of nosocomial infections caused by echovirus 11 in a neonatal intensive care unit.[221] In a 1-month-old premature infant with frequent apneic episodes, the CSF contained 2200 white blood cells per mm³, 89% of them polymorphonuclear cells, with a protein level of 280 mg/dl. The infant made a gradual recovery. Echovirus 11 was isolated from the CSF and the stool. In another premature infant, apneic episodes and bradycardia suddenly began on the 20th

TABLE 10–7
Neonatal Infection with Echovirus 9

AUTHOR	FINDING
Moskovici and Maisel[145]	Asymptomatic infection
Mirani et al.[367]	Meningitis (4 cases)
	Gastroenteritis (2 cases)
	Pneumonia (1 case)
Rawls et al.[315]	Hepatic necrosis
Cho et al.[354]	Severe generalized disease
Jahn and Cherry[197]	Mild febrile illness
Elchenwald and Kostevalov[146]	Aseptic meningitis
	Gastroenteritis (2 cases)
Haynes et al.[380]	Meningoencephalitis
Cheeseman et al.[150]	Fatal interstitial pneumonia
Krajden and Middleton[27]	Meningitis

TABLE 10–8
Neonatal Infection with Echovirus 11

AUTHOR	FINDING
Miller et al.[224]	Exanthem and pneumonia (1 case)
	Nonspecific febrile illness (1 case)
	Aseptic meningitis (1 case)
Sanders and Cramblett[229]	Gastroenteritis (2 cases)
Berkovich and Kibrick[228]	Gastroenteritis (1 case)
	Meningitis (1 case)
Cramblett et al.[221]	Meningitis (3 cases, 1 with rash)
	Severe nonspecific febrile illness (1 case)
Hercík et al.[225]	Respiratory illness (22 cases)
Hasegawa[238]	Fever (31 cases)
	Stomatitis (4 cases)
	Fever and stomatitis (6 cases)
Davies et al.[237]	Encephalopathy (1 case)
	Nonspecific febrile illness (1 case)
	Sepsis-like with cardiac failure (1 death)
	Lower respiratory infection (1 case)
Jones et al.[151]	Sepsis-like with hepatitis and rash (1 case)
Lapinleimu and	Aseptic meningitis (4 cases)
Hakulinen[239]	Gastroenteritis and/or respiratory distress (3 cases)
Nagington et al.[236]	Sepsis-like with shock, diffuse bleeding and renal hemorrhage (3 deaths)
Suzuki et al.[364]	Fever (100%); pharyngitis (7%) (42 cases)
Krous et al.[310]	Sepsis-like with disseminated intravascular coagulation, hepatic necrosis (1 death)
Modlin[240]	Sepsis-like with apnea, lethargy, poor feeding, jaundice, hepatitis, disseminated intravascular coagulation (4 deaths)
Drew[375]	Myocarditis (5 cases)
Piraino et al.[154]	Meningitis and rash (2 cases)
	Meningitis (4 cases)
	Fatal case with cardiac failure, interstitial pneumonia and interventricular cerebral hemorrhage
Krajden and Middleton[27]	Meningitis
Mertens et al.[243]	Fever (2 cases)
	Meningitis (4 cases)
Reyes et al.[153]	Fatal sepsis-like illness
Berry and Nagington[311]	Sepsis-like illness (11 deaths)
	Sudden death
Gh et al.[312]	Sepsis-like illness (5 deaths)
Bose et al.[152]	Sepsis-like illness (1 death, 1 survived)
Bowen et al.[387]	Meningitis (34 infants ≤4 mo old)
Halfon and Spector[313]	Sepsis-like illness (2 deaths)
Steinmann and Albrecht[245]	Sepsis-like illness with meningitis and apnea (5 cases)
	Meningitis (4 cases)
	Gastroenteritis (3 cases)
Gitlin et al.[314]	Sepsis-like illness with hepatic necrosis (4 deaths)
Kinney et al.[244]	Meningitis (8 cases with 1 death)
	Mild illness (4 cases)
	Inapparent infection (2 cases)
Rabkin et al.[248]	Sepsis-like illness (9 cases, 5 with meningitis)
	Inapparent infection (1 case)
Isaacs et al.[251]	Meningitis (2 cases, 1 with myocarditis)
	Pneumonia (1 case)
	Inapparent infection (7 cases)
	Apnea (1 case)

day of life. Fever developed, the apneic spells continued, and digitalis therapy was necessary because of congestive heart failure. Examination of the CSF revealed an aseptic meningitis, and echovirus 11 was recovered from the CSF, throat, and stool. A third child with aseptic meningitis had an exanthem as well. The disease began suddenly with shallow respirations and poor skin color. On the following day, generalized seizures occurred and a maculopapular rash developed on the trunk, extremities, and face. The patient made a gradual recovery. A fourth child had a severe nonspecific febrile illness.

A particularly noteworthy finding in neonatal echovirus 11 infection has been severe sepsis-like illness, with hepatitis or hepatic necrosis, disseminated intravascular coagulation, and extensive hemorrhagic manifestations.[151–153, 236, 237, 240, 310–314, 316] During the past 15 years, more than 40 such cases have been described, and most of the illnesses have been fatal.

Hercík and co-workers reported an epidemic of respiratory illness in 22 newborns.[225] Six of the infants were severely ill, and one subsequently died. The incubation period varied from 17 hours to 9 days, with an average of 3 days. Seven infants had an interstitial pneumonia, and all were reported to have rhinitis, pharyngitis, and vomiting. More recently, Toce and Keenan reported two newborns with respiratory distress and pneumonia at birth.[156] Both of these infants died of their echovirus 11 infections.

Echovirus 13. Echovirus 13 was isolated from one asymptomatic infant in a neonatal surveillance study.[164]

Echovirus 14. Hughes and colleagues reported an infant boy who became febrile (temperature 38° C) and had cyanotic episodes on the third day of life.[148] At 4 days of age, his temperature was 38.9° C, and he experienced recurrent apneic spells. Liver enlargement, hypothermia, bradycardia, periodic breathing, and spontaneous ecchymoses developed, and the infant died on the seventh day of life. Laboratory study revealed the presence of leukopenia and thrombocytopenia, and autopsy showed severe hepatic necrosis. Drouhet[399] described a child with aseptic meningitis and echovirus 14 infection, and Hinuma and associates[346] noted four newborns with apparent asymptomatic echovirus 14 infections.

Echovirus 16. In 1974, Hall and colleagues studied five neonates with echovirus 16 infections.[350] All five infants were admitted to the hospital because of suspicion of sepsis. Four of five were febrile, all were lethargic and irritable, and two had abdominal distention. Three of the neonates had erythematous maculopapular exanthems, and in two the rash appeared after or with defervescence. Leukocyte counts in four infants revealed an increased percentage of band form neutrophils. Two neonates had aseptic meningitis. Lake and associates[308] noted three infants with echovirus 16 infections; in their study, clinical findings were not itemized by virus type, but it is inferred that sepsis-like illnesses occurred.

Echovirus 17. Neonatal infection with echovirus 17 has been observed by three investigators. Cherry and co-workers reported on two ill infants.[132] One infant, 19 days old, developed otitis media 5 days after his mother had a flulike illness. Echovirus 17 was isolated from his feces, and serologic evidence of echovirus 17 infection was found in both the infant and the mother. The second child had a nonspecific febrile illness at the age of 4 weeks, which was severe enough to require hospitalization. Virus was isolated from the infant's throat, feces, and serum.

Sanders and Cramblett noted two neonates with exanthem associated with echovirus 17.[229] The first child, a 3-week-old girl, became drowsy, anorectic and febrile. She had a fine maculopapular rash on the trunk, a slightly injected pharynx, and a few petechiae on the soft palate. She remained febrile for 5 days. Echovirus 17 was recovered from the CSF and the feces. The second infant became ill at 3 weeks of age. His symptoms were mild rhinitis and cough followed by lethargy and refusal to eat. Four days after the onset of symptoms, his temperature was 39° C and his respiratory rate

was 60 breaths per minute. A fine maculopapular rash appeared on the trunk, and radiographs revealed an infiltrate in the right lung. The patient's course was uneventful, and he was much improved 12 days after the onset of symptoms.

Faulkner and van Rooyen described an outbreak of echovirus 17 infection with illness in a nursery in mid-August of 1971.[233] Seven infants were involved, including one with aseptic meningitis who was 7 weeks old. All the infants had fever, four had central nervous system signs, three had abdominal distention, four had diarrhea, and three had a rash. One other infant from another community was also studied by the authors. This child had a febrile pneumonitis at the age of 3½ weeks. The findings abated in 5 days, but the child suddenly died 6 days later. Autopsy revealed interstitial pneumonitis with extensive edema and scattered petechial hemorrhages of the viscera. Echovirus 17 was isolated from the liver, lung, spleen, and kidney.

Echovirus 18. In 1958, Eichenwald and colleagues described two neonates with epidemic diarrhea associated with echovirus 18 infections.[230] In a nursery unit of premature infants, 12 of 21 were mildly ill. Neither temperature elevation nor hypothermia occurred. Six infants were lethargic and listless, and two developed moderate abdominal distention. The diarrhea lasted from 1 to 5 days; there were five or six watery, greenish stools per day, occasionally expelled explosively. In two infants, a small amount of blood was noted in the stools, but no mucus or pus cells. Five other infants in another nursery also had similar diarrheal illness. Echovirus 18 was recovered from all ill infants.

Medearis and co-workers reported a 3-week-old girl with fever, irritability, lethargy, pharyngitis, and postnasal drainage.[365] Admitted to the hospital because of apneic spells, she developed a generalized erythematous blotchy macular rash and had frequent stools. The illness lasted about 7 days. Echovirus 18 was recovered from the blood, throat, and feces. Berkovich and Kibrick found echovirus 18 in the stool of a 12-day-old twin infant with fever and a red throat.[228] The relationship of the virus to the illness is uncertain because the patient's twin was infected with echovirus 11 and the patient also had serologic evidence of echovirus 11 infection. Wilfert and associates observed a 9-day-old infant with aseptic meningitis.[383]

Echovirus 19. Cramblett and co-workers noted two neonates with echovirus 19 infections.[363] One child had an upper respiratory infection, cough, and paroxysmal atrial tachycardia. The other child also had an upper respiratory infection, but, in addition to echovirus 19 infection, coxsackievirus B4 was recovered from the throat of this infant. Butterfield and associates isolated echovirus 19 post mortem from the brain, lung, heart, liver, spleen, lymph nodes, and intestine of a premature infant who had cystic emphysema.[231] The relationship between the generalized viral infection and the pulmonary disease is unknown.

Philip and Larson reported three catastrophic neonatal echovirus 19 infections, which resulted in hepatic necrosis and massive terminal hemorrhage.[149] One infant, infected in utero, was symptomatic at birth. The

Apgar score was 3, and multiple petechiae were observed. Generalized ecchymoses and apneic episodes occurred, and the infant died at 3½ hours of age. Thrombocytopenia was noted, and echovirus 19 was isolated from the brain, liver, spleen, and lymph nodes. The other two infants who died of echovirus 19 infection were twins. They were normal during the first 3 days of life but then became mildly cyanotic and lethargic. Shortly thereafter, apneic episodes occurred and jaundice and petechiae developed. Both twins became oliguric, and they died on the eighth and ninth days of life, with severe gastrointestinal bleeding. Both twins were thrombocytopenic, and virus was recovered from systemic sites in both. More recently, two similar catastrophic cases have been described.[370]

Purdham and associates reported an outbreak of echovirus 19 in a neonatal unit in which 12 infants were affected.[241] All but 1 infant were febrile, 10 were irritable, 7 had marked abdominal distention with decreased bowel sounds, and 5 had apneic episodes. Bacon and Sims noted two neonates with sepsis-like illness.[357] The infants were cyanotic with peripheral circulatory failure. In another study involving the same echovirus 19 epidemic, five infants younger than 3 months of age were reported.[355] All had sepsis-like illness with hypotonia and peripheral circulatory failure. Two infants had aseptic meningitis, and two others had diarrhea.

Echovirus 20. Eichenwald and Kostevalov[146] recovered echovirus 20 from four asymptomatic infants younger than 8 days of age (see earlier discussion of cloud baby under Respiratory Illness). Five neonates with severe illness due to echovirus 20 have also been described.[317, 318] All had hepatitis, and two died.

Echovirus 21. Jack and co-workers recovered echovirus 21 from the feces of a 7-day-old infant with jaundice and diarrhea.[222] No other details of the child's illness are available. Chonmaitree and associates[373] studied a 19-day-old infant with aseptic meningitis and rash, and Georgieff and colleagues[316] reported a newborn with fulminant hepatitis. Lake and colleagues[308] also mentioned one infected infant but presented no specific details.

Echovirus 22. Echovirus 22 has been associated with three epidemics of nursery infections. During a survey of perinatal virus infections, 44 infants were found to be infected with echovirus 22 during a study period from May to December 1966.[222] The virus prevalence and the incidence of new infections during this period were fairly uniform. No illness was attributed to echovirus 22 infection, and the virus disappeared from the nursery in mid-December of 1966. Berkovich and Pangan studied respiratory illnesses in premature infants and reported 64 infants with illness, 18 of whom had virologic or serologic evidence of echovirus 22 infection.[223] In addition, many had high but constant levels of serum antibody to echovirus 22. Some of these latter infants were probably also infected with echovirus 22. The children with proven echovirus 22 infections could not be clinically differentiated from those without evidence of echovirus 22 infection. Of 18 infants with documented echovirus 22 infections, 90% had coryza, 39% had pneumonia, and 11% had morbilliform rash and/or conjunctivitis. In contrast to the studies of Jack and co-workers,[222] only 3 of 35 asymptomatic infants were found to be infected with echovirus 22. Nakao and associates recovered echovirus 22 from 29 premature infants.[232] Many of the infected infants were asymptomatic, and those who were ill had only mild symptoms of coryza, cough, and diarrhea. Jenista and colleagues noted 17 echovirus 22 infections in nonhospitalized neonates.[164] Clinical details were not presented, but it appears that all of these infants were asymptomatic.

Echovirus 23. Ehrnst and Eriksson reported a 1-month-old girl with encephalopathy resulting from a nosocomial echovirus 23 infection.[394] No further details of this case were provided.

Echovirus 25. Linnemann and colleagues noted one neonate with echovirus 25 infection but gave no virus-specific details except that fever and irritability occurred.[348]

Echovirus 30. Matsumoto and associates described a nursery outbreak involving 11 infants during a 2-week period.[386] All the neonates had aseptic meningitis, and all recovered. Two symptomatic and six asymptomatic neonates were noted in the Rochester, New York, surveillance study.[164]

Echovirus 31. McDonald and associates reported three neonates in an intensive care nursery with echovirus 31 infections.[242] One infant had a fatal encephalitis-like illness, with hypertonicity, hyperreflexia, and apneic spells. The other two infants also experienced apneic spells, and, in addition, one had pneumonia and meningitis.

Echovirus 33. In a study of epidemic illness related to echovirus 33 disease in the Netherlands, Kapsenberg stated that 7- to 8-day-old neonates in a maternity ward had a febrile illness.[235] No further data were presented.

Enterovirus 71

Schmidt and colleagues mentioned one 3-week-old infant with meningitis and enterovirus 71 infection.[384] Chonmaitree and colleagues noted one 9-day-old neonate with aseptic meningitis and one 14-day-old infant with gastroenteritis from enterovirus 71.[369]

DIAGNOSIS AND DIFFERENTIAL DIAGNOSIS

Clinical Diagnosis

The clinical differentiation of neonatal infectious diseases is frequently thought to be an impossible task. Although it is true that treatable bacterial and viral illnesses should always be considered and treated first, it is also true that, when all the circumstances of a particular neonatal illness are considered, enterovirus diseases can be suspected on clinical grounds. The most important factors in clinical diagnosis are season of the year, geographic location, exposure, incubation period, and clinical symptoms.

In temperate climates, enteroviral prevalence is distinctly seasonal, so disease is usually seen in the summer and fall. Neonatal enterovirus disease is unlikely in the winter. In the tropics, enteroviruses are prevalent throughout the year, and season, therefore, is not helpful diagnostically.

As with all infectious illnesses, the knowledge of exposure and incubation time is important. A careful history of maternal illness is vitally important, particularly the symptoms of maternal illness. For example, nonspecific mild febrile illness in the mother that occurs in the summer and fall should warn of the possibility of more severe neonatal illness. More specific findings in the mother (i.e., aseptic meningitis, pleurodynia, herpangina, pericarditis, myocarditis) should alert the clinician to more specific enteroviral illnesses. Minor illness in nursery personnel during enteroviral seasons should also be kept in mind. The short incubation period of enteroviral infections should be taken into consideration. Manifestations of neonatal nonpolio enteroviral infections are presented in Table 10–3.

Laboratory Diagnosis

VIRUS ISOLATION

Most viral diagnostic laboratories have facilities for the recovery of the majority of enteroviruses that cause congenital and neonatal illness. Three tissue culture systems—primary rhesus, cynomolgus, or African green monkey kidney tissue culture; a diploid, human embryonic lung fibroblast cell strain; and the RD cell line—allow the isolation of all polioviruses, coxsackieviruses B, echoviruses, newer enteroviruses, and many coxsackieviruses A. In a 1988 study in which Buffalo green monkey kidney cells and subpassages of primary human embryonic kidney cells were used in addition to primary monkey kidney and human diploid fibroblast (MRC-5) cells, it was found that the enterovirus recovery rate was increased 11%.[400] For a complete diagnostic isolation spectrum, suckling mouse inoculation should also be performed. Optimally, at least one blind passage should be carried out in each of the culture systems.

Proper selection and handling of specimens are most important in the isolation of viruses from ill neonates. Infection in neonates tends to be generalized, so collection of material from multiple sites is important; specimens should be taken from any or all of the following: nose, throat, stool, blood, urine, CSF, and any other body fluids that are available. Swabs from the nose, throat, and rectum should be placed in a transport medium.

The primary purpose of a transport medium is to provide a protective protein, neutral pH, and antibiotics for control of microbial contamination and, most importantly, to prevent desiccation. Many viral transport and storage media are commercially available or are prepared readily in the laboratory; their utility has been reviewed.[401] Convenient and practical collection devices, such as the Culturette (Becton-Dickinson, Cockeysville, Md) or Virocult (Medical Wire and Equipment Co., Victory Gardens, NY), consist of a swab, usually Dacron or rayon, on a plastic or aluminum shaft accompanied by a self-contained transport medium (Stuart or Amies)

and are routinely available in most hospitals for bacteriologic culture. Calcium alginate swabs, which are toxic to herpes simplex virus and wooden shafts, which may be toxic for viruses as well as the cell culture system itself, should not be used. Saline or holding media that contain serum also should be avoided. Useful liquid transport media (2-mL aliquots in screw-capped vials) consist of tryptose phosphate broth with 0.5% bovine albumin; Hanks balanced salt solution with 5% gelatin or 10% bovine albumin; or buffered sucrose phosphate (0.2 M, 2-SP),[401, 402] which has been used as a combined transport for viral, chlamydial, and mycoplasmal culture requests and is appropriate for long-term frozen storage of specimens and isolates.[403]

Fluid specimens should be collected in sterile vials; specimens of autopsy material are best collected in vials that contain transport medium. In general, specimens should be refrigerated immediately after collection and during transportation to the laboratory. It is important not to expose specimens to sunlight during transportation. If it is known that an extended period of time will elapse before a specimen will be processed in the laboratory, it is advisable to ship and store it frozen.

Contrary to popular belief, evidence of enteroviral growth from tissue cultures takes only a few days in many cases and less than a week in most.[404] The use of the spin amplification, shell viral technique, and monoclonal antibodies has been shown to significantly reduce the time of detection in enteroviral cultures.[59, 405] After isolation of an enterovirus, its identification as to type is conventionally done by neutralization, and this process, unfortunately, is expensive and frequently takes an extended period of time.

RAPID VIRUS IDENTIFICATION

Because of the number of different serotypes of enteroviruses, the use of immunofluorescence, agglutination, counterimmunoelectrophoresis, and enzyme-linked immunosorbent assay (ELISA) techniques for the direct detection of antigen in suspected enteroviral infections has not been useful.

Nucleic acid techniques with complementary DNA and RNA probes have been shown to be useful for the direct identification of enteroviruses.[406–408] Of most importance today, however, has been the development of a number of PCR techniques. During the past decade there have been innumerable reports that describe enteroviral PCR methods and the use of PCR in identifying enterovirus RNA in clinical specimens.[48–62, 409, 410] PCR has proven most useful for the direct identification of enteroviruses in the CSF of patients with meningitis. In comparison with culture of CSF specimens, PCR is more rapid and sensitive and the specificity is equal. The short-coming of PCR is that enterovirus RNA is identified but the specific enteroviral type is not determined.

PCR has also proven useful in the identification of enteroviruses in blood, urine, and throat specimens and in frozen and formalin-fixed biopsy and autopsy specimens of myocardium.[51, 56, 58, 410a, 410b] In one study enteroviruses were identified in myocardial tissue from four neonates who died of myocarditis.[410b] In one case the specimen was obtained during life by a right ventricular endomyocardial biopsy and in the other three on frozen or formalin-fixed autopsy samples. Most PCR methods available today will detect 1 tissue culture infective dose of enterovirus in cerebrospinal fluid, stool, or throat specimen.[410a] Polioviruses can be separated from other enteroviruses, and poliovirus vaccine strains can be rapidly identified by PCR.[411–413]

SEROLOGY

Except in special circumstances, the use of serologic techniques in the primary diagnosis of suspected neonatal enterovirus infections is impractical. Standard serologic study depends on the demonstration of an antibody titer rise to a specific virus as an indication of infection with that agent. Although hemagglutination-inhibition, ELISA and complement fixation tests take only a short time to perform, these tests can be done only after the collection of a second, convalescent-phase blood specimen. These tests are also impractical in searching for the cause of a specific illness in a child because there are so many antigenically different enteroviruses; there are no common group antigens, and thus the identification of a particular illness might require the performance of more than 60 individual specific serologic tests.

In the evaluation of an infant with a suspected enterovirus infection, serum should be collected as soon as possible after the onset of illness and then again 2 to 4 weeks later. This serum should be stored frozen. In most clinical situations, it is not necessary to carry out serologic tests on the collected serum because demonstration of an antibody titer rise in the serum of an infant from whom a specific virus has been isolated from a body fluid is obviously superfluous. However, collected serum can be useful diagnostically if the prevalence of specific enteroviruses in a community is known. In this situation, it is relatively easy to look for antibody titer changes to a selected number of viral types. More rapid diagnosis utilizing a single serum sample is possible if a search for specific IgM enteroviral antibody is made.[193, 414–422]

Unfortunately there are presently no commercially available enterovirus IgM antibody tests. Commercial laboratories do offer enteroviral complement fixation antibody panels. However, the results of these tests in the clinical setting are almost always meaningless unless acute and convalescent-phase sera are analyzed.

HISTOLOGY

There are no specific histologic findings in enteroviral infections, such as those seen in cytomegalovirus or herpes simplex viral infections. However, tissues can be examined for specific enteroviral antigens by immunofluorescent study and by PCR.[139, 409]

Differential Diagnosis

The differential diagnosis of congenital and neonatal enterovirus infections depends on the clinical manifesta-
tions. In general, the most important illness categories are generalized bacterial sepsis or meningitis, congenital heart disease, and congenital and neonatal infections with other viruses.

Hypothermia and hyperthermia in association with such nonspecific signs as lethargy and poor appetite are common in neonatal enteroviral infections; they are also the presenting manifestations in bacterial sepsis. Proper bacterial cultures are essential. The differentiation between congenital heart disease and neonatal myocarditis is frequently difficult. However, the occurrence of fever or hypothermia, generalized lethargy and weakness, and characteristic electrocardiographic changes should suggest the viral etiology.

Congenital infections with rubella virus, cytomegalovirus, *Toxoplasma gondii*, or *Treponema pallidum* are frequently associated with intrauterine growth retardation; this is not usual with enterovirus infections. Generalized herpes simplex infections are clinically similar to severe infections with several enteroviruses; in herpes infections, skin lesions are common, and a scraping of a lesion and a culture should allow a rapid diagnosis. In infants with signs of central nervous system involvement, it is particularly important to consider herpes simplex virus infection as a possible cause because infection with this agent is treatable and early treatment is essential. In infants with meningitis, proper cultures are essential because the CSF findings in bacterial and viral illnesses are frequently similar.

PROGNOSIS

Polioviruses

As noted in the review by Bates[101] and the summary in Table 10–5, poliovirus infections in neonates are generally severe. Of the 44 cases with available follow-up data, there were 21 deaths; of the survivors, 12 had residual paralyses. Infant survivors of poliomyelitis are susceptible to infection by the other two types of poliovirus, so these infants should receive attenuated polio vaccine.

Nonpolio Enteroviruses

It is apparent that the immediate prognosis in coxsackievirus and echovirus infections is related to the specific manifestations. Mortality is greatest in infants with myocarditis, encephalitis, or sepsis-like illness with liver involvement. There are apparent differences in the severity of illness, depending on viral type, as well as differences, probably more subtle, related to strain variations. In general, infections with coxsackieviruses B1 to B4 and, more recently, echovirus 11 appear to carry the most ominous initial prognoses.

There is a surprising dearth of information related to long-term sequelae of neonatal coxsackievirus and echovirus infections. Gear, in a 4-year follow-up study, found no evidence of permanent cardiac damage in several children who had coxsackievirus B myocarditis.[181] In children with aseptic meningitis, there is little available evidence of neurologic damage. One of five infants studied by Nogen and Lepow,[198] from whom virus was recovered from the CSF, was suspected of having possible brain damage. Cho and colleagues noted that a child who had had severe neonatal echovirus 9 disease was developing normally at 1 year of age.[354] Tuuteri and associates reported that two children who had had clinically mild neonatal coxsackievirus B3 infections were thriving when seen at 1 year of age.[215] After an epidemic of mild febrile disease related to echovirus 5, 51 children were examined at 1 year of age and found to be normal.[226]

Farmer and colleagues did a careful follow-up study of 15 children who had meningoencephalitis related to coxsackievirus B5 during the neonatal period.[381] At 6 years of age, 2 of the children were found to have developed spasticity, and their intelligence was below the mean for the study group as a whole and also below the mean of a carefully selected control group. Three children who had myocarditis as well as meningoencephalitis had no cardiac sequelae at the age of 6 years. Sells and associates noted neurologic impairment at later follow-up in some children who had central nervous system enteroviral infections during the first year of life.[385]

In a study in which nine children with enteroviral meningitis during the first 3 months of life were compared with nine matched control children, Wilfert and associates noted that the receptive language functioning of patients was significantly less than that of the controls.[390] Head circumference, hearing, and intellectual function were similar between the patients and the controls. Bergman and colleagues reported an extensive study in which 33 survivors of enteroviral meningitis during infancy were compared with their siblings.[389] In this comprehensive study, none of the survivors had major neurologic sequelae, and they performed as well as their siblings on a large number of cognitive, achievement, perceptual-motor skills, and language tests. Rantakallio and co-workers noted that 16 of 17 patients with neonatal meningitis related to coxsackievirus B5 had normal neurologic development on follow-up.[374] The one exception was a child with suspected intrauterine myocarditis. In another study, 16 newborns with meningitis related to coxsackievirus A14 were normal 2½ years later.

The most alarming report is that of Eichenwald,[423] who presented a 5-year follow-up study of infants who had had neonatal diarrhea associated with echovirus 18 infection.[230] Thirteen of 16 infants who had had an echovirus 18 infection during the neonatal period showed neurologic damage; these children had an IQ of less than 70, spasticity, deafness, blindness, or a combination of these effects.

In most instances, the antibody response of neonates after enterovirus infection is good. It is therefore to be expected that one attack of infection with a particular viral type provides immunity to the specific agent in the future. From the evidence derived from polio vaccine studies, it is probable that reinfection with all enteroviruses is common but that after an initial antibody response a secondary inapparent infection occurs and is confined to the gastrointestinal tract.

THERAPY

Specific Therapy

No specific therapy for any enterovirus infection is available. In severe, catastrophic and generalized neonatal infection, it is likely that the infant received no specific antibody for the particular virus from the mother. In this situation, it is probably advisable to administer human immune serum globulin to the infant. Dagan and associates examined three lots of human serum globulin and noted the presence of neutralizing antibodies to several commonly circulating and infrequently circulating enteroviruses.[424] Although there is at present no evidence that this therapy is beneficial in treating acute neonatal infections, there is evidence of some success in the treatment of chronic enteroviral infections in agammaglobulinemic patients.[425] Because it was found by Hammond and co-workers[426] that a single dose of intramuscular immune globulin resulted in little change in circulating neutralizing antibodies to coxsackievirus B4 and echovirus 11 in seven infants, it would seem advisable when therapy is decided on to use high-dose intravenous immune globulin. A neonate with disseminated echovirus 11 infection with hepatitis, pneumonitis, meningitis, disseminated intravascular coagulation, decreased renal function, and anemia who survived after receiving a large dose of intravenous immune globulin and supportive care has been described.[427]

Abzug and colleagues performed a small but controlled study in which nine enterovirus-infected neonates received intravenous immune globulin and seven similarly infected infants received supportive care.[428] In this study, there was no significant difference in clinical scores, antibody values, or magnitude of viremia and viruria in those treated compared with the control infants. However, five infants received IGIV with a high neutralizing antibody titer ($\geq$ 1:800) to their individual viral isolates and they were noted to have a more rapid cessation of viremia and viruria.

Jantausch and associates reported an infant with a disseminated echovirus 11 infection who survived after maternal plasma transfusions.[429] A neonate with a fulminant echovirus 11 infection survived after an orthotopic liver transplant.[430]

A number of antipicornavirus drugs and biologicals have been studied during the past 25 years.[63, 64] Studies with pleconaril (a capsid-binding compound) has shown promise in the treatment of enteroviral meningitis.[63] Further studies, including those in neonatal sepsis-like illnesses, are in progress.

In severe illnesses, such as neonatal myocarditis or encephalitis, it is frequently tempting to administer corticosteroids. Although some authors have thought that this therapy has been beneficial in coxsackievirus myocarditis, I believe that corticosteroids should not be given during acute enterovirus infections. The deleterious effects of these agents in coxsackievirus infections of mice[431] are particularly persuasive factors in this opinion.

Because the possibility of bacterial sepsis cannot be ruled out in most instances of neonatal enteroviral infections, antibiotics should be administered for the most likely potential pathogens. Care in antibiotic selection and administration is urged so that drug toxicity is not added to the problems of the patient. In neonates with meningitis or meningoencephalitis as well as in some infants with sepsis-like illnesses, the possibility of herpes simplex virus infections should be strongly considered and empirical treatment with intravenous acyclovir instituted after obtaining appropriate viral cultures.

Nonspecific Therapy

MILD NONSPECIFIC FEBRILE ILLNESS

In infants in whom fever is the only symptom, careful observation is most important. Many infants who eventually become severely ill have 2 to 3 days of fever initially without other localized findings. Care should be taken to administer adequate fluids to febrile infants, and excessive elevation of temperature should be prevented if possible.

SEPSIS-LIKE ILLNESS

In infants with severe sepsis-like illness, the major problems are shock, hepatitis and hepatic necrosis, and disseminated intravascular coagulation. For shock, attention should be directed toward treating hypotension and acidosis and ensuring adequate oxygenation.

For hepatitis, oral neomycin (25 mg/kg every 6 hours) or other nonabsorbable antibiotics to suppress intestinal bacterial flora may be helpful. The administration of blood (exchange transfusion) as well as vitamin K may be useful when bleeding occurs owing to liver dysfunction. Heparin therapy should be considered when disseminated intravascular coagulation occurs.

MYOCARDITIS

There is no specific therapy for myocarditis. However, congestive heart failure and arrhythmias should be treated by the usual methods. In administering digitalis to infants with enteroviral myocarditis, careful attention to the initial dosage is most important because the heart is often extremely sensitive; frequently, only small amounts of digoxin are necessary.

MENINGOENCEPHALITIS

In patients with meningoencephalitis, convulsions, cerebral edema, and disturbances of fluid and electrolyte balance all occur frequently and respond to treatment. Seizures are best treated with phenobarbital, phenytoin (Dilantin), or lorazepam. Cerebral edema can be treated with urea, mannitol, or large doses of corticosteroids. As already stated, it seems unwise to use corticosteroids in active enterovirus infections because the local benefit might be outweighed by the overall deleterious effects. Fluids should be monitored closely, and frequent determinations of serum electrolyte levels should be made because inappropriate antidiuretic hormone secretion is common.

PARALYTIC POLIOMYELITIS

Infants should be observed carefully for evidence of respiratory paralysis. If respiratory failure occurs, the early use of a positive-pressure ventilator is essential. In newborns, this is better performed without tracheotomy. Careful attention to pooling of secretions is important. Blood gas levels should be monitored frequently.

Passive exercises of all involved extremities should be started if the infant has been afebrile for 3 days.

PREVENTION

Immunization

Congenital and neonatal poliomyelitis should be illnesses of historical interest only. However, because large segments of populations throughout the world have not been immunized with attenuated polioviral vaccines, clinical poliomyelitis will continue to occur. In adequately immunized populations, congenital and neonatal poliomyelitis has been eliminated.

Attenuated viral vaccines for other enteroviruses are not available. However, if a virulent enteroviral type became prevalent, it is probable that a specific attenuated virus for active immunization could be developed. Because of the considerable morbidity and mortality associated with coxsackieviruses B in neonates and older persons as well, I believe that these agents should be candidates for vaccine development. Unfortunately, only a very small fraction of the severe illnesses related to these viruses ever receive proper diagnosis, so most physicians and lay persons are unaware of the magnitude of the problem.

Passive protection with intramuscular immune globulin (0.15 to 0.5 ml/kg) or perhaps intravenous immune globulin can be useful in preventing disease.[426, 432–434] In practice, however, this would seem to be worthwhile only in sudden and virulent nursery outbreaks. For example, if several cases of myocarditis occurred in a nursery, it would seem wise to administer immune globulin to all infants in the nursery. Pooled human immune globulin in most instances can be expected to contain antibodies against coxsackievirus types B1 through B5 and echovirus 11. Therefore, this procedure would offer protection to those infants without transplacentally acquired specific antibody who had not yet become infected.

Other Measures

Careful attention to routine nursery infection control procedures is important in preventing and controlling epidemics of enteroviral diseases. Nursery personnel should exercise strict care in washing their hands after handling each infant. It is also important to restrict the nursery area to personnel who are free of even minor illnesses.

Nursery infection, when it occurs, is best controlled in units that follow a cohort system. When illness occurs, the infant in question should be immediately isolated and the nursery should be closed to all new admissions.

References

1. Cherry JD, Nelson DB. Enterovirus infections: their epidemiology and pathogenesis. Clin Pediatr 5:659, 1966.
2. Bodian D, Horstmann DM. Polioviruses. *In* Horsfall FL Jr, Tamm I (eds). Viral and Rickettsial Infections of Man, 4th ed. Philadelphia, JB Lippincott, 1965, p 430.
3. Dalldorf G, Melnick JL. Coxsackie viruses. *In* Horsfall FL Jr, Tamm I (eds). Viral and Rickettsial Infections of Man, 4th ed. Philadelphia, JB Lippincott, 1965, p 474.
4. Melnick JL. Echoviruses. *In* Horsfall FL Jr, Tamm I (eds). Viral and Rickettsial Infections of Man, 4th ed. Philadelphia, JB Lippincott, 1965, p 513.
5. Kibrick S. Current status of coxsackie and ECHO viruses in human disease. Prog Med Virol 6:27, 1964.
6. Morens DM, Zweighaft RM, Bryan JM. Nonpolio enterovirus disease in the United States, 1971–1975. Int J Epidemiol 8:49, 1979.
7. Wenner, HA, Behbehani, AM. Echoviruses. *In* Gard S, Hallaner C, Meyer KF (eds). Virology Monographs, vol. 1. New York, Springer-Verlag, 1968, p 1.
8. Scott TFM. Clinical syndromes associated with entero virus and REO virus infections. Adv Virus Res 8:165, 1961.
9. Cherry JD. Enteroviruses: coxsackieviruses, echoviruses, and polioviruses. *In* Feigin RD, Cherry JD (eds). The Textbook of Pediatric Infectious Diseases, 4th ed. Philadelphia, WB Saunders, 1998, p 1787.
10. Grist NR, Bell EJ, Assaad F. Enteroviruses in human disease. Prog Med Virol 24:114, 1978.
11. Melnick JL. Enteroviruses. *In* Evans AS (ed). Viral Infections of Humans: Epidemiology and Control, 3rd ed. New York, Plenum Publishing, 1989, p 191.
12. Gear JHS, Measroch V. Coxsackievirus infections of the newborn. Prog Med Virol 15:42, 1973.
13. Melnick JL. Enteroviruses: polioviruses, coxsackieviruses, echoviruses, and newer enteroviruses. *In* Fields BN (ed). Virology, 2nd ed. New York, Raven Press, 1990, p 549.
14. Rueckert RR. Picornaviruses and their replication. *In* Fields BN (ed). Virology. New York, Raven Press, 1985, p 705.
15. Zeichhardt H. Enteroviruses. *In* Specter S, Lancz GJ (eds). Clinical Virology Manual. New York, Elsevier, 1986, p 283.
16. Melnick JL, Dalldorf G, Enders JF, et al. The enteroviruses. Am J Public Health 47:1556, 1957.
17. Overall JC Jr, Glasgow LA. Virus infections of the fetus and newborn infant. J Pediatr 77:315, 1970.
18. Monif GRG. Viral Infections of the Human Fetus. Toronto, Macmillan, 1969.
19. Kibrick S. Viral infections of the fetus and newborn. Perspect Virol 2:140, 1961.
20. Eichenwald HF, McCracken GH, Kindberg SJ. Virus infections of the newborn. Prog Med Virol 9:35, 1967.
21. Blattner RJ, Heys FM. Role of viruses in the etiology of congenital malformations. Prog Med Virol 3:311, 1961.
22. Hardy JB. Viral infection in pregnancy: A review. Am J Obstet Gynecol 93:1052, 1965.
23. Horstmann DM. Viral infections in pregnancy. Yale J Biol Med 42:99, 1969.
24. Hardy JB. Viruses and the fetus. Postgrad Med 43:156, 1968.
25. Plotz EJ. Virus disease in pregnancy. NY J Med 65:1239, 1965.
26. Hanshaw JB, Dudgeon JA. Viral Diseases of the Fetus and Newborn. Philadelphia, WB Saunders, 1978.
27. Krajden S, Middleton PJ. Enterovirus infections in the neonate. Clin Pediatr 22:87, 1983.
28. Kaplan MH, Klein SW, McPhee J, et al. Group B coxsackievirus infections in infants younger than three months of age: a serious childhood illness. Rev Infect Dis 5:1019, 1983.
29. Modlin JF. Perinatal echovirus infection: insights from a literature review of 61 cases of serious infection and 16 outbreaks in nurseries. Rev Infect Dis 8:918, 1986.
30. Paul JR. A History of Poliomyelitis. New Haven, Conn, Yale University Press, 1971.
31. Horstmann DM. The poliomyelitis story: a scientific hegira. Yale J Biol Med 58:79, 1985.
32. Melnick JL. Portraits of viruses: the picornaviruses. Intervirology 20:61, 1983.
33. Underwood M. A Treatise on the Diseases of Children, 2nd ed. London, J Mathews, 1789.
34. Wickman I. On the epidemiology of Heine-Medin's disease. Rev Infect Dis 2:319, 1980.
35. Landsteiner K, Popper E. Übertragung der Poliomyelitis acuta auf Affen. Z. Immun Forsch 2:377, 1909.
36. Hannaeus G. Dissertation. Copenhagen, 1735.
37. Dalldorf G, Sickles GM. An unidentified, filtrable agent isolated from the feces of children with paralysis. Science 108:61, 1948.
38. Enders JF, Weller TH, Robbins FC. Cultivation of the Lansing strain of poliomyelitis virus in cultures of various human embryonic tissues. Science 109:85, 1949.
39. Hogle JM, Chow M, Filman DJ. Three-dimensional structure of poliovirus at 2.9 NA resolution. Science 229:1358, 1985.
40. Hull HF, Birmingham ME, Melgaard B, et al. Progress toward global polio eradication. J Infect Dis 175:S4–9, 1997.
41. Robbins FC, de Quadros CA. Certification of the eradication of indigenous transmission of wild poliovirus in the Americas. J Infect Dis 175:S281–S285, 1997.
43. Cochi SL, Hull HF, Sutter RW, et al. Commentary: The unfolding story of global poliomyelitis eradication. J Infect Dis 175:S1–S3, 1997.
43. Centers for Disease Control and Prevention: Progress toward global poliomyelitis eradication, 1985–1994. MMWR 44:273–281, 1995.
44. Hull HF, Ward NA, Hull BP, et al. Paralytic poliomyelitis: seasoned strategies, disappearing disease. Lancet 343:1331–1337, 1994.
45. Romero JR, Rotbart HA. Sequence diversity among echoviruses with different neurovirulence phenotypes. Pediatr Res 33:181A, 1993.
46. Sawyer MH, Aintablian N, Keyser EF, et al. Detection of enterovirus RNA in the CSF of patients with both aseptic meningitis and generalized infection by polymerase chain reaction. Pediatr Res 33:182A, 1993.
47. Schlesinger Y, Sawyer MH, Camou M, et al. Use of PCR to investigate the roles of enteroviruses and herpes simplex virus in central nervous system infections of infants. Pediatr Res 33:182A, 1993.
48. Rotbart HA, Kinsella JP, Wasserman RL. Persistent enterovirus infection in culture-negative meningoencephalitis: demonstration by enzymatic RNA amplification. J Infect Dis 161:787, 1990.
49. Schlesinger Y, Sawyer MH, Storch GA. Enteroviral meningitis in infancy: Potential role for polymerase chain reaction in patient management. Pediatrics 94:157–162, 1994.
50. Sawer MH, Holland D, Aintablian N, et al. Diagnosis of

enteroviral central nervous system infection by polymerase chain reaction during a large community outbreak. Pediatr Infect Dis J 13:177–182, 1994.

51. Abzug MJ, Loeffelholz M, Rotbart HA. Clinical and laboratory observations. J Pediatr 126:447–450, 1995.

52. Andréoletti L, Blassel-Damman N, Dewilde A, et al. Comparison of use of cerebrospinal fluid, serum, and throat swab specimens in the diagnosis of enteroviral acute neurological infection by a rapid RNA detection PCR assay. J Clin Microbiol 36:589–591, 1998.

53. Rotbart HA. Reproducibility of AMPLICOR enterovirus PCR test results. J Clin Microbiol 35:3301–3302, 1997.

54. Marshall GS, Hauck MA, Buck G, et al. Potential cost savings through rapid diagnosis of enteroviral meningitis. Pediatr Infect Dis J 16:1086–1087, 1997.

55. Yerly S, Gervaix A, Simonet V, et al. Rapid and sensitive detection of enteroviruses in specimens from patients with aseptic meningitis. J Clin Microbiol 34:199–201, 1996.

56. Sharland M, Hodgson J, Davies EG, et al. Enteroviral pharyngitis diagnosed by reverse transcriptase-polymerase chain reaction. Arch Dis Child 74:462–463, 1996.

57. Tanel RE, Kao S, Niemiec TM, et al. Prospective comparison of culture vs genome detection for diagnosis of enteroviral meningitis in childhood. Arch Pediatr Adolesc Med 150:919–924, 1996.

58. Nielsen LP, Modlin JF, Rotbart HA. Detection of enteroviruses by polymerase chain reaction in urine samples of patients with aseptic meningitis. Pediatr Infect Dis J 15:125–627, 1996.

59. Klespies SL, Cebula DE, Kelley CL, et al. Detection of enterovirus from clinical specimens by spin amplification shell vial culture and monoclonal antibody assay. J Clin Microbiol 34:1465–1467, 1996.

60. Uchio E, Yamazaki K, Aoki K, et al. Detection of enterovirus 70 by polymerase chain reaction in acute hemorrhagic conjunctivitis. Am J Ophthalmol 122:273–275, 1996.

61. Andréoletti L, Hober D, Belaich S, et al. Rapid detection of enterovirus in clinical specimens using PCR and microwell capture hybridization assay. J Virol Meth 62:1–10, 1996.

62. Lina B, Pozzetto B, Andréoletti L, et al. Multicenter evaluation of a commercially available PCR assay for diagnosing enterovirus infection in a panel of cerebrospinal fluid specimens. J Clin Microbiol 34:3002–3006, 1996.

63. Rotbart HA, O'Connel JF, McKinlay MA. Treatment of human enterovirus infections. Antivir Res 38:1–4, 1998.

64. Diana GD, Pevear DC. Antipicornavirus drugs: current status. Antivir Chem Chemother 8:401–408, 1997.

65. Fenner F. Classification and nomenclature of viruses: second report of the International Committee on Taxonomy of Viruses. Intervirology 7:1, 1976.

66. Melnick JL, Wenner HA. Enteroviruses. In Lennette EH, Schmidt NJ (eds). Diagnostic Procedures for Viral and Rickettsial Infections, 4th ed. New York, American Public Health Association, 1969.

67. Rueckert RR. Picornaviridae and their replication. In Fields BN, Knipe DM (eds). Virology, 2nd ed. New York, Raven Press, 1990, p 507.

68. Pöyry T, Kinnunen L, Hyypiä T, et al. Genetic and phylogenetic clustering of enteroviruses. J Gen Virol 77:1699–1717, 1996.

69. Diedrich S, Driesel G, Schreier E. Sequence comparison of echovirus type 30 isolates to other enteroviruses in the 5' noncoding region. J Med Virol 46:148–152, 1995.

70. Kew OM, Mulders MN, Lipskaya GY, et al. Molecular epidemiology of polioviruses. Virology 6:401–414, 1995.

71. Pöyry T, Hyypiä T, Horsnell C, et al. Molecular analysis of coxsackievirus A16 reveals a new genetic group of enteroviruses. Virology 202:962–967, 1994.

72. Pulli T, Koskimies P, Hyypiä T. Molecular comparison of coxsackie A virus serotypes. Virology 212:30–38, 1995.

73. Bryden AS. Isolation of enteroviruses and adenoviruses in continuous simian cell lines. Med Lab Sci 49:60–65, 1992.

74. Hatch MH, Marchetti GE. Isolation of echoviruses with human embryonic lung fibroblast cells. Appl Microbiol 22:736, 1971.

75. Kelen AE, Lesiak JM, Labzoffsky NA. An outbreak of aseptic meningitis due to ECHO 25 virus. Can Med Assoc J 90:1349, 1964.

76. Cherry JD, Bobinski JE, Horvath FL, et al. Acute hemangiomalike lesions associated with ECHO viral infections. Pediatrics 44:498, 1969.

77. Bell EJ, Cosgrove BP. Routine enterovirus diagnosis in a human rhabdomyosarcoma cell line. Bull WHO 58:423, 1980.

78. Gelfand HM. The occurrence in nature of the coxsackie and ECHO viruses. Prog Med Virol 3:193, 1961.

79. Keswick BH, Gerba CP, Goyal SM. Occurrence of enteroviruses in community swimming pools. Am J Public Health 71:1026, 1981.

80. Johnson I, Hammond GW, Verma MR. Nosocomial coxsackie B4 virus infections in two chronic-care pediatric neurological wards. J Infect Dis 151:1153, 1985.

81. Downey TW. Polioviruses and flies: studies on the epidemiology of enteroviruses in an urban area. Yale J Biol Med 35:341, 1963.

82. Melnick JL, Emmons J, Coffey JH, et al. Seasonal distribution of coxsackie viruses in urban sewage and flies. Am J Hyg 59:164, 1954.

83. Melnick JL, Dow RP. Poliomyelitis in Hidalgo County, Texas 1948: poliomyelitis and coxsackie viruses from flies. Am J Hyg 58:288, 1953.

84. Horn P. Poliomyelitis in pregnancy: a twenty-year report from Los Angeles County, California. Obstet Gynecol 6:121, 1955.

85. Gresser I, Chany C, Enders JF. Persistent polioviral infection of intact human amniotic membrane without apparent cytopathic effect. J Bacteriol 89:470, 1965.

86. Blattner RJ. Intrauterine infection with poliovirus, type I. J Pediatr 62:625, 1963.

87. Aycock WL. The frequency of poliomyelitis in pregnancy. N Engl J Med 225:405, 1941.

88. Shelokov A, Habel K. Subclinical poliomyelitis in a newborn infant due to intrauterine infection. JAMA 160:465, 1956.

89. Schaeffer M, Fox MJ, Li CP. Intrauterine poliomyelitis infection. JAMA 155:248, 1954.

90. Shelokov A, Weinstein L. Poliomyelitis in the early neonatal period: report of a case of possible intrauterine infection. J Pediatr 38:80, 1951.

91. Lance M. Paralysis infantile (poliomyelité) constatée des la naissance. Bull Soc Pediatr (Paris) 31:2297, 1933.

92. Severin G. Case of poliomyelitis in newborn. Nord Med 1:55, 1939.

93. Baskin JL, Soule EH, Mills SD. Poliomyelitis of the newborn: pathologic changes in two cases. Am J Dis Child 80:10, 1950.

94. Kreibich H, Wold W. Ueber einen Fall von diaplazenter poliomyelitis Infektion des Feten in 9 Schwangerschaftsmonat. Zentralbl Gynaekol 72:694, 1950.

95. Johnson JF, Stimson PM. Clinical poliomyelitis in the early neonatal period. J Pediatr 40:733, 1956.

96. Carter HM. Congenital poliomyelitis. Obstet Gynecol 8:373, 1956.

97. Jackson AL, Louw JX. Poliomyelitis at birth due to transplacental infection. S Afr Med J 33:357, 1959.

98. Wingate MB, Meller HK, Ormiston G. Acute bulbar poliomyelitis in late pregnancy. Br Med J 1:407, 1961.

99. Abramson H, Greenberg M, Magee MC. Poliomyelitis in the newborn infant. J Pediatr 43:167, 1953.

100. Swarts CL, Kercher EF. A fatal case of poliomyelitis in a newborn infant delivered by cesarean section following maternal death due to poliomyelitis. Pediatrics 14:235, 1954.

101. Bates T. Poliomyelitis in pregnancy, fetus, and newborn. Am J Dis Child 90:189, 1955.

102. Elliott GB, McAllister JE, Alberta C. Fetal poliomyelitis. Am J Obstet Gynecol 72:896, 1956.

103. Siegel M, Greenberg M. Poliomyelitis in pregnancy: effect on fetus and newborn infant. J Pediatr 49:280, 1956.

104. Barsky P, Beale AJ. The transplacental transmission of poliomyelitis. J Pediatr 51:207, 1957.

105. Lycke E, Nilsson LR. Poliomyelitis in a newborn due to intrauterine infection. Acta Paediatr 51:661, 1962.

106. Winsser J, Pfaff ML, Seanor HE. Poliomyelitis viremia in a newborn infant. Pediatrics 20:458, 1957.

107. Wyatt HV. Poliomyelitis in the fetus and the newborn: a comment on the new understanding of the pathogenesis. Clin Pediatr 18:33, 1979.

108. Pearson RJC, Miller DG, Palmier ML. Reactions to the oral vaccine. Yale J Biol Med 34:498, 1962.

109. Prem KA, Fergus JW, Mathers JE, et al. Vaccination of pregnant women and young infants with trivalent oral attenuated live poliomyelitis vaccine. In Second International Conference on Live Poliovirus Vaccines, Washington, D.C., June 6–10, 1960. Washington, D.C., Pan American Sanitary Bureau, 1960.

110. Prem KA, McKelvey, JL. Immunologic response of pregnant women to oral trivalent poliomyelitis vaccine. In First International Conference on Live Poliovirus Vaccines, Washington, D.C., June 22–26, 1959. Washington, D.C., Pan American Sanitary Bureau, 1959.

111. McKay HW, Fodor AR, Kokko UP. Viremia following the administration of live poliovirus vaccines. Am J Public Health 53:274, 1963.

112. Horstmann DM, Opton EM, Klemperer R, et al. Viremia in infants vaccinated with oral poliovirus vaccine (Sabin). Am J Hyg 79:47, 1964.

113. Melnick JL, Proctor RO, Ocampo AR, et al. Free and bound virus in serum after administration of oral poliovirus vaccine. Am J Epidemiol 84:329, 1966.

114. Cabasso VJ, Jungherr EL, Moyer AW, et al. Oral poliomyelitis vaccine, Lederle: thirteen years of laboratory and field investigation. N Engl J Med 263:1321, 1960.

115. Katz SL. Efficacy, potential and hazards of vaccines. N Engl J Med 270:884, 1964.

116. Payne AMM. Summary of the conference. In Second International Conference on Live Poliovirus Vaccines, Washington, D.C., June 6–10, 1960. Washington, D.C., Pan American Sanitary Bureau, 1960.

117. White LR. Comment. In Viral Etiology of Congenital Malformations, May 19–20, 1967. Washington, D.C., U.S. Government Printing Office, 1968.

118. Horstmann DM. Epidemiology of poliomyelitis and allied diseases—1963. Yale J Biol Med 36:5, 1963.

119. Dalldorf G, Gifford R. Susceptibility of gravid mice to coxsackie virus infection. J Exp Med 99:21, 1954.

120. Berger E, Roulet F. Beitrage zur Ausscheidung und Tier-pathogenitüt des Coxsackie-virus. Schweiz Z Allg Pathol 15:462, 1952.

121. Selzer G. Transplacental infection of the mouse fetus by Coxsackie viruses. Israel J Med Sci 5:125, 1969.

122. Soike K. Coxsackie B-3 virus infection in the pregnant mouse. J Infect Dis 117:203, 1967.

123. Modlin JF, Crumpacker CS. Coxsackievirus B infection in pregnant mice and transplacental infection of the fetus. Infect Immun 37:222, 1982.

124. Flamm H. Some considerations concerning the pathogenesis of prenatal infections. In Eichenwald HC (ed). The Prevention of Mental Retardation Through Control of Infectious Diseases. Washington, D.C., U.S. Government Printing Office, 1966.

125. Flamm H. Untersuchungen über die diaplazentare Übertragung des Coxsackievirus. Schweiz Z Allg Pathol 18:16, 1955.

126. Palmer AL, Rotbart HA, Tyson RW, et al. Adverse effects of maternal enterovirus infection on the fetus and placenta. J Infect Dis 176:1437–1444, 1997.

127. Abzug MJ. Maternal factors affecting the integrity of the late gestation placental barrier to murine enterovirus infection. J Infect Dis 176:41–49, 1997.

128. Benirschke K. Viral infection of the placenta. In Viral Etiology of Congenital Malformations, May 19–20, 1967. Washington, D.C., U.S. Government Printing Office, 1968.

129. Kibrick S, Benirschke K. Acute aseptic myocarditis and meningoencephalitis in the newborn child infected with Coxsackie virus group B, type 3. N Engl J Med 255:883, 1956.

130. Brightman VJ, Scott TFM, Westphal M, et al. An outbreak of coxsackie B-5 virus infection in a newborn nursery. J Pediatr 69:179, 1966.

131. Makower H, Skurska Z, Halazinska L. On transplacental infection with Coxsackie virus. Texas Rep Biol Med 16:346, 1958.

132. Cherry JD, Soriano F, Jahn CL. Search for perinatal viral infection: a prospective, clinical, virologic and serologic study. Am J Dis Child 116:245, 1968.

133. Puschak RB. Coxsackie virus infection in the newborn with case report. Harrisburg Polyclinic Hosp J 1962, p 14.

134. Basso NGS, Fonseca MEF, Garcia AGP, et al. Enterovirus isolation from foetal and placental tissues. Acta Virol 34:49, 1990.

135. Bates HR. Coxsackie virus B3 calcific pancarditis and hydrops fetalis. Am J Obstet Gynecol 106:629, 1970.

136. Hanson L, Lundgren S, Lycke E, et al. Clinical and serological observations in cases of Coxsackie B3 infections in early infancy. Acta Paediatr Scand 55:577, 1966.

137. Benirschke K, Pendleton ME. Coxsackie virus infection: an important complication of pregnancy. Obstet Gynecol 12:305, 1958.

138. McLean DM, Donohue WL, Snelling CE, et al. Coxsackie B5 virus as a cause of neonatal encephalitis and myocarditis. Can Med Assoc J 85:1046, 1961.

139. Burch GE, Sun SC, Chu KC, et al. Interstitial and coxsackievirus B myocarditis in infants and children. JAMA 203:1, 1968.

140. Plager H, Beeve R, Miller JK. Coxsackie B-5 pericarditis in pregnancy. Arch Intern Med 110:735, 1962.

141. Yoshioka I, Horstmann DM. Viremia in infection due to ECHO virus type 9. N Engl J Med 262:224, 1960.

142. Rantasalo I, Penttinen K, Saxen L, et al. ECHO 9 virus antibody status after an epidemic period and the possible teratogenic effect of the infection. Ann Paediatr Fenn 6:175, 1960.

143. Kleinman H, Prince JT, Mathey WE, et al. ECHO 9 virus infection and congenital abnormalities: a negative report. Pediatrics 29:261, 1962.

144. Landsman JB, Grist NR, Ross CAC. Echo 9 virus infection and congenital malformations. Br J Prev Soc Med 18:152, 1964.

145. Moscovici C, Maisel J. Intestinal viruses of newborn and older prematures. Am J Dis Child 101:771, 1961.

146. Eichenwald HF, Kostevalov O. Immunologic responses of premature and full-term infants to infection with certain viruses. Pediatrics 25:829, 1960.

147. Berkovich S, Smithwick EM. Transplacental infection due to ECHO virus type 22. J Pediatr 72:94, 1968.

148. Hughes JR, Wilfert CM, Moore M, et al. Echovirus 14 infection associated with fatal neonatal hepatic necrosis. Am J Dis Child 123:61, 1972.

149. Philip AGS, Larson EJ. Overwhelming neonatal infection with ECHO 19 virus. J Pediatr 82:391, 1973.

150. Cheeseman SH, Hirsch MS, Keller EW, et al. Fatal neonatal pneumonia caused by echovirus type 9. Am J Dis Child 131:1169, 1977.

151. Jones MJ, Kolb M, Votava HJ, et al. Intrauterine echovirus type 11 infection. Mayo Clin Proc 55:509, 1980.

152. Bose CL, Gooch WM III, Sanders GO, et al. Dissimilar manifestations of intrauterine infection with echovirus 11 in premature twins. Arch Pathol Lab Med 107:361, 1983.

153. Reyes MP, Ostrea EM Jr, Roskamp J, et al. Disseminated neonatal echovirus 11 disease following antenatal maternal infection with a virus-positive cervix and virus-negative gastrointestinal tract. J Med Virol 12:155, 1983.

154. Piraino FF, Sedmak G, Raab K. Echovirus 11 infections of newborns with mortality during the 1979 enterovirus season in Milwaukee, Wisc. Public Health Rep 97:346, 1982.

155. Nielsen JL, Berryman GK, Hankins GD. Intrauterine fetal death and the isolation of echovirus 27 from amniotic fluid. J Infect Dis 158:501, 1988.

156. Toce SS, Keenan WJ. Congenital echovirus 11 pneumonia in association with pulmonary hypertension. Pediatr Infect Dis J 7:360, 1988.

157. Kleger B, Prier JE, Rosato DJ, et al. Herpes simplex infection of the female genital tract: I. Incidence of infection. Am J Obstet Gynecol 102:745, 1968.

158. Montgomery R, Youngblood L, Medearis DN Jr. Recovery of cytomegalovirus from the cervix in pregnancy. Pediatrics 49:524, 1972.

159. Reyes MP, Zalenski D, Smith F, et al. Coxsackievirus-positive cervices in women with febrile illnesses during the third trimester in pregnancy. Am J Obstet Gynecol 155:159, 1986.

160. Cole RM, Bell JA, Beeman EA, et al. Studies of Coxsackie viruses: observations on epidemiologic aspects of group A viruses. Am J Public Health 41:1342, 1951.

161. Ramos-Alvarez M, Sabin AB. Intestinal viral flora of healthy children demonstrable by monkey kidney tissue culture. Am J Public Health 46:295, 1956.

162. Vandeputte M. L'endémicité des virus entériques à Léopoldville. Congo Bull WHO/OMS 22:313, 1960.

163. Katz SL. Case records of the Massachusetts General Hospital. Case 20-1965. N Engl J Med 272:907, 1965.

164. Jenista JA, Powell KR, Menegus MA. Epidemiology of neonatal enterovirus infection. J Pediatr 104:685, 1984.

165. Pagano JS, Plotkin SA, Cornely D. The response of premature infants to infection with type 3 attenuated poliovirus. J Pediatr 65:165, 1964.

166. Pagano JS, Plotkin SA, Koprowski H. Variations in the response of infants to living attenuated poliovirus vaccines. N Engl J Med 264:155, 1961.

167. Pagano JS, Plotkin SA, Cornely D, et al. The response of premature infants to infection with attenuated poliovirus. Pediatrics 29:794, 1962.

168. Murphy W. Response of infants to trivalent poliovirus vaccine (Sabin strains). Pediatrics 40:980, 1967.

169. Lepow ML, Warren RJ, Gray N, et al. Effect of Sabin type 1 poliomyelitis vaccine administered by mouth to newborn infants. N Engl J Med 264:1071, 1961.

170. Sabin AB, Michaels RH, Krugman S, et al. Effect of oral poliovirus vaccine in newborn children: I. Excretion of virus after ingestion of large doses of type 1 or of mixture of all three types, in relation to level of placentally transmitted antibody. Pediatrics 31:623, 1963.

171. Sabin AB, Michaels RH, Ziring P, et al. Effect of oral poliovirus vaccine in newborn children: II. Intestinal resistance and antibody response at 6 months in children fed type 1 vaccine at birth. Pediatrics 31:641, 1963.

172. Warren RJ, Lepow ML, Bartsch GE, et al. The relationship of maternal antibody, breast feeding, and age to the susceptibility of newborn infants to infection with attenuated polioviruses. Pediatrics 34:4, 1964.

173. Lepow ML, Warren RJ, Ingram VG, et al. Sabin type 1 (LSc2ab) oral poliomyelitis vaccine. Am J Dis Child 104:67, 1962.

174. Keller R, Dwyer JE, Oh W, et al. Intestinal IgA neutralizing antibodies in newborn infants following poliovirus immunization. Pediatrics 43:330, 1969.

175. Földes P, Bános A, Bános Z, et al. Vaccination of newborn children with live poliovirus vaccine. Acta Microbiol Acad Sci Hung 9:305, 1962.

176. Plotkin SA, Katz M, Brown RE, et al. Oral poliovirus vaccination in newborn African infants. Am J Dis Child 111:27, 1966.

177. Katz M, Plotkin SA. Oral polio immunization of the newborn infant: a possible method of overcoming interference by ingested antibodies. J Pediatr 73:267, 1968.

178. Bergeisen GH, Bauman RJ, Gilmore RL. Neonatal paralytic poliomyelitis: a case report. Arch Neurol 43:192, 1986.

179. Javett SN, Heymann S, Mundel B, et al. Myocarditis in the newborn infant. J Pediatr 48:1, 1956.

180. Kipps A, Naudé WDT, Don P, et al. Coxsackie virus myocarditis of the newborn. Med Proc 4:401, 1958.

181. Gear JHS. Coxsackie virus infection of the newborn. Prog Med Virol 1:106, 1958.

182. Montgomery J, Gear J, Prinsloo FR, et al. Myocarditis of the newborn: an outbreak in a maternity home in Southern Rhodesia associated with Coxsackie group-B virus infection. S Afr Med J 29:608, 1955.

183. Winsser J, Altieri RH. A three-year study of coxsackie virus, group B, infection in Nassau County. Am J Med Sci 247:269, 1964.

184. Artenstein MS, Cadigan FC, Buescher EL. Epidemic coxsackie virus infection with mixed clinical manifestations. Ann Intern Med 60:196, 1964.

185. Farber S, Vawter GF. Clinical pathological conference. J Pediatr 62:786, 1963.

186. Koch VF, Enders-Ruckle G, Wokittel E. Coxsackie B5-Infektionen mit signifikanter Antikörperentwicklung bei Neugeborenen. Arch Kinderheilkd 165:245, 1962.

187. Moossy J, Geer JC. Encephalomyelitis, myocarditis and adrenal cortical necrosis in coxsackie B3 virus infection. Arch Pathol 70:614, 1960.

188. Sussman ML, Strauss L, Hodes HL. Fatal Coxsackie group B infection in the newborn. Am J Dis Child 97:483, 1959.

189. Hosier DM, Newton WA. Serious Coxsackie infection in infants and children. Am J Dis Child 96:251, 1958.

190. Fechner RE, Smith MG, Middelkamp JN. Coxsackie B virus infection of the newborn. Am J Pathol 42:493, 1963.

191. Verlinde JD, Van Tongeren HAE, Kret A. Myocarditis in newborns due to group B Coxsackie virus: virus studies. Ann Pediatr 187:113, 1956.

192. Van Creveld S, De Jager H. Myocarditis in newborns, caused by Coxsackie virus: clinical and pathological data. Ann Pediatr 187:100, 1956.

193. Sieber OF, Kilgus AH, Fulginiti VA, et al. Immunological response of the newborn infant to Coxsackie B-4 infection. Pediatrics 40:444, 1967.

194. Butler N, Skelton MO, Hodges GM, et al. Fatal Coxsackie B3 myocarditis in a newborn infant. BMJ 1:1251, 1962.

195. Robino G, Perlman A, Togo Y, et al. Fatal neonatal infection due to Coxsackie B2 virus. J Pediatr 61:911, 1962.

196. Jack I, Townley RRW. Acute myocarditis of newborn infants, due to Coxsackie viruses. Med J Aust 2:265, 1961.

197. Jahn CL, Cherry JD. Mild neonatal illness associated with heavy enterovirus infection. N Engl J Med 274:394, 1966.

198. Nogen AG, Lepow ML. Enteroviral meningitis in very young infants. Pediatrics 40:617, 1967.

199. Kibrick S, Benirschke, K. Severe generalized disease (encephalohepatomyocarditis) occurring in the newborn period and due to infection with Coxsackie virus, group B. Pediatrics 22:857, 1958.

200. McLean DM, Coleman MA, Larke RPB, et al. Viral infections of Toronto children during 1965: I. Enteroviral disease. Can Med Assoc J 94:839, 1966.

201. Rapmund G, Gauld JR, Rogers NG, et al. Neonatal myocarditis and meningoencephalitis due to Coxsackie virus group B, type 4: Virologic study of a fatal case with simultaneous aseptic meningitis in the mother. N Engl J Med 260:819, 1959.

202. Wright HT Jr, Okuyama K, McAllister RM. An infant fatality associated with Coxsackie B1 virus. J Pediatr 63:428, 1963.

203. Gear J. Coxsackie virus infections in Southern Africa. Yale J Biol Med 34:289, 1961.

204. Volakova N, Jandasek L. Epidemic of myocarditis in newborn infants caused by Coxsackie B1 virus. Cesk Epidemiol 13:88, 1963.

205. Cherry JD, Lerner AM, Klein J, et al. Unpublished data, 1962.

206. Gear J, Measroch V, Prinsloo FR. The medical and public health importance of the coxsackie viruses. S Afr Med J 30:806, 1956.

207. Woodward TE, McCrumb FR Jr, Carey TN, et al. Viral and rickettsial causes of cardiac disease, including the Coxsackie virus etiology of pericarditis and myocarditis. Ann Intern Med 53:1130, 1960.

208. Hurley R, Norman AP, Pryse-Davies J. Massive pulmonary hemorrhage in the newborn associated with coxsackie B virus infection. BMJ 3:636, 1969.

209. Suckling PV, Vogelpoel L. Coxsackie myocarditis of the newborn. Med Proc 4:372, 1958.

210. Cherry JD, Jahn CL. Virologic studies of exanthems. J Pediatr 68:204, 1966.

211. Jennings RC. Coxsackie group B fatal neonatal myocarditis associated with cardiomegaly. J Clin Pathol 19:325, 1966.

212. Johnson WR. Manifestations of Coxsackie group B infections in children. Delaware Med J 32:72, 1960.

213. Delaney TB, Fakunaga FH. Myocarditis in a newborn with encephalomeningitis due to Coxsackie virus group B, type 5. N Engl J Med 259:234, 1958.

214. Dömök I, Molnár E. An outbreak of meningoencephalomyocarditis among newborn infants during the epidemic of Bornholm disease of 1958 in Hungary: II. Aetiological findings. Ann Pediatr 194:102, 1960.

215. Tuuteri L, Lapinleimu K, Meurman L. Fatal myocarditis associated with coxsackie B3 infection in the newborn. Ann Paediatr Fenn 9:56, 1963.

216. Archibald E, Purdham DR. Coxsackievirus type A16 infection in a neonate. Arch Dis Child 54:649, 1979.

217. Rantakallio P, Lapinleimu K, Mäntyjärvi R. Coxsackie B5 outbreak in a newborn nursery with 17 cases of serious meningitis. Scand J Infect Dis 2:17, 1970.

218. Lapinleimu K, Kaski U. An outbreak caused by coxsackievirus B5 among newborn infants. Scand J Infect Dis 4:27, 1972.

219. Isacsohn M, Eidelman AI, Kaplan M, et al. Neonatal coxsackievirus group B infections: experience of a single department of neonatology. Israel J Med Sci 30:371–374, 1994.

220. Swender PT, Shott RJ, Williams ML. A community and intensive care nursery outbreak of coxsackievirus B5 meningitis. Am J Dis Child 127:42, 1974.

221. Cramblett HG, Haynes RE, Azimi PH, et al. Nosocomial infection with echovirus type 11 in handicapped and premature infants. Pediatrics 51:603, 1973.

222. Jack I, Grutzner J, Gray N, et al. A survey of prenatal virus disease in Melbourne. Personal communication, July 21, 1967.

223. Berkovich S, Pangan J. Recoveries of virus from premature infants during outbreaks of respiratory disease: the relation of ECHO virus type 22 to disease of the upper and lower respiratory tract in the premature infant. Bull NY Acad Med 44:377, 1968.

224. Miller DG, Gabrielson MO, Bart KJ, et al. An epidemic of aseptic meningitis, primarily among infants, caused by echovirus 11-prime. Pediatrics 41:77, 1968.

225. Hercík L, Huml M, Mimra J, et al. Epidemien der Respirationstrakterkrankunger bei Neugeborenen durch ECHO 11-Virus. Zentrabl Bakteriol 213:18, 1970.

226. German LJ, McCracken AW, Wilkie KM. Outbreak of febrile illness associated with ECHO virus type 5 in a maternity unit in Singapore. BMJ 1:742, 1968.

227. Hart EW, Brunton GB, Taylor CED, et al. Infection of newborn babies with ECHO virus type 5. Lancet 2:402, 1962.

228. Berkovich S, Kibrick S. ECHO 11 outbreak in newborn infants and mothers. Pediatrics 33:534, 1964.

229. Sanders DY, Cramblett HG. Viral infections in hospitalized neonates. Am J Dis Child 116:251, 1968.

230. Eichenwald HF, Ababio A, Arky AM, et al. Epidemic diarrhea in premature and older infants caused by ECHO virus type 18. JAMA 166:1563, 1958.

231. Butterfield J, Moscovici C, Berry C, et al. Cystic emphysema in premature infants: a report of an outbreak with the isolation of type 19 ECHO virus in one case. N Engl J Med 268:18, 1963.

232. Nakao T, Miura R, Sato M. ECHO virus type 22 in a premature infant. Tohoku J Exp Med 102:61, 1970.

233. Faulkner RS, van Rooyen CE. Echovirus type 17 in the neonate. Can Med Assoc J 108:878, 1973.

234. Eichenwald HF, Kostevalov O, Fasso LA. The "cloud baby": an example of bacterial-viral interaction. Am J Dis Child 100:161, 1960.

235. Kapsenberg JG. ECHO virus type 33 as a cause of meningitis. Arch Ges Virusforsch 23:144, 1968.

236. Nagington J, Wreghitt TG, Gandy G, et al. Fatal echovi-

rus 11 infections in outbreak in special-care baby unit. Lancet 2:725, 1978.

237. Davies DP, Hughes CA, MacVicar J, et al. Echovirus-11 infection in a special-care baby unit. Lancet 1:96, 1979.

238. Hasegawa A. Virologic and serologic studies on an outbreak of echovirus type 11 infection in a hospital maternity unit. Jpn J Med Sci Biol 28:179, 1975.

239. Lapinleimu K, Hakulinen A. A hospital outbreak caused by ECHO virus type 11 among newborn infants. Ann Clin Res 4:183, 1972.

240. Modlin JF. Fatal echovirus 11 disease in premature neonates. Pediatrics 66:775, 1980.

241. Purdham DR, Purdham PA, Wood BSB, et al. Severe ECHO 19 virus infection in a neonatal unit. Arch Dis Child 51:634, 1976.

242. McDonald LL, St. Geme JW, Arnold BH. Nosocomial infection with ECHO virus type 31 in a neonatal intensive care unit. Pediatrics 47:995, 1971.

243. Mertens T, Hager H, Eggers HJ. Epidemiology of an outbreak in a maternity unit of infections with an antigenic variant of echovirus 11. J Med Virol 9:81, 1982.

244. Kinney JS, McCray E, Kaplan JE, et al. Risk factors associated with echovirus 11 infection in a hospital nursery. Pediatr Infect Dis 5:192, 1986.

245. Steinmann J, Albrecht K. Echovirus 11 epidemic among premature newborns in a neonatal intensive care unit. Zentralbl Bakteriol Mikrobiol Hyg 259:284, 1985.

246. Modlin JF. Perinatal echovirus infection: insights from a literature review of 61 cases of serious infection and 16 outbreaks in nurseries. Rev Infect Dis 8:918, 1986.

247. Modlin JF. Echovirus infections of newborn infants. Pediatr Infect Dis 7:311, 1988.

248. Rabkin CS, Telzak EE, Ho MS, et al. Outbreak of echovirus 11 infection in hospitalized neonates. Pediatr Infect Dis J 7:186, 1988.

249. Wreghitt TG, Sutehall GM, King A, et al. Fatal echovirus 7 infection during an outbreak in a special care baby unit. J Infect 19:229, 1989.

250. Wilson CW, Stevenson DK, Arvin AM. A concurrent epidemic of respiratory syncytial virus and echovirus 7 infections in an intensive care nursery. Pediatr Infect Dis J 8:24, 1989.

251. Isaacs D, Wilkinson AR, Eglin R, et al. Conservative management of an echovirus 11 outbreak in a neonatal unit. Lancet 1:543, 1989.

252. Verlinde JD, Versteeg J, Beeuwkes H. Mogelijkheid van een besmetting van de mens door varkens lijdende aan een Coxsackievirus pneumonie. Ned Tijdschr Geneeskd 102:1445, 1958.

253. Moscovici C, Ginevri A, Felici A, et al. Virus 1956 R.C. 1st suppl. Sanita 20:1137, 1957.

254. Lundgren DL, Clapper WE, Sanchez A. Isolation of human enteroviruses from beagle dogs. Proc Soc Exp Biol Med 128:463, 1968.

255. Lundgren DL, Sanchez A, Magnuson MG, et al. A survey for human enteroviruses in dogs and man. Arch Ges Virusforsch 32:229, 1970.

256. Koprowski H. Counterparts of human viral disease in animals. Ann NY Acad Sci 70:369, 1958.

257. Sommerville RG. Type I poliovirus isolated from a budgerigar. Lancet 1:495, 1959.

258. Makower H, Skurska Z. Badania nad wirusami Coxsackie. Doniesienie III. Izolacja wirusa Coxsackie z mózgu lisa. Arch Immunol Ter Dosw 5:219, 1957.

259. Bendinelli M, Ruschi A. Isolation of human enterovirus from mussels. Appl Microbiol 18:531, 1969.

260. Metcalf TG, Stiles WC. Enterovirus within an estuarine environment. Am J Epidemiol 88:379, 1968.

261. Horstmann DM, Manuelidis EE. Russian Coxsackie A-7 virus ("AB IV" strain)—neuropathogenicity and comparison with poliovirus. J Immunol 81:32, 1958.

262. Bartell P, Klein M. Neutralizing antibody to viruses of poliomyelitis in sera of domestic animals. Proc Soc Exp Biol Med 90:597, 1955.

263. Morris JA, O'Connor JR. Neutralization of the viruses of the Coxsackie group by sera of wild rabbits. Cornell Vet 42:56, 1952.

264. Chang PW, Liu OC, Miller LT, et al. Multiplication of human enteroviruses in northern quahogs. Proc Soc Exp Biol Med 136:1380, 1971.

265. Metcalf TG, Stiles WC. Accumulation of enteric viruses by the oyster, *Crassostrea virginica*. J Infect Dis 115:68, 1965.

266. Liu OC, Seraichekas HR, Murphy BL. Viral depuration of the Northern quahaug. Appl Microbiol 15:307, 1967.

267. Duff MF. The uptake of enteroviruses by the New Zealand marine blue mussel *Mytilus edulis aoteanus*. Am J Epidemiol 85:486, 1967.

268. Atwood RP, Cherry JD, Klein JO. Clams and viruses. Hepatitis Surveillance Rep 20:26, 1964.

269. Lynt RK. Survival and recovery of enterovirus from foods. Appl Microbiol 14:218, 1966.

270. Kalter SS. A serological survey of antibodies to selected enteroviruses. Bull World Health Organ 26:759, 1962.

271. Fox JP. Epidemiological aspects of coxsackie and ECHO virus infections in tropical areas. Am J Public Health 54:1134, 1964.

272. Centers for Disease Control. Enterovirus Surveillance, Summary 1970–1979. Issued November 1981.

273. Bodian D, Horstmann DM. Poliomyelitis. *In* Horsfall FL, Tamm I (eds). Viral and Rickettsial Infections of Man, 4th ed. Philadelphia, JB Lippincott, 1965, p 430.

274. Christie AB. Acute poliomyelitis. *In* Infectious Diseases: Epidemiology and Clinical Practice. Edinburgh, Churchill Livingstone, 1974, p 567.

275. Assaad F, Ljungars-Esteves K. World overview of poliomyelitis: regional patterns and trends. Rev Infect Dis 6:S302, 1984.

276. Phillips CA, Aronson MD, Tomkow J, et al. Enteroviruses in Vermont, 1969–1978: an important cause of illness throughout the year. J Infect Dis 141:162, 1980.

277. Drebit MA, Nguan CY, Campbell JJ, et al. Molecular epidemiology of enterovirus outbreaks in Canada during 1991–1992: identification of echovirus 30 and coxsackievirus B1 strains by amplicon sequencing. J Med Virol 44:340–347, 1994.

278. Ishiko H, Takeda N, Miyanura K, et al. Phylogenetic analysis of a coxsackievirus A24 variant: the most recent worldwide pandemic was caused by progenies of a virus prevalent around 1981. Virology 187:748–759, 1992.

279. Lin KH, Wang HL, Sheu MM, et al. Molecular epidemiology of a variant of coxsackievirus A24 in Taiwan: two epidemics caused by phylogenetically distinct viruses from 1985 to 1989. J. Clin. Microbiol. 31:1160–1166, 1993.

280. Mulders MN, Lipskaya GY, van der Avoort HGAM, et al. Molecular epidemiology of wild poliovirus type 1 in Europe, the Middle East, and the Indian subcontinent. J Infect Dis 171:1399–1405, 1995.

281. Strikas RA, Anderson LJ, Parker RA. Temporal and geographic patterns of isolates of nonpolio enterovirus in the United States, 1970–1983. J Infect Dis 153:346, 1986.

282. Center for Disease Control. Neurotropic Diseases Surveillance. No. 3, Annual Summary, U.S. Department of Health, Education, and Welfare, 1970.

283. Communicable Disease Center. Poliomyelitis Surveil-

lance, No. 274. U.S. Department of Health, Education, and Welfare, 1963.

284. Horstmann DB, Emmons J, Gimpel L, et al. Enterovirus surveillance following a community-wide oral poliovirus vaccination program: a seven-year study. Am J Epidemiol 97:173, 1973.

285. Batcup G, Holt P, Hambling MH, et al. Placental and fetal pathology in coxsackie virus A9 infection: a case report. Histopathology 9:1227, 1985.

286. Heineberg H, Gold E, Robbins FC. Differences in interferon content in tissues of mice of various ages infected with coxsackie B1 virus. Proc Soc Exp Biol Med 115:947, 1964.

287. Behbehani AM, Sulkin SE, Wallis C. Factors influencing susceptibility of mice to coxsackie virus infection. J Infect Dis 110:147, 1962.

288. Boring WD, Angevine DM, Walker DL. Factors influencing host-virus interactions: I. A comparison of viral multiplication and histopathology in infant, adult, and cortisone-treated adult mice infected with the Conn-5 strain of coxsackie virus. J Exp Med 102:753, 1955.

289. Kunin CW. Cellular susceptibility to enteroviruses. Bacteriol Rev 28:382, 1964.

290. Kunin CM. Virus-tissue union and the pathogenesis of enterovirus infections. J Immunol 88:556, 1962.

291. Teisner B, Haahr S. Poikilothermia and susceptibility of suckling mice to coxsackie B1 virus. Nature 247:568, 1974.

292. Arola A, Kalimo H, Ruuskanen O, et al. Experimental myocarditis induced by two different coxsackievirus B3 variants: aspects of pathogenesis and comparison of diagnostic methods. J Med Virol 47:251–259, 1995.

293. Gauntt CJ, Arizpe HM, Higdon AL, et al. Molecular mimicry, anti-coxsackievirus B3 neutralizing monoclonal antibodies, and myocarditis. J Immunol 154:2983–2995, 1995.

294. Gauntt CJ, Higdon AL, Arizpe HM, et al. Epitopes shared between coxsackievirus B3 (CVB3) and normal heart tissue contribute to CVB3-induced murine myocarditis. Clin Immunol Immunopathol 68:129–134, 1993.

295. Henke A, Huber S, Stelzner A, et al. The role of CD8 + T lymphocytes in coxsackievirus B3-induced myocarditis. J Virol 69:6720–6728, 1995.

296. Hosier DM, Newton WA Jr. Serious coxsackie infection in infants and children: myocarditis, meningoencephalitis, and hepatitis. Am J Dis Child 96:251–267, 1958.

297. Pague RE. Role of anti-idiotypic antibodies in induction, regulation, and expression of coxsackievirus-induced myocarditis. Prog Med Virol 39:204–227, 1992.

298. Rabausch-Starz I, Scwaiger A, Grünewald K, et al. Persistence of virus and viral genome in myocardium after coxsackievirus B3-induced murine myocarditis. Clin Exp Immunol 96:69–74, 1994.

299. Seko Y, Yoshifumi E, Yagita H, et al. Restricted usage of T-cell receptor Va genes in infiltrating cells in murine hearts with acute myocarditis caused by coxsackie virus B3. J Pathol 178:330–334, 1996.

300. Neu N, Beisel KW, Traystman MD, et al. Autoantibodies specific for the cardiac myosin isoform are found in mice susceptible to coxsackievirus B3-induced myocarditis. J Immunol 183:2488, 1987.

301. Herskowitz A, Beisel KW, Wolfgram LJ, et al. Coxsackievirus B3 murine myocarditis: wide pathologic spectrum in genetically defined inbred strains. Hum Pathol 16:671, 1985.

302. Wolfgram LJ, Rose NR. Coxsackievirus infection as a trigger of cardiac autoimmunity. Immunol Res 8:61, 1989.

303. McManus BM, Chow LH, Wilson JE, et al. Direct myocardial injury by enterovirus: a central role in the evolution of murine myocarditis. Clin Immunol Immunopathol 68:159–169, 1993.

304. Balduzzi PC, Greendyke RM. Sudden unexpected death in infancy and viral infection. Pediatrics 38:201, 1966.

305. Gold E, Carver DH, Heineberg H, et al. Viral infection: a possible cause of sudden, unexpected death in infants. N Engl J Med 264:53, 1961.

306. Baker DA, Phillips CA. Maternal and neonatal infection with coxsackievirus. Obstet Gynecol 55:12S, 1980.

307. Estes ML, Rorke LB. Liquefactive necrosis in coxsackie B encephalitis. Arch Pathol Lab Med 110:1090, 1986.

308. Lake AM, Lauer BA, Clark JC, et al. Enterovirus infections in neonates. J Pediatr 89:787, 1976.

309. Iwasaki T, Monma N, Satodate R, et al. An immunofluorescent study of generalized coxsackie virus B3 infection in a newborn infant. Acta Pathol Jpn 35:741, 1985.

310. Krous HF, Dietzman D, Ray CG. Fatal infections with echovirus types 6 and 11 in early infancy. Am J Dis Child 126:842, 1973.

311. Berry PJ, Nagington J. Fatal infection with echovirus 11. Arch Dis Child 57:22, 1982.

312. Gh MM, Lack EE, Gang DL, et al. Postmortem manifestations of echovirus 11 sepsis in five newborn infants. Hum Pathol 14:818, 1983.

313. Halfon N, Spector SA. Fatal echovirus type 11 infections. Am J Dis Child 135:1017, 1981.

314. Gitlin N, Visveshwara N, Kassel SH, et al. Fulminant neonatal hepatic necrosis associated with echovirus type 11 infection. West J Med 138:260, 1983.

315. Rawls WE, Shorter RG, Herrmann EC Jr. Fatal neonatal illness associated with ECHO 9 (coxsackie A-23) virus. Pediatrics 33:278, 1964.

316. Georgieff MK, Johnson DE, Thompson TR, et al. Fulminant hepatic necrosis in an infant with perinatally acquired echovirus 21 infection. Pediatr Infect Dis 6:71, 1987.

317. Chambon M, Delage C, Bailly J, et al. Fatal hepatitis necrosis in a neonate with echovirus 20 infection: use of the polymerase chain reaction to detect enterovirus in the liver tissue. Clin Infect Dis 24:523–524, 1997.

318. Verboon-Maciolek MA, Swanink CM, Krediet TG, et al. Severe neonatal echovirus 20 infection characterized by hepatic failure. Pediatr Infect Dis J 16:524–527, 1997.

319. Wreghitt TG, Gandy GM, King A, et al. Fatal neonatal echo 7 virus infection. Lancet 2:465, 1984.

320. Boyd MT, Jordan SW, Davis LE: Fatal pneumonitis from congenital echovirus type 6 infection. Pediatr Infect Dis J 6:1138, 1987.

321. Aycock WL, Ingalls TH. Maternal disease as a principle in the epidemiology of congenital anomalies. Am J Med Sci 212:366, 1946.

322. Bowers VM Jr, Danforth DN. The significance of poliomyelitis during pregnancy—an analysis of the literature and presentation of twenty-four new cases. Am J Obstet Gynecol 65:34, 1953.

323. Schaefer J, Shaw EB. Poliomyelitis in pregnancy. Calif Med 70:16, 1949.

324. Anderson GW, Anderson G, Skaar A, et al. Poliomyelitis in pregnancy. Am J Hyg 55:127, 1952.

325. Kaye BM, Rosner DC, Stein I Sr. Viral diseases in pregnancy and their effect upon the embryo and fetus. Am J Obstet Gynecol 65:109, 1953.

326. Harjulehto-Mervaala T, Aro T, Hiilesmaa VK, et al. Oral polio vaccination during pregnancy: lack of impact on fetal development and perinatal outcome. Clin Infect Dis 18:414–420, 1994.

327. Frisk G, Diderholm, H. Increased frequency of coxsackie B virus IgM in women with spontaneous abortion. J Infect 24:141–145, 1992.

328. Axelsson C, Bondestam K, Frisk G, et al. Coxsackie B virus infections in women with miscarriage. J Med Virol 39:282–285, 1993.

329. Berendes HW, Weiss W, Miller RW. Presented at Third International Conference on Congenital Malformations, The Hague, Netherlands, 1969.

330. News and Notes. Polio vaccine and congenital defects. BMJ 1:510, 1967.

331. Connelly JP, Reynolds S, Crawford JD, et al. Viral and drug hazards in pregnancy. Clin Pediatr 3:587, 1964.

332. Harjulehto T, Hovi T, Aro T, et al. Congenital malformations and oral poliovirus vaccination during pregnancy. Lancet 1:771, 1989.

333. Brown GC. Maternal virus infection and congenital anomalies. Arch Environ Health 21:362, 1970.

334. Brown GC. Recent advances in the viral aetiology of congenital anomalies. Adv Teratol 1:55, 1966.

335. Brown GC. Coxsackie virus infections and heart disease. Am Heart J 75:145, 1968.

336. Evans TN, Brown GC. Congenital anomalies and virus infections. Am J Obstet Gynecol 87:749, 1963.

337. Brown GC, Evans TN. Serologic evidence of coxsackievirus etiology of congenital heart disease. JAMA 199:183, 1967.

338. Brown GC, Karunas RS. Relationship of congenital anomalies and maternal infection with selected enteroviruses. Am J Epidemiol 95:207, 1972.

339. Elizan TS, Ajero-Froehlich L, Fabiyi A, et al. Viral infection in pregnancy and congenital CNS malformations in man. Arch Neurol 20:115, 1969.

340. Gauntt CJ, Gudvangen RJ, Brans YW, et al. Coxsackievirus group B antibodies in the ventricular fluid of infants with severe anatomic defects in the central nervous system. Pediatrics 76:64, 1985.

341. Aycock WL. Acute poliomyelitis in pregnancy: its occurrence according to month of pregnancy and sex of fetus. N Engl J Med 235:160, 1946.

342. Freedman PS. Echovirus 11 infection and intrauterine death. Lancet 1:96, 1979.

343. Morens DM. Enteroviral disease in early infancy. J Pediatr 92:374, 1978.

344. Barton LL. Febrile neonatal illness associated with echo virus type 5 in the cerebrospinal fluid. Clin Pediatr 16:383, 1977.

345. Farmer K, Patten PT. An outbreak of coxsackie B5 infection in a special care unit for newborn infants. NZ Med J 68:86, 1968.

346. Hinuma Y, Murai Y, Nakao, T. Two outbreaks of echovirus 14 infection: a possible interference with oral poliovirus vaccine and a probable association with aseptic meningitis. J Hyg (London) 63:277, 1965.

347. Eilard T, Kyllerman M, Wennerblom I, et al. An outbreak of coxsackie virus type B2 among neonates in an obstetrical ward. Acta Paediatr Scand 63:103, 1974.

348. Linnemann CC Jr, Steichen J, Sherman WG, et al. Febrile illness in early infancy associated with ECHO virus infection. J Pediatr 84:49, 1974.

349. News and Notes. Coxsackie B virus infections in 1971. BMJ 1:453, 1972.

350. Hall CB, Cherry JD, Hatch MH, et al. The return of Boston exanthem. Am J Dis Child 131:323, 1977.

351. Abzug MJ, Levin MJ, Rotbart HA. Profile of enterovirus disease in the first two weeks of life. Pediatr Infect Dis J 12:820–824, 1993.

352. Haddad J, Gut JP, Wendling MJ, et al. Enterovirus infections in neonates: a retrospective study of 21 cases. Eur J Med 2:209–214, 1993.

353. Barre V, Marret S, Mendel I, et al. Enterovirus-associated haemophagocytic syndrome in a neonate. Acta Paediatr 87:467–471, 1998.

354. Cho CT, Janelle JG, Behbehani A. Severe neonatal illness associated with ECHO 9 virus infection. Clin Pediatr 12:304, 1973.

355. Codd AA, Hale JH, Bell TM, et al. Epidemic of echovirus 19 in the northeast of England. J Hyg (London) 76:307, 1976.

356. Marier R, Rodriguez W, Chloupek RJ, et al. Coxsackievirus B5 infection and aseptic meningitis in neonates and children. Am J Dis Child 129:321, 1975.

357. Bacon CJ, Sims DG. Echovirus 19 infection in infants under six months. Arch Dis Child 51:631, 1976.

358. Grossman M, Azimi P. Fever, hepatitis and coagulopathy in a newborn infant. Pediatr. Infect Dis J 11:1069, 1992.

359. Wong SN, Tam AYC, Ng THK, et al. Fatal coxsackie B1 virus infection in neonates. Pediatr Infect Dis J 8:638, 1989.

360. Chawareewong S, Kiangsiri S, Lokaphadhana K, et al. Neonatal herpangina caused by coxsackie A-5 virus. J Pediatr 93:492, 1978.

361. Murray D, Altschul M, Dyke J. Aseptic meningitis in a neonate with an oral vesicular lesion. Diagn Microbiol Infect Dis 3:77, 1985.

362. Nakayama T, Urano T, Osano M, et al. Outbreak of herpangina associated with coxsackievirus B3 infection. Pediatr Infect Dis J 8:495, 1989.

363. Cramblett HG, Moffet HL, Middleton GK Jr, et al. ECHO 19 virus infections. Arch Intern Med 110:574, 1962.

364. Suzuki N, Ishikawa K, Horiuchi T, et al. Age-related symptomatology of ECHO 11 virus infection in children. Pediatrics 65:284, 1980.

365. Medearis DN Jr, Kramer RA. Exanthem associated with ECHO virus type 18 viremia. J Pediatr 55:367, 1959.

366. Eckert HL, Portnoy B, Salvatore MA, et al. Group B, Coxsackie virus infection in infants with acute lower respiratory disease. Pediatrics 39:526, 1967.

367. Mirani M, Ogra PL, Barron AL. Epidemic of echovirus type 9 infection: certain clinical and epidemiologic features. NY J Med 73:403, 1973.

368. Ramos-Alvarez M. Cytopathogenic enteric viruses associated with undifferentiated diarrheal syndromes in early childhood. Ann NY Acad Sci 67:326, 1957.

369. Chonmaitree T, Menegus MA, Schervish-Swierkosz EM, et al. Enterovirus 71 infection: report of an outbreak with two cases of paralysis and a review of the literature. Pediatrics 67:489, 1981.

370. Arnon R, Naor N, Davidson S, et al. Fatal outcome of neonatal echovirus 19 infection. Pediatr Infect Dis J 10:788, 1991.

371. Talsma M, Vegting M, Hess J. Generalised coxsackie A9 infection in a neonate presenting with pericarditis. Br Heart J 52:683, 1984.

372. Barson WJ, Craenen J, Hosier DM, et al. Survival following myocarditis and myocardial calcification associated with infection by coxsackie virus B4. Pediatrics 68:79, 1981.

373. Chonmaitree T, Menegus MA, Powell KR. The clinical relevance of "CSF viral culture." A two-year experience with aseptic meningitis in Rochester, N. Y. JAMA 247:1843, 1982.

374. Rantakallio P, Saukkonen AL, Krause U, et al. Follow-up study of 17 cases of neonatal coxsackie B5 meningitis

and one with suspected myocarditis. Scand J Infect Dis 2:25, 1970.

375. Drew JH. ECHO 11 virus outbreak in a nursery associated with myocarditis. Aust Paediatr J 9:90, 1973.

376. Cherry JD, Lerner AM, Klein JO, et al. Coxsackie B5 infections with exanthems. Pediatrics 31:445, 1963.

377. Chesney PJ, Quennec P, Clark C. Hypoglycorrhachia and coxsackie B3 meningoencephalitis. Am J Clin Pathol 70:947, 1978.

378. Johnson RT, Shuey HE, Buescher EL. Epidemic central nervous system disease of mixed enterovirus etiology: I. Clinical and epidemiologic description. Am J Hyg 71:321, 1960.

379. Haynes RE, Cramblett HG, Hilty MD, et al. ECHO virus type 3 infections in children: clinical and laboratory studies. J Pediatr 80:589, 1972.

380. Haynes RE, Cramblett HG, Kronfol HJ. Echovirus 9 meningoencephalitis in infants and children. JAMA 208:1657, 1969.

381. Farmer K, MacArthur BA, Clay MM. A follow-up study of 15 cases of neonatal meningoencephalitis due to coxsackie virus B5. J Pediatr 87:568, 1975.

382. Helin I, Widell A, Borulf S, et al. Outbreak of coxsackievirus A-14 meningitis among newborns in a maternity hospital ward. Acta Paediatr Scand 76:234, 1987.

383. Wilfert CM, Lauer BA, Cohen M, et al. An epidemic of echovirus 18 meningitis. J Infect Dis 131:75, 1975.

384. Schmidt NJ, Lennette EH, Ho HH. An apparently new enterovirus isolated from patients with disease of the central nervous system. J Infect Dis 129:304, 1974.

385. Sells CJ, Carpenter RL, Ray CG. Sequelae of central-nervous-system enterovirus infections. N Engl J Med 293:1, 1975.

386. Matsumoto K, Yokochi T, Matsuda S, et al. Characterization of an echovirus type 30 variant isolated from patients with aseptic meningitis. Microbiol Immunol 30:333, 1986.

387. Bowen GS, Fisher MC, Deforest A, et al. Epidemic of meningitis and febrile illness in neonates caused by echo type 11 virus in Philadelphia. Pediatr Infect Dis 2:359, 1983.

388. Sumaya CV, Corman LI. Enteroviral meningitis in early infancy: significance in community outbreaks. Pediatr Infect Dis 1:151, 1982.

389. Bergman I, Painter, MJ, Wald ER, et al. Outcome in children with enteroviral meningitis during the first year of life. J Pediatr 110:705, 1987.

390. Wilfert CM, Thompson RJ Jr, Sunder TR, et al. Longitudinal assessment of children with enteroviral meningitis during the first three months of life. Pediatrics 67:811, 1981.

391. Schurmann W, Statz A, Mertens T, et al. Two cases of coxsackie B2 infection in neonates: clinical, virological, and epidemiological aspects. Eur J Pediatr 140:59, 1983.

392. Barson WJ, Reiner CB. Coxsackievirus B2 infection in a neonate with incontinentia pigmenti. Pediatrics 77:897, 1986.

393. Blokziji ML, Koskiniemi M. Echovirus 6 encephalitis in a preterm baby. Lancet 2:164, 1989.

394. Ehrnst A, Eriksson M. Echovirus type 23 observed as a nosocomial infection in infants. Scand J Dis 28:205–506, 1996.

395. Grangeot-Keros L, Broyer M, Briand E, et al. Enterovirus in sudden unexpected deaths in infants. Pediatr Infect Dis J 15:123–128, 1996.

396. Paul JR. Epidemiology of poliomyelitis. World Health Organ Monogr Ser 26:9, 1955.

397. Weibel RE, Benor DE. Reporting vaccine-associated paralytic poliomyelitis: concordance between the CDC and the National Vaccine Injury Compensation Program. Am J Public Health 86:734–737, 1996.

398. Sabin AB, Krumbiegel ER, Wigand R. ECHO type 9 virus disease. Am J Dis Child 96:197, 1958.

399. Drouhet V. Enterovirus infection and associated clinical symptoms in children. Ann Inst Pasteur 98:562, 1960.

400. Chonmaitree T, Ford C, Sanders C, et al. Comparison of cell cultures for rapid isolation of enteroviruses. J Clin Microbiol 26:2576, 1988.

401. Johnson FB. Transport of viral specimens. Clin Microbiol Rev 3:120–131, 1990.

402. Howell CL, Miller MJ. Effect of sucrose phosphate and sorbitol on infectivity of enveloped viruses during storage. J Clin Microbiol 18:658–662, 1983.

403. August MJ, Warford AL. Evaluation of a commercial monoclonal antibody for detection of adenovirus antigen. J Clin Microbiol 25:2233–2235, 1987.

404. Herrmann EC Jr. Experience in providing a viral diagnostic laboratory compatible with medical practice. Mayo Clin Proc 42:112, 1967.

405. Trabelsi A, Grattard F, Nejmeddine M, et al. Evaluation of an enterovirus group-specific anti-VPI monoclonal antibody, 5-D8/1, in comparison with neutralization and PCR for rapid identification of enteroviruses in cell culture. J Clin Microbiol. 33:2454–1457, 1995.

406. Carstens JM, Tracy S, Chapman NM, et al. Detection of enteroviruses in cell cultures by using in situ transcription. J Clin Microbiol 30:25–35, 1992.

407. De L, Nottay B, Yang CF, et al. Identification of vaccine-related polioviruses by hybridization with specific RNA probes. J Clin Microbiol 33:562–571, 1995.

408. Rotbart HA. Nucleic acid detection systems for enteroviruses. Clin Microbiol Rev 4:156–168, 1991.

409. Redline RW, Genest DR, Tycko B. Detection of enteroviral infection in paraffin-embedded tissue by the RNA polymerase chain reaction technique. Am J Clin Pathol 96:568, 1991.

410. Muir P, Nicholson F, Jhetam M, et al. Rapid diagnosis of enterovirus infection by magnetic bead extraction and polymerase chain reaction detection of enterovirus RNA in clinical specimens. J Clin Microbiol 31:31, 1993.

410a. Muir P, Ras A, Klapper PE, et al. Multicenter quality assessment of PCR methods for detection of enteroviruses. J Clin Microbiol 37:1409, 1999.

410b. Martin AB, Webber S, Fricker FJ, et al. Acute myocarditis: rapid diagnosis by PCR in children. Circulation 90:330, 1994.

411. Abraham R, Chonmaitree T, McCombs J, et al. Rapid detection of poliovirus by reverse transcription and polymerase chain amplification: application for the differentiation between poliovirus and nonpoliovirus enteroviruses. J Clin Microbiol 31:295–399, 1993.

412. Chezzi C. Rapid diagnosis of poliovirus infection by PCR amplification. J Clin Microbiol 34:1722–1725, 1996.

413. Egger D, Pasamontes L, Ostermayer M, et al. Reverse transcription multiplex PCR for differentiation between polio and enteroviruses from clinical and environmental samples. J Clin Microbiol 33:1442–1447, 1995.

414. Chan D, Hammond GW. Comparison of serodiagnosis of group B coxsackievirus infections by an immunoglobulin M capture enzyme immunoassay versus microneutralization. J Clin Microbiol 21:830, 1985.

415. Chomel JJ, Thouvenot D, Fayol V, et al. Rapid diagnosis of echovirus type 33 meningitis by specific IgM detection using an enzyme linked immunosorbent assay (ELISA). J Virol Methods 10:11, 1985.

416. Gong CM, Ho DWT, Field PR, et al. Immunoglobulin responses to echovirus type 11 by enzyme linked immunosorbent assay: single-serum diagnosis of acute infection by specific IgM antibody. J Virol Methods 9:209, 1984.

417. Pozzetto B, LeBihan JC, Gaudin OG. Rapid diagnosis of echovirus 33 infection by neutralizing specific IgM antibody. J Med Virol 18:361, 1986.

418. McCartney RA, Banatvala JE, Bell EJ. Routine use of m-antibody-capture ELISA for the serological diagnosis of Coxsackie B virus infections. J Med Virol 19:205, 1986.

419. Dorries R, Ter Meulen V. Specificity of IgM antibodies in acute human coxsackievirus B infections, analysed by indirect solid phase enzyme immunoassay and immunoblot technique. J Gen Virol 64:159, 1983.

420. Bell EJ, McCartney RA, Basquill D, et al. m-Antibody capture ELISA for the rapid diagnosis of enterovirus infections in patients with aseptic meningitis. J Med Virol 19:213, 1986.

421. Glimaker M, Ehrnst A, Magnius L, et al. Early diagnosis of enteroviral meningitis by a solid-phase reverse immunosorbent test and virus isolation. Scand J Infect Dis 22:519, 1990.

422. Gaudin O-G, Pozzetto B, Aouni M, et al. Detection of neutralizing IgM antibodies in the diagnosis of enterovirus infections. J Med Virol 28:200, 1989.

423. Eichenwald HC (ed). The Prevention of Mental Retardation Through Control of Infectious Diseases. Washington, D.C., U.S. Government Printing Office, 1966, p 31.

424. Dagan R, Prather SL, Powell KR, et al. Neutralizing antibodies to non-polio enteroviruses in human immune serum globulin. Pediatr Infect Dis 2:454, 1983.

425. McKinney RE Jr, Katz SL, Wilfert CM. Chronic enteroviral meningoencephalitis in agammaglobulinemic patients. Rev Infect Dis 9:334, 1987.

426. Hammond GW, Lukes H, Wells B, et al. Maternal and neonatal neutralizing antibody titers to selected enteroviruses. Pediatr Infect Dis 4:32, 1985.

427. Johnston JM, Overall JC Jr. Intravenous immunoglobulin in disseminated neonatal echovirus 11 infection. Pediatr Infect Dis J 8:254, 1989.

428. Abzug MJ, Keyerling HL, Lee ML, et al. Neonatal enterovirus infection: Virology, serology, and effects of intravenous immune globulin. Clin Infect Dis 20:1201–1206, 1995.

429. Jantausch BA, Luban NLC, Duffy L, et al. Maternal plasma transfusion in the treatment of disseminated neonatal echovirus 11 infection. Pediatr Infect Dis J 14:154–155, 1995.

430. Chuang E, Maller ES, Hoffman MA, et al. Successful treatment of fulminant echovirus 11 infection in a neonate by orthotopic liver transplantation. 17:211–214, 1993.

431. Kilbourne ED, Wilson CB, Perrier D. The induction of gross myocardial lesions by a Coxsackie (pleurodynia) virus and cortisone. J Clin Invest 35:367, 1956.

432. Carolane DJ, Long AM, McKeever PA, et al. Prevention of spread of echovirus 6 in a special care baby unit. Arch Dis Child 60:674, 1985.

433. Nagington J, Walker J, Gandy G, et al. Use of normal immunoglobulin in an echovirus 11 outbreak in a special-care baby unit. Lancet 2:443, 1983.

434. Pasic S, Jankovic B, Abinun M, et al. Intravenous immunoglobulin prophylaxis in an echovirus 6 and echovirus 4 nursery outbreak. Pediatr Infect Dis J 16:718–719, 1997.

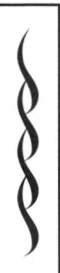

Lyme Disease

TESSA GARDNER, M.D.

Lyme disease, or Lyme borreliosis, is a tickborne zoonosis of both children and adults caused by the spirochete *Borrelia burgdorferi*.[1, 2] It has a worldwide geographic distribution and has been reported from more than 40 countries and 6 continents; the geographic distribution and number of cases reported continue to increase (Figs. 11–1 and 11–2). It is now the most common tickborne infection in the United States,[3–6] where 16,800 cases were reported to the Centers for Disease Control and Prevention (CDC) in 1998 (Fig. 11–3); in Europe,[8–10] where 2100 cases were reported to the European Union Concerted Action of Risk Assessment in Lyme Borreliosis (EUCALB) in 1994, and more than 60,000 cases were estimated to occur annually as of 1998[9]; and possibly in the world.[11–13]

Lyme borreliosis is a fairly recently recognized infection, although erythema migrans (EM), the characteristic skin lesion of early Lyme borreliosis, was first described in a Swedish woman in 1909 by Afzelius, who proposed that it was related to a zoonosis transmitted by a tick bite.[14] In 1975, Steere and associates recognized an outbreak of infectious arthritis and unusual rash similar to European EM in Old Lyme, Connecticut; they proposed that transmission occurred via an arthropod

vector and named the disease Lyme arthritis.[15] Eventually, it was found to be associated with ixodid tick bites and later, when its multisystem involvement was recognized, became known as Lyme disease.

In 1981, Burgdorfer and colleagues discovered a new species of *Borrelia* in *Ixodes* ticks associated with Lyme disease, and this became known as *Borrelia burgdorferi*.[1, 16, 17] This spirochete was found to be the causative agent of North American Lyme disease[18] and of European EM,[19] as well as other European syndromes such as acrodermatitis chronica atrophicans (ACA),[20] Bannwarth's syndrome,[21] and lymphadenosis benigna cutis[22]; the entire disease complex is now known as Lyme borreliosis.

As worldwide reporting of Lyme borreliosis increases, a geographically defined "Lyme Belt" is emerging between 30 and 65 degrees North latitude in the Eastern Hemisphere, and between 25 and 50 degrees North latitude in the Western Hemisphere; there may also be a belt developing between 30 and 40 degrees South latitude in the Eastern Hemisphere. This is reminiscent of the "Malaria Belt," which has been defined by climatic conditions and the distribution of another major arthropod vector of human disease, the *Anopheles* mosquito.

COUNTRIES IN EUROPE FROM WHICH LYME DISEASE HAS BEEN REPORTED

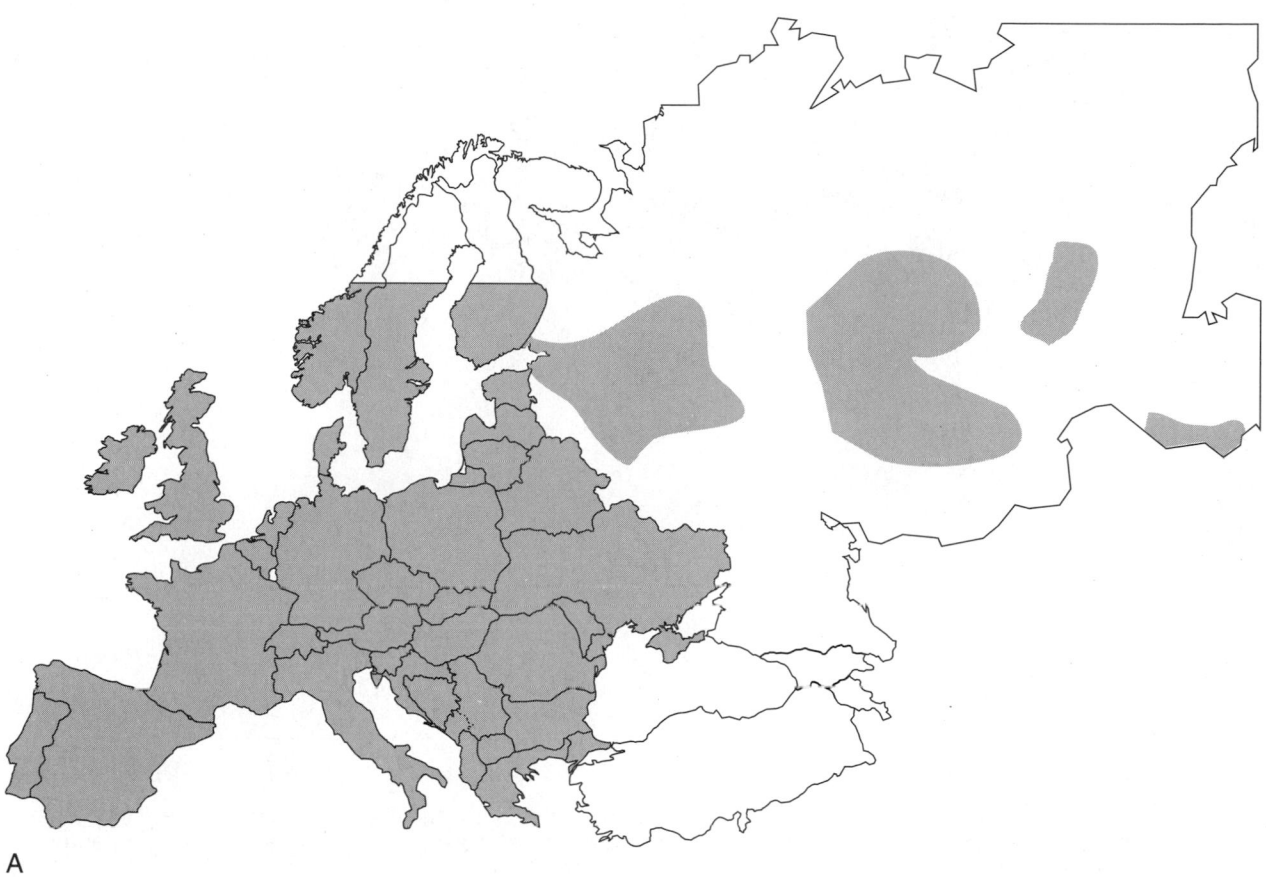

A

FIGURE 11–1 *A,* The geographic distribution of Lyme borreliosis in Europe. Europe is the main area outside North America from which Lyme borreliosis has been reported. This map shows European countries from which cases of Lyme borreliosis have been reported either to the World Health Organization,[501] to the European Union Concerted Action on Risk Assessment in Lyme Borreliosis,[9, 10] or in the medical literature.[11, 12, 41–44, 48, 83, 85–87, 90, 162, 251, 268, 275, 276, 305, 310, 352, 370, 371, 381, 387, 389, 402–405, 409, 422, 432–435, 448, 503, 504, 507–523, 525–537, 539–550, 552, 553] Reliable statistics on incidence by country are not available, as reporting of cases is voluntary in most countries. The highest incidences (either 1000–20,000 cases/country or 15–140 cases/100,000 population annually) of European Lyme borreliosis have been reported from Austria, Slovenia, Poland, Sweden, Bulgaria, Denmark, Hungary, the Netherlands, Finland, the Czech Republic, Switzerland, Germany, Italy, and France; lower incidences (either <500 cases/country, or <5 cases/100,000 population annually) have been reported from Belgium, Croatia, Estonia, Greece, Ireland, Latvia, Lithuania, Luxembourg, Moldavia, Norway, Romania, Russia, Spain, the United Kingdom, and the former Yugoslavia.

Illustration continued on following page

Lyme borreliosis is a multisystem infection that initially emerged as a new "great imitator"[14] because of the diversity of its clinical presentations, which comprise both early and late stages and include dermatologic, cardiac, neurologic, arthritic, and ocular manifestations.[23] However, more than 20 years since its recognition as a new disease,[15] the spectrum of its clinical manifestations has been extensively characterized, resulting in gradual loss of this reputation.[24] The existence of congenital borreliosis was suspected because of clinical similarities between the two spirochetoses Lyme borreliosis and the classic "great imitator" syphilis,[599] and the well-known association of gestational syphilis with mis-

carriage, early congenital infection, and late congenital infection.

Maternal-fetal transmission of *B. burgdorferi* was first reported in 1985 by Schlesinger and co-workers.[25] As the number of reported cases of Lyme disease continues to increase, there have been increasing reports of gestational Lyme disease associated with adverse outcomes and suspected congenital Lyme borreliosis.[25–48] Although a homogeneous congenital Lyme borreliosis syndrome has not yet emerged, there are several features that are common among the 66 adverse outcomes of pregnancies complicated by gestational Lyme borreliosis reviewed later in this chapter (including miscarriage during the

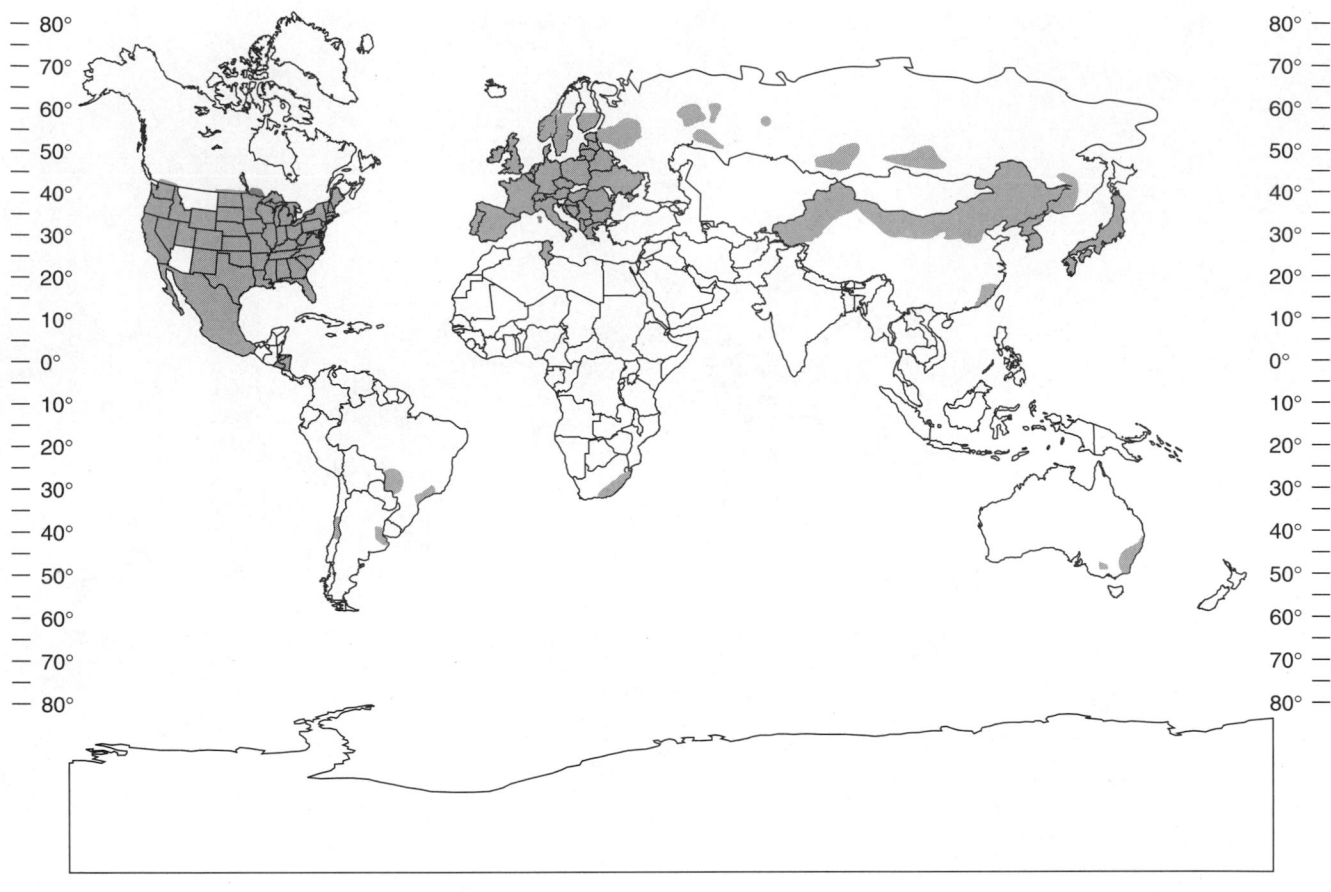

B

FIGURE 11–1 *Continued. B,* The worldwide geographic distribution of Lyme disease in temperate zone "Lyme Belts." In addition to North America and Europe, Lyme borreliosis is also endemic in Asia, mainly in China and Japan, and it has been reported from countries on three other continents and the Caribbean, including Argentina, Australia, Brazil, Chile, Egypt, Honduras, Israel, Mexico, Mozambique, Puerto Rico, South Africa, Taiwan, and Tunisia, although some of these cases may not have been indigenously acquired. The existence of indigenous cases in Central and South America, the Caribbean, Australia, and central and southern Africa is still uncertain.[164, 165, 303, 344, 349–351, 374, 388, 439, 448, 449, 451–453, 455, 456, 506, 554–561, 563, 566–569] Ixodid ticks infected with *Borrelia burgdorferi* have been found in Korea, and in several subarctic and subantarctic circumpolar islands (Egg and St. Lazaria Islands of Alaska, Flatey Island of Iceland, Campbell Island of New Zealand, and the Crozet Islands), but no cases of Lyme borreliosis have been reported yet from these areas.[165, 555] The geographic distribution of Lyme disease cases forms two belts—a 35-degree-wide northern temperate zone belt between 30 and 65 degrees North latitude in the Eastern Hemisphere, and another one slightly more southerly between 15 and 50 degrees North latitude in the Western Hemisphere. These include the majority of the Asian, European, North African, and North American cases. In addition, the cases from Australia, southern Africa, and South America appear to be clustered in a temperate zone belt between 10 and 40 degrees South latitude, but more cases are needed to determine if this is a true Southern Hemisphere "Lyme Belt."

first 20 weeks of gestation with a high frequency of fetal cardiac abnormality; severe early congenital infection with fulminant neonatal sepsis and meningoencephalitis and a high frequency of cardiac abnormality; mild early congenital infection with growth retardation and mild cardiac abnormality; and late congenital infection with growth retardation, developmental delay, and neurologic, cutaneous, dental, and skeletal involvement).

THE ORGANISM

Borrelia organisms are arthropod-borne spirochetes that infect birds, domestic and wild animals, and humans.[49,]

[50, 52] It is now recognized that *B. burgdorferi* is a phenotypically and genotypically heterogeneous genospecies complex, and the name has been modified to *Borrelia burgdorferi sensu lato* to reflect this. There are several genospecies of *Borrelia burgdorferi sensu lato: Borrelia burgdorferi sensu stricto, Borrelia andersonii, Borrelia garinii, Borrelia afzelii, Borrelia valaisiana, Borrelia lusitaniae, Borrelia japonica, Borrelia tanukii, Borrelia turdae,* and several genetically distinct genomic groups that have not yet achieved genospecies status.[51–71, 884] *B. burgdorferi sensu stricto, garinii,* and *afzelii* have been associated with human Lyme borreliosis[55]; *B. valaisiana* DNA has been found in EM lesions of two patients by polymerase chain reaction (PCR)[72]; and strains similar to strain 25015 in

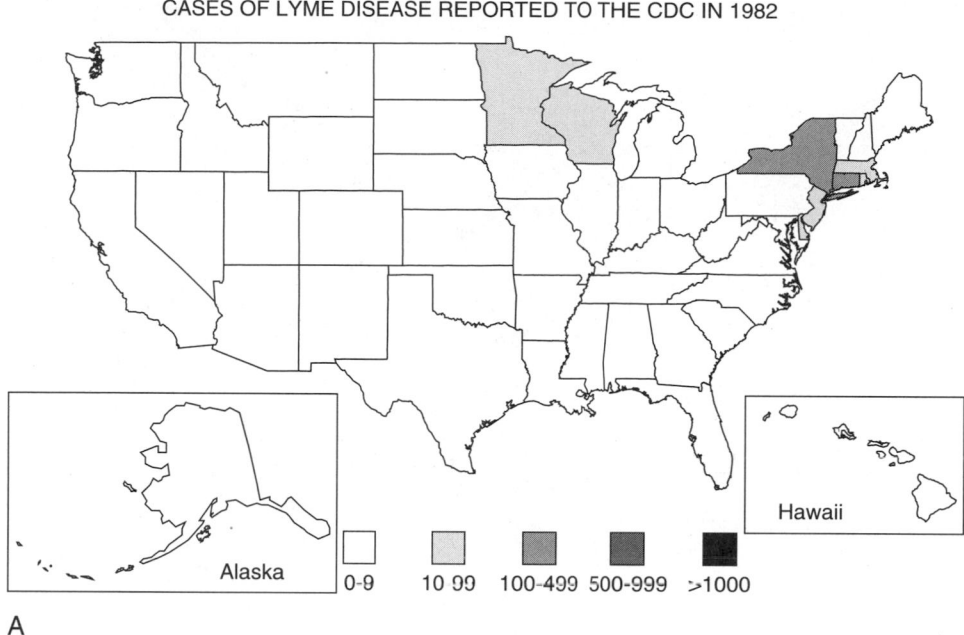

CASES OF LYME DISEASE REPORTED TO THE CDC IN 1982

A

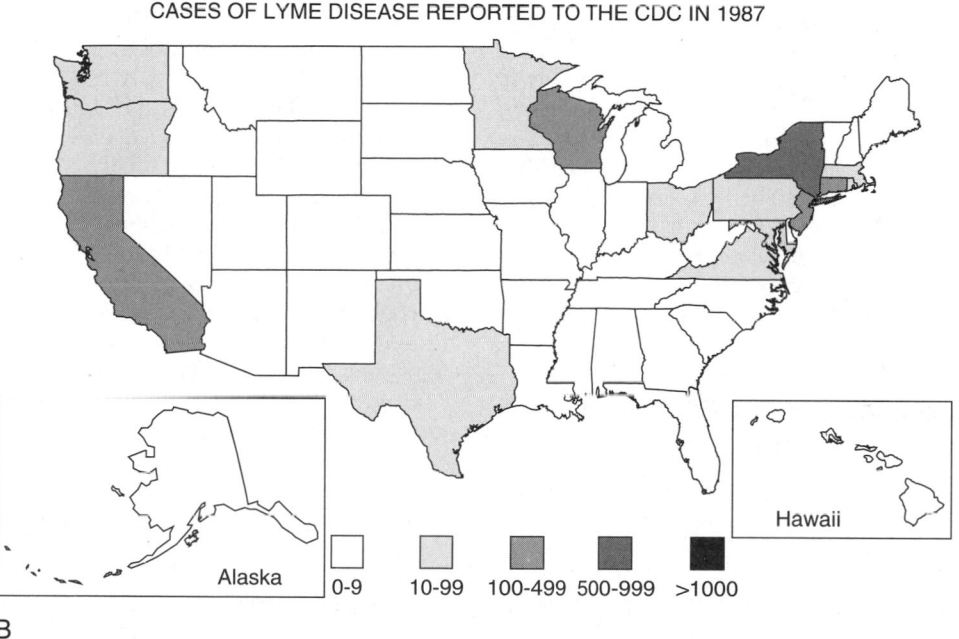

CASES OF LYME DISEASE REPORTED TO THE CDC IN 1987

B

FIGURE 11–2 The increase in the number of cases and expansion of the geographic distribution of Lyme disease in the United States from 1982 through 1998. The number of cases of Lyme disease reported to the Centers for Disease Control and Prevention (CDC) by state health departments in (A) 1982, (B) 1987, and (C) 1998.[4, 461] National surveillance began in 1982, and Lyme disease became a notifiable disease in 1990.[3] Cases of Lyme disease have also been reported to the Canadian Laboratory Centre for Disease Control (LCDC), mostly from southern areas that border Lyme-endemic areas of the northeastern, upper midwestern, and northwestern United States.[479]

Illustration continued on following page

CASES OF LYME DISEASE REPORTED TO THE CDC IN 1998

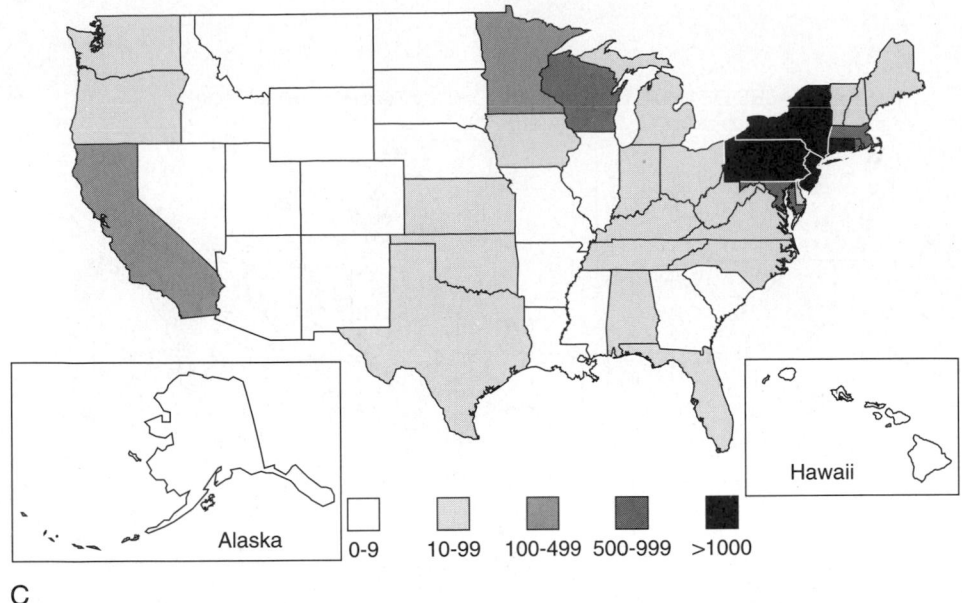

| | 0-9 | 10-99 | 100-499 | 500-999 | >1000 |

FIGURE 11–2 *Continued*

genomic group DN127 occasionally have been associated with Lyme disease.[83, 865] The other genospecies are involved in enzootic cycles of maintenance of *B. burgdorferi* in nature, but have not yet been isolated from patients with Lyme borreliosis.[55, 56] There is a newly described uncultivable *Borrelia* species, *Borrelia lonestarii*, which has been found in the Lone Star tick, *Amblyomma americanum*, and may be associated with Lyme-like disease in the southern United States.[73] Certain genospecies have been associated more frequently with certain clinical manifestations.[10, 74–76] *B. lonestarii* and a new species, *Borrelia miyamotoi*,[77] may be more closely related to the relapsing fever borreliae than to *B. burgdorferi sensu lato*.[73, 77]

Borrelia burgdorferi as the Etiologic Agent of Lyme Borreliosis

In 1981, Burgdorfer and associates discovered (isolated) a new species of *Borrelia* in *Ixodes dammini* (later re-named *Ixodes scapularis*[78]) ticks from a Lyme-endemic area in New York, demonstrated elevated antibody titers to this spirochete in convalescent sera of patients with Lyme disease, and proposed that this spirochete was involved in the etiology of Lyme disease.[1, 17]

In 1982, Berger and colleagues demonstrated rare spirochetes, similar to the *I. dammini (scapularis)* spirochete, by Warthin-Starry silver stain in skin biopsy specimens of untreated patients with EM skin lesions; they were able to isolate spirochetes from one specimen, thus supporting a spirochetal etiology for EM.[79] In 1985, Berger and co-workers grew the *I. dammini (scapularis)* spirochete from several skin biopsy specimens of EM lesions[79] and thus confirmed this spirochete as the etiologic agent of North American EM.

In 1983, Steere and associates isolated the new spirochete, which was subsequently named *Borrelia burgdorferi*, from blood, spinal fluid, and joint fluid of American Lyme disease patients and from *I. dammini (scapularis)* ticks in a Lyme-endemic area of Connecticut; they

CASES OF LYME DISEASE REPORTED TO THE CDC, 1982–1998, UNITED STATES

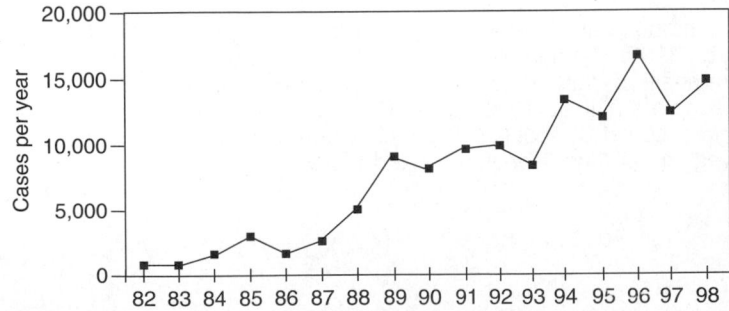

FIGURE 11–3 The number of cases of Lyme disease in the United States reported to the CDC by the individual state health departments has increased steadily from 1982 to 1998.[4, 461] Lyme disease became a reportable disease in 1990.[3]

demonstrated serum IgM and IgG antibody titer increases in these patients directed against this spirochete.[18] Simultaneously in 1983, Benach and colleagues isolated the same spirochete from the blood of patients with American Lyme disease and demonstrated similar seropositivity in these patients.[80] Both groups proposed the *I. dammini (scapularis)* spirochete as the etiologic agent of Lyme disease.[18, 80] In the same year, Barbour and co-workers, including Burgdorfer, isolated a new spirochete, similar to the *I. dammini (scapularis)* spirochete, from *Ixodes ricinus* ticks from an EM-endemic area of Switzerland.[81]

Ryberg and associates, including Burgdorfer, in 1983 demonstrated significant levels of IgM and IgG serum antibodies against the North American Lyme disease spirochete in sera of European patients with lymphocytic meningoradiculitis (Bannwarth's syndrome); they proposed the Lyme disease spirochete as the etiologic agent of Bannwarth's syndrome.[21]

In 1984 and 1985, Asbrink, Hovmark, and colleagues isolated the *I. ricinus* spirochete from skin biopsy specimens of European patients with EM,[19] acrodermatitis chronica atrophicans,[19, 20] and lymphadenosis benigna cutis[22]; antibody titer elevations against this spirochete were demonstrated in these patients, thus confirming the spirochetal etiology of these European skin diseases. In 1987, de Koning and co-workers demonstrated spirochetes, morphologically consistent with *B. burgdorferi*, in European EM and lymphadenosis benigna cutis skin lesions, in synovia of patients with European Lyme arthritis, and in spinal fluid of a patient with European Bannwarth's syndrome, and thus confirmed the spirochetal etiology of these additional European diseases.[82]

Some genospecies, such as *B. burgdorferi sensu stricto*, *garinii*, and *afzelii*, have been associated with human Lyme borreliosis, and others, such as *B. japonica*, only with tick vectors and reservoir hosts but not yet with human disease.[55, 56] *B. valaisiana* DNA has been found in EM lesions of two patients by PCR[72]; *B. burgdorferi sensu lato* isolates similar to strain 25015 of group DN127 were found in the cerebrospinal fluid (CSF) and EM of nine Slovenian patients[83, 884]; and *B. burgdorferi* genospecies DN127 was isolated from one patient with borrelial lymphocytoma.[74]

There is clustering of genospecies from patients with different clinical manifestations, such as EM, ACA, neuroborreliosis, arthritis, and carditis[55, 67, 74–76, 84–89]; this clustering suggests the possibility of differences in pathogenicity and organotropism of strains of different phenotypes and genotypes, which may be related to differences in clinical syndromes associated with these strains.[51–53]

In North America, where ACA does not occur, *B. burgdorferi sensu stricto* is the only agent of human Lyme disease, and is associated with all North American manifestations of Lyme disease, EM, neuroborreliosis, arthritis, and carditis.[5] In Europe, ACA is associated predominantly with *B. afzelii*, and occasionally with *garinii* or *sensu stricto*[67, 74–76, 85–87, 89]; EM with all three genospecies (*B. burgdorferi sensu stricto, garinii, afzelii*)[74–76, 85, 89]; neuroborreliosis predominantly but not exclusively with *B. garinii*[74–76, 85, 87, 88]; arthritis predominantly with *sensu*

stricto and sometimes with *garinii*[75, 76]; and carditis with *sensu stricto* and occasionally with *garinii*.[75, 76]

Within genospecies, there may be strains that are more pathogenic than others, as may be involved in the clustering of strains isolated from European patients with disseminated Lyme borreliosis in one sub-branch of *B. garinii*,[55] the clustering of *B. garinii* strains associated with adult neuroborreliosis in Osp A serotype 4, and the clustering of *garinii* associated with pediatric neuroborreliosis in Osp A serotype 6.[88]

A large study by the EUCALB, of over 2000 patients with Lyme borreliosis in 15 European countries during 12 months in 1994, found that the incidence of Lyme borreliosis per 100,000 population increased from Western to Eastern Europe, with higher incidences east of the Netherlands, France, and Italy.[10]

Morphology

Borrelia burgdorferi[56, 81, 91–98, 218] is a long (10 to 30 micrometers in length), narrow (0.18 to 0.25 micrometer in diameter), irregularly and loosely coiled, helical, motile, flexible spirochete with tapered ends and sheathed flagellae.

It has an inner and an outer cell membrane and four to eight flagellae, located in the periplasmic space between the inner and outer trilaminar cell membranes. These membranes, which are inserted at each end and extend toward the middle of the spirochete, allow it to move efficiently through viscous solutions and presumably enhance its ability to disseminate in body tissues. The trilaminar outer membrane structure is similar to, but more fluid than, that of gram-negative bacteria, and it contains the embedded outer surface membrane lipoproteins and a lipopolysaccharide with weak endotoxin-like activity.[100] The flexible cell wall is located just outside the cytoplasmic membrane.[99] In addition to the typical *B. burgdorferi* morphology, morphologic variants have been found in tissue biopsies.[101–103]

Molecular Biology

B. burgdorferi has several major antigens that can be separated by polyacrylamide gel electrophoresis and characterized antigenically by reactivity in Western blots with *B. burgdorferi*-specific polyclonal and monoclonal antibodies.[51, 52, 92, 93, 104, 105]

The 83- to 100-kilodalton (kd) antigen p83/100 is *Borrelia* genus-specific,[51, 106, 107] cross reacts minimally with other bacteria,[104] is associated with either the flagella or the protoplasmic cylinder, and is a chromosomally encoded immunodominant antigen of *B. burgdorferi sensu lato*, which has minor homology with the muscle and cytoskeletal proteins myosin and troponin, and contains an amino acid sequence that is a common cell recognition signal of integrins and may be involved in spirochetal attachment to cells.[106] The constant-molecular-weight, major immunodominant 60-kd common antigen HSP60, and the 70-kd antigen HSP70 are heat shock proteins that function as flagellin chaperones, are encoded by chromosomal genes, and cross react broadly with other bacteria.[104, 109, 882] The 35-kd protein, a *B.*

burgdorferi sensu lato–specific lipoprotein encoded by a chromosomal gene, is expressed early in human infection and is an important immunodominant marker for early human infection.[110] There are several other significant antigens, including the 39-kd molecular weight protein, some encoded by chromosomal and some by plasmid genes.[882]

The 41-kd flagellar antigen p41 is the other major protein of the organism[51, 52]; it has a uniform molecular weight in all *B. burgdorferi* strains,[51] is encoded by a highly conserved gene (with 96–97% sequence homology between strains) located on the main chromosome,[111] and is the antigen most often recognized in Lyme borreliosis patient sera.[112] *B. burgdorferi* flagellin has an epitope that shares amino acid homology with the N-terminal amino acid sequences of human chaperonin, a 60-kd heat shock protein,[113] and has some cross-reactivity with other spirochetes.

B. burgdorferi has several major outer surface lipoproteins—Osp A,[114] Osp B,[114] Osp C,[114, 116] Osp D,[117] Osp E,[118] Osp F,[118] and pG[119]—that are encoded by plasmids.[114, 120, 882] The 18-kd EppA protein (exported plasmid protein A) is thought to be either an outer membrane or a secreted protein.[121] Osp A has the least variability and the greatest homology (77–83%) of the three major *B. burgdorferi* genospecies[108, 114, 122]; Osp B has high variability[114]; and Osp C has the highest variability and exhibits polymorphism of its amino acid sequences and Osp C–encoding gene sequences.[114, 120, 123] Osp C is expressed early in infection,[124, 125] and, despite this heterogeneity, the three major genospecies have common as well as genospecies-specific Osp C immunogenic epitopes recognized by patient sera.[108, 125] Osp A has an immunodominant epitope that shares amino acid sequence homology and encoding DNA sequence homology with human leukocyte function–associated antigen-1 (LFA-1), which is a candidate arthritogenic autoantigen that may be involved in the immunopathogenesis of Lyme arthritis.[126]

The smaller, variable-molecular-weight outer surface membrane lipoproteins of *B. burgdorferi* are species-specific, and antigenic modulation, variation in size, antigenicity, and expression of these outer surface proteins have been found.[51, 52, 92, 93, 129, 130] In 1998, Kawabata and associates reported that *B. burgdorferi sensu stricto* strain 297 has VMP-like proteins coded by VMP-like sequences (Vls) located in multiple copies on the 20 kilobase pair plasmid.[130] In 1997, Zhang and colleagues described a system in *B. burgdorferi sensu stricto* strain B31 that produces extensive antigenic variability in a surface lipoprotein.[131] *B. burgdorferi* Vls is expressed in patients with Lyme borreliosis,[130] and the system of antigenic variability may enhance evasion of the host immune response.[130, 131]

B. burgdorferi also has nonprotein antigens, composed of lipid-carbohydrate-, and phosphorus-containing compounds, which react with Lyme disease patient sera but are of unknown significance.[132]

The genome of *B. burgdorferi* has been sequenced.[133, 882] *B. burgdorferi sensu stricto* strain B31 has a large linear chromosome of 910, 725 base pairs (about 900 kbp) and at least 17 plasmids (10 linear plasmids ranging in size from 17 to 56 kbp, and 7 circular plasmids ranging from 9 to 32 kbp) with a combined total of 533,000 base pairs (about 500 kbp) of double-stranded DNA with an average G plus C content of 28.6%.[882] The linear chromosome has been sequenced and contains 853 genes that encode proteins needed for DNA replication, transcription, translation, energy metabolism, and solute transport, but not for cellular biosynthesis. Eleven of the plasmids (ranging from about 9 to 54 kbp in size), containing 430 genes, have been sequenced. The functions of most of these genes are unknown, but they may be involved in antigenic variation and immune evasion; some, such as the 53- to 58-kbp linear plasmid in *B. burgdorferi sensu stricto*, *garinii*, and *afzelii*, and the 90- to 105-kbp linear plasmid in *B. japonica*, encode outer surface proteins A and B. Others, such as the 26- to 27-kbp circular plasmid, encode Osp C. Fifty-nine percent of the chromosomal genes have known biologic roles, 12% match genes in other organisms with unknown roles, and 29% are new genes; these percentages for plasmid genes are 16, 26, and 58, respectively.[882] Almost all of the membrane proteins of *B. burgdorferi* are lipoproteins, and 8% of its genes encode 105 putative lipoproteins, which is a much greater percentage than occurs with most other bacteria; six percent of the genes encode proteins involved in spirochetal motility and chemotaxis.[882]

Although North American and European *B. burgdorferi sensu stricto* isolates tend to cluster into separate subbranches by DNA analysis,[55] there are genetic similarities between some isolates from the two continents, suggesting some previous interchange of strains between the two continents.[62]

Among the different genospecies,[657, 117, 134] there are differences in the number, size, and sequences of the linear and circular plasmids, as well as their presence or absence, which correlate with the expression of the outer surface proteins they encode. The Osp A– and Osp B–encoding linear plasmid is present in all *B. burgdorferi sensu lato* genospecies (although some individual isolates may lack the Osp B gene, and this plasmid may be lost in culture). Almost all North American and European strains express Osp A and it shows the least antigenic variability between genospecies[120]; Osp A serotyping has been used to divide *B. burgdorferi sensu lato* into different phenotypes,[105] which correlate with different genotypes by Osp A gene sequencing. The Osp C gene is located on a 26-kbp circular plasmid that is present in all genospecies, but its expression, both qualitatively and quantitatively, is variable; most European strains express Osp C, but Osp C has been found to be cryptic in North American strains, where it is expressed only in strains that have lost all plasmids other than the Osp C–encoding and Osp AB–encoding plasmids.[116] The Osp D gene is highly conserved and is present in 24, 50, and 90%, respectively, of isolates of *B. burgdorferi sensu stricto*, *afzelii*, and *garinii*; its encoding plasmid has significant size variability, ranging from 36 to 40 kbp, and contains varying numbers of copies of a 17-kbp repeating sequence bordering a variable region with evidence of homologous recombinational events.[117] The Osp E and Osp F genes are located in tandem on the

45-kbp linear plasmid.[118] The pG gene is located on a 48-kbp linear plasmid that has some sequence homology to the Osp EF gene and is detectable in most strains of *B. burgdorferi sensu stricto* and *B. afzelii*, but not in *B. garinii* or *B. japonica*.[119] There is p83/100 gene heterogeneity in *B. garinii*, but not in either *B. burgdorferi sensu stricto* or *B. afzelii*; *B. garinii* strains could be separated into two major subtypes on the basis of p83/100 gene sequence variation, one corresponding to Osp A serotype 4 and the other to serotypes 3, 5, 6, and 7.[106] The EppA protein gene is located on the 9-kbp circular plasmid, and loss of this plasmid has been associated with loss of virulence during passage of *B. burgdorferi* in culture.[121]

It has been proposed that the high level of variability of Osp C[115] and D,[117] and the existence of a VMP-like system[130, 131] may be involved in immune evasion by *B. burgdorferi*. Evasion of the immune response by a *B. burgdorferi* strain expressing a truncated Osp B also raised this as a possible immune escape mechanism.[135, 136]

Differential gene expression, which has been found in *B. burgdorferi*, has also been suspected to be involved in infectivity, invasion, and dissemination, and in evasion of the host immune response to the infection[120, 137]; it may also have a role in differential organotropism. Abundant Osp A and Osp B, and no Osp C, are expressed by *B. burgdorferi* in unfed tick midguts. The beginning of tick feeding and the arrival of the blood meal in the tick midgut trigger downregulation of Osp A and B, and upregulation of Osp C expression of *B. burgdorferi* in the engorged tick midgut.[138–140] Although Osp A and B are not expressed initially after infection, they are eventually expressed, in particular in patients with chronic Lyme arthritis. Although Osp E and Osp F are expressed by *B. burgdorferi* in ticks and in the mammalian host, it appears that the Osp E and F homologues, the Erp proteins (Osp EF–related proteins), form a gene group that is differentially expressed at different stages of the spirochete's life cycle; the Osp E homologue, p21, which has 70% amino acid homology with Osp E, and the Osp F homologues, pG, bbk2.10, and bbk2.11, are expressed only in the mammalian host and not in the spirochete in culture or in ticks.[119, 127, 141] Expression of p21 does not occur even in engorged ticks, only in the mammalian host; antibody to p21 is found in 28 to 33% of patients with early or late Lyme disease, including Lyme arthritis, indicating its expression during Lyme disease.[127] Confirmation of differential gene expression during Lyme disease was first reported in 1998, when p35 (the 35-kd protein) and p37 (the 37-kd protein) messenger RNA (mRNA), but not Osp A mRNA, was found in EM skin biopsies and Lyme arthritis synovium, consistent with upregulation of p35 and p37 and the downregulation of Osp A.[141] The protein EppA (exported plasmid protein A) is downregulated at the transcriptional level in cultured *B. burgdorferi*, is expressed only in the mammalian host, and is associated with virulent strains of *B. burgdorferi*.[121] Temperature increases, as occur with ingestion of the blood meal by the tick, and even increases in culture temperature from 23° C to 35° C, induce downregulation of Osp A expression, and upregulation of Osp C, Osp E, Osp F, and of

the Osp EF homologues, the Erp proteins.[128, 140, 142] As Osp A is downregulated and disappears, the spirochete becomes resistent to antibody against Osp A; this is important in vaccine development, as is discussed in the section Prevention: Vaccine Development.

B. burgdorferi produces none of its own proteolytic enzymes. It acquires a host-derived activated proteolytic complex consisting of plasmin, plasminogen, and a urokinase-type plasminogen activator, which arrives at the tick midgut in the blood meal, binds to Osp A while it is still expressed, and coats the spirochete; this complex is presumably able to dissolve extracellular matrix, facilitate dissemination of the spirochete to the tick salivary glands for transmission to the host, and then enhance spirochete dissemination in host tissues, where the host-derived antigens cause the spirochete to be invisible immunologically to the host.[143–146] Surface antigens of *B. burgdorferi*, particularly Osp A, are also involved in binding of the spirochete to collagen fibers, vascular endothelium, and other cells,[147] including antigen-presenting cells,[148] and in triggering a variety of events in host cells, ranging from expression of adhesion molecules to production of cytokines and other factors involved in the immunopathogenesis of the infection,[149, 150] as is discussed in the section Pathology and Pathogenesis.

Some antigens of *B. burgdorferi* have epitopes that share homology and cross react with host epitopes, leading to molecular mimicry,[151] such as *B. burgdorferi* Osp A and human leukocyte function–associated antigen-1 (LFA-1),[126] and possibly p83/100 and the human muscle and cytoskeletal proteins myosin and troponin,[106] *B. burgdorferi* flagellin, and human axonal heat shock protein 60.[113] This is discussed further in the sections Pathology and Pathogenesis, and Interactions with the Immune System: Correlation of Clinical Manifestations with HLA Type.

Taxonomy

Borrelia burgdorferi,[51, 94] the etiologic agent of Lyme borreliosis, is a member of the order Spirochaetales, the family Spirochaetaceae, the genus *Borrelia*, and the species *burgdorferi*. Borreliae are more closely related genetically to *Spirochaeta* than to *Treponema*, and all borreliae are transmitted by arthropods.[99]

B. burgdorferi was initially divided into four phenotypes,[92] and later into eight serotypes[51, 52, 105, 259] on the basis of antigenic diversity of Osp A as determined by reactivity with various monoclonal antibodies and by Osp A gene sequencing.[105] It was also initially divided into three genotype subspecies, based on DNA homology and ribosomal RNA restriction endonuclease pattern analysis,[50, 53] and corresponding to phenotypes based on major protein antigenicity, with 76 to 100% DNA homology within groups, and 46 to 74% between groups.[53]

As more isolates of *B. burgdorferi* have been studied by various methods, it has become clear that *B. burgdorferi* has phenotypic and genotypic heterogeneity.* On the basis of phenotypic and genotypic differences from

---

*See references 13, 51–66, 68, 70, 100, 105, 115, 117, 123, and 884.

B. burgdorferi sensu stricto and from each other, further subdivision into additional subbranches was done, dendrograms of genetic relatedness were constructed,* and some of the subbranches were designated as new genospecies—*Borrelia garinii* (formerly 20047),[53] *B. afzelii* (formerly VS461),[53, 67] *B. andersonii* (includes former groups 21038 and 21123),[56, 59, 66, 70, 100] *B. valaisiana* (formerly VS116 and M19),[61] *B. lusitaniae* (formerly PotiB2),[65] *B. japonica* (formerly HO14),[66, 69] *B. tanukii* (formerly Hk501),[58, 68] *B. turdae* (formerly Ya501),[58, 68] and *B. miyamotoi* (formerly HT31).[77] There is also a genomic group DN127, which includes strain CA55 and sometimes strain 25015, and which is distinct from the other genospecies.[55, 57, 64, 123, 884]

In 1998, isolation of an unusual strain of *B. burgdorferi sensu lato* was reported from *Ixodes dentatus* and *A. americanum* in southeastern Missouri, which is similar to strains isolated from *I. dentatus* in New York and Georgia, but different from *B. burgdorferi sensu stricto*.[153] Also, an uncultivable borrelia, *Borrelia lonestarii*, was found in *A. americanum* from New York, New Jersey, Missouri, and North Carolina,[73] which may be related to the Lyme-like disease in the southern states. A borrelia identified as *B. burgdorferi* has been found in *A. americanum* in New Jersey, Missouri, Texas, Oklahoma, Virginia, North Carolina, and Alabama.[154–158]

There is clustering of *B. burgdorferi* genospecies from different geographic areas, such as North America, Europe, Asia, and the circumpolar arctic and subantarctic regions, and from different tick vectors.[10, 13, 51–57, 59, 62, 71, 74] *B. garinii*, *afzelii*, *sensu stricto*, *valaisiana*, and *lusitaniae* accounted for 39.7, 37.1, 15.9, 6.7, and 0.6% of *B. burgdorferi sensu lato* genospecies isolated from arthropod vectors, animal hosts, and human patients in Europe.[54] *B. burgdorferi sensu stricto* is found in *I. scapularis* and *I. pacificus* in North America.[55, 56, 59, 63, 70, 100, 123, 159] *B. andersonii* is found in *I. dentatus*,[59, 100] and *I. scapularis* in North America.[64] *B. bissettii* is found in *I. pacificus*[55–57, 59, 123] and group CA55 in *Ixodes neotomae* in the western United States,[57, 59, 884] and group 25015 in *I. scapularis* from New York.[55–57, 123, 884] *B. bissettii* represents the only strain other than *sensu stricto* to be present in both Europe and North America.[83, 884] Four genospecies—*B. burgdorferi sensu stricto*, *B. afzelii*, *B. garinii*, and *B. valaisiana*—are found in *I. ricinus* in central Europe.[61, 74] Human co-infections[74, 84] and *I. ricinus* co-infections[83, 85, 160–162] with different genospecies have been reported. *B. afzelii* and *B. garinii* have been found in *Ixodes persulcatus* in eastern Europe and in Asia, including Japan, and *B. burgdorferi sensu stricto* has not been found.[67, 74, 163, 164] *B. japonica* is found in *Ixodes ovatus* in Japan[66, 69, 163]; *B. garinii*, and no other genospecies, is found in *Ixodes uriae* and *I. ricinus* in the far northern subarctic latitudes,[152, 165, 166] and in *I. uriae* in the far southern subantarctic latitudes; genetically heterogeneous *B. burgdorferi sensu stricto*, *B. garinii*, and *B. afzelii* occur in migratory passerine (perching) birds in Sweden.[13]

Hypotheses about the phylogenetic origins and historical patterns of global migration of the different *B. burgdorferi* genospecies have been developed, based on genetic analysis of the different strains. Initially, it was thought that there was greater diversity of genospecies in Europe,[53] with *B. garinii*, *afzelii*, and *sensu stricto*, and in Asia, with *B. garinii*, *afzelii*, and *japonica*, than in North America, where only *B. burgdorferi sensu stricto* was thought to occur; this led to hypotheses that *B. burgdorferi* was introduced into North America from Europe, possibly by migratory birds or small mammalian hosts of infected ticks.[13, 157, 165, 167–171] The initial genetic studies were done mainly on isolates from the restricted hyperendemic areas of the Northeast and Upper Midwest; later, when isolates from the South and West were studied, more genetic heterogeneity was found,[62, 63] raising the reverse hypothesis—that introduction was from North America into Europe. The similarity in Osp A phenotype of a few west central European strains and the North American strains raises the possibility that the *B. burgdorferi* originally introduced into the United States came from west central Europe,[92] or that North American strains were introduced into Europe. The differences in DNA sequences for outer surface proteins of North American and European strains of *B. burgdorferi* suggest that these strains may have diverged long ago and may be pathogenically different.

B. burgdorferi is clonal, and widespread genetic exchange between chromosomal genes is thought not to occur.[57, 60] The order of occurrence of genes is the same across different genospecies, and there is no evidence of chromosomal rearrangements since the evolutionary divergence of the different genospecies from a common ancestor.[57, 60] Genetic exchange between plasmid genes, such as the Osp A and Osp B linear plasmid genes, has been found[80] but is thought to be rare[57, 60]; there is evidence of exchange with other plasmid genes, such as the Osp D–encoding plasmid, which suggests that *B. afzelii* and *garinii* are closely related and that *B. burgdorferi sensu stricto* only recently acquired the Osp D gene.[117]

There are differences in vector competence of *I. ricinus* and *I. scapularis* for three genospecies of *B. burgdorferi sensu lato*, which correlates with the known geographic association of these vectors and genospecies: Acquisition of infection by *I. scapularis* was 83 to 90, 87, 10, and 5% for *B. burgdorferi sensu stricto*, *afzelii*, *garinii* VS286, and *garinii* VSBP, compared with acquisition of infection by *I. ricinus* of 3, 90, 5, and 3%, respectively.[878] Other genospecies are associated with some tick species and have not been found in others.[68, 69]

There is clustering of *B. burgdorferi* genospecies from different reservoir host species[74] and some host species, which may act as biologic filters.[172, 173]

Isolation and Cultivation

B. burgdorferi lives in hosts such as vertebrates or hematophagous arthropods and is not found living free in the environment. In 1981, it was first isolated by Burgdorfer and associates from the midgut and other tissues dissected from *Ixodes scapularis (dammini)* ticks from Shelter Island, a Lyme-endemic area of New York, and was cloned to become the B31 strain of *B. burgdorferi*.[1] In 1983, Burgdorfer and colleagues also first isolated a similar spirochete from *Ixodes ricinus* ticks from the Seo-

---

*See references 55–57, 59–63, 65, 66, 68, 76, 77, and 117.

wald Forest, a Lyme-endemic area of Switzerland, and showed it to be morphologically and antigenically similar to the *I. dammini* spirochete.[81] Since then, it has been isolated from several species of ticks, vertebrate hosts, and humans; this is described in the section Epidemiology and Transmission.

B. burgdorferi is fastidious and microaerophilic and grows best in a liquid medium, modified Barbour-Stoenner-Kelly medium (BSK II), at 33° C to 35° C.[50, 81, 91] It has an 11- to 24-hour doubling time, which may be shortened to 11 to 12 hours under ideal conditions, but it still may take 3 weeks or longer to grow sufficiently in culture to become detectable by microscopy.[18, 50, 91, 174] However, the use of *B. burgdorferi*–specific PCR has shortened the time for detection in culture media.[175] It can also grow anaerobically, and has even been grown aerobically in the presence of 1 to 5% carbon dioxide.[99]

Unlike other spirochetes, *B. burgdorferi* can be grown in solid media.[97] It has been found to produce colonies of several types, including a compact 0.43-mm round colony at the agarose surface, and three types of colonies that penetrated into the agarose—a 1.43-mm colony with a raised center surrounded by a diffuse ring, a colony composed of many small aggregations, and a diffuse 1.8-mm colony. It was also found to cause intense hemolysis on solid BSK II medium with horse blood.[879] More recently, *B. burgdorferi* has been found to have shorter doubling times of even 7 hours, when grown in solid media under strict anaerobic conditions, and it may be considered an obligate anaerobe.[176]

B. burgdorferi can be seen in cultures by dark-field or phase-contrast microscopy. It stains with acridine orange, Giemsa, and silver stains such as Warthin-Starry or Dieterle's[25] or Bosma-Steiner stain,[82] and can be identified with immunofluorescence techniques using *B. burgdorferi*–specific polyclonal or monoclonal antibodies[177] or *B. burgdorferi*–specific PCR.[175]

Transformation of *B. burgdorferi* from typical motile spirochetes to immotile cystic spheroplast L-forms occurs when *B. burgdorferi* is grown in culture in the presence of antibiotics, *B. burgdorferi*–specific antibody, or normal CSF.[102] The conversion to spheroplast forms may be related to the ability of the spirochete to persist in tissues without elimination by the host immune response.

B. burgdorferi shows antigenic variation and loss of pathogenicity after 10 to 15 passages in culture, and becomes noninfectious; this correlates with loss of plasmids.[129, 133, 134, 178, 882] Loss of several outer surface proteins and their encoding plasmid genes, including Osp B, C, and D, with passage has been noted; there is a suggestion that linear plasmid of 24.7 kbp (1p24.7) is required for infectivity of *B. burgdorferi sensu stricto, garinii,* and *afzelii,* and that 1p38 (which encodes Osp D) is not required. Loss of 1p27.5 may increase infectivity, but correlation of individual plasmids with infectivity has been inconsistent.[117, 134, 178] High-passage strains of *B. burgdorferi* have also been found to decrease both invasiveness and cytopathic killing of B and T lymphocytes.[179]

B. burgdorferi is relatively easily isolated and grown from midgut and other tissues dissected from infected *Ixodes* ticks,[50, 74, 174, 180, 181] from which the isolation rate depends on the incidence of infection within the tick population (see section Epidemiology and Transmission: *B. burgdorferi* Tick Infection Rates); from blood and organ cultures of infected reservoir-competent host animals[167, 182] (see section Epidemiology and Transmission: *B. burgdorferi* Reservoir Animal Infection Rates); and from biopsy specimens of the leading edge of EM skin lesions, from which the isolation rate is usually 28 to 86% (it may be higher in disseminated infection).[183, 184] It has been isolated occasionally from blood, CSF, and ACA skin biopsy specimens, and rarely from borrelial lymphocytoma skin biopsies, synovium and synovial fluid, myocardium and heart valves, the iris, ligamentous tissue, placenta, fetal tissues, or other tissues because the organism density is low[50] (see section Diagnosis and Differential Diagnosis: Diagnostic Tests: Culture).

The *B. burgdorferi*–specific PCR[185–187] increases the sensitivity of detection of *B. burgdorferi* in body fluids and tissues by using DNA target sequences that are unique to *B. burgdorferi*, are not present in other closely related *Borrelia* species or other spirochetes, and are highly conserved among *B. burgdorferi* strains. PCR has been used to demonstrate the spirochetes in EM, ACA, and borrelial lymphocytoma skin biopsy specimens; serum, plasma, and bone marrow; CSF, brain biopsy, sural nerve biopsy, and vitreous fluid; synovial fluid and membrane; urine; breast milk; placental tissue; and various animal hosts and tick vectors (see section Diagnosis and Differential Diagnosis: Diagnostic Tests: Polymerase Chain Reaction).

Antibiotic Susceptibility

Isolates of *B. burgdorferi* from humans and ticks from different geographic areas, including the United States and Europe, generally have similar antimicrobial susceptibility patterns,[50, 174, 100–190, 192, 196–198] as is shown in Table 11–1. *B. burgdorferi* antibiotic susceptibility can be assessed in vitro by comparison of the minimal inhibitory concentrations (either mean MIC or MIC 50%) and the minimal bacteriocidal concentrations (either mean MBC or MBC 50%) for various antibiotics, and in vivo by comparison of the antibiotic dose required to cure 50% of infected animals of their infection (CD_{50}). However, there is one report[196] of lower doxycycline MIC values for cutaneous isolates than for CSF isolates.

B. burgdorferi was the most susceptible in vitro to the macrolides erythromycin, azithromycin, clarithromycin, and roxithromycin (MIC, 0.01 to 0.17 μg/ml); the penicillins penicillin, amoxicillin, ampicillin, amoxicillin–clavulanic acid, mezlocillin, azlocillin, and oxacillin (MIC, 0.02 to 1.1 μg/ml); the second- and third-generation cephalosporins ceftriaxone, cefotaxime, cefuroxime, ceftizoxime, and cefixime (MIC, 0.02 to 0.8 μg/ml); and the tetracyclines doxycycline, minocycline, and tetracycline (MIC, <0.13 to 0.79 μg/ml). Isolates were also susceptible to imipenem (MIC, 0.12 μg/ml) and chloramphenicol (MIC, 2 μg/ml). The mean MIC (or MIC 50%) value for penicillin was 0.02 to 1.1 μg/ml, but the range was wide (up to 8 μg/ml). According to MIC values, the aminoglycosides, sulfonamides, metronida-

☐ **TABLE 11-1**
In Vitro and In Vivo Antimicrobial Susceptibilities of *Borrelia burgdorferi*

ANTIMICROBIAL AGENT	MEAN[a] (RANGE[b]) MIC (μg/ml)	MEAN[c] (RANGE[d]) MBC (μg/ml)	SUSCEP-TIBILITY[e] IN VITRO	CD_{50}[f] (mg/kg/day)	SUSCEP-TIBILITY IN VIVO
Penicillin	0.02–1.1(0.003–8)	1.08–8.7(0.1–50)	S-MS-R	>320->1975	R
Amoxicillin	<0.03–0.25(<0.03–1)	0.06–1.9(<0.03–3.2)	S	50	S
Ampicillin	<0.25–0.47(<0.25–1)		S		
Amox/clav[g]	0.12(0.12–5)		S	25	S
Mezlocillin	0.5(0.25–1)		S		
Oxacillin	0.5(0.25–2)		S		
Cefaclor	(23–128)	(64->256)	MS		
Cefadroxil	(11–128)	(32->128)	MS		
Cefalexin	(16–32)	(32->256)	MS		
Cefixime	0.8(0.8)	(0.8–1.6)	S		
Cefotaxime	<0.03–0.45(<0.03–1)	<0.03–0.17(<0.03–0.8)	S	50	S
Ceftizoxime	0.125(0.06–.5)	0.5(0.25–1)	S		
Ceftriaxone	0.02–0.06(0.006–1)	0.04–3.8(0.02–50)	S	50–240	S
Cefuroxime	(0.06–0.5)	(0.25–0.75)	S		
Doxycycline	0.125–1(0.1–2)	0.71–2(0.2–6.4)	S		
Minocycline	<0.13(<0.12–0.25)	2.3	S		
Tetracycline	0.14–0.79(0.01–2)	0.8–4(0.8–6)	S	50–287	S
Azithromycin	0.01–0.017(0.003–0.03)		S	8	S
Clarithromycin	0.01(0.003–0.06)	0.13(0.06–0.25)	S	>50	R
Erythromycin	0.03–0.15(0.007–1)	0.05–2.17(0.04–10)	S	400–2353	R
Roxithromycin	0.02–1.05(0.02–1.6)	1.1(0.02–1.6)	S	>50	R
Ciprofloxacin	1(0.25–4)	2–4(0.5–16)	MS		
Ofloxacin	2(0.5–8)	2(1–8)	MS		
Gentamicin	>16		R		
Amikacin	>32		R		
Chloramphenicol	2(1–3)		S		
Imipenem	0.12(0.06–1)		S		
Rifampin	>16		R		
Trimethoprim-sulfamethoxazole	>256		R		

[a]MIC = minimal inhibitory concentration (either mean MIC or MIC 50%).
[b]MIC Range, minimum and maximum MIC values reported.
[c]MBC = minimal bactericidal concentration (either mean MBC or MBC 50%).
[d]MBC Range, minimum and maximum MBC values reported.
[e]S = susceptible to antimicrobial agent; MS = moderately susceptible to antimicrobial agent; R = resistant to antimicrobial agent.
[f]CD_{50} = dose of antimicrobial agent required to cure 50% of infected animals in animal model.
[g]Amox/clav = amoxicillin-clavulanic acid.
Data obtained from references 50, 79, 174, 188, 189, 191, 192, 194–200, and 621.

zole, rifampin, and quinolones were not useful for *B. burgdorferi*. Although *B. burgdorferi* is resistant to co-trimoxazole in vitro, a minor synergistic decrease in the roxithromycin MIC from 0.031 to 0.015 μg/ml and a significant decrease in spirochetal motility were reported to occur in combination with co-trimoxazole.[199]

For the various antibiotics, the in vitro MIC efficacy and the in vivo CD_{50} efficacy were in agreement except for penicillin, erythromycin, clarithromycin, and roxithromycin. For erythromycin, clarithromycin, and roxithromycin, evaluation of the CD_{50} showed that despite excellent MIC values, they were poorly active in vivo in the animal models. For penicillin, the poor in vivo efficacy may be due to strains of *B. burgdorferi* with high MIC values.

B. burgdorferi is killed slowly even by antibiotics to which it is sensitive, and prolonged exposure of the spirochetes to the antibiotics is necessary to achieve adequate killing.[188, 192, 200] In one study,[188] the length of time required to kill 99% of *B. burgdorferi* exposed to twice the MIC of antibiotic ranged from 72 hours for ceftriaxone and cefuroxime to 96 hours for cefixime. In another study,[192] the length of time needed to kill 99% of *B. burgdorferi* was 72 hours for 0.1 μg/ml and 48 hours for 1.0 μg/ml of both penicillin and ceftriaxone, and 72 hours for 1.0 μg/ml of tetracycline. Low concentrations of tetracycline (0.1 and 1.0 μg/ml) allowed regrowth of organisms after prolonged incubation for 96 hours or longer, but no such regrowth occurred with low concentrations of penicillin or ceftriaxone, or higher concentrations of tetracycline (above 10 μg/ml). In one study,[200] some differences in the kinetics of killing of different *B. burgdorferi* strains by different antibiotics were found after 48 hours, but all strains were effectively killed by antibiotics to which they were susceptible after 72 hours.

Results of the animal model efficacy studies show better correlation for some antibiotics than others with clinical human patient results. For example, Steere and colleagues reported[201] that, of the oral antibiotics, tetracycline was most effective, penicillin was next most effective, and erythromycin was least effective for treatment of early Lyme disease. Clarithromycin[202] and azithromycin[193, 203] have been found to be equally or almost equally as efficacious as amoxicillin and doxycycline in the treatment of EM. Several factors, in addition to the MIC of the antibiotic, play a role in determining whether an antibiotic will be clinically effective in the elimination of *B. burgdorferi* infection; these include the duration of adequate serum, spinal fluid, intraocular, intrasynovial, and tissue antibiotic concentrations; the efficacy of the host immune response; and the potential sequestration of organisms in protected sites.

Interactions with the Immune System

B. burgdorferi infection triggers a sequence of immunologic and other cellular events that are involved in the local and systemic dissemination of the infection, the immunopathogenesis of the various manifestations of the infection, and the host elimination of the infection, as well as in the ability of the spirochete to evade host defenses.[148, 149, 151, 204–207] A discussion of the immunopathogenesis of Lyme borreliosis is provided in the section Pathology and Pathogenesis.

T LYMPHOCYTE REACTIVITY

B. burgdorferi antigen–triggered T cell activation occurs within a few days of the tick bite, develops before the B cell antibody response, rises during infection, is directed initially against the 41-kd flagellar and the 31-kd Osp A antigens, and is directed later against additional outer surface membrane proteins.[208, 209, 211, 212] *B. burgdorferi* spirochetes, Osp A, and Osp B have been reported to induce specific proliferation in T lymphocytes from Lyme disease patients[213, 214]; the response is predominantly due to CD4+ and CD8+ T lymphocytes,[214] and there is also a response due to CD56+ NK (natural killer) cells.[213] *B. burgdorferi*, Osp A, Osp B, and even Osp-containing membrane blebs have been found to possess nonspecific B lymphocyte proliferative activity.[215, 216] However, *B. burgdorferi*–induced nonspecific T lymphocyte or mononuclear cell proliferation has been found by some groups[217] and not by others.[213]

B. burgdorferi antigen–specific T lymphocyte reactivity, measured by the *B. burgdorferi*–specific lymphocyte proliferative assay, is long lasting, and may persist even in seronegative patients with Lyme borreliosis.[208, 214, 218, 219] The lymphoproliferative response may be greater in spinal fluid and synovial fluid than in peripheral blood in some patients with neurologic or arthritic manifestations of Lyme borreliosis.[214, 220, 221] There is *B. burgdorferi*–specific synovial fluid T lymphocyte production of Th1-type cytokines interferon-gamma (IFN-γ) and tumor necrosis factor-alpha (TNF-α).[393] There is peripheral blood and intrathecal *B. burgdorferi*–specific T lymphocyte production of the Th1-type cytokine IFN-γ, as well as specific B lymphocyte production of IgG antibody, all of which persist for several months after clinical recovery from treated neuroborreliosis.[214] After successful antibiotic therapy of Lyme disease, the reactivity may decrease somewhat but is usually still detectable if the most sensitive assay methods are used.[208–210, 212, 213, 231]

DEVELOPMENT OF SERUM ANTIBODY

The antibody response to *B. burgdorferi* infection begins to develop a few days after the tick bite, after the development of the T lymphocyte response,[211] and there are several studies of the temporal evolution of serum IgG and IgM antibody responses to the infection in North American[222, 226, 232] and European[227, 228] patients. *B. burgdorferi sensu stricto* is the only major genospecies causing Lyme disease in North America; all three of the major genospecies, *B. burgdorferi sensu stricto*, *B. garinii*, and *B. afzelii*, cause Lyme borreliosis in Europe, resulting in some differences between the antibody responses of North American and European patients. Because of these differences, distinct criteria for Western blot positivity for each of the three genospecies in European patient sera, and for *B. burgdorferi sensu stricto* in North American patient sera, have been recommended.[233, 234, 237, 238] In both North American and European patients, the initial polyvalent antibody response to *B. burgdorferi* infection is directed primarily against the 24-kd Osp C[223, 235, 239, 240] and the 41-kd flagellar antigen. The early response to the 39-kd antigen is more common in North American than European patients,[233, 237] and the late antibody response is more often directed primarily against the outer surface membrane proteins, that is, 31-kd Osp A and 34-kd Osp B, in North American than in European patients.[234, 237, 241, 242]

The *B. burgdorferi*–specific IgM response develops in 1 to 2 weeks, peaks at 2 to 8 weeks, and usually disappears after several months in uncomplicated treated patients but may persist in patients with disseminated rather than localized infection, patients with persistent infection, some with late chronic infection,[18, 222, 226, 240, 243] patients with initially delayed antibiotic therapy (even after clinical recovery),[226, 244] and some patients with promptly and successfully treated EM and neuroborreliosis.[226, 227, 233] Although comparisons of the temporal evolution of antibodies detectable by Western blots to individual *B. burgdorferi* antigens are often difficult because of lack of standardization of band and molecular weight nomenclature, a general pattern of progressive expansion of the antibody repertoire after infection emerges. There is general agreement that the initial specific IgM response is made to the 24-kd Osp C antigen and to the 41-kd flagellar antigen. Several investigators describe early development of IgM antibody and other antigens as well. After recovery, Western blot IgM antibody reactivity to several antigens declines after 1 month and usually disappears after several months. IgM reactivity to the 24-kd Osp C and 41-kd flagellin may persist,[226, 240, 247, 248] and is even still detectable in 38% of patients with successfully treated EM 1 year later[226]; IgM antibody to Osp C is detectable in 45% of patients with chronic arthritis for months to years, and in 20% of those with chronic neuroborreliosis.[240] However, in a follow-up study of resolved pediatric Lyme arthritis, only 5% had any IgM Western blot reactivity at a mean of 10 months after treatment, and this was only to the 41-kd flagellar antigen.[229] In very early infection, in both North American and European patients, IgM antibody to Osp A may be bound in immune complexes, and may be detectable only when these are dissociated.[246] The acute IgM response during EM in North American patients who progress to severe persistent Lyme disease includes the 83-kd and 34-kd antigens, and these responses persist into chronic disease.[222] In North American patients, the IgM Osp C antibody response is greatest in patients with EM and meningitis, early in the course of infection, and decreases to low levels in those who develop chronic neuroborreliosis.[240]

In North America, the CDC criteria for a positive IgM Western immunoblot are the presence of two of the following three bands in early disease: 24-kd Osp C, 39-kd Bmp A, and 41-kd Fla.[238] In Europe, proposed criteria for IgM Western blot positivity include the following: for *B. burgdorferi sensu stricto* IgM, at least one of 39, Osp C, and 17a or a strong 41; for *B. afzelii* IgM, at least one of 39, Osp C, and 17 or a strong 41; and for *B. garinii* IgM, at least one of 39 and Osp C or a strong 41.[237]

A delay in initial antibiotic therapy appears to be associated with increased dissemination, with development of higher polyvalent enzyme-linked immunosorbent assay (ELISA) titers and greater numbers of Western blot IgM bands, and with persistence of IgM positivity even after clinically successful treatment[226, 232, 244]; however, prompt antibiotic treatment of early Lyme disease appears to be associated with disappearance of IgM positivity within several months.[226, 229, 248] Longer disease duration is associated with a higher incidence of IgM seropositivity.[124] The IgM ELISA antibody is higher in neuritis and arthritis patients with early Lyme disease than in patients with only EM.[124] In late chronic Lyme borreliosis, such as arthritis, neuroborreliosis, and sometimes even in acrodermatitis chronica atrophicans, the specific IgM is often persistently positive by immunofluorescent assay (IFA), ELISA, or Western blot assays.[18, 209, 222, 223, 241, 242, 244, 249–252]

The *B. burgdorferi*–specific IgG response develops at 2 to 8 weeks, peaks at 4 to 6 months, and in uncomplicated treated patients, usually gradually declines and sometimes eventually disappears after several months, but it may persist for years in persistent infection, sometimes even after successful antibiotic therapy.[18, 222, 226–228] This response may be aborted by early antibiotic therapy.[226, 253] Delays in initial antibiotic therapy are associated with a higher incidence of dissemination, progression to later stages of infection, strongly positive IgG responses, higher polyvalent ELISA antibody titers, and increased numbers of IgG Western blot bands.[222, 226, 234, 235, 254] In one study, the number of Western blot bands reacting with serum IgG antibody decreased after successful treatment of pediatric Lyme arthritis, and no new ones appeared.[229] As is the case for IgM Western blot bands, direct comparison of IgG bands from different studies is not always possible. However, general patterns of the temporal evolution of the IgG antibody response to infection emerge. The initial IgG response

is made to the 41-kd flagellar and the 24-kd Osp C antigens; it progressively expands to include additional antigens, such as the 26-kd Osp F,[245] and eventually, within the first month after successful treatment, it includes many additional antigens.[211, 222, 223, 226, 235, 240, 245] In very early infection, in both European and North American patients, IgG antibody to Osp A is often present in immune complexes, but may be detectable only if these are dissociated.[246] In persistent infection, the IgG response expands over months to years.[211, 222, 255, 256] In late European Lyme borreliosis, IgG antibody is almost always directed toward the 41-kd flagellin, and the 58-kd and 83/100-kd antigens.[107, 108, 237, 247, 257] The progressive expansion of the IgG antibody response develops regardless of whether the late manifestations are arthritic, neurologic, or cardiac,[279] although the Western blot antibody patterns may differ with various late manifestations.[234, 237, 247, 257]

In North America, the CDC criteria for a positive IgG Western immunoblot are the presence of five of the ten most common bands after the first few weeks of disease.[238] The proposed criteria for IgG Western blot positivity in Europe can be seen in reference 237.

The development of IgM and IgG antibody to new antigens months to years after onset of infection suggests either the persistence of viable *B. burgdorferi* throughout the illness, or reinfection.[222, 226, 228] There are varying opinions regarding the significance of positive IgM antibody in Lyme disease of more than 1 month's duration, but there is agreement that a diagnosis of active Lyme disease should not be made on this basis alone.[24, 226–228, 233, 244, 254]

Patients with neuroborreliosis usually have higher polyvalent *B. burgdorferi* antibody in spinal fluid than in serum,[258, 259] and some may have spinal fluid antibody in the absence of serum antibody.[253, 260, 261] Patients with arthritis usually have higher polyvalent specific antibody in synovial fluid than in serum.[262]

Highly specific antibody capable of killing *B. burgdorferi* in culture and of passively protecting mice against experimental *B. burgdorferi* challenge develops during infection and quantitatively increases with increasing severity and duration of the infection.[230] In one study, the seroprotective and borreliacidal activity occurring in patient sera from late but not early Lyme borreliosis correlated with the presence of reactivity to Osp A and Osp B.[230] Borreliacidal antibody is seroprotective against the homologous strain, and sometimes against heterologous strains.[263]

INDUCTION OF OTHER ANTIBODIES

The *B. burgdorferi*–specific IgM antibody rise during infection is also associated with polyclonal B lymphocyte activation that peaks 3 to 6 weeks after onset of infection and corresponds to the time of maximal total and *B. burgdorferi*–specific IgM antibody.[243, 264] This B cell hyperactivity leads to the development of several antibodies that are not specific for *B. burgdorferi* and are directed against host tissues, such as rheumatoid factor,[211, 243, 264] antinuclear antibody,[211, 243] anti-cardiolipin antibody,[211, 243] antibody to fibronectin-binding protein,[255] antibody to neuronal axons,[151, 265] antibodies to myelin basic proteins,[266] and antibody to neurofilament proteins[266] and oligoclonal bands.[258, 267, 268] False-positive Venereal Disease Research Laboratory (VDRL) antibody,[211] cryoglobulins,[211, 243] and circulating immune complexes[211, 243, 264] are also found during this time. In patients with Lyme arthritis, the circulating immune complexes disappear from serum in 3 months but increase in synovial fluid; in patients with cardiac or neurologic involvement, the immune complexes persist in the serum.[262, 269]

Induced low levels of rheumatoid factor are detectable in 32% of Lyme patients by ELISA IgM and in 4% by latex agglutination assay.[264] Serum IgM antibodies to neuronal axons were found in all patients with neuroborreliosis in one study[151]; autoantibodies were found in the spinal fluid of 20% of patients with neuroborreliosis in another study.[266] B. burgdorferi–specific oligoclonal bands were found in the spinal fluid of 40 to 100% of patients with neuroborreliosis.[258, 267]

Anti–tick saliva antibody (ATSA) develops after a tick bite in response to the bolus of tick saliva injected, peaks at 3 to 5 weeks, persists for weeks to months, and subsequently decreases.[270] This antibody is a good biologic marker for tick exposure and may be useful in confirming tick exposure in seronegative patients with suspected Lyme borreliosis.

FAILURE TO DEVELOP SERUM ANTIBODY

Early antibiotic therapy may attenuate or eliminate the B. burgdorferi–specific antibody response.[18, 208, 209, 218, 225, 253, 273] Normally, B. burgdorferi antigen triggers B lymphocyte as well as T lymphocyte responses, but if antigen is removed by early antibiotic therapy, the antigen-dependent T cell stimulation of B cell maturation does not occur, and the mature antibody response does not develop.[253] Thus, if antibiotic therapy is given before the development of the mature IgG antibody response, this response may be aborted even though the infection may not be fully eradicated, and the patient may be seronegative. If antibiotic therapy is given after the development of the mature IgG response, the antibody response may eventually decrease, disappear, or persist, even after successful eradication of the infection.[274–277] The longer the Lyme disease persists before antibiotic therapy is begun, the more B. burgdorferi–specific antibody bands develop by Western blot assay.[208, 226, 244] Persistent B. burgdorferi infection may also occur in sequestered sites such as the central nervous system, inducing local CSF but not systemic antibody responses. Seronegative patients usually still have detectable T lymphocyte proliferative responses.[208, 218, 219, 234, 269, 277, 278] Seropositivity or seronegativity alone is not always a reliable indicator of cure.

Steere and colleagues[279] reported the incidence of true seronegative Lyme disease to be 4% in a large study of 180 patients with confirmed North American Lyme disease; they noted that all were EM history–positive, 75% had B. burgdorferi–specific T lymphocyte reactivity, and manifestations were usually neurologic or musculoskeletal. In seronegative patients, clinical manifestations were attenuated compared with those in seropositive patients; in seronegative patients with symptoms of significant arthritis, the term seronegative Lyme arthritis is contradictory, as the B. burgdorferi antibody response is considered to be involved in the pathogenesis of the arthritis, and these patients are unlikely to have Lyme disease.

In some patients, apparent seronegativity is due to testing by standard ELISA and Western blot assays, which detect free antibody, and specific antibody may be detected by using methods that dissociate immune complexed antibody.[278]

Failure to develop B. burgdorferi serum antibody in patients with confirmed Lyme borreliosis may be due to serologic testing done very early after onset of infection, during the spirochetemic phase, before the development of even a very early antibody response. Thirty-five to 100% of early Lyme borreliosis patients with B. burgdorferi detectable in plasma or serum by PCR were seronegative,[280, 281] and 53% of seronegative Lyme borreliosis patients had B. burgdorferi DNA detectable in serum by PCR, compared with none of the seropositive patients.[281]

DEVELOPMENT OF CEREBROSPINAL FLUID ANTIBODY

B. burgdorferi invasion of the central nervous system (CNS) occurs early in two thirds of patients with disseminated infection even in the absence of neurologic symptoms; this has been reported from both North America[282, 283] and Europe.[284] Patients who develop either acute or chronic neurologic involvement may have intrathecal production of specific IgG, IgM, or IgA antibodies to B. burgdorferi demonstrable by IFA, ELISA (standard, antibody capture, or immune-complex ELISA), or Western blot assay.*

Intrathecal production of B. burgdorferi–specific antibody confirms neuroborreliosis. Patients with late neuroborreliosis may be seronegative and still have intrathecal specific antibody production, presumably because oral antibiotic therapy eradicates the majority of organisms systemically, but it may fail to achieve adequate MICs in the CSF, thus allowing persistence of the organism in this privileged site.[253] Some patients with early neuroborreliosis may also have specific intrathecal antibody production, as has been observed with B. burgdorferi IgM antibody, without seropositivity.[253, 260, 261] Early in CNS invasion, B. burgdorferi–specific CSF antibody may be located in immune complexes, which are not detected by free antibody assays.[283]

There are some differences in intrathecal B. burgdorferi antibody between North American and European patients.[259, 290, 293] Polyclonal intrathecal B. burgdorferi–specific antibody was found in almost all North American patients with early Lyme meningitis, and in almost half of those with late central nervous system borreliosis, but not in those with late peripheral nervous system borreliosis. Polyclonal intrathecal B. burgdorferi–specific antibody was found in almost all European patients with either early or late neuroborreliosis. In one study of North American Lyme disease,[292] there was intrathecal

*See references 211, 253, 259, 260, 265, 267, 268, 283, and 285–292.

B. burgdorferi–specific ELISA IgM in 100% and IgG in 40% of patients with meningitis, as well as ELISA IgM and IgG in 26 to 30% of patients with encephalitis; in another study of North American early and late neuroborreliosis, intrathecal free antibody detectable by ELISA was found in 48% and specific immune complex–associated IgG and IgM antibody in 43%.[283]

B. burgdorferi–specific CSF antibody was directed primarily against the 41-kd flagellar antigen, and also against the 33-kd Osp A and 17-kd antigens.[258, 260, 283, 293] CSF ELISA antibody levels were higher than serum antibody levels,[259] but IFA antibody levels were higher in serum than in CSF.

INTERACTIONS WITH COMPLEMENT

B. burgdorferi activates the alternate and classic complement pathways but is resistant to the nonspecific bactericidal activity of normal human serum. However, in the presence of *B. burgdorferi* immune serum, it is sensitive to serum and is killed via the classic pathway.[96] Host-specific differential transmission of different *B. burgdorferi sensu lato* genospecies by ticks has been found to correlate with the differential susceptibility of the genospecies to bacteriolysis by serum complement, including via the alternate pathway, of the different host species.[294]

INTERACTIONS WITH PHAGOCYTES

Peripheral blood polymorphonuclear and mononuclear phagocytes and macrophages are able to phagocytose opsonized and nonopsonized *B. burgdorferi*.[295, 296] *B. burgdorferi* binds to polymorphonuclear phagocytes via integrin $\alpha_m\beta_2$, the CR3 complement receptor, during nonimmune phagocytosis.

B. burgdorferi stimulates human endothelial cells to express the neutrophil adhesion molecule, E-selectin, and the neutrophil chemotactic agent, interleukin-8 (IL-8), both of which are probably involved in recruitment of neutrophils to sites of *B. burgdorferi*–induced inflammation, and in transmigration of neutrophils across the endothelium.[150, 297] Whole *B. burgdorferi* spirochetes were demonstrated to be strong inducers, equivalent to or more potent than lipopolysaccharide (LPS), of chemoattractant cytokine production by human monocytes, including MIP-1α (macrophage inflammatory protein-1α), MCP-1 (monocyte chemotactic protein-1), and RANTES (regulated upon activation, normal T cell expressed and secreted), which attract monocytes and lymphocytes, and IL-8 (interleukin-8) and GRO-α (melanoma growth–stimulatory activity), which attract neutrophils and contribute to tissue inflammation and damage.[298]

Recombinant lipidated, but not unlipidated, *B. burgdorferi* Osp A, even in minute amounts, is a potent human neutrophil activator that induces neutrophil responses similar to those induced by bacterial LPS. Neutrophils are the main cell type in Lyme arthritic joints; they are involved both in maintaining an inflammatory response and in the destruction of opsonized *B. burgdorferi*, presumably via a combination of reactive oxygen intermediates and lysosomal products, including the proteolytic enzyme elastase.[299] Elastase has been demonstrated to be the main borreliacidal factor in human neutrophils.[300]

A possible additional mechanism by which the spirochete might evade borreliacidal antibody and temporarily persist in a protected niche is by invasion and killing of both B and T lymphocytes.[179]

EVASION OF HOST DEFENSES AND PERSISTENCE IN TISSUE

B. burgdorferi has the unusual, but fortunately uncommon, ability to evade the host immune response and persist in tissues for months to years, sometimes even after antibiotic therapy, and sometimes even after intravenous antibiotic therapy.* When it occurs, this persistence is usually either in immunologically privileged sites inaccessible to host defenses, after local or systemic steroid therapy, after initially delayed or inadequate antibiotic therapy, or in patients with risk factors such as HLA-DR4 specificity, and may occur in the presence or absence of seropositivity.[306, 307]

B. burgdorferi has been isolated, months to several years after oral or intravenous (IV) antibiotic therapy, from CSF[284, 302]; synovial fluid[200]; EM skin lesions[83, 200, 302, 303]; mitral valve tissue[200]; ligamentous tissue[304]; and iris biopsy tissue.[284] It has also been isolated, 1 month to 10 years after onset, without preceding antibiotic therapy, from CSF[302]; synovial fluid[301]; EM skin biopsy[305–307]; ACA skin lesions[19, 20]; and myocardium.[308] Its presence has been demonstrated, months to 27 years after antibiotic therapy, by *B. burgdorferi*–specific PCR or antigen capture ELISA in CSF[269, 283, 287, 309–311]; brain[311]; synovial fluid and membrane[312–314]; ACA skin biopsy[315]; and serum, blood, plasma, and bone marrow.[281, 311] Persistence for 1 month to 10 years without antibiotic therapy has also been demonstrated by PCR or antigen-detection methods in CSF and ACA skin biopsy.[143, 316, 317] The development of *B. burgdorferi*–specific IgM antibody responses to new spirochetal antigens late in the course of Lyme disease also indicates long-term persistence of live organisms in these patients.[222]

Differential gene expression of *B. burgdorferi* antigens, which results in variation in antigenicity of the spirochete during different stages of infection, is thought to be involved in evasion of the immune response.[120, 137, 142]

It has been proposed that the spirochete may be able to evade the host immune response while still inducing the inflammatory pathology characteristic of the various manifestations of Lyme disease. Differential expression of surface lipoproteins during various stages of infection allows the spirochete to vary its antigenicity[120, 130, 131, 135–137, 141, 142] while maintaining its ability to activate cells because the lipid moiety of the lipoproteins is responsible for cell activation.[147]

The use of the host's own fibrinolytic enzymes for invasion, while eliciting minimal immunologic response by the host, is an immunologically silent method of invasion called "stealth pathogenesis,"[144] which may ex-

---

*See references 19, 20, 206, 269, 281, 283, 284, 287, 302–308, and 311–318.

plain the long-term persistence of *B. burgdorferi* in host tissues with only minimal mononuclear cell infiltration. *B. burgdorferi* invasion of epidermal dendritic Langerhans' cells induces downregulation of major histocompatibility class II (MHC II) molecules on this major antigen-presenting cell, and may result in inability of Langerhans' cells to eliminate the spirochete and long-term *B. burgdorferi* persistence in the skin.[148]

The immunosuppressive and immunomodulatory properties of *B. burgdorferi* may also be involved in its ability to evade the host immune response. The addition of *B. burgdorferi* to lymphocyte proliferative assays reduces the proliferative responses of human peripheral blood lymphocytes to concanavalin A and phytohemagglutinin. It has been proposed that this immunosuppressive effect may allow the spirochete to rapidly disseminate from the skin inoculation site and persist in the host; it could also explain the better efficacy of prompt antibiotic therapy in elimination of the spirochete.[217]

Another mechanism by which the spirochete might evade borreliacidal antibody is by entering a protected niche such as an intracellular or other environment that is inaccessible to either a borreliacidal immune response or antibiotic therapy. Proposed potential sites for such persistence include the central nervous system, the eye, and the joints.[179, 320, 321] Temporarily, persistence in a protected niche occurs by invasion of B and T lymphocytes. *B. burgdorferi* persistence in ligamentous tissue, the iris, synovium, and the central nervous system may also represent the use of a protected niche.

Several antigens of *B. burgdorferi* have portions that share amino acid homology with human cellular proteins; molecular mimicry may also be involved in immune evasion.[113, 126, 151, 204, 205, 256, 265, 323]

CORRELATION OF CLINICAL MANIFESTATIONS WITH HLA TYPE

Differences in HLA specificities may determine *B. burgdorferi* antigen binding and presentation to T cells and the composition of the T cell response, and may be related to susceptibility to infection.[256]

Several studies by Steere and colleagues and others reported that HLA-DR4 specificity and Osp A or Osp B IgG seropositivity are associated with chronic antibiotic-resistant Lyme arthritis but not with EM or acute or chronic neuroborreliosis.[256, 312, 324, 325] Long-duration chronic Lyme arthritis patients had high frequencies of HLA-DR4 or -DR2 positivity (89%) compared with those with short-duration Lyme arthritis (27%), and HLA-DR4 positivity but not -DR2 positivity correlated with lack of response to antibiotic therapy.

Correlation of HLA specificity with outcome of antibiotic therapy of Lyme arthritis is discussed in the section Therapy: Predictors of Antibiotic Therapy Cure.

EPIDEMIOLOGY AND TRANSMISSION

World Wide Web sites for the Centers for Disease Control and Prevention (CDC), http://www.cdc.gov/ ncidod/dvbid/lymegen.htm, and the European Union Concerted Action of Risk Assessment in Lyme Borreliosis (EUCALB), http://www.dis.strath.ac.uk/vie/LymeEU,[326] have updated Lyme borreliosis epidemiologic and clinical information.

Historical Review

In 1909, Afzelius described a migrating annular skin lesion in a Swedish woman at the site of an *Ixodes ricinus* sheep tick bite, called it erythema chronicum migrans (ECM), and proposed that it was a zoonosis transmitted by a tick from an animal reservoir to humans.[14, 17] ECM became a well-recognized European disease thought initially to be caused by either a tick-associated toxin or an infectious agent.[17]

Another European disease, acrodermatitis chronica atrophicans (ACA), which had first been described by Buchwald in 1883 in Germany,[327] was noted to be preceded frequently by ECM and was named ACA Herxheimer by Herxheimer and Hartman in 1902. In 1922, Garin and Boujadoux described cutaneous lesions and paralysis after a tick bite and suspected a spirochetal etiology,[328] and in 1944, Bannwarth described chronic lymphocytic meningitis after European ECM; this became known as Garin-Boujadoux-Bannwarth syndrome, or simply Bannwarth's syndrome.[17, 329]

In 1948, Lennhoff reported spirochetes in ECM skin biopsy specimens,[17, 330] but this finding could not be confirmed by others and was essentially forgotten. By 1949, there were suggestions in Europe that penicillin therapy was beneficial in ECM,[17, 331] and between 1948 and 1957, Hollstrom found that most European ECM cleared within 2 weeks after intramuscular penicillin therapy.[79, 331] In 1949, Thyresson successfully treated patients with ACA with penicillin, and in 1952, Gruneberg considered spirochetes as possible etiologic agents.[20]

In 1955, Binder and associates, in Europe, transplanted skin biopsy specimens from the rim of an ECM lesion from a patient to three scientist-volunteers who then developed ECM lesions within 3 weeks. They established that ECM was caused by a penicillin-susceptible infectious agent transmitted by the *Ixodes ricinus* tick.[17] In 1955, Gotz transmitted ACA from patient to patient by transplantation of ACA skin biopsy specimens[20] and thus confirmed ACA as an infectious disease. Both ECM and ACA became well-known European skin diseases.

The first report in the medical literature of North American erythema migrans (EM), as ECM was eventually called, was from Wisconsin in 1970 by Scrimenti,[333] although retrospective studies have found that it existed in small foci in New England as early as 1962 and 1965.[334, 335]

The recognition of Lyme arthritis as a distinct disease came in 1975, when two mothers from the small village of Old Lyme, Connecticut, brought the existence of an epidemic of children diagnosed as having juvenile rheumatoid arthritis to the attention of the state health department and the Yale Rheumatology Clinic. Steere and colleagues investigated and recognized an outbreak of infectious arthritis, noted that many patients had an unusual rash similar to European EM, proposed that transmission occurred via an arthropod vector, and named the disease Lyme arthritis.[15] By 1980, it became known as Lyme disease because meningoencephalitis and myocarditis were also recognized as part of the disease.

In 1980, Steere and co-workers[339] found that penicillin or tetracycline therapy shortened the duration of EM and reduced the severity and frequency of subsequent arthritis. They concluded that antibiotic therapy was useful and that the disease was caused by a penicillin-sensitive bacterium such as a spirochete.

In 1981, a new spirochete was accidentally discovered by Burgdorfer in *I. dammini* ticks (now renamed *I. scapularis*) collected for a rickettsial study from Shelter Island, New York, a highly Lyme-endemic focus.[1, 17] It induced EM lesions in rabbits, and convalescent sera from Lyme patients reacted with it.[1, 17] In 1983, two groups of investigators, Steere and associates[18] and Benach and colleagues,[80] isolated the same spirochete from patients with Lyme disease, found specific antibody titers against this spirochete in convalescent sera of Lyme disease patients, and concluded that the *I. dammini* spirochete was the etiologic agent of Lyme disease. In 1984, it was named *B. burgdorferi* when it was confirmed to be a new species.[16]

In 1983, Barbour, Burgdorfer, and co-workers isolated a spirochete similar to the *I. dammini* spirochete from *Ixodes ricinus* ticks[81]; it was indistinguishable from *B. burgdorferi* and was also confirmed to be the etiologic agent of European ECM,[19] European ACA,[19, 20] European Bannwarth's syndrome,[21, 302] and European borrelial lymphocytoma.[22]

The recent application of new molecular biologic techniques such as the polymerase chain reaction (PCR) to the historical study of *B. burgdorferi* in museum specimens of ticks and animals has made it possible to retrospectively document its presence in Europe in museum tick specimens as early as 1882 to 1897,[340] and in North America in museum mouse specimens as early as 1894. This dates the presence of the spirochete in Europe to the times of the earliest clinical descriptions of Lyme borreliosis.

The first case of congenitally transmitted Lyme borreliosis was described by Schlesinger and associates in 1985 after gestational Lyme disease acquired in Wisconsin.[25] Since then, several additional cases have been reported, and it has become clear that gestational Lyme borreliosis carries a low but serious risk of congenital infection.

Tick (and Other Arthropod) Vectors

Epidemiologic studies have indicated that Lyme borreliosis is caused by *B. burgdorferi sensu lato* transmitted from animals to humans by ixodid ticks that are members of the *Ixodes ricinus* complex,[167, 336] and that this transmission occurs during tick feeding because of either tick salivation or regurgitation of organisms.[341, 342] Ticks that are members of the *I. ricinus* complex and have been associated with human Lyme borreliosis transmission are

the deer tick *Ixodes dammini/scapularis* in the northeastern and upper midwestern United States,[335, 337] the black-legged tick *Ixodes pacificus* in the western United States,[2, 180, 335, 337, 343] the sheep tick *Ixodes ricinus* in Europe,[11, 81] and the *Ixodes persulcatus* tick in Asia.[163, 344] Other ticks that are not members of the *I. ricinus* complex are also associated with enzootic *B. burgdorferi* cycles, but either are not or are rarely involved in human Lyme borreliosis transmission and may be involved in bridging between separate enzootic cycles.[13] (In this chapter, the name *I. scapularis* is used to indicate both northern and southern ticks.[346, 348])

B. burgdorferi is often found in nymphal and adult stages of *Ixodes scapularis*, *pacificus*, *ricinus*, and *persulcatus*, but rarely in unfed larvae, because infection is acquired by larvae feeding on *B. burgdorferi*–infected animal reservoirs, is passed transstadially (between stages) from larvae to nymphs to adults, and is rarely passed transovarially from infected female ticks to less than 1% of eggs and larvae.[18, 154, 167, 182, 352–356] However, because occasional female ticks may produce progeny with high infection rates, rare transovarial transmission may be important for establishment of new endemic foci of Lyme disease in instances in which an infected tick is transported by birds or other methods into a new, previously nonendemic area. Partially fed larval ticks (in which feeding on infected hosts was interrupted) are able to transmit *B. burgdorferi* during refeeding, which may explain some larval positivity.[357]

In North America, most Lyme disease transmission is due to northern *I. scapularis*[348] and *I. pacificus* tick vectors,[180, 348] which frequently bite humans, but several other species of ticks have been thought to be vectors in some geographic areas, particularly in areas where northern *I. scapularis* and *I. pacificus* are not prevalent[348]; the southern *I. scapularis* has been considered a Lyme disease vector in parts of the southern United States.[358–361] In the western United States, *I. neotomae* and *Ixodes spinipalpus* are involved in *B. burgdorferi* enzootic cycles, and *I. pacificus* serves as a bridge vector to man[361]; in the eastern United States, *I. dentatus* and *Ixodes minor* are also involved in *B. burgdorferi* enzootic cycles, and *I. scapularis* may be involved as a bridge vector.[361] Although infrequent, human bites have been documented for *I. spinipalpus*[362] and *I. dentatus*,[70, 363] and for two other ticks that are not members of the subgenus *Ixodes*—*Ixodes angustus*[364] and *Ixodes cookei*[363]; rare cases of possible EM have been reported after human bites by *I. angustus* in Washington state[364] and *I. cookei* in West Virginia.[363]

Other ticks in North America commonly biting humans are the dog tick *Dermacentor variabilis*, and the Pacific Coast tick *Dermacentor occidentalis*[348, 365]; *D. variabilis* in Kentucky[366] has been considered a possible secondary human Lyme disease vector. The Lone Star tick *Amblyomma americanum*, which is the most common tick biting humans in the southeastern and south central United States,[367] has been considered a potentially important alternate human vector in New Jersey,[155] southeastern Missouri,[153, 367, 368] North and South Carolina,[359, 360] Kentucky,[366] Alabama,[156] and Texas.[369] *B. burgdorferi sensu lato*[153] and *Borrelia lonestari*,[73] a noncultivable *Borrelia* possibly related to Lyme-like disease in the South, have been found in *A. americanum. H. leporispalustri* and *Dermacentor parumapertus* rarely bite humans.[336] There have been occasional reports of suspected Lyme borreliosis transmission by other hematophagous arthropods such as mosquitoes[370] and tabanid flies (deer and horseflies) in North America and Europe.[371, 372] Figure 11–4 shows different stages of three common North American ticks: *I. scapularis, A. americanum,* and *D. variabilis.*

In South America, the *Ixodes affinis* and *Ixodes pararicinus* ticks from Peru are also members of the *Ixodes ricinus* complex and are considered potential vectors of *B. burgdorferi.*[373] In Asia, although the *Ixodes ovatus* tick in Japan frequently bites humans and has been found to harbor *B. japonica,* this has not been found to be associated with human Lyme borreliosis.[163, 374] The *Ixodes holo-*

cyclus tick in Australia is the tick most often biting humans, but it has not been found to harbor *B. burgdorferi.*[375]

In addition to *Ixodes scapularis, pacificus, ricinus,* and *persulcatus* ticks,[336] *B. burgdorferi* has been isolated from ticks of other *Ixodes* species and of four additional genera (Table 11–2).

For a tick to be vector-competent for *B. burgdorferi,* it must be able to become and remain infected, pass the infection transstadially, and transmit the infection to a host. *Ixodes scapularis, pacificus, ricinus, persulcatus, dentatus, neotomae,* and *hexagonus* are efficient and competent *B. burgdorferi* vectors,[170, 336, 355, 357, 365, 378, 390] and *I. uriae,*[165, 166] and *I. spinipalpus*[362] are probably efficient and competent vectors.

It has been recognized that there are significant differ-

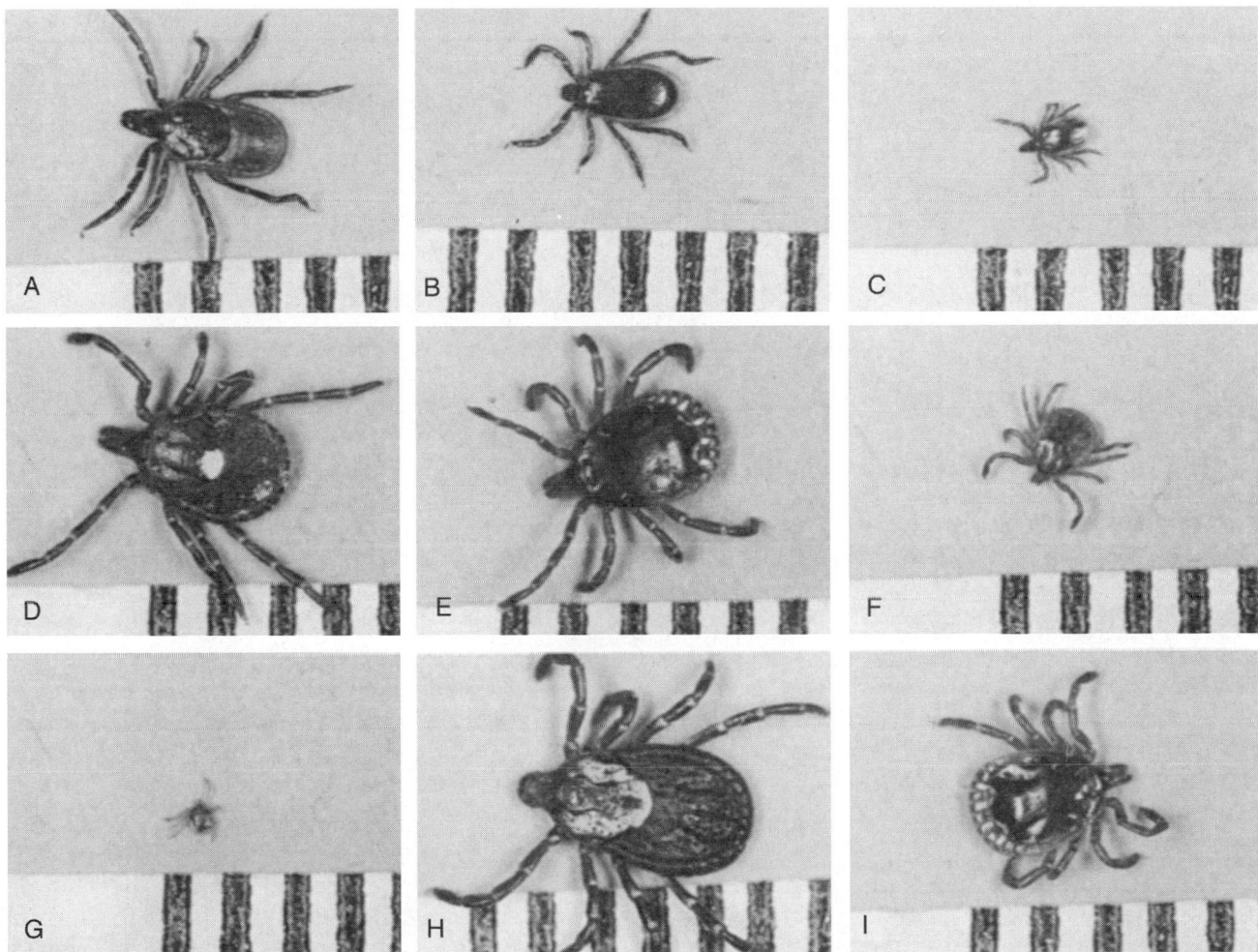

FIGURE 11–4 Common species of ticks. *Ixodes ricinus* complex ticks are vectors of transmission of the Lyme disease spirochete, *Borrelia burgdorferi,* to humans. *A, Ixodes dammini/scapularis* (northern species) adult female. *B,* Adult male. *C,* Nymph. The North American deer tick *Ixodes dammini* (the same species as the black-legged tick *Ixodes scapularis*) is the vector in the northeastern and north central, and possibly in southeastern and south central, United States. Other *Ixodes* ticks are similar in appearance, such as the western black-legged tick *Ixodes pacificus* (the vector in the northwestern United States), the European wood or sheep tick *Ixodes ricinus* (the vector in Europe), and the taiga tick *Ixodes persulcatus* (the vector in Eurasia). Some non-*Ixodes* ticks have been suspected but not proved to be associated with transmission of the Lyme disease spirochete to humans. *(D) Amblyomma americanum* adult female, *(E)* adult male, *(F)* nymph, and *(G)* larva. The Lone Star tick *A. americanum* may be a vector in the southeastern and south central United States. *H, Dermacentor variabilis* adult female. *I,* Adult male. The American dog tick *Dermacentor variabilis* and the Rocky Mountain wood tick *Dermacentor andersoni* may be occasional vectors and are similar in appearance.

TABLE 11–2
Arthropod Species in Which *Borrelia burgdorferi sensu lato* Has Been Confirmed

SPECIES	GEOGRAPHIC LOCATION	COMMON NAME	Bb SENSU LATO GENOSPECIES ISOLATED	VECTOR COMPETENCE FOR B. BURGDORFERI
Ixodes scapularis	N. America	Deer tick	*B.b.s.s., B. andersonii B. bissettii*	Efficient
Ixodes pacificus	N. America	Western black-legged tick	*B.b.s.s., B. andersonii, B. bissettii*	Efficient
Ixodes ricinus	Europe	Sheep tick	*B. garinii, B. afzelii, B.b.s.s., B. valaisiana, B. lusitaniae*	Efficient
Ixodes persulcatus	Asia	Taiga tick	*B. garinii, B. afzelii, B. valaisiana, B. lusitaniae, B. miyamotoi*	Efficient
Ixodes dentatus	N. America	Rabbit tick	*B.b.s.l., B. andersonii*	Efficient
Ixodes neotomae	N. America	Woodrat tick	*B.b. B. bissettii, B.b.s.l.*	Efficient
Ixodes angustus	N. America		*B.b.*	
Ixodes cookei	N. America		*B.b.*	Poor
Ixodes spinipalpis	N. America	Mexican woodrat tick	*B.b.*	Efficient
Ixodes hexagonus	Europe	Hedgehog and fox tick	*B.b.s.l.*	Efficient
Ixodes canisuga	Europe	Fox tick	*B.b.s.l.*	?
Ixodes frontalis	Europe	Bird tick	*B.b.s.l.*	?
Ixodes ovatus	Asia	Oriental and Palearctic tick	*B. japonica*	?
Ixodes granulatus	Asia		*B.b.*	?
Ixodes uriae	Subarctic and subantarctic islands	Seabird tick	*B. garinii*	Efficient
Ixodes rangtangensis	Asia		*B.b.*	?
Ixodes columnae	Asia		*B.b.* Am501	?
Ixodes tanuki	Asia		*B. tanukii*	
Ixodes turdus	Asia		*B. turdae*	
Amblyomma americanum	N. America	Lone Star tick	*B.b.s.s., B.b.s.l., B. lonestarii*	Poor
Amblyomma maculatum	N. America	Gulf Coast tick	*B.b.*	?
Dermacentor variabilis	N. America	Dog tick	*B.b.*	Poor
Dermacentor albipictus	N. America		*B.b.*	
Dermacentor occidentalis	N. America	Pacific Coast tick	*B.b.*	Poor
Dermacentor parumapertus	N. America	Rabbit tick	*B.b.*	?
Dermacentor marginatus	Europe		*B.b.*	?
Rhipicephalus sanguineus	N. America	Dog tick	*B.b.*	?
Haemaphysalis leporispalustris	N. America	Rabbit tick	*B.b.*	?
Haemaphysalis punctata	Europe		*B.b.*	?
Haemaphysalis concinna	Asia		*B.b.s.l.*	?
Haemaphysalis bispinosa	Asia		*B.b.s.l.*	?
Haemaphysalis longicornis	Asia		*B.b.s.l.*	?
Ctenocephalides felis	N. America	Cat flea	*B.b.*	?
Chrysops and *Hybomitra* spp.	N. America	Tabanid (Deer and horse) flies	*B.b.*	Poor
Aedes spp. and *Culex* spp.	N. America, Europe	Mosquitoes	*B.b.*	Poor

Data obtained from references 53, 59, 61, 64–70, 73, 74, 77, 100, 153–158, 163–166, 170, 180, 336, 344, 350, 351, 355, 362, 365, 376–381, 382–389, 405, 412, 420, 438, 449, 621, 878, 884, and additional references noted in text.

ences in vector competence of *I. scapularis* and *I. ricinus* for different genospecies of *B. burgdorferi*, and even for different strains within the same genospecies,[878] which may be related to differential susceptibility to bacteriolysis of various *B. burgdorferi* genospecies by complement of different host species.[294]

In North America, *I. scapularis* has also been reported to be the vector of the agent of human babesiosis, *Babesia microti*,[394] and of the agent of human granulocytic ehrlichiosis (HGE) (which is closely related to *Ehrlichia equi/phagocytophila*)[395–398]; presumably, *I. pacificus* in the western United States[398] and *I. ricinus* in Europe[398–400] act in the same capacity. In North America, *Amblyomma americanum* is the vector of the agent of human monocytic ehrlichiosis (HME), *Ehrlichia chaffeensis* (initially incorrectly reported as *Ehrlichia canis*), and has also been considered a possible secondary vector of *B. burgdorferi*; the European vector of HME is not known. The vector of the *Babesia* species piroplasm WA1, which causes human infection in California, is not known.[401] Co-infections of ticks with *B. burgdorferi* and *Ehrlichia* or *Babesia* have been reported.

Enzootic Cycles: Tick Vector Life Cycles and Reservoir Animal Hosts

The *Ixodes ricinus* complex ticks are all three-host ticks with a 2- to 3-year life cycle, and each of the three stages of the tick feeds once (Table 11–3): Larvae feed on small rodents, reptiles, and birds; nymphs feed on small or medium-sized mammals; and adults feed on large mammals.* Eggs laid by infected adult female ticks usually hatch into uninfected larvae, as the rate of transovarial transmission of the spirochete is very low,[352–356] and larvae acquire the spirochete by feeding on *B. burgdorferi* spirochetemic–competent reservoir hosts. The infection is maintained in the larvae through the transstadial molt and is passed from the larval to the nymphal stage. The infected nymphs transmit the infection to reservoir-competent hosts by feeding, maintain the infection through the transstadial molt, and pass it to the

*See references 138, 167, 168, 182, 336, 346, 347, 390, 407, and 408.

adult stage of the tick, which then mates while feeding on a large mammalian host. The prevalence of *B. burgdorferi* infection in a tick population is determined by the frequency of feeding of larvae and nymphs on infected reservoir-competent hosts. The infection rate in adult ticks is higher than in nymphal ticks.[161, 396, 409, 410] Larval ticks have been found to acquire *B. burgdorferi* even after only partial feeding.[357]

For *B. burgdorferi* infection to be maintained in nature, there must be horizontal transmission of infection from infected nymphs to a competent reservoir host to larvae, which requires that nymphs feed before larvae on the same reservoir-competent host.[347] The white-footed mouse, *Peromyscus leucopus*, and other *Peromyscus* species mice are reservoir-competent for *B. burgdorferi*, are easily infected by a single infected tick bite, develop persistent spirochetemia, are able to infect feeding ticks, and are almost universally infected in endemic areas.[411] Humans are accidental hosts of all stages of *I. scapularis* and *I. ricinus*, and of the adult ticks of *I. pacificus*, *I. persulcatus*, and *I. ovatus*. Some animal hosts of *I. ricinus* complex ticks, such as North American catbirds, western fence lizards, and European blackbirds, have a zooprophylactic effect, and decrease the force of *B. burgdorferi* transmission by eliminating infectious spirochetes within feeding ticks, thus removing these ticks from the enzootic cycle.[173]

The life cycle of *I. scapularis* has been the most extensively studied.[138, 154, 167, 168, 182, 390, 407, 408] Eggs laid on the ground in the spring hatch into larvae in mid- to late summer. In late summer, July and August, larvae become

TABLE 11–3
Preferred Hosts for Different Stages of *Ixodes ricinus* Complex Ticks That Transmit Lyme Borreliosis to Humans[a, b]

TICK	LARVAL AND NYMPHAL STAGES	ADULT STAGE	TOTAL NO. HOSTS			
			Mammal	Bird	Reptile	All
I. scapularis						
(northern U.S.)	White-footed mouse, *Peromyscus leucopus*	White-tailed deer, *Odocoileus virginianus*	31	49	0	80
(southern U.S.)	Lizards and skinks Cotton mouse, *Peromyscus gossypinus* Cotton rat, *Sigmodon hispidus*	White-tailed deer, *Odocoileus virginianus* Black-tailed deer, *Odocoileus hemionus columbianus*	39	11	6	53
I. pacificus	Fence lizard, *Sceloporus occidentalis*	Black-tailed deer, *Odocoileus hemionus columbianus*, cattle, horses, bears	54	19	7	80
I. ricinus	Woodmouse, *Apodemus sylvaticus*, and Yellow-necked mouse, *Apodemus flavicolus* Bank vole, *Clethrionomys glareolus* Black rat, *Rattus rattus*, and Norway rat, *Rattus norvegicus*	Deer, *Capreolus capreolus* Deer, canids, cattle, hares, sheep	91	132	14	237
I. persulcatus	Woodmouse, *Apodemus speciosus* Red-backed vole, *Clethrionomys rutilus* Black-faced bunting, *Emberiza spodocephala* Red-bellied thrush, *Turdus chrysolaus*	Deer, canids, cattle, hares	89	121	2	212

[a]Data from references 163, 164, 167–169, 182, 336, 348, 378, 413, and 419–421.
[b]Humans are incidental hosts of all stages of the ticks.

infected with *B. burgdorferi* by feeding for 3 to 5 days on small rodents such as the white-footed mouse, which are amplifying reservoirs for *B. burgdorferi* infection; the fed larvae then fall to the ground. The infection persists in the larvae throughout the winter and through the transstadial molt the following spring into the nymphal stage. The nymphs are voracious and feed in the spring and early summer (May, June, and early July) for 4 to 7 days on a variety of hosts, including small rodents such as the white-footed mouse, birds, wild and domestic animals, and occasionally, humans; the fed nymphs fall to the ground. Because transovarial passage of *B. burgdorferi* infection is rare, horizontal transmission is necessary to maintain the tick infection, and it occurs because infected nymphs feed earlier in the season on the same hosts as the larvae and infect the hosts, which then infect the larvae. The nymphs molt into adults by late summer or fall, and the spirochete is passed transstadially to the adult form. The adults quest for vegetation, especially at edges between lawns and forests,[336] and for medium-sized to large mammalian hosts, such as white-tailed deer, in the fall (mid-October through November), warm days in winter, and the following spring (April and early May); they mate while the females are feeding on these hosts. Questing adult field-collected infected ticks contain a median of 1500 to 1900 spirochetes per tick.[412] Because tick mating occurs on these large mammalian hosts, particularly deer, these hosts are needed for tick survival but not for maintenance of the *B. burgdorferi* infection.[411] The females then feed for 8 to 11 days, fall to the ground, lay eggs in the spring, and die; the eggs hatch in 45 to 53 days into larvae in the summer. The prevalence of *B. burgdorferi* infection increases from the nymphal to the adult stage because the ticks feed on amplifying reservoir-competent hosts.

In northeastern and upper midwestern North America, the preferred small rodent host of *I. scapularis* is the white-footed mouse, *Peromyscus leucopus*, which is also the primary reservoir of *B. burgdorferi* infection in nature,[167, 182, 346, 411] and the preferred large mammal host is the white-tailed deer, *Odocoileus virginianus*, which is the host of the reproductive stage of the tick[346, 408]; however, larvae and nymphs have been found attached to 80 different species of mammals and birds, but not reptiles, and adult ticks to 13 species of medium-sized to large mammals.[167, 168, 336, 337, 413] The mice remain chronically spirochetemic but asymptomatic. The deer are occasionally spirochetemic with *B. burgdorferi* but are also asymptomatic.[169, 407, 408, 413] The deer are responsible for the geographic expansion of Lyme-endemic areas because the infected *I. scapularis* adult females overwinter and mate on the deer, and the deer travel widely but are not considered reservoirs for *B. burgdorferi* maintenance in nature. The geographic distribution of North American Lyme disease and *I. scapularis* correlates with that of the white-tailed deer.[408]

Other reservoir-competent small mammal hosts may be involved in the maintenance of *B. burgdorferi* infection in nature[182] in certain geographic areas, or at times in which the population of the usual reservoir host, the white-footed mouse, is low or absent. The deer mouse, *Peromyscus maniculatus*, has been shown to be a compe-

tent reservoir host for *I. scapularis* on an offshore island in Maine with no resident *P. leucopus*, and may also be an important alternate reservoir host in the northern forests of Maine.[414] The eastern chipmunk, *Tamias striatus*, is an important reservoir-competent alternate host for immature *I. scapularis*, which can feed on either mice or chipmunks in hardwood forests of the Upper Midwest, including Wisconsin[416] and northwestern Illinois[417]; the meadow vole *Microtus pennsylvanicus* is a secondary, less important, small mammal reservoir host of *I. scapularis* in some areas of eastern North America.[168] A parallel cycle involving the cottontail rabbit, *Sylvilagus floridanus*, *I. scapularis*, and the rabbit tick *Ixodes dentatus*[169, 170] occurs either in areas where the enzootic *I. scapularis*–white footed mouse cycle of maintenance of *B. burgdorferi* infection is inefficient or does not occur, or in areas such as Nantucket Island, Massachusetts, New York,[100] and other parts of the northeastern United States[70] where the *I. scapularis*–mouse cycle occurs but the *I. dentatus*–rabbit cycle functions as an independent complementary cycle.[170] The *I. dentatus*–rabbit cycle is silent with respect to human Lyme disease as *I. dentatus* rarely bites humans; *I. scapularis* rarely feeds on rabbits,[170] but may be important in the spread of *B. burgdorferi* to new geographic areas because immature *I. dentatus* also feeds on birds.[157]

In some parts of North America, *B. burgdorferi* is present in areas that are not endemic for human Lyme disease because *B. burgdorferi* is maintained in nature by enzootic cycles that produce endemic foci that are silent with respect to human transmission of Lyme disease. One such cycle is the *I. spinipalpus*–*Mexican woodrat* cycle in Colorado; this tick has a broad host range, including rodents, rabbits, and ground-dwelling birds, but humans are rarely bitten because questing ticks are found only in woodrat nests; therefore, this cycle does not contribute to transmission of human Lyme disease.[362]

In the southern United States, the enzootic cycles that maintain *B. burgdorferi* in nature have been less fully described, are more complex and less efficient than those in the North, and result in lower *B. burgdorferi* tick infection rates.[156, 167, 361] The most common reservoir hosts for maintenance of *B. burgdorferi* infection in nature are the cotton mouse, *Peromyscus gossypinus*, and the cotton rat, *Sigmodon hispidus*; however, the life cycle of southern *I. scapularis* is less synchronized, so that nymphal feeding does not always precede larval feeding, thereby reducing the acquisition of infection by feeding larvae.[361] The southern *I. scapularis* is able to feed on 53 species of hosts, including mammals, birds, and reptiles, but the preferred hosts for immature *I. scapularis* are lizards and skinks (which are incompetent hosts incapable of maintaining and amplifying *B. burgdorferi* infection)[336, 348, 418]; the large mammal hosts for adult *I. scapularis* are white- and black-tailed deer, *Odocoileus virginianus* or *hemionus columbianus*. Reptiles exert a zooprophylactic effect on Lyme disease transmission, with a decrease in transmission in areas where reptiles predominate: South of the 38 degrees North latitude boundary, which runs from Virginia through Missouri, reptiles make up over 10% of the total *I. scapularis* hosts available (reptile index is greater than 10), and questing ticks are significantly diverted away from reservoir-competent amplifying hosts, such as the cotton mouse and the cotton rat, leading to lower tick infection rates.[156, 348, 418] B. burgdorferi in Missouri, and probably in Georgia, appears to be maintained in a cottontail rabbit–I. dentatus enzootic cycle, and I. scapularis and possibly A. americanum have been proposed as bridge vectors from rabbits to humans.[153, 361] I. cookei has been reported to bite humans in West Virginia, where it is considered a possible human Lyme disease vector; its immature forms feed on small and medium-sized carnivores, and its adults only on medium-sized carnivores.[363] I. affinis may enhance enzootic I. scapularis–cotton mouse/rat cycles, and I. minor may be involved in parallel enzootic cycles with the eastern woodrat, Neotoma floridana, or birds; these cycles maintain B. burgdorferi infection in nature in Georgia and South Carolina.[361]

Ixodes pacificus,[167, 180, 182, 336, 419, 420] in the far western United States, has a life cycle similar to that of I. scapularis but with some differences in hosts, reservoirs, and seasonality of feeding. Although I. pacificus is able to feed on a wide variety of hosts, including 80 different species of mammals, birds, and reptiles, its immature stages feed preferentially on lizards,[421] which are not competent B. burgdorferi reservoirs and cannot infect feeding ticks[336, 347, 348]; its larval feeding peaks before nymphal feeding,[336, 421] leading to the relatively low tick infection rates reported for adult ticks.[420] The black-tailed deer, Odocoileus hemionus columbianus, is the host of the adult tick, which feeds mostly in fall and winter, and to a lesser degree of the immature stages; in one study, all three stages were present simultaneously on deer.[421] B. burgdorferi infection is maintained in nature by a parallel enzootic cycle involving the competent reservoir host, the dusky-footed woodrat Neotoma fuscipes, and a non–I. ricinus complex tick, I. neotomae (now I. spinipalpis),[378] which rarely bites humans. I. pacificus is responsible for human transmission and acts as a bridging vector between the I. neotomae–woodrat cycle and man. In 1995, in California, the nymphal tick infection rate was found to be 14%, compared with the adult rate of 4%, and the possibility of a borreliacidal factor in lizard hosts was raised.[173, 180]

There are some differences between the life cycles of European I. ricinus and North American I. scapularis ticks.[167–169, 182, 336] I. ricinus has a 2- to 3-year life cycle (occasionally, 5 to 6 years in far northern latitudes), less coherent seasonal activity, and all three tick stages have feeding activity at the same time, particularly from mid-May to early July[181]; it has a broader host range, which includes 237 to 317 species of mammals, birds, and reptiles. I. ricinus abundance correlates with that of deer,[181] but I. ricinus occurs in some geographic areas even in the absence of deer because it can use cattle as well as deer as the large mammalian host.[168] The geographic distribution of Lyme borreliosis in Europe correlates with the geographic distribution of I. ricinus ticks,[11] particularly the distribution of B. burgdorferi–infected ticks,[181, 402] and even more with the distribution of highly infected ticks[422] and of deer,[168, 181] as in North America. The hedgehog Erinaceus europaeus–I. hexagonus cycle is involved in maintenance of B. burgdorferi infec-

tion in nature in Europe and Asia, but I. hexagonus rarely bites humans and is not considered important in the transmission of human Lyme disease.[182] In some areas, such as an urban park in Magdeburg, Germany, Norway rats, Rattus norvegicus, and I. ricinus are involved in maintenance of B. burgdorferi in nature in a cycle that occurs in addition to the mouse cycle.[423]

I. persulcatus[167, 169, 182] is responsible for human Lyme disease transmission in Asia; it has a similar life cycle to I. ricinus but a greater host range, which includes 212 to 241 different species of mammals, birds, and reptiles, although deer, canids, cattle, and hares are particularly important hosts.[344] The life cycle is usually 2 to 3 years, but in extreme northern latitudes it may be 5 to 6 years. The geographic distribution of Lyme disease and the genospecies of B. burgdorferi isolated from human Lyme disease patients in China, Japan, and eastern Russia correlate with the geographic distribution of, and genospecies isolated from, I. persulcatus.[163, 164, 374] There appear to be two separate enzootic cycles involving larvae and nymphs in Japan—the I. persulcatus–rodent cycle involving mainly the woodmouse (and sometimes the vole), and the I. persulcatus–bird cycle[163]; adult ticks feed mainly on large animals.

I. holocyclus, the most common tick in Australia, is not competent for B. burgdorferi.[392] So far, no competent vector or reservoir host has been identified in Australia. The mammalian hosts of B. burgdorferi in the northern hemisphere are all placental animals, and none of these are present in Australia, where the small mammals are mostly marsupial.[375]

A migratory seabird–I. uriae enzootic cycle has been described in high-latitude subarctic and subantarctic circumpolar areas, in which the seabirds maintain B. burgdorferi (B. garinii) infection in nature without the involvement of mammalian hosts.[152, 165, 166] The geographic distributions of I. uriae and I. ricinus overlap on islands in the Bothnian Gulf at the northern end of the Baltic Sea, and bridging may occur between the two enzootic cycles.[13, 152] It has been proposed that the migratory seabird is the reservoir for B. burgdorferi in the southern hemisphere, is responsible for the transhemispheric and global spread of B. burgdorferi, and may be important for the spread of Lyme disease to Australia and South Africa.[165]

In addition to I. uriae, other ixodid ticks, including the human Lyme disease vectors, I. ricinus, I. scapularis, I. pacificus, and I. persulcatus, and the rabbit-feeding ticks, I. dentatus, I. spinipalpus, and H. leporispalustris, are able to feed on birds as alternate hosts in addition to mammalian hosts[157, 163, 167, 182, 362]; therefore, they presumably have an opportunity to be transported by migratory birds to new geographic areas,[425, 426] and also to acquire B. burgdorferi from birds that may be reservoir-competent. The potential epidemiologic impact of migratory birds as transporters of infected ticks is great because an estimated 100 million birds migrate into Sweden each spring, carrying 6.8 million new ticks, 1.8 million of which carry B. burgdorferi; also, 4.7 million ticks, 1.3 million of which harbor B. burgdorferi, are transported out of Sweden toward the South every fall.

Small mammals, including mice and rabbits, and their

ticks may be important in establishment and maintenance of new cryptic *B. burgdorferi* endemic foci in nature by providing reservoir-competent hosts for infected ticks carried to new sites by migratory birds.[170, 171]

Seasonality of Human Tick Bites/Transmission of *Borrelia burgdorferi* Infection

Humans acquire Lyme borreliosis by being used as the incidental host of a *B. burgdorferi*–infected tick. Table 11–4 shows the seasonality of human tick bites and the time of onset of Lyme borreliosis by geographic region.

In North America, humans are incidental hosts of all stages of *I. scapularis*,[337] and in the Northeast and Upper Midwest, they are usually infected by voracious host-seeking *I. scapularis* nymphs during the spring and early summer (in May and June); the peak incidence of Lyme disease with erythema migrans occurs 1 month later during June and July.[336, 428] In mid-Atlantic states such as Maryland, the onset of most cases of Lyme disease is from May through September.[429] Epidemiologic studies have found that the tick infectivity rate increases from less than 1% of larvae, to 20 to 74% of nymphs, to 57 to 87% of adult ticks.[411] Nymphs are responsible for transmission of almost 90% of cases of Lyme disease.[347] Because the nymphs are so small, and because the tick injects saliva containing anti-inflammatory, analgesic, antihemostatic, and immunosuppressive components while feeding,[168] the bites are not painful and often go unnoticed long enough to allow *B. burgdorferi* transmission, which usually takes 2 to 3 days.[430] However, there are rare European reports of transmission after less than 24 hours[430, 431] and within 2 hours.[9] Human infection is less often caused by adult female *I. scapularis*, which feeds in late fall through early winter (from October through May), with a peak in October, even though *B. burgdorferi* infection rates among adults are higher than for nymphs, because the adults are larger and more easily detected and can be removed before transmission of *B. burgdorferi* infection occurs.[336, 430]

The *I. scapularis* tick takes a long time to feed; during a 5-day feeding period, the female tick ingests 3.5 ml of blood and injects or regurgitates 2.5 ml of fluid secretions into the host.[270] The blood meal triggers multiplication of the *B. burgdorferi* associated with the tick's gastrointestinal tract, which disseminate to the hemolymph by the third day of feeding and then spread to the host either by injection of *B. burgdorferi*–containing tick saliva or by regurgitation of *B. burgdorferi*–containing tick gut contents into the dermal feeding cavity created by the tick.[341, 342] These immunosuppressive salivary secretions and other factors related to the spirochete and its acquisition of host extracellular matrix digestive enzymes[144] result in host-specific immune evasion by the tick, which modifies the tick attachment site so that *B. burgdorferi* deposited in the skin may be in an immunologically privileged site and may be protected against attack by the host immune system.[168]

In the Pacific Northwest, along the Pacific Coast, humans are also incidental hosts of both the adult and immature stages of *I. pacificus*, which is one of the most common ticks biting humans[336, 420]; it is responsible for 59% of human tick bites[180] (66% of bites by adult ticks, and 44% by nymphs). The incidence of *B. burgdorferi* infection in nymphal ticks is much higher than in adult ticks, possibly because of the zooprophylactic effect of the reptile hosts of the immature stages.[180] The peak onset of Lyme disease with EM (March through August) corresponds to the nymphal feeding season (March through September), rather than to the adult tick feeding season (October through June, with peaks in December and March).[180] Because the incidence of *B. burgdorferi* infection of *I. pacificus* is lower than that of the northeastern *I. scapularis*, the rate of human infection following *I. pacificus* bites is also lower.[378, 420]

In Europe, humans are incidental hosts for all stages of the *I. ricinus* tick—which is the most common tick in Europe,[336] the most frequent cause of human tick bites in Central Europe, and the main vector for *B. burgdorferi* transmission to humans in Europe.[181, 336] The feeding activities of the three stages of *I. ricinus* overlap throughout Europe, especially from April through July,[181, 409, 422,]

TABLE 11–4
Seasonal Risk of Human Tick Bites and Development of Lyme Borreliosis (LB[a])

GEOGRAPHIC LOCATION	*B. BURGDORFERI* TICK VECTOR	MONTHS OF TICK FEEDING ACTIVITY, BY STAGE			MOST COMMON MONTHS OF ONSET OF LB
		Larvae	Nymphs	Adults	
North America					
Northeast, Atlantic, Midwest	*I. dammini/scapularis*	July–Sept.	May–July[b]	Oct.–May	May–Sept. (peak June–July)
Pacific Northwest	*I. pacificus*	Mar.–Sept.	Mar.–Sept.[b]	Oct.–June (peaks Dec. and Mar.)	Mar.–Aug.
Europe	*I. ricinus*	Mar.–Nov.	Mar.–Nov.	Mar.–Nov.	May–Oct.
Asia	*I. persulcatus*			May–June[c]	May–June

[a]Data from references 23, 180, 243, 251, 336, 344, 347, 358, 371, 428, 434, 460, 463, 464, 466–469, 596, and 637.
[b]Nymphal ticks feeding during this time are responsible for most *B. burgdorferi* transmission to humans.
[c]Adult ticks feeding during this time are responsible for most *B. burgdorferi* transmission to humans.

[432, 433] and the peak incidence of Lyme borreliosis occurs between May and October.[251, 371, 405, 409, 422, 432, 434–436] Similar seasonality has been demonstrated historically in a retrospective study of museum ticks from Great Britain over the past 100 years, in which *B. burgdorferi* PCR–positive museum specimens of *I. ricinus* ticks were found mainly from May through October, the overall PCR positivity rate was 20%, and the nymphal positivity rate was 38%.[340] The seasonality was particularly well defined in the migratory seabird tick, *I. uriae*, because ticks of this species were found only from April through August, and the PCR positivity rate was 98%.[340] The frequency with which *I. uriae* bites humans is not known, but one of the British museum *I. uriae* was involved in a human bite.[340]

In Asia, the adult stage of *I. persulcatus*, the most common tick in the Lyme-endemic areas of China and Japan, feeds in May and June and commonly bites humans, but larvae and nymphs rarely bite humans. The *B. burgdorferi* infection rate of the adult ticks is high in endemic regions, and the seasonality of EM, which peaks in May and June, correlates with that of human *I. persulcatus* tick bites.[344, 351, 374, 437, 438] *I. ovatus* is also frequently found in Japan, and has been demonstrated to be infected with *B. japonicus*, but no human cases of Lyme disease have been associated with it[163, 374]; *B. burgdorferi* isolates from Japanese patients with EM have been strains transmitted by *I. persulcatus* ticks.[164, 374, 439]

The risk of transfusion-acquired Lyme borreliosis was zero in a large study of 149 recipients of 601 units of packed red blood cells, and 48 recipients of 371 units of platelets, in a Lyme-endemic area of Connecticut; one patient developed transfusion-acquired babesiosis during this study.[440]

In North America, seasonal peaks of other tickborne infections that share vectors with Lyme disease are similar to those of Lyme disease: HME peaks in May through July,[398] HGE in May through July and in October through December,[397, 398] and babesiosis in the summer.[394] In Europe, the seasonality of tickborne encephalitis (TBE) is similar to that of Lyme borreliosis, which shares tick vectors.[402]

Geographic Distribution of Tick Vectors

The focus here is on the vectors involved in human transmission. The *Ixodes ricinus* complex ticks are widely distributed in the northern hemisphere,[182] require an environment with high humidity and temperature between −10° C and 35° C, and are therefore not found at high elevations because they are susceptible to the desiccation that occurs in unprotected, high windy areas.[181, 336] *I. scapularis* inhabits heavily forested and brushy areas, particularly the brushy areas at junctions between cleared and forested areas,[336, 407] but it has also been found on well-manicured lawns in hyperendemic areas such as Westchester County, New York, at densities as high as one tick per square meter of lawn.[441] *I. pacificus* is found only at elevations less than 2100 feet in coastal California.[420] *I. ricinus* inhabits dense heterogeneous deciduous forests with dense undergrowth,[181] as well as pastures below 1000 meters of elevation, is rare between 1000 and 1500 meters, and is not found above 1500 meters of elevation.[167, 336, 352] There is uneven distribution of these ticks even within their geographic range as a result of local microniche differences in elevation, foliage, humidity, temperature, and host populations.[181]

The evolution of distinct tick species and their *B. burgdorferi* genospecies has resulted in unique geographic ranges of both ticks and *B. burgdorferi* genospecies.[7, 13, 54, 63, 74]

The geographic distribution of the northern *I. scapularis* includes the northeastern and upper midwestern United States from Maine to Virginia, from the Atlantic Coast to Minnesota and Iowa, and from southern Ontario along coastal Lake Erie through Illinois and Indiana; small numbers of *I. scapularis* have also been found in Canada as far north as 50 degrees North latitude in Ontario, and in all provinces from Manitoba east to the Gulf of St. Lawrence and the Atlantic coast; the southern *I. scapularis* is found in the Southeast from Virginia to Florida, from the Atlantic coast to Texas and Oklahoma, and from the Midwest to the Gulf Coast.[167, 182, 348, 419, 445, 447] These areas include most of the Atlantic and Gulf Coasts, the Mississippi Valley, and forested areas of Missouri, Arkansas, Louisiana, Oklahoma, and Texas; *I. scapularis* is not found west of the 100th meridian, which runs midway through Texas and beyond which annual rainfall decreases.[348]

The distribution of *I. pacificus* extends from British Columbia to Baja California, from the Pacific coast to the Cascade and Sierra Nevada Mountains, and from Nevada to the Wasatch Range in Utah; it also includes some pockets of higher humidity within arid regions in eastern Oregon, northwestern Arizona, southern Nevada and Utah, and Idaho.[167, 348, 419] *I. pacificus* is well established in localized areas of southern British Columbia around the Fraser Delta, the Gulf Islands, and Vancouver Island.[445] *Ixodes angustus*, also suspected to be a potential *B. burgdorferi* vector for humans in Washington State,[364] has a wide geographic range that overlaps with that of *I. pacificus* and extends along the Pacific from California to Alaska[336, 364]; *B. burgdorferi* has also been found in *I. angustus* in British Columbia. It is the most common tick in some parts of coastal Oregon.[364]

Several tick species involved in enzootic cycles also overlap geographically with human Lyme disease tick vectors but are rarely or never related to human Lyme disease transmission as they rarely bite humans.[348, 378] These include *I. neotomae*,[348, 378] *I. dentatus*,[100, 170, 348, 363] *I. cookei*,[129] *I. affinis*, and *I. minor*;[361] as well as *I. spinipalpis*[362] in North America, and *I. hexagonus*[182, 381] in Europe and Asia.

Although the status of *A. americanum* as a human vector of Lyme disease has not been proved, it has been suspected as a secondary vector in some mid-Atlantic, southeastern, and southern states[153–155, 158, 359, 360, 366–369]; it occurs from Rhode Island to Florida, and from the Atlantic Coast to central Texas.[73] A *Borrelia* identified as *B. burgdorferi* has been found in *A. americanum* in New Jersey, Missouri, Texas, Oklahoma, Virginia, North Carolina, and Alabama.[153–158, 386] Also, an uncultivable *Borrelia*, *Borrelia lonestarii*, which may be related to the

Lyme-like disease in the southern states,[73] was found in *A. americanum* from New York, New Jersey, Missouri, and North Carolina.

The geographic distribution of *I. ricinus* extends from Algeria, Tunisia, and Egypt in North Africa to 65 degrees North latitude in Europe to southern Norway, Sweden, and Finland, and from the United Kingdom to 50 to 55 degrees East longitude in Turkey, Iran, and Russia to the Caspian Sea west of the Ural Mountains.[11, 167, 181, 182, 336, 448] It also includes southern Italy, the Balkans, and subtropical Madeira Island. *I. ricinus* is the most common tick in Europe.[336] *I. ricinus* occurs in northern but not southern Spain.[90]

The distribution of *I. persulcatus* extends east from the Ural Mountains[448] in eastern Europe to Asia and Japan and, at its western margin, overlaps somewhat with that of *I. ricinus*[167, 344]; it extends south to include the Hokkaido and Nagano districts in northern Japan, but does not occur in southern Japan.[351] *I. persulcatus* was the predominant tick in the Lyme-endemic areas of northeastern (Heilongjiang, Jilin, Liaoning, and Hebei Provinces), north central (Inner Mongolia), and northwestern (Xinjiang Province) China,[344, 350, 437, 438, 449] and in the Lyme-endemic areas, Hokkaido and Nagano districts, and Saitama Prefecture of Japan.[163, 351, 450]

So far, no ticks of the *I. ricinus/persulcatus* complex have been found to occur in Australia.[375]

In South America, there are ixodid ticks but it is unknown whether they harbor *B. burgdorferi*[453]; there are no *Ixodes* ticks in Chile.[454]

I. ricinus is prevalent in northern Africa, including Tunisia,[455] but does not occur farther south. In most of Africa, the Middle East, Asia, South America, and Central America, there are ticks that transmit human non-Lyme borrelial relapsing fever.[342]

I. uriae has a large high-latitude bi- and circumpolar marine ecologic geographic distribution[13, 152, 165, 166]; migratory seabirds congregate to breed on subarctic and subantarctic islands and peninsulas; they make transequatorial migrations to overwinter in northern parts of the Atlantic and Pacific, and in southern waters around South America and South Africa.[165, 166] Migratory seabirds and their *I. uriae* ticks are thought to be involved in transhemispheric spread of *B. burgdorferi* to the southern hemisphere, and possibly to be involved in the occurrence of Lyme disease in the southern hemisphere in areas without known *I. ricinus* complex vector ticks, such as Australia and South Africa. *I. uriae* have occasionally been found to bite humans.[165, 340] Migratory birds are able to bring potentially *B. burgdorferi*–infected ticks into contact with humans in geographic areas in which they would otherwise have no tick contact.[182, 425]

Geographic Distribution of Lyme Borreliosis

GEOGRAPHIC DISTRIBUTION OF LYME DISEASE IN NORTH AMERICA

The earliest cases of Lyme disease in the United States were recognized retrospectively to have occurred in the small New England communities of Great Island, Massachusetts, in 1962[334] and in and around Lyme, Connecticut, in 1965.[335] The earliest recognized case of EM in the United States occurred in 1969 in the Upper Midwest, in north central Wisconsin,[333] and the earliest recognized case in the Pacific Northwest, which followed an *I. pacificus* tick bite,[343] was reported in 1978 from Sonoma County, California.

To monitor trends and determine endemic geographic areas, the CDC and the Council of State and Territorial Epidemiologists began a national Lyme disease surveillance program in 1982 and established Lyme disease as a nationally notifiable disease in 49 states and the District of Columbia in 1990.[3] In addition to the increased reporting of cases of Lyme disease since then, there has been a true increase in the incidence of Lyme disease because of spread of the *I. scapularis* tick vector and its large mammalian host, the white-tailed deer, into larger geographic areas. If nymphal tick infection rates are high, as in some endemic areas of the northeastern United States, small variations in the tick population can significantly change the risk of Lyme disease exposure, and this will be reflected in the annual incidence of Lyme disease cases.[459]

A comparison of Lyme disease cases reported to the CDC from 1982 through 1998 shows impressive increases in both the number of cases reported (see Fig. 11–3) and the number of states reporting cases (see Fig. 11–2).[460, 461] The original northeastern focus of endemic Lyme disease in Connecticut[15] and Massachusetts[334, 462] in the late 1970s progressively expanded[463] to the mid-Atlantic states, and by 1982 it included Rhode Island, New York,[464–466] and New Jersey[155, 467, 468]; by 1987, Ohio, Pennsylvania, Maryland,[469, 470] and Virginia[358]; by 1992, New Hampshire; and by 1998, it extended to Vermont.[4] The original upper midwestern focus in Wisconsin[271, 471–473] expanded to include Minnesota[272] by 1982. By 1987, cases of Lyme disease were reported from Texas,[382] and by 1992, from the majority of the southeastern,[359, 360, 474] south central,[369] and midwestern[366, 368, 473, 475, 476] states. In the northwestern states between 1982 and 1987, Lyme disease began to be reported from California, Oregon, and Washington State.[364] As of 1998, ten states—New York, Connecticut, New Jersey, Pennsylvania, Wisconsin, Rhode Island, Maryland, Massachusetts, California, and Minnesota—accounted for 90%, and the first four states accounted for 75%, of all cases of Lyme disease reported to the CDC from 1982 through 1998.[4, 461] Endemic areas have become established in many other states.

Although Lyme disease now has been reported from all states except Montana,[3, 4, 461] some states such as the Mountain states (Montana, Idaho, Wyoming, Colorado, New Mexico, Arizona, Utah, and Nevada), the Dakotas, Louisiana, Mississippi, South Carolina, Maine, Vermont, Hawaii, and Alaska reported very few or no cases in 1992, and most cases continue to be reported from the highly endemic areas of the northeastern, mid- and south Atlantic, and upper midwestern states. By region, in 1992 and 1998, there were approximately 5300 and 6900 cases of Lyme disease reported from the mid-Atlantic states, 2300 and 4500 from the northeastern states, 1100 and 1165 from the north central states, 700 and 900 from the south Atlantic states (over 75% from the northern part of this area—Maryland, Delaware, and Virginia), 200 and 100 from the south central states, 300 and 200 from the Pacific states, and only 16 and 25 cases from the Mountain states. Cases reported from nonendemic areas but acquired in endemic areas may explain the reporting of some cases from nonendemic states. Variation in tick and reservoir host population density, application of more stringent case definitions, and Lyme disease educational programs may be related to decreases in incidence of cases in some areas in 1998 compared with 1992.

The existence of Lyme disease in southern United States has been controversial,[361, 477] although there is general agreement about the existence of a Lyme-like illness with erythema migrans in the South.[367, 368, 477] The presence of B. burgdorferi in I. scapularis and small mammals in the South has been established,[386, 477] but it has been suggested that genospecies of B. burgdorferi other than sensu stricto and tick vectors other than I. scapularis, such as I. dentatus or A. americanum, might be involved in enzootic cycles in nature and in transmission of this disease to humans.[153, 158, 359, 360, 366–368] This issue has been complicated by misdiagnosis, as was the case in Georgia in 1989 when more than 700 cases were suddenly reported in 1 year, the majority of which were later considered not to be Lyme disease.[461]

Yearly incidences of Lyme disease cases occurring per 100,000 population have been calculated for different geographic areas of the United States, and are designated as follows: low incidence, 10 cases per 100,000 population (0.01% annually); moderate, 100 cases per 100,000 (0.1% annually); high, 1000 cases per 100,000 (1% annually); and very high, 3000 cases per 100,000 (3% annually).[478] Very high, hyperendemic areas are Westchester County, New York, with a 2.6 to 3% annual incidence and a 17% cumulative incidence; Great Island, Massachusetts, with a 3% annual incidence and a 16% cumulative incidence; and Fire Island, New York, with a 1 to 3% annual incidence and a 7.5% cumulative incidence.[478]

In Canada, southern British Columbia (the Fraser Delta area, Vancouver Island, and the Gulf Islands) and Ontario (Long Point Peninsula and coastal areas of Lake Erie) are now considered Lyme-endemic areas,[376, 445, 479] with established tick vector populations (I. pacificus and I. angustus in British Columbia, and I. scapularis in Ontario)[376, 445]; there are limited focal, established populations of I. scapularis and I. pacificus in other areas of Canada at risk to become endemic foci if B. burgdorferi is introduced into these populations.[445] I. pacificus is established in southern British Columbia in the Fraser Delta area, the Gulf Islands, and Vancouver Island; I. scapularis is established in Ontario in coastal Lake Erie, and has also been reported in Manitoba, Quebec, Nova Scotia, New Brunswick, Newfoundland, and Prince Edward Island; its occasional appearance in other provinces has been thought to be due to introduction by migratory birds.[445] Between 1977 and 1989, 30 cases of Lyme disease were reported to the Canadian Laboratory Centre for Disease Control; Lyme disease is now notifiable

in 8 of 12 provinces; between 1987 and 1997, 333 cases were reported, half acquired in Canada, mostly from southern Ontario (71% of autochthonous cases), British Columbia, Ontario, Quebec, Manitoba, and New Brunswick near Lyme-endemic areas in the United States.[479] In 1993, B. burgdorferi was found in I. pacificus and I. angustus, as well as deer mice, in British Columbia.[376] A serosurvey of residents of Alberta, Canada, in 1993 found no seropositivity by ELISA or Western blot assays, and a tick survey found I. angustus and H. leporispalustris but no I. scapularis[479]; in 1995, B. burgdorferi was isolated from an H. leporispalustris tick removed from a rabbit in Alberta, near the border with British Columbia, establishing its presence in Alberta.[479] In 1993, B. burgdorferi was found in I. scapularis from a dog in Ontario, at 50 degrees North latitude near the Manitoba border, just north of the endemic areas of Minnesota.[446]

EXPANSION OF LYME-ENDEMIC AREAS IN NORTH AMERICA

B. burgdorferi–infected ticks may be transported from Lyme-endemic areas into nonendemic areas, which may establish new Lyme-endemic foci.[165, 168, 169, 336, 408, 462, 490] Infected I. ricinus complex ticks (including I. scapularis) and infected I. uriae have been found on migratory birds and along migratory "flyways"; they may be transported into new areas by these birds as they travel between endemic and nonendemic areas, including counties, states, countries, continents, and even hemispheres.[13, 63, 157, 165, 167–169, 171, 376] Rodents, hunting dogs, household pets,[454] domestic animals, wide-ranging wild animals such as coyotes and foxes, and campers, hunters, and other people[13] traveling between endemic and nonendemic areas may also transport infected ticks from one area to another; deer hunters may transport deer or other game animals[63] with infected ticks still attached. If the newly arrived tick finds its necessary hosts, or if it arrives together with a population of its hosts, a new endemic focus of infected ticks and Lyme disease will be established.[460, 470, 492] I. scapularis and other I. ricinus complex ticks, along with the rabbit ticks I. dentatus and H. leporispalustris, are able to feed on birds as well as mammals,[157, 163, 167, 362] and could provide a bridging vector between hosts.[167]

In North America, the incidence of Lyme disease has been found to correlate with the population density and geographic distribution of I. scapularis[335, 442, 443, 490, 491] and white-tailed deer.[335] Because deer are the reproductive hosts of adult I. scapularis and they determine the success rate of tick mating, the population density of I. scapularis correlates with the population density of deer, and an I. scapularis focus may enlarge geographically as the geographic distribution of deer expands.[408] Even infrequent visits by deer to an area may be sufficient to sustain a small population of I. scapularis.[492]

The deer populations in North America have changed dramatically over the past 400 years.[168, 394] Particularly since the 1970s, there has been a deer population explosion, and deer have regained their original widespread North American distribution as forests have replaced farmland and federal programs have protected deer. Human contact with deer has been increasing as residence or recreation in rural and suburban forested areas has become increasingly popular.[6, 7, 168, 336, 390, 394]

The expansion of the Lyme-endemic areas has been particularly impressive in New England, the mid-Atlantic states, and Wisconsin, where this has been extensively studied epidemiologically. In Ipswich, Massachusetts, the emergence of a new focal epidemic of Lyme disease was associated with a 35% Lyme disease attack rate overall for residents living near the deer-populated nature preserve considered to be the focus, and 66% for those living closest to the preserve.[462] Among permanent residents of Great Island, Massachusetts, the Lyme seropositivity rate was 8%, the history positivity rate was 16%, and the incidence of Lyme disease was 7% over a 2-year period.[334] Among middle and high school students in an endemic area of Connecticut, the physician-diagnosed Lyme disease history positivity and seropositivity rates were 7 and 3%, respectively; during the 1990–1992 tick season, 2% developed clinical physician-diagnosed Lyme disease and 1% experienced asymptomatic seroconversion.[493] The incidence of Lyme disease increased steadily between 1991 and 1996 from rates of 36 to 94 cases per 100,000 population annually overall for Connecticut, and from 340 to 450 cases per 100,000 annually for a hyperendemic 12-town area along the Connecticut River and the Atlantic Coast; the increase in the 12-town area was found to correlate with the abundance and B. burgdorferi infection rate of I. scapularis in this area; nymphal tick infection rates increased from 14 to 24% during this time in the 12-town area.[490]

In the mid-Atlantic United States, in New York and New Jersey, the geographic distribution of the I. scapularis tick vector has expanded annually outside of the original Long Island focus, and there has been a corresponding increase in both the number of counties reporting Lyme disease and the number of cases reported per county.[465, 494–497]

In Wisconsin, the Lyme-endemic area has expanded southward from the original northwestern region,[271, 416] and the seropositivity rate is 6 to 11%,[471, 473] which is similar to the 7% seropositive rate in Minnesota. In southern and southwestern United States, where the reported incidence of Lyme disease is low, seroprevalence studies have been less frequent; the rate of seropositivity was 23 to 26% in Texas,[382] and 0% in a nonendemic area of Arizona.[473] In western United States, the deer population is more stable than in eastern United States and in Europe, and apparent increases in Lyme disease may be related more to reporting than to actual increased incidence.[394]

Studies of the seroprevalence of antibody to B. burgdorferi, Babesia microti, E. chaffeensis, and the agent of HGE have been done in various geographic areas. In Wisconsin, the frequency of co-infection in patients with Lyme disease was 5.2% for HGE, 2.1% for B. microti, and 2.1% for both; the frequency of co-infection in patients with HGE was 5.3% for B. burgdorferi, 5.3% for B. microti, and 5.3% for both.[486] In Minnesota, one third of HGE patients had seropositivity to B. burgdorferi.[498] In Westchester County, New York, 22% of HGE patient sera were also seropositive for B. burgdorferi.[488]

Twenty percent of patients from Minnesota, New York, New Jersey, and Connecticut with early Lyme disease had serologic evidence of previous or current HGE.[498] In Rhode Island and Connecticut, 11% of patients with Lyme disease were co-infected with B. microti, 72% of patients with babesiosis were co-infected with B. burgdorferi, and seroprevalence was 7% for B. burgdorferi compared with 5% for B. microti.[481] In Connecticut in 1994, the rates of co-infection with other tickborne infections in patients with serologically confirmed Lyme disease were 10% for HME, 7.5% for HGE, 7.5% for babesiosis, and 5% for more than two infections.[487] In eastern Long Island, 66% of Lyme disease sera were also positive for B. microti antibody, and 54% of babesiosis sera were positive for B. burgdorferi antibody.[485]

The earliest reported major inland focus of I. scapularis was on Long Point Peninsula, which extends into Lake Ontario from the southern coast of Ontario.[394] Lyme disease is notifiable in 8 of 12 provinces in Canada, and its incidence has gradually increased from 30 cases reported to the Canadian Laboratory Centre for Disease Control between 1977 and 1989, predominantly from southern parts of the provinces Ontario and Manitoba (with single cases reported from the provinces of Alberta, British Columbia, and Quebec), to 333 cases (half acquired within Canada) between 1987 and 1997,[479] predominantly from the endemic areas in southern British Columbia, Vancouver Island, the Gulf Islands, Ontario along coastal Lake Erie, and other provinces such as Manitoba, Quebec, and New Brunswick, which are near Lyme-endemic areas of the United States. The presence of B. burgdorferi has been confirmed in ticks in the endemic provinces[376, 446] and Alberta,[479] but because of the existence of established vector tick populations in other parts of Canada, spread to these areas may occur if B. burgdorferi is introduced into these tick populations by dog and human travelers, or by migratory birds.[445]

Several studies have been done[442, 443, 491, 499] to try to develop predictors of geographic risk by using satellite photographs of vegetation, as well as data on I. scapularis population density and infection rate (acarologic index), deer population density, mouse reservoir population density, B. burgdorferi seroprevalence in resident dog populations, and human Lyme disease incidence; correlations have been found with vegetation, wetness, residence in less developed areas outside of towns, deer density, tick density, tick infection rates, mouse population density, dog seroprevalence rates, and even with the abundance of acorns. The abundance of acorns as a food source for white-footed mice determines their survival through the winter and resulting mouse population density; abundant acorns also attract deer, resulting in increased I. scapularis population density brought by the deer; the combination of increases in mouse, deer, and tick population densities is expected to increase the risk of Lyme disease acquisition about 2 years after a bumper crop of acorns.[500]

GEOGRAPHIC DISTRIBUTION OF LYME BORRELIOSIS IN EUROPE, ASIA, AND OTHER CONTINENTS

The true worldwide country-by-country incidence of Lyme borreliosis is impossible to determine because only a few countries other than the United States have mandatory reporting of Lyme borreliosis, and because clinical and serologic criteria for definition and reporting of the disease vary in different countries.[11, 12, 501] Efforts are being made by the EUCALB to improve reporting and to standardize European case definitions.[8, 10, 502]

Lyme borreliosis has been reported from six continents—North and South America, Europe, Asia, northern Africa, and Australia—but the majority of cases have originated in North America, Central Europe, and Asia (see Fig. 11–1; Table 11–5).[4, 8–13, 504] The existence of indigenous Lyme borreliosis in South America[452, 453, 505, 506] and Australia is still uncertain.[391, 392]

In Europe, as of 1998, *B. burgdorferi sensu lato* had been isolated from either arthropod vectors, animal hosts, or human patients in the following European countries (Table 11–6): Austria, Belarus, Belgium, Croatia, the Czech Republic, Denmark, Estonia, Finland, France, Germany, Great Britain, Hungary, Iceland, Ireland, Italy, Latvia, Lithuania, Moldavia, the Netherlands, Norway, Poland, Portugal, Russia, Slovakia, Slovenia, Spain, Sweden, Switzerland, and the Ukraine.[10, 54, 405] A large study by the EUCALB of over 2000 pa-

tients with Lyme borreliosis in 15 European countries during 12 months in 1994 found that the incidence of Lyme borreliosis per 100,000 population increased from western to eastern Europe, with higher incidences east of the Netherlands, France, and Italy.[10]

The number of European cases of Lyme borreliosis (LB) through 1998, since reporting has improved, has been estimated to be over 60,000 annually, based on *B. burgdorferi*–seropositive cases reported voluntarily to the World Health Organization (WHO) by Public Health Administrations of WHO European Region countries, and to the EUCALB by member countries, as well as cases reported in the medical literature through 1998.[9] Most of these cases were from central Europe (see Table 11–5).

In Asia, cases have been reported from China and Japan, as well as from eastern parts of Russia. In 1981, one case of EM was reported from Japan following an *Ixodes persulcatus* bite in the mountainous district of the Nagano Prefecture, across the Sea of Japan from Vladivostock, and as of 1998, 100 cases of Lyme disease had been reported, mainly from Hokkaido and Nagano Prefectures.[164, 374, 439] *I. persulcatus* is considered the major

TABLE 11–5
Incidence of Lyme Borreliosis (LB) in Europe, by Country[a]

RELATIVE RISK[b]	COUNTRY	LB/100,000 POPULATION PER YEAR	LB/YEAR	REGION
High	Austria	150	14,000	
	Slovenia	120	2000	Central
	Poland	120		
	Sweden	69	>2000	South, Southeast
	Bulgaria	50–55	3500	
Medium	Denmark[c]	50		
	Hungary	50	1000	
	Netherlands	43	6500	North, East, Coast
	Czech Republic	40	6300	
	Finland	40	2000	Southeast, Southwest, Aland Islands
	France	40	7200	Northwest, East
	Switzerland	30	2000	
	Germany	25	20,000	
	Italy	17		North, North Central
Low	Belgium	<5	50–100	East
	Yugoslavia (former)		400	
	Croatia		200	Northwest
	U.K.		200	South, Southwest England, Scottish Highlands
	Lithuania		350	
	U.S.S.R. (former)		6000–11,000	Kaliningrad, Leningrad, Kirov, Perm, Kurgan, Omsk, Tomsk, Khabarovsk, and Northwestern areas
Very low	Norway		<50	
	Ireland		<50	
	Spain		<50	North, Northeast
	Luxembourg		<100	
	Greece		~0	
	Romania		<100	

[a]Estimated or reported LB cases.
[b]LB/100,000 population/year: High: >50; Medium: 5–50; Low: <5; Very low: Only a few cases reported.
[c]As only neuroborreliosis is reported in Denmark, this is an underestimate of total LB cases in Denmark.
Data obtained from 9–12, 90, 162, 251, 268, 352, 370, 371, 402, 404, 405, 409, 432–434, 448, 501, 503, 504, 507, 511, 515, 517, 519, 525, 532, 534, 535, 539, 544–548, 550, 552, 621, and 881.

TABLE 11–6

Borrelia burgdorferi (Bb) Tick Infection Rates, by Country and Tick Species

COUNTRY	REGION	TICK SPECIES	% OF TICKS POSITIVE FOR *Bb*[a]
U.S.	Northeast and Mid-Atlantic	*I. scapularis*[b, c]	24–61
	Northeast	*I. dentatus*	32
	Mid-Atlantic	*A. americanum*	6–22
	Mid-Atlantic	*I. cookei*	22
	Upper Midwest	*I. scapularis*	38–40
	South and Southeast	*A. americanum*	4
	South	*I. scapularis*	0–3
	West	*I. neotomae*	15
	West	*I. spinipalpis*	50–66
	West and Pacific Northwest	*I. pacificus*	1–14
Austria		*I. ricinus*	4–40
Belgium		*I. ricinus*	10–50
Bulgaria		*I. ricinus*	17
Bulgaria		*D. marginatus*	4
China	North Inner Mongolia, Heilongjiang, Jilin, Liaoning, Hebei, Xinjiang	*I. persulcatus*	20–40
Croatia		*I. ricinus*	45
Czech Republic	South Moravia	*I. ricinus*	15–23
Finland	Coastal islands	*I. ricinus*	40
France		*I. ricinus*	7
Germany		*I. ricinus*	19–44
Germany		*I. hexagonus*	12
Ireland	National parks (greatest in South)	*I. ricinus*	4–27
Japan	North to Central (Hokkaido, Nagano)	*I. persulcatus*	7–22
Japan	North (Hokkaido)	*I. ovatus*	10
Japan	Central to South (Nagano, Fukushima)	*I. ovatus*	26–27
Lithuania		*I. ricinus*	10
Netherlands		*I. ricinus*	2–27
Poland		*I. ricinus*	10–23
Russia		*I. ricinus*	4–27
Russia		*I. persulcatus*[d]	30
Slovenia		*I. ricinus*	>40
Spain	La Rioja	*I. ricinus*	11
Sweden	North	*I. ricinus*	3
Sweden	Northern Baltic Islands	*I. ricinus*	8–19
Sweden	South and Liso Peninsula	*I. ricinus*	23–30
Switzerland		*I. ricinus*	10–50
U.K.		*I. ricinus*	8
Yugoslavia (former)		*I. ricinus*	29
—	Eastern Europe	*I. ricinus*	0–50
—	Eastern Europe	*I. persulcatus*	21–58
—	Subarctic islands	*I. ricinus*	5
—	Subarctic islands	*I. uriae*[e]	2–6

[a] *Bb* positivity determined by microscopy, polymerase chain reaction, immunofluorescence, or other assay. Tick infection rates of adult ticks are generally higher than those of nymphal ticks,[181] with the exception of *I. pacificus.*

[b] *I. scapularis* from Lyme-endemic areas contains a median of 1900 *Bb* per tick.[412]

[c] *I. scapularis* from some Lyme-endemic areas may also contain *Babesia microti* and/or the agent of human granulocytic ehrlichiosis, in addition to *Bb*.[395, 396, 497]

[d] Co-infection of ticks with *Bb* and tick-borne encephalitis virus may occur.[405]

[e] 98% of museum specimens of British *I. uriae* were positive for *Bb*.[340]

Data from references 1, 123, 154–157, 161, 162, 170, 180, 181, 336, 344, 350, 351, 356, 362, 371, 378, 387, 394, 395, 403, 405, 409, 410, 412, 416, 420, 422, 424, 438, 449, 497, 503, 508, 513–515, 517, 522, 528, 535, 540, 549, and 579.

vector and *I. ovatus* another potential vector,[164, 351, 357, 374] although human Lyme disease has not been associated with *B. burgdorferi* strains from *I. ovatus*.[163, 374]

Lyme disease was first recognized in China in 1985, and in 1990, 132 cases of EM were reported from Hailin County in the Heilongjiang Province of northeastern China,[12, 344] adjacent to the Vladivostock focus of Lyme borreliosis in southeastern Russia.[448] Since then, it has become the most common tickborne disease in China, and hundreds of additional cases have been recognized. It has been reported from ten provinces and two autonomous areas, predominantly from the northeastern and northwestern regions, including the Heilonjiang, Jilin, Liaoning, Hebei, Inner Mongolia, Xinjiang, and Mudanjiang provinces[344, 349, 350, 449, 554] and the Beijing area.[388] *I. persulcatus* is the vector in most of these areas, but

Haemaphysalis longicornis has also been identified as a vector in the Beijing area.[388]

In 1998, the first case of Lyme disease, serologically confirmed but not culture-confirmed, was reported from Taiwan; although several strains of *Borrelia* have been isolated from indigenous rodents, and *I. ovatus* and *I. granulatus* occur locally, the vector has not been identified.[451] *B. burgdorferi* has been isolated from *Ixodes* ticks and rodents in Korea; Korea would therefore be considered an endemic area.[555]

In Central and South America, rare cases, not culture-confirmed, have been reported from Mexico,[556] Chile,[557] Brazil,[558] Argentina,[559] Puerto Rico, and Honduras.[560] In Chile, a case of confirmed Lyme neuroborreliosis was not considered autochthonous, and was attributed to imported German hamsters.[454] There are no ixodid ticks in Chile, and a large study of Chilean patients with suspected Lyme disease could not confirm any cases by either culture or Western blot; ELISA seropositivity in 5 patients was attributed to cross-reactivity, possibly with non-Lyme *Borreliae*.[505] Thirty-three clinical Lyme disease cases, most with serologic confirmation (including Western blot confirmation), have been reported from Rio de Janeiro and the nearby Cotia/Itapevi region of Brazil,[452, 506, 558] where several species of ixodid ticks occur; seroprevalence in blood donors was 3% in a low-risk area and 6.7% in the Cotia area; *Borreliae* were isolated by culture from human, tick, and wild animal sources in the Cotia region, but PCR could not confirm identity with either *B. burgdorferi sensu stricto*, *B. garinii*, or *B. afzelii*. Three patients with serologically confirmed suspected Lyme disease were reported from Mato Grosso do Sul, Brazil.[506] In Argentina, one clinical case has been reported,[559] and no culture-confirmed cases have been reported; three farm workers with arthritis were found to be seropositive.[453] It is uncertain whether reports of Lyme disease from Haiti,[560] Jamaica,[560] Peru,[373] and India[561] were due to cross-reacting non-Lyme *Borrelia* species such as those that cause relapsing fever, or to Lyme borreliosis originally acquired in an endemic country outside the country of reporting.

In northern Africa, 21 cases of serologically confirmed Lyme disease, with arthritis, lymphocytic meningitis, facial palsy, or pericarditis, were reported from Tunisia in 1998.[455] In South Africa, rare cases of Lyme disease[456, 562] have been reported, four potential tick vectors occur, and at least one has been found to be competent for *B. burgdorferi*.[456] From the rest of Africa, only sporadic cases have been reported, without culture confirmation, and several serosurveys have been done; it is uncertain whether these represent locally or non–locally acquired Lyme borreliosis, infection with other *Borreliae* producing Lyme-like illness, or cross-reacting infection with other prevalent bacteria. In southeastern Africa, a serosurvey in Zimbabwe found ELISA seropositivity rates of 1.6 to 5% in blood donors and healthy villagers, and 0% in dogs, cattle, and horses, and concluded that Lyme borreliosis was absent there[458]; a case of serologically confirmed probable Lyme disease with EM at a tick bite site from an autochthonous tick bite in Mozambique was reported in 1993,[563] but a serosurvey in Mozambique, reported in 1997, attributed 11% ELISA positivity in febrile patients to serologic cross-reactivity with leptospira, *Borrelia crocidurae*, and syphilis[564]; a serosurvey in Tanzania found very high ELISA seropositivity rates in blood donors, pregnant women, and arthritis and syphilis patients (30 to 55%) and noted that Lyme-like illness and tick bites occur, but that the seropositivity probably represents cross-reactions with leptospira, relapsing fever, and syphilis, which are prevelent.[565] A serosurvey of rural residents in Mali found no seropositivity by ELISA, but a survey of patients with neurologic disease identified six patients who were seropositive by both ELISA and Western blot; no ixodes ticks occur in Mali, and the authors conclude that *B. burgdorferi* does not exist in Mali, but that other cross-reacting *Borreliae*, such as *B. crocidurae*, transmitted by the soft tick *Alectorobius sonraai*, which causes tickborne meningoencephalitis in nearby Senegal, might cause a Lyme-like illness.[457]

From the Middle East, two serologically confirmed (IFA, ELISA, and/or Western blot), but not culture-confirmed, cases have been reported from Israel,[566, 567] but none has occurred in the absence of previous travel to known endemic areas. *B. burgdorferi* IFA and Western blot seropositivity of uncertain etiology have been reported from Fayoum, Egypt, and four ELISA serologically confirmed, but not culture-confirmed, cases have been reported from Alexandria, Egypt[568]; no information about travel to endemic areas was given. *I. ricinus* ticks have been found on migratory birds resting in Egypt during their fall migration from Europe and Asia to Africa.[376]

In southeastern Australia, between 1982 and 1986, nine cases of erythema migrans–like rashes were reported from the Hunter Valley and the New South Wales coast near Sydney; this area was initially considered a possible newly recognized endemic area.[391] In 1994, a case of ACA was reported in an Australian resident who had immigrated from Europe 25 years earlier, but it could not be considered an autochthonous case.[569] In 1998, the first case of an Australian patient with *B. garinii* culture–positive Lyme borreliosis (erythema migrans–like rash) associated with a locally acquired tick bite (from the New South Wales coastal area near Sydney) was reported[303]; however, because this patient had traveled to European endemic areas 17 months earlier, it could not be definitely proven that the case was acquired in Australia. Proof of Lyme endemicity will require additional culture-confirmed, locally acquired cases without previous travel to endemic areas.[391-392]

In the northern hemisphere, the Lyme borreliosis endemic and hyperendemic areas of Europe and Asia cluster in a definite band, which could be called the "Lyme Belt" (see Fig. 11–1); it is located approximately between 30 degrees North latitude and the Arctic Circle at 65 degrees North latitude (65° N). This region includes the majority of cases from Central Europe, Scandinavia, the former USSR, China, Japan, and northern Africa (Tunisia and Alexandria, Egypt). Israel is also located within this belt. In the western part of the northern hemisphere, the "Lyme Belt" extends from approximately 15° N to 50° N and includes the endemic areas of the United States and southern Canada, as well as the cases from Mexico and the Caribbean. In the southern hemisphere, the cluster of Lyme or Lyme-like cases from southeastern Australia and Rio de Janeiro, Brazil, the cases from South Africa and Mozambique, and the *B. burgdorferi* seropositivity noted near Buenos Aires, Argentina, are all between 10 degrees South latitude (10° S) and approximately 40° S, but insufficient cases have been reported from the southern hemisphere to determine whether there is a similar southern hemisphere "Lyme belt." The presence of the migratory bird *B. burgdorferi* tick vector, *I. uriae*, has been demonstrated in the Falkland Islands at 51° S; the presence of this vector and *B. burgdorferi* has been demonstrated in Crozet Island at 46° S and in Campbell Island, New Zealand, between 45° S and 55° S in the southern hemisphere, placing the southern margin of the range of *B. burgdorferi* at least to the subantarctic region,[165] although no human Lyme disease cases have been reported from these islands.

EXPANSION OF LYME-ENDEMIC AREAS IN EUROPE, ASIA, AND OTHER CONTINENTS

In Europe, the geographic distribution of Lyme borreliosis correlates with the distribution of *I. ricinus*[4, 125] and the distribution of the deer population, and the number of deer has increased dramatically, as in North America.[144] Deer were initially abundant in Central Europe, but in the 1940s during and after World War II, deer were used for food and forests for fuel, resulting in almost complete destruction of the deer population and partial deforestation of the region. In the 1960s, regrowth of forests and return of deer began, and there has since been a deer population explosion, which has coincided with the increase in Lyme borreliosis in Central Europe. *B. burgdorferi* has been found in museum specimens of European ticks from the late nineteenth century.[340]

Several seroepidemiologic studies have reported the rates of *B. burgdorferi* seropositivity in the general population in Europe and Asia (Table 11–7).

The existence of Lyme borreliosis in South America is uncertain, although its presence has been suspected. A 2% seropositivity rate was reported in agricultural workers in Peru, but this may be due to cross-reacting relapsing fever *Borrelia* organisms[373]; seropositive farmers with arthritis have been reported from Argentina,[453] and 7% seropositivity was reported in residents of Cotia, Brazil, which is suspected to be an endemic area.[452]

Lyme disease has been reported from northern Africa, where *I. ricinus* is prevalent, including Tunisia[455] and Egypt,[568] but its presence in the rest of Africa is uncertain, although suspected. An 11% seropositivity rate found in patients with nonspecific febrile illness in Mozambique, Africa, was considered due to cross-reactions with leptospirosis, non-Lyme borrelial relapsing fever, and syphilis.[564] However, one serologically confirmed case of Lyme disease with EM acquired from a Mozambique tick has been reported,[563] and its presence is suspected in South Africa.[456]

TABLE 11–7
Borrelia burgdorferi (Bb) Seropositivity Rates in Europe and Asia, by Country

COUNTRY	% OF PERSONS SEROPOSITIVE	
	General Population	High-Risk Population[a]
Austria	4–8	
Bulgaria		15–35 (forest workers, animal farmers)
China	1–12	26–53 (forest workers and rural northeastern residents)
Croatia	7	
Finland	3–6	12 (military recruits in Southwestern archipelago)
France		18–26 (forest workers)
Germany	5	18–34 (forest workers)
Greece	1	
Hungary	2–5	
Italy	0–13	8–18 (forest workers)
Ireland	5–15	
Japan	1	6–20 (forest workers)
Lithuania	4	14–32 (forest/field workers, veterinarians)
Netherlands	2–17	15 (hunters, military recruits)
Poland	19–24	50–71 (outdoor workers)
Russia	9	
Spain	3–13	31 (forest workers, farmers, cattle raisers)
Sweden	2–9	26–30 (Liso peninsula/Aspo Island residents)
Switzerland	4–6	19–60 (orienteers, sportsmen, forest workers, rural residents)
U.K./England	0–4	14–55 (forest workers, farmers, game keepers)
U.K./Scotland		16–27 (nature conservancy workers, Highlands residents)
Yugoslavia (former)	5	

[a]Persons with high frequencies of occupational, recreational, or residential exposure to tick-infested *Bb*-endemic geographic areas within these countries. Seropositivity rates increased with age and length of exposure in several longitudinal studies.

Data from references 162, 305, 344, 349, 388, 405, 406, 409, 437, 438, 450, 504, 508–510, 512, 514, 516, 517, 521–524, 526, 527, 529, 532, 533, 538, 539, 541–543, 548, 549, 551, 553, 554, 570, 571, and 573.

Lyme Borreliosis in Travelers to Endemic Areas

There are increasing reports of Lyme borreliosis in individuals who have acquired the infection during travel, often international, to Lyme-endemic areas in the recent or remote past.[9, 75, 454, 482, 569, 574-576] This may explain some of the cases that have been reported from areas such as Australia, which lack either the necessary tick vectors or *B. burgdorferi*.[303, 392, 566, 567] In Canada, where the incidence of Lyme disease is relatively low, half of all cases reported to the Laboratory Centre for Disease Control were acquired outside of Canada.[429] Pets that travel from endemic to nonendemic areas could be potential vehicles of transfer of infected ticks to their owners.[454]

Presentation with Lyme borreliosis in a nonendemic region may increase the risk of delayed diagnosis because the clinical presentations, although easily recognized by physicians in the endemic area, may be unrecognized by physicians in the nonendemic area who have little experience with the infection, or with its possibly different clinical manifestations in the area of acquisition.[482]

Travelers from nonendemic areas who engage in outdoor activities such as hiking, mountaineering, orienteering, or camping in endemic areas are at increased risk as they may be unaware of the local risk of tickborne infections, including the higher risk in hyperendemic areas, and may be less likely to use appropriate precautions, to recognize a tick bite, or to recognize early symptoms of infection. Vacationers, even when residing in endemic areas and knowledgeable about Lyme disease, are less likely to engage in tick-avoidance behaviors while on vacation.[577]

Borrelia burgdorferi Tick Infection Rates

In the United States, rates of *B. burgdorferi* infection of *I. scapularis* and *I. pacificus* in North America, and of *I. ricinus* and *I. persulcatus* in Europe and Asia, vary with geographic region, elevation, season, and stage of the tick, and are highest in the hyperendemic areas during early summer.[181, 411] *I. ricinus* infection rates were noted to increase significantly from Western to Eastern Europe.[181]

The distribution of the different genospecies of *B. burgdorferi sensu lato* in *I. ricinus* complex ticks varies with the global geographic location, and is more fully characterized in the northern hemisphere than the southern hemisphere. In Central Europe, the diversity is greatest, with four genospecies—*B. burgdorferi sensu stricto*, *B. garinii*, *B. afzelii*, and *B. valaisiana*—found in ticks.[53, 74] At the far western margin, in North America, only *B. burgdorferi sensu stricto* is indigenous.[53] At the far eastern margin of the range of its geographic distribution, in far eastern Russia and Japan, *B. burgdorferi sensu stricto* is absent but *B. garinii*, *B. afzelii*, and *B. japonica* are found[67, 69, 74, 163, 164]; in Japan, *B. tanukii* and *B. turdae* are also found.[58, 68] At the far northern, subarctic edge of the range in the northern hemisphere, only *B. garinii* has been found.[13, 152, 165] Co-infection of ticks with more

than one genospecies has been reported from areas in which several genospecies occur.[74, 84, 160]

Borrelia burgdorferi Reservoir Animal Infection Rates

North American epidemiologic studies indicate that the white-footed mouse, *Peromyscus leucopus*, is reservoir-competent for *B. burgdorferi*[580] and is in fact the most important reservoir for *B. burgdorferi* infection in nature,[167, 182] and that the white-tailed deer *Odocoileus virginianus* is the reproductive host of the *I. scapularis* tick vector and is necessary for the maintenance of the tick, but not the spirochete, in nature.[411]

In the northeastern part of the United States, the enzootic cycle that maintains *B. burgdorferi* infection in nature is the white-footed mouse–*I. scapularis* cycle. The mice are reservoir-competent for *B. burgdorferi*[336, 378, 578, 580] because they have a high rate of infection, remain spirochetemic and highly infectious for all stages of *I. scapularis* ticks throughout the tick feeding season, do not develop immunity to the tick vector and therefore do not reject the tick, and serve as the reservoir of *B. burgdorferi* that infects the next cycle of ticks and results in high tick infection rates.

The white-footed mouse is the most important reservoir for *B. burgdorferi* infection in nature, and it maintains the horizontal transmission of infection from nymphal to larval ticks. Because ticks are already infected with *B. burgdorferi* before deer attachment, the white-tailed deer does not appear to be important for transmission and maintenance of *B. burgdorferi* infection in nature, although they are important for maintenance and geographic dissemination of the tick.[167]

B. burgdorferi has been isolated from the blood of asymptomatic, wild, white-footed mice and white-tailed deer from the Lyme-endemic coastal islands of northeastern United States.[413, 578] The geographic distribution of infected mice has been noted to correlate with the areas of Lyme endemicity.[384] Mice were found to be chronically spirochetemic in nature during the spring, summer, and fall,[578] and were spirochetemic and infectious for ticks for more than 200 days after experimental infection with *B. burgdorferi*.[580] Deer were heavily infested by adult but not immature *I. scapularis* during the winter, suggesting that deer were important wintertime hosts for adult *I. scapularis*.[578] Although the deer were spirochetemic during summer, fall, and winter, and may be reservoirs for *B. burgdorferi*,[578] they are not major reservoirs for maintenance of *B. burgdorferi* in nature because they host mainly adult ticks that have a very low rate of transovarial transmission of the spirochete.[154, 167, 354]

In northwestern United States, the *I. pacificus* tick transmits Lyme borreliosis to humans, but the enzootic transmission cycle is different from that in northeastern United States.[378, 420] Because the preferred host of immature *Ixodes pacificus* is the fence lizard, which is not a competent reservoir for *B. burgdorferi*, the infection rate of *I. pacificus* is low (1 to 2%) and the *I. pacificus–Peromyscus* mouse cycle is unable to maintain transmission of the *B. burgdorferi* infection in nature; this is accomplished instead by *Ixodes neotomae*, a non–*ricinus* complex tick that has a 15% infection rate, and the dusky-footed woodrat, *Neotoma fuscipes*. *I. neotomae* and *I. pacificus* are both competent vectors for *B. burgdorferi*, but *I. neotomae* rarely bites humans and is needed only for maintenance of *B. burgdorferi* infection in the woodrat reservoir, which remains spirochetemic and is able to infect feeding ticks. *I. pacificus* nymphs and adult ticks are commonly associated with human tick bites, and they are needed to transfer infection from the woodrat to humans. These two ticks and the woodrat have the same geographic distribution, which extends from Oregon to Southern California and into the Sierra Nevada foothills, from sea level to 2100 meters elevation, where Lyme disease is endemic. The infection rate in woodrats in California was 44% and in *I. neotomae* was 15%.[378]

In some geographic areas of North America, other mammalian reservoir-tick cycles in addition to or instead of the mouse–*I. scapularis* cycle may contribute to maintenance of *B. burgdorferi* infection in nature, such as the cottontail rabbit–*I. dentatus* cycle in Nantucket[170] and New York,[100] the Norway rat–*I. scapularis* cycle on Monhegan Island, Maine (where no mice occur),[415] the *Peromyscus maniculatus*–*I. scapularis* cycle on Isle au Haut, Maine (where no *P. leucopus* occur),[414] the chipmunk–*I. scapularis* cycle in Wisconsin and Illinois,[416, 417] the squirrel–*I. scapularis* cycle in Connecticut and Wisconsin,[416] the woodrat–*I. neotomae* cycle in California,[378] the Mexican woodrat–*I. spinipalpis* cycle in Colorado,[362] the meadow vole–*I. scapularis* cycle in the Northeast,[168] and the cotton mouse–*Peromyscus gossypinus* cycle on Sapelo Island, Georgia.[361] The *B. burgdorferi* infection rate in some of these reservoir hosts may be as high as 90 to 100%, depending on the host species and geographic location. Seroepidemiologic studies found the rates of *B. burgdorferi* seropositivity in wild and domestic host animals in various geographic areas of the United States to be 10 to 100% in the northeastern states,[154, 169, 578] 5 to 60% in Wisconsin,[169, 416] 11% in North Carolina,[169] and 14 to 99% in Texas.[169, 382]

In Europe, in addition to the woodmouse–and yellow-necked mouse–*I. ricinus* cycle, which is considered to maintain *B. burgdorferi* infection in nature, other cycles such as the edible dormouse *Glis glis*–*I. ricinus* cycle in Germany,[581] the hedgehog–*I. hexagonus* cycle in Germany,[336] and the mouse–*I. trianguliceps* cycle in Central Europe[168] may be important. In a highly Lyme-endemic area of Germany, the edible dormouse is the preferred host of *I. ricinus*, even though the woodmouse and yellow-necked mouse are abundant, and it is considered more important in amplification of the human Lyme disease risk because these mice have a peridomestic rather than sylvan habitat.[581]

In Japan, the *I. persulcatus*–rodent (woodmouse and vole) and *I. persulcatus*–migratory bird enzootic cycles are responsible for maintenance of the *B. burgdorferi* infection in nature; *B. burgdorferi* has been isolated from woodmice[163] and voles,[68, 163] and from larval ticks that fed on migratory birds of the genera *Emberiza* and *Turdus*.[163]

B. burgdorferi infection has been demonstrated in 24 different species of mammals and birds.[167] It has even been found in migratory European seabirds, which may play a role both in transhemispheric transfer of infection and in maintenance of *B. garinii* in enzootic cycles of remote high-latitude northern and southern hemisphere islands and peninsulas.[165]

Serosurveys for the presence of *B. burgdorferi* antibody in sentinel animals such as white-tailed deer,[154, 578, 582] which usually have a travel range of less than 10 kilometers, and cattle[583] are useful in the definition of geographic areas of *I. scapularis* occurrence and *B. burgdorferi* endemicity.

PATHOLOGY AND PATHOGENESIS

Immunopathogenesis

Tissue damage or dysfunction is the result of either direct tissue invasion by *B. burgdorferi* or the immunopathologic immune response to the infection.[148, 149, 151, 204–207] Infection elicits a sequence of immunologic, B and T lymphocyte, and other cellular responses in activated antigen-presenting cells, and in various host tissues and organs, as is discussed in the section on Interactions with the Immune System, earlier in this chapter. These responses are the reaction to either live *B. burgdorferi*, degenerated dead organisms, degraded antigens, or even membrane-bound blebs (containing *B. burgdorferi* antigens on their surfaces and DNA fragments inside),[102, 103, 215] and they result in characteristic histopathologic findings.

Adhesion of *B. burgdorferi* to different host tissues and cells may be involved in tropism for various tissues and organs, and in the pathogenesis of the manifestations of Lyme disease in various organs.[150, 204, 297, 298, 585–587] Several different strains of all three genospecies, *B. burgdorferi sensu stricto*, *B. garinii*, and *B. afzelii*, bind to at least one of three mammalian cell integrins, $\alpha_{IIb}\beta_3$ (the fibrinogen receptor located on platelets), $\alpha_V\beta_3$ (the vitronectin receptor located on platelets, osteoclasts, smooth muscle, endothelial cells, and some lymphocytes), and $\alpha_5\beta_1$ (the fibronectin receptor located on epithelial cells, endothelial cells, fibroblasts, lymphocytes, and platelets); each strain has a distinct integrin recognition pattern.[585]

B. burgdorferi, Osp A, and even *B. burgdorferi* membrane blebs induce T lymphocyte proliferation in immune individuals,[208, 209, 211–213] and some groups have reported a nonspecific T lymphocyte proliferative effect, even in nonimmune individuals.[217] T lymphocyte populations in peripheral blood, synovial fluid, and CSF of patients with Lyme borreliosis are mainly of the type 1 helper (Th1) subset.[205, 214, 393] The responding T lymphocytes form inflammatory infiltrations in the synovium,[323, 370, 372, 393] central nervous system,[295, 592] and other tissues.

B. burgdorferi, Osp A, and membrane blebs also induce polyclonal B lymphocyte stimulation in immune and even in nonimmune individuals.[215, 216] The responding B lymphocytes differentiate into plasma cells and produce perivascular lymphoplasmacytic infiltrations and hypercellular vascular occlusive damage, resembling syphilitic endarteritis obliterans, in many involved tissues but primarily in the skin and soft tissues, heart, synovium, reticuloendothelial system, and peripheral nervous system. *B. burgdorferi* also induces macrophage production of cytokines (IL-6 and TNF-α)[216] and nitric oxide,[216, 296] as well as peripheral blood mononuclear cell production of IL-10.[217] The histopathology of Lyme borreliosis includes inflammatory infiltrates consisting of neutrophils, lymphocytes, plasma cells, and macrophages.

Changes in the expression of *B. burgdorferi* outer surface proteins (such as the downregulation of Osp A and B expression and the upregulation of Osp C, E, and F) and in Erp protein expression that occur either during tick feeding, with transmission of the spirochete to the bite site, or after entry of the spirochete into the mammalian host are important in the pathogenesis of the infection.[119, 121, 127, 128, 138–142] *B. burgdorferi* does not produce proteolytic enzymes, but its outer surface protein A is able to bind host blood meal–derived plasmin, plasminogen, and urokinase-type plasminogen activator, creating a host-derived bioactive surface protease, which is involved in dissemination of *B. burgdorferi* from the tick midgut to the tick salivary glands for transmission, and which is necessary for spirochetemia in mice after tick-transmitted infection.[146] It also presumably digests extracellular matrix and facilitates spirochetal spread in the skin after inoculation by the tick. Because of these bound host-derived enzymes, the spirochete is invisible to, and able to evade, the host immune response, in a mechanism referred to as "stealth pathogenesis."[144–146] This may explain the paradox of the ability of *B. burgdorferi* to persist in skin or other tissues for long periods of time with only minimal mononuclear cell infiltration, despite eliciting a strong immune response that, in vitro, is capable of killing it.

B. burgdorferi is introduced into the deep dermis via the bite of an infected tick, which produces a "tick papule" at the bite site. The spirochete induces expression of adhesion molecules by endothelial cells, which facilitate the spirochete's ability to cross endothelial cell layers and extravasate into tissues; this also leads to recruitment of inflammatory cells to areas of spirochetal infection.[145] Within several days to a few weeks, the organism migrates centrifugally in the skin, produces a local skin lesion (EM), and also enters the skin vasculature and disseminates hematogenously[280, 591] throughout the body to the skin, where it may produce secondary EM lesions, and to the organs and reticuloendothelial system, where it may produce a generalized flulike illness with fever, headache, myalgias, arthralgias, conjunctivitis, pharyngitis, adenopathy, tender hepatosplenomegaly, pneumonitis, and orchitis.[145, 393, 592] Some of the nonspecific symptoms occuring during infection, such as myalgia, arthralgia, fatigue, malaise, and fever, may be due to spirochetal triggering of host cell cytokine release.[151] Four to nine weeks after the initial hematogenous dissemination, spirochetal invasion of heart, central nervous system (CNS), and presumably peripheral nervous system may occur, producing myocarditis, meningoencephalitis, cranial nerve paresis, stupor, and personality changes.[588, 592] Months to years after infection, late manifestations of *B. burgdorferi* infection may develop as a result of the initial dissemination of *B. burgdorferi* to various organs, especially the skin, eye, joints, and nervous system.[592]

The manifestations of acute Lyme borreliosis are related to direct spirochetal invasion of the involved tissues and the resulting local immunohistopathologic response, and they are generally responsive to antibiotic therapy. The manifestations of late disease, if not previously treated with adequate antibiotic therapy, may be related to a combination of persistence of infection and the host immunohistopathologic response; these may respond to antibiotic therapy if the presence of active ongoing infection is the essential trigger of the pathologic response. The manifestations of late chronic disease, if resistant to repeated courses of antibiotic therapy considered adequate by current standards, are considered related to previous damage or to ongoing autoimmune immunopathologic responses induced by the initial infection.

Immunopathologic mechanisms, based on autoimmunity and molecular mimicry, may be involved in the pathogenesis of Lyme peripheral neuropathy and chronic Lyme arthritis, even after elimination of active *B. burgdorferi* infection.[126, 151, 204, 256, 323, 587, 589] An epitope of flagellin that cross reacts with an epitope at the N-terminal end of human axonal HSP 60 may be involved in the immunopathogenesis of peripheral nerve damage.[113, 151, 265] An arthritogenic epitope of Osp A, which cross reacts and shares homology with an epitope of human leukocyte function–associated antigen-1 (LFA-1), is a candidate autoantigen for chronic treatment-resistant Lyme arthritis in patients with HLA-DR4 specificity.[126, 323, 593] The phenomenon of epitope spreading, in which T cells initially recognize a single immunodominant epitope, and then progressively recognize an increasing number of nearby epitopes, could play a role in the immunopathogenesis of Lyme arthritis, if an arthritogenic epitope is eventually recognized, which results in overcoming of self-tolerance.[323]

Small numbers of *B. burgdorferi* may be visualized in some infected tissue samples, particularly skin biopsy specimens. Organisms are most easily found in early infection, but persistence of live *B. burgdorferi* for several years after onset of infection has also been demonstrated.[19, 200, 284, 304, 306, 594] *B. burgdorferi* PCR has also demonstrated *B. burgdorferi* DNA in tissue samples and body fluids but does not confirm the presence of viable spirochetes, as PCR will detect even *B. burgdorferi* DNA fragments in cystic blebs arising from spirochetal outpouchings.[102, 103, 186]

The histopathology of the various manifestations of Lyme borreliosis has been extensively studied, but only sparse data are available on the histopathology of congenital Lyme borreliosis. This section includes a description of the pathology of Lyme borreliosis by organ system, followed by a discussion on the pathology of the placenta and the congenitally infected fetus or infant.

Lyme Borreliosis in Pregnant and Nonpregnant Women

CUTANEOUS

A "tick papule" develops at the tick bite site, which consists of an ulcerated papule of partially denuded hyperplastic epithelium above a lymphocytic, plasmacytic, macrophage, and mast cell inflammatory infiltrate.[590] During an ixodid (hard) tick bite, the tick's salivary glands secrete a latex-like material that hardens to a tough tissue-like material and cements the mouthparts to the skin; the mouthparts have rows of "teeth" called *denticles*, which become embedded in the skin and the cement.[880] *B. burgdorferi* spirochetes have been detected in skin surrounding the bite site.

Erythema migrans (EM)[82, 148, 338, 592, 596, 597] occurs during early infection as either single (localized) or multiple (disseminated) skin lesions. The skin lesion contains upper and deep dermal perivascular and interstitial mononuclear cell infiltration. Spirochetes are found most often in the peripheral advancing edge of the EM lesion in areas with plasma cell infiltration, around and in small vessels, in collagen fibers, in the upper dermis, or at the dermal-epidermal junction.

Borrelial lymphocytoma (BL),[82, 592, 597] also known as lymphadenosis benigna cutis or B cell pseudolymphoma, occurs during early infection as either single (solitaria) or multiple (dispersa) skin lesions, usually on the earlobe or areola, and more often in Europe than the United States. The histopathology consists of hyperplastic and crowded, well-defined lymphoid follicles composed of dense, diffuse polyclonal lymphocytic (polyclonal B cells, helper T cells, or suppressor T cells), plasmacytic, macrophage, and occasionally eosinophilic infiltration in the dermis or subcutaneous tissue (sometimes with formation of germinal centers) that is similar in appearance to tonsillar tissue. Spirochetes are found in the subepidermal zone, in and around small blood vessels, and in collagen fibers in areas of inflammatory infiltration.

Acrodermatitis chronica atrophicans (ACA)[148, 592, 600–602] occurs during late chronic infection as either unilateral or symmetrical bilateral distal extremity skin lesions, more often in Europe than in the United States. The histopathology in the infiltrative phase shows epidermal loss of rete ridges, a subepidermal bandlike infiltrate, a dense patchy or interstitial mononuclear infiltration of the dermis and subcutaneous fat around and between blood vessels and skin appendages, a small fibrotic zone between the epidermis and the infiltrate, panniculitis, prominent dilated dermal blood vessels, endothelial proliferation, telangiectasia, and disappearance of elastin fibers; this progresses to eventual epidermal atrophy. Spirochetes can be found easily in these nodules and sparsely in ACA skin lesions.

RETICULOENDOTHELIAL

Splenitis,[590, 592, 604] hepatitis,[590, 605] and lymphadenitis[590, 592, 606] may occur during early infection.

Lymphadenopathy occurs in early infection, and lymph node histopathology ranges from perifollicular mononuclear cell (lymphocytic, plasmacytic, macrophage, and occasionally eosinophilic) infiltration and follicular hypertrophy, to focal necrotizing microabscesses with thrombosed capillaries; rare spirochetes may be seen.

Splenomegaly occurs in early infection, and splenic histopathology ranges from perifollicular lymphoplas-macytic infiltration with prominent germinal centers, to necrotizing splenitis with patchy subcapsular inflammation and suppuration, inflammation and acute central necrosis of splenic follicles, occasional destruction of blood vessels, and the presence of many spirochetes.

Hepatomegaly and hepatitis may occur in early infection and may be either transient or severe. Histopathology ranges from mild granulomatous hepatitis or lymphocytic portal triaditis to severe hepatocellular damage with ballooned hepatocytes, fat microvesicles, mononuclear (including plasmacytic) and granulocytic sinusoidal infiltration, Kupffer cell hyperplasia, marked hepatocyte mitotic activity, and sparse spirochetes in the hepatic sinusoids and parenchyma.

CARDIAC

Cardiac involvement[590, 592, 607] in early disseminated infection consists of tachycardia, varying degrees of heart block, or myocarditis. Histopathologic examination of endomyocardial biopsy (or autopsy) specimens shows perivascular and interstitial mononuclear cell (lymphocytic, plasmacytic, and macrophage) bandlike endocardial infiltration, myocardial infiltration, and occasionally pericardial infiltration, as well as vascular changes suggestive of early obliterative vasculopathy. Spirochetes may be seen in endocardium and myocardium near interstitial infiltrations and in intramyocardial vessels.[308]

NEUROLOGIC

The meningoencephalitis and meningoradiculoneuritis of early infection, which include meningitis, encephalopathy, psychoneurosis, cranial neuritis, radiculoneuritis, and the triad of cranial neuritis–meningitis–radiculoneuritis (Bannwarth's syndrome), have a common basic histopathology consisting of lymphoplasmacytic infiltration around epineural blood vessels,[82, 311, 590, 592, 609–611] which suggests vasculitis as a major pathophysiologic mechanism in neuroborreliosis. Rare spirochetes may be seen in brain tissue. Demonstration of spirochetes in CSF is very unusual.

The peripheral neuropathy of late chronic borreliosis[590, 592, 612] is more common in Europe than in the United States and is often associated with ACA. The histopathology of chronic peripheral neuropathy is similar to that of acute meningoradiculoneuritis but is more severe. Spirochetes have not been demonstrated in these biopsy specimens.

Acute focal encephalitis[267, 311, 610] with focal contrast-enhancing central nervous system lesions may develop during either early disseminated or late chronic infection. The histopathology of brain biopsy or autopsy specimens shows sharply demarcated areas of lymphocytic (and occasionally eosinophilic) perivascular cuffing, increased cellularity as a result of foamy macrophages and astrocytes, spongiform change with reactive astrocytes, and areas of necrosis and subcortical and periventricular loss of myelinated fibers, similar to an acute demyelinating process; only rare spirochetes are seen.

The pathogenesis of neuroborreliosis probably involves a small number of spirochetes, adhering to oligodendroglia in neural tissue, which elicit an intense local inflammatory immune response that produces the actual tissue damage; molecular mimicry may also be involved, as *B. burgdorferi* and axonal proteins have cross-reactive epitopes.[113, 151, 265]

Vasculitis is one of the major mechanisms involved in the pathogenesis of central nervous system neuroborreliosis.[311]

MUSCULOSKELETAL

Myositis,[592, 614–616] especially of proximal muscles, may occur in early disseminated infection, and localized myositis may occur adjacent to areas of cutaneous, articular, or neuropathic involvement.

Arthritis[82, 177, 205, 590, 618, 620] may be a manifestation of either early or late chronic infection. Histopathology consists of hypertrophy and hyperplasia of synovial lining cells; deposition of fibrin and neutrophils on synovial surfaces and villous stroma; synovial villous hypertrophy; diffuse or perivascular subsynovial mononuclear cell infiltration; subsynovial vascular proliferation; endarteritis obliterans; and even synovial pannus formation and cartilage erosion. Rare spirochetes are found in areas of heavy perivascular and subsynovial inflammatory infiltration but not in synovial fluid. The small number of spirochetes present is similar to tertiary syphilis or tuberculoid leprosy, in which a small number of organisms elicit an intense immunologic response.

The synovial histopathology of Lyme arthritis and other chronic inflammatory arthritides, including rheumatoid arthritis, is similar, but endarteritis obliterans is seen only in Lyme arthritis and syphilis, and not in other non-Lyme arthritis synovial biopsy specimens. There has also been evidence of active vascular injury consistent with repeated microvascular injuries, probably occurring with each episode of arthritis.[620]

The histopathology of the chronic arthritis associated with ACA[600] shows degenerative arthritis, joint capsule atrophy, bony atrophy, and cortical thickening.

Lyme Borreliosis in the Fetus and Newborn Infant

Although there have been a relatively small number (only 66) of reported cases that could be considered congenital Lyme borreliosis,[25, 27, 29–38, 41–48, 621] there are several reports of the pathologic findings. There are 13 descriptions of pathologic or culture findings in gestational Lyme disease placentas or decidua,[33–36, 41, 690, 622, 623] 19 descriptions of fetal or neonatal pathologic findings in congenital Lyme borreliosis, 2 descriptions of skin biopsies in congenital Lyme borreliosis, and 2 descriptions of brain pathologic and culture findings in sudden infant death syndrome of suspected Lyme borrelial etiology. Spirochetes have been found by culture, silver stain, or *B. burgdorferi*–specific IFA in autopsied organs (liver, spleen, bone marrow, heart, brain, kidney) of congenitally infected fetuses and neonates by Schlesinger and associates,[25] MacDonald and colleagues,[33–35] Lavoie and co-workers,[32] and Weber and associates,[38, 39] as well as in the skin biopsy of a congenitally infected infant by Trevisan and colleagues.[43]

It is striking that many of the late stillbirths and perinatal deaths occurred in infants with cardiac abnormalities and generalized spirochetosis involving the kidneys, reticuloendothelial system, and central nervous system, after first-trimester gestational Lyme disease, and that most of the miscarriages studied pathologically occurred late, between 15 and 25 weeks. The lack of inflammatory findings even when spirochetes were present has been remarkable, and could be related to the immunopathogenetic features of *B. burgdorferi* infection, in which the spirochete is able to spread and persist in tissues without eliciting a prominent host immune response (discussion of this is in the sections Pathology and Pathogenesis: Immunopathogenesis, and The Organism: Interactions with the Immune System: Evasion of Host Defenses and Persistence in Tissue).

Although relatively few cases of congenital Lyme borreliosis have been studied pathologically, comparisons with congenital syphilis may be appropriate, particularly as congenital syphilis causes late abortion, stillbirth, and early perinatal death, and the histopathology shows perivascular and interstitial inflammation, including endarteritis obliterans, of the reticuloendothelial system, nervous system, skeletal system, and placenta.

The histopathologic findings of patients with congenital Lyme borreliosis listed in Table 11–8 in the section Clinical Manifestations are described by organ system in Table 11–9.

CUTANEOUS

There are no reports on the histopathology of the skin of fatal cases of early congenital Lyme disease, but skin biopsy of a patient with infantile multisystem inflammatory disease who was considered to have congenital Lyme disease showed vasculitis with stromal edema and marked eosinophilia (patient 40, see Table 11–8).[31] Biopsy of a skin lesion of a 9-year-old child with congenital Lyme borreliosis (patient 51, see Table 11–8), with a history of recurrent multiple EM lesions since 3 weeks of age, showed a normal epidermis; superficial and deep perivascular, periadnexal, and interstitial lymphocytic infiltrates with sparse plasma cells and some neutrophils; and numerous *Borreliae* by Warthin-Starry silver stain visible in the epidermis and dermis; *B. burgdorferi* PCR of the biopsy material was positive.[43]

RETICULOENDOTHELIAL

Spirochetes have been found in liver, spleen, or bone marrow of six fetuses or infants with congenital Lyme borreliosis in the absence of inflammation, necrosis, or granuloma formation. Spirochetes were seen by silver stain, *B. burgdorferi*–specific IFA stain, or culture in the livers of two term infants (patients 2 and 22, see Table 11–8) and in the spleen and bone marrow of one 35-week, slightly premature infant (patient 1, see Table 11–8) with severe fatal early congenital Lyme borreliosis after first-trimester gestational Lyme disease.[25, 33–35, 38, 39] The spirochetes were seen in the lumen of a large

Text continued on page 561

TABLE 11–8

Congenital Lyme Borreliosis: 66 Adverse Outcomes of Pregnancies Complicated by Lyme Borreliosis (LB)

| PATIENT NO. | MATERNAL GESTATIONAL | | | | FETAL/NEONATAL | | | | |
	Trimester of LB	Clinical History[b]	Antibiotic Therapy No. Days[c]	LB Serology[d]	Gestational Age (wk)	Weight (g)	Antibiotic Therapy No. Days[c]	LB Serology[d]	Tissue Borrelia[f]
1	1	EM,Fl,Ar	−	+	35	3000	−		+H,S,K,BM
2	1	EM,Ar	−	+	40	2500			+L,H,K,AB
3	≤2	Tx	−	−	19	514			+L,P
4	≤2	Tx,Ar	−	−	23	490			+L,K
5	≤2	O	−	−	15	85			+L,P
6	≤1	VB	NA[a]	NA	39	2250	NA		+F
7	NA	O	NA	NA	40	1950	NA		+F
8	≤2	VB	NA	−	17	30			+B
9	≤2	VB	NA	−	16	150			+B
10	≤1	O	NA	NA	12	294			+K
11	≤2	Ar	−	−	25	NA			+F
12	NA	O	−	NA	~40	3746	+ IV		+P
13	NA	Tx	−	NA	37	2157	+ IVPN, IVMT		+P
14	1	EM,Ar	+ PO PN 10 d	+	20	NA			−
15	1	BP,Ar	−	NA	36	2100	NA		
16	2	EM,Ar	+ PO ER 10 d PO PN 10 d	NA	NA	NA	NA		
17	2	EM	+ PO PN 10 d	NA	40	NA	NA	−	
18	3	EM,Me	−	NA	40	NA	+ IVPN 10 d		
19	1	LB	+	+	13	NA			−
20	1	LB	+	+	NA	NA	NA		
21	≤1	Ar	−	−	~40	NA	NA		+B,H
22	1	EM	+ PO PN 7 d	+	40	3400	NA		+L,B
23	1	EM,Fl	+ IV CTX 2 d, PO PN 12 d	+(+LPA[e])	40	3461	+ IVCTX 14 d	−(+LPA)[e]	
24	2	Fl	+ PO AM 10 d	−(−LPA[e])	34	1050	+ IVAM 6 d, IVCTX 7 d	+(+LPA)[e]	
25	1	EM,Pn,Ar	+ PO ER 10 d, IV CFX 5 d, PO CFC/CEP/ CFM 39 d	+(+LPA[e])	37	3490	+ IVAM 5 d, IVCFT/CTX 3 d	−(+LPA)[e]	
26	2	EM,Ar	+ PO ER 10 d, PO CFM 49 d	−(+LPA[e])	40	3461	+ IVCTX 28 d	−(+LPA)[e]	
27	1	EM,Ar	−	+	NA	NA	NA	−	
28	NA	NA	NA	+	NA	NA	NA	−	
29	NA	NA	NA	+	NA	NA	NA	−	
30	NA	NA	NA	+	NA	NA	NA	−	
31	NA	NA	NA	+	NA	NA	NA	−	
32	NA	NA	NA	+	NA	NA	NA	−	
33	NA	NA	NA	+	NA	NA	NA	−	

[a]NA, information not available.

[b]O = unremarkable; EM = erythema migrans; Fl = flulike illness; Ar = arthralgia/arthritis; BP = Bell's palsy; Me = meningoencephalitis; Cr = cranial neuritis; Ra = radiculitis; HA = headache; LB = Lyme borreliosis, unspecified; Pn = pneumonia; Tx = toxemia; VB = vaginal bleed.

[c]PO = oral; IV = intravenous; PN = penicillin; ER = erythromycin; CTX = ceftriaxone; CFX = cefuroxime; CFC = cefaclor; CEP = cephalexin; CFM = cefixime; CFT = cefotaxime; CDX = cefadroxil; MT = metronidazole; AM = ampicillin; NA = not available (use of antibiotic therapy could not be definitively established for the individual patient, although in some reports, some patients in the group may have been treated).

[d]Borrelia burgdorferi antibody detected either by IFA (immunofluorescence assay), ELISA (enzyme-linked immunosorbent assay), or WB (Western immunoblot).

[e]LPA = in vitro lymphocyte proliferative assay for B. burgdorferi.

[f]Borrelia detected in tissue samples by IFA, silver stain, culture, or PCR (polymerase chain reaction); H = heart; S = spleen; K = kidney; BM = bone marrow; L = liver; A = adrenal; B = brain; Sk = skin; P = placenta; F = fetal tissue unspecified; D = decidua.

[g]CoA = coarctation aorta; EFE = endocardial fibroelastosis; AS = aortic stenosis; LSVC = left superior vena cava; PDA = patent ductus arteriosus; VSD = ventricular septal defect; ASD = atrial septal defect; RD = respiratory distress; IUGR = intrauterine growth retardation; GR = growth retardation; DD = developmental delay; GER = gastroesophageal reflux; TEF = tracheoesophageal fistula; BIH = bilateral inguinal hernia.

[h]21 of 23 (91.3%) of patients with LB in this subgroup received antibiotic therapy, but individual outcomes of the two untreated pregnancies were not specifically identified.

CLINICAL OUTCOME[g]	REFERENCE
CoA, EFE, AS, LSVC, PDA, cardiac dysfunction, RD, death 39 hours	25, 33
IUGR, VSD, stillbirth	33–35
ASD, stillbirth	33, 34
CoA, stillbirth	33, 34
Miscarriage	33, 34
VSD, hydrocephalus, omphalocele, clubfoot, meningomyelocele, RD, death 4 hours	33
IUGR, absent hemidiaphragm, RD, cardiac dysfunction, VSD, death 30 min	33
Hydrocephalus, miscarriage	33
Miscarriage	33
Miscarriage	33
VSD, miscarriage	33
R/O sepsis, RD	33
R/O sepsis, RD, hypoglycemia, fever	33
Miscarriage	36
Prematurity, hyperbilirubinemia	36
Syndactyly	36
DD, cortical blindness	28, 36
Rash, hyperbilirubinemia	36
Miscarriage	29
Syndactyly	29
Cardiac dysfunction, aortic thrombosis, lethargy, hypertension, acidosis, death 8 days	32
RD, death 23 hours	38, 39
Rash, adenopathy	621
IUGR, cardiomyopathy, PDA, R/O sepsis, RD, rash, adenopathy, hepatomegaly, hyperbilirubinemia, meconium ileus, metaphyscal bands, joint contractures, R/O encephalitis	621
R/O sepsis, rash, hepatomegaly, hyperbilirubinemia, metaphyseal bands, pectus excavatum, R/O encephalitis, hypotonia, hemiparesis, eso/exotropia, dysphagia, GER, BIH, facial/ear dysmorphia, unilateral simian crease, GR, DD, dental anomalies	621
Hyperbilirubinemia, retinal lesions, R/O meningoencephalitis	621
VSD	37
Hyperbilirubinemia	37
Hyperbilirubinemia	37
Hypotonia	37
IUGR	37
Macrocephaly	37
Supraventricular extrasystoles	37

Table continued on following page

TABLE 11–8

Congenital Lyme Borreliosis: 66 Adverse Outcomes of Pregnancies Complicated by Lyme Borreliosis (LB) *Continued*

| PATIENT NO. | MATERNAL GESTATIONAL | | | | FETAL/NEONATAL | | | | |
	Trimester of LB	Clinical History[b]	Antibiotic Therapy No. Days[c]	LB Serology[d]	Gestational Age (wk)	Weight (g)	Antibiotic Therapy No. Days[c]	LB Serology[d]	Tissue *Borrelia*[f]
34	≤1	NA	–	+	11	NA			
35	≤1	NA	+	+	9	NA			
36	≤1	NA	–	+	9	NA			
37	≤1	NA	NA	+	10	NA			
38	≤1	NA	–	+	10	NA			
39	≤1	NA	NA	+	8	NA			
40	NA	NA	NA	NA	37	2150	NA	+	
41	NA	O	–	+	NA	NA			
42	≤1	LB	NA[h]	NA	NA	NA	NA	–	
43	≤1	LB	NA[h]	NA	NA	NA	NA	–	
44	NA	LB	+	NA	NA	NA	NA	–	
45	NA	O	NA	NA	NA	NA	NA	+	
46	2	EM,Ar	+	+	33	1450	NA	–	–
47	NA	NA	NA	+	NA	NA	NA	+	
48	NA	NA	NA	+	NA	NA	NA	+	
49	NA	NA	NA	+	NA	NA	NA	+	
50	NA	O	–	+	39	NA	–	–	+Sk
51	1	EM	NA	–	40	3160	–	–	
52	2	EM	+ IV PNx14 d	–	40	2700	–	NA	
53	2	EM	+ IV PNx14 d	–	40	3500	–	–	
54	3	EM,Fl	+ IV PNx14 d	+	40	3650	–	+	
55	2	EM	+ IV PNx14 d	+	40	2920	–	–	
56	NA	EM,Fl,Ar, Cr,Ra	–	+	NA	NA	NA	+	
57	≤2	O	–	+	28	1030	NA		
58	NA	O	–	+	37	2125	NA		
59	2	EM	+ IV CTXx14 d	NA	26	840	NA		
60	2	EM,Ar	+ IV CTXx14 d	NA	36	2940	NA		
61	3	persistent EM	+ PO CDXx14 d, IV CTXx13 d	NA	40	NA	NA		
62	1	EM,Fl,HA, Ar	+ IV CTXx14 d	–	9	NA	NA		
63	NA	EM	NA						
64	NA	EM	NA						
65	≤2	EM	NA	+	15	NA			+D
66	≤2	EM	NA	+	18	NA			

CLINICAL OUTCOME[g]	REFERENCE
Miscarriage	27
Miscarriage	27
Miscarriage	27
Miscarriage	27
Miscarriage	27
Miscarriage	27
Cardiac hypertrophy, fever, rash, adenopathy, hepatosplenomegaly, chronic arthritis, chronic meningoencephalitis, macrocephaly, exophthalmos, blepharitis, GR, DD	31
Miscarriage	30
Neonatal death, multiple congenital cardiac defects	46
Hydrocele, laryngomalacia	46
Hypospadias	46
Cryptorchidism	46
RD, anemia	26
Metatarsus adductus	45
GER	45
Multiple major anomalies (vertebral defects, radial dysplasia, imperforate anus, TEF, renal dysplasia)	45
Chronic relapsing multiple annular erythema, fever, generalized lymphadenopathy	43
PDA at 1 year	41, 42
Cryptorchidism	42
Hypoplastic dental enamel	41, 42
Hypoplastic dental enamel	41, 42
DD	42
Huge sacral hemangioma, gluteal atrophy, general weakness, recurrent fever, minor mental abnormalities	44
Preterm, acute chorioamnionitis and funisitis, 5 min Apgar 7 (+ *Staphylococcus aureus* on fetal placental surface)	47
IUGR, 5 min Apgar 5 (+maternal drug abuse)	47
RD	48
RD, pneumothorax, ASD, VSD	48
Bilateral ureteral stenosis and hydronephrosis	48
Missed abortion	48
Hyperbilirubinemia	41
Hypotrophic infant	41
Fetal death at 15 weeks	41
Induced abortion; hydrocephalus and spina bifida	41

TABLE 11–9
Clinical Symptoms of Lyme Borreliosis, by Organ System Involved

SITE	CLINICAL DIAGNOSIS	SYMPTOMS
Systemic	Dissemination of spirochetes	Fever, sore throat, conjunctival injection, malaise, fatigue, myalgias, arthralgias, headache, meningismus, generalized adenopathy
Skin	Erythema migrans (single or multiple)	Expanding erythematous bull's-eye, or diffuse maculopapular rash
	Borrelial lymphocytoma (single or multiple)	Bluish nodule on earlobe or areola
	Acrodermatitis chronica atrophicans	Violaceous doughy distal extremity rash, later atrophic skin overlying subluxed joint with associated peripheral neuropathy and chronic arthritis
	Septal panniculitis	Skin lesions resembling erythema nodosum
Heart	Fluctuating heart block	Syncope, dizziness, chest pain, palpitations
	Myopericarditis, pancarditis	Arrhythmia, chest pain, acute heart failure
	Chronic cardiomyopathy	Chronic heart failure
Nervous system	Meningitis (acute or chronic)	Headache, meningismus
	Cranial and peripheral neuropathy (acute or chronic) and Bannwarth's syndrome (meningopolyneuritis)	Facial palsy (Bell's), other cranial nerve palsy, paresthesia/hyperesthesia, paresis, radicular pain, carpal tunnel syndrome
	Encephalopathy (acute or chronic)	Disturbance of sleep, mood, memory, or personality; neuropsychiatric disorders, including psychosis, schizophrenia, paranoia, depression, anorexia
	Multifocal encephalomyelitis (acute or chronic)	Spastic paraparesis, hemiparesis, ataxia, aphasia, apraxia, dementia, focal neurologic deficits, meningovasculitis, leukoencephalitis, mononeuritis multiplex, cerebellar ataxia, Guillain-Barré, transverse myelitis
Musculoskeletal system	Arthralgia/arthritis	Intermittent monarticular or oligoarticular asymmetrical migratory joint pain, with swelling and warmth, but no erythema; may become chronic with joint space narrowing, bone cysts, cartilage loss, bone erosion
	Ruptured Baker's cyst	Sudden popliteal pain and swelling
	Temporomandibular joint arthritis	Temporomandibular joint syndrome
	Myositis	Muscle pain, swelling
Reticuloendothelial system	Lymphadenitis (regional or generalized)	Lymphadenopathy
	Hepatitis	Tender hepatomegaly, elevated hepatocellular enzymes
	Splenitis	Tender splenomegaly
Genitourinary system	Bladder neuropathy	Urinary retention, hydronephrosis
Eye	Conjunctivitis, interstitial keratitis, nodular episcleritis, panophthalmitis, uveitis, pars planitis, iridocyclitis, choroiditis, vitritis, retinitis, cranial and peripheral nerve palsies, pseudotumor cerebri, papilledema, optic neuritis/atrophy, orbital myositis	Conjunctival injection, visual disturbances, ocular pain, decreased vision/blindness, Horner's syndrome, Argyll Robertson pupil, extraocular muscle paresis
Ear	Auditory neuritis	Otalgia; tinnitus; acute, intermittent, or progressive neuronal hearing loss

hepatic vein in one case. *B. burgdorferi* was also found by IFA in the livers of three fetuses miscarried at 15, 19, and 23 weeks, respectively (patients 5, 3, and 4, see Table 11–8), without definite histories of gestational Lyme disease.[33, 34] The histopathology of a lymph node biopsy of a patient with infantile multisystem inflammatory disease considered to have congenital Lyme borreliosis (patient 40, see Table 11–8) showed acute lymphadenitis with follicle hyperplasia.[31]

PULMONARY

Histopathologic examination of the lungs in one term baby with severe fatal early congenital Lyme borreliosis after first-trimester gestational Lyme disease showed microscopic edema and extreme congestion but no inflammation, and no spirochetes were seen (patient 22, see Table 11–8).[38, 39]

CARDIAC

Cardiac histopathology has been reported for 11 infants or fetuses with congenital Lyme borreliosis. Major cardiac malformations were found in 12 infants, and spirochetes were found in the heart in 3, and in other or unspecified fetal tissues in 4 of these cases, in the absence of associated inflammatory findings.

Major cardiac malformations were seen in seven term or near-term infants with congenital Lyme borreliosis (four fatal and three nonfatal) following first-trimester, or in one case, early second-trimester (15 to 19 weeks) gestational Lyme disease during the period of cardiac organogenesis (patients 1, 2, 6, 27, 42, 51, and 60, see Table 11–8),[25, 33–35, 37, 42, 46, 48] and *B. burgdorferi* spirochetes were found by IFA in the myocardium of two of these infants (patients 1 and 2).[33, 35] The malformations consisted of aortic coarctation, endocardial fibroelastosis, persistent left superior vena cava, patent ductus arteriosus, and aortic stenosis in one 35-week, slightly premature infant (patient 1)[25, 33]; ventriculoseptal defects in three term infants (patients 2, 6, and 27)[33–35, 37]; a persistent patent ductus arteriosus in one term infant (patient 51)[41, 42]; atrial and ventricular septal defects in a 36-week, slightly premature infant (patient 60)[48]; and multiple unspecified fatal congenital cardiac defects in another infant (patient 42).[40, 46]

Spirochetes were found in either the myocardium or unspecified tissue of two additional term babies who died of early congenital Lyme borreliosis. One had a large ventriculoseptal defect and no known history of gestational Lyme disease (patient 7),[33] and the other had myocardial dysfunction but no malformation, following gestational Lyme disease of unspecified trimester (patient 21).[32]

Cardiac malformations were also found in three fetuses miscarried at 15, 23, and 25 weeks, respectively, with congenital Lyme borreliosis but no definite history of gestational Lyme disease (patients 3 and 4),[33, 34] although one mother had arthritis (patient 11),[33] and in one 34-week infant with nonfatal congenital Lyme borreliosis after second-trimester gestational Lyme disease (patient 24)[621]; these consisted of an atrial septal defect (patient 3), aortic coarctation (patient 4), a ventriculoseptal defect (patient 11), and patent ductus arteriosus (patient 24).

NEUROLOGIC

Neuropathology has been described in seven fetuses or infants with fatal congenital Lyme borreliosis, and spirochetes were found in the brain tissue of five of these and in unspecified fetal tissue in one, using silver staining, IFA staining, or culture, without evidence of inflammation even in areas where spirochetes were found. *B. burgdorferi* was found in the brain parenchyma, meninges, or subarachnoid space in two term infants after first-trimester gestational Lyme disease (patients 2 and 22),[33–35, 38, 39] in the frontal cerebral cortex of another term infant after gestational Lyme disease of unspecified trimester (patient 21),[32] and in the brain of a 16-week miscarried fetus with no history of gestational Lyme disease (patient 9).[33]

Three infants had either structural or histopathologic abnormalities. Patient 22 had minor histopathologic findings that could have been related to either the congenital infection or birth trauma; these consisted of small perivenous hemorrhages with aggregates of leukocytes in the pons, small infratentorial hemorrhages, and cerebral edema and congestion, with no significant inflammation.[38, 39] One term infant had hydrocephalus and spirochetes in unspecified fetal tissue following probable first-trimester infection (patient 6),[33] one 17-week miscarried fetus had hydrocephalus and *B. burgdorferi* in fetal brain tissue (patient 8),[33] and one 18-week fetus had hydrocephalus and spina bifida.[41]

MacDonald retrospectively described spirochetes consistent with *B. burgdorferi* in autopsy sections of brain from 2 of 10 infants who died of sudden infant death syndrome in a highly Lyme-endemic area; there was no inflammation in the tissues containing the spirochetes.[33]

MUSCULOSKELETAL

Musculoskeletal abnormalities have been found in five term or near-term infants with congenital Lyme borreliosis. Abnormalities in two term infants with fatal congenital Lyme borreliosis but no definite history of gestational Lyme disease consisted of clubfoot, spina bifida with meningomyelocele, and omphalocele in one (patient 6),[33] and absent left hemidiaphragm in the other (patient 7)[33]; spirochetes were seen in unspecified fetal tissues. In addition, syndactyly has been reported in two term infants who survived after first- or second-trimester gestational Lyme disease (patients 16 and 20)[29, 36]; metatarsus adductus (patient 47)[45] and multiple major anomalies, including vertebral defects and radial dysplasia (patient 49),[45] have been reported in infants of seropositive mothers without histories of previous Lyme disease.[45] An infant (patient 56),[44] born after severe gestational Lyme disease (trimester unspecified but of long duration, with progression from EM to arthritis and neuroborreliosis), had a sacral hemangioma, gluteal atrophy, and general weakness; another infant (patient 25),[621] born after prolonged gestational Lyme disease (first-trimester EM with progression to arthritis), had pectus excavatum and hypotonia. Another (patient 24),[621] born after early second-trimester infection, had joint contractures.

GENITOURINARY

Renal histopathology has been reported in five fetuses or infants with fatal congenital Lyme borreliosis. Spirochetes were found by silver staining, IFA staining, or culture (without inflammation) in the kidney in all five, including two term infants (patients 2 and 22)[33–35, 38, 39] and one 35-week premature infant (patient 1),[25] born after first-trimester gestational Lyme disease, as well as two fetuses who were miscarried or stillborn at 12 weeks (patient 10)[33] and 23 weeks (patient 4),[33, 34] with no definite history of gestational Lyme disease. Spirochetes were also found in the neonatal adrenal in one of the term infants (patient 2). Renal dysplasia was reported in an infant (patient 49) with other major congenital anomalies, born to a seropositive asymptomatic mother. Inguinal hernias were found in a 37-week infant who survived following first-trimester gestational Lyme disease (patient 25).[621] Bilateral ureteral stenosis and hydronephrosis were reported in an infant (patient 61)[48] after third-trimester gestational Lyme borreliosis with persistent EM. Cryptorchidism was found in two infants (patients 45 and 52)[42, 46]—one born after second-trimester gestational Lyme disease, and the other to an asymptomatic seropositive mother. Hypospadias was found in one infant (patient 44),[46] born after gestational Lyme disease of unspecified trimester, and hydrocele was found in another (patient 43),[46] born after first-trimester Lyme disease.

INFANTILE MULTISYSTEM INFLAMMATORY DISEASE

Although the etiology of neonatal or infantile multisystem inflammatory disease[624] (a persistent inflammation of skin, synovia, lymph nodes, eyes, and the central nervous system) is unclear, 1 of 14 reported patients with this syndrome has been considered most likely to have congenital Lyme disease.[31] The histopathology[625] of skin, lymph nodes, and synovia has been reported in several of these patients and consists of chronic perivascular granulocytic, mast cell, and especially eosinophilic, inflammatory infiltration of skin, lymph nodes, synovia, and muscle, and granulocytic (including eosinophilic) meningeal inflammation. Muscle atrophy associated with the inflammatory infiltration has also been seen.

PLACENTA

The placental histopathology associated with gestational Lyme borreliosis has been reported only occasionally.[33–36, 590, 622, 623] Some of the placentas described were associated with normal fetal and neonatal outcomes; others were associated with infants with congenital Lyme borreliosis (included in Table 11–14 in the section Clinical Manifestations).

MacDonald and colleagues[33–35] described seven placentas associated with gestational Lyme borreliosis. Spirochetes were grown from one placenta and were seen by silver staining or identified as B. burgdorferi by IFA staining in placental tissues or villi from six placentas, in the absence of inflammation or other placental abnormalities (except for rare plasma cells in the placental villi of one placenta); this lack of inflammation despite the presence of spirochetes was remarkable. Spirochetes were demonstrated in the placentas of two women with 15-week and 19-week miscarriages with no history of gestational Lyme disease (patients 3 and 5, see Table 11–8), in one woman with a term stillbirth after untreated first-trimester gestational Lyme disease (patient 2, see Table 11–8), in two women with term or near-term infants with severe early congenital Lyme disease with no history of gestational Lyme disease (patients 12 and 13, see Table 11–8), and in one woman with treated second-trimester and untreated third-trimester Lyme disease who delivered a normal term infant, who was treated with antibiotics after delivery. A term placenta, from a gestation complicated by second-trimester Lyme disease and treated with intravenous antibiotic therapy, had no spirochetes detectable.

Markowitz and colleagues[36] described a placenta with hypoperfusion, immaturity, syncytial and cytotrophoblastic features, and autolytic membrane changes (but no inflammation or nodularity), associated with a 20-week miscarriage following first-trimester–treated gestational Lyme disease (patient 14, see Table 11–8), but found no spirochetes by either culture or IFA. Duray and Steere[590] reported that in maternal gestational Lyme disease, the placental chorionic villi had increased Hofbauer cells as in syphilitic placentitis. Mikkelsen and Palle[622] reported a normal placenta following last-trimester–treated gestational Lyme disease.

Placental histopathology of two of my cases of congenital Lyme borreliosis consisted of focal acute chorioamnionitis, focal calcification, marked congestion, and a 2.5-cm subchorionic nodular infarct in one term placenta following first-trimester–treated Lyme disease (patient 23, see Table 11–8), as well as focal chorionic villous edema, chronic fibrosing villitis, fibrin deposition between villi, syncytial knots, and marked congestion in the other 34-week placenta following second-trimester–treated gestational Lyme disease (patient 24, see Table 11–8).

The histopathology of one placenta associated with neonatal multisystem inflammatory disease[626] showed thickened thrombotic vessels and subchorionic and intrachorionic calcification; this is of interest because 1 of 14 patients with this syndrome was considered to have congenital Lyme borreliosis.[31]

Hercogova and colleagues[41] reported that Borrelia-like spirochetes, visualized by staining with specific monoclonal antibody against B. burgdorferi flagellin, were found in a placenta evaluated after an intrauterine fetal death at 15 weeks in a pregnancy complicated by EM, but no description of the histopathology was given. Figueroa and colleagues[623] reported that spirochetes were demonstrated in the villi and intervillous maternal space in 3 of 60 placentas of asymptomatic B. burgdorferi ELISA–seropositive/equivocal, syphilis-negative women;

spirochetes in two of these placentas were identified as *B. burgdorferi* by PCR, and identification was not done in the other. There was no correlation of pregnancy outcome with presence or absence of these spirochetes, and no information was given regarding any antibiotic therapy; therefore, the significance of this observation is uncertain.

Thus, in the small number of gestational Lyme borreliosis placentas described, rare spirochetes may be found, and the histopathology may be either normal or abnormal. The focal chronic fibrosing villitis, nodular subchorionic infarcts, focal calcification, fibrin deposition between chorionic villi, syncytial and trophoblastic features, and the suggestion of perivascular lymphoplasmacytic infiltrations are reminiscent of the pathology of syphilitic placentitis, just as the basic histopathologic lesion of Lyme disease, lymphoplasmacytic perivascular infiltration with vasculopathic damage, shows similarities with syphilis. A larger number of placentas must be studied histologically, using silver and *B. burgdorferi*-specific IFA stains, and possibly with PCR and culture, before a definitive description of placental pathology in gestational Lyme borreliosis is to emerge.

Other Congenital Borrelial Infections

RELAPSING FEVER

The other human borrelioses, tickborne and louseborne gestational relapsing fever, caused by *B. hermsii*, *B. duttonii*, and related *Borrelia* strains, may also result in congenital infection[627, 628] and have been described more extensively than congenital Lyme borreliosis.

The placental histopathology in congenital relapsing fever has only rarely been reported[627] and consists of abundant spirochetes seen in placental villous capillaries, both on the fetal side of the circulation and in the umbilical vessels. The histopathology of the congenitally infected fetus has also rarely been reported[628] and shows mononuclear and occasional neutrophil inflammatory infiltration of the meninges, miliary splenic lesions consisting of liquefaction necrosis of the white pulp, hypertrophy of Kupffer cells in the liver, and hemorrhagic lesions in the skin, subepicardium, and brain. Abundant spirochetes have been found in spleen, liver, and brain.

Leptospirosis, although not tickborne or borrelial, is another nonsyphilitic spirochetosis capable of causing occasional congenital infection with some similarities to Lyme borreliosis. Sixteen cases, many with fetal and placental histopathology, are summarized in an excellent review.[629]

CLINICAL MANIFESTATIONS

Lyme borreliosis is a multisystem infection with a variety of clinical manifestations that may change with time as the infection progresses; these may be modified by antibiotic therapy and by patient immune responses. It has many similarities to another human spirochetosis—syphilis—because of its ability to persist in body tissues for long periods of time, its association with both early and late stages of infection, including neuroborreliosis, and its ability to produce a wide range of symptoms.[98, 206, 290]

Case Definition and Classification of Stages of Lyme Borreliosis

The case definitions of Lyme borreliosis used by the CDC[633] for epidemiologic purposes to follow the geographic spread of the infection in the United States are given in Table 11–10; although they were not initially intended for use in patient care situations, they have proven useful in standardizing criteria for the disease. Clinical case definitions of the main presentations of European Lyme borreliosis were developed by the European Union Concerted Action of Risk Assessment in Lyme Borreliosis (EUCALB)[8, 502] by consensus agreement of representatives from many European countries, to standardize criteria for reporting of Lyme borreliosis, to facilitate clinical management of Lyme borreliosis, and to more fully define the broad spectrum of the disease in different European countries (Table 11–11).

TABLE 11–10
CDC Lyme Disease Case Definition for Public Health Surveillance Purposes[a]

ERYTHEMA MIGRANS

Single primary red macule or papule, expanding for days to weeks to large round lesion ≥5 cm diameter (physician-confirmed), +/− central clearing, +/− secondary lesions, +/− systemic symptoms (fever, fatigue, headache, mild neck stiffness, arthralgia, myalgia)

plus

Known exposure ≤30 days before onset to an endemic area (in which ≥2 confirmed cases have been acquired, or in which *B. burgdorferi*-infected tick vectors are established)

or

One or more late manifestations without other etiology:

1. Musculoskeletal
   —Recurrent brief episodes of monarticular or pauciarticular arthritis with objective joint swelling, +/− chronic arthritis
2. Neurologic
   —Lymphocytic meningitis, facial palsy, other cranial neuritis, radiculoneuropathy, encephalomyelitis (confirmed by CSF *B. burgdorferi* antibody > serum *B. burgdorferi* antibody)
3. Cardiovascular
   —Acute second- or third-degree atrioventricular conduction defects, lasting days to weeks, +/− myocarditis

plus

Laboratory confirmation by either:

1. Isolation of *B. burgdorferi* from patient specimen
2. Diagnostic levels of *B. burgdorferi* IgM or IgG antibodies in serum or CSF (initial ELISA or IFA screen followed by Western blot of positive or equivocal results)

CSF = cerebrospinal fluid; ELISA = enzyme-linked immunosorbent assay; IFA = immunofluorescence assay.
[a]Adapted from Centers for Disease Control. MMWR 46(RR):20–21, 1997.[633]

TABLE 11–11
EUCALB Lyme Borreliosis Clinical Case Definitions[a]

Erythema migrans
Macule or papule, expanding for days to weeks to a red or blue-red patch, usually but not always ≥5 cm diameter, +/− central clearing, +/− secondary lesions, +/− systemic symptoms of fever, fatigue, headache, mild neck stiffness, arthralgia, myalgia (laboratory confirmation not required)[b]

or

Borrelial lymphocytoma
Blue-red painless nodule or plaque, usually on earlobe/pinna, nipples, or scrotum (confirmed by diagnostic change of *Bb*[c] serum antibody)[b]

or

Acrodermatitis chronica atrophicans
Chronic red or blue-red lesion, +/− initial doughy swelling, eventual atrophy, usually on extensor surface of distal extremity, +/− induration over bony prominences (confirmed by high *Bb* serum IgG antibody)[b]

or

Early neuroborreliosis
Painful meningoradiculoneuritis (Garin-Bujardoux-Bannwarth syndrome), lymphocytic meningitis, facial palsy, other cranial neuritis (confirmed by cerebrospinal fluid (CSF) lymphocytic pleocytosis and CSF *Bb* antibody >serum *Bb* antibody)[b]

or

Chronic neuroborreliosis
Chronic encephalitis, encephalomyelitis, meningoencephalitis, radiculomyelitis (confirmed by CSF lymphocytic pleocytosis and CSF *Bb* antibody >serum *Bb* antibody and diagnostic *Bb* serum IgG antibody)[b]

or

Lyme arthritis
Recurrent brief episodes of monarticular or pauciarticular arthritis with objective joint swelling, +/− chronic arthritis (confirmed by high *Bb* serum IgG antibody)[b]

or

Lyme carditis
Acute second- or third-degree atrioventricular conduction defects, lasting days to weeks, +/− myocarditis or pericarditis (confirmed by diagnostic change in *Bb* serum IgG antibody)[b]

---

[a]Adapted from Stanek, G, et al. European Union Concerted Action on Risk Assessment in Lyme Borreliosis: Clinical case definitions for Lyme Borreliosis. Wien Klin Wochenschr 108:741–747, 1996[502] and Cimmino, M, et al. European Lyme Borreliosis Clinical Spectrum. Zentralbl Bakteriol 287:248–252, 1998.[8]
[b]*Borrelia burgdorferi* may also be isolated from patient specimen.
[c]*Bb* = *Borrelia burgdorferi*.

Initial classification of Lyme borreliosis as stage 1, 2, or 3 proved to be confusing because the stages did not necessarily develop sequentially. A more useful clinical classification of the infection into three stages according to different clinical manifestations has been agreed upon by many European and North American clinicians and consists of division of the infection into early localized, early disseminated, and late chronic Lyme borreliosis[8, 24, 502, 633–635] (Table 11–12). Early localized Lyme borreliosis includes solitary EM and solitary borrelial lymphocytoma, without significant constitutional symptoms, although mild regional adenopathy and mild constitu-

tional symptoms may be present. Early disseminated Lyme borreliosis includes multiple EM and multiple borrelial lymphocytomas, as well as other manifestations of systemic spread of the spirochete such as neurologic, arthritic, cardiac, or other organ involvement. Early Lyme borreliosis has also been clearly shown to present occasionally as a flulike illness[636] without the pathognomonic erythema migrans lesion; it is characterized by fever, fatigue, and headache, and sometimes by neck pain, anorexia, and arthralgia, lasting 5 to 21 days if untreated. Late Lyme borreliosis consists of cutaneous, neurologic, or arthritic manifestations that persist either constantly or intermittently for at least 6 to 12 months.

Incidence of Lyme Borreliosis in Women of Childbearing Age

It is estimated that between 7 and 20% of patients with North American Lyme borreliosis and 18 to 34% of patients with European Lyme borreliosis are women 20 to 49 years old, and therefore in the major childbearing years. This is based on data from reports of patients with Lyme borreliosis from various geographic areas in the United States* and Europe[162, 344, 371] that note the age and sex of the patients. Lyme borreliosis may affect patients of all ages, from the infant to the elderly, but the majority of cases occur in patients younger than 40 years of age. In large studies by the CDC of over 4500 patients, the highest incidence was in those younger than 15 years and between 24 and 44 years old. The percentage of female patients with Lyme borreliosis acquired in different states of the United States usually ranges from 44 to 51%, but it may be as low as 22 to 36% in some groups studied. The percentage of female patients in several European studies was slightly higher than in the United States and ranged between 40 and 63%.

Clinical Manifestations of Gestational and Nongestational Lyme Borreliosis

Initial consideration of the diagnosis of congenital Lyme borreliosis and therefore initiation of prompt antibiotic therapy of the congenitally infected infant usually depend on suspicion or confirmation of Lyme borreliosis in the mother. Therefore, in order for infants with congenital Lyme borreliosis to be recognized, it is essential for clinicians caring for newborns and infants to become familiar with the various manifestations of Lyme borreliosis in the adult, as well as in the congenitally infected infant. The symptoms of Lyme borreliosis in pregnant women are the same as those in nonpregnant patients, and the clinical manifestations of Lyme borreliosis are shown in Table 11–9.

Diagnostic tests and differential diagnosis of both gestational and congenital Lyme borreliosis are discussed in the section Diagnosis and Differential Diagnosis. All stages of Lyme borreliosis respond to antibiotic therapy, but it is important to select therapy appropriate for the

---

*See references 243, 271, 272, 359, 360, 460, 463, 464, 466–469, 471, and 637.

TABLE 11–12
Clinical Classification of Lyme Borreliosis (LB)[a]

Early localized LB (≤1 month after bite by infected tick)	Solitary erythema migrans or Borrelia lymphocytoma +/− regional lymphadenopathy or minor constitutional symptoms (fatigue, malaise, lethargy, headache, myalgia, arthralgia)
Early disseminated LB (days to months after bite by infected tick)	Multiple erythema migrans or early neurologic (lymphocytic meningitis; cranial neuritis; radiculoneuritis; encephalitis), musculoskeletal (migratory arthralgia; myalgia; polyarthritis), cardiac (myocarditis; brief atrioventricular block), or other organ involvement (ophthalmic, hepatic, renal, etc.). Lymphocytoma is sometimes considered disseminated LB
Late chronic LB (months to years after bite by infected tick)	Acrodermatitis chronica atrophicans or persisting/remitting neurologic (chronic encephalitis; chronic neuropathy), musculoskeletal (migratory polyarthritis; chronic arthritis), or other organ involvement for over 6–12 months

[a]Adapted from Rahn DW, Felz MW. Lyme disease update. Current approach to early, disseminated, and late disease. Postgrad Med 103:51, 1998,[635] and Asbrink E, Hovmark A. Comments on the course and classification of Lyme borreliosis. Scand J Infect Dis Suppl 77:41, 1991.[634]

stage of the infection, and this is discussed in the section Therapy. Because decisions regarding antibiotic therapy of infants with gestational Lyme exposure depend on the adequacy of previous antibiotic therapy of the mother's Lyme borreliosis, it is also important for the clinician managing these infants to be familiar with recommended antibiotic therapy for adults with Lyme borreliosis.

ERYTHEMA MIGRANS

The EM skin lesion is common in both Eurasian and North American Lyme borreliosis. About half of patients with Lyme borreliosis recall a preceding tick bite, but the range is 21 to 80%. EM is reported in 45 to 87% of patients with Lyme borreliosis from Eurasia and North America.*

The spirochete is transmitted to the skin by the bite of a *B. burgdorferi*–infected tick, and a small papule develops at the bite site. After an average interval of 10 days (1 to 4 weeks), with a range of 1 day to 4 months,[434, 467, 596, 640] the skin lesion of EM develops as an initially erythematous patch at the bite site that slowly expands over a period of several days to several weeks and may reach a diameter of 40 to 73 cm[338, 596, 638, 640] before spontaneously resolving, unless antibiotic therapy interrupts the course and causes more rapid resolution of the lesion.

EM (Fig. 11–5A to C) is usually erythematous but may be purplish or brownish; is usually round but may be elongated or triangular; is usually smooth but may be stippled, bumpy, or even vesicular, necrotic, hemorrhagic, crusty, or scaly; usually shows central clearing as it expands (if duration is longer than 3 weeks) but may be homogeneous (if duration is short) or have secondary concentric annuli ("bull's-eye" appearance) in the center; and is usually asymptomatic but may be associated with minimal pruritus, burning, dysesthesia, and regional adenopathy.[338, 502, 596, 599, 640] Some lesions have recurred over as long as 1 year,[599] and these probably represent hematogenous spread (Fig. 11–5D). In China, EM lesions are usually indurated, less often show annular erythema, and sometimes have central necrosis or vesiculation.[438]

Although solitary EM with only very mild associated flulike symptoms is considered early localized infection, the development of significant systemic symptoms of fatigue, arthralgia, myalgia, headache, fever, chills, meningismus, anorexia, dysesthesia, dizziness, nausea, vomiting, difficulty concentrating, pharyngitis, regional or generalized adenopathy, conjunctivitis, and malaise, either alone or associated with single or multiple EM, occurs in about half to two thirds of patients, indicates systemic hematogenous spread of the spirochete, and is considered early disseminated infection.[338, 434, 502, 638, 640, 642]

Multiple EM (Fig. 11–6) indicates early disseminated Lyme borreliosis with hematogenous spread and occurs in 13 to 50% of North American patients[232, 243, 463, 596, 638, 640, 643] with EM, 23% of Russian patients with EM,[546] only 4 to 10% of other European patients[434, 448] with EM, and is becoming less common owing to prompt diagnosis and antibiotic therapy of solitary EM before dissemination occurs.[639, 640] The skin lesions are smaller than the initial EM lesion and presumably arise from hematogenous spread.[460, 467] A maculopapular rash (Fig. 11–7) rather than multiple EM lesions has been reported in some patients, and also indicates early disseminated infection. Presentation of Lyme disease as multiple erythema multiforme lesions has also been reported.[277]

Dissemination of infection may lead to severe complications of early infection of various organs, such as meningitis, myocarditis, hepatitis, myositis, and arthritis. Dissemination to organs without successful eradication of infection by antibiotic therapy may lead to late chronic manifestations of infection such as acrodermatitis chronica atrophicans, chronic neuroborreliosis, and chronic Lyme arthritis.

Seropositivity correlates with the duration of EM; usually, one third of patients with EM are seropositive at presentation, and 88% are seropositive during the first month after EM, using the standard polyvalent ELISA assay.[640]

BORRELIAL LYMPHOCYTOMA

Borrelial lymphocytoma (BL),[22, 434, 502, 644–646, 865] a B cell pseudolymphoma, is also called lymphadenosis cutis benigna, and is reported predominantly from Europe, where it occurs in 1 to 5% of European patients with

---

*See references 2, 98, 251, 334, 352, 374, 432, 434, 437, 460, 463, 471, 511, 546, 638, and 640.

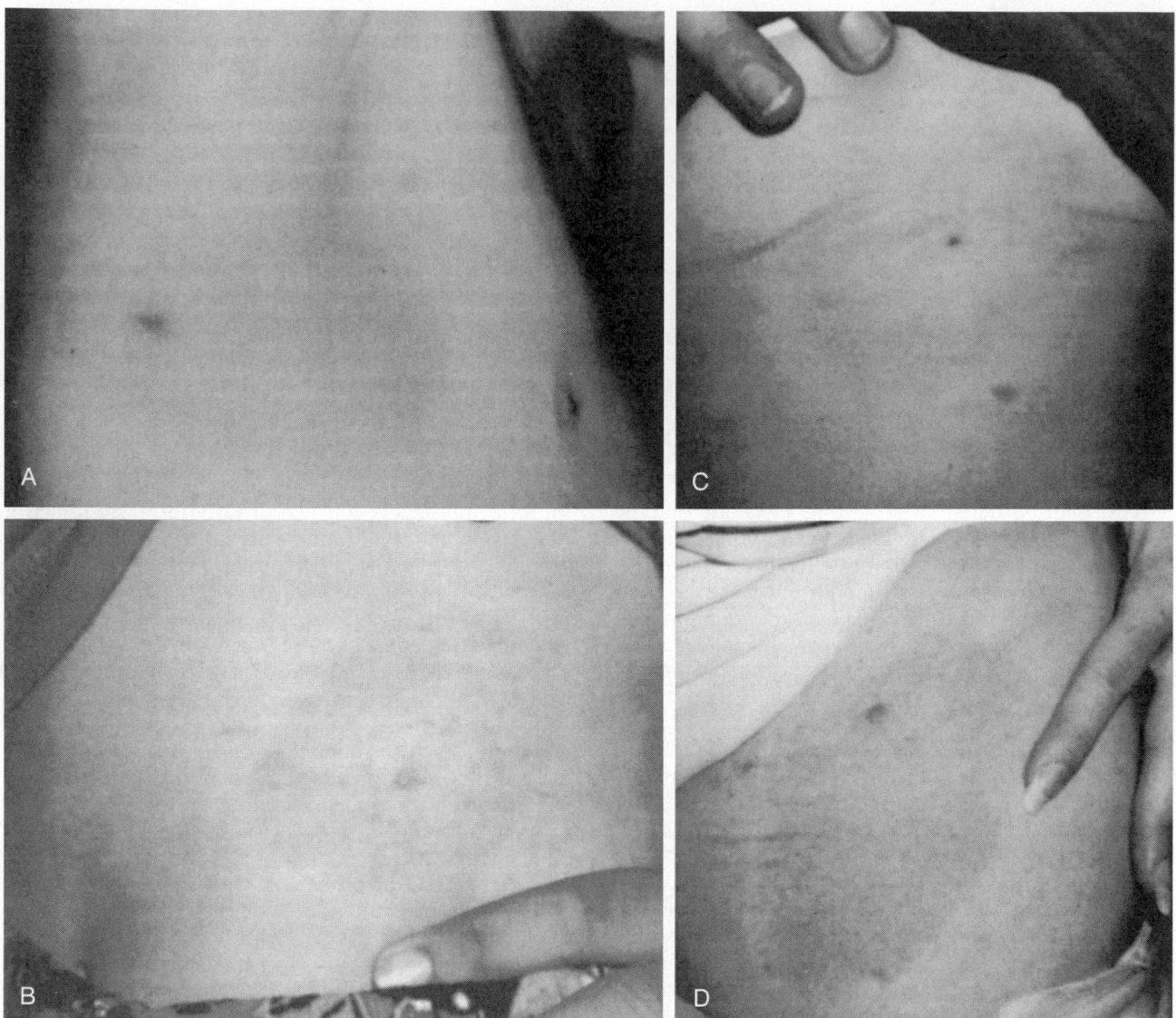

FIGURE 11–5 The pathognomonic skin lesion of Lyme disease, the "bull's-eye" or erythema migrans (EM) lesion. *A* to *C*, EM lesion of early Lyme disease, which is a large, expanding, round or oval, smooth or stippled, erythematous annular rash with central clearing located around a central or eccentric erythematous papule at a tick bite site. *D*, EM lesion of late Lyme disease, which is similar in appearance but develops around an erythematous papule that arises from hematogenous spread and not at a tick bite site. This photograph was taken 4 months post partum and shows an EM lesion on the thigh of a woman who had similar lesions since the first trimester of pregnancy (patient 25 in Table 11–8).

Lyme borreliosis, either at the time of EM or within 10 months after onset of infection, although it has also been reported from Wisconsin[257] and China.[438] It presents as a bluish red, tumor-like or nodular swelling, 1 to 5 cm in diameter, more often occurring in children, usually of the earlobe, nipple, or areola (less often of the nose, scrotum, or other sites), with minimal or no local symptoms such as pruritus or tenderness; two thirds have regional lymphadenopathy, and half have constitutional symptoms. A history of tick bite 4 to 6 weeks previously is reported in 40 to 80% of patients, and a history of previous or concomitant EM in 50 to 70%.[22, 644] The BL usually occurs at the site of the EM lesion if EM is present, but it may also occur at a distant site; if untreated, it may last weeks to months. One third of patients are seropositive for specific IgM antibody, and

one half to three quarters for specific IgG at presentation.[22, 644, 646] Antibiotic therapy usually results in full resolution within 3 to 8 weeks of initiation of therapy.[22, 644, 646] Lymphocytoma solitaria, a single lesion, is considered to be early localized Lyme borreliosis; lymphocytoma dispersa (multiple lesions) represents disseminated infection.[22, 501, 599, 644, 645] A true B cell cutaneous lymphoma, of low-grade malignancy, has also been associated occasionally with *B. burgdorferi*–induced ACA.[647]

ARTHRITIS

In the early years after recognition of Lyme disease, and before routine use of antibiotic therapy for its treatment, approximately 20% of patients with Lyme borreliosis presented with arthritis or arthralgia without preceding

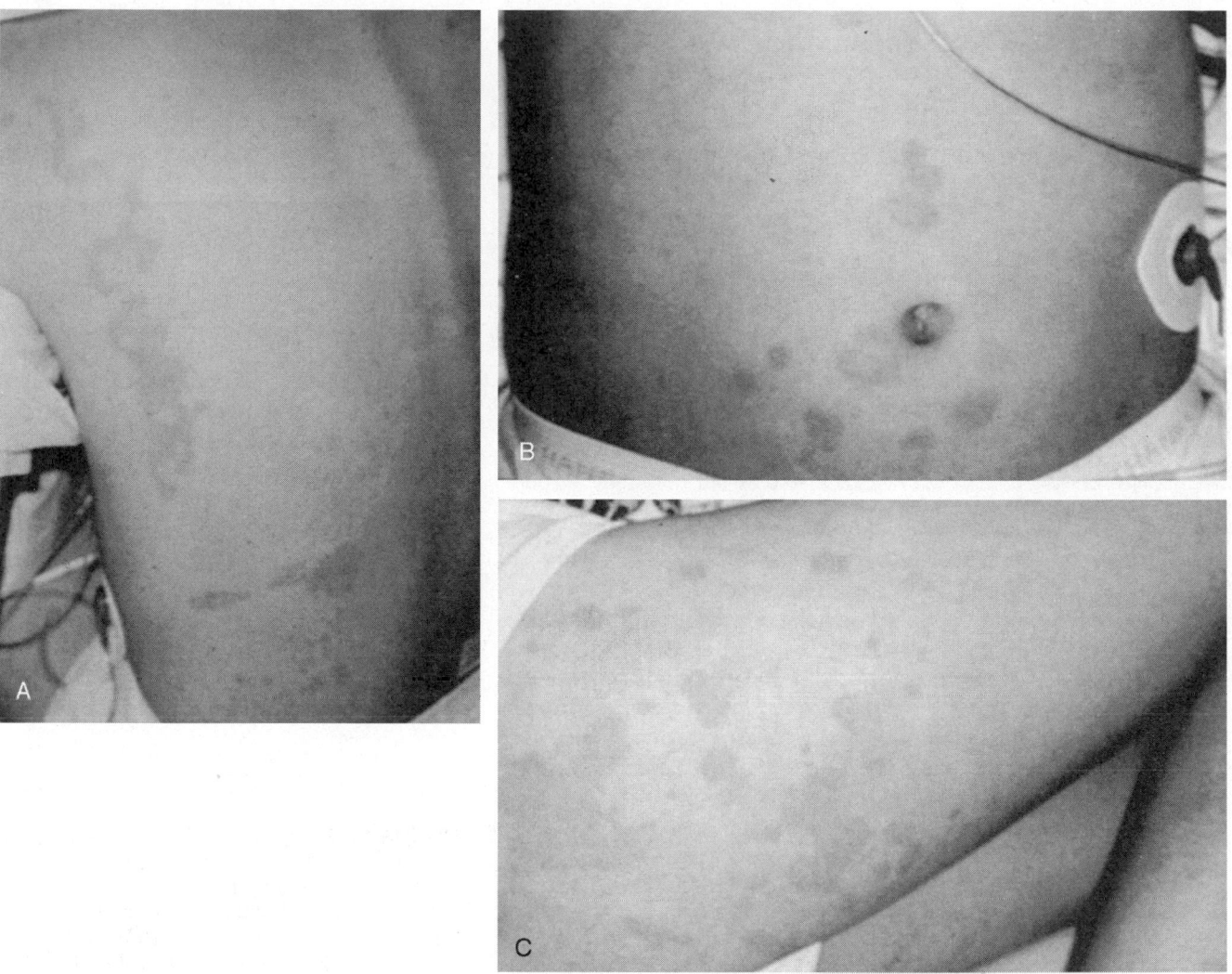

FIGURE 11–6 The rash of early disseminated Lyme disease. *A* to *C,* Extensive distribution of the rash, which consists of erythematous macular lesions with central clearing that range from one to several centimeters in diameter. This patient also had a simultaneous large (>15 cm in diameter) erythema migrans lesion covering most of the right upper arm, and smaller erythematous maculopapular lesions at many tick bite sites.

skin lesions.[464] Since antibiotic treatment of EM has become routine, with the resulting decrease in progression to late sequelae such as arthritis, 75 to 82% of patients with Lyme arthritis in the United States present with negative histories of EM.[274, 324, 648] Eighty percent of untreated North American patients with Lyme borreliosis develop arthralgias within 2 months, and 40 to 60% develop arthritis, usually 4 to 6 weeks to 2 years after the initial infection.[325, 338, 637, 648, 651, 652] The arthritis usually begins as intermittent asymmetrical arthralgias, each lasting about 1 week, and then progresses to intermittent episodes of monarticular or oligoarticular frank arthritis, especially of the large joints, which become markedly swollen, hot, and tender, but not red.[15, 338] The development of Baker's cysts that may rupture is not infrequent,[338, 641] and quadriceps femoris muscle atrophy resulting in knee instability and patellofemoral syndrome with joint dysfunction and pain is an uncommon but characteristic sequela of North American chronic Lyme arthritis.[206, 325] About 10 to 20% of patients with

arthritis experience spontaneous resolution each year, about 10% eventually progress to severe destructive chronic arthritis with longer episodes of arthritis by the second or third year, and about 2% develop joint space narrowing, bone cysts, cartilage loss, osteopenia, and erosive bone disease.[641, 651]

The most common joint involved is the knee, but other commonly involved joints include the wrist, elbow, shoulder, ankle, hip, temporomandibular joint, and even the heel and fingers.[460, 463, 641, 652] Synovial fluid shows 500 to 100,000 white blood cells per mm^3, usually with a predominance of polymorphonuclear leukocytes, and an elevated protein of 5 g/dl.[324, 338, 648, 649, 653] Sedimentation rates are mildly elevated. Most patients with Lyme arthritis have *B. burgdorferi* IgG antibody, and particularly Osp A antibody in chronic Lyme arthritis, detectable by ELISA and Western blot, and *B. burgdorferi* DNA may often be detectable in synovial fluid by PCR.[312, 314, 652] Persistent *B. burgdorferi* PCR positivity in synovial fluid correlates with active infection[312, 314] and

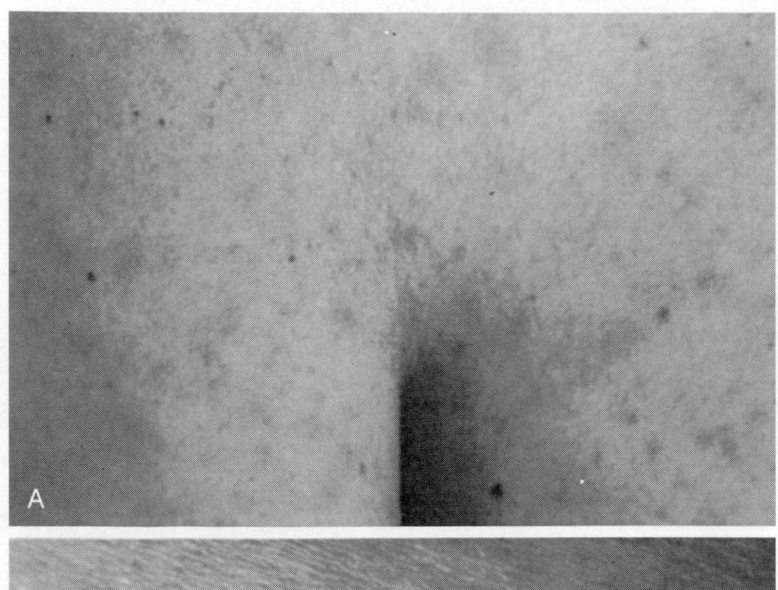

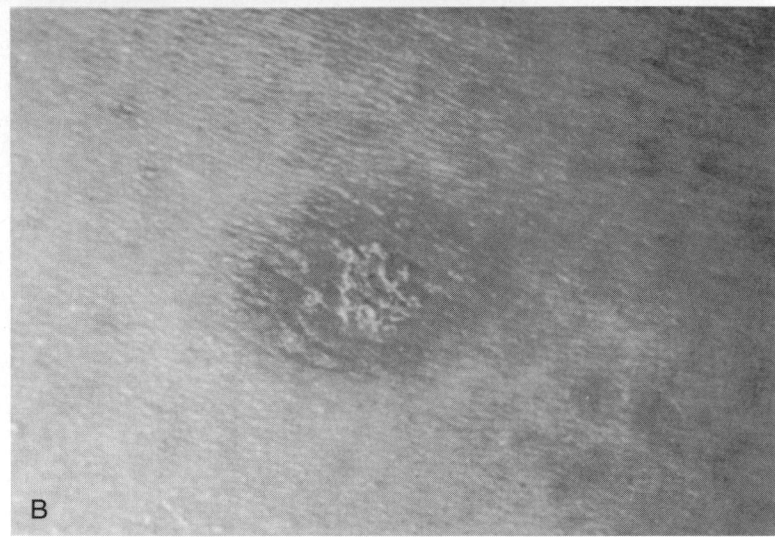

FIGURE 11–7 The rash of early disseminated Lyme disease. Dense erythematous maculopapular rash on the chest *(A)* and an erythematous oval expanding erythema migrans lesion on the buttock *(B)* in a first-trimester pregnant woman (patient 23 in Table 11–8).

indicates a need for antibiotic therapy; PCR negativity in chronic Lyme arthritis is consistent with an immunopathologic process likely to be antibiotic-unresponsive.[312]

It was initially thought that Lyme arthritis was found only in North American patients with Lyme borreliosis; however, once it was recognized, it was subsequently also found in European[39, 502, 511, 546, 649, 650, 652] and Asian patients.[374, 438]

NEUROBORRELIOSIS

Before the routine use of antibiotic therapy for early Lyme disease, about 4% of patients with Lyme borreliosis presented with neurologic symptoms without any preceding skin lesions.[464] Because routine antibiotic therapy of early Lyme borreliosis has become standard, especially when associated with the pathognomonic EM lesion, fewer patients with neuroborreliosis present with a history of EM; 10 to 64% of patients with neuroborreliosis report a history of EM, and 10 to 65% a history of tick bite.[268, 289, 290, 310, 404, 435] Approximately 5 to 17% of untreated patients develop neurologic abnormalities,

usually 2 to 4 weeks to several months after the initial infection.[268, 325] Two thirds of patients with early disseminated Lyme borreliosis even without symptoms of central nervous system involvement had evidence of spread of the spirochete to the central nervous system by PCR assay for *B. burgdorferi* DNA.[282] Chronic peripheral nervous system manifestations develop over a median of 16 months, and chronic central nervous system manifestations over a median of 26 months after initial infection.[655]

It was initially thought that neuroborreliosis was primarily a European* manifestation of Lyme borreliosis, but it is now recognized to occur in North America and Asia as well.[288, 291, 292, 437] The reported incidence of neuroborreliosis is higher in Europe than in North America, and there is a suggestion that it is higher in the northern European countries, particularly Scandinavia, than in the southern, central, and eastern European countries.[11, 12, 501, 532] Involvement of the peripheral nervous system is more frequent than that of the central

---

*See references 90, 162, 268, 290, 404, 435, 502, 511, 516, 546, and 550.

nervous system[265]; the incidence of central nervous system infection may be higher in North America than Europe, and the incidence of peripheral neuropathy may be higher in Europe,[268, 532] although severe and even fatal central nervous system neuroborreliosis has been reported from Europe.[311]

Patients with Lyme borreliosis may develop either central or peripheral nervous system involvement at any stage of the infection.[265, 286–292, 435, 655–657] The early neurologic syndromes (meningitis, cranial neuropathy, and radiculoneuropathy) usually develop a median of 1 month after EM, the chronic peripheral nervous system syndromes (polyradiculopathies) develop over a median of 16 months, and the central nervous system syndromes (encephalopathy and leukoencephalitis) a median of 26 months after EM.[291] The diversity of clinical manifestations is great and includes central nervous system infection (including acute or chronic lymphocytic meningitis, acute or chronic mild encephalopathy, and acute multifocal or chronic progressive multifocal encephalomyelitis),[267, 286, 292, 311, 516, 655, 657] cranial neuropathy (including Bell's palsy),[90, 659, 660] peripheral neuropathy,[291, 656, 662] and painful meningopolyneuritis with peripheral extremity paresis (Bannwarth's syndrome),[516, 572] neuropsychiatric disorders,[663–665] transverse myelitis,[668, 669] acute focal meningoencephalitis, Guillain-Barré syndrome,[265, 289, 530] acute cerebellar ataxia,[261, 311, 530] and chorea.[90] Peripheral nervous system manifestations are grouped under the designation of mononeuropathy multiplex, with perivascular inflammation and axonal loss.[265]

Acute lymphocytic meningitis may occur as a manifestation of early disseminated Lyme borreliosis, with or without radiculitis or cranial neuritis[290–292, 657, 658]; it occurs in up to 15% of patients with other manifestations of Lyme borreliosis.[657] Spinal fluid of patients with acute neuroborreliosis shows a lymphocytic pleocytosis of approximately 100 to 250 cells per mm³; slightly elevated protein, normal glucose, and sometimes oligoclonal bands; and intrathecal production of *B. burgdorferi*–specific antibody.[260, 265, 268, 287, 290–292] In some patients with neuroborreliosis, particularly those with very early infection, spinal fluid *B. burgdorferi* antigen-detection methods such as PCR[282, 309] or antigen capture ELISA[283] may be positive before the development of specific intrathecal antibody, and even without evidence of inflammation.[283]

One of the more common neurologic manifestations of early Lyme disease in both North American and European patients is cranial neuropathy, especially unilateral (Fig. 11–8) or bilateral Bell's palsy, which develops in about 10% of patients with Lyme borreliosis, and in 50 to 75% of patients with early neuroborreliosis, within 4 weeks of EM.[659, 660] Because Bell's palsy may also be the initial presentation, without preceding tick bite or EM, the possibility of Lyme borreliosis should be considered as a potential etiology for idiopathic Bell's palsies in Lyme-endemic areas.[661] Sixth nerve palsy is reported in 1 to 2% of pediatric neuroborreliosis patients in North America[289] and Europe.[435] In a large study of North American pediatric Lyme facial palsy patients, the incidence of CSF pleocytosis, increased CSF protein, intrathecal specific antibody, and neuroborreliosis was 55, 45, 82, and 92%, respectively.[289, 661] In patients with isolated cranial neuropathy, CSF evaluation for pleo-

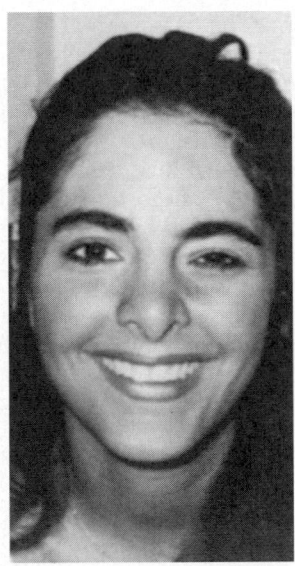

FIGURE 11–8 Bell's palsy. Persistence of residual left facial weakness 2½ years after the onset of last-trimester gestational Bell's palsy in a young woman who was later diagnosed as having Lyme disease (clinical case described in asymptomatic infant with gestational Lyme exposure).

cytosis, *B. burgdorferi* antibody, and PCR, is helpful in determining the presence of CNS spread, as this has therapeutic implications.[291, 654, 657, 661]

Bannwarth's syndrome,[502, 572] also known as Garin-Boujadoux-Bannwarth syndrome, tickborne meningopolyneuritis, meningoradiculoneuritis, or lymphocytic meningoradiculitis, occurs in 10 to 15% of patients with North American Lyme borreliosis,[265] is the most common manifestation of European neuroborreliosis, and occurs in 75% of patients with European neuroborreliosis[288, 290]; it occurs infrequently in pediatric neuroborreliosis,[289, 435] with a reported incidence of 4% in a large European study[435] and 1% in a large North American study.[289] Symptoms and signs consist of intense radicular pain with paresthesias or hyperesthesias, progressing to asymmetrical polyneuritis, with sensory loss, weakness, or hyporeflexia, often with cranial nerve palsy (particularly unilateral or bilateral facial palsy), and sometimes with transverse myelitis and lymphocytic meningitis that develops within a few days to weeks after the initial EM or tick bite and lasts approximately 3 to 5 months if untreated. Manifestations of progressive peripheral nervous system involvement (mononeuritis multiplex) are cranial neuropathy, radiculoneuropathy, brachial or lumbosacral plexopathy, distal axonopathy, acute disseminated neuropathy (Guillain-Barré–like), and motor neuropathy.[265] Most patients with Lyme radiculoneuritis are *B. burgdorferi*–seropositive and have CSF pleocytosis and specific CSF *B. burgdorferi* antibody, some have CSF culture or PCR positivity, and some (European patients) have CSF oligoclonal bands.[290–292]

Manifestations of late parenchymal central nervous system and spinal cord neuroborreliosis include progressive encephalomyelitis,[265, 292, 657] with cranial and peripheral neuropathies, myelitis, meningitis, and multifocal encephalitis[265, 286, 311]; spastic paraparesis or quadriparesis, bladder dysfunction, ataxia, cranial nerve deficits, and dementia[98, 311]; seizures[311, 325]; and chronic encephalopathy and leukoencephalitis.[655] The incidence of Lyme encephalomyelitis is estimated to be 0.1% of cases of untreated Lyme borreliosis[265, 292, 657]; most patients have intrathecal *B. burgdorferi* antibody, some (European patients) have oligoclonal bands, and some have CSF PCR positivity.[290, 657] Late neuroborreliosis manifestations may also include distal limb paresthesias, carpal tunnel syndrome, painful radiculopathy, Bell's palsy, and disseminated multifocal patchy axonal neuropathy similar to mononeuritis multiplex.[289] Spinal fluids of patients with chronic neuroborreliosis show slight lymphocytic pleocytosis of approximately 150 to 200 cells per mm³, slightly elevated protein, and usually *B. burgdorferi*–specific intrathecal antibody production.[290, 655, 656] Spinal fluid and lesion brain biopsy[311] may also be positive for *B burgdorferi*–specific antigen by PCR.[287, 309, 311]

Neuropsychiatric disorders have been reported.[664, 665, 682–684] Encephalopathy, or neurocognitive dysfunction, particularly subjective perception of memory deficits, may occur during or after Lyme borreliosis, with and even without evidence of invasive inflammatory neurologic infection; it was initially thought to occur only in North American patients, but is now recognized in European patients as well.[265, 681]

Magnetic resonance imaging (MRI) of the brain may be useful in evaluation of central nervous system neuroborreliosis,[311, 610, 671, 672, 685] including meningitis, encephalitis, acute or indolent multifocal encephalitis, chronic neuroborreliosis with encephalopathy and leukoencephalitis, and even facial palsy, as well as other manifestations of Lyme borreliosis that may also involve the central nervous system,[679] including neuro-ophthalmic manifestations; it has demonstrated focal nodular areas or large patchy areas of hyperintense T₂ signal in deep or periventricular white matter, sometimes with ringlike enhancement with gadolinium contrast suggestive of demyelination, perivascular inflammation, or even pontine, frontal, or parietal mass lesions, and occasionally lesions in cortical or subcortical gray matter. MRI imaging has also demonstrated T₂ hyperintense areas with gadolinium contrast enhancement of the nerve roots and cauda equina in Bannwarth's syndrome.[680]

Functional brain imaging, by single photon emission computed tomography (SPECT) or positron emission tomography (PET), may be useful in determination of whether there are objective abnormalities in patients with subjective neuropsychiatric complaints in late Lyme encephalopathy; in some of these patients, including some with normal brain MRI imaging,[666, 667] it has demonstrated multifocal areas of diminished perfusion in the cortex and subcortical white matter, including the frontal white matter, basal ganglia, and medial cortex.

CARDITIS

About 2 to 8% of patients with North American Lyme borreliosis present with carditis initially and 4 to 10% develop it if untreated, usually within 2 to 4 weeks but up to 3 months after the initial infection.[325, 643, 686–688] Although Lyme carditis was initially thought to occur

only in North American patients, it has now been reported, with a lower rate of 0.3 to 4%, from Europe as well,[10, 435, 502, 516, 546, 689] and has also been occasionally reported in Asia.[374, 438]

The most common findings are conduction disturbances,[689–986] including mild transient fluctuating first- and second-degree atrioventricular block, Wenckebach periodicity, intraventricular conduction disturbances, and bundle branch block, but complete heart block may also occur and may manifest as syncopal episodes, seizure-like episodes, dizziness, chest pain, and fatigue,[686, 687, 689, 890] although other manifestations also have been reported.[607, 691–693] Electrocardiograms commonly show atrioventricular block or other conduction defects, ST changes, T wave flattening or inversion, intraventricular conduction defects, or occasional premature ventricular contractions. Because carditis is usually a complication of early Lyme borreliosis, specific *B. burgdorferi* antibody is not always detectable at the time of presentation, but it develops later.

The prognosis of acute Lyme carditis is usually good, and it usually resolves spontaneously within 3 days to 6 weeks.[687]

ACRODERMATITIS CHRONICA ATROPHICANS

ACA is a late chronic cutaneous manifestation of Lyme borreliosis that occurs in 2 to 16% of European patients with Lyme borreliosis,[39, 251, 352, 404, 502, 525, 532, 546, 641] 6 months to 10 years after initial infection.[600] Although this is rare in North America, is more common in the elderly, and is rare in childhood, it has been reported in both a child and two young women in the United States,[695] and occasionally in European children.[435, 530] Progression of erythema migrans skin lesions to ACA skin lesions in the same patient over time has been demonstrated.[696] There is an initial inflammatory phase that manifests as insidious onset of bluish red discoloration and doughy induration of the skin on the distal extremities at the site of a previous EM lesion, followed by the atrophic phase, which produces atrophic skin changes in the previously affected areas of skin.[501, 599, 600, 612] Patients may have periarticular bursitis, Achilles tendinitis and epicondylitis, juxta-articular fibrotic nodules, peripheral neuropathies, and joint deformities, including subluxation and degenerative arthritis.[600, 612, 670, 697] Most patients with ACA are seropositive by IgG antibody assay and by the lymphocyte proliferative assay.[219] Antibiotic therapy has resulted in improvement of the inflammatory component but not the permanent atrophic component of ACA.

OTHER ORGAN INVOLVEMENT IN DISSEMINATED INFECTION

During the dissemination phase of the infection, there have also been reports of hepatitis,[243, 698] necrotizing splenitis,[604] eosinophilic lymphadenitis,[606] localized or generalized myositis,[616, 617] eosinophilic fasciitis,[603] panniculitis resembling erythema nodosum,[598] tenosynovitis with ligament involvement,[304] multifocal osteomyelitis (in distal tibial and femoral metaphyses),[699] and rarely hematologic abnormalities.[711, 712]

Ophthalmologic manifestations of Lyme borreliosis may occur alone or in combination with other manifestations of Lyme borreliosis.[320, 702] These include cranial nerve palsies affecting extraocular movements[643]; conjunctivitis, nodular episcleritis, and keratitis[284, 325]; and orbital myositis,[703] optic neuritis,[704] retinitis, and panophthalmitis. The incidence of otologic complications, other than facial nerve palsy, is less than 12%; these include vestibular neuronitis, moderate hearing loss, tinnitus, otalgia, and temporomandibular joint pain.[284, 707]

Post-Lyme Syndromes

The post-Lyme syndrome (PLS), which includes persistence of fatigue and arthralgia for longer than 6 months after adequate antibiotic therapy of confirmed Lyme disease, has been reported to be associated with objective neuropsychiatric and neurocognitive abnormalities,[682, 683, 713, 714] and with delayed initial antibiotic therapy.[683, 714]

Fibromyalgia has been reported in 8 to 10% of patients with Lyme borreliosis, but it persisted after resolution of the symptoms of Lyme disease and was not considered to be related to active Lyme disease.[279, 715]

REINFECTION WITH *BORRELIA BURGDORFERI*

Reinfection rates as high as 5 to 21%, based on clinical histories, have been reported in some highly endemic areas in both North America and Europe.[522, 683, 714, 716] Reinfection with different strains of *B. burgdorferi* has been confirmed serologically and by culture[717, 718] in both North America and Europe; these patients developed seropositivity after the initial episode, but some became seronegative before the second episode and others remained seropositive between episodes. Serologic evaluation by IgG as well as IgM *B. burgdorferi* assays is recommended in patients suspected of having reinfection, as some have only an IgG response.[233]

CO-INFECTION WITH *BABESIA* OR *EHRLICHIA*

Babesiosis, caused by the protozoan *Babesia microti* in the United States, and *Babesia divergens* and *Babesia bovis* in Europe, is another tickborne infection of increasing prevalence and significance, which is co-vectored by the ticks that transmit Lyme borreliosis and human granulocytic ehrlichiosis and shares the same geographic distribution. There are two reports of infants with probable transplacental acquisition of babesiosis.[630]

HGE shares tick vectors and some geographic distribution with Lyme borreliosis. Co-infections with Lyme disease and ehrlichiosis are being increasingly reported, including one case in pregnancy,[632] and there is one report of probable transplacental transmission of HGE.[631]

Clinically symptomatic as well as asymptomatic past or recent co-infection with Lyme borreliosis and babesiosis[481–483] or ehrlichiosis[484] has been reported,[397, 400, 401, 481, 485–488, 498] although some seropositivity to more than one agent may be due to cross-reactivity. There is recent concern because of accumulating evidence for increased severity of Lyme disease in patients with concurrent babesiosis,[481] and it is uncertain if this occurs also with ehrlichiosis and Lyme borreliosis.

Insufficient data are available so far to determine the frequency of transplacental transmission of babesiosis or ehrlichiosis, or the optimal antibiotic therapy of either gestational or neonatal infection.

The possibility that co-infection with *B. burgdorferi* and tickborne encephalitis (TBE) may increase the severity of TBE has been raised.

Clinical Manifestations of Congenital Lyme Borreliosis

CONGENITAL AND GESTATIONAL LYME BORRELIOSIS

A review of the congenital and gestational Lyme borreliosis literature yielded 259 reported cases for which the outcome of the individual episode of gestational Lyme borreliosis was noted,* and addition of four of the author's cases brought the total to 263 cases. A total of 66 cases of the 263 were found that the author considers to represent an adverse event at least associated with an episode of gestational Lyme borreliosis,[25, 26, 28–48] including miscarriage, stillbirth, perinatal death, congenital anomalies, systemic illness, early-onset fulminant sepsis, and later-onset chronic progressive infection (Tables 11–8, 11–13, and 11–14). These 66 cases have been divided into logical groups (Table 11–15) based on an understanding of the pathophysiology and clinical course of Lyme borreliosis in older patients, and on inescapable similarities of Lyme borreliosis to syphilis. Many of the calculations of rates of adverse outcomes became apparent only when all of the available case information was compared, as each individual report of one or several cases represented too few cases from which to draw conclusions; in the larger, population-based studies or serologic surveys, individual outcomes of gestational Lyme disease were not provided for all patients, which made difficult the recognition of a small number of individual adverse outcomes associated with gestational Lyme disease. The reader is directed to additional information about these cases of congenital Lyme borreliosis, which are discussed in the individual sections of Pathology and Pathogenesis, Diagnosis and Differential Diagnosis, Therapy, Prevention, and Prognosis, in this chapter.

In some of these reports, the gestational trimester of onset of Lyme borreliosis, the clinical manifestation of Lyme borreliosis, the gestational antibiotic therapy, the *B. burgdorferi* serologic status of the mother, and details about the specific type of fetal or neonatal abnormality that may have occurred, including specific malformations, birth weight, prematurity, serologic status of the infant, trimester of miscarriage, antibiotic therapy of the infant, and placental and autopsy pathologic information, are indicated; in others, this information is missing.

Several reports that involved serologic screening of

---

*See references 25–39, 42–48, 531, 536, 537, 622, 632, and 719–723.

TABLE 11–13
Frequency of Specific Adverse Outcomes[a] of 66 Pregnancies Complicated by Gestational Lyme Borreliosis (GLB) and Adverse Clinical Outcome

FETAL/NEONATAL ABNORMALITY	NO. WITH FINDING[b]	% WITH FINDING	REFERENCE
Cardiac	15/66	22.7%	
Myocardial dysfunction	5/66	7.6%	25, 31–33, 621
VSD	6/66	9.1%	33–35, 37, 48
PDA	3/66	4.5%	25, 33, 42, 621
Coarctation aorta	2/66	3.0%	25, 33, 34
ASD	2/66	3.0%	33, 34, 48
Other[d]	4/66	6.1%	25, 32, 33, 37, 46, 621
Neurologic	10/66	15.2%	
Developmental delay/mental abnormalities	5/66	7.6%	31, 36, 42, 44, 621
Hydrocephalus/macrocephaly	5/66	7.6%	31, 33, 37, 41
Hypotonia/lethargy	3/66	4.5%	32, 37, 621
Meningoencephalitis[e]	4/66	6.1%	31, 621
CNS lesions on scan[f]	2/66	3.0%	31, 621
Cortical blindness	1/66	1.5%	36
Hemiparesis	1/66	1.5%	621
Meningomyelocele	1/66	1.5%	33
Orthopedic	8/66	12.1%	
Syndactyly/clubfoot/metatarsus adductus	4/66	6.1%	29, 33, 36, 45
Arthritis/contractures	2/66	3.0%	31, 621
Long bone metaphyseal bands	2/66	3.0%	621
Pectus excavatum	1/66	1.5%	621
Vertebral defects	3/66	4.5%	33, 41, 45
Radial dysplasia	1/66	1.5%	45
Dermatologic	6/66	9.1%	
Rash	6/66	9.1%	31, 36, 43, 621
Ophthalmic	3/66	4.5%	
Blepharitis/exophthalmos	1/66	1.5%	31
Punctate retinal lesions	1/66	1.5%	621
Eso- /exotropia	1/66	1.5%	621
Genitourinary	7/66	10.6%	
Cryptorchidism	2/66	3.0%	42, 46
Hypospadias	1/66	1.5%	46
Inguinal hernia, bilateral	1/66	1.5%	621
Hydrocele	1/66	1.5%	46
Renal dysplasia	1/62	1.5%	45
Ureteral stenosis with hydronephrosis, bilateral	1/66	1.5%	48
Miscellaneous anomalies	8/66	12.1%	
Pilonidal dimple	2/66	3.0%	621
Sacral hemangioma with gluteal atrophy	1/66	1.5%	44
Facial/ear dysmorphia	1/66	1.5%	621
Simian crease, unilateral	1/66	1.5%	621
Absence of hemidiaphragm	1/66	1.5%	33
Omphalocele	1/66	1.5%	33
Laryngomalacia	1/66	1.5%	46
Tracheoesophageal fistula	1/66	1.5%	45
Imperforate anus	1/66	1.5%	45
Hypoplastic dental enamel/dental anomalies	3/66	4.5%	42

Table continued on opposite page

large populations of obstetric patients, but provided no information about the occurrence, treatment, or specific outcomes of any clinically symptomatic cases of gestational Lyme borreliosis, could not be used in evaluation of outcomes of gestational Lyme borreliosis; however, they provided data on seroprevalence in the obstetric patient population.[530, 724] In Germany, the seroprevalence of *B. burgdorferi*–specific IgM and IgG antibody was 0.8 and 7%, respectively, in 2600 patients in obstetric clinics, and pregnancy outcomes were considered the same in seropositive and seronegative groups of patients.[530] A large *B. burgdorferi* antibody serosurvey of 1039 preg-

TABLE 11–13

Frequency of Specific Adverse Outcomes[a] of 66 Pregnancies Complicated by Gestational Lyme Borreliosis (GLB) and Adverse Clinical Outcome *Continued*

FETAL/NEONATAL ABNORMALITY	NO. WITH FINDING[b]	% WITH FINDING	REFERENCE
Miscellaneous abnormalities			
Neonatal sepsis/DIC/respiratory distress	11/66	16.7%	25, 26, 33, 38, 39, 47, 48, 621
Hyperbilirubinemia	8/66	12.1%	36, 37, 41, 621
Growth retardation[g]	8/66	12.1%	31, 33–35, 37, 41, 47, 621
Hepatomegaly/splenomegaly	3/66	4.5%	31, 621
Adenopathy	4/66	6.1%	31, 43, 621
Recurrent fever	2/66	3.0%	43, 44
Recurrent infections	2/66	3.0%	31, 621
Dysphagia/GE reflux/aspiration	2/66	3.0%	31, 45
Meconium ileus	1/66	1.5%	621
Fetal/Neonatal demise	26/66	39.4%	
GLB prior to conception or first prenatal visit	10/66	15.2%	27, 32, 33
GLB in first trimester	5/66	7.6%	25, 29, 33–36, 38, 39, 42
GLB in second trimester	8/66	12.1%	33, 34
GLB in third trimester	0/66	0.0%	
GLB in unspecified trimester	2/66	3.0%	30, 33, 41, 46

[a]Underestimate of incidence of findings, as autopsies not done on all fetal deaths.
[b]Number with finding/total number.
[c]Author's patients.
[d]Endocardial fibroelastosis, aortic stenosis, left superior vena cava, multiple congenital heart defects, aortic thrombosis, or arrhythmia.
[e]Chronic meningitis, or CSF pleocytosis/elevated protein.
[f]Cortical atrophy on CT or white matter lesions on MRI.
[g]Intrauterine or postnatal.
ASD = atrial septal defect; CNS = central nervous system; DIC = disseminated intravascular coagulation; GE = gastroesophageal; GLB = gestational Lyme borreliosis; PDA = patent ductus arteriosus; VSD = ventricular septal defect.

nant women in the Perm area of Russia from 1992 to 1994 found a 5.5% seropositivity rate (57 of 1039) and noted that their data indicated that Lyme borreliosis is a serious risk factor for miscarriage and perinatal death, but provided no information on individual outcomes of gestational Lyme borreliosis.[721] Some reports note the occurrence of adverse effects of gestational Lyme borreliosis such as stillbirth and congenital defects but provide no details.[725]

In 1989, Nadal and associates[37] reported a large serosurvey of 1416 mothers and their infants at the time of delivery, from 1986 to 1987, in a Lyme-endemic area of Switzerland, and found a *B. burgdorferi*–specific seropositivity rate of 0.85% (12 of 1416) in maternal sera. Of the seropositive mothers, one had a history of first-trimester tick bite and Lyme borreliosis and her infant had a congenital ventricular septal defect (VSD); five mothers had histories of pre-gestational Lyme borreliosis, one had a history of pre-gestational tick bite, and five were asymptomatic; 6 of their infants had minor problems that resolved.

Bracero and colleagues,[47] in a serosurvey of pregnant women at the first prenatal visit in an endemic area of New York from 1988 to 1989, found a seropositivity rate of 1.1% (7 of 638), and noted non–statistically significant but interesting differences in the pregnancy outcomes of seropositive and seronegative women: The frequencies of low birth weight, birth size small for gestational age, and Apgar less than 7 were 28.6, 14.3, and 14.3% for seropositive women, and 16.4, 2.6, and 5.2% for seronegative women.

In 1993, Strobino and co-workers[45] reported a prospective *B. burgdorferi* serosurvey of 2000 pregnant women from areas of high and low Lyme endemicity in New York, from 1988 to 1990, at the first prenatal visit and at delivery; pregnancy outcomes were available for 96%. Eleven patients were seropositive at the first visit (rate 0.7%); only one patient seroconverted by delivery, and this patient had an untreated second-trimester flu-like illness and delivered a normal infant; the seropositive mothers delivered live-born infants, one with gastroesophageal reflux, one with metatarsus adductus, and one with multiple major anomalies. Fifteen developed Lyme disease during the pregnancy, but the specific outcomes of these pregnancies were not provided. They concluded that gestational Lyme disease or *B. burgdorferi* exposure was not associated with an overall increase in fetal death, prematurity, or congenital malformations, but noted that the incidence of cardiac defects was two times higher in infants born to mothers in high versus low endemicity areas, and that there was an association of minor malformations with a history of maternal tick bite less than 3 years before conception. The frequencies of total, major, and minor malformations in the infants born to these mothers were 24, 7, and 17% for those with a history of previous Lyme disease at any time; 19, 3 to 7, and 15 to 16% for those with a history of tick bite within 3 years; 16, 5, and 10% for those with no history of previous Lyme disease; and 15, 5, and 10% for those with no history of tick bite. They qualified their conclusions by noting that the miscarriage rate in this study was 8%, which is lower than the usual rate of

TABLE 11–14
Outcomes of 263 Pregnancies Complicated by Lyme Borreliosis (LB)[a]

TRIMESTER OF LB[b]	ANTIBIOTIC THERAPY OF LB[c]	NO. PATIENTS	NO. FETAL DEATHS[d]	NO. NEONATAL DEATHS[e]	NO. LIVEBORN, ILL, OR ABNORMAL[f]	NO. LIVEBORN, NORMAL	NO. TOTAL ADVERSE OUTCOMES[g,h]	NO. TOTAL NORMAL OUTCOMES[h]
≤1[i]	yes	57[i]	4	1	5	47	10 (17.5%)	47 (82.5%)
	no	11	4	2	2	3	8 (72.7%)	3 (27.3%)
	unknown	6	3	2	1	0	6 (100.0%)	0 (0.0%)
	Total	**74**	**11**	**5**	**8**	**50**	**24 (32.4%)**	**50 (67.6%)**
2	yes	56	0	0	9	47	9 (16.1%)	47 (83.9%)
	no	6	4	0	0	2	4 (66.7%)	2 (33.3%)
	unknown	6	4	0	0	2	4 (66.7%)	2 (33.3%)
	Total	**68**	**8**	**0**	**9**	**51**	**17 (25.0%)**	**51 (75.0%)**
3	yes	32	0	0	3	29	3 (9.4%)	29 (90.6%)
	no	6	0	0	3	3	3 (50.0%)	3 (50.0%)
	unknown	0	0	0	0	0	0 (0.0%)	0 (0.0%)
	Total	**38**	**0**	**0**	**6**	**32**	**6 (15.8%)**	**32 (84.2%)**
Unknown	yes	12	0	0	1	11	1 (8.3%)	11 (91.7%)
	no	7	1	0	4	2	5 (71.4%)	2 (28.6%)
	unknown	64[k]	0	1	12	51[k]	13 (20.3%)	51 (79.7%)
	Total	**83**	**1**	**1**	**17**	**64**	**18 (21.7%)**	**64 (77.1%)**
Total	yes	157	4	1	18	134	23 (14.6%)	134 (85.4%)
	no	30	9	2	9	10	20 (66.7%)	10 (33.3%)
	unknown	76	7	3	13	53	23 (30.3%)	53 (69.7%)
	Total	**263**	**20**	**6**	**40**	**197**	**66 (25.1%)**	**197 (74.9%)**

[a]Data from cases reported in references 25–39, 41–48, 531, 536, 537, 621, 622, 632, 719–723.
[b]LB either by clinical history or positive *Borrelia burgdorferi* assay.
[c]Antibiotic therapy given for the episode of LB.
[d]Miscarriages or stillbirths.
[e]Four neonatal deaths occurred before 2 days of age, and one at 8 days.
[f]Includes nonfatal congenital anomalies, growth retardation, developmental delay, and neonatal illness (see Table 11–8).
[g]Includes miscarriages, stillbirths, neonatal deaths, illness, or abnormality.
[h]Percentage of total in treatment category is included despite small numbers in some categories.
[i]Trimester ≤1 indicates LB in first trimester, or prior to conception or first prenatal care visit.
[j]2 of 23 patients in one group in this category were not treated with antibiotics but, as specific outcomes were not separated out from their group, these were placed in the treated group and considered as Live Born, Normal, for use in this table to avoid overestimation of adverse outcome risk.
[k]Unspecified outcome for two pregnancies was considered as Live Born, Normal, for use in this table.

TABLE 11-15
Clinical Manifestations of Congenital Lyme Borreliosis (CLB)[a]

Fetal Death[b]

30% (9/30) risk after untreated GLB[c]

2.5% (4/157) risk after treated GLB

8% (20/263) risk after any GLB (9/20+)[d]

Most (75%, 15/20) occur at ≤20 weeks of gestation (range, 8–40 weeks) and may present with
- High frequency of
  - Cardiac anomaly/abnormality (40%, 4/9, of fetal deaths after untreated GLB; 0%, 0/4, of fetal deaths after treated GLB)

Most occur after first- or second-trimester GLB (95%, 19/20), with variable interval between GLB and fetal demise.

Early Congenital, Severe

20% (6/30) risk after untreated GLB

4% (6/157) risk after treated GLB

6% (16/263) risk after any GLB (7/16+)[e]

Present in first week of life with acute suspected sepsis
- High frequency of
  - Mortality (36%, 6/16)
  - Cardiac anomaly or abnormality (56%, 9/16, overall; 85%, 5/6, in fatal cases)
  - Respiratory distress (50%, 8/16)
  - Prematurity (50.0%, 8/16, most ≤5 wks premature)
- May also have
  - Intrauterine growth retardation
  - Skeletal anomaly/abnormality/metaphyseal bands
  - Neurologic abnormality/meningoencephalitis
  - Fever
  - Hepatosplenomegaly
  - Hyperbilirubinemia
  - Adenopathy
  - Rash
  - Lethargy/meningoencephalitis
  - Miscellaneous anomalies

Most occur after first- or second-trimester GLB (63%, 10/16, overall; 100%, 10/10, when trimester of GLB is known).

Early Congenital, Mild

10% (3/30) risk after untreated GLB

4% (6/157) risk after treated GLB

8% (22/263) risk after any GLB

Present in first 2 weeks of life with mild illness
- Moderate frequency of
  - Hyperbilirubinemia (32%, 7/22)
- May also have
  - Genitourinary anomaly/abnormality
  - Skeletal anomaly
  - Cardiac abnormality/anomaly
  - Rash
  - Neurologic abnormality/meningoencephalitis/hypotonia
  - Prematurity (all ≤4 weeks premature)
  - Suspected sepsis
  - Intrauterine growth retardation
  - Adenopathy
  - Miscellaneous anomalies

Most occur after first- or second-trimester GLB (41%, 9/22, overall; 90%, 9/10, when trimester of GLB is known).

Late Congenital

7% (2/30) risk after untreated GLB

4% (7/157) risk after treated GLB

4% (10/263) risk after any GLB (1/10+)[f]

Risk is a minimum estimate as long-term follow-up unavailable for most patients. 70% (7/10) of cases of late CLB occurred after treated GLB.

Present after 2 weeks of life, usually within first 2 years, with subacute illness
- High frequency of
  - Developmental delay/meningoencephalitis (50%, 5/10)
- Moderate frequency of
  - Genitourinary anomaly/abnormality (30%, 3/10)
- May also have
  - Skeletal abnormality/metaphyseal bands
  - Rash
  - Prematurity
  - Adenopathy
  - Hepatosplenomegaly
  - Fever
  - Growth retardation/failure to thrive
  - Miscellaneous anomalies

Potential progression to chronic neurologic, cardiac, skeletal, cutaneous, ocular involvement should be considered.

Most occur after second- or third-trimester GLB (60%, 6/10, overall; 86%, 6/7, when trimester of GLB is known).

[a]Data from Tables 11–8, 11–13, and 11–14, summaries of 66 adverse outcomes of gestational Lyme borreliosis.

[b]Miscarriages (including one induced abortion with congenital anomalies) or stillbirths. This represents a minimum estimate, as many of the published reports included patients enrolled only at the first prenatal visit or at delivery, and therefore did not include early miscarriage data.

[c]GLB-gestational Lyme borreliosis; treated/untreated refers to gestational antibiotic therapy.

[d]9 positive for borreliae in tissue samples.

[e]7 positive for borreliae in tissue samples.

[f]1 positive for borreliae in tissue samples.

10 to 15%; however, they indicated that enrollment at the first prenatal visit would have missed miscarriages that occurred before that visit. They also noted that if *B. burgdorferi* were to have very specific fetal teratogenic effects, if the period of fetal susceptibility to such effects were narrow, and if successful antibiotic therapy were to decrease the risk of such teratogenesis, a much larger study would be needed to determine a teratogenic effect.

In 1995, Williams and associates,[46] from the same group, reported a large cord blood serosurvey of 2500 infants in a Lyme-endemic and 2500 in a nonendemic area from 1986 to 1988 in New York; clinical informa-

tion regarding congenital malformations was available for 95% of endemic and 97% of nonendemic area infants. Maternal *B. burgdorferi* exposure was 5 to 10 times higher in mothers from endemic than from nonendemic areas, and infants from endemic areas had a (significantly higher) 13% incidence of congenital cardiac defects and murmurs compared with a 5% incidence in those from nonendemic areas; there was no increase in the incidence of other malformations. Of cardiac malformations, VSD was the most common in both endemic and nonendemic infants; other defects in the endemic infants included tetralogy of Fallot, atrial septal defect, patent ductus arteriosus, pulmonic stenosis, cyanotic congenital heart disease, multiple cardiac defects, hypoplastic right heart, and dextrocardia. Among endemic area infants, major malformations occurred in 17, 9, and 5% of infants born after gestational Lyme disease, pre-gestational Lyme disease, and gestational tick bite, compared with 3% born after neither maternal Lyme disease nor tick bite. Six infants, all from the endemic area, had histories of antibiotic-treated gestational Lyme disease, and one had had hypospadias. The authors note that late developmental sequelae would not be detected by this study owing to absence of long-term follow-up, and that a larger study would be needed to address the question of cardiac teratogenicity.

Two retrospective studies assessed the possible association of late neurologic or cardiac sequelae in infants with histories of gestational Lyme disease exposure.[727, 728] Gerber and Zalneraitis[727] surveyed 162 of 176 listed pediatric neurologists in Lyme-endemic areas of the northeastern and upper midwestern United States, as well as a random subset of adult neurologists in Connecticut, from 1989 to 1990, for possible cases of congenital Lyme disease in their practices. Only three children with a diagnosis of congenital Lyme disease were found, but the clinical histories were not considered by the study authors to meet criteria for gestational Lyme disease, and they concluded that one of the following is true: (1) congenital Lyme disease with neurologic sequelae is very rare; (2) it may involve sequelae not recognized as related; (3) the association of sequelae with congenital Lyme disease may be underrecognized because the association between the child's neurologic disorder and maternal Lyme disease was not made; or (4) neurologic sequelae could be too subtle to result in pediatric neurology consultation. Additionally, they note that the incidence of gestational Lyme disease is low in these areas because pregnant women commonly avoid tick exposure, because women with recent Lyme disease commonly delay pregnancy until after full recovery, because antibiotic prophylaxis of gestational tick bites by obstetricians in these areas is routine, and because prompt antibiotic therapy of gestational Lyme disease occurs. They note that a larger study would be needed to determine any association between subtle neurologic sequelae and congenital Lyme disease.

Strobino and colleagues[728] conducted a retrospective case-control study of 796 children who were followed by pediatric cardiologists for congenital cardiac anomalies (and 705 controls evaluated by those cardiologists for possible cardiac disease and found to have none), from 1985 to 1995, in a Lyme-endemic area in New York; they found no association of the occurrence of congenital cardiac anomalies with histories of maternal gestational or pre-gestational Lyme disease or tick bite, based on maternal retrospective questionnaires. Only four patients in each group had histories of maternal Lyme disease within 3 months before or during the pregnancies with these patients. Because the enrollment population included only children with congenital cardiac anomalies who survived to be referred to pediatric cardiologists, no conclusions could be made regarding any association of gestational or pre-gestational Lyme

disease with cardiac anomalies that might have resulted in miscarriage, stillbirth, or early infant death.

Sigal suggests that because organogenesis is complete by the end of the second trimester, the risk of congenital anomaly should be very low in the late second and third trimesters.[729] It is generally agreed that the incidence of adverse outcomes of gestational Lyme borreliosis is low,[435, 530, 729–732] probably because of prompt antibiotic therapy for early gestational Lyme borreliosis, particularly when it presents with its easily recognized and most common manifestation, erythema migrans. Shapiro suggests that the existence of congenital Lyme borreliosis has not been ruled out, but it must be very rare.[733]

REVIEW OF 66 CASES OF ADVERSE OUTCOMES OF GESTATIONAL LYME BORRELIOSIS

Table 11–8 lists 66 individual cases of adverse outcomes of gestational Lyme borreliosis. Only five groups—Schlesinger and co-workers,[25] MacDonald,[33–35] Lavoie and associates,[32] Weber and colleagues,[38, 39] and Hercogova and co-workers[41]—have had any success in demonstrating spirochetes in either fetal autopsy or placental tissues, and only Trevisan and associates have confirmed spirochetes in a tissue biopsy.[43] Only one infant was found to be seropositive for *B. burgdorferi* antibody (patient 24), and this was transient; therefore, this does not appear to be a sensitive method of diagnosis, and reliance on seropositivity leads to misdiagnosis of the majority of congenitally infected infants. The poor protection provided by short courses of oral antibiotic therapy against the development of serious adverse complications of gestational Lyme borreliosis is evident from this table; this is discussed in detail in the section on Therapy.

Of the 20 fetal deaths among the 66 patients with adverse outcomes after gestational Lyme borreliosis, 95% (19 of 20) of the fetal deaths occurred after first- or second-trimester infection, 75% (15 of 20) of these fetal deaths occurred before 20 weeks of gestational age, and the incidence of cardiac anomaly or abnormality in fetal deaths after untreated and treated gestational Lyme borreliosis was 40% (4 of 9) and 0% (0 of 4), respectively. Information from fetal autopsies was available only for fetuses over 25 weeks' gestation, and all three stillborn infants and the 25-week miscarried fetus had significant cardiac anomalies.

Of the 16 infants with an early severe presentation among the 66 patients with adverse outcomes after gestational Lyme borreliosis, 100% (10 of 10) in whom the trimester of gestational Lyme disease was known occurred after first- or second-trimester infection; the incidence of cardiac anomaly or abnormality was 56% (9 of 16) overall and 85% (5 of 6) in fatal cases.

Currently, it is uncertain whether or not *B. burgdorferi* is teratogenic, although there is an indication that there may be, as noted earlier, an increased risk of congenital cardiac malformations after first- and early second-trimester gestational Lyme borreliosis, which is decreased by antibiotic therapy for the gestational episode. It is also possible that *B. burgdorferi* gestational infection with transplacental dissemination could cause fetal pathology simply by causing Lyme borreliosis with the same manifestations (cutaneous, musculoskeletal, neurologic, neuropsychiatric, neurocognitive, and urologic) that it produces in children and adult patients, which could explain some of the adverse events noted in Table 11–8.

It is likely that prompt and adequate antibiotic therapy of gestational Lyme borreliosis may attenuate its potential adverse fetal effects, and may shift the clinical manifestations away from the more severe presentations such as miscarriages, stillbirths, perinatal deaths, and cardiac anomalies. This could result in higher infant survival rates, with an increased incidence of presentation with late sequelae, which would be expected to exhibit features similar to those of late Lyme borreliosis as described in the section Clinical Manifestations. It is also likely that neonates or infants with undiagnosed congenitally acquired *B. burgdorferi* infection who have received antibiotic therapy for bacterial culture–negative presumed sepsis may not be seropositive for *B. burgdorferi* antibody because of attenuation or prevention of seroconversion by early antibiotic therapy. If the antibiotic therapy has been inadequate to eliminate *B. burgdorferi* infection, these infants may present the dilemma of seronegative late Lyme borreliosis.

It is anticipated that more infants and fetuses with complications related to gestational Lyme borreliosis will be diagnosed in the future as the diagnosis is more frequently considered; it eventually will be possible to better describe the various clinical manifestations of congenital Lyme borreliosis. Large-scale prospective studies of sufficient numbers of patients with gestational Lyme borreliosis, with follow-up to determine the pregnancy outcome of each enrolled patient; *B. burgdorferi*–specific evaluation of any fetal or neonatal demise; and long-term follow-up of each infant born to determine the occurrence of possible early and late sequelae are needed.

FREQUENCY OF SPECIFIC ADVERSE OUTCOMES OF GESTATIONAL LYME BORRELIOSIS

Table 11–13 shows the frequency of occurrence of various types of fetal or neonatal adverse outcomes after gestational Lyme borreliosis.

The 23% incidence of cardiac malformation is strikingly high and includes significant abnormalities such as ventricular septal defect, coarctation of the aorta, and myocardial dysfunction, as well as less severe abnormalities such as patent ductus arteriosus and atrial septal defect; it is reminiscent of the ability of the spirochete to cause carditis, including cardiomyopathy and pancarditis, in older patients.

The 15% incidence of neurologic abnormalities is also high, and includes meningoencephalitis, hydrocephalus, and developmental delay; this would also be consistent with the neurotropic nature of the infection in older patients. One infant (patient 24) had focal parenchymal brain lesions with increased T_2 signal demonstrated by MRI scan that were similar to those reported in the literature in adult patients with chronic meningoencephalomyelitis.

The incidence of orthopedic abnormalities was 12%, but there were some unique features of this involvement, including 4 patients of the 66 with syndactyly or clubfoot, 2 with significant joint contractures, and 2 with a new finding of transverse metaphyseal bands.

The incidence of genitourinary abnormalities was 11%; these included cryptorchidism, inguinal hernia, hydrocele, hypospadias, renal dysplasia, and ureteral stenosis with hydronephrosis.

The incidence of maculopapular erythematous rash was 9%, which would be consistent with disseminated spirochetosis, and many of these rashes increased or developed during the first few days of antibiotic therapy and resembled Jarisch-Herxheimer reactions. The one infant (case 25) with chronic distal extremity rash that resolved after prolonged antibiotic therapy raises the possibility that this was similar to the rash of secondary syphilis or disseminated Lyme borreliosis in older patients.

Among the miscellaneous abnormalities reported were three patients (4.5%) with dental anomalies, including two with hypoplastic enamel and one with structural anomalies.

Hepatosplenomegaly and inguinal adenopathy were also seen in several patients and probably represent disseminated spirochetal infection, as these findings resolved with antibiotic therapy.

Congenital Lyme borreliosis presenting as manifestations that are not specific for *B. burgdorferi*, such as the 17% incidence of presentation as fulminant early sepsis, the 12% presentation with hyperbilirubinemia, and the 12% presentation with growth retardation, may be missed unless careful maternal gestational and pre-gestational histories are obtained.

Thirty percent (20 of 66) of the total number of adverse outcomes were miscarriages (including one aborted fetus with congenital anomalies), 9% (6 of 66) were neonatal deaths, and 39% (26 of 66) were either fetal or neonatal deaths.

FREQUENCY OF ADVERSE OUTCOMES OF 263 CASES OF GESTATIONAL LYME BORRELIOSIS

Table 11–14 shows the fetal and neonatal mortality rates, and the total fetal and neonatal adverse outcome rates divided by trimester and according to whether or not gestational antibiotic therapy was given. Those considered treated or untreated were patients in whom antibiotic therapy was specifically reported as having been specifically given or not given to the individual patient, and those considered as having unknown treatment were those in whom statements about treatment could not be correlated with the individual patient.

Effect of Trimester of Infection

Lyme borreliosis in the first trimester carried an overall 32% (24 of 74 patients) risk of adverse outcome. In the second trimester, the risk was 25% (17 of 68); in the third trimester, it was 16% (6 of 38); in gestational Lyme borreliosis with trimester unspecified, it was 22% (18 of 83); the overall risk in all trimesters was 25% (66 of 263).

Effect of Gestational Antibiotic Therapy

Gestational antibiotic therapy had a protective effect against adverse fetal or neonatal outcome, and the overall adverse outcome risk after treatment in all trimesters was 15% (23 of 157); after no treatment in all trimesters, it was 67% (20 of 30). This protective effect was apparent in all trimesters: 18 compared with 73% in the first trimester, 16 compared with 67% in the second trimester, and 9 compared with 50% in the third trimester.

Rate of Miscarriage and Stillbirth

The overall risk of miscarriage for any trimester of infection was 7.6% (20 of 263 patients). Antibiotic therapy showed a protective effect, with a rate of 2.5% (4 of 157) fetal loss after treated gestational Lyme borreliosis, compared with 30% (9 of 30) without antibiotic therapy.

Rate of Neonatal Death

The overall risk of neonatal death for any trimester of infection was 2% (6 of 263 patients); the rate was less than 1% (1 of 157) with antibiotic therapy, and 7% (2 of 30) without antibiotic therapy, for gestational Lyme borreliosis.

Rate of Neonatal Illness

The risk of nonfatal neonatal illness for any trimester of infection was 15% (40 of 263 patients); the risk was 11% (18 of 157) with antibiotic therapy compared with 30% (9 of 30) without antibiotic therapy for the gestational Lyme borreliosis episode.

Description of Congenital Lyme Borreliosis

Table 11–15 lists the incidence, time of presentation, and clinical manifestations of the various adverse outcomes associated with gestational Lyme borreliosis, including miscarriage, early severe congenital Lyme borreliosis, early mild congenital Lyme borreliosis, and late chronic congenital Lyme borreliosis.

Clinical case reports of mother-infant pairs who illustrate these various manifestations of congenital Lyme borreliosis are presented in the following sections.

ASYMPTOMATIC INFANT WITH GESTATIONAL LYME BORRELIOSIS EXPOSURE

CLINICAL CASE

Mother. A 26-year-old woman developed acute onset of hypertension of 160/140 and severe left facial pain, paresthesia, and paralysis in the thirty-eighth week of her third pregnancy in mid-March of 1991; because of the hypertension, she had a cesarean section for delivery of the infant 2 days later. A diagnosis of idiopathic Bell's palsy was made, and she was treated with prednisone, 40 to 60 mg daily, for less than 1 week, had partial return of motor function after 6 months, but still had residual discomfort, paresthesias, and mild to moderate left facial motor deficits 2 years later.

In 1992, during her next pregnancy, she was treated with oral cephalexin for a first-trimester urinary tract infection and gave birth at term to a second infant in October 1992.

In April 1993, during routine questioning about maternal gestational history because of hospitalization of her then 2-year-old child for gastroenteritis, she reported that ever since the Bell's palsy, she had persistent severe daily headaches; neck aches; intermittent left conjunctivitis; migratory polyarthralgias of the wrists, elbows, knees, and hips; infrequent 10- to 20-cm-diameter round erythematous rashes on her legs that spontaneously resolved; fatigue; and short-term memory deficits. She was an avid hiker and had an over-10-year history of multiple tick bites to her scalp, ears, and neck; she reported that many of these ticks had become fully engorged before removal. In April 1993, she was found to have specific B. burgdorferi antibody by polyvalent EIA and IgM Western blot assays.

Initially, she was treated with oral cefuroxime axetil (because of a history of penicillin allergy) for 6 weeks, had a mild Jarisch-Herxheimer reaction on the second day, and had resolution of fatigue and headache and improvement in the residual Bell's palsy symptoms by the end of therapy. She experienced relapse within 1 week of completion of the oral cefuroxime, with fatigue, headache, left eye conjunctivitis, and left facial weakness (the residual Bell's palsy of this patient at the time of this relapse is shown in Figure 11–8). She had a lumbar puncture (spinal fluid B. burgdorferi antibody negative, and spinal fluid normal); was treated over 3.5 weeks with intravenous ceftriaxone; had resolution of fatigue, headache, and conjunctivitis and marked improvement of the left facial weakness by the end of therapy; and remained well at 6-month follow-up.

Placenta. No pathologic testing was performed on either placenta.

Infant 1. The baby, who was delivered by cesarean section 2 days after onset of the maternal Bell's palsy at 38 weeks of gestation, was considered normal at birth. However, he was hospitalized at 5.5 months of age for fever, irritability, lethargy, full fontanelle, and the possibility of culture-negative (bacterial and viral) sepsis or meningitis (normal spinal fluid); responded clinically to intravenous cefotaxime over 3 days; and developed a maculopapular rash on the second day of the cefotaxime treatment that resolved despite continuation of the cefotaxime. He was treated by his pediatrician with oral amoxicillin several times during his first 2 years of life for upper respiratory infections. When the mother's Lyme borreliosis was diagnosed 2 years after the birth of this infant, he was tested and found to have no antibodies to B. burgdorferi; he has remained normal at 2.8-year follow-up.

Infant 2. A second baby born to this mother in

October 1992 after a term pregnancy was also normal at birth. At 7.5 months of age, this infant was treated by his pediatrician with oral amoxicillin–clavulanic acid for an upper respiratory infection and developed an erythematous maculopapular rash on the fourth day, which resolved despite continuation of the antibiotic. When the mother's Lyme borreliosis was diagnosed, he was tested and found to be seronegative for *B. burgdorferi* antibodies; he has remained normal at 1.3-year follow-up.

Comments. This mother gave birth to two infants before the diagnosis of Lyme borreliosis (during gestation for the first infant) was made retrospectively 2 years later; this followed routine questioning to obtain a gestational history because of hospitalization of one of the infants for an unrelated illness (bacterial gastroenteritis). Her *B. burgdorferi* seropositivity, Jarisch-Herxheimer reaction (refer to discussion of Jarisch-Herxheimer reaction in section Therapy) after initiation of antibiotic therapy, and impressive clinical response to antibiotic therapy all support the diagnosis of chronic Lyme borreliosis in this patient, although it was made retrospectively.

Fortunately, both infants were normal at birth and remained so. However, both had erythematous maculopapular rashes, possibly reminiscent of Jarisch-Herxheimer reactions, between 5.5 and 7.5 months of age within the first few days of either intravenous third-generation cephalosporin or oral amoxicillin therapy, which was given in one case for an episode of "rule out sepsis and meningitis" with negative viral and bacterial cultures, and in the other case for an upper respiratory infection. It is not known whether either of these infants ever acquired the spirochete gestationally, as both infants were *B. burgdorferi*–seronegative, but they were not tested by the in vitro lymphocyte proliferative assay, which may be more sensitive in detection of congenital Lyme borreliosis.

This mother-infant group illustrates the possibility that infants born after untreated gestational Lyme borreliosis may be normal. A possible explanation for this could be that transplacental spread of the spirochete is variable; that spirochetemia may not yet have occurred at the time the first infant was delivered, which was within 2 days of onset of the Bell's palsy; that the oral cephalosporin therapy during the first trimester of gestation of the second infant may have partially treated the Lyme borreliosis, sufficiently to prevent transplacental spread to the fetus; or that if transplacental spread of infection occurred in either of these two infants, the courses of antibiotic therapy given by the pediatrician for other illnesses during the first year of life may have been beneficial in prevention of symptomatic congenital Lyme borreliosis. ∎

MILD EARLY CONGENITAL LYME BORRELIOSIS

CLINICAL CASE (patient 23 in Table 11–8)

Mother. A 38-year-old woman visited a lake for 4 days in mid-April 1987, and the day after returning home, found and removed an engorged tick attached to her groin. A 1-cm indurated erythematous patch had developed at the bite site and resolved a few days after she applied topical Neosporin ointment. She conceived in mid-May 1987, developed a mild flulike illness 1 week later at 3 weeks of gestational age, developed an asymptomatic rash on her trunk at 4 weeks, and presented at 4.5 weeks with low-grade fever, a dense erythematous maculopapular rash of her trunk and proximal extremities (see Fig. 11–7*A*), and two larger (1- to 2-cm) erythematous patches with central clearing (see Fig. 11–7*B*).

She was referred for infectious disease evaluation for suspected rubella, but because of the appearance of the rash and the history of the tick bite, the diagnosis of Lyme borreliosis was considered; she was treated immediately at 4.5 weeks' gestation with intravenous ceftriaxone 2 g daily and showed improvement in the rash after 2 days; however, she developed severe watery diarrhea, which necessitated a change to penicillin 500 mg four times daily for the remainder of the 2-week course. The rash resolved completely after 8 days, and she remained well throughout the rest of the pregnancy, except for mild toxemia in the last trimester; she delivered a term infant by cesarean section because of nonprogression of labor. Maternal polyvalent ELISA serum antibody to *B. burgdorferi* was initially negative at presentation at 4.5 weeks' gestation, became positive at 5.5 weeks, remained positive through 12 weeks, and was negative at delivery. In vitro lymphocyte proliferative assay for *B. burgdorferi* was positive at 16 weeks' gestation, at delivery, and at 1 month post partum, but the level decreased with time. She has remained well after 6.5 years, as assessed by verbal follow-up.

Placenta. Focal chorioamnionitis and subchorionic nodules were found (refer to discussion of placental pathology in section Pathology and Pathogenesis).

Infant. The infant was normal at birth except for a sacral dimple and 0.5-cm bilateral inguinal adenopathy of initially unclear significance (patient 23 in Table 11–8). The child weighed 3461 g and had a normal pediatric ophthalmology examination, normal brain-stem auditory evoked response evaluation, normal head ultrasound, normal electrocardiogram, normal chest and long bone x-rays, and normal complete blood count. Spinal fluid included three mononuclear cells, protein 53 mg/dl, glucose 37 mg/dl; both blood and spinal fluid were negative for polyvalent EIA *B. burgdorferi* antibody. In vitro lymphocyte proliferative assay for *B. burgdorferi* was positive on both cord blood and infant blood at 1 month of age but was lower at 1 month.

After the result of the proliferative assay was obtained, the infant was treated with intravenous ceftriaxone 100 mg/kg daily for 2 weeks and developed an intensely erythematous generalized maculopapular rash on the sixth day of treatment, which resolved despite continuation of the antibiotic. The inguinal adenopathy resolved by the end of the antibiotic therapy; the infant remained clinically well at 15 months, and by verbal report continued to be well at almost 6 years of age. ∎

CLINICAL CASE (case 26 in Table 11–8)

Mother. In early April 1989, a 29-year-old woman in the seventeenth week of pregnancy camped in a wooded area frequented by deer and had several small tick bites, including one that was deeply embedded in her scalp. At 18 weeks' gestation, she developed on her thigh at one of the tick bite sites a 10 × 5-cm-diameter erythematous oval "bull's-eye" rash that lasted 3 weeks and then spontaneously resolved. Between 20 and 28 weeks' gestation, she experienced low-grade fever, myalgias, fatigue, stiff neck, dizziness, photophobia, and migratory polyarthralgias, especially of the knees, and between 23 and 26 weeks, she had recurrence of the rash.

At 28 weeks, she took oral erythromycin 250 mg four times daily for 10 days, and her symptoms resolved. She then heard about Lyme disease, obtained and began oral cefuroxime axetil 1 g twice daily from 33 weeks to the time of delivery, and remained well except for mild knee arthralgias. She reported that her urine had been positive for Lyme antigen at a commercial laboratory at 32 weeks.

At delivery, maternal blood was negative for polyvalent EIA *B. burgdorferi* antibody, but blood obtained 1 day post partum was positive by the *B. burgdorferi* in vitro lymphocyte proliferative assay (LPA). After delivery, because of recurrence of headache, photophobia, flulike symptoms, and knee arthralgias, she was treated with oral doxycycline 100 mg twice daily for 1 month, improved within 24 hours, and recovered by the end of therapy. Long-term follow-up information is unavailable.

Infant. The infant was normal at birth except for diffuse small retinal hemorrhages with white centers; weighed 3461 g; and had a normal brain-stem auditory evoked response evaluation, normal electrocardiogram and two-dimensional echocardiogram, and normal complete blood count and liver enzyme panel. Cord blood and infant's blood on the first day, at 2.5 weeks, and at 7 weeks were all seronegative for polyvalent EIA *B. burgdorferi* antibody, but blood from the first day was positive by the in vitro LPA for *B. burgdorferi*.

By 2.5 weeks, the infant had become somewhat listless and slept more than expected; spinal fluid showed a slight lymphocytic pleocytosis, slightly elevated protein, and normal glucose. MRI scan of the brain was normal, complete blood count was normal, liver enzymes were normal, and there was slight hyperbilirubinemia, but the retinal lesions had spontaneously resolved. The infant was treated with intravenous ceftriaxone 75 mg/kg daily for 4 weeks, developed a "pale spell" on the second day of therapy, became more active and alert after 3 days of therapy, and was completely well by completion of antibiotic therapy. A repeat lumbar puncture was performed at the end of the antibiotic therapy but was traumatic; long-term follow-up is unavailable.

Comments. The preceding two mothers both had gestational erythema migrans with systemic symptoms, both were treated with antibiotic therapy during pregnancy, and both delivered infants who were clinically normal at birth except for minor manifestations of early congenital Lyme borreliosis. The infant born to the mother with gestational Lyme borreliosis treated within 2 weeks of onset had only inguinal adenopathy, rash, and a sacral dimple (dimple is of unclear significance); the one born to the mother with symptoms of gestational Lyme borreliosis persisting for 10 weeks before antibiotic therapy had evidence of mild neurologic symptoms, transient retinal lesions, mild lymphocytic meningitis, and mild hyperbilirubinemia. Both infants had episodes resembling Jarisch-Herxheimer reactions shortly after initiation of ceftriaxone therapy at 2 weeks of age; both had resolution of their manifestations of early congenital Lyme borreliosis by the end of antibiotic therapy. Both infants and mothers were seronegative for polyvalent EIA *B. burgdorferi* antibody at delivery and positive by the *B. burgdorferi*–specific in vitro LPA.

These mother-infant groups illustrate the observation that infants with congenital Lyme borreliosis and mothers who have been treated with antibiotics for gestational Lyme borreliosis may be seronegative by antibody assays at delivery or in the peripartum period, and they may be positive by the *B. burgdorferi*–specific LPA.

These cases illustrate the importance of prompt and aggressive antibiotic therapy for gestational Lyme borreliosis. In one of these cases, the intravenous ceftriaxone had to be discontinued because of severe diarrhea and therapy was completed with high-dose penicillin; in the other case, the mother was treated with prolonged oral cefuroxime axetil through the time of delivery. Longer courses of intravenous antibiotic therapy have been more effective in the treatment of other manifestations of Lyme borreliosis. Recommendations for optimal antibiotic therapy of gestational Lyme borreliosis, for mild symptoms of congenital Lyme borreliosis such as inguinal adenopathy and mild lethargy as well as for the more obvious symptoms of severe congenital Lyme borreliosis are discussed in the section on gestationally exposed newborn infants; also, recommendations are made to begin antibiotic therapy promptly after birth to prevent later clinical sequelae. ∎

SEVERE EARLY CONGENITAL LYME BORRELIOSIS

CLINICAL CASE (patient 24 in Table 11–8)

Mother. A 34-year-old woman had a tick bite between mid-April and late May 1987 at 6.5 to 12.5 weeks' gestation; she was treated with oral amoxicillin 250 mg three times daily for 10 to 14 days for sinusitis and flulike symptoms at 5 to 7 weeks', and at 20 to 22 weeks' gestation. A routine fetal sonogram performed at 17 weeks was normal, but another done at 24 weeks because of decreased amniotic fluid showed marked intrauterine growth retardation. Fetal blood sampling at 24.5 weeks showed normal chromosomes and no evidence of intrauterine viral infection; the infant was delivered by cesarean section at 34 weeks' gestation. The mother remained clinically well following delivery and was seronegative for polyvalent EIA *B. burgdorferi* antibody at 1 week, 9 months, and 10 months after delivery; she was also negative by the *B. burgdorferi* LPA at 9 and 10 months.

Placenta. Pathologic evaluation showed chronic fibrosing villitis, which is described in the section on the placenta in Pathology and Pathogenesis.

Infant. The infant was small for gestational age (1050 g, 34 weeks) and had a low Apgar score; a "blueberry muffin" rash and profound thrombocytopenia that required platelet transfusions; hepatomegaly and hyperbilirubinemia; meconium ileus that required enemas; severe dilated cardiomyopathy with biventricular dysfunction and low voltage on electrocardiogram that required intensive cardiopulmonary support with intubation, mechanical ventilation, and pressors; and a transient patent ductus arteriosus. Several additional abnormalities were noted, including a pilonidal dimple, flexion contractures of the large joints (hips, knees, and elbows), longitudinal striations and dense sclerotic transverse metaphyseal bands of the long bones, a large forehead and split sutures, a full fontanelle, and bilateral inguinal adenopathy. Head ultrasound showed diffuse punctate increased parenchymal echogenicity, skull x-rays showed no calcifications, liver enzymes were normal, brain-stem auditory evoked response evaluation was normal, and ophthalmologic examination was normal. Figure 11–9 shows the meconium ileus, cardiomegaly, and sclerotic metaphyseal bands of this patient.

This infant was initially considered to have culture-negative bacterial sepsis and was treated with intravenous ampicillin and gentamicin for 6 days, but failed to improve and continued to require platelet transfusions and intensive cardiovascular support. Because of the maternal gestational history of tick bite, the possibility of congenital Lyme borreliosis was raised, and intravenous ceftriaxone (100 mg/kg per day) was added on the seventh day and continued for 1 week; within 24 hours, the platelet count stabilized, the pressors were able to be discontinued, and the infant began to recover. Spinal fluid on the sixth day showed an elevated protein but no pleocytosis. The dense sclerotic transverse metaphyseal bands present in all of the long bones during the first week gradually resolved during ceftriaxone therapy. Extensive evaluation for bacterial and viral causes of this fulminant sepsis was unrevealing; neither did the infant have detectable polyvalent EIA *B. burgdorferi* antibody. The infant was eventually discharged from the hospital at 2 months of age in good condition.

By 9 months, she demonstrated growth retardation, mild developmental delay, mild lower extremity spasticity, and persistently small head circumference; the possibility of congenital Lyme borreliosis was reconsidered. At 9 but not at 10 months, she was found to have polyvalent EIA *B. burgdorferi* antibody; at 9 and 10 months, she had a positive *B. burgdorferi* in vitro LPA; and between 9 and 10 months, further evaluation included a normal spinal fluid with no

detectable *B. burgdorferi* antibody, a normal electrocardiogram, normal complete blood count, slightly elevated liver enzymes, and MRI scan of the brain that showed left parietal parenchymal lesions of increased T_2 signal. She was treated with intravenous ceftriaxone (75 mg/kg daily) for 3 weeks for neuroborreliosis. She subsequently improved and exhibited normal growth and development at follow-up at 2.5 years of age.

Comments. This mother-infant pair illustrates the presentation of severe early congenital Lyme borreliosis as fulminant neonatal sepsis; the need to consider Lyme borreliosis in the differential diagnosis of culture-negative sepsis; and the need to include optimal intravenous antibiotic therapy for Lyme borreliosis, such as third-generation cephalosporins, if Lyme disease is considered. This case also indicates the failure of short oral courses of antibiotic therapy in the prevention of severe congenital Lyme borreliosis and the need for more aggressive antibiotic therapy of gestational Lyme disease.

The unusual finding of sclerotic transverse metaphyseal bands in the long bones, which faded during the ceftriaxone therapy in this infant and in one other infant (case 25 in Table 11–8) with congenital Lyme borreliosis, may eventually prove to be a useful diagnostic finding in severe congenital Lyme borreliosis.

The initial clinical presentation of this infant resembles the description by Lampert[31] of the infant with infantile multisystem inflammatory syndrome who was later found to have chronic Lyme borreliosis, as well as the description of some reported infants who had fulminant early congenital Lyme sepsis,[26, 32, 33, 38, 39] although this infant did not have the severe cardiac malformations found in some of these patients. ∎

LATE CONGENITAL LYME BORRELIOSIS

CLINICAL CASE (patient 25 in Table 11–8)

Mother. A 35-year-old mother of five children visited a tick-infested farm with her entire family for 2 weeks every summer from 1988 through 1990, and she and several family members had occasional tick bites during this time. During the first 6 weeks of her next pregnancy, between mid-March and late April 1990, she developed a flulike illness that progressed to pneumonia and was associated with unusually large nonpruritic, nontender, vesiculobullous, and even purulent round or oval skin lesions on her legs. She was treated with almost continuous antibiotic therapy for the first 10 weeks of gestation, initially oral erythromycin (333 mg three times daily) for 7 weeks; followed by cefaclor (250 mg three times daily) for 3 days, intravenous cefuroxime (750 mg three times daily) for 4 days, and oral cephalexin (500 mg four times daily) for 2 weeks; and then oral cefixime (100 mg daily) for 10 days at 12 to 13 weeks. The large erythematous skin lesions intermittently reappeared during the second and third trimesters, and she

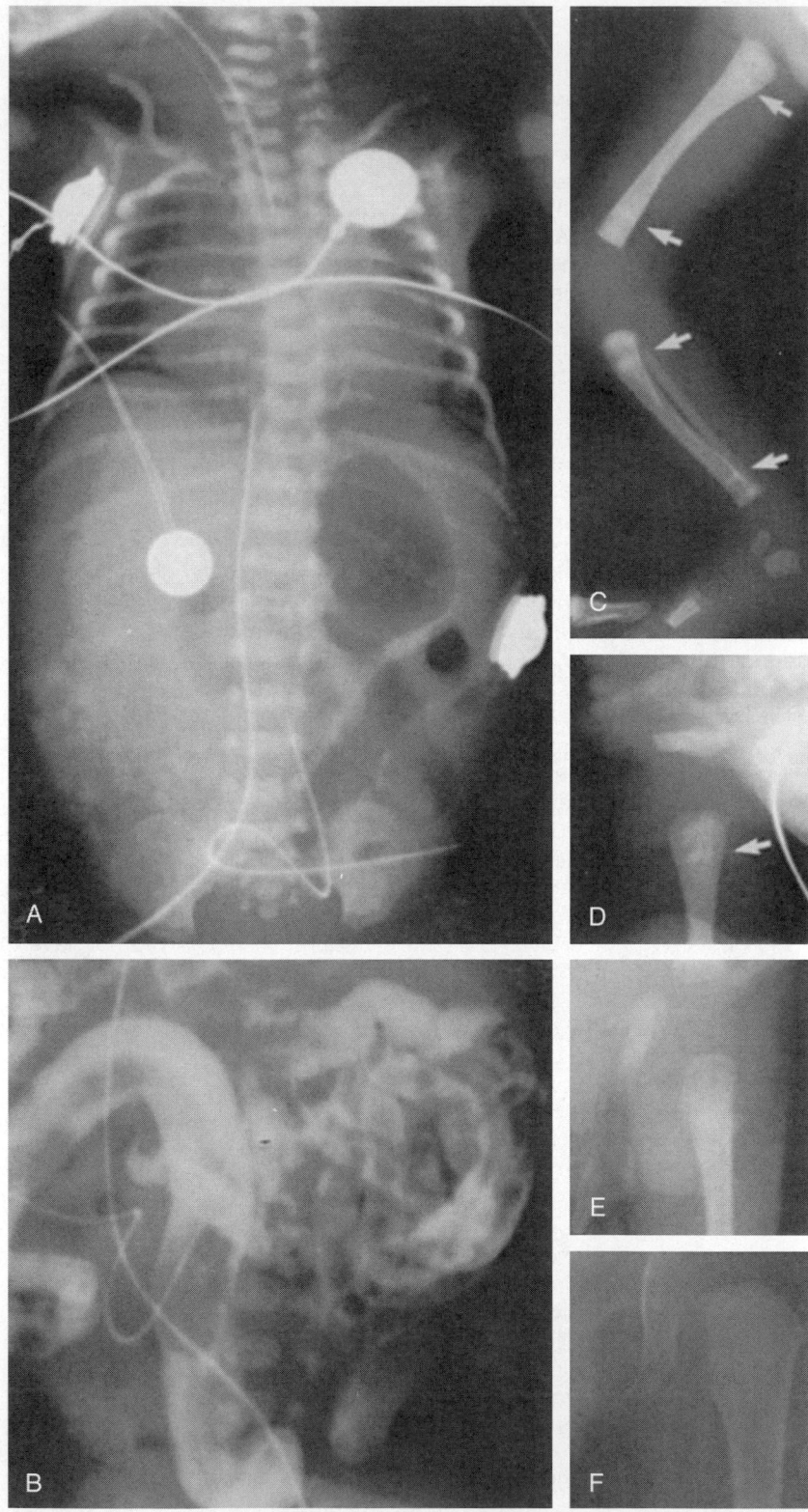

FIGURE 11–9 Congenital Lyme disease. An infant presented at birth with thrombocytopenia, cardiomyopathy, meconium ileus equivalent, and intrauterine growth retardation. *A,* Chest and abdominal radiograph at 1 day of age show cardiomegaly and mottled increased density in the right lower quadrant from inspissated meconium. *B,* Lower GI study at 1 day of age demonstrates impacted meconium in the distal ileum. Bone radiographs show *(C)* sclerotic transverse metaphyseal bands at birth (arrows), *(D)* fading metaphyseal bands after antibiotic therapy for 5 days (arrow), *(E)* further fading of the metaphyseal bands after antibiotic therapy for 16 days, and *(F)* resolution of the metaphyseal bands by 7 months (patient 24 in Table 11–8).

developed progressive arthralgias and arthritis of her hips, knees, and lower back; by the time of delivery, in December 1990, she was unable to walk without stooping over. The skin lesions, polyarthralgias, and polyarthritis recurred after delivery and continued intermittently for 4 months post partum; she also noted headaches, fatigue, and short-term memory lapses.

In March 1991, the history of this maternal gestational illness and tick exposure was discovered on routine questioning during hospitalization of the then 3-month-old infant for severe failure to thrive. As part of the evaluation of the infant for possible congenital infection, maternal blood was sent and found to be seropositive for polyvalent EIA *B. burgdorferi* antibody. Figure 11–5D shows one of the mother's recurrent skin lesions, and a skin biopsy of this lesion showed the superficial and deep dermal perivascular lymphocytic inflammatory infiltrates commonly seen in erythema migrans lesions, but no spirochetes were seen.

She was treated with oral doxycycline 100 mg twice daily and showed initial improvement of the lesions, was changed to intravenous ceftriaxone 1 week later because of subsequent intensification of the skin lesions and recurrence of fever and arthralgias, and was changed back to oral doxycycline after 3 days of ceftriaxone because of development of a generalized erythematous nonpruritic maculopapular rash that was considered by her physicians to be an allergic reaction. The headache, memory loss, fatigue, and skin lesions resolved after 6 weeks of doxycycline, but the right hip arthritis and polyarthralgias persisted, and 1.5 years later, she developed chronic palpebral conjunctivitis and distal paresthesias of her hands and was treated with several weeks of intravenous ceftriaxone with good clinical improvement.

Placenta. No placental pathologic examination was performed.

Infant. The infant was born after 37 weeks' gestation, had birth weight of 3490 g, and was considered normal at birth, but developed neonatal hyperbilirubinemia and nursed poorly. He was treated with intravenous ampicillin and a third-generation cephalosporin for suspected sepsis and urinary tract infection at 1 week of age, and developed a generalized erythematous maculopapular rash thought to be an allergic reaction. Bilateral inguinal hernias were repaired at 1 month of age, and he received a short course of oral cefaclor for otitis media at 2 months of age.

His very experienced mother noted that he became increasingly limp and listless, held his head and neck to the right, slept almost all day, and fed poorly. He presented at 2.5 months of age for infectious disease evaluation to look for possible congenital infection because of severe failure to thrive, developmental delay, growth retardation, and gastroesophageal reflux with recurrent vomiting and recurrent aspiration pneumonias; he was found to have hepatomegaly, erythematous abdominal and distal extremity rough maculopapular rash, lethargy, marked proximal hypotonia, distal hyperreflexia and hypertonia, jitteriness, alternating exotropia, and some dysmorphic

features consisting of cupped ears, upturned nose, small chin, a unilateral simian crease, and pectus excavatum. The collecting system was slightly dilated and the kidneys slightly small; there were dense transverse metaphyseal bands in the long bones, an MRI scan of the brain was normal, brain-stem auditory evoked response evaluation was normal, spinal fluid was unremarkable, and chromosome analysis was normal. He underwent fundoplication and feeding gastrotomy because of inability to swallow without aspiration, and the exotropia was surgically corrected.

Evaluation for possible congenital infection was initially unrevealing, and the spinal fluid and serum were both negative for polyvalent EIA antibody to *B. burgdorferi*. However, because of the presence of metaphyseal bands (which were reminiscent of those in an earlier infant with congenital Lyme borreliosis), the maternal gestational history, and the maternal Lyme seropositivity, the diagnosis of late congenital Lyme borreliosis was still considered, and both the infant and mother were found to have positive responses in the *B. burgdorferi* in vitro LPA.

The child received a total of 7 weeks of intravenous ceftriaxone (100 mg/kg daily) between 2.5 and 7 months and showed dramatic improvement in neurologic function. When initial attempts were made to use a less aggressive and shorter course of intravenous ceftriaxone, he experienced relapse with evidence of loss of developmental milestones; finally, after a total of 7 weeks of intravenous ceftriaxone followed by a 1-year course of oral amoxicillin (40 mg/kg daily) from 7 months to 19 months of age, he remained clinically well and continued to progress to essentially normal neurologic status by 3 years of age. He had gradual resolution of the scaly erythematous maculopapular abdominal and distal extremity rash by the completion of the ceftriaxone therapy. He gradually improved neurologically, regained lost developmental milestones, and resolved the majority of his focal neurologic findings, including the subtle right hemiparesis, mild proximal hypotonia, and distal hyperreflexia, by 2 years of age. At follow-up at 3 years of age, he remained well, was at an appropriate developmental level, and was slowly learning to take food by mouth. At 8 years of age, he had reached an almost age-appropriate developmental and intellectual level, but developed regression of reading, spelling, and vocabulary skills, a seizure disorder, and episodic unilateral knee and ankle arthritis, with no additional *B. burgdorferi* exposure; the arthritis and deterioration of language skills responded to intravenous ceftriaxone therapy. At 9 years of age, he has regained almost all of the lost language skills, but exhibits delayed dentition and structural dental anomalies.

Figure 11–10A to J shows the gastroesophageal reflux, aspiration, strabismus, facial dysmorphia, severe hypotonia, rash, and metaphyseal bands in the first few months of life; Figure 11–10K shows the patient at 2 years of age.

Comments. This mother-infant pair illustrates the ability of *B. burgdorferi* to cause severe progressive neurologic deficits consistent with chronic

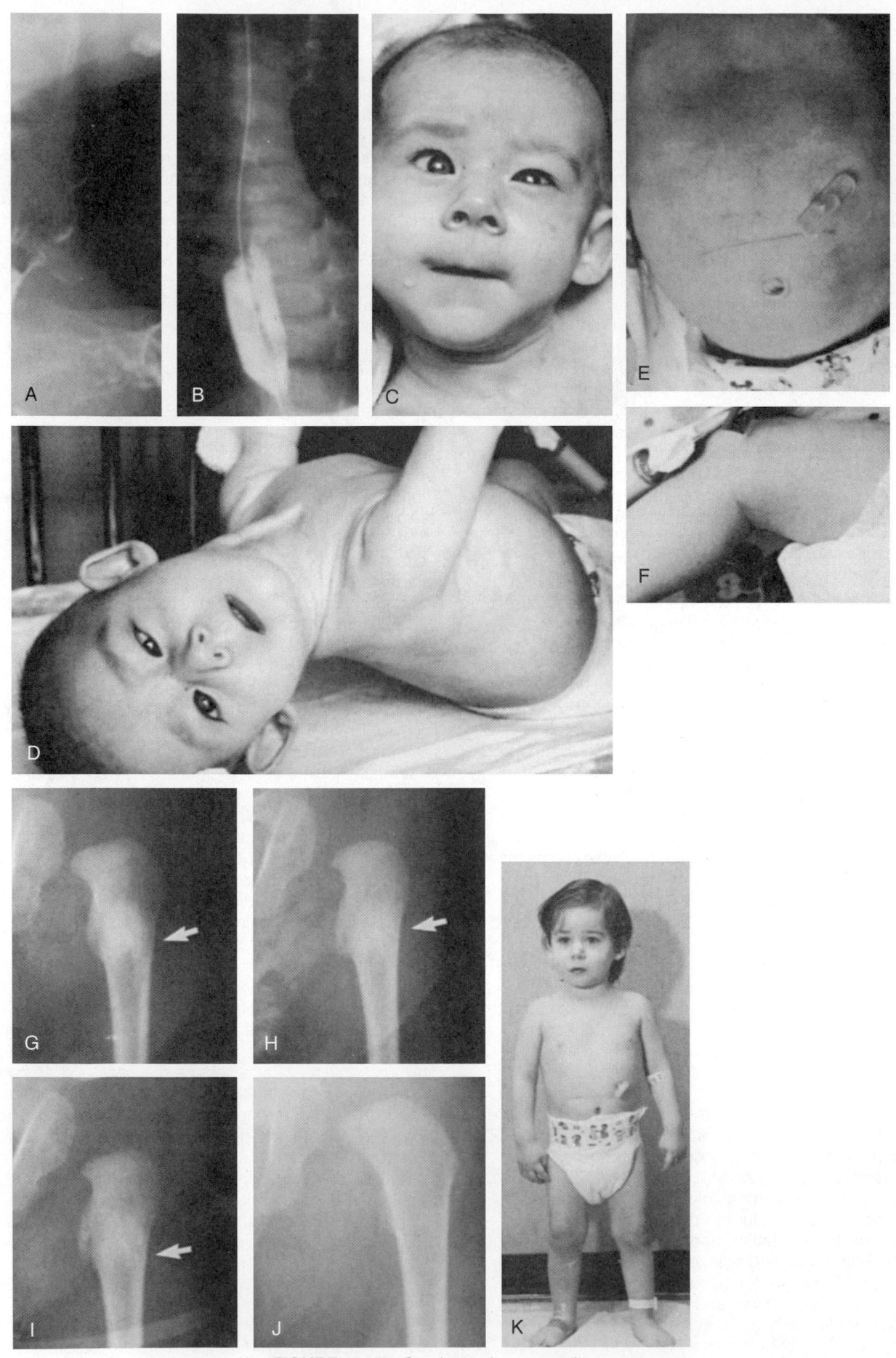

FIGURE 11–10 *See legend on opposite page*

neuroborreliosis, and the failure of oral erythromycin and oral cephalosporins to prevent these complications. However, the prolonged first-trimester courses of oral antibiotics may have sufficiently stabilized the gestational spirochetal infection to allow the pregnancy to be carried almost to term. Although there were several dysmorphic features in this infant, the significance of the cupped ears is unclear, as there were two other siblings with slightly "lop" ears.

The neurologic recovery of this patient during the prolonged course of antibiotic therapy and the near-normalization of his developmental level by 3 years of age lend support for such prolonged therapy until it appears that maximum recovery of neurologic function has occurred. The later development of arthritis, seizure disorder, and deterioration of language skills with no additional B. burgdorferi exposure, and improvement after antibiotic therapy are suggestive of a relapse of Lyme disease, and provide support for the use of additional antibiotic therapy for such relapses. The infant reported by Markowitz and colleagues who was normal at birth and later developed cortical blindness may represent this type of clinical manifestation of congenital Lyme borreliosis.[36]   ■

DIAGNOSIS AND DIFFERENTIAL DIAGNOSIS

The demand for diagnostic testing for Lyme disease is great, particularly in Lyme-hyperendemic areas.[734–737]

False-positive serologic results for Lyme disease may occur because of cross-reactivity with other bacteria, particularly other spirochetes (Table 11–16); because of intra- or interlaboratory variability of assay results[529, 738, 739, 741]; or because of cross-reactivity seen in other diseases, including autoimmune disorders[224, 233, 236, 252, 742, 743] such as systemic lupus erythematosus, rheumatoid arthritis, and Reiter's disease; peridontal disease[245]; viral infections[233, 744–746] such as Epstein-Barr Virus (EBV), varicella zoster Virus (VZV), and parvovirus B19; and non-Lyme meningoencephalitis or other neurologic diseases.[223, 233] Another problem is that seropositivity in residents of Lyme-endemic areas reflects the frequency of seropositivity of the area and may be unrelated to clinical illness.[254] Because ehrlichiosis and babesiosis occur in the same geographic distribution as Lyme borreliosis, and share many of the same tick vectors, seropositivity for these agents may reflect true exposure rather than cross-reactivity with B. burgdorferi[481–484, 486]; how-

ever, some cross-reactivity may be due to a heat shock protein of B. burgdorferi and the agent of human granulocytic ehrlichiosis (HGE) that shares amino acid sequence homology. Cross-reactivity is greatest, even by Western blot assay, between relapsing fever Borreliae and B. burgdorferi, which are usually distinguishable clinically, and are vectored by different tick species that do not share the same habitat niches; however, the geographic distribution of the tick vectors may overlap in some areas of the south central and southwestern United States.[477] Recognition that cross-reactivity may produce false-positive B. burgdorferi seroprevalence data in non–Lyme-endemic countries without known tick vectors is important.

False-negative serologic results may occur either because the sample was obtained early in the course of the Lyme disease before development of detectable B. burgdorferi immune responses,[222, 254] because early antibiotic therapy eliminated or blunted the B. burgdorferi immune response,[208, 209, 218, 232, 233, 254, 271, 272, 275] because of intra- or interlaboratory variability of assay results,[529, 738, 739, 741] because of regional antigenic strain variability, or because a low-level true-positive result is masked by cross-reacting antibody that necessitates a high "cut-off" for positivity.[739] Some patients reinfected with B. burgdorferi may have only an IgG response, and seropositivity may not be detected if only IgM assays are done in early reinfection.[233]

The practical ability to confirm or exclude Lyme disease by diagnostic assays remains a complicated and controversial problem. Continued development and clinical correlation of new diagnostic assays using increasingly sophisticated molecular biologic tools have improved diagnostic sensitivity and specificity, but the diagnosis of Lyme disease cannot be either made or excluded solely on the basis of these assays. Lyme disease must remain a clinical diagnosis, based on clinical and epidemiologic history, physical findings, and laboratory data other than B. burgdorferi serologic tests; the serologic test results may be considered either supportive or nonsupportive of the diagnosis, according to accepted guidelines.[238, 254, 478, 633, 748–750]

Diagnostic Tests

Diagnostic tests for Lyme disease are divided into several categories and are listed in Table 11–16. Practical problems with these tests are low sensitivity or low specificity, wide intra- and interlaboratory variability of the most common commercially available antibody de-

---

FIGURE 11–10 Congenital Lyme disease. An infant presented at 2½ months of age with developmental delay, hypotonia, failure to thrive, and recurrent aspiration pneumonia. A, Barium swallow at 2½ months shows aspiration of barium into the trachea. B, Esophagram shows reflux of barium from the stomach into the distal esophagus. C and D, At 5 months, the patient shows strabismus, a foreshortened nasal bridge, cupped ears, a small mouth and chin, and severe hypotonia. E and F, At 5 months, the patient had a persistent erythematous, maculopapular rash, most prominent on the trunk and proximal extremities, which faded with antibiotic therapy. Bone radiographs show (G) sclerotic metaphyseal bands at 2½ months of age (arrow), (H) fading metaphyseal bands after antibiotic therapy for 5 days (arrow), (I) further fading of the metaphyseal bands after antibiotic therapy for 6 days (arrow), and (J) resolution of the metaphyseal bands by 5 months of age. K, The patient at 25 months (patient 25 in Table 11–8).

TABLE 11–16
Cross-Reactivity Between *Borrelia burgdorferi* and Other Spirochetes, *Babesia*, and *Ehrlichia*

DIAGNOSTIC TEST	Lyme	Syphilis	Yaws, Pinta	Borrelial Relapsing Fever[a]	Borrelia coriaceae[b]	Leptospirosis	Babesiosis[c] B.m.	Babesiosis[c] WA1	Ehrlichiosis[d] HGE	Ehrlichiosis[d] HME
Bb IFA[e]		13–61	28–40	50	63	0–14			36	2
Bb ELISA[f]		20–100	40–43	45–100[g]		0–23	0	0	0–86[h]	0
ELISA-AC		0–4				5				
Bb WB[i]		0–50		64–100[g]		5–17	0	0	23–90[h]	0
WB (stringent)		0–9								
FTA-Abs[j]	6–43									
MHA-TP[k]	0									
RPR[l]	0									
VDRL[m]	0									
TP WB[n]	0–67									
Other borreliae[o], IFA	54–85									
Leptospira MA[p]	0									
B. microti IFA	0	0						0	0	0
B. microti ELISA	0									
B. microti WB	0									
WA1	0									<10
HGE IFA	0–6	0		0			0	0		0
HGE ELISA	4–26	0		0						0
HGE WB	4–13	0		0						0
HME IFA	0	0					0	3	11–56	
HME WB									0	

[a]*B. hermsii* and *B. recurrentis*, as well as many other borreliae, are the major causes of relapsing fever.
[b]*B. coriaceae* is endemic in soft ticks in California but rarely causes human illness.
[c]*B.m.* = *Babesia microti*; WAI = *Babesia* species WA1.
[d]HGE = human granulocytic ehrlichiosis; HME = human monocytic ehrlichiosis.
[e]*Bb* IFA = *B. burgdorferi* immunofluorescence assay.
[f]ELISA = enzyme-linked immunosorbent assay; ELISA-AC = antibody capture ELISA.
[g]This represents only two patients in one group of two.
[h]Some of these results may represent past or current co-infection rather than cross-reactivity.
[i]WB = Western blot, results from all references listed; WB (stringent) = results from references 233–236, using stringent criteria for positivity.
[j]FTA-Abs = fluorescent treponemal antibody absorption test.
[k]MHA-TP = microhemagglutination assay for antibodies to *Treponema pallidum*.
[l]RPR = rapid plasma reagin test.
[m]VDRL = Venereal Disease Research Laboratory test.
[n]TP WB = *Treponema pallidum* WB.
[o]Other borreliae, IFA = immunofluorescence assay for other borreliae, including *B. hermsii*, a major cause of relapsing fever, and *B. coriaceae*.
[p]MA = microhemagglutination assay for antibodies to *Leptospira*.
Data obtained from references 20, 112, 233–236, 245, 401, 485, 487, 488, 498, 621, 746, 747, 757, 758, and 762.

tection tests,[529, 738, 739, 741, 750] and lack of availability of some of the better research laboratory tests.

CULTURE

The organism grows best in liquid Barbour-Stoenner-Kelly medium II (BSK II)[81, 91] at 35° C, usually takes 2 to 6 weeks to grow, is usually detected by dark-field examination of culture medium every 1 to 2 weeks, and is confirmed as *B. burgdorferi* by IFA with *B. burgdorferi*-specific monoclonal or other antibody, or by *B. burgdorferi*-specific PCR.[175] Use of PCR analysis to detect *B. burgdorferi* growth in culture fluids has produced more rapid detection of positive cultures, with detection of 95% of positive cultures 2 weeks after inoculation, compared with 70% by microscopic examination.[175] Culture is the "gold standard" for confirmation of Lyme disease, but disadvantages of culture are that generally it is not available outside of research institutions, it is cumber-

some and time-consuming and is often positive only very early in untreated infection, and the overall yield is quite low.

Under optimal conditions, isolation rates from biopsies of active untreated EM skin lesions usually range from 28 to 86%[19, 79, 175, 183, 184] ACA lesions from 10 to 26%[19, 20, 436]; rates are much lower from other sites. Isolation rates from antibiotic-treated or partially treated EM lesions are 0 to 8%,[175, 183, 436] from normal-appearing skin after spontaneous resolution of EM lesions 8%,[436] and from partially treated ACA lesions 0%.[436] Berger and associates achieved an isolation rate of 86% by biopsy inside the peripheral border of the lesion,[183] and 57% by biopsy of perilesional skin just outside the peripheral border; the isolation rate was higher in EM from disseminated infection (88%), than from localized infection (71%); it was 100% in untreated disseminated infection.[183]

The rate of isolation of *B. burgdorferi* from blood

cultures has usually been 1 to 6%[80, 591, 751] in Lyme borreliosis even though hematogenous dissemination occurs clinically. In 1998, Wormser and colleagues[591] found that by using 3 ml of serum instead of 3 ml of whole blood, and inoculating samples within 3 hours of collection, positive cultures were detectable in 2.7 rather than 7.7 weeks, and positive cultures could be obtained in 20% of untreated early EM patients with solitary EM, 50% of untreated early multiple EM patients, and 25% overall of untreated early EM patients. Culturing a larger volume of serum by obtaining six simultaneously drawn 3-ml serum samples increased the yield, especially in patients with solitary EM. Patients with multiple EM had more positive blood cultures than those with single EM, indicating a higher level of spirochetemia. Goodman and co-workers[280] found higher rates of both culture and PCR positivity from plasma than from whole blood, and of PCR positivity from plasma than from serum, indicating possible concentration of spirochetes in plasma.

B. burgdorferi has been successfully grown from skin biopsy specimens of EM,[18, 79, 183, 184, 432] BL,[22] cutaneous B cell lymphoma,[647] ACA,[20, 436] and tick bite site skin biopsies,[307, 752] and of blood,[80, 591] CSF,[95] iris,[284] synovium or joint fluid,[200] ligamentous tissue,[304] bone,[699] myocardium,[607] and placental and fetal tissues.[32–35]

SILVER AND IMMUNOFLUORESCENT STAINS

B. burgdorferi spirochetes may be visualized by Dieterle,[16] Warthin-Starry,[33–35, 79] or Bosma-Steiner[94] silver staining, or by B. burgdorferi–specific immunohistochemical monoclonal or polyclonal antibody staining of tissue, or immuno-electron microscopy of blood or CSF.[620] The Bosma-Steiner modification of the Warthin-Starry stain has resulted in much improved sensitivity for demonstration of B. burgdorferi.[94]

B. burgdorferi has a characteristic morphology by silver staining that is distinct from that of other spirochetes and even other Borrelia species; they are sharply demarcated, short or long, coiled, undulating, or elongated straight forms, of equal thickness, with no irregularities or granularity, and they are found sparsely in tissues, in the superficial dermal papillae, often between collagen fibers, or in vessel walls.[597] B. burgdorferi spirochetes have also been found in the endomysial space in a myocardial biopsy by silver staining.[308] Its morphologic appearance may vary in different tissues and with the serologic status of the patient.

The specificity of immunohistochemical staining, including immunogold silver staining, is greater than that of silver staining alone. The sensitivity of detection of B. burgdorferi by staining ranges from 25 to 100%.

Spirochetes have been demonstrated in multiple tissues.*

DARK-FIELD EXAMINATION

Dark-field microscopy is not a sensitive method for visualization of B. burgdorferi because the number of

organisms in infected tissues is very small and the yield is essentially zero, with occasional rare exceptions.[18]

POLYMERASE CHAIN REACTION

PCR is generally considered more sensitive than either culture or special stains for detection of B. burgdorferi in multiple tissues or body fluids; it is much faster than culture, providing results in a few days rather than the several weeks required for culture detection of B. burgdorferi.[185–187, 317] The sensitivity of PCR for detection of B. burgdorferi is highest in fresh or fresh-frozen specimens,[187] but PCR, using short DNA segments to detect DNA degraded by fixation, has even detected B. burgdorferi DNA extracted from 67% of de-paraffinized formalin-fixed, paraffin-embedded EM skin biopsies.[753]

Different PCR target gene sequences have been used to detect B. burgdorferi.[187] Use of sequences for the 41-kd flagellar antigen and 34-kd Osp B in PCR improved the sensitivity of detection of B. burgdorferi in CSF to 67% of patients with very early disseminated Lyme disease, even when CSF B. burgdorferi antibody was still negative.[282] Use of an Osp A gene sequence and use of a B. burgdorferi RNA polymerase gene sequence detected B. burgdorferi DNA in serum and plasma, respectively, of early Lyme disease patients, even before seropositivity developed.[280, 281]

In a comparative study that used a sequence from the B. burgdorferi RNA polymerase C gene, PCR was more sensitive than culture for detection of spirochetemia.[280] Other studies, however, have achieved higher culture positivity but did not directly compare PCR.[591]

The B. burgdorferi PCR is 100% specific if performed in a reliable laboratory without cross-contamination because the DNA target sequences are selected specifically for lack of cross-reactivity with other spirochetes.[143, 185, 753] These sequences are not present in other closely related Borrelia species or other spirochetes, and they are highly conserved among B. burgdorferi strains. PCR is generally considered to be useful in the detection of small numbers of B. burgdorferi in tissue or body fluid samples,[280–282, 591, 755] is particularly useful in the diagnosis of very early Lyme disease before standard serologic assays become positive,[280, 281] and may be more sensitive and less cumbersome than culture, but its use is limited to research facilities. Although reports of B. burgdorferi CSF, plasma, synovial fluid, or skin biopsy, or of urine PCR positivity converting to negativity after antibiotic therapy of neuroborreliosis,[287, 309–311] arthritis,[312, 314] EM,[316, 754] ACA,[143, 316] and BL,[754] suggest a correlation of PCR positivity with active infection, the role of PCR in decisions about antibiotic therapy has not been definitively established[186, 187, 324]; a positive B. burgdorferi PCR indicates presence of B. burgdorferi antigens; this may be due to either past or present B. burgdorferi infection, but it provides no information on organism viability or persistence of active infection because it detects even degraded DNA or residual DNA fragments present inside membrane bound blebs[102, 103] produced by B. burgdorferi.[186, 187] PCR has often been noted to have increased sensitivity for the detection of B. burgdorferi in clinical specimens obtained from patients after a few

---

*See references 25, 32–35, 38, 41, 43, 82, 267, 596, 597, 605, 607, 617, 618, 620, 623, and 695.

days of antibiotic therapy, which possibly is related to the release of spirochetal antigens into body fluids as spirochetes are killed by antibiotic therapy.[187]

IMMUNOFLUORESCENT ASSAY

Immunofluorescent assay (IFA) uses fluorescein-tagged antihuman immunoglobulin to detect serum, CSF, or synovial fluid IgG, IgM, or IgA antibody binding specifically to whole *B. burgdorferi* fixed on a slide.[1, 10]

The range of sensitivity of the polyvalent IFA is 13 to 100% in early Lyme disease, and 64 to 100% in late Lyme disease. With IFA, IgM antibody is detectable earlier in infection than IgG antibody; thus, it is more sensitive in the diagnosis of early Lyme disease, and it generally disappears by convalescence except in patients with persistently active Lyme disease. Under ideal circumstances, IFA may detect *B. burgdorferi*–specific IgM antibody in 100% of patients with early culture-positive erythema migrans on the day of presentation.[756] The specificity of Lyme IFA is low in patients with other spirochetal infections because of cross-reactivity between *B. burgdorferi* and other spirochetes, especially syphilis, but it is good in rapid plasma reagin (RPR)-negative patients (see Table 11–16). Major disadvantages of the IFA—subjective test reading, the need for highly trained personnel for test performance, lack of test automation, and unsuitability for high volume use—have resulted in its replacement by the ELISA in most laboratories.[250, 252, 750]

ENZYME-LINKED IMMUNOSORBENT ASSAY

The standard indirect enzyme-linked immunosorbent assay (ELISA) uses enzyme-tagged antihuman immunoglobulin to detect serum, CSF, or synovial fluid IgG, IgM, or IgA antibody binding specifically to either whole disrupted (sonicated) *B. burgdorferi* or specific *B. burgdorferi* components (antigens) bound to multi-well ELISA plates.[224, 252]

The ELISA is 13 to 92% sensitive in early Lyme disease and 89 to 100% sensitive in late Lyme disease. IgM antibody is detectable earlier in infection than IgG, and it generally decreases during convalescence except in patients with persistently active infection, although ELISA IgM antibody positivity has been found even in some successfully treated patients.[244]

The ELISA is more efficient and reproducible than the IFA.[224, 252] Comparisons of IFA and ELISA generally have shown that ELISA is also more sensitive and specific than IFA,[98, 224] although some reports have found them to be comparable.[250, 252] In RPR-negative patients, the sensitivity of IFA and ELISA is high for detection of late Lyme disease, when *B. burgdorferi* antibody levels are high, but lower for detection of early Lyme disease, when there is a high false-negative rate because of the combination of low *B. burgdorferi* antibody in the first few weeks and high background as a result of cross-reactive antibody.[222]

Cross-reactivity in both ELISA and IFA assays occurs between *B. burgdorferi* and other spirochetes (see Table 11–16). Because of the high cross-reactivity with syphi-

lis, it is essential that an RPR test be performed on all Lyme-positive sera to exclude syphilis (as RPR does not cross react and should be negative in Lyme disease.[252] Only a low rate of cross-reactivity occurs with *Leptospira*[252, 746, 758] and *Rickettsia*.[252, 758] Cross-reactivity with *B. coriacea* may lead to confusion, as this infection is endemic in *Ornithodoros coriaceus* ticks in California's Mendocino County, and humans are an occasional host for this tick.

Other causes of false-positive Lyme ELISA or IFA results are normal spirochetal oral flora,[245] viral infections such as varicella-zoster virus (VZV), Epstein-Barr virus (EBV), or parvovirus,[18, 74, 224, 746] other bacterial infections such as subacute bacterial endocarditis,[745] and autoimmune diseases such as systemic lupus erythematosus, rheumatoid arthritis, and Reiter's disease.[224, 252, 743] Lyme Western blot appears to be more useful than ELISA for evaluation of Lyme serologic status in patients with certain of the illnesses listed here. The significant problem of false Lyme seropositivity by ELISA or IFA testing should serve as a reminder that serologic data should be judiciously interpreted in the context of both the clinical illness and epidemiologic data.

The sensitivity and specificity of the standard whole-cell ELISA sometimes have been increased by using either purified or recombinant components of the organism such as outer surface membrane lipoproteins,[124, 239, 241, 245] the 41-kd flagellar antigen[241, 242, 746] combinations of recombinant Osp C with a recombinant flagellin fragment,[125] or synthetic, non–cross-reactive, immunodominant peptide sequences of the flagellar antigen as antigens. Some Lyme disease patient sera may react with individual antigens present in whole-cell antigen preparations but not with recombinant preparations of the same antigens, possibly because the immunogenic epitopes are presented differently in the recombinant antigens.[108, 124] *B. burgdorferi* loses Osp C during repeated passage in culture; these strains are often used to produce antigens for ELISA assays, which do not detect the early IgM antibody response that is mainly directed toward Osp C. The use of either recombinant Osp C or Osp C–positive strains in ELISA assays has increased the sensitivity of detection of specific IgM antibody in early Lyme disease.[239]

ANTIBODY CAPTURE ELISA, IMMUNE-COMPLEX ELISA, AND ANTIBODY CAPTURE IMMUNE-COMPLEX BIOTINYLATED ELISA

The antibody capture ELISA (ELISA-AC),[757] which reduces competition between IgG and IgM for the same antigenic sites in the assay and false positivity due to rheumatoid factor, increased the sensitivity of detection of IgM and IgG in early Lyme disease so that diagnosis could be confirmed in 67% of acute patient sera and in 93% of convalescent sera. The IgM ELISA-AC was particularly useful in disseminated disease, where the rate of positivity was 71 to 100% and 93 to 100%, respectively, of acute and convalescent sera, compared with 25% and 75%, respectively, in localized Lyme disease. The ELISA-AC assay with flagellar antigen, using the biotin–avidin peroxidase method for demonstration of IgM, increased the sensitivity and specificity of detection of IgM antibody compared with the standard indirect IgM ELISA with flagellar antigen.[746]

The sensitivity of the ELISA for detection of IgG antibody in early Lyme disease was increased by using a polyethylene glycol (PEG) precipitation method to dissociate the antibody sequestered in circulating immune complexes (IC) before performing the ELISA.[278] This PEG ELISA-IC assay detected IgG antibody in 100% of patients with histories of recent erythema migrans who were seronegative by the standard ELISA assay, and 95% of patients with seropositive Lyme disease; the false positivity rate was zero.

The antibody capture immune-complex biotinylated ELISA (EMIBA)[756] was able to detect specific IgM seropositivity in culture-positive EM patients, as early as the day of lesion biopsy in 100% of disseminated EM patients and in 73% of localized EM patients, including some who were IgM-seronegative by standard IgM or polyvalent ELISA, IgM Western blot, IgM IFA, and IgM ELISA-AC. For localized EM patients, the rate of IgM seropositivity was 36% by the ELISA-AC assay for free serum antibody, 55% by the EMIBA assay with whole B. burgdorferi antigen, and 73% with the addition of the flagellar peptide. The false positivity rate was zero. The EMIBA assay is specific and sensitive, particularly for serologic confirmation of early disseminated EM. It is less cumbersome than the lymphocyte proliferative assay and may be useful in the evaluation of seronegative Lyme patients, but it is not widely available.

WESTERN BLOT (IMMUNOBLOT)

This method detects serum, CSF, or synovial fluid IgG or IgM antibodies to many of the over 30 individual B. burgdorferi protein antigens,[120, 223, 232, 241, 249, 742] including major outer surface proteins, flagellar antigen, and heat shock proteins. The pattern of antibody to these specific B. burgdorferi antigens, demonstrated by the pattern of bands seen in the Western blot assay, is characteristic of Lyme disease and shows temporal evolution with initial expansion of the antibody repertoire and increasing disease duration.[222, 232–234]

The Western blot test is currently recommended as the second test in a two-step serologic testing algorithm, in which ELISA or IFA is used as the highly sensitive initial test, and positive or equivocal ELISA or IFA results are then evaluated by a highly specific Western blot test to exclude false positivity.[236, 478, 748] The Western blot is generally considered more sensitive and more specific than ELISA or IFA, but because of its complexity, it has been plagued by lack of standardization. Efforts are under way to reduce interlaboratory variability in the definition of Western blot positivity.[225, 254, 741, 749, 766]

CDC criteria for positive Western blots[238] are based on studies by Dressler and associates[234] and Engstrom and colleagues.[233] CDC criteria for a positive IgM Western immunoblot are the presence of two of the following three bands in early disease: 24-kd Osp C, 39-kd Bmp A, and 41-kd Fla. For a positive IgG Western immunoblot, five of the ten most common bands must be present after the first few weeks of disease: 18-kd, 21-kd Osp C, 28-kd, 30-kd, 39-kd Bmp A, 41-kd Fla, 45-kd, 58-kd, 66-kd, and 93-kd bands. A dissenting opinion[759] regarding the CDC criteria[238] for Western blot positivity recommends inclusion of IgG antibody to 31-kd Osp A and 34-kd Osp B in the criteria because of concern that serologic confirmation in some patients would not be possible without these inclusions.

Although European criteria for Western blot positivity have not been officially standardized,[738] in 1997, Hauser and co-workers[237] proposed such criteria, based on extensive studies of over 500 European sera (from patients with early and late Lyme borreliosis and controls) tested in IgG and IgM Western blots prepared with antigens from the three major European genospecies: B. burgdorferi sensu stricto, B. afzelii, and B. garinii. The proposed criteria for positivity, with over 96% specificities, are: for sensu stricto IgG, at least one band of molecular weight 83/100, 58, 56, Osp C, 21, and 17a, and for IgM, at least one of 39, Osp C, and 17a or a strong 41; for afzelii IgG, at least two bands of 83/100, 58, 43, 39, 30, Osp C, 21, 17, and 14, and for IgM, at least one of 39, Osp C, and 17 or a strong 41; and for garinii IgG, at least one of 83/100, 39, Osp C, 21, and 17b, and for IgM, at least one of 39 and Osp C or a strong 41-kd band.

Because of B. burgdorferi strain variability, both between genospecies and within genospecies, the molecular weights of several B. burgdorferi protein antigens may vary, and some antigens may be variably expressed, resulting in apparent differences in antibody patterns if different strains are used as antigen sources in preparation of Western blots[108, 529]; use of monoclonal antibodies for identification of the protein bands is important for Western blot standardization to allow comparisons between different laboratories.[232, 233, 237]

The Western blot reactivity pattern differs slightly in sera of patients infected with different strains and genospecies of B. burgdorferi sensu lato from the United States, Europe, and Asia,[237, 760, 761] and, because of antigenic heterogeneity, differs slightly to moderately in sera reacting in Western blots prepared with different strains and genospecies.[108, 231, 257, 529, 760, 761] Lyme borreliosis patient sera are usually more reactive in Western blot assays prepared with strains homologous to the infecting strains or from the same endemic area.[760, 761] In Europe, where the three major B. burgdorferi genospecies all cause Lyme borreliosis, because of the more frequent association of certain clinical manifestations with some genospecies than with others, sera of patients with different clinical manifestations may show different reactivity patterns in Western blots prepared with the different genospecies.[257]

In early Lyme disease, when ELISA and IFA antibody responses are low, Western blot may be more sensitive and specific, particularly during the first 4 weeks of illness.[223, 232, 233, 236, 757] Sera from early Lyme disease of less than 1 week's duration were positive in 79% by Western blot, compared with 71% by the two-step test using ELISA as the initial test followed by Western blot testing only of positives by ELISA.[236] Sensitivity of the polyvalent Western blot is 53 to 92% in early Lyme disease and 100% in late chronic Lyme disease. Use

Text continued on page 594

TABLE 11–17
Laboratory Diagnosis of Lyme Borreliosis (LB)

ASSAY FOR *B. BURGDORFERI* (*Bb*)	*B. BURGDORFERI* COMPONENT DETECTED BY OR USED IN ASSAY	TIME COURSE OF POSITIVE RESULT (% PATIENTS WITH POSITIVE ASSAY RESULT DURING DIFFERENT STAGES OF LB)			ASSAY SPECIFICITY FOR *B. BURGDORFERI*[a]	ASSAY COMMERCIALLY AVAILABLE
		Early Localized LB	Early Disseminated LB	Late LB		
Culture of biopsy (bx) or fluid	Whole *Bb*, live	46–71% ac	71–88% ac	10–26% ACA[c] bx low % Snv[e] bx low % CSF[f]	++++	no
Silver stain or FA stain[g] of biopsy[h]	Whole spirochetes	20% ac	50% ac	low % ACA bx 25–100% Snv bx	++++	no
PCR[h]	*Bb* DNA sequences	29–100% EM[b] bx 100% BL[b] bx 25–80% EM bx ac 7% whole blood ac 18% plasma ac 40–59% serum ac 45–90% urine ac	79% ac 30% ac	16–71% ACA bx 80–85% Snv fluid[i] 100% Snv bx[j]	++++	no
IFA[j] IgG	Whole *Bb*	25–58% ac 58–100% cv[k]		80–100%	+++	yes
IFA IgM	Whole *Bb*	20–94% ac 0–14% cv	100% ac	64–80%	+++	yes
IFA Polyvalent (IgG + IgM)	Whole *Bb*	13–100% ac 53–100% cv		94–100%	+++	yes
ELISA[k] IgG	Whole *Bb*	0–35% ac 8–100% cv 8% late cv	34–79% ac 60–62% cv	41–100% Ar[l] 90–92% NB[m] 90% ACA	+++	yes
	p83/100	14%	37%	86–100% Ar, NB, ACA	++++	no
	Flagellin	0–31% ac 26–88% cv 37–46% late cv	55–70% ac 81% cv 63–100% late cv	68–100% Ar 95% ACA	+++	no
	Osp A[n]	33% ac	34% ac	42% Ar	++++	no
	Osp B[o]	49% cv	51% cv	42% Ar	++++	no
	Osp C[p]		65% NB	84% Ar 36% NB	++++	no
ELISA IgM	Whole *Bb*	9–58% ac 21–67% cv	34–89% ac 35–44% cv	36–64% Ar 10% ACA	+++	yes
	p83/100	7%	0%	12% Ar 100% NB 5% ACA	++++	no
	Flagellin	18–50% ac 41–100% cv 23–44% late cv	43% ac 45% cv 17–53% late cv	68% 5% ACA	+++	no
	Osp C[s]	25% ac 50% cv	61% ac 72–80% cv	20–45% Ar, NB	++++	no

Test	Antigen						
ELISA Polyvalent (IgG + IgM)	Whole Bb	12–27% ac, 52–60% cv	13–56% ac, 19–98% cv	29–100%, 77–96% cv	89–100% Ar, NB, ACA	+++	yes
	Flagellin	13–44% ac, 53–54% cv	44% ac, 53–65% cv	21–100% ac, 83–100% cv	89–100% Ar, NB, ACA	+++	no
ELISA-AC^q IgG	Whole Bb	0% ac, 13% ac	13% ac, 30% cv	0–50% ac, 21–63% cv		+++	no
ELISA-AC IgM	Whole Bb	25–36% ac, 75% cv	46–67% ac, 90–100% cv	50–100% ac, 60–100% cv	47%	++++	no
	Flagellin		50% ac, 44% cv	65% ac, 60% cv	12%	+++	no
ELISA-AC Polyvalent (IgG + IgM)	Whole Bb	25% ac	57% ac	54% late cv, 47% late cv, 71% ac		+++	no
ELISA-IC^r IgG	Whole Bb		93% ac, 33–100%	93–100% cv	95–100%	+++	no
	Osp A		36% ac				
ELISA-IC IgM	Osp A		73% ac				
ELISA-AC/IC (EMIBA) IgM	Whole Bb	55% ac	70% ac	89% ac		++++	no
Western blot^s IgG	Whole Bb + Flagellin	73% ac	85% ac	100% ac	70–100% Ar, NB, ACA	++++	no
	Whole Bb	0–6% ac, 13–16% cv	0–48% ac, 16–80% cv, 49–50% late cv	17–72% ac, 25–71% cv		++++	yes
	83–100 kd		23% ac, 3–35% cv	28–29% ac, 83% cv	76–100% Ar, NB, ACA		
	66 kd HSP		7% cv	56–83% cv	72–92% Ar, NB		
	58–60 kd HSP		0–54% ac, 9–70% cv	84%	92–100% Ar, NB		
	41 kd Flagellin	0% ac, 25% cv, 0% late cv	57–85% ac, 87–100% cv	92–100%	83–100% Ar, NB, ACA		
	31–33 kd Osp A		0–20% ac, 5–7% cv	0–4%	40–100% Ar, NB, 0–15% ACA		
	34–35 kd Osp B		0–5% ac, 0–8% cv	0%	36–100% Ar, NB		
	20–25 kd Osp C		47–77% ac, 19–83% cv	10–28%	48–95% Ar, NB, 0–19% ACA		
	28–30 kd ?Osp D^t / 17–19 kd ?Osp E^u / 25–27 kd ?Osp F^v		0%	28–44%, 84%	72–100% Ar, NB / 80–100% Ar, NB		
	45–46 kd		0–5%	50% cv	49% Ar / 46% Ar		
	39 kd		100% ac, 70% cv, 85% ac	80%, 20%	72–84% Ar, NB / 88–97% Ar, NB		
	37 kd / 35 kd		14–91% cv, 46% ac, 57% cv	4%	44% Ar, NB		
Western blot IgM	Whole Bb	24–36% ac, 44–60% cv, 33% cv	23–87% ac, 27–86% cv	31–76% ac, 36–96% cv		++++	yes
	83–100 kd		8–42% ac, 5–49% cv	7–25% ac, 7–10% cv	14% ACA		
	66 kd HSP		4–68% ac, 8–80% cv	24%			
	58–60 kd HSP		28–58% ac, 22–87% cv	36%			

Table continued on following page

TABLE 11–17
Laboratory Diagnosis of Lyme Borreliosis (LB) Continued

ASSAY FOR B. BURGDORFERI (Bb)	B. BURGDORFERI COMPONENT DETECTED BY OR USED IN ASSAY	TIME COURSE OF POSITIVE RESULT (% PATIENTS WITH POSITIVE ASSAY RESULT DURING DIFFERENT STAGES OF LB)			ASSAY SPECIFICITY FOR B. BURGDORFERI[a]	ASSAY COMMERCIALLY AVAILABLE
		Early Localized LB	Early Disseminated LB	Late LB		
	41 kd Flagellin	33–65% ac / 73–90% cv	39–100% ac	33–40% Ar, NB / 19% ACA		
	31–33 kd Osp A	0% ac / 5–11% cv	0–12% ac	0–4% ACA		
	34–35 kd Osp B	0% cv / 0% cv	0–12% ac / 0%	20–100% Ar		
	20–25 kd Osp C	0–4% cv	37–68% ac	19% ACA		
	45–46 kd	44–84% ac / 52–91% cv	28%			
	39 kd	32–74% ac / 20–83% cv	0% ac			
	37 kd	4–84% ac / 8–94% cv	28% ac			
	35 kd	24–53% ac / 32–80% cv / 47% ac / 13–63% cv				
Western blot Polyvalent (IgG + IgM)	Whole Bb	25–55% ac / 14–86% cv	83–100% ac	100% Ar / 100% NB	++++	yes
	Flagellin	75% ac / 100% cv		83–100% Ar		
	Osp A	0% ac / 0% cv		50% Ar		
	Osp B	0% av / 0% cv		50% Ar		
LPAv	Whole Bb, killed or sonicated	0–36%		45–100%	+++	no
	Whole Bb, live	50–91%		82–100%	+++	no
	66 kd HSP			36%		no
	58 kd HSP			14%	+++	no
	Flagellin	82%		21–68%	++++	no
	Osp A	82%		29–76%	++++	no
	Osp B			14%	++++	no
	Osp C			29%	++++	no
PCR	Bb DNA sequence		25–100% CSF		++++	no
IFA	Whole Bb		92% CSF		+++	yes
Antigen-capture ELISA	Whole Bb		49% CSF		++++	no
	Osp A		24–100% CSF			
	Osp B		27% CSF			
	Flagellin		30% CSF			

Assay	Antigen	Value	Specificity[a]	LPA/WB
ELISA IgG	Whole *Bb* or Flagellin	10–100% CSF	yes	
ELISA IgM	Whole *Bb* or Flagellin	19–100% CSF	yes	
	Osp A	20–100% CSF		
	Osp B	20–100% CSF		
	Osp C	50–100% CSF		
ELISA Polyvalent	Whole *Bb*	48–100% CSF	yes	
ELISA-AC Polyvalent	Whole *Bb*	42–100% CSF	no	
IgM Polyvalent	Whole *Bb*	40–100% CSF		
ELISA-IC Polyvalent	Whole *Bb*	38–43% CSF	no	
IgG		47% CSF		
IgM		64% CSF		
Western blot	Whole *Bb*	92% CSF	yes	+++
LPA	Whole *Bb*, sonicated	100% CSF	no	+++
	Whole *Bb*	100% CSF	no	+++

Culture data obtained from references 18–20, 22, 79, 80, 95, 183, 184, 260, 267, 280, 301, 302, 374, 434, 436, 439, 591, 595, 621, and 751.

Stain data obtained from references 82, 177, 596, 618, 621, and 695.

PCR data obtained from references 143, 280, 282, 287, 312, 313, 315–317, 436, 439, 595, 753, 754, and 755.

IFA data obtained from references 1, 18, 20, 39, 209, 235, 250–252, 466, 600, 621, 638, 644, 756, and 869.

ELISA data obtained from references 107, 124, 223, 224, 226, 232–236, 239–242, 246, 247, 251, 252, 267, 278, 621, 746, 756, and 757.

Western blot data obtained from references 108, 124, 222, 223, 225, 226, 229, 232–237, 239–241, 247, 249, 621, and 756.

LPA data obtained from references 208–210, 212, 213, 218, 219, 221, 267, 621, and 765.

CSF data obtained from references 214, 259, 260, 267, 282, 283, 285–287, 293, 309, 621, 654, 661, and 755.

[a]Estimation of specificity is given for RPR-negative sera (see Table 11–15).

[b]EM = erythema migrans skin lesion.

[c]ACA = acrodermatitis chronicam atrophicans skin lesion.

[d]BL = borrelial lymphocytoma skin lesion.

[e]Snv = synovial.

[f]CSF = cerebrospinal fluid.

[g]Warthin-Starry, Bosma-Steiner, or Dieterle silver stains, or *B. burgdorferi*–specific polyclonal or monoclonal FA (fluorescent antibody) stains.

[h]PCR = polymerase chain reaction.

[i]Excluding patients with antibiotic-resistant chronic arthritis, in whom a 96% polymerase chain reaction–positivity rate is found.

[j]IFA = immunofluorescence assay.

[k]ELISA = enzyme-linked immunosorbent assay.

[l]Ar = arthritis.

[m]NB = neuroborreliosis.

[n]Osp A = outer surface protein A.

[o]Osp B = outer surface protein B.

[p]Osp C = outer surface protein C.

[q]ELISA-AC = ELISA-antibody capture.

[r]ELISA-IC = ELISA-immune complex.

[s]Western blot: kd-kilodalton size of individual *B. burgdorferi* antigens.

[t]Osp D = outer surface protein D.

[u]Osp E = outer surface protein E.

[v]Osp F = outer surface protein F.

[w]LPA = lymphocyte proliferative assay.

of both immune-complex dissociation techniques and biotin-avidin Western blots has increased the sensitivity of detection of IgM and IgG Osp A antibody early in infection, when it may be located in immune complexes.[246]

Cross-reactivity with other spirochetes and the presence of low levels of positivity in control sera from endemic areas make it difficult to estimate the true incidence of false-positive Western blot assays, but it is considered to be low.

Patients with a strong clinical history of objective symptoms of Lyme disease and seropositivity by both ELISA and Western blot[279, 742, 763, 764] usually improve clinically with antibiotic therapy[742]; however, patients with only subjective symptoms, with either negative ELISA and negative Western blot or positive ELISA but negative Western blot, usually have some other inflammatory or rheumatologic disease instead of Lyme disease[279, 742, 763, 764] and do not improve with antibiotic treatment. Most patients with late Lyme borreliosis, such as arthritis, chronic neuroborreliosis, and ACA, who are seropositive by ELISA are also seropositive by Western blot.[223, 234–236]

LYMPHOCYTE PROLIFERATIVE ASSAY

Lymphocyte proliferative assay (LPA) determines specific reactivity of viable peripheral blood, CSF, or synovial fluid lymphocytes to whole *B. burgdorferi*, whole disrupted (sonicated) *B. burgdorferi*, or individual *B. burgdorferi* antigens incubated with these lymphocytes in vitro.[208, 209, 213, 218–221, 765] Some assays use peripheral blood mononuclear cells.

The development of the T cell response to Lyme disease precedes the antibody response, and the LPA may be positive in IFA- and ELISA-seronegative patients with early Lyme disease.[208, 219] After successful antibiotic therapy of Lyme disease, there may be some decrease in the level of LPA positivity.[213, 221]

The LPA may be positive in other patients who are IFA- and ELISA-seronegative as a result of prompt antibiotic therapy of early Lyme disease. The LPA was positive in all of 40 chronic Lyme disease patients in six studies, who were IFA- and ELISA-seronegative because of early antibiotic therapy.[208–210, 218]

In some patients, CSF[214, 220] and synovial fluid[221] lymphocytes are more reactive in the LPA than are peripheral blood lymphocytes; therefore, sensitivity may be increased by using these fluids.

The sensitivity of LPA is 50 to 91% in early Lyme disease, and 82 to 100% in late Lyme disease. Cross-reactions occur with other spirochetes, and the LPA positivity rate in healthy controls is 0 to 5%; in patients with non-Lyme inflammatory diseases, it is 5 to 11%.[210, 214, 218]

Although the LPA is more sensitive than antibody assays in certain patients, it requires use of live lymphocytes and whole *B. burgdorferi* or *B. burgdorferi* antigens, and is available only in research laboratories. The LPA therefore should be reserved for the diagnosis of Lyme disease in seronegative patients with good clinical objective evidence of Lyme disease, or for babies with potential congenital Lyme disease; it is not considered useful in following patient immune responses sequentially.

ANTIGEN CAPTURE ELISA ASSAY

The antigen capture ELISA, using either antibody against whole, sonicated *B. burgdorferi* or monoclonal antibodies against individual antigens such as recombinant outer surface proteins and flagellin, has been used to detect specific *B. burgdorferi* antigens in CSF.[283] In very early Lyme disease with neurologic involvement, this method detected specific antigen in CSF even before the development of specific CSF antibody. The Western blot method has also been used to determine the presence of specific antigens in CSF.[283] However, neither of these methods is commercially available.

Laboratory Variability and Efforts at Serodiagnostic Standardization

One of the major problems with laboratory diagnosis of Lyme disease is the wide intra- and interlaboratory variability of results both in the United States[739, 740, 750] and in Europe.[529, 738] Several comparisons in which standard Lyme disease case or control sera were sent simultaneously to different commercial, hospital, state, and national reference or research laboratories for *B. burgdorferi* antibody testing, usually ELISA or IFA, with or without Western blot testing, demonstrated that the percentage of laboratories that reported concordant results ranged from 10 to 93%, and the reproducibility of results within the same laboratory ranged from 27 to 96%. Agreement among laboratories was greatest for sera with high positive titers to *B. burgdorferi*, and least for sera with low positive titers.

There has been concern that *B. burgdorferi* strain heterogeneity in Europe may be responsible for variability in serologic results, but this may be more significant in Western blot assays than in ELISA assays.[257, 529]

Because of the problem of interlaboratory variability, proficiency testing programs have been recommended[478] for laboratories that perform *B. burgdorferi* testing, and these have been implemented in several areas.[739, 740] A study of a proficiency testing program in New York State, implemented in 1989 for clinical laboratories applying for *B. burgdorferi* antibody testing permits, found that performance improved during the study, partially because laboratories that initially used poorly performing test kits tended to change to better-performing kits, and overall sensitivity of ELISA, IFA, or solid-phase IFA assays was 95.4%; overall specificity 98.9%.[740]

Variability in results may therefore be due to differences in strains of *B. burgdorferi* used for preparation of the diagnostic kits, differences in the methods of kit preparation, use of different assays by different laboratories, differences in definitions of negative and positive results, geographic differences in the incidence of background Lyme seropositivity, and differences in quality control within individual laboratories. Better standardization of commercially available assays for Lyme disease is needed because the more specific, sensitive, and reproducible research laboratory tests generally are not available.

Avoidance of Over- or Underdiagnosis

Establishment of a correct diagnosis of Lyme disease, with avoidance of over- or underdiagnosis,[24, 279, 763, 767, 768] allows selection of antibiotic therapy that is adequate and appropriate for the specific clinical presentation, as well as avoidance of over- or undertreatment, which is important for achieving maximal therapeutic efficacy with minimal adverse effects, both in the individual patient and in the population as a whole.

Between 38 and 79% of patients referred to Lyme disease or rheumatology specialty clinics for Lyme disease in endemic areas had been overdiagnosed and did not have active Lyme disease, and between 38 and 57% had alternate diagnoses made. Patients with only vague persisting symptoms, such as fatigue, headache, myalgia, and arthralgia, rarely had active Lyme disease and usually had fibromyalgia or fatigue syndrome (with or without previous Lyme disease); improvement in these patients did not correlate with antibiotic therapy.[279, 715, 763, 764, 767, 768, 770]

Although long-term persistence of active *B. burgdorferi* infection has been confirmed by culture,[200, 304, 306–308] and suggested by PCR,[312, 314] it is rare, particularly after adequate antibiotic therapy. Demonstration of objective evidence of persistent infection, preferably by culture positivity, but at least by PCR or diagnostic changes in specific *B. burgdorferi* antibody, is important because retreatment of true persistent infection is usually successful.[312, 314] Failure of a patient with a diagnosis of Lyme disease to respond to appropriate antibiotic therapy should raise the possibility that the initial diagnosis of Lyme disease may be incorrect, or that symptoms are not due to active *B. burgdorferi* infection.[24, 279, 767]

Alternately, underdiagnosis is also a potential problem, particularly after acquisition of the infection during travel to an endemic area and presentation with the clinical illness after return to a nonendemic area where the diagnosis may not be initially, or ever, considered. (See section Lyme Borreliosis in Travelers to Endemic Areas.)

Recommendations for Diagnostic Testing for Evaluation of Nongestational, Gestational, and Congenital Lyme Borreliosis

Because of wide variability in clinical case definitions used in the diagnosis of Lyme borreliosis, as well as in performance and interpretation of supportive *B. burgdorferi* diagnostic tests, there have been ongoing efforts in North America[238, 254, 478, 633, 741, 748] and Europe[8, 502, 738] to standardize clinical case definitions, as well as laboratory testing guidelines. The European Union Concerted Action on Lyme Borreliosis (EUCALB) has developed standardized European clinical case definitions[8, 502] (see Table 11–11), but serodiagnostic guidelines are not yet available.[738] Current CDC clinical case definitions of Lyme disease[633] (see Table 11–10) are intended for use in combination with CDC and FDA laboratory diagnostic test guidelines in the United States[238, 254, 633]; although they were initially designed for epidemiologic surveillance purposes, they have found widespread acceptance as a way to standardize the diagnosis of Lyme disease.

Several studies, including predictive statistical models[734–736] as well as prospective[767] and retrospective[279, 763, 768] clinical laboratory studies, have evaluated various approaches to the problem of how, when, and in whom to do diagnostic testing for Lyme disease. The American College of Physicians recently developed guidelines describing indications for diagnostic evaluation for Lyme disease.[478, 748]

The diagnosis of Lyme borreliosis in the nonpregnant patient should be a clinical diagnosis, made according to accepted case definitions, and supported by appropriate laboratory confirmation when needed, interpreted according to accepted criteria. According to the CDC case definition of Lyme disease (see Table 11–10), classic physician-diagnosed erythema migrans with endemic area exposure does not require laboratory confirmation, but other acute, early disseminated manifestations, including acute neuroborreliosis and carditis, or late manifestations require either positive culture or serologic confirmation by diagnostic CSF or serum levels of *B. burgdorferi* IgM or IgG antibody, according to the two-step method (by ELISA or IFA), followed by retesting of all positive or equivocal results by Western blot.[238, 254, 633] The EUCALB case definitions of Lyme borreliosis (see Table 11–11), similarly, do not require laboratory confirmation for classic erythema migrans, but do for other acute early manifestations, including borrelial lymphocytoma, acute neuroborreliosis, and carditis, and for late manifestations.[8, 502] There has been no standardization of diagnostic CSF *B. burgdorferi* antibody levels required for confirmation of neuroborreliosis,[178] but CSF IgM or IgG *B. burgdorferi* antibody levels exceeding serum levels are usually considered to indicate intrathecal antibody production.

The ELISA test, either polyvalent or IgM and IgG, is the most widely available assay for serodiagnosis of Lyme borreliosis; it is often preferred over the IFA for use as the initial test because of its suitability for large-volume testing. Antibody capture ELISA may have increased sensitivity and specificity but is not as widely available. Using Western blot retesting of sera that are positive or equivocal by initial ELISA or IFA tests increases specificity. Both IgM and IgG testing is recommended for evaluation during the first 4 weeks of early Lyme disease. Because negative serologic results during the first 2 weeks of illness are not sufficient to exclude Lyme disease, if early Lyme disease is strongly suspected and the first sample is negative, testing a 2- to 4-week convalescent sample is recommended. Although current CDC guidelines recommend only Western blot testing of ELISA-positive or equivocal sera, the Western blot may be useful in initial evaluation of early Lyme disease because its increased sensitivity may allow detection of more cases than ELISA during the first and second weeks of illness.[232, 233, 236] The Western blot may also provide additional information regarding the time course of the infection.[233] Criteria for Western blot positivity are stringently defined in the CDC recommendations.[233, 234, 238] Use of IgM testing alone after the first 4 weeks of illness is not recommended, as a diagnosis of active Lyme disease should not be made on this basis alone. Use of IgM testing alone even for evaluation of early infection is not recommended, because some patients who have been reinfected with *B. burgdorferi* may have only an IgG response, which would be missed if IgG testing were not done.[233]

The lymphocyte proliferative assay is useful for diagnosis of seronegative patients with suspected Lyme borreliosis but is not generally available commercially. Biopsies of involved tissues for histopathology, culture, PCR, or silver or IFA staining are usually best reserved for special clinical circumstances, when serologic diagnosis is insufficient; culture of more readily accessible sites such as the CSF, blood, synovial fluid, or skin may be useful, but yields are low, except from erythema migrans lesions, and culture is not widely available. PCR is usually reserved for research purposes, but culture or PCR is useful when identification of the *B. burgdorferi* strain is needed. Although PCR provides evidence for the presence of *B. burgdorferi* DNA, it does not indicate the presence of viable spirochetes; culture of *B. burgdorferi* remains the only definitive proof of active ongoing infection.

The diagnosis of Lyme borreliosis in a pregnant woman should also be made according to the currently accepted CDC or EUCALB case definitions (see Tables 11–10 and 11–11 and section on Clinical Manifestations), with the additional recommendation that laboratory confirmation of the diagnosis is advisable, even for the clinical presentation as classic erythema migrans, to avoid later uncertainty, which might arise if only a clinical diagnosis were made. Because specific IgM seropositivity may be transient and development of specific IgG seropositivity may be prevented by early antibiotic therapy, immediate acute serum and several convalescent sera should be collected at approximately 2-week intervals over a period of approximately 8 weeks and at delivery. The initial acute sera should be sent for polyvalent or IgM and IgG Lyme ELISA, and also IgM and IgG Western blot; the remaining convalescent sera may be sent if no confirmation is obtained with the first sera. It is advisable to save aliquots of sera for possible future testing with more sensitive assays if they become available. The Western blot is advisable in evaluation of pregnant women with early Lyme disease, in whom early serologic confirmation is preferable, because of its increased sensitivity during the first 2 weeks of illness,[232, 233, 236] and because it may provide useful information regarding the time course of the infection.[232, 233] Although it is not recommended that biopsies of involved tissues be performed routinely in pregnancy, this could be done for diagnostic confirmation if clinically indicated. It is important to determine whether dissemination has occurred as this influences selection of antibiotic therapy and may affect pregnancy outcome; blood evaluation for evidence of spirochetemia, by culture, or possibly PCR, and CSF examination for evidence of early neuroborreliosis may be indicated for this purpose in some pregnant women.

There is no basis for routine *B. burgdorferi* antibody screening of asymptomatic healthy persons, because the incidence of false positivity exceeds the incidence of active Lyme disease in this group.[748] For the same reason, in the absence of studies indicating otherwise, there is no indication for routine prenatal *B. burgdorferi* antibody screening of asymptomatic healthy women. *B. burgdorferi* antibody serosurveys have demonstrated that seroprevalence in pregnant women[27, 37, 40, 45–47] reflects community seroprevalence; the rate of asymptomatic seroconversion was only 0.8% in one study during pregnancy.[45]

Any infant with possible congenital Lyme borreliosis should undergo evaluation by *B. burgdorferi* IgM and IgG ELISA and IgM and IgG Western blot on paired maternal and cord blood at delivery, and on the infant's blood and preferably CSF after birth, and if possible, *B. burgdorferi* culture and PCR as well on these samples. If the index of suspicion is high for congenital Lyme borreliosis and these assays are negative, the LPA should be performed (at a research center), as it appears to be more sensitive than serologic testing for confirmation of Lyme borreliosis in congenitally infected patients. Histopathology, Bosma-Steiner or Warthin-Starry silver stains, *B. burgdorferi*–specific antibody stains, culture, and PCR of the placenta are recommended. If biopsy specimens of involved tissues, such as skin, are obtained, they should be sent for the same studies, as these may be useful in diagnosis. Cardiac and neurologic evaluation should be obtained if there is a clinical suspicion of congenital heart disease or neurologic involvement. It is also advisable to store samples of sera, CSF, or tissues for possible additional future testing.

A full histopathologic evaluation is recommended of any placenta, miscarriage, stillbirth, or perinatal death from a pregnancy complicated by Lyme borreliosis. In addition, Bosma-Steiner or Warthin-Starry silver stains, *B. burgdorferi*–specific antibody stains, culture and PCR of the brain, heart, lungs, kidneys, liver, spleen, lymph nodes, bone marrow, synovium, and any other histologically abnormal tissues, and antibody assays, PCR, and culture of any blood or CSF available are recommended. Serum, CSF, and other samples should also be stored for future diagnostic tests.

Because the incidence of congenital Lyme disease is quite low, and needs more complete characterization, it is important to evaluate any suspected cases as fully as possible. The physician may wish to contact a center engaged in Lyme research for help in processing of these samples. The author has agreed to be available, by prearrangement, for discussion of infants suspected of having congenital Lyme borreliosis: Tessa Gardner, M.D., 314–727–9101.

Differential Diagnosis of Lyme Borreliosis

The differential diagnosis of Lyme borreliosis (Table 11–18), including gestational Lyme borreliosis, is extensive and depends on the particular stage and manifesta-

TABLE 11–18
Differential Diagnosis of Lyme Borreliosis[a] (LB)

DISEASE	RASH	FLULIKE ILLNESS	MUSCULOSKELETAL SYMPTOMS	CARDIAC SYMPTOMS	NEUROLOGIC SYMPTOMS	REFERENCES
Granuloma annulare	+					596, 639
Ringworm	+					599, 639, 763, 768, 870
Cellulitis	+					595, 599, 639, 767, 768, 870
Impetigo	+					595
Pityriasis rosea	+					763
Contact/atopic dermatitis	+					595, 639, 763, 768, 870
Erythema annulare centrifugum	+					639
Tick/insect bite reaction	+					595, 599, 639, 768, 870
Cutaneous malignancy	+					599, 644
Circulatory insufficiency[b]	+					599
Brown recluse spider bite	+	+				871
Serum sickness	+	+	+			243, 768, 870
Erythema nodosum	+					596, 598, 599
Erythema multiforme/urticaria	+	+	+			243, 274, 277, 279, 639, 763, 767, 768
Henoch-Schönlein purpura	+					596
JRA/RA[c]	+	+	+	+		274, 279, 651, 763, 767, 768
Lupus	+	+	+		+	243, 599
Dermatomyositis	+	+	+			599, 617
Scleroderma	+				+	596
Reiter's syndrome			+			651
Fibromyalgia		+	+		+	279, 715, 763, 767, 769, 770
Chronic fatigue syndrome		+	+			279, 763, 767, 768
Inflammatory bowel disease		+	+			279
Rheumatic fever	+	+	+	+	+	243, 687, 872
Bacterial endocarditis		+	+	+		693, 745
Acute myocarditis		+		+		279, 687, 785
Chronic cardiomyopathy				+		368, 607, 692
Syphilis	+		+	+	+	286
Relapsing fever		+				873
Sarcoidosis		+			+	211, 599
Mycoplasma pneumoniae infection	+	+	+	+	+	
Urinary retention, bladder neuropathy					+	669, 678
Diaphragmatic paralysis					+	679
Epstein-Barr virus mono	+	+	+	+	+	243, 763
Cytomegalovirus mono	+	+	+	+	+	763
Echo/coxsackievirus infection	+	+	+	+	+	687

Table continued on following page

TABLE 11–18
Differential Diagnosis of Lyme Borreliosis[a] (LB) *Continued*

DISEASE	RASH	FLULIKE ILLNESS	MUSCULOSKELETAL SYMPTOMS	CARDIAC SYMPTOMS	NEUROLOGIC SYMPTOMS	REFERENCES
Rubella	+	+	+		+	
Rubeola	+	+	+		+	
Hepatitis	+	+	+			698
Mumps		+	+	+	+	687
Rocky Mountain spotted fever	+	+	+		+	639
Babesiosis		+	+		+	639
Ehrlichiosis	+	+	+		+	639
Influenza		+	+	+		687
Adenoviral infection	+	+	+	+	+	687
Fifth disease (parvovirus)	+	+	+	+		744, 763
Arboviral infection		+			+	874
Herpes simplex	+	+			+	595
Zoster	+	+	+		+	338
Osteomyelitis			+			699, 763
Gonococcal arthritis			+			
Yersinia arthritis			+	+		687
Septic arthritis			+			653
Traumatic arthritis			+			768
Gout			+			279, 637
Temporomandibular joint disorder			+			875
Vertebral disk herniation			+		+	876
Vestibular neuronitis					+	518, 708
Meniere's disease					+	518
Orbital myositis					+	703
Retinal detachment					+	705
Papilledema, pseudotumor cerebri					+	289, 435, 530
Temporal arteritis					+	706
Aseptic meningitis	+	+			+	243, 530, 663, 763, 767
Idiopathic cranial/peripheral neuropathy[d]					+	279, 659, 662, 763, 767, 768
European tick-borne encephalitis					+	639
Myasthenia gravis					+	767
Behçet's disease	+	+	+		+	211
Mollaret's meningitis		+			+	211
Multiple sclerosis		+			+	279, 608, 663
Amyotrophic lateral sclerosis					+	211, 279, 663, 677
Guillain-Barré syndrome, transverse myelitis		+			+	289, 530, 663, 669
Migraine					+	763, 768
Seizure disorder					+	279, 311, 325, 655, 663
Stroke, paresis, cerebral vasculitis, focal encephalitis					+	286, 292, 311, 663, 668, 672–676

TABLE 11–18
Differential Diagnosis of Lyme Borreliosis[a] (LB) *Continued*

DISEASE	RASH	FLULIKE ILLNESS	MUSCULOSKELETAL SYMPTOMS	CARDIAC SYMPTOMS	NEUROLOGIC SYMPTOMS	REFERENCES
Dementia					+	613, 663, 767
Catatonia, psychosis					+	663, 664
Brain tumor					+	279, 311, 610, 671
Meningeal lymphoma					+	768
Narcolepsy					+	289
Depression					+	767
Anorexia nervosa					+	663
Cryptococcal meningitis					+	
Severe pain syndrome[e]					+	279, 680

[a]Disease that, on clinical presentation, either could be misdiagnosed instead of LB or could be misdiagnosed as LB.
[b]Acrodermatitis chronica atrophicans may be confused with circulatory insufficiency of the extremities.
[c]Juvenile rheumatoid arthritis, rheumatoid arthritis, spondyloarthropathy.
[d]Including postvaricella peripheral neuropathy and reflex sympathetic dystrophy.
[e]Severe radicular pain may be confused with gastric ulcer, cholelithiasis, renal calculi, myocardial infarction, zoster, or herniated vertebral disk.

tion of infection, as described in the section Clinical Manifestations. Because Lyme borreliosis may manifest with symptoms relating to almost any organ system, a pregnant woman with Lyme disease may seek medical care from physicians in diverse medical or surgical specialties. Familiarity with the various clinical manifestations of Lyme borreliosis and a careful clinical and epidemiologic history, including history of tick bite or exposure to endemic areas, are necessary to allow correct diagnosis, especially when the clinical presentation is unusual. If the initial diagnosis of gestational Lyme borreliosis is not made, the neonatologist, pediatrician, or family practitioner may be presented with either a miscarriage, stillbirth, or congenitally infected infant and may need to make a retrospective diagnosis of maternal gestational Lyme borreliosis.

The characteristic rash of EM is usually easily recognized but may be misdiagnosed if it is vesicular, necrotic, or otherwise unusual in appearance. Usually, a careful clinical history of the rash will lead to the correct diagnosis, which may be confirmed by serologic testing, by biopsy, or by response to antibiotic therapy. Borrelial lymphocytoma is less widely recognized in the United States than in Europe and may therefore be mistaken for cellulitis or cutaneous malignancy, but a careful clinical history and serologic or biopsy confirmation usually lead to the correct diagnosis. A common error is to misdiagnose the initial presentation of ACA, a swollen painful bluish red leg, as circulatory insufficiency, even in Europe where ACA is prevalent; the diagnosis of ACA may be missed because it may present in a patient living in a nonendemic area, years after the initial infection was acquired in an endemic area. Nearly all patients with ACA are *B. burgdorferi* IgG–seropositive.[529]

The flulike illness associated with early Lyme borreliosis may be indistinguishable from that caused by other generalized infections or inflammatory illnesses, such as viral infections, connective tissue disorders, and drug hypersensitivity reactions. The correct diagnosis usually can be made by clinical and epidemiologic history, confirmation of Lyme seropositivity, and, when necessary, serologic exclusion of the other causes. It is important to consider Lyme borreliosis in patients with even fleeting objective signs, such as arthritis, meningitis, or neurologic symptoms, in Lyme-endemic areas.[636, 768]

The cardiac manifestations of Lyme disease initially may be misdiagnosed as acute or chronic viral myocarditis or even myocardial infarction because of the presence of arrhythmias and myocardial dysfunction; establishment of the correct diagnosis is based on Lyme seropositivity and exclusion of the other causes by appropriate testing. Rheumatic fever and bacterial endocarditis also may be confused initially with Lyme carditis but are usually excluded because of valvular involvement, which is absent in Lyme carditis; in addition, complete heart block is more characteristic of Lyme disease than of rheumatic fever or bacterial endocarditis.

When the presenting symptoms are acute and neurologic, without antecedent EM, the diagnosis of Lyme borreliosis may be difficult to make. In acute neuroborreliosis, cranial nerve palsies, such as Bell's palsy, Horner's syndrome, or Argyll Robinson pupil, may be misdiagnosed as idiopathic rather than Lyme-related; radiculitis may produce localized pain severe enough to be mistaken initially for an acute abdominal emergency, cholecystitis or cholelithiasis, ulcer, nephrolithiasis, vertebral disk herniation, myocardial infarction, or zoster, but these usually may be excluded by the absence of the expected abnormalities by appropriate radiographic, sonographic, or other diagnostic tests, and by Lyme seropositivity, as most patients with acute neuroborreliosis[234, 236, 529] are *B. burgdorferi*–seropositive by sensitive and specific assays. The central nervous system manifestations of neuroborreliosis initially may be mistaken for viral meningoencephalitis, stroke, multiple sclerosis, brain tumors, or even dementia or psychiatric disorders, but the correct diagnosis can usually be established by serologic testing for Lyme borreliosis, as most patients with chronic neuroborreliosis[234, 236] are *B. burgdorferi*–seropositive and have diagnostic levels of CSF antibody, and by appropriate testing to exclude the other diagnoses. When the presentation mimics brain tumor, a biopsy is indicated, and if Lyme borreliosis is in the differential diagnosis, the specimen should be sent for *B. burgdorferi* culture, staining, and possibly PCR, as well as for histopathologic examination.

The musculoskeletal manifestations of Lyme borreliosis, particularly Lyme arthritis, initially may be confused with rheumatoid arthritis and occasionally with septic arthritis, but the diagnosis of Lyme disease usually may be made by clinical history, negative rheumatoid factor, negative joint fluid cultures for standard bacteria, and Lyme seropositivity, as most Lyme arthritis patients are IgG *B. burgdorferi*–seropositive at presentation.[234-236] There may be slight increases in rheumatoid factor during Lyme arthritis, but these should be transient. Presentation with a ruptured Baker's cyst or with quadriceps femoris muscle atrophy, with resultant patellofemoral joint dysfunction, is characteristic for late complications of Lyme arthritis.[318]

Other spirochetal infections, such as leptospirosis and syphilis, and other tickborne infections, such as ehrlichiosis and babesiosis, may result in false seropositivity for *B. burgdorferi* by some screening tests, but usually can be distinguished from Lyme disease by Western blot testing and by careful clinical and epidemiologic evaluation. False seropositivity is also a problem with non-Lyme borrelial relapsing fever, and distinguishing the two diseases can be difficult serologically even with Western blot testing[233, 236]; however, the clinical presentations and epidemiologic niches of the diseases are quite different and are usually helpful in diagnosis.

Differential Diagnosis of Congenital Lyme Borreliosis

The differential diagnosis of congenital Lyme borreliosis (Table 11–19) includes bacterial and viral sepsis and meningoencephalitis, toxoplasmosis, syphilis, leptospirosis, relapsing fever, ehrlichiosis, babesiosis, idiopathic congenital heart disease, immunodeficiency and recurrent infections, infantile multisystem inflammatory disease, and even sudden infant death syndrome. Early severe congenital Lyme borreliosis may be misdiagnosed as acute fulminant sepsis and meningoencephalitis or severe congenital heart disease, because of its similar presentation. Early mild congenital Lyme borreliosis may be mistaken for viral meningitis or sepsis because standard bacterial cultures are negative; as a result, the clinical improvement resulting from intravenous antibiotic therapy (commonly with antibiotics that also treat *B. burgdorferi*) given for the possibility of bacterial sepsis is attributed to spontaneous resolution of the presumed viral infection rather than to treatment of the *B. burgdorferi* infection. Late congenital Lyme borreliosis may manifest with symptoms of a more chronic congenital infection, such as failure to thrive, developmental delay, hypotonia, or recurrent infection. It is possible that neurocognitive abnormalities may be currently underrecognized sequelae of late congenital Lyme borreliosis, similar to recent reports of neurocognitive abnormalities related to chronic Lyme encephalopathy in older patients (discussed in the section Clinical Manifestations: Neuroborreliosis).

The diagnosis of congenital Lyme borreliosis may be made in infants with these presentations by obtaining a history of maternal gestational illness compatible with Lyme disease (see earlier section Differential Diagnosis); by serologic, culture, or PCR confirmation of maternal gestational Lyme disease; by exclusion of the other causes by serologic and/or culture evaluation of the infant; and, if possible, by serologic, culture, PCR, or lymphocyte proliferative assay confirmation of *B. burgdorferi* infection of the infant. If placental tissue is available, histopathology, culture, PCR, and special stains for *B. burgdorferi* spirochetes may confirm the diagnosis.

Because of histopathologic similarities between con-

TABLE 11–19
Differential Diagnosis of Congenital Lyme Borreliosis (CLB)[a]

EARLY CLB	LATE CLB
Acute bacterial sepsis/meningoencephalitis	Subacute bacterial sepsis/meningoencephalitis
Congenital viral sepsis/meningoencephalitis	Congenital viral sepsis/meningoencephalitis
Enterovirus	Enterovirus
Cytomegalovirus	Cytomegalovirus
Herpes simplex	Herpes simplex
Rubella	Rubella
Hepatitis A/B/C	Hepatitis A/B/C
? Parvovirus or other	? Parvovirus or other
Congenital toxoplasmosis	Congenital toxoplasmosis
Congenital syphilis, early onset	Congenital syphilis, late onset
Congenital leptospirosis	Failure to thrive or developmental delay due to noninfectious etiologies
Congenital relapsing fever	Congenital hypotonia
Congenital ehrlichiosis	Idiopathic congenital heart disease
Congenital babesiosis	Immunodeficiency and recurrent infections
Idiopathic congenital heart disease	Infantile multisystem inflammatory disease
	Sudden infant death syndrome

[a]Diseases that, on clinical presentation or epidemiologic history, either could be misdiagnosed instead of CLB or could be misdiagnosed as CLB.

genital and placental Lyme borreliosis and syphilis, it is advisable to rule out syphilis serologically in infants with suspected congenital Lyme borreliosis. Because Lyme borreliosis, ehrlichiosis, and babesiosis often share tick vectors and geographically endemic areas, it is also advisable to evaluate infants with suspected congenital Lyme borreliosis for ehrlichiosis and babesiosis, and to consider the possibility that these co-infections may require additional antibiotic coverage or may increase the severity of illness. Congenital Lyme disease should also be considered as a possible cause of some cases of infantile multisystem inflammatory disease, a chronic progressive inflammatory disease of so far undetermined etiology, with cutaneous, neurologic, ophthalmologic, lymphoreticular, and joint involvement, particularly as one of these patients was considered to have congenital Lyme disease.[624, 625] Lyme borreliosis also appears to be involved in some instances of sudden infant death syndrome and should therefore be considered in infants with missed sudden infant death syndrome.[33]

THERAPY

Antibiotic therapy has been used for treatment of Lyme borreliosis since 1958 when Hollstrom found that penicillin cured the skin lesions of European EM.[331] Between 1977 and 1979, following the initial description of North American Lyme disease and EM by Steere and associates,[15] it was unclear whether antibiotic therapy was beneficial in Lyme disease. However, because of the similarities between Lyme disease and European EM, the improvement of European EM with penicillin therapy, and the suspicion that the etiology of both was spirochetal, trials of antibiotic therapy for Lyme disease were conducted between 1977 and 1983 by Steere and colleagues, and a definite response to antibiotic therapy of the cutaneous, arthritic, and neurologic manifestations was found.[201, 339, 619, 771] It is currently accepted that delayed or inadequate antibiotic therapy of early Lyme borreliosis may increase the risk of dissemination and long-term sequelae.[206, 308, 312, 314, 325, 683, 714]

Clinical antibiotic therapy trials are discussed in the remainder of the subsections of the section Therapy; recommendations for antibiotic therapy are discussed and provided in the subsection Recommendations for Antibiotic Therapy of Gestational, Nongestational, and Congenital Lyme Borreliosis, and in Tables 11–20 and 11–21.

Antibiotic Therapy Efficacy Trials

Early antibiotic therapy trials by Steere and co-workers[201, 339] between 1976 and 1981 demonstrated that low-dose, short (7- to 10-day) courses of oral penicillin or tetracycline for treatment of EM led to more rapid resolution of EM than did erythromycin. Tetracycline prevented development of major late manifestations, penicillin decreased this incidence to 8%, and erythromycin to 14%.[201] Penicillin decreased the incidence of later development of Lyme arthritis from 74% to 35% and shortened the duration of Lyme arthritis from 17

weeks to 4 weeks when it occurred, but it did not affect the incidence of later cardiac (4%) or neurologic (14%) involvement.[201, 339] The severity of the minor late systemic symptoms of headache and musculoskeletal pain correlated with the severity of the initial presentation. Patients who were seen more than 2 weeks after the onset of symptoms of early Lyme disease had evidence of clinical dissemination.[757]

Further trials by the same group in 1983[619, 771] showed that high-dose intravenous penicillin (20 million units daily for 10 days) was effective for treatment of chronic Lyme arthritis and acute Lyme meningitis. The possibility was raised that penicillin treatment failures,[79, 619, 771] with progression of early EM to later complications, could be due to failure to eradicate spirochetes in the central nervous system or synovia or other immunologically protected sites, either because of the short penicillin half-life, the relatively high and variable penicillin MIC of B. burgdorferi (see Table 11–1), or the failure to achieve and maintain spinal fluid or synovial fluid levels above the MIC of the spirochete. Inadequate antibiotic therapy may be due to inappropriate choice of antibiotic, route, dose, or duration of therapy.

It was proposed that cephalosporins with longer half-lives, lower MICs, and greater penetration into the central nervous system or synovia than penicillin might achieve better cure rates than penicillin. Because ceftriaxone and cefotaxime have long half-lives, achieve sustained high serum and spinal fluid levels, and have a low MIC for B. burgdorferi, clinical efficacy trials of these antibiotics were performed.

Intravenous ceftriaxone was found to be more effective than intravenous penicillin by Dattwyler and associates,[775] and it cured approximately 90% of refractory patients with late chronic Lyme disease, including arthritis and peripheral neuropathy of over 1 year's duration. Hassler and colleagues[776] found intravenous cefotaxime to be more effective than intravenous penicillin for treatment of late European Lyme borreliosis, including patients with oligoarthritis, peripheral neuropathies, radicular pain, ACA, and borrelial lymphocytoma. They proposed that success with cefotaxime was related to high tissue antibiotic concentrations above the MIC of B. burgdorferi during the entire dose interval and to excellent CSF penetration, and that high sustained levels above the MIC are needed because of reduced tissue permeability that may occur in late Lyme borreliosis as a result of microangiopathic changes in the synovia and nervous system.

If antibiotic therapy of the initial early Lyme disease has been inadequate for eradication of the spirochete but has been given promptly enough to attenuate or eliminate the B. burgdorferi antibody response,[18, 208, 209, 218, 272] seronegative late chronic Lyme borreliosis may develop.

Because rates of cure for late chronic Lyme borreliosis were less than 100%, even with high-dose intravenous cefotaxime or ceftriaxone therapy,[200, 269, 281, 283, 287, 304, 311–315] several studies were done to determine whether longer courses of therapy or use of different antibiotics was indicated to eliminate the spirochete in potentially se-

TABLE 11–20
Treatment of Lyme Borreliosis

CLINICAL CLASSIFICATION	ADULT, NONPREGNANT	CHILD, NON–CONGENITALLY INFECTED[a]	ADULT, PREGNANT[b]
Early localized[c] (Erythema migrans; borrelial lymphocytoma) *or* Early disseminated, mild[c] (Multiple erythema migrans; isolated cranial neuropathy; mild arthritis; mild cardiac, or other organ involvement; no evidence of central nervous system (CNS) involvement)	Doxycycline[d] 100 mg PO bid × 14–30 d *or* Amoxicillin[e] 500 mg PO tid–qid × 14–30 d *or* Cefuroxime axetil 500 mg PO bid × 14–30 d	Doxycycline[d] (for >8 yrs old) 2–4 mg/kg/day PO bid × 14–30 d *or* Amoxicillin[e] 50 mg/kg/day PO bid-tid × 14–30 d *or* Cefuroxime axetil 40 mg/kg/day PO bid × 14–30 d	Ceftriaxone 2 g IV QD × 14 d *or* Cefotaxime 6 g/day IV tid × 14 d *or* Penicillin G[f] 20–24 × 10⁶ units/day IV q4h × 14 d
Early disseminated, serious (Severe arthritis[g], CNS or severe neurologic[h] involvement; severe cardiac, or other organ involvement) *or* Late disseminated (Chronic arthritis[g]; chronic meningitis, encephalitis, peripheral neuropathy[h], chronic cardiac, or other organ involvement; >6–12 months)	Ceftriaxone 2 g IV QD × 14–30 d *or* Cefotaxime 6 g/day IV tid × 14–30 d *or* Penicillin G[f] 20–24 × 10⁶ units/day IV q4h × 14–30 d Doxycycline, amoxicillin, or cefuroxime axetil PO × 30–60 d alternative for arthritis[g]	Ceftriaxone 50–100 mg/kg/day IV qd × 14–30 d *or* Cefotaxime 150 mg/kg/day IV tid × 14–30 d *or* Penicillin G[f] 300,000 units/kg/day IV q4h × 14–30 d Doxycycline, amoxicillin, or cefuroxime axetil PO × 30–60 d alternative for arthritis[g]	Ceftriaxone 2 g IV QD × 14–30 d *or* Cefotaxime 6 g/day IV tid × 14–30 d *or* Penicillin G[f] 20–24 × 10⁶ units/day IV q4h × 14–30 d

Recommendations for children and nonpregnant adults are adapted from references 265, 291, 635, 639, 642, 652, 657, 784, 786, 877, 887, and 888, and recommendations for pregnant women are based on limited data from Tables 11–8 and 11–13 of adverse outcomes of gestational Lyme borreliosis following oral antibiotic therapy. Lengths of therapy are not well established. The author prefers consideration of the higher and longer dosages and lengths of therapy, and recommends cerebrospinal fluid evidence of absence of CNS involvement if isolated cranial neuritis is to be treated orally.

[a]Pediatric antibiotic doses should not exceed adult doses. Doxycycline (or tetracycline) should not be used in children <8 years of age.

[b]Doxycycline (or tetracycline) should not be used in pregnant or lactating women. The author prefers to recommend intravenous therapy, but if this is not feasible, amoxicillin 500 mg tid–qid, or cefuroxime axetil 500 mg bid, may be used for a prolonged period, not shorter than for nonpregnant patients, ranging from 21–30 days to the duration of pregnancy.

[c]Erythromycin 250–500 mg (30–50 mg/kg/day, pediatric) PO tid–qid is less effective but may be used in penicillin-, cephalosporin-, or tetracycline-allergic patients with early localized or early mild disseminated infection. It is not a first-line choice, and if used in pregnancy, it should be discontinued 1 week prior to delivery. Clarithromycin (500 mg PO bid × 10–30 d) is an alternative, but not in pregnancy,[255] and no data are available on its use for treatment of pediatric Lyme borreliosis.

[d]Tetracycline 500 mg PO qid (25–50 mg/kg/day qid for >9 years of age) is considered a doxycycline alternative by some.

[e]Addition of probenecid 500 mg (50 mg/kg/day, pediatric) PO tid–qid to enhance serum antibiotic levels is optional. Phenoxymethylpenicillin 500 mg (50 mg/kg/day pediatric) PO qid is considered an amoxicillin alternative by some.

[f]Ampicillin 8 g/day (200 mg/kg/day, pediatric) IV qid is considered a penicillin alternative.

[g]Oral alternative for arthritis in nonpregnant patients, in the absence of CNS involvement: doxycycline 100 mg (2–4 mg/kg/day, pediatric, for >8 yrs of age) PO bid, or amoxicillin 500 mg (50 mg/kg/day, pediatric) (+ optional probenecid) PO tid–qid or (for doxycycline- or penicillin-allergic patients) cefuroxime axetil 500 mg (40 mg/kg/day, pediatric) PO bid × 30–60 d. Doxycycline (or tetracycline) should not be given to pregnant or lactating women. In some antibiotic-refractory chronic Lyme arthritis patients, arthroscopic synovectomy may be considered.

[h]Some recommend longer, up to 42-d treatment for encephalomyelitis. Ceftriaxone 2 g IV qd × 30 d is recommended for treatment of late Lyme encephalopathy. Possible alternative for neuroborreliosis in penicillin- or cephalosporin-allergic nonpregnant patients: doxycycline 100 mg IV or 100–200 mg PO q12h × 30 d,[190, 275, 883] or chloramphenicol 1 g IV q6h × 14–30 d,[795] although insufficient data are available on long-term outcomes with doxycycline, and failures have been reported with chloramphenicol.[676]

questered sites that were less accessible to the immune response or antibiotic therapy.[199, 208, 265, 269, 273, 276, 310, 667]

Between the mid-1980s and the present, many antibiotic efficacy trials, ranging from small, open-label pilot studies to large, comparative, randomized, double-blind multicenter studies, were done to determine the optimal antibiotic, route of administration, and duration of therapy for the various clinical manifestations of Lyme borreliosis, predominantly in North America and Europe. Optimal therapeutic regimens should not only treat the existing Lyme borreliosis, but should ideally prevent development of later manifestations of Lyme disease, such as meningoencephalitis, myocarditis, and arthritis.

The question has arisen regarding management of asymptomatic persons with histories of previous untreated Lyme borreliosis; one group has recommended oral doxycycline (100 mg twice daily for 1 month), if not contraindicated, for such individuals to reduce the likelihood of development of late Lyme disease.[777]

ERYTHEMA MIGRANS, BORRELIAL LYMPHOCYTOMA, AND ACRODERMATITIS CHRONICA ATROPHICANS

Data from several antibiotic therapy trials indicate that prompt antibiotic therapy of early EM results in cure

TABLE 11–21
Treatment of Congenital Lyme Borreliosis (CLB)[a]

CLINICAL CLASSIFICATION OF CLB	AGE AT TIME OF ANTIBIOTIC THERAPY		
	Neonate, <1 Week	Neonate, 1–4 Weeks	Infant >4 Weeks
Gestational LB exposure: Asymptomatic infant, born to adequately treated mother[b]	No antibiotic *or* Amoxicillin 40 mg/kg/day PO tid × 10–30 d	No antibiotic *or* Amoxicillin 50 mg/kg/day PO tid × 10–30 d	No antibiotic *or* Amoxicillin 50 mg/kg/day PO tid × 10–30 d
Gestational LB exposure: Asymptomatic infant, born to inadequately treated mother[c] *or* Early CLB: Infant symptomatic in first 2 weeks of life[cf]	Ceftriaxone 50 mg/kg/day IV/IM q24h × 14–30 d *or* Cefotaxime 100 mg/kg/day IV/IM q12h × 14–30 d	Ceftriaxone[d] 75 mg/kg/day IV/IM q24h × 14–30 d *or* Cefotaxime[e] 150 mg/kg/day IV/IM q8h × 14–30 d	Ceftriaxone 100 mg/kg/day IV/IM q12h × 14–30 d *or* Cefotaxime[e] 150 mg/kg/day IV/IM q8h × 14–30 d
Late CLB: Infant symptomatic after first 2 weeks of life[cf]		Ceftriaxone[d] 75 mg/kg/day IV/IM q24h × 14–42 d[f] *or* Cefotaxime[e] 150 mg/kg/day IV/IM q8h × 14–42 d[f]	Ceftriaxone[d] 100 mg/kg/day IV/IM q12h × 14–42 d[f] *or* Cefotaxime[e] 150 mg/kg/day IV/IM q8h × 14–42 d[f]

Recommendations are based on limited data, and lengths of therapy are not well established.

[a]Different age-appropriate doses are shown, but treatment is recommended as soon as possible after birth.

[b]Because there is a wide range in what is considered adequate therapy, the alternative of oral amoxicillin therapy to be given pending further evaluation of the neonate for CLB is offered.

[c]Because ceftriaxone should not be used if hyperbilirubinemia is present, cefotaxime is offered as an alternative, although clinical experience in therapy of Lyme borreliosis is not as extensive as with ceftriaxone.

[d]Ceftriaxone dose 50 mg/kg/day IV/IM q24h if weight <2000 g.

[e]Cefotaxime dose 100 mg/kg/day IV/IM q12h if weight <1200 g.

[f]Prolonged oral amoxicillin (40 mg/kg/day) after the course of IV antibiotic therapy may be considered, depending on the clinical course of the infant.

rates of 76 to 92% with oral penicillin 10 to 12 days,[201, 785] 87 to 95% with oral amoxicillin plus probenecid for 10 to 21 days,[193, 782] 88 to 98% with oral doxycycline for 10 to 21 days,[193, 782, 784] 93 to 95% with oral cefuroxime axetil for 20 days,[783, 784] and 76 to 98% with oral azithromycin for 5 to 7 days,[193, 203] but that more severe early disseminated infection with multiple EM, arthralgia, or subtle neurologic symptoms is associated with increased risk of treatment failure, including late symptoms, and requires more aggressive antibiotic therapy.[643, 719, 720, 784, 786, 789]

Several European studies have demonstrated efficacy of antibiotic therapy for European borrelial lymphocytoma and ACA.[315, 316, 645, 646, 697]

B. burgdorferi PCR of skin biopsies of EM and ACA lesions has been reported to be useful in determining cure after antibiotic therapy.[143, 316]

LYME ARTHRITIS

Several studies have found that antibiotic therapy of chronic Lyme arthritis results in cure rates of 28 to 55% with intravenous penicillin,[619, 775, 776] and 81 to 100% with intravenous ceftriaxone,[775] intravenous cefotaxime,[776] oral doxycycline,[324] or oral amoxicillin and probenecid for periods of 10 to 30 days.[274, 424, 652, 775, 776] The major disadvantage of oral therapy for Lyme arthritis is that, in one large study, 12% developed later neuroborreliosis[324]; these patients all had subtle neurologic symptoms initially. It is now recognized that oral therapy should not be used in patients with even subtle neurologic involvement; they should be treated with IV ceftriaxone for at least 30 days.[652]

Because several studies have found that intra-articular or systemic steroid therapy of patients with Lyme disease is associated with lack of response to antibiotic therapy, including intravenous penicillin and ceftriaxone treatment of late Lyme arthritis, steroid therapy is not currently recommended in the initial routine treatment of Lyme arthritis.[620, 775] Steere and co-workers recommend intra-articular steroids only once or twice for antibiotic-unresponsive patients with negative synovial fluid PCR and persistent arthritis despite anti-inflammatory agents.[652]

Arthroscopic synovectomy has been successful in treating patients with chronic Lyme arthritis who had failed to respond to appropriate antibiotic therapy or intra-articular steroids.[652, 792] It has been suggested that PCR positivity of synovial fluid could be used to indicate the need for intravenous antibiotic therapy, and PCR negativity the need for anti-inflammatory agents (including hydroxychloroquine or intra-articular steroids) and possibly synovectomy.[312, 324, 652]

LYME CARDITIS

A 94% recovery rate was reported for 105 North American and European patients with Lyme carditis who were treated with various therapies, including penicillin, tetracycline, third-generation cephalosporins, steroids, and nonsteroidal anti-inflammatory agents.[689] A temporary pacemaker was required in 28% of these patients.[689] Improvement in patients with *B. burgdorferi*–associated chronic dilated cardiomyopathy has also been reported with intravenous ceftriaxone.[692]

Intravenous ceftriaxone or high-dose penicillin is preferable for treatment of serious carditis, although oral antibiotic therapy may be acceptable for mild carditis such as first-degree heart block (see Table 11–20). Systemic steroid therapy (1 to 2 mg/kg per day prednisone) may also be indicated for severe carditis if it is unresponsive to initial antibiotic therapy,[98, 687, 689, 793] and temporary pacemaker placement may be needed for complete heart block.[98, 689]

NEUROBORRELIOSIS

Clinical trials of antibiotic therapy of neuroborreliosis have reported cure rates of 66 to 100% with intravenous penicillin for 10 days,[275, 775, 776] 63 to 100% with intravenous ceftriaxone for 10 to 14 days,[291, 655, 662] and 60 to 90% with intravenous cefotaxime for 10 to 14 days.[776, 794]

Some recent studies of oral antibiotic therapy for the treatment of mild European neuroborreliosis have found over 90% efficacy with oral doxycycline for 10 to 20 days,[190, 191, 275, 883] and 80 to 93% efficacy with intravenous ceftriaxone for 14 days followed by oral amoxicillin or cefadroxil plus probenecid for 100 days, or with oral cefixime alone for 100 days.[276, 310]

Most studies have found ceftriaxone and cefotaxime superior to penicillin,[776] and longer courses of antibiotic therapy more efficacious for treatment of neuroborreliosis.[287, 291, 310, 324, 684]

B. burgdorferi has been demonstrated by PCR to invade the central nervous system (CNS) early in Lyme disease, even in the absence of CNS symptoms.[282] This has significant therapeutic implications and lends support to the concept that maintenance of high spinal fluid antibiotic levels during treatment of disseminated Lyme borreliosis is essential in order to eradicate the spirochete in the CNS, where it is in a relatively protected environment. Antibiotic therapy for disseminated Lyme disease, with or without cranial neuritis, should be selected to achieve high spinal fluid levels.

It has been suggested that PCR might be useful in therapeutic decisions: A positive CSF PCR in an untreated or an inadequately treated patient probably indicates that treatment or retreatment is indicated, and conversion of a CSF PCR from positive to negative probably indicates that therapy has been successful.[186, 287, 309]

The optimal duration and choice of antibiotic therapy for neuroborreliosis are still not well defined, although most sources currently recommend 2 to 4 weeks of intravenous ceftriaxone or cefotaxime for both early disseminated and late chronic neuroborreliosis with CNS involvement[657, 797]; longer courses are being evaluated.[265] Several sources note that treatment of isolated cranial neuropathy without CSF abnormalities with oral doxycycline or oral amoxicillin for 2 to 4 weeks is acceptable.[291, 654, 657, 661, 797] Four- to 6-week courses of intravenous antibiotic therapy may be needed for parenchymal brain neuroborreliosis,[292, 657] and it may be advisable to reevaluate CSF after the first 2 weeks to assess the need for further antibiotic therapy.[657] Steroid therapy is not recommended for neuroborreliosis,[657] and has been reported to be adversely associated with the course of neuroborreliosis.[674, 676]

Although optimal antibiotic therapy for ophthalmic Lyme borreliosis has not been determined, several sources currently recommend more aggressive antibiotic therapy than for other manifestations of early localized Lyme borreliosis, such as 30 days of oral antibiotic therapy for early disease (conjunctivitis, Bell's palsy, keratitis, and episcleritis), and 14 to 30 days of intravenous antibiotic therapy for more serious or late disease (optic nerve, posterior segment, or neuro-ophthalmic disease).[320, 702] Systemic steroid therapy in the absence of antibiotic therapy is not recommended[702] because of reports of adverse effects on the course of ophthalmic Lyme borreliosis.

Achievement of Serum and CSF Antibiotic Levels Above the *Borrelia burgdorferi* Minimal Inhibitory Concentration

European and North American *B. burgdorferi* isolates from patients as well as from ticks have all been found to demonstrate similar antibiotic susceptibility patterns (see Table 11–1), so that recommendations regarding antibiotic therapy are applicable to all geographic areas from which Lyme borreliosis has been reported.

Early comparisons of the clinical efficacy of various antibiotics in the treatment of Lyme disease demonstrated that tetracycline was best, penicillin next best, and erythromycin worst[201]; these results correlated with efficacy studies in animal models. The cephalosporins ceftriaxone, cefotaxime, cefuroxime, and cefixime all had good activity against *B. burgdorferi* by both in vitro MIC and in vivo animal model efficacy studies.[188, 195]

B. burgdorferi is killed slowly by antibiotics and requires prolonged levels above the MIC of the organism for cure,[192] suggesting the possible need for longer than 10 days of high-dose antibiotic therapy to kill *B. burgdorferi* in the spinal fluid.

Several studies correlating CSF antibiotic levels with clinical outcome of neuroborreliosis treated with oral or intravenous doxycycline,[190, 191, 194, 779] intravenous ceftriaxone,[194, 319, 778] intravenous cefotaxime,[190, 319] and intravenous penicillin[194, 778, 779] have been done.

Ceftriaxone, cefotaxime, or doxycycline may be preferable to penicillin for therapy of Lyme borreliosis because their longer half-lives allow maintainance of tissue antibiotic concentrations above the MIC for *B. burgdorferi* during the entire course of therapy.

Jarisch-Herxheimer Reaction and Other Antibiotic Therapy Side Effects

Symptoms of the Jarisch-Herxheimer reaction, which may occur in 7 to 50% of patients treated with antibiotics for Lyme borreliosis, are most likely due to antibiotic-induced spirochetal lysis, which releases lipoproteins capable of inducing tumor necrosis factor and other cytokines, and produces cytokine-mediated responses.[781] Typical symptoms initially consist of vasoconstriction with hypertension, pallor, and chills in the first 6 to 18 hours, followed by vasodilation with hypotension, headache, flushing, and exacerbation of arthralgias, myalgias, rash, and fever for 24 to 48 hours.[776] Development of the Jarisch-Herxheimer reaction is more common if the Lyme borreliosis is severe,[201] disseminated,[719] or chronic,[269, 704, 776] presumably because the spirochetal burden is high, but this may also occur with treatment of uncomplicated solitary erythema migrans.[781] In unusual instances, Jarisch-Herxheimer reactions in patients with chronic neuroborreliosis have been reported to be associated with transient visual deterioration, confusion, stupor, dysarthria, myoclonic jerks, or dense hemiparesis[269, 704]; similar observations have been made in occasional patients with ophthalmic syphilis.[704]

The incidence of occurrence of a Jarisch-Herxheimer reaction within 24 hours after initiation of antibiotic therapy of Lyme borreliosis is 10 to 50% with penicillin or amoxicillin,[201, 435, 719, 771, 776, 782] 0 to 16% with tetracycline,[201, 719] 8 to 12% with doxycycline,[782–784] 7% with erythromycin,[201] 12 to 29% with cefuroxime axetil,[783, 784] and 22 to 40% with cefuroxime, cefotaxime, or ceftriaxone.[775, 776, 783] Development of a Jarisch-Herxheimer reaction may be considered evidence of a response to antibiotic therapy. It is important to recognize this reaction, including the increased rash that may occur, as a Jarisch-Herxheimer reaction rather than an allergic reaction to the antibiotic, in order to prevent unnecessary discontinuation of the antibiotic therapy. Treatment of Jarisch-Herxheimer reactions consists of supportive management until the self-limited symptoms resolve. Symptoms may be prevented if desired by prophylactic treatment with 80 mg of triamcinolone acetonide intravenously 30 minutes before the start of antibiotic therapy.[776]

Frequently overlooked adverse side effects of the incorrect overdiagnosis of Lyme disease[24, 787] include the monetary costs[734–736, 767] of overdiagnosis and overtreatment, including the cost of intravenous antibiotic therapy and management of any adverse effects of antibiotic therapy[734–736, 767, 787]; the effects of failure to diagnose and treat the real illness, with its likely continuation and progression[279, 763, 767]; and the emotional burden of a disabled self-image resulting from the perception by misdiagnosed patients that they have a chronic, debilitating, incurable disease.[767]

Because complications of antibiotic therapy, particularly of intravenous therapy, have been reported in patients being treated for Lyme disease who did not meet diagnostic case definitions,[767, 788] it continues to be important to avoid overdiagnosis and overtreatment of Lyme disease, and to follow accepted guidelines for antibiotic therapy.

Correlation Between Antibiotic Therapy and Outcome of Gestational and Congenital Lyme Borreliosis

Table 11–14 shows the frequency of adverse outcomes of 263 pregnancies complicated by Lyme borreliosis reported in the literature, including four of my cases. Although there are relatively small numbers of patients in each trimester who were either treated or not treated with antibiotic therapy, the overall adverse outcome rate for all trimesters was 67% for untreated and 15% for treated gestational Lyme borreliosis. This protective effect of antibiotic therapy was seen in each trimester, so that the incidence of adverse outcomes of pregnancy decreased from 73% to 18% for first-trimester Lyme borreliosis, from 67% to 16% for second-trimester infection, and from 50% to 9% for third-trimester infection.

Antibiotic therapy for gestational Lyme borreliosis may be successful, partially successful, or unsuccessful in preventing congenital Lyme borreliosis; outcome probably depends on the choice, dose, route of administration, and duration of antibiotic therapy, as well as the trimester of the gestational Lyme borreliosis and the duration of infection before initiation of antibiotic therapy.

There are several reports of antibiotic therapy of gestational Lyme borreliosis that was associated with normal outcomes of pregnancies[33, 42, 47, 48, 536, 622, 719–723, 798]; most of these successful antibiotic regimens consisted of either prolonged oral penicillin for 2 to 4 weeks, or intravenous penicillin or third-generation cephalosporins. In 1986 and 1988, Berger[719, 720, 798] reported four patients with 12-, 14-, 22-, and 24-week gestational Lyme borreliosis that was treated promptly (within 4 to 10 days of onset of early localized EM) with oral penicillin (500 mg four times daily) for 3 to 4 weeks who all delivered normal infants. In 1987, Mikkelsen and Palle[622] reported a patient with third-trimester gestational EM who was treated with phenoxymethyl penicillin (3 million units daily) for 10 days and delivered a normal infant. In 1989, MacDonald[33] reported a patient with second-trimester gestational EM and neuroborreliosis who was treated with intravenous penicillin for 10 days and delivered a normal infant with no evidence of spirochetes in the placenta. In 1990, Luger[721] noted five patients with gestational Lyme borreliosis, including five with EM, carditis, facial palsy, and temporomandibular arthritis, who were treated with unspecified regimens of intravenous antibiotics and who all delivered normal infants. Also in 1990, Stiernstedt[723] reported three patients with gestational Lyme borreliosis who all were treated with antibiotic therapy and all delivered normal infants: One with localized EM was treated with oral penicillin of unspecified duration; one with disseminated EM was treated with intravenous penicillin for 4 days and then with oral penicillin for 10 days; and one with neuroborreliosis was treated with intravenous cefuroxime for 14 days. In 1991, Schutzer[722] and associates noted a patient with 27-week gestational EM treated within 3 days with intravenous ceftriaxone (2 g daily) for 3 weeks who delivered a normal infant. In 1992, Bracero and colleagues[47] reported three patients with symptomatic B. burgdorferi seropositivity in the first or early second trimester who all were treated with antibiotic therapy (noted as either amoxicillin or erythromycin 500 mg qid, or IV penicillin 20 million units per day, or ceftriaxone 2 g per day) for 14 days and delivered normal infants. In 1993, Isailovic and co-workers[536] reported a patient with first-trimester gestational EM treated with intramuscular jugocillin 800,000 units per day for 20 days, who delivered a normal infant.

In 1993, Hercogova and associates[42] reported a series of 15 patients treated prospectively for gestational Lyme borreliosis with EM. Ten patients had normal pregnancy outcomes after treatment (four in the first, three in the late second, and three in the third trimester) with either PO penicillin for 10 to 16 days, or IV penicillin or ampicillin for 14 to 21 days (one first- and one second-trimester patient); two of these patients also received benzathine penicillin of unspecified duration. However, in the same series, similar treatment resulted in five adverse outcomes: Treatment of four patients with early second- and third-trimester infection with PO penicillin for 14 days (and one additionally with benzathine penicillin of unspecified duration), and treatment of one with first-trimester infection with PO penicillin for 24 days, resulted in live-born term infants who were found later to have abnormalities, including persistent PDA (patient 51, Table 11–8), cryptorchidism (patient 52, Table 11–8), developmental delay (patient 55, Table 11–8), and hypoplastic dental enamel (patients 53 and 54, Table 11–8).

In 1996, Maraspin and colleagues,[48] reported a large prospective study from 1990 to 1994 of antibiotic therapy (2 with PO penicillin 1 million units tid, 3 with IM benzylpenicillin 10 million units bid, and 53 with IV ceftriaxone 2 g daily) for 14 days of 58 consecutive patients with gestational EM (13, 27, and 18 in the first, second, and third trimesters). Fifty-one of the pregnancies resulted in normal term infants who remained normal at follow-up (including all of those treated with either PO or IM penicillin); three infants were born with slight prematurity at 36 to 37 weeks and remained well at later follow-up; one pregnancy miscarried (patient 62, Table 11–8) at 9 weeks after severe gestational Lyme borreliosis at 6 weeks (of 1 week's duration before ceftriaxone); one 26-week premature infant (patient 59, Table 11–8) born after early second-trimester EM (of 1 week's duration before ceftriaxone) had respiratory distress and survived; another 36-week premature infant (patient 60, Table 11–8) born after severe early second-trimester Lyme borreliosis (of 1 week's duration before ceftriaxone) had major cardiac anomalies and respiratory distress and survived; and one infant (patient 61, Table 11–8) born after prolonged gestational EM throughout

the third trimester (treated initially with PO cefadroxil 500 mg tid for 14 days, and then with ceftriaxone for 13 days) was normal at birth but was found at 7 months to have ureteral stenosis and hydronephrosis.

There are also several reports of antibiotic therapy for gestational Lyme borreliosis that did not prevent adverse fetal outcomes[26–29, 36, 38, 39, 42]; most of these "unsuccessful" antibiotic regimens consisted of short (7- to 14-day) courses of oral penicillin or erythromycin or unspecified oral antibiotics. However, in one series, treatment consisted of 14 days of IV ceftriaxone.[48] In 1986 and 1988, Weber and associates[38, 39] reported on a patient with first-trimester gestational EM treated with oral penicillin (3 million units daily) for 1 week who delivered an infant (patient 22 in Table 11–8) with severe fatal early congenital Lyme borreliosis. In 1986, Markowitz and colleagues[36] and the CDC[28] reported on three patients with gestational EM treated with oral antibiotic therapy who had adverse fetal outcomes: One patient with 6-week gestational EM with associated headache, stiff neck, and arthritis was treated with oral penicillin for 10 days and had a fetal death at 20 weeks (patient 14 in Table 11–8); one patient with 20-week gestational EM associated with headache, stiff neck, and arthralgia was treated with oral erythromycin for 10 days and then with oral penicillin of unspecified duration at 27 weeks and delivered an infant with syndactyly (patient 16 in Table 11–8); and one patient with 27-week gestational EM treated with oral penicillin for 10 days delivered an infant who developed cortical blindness and developmental delay (patient 17 in Table 11–8). In 1987, Cieszelski and co-workers[29] reported on two patients with first-trimester gestational Lyme borreliosis treated with unspecified antibiotics: One patient with 4-week gestational infection had a miscarriage at 13 weeks (patient 19 in Table 11–8), and the other with 7-week gestational infection delivered an infant with syndactyly (patient 20 in Table 11–8). In 1988, Carlomagno and associates[27] noted a B. burgdorferi–seropositive patient who had a tick bite; she was treated with unspecified antibiotic therapy before pregnancy and had a miscarriage at 9 weeks of gestation (patient 35 in Table 11–8).

If the episode of maternal gestational Lyme borreliosis is untreated and if the fetus survives and is born alive, prompt antibiotic therapy is beneficial. There are reports of three infants born with early congenital Lyme borreliosis after undiagnosed and/or untreated gestational Lyme borreliosis who responded to prompt antibiotic therapy at birth.[28, 33, 36] In 1986, Markowitz and colleagues[36] reported on an infant with mild early illness following untreated gestational Lyme borreliosis 1 week before delivery, who recovered after 10 days of intravenous penicillin (patient 18 in Table 11–8). In 1989, MacDonald[33] reported on an infant with severe early congenital infection after an unremarkable gestation who recovered after treatment with unspecified intravenous antibiotic therapy (patient 12 in Table 11–8), and another infant with severe early congenital infection after a toxemic gestation who recovered after being treated with intravenous penicillin (patient 13 in Table 11–8).

Antibiotic therapy for gestational Lyme disease may

still attenuate the severity of congenital Lyme borreliosis, even if it does not prevent it completely. MacDonald[33] has described one infant and I have described four additional infants born after antibiotic-treated gestational Lyme borreliosis, who had evidence of symptomatic congenital Lyme borreliosis and who responded to intravenous antibiotic therapy either in the neonatal period or during the first year of life (patients 23, 24, 25, and 26 in Table 11–8).

One mother had 4-week gestational disseminated EM treated within 4 days with intravenous ceftriaxone (2 g daily) for 2 days, followed by oral penicillin (500 mg four times daily) for 12 days; she delivered an infant with very mild early congenital Lyme borreliosis (patient 23 in Table 11–8), who recovered with a 2-week course of intravenous ceftriaxone (100 mg/kg per day).

A second mother had flulike illnesses at 5 weeks and 20 weeks of gestation, was treated with amoxicillin (250 mg three times daily) for 10 to 14 days each time, and delivered an infant with severe early congenital Lyme borreliosis (patient 24 in Table 11–8); the child initially failed to improve but did not further deteriorate with intravenous ampicillin (100 mg/kg per day) for 6 days, and recovered when intravenous ceftriaxone (100 mg/kg per day) was added for the next 7 days. This infant required retreatment with intravenous ceftriaxone (75 mg/kg daily for 3 weeks) at 10 months for neuroborreliosis and subsequently remained well.

A third mother had intermittent disseminated EM with flulike symptoms and polyarthralgias; was treated with almost continuous antibiotic therapy for the first 10 weeks of gestation, initially erythromycin (333 mg three times daily) for about 7 weeks, followed by cefaclor (250 mg three times daily) for 3 days, intravenous cefuroxime (750 mg three times daily) for 4 days, oral cephalexin (500 mg four times daily) for 2 weeks, and then oral cefixime (100 mg daily) for 10 days at 12 to 13 weeks; she delivered an infant with moderate early congenital Lyme borreliosis (patient 25 in Table 11–8) who responded to intravenous antibiotic therapy for 6 days (including ampicillin for 5 days and ceftriaxone/cefotaxime for 3 days). This infant later presented with late chronic congenital Lyme borreliosis that required retreatment with a total of 7 weeks of intravenous ceftriaxone (100 mg/kg daily) between 2.5 and 7 months, and prolonged oral antibiotic therapy with amoxicillin (40 mk/kg daily) for 1 year from 7 to 19 months of age. Each time either a less aggressive course of oral cefaclor or a shorter course of intravenous ceftriaxone was given, a relapse consisting of loss of developmental milestones occurred. Finally, after a total of 7 weeks of intravenous ceftriaxone followed by a 1-year course of oral amoxicillin, the infant remained clinically well and continued to progress to essentially normal neurologic status by 8 years of age; at 9 years of age, he had an episode of arthritis associated with neurologic symptoms, which responded to retreatment with ceftriaxone. Patient 56[44] also had musculoskeletal and neurologic abnormalities considered to be late Lyme borreliosis of many years' duration since birth, after prolonged untreated maternal gestational Lyme borreliosis (EM, arthritis, and neuro-

borreliosis), and was noted to have a good response to treatment with oral roxithromycin and co-trimoxazole.

A fourth mother had second- and third-trimester EM associated with flulike illness, polyarthralgias, stiff neck, and dizziness, and was treated with oral erythromycin (250 mg four times daily) for 10 days at about 28 weeks, followed by oral cefuroxime axetil (2 g daily) from 33 weeks through delivery; she delivered an infant with mild early Lyme borreliosis (patient 26 in Table 11–8) who recovered with intravenous ceftriaxone (75 mg/kg daily) for 4 weeks. Two of these infants (cases 25 and 26) had episodes resembling Jarisch-Herxheimer reactions within 2 to 5 days of the start of initial antibiotic therapy.

MacDonald[33] reported on an infant whose placenta grew spirochetes following second-trimester gestational EM treated with oral penicillin (500 mg four times daily) for 15 days and untreated gestational EM 2 weeks before delivery, who was well at birth and was treated promptly with oral penicillin and probenecid and who remained well.

Review of Recommendations for Antibiotic Therapy of Gestational Lyme Borreliosis

Because there has been previous uncertainty about the true incidence of fetal risk associated with gestational Lyme borreliosis, there has been great diversity among recommendations for the management of gestational tick bites and gestational Lyme borreliosis; there are four basic approaches recommended in the medical literature. Prenatal screening for Lyme seropositivity to detect and treat seropositive patients with evidence of active Lyme borreliosis is recommended by some investigators.[27, 189, 799] Some recommend antibiotic prophylaxis of all Ixodes tick bites in pregnancy because of evidence that this is successful in the prevention of development of Lyme borreliosis following the bite of an infected tick, and because of concern that early dissemination to the placenta and fetus may occur before initiation of antibiotic therapy if Lyme borreliosis does develop.[211, 799–801] Some recommend antibiotic therapy of gestational Lyme borreliosis determined by the clinical stage and severity of the infection (which usually consists of oral antibiotic therapy for early localized infection and intravenous antibiotic therapy for early disseminated or late infection) because of their impression that the actual risk of development of congenital Lyme borreliosis is exceedingly low, and that there is no need for more aggressive treatment of gestational Lyme borreliosis,* although some of the lengths of therapy recommended are at the longer range of current recommendations. Others recommend longer duration of antibiotic therapy in gestational Lyme borreliosis because of concern about transplacental spread.[731] Yet other investigators recommend more aggressive therapy, such as intravenous antibiotic therapy for all cases of gestational Lyme borreliosis because of concern that there is a significant potential risk to the fetus, which is not yet fully appreciated, following any gestational Lyme borrel-

---

*See references 27, 36, 189, 723, 729, 730, 783, 793, and 799–806.

iosis infection; also, they believe that high-dose intravenous antibiotic therapy is more successful at achieving antibiotic levels above the MIC of the spirochete on both the maternal and fetal sides of the placenta,[38, 48, 211, 225, 530, 725, 804] and that parenteral antibiotic therapy[435] should be considered for some patients with gestational Lyme borreliosis, particularly in those with first- or early second-trimester or disseminated gestational Lyme borreliosis.[23, 731, 791, 807] Others say it is unclear how best to treat gestational Lyme borreliosis.[808]

Some reports favor prenatal screening. Carlomagno and colleagues[27] and Cryan and Wright[189] recommended prenatal screening for B. burgdorferi seropositivity, and treatment of all seropositive patients, even those with asymptomatic gestational B. burgdorferi seropositivity, with oral or intramuscular penicillin or with intravenous ceftriaxone. Williams and Strobino[799] also recommended prenatal screening but advised use of antibiotic treatment only for those with evidence of active infection. Bracero and associates[47] recommend antibiotic therapy according to the stage of the disease for all seropositive and symptomatic pregnant women. Some recommend against prenatal screening,[530] and others recommend no antibiotic therapy for asymptomatic seropositive patients during pregnancy.[804]

Some reports favor antibiotic prophylaxis of gestational B. burgdorferi vector tick bites. Edly[801] recommended prophylaxis for bites only in the first half of pregnancy during the period of maximum susceptibility to teratogens; Williams and Strobino,[799] Ostrov and Athreya,[211] and the American College of Obstetricians and Gynecologists[800] recommended prophylaxis of all gestational bites in endemic areas. Segura-Porta and co-workers recommend amoxicillin orally for 10 days in certain situations wherein Lyme borreliosis risk is high and follow-up is difficult, or patient anxiety is high.[804] When specified, the most commonly recommended prophylactic regimens consisted of oral amoxicillin 500 mg three times daily, or oral penicillin 500 mg four times daily, for 3 weeks.

Other reports favor antibiotic therapy of gestational Lyme disease based on guidelines for nonpregnant patients, with no special modifications for pregnancy other than not using doxycycline or probenecid. Markowitz and colleagues favor oral penicillin (500 mg four times daily for 10 to 20 days) for early infection and consideration of intravenous penicillin for late infection.[36] Stiernstedt,[723] Williams and Strobino,[799] and Segura-Porta[804] suggested oral penicillin or amoxicillin for 2 to 3 weeks for localized EM, and intravenous penicillin or cephalosporin therapy for 2 to 3 weeks for disseminated EM or neuroborreliosis. Carlomagno and colleagues,[27] Cartter and colleagues,[802] Smith and colleagues,[793] Nocton and Steere,[730] and the American Academy of Pediatrics[803] recommended treatment for gestational Lyme borreliosis but made no special modifications in the recommendations for more aggressive therapy of gestational infection. Nocton and Steere,[730] however, recommend that normal infants born to mothers with untreated gestational Lyme borreliosis should be evaluated with a higher level of suspicion, and that treatment may be considered; they also advise that in treatment of ill newborns, consideration should be given to use of antibiotics known to treat B. burgdorferi, and that in any of these infants, cord blood or serum B. burgdorferi IgM antibodies may be helpful.

There are investigators who favor more aggressive therapy for gestational Lyme disease. The National Institute of Arthritis and Musculoskeletal and Skin Diseases and the National Institute of Allergy and Infectious Diseases[791] recommended consideration of intravenous antibiotic therapy for first-trimester gestational Lyme borreliosis, and routine therapy according to guidelines for the clinical stage of disease for other trimesters. Podolsky[23] suggests that intravenous ceftriaxone may provide greater protection for the fetus than oral penicillin. MacDonald and colleagues,[35] Weber and associates,[38] and Ostrov and Athreya[211] favor intravenous penicillin therapy (20 million units daily for 10 to 14 days) and possibly intravenous ceftriaxone (2 to 4 g daily for 10 to 14 days)[211] for all gestational Lyme borreliosis cases. Dattwyler and co-workers[225] recommend antibiotic therapy of gestational Lyme borreliosis to achieve eradication of spirochetes on both the maternal and fetal sides of the placenta, and imply that this is best accomplished by high-dose intravenous therapy. Rahn and Malawista[807] recommend intravenous penicillin (20 million units daily) for 14 to 21 days for all cases of gestational Lyme borreliosis except single localized EM with no associated systemic symptoms, for which they recommend oral amoxicillin (500 mg three times daily) for 21 days. Christen and colleagues recommend intravenous penicillin G (500,000 IU/kg/day with a maximum of 20 megaunits daily) for 10 to 14 days for all pregnant women with Lyme borreliosis, but note that amoxicillin or azithromycin might be effective.[435, 530] Maiwald[809] recommends a slightly longer duration of antibiotic therapy for gestational Lyme borreliosis: 21 days of amoxicillin (500 mg three times daily) for early localized Lyme borreliosis, and 14 to 21 days of intravenous ceftriaxone (4 g daily) or cefotaxime (3 g twice daily) for early disseminated or late Lyme borreliosis. Sicuranza and Baker[731] recommend treatment of uncomplicated EM with amoxicillin (or erythromycin 250 mg four times daily), and treatment of disseminated or late Lyme disease or first-trimester gestational Lyme disease with intravenous penicillin G (20 million IU daily) or ceftriaxone (2 g daily). In 1996, Maraspin and colleagues[48] recommended intravenous antibiotic therapy, preferably with ceftriaxone 2 g daily for 14 days, for all gestational Lyme borreliosis, based on their large prospective study of 58 consecutively enrolled patients treated for gestational EM; this advice is offered out of concern that neither the occurrence of transplacental dissemination nor the timing of such occurrence during the acute infection can be accurately assessed.

Recommendations for Antibiotic Therapy of Gestational, Nongestational, and Congenital Lyme Borreliosis

Tables 11–20 and 11–21 show antibiotic regimens recommended for different stages of Lyme borreliosis, which have been developed based on the literature* and my own experience; these include specific recommendations for gestational and congenital Lyme borreliosis.

It should be emphasized that the best time to treat Lyme borreliosis successfully is at the onset of the early infection, as treatment of late chronic infection is more difficult and has a higher failure rate. The goal of antibiotic therapy ideally should be eradication of the spirochete from all sites, including potentially immunologically privileged sites such as the eye, the joints, the central nervous system, and, in pregnancy, the fetal side of the placenta. The lengths of therapy are not well established; because of concern regarding the need to maintain serum, synovial fluid, and spinal fluid levels above the MIC of the spirochete, I prefer to recommend the longer (4-week) durations of antibiotic therapy. There are no current recommendations regarding whether prolongation of oral antibiotic therapy for several months is beneficial, although this could be considered in individual unique clinical situations. However, an open mind must be maintained regarding any recommendations for antibiotic therapy for Lyme borreliosis because several Lyme research centers have modified their treatment recommendations over the past several years. Recommendations most likely will require further modification as additional data on clinical efficacy trials become available.

For treatment of nongestational, nonlactating, and noncongenital early localized or mild disseminated Lyme borreliosis without CNS involvement (see Table 11–20), 14- to 30-day courses of oral doxycycline (100 mg twice daily, or 2–4 mg/kg per day twice daily for children older than 8 years) or oral amoxicillin (500 mg three to four times daily, or 50 mg/kg per day two or three times daily for children) are the regimens of choice. Many recent sources prefer 21- to 30-day courses, and the durations of therapy are not well defined. Doxycycline should not be used either in pregnant or lactating women, or in children younger than 8 years of age. Oral probenecid (500 mg three to four times daily, or 50 mg/kg per day for children) may be given optionally with amoxicillin to increase serum antibiotic concentrations. Oral cefuroxime axetil (500 mg twice daily, or 40 mg/kg per day for children) is an effective alternative. Oral erythromycin (250–500 mg three to four times daily, or 30–50 mg/kg per day for children) has been associated with frequent treatment failures; its use should be reserved for patients in whom no other acceptable therapy is possible. Clarithromycin has been found to be as efficacious as amoxicillin and is a good alternative for penicillin- or cephalosporin-allergic patients, but it should not be used in pregnancy. Azithromycin is slightly less efficacious and has a slightly higher relapse rate than amoxicillin for treatment of EM. There are no data on the efficacy of clarithromycin or azithromycin for treatment of pediatric Lyme borreliosis. There are differing opinions regarding whether oral antibiotic therapy of isolated cranial neuritis, including facial palsy, requires confirmation of a negative CSF evaluation for neuroborreliosis; however, because of the

frequency of abnormal CSF in such patients, many recent recommendations favor CSF evaluation in this situation,[291, 657, 661] along with the use of intravenous ceftriaxone (2 g daily) or cefotaxime (6 g daily), as for CNS neuroborreliosis if CSF abnormalities such as pleocytosis, elevated protein, intrathecal specific antibody, or PCR positivity are found.

For treatment of gestational early localized or mild early disseminated Lyme borreliosis, as well as more serious disseminated Lyme borreliosis (see Table 11–20), intravenous antibiotic therapy is preferred because of reported failures of oral antibiotic therapy to reliably prevent the development of congenital Lyme borreliosis, including miscarriage, stillbirth, and early or late congenital infection. The drugs of choice are ceftriaxone (2 g daily), cefotaxime (6 g daily), and penicillin (24 million units daily) for 2 weeks for mild localized Lyme borreliosis without neurologic manifestations, and for longer durations for early disseminated and late Lyme borreliosis. Ampicillin (8 g daily) is considered an acceptable alternative to penicillin. If antibiotic-induced gastroenteritis develops because of an intravenous cephalosporin, either a change to penicillin or treatment of the diarrhea with oral vancomycin is indicated; if other serious complications of intravenous antibiotic therapy develop, a change of antibiotic or route is indicated. Intravenous antibiotic therapy is preferable. However, because oral antibiotic therapy has also been associated with a decreased incidence of adverse outcomes of gestational Lyme borreliosis, if intravenous antibiotic therapy is not feasible, reasonable oral alternatives would be amoxicillin (500 mg four times daily) or possibly cefuroxime axetil (500 mg twice daily) for 3 to 4 weeks; a prolonged course during gestation could be considered. The use of erythromycin for treatment of gestational Lyme borreliosis is to be discouraged unless no other options are possible, as it has been associated with failure to prevent congenital infection. If it is used, a prolonged course should probably be considered, and it should be discontinued at least 1 week before delivery to avoid neonatal hyperbilirubinemia.

For treatment of more severe nongestational early disseminated or late Lyme borreliosis (see Table 11–20), 14- to 30-day courses of intravenous antibiotic therapy with either ceftriaxone 2 g (or 50–100 mg/kg per day for children) daily, cefotaxime 6 g (or 150 mg/kg per day for children) daily, or penicillin 24 million units (or 300,000 units/kg per day for children) daily given every 4 hours are the regimens of choice. For arthritis without neurologic manifestations, oral amoxicillin (500 mg PO tid–qid, or 50 mg/kg per day for children) or doxycycline (100 mg PO bid, or 2–4 mg/kg daily for children over 8 years) for 30 to 60 days is an acceptable alternative. However, if even subtle neurologic manifestations are present, oral therapy increases the risk of later neuroborreliosis; in such instances, CSF evaluation is advisable, and intravenous antibiotic therapy should be used if CSF is abnormal. Higher daily pediatric doses, 100 mg/kg of ceftriaxone, 180 mg/kg of cefotaxime, and 400,000 units/kg of penicillin, may be needed for the most serious manifestations of Lyme disease. Current evidence supports ceftriaxone, or cefotaxime, as the first-choice drug;

---

*See references 24, 98, 190, 202, 203, 275, 324, and 795, in addition to those in Table 11–20.

clinical efficacy has been greater than with penicillin, although there is less difference in efficacy when longer durations of antibiotic therapy are used. Although the durations of therapy are not well defined, many sources recommend a longer treatment duration—30 days for severe, chronic, late, recurrent, or persistent infection, including neuroborreliosis, severe arthritis, significant neuro-ophthalmic or neuro-otologic involvement, severe carditis, myositis, and late chronic Lyme disease, including ACA. Some sources also recommend durations of 42 days for severe, progressive meningoencephalomyelitis. Although intravenous therapy is preferable, if this is impossible, alternatives include amoxicillin and optional probenecid (500 mg of each three to four times daily, or 50 mg/kg daily for children) or cefuroxime axetil (500 mg three times daily, or 40 mg/kg daily for children) for 30 days or, for nonpregnant and nonlactating patients older than 8 years of age, oral doxycycline 100 mg twice daily for 30 days. Although chloramphenicol was found to be effective in some cases, it has failed in others, and its use for the treatment of Lyme disease cannot be advocated unless no other antibiotic alternatives are possible; it should not be used in pregnant or lactating women.

Treatment of congenital Lyme borreliosis is summarized in Table 11–21; antibiotic dosages and intervals vary according to the age of the infant to be treated. For treatment of asymptomatic infants born to mothers who had adequate treatment of their pregestational or gestational Lyme borreliosis, no antibiotic therapy is necessary. However, if there is any question of adequacy of maternal treatment, the infant could be treated with oral amoxicillin for 10 to 30 days while evaluation is pending. If maternal Lyme borreliosis was inadequately treated, even an infant who is asymptomatic at birth may be at risk for congenital Lyme infection, and prompt antibiotic therapy should be started at birth with either intravenous cefotaxime or ceftriaxone for 2 to 4 weeks. If the infant is already symptomatic at birth, this indicates more severe infection, and prompt antibiotic therapy is essential and may be lifesaving; the longer duration of 4 weeks may be preferable because of concern regarding the risk of late chronic Lyme borreliosis with its associated developmental and neurologic deterioration. For the infant who either presents with or later develops signs of late congenital infection, intravenous therapy with ceftriaxone or cefotaxime for 4 to 6 weeks is recommended.

Intravenous ceftriaxone or cefotaxime is preferred to penicillin for treatment of congenital Lyme borreliosis because of lower *B. burgdorferi* MICs, higher cure rates of late chronic Lyme borreliosis,[775] and some reports of possible clinical resistance of neuroborreliosis to penicillin therapy.[794, 795] However, if intravenous penicillin or ampicillin has been used rather than ceftriaxone or cefotaxime for initial therapy of congenital Lyme borreliosis because of treatment of an initially different diagnosis, and if there is no clinical improvement, the patient should be changed to intravenous ceftriaxone or cefotaxime. This was done in one infant with severe early congenital infection (patient 24 in Table 11–8), and it resulted in dramatic clinical improvement.

If clinical relapse occurs after initial treatment of either gestational or congenital Lyme borreliosis, retreatment with a more aggressive antibiotic regimen such as a longer course of intravenous ceftriaxone or cefotaxime is indicated. Prolonged oral antibiotic therapy following this retreatment should be considered either for the duration of the pregnancy in gestational infection or, in the case of congenitally infected infants, until growth and developmental and neurologic assessment indicate that no further improvement is expected.

Clinical studies of antibiotic prophylaxis for tick bites are discussed in the section on prophylaxis, and recommendations are given in Table 11–22. The author prefers to recommend gestational antibiotic prophylaxis of *B. burgdorferi* vector tick bites in endemic areas because of the established success of antibiotic therapy in the prevention of Lyme borreliosis, and because some cases of congenital Lyme borreliosis have occurred in the absence of clinical symptoms of gestational Lyme borreliosis. Oral amoxicillin 500 mg three times daily for 10 days would be the first choice; a possible alternative includes cefuroxime axetil 500 mg twice daily or erythromycin 500 mg four times daily for 10 days. Antibiotic prophylaxis for tick bites of infants and children with histories of previous congenital Lyme borreliosis is also recommended because of concern that reinfection with *B. burgdorferi* may lead to unusual, possibly immunologically mediated, manifestations of infection. Antibiotic prophylaxis of tick bites of nonpregnant and noncongenitally infected individuals is not routinely recommended but may be considered if the estimated risk of acquisition of Lyme borreliosis from the bite exceeds 1%, or if unusual circumstances exist.

In general, with antibiotic therapy of either early localized or early disseminated Lyme borreliosis, EM skin lesions begin to improve within 2 to 3 days and resolve within a few weeks; the mild, associated flulike symptoms improve within a few days and resolve within a few weeks. Arthralgias should improve within a few days but may take a few months to fully resolve. Improvement is generally gradual in patients with chronic borreliosis who respond to antibiotic therapy. Subjective improvement usually becomes noticeable several weeks after the start of antibiotic therapy, and objective improvement is seen months later.[208, 775] Symptoms of arthritis improve within a few weeks and resolve by 3 months; symptoms of neuroborreliosis, including neuropathies, show initial improvement within a few weeks but may take as long as 24 months to resolve.

Documented clinical relapses or treatment failures after therapy of any patients with confirmed Lyme borreliosis with established antibiotic therapy regimens should be retreated with longer, more aggressive regimens.

Empirical intravenous antibiotic therapy of patients with fatigue syndromes without convincing clinical and epidemiologic evidence of Lyme borreliosis is not advocated, whether or not they are Lyme-seropositive.

Predictors of Antibiotic Therapy Cure

Cure rates following antibiotic therapy of Lyme borreliosis are generally highest for early localized infection and lowest for disseminated and late chronic infection.

TABLE 11–22
Recommendations for Use of Recombinant Osp A Lyme Vaccine[a]

Should consider for:	Persons (15 to 70 years of age) who reside, work, or engage in recreation in high[b] or moderate[c] Lyme disease risk areas, and have frequent or prolonged tick exposure
	Travelers (15 to 70 years of age) to high or moderate Lyme disease risk areas, with expected frequent or prolonged tick exposure
	Persons (15 to 70 years of age) with prior uncomplicated Lyme disease, with continued high Lyme disease risk
May consider for:	Persons (15 to 70 years of age) who reside, work, or engage in recreation in high or moderate Lyme disease risk areas, but have only infrequent and brief tick exposure
Not recommended for:	Persons who reside, work, or engage in recreation in low or no Lyme disease risk areas
	Persons younger than 15 years or older than 70 years of age
	Persons with treatment-resistant Lyme arthritis
	Pregnant women[d]
No recommendations available for[e]:	Persons with immunodeficiency, musculoskeletal disease[f], Lyme-related chronic arthritis or neurologic disease, second- or third-degree AV block
Vaccine schedules:	Initial dose, IM
	Second dose, IM, 1 month after first, several weeks before Lyme disease transmission season
	Third dose, IM, 12 months after first, several weeks before Lyme disease transmission season
	Boosters may be needed, but no recommendations available yet
	If administration simultaneously with other vaccines is necessary, requires separate syringe and injection site

[a]Adapted from Centers for Disease Control and Prevention Recommendations for the Use of Lyme Disease Vaccine: Recommendations of the Advisory Committee on Immunization Practices (ACIP). MMWR 48(RR7):1–25, 1999.[418]

[b]High predicted Lyme disease risk occurs in some or all areas in northeastern United States (Maine, New Hampshire, Massachusetts, Rhode Island, Connecticut, New York, New Jersey, Pennsylvania, Delaware, and Maryland) and upper midwestern United States (Minnesota and Wisconsin).

[c]Moderate predicted Lyme disease risk occurs in some or all areas in the above states, plus Vermont, Michigan, Indiana, Illinois, Iowa, and California.

[d]Registration of inadvertent vaccination of pregnant women is encouraged (SmithKline Beecham, 1-800-366-8900, ext. 5231).

[e]Limited or no data available to allow recommendations to be made.

[f]Arthritis, including rheumatoid arthritis, or diffuse musculoskeletal pain.

Most patients treated promptly with antibiotic therapy appropriate for the clinical stage and severity of the infection have good outcomes.[206, 274, 324, 594, 643, 648, 716, 790, 810] Delay in therapy, or therapy inadequate for the initial presentation of the infection, may be associated with a higher incidence of dissemination and the development of long-term sequelae.[206, 308, 312, 314, 325, 683, 714, 756, 757] Dissemination is a risk factor for late relapse. After adequate antibiotic therapy, most symptoms resolve within weeks to months: erythema migrans within 3 to 5 weeks,[202, 203,] borrelial lymphocytoma within 3 to 8 weeks,[644, 646, 865] meningitis within 4 weeks,[643] facial palsy within 4 to 8 weeks,[643, 654] carditis including AV block within 1 to 4 weeks,[643, 687] acute arthritis within 1 to 3 months,[256, 274, 324, 643] retreated antibiotic-responsive, persistent arthritis within 4 to 12 months,[314, 324] early neuroborreliosis (meningoencephalitis/radiculitis, polyneuritis) by 1 to 9 months,[520] peripheral neuropathy and radiculitis within 3 to 6 (possibly up to 24) months,[275, 291] and late chronic neuroborreliosis within 1 to 3 years.[520] The edema of ACA resolved within 2 weeks, the erythema within 2 to 10 weeks,[316] the arthritis of ACA within 1 to 3 months,[697] and other symptoms of ACA within several months, but atrophic changes tended to persist. Most of the nonspecific symptoms of early disseminated European Lyme borreliosis usually resolve within 2 weeks to 3 months—fever, nausea, vomiting, weight loss, headache, neurocognitive deficits, and arthralgia within 2 weeks, and malaise and fatigue within 3 months.[275]

Persistence or relapse of symptoms of Lyme borreliosis after antibiotic therapy,[269, 312, 318] beyond expected times of resolution, is due either to persistent *B. burgdorferi* infection because of use of an inadequate antibiotic regimen or survival of the spirochete in privileged sites inaccessible to antibiotics or the immune response; autoimmune phenomena related to *B. burgdorferi* molecular mimicry and HLA-DR specificity; *B. burgdorferi*-induced cytokine-mediated inflammatory reactions; post-Lyme fibromyalgia syndrome or other intercurrent non-Lyme illnesses; an incorrect initial diagnosis of Lyme disease; or residual *B. burgdorferi*-induced damage. Increased duration and severity of Lyme borreliosis increase the risk of irreversible damage; antibiotic therapy is able to halt further damage but does not alter irreversible damage.[206, 308, 311, 324, 786]

Inadequate antibiotic therapy of Lyme borreliosis is a risk factor for development of persistent, relapsing, or new symptoms, and *B. burgdorferi* persistence, and may be due to lack of antibiotic treatment; treatment with an ineffective antibiotic; or treatment with an inadequate dose, duration, or route of delivery of an adequate antibiotic, as occurred in some early clinical trials before the development of currently recommended antibiotic regimens.[325, 522, 648, 681, 683, 684] Some antibiotic regimens may not achieve or maintain adequate CSF levels[269, 778, 779] to eliminate early CNS dissemination, which may progress to neuroborreliosis with persistence of *B. burgdorferi*.[206, 253, 284, 311, 319, 324] Predictors of failure of antibiotic treatment, which correlate with the development of late manifestations, include persistence or recurrence of the skin lesions, survival of *B. burgdorferi* organisms in biopsies,[811] persistence of *B. burgdorferi* antigen positivity after antibiotic therapy,[253, 269, 283, 287, 311, 312, 314] progression of arthritis after the first week of antibiotic therapy or beyond one month after the end of antibiotic therapy,[274, 324] and development of new CNS vasculitic lesions detectable by MRI.[311] Persistence of facial nerve palsy longer than 3 months after antibiotic therapy suggests that there may be permanent damage.[786]

Persistent infection should be confirmed. If previous antibiotic therapy was inadequate, retreatment with an adequate course is indicated; if previous treatment was considered adequate, retreatment should be done with a different antibiotic, or with a higher dose and a longer duration of the same antibiotic. Retreatment is usually but not always effective when adequate antibiotic therapy regimens are used.[206, 269, 274, 287, 310–312, 314, 324, 790] Although demonstration of culture positivity is the definitive proof of persistence of active infection, the sensitivity of antigen-detection methods such as PCR and antigen capture ELISA is greater. Demonstration of *B. burgdorferi*–specific antigens in tissues or fluids is usually predictive of antibiotic responsiveness.[186, 187, 283, 287, 310, 312, 314]

Reduction of *B. burgdorferi* antibody titers has been reported following successful antibiotic therapy of Lyme disease,[274–277, 776] but Lyme seropositivity or seronegativity is not always a reliable indicator of antibiotic cure.[225, 244, 318] Patients may be seronegative even though inadequate antibiotic therapy may have failed to eradicate the infection because early antibiotic therapy aborts the development of the mature IgG antibody response to *B. burgdorferi* infection.[18, 208, 209, 273] Patients may be IgG-seropositive even though antibiotic therapy has successfully eradicated the infection if the antibiotic therapy was given later in infection, after the mature IgG antibody has already developed.[244] Persistence of *B. burgdorferi*–specific IgM antibody beyond the first few weeks after early treatment of infection, and particularly years after infection,[325] significant and sustained antibody titer increases (in IgG as well as IgM antibody),[325, 811] and expansion of the antibody repertoire by Western blot evaluation accompanied by persisting or relapsing symptoms of Lyme disease[206, 318, 324] are also predictors of possible persistent infection and appear to correlate with increased severity and dissemination of the initial Lyme borreliosis and with the development of late complications.

Early Lyme borreliosis without a history of either tick bite or EM is a risk factor for progression to late manifestations because the initial infection is often undiagnosed and therefore remains inadequately treated.[274, 648]

The routine use of intra-articular or systemic steroid therapy of Lyme disease has been associated with an increased risk of dissemination; development of chronic complications such as persistent arthritis, meningitis, and multifocal encephalitis; neuro-ophthalmic or neuro-otologic disorders; cardiac sequelae; and lack of responsiveness to antibiotic therapy, including high-dose penicillin or ceftriaxone.*

HLA-DR4 specificity and Osp A or Osp B IgG seropositivity are strong risk factors for the development of chronic Lyme arthritis[256, 324, 325] and are predictive of poor antibiotic response[256, 324, 325] if antibiotic therapy is delayed in patients with chronic Lyme arthritis.

Presentation with neurocognitive or neurologic symptoms during or shortly after an initial episode of Lyme disease was found to be associated with an increased risk of development of late neuroborreliosis in patients treated with delayed or inadequate antibiotic therapy.[324, 681, 683, 684]

Overdiagnosis of Lyme disease[24, 279] in patients who do not meet diagnostic criteria, which occurs in 38 to 79% of patients referred to Lyme disease clinics for evaluation,[763, 767, 768] is a major reason for apparent failure of response to antibiotic therapy, although some of these patients may show either a placebo effect or a response to antibiotic therapy of an unrecognized non-Lyme infectious disease. Many studies indicate that prompt treatment of correctly diagnosed Lyme borreliosis with antibiotic therapy considered adequate, in choice of drug, duration of therapy, and route of administration, for the stage and severity of the presentation, is a predictor of complete recovery without sequelae.[274, 643, 716, 764, 790]

PREVENTION

Methods to reduce the risk of development of Lyme borreliosis include attempts at reducing the population density, geographic distribution, and incidence of *B. burgdorferi* infection of the tick vectors and their animal hosts; development of animal and human *B. burgdorferi* vaccines; use of personal protective clothing and other methods to reduce the risk of tick bite and *B. burgdorferi* transmission; use of prophylactic antibiotic therapy for tick bites in endemic areas; and development of educational programs to increase awareness of Lyme disease risk and to promote early diagnosis and treatment of cases in the early stage to reduce the incidence of late manifestations.

Tick Vector and Animal Reservoir/ Host Control Measures

The large mammalian hosts of the adult *Ixodes ricinus* complex ticks determine the geographic distribution and population density of the larval and adult stages of the tick vectors; the small mammalian or other small reservoir hosts of *B. burgdorferi* determine the infection rate in the tick population.[347, 407, 408, 812] In hyperendemic areas, almost all of the nymphs and reservoir mice may be infected. In areas where the tick infection rate is very high, even small changes in tick density may significantly change the risk of Lyme disease exposure and the incidence of Lyme disease.[559]

When deer are the only large mammalian host, as in hyperendemic coastal islands of the northeastern United States, elimination or reduction of the deer population results in reduction of the *I. scapularis* tick population and of the incidence of Lyme disease.[407] Use of deer fencing, either electrified or 8 feet tall, for at least 2 years, decreases the nymphal tick density by up to 80% and reduces the incidence of Lyme disease; however, it is difficult to maintain and expensive,[6, 347, 812] and it must completely exclude deer from an area to be effective, as even small deer populations can support an infected tick population.[492, 812] When domestic animals such as cattle or sheep are the only large mammalian host, as in some endemic areas in Europe, pasture rotation results in

---

*See references 284, 309, 311, 314, 324, 619, 620, 674, 676, 709, 771, and 775.

reduction in the *I. ricinus* tick population and is more effective than acaricides.[407]

Rodent reservoir control is difficult and not necessarily effective,[6, 812] but elimination of bird feeders on residential property eliminates the attraction of rodents and other small mammalian reservoirs capable of transporting ticks onto the property.[347]

Because ticks inhabit humid areas of dense vegetation, tick populations may be reduced by habitat control measures[407, 812] or by changes in climatic conditions. Dry springtime weather conditions and light snowfall may temporarily decrease tick densities. Methods such as springtime burning and mowing of brushy areas in the northeastern United States reduce the questing nymph population and therefore the subsequent adult tick population by 70 to 88% for approximately 1 year, but the effects of such drastic measures on the risk of human Lyme disease are not known. Mowing of lawns reduces the adult tick population by 70% but does not eliminate nymphal ticks in hyperendemic areas. Removal of leaf litter, underbrush, and shrubs from the edges between lawns and forests, use of fences or dry border material between lawns and forests, and use of deer-proof fencing have had some success in reducing tick populations when these measures are sustained.

Chemical control of the tick population has been attempted using acaricides applied to small mammalian reservoirs, large mammalian hosts, or the environment.[407, 812, 813] Early studies found acaricide treatment of deer unsuccessful in reducing the number of ticks feeding on deer, but future efforts to apply acaricides to deer at feeding stations are planned. Acaricide applied to mice by distribution of permethrin-treated rodent nest materials in early spring and mid-summer, to kill nymphs and larvae, showed early promise in reducing the tick population and the incidence of Lyme disease, but it was not found to be successful in other tests.[347, 407]

Various acaricides, such as carbaryl, chlorpyrifos, diazinon, and cyfluthrin, have been applied to the environment in high-risk residential areas for immediate 97 to 100% reduction of the *Ixodes* tick populations within 3 days, but these measures only temporarily reduce the tick population for up to 1 year and are most useful for treatment of well-maintained lawns—not for wooded areas.[6, 407] Granular preparations of these acaricides target ticks in the soil before host seeking, and are easier to apply than liquids.[347] Single applications of granular carbaryl even to forested residential areas have achieved 70 to 90% reductions in nymphal ticks on host mice and are expected to decrease subsequent adult tick density.[813] Biologic tick attractants, such as *Ixodes* species pheromones, may be useful in the future to attract ticks to acaricide-containing traps.[407]

Efforts are being made to limit the spread of Lyme disease at the margins of endemic areas; mouse immunization via distribution of vaccine-containing food, to reduce acquisition of spirochetemia by uninfected young mice during infected tick feeding, and therefore remove these mice from the enzootic cycle, has been proposed.[812]

Biologic control of ticks has been attempted by introduction of a wasp species that lays eggs in *I. scapularis*

larvae into two northeastern coastal islands, but this was unsuccessful in one island and reduced the *I. dammini* population by only 50% in the other.[407]

The combination of annual environmental acaricide application in the spring for nymph tick control, and in the fall if adult tick control is desired, and deer management methods for overall reduction of tick population density appears to achieve the best reduction in human risk of acquisition of Lyme disease in endemic areas of North America.

Animal Models

Animal models of Lyme borreliosis have been of value in evaluating vaccine efficacy[814, 822–828] and in investigating the pathogenesis of Lyme disease.[815–821]

Transplacental transmission in mice has been investigated in several models.[732, 830] Two pregnant mice collected in the wild, *P. leucopus* and *Mus musculus*, were found to have *B. burgdorferi* in fetal tissues by culture.[831] Mice experimentally infected intradermally with *B. burgdorferi* developed arthritis 2 weeks later. Mice infected 5 days before or 4 days after mating, with gestation coinciding with acute infection, had a fetal death rate of 12 to 14% at 2 weeks of gestation; *B. burgdorferi* PCR showed that all uteri were positive, one placenta was faintly positive, all fetuses were negative, and 46% of the mice had litters with at least one fetal death. In contrast, mice infected 3 weeks before mating, with gestation coinciding with chronic rather than acute infection, had no fetal deaths and no PCR-positive uteri, placentas, or fetuses despite development of severe chronic arthritis. Fetal death was not associated with an inflammatory infiltrate, transplacental transmission occurred rarely and was not required for fetal death, and the increased rate of fetal death was thought to be due to a maternal response to infection rather than to fetal infection. Uterine persistence of *B. burgdorferi* was necessary for fetal loss to occur, consistent with production of intrauterine inflammatory mediators such as IL-1 and TNF in response to *B. burgdorferi* outer response to infection and the mechanism of *B. burgdorferi*–induced surface proteins. This model should prove useful in evaluation of intrauterine fetal death. Transplacental transmission has not been found in rats.[832]

B. burgdorferi causes arthritis and spontaneous abortion in horses[833] and cows, and transplacental infection has been demonstrated in one aborted calf and one newborn calf.[833] A closely related species, *Borrelia coriaceus*, transmitted by the soft tick *Ornithodoros coriaceus*, has been suspected to be the cause of epizootic bovine abortion in California.

Transplacental *B. burgdorferi* infection has been documented in beagle dogs.[834] Dogs were experimentally infected intradermally with *B. burgdorferi* on the first day of estrus and at two weekly intervals during pregnancy. All infected dogs delivered litters with at least some infected pups (either positive PCR or culture), and four pups had documented infection at younger than 2 days of age, supporting the transplacental route of infection. Infected pups had no increased mortality rate and showed no evidence of inflammation when sacrificed at

6 weeks for autopsy. Pups had evidence of passive maternal IgG antibody, which declined by 6 weeks; three had evidence of positive IgM response at 6 weeks, which persisted in two pups, and the possibility of tolerance was raised.

Vaccine Development

Lyme disease is a major worldwide public health problem, and fear of acquisition of Lyme borreliosis has interfered with outdoor activities and led to loss of real estate value in hyperendemic regions.[120] In addition, pets and domestic animals in endemic areas have also been affected by B. burgdorferi infection. Because elimination of wildlife reservoirs has been impractical, and reduction of vector ticks has not been completely successful, there has been and continues to be intense interest in the development of vaccines for wildlife, domestic animals, and humans.[120] Extensive animal model immunization studies,[120, 139, 140, 814, 822–827] and human clinical trials[835–841] have led to the development of two lipidated Osp A human Lyme disease vaccines, LYMErix, licensed by the U.S. Food and Drug Administration in January 1999,[418, 842–845] and ImuLyme,[418, 844] for which licensing is still pending as of the time of this writing. These vaccines are unique among all human vaccines because they are arthropod-specific transmission-blocking vaccines, which act primarily in the tick to inactivate the spirochete before it is transmitted during the tick bite.[139, 140]

Currently, selective rather than widespread vaccination with LYMErix, the recently licensed vaccine, based on a combination of individual risk and geographic risk in specific groups, is recommended (see Table 11–22).[120, 418, 842, 845] Maes and colleagues[846] also recommend targeting of selected groups for vaccination, based on cost-of-illness estimations.

Pregnant women were excluded from the vaccine trials, and Lyme disease vaccine is not currently recommended for use in pregnancy. However, because inadvertent vaccination may occasionally occur, the manufacturer has created a registry for such patients (1–800–366–8900, ext. 5231), and registration is encouraged.[843] Women contemplating pregnancy should be given the Lyme vaccine according to CDC guidelines based on geographic and individual Lyme disease risk, ideally with all three vaccine doses given before pregnancy to provide adequate protection throughout pregnancy.

A significant concern regarding the Lyme vaccine is that it may provide a false sense of security and result in the reduced use of other very important protective methods against tick bites, including personal protective methods, which would place vaccine recipients with inadequate immunity at risk for acquisition of Lyme disease.[842] In addition, Lyme vaccine recipients remain susceptible to other tickborne pathogens, including ehrlichiosis and babesiosis, which require continued tick bite precautions, and both of which have been associated with rare cases of transplacental transmission.[396, 630–632]

Borrelia burgdorferi subunit antigens have been considered better human vaccine candidates[120, 145, 814] than whole inactivated spirochetes because of concerns that some B. burgdorferi antigens such as flagellin and the heat shock proteins may induce cross-reactive antibodies to human tissues such as synovia, axons, liver, heart, and skeletal muscle. Osp A, which is highly immunogenic in animal models and has minimal strain variation among U.S. strains, has been the major human vaccine candidate; Osp B and Osp C are also highly immunogenic but have been less promising human vaccine candidates because they have greater strain heterogeneity. The lipid moiety of Osp A enhances its immunogenicity even without potent and potentially toxic adjuvants. Patients with Lyme disease have minimal or no early Osp A antibody response because Osp A expressed by B. burgdorferi inside of ticks is suppressed during tick feeding[828] and further suppressed after spirochete entry into the host.[844] Osp A vaccine has a unique dual mode of action—direct neutralization of the spirochete immediately after transmission when small amounts of Osp A are still expressed, but, more importantly, inactivation of the spirochete in the tick before transmission when it actively expresses Osp A.[139, 140, 826–828, 843, 844] Mouse immunization studies indicating protection by Osp A and Osp B vaccines against heterologous as well as homologous tick-transmitted strains[827] raise the possibility that monoclonal human Osp A vaccine may be effective against more diverse strains than was initially expected, in the actual clinical setting of human tick-transmitted infection.

The current Lyme disease vaccine is a recombinant lipidated Osp A subunit vaccine derived from the German ZS7 B. burgdorferi sensu stricto isolate adsorbed onto aluminum hydroxide adjuvant.[843] In 1994, Keller and colleagues published the first human clinical trial,[835] which demonstrated safety and immunogenicity of two 10-microgram doses of either aluminum-adsorbed or -unadsorbed recombinant Osp A vaccine in normal human volunteers. In 1995, Schoen and associates, in a clinical trial of an aluminum hydroxide–adsorbed vaccine in persons with previous histories of Lyme disease,[836] also demonstrated safety, and found that immunogenicity was greatest when three 30-microgram vaccine doses were used. Because of reports of the association of high Osp A antibody levels and treatment-resistant chronic Lyme arthritis,[255, 256, 587] the vaccine was not studied in persons with treatment-resistant chronic arthritis. Van Hoecke and co-workers[838, 839] compared several vaccine formulations and found that lipidated Osp A given on a 0-, 1-, 2-, and 12-month vaccination schedule produced the best Osp A antibody and Osp A protective epitope antibody responses in human volunteers.

The safety, efficacy, and immunogenicity of LYMErix, an aluminum hydroxide–adsorbed recombinant lipidated Osp A Lyme disease vaccine, were evaluated in a large multicenter, double-blind, randomized, placebo-controlled study at 31 U.S. sites in ten highly Lyme-endemic areas by Steere and colleagues,[841] which led to licensing of this vaccine in January 1999. In the winter of 1995, before the start of the spring tick feeding season, 5469 vaccinees and 5467 controls, aged 15 to 70 years, were enrolled and followed clinically and serologically for 20 months. High levels of protection were found against clinical Lyme disease and asymptomatic seroconversion after three 30-microgram doses of recombinant lipidated Osp A vaccine with aluminum hydroxide adjuvant, at 0, 1, and 12 months. After two doses, during the first year of Lyme disease exposure, the vaccine was 49% effective in prevention of clinical disease and 83% effective in prevention of asymptomatic seroconversion; after three doses, during the second year of Lyme disease exposure, it was 76% and 100% effective, respectively. Lower levels of antibody against the protective epitope of Osp A correlated with breakthrough Lyme disease. Mild to moderate local injection-site reactions occurred in 24.1% of vaccinees and 7.6% of controls, and brief mild flulike systemic reactions occurred in 19.4% of vaccinees and 15.1% of controls. Pregnant or lactating women, and persons with recent Lyme disease, long-term antibiotic therapy, arthritis, musculoskeletal pain, or AV block were excluded from the study.

The safety and efficacy of ImuLyme™, a recombinant lipidated Osp A vaccine without aluminum hydroxide adjuvant, were evaluated in a multicenter, double-blind, randomized, placebo-controlled study at 14 U.S. sites in highly Lyme-endemic areas by Sigal and colleagues,[840] but it has not yet been licensed. In the spring of 1994, 5149 vaccinees and 5156 controls, older than 18 years of age, were enrolled and followed clinically for two Lyme disease transmission seasons. Three doses of 30 micrograms of vaccine were given at 0, 1, and 12 months. After two doses, the vaccine was 68% effective in the prevention of clinical Lyme disease during the first year after vaccination; it was 92% effective in the second year among recipients of all three vaccine doses. Although volunteers were not followed serologically for asymptomatic seroconversion, none who were asymptomatic during the trial have so far developed late Lyme disease, supporting the absence of asymptomatic infection. Mild brief local reaction at the injection site was the most common adverse reaction, and adverse reactions were reported in 32 to 36% of vaccinees and 28 to 32% of controls. Persons with recent Lyme disease, previous Lyme vaccination within 18 months, or long-term antibiotic therapy were excluded from the study. The vaccine was found to have a lower efficacy of uncertain etiology, 40% in the first year and 37% in the second, in a subset of 1634 of these volunteers enrolled at a single site in Westchester County, New York.[857]

There are several areas of concern regarding LYMErix immunization that still require further study.[418, 842, 844, 845] The duration of protection and the need for booster immunization need to be determined. Optimal dosing schedules to achieve adequate protection in a single tick feeding season are needed, as the present schedule provides only 49% protection during the first season, and Osp A antibody must be present before *B. burgdorferi* exposure to be effective.[841, 843, 844] Vaccine evaluation in adults older than age 70 years and in children is needed, particularly because children have a higher incidence of tick exposure. Because of exclusions from the clinical vaccine trials, little or no information is available on safety and efficacy in pregnant, lactating, or immunocompromised persons, or persons with chronic arthritis, musculoskeletal conditions, treatment-resistant Lyme arthritis, Lyme-related chronic arthritic or neurologic illness, or second- or third-degree AV block. Long-term surveillance for assessment of infrequent or late adverse vaccine events is needed, as is further evaluation of the theoretical possibility of vaccine-induced immunopathogenicity related to molecular mimicry of Osp A and the role of Osp A antibody in treatment-resistant Lyme arthritis. Because Osp A antibody in vaccinees results in positive standard ELISA assays, serologic evaluation for Lyme disease in vaccinees currently requires the more expensive Western blot; additional serologic screening tests such as ELISA assays using Osp A–negative *B. burgdorferi* strains are needed to distinguish natural infection from vaccine immunity.[847] The efficacy of the current vaccine for prevention of Eurasian Lyme borreliosis is unknown, and clinical trials of vaccines designed for Eurasian use are needed. Ongoing post-licensing studies of vaccine safety, efficacy, and cost effectiveness are needed.

A canine *B. burgdorferi* bactericin vaccine, licensed by the U.S. Department of Agriculture in 1992,[584, 814] requires two initial doses, separated by 2 to 3 weeks, and yearly boosters; induces antibodies to Osp A and Osp B; and is protective against homologous or closely related heterologous *B. burgdorferi* strains. Additional vaccines for household and domestic animals are being developed. Many veterinarians in Lyme-endemic areas recommend vaccination of dogs.

Recreational and Occupational Lyme Borreliosis Risk, and Methods for Individual Protection Against Tick Bites

One of the most important methods of protection against the development of Lyme borreliosis is avoidance of exposure to tick-infested endemic areas during the seasons of maximal tick feeding activity, and this is strongly recommended during pregnancy[76]; however, if such exposure is unavoidable, as is the case with individuals who live or work in endemic areas, there are additional effective precautions that are recommended.[7, 305, 347, 407, 418, 459, 848]

Particularly high-risk recreational and residential activities include residential property maintenance such as landscaping and clearing leaf litter, underbrush, or wood piles; and outdoor activities such as hunting (Dutch hunters[514]), fishing, camping, hiking, orienteering (Swiss orienteers and sportsmen[521, 522, 572]), and other outdoor activities in endemic areas (see Table 11–7).

Particularly high occupational risk includes work in forestry*; wildlife management and game keeping[541, 542]; zookeeping[470]; park management[543]; nature conservancy[538, 539]; farming and cattle raising[541, 542, 409, 504, 512, 549]; veterinary medicine[409]; the military[305, 517, 576]; and other outdoor occupations.[495, 504] Relatives of military personnel stationed in Lyme-endemic areas are at risk to ac-

---

*See references 344, 346, 409, 433, 450, 504, 512, 523, 524, 527, 529, 533, 541, 542, 549, 554, and 573.

quire Lyme borreliosis during recreational activities in these areas[576] (see Table 11–7).

It is best to remain on trails and avoid leaf litter, tall grass, and low-lying vegetation in wooded and brushy areas frequented by deer and rodents. Use of hats and light-colored, long-sleeved, long-legged, smooth-fabric clothing, with pants tucked into socks and shirts tucked into pants, reduces the risk of tick attachment. One study[305] of Dutch military personnel, training in a hyperendemic forest, found that use of protective clothing reduced the incidence of tick bites to 6.4% compared with previously reported rates of 55 to 78% in Swiss orienteers and Dutch forestry workers.

Clothing, shoes, and socks may be treated with chemical tick repellents[7, 347, 459, 848] such as N-diethyltoluamide (DEET), or acaricides such as permethrin, which discourage ticks from adhering to clothing; DEET may be applied to exposed skin according to the manufacturer's directions and U.S. Environmental Protection Agency guidelines.[848] Permethrin tick repellent kills ticks on contact but is not indicated for skin application, although other permethrin preparations are approved for treatment of scabies mites and head lice.[848] Tick repellents containing 0.5% permethrin are 100% protective, and mosquito repellents containing 30% DEET are 92% protective against all stages of Lyme disease vector ticks.[848, 849] However, these may be toxic or teratogenic, and there is concern regarding their use in pregnant women; one report urges use of DEET in pregnancy only if clearly indicated.[799]

Prompt and proper tick removal reduces the risk of transmission of the spirochete because B. burgdorferi is transmitted most often after 48 to 72 hours of feeding.[341, 342, 347, 430] In a study in a highly endemic area of New York, transmission was between 18 and 25% after nymphal and female tick attachment for over 72 hours, compared with 1% for less than 72 hours.[430] Because of some recent reports of transmission of Lyme borreliosis after tick attachment of less than 24 hours,[9, 430–432] and even less than 2 hours,[9] frequent inspection every few hours for tick attachment and immediate tick removal are recommended during exposure to tick-infested areas.[407] Shower, shampoo, and total body tick checks are recommended on return from tick-infested areas, and also 1 to 2 days later, as small nymphal or larval ticks may be detected more easily after they engorge. Clothing worn into tick-infested endemic areas should be placed into sealed plastic bags until washed in hot water, and cars and camping equipment should be inspected for ticks that may be seeking hosts.

At present, tick removal using tweezers without pressure on the tick's body is recommended, but further evaluation of removal methods is needed. Needham[347, 880] evaluated several methods of removal of both hard (ixodid) and soft (argasid) ticks and found that the best method for complete removal of the intact tick was to grasp it near the skin surface with forceps or protected fingers and pull steadily upward without squeezing, puncturing, or crushing the tick, and without twisting or jerking it so that the mouth parts did not break off. The possibility that inexperienced tick removal with tweezers might cause regurgitation of midgut Borrelia and lead to increased Borrelia transmission was raised by Hassler[850] because the incidence of Lyme disease in a German hyperendemic region decreased over threefold after the method of tick removal changed from self-removal using tweezers to physician office removal using scalpels to avoid pressure on the ticks' bodies. It is also important to remove the latex-like cement secreted by the tick around the attachment site. The bite site should be disinfected afterward, and the tick disposed of in alcohol or saved in an airtight container with a moist cotton-tipped swab, if analysis for presence of B. burgdorferi is desired. The tick may continue to salivate for several minutes after removal, so care must be taken to avoid direct contact with this potentially infectious fluid. Ticks should not be squashed because this increases the risk of exposure to infectious tick body fluids; transmission of Lyme borreliosis has been reported after conjunctival contact with squashed tick intestinal contents.[851]

The body site location of any tick bite should be noted, the site observed for 1 month, and prompt antibiotic therapy instituted if any evidence of EM or other illness consistent with Lyme borreliosis develops. In some geographic areas, and particularly for tick bites in pregnancy, antibiotic prophylaxis is indicated and is reviewed in the following section.

It is advisable to keep pets away from endemic tick-infested areas if possible, but if this is unavoidable, they should be checked for ticks and the ticks removed before the pets are allowed into the home. Gloves and tweezers should always be used for removal of ticks from pets.

Antibiotic Prophylaxis of Tick Bites in Pregnant and Nonpregnant Patients

For nonpregnant patients, there is controversy over whether antibiotic prophylaxis is indicated for tick bites in Lyme-endemic areas; the risks and benefits of both prophylaxis and no prophylaxis should be weighed. Several reports discuss the pros and cons of prophylaxis.[430, 431, 752, 806, 852–857] For pregnant patients, many groups,[211, 799, 801, 858] including the American College of Obstetricians and Gynecologists,[800] recommend antibiotic prophylaxis (some consider it specifically for embedded or engorged ticks in endemic areas),[859] and others recommend against it.[189, 802]

The approach to tick bite antibiotic prophylaxis taken by many physicians practicing in Lyme-endemic areas of North America is often in disagreement with that recommended by researchers. Fix and colleagues[737] found that physicians practicing in 1995 in the Eastern Shore of Maryland, a Lyme-hyperendemic area with an annual incidence of 86 cases per 100,000, prescribed prophylactic antibiotic therapy for 55% of tick bites.[737] Twenty to nearly 50% of physicians practicing in endemic areas of the eastern and northeastern United States routinely prescribed prophylactic antibiotics for tick bites, and an additional 33% sometimes did.[772–774] A more conservative approach recommended by many researchers studying the epidemiology of the disease is to reserve antibiotic prophylaxis for bites with high

TABLE 11–23
Antibiotic Prophylaxis of *Borrelia burgdorferi* Vector Tick Bites in Lyme-Endemic Areas

CLINICAL SITUATION	LYME BORRELIOSIS SYMPTOMS	ANTIBIOTIC PROPHYLAXIS RECOMMENDED[a]
Tick bite, pregnant woman	Asymptomatic	Yes, amoxicillin 500 mg PO tid × 10–21 d[b, c]
	Symptomatic	No, full antibiotic therapy for active Lyme borreliosis instead, according to clinical stage of the infection
Tick bite, infant or child with history of congenital Lyme borreliosis	Asymptomatic	Yes, amoxicillin 50 mg/kg/day PO tid × 10 d[d]
	Symptomatic	No, full antibiotic therapy for active Lyme borreliosis instead, according to clinical stage of the infection
Tick bite, nonpregnant and non–congenitally infected person, with <1% risk of development of Lyme borreliosis	Asymptomatic	No, not routinely recommended
	Symptomatic	No, full antibiotic therapy for active Lyme borreliosis instead, according to clinical stage of the infection
Tick bite, nonpregnant and non–congenitally infected person, with >1%[e] risk of development of Lyme borreliosis	Asymptomatic	Possibly, doxycycline 100 mg PO bid or amoxicillin 500 mg PO tid × 3–10 d[f]
	Symptomatic	No, full antibiotic therapy for active Lyme borreliosis instead, according to clinical stage of the infection

Based on data from references 211, 430, 431, 752, 799–801, 852–854, and 856–859.

[a]Antibiotic prophylaxis would not be recommended for persons who have adequate immunity due to Lyme vaccination.

[b]Possible alternatives are cefuroxime axetil 500 mg PO bid × 10 d, or erythromycin 500 mg PO qid × 10 d, but the efficiency of these for prophylaxis has not been tested in large clinical trials. Erythromycin should not be given during the week before delivery, and tetracycline or doxycycline should not be given to pregnant women.

[c]American College of Obstetricians and Gynecologists recommends 21 days.

[d]Possible alternatives are cefuroxime axetil 40 mg/kg/day PO bid × 10 d, or erythromycin 30 mg/kg/day PO tid × 10 d. Tetracycline or doxycycline should not be given to children <9 years of age, and doses of other antibiotics should not exceed adult doses.

[e]Factors increasing this risk include tick-engorged, nymphal, or adult; tick attached >48 to 72 hours; tick confirmed to contain spirochetes or from a tick population with *B. burgdorferi* infection rate >10%; tick removal by a method that increases transmission risk; multiple tick bites.

[f]Alternatives include penicillin or tetracycline at standard PO doses × 3–10 d, or possibly cefuroxime axetil PO or erythromycin PO at above doses × 3–10 d.

Lyme disease transmission risk, and to withhold it from those with low risk and treat the infection if it develops.[860] Although serologic screening of patients with tick bites for *B. burgdorferi* antibody has been found to be frequent in hyperendemic areas,[737] there is general agreement that this is not recommended, but that if done, is appropriate only if antibiotic prophylaxis is to be withheld and if both short-term and later follow-up serologic testing is done.[238, 860]

In some hyperendemic areas such as southwestern Finland where the incidence of tick bites ranges from 26.9% of army recruits in a single summer to 85% of the overall population, with 28% reporting multiple bites, antibiotic prophylaxis of tick bites has been considered impractical. It has been recommended that education of at-risk individuals about tick recognition and removal, and use of protective clothing, is preferable.[516, 517]

Data regarding risk of infection after single tick bites in nonpregnant individuals suggest that it is reasonable to use antibiotic prophylaxis in carefully selected subgroups in whom the chance of development of Lyme disease is predictably high, but that routine antibiotic prophylaxis of all *B. burgdorferi* vector (*I. scapularis, pacificus, ricinus, persulcatus*) tick bites in endemic areas is not indicated (Table 11–23). There are several factors that should be considered in making this decision. The risk of development of Lyme borreliosis increases if the tick is a nymph or an adult rather than a larva, if the

B. burgdorferi infection rate in the endemic tick vector population is over 10%, if the tick is shown to be infected, if there are multiple tick bites, if the duration of tick attachment before removal is longer than 48 to 72 hours, or if the tick is engorged and the method of tick removal used was likely to have caused injection of tick contents into the bite site. In addition, if the likelihood of good patient follow-up is low, and therefore adequate treatment of Lyme disease, if it were to develop, would be impossible, it is advisable to use antibiotic prophylaxis for the bite at the time the patient seeks medical attention. In occasional cases, if patient anxiety is high, and if there are significant valid concerns about the potential risk of development of late chronic Lyme borreliosis without the initial EM lesion, it would not be unreasonable to use prophylaxis. Close follow-up for clinical signs of Lyme disease and treatment of diagnosed cases is important for all patients in endemic areas with vector tick bites, even after short-duration attachment, because there are some reports of transmission with attachments of less than 24 hours,[9, 430–432] but routine serologic screening is not necessary.

In pregnant women, antibiotic prophylaxis of all *B. burgdorferi* vector tick bites in known endemic areas is indicated (see Table 11–23) because of the potential risk of congenital Lyme borreliosis following maternal gestational Lyme borreliosis. In lactating women, antibiotic prophylaxis could also be considered because only insufficient data are so far available regarding the potential risk of transmission to the infant by nursing, although there have been no reports of documented transmission by this route. There are no recommendations to support routine treatment of asymptomatic pregnant women with histories of remote pre-gestational tick bite who have no evidence of active Lyme disease and who have serologic responses consistent with previously resolved Lyme borreliosis. The antibiotic regimen of choice for prophylaxis of tick bites in pregnant women is amoxicillin 500 mg by mouth three times daily for at least 10 days; acute and convalescent sera are indicated if there is any suspicion that asymptomatic infection has occurred following the bite. In penicillin-allergic patients, cefuroxime axetil 500 mg orally twice a day (if the patient has no cross-reacting hypersensitivity) or erythromycin 500 mg orally four times daily for at least 10 days may be used. Doxycycline or tetracycline should not be used in pregnant or lactating women.

No data exist regarding whether antibiotic therapy should be given for tick bite prophylaxis of congenitally infected infants or children because so few of these infants have been recognized. Because some of the chronic complications of Lyme borreliosis may be immunologically mediated and the immune response of congenitally infected infants to future B. burgdorferi infection is unknown, the author currently favors use of antibiotic prophylaxis for congenitally infected children, although these recommendations may change as further data become available (see Table 11–23).

Educational Programs to Increase Lyme Disease Awareness

Educational campaigns to increase awareness of Lyme disease and methods of reduction of human risk are widespread in many hyperendemic areas of North America. The European Union Concerted Action on Risk Assessment in Lyme Borreliosis (EUCALB) has prepared a pamphlet[861] that reviews Lyme borreliosis and risk reduction methods, is available via the EUCALB web site,[862] is intended for use in every European country to increase knowledge about Lyme borreliosis in low-awareness groups, and may also be used to educate tourists to Lyme-endemic areas.

However, even in areas where knowledge of Lyme disease is high, tick-avoidance behavior has often been found to be inadequate, particularly among visitors.[577, 863] A survey of 100 women in a Lyme-endemic area of Connecticut, at either prenatal or postnatal visits, found that although almost all would be concerned about tick bites or Lyme disease, and half reported they were concerned about effects on pregnancy, one fourth had misconceptions about Lyme disease transmission and were concerned about exposure to a person with Lyme disease but were unconcerned about working or playing on their lawns.[864] In a hyperendemic area of New Jersey, a survey of over 300 tick bite victims[863] found that only 58% used proper tick removal methods, only 16% treated their residential property with acaricides for tick control, only 0.6% cleared brush or vegetation from near their residences, and 84% of dog and cat owners allowed their pets to roam outdoors and indoors. Eighty-six percent took personal precautions against tick bites as a result of the bite, compared with estimates of 43% of visitors to recreational areas in New Jersey. A case-control study[496] in Hunterdon County, New Jersey, a hyperendemic area with an incidence of 193 cases per 100,000, found that only 55% of patients with Lyme disease did routine tick checks, 47% wore protective clothing, and 16% used tick repellents. A survey[577] of 304 ferry passengers leaving Martha's Vineyard in 1992, an endemic area with an incidence of over 30 cases per 100,000 and 180,000 visitors annually, found that despite a very good level of knowledge about Lyme disease in 73%, only 58 to 59% limited tick exposure or wore protective clothing, 66% did tick checks, and 40% used tick repellent. Visitors followed tick-avoidance and tick-checking recommendations less often than residents. In a hyperendemic area in the Czech Republic, another study[519] found that despite high awareness of ticks and Lyme disease, 87% of people, including both residents and visitors, had a history of tick bite, and few people used proper tick removal methods. A survey of visitors to the endemic Thetford Forest in southeastern Great Britain, which has 1.5 million visitors per year, found that less than half knew that Lyme disease was transmitted by tick bites, and only 13% recognized an unfed nymphal I. ricinus tick.[544] There are a million visitors annually to the Aland Islands of Finland, another highly endemic area.[516] Many popular tourist resorts worldwide are in Lyme-endemic areas, and Lyme disease educational programs in these areas are needed.

Although educational campaigns to increase knowledge about Lyme disease and risk-reduction methods are important, it is also necessary to increase actual observance of risk-reduction methods among both residents of, and visitors to, endemic areas by provision of information that convinces individuals at risk that risk-reduction methods are effective and worthwhile. A dramatic reduction in the incidence of seroconversion of New Jersey outdoor workers occurred after 3 years of educational tick bite recognition programs, although climatic factors may also have played a role.[495] Specific programs targeting tourists and visitors to these areas are needed.[577, 861]

As discussed in the Vaccine section previously, it is essential to educate all recipients of the Lyme vaccine, including women who plan to become pregnant, that continued use of protective methods against tick bites, including personal protective methods, is extremely important because of possible waning of effective vaccine-induced immunity. Such precautions are also essential to decrease risk of acquisition of other tickborne pathogens, including ehrlichiosis and babesiosis, and in some areas of Europe, tickborne encephalitis.

PROGNOSIS

Data indicate that the prognosis of gestational Lyme borreliosis is good if the infection is recognized promptly and treated aggressively with antibiotic therapy aimed at crossing the placental barrier. The prognosis is unknown in gestational Lyme borreliosis that lacks the typical history of tick bite followed by EM or other symptoms that lead to its recognition. It is uncertain how many episodes of gestational toxemia, spontaneous miscarriage, spontaneous abortion, stillbirth, culture-negative neonatal sepsis, failure to thrive, developmental delay, congenital heart disease, or sudden infant death syndrome may be due to unrecognized gestational Lyme borreliosis. Most studies addressing the issue of gestational and congenital Lyme borreliosis have evaluated pregnancy outcomes after the first prenatal visit or at delivery; although they provide useful data, they may either miss adverse events in early pregnancy or underestimate the fetal mortality rate. Determination of true risk to the fetus and infant of maternal gestational Lyme disease requires prospective studies of all pregnancy outcomes of gestational Lyme disease, long-term follow-up of live-born products of these pregnancies, and improved diagnosis of Lyme disease in affected fetuses, placentas, and infants.

The prognosis for immediate survival of infants who present with fulminant early congenital Lyme borreliosis depends on recognition of the disease and institution of prompt aggressive intravenous antibiotic therapy appropriate for B. burgdorferi sepsis, as discussed in the section Therapy. It should be stressed that maximal supportive management alone, including supportive measures for management of severe septic shock and respiratory distress, without appropriate antibiotic therapy, is not sufficient and may result in death of the infant.

The prognosis of infants who present with late congenital Lyme borreliosis depends on the extent of any irreversible damage already present at the time of diagnosis and institution of appropriate antibiotic therapy. It is my opinion that aggressive intravenous antibiotic therapy initially, followed by prolonged oral antibiotic therapy, as discussed in the section Therapy, should at least prevent further clinical deterioration and may lead to improvement in any reversible damage.

Because long-term chronicity of Lyme borreliosis with persistence of spirochetes in immunologically protected sites has been reported in older patients, because it is not known whether fetally acquired B. burgdorferi infection may result in similar persistence of the organism in some immunologically protected site, and because the effect of this fetally acquired infection on the way a congenitally infected infant will respond to future B. burgdorferi infection is unknown, any evidence of clinical deterioration, particularly in growth and development, hearing, or neurologic status, should be closely reevaluated for possible relation to B. burgdorferi relapse or reinfection. If the deterioration is considered to be due to B. burgdorferi infection, aggressive antibiotic therapy should be instituted to prevent future clinical deterioration, as reviewed in the sections Diagnosis and Differential Diagnosis, and Therapy.

Because there are insufficient data to allow prognostic predictions of long-term outcome of infants treated for early or late congenital Lyme borreliosis, close follow-up is required for these infants and should include at least pediatric neurology, ophthalmology, otolaryngology, and infectious disease evaluations. Other specialties such as pediatric cardiology, cardiac surgery, gastro-enterology, orthopedics, or rheumatology may be indicated, depending on the extent of involvement of these systems.

The index of suspicion should be high that any illness consistent with the late manifestations of Lyme borreliosis reported in children or adults may also theoretically occur in the congenitally infected infant. It will continue to be most important to recognize, treat, and evaluate infants with suspected congenital Lyme borreliosis in order for a more complete description of the syndrome to evolve.

References

1. Burgdorfer W, Barbour AG, Hayes SF, et al. Lyme disease—a tick-borne spirochetosis? Science 216:1317, 1982.
2. Steere AC, Broderick TF, Malawista SE. Erythema chronicum migrans and Lyme arthritis: epidemiologic evidence for a tick vector. Am J Epidemiol 108:312, 1978.
3. Centers for Disease Control. Lyme disease—United States, 1991–1992. MMWR 42:345, 1993.
4. Centers for Disease Control and Prevention. Provisional cases of selected notifiable diseases, United States. MMWR 48(51):1183–1190, 2000.
5. Evans J. Lyme disease. Curr Opin Rheumatol 10(4):339–346, 1998.
6. Barbour AG, Fish D. The biological and social phenomenon of Lyme disease. Science 260(5114):1610–1616, 1993.
7. Steere AC. Lyme disease: a growing threat to urban populations. Proc Natl Acad Sci U S A 91(7):2378–2383, 1994.
8. Cimmino M, Granstrom M, Gray JS, et al. European Lyme borreliosis clinical spectrum. Zentralbl Bakteriol 287(3):248–252, 1998.
9. O'Connell S, Granstrom M, Gray JS, Stanek G. Epidemiology of European Lyme borreliosis. Review. [54 refs] Zentralbl Bakteriol 287(3):229–240, 1998.
10. Cimmino MA. Relative frequency of Lyme borreliosis and of its clinical manifestations in Europe. European Community Concerted Action on Risk Assessment in Lyme Borreliosis. Infection 26(5):298–300, 1998.
11. Schmid GP. The global distribution of Lyme disease. Rev Infect Dis 7:41, 1985.
12. Sigal LH. Lyme disease: a world-wide borreliosis. Clin Exp Rheumatol 6:411, 1988.
13. Barthold SW. Globalisation of Lyme borreliosis. Lancet 348(9042):1603, 1996.
14. Afzelius A. Report to Verhandlungen der dermatologischen Gesellschaft zu Stockholm on December 16, 1909. Arch Fuer Dermatol Syph 101:405, 1910.
15. Steere AC, Malawista SE, Snydman DR, et al. Lyme arthritis: an epidemic of oligoarticular arthritis in children and adults in three Connecticut communities. Arthritis Rheum 20:7, 1977.
16. Johnson RC, Schmid GP, Hyde FW, et al. Borrelia burgdorferi sp. nov.: etiologic agent of Lyme disease. Int J Syst Bacteriol 34:496, 1984.
17. Burgdorfer W. How the discovery of Borrelia burgdorferi came about. Clin Dermatol 11(3):335–338, 1993.
18. Steere AC, Grodzicki RL, Kornblatt AN, et al. The spirochetal etiology of Lyme disease. N Engl J Med 308:733, 1983.
19. Asbrink E, Hovmark A. Successful cultivation of spirochetes from skin lesions of patients with erythema chron-

icum migrans Afzelius and acrodermatitis chronica atrophicans. Acta Pathol Microbiol Scand 93:161, 1985.

20. Asbrink E, Hovmark A, Hederstedt B. The spirochetal etiology of acrodermatitis chronica atrophicans Herxheimer. Acta Derm Venereol 64:506, 1984.

21. Ryberg B, Nilsson B, Burgdorfer W, Barbour A. Antibodies to Lyme disease spirochete in European lymphocytic meningoradiculitis (Bannwarth's syndrome). Lancet 2:519, 1983.

22. Hovmark A, Asbrink E, Olsson I. The spirochetal etiology of lymphadenosis benigna cutis solitaria. Acta Derm Venereol Suppl (Stockh) 66:479, 1986.

23. Podolsky ML. Lyme disease in pregnancy: the new great imitator. Clin Adv Treat Infect 5(5):1, 1991.

24. Sigal LH. Pitfalls in the diagnosis and management of Lyme disease. Arthritis Rheum 41(2):195–204, 1998.

25. Schlesinger PA, Duray PH, Burke BA, et al. Maternal-fetal transmission of the Lyme disease spirochete, *Borrelia burgdorferi*. Ann Intern Med 103:67, 1985.

26. Andrasova V, Svarovsky J, Matousek B. Lyme disease in pregnancy. Ceska Gynekol 53:39, 1988.

27. Carlomagno G, Luksa V, Candussi G, et al. Lyme borrelia positive serology associated with spontaneous abortion in an endemic Italian area. Acta Eur Fertil 19:279, 1988.

28. Centers for Disease Control. Update: Lyme disease and cases occurring during pregnancy—United States. MMWR 34:376, 1985.

29. Cieszelski CA, Russell H, Johnson S, et al. Prospective study of pregnancy outcomes in women with Lyme disease. Twenty-seventh Interscience Conference on Antimicrobial Agents and Chemotherapy, New York, NY, Oct 4, 1987 (abstract No 39).

30. Dlesk A, Broste SK, Harkins PG, et al. Lyme seropositivity and pregnancy outcome in the absence of symptoms of Lyme disease. Abstract. Arthritis Rheum 32:S46, 1989.

31. Lampert F. Infantile multisystem inflammatory disease: another case of a new syndrome. Eur J Pediatr 144:593, 1986.

32. Lavoie PE, Lattner BP, Duray PH, et al. Culture positive, seronegative, transplacental Lyme borreliosis infant mortality. Abstract. Arthritis Rheum 3:S50, 1987.

33. MacDonald AB. Gestational Lyme borreliosis: implications for the fetus. Rheum Dis Clin North Am 15:657, 1989.

34. MacDonald AB. Human fetal borreliosis, toxemia of pregnancy, and fetal death. Zentralbl Bakteriol Mikrobiol Hyg A 263:189, 1986.

35. MacDonald AB, Benach JL, Burgdorfer W. Stillbirth following maternal Lyme disease. N Y State J Med 87:615, 1987.

36. Markowitz LE, Steere AC, Benach JL, et al. Lyme disease during pregnancy. JAMA 255:3394, 1986.

37. Nadal D, Hunziker UA, Bucher HU, et al. Infants born to mothers with antibodies against *Borrelia burgdorferi* at delivery. Eur J Pediatr 148:426, 1989.

38. Weber K, Bratzke H-J, Neubert U, et al. *Borrelia burgdorferi* in a newborn despite oral penicillin for Lyme borreliosis during pregnancy. Pediatr Infect Dis J 7:286, 1988.

39. Weber K, Neubert U. Clinical features of early EM disease and related disorders. Zentralbl Bakteriol Mikrobiol Hyg A 263:209, 1986.

40. Williams CL, Benach JL, Curran AS, et al. Lyme disease during pregnancy: a cord blood serosurvey. Ann N Y Acad Sci 539:504, 1988.

41. Hercogova J, Moidlova M, Zirny J, et al. Could borrelia found in the placenta influence the fetus? Study of 19 women with erythema migrans during pregnancy. *In* Program and Abstracts of the 6th International Conference on Lyme Borreliosis. Bologna, Italy, Societa Editrice Esculapio, 1994, p 76 (abstract No PO 06T).

42. Hercogova J, Tomankova M, Frosslova D, Janovska D. Early-stage lyme borreliosis during pregnancy: treatment in 15 women with erythema migrans. Ceska Gynekol 58(5):229–232, 1993.

43. Trevisan G, Stinco G, Cinco M. Institute of Dermatology. Neonatal skin lesions due to a spirochetal infection: a case of congenital Lyme borreliosis? Int J Dermatol 36(9):677–680, 1997.

44. Gasser R, Dusleag J, Reisinger E, et al. A most unusual case of a whole family suffering from late Lyme borreliosis for over 20 years. Angiology 45(1):85–86, 1994.

45. Strobino BA, Williams CL, Abid S, et al. Lyme disease and pregnancy outcome: a prospective study of two thousand prenatal patients. Am J Obstet Gynecol 169(2 Pt 1):367–374, 1993.

46. Williams CL, Strobino B, Weinstein A, et al. Maternal Lyme disease and congenital malformations: a cord blood serosurvey in endemic and control areas. Paediatr Perinat Epidemiol 9(3):320–330, 1995.

47. Bracero LA, Wormser GP, Leikin E, Tejani N. Prevalence of seropositivity to the Lyme disease spirochete during pregnancy in an epidemic area. A preliminary report. J Matern Fetal Invest 2:265–268, 1992.

48. Maraspin V, Cimperman J, Lotric-Furlan S, et al. Treatment of erythema migrans in pregnancy. Clin Infect Dis 22(5):788–793, 1996.

49. Burgdorfer W. The enlarging spectrum of tick-borne spirochetoses: R. R. Parker Memorial Address. Rev Infect Dis 8:932, 1986.

50. Johnson RC. Isolation techniques for spirochetes and their sensitivity to antibiotics in vitro and in vivo. Rev Infect Dis 11:S1505, 1989.

51. Wilske B, Anderson JF, Baranton G, et al. Taxonomy of *Borrelia* spp. Scand J Infect Dis Suppl 77:108, 1991.

52. Wilske B, Preac-Mursic V, Schierz G, et al. Antigenic variability of *Borrelia burgdorferi*. Ann N Y Acad Sci 539:126, 1988.

53. Baranton G, Postic D, Saint Girons I, et al. Delineation of Borrelia burgdorferi sensu stricto, *Borrelia garinii* sp. nov., and Group VS461 associated with Lyme borreliosis. Int J Syst Bacteriol 42:378, 1992.

54. Hubalek Z, Halouzka J. Distribution of *Borrelia burgdorferi* sensu lato genomic groups in Europe, a review. Eur J Epidemiol 13(8):951–957, 1997.

55. Wang G, van Dam AP, Spanjaard L, Dankert J. Molecular typing of *Borrelia burgdorferi* sensu lato by randomly amplified polymorphic DNA fingerprinting analysis. J Clin Microbiol 36(3):768–776, 1998.

56. Balmelli T, Piffaretti JC. Analysis of the genetic polymorphism of *Borrelia burgdorferi* sensu lato by multilocus enzyme electrophoresis. Int J Syst Bacteriol 46(1):167–172, 1996.

57. Casjens S, Delange M, Ley HL III, et al. Linear chromosomes of Lyme disease agent spirochetes: genetic diversity and conservation of gene order. J Bacteriol 177:2769–2780, 1995.

58. Fukunaga M, Hamase A, Okada K, Nakao M. *Borrelia tanukii* sp. nov. and *Borrelia turdae* sp. nov. found from *Ixodes* ticks in Japan: rapid species identification by 16S rRNA gene-targeted PCR analysis. Microbiol Immunol 40:877–881, 1996.

59. Assous MV, Postic D, Paul G, et al. Individualisation of two new genomic groups among American *Borrelia*

burgdorferi sensu lato strains. FEMS Microbiol Lett 121(1):93–98, 1994.

60. Dykhuizen DE, Polin DS, Dunn JJ, et al. *Borrelia burgdorferi* is clonal: implications for taxonomy and vaccine development. Proc Natl Acad Sci U S A 90(21):10163–10167, 1993.

61. Wang G, van Dam AP, Le Fleche A, et al. Genetic and phenotypic analysis of *Borrelia valaisiana* sp. nov. (Borrelia genomic groups VS116 and M19). Int J Syst Bacteriol 47:926–932, 1997.

62. Foretz M, Postic D, Baranton G. Phylogenetic analysis of *Borrelia burgdorferi* sensu stricto by arbitrarily primed PCR and pulsed-field gel electrophoresis. Int J Syst Bacteriol 47(1):11–18, 1997.

63. Mathiesen DA, Oliver JH Jr, Kolbert CP, et al. Genetic heterogeneity of *Borrelia burgdorferi* in the United States. J Infect Dis 175(1):98–107, 1997.

64. Anderson JF, Magnarelli LA, McAninch JB. New *Borrelia burgdorferi* antigenic variant isolated from *Ixodes dammini* from upstate New York. J Clin Microbiol 26:2209–2212, 1988.

65. Le Fleche A, Postic D, Girardet K, et al. Characterization of *Borrelia lusitaniae* sp. nov. by 16S ribosomal DNA sequence analysis. Int J Syst Bacteriol 47:921–925, 1997.

66. Marconi RT, Liveris D, Schwartz I. Identification of novel insertion elements, restriction fragment length polymorphism patterns, and discontinuous 23S rRNA in Lyme disease spirochetes: phylogenetic analysis of rRNA genes and their intergenic spacers in *Borrelia japonica* sp. Nov. and genomic group 21038 (*Borrelia andersonii* sp. Nov.) isolates. J Clin Microbiol 33(9):2427–2434, 1995.

67. Canica MM, Nato F, du Merle L, et al. Monoclonal antibodies for identification of *Borrelia afzelii* sp. Nov. associated with late cutaneous manifestations of Lyme borreliosis. Scand J Infect Dis 25(4):441–448, 1993.

68. Fukunaga M, Hamase A, Okada K, et al. Characterization of spirochetes isolated from ticks (*Ixodes tanuki, Ixodes turdus,* and *Ixodes columnae*) and comparison of the sequences with those of *Borrelia burgdorferi* sensu lato strains. Appl Environ Microbiol 62:2338–2344, 1996.

69. Kawabata H, Masuzawa T, Yanagihara Y. Genomic analysis of *Borrelia japonica* sp. nov. isolated from *Ixodes ovatus* in Japan. Microbiol Immunol 37:843–848, 1993.

70. Anderson JF, Flavell RA, Magnarelli LA, et al. Novel *Borrelia burgdorferi* isolates from *Ixodes scapularis* and *Ixodes dentatus* ticks feeding on humans. J Clin Microbiol 34(30):524–529, 1996.

71. Peter O, Bretz AG, Bee D. Occurrence of different genospecies of *Borrelia burgdorferi* sensu lato in Ixodid ticks of Valais, Switzerland. Eur J Epidemiol 11(4):463–467, 1995.

72. Rijpkema SG, Tazelaar DJ, Molkenboer MJ, et al. Detection of *Borrelia afzelii, Borrelia burgdorferi sensu lato, Borrelia garinii* and group VS116 by PCR in skin biopsies of patients with erythema migrans and acrodermatitis chronica atrophicans. Clin Microbiol Infect 3:109–116, 1997.

73. Barbour AG, Maupin GO, Teltow GJ, et al. Identification of an uncultivable Borrelia species in the hard tick *Amblyomma americanum*: possible agent of a Lyme disease–like illness. J Infect Dis 173:403–409, 1996.

74. Saint Girons I, Gern L, Gray JS, et al. Identification of *Borrelia burgdorferi* sensu lato species in Europe. Zentralbl Bakteriol 287(3):190–195, 1998.

75. Van Dam AP, Kuiper H, Vos K, et al. Different genospecies of *Borrelia burgdorferi* are associated with distinct clinical manifestations of Lyme borreliosis. Clin Infect Dis 17(4):708–717, 1993.

76. Balmelli T, Piffaretti JC. Association between different clinical manifestations of Lyme disease and different species of *Borrelia burgdorferi* sensu lato. Res Microbiol 146(4):329–340, 1995.

77. Fukunaga M, Takashi Y, Tsuruta Y, et al. Genetic and phenotypic analysis of *Borrelia miyamotoi* sp. nov., isolated from the Ixodid tick, *Ixodes persulcatus,* the vector for Lyme disease in Japan. Int J Syst Bacteriol 45:804–810, 1995.

78. Oliver JH Jr, Owsley MR, Hutcheson HJ, et al. Conspecificity of the ticks *Ixodes scapularis* and *I. dammini* (Acari: Ixodidae). J Med Entomol 30:54, 1993.

79. Berger BW, Kaplan MH, Rothenberg IR, Barbour AG. Isolation and characterization of the Lyme disease spirochete from the skin of patients with erythema chronicum migrans. J Am Acad Dermatol 13:444, 1985.

80. Benach JL, Bosler EM, Hanrahan JP, et al. Spirochetes isolated from the blood of two patients with Lyme disease. N Engl J Med 308:740, 1983.

81. Barbour AG, Burgdorfer W, Hayes SF, et al. Isolation of a cultivable spirochete from *Ixodes ricinus* ticks of Switzerland. Curr Microbiol 8:123, 1983.

82. de Koning J, Bosma RB, Hoogkamp-Korstanje JA. Demonstration of spirochetes in patients with Lyme disease with a modified silver stain. J Med Microbiol 23:261, 1987.

83. Strle F, Picken RN, Cheng Y, et al. Clinical findings for patients with Lyme borreliosis caused by *Borrelia burgdorferi* sensu lato with genotypic and phenotypic similarities to strain 25015. Clin Infect Dis 25(2):273–280, 1997.

84. Demaerschalck I, Ben Messaoud A, De Kesel M, et al. Simultaneous presence of different *Borrelia burgdorferi* genospecies in biological fluids of Lyme disease patients. J Clin Microbiol 33(3):602–608, 1995.

85. Ohlenbusch A, Matuschka FR, Richter D, et al. Etiology of the acrodermatitis chronica atrophicans lesion in Lyme disease. J Infect Dis 174(2):421–423, 1996.

86. Picken RN, Strle F, Picken MM, et al. Identification of three species of *Borrelia burgdorferi* sensu lato (*B. burgdorferi* sensu stricto, *B. garinii,* and *B. afzelii*) among isolates from acrodermatitis chronica atrophicans lesions. J Invest Dermatol 110(3):211–214, 1998.

87. Anthonissen FM, de Kesel M, Hoet PP, Bigaignon GH. Evidence for the involvement of different genospecies of *Borrelia* in the clinical outcome of Lyme disease in Belgium. Res Microbiol 145(4):327–331, 1994.

88. Busch U, Hizo-Teufel C, Boehmer R, et al. Three species of *Borrelia burgdorferi* sensu lato (*B. burgdorferi* sensu stricto, *B. afzelii,* and *B. garinii*) identified from cerebrospinal fluid isolates by pulsed-field gel electrophoresis and PCR. J Clin Microbiol 34(5):1072–1078, 1996.

89. Busch U, Hizo-Teufel C, Bohmer R, et al. *Borrelia burgdorferi* sensu lato strains isolated from cutaneous Lyme borreliosis biopsies differentiated by pulsed-field gel electrophoresis. Scand J Infect Dis 28(6):583–589, 1996.

90. Anda P, Rodriguez I, de la Loma A, et al. A serological survey and review of clinical Lyme borreliosis in Spain. Clin Infect Dis 16(2):310–319, 1993.

91. Barbour AG. Isolation and cultivation of Lyme disease spirochetes. Yale J Biol Med 57:521, 1984.

92. Barbour AG. The molecular biology of *Borrelia*. Rev Infect Dis 11(Suppl 6):S1470, 1989.

93. Bergstrom S, Barbour AG, Garon CF, et al. Genetics of *Borrelia burgdorferi*. Scand J Infect Dis Suppl 77:102, 1991.

94. Johnson RC, Hyde FW, Rumpel CM. Taxonomy of the Lyme disease spirochetes. Yale J Biol Med 57:529, 1984.

95. Karlsson M, Hovind-Hougen K, Svenungsson B, Stiernstedt G. Cultivation and characterization of spirochetes from cerebrospinal fluid of patients with Lyme borreliosis. J Clin Microbiol 28:473, 1990.

96. Kochi SK, Johnson RC. Role of immunoglobulin G in killing of *Borrelia burgdorferi* by the classical complement pathway. Infect Immun 56:314, 1988.

97. Kurtti TJ, Munderloh UG, Johnson RC, Ahlstrand GG. Colony formation and morphology in *Borrelia burgdorferi*. J Clin Microbiol 25:2054, 1987.

98. Steere AC. Lyme disease. N Engl J Med 321:586, 1989.

99. Rosa PA. Microbiology of *Borrelia burgdorferi*. Semin Neurol 17(1):5–10, 1997.

100. Anderson JF, Magnarelli LA, LeFebvre RB, et al. Antigenically variable *Borrelia burgdorferi* isolates from cottontail rabbits and *Ixodes dentatus* in rural and urban areas. J Clin Microbiol 27:13–20, 1989.

101. Aberer E, Kersten A, Klade H, et al. Heterogeneity of *Borrelia burgdorferi* in the skin. Am J Dermatopathol 18(6):571–579, 1996.

102. Brorson O, Brorson SH. In vitro conversion of *Borrelia burgdorferi* to cystic forms in spinal fluid, and transformation to mobile spirochetes by incubation in BSK-H medicine. Infection 26(3):144–150, 1998.

103. Garon C, Dorward DW, Corwin DMD. Structural features of *Borrelia burgdorferi*—the Lyme disease spirochete: silver staining for nucleic acids. Scanning Microsc Suppl 3:109–115, 1989.

104. Bruckbauer HR, Preac-Mursic V, Fuchs R, Wilske B. Cross-reactive proteins of *Borrelia burgdorferi*. Eur J Clin Microbiol Infect Dis 11:224, 1992.

105. Wilske B, Preac-Mursic V, Gobel UB, et al. An OspA serotyping system for *Borrelia burgdorferi* based on reactivity with monoclonal antibodies and OspA sequence analysis. J Clin Microbiol 31(2):340–350, 1993.

106. Rossler D, Eiffert H, Jauris-Heipke S, et al. Molecular and immunological characterization of the p83/100 protein of various *Borrelia burgdorferi* sensu lato strains. Med Microbiol Immunol 184(1):23–32, 1995.

107. Rauer S, Kayser M, Neubert U, et al. Establishment of enzyme-linked immunosorbent assay using purified recombinant 83-kilodalton antigen of *Borrelia burgdorferi* sensu stricto and *Borrelia afzelii* for serodiagnosis of Lyme disease. J Clin Microbiol 33(10):2596–2600, 1995.

108. Wilske B, Fingerle V, Preac-Mursic V, et al. Immunoblot using recombinant antigens derived from different genospecies of *Borrelia burgdorferi* sensu lato. Med Microbiol Immunol 183(1):43–59, 1994.

109. Scorpio A, Johnson P, Laux DC, Nelson DR. Chaperone activities and subcellular localization of *Borrelia burgdorferi* HSP60 and HSP70. Proceedings of the VI International Conference on Lyme Borreliosis. Bologna, Italy, June 19–22, 1994, pp 47–50.

110. Gilmore RD Jr, Kappel KJ, Johnson BJ. Molecular characterization of a 35-kilodalton protein of *Borrelia burgdorferi*, an antigen of diagnostic importance in early Lyme disease. J Clin Microbiol 35(1):86–91, 1997.

111. Jauris-Heipke S, Fuchs R, Motz M, et al. Genetic heterogeneity of the genes coding for the outer surface protein C (OspC) and the flagellin of *Borrelia burgdorferi*. Med Microbiol Immunol 182(1):37–50, 1993.

112. Luft BJ, Dunn JJ, Dattwyler RJ, et al. Cross-reactive antigenic domains of the flagellin protein of *Borrelia burgdorferi*. Res Microbiol 144(4):251–257, 1993.

113. Sigal LH, Williams S. A monoclonal antibody to *Borrelia burgdorferi* flagellin modifies neuroblastoma cell neurito-genesis in vitro: a possible role for autoimmunity in the neuropathy of Lyme disease. Infect Immun 65(5):1722–1728, 1997.

114. Bergstrom S, Bundoc VG, Barbour A. Molecular analysis of linear plasmid-encoded major surface proteins, OspA and OspB, of the Lyme disease spirochaete *Borrelia burgdorferi*. Mol Microbiol 3:479–486, 1989.

115. Masuzawa T, Komikado T, Yanagihara Y. PCR–restriction fragment length polymorphism analysis of the ospC gene for detection of mixed culture and for epidemiological typing of *Borrelia burgdorferi* sensu stricto. Clin Diagn Lab Immunol 4(1):60–63, 1997.

116. Sadziene A, Wilske B, Ferdows MS, Barbour A. The cryptic ospC gene of *Borrelia burgdorferi* B31 is located on a circular plasmid. Infect Immun 61:2192–2195, 1993.

117. Marconi RT, Samuels DS, Landry RK, Garon CF. Analysis of the distribution and molecular heterogeneity of the ospD gene among the Lyme disease spirochetes: evidence for lateral gene exchange. J Bacteriol 176(15):4572–4582, 1994.

118. Lam TT, Nguyen TP, Montgomery RR, et al. Outer surface proteins E and F of *Borrelia burgdorferi*, the agent of Lyme disease. Infect Immun 62(1):290–298, 1994.

119. Wallich R, Brenner C, Kramer MD, Simon MM. Molecular cloning and immunological characterization of a novel linear-plasmid-encoded gene, pG, of *Borrelia burgdorferi* expressed only in vivo. Infect Immun 63(9):3327–3335, 1995.

120. Sadziene A, Barbour AG. Experimental immunization against Lyme borreliosis with recombinant Osp proteins: an overview. Infection 24(2):195–202, 1996.

121. Champion CI, Blanco DR, Skare JT, et al. A 9.0-kilobase-pair circular plasmid of *Borrelia burgdorferi* encodes an exported protein: evidence for expression only during infection. Infect Immun 62(7):2653–2661, 1994.

122. Zumstein G, Fuchs R, Hofmann A, et al. Genetic polymorphism of the gene encoding the outer surface protein A (OspA) of *Borrelia burgdorferi*. Med Microbiol Immunol 181:57–70, 1992.

123. Picken RN, Cheng Y, Han D, et al. Genotypic and phenotypic characterization of *Borrelia burgdorferi* isolated from ticks and small animals in Illinois. J Clin Microbiol 33(9):2304–2315, 1995.

124. Padula SJ, Dias F, Sampieri A, et al. Use of recombinant OspC from *Borrelia burgdorferi* for serodiagnosis of early Lyme disease. J Clin Microbiol 32(7):1733–1738, 1994.

125. Rauer S, Spohn N, Rasiah C, et al. Enzyme-linked immunosorbent assay using recombinant OspC and the internal 14-kDa flagellin fragment for serodiagnosis of early Lyme disease. J Clin Microbiol 36(4):857–861, 1998.

126. Gross DM, Frosthuber T, Tary-Lehmann M, et al. Identification of LFA-1 as a candidate autoantigen in treatment-resistant Lyme arthritis. Science 281(5377):703–706, 1998.

127. Das S, Barthold SW, Giles SS, et al. Temporal pattern of *Borrelia burgdorferi* p21 expression in ticks and the mammalian host. J Clin Invest 99(5):987–995, 1997.

128. Stevenson B, Bono JL, Schwan TG, Rosa P. *Borrelia burgdorferi* erp proteins are immunogenic in mammals infected by tick bite, and their synthesis is inducible in cultured bacteria. Infect Immun 66(6):2648–2654, 1998.

129. Schwan TG, Burgdorfer W. Antigenic changes of *Borrelia burgdorferi* as a result of in vitro cultivation. J Infect Dis 156:852, 1987.

130. Kawabata H, Myouga F, Inagaki Y, et al. Genetic and immunological analyses of V1s (VMP-like sequences) of *Borrelia burgdorferi*. Microb Pathog 24(3):155–166, 1998.

131. Zhang J-R, Hardham JM, Barbour AG, Norris SJ. Antigenic variation in Lyme disease *Borrelia* by promiscuous recombination of VMP-like sequence cassettes. Cell 89:275–285, 1997.

132. Wheeler CM, Garcia Monco JC, Benach JL, et al. Nonprotein antigens of *Borrelia burgdorferi*. J Infect Dis 167(3):665–674, 1993.

133. Casjens S, Huang WM. Linear chromosomal physical and genetic map of *Borrelia burgdorferi*, the Lyme disease agent. Mol Microbiol 8(5):967–980, 1993.

134. Xu Y, Kodner C, Coleman L, Johnson RC. Correlation of plasmids with infectivity of *Borrelia burgdorferi sensu stricto* type strain B31. Infect Immun 64:3870–3876, 1996.

135. Fikrig E, Tao H, Kantor FS, et al. Evasion of protective immunity by *Borrelia burgdorferi* by truncation of outer surface protein B. Proc Natl Acad Sci U S A 90(9):4092–4096, 1993.

136. Sadziene A, Barbour AG, Rosa PA, Thomas DD. An OspB mutant of *Borrelia burgdorferi* has reduced invasiveness in vitro and reduced infectivity in vivo. Infect Immun 61(9):3590–3596, 1993.

137. De Silva AM, Fikrig E. Arthropod- and host-specific gene expression by *Borrelia burgdorferi*. J Clin Invest 99(3):377–379, 1997.

138. Schwan TG. Ticks and *Borrelia*: model systems for investigating pathogen-arthropod interactions. Infect Agents Dis 5(3):167–181, 1996.

139. De Silva AM, Telford SR, Brunet LR, et al. *Borrelia burgdorferi* OspA is an arthropod-specific transmission-blocking Lyme disease vaccine. J Exp Med 183:271–275, 1996.

140. De Silva AM, Zeidner NS, Zhang Y, et al. Influence of outer surface protein A antibody on *Borrelia burgdorferi* within feeding ticks. Infect Immun 67:30–35, 1999.

141. Fikrig E, Feng W, Aversa J, et al. Differential expression of *Borrelia burgdorferi* genes during erythema migrans and Lyme arthritis. J Infect Dis 178(4):1198–1201, 1998.

142. Stevenson B, Schwan TG, Rosa P. Temperature-related differential expression of antigens in the Lyme disease spirochete, *Borrelia burgdorferi*. Infect Immun 63:4535–4539, 1995.

143. Von Stedingk LV, Olsson I, Hanson HS, et al. Polymerase chain reaction for detection of *Borrelia burgdorferi* DNA in skin lesions of early and late Lyme borreliosis. Eur J Clin Microbiol Infect Dis 14(1):1–5, 1995.

144. Klempner MS, Noring R, Epstein MP, et al. Binding of human plasminogen and urokinase-type plasminogen activator to the Lyme disease spirochete, *Borrelia burgdorferi*. J Infect Dis 171(5):1258–1265, 1995.

145. Kramer MD, Wallich R, Simon MM. The outer surface protein A (OspA) of *Borrelia burgdorferi*: a vaccine candidate and bioactive mediator. Infection 24(2):190–194, 1996.

146. Coleman JL, Gebbia JA, Piesman J, et al. Plasminogen is required for efficient dissemination of *B. burgdorferi* in ticks and for enhancement of spirochetemia in mice. Cell 89(7):1111–1119, 1997.

147. Wooten RM, Morrison TB, Weis JH, et al. The role of CD14 in signaling mediated by outer membrane lipoproteins of *Borrelia burgdorferi*. J Immunol 160(11):5485–5492, 1998.

148. Aberer E, Koszik F, Silberer M. Why is chronic Lyme borreliosis chronic? Clin Infect Dis 25(Suppl 1):S64–S70, 1997.

149. Hu LT, Klempner MS. Host-pathogen interactions in the immunopathogenesis of Lyme disease. J Clin Immunol 17(5):354–365, 1997.

150. Sellati TJ, Abrescia LD, Radolf JD, Furie MB. Outer surface lipoproteins of *Borrelia burgdorferi* activate vascular endothelium in vitro. Infect Immun 64(8):3180–3187, 1996.

151. Sigal LH. Immunologic mechanisms in Lyme neuroborreliosis: the potential role of autoimmunity and molecular mimicry. Semin Neurol 17(1):63–68, 1997.

152. Bunikis J, Olsen B, Fingerle V, et al. Molecular polymorphism of the Lyme disease agent *Borrelia garinii* in northern Europe is influenced by a novel enzootic *Borrelia* focus in the North Atlantic. J Clin Microbiol 34(2):364–368, 1996.

153. Oliver JH Jr, Kollars TM Jr, Chandler FW Jr, et al. First isolation and cultivation of *Borrelia burgdorferi* sensu lato from Missouri. J Clin Microbiol 36(1):1–5, 1998.

154. Magnarelli LA, Anderson JF, Apperson CS, et al. Spirochetes in ticks and antibodies to *Borrelia burgdorferi* in white-tailed deer from Connecticut, New York State, and North Carolina. J Wildl Dis 22:178, 1986.

155. Schulze TL, Bowen GS, Bosler EM, et al. *Amblyomma americanum*: a potential vector of Lyme disease in New Jersey. Science 224:601, 1984.

156. Luckhart S, Mullen GR, Wright JC. Etiologic agent of Lyme disease, *Borrelia burgdorferi*, detected in ticks (Acari: Ixodidae) collected at a focus in Alabama. J Med Entomol 28:652, 1991.

157. Levine JF, Sonenshine DE, Nicholson WL, Turner RT. *Borrelia burgdorferi* in ticks (Acari: Ixodidae) from coastal Virginia. J Med Entomol 28:668, 1991.

158. Teltow GJ, Fournier PV, Rawlings JA. Isolation of *Borrelia burgdorferi* from arthropods collected in Texas. Am J Trop Med Hyg 44:469, 1991.

159. Liveris D, Wormser GP, Nowakowski J, et al. Molecular typing of *Borrelia burgdorferi* from Lyme disease patients by PCR–restriction fragment length polymorphism analysis. J Clin Microbiol 34(5):1306–1309, 1996.

160. Pichon B, Godfroid E, Hoyois B, et al. Simultaneous infection of Ixodes ricinus nymphs by two *Borrelia* sensu lato species: possible implications for clinical manifestations. Emerg Infect Dis 1(3):89–90, 1995.

161. Kirstein F, Rijpkema S, Molkenboer M, Gray JS. The distribution and prevalence of *B. burgdorferi* genomospecies in Ixodes ricinus ticks in Ireland. Eur J Epidemiol 13:67–72, 1997.

162. Golubic D, Rijpkema S, Tkalec-Makovec N, Ruzic E. Epidemiologic, ecologic and clinical characteristics of Lyme borreliosis in northwest Croatia. Acta Med Croatica 52(1):7–13, 1998.

163. Nakao M, Fukunaga M, Miyamoto K. Lyme disease spirochetes in Japan: enzootic transmission cycles in birds, rodents, and *Ixodes persulcatus* ticks. J Infect Dis 170:878–882, 1994.

164. Masuzawa T, Wilske B, Komikado T, et al. Comparison of OspA serotypes for *Borrelia burgdorferi* sensu lato from Japan, Europe and North America. Microbiol Immunol 40(8):539–545, 1996.

165. Olsen B, Duffy DC, Jaenson TGT, et al. Transhemispheric exchange of Lyme disease spirochetes by seabirds. J Clin Microbiol 33:3270–3274, 1995.

166. Olsen B, Jaenson TGT, Noppa L, et al. A Lyme borreliosis cycle in seabirds and *Ixodes uriae* ticks. Nature 362:340–342, 1993.

167. Anderson JF. Epizootiology of Lyme borreliosis. Scand J Infect Dis Suppl 77:23, 1991.

168. Matuschka FR, Spielman A. The emergence of Lyme disease in a changing environment in North America and central Europe. Exp Appl Acarol 2:337, 1986.

169. Anderson JF. Mammalian and avian reservoirs for *Borrelia burgdorferi*. Ann N Y Acad Sci 539:180, 1988.
170. Telford SR, Spielman A. Enzootic transmission of the agent of Lyme disease in rabbits. Am J Trop Med Hyg 41:482, 1989.
171. Rand PW, Lacombe EH, Smith RP Jr, Ficker J. Participation of birds (Aves) in the emergence of Lyme disease in southern Maine. J Med Entomol 35(3):270–276, 1998.
172. Humair PF, Postic D, Wallich R, Gern L. An avian reservoid (*Turdus merula*) of the Lyme borreliosis spirochetes. Zentralbl Bakteriol 287(4):521–538, 1998.
173. Lane RS, Quistad GB. Borreliacidal factor in the blood of the western fence lizard (*Sceloporus occidentalis*). J Parasitol 84:29–34, 1998.
174. Preac-Mursic V, Wilske B, Schierz G. European *Borrelia burgdorferi* isolated from humans and ticks: culture conditions and antibiotic susceptibility. Zentralbl Bakteriol Mikrobiol Hyg A 263:112, 1986.
175. Schwartz I, Bittker S, Bowen SL, et al. Polymerase chain reaction amplification of culture supernatants for rapid detection of *Borrelia burgdorferi*. Eur J Clin Microbiol Infect Dis 12(11):879–882, 1993.
176. Preac-Mursic V, Wilske B, Reinhardt S. Culture of *Borrelia burgdorferi* on six solid media. Eur J Clin Microbiol Infect Dis 10:1076, 1991.
177. Steere AC, Duray PH, Butcher EC. Spirochetal antigens and lymphoid cell surface markers in Lyme synovitis: comparison with rheumatoid synovium and tonsillar lymphoid tissue. Arthritis Rheum 31:487, 1988.
178. Norris SJ, Howell JK, Garza SA, et al. High- and low-infectivity phenotypes of clonal populations of in vitro–cultured *Borrelia burgdorferi*. Infect Immun 63:2206–2212, 1995.
179. Dorward DW, Fischer ER, Brooks DM. Invasion and cytopathic killing of human lymphocytes by spirochetes causing Lyme disease. Clin Infect Dis 25(Suppl 1):S2–S8, 1997.
180. Clover JR, Lane RS. Evidence implicating nymphal *Ixodes pacificus* (Acari:Ixodidae) in the epidemiology of Lyme disease in California. Am J Trop Med Hyg 53(3):237–240, 1995.
181. Gray JS, Kahl O, Robertson JN, et al. Lyme borreliosis habitat assessment. Zentralbl Bakteriol 287(3):211–228, 1998.
182. Anderson JF, Magnarelli LA. Epizootiology of Lyme disease–causing borreliae. Clin Dermatol 11(3):339–351, 1993.
183. Berger BW, Johnson RC, Kodner C, Coleman L. Cultivation of *Borrelia burgdorferi* from erythema migrans lesions and perilesional skin. J Clin Microbiol 30:359–361, 1992.
184. Jurca T, Ruzic-Sabljic E, Lotric-Furlan S, et al. Comparison of peripheral and central biopsy sites for the isolation of *Borrelia burgdorferi* sensu lato from erythema migrans skin lesions. Clin Infect Dis 27(3):636–638, 1998.
185. Rosa PA, Schwan TG. A specific and sensitive assay for the Lyme disease spirochete *Borrelia burgdorferi* using the polymerase chain reaction. J Infect Dis 160:1018, 1989.
186. Sigal L. The role of the *Borrelia burgdorferi* polymerase chain reaction in the diagnosis of Lyme disease. Am Intern Med 120:520–521, 1994.
187. Schmidt BL. PCR in laboratory diagnosis of human *Borrelia burgdorferi* infections. Clin Microbiol Rev 10(1):185–201, 1997.
188. Agger WA, Callister SM, Jobe DA. In vitro susceptibilities of *Borrelia burgdorferi* to five oral cephalosporins and ceftriaxone. Antimicrob Agents Chemother 36:1788, 1992.
189. Cryan B, Wright DJM. Antimicrobial agents in Lyme disease. J Antimicrob Chemother 25:187, 1990.
190. Dotevall L, Alestig K, Hanner P, et al. The use of doxycycline in nervous system *Borrelia burgdorferi* infection. Scand J Infect Dis Suppl 53:74, 1988.
191. Dotevall L, Hagberg L. Penetration of doxycycline into cerebrospinal fluid in patients treated for suspected Lyme neuroborreliosis. Antimicrob Agents Chemother 33:1078, 1989.
192. Luft BJ, Volkman DJ, Halperin JJ, Dattwyler RJ. New chemotherapeutic approaches in the treatment of Lyme borreliosis. Ann N Y Acad Sci 539:352, 1988.
193. Massarotti EM, Luger SW, Rahn DW, et al. Treatment of early Lyme disease. Am J Med 92:396, 1992.
194. Philipson A. Antibiotic treatment in Lyme borreliosis. Scand J Infect Dis Suppl 77:145, 1991.
195. Preac-Mursic V, Wilske B, Schierz G, et al. In vitro and in vivo susceptibility of *Borrelia burgdorferi*. Eur J Clin Microbiol 6:424, 1987.
196. Baradaran-Dilmaghani R, Stanek G. In vitro susceptibility of thirty *Borrelia* strains from various sources against eight antimicrobial chemotherapeutics. Infection 24(1):60–63, 1996.
197. Levin JM, Nelson JA, Segreti J, et al. In vitro susceptibility of *Borrelia burgdorferi* to 11 antimicrobial agents. Antimicrob Agents Chemother 37(7):1444–1446, 1993.
198. Dever LL, Jorgensen JH, Barbour AG. Comparative in vitro activities of clarithromycin, azithromycin, and erythromycin against *Borrelia burgdorferi*. Antimicrob Agents Chemother 37(8):1704–1706, 1993.
199. Gasser R, Wendelin I, Reisinger E, et al. Roxithromycin in the treatment of Lyme disease—update and perspectives. Infection 23(Suppl 1):S39–S43, 1995.
200. Preac-Mursic V, Marget W, Busch U, et al. Kill kinetics of *Borrelia burgdorferi* and bacterial findings in relation to the treatment of Lyme borreliosis [published erratum appears in Infection 1997 March–April; 24(2):169]. Infection 24(1):9–16, 1996.
201. Steere AC, Hutchinson GJ, Rahn DW, et al. Treatment of the early manifestations of Lyme disease. Ann Intern Med 99:22, 1983.
202. Dattwyler RJ, Grunwaldt E, Luft BJ. Clarithromycin in treatment of early Lyme disease: a pilot study. Antimicrob Agents Chemother 40(2):468–469, 1996.
203. Luft BJ, Dattwyler RJ, Johnson RC, et al. Azithromycin compared with amoxicillin in the treatment of erythema migrans. Ann Intern Med 124:785–791, 1996.
204. Garcia-Monco JC, Benach JL. Mechanisms of injury in Lyme neuroborreliosis. Semin Neurol 17(1):57–62, 1997.
205. Lahesmaa R, Shanafelt MC, Steinman L, Peltz G. Immunopathogenesis of human inflammatory arthritis: lessons from Lyme and reactive arthritis. J Infect Dis 170(4):978–985, 1994.
206. Sigal LH. Management of Lyme disease refractory to antibiotic therapy. Rheum Dis Clin North Am 21(1):217–230, 1995.
207. Sigal LH. Lyme disease: a review of aspects of its immunology and immunopathogenesis. Ann Rev Immunol 15:63–92, 1997.
208. Dattwyler RJ, Volkman DJ, Luft BJ, et al. Seronegative Lyme disease: dissociation of specific T- and B-lymphocyte responses to *Borrelia burgdorferi*. N Engl J Med 319:1441, 1988 (reply to letters: N Engl J Med 320:1280, 1989).
209. Krause A, Burmester GR, Rensing A, et al. Cellular immune reactivity to recombinant OspA and flagellin from *Borrelia burgdorferi* in patients with Lyme borrel-

iosis: complexity of humoral and cellular immune responses. J Clin Invest 90:1077, 1992.

210. Krause A, Brade V, Schoerner C, et al. T cell proliferation induced by *Borrelia burgdorferi* in patients with Lyme borreliosis: autologous serum required for optimum stimulation. Arthritis Rheum 34:393, 1991.

211. Ostrov BE, Athreya BH. Lyme disease: difficulties in diagnosis and management. Pediatr Clin North Am 38:535, 1991 (erratum 38:viii, 1991).

212. Yoshinari NH, Reinhardt BN, Steere AC. Components of *B. burgdorferi* causing T-cell proliferative responses in patients with Lyme arthritis. Abstract. Arthritis Rheum 32:S46, 1989.

213. Rutkowski S, Busch DH, Huppertz HI. Lymphocyte proliferation assay in response to *Borrelia burgdorferi* in patients with Lyme arthritis: analysis of lymphocyte subsets. Rheumatol Int 17(4):151–158, 1997.

214. Wang WZ, Fredrikson S, Sun JB, Link H. Lyme neuroborreliosis: evidence of persistent up-regulation of *Borrelia burgdorferi*–reactive cells secreting interferon-gamma. Scand J Immunol 42(6):694–700, 1995.

215. Whitmire WM, Garon CF. Specific and nonspecific responses of murine B cells to membrane blebs of *Borrelia burgdorferi*. Infect Immun 61:1460–1467, 1993.

216. Weis J, Ma Y, Erdile LF. Biological activities of native and recombinant *Borrelia burgdorferi* outer surface protein A: dependence on lipid modification. Infect Immun 62:4632–4636, 1994.

217. Giambartolomei GH, Dennis VA, Phillip MT. *Borrelia burgdorferi* stimulates the production of interleukin-10 in peripheral blood mononuclear cells from uninfected humans and rhesus monkeys. Infect Immun 66(6):2691–2697, 1998.

218. Dressler F, Yoshinari NH, Steere AC. The T-cell proliferative assay in the diagnosis of Lyme disease. Ann Intern Med 115:533, 1991.

219. Buechner SA, Lautenschlager S, Itin P, et al. Lymphoproliferative responses to *Borrelia burgdorferi* in patients with erythema migrans, acrodermatitis chronica atrophicans, lymphadenosis benigna cutis, and morphea. Arch Dermatol 131(6):673–677, 1995.

220. Pachner AR, Steere AC, Sigal LH, Johnson CJ. Antigen-specific proliferation of CSF lymphocytes in Lyme disease. Neurology 35:1642, 1985.

221. Sigal LH, Steere AC, Freeman DH, Dwyer JM. Proliferative responses of mononuclear cells in Lyme disease: reactivity to *Borrelia burgdorferi* antigens is greater in joint fluid than in blood. Arthritis Rheum 29:761, 1986.

222. Craft JE, Fischer DK, Shimamoto GT, Steere AC. Antigens of *Borrelia burgdorferi* recognized during Lyme disease: appearance of a new immunoglobulin M response and expansion of the immunoglobulin G response late in the illness. J Clin Invest 78:934, 1986.

223. Karlsson M, Mollegard I, Stiernstedt G, Wretlind B. Comparison of Western blot and enzyme-linked immunosorbent assay for diagnosis of Lyme borreliosis. Eur J Clin Microbiol Infect Dis 8:871, 1989.

224. Craft JE, Grodzicki RL, Steere AC. Antibody response in Lyme disease: evaluation of diagnostic tests. J Infect Dis 149:789, 1984.

225. Dattwyler RJ, Volkman DJ, Luft BJ. Immunologic aspects of Lyme borreliosis. Rev Infect Dis 11:S1494, 1989.

226. Aguero-Rosenfeld ME, Nowakowski J, Bittker S, et al. Evolution of the serologic response to *Borrelia burgdorferi* in treated patients with culture-confirmed erythema migrans. J Clin Microbiol 34(1):1–9, 1996.

227. Hammers-Berggren S, Lebech AM, Karlsson M, et al. Serological follow-up after treatment of patients with erythema migrans and neuroborreliosis. J Clin Microbiol 32(6):1519–1525, 1994.

228. Hammers-Berggren S, Lebeech AM, Karlsson M, et al. Serological follow-up after treatment of *Borrelia* arthritis and acrodermatitis chronica atrophicans. Scand J Infect Dis 26(3):339–347, 1994.

229. Rose CD, Fawcett PT, Gibney KM, Doughty RA. Residual serologic reactivity in children with resolved Lyme arthritis. J Rheumatol 23(2):367–369, 1996.

230. Pavia CS, Wormser GP, Norman GL. Activity of sera from patients with Lyme disease against *Borrelia burgdorferi*. Clin Infect Dis 25(Suppl 1):S25–S30, 1997.

231. Batsford S, Rust C, Neubert U. Analysis of antibody response to the outer surface protein family in Lyme borreliosis patients. J Infect Dis 178(6):1676–1683, 1998.

232. Aguero-Rosenfeld ME, Nowakowski J, McKenna DF, et al. Serodiagnosis in early Lyme disease [published erratum appears in J Clin Microbiol 1994 Mar; 32(3):860]. J Clin Microbiol 31(12):3090–3095, 1993.

233. Engstrom SM, Shoop E, Johnson RC. Immunoblot interpretation criteria for serodiagnosis of early Lyme disease. J Clin Microbiol 33(2):419–427, 1995.

234. Dressler F, Whalen JA, Reinhardt BN, Steere AC. Western blotting in the serodiagnosis of Lyme disease. J Infect Dis 167(2):392–400, 1993.

235. Kowal K, Weinstein A. Western blot band intensity analysis. Application to the diagnosis of Lyme arthritis. Arthritis Rheum 37:1206–1211, 1994.

236. Johnson BJ, Robbins KE, Bailey RE, et al. Serodiagnosis of Lyme disease: accuracy of a two-step approach using a flagella-based ELISA and immunoblotting. J Infect Dis 174(2):346–353, 1996.

237. Hauser U, Lehnert G, Wilske B. Interpretation criteria for standardized Western blots (Immunoblots) for serodiagnosis of Lyme borreliosis based on sera collected throughout Europe. J Clin Microbiol 37:2241–2247, 1999.

238. Centers for Disease Control and Prevention. Recommendations for test performance and interpretation from the Second National Conference on Serologic Diagnosis of Lyme Disease. MMWR Morb Mortal Wkly Rep 44(31):590–591, 1995.

239. Gerber MA, Shapiro ED, Bell GL, et al. Recombinant outer surface protein C ELISA for the diagnosis of early Lyme disease. J Infect Dis 171(3):724–727, 1995.

240. Fung BP, McHugh GL, Leong JM, Steere AC. Humoral immune response to outer surface protein C of *Borrelia burgdorferi* in Lyme disease: role of the immunoglobulin M response in the serodiagnosis of early infection. Infect Immun 62(8):3213–3221, 1994.

241. Fikrig E, Huguenel ED, Berland R, et al. Serologic diagnosis of Lyme disease using recombinant outer surface proteins A and B and flagellin. J Infect Dis 165:1127, 1992.

242. Hansen K, Asbrink E. Serodiagnosis of EM and acrodermatitis chronica atrophicans by the *Borrelia burgdorferi* flagellum enzyme-linked immunosorbent assay. J Clin Microbiol 27:545, 1989.

243. Steere AC, Bartenhagen NH, Craft JE, et al. The early clinical manifestations of Lyme disease. Ann Intern Med 99:76, 1983.

244. Hilton E, Tramontano A, De Voti J, Sood SK. Temporal study of immunoglobin M seroreactivity to *Borrelia burgdorferi* in patients treated for Lyme borreliosis. J Clin Microbiol 35(3):774–776, 1997.

245. Magnarelli LA, Fikrig E, Padula SJ, et al. Use of recombinant antigens of *Borrelia burgdorferi* in serologic tests for diagnosis of Lyme borreliosis. J Clin Microbiol 34(2):237–240, 1996.

246. Schutzer SE, Coyle PK, Dunn JJ, et al. Early and specific antibody response to OspA in Lyme disease. J Clin Invest 94(1):454–457, 1994.

247. Hofmann H. Lyme borreliosis—problems of serological diagnosis. Infection 24(6):470–472, 1996.

248. Jain VK, Hilton E, Maytal J, et al. Immunoglobulin for diagnosis of Borrelia burgdorferi infection in patients with acute facial palsy. J Clin Microbiol 34(8):2033–2035, 1996.

249. Barbour AG, Burgdorfer W, Grunwaldt E, Steere AC. Antibodies of patients with Lyme disease to components of the Ixodes dammini spirochete. J Clin Invest 72:504, 1983.

250. Magnarelli LA, Meegan JM, Anderson JF, Chappell WA. Comparison of an indirect fluorescent-antibody test with an enzyme-linked immunosorbent assay for serological studies of Lyme disease. J Clin Microbiol 20:181, 1984.

251. Stanek G, Flamm H, Groh V, et al. Epidemiology of Borrelia infections in Austria. Zentralbl Bakteriol Mikrobiol Hyg A 263:442, 1986.

252. Russell H, Sampson JS, Schmid GP, et al. Enzyme-linked immunosorbent assay and indirect immunofluorescence assay for Lyme disease. J Infect Dis 149:465, 1984.

253. Logigian EL, McHugh GL, Steere AC. Antibiotics for early Lyme disease may prevent full seroconversion but not CNS infection. Neurology 48:A388–A389, 1997.

254. Food and Drug Administration. FDA Public Health Advisory: Assays for Antibodies to Borrelia burgdorferi: Limitations, Use, and Interpretation for Supporting a Clinical Diagnosis of Lyme Disease. July 7, 1997.

255. Akin E, McHugh GL, Flavell RA, et al. Immunoglobulin (IgG) antibody response to OspA and OspB correlates with severe and prolonged Lyme arthritis and the IgG response to P35 correlates with mild and brief arthritis. Infect Immun 67:173–181, 1999.

256. Kalish RA, Leong JM, Steere AC. Association of treatment-resistant chronic Lyme arthritis with HLA-DR4 and antibody reactivity of OspA and OspB or Borrelia burgdorferi. Infect Immun 61(7):2774–2779, 1993.

257. Dressler F, Ackermann R, Steere AC. Antibody responses to the three genomic groups of Borrelia burgdorferi in European Lyme borreliosis. J Infect Dis 169(2):313–318, 1994.

258. Hansen K, Cruz M, Link H. Oligoclonal Borrelia burgdorferi–specific IgG antibodies in cerebrospinal fluid in Lyme neuroborreliosis. J Infect Dis 161:1194, 1990.

259. Steere AC, Berardi VP, Weeks KE, et al. Evaluation of the intrathecal antibody response to Borrelia burgdorferi as a diagnostic test for Lyme neuroborreliosis. J Infect Dis 161:1203, 1990.

260. Schutzer SE, Coyle PK, Krupp LB, et al. Simultaneous expression of Borrelia OspA and OspC and IgM response in cerebrospinal fluid in early neurologic Lyme disease. J Clin Invest 100(4):763–767, 1997.

261. Neophytides A, Khan S, Louie E. Subacute cerebellitis in Lyme disease. Int J Clin Pract 51(8):523–524, 1997.

262. Hardin JA, Steere AC, Malawista SE. Immune complexes and the evolution of Lyme arthritis: dissemination and localization of abnormal C1q binding activity. N Engl J Med 301:1358, 1979.

263. Lovrich SD, Callister SM, Lim LC, et al. Seroprotective groups of Lyme borreliosis spirochetes from North America and Europe. J Infect Dis 170(1):115–121, 1994.

264. Kujala GA, Steere AC, Davis JS IV. IgM rheumatoid factor in Lyme disease: correlation with disease activity, total serum IgM, and IgM antibody to Borrelia burgdorferi. J Rheumatol 14:772, 1987.

265. Halperin JJ. Nervous system Lyme disease. J Neurol Sci 153(2):182–191, 1998.

266. Kaiser R. Intrathecal immune response in patients with neuroborreliosis: specificity of antibodies for neuronal proteins. J Neurol 242(5):319–325, 1995.

267. Pachner AR, Duray P, Steere AC. Central nervous system manifestations of Lyme disease. Arch Neurol 46:790, 1989.

268. Hansen K. Lyme neuroborreliosis: improvements of the laboratory diagnosis and a survey of epidemiological and clinical features in Denmark 1985–1990. Acta Neurol Scand Suppl 151:1–44, 1994.

269. Lawrence C, Lipton RB, Lowy FD, Coyle PK. Seronegative chronic relapsing neuroborreliosis. Eur Neurol 35(2):113–117, 1995.

270. Schwartz BS, Ford DP, Childs JE, et al. Anti–tick saliva antibody: a biologic marker of tick exposure that is a risk factor for Lyme disease seropositivity. Am J Epidemiol 134:86, 1991.

271. Davis JP, Schell WL, Amundson TE, et al. Lyme disease in Wisconsin: epidemiologic, clinical, serologic, and entomologic findings. Yale J Biol Med 57:685, 1984.

272. Osterholm MT, Forfang JC, White KE, Kuritsky JN. Lyme disease in Minnesota: epidemiologic and serologic findings. Yale J Biol Med 57:677, 1984.

273. Donta ST. Tetracycline therapy for chronic Lyme disease. Clin Infect Dis 25(Suppl 1):S52–S56, 1997.

274. Rose CD, Fawcett PT, Eppes SC, et al. Pediatric Lyme arthritis: clinical spectrum and outcome. J Pediatr Orthop 14(2):238–241, 1994.

275. Karlsson M, Hammers-Berggren S, Lindquist L, et al. Comparison of intravenous penicillin G and oral doxycycline for treatment of Lyme neuroborreliosis. Neurology 44(7):1203–1207, 1994.

276. Wahlberg P, Granlund H, Nyman D, et al. Treatment of late Lyme borreliosis. J Infect 29(3):255–261, 1994.

277. Schuttelaar ML, Laeijendecker R, Heinhuis RJ, Van Joost T. Erythema multiforme and persistent erythema as early cutaneous manifestations of Lyme disease. J Am Acad Dermatol 37(5 Pt 2):873–875, 1997.

278. Schutzer SE, Coyle PK, Belman AL, et al. Sequestration of antibody to Borrelia burgdorferi in immune complexes in seronegative Lyme disease. Lancet 335:312, 1990.

279. Steere AC, Taylor E, McHugh GL, Logigian EL. The overdiagnosis of Lyme disease. JAMA 269(14):1812–1816, 1993.

280. Goodman JL, Bradley JF, Ross AE, et al. Bloodstream invasion in early Lyme disease: results from a prospective, controlled, blinded study using the polymerase chain reaction [published erratum appears in Am J Med 1996 Aug; 101(2):239]. Am J Med 99(1):6–12, 1995.

281. Mouritsen CL, Wittwer CT, Litwin CM, et al. Polymerase chain reaction detection of Lyme disease: correlation with clinical manifestations and serologic responses. Am J Clin Pathol 105(5):647–654, 1996.

282. Luft BJ, Steinman CR, Neimark HC, et al. Invasion of the central nervous system by Borrelia burgdorferi in acute disseminated infection. JAMA 267:1364, 1992.

283. Coyle PK, Schutzer SE, Deng Z, et al. Detection of Borrelia burgdorferi–specific antigen in antibody-negative cerebrospinal fluid in neurologic Lyme disease. Neurology 45(11):2010–2015, 1995.

284. Preac-Mursic V, Pfister HW, Spiegel H, et al. First isolation of Borrelia burgdorferi from an iris biopsy. J Clin Neuro-Ophthalmol 13(3):155–161; discussion 162, 1993.

285. Wilske B, Schierz G, Preac-Mursic V, et al. Intrathecal production of specific antibodies against Borrelia burg-

dorferi in patients with lymphocytic meningoradiculitis (Bannwarth's syndrome). J Infect Dis 153:304, 1986.

286. Ackermann R, Rehse-Kupper B, Gollmer E, Schmidt R. Chronic neurologic manifestations of EM borreliosis. Ann N Y Acad Sci 539:16, 1988.

287. Nocton JJ, Bloom BJ, Rutledge BJ, et al. Detection of *Borrelia burgdorferi* DNA by polymerase chain reaction in cerebrospinal fluid in Lyme neuroborreliosis. J Infect Dis 174(3):623–627, 1996.

288. Haass A. Lyme neuroborreliosis. Curr Opin Neurol 11(3):253–258, 1998.

289. Belman AL, Iyer M, Coyle PK, Dattwyler R. Neurologic manifestations in children with North American Lyme disease. Neurology 43(12):2609–2614, 1993.

290. Oschmann P, Dorndorf W, Hornig C, et al. Stages and syndromes of neuroborreliosis. J Neurol 245(5):262–272, 1998.

291. Logigian EL. Peripheral nervous system Lyme borreliosis. Semin Neurol 17(1):25–30, 1997.

292. Halperin JJ. Neuroborreliosis: central nervous system involvement. Semin Neurol 17(1):19–24, 1997.

293. Coyle PK. *Borrelia burgdorferi* infections. Clinical diagnostic techniques. Immunol Invest 26(1–2):117–128, 1997.

294. Kurtenbach K, Sewell HS, Ogden NH, et al. Serum complement sensitivity as a key factor in Lyme disease ecology. Infect Immun 66(3):1248–1251, 1998.

295. Suhonen J, Hartiala K, Viljanen MK. Tube phagocytosis, a novel way for neutrophils to phagocytize *Borrelia burgdorferi*. Infect Immun 66(7):3433–3435, 1998.

296. Modolell M, Schaible UE, Rittig M, Simon MM. Killing of *Borrelia burgdorferi* by macrophages is dependent on oxygen radicals and nitric oxide and can be enhanced by antibodies to outer surface proteins of the spirochete. Immunol Lett 40:139–146, 1994.

297. Burns MJ, Sellati TJ, Teng EI, Furie MB. Production of interleukin-8 (IL-8) by cultured endothelial cells in response to *Borrelia burgdorferi* occurs independently of secreted [corrected] IL-1 and tumor necrosis factor alpha and is required for subsequent transendothelial migration of neutrophils [published erratum appears in Infect Immun 1997 June; 65(6):2508]. Infect Immun 65(4):1217–1222, 1997.

298. Sprenger H, Krause A, Kaufmann A, et al. *Borrelia burgdorferi* induces chemokines in human monocytes. Infect Immun 65(11):4384–4388, 1997.

299. Morrison TB, Weis JH, Weiss JJ. *Borrelia burgdorferi* outer surface protein A (OspA) activates and primes human neutrophils. J Immunol 158(10):4838–4845, 1997.

300. Garcia R, Gusmani L, Murgia R, et al. Elastase is the only human neutrophil granule protein that alone is responsible for in vitro killing of *Borrelia burgdorferi*. Infect Immun 66(4):1408–1412, 1998.

301. Snydman DR, Schenkein DP, Berardi VP, et al. *Borrelia burgdorferi* in joint fluid in chronic Lyme arthritis. Ann Intern Med 104:798, 1986.

302. Preac-Mursic V, Weber K, Pfister HW, et al. Survival of *Borrelia burgdorferi* in antibiotically treated patients with Lyme borreliosis. Infection 17:355, 1989.

303. Hudson BJ, Stewart M, Lennox VA, et al. Culture-positive Lyme borreliosis. Med J Aust 168(10):500–502, 1998.

304. Haupl T, Hahn G, Rittig M, et al. Persistence of *Borrelia burgdorferi* in ligamentous tissue from a patient with chronic Lyme borreliosis. Arthritis Rheum 36(11):1621–1626, 1993.

305. Vos K, Van Dam AP, Kuiper H, et al. Seroconversion for Lyme borreliosis among Dutch military. Scand J Infect Dis 26(4):427–434, 1994.

306. Strle F, Cheng Y, Cimperman J, et al. Persistence of *Borrelia burgdorferi* sensu lato in resolved erythema migrans lesions. Clin Infect Dis 21(2):380–389, 1995.

307. Kuiper H, van Dam AP, Spanjaard L, et al. Isolation of *Borrelia burgdorferi* from biopsy specimens taken from healthy-looking skin of patients with Lyme borreliosis. J Clin Microbiol 32(3):715–720, 1994.

308. Stanek G, Klein J, Bittner R, Glogar D. Isolation of *Borrelia burgdorferi* from the myocardium of a patient with longstanding cardiomyopathy. N Engl J Med 322:249–252, 1990.

309. Keller TL, Malperin JJ, Whitman M. PCR detection of *Borrelia burgdorferi* DNA in cerebrospinal fluid of Lyme neuroborreliosis patients. Neurology 42:32–42, 1992.

310. Oksi J, Nikoskelainen J, Viljanen MK. Comparison of oral cefixime and intravenous ceftriaxone followed by oral amoxicillin in disseminated Lyme borreliosis. Eur J Clin Microbiol Infect Dis 17(10):715–719, 1998.

311. Oksi J, Kalimo H, Marttila RJ, et al. Inflammatory brain changes in Lyme borreliosis. A report on three patients and review of literature. Brain 119(Pt 6):2143–2154, 1996.

312. Nocton JJ, Dressler F, Rutledge BJ, et al. Detection of *Borrelia burgdorferi* DNA by polymerase chain reaction in synovial fluid from patients with Lyme arthritis. N Engl J Med 330(4):229–234, 1994.

313. Bradley JF, Johnson RC, Goodman JL. The persistence of spirochetal nucleic acids in active Lyme arthritis. Ann Intern Med 120(6):487–489, 1994.

314. Priem S, Burmester GR, Kamradt T, et al. Detection of *Borrelia burgdorferi* by polymerase chain reaction in synovial membrane, but not in synovial fluid from patients with persisting Lyme arthritis after antibiotic therapy. Ann Rheum Dis 57(2):118–121, 1998.

315. Aberer E, Breier F, Stanek G, Schmidt B. Success and failure in the treatment of acrodermatitis chronica atrophicans. Infection 24(1):85–87, 1996.

316. Muelleger R, Zoechling N, Schluepen EM, et al. Polymerase chain reaction control of antibiotic treatment in dermatoborreliosis. Infection 24(1):76–79, 1996.

317. Melchers W, Meis J, Rosa P, et al. Amplification of *Borrelia burgdorferi* DNA in skin biopsies from patients with Lyme disease. J Clin Microbiol 29(11):2401–2406, 1991.

318. Sigal LH. Persisting complaints attributed to chronic Lyme disease: possible mechanisms and implications for management. Am J Med 96(4):365–374, 1994.

319. Pfister H-W, Preac-Mursic V, Wilske B, et al. Randomized comparison of ceftriaxone and cefotaxime in Lyme neuroborreliosis. J Infect Dis 163:311, 1991.

320. Balcer LJ, Winterkorn JM, Galetta SL. Neuro-ophthalmic manifestations of Lyme disease. J Neuroophthalmol 17(2):108–121, 1997.

321. Girschick HJ, Huppertz HI, Russmann H, et al. Intracellular persistence of *Borrelia burgdorferi* in human synovial cells. Rheumatol Int 16(3):125–132, 1996.

322. Klempner MS, Noring R, Rogers RA. Invasion of human skin fibroblasts by the Lyme disease spirochete, *Borrelia burgdorferi*. J Infect Dis 167(5):1074–1081, 1993.

323. Kamradt T, Lengl-Janssen B, Strauss AF, et al. Dominant recognition of a *Borrelia burgdorferi* outer surface protein A peptide by T helper cells in patients with treatment-resistant Lyme arthritis. Infect Immun 64(4):1284–1289, 1996.

324. Steere AC, Levin RE, Molloy PJ, et al. Treatment of Lyme arthritis. Arthritis Rheum 37(6):878–888, 1994.

325. Szer IS, Taylor BA, Steere AC. The long-term course of Lyme arthritis in children. N Engl J Med 325:159–163, 1991.

326. Smith M, Gettinby G, Granstrom M, et al. The European Union Concerted Action World Wide Web site for Lyme borreliosis. Zentralbl Bakteriol 287(3):266–269, 1998.

327. Buchwald A. Ein Fall von diffuser idiopathischer Haut-Atrophie. Arch Dermatol Syph 10:553–556, 1883.

328. Garin CH, Boujadoux C. Paralysie par les tiques. J Med Lyon 71:765, 1922.

329. Bannwarth A. Chronische lymphocytare meningitis entzundliche polyneuritis und "rheumatismus." Arch Psychiatr Nervenkr 113:284, 1941.

330. Lennhoff C. Spirochaetes in aetiologically obscure disease. Acta Dermatol Venereol 28:295, 1948.

331. Hollstrom E. Penicillin treatment of erythema chronicum migrans Afzeli. Acta Dermatol Venereol 38:285, 1958.

332. Binder E, Doepfmer R, Hornstein O. Experimental transmission of erythema chronicum migrans from man to man. Hautarzt 6:494, 1955.

333. Scrimenti RJ. Erythema chronicum migrans. Arch Dermatol 102:104, 1970.

334. Steere AC, Taylor E, Wilson ML, et al. Longitudinal assessment of the clinical and epidemiologic features of Lyme disease in a defined population. J Infect Dis 154:295, 1986.

335. Steere AC, Malawista SE. Cases of Lyme disease in the United States: locations correlated with distribution of *Ixodes dammini*. Ann Intern Med 91:730, 1979.

336. Lane RS, Piesman J, Burgdorfer W. Lyme borreliosis: relation of its causative agent to its vectors and hosts in North America and Europe. Annu Rev Entomol 36:587, 1991.

337. Wallis RC, Brown SE, Kloter KO, Main AJ. Erythema chronicum migrans and Lyme arthritis: field study of ticks. Am J Epidemiol 108:322, 1978.

338. Steere AC, Malawista SE, Hardin JA, et al. Erythema chronicum migrans and Lyme arthritis: the enlarging clinical spectrum. Ann Intern Med 86:685, 1977.

339. Steere AC, Malawista SE, Newman JH, et al. Antibiotic therapy in Lyme disease. Ann Intern Med 93:1, 1980.

340. Hubbard MJ, Baker AS, Cann KJ. Distribution of *Borrelia burgdorferi* s.l. spirochaete DNA in British ticks (Argasidae and Ixodidae) since the 19th century, assessed by PCR. Med Vet Entomol 12(1):89–97, 1998.

341. Benach JL, Coleman JL, Skinner RA, Bosler EM. Adult *Ixodes dammini* on rabbits: a hypothesis for the development and transmission of *Borrelia burgdorferi*. J Infect Dis 155:1300, 1987.

342. Burgdorfer W, Hayes SF, Corwin D. Pathophysiology of the Lyme disease spirochete, *Borrelia burgdorferi*, in Ixodid ticks. Rev Infect Dis 11:S1442, 1989.

343. Naversen DN, Gardner LW. Erythema chronicum migrans in America. Arch Dermatol 114:253, 1978.

344. Ai CX, Hu RJ, Hyland KE, et al. Epidemiological and aetiological evidence for transmission of Lyme disease by adult *Ixodes persulcatus* in an endemic area in China. Int J Epidemiol 19:1061, 1990.

345. Cooley RA, Kohls GM. The genus *Ixodes* in North America. NIH Bulletin No. 184. Bethesda, Md, National Institutes of Health, 1945, 1–246.

346. Dammin GJ. Lyme disease: its transmission and diagnostic features. Lab Manage 24:33, 1986.

347. Fish D. Environmental risk and prevention of Lyme disease. Am J Med 98(4A):2S–8S; discussion 8S–9S, 1995.

348. Dennis DT, Nekomoto TS, Victor JC, et al. Reported distribution of *Ixodes scapularis* and *Ixodes pacificus* (Acari: Ixodidae) in the United States. J Med Entomol 35:629–638, 1998.

349. Zhang Z. Investigation of Lyme disease in northeast of China. Chung Hua Liu Hsing Ping Hsueh Tsa Chih (Chinese J Epidemiol) 10:261, 1989.

350. Zhang Z. Survey on tick vectors of Lyme disease spirochetes in China. Chung Hua Liu Hsing Ping Hsueh Tsa Chih (Chinese J Epidemiol) 13:271, 1992.

351. Miyamoto K, Nakao M, Uchikawa K, Fujita H. Prevalence of Lyme borreliosis spirochetes in ixodid ticks of Japan, with special reference to a new potential vector Ixodes ovatus (Acari: Ixodidae). J Med Entomol 29:216, 1992.

352. Aeschlimann A, Chamot E, Gigon F, et al. *B. burgdorferi* in Switzerland. Zentralbl Bakteriol Mikrobiol Hyg A 263:450, 1986.

353. Burgdorfer W, Barbour AG, Hayes SF, et al. Erythema chronicum migrans—a tick-borne spirochetosis. Acta Trop 40:79, 1983.

354. Magnarelli LA, Anderson JF, Fish D. Transovarial transmission of *Borrelia burgdorferi* in *Ixodes dammini* (Acari: Ixodidae). J Infect Dis 156:234, 1987.

355. Lane RS, Burgdorfer W. Transovarial and transstadial passage of *Borrelia burgdorferi* in the Western black-legged tick, *Ixodes pacificus* (Acari: Ixodidae). Am J Trop Med Hyg 37:188, 1987.

356. Sinski E, Karbowiak G, Siuda K, et al. *Borrelia burgdorferi* infection of ticks in some regions of Poland. Przegl Epidemiol 48(4):461–465, 1994.

357. Nakao M, Sato Y. Refeeding activity of immature ticks of *Ixodes persulcatus* and transmission of Lyme disease spirochete by partially fed larvae. J Parasitol 82(4):669–672, 1996.

358. Heimberger T, Jenkins S, Russell H, Duma R. Epidemiology of Lyme disease in Virginia. Am J Med Sci 300:283, 1990.

359. Levine JF, Apperson CS, Spiegel RA, et al. Indigenous cases of Lyme disease diagnosed in North Carolina. South Med J 84:27, 1991.

360. Rumpel C, Jones JL. Lyme disease in South Carolina. J South Carolina Med Assoc 87:420, 1991.

361. Oliver JH Jr. Lyme borreliosis in the southern United States: a review. J Parasitol 82(6):926–935, 1996.

362. Maupin GO, Gage KL, Piesman J, et al. Discovery of an enzootic cycle of *Borrelia burgdorferi* in *Neotoma mexicana* and *Ixodes spinipalpis* from northern Colorado, an area where Lyme disease is nonendemic. J Infect Dis 170(3):636–643, 1994.

363. Hall JE, Amrine JW Jr, Gais RD, et al. Parasitization of humans in West Virginia by *Ixodes cookei* (Acari: Ixodidae), a potential vector of Lyme borreliosis. J Med Entomol 28:186, 1991.

364. Damrow T, Freedman H, Lane RS, Preston KL. Is *Ixodes (Ixodiopsis) augustus* a vector of Lyme disease in Washington state? West J Med 150:580, 1989.

365. Lane RS, Brown RN, Piesman J, Peavey CA. Vector competence of *Ixodes pacificus* and *Dermacentor occidentalis* (Acari: Ixodidae) for various isolates of Lyme disease spirochetes. J Med Entomol 31(3):417–424, 1994.

366. Pelletier AR, Finger RF, Sosin DM. The epidemiology of Lyme disease in Kentucky, 1985–1990. Kentucky Med Assoc J 89:266, 1991.

367. Campbell GL, Paul WS, Schriefer ME, et al. Epidemiologic and diagnostic studies of patients with suspected early Lyme disease, Missouri, 1990–1993. J Infect Dis 172(2):470–480, 1995.

368. Masters E, Granter S, Duray P, Cordes P. Physician-diagnosed erythema migrans and erythema migrans–like rashes following Lone Star tick bites. Arch Dermatol 134:955–960, 1998.

369. Reiner KL, Huycke MM, McNabb SJN. The descriptive epidemiology of Lyme disease in Oklahoma. J Oklahoma State Med Assoc 84:503, 1991.

370. Bozsik BP, Lakos A, Budai J, et al. Occurrence of Lyme borreliosis in Hungary. Zentralbl Bakteriol Mikrobiol Hyg A 263:466, 1986.

371. Bigaignon G, Tomasi J-P, Goubau P, et al. A clinical and sero-epidemiological study of 190 Belgian patients suffering from Lyme borreliosis. Acta Clin Belg 44:174, 1989.

372. Luger SW. Lyme disease transmitted by a biting fly. N Engl J Med 322:1752, 1990.

373. Need JT, Escamilla J. Lyme disease in South America? J Infect Dis 163:681, 1991.

374. Hashimoto Y, Kawagishi N, Sakai H, et al. Lyme disease in Japan. Analysis of *Borrelia* species using rRNA gene restriction fragment length polymorphism. Dermatology 191(3):193–198, 1995.

375. Russell RC, Doggett SL, Munro R, et al. Lyme disease: a search for a causative agent in ticks in south-eastern Australia. Epidemiol Infect 112(2):375–384, 1994.

376. Banerjee SN, Banerjee M, Smith JA, et al. Lyme disease in British Columbia—an update. British Columbia Med J 36:540 541, 1994.

377. Ryder JW, Pinger RR, Glancy TG. Inability of *Ixodes cookei* and *Amblyomma americanum* nymphs (Acari: Ixodidae) to transmit *Borrelia burgdorferi*. J Med Entomol 29:525, 1992.

378. Brown RN, Lane RS. Lyme disease in California: a novel enzootic transmission cycle of *Borrelia burgdorferi*. Science 256:1439, 1992.

379. Schwan TG, Schrumpf ME, Karstens RH, et al. Distribution and molecular analysis of Lyme disease spirochetes, *Borrelia burgdorferi*, isolated from ticks throughout California. J Clin Microbiol 31(12):3096–3108, 1993.

380. Gern L, Toutoungi LN, Hu CM, et al. *Ixodes (Pholeoxodes) hexagonus*, an efficient vector of *Borrelia burgdorferi* in the laboratory. Med Vet Entomol 5:431–435, 1991.

381. Estrada-Pena A, Oteo JA, Estrada-Pena R, et al. *Borrelia burgdorferi* sensu lato in ticks (Acari: Ixodidae) from two different foci in Spain. Exp Appl Acarol 19(3):173–180, 1995.

382. Rawlings JA. Lyme disease in Texas. Zentralbl Bakteriol Mikrobiol Hyg A 263:483, 1986.

383. Piesman J, Sinsky RJ. Ability of *Ixodes scapularis*, *Dermacentor variabilis*, and *Amblyomma americanum* (Acari: Ixodidae) to acquire, maintain, and transmit Lyme disease spirochetes (*Borrelia burgdorferi*). J Med Entomol 25:336, 1988.

384. Anderson JF, Johnson RC, Magnarelli LA, Hyde FW. Identification of endemic foci of Lyme disease: isolation of *Borrelia burgdorferi* from feral rodents and ticks (Dermacentor variabilis). J Clin Microbiol 22:36, 1985.

385. Magnarelli LA, Anderson JF. Ticks and biting insects infected with the etiologic agent of Lyme disease, *Borrelia burgdorferi*. J Clin Microbiol 26:1482, 1988.

386. Kocan AA, Mukolwe SW, Murphy GL, et al. Isolation of *Borrelia burgdorferi* (Spirochaetales: Spirochaetaceae) from *Ixodes scapularis* and *Dermacentor albipictus* ticks (Acari: Ixodidae) in Oklahoma. J Med Entomol 29:630–633, 1992.

387. Angelov L, Dimova P, Berbencova W. Clinical and laboratory evidence of the importance of the tick *D. marginatus* as a vector of *B. burgdorferi* in some areas of sporadic Lyme disease in Bulgaria. Eur J Epidemiol 12(5):499–502, 1996.

388. Feng FP, Zhang W, Zhou G. Discovery and clinical investigation of Lyme disease in Beijing area. Chung Hua Liu Hsing Ping Hsueh Tsa Chih 15(1):10–13, 1994.

389. Halouzka J, Postic D, Hubalek Z. Isolation of the spirochaete *Borrelia afzelii* from the mosquito *Aedes vexans* in the Czech Republic. Med Vet Entomol 12(1):103–105, 1998.

390. Spielman A, Levine JF, Wilson ML. Vectorial capacity of North American *Ixodes* ticks. Yale J Biol Med 57:507, 1984.

391. Nash PT. Does Lyme disease exist in Australia? Med J Aust 168(10):479–480, 1998.

392. Russell RC. Lyme disease in Australia—still to be proven. Emerg Infect Dis 1(1):29–31, 1995.

393. Yin Z, Braun J, Neure L, et al. T cell cytokine pattern in the joints of patients with Lyme arthritis and its regulation by cytokines and anticytokines. Arthritis Rheum 40(1):69–79, 1997.

394. Spielman A. The emergence of Lyme disease and human babesiosis in a changing environment. Ann N Y Acad Sci 740:146–156, 1994.

395. Chang YF, Novosel V, Chang CF, et al. Detection of human granulocytic ehrlichiosis agent and *Borrelia burgdorferi* in ticks by polymerase chain reaction. J Vet Diagn Invest 10(1):56–59, 1998.

396. Schwartz I, Fish D, Daniels TJ. Prevalence of the rickettsial agent of human granulocytic ehrlichiosis in ticks from a hyperendemic focus of Lyme disease. N Engl J Med 337:49–50, 1997.

397. Dumler JS. Is human granulocytic ehrlichiosis a new Lyme disease? Review and comparison of clinical, laboratory, epidemiological, and some biological features. Clin Infect Dis 25(Suppl 1):S43–S47, 1997.

398. Walker DH, Dumler JS. Emergence of the ehrlichioses as human health problems. Emerg Infect Dis 2:18–29, 1996.

399. Gorenflot A, Moubri K, Precigout E, et al. Human babesiosis. Ann Trop Med Parasitol 92(4):489–501, 1998.

400. Dumler JS, Dotevall L, Gustafson R, Granstrom M. A population-based seroepidemiologic study of human granulocytic ehrlichiosis and Lyme borreliosis in the west coast of Sweden. J Infect Dis 175:720–722, 1997.

401. Fritz CL, Kjemtrup AM, Conrad PA, et al. Seroepidemiology of emerging tickborne infectious diseases in a northern California community. J Infect Dis 175:1432–1439, 1997.

402. Zeman P. Objective assessment of risk maps of tickborne encephalitis and Lyme borreliosis based on spatial patterns of located cases. Int J Epidemiol 26(5):1121–1129, 1997.

403. Gilot B, Degeilh B, Pichot J, et al. Prevalence of *Borrelia burgdorferi* (sensu lato) in *Ixodes ricinus* (L.) populations in France, according to a phytoecological zoning of the territory. Eur J Epidemiol 12(4):395–401, 1996.

404. Pal E, Barta Z, Nagy F, et al. Neuroborreliosis in county Baranya, Hungary. Funct Neurol 13(1):37–46, 1998.

405. Korenberg EI, Kryuchechnikov VN, Kovalevsky YV. Advances in investigations of Lyme borreliosis in the territory of the former USSR. Eur J Epidemiol 9(1):86–91, 1993.

406. Pierer K, Kock T, Freidl W, et al. Prevalence of antibodies to *Borrelia burgdorferi* flagellin in Styrian blood donors. Zentralbl Bakteriol 279(2):239–243, 1993.

407. Jaenson TG, Fish D, Ginsberg HS, et al. Methods for control of tick vectors of Lyme borreliosis. Scand J Infect Dis Suppl 77:151, 1991.

408. Wilson ML, Adler GH, Spielman A. Correlation between abundance of deer and that of the deer tick, *Ixodes dammini* (Acari: Ixodidae). Ann Entomol Soc Am 78:172, 1985.

409. Motiejunas L, Bunikis J, Barbour AG, Sadziene A. Lyme borreliosis in Lithuania. Scand J Infect Dis 26(2):149–155, 1994.

410. Gustafson R, Jaenson TG, Gardulf A, et al. Prevalence of *Borrelia burgdorferi* sensu lato infection in *Ixodes ricinus* in Sweden. Scand J Infect Dis 27(6):597–601, 1995.

411. Levine JF, Wilson ML, Spielman A. Mice as reservoirs of the Lyme disease spirochete. Am J Trop Med Hyg 34:355, 1985.

412. Brunet LR, Spielman A, Telford SR 3rd. Short report: density of Lyme disease spirochetes within deer ticks collected from zoonotic sites. Am J Trop Med Hyg 53(3):300–302, 1995.

413. Bosler EM, Coleman JL, Benach JL, et al. Natural distribution of the *Ixodes dammini* spirochete. Science 220:321, 1983.

414. Rand PW, Lacomb EH, Smith RP, et al. Competence of *Peromyscus maniculatus* (Rodentia: Cricetidae) as a reservoir host for *Borrelia burgdorferi* (Spirochaetares: Spirochaetaceae) in the wild. J Med Entomol 30:614–618, 1993.

415. Smith RP Jr, Rand PW, Lacombe EH, et al. Norway rats as reservoir hosts for Lyme disease spirochetes on Monhegan Island, Maine. J Infect Dis 168(3):687–691, 1993.

416. Godsey MS, Jr, Amundson TE, Burgess EC, et al. Lyme disease ecology in Wisconsin: distribution and host preferences of *Ixodes dammini*, and prevalence of antibody to *Borrelia burgdorferi* in small mammals. Am J Trop Med Hyg 37:180, 1987.

417. Mannelli A, Kitron U, Jones CJ, Slajchert TL. Role of the eastern chipmunk as a host for immature *Ixodes dammini* (Acari: Ixodidae) in northwestern Illinois. J Med Entomol 30:87–93, 1993.

418. Centers for Disease Control and Prevention. Recommendations for the Use of Lyme Disease Vaccine: Recommendations of the Advisory Committee on Immunization Practice (ACIP). MMWR 48(RR7):1–25, 1999.

419. Burgdorfer W, Keirans JE. Ticks and Lyme disease in the United States. Ann Intern Med 99:122, 1983.

420. Burgdorfer W, Lane RS, Barbour AG, et al. The Western black-legged tick, *Ixodes pacificus*: a vector of *Borrelia burgdorferi*. Am J Trop Med Hyg 34:925, 1985.

421. Westrom DR, Lane RS, Anderson JR. *Ixodes pacificus* (Acari: Ixodidae): population dynamics and distribution on Columbian black-tailed deer (*Odocoileus hemionus columbianus*). J Med Entomol 22:507–511, 1985.

422. Hubalek Z, Halouzka J, Juricova Z. A simple method of transmission risk assessment in enzootic foci of Lyme borreliosis. Eur J Epidemiol 12(4):331–333, 1996.

423. Matuschka FR, Endepols S, Richter D, et al. Risk of urban Lyme disease enhanced by the presence of rats. J Infect Dis 174(5):1108–1111, 1996.

424. Jaenson TG, Talleklint L. Lyme borreliosis spirochetes in *Ixodes ricinus* (Acari:Ixodidae) and the varying hare on isolated islands in the Baltic Sea. J Med Entomol 33(3):339–343, 1996.

425. Hoogstraal H, Kaiser MN, Traylor MA, et al. Ticks (Ixodidae) on birds migrating from Europe and Asia to Africa, 1959–61. Bull World Health Organ 28:235–262, 1963.

426. Olsen B, Jaenson TG, Bergstrom S. Prevalence of *Borrelia burgdorferi* sensu lato–infected ticks on migrating birds. Appl Environ Microbiol 61(8):3082–3087, 1995.

427. Kurtenbach K, Peacey M, Rijpkema SG, et al. Differential transmission of the genospecies of *Borrelia burgdorferi* sensu lato by game birds and small rodents in England. Appl Environ Microbiol 64(4):1169–1174, 1998.

428. Piesman J, Mather TN, Dammin GJ, et al. Seasonal variation of transmission risk of Lyme disease and human babesiosis. Am J Epidemiol 126:1187, 1987.

429. Maryland Department of Health and Mental Hygiene, Epidemiology and Disease Control Program. Selected communicable diseases in Maryland in 1995. Maryland Med J 45:715–718, 1996.

430. Sood SK, Salzman MB, Johnson BJ, et al. Duration of tick attachment as a predictor of the risk of Lyme disease in an area in which Lyme disease is endemic. J Infect Dis 175(4):996–999, 1997.

431. Korenberg EI, Vorobyeva NN, Moskvitina HG, Gorban LY. Prevention of borreliosis in persons bitten by infected ticks. Infection 24:187–189, 1996.

432. Strle F, Nelson JA, Ruzic-Sabljic E, et al. European Lyme borreliosis: 231 culture-confirmed cases involving patients with erythema migrans [published erratum appears in Clinical Infectious Diseases 1996 November; 23(5):1202]. Clin Infect Dis 23(1):61–65, 1996.

433. Zhioua E, Rodhain F, Binet P, Perez-Eid C. Prevalence of antibodies to *Borrelia burgdorferi* in forestry workers of Ile de France, France. Eur J Epidemiol 13(8):959–962, 1997.

434. Asbrink E, Olsson I, Hovmark A. Erythema chronicum migrans Afzelius in Sweden. A study of 231 patients. Zentralbl Bakteriol Mikrobiol Hyg A 263:229, 1986.

435. Christen HJ, Hanefeld F, Eiffert H, Thomssen R. Epidemiology and clinical manifestations of Lyme borreliosis in childhood. A prospective multicentre study with special regard to neuroborreliosis. Acta Paediatr Suppl 386:1–75, 1993.

436. Picken MM, Picken RN, Han D, et al. A two year prospective study to compare culture and polymerase chain reaction amplification for the detection and diagnosis of Lyme borreliosis. Mol Pathol 50(4):186–193, 1997.

437. Ai CX, Zhang WF, Zhao JH. Sero-epidemiology of Lyme disease in an endemic area in China. Microbiol Immunol 38(7):505–509, 1994.

438. Ai C, Wen Y, Zhang Y, et al. Clinical manifestations and epidemiological characteristics of Lyme disease in Hailin Country, Heilongjiang Province, China. Ann N Y Acad Sci 539:302–313, 1988.

439. Hashimoto Y, Takahashi H, Kishiyama K, et al. Lyme disease with facial nerve palsy: rapid diagnosis using a nested polymerase chain reaction–restriction fragment length polymorphism analysis. Br J Dermatol 138(2):304–309, 1998.

440. Gerber MA, Shapiro ED, Krause PJ, et al. The risk of acquiring Lyme disease or babesiosis from a blood transfusion. J Infect Dis 170(1):231–234, 1994.

441. Falco RC, Fish D. Prevalence of *Ixodes dammini* near the homes of Lyme disease patients in Westchester County, New York. Am J Epidemiol 127:826, 1988.

442. Dister SW, Fish D, Bros SM, et al. Landscape characterization of peridomestic risk for Lyme disease using satellite imagery. Am J Trop Med Hyg 57(6):687–692, 1997.

443. Kitron U, Kazmierczak JJ. Spatial analysis of the distribution of Lyme disease in Wisconsin. Am J Epidemiol 145(6):558–566, 1997.

444. Schutze TL, Bowen GS, Lakat MF, et al. Geographical distribution and density of *Ixodes dammini* (Acari: Ixodidae) and relationship to Lyme disease transmission in New Jersey. Yale J Biol Med 57:669, 1984.

445. Lindsay R, Artsob H, Barker I. Distribution of *Ixodes pacificus* and *Ixodes scapularis* re concurrent babesiosis and Lyme disease. Can Commun Dis Rep 24(15):121–122, 1998.

446. Banerjee SN, Banerjee M, Fernandeo K, et al. Isolation of *Borrelia burgdorferi*, the Lyme disease spirochete, from rabbit ticks, *Haemaphysalis leporispalustris*—Alberta. Can Commun Dis Rep 21(10):86–88, 1995.

447. Rawlings JA, Teltow GJ. Prevalence of *Borrelia* (Spirochaetaceae) spirochetes in Texas ticks. J Med Entomol 31:297–301, 1994.

448. Dekonenko EJ, Steere AC, Berardi VP, Kravchuk LN. Lyme borreliosis in the Soviet Union: a cooperative US-USSR report. J Infect Dis 158:748, 1988.

449. Zhang Z. Investigation of Lyme disease in Xinjiang. Chin Med J 104:244, 1991.

450. Ikushima M, Kawahashi S, Okuyama Y, et al. The survey of prevalence of Lyme borreliosis in forestry workers in Saitama prefecture. Kansenshogaku Zasshi 69(2):139–144, 1995.

451. Shih CM, Wang JC, Chao LL, Wu TN. Lyme disease in Taiwan: first human patient with characteristic erythema chronicum migrans skin lesion. J Clin Microbiol 36(3):807–808, 1998.

452. Yoshinari NH, de Barros PJ, Bonoldi VL, et al. Outline of Lyme borreliosis in Brazil. Rev Hosp Clin Fac Med Sao Paulo 52(2):111–117, 1997.

453. Stanchi NO, Balague LJ. Lyme disease: antibodies against *Borrelia burgdorferi* in farm workers in Argentina. Rev Saude Publica 27(4):305–307, 1993.

454. Abarca K, Ribera M, Prado P, et al. Neuroborreliosis in Chile. Report of a child probably infected by imported pets. Rev Med Chil 124(8):975–979, 1996.

455. Aoun K, Kechrid A, Lagha N, et al. Lyme disease in Tunisia, results of a clinical and serological study (1992–1996). Sante 8(2):98–100, 1998.

456. Strijdom SC, Berk M. Lyme disease in South Africa. S Afr Med J 86(6 Suppl):741–744, 1996.

457. Marjolet M, Gueglio B, Traore M. Does Lyme disease (or an analogous disease) exist in Mali, West Africa? Trans R Soc Trop Med Hyg 89(4):387, 1995.

458. Mason PR, Kelly PJ, Nilsson I, Wadstrom T. Apparent absence of Lyme borreliosis in Zimbabwe. Trans R Soc Trop Med Hyg 88(4):412, 1994.

459. Centers for Disease Control and Prevention. Lyme disease—United States, 1994. MMWR 44(24):459–462, 1995.

460. Schmid GP, Horsley R, Steere AC, et al. Surveillance of Lyme disease in the United States, 1982. J Infect Dis 151:1144, 1985.

461. Centers for Disease Control and Prevention. Lyme Disease Cases Reported to CDC by State Health Departments, 1982–1997. http://www.cdc.gov/epo/mmwrhtml/00056949.htm

462. Lastavica CC, Wilson ML, Berardi VP, et al. Rapid emergence of a focal epidemic of Lyme disease in coastal Massachusetts. N Engl J Med 320:133, 1989.

463. Petersen LR, Sweeney AH, Checko PJ, et al. Epidemiological and clinical features of 1,149 persons with Lyme disease identified by laboratory-based surveillance in Connecticut. Yale J Biol Med 62:253, 1989.

464. Benach JL, Coleman JL. Clinical and geographic characteristics of Lyme disease in New York. Zentralbl Bakteriol Mikrobiol Hyg A 263:477, 1986.

465. White DJ, Chang H-G, Benach JL, et al. The geographic spread and temporal increase of the Lyme disease epidemic. JAMA 266:1230, 1991.

466. Williams CL, Curran AS, Lee AC, Sousa VO. Lyme disease: Epidemiologic characteristics of an outbreak in Westchester County, N Y Am J Public Health 76:62, 1986.

467. Bowen GS, Griffin M, Hayne C, et al. Clinical manifestations and descriptive epidemiology of Lyme disease in New Jersey, 1978 to 1982. JAMA 251:2236, 1984.

468. Goldoft MJ, Schulze TL, Parkin WE, Gunn RA. Lyme disease in New Jersey. N J Med 87:579, 1990.

469. Mitchell CS, Cloeren M, Israel E, et al. Lyme disease in Maryland: 1987–1990. Maryland Med J 41:391, 1992.

470. Schwartz BS, Hofmeister E, Glass GE, et al. Lyme borreliosis in an inner-city park in Baltimore. Am J Public Health 81:803, 1991.

471. Agger W, Case KL, Bryant GL, Callister SM. Lyme disease: clinical features, classification, and epidemiology in the upper Midwest. Medicine 70:83, 1991.

472. Dryer RF, Goellner PG, Carney AS. Lyme arthritis in Wisconsin. JAMA 241:498, 1979.

473. Huycke MM, D'Alessio DD, Marx JJ. Prevalence of antibody to *Borrelia burgdorferi* by indirect fluorescent antibody assay, ELISA, and Western immunoblot in healthy adults in Wisconsin and Arizona. J Infect Dis 165:1133, 1992.

474. McBryde RR. Lyme disease in Alabama. Ala Med 59:24, 1990.

475. Dryer RF, Buckwalter JA, Carney AS, Weinstein SL. Lyme arthritis in the Midwest: a diagnostic challenge. J Iowa Med Soc 71:249, 1981.

476. Stobierski MG, Bidol SA, Hall WN. Lyme disease in Michigan: an update. Mich Med 91:41, 1992.

477. Barbour AG. Does Lyme disease occur in the South?: a survey of emerging tick-borne infections in the region. Am J Med Sci 311(1):34–40, 1996.

478. Tugwell P, Dennis DT, Weinstein A, et al. Laboratory evaluation in the diagnosis of Lyme disease. Ann Intern Med 127(12):1109–1123, 1997.

479. Laboratory Centre for Disease Control. Lyme Disease by Province/Territory 1987–1997, personal communication.

480. Bakken JS, Krueth J, Wildon-Nordskog C, et al. Clinical and laboratory characteristics of human granulocytic chrlichiosis. JAMA 275:199–205, 1996.

481. Krause PJ, Telford SR 3rd, Spielman A, et al. Concurrent Lyme disease and babesiosis. Evidence for increased severity and duration of illness. JAMA 275(21):1657–1660, 1996.

482. dos Santos C, Kain K. Concurrent babesiosis and Lyme disease diagnosed in Ontario. Can Commun Dis Rep 24(12):97–101, 1998.

483. Sweeney CJ, Ghassemi M, Agger WA, Persing DH. Coinfection with *Babesia microti* and *Borrelia burgdorferi* in a western Wisconsin resident. Mayo Clin Proc 73(4):338–341, 1998.

484. Nadelman RB, Horowitz HW, Hsieh TC, et al. Simultaneous human granulocytic ehrlichiosis and Lyme borreliosis. N Engl J Med 337(1):27–30, 1997.

485. Benach JL, Coleman JL, Habicht GS. Serologic evidence for simultaneous occurrences of Lyme disease and babesiosis. J Infect Dis 144:473–477, 1981.

486. Mitchell PD, Reed KD, Hofkes JM. Immunoserologic evidence of coinfection with *Borrelia burgdorferi*, Babesia microti, and human granulocytic *Ehrlichia* species in residents of Wisconsin and Minnesota. J Clin Microbiol 34(3):724–727, 1996.

487. Magnarelli LA, Dumler JS, Anderson JF, et al. Coexistence of antibodies to tick-borne pathogens of babesiosis, ehrlichiosis, and Lyme borreliosis in human sera. J Clin Microbiol 33:3054–3057, 1995.

488. Wong SJ, Brady GS, Dumler JS. Serological responses

to *Ehrlichia equi, Ehrlichia chaffeensis,* and *Borrelia burgdorferi* in patients from New York State. J Clin Microbiol 35(9):2198–2205, 1997.

489. Anderson JF, Johnson RC, Magnarelli LA, et al. *Peromyscus leucopus* and *Microtus pennsylvanicus* simultaneously infected with *Borrelia burgdorferi* and *Babesia microti.* J Clin Microbiol 23:135–137, 1986.

490. Stafford KC III, Cartter ML, Magnarelli LA, et al. Temporal correlations between tick abundance and prevalence of ticks infected with *Borrelia burgdorferi* and increasing incidence of Lyme disease. J Clin Microbiol 36(5):1240–1244, 1998.

491. Mather TN, Nicholson MC, Donnelly EF. Matyas BT. Entomologic index for human risk of Lyme disease. Am J Epidemiol 144(11):1066–1069, 1996.

492. Daniels TJ, Falco RC, Schwartz I, et al. Deer ticks (Ixodes scapularis) and the agents of Lyme disease and human granulocytic ehrlichiosis in a New York City park. Emerg Infect Dis 3(3):353–355, 1997.

493. Feder HM Jr, Gerber MA, Cartter ML, et al. Prospective assessment of Lyme disease in school-aged population in Connecticut. J Infect Dis 171(5):1371–1374, 1995.

494. Falco RC, Daniels TJ, Fish D. Increase in abundance of imature *Ixodes scapularis* (Acari: Ixodidae) in an emergent Lyme disease endemic area. J Med Entomol 32(4):522–526, 1995.

495. Schwartz BS, Goldstein MD, Childs JE. Longitudinal study of *Borrelia burgdorferi* infection in New Jersey outdoor workers, 1988–1991. Am J Epidemiol 139(5):504–512, 1994.

496. Orloski KA, Campbell GL, Genese CA, et al. Emergence of Lyme disease in Hunterdon County, New Jersey, 1993: a case-control study of risk factors and evaluation of reporting patterns. Am J Epidemiol 147(4):391–397, 1998.

497. Varde S, Beckley J, Schwartz I. Prevalence of tick-borne pathogens in Ixodes scapularis in a rural New Jersey county. Emerg Infect Dis 4(1):97–99, 1998.

498. Ravyn MD, Goodman JL, Kodner CB, et al. Immunodiagnosis of human granulocytic ehrlichiosis by using culture-derived human isolates. J Clin Microbiol 36(6):1480–1488, 1998.

499. Cromley EK, Cartter ML, Mrozinski RD, Ertel SH. Residential setting as a risk factor for Lyme disease in a hyperendermic region. Am J Epidemiol 147(5):472–477, 1998.

500. Jones CG, Ostfeld RS, Richard MP, et al. Chain reactions linking acorns to gypsy moth outbreaks and Lyme disease risk. Science 279(5353):1023–1026, 1998.

501. World Health Organization unpublished document. Report on an International Meeting, "EURO Workshop on Lyme Borreliosis," held in Baden (Vienna), Austria, 4 June 1987 (EUR/ICP/CDS 011 1989).

502. Stanek G, O'Connell S, Cimmino M, et al. European Union Concerted Action on Risk Assessment in Lyme Borreliosis: clinical case definitions for Lyme borreliosis. Wien Klin Wochenschr 108(23):741–747, 1996.

503. Strle F, Stantic-Pavlinic M. Lyme disease in Europe. N Engl J Med 334:803, 1996.

504. Flisiak R, Zabicka J. Epidemiologic situation of Lyme borreliosis in Europe. Przegl Epidemiol 49(4):375–379, 1995.

505. Neira O, Cerda C, Alvarado MA, et al. Lyme disease in Chile. Prevalence study in selected groups. Rev Med Chil 124(5):537–544, 1996.

506. Costa IP, Yoshinari NH, Barros PJ, et al. Lyme disease in Mato Grosso do Sul State, Brazil: report of three clinical cases. Including the first of Lyme meningitis in Brazil. Rev Hosp Clin Fac Med Sao Paulo 51(6):253–257, 1996.

507. Ellert-Zygadlowska J, Radowska D, Orlowski M, et al. Borreliosis—Lyme disease—a growing clinical problem. Przegl Lek 53(8):587–591, 1996.

508. Pancewicz SA, Januszkiewicz A, Hermanowska-Szpakowicz T. Detection of antibodies of *Borrelia burgdorferi* among inhabitants of north-eastern Poland. Przegl Epidemiol 50(4):375–381, 1996.

509. Gustafson R, Svenungsson B, Gardulf A, et al. Prevalence of tick-borne encephalitis and Lyme borreliosis in a defined Swedish population. Scand J Infect Dis 22:297, 1990.

510. Berglund J, Eitrem R, Norrby SR. Long-term study of Lyme borreliosis in a highly endemic area in Sweden. Scand J Infect Dis 28(5):473–478, 1996.

511. Berglund J, Eitrem R, Ornstein K, et al. An epidemiologic study of Lyme disease in southern Sweden. N Engl J Med 333(20):1319–1327, 1995.

512. Angelov L, Aeshliman A, Korenberg E, et al. Data on the epidemiology of Lyme disease in Bulgaria. Med Parazitol (Mosk) 4:13, 1990.

513. Christova I, Hohenberger S, Zehetmeier C, Wilske B. First characterization of *Borrelia burgdorferi* sensu lato from ticks and skin biopsy in Bulgaria. Med Microbiol Immunol 186(4):171–175, 1998.

514. Blaauw I, Nohlmans L, van den Bogaard T, van der Linden S. Diagnostic tools in Lyme borreliosis: clinical history compared with serology. J Clin Epidemiol 45:1229, 1992.

515. De Mik EL, Van Pelt W, Docters-van Leeuwen BD, et al. The geographical distribution of tick bites and erythema migrans in general practice in The Netherlands. Int J Epidemiol 26(2):451–457, 1997.

516. Wahlberg P, Granlund H, Nyman D, et al. Late Lyme borreliosis: epidemiology, diagnosis and clinical features. Ann Med 25(4):349–352, 1993.

517. Oksi J, Viljanen MK. Tick bites, clinical symptoms of Lyme borreliosis, and *Borrelia* antibody responses in Finnish army recruits training in an endemic region during summer. Mil Med 160(9):453–456, 1995.

518. Ishizaki H, Pyykko I, Nozue M. Neuroborreliosis in the etiology of vestibular neuronitis. Acta Oto-Laryngol Suppl 503:67–69, 1993.

519. Basta J, Janovska D, Daniel M. Educational status of the Czech population about Lyme borreliosis and experience with tick bites—pilot study. Epidemiol Mikrobiol Imunol 47(2):52–55, 1998.

520. Rohacova H, Hancil J, Hulinska D, et al. Ceftriaxone in the treatment of Lyme neuroborreliosis. Infection 24(1):88–90, 1996.

521. Fahrer H, van der Linden SM, Sauvain MJ, et al. The prevalence and incidence of clinical and asymptomatic Lyme borreliosis in a population at risk. J Infect Dis 163:305, 1991.

522. Fahrer H, Sauvain MJ, Zhioua E, et al. Longterm survey (7 years) in a population at risk for Lyme borreliosis: what happens to the seropositive individuals? Eur J Epidemiol 14(2):117–123, 1998.

523. Nadal D, Wunderli W, Briner H, Hansen K. Prevalence of antibodies to *Borrelia burgdorferi* in forest workers and blood donors from the same region in Switzerland. Eur J Clin Microbiol Infect Dis 8:992–995, 1989.

524. Neubert U, Munchhoff P, Volker B, et al. *Borrelia burgdorferi* infections in Bavarian forest workers. Ann N Y Acad Sci 539:476, 1988.

525. Schmidt R, Kabatzki J, Hartung S, Ackermann R. Erythema chronicum migrans disease in the Federal Repub-

lic of Germany. Zentralbl Bakteriol Mikrobiol Hyg A 263:435, 1986.

526. Sticht-Groh V, Martin R, Schmidt-Wolf I. Antibody titer determination against *Borrelia burgdorferi* in blood donors and in two different groups of patients. Ann N Y Acad Sci 539:497, 1988.

527. Rath PM, Ibershoff B, Mohnhaupt A, et al. Seroprevalence of Lyme borreliosis in forestry workers from Brandenburg, Germany. Eur J Clin Microbiol Infect Dis 15(5):372–377, 1996.

528. Maiwald M, Petney TN, Bruckner M, et al. Natural epidemiology of Lyme borreliosis with reference to clustered incidence of illnesses in the suburbs of a North Baden community. Gesundheitswesen 57(7):419–425, 1995.

529. Hauser U, Krahl H, Peters H, et al. Impact of strain heterogeneity on Lyme disease serology in Europe: comparison of enzyme-linked immunosorbent assays using different species of *Borrelia burgdorferi* sensu lato. J Clin Microbiol 36(2):427–436, 1998.

530. Christen HJ, Hanefeld F. Lyme borreliosis in childhood and pregancy. *In* Weber K, Burgdorfer W (eds). Aspects of Lyme borreliosis. Berlin, Springer-Verlag, 1993, pp 228–239.

531. Bussen S, Steck T. Manifestation of Lyme arthritis in the puerperal period. Z Geburtshilfe Perinatol 198(4):150–152, 1994.

532. Cimmino MA, Fumarola D, Sambri V, Accardo S. The epidemiology of Lyme borreliosis in Italy. Microbiologica 15:419, 1992.

533. Nuti M, Amaddeo D, Crovatto M, et al. Infections in an Alpine environment: antibodies to hantaviruses, leptospira, rickettsiae, and *Borrelia burgdorferi* in defined Italian populations. Am J Trop Med Hyg 48(1):20–25, 1993.

534. Petrovic M, Vogelaers D, Van Renterghem L, et al. Lyme borreliosis—a review of the late stages and treatment of four cases. Acta Clin Belg 53(3):178–183, 1998.

535. Dmitrovic R, Djordjevic D, Djerkovic V, et al. Epidemiology of Lyme borreliosis. Glas Srp Akad Nauka [Med] (43):11–21, 1993.

536. Isailovic G, Veljkovic M, Soc N, et al. Erythema migrans after a tick bite in a pregnant woman. Glas Srp Akad Nauka [Med] (43):173–175, 1993.

537. Jovanovic R, Hajric A, Cirkovic A, et al. Lyme disease and pregnancy. Glas Srp Akad Nauka [Med] (43):169–172, 1993.

538. Hamlet N, Nathwani D, Ho-Yen DO, Walker E. *Borrelia burgdorferi* infections in U.K. workers at risk of tick bites. Lancet 1:789, 1989.

539. Ho-Yen D, Bennet AJ, Chisholm S, Deacon AG. Lyme disease in the highlands. Scot Med J 35:168, 1990.

540. Muhlemann MF, Wright DJM. Emerging pattern of Lyme disease in the United Kingdom and Irish Republic. Lancet (Jan. 31):260, 1987.

541. Guy EC, Bateman DE, Martyn CN, et al. Lyme disease: prevalence and clinical importance of *Borrelia burgdorferi* specific IgG in forest workers. Lancet 1:484, 1989.

542. Morgan-Capner P, Cutler SJ, Wright DJM. *Borrelia burgdorferi* infection in U.K. workers at risk of tick bites. Lancet 1:789, 1989.

543. Rees DH, Axford JS. Evidence for Lyme disease in urban park workers: a potential new health hazard for city inhabitants. Br J Rheumatol 33(2):123–128, 1994.

544. Mawby TV, Lovett AA. The public health risks of Lyme disease in Breckland, U.K.: an investigation of environmental and social factors. Soc Sci Med 46(6):719–727, 1998.

545. O'Connell S. Lyme disease in the United Kingdom. BMJ 310(6975):303–308, 1995.

546. Ananjeva LP, Skripnikowva IA, Barskova VG, Steere AC. Clinical serologic features of Lyme borreliosis in Russia. J Rheumatol 22(4):689–694, 1995.

547. Jenum PA, Mehl R, Hasseltvedt V, Bjark P. Lyme borreliosis. Tidsskr Nor Laegeforen 114(17):1968–1973, 1994.

548. Cryan B, Cutler S, Wright DJM. Lyme disease in Ireland. Irish Med J 85:65, 1992.

549. Oteo JA, Martinez de Artola V, Casas J, et al. Epidemiology and prevalence of seropositivity against *Borrelia burgdorferi* antigen in La Rioja, Spain. Rev Epidemiol Sante Publique 40:85, 1992.

550. Guerrero A, Escudero R, Marti-Belda P, Quereda C. Frequency of the clinical manifestations of Lyme borreliosis in Spain. Enferm Infecc Microbiol Clin 14(2):72–79, 1996.

551. Saz JV, Merino FJ, Beltran M. Current status of Lyme disease in Spain: clinical and epidemiological aspects. Rev Clin Esp 195(1):44–49, 1995.

552. Chatzipanagiotou S, Papandreou-Rakitzis P, Malamou-Ladas H, Antoniou P. Determination of antibody titres for *Borrelia burgdorferi* in the serum of gipsies living in Attika, Greece. Eur J Clin Microbiol Infect Dis 11:477, 1992.

553. Santino I, Dastoli F, Lavorino C, et al. Determination of antibodies to *Borrelia burgdorferi* in the serum of patients living in Calabri, southern Italy. Panminerva Med 38(30):167–172, 1996.

554. Zhang Z. Geographic distribution of Lyme disease in Madanjiang. Chung Hua Liu Hsing Ping Hsueh Tsa Chih (Chinese J Epidemiol) 12:154, 1991.

555. Park KH, Chang WH, Schwan TG. Identification and characterization of Lyme disease spirochetes, *Borrelia burgdorferi* sensu lato, isolated in Korea. J Clin Microbiol 31:1831, 1993.

556. Maradiaga-Cecena MA, Llausas-Vargas A, Baguera-Heredia J, et al. Eritema cronico migratorio asociado a artritis. Enfermedad de Lyme o una variante. Rev Mex Reumatol 6:61, 1991.

557. Guzman L, Neira O. Lyme disease in Chile. J Rheumatol 20:774, 1993.

558. Azulay RD, Azulay-Abulafia L, Tavares-Sodre C, et al. Lyme disease in Rio de Janeiro, Brazil. Int J Dermatol 30:569, 1991.

559. Vasquez L, Couto C, Mato OL. Lyme disease: first case in Argentina. Prensa Med Argent 79:584, 1992.

560. Winward KE, Smith JL. Ocular disease in Caribbean patients with serologic evidence of Lyme borreliosis. J Clin Neuro-Ophthalmol 9:65, 1989.

561. Patial RK, Kashyap S, Bansal SK, Sood A. Lyme disease in a Shimla boy. J Assoc Physicians India 38:503, 1990.

562. Stanek G, Hirschl A, Stemberger H, et al. Does Lyme borreliosis also occur in tropical and subtropical areas? Zentralbl Bakteriol Mikrobiol Hyg A 263:491, 1986.

563. Nozais JP, Assous M, Cordier F, Gentilini M. A probable case of Lyme disease contracted in Mozambique. Bull Soc Pathol Exot 86(5):345–346, 1993.

564. Collares-Pereira M, Gomes AC, Prassad M, et al. Preliminary survey of leptospirosis and Lyme disease amongst febrile patients attending community hospital ambulatory care in Maputo, Mozambique. Cent Afr J Med 43(8):234–238, 1997.

565. Mhalu FS, Matre R. Serological evidence of Lyme borreliosis in Africa: results from studies in Dar es Salaam, Tanzania. East Afr Med J 73(9):583–585, 1996.

566. Abraham Z, Feuerman EJ, Rozenbaum M, Gluck Z.

Lyme disease in Israel. J Am Acad Dermatol 25:729, 1991.

567. Berger SA, Samish M, Klette RY, et al. Lyme disease acquired in Israel: report of a case and studies of serological cross reactivity in relapsing fever. Isr J Med Sci 29(8):464–465, 1993.

568. Hammouda NA, Hegazy IH, el-Sawy EH. ELISA screening for Lyme disease in children with chronic arthritis. J Egypt Soc Parasitol 25(2):525–533, 1995.

569. McColl GJ, Frauman AG, Dowling JP, Varigos GA. A report of Lyme disease in Victoria. Aust N Z J Med 24(3):324–325, 1994.

570. Santino I, Dastoli F, Sessa R, Del Piano M. Geographical incidence of infection with Borrelia burgdorferi in Europe. Panminerva Med 39(3):208–214, 1997.

571. Nidzovic Z, Stajkovic N, Bodiroga T. Use of repellents for protection against vectors of Lyme borreliosis. Glas Srp Akad Nauka [Med] (43):107–113, 1993.

572. Ackermann R, Horstrup P, Schmidt R. Tick-borne meningopolyneuritis (Garin-Bujadoux-Bannwarth). Yale J Biol Med 57:485, 1984.

573. Nakama H, Muramatsu K, Uchikama K, Yamagishi T. Possibility of Lyme disease as an occupational disease—seroepidemiological study of regional residents and forestry workers. Asia Pac J Public Health 7(4):214–217, 1994.

574. DiCaudo DJ, Su WP, Marshall WF, et al. Acrodermatitis chronica atrophicans in the United States: clinical and histopathologic features of six cases. Cutis 54(2):81–84, 1994.

575. Rees DH, O'Connell S, Brown MM, et al. The value of serological testing for Lyme disease in the UK. Br J Rheumatol 34(2):132–136, 1995.

576. Gregory RP, Green AD, Merry RT. Lyme disease in military personnel. J R Army Med Corps 139(1):11–13, 1993.

577. Shadick NA, Daltroy LH, Phillips CB, et al. Determinants of tick-avoidance behaviors in an endemic area for Lyme. Am J Prev Med 13(4):265–270, 1997.

578. Bosler EM, Ormiston BG, Coleman JL, et al. Prevalence of the Lyme disease spirochete in populations of white-tailed deer and white-footed mice. Yale J Biol Med 57:651, 1984.

579. Wegner Z, Racewicz M, Kubica-Biernat B, et al. The prevalence of Ixodes ricinus ticks (Acari, Ixodidae) in the forested areas of Gdansk, Sopot, and Gdynia and their infection rate with Borrelia burgdorferi spirochetes. Przegl Epidemiol 51(1–2):11–20, 1997.

580. Donahue JG, Piesman J, Spielman A. Reservoir competence of white-footed mice for Lyme disease spirochetes. Am J Trop Med Hyg 36:92, 1987.

581. Matuschka FR, Eiffert H, Ohlenbusch A, Spielman A. Amplifying role of edible dormice in Lyme disease transmission in central Europe. J Infect Dis 170(1):122–127, 1994.

582. Gill JS, McLean RG, Shriner RB, Johnson RC. Serologic surveillance for the Lyme disease spirochete, Borrelia burgdorferi, in Minnesota by using white-tailed deer as sentinel animals. J Clin Microbiol 32(2):444–451, 1994.

583. Ji B, Collins MT. Seroepidemiologic survey of Borrelia burgdorferi exposure of dairy cattle in Wisconsin. Am J Vet Res 55(9):1228–1231, 1994.

584. Levy SA, Lissman BA, Ficke CM. Performance of Borrelia burgdorferi bacterin in borreliosis-endemic areas. JAM Vet Med Assoc 202:1834–1838, 1993.

585. Coburn J, Magoun L, Bodary SC, Leong JM. Integrins $\alpha_v\beta_3$ and $\alpha_5\beta_1$ mediate attachment of Lyme disease spiro-

chetes to human cells. Infect Immun 66(5):1946–1952, 1998.

586. Leong JM, Wang H, Magoun L, et al. Different classes of proteoglycans contribute to the attachment of Borrelia burgdorferi to cultured endothelial and brain cells. Infect Immun 66(3):994–999, 1998.

587. Gross DM, Steere AC, Huber BT. T helper 1 response is dominant and localized to the synovial fluid in patients with Lyme arthritis. J Immunol 160(2):1022–1028, 1998.

588. Halperin J, Heyes MP. Neuroactive kynurenines in Lyme borreliosis. Neurology 42:43–50, 1992.

589. Roessner K, Trivdedi H, Gaur L, et al. Biased T-cell antigen receptor repertoire in Lyme arthritis. Infect Immun 66(3):1092–1099, 1998.

590. Duray PH, Steere AC. Clinical pathologic correlations of Lyme disease by stage. Ann N Y Acad Sci 539:65, 1988.

591. Wormser GP, Nowakowski J, Nadelman RB, et al. Improving the yield of blood cultures for patients with early Lyme disease. J Clin Microbiol 36(1):296–298, 1998.

592. Duray PH. Clinical pathologic correlations of Lyme disease. Rev Infect Dis 11(Suppl 6):S1487, 1989.

593. Persing DH, Rutledge BJ, Rys PN, et al. Target imbalance: disparity of Borrelia burgdorferi genetic material in synovial fluid from Lyme arthritis patients. J Infect Dis 169(3):668–672, 1994.

594. Hulshof MM, Vandenbroucke JP, Nohlmans LM, et al. Long-term prognosis in patients treated for erythema chronicum migrans and acrodermatitis chronica atrophicans. Arch Dermatol 133(1):33–37, 1997.

595. Goldberg NS, Forseter G, Nadelman RB, et al. Vesicular EM. Arch Dermatol 128:1495, 1992.

596. Berger BW. Dermatologic manifestations of Lyme disease. Rev Infect Dis 11(Suppl 6):S1475, 1989.

597. De Koning J. Histopathologic patterns of erythema migrans and borrelial lymphocytoma. Clin Dermatol 11(3):377–383, 1993.

598. Kramer N, Rickert RR, Brodkin RH, Rosenstein ED. Septal panniculitis as a manifestation of Lyme disease. Am J Med 81:149, 1986.

599. Asbrink E. Cutaneous manifestations of Lyme borreliosis: clinical definitions and differential diagnosis. Scand J Infect Dis Suppl 77:44, 1991.

600. Asbrink E, Brehmer-Andersson E, Hovmark A. Acrodermatitis chronica atrophicans—a spirochetosis. Am J Dermatopathol 8:209, 1986.

601. Buechner SA, Rufli T, Erb P. Acrodermatitis chronic atrophicans: a chronic T-cell–mediated immune reaction against Borrelia burgdorferi? Clinical, histologic, and immunohistochemical study of five cases. J Am Acad Dermatol 28(3):399–405, 1993.

602. De Koning J, Tazelaar DJ, Hoogkamp-Korstanje JA, Elema JD. Acrodermatitis chronica atrophicans: a light and electron microscopic study. J Cutan Pathol 22(1):23–32, 1995.

603. Granter SR, Barnhill RL, Hewins ME, Duray PH. Identification of Borrelia burgdorferi in diffuse fasciitis with peripheral eosinophilia: borrelial fasciitis. JAMA 272(16):1283–1285, 1994.

604. Rank EL, Dias SM, Hasson J, et al. Human necrotizing splenitis caused by Borrelia burgdorferi. Am J Clin Pathol 91:493, 1989.

605. Goellner MH, Agger WA, Burgess JH, Duray PH. Hepatitis due to recurrent Lyme disease. Ann Intern Med 108:707, 1988.

606. Ramakrishnan T, Gloster E, Bonagura VR, et al. Eosinophilic lymphadenitis in Lyme disease. Pediatr Infect Dis J 8:180, 1989.

607. Stanek G, Klein J, Bittner R, Glogar D. Borrelia burgdorf-

eri as an etiologic agent in chronic heart failure? Scand J Infect Dis Suppl 77:85, 1991.

608. Heller J, Holzer G, Schimrigk K. Immunological differentiation between neuroborreliosis and multiple sclerosis. J Neurol 237:465, 1990.

609. Meurers B, Kohlhepp W, Gold R, et al. Histopathological findings in the central and peripheral nervous systems in neuroborreliosis. J Neurol (Springer-Verlag) 237:113, 1990.

610. Murray R, Morawetz R, Kepes J, et al. Lyme neuroborreliosis manifesting as an intracranial mass lesion. Neurosurgery 30:769, 1992.

611. Maimone D, Villanova M, Stanta G, et al. Detection of *Borrelia burgdorferi* DNA and complement membrane attack complex deposits in the sural nerve of a patient with chronic polyneuropathy and tertiary Lyme disease. Muscle Nerve 20(8):969–975, 1997.

612. Kristoferitsch W, Sluga E, Graf M, et al. Neuropathy associated with acrodermatitis chronica atrophicans. Ann N Y Acad Sci 539:35, 1988.

613. Waniek C, Prohovnik I, Kaufman MA, Dwork AJ. Rapidly progressive frontal-type dementia associated with Lyme disease. J Neuropsychiatry Clin Neurosci 7(3):345–347, 1995.

614. Muller-Felber W, Reimers DC, de Koning J, et al. Myositis in Lyme borreliosis: an immunohistochemical study of seven patients. J Neurol Sci 118(2):207–212, 1993.

615. Callister SM, Schell RF, Lim LC, et al. Detection of borreliacidal antibodies by flow cytometry. An accurate, highly specific serodiagnostic test for Lyme disease. Arch Intern Med 154(14):1625–1632, 1994.

616. Ilowite NT. Muscle, reticuloendothelial, and late skin manifestations of Lyme disease. Am J Med 98(4A):63S–68S, 1995.

617. Hoffmann JC, Stichtenoth DO, Zeidler H, et al. Lyme disease in a 74-year-old forest owner with symptoms of dermatomyositis. Arthritis Rheum 38(8):1157–1160, 1995.

618. Johnston YE, Duray PH, Steere AC, et al. Lyme arthritis: spirochetes found in synovial microangiopathic lesions. Am J Pathol 118:26, 1985.

619. Steere AC, Green J, Schoen RT, et al. Successful parenteral penicillin therapy of established Lyme arthritis. N Engl J Med 312:869, 1985.

620. Nanagara R, Duray PH, Schumacher HR Jr. Ultrastructural demonstration of spirochetal antigens in synovial fluid and synovial membrane in chronic Lyme disease: possible factors contributing to persistence of organisms. Hum Pathol 27(10):1025–1034, 1996.

621. Gardner T. Lyme disease. *In* Infectious Diseases of the Fetus and Newborn Infant. Remington J, Klein JO (eds). Philadelphia, WB Saunders, 1995, pp 489–493.

622. Mikkelsen AL, Palle C. Case report: Lyme disease during pregnancy. Acta Obstet Gynecol Scand 66:477, 1987.

623. Figueroa R, Bracero LA, Aguero-Rosenfeld M, et al. Confirmation of *Borrelia burgdorferi* spirochetes by polymerase chain reaction in placentas of women with reactive serology for Lyme antibodies. Gynecol Obstet Invest 41(4):240–243, 1996.

624. Hashkes PJ, Lovell DJ. Recognition of infantile-onset multisystem inflammatory disease as a unique entity. J Pediatr 130(4):513–515, 1997.

625. Yarom A, Rennebohm RM, Levinson JE. Infantile multisystem inflammatory disease: a specific syndrome? J Pediatr 106:390, 1985.

626. Prieur HM, Griscelli C. Arthropathy with rash, chronic meningitis, eye lesions, and mental retardation. J Pediatr 99:79, 1981.

627. Steenbarger JR. Congenital tick-borne relapsing fever: report of a case with first documentation of transplacental transmission. March of Dimes Birth Defects Foundation, Birth Defects: Original Article Series 18:39, 1982.

628. Yagupsky P, Shimon M. Neonatal Borrelia species infection (relapsing fever). Am J Dis Child 139:74, 1985.

629. Shaked Y, Shpilberg O, Samra D, Samra Y. Leptospirosis in pregnancy and its effect on the fetus: case report and review. Clin Infect Dis 17(2):241–243, 1993.

630. New DL, Quinn JB, Qureshi MZ, Sigler SJ. Vertically transmitted babesiosis [letter; comment]. J Pediatr 131(1 Pt 1):163–164, 1997.

631. Horowitz HW, Kilchevsky E, Haber S, et al. Perinatal transmission of the agent of human granulocytic ehrlichiosis. N Engl J Med 339(6):375–378, 1998. (Reply to letter. N Engl J Med 339(26):1942–1943, 1998.)

632. Buitrago MI, Ijdo JW, Rinaudo P, et al. Human granulocytic ehrlichiosis during pregnancy treated successfully with rifampin. Clin Infect Dis 27(1):213–215, 1998.

633. Centers for Disease Control and Prevention. Lyme disease—diagnostic criteria. MMWR 46(RR):20–21, 1997.

634. Asbrink E, Hovmark A. Comments on the course and classification of Lyme borreliosis. Scand J Infect Dis Suppl 77:41, 1991.

635. Rahn DW, Felz MW. Lyme disease update. Current approach to early, disseminated, and late disease. Postgrad Med 103(5):51–54, 57–59, 63–64 passim, 1998.

636. Feder HM Jr, Gerber MA, Krause PJ, et al. Early Lyme disease: a flu like illness without erythema migrans. Pediatrics 91(2):456–459, 1993.

637. Steere AC, Schoen RT, Taylor E. The clinical evolution of Lyme arthritis. Ann Intern Med 107:725, 1987.

638. Williams CL, Strobino B, Lee A, et al. Lyme disease in childhood: clinical and epidemiologic features of ninety cases. Pediatr Infect Dis J 9:10, 1990.

639. Nadelman RB, Wormser GP. Erythema migrans and early Lyme disease. Am J Med 98(4A):15S–23S; discussion 23S–24S, 1995.

640. Nadelman RB, Nowakowski J, Forseter G, et al. The clinical spectrum of early Lyme borreliosis in patients with culture-confirmed erythema migrans. Am J Med 100(5):502–508, 1996.

641. Herzer P. Joint manifestations of Lyme borreliosis in Europe. Scand J Infect Dis Suppl 77:55, 1991.

642. Berger BW. Current aspects of Lyme disease and other *Borrelia burgdorferi* infections. Dermatol Clin 15(2):247–255, 1997.

643. Gerber MA, Shapiro ED, Burke GS, et al. Lyme disease in children in southeastern Connecticut. Pediatric Lyme Disease Study Group. N Engl J Med 335(17):1270–1274, 1996.

644. Strle F, Pleterski-Rigler D, Stanek G, et al. Solitary borrelial lymphocytoma: report of 36 cases. Infection 20:201, 1992.

645. Pohl-Koppe A, Wilske B, Weiss M, Schmidt H. *Borrelia* lymphoctyoma in childhood. Pediatr Infect Dis J 17(5):423–426, 1998.

646. Strle F, Maraspin V, Pleterski-Rigler D, et al. Treatment of borrelial lymphocytoma. Infection 24(1):80–84, 1996.

647. Kutting B, Bonsmann G, Metze D, et al. *Borrelia burgdorferi*–associated primary cutaneous B cell lymphoma: complete clearing of skin lesions after antibiotic pulse therapy or intralesional injection of interferon alfa-2a. J Am Acad Dermatol 36(2 Pt 2):311–314, 1997.

648. Gerber MA, Zemel LS, Shapiro ED. Lyme arthritis in children: clinical epidemiology and long-term outcomes. Pediatrics 102(4 Pt 1):905–908, 1998.

649. Huppertz HI, Karch H, Suschke HJ, et al. Lyme arthritis in European children and adolescents. The Pediatric Rheumatology Collaborative Group. Arthritis Rheum 38(3):361–368, 1995.

650. Huppertz HI, Bentas W, Haubitz I, et al. Diagnosis of paediatric Lyme arthritis using a clinical score. Eur J Pediatr 157(4):304–308, 1998.

651. Steere AC. Clinical definitions and differential diagnosis of Lyme arthritis. Scand J Infect Dis Suppl 77:51, 1991.

652. Steere AC. Diagnosis and treatment of Lyme arthritis. Med Clin North Am 81(1):179–194, 1997.

653. Miller A, Stanton RP, Eppes SC. Acute arthritis of the hip in a child infected with the Lyme spirochete. Clin Orthop Rel Res (286):212–214, 1993.

654. Albisetti M, Schaer G, Good M, et al. Diagnostic value of cerebrospinal fluid examination in children with peripheral facial palsy and suspected Lyme borreliosis. Neurology 49(3):817–824, 1997.

655. Logigian EL, Kaplan RF, Steere AC. Chronic neurologic manifestations of Lyme disease. N Engl J Med 323:1438, 1990.

656. Halperin JJ. North American Lyme neuroborreliosis. Scand J Infect Dis Suppl 77:74, 1991.

657. Halperin JJ, Logigian EL, Finkel MF, Pearl RA. Practice parameters for the diagnosis of patients with nervous system Lyme borreliosis (Lyme disease). Quality Standards Subcommittee of the American Academy of Neurology. Neurology 46(3):619–627, 1996.

658. Pachner AR. Early disseminated Lyme disease: Lyme meningitis. Am J Med 98(4A):30S–37S; discussion 37S–43S, 1995.

659. Clark JR, Carlson RD, Sasaki CT, et al. Facial paralysis in Lyme disease. Laryngoscope 95:1341, 1985.

660. Cook SP, Macartney KK, Rose CD, et al. Lyme disease and seventh nerve paralysis in children. Am J Otolaryngol 18(5):320–323, 1997.

661. Belman AL, Reynolds L, Preston T, et al. Cerebrospinal fluid findings in children with Lyme disease–associated facial nerve palsy. Arch Pediatr Adolesc Med 151(12):1224–1228, 1997.

662. Logigian EL, Steere AC. Clinical and electrophysiologic findings in chronic neuropathy of Lyme disease. Neurology 42:303, 1992.

663. Fallon BA, Nields JA, Burrascano JJ, et al. The neuropsychiatric manifestations of Lyme borreliosis. Psychiatr Q 63:95, 1992.

664. Pfister HW, Preac-Mursic V, Wilske B, et al. Catatonic syndrome in acute severe encephalitis due to *Borrelia burgdorferi* infection. Neurology 43(2):433–435, 1993.

665. Kaplan RF, Jones-Woodward L. Lyme encephalopathy: a neuropsychological perspective. Semin Neurol 17(1):31–37, 1997.

666. Fallon BA, Das S, Plutchok JJ, et al. Functional brain imaging and neuropsychological testing in Lyme disease. Clin Infect Dis 25(Suppl 1):S57–S63, 1997.

667. Logigian EL, Johnson KA, Kijewski MF, et al. Reversible cerebral hypoperfusion in Lyme encephalopathy. Neurology 49(6):1661–1670, 1997.

668. Salonen R, Rinne JO, Halonen P, et al. Lyme borreliosis associated with complete flaccid paraplegia. J Infect 28(2):181–184, 1994.

669. Olivares JP, Pallas F, Ceccaldi M, et al. Lyme disease presenting as isolated acute urinary retention caused by transverse myelitis: an electrophysiological and urodynamical study. Arch Phys Med Rehabil 76(12):1171–1172, 1995.

670. Kindstrand E, Nilsson BY, Hovmark A, et al. Peripheral neuropathy in acrodermatitis chronica atrophicans—a late Borrelia manifestation. Acta Neurol Scand 95(6):338–345, 1997.

671. Curless RG, Schatz NJ, Bowen BC, et al. Lyme neuroborreliosis masquerading as a brainstem tumor in a 15-year-old. Pediatr Neurol 15(3):258–260, 1996.

672. Oksi J, Kalimo H, Martila RJ, et al. Intracranial aneurysms in three patients with disseminated Lyme borreliosis: cause or chance association? J Neurol Neurosurg Psychiatr 64(5):636–642, 1998.

673. Feder HM, Jr, Zalneraitis EL, Reik L, Jr. Lyme disease: acute focal meningoencephalitis in a child. Pediatrics 82:931, 1988.

674. Reik L Jr. Stroke due to Lyme disease. Neurology 43(12):2705–2707, 1993.

675. Broderick JP, Sandok BA, Mertz LE. Focal encephalitis in a young woman 6 years after the onset of Lyme disease: tertiary Lyme disease? Mayo Clin Proc 62:313, 1987.

676. Chehrenama M, Zagardo MT, Koski CL. Subarachnoid hemorrhage in a patient with Lyme disease. Neurology 48(2):520–523, 1997.

677. Hemmer B, Glockner FX, Kaiser R, et al. Generalized motor neuron disease as an unusual manifestation of *Borrelia burgdorferi* infection. J Neurol Neurosurg Psychiatr 63:257–258, 1997.

678. Chancellor MB, McGinnis DE, Shenot PJ, et al. Urinary dysfunction in Lyme disease. J Urol 149(1):26–30, 1993.

679. Sigler S, Kershaw P, Scheuch R, et al. Respiratory failure due to Lyme meningoradiculitis. Am J Med 103(6):544–547, 1997.

680. Demaerel P, Crevits I, Casteels-Van Daele M, Baert AL. Meningoradiculitis due to borreliosis presenting as low back pain only. Neuroradiology 40(2):126–127, 1998.

681. Benke T, Gasse T, Hittmair-Delazer M, Schmutzhard E. Lyme encephalopathy: long-term neuropsychological deficits years after acute neuroborreliosis. Acta Neurol Scand 91(5):353–357, 1995.

682. Ravdin LD, Hilton E, Primeau M, et al. Memory functioning in Lyme borreliosis. J Clin Psychiatr 57(7):282–286, 1996.

683. Shadick NA, Phillips CB, Logigan EL, et al. The long-term clinical outcomes of Lyme disease. A population-based retrospective cohort study. Ann Intern Med 121(8):560–567, 1994.

684. Bloom BJ, Wyckoff PM, Meissner HC, Steere AC. Neurocognitive abnormalities in children after classic manifestations of Lyme disease. Pediatr Infect Dis J 17(3):189–196, 1998.

685. Fernandez RE, Rothberg M, Ferencz G, Wujack D. Lyme disease of the CNS: MR imaging findings in 14 cases. AJNR 11:479, 1990.

686. Rubin DA, Sorbera C, Nikitin P, et al. Prospective evaluation of heart block complicating early Lyme disease. Pacing Clin Electrophysiol 15:252, 1992.

687. Steere AC, Batsford WP, Weinberg M, et al. Lyme carditis: cardiac abnormalities of Lyme disease. Ann Intern Med 93:8, 1980.

688. Sigal LH. Early disseminated Lyme disease: cardiac manifestations. Am J Med 98(4A):25S–28S; discussion 28S–29S, 1995.

689. van der Linde MR. Lyme carditis: clinical characteristics of 105 cases. Scand J Infect Dis Suppl 77:81, 1991.

690. Robinson TT, Herman L, Birrer RB, et al. Lyme carditis: a rare presentation in an unexpected setting. Am J Emerg Med 16(3):265–269, 1998.

691. Bruyn GA, De Koning J, Reijsoo FJ, et al. Lyme pericarditis leading to tamponade. Br J Rheumatol 33(9):862–866, 1994.

692. Gasser R, Fruhwald F, Schumacher M, et al. Reversal of *Borrelia burgdorferi* associated dilated cardiomyopathy by antibiotic treatment? Cardiovasc Drugs Ther 10(3):351–360, 1996.

693. Anish SA. Case report: possible Lyme endocarditis. N J Med 90(8):599–601, 1993.

694. Sangha O, Phillips CB, Fleischmann KE, et al. Lack of cardiac manifestations among patients with previously treated Lyme disease. Ann Intern Med 128(5):346–353, 1998.

695. Gellis SE, Stadecker MJ, Steere AC. Spirochetes in atrophic skin lesions accompanied by minimal host response in a child with Lyme disease. J Am Acad Dermatol 25:395, 1991.

696. Patmas MA. Lyme disease: the evolution of erythema chronicum migrans into acrodermatitis chronica strophicans. Cutis 52(3):169–170, 1993.

697. Gerster JC, et al. Rheumatic manifestations related to acrodermatitis chronica atrophicans. A review of four cases. Rev Rhum Engl Ed 65(10):567–570, 1998.

698. Edwards KS, Kanengiser S, Li KI, et al. Lyme disease presenting as heptatitis and jaundice in a child. Pediatr Infect Dis J 9:592, 1990.

699. Oksi J, Mertsola J, Reunanen M, et al. Subacute multiple-site osteomyelitis caused by *Borrelia burgdorferi*. Clin Infect Dis 19(5):891–896, 1994.

700. Horowitz HW, Dworkin B, Forseter G, et al. Liver function in early Lyme disease. Hepatology 23(6):1412–1417, 1996.

701. Lesser RL. Ocular manifestations of Lyme disease. Am J Med 98(4A):60S–62S, 1995.

702. Bergloff J, Gasser R, Feigl B. Ophthalmic manifestations in Lyme borreliosis. A review. J Neuro-Ophthalmol 14(1):15–20, 1994.

703. Seidenberg KB, Leib ML. Orbital myositis with Lyme disease. Am J Ophthal 109:13–16, 1990.

704. Strominger MB, Slamovits TL, Herskovitz S, Lipton RB. Transient worsening of optic neuropathy as a sequela of the Jarisch-Herxheimer reaction in the treatment of Lyme disease. J Neuro-Ophthalmol 14(2):77–80, 1994.

705. Koch F, Augustin AJ, Boker T. Neuroborreliosis with retinal pigment epithelium detachments. Ger J Ophthalmol 5(1):12–15, 1996.

706. Pizzarello LD, MacDonald AB, Semlear R, et al. Temporal arteritis associated with Borrelia infection: a case report. J Clin Neuroophthalmol 9:3–6, 1989.

707. Moscatello AL, Worden DL, Nadelman RB, et al. Otolaryngologic aspects of Lyme disease. Laryngoscope 101:592, 1991.

708. Scasso CA, Bruschini L, Berrettini S, Bruschini P. Progressive sensorineural hearing loss from infectious agents. Acta Otorhinolaryngol Ital 18(4 Suppl 59):51–54, 1998.

709. Quinn SJ, Boucher BJ, Booth JB. Reversible sensorineural hearing loss in Lyme disease. J Laryngol Otol 111(6):562–564, 1997.

710. Heir GM, Fein LA. Lyme disease awareness for the New Jersey dentist. A survey of orofacial and headache complaints associated with Lyme disease. J N J Dent Assoc 69(1):19, 21, 62–63 passim, 1998.

711. Gunthard HF, Peter O, Gubler J. Leukopenia and thrombocytopenia in a patient with early Lyme borreliosis. Clin Infect Dis 22(6):1119–1120, 1996.

712. Cantero-Hinojosa J, Diez-Ruiz A, Santos-Perez JL, et al. Lyme disease associated with hemophagocytic syndrome. Clin Invest 71(8):620, 1993.

713. Gaudino EA, Coyle PK, Krupp LB. Post-Lyme syndrome and chronic fatigue syndrome. Neuropsychiatric

714. Bujak DI, Weinstein A, Dornbush RL. Clinical and neurocognitive features of the post Lyme syndrome. J Rheumatol 23(8):1392–1397, 1996.

715. Dinerman H, Steere AC. Lyme disease associated with fibromyalgia. Ann Intern Med 117:281, 1992.

716. Salazar JC, Gerber MA, Goff CW. Long-term outcome of Lyme disease in children given early treatment. J Pediatr 122(4):591–593, 1993.

717. Nowakowski J, Schwartz I, Nadelman RB, et al. Culture-confirmed infection and reinfection with *Borrelia burgdorferi*. Ann Intern Med 127(2):130–132, 1997.

718. Golde WT, Robinson-Dunn B, Stobierski MG, et al. Culture-confirmed reinfection of a person with different strains of *Borrelia burgdorferi* sensu stricto. J Clin Microbiol 36(4):1015–1019, 1998.

719. Berger BW. Treatment of erythema chronicum migrans of Lyme disease. Ann N Y Acad Sci 539:346, 1988.

720. Berger BW. Treating erythema chronicum migrans of Lyme disease. J Am Acad Dermatol 15:459, 1986.

721. Luger SW. Active Lyme borreliosis in pregnancy: outcomes of six cases with stage 1, stage 2, and stage 3 disease. Fourth International Conference on Lyme Borreliosis, Stockholm, Books A and B abstracts, 1990.

722. Schutzer SE, Janniger CK, Schwartz RA. Lyme disease in pregnancy. Cutis 47:267, 1991.

723. Stiernstedt G. Lyme borreliosis during pregnancy. Scand J Infect Dis Suppl 71:99, 1990.

724. Elsukova LV, Korenberg EI, Kozin GA. Pathology of pregnancy and the fetus in Lyme disease. Med Parazitol (Mosk) (4):59–62, 1994.

725. Neubert U. Clinical aspects of *Borrelia burgdorferi* infections. Z Hautkr 64(8):649–652, 655–656, 1989.

726. Lakos A. Lyme borreliosis and pregnancy [abstract no. P11]. *In* Symposium on the therapy and prophylaxis for Lyme borreliosis. Portoroz, Slovenia, Austrian Society for Hygiene and Slovenian Society for Infectious Diseases, 1995, p 43.

727. Gerber MA, Zalneraitis EL. Childhood neurologic disorders and Lyme disease during pregnancy. Pediatr Neurol 11(1):41–43, 1994.

728. Strobino B, et al. Maternal Lyme disease and congenital heart disease: A case-control study in an endemic area. Am J Obstet Gynecol 180(3 Pt 1):711–716, 1999.

729. Sigal LH. Lyme disease: testing and treatment. Who should be tested and treated for Lyme disease and how? Rheum Dis Clin North Am 19(1):79–93, 1993.

730. Nocton JJ, Steere AC. Lyme disease. Adv Intern Med 40:69–117, 1995.

731. Sicuranza G, Baker DA. Lyme disease in pregnancy. *In* Coyle PK (ed). Lyme Disease. St. Louis, Mosby-Year Book, 1993, pp 184–186.

732. Silver RM, Yang L, Daynes RA, et al. Fetal outcome in murine Lyme disease. Infect Immun 63(1):66–72, 1995.

733. Shapiro ED. Lyme disease. Pediatr Rev 19(5):147–154, 1998.

734. Eckman MH, Steere AC, Kalish RA, Pauker SG. Cost effectiveness of oral as compared with intravenous antibiotic therapy for patients with early Lyme disease or Lyme arthritis. N Engl J Med 337(5):357–363, 1997.

735. Nichol KG, Dennis DT, Steere AC, et al. Test-treatment strategies for patients suspected of having Lyme disease: a cost-effectiveness analysis. Ann Intern Med 128(1):37–48, 1998.

736. Lightfoot RW Jr, Luft BJ, Rahn DW, et al. Empiric parenteral antibiotic treatment of patients with fibromyalgia and fatigue and a positive serologic result for Lyme

disease. A cost-effectiveness analysis. Ann Intern Med 119(6):503–509, 1993.

737. Fix AD, Strickland GT, Grant J. Tick bites and Lyme disease in an endemic setting: problematic use of serologic testing and prophylactic antibiotic therapy. JAMA 279(3):206–210, 1998.

738. Guy EC, Robertson JN, Cimmino M, et al. European interlaboratory comparison of Lyme borreliosis serology. Zentralbl Bakteriol 287(3):241–247, 1998.

739. Bakken LL, Callister SM, Wand PJ, Schell RF. Interlaboratory comparison of test results for detection of Lyme disease by 516 participants in the Wisconsin State Laboratory of Hygiene/College of American Pathologists Proficiency Testing Program. J Clin Microbiol 35(3):537–543, 1997.

740. Dayian G, Morse DL, Schryver GD, et al. Implementation of a proficiency testing program for Lyme disease in New York State. Arch Pathol Lab Med 118(5):501–505, 1994.

741. Craven RB, Quan TJ, Bailey RE, et al. Improved serodiagnostic testing for Lyme disease: results of a multicenter serologic evaluation. Emerg Infect Dis 2(2):136–140, 1996.

742. Rose CD, Fawcett PT, Singsen BH, et al. Use of Western blot and enzyme-linked immunosorbent assays to assist in the diagnosis of Lyme disease. Pediatrics 88:465, 1991.

743. Weiss NL, Sadock VA, Sigal LH, et al. False positive seroreactivity to Borrelia burgdorferi in systemic lupus erythematosus: the value of immunoblot analysis. Lupus 4(2):131–137, 1995.

744. Fatehnejad S, Fikrig MK, Rahn DW, Malawista SE. Parvovirus arthritis mistaken for Lyme arthritis. J Rheumatol 19:1002, 1992.

745. Kaell AT, Redecha PR, Elkon KB, et al. Occurrence of antibodies to Borrelia burgdorferi in patients with nonspirochetal subacute bacterial endocarditis. Ann Intern Med 119(11):1079–1083, 1993.

746. Hansen K, Pii K, Lebech A-M. Improved immunoglobulin M serodiagnosis in Lyme borreliosis by using a μ-capture enzyme-linked immunosorbent assay with biotinylated Borrelia burgdorferi flagella. J Clin Microbiol 29:166–173, 1991.

747. Wormser GP, Horowitz HW, Nowakowski J, et al. Positive Lyme disease serology in patients with clinical and laboratory evidence of human granulocytic ehrlichiosis. Am J Clin Pathol 107(2):142–147, 1997.

748. Tugwell P, Dennis DT, Weinstein A, et al. Guidelines for laboratory evaluation in the diagnosis of Lyme disease. American College of Physicians. Ann Intern Med 127(12):1106–1108, 1997.

749. Association of State and Territorial Public Health Laboratory Directors and the Centers for Disease Control and Prevention. Recommendations. In Proceedings of the Second National Conference on Serologic Diagnosis of Lyme Disease (Dearborn, MI). Washington, DC, Association of State and Territorial Public Health Laboratory Directors, 1995, pp 1–5.

750. Golightly MG. Lyme borreliosis: laboratory considerations. Semin Neurol 17(1):11–17, 1997.

751. Steere AC, Grodzicki RL, Craft JE, et al. Recovery of Lyme disease spirochetes from patients. Yale J Biol Med 57:557, 1984.

752. Berger BW, Johnson RC, Kodner C, Coleman L. Cultivation of Borrelia burgdorferi from human tick bite sites: a guide to the risk of infection. J Am Acad Dermatol 32(2 Pt 1):184–187, 1995.

753. Wienecke R, Neubert U, Volkenandt M. Molecular detection of Borrelia burgdorferi in formalin-fixed, paraffin-embedded lesions of Lyme disease. J Cutan Pathol 20(5):385–388, 1993.

754. Schmidt BL, Aberer E, Stockenhuber D, et al. Detection of Borrelia burgdorferi DNA by polymerase chain reaction in the urine and breast milk of patients with Lyme borreliosis. Diagn Microbiol Infect Dis 21(3):121–128, 1995.

755. Priem S, Rittig MG, Kamradt T, et al. An optimized PCR leads to rapid and highly sensitive detection of Borrelia burgdorferi in patients with Lyme borreliosis. J Clin Microbiol 35(3):685–690, 1997.

756. Brunner M, Stein S, Mitchell PD, Sigal LH. Immunoglobulin M capture assay for serologic confirmation of early Lyme disease: analysis of immune complexes with biotinylated Borrelia burgdorferi sonicate enhanced with flagellin peptide epitope. J Clin Microbiol 36(4):1074–1080, 1998.

757. Berardi VP, Weeks KE, Steere AC. Serodiagnosis of early Lyme disease: analysis of IgM and IgG antibody responses by using an antibody-capture enzyme immunoassay. J Infect Dis 158:754, 1988.

758. Magnarelli LA, Anderson JF, Johnson RC. Cross-reactivity in serological tests for Lyme disease and other spirochetal infections. J Infect Dis 156:183, 1987.

759. Hilton E, Devoti J, Sood S. Recommendation to include OspA and OspB in the new immunoblotting criteria for serodiagnosis of Lyme disease [published erratum appears in J Clin Microbiol 1997 October; 35(10):2713]. J Clin Microbiol 34(6):1353–1354, 1996.

760. Bunikis J, Olsen B, Westman G, Bergstroom S. Variable serum immunoglobulin responses against different Borrelia burgdorferi sensu lato species in a population at risk for and patients with Lyme disease. J Clin Microbiol 33(6):1473–1478, 1995.

761. Norman GL, Antig JM, Bigaignon G, Hogrefe WR. Serodiagnosis of Lyme borreliosis by Borrelia burgdorferi sensu stricto, B. garinii, and B. afzelii western blots (immunoblots). J Clin Microbiol 34(7):1732–1738, 1996.

762. Rath PM, Marsch WC, Brade V, Fehrenbach F. Serological distinction between syphilis and Lyme borreliosis. Zentralbl Bakteriol 280(3):319–324, 1994.

763. Rose CD, Fawcett PT, Gibney KM, Doughty RA. The overdiagnosis of Lyme disease in children residing in an endemic area. Clin Pediatr 33(11):663–668, 1994.

764. Fawcett PT, Rose CD, Gibney KM, Doughty RA. Correlation of seroreactivity with response to antibiotics in pediatric Lyme borreliosis. Clin Diagn Lab Immunol 4(1):85–88, 1997.

765. Huppertz HI, Mosbauer S, Busch DH, Karch H. Lymphoproliferative responses to Borrelia burgdorferi in the diagnosis of Lyme arthritis in children and adolescents. Eur J Pediatr 155(4):297–302, 1996.

766. Quan TJ, Wilmoth BA, Carter LG, Bailey RE. A comparison of some commercially available serodiagnostic kits for Lyme disease. In Proceedings of the First National Conference on Lyme Disease Testing (Dearborn, MI). Washington, DC, Association of State and Territorial Public Health Laboratory Directors, 1991, pp 61–73.

767. Reid MC, Schoen RT, Evans J, et al. The consequences of overdiagnosis and overtreatment of Lyme disease: an observational study. Ann Intern Med 128(5):354–362, 1998.

768. Feder HM Jr, Hunt MS. Pitfalls in the diagnosis and treatment of Lyme disease in children. JAMA 274(1):66–68, 1995.

769. Hsu VM, Patella SJ, Sigal LH. "Chronic Lyme disease" as the incorrect diagnosis in patients with fibromyalgia. Arthritis Rheum 36(11):1493–1500, 1993.

770. Sigal LH. Summary of the first 100 patients seen at a Lyme referral center. Am J Med 88:577–581, 1990.

771. Steere AC, Pachner AR, Malawista SE. Neurologic abnormalities of Lyme disease: successful treatment with high-dose intravenous penicillin. Ann Intern Med 99:767, 1983.

772. Jung PI, Nahas JN, Strickland GT, et al. Maryland physicians' survey on Lyme disease. Maryland Med J 43(5):447–450, 1994.

773. Eppes SC, Klein JD, Caputo GM, et al. Physician beliefs, attitudes, and approaches toward Lyme disease in an endemic area. Clin Pediatr 33(3):130–134, 1994.

774. Ziska MH, Donta ST, Demarest FC. Physician preferences in the diagnosis and treatment of Lyme disease in the United States. Infection 24(2):182–186, 1996.

775. Dattwyler RJ, Halperin JJ, Volkman DJ, Luft BJ. Treatment of late Lyme borreliosis–randomised comparison of ceftriaxone and penicillin. Lancet 1:1191, 1988.

776. Hassler D, Zoller L, Haude M, et al. Cefotaxime versus penicillin in the late stage of Lyme disease—prospective, randomized therapeutic study. Infection 18:16, 1990.

777. Cooper JD, Schoen RT, Malawista SE. Treatment of asymptomatic, retrospectively diagnosed Lyme disease: comment on the report by Christian. Arthritis Rheum 36:1637–1638, 1993.

778. Millner MM, Thalhammer GH, Dittrich P, et al. Beta-lactam antibiotics in the treatment of neuroborreliosis in children: preliminary results. Infection 24(2):174–177, 1996.

779. Karlsson M, Hammers S, Nilsson-Ehle I, et al. Concentrations of doxycycline and penicillin G in sera and cerebrospinal fluid of patients treated for neuroborreliosis. Antimicrob Agents Chemother 40(5):1104–1107, 1996.

780. Wormser GP. Treatment and prevention of Lyme disease, with emphasis on antimicrobial therapy for neuroborreliosis and vaccination. Semin Neurol 17(1):45–52, 1997.

781. Maloy AL, Black RD, Segurola RJ, Jr. Lyme disease complicated by the Jarisch-Herxheimer reaction. J Emerg Med 16(3):437–438, 1998.

782. Dattwyler RJ, Volkman DJ, Conaty SM, et al. Amoxycillin plus probenecid versus doxycycline for treatment of EM borreliosis. Lancet 336:1404, 1990.

783. Nadelman RB, Luger SW, Frank E, et al. Comparison of cefuroxime axetil and doxycycline in the treatment of early Lyme disease. Ann Intern Med 117:273, 1992.

784. Luger SW, Paparone P, Wormser GP, et al. Comparison of cefuroxime axetil and doxycycline in treatment of patients with early Lyme disease associated with erythema migrans. Antimicrob Agents Chemother 39(3):661–667, 1995.

785. Weber K, Preac-Mursic V, Wilske B, et al. A randomized trial of ceftriaxone versus oral penicillin for the treatment of early European Lyme borreliosis. Infection 18:91, 1990.

786. Dattwyler RJ, Luft BJ, Kunkel MJ, et al. Ceftriaxone compared with doxycycline for the treatment of acute disseminated Lyme disease. N Engl J Med 337(5):289–294, 1997.

787. Genese C, Fineli L, Parkin W, Spitalny KC. From the Centers for Disease Control and Prevention. Ceftriaxone-associated biliary complications of treatment of suspected disseminated Lyme disease—New Jersey, 1990–1992. JAMA 269(8):979–980, 1993.

788. Ettestad PJ, Campbell GL, Welbel SF, et al. Biliary complications in the treatment of unsubstantiated Lyme disease. J Infect Dis 171(2):356–361, 1995.

789. Kuiper H, de Jongh BM, van Dam AP, et al. Evaluation of central nervous system involvement in Lyme borreliosis patients with a solitary erythema migrans lesion. Eur J Clin Microbiol Infect Dis 13(5):379–387, 1994.

790. Wang TJ, Sangha O, Phillips CB, et al. Outcomes of children treated for Lyme disease. J Rheumatol 25(11):2249–2253, 1998.

791. National Institute of Arthritis and Musculoskeletal and Skin Disease, and National Institute of Allergy and Infectious Disease. Diagnosis and treatment of Lyme disease, N.I.H. State-of-the-Art Conference. Clin Courier 9(5):1, 1991.

792. Schoen RT, Aversa JM, Rahn DW, Steere AC. Treatment of refractory chronic Lyme arthritis with arthroscopic synovectomy. Arthritis Rheum 34:1056, 1991.

793. Smith LG, Jr, Pearlman M, Smith LG, Faro S. Lyme disease: a review with emphasis on the pregnant woman. Obstet Gynecol Surv 46:125, 1991.

794. Pal GS, Baker JT, Wright DJM. Penicillin-resistant Borrelia encephalitis responding to cefotaxime. Letter. Lancet 1:50, 1988.

795. Diringer MN, Halperin JJ, Dattwyler RJ. Lyme meningoencephalitis: report of a severe, penicillin-resistant case. Arthritis Rheum 30:705, 1987.

796. Hassler D, Riedel K, Zorn J, Preac-Mursic V. Pulsed high-dose cefotaxime therapy in refractory Lyme borreliosis. Lancet 338:193, 1991.

797. American Academy of Neurology. Practice parameter: Diagnosis of patients with nervous system Lyme borreliosis (Lyme disease)—Summary statement. Report of the Quality Standards Subcommittee of the American Academy of Neurology. Neurology 46(3):881–882, 1996.

798. Berger BW. Antibiotic treatment for pregnant victims of Lyme disease. J Am Acad Dermatol 24:663, 1991.

799. Williams CL, Strobino BA. Lyme disease transmission during pregnancy. Contemp Obstet Gynecol 6:48, 1990.

800. American College of Obstetricians and Gynecologists (ACOG). Lyme disease during pregnancy. ACOG Committee Opinion: Committee on Obstetrics: Maternal and Fetal Medicine. Int J Gynaecol Obstet 39:59, 1992.

801. Edly SJ. Lyme disease in pregnancy. N J Med 87:557, 1990.

802. Cartter ML, Hadler JL, Gerber MA, Mofenson L. Lyme disease and pregnancy. Conn Med 53:341, 1989.

803. Plotkin SA, Peter G, Easton JG, et al. Treatment of Lyme borreliosis. Pediatrics 88:176, 1991.

804. Segura-Porta F, Fernandez MM. Treatment of borreliosis. Enferm Infecc Microbiol Clin 16(5):239–244, 1998.

805. Silver HM. Lyme disease during pregnancy. Infect Dis Clin North Am 11(1):93–97, 1997.

806. Nadelman RB, Wormser GP. Lyme borreliosis. Lancet 352(9127):557–565, 1998.

807. Rahn DW, Malawista SE. Lyme disease: recommendations for diagnosis and treatment. Ann Intern Med 114:472, 1991.

808. Kramer MD, Hassler D, Hofmann H, et al. Therapy of Lyme borreliosis. Dtsch Med Wochenschr 118(13):469–473, 1993.

809. Maiwald M. Lyme borreliosis—an infectious disease with interdisciplinary demands. Tierarztl Prax 22(4):301–308, 1994.

810. Adams WV, Rose DC, Eppes SC, Klein JD. Cognitive effects of Lyme disease in children. Pediatrics 94(2 Pt 1):185–189, 1994.

811. Weber K. Treatment failure in erythema migrans: a review. Infection 24:73–75, 1996.

812. Caraco T, Gardner G, Maniatty W, et al. Lyme disease: self-regulation and pathogen invasion. J Theor Biol 193(4):561–575, 1998.

813. Schulze TL, Jordan RA, Vasvary LM, et al. Suppression of *Ixodes scapularis* (Acari: Ixodidae) nymphs in a large residential community. J Med Entomol 31(2):206–211, 1994.

814. Wormser GP. Prospects for a vaccine to prevent Lyme disease. Clin Infect Dis 21(5):1267–1274, 1995.

815. Foley DM, Wang YP, Wu XY, et al. Acquired resistance to *Borrelia burgdorferi* infection in the rabbit. Comparison between outer surface protein A vaccine- and infection-derived immunity. J Clin Invest 99(8):2030–2035, 1997.

816. Gondolf KB, Mihatsch M, Curschellas E, et al. Induction of experimental allergic arthritis with outer surface proteins of *Borrelia burgdorferi*. Arthritis Rheum 37:1070–1077, 1994.

817. Preac-Mursic V, Patsouris E, Wilske B, et al. Persistence of Borrelia burgdorferi and histopathological alterations in experimentally infected animals. A comparison with histopathological findings in human disease. Infection 18:332, 1990.

818. Johnson RC, Kodner C, Russell M. Passive immunization of hamsters against experimental infection with Lyme disease spirochete. Infect Immun 53:713–714, 1986.

819. Sonnesyn SW, Manivel JC, Johnson RC, Goodman JL. A guinea pig model for Lyme disease. Infect Immun 61:4777–4784, 1993.

820. England JD, Bohm RP Jr, Roberts ED, Philipp MT. Lyme neuroborreliosis in the rhesus monkey. Semin Neurol 17(1):53–56, 1997.

821. Pachner AR, Delaney E, O'Neill T. Neuroborreliosis in the nonhuman primate: *Borrelia burgdorferi* persists in the central nervous system. Ann Neurol 38:667–669, 1995.

822. Fikrig E, Barthold SW, Kantor FS, Flavell RA. Protection of mice against the Lyme disease agent by immunizing with recombinant OspA. Science 250:553, 1990.

823. Fikrig E, Barthold SW, Kantor FS, Flavell RA. Protection of mice from Lyme borreliosis by oral vaccination with *Escherichia coli* expressing OspA. J Infect Dis 164:1224, 1991.

824. Nguyen TP, Lam TT, Barthold SW, et al. Partial destruction of *Borrelia burgdorferi* within ticks that engorged on OspE- or OspF-immunized mice. Infect Immun 62(5):2079–2084, 1994.

825. Probert WS, Lefebvre RB. Protection of C3H/HeN mice from challenge with *Borrelia burgdorferi* through active immunization of OspA, OspB, or OspC, but not with OspD or the 83-kilodalton antigen. Infect Immun 62:1920–1926, 1994.

826. Telford SR 3rd, Kantor FS, Lobet Y, et al. Efficacy of human Lyme disease vaccine formulations in a mouse model. J Infect Dis 171(5):1368–1370, 1995.

827. Fikrig E, Telford SR III, Wallich R, et al. Vaccination against Lyme disease caused by diverse *Borrelia burgdorferi*. J Exp Med 181:215–221, 1995.

828. Shih CM, Liu LP. Differential efficacy of passive immunization against infection by Lyme disease spirochaetes transmitted by partially fed vector ticks. J Med Microbiol 47(9):773–779, 1998.

829. Gern L, Schaible UE, Simon MM. Mode of inoculation of the Lyme disease agent *Borrelia burgdorferi* influences infection and immune responses in inbred strains of mice. J Infect Dis 167:971–976, 1993.

830. Mather TN, Telford SR III, Adler GH. Absence of transplacental transmission of Lyme disease spirochetes from reservoir mice (*Peromyscus leucopus*) to their offspring. J Infect Dis 164:564, 1991.

831. Burgess EC, Wachal MD, Cleven TD. *Borrelia burgdorferi* infection in dairy cows, rodents, and birds from four Wisconsin dairy farms. Vet Microbiol 35(1–2):61–77, 1993.

832. Moody KD, Barthold SW. Relative infectivity of *Borrelia burgdorferi* in Lewis rats by various routes of inoculation. Am J Trop Med Hyg 44:135, 1991.

833. Burgess EC. *Borrelia burgdorferi* infection in Wisconsin horses and cows. Ann N Y Acad Sci 539:235, 1988.

834. Gustafson JM, Burgess EC, Wachal MD, Steinberg H. Intrauterine transmission of *Borrelia burgdorferi* in dogs. Am J Vet Res 54(6):882–890, 1993.

835. Keller D, Koster FT, Marks DH, et al. Safety and immunogenicity or a recombinant outer surface protein A Lyme vaccine. J Am Med Assoc 271:1764–1768, 1994.

836. Schoen RT, Meurice F, Brunet CM, et al. Safety and immunogenicity of an outer surface protein A vaccine in subjects with previous Lyme disease. J Infect Dis 172(5):1324–1329, 1995.

837. Wormser GP, Nowakowski J, Nadelman RB, et al. Efficacy of an OspA vaccine preparation for prevention of Lyme disease in New York State. Infection 26(4):208–212, 1998.

838. Van Hoecke C, Comberbach M, De Grave D, et al. Evaluation of the safety, reactogenicity and immunogenicity of three recombinant outer surface protein (OspA) Lyme vaccines in healthy adults. Vaccine 14(17–18):1620–1626, 1996.

839. Van Hoecke C, Fu D, De Grave D, et al. Clinical and immunological assessment of a candidate Lyme disease vaccine in healthy adults: antibody persistence and effect of a booster dose at month 12. Vaccine 16(17):1688–1692, 1998.

840. Sigal LH, Zahradnik JM, Lavin P, et al. A vaccine consisting of recombinant *Borrelia burgdorferi* outer-surface protein A to prevent Lyme disease. Recombinant Outer-Surface Protein A Lyme Disease Vaccine Study Consortium. N Engl J Med 339(4):216–222, 1998 [erratum 339(8):571, 1998].

841. Steere AC, Sikand VK, Meurice F, et al. Vaccination against Lyme disease with recombinant *Borrelia burgdorferi* outer-surface lipoprotein A with adjuvant. Lyme Disease Vaccine Study Group. N Engl J Med 339(4):209–215, 1998.

842. Centers for Disease Control and Prevention. Availability of Lyme disease vaccine. MMWR 48(2):35–36, 43, 1999.

843. SmithKline Beecham Biologicals. LYMErix product label. Rixensart, Belgium, SmithKline Beecham Biologicals, December 1998.

844. Steigbigel RT, Benach JL. Immunization against Lyme disease—an important first step. N Engl J Med 339(4):263–264, 1998.

845. Marwick C. Guarded endorsement for Lyme disease vaccine. JAMA 279(24):1937–1938, 1998.

846. Maes E, Lecomte P, Ray N. A cost-of-illness study of Lyme disease in the United States. Clin Ther 20(5):993–1008; discussion 992, 1998.

847. Zhang YQ, Mathiesen D, Kolbert CP, et al. *Borrelia burgdorferi* enzyme-linked immunosorbent assay for discrimination of OspA vaccination from spirochete infection. J Clin Microbiol 35(1):233–238, 1997.

848. Brown M, Hebert AA. Insect repellents: an overview. J Am Acad Dermatol 36:243–249, 1997.

849. Schwartz B, Warren D. Ticks carrying Lyme disease repelled with two sprays. NEWS US Dept Agriculture, April 29, 1985.

850. Hassler D, Maiwald M, Petney TN. Diagnosis, treatment, and prevention of Lyme disease. JAMA 280(12):1049–1050; discussion 1051, 1998.

851. Angelov L. Unusual features in the epidemiology of Lyme borreliosis. Eur J Epidemiol 12(1):9–11, 1996.

852. Costello CM, Steere AC, Pinkerton RE, Feder HM. A prospective study of tick bites in an endemic area for Lyme disease. J Infect Dis 159:136, 1989.

853. Magid D, Schwartz B, Craft J, Schwartz JS. Prevention of Lyme disease after tick bites: a cost-effectiveness analysis. N Engl J Med 327:534, 1992.

854. Shapiro ED, Gerber MA, Holabird NB, et al. A controlled trial of antimicrobial prophylaxis for Lyme disease after deer-tick bites. N Engl J Med 327:1769, 1992.

855. Dennis DT, Meltzer MI. Antibiotic prophylaxis after tick bites. Lancet 350(9086):1191–1192, 1997.

856. Agre F, Schwartz R. The value of early treatment of deer tick bites for the prevention of Lyme disease. Am J Dis Child 147(9):945–947, 1993.

857. Warshafsky S, Nowakowski J, Nadelman RB, et al. Efficacy of antibiotic prophylaxis for prevention of Lyme disease. J Gen Intern Med 11(6):329–333, 1996.

858. Dhote R, Basse-Guerineau AL, Bachmeyer C, et al. Lyme borreliosis: therapeutic aspects. Presse Med 27(39):2043–2047, 1998.

859. Melski JW. The many faces and phases of borreliosis. I. Lyme disease. J Am Acad Dermatol 24(5 Pt 1):799–801, 1991.

860. Barbour AG. Expert advice and patient expectations: laboratory testing and antibiotics for Lyme disease. JAMA 279(3):239–240, 1998.

861. Gray JS, Granstrom M, Cimmino M, et al. Lyme borreliosis awareness. Zentralbl Bakteriol 287(3):253–265, 1998.

862. European Union Concerted Action on Lyme Borreliosis. http://www.dis.strath.ac.uk/vie/LymeEU

863. Smith-Fiola DC, Hallman WK. Tick bite victims and their environment: the risk of Lyme disease. N J Med 92(9):601–603, 1995.

864. Curi MB. Public awareness of Lyme disease in obstetric, pediatric, and student settings in northwestern Connecticut. Conn Med 57(10):661–663, 1993.

865. Picken RN, Strle F, Ruzic-Sabljic E, et al. Molecular subtyping of Borrelia burgdorferi sensu lato isolates from five patients with solitary lymphocytoma. J Invest Dermatol 108(1):92–97, 1997.

866. Kondrat'ev VG, Bykova LA, Poltoratskaia TN, Istratkina SV. The epidemic situation of tick-borne encephalitis and Lyme disease in the city of Tomsk. Med Parazitol (Mosk) (1):52–53, 1998.

867. Bondarenko AL, Abbasova SV, Tikhomolova EG, et al. The clinico-epidemiological and laboratory characteristics of the early period of Lyme borreliosis in Kirov Province. Med Parazitol (Mosk) (4):18–21, 1997.

868. Matushchenko AA, Rudakova SA, Korenberg EI. The preliminary results of an ecological epidemiological study of Lyme disease in western Siberia. Med Parazitol (Mosk) (4):27–29, 1993.

869. Mitchell PD, Reed KD, Aspeslet TL, et al. Comparison of four immunoserologic assays for detection of antibodies to Borrelia burgdorferi in patients with culture-positive erythema migrans [published erratum appears in 1994 Sept;32(9):2343]. J Clin Microbiol 32(8):1958–1962, 1994.

870. Feder HM Jr, Whitaker DL. Misdiagnosis of erythema migrans. Am J Med 99:412–419, 1995.

871. Masters EJ, King LE. Differentiating Loxoscelism from Lyme disease. Emerg Med 26(10):47–49, 1994.

872. Dlesk A, Balian AA, Sullivan BJ, et al. Diagnostic dilemma for the 1990s: Lyme disease versus rheumatic fever. Wisconsin Med J 90:632, 1991.

873. Rath P-M, Rogler G, Schonberg A, et al. Relapsing fever and its serological discrimination from Lyme borreliosis. Infection 20:283, 1992.

874. Edlinger E, Rodhain F, Perez C. Lyme disease in patients previously suspected of arbovirus infection. Lancet 2:93, 1985.

875. Lader E. Lyme disease misdiagnosed as a temporomandibular joint disorder. J Prosthet Dent 63:82, 1990.

876. Meier C, Reulen HJ, Huber P, Mumenthaler M. Meningoradiculoneuritis mimicking vertebral disc herniation. A "neurosurgical" complication of Lyme-borreliosis. Acta Neurochir 98:42, 1989.

877. Anonymous. Treatment of Lyme disease. Med Lett Drugs Ther 39(1000):47–48, 1997.

878. Dolan MC, Piesman J, Mbow ML, et al. Vector competence of Ixodes scapularis and Ixodes ricinus (Acari: Ixodidae) for three genospecies of Borrelia burgdorferi. J Med Entomol 35(4):465–470, 1998.

879. Williams LR, Austin FE. Hemolytic activity of Borrelia burgdorferi. Infect Immun 60:3224, 1992.

880. Needham GR. Evaluation of five popular methods for tick removal. Pediatrics 75:997, 1985.

881. Angelov L, Rakadieva T, Kostova E, Liptchev G. Epidemiology, diagnostics, clinical manifestations, prophylaxis and fight against Lyme borreliosis in Bulgaria. Folia Med 37(4A Suppl):94–95, 1995.

882. Fraser CM, Casjens S, Huang WM, et al. Genomic sequence of a Lyme disease spirochaete, Borrelia burgdorferi. Nature 390:580–586, 1997.

883. Dotevell L, Hagberg L. Successful oral doxycycline treatment of Lyme disease-associated facial palsy and meningitis. Clin Infect Dis 28:569–574, 1999.

884. Wang G, van Dam AP, Schwartz I, Dankert J. Molecular typing of Borrelia burgdorferi sensu lato: Taxonomic, epidemiological, and clinical implications. Clin Microbiol Rev 12(4):633–653, 1999.

885. Van Hoecke C, Lebacq E, Beran J, Parenti D. Alternative vaccination schedules (0, 1, and 6 months) for a recombinant Osp A Lyme disease vaccine. Clin Infect Dis 28:1260–1264, 1999.

886. Feder HM, Beran J, Van Hoecke C, et al. Immunogenicity of a recombinant Borrelia burgdorferi outer surface membrane protein A vaccine against Lyme disease in children. J Pediatr 135:575–579, 1999.

887. American Academy of Pediatrics. Lyme Disease. In: Pickering LK (ed). 2000 Red Book: Report of the Committee on Infectious Diseases, 25th ed. Elk Grove Village, Ill, Amer Acad Pediatr, 2000, 374–379.

888. Logigian EL, Kaplan RF, Steere AC. Successful treatment of Lyme encephalopathy with intravenous ceftriaxone. J Infect Dis 180:377–383, 1999.

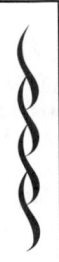

CHAPTER 12

Syphilis

DAVID INGALL, M.D., and PABLO J. SÁNCHEZ, M.D.

"Foetal syphilis is the malady that most medical men think of when reference is made to foetal disease. It has been studied in all its aspects and at very considerable length by a multitude of careful observers. It has been taken as the type of antenatal maladies, as the typical disease of the foetus; it may almost be said that, to some investigators, foetal pathology and foetal syphilis have been synonymous terms." Times have changed since Ballantyne wrote his treatise in 1902,[1] but in spite of the availability of preventive and therapeutic approaches, congenital syphilis remains a challenging problem.

The first major work on syphilis, written by Francisco Lopez de Villalobos, appeared in 1498.[2, 3] In 1530, Hieronymus Fracastorius[3, 4] wrote an epic poem that featured a shepherd named Syphilus and described the disease: one generation later, Gale[5] introduced the word syphilis into the English language. Both Lopez and Fracastorius mentioned syphilis of the newborn, but they and others[2, 5, 6] of their time thought that infants became infected by ingestion of infected milk or through contact with the infection at birth. Because all mothers did not have obvious signs of infection, some investigators believed that congenital disease was transmitted by the father.

Nevertheless, by 1850, it was believed that an infant could not have syphilis unless the mother had acquired the infection.

A lengthy account of the signs and symptoms of syphilis in infants was published in 1854 by Diday, but he failed to recognize that children who were without symptoms by 6 months of age could still be infected.[5] In 1858, Sir Jonathan Hutchinson described the famous triad of signs of late congenital syphilis: notched incisor teeth, interstitial keratitis, and eighth cranial nerve deafness.[7] Rosebury has provided an eminently readable account of the history of syphilis and other venereal diseases.[8]

THE ORGANISM

Treponema constitutes one of the five genera in the order Spirochaetales, the others being *Borrelia*, *Spirochaeta*, *Leptospira*, and *Cristispira*. Pathogenic treponemes that cause syphilis and yaws have been designated as subspecies of *Treponema pallidum* because no differences have been detected by electron microscopy, analysis of DNA homology, or polyacrylamide gel electrophoresis of outer membrane proteins; these subspecies designations are *T. pallidum* subsp. *pallidum* and *T. pallidum* subsp. *pertenue*.[9–14] Moreover, because the etiologic agent of

Supported in part by Public Health Service grant 1R29 AI 34932-01 from the National Institute of Allergy and Infectious Diseases and by Centers for Disease Control and Prevention contract C1000 689.

endemic (nonvenereal) syphilis is a variant of *T. pallidum*, it has been designated *T. pallidum* subsp. *endemicum*. The designation for the causative agent of pinta remains *Treponema carateum*. Only *T. pallidum*, and possibly *T. pertenue*,[15] can cause congenital infection.[16–18] None of these organisms has been cultivated successfully in vitro, although the viability and virulence of *T. pallidum* can be maintained for days to weeks in artificial media; and a limited degree of replication has been documented, especially in the presence of mammalian cells.[19–21]

The fact that these virulent treponemes are not readily cultivated in vitro is, to a great extent, responsible for our incomplete understanding of their properties. The problem of understanding more thoroughly the biology of *T. pallidum* is further compounded by the relative unavailability of good animal models to study syphilitic infection in the laboratory. Guinea pigs develop atypical lesions after challenge with *T. pallidum*,[16] and vigorously immunosuppressed mice may also be susceptible to infection.[22] However, aside from primates, only the rabbit is readily infected with *T. pallidum* and develops lesions that resemble those seen in humans and even progressing to a secondary infection. There is no animal model for tertiary syphilis. Recently, a nonhuman primate model of central nervous system (CNS) invasion by *T. pallidum* was developed for elucidation of the immune mechanisms responsible for clearance of the organism from the CNS.[23] Initial results demonstrated the participation of locally produced interferon-γ in this process. Rabbit,[24] guinea pig,[25] and hamster[26] models for congenital infection have been described, but the relevance to human congenital syphilis is not yet defined. Vertical transmission of *T. pallidum* to various litters and generations of guinea pigs has been recently reported,[26a] supporting the observation that an untreated female congenitally infected with syphilis is able to transmit the disease to her fetus (third-generation syphilis).

Morphology

The pathogenic treponemes are so narrow ($< 0.15 \mu m$) that they are below the resolution of the light microscope. They can be detected by darkfield microscopy, which reveals a characteristic pattern of motion.[27] Electron microscopy shows them to be wavelike organisms with tapered ends. They have tight, regular spirals with a wavelength of $1.1 \mu m$ and amplitude of 0.2 to $0.3 \mu m$; their length ranges from 6 to $15 \mu m$, usually being 10 to $13 \mu m$.[9, 10]

T. pallidum morphologically consists of an outer membrane that surrounds the endoflagella, cytoplasmic membrane, and protoplasmic cylinder of the organism.[28, 29] Three sheathed flagella or axial fibrils emerge from each end of the organism. Although it might seem reasonable to assume that, by analogy to bacterial flagella, the axial fibrils are responsible for motility, their location within the outer membrane and the failure of antiflagellar antibody to immobilize certain spirochetes make this less certain. Ruthenium red staining has demonstrated an amorphous outer layer in *T. pallidum* isolated from infected tissue and in situ in the infected tissues themselves

in some studies,[30–32] although other investigators (K Hovind-Hougen, personal communication to Dr. Daniel Musher, 1983) believe that artifacts may be responsible. A glycosaminoglycan layer that has been demonstrated in vitro[19, 33, 34] may function as an antiphagocytic capsule. Intracytoplasmic tubules are present, but their characteristics and function are as yet undefined.

Composition

The advent of polyacrylamide gel electrophoresis techniques has allowed characterization of some of the major constituent proteins of *T. pallidum*; 16 major proteins have been described.[35–37] By phase partitioning analysis utilizing the nonionic detergent Triton X-114, integral membrane proteins with apparent molecular masses of 47, 38, 36, 34, 32, 17, and 15 kDa have been identified.[38–45] It has been determined that these proteins, particularly the 47-, 34- and 17-kDa antigens, are proteolipids containing covalently linked fatty acids.[40–42] Recent work using cell fractionation has demonstrated that the *T. pallidum* outer membrane consists of a lipid bilayer with a paucity of proteins.[38] Freeze-fracture and freeze-etch electron microscopy studies have provided more direct support for this contention.[43, 44] However, the demonstration that a number of the abundant membrane immunogens are proteolipids complicates interpretation of these data because proteins presumably anchored to membranes solely by lipid moieties would not be detected by freeze-fracture methods. The precise cellular locations for the protein components of these antigens, therefore, require further elucidation. The nonprotein constituents remain a controversial area of study, as exemplified by diphosphatidylglycerol (cardiolipin), the antigen that stimulates production of Venereal Disease Research Laboratory (VDRL) antibody (see later part of chapter). This substance comprises a small proportion of the lipids of *T. pallidum*, but these organisms may be unable to synthesize it; and it is possible that they instead incorporate it from damaged host tissues.

Recently, the complete genome of *T. pallidum* subsp. *pallidum* (Nichols) was sequenced by the whole genome random sequencing method.[46–50] The *T. pallidum* genome is a circular chromosome containing 1,138,006 base pairs with 1041 predicted coding sequences (open reading frames). Systems for DNA replication, transcription, translation, and repair are intact, but catabolic and biosynthetic activities are minimized. Potential virulence factors include a family of 12 potential membrane proteins and several putative hemolysins. This exciting, technologic accomplishment has led to rapid advances in the development of approaches to identifying strains or subtypes of *T. pallidum* that will aid in epidemiologic studies of syphilis. It also should lead to a greater understanding of the biologic mechanisms of the organism, leading to its in vitro cultivation, to improved diagnostic and treatment advances, and, ultimately, to development of an effective vaccine.

Metabolism

In the past, *T. pallidum* was regarded as an anaerobe; however, this organism takes up oxygen[51] and degrades glucose aerobically to carbon dioxide and acetate as well as anaerobically to pyruvate and lactate.[52] Of 22 carbon sources studied, only glucose and pyruvate were metabolized aerobically.[53] T. pallidum is better able to incorporate amino acids into proteins in the presence of 10% oxygen under anaerobic conditions.[53] The aerobic capabilities of T. pallidum have been substantiated by finding a functional flavoprotein-cytochrome electron transport system[54] and by demonstrating oxygen consumption with oxidative phosphorylation.[55] Studies of in vitro growth of T. pallidum have generally found best survival or slight replication or both at oxygen atmospheres of 3 to 6%.[56, 57]

Immunity

Humoral immunity in syphilis has been a subject of study in syphilis since the serendipitous discovery of antibody to cardiolipin by Wassermann early in this century. By the time patients seek medical attention for primary syphilis, antibodies to T. pallidum can be detected by immunofluorescent and hemagglutination techniques in 90% of cases and antibody to cardiolipin in 75% of cases.[58] Western blot techniques show both IgM and IgG class antibody responses to a wide repertoire of T. pallidum proteins,[37] with the 47-kDa antigen being the most immunogenic.[45] A small percentage of patients have antibodies that, together with complement, inhibit motility and eliminate infectivity of the organism (T. pallidum–immobilizing antibodies).[59, 60] Despite this ample evidence for an immune response, syphilis progresses and secondary lesions develop in nearly all patients unless specific therapy is given. T. pallidum–immobilizing antibody is present in the majority of patients who have active secondary syphilis,[59] and one could argue either that this antibody is protective, being just about able to bring the disease under control, or that it is not protective because active disease is still present. After 1 to 3 months of secondary lesions, spontaneous remission occurs; this is called latency because the organism persists in lymph and other tissues and tertiary syphilis may appear at a later date. Moreover, in the preantibiotic era, relapse to active infection occurred in up to 25% of untreated subjects after their infection had become latent.[61] Most recurrences occur toward the end of the first year after infection, are rare after 2 years, and presumably do not occur after 4 years. This has led to the designation of early latent syphilis as being of 1 year or less in duration and that of late latent syphilis as being greater than 1 year in duration. Passive immunization with huge amounts of serum from rabbits that have recovered from experimental infection and are immune to rechallenge with T. pallidum delays and attenuates infection but does not prevent the ultimate development of syphilitic lesions.[62–65] Immune serum facilitates uptake of T. pallidum by human polymorphonuclear leukocytes.[66] What remains unclear is why the disease progresses despite abundant evidence for antibody responses; these observations all suggest that humoral immunity is insufficient and that cellular mechanisms play a significant role.

Although the overwhelming majority of treponemes in syphilitic lesions are found in extracellular spaces, treponemes have occasionally been found within macrophages and other cells.[67] Radolf and associates[68] have shown that T. pallidum lipoproteins induce macrophages to secrete tumor necrosis factor by a mechanism distinct from that of lipopolysaccharide. The direct interaction of T. pallidum with vascular endothelium may be an important early event in the initiation of the host immune response to syphilitic infection[69]; purified 47-kDa lipoprotein can activate human vascular endothelial cells to upregulate the expression of intercellular adhesion molecule-1 and procoagulant activity on its surface.[70] This may result in the perivasculitis and fibrin deposition that are characteristic histopathologic findings in syphilis.

Delayed-type hypersensitivity to treponemal antigens appears late in secondary syphilis and might be related to the onset of latency. Although infection with T. pallidum stimulates acquired cellular resistance,[71] infection with unrelated organisms such as Mycobacterium bovis (bacille Calmette-Guérin) or Propionibacterium acnes does not protect animals against challenge with T. pallidum.[72–74] However, Schell and associates have transferred resistance to infection with T. pallidum strain Bosnia by transfusing T cells from immune hamsters.[75] T lymphocytes responsive to T. pallidum appear in syphilitic lesions as the number of treponemes decreases,[76] which gives further evidence, albeit circumstantial, for a role of cellular immunity in controlling infection.

Some findings suggest that immune responses may be impaired early in syphilis. In early syphilis (1) in vitro blastogenic transformation of lymphocytes after stimulation with a variety of antigens is depressed[67]; (2) paracortical (thymus-dependent) areas of lymph nodes are depleted[77, 78]; (3) delayed hypersensitivity to several antigens may be depressed[79, 80]; and (4) ability to produce IgG in response to sensitization with sheep red blood cells (a T cell–dependent antigen) is markedly inhibited.[81, 82] Other authorities believe that the evolution of immunity is slow, albeit for unknown reasons, but that suppression of immunity is not responsible.[36]

It is even possible that true immunity to T. pallidum does not exist. Active lesions may be brought under control and animals may become resistant to rechallenge with T. pallidum, but the host is unable to rid itself completely of the infecting organism, which persists in lymph nodes. Premunition, resistance to rechallenge, or, in the case of syphilis, a "chancre-fast" state without biologic cure may best describe this situation. It is known that individuals with untreated secondary syphilis or true latent infection are resistant to rechallenge with T. pallidum, as are those with untreated congenital syphilis.[83]

Some observations on congenital syphilis helped to contribute to the understanding of immunity. That a degree of maternal immunity is acquired during infection was known to nineteenth century physicians. Colles[84] observed that an infected infant did not infect the mother's breast, although he would not have disagreed with Paré that if an infant has acquired the infection from a syphilitic wet nurse it could pass infection to the mother.[3] In 1846, Kassowitz observed that the longer syphilis exists untreated in a woman before pregnancy occurs, the more likely it is that when she does become pregnant her treponemes will be held in check and the less likely it is that her fetus will die in utero or be born with congenital syphilis; this observation is called Kassowitz's law.[8, 84]

It remains unclear what factors determine which mothers, particularly those in the latent stage of infection, will pass disease to their fetuses. It is also not clear why some infants who are infected in utero are born without any clinical manifestations but develop overt disease in the first weeks or months of life or even at puberty.

Modern immunology has only recently started to pay attention to the problem of congenital syphilis. As would be suspected by transplacental transfer of immunoglobulin, the IgG levels of infected infants largely match those of the mother. Moreover, by immunoblotting, the IgG reactivity of infant sera is indistinguishable from that of the mother, again indicating the transplacental nature of the IgG antibodies.[85–88] The range of IgM antibody responses to the proteins of *T. pallidum* in the sera of overtly infected newborns is comparable to that of disseminated (secondary) infection in adults.[85] However, the IgM response of the infant is distinct from that of the mother and is uniformly directed against the 47-kDa membrane lipoprotein antigen.[85, 86, 88]

TRANSMISSION

Humans are the natural host of *T. pallidum* and also serve as the vector. Sexual contact provides the usual means of transmission between adults. Rarely is the disease passed to health care personnel or others who accidentally touch infectious lesions or to laboratory workers who handle infected animals. The infant is usually infected in utero presumably by transplacental passage of *T. pallidum* from an infected mother. In utero transmission has been supported by isolation of the organism from umbilical cord blood and amniotic fluid,[88–90] detection of spirochetes in the placenta and umbilical cord in association with typical histopathologic changes,[91, 92] and detection of specific IgM antibody to *T. pallidum* in neonatal serum obtained at birth.[85–88] Lucas and associates[90] have found that *T. pallidum* can be isolated from approximately 74% of amniotic fluid samples from women with early syphilis; it is possible that *T. pallidum* may infect the fetus by traversing the fetal membranes, thereby gaining access to the amniotic fluid and resulting in fetal infection. Alternatively, infection may occur from contact with an infectious lesion during passage through the birth canal.[1, 84] When it was commonplace for infants to be fed by a wet nurse, small epidemics of syphilis among groups of infants were sometimes caused by an infectious lesion on the nipple of the woman serving as wet nurse. There are no recent data to suggest that breast milk alone is associated with transmission of syphilis.

The risk to the fetus or infant appears to vary considerably according to the stage of untreated syphilis in the mother, although there is controversy about the incidence of morbidity and mortality.[93–95] Paley[93] reported that approximately 50% of the pregnancies in which the untreated syphilitic infection was of less than 2 years' duration resulted in living nonsyphilitic infants. In 1951, Ingraham reported that for 220 women who had untreated early syphilis (up to 4 years duration), 41% of their infants were liveborn and had congenital syphilis, 25% were stillborn, 14% died in the neonatal period, 21% were premature (defined as birth weight less than 5 lb) but had no evidence of congenital syphilis, and only 18% were normal, full-term infants.[95] These outcomes were all significantly different from those observed among nonsyphilitic women. In contrast, only 2% of infants born to 82 mothers with untreated late syphilis (over 4 years' duration) had congenital syphilis. Subsequently, Fiumara and colleagues[94] stated that when primary or secondary syphilis went untreated, half of the infants were premature, stillborn, or died as neonates and the other half developed congenital syphilis; there was little chance of the mother giving birth to a normal full-term infant. In the case of early latent syphilis, 20 to 60% of the infants were normal, 20% were premature, and 16% were stillborn; 4% died as neonates, and 40% had congenital syphilis. In the case of untreated late syphilis, about 70% of the infants were healthy, 10% were stillborn, and, as in normal pregnant women, about 9% were premature and about 1% died as neonates; 10% had congenital syphilis.[94]

Recent data from Sheffield and associates[96] on the influence of maternal stage of syphilis on vertical transmission have supported the fact that untreated maternal syphilis results in significant adverse pregnancy outcomes and neonatal morbidity with high rates of stillbirths (12%) and live births (29%) with congenital infection. In a prospective cohort analysis of 428 women with untreated syphilis from 1988 to 1998, untreated primary syphilis at delivery resulted in a transmission rate of 29% (3% stillbirths and 26% live births with congenital syphilis). Untreated secondary syphilis at delivery resulted in 59% of infants having congenital infection (20% stillborn, 39% live born), whereas with early latent disease, the transmission rate was 50% (17% stillborn, 33% live born). On the other hand, maternal late latent infection resulted in 5% stillbirths and only 8% live births with congenital syphilis.

These statistical estimates put Kassowitz's law into epidemiologic terms. An interesting family study illustrating this "law" described a syphilitic mother who had five pregnancies resulting in eight children.[97] The first pregnancy produced a stillborn child; the second a full-term infant with congenital syphilis; the third, triplets, two of whom had congenital syphilis; the fourth, twins, one of whom had congenital syphilis; and the fifth, a normal full-term infant. Although this illustrates the law in operation to the extent that with each succeeding pregnancy the effect of syphilis on the fetus was less severe, the sobering point was made that the mother, whose case had somehow escaped detection and treatment during the time she was delivering the syphilitic infants, was able to transmit congenital syphilis over a span of 10 years. Two unusual aspects of this report are the unavailability of data to identify when and during which pregnancy the mother became infected and the disturbing fact that the diagnosis of infection in the parents occurred 4 years after the fifth pregnancy.

The majority of infants born to mothers with untreated or inadequately treated syphilis have no clinical or laboratory evidence of infection at birth. These infants may later develop manifestations of disease at several months or years of age if left untreated. The exact pathogenesis of this "late-onset" type of infection is not known. Nasopharyngeal or gastrointestinal colonization, or both, with *T. pallidum* from in utero exposure to infected amniotic fluid may play a role in the later development of symptomatic infection in these infants if they are not treated appropriately in the newborn period.

The effect of concurrent maternal infection with *T. pallidum* and human immunodeficiency virus (HIV) on the risk of fetal infection with *T. pallidum* and HIV is not fully known.[98–100] The cellular immune dysfunction associated with HIV infection may permit a greater degree of treponemal proliferation and lead to a higher rate of fetal infection. HIV-infected women who acquire syphilis during pregnancy may not respond adequately to currently recommended benzathine penicillin therapy, thereby increasing the risk of fetal infection with *T. pallidum*.[101] Preliminary studies by Sánchez[98] indicate that infants born to co-infected mothers with early syphilis were significantly more likely to have clinical or laboratory evidence of congenital syphilis at delivery than infants delivered of women with early syphilis but who lacked antibody to HIV. Alternatively, untreated syphilis during a pregnancy complicated by maternal HIV may result in an increased risk of fetal HIV infection by producing a placentitis and allowing transmission of the virus from the maternal to the fetal circulation.[99] The finding by Theus and colleagues[102] that virulent *T. pallidum* can directly promote the induction of HIV gene expression in macrophages and possibly result in increased systemic HIV levels and more rapid progression of the HIV infection supports the possible increased vertical transmission of HIV from a co-infected mother to the fetus.

T. pallidum is present in mucocutaneous lesions as well as in body fluids such as blood and cerebrospinal fluid (CSF) of infected infants. Health personnel should observe blood and fluid (standard) precautions when caring for infected individuals; moreover, infants and adults with infectious lesions should be placed in contact isolation for the first 24 hours of therapy. Once antibiotic therapy has been given, the risk of further transmission is virtually nonexistent because penicillin in sufficient dosage causes a complete disappearance of viable treponemes from syphilitic lesions within a few hours.[103] *T. pallidum* does not survive well outside the host and is easily destroyed by heat, drying, and soap and water.[104, 105]

The existence of *third-generation syphilis*,[106, 107] a term used to define transmission from a congenitally syphilitic mother to her fetus, is difficult to prove. There are families in which three generations have had syphilis, but it is difficult to determine whether the congenitally syphilitic mother had only that infection or whether, as

an adult, she contracted a new infection that was then transmitted to her fetus.

Limited data suggest that untreated mothers with yaws may give birth to infants with congenital infection.[15]

EPIDEMIOLOGY

Because of the exquisite susceptibility of *T. pallidum* to penicillin, it was thought that the widespread use of this antibiotic after World War II would lead to the virtual disappearance of syphilis. Indeed, a dramatic decline in the number of cases did occur, reaching a low point about 1956. Unfortunately, there is truth in the observation that as the control program for a disease approaches eradication of that disease, the control program rather than the disease may be eradicated. As the incidence of syphilis decreased remarkably, there were drastic reductions in the funds and personnel allocated for syphilis control. By the early 1960s, the disease was again clearly resurgent, and more resources were again committed to control efforts. Syphilis subsequently declined in the 1970s, only to have a dramatic resurgence in the 1980s.[108, 109] From 1986 to 1991, there was a steady increase in the incidence of primary and secondary syphilis among females in the United States (Fig. 12–1).[98] This increase was greatest among blacks and Hispanics in large urban centers such as New York City, Detroit, Miami, and Los Angeles.[108, 110–112] The exchange of illegal drugs, particularly crack cocaine, for sex with multiple partners appears to play a major role in the transmission of syphilis.[108, 110, 113–115] Because the identities of sexual partners are often unknown among persons trading sex for drugs, partner notification, a traditional syphilis-control strategy, is virtually impossible. Other factors implicated in the dramatic increase of syphilis include a reduction in resources for syphilis control programs that are coordinated in sexually transmitted disease clinics of

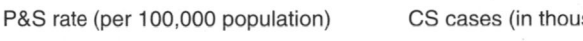

CONGENITAL SYPHILIS—REPORTED CASES FOR INFANTS <1 YEAR OF AGE AND RATES OF PRIMARY AND SECONDARY SYPHILIS AMONG WOMEN: UNITED STATES, 1970–1998

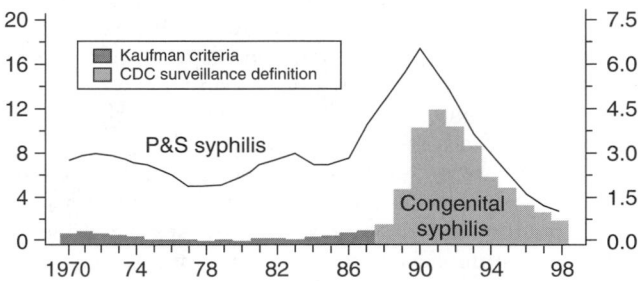

FIGURE 12–1 Case rates of primary and secondary (P&S) syphilis among females and congenital syphilis among infants younger than 1 year of age in the United States, 1970 to 1998. The surveillance case definition for congenital syphilis changed in 1988. (From Statistical Branch, Sexually Transmitted Diseases, Centers for Disease Control and Prevention.)

local public health departments[116, 117] as well as the use of spectinomycin for treatment of penicillinase-producing *Neisseria gonorrhoeae* because spectinomycin is not effective against incubating syphilis.[118, 119]

Since 1990, there has been an 86% decrease in the incidence of primary and secondary syphilis in the United States (see Fig. 12–1). Several factors have contributed to this significant decrease.[120–126] The awareness of the syphilis epidemic of the late 1980s has led to wider screening practices and identification of infected individuals. Increased state and federal resources were invested in syphilis control programs for traditional (e.g., partner notification and clinical services) and nontraditional (e.g., community-based screening and outreach and risk-reduction counseling) activities.[121, 122] These programs helped identify particular locations with a high prevalence of syphilis and with core populations at high risk for infection.[121, 122] The recognition of these demographics has allowed presumptive treatment of syphilis based on epidemiologic indications. Other reasons for the recent decline include a decrease in crack cocaine use and exchange of sex for drugs, major contributors to the epidemic, as well as the introduction of HIV prevention programs that target prevention of other sexually transmitted diseases. The development of acquired immunity to syphilis that occurred among high-risk populations when syphilis was more prevalent may also have played a role. In addition, changing the treatment protocol from spectinomycin or ampicillin to ceftriaxone may have treated incubating syphilis.[124]

Despite this decline, syphilis remains endemic in the United States.[123, 124] Syphilis is a reportable disease; the number of reported cases of primary and secondary syphilis has varied between 6999 and more than 45,000 cases per year,[125, 126] although it is estimated that only about 1 of every 3 cases is reported.[127] Syphilis in the United States is currently found among racial and ethnic minorities who live in poverty and whose medical care is poor.[128] In 1998, the rate (number of cases per 100,000 population) of primary and secondary syphilis was substantially higher in blacks (17.1) than in American Indians/Alaskan natives (2.8), Hispanics (1.5), non-Hispanic whites (0.5), and Asian/Pacific Islanders (0.4).[126] People who live in the inner cities on the East Coast and in the rural South[130] bear a disproportionate burden. In 1998, the rate of primary and secondary syphilis was higher in the South (5.1) than in the Midwest (1.9), West (1.0), and Northeast (0.8).[126] In fact, the majority of the total reported cases of primary and secondary syphilis occurred in the southeastern United States, which contains only 19% of the total U.S. population.[120]

Moreover, focal outbreaks of primary and secondary syphilis continue to occur, and these have been associated with illicit drug use, exchange of sex for drugs or money, and homosexual activity.[126, 129] Attention also has focused on the induced migration that results when public housing projects are dismantled and infected individuals move to less impoverished areas that surround the inner city; this results in infection of new sexual partners, who often lack a history of drug use. These continuing outbreaks are disconcerting because cyclic national epidemics have occurred every 7 to 10 years;

they underscore the need for syphilis elimination rather than enhanced control.[128]

Worldwide, syphilis remains a considerable public health problem, particularly in Eastern Europe and in the developing countries of Africa and Latin America.[131] In countries such as those of the former Soviet Union, the occurrence of syphilis has been related to changes in sexual behavior and in the patterns of provisions, use, and effectiveness of diagnostic treatment and contact tracing services.[132] In South America, the problem of syphilis and congenital syphilis is only now being unraveled. In a study in Buenos Aires, 10% of women with reactive serologic tests for syphilis had a history of stillbirth that was believed to be secondary to syphilis.[133] In 1996 in Bolivia, 26% of women who delivered stillborn infants had syphilis, compared with only 4% of mothers of liveborn infants.[134]

Nonetheless, in the United States, there are currently heightened expectations for the possibility of the eventual control and elimination of endemic syphilis.[128] In 1998, primary and secondary syphilis declined to 2.6 cases per 100,000 population, the lowest rate ever reported in the United States.[126] There were no reported cases in 78% of U.S. counties, and 90% of U.S. counties had 4 or fewer cases per 100,000 population, the Healthy People 2000 national objective rate. Moreover, syphilis today is occurring in fewer geographic areas, with 50% of new syphilis cases reported from less than 1% of U.S. counties that are disproportionately clustered in the southeastern United States (Fig. 12–2). Because of these findings, the Centers for Disease Control and Prevention (CDC) has developed a National Plan for Elimination of Syphilis from the United States.[126, 128] The CDC has defined syphilis elimination as the absence of sustained transmission. The national goal for syphilis elimination is to reduce primary and secondary syphilis cases to 1000 or less (rate: 0.4 per 100,000 population) and to increase the number of syphilis-free counties to 90% by 2005. The five key strategies of the plan focus on (1) enhanced community involvement and partnerships at local, state, and national levels; (2) intensified surveillance; (3) rapid outbreak response; (4) expanded access to health care for those infected or exposed to syphilis; and (5) improved health promotion.

Gestational syphilis primarily affects women who are young, unmarried, and from a low socioeconomic background and who receive inadequate prenatal care.[112, 135] The incidence of congenital syphilis closely correlates with that of primary and secondary disease in women (see Fig. 12–1); it is not surprising that the incidence of congenital syphilis increased dramatically in the late 1980s coincident with the rise in early syphilis among women of childbearing age. With the recent decline in syphilis, the number of cases of congenital syphilis in 1992 decreased for the first time since 1980.

The dramatic increase in the number of cases of congenital syphilis was due to both an increase in actual cases and the use of revised reporting guidelines beginning in 1989, which broadened the surveillance definition for congenital syphilis.[108, 136, 137] Previous criteria for reporting cases of congenital syphilis were based on a clinical case definition.[138] A confirmed case was that of

PRIMARY AND SECONDARY SYPHILIS
UNITED STATES, 1998*

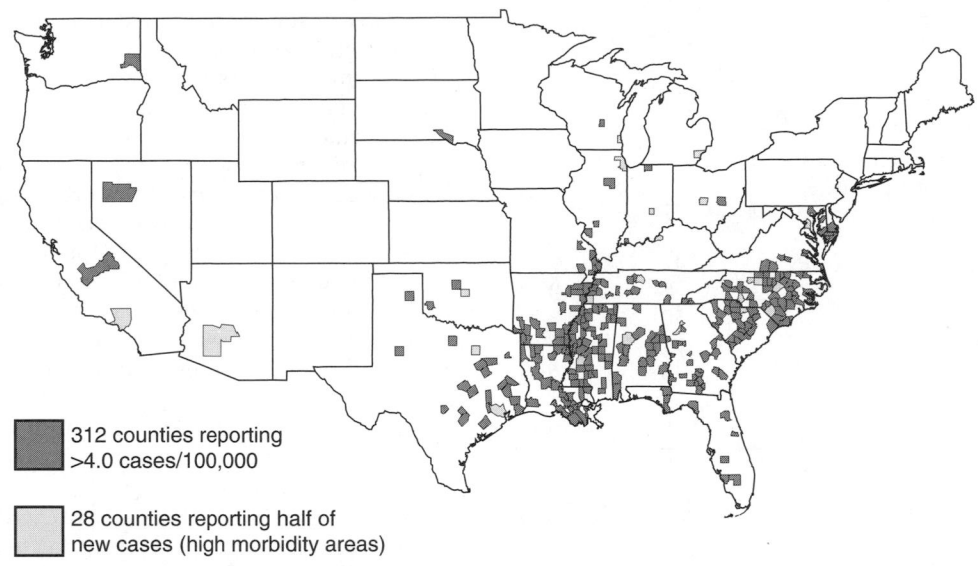

312 counties reporting
>4.0 cases/100,000

28 counties reporting half of
new cases (high morbidity areas)

* Note: 1998 P&S rate for the U.S. is 2.6 per 100,000

FIGURE 12–2 Counties with primary and secondary syphilis rates above the national health objective for 2000 of four cases per 100,000 population—United States, 1998. (From Centers for Disease Control and Prevention. Primary and secondary syphilis—United States, 1998. MMWR Morb Mortal Wkly Rep 48:876, 1999.)

an infant or stillbirth in whom *T. pallidum* was identified with dark-field microscopy or specific stains in specimens from lesions. A presumptive case was that of an infant or a stillborn infant who had a reactive test for syphilis and an abnormal physical examination, an abnormal long bone radiograph result, a reactive CSF VDRL test, an elevated CSF cell count or protein without other cause, a nontreponemal serologic titer that was fourfold higher than that of the mother's, or the persistence of a reactive treponemal test beyond 1 year of age. In 1989, a new surveillance case definition for reporting cases of congenital syphilis was approved by the CDC (Table 12–1).[108] It includes all infants with clinical evidence of active syphilis as well as infants without clinical findings and stillborn infants born to women with untreated or inadequately treated syphilis. Use of these guidelines increases the number of reported cases labeled as congenital syphilis by almost fourfold,[98, 139, 140] although clearly some cases will be reported that are actually not infections. The surveillance case definition thus reflects the public health burden of the disease because these infants require medical and public health interventions. However, it does not represent diagnostic criteria.

The persistence of congenital syphilis despite the wide availability of effective penicillin therapy has prompted close scrutiny of those cases still occurring. Mascola and associates[141] reviewed 50 cases of congenital syphilis reported during 1 year in Texas for epidemiologic characteristics that might have led to their prevention. Their findings, including unpublished observations of 659 cases (C Beck-Sague, A Hadgu, L Frau, et al, unpublished data), are summarized in Table 12–2. Similar data have been reported from Miami,[110] Detroit,[111] and New

TABLE 12–1
Surveillance Case Definition for Congenital Syphilis

A *confirmed case* of congenital syphilis is an infant in whom *Treponema pallidum* is identified by dark-field microscopy, fluorescent antibody, or other specific stains in specimens from lesions, placenta, umbilical cord, amniotic fluid, or autopsy material.

A *presumptive case* of congenital syphilis is either of the following:

A. Any infant whose mother had untreated or inadequately treated[a] syphilis at delivery, regardless of findings in the infant; or

B. Any infant or child who has a reactive treponemal test for syphilis and any one of the following:
  1. Any evidence of congenital syphilis on physical examination; or
  2. Any evidence of congenital syphilis on long-bone radiograph; or
  3. Reactive cerebrospinal fluid VDRL; or
  4. Elevated cerebrospinal fluid cell count or protein (without other cause); or
  5. Quantitative nontreponemal serologic titers that are fourfold higher than the mother's (both drawn at birth).

A *syphilitic stillbirth* is defined as a death of a fetus weighing > 500 g or having a gestational age > 20 weeks in which the mother had untreated or inadequately treated syphilis at delivery.

[a]Inadequate treatment consists of any nonpenicillin therapy or penicillin given < 30 days before delivery.
From Sánchez PJ. Congenital syphilis. *In* Aranoff SC (ed): Advances in Pediatric Infectious Diseases, vol 7. St. Louis, Mosby–Year Book, 1992, p 31, with permission. Adapted from Centers for Disease Control. Congenital syphilis, New York City, 1986–1988. MMWR Morb Mortal Wkly Rep 38:825, 1989.

TABLE 12–2
Factors Contributing to the Occurrence of Congenital Syphilis

FACTOR	NO. OF CASES	% OF TOTAL
No prenatal care, STS positive at delivery	301	46
Prenatal care received, STS negative at first trimester, not repeated	96	15
No STS performed during prenatal care	27	4
Negative maternal STS at delivery	44	7
Laboratory error	2	0.3
Delay in treatment	50	8
Prenatal treatment failures	95	14
Insufficient data	36	6
Other	8	1
Total	659	

STS = serologic test for syphilis.

Modified from Mascola L, Pelosi R, Blout JH, et al. Congenital syphilis. Why is it still occurring? JAMA 252:1719–1722. Copyright 1984, American Medical Association; and Beck-Sague C, Hadgu A, Frau L, et al. Unpublished observations.

York.[142, 143] Lack of prenatal care was, by far, the single most important cause. Congenital syphilis is preventable, but only if prenatal care is accessible to, as well as sought by, those often hard-to-reach groups that are most at risk, such as teenage and/or unwed mothers, drug users, women who are sexually promiscuous, and members of disadvantaged minority groups (Table 12–3). Syphilis needs to be considered and ruled out with serologic tests in the first trimester of all pregnancies and with additional screenings at the beginning of the third trimester (28 weeks) and at delivery for mothers who live in areas with high incidences of infection.[108, 112, 135, 139, 144, 145]

Data from the CDC identify changing percentages of the factors contributing to the occurrence of congenital syphilis in 1998.[146] Six hundred fifty-one (81%) of 801 reported cases occurred because the mother received either no penicillin or inadequate treatment before or during pregnancy. In 223 (36%) of these cases, the mother had no prenatal care. Infants of mothers who

TABLE 12–3
Epidemiologic Factors Suggesting High Risk for Syphilis Exposure

Being unmarried mother or teenage mother
Inadequate prenatal care
Drug use (esp. cocaine) in mother or sexual partner
Sexual promiscuity
Sexual contact with anyone known to have a sexually transmitted disease[a]
History of sexually transmitted disease[a]
Disadvantaged racial/ethnic minorities (esp. African-American race)
Residence in the southeastern United States

[a]Including human immunodeficiency virus infection.

had an unknown or equivocal response to therapy accounted for 91 (11%) of all cases. The remaining 59 (7%) cases were due to inappropriate serologic response to therapy in the mother, evidence of treatment failure, or re-infection or other reasons.

Other investigators have called attention to problems with antenatal management and communication.[147–149] These include failure to (1) obtain an appropriate and complete maternal history, (2) perform routine screening at appropriate times during the pregnancy, (3) correctly interpret serologic results, (4) recognize signs of maternal syphilis, (5) treat the pregnant sexual partner of an acutely infected man, and (6) communicate pertinent maternal history and results of screening tests to the infant's health care practitioner. Local health departments and clinicians must improve the exchange of information between obstetric and pediatric services. These issues further underscore the need for education of health care providers on the management of sexually transmitted diseases.

Sexually transmitted diseases potentially threaten everyone regardless of demographic probabilities. As shown in Table 12–2, 44 cases occurred in women who were incubating syphilis at the time of delivery, which highlights the limitation of the screening serologic tests to detect early cases. Serologic tests are poor diagnostic tools during the incubation or early primary stage of syphilis. During those times, results of the nontreponemal (rapid plasma reagin or VDRL) tests may not show reactivity because reactivity occurs 4 to 8 weeks after the infection is acquired and several days to 1 week after the development of a chancre.[150, 151] In primary syphilis, nonreactivity to nontreponemal tests is reported to occur in one fourth to one third of cases.[152, 153] Nonreactivity of the microhemagglutination–T. pallidum (MHA-TP) assay and the fluorescent treponemal antibody (FTA) test occurs in as many as 36% and 18% of cases of primary syphilis, respectively.[155] A prenatal prevention strategy that uses only currently available serologic tests, therefore, cannot eliminate all congenital syphilis,[155] and reliance must still be placed on contact tracing of sexual partners, careful physical examination of women in labor for evidence of primary syphilis, and additional testing of postpartum women at 4 weeks after delivery.[98, 120, 156, 157] Moreover, if a woman with a child younger than 1 year is diagnosed to have early syphilis, that child should be evaluated for signs of congenital syphilis, tested serologically, and treated accordingly.

PATHOLOGY AND PATHOGENESIS

Controversy remains about the pathogenesis of congenital syphilis. It was believed that infection of the fetus by a syphilitic mother does not occur before the fifth month of pregnancy because pathologic changes in fetal tissue could not be demonstrated before this time. It was thought that the Langhans' cell layer of the cytotrophoblast formed a placental barrier against treponemal invasion of the fetus.[158, 159] This theory, however, has been disproved by the demonstration, with electron microscopy, of the persistence of the Langhans' cell layer throughout pregnancy.[160] Moreover, using silver stains and immunofluorescence techniques, Harter and Benirschke demonstrated spirochetes in fetal tissue from spontaneous abortions at 9 and 10 weeks of gestation.[161] However, infectivity testing that would have proved the presence of *T. pallidum* conclusively was not done. The lack of pathologic changes in fetal tissues earlier than the fifth month of pregnancy may be a result of fetal immunoincompetence during early gestation.[162] Moreover, viable spirochetes in amniotic fluid obtained by amniocentesis from a woman with early syphilis have been demonstrated as early as at 14 weeks of gestation, thus clearly proving that the fetus can be exposed to *T. pallidum* early in pregnancy.[163]

Pathologic changes in congenital syphilis are similar to those that occur in acquired syphilis, except that there is no primary or chancre stage. Because the infection involves the placenta[164] and spreads hematogenously to the fetus, widespread involvement is characteristic. No matter which organ is involved, the essential microscopic appearance of the lesion is that of perivascular infiltration of lymphocytes, plasma cells, and histiocytes, with obliterative endarteritis and extensive fibrosis.[165–167] This typical histopathology of the inflammatory response to invasion by *T. pallidum* in tissues and blood vessels suggests an important role for cytokines as mediators of immunopathogenesis during syphilis.[68] Radolf and associates[68] have shown that *T. pallidum* lipoproteins induce macrophages to secrete tumor necrosis factor as well as activate vascular endothelium.

In addition, Brightbill and colleagues[168] have shown that the 47-kDa lipoprotein of *T. pallidum* induced production of IL-12 mRNA from human macrophages, a key signal of the innate immune system. The spirochete also has been shown to activate human promyelomonocytic cell line THP-1 cells in a CD14-dependent manner.[169] These findings lend further support to the concept that lipoproteins are the principal components of intact spirochetes that are responsible for monocyte activation, and they indicate that surface exposure of lipoproteins is an important determinant of a spirochetal pathogen's proinflammatory capacity.

Placenta

The infected placenta is paler, thicker, and larger than normal.[170] Histopathologic examination of the placenta, especially if unexpectedly large, and of the umbilical cord is a useful adjunct for the diagnosis of congenital syphilis.[112, 170–175] The histologic findings consist of focal villositis with endovascular and perivascular proliferation and relative immaturity of the villi, which become enlarged and hypercellular and have bullous projections[171, 172]; these larger villi in relation to the amount of blood in the capillaries are the cause of the pallor. Rogers and colleagues[176] have correlated villous enlargement as well as placental erythroblastosis with stillbirth due to congenital syphilis. In addition, an increased amount of connective tissue surrounds the capillaries and also makes up the stroma. Treponemes are demonstrable with silver stains,[164, 171, 172] although tissue membrane artifacts may in fact be difficult to distinguish from treponemes (T Turner, personal communication to Dr.

Daniel Musher, 1977). Necrotizing funisitis, a deeply seated inflammatory process within the matrix of the umbilical cord, has been associated with congenital syphilis and may provide a diagnostic clue to its diagnosis at birth.[173, 175] Spirochetes have been identified within the umbilical cord lesions by silver stain. Bromberg and co-workers[174] have detected *T. pallidum* in umbilical specimens by an immunofluorescent antigen detection assay (IFA). Using polymerase chain reaction (PCR) to detect *T. pallidum* DNA, Genest and colleagues[91] confirmed the strong association between the placental histopathologic features (enlarged hypercellular villi, proliferative fetal vascular changes, and acute or chronic villitis) and congenital syphilis and suggested that PCR may identify additional cases of histologically unidentified congenital syphilis.

The Fetus and Newborn

A stillborn syphilitic fetus often has a macerated appearance, with a collapsed skull and protuberant abdomen. The skin shows vesicular or bullous lesions, which have a fluid rich in treponemes. Guarner and associates[177] reported that a constant feature throughout the tissues was concentric macrophage (CD68-positive) infiltrate around vessels, giving an onion-skin appearance. Immunohistochemical analysis identified the macrophages as the prime immune response in congenital syphilis. The liver and spleen are enlarged and show fibrosis and extramedullary hematopoiesis.[178] Roentgenographs of long bones show evidence of osteochondritis and periostitis.[179]

Liver. There is a divergence of opinion on the nature and extent of hepatic involvement in congenital syphilis. The traditional view has been that diffuse interstitial inflammation is present that may progress to disrupt the normal hepatic architecture by extensive scarring.[180, 181] Oppenheimer and Hardy found 15 of 16 livers from children who died when younger than 9 weeks of age to be abnormal; lesions varied considerably in severity and included inflammation in the interstitial stroma and perivascular network, especially in the area of the portal triads, with diffuse hepatitis and excessive extramedullary hematopoiesis.[178] When Wright and Berry[182] reviewed liver sections from which Nabarro[84] had previously described intercellular fibrosis, they found that 50 of 59 sections stained with hematoxylin and eosin were histologically normal, although silver stains revealed heavy infiltration with treponemes. The discrepancies in the observations of these workers may be related to the different ages of the patients and the severity of the infections. The patients described by Wright and Berry were up to 1 year of age. Rarely, gummas have been described in the liver in infants with congenital syphilis, and cirrhosis appears to be an uncommon complication.[178]

Spleen. The spleen is enlarged because of an extensive nonspecific inflammatory reaction[183] as well as extramedullary hematopoiesis.

Lung. The "pneumonia alba" of congenital syphilis is characterized grossly by yellowish white, heavy, firm, and grossly enlarged lungs.[167, 183] Histologically, a marked increase in the amount of connective tissue in the interalveolar septa and the interstitium associated with collapse and loss of alveolar spaces explains the increased weight and density of the lung. This obliterative fibrosis of the lung is now reported only rarely.[178]

Stomach and Intestine. Attention has been called to the unique submucosal inflammation and fibrosis of the gastrointestinal tracts of patients who died in the first 2 months of life.[178] An initial mucosal and submucosal infiltration with mononuclear cells is associated with a striking submucosal fibroblastic proliferation, resulting in a remarkable increase in the width of the submucosa. These changes are found more often in the small intestine than in the colon and stomach.[177, 184]

Pancreas. An intense pancreatitis[178] is present with a perivascular inflammatory infiltrate, obliteration of ductules and acini, reduction in the number of islets, and extensive fibrosis.

Kidneys. Renal involvement appears to be the consequence of injury to the glomeruli by immune complex deposition,[185] just as has been described for the glomerulitis of secondary syphilis in adults.[186] An epimembranous glomerulopathy[187] is common and is associated with two different forms of immune complex injury, one involving complement deposition in addition to IgA, IgM, and IgG and the other involving immune complexes without complement deposition along the basement membrane.[185] A perivascular inflammatory infiltrate, consisting of plasma cells and lymphocytes involving the interstitial tissues, is prominent. The visceral and parietal epithelial cells of the glomeruli are swollen and increased in number. Increased matrix, collagen, and cells broaden axial regions in each tuft. Numerous electron-dense nodular deposits are noted on the epithelial aspect of the thickened glomerular basement membrane.[185, 187] Elution studies have demonstrated the presence of antitreponemal antibodies in the eluate and of treponemal antigen in the eluted sections.[188] A seemingly rarer proliferative glomerulonephritis has also been described with mesangioendothelial proliferation and crescent formation.[189]

Nervous System. The neuropathology of congenital syphilis is comparable to that of acquired syphilis except that the parenchymatous processes (general paresis, tabes dorsalis) that were described infrequently in the older literature on congenital syphilis are now extremely rare.[190] Meningeal involvement is apparent as a discoloration and thickening of the basilar meninges,[167, 190] especially around the brain stem and the optic chiasm. Microscopically, endarteritis is usually present; and, depending on the severity and chronicity of the infection as well as on the blood vessels involved, various degrees of neuronal injury may ensue. As the infection resolves, fibrosis may occur, causing adhesions that obliterate the subarachnoid space and leading in turn to an obstructive hydrocephalus or to a variety of cranial nerve palsies.[190]

Pituitary. Interstitial inflammation and fibrosis of the anterior lobe of the pituitary gland, at times accompanied by focal necrosis, also have been reported among infants with congenital syphilis.[191] The posterior lobe remains intact. An evolving anterior pituitary gumma

has been noted at autopsy in a 3-day-old patient with congenital syphilis after failed maternal treatment.[192]

Skeletal System. Widespread involvement of bones is characteristic of congenital syphilis. Osteochondritis, periostitis, and osteomyelitis are present, especially in the long bones and ribs. The osteochondritis is recognized grossly by the presence of a moderate and irregular yellow line in the zone of provisional calcification.[193] The trabeculae are irregular, discontinuous, and variable in size and shape. The excessive fibrosis occurring at the osseous-cartilaginous junction is referred to as syphilitic granulation tissue and contains numerous blood vessels surrounded by the inflammatory infiltrate.[167, 194, 195] The characteristic saw-toothed appearance is now seen uncommonly on radiographs[196]; however, xeroradiography of long bones of stillborn infants with congenital syphilis often demonstrates this classic pattern,[179] which is produced by irregularity in the provisional zone of calcification, corresponding to an irregular ingrowth of capillaries. Small islands of cartilage may persist in the ossified bone.[178]

A subperiosteal deposit of osteoid, which may completely encircle the shaft of the long bone, is a feature of the periostitis.[84, 197] An associated osteomyelitis (osteitis) is usually present and, when it involves the large bones, is called diaphysitis.[196] Microscopically, there is an inflammatory infiltrate with erosion of the trabeculae and prominent fibrosis.[196] In the skull, the periosteal reaction may eventually lead to the radiographic finding known as frontal bossing.

The basic process of the osseous disturbance seems to involve a failure to convert cartilage in the normal sequence to mature bone. For years there has been controversy about the pathogenesis of these bony changes.[186, 198] One view is that they are specific results of local infection by the spirochete; the other is that they represent nonspecific trophic changes on endochondral bone formation caused by severe generalized disease. The fact that they heal without specific antibiotic therapy tends to favor the latter view.

Blood and Blood-Forming Tissues. Pathologic observations do not provide a basis for hematologic manifestations of congenital syphilis, which are thought to reflect physiologic changes of unknown pathogenesis (see later). Adequate numbers of megakaryocytes are present.[199] Severe anemia is initially an acute hemolytic process, compounded by the finding of splenomegaly. This is followed by a chronic progressive anemia, accentuated by physiologic marrow hypoplasia.[200]

CLINICAL MANIFESTATIONS

General Considerations

The spectrum of perinatal syphilis is similar in many ways to that of other infections in which the infecting organism spreads hematogenously from the mother to involve the placenta and infect the fetus. Damage to the fetus presumably depends on the stage of development at which infection has taken place and the time that has elapsed before treatment. With early infection and in the absence of therapy, miscarriage, stillbirth, premature delivery, or neonatal death may occur.[84, 94, 95, 164, 170, 201–203] Infection may be clinically recognizable or silent and may be present at birth; if this infection is left untreated, its expression is delayed for several months to years.[159, 204, 205]

Congenital syphilis has traditionally been divided somewhat arbitrarily into early and late stages.[166] Clinical manifestations appearing within the first 2 years of life are designated early, and those occurring after this time are called late. The clinical manifestations of early congenital syphilis are a direct result of active infection and inflammation. The clinical manifestations of late congenital syphilis are malformations or stigmata that represent the scars induced by initial lesions of early congenital syphilis or reactions to persistent and ongoing inflammation. The so-called stigmata of late congenital syphilis clearly reflect the delayed expression of a prenatal insult in a fashion comparable to the occurrence of deafness beyond infancy that is related to congenital rubella.[206]

Syphilis in the Pregnant Woman

Clinical manifestations of acquired syphilis[131, 135] are not apparently altered by pregnancy. Genital chancres, the principal manifestation of primary infection, occur about 3 weeks after contact. They are often unrecognized in women because they are asymptomatic, and their location within the vagina or on the cervix, the labia, or the perineum discourages detection. Extragenital chancres may occur in other locations, such as lips, tongue, tonsil, nipple, finger, and anus. Syphilitic chancres are painless, clearly demarcated ulcers 0.5 to 2 cm in diameter and are generally associated with enlargement of the regional lymph nodes. Multiple lesions occur more commonly than was once believed.[207] Because these lesions are painless and are often hidden, the diagnosis of active syphilis in women is usually not made until the secondary or latent stage. Accordingly, ulcerating lesions at these sites warrant evaluation with dark-field microscopy and serologic tests. If untreated, syphilitic chancres heal spontaneously 3 to 8 weeks after their appearance. The mechanism for healing is obscure; some kind of local immunity is partly responsible because secondary lesions appear during or after the regression of the primary one(s).

Lesions of secondary syphilis result from the dissemination of treponemes from syphilitic chancres, and the term *disseminated syphilis* is probably more appropriate.[19, 208] More than 3 weeks elapse between the deposition of *T. pallidum* in the dermis and emergence of these lesions; this delay in development and the failure of the affected sites to develop into lesions that resemble primary chancres probably reflect a degree of humoral or cellular immunity, or both, that modifies the evolution of infection. Thus, secondary syphilis appears 4 to 10 weeks after the initial appearance of primary lesions; however, in some patients who present with disseminated lesions, a careful search leads to discovery of the primary chancre. The rash may be macular, papular, follicular, papulosquamous, or pustular[166, 209]; the vesiculobullous eruption that is common in congenital syphilis rarely occurs in adults. Lesions are symmetrical and generally involve the trunk, where they tend to follow skin lines and the palms and soles. The rash may be misidentified as an allergic reaction even though it is seldom pruritic. Mucus patches that appear as white plaques on erythematous bases represent superficial mucosal erosions and may involve the oral cavity, vulva, vagina, or cervix.[166] In warm, moist areas of the body such as the anogenital region and intertriginous surfaces, the papules enlarge and become exuberant, raised, wartlike lesions that are highly infectious[209]; these are called condylomata lata.

Secondary syphilis is a systemic disease, and interest in the dermatologic manifestations should not prevent the physician from recognizing the presence of constitutional symptoms such as fever, weight loss, anorexia, headache, fatigue, and arthralgia that may precede or accompany the dermatologic manifestations. Generalized nontender lymphadenopathy is usually present. A variety of other complications occur, including hepatitis,[210, 211] glomerulonephritis or nephrotic syndrome,[212–215] osteitis,[216–218] iritis, and meningitis (Table 12–4).[208] *T. pallidum* has been isolated from the CSF of 30% of adults with untreated primary and secondary syphilis.[101] Either with or without treatment, the lesions of secondary syphilis heal, and the infection enters a subclinical latent phase that lasts for years and can only be diagnosed by serologic testing.[219, 220] Too often its protean clinical manifestations are overlooked and misdiagnosed.[221–223]

Latent syphilis is subdivided into early (≤ 1 year from onset of infection) and late (> 1 year) latent stages based on the time when mucocutaneous lesions may still recur and the infection may still be transmitted.[156, 166] Patients are diagnosed with early latent syphilis if, within the year preceding the evaluation, they had a documented seroconversion, symptoms of primary or secondary syphilis, or a sexual partner who had primary, secondary, or early latent syphilis. If the time of infection cannot be ascertained, then a diagnosis of syphilis of unknown duration is made and the patient is managed as if she had late latent syphilis.

TABLE 12–4

Clinical Manifestations of Early Syphilis in the Pregnant Woman

Asymptomatic
Symptomatic
    Chancre(s), genital and extragenital
    Mucocutaneous lesions
    Macular, papular, follicular, papulosquamous, pustular
    Condylomata lata
    Mucus patches
    Lymphadenopathy
    Constitutional symptoms
    Less common manifestations (alopecia, hepatitis, glomerulonephritis or nephrotic syndrome, osteitis, iritis, meningitis)
    Preterm labor (spontaneous abortion, stillbirth, preterm delivery)

A high index of suspicion (see Table 12–3) is needed by the obstetrician or perinatologist to consider the diagnosis of syphilis in pregnancy and prevent adverse outcomes. Two caveats should be heeded. Any ulcerated lesion, regardless of location, that is painless, indurated, and indolent and that fails to heal within 2 weeks warrants exclusion of this diagnosis. Similarly, any generalized eruption, regardless of its morphology, should be viewed as secondary (disseminated) syphilis until proven otherwise. One of the most common sequelae of untreated syphilis during pregnancy that is recognized worldwide is spontaneous abortion during the second and early third trimesters.[92] Moreover, untreated maternal syphilis can result in preterm delivery, perinatal death, and congenital infection. Antenatal ultrasonography may be helpful in diagnosis of fetal syphilis; hydramnios, fetal hydrops, as well as placentomegaly, hepatosplenomegaly, and bowel dilation have been described.[224, 225] Ultrasonography performed on pregnant women with early syphilis has suggested that fetal hepatosplenomegaly may be an important early indicator of congenital infection.[225]

Early Congenital Syphilis

The diagnosis of early congenital syphilis should be entertained in any infant who is born prematurely if another explanation of prematurity is not forthcoming or if unexplained hydrops fetalis or an enlarged placenta is present. In infancy, failure to thrive, persistent rhinitis, an intractable diaper rash, unexplained jaundice or hepatosplenomegaly, or an anemia or thrombocytopenia of uncertain cause should raise consideration of congenital syphilis (Table 12–5).

Hepatosplenomegaly. Hepatomegaly is present in nearly all infants with congenital syphilis and may occur in the absence of splenomegaly, although the reverse is not true.[226] Jaundice, which has been recorded in 33% of patients,[226] may be caused by syphilitic hepatitis (with elevated direct and indirect bilirubin levels) or by the hemolytic component of the disease. It may be the only manifestation of the disease. Hepatic dysfunction in the form of elevated aminotransferases, alkaline phosphatase,[227] and direct bilirubin[227–229] may initially worsen with initiation of penicillin therapy and may persist for several months.[228, 229]

Generalized Lymphadenopathy. Generalized lymphadenopathy usually occurs in association with hepatosplenomegaly and has been described in 50% of patients.[226] The nodes themselves may be as large as 1 cm and are usually nontender. Generalized enlargement of the lymph nodes may occur in a variety of systemic illnesses but is certainly uncommon in early infancy. In the presence of enlarged epitrochlear nodes, the diagnosis of syphilis must receive special consideration.

Hematologic Manifestations. Major findings include anemia, jaundice, leukopenia or leukocytosis, and thrombocytopenia. A characteristic feature in the immediate newborn period is that of a Coombs-negative hemolytic anemia. After the neonatal period, chronic nonhemolytic anemia may occur, accentuated by the usual physiologic anemia of infancy.[199, 200] The pathogenesis of

TABLE 12–5
Clues That Suggest a Diagnosis of Congenital Syphilis[a]

EPIDEMIOLOGIC BACKGROUND	CLINICAL FINDINGS
Untreated early syphilis in the mother	Osteochondritis, periostitis
Untreated latent syphilis in the mother	Snuffles, hemorrhagic rhinitis
An untreated contact of mother to a known syphilitic during pregnancy	Condylomata lata
	Bullous lesions, palmar/plantar rash
	Mucus patches
Mother treated for syphilis during pregnancy with a drug other than penicillin	Hepatomegaly, splenomegaly
	Jaundice
	Nonimmune hydrops fetalis
	Generalized lymphadenopathy
Mother treated for syphilis during pregnancy and not followed to delivery	Central nervous system signs; elevated cell count or protein in cerebrospinal fluid
Any high-risk factor given in Table 12–3	Hemolytic anemia, diffuse intravascular coagulation, thrombocytopenia
	Pneumonitis
	Nephrotic syndrome
	Placental villitis or vasculitis (unexplained enlarged placenta)
	Intrauterine growth retardation; failure to thrive

[a]Arranged in decreasing order of confidence of diagnosis.
Adapted from Rathbun KC. Congenital syphilis: A proposal for improved surveillance, diagnosis and treatment. Sex Transm Dis 10:102, 1983, with permission.

these anemias is not known. Other findings include polychromasia and erythroblastemia with up to 500 nucleated red blood cells per 100 leukocytes. This pattern of anemia and erythropoietic response has led to confusion with erythroblastosis fetalis.[84] Although the leukocyte count usually falls within the normal range,[199] leukopenia, leukocytosis, or a leukemoid reaction[226] has been described. Lymphocytosis and monocytosis may occur. Thrombocytopenia, related to decreased platelet survival rather than to insufficient production of platelets, is often present and may be the only manifestation of congenital infection. Hemophagocytosis has been described and may play an important role in the pathogenesis of anemia and thrombocytopenia.[230]

Hydrops fetalis may also be a manifestation of congenital syphilis in newborns.[231] A negative Coombs' test result in a hydropic infant with hemolytic anemia should suggest this diagnosis. A few patients with congenital syphilis develop paroxysmal cold hemoglobinuria, a disease mediated by an antibody to erythrocytes that meets even the most rigorous definition of an autoantibody.[232, 233]

Mucocutaneous Manifestations. Mucocutaneous manifestations occur in 15 to 60% of infected infants.[226, 234] Rhinitis (snuffles) may be an early feature, developing after the first week of life and usually before the end of the third month. It was reported in two thirds of patients in the older literature[234] but is now thought to be less common.[226] A mucus discharge develops similar to that occurring in upper respiratory tract infections. The discharge, which is teeming with spirochetes and is highly infectious, can become progressively more profuse and occasionally is blood tinged. Secondary bacterial infection may occur, causing the discharge to become purulent. If ulceration of the nasal mucosa is sufficiently deep and involves the nasal cartilage, a "saddle nose" deformity, one of the later stigmata of the disease, may develop. Snuffles have also been associated with laryngitis and an aphonic cry.[234] Mucus patches may appear in the mouth and are more prevalent in infants with severe systemic disease.

The most common cutaneous lesion is a maculopapular one that is oval and pink or red, subsequently becoming coppery brown.[235] As the rash changes color, very fine superficial desquamation or scaling may occur, particularly on the palms and soles. The lesions are more common on the posterior portion of the body (especially the buttocks, back, thighs, and soles) than on the anterior surface, and they may also involve the perioral area and the palms. Other maculopapular types of eruptions are seen uncommonly in early congenital syphilis. They may be annular or circinate or may have the appearance of any other kind of lesion seen in acquired secondary syphilis.[209]

Pemphigus syphiliticus occurs most commonly in the neonatal period and is characterized by a widely disseminated vesicular bullous eruption that also involves the palms and soles.[235] The lesions vary in size and may contain a cloudy hemorrhagic fluid that teems with organisms. When they rupture, they leave a denuded area that can undergo extensive maceration and crusting.

After the first 2 or 3 months of age, the perioral area, especially the nares and the angles of the mouth, and the perianal area may be affected by condylomata lata.[202, 235] These highly infected areas are flat or wartlike and moist. The condylomata may be single or multiple and are frequently asymptomatic. They may lead to deep fissures radial to the affected orifices and may result in fine scars called rhagades. Comparable eruptions may also be found in other body folds or intertriginous zones but are considered to be more characteristic of the later stage of early congenital syphilis.

There are other dermatologic manifestations of congenital syphilis. Petechial lesions may reflect the presence of thrombocytopenia; jaundice may last for several months, and generalized edema may be present[199, 226] as a consequence of hypoproteinemia related to renal or hepatic disease.

Bony Lesions. Bony lesions are perhaps the most frequently encountered abnormalities in untreated early congenital syphilis. Most of these are discussed in the Roentgenologic Diagnosis section because, except for pseudoparalysis, there are usually no clinical signs to suggest osseous involvement.[236, 237] Pseudoparalysis of Parrot, a syndrome in which pain is associated with a bony lesion or a superimposed fracture, or both, occurs infrequently.[238] Clinically, it may be manifest as irritability in an infant who does not move one of the limbs.[239] The upper extremities are more frequently affected, and

unilateral involvement predominates. This clinical picture may mimic Erb's palsy but is rarely manifest at birth. The correlation between the clinical and the radiologic findings is poor, inasmuch as other areas of bony involvement may look more severe on the film even though no clinical symptoms or signs suggest their presence.

Renal Manifestations. The clinical picture of a nephrotic syndrome usually appears at 2 or 3 months of age, the predominant manifestation being generalized edema, including pretibial, scrotal, and periorbital areas together with ascites.[240–244] Rarely, the infant may have hematuria with less severe proteinuria but more profound azotemia, which suggests that a glomerulitis predominates.

Central Nervous System Manifestations. According to Platou in 1949, clinically inapparent involvement of the brain and spinal cord as assessed by CSF abnormalities occurred in 60% of infants with congenital syphilis.[234] However, he empirically defined an abnormal CSF as having greater than 5 white blood cells per mm^3 and a protein content greater than 45 mg/dl. The overall incidence of neurosyphilis by these criteria could be challenged because in CSF of neonates up to 25 white blood cells per mm^3 and a protein content as high as 150 mg/dl in full-term infants and 170 mg/dl in preterm infants may be considered normal.[245] Furthermore, the significance of a reactive CSF VDRL in the absence of other diagnostic evidence of congenital syphilis is suspect, inasmuch as nontreponemal IgG can pass from the serum to the CSF.[246] Recent work using rabbit inoculation of CSF from infants born to mothers with untreated early syphilis documented a prevalence of spirochetal invasion of the CSF of 86% (6 of 7 infants) in infants with clinical and laboratory evidence of congenital syphilis, but only 8% (1 of 12) among infants born to mothers with untreated early syphilis and whose physical examination and laboratory evaluation were normal.[88] Neurologic manifestations, although well documented in the older literature,[190] have been reported infrequently in recent papers. The clinical types of CNS involvement have been separated arbitrarily into supposedly well-defined groups, but in fact there is frequent overlapping.

Acute syphilitic leptomeningitis appears during the first year of life, usually between 3 and 6 months of age. Symptoms and signs may suggest acute bacterial meningitis, including a stiff neck, progressive vomiting, a positive Kernig sign, bulging of the fontanelles, separation of the suture, and hydrocephalus.[247] In contrast to the clinical picture, CSF shows changes that suggest an aseptic meningitis, with up to 200 mononuclear cells per mm^3, a modest increase in protein (50 to 200 mg/dl), and a normal glucose level. The CSF VDRL test is positive. This is the one form of CNS involvement that clearly responds to antisyphilitic therapy.[234]

Chronic meningovascular syphilis may have a protracted course, resulting in progressive hydrocephalus, cranial nerve palsies or vascular lesions of the brain, and gradual intellectual deterioration.[247] This usually develops toward the end of the first year. The hydrocephalus is low grade, progressive, and communicating because of obstruction in the basilar cisterns. Cranial nerve palsies may complicate the picture.[190] The seventh nerve is involved most often, but the third, fourth, and sixth cranial nerves can also be affected. Optic atrophy may be preceded by papilledema.

A variety of cerebrovascular syndromes have been described, but they are uncommon.[190] Cerebral infarction results from syphilitic endarteritis and may occur between the first and second years of life, commonly presenting as acute hemiplegia. Convulsions frequently complicate the picture.

Ocular Manifestations. The occurrence of syphilitic involvement of the eye in early congenital syphilis is rare. Chorioretinitis, salt-and-pepper fundus, glaucoma, uveitis, cataract,[248] and chancres of the eyelid have been described.[84] Involvement by syphilis leads to a granular appearance of the fundus on which can be seen pigmentary patches of various shapes and colors[84] in the periphery of the retina. The young infant rarely manifests the signs of photophobia and diminution in vision that occur in older patients. Congenital glaucoma can occur[84] and should be considered in the presence of blepharospasm, cloudy cornea, enlarged cornea (diameter exceeding 12 mm), and excessive tearing.

Inflammation of the uveal tract (including the iris and ciliary body anteriorly and the choroid posteriorly) affects the retina because of the close anatomic relationship of the cornea to the structures of the uveal tract. Consequently, chorioretinitis rather than uveitis is the more commonly diagnosed ocular problem in infancy. However, a recent pathologic report of an eye from a 3-day-old infant who died of congenital syphilis revealed a focal granulomatous reaction involving the anterior uvea and lens.[248] Rarely, a chancre of the eyelid appears 4 weeks after birth, apparently resulting from recently developed syphilitic lesions of the maternal genitalia.[84]

Intrauterine Growth Retardation. The effect of syphilis on the growth of the fetus in utero could be related to the timing and severity of the fetal infection. In a carefully performed quantitative morphologic study, Naeye demonstrated that syphilitic infection in utero did not seem to have a significant effect on the growth of the fetus, as manifested by a study of 36 perinatal deaths.[249] This finding was similar to his previous results,[250] which showed a relative lack of effect of toxoplasmosis on fetal growth in contrast to the intrauterine growth retardation associated with rubella and cytomegalovirus infections. On the other hand, case reports have shown that, at birth, the infected newborns were small for their gestational age.[239] Whether this growth retardation is the result of syphilitic infection or other factors, such as maternal use of intravenous drugs,[251] that affect fetal growth is not known.

Other Findings. The classic description of the congenital syphilitic patient is a severely infected premature infant with marasmus, a pot belly, "old man" facies, and withered skin.[84, 235] The clinical state of failure to thrive may be correlated with the frequently encountered pathologic finding of intense pancreatitis[178] and inflammation of the gastrointestinal tract.[178] Rectal bleeding due to syphilitic ileitis with ulcer formation and associated with intestinal obstruction has been re-

ported.[185] Involvement of the anterior pituitary gland in congenital syphilis is manifested by persistent hypoglycemia beyond the early neonatal period.[191] Evaluation of pituitary function, including tests for thyroid function and growth hormone and cortisol levels, combined with magnetic resonance imaging of the pituitary, confirms the diagnosis of hypopituitarism.[191]

Other uncommon manifestations of congenital syphilis include pneumonia alba, or syphilitic pneumonitis, which produces an obliterative fibrosis of the lung tissue. Myocarditis[178] also has been reported at autopsy in approximately 10% of affected infants, although the clinical significance of this finding is unclear. Fever has been reported among infants who present beyond the newborn period with clinical signs of congenital syphilis.[111, 227]

Late Congenital Syphilis

The clinical manifestations of late congenital syphilis are malformations or stigmata that represent scars induced by initial lesions of early congenital syphilis or reactions to persistent and ongoing inflammation. In patients older than 2 years of age, late congenital syphilis may be manifest by (1) the stigmata of the disorder that represent the scars of initial lesions or developmental changes induced by the early infection; (2) ongoing inflammation that causes interstitial keratitis, nerve deafness, and Clutton's joints (although treponemes are not demonstrable); or (3) a persistently positive treponemal serologic test for syphilis in the absence of apparent disease.[166] In reviewing the manifestations of late congenital syphilis (Table 12–6), Fiumara and Lessel concluded that only Hutchinson's triad (Hutchinson's teeth, interstitial keratitis, and eighth nerve deafness), mulberry molars, or Clutton's joints are specific enough to lead to the diagnosis.[252]

Dentition. Vasculitis that occurs around the time of birth damages the developing tooth bud, which leads to a number of dental abnormalities that appear in late congenital syphilis. The deciduous teeth do not seem to be affected except for a possible increase in the incidence of dental caries.[84] Hutchinson's teeth are abnormalities of the permanent upper central incisors; these teeth are

---

TABLE 12–6
Clinical Manifestations of Late Congenital Syphilis

Dentition: Hutchinson's teeth, mulberry molars (Moon's, Fournier's)
Eye: interstitial keratitis, healed chorioretinitis, secondary glaucoma (uveitis), corneal scarring
Ear: eighth nerve deafness
Nose and face: "saddle nose," protuberant mandible
Skin: rhagades
Central nervous system: mental retardation, arrested hydrocephalus, convulsive disorders, optic nerve atrophy, juvenile general paresis, cranial nerve palsies
Bones and joints: saber shins, Higouménakis' sign, Clutton's joints

peg shaped and notched, usually with obvious thinning and discoloration of enamel in the area of the notching. The teeth are widely spaced and shorter than the lateral incisors. The width of the biting surface is less than that of the gingival margin.[252]

A diagnostic lesion, the mulberry molar (also known as Moon's or Fournier's molar) is seen in the first lower molar.[252] Characteristically, the tooth's grinding surface, which is narrower than that at the gingival margin, has many small cusps instead of the usual four well-formed cusps. The enamel itself tends to be poorly developed.

Putkonen examined 30 children whose infected mothers had received penicillin during the latter half of pregnancy and an additional 36 children whose initial therapy for congenital syphilis was started during the first few months of life.[253] He noted distinct syphilitic dental changes in 7 of 15 children whose treatment began during the fourth month of life or after but none in children whose mothers had received treatment during the last half of pregnancy or the first 3 months of life. He thus concluded that early treatment prevented the dental changes of syphilis.

Eye. Interstitial keratitis is the second manifestation of Hutchinson's triad. This lesion may be detected in patients between 5 and 20 years of age. A severe inflammatory reaction begins in one eye, generally becoming bilateral during the ensuing weeks or months. Spirochetes have not been found to be present.[201] Symptoms include photophobia, pain, excessive lacrimation, and blurred vision. On physical examination, patients may have conjunctival injection, miosis, keratitis, or anterior uveitis, or a combination of these. Interstitial keratitis is considered preventable if treatment is given before the age of 3 months.[253] Buphthalmos has rarely been described.

Interstitial keratitis usually appears at puberty and is not affected by penicillin therapy but responds transiently to corticosteroid treatment.[254] Keratitis often has a relapsing course that may result in secondary glaucoma or corneal clouding.

Ear. Eighth nerve deafness is the least common component of Hutchinson's triad, occurring in only 3% of patients with late congenital syphilis.[252, 255, 256] The pathology of luetic involvement of the temporal bone is that of mononuclear leukocytic infiltration and obliterative endarteritis. The periosteal, endochondral, and endosteal layers of bone are also involved. Osteochondritis affecting the otic capsule may lead to cochlear degeneration and fibrous adhesions, resulting in eighth nerve deafness along with vertigo. Although the deafness usually occurs in the first decade, it may not appear until the third or fourth decade of life. The initial involvement may be unilateral or bilateral; the deafness initially involves the higher frequencies, and normal conversational tones are affected later. It may be responsive to long-term corticosteroid therapy.

Nose and Face. The sequelae of syphilitic rhinitis include failure of the maxilla to grow fully, resulting in a concave configuration in the middle section of the face with relative protuberance of the mandible and an associated high palatal arch. Inflammation of the nasal mucosa may affect the cartilage and lead to destruction of the underlying bone and perforation of the nasal septum. The resulting depression of the roof of the nose gives the appearance of a "saddle nose."

Skin. An infrequent sign of late congenital syphilis consists of early linear scars that become fissured or ulcerated, resulting in deeper scars called rhagades that are located around the body orifices, including the mouth, nostrils, and anus.[84]

Central Nervous System. The reported incidence of neurologic involvement in late congenital syphilis varies considerably according to different authors. Some report that as many as one third of patients more than 2 years of age have CSF abnormalities that would justify a diagnosis of late asymptomatic neurosyphilis.[234] The neurologic manifestations may include mental retardation, arrested hydrocephalus, convulsive disorders, juvenile general paresis, and cranial nerve abnormalities, including deafness and blindness, which is due to optic nerve atrophy.[190, 247] These findings are now uncommon.[252] Use of single photon emission computed tomography (SPECT) in a 5-year-old patient with late neurosyphilis manifested as seizures demonstrated areas of hypoperfusion that closely agreed with abnormalities seen in the electroencephalogram.[257] Cranial computed tomography, magnetic resonance imaging, and cerebral angiography were normal.

Bones and Joints. Bony involvement in late congenital syphilis is relatively infrequent in comparison with its involvement in early congenital syphilis.[84] The sequelae of periosteal reactions may involve the skull, resulting in frontal bossing; the tibia, resulting in saber shin; or the sternoclavicular portion of the clavicle, resulting in a deformity called Higouménakis' sign.[252] For unknown reasons, the last-named finding tends to occur only on the side of dominant handedness.

Joint involvement is even less common. Clutton's joints were found in only 1 of 271 patients.[252] In this condition, synovitis occurs with hydrarthrosis, local tenderness, and limitation of motion[258]; the knee joint is most commonly affected. Roentgenograms do not show involvement of the bones, and examination of the joint fluid reveals a few mononuclear cells.

DIAGNOSIS

The ideal for diagnosis would be to identify easily and accurately the five following groups: (1) infected mothers giving birth to clinically recognized infected infants, (2) infected mothers giving birth to infected infants without clinically manifest signs, (3) infected mothers giving birth to uninfected infants without clinical findings, (4) infected but seronegative mothers giving birth to infected infants without clinical manifestations, and (5) uninfected mothers. The problem of distinguishing among the latter four groups is a recurring theme in discussing identification of the infected infant and underscores the need for a "safety first" approach to investigation and treatment.

A definitive diagnosis of congenital syphilis can be made in the unusual situation in which the organism can be identified by dark-field or pathologic examination of specimens from suspicious lesions or amniotic fluid.[89, 92, 156, 163, 225, 259] Seroconversion or a fourfold rise in the rapid plasma reagin (RPR) (or VDRL) test with a positive treponemal test (fluorescent treponemal antibody absorption [FTA-ABS] test or hemagglutination tests) is sufficient for a definitive diagnosis to be made.[88]

In most patients, the presence of one or more clinical findings of congenital syphilis together with laboratory findings leads to a diagnosis (Table 12–7).[260] The finding of other early manifestations (e.g., hepatosplenomegaly with or without jaundice, generalized lymphadenopathy), hematologic manifestations (i.e., hemolytic anemia or thrombocytopenia), nonimmune hydrops fetalis, mucocutaneous manifestations (vesiculobullous rash, snuffles, condylomata lata), bony involvement, pseudoparalysis of Parrot, renal manifestations, or CNS or CSF abnormalities leads to a probable diagnosis. The diagnosis of possible syphilis is made when the serologic test is positive but clinical evidence of disease is absent. The diagnosis can be excluded if both the RPR and FTA-ABS tests become nonreactive in less than 6 months in an untreated infant or are nonreactive in the mother and infant, barring the situation in which the mother is seronegative but in the incubation period of syphilis and still able to transmit the infection to the fetus.[157, 227]

Because of the infrequent occurrence of congenital syphilis and its protean manifestations, it is essential for the physician to remain alert to the possibility of this diagnosis. This is especially true because the diagnosis of syphilis in the mother may also be difficult. A serologic test for syphilis must be done routinely in the first trimester of pregnancy[144, 145] and again at the beginning of the third trimester and at delivery in areas where congenital syphilis is still occurring (see Table 12–3).[108, 135, 156] The diagnosis of syphilis in the early weeks of life

thus depends on epidemiologic evidence, observation of the more common clinical presentations, documentation of radiologic abnormalities consistent with the diagnosis, and confirmation of these factors by serologic tests or, rarely, the demonstration of spirochetes by dark-field microscopic examination or immunofluorescent staining of appropriate lesions or amniotic fluid.[89, 156, 163, 225, 259, 261, 262]

Roentgenologic Diagnosis

Bony involvement, the most common and frequent manifestation of congenital syphilitic infection,[234, 263] tends to be multiple and symmetrical. The metaphyses and diaphyses are most often involved, especially in the long bones (tibia, humerus, and femur). The lesions include osteochondritis (metaphyseal dystrophy), osteomyelitis (osteitis-like dystrophy), and periostitis (periosteal dystrophy).

Characteristically, bony involvement is widespread and includes the long bones, cranium, spine, and ribs. The earliest and most characteristic changes occur in the metaphysis, with sparing of the epiphysis.[198] The changes are nonspecific and vary from radiopaque bands to actual fragmentation and apparent destruction with mottled areas of radiolucency. Frequently, an enhanced zone of provisional calcification (radiopaque band) is associated with osteoporosis immediately beneath the dense zone. Variations of these porotic changes occur, including peripheral (lateral) porosis only and alternating bands of density sandwiching a porotic zone (Fig. 12–3).[196] The classic saw-toothed appearance of the bone is now an uncommon finding, although it can be seen on xeroradiographs from stillborn infants with congenital syphilis.[179] Metaphysitis or metaphyseal dystrophy (the choice of terms depends on the concept of pathogenesis) of the long bones may be present at birth or may first appear after the first or second month of life.

In many of the long bones, the lesions are located on the lateral aspects of the metaphyses.[198] The tibia, however, shows similar metaphyseal defects on its upper medial aspect. When this defect occurs bilaterally, it is called Wimberger's sign (Fig. 12–4). Rarely, similar changes may occur at the upper ends of the humeri. Although Wimberger's sign was formerly thought to be pathognomonic of congenital syphilis,[264] it was later described[265] in other disease states, including osteomyelitis, hyperparathyroidism, and infantile generalized fibromatosis.

Focal areas of patchy cortical radiolucency with spreading of the medullary canal and irregularity of the endosteal and periosteal aspects of the cortex may be found. In severe cases, the radiolucent areas may appear as columns, giving a "celery stick" appearance of alternating bands of longitudinal translucency and relative density, a finding also seen in rubella and cytomegalovirus infection.[196]

The inflammatory reaction in the diaphysis stimulates the periosteum to lay down new bone. The single or multiple layers of periosteal new bone formation extend along the cortex of the entire diaphysis. Unlike the other two forms of osseous involvement (metaphyseal

---

TABLE 12–7
Suggested Diagnostic Categories of Congenital Syphilis Relative to Confidence of Diagnosis

DEFINITE DIAGNOSIS
1. Confirmation of presence of *T. pallidum* by dark-field microscopic or histologic examination or rabbit infectivity test (RIT)
2. STS (RPR, VDRL) increased fourfold or greater than maternal STS (both drawn at time of evaluation)

PROBABLE DIAGNOSIS
1. STS (RPR or VDRL) reactive in presence of snuffles, condylomata lata, pemphigus syphiliticus, hepatosplenomegaly or osseous lesions
2. STS (RPR or VDRL) reactive in presence of other clinical manifestations given in Table 12–5
3. STS (VDRL) reactive in cerebrospinal fluid
4. Reactive treponemal antibody test after 15 months of age

POSSIBLE DIAGNOSIS
STS (RPR or VDRL, FTA-ABS) reactive in absence of clinical disease

UNLIKELY DIAGNOSIS
STS nonreactive when < 6 months of age

FTA-ABS = fluorescent treponemal antibody absorption test; RPR = rapid plasma reagin; STS = serologic test for syphilis; VDRL = Venereal Disease Research Laboratory.

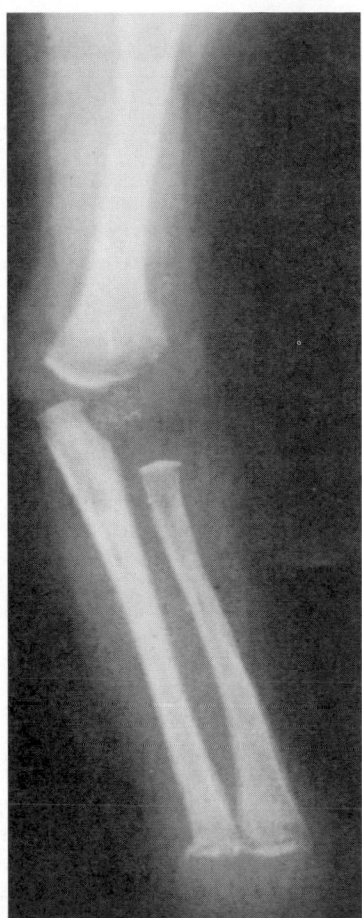

FIGURE 12–3 A 1-month-old male infant presented with a respiratory illness and a positive VDRL test. The radiograph of the forearm and distal humerus shows evidence of irregular metaphyseal demineralization associated with periosteal new bone formation. There is minimal soft tissue swelling. The changes are most marked in the distal radius and ulna, but the radial aspect of the distal humerus is also involved. The dense bands in the distal metaphysis of the radius and ulna as well as the distal humerus are also present but are nonspecific findings. Although these metaphyseal bands of density are seen in a significant number of patients with congenital syphilis, they are not diagnostic. The presence of symmetrical metaphyseal lesions is more typical and helps to separate the lesions of congenital syphilis from other causes of osteomyelitis or osseous dysplasia associated with disseminated infection.

dystrophy and osteitis-like dystrophy), it is less commonly present at birth. Osteochondritis is evident radiographically 5 weeks after fetal infection has occurred; periostitis requires 16 weeks for radiographic diagnosis.[266] Obstetric radiography[267] allows for the in utero diagnosis of fetal syphilis by demonstrating periosteal cloaking. Although maternal treatment has been associated with radiologic resolution of these lesions, the radiographic signs of congenital syphilis will resolve spontaneously even without therapy. Periostitis usually occurs during the early months of life and must be distinguished from that seen in healing rickets, battered child

syndrome, infantile cortical hyperostosis, a variety of poorly understood disorders presumed to be related to nutritional deficiencies, occasionally pyogenic osteomyelitis,[198] and prostaglandin-induced periostitis.[268]

Involvement of the metacarpals, metatarsals, or proximal phalanges of the hand is rarely seen. Dactylitis appears radiologically as a spindle-shaped enlargement of the bone and may occur between the third month of life[198] and the end of the second year. Unusual osseous manifestations have been reported. A case of syphilitic arthritis of the hip and elbow in association with osteomyelitis of the femur and humerus has been described[269, 270] in the immediate newborn period. Single bone involvement is unique, but, in a brief case report, solitary involvement of the radius was described.[271] Solomon and Rosen interpreted more than one third of their radiologic findings in 112 children with congenital syphilis to be more consistent with trauma occurring in bone made more fragile by syphilitic infection.[272, 273] Bone scans have been performed in very few patients; although they have been diffusely abnormal when conducted,[274–276] they are not needed for diagnosis.

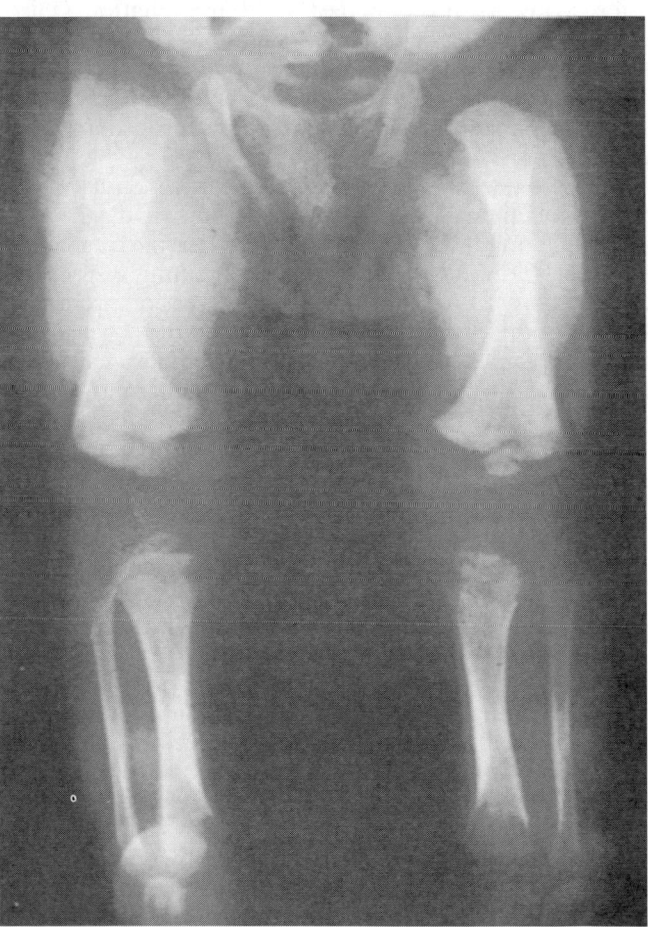

FIGURE 12–4 An anteroposterior film of both lower extremities of the same patient as shown in Figure 12–3 demonstrates demineralization and osseous destruction of the proximal medial tibial metaphysis. These lesions are typical of Wimberger's sign. Note the diffuse symmetrical periostitis and irregular demineralization of the metaphyses of the distal tibias and femurs.

Examination of the Placenta

See Pathology and Pathogenesis section.

Demonstration of the Organism

The current reference standard for the identification of *T. pallidum* in clinical specimens is by inoculation into rabbits (rabbit infectivity test [RIT])[88, 89, 101, 277, 278]; RIT has a sensitivity of 5 to 10 organisms. Within 30 to 60 minutes of collection, the clinical sample (serum, blood, CSF, or amniotic fluid) is injected intratesticularly into a seronegative adult male rabbit. While housed at 10° C to 20° C, each animal is regularly examined over 3 months for evidence of infection by *T. pallidum* (orchitis) and also by serologic testing (RPR and treponemal tests). If at 3 months there is no evidence of orchitis and the serologic test results are nonreactive, the rabbit is considered to be noninfected and thus the specimen negative for viable *T. pallidum*. When treponemal infection is suspected by seroconversion or development of orchitis, the rabbit is sacrificed, popliteal lymph nodes and testicular tissue are removed and minced in sterile saline, and the tissue extract is examined by dark-field microscopy. A positive dark-field examination (spirochetes visualized) of testicular extract is confirmatory. If the dark-field examination again is negative, 2 ml of the testicular homogenate is then injected into a second seronegative rabbit and the previous procedure is repeated.

RIT, however, is performed only in research laboratories; in clinical situations, the definitive diagnosis of syphilis is made by detecting characteristic treponemes by dark-field microscopy.[27] While obtaining a specimen, the examiner should wear rubber gloves for protection. Bullae should be aspirated with a sterile syringe and needle. Papules or condylomas may be abraded with a gauze square until oozing occurs. A sterile glass slide is applied to the exudate, which is then covered by a drop of normal saline and a coverslip and is promptly examined. A negative examination does not exclude the diagnosis of syphilis, and examinations should be repeated if the clinical findings are suggestive. The scaly eruption is not a good source of such material.

Hematology

Blood should be obtained for determination of hematocrit and hemoglobin, red blood cell count, reticulocyte count, platelet count, and white blood cell count, as well as for a differential smear, direct Coombs' test, and serologic testing (RPR/VDRL). Performance of a serum treponemal test such as the FTA-ABS test is not necessary in the newborn period if the mother is known to have a reactive result (see later).

Serology

GENERAL CONSIDERATIONS

Serologic tests[155] have played a prominent role in the clinical diagnosis of syphilis since the early part of this century, when antibody to the mammalian membrane

---

TABLE 12–8
Serologic Tests for Syphilis

TESTS TO DETECT ANTIBODIES TO CARDIOLIPIN

1. VDRL (Venereal Disease Research Laboratory): usually done by reference laboratories
2. RPR (rapid plasma reagin): now used in offices and small laboratories

TESTS TO DETECT ANTIBODY TO *T. PALLIDUM*

1. TPI (*T. pallidum*–immobilizing test): no longer available for diagnostic purposes
2. FTA-ABS (fluorescent treponemal antibody, absorbed with nonpallidum treponemes [*T. phagedenis*])
3. TP-PA (*T. pallidum* particle agglutination test): hemagglutination test that detects antibody to *T. pallidum* components; hemagglutination assays have largely replaced FTA-ABS; MHA-TP (microhemagglutination–*T. pallidum*): no longer commercially available.
4. ELISA (enzyme-linked immunosorbent assay): IgG and IgM antibody tests
5. FTA-ABS-IgM (fluorescent *T. pallidum* antibody-absorbed-IgM test): not recommended (see text)
6. Immunoblotting (IgG, IgM, IgA): not yet adapted for clinical use in diagnosing syphilis

---

lipid cardiolipin (diphosphatidylglycerol) was serendipitously detected by Wassermann in the serum of patients with active syphilis (Table 12–8). The test used to detect this antibody went through a number of modifications (by Kolmer, Kahn, and Mazzini, for example), culminating in that of the Venereal Disease Research Laboratory (VDRL) of the Communicable Disease Center (as the CDC was then known). This antibody was also called reagin, a term that by now should have been abandoned because of confusion with IgE but one that has remained in use to describe a simplified, rapid test to detect antibody to cardiolipin, the RPR test, which has replaced the VDRL in many laboratories because of the ease of performing the test. Results are reported with dilutions (titers) so that the degree of reactivity can be determined; a high titer in the absence of treatment and especially a rising titer (fourfold increase) indicate the presence of active disease. The RPR titer is often one to two dilutions higher than results obtained from the VDRL test; therefore, caution must be exercised when making clinical decisions on the basis of results of these two tests on the same patient. For similar reasons, in order that appropriate comparisons can be made, the same nontreponemal test should be performed on the mother and infant.[156] Because the RPR test is generally more sensitive than the VDRL test, it is the preferred test for screening pregnant women. The VDRL test, however, is recommended for use on CSF.

Infection with *T. pallidum* also causes the host to produce antitreponemal antibodies that are detected by using the FTA test. More recently developed *T. pallidum* hemagglutination tests (*T. pallidum* particle agglutination [TP-PA] test and the microhemagglutination assay for *T. pallidum* antibody [MHA-TP]) are easier to carry out and can be done with small volumes of serum in an automated system. These tests appear to provide results that are comparable to those of the FTA, although the FTA is slightly more sensitive and specific.[279] When syphilis is suspected in a patient who has a reactive RPR but negative TP-PA test, an FTA should be performed to rule out early syphilis.

Nontreponemal Antibody Tests (RPR and VDRL Tests). The VDRL and RPR tests are often called nontreponemal antibody tests. Actually, the antigenic stimulus is uncertain. Diphosphatidylglycerol comprises a small proportion of the lipids of *T. pallidum*[280]; but these organisms may be unable to synthesize this substance, and it is possible that, instead, they incorporate it from damaged host tissues. Thus, the production of RPR antibody could reflect an autoimmune host response to a slightly altered and/or a differently presented cardiolipin. In this context, it is interesting that anticardiolipin antibody reflects ongoing tissue damage, its detection correlating closely with the level of activity in the early stages of syphilis. These observations may explain why patients with autoimmune diseases, such as systemic lupus erythematosus, characteristically have positive RPR reactions. The RPR may also be reactive, generally not exceeding a 1:8 dilution, in nonsyphilitic patients who have infections caused by viruses (especially infectious mononucleosis and hepatitis viruses), *Mycoplasma*, or protozoa.[67, 150, 281, 282] A reactive RPR is also seen in the absence of syphilis in heroin addicts, in elderly subjects, and in patients with cirrhosis, malignancy (especially if associated with production of excess globulin), and autoimmune disease or, rarely, in pregnancy itself.[67, 150, 283–287] VDRL reactivity in these conditions has acquired the unfortunate designation of biologic false positive to indicate an etiology other than *T. pallidum* infection.

The VDRL is reactive in about 75% of adult patients at the time they seek medical attention for primary syphilis (Table 12–9). Secondary syphilis is always characterized by a reactive VDRL, usually in a dilution greater than 1:16.[58, 279] Persistence of VDRL antibody after appropriate antibiotic therapy, sometimes called a sero-fast state, is apparently uncommon; studies have shown that the VDRL usually becomes negative within 2 years of treatment.[155, 288, 289] Even in the absence of treatment, the VDRL slowly returns toward a nonreactive state and is, in fact, negative in one third of patients with late syphilis.[58]

One to 2% of sera from patients with secondary syphilis will exhibit a prozone phenomenon.[150–153] This is due to an excess amount of reagin antibody present in the patient's undiluted serum, which prevents flocculation and results in a false-negative reaction. The prozone effect can be overcome by diluting the serum before testing, after which the serum will usually exhibit titers of 1:16 or greater. Failure to detect a prozone effect in maternal serum tested during pregnancy has resulted in failure to diagnose congenital syphilis, with devastating results.[153]

Treponemal Antibody Tests. Other serologic tests detect an interaction between serum immunoglobulins and surface antigens of *T. pallidum*; these tests are distinguished from those for cardiolipin antibody, being called treponemal antibody tests. The *T. pallidum*–immobilizing test was, for many years, foremost among these, being used as the gold standard to determine whether someone had been infected with *T. pallidum*. This test was difficult to perform, requiring a source of viable organisms (usually obtained from an infected rabbit), a dark-field microscope, and a substantial investment of time, and it is no longer available except in the few research laboratories that have a special interest in syphilis immunology.

Antibody to treponemal antigens from lyophilized *T. pallidum* was also detected by the FTA test. Because all of the antigens of *T. pallidum* are not unique and antibody reactivity with some of them may exist in normal serum, an absorption step was added using a nonpathogenic treponeme (*Treponema reiteri*, now called *Treponema phagedenis*), giving rise to the more specific FTA-ABS test. Except for the rare instance in which antibody to DNA caused a positive FTA-ABS reaction in serum from a patient with lupus erythematosus or rheumatoid arthritis, this test was regarded as specific, and it essentially replaced the *T. pallidum*–immobilizing test as the standard for determining whether prior infection with *T. pallidum* had ever occurred.[287] However, the FTA-ABS test requires a fluorescence microscope and a highly trained technician.

The development of hemagglutination tests, for example, the TP-PA and MHA-TP tests, has provided specific tests that are performed easily in most laboratories and require less specialized equipment. These tests use a lysate of pathogenic *T. pallidum*. These tests yield results that are very similar to those obtained by the FTA-ABS, and they have largely replaced the FTA-ABS as the most efficient specific test for antibody to *T. pallidum*.[60, 286, 290–293] The MHA-TP test, however, is no longer commercially available. The TP-PA test uses the same treponemal antigen as the MHA-TP test but uses gelatin particles rather than sheep red blood cells, which may eliminate nonspecific reactions with serum/plasma samples. The TP-PA test was developed in Japan; its performance has been comparable to that of the MHA-TP and FTA-ABS tests.[294] Physicians, however, continue to request an FTA-ABS out of habit, although at present most laboratories perform hemagglutination tests; these terms (FTA-ABS and hemagglutination reaction) are used interchangeably throughout this chapter. Immunoblotting has been used by several investigators to detect IgG and IgM antibodies to specific *T. pallidum* proteins in sera of adults with syphilis.[35, 37, 45] The sensitivity and specificity are excellent; however, immu-

| **TABLE 12–9** |
| Seroreactivity of More Common Tests for |
| Untreated Syphilis |

TEST[a]	% POSITIVE			
	Primary Stage	Secondary Stage	Latent Stage	Tertiary Stage
VDRL or RPR	75	100	75	75
FTA-ABS, TP-PA, MHA-TP	90	100	100	100

[a]See Table 12–8 for full test names.

noblotting for syphilis diagnosis has not been feasible in the clinical laboratory.[295] Enzyme-linked immunosorbent assays[295–300] are under study; some of them use *T. pallidum* outer membrane proteins that have been generated by recombinant techniques. These tests ultimately will be helpful if their sensitivity is such as to detect early syphilis cases, where the currently used tests may still be nonreactive.

About 90% of patients with a primary syphilitic chancre have a positive hemagglutination test result by the time they seek medical attention.[60, 279, 285, 286, 288] All patients with disseminated and late infection have a positive reaction. These tests are highly specific as well as being extremely sensitive. A few disease states, such as systemic lupus erythematosus, polyarteritis or related conditions, and, in one report, even pregnancy, are said to cause a false-positive FTA-ABS result, but these diagnoses should be apparent, and the sophisticated observer can often detect a distinctive beaded pattern of fluorescence in these reactions.[67] It has traditionally been felt that, once positive, these tests usually remain so for life, even if the infection has been cured. However, Romanowski and co-workers[301] found that 24% of first-episode primary syphilis patients seroconverted to nonreactivity by the FTA-ABS test and 13% were nonreactive by the MHA-TP test after 36 months after treatment. Nevertheless, positive reactions are not helpful in determining whether active infection is present. As a result, despite their exquisite sensitivity and specificity, a positive test result may not be helpful diagnostically in an individual patient; a negative result excludes a diagnosis of all but early primary infection.

SEROLOGIC DIAGNOSIS IN THE INFANT

RPR and FTA-ABS Tests. Maternal RPR and FTA-ABS test reactivity can be found in both IgG and IgM antibody classes.[37, 302–304] If the placenta is intact, IgG is passively transferred to the newborn. Thus, a reactive serology in the neonate could be due to maternally derived IgG and does not necessarily indicate that the infant is actively infected. Furthermore, the maternal antibody could have arisen from untreated, inadequately treated, or adequately treated disease. If the antibody titer is higher in the infant than in the mother when the same nontreponemal test is performed on both of them (a fourfold or greater difference is generally required to exclude laboratory error), this would signify congenital infection.[88] If the infant's reactive RPR test is caused by passively transferred antibody, the reactivity progressively declines as time passes and should disappear by 6 to 12 months of age. A persistently reactive RPR test in the infant beyond 12 to 15 months of age suggests an active infection, and a rising titer makes this diagnosis virtually certain.

The CDC has recommended that serum from the infant, rather than from umbilical cord blood obtained at birth, be used for serologic testing because the rates of false-positive and false-negative results are lower.[156] However, owing to its ease of collection, umbilical cord blood continues to be a readily available specimen. Appropriate care in collection of umbilical cord blood

should be taken to avoid contamination with maternal blood. Serologic testing of umbilical cord blood may be performed with either the RPR or VDRL test. The RPR test is more sensitive,[305] although false-positive reactions secondary to contamination of the sample with Wharton's jelly may occur. Both tests, however, may be nonreactive when the maternal serologic titer is low. It is therefore best to screen the mother rather than the newborn[306]; routine screening of umbilical cord blood is discouraged.[307]

If the mother has a false-positive RPR test, this antibody can be passively transferred to the infant. Naturally, in such a case, neither the mother nor the infant will have a reactive treponemal test. If the mother has a reactive treponemal test because of untreated or previously treated syphilis, this antibody also appears in the newborn by passive transfer. Thus, detection of such reactivity in the newborn indicates that the mother had at some point encountered *T. pallidum*, but it does not indicate whether her infection was treated, and it certainly does not diagnose active infection of the infant. Because the FTA-ABS test is conventionally performed without dilutions in the United States, it is not useful to use it sequentially to study infants suspected of having syphilis. Eventually, of course, any passively transferred maternal IgG antibody causing reactivity in a normal infant is catabolized until it is no longer detectable. Persistence of antibody beyond 15 to 18 months of age can be considered a reliable, but often retrospective, diagnostic test, which is seen in 50 to 70% of infants with congenital syphilis.[308, 309]

FTA IgM Test. Detection of IgM by FTA-ABS theoretically should be helpful in distinguishing congenital infection because IgM is not transferred across the placenta. However, in clinical studies of this antibody, false-negative results have been obtained in 20 to 39% of cases, and false-positive results, perhaps related to rheumatoid factor[310] (also, S Dobson, unpublished data), in up to 10%. Definitive prospective clinical investigations using rigorous case definitions and standardized methodology have not been done, and the place of this test in the clinical practice of pediatrics remains in question.[311] Stoll and associates[312] modified the original FTA-ABS IgM test by using the IgM fraction of neonatal serum. This FTA-ABS 19S IgM test had a sensitivity of 73% and a specificity of 100% among at-risk infants.

Enzyme-Linked Immunosorbent Assay (ELISA). IgM ELISA tests have been developed to detect both nontreponemal[87, 313] and treponemal antibodies.[174, 312, 313] As currently marketed, these are of limited usefulness in diagnosis of congenital syphilis, owing to less than optimal sensitivity and specificity. Stoll and associates[312] used an IgM capture ELISA for *T. pallidum* and found a sensitivity of only 88% among infants with clinical and laboratory findings of congenital syphilis. Further refinement and evaluation of these assays will be important because the ELISA has the potential for rapid diagnosis of congenitally infected infants. Moreover, many clinical laboratories already are experienced with this technique.

IgM and IgA Immunoblotting. Immunoblotting has been used to detect and characterize the specific neonatal IgM and IgA[314] antibody responses to *T. pallidum*.

Specific IgM antibody directed against *T. pallidum* membrane lipoprotein antigens with apparent molecular masses of 72, 47, 45, 42, 37, 17, and 15 kDa has been detected among sera of infants with clinical findings of congenital syphilis; reactivity against the 47-kDa antigen was uniformly present in all of the positive neonatal serum IgM immunoblots.[85-88, 315, 316] Fractionation of sera into IgG and IgM components by high-performance liquid chromatography confirmed that serum reactivity to these treponemal antigens was not due to rheumatoid factors.[86] Similar IgA reactivity to a variety of *T. pallidum* antigens has been detected by immunoblotting in infants with possible congenital syphilis.[314]

IgM reactivity to the 47-kDa antigen also has been found in sera of 20 to 42% of subclinically infected infants delivered of mothers with untreated syphilis.[88, 316] It also has been detected in fetal blood obtained by cordocentesis at 24 weeks of gestation; the positive serum IgM immunoblot was validated by the simultaneous detection of viable spirochetes in the blood of this hydropic fetus by RIT.[89] Moreover, 14 weeks later at delivery, after appropriate maternal therapy, the neonatal serum lacked IgM reactivity, suggesting that the fetus also had been successfully treated in utero. Dobson and colleagues[85] also have reported disappearance of neonatal IgM reactivity to *T. pallidum* 1 to 3 months after appropriate treatment.

The ability to detect IgM reactivity in neonatal sera has been enhanced when the antigen source for immunoblotting comprised the subset of membrane proteins selectively extracted by Triton X-114 phase partitioning (detergent-phase proteins) rather than whole cell lysates of *T. pallidum*.[88] This was particularly evident when evaluating IgM reactivities to the 15- and 17-kDa immunogens, which are known to be present in *T. pallidum* in relatively low abundance. Recently, Sánchez and coworkers showed that immunoblot analysis with a recombinant form of the highly immunogenic 47-kDa lipoprotein of *T. pallidum* appeared to be even more sensitive than immunoblotting with native *T. pallidum* antigens.[317] In some infants with congenital syphilis, IgM reactivity was apparent only when the recombinant 47-kDa lipoprotein was used as the antigen source.

Similarly, IgM reactivity to the 47-kDa antigen also has been found in CSF of infants with congenital syphilis.[88, 316, 318] Lewis and associates[316] found 82% reactive CSF IgM immunoblots in infants with clinical and laboratory evidence of congenital syphilis, but 4% reactivity among infants at risk of having congenital infection with *T. pallidum* but whose clinical and laboratory evaluations were normal. Sánchez and co-workers[88] detected IgM reactivity to the 47-kDa antigen in CSF of two of seven infants whose physical and laboratory examinations were consistent with a diagnosis of congenital syphilis; the significance of the positive IgM immunoblot was confirmed by the finding of viable *T. pallidum* in the CSF by RIT.

Polymerase Chain Reaction. PCR for detection of specific *T. pallidum* DNA in tissues and body fluids has been developed.[319-324] PCR is said to be capable of detecting an amount of purified treponemal DNA equivalent to that of only a few organisms (about 0.01

pg).[319] Sánchez and co-workers[88] have reported on the use of PCR for congenital syphilis diagnosis; they have compared results of PCR on neonatal serum and CSF to those obtained by RIT, the current reference standard.[88, 324] Five CSF samples from 19 infants born to mothers with untreated early syphilis were positive by both PCR and RIT, 12 were negative by both tests, 2 were positive by RIT but negative by PCR, and none was positive by PCR and negative by RIT. Thus, the sensitivity of PCR relative to RIT was 71% for CSF, and the specificity was 100%. When the results of PCR and RIT on 29 serum and CSF samples were combined, 9 were positive by both tests, 17 were negative by both tests, 3 were positive by RIT but negative by PCR, and none that was negative by RIT was positive by PCR. Similarly, for amniotic fluid obtained from 12 pregnant women with early syphilis, 7 of 7 samples were positive by both tests and all 5 that were negative by RIT were negative by PCR. The excellent agreement between RIT and PCR substantiates the future use of PCR as a surrogate for RIT.

Cerebrospinal Fluid Examination

Using RIT of neonatal CSF, Sánchez and co-workers[88] studied the prevalence of CNS invasion by *T. pallidum* among 19 infants born to mothers with early syphilis. Seven of the infants had clinical and laboratory evidence of congenital syphilis, and 12 had no clinical or laboratory findings suggestive of congenital infection. They found the prevalence of spirochetal invasion of the CSF to be 86% (6 of 7) in infants with clinically recognizable congenital syphilis, but only 8% (1 of 12) among infants who lacked clinical and laboratory findings. The sensitivity and specificity of a reactive CSF VDRL, pleocytosis and elevated CSF protein content were 71% and 92%, 43% and 92%, and 43% and 92%, respectively. All infants with a positive CSF RIT had a reactive serum IgM immunoblot (100% sensitivity) and a positive serum PCR (100% sensitivity). No infant with a negative serum IgM immunoblot and a negative serum PCR had a positive CSF RIT, leading these investigators to conclude that the diagnosis of congenital syphilis, particularly in the infant without clinical and laboratory findings, will ultimately require a comprehensive approach using assays for both specific neonatal IgM and *T. pallidum* DNA in serum and CSF.

Using currently available methodologies, leukocytosis ($\geq$ 25 white blood cells/mm^3) and elevated protein content ($>$ 150 mg/dl in full-term and $>$ 170 mg/dl in preterm infants) in the CSF in an infant who has any suggestion of congenital syphilis should be regarded as supportive of the diagnosis. Also, an infant with a reactive CSF VDRL should be treated as if neurosyphilis were present, although a reactive CSF VDRL in the absence of other evidence of congenital syphilis is suspect, inasmuch as nontreponemal IgG can pass from serum to the CSF in neonates.[246]

An unsettling element has been introduced by the use of various modifications of the serum FTA technique to study CSF from syphilitic patients. Conflicting results have been obtained in adults,[325-329] and systematic studies have yet to be done for congenital syphilis. Thus, at present, the FTA-ABS and hemagglutination tests should not be done using the CSF in infants suspected of having congenital syphilis; the results cannot be interpreted properly, and other means must be used to establish or exclude the diagnosis.

DIFFERENTIAL DIAGNOSIS

Syphilitic infection is highly suspect in the presence of snuffles, a vesiculobullous eruption, hepatosplenomegaly, generalized lymphadenopathy, condylomata lata, symmetrical metaphyseal lesions, and a positive RPR or VDRL test.

Dermatologic Manifestations

The vesiculobullous manifestations of congenital syphilis may be confused with other infections or with congenital disorders of the skin that may be manifest in infancy as vesiculobullous eruptions.[330] Infection caused by *Staphylococcus aureus* may produce vesicles or bullae on any part of the body. Severe infection may result in confluent bullae with erythema and desquamation (Ritter's disease). Examination of aspirated fluid reveals many polymorphonuclear leukocytes and, on occasion, gram-positive cocci in clusters.

Pseudomonas aeruginosa septicemia may be accompanied by a cutaneous eruption consisting of clustered pearly vesicles on an erythematous background, which rapidly becomes purulent green or hemorrhagic.[331] When the lesion ruptures, a circumscribed ulcer with a necrotic base appears and may persist, surrounded by a purplish cellulitis. Culture of the lesion and the blood confirms the diagnosis.

In the septicemic form of listeriosis, a cutaneous eruption consisting of miliary abscesses resembling papules, pustules, or papulopustules may occur over the entire body, with a predilection for the back.[332] Culture of these lesions, the blood, or the CSF usually reveals *Listeria monocytogenes* as the offending agent. Newer reported causes for vesicular or bullous lesions of the skin of the newborn include group B streptococci,[333] *Haemophilus influenzae* type B,[334] *Mycobacterium tuberculosis*,[335] and cytomegalovirus.[336]

In viral-induced eruptions, the vesicles are located in the mid epidermis. In herpesvirus infection, vesicles are the most common dermatologic manifestation. They tend to be sparsely disseminated throughout the body, or they may occur in crops or clusters. Involvement of the palms and soles has been recorded, and bullous formations may occur. Recurrence of these skin lesions is not unusual. Scrapings from the base of these lesions, when fixed in alcohol and stained with Papanicolaou stain, may show intranuclear inclusions or multinucleated giant cells compatible with the diagnosis of herpes simplex or varicella-zoster infection, and cultures may yield the offending virus. The latter infection rarely occurs in the newborn period, and the diagnosis may be discarded on epidemiologic or clinical grounds. Variola and vaccinia may affect the fetus or newborn and cause vesicular eruptions. Appropriate epidemiologic evidence should be sought to exclude these diagnoses.

Mucocutaneous candidiasis may present as a vesicular dermatitis at the end of the first week of life. The vesicles usually become confluent and rupture, leaving a denuded area surrounded by satellite vesicles or pustules. Congenital candidiasis with skin manifestations has also been described, and severe systemic involvement may accompany this intrauterine infection.[337]

A variety of hereditary disorders of the skin appears at birth or in early infancy as vesiculobullous eruptions.[330] Epidermolysis bullosa constitutes a group of specific genetic disorders. Erythema toxicum, miliaria rubra, incontinentia pigmenti, urticaria pigmentosa, epidermolytic hyperkeratosis, acrodermatitis enteropathica, histiocytosis X, transient neonatal pustular melanosis, infantile acropustulosis, and aplasia cutis congenita must also be included in the differential diagnosis.[338]

Hepatosplenomegaly

When the clinical presentation is that of hepatosplenomegaly with or without jaundice, the differential diagnosis is extensive and includes all causes of elevated direct and indirect bilirubin. Thus, one should consider isoimmunization problems (e.g., Rh incompatibility), other infectious diseases (bacterial sepsis, cytomegalovirus infection, rubella, herpes simplex infection, coxsackievirus B infection, varicella-zoster infection, toxoplasmosis), neonatal hepatitis, diseases of the biliary tract (such as extrahepatic biliary atresia and choledochal cyst), and metabolic disorders (such as cystic fibrosis, galactosemia, and α_1-antitrypsin deficiency).[339]

Hydrops Fetalis

Hydrops fetalis may be caused by chronic anemia (isoimmunization disorder, homozygous alpha-thalassemia, fetomaternal or fetofetal transfusions), cardiac or pulmonary failure owing to causes other than anemia (large arteriovenous malformations, premature closure of the foramen ovale, cystic adenomatoid malformation, pulmonary lymphangiectasia), perinatal tumors (neuroblastoma, chorioangioma), achondroplasia, renal disorders (congenital nephrosis, renal vein thrombosis), and infections such as cytomegalic inclusion disease, toxoplasmosis, congenital parvovirus infection,[340] and congenital hepatitis.[339]

Most cases of hydrops are caused by isoimmunization disorders, which can be ruled out by a negative direct Coombs' test result. A normal hemoglobin electrophoresis pattern excludes the diagnosis of alpha-thalassemia. The Kleihauer-Betke technique of acid elution for identifying fetal cells in the maternal circulation may aid in rejecting the diagnosis of fetomaternal transfusion. The other diagnostic considerations may be discarded on the basis of appropriate roentgenograms, placental examination, urinalysis, biopsy, and immunologic studies.

Renal Disease

In the neonatal period and early infancy, the nephrotic syndrome and acute nephritis occur infrequently. The former is more often associated with infantile microcystic disease, minimal lesion nephrotic syndrome, or renal vein thrombosis than with congenital syphilis. Neonatal nephritis may occur as a manifestation of congenital syphilis, hereditary nephritis, hemolytic-uremic syndrome, and, rarely, pyelonephritis. The clinical signs that distinguish syphilitic renal involvement from the other conditions mentioned include the presence of other manifestations of early congenital syphilis, a positive serologic test for syphilis, elevated levels of IgG (in the more common infantile microcystic disease the levels of IgG are low), and the response to specific antisyphilitic therapy.

Ophthalmologic Involvement

Neonatal buphthalmos occurs as an isolated genetic disorder and may be associated with a variety of syndromes (e.g., aniridia, Hallermann-Streiff syndrome, Reiger's anomaly, Lowe's syndrome, Sturge-Weber syndrome, oculodentodigital syndrome, Pierre Robin syndrome); it is also associated with rubella.[341] Nasolacrimal duct obstruction is a more frequent cause of excessive lacrimation in the newborn period and early infancy.

THERAPY

The Pregnant Woman

A pregnant woman who has a suspicious lesion and a negative RPR test result may be in an early stage of infection. Detection of treponemes by dark-field microscopy should lead to therapy without regard to results of serologic tests; a repeat RPR test should be done in 3 to 6 weeks (Table 12–10). A patient who has neither lesions nor a positive serology but who has been exposed sexually to a person who has syphilis should be treated for syphilis on the 25 to 50% likelihood that she has acquired syphilis and is in the early phase of the infection and able to infect the fetus.[157, 227]

The finding of a positive RPR reaction should lead to a careful and complete evaluation of the pregnant patient for evidence of primary or secondary syphilis. If signs of active disease are not found and the treponemal test result is also reactive, then a diagnosis of latent syphilis is made, with the diagnosis being early latent disease if she was known to have a negative RPR within the previous 1 to 2 years.

Failure of nontreponemal serologic titers to decrease appropriately is reason for CSF examination and retreatment unless reinfection can be established as the cause.[116] Moreover, such persons should be reevaluated for HIV infection. In late latent syphilis or syphilis of unknown duration, a lumbar puncture is generally recommended in patients who are positive for antibody to HIV to exclude neurosyphilis.[156]

If the pregnant woman had a positive RPR and treponemal tests before this pregnancy and it is certain that she received appropriate treatment, observation during the pregnancy is allowed with clinical evaluation and RPR testing repeated in the third trimester and at delivery. Serologic titers may be checked monthly in women at high risk for reinfection or in geographic areas in which the prevalence of syphilis is high.[156, 342] Although it is expected that the nontreponemal test will eventually become nonreactive after appropriate treatment, some patients may have persistence of nontreponemal antibodies at a low titer for an extended period of time. This response is referred to as the serofast reaction, and the patient is not infectious.

If the pregnant woman has a positive RPR result but a nonreactive treponemal test result, then this situation is referred to as a "biologically false-positive" result. Caution must be exercised that the patient does not have early syphilis, because the RPR test becomes positive earlier than the treponemal tests. In such cases of early syphilis, a repeat treponemal test 3 to 6 weeks later will be reactive, and the patient should be treated as noted earlier.

PENICILLIN

Parenteral penicillin G remains the drug of choice in the treatment of syphilis (Table 12–11).[156, 343–345] A regi-

---

TABLE 12–10	
Therapeutic Decisions Involving the Pregnant Woman in Relation to RPR Status[a, b, c]	

RPR STATUS	DECISION
Negative RPR	
Signs of clinical disease	Treat[d, e]
No signs of clinical disease	High risk
	Repeat RPR at 28 wk and at term
	Low risk
	Repeat RPR at term
Positive RPR	
Signs of clinical disease[e]	Treat
No signs of clinical disease	
Known positive syphilis tests in past[e]	
Adequate Rx	Observe[f]
Untreated	Treat
New positive TP-PA test	
If positive[e]	Evaluate and treat
If negative	Perform FTA-ABS
	If positive—evaluate and treat[e]
	If negative—observe[g] and repeat TP-PA in 3 wk, and if positive, evaluate and treat[e]; if negative, observe[g]

[a]RPR most common reason for medical evaluation.
[b]See text.
[c]See Table 12–8 for full test names.
[d]Test for possible prozone effect.
[e]Test for HIV-antibody.
[f]Treat if RPR > 1:4 (VDRL > 1:2) in woman with a history of prepregnancy therapy—possible reinfection.
[g]Assume biologically false-positive result (see text).

TABLE 12–11
Recommended Treatment of Pregnant Patient[a]

STAGES OF SYPHILIS	DRUG (PENICILLIN)	ROUTE	DOSE (UNITS)
Early (<1 yr duration)	*Recommended*		
Primary, secondary, or early latent			
HIV antibody-negative	Benzathine	IM	2.4 million single dose; possibly repeat in 1 wk
HIV antibody-positive[b]	Benzathine	IM	2.4 million single dose; possibly repeat weekly × 2
	Alternative		
	Penicillin desensitization[c]		
Latent (>1 yr duration)[d]	*Recommended*		
	Benzathine	IM	2.4 million weekly × 3 wk
	Alternative		
	Penicillin desensitization		
Neurosyphilis	*Recommended*		
	Aqueous	IV	3–4 million every 4 hr × 10–14 days
	Alternative		
	Procaine[e]	IM	2.4 million daily × 10–14 days

[a]See text.
[b]With normal cerebrospinal fluid findings, if performed.
[c]For details, see MMWR Morb Mortal Wkly Rep 47:28, 1998.
[d]Lumbar puncture to exclude neurosyphilis is recommended for HIV-antibody positive patients.
[e]Probenecid, 500 mg orally QID × 10–14 days, should also be prescribed.
HIV = human immunodeficiency virus; IM = intramuscular; IV = intravenous.

men of benzathine penicillin G (2.4 million units given as 1.2 million units in each buttock) appropriate for the stage of syphilis cures maternal infection and prevents or cures fetal infection.[156, 343] For women with early syphilis, a second dose of benzathine penicillin (2.4 million units intramuscularly) administered 1 week after the initial dose has been recommended in order to minimize the occurrence of a fetal treatment failure.[156]

Failure rates for prevention of fetal infection from 2%[270] to as high as 14% (see Table 12–2) have been reported. The majority of fetal treatment failures seem to occur after maternal treatment for secondary syphilis.[346] This may be explained, in part, by the marked spirochetemia that occurs during secondary syphilitic infection. Other reasons for the presumptive treatment failures have been related to possibly altered penicillin pharmacokinetics in pregnancy[347] or to advanced fetal disease.[348] Problems exist in the interpretation of these data because, by currently available methodologies, the accurate identification of an infected newborn is problematic at best. The clinical and laboratory manifestations of congenital syphilis may require several weeks to months for resolution despite adequate penicillin therapy. Likewise, the fetus may be adequately treated in utero by maternal penicillin therapy yet have persistent abnormalities that are detected at birth because insufficient time has elapsed for complete disappearance of the physical and laboratory abnormalities. Such a case would be erroneously classified as a treatment failure. Moreover, the improper use of the new CDC surveillance case definition as diagnostic criteria for congenital syphilis has led to the misclassification of infants as infected when the diagnosis is not certain.

Invasion of the CNS by *T. pallidum* can occur during any stage of syphilis.[101] Currently recommended therapy for neurosyphilis is aqueous crystalline penicillin G, 18 to 24 million units daily, administered as 3 to 4 million units intravenously every 4 hours for 10 to 14 days. If compliance can be ensured, an alternative regimen consists of procaine penicillin G, 2.4 million units intramuscularly daily, plus probenecid, 500 mg orally four times a day, both given for 10 to 14 days.[208, 293] Benzathine penicillin G, 2.4 million units intramuscularly, is often provided after completion of either of these two neurosyphilis treatment regimens.[156]

Syphilis may be more difficult to eradicate in the presence of concurrent HIV infection.[101, 344, 349] Nevertheless, current recommendations include a regimen similar to that for patients who lack HIV antibody (see Table 12–11), along with careful and frequent clinical and serologic follow-up.[156] For HIV-infected patients with primary or secondary syphilis, some authorities recommend up to three weekly doses of 2.4 million units of benzathine penicillin G or other supplemental antibiotics[156] in addition to a single intramuscular dose of benzathine penicillin G. HIV-infected patients who have either late latent syphilis or syphilis of unknown duration should have a CSF examination before treatment. If nontreponemal antibody titers have not declined fourfold by 6 months with primary or secondary syphilis, or by 6 to 12 months in early latent syphilis, or if the titer has increased fourfold at any time, a CSF examination should be performed and the patient retreated with 7.2 million units of benzathine penicillin G (administered as three weekly doses of 2.4 million units each) if CSF examination is normal. Patients who have CSF abnormalities consistent with neurosyphilis should be treated for neurosyphilis as described earlier (see Table 12–11).

ALTERNATIVE DRUGS

The pregnant syphilitic patient who has a history of penicillin allergy should be skin tested and, if necessary, desensitized according to the protocol by Wendel and co-workers.[350] This can be accomplished by providing the patient with gradually increasing doses of oral or intravenous penicillin during several hours until the objective of full tolerance is achieved. Such an approach must be performed only under expert guidance and under circumstances in which emergency treatment is available.[156]

Cephalosporins may represent an alternative to penicillin. Transplacental levels of cephaloridine were said to reach 60% of maternal blood levels,[351] and no treatment failures (in 23 patients) were recorded with a dose of 0.5 g daily for 10 days. This cephalosporin is no longer in use. Multiple-dose regimens of ceftriaxone for treatment of primary and secondary syphilis as well as neurosyphilis have been efficacious in limited studies.[352–357] A 10-day course of ceftriaxone (250 mg intramuscularly daily) may be an alternative regimen for the penicillin-allergic patient with early syphilis; careful serologic follow-up is mandatory. In rabbits, a 7- to 10-day course of ceftriaxone failed to clear CNS infection with *T. pallidum* in a consistent fashion.[358] An occasional patient who is allergic to penicillin is also allergic to the cephalosporins, and cephalosporins should not be used if the penicillin allergy is potentially life threatening.[156, 352–357]

Erythromycin, which is effective in syphilis,[343, 359] crosses the placenta in an unpredictable fashion, often poorly.[345] Although pregnant women with syphilis have been treated successfully with erythromycin, 40 mg/kg per day orally for 10 to 14 days (maximum 500 mg qid), failure to cure the fetus has been reported, and its use is strongly discouraged.[360]

Tetracycline given in a dosage of 30 g orally over a 10- to 14-day period (approximately 30 to 60 mg/kg per day in four doses, not to exceed 2 g per day) compares favorably in effectiveness with penicillin,[361] but its potential for damage to the liver of the pregnant woman[362, 363] and its adverse effects on the teeth and long bones of the fetus[364, 365] when administered in the last trimester are deterrents to its use in pregnancy.

Although chloramphenicol has had wide acceptance as a penicillin substitute and was shown to be effective in doses comparable to those of tetracycline,[343] its use has been discouraged because of the risks of aplastic anemia and inactivation of hepatic conjugating enzymes in the mother and because of the immature renal function in the fetus.[366]

Preliminary data on the use of azithromycin for treatment of syphilis in nonpregnant adults have shown efficacy.[367, 368] No data, however, are available for its use in pregnancy for treatment of maternal syphilis and prevention and/or treatment of fetal syphilis.

With the recent shortage of intravenous aqueous penicillin G in the United States,[369] the CDC has recommended that for treatment of neurosyphilis, procaine penicillin G plus probenecid (see Table 12–11) be administered when intravenous penicillin is not available.[370] For persons with neurologic involvement with syphilis who do not tolerate intramuscular procaine penicillin G, intravenous ampicillin (12–16 g per day in four divided doses for 10 to 14 days) or, alternatively, intravenous ceftriaxone (2 g per day as a single dose for 10 to 14 days) may be considered with careful clinical and serologic follow-up. Consultation with an expert in the treatment of persons who have neurologic involvement with syphilis is also recommended. For persons with neurosyphilis who are allergic to penicillin, desensitization to penicillin and treatment with procaine penicillin is preferred. These regimens for neurosyphilis may be followed by a single dose of benzathine penicillin G (see Table 12–11).

The Infant

Treatment of newborns with a reactive serologic test for syphilis is required in the following situations: (1) the infant has clinical, laboratory, or radiographic findings, or a combination of these, compatible with congenital syphilis; (2) there is no documented maternal treatment before delivery; (3) maternal treatment was inadequate or unknown; (4) the mother was treated with drugs other than penicillin; (5) the mother was treated within 4 weeks of delivery; (6) the mother was treated for early syphilis during the pregnancy with the appropriate penicillin regimen, but nontreponemal antibody titers did not decrease at least fourfold; (7) the mother had serologic evidence of relapse or reinfection after treatment (a fourfold or greater increase in nontreponemal antibody titer); or (8) adequate follow-up of the infant is uncertain (Table 12–12).[156, 371, 372]

A practical approach is to treat all newborns who have a positive RPR test result as if they have congenital syphilis even if the mother is not thought to have an active infection. This recommendation is based on a number of pragmatic considerations: (1) it may be difficult to document that the mother received adequate therapy and has a falling RPR titer; (2) a low-titer RPR test may be compatible with untreated latent maternal syphilis; (3) the newborn, if infected, may not have any clinical manifestations at birth; and (4) compliance with follow-up visits is a monumental problem. Clearly, if the infant has a positive RPR test result and any signs consistent with congenital syphilis, treatment should be administered. However, if no clinical findings are present, a quantitative RPR test should be performed on the mother and her newborn. Treatment is indicated if the infant has a titer four times or higher than that of the mother.

In infants who have a normal physical examination result and the quantitative RPR test is not significantly higher in the infant than in the mother, the maternal history of infection with *T. pallidum* and treatment for syphilis must be considered when evaluating and treating the infant. If the possibility exists that the infant may be infected, then hematologic investigation, skeletal radiographs, and lumbar puncture should be performed. If any of these reveal abnormalities that are consistent with the diagnosis of congenital syphilis, the infant must be treated.[156, 372]

In recent years, the need for performing a lumbar

TABLE 12–12
Therapeutic Decisions Involving the Infant in Relation to Rapid Plasma Reagin (RPR) Status*

RPR STATUS	DECISION
Negative RPR	
Early disease	
Without clinical findings	Treat
With clinical findings	Reevaluate for other congenital infection; if none apparent, treat
Positive RPR	
With clinical manifestations	Treat
Without clinical manifestations, perform the following:	
1. Quantitative RPR on mother and infant— if infant titer fourfold higher	Treat
2. Hematologic studies— if abnormal	Treat
3. Bone radiography— if abnormal	Treat
4. Liver function tests— if abnormal	Treat
5. Lumbar puncture— if abnormal	Treat
6. If mother	
a. Has no, inadequate, or undocumented treatment	Treat
b. Was treated with nonpenicillin	Treat
c. Was treated within 4 wk of delivery	Treat
d. Or if adequate follow-up of newborn in doubt	Treat

*See text.

puncture and bone radiographs has been questioned.[373, 374] Beeram and colleagues[373] have reported that in infants who had a normal physical examination result but who were born to mothers with untreated or inadequately treated syphilis, a reactive CSF VDRL test occurred in only 0.6% of evaluated infants. Mean CSF white blood cell counts and protein content did not differ significantly from a control population of normal infants who had negative evaluations for bacterial disease, including sterile cultures of blood and CSF. Using the stricter criteria of Platou (white blood cell count > 5 cells/mm^3; protein content > 40 mg/dl) in determination of abnormal CSF indices, 44% and 95% of control infants had CSF pleocytosis and elevated protein contents, respectively. This study supports the recent recommendation by the CDC (see later) that if treatment for possible neurosyphilis is provided to infants at risk of being infected with *T. pallidum*, performance of a lumbar puncture is not necessary.[156] This study also highlights the need to use appropriate reference values in the evaluation of neonatal CSF.

Similarly, long-bone radiograph results are frequently abnormal among infants with clinical signs of congenital syphilis.[374] These infants require prolonged penicillin therapy irrespective of the results of the skeletal survey, and both the CDC and American Academy of Pediatrics no longer require that they be routinely performed in these circumstances.[156, 372] However, because as many as 6% of normal infants born to mothers with untreated syphilis may have bony abnormalities as the sole manifestation of possible congenital syphilis,[374] radiography should be performed before at-risk infants receive only a single dose of benzathine penicillin therapy.[156]

If there is doubt about the meaning of a positive RPR test result in an otherwise normal infant and all other tests are negative, repeated quantitative RPR testing should be done. When antibody is passively acquired from the mother, serial quantitative tests show a declining titer. A falling titer suggests that the infant is free of infection; on the other hand, a stable or rising titer implies the presence of infection. The decision concerning treatment or observation of such a newborn depends on the clinical setting; whether the mother has received antibiotic therapy; the results of other tests such as skeletal radiographs, liver function tests, and hematologic studies; and the opportunity for adequate follow-up. Antisyphilitic therapy is indicated in any circumstance in which the mother is unreliable and compliance with the therapeutic regimen and adequate follow-up care cannot be ensured.

It should not be forgotten that in the newborn a negative RPR test result may not exclude incubating syphilis if maternal infection was in the earliest clinical stage and antibodies had not reached detectable levels.[157, 227] Thus, such an infant without clinical findings should have a second RPR test within 3 to 4 weeks. If the risk of exposure to the infant is considerable (e.g., born to a known syphilitic with no documented treatment history), a reasonable case can be made for immediate penicillin therapy. If the newborn has clinical manifestations that are thought to be consistent with the diagnosis of congenital syphilis, a negative RPR test makes this clinical diagnosis highly questionable; reevaluation of the entire case is indicated. Finally, the appearance of secondary or tertiary syphilis in the mother within the year after delivery should prompt a thorough reevaluation of the infant for the possibility of congenital syphilis.

PENICILLIN

Penicillin remains the drug of choice for congenital syphilis (Table 12–13).[88, 98, 136, 156, 359, 371, 372, 375] Infants who are 4 weeks of age or younger and who have proved or highly probable disease are likely to have CNS invasion by *T. pallidum*.[88] These include (1) infants with physical findings compatible with congenital syphilis; (2) infants who lack physical findings but have an abnormal CSF examination, abnormal bone radiographs, or laboratory evaluation; (3) infants who have a serum quantitative nontreponemal serologic titer that is fourfold greater than the mother's titer; or (4) infants who have a positive

TABLE 12–13
Recommended Treatment of the Newborn[a, b]

MATERNAL RX[c]	CLINICAL FINDINGS IN NEWBORN	DRUG (PENICILLIN G)	ROUTE	DOSE (50,000 UNITS/KG)
None or inadequate[d]	Present	Aqueous *or*	IM or IV	Daily × 10–14 days in two (<7 days), three (8–30 days), or four (>1 mo) doses
		Procaine	IM	Daily dose × 10–14 days
None or inadequate[d]	Absent	Aqueous *or*	IM or IV	Daily × 10–14 days in two (<7 days), three (8–30 days), or four (>1 mo) doses
		Procaine *or*	IM	Daily dose × 10–14 days
		Benzathine	IM	Single dose
Adequate (during pregnancy)	Absent	Benzathine (CDC) *or* Follow-up only (AAP)	IM	Single dose
Adequate (before pregnancy)	Absent	Follow-up only *or* Benzathine (only if follow-up cannot be ensured)	IM	Single dose

[a]See text.
[b]Close and frequent follow-up, including serologic test for syphilis, is essential.
[c]Test mother for HIV-antibody.
[d]Inadequate maternal treatment: Rx not documented; Rx within 4 weeks of delivery; Rx with erythromycin or nonpenicillin drug; or serologic antibody titers do not fall appropriately (see text).
IM = intramuscular; IV = intravenous.

result on dark-field or fluorescent antibody test of body fluids. The evaluation[156, 372] of these infants should consist of CSF analysis to detect evidence of possible neurosyphilis and establish a baseline for follow-up. Moreover, they should have a complete blood cell count and platelet count performed because anemia and thrombocytopenia may not be readily detected by physical examination only. Other tests such as bone and chest radiographs, liver function tests, cranial ultrasound, ophthalmologic examination, and auditory brain-stem response should be performed as clinically indicated. Although bone radiographs are frequently abnormal in infants with physical findings consistent with a diagnosis of congenital syphilis, the finding of radiographic abnormalities does not change the recommended therapy for these infants.

Infants with proved or highly probable disease should be treated for 10 days with either (1) aqueous crystalline penicillin G, 50,000 units/kg intravenously every 12 hours for the first week of life and every 8 hours beyond 1 week of age or (2) aqueous procaine penicillin G, 50,000 units/kg administered intramuscularly once daily.[156, 372] If more than 1 day of therapy is missed, the CDC recommends that the entire course of penicillin be restarted.[156] Although the CSF levels of penicillin are higher in infants who receive intravenous aqueous penicillin G than in those treated with procaine penicillin IM, the significance of this finding remains unclear, since both therapies have resulted in clinical and laboratory cure.[376] Similarly, infants and children who are identified as having congenital syphilis after the neonatal period (at > 4 weeks of age) should receive aqueous

penicillin G, 50,000 units/kg intravenously every 6 hours for 10 days.[156] For older children, the amount of penicillin should not exceed that recommended for adults (see Table 12–11). The short-term efficacy of a 10-day course of penicillin for eradication of spirochetes from neonatal CSF has been documented by RIT.[88]

For infants who have a normal physical examination and a serum quantitative nontreponemal serologic titer that is the same or less than fourfold the maternal titer, the evaluation is dependent on the maternal treatment history, maternal stage of infection, and planned infant treatment (see Table 12–13).[156] If maternal treatment for syphilis was not given, was undocumented, was a nonpenicillin regimen, or was administered 4 weeks or less before delivery, or the adequacy of maternal treatment for early syphilis cannot be evaluated because the nontreponemal serologic titer has not decreased fourfold, or relapse or reinfection is suspected because of a fourfold increase in the maternal nontreponemal serologic titer, then the infant should receive the following treatment: (1) aqueous penicillin G or procaine penicillin G for 10 days or (2) benzathine penicillin G, 50,000 units/kg (single dose intramuscularly) with close serologic follow-up.[156, 372] If the infant receives a 10-day course of parenteral penicillin, then a complete evaluation consisting of a lumbar puncture, complete blood cell count and platelet count, and bone radiographs may not be necessary because the infant will receive adequate therapy for proved or highly probable disease (see earlier), including possible neurosyphilis.[116] Nevertheless, abnormalities found on these tests may further support a diagnosis of congenital syphilis, and performance of a lumbar puncture may document CSF abnormalities that would prompt close follow-up. On the other hand, if the infant is to receive a single intramuscular injection of benzathine penicillin G, then a complete evaluation (lumbar puncture, complete blood cell count with platelet count, and bone radiographs) is mandatory.[156, 372] If any part of the infant's evaluation is abnormal or not done, then a 10-day course of penicillin is recommended.

The decision by both the CDC[116] and the American Academy of Pediatrics[372] to allow the expanded use of a single intramuscular dose of benzathine penicillin G is based on the finding that, in contrast to the infant with clinical manifestations of congenital syphilis, the prevalence of CNS invasion by *T. pallidum* as documented by RIT is very low in infants who lack physical, radiographic, or laboratory evidence of congenital infection.[88] Single-dose benzathine penicillin therapy has been widely used in the past, and its use today would allow earlier discharge of the infant with subsequent improved maternal-infant interaction and decrease in hospital costs.[377] This regimen has been supported by two recent small clinical studies.[378, 379]

Nonetheless, failure of a single injection of benzathine penicillin G administered to three infants has been reported.[380, 381] These infants were delivered of mothers with early syphilis and were not fully evaluated for evidence of congenital syphilis at delivery. These treatment failures have been attributed to the inability of benzathine penicillin G to adequately penetrate and achieve treponemicidal concentration in certain sites, such as the aqueous humor and CNS.[382, 383] Sánchez and colleagues have documented the presence of spirochetes in the CSF of three infants without clinical manifestations who received a single injection of benzathine penicillin; on follow-up, all three infants had CSF examinations that were normal and negative for spirochetes by RIT (unpublished observation, 1993).

For infants who have a normal result on physical examination and a serum quantitative nontreponemal serologic titer that is the same or less than fourfold the maternal titer, evaluation is unnecessary if the maternal treatment was during pregnancy, appropriate for the stage of infection, and (1) more than 4 weeks before delivery; (2) was for early syphilis and the nontreponemal serologic titers decreased fourfold after appropriate therapy; or (3) was for late latent syphilis, the nontreponemal titers remained stable and low, and there is no evidence of maternal reinfection or relapse.[156] The CDC recommends that in these situations, a single intramuscular dose of benzathine penicillin G 50,000 units/kg be administered.[156] Some experts, however, would not treat these infants but would provide close serologic follow-up only.[156, 372]

For infants who have normal findings on physical examination and a serum quantitative nontreponemal serologic titer that is the same or less than fourfold the maternal titer, evaluation and treatment are unnecessary if the maternal treatment was before pregnancy and the nontreponemal serologic titers remained low and stable before and during the pregnancy and at delivery.[156] If

follow-up is uncertain, a single intramuscular dose of benzathine penicillin G, 50,000 units/kg, may be given.

Infants born to mothers co-infected with syphilis and HIV do not require different evaluation or therapy for syphilis than is recommended for all infants.[156] These infants born to co-infected women may be at higher risk of infection with *T. pallidum*[98, 100]; however, it is not known whether co-infected infants respond to treatment for congenital syphilis differently from infants uninfected with HIV. Close serologic follow-up of these infants is mandatory.

ALTERNATIVE DRUGS

There are very few reports on alternative regimens when penicillin is contraindicated in children with congenital syphilis. Clinical studies of the treatment of congenital syphilis with ampicillin or ceftriaxone and other new cephalosporins that readily penetrate the blood-brain barrier have not been reported, although these drugs should be effective.[384] Consequently, it is emphasized that follow-up is of paramount importance if a new cephalosporin derivative is administered.

With the recent shortage of intravenous aqueous penicillin G in the United States,[369] the CDC has recommended that infants with congenital syphilis receive procaine penicillin or benzathine penicillin G whenever possible. Alternative therapy for those who may not tolerate repeated intramuscular injections of procaine penicillin consists of intravenous ampicillin or, alternatively, ceftriaxone with careful clinical and serologic follow-up.[370]

The lack of adequate CNS penetration by erythromycin or oral tetracycline makes these drugs inadequate for the treatment of congenital syphilis. In addition, tetracycline and doxycycline are not advised for children younger than 8 years of age because they may stain the teeth and cause possible bone toxicity.

Jarisch-Herxheimer Reaction

The Jarisch-Herxheimer reaction, a common occurrence in the treatment of acquired early syphilis in adults,[385] consists of chills, fever, generalized malaise, hypotension, tachycardia, tachypnea, accentuation of the cutaneous lesions, leukocytosis, and, exceedingly rarely, death. It begins within 2 hours of treatment, peaks at about 8 hours, and disappears in 24 to 36 hours. The cause of the reaction is not known,[386] although release of *T. pallidum* membrane lipoproteins that possess inflammatory activities likely induces this clinical phenomenon.[387]

Approximately 40% of pregnant women treated for syphilis will develop a Jarisch-Herxheimer reaction.[388, 389] In addition, these women may experience the onset of uterine contractions and preterm labor, with decreased fetal activity and fetal heart rate changes, including late decelerations, which last up to 24 to 48 hours and may lead to fetal death. These manifestations of the Jarisch-Herxheimer reaction in pregnancy may possibly be mediated secondarily by prostaglandins. No prophylactic measure or treatment is currently available. Abnormal ultrasonographic evaluation of the fetus as well as fetal monitoring for 24 hours may identify pregnancies at highest risk.

In congenital syphilis, the incidence of the Jarisch-Herxheimer reaction is low in the immediate newborn period, although it may be more common when treatment occurs later in infancy[227]; when it does occur, it varies from fever to cardiovascular collapse and seizures.[88] In Platou's series,[234] almost half of the infants sustained a febrile reaction during the first 36 hours after penicillin injection. There was no relationship between the severity or the outcome of the infection and this temperature elevation.

Post-treatment Follow-up

Recommendations for follow-up are summarized in Table 12–14. It is advisable to monitor the outcome of

---

TABLE 12–14
Follow-up After Treatment or Prophylaxis for Congenital Syphilis

PATIENT CATEGORY	FOLLOW-UP PROCEDURES
Patients diagnosed as having congenital syphilis	1. RPR testing every 2–3 mo until negative or decreased fourfold. If RPR is stable or increasing after 6–12 months after treatment, reevaluate and re-treat. 2. Treponemal antibody test after 15 mo of age 3. If initial CSF was abnormal or infant showed signs of central nervous system disease, repeat CSF evaluation every 6 mo until normal. If repeat CSF is abnormal and not due to intercurrent illness, then re-treat. 4. Careful developmental evaluation, vision testing, and hearing testing
Patients treated in utero or at birth because of maternal syphilis	1. RPR testing at birth and then every 3 mo until test is negative 2. Treponemal antibody test after 15 mo of age
Women treated for syphilis during pregnancy	1. RPR testing as often as monthly until delivery, then every 6 mo until negative or decreased fourfold 2. Re-treatment any time there is a fourfold rise in RPR titer

CSF = cerebrospinal fluid; RPR = rapid plasmid reagin.
Modified from Rathbun KC. Congenital syphilis: a proposal for improved surveillance, diagnosis and treatment. Sex Transm Dis 10:102, 1983, with permission; and MMWR Morb Mortal Wkly Rep 47:45, 1998.

---

therapy by repeated RPR testing. Patients responding to therapy should have falling titers ($\geq$ fourfold decrease), and as many as 70 to 93% should become negative within 1 year.[234, 309] Re-treatment should be considered if signs persist or recur, if there is any increase in the titer of a nontreponemal test, if an initially high-titer nontreponemal test fails to decrease fourfold in the first year, or if the repeat spinal tap at 6 months shows persistent abnormalities, including a positive VDRL result.[156] The recommendation of a second treponemal test beyond 15 months as a way of retrospectively diagnosing a child as having had congenital syphilis at birth[308] is not merely for epidemiologic use but because an established diagnosis can help in the medical and developmental follow-up of the child.

PROGNOSIS

Although treatment may cure the infection, the prognosis in treated congenital syphilis depends on the degree of damage that has already been done. In general, the earlier treatment is initiated, the more likely it is that a satisfactory response can be obtained.[390] If marked damage to the fetus has occurred, treatment in utero may not prevent abortion, stillbirth, or neonatal death, and even if treatment keeps the newborn infant alive, stigmata that have already appeared will remain. If the treatment is provided prenatally or within the first 3 months of life, and the stigmata have not yet become apparent, they can be prevented,[253] although the relation between the adequate treatment of early congenital syphilis and the long-term outcome is inadequately documented in the literature. Interstitial keratitis is an exception; this complication does not seem to be responsive to specific antibiotic therapy. On occasion, dramatic relief has been afforded by the use of corticosteroids and mydriatics, although relapses have occurred with cessation of corticosteroid therapy. As pointed out previously, the osseous lesions seem to heal independently of specific therapy. Treatment of congenital syphilis in the late stage does not reverse the stigmata.[194]

A number of reports described the persistence of treponemes after therapy for syphilis in both humans and experimental animals.[391–394] Although some of these observations were found to have been based on artifact, T. pallidum has been shown to survive in the lymph nodes, eye, and CSF after doses of penicillin that are presumed to be adequate to destroy it. Thus, Silverstein observed that monkeys inoculated in utero with T. pallidum had a significant number of viable treponemes in the aqueous humor of their clinically normal eyes 6 months after birth.[162, 395] Hardy and associates[396] reported the case of a penicillin-treated newborn with congenital syphilis in whom the aqueous humor contained virulent treponemes, and a number of cases of recrudescence of neurosyphilis in adults have been described after treatment with recommended doses of penicillin.[397–399] Survival of these organisms in the eye or CSF is thought to be related to inadequate penetration of antibiotic, but this would not explain the observed persistence of treponemes in the lymph nodes after treatment.[16] Although experts in the field continue to treat congenital syphilis in accord with the guidelines that were outlined previously, there is always a nagging thought that it is not really known what happens to such patients in later life, particularly if they are subjected to immunosuppressive therapy or to any other procedure that might abrogate body defenses necessary to prevent recrudescence.

PREVENTION

Congenital syphilis is an eminently preventable disease. To minimize the likelihood of its occurrence, every woman who becomes pregnant should have at least one serologic test for syphilis performed during the first trimester.[112, 144, 307, 400] For communities and populations in which the prevalence of syphilis is high or for women in high-risk groups (see Table 12–3), repeated testing at the beginning of the third trimester (28 weeks)[135, 139, 401] and at delivery should be done.[156, 342] Sánchez and associates[139] have reported on the importance of maternal serologic screening for syphilis at delivery among a high-risk inner-city population. During the years 1987 to 1990, approximately 3% of 58,387 pregnant women had reactive serologic tests for syphilis; 5% of these women had had a nonreactive antepartum RPR test, which subsequently became reactive at delivery. There were 13 cases of congenital syphilis documented among these women who seroconverted during the pregnancy.

Moreover, screening tests at delivery should be performed on mothers and not on infants.[112, 156, 306] An infant's serologic titer is often one to two dilutions less than that of the mother's serum; thus, an infant may have a nonreactive umbilical cord VDRL test result but have a mother with a reactive serologic test for syphilis at delivery. From 1987 to 1990, Sánchez and co-workers[139] compared results of maternal serology at delivery to those obtained from VDRL testing of umbilical cord blood. There were 534 cases of reactive maternal serologic test results at delivery but negative umbilical cord blood VDRL test results. Eighty-seven, or 16%, of these infants were delivered of mothers with untreated syphilis at delivery and were therefore at risk of developing clinical evidence of infection if left untreated. It is clear that these infants would not have been identified if only the umbilical cord blood were screened. Moreover, no infant should be discharged to home from the nursery before results of maternal serologic screening has been documented at least once during the pregnancy. With the practice of early discharge at 24 hours or less becoming more common, it becomes the responsibility of the infant's health care provider to have adequate follow-up arrangements for infants who are discharged before the result of the maternal serologic test is known.

In most facilities, prenatal testing is required by law or as a matter of institutional procedure. Some states also mandate serologic screening at delivery for all women. Printed requirements do not eliminate human error, and prenatal testing requirements are not applicable to a woman who does not enter the medical care system until the moment before delivery.

The case of a woman who is incubating syphilis at delivery and whose serologic tests are nonreactive is, by current methodologies, impossible to prevent.[157, 227] In areas with a high incidence of congenital syphilis, a postpartum serologic test for syphilis at 6 weeks may be beneficial to detect this high-risk group.

Reporting of cases to the local health department will allow rapid contact investigation of named sexual partners and appropriate follow-up of infected individuals. Individuals who have had sexual contact with an untreated person should have clinical evaluation, serologic testing, and treatment. The time periods before treatment used for identifying at-risk sexual partners are (1) 3 months plus duration of symptoms for primary syphilis; (2) 6 months plus duration of symptoms for secondary syphilis, and (3) 1 year for early latent syphilis.[156] Persons who were exposed within 90 days preceding the diagnosis of primary, secondary, or early latent syphilis in a sexual partner might be infected even if seronegative and should be treated presumptively.

As partner notification has become more challenging because of anonymous sex and the inability to locate sexual partners, attention has focused on identifying core environments and populations in which syphilis transmission is occurring.[402] Such knowledge has resulted in provision of prophylactic syphilis treatment to groups of people in high-risk populations. Recently, the CDC has designed a strategy to assist public health providers at both the state and local level to design interventions for targeted at-risk populations that are locally identified.[403] Called the rapid ethnographic community assessment process (RECAP), the assessment is a package of activities and tools designed to use ethnographic methods for improving community involvement, as well as developing interventions that fit a population's social and behavioral context. It has been used in North Carolina with success.[403] Ultimately, prevention of congenital syphilis will only be accomplished if elimination of syphilis becomes a reality.

ACKNOWLEDGMENTS

The authors acknowledge the previous contributions to this chapter of Dr. Daniel Musher.

References

1. Ballantyne JW. Manual of Antenatal Pathology and Hygiene. Edinburgh, William Green & Son Publishers, 1902.
2. Goodman H. Notable Contributions to the Knowledge of Syphilis. New York, Froben Press, 1943.
3. Dennis CC. A History of Syphilis. Springfield, Ill, Charles C Thomas, 1962.
4. Truffi M. Hieronymous Fracastor's Syphilis: A Translation in Prose, 2nd ed. St. Louis, Urologic and Cutaneous Press, 1931.
5. Pusey WA. The History and Epidemiology of Syphilis. Springfield, Ill, Charles C Thomas, 1933.
6. Brown WJ, Donohue JF, Axnick NW, et al. Syphilis and Other Venereal Diseases. Cambridge, Mass, Harvard University Press, 1970.
7. Hutchinson J. On the different forms of the inflamma-

tion of the eye consequent on inherited syphilis. Ophthalmol Hosp Rev 1:191, 1858.

8. Rosebury T. Microbes and Morals: The Strange Story of Venereal Disease. New York, Viking Press, 1971.

9. Hovind-Hougen K. Determination by means of electron microscopy of morphological criteria of value for classification of some spirochetes in particular treponemes. Acta Pathol Microbiol Scand B Suppl 225, 1976.

10. Canale-Parola E. Physiology and evolution of spirochetes. Bacteriol Rev 41:181, 1977.

11. Fieldsteel AH. Genetics of treponema. In Schell RF, Musher DM (eds). Pathogenesis and Immunology of Treponemal Infection. New York, Marcel Dekker, 1982, p 39.

12. Hovind-Hougen K. Morphology. In Schell RF, Musher DM (eds). Pathogenesis and Immunology of Treponemal Infection. New York, Marcel Dekker, 1982, p 3.

13. Fohn MJ, Wisnall S, Baker-Zander SA, et al. Specificity of antibodies from patients with pinta for antigens of Treponema pallidum subspecies pallidum. J Infect Dis 157:32, 1988.

14. Krieg NR, Holt JG (eds). Bergey's Manual of Systematic Bacteriology, vol 1. Baltimore/London, Williams & Wilkins, 1984, p 50.

15. Román GC, Román LN. Occurrence of congenital, cardiovascular, visceral, neurologic, and neuro-opthalmologic complications in late yaws: a theme for future research. Rev Infect Dis 8:760, 1986.

16. Turner TB, Hollander DH. Biology of the Treponematoses. WHO Monogr Ser 35:1, 1957.

17. Wilcox RR, Guthe T. Treponema pallidum: a bibliographical review of the morphology, culture and survival of T. pallidum and associated organisms. Bull WHO 35:1, 1966.

18. Turner TB. Syphilis and the treponematoses. In Mudd S (ed). Infectious Agents and Host Reactions. Philadelphia, WB Saunders, 1970, p 346.

19. Jenkin HM, Banook PC. In vitro cultivation of treponemal infections. In Schell RF, Musher DM (eds). Pathogenesis and Immunology of Treponemal Infections. New York, Marcel Dekker, 1982, p 71.

20. Fieldsteel AH, Becker FA, Stout JG. Prolonged survival of virulent Treponema pallidum (Nichols strain) in cell-free and tissue culture systems. Infect Immun 18:173, 1977.

21. Fieldsteel AH, Cox DL, Moeckli RA. Cultivation of virulent Treponema pallidum in tissue culture. Infect Immun 32:908, 1981.

22. Klein JR, Monjan AA, Hardy PH Jr, et al. Abrogation of genetically controlled resistance of mice to Treponema pallidum by irradiation. Nature 283:572, 1980.

23. Marra CM, Castro CD, Kuller L, et al. Mechanisms of clearance of Treponema pallidum from the CSF in a nonhuman primate model. Neurol 51:957–961, 1998.

24. Fitzgerald TJ. Experimental congenital syphilis in rabbits. Can J Microbiol 31:757, 1985.

25. Wicher K, Baughn RE, Wicher V, et al. Experimental congenital syphilis: guinea pig model. Infect Immun 60:271, 1992.

26. Kajdacsy-Balla A, Howeedy A, Bagasra O. Experimental model of congenital syphilis. Infect Immun 61:3559, 1993.

26a. Wicher K, Baughn RE, Abbruscato F, Wicher V. Vertical transmission of Treponema pallidum to various litters and generations of guinea pigs. J Infect Dis 179:1206, 1999.

27. Clarkson KA. Technique of darkfield examination. Med Tech Bull 7:199, 1956.

28. Holt SC. Anatomy and chemistry of spirochetes. Microbiol Rev 42:114, 1978.

29. Johnson RC, Wachter MS, Ritzi DM. Treponeme outer cell envelope: solubilization and reaggregation. Infect Immun 7:249, 1973.

30. Zeigler JA, Jones AM, Jones RH, et al. Demonstration of extracellular material at the surface of pathogenic T. pallidum cells. Br J Vener Dis 52:1, 1976.

31. Fitzgerald TJ, Cleveland P, Johnson RC, et al. Scanning electron microscopy of Treponema pallidum (Nichols strain) attached to cultured mammalian cells. J Bacteriol 130:1333, 1977.

32. Fitzgerald TJ, Johnson RC, Wolff ET. Mucopolysaccharide material resulting from the interaction of Treponema pallidum (Nichols strain) with cultured mammalian cells. Infect Immun 22:575, 1978.

33. Fitzgerald TJ, Johnson RC. Surface mucopolysaccharides of Treponema pallidum. Infect Immun 24:244, 1979.

34. Fitzgerald TJ, Johnson RC, Ritzi D. Relationship of Treponema pallidum to acidic mucopolysaccharides. Infect Immun 24:252, 1979.

35. Norris SJ, Alderete JF, Axelson NH, et al. Identity of Treponema pallidum subsp. pallidum polypeptides: correlation of sodium dodecyl sulfate-polyacrylamide gel electrophoresis results from different laboratories. Electrophoresis 8:77, 1987.

36. Hanff PF, Fehniger TE, Miller JN, et al. Humoral immune response in human syphilis to polypeptides of Treponema pallidum. J Immunol 129:1287, 1982.

37. Baker-Zander SA, Hook EW III, Bonin P, et al. Antigens of Treponema pallidum recognized by IgG and IgM antibodies during syphilis in humans. J Infect Dis 151:264, 1985.

38. Radolf JD, Chamberlain NR, Clausell A, et al. Identification and localization of integral membrane proteins of virulent Treponema pallidum subsp. pallidum by phase partitioning with the nonionic detergent Triton X-114. Infect Immun 56:490, 1988.

39. Radolf JD, Norgard MV. Pathogen specificity of Treponema pallidum integral membrane proteins identified by phase partitioning with Triton X-114. Infect Immun 56:1825, 1988.

40. Cunningham TM, Walker EM, Miller JN, et al. Selective release of the Treponema pallidum outer membrane and associated polypeptides with Triton X-114. J Bacteriol 170:5789, 1988.

41. Chamberlain NR, Brandt ME, Erwin AL, et al. Major integral membrane protein immunogens of Treponema pallidum are proteolipids. Infect Immun 57:2872, 1989.

42. Swancutt MA, Radolf JD, Norgard MV. The 34-kilodalton membrane immunogen of Treponema pallidum is a lipoprotein. Infect Immun 58:384, 1990.

43. Walker EM, Zampighi GA, Blanco DR, et al. Demonstration of rare protein in the outer membrane of Treponema pallidum subsp. pallidum by freeze-fracture analysis. J Bacteriol 171:5005, 1989.

44. Radolf JD, Norgard MV, Schulz WW. Outer membrane ultrastructure explains the limited antigenicity of virulent Treponema pallidum. Proc Natl Acad Sci U S A 86:2051, 1989.

45. Jones SA, Marchitto KS, Miller JN, et al. Monoclonal antibody with hemagglutination, immobilization, and neutralization activities defines an immunodominant, 47,000 mol wt, surface-exposed immunogen of Treponema pallidum (Nichols). J Exp Med 160:1404, 1984.

46. Fraser CM, Morris SJ, Weinstock GM, et al. Complete genome sequence of Treponema pallidum, the syphilis spirochete. Science 281:375, 1998.

47. Pennisi E. Genome reveals wiles and weak points of syphilis. Science 281:324, 1998.
48. Weinstock GM, Hardham JM, McLeod MP, et al. The genome of *Treponema pallidum*: new light on the agent of syphilis. FEMS Microbiol Rev 22:323, 1998.
49. Norris SJ, Fraser CM, Weinstock GM. Illuminating the agent of syphilis: the *Treponema pallidum* genome project. Electrophoresis 19:551, 1998.
50. Radolf JD, Steiner B, Shevchenko D. *Treponema pallidum*: doing a remarkable job with what it's got. Trends Microbiol 7:7, 1999.
51. Cox CD, Barber MK. Oxygen uptake by *Treponema pallidum*. Infect Immun 10:123, 1974.
52. Baseman JB, Nichols JC, Hayes NS. Virulent *Treponema pallidum*: aerobe or anaerobe. Infect Immun 13:704, 1976.
53. Nichols JC, Baseman JB. Carbon sources utilized by virulent *Treponema pallidum*. Infect Immun 12:1044, 1975.
54. Lysko PG, Cox CD. Terminal electron transport in *Treponema pallidum*. Infect Immun 16:885, 1977.
55. Lysko PG, Cox CD. Respiration and oxidative phosphorylation in *Treponema pallidum*. Infect Immun 21:462, 1978.
56. Norris SJ, Miller JN, Sykes JA, et al. Influence of oxygen tension, sulfhydryl compounds, and serum on the motility and virulence of *Treponema pallidum* (Nichols strain) in a cell-free system. Infect Immun 22:689, 1978.
57. Graves S, Billington T. Optimum concentrations of dissolved oxygen for the survival of virulent *Treponema pallidum* under conditions of low oxidation-reduction potential. Br J Vener Dis 55:387, 1979.
58. Olansky S, Norins LC. Current serodiagnosis and treatment of syphilis. JAMA 198:165, 1966.
59. Turner TB, Kluth FC, McLeod C, et al. Protective antibodies in the serum of syphilitic patients. Am J Hyg 48:173, 1948.
60. Garner MF, Backhouse JL, Daskalopoulos G, et al. *Treponema pallidum* haemagglutination test for syphilis: comparison with the TPI and FTA-ABS tests. Br J Vener Dis 48:470, 1972.
61. Clark EG, Danbolt N. The Oslo study of the natural course of untreated syphilis: an epidemiologic investigation based on a re-study of the Boeck-Bruusgaard material. Med Clin North Am 48:613, 1964.
62. Turner TB, Hardy PH, Newman B, et al. Effects of passive immunization on experimental syphilis in the rabbit. Johns Hopkins Med J 133:241, 1973.
63. Weiser RS, Erickson D, Perine PL, et al. Immunity to syphilis: passive transfer in rabbits using serial doses of immune serum. Infect Immun 13:1402, 1976.
64. Bishop NH, Miller JN. Humoral immunity in experimental syphilis: I. The demonstration of resistance conferred by passive immunization. J Immunol 117:191, 1976.
65. Graves S, Alden J. Limited protection of rabbits against infection with *Treponema pallidum* by immune rabbit sera. Br J Vener Dis 55:399, 1979.
66. Musher DM, Hague-Park M, Gyorkey F, et al. The interaction between *Treponema pallidum* and human polymorphonuclear leukocytes. J Infect Dis 147:77, 1983.
67. Musher DM, Baughn RE. Syphilis. *In* Samter M (ed). Immunologic Diseases, 3rd ed. Boston, Little, Brown, 1978, p 639.
68. Radolf JD, Norgard MY, Brandt ME, et al. Lipoproteins of *Borrelia burgdorferi* and *Treponema pallidum* activate cachectin/tumor necrosis factor synthesis: analysis using a CAT reporter construct. J Immunol 147:1968, 1991.
69. Thomas DD, Navab M, Haake DA, et al. *Treponema pallidum* invades intercellular junctions of endothelial cell monolayers. Proc Natl Acad Sci U S A 85:3608, 1988.
70. Riley BS, Oppenheimer-Marks N, Hansen EJ, et al. Virulent *Treponema pallidum* activates human vascular endothelial cells. J Infect Dis 165:484, 1992.
71. Schell RF, Musher DM, Jacobson K, et al. Induction of acquired cellular resistance following transfer of thymus-dependent lymphocytes from syphilitic rabbits. J Immunol 114:550, 1975.
72. Schell R, Musher D, Jacobson K, et al. Effect of macrophage activation on infection with *Treponema pallidum*. Infect Immun 12:505, 1973.
73. Graves SR, Johnson RC. Effect of pretreatment with *Mycobacterium bovis* (strain BCG) and immune syphilitic serum on rabbit resistance to *Treponema pallidum*. Infect Immun 12:1029, 1975.
74. Baughn RE, Musher DM, Knox JM. Effect of sensitization with *Propionibacterium acnes* on the growth of *Listeria monocytogenes* and *Treponema pallidum* in rabbits. J Immunol 118:109, 1977.
75. Schell RF, Chan JK, LeFrock JL, et al. Endemic syphilis: transfer of resistance to *Treponema pallidum* strain Bosnia A in hamsters with a cell suspension enriched in thymus-derived cells. J Infect Dis 141:752, 1980.
76. Lukehart SA, Baker-Zander SA, Lloyd RMC, et al. Characterization of lymphocyte responsiveness in early experimental syphilis: II. Nature of cellular infiltration and *Treponema pallidum* distribution in testicular lesions. J Immunol 124:461, 1980.
77. Festenstein HC, Abrahams C, Bokkenheuser V. Runting syndrome in neonatal rabbits infected with *Treponema pallidum*. Clin Exp Immunol 2:311, 1967.
78. Turner DR, Wright DJM. Lymphadenopathy in early syphilis. J Pathol 110:304, 1973.
79. From E, Thestrup-Pedersen K, Thulin H. Reactivity of lymphocytes from patients with syphilis towards *T. pallidum* antigen in the lymphocyte migration and lymphocyte transformation tests. Br J Vener Dis 56:224, 1976.
80. Wicher V, Wicher K. In vitro cell response to *Treponema pallidum*-infected rabbits: III. Impairment in production of lymphocyte mitogenic factor. Clin Exp Immunol 24:496, 1977.
81. Baughn RE, Musher DM. Altered immune responsiveness associated with experimental syphilis in the rabbit: elevated IgM and depressed IgG responses to sheep erythrocytes. J Immunol 120:1691, 1978.
82. Baughn RE, Musher DM. Aberrant secondary antibody responses to sheep erythrocytes in rabbits with experimental syphilis. Infect Immun 25:133, 1979.
83. Magnuson HJ, Thomas EW, Olansky S, et al. Inoculation syphilis in human volunteers. Medicine 35:33, 1956.
84. Nabarro D. Congenital Syphilis. London, E Arnold, 1954.
85. Dobson SRM, Taber LH, Baughn RE. Recognition of *Treponema pallidum* antibodies in congenitally infected newborns and their mothers. J Infect Dis 157:903, 1988.
86. Sánchez PJ, McCracken GH, Wendel GD, et al. Molecular analysis of the fetal IgM response to *Treponema pallidum* antigens: implications for improved serodiagnosis of congenital syphilis. J Infect Dis 159:508, 1989.
87. Lewis LL. Congenital syphilis: serologic diagnosis in the young infant. Infect Dis Clin North Am 6:31, 1992.
88. Sánchez PJ, Wendel GD, Grimprel K, et al. Evaluation of molecular methodologies and rabbit infectivity testing for the diagnosis of congenital syphilis and neonatal central nervous system invasion by *Treponema pallidum*. J Infect Dis 167:148, 1993.

89. Wendel GD, Sánchez PJ, Peters MT, et al. Identification of *Treponema pallidum* in amniotic fluid and fetal blood from pregnancies complicated by congenital syphilis. Obstet Gynecol 78:890, 1991.

90. Lucas MJ, Theriot SK, Wendel GD. Doppler systolic-diastolic ratios in pregnancies complicated by syphilis. Obstet Gynecol 77:217, 1991.

91. Genest DR, Choi-Hong SR, Tate JE, et al. Diagnosis of congenital syphilis from placental examination. Hum Pathol 27:366, 1996.

92. Rawstron SA, Vetrano J, Tannis G, Bromberg K. Congenital syphilis: detection of *Treponema pallidum* in stillborns. Clin Infect Dis 24:24, 1997.

93. Paley SS. Syphilis in pregnancy. NY J Med 37:585, 1937.

94. Fiumara NJ, Fleming WL, Downing JG, et al. The incidence of prenatal syphilis at the Boston City Hospital. N Engl J Med 247:48, 1952.

95. Ingraham NR. The value of penicillin alone in the prevention and treatment of congenital syphilis. Acta Derm Venereol 31(Suppl 24):60, 1951.

96. Sheffield JS, Wendel GD Jr, Zeray F, et al. Congenital syphilis: the influence of maternal stage of syphilis on vertical transmission. Am J Obstet Gynecol 180:S85, 1999 (abstract).

97. Fiumara NJ. A legacy of syphilis. Arch Dermatol 92:676, 1965.

98. Sánchez PJ. Congenital syphilis. *In* Aronoff SC (ed). Advances in Pediatric Infectious Diseases. St. Louis, Mosby–Year Book, 1992, p 161.

99. Pollack M, Borkowsky W, Krasinski K. Maternal syphilis is associated with enhanced perinatal HIV transmission. *In* Program and Abstracts, 30th Interscience Conference on Antimicrobial Agents and Chemotherapy, Atlanta. American Society for Microbiology, Washington, DC, 1990, p 1274.

100. Chadwick, EG, Millard DD, Rowley AH. Congenital syphilis in HIV-infected and uninfected children in Chicago 1989–1991. Pediatr Res 31:89A, 1992.

101. Lukehart SA, Hook EW III, Baker-Zander SA, et al. Invasion of the central nervous system by *Treponema pallidum*: implications for diagnosis and treatment. Ann Intern Med 1:855, 1988.

102. Theus SA, Harrich DA, Gaynor R, et al. *Treponema pallidum*, lipoproteins, and synthetic lipoprotein analogues induce human immunodeficiency virus type 1 gene expression in monocytes via NF-kB activation. J Infect Dis 177:941–950, 1998.

103. Tucker HA, Robinson RCV. Disappearance time of *T. pallidum* from lesions of early syphilis following administration of crystalline penicillin G. Bull Johns Hopkins Hosp 80:169, 1947.

104. Turner TB, Bauer JA, Kluth FC. The viability of the spirochetes of syphilis and yaws in desiccated blood serum. Am J Med Sci 202:416, 1941.

105. Keller R, Morton HE. The effect of a hand soap and a hexachlorophene soap on the cultivatable treponemata. Am J Syph 36:524, 1952.

106. McIntosh J, Fildes P. Syphilis from the Modern Standpoint. London, E Arnold, 1911.

107. Singh R, Sharma RC, Barvah MC. Third generation infantile syphilis: an unusual presentation. Acta Derm Venereol 58:181, 1978.

108. Centers for Disease Control. Congenital syphilis, New York City, 1986–1988. MMWR Morb Mortal Wkly Rep 38:825, 1989.

109. Rolfs RT, Nakashima AK. Epidemiology of early syphilis in the United States, 1981–89. JAMA 264:1432, 1990.

110. Ricci JM, Fojaco RM, O'Sullivan MJ. Congenital syphilis: the University of Miami/Jackson: Memorial Medical Center experience, 1986–1988. Obstet Gynecol 74:687, 1989.

111. Berry MC, Dajani AS. Resurgence of congenital syphilis. Infect Dis Clin North Am 6:19, 1992.

112. Reyes MP, Hunt N, Ostrea EM Jr, George D. Maternal/congenital syphilis in a large tertiary-care urban hospital. Clin Infect Dis 17:1041, 1993.

113. Rolfs RT, Goldberg M, Sharrar RG. Risk factors for syphilis: cocaine use and prostitution. Am J Public Health 80:853, 1990.

114. Klass PE, Brown ER, Pelton SL. The incidence of prenatal syphilis at the Boston City Hospital: a comparison across four decades. Pediatrics 94:24, 1994.

115. Sison CG, Ostrea EM Jr, Reyes MP, Salari V. The resurgence of congenital syphilis: a cocaine-related problem. J Pediatr 130:289, 1997.

116. Rathbun KC. Congenital syphilis: a proposal for improved surveillance, diagnosis, and treatment. Sex Transm Dis 10:102, 1983.

117. Centers for Disease Control. Impact of closure of a sexually transmitted disease clinic on public health surveillance of sexually transmitted diseases—Washington, D.C., 1995. MMWR Morb Mortal Wkly Rep 47:1067, 1998.

118. Petzoldt D. Effect of spectinomycin on *T. pallidum* in incubating syphilis. Br J Vener Dis 51:305, 1975.

119. Schroeter AL, Turner RH, Lucas JB, et al. Therapy for incubating syphilis: effectiveness of gonorrhea treatment. JAMA 218:711, 1971.

120. Nakashima AK, Rolfs RT, Flock ML, et al. Epidemiology of syphilis in the United States, 1941–1993. Sex Transm Dis 23:16, 1996.

121. Centers for Disease Control. Alternative case-finding methods in a crack-related syphilis epidemic—Philadelphia. MMWR Morb Mortal Wkly Rep 40:77, 1991.

122. Centers for Disease Control. Selective screening to augment syphilis case-finding—Dallas, 1991. MMWR Morb Mortal Wkly Rep 42:424, 1993.

123. Centers for Disease Control. Primary and secondary syphilis. MMWR Morb Mortal Wkly Rep 47:493, 1998.

124. Risser JMH, Hwang L, Risser WL et al. The epidemiology of syphilis in the waning years of an epidemic: Houston, Texas 1991–1999. Sex Transm Dis 26:121, 1999.

125. US Department of Health, Education and Welfare, Public Health Service. VD Fact Sheet. Washington, DC, U.S. Government Printing Office, 1974.

126. Centers for Disease Control. Primary and secondary syphilis—United States, 1998. MMWR Morb Mortal Wkly Rep 48:873, 1999.

127. Centers for Disease Control. Epidemic of congenital syphilis—Baltimore, 1996 – 1997. MMWR Morb Mortal Wkly Rep 47:904, 1998.

128. Fleming WL, Brown WN, Donohue JF, et al. National survey of venereal disease treated by physicians in 1968. JAMA 211:11, 1970.

129. St. Louis ME, Wasserheit JM. Elimination of syphilis in the United States. Science 281:353, 1998.

130. Mobley JA, McKeown RE, Jackson KL, et al. Risk factors for congenital syphilis in infants of women with syphilis in South Carolina. Am J Public Health 88:597, 1998.

131. Report of WHO Scientific Group. Treponemal infections. WHO Tech Rep Ser G74, 1982.

132. Tichonova L, Borisenko K, Ward H, et al. Epidemics of syphilis in the Russian Federation: trends, origins, and priorities for control. Lancet 350:210, 1997.

133. Pereyra N, Parisi A, Baptista G. Situación de la sífilis

congénita en un municipio del gran Buenos Aires tres años de evaluación 1994–97, San Isidro. *In* Program and Abstracts of the XI Latin American Congress on Sexually Transmitted Diseases/V Pan-American Congress on AIDS, 1997, p 187.

134. Southwick K, Blanco S, Santander A, et al. Rapid assessment of maternal and congenital syphilis in Bolivia, 1996. *In* Program and Abstracts of the International Congress of Sexually Transmitted Diseases, 1997, p 96.

135. Wendel GD. Gestational and congenital syphilis. Clin Perinatol 15:287, 1988.

136. Zenker PN, Berman SM. Congenital syphilis: trends and recommendations for evaluation and management. J Pediatr Infect Dis 10:516, 1991.

137. Ikeda MK, Jenson HB. Evaluation and treatment of congenital syphilis. J Pediatr 117:843, 1990.

138. Mascola L, Pelosi R, Blount JH, et al. Congenital syphilis revisited. Am J Dis Child 139:575, 1985.

139. Sánchez PJ, Wendel GD, Hall M, et al. Congenital syphilis: the Dallas experience. Pediatr Res 29:286A, 1991.

140. Cohen DA, Boyd D, Pabhudas I, et al. The effects of case definition, maternal screening, and reporting criteria on rates of congenital syphilis. Am J Public Health 80:316, 1990.

141. Mascola L, Pelosi R, Blount JH, et al. Congenital syphilis. Why is it still occurring? JAMA 252:1729, 1984.

142. Rawstron SA, Jenkins S, Blanchard S, et al. Maternal and congenital syphilis in Brooklyn, NY: epidemiology, transmission and diagnosis. Am J Dis Child 146:727, 1993.

143. Webber MP, Lambert G, Bateman DA, Hauser WA. Maternal risk factors for congenital syphilis: a case-control study. Am J Epidemiol 137:415, 1993.

144. Monif GRG, Williams BR Jr, Shulman ST, et al. The problem of maternal syphilis after serologic surveillance during pregnancy. Am J Obstet Gynecol 117:268, 1973.

145. Bellingham FR. Syphilis in pregnancy: transplacental infection. Med J Aust 2:647, 1973.

146. Centers for Disease Control. Congenital syphilis— United States, 1998. MMWR Morb Mortal Wkly Rep 48:757, 1999.

147. Knight J, Richardson S, Petric M, et al. Contributions of suboptimal antenatal care and poor communication to the diagnosis of congenital syphilis. Pediatr Infect Dis 14:238, 1995.

148. Finelli L, Crayne EM, Spitalny KC. Treatment of infants with reactive syphilis serology, New Jersey: 1992 to 1996. Pediatrics 102:394, 1998.

149. Lackmann FM, Willnow V, Wahn V, Schroten H. The importance of reading test results. Lancet 353:290, 1999.

150. Felman Y. How useful are the serologic tests for syphilis? Int J Dermatol 21:79, 1982.

151. Spangler AS, Jackson JH, Fiumara NJ, et al. Syphilis with a negative blood test reaction. JAMA 189:113, 1964.

152. Sparling PF. Diagnosis and treatment of syphilis. N Engl J Med 284:642, 1971.

153. Levine Z, Sherer DM, Jacobs A, Rotenberg O. Nonimmune hydrops fetalis due to congenital syphilis associated with negative intrapartum maternal serology screening. Am J Perinatol 15:233, 1998.

154. Larsen SA, Hambie EA, Pettit DE, et al. Specificity, sensitivity, and reproducibility among the fluorescent treponemal antibody-absorption test, the microhemagglutination assay for *Treponema pallidum* antibodies, and the hemagglutination treponemal test for syphilis. J Clin Microbiol 14:441, 1981.

155. Larsen SA, Steiner BM, Rudolph AH. Laboratory diagnosis and interpretation of tests for syphilis. Clin Microbiol Rev 8:1, 1995.

156. Centers for Disease Control and Prevention. 1998 Guidelines for treatment of sexually transmitted diseases. MMWR Morb Mortal Wkly Rep 47:28, 1998.

157. Sánchez PJ, Wendel GD, Norgard MV. Congenital syphilis associated with negative results of maternal serologic tests at delivery. Am J Dis Child 145:967, 1991.

158. Dippel AL. The relationship of congenital syphilis to abortion and miscarriage, and the mechanism of intrauterine protection. Am J Obstet Gynecol 47:369, 1944.

159. Fiumara NJ. Venereal disease. *In* Charles D, Finland M (eds). Obstetric and Perinatal Infections. Philadelphia, Lea & Febiger, 1973.

160. Benirschke K. Syphilis—the placenta and the fetus. Am J Dis Child 128:142, 1974.

161. Harter CA, Benirschke K. Fetal syphilis in the first trimester. Am J Obstet Gynecol 124:705, 1976.

162. Silverstein AM. Congenital syphilis and the timing of immunogenesis in the human fetus. Nature 194:196, 1962.

163. Nathan L, Bohman VR, Sánchez PJ, et al. In utero infection with *Treponema pallidum* in early pregnancy. Prenat Diag 17:119, 1997.

164. Dorman HG, Sahyun PF. Identification and significance of spirochetes in the placenta: a report of 105 cases with positive findings. Am J Obstet Gynecol 33:954, 1937.

165. Turner TB. The spirochaetes. *In* Dubos RJ, Hirsch JG (eds). Bacterial and Mycotic Infection of Man, 4th ed. Philadelphia, JB Lippincott, 1965.

166. Syphilis: a synopsis. US Public Health Service Publication No. 1660. Washington, DC, U.S. Government Printing Office, 1968.

167. Robbins SL. Pathologic Basis of Disease. Philadelphia, WB Saunders, 1974.

168. Brightbill HO, Libraty DH, Krutzik SR. Host defense mechanisms triggered by microbial lipoproteins through toll-like receptors. Science 285:732, 1999.

169. Sellati TJ, Bouis DA, Caimano MJ, et al. Activation of human monocytic cells by *Borrelia burgdorferi* and *Treponema pallidum* is facilitated by CD14 and correlates with surface exposure of spirochetal lipoproteins. J Immunol 163:2049, 1999.

170. Whipple DV, Dunham EC. Congenital syphilis: I. Incidence, transmission and diagnosis. J Pediatr 12:386, 1938.

171. Russell P, Altschuler G. Placental abnormalities of congenital syphilis. Am J Dis Child 128:160, 1974.

172. Qureshi F, Jacques SM, Reyes MP. Placental histopathology in syphilis. Hum Pathol 24:779, 1993.

173. Fojaco RM, Hensley GT, Moskowitz L. Congenital syphilis and necrotizing funisitis. JAMA 261:1788, 1989.

174. Bromberg K, Rawstron S, Tannis G. Diagnosis of congenital syphilis by combining *Treponema pallidum*–specific IgM detection with immunofluorescent antigen detection for *T. pallidum*. J Infect Dis 168:238, 1993.

175. Jacques SM, Qureshi F. Necrotizing funisitis: a study of 45 cases. Hum Pathol 23:1278, 1992.

176. Rogers B, Sheffield J, Margraf L, et al. Placental villous enlargement correlates with poor pregnancy outcome in congenital syphilis. New Orleans, Society for Pediatric Pathology, March 1999 (abstract).

177. Guarner J, Greer PW, Bartlett J, et al. Congenital syphilis in a newborn: an immunopathologic study. Mod Pathol 12:82, 1999.

178. Oppenheimer EH, Hardy JB. Congenital syphilis in the newborn infant: clinical and pathological observations in recent cases. Johns Hopkins Med J 129:63, 1971.

179. Cox SM, Wendel GD. Xeroradiography and skeletal survey in the diagnosis of congenital syphilis following fetal death. Presented before the Society of Perinatal Obstetricians, February 1987 (abstract).

180. Stowens D. Pediatric Pathology, 2nd ed. Baltimore, Williams & Wilkins, 1966.

181. Kissane JM, Smith MG. Pathology of Infancy and Childhood. St. Louis, CV Mosby, 1967.

182. Wright DJM, Berry CL. Liver involvement in congenital syphilis. Br J Vener Dis 50:241, 1974.

183. Morison JE. Foetal and Neonatal Pathology. New York, Appleton-Century-Crofts, 1970.

184. Ajayi NA, Marven S, Kaschula RO, et al. Intestinal ulceration, obstruction and hemorrhage in congenital syphilis. Pediatr Surg Int 15:391, 1999.

185. Kaplan BS, Wiglesworth FW, Marks MI, et al. The glomerulopathy of congenital syphilis—an immune deposit disease. J Pediatr 81:1154, 1972.

186. Gamble CN, Reardon JB. Immune pathogenesis of syphilitic glomerulonephritis. N Engl J Med 292:449, 1975.

187. Hill LL, Singer DB, Falletta J, et al. The nephrotic syndrome in congenital syphilis: an immunopathy. Pediatrics 49:260, 1972.

188. Losito A, Cucciarelli E, Massi-Benedetti F, et al. Membranous glomerulonephritis in congenital syphilis. Clin Nephrol 12:32, 1979.

189. Wiggelinkhuizen J, Kaschula ROC, Uys CJ, et al. Congenital syphilis and glomerulonephritis with evidence for immune pathogenesis. Arch Dis Child 48:375, 1973.

190. Ford FR. Diseases of the Nervous System in Infancy, Childhood, and Adolescence. Springfield, Ill, Charles C Thomas, 1973.

191. Daaboul JJ, Kartchner W, Jones KL. Neonatal hypoglycemia caused by hypopituitarism in infants with congenital syphilis. J Pediatr 123:983, 1993.

192. Benzick AE, Wirthwein DP, Weinberg A, et al. Pituitary gland gumma in congenital syphilis after failed maternal treatment: a case report. Pediatrics 104:102, 1999.

193. Turnbull HM. Recognition of congenital syphilitic inflammation of the long bones. Lancet 1:1239, 1922.

194. Pendergrass EP, Bromer RS. Congenital bone syphilis: preliminary report: roentgenologic study with notes on the histology and pathology of the condition. AJR Am J Roentgenol 22:1, 1929.

195. Park EA, Jackson DA. The irregular extensions of the end of the shaft in the x-ray photograph in congenital syphilis, with pertinent observations. J Pediatr 13:748, 1938.

196. Cremin BJ, Fisher RM. The lesions of congenital syphilis. Br J Radiol 43:333, 1970.

197. Caffey J. Syphilis of the skeleton in early infancy: the nonspecificity of many of the roentgenographic changes. AJR Am J Roentgenol 42:637, 1939.

198. Caffey J. Pediatric X-ray Diagnosis. Chicago, Year Book Medical Publishers, 1973.

199. Whitaker JA, Sartain P, Shaheedy MD. Hematological aspects of congenital syphilis. J Pediatr 66:629, 1965.

200. Sartain P. The anemia of congenital syphilis. South Med J 58:27, 1965.

201. Thomas E. Syphilis: Its Course and Management. New York, Macmillan, 1949.

202. Willcox RR. A Text-Book of Venereal Disease. New York, Grune & Stratton, 1950.

203. Fiumara NJ. Congenital syphilis in Massachusetts. N Engl J Med 245:634, 1951.

204. Brown WJ, Moore MB Jr. Congenital syphilis in the United States. Clin Pediatr (Phila) 2:220, 1963.

205. Sever JL. Effects of infection on pregnancy risk. Clin Obstet Gynecol 16:225, 1973.

206. Sheridan MD. Final report of a prospective study of children whose mothers had rubella in early pregnancy. BMJ 2:536, 1964.

207. Chapel TA. The variability of syphilitic chancres. Sex Transm Dis 5:68, 1978.

208. Musher DM. Syphilis. Infect Dis Clin North Am 1:83, 1987.

209. Olansky S, Norins LC. Syphilis and other treponematoses. In Fitzpatrick TB, Arndt K, Clark WH, et al (eds). Dermatology in General Medicine. New York, McGraw-Hill, 1971, p 1955.

210. Feher J, Somogyi T, Timmer M, et al. Early syphilitic hepatitis. Lancet 2:896, 1975.

211. Jozsa L, Timmer M, Somogyi T, et al. Hepatitis syphilitica: a clinico-pathological study of 25 cases. Acta Hepatogastroenterol 24:344, 1977.

212. Brophy EM, Ashworth CT, Aries M, et al. Acute syphilitic nephrosis in pregnancy. Obstet Gynecol 24:930, 1964.

213. Falls WF Jr, Ford KL, Answorth CT. The nephrotic syndrome in secondary syphilis: report of a case with renal biopsy findings. Ann Intern Med 63:1047, 1965.

214. Braunstein GD, Lewis EJ, Galvanek EG, et al. The nephrotic syndrome associated with secondary syphilis. Am J Med 48:643, 1970.

215. Bhorade MS, Carag IIB, Lee IIJ, et al. Nephropathy of secondary syphilis: a clinical and pathological spectrum. JAMA 216:1159, 1971.

216. Dismukes WE, Delgado DG, Mallernee SV, et al. Destructive bone disease in early syphilis. JAMA 236:2646, 1976.

217. Tight RR, Warner JF. Skeletal involvement in secondary syphilis detected by bone scanning. JAMA 235:2326, 1976.

218. Shore RN, Kiesel HA, Bennett HD. Osteolytic lesions in secondary syphilis. Arch Intern Med 137:1465, 1977.

219. Sánchez PJ, Wendel GD. Syphilis in pregnancy. Clin Perinatol 24:71, 1997.

220. Holder NR, Knox JM. Syphilis in pregnancy. Med Clin North Am 56:1153, 1972.

221. Blair EK, Lawson JM. Unsuspected syphilitic hepatitis in a patient with low-grade proteinuria and abnormal liver function. Mayo Clin Proc 65:1365, 1990.

222. Drusin LM, Topf-Olstein B, Levy-Zombek E. Epidemiology of infectious syphilis at a tertiary hospital. Arch Intern Med 139:901, 1979.

223. Scully RE, Mark EJ, McNeely WF, et al. Case records of the Massachusetts General Hospital. N Engl J Med 325:414, 1991.

224. Hill LM, Maloney JB. An unusual constellation of sonographic findings associated with congenital syphilis. Obstet Gynecol 78:895, 1991.

225. Nathan L, Twickler DM, Peters MT, et al. Fetal syphilis: correlation of sonographic findings and rabbit infectivity testing of amniotic fluid. J Ultrasound Med 2:97, 1993.

226. Saxoni F, Lapatsanis P, Pantelakis SN. Congenital syphilis: a description of 18 cases and re-examination of an old but ever-present disease. Clin Pediatr (Phila) 6:687, 1967.

227. Dorfman DH, Glaser JH. Congenital syphilis presenting in infants after the newborn period. N Engl J Med 323:1299, 1990.

228. Shah MC, Barton LL. Congenital syphilis hepatitis. Pediatr Infect Dis J 8:891, 1989.

229. Long WA, Ulshen MA, Lawson EE. Clinical manifestations of congenital syphilitic hepatitis: implications for pathogenesis. J Pediatr Gastroenterol Nutr 3:551, 1984.

230. Pohl M, Niemeyer CM, Hentschel R, et al. Hemophago-cytosis in early congenital syphilis. Eur J Pediatr 158:553, 1999.
231. Bulova SI, Schwartz E, Harrer WV. Hydrops fetalis and congenital syphilis. Pediatrics 49:285, 1972.
232. Levine P, Celano MJ, Falkowski F. The specificity of the antibody in paroxysmal cold hemoglobinuria (P.C.H.) Ann NY Acad Sci 124:456, 1965.
233. Shah AA, Desai AB. Paroxysmal cold hemoglobinuria (case report). Indian Pediatr 14:219, 1977.
234. Platou RV. Treatment of congenital syphilis with penicillin. Adv Pediatr 4:35, 1949.
235. King A, Nicol C. Venereal Diseases. Philadelphia, FA Davis, 1964.
236. Wilkinson RH, Heller RM. Congenital syphilis: resurgence of an old problem. Pediatrics 47:27, 1971.
237. Brion LP, Manuli M, Rai B, et al. Long bone radiographic abnormalities as a sign of active congenital syphilis in asymptomatic newborns. Pediatrics 88:1037, 1991.
238. Seckler AB, Kliner MM, Tunnessen W Jr. Pediatric Puzzler: play it again Sam. Contemp Pediatr 12:135, 1995.
239. Teberg A, Hodgman JE. Congenital syphilis in newborn. Calif Med 118:5, 1973.
240. Papaioannou AC, Asrow GG, Schuckmell NH. Nephrotic syndrome in early infancy as a manifestation of congenital syphilis. Pediatrics 27:636, 1961.
241. Pollner P. Nephrotic syndrome associated with congenital syphilis. JAMA 198:263, 1966.
242. Rosen EU, Abrahams C, Rabinowitz L. Nephropathy of congenital syphilis. S Afr Med J 47:1606, 1973.
243. Yuceoglu AM, Sagel I, Tresser G, et al. The glomerulopathy of congenital syphilis: a curable immune-deposit disease. JAMA 229:1085, 1974.
244. McDonald R, Wiggelinkhuizen J, Kaschula RO. The nephrotic syndrome in very young infants. Am J Dis Child 122:507, 1971.
245. Ahmed A, Hickey SM, Ehrett S, et al. Cerebrospinal fluid values in the term neonate. Pediatr Infect Dis J 15:298, 1996.
246. Thorley JD, Holmes RK, Kaplan JM, et al. Passive transfer of antibodies of maternal origin from blood to cerebrospinal fluid in infants. Lancet 1:651, 1975.
247. Wolf B, Kalangu K. Congenital neurosyphilis revisited. Eur J Pediatr 152:493, 1993.
248. Contreras F, Pereda J. Congenital syphilis of the eye with lens involvement. Arch Ophthalmol 96:1052, 1978.
249. Naeye RL. Fetal growth with congenital syphilis. Am J Clin Pathol 55:228, 1971.
250. Naeye RL. Judgment of fetal age: III. The pathologist's evaluation. Pediatr Clin North Am 13:849, 1966.
251. Bateman DA, Ng SKC, Hansen CA, et al. The effects of intrauterine cocaine exposure in newborns. Am J Public Health 83:190, 1993.
252. Fiumara NJ, Lessell S. Manifestations of late congenital syphilis: an analysis of 271 patients. Arch Dermatol 102:78, 1970.
253. Putkonen T. Does early treatment prevent dental changes in congenital syphilis? Acta Derm Venereol 43:240, 1963.
254. Azimi PH. Interstitial keratitis in a five-year old. Pediatr Infect Dis 18:299, 1999.
255. Hendershot EL. Luetic deafness. Otolaryngol Clin North Am 11:43, 1978.
256. Rothenberg R. Syphilitic hearing loss. South Med J 72:118, 1979.
257. Lapunzina PD, Alteca JM, Fuchman JC, Freilij H. Neurosyphilis in an eight-year old child: usefulness of the SPECT study. Pediatr Neurol 18:81, 1998.
258. Borella L, Goobar JE, Clark GM. Synovitis of the knee joints in late congenital syphilis. JAMA 180:84, 1962.
259. Wendel GD, Maberry MC, Christmas JT, et al. Examination of amniotic fluid in diagnosing congenital syphilis with fetal death. Obstet Gynecol 74:967, 1989.
260. Rathbun KC. Congenital syphilis: a proposal for improved surveillance, diagnosis and treatment. Sex Transm Dis 10:102, 1983.
261. Jensen HB. Congenital syphilis. Semin Pediatr Infect Dis 10:183, 1999.
262. Sánchez PJ. Laboratory tests for congenital syphilis. Pediatr Infect Dis J 17:70, 1998.
263. Hira SK, Bhat GJ, Patel JB, et al. Early congenital syphilis: clinicoradiologic features in 202 patients. Sex Transm Dis 12:77, 1985.
264. Woody NC, Sistrunk WF, Platou RV. Congenital syphilis: a laid ghost walks. J Pediatr 64:63, 1964.
265. Swischuk LE. Radiology of the Newborn and Young Infant. Baltimore, Williams & Wilkins, 1973.
266. Ingraham NR. The lag phase in early congenital osseous syphilis: a roentgenographic study. Am J Med Sci 191:819, 1936.
267. Cremin BJ, Shaff MI. Congenital syphilis diagnosed in utero. Br J Radiol 48:939, 1975.
268. Ringel RE, Brenner JI, Haney PJ, et al. Prostaglandin-induced periostitis: a complication of long-term PGE, infusion in an infant with congenital heart disease. Radiology 142:657, 1982.
269. Harris VJ, Jiminez CA, Vidyasager D. Congenital syphilis with syphilitic arthritis. Radiology 123:416, 1977.
270. Harris VJ, Jiminez CA, Vidvasager D. Congenital syphilis with unusual clinical presentations. Ill Med J 151:371, 1977.
271. Chipps BE, Swischuk LE, Voelter WW. Single bone involvement in congenital syphilis. Pediatr Radiol 5:50, 1976.
272. Solomon A, Rosen E. The aspect of trauma in the bone change of congenital lues. Pediatr Radiol 3:176, 1975.
273. Solomon A, Rosen E. Focal osseous lesions in congenital lues. Pediatr Radiol 7:36, 1978.
274. Heyman S, Mandell GA. Skeletal scintigraphy in congenital syphilis. Clin Nucl Med 8:531, 1983.
275. Wolpowitz A. Osseous manifestations of congenital lues. S Afr Med J 50:675, 1976.
276. Siegel D, Hirschman SZ. Syphilitic osteomyelitis with diffusely abnormal bone scan. Mt Sinai J Med 46:320, 1979.
277. Magnuson HJ, Eagle H, Fleischman R. The minimal infectious inoculum of Spirochaeta pallida (Nichols strain), and a consideration of its rate of multiplication in vivo. Am J Syph Gon Vener Dis 32:1, 1948.
278. Turner TB, Hardy PH, Newman B. Infectivity tests in syphilis. Br J Vener Dis 45:183, 1969.
279. Moore MB Jr, Knox JM. Sensitivity and specificity in syphilis serology: clinical implications. South Med J 48:963, 1965.
280. Matthews HM, Yang TK, Jenkin HM. Unique lipid composition of Treponema pallidum (Nichols virulent strain). Infect Immun 24:713, 1979.
281. Catterall RD. Systemic disease and the biological false positive reaction. Br J Vener Dis 48:1, 1972.
282. Boak RA, Carpenter CM, Miller JN, et al. Biologic false-positive reactions for syphilis in pregnancy as determined by the Treponema pallidum immobilization test. Surg Gynecol Obstet 101:751, 1955.
283. Buchanan CS, Haserick JR. FTA-ABS test in pregnancy: a probable false-positive reaction. Arch Dermatol 102:322, 1970.

284. Kostant GH. Familial chronic biologic false-positive seroreactions for syphilis: report of two families, one with three generations affected. JAMA 219:45, 1972.

285. Duncan WC, Knox JM, Wende RD. The FTA-ABS test in darkfield-positive primary syphilis. JAMA 228:859, 1974.

286. Rudolph AH. The microhemagglutination assay for *Treponema pallidum* antibodies (MHA-TP), a new treponemal test for syphilis: where does it fit? J Am Vener Dis Assoc 3:3, 1976.

287. Goodhard GL, Brown ST, Zaidi AA, et al. Blinded proficiency testing of the FTA-ABS test. Arch Intern Med 141:1245, 1981.

288. Schroeter AL, Lucas JB, Price EV, et al. Treatment for early syphilis and reactivity of serologic tests. JAMA 221:471, 1972.

289. Fiumara NJ. Treatment of primary and secondary syphilis: serological response. JAMA 243:2500, 1980.

290. O'Neill P, Warner RW, Nicol CS. *Treponema pallidum* haemagglutination assay in the routine serodiagnosis of treponemal disease. Br J Vener Dis 49:427, 1973.

291. Lesinski J, Krauch J, Kadziewicz E. Specificity, sensitivity and diagnostic value of the TPHA test. Br J Vener Dis 50:334, 1974.

292. Larsen SA, McCrew BE, Hunter EF, et al. Syphilis serology and dark field microscopy. *In* Holmes KK, Mardh PA, Sparling PF, et al (eds). Sexually Transmitted Diseases. New York, McGraw-Hill, 1984, p 875.

293. Musher DM. A positive VDRL reaction in an asymptomatic patient. *In* Remington JS, Swartz MN (eds). Current Clinical Topics in Infectious Diseases, no. 9. New York, McGraw-Hill, 1988, p 147.

294. Deguchi M, Hosotsubo H, Yamashita N, et al. Evaluation of gelatin particle agglutination method for detection of *Treponema pallidum* antibody. J Jpn Assoc Infect Dis 68:1271–1277, 1994.

295. Norgard MV. Clinical and diagnostic issues of acquired and congenital syphilis encompassed in the current syphilis epidemic. Curr Opin Infect Dis 6:9, 1993.

296. Young H, Moyes A, McMillan A, Robertson DH. Screening for treponemal infection by a new enzyme immunoassay. Genitourin Med 65:72, 1989.

297. Lefevre JC, Bertrand MA, Bauriaud R. Evaluation of the Captia enzyme immunoassays for detection of immunoglobulins G and M to *Treponema pallidum* in syphilis. J Clin Microbiol 28:1704, 1990.

298. Young H, Moyes A, McMillan A, Patterson J. Enzyme immunoassay for antitreponemal IgG: screening or confirmatory test? J Clin Pathol 45:37, 1992.

299. Ross J, Moyes A, Young H, McMillan A. An analysis of false positive reactions occurring with the Captia Syph-G EIA. Genitourin Med 67:408, 1991.

300. Lefevre JC, Bertrand MA, Bauriaud R, Lareng MB. False positive reactions occurring with the Captia Syphilis-G EIA, in sera from patients with Lyme disease. Genitourin Med 68:142, 1992.

301. Romanowski B, Sutherland R, Fick GH, et al. Serologic response to treatment of infectious syphilis. Ann Intern Med 114:1005, 1991.

302. Julian AJ, Logan LC, Norms LC, et al. Latent syphilis: immunoglobulins reactive in immunofluorescence and other serologic tests. Infect Immunol 3:559, 1971.

303. Moskophidis M, Muller F. Molecular analysis of immunoglobulins M and G immune response to protein antigens of *Treponema pallidum* in human syphilis. Infect Immun 43:127, 1984.

304. Muller F. Specific immunoglobulin M and G antibodies in the rapid diagnosis of human treponemal infections. Diagn Immunol 4:1, 1986.

305. Sánchez PJ, Leos NK, Osorio MA, et al. Umbilical cord blood VDRL or RPR: what's the difference? Pediatr Res 35:303A, 1994.

306. Rawstron SA, Bromberg K. Comparison of maternal and newborn serologic tests for syphilis. Am J Dis Child 145:1383, 1991.

307. Chhabra RS, Brion LP, Castro M, et al. Comparison of maternal sera, cord blood and neonatal sera for detecting presumptive congenital syphilis: relationship with maternal treatment. Pediatrics 91:88, 1993.

308. Taber L, Baughn B. Long term follow-up of infants born of mothers with past or active infection with *T. pallidum.* 31st Interscience Conference on Antimicrobial Reagents and Chemotherapy, September 29–October 2, 1991, Chicago, p 155 (abstract 337).

309. Sánchez PJ, Wendel GD, Zeray F, et al. Serologic follow-up in congenital syphilis: what's the point? Program and Abstracts of the 34th Interscience Conference on Antimicrobial Agents and Chemotherapy, Orlando, Fla, 1994.

310. Reimer CG, Black CM, Phillips DJ, et al. The specificity of fetal IgM: Antibody or anti-antibody? Ann NY Acad Sci 254:77, 1975.

311. Kaufman RE, Olansky DC, Wiesner PJ. The FTA-ABS (IgM) test for neonatal congenital syphilis: a critical review. J Am Vener Dis Assoc 1:79, 1974.

312. Stoll BJ, Lee FK, Larsen S, et al. Clinical and serologic evaluation of neonates for congenital syphilis: a continuing diagnostic dilemma. J Infect Dis 167:1093, 1993.

313. Pedersen NS, Sheller JP, Ratnam AV, et al. Enzyme-linked immunosorbent assays for detection of immunoglobulin M to nontreponemal and treponemal antigens for the diagnosis of congenital syphilis. J Clin Microbiol 27:1835, 1989.

314. Schmitz JL, Gertis KS, Mauney C, et al. Laboratory diagnosis of congenital syphilis by immunoglobulin M (IgM) and IgA immunoblotting. Clin Diag Lab Immunol 1:32, 1994.

315. Meyer MP, Eddy T, Baughn RE. Analysis of western blotting (immunoblotting) technique in diagnosis of congenital syphilis. J Clin Microbiol 32:629, 1994.

316. Lewis LL, Taber LH, Baughn RE. Evaluation of immunoglobulin M Western blot analysis in the diagnosis of congenital syphilis. J Clin Microbiol 28:296, 1990.

317. Sanchez PJ, Wendel GD Jr, Leos NK, et al. IgM immunoblotting utilizing recombinant 47- and 17-kDa antigens for the diagnosis of congenital syphilis. Presented before the 35th Interscience Conference on Antimicrobial Agents and Chemotherapy, San Francisco, Calif.

318. Sánchez PJ, Wendel GD, Norgard MV. IgM antibody to *Treponema pallidum* in cerebrospinal fluid of infants with congenital syphilis. Am J Dis Child 146:1171, 1992.

319. Burstain JM, Grimprel E, Lukehart SA, et al. Sensitive detection of *Treponema pallidum* by using the polymerase chain reaction. J Clin Microbiol 29:62, 1991.

320. Wicher K, Noordhoek GT, Abbruscato F, et al. Detection of *Treponema pallidum* in early syphilis by DNA amplification. J Clin Microbiol 30:497, 1992.

321. Hay PE, Clarke JR, Strugnell RA, et al. Use of the polymerase chain reaction to detect DNA sequences specific to pathogenic treponemes in cerebrospinal fluid. FEMS Microbiol Lett 68:233, 1990.

322. Hay PE, Clarke JR, Taylor-Robinson D, et al. Detection of treponemal DNA in the CSF of patients with syphilis and HIV infection using the polymerase chain reaction. Genitourin Med 66:428, 1990.

323. Noordhoek GT, Wolters EC, DeJonge MEJ, et al. De-

tection by polymerase chain reaction of *Treponema pallidum* in cerebrospinal fluid from neurosyphilis patients before and after antibiotic treatment. J Clin Microbiol 29:1976, 1991.

324. Grimprel E, Sánchez PJ, Wendel GD, et al. Use of the polymerase chain reaction and rabbit infectivity testing to detect *Treponema pallidum* in amniotic fluid, fetal and neonatal sera, and cerebrospinal fluid. J Clin Microbiol 29:1711, 1991.

325. Escobar MR, Dalton HP, Allison MJ. Fluorescent antibody tests for syphilis using cerebrospinal fluid: clinical correlation in 150 cases. Am J Clin Pathol 53:88, 1976.

326. Jaffe HW, Larsen SA, Peters M, et al. Tests for treponemal antibody in CSF. Arch Intern Med 138:22, 1978.

327. LeClerc G, Giroux M, Birry A, et al. Study of fluorescent treponemal antibody test on cerebrospinal fluid using nonspecific anti-immunoglobulin conjugates IgG, IgM and IgA. Br J Vener Dis 54:303, 1978.

328. Muller F, Moskophidis M, Pranse HW. Demonstration of locally synthesized immunoglobulin M antibodies to *Treponema pallidum* in the central nervous system of patients with untreated syphilis. J Neuroimmunol 7:43, 1984.

329. Lee JB, Farshy CE, Hunter EF, et al. Detection of immunoglobulin M in cerebrospinal fluid for syphilis patients by enzyme-linked immunosorbent assay. J Clin Microbiol 47:736, 1986.

330. Esterly NB, Solomon LM. Neonatal dermatology: II. Blistering and scaling dermatoses. J Pediatr 77:1075, 1970.

331. Geppert LJ, Baker HJ, Copple BI, et al. *Pseudomonas* infections in infants and children. J Pediatr 41:555, 1952.

332. Ray CG, Wedgewood RJ. Neonatal listeriosis. Pediatrics 34:378, 1964.

333. Lopez JB, Gross P, Boggs TR. Skin lesions in association with β hemolytic *Streptococcus* group B. Pediatrics 58:859, 1976.

334. Halal F, Delorme L, Brazeau M, et al. Congenital vesicular eruption caused by *H. influenzae* type B. Pediatrics 62:494, 1978.

335. Hageman J, Shulman S, Schreiber M, et al. Congenital tuberculosis: critical reappraisal of clinical findings and diagnostic procedures. Pediatrics 66:980, 1980.

336. Blatt J, Kastner D, Hodes DS. Cutaneous vesicles in congenital cytomegalovirus infection. J Pediatr 92:509, 1978.

337. Dvorak AM, Gavaller B. Congenital systemic candidiasis. N Engl J Med 274:540, 1966.

338. Esterly NB, Spraker MK. Neonatal skin problems. *In* Moschella SL, Hurley HJ (eds). Dermatology. Philadelphia, WB Saunders, 1985, p 1882.

339. Oski FA, Naiman JL. Hematologic Problems in the Newborn. Philadelphia, WB Saunders, 1972.

340. Anand A, Gray ES, Brown T, et al. Human parvovirus infection in pregnancy and hydrops fetalis. N Engl J Med 316:183, 1987.

341. Weiss DI, Cooper LZ, Green RH. Infantile glaucoma. JAMA 195:105, 1966.

342. Coles FB, Hipp SS, Silberstein GS, Chen J. Congenital syphilis surveillance in upstate New York, 1989–1992: implications for prevention and clinical management. J Infect Dis 171:732, 1995.

343. Idsoe O, Guthe T, Willcox RR. Penicillin in the treatment of syphilis: the experience of three decades. Bull WHO 47(Suppl):5–68, 1972.

344. Augenbraun MH, Rolfs R. Treatment of syphilis, 1998: nonpregnant adults. Clin Infect Dis 28(Suppl):S21, 1999.

345. Musher DM. How much penicillin cures early syphilis? Ann Intern Med 109:849, 1988.

346. Alexander JM, Sheffield JS, Sánchez PJ, et al. Efficacy of treatment for syphilis in pregnancy. Obstet Gynecol 93:5, 1999.

347. Conover CS, Reno CA, Miller GB Jr, Schmid GP. Congenital syphilis after treatment of maternal syphilis with a penicillin regimen exceeding CDC guidelines. Infect Dis Obstet Gynecol 6:134–137, 1998.

348. Nathan L, Bawdon RE, Sidawi JE, et al. Penicillin levels following administration of benzathine penicillin G in pregnancy. Obstet Gynecol 82:338, 1993.

349. Rolfs RT, Joesoef JR, Hendershot EF, et al. A randomized trial of enhanced therapy for early syphilis in patients with and without human immunodeficiency virus infection. N Engl J Med 337:307, 1997.

350. Wendel GD Jr, Stark BJ, Jamison RB, et al. Penicillin allergy and desensitization in serious infections during pregnancy. N Engl J Med 312:1229, 1985.

351. Barr W. Placental transmission of cephaloridine. J Obstet Gynaecol Br Commonw 74:739, 1967.

352. Hook EW III, Roddy RE, Handsfield HH. Ceftriaxone therapy for incubating and early syphilis. J Infect Dis 158:881, 1988.

353. Moorthy TT, Lee CT, Lim KB, et al. Ceftriaxone for treatment of primary syphilis in men: a preliminary study. Sex Transm Dis 14:116, 1987.

354. Schöfer H, Vogt HJ, Milbradt R. Ceftriaxone for the treatment of primary and secondary syphilis. Chemotherapy 35:140, 1989.

355. Vignale R, Burno J, Gibert P. Ceftriaxone in the treatment of primary and secondary syphilis: a comparative study with benzathine penicillin. *In* Hall TC (ed). Prediction of Response to Cancer Therapy. Proceedings of the 15th International Chemotherapy Congress, Istanbul, Turkey, July 19–24, 1987. New York, Alan R Liss, 1988, p 75.

356. Hook EW III, Baker-Zander SA, Moskovitz BL, et al. Ceftriaxone therapy for asymptomatic neurosyphilis: case report and Western blot analysis of serum and cerebrospinal fluid IgG response to therapy. Sex Transm Dis 13:185, 1986.

357. Dowell ME, Ross PG, Musher DM, et al. Response of latent syphilis or neurosyphilis to ceftriaxone therapy in persons infected with human immunodeficiency virus. Am J Med 93:481, 1992.

358. Marra C, Slatter V, Tartaglione T, et al. Comparison of ceftriaxone and aqueous crystalline penicillin G for central nervous system syphilis in an experimental model. 30th Interscience Conference on Antimicrobial Agents and Chemotherapy, Atlanta, Georgia, October 21–24, 1990, p 101 (abstract 87).

359. Philipson A, Sabath LD, Charles D. Transplacental passage of erythromycin and clindamycin. N Engl J Med 288:1219, 1973.

360. South MA, Short DH, Knox JM. Failures of erythromycin estolate therapy in in utero syphilis. JAMA 199:70, 1964.

361. Montgomery CH, Knox JM. Antibiotics other than penicillin in the treatment of syphilis. N Engl J Med 261:277, 1959.

362. Schultz JC, Adamson JS Jr, Workman WW, et al. Fatal liver disease after intravenous administration of tetracycline in high doses. N Engl J Med 269:999, 1963.

363. Tetracycline in pregnancy. Editorial. BMJ 1:743, 1965.

364. Demers P, Fraser RB, Goldbloom J, et al. Effects of tetracycline on skeletal growth dentition: a report to the

Nutrition Committee of the Canadian Pediatric Society. Can Med Assoc J 99:849, 1968.

365. Condue JM, Munroe JD, Anderson DO. The incidence of staining of permanent teeth by the tetracyclines. Can Med Assoc J 103:351, 1970.

366. Ingall D, Sherman J. Chloramphenicol. *In* Kagan BM (ed). Antimicrobial Therapy. Philadelphia, WB Saunders, 1970, p 61.

367. Verdon MS, Handsfield HH, Johnson RB. Pilot study of azithromycin for the treatment of primary and secondary syphilis. Clin Infect Dis 19:486, 1994.

368. Mashkilleyson AL, Gomberg MA, Mashkilleyson N. Treatment of syphilis with azithromycin. Int J STD AIDS 7:13, 1996.

369. Notice to Readers: Shortage of Intravenous Penicillin G—United States. MMWR Morb Mortal Wkly Rep 48:974, 1999.

370. Alternatives to intravenous penicillin G for specific infections. http://www.cdc.gov/nchstp/dstd/penicilllinG.htm

371. Sánchez PJ. Syphilis. *In* Burg FD, Ingelfinger JR, Wald ER (eds). Gellis and Kagan's Current Pediatric Therapy 14. Philadelphia, WB Saunders, 1993, p 590.

372. American Academy of Pediatrics. Syphilis. *In* Report of the Committee on Infectious Diseases (Red Book), 24th ed. Elk Grove Village, Ill, American Academy of Pediatrics, 1997, p 504.

373. Beeram MR, Chopde N, Dawood Y, et al. Lumbar puncture in the evaluation of possible asymptomatic congenital syphilis in neonates. J Pediatr 128:125, 1996.

374. Moyer VA, Schneider V, Yetman R, et al. Contribution of long-bone radiographs to the management of congenital syphilis in the newborn infant. Arch Pediatr Adolesc Med 152:353, 1998.

375. Centers for Disease Control. 1993 Sexually transmitted diseases treatment guidelines. MMWR Morb Mortal Wkly Rep 42(No. RR-14):40, 1993.

376. Azimi PH, Janner D, Berne P, et al. Concentrations of procaine and aqueous penicillin in the cerebrospinal fluid of infants treated for congenital syphilis. J Pediatr 124:649, 1994.

377. Bateman DA, Phibbs CS, Joyce T, Heagarty MC. The hospital cost of congenital syphilis. J Pediatr 130:752, 1997.

378. Paryani SG, Vaughn AJ, Crosby M, Lawrence S. Treatment of asymptomatic congenital syphilis: Benzathine versus procaine penicillin G therapy. J Pediatr 125:471, 1994.

379. Radcliffe M, Meyer M, Roditi D, et al. Single-dose benzathine penicillin in infant's at risk of congenital syphilis: results of a randomized study. S Afr Med J 87:62, 1997.

380. Beck-Sague C, Alexander ER. Failure of benzathine penicillin G treatment in early congenital syphilis. Pediatr Infect Dis J 6:1061, 1987.

381. Woolf A, Wilfert C, Kelsey D, et al. Childhood syphilis in North Carolina. NC Med J 41:443, 1980.

382. McCracken GH, Kaplan JM. Penicillin treatment for congenital syphilis: a critical reappraisal. JAMA 228:855, 1974.

383. Speer ME, Taber LH, Clark DB, et al. Cerebrospinal fluid levels of benzathine penicillin G in the neonate. J Pediatr 91:966, 1977.

384. Norris SJ, Edmondson DG. In vitro culture system to determine MICs and MBCs of antimicrobial agents against *Treponema pallidum* subsp. *pallidum* (Nichols strain). Antimicrob Agents Chemotherapy 32:68, 1988.

385. Gelfano JA, Elin RJ, Berry FW Jr, et al. Endotoxemia associated with the Jarisch-Herxheimer reaction. N Engl J Med 295:211, 1976.

386. Young EJ, Weingarten NM, Baughn RE, et al. Studies on the pathogenesis of the Jarisch-Herxheimer reaction: development of animal model and evidence against a role for classical endotoxin. J Infect Dis 146:606, 1982.

387. Radolf JD, Norgard MV, Brandt ME, et al. Lipoproteins of *Borrelia burgdorferi* and *Treponema pallidum* activate cachectin/tumor necrosis factor synthesis: analysis using a CAT reporter construct. J Immunol 147:1968, 1991.

388. Klein VR, Cox SM, Mitchell MD, Wendel GD Jr. The Jarisch-Herxheimer reaction complicating syphilotherapy in pregnancy. Obstet Gynecol 75:375–380, 1990.

389. Myles TD, Elan G, Parik-Hwang E, Nguyen T. The Jarisch-Herxheimer reaction and fetal monitoring changes in pregnant women treated for syphilis. Obstet Gynecol 92:859, 1998.

390. Tan KL. The re-emergence of early congenital syphilis. Acta Paediatr Scand 62:661, 1973.

391. Goldman JN, Girard KF. Intraocular treponemes in treated congenital syphilis. Arch Ophthalmol 78:47, 1967.

392. Dunlop EMC, King AJ, Wickinson AE. Study of late ocular syphilis: demonstration of treponemes in aqueous humour and cerebrospinal fluid. 3. General and serological findings. Trans Ophthalmol Soc UK 88:275, 1969.

393. Dunlop EMC. Persistence of treponemes after treatment. BMJ 2:577, 1972.

394. Ryan SJ, Hardy PH, Hardy JM, et al. Persistence of virulent *Treponema pallidum* despite penicillin therapy in congenital syphilis. Am J Ophthalmol 73:259, 1972.

395. Report of the World Health Organization Expert Committee on Venereal Infections and Treponematoses. WHO Tech Rep Ser 674:27, 1982.

396. Hardy JB, Hardy PH, Oppenheimer EH. Failure of penicillin in a newborn with congenital syphilis. JAMA 212:1345, 1970.

397. Bayne LL, Schmidley JW, Goodwin DS. Acute syphilitic meningitis: its occurrence after clinical and serologic cure of secondary syphilis with penicillin G. Arch Neurol 43:137, 1986.

398. Jorgensen J, Tikjob G, Weisman K. Neurosyphilis after treatment of latent syphilis with benzathine penicillin. Genitourin Med 62:129, 1986.

399. Markovitz DM, Beutner KR, Maggio RR, et al. Failure of recommended treatment for secondary syphilis. JAMA 256:1767, 1986.

400. Hurtig AK, Nicoll A, Carne C, et al. Syphilis in pregnant women and their children in the United Kingdom: results from national clinician reporting surveys, 1994–97. BMJ 317:1617, 1998.

401. Southwick KL, Guidry HM, Weldon MM, et al. An epidemic of congenital syphilis in Jefferson County, Texas, 1994–1995: inadequate prenatal syphilis testing after an outbreak in adults. Am J Public Health 89:557, 1999.

402. Williams LA, Klausner JD, Whittington AB, et al. Elimination and reintroduction of primary and secondary syphilis. Am J Public Health 89:1093, 1999.

403. Centers for Disease Control. Outbreak of primary and secondary syphilis—Guilford County, North Carolina, 1996–1997. MMWR Morb Mortal Wkly Rep 47:1070, 1998.

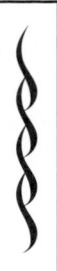

Chickenpox, Measles, and Mumps

ANNE A. GERSHON, M.D.

The viruses that cause varicella, zoster, measles, and mumps may adversely affect a fetus or newborn when a maternal infection with one of these agents occurs during pregnancy or at term. In the United States, because most women of childbearing years are immune to measles and mumps and because there is little opportunity for exposure to these infections since the population is currently highly immunized, these diseases now pose fewer practical problems during pregnancy than they did during the first half of the twentieth century. Now that there is a licensed varicella vaccine, moreover, varicella can be expected to decrease in incidence in women of childbearing age. The varicella-zoster virus (VZV), however, still inflicts a significant amount of fetal damage as the cause of the congenital varicella syndrome in which infants manifest cicatricial skin scars, eye and brain damage, and hypoplastic limbs. Improved methods for control of this virus, including improved diagnostic methods, antiviral therapy with acyclovir (ACV), passive immunization with varicella-zoster immune globulin (VZIG), and use of live attenuated varicella vaccine, have decreased both prenatal and postnatal morbidity from this virus. In addition, understanding of this viral infection at the molecular level, including clarification of the cause of zoster by molecular studies of viral DNA, RNA, and proteins in latency, and study of specific viral glycoproteins (gps) and their importance in the immune response have advanced our knowledge and can be expected to lead to improved therapeutic measures.

CHICKENPOX AND ZOSTER

Chickenpox (varicella) is an acute, contagious disease that most commonly occurs in childhood. It is characterized by a generalized exanthem consisting of vesicles that develop in successive crops and that rapidly evolve to pustules, crusts, and scabs. Zoster (herpes zoster, shingles) occurs in persons who have previously had chickenpox. It is typified by a painful vesicular eruption usually restricted to one or more segmental dermatomes. An abundance of virologic, epidemiologic, and immunologic evidence has now been amassed, indicating that these two illnesses are caused by the same etiologic agent,[1] which therefore was designated VZV. Chickenpox is a manifestation of primary infection with VZV. After the acute infection subsides, VZV, like other herpesviruses, may persist in a latent form. For VZV, the site of latent infection is in the dorsal root ganglia, where certain early viral genes and proteins are expressed.[2–4] VZV may subsequently be reactivated with expression of all of its genes as immunity wanes. The reactivated infection assumes the segmental distribution of the nerve cells in which latent virus resided, giving rise to zoster. A description of the historical recognition of disease caused by VZV follows.

Varicella is a modernized Latin word used since at least 1764 and intended to connote a diminutive of the more serious variola (smallpox).[5] The etymology of chicken in chickenpox is less clear. It, too, may be a diminutive derived from the French *pois chiche*, or chick pea, a dwarf species of pea *(Cicer arietinum)*.[5] Other workers doubt this Latin origin and conjecture that the word originated from the farmyard fowl, in which case it has a Teutonic ancestry in the Old English *cicen* and the Middle High German *kuchen*.[6] Herpes has been used to designate a malady since 1398 ("this euyll callyd Herpes")[7] but derives from the Greek word meaning to creep; *zoster* is the Greek and Latin word meaning girdle or belt. Shingles, from the Latin *cingulus*, or girdle, was also used in the fourteenth century as *schingles* to describe "icchynge and scabs wett and drye."[7]

The Organism

CLASSIFICATION AND MORPHOLOGY

The VZV, or *Herpesvirus varicellae*, is a member of the herpesvirus family. In addition to a burgeoning number of animal herpesviruses, this group includes eight additional closely related viruses that infect humans: herpes simplex viruses (HSV) types 1 and 2 *(Herpesvirus hominis)*, cytomegalovirus (CMV), Epstein-Barr virus (EBV), and human herpesviruses 6, 7, and 8. Only one antigenic type of VZV has been identified, but restriction endonuclease studies have revealed some minor differences in VZV.[8] Common properties of the family include a DNA genome and enveloped virions exhibiting icosahedral symmetry with a diameter of 180 to 200 nm.[1] Nucleocapsids, which are assembled in the nucleus, have a diameter of about 100 nm and consist of a DNA core surrounded by 162 identical subunits, or capsomeres. Nucleocapsids acquire a temporary envelope at the nuclear membrane; they are further transported by means of the endoplasmic reticulum to the Golgi, where they receive a final envelope. In cell cultures, virions are packaged in vesicles identified as endosomes, which are acidic.[9, 10] Virus particles are released from these structures at the cell surface by exocytosis. Extracellular virions are extremely pleomorphic compared with those of HSV. This pleomorphism, presumably reflecting injury to the envelope possibly caused by exposure to acid or enzymes in endosomes, is believed to account for the lability and lack of cell-free virus that characterizes VZV in tissue culture and also distinguishes it from HSV.[9–11] In vivo, VZV is released from skin cells in highly infectious form, leading to a high degree of communicability.

PROPAGATION

VZV grows readily in diploid human fibroblasts such as WI 38 cells, the most commonly used cell type for virus isolation. VZV also can be propagated in certain epithelial cells, such as human embryonic kidney, primary human amnion cells, primary human thyroid cells and Vero (African green monkey kidney) cells. Like CMV, the cytopathic effect of VZV is focal in cell culture owing to its cell-associated character, and cytopathic effects develop more slowly (3 to 7 days) than with HSV. An animal model for varicella (the guinea pig)[12] and for zoster (the rat)[13] has been described.

SEROLOGIC TESTS AND ANTIGENIC PROPERTIES OF VARICELLA-ZOSTER VIRUS

A number of serologic tests are available to measure antibodies to VZV. These include indirect immunofluorescence, often termed *fluorescent antibody to membrane antigen* (FAMA),[14, 15] latex agglutination (LA),[16] enzyme-linked immunosorbent assay (ELISA),[17–20] radioimmunoassay,[21] immune adherence hemagglutination,[22] neutralization,[17, 23] and complement-enhanced neutralization.[24] All of these methods are more sensitive than the complement fixation (CF)[25] assay. Based on data gathered from these assays, it is clear that antibody to VZV develops within a few days after onset of varicella, persists for many years, and is often present before onset of zoster.

Serologic cross-reactions between HSV and VZV have been described.[26, 27] HSV and VZV share common antigens, and similar polypeptides and gps have been identified for both viruses, although cross-protection has not been observed.[28–30] In addition, rare simultaneous infections with one or more human herpesviruses have been reported.[31, 32] Thus, rises in hetcrologous antibody titers in apparent HSV or VZV infections may be due to cross-reactions of the viruses but also may indicate simultaneous infection by both viruses.

VZV produces at least six major gp antigens—called E, B, H, I, C, and L—all of which are present on the envelope of the virus and on the surface of infected cells. The gps stimulate production of neutralizing and other types of antibodies as well as cellular immunity.[33, 34] Antibodies elaborated in both varicella and zoster are of the IgG, IgA, and IgM classes.[35, 36]

Epidemiology and Transmission

Chickenpox ranks as one of the most communicable of human diseases. No extrahuman reservoir of VZV is known. Because the supply of susceptible persons, especially in the era before the urbanization of society, would be rapidly exhausted by so contagious a disease, virus latency may have adaptive evolutionary significance in perpetuating this disease. In isolated communities, cases of zoster would be responsible for the reintroduction of VZV and its transmission to new generations of susceptible individuals.[1, 37]

COMMUNICABILITY BY DROPLETS AND CONTACT

The transmission of chickenpox is not completely understood, and the vehicle by which it occurs is poorly documented. Historically, transfer of VZV has been believed to occur by way of respiratory droplets, and epidemiologic evidence suggests that transmission can occur before onset of rash.[38–40] It is extremely rare, however, to isolate VZV from the pharynx of infected patients. A study using polymerase chain reaction (PCR) has demonstrated that VZV DNA is present in the nasopharynx of a high percentage of children during the early stages of clinical varicella,[41] but PCR does not necessarily indicate the presence of infectious virus. In contrast, the vesicular lesions in both varicella and zoster are full of infectious VZV that can readily be cultured. In a study of leukemic recipients of live attenuated varicella vaccine, moreover, only those with skin lesions as a side effect of varicella vaccination spread vaccine-type virus to varicella-susceptible close contacts.[42] Thus, it appears that a major source of infectious VZV is the skin, but it seems likely that transmission from both the respiratory tract and skin occurs.

Airborne spread of varicella has been documented,[43, 44] but indirect transfer by fomites has not. VZV DNA has been detected in air samples for many hours in hospitals,[45] but again the relationship to infectivity of the virus is unclear. Varicella is most contagious at the time of onset of rash and for 1 to 2 days afterward,[46] but the period of infectivity probably encompasses 1 to 2 days before until 5 days after the onset of rash.

INCUBATION PERIOD

The usual incubation period for chickenpox is 13 to 17 days, with a mean of 15 days. The extremes are 10 and 21 days, unless passive immunization has been given, in which the incubation period may be prolonged.[40, 47]

RELATIONSHIP BETWEEN VARICELLA AND ZOSTER

It is amply documented that exposure of susceptible persons to zoster may result in chickenpox. Vesicular fluid from patients with zoster produced chickenpox when inoculated into susceptible children.[48, 49] Other studies have confirmed that a similar relationship exists under conditions of natural exposure.[50] Claims to the contrary notwithstanding,[51, 52] it has not been documented that zoster is acquired from other patients with zoster or chickenpox. Instances that have been reported do not exclude the chance sporadic occurrence of zoster in persons who happen to have been exposed to chickenpox or zoster. Furthermore, it is difficult to reconcile this postulated mode of transmission with current concepts of the pathogenesis of zoster, particularly the strict segmental distribution of lesions and the demonstrated presence of VZV DNA, RNA, and certain proteins in ganglia during latency.[2, 53] Studies have also determined that the VZV DNA from zoster isolates is similar to that which caused the primary infection, proving that zoster is due to reactivation of latent VZV.[54-56]

TRANSPLACENTAL TRANSMISSION

In pregnancy, VZV may be transmitted across the placenta, resulting in congenital or neonatal chickenpox.[57] The consequences of transplacental infection are discussed in a later section.

INCIDENCE AND DISTRIBUTION OF CHICKENPOX

Chickenpox is worldwide in distribution and, until vaccination becomes universally used, can be expected to remain endemic in the United States. Outbreaks occur each year without major fluctuations between years.[58] Although the disease is seen in all months, more cases occur in the winter and early spring. This seasonal variation is attributed primarily to the gathering of children in school but may also be related to changes in environmental temperature. Chickenpox is more contagious than mumps but less so than measles.[47, 59] After exposure within households, 61% of susceptible persons of all age groups (those without a history of previous disease) developed chickenpox, compared with 76% for measles and 31% for mumps.[47] Compared with measles, chickenpox is about 80% as infectious in the household but only 35 to 65% as infectious in society. The reason is believed to be that chickenpox requires relatively intimate contact for transmission, such as that occurring in the household, whereas in society there are more casual contacts. Measles, on the other hand, may infect efficiently even through casual contacts.[59]

About 4 million cases of chickenpox are estimated to occur yearly in the United States. The disease affects both sexes equally and is most commonly seen in children of early school age. Increasing urbanization has been associated with acquisition of the disease at younger ages. In Massachusetts between 1952 and 1961, 29% of children reported with chickenpox were younger than 4 years old, 62% were age 5 to 9, 7% were age 10 to 14, and less than 3% were older than age 15.[60] More recent data continue to indicate that varicella is primarily a disease of young children.[61] Seventy to 80% of young adults report a history of varicella.[60, 62] This compares with histories in the same age group in the prevaccine era of 92% for measles, 45% for mumps, and 31% for rubella. Subclinical varicella is believed to be uncommon. Data from family studies indicate that only 8% of adults without a history of varicella develop clinical disease when exposed to their own infected children.[63] The relative importance of faulty memory or subclinical infection in this low secondary attack rate is uncertain.

With the use of sensitive assays for the measurement of antibodies to VZV, it appears that less than 25% of adults with no history of chickenpox are actually susceptible.[64] Based on a population of adults in which 90% are immune, this suggests a subclinical attack rate of varicella of roughly 7%.

INCIDENCE OF CHICKENPOX, MUMPS, AND MEASLES IN PREGNANCY

Few studies have been addressed to determine the incidence of chickenpox, mumps, and measles during pregnancy. In these studies, two questions are posed: (1) Of all pregnancies, how many are complicated by measles, mumps, or chickenpox? (2) Among all reported cases of those diseases, how many occur in pregnant women? In a prospective study of clinically recognized infections that occurred during 30,059 pregnancies between 1958 and 1964, the Collaborative Perinatal Research Study identified approximately 1600 women with presumed viral infections (excluding the common cold).[65] Serologic testing was used to confirm the diagnoses of measles, varicella, and mumps. Taking into account the many possible inaccuracies in such a study, the minimum frequency per 10,000 pregnancies of confirmed cases was 0.6 case for measles, 5 cases for varicella, and 10 cases for mumps.

In another study of maternal virus diseases in New York City between 1957 and 1964, Siegel and Fuerst followed pregnant women in whom a clinical diagnosis of measles, mumps, chickenpox, or other viral infection had been made.[66] Of the 826 virus-infected pregnant women who were identified, 417 were infected with rubella (50.5%), 150 with chickenpox (18.1%), 128 with mumps (15.5%), and 66 with measles (8.0%). Approximately 190,000 pregnancies per year were reported in this population. The data in these studies are undoubtedly inaccurate because of incorrect clinical diagnoses, under-reporting of mild or subclinical infections, and other factors. The calculated attack rates of varicella, mumps, and measles are shown in Table 13-1. It should be remembered that these figures reflect the prevaccine era. It seems likely that measles occurred less frequently during pregnancy than either mumps or chickenpox. The probable explanation for this is that in unvaccinated populations the greater communicability of measles results in fewer females reaching childbearing age without already having been infected. In highly immunized populations such as exist today in the United States, an even lower incidence of infection during pregnancy would be predicted for measles and mumps. It may be that the incidence of varicella in pregnant women in the United States is increasing, owing to an influx of varicella-susceptible immigrants from countries with tropical climates. One calculation projected an incidence of 7 cases of varicella per 10,000 pregnancies.[67] Even these crude data, however, indicate that varicella, mumps, and measles are unusual during pregnancy.

The relative rarity of the association of each of these diseases with pregnancy as indicated by these studies highlights the difficulties involved in obtaining data on their effect on the outcome of pregnancy when compared with a disease with a higher incidence during pregnancy such as was once true for rubella. Clearly, the

TABLE 13–1
Attack Rates of Various Viral Infections During Pregnancy[a]

STUDY	MEASLES	VARICELLA-ZOSTER	MUMPS
Cases per 10,000 Pregnancies			
Collaborative[65]	0.6	5	10
New York[66]	0.4	0.8	1
Connecticut[67]	—	7	—
Predicted Cases per Year in the United States During Pregnancy			
	120–180	240–2450	300–3000

[a]Reflects mainly prevaccine era for measles and mumps, based on 3.5 million U.S. births yearly.

answers can only come from uniform national reporting policies involving many collaborating agencies.

INCIDENCE AND DISTRIBUTION OF ZOSTER

In contrast to chickenpox, zoster is primarily a disease of adults, especially older adults or immunosuppressed patients. Hope-Simpson, describing patients of all ages in a general practice observed during a 16-year period, found an incidence of 3.4 cases per thousand per year.[37] Zoster occurs with approximately the same frequency each month, a fact compatible with the hypothesis that it results from reactivation of latent infection rather than exogenous reinfection after exposure to VZV. In the household or hospital, persons exposed to zoster are not at increased risk of developing zoster but are likely to develop chickenpox in the absence of a previous history of varicella. Zoster "epidemics" have been claimed under special circumstances, such as in a hospitalized leukemic population,[51] but their documentation is not convincing.

Adults and children older than 2 years of age who have zoster usually give a history of a previous attack of varicella, whereas in younger infants a history of intrauterine exposure to VZV can often be elicited.[37] The latency period between primary infection and zoster is shorter if varicella occurs in prenatal rather than in postnatal life.[68] Chickenpox in the first year of life also increases the risk of childhood zoster, by a relative risk between roughly 3 and 21.[69, 70] Possibly this phenomenon is due to immaturity of the immune response during chickenpox in young infants, permitting early viral reactivation.[71]

After infancy, the incidence of zoster rises progressively with age. The attack rate in octogenarians was 14 times that of children in Hope-Simpson's series.[37] Second attacks of zoster are unusual; 8 were observed among 192 cases in the previously cited series.[37] Four of those attacks involved the same dermatome as the first attack, suggesting a tendency for reactivation of VZV from the same ganglion cells in which they were dormant. Some of these cases, however, may have been due to reactivation of HSV; in one study, HSV was isolated from 13% of a series of 47 immunocompetent patients with clinically diagnosed zoster.[72] Zoster in adults and children occurs with increased frequency in patients with malignant hematopoietic neoplasms, especially Hodgkin's disease, after organ transplantation, and with infection with human immunodeficiency virus (HIV).[73–75]

Spinal trauma, irradiation, and corticosteroid therapy may also be precipitating factors. The distribution of lesions in chickenpox, which primarily affects the trunk, head, and neck, is reflected in a proportionately greater representation of these regions in the segmental lesions of zoster.[37]

INCIDENCE OF ZOSTER IN PREGNANCY

Several reports describe the occurrence of zoster during pregnancy, but adequate statistics from which to calculate attack rates during pregnancy are not available. Brazin and associates have projected an incidence of 6000 cases annually in pregnant women,[76] which would mean that gestational zoster is more common than gestational chickenpox. Assuming that there are 3.5 million pregnant women yearly in the United States, this calculates to a rate of 20 cases per 10,000 pregnant women per year. Prospective studies of pregnant women in Sweden, however, have suggested that zoster is less common in pregnancy than varicella.[77] The severity or natural history of zoster does not appear to be worse in pregnant women than in the population at large. Implications of gestational zoster for the fetus are discussed in a subsequent section.

NOSOCOMIAL CHICKENPOX IN THE NURSERY

The precise risk of horizontal transmission in maternity wards or the newborn nursery after the virus has been introduced is unclear, but apparently it is low. This is in part because about 70% of persons give a history of chickenpox by age 20 and still others are immune in the absence of a positive history, so that most mothers and hospital personnel are not at risk. It seems generally agreed that only 5 to 10% of women born in the United States are susceptible to varicella and that more than 75% of those with no history of chickenpox are immune.[64, 78–81] The percentage of susceptible persons among women raised in tropical climates is somewhat higher, probably because viral spread is impeded by high temperatures and/or lack of urbanization.[78, 82–85] Because IgG antibodies to VZV cross the placenta,[78, 86] the newborns of immune mothers should likewise be at least partially protected. With the use of the sensitive FAMA assay to measure antibodies to VZV, it was found in a study of 67 infants that even by 5 months of age 50% still had detectable VZV antibodies.[78] Even in premature and low-birth-weight infants, antibodies to VZV are likely to be detectable.[87-89] Nevertheless, perinatal chickenpox has been reported in infants born to women with positive histories of chickenpox.[90-94] In Newman's study, varicella developed in a mother and her baby after exposure to a student midwife with chickenpox. The mother had experienced varicella as a child and had a few old remaining skin scars; apparently she had developed a second attack as an adult.[93] In addition, Readett and McGibbon reported two cases of extrauterine infection in neonates whose mothers had histories of chickenpox.[94] After delivery at home, each of these infants was exposed within 24 hours of birth to a sibling with chickenpox and subsequently developed skin lesions at ages 12 and 14 days, respectively. Their mothers did not develop chickenpox in the perinatal period and were found to have serum neutralizing antibodies to VZV. In the literature before 1975, VZV antibody titers were not often reported because sensitive tests for measuring these antibodies were not readily available. Since that time, however, infection of a few seropositive infants after postnatal exposure to VZV has been documented.[90, 91] These infants have had mothers with a history of varicella, and the VZV antibody in the infants' blood was transplacentally acquired. In one instance, mild varicella developed in a 2-week-old, 1040-g infant who was seropositive at exposure and was also passively immunized with VZIG 72 hours after the exposure.[91] In another study, five infants younger than 2 months old, all of whom were seropositive at exposure, developed varicella in a children's custodial institution.[90] Varicella developing in the presence of maternal antibodies appears to be modified, and in some instances protection may also be conferred by maternal antibodies. Absolute protection of the neonate against chickenpox, however, is clearly not guaranteed by apparent immunity in the mother.

Notwithstanding this lack of protection, horizontal transmission of chickenpox in maternity wards and newborn nurseries seems to be an uncommon event. Newman reported two cases of varicella that occurred in mothers in the same prenatal ward 18 to 19 days after exposure to the index-infected infant and its mother.[93] One mother developed chickenpox 7 days ante partum, and the other developed it 3 days post partum. Each mother was immediately isolated from the ward but not from her own infant; neither of the infants developed chickenpox. In all, 139 mothers, excluding the index case, were exposed, and 8 developed infection. Three of the 42 staff members also became infected. Remarkably, the index infant was the only neonate infected; all other infants, including those born to the 8 infected mothers, remained free of disease. Gershon and co-workers described an outbreak in which a woman developed varicella post partum and exposed 10 mothers, their infants, 1 antepartum woman, and approximately 25 staff members during a brief period while she was waiting in the hospital corridor.[78] Her infant developed varicella 10 days afterward. About 2 weeks later, three cases of varicella developed in the exposed persons: a hospital employee and a postpartum woman and her infant. Gustafson and colleagues described another mini-outbreak that

took place during a 2-month period in a neonatal intensive care unit in which two infants whose mothers gave a history of previous varicella developed chickenpox after exposure to two hospital employees who had been infected nosocomially.[91] A total of 29 infants had been exposed.

Other reports largely confirm the low rate of transmissibility of chickenpox in neonates. Freud described an infant who had transplacentally acquired disease and developed lesions on the second day of life. None of the other 17 neonates in the nursery became infected, but the index infant had been isolated immediately, so exposure had been very brief.[95] When transferred to another ward, this same infant transmitted the disease to two older children, aged 4 and 7 years. Odessky reported three instances of congenital varicella: two infants were immediately isolated, but the third was not recognized as having chickenpox and exposed other neonates for 4 days.[96] The number at risk is not stated, but no instances of transmission were observed. In the report of Harris, a total of 35 infants were exposed to two infants with congenital chickenpox for periods of 18 and 10 hours before isolation.[97] None subsequently became infected, possibly because all the mothers had positive histories of chickenpox. In an additional case described by Matseoane and Abler, an infant developed transplacentally acquired chickenpox at the age of 9 days and exposed 13 other neonates in the nursery for periods of 2 to 10 hours before isolation.[98] The history of their mothers for varicella was positive in six, negative in three, and unknown in four. None of the exposed mothers or infants developed chickenpox. Lack of transmission despite hospital exposure to an adult with varicella in neonatal intensive care nurseries was also reported by Wang and associates (32 infants),[89] Lipton and Brunell (22 infants),[99] Patou and co-workers (15 infants),[100] Mendez and associates (16 infants),[87] and Gold and co-workers (29 infants).[101]

One experience in a neonatal intensive care unit in Mississippi is of note.[102] After the development of hemorrhagic varicella in a 25-week gestation infant whose mother had varicella 2 weeks previously, 14 infants in the unit were exposed over a period of several days. None of the infants in isolettes became ill, but 4 who were in open warming units at exposure developed varicella 10 days later. All had received VZIG, and in each instance the mother gave a past history of varicella. The illnesses were mild with only a few papular skin lesions, but 3 of the 4 infants were positive for VZV on immunofluorescence testing of skin scrapings. Each child with varicella was treated with intravenous ACV. The incidence of disease was higher in infants younger than 29 weeks' gestation than in older infants.

Of historical interest is an extensive epidemic lasting 5 months described by Apert in 1895.[103] Two infants in a newborn nursery developed chickenpox on January 7 and 8. They were immediately transferred with their mothers to another ward where they were isolated, but a third infant (second generation of chickenpox) developed disease on January 24 and was likewise isolated with its mother. A fourth infant (third generation) developed varicella on February 7 but was not isolated until

February 13 because the mother deliberately obscured the fact that the infant had lesions. Subsequently, a fifth infant (fourth generation) developed chickenpox on February 21. Because the number of infants exposed and the maternal histories of varicella are not stated, the attack rates are unclear. Although this was the last case of chickenpox in the newborn nursery, one of the infected neonates introduced the virus to another ward of 40 to 45 debilitated infants. Before the epidemic was over in May, nine generations of chickenpox separated with mathematical precision by 14 days had occurred. In all, 19 infants, 12 younger than 6 six months old, were infected, as well as two mothers.

These experiences with nosocomial chickenpox in the newborn nursery are summarized in Table 13–2. In the twentieth century, in those reports in which the number of neonates exposed is explicitly stated, a total of 218 exposures resulted in only seven instances of transmission to infants. Most of the mothers had histories of varicella, although in many the history was unknown. Several factors undoubtedly contribute to the low rate

of transmission of disease to neonates: (1) passive immunity in some; (2) relatively brief exposure compared with that in the household setting, where 80 to 90% of susceptibles become clinically infected[37, 63]; and (3) relative lack of intimacy of contact in the nursery, particularly for infants in isolettes.

Pathogenesis of Varicella and Zoster

In the usual case of chickenpox, the portal of entry and initial site of virus replication is probably the oropharynx, but attempts to demonstrate this directly have been surprisingly unrewarding. In five patients whose blood, throat secretions, and skin were cultured repeatedly during the prodromal period as well as after the appearance of cutaneous lesions, VZV was recovered from a throat swab in only one instance and from the blood in none. In contrast, vesicle fluid from these patients yielded VZV in all instances.[104] Attempts to isolate the virus from the blood of six additional patients were positive in only one instance, this being on the second day of

TABLE 13–2
Nosocomial Chickenpox Infections in the Nursery

REFERENCE NO. (YEAR)	CASE NO.	PERIOD OTHERS EXPOSED AFTER ONSET OF RASH	PRIOR HISTORY OF VARICELLA IN MOTHERS OF INFANTS EXPOSED			NO. OF PERSONS EXPOSED	NO. SUBSEQUENTLY INFECTED
			Yes	No	Unknown		
103 (1895)	1	Variable[a]		No data		<40 young infants	19
96 (1954)	2	4 days		No data		Not stated	0
	3	0 (immed. isolation)		No data		Not stated	0
	4	0 (immed. isolation)		No data		Not stated	0
95 (1958)	5	0 (immed. isolation in nursery)	0	0	17	17 neonates	0
		3 days (other ward)		No data		Not stated	2[b]
97 (1963)	6	18 hours					
	7	10 hours	35	0	0	35 neonates	0
98 (1965)	8	2, 3, 8, 10 hr in susceptible neonates	6	3	4	13 neonates 13 mothers	0
93 (1965)	9	Variable	1	7	132?	139 mothers ?139 neonates	8 0[c]
78 (1976)	10	Brief	0	2	9	11 mothers 10 infants 25 staff	2 1 1
89 (1983)	11	Brief		No data		32 infants	0
91 (1984)	12	Variable	8	0	21	29 infants	2[d]
99 (1989)	13	Brief, intimate	22			22 infants	0
100 (1990)	14	Brief[d, e]	13	1	1	15 infants	0
87 (1992)	15	Brief[d, e]		No data		16 infants	0
101 (1993)	16	1 hr. on each of 3 days		No data		29 infants	0
102 (1994)	17	Intimate	10		4	14 infants	4
Total since 1900						218 infants	7 infants

[a]See text.

[b]Infected infant transferred to another ward, where two older children (ages 4 and 7) later developed chickenpox.

[c]No cases of chickenpox in neonates, despite appearance of chickenpox in eight mothers from 34 days ante partum to 14 days post partum.

[d]In neonatal intensive care unit.

[e]Exposure 1–2 days before rash in index case.

rash in an immunosuppressed host. Other, more extensive searches for VZV in throat secretions of patients with varicella, even during the incubation period, proved essentially negative.[105, 106] However, in one report VZV was isolated from nasal swabs in 4 of 11 children on days 2 through 4 after onset of the rash. VZV could not be isolated during the incubation period or even during the first day of the rash. It was not clear whether the virus was actually multiplying in the nasal mucosa.[107]

More recently, it has been possible to isolate VZV from blood obtained from patients with varicella. Ozaki and colleagues cultured blood from seven immunocompetent children; VZV was isolated either a few days before onset of rash or within 1 day after onset.[108] Asano and co-workers similarly isolated VZV from the blood of 7 of 12 otherwise healthy patients with early varicella.[109] Those from whom virus could not be isolated had been studied after they had the rash for more than 4 days. Both of these investigators introduced an additional technical step into the blood culture process that may explain why they were successful in isolating VZV while many others before had not been. The white blood cells were separated on Ficoll-Hypaque gradients and added to cell cultures. Although there was no evidence of viral growth in these cultures, they were blindly passaged onto new cell cultures. Evidence of growth of VZV was present in these second cultures after the blind passage within 2 to 5 days. Before these studies, VZV had been isolated only from blood obtained from immunocompromised patients with varicella or zoster.[105, 110, 111] The white blood cell infected with VZV is a mononuclear cell, but it is uncertain whether monocytes or lymphocytes (or both) are actually involved.[108, 109] Experiments in the SCID-hu mouse model have shown that VZV is lymphotropic for human CD4$^+$ and CD8$^+$ T lymphocytes and that human T cells release infectious virus.[112]

Data from PCR studies of patients with varicella are of interest, although they have yielded differing results. In the study of Koropchak and colleagues, performed 24 hours after rash onset in 12 patients, 3.3% of oropharyngeal samples, 67% of mononuclear cells, and 75% of skin vesicles were positive for VZV DNA.[113] In the study by Ozaki and co-workers of pharyngeal secretions of chickenpox patients, 26% and 90% were positive during the incubation period and after clinical onset, respectively.[114]

Virus is readily recovered from cutaneous lesions soon after the onset of chickenpox. Isolation of VZV was successful in 23 of 25 cases in which vesicle fluid was cultured within 3 days after the onset of the rash, but in only one of seven specimens collected between 4 and 8 days after onset.[104] In contrast, the virus apparently persists longer in vesicles of zoster patients, in whom 7 of 10 specimens collected later than 3 days after onset were positive.[104] As might be predicted, PCR is more sensitive than virus culture. In the study of Koropchak and co-workers, for example, VZV was recovered from only 21% of skin lesions, but 75% were positive by PCR.[113] Unlike smallpox, chickenpox is no longer communicable by the time the lesions have crusted and scabbed.

The pathogenesis of chickenpox, therefore, appears to be as follows. Transmission is probably effected by airborne spread of virus from respiratory droplets or cutaneous vesicles from patients with varicella or zoster. After an initial period of virus replication in the oropharynx, there is invasion of the local lymph nodes and then a primary viremia of low magnitude, delivering virus to the viscera.[115] After several more days of virus multiplication, a secondary viremia of greater magnitude occurs, resulting in widespread cutaneous dissemination and rash. Cropping of the vesicles is thought to represent several viremic phases. Crusting and scabbing of the vesicles and pustules occur as host defense mechanisms, particularly as various forms of cell-mediated immunity (CMI) become active.

The pathogenesis of zoster is different from that of varicella. Before development of zoster, latent VZV begins to multiply in the dorsal root ganglion (or ganglia) because of unknown local factors.[2] The virus then travels down the sensory nerve of the ganglion to the skin supplied by that nerve. Development of a localized rash occurs if there is a deficiency in CMI to VZV.[116–119] This compromise in CMI may be obvious, as in patients who have had transplantation, therapy for malignant disease, or HIV infection[120]; or presumably it may be transient, as in normal persons who develop zoster for no apparent reason. In immunosuppressed patients, a viremic phase with zoster has been documented on occasion[121, 122]; this probably happens after skin involvement has occurred, especially if there continues to be an inadequate immune response to VZV after the virus has reached the skin. The clinical manifestation of this viremia is disseminated zoster, in which vesicular lesions develop outside the original dermatome. A viremic phase in pregnant patients with disseminated zoster has not been documented, but it seems logical to assume that viremia would be a prerequisite for dissemination.

Pathology

CUTANEOUS LESIONS

Histologic changes in the skin leading to the formation of vesicles are essentially identical for chickenpox, zoster, and HSV infection. The hallmark of each is the presence of multinucleated giant cells and intranuclear inclusions, changes that are not found in the vesicular lesions caused by vaccinia virus and coxsackieviruses. The lesion is primarily localized in the epidermis, where ballooning degeneration of cells in the deeper layers is accompanied by intercellular edema. As edema progresses, the cornified layers are separated from the more basal layers to form a delicate vesicle with a thin roof. An exudate consisting primarily of mononuclear cells is seen in the dermis, but the characteristic nuclear changes of epithelial cells are absent in this region.

The predominant cell in vesicular lesions is the polymorphonuclear leukocyte. These cells may play a role in generating interferon in vesicular lesions, which may be important in recovery from the disease.[123] In vitro data also suggest that the polymorphonuclear leukocyte plays a role in host defense against VZV, possibly by mediating antibody-dependent cell-mediated cytotoxicity (ADCC).[124–126]

VISCERAL LESIONS IN THE FETUS AND PLACENTA

There are few reports describing the appearance of the placenta in cases of congenital chickenpox with or without survival. Garcia noted grossly visible necrotic lesions of the placenta in a case of chickenpox occurring in the fourth month of pregnancy that resulted in spontaneous abortion.[127] Microscopically, central areas of necrosis were surrounded by epithelioid cells and rare giant cells of the foreign body type, thus giving a granulomatous appearance. Peripherally, these lesions in the villi were accompanied by an exudate of necrotic material, nuclear fragments, and leukocytes filling the intervillous spaces. Some decidual cells had typical intranuclear inclusions.

Descriptions of the pathology of visceral lesions in fetal or neonatal chickenpox are necessarily restricted to autopsies in fatal cases.[127–132] Grossly, the lesions are small, punctate, white or yellow, and resemble miliary tuberculosis. Microscopically, their appearance resembles that of the lesions of the placenta: central necrotic areas, often resembling fibrinoid necrosis, surrounded by a few epithelioid cells and a scant infiltrate of mononuclear cells. Intranuclear inclusions are present. The skin, lungs, and liver are uniformly involved (Table 13–3). Slightly less frequently, the adrenals, gastrointestinal tract mucosa, and thymus are also involved. Less often, lesions appear in the kidneys, spleen, pancreas, and heart. Only one report describes necrotic foci in the brain.[127] In this case, the cortical, subependymal, and basilar structures of the cerebrum were totally destroyed and accompanied by extensive calcification. Although a search for *Toxoplasma* was negative, serologic data to rule out dual infection are lacking in the report. The gross and microscopic lesions of fatal perinatal chickenpox resemble those of disseminated HSV infection, including a preference for the liver and adrenal gland, but the data just given suggest that involvement of the brain is more common in neonatal HSV infection than it is in fatal neonatal chickenpox. A neonate with fatal hemorrhagic varicella with pneumonia and hepatitis is shown in Figure 13–1.

VISCERAL LESIONS IN THE MOTHER

In fatal cases of chickenpox in pregnant women, maternal death is almost always caused by pulmonary involvement. The pathologic course of chickenpox pneumonia in pregnant women is identical to that in nonpregnant women and in children.[133, 134] The lungs are usually edematous and congested. Interstitial pneumonitis may follow a peribronchiolar distribution of disease. Edema, septal cell proliferation, and infiltration of the alveolar septa by mononuclear leukocytes occur. Intranuclear inclusions may be found in alveolar lining cells, macrophages, capillary endothelium, and tracheobronchial mucosa. Necrotic foci may be accompanied by hemorrhage, and hyaline membranes lining the alveoli are often prominent.

ZOSTER

The pathologic picture of cutaneous lesions in zoster is indistinguishable from that of chickenpox lesions. In addition, the dorsal root ganglion of the affected dermatome exhibits a mononuclear inflammatory infiltrate. There may also be necrosis of ganglion cells and demyelination of the corresponding axon. There are no descriptions of these lesions in pregnant women or in neonates specifically.

Clinical Manifestations

CHICKENPOX RASH

After an incubation period of usually 13 to 17 days,[37, 60] chickenpox is heralded by the approximately simultaneous occurrence of fever and rash. In adults, the exanthem is often preceded by a prodromal fever and constitutional symptoms lasting 2 or 3 days.[6] Occasionally one or more isolated vesicles may precede a generalized exanthem by 1 or 2 days. The rash is characteristically centripetal, beginning on the face or scalp and spreading rapidly to the trunk, but with relative sparing of the extremities. The lesions begin as red macules but progress quickly to vesicles and crusts. Itching is the rule. There is a tendency for new lesions to occur in crops. Unlike smallpox, all stages of lesions—vesicles, pustules, and scabs—may be present simultaneously in the same anatomic region. New crops often continue to appear over a 2- to 5-day period. Lesions may be more numerous in skin folds or in the diaper area. The total number of vesicles varies from only two or three in very mild cases, especially in infants, to thousands of lesions that border on confluence, especially in adults.[6] In many cases, one or two mucosal lesions may be present in the mouth or, less commonly, in the vulva. Occasionally the

---

TABLE 13–3
Frequency of Gross and Microscopic Lesions in Seven Autopsies in Cases of Fetal and Neonatal Chickenpox

ORGAN	NO. OF CASES/ NO. EXAMINED	%	REFERENCES
Skin	7/7	100	127–132
Lungs	7/7	100	127–132
Liver	7/7	100	127–132
Adrenals	6/7	86	127, 128, 130–132
Esophagus or	5/6	83	127–132
intestines	4/5	80	
Thymus	5/7	71	127, 128, 130, 132
Kidneys	4/7	56	127, 128, 130, 132
Spleen	3/7	43	127, 130–132
Pancreas	2/7	29	127, 128, 130
Heart	1/5	20	127, 131
Brain[a]			127
Miscellaneous			
Ovaries	1		128
Bone marrow	1		130
Placenta	1		127

[a]Not well documented; possibility of concomitant toxoplasmosis not definitely excluded.

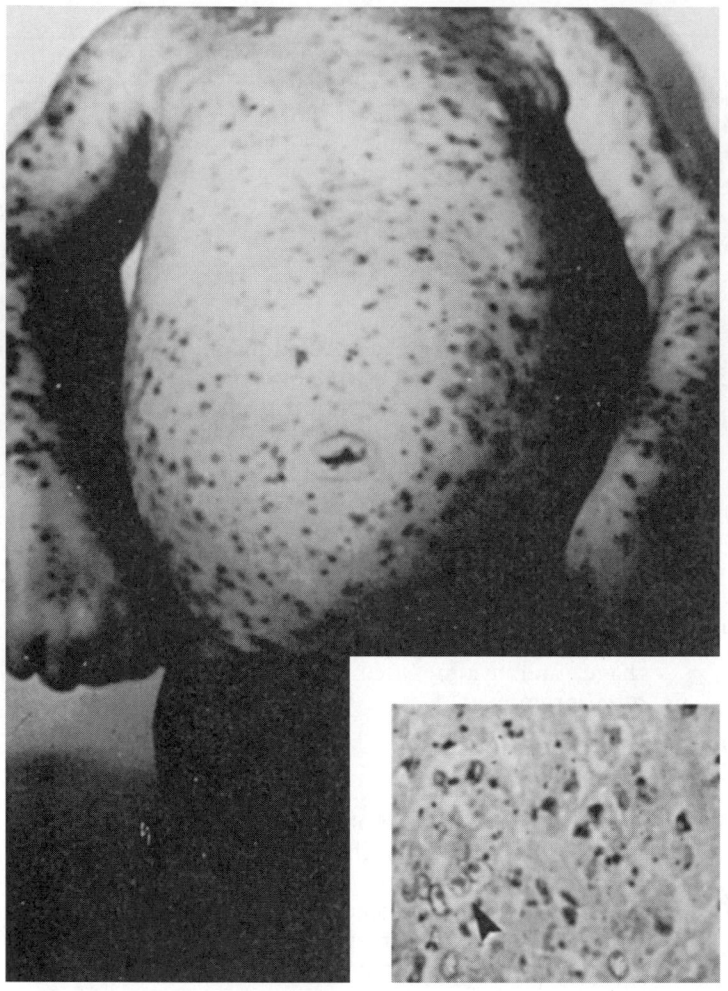

FIGURE 13–1 Congenital hemorrhagic varicella complicated by pneumonia and hepatitis. The mother of this infant developed varicella a few days before delivery. Zoster immune globulin was not available at that time. Inset shows a section of liver with intranuclear inclusion bodies obtained at autopsy.

lesions may be bullous or hemorrhagic. Residual scarring is exceptional. Constitutional symptoms tend to be mild even in the presence of an extensive exanthem.

COMPLICATIONS OF CHICKENPOX

The most common complication is secondary bacterial infection, usually caused by streptococci or staphylococci. Skin infections may lead to severe sequelae such as toxic shock syndrome and necrotizing fasciitis.[135–143] Septicemia was observed in 0.5% of 2534 cases seen at the Willard Parker Hospital from l929 to l934.[144] Central nervous system complications, which are uncommon, include encephalitis, cerebellar ataxia, aseptic meningitis, and myelitis.[145, 146] Glomerulonephritis,[147, 148] myocarditis,[149, 150] and arthritis[151, 152] have also been reported.

CHICKENPOX IN IMMUNOCOMPROMISED CHILDREN

It is widely appreciated that varicella may be severe and even fatal in children with an underlying malignancy, those with congenital deficits in cellular immunity or those receiving high doses of corticosteroids for any reason,[153] and children with underlying infection with HIV and the acquired immunodeficiency syndrome

(AIDS).[75, 154] Leukemic children have a mortality rate approaching 10% if untreated[155] and may develop what has been termed progressive varicella. Instead of developing new vesicular lesions for several days, they continue to have fever and new lesions for as long as 2 weeks after the onset of illness. Frequently, their skin lesions become hemorrhagic as well as large and umbilicated. Often varicella pneumonia ensues and is a major factor contributing to the death of a child. It is believed that this abnormal response to VZV represents a failure of the normal CMI response to eliminate the virus.[155] The CMI response to VZV includes antibody-dependent cell-mediated cytotoxicity, natural killer cells, and cytotoxic T cells, including CD4 and CD8 cells.[33, 124–126, 156–158]

CHICKENPOX PNEUMONIA

Primary varicella pneumonia is a dreaded complication of chickenpox and is responsible for most fatalities. It is most common in immunocompromised patients, in adults, and in most fatal cases of neonatal chickenpox,[127–129, 159] but it is rarely seen in otherwise healthy children. It has been suggested that the incidence is about 15% in adults and that 90% of cases have occurred in persons older than 19 years old.[159, 160] The true incidence is difficult to determine because chest roentgenograms are not performed in most cases of chickenpox and extensive radiographic evidence of disease may be present when pulmonary symptoms are only minimal. In male military recruits with varicella, virtually all of whom had been hospitalized and had chest roentgenograms, radiographic evidence of pneumonia was found in 16.3% of 110 cases.[161]

Two reviews of chickenpox pneumonia in adults outline the major features.[134, 162] The onset of pneumonia occurs generally 2 to 4 days but sometimes as long as 10 days after the appearance of the exanthem. Fever and cough are present in 87 to 100% of cases, and dyspnea occurs in 70 to 80%. Other symptoms and signs include cyanosis (42 to 55%), rales (55%), hemoptysis (35 to 38%), and chest pain (21%). Radiographic changes seem to correlate best with the severity of the rash rather than with the physical examination of the lungs. The roentgenogram typically reveals a diffuse nodular or miliary pattern, most pronounced in the perihilar regions. The radiographic appearance changes rapidly. The white blood cell count varies between 5000 and 20,000 per mm³ and is of little help in differentiating viral from secondary bacterial pneumonia. Pneumonia is usually self-limiting, and recovery is temporally correlated with clearing of skin lesions. The fatality rate has been variously estimated at 10 to 30% but most probably approximates the lower of these values if immunocompromised hosts are excluded.[134, 162] Blood gas analyses and pulmonary function tests indicate a significant diffu-sion defect that may persist in some cases for months after clinical recovery.[163] The introduction of antiviral chemotherapy has greatly improved the outcome in this disease.

MATERNAL EFFECTS OF CHICKENPOX

Early reports suggested that if chickenpox occurred during pregnancy, it was a highly lethal disease. Deaths usually resulted from varicella pneumonia, in some cases accompanied by glomerulitis and renal failure or myocarditis, occurring after the fourth month of gestation.[164, 165] Harris and Rhoades reviewed the literature to 1963 and found a reported mortality of 41% for 17 pregnant women with chickenpox pneumonia compared with 11% for 236 nonpregnant adults with chickenpox pneumonia.[166] Other reports, however, question whether varicella, especially in the absence of pneumonia, is more serious in pregnant women than in the adult population at large.[131, 167, 168] Because most cases of gestational varicella with an uncomplicated course are undoubtedly not reported, the denominator of the case:fatality ratio is unknown. In a prospective study of 150 cases of chickenpox in pregnancy in 1966, only one maternal death related to chickenpox pneumonia was recorded.[169] It is probable that the mortality figures even for chickenpox pneumonia occurring in pregnancy are biased by selective reporting of fatal cases.

To a review of the literature on varicella pneumonia in pregnancy before 1964,[166] Table 13–4 adds data from

TABLE 13–4
Maternal Mortality Associated with Gestational Varicella[a]

REFERENCE	YEAR	NO. OF CASES	NO. WITH VARICELLA PNEUMONIA	NO. OF DEATHS	ONSET OF RASH[b]			
					0–3 mo	4–6 mo	7–9 mo	Immediately Postpartum
127	1963	2	0	0	0	1	1	0
170	1964	18	0	0	0	0	15	3
131	1964	16	1	1	0	0	16 (1)[c]	0
93	1965	9	0	0	0	0	5	4
171	1966	11[d]	0	0	0	4	7	0
166	1965[e]	17	17	7	2 (1)[e]	3 (2)	11 (4)	1 (0)
479	1968	1	1	1	0	1 (1)	0	0
173	1969	2	2	1	0	0	2 (1)	0
174	1971	1	1	0	0	0	1	1
175	1986	43	4	1	11	11 (1)	21	0
176	1989	3	3	1	0	1	2 (1)	0
178	1990	5	5	1	3	0	2 (1)	0
188	1991	1	1	0	0	2	0	0
179[f]	1991	21	21	3	0	7	14 (3)	0
158[g]	1996	28	1	0	7	7	11	0
177	1997	22	0	0	3	9	0	0
Totals		198	57 (16) (28%)	16	26 (1) (4%)	46 (4) (9%)	108 (11) (10%)	0

[a]The antiviral therapy era is considered to have begun after 1985.
[b]If specified.
[c]Numbers in parentheses give deaths at indicated gestational period.
[d]Includes one patient with zoster whose gestational dates are not given.
[e]Includes review of literature before 1963.
[f]Reports 5 new cases with review of additional case reports in the literature.
[g]In a series of 28 pregnant women with varicella, 1 (3.6%) had pneumonia.

subsequent case reports of gestational varicella, with and without pneumonia, as well as reports of perinatal varicella in which the outcome in the mother is described.[93, 127, 131, 166, 168, 170–179] Among 198 cases of chickenpox in pregnant women, there were 16 deaths (8%). All of the deaths occurred among the 57 women who had chickenpox pneumonia (28% fatality rate for pneumonia). One of 26 women whose disease occurred during the first trimester died (4%), as did 4 of 46 women with disease in the second trimester (9%) and 11 of 108 women (10%) who became ill in the third trimester. No deaths occurred among 8 women who were exposed to chickenpox in late pregnancy but did not develop an exanthem until the first few days post partum. In summary, it remains uncertain whether chickenpox pneumonia has a graver prognosis if it occurs during pregnancy. There is no definitive evidence that chickenpox in the absence of pneumonia is a more serious illness in pregnant women than in other adults; however, the risk of maternal death may be increased after the sixteenth week of pregnancy.

A number of patients with varicella during pregnancy who were treated with ACV have been reported.[168, 176, 178–189] These reports suggest that ACV has improved the outcome of this complication of varicella, although controlled studies have not been performed. Although a wide variety of dosages has been used, the standard dosage of 30 mg/kg per day intravenously would seem to make most sense for treatment of pregnant women with varicella pneumonia. It is not know whether all pregnant women who develop varicella should be treated with ACV and whether oral ACV has merit. Congenital abnormalities from administration of ACV to women during pregnancy have not been observed.[190, 191]

Controlled studies of the value of corticosteroids in pregnant women with varicella pneumonia have not been performed. Two of 6 reported pregnant women treated with corticosteroids died, whereas 8 of 17 pregnant women given supportive therapy without corticosteroids died.[166, 172–174, 192] It would seem that administration of an antiviral drug would be of greater importance than administration of corticosteroids. Passive immunization with VZIG may be administered to seronegative women after close exposure to VZV to attempt to modify the infection; although it is not certain whether this will prevent fetal infection, it is possible that it may.[193, 194] In a study from 1994, of 97 women who developed varicella after receiving VZIG, there were no observed cases of the congenital varicella syndrome.[194] One would usually expect about two abnormal infants from a series of this magnitude, but obviously the number of women followed is too low to achieve statistical significance.

EFFECTS OF GESTATIONAL VARICELLA ON THE FETUS

Chromosomal Aberrations

VZV has been shown to induce chromosomal abnormalities both in vitro and in vivo. When human diploid fibroblasts are infected with the virus, a high proportion of cells are observed in metaphase arrest as if they were under the influence of colchicine.[195] Twenty-four hours after infection, the incidence of chromatid and chromosome breaks ranges from 26 to 45%, compared with 2% for control cultures. In the acute phase of chickenpox, up to the fifth day of rash, peripheral blood leukocytes show a 17 to 28% incidence of chromosome breaks compared with 6% in controls, but 1 month after infection these abnormalities have disappeared.[196] A single case report suggests the possibility that when chickenpox is acquired in utero, chromosomal damage may be more lasting. A boy with bird-headed dwarfism, born to a mother who contracted chickenpox in the sixth month of pregnancy, had a 26% incidence of chromosomal breakage in peripheral blood leukocytes when he was examined at 2 years of age.[197] Interestingly, however, chromosomal analysis in four infants with the congenital varicella syndrome, whose mothers had chickenpox at the eighth, fourteenth, sixteenth, and twentieth week of gestation, respectively, was reported as normal.[198–201] Information on chromosomal aberrations in infants who have no congenital anomalies and are the offspring of mothers with gestational varicella is unfortunately lacking. Further concern about the possibility of persistent chromosomal abnormalities after intrauterine exposure to VZV is suggested by a prospective survey of deaths among children born in England and Wales between 1950 and 1952 whose mothers had chickenpox in pregnancy. Two deaths, both from acute leukemia, were reported among the offspring of 270 women; the two children developed acute leukemia at the ages of 3 and 4 years after intrauterine exposure at 25 and 23 weeks' gestation, respectively.[202] In view of the absence of confirmation of these data, it remains questionable as to whether exposure to chickenpox in utero is a risk factor for leukemia or other malignancies.

Abortion and Prematurity

Several studies have addressed the question of whether gestational chickenpox and other viral diseases result in an increased incidence of spontaneous abortion or prematurity. In a retrospective study in 1948, only four cases of chickenpox were identified among 26,353 pregnant women.[203] No stillbirths occurred among these four. Prospective studies have tended to confirm that maternal chickenpox during pregnancy is not associated with a significant excess of either prematurity[169] or fetal death.[171] Among 826 virus-infected pregnant subjects observed in New York City from 1957 to 1964, 150 women with cases of chickenpox were followed to term. After exclusion of fetal deaths and multiple births, 5 of 135 live-born infants were found to have birth weights of less than 2500 g. This incidence of prematurity was actually lower than that in the control group of non–virus-infected pregnant women (Table 13–5). Similarly, in the study of Paryani and Arvin, premature delivery occurred in 2 of 42 (5%) pregnancies, with delivery at 31 and 35 weeks' gestation.[175] In a prospective study involving 194 women with gestational varicella and 194 control women, the rate of spontaneous abortion was 3% and 7%, respectively, in the first 20 weeks.[204] In the

TABLE 13–5
Frequency of Low Birth Weight Among Infants Born to Mothers with Selected Virus Infections During Pregnancy

DISEASE	VIRUS-INFECTED GROUP			CONTROL GROUP[a]		
	No. of Live Births	No. with Low Birth Weight[b]	%	No. of Live Births	No. with Low Birth Weight[b]	%
Rubella	359	50	13.9	402	21	5.2
Chickenpox	135	5	3.7	146	13	8.9
Mumps	117	9	7.7	122	4	3.3
Measles	60	10	16.7	62	2	3.3

[a]Control group was matched for age, race, and parity of the mother and type of obstetric service.
[b]Low birth weight was defined as less than 2500 g.
Table modified from data of Siegel M, Fuerst HT. Low birth weight and maternal virus diseases: a prospective study of rubella, measles, mumps, chickenpox, and hepatitis. JAMA 197:88, 1966. Fetal deaths and multiple births were excluded from the analysis.

large prospective series of Enders and associates of 1330 women in England and Germany who developed varicella, 36 (3%) experienced spontaneous abortions after varicella in the first 16 weeks.[194] However, in the prospective study of Pastuszak and co-workers involving 106 women with varicella in the first 20 weeks of pregnancy, there were more premature births (14.3%) among women with varicella than among controls (5.6%; $p = 0.05$).[205] There is no question, however, that the congenital varicella syndrome is associated with low birth weight. Approximately one third of reported cases of the syndrome have been premature, of low birth weight, or small for dates.

An accurate assessment of the incidence of fetal mortality after maternal chickenpox is difficult to obtain. Fetal wastage is probably unreported, in part because some spontaneous abortions occur before prenatal care is sought. In the prospective study of maternal viral diseases in New York City referred to earlier,[171] nine fetal deaths were observed among 144 instances of maternal chickenpox. Five fetal deaths occurred among 32 pregnancies in the first trimester, four among 60 second-trimester pregnancies and none among 52 third-trimester pregnancies (Table 13–6). These do not represent significant increases in fetal wastage associated with chickenpox infection compared with control groups in which no maternal viral infection occurred. Only for mumps was there a significant excess of fetal deaths, with these occurring primarily in the first trimester. Only three of the nine fetal deaths associated with maternal chickenpox occurred within 2 weeks of the onset of the mother's illness, and two of these were in the first trimester. Two additional deaths occurred 2 to 4 weeks after the onset of maternal chickenpox, two after 5 to 9 weeks, and two 10 or more weeks after the onset of maternal illness. The absence of a close temporal relationship between most fetal deaths and maternal disease also provides further support for the concept that maternal chickenpox during pregnancy does not commonly result in fetal mortality.

Although the incidence of fetal death is not increased by maternal varicella, fetal deaths have been associated with maternal varicella. Deaths in utero may result from direct invasion of the fetus by VZV[127, 194, 206–208]

or from a presumed "toxic" effect of high fever, anoxia, or metabolic changes caused by maternal disease.[171] The precise pathogenesis of the second mechanism has not been elucidated. When maternal disease is unusually severe, particularly in cases of chickenpox pneumonia, fetal death may also result from premature onset of labor or death in utero secondary to maternal death.[131, 166, 172, 173, 178, 207]

Congenital Malformations

Two types of investigations have been carried out in an attempt to discover whether chickenpox during pregnancy is a cause of congenital malformations. The first

TABLE 13–6
Fetal Deaths in Relation to Gestational Age After Selected Virus Infections During Pregnancy

	WEEKS OF GESTATION		
	0–11	12–27	>28
Mumps			
No. of cases	33	51	43
No. of fetal deaths	9	1	0
%	27.3	2.0	—
Measles			
No. of cases	19	29	17
No. of fetal deaths	3	1	1.9
%	15.8	3.4	5.9
Chickenpox			
No. of cases	32	60	52
No. of fetal deaths	5	4	0
%	15.6	4.7	—
Controls			
No. of cases	1010[a]	392[b]	152[b]
No. of fetal deaths	131	15	1
%	13.0	3.8	0.7

[a]Subjects were attending prenatal clinic in first trimester without virus infections.
[b]Controls were matched for age, race, and parity of the mother and type of obstetric service.
Table modified from Siegel M, Fuerst HT, Peress NS. Comparative fetal mortality in maternal virus diseases: a prospective study on rubella, measles, mumps, chickenpox, and hepatitis. N Engl J Med 274:768, 1966.

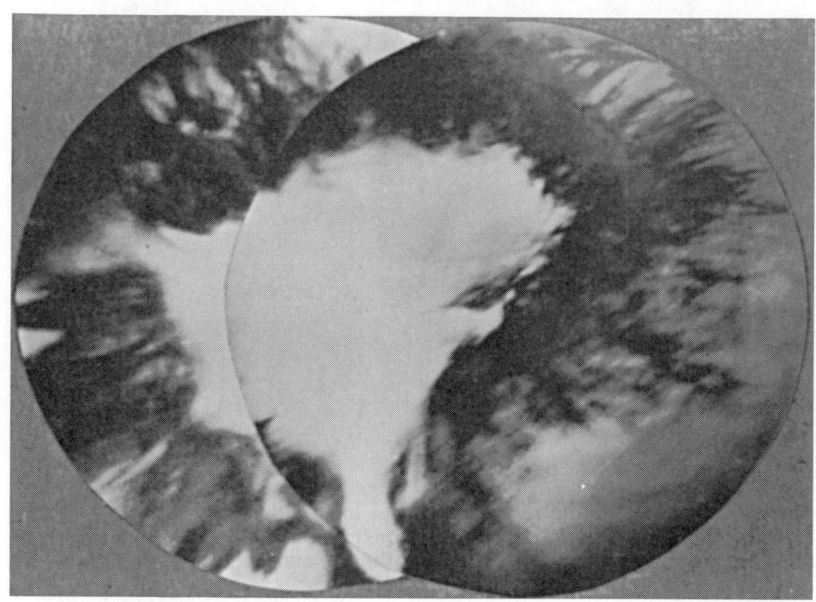

FIGURE 13–2 Fundus photograph of right eye of patient at age 13 months, showing central gliosis with surrounding ring of black pigment. The child's mother had varicella during the early fourth month of pregnancy.[235, 246] (From Charles N, Bennett TW, Margolis S. Ocular pathology of the congenital varicella syndrome. Arch Ophthalmol 95:2034–2037, 1977. Copyright 1977, American Medical Association.)

consists of retrospective analyses or case reports describing specific anomalies that have occurred in the offspring of mothers who had gestational varicella. These reports are necessarily highly selective and do not define the incidence of such anomalies. They do, however, consistently describe a syndrome of skin scarring, eye and brain damage, and limb hypoplasia that is related to intrauterine varicella.

The second type of analysis consists of prospective studies of pregnant women followed throughout pregnancy and afterward. Here the problem is to delineate the coincidence of two events, each of which is itself uncommon—gestational chickenpox and congenital malformations—to determine the risk to the fetus after maternal varicella. Siegel, despite an 8-year observation period encompassing approximately 190,000 pregnancies annually in New York City, was able to identify only four malformations among infants born to 135 mothers who had chickenpox during pregnancy, compared with five malformations among 146 matched controls.[66] The follow-up period was 5 years and included psychomotor and audiometric tests. Only 27 of the pregnancies complicated by chickenpox occurred during the first trimester, and of these 2 were associated with congenital anomalies (7.4%), compared with three anomalies among 87 pregnancies in the control population (3.4%). Since this series of Siegel, the largest single prospective series to date comes from Enders and associates.[194] In a joint prospective study in Germany and the United Kingdom between 1980 and 1993, Enders and associates followed 1373 women with varicella and 366 with zoster during pregnancy. Of the women with varicella, 1285 continued to term, and 9 had defects attributed to the congenital varicella syndrome.[194] The incidence was 2/472 (0.4%) for infections between 0 and 12 weeks and 7/351 (2%) for infections between 13 and 20 weeks. Only very recently has it become possible to make a tissue diagnosis of the congenital varicella syndrome, because affected infants do not chronically shed virus as is seen in congenital infections with rubella virus and CMV.[194, 206,]

[208–210] That the congenital varicella syndrome is a reality has now been proven. Hopefully it may be prevented in the future by widespread use of varicella vaccine, analogous to the situation for congenital rubella.

The constellation of developmental abnormalities described in individual case reports of infants born to mothers who had varicella in early pregnancy and in prospective series is sufficiently distinctive to indicate that VZV is a teratogen. LaForet and Lynch in 1947 described an infant with multiple congenital anomalies after maternal chickenpox in early pregnancy.[211] The infant had hypoplasia of the entire right lower extremity, talipes equinovarus, and absent deep tendon reflexes on the right. In addition, there were cerebral cortical atrophy, cerebellar aplasia, chorioretinitis, right torticollis, insufficiency of the anal and vesical sphincters, and cicatricial cutaneous lesions of the left lower extremity. In 1974, Srabstein and co-workers rekindled interest in the subject, reported another case, and reviewed the literature, concluding that although the virus could not be isolated from the infants, the congenital syndrome typically consisted of some combination of cicatricial skin lesions, ocular abnormalities, limb deformities, mental retardation, and early death after maternal varicella in early pregnancy (Figs. 13–2 to 13–4).[212] There have now been numerous additional reports in the literature of the syndrome, encompassing over 75 cases, indicating that there is a wide spectrum of manifestations.*

Whereas at one time it was thought that the syndrome occurred after maternal VZV infection in the first trimester of pregnancy, current evaluation of the data indicates that cases clearly occur in the second trimester as well. Of 69 cases in which data are available, 28 (40%) occurred after maternal varicella that developed before the 13th week,† 40 (58%) occurred between weeks 13

---

*See references 68, 175, 177, 194, 201, 204, 205, 208–210, and 213–255.

†See references 66, 175, 194, 201, 204–206, 209, 211, 214–216, 219–221, and 223–230.

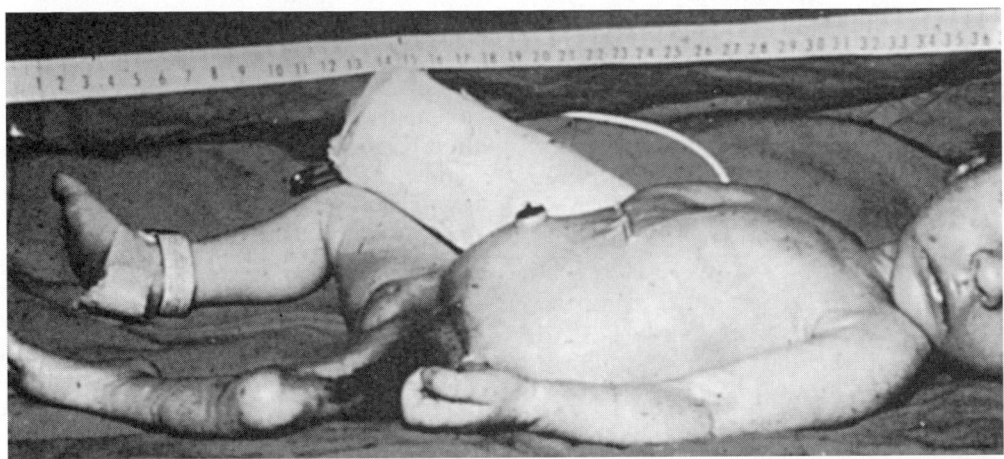

FIGURE 13–3 This infant, whose mother had varicella during the thirteenth to fifteenth weeks of pregnancy, had bilateral microphthalmia with cataracts and an atrophic left leg. The infant died of bronchopneumonia at age 6½ months. (From Srabstein JC, Morris N, Larke RPB, et al. Is there a congenital varicella syndrome? J Pediatr 84:239, 1974, with permission.)

and 26,* and 1 (1%)[242] occurred in the twenty-eighth week. The average gestation when maternal varicella occurred was 15 weeks. Five cases occurring after maternal zoster have been reported[243, 244, 258, 259]; four occurred after maternal zoster in the first trimester and one followed zoster in the second trimester.[258] A total of 77

*See references 68, 194, 198–200, 204–206, 209, 210, 212, 217, 218, 222, 231–241, 247, and 250–257.

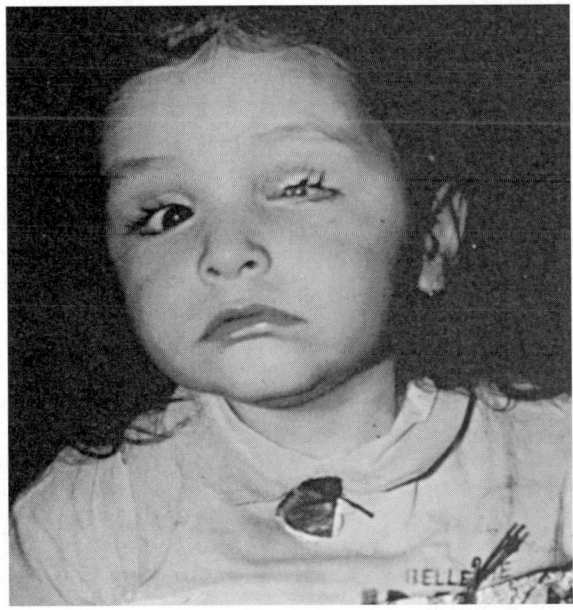

FIGURE 13–4 A child whose mother had varicella during the sixteenth week of pregnancy. There was atrophy of the left orbit with blindness that required cosmetic enucleation. Severe choreoretinitis occurred in the right eye. Except for blindness, the child developed normally. She died at approximately 4 years of age of pneumonia. (From Frey HM, Bialkin G, Gershon A. Congenital varicella: case report of a serologically proved long-term survivor. Pediatrics 59:110, 1977, with permission.)

affected infants have been described: 72 cases followed maternal varicella (93%) and 5 followed maternal zoster (disseminated in one instance) (7%).

Scars of the skin, usually cicatricial lesions, were the most prominent stigmata, reported in 47 infants (61%).* Eye abnormalities (chorioretinitis, microphthalmia, Horner's syndrome, cataract, and nystagmus) are similarly common; other essential features include a hypoplastic limb, cortical atrophy and mental retardation, and early death. The features of the syndrome are summarized in Table 13–7.

Cutaneous scars were usually overlying a hypoplastic limb but also have been seen in the contralateral limb.[211] Characteristically, the skin scars were cicatricial, depressed, and pigmented and often had a zigzag configuration. Such scars are thought to be the result of zoster that occurred before birth. In some patients, large areas of scarred skin have required skin grafting.[224, 232] In other patients, the rash was bullous[231] or consisted of multiple scattered depressed white scars.[235, 239, 252] In one reported infant, healing zoster was present at the T11 dermatome at birth; there was also spinal cord atrophy at the same level, and aganglionosis of the intestine.[251]

Ocular abnormalities were noted in 43 patients (56%). These included chorioretinitis in 21 (27%),† Horner's syndrome or anisocoria in 12 (16%),[204, 213–216, 218, 220–222, 231, 241, 243] microphthalmia in 15 (19%),‡ cataract in 15 (19%),§ and nystagmus in 10 (13%).¶ In five cases, including one that occurred after maternal zoster, the major abnormalities were confined to the eye, suggesting the possibility of formes frustes of the syndrome, perhaps associated with more limited viral replication.

*See references 68, 175, 204–206, 208, 211–224, 227, 228, 230–239, 241, 242, 245, 251, 252, and 256.
†See references 68, 175, 199, 204, 208, 210–212, 219, 220, 226, 229, 235, 237–239, 241, and 246–248.
‡See references 68, 194, 198, 201, 208, 209, 212, 223, 233, 235, 241, 246, 248, 258, and 260.
§See references 66, 194, 198, 201, 209, 212, 223, 233, 235, 241, 246, 248, 257, 258, and 260.
¶See references 68, 175, 201, 204, 211, 219, 220, 235, 241, and 258.

TABLE 13–7
Clinical Data in 77 Infants with Developmental Defects Born to Women with VZV Infections in Pregnancy (1947–1998)

DEFECT	NO. OF CASES[a]	%
Skin scars[b]	47	61
Eye abnormalities	43	56
Chorioretinitis	21	27
Horner's/anisocoria	12	16
Microphthalmia	15	19
Cataract	15	19
Nystagmus	10	13
Abnormal limb[c]	36	47
Hypoplasia	28	36
Equinovarus	11	14
Abnormal/absent digits	8	10
Cortical atrophy/mental retardation	31	40
Prematurity/low birth weight	28	36
Early death	20	26
Dysphagia/aspiration	15	19
Gastrointestinal tract abnormalities	9	12
Urinary tract abnormalities	8	10

[a]For specific references, see text.
[b]Cicatricial in 37 (79%).
[c]11/28 (39%) with hypoplastic limb had mental retardation or early death.

There was no apparent effect of timing of maternal varicella during gestation because the times of infection varied from 9 to 23 weeks in these infants.[66, 235, 240, 246, 247, 258] Figure 13–2 is a photograph showing retinal involvement in one of these patients.[235, 246]

Abnormalities of the limbs were reported in 36 (47%) patients. Hypoplasia of a limb, most commonly unilateral involvement of a leg or arm, was seen in 28 (36%) patients (see Table 13–7).* Hypoplasia or absence of digits was reported in 8 patients (10%).[211, 213, 216, 217, 220–222] Talipes equinovarus or a calcaneovalgus deformity was noted in 11 cases (14%).† This complex of abnormalities in the limbs, including the bony abnormalities, is probably attributable to a neuropathy caused by direct viral invasion of the ganglia and spinal cord.

Thirty-one (40%) patients showed cerebral cortical atrophy, diffuse brain involvement, or mental retardation,‡ frequently accompanied by abnormal electroencephalograms and seizures or myoclonic jerks.[211, 212, 219–221, 254] In a few patients, cerebrospinal fluid findings were normal[68, 212, 221, 248]; in others there were increased numbers of leukocytes or protein levels.[211, 218, 220] Bulbar palsy is suspected to have resulted in dysphagia and bouts of aspiration pneumonia in 15 (19%) infants.§ Deep tendon reflexes were reported as normal in 1 infant[220] and

diminished to absent in 6,[200, 201, 211, 212, 216, 217] and were in some cases accompanied by sensory deficits.[68, 212, 217, 221, 248] Electromyography in some patients revealed a denervation pattern with loss of motor units.[212, 221, 222, 244, 248] Biopsy in one instance showed replacement of muscle bundles by fat.[212] One child with vocal cord paralysis has been reported.[254]

Eighteen (24%) infants died within the first 14 months of life.* One child with the obvious syndrome was stillborn.[208] In one who died at 6 months, autopsy revealed a necrotizing encephalitis with varying degrees of gliosis and inflammatory infiltrates. Focal calcification was observed in white and gray matter of the cerebrum, brain stem, and cerebellum. Atrophy of the anterior columns of the spinal cord and scarring in the ganglion corresponding to the distribution of the skin lesions, and atrophic limb was also present. No inclusion bodies were identified.[212] Of 28 reported infants with a hypoplastic limb, 11 (39%) were described to have had evidence of mental retardation or died early.

Twenty-eight (36%) infants also were described as premature or had low birth weight for their gestational ages.†

Nine infants (12%) have had various abnormalities of the gastrointestinal tract, including reflux, duodenal stenosis, jejunal dilatation, microcolon, atresia of the sigmoid colon, and sphincter malfunction.[65, 210, 211, 218, 232, 247, 250, 253, 261] Eight children (10%) have had abnormalities of the urinary tract, often due to poor or absent bladder sphincter function.[68, 175, 211, 212, 215, 230, 243, 248, 251] Involvement of the cervical or lumbar spinal cord and the autonomic nervous system is thought to account for the observed hypoplasia or aplasia of limbs and digits, motor and sensory defects, decrease or absence of deep tendon reflexes, Horner's syndrome, and gastrointestinal and urinary tract abnormalities.[262]

Figures 13–3 and 13–4 depict two children with stigmata of the congenital varicella syndrome, one with severe[212] and one with relatively mild involvement.[235, 246]

Zoster After the Congenital Varicella Syndrome. Fourteen patients (18%) with the congenital varicella syndrome have been reported to have developed clinical zoster in infancy or early childhood: 11 in the first year of life, 1 at 13 months, 1 at 3 years, and 1 at 41 months of age.‡ This is of particular interest because CMI to VZV in 2 of 10 of children with the syndrome has been reported to be absent as determined by lymphocyte transformation.[175, 199] It is also of note that in Enders' series of 1291 live births of whom conservatively perhaps 25% were infected with VZV, the rate of zoster was 10/322 (3%). It appears that zoster is even more common in children with the congenital syndrome than in infants who were infected with VZV in utero but were asymptomatic at birth.

Diagnosis of the Congenital Varicella Syndrome. During the neonatal period or infancy, attempts to iso-

---

*See references 68, 175, 194, 209, 211–224, 227, 236, 244, 248, 256, and 257.

†See references 68, 200, 201, 205, 209, 211, 220, 228, 242, 244, 248, and 258.

‡See references 66, 194, 199–201, 206, 211, 212, 215, 216, 218–220, 223, 225, 228–230, 234, 236, 241, 243, 244, 250, 251, 253–255, 258, 259, and 261.

§See references 68, 175, 212, 216, 218, 221, 228, 229, 234, 236, 238, 241, 248, and 254–256.

---

*See references 175, 194, 199, 200, 205, 206, 212, 218, 219, 221, 223, 225, 228–231, 234, and 250.

†See references 66, 68, 198, 200, 205, 211, 212, 215–221, 223, 229–231, 233, 235, 239, 241, 248, 250, 255, and 256.

‡See references 68, 194, 209, 210, 215, 229, 234, 239, 240, 248, 252, 254, and 255.

late VZV from the skin, cerebrospinal fluid, eye, and other tissues in infants with developmental defects were negative.[68, 198, 212, 220, 228, 229, 234, 235] Although rubella virus and CMV are commonly isolated from young infants afflicted by these viruses, failure to isolate VZV in these cases is probably explained by the fact that the period of viral replication took place during early gestation and no replicating virus persisted by the time of birth. In children who developed zoster at an early age, it has been possible to isolate VZV from the rash.[210, 229, 254] In seven infants who died, there was at autopsy apparent dissemination of VZV with varicella-like involvement of the lungs, liver, spleen, adrenals, and/or pancreas.[206–208, 212, 228–231]

Total IgM concentrations in the serum or cord blood of six infants were measured.[198, 212, 221, 233–235] In three instances, the levels were 48 to 100 mg/dl at 1.5 to 6 weeks of age. Specific VZV antibodies in the IgM fraction were not detected in seven cases in which they were sought,[175, 221, 235, 241, 263] but they were detectable in six other cases.[194, 199, 200, 225, 233] In one of these cases, VZV IgM was detected prenatally, by obtaining blood by cordocentesis.[264] In most infants, a decline of antibodies in the serum was observed, a finding compatible with either a fetal or a maternal origin. In 10 instances, however, persistence of, or an increase in, antibodies in the infant supported a presumption of intrauterine infection.[68, 198, 214, 219, 227, 234, 235, 246, 248]

Thus, it has been possible to document some reported cases of the congenital varicella syndrome but not all of them, because antibody titers may be inconclusive even in children with the apparent full-blown and rather distinctive constellation of abnormalities. The development of zoster at an early age can be interpreted as substantiating VZV infection in utero. Although many of the cases reported as the congenital varicella syndrome lack proof, it has been possible to show that some infants with characteristic stigmata were infected in utero with VZV, although an active chronic infection does not occur. Modern molecular methods such as PCR and in situ hybridization have been useful for proving the congenital syndrome in a few reported infants and will undoubtedly be used to prove future cases.[194, 206, 208–210, 254] It is expected that these will become the methods of choice in the future rather than antibody testing.

Management of Pregnant Women with Varicella Zoster Virus Infection with Regard to Fetal Malformations

In the decade of the 1990s, the incidence of fetal malformations after maternal VZV infection has been clarified. Varicella is a significantly greater threat than zoster; 93% of reported cases of the congenital varicella syndrome have followed maternal chickenpox. Furthermore, in Enders' series of 366 women with zoster in pregnancy, there were no cases of the congenital syndrome.[194] This outcome is not unexpected because, as already mentioned, zoster is probably less likely to be accompanied by a viremia than is varicella; thus, many fetuses may escape VZV infection from maternal zoster. In addition, because zoster is a secondary infection,

residual maternal immunity to VZV may at least partially protect the fetus from damage, analogous to that seen when congenital CMV infection is due to reactivation rather than to primary CMV infection.[265]

The time at which maternal VZV infection occurs during gestation also influences whether the infant is likely to be severely damaged. Infection during the first and early second trimester appears to be the most critical. Most of the reported cases of the congenital syndrome have occurred when the onset of maternal infection was before the 20th week of pregnancy. Only five infants (7%) with some of the stigmata have been recorded as the result of maternal varicella after the twentieth week.[206, 240–242, 250] When maternal varicella occurs after the twentieth week, the infant may be infected but usually the only evidence is a positive VZV antibody titer when the infant is more than 1 year old and, in some cases, development of zoster at an early age.

Ten prospective studies of the incidence of the congenital varicella syndrome have now been published. Data from these studies are presented in Table 13–8. There were a total of 13 cases of the congenital varicella syndrome in 718 (1.8%) women who developed varicella in the first 20 weeks of pregnancy. If the entire gestational period is considered, 1898 women who had varicella during pregnancy were delivered of live-born infants; the overall incidence of the congenital syndrome was 0.6%. These data indicate that the risk for development of the congenital varicella syndrome is mostly confined to the first 20 weeks of pregnancy and even the risk after maternal varicella in the first 20 weeks of pregnancy is extremely low, on the order of 2%. Weeks 7 to 20 are the time of the greatest risk.[194] The tendency to develop overwhelming forms of VZV infection in the fetus indicates the increased ability of VZV to multiply in fetal tissues, which is similar to that of other viruses such as rubella virus and CMV.

Counseling of pregnant women who have acquired varicella during pregnancy can be very difficult. Because

TABLE 13–8
Incidence of the Congenital Varicella Syndrome: Results of Prospective Studies 1960–1997

REFERENCE NO.	YEAR	First Trimester/ First 20 Weeks	Total Gestation
462	1960	0/70	0/288
66	1973	2/27	2/135
224	1984	0/23	
175	1986	1/11	1/38
67	1992	0/40	
205	1994	1/49	
194	1994	7/351	7/1291
204	1994	2/99	2/146
168	1996	0/26	
177	1997	0/22	
Total reported		13/718 (1.8%)	13/1898 (0.6%)

INCIDENCE OF SYNDROME

the congenital syndrome is so rare, termination of pregnancy is not routinely recommended, in contrast to recommendations for gestational rubella. When the syndrome does occur, however, it is likely to be extremely severe. It would be helpful if prenatal diagnosis were available, but diagnostic attempts such as measurement of maternal antibody titers and amniocentesis have not proved useful. Although blood may be obtained by cordocentesis for antibody testing, even the presence of fetal VZV IgM does not mean that the infant has the congenital varicella syndrome but only that infection with VZV has taken place. Similarly, PCR may identify an infected fetus but not necessarily one with malformations.[266]

Ultrasound has been used successfully in nine infants to identify the following fetal abnormalities after maternal varicella: hydrocephalus 12 weeks later,[199] clubfeet and hydrocephalus 13 weeks later,[228] a large bullous skin lesion originally believed to be a meningocele 15 weeks later,[231] calcifications in the liver and other organs 9, 15, and 18 weeks later,[209, 229, 256] a hypoplastic limb and clubfoot 11 and 16 weeks later,[194, 209] and a lacuna of the skull 25 weeks later.[225] In two instances, ultrasound was normal 3 weeks after maternal varicella, but the fetus was later diagnosed as having the congenital varicella syndrome.[200, 228] One infant was diagnosed with liver calcifications by ultrasonography at 27 weeks and a positive PCR for VZV; his mother had varicella at 12.5 weeks. At birth, no obvious anomalies were present and the infant did well except for development of zoster at age 8 months.[267] Thus, even defects detected by ultrasonography must be interpreted with caution.

Because 39% of patients with a hypoplastic limb also sustained brain damage and/or died in early infancy, the presence of a limb abnormality on ultrasound would seem to suggest a poor overall prognosis for the fetus. Two women were reported to have terminated their pregnancies after the diagnosis of the congenital varicella syndrome was made based on abnormal limbs at ultrasound. At physical examination the infants were found to be severely affected.[194, 268] Because abnormalities may not be expected to be detected by ultrasound immediately after maternal varicella, by the time any might be noted it may be too late to consider interruption of pregnancy, depending on the time of onset of maternal varicella.

Although it has been observed that the congenital varicella syndrome seems to represent a spectrum of involvement, most cases are in the severe range, and therefore it would be most helpful clinically if an affected fetus could be identified early. It is not known whether administration of VZIG or ACV to a pregnant woman will prevent her fetus from developing the congenital varicella syndrome. In Enders' study, there were no cases of the congenital syndrome in 97 women who were given VZIG on exposure; unfortunately, it is not known how many of these women were in the first 20 weeks of pregnancy.[194] It is hoped that after use of live attenuated varicella vaccine becomes widespread, most varicella-susceptible women will have been immunized before they become pregnant so that the syndrome will become even more rare.

PERINATAL CHICKENPOX

Perinatal chickenpox includes disease that is (1) acquired postnatally by droplet infection and (2) transplacentally transmitted or congenital. Chickenpox is considered to be transplacentally transmitted when it occurs within 10 days of birth.

Postnatally Acquired Chickenpox

Postnatally acquired chickenpox, which begins between 10 and 28 days after birth, is generally mild.[269] The experiences with nosocomial chickenpox infections in the newborn nursery that were described in a previous section further corroborate the benign nature of the disease and the fact that transmission to neonates in this environment is inefficient and rarely reaches epidemic proportions.

Deaths among neonates caused by postnatally acquired disease are very rare. There are data indicating an appreciably higher incidence of complications or deaths in neonates than in older children.[91, 96–98, 103, 269, 270] Preblud and associates found that of 92 reported deaths caused by varicella from 1968 to 1978 in children younger than 1 year of age, only 5 occurred in newborns (age 8 hours to 19 days). Although mortality was increased by a factor of 4 in infants younger than 1 year of age compared with older children, there was a low calculated death rate for varicella throughout childhood (8 in 100,000 patients if younger than 1 year old and 2 in 100,000 patients aged 1 to 14 years).[269] One 15-day-old infant with severe disseminated chickenpox born to a woman who developed varicella 7 days after delivery has been described.[270] The child survived; ACV was administered for 10 days. The only other report in the English literature of severe postnatally acquired varicella in an infant younger than 1 month old is that of Gustafson and colleagues.[91] This full-term infant with Turner's syndrome was exposed to varicella at 7 days of age, developed more than 200 vesicles, and died of pneumonia; however, the role of VZV in the child's death was unclear because no autopsy was performed.

Congenital Chickenpox

Congenital chickenpox is not inevitable when maternal chickenpox occurs in the 21 days preceding parturition. In 8 of 34 reported cases (24%) of maternal disease with onset during this period did chickenpox develop in the neonate within the first 10 days of life.[93, 131, 167, 169] An identical attack rate of 24% for congenital varicella after the occurrence of maternal varicella within 17 days preceding delivery was arrived at by Meyers, who reviewed many cases in the literature and 14 examples reported to the Centers for Disease Control in 1972 to 1973.[271] However, higher attack rates, on the order of 50%, were reported in two studies on the efficacy of passive immunization to prevent severe neonatal varicella.[272, 273] In Meyers' study, there was no statistically significant relationship between day of onset of the rash in the mother and subsequent attack rates of congenital varicella.[271] Seven of 22 neonates born to mothers whose rash appeared less than 5 days ante partum ultimately developed congenital chickenpox, whereas 4 of 24 infants born to mothers whose rash began 5 to 14 days ante partum had congenital disease.[271] These data indicate that the attack rate in congenital varicella (25–50%) is lower than that following household exposure to VZV (90%) and suggest that blood-borne transmission is less efficient than by the skin and respiratory routes.

The incubation period in congenital varicella, defined as the interval between onset of rash in the mother and onset in the fetus or neonate, is usually 9 to 15 days.[274] This interval is slightly shorter than the normal postnatal incubation period, possibly because fetal tissues are more susceptible to VZV than more mature tissues. Very rarely, presumably when fetal infection is due to the primary maternal viremia, the exanthem appears in the mother and neonate within 3 days of each other[96] or even simultaneously.[274] The average incubation period in 36 cases reported in the literature was 11 days, with a maximum of 16 days. In only three instances was the incubation period less than 6 days.[271]

In contrast to postnatally acquired neonatal chickenpox, congenital chickenpox can be associated with significant mortality. Severe cases clinically resemble varicella in the immunocompromised host. A child who died of hemorrhagic varicella with pulmonary and liver involvement is shown in Figure 13–1. The spectrum of illness also includes extremely mild infections with only a handful of vesicles. Erlich and co-workers first observed that infants born with the rash or who had an early onset of rash survived, whereas those who died had a relatively late onset of rash.[128] It was hypothesized that in those neonates with early onset, maternal illness had occurred long enough before parturition to allow antibodies to be elaborated by the mother and to cross the placenta. Subsequent reports offer strong confirmation of these observations. There were no deaths among 22 infants with congenital chickenpox (reviewed by Meyers) whose onset of rash occurred between birth and 4 days of age. In contrast, 4 of 19 (21%) neonates in whom the rash began at 5 to 10 days of age died (Table 13–9).[271] These four deaths occurred among 13 neonates (31%)

whose mothers' exanthems developed within 4 days before birth, but no deaths were observed among 23 neonates with congenital chickenpox whose mothers developed a rash 5 or more days before birth.

Further support for the protective or modifying effect of maternal antibody has come from measurements of placental transfer of IgG to VZV.[86] When varicella occurred more than 1 week before delivery, complement-fixing antibody titers in maternal and cord blood were similar. In contrast, when infection occurred 3 to 5 days before delivery, maternal antibody was present at parturition and antibodies to VZV in the neonate were absent or at least eightfold lower. These data suggest that a lag of several days occurs before IgG antibodies to VZV cross the placenta and equilibrate with the fetal circulation. The development of mild congenital varicella in the presence of placentally transferred maternal antibody has also been demonstrated using the more sensitive FAMA test.[57] The neonate may be at risk to develop severe varicella because the immune system is immature, as has been demonstrated by Kohl with regard to host defense against HSV.[275]

ZOSTER IN NEONATES AND OLDER CHILDREN

The most characteristic feature of zoster is the localization of the rash. It is nearly always unilateral, does not cross the midline, and is typically limited to an area of skin served by one to three sensory ganglia. In children, prodromata of malaise, fever, headache, and nausea may be observed. Pain and paresthesias in the involved dermatome may precede the exanthem by 4 or 5 days. Involvement of the dermatomes of the head, neck, and trunk is more common than involvement of the extremities, a distribution that also reflects the density of lesions in chickenpox.[37] Erythematous papules give rise to grouped vesicles, which progress to pustules in 2 to 4 days. New crops of vesicles may keep appearing for a week. Pain may be associated with the exanthem and usually abates as the skin lesions scab; in elderly adults, severe and incapacitating neuralgia of the involved nerve may persist for months. Cutaneous dissemination of vesicles to sites distant from the involved dermatome is observed uncommonly and is more frequent in compromised hosts such as patients with lymphoma or immunologic deficiencies.

Zoster occurs as host defense mechanisms against VZV wane in a person who has previously experienced chickenpox. Because most children develop chickenpox during the school years and immunity is relatively durable, this hypothesis presumes that zoster will occur predominantly in the aged and will be rare in neonates. Among 192 patients with zoster in a general practice, the attack rate increased progressively with age.[37] Only six patients were younger than 10 years old, the youngest being 2 years of age. In two reported series describing zoster in a total of 22 children, only two cases occurred in children younger than 2 years old.[167, 276] These reports confirm the rarity of zoster among infants. When zoster occurs in children who have not previously had chickenpox, there is often a history of intrauterine exposure

TABLE 13–9
Deaths from Congenital Varicella in Relation to Date of Onset of Rash in Mother or Neonate

	NEONATAL DEATHS	NEONATAL CASES	%
Day of onset of rash in neonate			
0–4	0	22	0
5–10	4	19	21
Onset of maternal rash, days ante partum			
≥5	0	23	0
0–4	4	13	31

Modified from Meyers JD. Congenital varicella in term infants: risk reconsidered. J Infect Dis 129:215, 1974, with permission from the University of Chicago.

to VZV. In these reports, the mothers contracted chickenpox during gestation but gave birth to normal infants who, without ever developing chickenpox despite frequent childhood exposure, developed typical zoster at a young age, many in the first few months of life.[68, 255, 277–281] In most of these infants, the course of zoster was benign. One child developed a second attack of zoster at 10 months of age, the first having occurred at age 4 months.[277] Another developed zoster at the age of 18 days. The mother had varicella during her fourteenth week of pregnancy. The infant had no characteristic stigmata of the congenital varicella syndrome such as skin scarring, eye involvement, or limb hypoplasia, but he had encephalitis with bulbar paralysis and frequent aspiration.[255]

Although there are six reports of zoster during the neonatal period,[282–287] it is doubtful whether any of these cases diagnosed on clinical grounds are authentic examples of zoster. HSV may produce a vesicular exanthem in the newborn that appears to have a dermatomal distribution. Therefore, virus isolation (or demonstration of VZV antigen from skin lesions) is required before a diagnosis of zoster can be accepted. Serologic studies are not useful in differentiating these diseases.

Diagnosis and Differential Diagnosis

CHICKENPOX

In a neonate with a widespread, generalized vesicular exanthem and a history of either recent maternal varicella or postnatal exposure, a diagnosis of chickenpox can usually be made with confidence on clinical grounds alone. Greater difficulty is encountered when lesions are few or when there is no history of exposure.

Diagnostic Techniques

If laboratory diagnosis is required, it is best accomplished by demonstration of VZV antigen or DNA in skin lesions or isolation of virus from vesicular fluid. VZV antigen may be demonstrated by using immunofluorescence, employing a monoclonal antibody to VZV that is conjugated to fluorescein and is commercially available.[288, 289] For virus isolation, fluid should be promptly inoculated onto tissue cultures because VZV is rather labile. PCR has proven extremely sensitive and accurate for diagnosis of VZV infections, although it remains a research test in most locations.[113, 290–296] In situ hybridization is also a useful diagnostic technique.[210, 297, 298]

VZV infections may also be documented by demonstration of a fourfold or greater rise in VZV antibody titer, by using a sensitive test such as FAMA or ELISA. The presence of specific IgM in one serum specimen suggests recent VZV infection.[35, 36, 299] Persistence of VZV antibody beyond 8 months of age is highly suggestive of intrauterine varicella, providing there is no history of clinical varicella after birth.[22] Persistence of VZV antibody with no fall in titer over several months in a young infant (as long as all sera are tested simultaneously) is highly suggestive of intrauterine infection. An FAMA or LA antibody titer of 1:4 or greater beyond 8 months of life is suggestive of immunity to varicella, provided that the patient has not received gamma globulin or other blood products in the previous 3 to 4 months. Physicians do need to be aware, however, that no serologic test is 100% accurate for identifying individuals immune to varicella, although in general these antibody tests are quite reliable.[300]

Differential Diagnosis

Several diseases may be considered in the differential diagnosis of varicella in the newborn:

1. *Neonatal Herpes Simplex Virus.* Cutaneous lesions may be relatively sparse and may be absent altogether despite widespread visceral dissemination. Vesicles tend to occur in clusters rather than in the more even distribution seen in chickenpox. Fever, marked toxicity, and encephalitis are more common in neonates with HSV. Stained smears of vesicle fluid (Tzanck preparation) are of no help in differentiating HSV from varicella because both are characterized by multinucleated giant cells and intranuclear inclusion bodies. In cell cultures, HSV typically produces a widespread cytopathic effect in 24 to 48 hours, whereas the cytopathic effect caused by VZV is cell associated and focal and develops more slowly. Indirect immunofluorescence using monoclonal antibodies conjugated to fluorescein can be performed on smears of skin scrapings, which, if positive, can identify VZV, HSV 1, and HSV 2 within several hours. Paired serum samples can be examined for rising antibody titers to both HSV and VZV antigens. It is exceedingly rare for varicella to develop in a newborn in the absence of any (i.e., infant or mother) exposure to varicella or zoster. In contrast, most infants with neonatal HSV have no recognized exposure to the virus.

2. *Smallpox.* Smallpox is traditionally part of the differential diagnosis of vesicular lesions in neonates. At present, however, smallpox has been eradicated, so that the following discussion is mainly of academic interest. Smallpox modified by exposure to vaccinia in the distant past and alastrim (variola minor) may be particularly difficult to distinguish from chickenpox. Classically, the vesicles of smallpox appear to be at the same stage of development instead of showing the pattern of crops over a period of several days. A centrifugal distribution is common. Accurate diagnosis may be achieved in a matter of hours by electron microscopy of the vesicle fluid or crusts; such microscopic examination reveals virus particles whose morphology is very different from that of viruses of the herpes family.

3. *Disseminated Vaccinia.* This disease is extremely rare today because smallpox vaccine (vaccinia virus) is not used. Vaccinia can be considered in a neonate exposed postnatally to a person who has been recently vaccinated. The lesions resemble those of smallpox. Impression smears of vesicle fluid do not show intranuclear inclusions or giant cells. Laboratory diagnosis may be achieved by electron microscopy and immunofluorescence.

4. *Contact Dermatitis.* After exposure to specific chemi-

cal irritants, papules and vesicles may appear. Typically, these appear on exposed body surfaces and do not have the characteristic distribution of chickenpox or smallpox.

5. *Hand-Foot-and-Mouth Syndrome.* A vesicular exanthem usually caused by coxsackievirus A16 or A5 may be observed during the enterovirus season (summer or early autumn). Vesicles rarely exceed a dozen in number and typically occur on the distal extremities, especially the palms and soles. Vesicular lesions that ulcerate quickly may also be seen in the oropharynx. The causative virus is readily isolated from vesicle fluid or from feces.

6. *Impetigo.* Impetigo may be seen in neonates. In bullous impetigo (pemphigus neonatorum), large blebs are present instead of the smaller vesicles of chickenpox. This disease, which is caused by *Staphylococcus aureus*, may be associated with high fever, toxicity, septicemia, and death.

ZOSTER

Zoster is usually easily recognized by the typical dermatomal distribution of the vesicular lesions. In the differential diagnosis, the main entity to be distinguished in the neonatal period is HSV appearing in a linear pattern. Identification of VZV or HSV antigen by immunofluorescence or virus isolation is the only reliable means of differentiating these entities when the distribution of the exanthem is linear. Contact dermatitis should also be considered in the differential diagnosis of zosteriform lesions in the neonatal period.

Therapy

ANTIVIRAL CHEMOTHERAPY

The antiviral drug ACV is the drug of choice for treatment of potentially severe or severe VZV infections.[301, 302] ACV itself has no antiviral action; however, when it is phosphorylated by enzymes produced by cells infected with VZV, it is incorporated as a DNA chain terminator and it also inhibits viral DNA polymerase. Because these actions occur only in virus-infected cells, ACV is well tolerated and associated with little toxicity. The drug is available in topical, oral, and intravenous formulations.

Because most VZV infections in normal hosts are self-limited, and long-term toxicity of ACV in the fetus is unknown, ACV is not usually recommended for use during pregnancy. However, pregnant women with severe varicella, especially if accompanied by pneumonia, should be treated. ACV crosses the placenta,[303] and a registry of patients (and their offspring) who have received ACV during pregnancy has been established.[190, 191] Supportive respiratory therapy (nasal oxygen, tracheostomy, ventilatory assistance) should be used as needed. Controlled studies of corticosteroids for varicella pneumonia are not available; therefore, steroids are not recommended. Antibiotics should be given if there is evidence of bacterial superinfection. As mentioned in a previous section, anecdotal reports on the apparently successful use of ACV in pregnant women with varicella have been published, although controlled studies have not been performed. There is no information on the use of ACV for pregnant women with zoster. Presumably because zoster would be expected to be self-limited in most women of childbearing age, there would be little need for antiviral therapy in this situation.

ACV has been most effective when it is administered within 3 days after the onset of varicella or zoster. The usual adult dose for intravenous ACV is 10 mg/kg, given three times a day. Orally administered ACV has been found to have a modest effect on the fever and rash of varicella in otherwise healthy populations. A multicenter double-blind placebo-controlled collaborative study involving 815 similarly treated children, given 20 mg/kg of ACV four times per day, shortened the course of illness by about 1 day.[304] The benefit to secondary household cases was not increased beyond that of primary cases. Similar results emerged from a study involving adolescents with varicella.[305] The modest benefit conferred by oral ACV therapy is not surprising in view of the self-limited nature of chickenpox in children and the poor oral absorption of ACV. There is a similar small benefit for adults with varicella, who were given oral ACV 800 mg five times a day for 5 days, within 24 hours of onset of rash.[306, 307] In the double-blind placebo-controlled study of Wallace and associates, involving 76 military recruits, the duration of illness was shortened by about 1 day and the personnel were able to return to work 1 day sooner on average, if they received ACV.[307]

Although there is little information on the use of ACV in newborns, it has been used to treat a great many infants with neonatal HSV infection. In a study in which 95 infants received ACV (30 mg/kg per day intravenously), no short- or long-term toxicity was observed.[302, 308, 309] There is little information, however, on the use of the larger dose usually employed to treat VZV infections in newborns (a dose of 1500 mg/m^2 per day is about three times that of the dose for neonatal HSV infection). For infants with severe disease, however, this dosage has been employed without obvious difficulties, although there are no controlled studies. Pharmacokinetic studies have indicated that dose adjustments may be necessary in premature infants and/or those with hepatic or renal dysfunction.[310] There are no data with regard to use of oral ACV for neonatal infections caused by VZV, and, in addition, ACV is poorly absorbed when given by the gastrointestinal route. Therefore, only intravenous ACV can be recommended for treatment of severe varicella in the neonate.

Prevention

IMMUNITY TO VARICELLA-ZOSTER VIRUS

It is gradually becoming clear that immunity to VZV is often incomplete in some persons. Although it was recognized years ago that waning of immunity to VZV might predispose one to zoster,[37] that immunity to varicella may also wane on rare occasion has been recognized only fairly recently. Immunologic evidence of reinfection with VZV, manifested by an increase in specific IgG or IgA concentration, or the presence of IgM, as well as an increase in the CMI response to VZV, presumably due to asymptomatic reinfection, has been documented in adults with a household exposure to varicella.[311, 312] In addition, clinical reinfection with VZV has been observed in some persons despite a positive antibody titer at exposure.[313–316] Most clinical reinfections are mild, however, which suggests that partial immunity to the virus may be present. It has also been suggested that cellular immunity at the mucosal level may play an important role in protection against clinical varicella. In one study by Bogger-Goren and co-workers, children with positive responses were likely to be protected against varicella after household exposure even if they were seronegative; in contrast, children with negative responses became infected.[317] Secretory IgA against VZV has also been demonstrated after chickenpox.[318]

Incomplete immunity to VZV is associated with development of zoster as well as reinfection with the virus. In addition to clinical zoster, silent reactivation of latent VZV in those who have had previous varicella probably also occurs; this may be detected immunologically by an increase in antibody titer or the transient appearance of specific IgM.[36, 319–321] At times, clinical manifestations of zoster such as pain may occur in the absence of a rash, so-called zoster sine herpete. Silent reactivation of VZV in bone marrow transplant patients has been demonstrated by PCR.[322] Zoster results in patients who have latent VZV infection when specific CMI is depressed.[116, 118, 119, 323] Defective antibody responses to VZV gps have not been associated with development of zoster in immunocompromised persons.[324] In the elderly, an increased incidence of zoster has been associated with loss of CMI to VZV.[325, 326] Antibody to VZV does not wane with age but rather tends to increase.[327] Thus immunity to VZV may be seen as a complex interaction between humoral and CMI responses, with the possibility of partial as well as complete immunity to the virus. It is possible to provide humoral immunity to persons at high risk to develop severe varicella by passive immunization with VZIG. Although used successfully to prevent severe varicella, passive immunization has not prevented zoster in those at high risk to develop it,[328] nor is it believed to be useful to treat patients with varicella or zoster.[329] Passive immunization should therefore not be employed to try to prevent development of varicella pneumonia in the pregnant woman with chickenpox or dissemination in an already infected infant. It is uncertain whether passive immunization of a woman with varicella will prevent infection of her fetus or development of the congenital varicella syndrome. It is possible to increase CMI to VZV by immunization, and whether this approach can prevent or modify zoster is being explored.[330–332]

PASSIVE IMMUNIZATION: ZOSTER IMMUNOGLOBULIN AND VARICELLA-ZOSTER IMMUNE GLOBULIN

Controlled studies have indicated that (1) pooled immunoglobulin (IG) attenuates but does not prevent chickenpox when administered to susceptible family contacts[63] and (2) zoster immunoglobulin (ZIG) prevents clinical chickenpox when given to susceptible healthy children within 72 hours of household exposure.[333] Additional uncontrolled studies in immunocompromised children, such as leukemics receiving maintenance chemotherapy, at high risk to develop severe or fatal varicella have indicated that ZIG administered within 3 to 5 days of a household exposure usually modifies varicella so that the infection is mild or subclinical.[334–336] ZIG that was prepared from plasma from donors with zoster has now been supplanted by VZIG, which is prepared from normal donors with high antibody titers to VZV. The antibody content of the two preparations is similar,[337] and the protective efficacy is also similar.[338] VZIG is potentially more widely available than ZIG. VZIG is licensed in the United States, and it is commercially available through the American Red Cross and local blood centers.[193] Administration of VZIG may prolong the incubation period of varicella.[335]

Passive immunization has also been studied for its possible efficacy in modifying severe congenital varicella that may occur in the infant of a woman who develops chickenpox close to term. Infants born to women with the onset of varicella more than 5 days before delivery can be expected to have mild infection,[57, 128, 271, 339, 340] and these infants do not require passive immunization. In contrast, infants born to women who develop varicella 5 days or less before delivery are at risk to develop disseminated or fatal varicella, and these infants can be expected to benefit from passive immunization. In an uncontrolled study by Hanngren and co-workers, of 41 neonates born to women who developed varicella between 4 days before and 2 days after delivery, the illness appeared to be modified.[272] These infants received 1 ml of ZIG. Although there was an attack rate of 51% and the incubation period averaged 11 days, instead of the expected mortality rate of about 30% there were no fatalities and 13 of 21 (62%) had fewer than 20 vesicles with no fever. Two (10%) infants had rather severe infections, and 1 was treated with interferon. In a similar study of VZIG by Preblud and colleagues, in 132 infants, a similar attack rate of varicella of 45% was observed.[273] In this study, 125 units (1.25 ml) of VZIG was administered. The illness also appeared to be modified in that of 53 infants with varicella, 74% had fewer than 50 vesicles and only 10% had more than 100 vesicles. No antiviral therapy was given; there was one death in the group, but it was not clear that it was due to varicella. The high attack rates of varicella in these studies in comparison with historical data have not been explained. In previous studies, attack rates in similar infants of 24% in both late[271] and overall[175] pregnancy have been reported. Successful passive immunization would, if anything, be expected to decrease the attack rate rather than increase it. Nevertheless, the mildness of the illness and absence of mortality in these two studies are suggestive if not proof positive of successful passive immunization of infants born to women with varicella at term.

It is therefore recommended that VZIG be administered to infants whose mothers have the onset of varicella 5 days or less before delivery or in the first 48 hours after delivery.[193, 341] A dose of 125 units (1.25 ml or one vial) should be administered intramuscularly as soon as possible after birth. Administration of VZIG to the mother before delivery of the infant is not recommended because a larger dose will be required to passively immunize the infant and no benefit to the mother will result. Early delivery of the infant of a mother with active varicella is also not recommended; the longer the infant remains in utero, the more likely there will be transplacental transfer of maternal antibody. A diagram of the relationship between maternal and infant varicella, development of maternal antibodies, and transplacental transfer of these antibodies is shown in Figure 13–5. Because women with zoster near term have high antibody titers to VZV, it is not necessary to administer VZIG to their infants.

A number of infants who developed severe or fatal congenital varicella despite prompt administration of VZIG in adequate dosage have been reported.[342–347] The reason for the severity of these cases has not been explained adequately; presumably, they were immunologically normal infants. Many of these children were reported from the United Kingdom, and it may be that VZIG used there is less potent than that produced in the United States. The antibody titers of the two preparations have never been compared. It seems obvious, however, that passively immunized infants need to be observed carefully for the rare instance in which antiviral therapy may also be required. Rapid evolution of large numbers of vesicles, hemorrhagic manifestations, and respiratory involvement would indicate use of ACV. Some investigators have recommended prophylactic use of intravenously administered ACV in any infant who develops varicella despite passive immunization[343, 344, 348, 349]; however, this strategy has not been formally studied. Based on the studies cited previously, the overwhelming majority of passively immunized infants who develop clinical illness will have mild or moderate infections. Administration of ACV to all such infants who develop clinical illness would result in needless hospitalization of many infants and potential iatrogenic problems and would not be cost-effective. Unless further data become available, ACV should be given only to infants who manifest early signs of potentially severe varicella.

Although it is recommended that VZIG be administered to infants born to women who develop varicella in the first 2 days after delivery, there are few reports to indicate that this timing of birth at onset of maternal varicella is associated with increased risk to the infant. One of the reported infants with fatal varicella despite passive immunization was born to a woman who developed chickenpox on the second postpartum day.[345] A child with severe varicella whose mother developed chickenpox 3 days after delivery has also been reported.[350] This child was treated with a leukocyte transfusion from her mother and thymic hormone and survived. In view of the absence of data indicating efficacy, and the potential danger of graft-versus-host reaction after leukocyte transfusion in immunocompromised patients,[351] this therapy cannot be recommended.

To minimize the possibility of infection of the infant, mother and infant should be separated until the mother's chickenpox vesicles have dried, even if the infant has been passively immunized. Normally, this will be 5 to 7 days after onset of maternal rash. Should the infant develop clinical varicella, the mother may continue to care for the infant.

Pregnant women who are closely exposed to persons with varicella or zoster and who have no history of varicella and are also seronegative may be passively immunized with VZIG.[193] Although precise information regarding dosage is not available, a dose of 5 ml (625 units) is usually recommended for adults. The rationale for passive immunization of the mother is to protect her from developing severe chickenpox.

Because some low-birth-weight infants may have low or absent levels of transplacentally acquired maternal VZV antibody, it is recommended that infants of less than 28 weeks' gestation and/or who weighed less than 1000 g at birth be passively immunized with VZIG after close exposure.[193, 341] Administration of VZIG to infants who are 2 to 7 days old at the time of exposure is not recommended but may be done optionally to decrease morbidity from varicella in this age group.[352] VZIG should not be used to try to control nosocomial varicella

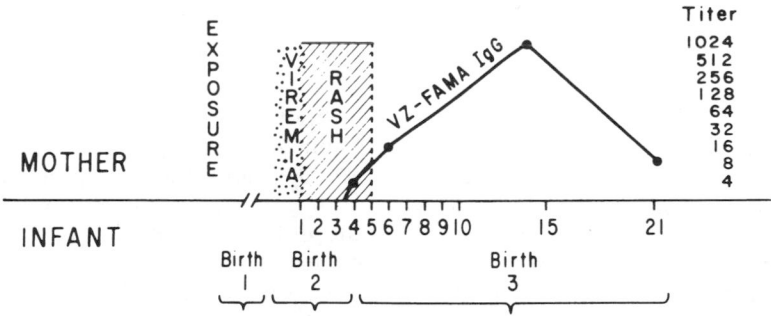

FIGURE 13–5 Diagrammatic representation of transmission of varicella-zoster virus (VZV) and VZV antibody to the fetus in maternal varicella near term. When the infant is born during the maternal incubation period (1), no varicella occurs unless the infant is exposed postnatally to the infection. When the infant is born 0 to 4 days after onset of maternal varicella (2), disseminated varicella may develop because the infection will not be modified by maternal antibody. The onset of the varicella occurs between 5 and 10 days of age. Infants born 5 days or more after maternal varicella (3) receive maternal antibody, which leads to mild infection. This diagram is based on 50 newborn infants with varicella. (From Gershon A. Varicella in mother and infant: problems old and new. *In* Krugman S, Gershon A [eds]. Infection of the Fetus and Newborn Infant, New York, Alan R Liss, 1975, pp 79–95, with permission.)

because it does not necessarily prevent varicella but rather modifies it.

GUIDELINES FOR PREVENTIVE MEASURES AND ISOLATION PROCEDURES IN THE NURSERY

In contrast to transplacentally transmitted chickenpox, there is little evidence that postnatally acquired chickenpox (defined as disease beginning after 10 days of age) is significantly more serious in infants than in older children (see preceding section). Nevertheless, despite evidence cited previously indicating that nosocomial chickenpox among infants in the nursery is relatively uncommon, it is desirable to institute preventive measures to minimize the possibility of transmission of infection to other neonates, mothers, and hospital personnel. Any hospital patient isolated because of chickenpox or zoster should be in a separate room with the door closed, preferably in a room with air pressure negative to that in the corridor. Visitors and staff should be limited to persons immune to varicella. They should wear a new gown for each entry and wash their hands when leaving. Bedding and tissues soiled with respiratory excreta of the patient should be bagged and autoclaved. Special precautions for feces, urine, and needles or blood products are not required. Terminal disinfection of the room is likewise unnecessary.

Guidelines for isolation procedures and other measures are summarized in Table 13–10. If at the time mother and infant are ready for discharge from the hospital there are siblings or others at home with active VZV infections, one of the following alternatives is recommended: (1) the mother and neonate may be sent home after boarding the older siblings with immune relatives until they are no longer infectious, generally when no new vesicles have appeared for 72 hours and all lesions have progressed to the stage of crusts; (2) the mother can return home while the neonate remains in the nursery; (3) the neonate can be boarded with a surrogate mother until the siblings are no longer infectious; or (4) VZIG may be given to the newborn. If siblings at home develop chickenpox at the time of delivery or shortly after birth and the mother lacks a definite history of previous chickenpox, the first or last alternative is recommended. Serologic determination of the mother's immune status to varicella is recommended. Women with detectable VZV antibodies may be discharged home. Those who are seronegative should be offered varicella vaccine. Theoretically, if a woman has a history of varicella, her newborn should be at least partially protected from varicella. It seems prudent, however, to use a conservative approach, such as outlined here, because the real risk of varicella to the newborn is unknown.

When a mother with a negative history is exposed to chickenpox or zoster 6 to 20 days ante partum, she may become infectious before the onset of exanthem, during hospitalization for labor and the puerperium, assuming an average stay of 72 hours. This calculation is based on a minimum incubation period (exposure until onset of rash) of 10 days and a period of communicability preceding the exanthem by 3 days. On the other hand, when maternal exposure occurs less than 6 days before the onset of labor, the mother is unlikely to become infectious until after she has returned home. In either case, if the mother is exposed to chickenpox during the 20-day period ante partum, it is advisable to send both the mother and infant home at the earliest possible date.

No special management is necessary for other mothers and infants in the nursery, or for physicians and nurses potentially exposed in either the delivery room or the nursery if they have previously had chickenpox. In the absence of a positive history, immediate serologic testing to determine the immune status of exposed hospital personnel may be performed when diagnostic facilities are available. Exposed personnel with negative histories may continue to work in the nursery for a period of 8 days after exposure pending serologic results because they are not potentially infectious during this period. Personnel with positive VZV antibody titers in serum are probably immune. Nonimmune (seronegative) nursery and delivery personnel should be excluded from patient care activities between days 8 and 21 after exposure. Subsequently, they should be strongly encouraged to be immunized against varicella.

The greatest risk of nosocomial chickenpox exists when a mother develops chickenpox lesions less than 5 days before delivery or in the immediate postpartum period. If the neonate is born with lesions (congenital chickenpox), the mother and her newborn should be isolated together and sent home as soon as they are clinically stable. Other exposed mothers and infants in the nursery may also be sent home at the earliest date possible. Restriction of patient care activities and serologic testing of exposed delivery and nursery personnel as described earlier should be instituted. Passive immunization of exposed infants is optional considering the usually benign course of postnatally acquired chickenpox.

When maternal chickenpox occurs within approximately 5 days of delivery or immediately post partum and no lesions are present in the neonate, the mother and the infant should be isolated separately. Transplacentally acquired chickenpox, beginning 7 to 15 days after disease appears in the mother, will ultimately develop in about half of these neonates despite administration of VZIG. The remainder will be at risk of postnatally acquired chickenpox unless isolated from their mothers. If no lesions develop in the neonate by the time its mother is noninfectious, both may be sent home. Guidelines for exposed hospital personnel and patients are like those described previously.

In congenital chickenpox, lesions may be absent in the mother at the time of delivery but present in the neonate. This may occur either after rare subclinical infection in the mother[93] or because the onset of the exanthem in the infant occurs after the lesions in the mother have already healed. In either circumstance, the mother is not at risk and may be isolated with her newborn infant.

ACTIVE IMMUNIZATION AGAINST CHICKENPOX

A live attenuated varicella vaccine was developed in Japan by Takahashi and colleagues.[353] This vaccine was

⬜ **TABLE 13–10**
Guidelines for Preventive Measures After Exposure to Chickenpox in the Nursery or Maternity Ward

TYPE OF EXPOSURE OR DISEASE	CHICKENPOX LESIONS PRESENT		DISPOSITION
	Mother	Neonate	
A. Siblings at home have active chickenpox when neonate and mother are ready for discharge from hospital	No	No	1. *Mother:* if she has a history of chickenpox, she may return home. Without a history, she should be tested for VZV antibody titer.[a] If test is positive, she may return home. If test is negative, VZIG[b] may be administered and she is discharged home. If she is antibody negative, 3 months after VZIG she should be immunized. 2. *Neonate:* may be discharged home with mother if mother has history of varicella or is VZV antibody positive. If mother is susceptible, administer VZIG to infant and discharge home or place in protective isolation (see text).
B. Mother with no history of chickenpox; exposed during period 6–20 days ante partum[d]	No	No	1. *Exposed mother and infant:* send home at earliest date unless siblings at home have communicable chickenpox.[c] If so, may administer VZIG and discharge home, as above (see text). 2. *Other mothers and infants:* no special management indicated. 3. *Hospital personnel:* no precautions indicated if there is a history of previous chickenpox or zoster. In absence of history, immediate serologic testing is indicated to determine immune status.[a] Nonimmune personnel should be excluded from patient contact until 21 days after an intimate exposure. Vaccination of nonimmune personnel should be encouraged. Immunized personnel who develop a vaccine-associated rash should be excluded from work until rash has healed. 4. If mother develops varicella 1 to 2 days post partum, infant should be given VZIG.
C. Onset of maternal chickenpox ante partum[d] or post partum	Yes	No	1. *Infected mother:* isolate until no longer clinically infectious. If seriously ill, treat with ACV.[e] 2. *Infected mother's infant:* administer VZIG[b] to neonates born to mothers with onset of chickenpox <5 days before delivery and isolate separately from mother. Send home with mother if no lesions develop by the time mother is noninfectious. 3. *Other mothers and infants:* send home at earliest date. VZIG may be given to exposed neonates. 4. *Hospital personnel:* same as B-3.
D. Onset of maternal chickenpox ante partum[c]			1. *Mother:* isolation unnecessary. 2. *Infant:* isolate from other infants but not from mother. 3. *Other mothers and infants:* same as C-3 (if exposed). 4. *Hospital personnel:* same as B-3.
E. Congenital chickenpox	No	Yes	1. *Infected infant and mother:* same as D-1 and 2. 2. *Other mothers and infants:* same as C-3. 3. *Hospital personnel:* same as B-3.

[a]Send serum to virus diagnostic laboratory for determination of antibodies to VZV by a sensitive technique such as FAMA, LA, or ELISA (see text). Personnel may continue to work for 8 days after exposure pending serologic results because they are not potentially infectious during this period. Antibodies to VZV >1:4 probably are indicative of immunity.

[b]VZIG is available through the American Red Cross (see text). The dose for a newborn is 1.25 ml (1 vial). The dose for a pregnant woman is conventionally 6.25 ml (5 vials).

[c]Considered noninfectious when no new vesicles have appeared for 72 hours and all lesions have crusted.

[d]If exposure occurred less than 6 days ante partum, mother would not be potentially infectious until at least 72 hours post partum.

[e]Dosage of ACV for pregnant woman is 30 mg/kg per day; for seriously ill infant with varicella 750–1500 mg/m^2 per day.

licensed by the Food and Drug Administration in the United States for varicella-susceptible healthy children older than 1 year of age, adolescents, and adults in 1995. The vaccine is also licensed for routine use in a number of countries in Europe and in Asia, including Japan. The vaccine has proved to be safe and highly effective,[354, 355] and it is recommended for routine use by the American Academy of Pediatrics[341, 356] and the Centers for Disease Control and Prevention.[193] The vaccine not only protects against varicella in about 90% of those vaccinated but also decreases the incidence of zoster in immunocompromised patients and presumably in healthy vaccinees as well.[323, 354, 357]

The major adverse effect of vaccination is development of a mild transient rash about 1 month (range from a few days to up to 6 weeks) after immunization. The main concern about the rash is the possibility of spread of the vaccine-type virus to varicella-susceptibles intimately exposed to a vaccinee with a rash. Contagion has not been reported in the absence of rash, and contact cases have uniformly been mild. There is no evidence of clinical reversion to wild type VZV.[42, 153, 354] The vaccine-type virus spreads less efficiently than the wild-type virus, by a factor of about 4 in children with leukemia who were immunized.[42] Furthermore, there is a much greater tendency to develop rash and also to transmit vaccine-type VZV from immunocompromised vaccinees than from healthy vaccinated individuals. A quantitative comparison is difficult to make, but in household contacts of leukemic vaccinees with rash, transmission occurred in about 25%.[42] In contrast, since the licensure of vaccine in the United States, about 15 million doses of vaccine have been distributed by the manufacturer, with only 3 reported instances of spread. (There is one additional recorded instance of spread of varicella vaccine from a healthy vaccinee involving an experimental vaccine.[358]) Unfortunately one instance occurred when a healthy child was immunized and his pregnant mother developed mild varicella from which the vaccine-type virus was identified by PCR.[359] The mother terminated the pregnancy, but the products of conception were negative for VZV by PCR. At this point it is important to immunize susceptible women of childbearing age before they become pregnant. The risk of immunizing healthy toddlers is calculated to be lower than not immunizing them and risking their development of natural varicella that would expose a pregnant varicella-susceptible pregnant mother to the fully virulent virus.[360] Hopefully, widespread use of vaccine in the United States will decrease or even eliminate the problems of congenital malformations and severe varicella in the neonatal period, as has occurred with rubella. Although varicella vaccine-type virus has not been shown to cause the congenital varicella syndrome, immunization during pregnancy is contraindicated. It is also recommended that immunized women refrain from becoming pregnant for at least 3 months after receipt of vaccine.[193, 341, 356] Individuals older than 13 years of age are recommended to receive two doses of vaccine 4 to 8 weeks apart. The reported seroconversion rate after two doses of vaccine in healthy adults is about 90%.[153, 354] Ideally, women should have serologic testing for immunity after immunization, but at present a negative antibody titer after immunization does not necessarily indicate vaccine failure since commercially available ELISA antibody tests may fail to identify some individuals who have responded to the vaccine.[361]

MEASLES

Measles (rubeola) is a highly communicable childhood disease whose hallmarks are fever, coryza, conjunctivitis, cough, and a generalized maculopapular rash that usually appears 1 to 2 days after a specific enanthem (Koplik's spots). The word *measles* means "little spots" and is derived from the Dutch word for the disease, *maeselen*, a diminutive of *maese*, meaning "spot" or "stain."[362] Although measles was described in medieval times, it was not until the seventeenth century that Sydenham clearly differentiated the disease from smallpox and scarlet fever.

The Organism

CLASSIFICATION AND MORPHOLOGY

Measles virus is a paramyxovirus, but some of its properties, such as the lack of neuraminidase, are distinct from those of other members of this family. Like paramyxoviruses, measles virions have a diameter of 100 to 250 nm and consist of a helical ribonucleoprotein core surrounded by a lipid envelope.

In cell culture, virions replicate predominantly in the cytoplasm and are released from the cell surface by budding. The envelope of the virion is composed of at least two gps: E, which causes membrane fusion and is crucial for infectivity, and H, the hemagglutinin. A nonglucosylated matrix protein, M, is also present on the envelope. Antibodies to gpF inhibit viral infectivity.[363] Other internal structural proteins are the large protein (L), the phosphoprotein or polymerase (P), and the nucleocapsid protein (N).

Measles virus has been fully sequenced. Recent genomic data indicate that the viruses that caused the resurgence of measles between 1989 and 1992 were not new strains, that most of the reported cases in 1994 and 1995 were the result of international importation of virus, and that aggressive control measures in 1992 resulted in control of the viruses circulating at that time.[364]

PROPAGATION OF MEASLES VIRUS

Primary cultures of human embryonic kidney and rhesus monkey kidney cells have proved to be superior to all others for the isolation of measles virus, although the agent has been adapted after several passages to a number of continuous cell lines.[365] Cytopathic effect on primary isolation is not generally detected before 5 to 10 days. Rapid identification may be accomplished by use of immunofluorescent staining using monoclonal antibodies.

ANTIGENIC PROPERTIES AND SEROLOGIC TESTS

Measles virus isolates are antigenically homogeneous. Some cross-reactivity of both soluble ribonucleoprotein antigens and hemagglutinins has been observed among measles and the related viruses of rinderpest and canine distemper but not with other paramyxoviruses. The hemagglutination inhibition (HI) test has essentially been replaced with more modern assays for antibodies.

ELISA has emerged as the most useful and sensitive method for measuring antibodies to measles virus.[366] A similar test that identifies specific IgM antibody and is useful diagnostically when only one serum specimen is available has also been developed.[367, 368]

Transmission and Epidemiology

TRANSMISSION BY DROPLETS AND FOMITES

Measles is the most communicable of the childhood exanthems.[47, 59] The virus is spread chiefly by droplets expectorated by an infected subject in proximity to susceptible persons. Rarely, transmission may occur by means of articles soiled by respiratory secretions. There is some uncertainty concerning the precise portal of entry of the virus. Although the virus may gain access through the nose or the oropharynx, the work of Papp suggests that the conjunctival mucosa is at least a possible portal of entry.[369]

Measles occurs worldwide in temperate, tropical, and Arctic climates. Before the introduction of live measles vaccines, urban areas of the United States typically experienced epidemics at intervals of 2 to 3 years. In interepidemic years, few cases of measles occur, probably because the supply of susceptible persons has been exhausted. Additional births add to this pool, again permitting epidemic transmission when the pool is sufficiently large. In the United States, the disease had a peak incidence between March and May. Seasonal variation is attributed to the crowding of children indoors and in schools in the winter, resulting in increased transmission. Amplification of each cycle leads to a progressively larger number of cases of measles by the end of the winter. Attack rates are highest among the lowest socioeconomic populations.

Patterns of disease vary strikingly with respect to age, incidence, and severity in different geographic regions. In urban areas of industrialized countries, measles infects predominantly children between the ages of 2 and 6 years and the disease is relatively mild. In rural areas of the same countries, children are characteristically older when they contract the disease and may reach adulthood without becoming infected. For this reason, measles in pregnant women may be observed more often among women from rural or otherwise geographically isolated localities (see later discussion). A different pattern of disease is seen in less developed areas, such as equatorial Africa, where measles occurs predominantly in children younger than 2 years old and has a high fatality rate.[370] Protein deficiency is associated with an increased incidence of complications, such as bronchopneumonia and death. Still another pattern of infection has been observed in extremely isolated regions of the world, where whole populations may never have experienced measles before its exogenous introduction. In a classic description of such an epidemic in the Faroe Islands in 1846, measles was observed to spread rapidly through an entire population, irrespective of age, with an attack rate of virtually 100%.[371] Mortality rates tend to be higher in populations having little experience with measles. An extreme example is the Fiji Islands epidemic of 1875, in which 20,000 people, or about one fourth of the population, are said to have died.[371]

The use of live attenuated measles vaccine in the United States since 1963 has decreased the incidence of measles to less than 1% of its former incidence. Before 1963, there were about 400,000 reported cases of measles annually; a record low of 1497 cases was reported in 1983, but in the late 1980s and early 1990s there was an increase in the incidence of measles that has now come under control.[372] From 1989–1991, there were more than 55,000 reported cases with over 120 measles-associated deaths reported to the Centers for Disease Control and Prevention, but in 1991, the number of reported cases dropped significantly.[372] Measles today is seen primarily in preschoolers, many of whom are too young to have been vaccinated.[372] Measles also occurs, but to a lesser extent, in schoolchildren who were vaccinated. About half of the reported schoolchildren who have developed measles have a history of prior receipt of measles vaccine. At present, it is believed that these cases are the result of primary vaccine failure, a no "take" for the vaccine, rather than secondary vaccine failure because of loss of immunity to measles after vaccination.[373, 374] There is little evidence that immunity induced by measles wanes with time.[373-376] Since the requirement for two doses of measles vaccine in childhood in 1993, the number of annual cases of measles has fallen to an all-time low. In 1995, 309 cases were reported, and in 1996, 508 cases were reported to the Centers for Disease Control and Prevention.[372]

INCIDENCE OF MEASLES IN PREGNANT WOMEN

Because measles is currently well controlled in the United States by immunization it occurs less frequently during pregnancy than chickenpox.

Pathogenesis

By analogy with other viral infections whose pathogenesis has been better delineated, the initial multiplication of measles virus is believed to occur in epithelial and lymphoid cells near the portal of entry. A transient viremia then delivers virus to the reticuloendothelial system, where further replication occurs. A second viremia, more severe and more sustained, disseminates virus to the skin, gut, respiratory tract, and other affected organs. In monkeys, this viremia may occur over a period as long as 1 week before the appearance of the prodrome or exanthem. Measles virus replicates in and probably destroys lymphocytes in the peripheral blood,[377] giving rise to a circulating lymphopenia. The symptoms of measles are probably attributable to inflammation accompanying necrosis of cells in which the virus is replicating. By the time the exanthem appears, 13 to 14 days after infection, measles virus is actively replicating in the skin, gut, and respiratory mucosa. Electron microscopy of biopsies of Koplik's spots and cutaneous lesions reveals syncytial giant cells whose nuclear and cytoplasmic inclusions contain aggregates of microtubules, 15 to 20 nm in diameter, which are characteristic of paramyxovirus infection.[378] This finding and the observation that convalescent measles serum injected into the skin will prevent the local development of the exanthem[379] suggest that replication of virus per se is directly responsible for the lesions. Nevertheless, it is possible that an interaction between viral antigen and antibody is required. The latter hypothesis is supported by the observation that immunosuppressed children who develop giant cell pneumonia caused by measles virus do not develop a rash and do not elaborate antibodies.[380, 381] Furthermore, virus titers in the viscera have already diminished considerably by the time the exanthem appears, and serum antibodies are readily detectable within 24 hours. There is, in addition, experimental evidence that T lymphocytes are important in the development of some symptoms of measles such as the rash, as well as in recovery from the disease.[382]

INCUBATION PERIOD FOR MEASLES ACQUIRED BY DROPLET INFECTION

In general, the usual interval between exposure to measles and onset of first symptoms (prodrome) is about 10 days; 12 to 14 days usually elapse before onset of rash. However, considerable variation may be observed.[383] The incubation period in modified measles may last as long as 17 to 21 days, owing to the presence of low levels of measles antibodies.[383]

INCUBATION PERIOD FOR HEMATOGENOUSLY ACQUIRED MEASLES

It has been claimed that infantile measles may be acquired by transfusion of maternal blood presumably containing measles virus.[384] Two infants developed typical enanthems and exanthems 13 and 14 days after transfusion, and their mothers developed measles exanthems 4 and 2 days, respectively, after blood donation. The infants had not been visited by their mothers for 4 days and 1 day, respectively, before transfusion. Hematogenous transmission may not have occurred, however, because the mothers may well have been shedding virus from the respiratory tract at the time they last handled their infants.

Intrauterine hematogenous transmission, on the other hand, is well documented and is discussed in a subsequent section. In these cases, onset of disease in the infant may occur almost simultaneously with that in the mother or after a variable interval that is less than the minimum time required for extrauterine infection by the respiratory route.

PERIOD OF COMMUNICABILITY

Measles is more communicable during the prodrome and catarrhal stage of infection than during the period of the exanthem. Dramatic corroboration of this observation was provided during an epidemic in Greenland in 1962.[385] Deliberate exposure of 400 susceptible persons to disease was achieved by having a patient on the first day of appearance of the exanthem cough twice in the face of each. Not a single transmission resulted. When the experiment was repeated with a patient during the pre-exanthematous period, measles was readily transmitted.

Patients with measles should be considered infectious from the onset of the prodrome (about 4 days before the appearance of the exanthem) until 3 days after the onset of the exanthem, although the risk of contagion abruptly diminishes 48 hours after the rash appears, concomitant with the appearance of circulating neutralizing antibodies. Measles virus is most readily recovered from respiratory secretions from 2 days before until 1 or 2 days after the onset of the rash.

Pathology

The replication of measles virus in epithelial cells of the mucous membranes and skin leads to the formation of intranuclear inclusions and syncytial giant cells with up to 100 nuclei per cell (Warthin-Finkeldey cells).[386] Focal hyaline necrosis of epithelial cells is accompanied by a subepithelial exudate containing predominantly mononuclear leukocytes. The pathology of cutaneous lesions and Koplik's spots is essentially similar.[378] It is likely that virus replicates simultaneously in the skin and mucous membranes, but Koplik's spots are detected earlier than the exanthem, probably because the epithelium that forms the roof of the lesions is thinner and more translucent in the mucous membranes.

Similar lesions containing the characteristic multinucleated giant cells may be widespread throughout the respiratory and gastrointestinal tracts. The pharynx, tonsils, bronchial epithelium, appendix, colon, and lymph nodes have all been reportedly involved. Viral bronchitis occurs in most cases of measles. Necrotic columnar epithelial cells and giant cells are sloughed into the lumen of the bronchi and bronchioles. When this damage is extensive, the regenerating epithelium frequently undergoes squamous metaplasia and is accompanied by bronchial and peribronchial inflammation. Extension of the process into the alveolar septa results in interstitial pneumonitis. Secondary bacterial infection commonly supervenes, leading to a bronchopneumonia with purulent exudate.

Measles virus has been demonstrated, using immunofluorescence and immunoperoxidase methodology in the placental syncytial trophoblastic cells and decidua, in a 25-week fetus of a woman who developed gestational measles. Interestingly, the fetus was spared. It was postulated that placental damage induced by the virus, leading to hypoxia, is responsible for fetal death during maternal measles.[387]

The pathologic signs of measles encephalitis are not

readily distinguishable from those of other postinfectious encephalitides, such as those caused by vaccinia, chickenpox, and rubella. The characteristic lesion is perivenous demyelination, often accompanied by mild perivascular infiltrates of mononuclear leukocytes, petechial hemorrhages, and microglial proliferation. Neuronal damage and meningeal inflammation are not prominent. Nuclear or cytoplasmic inclusions and giant cells are inconstant. Measles virus has been isolated only infrequently from the brain or spinal cord, and it remains unclear whether the pathologic changes in the brain are a direct result of measles virus or an allergic response to a virus-induced product or antigen-antibody complexes.[388, 389] Owing to the spectrum of pathology, including acute demyelinating encephalitis and acute hemorrhagic leukoencephalitis, it has been postulated that measles encephalitis is an autoimmune process. Myelin basic protein has been demonstrated in the cerebrospinal fluid of patients with measles encephalitis, and the pathologic process has been likened to experimental allergic encephalitis as produced in animal models.[390] One theory regarding pathogenesis is that measles virus has an epitope similar to that of the encephalitogenic sequence in central nervous system myelin (i.e., an instance of molecular mimicry leading to disease).[391] A second form of encephalitis, due to continued replication of measles virus in the brain, occurring in immunocompromised patients has also been described.[392]

Clinical Manifestations

PRODROME AND RASH

The prodrome typically begins 10 to 11 days after exposure, with fever and malaise, followed within 24 hours by coryza, sneezing, conjunctivitis, and cough. During the next 2 to 3 days, this catarrhal phase is accentuated, with markedly infected conjunctivae and photophobia. Toward the end of the prodrome, Koplik's spots appear. These are tiny (no larger than a pinhead), granular, slightly raised, white lesions surrounded by a halo of erythema. Beginning with less than a dozen specks on the lateral buccal mucosa, Koplik's spots may multiply during a 24-hour period to affect virtually all the mucous membranes of the cheeks and may also extend to the lips and eyelids. Hundreds of spots may be present. At this stage, the lesions may be said to resemble grains of salt on a wet background. Koplik's spots appear 1 to 2 days before the exanthem.

The rash, which appears 12 to 14 days after exposure, begins on the head and neck, especially behind the ears and on the forehead. At first the lesions are red macules 1 to 2 mm in diameter, but during a period of 2 or 3 days they enlarge and coalesce. By the second day, the exanthem has spread to the trunk and upper extremities. The lower extremities are involved by the third day. The lesions are most prominent in those regions where the exanthem appears first, namely, the face and upper trunk. By the third or fourth day, the exanthem begins to fade in the order of its appearance. A brown staining of the lesions often persists for 7 to 10 days and is followed by fine desquamation.

The clinical course of measles may be greatly altered by administration of IG during the incubation period. In modified measles, the catarrhal phase may be completely suppressed and the exanthem limited to a few macules on the trunk.

COMPLICATIONS AND MORTALITY

The most frequent complications of measles involve the respiratory tract. Otitis media and mild croup are common in young children during the catarrhal phase, but bacterial pneumonia is the complication that results in death most frequently. If carefully sought, fine rales and radiologic evidence of bronchopneumonia can be found during the early exanthematous phase in most patients. Cough may persist beyond the peak of the exanthem in uncomplicated measles, but when the fever fails to decline or recurs as the rash is fading, a bacterial superinfection is usually present. The chest roentgenogram may show consolidation. A peripheral blood polymorphonuclear leukocytosis is present. When bacterial superinfection occurs, antimicrobial therapy is indicated and should be directed against the most likely etiologic agents: *Streptococcus pneumoniae*, *S. aureus*, and *Streptococcus pyogenes*. Smears and cultures of sputum should be obtained, but in young infants it may be necessary to treat bacterial superinfection without a specific etiologic diagnosis because of the difficulty in obtaining adequate sputum and the potential gravity of the illness (see Therapy later).

After otitis and pneumonia, encephalitis is the most frequent serious complication of measles. It is far less common than pneumonia. Encephalitis, including coma and gross cerebral dysfunction, is estimated to occur with a frequency of 1 per 1000 cases[388] but is probably more common if drowsiness, irritability, and transient electroencephalographic changes are accepted as evidence of encephalitis. This complication occurs in all age groups, including the neonatal period. A fatal outcome has been recorded in an infant, born in the hospital, who developed measles with encephalitis at 27 days of age.[389] Measles encephalitis may occur at any stage of the illness but appears most commonly 3 to 7 days after the onset of the exanthem. The initial symptoms are drowsiness and irritability, followed by lethargy, convulsions, and coma. The cerebrospinal fluid changes are those of a mild aseptic meningitis. Mental obtundation may clear over a period of 1 to 4 days or may assume a more protracted course that is associated with a higher incidence of such sequelae as severe behavioral abnormalities and mental retardation. Death occurs in about 11% of cases.[388] Other complications of measles have been described. These include thrombocytopenic purpura, appendicitis, myocarditis, subacute sclerosing panencephalitis, and reactivation or exacerbation of previously acquired tuberculosis. In a study of 3220 U.S. Air Force recruits with measles, whose mean age was 19 years, between 1976 and 1979, bacterial superinfection and elevated serum transaminase levels were observed in 30%, otitis in 29%, sinusitis in 25%, bronchospasm in 17%, and pneumonia in 3%.[393]

The precise case:fatality ratio in measles is highly

variable among different populations and at different periods in the history of the same population. Between 1920 and 1950 in Massachusetts, deaths caused by measles declined progressively during each successive 5-year period from 7.6 to 0.28 per 100,000 population, despite an approximately constant morbidity related to measles.[371] Since the decline preceded the widespread use of antibiotics, much of the change is attributed to improved social conditions, less crowding, improved nutrition, and medical care. In the United States since 1963 the case:fatality ratio has averaged about 0.1% based on reported cases, but it may be closer to 0.01% if estimated unreported cases of measles are included in the calculation.[394] However, the risk is considerably greater in children younger than 1 year old. The age-specific death rates for measles in the United States reported in 1949 (per 100,000 population) were 7.8 when younger than 1 year of age, 2.8 at 1 to 4 years of age, 1.3 at 5 to 9 years of age, and 0.4 at 10 to 14 years of age. That death rates are higher in infants is confirmed by data obtained during an epidemic in Greenland in 1951, in which the age-specific death rates, per 1000 population, were 26 for infants younger than 1 year old and 15 for infants 1 to 2 years old; no deaths were recorded in children between 2 and 14 years of age.[395] In those cases in which adequate information was available, apparently all deaths in children younger than 1 year old were caused by pneumonia, which appeared either during the prodrome or shortly after the onset of the exanthem.

Children with underlying infection with HIV have been reported to be at risk to develop severe measles, and fatalities have been reported, especially in children who have developed AIDS.[396] In Africa, it has been observed that infants born to HIV-infected women have lower titers of measles antibodies in cord sera than infants from women not infected with HIV. The outcome has been that these infants are at greater risk to develop measles early in infancy.[397] One adolescent with HIV infection who had previously received measles vaccine developed fatal measles pneumonia after the second dose. Because the infection was proven to be from the vaccine virus, measles vaccine is no longer recommended for HIV-infected children who have developed AIDS or evidence of severe immunosuppression.[372]

Immunocompromised children with underlying malignant diseases who have not been immunized are also at risk to develop severe and even fatal measles.[398–400]

MATERNAL EFFECTS OF MEASLES

Is the pregnant woman with measles at greater risk of serious complications and death than other adults with this disease? The answer is probably yes. Some of the published experiences leading to this conclusion are summarized in the following paragraphs.

In the early part of the twentieth century, fatality rates for pregnant women with measles were reported to be approximately 15%, mostly caused by pneumonia in the puerperium.[401, 402] In the 1951 Greenland epidemic, four deaths occurred among 83 women (4.9%) who had measles during pregnancy or the puerperium. In contrast, there were 19 deaths among 1099 nonpregnant women

(1.7%) between the ages of 15 and 54.[395] This difference is probably significant (χ^2 3.9, $p = 0.05$). There was no significant difference in the frequency of pneumonia as a complication of measles among pregnant and nonpregnant women in the same age group, but heart failure was observed far more often in pregnant women with measles. Heart failure was observed in a total of seven patients with gestational measles. Of these, three were in the second half of pregnancy and four were puerperal. Although in some patients heart failure occurred during the prodrome, in most women it occurred within 2 weeks after onset of the exanthem.

Additional experience in the United States and Australia since 1940 supports the concept that measles during pregnancy is only rarely catastrophic. Among 24 women with gestational measles in an outbreak in rural Oklahoma, no deaths occurred and serious morbidity was likewise not increased.[403] In another epidemic, reported in 1950 from Australia, 18 cases of gestational measles were observed. In only 1, which occurred in a woman in the third trimester with measles pneumonia, were complications reported.[404]

During the recent period in the United States, 1988 to 1992, when there was a resurgence of measles, a number of pregnant women developed this infection. Thirteen such women who were hospitalized in Houston, Texas, were reported because 7 (54%) had respiratory complications that were the basis for their hospitalization. They required supplemental oxygen and monitoring in the intensive care unit, and 1 woman died.[405] These women appeared to have primary measles pneumonia rather than bacterial superinfection. Nine of these 13 women were treated with aerosolized ribavirin administered by face mask. Hepatitis, demonstrated by elevations of transaminases, also occurred frequently in these women, but this is also a common finding in nonpregnant adults with hepatitis that seems to be of little clinical importance. During this same time period, medical records from 58 women from Los Angeles with measles were reviewed. Thirty-five (60%) were hospitalized for measles, 15 (26%) developed pneumonia, and 2 (3%) died.[406] Although it is difficult to prove that measles is more severe in pregnant than nonpregnant women, it seems likely to be so.

EFFECTS OF GESTATIONAL MEASLES ON THE FETUS

Chromosomal Aberrations

The possibility that measles occurring in pregnancy may potentially damage the fetus is suggested by the observation that there is a high frequency of chromosome breaks in leukocyte metaphase preparations between the second and fifth day of the exanthem.[407] Other reports, however, have not fully confirmed the preceding observations. Miller found no chromosome breaks in leukocytes of patients with measles who were examined 1 to 12 days after onset of the rash, but he attributed this discrepancy to methodologic differences involving more gentle treatment of the leukocytes.[408] A report from Japan also failed to show an increased frequency of chromosome breaks per cell in patients with measles compared with those in normal subjects. However, a significant increase in chromosome breaks was observed in patients with Down syndrome who had measles and it was inferred that their chromosomes were more sensitive to measles infection.[409]

These chromosomal abnormalities are transient and disappear during convalescence. No studies have examined whether intrauterine exposure of the fetus to measles results in more lasting chromosomal aberrations.

Abortion and Prematurity

The consensus of several reports dealing with the frequency of premature births is that this untoward event occurs more often in association with measles during pregnancy than in the pregnant population at large. In contrast to rubella, in which there is retarded intrauterine development, prematurity caused by measles is associated with normal intrauterine development but premature expulsion of the fetus. Although there is no statistically valid proof that gestational measles also causes a higher rate of abortion, it seems probable that measles is responsible for some specific instances of abortion.

Among the retrospective studies is that of Dyer, who reported 24 cases of gestational measles from rural Oklahoma in 1938 and 1939.[403] Uterine contractions, which typically occurred during the illness, were noted in 11 of the 24 women and caused premature delivery of the fetus in 9 (38%). In one woman, in whom measles occurred at 18 weeks' gestation, the exanthem was followed by spontaneous abortion 7 days later. Two additional pregnancies were associated with premature births at 33 weeks' gestation. No abortions were associated with eight cases of measles occurring in the first trimester.

Adverse outcomes of gestational measles on the fetus involving 18 pregnant women with measles were reported in the epidemic in South Australia in 1950.[404] There were three spontaneous abortions (17%), which occurred in one of seven women who had measles in the first trimester, one of eight in the second trimester, and one of three in the third trimester. Abortions followed the onset of the exanthem by 2 to 3 weeks in the patients who became ill in the first and second trimesters. The patient with measles in the third trimester had severe measles pneumonia and expelled a macerated fetus 7 weeks later. One live premature birth was recorded in the third trimester.

In the 1951 Greenland epidemic, birth or abortion occurred in 26 of the 76 pregnant women while they had measles.[395] Thirteen were term pregnancies. Of the remainder, spontaneous abortion at 3 to 5 months' gestation occurred in seven women (9%). There were six instances of premature delivery (8%), and perinatal death ensued in three. A retrospective analysis of 51 women in Greenland who developed measles during the first 3 months of pregnancy between 1951 and 1962 also suggested a high fetal death rate. One half with measles in the first 2 months and one fifth with measles in the third month had a spontaneous abortion.[410] Five infants

born to women with measles during an outbreak in 1981 and 1982 in Israel have been reported.[411] All were born prematurely (range, 28 to 34 weeks) with a mean duration between maternal onset of illness and delivery of 3.5 days and a mean birth weight of 1496 g. None had any signs of measles at birth or in the neonatal period.

Controlled prospective studies carried out in New York City during the period from 1957 to 1964 demonstrated a significant association between maternal measles and prematurity but not between maternal measles and abortion. Low birth weight (< 2500 g) was identified in 10 of 60 (16.7%) infants born to measles-infected mothers, compared with 2 of 62 (3.3%) matched controls (χ^2 6.2, $p < 0.025$) (see Table 13–5).[171] When fetal mortality was examined in relation to gestational age (see Table 13–6), it was found that three deaths occurred in 19 (15.8%) cases of measles in the first trimester, one in 29 (3.4%) in the second trimester, and one in 17 (5.9%) in the third trimester.[171] These figures were not significantly different from those for fetal deaths in control pregnancies not involving measles. Of the total of five fetal deaths that occurred in pregnant women with measles, fewer than half the deaths occurred within 2 weeks of maternal disease.

The resurgence of measles from 1989 to 1991 resulted in measles in a number of pregnant women. In the experience of Atmar and associates, there was an adverse fetal outcome in 4 of 13 pregnancies (31%) complicated by maternal measles. Two women gave birth in the 34th and 35th weeks, and one spontaneously aborted at 16 weeks during measles. One additional woman and her fetus died at 20 weeks.[405] In a report from Los Angeles of 58 women, the incidence of abortion was 5 (9%) and/or prematurity was 13 (22%).[406]

Congenital Defects

The teratogenic potential of gestational measles for the fetus has been neither proved nor refuted because of the rarity of the infection during pregnancy, particularly during the first trimester when the process of organogenesis is most active. It seems clear, however, that if measles causes congenital malformations, it does so far less frequently than does rubella. Furthermore, unlike gestational chickenpox, no particular constellation of abnormalities has been found among the sporadic instances of congenital defects that have occurred as a result of measles in the mother during pregnancy.

Isolated instances of buphthalmos,[412] congenital heart disease,[413] harelip,[203] pyloric stenosis,[413] genu valgum,[412] cerebral leukodystrophy,[410] and cyclopia[410] have been reported in infants born to mothers with diagnosed measles during the organogenic period. In these and other cases, documentation that the maternal illness was measles and not rubella or other exanthems is often lacking.

No congenital malformations were noted among four infants born to mothers who had measles during the first 4 months of pregnancy in the Oklahoma outbreak.[403] Similarly, in the 1951 Greenland epidemic, there were no congenital malformations among the infants of 76 mothers with gestational measles, although the number of cases that occurred in the first trimester is unclear.[395]

After the epidemic in South Australia,[404] two infants with congenital defects (one each with Down syndrome and partial deafness) were recorded among those whose mothers had measles during the first trimester. No birth defects occurred in infants born to eight mothers with measles in the second trimester and three mothers who had been ill in the third trimester. Although one of the five infants born during the outbreak in 1981 and 1982 in Israel was severely malformed, this was obviously not secondary to maternal measles, which had begun only a few days before birth. Five additional reported Israeli infants had no congenital anomalies, but all their mothers had measles just before delivery.[411] In the Houston report of 13 pregnant women, the fetal gestational age at onset of maternal measles ranged from 16 to 35 weeks (mean 27). Follow-up of eight of these infants, delivered a mean of 12 weeks later (range 1 to 24 weeks), revealed that no infants had congenital malformations.[405] These analyses are incapable of establishing whether the incidence of congenital defects is increased as a result of gestational measles because they were uncontrolled. One controlled prospective study is inconclusive because only small numbers of pregnant women with measles could be studied. Among 60 children who were born to mothers who had gestational measles and were followed to the age of 5 years, only one congenital malformation was identified, compared with a virtually identical incidence of one defect among 62 controls.[169] The defect in the infected group was bilateral deafness in an infant weighing 1990 g born to a mother who had measles at 6 weeks' gestation. In summary, if there is any increased risk of malformations from gestational measles, this risk appears to be small if it exists at all.

PERINATAL MEASLES

As in chickenpox, perinatal measles includes transplacental infection as well as disease acquired postnatally by the respiratory route. Because the usual incubation period from infection to the first appearance of the exanthem is 13 to 14 days, measles exanthems acquired in the first 10 days of life may be considered transplacental in origin, whereas those appearing at 14 days or later are probably acquired outside the uterus.

Postnatally Acquired Measles

Several reports describe cases of measles in which the onset of the exanthem occurred at 14 to 30 days of age. The course of the disease in these cases was generally mild.[403, 414, 415] In one infant with notably mild illness and little fever, the illness began at the age of 14 days. This neonate had been suckled by the mother, in whom the prodrome of measles developed on the first postpartum day. Because circulating and presumably also secretory antibodies appear within 48 hours of the onset of the exanthem, it is possible that the neonate's illness was modified by measles-specific IgA antibodies present in the mother's milk.[403, 414, 415] A report from Japan in 1997 described 7 cases of measles in infants during the first month of life. No case was believed to be severe, although there were three infants with pneumonia, two of

whom had received IG at exposure.[416] Measles acquired postnatally may also cause more severe illness; when a mother developed the disease 20 days post partum, her infant was quite sick with measles 10 days later but complications such as pneumonia or otitis apparently did not develop.[417]

Outbreaks of nosocomial measles in the newborn nursery apparently have not been recorded in the twentieth century, probably because of the low incidence of measles in the United States and other developed countries, nearly universal immunity in mothers in urban areas, and corresponding protection of the newborn by passive antibodies.

Congenital Measles

Congenital measles includes cases in which the exanthem is present at birth and also infections acquired in utero in which the rash appears during the first 10 days of life. In congenital measles, the incubation period, defined as the interval between onset of exanthem in the mother and in the infant, varies between 2 days[403] and 10 days,[418] with a mean of 6 days. A nearly simultaneous onset in mother and neonate implies that measles virus in the maternal bloodstream may sometimes cross the placenta in sufficient quantity to cause disease in the fetus without the need for many additional cycles of replication. However, the placenta may act as a barrier of limited effectiveness, as suggested by those instances in which disease does not appear in the fetus until 10 days after its appearance in the mother. Even more cogent is the fact that maternal measles immediately preceding parturition by no means invariably involves the fetus. Thus, of 44 pregnancies in which a maternal rash was present at delivery, only in 13 (30%) was exanthematous measles reported in the neonate.[402] More recent reports include 13 instances in which maternal rashes with onsets ranging from 7 days ante partum to 3 days post partum were associated with clinically apparent measles in the infant in only 3 (23%).[403, 411, 417, 419] However, eight of these children received IG, 0.25 ml/kg, at birth, including the three who developed measles.[411, 419] During the Greenland epidemic of 1951, no examples of congenital measles were observed among infants born to 13 women who had measles at parturition.[395] It appears that most of these neonates do not experience subclinical measles without exanthem but simply are not infected. This conclusion is supported by the observation that infants whose mothers had measles late in the third trimester are fully susceptible to infection later in childhood.[402] During the Faroe Islands epidemic of 1846, many pregnant women had measles, but 36 years later their infants were infected as adults in a new epidemic in 1882.[417]

As in congenital chickenpox, the spectrum of illness in congenital measles varies from a mild illness, in which the rash is transient and Koplik's spots may be absent, to rapidly fatal disease. The precise case:fatality ratio is uncertain because the course of measles in different populations has been so variable, even in older children and adults. Among 22 cases of congenital measles culled from the literature in which IG prophylaxis was not given,

TABLE 13–11
Deaths in Neonates Whose Mothers Had Measles at Parturition

EXANTHEM IN NEONATE	NEONATAL DEATHS[a]	NEONATAL CASES	%
Present at birth	4	12	33
Appeared after birth	3	10	30
Did not appear	7[b]	16	44

[a]Stillborns excluded.
[b]All of these were premature infants reported in a single series.[402]

there were seven deaths (Table 13–11).[402, 403, 417, 418] Approximately the same case:fatality ratio (30 to 33%) was observed whether the rash was present at birth or appeared subsequently. Although the number of observations is small, it appears that in premature infants with congenital measles the death rate is higher (5 of 9) than in infants with congenital measles delivered at term (2 of 10). The death rate has also been high among premature infants born to women who had measles at parturition even when the infant never developed clinically apparent measles (see Table 13–11).[395, 402]

Insufficient data are available to evaluate whether transplacentally acquired antibodies to measles virus may diminish the case:fatality ratio in congenital measles when the mother's exanthem appears more than 48 hours ante partum. The death rate from congenital measles does not appear to differ appreciably whether the maternal rash appears ante partum or post partum (Table 13–12), but more precise information on the time of appearance of the maternal rash is needed to answer this question definitively. Although firm data are not available, administration of IG at birth may also decrease mortality.[405, 411, 419]

Most reports of death related to congenital measles do not specify the immediate cause, but pneumonia is among the leading complications.[402, 403, 405, 411, 419, 420] Because nearly all reports of deaths preceded the antibiotic era, the present case:fatality ratio may be significantly lower than it was previously because of improved supportive care and appropriate antimicrobial therapy of bacterial superinfections.

Diagnosis and Differential Diagnosis

The diagnosis of measles is easy when there is a history of recent exposure and the typical catarrhal phase is followed by Koplik's spots and a maculopapular exanthem in the characteristic distribution. Indeed, Koplik's spots are pathognomonic. However, the diagnosis is more difficult during the prodrome (when the illness is maximally communicable) or when the illness and the exanthem are attenuated by passively acquired measles antibodies. Measles antibodies may be contained in transfused plasma or IG, or they may cross the placenta to the neonate if the mother develops measles shortly before parturition. The atypical exanthem of measles in subjects who have been previously immunized with inactivated measles vaccine may potentially also cause diagnostic difficulties. In situations in which the diagnosis cannot be made confidently on clinical and epidemiologic grounds, laboratory confirmation is indicated so that appropriate measures can be taken to prevent the occurrence of nosocomial measles among susceptible persons. Aids to rapid diagnosis include examination of exfoliated cells from the pharynx, nasal and buccal mucosa, conjunctiva, or urinary tract by direct staining for epithelial giant cells[421, 422] or identification of measles antigens by direct immunofluorescence.[423–425] These tests are positive in more than 90% of patients during the prodrome and the period of the early exanthem. At later stages of the illness, the diagnosis may be confirmed by detecting measles-specific IgM antibodies in serum and/or rising antibody titers in acute and convalescent sera.[366, 367, 426] Because serum antibodies appear within 48 hours of the exanthem, it is important that the acute-phase serum be collected at the onset of the rash or earlier.

Among the diseases and conditions to be considered in the differential diagnosis of measles are the following. None is likely to occur in the newborn.

1. *Drug eruptions and other allergies.* Maculopapular exanthems may be caused by a variety of drugs and chemicals in susceptible persons. A history of exposure is of paramount importance in distinguishing these from measles. An urticarial component may be seen in some instances of drug hypersensitivity but is not present in measles.

2. *Kawasaki's disease.* This illness is often confused with measles and vice versa in children younger than age 5 years. Classic signs include conjunctivitis, red cracked lips, strawberry tongue, morbilliform or scarlatiniform rash, induration of the hands and feet, and usually a solitary enlarged cervical lymph node. In confusing cases, viral diagnostic procedures may be necessary to rule measles in or out.

3. *Rubella.* The maculopapular exanthem of rubella is finer and more transient. It undergoes a more rapid evolution and does not assume the blotchy configuration often seen in measles. The posterior cervical and postauricular lymphadenopathies of rubella are not present in measles, and conversely the prominent catarrhal symptoms in the prodrome of measles are not a feature of rubella.

4. *Scarlet fever.* The rash of scarlet fever is punctate and extremely fine rather than papular. It blanches on pressure and is accentuated in skin folds. The onset is typically abrupt without a prodrome. There is an accompanying sore throat, and the cheeks are flushed.

TABLE 13–12
Deaths from Congenital Measles in Relation to Date of Onset of Rash in Mothers

ONSET OF MATERNAL RASH	NEONATAL DEATHS	NEONATAL DEATHS	%
Antepartum	4	15	27
Postpartum	3	11	27

Peripheral blood leukocytosis is usual, in contrast to the leukopenia of measles.

5. *Meningococcemia.* When the early rash of meningococcemia is maculopapular rather than petechial, it may be confused with measles. Unlike measles, it has no characteristic distribution.

6. *Roseola.* The exanthem of roseola, which usually appears when the patient's temperature drops to normal, typically appears on the trunk before it is evident on the head. It lasts only 1 or 2 days. Roseola, which is caused by human herpesvirus type 6, is seen most often in children younger than 3 years old and is almost never noted in adults.

7. *Atypical measles.* This is a hypersensitivity disease, related to infection with measles virus in persons who received killed measles vaccine years ago. Killed measles vaccine was removed from the U.S. market in 1968. Extremely high measles HI antibody titers (e.g., 1:1 million) have been observed in patients with this disease.

8. *Other infections.* Rocky Mountain spotted fever, toxoplasmosis, enterovirus infections, and infectious mononucleosis all may cause maculopapular exanthems resembling measles.

Therapy

The treatment of uncomplicated measles is symptomatic. IG has no proven value in established disease. Antibiotics are not indicated for prophylaxis of bacterial superinfections (otitis and pneumonia). When these complications develop, antimicrobial therapy should be selected on the basis of Gram's stain and culture of appropriate body fluids, such as sputum. If culture specimens cannot be obtained or if the illness is grave, broad-spectrum antibiotics may be selected on the basis of the most likely offending pathogens. The antibiotic regimen for pneumonia, most commonly caused by *S. pneumoniae* or *S. aureus*, should include a penicillinase-resistant penicillin; the drug of choice for otitis media, which is usually caused by *S. pneumoniae* or *Haemophilus influenzae*, is amoxicillin. Vitamin A, 200,000 IU orally for 2 days, has been used to treat infants with measles and seems to decrease the severity of the infection.[427–429] The drug ribavirin has been used experimentally to treat severe measles in immunocompromised and other high-risk patients.[430, 431]

Prevention

PASSIVE IMMUNIZATION

Passive immunization is recommended for the prevention of measles in exposed, susceptible pregnant women, neonates, and their contacts in the delivery room or newborn nursery (see later section Nosocomial Measles in the Nursery). Therapy with intramuscularly administered IG should be given as soon as possible after exposure. A dose of 0.25 ml/kg given within 72 hours of exposure is a reliable means of prevention of clinical measles, although IG given later (up to 7 days after exposure) or in smaller doses (0.04 ml/kg) may also prevent or at least modify the infection. It is recommended that passive prophylaxis be followed in 5 months or more by administration of live measles vaccine in those old enough to receive it.[341]

ACTIVE IMMUNIZATION

Live measles vaccines currently recommended are derivatives of the Edmonston B strain that have been further attenuated. They produce a noncommunicable infection, which is mild or inapparent. Fever occurs in about 5% of susceptible recipients. A mild rash is observed in 10 to 20% of susceptible recipients 5 to 10 days after administration. The vaccines induce seroconversion in 95% and prevent clinical disease in more than 90% of exposed susceptible recipients.

Live attenuated measles vaccines are contraindicated in pregnant women.[341] In one small series, Edmonston B measles vaccine and gamma globulin were administered to seven pregnant women, 18 to 34 years of age, who were in the second to eighth months of pregnancy. There were no serologic data. Three of the seven developed fever (> 38.5° C) and rash. All were delivered of healthy infants at term.[432] Vaccination is likewise not usually recommended for infants younger than 12 months of age because the induction of immunity and the elaboration of antibodies may be suppressed by residual transplacentally acquired antibodies in the fetal circulation or other mechanisms. In exposed populations having little experience with measles, or in populations in which the incidence of natural measles before the age 1 year is high, live vaccines may be given at 6 to 9 months of age but should be followed by a second dose at 15 months to increase the seroconversion rate.[341] There are increasing data to indicate that measles antibody titers are lower in women vaccinated as children than in women who have previously had natural measles, and that the offspring of vaccinated women lose transplacentally acquired measles antibodies before 1 year of age.[433, 434] It is therefore predicted that routine vaccination against measles may be recommended at 12 rather than 15 months. Nevertheless, passive immunization should be given to protect young infants exposed during an epidemic.

NOSOCOMIAL MEASLES IN THE NURSERY: GUIDELINES FOR PREVENTION

Most women of childbearing age in urban areas are immune to measles because of previous natural infection or vaccination. Because it is amply documented that infants born to immune mothers are usually protected by transplacentally acquired antibodies, measles outbreaks in newborn nurseries are extraordinarily rare. Studies by Krugman and colleagues have indicated that before the introduction of live attenuated measles vaccine, 94% of infants had passive HI antibodies at 1 month of age, 47% had them at 4 months, and 26% had them at 6 months.[435] The rarity of measles among mothers, newborns, and hospital staff in the newborn nursery makes it difficult to assess the precise risk once the virus has been introduced. Nonetheless, the fact that age-specific mortality rates related to measles are highest in the first year of life (see previous discussion) justifies instituting measures designed to prevent disease in those exposed and the spread of infection to neonates of uncertain immune status (Table 13–13).

Infants born to mothers with an unequivocal history of either previous natural measles or vaccination with live attenuated measles virus are assumed not to be at risk when exposed to measles in the neonatal period. Therefore, if siblings at home have measles in a communicable stage, neonates born to immune mothers may be discharged from the hospital with no treatment. In the absence of a maternal history of measles or measles vaccine, the mother's serum should be tested for the presence of antibodies to measles. If the mother's serum contains detectable levels of measles antibodies by a reliable method, both mother and baby may be sent home. If specific antibodies are not detected in the mother's serum, the neonate and mother should not have contact with the older siblings until they are no longer infectious. In addition, both mother and neonate, as well as any nonimmune older siblings without disease, should receive IG, 0.25 mg/kg intramuscularly, to prevent or modify subsequent measles infection that might have been incubating at the time of delivery.

If a mother without a history of previous measles or measles vaccination is exposed 6 to 15 days ante partum,

TABLE 13–13
Guidelines for Preventive Measures After Exposure to Measles in the Nursery or Maternity Ward

| TYPE OF EXPOSURE OR DISEASE | MEASLES PRESENT (PRODROME OR RASH)[a] | | DISPOSITION |
	Mother	Neonate	
A. Siblings at home with measles[a] when neonate and mother are ready for discharge from hospital	No	No	1. *Neonate:* protective isolation and IG indicated unless mother had unequivocal history of previous measles or measles vaccination.[b] 2. *Mother:* with history of previous measles or measles vaccination, she may either remain with neonate or return to older children. Without previous history she may remain with neonate until older siblings are no longer infectious, or she may receive IG prophylactically and return to older children.
B. Mother without history of measles or measles vaccination exposed during period 6–15 days ante partum[c]	No	No	1. *Exposed mother and infant:* administer IG to each and send home at earliest date unless there are siblings at home with communicable measles. Test mothers for susceptibility if possible. If susceptible, administer live measles vaccine 5 months after IG (see text). 2. *Other mothers and infants:* same unless clear history of previous measles or measles vaccination in the mother. 3. *Hospital personnel:* unless clear history of previous measles or measles vaccination administer IG within 72 hours of exposure. Vaccinate 5 months or more later.
C. Onset of maternal measles ante partum or post partum[d]	Yes	Yes	1. *Infected mother and infant:* isolate together until clinically stable, then send home. 2. *Other mothers and infants:* same as B-3 except infants should be vaccinated at 15 months of age. 3. *Hospital personnel:* same as B-3.
D. Onset of maternal measles ante partum or post partum[d]	Yes	No	1. *Infected mother:* isolate until no longer infectious.[d] 2. *Infected mother's infant:* isolate separately from mother. Administer IG immediately. Send home when mother is no longer infectious. Alternatively, observe in isolation for 18 days for modified measles,[e] especially if IG administration was delayed more than 4 days. 3. *Other mothers and infants:* same as C-2. 4. *Hospital personnel:* same as B-3.

[a]Catarrhal stage or less than 72 hours after onset of exanthem.
[b]Vaccination with live attenuated measles virus (see text).
[c]With exposure less than 6 days ante partum, mother would not be potentially infectious until at least 72 hours post partum.
[d]Considered infectious from onset of prodrome until 72 hours after onset of exanthem.
[e]Incubation period for modified measles may be prolonged beyond the usual 10 to 14 days.

she may be in the incubation period and capable of transmitting measles infection during the postpartum period before discharge from the hospital. In such a situation, it is optimal to test the mother for measles antibodies. If no antibodies are detected (or the test cannot be performed), and if she had been exposed less than 6 days ante partum, she could not transmit measles by the respiratory route until at least 72 hours post partum. By this time in most instances, the mother would have been discharged from the hospital and potential nosocomial transmission would not be a problem. In either event (exposure from 0 to 5 days or from 6 to 15 days ante partum), both the exposed susceptible mother and her neonate should receive IG and be sent home as soon as possible unless siblings at home have measles in a communicable stage. If the mother's exposure occurred 6 to 15 days ante partum, prophylaxis with IG should also be administered to the other mothers, neonates, and hospital personnel in the delivery room and nursery except those with a history of natural measles or vaccination with live attenuated measles virus or who have detectable antibodies to measles virus. Globulin prophylaxis given within 72 hours of exposure prevents infection in nearly all instances, and in many cases it is effective for as long as 7 days.[371, 436] IG given after this period but before the prodrome usually results in modified measles infection with diminished morbidity.[371, 436] Those patients to whom IG had to be given should later be vaccinated, after allowing an interval of at least 5 months so that residual measles antibody does not interfere with the immune response to the vaccine.[341]

If a mother develops measles immediately ante partum or post partum and her infant is born with congenital measles, the mother and infant should be isolated together until 72 hours after the appearance of the exanthem. Close observation of the neonate for signs of bronchopneumonia and other complications is warranted. Other susceptible mothers, neonates, and hospital personnel should receive immediate prophylaxis with IG as outlined previously, followed by vaccination at a later date.

If a mother develops perinatal measles but her infant is born without signs of infection, each should be isolated separately. The infant may be incubating transplacentally acquired measles or may be at risk of postnatally acquired droplet infection. In either case, the infant should receive IG. The mother may be discharged with her infant after the third day of exanthem. The neonate should be followed closely and observed for signs of modified measles, which may require up to 18 days' observation because of the abnormally long incubation period of modified measles.[371]

The availability of virus diagnostic facilities varies, and the approach to potential nosocomial spread of measles therefore may differ from place to place. If serologic testing is expensive or unavailable, it may be simpler to administer IG to all exposed persons who do not have an unequivocal history of previous measles or previous vaccination with live attenuated measles virus vaccine. On the other hand, serologic testing of those exposed who are thought to possibly be susceptible to measles, with administration of IG to those exposed who are truly susceptible, would seem to be the ideal management for prevention of nosocomial measles.

Neonates or mothers isolated because of measles require a separate room with the door closed. Only immune visitors and staff should enter the room. Gown and hand washing precautions must be observed, and containment of bedding and tissues soiled with respiratory excreta by double bagging and autoclaving is indicated. Because measles virus is excreted in the urine during the early exanthematous phase, it is also advisable to treat the urine as potentially infectious and to disinfect bedpans. Terminal disinfection of the room is recommended.

MUMPS

Mumps is an acute, generalized, communicable disease whose most distinctive feature is swelling of one or both parotid glands. Involvement of other salivary glands, the meninges, the pancreas, and the testes of postpubertal males is also common. The origin of the name is obscure but probably is related to the Old English verb "to mump," meaning to sulk, or to the Scottish verb meaning to speak indistinctly.

The Organism

PROPERTIES AND PROPAGATION

Mumps virus is a member of the paramyxovirus family and therefore has most of the morphologic and physicochemical properties described earlier for measles. Five antigens have been described: two envelope gps, a hemagglutinin-neuraminidase (H-N) and a hemolysis cell fusion (F) gp antigen, and a matrix envelope protein. There are two internal antigens: a nucleocapsid protein (NP) and an RNA polymerase protein (P).[437]

Mumps virus is readily isolated after inoculation of appropriate clinical specimens into a variety of host systems. Rapid identification may be accomplished by use of cells grown in shell vials and use of fluorescein-labeled monoclonal antibodies.

The virus may be recovered during the first few days of illness from saliva, throat washings, and urine and from the cerebrospinal fluid of patients with mumps meningitis. Shedding of virus in the urine may persist longer, sometimes up to 2 weeks. Less commonly, the virus is present in blood, milk, and testicular tissue.[438]

A highly sensitive ELISA useful for diagnosing and determining susceptibility to mumps has been described. This assay has also been used to diagnose acute mumps in one serum specimen by the presence of specific IgM.[438] The diagnosis may also be established by demonstrating a rising antibody titer in paired acute and convalescent sera.

Epidemiology and Transmission

PERIOD OF COMMUNICABILITY

Mumps occurs worldwide and is endemic in most urban areas where routine vaccination is not practiced. In the

United States, before widespread vaccination against mumps, the incidence was highest in the winter, reaching a peak in March and April. Mumps was principally a disease of childhood, with most infections occurring between the ages of 5 and 15 years. Mumps in infancy is very uncommon (see later discussion). In the prevaccine era, approximately one third of infections were subclinical. Epidemics tended to occur in confined populations such as those in boarding schools, the military, and other institutions. Since the introduction of mumps vaccine in 1967, the incidence of clinical mumps has declined dramatically in the United States and mumps has become an extremely unusual disease.

INCUBATION PERIOD

The usual incubation period, measured between exposure to infection and onset of parotitis, is 14 to 18 days, with extremes between 7 and 23 days. However, because the contact may be shedding virus before the onset of clinical disease or may have subclinical infection and therefore be unrecognizable, the incubation period in individual cases is often uncertain.

INCIDENCE OF MUMPS IN PREGNANCY

The incidence of mumps in pregnancy today is unknown. Presumably because there is now little opportunity for exposure to mumps and many women are immune, the incidence would be expected to be low. The incidence in prospective studies has been variously estimated as between 0.8 and 10 cases per 10,000 pregnancies.[65, 169]

Pathogenesis

Mumps is transmitted by droplet nuclei, saliva, and fomites. The precise pathogenesis of infection has not been established because, although experimentally infected monkeys may develop parotitis, no animal model closely resembles human disease. After entry into the host, the virus initially replicates in the epithelium of the upper respiratory tract. A viremia ensues, after which there is localization in glandular or central nervous system tissues. Parotitis is believed to occur as a result of viremia rather than the reverse, because in many instances generalized disease precedes involvement of the parotid gland, which indeed may not be involved at all.

Pathology

Studies of the pathology of mumps are few because the disease is rarely fatal. The histologic changes that have been observed in the parotid gland and the testis are similar. The inflammatory exudate consists of perivascular and interstitial infiltrates of mononuclear cells accompanied by prominent edema. There is necrosis of acinar and duct epithelial cells in the salivary glands and of the germinal epithelium of the seminiferous tubules.

There are few reports of placental pathology in gestational mumps. Garcia and associates described a 29-year-old Brazilian woman with a history of two bleeding episodes during pregnancy who developed mumps in her fifth month. A hysterotomy was subsequently performed, yielding a macerated 90-g fetus. Necrotizing villitis and accumulation of necrotic material, mononuclear cells, and nuclear fragments were found in the intervillous spaces of the placenta. Necrotizing granulomas and cytoplasmic inclusions consistent with mumps virus infection were also noted. Two additional women with mumps in the 10th week and second month of pregnancy underwent therapeutic abortions. Typical inclusion bodies were noted in both placentas and in the adrenal cortex of one fetus.[439] No serologic data were available on these three women, however, so that it is possible that their parotitis was caused by an agent other than mumps virus.

Clinical Manifestations

The prodrome of mumps consists of fever, malaise, myalgia, and anorexia. Parotitis, when present, usually appears within the next 24 hours but may be delayed for a week or even more. Swelling of the gland is accompanied by tenderness to palpation and obliteration of the space between the earlobe and the angle of the mandible. The swelling progresses for 2 to 3 days, then gradually subsides, disappearing in 1 week or less. The orifice of Stenson's duct is commonly red and swollen. In most cases, parotitis is bilateral, although the onset in each gland may be asynchronous by 1 or more days. The submaxillary glands are involved less often than the parotid and almost never by themselves. The sublingual glands are only rarely affected.

Orchitis is the most common manifestation other than parotitis in postpubertal males; it affects about 20% of this group of patients. Orchitis in infancy has been described but is not well documented.[440] Oophoritis is far less common. It is associated with lower abdominal pain, and rarely the ovaries may be palpable. Oophoritis does not lead to sterility.

Aseptic meningitis may occur in children and adults of either sex but is more common in males. Although pleocytosis of the cerebrospinal fluid may occur in up to 50% of cases of clinical mumps, signs of meningeal irritation occur in a smaller proportion of cases, variably estimated at 5 to 25%. The cerebrospinal fluid contains up to 1000 cells per mm^3. Within the first 24 hours, polymorphonuclear leukocytes may predominate, but by the second day nearly all the cells are lymphocytes. In the absence of parotitis, the syndrome of aseptic meningitis in mumps is indistinguishable clinically from that caused by enteroviruses and other viruses. The course is almost invariably self-limited. Rarely, cranial nerve palsies have led to permanent sequelae, of which deafness is the most common.

Mumps pancreatitis may cause abdominal pain. The incidence of this manifestation is unclear because reliable diagnostic criteria are difficult to obtain. An elevated serum amylase level may be present in either parotitis or pancreatitis. The character of the abdominal pain is rarely sufficiently distinctive to permit unequivocal diagnosis. Other complications of mumps include mastitis, thyroiditis, myocarditis, nephritis, and arthritis.

The peripheral blood cell count in mumps is not characteristic. The white blood cell count may be elevated, normal, or depressed; and the differential count may reveal either a mild lymphocytosis or a polymorphonuclear leukocytosis.

MATERNAL EFFECTS OF MUMPS

Unlike varicella and measles, when mumps occurs in pregnant women the illness is generally benign and is not appreciably more severe than it is in other adult women.[440-449] In a 1957 "virgin soil" epidemic of mumps among the Inuit, 20 infections were observed in pregnant women. Of these, only 8 (40%) were clinically apparent, compared with an incidence of 57 clinically apparent cases among 92 nonpregnant women (62%). Overt disease, therefore, does not appear to be more common during pregnancy.[446] Some complications such as mastitis and perhaps thyroiditis are more frequent in postpubertal women than in men but probably do not occur more commonly in pregnant women than in other adult women.[446] Mumps virus has been isolated on the third postpartum day from the milk of a woman who developed parotitis 2 days ante partum.[450] Her baby, who was not breast-fed, did not develop clinically apparent mumps. Aseptic meningitis, apparently without unduly high incidence or severity, has also been reported in pregnant women.[441] In pregnant women, as well as in the population as a whole, deaths from mumps are exceedingly rare. One death has been reported in a woman who developed mumps complicated by glomerulonephritis at 8 months' gestation.[451]

EFFECTS OF GESTATIONAL MUMPS ON THE FETUS

Abortion

An excessive number of abortions is associated with gestational mumps when the disease occurs during the first trimester. In prospective studies of fetal mortality in virus diseases, Siegel and associates observed 9 fetal deaths among 33 first-trimester pregnancies complicated by mumps (27%), compared with 131 of 1010 (13%) matched uninfected controls (see Table 13–6). This difference is significant (χ^2 5.6, $p < .02$). Mumps-associated fetal deaths occurred in only 1 of 51 second-trimester pregnancies and none of 43 third-trimester pregnancies. Unlike fetal deaths associated with measles, those associated with mumps were closely related temporally to maternal infection: 6 of the 10 deaths occurred within 2 weeks after the onset of maternal mumps.[171]

Many other reports describe isolated cases of abortion associated with gestational mumps. Nearly all of these occurred in the first 4 months of pregnancy.[441, 445, 447, 449, 452-454] In one instance, mumps virus was isolated from a 10-week fetus spontaneously aborted 4 days after the mother developed clinical mumps.[454]

Prematurity

In the only prospective study of low birth weight in relation to maternal mumps infection, no significant association was found.[171] Nine of 117 (7.7%) pregnant women with mumps gave birth to infants with birth weights of less than 2500 g, compared with 4 of 122 (3.3%) uninfected pregnant women in a control group (see Table 13–5).

Congenital Malformations

In experimentally infected animals, mumps virus may induce congenital malformations.[455-457] Definitive evidence of a teratogenic potential for mumps virus in humans, however, has not been shown. Many reports describe the occurrence of congenital malformations after gestational mumps, but no data are available in most of these studies regarding the incidence of anomalies in uninfected matched control pregnancies. Thus, Swan reviewed the literature in 1951 and found 18 anomalies in the offspring of 93 pregnancies complicated by mumps.[452] These included four malformations originating in the first trimester (cutaneous nevus, imperforate anus, spina bifida, and Down syndrome) and nine originating in the second trimester (four of these infants had Down syndrome and miscellaneous other malformations). Other reports have described malformation of the external ear,[442] intestinal atresia,[449] chorioretinitis and optic atrophy in the absence of evidence of congenital toxoplasmosis,[458] corneal cataracts,[413] and urogenital abnormalities.[459] One case of hydrocephalus caused by obstruction of the foramen of Monro in an infant whose mother had serologically proven mumps during the fifth month of pregnancy has been described.[460] A similar phenomenon has been noted after extrauterine mumps with encephalitis[461] and in an animal model.[457] In the only controlled prospective study, the rate of congenital malformations in children whose mothers had mumps during pregnancy (2 of 117) was essentially identical to the rate of those in infants born to uninfected mothers (2 of 123).[66] Furthermore, neither of these affected infants, both of whom were mentally retarded, was born to any of the 24 pregnant women who had mumps in the first trimester. Similarly, no association between gestational mumps and fetal malformations was reported by British investigators, who evaluated the outcomes of 501 pregnancies complicated by maternal mumps and found no significant differences compared with a control series.[462]

Endocardial Fibroelastosis

A postulated association between gestational mumps infection and endocardial fibroelastosis in the offspring was at one time the subject of much debate.[463] An extensive review of evidence for and against an etiologic role for mumps virus in this condition has been made by Finland.[464] The issue remains unresolved. The rarity of mumps during pregnancy and the rarity of endocardial fibroelastosis as a possible sequel in the fetus make it unlikely that conclusive data will ever be obtained.

PERINATAL MUMPS

In contrast to congenital chickenpox and measles, congenital mumps or even postnatally acquired perinatal mumps has rarely been documented virologically or serologically. Although several cases of parotitis have been reported in women near delivery and their neonates and infants,[446, 465–468] the significance of these reports is often uncertain, especially when clinically apparent mumps only is present in the mother. Other viral, bacterial, and noninfectious causes are difficult to exclude without laboratory evidence of mumps infection.

Among the possible explanations for the rarity of transplacental and postnatally acquired mumps in neonates are (1) the rarity of mumps today, (2) protection of the neonate by passive maternal antibodies, (3) exclusion of mumps virus from the fetus by a hypothetical placental barrier, (4) relative insusceptibility of fetal and neonatal tissues to infection by mumps virus, and (5) occurrence of infections that are predominantly subclinical.

Passage of mumps virus across the human placenta has occasionally been reported. Live attenuated mumps virus has been recovered from the placenta, but not from fetal tissues, of pregnant women who were vaccinated 10 days before undergoing saline-induced abortion.[469] Mumps virus was isolated from two infants whose mothers had mumps at delivery; one infant had parotitis and the other had pneumonia, so presumably transplacental transmission had occurred.[467] Mumps virus was also isolated from a fetus spontaneously aborted on the fourth day after onset of maternal mumps.[439] However, transplacental passage of virus should not be assumed to occur invariably because in several instances passage was specifically not documented.[439, 470, 471]

A differentiation between lack of susceptibility and subclinical infection as explanations for failure of the neonate to develop parotitis or other manifestations of mumps can be made only by adequate serologic investigations and viral isolation attempts. Unfortunately, these data are not available. A number of investigators have noted that clinically apparent mumps with parotitis[472, 473] or orchitis[440] during the first year of life tends to be a very mild disease and that age-specific attack rates for manifest disease related to mumps increase progressively until the age of 5 years.[474] Antibodies to mumps virus are known to cross the placenta and to persist for several months.[475]

Diagnosis and Differential Diagnosis

The diagnosis of mumps is easy when there is acute, bilateral, painful parotitis with a history of recent exposure. More difficulty is encountered when the disease is unilateral or when the manifestations are confined to organs other than the parotid gland. In these cases, laboratory confirmation by either virus isolation or demonstration of a rising antibody titer may be performed.

Among neonates, few conditions need be considered in the differential diagnosis. Clinical parotitis in this age group is exceedingly rare. Suppurative parotitis of the newborn, usually caused by S. aureus, is most often unilateral.[476] Pus can be expressed from the parotid duct, and there is a polymorphonuclear leukocytosis of the peripheral blood. Other diagnostic considerations in the neonate include infection with parainfluenza viruses and coxsackieviruses, drug-induced parotitis, and facial cellulitis.

In addition to these conditions in the neonate, the differential diagnosis in pregnant women includes anterior cervical lymphadenitis, idiopathic recurrent parotitis, salivary gland calculus with obstruction, sarcoidosis with uveoparotid fever, and salivary gland tumors.

Other entities should be considered when the manifestations appear in organs other than the parotid. Testicular torsion in infancy may produce a painful scrotal mass resembling mumps orchitis.[440] Aseptic meningitis related to mumps typically occurs in the winter and early spring, and enterovirus aseptic meningitis is most common in the summer and early autumn. Other viruses may also cause aseptic meningitis that is clinically indistinguishable from mumps.

Therapy

Treatment of parotitis is symptomatic. Analgesics and application of heat or cold to the parotid area may be helpful. Mumps immune globulin has no proven value in the prevention or treatment of mumps. Mastitis may be managed by the application of ice packs and breast binders. Testicular pain may be minimized by the local application of cold and gentle support for the scrotum. Severe cases of orchitis have in some instances appeared to respond to the systemic administration of corticosteroids.

Prevention

ACTIVE IMMUNIZATION

Live attenuated mumps virus vaccine induces antibodies that protect against infection in more than 95% of recipients. The subcutaneously administered vaccine may be given to children older than 1 year, but its use in infants younger than this is not recommended because of possible interference by passive maternal antibodies. Usually it is administered simultaneously with measles and rubella vaccines at age 15 months. The vaccine is recommended for older children and adolescents, particularly adolescent males who have not had mumps; it is not recommended for pregnant women, for patients receiving corticosteroids, or for other immunocompromised hosts.

PASSIVE IMMUNIZATION

Passive immunization for mumps is ineffective and unavailable.

PREVENTION OF NOSOCOMIAL MUMPS IN THE NEWBORN NURSERY

In contrast to chickenpox and measles, mumps does not appear to be a potentially serious hazard in the newborn nursery. No outbreaks of nosocomial mumps have been described in this setting, and transmission of mumps in a hospital setting is highly unusual.[477] Most mothers are immune, and even neonates born to nonimmune mothers rarely develop clinically apparent mumps. Prudence dictates that mothers who develop parotitis or other manifestations of mumps in the period immediately ante partum or post partum should be isolated from other mothers and neonates. The case is less strong for isolating the puerperal mother with mumps from her own newborn. Furthermore, in the hospital setting, isolation of patients with mumps from the time of onset of parotitis has proved to be ineffective in preventing the spread of disease.[478] Infected subjects shed mumps virus in respiratory secretions for several days before the onset of parotitis or other manifestations recognizable as mumps.

At one time, exposed hospital personnel, particularly postpubertal males, and mothers with a negative history of mumps could be given mumps IG, although the prophylactic effectiveness of this product was never established. This preparation is no longer available. Live attenuated mumps virus vaccine has not been evaluated for protection after exposure but may theoretically modify or prevent disease by inducing neutralizing antibodies before the onset of illness because of the long incubation period of mumps. It should be considered for exposed susceptible hospital personnel and puerperal mothers. Some hospitals have the facilities to test for susceptibility to mumps by measurement of antibody titers, whereas others do not. Testing for susceptibility could eliminate some use of vaccine for the just-described situation.

Isolation procedures for mumps include the use of a single room for the patient with the door closed at all times except to enter. Immune personnel caring for the patient should exercise gown and hand-washing precautions. Isolation is continued until parotid swelling has subsided. Terminal disinfection of the room is desirable.

References

1. Weller TH. Varicella and herpes zoster: changing concepts of the natural history, control, and importance of a not-so-benign virus. N Engl J Med 309:1362, 1983.
2. Lungu O, Annunziato P, Gershon A, et al. Reactivated and latent varicella-zoster virus in human dorsal root ganglia. Proc Natl Acad Sci U S A 92:10980, 1995.
3. Mahalingham R, Wellish M, Wolf W, et al. Latent varicella-zoster viral DNA in human trigeminal and thoracic ganglia. N Engl J Med 323:627, 1990.
4. Lungu O, Panagiotidis C, Annunziato P, et al. Aberrant intracellular localization of varicella-zoster virus regulatory proteins during latency. Proc Natl Acad Sci U S A 95:780, 1998.
5. Old English Dictionary. London, Oxford University Press, 1933.
6. Christie AB. Chickenpox. In Infectious Diseases: Epidemiology and Clinical Practice. Edinburgh, E & S Livingstone, 1969, p 238.
7. Angelicus B. De Propreitatibus Rerum. Liber septimus, vol xciii. London, Trevisa John, 1398.
8. Straus SE, Hay J, Smith H, Owens J. Genome differences among varicella-zoster isolates. J Gen Virol 64:1031, 1983.
9. Gabel C, Dubey L, Steinberg S, et al. Varicella-zoster virus glycoproteins are phosphorylated during posttranslational maturation. J Virol 63:4264, 1989.
10. Gershon A, Cosio L, Brunell PA. Observations on the growth of varicella-zoster virus in human diploid cells. J Gen Virol 18:21, 1973.
11. Cook ML, Stevens J. Labile coat: reason for noninfectious cell-free varicella zoster virus in culture. J Virol 2:1458, 1968.
12. Myers M, Connelly BL. Animal models of varicella. J Infect Dis 166:S48, 1992.
13. Sadzot-Delvaux C, Merville-Louis M-P, Delree P, et al. An in vivo model of varicella-zoster virus latent infection of dorsal root ganglia. J Neurosci Res 26:83, 1990.
14. Williams V, Gershon A, Brunell P. Serologic response to varicella-zoster membrane antigens measured by indirect immunofluorescence. J Infect Dis 130:669, 1974.
15. Zaia J, Oxman M. Antibody to varicella-zoster virus-induced membrane antigen: immunofluorescence assay using monodisperse glutaraldehyde-fixed target cells. J Infect Dis 136:519, 1977.
16. Gershon A, Steinberg S, LaRussa P. Measurement of Antibodies to VZV by Latex Agglutination. Anaheim, Calif, Society for Pediatric Research, 1992.
17. Forghani B, Schmidt N, Dennis J. Antibody assays for varicella-zoster virus: comparison of enzyme immunoassay with neutralization, immune adherence hemagglutination, and complement fixation. J Clin Microbiol 8:545 1978.
18. Gershon A, Frey H, Steinberg S, et al. Enzyme-linked immunosorbent assay for measurement of antibody to varicella-zoster virus. Arch Virol 70:169, 1981.
19. LaRussa P, Steinberg S, Waithe E, et al. Comparison of five assays for antibody to varicella-zoster virus and the fluorescent-antibody-to-membrane-antigen test. J Clin Microbiol 25:2059, 1987.
20. Shehab Z, Brunell P. Enzyme-linked immunosorbent assay for susceptibility to varicella. J Infect Dis 148:472, 1983.
21. Friedman MG, Leventon-Kriss S, Sarov I. Sensitive solid-phase radioimmunoassay for detection of human immunoglobulin G antibodies to varicella-zoster virus. J Clin Microbiol 9:1, 1979.
22. Gershon A, Kalter Z, Steinberg S. Detection of antibody to varicella-zoster virus by immune adherence hemagglutination. Proc Soc Exp Biol Med 151:762, 1976.
23. Caunt AE, Shaw DG. Neutralization tests with varicella-zoster virus. J Hyg (London) 67:343, 1969.
24. Grose C, Edmond BJ, Brunell PA. Complement-enhanced neutralizing antibody response to varicella-zoster virus. J Infect Dis 139:432, 1979.
25. Gold E, Godek G. Complement fixation studies with a varicella-zoster antigen. J Immunol 95:692, 1965.
26. Schmidt NJ, Lennette EH, Magoffin RL. Immunological relationship between herpes simplex and varicella-zoster viruses demonstrated by complement-fixation, neutralization and fluorescent antibody tests. J Gen Virol 4:321, 1969.
27. Schaap GJP, Huisman J. Simultaneous rise in complement-fixing antibodies against herpesvirus hominis and varicella-zoster virus in patients with chickenpox and shingles. Arch Ges Virusforsch 25:52, 1968.
28. Schmidt NJ. Further evidence for common antigens in herpes simplex and varicella-zoster virus. J Med Virol 9:27, 1982.
29. Shiraki K, Okuno T, Yamanishi K, Takahashi M. Polypeptides of varicella-zoster virus (VZV) and immunological relationship of VZV and herpes simplex virus (HSV). J Gen Virol 61:255, 1982.
30. Kitamura K, Namazue J, Campo-Vera H, et al. Induction of neutralizing antibody against varicella-zoster virus

(VZV) by gp 2 and cross-reactivity between VZV gp 2 and herpes simplex viruses gB. Virology 149:74, 1986.

31. Lemon SM, Hutt LM, Huang Y-T, et al. Simultaneous infection with multiple herpesviruses. Am J Med 66:270, 1979.

32. Landry ML, Hsiung GD. Diagnosis of dual herpesvirus infection: varicella-zoster virus (VZV) and herpes simplex viruses. In Nahmias AJ, Dowdle WR, Schinazi RF (eds). The Human Herpesviruses. New York, Elsevier, 652, 1981.

33. Arvin AM. Cell-mediated immunity to varicella-zoster virus. J Infect Dis 166:S35, 1992.

34. Davison A, Edson C, Ellis R, et al. New common nomenclature for glycoprotein genes of varicella-zoster virus and their products. J Virol 57:1195, 1986.

35. Brunell P, Gershon AA, Uduman SA, Steinberg S. Varicella-zoster immunoglobulins during varicella, latency, and zoster. J Infect Dis 132:49, 1975.

36. Gershon A, Steinberg S, Borkowsky W, et al. IgM to varicella-zoster virus: demonstration in patients with and without clinical zoster. Pediatr Infect Dis 1:164, 1982.

37. Hope-Simpson RE. The nature of herpes zoster: a long-term study and a new hypothesis. Proc R Soc Med 58:9, 1965.

38. Brunell PA. Transmission of chickenpox in a school setting prior to the observed exanthem. Am J Dis Child 143:1451, 1989.

39. Evans P. An epidemic of chickenpox. Lancet 2:339, 1940.

40. Gordon JE, Meader FM. The period of infectivity and serum prevention of chickenpox. JAMA 93:2013, 1929.

41. Kido S, Ozaki T, Asada H, et al. Detection of varicella-zoster virus (VZV) DNA in clinical samples from patients with VZV by the polymerase chain reaction. J Clin Microbiol 29:76, 1991.

42. Tsolia M, Gershon A, Steinberg S, Gelb L. Live attenuated varicella vaccine: evidence that the virus is attenuated and the importance of skin lesions in transmission of varicella-zoster virus. J Pediatr 116:184, 1990.

43. Gustafson TL, Lavely GB, Brauner ER, et al. An outbreak of nosocomial varicella. Pediatrics 70:550, 1982.

44. Leclair JM, Zaia J, Levin MJ, et al. Airborne transmission of chickenpox in a hospital. N Engl J Med 302:450, 1980.

45. Sawyer M, Chamberlin C, Wu Y, et al. Detection of varicella-zoster virus DNA in air samples from hospital rooms. J Infect Dis 169:91, 1993.

46. Moore DA, Hopkins RS. Assessment of a school exclusion policy during a chickenpox outbreak. Am J Epidemiol 133:1161, 1991.

47. Hope-Simpson RE. Infectiousness of communicable diseases in the household (measles, mumps, and chickenpox). Lancet 2:549, 1952.

48. Kundratitz K. Experimentelle Übertragung von Herpes Zoster auf den Menschen und die Beziehungen von Herpes Zoster zu Varicellen. Monatsschr Kinderheilkd 29:516, 1925.

49. Bruusgaard E. The mutual relation between zoster and varicella. Br J Dermatol Syph 44:1, 1932.

50. Seiler HE. A study of herpes zoster particularly in its relationship to chickenpox. J Hyg (London) 47:253, 1949.

51. Schimpff S, Serpick A, Stoler B, et al. Varicella-zoster infection in patients with cancer. Ann Intern Med 76:241, 1972.

52. Berlin BS, Campbell T. Hospital-acquired herpes zoster following exposure to chickenpox. JAMA 211:1831, 1970.

53. Mahalingham R, Kido S, Wellish M, et al. In situ polymerase chain reaction detection of varicella-zoster virus in infected cells in culture. J Virol Methods 52:21, 1995.

54. Hayakawa Y, Torigoe S, Shiraki K, et al. Biologic and biophysical markers of a live varicella vaccine strain (Oka): identification of clinical isolates from vaccine recipients. J Infect Dis 149:956, 1984.

55. Straus SE, Reinhold W, Smith HA, et al. Endonuclease analysis of viral DNA from varicella and subsequent zoster infections in the same patient. N Engl J Med 311:1362, 1984.

56. Williams DL, Gershon A, Gelb LD, et al. Herpes zoster following varicella vaccine in a child with acute lymphocytic leukemia. J Pediatr 106:259, 1985.

57. Gershon A. Varicella in mother and infant: problems old and new. In Krugman S, Gershon A (eds). Infections of the Fetus and Newborn Infant. New York, Alan R Liss, 1975, p 79.

58. London WP, Yorke JA. Recurrent outbreaks of measles, chickenpox and mumps: I. Seasonal variation in contact rates. Am J Epidemiol 98:453, 1973.

59. Yorke JA, London WP. Recurrent outbreaks of measles, chickenpox and mumps: II. Systematic differences in contact rates and stochastic effects. Am J Epidemiol 98:469, 1973.

60. Gordon JE. Chickenpox: An epidemiologic review. Am J Med Sci 244:362, 1962.

61. Preblud S, Orenstein W, Bart K. Varicella: clinical manifestations, epidemiology, and health impact on children. Pediatr Infect Dis 3:505, 1984.

62. Preblud SR, D'Angelo LJ. Chickenpox in the United States 1972–1977. J Infect Dis 140:257, 1979.

63. Ross AH, Lencher E, Reitman G. Modification of chickenpox in family contacts by administration of gamma globulin. N Engl J Med 267:369, 1962.

64. LaRussa P, Steinberg S, Seeman MD, Gershon AA. Determination of immunity to varicella by means of an intradermal skin test. J Infect Dis 152:869, 1985.

65. Sever J, White LR. Intrauterine viral infections. Ann Rev Med 19:471, 1968.

66. Siegel M. Congenital malformations following chickenpox, measles, mumps, and hepatitis: results of a cohort study. JAMA 226:1521, 1973.

67. Balducci J, Rodis JF, Rosengren S, et al. Pregnancy outcome following first-trimester varicella infection. Obstet Gynecol 79:5, 1992.

68. Brunell PA, Kotchmar GSJ. Zoster in infancy: failure to maintain virus latency following intrauterine infection. J Pediatr 98:71, 1981.

69. Baba K, Yabuuchi H, Takahashi M, Ogra P. Increased incidence of herpes zoster in normal children infected with varicella-zoster virus during infancy: community-based follow up study. J Pediatr 108:372, 1986.

70. Guess H, Broughton DD, Melton LJ, Kurland L. Epidemiology of herpes zoster in children and adolescents: a population-based study. Pediatrics 76:512, 1985.

71. Terada K, Kawano S, Yoshihiro K, Morita T. Varicella-zoster virus (VZV) reactivation is related to the low response of VZV-specific immunity after chickenpox in infancy. J Infect Dis 169:650, 1994.

72. Kalman CM, Laskin OL. Herpes zoster and zosteriform herpes simplex virus infections in immunocompetent adults. Am J Med 81:775, 1986.

73. Locksley RM, Flournoy N, Sullivan KM, Meyers J. Infection with varicella-zoster virus after marrow transplantation. J Infect Dis 152:1172, 1985.

74. Veenstra J, Krol A, van Praag R, et al. Herpes zoster, immunological deterioration and disease progression in HIV-1 infection. AIDS 9:1153, 1995.

75. Gershon A, Mervish N, LaRussa P, et al. Varicella-zoster

virus infection in children with underlying HIV infection. J Infect Dis 175:1496, 1997.

76. Brazin SA, Simkovich JW, Johnson WT. Herpes zoster during pregnancy. Obstet Gynecol 53:175, 1979.

77. Sterner G, Forsgren M, Enocksson E, et al. Varicella-zoster infections in late pregnancy. Scand J Infect Dis 71:30, 1990.

78. Gershon A, Raker R, Steinberg S, et al. Antibody to varicella-zoster virus in parturient women and their offspring during the first year of life. Pediatrics 58:692, 1976.

79. Shehab Z, Brunell P, Cobb E. Epidemiological standardization of a test for susceptibility to mumps. J Infect Dis 149:810, 1984.

80. Sirpenski SP, Brennan T, Mayo D. Determination of infection and immunity to varicella-zoster virus with an enzyme-linked immunosorbent assay. J Infect Dis 152:1349, 1985.

81. Steele R, Coleman MA, Fiser M, Bradsher RW. Varicella-zoster in hospital personnel: skin test reactivity to monitor susceptibility. Pediatrics 70:604, 1982.

82. Kjersem H, Jepsen S. Varicella among immigrants from the tropics, a health problem. Scand J Soc Med 18:171, 1990.

83. Longfield JN, Winn RE, Gibson RL, et al. Varicella outbreaks in army recruits from Puerto Rico. Arch Intern Med 150:970, 1990.

84. Maretic Z, Cooray MPM. Comparisons between chickenpox in a tropical and a European country. J Trop Med Hyg 66:311, 1963.

85. Sinha DP. Chickenpox—a disease predominantly affecting adults in rural west Bengal, India. Int J Epidemiol 5:367, 1976.

86. Brunell P. Placental transfer of varicella-zoster antibody. Pediatrics 38:1034, 1966.

87. Mendez D, Sinclair MB, Garcia S, et al. Transplacental immunity to varicella-zoster virus in extremely low birthweight infants. Am J Perinatol 9:236, 1992.

88. Raker R, Steinberg S, Drusin L, Gershon A. Antibody to varicella-zoster virus in low birth weight infants. J Pediatr 93:505, 1978.

89. Wang E, Prober C, Arvin AM. Varicella-zoster virus antibody titers before and after administration of zoster immune globulin to neonates in an intensive care nursery. J Pediatr 103:113, 1983.

90. Baba K, Yabuuchi H, Takahashi M, Ogra P. Immunologic and epidemiologic aspects of varicella infection acquired during infancy and early childhood. J Pediatr 100:881, 1982.

91. Gustafson TL, Shehab Z, Brunell P. Outbreak of varicella in a newborn intensive care nursery. Am Dis Child 138:548, 1984.

92. Hyatt HW. Neonatal varicella. J Natl Med Assoc 59:32, 1967.

93. Newman CGH. Perinatal varicella. Lancet 2:1159, 1965.

94. Readett MD, McGibbon C. Neonatal varicella. Lancet 1:644, 1961.

95. Freud P. Congenital varicella. Am J Dis Child 96:730, 1958.

96. Odessky L, Newman B, Wein GB. Congenital varicella. NY State J Med 54:2849, 1954.

97. Harris LE. Spread of varicella in nurseries. Am J Dis Child 105:315, 1963.

98. Matseoane SL, Abler C. Occurrence of neonatal varicella in a hospital nursery. Am J Obstet Gynecol 92:575, 1965.

99. Lipton S, Brunell PA. Management of varicella exposure in a neonatal intensive care unit. JAMA 261:1782, 1989.

100. Patou G, Midgley P, Meurisse EV, Feldman RG. Immunoglobulin prophylaxis for infants exposed to varicella in a neonatal unit. J Infect 20:207, 1990.

101. Gold WL, Boulton J, Goldman C, et al. Management of varicella exposures in the neonatal intensive care unit. Pediatr Infect Dis J 12:954, 1993.

102. Friedman CA, Temple DM, Robbins KK, et al. Outbreak and control of varicella in a neonatal intensive care unit. Pediatr Infect Dis J 13:152, 1994.

103. Apert ME. Une epidemic de varicelle dans une maternité. Bull Med (Paris) 9:827, 1985.

104. Gold E. Serologic and virus-isolation studies of patients with varicella or herpes zoster infection. N Engl J Med 274:181, 1966.

105. Myers MG. Viremia caused by varicella-zoster virus: association with malignant progressive varicella. J Infect Dis 140:229, 1979.

106. Nelson A, St. Geme J. On the respiratory spread of varicella-zoster virus. Pediatrics 37:1007, 1966.

107. Trlifajova J, Bryndova D, Ryc M. Isolation of varicella-zoster virus from pharyngeal and nasal swabs in varicella patients. J Hyg Epidemiol Microbiol Immunol 28:201, 1984.

108. Ozaki T, Ichikawa T, Matsui Y, et al. Lymphocyte-associated viremia in varicella. J Med Virol 19:249, 1986.

109. Asano Y, Itakura N, Hiroishi Y, et al. Viremia is present in incubation period in nonimmunocompromised children with varicella. J Pediatr 106:69, 1985.

110. Feldman S, Epp E. Isolation of varicella-zoster virus from blood. J Pediatr 88:265, 1976.

111. Feldman S, Epp E. Detection of viremia during incubation period of varicella. J Pediatr 94:746, 1979.

112. Moffat JF, Stein MD, Kaneshima H, Arvin AM. Tropism of varicella-zoster virus for human CD4+ and CD8+ T lymphocytes and epidermal cells in SCID-hu mice. J Virol 69:5236, 1995.

113. Koropchak C, Graham G, Palmer J, et al. Investigation of varicella-zoster virus infection by polymerase chain reaction in the immunocompetent host with acute varicella. J Infect Dis 163:1016, 1991.

114. Ozaki T, Miwata H, Asano Y, et al. Varicella-zoster virus DNA in throat swabs of vaccinees. Arch Dis Child 267:328, 1993.

115. Grose CH. Variation on a theme by Fenner. Pediatrics 68:735, 1981.

116. Arvin AM, Pollard RB, Rasmussen L, Merigan T. Selective impairment in lymphocyte reactivity to varicella-zoster antigen among untreated lymphoma patients. J Infect Dis 137:531, 1978.

117. Hardy IB, Gershon A, Steinberg S, et al. The incidence of zoster after immunization with live attenuated varicella vaccine: a study in children with leukemia. N Engl J Med 325:1545, 1991.

118. Rand KH, Rasmussen LE, Pollard RB, et al. Cellular immunity and herpesvirus infections in cardiac transplant patients. N Engl J Med 296:1372, 1977.

119. Ruckdeschel JC, Schimpff SC, Smyth AC, Mardiney MR. Herpes zoster and impaired cell-associated immunity to the varicella-zoster virus in patients with Hodgkin's disease. Am J Med 62:77, 1977.

120. Friedman-Kien A, Lafleur F, Gendler F, et al. Herpes zoster: a possible early clinical sign for development of acquired immunodeficiency syndrome in high-risk individuals. J Am Acad Dermatol 14:1023, 1988.

121. Feldman S, Chaudhary S, Ossi M, Epp E. A viremic phase for herpes zoster in children with cancer. J Pediatr 91:597, 1977.

122. Gershon A, Steinberg S, Silber R. Varicella-zoster viremia. J Pediatr 92:1033, 1978.

123. Stevens D, Ferrington R, Jordan G, Merigan T. Cellular events in zoster vesicles: relation to clinical course and immune parameters. J Infect Dis 131:509, 1975.

124. Szanton E, Sarov I. Interaction between polymorphonuclear leukocytes and varicella-zoster infected cells. Intervirology 24:119, 1985.

125. Ihara T, Starr S, Ito M, et al. Human polymorphonuclear leukocyte-mediated cytotoxicity against varicella-zoster virus–infected fibroblasts. J Virol 51:110, 1984.

126. Ihara T, Ito M, Starr SE. Human lymphocyte, monocyte and polymorphonuclear leucocyte mediated antibody-dependent cellular cytotoxicity against varicella-zoster virus-infected targets. Clin Exp Immunol 63:179, 1986.

127. Garcia AGP. Fetal infection in chickenpox and alastrim, with histopathologic study of the placenta. Pediatrics 32:895, 1963.

128. Erlich RM, Turner JAP, Clarke M. Neonatal varicella. J Pediatr 53:139, 1958.

129. Lucchesi PF, LaBoccetta AC, Peale AR. Varicella neonatorum. Am J Dis Child 73:44, 1947.

130. Oppenheimer EH. Congenital chickenpox with disseminated visceral lesions. Bull Johns Hopkins Hosp 74:240, 1944.

131. Pearson HE. Parturition varicella-zoster. Obstet Gynecol 23:21, 1964.

132. Steen J, Pederson RV. Varicella in a newborn girl. J Oslo City Hosp 9:36, 1959.

133. Ranney EK, Norman MG, Silver MD. Varicella pneumonitis. Can Med Assoc J 96:445, 1967.

134. Triebwasser JH, Harris RE, Bryant RE, Rhodes ER. Varicella pneumonia in adults: report of seven cases and a review of the literature. Medicine 46:409, 1967.

135. Bradley JS, Schlievert PM, Sample TG. Streptococcal toxic shock–like syndrome as a complication of varicella. Pediatr Infect Dis J 10:77, 1991.

136. Brogan TV, Niozet V, Waldhausen JHT, et al. Group A streptococcal necrotizing fasciitis complicating primary varicella: a series of fourteen patients. Pediatr Infect Dis J 14:588, 1995.

137. Centers for Disease Control. Outbreak of invasive group A Streptococcus associated with varicella in a childcare center—Boston, MA, 1997. MMWR Morb Mortal Wkly Rep 46:944, 1997.

138. Davies HD, McGeer A, Schwarts B, et al. Invasive group A streptococcal infections in Ontario, Canada. N Engl J Med 335:547, 1996.

139. Doctor A, Harper MB, Fleischer GR. Group A beta-hemolytic streptococcal bacteremia: historical review, changing incidence, and recent ssociation with varicella. Pediatrics 96:428, 1995.

140. Gonzalez-Ruiz A, Ridgway GL, Cohen SL, et al. Varicella gangrenosa with toxic shock–like syndrome due to group A Streptococcus infection in an adult. Clin Infect Dis 20:1058, 1995.

141. Mills WJ, et al. Invasive group A streptococcal infections complicating primary varicella. J Pediatr Orthop 16:522, 1996.

142. Peterson CL, Vugia D, Meyers H, et al. Risk factors for invasive group A streptococcal infections in children with varicella: a case-control study. Pediatr Infect Dis J 15:151, 1996.

143. Wilson G, Talkington D, Gruber W, et al. Group A streptococcal necrotizing fasciitis following varicella in children: case reports and review. Clin Infect Dis 20:1333, 1995.

144. Bullowa JGM, Wishik SM. Complications of varicella: I. Their occurrence among 2,534 patients. Am J Dis Child 49:923, 1935.

145. Johnson R, Milbourn PE. Central nervous system manifestations of chickenpox. Can Med Assoc J 102:831, 1970.

146. Jenkins RB. Severe chickenpox encephalopathy. Am J Dis Child 110:137, 1965.

147. Minkowitz S, Wenk R, Friedman E, et al. Acute glomerulonephritis associated with varicella infection. Am J Med 44:489, 1968.

148. Yuceoglu AM, Berkovich S, Minkowitz S. Acute glomerular nephritis as a complication of varicella. JAMA 202:113, 1967.

149. Morales A, Adelman S, Fine G. Varicella myocarditis. Arch Pathol 91:29, 1971.

150. Moore CM, Henry J, Benzing G, et al. Varicella myocarditis. Am J Dis Child 118:899, 1969.

151. Priest JR, Groth KE, Balfour HH. Varicella arthritis documented by isolation of virus from joint fluid. J Pediatr 93:990, 1978.

152. Ward JR, Bishop B. Varicella arthritis. JAMA 212:1954, 1970.

153. Gershon A. Varicella-zoster virus: prospects for control. Adv Pediatr Infect Dis 10:93, 1995.

154. Jura E, Chadwick E, Josephs SH, et al. Varicella-zoster virus infections in children infected with human immunodeficiency virus. Pediatr Infect Dis J 8:586, 1989.

155. Feldman S, Hughes W, Daniel C. Varicella in children with cancer: 77 cases. Pediatrics 80:388, 1975.

156. Ihara T, Kamiya H, Starr SE, et al. Natural killing of varicella-zoster virus (VZV)–infected fibroblasts in normal children, children with VZV infections, and children with Hodgkin's disease. Acta Pediatr Jpn 31:523, 1989.

157. Arvin A, Sharp M, Smith S, et al. Equivalent recognition of a varicella-zoster virus immediate early protein (IE62) and glycoprotein I by cytotoxic T lymphocytes of either CD4+ or CD8+ phenotype. J Immunol 146:257, 1991.

158. Cooper E, Vujic L, Quinnan G. Varicella-zoster virus-specific HLA-restricted cytotoxicity of normal immune adult lymphocytes after in vitro stimulation. J Infect Dis 158:780, 1988.

159. Krugman S, Goodrich C, Ward R. Primary varicella pneumonia. N Engl J Med 257:843, 1957.

160. Mermelstein RH, Freireich AW. Varicella pneumonia. Ann Intern Med 55:456, 1961.

161. Weber DM, Pellecchia JA. Varicella pneumonia: study of prevalence in adult men. JAMA 192:572, 1965.

162. Sargent EN, Carson MJ, Reilly ED. Varicella pneumonia: a report of 20 cases with postmortem examination in 6. Calif Med 107:141, 1967.

163. Bocles JS, Ehrenkranz NJ, Marks A. Abnormalities of respiratory function in varicella pneumonia. Ann Intern Med 60:183, 1964.

164. Fish SA. Maternal death due to disseminated varicella. JAMA 173:978, 1960.

165. Hackel DB. Myocarditis in association with varicella. Am J Pathol 29:369, 1953.

166. Harris RE, Rhoades ER. Varicella pneumonia complicating pregnancy: report of a case and review of the literature. Obstet Gynecol 25:734, 1965.

167. Brunell PA. Varicella-zoster infections in pregnancy. JAMA 199:315, 1967.

168. Baren J, Henneman P, Lewis R. Primary varicella in adults: pneumonia, pregnancy, and hospital admission. Ann Emerg Med 28:165, 1996.

169. Siegel M, Fuerst HT. Low birth weight and maternal virus diseases: a prospective study of rubella, measles, mumps, chiockenpox, and hepatitis. JAMA 197:88, 1966.

170. Abler C. Neonatal varicella. Am J Dis Child 107:492, 1964.

171. Siegel M, Fuerst HT, Peress NS. Comparative fetal mortality in maternal virus diseases: a prospective study on rubella, measles, mumps, chickenpox, and hepatitis. N Engl J Med 274:768, 1966.

172. Pickard RE. Varicella pneumonia in pregnancy. Am J Obstet Gynecol 101:504, 1968.

173. Mendelow DA, Lewis GC. Varicella pneumonia during pregnancy. Obstet Gynecol 33:98, 1969.

174. Geeves RB, Lindsay DA, Robertson TI. Varicella pneumonia in pregnancy with varicella neonatorum: report of a case followed by severe digital clubbing. Aust NZ J Med 1:63, 1971.

175. Paryani SG, Arvin AM. Intrauterine infection with varicella-zoster virus after maternal varicella. N Engl J Med 314:1542, 1986.

176. Esmonde TF, Herdman G, Anderson G. Chickenpox pneumonia: an association with pregnancy. Thorax 44:812, 1989.

177. Figueroa-Damian R, Arrendondo-Garcia JL. Perinatal outcome of pregnancies complicated with varicella infection during the first 20 weeks of gestation. Am J Perinatol 14:411, 1997.

178. Cox SM, Cunningham FG, Luby J. Management of varicella pneumonia complicating pregnancy. Am J Perinatol 7:300, 1990.

179. Smego RA, Asperilla MO. Use of acyclovir for varicella pneumonia during pregnancy. Obstet Gynecol 78:1112, 1991.

180. Landsberger EJ, Hager WD, Grossman JH. Successful management of varicella pneumonia complicating pregnancy: a report of 3 cases. J Reprod Med 31:311, 1986.

181. Lotshaw RR, Keegan JM, Gordon HR. Parenteral and oral acyclovir for management of varicella pneumonia in pregnancy: A case report with review of literature. WV Med J 87:204, 1991.

182. Hockberger RS, Rothstein RJ. Varicella pneumonia in adults: a spectrum of disease. Ann Emerg Med 115:931, 1986.

183. Hollingsworth HM, Pratter MR, Irwin RS. Acute respiratory failure in pregnancy. J Intensive Care Med 4:11, 1089.

184. Hankins GDV, Gilstrap LC, Patterson AR. Acyclovir treatment of varicella pneumonia in pregnancy. Letter. Crit Care Med 15:336, 1987.

185. Glaser JB, Loftus J, Ferragamo V, et al. Varicella in pregnancy. Letter. N Engl J Med 315:1416, 1986.

186. Boyd K, Walker E. Use of acyclovir to treat chickenpox in pregnancy. BMJ 296:393, 1988.

187. White RG. Chickenpox in pregnancy. Letter. BMJ 196:864, 1988.

188. Broussard OF, Payne DK, George RB. Treatment with acyclovir of varicella pneumonia in pregnancy. Chest 99:1045, 1991.

189. Eder SE, Apuzzio JA, Weiss G. Varicella pneumonia during pregnancy: treatment of 2 cases with acyclovir. Am J Perinatol 5:16, 1988.

190. Andrews EB, Tilson HH, Hurn BAL, Cordero JF. Acyclovir in pregnancy registry. Am J Med 85:123, 1988.

191. Centers for Disease Control. Acyclovir Registry. MMWR Morb Mortal Wkly Rep 42:806, 1993.

192. Pearse BM. Characterization of coated-vesicle adaptors: their reassembly with clathrin and with recycling receptors. Methods Cell Biol 31:229, 1989.

193. Centers for Disease Control. Prevention of varicella: recommendations of the Advisory Committee on Immunization Practices (ACIP). MMWR Morb Mortal Wkly Rep 45:1, 1996.

194. Enders G, Miller E, Cradock-Watson J, et al. Consequences of varicella and herpes zoster in pregnancy: prospective study of 1739 cases. Lancet 343:1548, 1994.

195. Benyesh-Melnick M, Stich HF, Rapp F, et al. Viruses and mammalian chromosomes: III. Effect of herpes zoster virus on human embryonal lung cultures. Proc Soc Exp Biol Med 117:546, 1964.

196. Aula P: Chromosomes and virus infections. Lancet 1:720, 1964.

197. Massimo I, Vianello MG, Dagna-Bricarelli F, et al. Chickenpox and chromosome aberrations. BMJ 2:172, 1965.

198. Collier E. Congenital varicella cataract. Am J Ophthalmol 86:627, 1978.

199. Cuthbertson G, Weiner CPW, Giller RH, Grose C. Prenatal diagnosis of second-trimester congenital varicella syndrome by virus-specific immunoglobulin M. J Pediatr 111:592, 1987.

200. Harding B, Bonner JA. Congenital varicella-zoster: a serologically proven case with necrotizing encephalitis and malformations. Acta Neuropathol 76:311, 1988.

201. Hammad E, Helin I, Pasca A. Early pregnancy varicella and associated congenital anomalies. Acta Paediatr Scand 78:963, 1989.

202. Adelstein AM, Donovan JW. Malignant disease in children whose mothers had chickenpox, mumps, or rubella in pregnancy. BMJ 2:629 1972.

203. Fox MJ, Krumpiegel ER, Teresi JL. Maternal measles, mumps, and chickenpox as a cause of congenital anomalies. Lancet 1:746, 1948.

204. Jones KL, Johnson KA, Chambers CD. Offspring of women infected with varicella during pregnancy: a prospective study. Teratology 49:29, 1994.

205. Pastuszak A, Levy M, Schick B, et al. Outcome after maternal varicella infection in the first 20 weeks of pregnancy. N Engl J Med 330:901 1994.

206. Michie CA, Acolet D, Charlton R, et al. Varicella-zoster contracted in the second trimester of pregnancy. Pediatr Infect Dis J 10:1050, 1992.

207. Connan L, Ayoubi J, Icart J, et al. Intra-uterine fetal death following maternal varicella infection. Eur J Obstet Gynecol 68:205, 1996.

208. Sauerbrai A, Muller D, Eichhorn U, Wutzler P. Detection of varicella-zoster virus in congenital varicella syndrome: a case report. Obstet Gynecol 88:687 1996.

209. Mouly F, Mirlesse V, Meritet JF, et al. Prenatal diagnosis of fetal varicella-zoster virus infection with polymerase chain reaction of amniotic fluid in 107 cases. Am J Obstet Gynecol 177:894, 1997.

210. Ussery XT, Annunziato P, Gershon A, et al. Congenital varicella-zoster infection and Barrett's esophagus. J Infect Dis 178:539, 1998.

211. LaForet EG, Lynch LL. Multiple congenital defects following maternal varicella. N Engl J Med 236:534, 1947.

212. Srabstein JC, Morris N, Larke B, et al. Is there a congenital varicella syndrome? J Pediatr 84:239, 1974.

213. Alfonso I, Palomino JA, DeQuesada G, et al. Picture of the month: congenital varicella syndrome. Am J Dis Child 138:603, 1984.

214. Alkalay AL, Pomerance JJ, Yamamura JM, et al. Congenital anomalies associated with maternal varicella infections during early pregnancy. J Perinatol 7:69, 1987.

215. Borzykowski M, Harris RF, Jones RWA. The congenital varicella syndrome. Eur J Pediatr 137:335, 1981.

216. Dietzsch H, Rabenalt P, Trlifajova J. Varizellen-Embryopathie: Kliniche und serologische verlaufsbeobachtungen. Kinderarztl Prax 3:139, 1980.

217. Fuccillo DA. Congenital varicella. Teratology 15:329, 1977.

218. Hajdi G, Meszner Z, Nyerges G, et al. Congenital varicella syndrome. Infection 14:177, 1986.

219. McKendry JBJ. Congenital varicella associated with multiple defects. Can Med Assoc J 108:66, 1973.

220. Rinvik R. Congenital varicella encephalomyelitis in surviving newborn. Am J Dis Child 117:231, 1969.

221. Savage MO, Moosa A, Gordon RR. Maternal varicella infection as a cause of fetal malformations. Lancet 1:352, 1973.

222. Schlotfeld-Schafer I, Schafer P, Llatz S, et al. Congenitales Varicellensyndrom. Monatsschr Kinderheilkd 131:106, 1983.

223. Broomhead. Cited in Dudgeon HA (ed): Viral Diseases of the Fetus and Newborn. Philadelphia, WB Saunders, 1982, p 161.

224. Enders G. Varicella-zoster virus infection in pregnancy. Prog Med Virol 29:166, 1984.

225. Essex-Cater A, Heggarty H. Fatal congenital varicella syndrome. J Infect 7:77, 1983.

226. Lamy M, Minkowski A, Choucroun J. Embryopathie d'origine infectieuse. Semaine Med 72, 1951.

227. Konig R, Gutjahr P, Kruel R, et al. Konnatale varizellen-embryo-fetopathy. Helv Paediatr Acta 40:391, 1985.

228. Scharf A, Scherr O, Enders G, Helftenbein E. Virus detection in the fetal tissue of a premature delivery with a congenital varicella syndrome. J Perinat Med 18:317, 1990.

229. DaSilva O, Hammerberg O, Chance GW. Fetal varicella syndrome. Pediatr Infect Dis J 9:854, 1990.

230. Magliocco AM, Demetrick DJ, Sarnat HB, Hwang WS. Varicella embryopathy. Arch Pathol Lab Med 116:181, 1992.

231. Alexander I. Congenital varicella. BMJ 2:1074, 1979.

232. Bailie FB. Aplasia cutis congenita of neck and shoulder requiring a skin graft: a case report. Br J Plastic Surg 36:72 1983.

233. Brice JEH. Congenital varicella resulting from infection during second trimester at pregnancy. Arch Dis Child 51:474, 1976.

234. Dodion Fransen J, Dekegel D, Thiry L. Maternal varicella infection as a cause of fetal malformations. Scand J Infect Dis 5:149, 1973.

235. Frey H, Bialkin G, Gershon A. Congenital varicella: case report of a serologically proved long-term survivor. Pediatrics 59:110, 1977.

236. Pettay O. Intrauterine and perinatal viral infections. Ann Clin Res 11:258, 1979.

237. Taranger J, Blomberg J, Strannegard O. Intrauterine varicella: a report of two cases associated with hyper-A-immunoglobulinemia. Scand J Infect Dis 13:297, 1981.

238. Unger-Koppel J, Kilcher P, Tonz O. Varizellenfetopathie. Helv Paediatr Acta 40:399, 1985.

239. White MI, Daly BM, Moffat MA, Rankin R. Connective tissue naevi in a child with intra-uterine varicella infection. Clin Exp Dermatol 15:149, 1990.

240. Palmer CGS, Pauli RM. Intrauterine varicella infection. J Pediatr 112:506, 1988.

241. Lambert SR, Taylor D, Kriss A, et al. Ocular manifestations of the congenital varicella syndrome. Arch Ophthalmol 107:52, 1989.

242. Bai PVA, John TJ. Congenital skin ulcers following varicella in late pregnancy. J Pediatr 94:65, 1979.

243. Klauber GT, Flynn FJ, Altman BD. Congenital varicella syndrome with genitourinary anomalies. Urology 8:153, 1976.

244. Michon L, Aubertin D, Jager-Schmidt G. Deux observations de malformations congenitales paraissant relever d'embryopathies zosteriennes. Arch Fr Pediatr 16:695, 1959.

245. Enders G. Serodiagnosis of varicella-zoster virus infection in pregnancy and standardisation of the ELISA IgG and IgM antibody tests. Dev Biol Stand 52:221, 1982.

246. Charles N, Bennett TW, Margolis S. Ocular pathology of the congenital varicella syndrome. Arch Ophthalmol 95:2034, 1977.

247. Andreou A, Basiakos H, Hatsikoumi I, Lazarides A. Fetal varicella syndrome with manifestations limited to the eye. Am J Perinatol 12:347, 1995.

248. Kotchmar G, Grose C, Brunell P. Complete spectrum of the varicella congenital defects syndrome in 5-year-old child. Pediatr Infect Dis 3:142, 1984.

249. Grose C. Congenital varicella-zoster virus infection and the failure to establish virus-specific cell-mediated immunity. Mol Biol Med 6:453, 1989.

250. Salzman MB, Sood SK. Congenital anomalies resulting from maternal at 25 and a half weeks of gestation. Pediatr Infect Dis J 11:504, 1992.

251. Hitchcock R, Birthistle K, Carrington D, et al. Colonic atresia and spinal cord atrophy associated with a case of fetal varicella syndrome. J Pediatr Surg 30:1344, 1995.

252. Lloyd KM, Dunne JL. Skin lesions as the sole manifestation of the fetal varicella syndrome. Clin Exp Dermatol 15:149, 1990.

253. Scheffer IE, Baraitser M, Brett EM. Severe microcephaly associated with congenital varicella infection. Dev Med Child Neurol 33:916, 1991.

254. Randel R, Kearns DB, Sawyer MH. Vocal cord paralysis as a presentation of intrauterine infection with varicella-zoster virus. Pediatrics 97:127, 1996.

255. Bennet R, Forsgren M, Herin P. Herpes zoster in a 2-week-old premature infant with possible congenital varicella encephalitis. Acta Pediatr Scand 74:979, 1985.

256. Byrne JLB, Ward K, Kochenour NK, Dolcourt JL. Prenatal sonographic diagnosis of fetal varicella syndrome. Am J Hum Genet 47:A470, 1990.

257. Sauerbrai A, Prager J, Hengst U, et al. Varicella vaccination in children after bone marrow transplantation. Bone Marrow Transplant 20:381, 1997.

258. Duehr PA. Herpes zoster as a cause of congenital cataract. Am J Ophthalmol 39:157, 1955.

259. Webster MH, Smith CS. Congenital abnormalities and maternal herpes zoster. BMJ 4:1193, 1977.

260. Webster CB, Chen D, Horgan M, Olivo PD. The varicella-zoster virus origin-binding protein can substitute for the herpes simplex virus origin-binding protein in a transient origin-dependent DNA replication assay in insect cells. Virology 206:655, 1995.

261. Paryani SG, Arvin AM, Koropchak C, et al. Varicella zoster antibody titers after the administration of intravenous immune serum globulin or varicella zoster immune globulin. Am J Med 76:124, 1984.

262. Grose C, Itani O, Weiner C. Prenatal diagnosis of fetal infection: advances from amniocentesis to cordocentesis—congenital toxoplasmosis, rubella, cytomegalovirus, varicella virus, parvovirus and human immunodeficiency virus. Pediatr Infect Dis J 8:459, 1989.

263. Alkalay AL, Pomerance JJ, Rimoin D. Fetal varicella syndrome. J Pediatr 111:320, 1987.

264. Culbertson W, Blumenkranz M, Pepse J, et al. Varicella zoster virus is a cause of the acute retinal necrosis syndrome. Ophthalmology 93:559, 1986.

265. Fowler KB, Stagno S, Pass RF, et al. The outcome of congenital cytomegalovirus infection in relation to maternal antibody status. N Engl J Med 326:663, 1992.

266. Isada NB, Paar DP, Johnson M, et al. In utero diagnosis

of congenital varicella zoster infection by chorionic villus sampling and polymerase chain reaction. Am J Obstet Gynecol 165:1727, 1991.

267. Lecuru F, Taurells R, Bernard JP, et al. Varicella-zoster virus infection during pregnancy: the limits of prenatal diagnosis. Eur J Obstet Gynecol Reprod Biol 56:67, 1994.

268. Hofmeyer GJ, Moolla S, Lawrie T. Prenatal sonographic diagnosis of congenital varicella infection—a case report. Prenat Diagn 16:1148, 1996.

269. Preblud S, Bregman DJ, Vernon LL. Deaths from varicella in infants. Pediatr Infect Dis 4:503, 1985.

270. Rubin L, Leggiadro R, Elie MT, Lipsitz P. Disseminated varicella in a neonate: implications for immunoprophylaxis of neonates postnatally exposed to varicella. Pediatr Infect Dis 5:100, 1986.

271. Meyers J. Congenital varicella in term infants: risk reconsidered. J Infect Dis 129:215, 1974.

272. Hanngren K, Grandien M, Granstrom G. Effect of zoster immunoglobulin for varicella prophylaxis in the newborn. Scand J Infect Dis 17:343, 1985.

273. Preblud S, Nelson W L, Levin M, Zaia J. Modification of congenital varicella infection with VZIG, Interscience Conference on Antimicrobial Agents and Chemotherapy, New Orleans, 1986.

274. Nankervis GA, Gold E. Varicella-zoster viruses. In Kaplan AS (ed). The Herpesviruses. New York, Academic Press, 1973, p 327.

275. Kohl S. The neonatal human's immune response to herpes simplex virus infection: a critical review. Pediatr Infect Dis J 8:67, 1989.

276. Winkelman RK, Perry HO. Herpes zoster in children. JAMA 171:876, 1959.

277. David T, Williams M. Herpes zoster in infancy. Scand J Infect Dis 11:185, 1979.

278. Dworsky M, Whitely R, Alford C. Herpes zoster in early infancy. Am J Dis Child 134:618, 1980.

279. Helander I, Arstila P, Terho P. Herpes zoster in a 6 month old infant. Acta Dermatol 63:180, 1982.

280. Lewkonia IK, Jackson AA. Infantile herpes zoster after intrauterine exposure to varicella. BMJ 3:149, 1973.

281. Lyday JH. Report of severe herpes zoster in a 13½ year old boy whose chickenpox infection may have been acquired in utero. Pediatrics 50:930, 1972.

282. Adkisson MA. Herpes zoster in a newborn premature infant. J Pediatr 66:956, 1965.

283. Bonar BE, Pearsall CJ. Herpes zoster in the newborn. Am J Dis Child 44:398, 1932.

284. Counter CE, Korn BJ. Herpes zoster in the newborn associated with congenital blindness: report of a case. Arch Pediatr 67:397, 1950.

285. Feldman GV. Herpes zoster neonatorum. Arch Dis Child 27:126, 1952.

286. Freud P, Rook GD, Gurian S. Herpes zoster in the newborn. Am J Dis Child 64:895, 1942.

287. Music SI, Fine EM, Togo Y. Zoster-like disease in the newborn due to herpes-simplex virus. N Engl J Med 284:24, 1971.

288. Gershon A, Steinberg S, LaRussa P. Varicella-zoster virus. In Lennette EH (ed). Laboratory Diagnosis of Viral Infections. New York, Marcel Dekker, 1992, p 749.

289. Rawlinson WD, Dwyer DE, Gibbons V, Cunningham A. Rapid diagnosis of varicella-zoster virus infection with a monoclonal antibody based direct immunofluorescence technique. J Virol Methods 23:13, 1989.

290. Hughes P, LaRussa PS, Pearce JM, et al. Transmission of varicella-zoster virus from a vaccinee with underlying leukemia, demonstrated by polymerase chain reaction. J Pediatr 124:932, 1994.

291. Ito M, Nishihara H, Mizutani K, et al. Detection of varicella zoster virus (VZV) DNA in throat swabs and peripheral blood mononuclear cells of immunocompromised patients with herpes zoster by polymerase chain reaction. Clin Diagn Virol 4:105, 1995.

292. LaRussa P, Lungu O, Hardy I, et al. Restriction fragment length polymorphism of polymerase chain reaction products from vaccine and wild-type varicella-zoster virus isolates. J Virol 66:1016, 1992.

293. LaRussa P, Steinberg S, Gershon A. Diagnosis and typing of varicella-zoster virus (VZV) in clinical specimens by polymerase chain reaction (PCR). Thirty-fourth International Conference on Antimicrobial Agents and Chemotherapy, Orlando, FL, September 1994.

294. Mahalingham R, Cohrs R, Dueland AN, Gilden DH. Polymerase chain reaction diagnosis of varicella-zoster virus. In Becker Y, Darai G (eds). Diagnosis of Human Viruses by Polymerase Chain Reaction Technology, vol 1. New York, Springer-Verlag, 1992, p 134.

295. Puchhammer-Stockl E, Kunz C, Wagner G, Enders G. Detection of varicella zoster virus (VZV) in fetal tissue by polymerase chain reaction. J Perinat Med 22:65, 1994.

296. Sawyer M, Wu YN. Detection of varicella-zoster virus DNA by polymerase chain reaction in CSF of patients with VZV-related central nervous system complications. International Conference on Antimicrobial Agents and Chemotherapy, New Orleans, September 1993.

297. Annunziato P, Lungu O, Gershon A, et al. In situ hybridization detection of varicella zoster virus in paraffin-embedded skin biopsy specimens. Clin Diagn Virol 7:69, 1997.

298. Silliman CC, Tedder D, Ogle JW, et al. Unsuspected varicella-zoster virus encephalitis in a child with acquired immunodeficiency syndrome. J Pediatr 123:418, 1993.

299. Gershon AA, LaRussa P. Varicella-zoster virus. In Donowitz LG (ed). Hospital-Acquired Infection in the Pediatric Patient. Baltimore, Williams & Wilkins, 1988, p 139.

300. Le CT, Lipson M. Difficulty in determining varicella-zoster immune status in pregnant women. Pediatr Infect Dis J 8:650–651, 1989.

301. Whitley RJ, Straus S. Therapy for varicella-zoster virus infections: where do we stand? Infect Dis Clin Pract 2:100, 1993.

302. Whitley RJ, Gnann JW. Acyclovir: a decade later. N Engl J Med 327:782, 1992.

303. Greffe BS, Dooley S, Deddish R, Krasny H. Transplacental passage of acyclovir. J Pediatr 108:1020, 1986.

304. Dunkel L, Arvin A, Whitley R, et al. A controlled trial of oral acyclovir for chickenpox in normal children. N Engl J Med 325:1539, 1991.

305. Balfour HH, Rotbart H, Feldman S, et al. Acyclovir treatment of varicella in otherwise healthy adolescents. J Pediatr 120:627, 1992.

306. Feder H. Treatment of adult chickenpox with oral acyclovir. Arch Intern Med 150:2061, 1990.

307. Wallace MR, Bowler WA, Murray NB, et al. Treatment of adult varicella with oral acyclovir: a randomized, placebo-controlled trial. Ann Intern Med 117:358, 1992.

308. Whitley RJ, Middlebrooks M, Gnann JW. Acyclovir: the past ten years. Adv Exp Med Biol 278:243, 1990.

309. Whitley R, Arvin A, Prober C, et al. A controlled trial comparing vidarabine with acyclovir in neonatal herpes simplex virus infection. N Engl J Med 324:444, 1991.

310. Englund J, Fletcher CV, Balfour HH. Acyclovir therapy in neonates. J Pediatr 119:129, 1991.

311. Gershon AA, Steinberg S, NIAID-Collaborative-Varicella-Vaccine-Study-Group. Live attenuated varicella vaccine: protection in healthy adults in comparison to leukemic children. J Infect Dis 161:661, 1990.

312. Arvin A, Koropchak CM, Wittek AE. Immunologic evidence of reinfection with varicella-zoster virus. J Infect Dis 148:200, 1983.

313. Gershon AA, Steinberg S, Gelb L, NIAID-Collaborative-Varicella-Vaccine-Study-Group. Clinical reinfection with varicella-zoster virus. J Infect Dis 149:137, 1984.

314. Junker AK, Angus E, Thomas E. Recurrent varicella-zoster virus infections in apparently immunocompetent children. Pediatr Infect Dis J 10:569, 1991.

315. Junker AK, Tilley P. Varicella-zoster virus antibody avidity and IgG-subclass patterns in children with recurrent chickenpox. J Med Virol 43:119, 1994.

316. Martin KA, Junker AK, Thomas EE, et al. Occurrence of chickenpox during pregnancy in women seropositive for varicella-zoster virus. J Infect Dis 170:991, 1994.

317. Bogger-Goren S, Bernstein JM, Gershon A, Ogra PL. Mucosal cell mediated immunity to varicella zoster virus: role in protection against disease. J Pediatr 105:195, 1984.

318. Bogger-Goren S, Baba K, Hurley P, et al. Antibody response to varicella-zoster virus after natural or vaccine-induced infection. J Infect Dis 146:260, 1982.

319. Ljungman P, Lonnqvist B, Gahrton G, et al. Clinical and subclinical reactivations of varicella-zoster virus in immunocompromised patients. J Infect Dis 153:840, 1986.

320. Weigle K, Grose C. Molecular dissection of the humoral immune response to individual varicella-zoster viral proteins during chickenpox, quiescence, reinfection, and reactivation. J Infect Dis 149:741, 1984.

321. Gilden DH, Wright R, Schneck S, et al. Zoster sine herpete, a clinical variant. Ann Neurol 35:530, 1994.

322. Wilson A, Sharp M, Koropchak C, et al. Subclinical varicella-zoster virus viremia, herpes zoster, and T lymphocyte immunity to varicella-zoster viral antigens after bone marrow transplantation. J Infect Dis 165:119, 1992.

323. Hardy IB, Gershon A, Steinberg S, et al. Incidence of zoster after live attenuated varicella vaccine. International Conference on Antimicrobial Agents and Chemotherapy, Chicago, September 1991.

324. LaRussa PL, Gershon AA, Steinberg S, Chartrand S. Antibodies to varicella-zoster virus glycoproteins I, II, and III in leukemic and healthy children. J Infect Dis 162:627, 1990.

325. Burke BL, Steele RW, Beard OW, et al. Immune responses to varicella-zoster in the aged. Arch Intern Med 142:291, 1982.

326. Miller AE. Selective decline in cellular immune response to varicella-zoster in the elderly. Neurology 30:582, 1980.

327. Gershon A, Steinberg S. Antibody responses to varicella-zoster virus and the role of antibody in host defense. Am J Med Sci 282:12, 1981.

328. Stevens D, Merigan T. Zoster immune globulin prophylaxis of disseminated zoster in compromised hosts. Arch Intern Med 140:52, 1980.

329. Gershon A. Immunoprophylaxis of varicella-zoster infections. Am J Med 76:672, 1984.

330. Levin M. Can herpes zoster be prevented? Eur J Clin Microbiol Infect Dis 15:1, 1996.

331. Levin M, Murray M, Rotbart H, et al. Immune response of elderly individuals to a live attenuated varicella vaccine. J Infect Dis 166:253, 1992.

332. Levin M, Murray M, Zerbe G, et al. Immune responses of elderly persons 4 years after receiving a live attenuated varicella vaccine. J Infect Dis 170:522, 1994.

333. Brunell P, Ross A, Miller L, Kuo B. Prevention of varicella by zoster immune globulin. N Engl J Med 280:1191, 1969.

334. Brunell P, Gershon A, Hughes W, et al. Prevention of varicella in high-risk children: a collaborative study. Pediatrics 50:718, 1972.

335. Gershon A, Steinberg S, Brunell P. Zoster immune globulin: a further assessment. N Engl J Med 290:243, 1974.

336. Orenstein W, Heymann D, Ellis R, et al. Prophylaxis of varicella in high risk children: response effect of zoster immune globulin. J Pediatr 98:368, 1981.

337. Zaia JA, Levin MJ, Wright GG, et al. A practical method for preparation of varicella-zoster immune globulin. J Infect Dis 137:601, 1978.

338. Zaia J, Levin M, Preblud S, et al. Evaluation of varicella-zoster immune globulin: protection of immunosuppressed children after household exposure to varicella. J Infect Dis 147:737, 1983.

339. Neustadt A. Congenital varicella. Am J Dis Child 106:391, 1963.

340. O'Neill RR. Congenital varicella. Am J Dis Child 104:391, 1962.

341. Committee on Infectious Diseases, American Academy of Pediatrics. Report of the Committee on Infectious Diseases. Elk Grove Village, Ill, American Academy of Pediatrics, 1997.

342. Bakshi S, Miller TC, Kaplan M, et al. Failure of VZIG in modification of severe congenital varicella. Pediatr Infect Dis 5:699, 1986.

343. Haddad J, Simeoni U, Willard D. Perinatal varicella. Lancet 1:494, 1986.

344. Holland P, Isaacs D, Moxon ER. Fatal neonatal varicella infection. Lancet 2:1156, 1986.

345. King S, Gorensek M, Ford-Jones EL, Read S. Fatal varicella-zoster infection in a newborn treated with varicella-zoster immunoglobulin. Pediatr Infect Dis 5:588, 1986.

346. Oglivie MM, Stephens JRD, Larkin M. Chickenpox in pregnancy. Lancet 1:915, 1986.

347. Williams H, Latif A, Morgan J, Ansari BM. Acyclovir in the treatment of neonatal varicella. J Infect 15:65, 1987.

348. Haddad J, Simeoni U, Messer J, Willard D. Acyclovir in prophylaxis and perinatal varicella. Lancet 1:161, 1987.

349. Sills J, Galloway A, Amegavie L, et al. Acyclovir in prophylaxis and perinatal varicella. Lancet 1:161, 1987.

350. Fried D, Hanukoglu A, Birk O. Leukocyte transfusion in severe neonatal varicella. Acta Pediatr Scand 71:147, 1982.

351. Betzhold J, Hong R. Fatal graft versus host reaction in a small leucocyte transfusion in a patient with lymphoma and varicella. Pediatrics 60:62–66, 1978.

352. Gershon A. Commentary on VZIG in infants. Pediatr Infect Dis J 6:469, 1987.

353. Takahashi M, Otsuka T, Okuno Y, et al. Live vaccine used to prevent the spread of varicella in children in hospital. Lancet 2:1288, 1974.

354. Arvin A, Gershon A. Live attenuated varicella vaccine. Annu Rev Microbiol 50:59, 1996.

355. White CJ. Varicella-zoster virus vaccine. Clin Infect Dis 24:753, 1997.

356. Committee-on-Infectious-Diseases. Live attenuated varicella vaccine. Pediatrics 95:791, 1995.

357. Broyer M, Tete MT, Guest G, et al. Varicella and zoster in children after kidney transplantation: long term results of vaccination. Pediatrics 99:35, 1997.

358. LaRussa P, Steinberg S, Meurice F, Gershon A. Trans-

mission of vaccine strain varicella-zoster virus from a healthy adult with vaccine-associated rash to susceptible household contacts. J Infect Dis 176:1072, 1997.

359. Salzman MB, Sharrar R, Steinberg S, LaRussa P. Transmission of varicella-vaccine virus from a healthy 12 month old child to his pregnant mother. J Pediatr 131:151, 1997.

360. Long S. Toddler-to-mother transmission of varicella-vaccine virus: how bad is that? J Pediatr 131:10, 1997.

361. Saiman L, Crowley K, Gershon A. Control of varicella-zoster infections in hospitals. In Abrutyn E, Goldmann DA, Scheckler WE (eds). Infection Control Reference Service. Philadelphia, WB Saunders, 1997, p 687.

362. Wain H. The Story Behind the Word. Springfield, Ill, Charles C Thomas, 1958, p 199.

363. Choppin P, Richardson C, Merz D, et al. The functions and inhibition of the membrane glycoproteins of paramyxoviruses and myxoviruses and the role of the measles virus M protein in subacute sclerosing panencephalitis. J Infect Dis 143:352, 1981.

364. Rota PA, Rota JS, Bellini WJ. Molecular epidemiology of measles virus. Semin Virol 6:379, 1995.

365. Matumoto M. Multiplication of measles virus in cell cultures. Bacteriol Rev 30:152, 1966.

366. Weigle K, Murphy D, Brunell P. Enzyme-linked immunosorbent assay for evaluation of immunity to measles virus. J Clin Microbiol 19:376, 1984.

367. Mayo DR, Brennan T, Cormier DP, et al. Evaluation of a commercial measles virus immunoglobulin M enzyme immunoassay. J Clin Microbiol 29:2865, 1991.

368. Lievens A, Brunell PA. Specific immunoglobulin M enzyme-linked immunosorbent assay for confirming the diagnosis of measles. J Clin Microbiol 24:391, 1986.

369. Papp K. Experiences prouvant que la voie d'infection de la rougeole est la contamination de la musqueuse conjunctivale. Rev Immunol 20:27, 1956.

370. Morley DC, Woodland M, Martin WJ. Measles in Nigerian children: a study of the disease in West Africa, and its manifestations in England and other countries during different epochs. J Hyg (London) 61:113, 1963.

371. Babbott FL Jr, Gordon JE. Modern measles. Am J Med Sci 225:334, 1954.

372. Centers for Disease Control. Measles, mumps, and rubella—vaccine use and strategies for elimination of measles, rubella, and congenital rubella syndrome and control of mumps. MMWR Morb Mortal Wkly Rep 47:1, 1998.

373. Frank J, Orenstein W, Bart K, et al. Major impediments to measles elimination. Am J Dis Child 139:881, 1985.

374. Markowitz LE, Preblud SR, Fine PE, et al. Duration of live measles vaccine-induced immunity. Pediatr Infect Dis J 9:101, 1990.

375. Krugman S. Further-attenuated measles vaccine: characteristics and use. Rev Infect Dis 5:477, 1983.

376. Mathias RG, Meekison WG, Arcand TA, et al. The role of secondary vaccine failures in measles outbreaks. Am J Public Health 79:475, 1989.

377. Berg RB, Rosenthal MS. Propagation of measles virus in suspensions of human and monkey leukocytes. Proc Soc Exp Biol Med 106:581, 1961.

378. Suringa DWR, Bank LJ, Ackerman AB. Role of measles virus in skin lesions and Koplik's spots. N Engl J Med 283:1139, 1970.

379. Debre R, Celers J. Measles: pathogenicity and epidemiology. In Debre R, Celers J (eds). Clinical Virology. Philadelphia, WB Saunders, 1970, p 336.

380. Enders J, McCarthy K, Mitus A, et al. Isolation of measles virus at autopsy in cases of giant cell pneumonia without rash. N Engl J Med 261:875, 1959.

381. Mitus A, Enders J, Crair JM, et al. Persistence of measles virus and depression of antibody formation in patients with giant cell pneumonia after measles. N Engl J Med 261:882, 1959.

382. Lachmann P. Immunopathology of measles. Proc R Soc Med 67:12, 1974.

383. Stillerman M, Thalhimer W. Attack rate and incubation period of measles. Am J Dis Child 67:15, 1944.

384. Baugess H. Measles transmitted by blood transfusion. Am J Dis Child 27:256, 1924.

385. Littauer J, Sorensen K. The measles epidemic at Umanak in Greenland in 1962. Dan Med Bull 12:43, 1965.

386. Warthin AS. Occurrence of numerous large giant cells in tonsils and pharyngeal mucosa in prodromal stage of measles: report of four cases. Arch Pathol 11:864, 1932.

387. Moroi K, Saito S, Kurata T, et al. Fetal death associated with measles virus infection of the placenta. Am J Obstet Gynecol 164:1107, 1991.

388. La Boccetta AC, Tornay AS. Measles encephalitis: report of 61 cases. Am J Dis Child 107:247, 1964.

389. Musser JH, Hauser GH. Encephalitis as a complication of measles. JAMA 90:1267, 1928.

390. Pearl PL, Abu-Farsakh H, Starke JR, et al. Neuropathology of two fatal cases of measles in the 1988–1989 Houston epidemic. Pediatr Neurol 6:126, 1990.

391. Jahnke U, Fischer EH, Alvord EC. Hypothesis—certain viral proteins contain encephalitogenic and/or neuritogenic sequences. J Neuropathol Exp Neurol 44:320, 1985.

392. Kipps A, Dick G, Moodie JW. Measles and the central nervous system. Lancet 2:1406, 1983.

393. Gremillion DH, Crawford GE. Measles penumonia in young adults: an analysis of 106 cases. Am J Med 71:539, 1981.

394. Centers for Disease Control. Measles surveillance. MMWR Morb Mortal Wkly Rep #9, 1973.

395. Christensen PE, Schmidt H, Bang HO, et al. An epidemic of measles in southern Greenland, 1951. Acta Med Scand 144:430, 1953.

396. Krasinski K, Borkowsky W. Measles and measles immunity in children infected with human immunodeficiency virus. JAMA 261:2512, 1989.

397. Embree JE, Datta P, Stackiw W, et al. Increased risk of early measles in infants of human immunodeficiency type 1–seropositive mothers. J Infect Dis 165:262, 1992.

398. Kaplan LJ, Daum RS, Smaron M, McCarthy C. Severe measles in immunocompromised patients. JAMA 267:1237, 1992.

399. Kernahan J, McQuillin J, Craft A. Measles in children who have malignant disease. BMJ 295:15, 1987.

400. Breitfeld V, Hashida Y, Sherman FE, et al. Fatal measles infection in children with leukemia. Lab Invest 28:279, 1973.

401. Greenhill JP. Acute (extragenital) infections in pregnancy, labor, and the puerperium. Am J Obstet Gynecol 25:760, 1933.

402. Nouvat JR. Rougeole et Grossesse. Bordeaux, 1904.

403. Dyer I. Measles complicating pregnancy: report of 24 cases with three instances of congenital measles. South Med J 33:601, 1940.

404. Packer AD. The influence of maternal measles (morbilli) on the newborn child. Med J Aust 1:835, 1950.

405. Atmar RL, Englund JA, Hammill H. Complications of measles during pregnancy. Clin Infect Dis 14:217, 1992.

406. Eberhart-Phillips JE, Fredrick PD, Baron RC, Mascola

L. Measles in pregnancy: a descriptive study of 58 cases. Obstet Gynecol 82:797, 1993.

407. Nichols WW, Levan A, Hall B, et al. Measles-associated chromosome breakage. Preliminary communication. Hereditas 48:367, 1962.

408. Miller ZB. Chromosome abnormalities in measles. Lancet 2:1070, 1963.

409. Higurashi M, Tamura T, Nakatake T. Cytogenic observations in cultured lymphocytes from patients with Down's syndrome and measles. Pediatr Res 7:582, 1973.

410. Jespersen CS, Littauer J, Sigild U. Measles as a cause of fetal defects. Acta Pediatr Scand 66:367, 1977.

411. Gazala E, Karplus M, Sarov I. The effect of maternal measles on the fetus. Pediatr Infect Dis 4:202, 1985.

412. Rones B. The relationship of German measles during pregnancy to congenital ocular defects. Med Ann DC 13:285, 1944.

413. Swan C, Tostevin AL, Moore B, et al. Congenital defects in infants following infectious diseases during pregnancy, with special reference to relationship between German measles and cataract, deaf mutism, heart disease and microcephaly, and to period in pregnancy in which occurrence of rubella was followed by congenital abnormalities. Med J Aust 2:201, 1943.

414. Canelli AF. Sur le comportement normal et pathologique de l'immunity antimorbilleuse chez le nourison jeune. Rev Fr Pediatr 5:668, 1929.

415. Ronaldson GW. Measles at confinement with subsequent modified attack in the child. Br J Child Dis 23:192, 1926.

416. Narita M, Togashi T, Kikuta H. Neonatal measles in Hokkaido, Japan. Pediatr Infect Dis J 16:908, 1997.

417. Kohn JL. Measles in newborn infants (maternal infection). J Pediatr 23:192, 1933.

418. Richardson DL. Measles contracted in utero. R I Med J 3:13, 1920.

419. Muhlbauer B, Berns LM, Singer A. Congenital measles—1982. Isr J Med Sci 19:987, 1983.

420. Noren GR, Adams P Jr, Anderson RC. Positive skin reactivity to mumps virus antigen in endocardial fibroelastosis. J Pediatr 62:604, 1963.

421. Abreo F, Bagby J. Sputum cytology in measles infection: A case report. Acta Cytol 35:719, 1991.

422. Lightwood R, Nolan R. Epithelial giant cells in measles as an aid in diagnosis. J Pediatr 77:59, 1970.

423. Llanes-Rodas R, Liu C. Rapid diagnosis of measles from urinary sediments stained with fluorescent antibody. N Engl J Med 275:516, 1966.

424. Minnich LL, Goodenough F, Ray CG. Use of immunofluorescence to identify measles virus infections. J Clin Microbiol 29:1148, 1991.

425. Smaron MF, Saxon E, Wood L, et al. Diagnosis of measles by fluorescent antibody and culture of nasopharyngeal secretions. J Virol Methods 33:223, 1991.

426. Rossier E, Miller H, McCulloch B, et al. Comparison of immunofluorescence and enzyme immunoassay for detection of measles-specific immunoglobulin M antibody. J Clin Microbiol 29:1069, 1991.

427. Arrieta C, Zaleska M, Stutman H, Marks M. Vitamin A levels in children with measles in Long Beach, California. J Pediatr 121:75, 1992.

428. Frieden TR, Sowell AL, Henning K, et al. Vitamin A levels and severity of measles. Am J Dis Child 146:182, 1992.

429. Hussey GD, Klein M. A randomized, controlled trial of vitamin A in children with severe measles. N Engl J Med 323:160, 1990.

430. Forni AL, Schluger NW, Roberts RB. Severe measles pneumonitis in adults: evaluation of clinical characteristics and therapy with intravenous ribavirin. Clin Infect Dis 19:454, 1994.

431. Mustafa MM, Weitman SD, Winick NJ, et al. Subacute measles encephalitis in the young immunocompromised host: report of two cases diagnosed by polymerase chain reaction and treated with ribavirin and review of the literature. Clin Infect Dis 16:654, 1993.

432. Gudnadottir M, Black FL. Measles vaccination in adults with and without complicating conditions. Arch Ges Virusforsch 16:521, 1965.

433. Chui LW-L, Marusyk RG, Pabst HF. Measles virus specific antibody in infants in a highly vaccinated society. J Med Virol 33:199, 1991.

434. Lennon J, Black F. Maternally derived measles immunity in sera of vaccine-protected mothers. J Pediatr 108:671, 1986.

435. Krugman S, Giles JP, Friedman H. Studies on immunity to measles. J Pediatr 66:471, 1965.

436. Stillerman M, Marks HH, Thalhimer W. Prophylaxis of measles with convalescent serum. Am J Dis Child 67:1, 1944.

437. Orvell C. The reactions of monoclonal antibodies with structural proteins of mumps virus. J Immunol 132:2622, 1984.

438. Lennette E. Laboratory diagnosis of viral infections. New York: Marcel Dekker, 1992.

439. Garcia A, Periera J, Vidigal N, et al. Intrauterine infection with mumps virus. Obstet Gynecol 56:756, 1980.

440. Connolly NK. Mumps orchitis without parotitis in infants. Lancet 1:69, 1953.

441. Bowers D. Mumps during pregnancy. West J Surg Obstet Gynecol 61:72, 1953.

442. Greenberg MW, Beilly JS. Congenital defects in the infant following mumps during pregnancy. Am J Obstet Gynecol 57:805, 1949.

443. Hardy JB. Viral infection in pregnancy: a review. Am J Obstet Gynecol 93:1052, 1965.

444. Homans A. Mumps in a pregnant woman. Premature labor, followed by the appearance of the same disease in the infant, twenty-four hours after its birth. Am J Med Sci 29:56, 1855.

445. Moore JH. Epidemic parotitis complicating late pregnancy: report of a case. JAMA 97:1625, 1931.

446. Philip RN, Reinhard KR, Lackman DB. Observations on a mumps epidemic in a "virgin" population. Am J Epidemiol 69:91, 1959.

447. Schwartz HA. Mumps in pregnancy. Am J Obstet Gynecol 60:875, 1950.

448. Siddall RS. Epidemic parotitis in late pregnancy. Am J Obstet Gynecol 33:524, 1937.

449. Ylinen O, Jervinen PA. Parotitis during pregnancy. Acta Obstet Gynecol Scand 32:121, 1953.

450. Kilham L. Mumps virus in human milk and in milk of infected monkey. Am J Obstet Gynecol 33:524, 1951.

451. Dutta PC. A fatal case of pregnancy complicated with mumps. J Obstet Gynaecol Br Emp 42:869, 1935.

452. Swan C. Congenital malformations associated with rubella and other virus infections. In Banks HS (ed). Modern Practice in Infectious Fevers. New York, PB Hoeber, 1951, p 528.

453. Hyatt H. Relationship of maternal mumps to congenital defects and fetal deaths, and to maternal morbidity and mortality. Am Pract Dig Treat 12:359, 1961.

454. Kurtz J, Tomlinson A, Pearson J. Mumps virus isolated from a fetus. BMJ 284:471, 1982.

455. Robertson GG, Williamson AP, Blattner RJ. Origin and development of lens cataracts in mumps-infected chick embryos. Am J Anat 115:473, 1964.

456. St. Geme JW Jr, Davis CWC, Peralta HJ, et al. The biologic perturbations of persistent embryonic mumps virus infection. Pediatr Res 7:541, 1973.

457. Johnson RT, Johnson KP, Edmonds CJ. Virus-induced hydrocephalus: development of aqueductal stenosis in hamsters after mumps infection. Science 157:1066, 1967.

458. Holowach J, Thurston DL, Becker B. Congenital defects in infants following mumps during pregnancy: a review of the literature and a report of chorioretinitis due to fetal infection. J Pediatr 50:689, 1957.

459. Grenvall H, Selander P. Some virus diseases during pregnancy and their effect on the fetus. Nord Med 37:409, 1948.

460. Baumann B, Danon L, Weitz R, et al. Unilateral hydrocephalus due to obstruction of the foramen of Monro: another complication of intrauterine mumps infection? Eur J Pediatr 139:158, 1982.

461. Timmons G, Johnson K. Aqueductal stenosis and hydrocephalus after mumps encephalitis. N Engl J Med 283:1505, 1970.

462. Manson MM, Logan WPD, Loy RM. Rubella and Other Virus Infections During Pregnancy. London, Her Majesty's Stationery Office, 1960.

463. St. Geme JW Jr, Noren GR, Adams P. Proposed embryopathic relation between mumps virus and primary endocardial fibroelastosis. N Engl J Med 275:339, 1966.

464. Finland M. Mumps. In Charles D, Finland M (eds). Obstetric and Perinatal Infections. Philadelphia, Lea & Febiger, 1973, p 333.

465. Zardini V. Eccezionale casso di parotite epidemica in neonato da madre convalescente della stessa malattia. Lattante 33:767, 1962.

466. Shouldice D, Mintz S. Mumps in utero. Can Nurse 51:454, 1955.

467. Jones JF, Ray G, Fulginiti VA. Perinatal mumps infection. J Pediatr 96:912, 1980.

468. Reman O, Freymuth F, Laloum D, et al. Neonatal respiratory distress due to mumps. Arch Dis Child 61:80, 1986.

469. Yamauchi T, Wilson C, St. Geme JW Jr. Transmission of live, attenuated mumps virus to the human placenta. N Engl J Med 290:710, 1974.

470. Chiba Y, Ogra PA, Nakao T. Transplacental mumps infection. Am J Obstet Gynecol 122:904, 1975.

471. Monif GR. Maternal mumps infection during gestation: observations on the progeny. Am J Obstet Gynecol 121:549, 1974.

472. Meyer MB. An epidemiologic study of mumps: its spread in schools and families. Am J Hyg 75:259, 1962.

473. Hoen E. Mumpsinfektion beim jungen Sugling. Kinderprtzl 36:27, 1968.

474. Harris RW, Turnball CD, Isacson P, et al. Mumps in a Northeast metropolitan community: epidemiology of clinical mumps. Am J Epidemiol 88:224, 1968.

475. Hodes D, Brunell P. Mumps antibody: placental transfer and disappearance during the first year of life. Pediatrics 45:99, 1970.

476. Sanford HN, Shmigelsky II. Purulent parotitis in the newborn. J Pediatr 26:149, 1945.

477. Wharton M, Cochi S, Hutcheson RH, Schaffner W. Mumps transmission in hospitals. Arch Intern Med 150:47, 1990.

478. Brunell PA, Brickman A, O'Hare D, et al. Ineffectiveness of isolation of patients as a method of preventing the spread of mumps. N Engl J Med 279:1357, 1968.

479. Picard O, Brunereau L, Pelosse B, et al. Cerebral infarction associated with vasculitis due to VZV in patients infected with HIV. Biomed Pharmacother 51:449, 1998.

C H A P T E R 1 4

Mycoplasmal Infections

GAIL H. CASSELL, Ph.D., KEN B. WAITES, M.D., and DENNIS T. CROUSE, M.D.*

The mycoplasmas are a unique group of microorganisms that are ubiquitous and can be found in humans, animals, plants and insects. They are the smallest free-living microorganisms. Individual mycoplasmal cells range from 100 to 300 nm in diameter, approximately the size of influenza viruses or poxviruses. They are unique among prokaryotes, differing by one or more characteristics from all other major groups of human

pathogens. Although mycoplasmas have evolved from gram-positive ancestors,[1] they lack a cell wall, which is their single most distinguishing feature and is responsible for their inclusion as a separate class, the Mollicutes. Many of the biologic properties of mycoplasmas are due to the absence of a rigid cell wall, including resistance to all β-lactam antibiotics and marked pleomorphism among individual cells. In contrast to L-phase variants of bacteria (bacterial variants that lack cell walls and replicate serially as nonrigid cells), mycoplasmas are unable to synthesize cell wall precursors under any condi-

*Material new to this edition in this chapter was prepared by the editors and is indicated in bracketed italic type.

tions. Bacterial L forms retain the capability of cell wall synthesis, and unstable strains may revert to the parent form. The mycoplasmal cell membrane contains phospholipids, glycolipids, sterols, and various proteins. The extremely small size of the mycoplasmal genome (approximately one sixth the size of *Escherichia coli*)[1] severely limits the biosynthetic capabilities of mycoplasmas, helps explain their complex nutritional requirements for cultivation, and necessitates a parasitic or saprophytic existence for most species. In mammals, mycoplasmas most commonly colonize mucosal surfaces, particularly those of the respiratory and genital tracts.

Within the class Mollicutes, there are three orders and four families consisting of six genera (*Mycoplasma, Ureaplasma, Spiroplasma, Acholeplasma, Anaeroplasma,* and *Asteroplasma*), which contain 150 distinct species.[2] Of these, 14 are known to infect humans (Table 14–1). *Ureaplasma urealyticum* and *Mycoplasma hominis* are the organisms most commonly isolated from the genital tract of females and are the only ones shown to be a cause of both maternal and fetal infection. For this reason, information provided in this chapter focuses on these two organisms and only on those aspects related to pregnancy outcome. Current evidence suggests that *Mycoplasma pneumoniae, M. genitalium,* and *M. fermentans* warrant further attention as potential causes of maternal and fetal infection. Thus, information is also included on these three organisms, with emphasis on future needs

in research. [*Articles of particular interest published between 1994 and January 2000 are referred to in the footnote commentaries by the editors.*]

UREAPLASMA UREALYTICUM AND *MYCOPLASMA HOMINIS* INFECTIONS: ADVERSE PREGNANCY OUTCOME AND PERINATAL MORBIDITY AND MORTALITY

Few areas of scientific investigation have been as controversial as that of the role of *U. urealyticum* as it relates to adverse pregnancy outcome.[3, 4] Over the years, ureaplasmas have been implicated in infertility, spontaneous abortion, stillbirth, premature birth, and perinatal morbidity and mortality.[4] Most available evidence indicates that if any microorganism causes adverse outcome of pregnancy, it most likely does so by infection of the chorioamnion and/or amniotic fluid and fetus. It is now clear that *U. urealyticum* can invade the upper genital tract but does so only in a subpopulation of individuals colonized with ureaplasmas in the lower genital tract.[3, 5–9] Herein lies the root of the controversy. Most of the earlier studies were limited to culture of the cervix and/or vagina. In contrast to studies limited to isolation of

---

☐ **TABLE 14–1**
Mycoplasma Species Isolated from Humans

SPECIES	PRIMARY SITE(S) OF COLONIZATION	ETIOLOGIC SIGNIFICANCE
Acholeplasma laidlawii	Oropharynx, skin	Unknown
M. buccale	Oropharynx	None
M. faucium	Oropharynx	None
M. fermentans	Urethra, oropharynx	Pneumonia in otherwise healthy individuals, and possibly nephropathy and disseminated disease in patients with acquired immunodeficiency syndrome
M. genitalium	Oropharynx, urethra	Implicated in pneumonia, urethritis, pelvic inflammatory disease
M. hominis	Urethra/cervix/vagina; oropharynx	Adults: pelvic inflammatory disease; amnionitis and postpartum infections; pyelonephritis; bacteremia, sternal wound infection, abscesses, and arthritis especially in immunosuppressed patients Newborns: pneumonia, meningitis, bacteremia, soft tissue abscesses
M. lipophilum	Oropharynx	None
M. orale	Oropharynx	None
M. penetrans	Unknown[a]	Unknown
M. pirum	Unknown[b]	Unknown
M. pneumoniae	Nasopharynx and oropharynx, lung	Pharyngitis, otitis, pneumonia and extrapulmonary complications
M. salivarium	Oropharynx	None
M. spermatophilum	Urethra	Unknown
Ureaplasma urealyticum	Urethra/cervix/vagina; nasopharynx and oropharynx of infants	Adults: urethritis; urinary calculi; chorioamnionitis; postpartum endometritis, bacteremia, abscesses, and arthritis in immunosuppressed patients Newborns: pneumonia, meningitis, bacteremia

[a] *M. penetrans* has been isolated from urine of HIV-infected patients.
[b] *M. pirum* has been isolated from peripheral blood lymphocytes purified from the blood of HIV-infected patients.

U. urealyticum from the lower genital tract or surface cultures of infants, most studies based on infection of the placenta indicate a strong association between isolation of *U. urealyticum* from the placenta and histologic chorioamnionitis[6, 8, 10–14] and premature birth.[12, 15, 16] Whereas most of the earlier studies either did not evaluate the contribution of other microorganisms or did not take into account membrane rupture, duration of labor or other demographic and obstetric confounding variables, results of more recent studies[15, 16] that have taken these factors into account still show a strong association of *U. urealyticum* infection of the chorioamnion with chorioamnionitis and prematurity. Individual case reports provide compelling evidence that, in at least some individuals, *U. urealyticum* alone plays a causal role in chorioamnionitis,[5, 17, 18] spontaneous abortion, and premature birth.[5, 17, 18]

Recent evidence indicates that *U. urealyticum* is the single most common organism isolated from the central nervous system (CNS)[19, 20] *[For further discussion see the section on Perinatal Morbidity and Mortality: Infections of the Central Nervous System. Some investigators were able to isolate* U. urealyticum[19, 21] *and* M. hominis[22] *from cerebrospinal fluid of neonates, but other investigators did not corroborate these findings.[23–25a] Heggie and colleagues[25a] isolated* U. urealyticum *from cerebrospinal fluid of 2 of 920 infants and* M. hominis *from none.]* and lower respiratory tract[21, 26] of newborns, particularly those born prematurely. Isolation of the organism in pure culture from pleural fluid,[27, 28] lung biopsy samples[28] and lung tissue obtained at autopsy from infants with pneumonia,[5, 21, 26, 27, 29, 30] and reproduction of similar histologic lesions in lungs of newborn mice[31] and prematurely born nonhuman primates[32] with these isolates prove that this organism is a cause of pneumonia in newborns. Prospective studies from nine different centers in four different countries now indicate a significant association between *U. urealyticum* in the lower respiratory tract and development of chronic lung disease (CLD) in low-birth-weight infants.[23, 26, 30, 33–41] Available data provide a cohesive argument that *U. urealyticum* is a risk factor for, and not only associated with, CLD. Whereas the occurrence of clinically significant hydrocephalus and meningitis is variable in ureaplasmal CNS infections, it is clear that in some cases it is causal.[19, 20, 42–44] Available evidence indicates that *U. urealyticum*–induced CNS and respiratory diseases are uncommon in full-term infants and that infants with birth weights of 1000 g or less are at greatest risk.[19, 24, 30, 45–48] These infants may be unprotected as a result of suboptimal transplacental acquisition of maternal IgG.[49] Children and adults with primary antibody deficiency disorders are uniquely susceptible to *U. urealyticum* extragenital infections, in particular chronic sinopulmonary disease and progressive lung failure.[50, 51]

M. hominis is a cause of pelvic inflammatory disease (PID), postpartum septicemia, and endometritis.[52] It is also a cause of septicemia, meningitis, pneumonia, pericarditis, adenitis, and abscesses of the subcutaneous tissue in newborns.[53, 54] Extragenital infections (including septicemia, pneumonia, and brain and soft tissue abscesses) due to *M. hominis* are being recognized with increasing frequency in normal and immunosuppressed children and adults.[55–58]

In summary, *U. urealyticum* and *M. hominis* appear to be commensals in the lower female genital tract. However, both have been convincingly shown to be a cause of invasive and destructive disease in immunocompromised children and adults. Given the immunocompromised state of pregnant women and of prematurely born infants, it should not be surprising that these two organisms are also important causes of invasive disease in these two populations. Experience with *U. urealyticum* and *M. hominis* in other types of immunocompromised patients indicates that these organisms, unlike many other bacteria, result in progressive and destructive disease, often with a paucity of systemic signs of infection. They are most often refractory to antibiotic therapy, requiring prolonged administration of a combination of intravenous antibiotics and intravenous immunoglobulin.[59] Little information is available concerning the efficacy of antibiotic treatment of *U. urealyticum* and *M. hominis* in infants.

UREAPLASMA UREALYTICUM AND MYCOPLASMA HOMINIS COLONIZATION OF THE UROGENITAL TRACT: EPIDEMIOLOGY AND DISEASES OF THE URINARY AND REPRODUCTIVE TRACTS IN ADULTS

Epidemiology

After puberty, colonization of the male and female lower urogenital tract by *U. urealyticum* and *M. hominis* usually occurs as a result of sexual activity. In fact, venereal transmission is the major mode of transmission of these organisms. Among sexually mature but inexperienced adults, colonization increases dramatically with increasing numbers of sexual partners.[60–62]

In the asymptomatic female, genital mycoplasmas may be found throughout the lower urogenital tract, including the external cervical os, vagina, labia, and urethra.[63, 64] The vagina yields the largest number of isolates, followed by the periurethral area and the cervix.[64] *U. urealyticum* is isolated less often from urine than from the cervix, but *M. hominis* is present in both the urine and the cervix with approximately the same frequency. In the asymptomatic adult male, mycoplasmas have been isolated from urine, semen, and the distal urethra.[65]

U. urealyticum can be found in the vagina of 40 to 80% of sexually mature, asymptomatic women, and *M. hominis* is found in 21 to 53%. The incidence of each is somewhat lower in males. In females, colonization is linked to younger age, lower socioeconomic status, sexual activity with multiple partners, black ethnicity, and oral contraceptive use.[62, 66] Colonization rates among women may vary somewhat depending on hormonal factors. Mycoplasmas are prevalent in the lower genital tract of pregnant women.[67, 68] When genital mycoplasmas are present at the first prenatal visit, they usually persist throughout the pregnancy. Studies of postmenopausal women suggest that they are infrequently colonized with genital mycoplasmas.[69]

Disease Associations

There has been speculation surrounding the possible etiologic significance of both *U. urealyticum* and *M. hominis* in a variety of disorders of the genitourinary tract since the first successful cultivation and identification of mycoplasmas from clinical specimens. Many important questions regarding epidemiology, disease associations, and causality remain unanswered primarily because of (1) the ubiquity of mycoplasmas in the lower genitourinary tract of asymptomatic persons; (2) the problem that cultural specimens from the affected site are often unavailable; (3) the fact that many of the diseases possibly due to mycoplasmas can be of multifactorial etiologies; (4) the limited availability of experienced laboratories sufficiently equipped to perform mycoplasmal cultures; and (5) the consideration of a mycoplasmal cause only after failure of other diagnostic efforts. Nonetheless, within the past decade, systematic clinical studies involving cultural and/or serologic methods, detailed case reports, controlled antibiotic treatment trials, and experimental animal inoculations have provided information that has clarified the role of *U. urealyticum* and *M. hominis* in a number of pathologic conditions.

Urinary Tract

Three conditions of the urinary tract shown to be caused by mycoplasmas are urethritis in males due to *U. urealyticum*, urinary calculi due to *U. urealyticum*, and pyelonephritis caused by *M. hominis*.[52] Although the exact proportion of cases of nongonococcal urethritis caused by *U. urealyticum* may still be debated, the ability of this organism to cause urethritis can no longer be disputed. Intraurethral inoculation of human volunteers and nonhuman primates produces urethritis.[52] Serologic and antibiotic treatment trials also support a causative role for urethritis.[52] The common occurrence of ureaplasmas in the urethra of asymptomatic men suggests either that only certain serovars of ureaplasmas are pathogenic or that predisposing factors, such as a lack of mucosal immunity, must exist in those individuals who do develop disease. Alternatively, disease may develop only on initial exposure to these organisms.

Urinary stones composed of struvite and carbonate-apatite account for 20% of all urinary tract stones and are induced by the enzymatic breakdown of urea by bacterial urease, which splits urea into ammonia and carbon dioxide. *Proteus* species and, to a lesser extent, *Klebsiella*, *Pseudomonas*, and *Staphylococcus* species are the usual causes in humans. However, *U. urealyticum* also produces urease and has been demonstrated to induce crystallization of struvite and calcium phosphates in vitro in artificial urine, although the formation of crystals is slower with this ureaplasma than with *Proteus mirabilis*, the most common cause of these stones in humans. Thus, the capability of *U. urealyticum* to induce stones

in the appropriate location is proved.[70, 71] Renal calculi have been induced experimentally in rats by inoculation of pure cultures of *U. urealyticum* directly into the bladder and renal pelvis. *U. urealyticum* has been isolated from stones recovered by surgery in 6 of 15 patients. In 4 of these 6, no other urease-producing organisms were isolated either in the stone or in urine sampled from the renal pelvis. The major remaining questions concerning the role of this organism in production of urinary calculi are the frequency with which the organism reaches the kidney, the predisposing factors that allow this to occur, and the relative frequency of renal calculi induced by this organism compared with that of those induced by other organisms.

Despite the high incidence of *M. hominis* in the lower urogenital tract, it has been isolated from the upper tract only in patients with symptoms of acute infection.[72] In two studies, *M. hominis* was recovered from samples of ureteral urine collected during surgery from 7 of 80 patients (4 in pure culture) with acute pyelonephritis and from 3 to 18 patients with acute exacerbation of chronic pyelonephritis. The organism was not found in the upper urinary tract of 22 patients with chronic pyelonephritis without acute exacerbation, or from 60 patients with noninfectious urinary tract disease. In another study based on cultural isolation and detection of antibodies in urine, *M. hominis* was isolated from the upper urinary tract in seven patients and overall was thought to be a cause of approximately 5% of the acute pyelonephritis cases.

Reproductive Tract

Only one entity of either the male or the female reproductive tract has been shown to be caused by mycoplasmas. Although the exact proportion of cases is unknown, *M. hominis* is considered to be a cause of PID.[73–76] Inoculation of *M. hominis* into fallopian tubes of monkeys induces parametritis and salpingitis within 3 days,[77] and inoculation of human fallopian tube explants produces ciliostasis.[78] The organism has been isolated in pure cultures from the fallopian tubes of approximately 8% of women with salpingitis as diagnosed by laparoscopy, compared with 0% of women without lesions.[73] The organisms can also be isolated from the endometrium. In addition, a role for these organisms in cases of PID not associated with either *Neisseria gonorrhoeae* or *Chlamydia trachomatis* is supported by significant increases in specific antibody.[75] Whereas *U. urealyticum* can be isolated directly from affected fallopian tubes,[76] it is usually found in the presence of other known pathogens.

Given that *M. hominis* is a cause of salpingitis, it is reasonable to assume that severe tubal infections with this organism may lead to occlusion and infertility. However, prospective studies are needed to prove this. Although the possibility that *U. urealyticum* may play a role in involuntary infertility in humans was first raised over 20 years ago, the association remains speculative.[9]

EXTRAGENITAL INFECTIONS IN IMMUNOCOMPROMISED CHILDREN AND ADULTS

U. urealyticum and *M. hominis* typically remain localized in the lower genital tract in a normal host, but both organisms can cause extragenital infections. These infections have been reported in patients of both sexes, with a broad range of ages (14 to 76 years) and underlying diagnoses. Extragenital infections due to *M. hominis* have been reported more frequently than those caused by *U. urealyticum*; however, this is probably a reflection of the growth of *M. hominis*, and not ureaplasmas, on some conventional bacteriologic media. In fact, most of the reported cases of extragenital infections have been discovered "by accident" as a result of the occasional growth of *M. hominis* on blood agar and in routine blood cultures or after specific mycoplasmal cultures were obtained following exclusion of other possible infectious causes. Thus, the true incidence of extragenital infections due to either ureaplasmas or *M. hominis* is not known because these organisms are not sought routinely. Prospective studies using methods specifically optimized for detection of *U. urealyticum* and *M. hominis* are needed to determine their precise incidence. Likewise, detailed epidemiologic studies are necessary to clarify the pathogenesis of these infections. Disseminated infection has been reported in otherwise healthy hosts, but most infections follow genitourinary manipulation or trauma of the genitourinary tract or occur in individuals with underlying immunosuppression and/or hypogammaglobulinemia.

A detailed discussion of *U. urealyticum* and *M. hominis* invasive disease in immunocompromised children and adults seems particularly relevant to understanding the invasive potential of these organisms and their impact on pregnancy and perinatal morbidity and mortality. In many respects, pregnancy is a state of immunosuppression. It is reasonable to assume that increased susceptibility of premature infants is most likely related to lack of significant transplacental transfer of antibody before 32 weeks' gestation as well as to other defects in both specific and nonspecific defense mechanisms.[49] Thus, a summary of extragenital infections produced by *M. hominis* and *U. urealyticum* in immunocompromised patients is given next.

Blood and Vascular Infections

U. urealyticum and *M. hominis* have been isolated from blood after trauma or surgical manipulation of the urogenital tract.[56, 57, 79–85] Prosthetic valve endocarditis has been reported.[86, 87] Persistent and fatal mycoplasmemia due to *M. hominis* has been reported in patients with immunosuppression or other underlying disease.[56, 57] *M. hominis* septic thrombophlebitis requiring surgical excision of the cephalic vein also has been reported.[87, 88] Isolation of *M. hominis* from blood is most often accompanied by a significant increase in specific antibody levels.

Wound Infections

The ability of *M. hominis* to infect surgical wounds or sites of trauma is well documented.[56–58, 80, 81, 89–94] Infected surgical wound sites most often include sternotomies and pelvic and inguinal wounds. Heart-lung transplant recipients commonly develop sternal wound infections

due to *M. hominis* with associated mediastinitis and empyema thoracis. These infections in particular are refractory to treatment and often require closure by muscle flaps after sternotomy. Peritonitis after organ transplantation and renal dialysis also has been reported.[95–97] *[A retroperitoneal abscess in a woman who had a cesarean section yielded pure growth of* M. hominis; *the patient recovered following use of oral doxycyline.[97a]]*

Wound infections due to *M. hominis* infections manifest with fever, leukocytosis, and wound drainage with or without tenderness and erythema. The wound drainage is often purulent but occasionally watery. Gram stain reveals numerous neutrophils with few or no bacteria. The etiologic significance of *M. hominis* in these cases is indicated by isolation of the organisms from deep tissue spaces or as a sole isolate in large numbers from purulent drainage. Significant increases in specific antibody provide ancillary evidence of infection.[57]

Joint Infections and Osteomyelitis

Approximately 20% of individuals with agammaglobulinemia develop "septic" joint inflammation.[50, 98] There is evidence to suggest that mycoplasmas may be responsible for the majority of these.[99] *U. urealyticum* and *M. hominis* can be isolated repeatedly from the joints in the absence of any other microbial agent.[51, 100–107] Both *U. urealyticum* and *M. hominis* are also a cause of arthritis in other types of immunosuppressed or otherwise compromised (i.e., those with prosthetic joints) patients.[56, 80, 108–114] In most of the reported cases, the arthritis has been persistent, lasting from several months to over a year. Aggressive, erosive arthritis that progresses in the face of anti-inflammatory therapy and gamma globulin replacement can occur. In some of the cases involving *U. urealyticum*, the arthritis is associated with subcutaneous abscesses, persistent urethritis, and chronic urethrocystitis/cystitis. Most of these cases have required massive and prolonged antibiotic therapy, but some of the strains involved are or have become resistant to multiple antibiotics.

Osteomyelitis has been reported in association with invasive infection with both *U. urealyticum* and *M. hominis*, with direct isolation of the organism from bone tissue.[101, 105, 107, 115, 116]

Infections of the Central Nervous System, Respiratory Tract, and Pericardium

M. hominis has been identified in several cases of meningitis after trauma and in brain abscesses of immunocompromised patients.[56, 58, 117] *U. urealyticum* is a cause of sinopulmonary disease and progressive lung failure in agammaglobulinemic patients, and in such cases it has been isolated directly from the bronchus.[50] *M. hominis* has been reported as a cause of lower respiratory tract infections and pneumonia in immunosuppressed and other compromised patients.[56–58, 118] In at least two cases, *M. hominis* was thought to contribute to the death of the patients.[56, 118] In both cases, the organism was directly isolated from lung tissue at autopsy; in one of the cases, from blood and pleural fluid pre mortem. No other infectious agent or cause of death was identified. Both *U. urealyticum* and *M. hominis* have been isolated from pericardial fluid and/or tissue of patients with large pericardial effusions requiring surgical drainage.[119] [*M. hominis has also been associated with life-threatening mediastinitis.[119a]*]

CHORIOAMNIONITIS, CLINICAL AMNIONITIS, AND MATERNAL SEPTICEMIA

Histologic Chorioamnionitis

Isolation of *U. urealyticum*, but not *M. hominis*, from the chorioamnion has uniformly shown a significant association with chorioamnionitis documented by histopathologic examination of the placenta.[3, 5, 10–14] Although some studies did not rigorously seek other infectious agents and did not take into account duration of labor and/or membrane rupture, recent studies that cultured extensively for other agents showed that women whose amniotic membranes were colonized with *U. urealyticum* were more likely to have histologic chorioamnionitis than were women without *U. urealyticum*, even after adjusting for duration of labor, premature rupture of membranes (PROM), duration of membrane rupture, and the presence of other bacteria.[11] In recent studies conducted in our laboratory, *U. urealyticum* in the chorioamnion was found to be significantly associated with chorioamnionitis even in the presence of intact membranes in women who delivered by cesarean section.[15] In some of these, *U. urealyticum* was the only organism isolated. Individual case reports[5, 17, 18] indicate that *U. urealyticum* can persist in the amniotic fluid as long as 7 weeks in the presence of intact membranes and an intense inflammatory response and in the absence of labor and other detectable microorganisms (Table 14–2; Fig. 14–1). Furthermore, in such cases, ureaplasmas can be demonstrated directly

---

TABLE 14–2
Chorioamnionitis and Congenital Pneumonia Due to *Ureaplasma urealyticum*: a Case History

17 weeks	*U. urealyticum* isolated from discolored amniotic fluid ($\geq 10^3$ color-changing units [ccu]/ml) obtained by amniocentesis 10^3 polymorphonuclear leukocytes/ml amniotic fluid No clinical signs of amnionitis Fetus normal by ultrasound
23 weeks	Vaginal bleeding
24 weeks	Onset of premature labor, and within 7 hr a 463-g male fetus delivered but died within 24 hr. *U. urealyticum* isolated in pure cultures from lungs, liver, spleen, kidney, peritoneal fluid and gallbladder ($\geq 10^3$ ccu/g of tissue). Severe chorioamnionitis, placental vasculitis, intervillositis, funisitis, and congenital pneumonia (see Fig. 14–1) determined by microscopic examination.

---

in the inflammatory infiltrates in the fetal membranes by immunofluorescence (see Fig. 14–1).[8] Taken together, these findings provide a convincing argument that ureaplasmas alone can actually produce chorioamnionitis.

Infection of the Amniotic Fluid and Clinical Amnionitis

Both *U. urealyticum* and *M. hominis* can invade the amniotic fluid as early as 16 to 20 weeks' gestation in the presence of intact membranes and in the absence of other microorganisms.[5, 17] These infections tend to be clinically silent and chronic. In one case, *U. urealyticum* was isolated from amniotic fluid over a period of 7 weeks[5] (see Table 14–2). Although there was an intense polymorphonuclear response in the amniotic fluid and fetal membranes (see Fig. 14–1), there were no clinical signs of amnionitis, i.e., fever and abdominal tenderness. This is consistent with other types of invasive infection due to these organisms, which normally produce a clinically silent infection. This may in part be due to the lack of a cell wall, which for other bacteria is the major pyrogenic factor.

Recent studies in our laboratory of women whose membranes are intact and who deliver by cesarean section indicate that ureaplasmal infection of the amniotic fluid occurs in less than half of those individuals with ureaplasmal infection of the chorioamnion (GH Cassell, unpublished observation). The lower isolation rate from amniotic fluid was not due to reduced sensitivity of cultures of the amniotic fluid, as was shown by analysis of the amniotic fluids by polymerase chain reaction (PCR).[120] *M. hominis*, as well as other bacteria, was also isolated at least twice as frequently from the chorioamnion as from amniotic fluid. Isolation of organisms from the chorioamnion and/or amniotic fluid was significantly associated with the presence of histologic chorioamnionitis, but the women did not have evidence of clinical amnionitis.

The role of *U. urealyticum* and *M. hominis* in clinical amnionitis after membrane rupture is not clear.[8] Ureaplasmas can be isolated from amniotic fluid in up to 50% of both asymptomatic and symptomatic individuals.[8] When blood and amniotic fluid from patients were cultured, *U. urealyticum* was the single most common microorganism isolated not only from amniotic fluid (65 of 125, 52%) but also from maternal blood (19 of 125, 15%). However, the isolation rate did not differ between symptomatic and asymptomatic individuals. This was also true for *M. hominis*. Serum antibody responses to *Ureaplasma* and *M. hominis* were more common in symptomatic women.

In summary, *U. urealyticum* causes histologic chorioamnionitis and amniotic fluid infection often in the absence of other infectious agents, even in the first trimester. Most often, these infections appear to be clinically silent. In contrast, *M. hominis* can commonly invade the chorioamnion and amniotic fluid, but it rarely occurs in the absence of other organisms, particularly ureaplasmas. Thus, it is unclear whether this organism alone is a cause of histologic chorioamnionitis or clinical amnionitis.

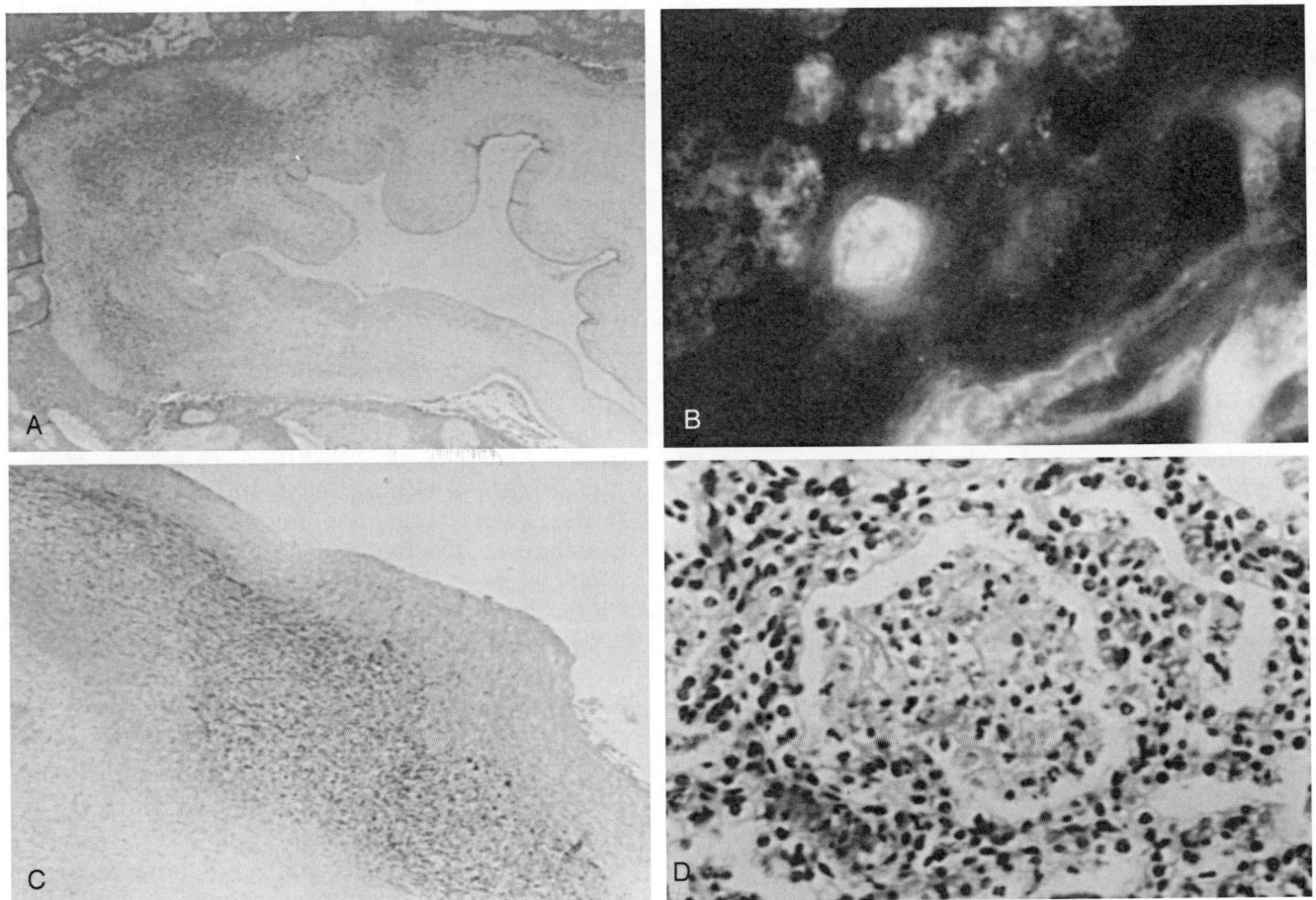

FIGURE 14–1 *A,* Section of placenta at 24 weeks' gestation showing extensive inflammation in the amnion and the chorion (H&E, 25×). *Ureaplasma urealyticum* was isolated in pure culture from the amniotic fluid 7 weeks before delivery and from multiple fetal organs at autopsy. *B,* Adjacent section of placenta stained with rabbit anti–*U. urealyticum* serovar 1 serum and reacted with affinity-purified, fluorescein-labeled goat anti–rabbit IgG. Ureaplasmas are present in the most intense areas of inflammation. Serial sections that reacted with normal rabbit serum and conjugate were negative. Brown-Brenn–stained adjacent sections of placenta were negative for bacteria (750×). *C,* Photomicrograph of umbilical cord from the same case as shown in *A* and *B.* Note extensive inflammation. *U. urealyticum* was isolated in pure culture from the amniotic fluid at 17 weeks' gestation and from lung tissue and spleen, kidney, liver, and peritoneal fluid post mortem (25×). *D,* Photomicrograph of lung tissue obtained at postmortem examination showing histologic evidence of pneumonia (50×).

Maternal Septicemia

M. hominis[121–124] and *U. urealyticum*[125, 126] have been isolated from cultures of blood of women with postpartum fever and septic abortion. Postpartum fever (>37.7° C) occurred in 9% of 535 women who delivered vaginally at Boston City Hospital; the most common cause of fever was infection caused by *M. hominis* (demonstrated by a fourfold or greater rise in mycoplasmacidal antibody titer).[127]

In another study at Boston City Hospital,[128] blood was obtained from 327 women shortly after vaginal delivery. Of these, 10 women had blood cultures that contained *M. hominis*; 15 women had blood cultures containing *U. urealyticum*; and both *M. hominis* and *U. urealyticum* were isolated from the blood of 1 woman. The frequency of *Mycoplasma* isolation was inversely related to the interval between delivery and the time that the blood was obtained for culture: 2 (15%) of 13 cultures obtained within 2 minutes of delivery were

positive, but only 1 (2%) of 42 cultures obtained more than 10 minutes after delivery yielded mycoplasmas. Twenty women whose blood contained mycoplasmas at the time of delivery were recultured 1 or more days later; only one woman had a second positive culture of blood. Pathogenic bacteria were isolated from the blood of 16 of the 327 women, including 4 of the 11 women whose blood contained *M. hominis* but none of the women whose blood contained *U. urealyticum*.

"Blind" plating of routine aerobic blood culture media resulted in isolation of *M. hominis* (seven isolates) and *U. urealyticum* (seven isolates) from 607 blood cultures of obstetric patients with postpartum or postoperative pelvic infection and from cultures from three neonates. These accounted for 35% of all positive cultures and for 4% of all positive neonatal blood cultures from among 1600 infants over a 22-month period.[129]

In a more recent prospective study of 620 blood specimens collected from febrile obstetric-gynecologic patients,[130] *U. urealyticum* was the second and *M. hominis* the third most common microorganisms isolated. All isolates were either post partum or post abortum. Genital mycoplasmas were isolated on a number of occasions from blood drawn more than 2 days after delivery or following curettage. Endometritis or histologically documented chorioamnionitis was present in half of the cases, and persistent fever occurred after delivery or abortion in many of the cases despite conventional administration of antibiotics. In these cases, fever abated after tetracycline therapy.

We have recently shown that colonization of the chorioamnion with *U. urealyticum* in women with intact membranes undergoing cesarean delivery is a significant and independent predictor of subsequent endometritis.[131] Endometritis occurred in 28% of women with ureaplasmas present in the chorioamnion at cesarean delivery, compared with only 8.4% if the culture was negative and 8.8% if only bacteria and no ureaplasmas were present.

Roberts and associates[132] found *U. urealyticum* to be the most common microorganism isolated from postcesarean wound infections. Of 47 cultures positive from 939 wounds, ureaplasmas were recovered from 29 (i.e., 62%). One third of the samples positive for ureaplasmas had no other microorganisms detected.

M. hominis was recovered from the joint fluid of two women at 3 weeks post partum. The organism was also isolated from the blood of one of the women. Both women had been febrile during the immediate postpartum period and developed signs of arthritis 7 days to 3 weeks after delivery.[133] The report of suppurative arthritis in postpartum women suggests that the organisms may localize in some tissues as a result of hematogenous dissemination. Cases of postpartum pneumonia with isolation of *M. hominis* from pleural fluid also have been reported, as have *M. hominis* wound infections after cesarean section.[134–137]

ADVERSE PREGNANCY OUTCOME

Spontaneous Abortion and Stillbirth

U. urealyticum and *M. hominis* can be isolated in pure culture from the endometria of asymptomatic, nonpregnant females, indicating that these organisms can be present at the time of implantation and thus could potentially be involved in early pregnancy losses.[6] *U. urealyticum* and *M. hominis* have been isolated from the lungs, brain, heart, and viscera of aborted fetuses and stillborn infants, in some cases in the presence of an inflammatory response and in the absence of other organisms.[5, 13, 138, 139] However, in these cases it was not clear whether death of the fetus occurred before infection. *U. urealyticum* has been isolated more frequently from the products of early abortions and midtrimester fetal losses than from products of induced abortions.[140, 141] Although rates of isolation of ureaplasmas from the lower genital tract of habitual aborters do not differ from those of normal controls, ureaplasmas are isolated more often from the endometria of habitual aborters.[140, 141] However, when only those patients with a positive cervical culture are considered, no higher endometrial colonization rate is found.[142] *U. urealyticum* is isolated more frequently from the placentas of aborted fetuses than from controls.[10, 13] Antibody titers to *U. urealyticum* are higher in mothers with a history of fetal wastage.[143] However, the results of all of these epidemiologic studies are difficult to interpret because comparability of the various groups of women is uncertain and the role of other potential infectious agents was not always assessed.

Isolation of *U. urealyticum* from amniotic fluid in pure culture from women with intact membranes and subsequent fetal loss in the presence of histologic chorioamnionitis has recently been reported by three different groups of investigators.[5, 18, 144] Unlike previous reports, it is clear in these cases that the fetus was alive before *U. urealyticum* infection and that there were no other apparent causes of abortion present. This indicates that in some cases the role of *U. urealyticum* is causal. Although *M. hominis* can be a cause of postabortal septicemia and fever,[122] direct evidence implicating this organism as a cause of abortion is lacking.

Premature Birth

The first suggestion that infection might be involved in prematurity and low birth weight resulted from studies in which tetracycline was administered to nonbacteriuric, pregnant women on a double-blind basis.[145] Women who were treated for 6 weeks during pregnancy gave birth to significantly fewer infants weighing 2500 g or less than did women given a placebo. Although no microbiologic investigations were conducted, it was postulated that tetracycline-sensitive microorganisms might be responsible, and mycoplasmas were considered among them.

Since 1970, approximately 13 studies involving almost 12,000 patients have been conducted to evaluate the role of cervical ureaplasmal infection in prematurity.[4, 146] The evidence suggests that no consistent relationship exists between the presence of *U. urealyticum* in the lower genital tract of the mother and prematurity or low birth weight. These studies have since been reviewed[4, 147] and are not discussed here.

Most available information indicates that if *U. urealyticum*, or for that matter any microorganism, causes premature birth, it most likely does so by infection of the chorioamnion with or without infection of the amniotic fluid and fetus.[4] Five prospective studies have evaluated the role of ureaplasmal infection of the amniotic fluid and prematurity. Two studies were designed to evaluate the presence of ureaplasmas at the time of genetic amniocenteses at 12 to 20 weeks' gestation, when membranes were intact and there was no labor.[5, 144] In neither study was there a difference in maternal age, indication for amniocentesis, percentage of chromosomal anomalies, or abnormal alpha-fetoprotein levels. However, marked differences were seen in adverse (fetal loss and premature delivery) versus normal (term delivery) outcome. In the study by Cassell and colleagues,[5] both infants from whom ureaplasmas were isolated from amniotic fluid were born prematurely, both infants died and both had evidence of pneumonia. *U. urealyticum* was isolated in pure culture at autopsy from both infants. In the study by Gray and co-workers,[144] 7 of 10 patients from whom ureaplasmas were isolated from the amniotic fluid subsequently aborted within 4 to 7 weeks after amniocentesis and at less than 25 weeks' gestation. The three remaining delivered prematurely, and two neonatal deaths resulted. Histologic evidence of chorioamnionitis was present in all 10 placentas, and histologic evidence of pneumonia was present in all eight fetuses. Placentas were culturally positive for *U. urealyticum* and negative for all other microorganisms in six of seven evaluated at delivery and from four of six fetal lungs evaluated.

In the remaining three studies designed to culture amniotic fluid of women admitted to the hospital with preterm labor and intact membranes, *U. urealyticum* in the amniotic fluid was not found to be consistently related to premature birth.[148–150] It is difficult to interpret these studies because chorioamnion infection was not assessed and the numbers of culture-positive patients were less than eight in each of the three studies. Another major limitation of the studies is that the mean week of gestation for women at the time of amniotic fluid culture was 31 to 32 weeks. Isolation of *U. urealyticum* from the chorioamnion is almost three times higher in infants who weigh less than 1500 g at birth and are born before 32 weeks' gestation compared with that in larger and older infants.[11, 12, 15]

Isolation of *U. urealyticum* from the chorioamnion with or without other bacteria is associated with chorioamnionitis and is a relatively consistent finding among studies.[4, 147] Furthermore, as already discussed, *U. urealyticum* in the absence of other microorganisms can be a cause of chorioamnionitis. Although numerous studies have shown a strong correlation between histologic chorioamnionitis and premature birth,[151] only three of six prospective studies have shown a significant association between isolation of *U. urealyticum* from the chorioamnion and premature birth.[10–12, 16, 152, 153] In contrast to amniotic fluid studies, these have included a larger number of patients, and some have specifically looked at infection related to birth at less than 34 weeks' gestation. However, most patients have had their membranes ruptured, which could lead to intrapartum microbial invasion of the chorioamnion and could thus confound results even if duration of membrane rupture is taken into account. In addition, these studies did not include a control group of women delivered at similar preterm gestational ages but who did not have the spontaneous onset of labor. Such a control group is essential to establish that microbial colonization of the chorioamnion is correlated independently and specifically with spontaneous preterm labor and not simply with a preterm gestational age alone.

As discussed earlier, prospective studies begun at 16 to 20 weeks' gestation indicate that, in at least some cases, *U. urealyticum* infection of the chorioamnion results in premature birth. If *U. urealyticum* is a significant cause of prematurity, one should be able to prove that it precedes onset of labor and rupture of membranes in other populations of women. Recent studies at the Uni-

versity of Alabama at Birmingham indicate that *U. urealyticum* is the single most common microorganism isolated from the chorioamnion of women with spontaneous labor delivering by cesarean section with intact membranes.[15] Furthermore, logistic regression analyses of demographic and obstetric variables indicate that *U. urealyticum* alone or in the presence of other bacteria in the chorioamnion is independently associated with birth at less than 37 weeks' gestation regardless of the duration of labor. The fact that isolation was three to five times more frequent in women with spontaneous labor compared with that in women with indicated deliveries and that isolation from those with indicated deliveries was not associated with premature birth provides compelling evidence for an important role of subclinical chorioamnion infection with *U. urealyticum* and preterm labor.

Even though risk factors for *U. urealyticum* colonization of the lower genital tract have been identified,[62, 66, 139] virtually nothing is known about potential risk factors for invasion of the upper tract. The presence of bacterial vaginosis (BV) may be one such risk factor.[4] The presence of BV is independently and significantly associated with birth at less than 37 weeks' gestation when cervical organisms and obstetric and demographic factors are taken into consideration.[11] However, it has not been determined whether BV is associated with premature delivery independent of chorioamnion infection (with organisms associated with BV or those that are not, i.e., *U. urealyticum*). Symptomatic BV is characterized by a watery discharge with a fishy odor. Patients with BV consistently have an increased prevalence of *Gardnerella vaginalis*, selected anaerobic bacteria (most notably *Bacteroides* and *Mobiluncus* species) and *M. hominis* and a decreased prevalence of facultative lactobacilli.[154] Although *U. urealyticum* is not independently associated with BV, the prevalence of vaginal colonization by *U. urealyticum* is increased about twofold and the intravaginal concentration of these organisms is increased 100-fold.[155] Some have postulated that the increased intravaginal concentrations of BV organisms may result in increases in the synthesis of phospholipase A_2 and the production of prostaglandins, which may lead to preterm labor or PROM.[154, 156] Alternatively, *Bacteroides* species in the lower genital tract could produce enough proteases to weaken the fetal membrane, causing PROM and invasion by other organisms.[154, 156] In addition, it is possible that certain BV-associated microorganisms, like *U. urealyticum*, may be more likely to invade the intact fetal membranes simply because they are present in larger numbers. However, this latter possibility cannot be the total explanation for *U. urealyticum* association with prematurity because intravaginal concentrations of *Peptococcus* species are also increased in BV but are found infrequently in the chorioamnion and amniotic fluid. Although *M. hominis* and *G. vaginalis* were the next most common organisms isolated from women with intact membranes in the University of Alabama at Birmingham study described earlier, they were not independently associated with birth at less than 37 weeks' gestation. A possibility based on current evidence is that both BV and *U. urealyticum* may be of etiologic significance independent of each other, yet when present simultaneously they may be additive.

TRANSMISSION OF *UREAPLASMA UREALYTICUM* AND *MYCOPLASMA HOMINIS* TO THE FETUS AND NEWBORN

U. urealyticum and *M. hominis* can be transmitted from an infected female to a fetus either in utero or at the time of delivery by passage through a colonized birth canal. Isolation of *U. urealyticum* in pure culture from the chorioamnion, amniotic fluid, and internal fetal organs in the presence of funisitis and pneumonia[5] and a specific IgM response[157] can be taken as strong evidence that fetal infection can occur in utero. Cassell and co-workers[26] found that up to 14% of *U. urealyticum* and 30% of *M. hominis* endotracheal isolates collected within the first 12 to 24 hours after birth from infants whose birth weight was less than 2500 g were from infants born by cesarean section with intact membranes, indicating that in utero transmission occurs rather commonly, at least in premature infants. Other investigators[21] have found that up to 48% of *U. urealyticum* isolates from endotracheal aspirates collected within 30 minutes of birth are from infants delivered by cesarean section with intact membranes. Acquisition of *U. urealyticum* and *M. hominis* can occur in utero either by an ascending route secondary to colonization of the mother's genital tract or transplacentally from the mother's blood. Both organisms have been isolated from maternal and umbilical cord blood at the time of delivery.[129, 130]

The rate of vertical transmission of *U. urealyticum* and *M. hominis* ranges from 18 to 55% among infants.[47,] [158–160] The number of infants found to be colonized in a particular neonatal population is reflective of the colonization rates of the maternal population, the number and location of body sites sampled in infants, the proportion of female infants included (due to the high colonization rate of the vagina), as well as the percentage of very low birth weight (<1000 g) infants.[161] Although it does not appear that preterm infants are consistently more likely to be colonized than term infants, those with birth weights less than 1000 g have the highest colonization rates (Fig. 14–2). The rate of vertical transmission is not affected by method of delivery but is significantly increased when chorioamnionitis or amniotic fluid infection is present. Nosocomial transmission of mycoplasmas in a newborn or intensive care nursery has not been reported, and whether it occurs is not known.

Colonization of healthy full-term infants is relatively transient, with a sharp drop in isolation rates after 3 months of age.[162] Long-term follow-up studies of premature infants have not been conducted. In premature infants with invasive ureaplasmal infection, persistence of the organism in the lower respiratory tract and cerebrospinal fluid (CSF) has been documented for weeks to months.[19, 21]

Less than 10% of older children and sexually inexperienced adults are colonized. As already discussed, colonization after puberty increases with sexual activity.

PERINATAL MORBIDITY AND MORTALITY

Several studies have shown a significant association between isolation of *U. urealyticum* from the chorioamnion and perinatal morbidity and mortality.[12, 13, 163, 164] How-

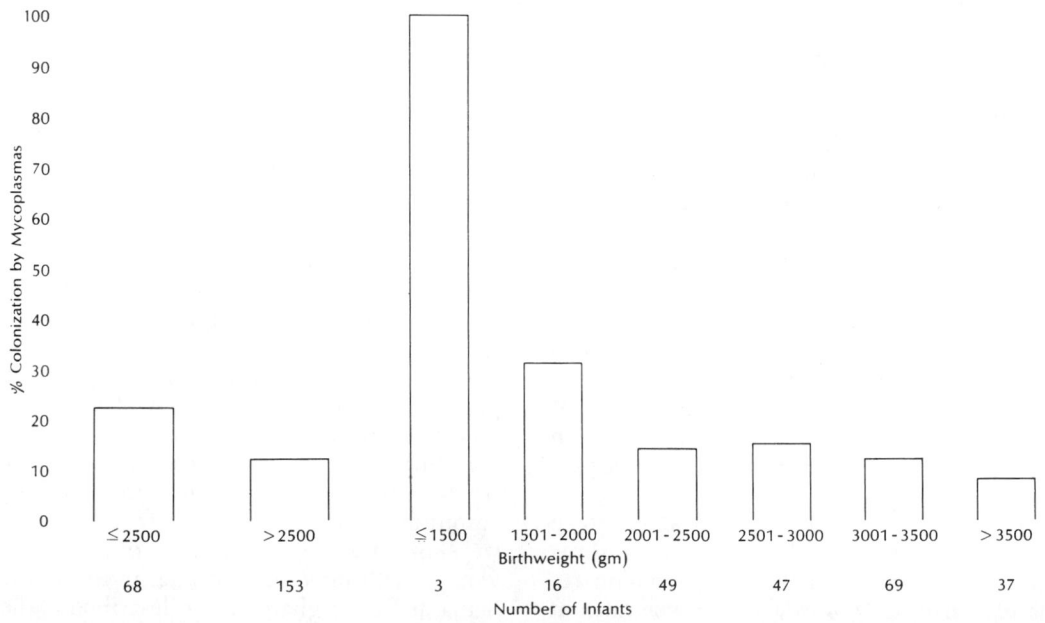

FIGURE 14–2 Relation of genital mycoplasma colonization to birth weight. Positive isolate from throat or nose or both. Mean weight of positive infants = 2605 g (*p*<0.01 [t test]). Mean weight of negative infants = 2952 g (*p*<0.01 [t test]). (From Klein JO. Mycoplasmas, genitourinary tract infections, and reproductive failure. Hosp Pract 6:127–133, 1971, with permission.)

ever, these investigators did not culture the affected infants. Thus, it is unclear whether the morbidity and mortality resulted from the direct effect of fetal and neonatal infection due to *U. urealyticum* or whether it was the result of the complications associated with premature birth. In assessing the role of intrauterine and perinatal infection, one must demonstrate the suspected organism at the affected site. Infection of the chorioamnion and/or amniotic fluid does not always necessarily result in infection of the fetus. Likewise, surface cultures alone (e.g., eyes, ears, nose, throat, gastric aspirates, vagina, urine) are not indicative of invasive infection of the blood, CSF, or lungs. A number of prospective studies based on direct culture of the affected site indicate that both *U. urealyticum* and *M. hominis* can cause invasive disease in infants and are a cause of perinatal morbidity and mortality, particularly in those infants born prematurely.

Congenital and Neonatal Pneumonia

Table 14–3 summarizes direct evidence that *U. urealyticum* is a cause of pneumonia in the fetus and the newborn. Retrospective[165] as well as prospective[5, 13, 17] studies indicate an association of *U. urealyticum* with congenital

---

TABLE 14–3

Findings That Suggest That *Ureaplasma urealyticum* Is a Cause of Pneumonia in the Fetus and the Newborn

---

1. *U. urealyticum* has been isolated from amniotic fluid over a 7-wk period (17–24 weeks' gestation) in the presence of intact membranes and the absence of other microorganisms. In some of these same cases, *U. urealyticum* has been isolated in pure culture from lung tissue at autopsy less than 24 hr after birth. Inflammatory changes compatible with a histologic diagnosis of congenital pneumonia were demonstrated in the lungs (see Fig. 14–1).[5] Organisms have been identified by immunofluorescence and electron microscopy directly in the areas of pulmonary inflammation, and, in the same infant, an increase in IgM antibody has been documented by metabolic inhibition.[154]

2. *U. urealyticum*, in the absence of other microorganisms, can be isolated from endotracheal aspirates at birth from infants with evidence of respiratory disease. In these same infants, it can also be isolated from pleural fluid before death and from lung tissue at autopsy in the absence of other microorganisms but in the presence of histologically proven pneumonia.[21, 23]

3. Isolation of *U. urealyticum* from endotracheal aspirates in the absence of other documented respiratory pathogens is significantly associated with radiographic evidence of pneumonia,[32] increased number of circulating white blood cells,[165] and increased numbers of neutrophils in the tracheal aspirate 2 days after birth.[36]

4. *U. urealyticum* can induce ciliostasis in human fetal tracheal organ cultures,[154] and isolates from lungs of human infants produce pneumonia in experimentally infected newborn mice[29] and premature baboons.[30] *U. urealyticum* can induce proinflammatory cytokine release in neonatal pulmonary fibroblasts. *U. urealyticum* induces a significant increase of interleukin-6 and a dramatic increase in interleukin-8.[167]

---

pneumonia. The organism has been isolated from affected lungs in the absence of chlamydiae, viruses, fungi, and bacteria and in the presence of chorioamnionitis and funisitis[5] and has been demonstrated within fetal membranes by immunofluorescence[5] and in lung lesions by electron and immunofluorescent microscopy.[157] A specific IgM response in the newborn has been demonstrated in individual cases with pneumonia, further documenting in utero infection.[157] A case of *U. urealyticum* congenital pneumonia is summarized in Table 14–2 and shown in Figure 14–1. Similar cases also have recently been described.[144]

We have found that *U. urealyticum* is the single most common microorganism isolated from endotracheal aspirates of infants with a birth weight of 2500 g or less and who have an oxygen requirement within the first 24 hours after birth.[26] Those infants weighing 1000 g or less from whom *U. urealyticum* was isolated from the endotracheal aspirate are twice as likely to die as infants of similar birth weight but who are uninfected and as infected or uninfected infants weighing more than 1000 g. These findings support the hypothesis that only a select group of infants (i.e., those with very low birth weights) is subject to disease due to *U. urealyticum*. This fact may account for the seeming disparities in conclusions regarding the role of *U. urealyticum* in neonatal respiratory disease reached in earlier prospective studies that failed to distinguish this high-risk subpopulation from the whole.[166, 167]

That the endotracheal isolations of *U. urealyticum* represent true infection of the lower respiratory tract is supported by initial isolation of ureaplasmas in numbers exceeding 1000, and in some cases exceeding 10,000, colony-forming units and by repeated isolations of the organism from tracheal aspirates for weeks and even months in some infants who continue to require mechanical ventilation. That the tracheal isolates are not merely a reflection of contamination from the nasopharynx is supported by the discrepancy in isolation rates between the two sites and recovery of *U. urealyticum* in pure culture from endotracheal aspirates in over 85% of the infants.[26] Concomitant recovery of the organism from blood in up to 26% of those with positive endotracheal aspirates and from the CSF of some infants indicates that in some infants the organism is invasive.[26] Other investigators[21] have recently shown, in a study of 98 infants, that respiratory distress syndrome, the need for assisted ventilation, severe respiratory insufficiency, and death are significantly more common among those infants younger than 34 weeks' gestational age from whom *U. urealyticum* is recovered from endotracheal aspirates at the time of delivery as compared with uninfected infants. *U. urealyticum* was isolated from 34% of blood cultures and also from 4 of 6 CSF samples and 6 of 11 postmortem brain and lung biopsy specimens. Eighty-two percent of the ureaplasma isolates were present in pure culture, and 48% of infants born by cesarean section with intact membranes had ureaplasmas isolated from one or more sites.

Individual case reports also provide evidence that *U. urealyticum* is a cause of pneumonia in newborns. Waites and associates[27] described a severely asphyxiated infant born after 33 weeks' gestation. At birth, *U. urealyticum* was isolated from blood and tracheal aspirate in the absence of other microorganisms. The organism was also isolated from blood, tracheal aspirate, and pleural fluid on day 4 and on day 6 and from brain and trachea at autopsy on day 6. At autopsy, severe bilateral pneumonia was confirmed, with a mixed cellular intra-alveolar inflammatory exudate and early fibrotic changes of bronchopulmonary dysplasia. The occurrence of histologically proven pneumonia in an infant from whom *U. urealyticum* was the only organism isolated from multiple sites before and after death proves unequivocally that this organism is capable of producing pneumonia in the newborn. Other individual case reports also document isolation of *U. urealyticum* from tracheal specimens before death and from lung tissue in pure culture at autopsy.[17, 29]

In a study of 292 infants with a birth weight of less than 2500 g who were followed for 28 days after birth, isolation of *U. urealyticum* from the endotracheal aspirate within the first 7 days of birth (average, 1.3 days) was significantly associated with radiographic evidence of pneumonia as compared with uninfected infants.[34] Precocious dysplastic changes also were significantly more common in infants with *U. urealyticum* than in those without this isolate. In this study, *U. urealyticum* was the single most common microorganism isolated (45 of 292 [15%]), and it was the only organism isolated 71% of the time.

Infants with a birth weight 1251 g or less from whom *U. urealyticum* is isolated from their endotracheal aspirate have greater than 2+ polymorphonuclear leukocytes in their aspirate at 2 ± 1 days of age, significantly more often than uncolonized infants. Aspirates from colonized infants are also more likely to have class II cytology than those from uncolonized patients on day 2.[41]

Other investigators have observed an association between colonization of the respiratory tract and elevation in the peripheral white blood cell count caused by an increase in the number of mature and immature neutrophils.[168] *U. urealyticum* can induce ciliostasis and mucosal lesions in human fetal tracheal organ cultures.[157] Furthermore, ureaplasmas isolated from the lungs of human infants with congenital and neonatal pneumonia produce a histologically similar pneumonia in newborn mice.[20] Even in this mouse model, age is a critical determinant of disease. Newborn mice are susceptible to colonization of the respiratory tract and development of pneumonia; 14-day-old mice are resistant.

The baboon as a model of prematurity is well established. At age 140 days, the animals demonstrate the same physiologic and pathologic characteristics as human neonates of 30 to 32 weeks' gestation (i.e., they have hyaline membrane disease).[169] Endotracheal inoculation of premature baboons with *U. urealyticum* isolated from human infants results in the development of pathologically recognizable pulmonary lesions, including acute bronchiolitis with epithelial ulceration and polymorphonuclear infiltration, which is distinguishable from hyaline membrane disease.[32] *U. urealyticum* can be isolated from blood, endotracheal aspirates, and pleural fluid and lung tissue 6 days after infection.

Taken together, the available evidence provides a strong argument that *U. urealyticum* is a common cause of pneumonia in newborns, particularly those born before 34 weeks' gestation. The organism can be isolated from endotracheal aspirates of up to 34% of infants with a birth weight of less than 2500 g, and radiographic evidence of pneumonia is twice as common in these infants than in *U. urealyticum*–negative infants (30% vs. 16%, $p = 0.03$). Many of these infections develop as a result of in utero exposure. Although cases of ureaplasmal pneumonia have been clearly documented in full-term infants, by comparison it occurs much less frequently. These findings in infants are consistent with the fact that *U. urealyticum* infection of the chorioamnion is also much more common before 34 weeks' gestation. Lack of transplacental passage of immunoglobulin before 32 weeks' gestation[49] may partially explain these findings. Experience from mycoplasmal respiratory diseases of animals indicates that preexisting antibody is protective, whereas antibody in the presence of an established infection is rarely effective in eradication of the organism.

Although individual case reports suggest that *M. hominis* also may be a cause of pneumonia in newborns, it has not been implicated as a common cause in prospective studies.

Chronic Lung Disease of Prematurity

Isolation of *U. urealyticum* from endotracheal aspirates of infants weighing 1250 g or less within the first 24 hours of birth is associated with an increased risk for development of bronchopulmonary dysplasia, or CLD of prematurity.[30, 37] This association is independent of birth weight, gender, and other known risk factors for development of CLD. The first three studies showing this association were concurrently conducted before the introduction of surfactant for treatment of hyaline membrane disease.[26, 37, 170] The next study, by Payne and associates,[41] was conducted 4 years later, when surfactant replacement was a widespread practice. Wang and co-workers[38] have performed a meta-analysis of these four studies. *[The authors subsequently expanded the meta-analysis to include 17 publications.[170a] They concluded that there was a significant association between* U. urealyticum *colonization and subsequent development of chronic lung disease.]* Although infants were enrolled in all studies soon after birth (in most cases within the first 12 to 24 hours of birth), before they had developed CLD, there were differences in patient population, the definition of colonization with *U. urealyticum*, neonatal management, and the definition of CLD of prematurity. Despite these differences, all four studies found an association between colonization and development of CLD of prematurity. A combined estimate of relative risk for the four studies was 1.91 (95% confidence interval, 1.54 to 2.37). When infants were categorized into groups by birth weight, the association was not observed in infants who weighed more than 1250 g. The association was also not observed in infants who weighed less than 750 g, but the risk of CLD in the uncolonized control group was already 82%, thus emphasizing that numerous factors may contribute to CLD in this birth weight group. Four subsequently published studies[23, 33, 35, 36] and others[39, 40] also have found the risk for CLD to be nearly double for those infants from whom *U. urealyticum* is isolated from the lower respiratory tract.

Several facts suggest that those infants who acquire *U. urealyticum* in utero may be the ones at greatest risk for development of CLD. Dyke and colleagues[35] found that *U. urealyticum* in the gastric aspirates of infants weighing 1000 g or less was associated with a significantly increased risk of CLD in those infants delivered by cesarean section but not in those delivered vaginally. This could result from a longer exposure to *U. urealyticum* as a result of in utero exposure, or it may be a reflection of differences in the virulence of those organisms found only in the cervix versus those that have invasive potential and that can cause an ascending infection from the vagina into the uterus. Along these lines, it is of interest that a recent study of 49 preterm infants, which included only 3 infants from whom *U. urealyticum* was recovered within 24 hours of birth, found no association with development of CLD.[171] The remaining 11 infants from whom *U. urealyticum* was recovered were not culture positive until 48 to 72 hours after birth, suggesting that only the 3 were infected in utero. In a study reported by Valencia and co-workers,[22] CLD was found in 26% of *U. urealyticum*–infected infants compared with only 4.7% of the noncolonized group. However, these results were not statistically significant, probably because of the small number of patients studied but also possibly because 22% of the patients included did not have cultures performed until between 2 days and 3 months of age.

Available evidence creates a cohesive argument that *U. urealyticum* infection of the lower respiratory tract is a risk factor for, and not only associated with, CLD. First, *U. urealyticum* is an organism that has only recently been suggested as a cause of pneumonia in newborns. Thus, the organism is not routinely sought by most hospital laboratories. Furthermore, the organism is not susceptible to those antibiotics that are used for presumptive therapy in very low birth weight infants with evidence of respiratory distress. Consequently, the infection (i.e., pneumonia) presently goes undetected and untreated. Isolation of *U. urealyticum* from endotracheal aspirates not only is a risk factor for development of pneumonia but has also been shown to be a risk factor for development of precocious dysplastic changes.[34] In this regard, one of the cases originally reported by Sanchez and Regan[170] is of interest. Of all infants who developed CLD in their study, 74% were colonized with *U. urealyticum*. Only one infant who developed CLD had no evidence of respiratory distress at birth. This infant was colonized with *U. urealyticum* within 24 hours of birth and developed clinical and radiographic evidence of pneumonitis at 1 week of age. Bacterial, viral, and chlamydial cultures were all negative in this patient. She was treated with erythromycin given intravenously, with subsequent improvement. Walsh and associates[28] isolated *U. urealyticum* directly from pleural fluid and tissue collected by open lung biopsy from four of eight infants cultured who had CLD. Cassell and colleagues[26] continued to recover ureaplasmas from endotracheal aspirates of infants with CLD for months after initial recovery of the organism from endotracheal aspirates within 12 hours of birth.

Current knowledge of the pathophysiology of CLD of prematurity would suggest that *U. urealyticum* produces pneumonia that goes undetected and untreated and results in an increased requirement for oxygen and subsequent development of CLD as a result of oxygen toxicity[30, 172] and/or a synergistic effect between the ureaplasmas and hyperoxia. Hyperoxia-induced lung injury is thought to contribute to development of CLD by means of stimulation of the proinflammatory cytokine interleukin (IL)-6.[173] *U. urealyticum* may also contribute to development of CLD by stimulation of proinflammatory cytokines. Infants from whom ureaplasmas are isolated from endotracheal aspirates within the first 24 hours of life are more likely to have neutrophils in their tracheal aspirates on day 2 than are those not colonized.[41] Aspirates from colonized infants are also more likely to have class II cytology than those from uncolonized patients on day 2 of life. This probably explains why *Ureaplasma*-infected infants respond to dexamethasone therapy.[41] These in vivo findings are consistent with the recent demonstration of *U. urealyticum* induction of IL-6 and IL-8 in human neonatal pulmonary fibroblasts even in the absence of hyperoxia.[173] Interestingly, ureaplasmas plus hyperoxia resulted in the greater stimulation of IL-6 and IL-8 than either alone. This is consistent with the synergism previously demonstrated in vivo between ureaplasmal infection and hyperoxia.[172]

U. urealyticum isolated from the endotracheal aspirate of an infant in the study of CLD by Cassell and colleagues[26] and from the lungs of an infant with proven congenital pneumonia[5] produced pneumonia in two different strains of newborn mice proven to be free of other known respiratory pathogens.[31] Furthermore, infection with *U. urealyticum* and exposure to 80% oxygen resulted in more severe lung lesions, organism persistence, and death than occurs in unexposed infected newborn mice or oxygen-exposed uninfected mice. These results suggest that increased oxygen requirements of very low birth weight infants might predispose them to lower respiratory tract infection or, alternatively, that *U. urealyticum* infection potentiates oxygen-induced injury. Exposure to oxidants is known to enhance respiratory disease and death in other mycoplasmal respiratory diseases.[174]

That *U. urealyticum* is a cause of pneumonia in newborns can no longer be questioned. The available data provide very strong evidence that *U. urealyticum* can actually be a primary cause or a contributing cofactor in development of CLD in humans, but the data are not definitive. Cohort studies allow follow-up of exposed individuals and thus reduce bias, but the designs of these studies cannot rule out the possibility that a third factor associated with *U. urealyticum* is not the true cause of CLD. A randomized trial of exposure to infection in humans is not ethical or practical. Although a randomized trial of antibiotic treatment could provide critical information related to patient management, it would still not bring us closer to proving causality. Even if treatment is found to be efficacious, conclusions about causation will be limited by the fact that the third factor might also be susceptible to the antibiotic chosen. Nevertheless, a treatment trial is urgently needed to determine whether appropriate therapy can reduce the incidence of morbidity and mortality associated with CLD. [The association of U. urealyticum with chronic pulmonary disease, including bronchopulmonary dysplasia, has been confirmed in recent studies[170a, 174a–174e] but not in others.[25a, 174f–174i] Documentation of a cause-and-effect relationship remains elusive. As an example of a negative study, Couroucli and colleagues[174b] obtained tracheal aspirates from infants within the first week of life and screened for the presence of adenovirus, cytomegalovirus, parvovirus, enteroviruses, U. urealyticum, M. hominis, M. pneumoniae, and Chlamydia species using PCR. Bronchopulmonary dysplasia was defined as persistent oxygen dependence at 28 days and 36 weeks postconceptional age. A significant increase in the frequency of the adenovirus genome was identified in patients with disease contrasted to controls (12/45 vs. 1/31). U. urealyticum was frequently identified in infants with disease (10/45) and controls (8/31). M. hominis was identified in only one control, and M. pneumoniae was not identified in either infants with disease or controls. In summary, U. urealyticum is a frequent colonizer of the upper respiratory tract but the role in causing chronic lung disease is uncertain. If a definitive role for Mycoplasma in neonatal pulmonary disease is established, pediatricians will need to reconsider initial therapy to include an active drug such as a macrolide. But the cause-and-effect relationship is still uncertain, and a therapeutic trial of erythromycin treatment of infants with positive ureaplasma culture did not alter the clinical outcome.[25a] The question of whether U. urealyticum causes or contributes to chronic lung disease in all infants, or only premature infants, may be answered only by microbiologic and therapeutic trials of sufficient sample size and appropriate attention to the many variables of the neonate.]

Pneumonia During Infancy

The preterm neonate constitutes a different host from the older, otherwise healthy infant who may be subject to development of pneumonitis. The fact that the majority of infants who present for medical care with respiratory illness never have a precise microbiologic diagnosis has led to a search for other fastidious organisms in addition to the usual bacterial and viral pathogens. Genital mycoplasmas represent only one group of organisms falling into this category.

Stagno and co-workers[175] performed a microbiologic study of 125 infants aged 2 to 12 weeks who were hospitalized with respiratory syndromes. Infants with CLD or acute pneumonia were excluded. The rate of isolation of U. urealyticum from nasopharyngeal aspirates of these infants was compared with that of hospitalized, age-matched controls without respiratory disease. Although the cervicovaginal isolation rate did not differ between mothers of the subjects and those of the controls, U. urealyticum was isolated significantly more often from nasopharyngeal aspirates of infants with pneumonitis than from those of controls, whereas M. hominis was isolated from comparable numbers of infants in each group. The majority of ureaplasmal isolates were

associated with other organisms, which makes the role of U. urealyticum, if any, in the clinical pneumonitis in this population unclear. Moreover, mere isolation from the upper respiratory tract may not accurately reflect the flora of the lower respiratory tract.

Syrogiannopoulos and associates[47] studied 108 full-term infants who were colonized with U. urealyticum at birth. They were monitored during the first 3 months of life. These researchers were unable to demonstrate an increased risk of lower respiratory illness during this period of early infancy in Ureaplasma-colonized infants compared with infants who were without pharyngeal ureaplasmal colonization.

Considering that there have been no prospective studies addressing the role of ureaplasmas in lower respiratory tract infections of infants outside the neonatal period that utilized direct cultures from the affected site (i.e., tracheal aspirates, lung biopsy samples, or autopsy material), no compelling evidence suggests that ureaplasmas are significant pathogens in lower respiratory tract infections in this population. Because of the well-documented difference in susceptibility of very low birth weight (i.e., extremely premature) infants versus older infants, we do not think that these organisms are likely to be a major cause of respiratory disease in otherwise healthy infants after the first month of life.

Bloodstream Infections

In the newborn, the factor most significantly associated with bloodstream invasion due to any microorganism is low birth weight. Other factors include prolonged ruptured membranes, traumatic delivery, maternal infection, chorioamnionitis, and fetal hypoxia. Preterm infants weighing 2500 g or less are nearly four times more likely to develop systemic infection than their full-term counterparts weighing more than 2500 g. U. urealyticum has been isolated from blood cultures from neonates and from cord blood.* Waites and associates[19] performed blood cultures for mycoplasmas in 43 newborns as part of a study of CSF infections. Two infants were positive for M. hominis, and two were positive for U. urealyticum. Cassell and colleagues[26] found that 26% of preterm infants with positive endotracheal aspirates had positive ureaplasmal blood cultures. These results suggest that bacteremia with ureaplasmas can be rather common in preterm infants. A case of M. hominis bacteremia, documented on two separate occasions at 20 hours and 11 days after birth in a full-term infant in association with respiratory distress and multiple systemic symptoms, was described by Unsworth and co-workers.[178] The infection was accompanied by an antibody response. Dan and colleagues[83] described a 10-month-old infant who received 70% surface-area burns and was later found to have M. hominis septicemia and fever documented on two separate occasions 11 days apart in association with an antibody response. Additional case reports have also described isolation of U. urealyticum from the bloodstream of neonates in association with pneumonia.[21, 29] Not all investigators have been successful in recovering

---

*See references 19, 21, 23, 26, 129, 130, 167, 176, and 177.

ureaplasmas or mycoplasmas from blood of infants.[22–24] This may be due to the age of infants cultured and/or the methods used. No mycoplasmas were isolated from blood cultures obtained within 30 minutes of birth from 146 preterm infants in Israel.[23] Investigators in Dallas, Texas,[24] failed to isolate mycoplasmas from the 191 blood specimens in a prospective study of older infants admitted to a hospital for suspected sepsis.

It is not known how often clinically significant illness occurs in neonates owing to the presence of *U. urealyticum* or *M. hominis* in the bloodstream, or how many naturally resolving cases may occur. Subclinical infections may be more prevalent than previously thought because mycoplasmas are so commonly isolated from mucosal surfaces of healthy women who then transmit them to their offspring.

Persistent Pulmonary Hypertension

Waites and associates[27] described a series of newborns in whom *U. urealyticum* was isolated from the blood and lower respiratory tract (endotracheal aspirate and lung tissue) in association with pneumonia and persistent pulmonary hypertension. Brus and co-workers[29] have also reported a fatal ureaplasmal pneumonia and sepsis in a newborn with persistent pulmonary hypertension. Postmortem examination revealed extensive hyaline membrane formation combined with inflammation in both lungs.

Infections of the Central Nervous System

The first cases of CNS infection due to an organism that was most likely *M. hominis* were reported as early as the 1950s. Since then, a series of cases of *M. hominis* meningitis in infants with spina bifida has been described[179] and there have been several case reports involving both full-term and preterm infants, with and without congenital malformations, and a patient with a cerebral abscess.[25, 53, 180–185] Persistence of *M. hominis* in CSF over several weeks before death in preterm infants with posthemorrhagic hydrocephalus has been reported.[53, 184]

Prior to 1986, there were no reports of isolation of *U. urealyticum* from the CNS. Since then, *U. urealyticum* has been shown to be one of the most common microorganisms isolated from the CSF of infants with suspected sepsis and meningitis in Birmingham, Alabama.[19, 20–22, 48, 62, 186] One hundred predominantly preterm infants undergoing lumbar puncture for suspected sepsis and/or meningitis or for treatment of posthemorrhagic hydrocephalus were cultured for conventional bacteria and mycoplasmas at the University of Alabama at Birmingham Hospital.[19] Infants were selected from a high-risk, university-based obstetric population. *U. urealyticum* was isolated from eight infants, and *M. hominis* was isolated from five. Only one other CSF infection, in an infant with *Escherichia coli* meningitis, was identified in this group of 100 infants, making ureaplasmas the most common organisms isolated. *U. urealyticum* was isolated from six infants with severe intraventricular hemorrhage and from three with hydrocephalus. *U. urealyticum* was isolated from the respiratory tracts of four of eight infants with CSF infections. One infant had clinical pneumonia with pleural effusions, from which the organism was also isolated. Four infants in whom multiple isolations of *U. urealyticum* were made over several weeks had each sustained an intraventricular hemorrhage at or shortly after birth and had large intraventricular blood clots, which may have sequestered organisms over long periods. Four *ureaplasma*-infected infants died. The most striking features of *M. hominis*–induced CNS infection occurred in a full-term infant in whom the clinical features of congenital infection (intracranial calcification) resembled those seen with viral or toxoplasmal infections and in whom major neurologic impairment was noted (Fig. 14–3).

Particular care was taken to ensure that the microbiologic results were valid. Lumbar skin cultures were taken from 80 newborns after the skin had been washed. No mycoplasmas were recovered from any infant. Multiple isolations from the CSF of the same infant over several weeks and the number of organisms (up to 10^5/ml) recovered also make it unlikely that the isolation of ureaplasmas reflects skin or laboratory contamination.

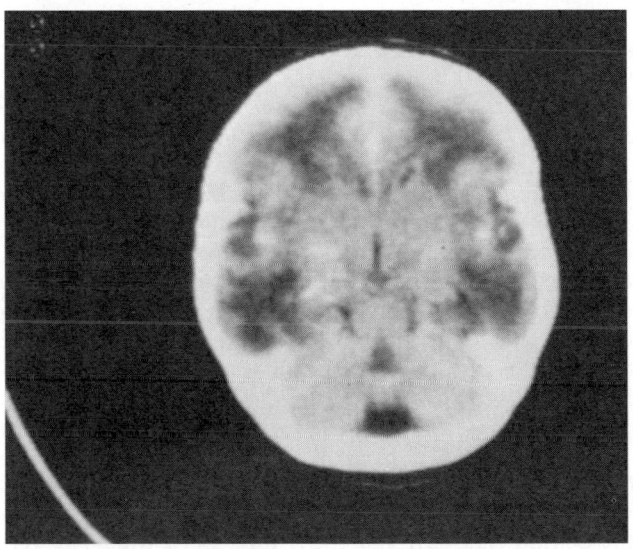

FIGURE 14–3 Cranial computed tomography (CT) scan from a full-term neonate delivered after 37 weeks' gestation by cesarean section. At 3 days of age, the infant was noted to be hypotonic, hypothermic, and lethargic. An electroencephalogram was consistent with diffuse encephalopathy. This CT scan showed decreased attenuation predominantly involving the supratentorial white matter symmetrically with a few punctate lesions of increased calcification suggestive of focal hemorrhage or early calcification, findings compatible with an intrauterine infection or a degenerative process. Congenital infections with herpes simplex virus, rubella, cytomegalovirus, bacteria, and toxoplasma were excluded. Cerebrospinal fluid (CSF) showed mononuclear pleocytosis. *Mycobacterium hominis* was isolated in pure culture from CSF at 6 days of age. CSF cultures were negative 5 days after doxycycline treatment was started. However, the infant later experienced convulsions, and spastic quadriplegia developed by 6 months of age.

The possibility that traumatic lumbar puncture with blood in the CSF specimen may have accounted for some positive cultures cannot be completely discounted. However, a number of isolations occurred in infants with few or no erythrocytes in the CSF and in some with no evidence of intraventricular hemorrhage.

A fundamental question that arose as a result of the study just described in a high-risk population was whether mycoplasmal CSF infections occur with the same frequency in patients of higher socioeconomic levels (i.e., those in private hospitals). CSF from an additional 318 infants delivered in three suburban community hospitals in Birmingham, Alabama,[44] was cultured. *M. hominis* was isolated from the CSF of nine of the infants, and *U. urealyticum* was cultured from five. With only three other verified CSF bacterial isolations in this population, mycoplasmas were again the most common microorganisms recovered, although the isolation rates were lower than in the original study.

In a study by Ollikainen and associates in Finland,[21] *U. urealyticum* was isolated from the CSF of four of six infants younger thatn 34 weeks' gestational age who were cultured within 30 minutes of birth. Although there was no pleocytosis or hypoglycorrhachia in the CSF, three had the organism also isolated from the blood and one from the tracheal sample; one died and also had a postmortem brain culture positive for *U. urealyticum.* None of these four infants had intracranial hemorrhages. This same group of investigators[177] reported isolation of *U. urealyticum* from the brain tissue at autopsy of premature twins who died on days 1 and 3 after birth and who had large intraventricular hemorrhages. The organism was isolated from endotracheal aspirate of one infant and from lung tissue at autopsy of this same infant, but blood samples of both infants were negative. Concurrent isolation of *U. urealyticum* from the CSF and endotracheal aspirate but not from blood in this and other infants suggests that the respiratory tract is the most common source of CNS infection.[19, 22, 179]

Valencia and co-workers[22] isolated *M. hominis* from 9 (13%) and *U. urealyticum* from 1 (1.5%) of 54 infants whose CSF was cultured within the first 24 hours of life and from 15 infants whose CSF was cultured between the second day and the third month of life. The biochemical findings, except for bloody specimens, were within normal limits for newborns. Only one of the infants with a positive CSF for *M. hominis* had clinical signs compatible with systemic bacterial infection. The rest were asymptomatic but were evaluated because of a maternal history of fever and prolonged rupture of membranes for more than 24 hours.

In other prospective studies, Likitnukul and colleagues[24] and Mardh[25] failed to recover mycoplasmas from CSF of infants. A possible explanation for these negative findings could be that the infants they studied were not really the population in whom mycoplasmal infection is most likely. The study by Likitnukul and colleagues involved primarily older term infants, all of whom had been previously discharged from the hospital and had returned because of suspected sepsis or meningitis.[24, 45] Mardh did not specify the ages and birth weights of infants in his study.[25] No mycoplasmas were recovered from the CSF of 47 preterm infants cultured within the first week of life by Izraeli and co-workers.[23]

Shaw and associates[187] performed a prospective study of 135 preterm infants undergoing lumbar puncture and found only one isolate of *U. urealyticum.* The reason for lumbar puncture was not stated. In some hospitals, it has been common practice to evaluate CSF of all infants weighing less than 2500 g regardless of clinical evidence of sepsis or meningitis. Thus, isolation rates for any microorganism would be significantly lower.

Shaw and associates[187] concluded that in their hospital the single isolation did not justify routine investigation of infants for mycoplasmal infection. This seems unjustified, because a similar or even lower bacterial isolation rate from CSF does not justify withholding diagnostic procedures to identify other bacterial infections. The attack rate of bacterial meningitis is greater in the neonatal period than in any other period in life, yet even in this select group the attack rate is less than 1%.[188]

Waites and colleagues[189] isolated *M. hominis* on two successive occasions in a 2-year-old girl with hydrocephalus undergoing a ventriculoperitoneal shunt revision, proving the ability of this organism to infect the CNS in older children. The source of the infection in this child was unclear. Cervicovaginal cultures were negative for mycoplasmas.

The clinical findings in infants with *U. urealyticum* and *M. hominis* infection of the CSF are variable. *U. urealyticum* and *M. hominis* may produce CSF pleocytosis, with either polymorphonuclear or mononuclear cells predominating, or the inflammatory reaction in CSF may be minimal or absent.[19, 21, 22, 25] In some patients, the organisms are eradicated spontaneously from the CSF, whereas in others, the organisms have been shown to persist in the CSF for weeks and even months even with antibiotic treatment.[44, 184, 190, 191]

Lack of inflammation in the CSF, when the presence of *U. urealyticum* or *M. hominis* has been verified in the CSF on multiple occasions, may logically lead to some skepticism about the significance of mycoplasmal CSF infection. However, it should be noted that early in the course of infection with a number of other proven bacterial pathogens, inflammatory reactions may be scant or absent. Visser and Hall[192] reported "normal" CSF (cell count less than 25, protein level less than 2000 mg/dl) in 6 of 39 (29%) infants with culture-proven meningitis. Subsequent examination of CSF identified an increase in number of cells and protein level. The magnitude of the inflammatory response depends on the type of pathogen, possibly related to differences in cell wall components. For example, the median number of cells per cubic millimeter in CSF of 98 infants with gram-negative meningitis was more than 2000, whereas that in 21 infants with group B streptococcal meningitis was less than 100.[193] The lack of a cell wall in mycoplasmas may be related to the inflammatory response to these organisms. Glucose and protein values found in the normal infant may overlap those of the infant with bacterial meningitis. The severely ill infant with meningitis may in fact represent only a fraction of the total number of *Ureaplasma*- or *Mycoplasma*-infected infants, with the majority experiencing only a mild, often subclinical infection that may resolve spontaneously. More work is needed to determine why ureaplasmas and *M. hominis* elicit inflammation only in some infants and not in others.

Prognosis and long-term neurodevelopmental outcomes of infants with mycoplasmal CSF infections have not been studied in depth. Knowledge is limited primarily to case reports and short-term observations from recent prospective studies.[19, 42, 43, 46] Infants have been described whose infections were either subclinical or in whom there was only moderate illness followed by complete recovery. A decrease in hydrocephalus in preterm infants with CNS infection caused by either *M. hominis* or *U. urealyticum* has been documented after antibiotic treatment. The relative contribution of mycoplasmas to demise in some infected infants has not always been clear, owing to the concurrent presence of other conditions, such as extreme immaturity, intraventricular hemorrhage, respiratory disease, and concomitant bacterial infection. Permanent neurologic handicaps in survivors ranging from mild hemiparesis to profound spastic quadriplegia have been described. Studies of additional infants with detailed case-controlled neurodevelopmental follow-up are needed to establish the characteristics and risk of long-term effects of mycoplasmal CSF infections during the perinatal period.

Most of the case reports of mycoplasmal CSF infections have involved symptomatic infants with CSF pleocytosis for which no bacterial cause could be ascertained, and a mycoplasmal infection was considered only as a last resort, often after suspicious colonies that did not Gram stain were identified on routine bacteriologic media or after failure of the child to respond to conventional chemotherapy. The prevalence, risk factors, typical manifestations, and long-term effects of mycoplasmal CNS infections in the newborn have remained an enigma until the recent publication of prospective studies that began to clarify these issues to some degree. Until there is widespread awareness of how common mycoplasmal infections of the CNS can be, knowledge of what group is at risk for infection, and development of improved diagnostic capabilities, it is likely that the majority of cases will not be identified. *[The role of mycoplasmas as a cause of CNS infections remains uncertain. Well-documented cases of meningitis due to* M. hominis *have been reported.[25, 53, 179–185] The reasons for the frequent isolation of* U. urealyticum *in some studies but not in others remain uncertain. Possible technical reasons are discussed by Waites and colleagues[193a] and Heggie and colleagues.[193b] Other perplexing issues associated with the isolation of* U. urealyticum *in CSF of neonates are absence of inflammatory reaction in CSF that yielded the organism (no pleocytosis, no increase in protein or decrease in glucose concentrations); and the fact that* U. urealyticum *was transient in some CSF (the organism disappeared from CSF without antibiotic intervention). These issues raise uncertainties about a cause-and-effect relationship of the* U. urealyticum *and neonatal meningitis.]*

Other Conditions in the Newborn Caused by Genital Mycoplasmas

M. hominis was isolated from the pericardial fluid of an infant born with respiratory distress related to cardiac tamponade.[54] A pericardial biopsy specimen revealed a chronic and subacute inflammatory reaction. The infant recovered after a pleuropericardial window was placed and sequential usage of intravenous erythromycin and clindamycin.

M. hominis in pure culture was isolated from subcutaneous abscesses in two infants.[194, 195] Both infants had been delivered by forceps, and abscesses developed in the area where the forceps were applied. The organisms were presumably present in the birth canal, colonized the skin of the infants, and were inoculated by the forceps during delivery. Submandibular adenitis related to *M. hominis* has been reported in a neonate.[196] The swollen node was noted on day 6 of life and incised and drained of 1 ml of nonputrid pus on day 9. *M. hominis* was isolated from the pus and from a throat swab. This suggests that lymphatic drainage from the oropharynx was the likely route of infection.

Abscess formation at the site of an internal fetal heart rate monitor was recently shown to be due to *U. urealyticum*.[197] The knowledge that many such abscesses are reported as sterile suggests that genital mycoplasmas may be a more important cause of this problem than previously appreciated. *U. urealyticum* has also been isolated from bronchial secretions, lung tissue, and brain tissue of a newborn with hydrops fetalis in which immunologic causes were excluded, as were anomalies and chromosomal aberrations and other potential infectious causes.[198] Infections are a rare but well-known cause of nonimmunologic hydrops fetalis. Infections explain 7% of all cases. Congenital viral, bacterial, and parasitic infections can lead to hydrops fetalis. This case suggests that *U. urealyticum* congenital infection may also lead to hydrops fetalis. Modern clinical and laboratory methods fail to reveal the etiology of hydrops fetalis in 25% of cases.[199]

Investigators in Dallas, Texas, collected 170 specimens of urine by suprapubic aspiration in a group of infants readmitted to the hospital for suspected sepsis.[24] *U. urealyticum* and *M. hominis* were isolated from four infants (two infected with both organisms) ranging in age from 3 days to 2 months. The clinical significance of mycoplasmas isolated from urine is uncertain. In the Dallas cases, the two infants with infection related to *U. urealyticum* improved without specific therapy; infection caused by *M. hominis* in two infants also was of uncertain pathogenicity.

Jones and Tobin[200] isolated *M. hominis* from the purulent drainage of 8 of 250 infants with conjunctivitis. Because *M. hominis* may be isolated from the conjunctivae of infants who have no signs of inflammation, the association of infection with disease is uncertain.

OTHER MYCOPLASMAS WITH POTENTIAL RELEVANCE TO MATERNAL AND FETAL INFECTIONS

Mycoplasma pneumoniae

Ten to 20% of all cases of pneumonia are due to *M. pneumoniae*.[201] In addition, this organism is a common cause of tracheobronchitis and other respiratory syndromes, such as bronchiolitis and pharyngitis. Less common manifestations include croup, conjunctivitis, and otitis.[202]

Severe and extensive pulmonary disease occurs occasionally in *M. pneumoniae* infections.[138, 203–209] Pleural effusions are common, and massive lobar pneumonia is occasionally observed. Adult respiratory distress syndrome has been reported, as well as interstitial pulmonary fibrosis. Bronchiectasis and lung abscesses also can occur. Symptoms can persist for several weeks and have been reported at least in one case for up to 8 months.[210]

Dermatologic, neurologic, cardiac, renal, and pulmonary complications occur in patients with *M. pneumoniae* infections, although data on their frequency are lacking.[138, 211] Exanthem is a common manifestation of *M. pneumoniae* infection. Although the cutaneous manifestations are varied, an erythematous maculopapular rash is most common. Erythema multiforme and Stevens-Johnson syndrome are the types most often reported and are the most serious.[212] Although uncommon, *M. pneumoniae* myocarditis and pericarditis are important causes of morbidity and mortality.[119] Subclinical anemia occurs in up to 50% of *M. pneumoniae*–infected individuals. Severe hemolytic anemia occurs less frequently and in general correlates with high titers of cold agglutinins. Clinically inapparent compensated hemolysis is common in association with *M. pneumoniae* pulmonary infections.[212] A large spectrum of neurologic manifestations are associated with *M. pneumoniae* infection and occur in 2.6 to 4.8% of infected patients.[213] Aseptic meningitis is the most commonly reported finding, but other, less common findings include poliomyelitis-like syndrome, transverse myelitis, Bell's palsy and Guillain-Barré syndrome. *M. pneumoniae* infection is occasionally associated with joint manifestations, including arthritis. Seventeen instances of illness suggestive of rheumatic fever have been described. In most of these, joint swelling was involved. About 25% of patients with *M. pneumoniae* infection have nausea, vomiting, and/or diarrhea.

Immunologic events related to respiratory infection have been proposed to explain the protean manifestations of *M. pneumoniae* infection, but evidence for this is lacking. However, *M. pneumoniae* has been recovered from blood, pericardial fluid, middle ear fluid, vesicular skin lesions, pleural fluid, kidney, brain, and CSF.[119, 212–219] Thus, extrapulmonary manifestations may result from dissemination of the organism.

Extrapulmonary complications generally occur between 3 and 21 days after onset of respiratory illness. However, some cases are preceded by no history of respiratory illness or only mild symptoms. Extrapulmonary manifestations have been reported in all age groups.

Although the frequency with which they occur is unknown, mixed infections with *M. pneumoniae* and parainfluenza, influenza, staphylococci, and pneumococci do occur. We have observed mixed infections with *M. pneumoniae* and *Chlamydia pneumoniae* in which the presence of both organisms was documented by culture. We have also observed concurrent outbreaks of *M. pneumoniae* and *Bordetella pertussis*.

M. pneumoniae is spread by aerosol from person to person. In contrast to other respiratory illnesses, such as influenza, spread is usually slow. The reported incubation period is from 1 to 3 weeks. The organism can persist for 4 to 6 weeks in the infected host.

In large urban areas, *M. pneumoniae* appears to be endemic and occurs throughout the year, although epidemics can occur every 3 to 7 years. Current evidence indicates an infection incidence rate of 20 to 30% per year. The incidence rate is highest among school children and second highest among children younger than 5 years of age.[220] In the 1960s, *M. pneumoniae* was thought to be rare among children younger than 5 years of age and was believed to cause only acute, self-limited respiratory disease. Recent studies indicate that the peak age incidence may actually be highest among 3 and 4 year olds and that there is a high rate of hospitalization for *M. pneumoniae* pneumonia among children younger than 5.[220–222] The popular belief that *M. pneumoniae* disease is rare in this age group has precluded most physicians from even considering it in the differential diagnosis.

One of the most comprehensive studies of the etiology of severe respiratory disease in children was performed by Kok and Marmion.[222] They performed bacterial, mycoplasmal, and viral cultures plus serologies on 1600 children younger than 15 years of age who were hospitalized with severe respiratory disease. Overall, 6% of the cases were culture positive for *M. pneumoniae*, and, of these patients, over half were younger than 5 years of age. Twenty percent of *M. pneumoniae* isolates were from children younger than 1 year of age. Seventy-two percent of patients from whom *M. pneumoniae* was isolated were suffering from pneumonia, whereas the remaining 28 percent (18 of 64) of isolates were from patients with croup, bronchiolitis, or upper respiratory symptoms. The reverse was true for those with evidence of viral infection. Sixty-four percent with evidence of viral infection had croup, bronchiolitis, or bronchitis, with the remainder having evidence of pneumonia.

Clearly, the role of *M. pneumoniae* in respiratory disease of newborns and infants needs to be reassessed in light of these recent findings. Many women in the childbearing age group have respiratory infections caused by *M. pneumoniae*. Yet there is little information about the effect of this agent on the course of pregnancy, the development of the fetus, or the health of the newborn. Investigators at Boston City Hospital cultured more than 1500 newborns and did not isolate *M. pneumoniae* from the nose, throat, external ear canal, external genitalia, conjunctivae, blood, urine, or CSF (Y-H Lee, WM McCormack, and JO Klein, unpublished observation).

Mycoplasma genitalium

M. genitalium occurs infrequently in the lower genital tract of healthy males and females. However, several groups of investigators have detected this organism in the urethra of 9 to 20% of men with nongonococcal urethritis and 6 to 20% of women attending a sexually transmitted disease clinic for urethritis or cervicitis.[223–227] Intraurethral inoculations of this organism into nonhu-

cal substrates from which they derive energy. *U. urealyticum* generates adenosine triphosphate by urea hydrolysis. *M. hominis* metabolizes arginine to ammonia. Although a variety of commercially prepared media are available, none have been rigorously evaluated in comparison to the individually prepared and tested broths and agars used by most reference laboratories. Mycoplasmal growth medium ordinarily contains animal serum, peptones, yeast extract, and metabolic substrates such as glucose, arginine, or urea. Shepard's 10B broth and A8 agar have been successfully employed for cultivation of both *M. hominis* and *U. urealyticum*. Antibiotics such as penicillin or nystatin are routinely incorporated into the media to inhibit bacterial and fungal contamination.

The relatively rapid growth rates of *M. hominis* and *U. urealyticum* make identification of most positive cultures possible within 2 to 5 days. Broth cultures may be incubated at 37°C under atmospheric conditions and agar plates under 95% nitrogen and 5% carbon dioxide. Ureaplasmas, in particular, are susceptible to a rapid, steep death phase in culture, which is likely to result from a combination of urea depletion, ammonia production, and elevated pH due to urease activity. The presence of growth in 10B medium is suggested by an alkaline shift due to the urease activity of ureaplasmas or arginine hydrolysis by *M. hominis*, causing the phenol red indicator to turn from yellow to pink. The presence of growth in SP4 broth is evident by a red to yellow (acidic) shift due to metabolism of glucose or red to deeper red (alkaline) shift due to arginine hydrolysis. Broth cultures showing color changes should be subcultured to agar immediately. This combination of broth-to-agar inoculation technique has been shown to be the most sensitive for recovery of genital mycoplasmas.

Colonies of *U. urealyticum* can be identified readily on A8 agar by urease production in the presence of calcium chloride indicator, following 24 to 72 hours of incubation. The colonies are often amorphous (Fig. 14–4). Colonies of other mycoplasmas are urease-negative and have a typical "fried egg" appearance (see Fig. 14–4). Unlike conventional bacteria, minute mycoplasmal colonies require a stereomicroscope to determine their presence and characterize their morphology.

In addition to *M. hominis*, other mycoplasmal species that may have similar growth requirements can also be present in clinical specimens and can be morphologically indistinguishable. Because there are no biochemical tests that can readily distinguish between the large-colony mycoplasmal species, serologic identification methods must be used. Due to increased specificity, sensitivity, and rapidity, immunoblotting with monoclonal antibodies and PCR are gradually replacing the other methods of speciation of large-colony mycoplasmas. A problem with any of these techniques, however, is the existence of multiple serovars and biovars of *M. hominis* and *U. urealyticum*.

Thus, any antibodies or PCR primers must react with all 14 reference serovars of ureaplasmas and members of both ureaplasma biovars and with the 7 reference strains of *M. hominis*.[120, 256] Also, before acceptance, reagents should be shown to react with large numbers of geographically diverse clinical isolates.

The development of invasive disease in only certain subpopulations of infected individuals has led to the hypothesis that only certain serovars or biovars may have invasive potential. However, definitive evidence for this is lacking, and the current methods for differentiating different serovars and biovars are not practically applied for routine use.[257]

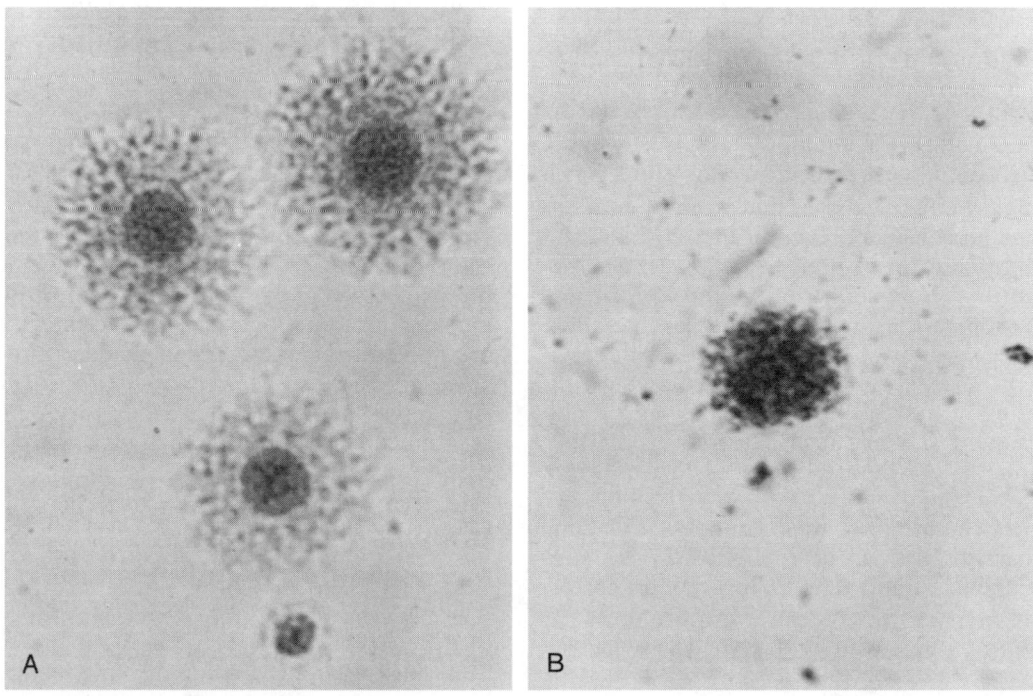

FIGURE 14–4 *A, Mycobacterium hominis* (original magnification 100×). *B, Ureaplasma urealyticum* (original magnification 1000×). (From Klein JO. Mycoplasmas, genitourinary tract infection, and reproductive failure. Hosp Pract 6:127–133, 1971, with permission.)

The MB antigen of *U. urealyticum* has been shown to be one of the most predominant antigens recognized by infected humans, and it has also been shown to undergo size variation that may be related to disease pathogenesis.[241, 242] The MB gene has recently been cloned and sequenced and shown to encode both serovar and biovar specificity.[258] Development of reagents should now be possible to address systematically the invasive potential to different serovars and biovars.

Nonculture Diagnostic Methods

PCR tests have been established for both *U. urealyticum*[120] and *M. hominis*.[256] The *U. urealyticum* assay appears to be as reliable as culture for detection of ureaplasmas in endotracheal aspirates and amniotic fluid and genital secretions. The *M. hominis* PCR remains to be evaluated for detection of organisms in clinical specimens, but in vitro data suggest that it should be comparable. Although the availability of these assays for rapid diagnosis (within 24 hours) is an important advance for diagnosis of invasive infections in newborns, cultures must still be performed on any positive specimen in order to assess accurately antibiotic susceptibility of the infecting organism. *[The latest techniques for PCR detection of* U. ureaplasma, M. hominis, *and* M. pneumoniae *are discussed by Couroucli and colleagues.[174b]]*

Serologic Diagnosis

The incidence of antibody to *M. hominis* or *U. urealyticum* is directly related to age: few prepubertal individuals have specific antibody, but the incidence rises sharply during adolescence, and 50 to 90% of adults have antibody to *U. urealyticum* or *M. hominis*.[232, 259–301]

Patients with invasive *M. hominis* infections almost without exception seroconvert or have a significant rise in existing antibody. This response can be measured by the metabolism-inhibition assay or enzyme-linked immunosorbent assay (ELISA).[8, 57, 115, 263] Both acute and convalescent sera should be evaluated, results based on single specimens being difficult or impossible to interpret. Owing to the ubiquity of most mycoplasmas in humans, it should be realized that detection of antibodies alone cannot be considered significant.

The ELISA has also been used to detect *U. urealyticum*–specific antibodies in sera from various female and infant patient populations.[8, 264, 265] Whereas the mere presence or absence of antibody agrees well with cervicovaginal isolation of *U. urealyticum*, particularly IgA, changes in antibody titer do not necessarily agree with cultural isolation of the organism from invasive sites. This may be due to the failure of the ELISA to detect serovar-specific antibody rises.

The unique susceptibility of hypogammaglobulinemic patients to chronic arthritis due to *U. urealyticum* suggests that antibody is important for protection against invasive disease due to this organism.[50] Increased susceptibility of infants younger than 30 weeks' gestational age to *U. urealyticum*–induced respiratory disease may be related to their hypogammaglobulinemia.[49]

A study of a hypogammaglobulinemic patient with arthritis provides evidence that serovar-specific antibody may be required for protection against invasive disease. We detected high levels of ureaplasma-specific antibodies by the nonserovar-specific ELISA in the serum of the patient as well as in that of two serum donors who served as sources of immunoglobulin replacement during the period of joint infection. However, by the serovar-specific metabolism inhibition (MI) assay, no antibodies to serovar 4, which was isolated from the joint and subcutaneous abscesses, were detected.[266] In another hypogammaglobulinemic patient with chronic arthritis due to an antibiotic-resistant strain of *U. urealyticum*, treatment with commercial immunoglobulin (Sandoz) was not effective, whereas arthritis and abscesses resolved when the patient was given infusions of goat hyperimmune *U. urealyticum* serum.[59, 267] Thus far, the serovars isolated from joints of hypogammaglobulinemic patients include 2, 4, 5, 7, 8, and an untypeable strain. Generally, these are not the more common serovars isolated from the patient and control populations that have been surveyed. Perhaps commercial immunoglobulin preparations contain antibodies to the more common serovars, such as 3 and 6.

That detection of serovar-specific *U. urealyticum* responses is clinically significant has also been demonstrated by Kass and co-workers.[268] They showed that women who experienced a fourfold or greater rise in antibody titer to any single strain of *U. urealyticum* had a low-birth-weight rate of 30%, whereas women who did not experience such a rise in antibody titer had a low-birth-weight rate of 7.3%. Correspondingly, the birth weight between the two groups differed by 230 g. In the majority of instances where there were significant rises in antibody titer, the titer rise was specific for a serologic type other than those for which the women had preexistent antibody, and the type-specific titer rose from undetectable levels. Data by Quinn and colleagues[269] also indicate selective antibody rises to certain serovars in women with pregnancy wastage and in infants with respiratory disease as compared to control patients.

Studies by Quinn and colleagues[269] and Gallo and associates[270] suggest that the presence of *U. urealyticum*–specific IgM antibody in infants is predictive of disease. However, more information is needed concerning the value of antibody detection and the incidence of antibodies in well-characterized, asymptomatic infants matched for gestational age. Furthermore, until methods are standardized and reagents made commercially available, serodiagnosis will remain limited mainly to specialized research or reference laboratories and cannot be recommended for routine diagnostic purposes.

Diagnosis of *Mycoplasma pneumoniae* and Other Mycoplasmal Infections

The carriage rate of *M. pneumoniae* is thought to be low (if it occurs at all).[220] The true frequency with which it causes disease in newborn and young infants is unknown. However, recent reports of severe disease in infants and children younger than 5 years old and in adults older than 21 emphasize the need for diagnostic consideration in all age groups, not just in patients between 6 and 21 years of age (as is the usual practice).[220]

M. pneumoniae infection is associated with diverse clinical illnesses that may lead to delay in definitive diagnosis. Although complications appear to be uncommon, their true incidence may have been underestimated. Because of the impression that severe pneumonia and extrapulmonary complications are inconsistent with *M. pneumoniae* disease, it is often not included in the differential diagnosis. The onset of extrapulmonary manifestations usually occurs from 1 to 21 days after that of the respiratory symptoms. However, some patients give no history of respiratory symptoms, and others report only upper respiratory tract infection. These patients present real diagnostic difficulties. The clinical manifestations and radiographic and laboratory findings in *M. pneumoniae* infection are not distinctive enough to allow an accurate diagnosis.

Isolation of *M. pneumoniae* from the upper respiratory tract usually indicates a current or recent infection. To enhance detection of the organism, it is best to evaluate multiple sites within the respiratory tract. Similar precautions should be followed for collection and processing of specimens as were already outlined for *U. urealyticum* and *M. hominis*. Nasopharyngeal and throat swabs and, if available, sputa and bronchoalveolar lavage fluid should all be evaluated for *M. pneumoniae*. SP4 broth is preferred for transport of specimens, and SP4 broth and agar are the preferred media for isolation of *M. pneumoniae*.[271] Growth of the organisms is not apparent until 3 to 7 days after incubation and may take as long as 21 days. After growth of the organism, species identification can be accomplished by epi-immunofluorescence on colonies grown on agar, by inhibition of growth by disks impregnated with homologous antisera, by immunoblotting with appropriate monoclonal antibodies, or by PCR. Such procedures are available only in specialized reference laboratories.

Because of the time and expense of culture, PCR and antigen detection assays are being used with increasing frequency for detection of *M. pneumoniae* infection.[272] All indications are that PCR is comparable to, if not even more reliable than, culture.[232, 272] Because of the persistence of *M. pneumoniae* within the respiratory tract for several weeks or months after resolution of clinical symptoms, serologic diagnosis may be required for proof of current infection.[272]

The immune response to *M. pneumoniae* infection may be demonstrated by indirect hemagglutination, growth inhibition, complement fixation, or ELISA, which provides separate detection of IgM and IgG antibodies. Cold agglutinins develop in approximately 50% of individuals infected with *M. pneumoniae*. Cold agglutinins appear during the second week of illness, disappear in 3 to 6 months, and are directly related to the severity of the respiratory infection, but they are nonspecific and can develop in patients with other diseases, including viral and other bacterial respiratory infections.[273] Growth-inhibiting antibodies are specific, rise within a few weeks after infection, peak at approximately 4 months, and persist for long periods. Complement-fixing antibodies rise rapidly, peak at 1 month after infection, and persist for a shorter time, but their analysis is satisfactory for routine diagnostic purposes. There is extensive cross-reactivity between *M. pneumoniae* and *M. genitalium* in each of these assays such that positives should be confirmed by immunoblotting.[274] Current research is directed toward identification of non–cross-reactive antigens that may be useful in the ELISA.

Because of the extreme fastidiousness and slow growth of *M. genitalium* and *M. fermentans*, PCR, in situ hybridization, and/or immunohistochemistry are recommended for detection of infection.[227, 232, 236] Currently, little information is available concerning the human immune response to these organisms.

IN VITRO ANTIBIOTIC SUSCEPTIBILITIES OF MYCOPLASMAS

Lack of on-site diagnostic facilities for mycoplasmas in many hospitals, coupled with the potentially serious nature of any systemic infection in a neonate, makes empirical treatment necessary in most cases. Thus, knowledge of susceptibility patterns is of considerable importance.

Absence of a cell wall and limited biosynthetic capabilities drastically limit the types of antibiotics potentially effective against mycoplasmas in general. Neither β-lactams, vancomycin, nor sulfonamides are useful. However, mycoplasmas may be susceptible to antibiotics that interfere with protein synthesis, such as tetracyclines, macrolides, aminoglycosides, or chloramphenicol, and to drugs that impair DNA replication, such as fluoroquinolones, but not predictably so. Lincosamides, including clindamycin, although active against *M. hominis*, are usually not effective against *U. urealyticum*. Aminoglycosides, commonly used against gram-negative infections, do not appear to be very active in vivo against *U. urealyticum* or *M. hominis* in neonates. We have isolated *U. urealyticum* numerous times from the lower respiratory tract, bloodstream, and CSF of neonates who have received 3 days or more of intravenous gentamicin for suspected bacterial sepsis. Chloramphenicol is not a popular drug for use in neonatal medicine, owing to bone marrow toxicity and the availability of alternative agents for most infections, but it generally has good in vitro activity against mycoplasmas.

Tetracycline resistance has been known to occur in *U. urealyticum* since the 1970s, when approximately 10% of the strains isolated from men with urethritis were found to be resistant.[275] Tetracycline resistance in *M. hominis* has been reported to occur in as many as 40% of clinical isolates and appears to be increasing.[276, 277] Furthermore, potential bone toxicities make this class of antibiotics undesirable for use in neonates except in some extreme circumstances such as CSF infection. Although the earlier fluoroquinolones, including ciprofloxacin, are not particularly active against *U. urealyticum*, in vitro studies of some of the newer investigational members of this class show promise. However, quinolones have not been recommended for use in neonates or other pediatric populations. Unlike with genital mycoplasmas, tetracycline and erythromycin resistance in *M. pneumoniae* has not been a problem thus far.

Over the past several years, dozens of publications have described the in vitro susceptibilities of *U. urealyticum* to existing and investigational antibiotics, often with conflicting and confusing results. Reasons for such discrepancies among published studies are multifactorial. Small sample sizes, samples collected in a nonrandom manner without regard to prior antibiotic exposure, sampling different populations from widely divergent geographic and socioeconomic strata, and the fact that resistance may change over time are among the many possible explanations. However, the most obvious and perhaps important reasons for the continuing controversy are the lack of uniform, standardized techniques and media formulations for performance of in vitro testing and of objective criteria for interpretation of results. The fastidious growth requirements of the organisms preclude application of most conventional and approved guidelines for bacteria to ureaplasmal testing procedures.[278–280] Influence of methodology on interpretation of erythromycin susceptibility data was evident when two techniques, microbroth and agar dilution, using known quantities of the same inoculum of organisms, showed differing results in strains whose minimal inhibitory concentrations (MICs) were near the defined breakpoints for resistance.[278, 281] Both agar dilution and microbroth dilution techniques are used in reference laboratories to determine drug susceptibilities for mycoplasmas.

A widespread misconception is that all mycoplasmal species are susceptible to erythromycin.[282] Although naturally occurring erythromycin-resistant strains of *M. pneumoniae* have not been documented, erythromycin resistance is universal in *M. hominis*. The majority of in vitro studies support the selection of erythromycin as the antibiotic of choice for pediatric ureaplasmal infections not involving the CSF.[279, 280] Some tetracycline-resistant strains of *U. urealyticum* may also be erythromycin-resistant, but high-level erythromycin resistance in *U. urealyticum* has been infrequently reported. Despite apparent in vitro susceptibility, either tetracycline or erythromycin treatment of vaginal mycoplasmas in women is not always successful. Treatment failure of infections due to infection with apparently susceptible organisms may be because of the inactivity of the drug at the site of infection due to pH or other variables.

In 1970, Braun and associates[275] reported initial MICs for erythromycin for 11 strains of *U. urealyticum* ranging from 0.8 to 1.6 μg/ml, similar results to those of Taylor-Robinson and Furr[283] 16 years later, clearly demonstrating in vitro susceptibility. More recently, Cassell and colleagues (unpublished observations), in a large multicenter study of adults with nongonococcal urethritis or cervicitis that encompassed several geographic locations (over 300 patients from 15 different geographic areas), reported MICs for erythromycin obtained by microbroth dilution ranging from 0.125 to 8 μg/ml, with the $MIC_{90} = 2$ μg/ml. Erythromycin susceptibility was defined as an MIC of 0.5 μg/ml or less, intermediate susceptibility as 1 to 4 μg/ml, and resis-

tance as 8 μg/ml or more. These standards were originally defined to apply to common aerobically growing bacteria and not to mycoplasmas. However, in the absence of other guidelines, they seem a reasonable means of classifying susceptibilities of ureaplasmal isolates until more specific recommendations are available, as they have been established by the National Committee for Clinical Laboratory Standards (NCCLS) according to rigid criteria, including achievable blood levels using approved dosages.

In vitro susceptibilities of 43 neonatal respiratory isolates of *U. urealyticum* obtained in Birmingham, Alabama, to erythromycin and five other antibiotics were determined by microbroth dilution. Resistance, as defined by the NCCLS,[284] was observed in one or more ureaplasmal strains for each of the antibiotics tested, except for erythromycin. In contrast to erythromycin MICs, values for doxycycline tend to be spread over a wider range, with clear separation of susceptible and resistant strains.

Newer macrolides, including clarithromycin and azithromycin, have a similar spectrum of in vitro activity to that of erythromycin against mycoplasmas and *U. urealyticum*, but there are as yet no published clinical data on their use specifically as treatment for ureaplasmal infections, and they are not yet approved in neonates. *[A review of the antibiotic susceptibilities of mycoplasmas and mycoplasmal infections includes data on the activity of newer macrolides, ketolides, and quinolones.[301a]]*

TREATMENT OF MYCOPLASMAL INFECTIONS

Ureaplasma urealyticum and *Mycoplasma hominis*

A positive culture for mycoplasmas, especially from a normally sterile site and particularly in the absence of other microorganisms, is sufficient justification for treatment of patients suffering from a condition known to be caused by or associated with mycoplasmas. However, the presence of mycoplasmas in clinical material obtained from patients without evidence of mycoplasma-associated disease does not warrant treatment. The limited availability of mycoplasmal diagnostic facilities and the impracticality of obtaining specimens for microbiologic study in some conditions make it necessary for clinicians to be familiar with the syndromes for which mycoplasmas may be responsible and to provide treatment that is likely to eliminate the organisms.

Antibiotics are used at some point in most admissions to neonatal intensive care units and almost universally in the low-birth-weight neonate owing to the inability to clinically distinguish nonspecific aspects of respiratory distress of prematurity from pulmonary infection.

Although systemic ureaplasmal and mycoplasmal infections have been described that probably contributed to morbidity and even death in a relatively small number of neonates studied to date, there is very little experience on which to base treatment indications, choice of drug, expected outcomes, or potential complications. The single most difficult issue to resolve is when antibiotics should be given to an infant from whom *U. urealyticum* or *M. hominis* has been isolated. It is not clear that treatment results in organism eradication or improved clinical outcome. No randomized clinical trials have been conducted to determine the efficacy of such treatment, and no guidelines can be put forward at this time as to empirical therapy or specific therapy once the organism has been isolated.

The proven ability of mycoplasmas to induce inflammation in the lung and CSF and the isolation from blood, CSF, pericardial fluid, and pleural fluid in pure culture are adequate justification for administering specific antimicrobial treatment in clinically ill neonates when the organisms are isolated from an affected site and when there are no other verifiable microbiologic etiologies of pneumonitis, meningitis, or nonspecific respiratory or other systemic problems typical of disseminated infection. Whether antibiotics should be administered to an infant with a positive CSF culture but in whom there is no evidence of inflammation (pleocytosis), progressive hydrocephalus, or other clinical illness is a contentious issue and probably should best be handled on a case-by-case basis. However, the finding of any microorganism in a sterile body fluid such as CSF is by definition abnormal, and the natural history and potential long-term effects of such infections, if left untreated, have not been adequately studied. There is evidence from one study[19] that some neonates, most of whom were near or at term when born, from whom *M. hominis* or *U. urealyticum* was isolated from CSF in the absence of pleocytosis may spontaneously clear the organisms without antimicrobial intervention. Whether this clearance occurs commonly in the low-birth-weight neonate has not been established. Because presumptive *M. hominis* and/or *U. urealyticum* infection can often be detected in the clinical laboratory within 24 to 48 hours following specimen collection, the neonatologist with mycoplasmal diagnostic facilities in-house may prefer to monitor the patient closely, repeat a lumbar puncture, and reculture and reexamine CSF for the presence of inflammation and organisms using DNA stains before committing to treatment with potentially toxic drugs in a neonate who is not clinically ill by the time initial culture results are known.

Clear-cut ureaplasmal pneumonia, with or without bloodstream infection, is adequate justification for therapeutic intervention, with appropriate microbiologic documentation whenever possible. Because of the problems in identifying pneumonia and in assigning a microbiologic cause with certainty in the early neonatal period, some physicians are taking a less conservative approach and treating low-birth-weight neonates from whom *U. urealyticum* is isolated from the lower respiratory tract and who have respiratory distress as evidenced by supplemental oxygen and/or ventilatory requirements. Such indiscriminate antibiotic use is without supportive data from large prospective studies to determine if there is a clear benefit in terms of either microbiologic efficacy in organism eradication or improved clinical outcome.

A few reports of clinical improvements have been described in critically ill infants infected with *U. urealyti-cum* who received antibiotics.[28, 33, 197] However, a number of cases had fatal outcomes despite treatment, suggesting that the mortality of symptomatic neonates with systemic ureaplasmal infection may be high.[27] The relative contribution of ureaplasmal infection to morbidity and/or mortality is difficult to interpret because most cases have been either very low birth weight infants with multiple complications or infants with other clinical problems that could likely contribute to the poor outcome.

The chronicity typical of ureaplasmal infections in other immunocompromised hosts suggests that prolonged treatment may be required to eradicate the organism.[50, 59] Indeed, the immune status of the host may be a major factor in a successful drug treatment of any ureaplasmal infection, particularly because the available antibiotics are only mycoplasmastatic and not mycoplasmacidal. Limited clinical experience suggests a minimum 10- to 14-day therapeutic regimen. Whether the intravenous or oral route is employed depends on the overall condition of the patient and the nature of the infection being treated, with the parenteral route being generally preferred in the preterm neonate. Patients treated for ureaplasmal infection should optimally have the isolates tested for drug susceptibility and should be followed for clinical response. Follow-up cultures are suggested in cases in which clinical improvement does not occur with treatment.

U. urealyticum has been successfully eradicated from amniotic fluid in pregnant women given erythromycin.[286, 287] Only a few cases of neonatal mycoplasmal or ureaplasmal infections successfully treated with antibiotics have been described. Garland and Murton[42] eradicated *U. urealyticum* from CSF by a combined 14-day regimen of intravenous erythromycin and chloramphenicol. Waites and associates[19] reported successful treatment of CSF infection with doxycycline alone in one infant. An additional infant was given erythromycin for 10 days after a 14-day treatment failure with doxycycline. A fourth infant with both a positive CSF culture and ureaplasmal pneumonia was successfully treated with intravenous erythromycin alone for 14 days. However, Shaw and colleagues[187] described an infant from whom *U. urealyticum* was persistently isolated from CSF over 16 weeks despite a protracted course of erythromycin. Eradication was finally achieved with doxycycline. Hentschel and co-workers[43] recently reported an erythromycin-resistant strain of *U. urealyticum* in the CSF of a premature infant with progressive hydrocephalus and successful eradication of the organism by treatment with chloramphenicol for 20 days. Whereas erythromycin is the first choice drug for ureaplasmal infections of the respiratory tract, it is not usually considered for infections involving the CNS because of poor penetration across the blood-brain barrier. Its initial selection in the previous cases was related to the undesirability of tetracycline use in neonates. In view of in vitro susceptibilities of neonatal ureaplasmal isolates[279] to chloramphenicol and the drug's ability to penetrate into CSF, further consideration of chloramphenicol as an alternative to tetracycline might be worthwhile.

Infants with meningitis caused by *M. hominis* have

been treated successfully with intravenous doxycycline or tetracycline.[46] In two cases of neonatal meningitis, treatment with chloramphenicol failed to eradicate the organism from the CSF.[52, 184] Eradication was accomplished by doxycycline in one infant and clindamycin in the other.

Clarithromycin and azithromycin have in vitro activities against *U. urealyticum* but not *M. hominis*.[279, 280, 288] No published data are available concerning clinical or in vivo microbiologic efficacy of clarithromycin against *U. urealyticum*. [*Azithromycin successfully eradicated* U. urealyticum *from the female genital tract after prior courses of doxycycline and ofloxacin had failed to eradicate the organism.[301b]*]

Data from the University of Alabama at Birmingham showed that *U. urealyticum* was eradicated at least transiently from the lower respiratory tract of 11 of 12 neonates suffering from respiratory disease when treated with 7 or more days of intravenous erythromycin lactobionate (25 to 40 mg/kg per day given in four divided doses) within 2 weeks of birth.[279] Only one tracheal aspirate was collected for culture 48 to 72 hours after completion of treatment. Whether subsequent cultures would have shown a recurrence of the organism is not known. Prior administration of gentamicin or other antibiotics in several participants makes interpretation of these findings more complex, and they should be confirmed by more rigorous testing in a larger population and by comparison with placebo controls. Other investigators have reported the reappearance of the organism in several weeks' time.

Most available information on appropriate dosages, pharmacologic behavior, safety, and tolerability of erythromycin in infants is limited to the oral estolate or ethylsuccinate forms, with very little data from low-birth-weight preterm subjects (see Chapter 35). Patamasucon and co-workers[289] performed a pharmacokinetic study in a group of infants younger than 4 months of age. They recommended that oral erythromycin estolate suspensions be given at 30 mg/kg per day in three divided doses or 20 mg/kg per day in two divided doses.

Serum levels of erythromycin, measured by liquid chromatography, after intravenous infusion of the lactobionate preparation were measured in a group of neonates of 1500 g or less birth weight and 2 weeks of age or younger in whom *U. urealyticum* was detected in the lower respiratory tract.[280] Subjects were given 25 to 40 mg/kg per day in four divided doses, scheduled for a total of 10 days. Among nine available neonates who received the 40-mg/kg/day dose, peak levels obtained at steady state exceeded the measured MIC of the corresponding *U. urealyticum* strain in eight cases. Trough levels met or exceeded the measured MIC of the corresponding *U. urealyticum* strains in seven of nine cases. One would expect the MIC in vivo under physiologic conditions in the respiratory tract to be lower, based on the earlier discussion regarding erythromycin activity in vitro at pH 6. Therefore, these preliminary findings, coupled with the earlier observations regarding ureaplasmal eradication in 11 of 12 neonates from this same group, suggest that erythromycin has favorable pharmacokinetic behavior in the preterm neonate and supports the use of this antibiotic as a therapeutic alternative in

clinically significant ureaplasmal infections. The fact that erythromycin concentrations in pulmonary secretions may exceed serum levels[293] suggests that adequate local concentrations of the drug for treatment of most *U. urealyticum* respiratory infections most likely occur, although much is yet to be learned regarding the pharmacologic behavior of erythromycin in the newborn.

Although erythromycin is generally considered a very safe drug, a study from 1963 addressed the question of toxicity in a group of 87 preterm infants who were given oral erythromycin estolate (40 mg/kg per day) for up to 14 days.[291] Infants were aged 1 to 43 days and weighed 860 to 2460 g. These investigators observed no evidence of toxicity or development of abnormal hepatic function and found satisfactory serum levels without accumulation of the drug. Birth weight and postnatal age did not affect the pattern of serum levels.

Ototoxicity has been associated with administration of erythromycin in adults with impaired renal and/or hepatic function who were receiving high intravenous doses.[292] There are no reported instances of erythromycin-associated ototoxicity in neonates.

Crouse and colleagues[293] evaluated hearing by auditory brain-stem–evoked potentials in 33 infants who received intravenous erythromycin for ureaplasmal infection and compared this with findings in 176 matched infants who did not receive the antibiotic. No difference in the occurrence of abnormal hearing screens was identified between the two groups, nor was there evidence of any other adverse effect related to administration of erythromycin, including hepatotoxicity, evaluated by measuring liver enzymes and bilirubin, and thrombophlebitis.

Farrar and co-workers[294] reported cardiac toxicity associated with intravenous erythromycin lactobionate in two premature infants treated for ureaplasmal infection. Obviously, much more information is needed regarding the safety and pharmacokinetics of the drug in newborns. [*Marked QT interval prolongation occurred in* term[301c] *and premature[301d] infants who received intravenous erythromycin lactobionate. The role of erythromycin lactobionate as an etiologic factor in neonatal arrhythmias is discussed by Gouyon.[301d] These cases raise concern about use of parenteral erythromycin for neonatal disease.*

An association of hypertrophic pyloric stenosis with therapeutic doses of erythromycin administered to infants after exposure to pertussis was documented in a Tennessee hospital.[301c] A cluster of seven cases of hypertrophic pyloric stenosis occurred among about 200 infants who were "advised to receive erythromycin." The authors hypothesize that erythromycin is a motilin antagonist that increases antral motility and contraction of the pyloric bulb (and is used in low doses to improve gastric emptying). The higher therapeutic doses may result in strong contractions of the musculature that could result in hypertrophy of the pyloris.]

Mycoplasma pneumoniae and Other Mycoplasmas

Controlled therapy trials in children and adults indicate that treatment with either erythromycin (30 to 60 mg/kg per day) or tetracycline (25 to 50 mg/kg per day) markedly reduces the duration of symptoms of the respiratory disease, although it does not always result in eradication of the organism. The effect of antibiotic therapy on extrapulmonary complications is debatable. Because most cases involving complications are not diagnosed until late in the course of disease, the benefit of early treatment is unknown.

All comparative in vitro studies to date have shown that macrolides are the most potent antimicrobial agents against *M. pneumoniae*.[300] MICs for erythromycin obtained in recent years have ranged from less than 0.004 to 8 μg/ml, with most reported values being several dilutions less than 1 μg/ml. Tetracycline MICs have recently been reported in the 0.06 to 1 μg/ml ranges.[300, 301] Norfloxacin and ciprofloxacin have MICs predominantly greater than 1 μg/ml, and the majority of strains would be designated as resistant.[301-304] Sparfloxacin, PD 127391, and WIN 57273 are the only quinolones that consistently have MICs less than 1 μg/ml (i.e., activity comparable to that of tetracycline).[300-304] Although naturally occurring strains of *M. pneumoniae* resistant to erythromycin or tetracycline have not been reported, the effectiveness of erythromycin may be limited because of dose-related nausea, vomiting, or diarrhea, especially after prolonged use. Use of tetracyclines is contraindicated in young children, owing to potential bone and tooth toxicities. A number of the new macrolides, such as clarithromycin, avoid these complications, have better pharmacokinetic properties, and have been shown to be effective both in vitro and in vivo against *M. pneumoniae*.[300, 302]

It has been noted that patients sometimes relapse after the 5- to 7-day courses of antibiotics that are commonly prescribed. This may be due to the continued presence of the mycoplasma; thus, 14 to 21 days of therapy is more appropriate. The newer macrolides, clarithromycin and azithromycin, show good in vitro activity against *M. pneumoniae*, but they are not currently approved for pediatric use and no clinical efficacy data in children or neonates are available.

Although indications for treatment have not been established, *M. genitalium* has basically the same antibiotic profile as *M. pneumoniae*.[305] In contrast, *M. fermentans* appears to be resistant to macrolides but sensitive to tetracyclines.[305]

References

1. Bove JM. Molecular features of Mollicutes. Clin Infect Dis 17(Suppl 1):S10–S31, 1993.
2. Tully JG. Current status of the Mollicute flora of humans. Clin Infect Dis 17(Suppl 1):S2–S9, 1993.
3. Cassell GH (ed). Proceedings of the International Symposium: Ureaplasmas of humans with emphasis on maternal and neonatal infections. Pediatr Infect Dis 5(Suppl 6), 1986.
4. Cassell GH, Waites KB, Watson HL, et al. *Ureaplasma urealyticum* intrauterine infection: role in prematurity and disease in newborns. Clin Microbiol Rev 6:69–87, 1993.
5. Cassell GH, Davis RO, Waites KB, et al. Isolation of *Mycoplasma hominis* and *Ureaplasma urealyticum* from amniotic fluid at 16–20 weeks gestation: potential effect on pregnancy outcome. Sex Transm Dis 10:294–302, 1983.
6. Cassell GH, Younger JB, Brown MB, et al. Microbiologic study of infertile women at the time of diagnostic laparoscopy. N Engl J Med 308:502–505, 1983.
7. Cassell GH, Clyde WA, Kenny GE, et al. Ureaplasmas of humans with emphasis on maternal and neonatal infections. Pediatr Infect Dis J 6(Suppl):S221–S354, 1986.
8. Cassell GH, Waites KB, Gibbs RS, et al. The role of *Ureaplasma urealyticum* in amnionitis. Pediatr Infect Dis J 5(Suppl):247–252, 1986.
9. Cassell GH. Future considerations: maternal and neonatal aspects. Pediatr Infect Dis J 5(Suppl):341–344, 1986.
10. Embree JE, Krause VW, Embil JA, et al. Placental infection with *Mycoplasma hominis* and *Ureaplasma urealyticum*: clinical correlation. Obstet Gynecol 56:475–481, 1980.
11. Hillier SL, Martius J, Krohn M, et al. A case-control study of chorioamnionic infection and histologic chorioamnionitis in prematurity. N Engl J Med 319:972–978, 1988.
12. Kundsin RB, Driscoll SG, Monson RR, et al. Association of *Ureaplasma urealyticum* in the placenta with perinatal morbidity and mortality. N Engl J Med 310:941–945, 1984.
13. Quinn PA, Butany J, Chipman M, et al. A prospective study of microbial infection in stillbirths and early neonatal death. Am J Obstet Gynecol 151:238–249, 1985.
14. Quinn PA, Butany J, Taylor J, et al. Chorioamnionitis: its association with pregnancy outcome and microbial infection. Am J Obstet Gynecol 156:379–387, 1987.
15. Cassell GH, Hauth J, Waites KB, et al. *Ureaplasma urealyticum* infection of the chorioamnion in the presence of intact membranes and in the absence of other microorganisms is significantly associated with premature birth. In preparation.
16. Hillier SL, Krohn MA, Kiviat NB, et al. Microbiologic causes and neonatal outcomes associated with chorioamnion infection. Am J Obstet Gynecol 165:955–961, 1991.
17. Gray DJ, Robinson HB, Malone J et al. Adverse outcome in pregnancy following amniotic fluid isolation of *Ureaplasma urealyticum*. Prenat Diagn 12:111–117, 1992.
18. Foulon W, Naessens A, Dewaele M, et al. Chronic *Ureaplasma urealyticum* amnionitis associated with abruptio placentae. Obstet Gynecol 68:280, 1986.
19. Waites KB, Rudd PT, Crouse DT, et al. Chronic *Ureaplasma urealyticum* and *Mycoplasma hominis* infections of central nervous systems in preterm infants. Lancet 2:17 21, 1988.
20. Waites KB, Cox NR, Crouse DT, et al. *Mycoplasma* infection of the central nervous system in humans and animals. Int J Med Microbiol 20(Suppl):379–386, 1990.
21. Ollikainen J, Heikkaniemi H, Korppi M, et al. *Ureaplasma urealyticum* infection associated with acute respiratory insufficiency and death in premature infants. J Pediatr 122:756–760, 1993.
22. Valencia GB, Banzon F, Cummings M, et al. *Mycoplasma hominis* and *Ureaplasma urealyticum* in neonates with suspected infection. Pediatr Infect Dis J 12:571–573, 1993.
23. Izraeli S, Samra Z, Sirota L, et al. Genital mycoplasmas in preterm infants: prevalence and clinical significance. Eur J Pediatr 150:804–807, 1991.
24. Likitnukul S, Kusmiesz H, Nelson JD, et al. Role of genital mycoplasmas in young infants with suspected sepsis. J Pediatr 109:971–974, 1986.
25. Mardh PA. *Mycoplasma hominis* infections of the central nervous system in newborn infants. Sex Transm Dis 10:331–334, 1983.
25a. *Heggie AD, Jacobs MR, Butler VT, et al. Frequency and significance of isolation of* Ureaplasma urealyticum *and* Mycoplasma hominis *from cerebrospinal fluid and tracheal aspi-*

rate specimens from low birth weight infants. J Pediatr 124:956–961, 1994.

26. Cassell GH, Waites KB, Crouse DT, et al. Association of *Ureaplasma urealyticum* infection of the lower respiratory tract with chronic lung disease and death in very low birthweight infants. Lancet 2:240–245, 1988.

27. Waites KB, Crouse DT, Phillips JB, et al. *Ureaplasma* pneumonia and sepsis associated with persistent pulmonary hypertension of the newborn. Pediatrics 83:84–89, 1991.

28. Walsh WF, Stanley S, Lally KP, et al. *Ureaplasma urealyticum* demonstrated by open lung biopsy in newborns with chronic lung disease. Pediatr Infect Dis J 10:823–827, 1991.

29. Brus F, van Waarde WM, Schoots C, et al. Fatal ureaplasmal pneumonia and sepsis in a newborn infant. Eur J Pediatr 150:782–783, 1991.

30. Cassell GH, Crouse DT, Waites KB, et al. Does *Ureaplasma urealyticum* cause respiratory disease in newborns? Pediatr Infect Dis J 7:535–541, 1988.

31. Rudd PT, Cassell GH, Waites KB, et al. Experimental production of *Ureaplasma urealyticum* pneumonia and demonstration of age-related susceptibility. Infect Immun 17:918–925, 1989.

32. Walsh WF, Butler J, Coalson J, et al. A primate model of *Ureaplasma urealyticum* infection in the premature infant with hyaline membrane disease. Clin Infect Dis 17(Suppl 1):S158–162, 1993.

33. Abele-Horn M, Hentschel J. *Ureaplasma urealyticum* bei Neu- und Fruhgeborenen. Dtsch Med Wochenschr 117:408–414, 1992.

34. Crouse DT, Odrezin GT, Cutter GR, et al. Radiographic changes associated with tracheal isolation of *Ureaplasma urealyticum* from neonates. Clin Infect Dis 17(Suppl 1):S122–S130, 1993.

35. Dyke MP, Grauaug A, Kohan R, et al. *Ureaplasma urealyticum* in a neonatal intensive care population. J Paediatr Child Health 29:295–297, 1993.

36. Horowitz S, Landau D, Shinwell ES, et al. Respiratory tract colonization with *Ureaplasma urealyticum* and bronchopulmonary dysplasia in neonates in southern Israel. Pediatr Infect Dis J 11:847–851, 1992.

37. Wang EE, Frayha H, Watts J, et al. The role of *Ureaplasma urealyticum* and other pathogens in the development of chronic lung disease of prematurity. Pediatr Infect Dis J 7:547–551, 1988.

38. Wang EL, Cassell GH, Sanchez P, et al. *Ureaplasma urealyticum* and chronic lung disease of prematurity: critical appraisal of the literature on causation. Clin Infect Dis 17(Suppl 1):S112–S115, 1993.

39. Wesenberg RL, Pillers DN, Gilhooly P, et al. *Ureaplasma* pneumonia in neonates: radiographic changes. Pediatr Res 29:239A, 1991.

40. Witman MN, Johnson GM, Holman M, et al. Pulmonary effects of the genital mycoplasmas in extremely low birth weight infants. Pediatr Res 29:336A, 1991 (abstract).

41. Payne NR, Steinberg S, Stefan H, et al. New prospective studies of the association of *Ureaplasma urealyticum* colonization and chronic lung disease. Clin Infect Dis 17(Suppl 1):S117–S121, 1993.

42. Garland S, Murton LJ. Neonatal meningitis caused by *Ureaplasma urealyticum*. Pediatr Infect Dis J 6:868–869, 1987.

43. Hentschel J, Abele-Horn M, Peters J. *Ureaplasma urealyticum* in the cerebrospinal fluid of a premature infant. Acta Paediatr Scand 82:690–693, 1993.

44. Shaw NJ, Pratt BC, Weindling AM. *Ureaplasma* and *Mycoplasma* infections of the central nervous system in preterm infants. Lancet 23:1530–1531, 1989.

45. Likitnukul S, Nelson JD, McCracken GH, et al. Role of genital *Mycoplasma* infection in young infants with aseptic meningitis. J Pediatr 110:998, 1987.

46. Mardh PA. *Mycoplasma hominis* infection of the central nervous system in newborn infants. Sex Transm Dis 10:332–334, 1983.

47. Syrogiannopoulos GA, Kapatais-Zoumbos K, Decavalas GO, et al. *Ureaplasma urealyticum* colonization of full term infants: perinatal acquisition and persistence during early infancy. Pediatr Infect Dis J 9:236–240, 1990.

48. Waites KB, Duffy LB, Crouse DT, et al. Mycoplasmal infection of cerebrospinal fluid in newborn infants from a community hospital population. Pediatr Infect Dis J 9:241–245, 1990.

49. Sidiropoulos D, Herrmann U, Morell A, et al. Transplacental passage of intravenous immunoglobulin in the last trimester of pregnancy. J Pediatr 109:505–508, 1986.

50. Gelfand EW. Unique susceptibility of patients with antibody deficiency to *Mycoplasma* infection. Clin Infect Dis 17(Suppl l):S250–S253, 1993.

51. Roifman CM, Rao CP, Lederman HM, et al. Increased susceptibility to *Mycoplasma* infection in patients with hypogammaglobulinemia. Am J Med 80:590–594, 1986.

52. Cassell GH, Davis JK, Waites KB, et al. Pathogenesis and significance of urogenital mycoplasmal infections. *In* Bondi A, Stieritz D, Campos J, et al (eds). Urogenital Infections. New Developments in Laboratory Diagnosis and Treatment. New York, Plenum Publishing, 1987, pp 93–115.

53. McDonald JC. *Mycoplasma hominis* meningitis in a premature infant. Pediatr Infect Dis J 7:795–798, 1988.

54. Miller TC, Baman SI, Albers WH. Massive pericardial effusion due to *Mycoplasma hominis* in a newborn. Am J Dis Child 136:271–272, 1982.

55. Meyer RD, Clough W. Extragenital *Mycoplasma hominis* infections in adults: emphasis on immunosuppression. Clin Infect Dis 17(Suppl 1):S243–S249, 1993.

56. McMahon D, Dummer JS, Pasculle AW, et al. Extragenital *Mycoplasma hominis* infections in adults. Am J Med 89:275–281, 1990.

57. Steffenson DO, Dummer JS, Granick MS, et al. Sternotomy infections with *Mycoplasma hominis*. Ann Intern Med 106:204–208, 1987.

58. Madoff S, Hooper DC. Nongenitourinary infections caused by *Mycoplasma hominis* in adults. Rev Infect Dis 10:602–613, 1988.

59. Taylor-Robinson D, Furr PM, Webster ADB. *Ureaplasma urealyticum* in the immunocompromised host. Pediatr Infect Dis J 5:S236–S238, 1986.

60. McCormack WM, Lee YH, Zinner SH. Sexual experience and urethral colonization with genital mycoplasmas. Ann Intern Med 78:696–698, 1973.

61. McCormack WM, Almeida PC, Bailey PE, et al. Sexual activity and vaginal colonization with genital mycoplasmas. JAMA 221:1375–1377, 1972.

62. McCormack WM. *Ureaplasma urealyticum*: ecologic niche and epidemiologic considerations. Pediatr Infect Dis J 5:S232–S233, 1986.

63. McCormack WM, Rankin JS, Lee YH. Localization of genital mycoplasmas in women. Am J Obstet Gynecol 112:920–923, 1972.

64. Braun P, Klein JO, Lee YH, et al. Methodologic investigations and prevalence of genital mycoplasmas in pregnancy. J Infect Dis 121:391–400, 1970.

65. Taylor-Robinson D, McCormack WM. The genital mycoplasmas. N Engl J Med 302:1003–1010, 1980.

66. McCormack WM, Rosner B, Alpert S, et al. Vaginal colonization with *Mycoplasma hominis* and *Ureaplasma urealyticum*. Sex Transm Dis 134:67–70, 1986.

67. McCormack WM, Rosner B, Lee YH. Colonization with genital mycoplasmas in women. Am J Epidemiol 97:240–245, 1973.

68. Braun P, Lee Y-H, Klein JO, et al. Birth weight and genital mycoplasmas in pregnancy. N Engl J Med 284:167–171, 1971.

69. Mardh PA, Westrom L. T-mycoplasmas in the genitourinary tract of the female. Acta Pathol Microbiol Scand 78B:367–374, 1970.

70. Becopoulos T, Tsagatakis E, Constantinides C, et al. *Ureaplasma urealyticum* and infected renal calculi. J Chemother 3:39–41, 1991.

71. Grenabo L, Hedelin H, Pettersson S. Urinary stones caused by *Ureaplasma urealyticum*: a review. Scand J Infect Dis Suppl 53:46–49, 1988.

72. Thomsen AC, Taylor-Robinson D, Hanson KB, et al. The infrequent occurrence of mycoplasmas in amniotic fluid from women with intact fetal membranes. Acta Obstet Gynecol Scand 3:425–429, 1983.

73. Mardh PA, Westrom L. Tubal and cervical cultures in acute salpingitis with special reference to *Mycoplasma hominis* and T-strain mycoplasmas. Br J Vener Dis 46:179–186, 1970.

74. Mardh PA. Mycoplasmal PID: a review of natural and experimental infections. Yale J Biol Med 56:529, 1983.

75. Miettinen A, Paavonen J, Jansson E, et al. Enzyme immunoassay for serum antibody to *Mycoplasma hominis* in women with acute pelvic inflammatory disease. Sex Transm Dis 10(Suppl):289, 1983.

76. Henry-Suchet J, Catalan F, Loffredo V, et al. Microbiology of specimens obtained by laparoscopy from controls and from patients with pelvic inflammatory disease or infertility with tubal obstruction. *Chlamydia trachomatis* and *Ureaplasma urealyticum*. Am J Obstet Gynecol 138:1022, 1980.

77. Moller BR, Freundt EA, Black FT, et al. Experimental infection of the genital tract of female grivet monkeys by *Mycoplasma hominis*. Infect Immun 20:248, 1978.

78. Mardh PA, Westrom L, Mecklenburg C. Studies on ciliated epithelia of the human genital tract: I. Swelling of the cilia of fallopian tube epithelium in organ cultures infected with *Mycoplasma hominis*. Br J Vener Dis 52:52, 1976.

79. Simberkoff MS, Toharsky B. Mycoplasmemia in adult patients. JAMA 236:2522–2524, 1976.

80. Ti TY, Dan M, Stemke GW, et al. Isolation of *Mycoplasma hominis* from the blood of men with multiple trauma and fever. JAMA 247:60–61, 1982.

81. Kailath EJ, Hrdy DB. Hematoma infected with *Mycoplasma hominis*. Sex Transm Dis 15:114–115, 1988.

82. DiGirolami P, Madoff S. *Mycoplasma hominis* septicemia. J Clin Microbiol 16:566–567, 1982.

83. Dan M, Tyrrel DL, Stemke GW, et al. *Mycoplasma hominis* septicemia in a burned infant. J Pediatr 99:743–744, 1981.

84. Burke D, Madoof S. Infection of a traumatic pelvic hematoma with *Mycoplasma hominis*. Sex Transm Dis 5:65–67, 1978.

85. Friis H, Plesner A, Scheibel J, et al. *Mycoplasma hominis* septicemia. BMJ 286:2013–2014, 1983.

86. DiSesa VJ, Sloss LJ, Cohn LH. Heart transplantation for intractable prosthetic valve endocarditis. J Heart Transplant 9:142–143, 1990.

87. Cohen JI, Sloss IJ, Kundsin R, et al. Prosthetic valve endocarditis caused by *Mycoplasma hominis*. Am J Med 86:819–821, 1989.

88. Martinez OV, Chan J, Cleary T, et al. *Mycoplasma hominis* septic thrombophlebitis in a patient with multiple trauma: a case report and literature review. Diagn Microbiol Infect Dis 12:193–196, 1989.

89. Shaw DR, Lim I. Extragenital *Mycoplasma hominis* infection: a report of two cases. Med J Aust 148:144–145, 1988.

90. Boyle EM, Burdine J, Bolman RM. Successful treatment of *Mycoplasma* mediastinitis after heart-lung transplantation. J Heart Lung Transplant 12:508–512, 1993.

91. Lee GH, Nersasian RR, Lan NK, et al. Wound infection with *Mycoplasma hominis*. JAMA 218:252–253, 1971.

92. Riccio JC, Evans DB, McKay D. *Mycoplasma hominis* sternal wound infection. Infect Med 3:83–85, 1986.

93. Wilson MAE, Dietze C. *Mycoplasma hominis* surgical wound infection: a case report and discussion. Surgery 103:257–260, 1988.

94. Dale BAS, McCormick JSC. *Mycoplasma hominis* wound infection following aortobifemoral bypass. Eur J Vasc Surg 5:213–214, 1992.

95. Mokhbat JE, Peterson PK, Sabath LD, et al. Peritonitis due to *Mycoplasma hominis* in a renal transplant patient. J Infect Dis 146:713, 1982.

96. Haller M, Forst H, Ruckdeschel G, et al. Peritonitis due to *Mycoplasma hominis* and *Ureaplasma urealyticum* in a liver transplant recipient. Eur J Clin Microbiol Infect Dis 10:172, 1991.

97. Miranda C, Carazo C, Banon R, et al. *Mycoplasma hominis* infection in three renal transplant patients. Diagn Microbiol Infect Dis 13:329–331, 1990.

97a. *Barbera J, Gasser I, Almirante B, Pigrau C. Postpartum retroperitoneal abscess due to* Mycoplasma hominis. *Clin Infect Dis 21:698–699, 1995.*

98. Lederman HM, Winkelstein JA. X-linked agammaglobulinemia: an analysis of 96 patients. Medicine (Baltimore) 64:145–156, 1985.

99. Furr PM, Taylor-Robinson D, Webster AD. Mycoplasmas and ureaplasmas in patients with hypogammaglobulinemia and their role in arthritis: microbiological observations over twenty years. Ann Rheum Dis 53:183–187, 1994.

100. Burdge DR, Reid GD, Reeve CE, et al. Septic arthritis due to dual infection with *Mycoplasma hominis* and *Ureaplasma urealyticum*. J Rheumatol 15:366 368, 1988.

101. Jorup-Ronstrom C, Ahl T, Hammarstrom L, et al. Septic osteomyelitis and polyarthritis with *Ureaplasma* in hypogammaglobulinemia. Infection 17:301–302, 1989.

102. Stuckey M, Quinn PA, Gelfand EW. Identification of *Ureaplasma urealyticum* (T-strain mycoplasma) in a patient with polyarthritis. Lancet 2:917–920, 1978.

103. Webster ADB, Taylor-Robinson DTR, Furr PM, et al. Mycoplasmal (ureaplasma) septic arthritis in hypogammaglobulinaemia. BMJ 1:478–479, 1978.

104. Kraus VB, Baraniuk JN, Hill GB, et al. *Ureaplasma urealyticum* septic arthritis in hypogammaglobulinemia. J Rheumatol 15:369–371, 1988.

105. Mohiuddin AA, Corren J, Harbeck RJ, et al. *Ureaplasma urealyticum* chronic osteomyelitis in a patient with hypogammaglobulinemia. J Allergy Clin Immunol 87:104–106, 1991.

106. Lee AH, Ramanujam T, Ware P, et al. Molecular diagnosis of *Ureaplasma urealyticum* septic arthritis in a patient with hypogammaglobulinemia. Arthritis Rheum 35:443–448, 1992.

107. Forgacs P, Kundsin RB, Margles SW, et al. A case of *Ureaplasma urealyticum* septic arthritis in a patient with

hypogammaglobulinemia. Clin Infect Dis 16:293–294, 1993.

108. McDonald MA, Moore JO, Harrelson JM, et al. Septic arthritis due to *Mycoplasma hominis*. Arthritis Rheum 26:1044–1047, 1983.

109. Verinder DGR. Septic arthritis due to *Mycoplasma hominis*: a case report and review of the literature. J Bone Joint Surg Br 60:224, 1978.

110. Taylor-Robinson D, Thomas BJ, Furr PM, et al. The association of *Mycoplasma hominis* with arthritis. Sex Transm Dis 10(Suppl):341–344, 1983.

111. Kim SK. *Mycoplasma hominis* septic arthritis. Ann Plast Surg 20:163–166, 1988.

112. Sneller M, Wellborne F, Barile MF, et al. Prosthetic joint infection with *Mycoplasma hominis*. J Infect Dis 153:174–175, 1986.

113. Nylander N, Tan M, Newcombe DS. Successful management of *Mycoplasma hominis* septic arthritis involving a cementless prosthesis. Am J Med 87:348–352, 1989.

114. Clough W, Cassell GH, Duffy LB, et al. Septic arthritis and bacteremia due to *Mycoplasma* resistant to antimicrobial therapy in a patient with systemic lupus erythematosus. Clin Infect Dis 15:402–407, 1992.

115. Hummel DS, Anderson SJ, Wright PF, et al. Chronic recurrent multifocal osteomyelitis: are mycoplasmas involved? N Engl J Med 317:510–511, 1987.

116. Gjuric G, Prislin-Muskic M, Zurga B, et al. *Ureaplasma urealyticum* infection in newborns: three case reports. Eur J Pediatr 152:599–600, 1993.

117. Payan DG, Seigal N, Madoff S. Infection of a brain abscess by *Mycoplasma hominis*. J Clin Microbiol 14:571–573, 1981.

118. Norton R. *Mycoplasma hominis* pneumonia. Med J Aust 158:361–362, 1993.

119. Kenney RT, Li JS, Clyde WA, et al. Mycoplasmal pericarditis: evidence of invasive disease. Clin Infect Dis 17(Suppl 1):S58–S62, 1993.

119a. *Mattila PS, Carlson P, Sivonen A, et al. Life-threatening* Mycoplasma hominis *mediastinitis. Clin Infect Dis 29:1529–1537, 1999.*

120. Blanchard A, Hentschel J, Duffy L, et al. Detection of *Ureaplasma urealyticum* by polymerase chain reaction in the urogenital tract of adults, in amniotic fluid, and in the respiratory tract of newborns. Clin Infect Dis 17(Suppl 1):S148–S153, 1993.

121. Stokes EJ. Human infection with pleuropneumonia-like organisms. Lancet 1:276–279, 1955.

122. Harwick HJ, Purcell RH, Iuppa JB, et al. *Mycoplasma hominis* and abortion. J Infect Dis 121:260–268, 1970.

123. Harwick HJ, Iuppa JB, Purcell RH, et al. *Mycoplasma hominis* septicemia associated with abortion. Am J Obstet Gynecol 99:725–727, 1967.

124. Tully JG, Brown MS, Sheagren JN, et al. Septicemia due to *Mycoplasma hominis* type 1. N Engl J Med 273:648–650, 1965.

125. Caspi E, Herczeg E, Solomon F, et al. Amnionitis and T strain mycoplasmemia. Am J Obstet Gynecol 111:1102–1106, 1971.

126. Sompolinsky D, Solomon F, Leiba H, et al. Puerperal sepsis due to T-strain mycoplasma. Isr J Med Sci 7:745–748, 1971.

127. Edelin KC, McCormack WM. Infection with *Mycoplasma hominis* in postpartum fever. Lancet 2:1217–1221, 1980.

128. McCormack WM, Rosner B, Lee YH, et al. Isolation of genital mycoplasmas from blood obtained shortly after vaginal delivery. Lancet 1:596–599, 1975.

129. Kelly VN, Garland SM, Gilbert GL. Isolation of genital mycoplasmas from the blood of neonates and women with pelvic infection using conventional SPS-free blood culture media. Pathology 19:277–280, 1987.

130. Neman-Simha V, Renaudin H, de Barbeyrac B, et al. Isolation of genital mycoplasmas from blood of febrile obstetrical-gynecologic patients and neonates. Scand J Infect Dis 24:317–321, 1992.

131. Andrews W, Shah S, Goldenberg R, et al. Post-cesarean endometritis: role of asymptomatic antenatal colonization of the chorioamnion with *Ureaplasma urealyticum*. Am J Obstet Gynecol 170:416, 1994.

132. Roberts S, Maccato M, Faro S, et al. The microbiology of post-cesarean wound morbidity. Obstet Gynecol 81:383–386, 1993.

133. *Mycoplasma hominis*. Newsnotes. BMJ 2:816, 1974.

134. Word BM, Baldridge A. *Mycoplasma hominis* pneumonia and pleural effusion in a postpartum adolescent. Pediatr Infect Dis J 9:295–296, 1990.

135. Young MJ, Cox RA. Near fatal puerperal fever due to *Mycoplasma hominis*. Postgrad Med J 66:147–149, 1990.

136. Phillips LE, Faro S, Pokorny S, et al. Postcesarean wound infection by *Mycoplasma hominis* in a patient with persistent post partum fever. Diagn Microbiol Infect Dis 7:193–197, 1987.

137. Maccato M, Faro S, Summers KL. Wound infections after cesarean section with *Mycoplasma hominis* and *Ureaplasma urealyticum*: a report of three cases. Diagn Microbiol Infect Dis 13:363–365, 1990.

138. Cassell GH, Cole BC. Mycoplasmas as agents of human disease. N Engl J Med 304:80–89, 1981.

139. McCormack WM, Taylor-Robinson D. The genital mycoplasmas. *In* Holmes KK, Mardh PA, Sparling PF, et al (eds). Sexually Transmitted Diseases. New York, McGraw-Hill, 1984, pp 408–419.

140. Sompolinsky D, Solomon F, Elkina L, et al. Infections with *Mycoplasma* and bacteria in induced midtrimester abortion and fetal loss. Am J Obstet Gynecol 121:610–616, 1975.

141. Stray-Pederson B, Engard J, Reikvam TM. Uterine T-*Mycoplasma* colonization in reproductive failure. Am J Obstet Gynecol 130:307, 1978.

142. Naessens A, Foulon W, Cammu H, et al. Epidemiology and pathogenesis of *Ureaplasma urealyticum* in spontaneous abortion and early preterm labor. Acta Obstet Gynecol Scand 66:513–516, 1987.

143. Quinn PA, Shewchuk AB, Shuber J, et al. Serologic evidence of *Ureaplasma urealyticum* infection in women with spontaneous pregnancy loss. Am J Obstet Gynecol 145:245–250, 1983.

144. Gray DJ, Robinson HB, Malone J, et al. Adverse outcome in pregnancy following amniotic fluid isolation of *Ureaplasma urealyticum*. Prenat Diagn 12:111–117, 1992.

145. Elder HA, Santa Maria BAG, Smithietal S. The natural history of asymptomatic bacteriuria during pregnancy: the effect of tetracycline on the clinical course and the outcome of pregnancy. Am J Obstet Gynecol 3:441–462, 1971.

146. Romero R, Mazor M, Oyarzun E, et al. Is genital colonization with *Mycoplasma hominis* or *Ureaplasma urealyticum* associated with prematurity/low birth weight? Obstet Gynecol 73:532–536, 1989.

147. Eschenbach DA. *Ureaplasma urealyticum* and premature birth. Clin Infect Dis 17(Suppl 1):S100–S106, 1993.

148. Gravett MG, Hummel D, Eschenbach D, et al. Preterm labor associated with subclinical amniotic fluid infection and with bacterial vaginosis. Obstet Gynecol 67:229–237, 1986.

149. Romero R, Sirtori M, Oyarzun E, et al. Infection and labor: V. Prevalence, microbiology, and clinical signifi-

cance of intraamniotic infection in women with preterm labor and intact membranes. Am J Obstet Gynecol 161:817–824, 1989.

150. Watts DH, Krohn MA, Hillier SL, et al. The association of occult amniotic fluid infection with gestational age and neonatal outcome among women in preterm labor. Obstet Gynecol 79:351–357, 1992.

151. Russell P. Inflammatory lesions of the human placenta: I. Clinical significance of acute chorioamnionitis. Am J Diagn Gynecol Obstet 2:127–137, 1979.

152. Naessens A, Foulon W, Breynaert J, et al. Postpartum bacteremia and placental colonization with genital mycoplasmas and pregnancy outcome. Am J Obstet Gynecol 160:647–650, 1989.

153. Zlatnik FJ, Gellhaus TM, Benda JA, et al. Histologic chorioamnionitis, microbial infection, and prematurity. J Obstet Gynaecol 76:355–359, 1990.

154. Martius J, Eschenbach DA. The role of bacterial vaginosis as a cause of amniotic fluid infection, chorioamnionitis and prematurity—a review. Arch Gynecol Obstet 247:1–13, 1990.

155. Gravett MG, Eschenbach DA. Possible role of Ureaplasma urealyticum in preterm premature rupture of fetal membranes. Pediatr Infect Dis J 5:S253–S257, 1986.

156. Eschenbach D. Bacterial vaginosis. Obstet Gynecol Clin North Am 16:593, 1989.

157. Quinn PA, Gillian JE, Markestad T, et al. Intrauterine infection with Ureaplasma urealyticum as a cause of fatal neonatal pneumonia. Pediatr Infect Dis J 4:538–543, 1985.

158. Sanchez P, Regan JA. Vertical transmission of Ureaplasma urealyticum in full term infants. Pediatr Infect Dis J 6:825–828, 1988.

159. Sanchez PJ, Regan JA. Vertical transmission of Ureaplasma urealyticum from mothers to preterm infants. Pediatr Infect Dis J 9:398–401, 1990.

160. Dinsmoor MJ, Ramamurthy RS, Gibbs RS. Transmission of genital mycoplasmas from mother to neonate in women with prolonged membrane rupture. Pediatr Infect Dis J 8:483–487, 1989.

161. Klein JO, Buckland DO, Finland M. Colonization of newborn infants by mycoplasmas. N Engl J Med 280:1025–1030, 1969.

162. Foy HM, Kenny GE, Levinsohn EM, et al. Acquisition of mycoplasmata and T-strains during infancy. J Infect Dis 121:579–587, 1970.

163. Madan E, Meyer MP, Amortegui AJ. Isolation of genital mycoplasmas and Chlamydia trachomatis in stillborn and neonatal autopsy material. Arch Pathol Lab Med 112:749–751, 1988.

164. Madan E, Meyer MP, Amortegui AJ. Histologic manifestations of perinatal genital mycoplasmal infection. Arch Pathol Lab Med 113:465–469, 1989.

165. Tafari N, Ross S, Naeye RL, et al. Mycoplasma "T" strains and perinatal death. Lancet 1:108–109, 1976.

166. Rudd PT, Carrington D. A prospective study of chlamydial, mycoplasmal and viral infections in a neonatal intensive care unit. Arch Dis Child 59:120–125, 1985.

167. Taylor-Robinson D, Furr PM, Liberman MM. The occurrence of genital mycoplasmas in babies with and without respiratory diseases. Acta Paediatr Scand 73:383–386, 1984.

168. Ohlsson A, Wang E, Vearncombe M. Leukocyte counts and colonization with Ureaplasma urealyticum in preterm neonates. Clin Infect Dis 17(Suppl 1):S144–S147, 1993.

169. Escobedo MB, Hilliard JL, Smith F, et al. A baboon model of bronchopulmonary dysplasia. Exp Mol Pathol 37:323–324, 1982.

170. Sanchez PJ, Regan JA. Ureaplasma urealyticum colonization and chronic lung disease in low birth weight infants. Pediatr Infect Dis J 78:542–546, 1988.

170a. Wang EEL, Ohlsson A, Kellner JD. Association of Ureaplasma urealyticum colonization with chronic lung disease of prematurity: results of a metaanalysis. J Pediatr 127:640–644, 1995.

171. Saxen H, Hakkarainen K, Pohjavuori M, et al. Chronic lung disease of preterm infants in Finland is not associated with Ureaplasma urealyticum colonization. Acta Paediatr 82:198–201, 1993.

172. Crouse DT, Cassell GH, Waites KB, et al. Hyperoxia potentiates Ureaplasma urealyticum pneumonia in newborn mice. Infect Immun 58:3487–3493, 1990.

173. Stancombe BB, Walsh WF, Derdak S, et al. Induction of human neonatal pulmonary fibroblast cytokines by hyperoxia and Ureaplasma urealyticum. Clin Infect Dis 17(Suppl 1):S154–S157, 1993.

174. Parker RF, Davis JK, Cassell GH, et al. Short-term exposure to nitrogen dioxide enhances susceptibility to murine respiratory mycoplasmosis and decreases intrapulmonary killing of Mycoplasma pulmonis. Am Rev Respir Dis 140:502–512, 1989.

174a. Garland SM, Bowman ED. Role of Ureaplasma urealyticum and Chlamydia trachomatis in lung disease in low birth weight infants. Pathology 28:266–269, 1996.

174b. Iles R, Lyon A, Ross P, McIntosh N. Infection with Ureaplasma urealyticum and Mycoplasma hominis and the development of chronic lung disease in pre-term infants. Acta Paediatr 85:482–484, 1996.

174c. Pacifico L, Panero A, Roggini M, et al. Ureaplasma urealyticum and pulmonary outcome in a neonatal intensive care population. Pediatr Infect Dis J 16:579–586, 1997.

174d. Perzigian RW, Adams JT, Weiner GM, et al. Ureaplasma urealyticum and chronic lung disease in very low birth weight infants during the exogenous surfactant era. Pediatr Infect Dis J 17:620–625, 1998.

174e. Abele-Horn M, Genzel-Boroviczeny O, Uhlig T, et al. Ureaplasma urealyticum colonization and bronchopulmonary dysplasia: a comparative prospective multicentre study. Eur J Pediatr 157:1004–1011, 1998.

174f. Da Silva O, Gregson D, Hammerberg O. Role of Ureaplasma urealyticum and Chlamydia trachomatis in development of bronchopulmonary dysplasia in very low birth weight infants. Pediatr Infect Dis J 16:364–369, 1997.

174g. Van Waarde WM, Brus F, Okken A, Kimpen JLL. Ureaplasma urealyticum colonization, prematurity and bronchopulmonary dysplasia. Eur Respir J 10:886–890, 1997.

174h. Couroucli XI, Welty SE, Ramsay PL, et al. Detection of microorganisms in the tracheal aspirates of preterm infants by polymerase chain reaction: association of adenovirus infection with bronchopulmonary dysplasia. Pedatr Res 47:225–232, 2000.

174i. Cordero L, Coley BD, Miller RL, Mueller CF. Bacterial and Ureaplasma colonization of the airway: radiologic findings in infants with bronchopulmonary dysplasia. J Perinatol 17:428–433, 1997.

175. Stagno S, Brasfield DM, Brown MB, et al. Infant pneumonitis associated with cytomegalovirus, Chlamydia, Pneumocystis, and Ureaplasma: a prospective study. Pediatrics 68:322–327, 1981.

176. Steytler JG. Statistical studies on mycoplasma-positive human umbilical cord blood cultures. S Afr J Obstet Gynecol 8:10–13, 1970.

177. Ollikainen J, Hiekkaniemi H, Korppi M, et al. Ureaplasma urealyticum cultured from brain tissue of preterm twins who died of intraventricular hemorrhage. Scand J Infect Dis 25:529–531, 1993.

178. Unsworth PF, Taylor-Robinson D, Shoo EE, et al. Neonatal mycoplasmemia: *Mycoplasma hominis* as a significant cause of disease? J Infect 10:163–168, 1985.

179. Wealthall SR. *Mycoplasma* meningitis in infants with spina bifida. Dev Med Child Neurol 17(Suppl 35):117–122, 1975.

180. Siber GR, Alpert S, Smith DL, et al. Neonatal central nervous system infection due to *Mycoplasma hominis*. J Pediatr 90:625–627, 1977.

181. Kirk N, Kovar I. *Mycoplasma hominis* meningitis in a preterm infant. J Infect 15:109–110, 1987.

182. Hjelm E, Jousell E, Linglof T, et al. Meningitis in a newborn infant caused by *Mycoplasma hominis*. Acta Paediatr Scand 69:415–418, 1980.

183. Gewitz M, Dinwiddle R, Rees L, et al. *Mycoplasma hominis*: a cause of neonatal meningitis. Arch Dis Child 54:231–233, 1979.

184. Gilbert GL, Law F, Macinnes SJ. Chronic *Mycoplasma hominis* infection complicating severe intraventricular hemorrhage, in a premature neonate. Pediatr Infect Dis J 7:817–818, 1988.

185. Boe O, Diderichsen J, Matre R. Isolation of *Mycoplasma hominis* from cerebrospinal fluid. Scand J Infect Dis 5:285–288, 1973.

186. Waites KB, Crouse DT, Cassell GH. Systemic neonatal infection due to *Ureaplasma urealyticum*. Clin Infect Dis 17(Suppl 1):S131–S135, 1993.

187. Shaw NJ, Pratt BC, Weindling AM. *Ureaplasma* and *Mycoplasma* infections of central nervous systems in preterm infants. Lancet 2:1530–1531, 1989.

188. Davies PA, Gothefors LA. Bacterial Infections in the Fetus and Newborn Infant. Philadelphia, WB Saunders, 1984, pp 112–142.

189. Waites KB, Duffy LB, Baldus K, et al. Mycoplasmal infections of cerebrospinal fluid in children undergoing neurosurgery for hydrocephalus. Pediatr Infect Dis J 10:952–953, 1991.

190. Waites KB, Brown M, Greenberg S, et al. Association of genital mycoplasmas with exudative vaginitis in a 10 year old: a case of misdiagnosis. Pediatrics 71:250–252, 1983.

191. Garland SM, Murton LJ. Neonatal meningitis caused by *Ureaplasma urealyticum*. Pediatr Infect Dis J 6:868–870, 1987.

192. Visser VE, Hall RT. Lumbar puncture in the evaluation of suspected neonatal sepsis. J Pediatr 96:1063, 1980.

193. Sarff LD, Platt LH, McCracken GHJ. Cerebrospinal fluid evaluation in neonates: comparison of high-risk infants with and without meningitis. J Pediatr 88:473, 1976.

193a. *Waites KB, Cassell GH, Duffey LB, Searcey KB. Isolation of* Ureaplasma urealyticum *from low birth weight infants. J Pediatr 126:502, 1995.*

193b. *Heggie AD, Jacobs MR, Butler VT, et al. Isolation of* Ureaplasma urealyticum *from low birth weight infants. J Pediatr 126:503–504, 1995.*

194. Glaser JB, Engelbert M, Hamerschlag M. Scalp abscess associated with *Mycoplasma hominis* infection complicating intrapartum monitoring. Pediatr Infect Dis J 2:468–470, 1983.

195. Sacker I, Brunell PA. Abscess in newborn infants caused by *Mycoplasma*. Pediatrics 46:303–304, 1970.

196. Powell DA, Miller K, Clyde WA Jr. Submandibular adenitis in a newborn caused by *Mycoplasma hominis*. Pediatrics 63:789–799, 1979.

197. Hamrick HJ, Mangum ME. *Ureaplasma urealyticum* abscess at site of an internal fetal heart rate monitor. Pediatr Infect Dis J 12:410–411, 1993.

198. Ollikainen J, Hiekkaniemi H, Korppi M, et al. Hydrops fetalis associated with *Ureaplasma urealyticum*. Acta Paediatr Scand 81:851–852, 1992.

199. Machin GA. Hydrops revisited: literature review of 1414 cases published in the 1980's. Am J Med Genet 34:366–390, 1992.

200. Jones DM, Tobin B. Neonatal eye infections due to *Mycoplasma hominis*. BMJ 2:467–468, 1968.

201. Foy HM, Kenny GE, McMahan R, et al. *Mycoplasma pneumoniae* pneumonia in an urban area: five years of surveillance. JAMA 214:1666–1672, 1970.

202. Clyde WA Jr. Clinical overview of typical *Mycoplasma pneumoniae* infections. Clin Infect Dis 17(Suppl 1):S32–S36, 1993.

203. Chusid MJ, Lachman BS, Lazerson J. Severe *Mycoplasma* pneumonia and vesicular eruption in SC hemoglobinopathy. J Pediatr 93:449–451, 1978.

204. Decancq HG, Lee FA. *Mycoplasma pneumoniae*: massive pulmonary involvement and pleural effusion. JAMA 194:1010–1011, 1965.

205. Fischman RA, Marschall KE, Kislak JW, et al. Adult respiratory distress syndrome caused by *Mycoplasma pneumoniae*. Chest 74:471–473, 1978.

206. Grix A, Giammona ST. Pneumonitis with pleural effusion in children due to *Mycoplasma pneumoniae*. Am Rev Respir Dis 109:665–671, 1974.

207. Gump DW, Hawley HB. Severe *Mycoplasma pneumoniae* pneumonia. Respiration 33:475–486, 1976.

208. Lewis JE, Sheptin C. Mycoplasmal pneumonia associated with abscess of the lung. Calif Med 117:69–72, 1972.

209. Meyers BR, Hirschman SZ. Fatal infections associated with *Mycoplasma pneumoniae*: discussion of three cases with necropsy findings. Mt Sinai J Med 39:258–264, 1972.

210. Mufson MA, Sanders V, Wood SC, et al. Primary atypical pneumonia due to *Mycoplasma pneumoniae* (Eaton agent): report of a case with a residual pleural abnormality. N Engl J Med 268:1109–1111, 1963.

211. Murray HW, Masur H, Senterfit LB, et al. The protean manifestations of *Mycoplasma pneumoniae* infection in adults. Am J Med 58:229–242, 1975.

212. Cherry JD. Anemia and mucocutaneous lesions due to *Mycoplasma pneumoniae* infection. Clin Infect Dis 17(Suppl 1):S47–S51, 1993.

213. Koskiniemi M. CNS manifestations associated with *Mycoplasma pneumoniae* infections: summary of cases at the University of Helsinki and review. Clin Infect Dis 17(Suppl 1):S52–S57, 1993.

214. Cassell GH, Hauth J, Cutter G, et al. *Ureaplasma urealyticum* chorioamnion infection and prematurity. Unpublished data.

215. Cherry JD. *Mycoplasma* and *Ureaplasma* infections. *In* Feigin RD, Cherry JD (eds). Textbook of Pediatric Infectious Diseases, 3rd ed. Philadelphia, WB Saunders, 1992, pp 1866–1890.

216. Kasahara I, Otsubu Y, Yanase T, et al. Isolation and characterization of *Mycoplasma pneumoniae* from cerebrospinal fluid of a patient with pneumonia and meningoencephalitis. J Infect Dis 152:823–825, 1985.

217. Koletsky RJ, Weinstein AJ. Fulminant *Mycoplasma pneumoniae* infection: report of a fatal case, and a review of the literature. Am Rev Respir Dis 122:491–496, 1980.

218. Naftalin JM, Wellisch G, Kahana Z, et al. *Mycoplasma pneumoniae* septicemia. JAMA 228:565, 1974.

219. Nakao T, Orii T, Umetsu M. *Mycoplasma pneumoniae* pneumonia with pleural effusion, with special reference to isolation of *Mycoplasma pneumoniae* from pleural fluid. Tohoku J Exp Med 104:13–18, 1971.

220. Foy HM. Infections caused by *Mycoplasma pneumoniae*

and possible carrier state in different populations of patients. Clin Infect Dis 17(Suppl 1):S37–S46, 1993.

221. Ruhrmann G, Holthusen W. *Mycoplasma* infection and erythromycin therapy in childhood. Scott Med J 22:401–403, 1977.

222. Kok T. Improved laboratory diagnosis of *Mycoplasma pneumoniae* infection. University of Adelaide, 1986.

223. Horner PJ, Gilroy CB, Thomas BJ, et al. Association of *Mycoplasma genitalium* with acute non-gonococcal urethritis. Lancet 342:582–589, 1993.

224. Jensen JS, Uldum SA, Sondergard-Anderson J, et al. Polymerase chain reaction for detection of *Mycoplasma genitalium* in clinical samples. J Clin Microbiol 29:46–50, 1991.

225. Jensen JS, Orsum R, Dohn B, et al. *Mycoplasma genitalium*: a cause of male urethritis? Genitourin Med 69:265–269, 1993.

226. Hooton TM, Roberts MC, Roberts PL, et al. Prevalence of *Mycoplasma genitalium* determined by DNA probe in men with urethritis. Lancet 1:266–268, 1988.

227. Blanchard A, Hamrick W, Duffy L, et al. Use of the polymerase chain reaction for detection of *Mycoplasma fermentans* and *Mycoplasma genitalium* in the urogenital tract and amniotic fluid. Clin Infect Dis 17(Suppl 1):S272–S279, 1993.

228. Tully JG, Taylor-Robinson D, Rose DL, et al. Urogenital challenge of primate species with *Mycoplasma genitalium* and characteristics of infection induced in chimpanzees. J Infect Dis 153:1046–1054, 1986.

229. Moller BR, Taylor-Robinson D, Furr PM. Serological evidence implicating *Mycoplasma genitalium* in pelvic inflammatory disease. Lancet 1:1102–1103, 1984.

230. Taylor-Robinson D, Gilroy CB, Hay PE. Occurrence of *Mycoplasma genitalium* in different patient populations and its clinical significance. Clin Infect Dis 17(Suppl 1):S66–S68, 1993.

231. Taylor-Robinson D, Furr PM, Tully JG, et al. Animal models of *Mycoplasma genitalium* urogenital infections. Isr J Med Sci 23:561–564, 1987.

232. de Barbeyrac B, Bernet-Poggi C, Febrer F, et al. Detection of *Mycoplasma pneumoniae* and *Mycoplasma genitalium* in clinical samples by polymerase chain reaction. Clin Infect Dis 17(Suppl 1):S83–S89, 1993.

233. Baseman JB, Dallo SF, Tully JG, et al. Isolation and characterization of *Mycoplasma genitalium* strains from the human respiratory tract. J Clin Microbiol 26:2266–2269, 1988.

234. Lo S-C. Mycoplasmas in AIDS. *In* Maniloff J, McElhaney R, Finch L, et al (eds). Mycoplasmas: Molecular Biology and Pathogenesis. Washington, DC, American Society for Microbiology, 1992, pp 525–545.

235. Lo S-C, Wear DJ, Green SL, et al. Adult respiratory distress syndrome with or without systemic disease associated with *Mycoplasma fermentans*. Clin Infect Dis 17(Suppl 1):S259–S263, 1993.

236. Lo S-C, Dawson MS, Wong DM, et al. Identification of *Mycoplasma incognitus* infection in patients with AIDS: an immunohistochemistry, in situ hybridization and ultrastructural study. Am J Trop Med Hyg 41:601–616, 1989.

237. Razin S, Jacobs E. *Mycoplasma* adhesion. J Gen Microbiol 138 (Part 3):407–422, 1992.

238. Taylor-Robinson D. Intracellular location of mycoplasmas in cultured cells demonstrated by immunocytochemistry and electron microscopy. Int J Exp Pathol 72:705, 1991.

239. Lo S-C. Newly discovered *Mycoplasma* isolated from patients with HIV. Lancet 338:1415, 1991.

240. Olson LD. Monoclonal antibodies to surface antigens of a pathogenic *Mycoplasma hominis* strain. Infect Immun 59:1683, 1991.

241. Watson HL, Blalock DK, Cassell GH. Variable antigens of *Ureaplasma urealyticum* containing both serovar-specific and serovar–cross-reactive epitopes. Infect Immun 58:3679–3688, 1990.

242. Zheng X, Watson H, Waites KB, et al. Serotype diversity and antigen variation among invasive isolates of *Ureaplasma urealyticum* from newborn infants. Infect Immun 60:3472–3474, 1992.

243. Cassell GH, Watson HL, Blalock DK, et al. Protein antigens of the genital mycoplasmas. Rev Infect Dis 10:S391–S398, 1988.

244. Thirkell D, Myles AD, Precious BL, et al. The urease of *Ureaplasma urealyticum*. J Gen Microbiol 135:315, 1989.

245. Blanchard A. Sequencing of *Ureaplasma urealyticum* urease genes: use of a UGA tryptophan codon. Mol Microbiol 4:669, 1990.

246. Blanchard A. Characteristics of *Ureaplasma urealyticum* urease. J Bacteriol 170:2692, 1988.

247. Kilian M. Immunoglobulin A1 protease activity in strains of *Ureaplasma urealyticum*. Acta Pathol Microbiol Immunol 92:61, 1984.

248. Spooner RK, Russell WC, Thirkell D. Characterization of the immunoglobulin A protease of *Ureaplasma urealyticum*. Infect Immun 60:2544, 1992.

249. Bejar R. Premature labour: bacterial sources of phospholipase. Obstet Gynecol 57:479, 1981.

250. DeSilva NS, Quinn PA. Endogenous activity of phospholipase A and C in *Ureaplasma urealyticum*. J Clin Microbiol 23:354–359, 1986.

251. DeSilva NS, Quinn PA. Localization of endogenous activity of phospholipases A and C in *Ureaplasma urealyticum*. J Clin Microbiol 29:1498–1503, 1991.

252. Cassell GH, Blanchard A, Duffy L, et al. Mycoplasmas. *In* Howard BJ, Klaas J III, Rubin SJ, et al (eds). Clinical and Pathogenic Microbiology. St. Louis, Mosby–Year Book, 1994, pp 491–502.

253. Shepard MC, Masover GK. Special features of ureaplasmas. *In* Barile MF, Razin S (eds). The Mycoplasmas I. Cell Biology. New York, Academic Press, 1979, pp 452–494.

254. Shepard MC. Culture media for ureaplasmas. *In* Razin S, Tully JG (eds). Methods in Mycoplasmology. New York, Academic Press, 1983.

255. Taylor-Robinson D, Chen TA. Growth inhibitory factors in animal and plant tissues. *In* Razin S, Tully JG (eds). Methods in Mycoplasmology. New York, Academic Press, 1983, pp 109–114.

256. Blanchard A, Yanez A, Dybvig K, et al. Evaluation of intraspecies genetic variation within the 16S rRNA gene of *Mycoplasma hominis* and detection by polymerase chain reaction. J Clin Microbiol 31:1358–1361, 1993.

257. Horowitz S, Duffy LB, Garrett B, et al. Can group- and serovar-specific proteins be detected in *Ureaplasma urealyticum*? Pediatr Infect Dis J 5:S325–S331, 1986.

258. Zheng X, Teng LJ, Glass JI, et al. Size variation of a major serotype-specific antigen of *Ureaplasma urealyticum*. Ann N Y Acad Sci 730:294–301, 1994.

259. Taylor-Robinson D, Ludwig WM, Purcell RH, et al. Significance of antibody to *Mycoplasma hominis* type 1 as measured by indirect hemagglutination. Proc Soc Exp Biol Med 118:1073–1083, 1965.

260. Taylor-Robinson D, Ludwig WM, Purcell RH, et al. Antibodies to *Mycoplasma hominis* in patients with genital infections and in healthy controls. Br J Vener Dis 46:390–397, 1970.

261. Purcell RH, Wong D, Chanock RM, et al. Significance

of antibody to *Mycoplasma* as measured by metabolic-inhibition techniques. Ann N Y Acad Sci 143:664–675, 1967.

262. Purcell RH, Taylor-Robinson D, Wong DC, et al. A color test for the measurement of antibody to the non–acid-forming human mycoplasma species. Am J Epidemiol 84:51–66, 1966.

263. Brown MB, Cassell GH, McCormack WM, et al. Measurement of antibody to *Mycoplasma hominis* by an enzyme-linked immunoassay and detection of class-specific antibody responses in women with postpartum fever. Am J Gynecol 56:701–708, 1987.

264. Brown MB, Taylor-Robinson D, Shepard MC, et al. Measurement of antibody to *Ureaplasma urealyticum* by an enzyme-linked immunosorbent assay and detection of antibody response in patients with non-gonococcal urethritis. J Clin Microbiol 17:288–295, 1983.

265. Dinsmoor MJ, Ramamurthy RS, Cassell GH, et al. Neonatal serologic response at term to the genital mycoplasmas. Pediatr Infect Dis J 8:487–491, 1989.

266. Vogler LB, Waites KB, Wright P, et al. *Ureaplasma urealyticum* polyarthritis in hypogammaglobulinemia. Pediatr Infect Dis J 6:687–691, 1985.

267. Webster ADB, Furr PM, Hughes-Jones NC, et al. Critical dependence on antibody for defense against mycoplasmas. Clin Exp Immunol 71:383–387, 1988.

268. Kass EH, Lin JS, McCormack WM. Low birth weight and maternal colonization with genital mycoplasmas. Pediatr Infect Dis J 5:S279–S281, 1986.

269. Quinn PA, Li HCS, Th'ng C, et al. Serological response to *Ureaplasma urealyticum* in the neonate. Infect Dis 17(Suppl 1):S136–S147, 1993.

270. Gallo D, Dupuis KW, Schmidt NJ, et al. Broadly reactive immunofluorescence test for measurement of immunoglobulin M and G antibodies to *Ureaplasma urealyticum* in infant and adult sera. J Clin Microbiol 17:614–618, 1983.

271. Tully JG, Taylor-Robinson D, Rose DL, et al. Evaluation of culture media for the recovery of *Mycoplasma hominis* from the urogenital tract. Sex Transm Dis 10(Suppl):256–260, 1983.

272. Marmion BP, Williamson J, Worswick DA, et al. Experience with newer techniques for the laboratory detection of *Mycoplasma pneumoniae* infection: Adelaide, 1978–1992. Clin Infect Dis 17(Suppl 1):S90–S99, 1993.

273. Sussman SJ, Magoffin RL, Lennette EH, et al. Cold agglutinins: Eaton agent and respiratory infections of children. Pediatrics 38:571–577, 1966.

274. Jacobs E. Serological diagnosis of *Mycoplasma pneumoniae* infections: critical review of current procedures. Clin Infect Dis 17(Suppl 1):S79–S80, 1993.

275. Braun P, Klein JO, Kass EH. Susceptibility of *Mycoplasma hominis* and T-strains to 14 antimicrobial agents. Appl Microbiol 19:62–70, 1970.

276. Koutsky LA, Stamm WE, Brunham RC, et al. Persistence of *Mycoplasma hominis* after therapy: importance of tetracycline resistance and of co-existing vaginal flora. Sex Transm Dis 10(Suppl):374–381, 1983.

277. Cummings MC, McCormack WM. Increase in resistance of *Mycoplasma hominis* to tetracyclines. Antimicrob Agents Chemother 34:2297–2299, 1990.

278. Waites KB, Figarola TA, Schmid T, et al. Comparison of agar versus broth dilution techniques for determining antibiotic susceptibilities of *Ureaplasma urealyticum*. Diagn Microbiol Infect Dis 14:265–271, 1991.

279. Waites KB, Crouse DT, Cassell GH. Antibiotic susceptibilities and therapeutic options for *Ureaplasma urealyticum* infections in neonates. Pediatr Infect Dis J 11:23–29, 1992.

280. Waites KB, Crouse DT, Cassell GH. Therapeutic consideration for *Ureaplasma urealyticum* infections in neonates. Clin Infect Dis 17(Suppl 1):S208–S214, 1993.

281. Kenny GE, Cartwright FD. Effect of pH, inoculum size, and incubation time on the susceptibility of *Ureaplasma urealyticum* to erythromycin *in vitro*. Clin Infect Dis 17(Suppl 1):S215–S218, 1993.

282. McCormack WM. Susceptibility of mycoplasmas to antimicrobial agents: clinical implications. Clin Infect Dis 17(Suppl 1):S200–S201, 1993.

283. Taylor-Robinson D, Furr PM. Clinical antibiotic resistance of *Ureaplasma urealyticum*. Pediatr Infect Dis J 5:S335–S337, 1986.

284. Thornsberry C, Barry AJ. Methods for dilution—antimicrobial susceptibility tests for bacteria that grow aerobically. *In* Tentative Standards, 2nd ed. NCCLS document M7-T2. Villanova, Pa, National Committee for Clinical Laboratory Standards, 1988.

285. Satow K, Groneck P, Schutt-Gerowitt H, et al. *Ureaplasma urealyticum*—ein neuer Problemkeim in der Neonatologie. Monatsschr Kinderheilkd 139:344–348, 1991.

286. Romero R, Hagay Z, Nores J, et al. Eradication of *Ureaplasma urealyticum* from the amniotic fluid with transplacental antibiotic treatment. Am J Obstet Gynecol 166:618–620, 1992.

287. Mazor M, Meril T, Horowitz S, et al. Eradication of *Ureaplasma urealyticum* from amniotic fluid. Isr J Med Sci 28:296–298, 1992.

288. Waites KB, Cassell GH, Canupp KC, et al. In vitro susceptibilities of mycoplasmas and ureaplasmas to new macrolides and aryl-fluoroquinolones. Antimicrob Agents Chemother 32:1500–1502, 1988.

289. Patamasucon P, Kaojarern S, Kusmiesz H, et al. Pharmacokinetics of erythromycin ethylsuccinate and estolate in infants under 4 months of age. Antimicrob Agents Chemother 19:736–739, 1981.

290. Waites KB, Sims PJ, Crouse DT, et al. Serum concentrations of erythromycin after intravenous infusion in preterm neonates treated for *Ureaplasma urealyticum* infection. Pediatr Infect Dis J 13:287–293, 1994.

291. Burns L, Hodgman J. Studies of prematures given erythromycin estolate. Am J Dis Child 10:280–288, 1963.

292. Gribble MJ, Chow AW. Erythromycin. Med Clin North Am 66:79–89, 1982.

293. Crouse DT, Waites KB, Geerts MH, et al. Parenteral erythromycin is not associated with hearing loss in preterm infants. Clin Res 39:832A, 1991 (abstract).

294. Farrar HC, Walsh-Sukys MC, Pharmd KK, et al. Cardiac toxicity associated with intravenous erythromycin lactobionate: two case reports and a review of the literature. Pediatr Infect Dis J 12:688–692, 1993.

295. Bebear C, Dupon M, Renaudin H, et al. Potential improvements in therapeutic options for mycoplasmal respiratory infections. Clin Infect Dis 17(Suppl 1):S202–S207, 1993.

296. Kenny GE, Cartwright FD. Susceptibility of *Mycoplasma pneumoniae* to several new quinolones, tetracycline, and erythromycin. Antimicrob Agents Chemother 32:587, 1991.

297. Cassell GH, Drnec J, Waites KB, et al. Efficacy of clarithromycin against *Mycoplasma pneumoniae*. J Antimicrob Chemother 27(Suppl A):47–59, 1991.

298. Cassell GH, Waites KB, Pate MS, et al. Comparative susceptibility of *Mycoplasma pneumoniae* to erythromycin, ciprofloxacin, and lomefloxacin. Diagn Microbiol Infect Dis 12:433–435, 1989.

299. Waites KB, Duffy LB, Schmid T, et al. In vitro susceptibilities of *Mycoplasma pneumoniae*, *Mycoplasma hominis* and

Ureaplasma urealyticum to investigational quinolones, sparfloxacin and PD 127391. Antimicrob Agents Chemother 35:1181–1185, 1991.

300. Renaudin H, Tully JG, Bebear C. In vitro susceptibilities of *Mycoplasma genitalium* to antibiotics. Antimicrob Agents Chemother 36:870–872, 1992.

301. Hayes MM, Wear DJ, Lo S-C. In vitro antimicrobial susceptibility testing for the newly identified AIDS-associated *Mycoplasma: Mycoplasma fermentans* (incognitus strain). Arch Pathol Lab Med 115:464–466, 1991.

301a. *Taylor-Robinson D, Bebear C. Antibiotic susceptibilities of mycoplasmas and treatment of mycoplasma infections. J Antimicrob Chemother 40:622–630, 1997.*

301b. *Kober MB, Mason BA. Colonization of the female genital tract by resistant* Ureaplasma urealyticum *treated successfully with azithromycin. Clin Infect Dis 278:401–402, 1998.*

301c. *Benoit A, Bodiou C, Villain E, et al. QT long et arret circulatoire après une injection d'erythromycine chez un nouveau-né. Arch Fr Pediatr 48:39–41, 1991.*

301d. *Gouyon JB, Benoit A, Betremieux P. Cardiac toxicity of intravenous erythromycin lactobionate in preterm infants. Pediatr Infect Dis J 13:840–841, 1994.*

301e. *Honein MA, Paulozzi LJ, Himmelright IM, et al. Infantile hypertrophic pyloric stenosis after pertussis prophylaxis with erythromycin: a case review and cohort study. Lancet 354:2101–2105, 1999.*

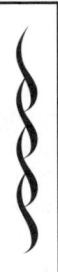

Chlamydia

JULIUS SCHACHTER, Ph.D., and MOSES GROSSMAN, M.D.

Chlamydia trachomatis is a common human pathogen.[1, 2] The organism was first seen in conjunctival scrapings taken from orangutans that had been infected with human trachomatous material and then in direct smears from patients with trachoma. Typical intracytoplasmic inclusions were then identified in infants with a nongonococcal form of ophthalmia neonatorum called inclusion conjunctivitis of the newborn (ICN) or inclusion blennorrhea. These latter studies, performed by Lindner and some of his colleagues in the first decade of this century, led to elucidation of the epidemiology of sexually transmitted chlamydial infections.[3] Thus, mothers of affected infants were found to have inclusions in their cervical epithelial cells and fathers of such infants had inclusions in their urethral cells.

For 50 years, cytology (the demonstration of chlamydial inclusions in epithelial cells) was the only diagnostic procedure available. When chlamydial isolation procedures were developed, first in the yolk sac of the embryonated hen's egg and then in tissue culture, the studies followed the same sequence. They started with an infant (or adult) with conjunctivitis as the index case and confirmed the genital tract reservoir of the agent.[4] Although ICN was studied for 60 years, it was not until the late 1970s, with the impetus of the report by Beem and Saxon,[5] that an appreciation evolved of the importance of extraocular chlamydial infections in infants. It is now clear that ICN is not a rarity but probably the most common form of conjunctivitis seen in the first month of life and that chlamydial pneumonia of infants is one of the relatively common causes of pneumonia in the first 6 months of life.

More rapid nonculture methods (direct fluorescent antibody and enzyme immunoassay) for the diagnosis of *C. trachomatis* infection have become commercially available. Although these methods are not as accurate as culture, they are less expensive and technically less demanding. They have made chlamydial diagnosis widely available.

THE ORGANISM

The chlamydiae are a group of obligate intracellular bacteria separated into their own order, Chlamydiales (with one family, Chlamydiaceae), on the basis of a growth cycle that distinguishes them from all other microorganisms. This cycle involves infection of a susceptible host cell by a *Chlamydia*-specified phagocytic process so that these organisms are preferentially ingested.[6] After attachment and ingestion, the chlamydiae remain in a phagosome throughout the growth cycle, but surface antigens of chlamydiae appear to inhibit phagolysosomal fusion.[7] These two virulence factors, enhanced ingestion and inhibition of phagolysosomal fusion, speak for an exquisitely adapted parasitism. Once in the cell, the chlamydial elementary body, which is the infectious particle, changes to a metabolically active replicating form called the reticulate body (initial body). This synthesizes its own macromolecules and divides by binary fission. The chlamydiae are energy parasites and do not synthesize their own adenosine triphosphate; thus, energy-rich compounds must be supplied to them by the host cell.[8] By the end of the growth cycle (approximately 48 hours), most initial bodies have reorganized into elementary bodies, and these particles are released to initiate new infectious cycles.

The structure of the organisms also reflects adaptation to this specialized life cycle. Chlamydiae lack a peptidoglycan layer. Structural rigidity is maintained by disulfide bonds between molecules of the major outer membrane protein (which constitutes 30 to 60% of the cell membrane's weight), as well as some other outer membrane proteins.[9, 10] Morphologic and permeability changes probably reflect reduction and oxidation of these disulfide bonds.[11]

Three species within the genus infect humans (Table 15–1). *Chlamydia psittaci* is the causative agent of psittacosis and is a common pathogen in avian species and lower mammals. *C. trachomatis* seems to be a specific pathogen for humans (except for a few strains of rodent origin). The two organisms are differentiated on the basis of glycogen-containing inclusions that stain with iodine (*C. trachomatis* is positive, whereas *C. psittaci* is negative in this test) and susceptibility to sulfonamides (*C. trachomatis* is sensitive whereas *C. psittaci* is resistant). *Chlamydia pneumoniae* is similar to *C. psittaci* in the iodine and sulfonamide tests. It can be identified by staining with specific monoclonal antibodies or by DNA hybridization. *C. pneumoniae* is only known to infect humans. It can cause primary atypical pneumonia and may cause coronary artery disease and asthma. It is not known to cause disease in infants and thus is not discussed further.

Genetic studies on chlamydiae have been limited because the organism's replicative cycle takes place in a protected intracellular site. However, the genome of *C. trachomatis* has been sequenced and this should lead to a better understanding of its biology.[12]

All chlamydiae share a common genus-specific antigen. The *C. trachomatis* strains also share species- and type-specific antigens to a varying degree. The chlamydial lipopolysaccharide is the genus-specific antigen, whereas many of the other, more specific antigens are found on the major outer membrane protein. There are 15 major serovars of *C. trachomatis*. Three of these serovars (L1, L2, and L3) represent the agents causing lymphogranuloma venereum (LGV). LGV strains appear to have different receptor sites and a much broader tissue spectrum in vivo and host spectrum in vitro than the other strains of *C. trachomatis*. The other serovars of *C. trachomatis* represent the agents causing endemic blinding trachoma (A, B, Ba, and C) and the sexually transmitted *C. trachomatis* strains (D through K), which cause inclusion conjunctivitis, urethritis, cervicitis, and so forth and may be capable of causing sporadic eye disease clinically indistinguishable from trachoma.[13]

Chlamydiae are also susceptible to the action of broad-spectrum antibiotics. Tetracyclines and erythromycin are generally considered the drugs of choice in treating chlamydial infections. Aminoglycosides and cephalosporins are inactive, and penicillins, which may have some in vitro activity, are not considered clinically useful.

EPIDEMIOLOGY AND TRANSMISSION

For purposes relevant to this chapter, the major method of transmission of *C. trachomatis* is sexual. The child-to-child and intrafamilial infecting patterns that predominate in trachoma endemic areas have not been proved to cause disease in newborns.[14] *C. trachomatis* is probably the most common sexually transmitted pathogen in Western industrialized society.[1] Chlamydiae cause between one third and one half of nongonococcal urethritis in men, and concomitant infections with gonococci are common in both men and women.[15, 16] Men who have gonorrhea and are being treated with a penicillin often develop postgonococcal urethritis related to the concomitant chlamydial infection.[15–17] Epididymitis is an important complication of chlamydial infection of the male urethra.[18] Rectal and pharyngeal infections occur in both sexes.[19, 20]

In the female, a number of clinical conditions can be attributed to *Chlamydia;* among these are cervicitis, urethral syndrome, salpingitis, and urethritis.[21–23] Unfortunately, there are no specific symptoms associated with the cervical infection, and many of the chlamydial infections of the cervix are clinically inapparent. The infant born to a woman with a chlamydial infection of the cervix is at 60 to 70% risk of acquiring the infection during passage through the birth canal.[24–27] Twenty to 50% of exposed infants develop conjunctivitis, and 10 to 20% develop pneumonia. In utero transmission is not definitively known to occur. Infants born by cesarean section are at very small risk of acquiring chlamydial infection unless there has been a premature rupture of the membranes. A number of such cases have been described. Other anatomic sites may also be infected after perinatal exposure, but a clear-cut relationship with

☐ **TABLE 15–1**
☐ Human Diseases Caused by *Chlamydia*

SPECIES	SEROVAR[a]	DISEASE
C. psittaci	Many unidentified serovars	Psittacosis
C. trachomatis	L1, L2, L3	Lymphogranuloma venereum
C. trachomatis	A, B, Ba, C	Hyperendemic blinding trachoma
C. trachomatis	D, E, F, G, H, I, J, K	Inclusion conjunctivitis (adult and newborn), nongonococcal urethritis, cervicitis, salpingitis, proctitis, epididymitis, pneumonia of newborn
C. pneumoniae	One serovar	Atypical pneumonia, perhaps asthma and coronary artery disease

[a]Predominant, but not exclusive, association of serovar with disease.
Adapted from Schachter J. Chlamydial infections. N Engl J Med 298:428, 1978, with permission.

disease in these sites has not yet been elucidated. For example, 25 to 50% of exposed infants will have infections of the upper respiratory tract (nasopharynx or pharynx), approximately 20% develop enteric infections and will shed the agent in their feces, and 10 to 20% of exposed female infants will have chlamydial infections detectable by culture of vaginal swabs.[27, 28]

ICN usually has an incubation period of 5 to 14 days, and rarely is it reported with an onset beyond 19 days after delivery.[2] The agent usually cannot be demonstrated in the conjunctiva within the first 24 hours of life. Because the organism has approximately a 48-hour growth cycle, it is unlikely that any conjunctivitis in the first day of life (except after prolonged labor following premature rupture of the membranes) can be attributed to chlamydiae. The great majority of pneumonia cases occur between age 2 weeks and 3 months.

Given the relative constancy of the attack rates that have been observed in a number of studies, it would appear that the determinant as to whether chlamydial infections of the newborn represent a major medical problem in a specific population group is the prevalence rate of chlamydial infections of the cervix.[29] This carriage rate can vary broadly.[1] Some investigators have found rates of infection of the cervix to be on the order of 1 to 2%. The consensus is that the national average of chlamydial infection of the cervix in the United States is probably closer to 4 to 5% of sexually active women. However, high-risk populations can be readily identified. A number of studies have shown that the same populations that are at high risk for other sexually transmitted infections are at highest risk for chlamydial infections. Thus, young unwed mothers are often found to have high rates of chlamydial infection of the cervix. Rates as high as 25 to 37% have been detected in screening and prospective studies.[30, 31]

The first prospective study that was aimed at determining the true incidence of these ocular infections was performed in Seattle. It was found that 12.7% of pregnant women carried *Chlamydia* in their cervices and half of the exposed infants developed conjunctivitis.[24] Thus, 6.3% (63 per 1000 live births) of the infants in this clinic developed conjunctivitis. Similar attack rates were found in other studies,[1, 25–27] and reported incidences for ICN in prospective studies have ranged from 10 to 63 per 1000 live births.[29] Prospective studies have

also revealed that the incidence of chlamydial pneumonia ranges from 3 to 10 per 1000 live births[29] (Table 15–2).

There is no evidence to suggest that infants with chlamydial infections should be isolated. Transmission of the organism to other infants in nurseries or intensive care units has not been reported. However, this subject has not been well studied. Because these infants shed large numbers of organisms in their nasal discharges and feces, rigorous hand washing and change of gowns between examinations of infants should suffice to prevent transmission.

PATHOGENESIS

Conjunctivitis

Chlamydiae replicate extensively in superficial epithelial cells of the conjunctiva and cause considerable cell damage. There is an exuberant inflammatory reaction involving largely polymorphonuclear leukocytes; pseudomembranes may form. (If they do, they may result in scar formation.) A marked lymphoid reaction is not noticed until the infant has had the disease for several weeks. This may reflect the immaturity of the lymphoid system of the newborn. Follicles such as are seen in adults or older children with chlamydial infection of the conjunctiva are not usually observed until the disease has been active for 1 or 2 months. Because in most infants the conjunctivitis spontaneously resolves by that time, lymphoid follicles are not commonly observed. Conjunctivitis in the majority of untreated infants resolves spontaneously during the first few months of life. Occasionally, infants maintain persistent conjunctivitis, and the pannus formation (neovascularization of the cornea) and scarring typical of trachoma have been reported.[4, 32] Loss of vision is rare. Micropannus and some scarring most likely occur in infants if they are not treated within the first 2 weeks of the disease.[33] If they are treated early, no ocular sequelae develop.

Pneumonia

Pneumonia may develop as a descending infection. Antecedent conjunctival infection is not required. Shortly

TABLE 15–2
Prospective Studies of Perinatal Chlamydial Infection

PREVALENCE OF MATERNAL INFECTION (%)	ATTACK RATE		CASES/1000 LIVE BIRTHS		REFERENCE NO.
	Conjunctivitis (%)	Pneumonia (%)	Conjunctivitis	Pneumonia	
12.7	50	NS	63	NS	24
8.8	44	11	40	10	25
5.0	40	NS	20	NS	1
4.7	18	17	8	8	27
2.0	33	16	7	3	26

NS = not studied.
Modified from Schachter J, Grossman M. Chlamydial infections. Annu Rev Med 32:45–61, 1981, with permission.

after chlamydial pneumonia of infants was first described, it was speculated that this disease might result from *C. trachomatis* draining into the respiratory tract from the involved conjunctiva.[34] Prospective studies have shown that conjunctivitis is not a prerequisite, and indeed prevention of conjunctivitis by appropriate ocular prophylaxis does not prevent respiratory tract infection and pneumonia.[27, 35] Although it seems likely that some respiratory tract infections may result from conjunctival seeding at birth, it is apparent that the respiratory tract can be directly infected during the birth process. *C. trachomatis* has been recovered from gastric aspirates from newborns.[36]

Because the pneumonia is rarely fatal and in most infants the course is relatively benign, there has been little occasion to obtain lung specimens. When such specimens have been obtained, *C. trachomatis* has been recovered from the lung, both as a single pathogen and together with other pathogens such as cytomegalovirus.[37, 38]

PATHOLOGY

In ICN the affected conjunctiva is highly vascularized and edematous. The agent is found only in the superficial levels, where inclusions can be demonstrated. There is a massive polymorphonuclear leukocyte infiltration, and pseudomembrane formation may occur. Lymphoid follicles are rarely seen, particularly in the early stages of the disease.

The pathology of the lung in chlamydial pneumonia of infants is not clear. Few specimens of proven pneumonia have come to pathologic study, and there are difficulties in dealing with the timing of the disease and the appropriateness of the sample to allow a firm presentation of the pathology. Interpretation of one of the published isolate-positive biopsies was complicated (as are many of these infections) by the presence of cytomegalovirus.[37]

In general, most reported histologic sections have yielded a picture of interstitial pneumonia. There has been a moderate inflammatory response of mixed cells, with mononuclear cells predominating in some instances. We have been able to isolate *Chlamydia* as a sole pathogen from the lungs of three infants. Although one specimen did show a pattern of interstitial pneumonia, another had a picture consistent with descending necrotizing bronchiolitis and there was complete obliteration of air spaces in the involved areas of the lung. Although the architecture of the lung was not destroyed, there was massive mixed cell (mononuclear and polymorphonuclear leukocytes) infiltration into the alveolar spaces.[38] Thus, there are no consistent markers recognized for the pathology of chlamydial pneumonia in infants.

CLINICAL MANIFESTATIONS

The principal clinical manifestations in infants are conjunctivitis, occurring in the first few weeks of life, and pneumonia, which occurs somewhat later.

Conjunctivitis

The acute conjunctivitis of infants, or ICN or inclusion blennorrhea, was first described some 70 years ago. We now know that it is the most common conjunctivitis in the first month of life.[39] Approximately one third of infants exposed to chlamydiae during vaginal delivery develop this disease.[1, 24–27] The incubation period is usually 5 to 14 days. Exceptionally, when amniotic membranes have been ruptured early, conjunctivitis has been described in the first few days of life, but the vast majority of cases occur after the fifth day of life. The disease often starts with a watery discharge from the eye, which rapidly and progressively becomes purulent. The eyelids are usually markedly swollen. The conjunctivae become red and somewhat thickened throughout. The follicular nature of the infection, so characteristic of trachoma, is missing because the conjunctiva of the neonate lacks lymphoid tissue; however, at times, "pseudomembrane" may be evident as inflammatory exudate adheres to the inflamed surface of the conjunctiva. "Sheet scarring," contrasted to the lineal scars typical of trachoma, may result. Except for micropannus formation, the cornea is usually spared.

Pneumonia

Chlamydial pneumonia was first reported in 1975, and the characteristic clinical picture was described in 1977.[5, 40] It has now become clear that this disease is very common; indeed, it is probably one of the three most common pneumonias seen in infancy. Most clinicians dealing with patients in this age group have learned to recognize the rather typical pattern of this illness; furthermore, they realize that they have often seen the identical illness in the past without understanding the etiology. Many case reports and the series described by Beem and Saxon,[5] by Tipple and associates,[41] and by Harrison and colleagues[42] have helped to delineate the clinical features of this infection (Table 15–3).

The illness in the vast majority of infants is recognized between weeks 4 and 11 of life; virtually all will be symptomatic before the eighth week, some will have symptoms as early as the second week, initially involving the upper respiratory tract. The infants are usually afebrile or have only a minimal fever. The upper respiratory tract symptoms are those of congestion and obstruction of the nasal passages without significant discharge. The finding of abnormal-appearing ear drums is common, occurring in more than half the cases described by Tipple and co-workers.[41] The history or presence of conjunctivitis can be elicited in half the cases. Lower respiratory tract symptoms consist of tachypnea and a very prominent staccato cough occurring in paroxysms. Some infants have apneic periods. Crepitant inspiratory rales are commonly heard; on the other hand, expiratory wheezes are distinctly uncommon. The paroxysmal cough often interferes with sleeping and eating and may be quite disturbing to the infant and parents. For the same reason, food intake drops and the child fails to gain weight.

Radiographic findings are those of hyperexpansion of the lungs with bilateral symmetrical interstitial infiltrates. The effects of this hyperexpansion on the diaphragm may result in an easily palpable liver and spleen.

TABLE 15–3
Selected Clinical Findings of Infants with Chlamydial Pneumonia

CLINICAL FINDINGS	PERCENTAGE WITH FINDINGS	
	Tipple et al. (N = 41)	Harrison et al. (N = 16)
Age at and Mode of Onset		
Presentation at wk 4–11	98	81
Onset <8 wk	93	
Prodrome >1 wk	78	81
Physical Findings		
Conjunctivitis	46	44
Eardrum findings	59	
Staccato cough	59	
Expiratory wheeze	12	25
Rales		87
Radiography		
Hyperinflation with infiltrates	81	87
Laboratory Values		
Eosinophils >300 per mm³	71	
Eosinophils >400 per mm³		75
Elevated IgM level	100	93
Elevated IgG level	93	87
Specific *C. trachomatis* antibody	98	94

Data from Tipple MA, Beem MO, Saxon EM. Clinical characteristics of the afebrile pneumonia associated with *Chlamydia trachomatis* infection in infants less than 6 months of age. Pediatrics 63:192–197, 1979; and Harrison HR, English MG, Lee CK, Alexander CR. *Chlamydia trachomatis* infant pneumonitis: comparison with matched controls and other infant pneumonitis. N Engl J Med 298:702–708, 1978.

Laboratory findings include a normal white blood cell count and an increase in the number of eosinophils (see Table 15–3). Blood gas analysis usually shows that many of the infants have a mild or moderate degree of hypoxemia, which may persist for weeks after the acute infection has subsided. Serum IgG and IgM levels are generally elevated.

Other Clinical Manifestations

There is suggestive evidence that chlamydiae play a role in causing disease in other sites of the respiratory tract as well. Their role in the etiology of otitis media is unclear. There is evidence in the findings of Tipple and co-workers suggestive of abnormal ear drums.[41] The study of Hammerschlag and co-workers did not support a significant role for chlamydiae, but the cultures in this study were performed after one or more courses of therapy.[43] Obstruction of nasal passages (stuffiness) and lower airway disease (bronchiolitis) in young infants have also been ascribed to chlamydiae. Many infants who ultimately develop pneumonia have a history of persistent rhinitis. Some infants with severe rhinitis, causing respiratory difficulty, have chlamydial infections of the nasopharynx.[44] In infants born prematurely, pneumonia tends to be a more serious illness. These infants are likely to have apneic spells with this infection, as they do with other respiratory infections. Additionally, premature infants are more likely to be left with residual airway disease. Respiratory distress syndrome may coexist with chlamydial pneumonia in this group of infants and contribute to these problems.[45, 46] Because chlamydial infection may result in nasopharyngeal obstruction and apnea, it is possible that some infants with sudden infant death syndrome have chlamydial infection. Our unpublished studies suggest that the contribution of chlamydiae to this syndrome is small (< 5% of cases). Furthermore, it is clear that many infants develop antibodies to *C. trachomatis* without having experienced a discrete and recognized infection, which suggests that there may be other, as yet undescribed clinical entities caused by this organism.

DIAGNOSIS

Conjunctivitis

The most widely used diagnostic tests for chlamydial infection are commercial nonculture methods to detect chlamydial antigen. Both the direct fluorescent antibody (DFA) method using fluorescein-conjugated monoclonal antibodies to stain chlamydial elementary bodies in a smear and enzyme immunoassays have been successfully used in diagnosis of ICN.[47–49] Highly sensitive nucleic acid amplification procedures are commercially available for diagnosis of genital chlamydial infection.[50–51] Although experience with these procedures is limited, they will probably be equally successful in diagnosis of *C. trachomatis* infection in infants.

For resource-poor settings, a useful diagnostic method is examination of Giemsa-stained conjunctival scrapings (particularly for severe cases of ICN).[49] This method also allows visualization of bacteria, such as gonococci, and of cytologic findings suggesting viral infection. The inclusion bodies that are diagnostic for ICN (Fig. 15–1) are located within the epithelial cells; thus, it is imperative to scrape rather than swab the lower conjunctiva to harvest epithelial cells with the inclusion bodies. Smears prepared from ocular discharges are not considered adequate. Isolation of the chlamydiae from conjunctival scrapings inoculated into tissue cell culture is a more reliable, although more costly, method of diagnosis. Serologic diagnosis of chlamydial conjunctivitis (in contrast to pneumonia) is not reliable because of the presence of maternally transmitted IgG antibody and the unreliable appearance of IgM antibody in this infection. Secretory IgA antibody appears in tears several weeks after onset of conjunctivitis.

Even if a firm diagnosis of chlamydial conjunctivitis is established, one must be mindful of the possibility of a double infection, particularly with *Neisseria gonorrhoeae*. For this reason, appropriate stain and culture of the conjunctival exudate should be obtained.

Pneumonia

The definitive diagnosis can be made either by culturing *C. trachomatis* from the respiratory tract (or lung) or by showing a significant rise in, or high levels of, IgM

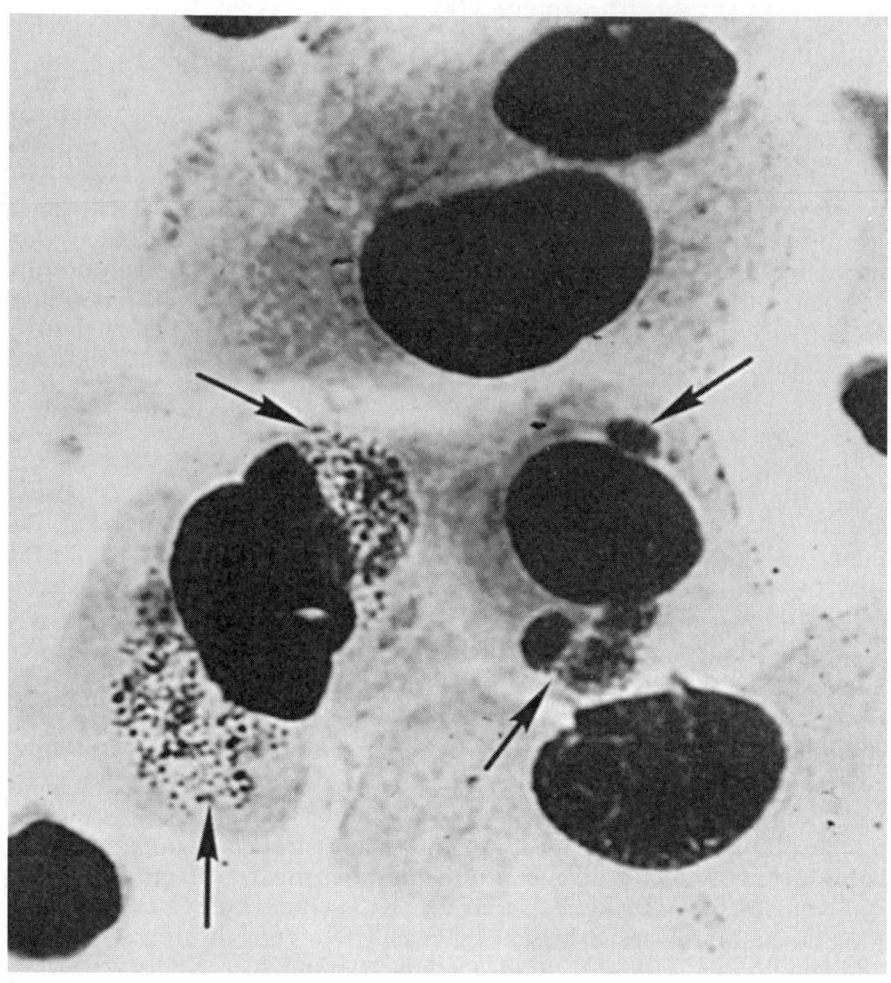

FIGURE 15–1 Chlamydial elementary body inclusions (arrows) in Giemsa-stained conjunctival scraping from a patient with inclusion conjunctivitis.

antibody to *C. trachomatis.*[52] DFA has also been successfully applied to nasopharyngeal specimens. The likelihood of obtaining a positive culture is enhanced by deep suction of the trachea or by collecting a nasopharyngeal aspirate rather than obtaining a specimen with a swab.[5, 42] In our hands, the serologic diagnosis of chlamydial pneumonia has been very successful. All the infants we have seen have had significantly elevated titers of specific IgM antibody (> 1:64 by microimmunofluorescence) by the time the pneumonia was apparent radiographically. Although at present it may be difficult to locate a laboratory able to perform these tests reliably, the physician can easily ship serum to regional laboratories.

The serologic test of choice is the microimmunofluorescent procedure of Wang and Grayston, in which elementary bodies are used as antigen.[53] Other indirect immunofluorescent antibody assays have been used that employ reticulate bodies or infected monolayers as antigens.[5] The important issue is that the presence of IgG antibody is not diagnostic. Maternal antibody may persist at high titers for months, and these antibodies are found at high rates (> 60%) in populations at high risk for sexually transmitted diseases. ICN does not regularly result in high titer of IgM antibody against *Chlamydia.* Infants with chlamydial pneumonia, at presentation, have geometric mean IgM antibody titers at least 10-

fold higher than the peak titers seen in uncomplicated ICN.[52] The great majority of pneumonia cases have IgM antichlamydial antibody levels greater than 1:64 by microimmunofluorescence. Rheumatoid factor does not seem to interfere with this assay.

The literature emphasizes the coexistence of several etiologic agents in young infants with pneumonia; this has been demonstrated both by lung culture and by serology.[54] Quite often chlamydiae and cytomegalovirus are found together, but the coexisting agent may be one of a variety of viruses. It is difficult to ascribe relative etiologic roles to the different agents in this setting. The clinical importance of these data is that the finding of a virus does not exclude the possibility that chlamydiae are also present and may in fact be playing the more important role. Beem and co-workers have found that when infants with such multiple infections are treated they usually improve at the same rate as those in whom chlamydiae are the only etiologic agent.[55]

DIFFERENTIAL DIAGNOSIS

Conjunctivitis

The differential diagnosis is important because it includes several serious infections. The principal entities to be considered are pyogenic infections, viral infections (primarily herpes simplex), and chemical conjunctivitis.

Of the pyogenic causes of conjunctivitis, gonococcal infection is the most threatening if not the most common (see Chapter 29). Like chlamydial conjunctivitis, it is acquired by passage through the infected birth canal, but it has a briefer incubation period; the disease usually makes its appearance between the second and the fifth day of life and is also characterized by marked reddening and a profuse purulent discharge, sometimes under pressure. Although the different time of onset is helpful in diagnosis, the two entities cannot be distinguished clinically. Gonococcal infection can be diagnosed presumptively by examination of the Gram-stained smear of the exudate and confirmed by culture of the exudate. It is important to keep this diagnosis in mind because unsuspected and untreated gonococcal eye infection may lead to blindness. Staphylococcal conjunctivitis (sometimes called "sticky eye") is usually acquired nosocomially from the nursery environment. It is characterized more by purulent discharge than by redness, with "golden crust" formation around the lids. This and other forms of pyogenic conjunctivitis—which may be due to pneumococci, *Haemophilus* species, or gram-negative bacteria such as *Pseudomonas aeruginosa*—can be easily diagnosed by Gram stain and culture of the exudate.

Of the viral infections, neonatal herpes simplex (see Chapter 8) is the most important. This disease is characterized by involvement of the skin as well as the eye, vesicle formation, and, at times, corneal involvement. Adenovirus infection of the newborn is very rare but has been described.

Chemical conjunctivitis related to instillation of silver nitrate at birth may also produce marked redness and a purulent discharge. However, these symptoms start on the first day of life and disappear after a few days, thus distinguishing this entity from a chlamydial infection. Therefore, conjunctivitis with a profuse mucopurulent discharge occurring around the second week of life is most likely related to chlamydial infection.

Pneumonia

The afebrile, tachypneic infant presenting with a paroxysmal cough and pneumonia in the first 4 months of life is very likely to have chlamydial disease. However, not all infants have a classic presentation, and other etiologic agents may cause an illness that mimics chlamydial infection. The second most common pneumonia in early infancy is due to respiratory syncytial virus (RSV). RSV usually occurs in late winter months and may be epidemic. RSV is the dominant cause of epidemics of pneumonia in a community. Chlamydial pneumonia occurs throughout the year. RSV is more likely to be associated with an expiratory wheeze and not to be associated with eosinophilia. The cough is usually not as paroxysmal. RSV infection can be rapidly diagnosed or ruled out by performing an immunofluorescent stain of the nasopharyngeal smear. Combined infections with RSV and *C. trachomatis* may also occur. Adenovirus or parainfluenza virus infection may also produce an interstitial pneumonia, again without the characteristic cough or eosino-

philia. Cytomegalovirus pneumonia may mimic the radiographic appearance of chlamydial disease but often has associated signs and symptoms in other organ systems, as do other pneumonias acquired in utero—those associated with rubella virus, herpes simplex virus, and *Toxoplasma gondii*. Many pyogenic bacteria may produce lower respiratory tract infections in infancy. Group B beta-hemolytic *Streptococcus*, *Streptococcus pneumoniae*, *Staphylococcus aureus*, *Haemophilus influenzae*, and the coliform group of bacteria are the most common. These patients are generally much sicker, are more toxic and febrile, and have pulmonary consolidation rather than an interstitial infiltrate. Pertussis caused by *Bordetella pertussis* is a classic cause of paroxysmal cough and may have pulmonary infiltrates. Infants with whooping cough are usually sicker and often have a very high absolute lymphocyte count as opposed to eosinophilia. *Pneumocystis carinii* pneumonia should also be considered in the differential diagnosis.

PROGNOSIS

Conjunctivitis

If untreated, ICN persists for many weeks or several months. In most instances, the inflammation clears without any complications; the scarring that occurs in trachoma that leads to lid deformities is not seen. However, several carefully documented series have demonstrated instances of superficial corneal vascularization and conjunctival scar formation.[2, 32, 33]

Pneumonia

If the pneumonia is untreated, infants are usually ill for several weeks; most of them cough a great deal, lose some weight or fail to gain weight, and are irritable but are not acutely or severely ill. A small number require oxygen and, exceptionally, even some ventilatory support. Beem and colleagues found in a series of 11 infants that the total course of illness is between 24 and 61 days, with an average of 43 days; mortality is exceptionally rare.[55]

Infants who develop chlamydial pneumonia are at risk of developing chronic respiratory deficits. Most of the original group of patients of Beem and Saxon had abnormal lung function tests 5 to 6 years after pneumonia had been diagnosed.[56] Reactive airway disease has been shown to follow early infancy infection with *Chlamydia*, as it has with other pathogens.[57]

THERAPY

Conjunctivitis

A 2-week course of oral therapy with erythromycin, 50 mg/kg per day, is recommended. Systemic treatment would be expected to eliminate the organism from the respiratory tract and thus prevent the occurrence of pneumonia, which may follow the conjunctivitis. In the past it was generally accepted that inclusion conjunctivitis responds to topically applied ophthalmic ointments or drops containing tetracycline, erythromycin, or sulfonamides. The ointment is applied four times a day for a 2-week period. Many infections, however, are slow to clear on this regimen; outright failures of treatment occur, possibly explained by the difficulty that parents have in getting ointment into their infant's eye or by reinfection from the nasopharynx. Failure rates greater than or equal to 50% have been reported.[39, 55] Because of such failures and because the infection usually extends beyond the anatomic reach of ointments, we see no reason to continue the use of topical regimens.

Pneumonia

The recommended treatment is a 2-week course of oral erythromycin, 50 mg/kg per day in divided doses.[58] There is convincing evidence that this treatment shortens clinical course significantly. The duration of nasopharyngeal shedding of *C. trachomatis* is also significantly decreased after a week of therapy. As noted earlier, the coexistence of a virus in the respiratory tract did not seem to alter the effectiveness of treatment. The standard regimen for a septic infant is likely to be an aminoglycoside and a penicillin analogue; although a controlled trial involving these drugs has not been reported, there is little reason to believe that they are effective in *C. trachomatis* infections. We have recovered chlamydiae from respiratory tracts of infants with pneumonia after courses of ampicillin and gentamicin. Because chlamydial pneumonia is so common, the routine practice of resorting to penicillin or ampicillin and aminoglycoside may be irrational for infants with pneumonia. Beyond the specific antimicrobial therapy, the infants require standard support measures, attention to nutrition and to fluid, and electrolyte balance and chest physical therapy. Oxygen and ventilatory therapy may be required in a minority of cases.

Diagnosis of any chlamydial infection in the infant signifies the presence of maternal infection. Thus, the mother and her sexual partner(s) should be treated for the infection. If untreated, chlamydial infections of the genital tract tend to persist and may do so for years. Second cases of chlamydial infection in newborns have been observed when the mothers were not treated. The mother is also at risk of developing upper genital tract disease.

PREVENTION

Given the morbidity associated with chlamydial infections, not only in infants but also in sexually active adults, it is clear that some control measures are indicated.[59] There are three general approaches that can be taken with our current technology. The first deals with efforts to reduce the reservoir.[58] The routine use of doxycycline (as recommended by the Centers for Disease Control and Prevention) as part of the treatment of gonorrhea would remove from the infective pool the approximately 20% of men and 30 to 40% of women with gonorrhea who also have chlamydial infection. Effective treatment of men with nongonococcal urethritis with doxycycline or azithromycin and routine treatment of their sexual contacts would also be appropriate. More widespread use of chlamydial diagnostic methods in screening high-risk populations would have the greatest impact.

Results from clinical trials had suggested that use of topical erythromycin or tetracycline for neonatal ocular prophylaxis would reduce rates of ICN. However, in routine use, the results have been disappointing; chlamydial eye infections were not prevented.[60–62]

There is a specific approach to prevent perinatal infections with *C. trachomatis*. It involves routine testing of pregnant women for chlamydial infection and treating those found to carry the organism. This can be an expensive undertaking. However, it can be justified as valid not only as a public health measure but also as cost effective in selected populations.[29] The remarkable constancy of attack rates observed in prospective studies allows reasonable certainty in predicting the outcomes of exposure to *Chlamydia* during vaginal deliveries. Thus, the crucial determinant in incidence of disease in infants will be the prevalence of chlamydial infection in the maternal cervix. The costs of managing conjunctivitis in the infant are relatively trivial. Chlamydial pneumonia is the condition that accrues the highest financial outlay. The majority of pneumonia cases can be managed on an outpatient basis. However, some of these infants are severely ill and, together with others who are very young, require hospitalization, some in an intensive care nursery. In our experience, approximately 25% of chlamydial pneumonia cases fall into these two groups. The reactive airway disease that may follow this infection,[56] with its attendant cost of visits and medication, further adds to the expense of treatment. When the cervical infection rate is above 6%, the costs of treating disease in these infants exceed the costs involved in identifying and treating the pregnant women to prevent perinatal exposure. Because infection rates of 15 to 30% are commonly reported in selected populations, routine screening for chlamydial infection should be initiated for these expectant mothers as an adjunct to obstetric management. The treatment of choice in managing chlamydial infection during pregnancy has not been clearly defined. Macrolides are the most likely candidates. Studies have shown the efficacy of erythromycin treatment in eradicating chlamydial infection in pregnant women and in preventing perinatal infection.[63] Amoxicillin may be used for those women who cannot tolerate erythromycin.[63, 64] Because of compliance advantages, efficacy, and fewer side effects, single-dose azithromycin will probably be a popular treatment.[65]

References

1. Schachter J. Chlamydial infections (third of three parts). N Engl J Med 298:540–549, 1978.
2. Schachter J, Dawson CR. Human Chlamydial Infections. Littleton, MA, PSG Publishing Co, 1978.
3. Lindner K. Gonoblennorrhoe, einschlussblennorrhoe und trachoma. Albrecht von Graefes Arch Ophthalmol 78:380, 1911.
4. Jones BR, Al-Hussaini MK, Dunlop EMC. Genital infec-

tion in association with TRIC virus infection of the eye: I. Isolation of virus from urethra, cervix, and eye: preliminary report. Br J Vener Dis 40:19–24, 1964.

5. Beem MO, Saxon EM. Respiratory-tract colonization and a distinctive pneumonia syndrome in infants infected with *Chlamydia trachomatis*. N Engl J Med 296:306–310, 1977.

6. Byrne GI, Moulder JW. Parasite-specified phagocytosis of *Chlamydia psittaci* and *Chlamydia trachomatis* by L and HeLa cells. Infect Immun 19:598–606, 1978.

7. Friis RR. Interaction of L cells and *Chlamydia psittaci*: entry of the parasite and host responses to its development. J Bacteriol 110:706–721, 1972.

8. Moulder JW. The relation of the psittacosis group (Chlamydiae) to bacteria and viruses. Annu Rev Microbiol 20:107–130, 1966.

9. Caldwell HD, Kromhout J, Schachter J. Purification and partial characterization of the major outer membrane protein of *Chlamydia trachomatis*. Infect Immun 31:1161–1176, 1981.

10. Newhall WJ, Jones RB. Disulfide-linked oligomers of the major outer membrane protein of chlamydiae. J Bacteriol 154:998–1001, 1983.

11. Stephens R, Kalman S, Fenner C, Davis R. *Chlamydia* Genome Project. http://chlamydia-www.berkeley.edu:4231/.

12. Bavoil P, Ohlin A, Schachter J. Role of disulfide bonding in outer membrane structure and permeability in *Chlamydia trachomatis*. Infect Immun 44:479–485, 1984.

13. Grayston JT, Wang S. New knowledge of chlamydiae and the diseases they cause. J Infect Dis 132:87–105, 1975.

14. Jones BR. The prevention of blindness from trachoma. Trans Ophthalmol Soc U K 95:16–33, 1975.

15. Holmes KK, Handsfield HH, Wang SP, et al. Etiology of nongonococcal urethritis. N Engl J Med 292:1199–1205, 1975.

16. Richmond SJ, Oriel JD. Recognition and management of genital chlamydial infection. BMJ 2:480–483, 1978.

17. Oriel JD, Reeve P, Thomas BJ, Nicol CS. Infection with *Chlamydia* group A in men with urethritis due to *Neisseria gonorrhoeae*. J Infect Dis 131:376–382, 1975.

18. Berger RE, Alexander ER, Monda GE, et al. *Chlamydia trachomatis* as a cause of acute "idiopathic" epididymitis. N Engl J Med 298:301, 1978.

19. Schachter J, Atwood G. Chlamydial pharyngitis? J Am Vener Dis Assoc 2:12, 1975.

20. Goldmeier D, Darougar S. Isolation of *Chlamydia trachomatis* from throat and rectum of homosexual men. Br J Vener Dis 53:184–185, 1977.

21. Mardh PA, Ripa T, Svensson L, Westrom L. *Chlamydia trachomatis* infection in patients with acute salpingitis. N Engl J Med 296:1377–1379, 1977.

22. Stamm WE, Wagner KF, Amsel R, et al. Causes of the acute urethral syndrome in women. N Engl J Med 303:409–415, 1980.

23. Brunham RC, Paavonen J, Stevens CE, et al. Mucopurulent cervicitis—the ignored counterpart in women of urethritis in men. N Engl J Med 311:1–6, 1984.

24. Chandler JW, Alexander ER, Pheiffer TA, et al. Ophthalmia neonatorum associated with maternal chlamydial infections. Trans Am Acad Ophthalmol Otolaryngol 83:302, 1977.

25. Frommell GT, Rothenberg R, Wang S, McIntosh K. Chlamydial infection of mothers and their infants. J Pediatr 95:28–32, 1979.

26. Hammerschlag MR, Anderka M, Semine DZ, et al. Prospective study of maternal and infantile infection with *Chlamydia trachomatis*. Pediatrics 64:142–148, 1979.

27. Schachter J, Grossman M, Sweet RL, et al. Prospective study of perinatal transmission of *Chlamydia trachomatis*. JAMA 255:3374–3377, 1986.

28. Schachter J, Grossman M, Holt J, et al. Infection with *Chlamydia trachomatis*: involvement of multiple anatomic sites in neonates. J Infect Dis 139:232–234, 1979.

29. Schachter J, Grossman M. Chlamydial infections. Annu Rev Med 32:45–61, 1981.

30. Lumicao GG, Gyves MT, Stuart LA, et al. Prospective study of perinatal infection with *Chlamydia trachomatis*. Abstract. Pediatr Res 13:464, 1979.

31. Hardy PH, Hardy JB, Nell EE, et al. Prevalence of six sexually transmitted disease agents among pregnant inner-city adolescents and pregnancy outcome. Lancet 2:333–337, 1984.

32. Mordhorst CH, Wang SP, Grayston JT. Childhood trachoma in a nonendemic area: Danish trachoma patients and their close contacts, 1963 to 1973. JAMA 239:1765–1771, 1978.

33. Mordhorst CH, Dawson C. Sequelae of neonatal inclusion conjunctivitis and associated disease in parents. Am J Ophthalmol 71:861–867, 1971.

34. Schachter J. The expanding clinical spectrum of infections with *Chlamydia trachomatis*. Sex Transm Dis 4:116–118, 1977.

35. Hammerschlag MR, Chandler JW, Alexander ER, et al. Erythromycin ointment for ocular prophylaxis of neonatal chlamydial infection. JAMA 244:2291–2293, 1980.

36. Moncada J, Strassburger J, Schachter J. Isolation of *Chlamydia trachomatis* from gastric aspirate of an infant. Pediatr Infect Dis 5:375–376, 1986.

37. Frommell GT, Bruhn FW, Schwartzman JD. Isolation of *Chlamydia trachomatis* from infant lung tissue. N Engl J Med 296:1150–1152, 1977.

38. Arth C, Von Schmidt B, Grossman M, Schachter J. Chlamydial pneumonitis. J Pediatr 93:447–449, 1978.

39. Rowe DS, Aicardi EZ, Dawson CR, Schachter J. Purulent ocular discharge in neonates: significance of *Chlamydia trachomatis*. Pediatrics 63:628–632, 1979.

40. Schachter J, Lum L, Gooding CA, Ostler B. Pneumonitis following inclusion blennorrhea. J Pediatr 87:779–780, 1975.

41. Tipple MA, Beem MO, Saxon EM. Clinical characteristics of the afebrile pneumonia associated with *Chlamydia trachomatis* infection in infants less than 6 months of age. Pediatrics 63:192–197, 1979.

42. Harrison HR, English MG, Lee CK, Alexander ER. *Chlamydia trachomatis* infant pneumonitis: comparison with matched controls and other infant pneumonitis. N Engl J Med 298:702–708, 1978.

43. Hammerschlag MR, Hammerschlag PE, Alexander ER. The role of *Chlamydia trachomatis* in middle ear effusions in children. Pediatrics 66:615–617, 1980.

44. Cohen SD, Azimi PH, Schachter J. *Chlamydia trachomatis* associated with severe rhinitis and apneic episodes in a one-month-old infant. Clin Pediatr (Phila) 21:498–499, 1982.

45. Sollecito D, Midulla M, Bavastrelli M, et al. *Chlamydia trachomatis* in neonatal respiratory distress of very preterm babies: biphasic clinical picture. Acta Paediatr 81:788–791, 1992.

46. Colarizi P, Chiesa C, Pacifico L, et al. *Chlamydia trachomatis*–associated respiratory disease in the very early neonatal period. Acta Paediatr 85:991–994, 1996.

47. Bell TA, Kuo CC, Stamm WE, et al. Direct fluorescent monoclonal antibody stain for rapid detection of infant *Chlamydia trachomatis* infections. Pediatrics 74:224–228, 1984.

48. Hammerschlag MR, Herrmann JE, Cox P, et al. Enzyme

immunoassay for diagnosis of neonatal chlamydial conjunctivitis. J Pediatr 107:741–743, 1985.

49. Schachter J, Stamm WE. Chlamydia. *In* Murray PR, Baron EJ, Pfaller MA, et al (eds). Manual of Clinical Microbiology, 7th ed. Washington, DC, American Society for Microbiology, 1998.

50. Schachter J, Stamm WE, Quinn TC, et al. Ligase chain reaction to detect *Chlamydia trachomatis* infection of the cervix. J Clin Microbiol 32:2540–2543, 1994.

51. Jaschek G, Gaydos CA, Welsh LE, Quinn TC. Direct detection of *Chlamydia trachomatis* in urine specimens from symptomatic and asymptomatic men by using a rapid polymerase chain reaction assay. J Clin Microbiol 31:1209–1212, 1993.

52. Schachter J, Grossman M, Azimi PH. Serology of *Chlamydia trachomatis* in infants. J Infect Dis 146:530–535, 1982.

53. Wang SP, Grayston JT, Alexander ER, Holmes KK. Simplified microimmunofluorescence test with trachoma-lymphogranuloma venereum (*Chlamydia trachomatis*) antigens for use as a screening test for antibody. J Clin Microbiol 1:250–255, 1975.

54. Paisley JW, Lauer BA, Melinkovich P, et al. Rapid diagnosis of *Chlamydia trachomatis* pneumonia in infants by direct immunofluorescence microscopy of nasopharyngeal secretions. J Pediatr 109:653–655, 1986.

55. Beem MO, Saxon E, Tipple M. Treatment of chlamydial pneumonia in infancy. Pediatrics 63:198–203, 1979.

56. Weiss SG, Newcomb RW, Beem MO. Pulmonary assessment of children after chlamydial pneumonia of infancy. J Pediatr 108(5 Pt 1):659–664, 1986.

57. Brasfield DM, Stagno S, Whitley RJ, et al. Infant pneumonitis associated with cytomegalovirus, *Chlamydia*, *Pneumocystis*, and *Ureaplasma*. Pediatrics 79:76, 1987.

58. Centers for Disease Control. 1998 Guidelines for Treatment of Sexually Transmitted Diseases. MMWR 47:vi, 118, 1997.

59. Schachter J. Why we need a program for the control of *Chlamydia trachomatis*. Editorial. N Engl J Med 320:802–804, 1989.

60. Bell TA, Sandstrom KI, Gravett MG, et al. Comparison of ophthalmic silver nitrate solution and erythromycin ointment for prevention of natally acquired *Chlamydia trachomatis*. Sex Transm Dis 14:195–200, 1987.

61. Hammerschlag MR, Cummings C, Roblin PM, et al. Efficacy of neonatal ocular prophylaxis for the prevention of chlamydial and gonococcal conjunctivitis. N Engl J Med 320:769–772, 1989.

62. Chen JY. Prophylaxis of ophthalmia neonatorum: comparison of silver nitrate, tetracycline, erythromycin and no prophylaxis. Pediatr Infect Dis J 11:1026–1030, 1992.

63. Schachter J, Sweet RL, Grossman M, et al. Experience with the routine use of erythromycin for chlamydial infections in pregnancy. N Engl J Med 314:276–279, 1986.

64. Alary M, Joly JR, Moutquin JM, et al. Randomised comparison of amoxycillin and erythromycin in treatment of genital chlamydial infection in pregnancy. Lancet 344:1461–1465, 1994.

65. Adair CD, Gunter M, Stovall TG, et al. Chlamydia in pregnancy: a randomized trial of azithromycin and erythromycin. Obstet Gynecol 91:165–168, 1998.

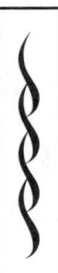

Human Parvovirus B19

THOMAS J. TÖRÖK, M.D.*

Human parvovirus B19 is a fairly recently recognized human pathogen, and the entire range of clinical manifestations caused by B19 has probably not been completely described. Despite this, the list of proven and suspected disease associations is already remarkable for its length and diversity (Table 16–1). In the normal host, the most widely recognized manifestation of B19 infection is the mild rash illness erythema infectiosum, also called fifth disease, but a self-limited symmetrical polyarthropathy is also common, especially in adults. Whether B19 is an important etiologic factor in the pathogenesis of chronic arthritis in some patients is an area of active research. B19 selectively infects and lyses human erythroblasts. In patients with hematologic disorders characterized by decreased red blood cell production (e.g., thalassemia) or increased red blood cell destruction or loss (e.g., sickle cell disease), B19 may cause an acute life-threatening red cell aplasia, commonly referred to as transient aplastic crisis. In immunocompromised patients, B19 infection may become persistent and cause chronic anemia. B19 infection has also been linked to sporadic cases of hemophagocytic syndrome, myocarditis, neurologic disease, and vasculitis, but an etiologic role for B19 has yet to be confirmed and host factors predisposing the patient to these disease processes have not yet been identified.

Fetal infection with B19 has been a special concern because many parvoviruses are known to cause reproductive failure and are teratogenic. Our understanding about the deleterious effects of B19 on the fetus is still fragmentary, but already B19 has been shown to cause nonimmune fetal hydrops and fetal death in some cases, and new data suggest that intrauterine B19 infection may sometimes cause birth defects with long-term disabilities among the survivors. Ultimately, it is likely that the magnitude of the impact B19 has on the fetus will be the most important factor shaping the public health response.

---

*Material new to this edition in this chapter was prepared by the editors and is indicated in bracketed italic type.

TABLE 16–1
Clinical Manifestations of B19 Infection

Normal Host
Asymptomatic or subclinical infection
Erythema infectiosum (fifth disease)
Arthropathy

Patients with Preexisting Anemia
Acute red blood cells aplasia (transient aplastic crisis)

Immunocompromised Patients
Chronic infection with anemia

Infection in the Fetus and Newborn
Anemia
Nonimmune fetal hydrops
Fetal death
Birth defects?

Other Conditions Associated with B19 Infection
Hemophagocytic syndrome
Myocarditis
Neurologic disease
Vasculitis

B19 was first identified in sera from healthy blood donors screened for hepatitis B surface antigen.[1] It appeared as an anomalous precipitin line by counterimmunoelectrophoresis. Its unusual name refers to the designation of the specimen containing the first isolate identified and carries no other special significance.[2] Specifically, there are no parvoviruses named B1 through B18. It was thought that using B19 would lead to less confusion than using HPV for human parvovirus, because HPV was already in widespread use to signify human papillomavirus.[3]

Within a few years after the first report from the United Kingdom in 1975, viruses indistinguishable from B19 were identified throughout the world[4–8] and seroprevalence studies demonstrated that exposure to B19 was extremely common. Still, it was not until 1981 that B19 was first directly linked to human disease. The virus was then discovered in acute serum samples collected from patients with sickle cell disease and transient aplastic crisis.[9, 10] Recovery was associated with the development of specific antibodies and disappearance of the virus. In 1983, serologic evidence of acute B19 infection was found in patients with recent onset of arthritis,[11, 12] and in schoolchildren with erythema infectiosum.[13] The first reports linking B19 to fetal disease came in 1984, when nonimmune hydrops[14] and fetal death[15] were reported after a community outbreak of erythema infectiosum. In 1987, ocular malformations were reported in an abortus after maternal infection, suggesting that B19 could have a teratogenic effect in humans.[15] Also in 1987, a patient with a congenital immunodeficiency syndrome was found to have chronic B19 infection and chronic anemia,[17] and the range of patients susceptible to chronic B19 infection has now grown to include patients with acquired immunodeficiency syndromes, patients immunosuppressed because of malignancy or drug therapy, and occasionally patients with no other evidence of immunodeficiency.[18] [*Articles of particular in-* *terest published between 1994 and 2000 are referred to in the italicized commentaries by the editors.*]

CHARACTERISTICS OF PARVOVIRUSES

Parvoviruses are nonenveloped single-stranded DNA viruses that infect animals.[19–22] The family Parvoviridae includes two genera whose members infect vertebrates—the genus *Parvovirus*, which includes the autonomously replicating parvoviruses; and the genus *Dependovirus*, whose members require a helper virus, such as adenovirus or herpesvirus, for replication. Members of the third genus, *Densovirus*, are pathogenic in arthropods. Many viruses belonging to the genus *Parvovirus* are important animal pathogens. Some important members of this genus are canine parvovirus, which can cause fatal myocarditis and enteritis in puppies; feline parvovirus, which can produce cerebellar hypoplasia and ataxia in perinatally infected kittens; and porcine parvovirus, which is an economically important cause of swine reproductive failure. So far, B19 is the only proven human pathogen in this genus, and none of the other autonomous parvoviruses are transmissible to humans. RA-1 has been previously reported as a possible human pathogen, but this has never been confirmed.[23, 24] Parvovirus-like particles have been found in stools of patients during some outbreaks of acute gastroenteritis, but they have not been fully characterized.[25–27] The genus Dependovirus includes the nonpathogenic human adeno-associated viruses. Serologic evidence of prior infection with adeno-associated viruses is present in the majority of adults.[28] These viruses can integrate into the host genome and are under active investigation as possible vectors for human gene therapy.[29–31]

Parvoviruses are 20 to 25 nm in diameter. The structure of canine parvovirus has been determined by x-ray crystallography, and the capsid consists of 60 copies of capsid proteins arranged with icosahedral symmetry.[32] A comparison with the protein sequences of the other parvoviruses suggests that they are structurally similar to canine parvovirus and may share important functional characteristics as well.[33] The capsid encloses a single copy of a linear, single-stranded DNA genome of approximately 5000 nucleotides. The left-hand of the positive sense strand contains the genes encoding the nonstructural proteins and the right-hand contains genes encoding the structural proteins. The genome contains inverted terminal repeats at each end, which form palindromic hairpins that are important in initiation of DNA replication by providing a segment of double-standed DNA of self-priming. Replication of parvoviruses is dependent on factors present during the DNA synthesis phase of host cell replication, and this limits productive viral infection to actively replicating host cells. Parviruses are among the most resistant viruses known to chemical and physical disinfection.

The genome of B19 has been sequenced in its entirety, and it consists of approximately 5600 nucleotides.[34–36] The genetic variability among strains of B19 has been investigated using restriction endonucleases and partial nucleotide sequencing.[37-41] Although differences have been noted between individual strains, similar strains can be found dispersed geographically and temporally and there is no evidence at this time linking differences at the nucleotide level to different clinical manifestations. For most parvoviruses, transcripts for the production of messenger RNA (mRNA) of nonstructural and structural proteins begin at different promoters. Structural gene expression is under control of early gene products that transactivate the late promoter. So far, the evidence suggests that B19 has only a single functional promoter located at map unit 6.[35, 42-44] A second promotor at map unit 44 has been proposed but not confirmed.[45] The importance of a single functional promoter is that, in contrast to other parvoviruses, structural gene expression in B19 would not be a function of promoter modulation. Nine mRNA transcripts have been identified, and the functional role of five has been determined.[46, 47] One codes for NS1, a nonstructural protein associated with cytotoxicity.[48] Two each code for the two structural proteins—VP1 (84 kDa) and VP2 (58 kDa). Both VP1 and VP2 are in the same reading frame, and the entire nucleotide sequence coding for VP2 is contained within that of VP1. VP2 is the major capsid protein and is 554 amino acids long; VP1 is 781 amino acids long.[48] Empty B19 capsids formed from recombinant VP2 protein have been analyzed, and the preliminary evidence suggests that B19 and canine parvovirus are structurally similar.[49] The minor capsid protein, VP1, is not required for capsid assembly but plays an important role in vivo in inducing neutralizing antibodies.[50] Studies using monoclonal antibodies have suggested some antigenic variability between strains, but the significance has not been determined.[51] Other studies have found conserved epitopes from strains collected over time and wide geographic regions.[52, 53]

EPIDEMIOLOGY AND TRANSMISSION

General Considerations

SOURCES AND LIMITATIONS OF DATA

Much of what is known about the epidemiology of B19 has been derived from studies of the B19-associated rash illness, erythema infectiosum, which was recognized as a distinct illnes beginning in the late 1800s.[54] In the nearly 100 years between the description of erythema infectiosum and the discovery of its etiologic agent in 1983,[13] many careful clinical and epidemiologic investigations of erythema infectiosum outbreaks have been reported,[55-64] and these descriptions continue to be an important source of epidemiologic information. Similarly, early studies of clusters of cases of transient aplastic crisis in patients with hemolytic anemia,[65] which predate the 1981 discovery of the etiologic link to B19 in 1981,[9, 10] also continue to be a source of invaluable information.

The epidemiology of B19 is incompletely understood, however. The application of serologic testing to outbreak investigations of erythema infectiosum and aplas-

tic crisis in the 1980s demonstrated the importance of clinically inapparent infection in these situations and the need to include laboratory diagnostic criteria to further our knowledge about B19 epidemiology. The varied clinical presentations associated with B19 infection in both normal and compromised hosts add to the difficulty in case recognition, and there is still relatively little known about the epidemiology of manifestations other than erythema infectiosum or aplastic crisis.

There are considerable laboratory obstacles as well. No practical system for culturing the virus exists at this time. Serologic tests have been developed that are sensitive and specific for the normal host but are still not widely available. The greatest morbidity and mortality associated with B19 infection occur in patients incapable of producing a normal immune response, and alternative methods, such as DNA or viral antigen assays, are required in conjunction with serology to characterize the epidemiology of infection in these populations.

GEOGRAPHIC AND TEMPORAL DISTRIBUTION

Infection with B19 occurs globally, and serologic evidence of B19 infection has been observed in all populations studied to date, including isolated island[66] and rural[8, 67, 68] populations. The clinical manifestations have been similar regardless of geographic location. Serologic assays are broadly reactive independent of the origin of the patient specimen or source of antigen used for testing, and so far there are no data suggesting clinically significant strain differences. Analyses of antigenic makeup[51-53] or nucleotide sequences[37-41] also show few differences between specimens dispersed widely geographically or temporally.

Transmission occurs year-round, but there are seasonal increases in reports of outbreaks of erythema infectiosum in winter and spring in temperate latitudes,* less commonly during fall and summer.[56, 59, 71] In institutional settings such as schools or day-care centers, outbreaks of erythema infectiosum may persist for months. Often these outbreaks begin in late winter and new cases are reported until school closes for summer vacation.

There have been few longitudinal studies of disease incidence to establish any general patterns in the periodicity of epidemics. Erythema infectiosum, the most commonly recognized clinical manifestation of B19 infection, is not a notifiable disease in most areas, and the sensitivity and specificity of clinical case reporting have not been determined. The best evidence for periodic epidemics followed by prolonged interepidemic periods with little or no disease activity comes from studies of island or isolated populations. In Jamaica, careful follow-up of patients with sickle cell disease has demonstrated epidemics of transient aplastic crises occurring at approximately 5-year intervals with little disease between outbreaks.[72] In Japan, age-specific seroprevalence studies of stored serum samples showed little evidence for widespread circulation during a 10-year interval.[73] The anti-B19 IgG seroprevalence among three tribes of Amerindians living in remote regions of Brazil was less than

---

*See references 6, 9, 55, 57, 58, 60–62, 64, 69, and 70.

11% overall, and in one tribe was zero for all persons tested younger than 30 years old.[68] Comparable serologic studies are not currently available from North America, but limited data suggest that in many communities endemic transmission and annual outbreaks do occur between years with recognized widespread epidemic activity. A review of school nursing records in Iowa over a 14-year period found that cases of erythema infectiosum were seen every year but one.[74] A better understanding of geographic and temporal patterns and the relative importance of endemic versus epidemic transmission may help us to better anticipate the needs of high-risk patient populations in the future.

PREVALENCE AND INCIDENCE

The seroprevalence of specific IgG antibodies increases with age.[1, 72, 75–80] Transplacentally acquired maternal antibodies are no longer detectable by 1 year of age and remain low in the preschool ages. In children younger than 5 years old, the prevalence of anti-B19 IgG antibodies is usually below 5%. The greatest increase in seroprevalence occurs between the ages of 5 and 20, when it increases from about 5% to nearly 40%. Afterward, the estimates increase slowly with increasing age. In adult blood donors, the seroprevalence of anti-B19 IgG antibodies ranges from 29 to 79% with a median of 45%.[81–87] By age 50, the seroprevalence may exceed 75%.

For most age groups, there are no significant differences between the sexes in the seroprevalence of specific IgG; however, some studies have shown an increase in the percentage of anti-B19 IgG among women of reproductive age compared with men and have attributed this to greater exposure to infected children because of child-rearing practices.[82, 88, 89] The proportion of women who were seropositive in one study of adult blood donors was 47.5%, nearly 1.5 times that of men. In a family study, the prevalence of anti-B19 IgG was greater for females of all ages and averaged 51% compared with 38% for males.[89] A difference in gender-specific seroprevalence has not been observed in other studies.[76]

The point prevalence of acute B19 infection can be estimated in cross-sectional studies by detection of viral antigens, DNA, or anti-B19 IgM antibodies. Blood donors have been the group most often studied because usually the principal objective of the investigators was to identify large volumes of virus-positive serum for use in diagnostic testing. Because of this bias, the true prevalence of acute infection in healthy adults and the difference between nonepidemic and epidemic periods are not known with certainty. The range of estimates using antigen detection tests is from 0 to 2.6 per 10,000, with a median of 1 per 10,000[5, 90–94]; using DNA detection methods, it is from 0 to 14.5 per 10,000, with a median of 2 per 10,000.[91, 92, 95, 96] In serologic studies of donors utilizing the most sensitive antibody assays, the seroprevalence of anti-B19 IgM antibodies has been zero, but all studies included fewer than 1000 patients.[81, 97, 98] The rates are slightly higher for specimens submitted to clinical laboratories but not selected for possible parvovirus infection. The proportion of specimens positive for viral antigens was 3.0 per 10,000,[99] and for DNA it was 8.9 per 10,000.[100]

RISK FACTORS FOR ACQUISITION

High rates of secondary transmission have been documented within households. Secondary attack rates based on clinical criteria have ranged from 17 to 30%.[63, 101] In serologic studies where immune household contacts can be excluded from consideration, the secondary attack rate has been shown to be as high as 50%.[102] The majority of secondary cases of erythema infectiosum or aplastic crisis in households occur 6 to 12 days after the index case.[53, 101, 103, 104] *[A serologic study of pregnant Danish women indicated that seropostivity was significantly correlated with increasing number of siblings, having a sibling of the same age, number of own children, and occupational exposure of children.[104a]]*

The peak incidence of infection occurs among school-aged children, and this is probably due in part to widespread transmission occurring at schools during community outbreaks. A review of nine investigations of school or classroom outbreaks of erythema infectiosum with at least one serologically confirmed case of acute B19 infection revealed student attack rates between 1 and 62% based on rash illnes surveys, with a median of 23%.[13, 105–112] Asymptomatic infection is common, and prodromal signs and symptoms may be mild and overlooked. Serologic studies of students during outbreaks have found that between 26 and 89% of infections may not be associated with rash illness and therefore go unrecognized.[106, 111, 112] Excluding students presumed to be immune before the outbreak (i.e., students who have anti-B19 IgG antibodies but lack IgM), the reported attack rates among susceptible students are still higher and vary from 34 to 72%.[106, 111, 112] Higher attack rates are generally reported in elementary schools and daycare centers compared with secondary schools, and in boarding students compared with day students.[63, 77, 110–112]

During school outbreaks, employees are at increased risk of infection compared with community controls. The attack rate based on detection of rash illness or arthropathy may be relatively low, and reported rates vary from 12 to 25%.[106, 110] However, the seroprevalence of anti-B19 IgG antibodies in school employees is as great or greater than adult community controls and ranges between 50 and 75%.[100, 109, 112–114] As a consequence, when serologic testing is used to help identify employees with asymptomatic infection and to exclude immune employees, the attack rate among the remaining susceptibles can actually be very high. In investigations of four school outbreaks where serologic criteria were used, the attack rate varied from 19 to 84% and the frequency of asymptomatic infection was greater than 50% in all but one outbreak.[106, 109, 112, 113] The highest infection rates were observed among susceptible elementary school teachers compared with middle and high school teachers, and this may reflect either exposure to more infected children or greater likelihood of contact with respiratory secretions in younger children.[112, 113] During a community-wide outbreak of erythema infectiosum in Connecticut in 1988, the infection rate among susceptible women was 16% for school teachers, 9% for day-care workers and homemakers, but only 4% for other women working outside the home.[119] The risk of infection may be increased for school employees even in the absence of recognized outbreaks of erythema infectiosum. In a longitudinal study of 927 susceptible school employees conducted during a 3.5-year period when no community outbreaks were detected, the annual incidence of specific IgG seroconversion was 2.9%, compared with 0.4% for a control population of 198 hospital employees.[114] The rates were higher—3.4%—for school employees with jobs involving direct contact with children, compared with only 0.6% observed for persons with other job classifications. Most of the individuals seroconverting did not recall an illness characterized by rash or arthropathy.

The possibility that health care workers are at increased risk of acquiring B19 infection is suggested by several reports describing probable transmission from patient to patient and patient to employee on hospital wards, and infections in persons working in diagnostic and research laboratories handling materials or specimens known to contain B19.[116–119] One patient with sickle cell anemia became ill with aplastic crisis 9 to 11 days after contact in the hospital with a patient with hereditary spherocytosis hospitalized for aplastic crisis; B19 infection was confirmed in both.[120] An outbreak of erythema infectiosum was described on a pediatric ward where 13 (26%) of 50 children developed a rash illness.[121] B19 seroconversion was demonstrated in 5 (71%) of 7 children with rash illness, and in 9 (35%) of 26 children without symptoms. Transmission from patient to health care worker was recognized on two occasions in one hospital after admission of patients with aplastic crisis.[116] In the first instance, 4 (36%) of 11 susceptible employees with close contact had anti-B19 IgM antibodies, indicating acute infection; in the second, 10 (48%) of 21 employees either had specific IgM or had recently seroconverted from IgG negative to positive. Eleven (79%) of 14 were symptomatic with rash or arthropathy. In another instance, an investigation of an outbreak of erythema infectiosum among health care workers on a pediatric ward revealed that 10 (33%) of 30 susceptible health care workers tested had serologic evidence of acute B19 infection, along with 2 (17%) of 12 immunocompromised patients being cared for on the ward.[117, 122] The source of the outbreak was not discovered. The two infected patients were not symptomatic, but analysis of preexisting serum samples demonstrated that they had acquired their infections while hospitalized. Onset of symptoms among the employees was not clustered in time, suggesting an ongoing source, or person-to-person transmission.

While the previously described studies demonstrate that there is a risk of nosocomial transmission, other studies suggest that the risk may be low overall. No evidence of transmission from patient to employee was identified among 10 susceptible health care workers with frequent contact with a chronically infected patient hospitalized for 24 days before institution of isolation precautions.[123, 124] *[Spread to hospital employees did not occur after exposure to a parvovirus B19 infected mother, her infected stillborn fetus, and contaminated fomites in the hospital room.[124a]]* During a community outbreak of B19, none of 17 susceptible pregnant health care workers with self-perceived exposure were anti-B19 IgM positive.[115] Two longitudinal studies from one institution help to define the incidence of infection in health care workers in the absence of epidemic disease. The first study followed 124 susceptible female health care workers an average of 1.7 years and found the annual seroconversion rate to be 1.4%. In a subsequent study of 198 susceptible hospital employees, the annual rate was 0.4%, compared with 2.9% for school employees.[114]

Female gender has been suggested as a possible risk factor for infection in some outbreaks of erythema infectiosum. During a community-wide outbreak of erythema infection in Port Angeles, Washington, the attack rate for women was 15.6%, more than twice the rate of 7.4% observed for men.[53] Crowding and low socioeconomic status have not been identified as risk factors for early exposure or acquisition of disease. However, the possibility was raised by a study in Rio de Janiero that found the seroprevalence of anti-B19 IgG antibodies to be 35% in children age 5 years or younger,[78] and in a study conducted in Niger where the seroprevalence was 90% at 2 years of age.[67] Host factors that place some patients at risk for more severe disease or complications from infection are considered in the sections describing clinical manifestations associated with B19 infection.

MODES OF TRANSMISSION

The principal mode of B19 transmission is presumed to be person-to-person through direct contact with respiratory secretions. Viral DNA is demonstrable in saliva[101, 104, 111, 125–127] at levels comparable with those found in blood, and from volunteer studies it has been demonstrated that the virus is infectious by intranasal inoculation.[125, 128] B19 has not been found in columnar epithelial cells lining large airways.[129] The evidence that B19 is not transmitted by aerosols is indirect. Cases of erythema infectiosum may occur over a time span of months in school outbreaks, suggesting that B19 transmission is relatively inefficient, and this is in marked contrast with the rapid dissemination of disease by airborne pathogens like measles and influenza virus. B19 DNA has also been found in urine.[104]

The only well-documented modes of transmission for B19 have been vertically from mother to fetus, and from parenteral transfusion with contaminated blood products or needles. Vertical transmission is discussed below. Transmission from contaminated single-donor blood products is rare because of the low prevalence of B19 viremia among donors; however, transmission may be common after treatment with pooled blood products.[116, 130–134] Parvovirus DNA is frequently found in clotting factor concentrates, including products treated with solvents and detergents, steam, or monoclonal antibodies, and even treated products may be infectious.[96, 131, 133–138] The seroprevalence of anti-B19 IgG among hemophiliacs is increased compared with age-matched controls,[132] is higher for patients with severe disease who have received more treatments, and is higher in patients receiving factors prepared from large compared with small donor pools.[88] Parenteral transmission has also been reported after tattooing.[127]

The autonomous parvoviruses, which include B19, are among the viruses most resistant to chemical inactivation, and environmental contamination plays an important role in transmission for many of these viruses.[22] After introduction of an infected animal, fecal contamination frequently results in prolonged epidemics of canine parvovirus in dog kennels, mink enteritis virus in mink sheds, or porcine parvovirus in pig herds. Environmental decontamination and eradication are difficult. Transmission of B19 has occurred in the hospital setting without recognized direct patient contact.[116] The possibility that B19 is also transmitted by fomites or through environmental contamination has not been evaluated, but considering the stability of related animal parvoviruses, this possibility deserves further investigation. Transmission by fomites might also explain in part the increased risk of transmission in households and daycare centers, where utensils and toys contaminated with saliva could be shared. *[The presence of parvovirus B19 DNA on fomites was identified in a study of a suspected nosocomial outbreak in a maternity ward.[124a] Surface swabs obtained from the hands of the mother of a stillborn infected fetus and the sink handles in her hospital room were positive for parvovirus B19 DNA by polymerase chain reaction (PCR). In addition, samples from countertops, an intravenous pump, and telephone were positive by a more-sensitive nested DNA technique. The study did not identify the transmissibility of the virus present on fomites. Heavily infected fetal tissues and placental or amniotic fluids are more likely sources of virus than fomites for health care workers.]*

Maternal Infection and Vertical Transmission

PREVALENCE AND INCIDENCE OF MATERNAL INFECTION

Many pregnant women do not have detectable anti-B19 IgG antibodies and may be susceptible to B19 infection. For pregnant women and women of reproductive age, the reported seroprevalence of anti-B19 IgG antibodies has varied between 16 and 72%, with the majority of estimates falling between 35% and 55%.[75, 80, 89, 115, 138–142] *[Among other serologic surveys: 65% of 31,000 pregnant Danish women had evidence of past infection[104a]; the seroprevalence of IgG antibody among 1610 pregnant women in Barcelona was 35.03%[142a]; and 81% of pregnant Swedish women had parvovirus antibodies.[142b]]* The prevalence of anti-B19 IgG antibodies in cord blood from normal newborns has also been used to estimate the level of maternal immunity and is in general agreement with the above, with estimates ranging from 50 to 75%.[138, 139, 143] There may be a considerable difference in susceptibility based on maternal age. In a study of pregnant women in Japan, the seroprevalence of anti-B19 IgG antibodies was 26% for women between the ages of 21 and 30, and 44% for women between the ages of 31 and 40.[80]

Surprisingly little is known about the incidence of acute B19 infection during pregnancy. There have been no studies, for example, that have attempted to follow a normal cohort of susceptible women from conception or diagnosis of pregnancy to term for evidence of acquisition of specific IgG. As a surrogate, one group conducted a longitudinal study of 235 susceptible women, most of whom were of reproductive age, and found that the annual seroconversion rate was 1.4% during a period when no outbreaks of erythema infectiosum were evident.[89] *[Seroconversion rates among susceptible pregnant Danish women during endemic and epidemic periods were 1.5% and 13%, respectively. Risk of acute infection increased with the number of children in the household and having children ages 6 to 7 years resulted in the highest rate of seroconversion. Nursery school teachers had a threefold increased risk of acute infection.[104a] Among Barcelona women surveyed beginning in the twenty-eighth week, 3.7% seroconverted during the pregnancy.[142a]]* Extrapolating to a 40-week period would place the infection rate during pregnancy among susceptible women at approximately 1.1%. A few studies have tried to estimate the infection rate with cross-sectional seroprevalence studies of specific IgM, in pregnancy or in women of reproductive age. Because specific IgM may persist for only a few months, this method would tend to underestimate the maternal infection rate. However, the representativeness of the available date is also a source of concern because the majority of studies have been conducted in high-risk populations—e.g., women with rash illness, possible exposure to cases of erythema infectiosum, or recent diagnosis of adverse reproductive outcomes—and this could markedly inflate the measured infection rate. For the few studies that have included a group of pregnant women or women of reproductive age, not otherwise selected because of signs or symptoms of acute infection or exposure to suspected cases of B19, the observed range of specific IgM is from 0 to 2.6%.[138, 139, 142] The proportion of susceptible women with specific IgM in populations recognized to be at increased risk has varied from 0 to 12.5%.[80, 115, 139, 140, 142]

RISK OF FETAL INFECTION

Transplacental transmission of B19 to the fetus has been well documented and may be common after maternal infection. However, the frequency with which intrauterine infection occurs in still uncertain, and whether the efficiency of transmission varies according to gestational age is completely unknown. The Public Health Laboratory Service (PHLS) Working Party on Fifth Disease conducted a prospective but uncontrolled study of 193 women with serologically confirmed B19 infection.[144] It estimated that the fetal infection rate was 33% based on a combination of DNA hybridization studies of a sample of abortuses, neonatal anti-B19 IgM determinations, and persistence of specific IgG at about 1 year of age. An important observation in that study was that screening the newborn for specific IgM antibodies was a very insensitive way of determining fetal infection, when compared with persistence of specific IgG beyond infancy. These investigators found that only 3 (17%) of 18 infants with persistence of specific IgG antibodies to approximately 1 year of age had been anti-B19 IgM positive in the newborn period. This confirms the observations of others who have demonstrated intrauterine B19 infection by detection of fetal IgM, viral particles, or DNA in prenatal specimens but have then been unable to find IgM in blood obtained at birth.[140, 145–150] Two infants in the PHLS study who were anti-B19 IgM positive in the neonatal period were found to lack specific IgM and IgG on follow-up at about 1 year. This finding has been confirmed by other investigators[151] and suggests there is no single, sensitive marker of intrauterine infection that can be used clinically in infancy to identify those who were infected in utero. *[Koch and colleagues[151a] followed 43 pregnant women with primary B19 infection to delivery. All of the women delivered healthy infants at term; none were hydropic or had other signs of congenital infection. Parvovirus B19 specific IgM was detected in 11, IgA in 10, and B19 DNA (by PCR) in 11 of the 43 infants. One infant was negative at birth but became positive for IgM, IgA, and PCR at 6 weeks of age. Intrauterine infection occurred in all trimesters. Results from serologic and DNA studies showed that 22 of the 43 (51%) infants born to acutely infected mothers developed infection. Among 56 infants born to infected women from Barcelona, all had IgG antibody but only 6 (10.7%) were also positive for IgM; none had congenital anomalies at follow-up at 1 year of age. Thus, many infants are infected in utero but are asymptomatic at birth.]*

ADVERSE REPRODUCTIVE OUTCOMES

Fetal Death

B19 was first recognized as a cause of intrauterine fetal death in 1984.[15] Its importance as a cause of fetal death has not been established with certainty, but the limited data available suggest that the overall contribution may be small. However, there are several important limitations to consider when interpreting these serologic studies. Because maternal anti-B19 IgM antibodies may not be detectable at the time of fetal death, serologic studies of maternal blood collected at diagnosis of death or at delivery may tend to underestimate the contribution of B19 to fetal mortality.[152] In a case-control study of 192 women with fetal deaths, half occurring before 20 weeks' gestation and half after, and controls matched by maternal age and timing of specimen collection in pregnancy, there was serologic evidence of acute B19 infection in 1% of both case and control groups.[139] The prevalence of IgG antibodies was also similar, suggesting that the failure to find a difference between the two groups was not a result of waning maternal IgM antibodies. The authors concluded that the proportion of fetal deaths attributed to B19 infection was unlikely to exceed 3% in cases not selected for parvovirus exposure.[130] In another study, 5 (6.3%) of 80 women with spontaneous abortions between 4 and 17 weeks' gestation had anti-B19 IgM antibodies, compared with 2 [2%] of 100 controls.[142] There were too few observations in the study for a small difference like this to reach statistical significance. Additionally, these investigators studied the products of conception for the five seropositive cases and found B19 DNA in only two, raising the question of whether B19 had caused the fetal deaths. Other studies attempting to look at the importance of B19 as a cause of fetal death have been even smaller or uncontrolled.[80, 152] Larger, controlled studies will be necessary to better define the role of B19 as a cause of fetal death and should also specifically evaluate its contribution in the setting of widespread community outbreak activity.

Most pregnancies complicated by maternal B19 infection result, however, in the delivery of a normal-appearing newborn at term, and the majority of intrauterine infections will probably go unrecognized. Early estimates of fetal mortality were unrealistically high because the studies failed to exclude women screened for B19 infection because of preexisiting fetal disease. The PHLS study was the first prospective study of pregnant women with laboratory-confirmed infection but no evidence of fetal disease at enrollment.[144] These investigators identified 193 anti-B19 IgM positive women and obtained outcome information on 190. Four pregnancies were terminated, and fetal death was reported in 30 (16%) of the remaining 186 pregnancies. Of 14 abortuses examined, viral DNA was detected by hybridization in 6, and the findings were equivocal in 2. Assuming that the findings were representative of all the fetal deaths and that the two equivocal cases were positive, the authors estimated that the B19-associated fetal mortality rate was 9%. In a prospective study of 39 pregnant women infected with B19 during a community-wide outbreak in Connecticut, there were two fetal deaths, and only one (3%) was attributable to B19 infection.[154] Preliminary data from studies in progress at the Centers for Disease Control and Prevention, and in Germany, are in agreement with these studies.[140, 155] *[Among women followed prospectively during pregnancy, there was no evidence of fetal damage in 43 Virginia infants and one fetal loss among 56 pregnancies in women from Barcelona.]*

Nonimmune Fetal Hydrops

B19 was first recognized as a cause of nonimmune fetal hydrops in 1984 when an asymptomatic woman was found to have a B19-infected hydropic fetus during the course of an evaluation of an elevated maternal serum alpha-fetoprotein level.[14] Subsequently, it has been recognized that B19 infection may be a common cause of nonimmune fetal hydrops, especially during community outbreaks of erythema infectiosum. Ten cases of B19-associated hydrops, representing 8% of all cases of nonimmune hydrops and 27% of anatomically normal cases of nonimmune hydrops, were seen in a 17-year period in one hospital series from England.[156] In a consecutive series of 72 patients with nonimmune hydrops from Germany, 3 (4.2%) had B19 infection.[157] In a series of 673 fetal and neonatal autopsies conducted in a 6-year period in Rhode Island, 32 (0.7%) cases of hydrops were identified, and 5 (16%) of these had histologic and laboratory evidence of B19 infection.[158, 159]

It does not follow, however, that intrauterine B19 infection frequently causes nonimmune hydrops. Despite early reports that gave the impression that nonimmune fetal hydrops was a common consequence of maternal B19 infections,[160] prospective studies have shown that it may not be very common. In the PHLS study, 1 of the 156 live-born infants had been diagnosed with intrauterine hydrops and recovered after intrauterine transfusion; and of the six fatal cases that were positive for B19 DNA, hydrops was present in one of three fatal cases with laboratory confirmed intrauterine infection.[144, 145] The adequacy of the postmortem examination to identify hydropic changes may be questionable in some cases of early fetal loss, but these data suggest that nonimmune hydrops is a less common outcome than had previously been thought.

Birth Defects

Experimental and natural infections with many of the animal parvoviruses are associated with birth defects.[161-164] In particular, central nervous system (CNS) malformations can be reproducibly induced in susceptible animals by inoculation in utero or in the perinatal period. Inoculation of newborn hamsters or rats with rat virus (RV) may result in infection and depletion of the external granular cell layer and produce cerebellar hypoplasia.[165] This animal system has been exploited by researchers studying the growth and development of the cerebellum. Infection of newborn kittens with the feline panleukopenia virus may also result in cerebellar hypoplasia and ataxia.

There is growing circumstantial evidence that intrauterine B19 infection may also be a cause of birth defects in some cases. The first convincing evidence that B19 could have a teratogenic effect in humans was presented in 1987.[16] An abortus at 11 weeks' gestation was described with striking ocular abnormalities including microphthalmia, aphakia and dysplatic changes of the cornea, sclera, and choroid of one eye, and retinal folds and degeneration of the lens in the other eye.[166, 167] Other pathologic findings were consistent with intrauterine B19 infection, and the mother had a history of a rash illness with arthropathy at 6 weeks that was serologically confirmed. Despite these suggestive findings, there have been few additional reports of malformations or developmental abnormalities in abortuses or live-born infants following intrauterine infection, and the few cases that have been described could not be unequivocally attributed to infection with B19.[144, 148, 150, 156, 158, 168-173]

However, there has been a preliminary report describing three live-born infants with severe central nervous system abnormalities after serologically confirmed maternal B19 infection.[174] This report raises the possibility of long-term neurologic sequelae in surviving infants that may not be clinically evident at birth in some cases. The most severely affected infant was born at term with arthrogryposis after a pregnancy complicated by a maternal rash illness at approximately 24 weeks and polyhydramnios at 29 weeks Neuroimaging studies showed cerebral atrophy, reduction in size of the brain stem and cerebellum, probable dysgenesis of the corpus callosum, uniform enlargement of the ventricles, and calcification of the basal ganglia and thalamus bilaterally (Fig. 16–1). The infant died in the first week, and histo-

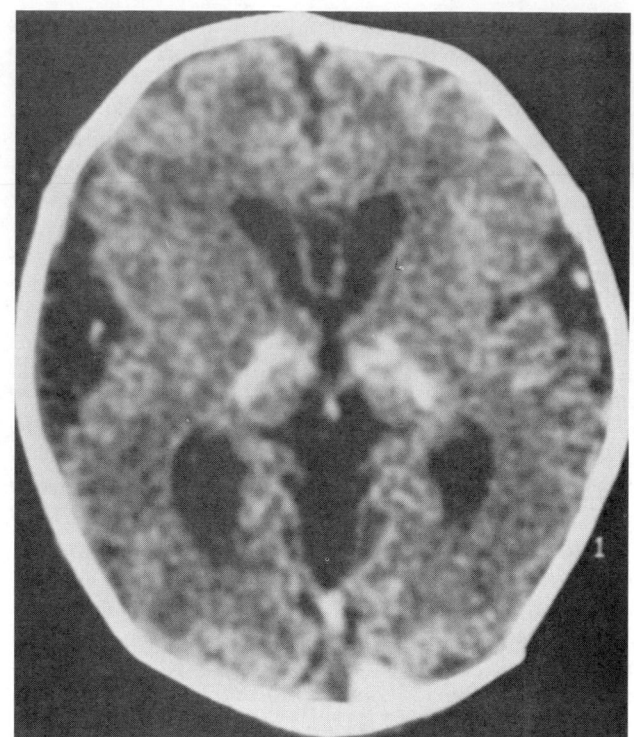

FIGURE 16–1 Computed tomography scan demonstrating atrophy, ventricular enlargement, and dense calcifications of the basal ganglia and thalami in a term infant with arthrogryposis and pregnancy complicated by maternal B19 infection.

pathologic examination showed atrophy, widespread dysplasia, extensive mineralization of the basal ganglia and thalami, and focal destruction of spinal cord anterior horn neurons. B19 DNA was present in tissue. In the second case, the pregnancy was complicated by a maternal illness within polyarthropathy at 18 weeks and fetal hydrops at 22 weeks, which spontaneously resolved; the infant was delivered at term. Neonatal hypotonia was the first neurologic abnormality noted, but the subsequent course has been complicated by cerebral palsy, developmental delay, and infantile spasms. Neuroimaging studies showed uniform enlargement of the ventricles, small periventricular calcifications, cortical dysplasia with pachygyria and polymicrogyria, and periventricular hypodensities (Fig. 16–2). In the third case, the patient had a febrile illness at 23 weeks' gestation, and a fetal ultrasound examination at 25 weeks showed hydrops with ascites, pleural effusions, and skin edema. The fetus was transfused in utero, recovered, and then was born at term. A neurologic examination was normal, but a computed tomographic scan of the brain showed periventricular calcifications (Fig. 16–3). On follow-up, the child had significant developmental delay and benign external hydrocephalus. These cases do not prove that B19 was the cause of the CNS defect; however, they should be the catalyst for additional studies, including those with longer, and more intensive, follow-up of live-born infants exposed in utero for developmental and late-onset manifestations.

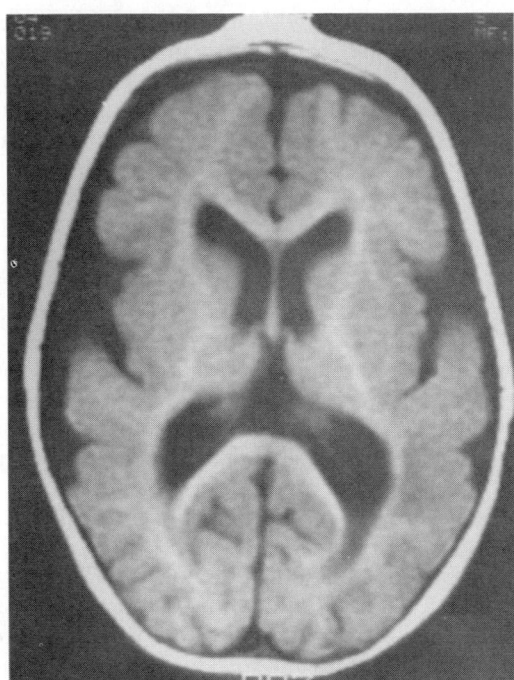

FIGURE 16–2 Magnetic resonance imaging scan demonstrating ventriculomegaly, diffuse cortical dysplasia (probable pachygyria and polymicrogyria), and myelination delay in a 7-month-old infant with cerebral palsy, infantile spasms, and developmental delay following B19-associated fetal hydrops.

There are currently no epidemiologic data available that show an association between intrauterine B19 infection and an increased risk of birth defects among live-born infants. There have been very few studies, and none of them have included enough patients to detect even modest increases in risk; and some are flawed because of failure to include a control population, absence of a comprehensive protocol to evaluate the newborn, and no long-term follow-up of children exposed in utero to identify delayed manifestations. Under the best of circumstances, this is currently a challenging problem to study because limited availability of diagnostic testing has made it difficult to identify a large group of B19-infected women, especially early in pregnancy when the risk of teratogenesis may be greatest. Additionally, the fetal infection rate after maternal infection is not well defined yet and, depending on the magnitude, many infants not exposed in utero could be incorrectly categorized in studies based on serologic evidence of maternal infection alone. This would tend to minimize the apparent risk. Finally, as noted previously, there are no sensitive laboratory markers that could be used to identify most children infected in utero at the time of delivery or in infancy.

With these major limitations in mind, there are currently no data suggesting that B19 is an important cause of birth defects in live-born infants. In an uncontrolled study of 243 infants younger than 4 months of age with birth defects, none had anti-B19 IgM antibodies detected.[138] In a controlled study of 57 infants with structural abnormalities or stigmata of congenital infec-

tion, specific IgM was not detected in cord blood of any of the affected infants or of the matched normal newborn controls.[139] Conversely, there are no data suggesting that structural defects are common in newborns after maternal B19 infection. After a large community-wide outbreak of erythema infectiosum, there was no increase in reports of congenital malformations compared with the pre-epidemic and postepidemic periods.[63] In the PHLS study, outcomes were available for 186 patients; anencephaly was reported in 1 of the 30 fatal cases but not attributed to B19 infection, and hypospadias was present in 2 of the 156 live-born infants.[144] No new anomalies or serious neurodevelopmental problems were detected in the 114 infants followed clinically for at least 1 year, although one had recurrent severe respiratory tract disease and a second had cystic fibrosis. In another prospective, but uncontrolled, study of 39 pregnancies complicated by maternal B19 infection, hypospadias was reported in 1 of the 37 live-born infants, and no abnormalities were reported in the one fatal case for which tissues were available.[154]

POSTNATAL INFECTION

Vertical transmission through breast-feeding has not been reported, and B19 excretion in human milk has not been studied. The autonomous parvovirus rat virus is shed in the milk of infected lactating rats.[175, 176] Whether the infant is at any increased clinical risk from B19 infection acquired in infancy has not been determined because so few cases have been recognized and reported.

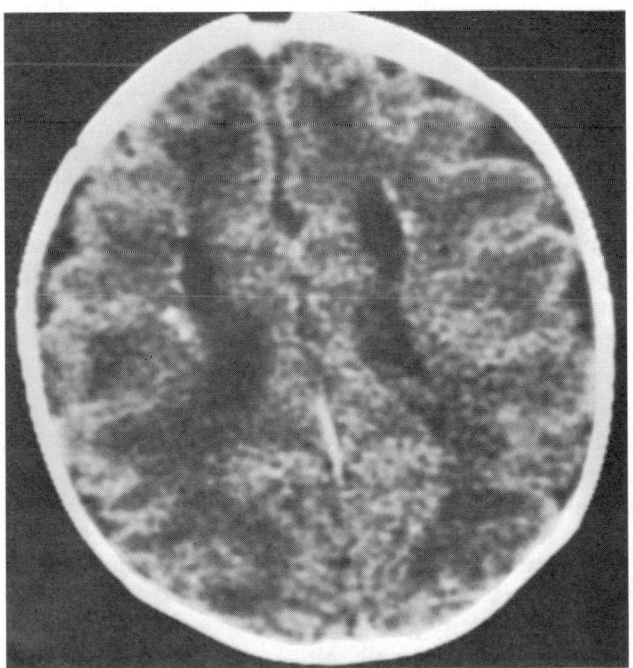

FIGURE 16–3 Computed tomography scan demonstrating periventricular calcifications in a neonate with developmental delay and benign external hydrocephalus following B19-associated fetal hydrops.

PATHOGENESIS AND IMMUNITY

General Considerations

Most of what is known about the pathogenesis of B19 infection comes from small studies of human volunteers and careful evaluation of selected patients.[65, 125, 128, 177, 178] The early events after natural infection are unknown. Entry into the host probably occurs through mucosal surfaces. B19 is found in the respiratory secretions of viremic patients,[101, 104, 111, 125–128] and infection follows intranasal inoculation experimentally.[125, 128] There is no known local replication within the mucosa or gut. Human erythroid progenitor cells in the bone marrow are the principal target cells, and infection results in lysis and aplasia. Most of the commonly recognized clinical manifestations associated with infection may be attributed directly to red cell aplasia or the immune response. In the normal host, B19 infection generally produces a transient decrease in red cell production that is not clinically recognizable. Instead, the illness is typically biphasic and begins with a mild nonspecific illness associated with the viremic phase. Subsequent onset of rash illness or arthropathy is coincident with detectable anti-B19 IgM and IgG antibodies in serum, which suggests that these symptoms are mediated immunologically. Severe symptomatic anemia, so-called aplastic crisis, occurs in persons with hematologic disorders characterized by decreased red cell production or increased red cell destruction. In immunodeficient patients, B19 infection can be persistent and produce chronic anemia. The special case of the fetus is considered in detail later in the chapter.

The time course of infection and host immune response has been characterized in volunteer studies.[125] Symptoms including fever, malaise, headache, coryza, and myalgias begin 5 to 7 days after intranasal inoculation. These prodromal symptoms peak about day 9 coincident with the peak in viremia, but they may be so mild that they are overlooked clinically. Specific IgM antibodies may be detected approximately 10 days after inoculation, and IgG is detectable 2 to 3 days later. Rash or arthropathy may develop at approximately 18 days after inoculation, and these symptoms usually resolve within several days of onset. In some cases, viral DNA can be detected in respiratory secretions for several days after rash onset by DNA hybridization studies or with the PCR assay, but the risk of infectivity is probably very low.[111, 127] Serum samples collected from infected volunteers were infectious in vitro for cultured erythrocyte precursor cells only from day 3 through 10 after intranasal inoculation, and the decrease in infectivity was associated with appearance of anti-B19 IgM antibodies.[178]

In convalescent sera, neutralizing antibodies to both VP1 and VP2 are found, but antibodies to VP2 predominate early after infection.[179] The subsequent appearance of neutralizing antibodies to VP1 is associated in vivo with protection. Antigenic sites of VP1 and VP2 have been characterized.[33, 51, 180–184] The presence of anti-B19 IgG antibodies is associated with clinical protection, and reinfection has been infrequently demonstrated.[122, 125, 185]

One human volunteer with low levels of specific IgG antibody developed a transient viremia and IgM response after intranasal inoculation; IgG levels increased by day 6 after inoculation, characteristic of a secondary response.[125] One woman with a B19-associated fetal loss had anti-B19 IgG antibodies detected in serum samples 24 months and 5 months before the abortion, suggesting the possibility of reinfection or chronic infection.[185] Asymptomatic reinfection was noted in a child after renal transplantation.[122] A serologically confirmed infection had been documented before transplantation, but at the time of exposure and reinfection, specific IgG antibodies were no longer detectable. During the convalescent phase, there was a brisk IgG response and low levels of IgM. Patients with chronic B19 infection presumably are unable to produce neutralizing antibody.[179] The importance of a cellular immune response is unclear.

In the peripheral blood, reticulocytes will decrease and disappear entirely 8 to 10 days after inoculation, with recovery and rebound reticulocytosis 1 to 2 weeks after the nadir. The hemoglobin may drop 2 to 3 g/dl over the course of the illness in the normal host, reaching its lowest point 2 to 3 weeks after inoculation and returning to normal levels within 2 months. Modest decreases in platelets, neutrophils, and lymphocytes occur, and the effect is maximal coincident with viremia; these values usually do not fall much below laboratory normals if at all. In the bone marrow, the earliest findings are macroerythroblastic changes beginning about day 6, with some cytoplasmic vacuolation. By day 10, there is a dramatic loss in erythroid cells at all stages of development. A few abnormally large proerythroblasts may be found. These cells may sometimes be greater than 100 μm in diameter and have prominent irregular nucleoli, and the cytoplasm may be vacuolated with pseudopod formation. Myeloid and megakaryocyte cell lines are generally normal. Hemophagocytosis by macrophages may be observed in some patients.[186] Bone marrow collected during the recovery phase is characterized by a rebound erythroblastosis.

In vitro cultivation studies originally suggested that the erythroid colony-forming unit and burst-forming unit cells were susceptible to productive infection.[104, 128, 187–189] More recently, co-labeling experiments of B19 cultured in vitro suggest that the majority of cells containing B19 nucleic acid express glycophorins A and C, CD43, and CD36, indicating that more mature cells, proerythroblasts, or erythroblasts are the principal site of B19 replication.[190] Two different cytopathic effects have been reported. The greatest concentration of viral nucleic acid is located in erythroblasts characterized by margination of chromatin with intranuclear viral inclusions; these cells resemble the typical inclusion-bearing cells found in hydropic fetuses. Giant proerythroblasts contain relatively little viral nucleic acid, suggesting that these cells display a toxic effect of infection and are not necessarily a site of viral replication.[190] Ultrastructure studies of erythroid cells infected in vitro show changes characteristic of apoptosis—programmed cell death—including viral crystalline arrays, nucleolar degeneration, margination of nuclear heterochromatin, and cytoplasmic vacuolation.[191]

The effect of B19 on nonerythroid cells and the reason for the other cytopenias are less certain. Several independent mechanisms may be responsible for the decrease in platelet count. A direct cytopathic effect is suggested by the finding of abnormally small, vacuolated megakaryocytes in some bone marrow samples.[192] Some studies, but not all, show that megakaryocyte colony formation is inhibited in vitro by B19 infection.[178, 190, 193, 194] Low levels of viral RNA are detectable, but the effect occurs in the absence of detectable viral DNA replication, and it can be reversed by mutation of the gene encoding NS1. Hypersplenism in patients with chronic hemolytic anemia could increase peripheral destruction of platelets. Finally, some reports suggest that platelet destruction may be mediated immunologically. There is evidence that B19 has an inhibitory effect on myeloid colony growth that is abolished by convalescent-phase serum or immunoglobulin.[194] Viral nucleic acids may be found in the cytoplasm of macrophages.[190]

Pathogenesis of Fetal and Congenital Disease

Infection of the fetus occurs through transplacental passage of infectious virus. B19 infection presents an extraordinary risk to the fetus. The fetus is particularly vulnerable to the effects of B19-associated red cell aplasia because it must increase its red cell mass greatly to meet growth requirements—about 34-fold between the third and sixth month—and fetal red cell survival is relatively short, with a life span of between 45 and 70 days.[195] These effects may be potentiated by the failure of the immature fetal immune system to clear the virus, which results in prolonged infection. Specific fetal IgM first becomes detectable in serum at approximately 18 weeks' gestation.[196] The importance of the fetal immune response is suggested by the finding of decreased rates of fetal death after 20 weeks and by demonstration that fetal serum collected at 21 weeks' gestational age is inhibitory in vitro.[144, 178] Finally, there is some evidence that other replicating cell populations may be susceptible to B19 infection. Virus has been demonstrated occasionally in situ in fetal myocytes, including myocardiocytes, along with inflammatory changes, but the clinical importance of fetal myocarditis is less certain.[129, 169, 197] Histologic studies have demonstrated evidence of vascular damage and perivascular infiltrates in some tissues. Whether this is a result of specific infection in endothelial cells or a nonspecific effect related to hypoxic damage is unclear. Similarly, the finding of dystrophic calcification in some organs and mineralization in the brain could be caused either indirectly by hypoxia or by direct tissue invasion.

Nonimmune hydrops is the best understood fetal complication of B19 infection. Several possible pathogenic mechanisms have been proposed, and more than one may contribute.[156] The most consistent finding, present in the majority of cases at the time of diagnosis, is severe fetal anemia. Hemoglobin levels below 2 g/dl have been found by cordocentesis of hydropic fetuses.[198, 199] Hypoxic injury to tissues may result in increased capillary permeability. Chronic, severe anemia may also increase cardiac output, as evidenced by increases in umbilical venous pressure, and subsequently result in high-output heart failure.[147] Alternatively, myocarditis may precipitate heart failure. Diminished fetal myocardial function has been demonstrated by echocardiography in some cases in association with fetal hydrops.[200] Regardless of the etiology, congestive heart failure could cause an increase in capillary hydrostatic pressure. Decreased venous return caused by massive ascites or organomegaly may lead to further cardiac decompensation. Hepatic function may be compromised by the extreme levels of extramedullary hematopoiesis, and lysis of B19-infected erythrocytes in the liver may cause hemosiderin deposition, fibrosis, and esophageal varices.[201, 202] Impaired production of albumin could lead to a decrease in colloid osmotic pressure with transfer of fluid to the extravascular compartment. Placental hydrops may further compromise oxygen delivery to the fetus.

PATHOLOGIC FINDINGS IN THE FETUS AND NEWBORN

There have only been a few reports of autopsy case series with detailed descriptions of the gross and microscopic findings associated with intrauterine B19 infection.[156, 158, 203, 204] Most of the available information comes from review of individual case reports of fetal or perinatal death.[170, 202, 205–209] Because of the well-documented association between B19, fetal anemia, and nonimmune hydrops, and the greater difficulty of diagnosing hydrops early in pregnancy, reports of late fetal deaths associated with hydrops are overrepresented in published accounts. The majority of B19-associated fetal deaths occur before 20 weeks' gestation.[140, 144, 155] Whether the pathologic findings or pathogenesis of fetal disease is different earlier in pregnancy is uncertain but needs further evaluation.

The most commonly reported abnormalities on external examination of the abortus include pallor, maceration, and subcutaneous edema. Foci of extramedullary hematopoiesis in the skin—so-called blueberry muffin rash—have been reported rarely.[149] Dysmorphic features have been reported only rarely and usually regarded as being incidental.[156, 173, 208, 210] Excess fluid in one or more body cavities is reported often and may be noted even in the absence of visible subcutaneous edema. Pallor of the viscera and organs and enlargement of the liver, spleen, and heart are the other most frequently reported internal abnormalities. The other organs are generally not increased in size, and some, like the thymus, may be abnormally small. Descriptions of some organs, especially the brain, have been very limited. This is because the number of samples suitable for study is decreased by the rapid rate of autolysis after fetal death; it is technically difficult to identify and interpret subtle fetal abnormalities; and there may be a reluctance of the pathologist to perform, or parents to permit, a complete autopsy. Considerable work remains to be performed before the complete range of pathologic manifestations associated with intrauterine infection has been catalogued.

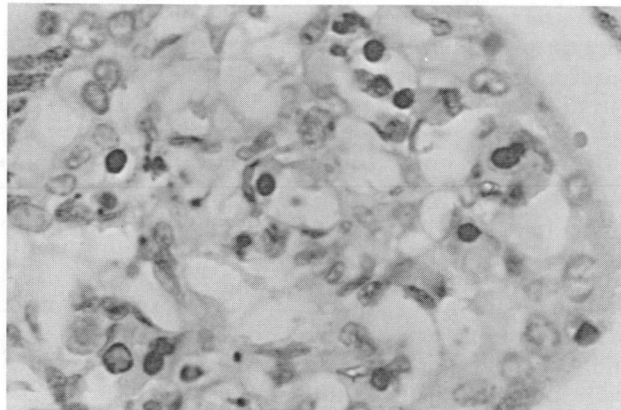

FIGURE 16–4 Placenta from a case of B19-associated nonimmune hydrops showing fetal capillaries filled with erythroblasts, most with marginated chromatin and typical amphophilic intranuclear inclusions. Hematoxylin and eosin stain.

The most characteristic and specific finding suggestive of B19 infection on histologic examination is the presence of nucleated red cells with amphophilic intranuclear inclusions (Figs. 16–4 and 16–5). Affected cells typically are found within the lumen of vessels in any organ, or in the parenchyma in sites of extramedullary hematopoiesis, chiefly in the liver.[129] With hematoxylin and eosin stain, the nuclei have a marginated, slightly irregular band of darkly staining chromatin, and the center of the nucleus is lighter in color and appears to have a smooth, glassy texture. The sensitivity of finding viral inclusions for diagnosis of fetal infection is unknown, but it is probably high when there are findings associated with anemia and hydrops. Cellular degenerative changes sometimes may be difficult to distinguish from the specific cytopathic effects caused by B19 by routine histologic examination. Uptake of stain by B19-affected cell nuclei may be relatively homogeneous and look like nonspecific pyknotic degeneration. Viral DNA

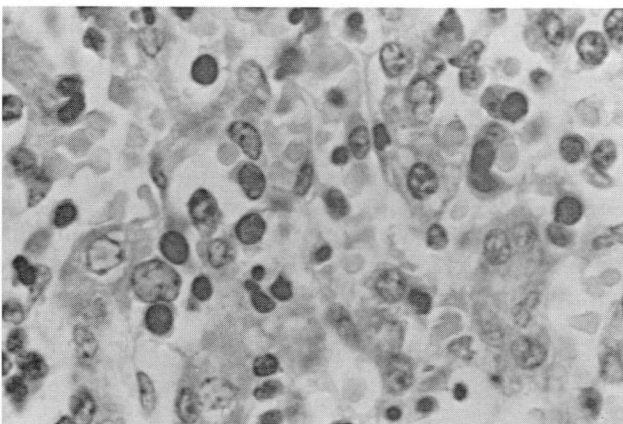

FIGURE 16–5 Fetal liver from a case of B19-associated nonimmune hydrops showing extramedullary hematopoiesis, intranuclear inclusions in erythroblasts, and focal areas with hemosiderin and fibrosis. Hematoxylin and eosin stain.

or inclusions have also been identified in tissue macrophages[129, 190] and myocytes.[169, 197]

A careful examination of the placenta is one of the most useful, but probably underappreciated and underutilized, procedures for the evaluation of a suspected case of intrauterine B19 infection. The placenta may be markedly enlarged with hydropic changes. In vascular spaces, nucleated red blood cells with typical intranuclear inclusions may be recognized by hematoxylin and eosin staining (see Fig. 16–4). Several planes should be examined because inclusion-bearing cells may not be distributed uniformly throughout. Placental erythroblastosis may be present and provide an important clue. Inflammatory changes of the placental vasculature, including the cord, have been reported in some cases.[156, 200, 208] Vasculitis of villous capillaries or stem arteries was present in 9 of 10 placentas reported in one series.[156] There was swelling of endothelial cells, fragmentation of endothelial cell nuclei, and fibrin thrombi, but so far B19 DNA has not been demonstrated to be in endothelial cells.[129] Perivascular infiltrates are composed predominantly of mononuclear cells. The number of inclusion-bearing cells or cells containing B19 DNA by in situ hybridization was found to be less in the placenta than in other organs in one study, but the availability and applicability to live-born infants with hydrops make the placental examination of unmatched value.[129]

The pathologic findings pertaining to the liver have been characterized the best.[129, 156, 170, 201, 202, 205, 211] It is generally enlarged and pale, extramedullary hematopoiesis may be markedly increased, and viral inclusions are usually found in nucleated red blood cells (see Fig. 16–5). Erythrophagocytosis by hepatic macrophages has been demonstrated in several cases. There may be considerable hemosiderin deposition, and hepatic stores of ferric iron may be increased, presumably because of hemolysis of B19-infected erythrocytes. Esophageal varices have been reported in some cases with severe liver disease.

Fetal anemia is a prominent finding in most fatal cases, but not in all.[169, 172, 198, 199, 201, 202, 207, 212, 213] The bone marrow generally shows marked erythroid hypoplasia or, less often, hyperplasia characteristic of recovery. The spleen may be enlarged and an important site of extramedullary hematopoiesis. The thymus has been infrequently described, but reported abnormalities include decreased organ size, cortical lymphocyte depletion consistent with severe intrauterine stress, and, correcting for gestational age, an increase in the number and size of Hassall's corpuscles.[129, 156, 205, 208] Cells containing viral DNA are located in the periphery of the lobules unrelated to Hassall's corpuscles.

The knowledge that canine parvovirus can cause acute and chronic myocarditis in puppies[214] and the early observation that cardiac enlargement was present in some B19-infected fetuses with hydrops have generated considerable interest in the pathologic findings in the heart.[129, 156, 158, 169, 170, 196, 197, 200, 215] The evidence collected so far suggests that B19-associated fetal heart disease may be caused by both direct and indirect mechanisms, with the latter predominating. Grossly, the heart may be normal or symmetrically enlarged and pale, suggesting biventricular congestive heart failure. Pericardial effusions are common. Myocytes with intranuclear inclusions have been identified in some cases but do not seem to be very common. Mononuclear cell infiltrates have been reported in some cases, either diffusely or perivascularly, and B19 DNA, not associated with cells, can be found in the lumen of large vessels. As a response to injury, focal areas with dystrophic calcification or fibroelastosis have been demonstrated. Anomalies of the heart, including conus defects, tricuspid valve dysplasia, and muscular ventricular septal wall defects, have been occasionally reported in association with B19 but have not been etiologically linked.

Descriptions of other organ systems are limited. Dystrophic calcification suggesting tissue injury has been reported in brain and adrenal glands.[170, 174, 205] Abnormalities of the CNS, including anencephaly, ventriculomegaly and motor developmental delay, have been reported but not clearly related to B19 infection.[144, 148, 168, 169] Pulmonary hypoplasia may result from accumulation of pleural fluid, and intranuclear inclusions may be found in red cells intravascularly.[205] Hypospadias and cleft lip have been reported occasionally.[144, 173] Meconium peritonitis has been reported in both fatal and surviving cases.[150, 171, 172]

CLINICAL FEATURES

The clinical expression of B19 infection is greatly modified in the presence of a variety of preexisting medical conditions. In the normal host, infection is self-limited and frequently asymptomatic, or associated with a rash illness or arthropathy. Patients with hematologic conditions characterized by decreased red cell production (e.g., thalassemia) or increased red cell destruction or loss (e.g., sickle cell disease) may be extremely vulnerable to the red cell aplasia caused by a self-limited B19 infection. They may present with signs and symptoms of severe anemia. Some patients (e.g., persons with lymphoproliferative and immunodeficiency disorders) may be unable to mount an effective immune response and may develop prolonged or chronic infections. The clinical presentation may be variable in this population, but chronic anemia is the problem most often recognized. The fetus suffers from both red cell aplasia and persistence. Finally, B19 has been linked to sporadic cases of hemophagocytic syndrome, myocarditis, central and peripheral nervous system disease, and systemic necrotizing vasculitis, although host factors that might predispose patients to these manifestations have not been defined.

Asymptomatic Infection

Most infections with B19 may not be clinically recognized. Investigations of school outbreaks of erythema infectiosum using anti-B19 IgM determinations have reported that from 26 to 89% of students, and that more than 50% of adult employees, may not be symptomatic with either rash or arthropathy.[106, 109, 111–113] In an outbreak of erythema infectiosum on a pediatric ward, 9

(64%) of 14 children with serologic evidence of acute infection did not have a rash illness.[117] Similar findings have been reported in studies of secondary transmission in households. In a study of household contacts of patients with erythema infectiosum, only 53% of anti-B19 IgM positive patients reported a rash illness and 33% had joint pains.[102]

Signs and symptoms of B19 infection may not be evident even in high-risk patients. In a cohort study of 114 patients with homozygous sickle cell disease and B19 infection diagnosed by seroconversion or detection of viral DNA, 91 (80%) developed typical aplastic crisis, but mild disease or asymptomatic infection was reported in 23 (20%).[72] The differences were not explained by prior transfusion or persistence of fetal hemoglobin.

Erythema Infectiosum (Fifth Disease) and Other Cutaneous Manifestations

The rash illness erythema infectiosum is the most frequently recognized manifestation of B19 infection. It was defined as a clinical entity, separate from scarlet fever, measles, or rubella, by the end of the nineteenth century,[54] and there are some descriptions of a compatible rash illness dating back to at least 1800.[216] Its unfortunate alias, fifth disease, refers to a schema established in the early 1900s to enumerate the rash illnesses of childhood.[217] In this system, the first two diseases were scarlet fever and measles (although many references disagree on the order of the first two), third disease was rubella, and fourth disease was subsequently shown to be nonexistent.[218, 219] Use of the term fifth disease has become more popular in recent years for reasons that are unclear. The etiologic link between erythema infectiosum and B19 infection was made in 1983 when serologic evidence of acute infection was reported from children with rash illness during a school outbreak.[13, 105] Subsequent investigations of erythema infectiosum outbreaks confirmed that B19 was the etiologic agent.[101]

The most distinctive feature of erythema infectiosum is an intensely erythematous maculopapular facial rash that affects the cheeks but generally spares the bridge of the nose and circumoral region. Erythema infectiosum is sometimes called "slapped cheek" disease because the flushed appearance of the cheeks looks as though they were just slapped. The trunk and extremities are affected with an erythematous maculopapular rash that becomes reticulated or lacelike as the central regions begin to fade. In some patients, either the facial rash or the body rash may be predominant, or be present in the absence of the other. Data from outbreak investigations suggest that the facial and trunk rashes develop concurrently.[220] The soles and palms are occasionally noted to be involved.[101] The rash may be intensely pruritic, but this seems to be a highly variable feature. Pruritus has been reported in as many as 70% of cases in some investigations.[63, 220] Another interesting feature of the rash is recurrence after exposure to heat or cold in the first few weeks after onset. Onset of the rash occurs coincident with production of B19-specific antibodies, suggesting that it is immune mediated. Biopsy findings have been infrequently described. Immune complex deposition was suggested in one case by the finding of C3 in blood vessel walls.[221] The duration of illness in most cases is less than 10 days.[63] In addition to the classic appearance of erythema infectiosum, a variety of other cutaneous manifestations of B19 infection have been well documented in laboratory-confirmed cases, including vesicular, petechial or purpuric, and desquamative rashes.[222–228] Many of these cases were detected during the course of outbreaks of erythema infectiosum, suggesting that the manifestations are not strain specific.

Arthropathy and Other Rheumatologic Manifestations

Arthralgias, sometimes accompanied by inflammatory changes of the symptomatic joints, are a common manifestation of acute B19 infection and frequently are reported in persons with erythema infectiosum.[229] An association between erythema infectiosum and acute joint disease had been suggested from outbreak investigations of erythema infectiosum, but the first reports providing laboratory confirmation of an etiologic link came in 1985, two years after B19 had been discovered to be the etiology of erythema infectiosum.[11, 12] The incidence of joint disease among adults with erythema infectiosum may exceed 50%, but it generally occurs in fewer than 10% of children.[63, 230] B19 infection may also be a common cause of acute arthropathy in adults and children and may be the sole manifestation of acute infection in many cases. In two studies, the proportion of adults with anti-B19 IgM antibodies presenting to an early synovitis clinic was 12%, and less than 25% had a concurrent rash illness.[11, 231] Twenty (19%) of 104 children presenting with new onset of joint complaints had serologic evidence of recent B19 infection, and only seven (35%) had a history of a concurrent rash illness.[232]

More females with arthropathy have been reported than men, but whether females are at increased risk of developing arthropathy, or are at increased risk of becoming infected or seeking medical care, has not been clearly established.[11, 12, 98] Other than age and possibly female gender, other risk factors for B19-associated arthropathy have not been established. HLA antigens have been studied in a small number of patients with B19-associated arthropathy. The HLA antigen DR4 was found in 12 (67%) of 18 patients with B19-associated arthropathy in one study,[233] but DR4 was found in only one of five patients in another study.[234] HLA B27 was associated with prolonged joint symptoms in a study of seven women.[235] The three women who were HLA-B27 positive had symptoms lasting for 9 months, compared with less than 2 weeks for the other four.

The most common clinical presentation in adults is a symmetrical polyarthropathy affecting the wrists, hands (metacarpophalangeal and proximal interphalangeal joints), and knees.[11, 12] Other joints may be affected but are reported in less than 50% of adults. In children, the knees are the joints most commonly affected and the disease is more likely to be pauciarticular, involving four or fewer joints.[232] The acute arthropathy may be mistaken for Lyme disease.[236] Four (10%) of 40 serum samples submitted from patients with suspected Lyme disease were anti-B19 IgM positive and had acute B19 infection.[237] In some cases, the rash and arthritis associated with B19 infection may resemble adult Still's disease or systemic lupus erythematosus, and this may be complicated by the effect of B19 on preexisting disease.[238–240] One patient with systemic lupus erythematosus had a flare-up after acute B19 infection,[241] and another patient with systemic lupus erythematosus and autoimmune hemolytic anemia developed aplastic crisis.[242]

Most patients note significant symptomatic improvement within 2 weeks and complete resolution within several months, but in some, arthralgias or arthritis may persist for many months to years, and these patients may meet criteria established by the American Rheumatism Association for diagnosis of juvenile rheumatoid arthritis, rheumatoid arthritis, or fibromyalgia.[11, 12, 98, 232, 243] Bone erosions are not evident even with chronic joint involvement. Some patients have been reported with acute B19 infection followed by rheumatoid factor positive rheumatoid arthritis, but no etiologic link has been clearly established and these findings may be coincidental.[231] In a serologic study of 55 HLA-identical, same-sexed sibling pairs, discordant for rheumatoid arthritis, the prevalence of anti-B19 IgG antibodies was not increased for those affected with rheumatoid arthritis.[244] The prevalence of anti-B19 IgG antibodies was similar in patients with rheumatoid arthritis compared with patients with other types of arthritis and normal controls.[245] A report suggesting that B19 DNA may be found in synovium of most patients with rheumatoid arthritis by using the very sensitive PCR technique has not been confirmed in other studies.[245]

Some patients are transiently positive for rheumatoid factor or antinuclear antibodies.[98, 228, 232, 246–249] Complement has been decreased in some patients.[11, 228, 232] Acute infection may be associated with positive laboratory tests for autoimmune disease.[250, 251] In a study of 48 anti-B19 IgM positive patients, 35 (73%) had anti-dsDNA, 28 (58%) had anti-ssDNA antibodies, and 43 (88%) had antilymphocyte IgM antibodies.[251] Joint fluid findings have been described infrequently but are consistent with inflammation.[238, 252–254] B19 DNA has been found in synovial fluid by dot-blot hybridization and in situ hybridization, but local replication has not been demonstrated and not shown to be a factor in pathogenesis.[255, 256]

Like the rash, onset of the arthropathy occurs coincident with the rise in anti-B19 antibodies, suggesting that the cause is related to the host immune response. Persistence of virus is one possible explanation for chronic arthropathy. B19 DNA sequences were detected by PCR in the bone marrow of four patients with arthropathy lasting longer than 2 years and in three patients with self-limited disease screened 2 to 18 months after disease onset.[257] B19 DNA was not found in seven anti-B19 IgG negative or in six anti-B19 IgG positive, IgM negative bone marrow donor controls. Other studies have not suggested an association between duration of symptoms and prolonged viremia or persistence of viral DNA in synovial membrane, cells, or fluid.[229] Attempts to culture B19 in synovial membrane cells have been unsuccessful.[258]

Acute Hematologic Complications

The first disease that was etiologically linked to B19 infection was aplastic crisis, a transient condition characterized by acute onset of anemia associated with pure red cell aplasia. In 1981, six children with sickle cell disease were described with aplastic crisis and laboratory evidence of acute B19 infection.[9] The association of aplastic crisis with B19 infection was quickly confirmed by demonstrating that B19 caused an outbreak of aplastic crisis among patients with sickle cell disease in Jamaica.[10] Subsequent studies have shown that B19 infection can cause aplastic crisis in all patients with chronic hemolytic anemia, regardless of etiology, as well as in patients with other hematologic disorders characterized by abnormally high rates of red cell destruction or decreased production.[259] Aplastic crisis is often the first indication of a disorder of erythropoiesis or red cell survival.[260–262] The proportion of cases of transient aplastic crisis attributable to B19 infection has been estimated to be between 68% and 100%.[72, 102, 263–266] In a study of 53 patients hospitalized with transient aplastic crisis, 36 (68%) had serologic or virologic evidence of acute B19 infection.[266] In the cohort study from Jamaica of 308 children with homozygous sickle cell disease, all 91 aplastic crises were attributable to B19 infection.[72] B19 infection may be subclinical in up to 20% of patients with sickle cell disease.[72]

The natural history of aplastic crisis was well characterized long before the discovery of B19. The term *aplastic crisis* was coined by Owren, who in 1948 meticulously described the clinical course of several affected family members with hereditary spherocytosis.[65] His report included the findings from serial bone marrow examinations and remains one of the best descriptions of the hematologic findings available. Patients with aplastic crisis present with a brief history of a mild upper respiratory tract infection, fever, headache, and malaise and on examination may be pale and tachycardic. Rash is very uncommon. The hemoglobin is significantly decreased compared with baseline values. Few or no reticulocytes are present in the peripheral blood smear. Mild thrombocytopenia and leukopenia are frequently reported. Early in the course, bone marrow examination shows a marked erythroid hypoplasia, and among the few erythroid precursors seen may be giant forms. Other cell lines are unaffected. During the recovery phase, which begins 10 to 12 days after the first onset of symptoms, the reticulocytes will be increased in the peripheral blood smear and there will be a rebound erythroid hyperplasia in the bone marrow. There may be significant morbidity and mortality associated with aplastic crisis. Extensive bone marrow necrosis has been reported,[267, 268] and B19-associated aplastic crises may sometimes precipitate strokes.[269] The mortality rate associated with aplastic crisis was 2.2% in the Jamaican cohort.[72]

A possible etiologic role for B19 has been investigated in patients with other hematologic disorders with mostly negative or inconclusive findings. One patient with aplastic anemia had anti-B19 IgM antibodies, suggesting recent infection; but in another study, none of 11 patients tested had B19 antigen in serum samples and 3 (11%) of 28 had low levels of IgM that were thought to be nonspecific.[270, 271] Because transient thrombocytopenia is frequently seen with acute B19 infection, a possible connection with idiopathic thrombocytopenic purpura has also been looked for. Three (5%) of 61 patients with idiopathic thrombocytopenic purpura had anti-B19 IgM antibodies in one study.[272] Additional sporadic cases have been reported, and whether there is a true association between B19 and idiopathic thrombocytopenic purpura is unresolved.[273–276] At most, it would probably play a minor role. Transient erythroblastopenia of childhood is a disease of unknown etiology and is the most common cause of red cell aplasia in childhood.[277] It has been reported occasionally in association with acute B19 infection.[194, 278, 279] However, in a series of 21 patients with transient erythroblastopenia of childhood, none had viral antigen or specific IgM antibodies, suggesting that B19 is not likely to be the etiology of this disorder.[271]

Chronic Infection

Parvovirus B19 may be an important opportunistic pathogen of patients with congenital[17, 124, 280–282] or acquired immunodeficiency syndromes,[126, 192, 283–293] organ transplant recipients,[1, 100, 119, 122, 294–297] patients with lymphoproliferative disorders,[4, 242, 298–314] and those with other malignancies.[4, 306] In these patients, B19 infection may be prolonged or chronic and signs and symptoms may wax and wane in response to changes in the underlying disease or therapy. Chronic anemia has been the finding reported most often, but pancytopenia is also common. It may be extremely difficult to distinguish the effects of the B19 infection from changes caused by the underlying disease or therapy. Diagnosis is difficult because serologic evidence of infection may be lacking, and even sensitive tests looking for viral DNA may be only intermittently positive, suggesting a low viral burden. Hematologic indices have been shown to improve in chronically infected patients treated with immune globulins.

There have been few epidemiologic studies to estimate the prevalence or incidence of chronic B19 infection in these high-risk patients, but there are some data suggesting that in patients infected with the human immunodeficiency virus (HIV) type 1, B19 may be an important cause of anemia and difficult to distinguish from the cytopenias associated with medications and concurrent illnesses. B19 DNA was not found by dot-blot hybridization in the sera of 50 patients with the acquired immunodeficiency syndrome (AIDS), or in the sera of 20 patients with lymphadenopathy.[315] In 55 HIV-infected patients, B19 DNA was found by dot-blot analysis in 1 (2%), anti-B19 IgM antibodies were found in 8 (15%), and anti-B19 IgG was detected in 33 (60%).[126] By using the more sensitive PCR assay, B19 DNA was found in the sera of 9 (64%) of 14 persons being treated with dideoxyinosine at one institution.[292] Four of the five patients switched from zidovudine to dideoxyinosine because of anemia were DNA positive. In another study of HIV-seropositive patients, B19 DNA was detected using the nested PCR in sera from 7 (26%) of 27 anti-B19 IgM positive patients but was not detected in any of 22 patients without IgM.[316] Dot-blot hybridization was negative for all 7 patients who had positive results by PCR. Further studies are necessary to define the epidemiology and natural history of disease in immunocompromised patients.

Other Conditions Associated with B19 Infection

HEMOPHAGOCYTIC SYNDROME

There are several reports of B19-associated hemophagocytic syndrome.[242, 317, 318] Virus-associated hemophagocytic syndrome is a severe, often life-threatening disease that may be difficult to distinguish from malignant histiocytosis.[319] Hemophagocytosis can also be observed in the bone marrow of patients with acute self-limited B19 infection[186] and in hepatic macrophages in fetal liver.[129, 211] The incidence of hemophagocytic syndrome in B19 infection and the etiologic fraction of virus-associated hemophagocytic syndrome attributable to B19 infection have not been determined.

MYOCARDITIS

Acute myocarditis is an important clinical manifestation of some animal parvovirus infections; and in the human fetus, B19 has been shown to infect myocardial cells in some cases.[129, 169, 197] Whether B19 infection may sometimes produce myocarditis in children or adults is still unclear, but several cases of acute B19 infection and myocarditis have been described. A fatal case of myocarditis was reported in a 1-year-old child after erythema infectiosum.[320, 321] At autopsy, both ventricles were dilated and there was a mononuclear cell infiltrate and myonecrosis. Anti-B19 IgM antibodies were present in the serum, and B19 capsid antigens were detected in myocardial tissue sections by immunocytochemistry, although the authors did not say if the antigens could be localized in situ within myocytes. Transient congestive heart failure was diagnosed in an adult with an acute rash illness and serologic evidence of acute B19 infection.[322]

NEUROLOGIC DISEASE

Neurologic abnormalities have been reported occasionally in children and adults with acute B19 infection, but a causal relationship has not been established with certainty. Peripheral nerve abnormalities, including brachial plexus neuropathies,[323, 324] ulnar nerve paralysis,[325] ophthalmoplegia,[326] and paresthesias and dysesthesias,[327, 328] have been described in conjunction with acute B19 infection. Paresthesias were reported in 5 (45%) of 11 B19-infected nurses with erythema infectiosum in a nosocomial outbreak, and an additional two had paresthesias as the sole manifestation.[327] Three of the infected nurses had paresthesias persisting for more than 1 year, and one had low levels of B19 DNA in serum samples for more than 3 years along with recurrent episodes of paresthesias.[329] Interestingly, the patient was not anemic

during this period. Onset of peripheral nerve signs and symptoms has been coincident with rash and joint pain onset, suggesting that the neurologic abnormalities are immunologically mediated. Aplastic crisis and erythema infectiosum have been associated with sporadic cases of meningitis, encephalopathy, and seizure disorders.[282, 330–334] B19 DNA was detected in cerebrospinal fluid from a patient with pancytopenia and meningitis.[185] Stroke may also complicate B19-associated aplastic crisis.[269]

VASCULITIS

There is increasing evidence of a link between B19 infection and systemic necrotizing vasculitis. Serologic evidence of acute B19 infection has been reported in patients with new onset of hypersensitivity vasculitis, Henoch-Schönlein purpura, polyarteritis nodosa, giant cell arteritis, and Wegener's granulomatosis.[224, 226, 335–340] Two serologic studies have not found anti-B19 IgM antibodies in patients with Kawasaki's disease,[341, 342] but a recurrence of Kawasaki's disease was reported in an HIV-infected infant during an acute B19 infection.[343] Chronic B19 infection was documented in one patient with polyarteritis nodosa, and signs and symptoms of vasculitis resolved following treatment with intravenous immunoglobulin.[338] There was laboratory evidence of B19 infection before treatment of the patient with immunosuppressive drugs, suggesting that infection was not a result of immunosuppressive therapy. A rash typical of erythema infectiosum and anemia were never documented during the course of the patient's illness. This case suggests that B19 has the potential to be an opportunistic pathogen in patients predisposed to systemic necrotizing vasculitis, or that chronic B19 infection may play an etiologic role in the development of vasculitis in some patients. Histologic studies have been infrequently reported, but a skin biopsy of a purpuric lesion in one case demonstrated a leukocytoclastic vasculitis with C3 deposition, suggesting that the findings may be a result of immune complex disease.[226]

INFECTION IN PREGNANCY AND EFFECTS ON THE FETUS AND NEWBORN

The clinical manifestations of B19 infection in the normal pregnant woman are the same as those observed in the normal host. Rash illness and arthropathy are the most commonly recognized manifestations, but most infected women may be asymptomatic or have mild nonspecific findings that are not attributed to B19 infection. There are no data suggesting that the clinical manifestation of B19 infection in the mother influences the pregnancy outcome. There is some evidence for an interaction between the B19-affected fetus and development of maternal hypertensive disorders. Pregnancy-induced hypertension, preeclampsia, and eclampsia have been reported in some women with B19-associated fetal hydrops,[148, 156, 157, 200, 201, 205] and improvement has been seen following spontaneous resolution of hydrops in one case.[200] The pathogenesis of hypertensive disorders of pregnancy is thought to be caused by poor fetoplacental perfusion, and there is an increased risk in pregnancies complicated by hydrops.[344] Controlled studies have not yet determined if there is an increased frequency of hypertensive disorders in B19-infected women compared with uninfected women or whether more careful monitoring of B19-infected women to detect findings of preeclampsia would be useful in identifying women at increased risk of B19-associated fetal hydrops.

Interpretation of data on adverse fetal outcomes after maternal infection with B19 is difficult because the intrauterine infection rate is not known with certainty, and whether the fetal infection rate changes depending on gestational age at the time of maternal infection is unknown. The crude fetal death rate, based on studies of women with serologic evidence of infection, is, as previously discussed, less than 10%.[140, 144, 154, 155] Although the majority of published accounts describe fetal morbidity and mortality occurring late in pregnancy, the fetus is probably most vulnerable early on. In the PHLS study, 93% of the fetal deaths occurred before 20 weeks' gestational age.[144] Fetal loss occurred up to 11 weeks after maternal symptom onset, but 70% occurred in the first 5 weeks. Most fetal losses reported by others have also occurred within 4 to 6 weeks after onset of maternal rash or arthropathy, and only rarely as late as 10 to 12 weeks.[152] Because the majority of cases included in the PHLS report were women identified because they were symptomatic with rash illness and had no evidence of rubella, the extent to which maternal symptoms may influence the outcome has not been determined. Other risk factors for fetal mortality have not been ascertained.

Nonimmune fetal hydrops is the adverse outcome that is most likely to be identified and reported, but the incidence after maternal B19 infection is probably low. In the PHLS study, clinical data were available for three fatal cases that were positive by DNA hybridization, and hydrops was reported in just one.[144] Among the 156 live-born infants, hydrops complicated one pregnancy only.[145] In the Connecticut study, in which 39 women were followed prospectively with ultrasound examinations at 1- to 2-week intervals, no cases of hydrops were detected, including the one fatal case attributed to B19 infection.[154] Both oligohydramnios and polyhydramnios may occur with B19-associated hydrops.[148, 200] There is a strong correlation between hydropic changes and severe fetal anemia as determined by cordocentesis, but not all cases are anemic.* This may reflect either sampling in the hematologic recovery phase or, alternatively, the importance of other mechanisms such as myocarditis in the pathogenesis of the hydrops. In addition to anemia, there may be moderate to severe thrombocytopenia, and this could increase the risk of morbidity associated with cordocentesis.[145, 147, 149, 169, 201, 207, 345, 346] Other causes of a decreased platelet count, such as immune thrombocytopenia, may coexist and should be excluded.[346] The white blood cell count has been reported infrequently in affected fetuses or newborns, but in most cases it has been normal or modestly decreased.[145, 147, 148, 169, 198, 201, 207, 346–348] Other laboratory parameters have been less well studied. Serum bili-

rubin and transaminase levels may be increased or normal.[147, 157, 200]

The natural history of B19-associated nonimmune hydrops is still incompletely characterized. Based on the first descriptions of cases of B19-associated nonimmune hydrops, the outcome was presumed to be uniformly fatal. In response, a number of investigators advocated early intervention with fetal blood sampling and intrauterine transfusion. More recently, however, a number of cases have been reported of hydrops associated with spontaneous recovery and delivery of a healthy appearing newborn at term.* The reported time course from detection of hydrops to spontaneous resolution has been between 1 and 7 weeks. The clinical features associated with spontaneous recovery or intrauterine death have not been studied, but the severity of anemia and gestational age at onset of hydrops are the two factors most likely to be of prognostic significance. The anemia may correlate best with severity of symptoms at presentation and gestational age with the ability of the fetus to clear the infection. Another factor that may ultimately prove to be important to survival includes susceptibility of other replicating cell populations, like myocytes, to infection. So far, there have been no controlled trials of expectant management compared with intrauterine transfusion, so it is unknown if survival is actually improved after transfusion. Recovery with survival to term has been the most common outcome reported after transfusion, but some fatal cases have also been reported and the treatment may have been a factor in some.[140, 145, 147, 157, 160, 196, 212, 345, 349] Intrauterine transfusion is known to be a high-risk procedure even in expert hands.

After intrauterine B19 infection, most of the morbidity reported in the newborn period has been a result of problems associated with prematurity, recovery from hydrops, or residual B19-associated hematologic abnormalities. Premature delivery has been reported in some cases, but only 6 (4%) of 156 live-born infants were born before 36 weeks in the PHLS study.[144] Small-for-gestational-age infants have also been reported in association with intrauterine B19 infection.[157, 347] In the PHLS study, 11 (8%) of 142 live-born infants, for whom data were available, were less than the third percentile of birth weight for gestational age.[144] Although the study was not controlled, the number of small-for-gestational-age infants was greater than expected. Pulmonary function may be decreased because of residual pleural or ascitic fluid. Laxity of the abdominal wall has been reported as a consequence of hydrops.[148, 348] Transfusions may be required for treatment of chronic anemia.

Data are sparse on B19 infection acquired in infancy. Erythroid hypoplasia lasting 5 months was reported in one infant.[350] The child had anti-B19 IgM antibodies, but specific IgG was low to undetectable. Remission occurred at 8 months, and subsequent evaluations and clinical course did not reveal evidence of an immunodeficiency disorder. There has been a preliminary report of a patient with intrauterine infection followed by persistent infection in infancy.[151] There are no data sug-

---

*See references 145–150, 157, 169, 172, 198–202, 207, 212, 213, and 345–348.

*See references 146, 148, 149, 150, 157, 196, 200, 215, 347, and 348.

gesting secondary transmission from infants infected in utero. One fetus had hydrops that resolved spontaneously. The child appeared healthy at birth but died suddenly at 7 weeks; unfortunately, no autopsy was performed.[215]

LABORATORY DIAGNOSIS

General Considerations

The greatest impediment to the study of human parvovirus B19 has been the limited access to sensitive and specific diagnostic tests. The fundamental problem is that the virus does not grow in any readily available continuous cell line, and, until fairly recently, viral capsid antigens needed for diagnostic tests were still derived primarily from asymptomatic viremic patients identified by screening thousands of blood donors. The situation has changed dramatically with the successful development of recombinant viral proteins that are immunologically similar to native virus, and with utilization of the PCR technique for detection of B19 DNA in clinical specimens. More widespread use of these tests in the near future should improve our understanding about the importance of B19 as a human pathogen. The application of these newer diagnostic methods to the diagnosis of B19 has been reviewed.[351]

Specific diagnosis of B19 infection can be made by detection of anti-B19 antibodies, viral proteins, or DNA. Histopathologic findings using routine stains may be sufficiently specific to provide strong presumptive evidence of B19 infection and may be refined with use of specific antibody or nucleotide probes. Electron microscopy may be useful in identifying virus particles and then confirmed by immune electron microscopy. The correct interpretation and use of the available laboratory diagnostic studies need to take into consideration the underlying clinical manifestations, the ability of the host to produce an immune response, and the experimental nature and limited clinical experience with some of the available assays.

ANTIGEN SOURCES

There are three sources of B19 antigens currently available for use in diagnostic assays: native virus recovered from serum or tissues, recombinant antigens, and synthetic peptides. The most commonly used source has been virus from sera of acutely infected persons.[352] Virus recovered from infected fetal liver has also been shown to be suitable for diagnostic assays.[353] The portion of the genome coding for the two capsid proteins VP1 and VP2 has been cloned and expressed in both prokaryotic[84, 354-361] and eukaryotic expression systems[50, 87, 362-364] by several groups and promises to serve as a renewable source of viral antigen.[365] A comparison between serum-derived and recombinant antigens shows excellent correlation in immunoassay tests.[366] Synthetic peptide antigens have also been used in serologic assays.[367-369]

CULTIVATION

Attempting to culture B19 in vitro is impractical for diagnosis because it has never been successfully grown in readily available continuous cell lines.[365, 370] The virus requires red cell precursors for productive infection, and originally they were obtained by bone marrow aspiration from human volunteers. Alternative sources have now been identified, including human cord blood,[371, 372] normal human adult peripheral blood,[373, 374] and fetal liver,[178, 375, 376] but none of these systems are practical for routine use in clinical laboratories. Established erythroleukemia cell lines have not been found to be permissive,[370] although B19 replication has been reported in fresh bone marrow leukemia cells obtained from a patient with chronic myeloid leukemia in erythroblastic crisis.[377] Low-level replication has been reported in UT-7, a continuous cell line derived from megakaryocytes adapted to grow in the presence of erythropoietin.[378] The cell line MB-02, derived from a patient with megakaryocytic leukemia, undergoes erythroid differentiation with erythropoietin treatment and becomes permissive for B19 replication, but at reduced levels of expression compared with normal bone marrow.[379] Cultivation of B19 is used primarily as a research tool by investigators studying the molecular biology, immunology, and pathogenesis of B19 infection.

ANTIBODY ASSAYS

Serologic assays are the mainstay for diagnosis of B19 infection.[95, 97, 352, 366, 367, 380, 381] In the normal host, acute B19 infection can be diagnosed by the presence of anti-B19 IgM antibodies in the serum. In the patient with erythema infectiosum or B19-associated arthropathy, sensitive capture radioimmunoassays[380] or enzyme immunoassays[352] become positive for IgM just before onset of symptoms, peak 2 to 3 weeks later, and then decline quickly over the next 2 to 3 months (Fig. 16–6, bottom).[104] However, specific IgM may be detectable for as long as 10 months in some patients.[266] The sensitivity of specific IgM determination is thought to be greater than 90% in the first month after symptom onset. In the immunocompromised host, the IgM response is unpredictable, but in practice, detection of anti-B19 IgM antibodies is a useful, if insensitive, indicator of recent or ongoing B19 infection. [About one fourth of infants infected in utero will have IgG but not IgA or IgM antibodies at 1 year of age.[142a, 142b] Identification of parvovirus B19 DNA by PCR may be positive in urine and saliva for 4 months.[151a]]

Specific IgG becomes positive within several days after IgM and persists for years in most cases (see Fig. 16–6, top). The presence of anti-B19 IgG antibodies is associated with protective immunity.[125] The sensitivity of specific IgG determinations as an indicator of recent or previous infection generally exceeds 90% in most reports.[102] However, in a study of 81 patients with sickle cell disease and B19-associated aplastic crisis diagnosed by detection of specific IgM or viral DNA, 17 (21%) never developed an IgG response.[72] There have been few longitudinal studies of anti-B19 IgG antibody persistence. In a study of 33 patients with B19-associated aplastic crisis, 15 (45%) had anti-B19 IgG antibodies for at least 5 years, 13 (39%) became seronegative, and 5 (15%) never had an increase in IgG.[72] Those patients in whom IgG levels became undetectable did not suffer

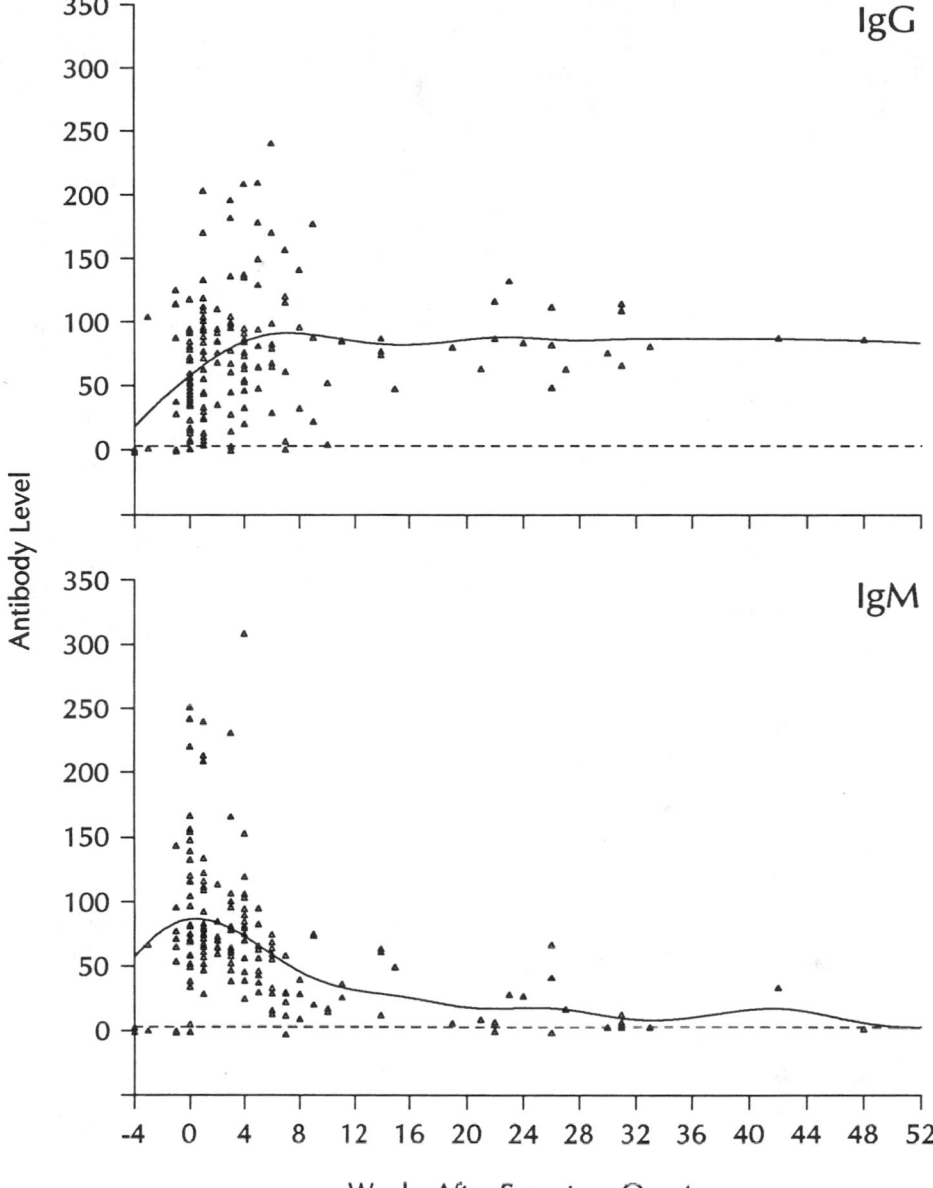

FIGURE 16–6 Time course of B19-specific IgG and IgM antibodies measured by capture enzyme immunoassay in 126 pregnant women (170 specimens) with rash illness or acute arthropathy and serologic evidence of acute infection. The antibody level is expressed as multiples of the standard deviation above the mean of replicates of pooled negative sera. The dashed line at three standard deviations is the cutoff; values above this line are considered positive. The curves representing antibody rise and decay were fit to the data by the distance-weighted least-squares method. (Source: CDC, unpublished data.)

recurrent aplasias, suggesting that protective immunity persisted. Anti-B19 IgG antibodies may also become undetectable in some patients receiving immunosuppressive therapy.[4, 306]

The data concerning the host IgA response to B19 are limited, but so far there are no data suggesting that anti-B19 IgA assays will be very helpful for serodiagnosis of B19 infection. Anti-B19 IgA may be present in serum for months to years, and about half of patients with specific IgG, not selected for recent B19 infection, are also IgA positive.[355]

The choice of assay, source of antigen, and choice of specimens included in test evaluation are all important variables to consider in evaluating the performance of a B19 immunoassay. Early reports using counterimmunoelectrophoresis to measure total anti-B19 antibody were insensitive.[76] Capture radioimmunoassays and enzyme immunoassays using native virus have been demonstrated to have great sensitivity and specificity and are the standards with which other assays should be compared. Recombinant antigens containing VP2, or a mixture of VP1 and VP2, self-assemble into empty capsids and are an excellent substitute for native virus. Synthetic peptide antigens have been used for serodiagnosis of B19, and test kits are commercially available in some countries.[382] However, both the sensitivity and specificity of assays using peptide antigens are significantly reduced compared with those using serum-derived or recombinant antigens.[185, 290, 368] The reported experience with immunoblot and immunofluorescence formats using native or recombinant antigens has been more limited, but some may prove to be clinically useful.[85]

DETECTION OF VIRAL ANTIGENS

Viral proteins can be detected transiently in the serum of acutely infected patients before the development of an antibody response. Counterimmunoelectrophoresis and enzyme immunoassays were developed to detect these antigens and used to screen for specimens with high titers of virus suitable for use in antibody assays.[81, 352] These assays are of limited use diagnostically because the overall sensitivity is low compared with tests for viral DNA and the sensitivity is reduced in the presence of circulating antibody.[91] The exception is in the case of immunohistochemistry, in which detection of specific staining of viral antigens in tissues in situ can provide unequivocal evidence of B19 infection.

DETECTION OF VIRAL DNA AND RNA

Assays to detect viral nucleotides, principally DNA, have proved invaluable for the diagnosis and characterization of some of the clinical manifestations of B19 infection. DNA hybridization assays may be positive during acute infection or in patients with chronic infection and are applicable to studies of tissues.[100, 382-384] False-positive results have been reported in up to 2% of blood donors using dot-blot DNA hybridization.[91, 385] The PCR has been widely used for testing for B19 DNA because of its increased sensitivity over blot hybridization methods.[127, 134, 159, 185, 195, 215, 316, 383, 386-395]

Viral DNA can be found in the majority of anti-B19 IgM positive patients presenting acutely with erythema infectiosum or arthropathy and may be detectable for 2 to 3 months after symptom onset.[287, 305] One study reported that 98% of serum specimens collected in the first month following onset of erythema infectiosum were B19 DNA positive by the PCR, and 67% were also positive during the second month; none of six specimens collected after 4 to 6 months were positive.[368] *[In a study of 80 cases of spontaneous abortions after fetal death or hydrops fetalis, amniotic fluid was the most common and reliable sample to assess for B19 DNA PCR diagnosis.[395a]]*

LIGHT AND ELECTRON MICROSCOPY

Routine histologic studies can play an important and practical role in the diagnosis of B19 infection. Finding the characteristic intranuclear inclusions in nucleated erythroid cells in formalin-fixed placenta or fetal tissues stained with hematoxylin and eosin provides strong presumptive evidence of intrauterine B19 infection (see Figs. 16–4 and 16–5). Inclusion-bearing cells may be found in blood of affected fetuses collected by cordocentesis.[212] The sensitivity is not known with any precision, but it is probably high in cases of B19-associated hydrops. The finding of giant proerythroblasts in bone marrow by Wright-Giemsa staining also is suggestive of acute B19 infection in a patient with a compatible clinical condition. In patients with chronic B19 infection and HIV, the frequency of giant proerythroblasts is low, constituting less than 1% of nucleated cells.[126, 192] Viral inclusions are less frequently identified in bone marrow, but one report suggests that detection may be facilitated by fixation with formalin before Wright-Giemsa or hematoxylin-eosin staining.[296] The possibility that this could be applied to fetal blood samples obtained prenatally deserves further study.

B19 proteins can be demonstrated in situ by immunohistochemistry, and this technique may prove to have widespread applicability in many clinical laboratories. All the necessary reagents, including anti-B19 antibodies, are currently available commercially, and good results have been reported using paraffin-embedded tissues.[52, 94, 396, 397] Not having to use frozen tissues should facilitate testing of routinely prepared placenta and fetal tissues. This technique has already proved valuable for diagnosis of fetal disease caused by B19.

The sensitivity of the histopathologic examination can also be improved with in situ hybridization studies.[156, 173, 210, 398-403] B19 DNA and RNA can also be visualized in tissues by in situ hybridization using DNA or RNA probes. In situ hybridization may become more clinically useful in the near future because nonisotopic methods applicable to paraffin-embedded tissues have been described, and the PCR technique has been used to generate probes for nucleotide detection.

Virus particles have been detected by electron microscopy in serum from patients in the prodromal phase of acute illness and in some patients with chronic infection.[285, 345] This method has also been used successfully to diagnose fetal infection prenatally by examination of fetal ascitic fluid, amniotic fluid, and fetal blood and in postmortem studies of fresh and fixed fetal tissues.*

Diagnosis During Pregnancy and the Newborn Period

The clinical manifestations of B19 infection during pregnancy are similar to the manifestations observed in the nonpregnant state. Acute maternal infection should be considered in any woman with new onset of a rash illness or arthropathy, and the diagnosis can be made by detection of anti-B19 IgM antibodies in a single serum sample. The presence of specific IgG and absence of IgM indicate prior infection and immunity, and the absence of both IgG and IgM indicates susceptibility to infection. Screening only symptomatic women would miss many and perhaps the majority of infected women, but routine prenatal screening for all is impractical at present. The yield from screening women with direct exposure to children with erythema infectiosum or aplastic crisis would be expected to be much higher and is currently recommended.[407]

Checking a maternal serum sample for anti-B19 IgM and IgG antibodies is also the best way to diagnose B19 infection in an affected fetus. Fetal hydrops or anemia along with specific IgM in maternal serum provides strong presumptive evidence of intrauterine B19 infection, and collection of fetal specimens may involve undue additional risk to the fetus without significantly increasing the diagnostic yield. Occasionally, anti-B19 IgM will not be detectable in maternal serum at the time

---

*See references 146, 147, 150, 152, 169, 198, 206, 209, 345, 347, 396, and 404–406.

of recognition of fetal disease, and additional diagnostic studies will be necessary to confirm the diagnosis if the mother is anti-B19 IgG positive and IgM negative.[145, 150, 152, 156, 196, 206, 348] On rare occasion, maternal serum has been negative for any specific anti-B19 antibodies when fetal specimens were positive.[196, 347]

Anti-B19 IgM is first detectable by capture enzyme immunoassay in fetal blood at approximately 18 weeks and has been used to diagnose infection prenatally, and in the infant in the neonatal period.* Finding specific IgM in the fetus is a highly specific method of diagnosing intrauterine infection, but the sensitivity may be very low. There have been a number of reports in which B19 infection has been confirmed by detection of viral DNA and by histologic criteria, yet fetal IgM was detected only transiently or not at all.[140, 145–148, 150, 395] Similarly, the sensitivity of anti-B19 IgM determinations is low in the neonatal period. There have been a number of reports of cases with proven intrauterine infection, or maternal infection with compatible fetal disease, yet no specific IgM was detectable in the neonatal period.[147, 149, 150, 185, 347] Total IgM may be increased in the fetus, but the sensitivity or applicability as a screening tool is unknown.[147]

A more sensitive way of documenting fetal infection prenatally is by demonstration of B19 DNA in amniotic fluid, fetal blood, or tissues. The PCR technique has been used by many investigators for the prenatal diagnosis of intrauterine infection.[196, 215, 348, 389, 395] There are insufficient data to determine the sensitivity by specimen source. In one report, three fetal but only one of the simultaneously collected amniotic fluid samples were positive by the PCR technique.[215] Viral DNA was detected in all 10 samples of amniotic fluid from affected fetuses of anti-B19 IgM positive women in another study,[196] suggesting that amniotic fluid may be the safest choice if fetal blood sampling or paracentesis is not required on other therapeutic grounds. B19 DNA may be detectable in fetal cord blood at a time when fetal IgM is negative.[212]

Although electron microscopy has been used to demonstrate fetal infection with B19, the sensitivity has not been established with any certainty and it may be too low to be very helpful for prenatal diagnosis compared with other methods like the PCR technique. In one study of intrauterine B19 infection, amniotic fluid was positive for B19 DNA by the PCR in 10 of 10 samples from B19-affected fetuses and negative by electron microscopy for all 10 cases.[196] The sensitivity of electron microscopy has been shown to be similar to that of dot-blot or in situ hybridization for fresh tissues but less so for formalin-fixed tissues.[405] Immune electron microscopy is more sensitive than direct electron microscopy for detection of virus in unfixed fetal tissues.

MANAGEMENT, PREVENTION, AND CONTROL

General Considerations

The majority of patients with B19 infection will either be asymptomatic or have mild self-limited symptoms

not requiring therapy. Severe pruritus may sometimes complicate the course of erythema infectiosum, and patients may benefit from treatment of symptoms. B19-associated arthropathy is generally self-limited and adequately controlled by short courses of analgesics or nonsteroidal anti-inflammatory agents. Patients with aplastic crisis may need red cell transfusions. Immunoglobulin therapy may improve hematologic indices in patients with chronic B19 infection.[126, 192, 242, 288, 291, 292, 408]

Interventions to prevent or control disease transmission in the community are of unproven value, and the options and recommendations are limited. In the setting of school or day-care center outbreaks of erythema infectiosum, the Centers for Disease Control and Prevention has recommended that parents and employees be informed of the outbreaks so that persons at risk for serious complications can be identified and referred to their physicians for close follow-up.[407] For example, in the case of a patient with sickle cell disease, early recognition by parents of signs or symptoms of B19-associated aplastic crisis may decrease the morbidity by shortening the time to seek medical care and initiate supportive therapy with red cell transfusions. Parental notification might also improve the likelihood that an exposure history would be obtained by health care providers, and contact isolation precautions would be instituted. In the immunocompromised patient with increased susceptibility to chronic B19 infection, some knowledge of B19 activity in the community could expedite the evaluation and initiation of specific or supportive therapy. The notification recommendation is limited to schools and day-care centers because the peak incidence of infection occurs in school-age children; most household transmission probably occurs after introduction by an infected child; and these are the only settings where an occupational risk has been clearly demonstrated. Advisories to the public at large would be expected to have a limited potential benefit.

Because the epidemiologic data suggest that direct contact with respiratory secretions is an important mode of transmission of B19, hand washing after contact with potentially infectious secretions and not sharing eating utensils have been suggested as common sense interventions to decrease the risk of infection in home and school settings.[407] The efficacy or practicality of either intervention has not been evaluated. The parvoviruses as a group are highly resistant to chemical disinfection and heat inactivation, and the limited data specifically available for B19 are consistent with the group characteristics.[409] Whether frequent cleaning or disinfection of toys likely to be placed in the mouth by infants and toddlers would decrease the risk of transmission at home or in day-care centers is unknown.

Contact isolation precautions have been recommended for potentially infectious patients admitted to the hospital.[407] These recommendations would apply to patients with suspected and proven transient aplastic crisis or chronic B19 infection but would not include patients with erythema infectiosum, who are not thought to be infectious by the time the disease becomes evident. Isolation of newborns after suspected intrauterine infection has been suggested,[410] but transmission from new-

---

*See references 15, 140, 144, 148, 160, 196, 200, 201, 213, and 347.

borns has not been demonstrated and routine isolation of infants with possible intrauterine infection is not currently recommended by the Centers for Disease Control and Prevention[407] or the American Academy of Pediatrics.[411] The issue of work restrictions for high-risk susceptible health care workers, including pregnant women, is more controversial. Restrictions have been recommended by the American Academy of Pediatrics[411] but not by the Centers for Disease Control and Prevention.[407] Work and visitation restrictions were implemented for anti-B19 IgG negative pregnant staff and parents during a hospital outbreak, but the impact on subsequent transmission was not determined.[119] Laboratories using infectious virus as a source of antigen for diagnostic studies can reduce the risk of laboratory-acquired infection by treating the antigen with gamma irradiation.[412]

Pre- or post-exposure prophylaxis of high-risk persons with immune globulin is an attractive option to consider because high-dose immunoglobulin therapy has proved to be beneficial in patients with chronic B19 infection. However, there are a number of concerns about generalizing observations about immunocompromised patients to other patient populations and other immune globulin preparations. Commercially available immunoglobulins contain anti-B19 antibodies but are not routinely screened to determine if they contain high titers of neutralizing antibodies.[300, 413, 414] Furthermore, the mechanism of action of immunoglobulins in the compromised patient may not be solely a matter of providing the patient with neutralizing antibodies to B19; rather, the immunoglobulins may be acting to enhance the patient immune response indirectly. The potential uses of immunoglobulin for prophylaxis and treatment are sufficiently great that development of a high-titer preparation should be a research priority, but use of any of the existing preparations may not be advisable outside of a specific research protocol.

Safe and effective vaccines for animal parvoviruses are widely used in veterinary medicine. Noninfectious B19 vaccine candidates have been developed using recombinant capsid proteins that self-assemble into empty capsids that are immunologically similar to native virus.[415] The empty capsids are immunogenic in mice and rabbits, and the proportions of VP1 and VP2 can be modified to enhance the production of neutralizing antibodies.[50, 51, 415] The development of a live attenuated B19 vaccine is not currently feasible because there is no experimental animal model for B19.

Pregnancy

Our knowledge about the optimal management of the pregnant woman with exposure to or infection with B19 during pregnancy currently lags considerably behind our understanding about the potential adverse consequences of fetal infection. As a result, there is great pressure on the clinician to diagnose, advise, and treat the patient, but there are little or no data demonstrating efficacy of any particular therapeutic approach or intervention. The majority of maternal infections with B19 during pregnancy are probably asymptomatic or at least not clinically recognized. Universal screening has not been recommended; however, because diagnostic testing is not widely available, many women would need to be screened for each acute infection identified, and there is no consensus on how to use the information obtained from mass screening to minimize fetal morbidity and mortality. The emphasis instead has been on identification of women at increased risk of B19 infection, including women with unexplained rash illness or arthropathy, women exposed to cases of erythema infectiosum or aplastic crisis, women with pregnancies complicated by nonimmune hydrops, and possibly women with unexplained fetal death or fetal anomalies. Women at increased risk of B19 infection should be screened for anti-B19 IgM and IgG antibodies to identify acute infection or immunity. Women who are anti-B19 IgG positive and IgM negative can be considered to be immune and at very low or no risk of a B19-related adverse event.

Management of susceptible women (i.e., women having no detectable specific IgG or IgM antibodies and ongoing exposure to cases) is problematic. For the most common clinically recognized B19-associated illness—erythema infectiosum—the greatest risk of transmission occurs in the prodromal phase before rash onset. This means that avoidance of persons with rash illness or exclusion of infected children from school or day care has little to offer in the way of decreasing the risk of transmission, and these actions are not recommended by the Centers for Disease Control and Prevention[407] or the American Academy of Pediatrics.[411] The more complicated issue concerns the situation in which ongoing exposure to patients incubating disease may occur, for example, the case of a pregnant teacher working in an elementary school with an outbreak of erythema infectiosum where the duration of the outbreak could be protracted. The risk to the teacher of becoming infected and losing the pregnancy because of an acute B19 infection has been estimated to be less than 1.5% in the situation of widespread disease activity at the school.[407] Some have recommended restricting women without anti-B19 IgG antibodies from working at schools with ongoing outbreaks.[160] Because a school outbreak may also be an indicator of epidemic transmission in the community, reassignment or taking leave from work cannot be assumed to produce a significant decrease in risk over background. Furthermore, no studies have been conducted to see if an individual's risk can be reduced in this manner. Considering the overall low level of risk of an adverse fetal outcome, the decision to try to limit exposure at work probably should be individualized.

Management of the pregnant woman with proven acute B19 infection is controversial. Numerous protocols have been suggested, but none has been evaluated in controlled studies. A baseline assessment of the fetus by ultrasound at the time of maternal diagnosis is appropriate; and if the examination is normal, the information is probably reassuring to most women. Because the peak in fetal morbidity and mortality occurs 4 to 6 weeks, but as late as 3 months, after onset of maternal symptoms, frequent fetal ultrasound examinations have been advocated by some as a way of identifying cases of fetal hydrops for early intervention.[157, 160, 348] However, in a study of 39 pregnancies complicated by maternal B19 infection, but otherwise uneventful, and followed with frequent fetal ultrasound examinations, none of the fetuses developed hydrops, although there were two fetal deaths and one of these was attributed to B19 infection.[154] This suggests that the yield from serial ultrasound examinations is too low to justify routine use at this time for all women testing anti-B19 IgM positive during pregnancy.

The prenatal diagnosis of intrauterine B19 infection can be made by laboratory analysis of amniotic fluid, fetal blood, and other fetal specimens. Because the frequency of hydrops is low after proven maternal infection, and a positive prenatal test in the absence of recognized fetal disease is of uncertain clinical importance, routine attempts to confirm intrauterine infection in women who are anti-B19 IgM positive are of questionable value at this time unless performed in the context of a controlled clinical study.

Maternal serum alpha-fetoprotein levels have been elevated in some B19-infected women with fetal disease or death, and some investigators have proposed performing serial determinations as a way of identifying a fetus at risk.[14, 170, 198, 205, 416] Levels also may be normal even in the presence of fetal disease.[146, 348] Because no one has yet demonstrated that serial testing is useful prospectively in the management of the B19-infected woman, it would be premature to recommend it at this time. Even if it is eventually shown to be useful in some studies, maternal serum alpha-fetoprotein levels are well standardized only for a narrow window in mid-pregnancy and the approach may not be applicable for many women anyway.

Pregnancy-associated hypertension, preeclampsia, and eclampsia have been reported in B19-infected women with fetal disease.[148, 156, 157, 200, 201, 205] Whether, applied prospectively, this would be helpful in identifying pregnancies at greater risk of B19-associated hydrops or death is unknown, but because these conditions are easily defined and monitored, they may be worth evaluating further as a screening tool.

The mortality rate is high for fetuses with ultrasonographic evidence of hydrops, and many will have evidence of severe anemia if fetal blood is sampled. However, the recognition that some of these cases of hydrops resolve spontaneously and then may result in the delivery of a healthy appearing infant greatly complicates the issue of when it is appropriate to intervene, and how.* Increased use of fetal blood sampling and intrauterine transfusion has been advocated, but they carry their own risks of fetal morbidity and mortality even in expert hands.[140, 145, 147, 157, 160, 196, 212, 345, 349] So far, there have been no controlled trials of expectant management compared with intrauterine transfusion, so it is unknown if survival is actually improved after transfusion, or if the long-term development of survivors is better following transfusion than without. Too often, intrauterine transfusion has been credited for the survival of a hydropic fetus in an uncritical manner, whereas fetal death after transfu-

sion or during expectant management has been blamed on intervening too late in the course of infection. The alternative hypothesis, that the fetus stable enough to reach the referral center capable of performing the procedure is in a favorable prognostic group, deserves fair consideration. Because intrauterine transfusion has not yet been shown to be beneficial in controlled studies for reducing B19-associated fetal morbidity or mortality, it should be regarded as experimental therapy. Maternal or fetal immunotherapy using commercially available immune globulin preparations has not been studied to see if there is a beneficial effect on fetal survival.

CONCLUSIONS

The data about B19 are still fragmentary, but it has been clearly demonstrated that intrauterine B19 infection is an important cause of nonimmune fetal hydrops and may result in fetal death. New observations also raise the possibility that B19 is teratogenic and may cause long-term sequelae in live-born infants. Progress has been restricted until now by the limited availability of specific diagnostic tests, but the development of recombinant antigens and molecular probes promises to greatly improve clinicians' access to diagnostic tests and facilitate research on the natural history and importance of fetal B19 infection. Important questions yet to be answered include how often intrauterine infection results in birth defects or significant developmental abnormalities among live-born infants, and how the exposed or infected pregnant woman and her fetus should be managed to reduce the risk of an adverse pregnancy outcome. Answering these questions will require better methods for identifying infants truly infected in utero, and larger controlled studies with longer and more intensive patient follow-up. Specific therapy or prophylaxis with high-titer immunoglobulins, and primary prevention with a B19 vaccine, may prove to be desirable and attainable goals for the near future.

ACKNOWLEDGMENTS

I am grateful to Drs. Larry J. Anderson and G. William Gary, Jr., for their advice and helpful comments.

References

1. Cossart YE, Field AM, Cant B, Widdows D. Parvovirus-like particles in human sera. Lancet 1:72, 1975.
2. Pattison JR. The discovery of human parvoviruses. *In* Pattison JR (ed). Parvoviruses and Human Disease. Boca Raton, Fla, CRC Press, 1988, pp 1–4.
3. Siegl G, Bates RC, Berns KI, et al. Characteristics and taxonomy of Parvoviridae. Intervirology 23:61, 1985.
4. Couroucé AM, Ferchal F, Morinet F, et al. Human parvovirus infections in France (letter). Lancet 1:160, 1984.
5. Couroucé AM, Ferchal F, Morinet F, et al. Parvovirus (SPLV) et antigène Aurillac. Rev Fr Transfus Immunohematol 27:5, 1984.
6. Okochi K, Mori R, Miyazaki M, et al. Nakatani antigen and human parvovirus (B19) (letter). Lancet 1:160, 1984.
7. de Miranda MFR, Linhares AC, Shirley JA. Fifth disease

---

*See references 146, 148–150, 157, 196, 200, 215, 347, and 348.

in children living in Belém, Brazil. Rev Inst Med Trop São Paulo 31:359, 1989.

8. Teuscher T, Baillod B, Holzer BR. Prevalence of human parvovirus B19 in sickle cell disease and healthy controls. Trop Geogr Med 43:108, 1991.

9. Pattison JR, Jones SE, Hodgson J, et al. Parvovirus infections and hypoplastic crisis in sickle-cell anaemia (letter). Lancet 1:664, 1981.

10. Serjeant GR, Topley JM, Mason K, et al. Outbreak of aplastic crises in sickle cell anaemia associated with parvovirus-like agent. Lancet 2:595, 1981.

11. White DG, Woolf AD, Mortimer PP, et al. Human parvovirus arthropathy. Lancet 1:419, 1985.

12. Reid DM, Reid TMS, Brown T, et al. Human parvovirus associated with arthritis: a clinical and laboratory description. Lancet 1:422, 1985.

13. Anderson MJ, Jones SE, Fisher-Hoch SP, et al. Human parvovirus, the cause of erythema infectiosum (fifth disease)? Letter to the editor. Lancet 1:1378, 1983.

14. Brown T, Anand A, Ritchie LD, et al. Intrauterine parvovirus infection associated with hydrops fetalis (letter). Lancet 2:1033, 1984.

15. Knott PD, Welply GAC, Anderson MJ. Serologically proved intrauterine infection with parvovirus (letter). BMJ 289:1960, 1984.

16. Weiland HT, Vermey-Keers C, Salimans MM, et al. Parvovirus B19 associated with fetal abnormality (letter). Lancet 1:682, 1987.

17. Kurtzman GJ, Ozawa K, Cohen B, et al. Chronic bone marrow failure due to persistent B19 parvovirus infection. N Engl J Med 317:287, 1987.

18. Frickhofen N, Young NS. Persistent parvovirus B19 infections in humans. Microbiol Pathogenesis 7:319, 1989.

19. Berns KI (ed). The Parvoviruses. New York, Plenum Press, 1984, p 410.

20. Berns KI. Parvoviridae and their replication. In Fields BN, Knipe DM (eds). Virology, vol 2. New York, Raven Press, 1990, pp 1743–1763.

21. Tijssen P (ed). Handbook of Parvoviruses, vol I. Boca Raton, Fla, CRC Press, 1990.

22. Tijssen P (ed). Handbook of Parvoviruses, vol II. Boca Raton, Fla, CRC Press, 1990.

23. Simpson RW, McGinty L, Simon L, et al. Association of parvoviruses with rheumatoid arthritis of humans. Science 223:1425, 1984.

24. Marx JL. First parvovirus linked to human disease. Science 223:152, 1984.

25. Paver WK, Clarke SKR. Comparison of human fecal and serum parvo-like viruses. J Clin Microbiol 4:67, 1976.

26. Appleton H, Pereira MS. A possible virus aetiology in outbreaks of food-poisoning from cockles. Lancet 1:780, 1977.

27. Turton J, Appleton H, Clewley JP. Similarities in nucleotide sequence between serum and faecal human parvovirus DNA. Epidemiol Infect 105:197, 1990.

28. Mayor HD, Drake S, Stahmann J, Mumford DM. Antibodies to adeno-associated satellite virus and herpes simplex in sera from cancer patients and normal adults. Am J Obstet Gynecol 126:100, 1976.

29. Srivastava CH, Samulski RJ, Lu L, et al. Construction of a recombinant human parvovirus B19: adeno-associated virus 2 (AAV) DNA inverted terminal repeats are functional in an AAV-B19 hybrid virus. Proc Natl Acad Sci U S A. 86:8078, 1989.

30. Nahreni P, Woody MJ, Zhou SZ, Srivastava A. Versatile adeno-associated virus 2–based vectors constructing recombinant virions. Gene 124:257, 1993.

31. Flotte TR. Prospects for virus-based gene therapy for cystic fibrosis. J Bioenerg Biomembr 25:37, 1993.

32. Tsao J, Chapman MS, Agbandje M, et al. The three-dimensional structure of canine parvovirus and its functional implications. Science 251:1456, 1991.

33. Chapman MS, Rossmann MG. Structure, sequence, and function correlations among parvoviruses. Virology 194:491, 1993.

34. Shade RO, Blundell MC, Cotmore SF, et al. Nucleotide sequence and genome organization of human parvovirus B19 isolated from the serum of a child during aplastic crisis. J Virol 58:921, 1986.

35. Blundell MC, Beard C, Astell CR. In vitro identification of a B19 parvovirus promoter. Virology 157:534, 1987.

36. Deiss V, Tratschin JD, Weitz M, Siegl G. Cloning of the human parvovirus B19 genome and structural analysis of its palindromic termini. Virology 175:247, 1990.

37. Morinet F, Tratschin JD, Perol Y, Siegl G. Comparison of 17 isolates of the human parvovirus B19 by restriction enzyme analysis. Arch Virol 90:165, 1986.

38. Mori J, Beattie P, Melton DW, et al. Structure and mapping of the DNA of human parvovirus B19. J Gen Virol 68:2797, 1987.

39. Umene K, Nunoue T. The genome type of human parvovirus B19 strains isolated in Japan during 1981 differs from types detected in 1986 to 1987: a correlation between genome type and prevalence. J Gen Virol 71:983, 1990.

40. Umene K, Nunoue T. Genetic diversity of human parvovirus B19 determined using a set of restriction endonucleases recognizing four or five base pairs and partial nucleotide sequencing: use of sequence variability in virus classification. J Gen Virol 72:1997, 1991.

41. Umene K, Nunoue T. Partial nucleotide sequencing and characterization of human parvovirus B19 genome DNAs from damaged human fetuses and from patients with leukemia. J Med Virol 39:333, 1993.

42. Ozawa K, Young N. Characterization of capsid and noncapsid proteins of B19 parvovirus propagated in human erythroid bone marrow cell cultures. J Virol 61:2627, 1987.

43. Doerig C, Beard P, Hirt B. A transcriptional promoter of the human parvovirus B19 active in vitro and in vivo. Virology 157:539, 1987.

44. Shimomura S, Wong S, Brown KE, et al. Early and late gene expression in UT-7 cells infected with B19 parvovirus. Virology 194:149, 1993.

45. Doerig C, Hirt B, Antonietti JP, Beard P. Nonstructural protein of parvovirus B19 and minute virus of mice controls transcription. J Virol 64:387, 1990.

46. Ozawa K, Ayub J, Hao YS, et al. Novel transcription map for the B19 (human) pathogenic parvovirus. J Virol 61:2395, 1987.

47. St. Amand J, Astell CR. Identification and characterization of a family of 11-kDa proteins encoded by the human parvovirus B19. Virology 192:121, 1993.

48. Ozawa K, Ayub J, Kajigava S, et al. The gene encoding the nonstructural protein of B19 (human) parvovirus may be lethal in transfected cells. J Virol 62:2884, 1988.

49. Agbandje M, McKenna R, Rossmann MG, et al. Preliminary x-ray crystallographic investigation of human parvovirus B19. Virology 184:170, 1991.

50. Kajigaya S, Fujii H, Field A, et al. Self-assembled B19 parvovirus capsids, produced in a baculovirus system, are antigenically and immunologically similar to native virus. Proc Natl Acad Sci U S A. 88:4646, 1991.

51. Brown CS, Jensen T, Meloen RH, et al. Localization of an immunodominant domain on baculovirus-produced

parvovirus B19 capsids: correlation to a major surface region on the native virus particle. J Virol 66:6989, 1992.

52. Morey AL, O'Neill HJ, Coyle PV, Fleming KA. Immunohistological detection of human parvovirus B19 in formalin-fixed, paraffin-embedded tissues. J Pathol 166:105, 1992.

53. Loughrey AC, O'Neill HJ, Coyle PV, DeLeys R. Identification and use of a neutralizing epitope of parvovirus B19 for the rapid detection of virus infection. J Med Virol 39:97, 1993.

54. Tschamer A. Ueber örtliche Rötheln. Jahrb Kinderheilkd 29:372, 1889.

55. Herrick TP. Erythema infectiosum: a clinical report of seventy-four cases. Am J Dis Child 31:486, 1926.

56. Lawton AL, Smith RE. Erythema infectiosum: a clinical study of an epidemic in Branford, Connecticut. Arch Intern Med 47:28, 1931.

57. Kerr PS, Marsh EH. Outbreak of erythema infectiosum in Elmsford, New York. Am J Public Health 23:1271, 1933.

58. Zuckerman SN. Erythema infectiosum, with report of an epidemic in San Francisco. Arch Pediatr 57:168, 1940.

59. Chargin L, Sobel N, Goldstein H. Erythema infectiosum: report of an extensive epidemic. Arch Dermatol Syphilol 47:467, 1943.

60. Epidemiological reports. Erythema infectiosum. Public Health Rep 66:1220, 1951.

61. Phillips IE. Erythema infectiosum: clinical and epidemiological observations. South Med J 47:253, 1954.

62. Auriemma PR. Erythema infectiosum: report on a familial outbreak. Am J Public Health 44:1450, 1954.

63. Ager EA, Chin TDY, Poland JD. Epidemic erythema infectiosum. N Engl J Med 275:1326, 1966.

64. Balfour HH Jr, May DB, Rotte TC, et al. A study of erythema infectiosum: recovery of rubella virus and echovirus-12. Pediatrics 50:285, 1972.

65. Owren PA. Congenital hemolytic jaundice: the pathogenesis of the "hemolytic crisis." Blood 3:231, 1948.

66. Schwarz TF, Gürtler LG, Zoulek G, et al. Seroprevalence of human parvovirus B19 infection in São Tomé and Principe, Malawi and Mascarene Islands. Int J Med Microbiol 271:231, 1989.

67. Jones PH, Pickett LC, Anderson MJ, Pasvol G. Human parvovirus infection in children and severe anaemia seen in an area endemic for malaria. J Trop Med Hyg 93:67, 1990.

68. de Freitas RB, Wong D, Boswell F, et al. Prevalence of human parvovirus (B19) and rubellavirus infections in urban and remote rural areas in northern Brazil. J Med Virol 32:203, 1990.

69. Hidano A, Ogihara Y, Oryu F, et al. Epidemiology of an outbreak of erythema infectiosum in Tokyo. Int J Dermatol 22:161, 1983.

70. Saburi Y, Takahashi T, Okuda K. Seasonal prevalence of erythema infectiosum. J Dermatol 12:375, 1985.

71. Galvon FAC. An outbreak of erythema infectiosum—Nova Scotia. Can Dis Wkly Rep 9:69, 1983.

72. Serjeant GR, Serjeant BE, Thomas PW, et al. Human parvovirus infection in homozygous sickle cell disease. Lancet 341:1237, 1993.

73. Yamashita K, Matsunaga Y, Taylor-Wiedeman J, Yamazaki S. A significant age shift of the human parvovirus B19 antibody prevalence among young adults in Japan observed in a decade. Jpn J Med Sci Biol 45:49, 1992.

74. Naides SJ. Erythema infectiosum (fifth disease) occurrence in Iowa. Am J Public Health 78:1230, 1988.

75. Cohen BJ, Buckley MM. The prevalence of antibody to human parvovirus B19 in England and Wales. J Med Microbiol 25:151, 1988.

76. Nascimento JP, Buckley MM, Brown KE, Cohen BJ. The prevalence of antibody to human parvovirus B19 in Rio de Janeiro, Brazil. Rev Inst Med Trop São Paulo 32:41.1990.

77. Edelson RN, Altman RA. Erythema infectiosum: a statewide outbreak. J Med Soc NJ 67:805, 1970.

78. Werner GH, Brachman PS, Ketler A, et al. A new viral agent associated with erythema infectiosum. Ann NY Acad Sci 67:338, 1957.

79. Greenwald P, Bashe WJ Jr. An epidemic of erythema infectiosum. Am J Dis Child 107:30, 1964.

80. Yaegashi N, Okamura K, Hamazaki Y, et al. Prevalence of anti-human parvovirus antibody in pregnant women. Nippon Sanka Fujinka Gakkai Zasshi 42:162, 1990.

81. Cohen BJ, Mortimer PP, Pereira MS. Diagnostic assays with monoclonal antibodies for the human serum parvovirus-like virus (SPLV). J Hyg (Lond) 91:113, 1983.

82. Schwarz TF, Roggendorf M, Deinhardt F. Häufigkeit der parovirus-B19-infektionen. Seroepidemiologishe untersuchungen. Dtsch Med Wochenschr 112:1526, 1987.

83. Bartolomei Corsi O, Assi A, Morfini M, et al. Human parvovirus infection in haemophiliacs first infused with treated clotting factor concentrates. J Med Virol 25:165, 1988.

84. Eiffert H, Köchel HG, Heuer M, et al. Expression of an antigenic polypeptide of the human parvovirus B19. Med Microbiol Immunol 179:169, 1990.

85. Brown CS, van Bussel MJAWM, Wassenaar ALM, et al. An immunofluorescence assay for the detection of parvovirus B19 IgG and IgM antibodies based on recombinant viral antigen. J Virol Methods 29:53, 1990.

86. Rollag H, Patou G, Pattison JR, et al. Prevalence of antibodies against parvovirus B19 in Norwegians with congenital coagulation factor defects treated with plasma products from small donor pools. Scand J Infect Dis 23:675, 1991.

87. Salimans MMM, van Bussel MJAWM, Brown CS, Spaan WJM. Recombinant parvovirus B19 capsids as a new substrate for detection of B19-specific IgG and IgM antibodies by an enzyme-linked immunosorbent assay. J Virol Methods 39:247, 1992.

88. Schwarz TF, Hottenträger B, Roggendorf M. Prevalence of antibodies to parvovirus B19 in selected groups of patients and healthy individuals. Int J Med Microbiol Virol Parasitol Infect Dis 276:437, 1992.

89. Koch WC, Adler SP. Human parvovirus B19 infections in women of childbearing age and within families. Pediatr Infect Dis J 8:83, 1989.

90. Cossart Y. Parvovirus B19 finds a disease (letter). Lancet 2:988, 1981.

91. Cohen BJ, Field AM, Gudnadottir S, et al. Blood donor screening for parvovirus B19. J Virol Methods 30:233, 1990.

92. da Silva Cruz A, Serpa MJA, Barth OM, Nascimento JP. Detection of the human parvovirus B19 in a blood donor plasma in Rio de Janeiro. Mem Inst Oswaldo Cruz 84:279, 1989.

93. Lefrère JJ, Couroucé AM, Bertrand Y, Soulier JP. Infections à parvovirus B19. Rev Fr Transfus Immunohematol 29:149, 1986.

94. O'Neill HJ, Coyle PV. Two anti-parvovirus B19 IgM capture assays incorporating a mouse monoclonal antibody specific for B19 viral capsid proteins VP1 and VP2. Arch Virol 123:125, 1992.

95. Schwarz TF, Roggendorf M. Diagnostic of parvovirus B19 infection. Behring Inst Mitt 85:35, 1990.

96. McOmish F, Yap PL, Jordan A, et al. Detection of parvovirus B19 in donated blood: a model system for screening by polymerase chain reaction. J Clin Microbiol 31:323, 1993.

97. Yaegashi N, Shiraishi H, Tada K, et al. Enzyme-linked immunosorbent assay for IgG and IgM antibodies against human parvovirus B19: use of monoclonal antibodies and viral antigen propagated in vitro. J Virol Methods 26:171, 1989.

98. Naides SJ, Scharosch LL, Foto F, Howard EJ. Rheumatologic manifestations of human parvovirus B19 infection in adults. Arthritis Rheum 33:1297, 1990.

99. Couroucé AM, Beaulieu MJ, Bouchardeau F, et al. Viraemia with human parvovirus (letter). Lancet 1:1218, 1985.

100. Zerbini M, Musiani M, Venturoli S, et al. Rapid screening for B19 parvovirus DNA in clinical specimens with a digoxigenin-labeled DNA hybridization probe. J Clin Microbiol 28:2496, 1990.

101. Plummer FA, Hammond GW, Forward K, et al. An erythema infectiosum-like illness caused by human parvovirus infection. N Engl J Med 313:74, 1985.

102. Chorba T, Coccia P, Holman RC, et al. The role of parvovirus B19 in aplastic crisis arid erythema infectiosum (fifth disease). J Infect Dis 154:383, 1986.

103. Mortimer PP. Hypothesis: the aplastic crisis of hereditary spherocytosis is due to a single transmissible agent. J Clin Pathol 36:445, 1983.

104. Saarinen UA, Chorba TL, Tattersall P, et al. Human parvovirus B19 induced epidemic red-cell aplasia in patients with hereditary hemolytic anemia. Blood 67:1411, 1986.

104a. *Valeur-Jensen A, Pedersen CB, Westergaard T, et al. Risk factors for parvovirus B19 infection in pregnancy. JAMA 281:1099–1105, 1999.*

105. Anderson MJ, Lewis E, Kidd IM, et al. An outbreak of erythema infectiosum associated with human parvovirus infection. J Hyg (Lond) 93:85, 1984.

106. Tuckerman JG, Brown T, Cohen BJ. Erythema infectiosum in a village primary school: clinical and virological studies. J R Coll Gen Pract 36:267, 1986.

107. Morgan-Capner P, Wright J, Longley JP, Anderson MJ. Sex ratio in outbreaks of parvovirus B19 infection (letter). Lancet 2:98, 1987.

108. Mansfield F. Erythema infectiosum: slapped face disease. Aust Fam Physician 17:737, 1988.

109. Woolf AD, Campion GV, Chishick A, et al. Clinical manifestations of human parvovirus B19 in adults. Arch Intern Med 149:1153, 1989.

110. Turner A, Olojugba O. Erythema infectiosum in a primary school: investigation of an outbreak in Bury. Public Health 103:391, 1989.

111. Grilli EA, Anderson MJ, Hoskins TW. Concurrent outbreaks of influenza and parvovirus B19 in a boys' boarding school. Epidemiol Infect 103:359, 1989.

112. Gillespie SM, Cartter ML, Asch S, et al. Occupational risk of human parvovirus B19 infection for school and day-care personnel during an outbreak of erythema infectiosum. JAMA 263:2061, 1990.

113. Anderson LJ, Gillespie SM, Török TJ, et al. Risk of infection following exposures to human parvovirus B19. Behring Inst Mitt 85:60, 1990.

114. Adler SP, Manganello AMA, Koch WC, et al. Risk of human parvovirus B19 infections among school and hospital employees during endemic periods. J Infect Dis 168:361, 1993.

115. Cartter ML, Farley TA, Rosengren S, et al. Occupational risk factors for infection with parvovirus B19 among pregnant women. J Infect Dis 163:282, 1991.

116. Bell LM, Naides SJ, Stoffman P, et al. Human parvovirus B19 infection among hospital staff members after contact with infected patients. N Engl J Med 321:485, 1989.

117. Pillay D, Patou G, Hurt S, et al. Parvovirus B19 outbreak in a children's ward. Lancet 339:107, 1992.

118. Cohen BJ, Couroucé AM, Schwarz TF, et al. Laboratory infection with parvovirus B19 (letter). J Clin Pathol 41:1027, 1988.

119. Shiraishi H, Sasaki T, Nakamura M, et al. Laboratory infection with human parvovirus B19 (letter). J Infect 22:308, 1991.

120. Evans JPM, Rossiter MA, Kumaran TO, et al. Human parvovirus aplasia: case due to cross infection in a ward. BMJ 288:681, 1984.

121. Ueda K, Akeda H, Tokugawa K, Nishima S. Human parvovirus infection (letter). N Engl J Med 314:645, 1986.

122. Pillay D, Patou G, Rees L, Griffiths PD. Secondary parvovirus B19 infection in an immunocompromised child. Pediatr Infect Dis J 10:623, 1991.

123. Koziol DE, Kurtzman G, Ayub JA, et al. Nosocomial human parvovirus B19 infection: lack of transmission from a chronically infected patient to hospital staff. Infect Control Hosp Epidemiol 13:343, 1992.

124. Kurtzman G, Frickhofen N, Kimball J, et al. Pure red-cell aplasia of 10 years' duration due to persistent parvovirus B19 infection and its cure with immunoglobulin therapy. N Engl J Med 321:519, 1989.

124a. *Dowell SF, Torok TJ, Thorp JA, et al. Parvovirus B19 infection in hospital workers: community or hospital acquisition? J Infect Dis 172:1076–1079, 1995.*

125. Anderson MJ, Higgins PG, Davis LR, et al. Experimental parvoviral infection in humans. J Infect Dis 152:257, 1985.

126. Frickhofen N, Abkowitz JL, Safford M, et al. Persistent B19 parvovirus infection in patients infected with human immunodeficiency virus type 1 (HIV-1): a treatable cause of anemia in AIDS. Ann Intern Med 113:926, 1990.

127. Patou G, Pillay D, Myint S, Pattison J. Characterization of a nested polymerase chain reaction assay for detection of parvovirus B19. J Clin Microbiol 31:540, 1993.

128. Potter CG, Potter AC, Hatton CSR, et al. Variation of erythroid and myeloid precursors in the marrow of volunteer subjects infected with human parvovirus (B19). J Clin Invest 79:1486, 1987.

129. Morey AL, Porter HJ, Keeling JW, Fleming KA. Non-isotopic in situ hybridisation and immunophenotyping of infected cells in investigation of human fetal parvovirus infection. J Clin Pathol 45:673, 1992.

130. Mortimer PP, Luban NLC, Kelleher JF, Cohen BJ. Transmission of serum parvovirus-like virus by clotting-factor concentrates. Lancet 2:482, 1983.

131. Lyon DJ, Chapman CS, Martin C, et al. Symptomatic parvovirus B19 infection and heat-treated factor IX concentrate (letter). Lancet 1:1085, 1989.

132. Williams MD, Cohen BJ, Beddall AC, et al. Transmission of human parvovirus B19 by coagulation factor concentrates. Vox Sang 58:177, 1990.

133. Morfini M, Longo G, Rossi Ferrini P, et al. Hypoplastic anemia in a hemophiliac first infused with a solvent/detergent treated factor VIII concentrate: the role of human B19 parvovirus (letter). Am J Hematol 39:149, 1992.

134. Zakrzewska K, Azzi A, Patou G, et al. Human parvovirus B19 in clotting factor concentrates: B19 DNA detection by the nested polymerase chain reaction. Br J Haematol 81:407, 1992.

135. Schwarz TF, Roggendorf M, Hottenträger B, et al. Re-

moval of parvovirus B19 from contaminated factor VIII during fractionation. J Med Virol 35:28, 1991.

136. Azzi A, Ciappi S, Zakrzewska K, et al. Human parvovirus B19 infection in hemophiliacs infused with two high purity, virally attenuated factor VIII concentrates. Am J Hematol 39:228, 1992.

137. Shneerson JM, Mortimer PP, Vandervelde EM. Febrile illness due to a parvovirus. BMJ 1:1580, 1980.

138. Mortimer PP, Cohen BJ, Buckley MM, et al. Human parvovirus and the fetus (letter). Lancet 2:1012, 1985.

139. Kinney JS, Anderson LJ, Farrar J, et al. Risk of adverse outcomes of pregnancy after human parvovirus B19 infection. J Infect Dis 157:663, 1988.

140. Enders G, Biber M. Parvovirus B19 infections in pregnancy. Behring Inst Mitt 85:74 1990.

141. Friese K, Beichert M, Hof H, et al. Untersuchung zur häufigkeit konnataler infektionen. Geburtshilfe Frauenheilkd 51:890, 1991.

142. Rogers BB, Singer DB, Mak SK, et al. Detection of human parvovirus B19 in early spontaneous abortuses using serology, histology, electron microscopy, in situ hybridization, and the polymerase chain reaction. Obstet Gynecol 81:402, 1993.

142a. *Gratacos E, Torres P-J, Vidal J, et al. The incidence of human parvovirus B19 infection during pregnancy and its impact on perinatal outcomes. J Infect Dis 171:1360–1363, 1995.*

142b. *Skjoldebrand-Sparre L, Fridell E, Nyman M, Wahren B. A prospective study of antibodies against parvovirus B19 in pregnancy. Acta Obstet Gynecol Scand 75:336–339, 1996.*

143. Wiersbitzky VS, Schwarz TF, Bruns R, et al. Seroprävalenz von Antikörpern gegen das humane parvovirus B19 (Ringelröteln/erythema infectiosum) in der DDR-Bevölkerung. Kinderärztl Prax 58:185, 1990.

144. Public Health Laboratory Service Working Party on Fifth Disease. Prospective study of human parvovirus (B19) infection in pregnancy. BMJ 300:1166, 1990.

145. Peters MT, Nicolaides KH. Cordocentesis for the diagnosis and treatment of human fetal parvovirus infection. Obstet Gynecol 75:501, 1990.

146. Morey AL, Nicolini U, Welch CR, et al. Parvovirus B19 infection and transient fetal hydrops (letter). Lancet 337:496, 1991.

147. Sahakian V, Weiner CP, Naides SJ, et al. Intrauterine transfusion treatment of nonimmune hydrops fetalis secondary to human parvovirus B19 infection. Am J Obstet Gynecol 164:1090, 1991.

148. Humphrey W, Magoon M, O'Shaughnessy R. Severe nonimmune hydrops secondary to parvovirus B-19 infection: spontaneous reversal in utero and survival of a term infant. Obstet Gynecol 78:900, 1991.

149. Glaser C, Tannenbaum J. Newborn with hydrops and a rash. Pediatr Infect Dis J 11:980, 984, 1992.

150. Zerbini M, Musiani M, Gentilomi G, et al. Symptomatic parvovirus B19 infection of one fetus in a twin pregnancy. Clin Infect Dis 17:262, 1993.

151. Adler SP, Harger J, Koch WC, et al. Intrauterine parvovirus B19 infection may cause a symptomatic chronic postnatal infection. Program and Abstracts of the 32nd Interscience Conference on Antimicrobial Agents and Chemotherapy, Anaheim, Calif, 1992, p 256 (abstract 875).

151a. *Koch WC, Harger JH, Barnstein B, Adler SP. Serologic and virologic evidence for frequent intrauterine transmission of human parvovirus B19 with a primary maternal infection during pregnancy. Pediatr Infect Dis 17:489–494, 1998.*

152. Bond PR, Caul EO, Usher J, et al. Intrauterine infection with human parvovirus (letter). Lancet 1:448, 1986.

153. Lefrere JJ, Dumez Y, Couroucé AM, Deschene G. Intrauterine infection with human parvovirus (letter). Lancet 1:449, 1986.

154. Rodis JF, Quinn DL, Gary GW Jr, et al. Management and outcomes of pregnancies complicated by human B19 parvovirus infection: a prospective study. Am J Obstet Gynecol 163:1168, 1990.

155. Török TJ, Anderson LJ, Gary GW Jr, Yodor CGT. Reproductive outcomes following human parvovirus B19 infection in pregnancy. Program and Abstracts of the 31st Interscience Conference on Antimicrobial Agents and Chemotherapy, Chicago, Ill, 1991, p 328 (abstract 1374).

156. Morey AL, Keeling JW, Porter HJ, Fleming KA. Clinical and histopathological features of parvovirus B19 infection in the human fetus. Br J Obstet Gynaecol 99:566, 1992.

157. Gloning KP, Schramm T, Brusis E, et al. Successful intrauterine treatment of fetal hydrops caused by parvovirus B19 infection. Behring Inst Mitt 85:79, 1990.

158. Rogers BB, Mark Y, Oyer CE. Diagnosis and incidence of fetal parvovirus infection in an autopsy series: I. Histology. Pediatr Pathol 13:371, 1993.

159. Mark Y, Rogers BB, Oyer CE. Diagnosis and incidence of fetal parvovirus infection in an autopsy series: II. DNA amplification. Pediatr Pathol 13:381, 1993.

160. Schwarz TF, Nerlich A, Roggendorf M. Parvovirus B19 infection in pregnancy. Behring Inst Mitt 85:69, 1990.

161. Cotmore SF, Tattersall P. The autonomously replicating parvoviruses of vertebrates. Adv Virus Res 33:91, 1987.

162. Margolis G, Kilham L. Problems of human concern arising from animal models of intrauterine and neonatal infections due to viruses: a review: II. Pathologic studies. Progr Med Virol 20:144, 1975.

163. Siegl G. The Parvoviruses. Vienna, Springer-Verlag, 1976, p 109.

164. Siegl G. Biology and pathogenicity of autonomous parvoviruses. *In* Berns KI (ed). The Parvoviruses. New York, Plenum Press, 1984, pp 297–362.

165. Jacoby RO. Parvovirus infection, rat. *In* Jones TC, Mohr U, Hunt RD (eds). Nervous System. Berlin, Springer-Verlag, 1988, pp 170–175.

166. Hartwig NG, Vermeij-Keers C, Van Elsacker-Niele AMW, Gleuren GJ. Embryonic malformations in a case of intrauterine parvovirus B19 infection. Teratology 39:295, 1989.

167. Hartwig NG, Vermeij-Keers C, Versteeg J. The anterior eye segment in virus induced primary congenital aphakia. Acta Morphol Neerl Scand 26:283, 1988–1989.

168. Rodis JF, Hovick TJ Jr, Quinn DL, et al. Human parvovirus infection in pregnancy. Obstet Gynecol 72:733, 1988.

169. Naides SJ, Weiner CP. Antenatal diagnosis and palliative treatment of non-immune hydrops fetalis secondary to fetal parvovirus B19 infection. Prenat Diagn 9:105, 1989.

170. Katz VL, Chescheir NC, Bethea M. Hydrops fetalis from B19 parvovirus infection. J Perinatol 10:366, 1990.

171. Bloom MC, Rolland M, Bernard JD, et al. Infection materno-foetale à parvovirus associée à une péritonite meconiale anétnatale. Arch Fr Pediatr 47:437, 1990.

172. Bernard JD, Berrebi A, Sarramon MF, et al. Infection materno-foetale à parvovirus humain B19: a propos de deux observations. J Gynecol Obstet Biol Reprod 20:855, 1991.

173. Schwarz TF, Nerlich A, Hottenträger B, et al. Parvovirus B19 infection of the fetus: histology and in situ hybridization. Am J Clin Pathol 96:121, 1991.

174. Conry JA, Török T, Andrews PI. Perinatal encephalopa-

thy secondary to in utero human parvovirus B-19 (HPV) infection (abstract 736S). Neurology 43(Suppl):A346, 1993.

175. Kilham L, Margolis G. Spontaneous hepatitis and cerebellar "hypoplasia" in suckling rats due to congenital infections with rat virus. Am J Pathol 49:457, 1966.

176. Kilham L, Margolis G. Transmission of rat virus in milk of rats. J Infect Dis 129:737, 1974.

177. Pattison JR. The pathogenesis of diseases associated with B19 virus. Behring Inst Mitt 85:55, 1990.

178. Morey AL, Patou G, Myint S, Fleming KA. In vitro culture for the detection of infectious human parvovirus B19 and B19-specific antibodies using foetal haematopoietic precursor cells. J Gen Virol 73:3313, 1992.

179. Kurtzman GJ, Cohen BJ, Field AM, et al. Immune response to B19 parvovirus and an antibody defect in persistent viral infection. J Clin Invest 84:114, 1989.

180. Sato H, Hirata J, Furukawa M, et al. Identification of the region including the epitope for a monoclonal antibody which can neutralize human parvovirus B19. J Virol 65:1667, 1991.

181. Sato H, Hirata J, Furukawa M, et al. Identification and mapping of neutralizing epitopes of human parvovirus B19 by using human antibodies. J Virol 65:5485, 1991.

182. Yoshimoto K, Rosenfeld S, Frickhofen N, et al. A second neutralizing epitope of B19 parvovirus implicates the spike region in the immune response. J Virol 65:7056, 1991.

183. Rosenfeld SJ, Yoshimoto K, Kajigaya S, et al. Unique region of the minor capsid protein of human parvovirus B19 is exposed on the virion surface. J Clin Invest 89:2023, 1992.

184. Saikawa T, Anderson S, Momoeda M, et al. Neutralizing linear epitopes of B19 parvovirus cluster in the VP1 unique and VP1–VP2 junction regions. J Virol 67:3004, 1993.

185. Cassinotti P, Weitz M, Siegl G. Human parvovirus B19 infections: routine diagnosis by a new nested polymerase chain reaction assay. J Med Virol 40:228, 1993.

186. Schaefer HE. Aplastic crisis in haemolytic anaemia due to infection parvovirus B19. Pathol Res Pract 188:817, 1992.

187. Mortimer PP, Humphries RK, Moore JG, et al. A human parvovirus-like virus inhibits haematopoietic colony formation "in vitro." Nature 302:426, 1983.

188. Young N, Harrison M, Moore J, et al. Direct demonstration of the human parvovirus in erythroid progenitor cells infected in vitro. J Clin Invest 74:2024, 1984.

189. Ozawa K, Kurtzman G, Young N. Productive infection of B19 parvovirus of human erythroid bone marrow cells in vitro. Blood 70:384, 1987.

190. Morey AL, Fleming KA. Immunophenotyping of fetal hematopoietic cells permissive for human parvovirus B19 replication in vitro. Br J Haematol 82:302, 1992.

191. Morey AL, Ferguson DJP, Fleming KA. Ultrastructural features of fetal erythroid precursors infected with parvovirus B19 in vitro: evidence of cell death by apoptosis. J Pathol 169:213, 1993.

192. Liesveld JL, Weissbach NE, Shafer JA, Abboud CN. In vitro erythroid effects of human stem cell factor in a case of human immunodeficiency virus-related chronic parvovirus B19 induced anemia. Hematol Pathol 7:23, 1993.

193. Srivastava A, Bruno E, Briddell R, et al. Parvovirus B19-induced perturbation of human megakaryocytopoiesis in vitro. Blood 10:1997, 1990.

194. Hanada T, Koike K, Takeya T, et al. Human parvovirus

195. Gray ES, Davidson RJL, Anand A. Human parvovirus and fetal anemia (letter). Lancet 1:1144, 1987.

196. Török TJ, Wang Q-Y, Gary GW Jr, et al. Prenatal diagnosis of intrauterine infection with parvovirus B19 by the polymerase chain reaction technique. Clin Infect Dis 14:149, 1992.

197. Porter HJ, Quantrill AM, Fleming KA. B19 parvovirus infection of myocardial cells (letter). Lancet 1:535, 1988.

198. Carrington D, Gilmore DH, Whittle MJ, et al. Maternal serum alpha-fetoprotein—a marker of fetal aplastic crisis during intrauterine human parvovirus infection. Lancet 1:433, 1987.

199. Anderson MJ, Khousam MN, Maxwell DJ, et al. Human parvovirus B19 and hydrops fetalis (letter). Lancet 1:535, 1988.

200. Pryde PG, Nugent CE, Pridjian G, et al. Spontaneous resolution of nonimmune hydrops fetalis secondary to human parvovirus B19 infection. Obstet Gynecol 79:859, 1992.

201. Metzman R, Anand A, DeGiulio PA, Knisely AS. Hepatic disease associated with intrauterine parvovirus B19 infection in a newborn premature infant. J Pediatr Gastroenterol Nutr 9:112, 1989.

202. Franciosi RA, Tattersall P. Fetal infection with human parvovirus B19. Hum Pathol 19:489, 1988.

203. Nerlich AG, Schwarz TF, Hillemanns P, et al. Pathomorphologie der fetalen parvovirus-B19-infektion. Pathologe 12:204, 1991.

204. Berry PJ, Gray ES, Porter HJ, Burton BA. Parvovirus infection of the human fetus and newborn. Semin Diagn Pathol 9:4, 1992.

205. Anand A, Gray ES, Brown T, et al. Human parvovirus infection in pregnancy and hydrops fetalis. N Engl J Med 316:183, 1987.

206. Caul EO, Usher MJ, Burton PA. Intrauterine infection with human parvovirus B19: a light and electron microscopy study. J Med Virol 24:55, 1988.

207. Maeda H, Shimokawa H, Satoh S, et al. Nonimmunologic hydrops fetalis resulting from intrauterine human parvovirus B-19 infection: report of two cases. Obstet Gynecol 72:482, 1988.

208. van Elsacker-Niele AMW, Salimans MMM, Weiland HT, et al. Fetal pathology in human parvovirus B19 infection. Br J Obstet Gynaecol 96:768, 1989.

209. Bonneau D, Berthier M, Maréchaud M, et al. L'infection à parvovirus B19 au cours de la grossesse. J Gynecol Obstet Biol Reprod 20:1109, 1991.

210. Hassam S, Briner J, Tratschin JD, et al. In situ hybridization for the detection of human parvovirus B19 nucleic acid sequences in paraffin-embedded specimens. Virchows Arch [B] 59:257, 1990.

211. Porter HJ, Heryet A, Quantrill AM, Fleming KA. Combined non-isotopic in situ hybridization and immunohistochemistry on routine clinical material: identification of cell type infected by human parvovirus and demonstration of CMV DNA and antigen in renal infection. J Clin Pathol 43:129, 1990.

212. Nerlich A, Schwarz TF, Roggendorf M, et al. Parvovirus B19-infected erythroblasts in fetal cord blood (letter). Lancet 337:310, 1991.

213. Sterniste W, Rosen A. Hydrops fetalis bedingt durch eine maternale parvovirus B19 infektion. Klin Wochenschr 69:46, 1991.

214. Pollock RVH, Carmichael LE. The canine parvoviruses. In Tijssen P (ed). CRC Handbook of Parvoviruses, vol II. Boca Raton, Fla CRC Press, 1990, pp 113–134.

215. Kovacs BW, Carlson DE, Shahbahrami B, Platt LD. Prenatal diagnosis of human parvovirus B19 in nonimmune hydrops fetalis by polymerase chain reaction. Am J Obstet Gynecol 167:461, 1992.

216. van Elsacker-Niele AMW, Anderson MJ. First picture of erythema infectiosum? Letter to the editor. Lancet 1:229, 1987.

217. Cheinisse L. Une cinquième maladie éruptive: le mégaléry-thème épidémique. Semaine Med 25:205, 1905.

218. Morens DM, Fifth disease: still hazy after all these years. JAMA 248:553, 1982.

219. Morens DM, Katz AR. The "fourth disease" of childhood: reevaluation of a nonexistent disease. Am J Epidemiol 134:628, 1991.

220. Lauer BA, MacCormack JN, Wilfert C. Erythema infectiosum: an elementary school outbreak. Am J Dis Child 130:252, 1976.

221. Veraldi S, Rizzitelli G, Lunghi G, Cardone R. Primary infection by human parvovirus B19. Dermatology 186:72, 1993.

222. Lefrere JJ, Couroucé AM, Muller JY, et al. Human parvovirus and purpura (letter). Lancet 2:730, 1985.

223. Mortimer PP, Cohen BJ, Rossiter MA, et al. Human parvovirus and purpura (letter). Lancet 2:730, 1985.

224. Lefrère JJ, Couroucé AM, Soulier JP, et al. Henoch-Schönlein purpura and human parvovirus infection (letter). Pediatrics 78:183, 1986.

225. Li Loong TC, Coyle PV, Anderson MJ, et al. Human serum parvovirus associated vasculitis. Postgrad Med J 62:493, 1986.

226. Lassen C, Bonneau D, Berthier M, Hoppeler A. Purpura vasculaire fébrile dû à un parvovirus (letter). Arch Fr Pediatr 44:619, 1987.

227. Naides SJ, Piette W, Veach LA, Argenyi Z. Human parvovirus B19-induced vesiculopustular skin eruption. Am J Med 84:968, 1988.

228. Dinerman JL, Corman LC. Human parvovirus B19 arthropathy associated with desquamation. Am J Med 89:826, 1990

229. Woolf AD. Human parvovirus B19 and arthritis. Behring Inst Mitt 85:64, 1990.

230. Joseph PR. Fifth disease: the frequency of joint involvement in adults. NY State J Med 86:560, 1986.

231. Taylor HG, Borg AA, Dawes PT. Human parvovirus B19 and rheumatoid arthritis. Clin Rheumatol 11:548, 1992.

232. Nocton JJ, Miller LC, Tucker LB, Schaller JG. Human parvovirus B19-associated arthritis in children. J Pediatr 122:186, 1993.

233. Klouda PT, Corbin SA, Bradley BA, et al. HLA and acute arthritis following human parvovirus infection. Tissue Antigens 28:318, 1986.

234. Dÿkmans BAC, Breedveld FC, de Vries, RRP. HLA antigens in human parvovirus arthropathy. J Rheumatol 13:1192, 1986.

235. Jawad ASM. Persistent arthritis after human parvovirus B19 infection (letter). Lancet 341:494, 1993.

236. Fatehnejad S, Fikrig MK, Rahn DW, Malawista SE. Parvovirus arthritis mistaken for Lyme arthritis (letter). J Rheumatol 19:1002, 1992.

237. Mayo DR, Vance DW Jr. Parvovirus B19 as the cause of a syndrome resembling Lyme arthritis in adults (letter). N Engl J Med 324:419, 1991.

238. Pouchot J, Ouakil H, Debin ML, Vinceneux P. Adult Still's disease associated with acute human parvovirus B19 infection (letter). Lancet 341:1280, 1993.

239. Kalish RA, Knopf AN, Gary GW, Canoso JJ. Lupus-like presentation of human parvovirus B19 infection. J Rheumatol 19:169, 1992.

240. Cope AP, Jones A, Brozovic M, et al. Possible induction of systemic lupus erythematosus by human parvovirus. Ann Rheum Dis 51:803, 1992.

241. Chassagne P, Mejjad O, Gourmelen O, et al. Exacerbation of systemic lupus erythematosus during human parvovirus B19 infection. Br J Rheumatol 32:158, 1993.

242. Koch WC, Massey G, Russell CE, Adler SP. Manifestations and treatment of human parvovirus B19 infection in immunocompromised patients. J Pediatr 116:355, 1990.

243. Leventhal LJ, Naides SJ, Freundlich B. Fibromyalgia and parvovirus infection. Arthritis Rheum 34:1319, 1991.

244. Deighton CM, Madeley CR, Walker DJ. Antiviral antibodies in rheumatoid arthritis discordant HLA-identical same-sexed sibling pairs (letter). Br J Rheumatol 31:357, 1992.

245. Saal JG, Steidle M, Einsele H, et al. Persistence of B19 parvovirus in synovial membranes of patients with rheumatoid arthritis. Rheumatol Int 2:147, 1992.

246. Cohen BJ, Buckley MM, Clewley JP, et al. Human parvovirus infection in an early rheumatoid and inflammatory arthritis. Ann Rheum Dis 45:832, 1986.

247. Naides SJ, Field EH. Transient rheumatoid factor positivity in acute human parvovirus B19 infection. Arch Intern Med 148:2587, 1988.

248. Sasaki T, Takahashi Y, Yoshinaga K, et al. An association between human parvovirus B-19 infection and autoantibody production (letter). J Rheumatol 16:708, 1989.

249. Luzzi GA, Kurtz JB, Chapel H. Human parvovirus arthropathy and rheumatoid factor (letter). Lancet 1:1218, 1993.

250. Soloninka CA, Anderson MJ, Laskin CA. Anti-DNA and antilymphocyte antibodies during acute infection with human parvovirus B19. J Rheumatol 16:777, 1989.

251. Soloninka CA, Anderson MJ, Laskin CA. Auto-antibodies in sera from patients with parvovirus B19 infection (letter). J Rheumatol 17:416, 1990.

252. Semble EL, Agudelo CA, Pegram PS. Human parvovirus B19 arthropathy in two adults after contact with childhood erythema infectiosum. Am J Med 83:560, 1987.

253. Aussedat R, Fener P, Pourel J. Coxite aiguë de l'adolescent, manifestation unique d'une infection par le parvovirus B19 (letter). Presse Med 16:1978, 1987.

254. Ueno Y, Umadome H, Shimodera M, et al. Human parvovirus B19 and arthritis (letter). Lancet 341:1280, 1993.

255. Dijkmans BAC, van Elsacker-Niele AMW, Salimans MMM, et al. Human parvovirus B19 DNA in synovial fluid. Arthritis Rheum 31:279, 1988.

256. Kandolf R, Kirschner P, Hofschneider PH, Vischer TL. Detection of parvovirus in a patient with "reactive arthritis" by in situ hybridization. Clin Rheumatol 8:398, 1989.

257. Foto F, Saag KG, Scharosch LL, et al. Parvovirus B19-specific DNA in bone marrow from B19 arthropathy patients: evidence for B19 virus persistence. J Infect Dis 167:744, 1993.

258. Miki NPH, Chantler JK. Non-permissiveness of synovial membrane cells to human parvovirus B19 in vitro. J Gen Virol 73:1559, 1992.

259. Török TJ. Parvovirus B19 and human disease. Adv Intern Med 37:431, 1992.

260. Green DH, Bellingham AJ, Anderson MJ. Parvovirus infection in a family associated with aplastic crisis in an affected sibling pair with hereditary spherocytosis. J Clin Pathol 37:1144, 1984.

261. Summerfield GP, Wyatt GP. Human parvovirus infection revealing hereditary spherocytosis (letter). Lancet 2:1070, 1985.

262. Lefrere JJ, Couroucé AM, Girot R, et al. Six cases of

hereditary spherocytosis revealed by human parvovirus infection. Br J Haematol 62:653, 1986.

263. Lefrere JJ, Courouce AM, Bertrand Y, et al. Human parvovirus and aplastic crisis in chronic hemolytic anemias: a study of 24 observations. Am J Hematol 23:271, 1986.

264. Gowda N, Rao SP, Cohen B, et al. Human parvovirus infection in patients with sickle cell disease with and without hypoplastic crisis. J Pediatr 110:81, 1987.

265. Goldstein AR, Anderson MJ, Serjeant GR. Parvovirus associated aplastic crisis in homozygous sickle cell disease. Arch Dis Child 62:585, 1987.

266. Rao SP, Miller ST, Cohen BJ. Transient aplastic crisis in patients with sickle cell disease. B19 parvovirus studies during a 7-year period. Am J Dis Child 146:1328, 1992.

267. Conrad ME, Studdard H, Anderson LJ. Case report: aplastic crisis in sickle cell disorders: bone marrow necrosis and human parvovirus infection. Am J Med Sci 295:212, 1988.

268. Godeau B, Galacteros F, Schaeffer A, et al. Aplastic crisis due to extensive bone marrow necrosis and human parvovirus infection in sickle cell disease. Am J Med 91:557, l991.

269. Balkran B, Char G, Morris JS, et al. Stroke in a cohort of patients with homozygous sickle cell disease. J Pediatr 120:360, 1992.

270. Hamon MD, Newland AC, Anderson MJ. Severe aplastic anaemia after parvovirus infection in the absence of underlying haemolytic anaemia. J Clin Pathol 41:1242, 1988.

271. Young NS, Mortimer PP, Moore JG, Humphries RK. Characterization of a virus that causes transient aplastic crisis. J Clin Invest 73:224, 1984.

272. Lefrere JJ, Courouce AM, Kaplan C. Parvovirus and idiopathic thrombocytopenic purpura (letter). Lancet 1:279, 1989.

273. Shirley JA, Revill S, Cohen BJ, Buckley MM. Serological study of rubella-like illnesses. J Med Virol 21:369, 1987.

274. Lefrere JJ, Got D. Peripheral thrombocytopenia in human parvovirus infection (letter). J Clin Pathol 40:469, 1987.

275. Foreman NK, Oakhill A, Caul EO. Parvovirus-associated thrombocytopenic purpura (letter). Lancet 2:1426, 1988.

276. Inoue S, Kinra NK, Mukkamala SR, Gordon R. Parvovirus B-19 infection: aplastic crisis, erythema infectiosum and idiopathic thrombocytopenic purpura. Pediatr Infect Dis J 10:251, 1991.

277. Glader BE. Red blood cell aplasias in children. Pediatr Ann 19:168, 1990.

278. Wodzinski MA, Lilleyman JS. Transient erythroblastopenia of childhood due to parvovirus B19 infection. Br J Haematol 73:127, 1989.

279. Nagai K, Morohoshi T, Kudoh T, et al. Transient erythroblastopenia of childhood with megakaryocytopenia associated with human parvovirus B19 infection. Br J Haematol 80:131, 1992.

280. Davidson JE, Gibson B, Gibson A, Evans TJ. Parvovirus infection, leukemia, and immunodeficiency (letter). Lancet 1:102, 1989.

281. Gahr M, Pekrun A, Eiffert H. Persistence of parvovirus B19-DNA in blood of a child with severe combined immunodeficiency associated with chronic pure red cell aplasia. Eur J Pediatr 150:470, 1991.

282. Zerbini M, Musiani M, Venturoli S, et al. Different syndromes associated with B19 parvovirus viraemia in paediatric patients: report of four cases. Eur J Pediatr 151:815, 1992.

283. de Mayolo JA, Temple JD. Pure red cell aplasia due to parvovirus B19 infection in a man with HIV infection. South Med J 83:1480, 1990.

284. Mitchell SA, Welch JM, Weston-Smith S, et al. Parvovirus infection and anaemia in a patient with AIDS: case report. Genitourin Med 66:95, 1990.

285. Chrystie IL, Almeida JD, Welch J. Case report: electron microscopic detection of human parvovirus (B19) in a patient with HIV infection. J Med Virol 30:249, 1990.

286. Bowman CA, Cohen BJ, Norfolk DR, Lacey CJN. Red cell aplasia associated with human parvovirus B19 and HIV infection: failure to respond clinically to intravenous immunoglobulin (letter). AIDS 4:1038, 1990.

287. Griffin TC, Squires JE, Timmons CF, Buchanan GR. Chronic human parvovirus B19-induced erythroid hypoplasia as the initial manifestation of human immunodeficiency virus infection. J Pediatr 118:899, 1991.

288. Taillan B, Heudier P, Ferrari E, et al. Pure red-cell aplasia due to parvovirus B19 infection in a patient with AIDS-related complex. Ann Med 24:137, 1992.

289. Nigro G, Gattinara GC, Mattia S, et al. Parvovirus-B19–related pancytopenia in children with HIV infection (letter). Lancet 340:115, 1992.

290. Nigro G, Luzi G, Fridell E, et al. Parvovirus infection in children with AIDS: high prevalence of B19-specific immunoglobulin M and G antibodies. AIDS 6:679, 1992.

291. Mitsuyasu RT, Lambertus M, Goetz MB. Transfusion-dependent anemia in a patient with AIDS. Clin Infect Dis 15:533, 1992.

292. Naides SJ, Howard EJ, Swack NS, et al. Parvovirus B19 infection in human immunodeficiency virus type 1-infected persons failing or intolerant to zidovudine therapy. J Infect Dis 168:101, l993.

293. García-Tapia AM, Fernández C, Bascuñana A. Infeccion persistente por parvovirus B19 en una paciente con sida (letter). Enferm Infecc Microbiol Clin 11:107, 1993.

294. Neild G, Anderson M, Hawes S, Colvin BT. Parvovirus infection after renal transplant (letter). Lancet 2:1226, 1986.

295. Marshall WF, Telenti A, Smith TF. Polymerase chain reaction detection of parvovirus B19 viremia after organ transplantation, abstract No. 1234. Program and Abstracts of the 30th Interscience Conference on Antimicrobial Agents and Chemotherapy, Atlanta, October 21–24, 1990, p 292.

296. Krause JR, Penchansky L, Knisely AS. Morphological diagnosis of parvovirus B19 infection. Arch Path Lab Med 116:178, 1992.

297. Corral DA, Darras FS, Jensen CWB, et al. Transplantation 55:427, 1993.

298. Van Horn DK, Mortimer PP, Young N, Hanson GR. Human parvovirus-associated red cell aplasia in the absence of underlying hemolytic anemia. Am J Pediatr Hematol Oncol 8:235, 1986.

299. Smith MA, Shah NR, Lobel JS, et al. Severe anemia caused by human parvovirus in a leukemia patient on maintenance chemotherapy. Clin Pediatr 27:383, 1988.

300. Kurtzman GJ, Cohen B, Meyers P, et al. Persistent B19 parvovirus infection as a cause of severe chronic anemia in children with acute lymphocytic leukemia. Lancet 2:1159, 1988.

301. Coulombel L, Morinet F, Mielot F, Tchernia G. Parvovirus infection, leukaemia, and immunodeficiency (letter). Lancet 1:101, 1989.

302. Carstensen H, Cohen BJ, Human parvovirus B19 infection associated with prolonged erythroblastopenia in a leukemic child (letter). Pediatr Infect Dis 8:56, 1989.

303. Weiland HT, Salimans MMM, Fibbe WE et al. Prolonged parvovirus B19 infection with severe anemia in a

bone marrow transplant recipient (letter). Br J Haematol 71:300, 1989.

304. Malarme M, Vandervelde D, Brasseur M. Parvovirus infection, leukemia, and immunodeficiency (letter). Lancet 1:1457, 1989.

305. Azzi A, Macchia PA, Favre C, et al. Aplastic crisis caused by B19 virus in a child during induction therapy for acute lymphoblastic leukemia. Haematologica (Pavia) 74:191, 1989.

306. Graeve JLA, de Alarçon PA, Naides SJ. Parvovirus B19 infection in patients receiving cancer chemotherapy: the expanding spectrum of disease. Am J Pediatr Hematol Oncol 11:441, 1989.

307. Niitsu H, Takatsu H, Miura I, et al. Pure red cell aplasia induced by B19 parvovirus during allogeneic bone marrow transplantation. Rinsho Ketsueki 31:1566, 1990.

308. Rao SP, Miller ST, Cohen BJ. Severe anemia due to B19 parvovirus infection in children with acute leukemia in remission. Am J Pediatr Hematol Oncol 12:194, 1990.

309. Takahashi M, Moriyama Y, Shibata A, et al. Anemia caused by parvovirus in an adult patient with acute lymphoblastic leukemia in complete remission (letter). Eur J Haematol 46:47, 1991.

310. Takahashi M, Nikkuni K, Tanaka I, et al. Serum erythropoietic inhibitors in patients with pure red cell aplasia. Ann Hematol 63:9, 1991.

311. Frickhofen N, Arnold R, Hertenstein B, et al. Parvovirus B19 infection and bone marrow transplantation. Ann Hematol 64(Suppl):A121, 1992.

312. Fisher D, Spencer D, Iland H, et al. Red cell aplasia caused by human parvovirus B19 in acute leukemia. Aust NZJ Med 22:303, 1992.

313. Fujita H, Takada K, Kuremoto K, et al. Human parvovirus B19 infection in patients with hematologic disorders on chemotherapy. Rinsho Ketsueki 34:28, 1993.

314. Hitchens R, Sloots TP. Another parvovirus B19 infection of a chronic lymphatic leukaemia patient (letter). Aust NZJ Med 23:217, 1993.

315. Anderson MJ, Kidd IM, Jones SE, et al. Parvovirus infection and the acquired immunodeficiency syndrome. Ann Intern Med 102:275, 1985.

316. Musiani M, Azzi A, Zerbini M, et al. Nested polymerase chain reaction assay for the detection of B19 parvovirus DNA in human immunodeficiency virus patients. J Med Virol 40.157, 1993.

317. Boruchoff SE, Woda BA, Pihan GA, et al. Parvovirus B19-associated hemophagocytic syndrome. Arch Intern Med 150:897, 1990.

318. Muir K, Todd WTA, Watson WH, Fitzsimons E. Viral-associated haemophagocytosis with parvovirus-B19-related pancytopenia. Lancet 339:1139, 1992.

319. Risdall RJ, McKenna RW, Nesbit ME, et al. Virus-associated hemophagocytic syndrome: a benign histiocytic proliferation distinct from malignant histiocytosis. Cancer 44:993, 1979.

320. Saint-Martin J, Choulot JJ, Bonnaud E, Morinet F. Myocarditis caused by parvovirus (letter). J Pediatr 116:1007, 1990.

321. Saint-Martin J, Bonnaud E, Morinet F, et al. Myocardité aiguë à parvovirus d'évolution Iétale. Pèdiatrie 46:597, 1991.

322. Malm C, Fridell E, Jansson K. Heart failure after parvovirus B19 infection (letter). Lancet 341:1408, 1993.

323. Denning DW, Amos A, Rudge P, Cohen BJ. Neuralgic amyotrophy due to parvovirus infection (letter). J Neurol Neurosurg Psychiatr 50:641, 1987.

324. Walsh KJ, Armstrong RD, Turner AM. Brachial plexus

325. Jacks TA. Pruritus in parvovirus infection. JR Coll Gen Pract 37:210, 1987.

326. Corridan PGJ, Laws DE, Morrell AJ, Murray PI. Tonic pupils and human parvovirus (B19) infection. J Clin Neuro Ophthalmol 11:109, 1991.

327. Faden H, Gary GW Jr, Korman M. Numbness and tingling of fingers associated with parvovirus B19 infection (letter). J Infect Dis 161:354, 1990.

328. Leray H, Canaud B, Cristol JP, et al. Infection à parvovirus B19 révélée par une insuffisance rénale aiguë. Néphrologie 13:123, 1992.

329. Faden H, Gary DW Jr, Anderson LJ. Chronic parvovirus infection in a presumably immunologically healthy woman. Clin Infect Dis 15:595, 1992.

330. Balfour HH Jr, Schiff GM, Bloom JE. Encephalitis associated with erythema infectiosum. JAMA 77:133, 1970.

331. Hall CB, Horner FA. Encephalopathy with erythema infectiosum. Am J Dis Child 131:65, 1977.

332. Brass C, Elliott LM, Stevens DA. Academy rash. A probable epidemic of erythema infectiosum ("fifth disease"). JAMA 248:568, 1982.

333. Lefrere JJ, Olivier C, Couroucé AM, Soulier JP. Erythroblastopénie et syndrome méningé fébrile dus as parvovirus chez un enfant drépanocytaire homozygote (letter). Presse Med 14:228, 1985.

334. Tsuji A, Uchida N, Asamura S, et al. Aseptic meningitis with erythema infectiosum. Eur J Pediatr 149:449, 1990.

335. Sørensen SF. Akut vasculitis og arthritis forårsaget af Parvovirus B 19 infektion. Ugeskr Læger 154:2032,1992.

336. Prato C, Paper T, Morinet F. Use of M13 single-stranded CNA digoxigenin labelled probe for detection of human parvovirus B19 viraemia. J Virol Methods 34:227, 1991.

337. Borreda D, Palomera S, Gilbert B, et al. A propos de vingt-quatre observations d'infections à parvovirus humain B19 chez l'enfant. Ann Pédiatr (Paris) 39:543, 1992.

338. Finkel TH, Gelfand F.W, Harbeck R, et al. Chronic parvovirus infection presenting as juvenile polyarteritis nodosum (abstract C167). Arthritis Rheum 33(Suppl):S132, 1990.

339. Corman LC, Dolson DJ. Polyarteritis nodosa and parvovirus B19 infection (letter). Lancet 339:491,1992.

340. Scholbach T. Nierenaffektion bei parvovirus B 19-infektion eines kindes. Kinderarztl Prax 60:156, 1992.

341. Rauch AM. Kawasaki syndrome: review of new epidemiologic and laboratory developments. Pediatr Infect Dis J 6:1016, 1987.

342. Okabe N, Koboyashi S, Tatsuzawa O, Mortimer PP. Detection of antibodies to human parvovirus in erythema infectiosum (fifth disease). Arch Dis Child 59:1016, 1984.

343. Nigro G, Pisano P, Krzysztofiak A. Recurrent Kawasaki disease associated with co-infection with parvovirus B19 and HIV-1 (letter). AIDS 7:288, 1993.

344. Roberts JM, Redman CWG. Pre-eclampsia: more than pregnancy-induced hypertension. Lancet 341:1447, 1993.

345. Soothill P. Intrauterine blood transfusion for non-immune hydrops fetalis due to parvovirus B19 infection (letter). Lancet 336:121, 1990.

346. Wright IMR, Williams ML, Cohen BJ. Congenital parvovirus infection. Arch Dis Child 66:253, 1991.

347. Weiner CP, Naides SJ. Fetal survival after human parvovirus B19 infection: spectrum of intrauterine response in a twin gestation. Am J Perinatol 9:66, 1992.

348. Sheikh AU, Ernest JM, O'Shea M. Long-term outcome in fetal hydrops from parvovirus B19 infection. Am J Obstet Gynecol 167:337, 1992.

349. Schwarz TF, Roggendorf M, Hottenträger B, et al. Hu-

man parvovirus B19 infection in pregnancy (letter). Lancet 2:566, 1988.

350. Belloy M, Morinet F, Blondin G, et al. Erythroid hypoplasia due to chronic infection with parvovirus B19 (letter). N Engl J Med 322:633, 1990.

351. Anderson LJ, Gary GW Jr, Young N. Human parvovirus B19. *In* Lennette EH (ed). Laboratory Diagnosis of Viral Infections, 2nd ed. New York, Marcel Dekker, 1992. pp 627–642.

352. Anderson LJ, Tsou C, Parker RA, et al. Detection of antibodies and antigens of human parvovirus B19 by enzyme-linked immunosorbent assay. J Clin Microbiol 24:522, 1986.

353. Westmoreland D, Cohen BJ. Human parvovirus B19 infected fetal liver as a source of antigen for a radioimmunoassay for B19 specific IgM in clinical samples. J Med Virol 33:1, 1991.

354. Cotmore SF, McKie VC, Anderson LJ, et al. Identification of the major structural and nonstructural proteins encoded by human parvovirus B19 and mapping of their genes by procaryotic expression of isolated genomic fragments. J Virol 60:548, 1986.

355. Morinet F, D'Auriol L, Tratschin JD, Galibert F. Expression of the human parvovirus B19 protein fused to protein A in *Escherichia coli*: recognition by IgM antibodies and IgG antibodies in human sera. J Gen Virol 70:3091, 1989.

356. Sisk WP, Berman ML. Expression of human parvovirus B19 structural protein in *E. coli* and detection of antiviral antibodies in human sera. Biotechnology 5:1077, 1987.

357. Morinet F, Couroucé AM, Galibert F, Perol Y. Development of an IgM antibody capture test using labelled fusion protein as antigen for diagnosis of B19 human parvovirus infections. Behring Inst Mitt 85:28, 1990.

358. Rayment FB, Crosdale E, Morris DJ, et al. The production of human parvovirus capsid proteins in *Escherichia coli* and their potential as diagnostic antigens. J Gen Virol 71:2665, 1990.

359. Söderlund M, Brown KE, Meurman O, Hedman K. Prokaryotic expression of a VP1 polypeptide antigen for diagnosis of a human parvovirus B19 antibody enzyme immunoassay. J Clin Microbiol 30:305, 1992.

360. Schwarz TF, Modrow S, Hottenträger B, et al. New oligopeptide immunoglobulin G test for human parvovirus B19 antibodies. J Clin Microbiol 29:431, 1991.

361. Morinet F, Couroucé AM, Galibert F, Perol Y. The use of labeled fusion protein for detection of B19 parvovirus IgM antibodies by an immunocapture test. J Virol Methods 32:21, 1991.

362. Brown CS, Salimans MMM, Noteborn MHM, Weiland HT. Antigenic parvovirus B19 coat proteins VP1 and VP2 produced in large quantities in a baculovirus expression system. Virus Res 15:197, 1990.

363. Kajigaya S, Shimada T, Fujita S, Young NS. A genetically engineered cell line that produces empty capsids of B19 (human) parvovirus. Proc Natl Acad Sci U S A 86:7601, 1989.

364. Brown CS, Van Lent JWM, Vlak JM, Spaan WJM. Assembly of empty capsids by using baculovirus recombinants expressing human parvovirus B19 structural proteins. J Virol 65:2702, 1991.

365. Clewley JP, Mori J, Turton J. Molecular approaches for production of B19 antigen. Behring Inst Mitt 85:14, 1990.

366. Erdman DD, Usher MJ, Tsou C, et al. Human parvovirus B19 specific IgG. IgA, and IgM antibodies and DNA in serum specimens from persons with erythema infectiosum. J Med Virol 35:110, 1991.

367. Fridell E, Trojnar J, Wahren B. A new peptide for human parvovirus B19 antibody detection. Scand J Infect Dis 21:597, 1989.

368. Fridell E, Cohen BJ, Wahren B. Evaluation of a synthetic-peptide enzyme-linked immunosorbent assay for immunoglobulin M to human parvovirus B19. J Clin Microbiol 29:1376, 1991.

369. Fridell E, Trojnar J, Mehlin H, Wahren B. A cyclized peptide for studies of human parvovirus B19 infection. J Immunol Methods 138:125, 1991.

370. Ozawa K, Kurtzman G, Young N. Replication of the B19 parvovirus in human bone marrow cell cultures. Science 233:883, 1986.

371. Sosa CE, Mahony JB, Luinstra KE, et al. Replication and cytopathology of human parvovirus B19 in human umbilical cord blood erythroid progenitor cells. J Med Virol 36:125, 1992.

372. Srivastava CH, Zhou S, Munshi NC, Srivastava A. Parvovirus B19 replication in human umbilical cord blood cells. Virology 189:456, 1992.

373. Serke S, Schwarz TF, Baurmann H, et al. Productive infection of in vitro generated haemopoietic progenitor cells from normal human adult peripheral blood with parvovirus B19: studies by morphology, immunocytochemistry, flow-cytometry and DNA-hybridization. Br J Haematol 79:6, 1991.

374. Schwarz TF, Serke S, Hottenträger B, et al. Replication of parvovirus B19 in hematopoietic progenitor cells generated in vitro from normal human peripheral blood. J Virol 1273, 1992.

375. Yaegashi N, Shiraishi H, Takeshita T, et al. Propagation of human parvovirus B19 in primary culture of erythroid lineage cells derived from fetal liver. J Virol 63:2422, 1989.

376. Brown KE, Mori J, Cohen BJ, Field AM. In vitro propagation of parvovirus B19 in primary foetal liver culture. J Gen Virol 72:741, 1991.

377. Takahashi T, Ozawa K, Mitani K, et al. B19 parvovirus replicates in erythroid leukemic cells in vitro (letter). J Infect Dis 160:548, 1989.

378. Shimomura S, Komatsu N, Frickhofen N et al. First continuous propagation of B19 parvovirus in a cell line. Blood 79:18, 1992.

379. Munshi NC, Zhou S, Woody MJ, et al. Successful replication of parvovirus B19 in the human megakaryocytic leukemia cell line MB-02. J Virol 67:562, 1993.

380. Anderson MJ, Davis LR, Jones SE, Pattison JR. The development and use of an antibody capture radioimmunoassay for specific IgM to a human parvovirus-like agent. J Hyg (Lond) 88:309, 1982.

381. Brown KE, Buckley MM, Cohen BJ, Samuel D. An amplified ELISA for the detection of parvovirus B19 IgM using monoclonal antibody to FITC. J Virol Methods 26:189, 1989.

382. Shattock RJ. Development of a gene probe assay suitable for use in routine diagnosis: a pilot study using a DNA probe for parvovirus B19. Med Lab Sci 47:97, 1990.

383. Salimans MMM. Detection of human parvovirus B19 DNA by dot-hybridization and the polymerase chain reaction: applications for diagnosis of infections. Behring Inst Mitt 85:39, 1990.

384. Musiani M, Zerbini M, Gibellini D, et al. Chemiluminescence dot blot hybridization assay for detection of B19 parvovirus DNA in human sera. J Clin Microbiol 29:2047, 1991.

385. Mori J, Field AM, Clewley JP, Cohen BJ. Dot blot hybridization assay of B19 virus DNA in clinical specimens. J Clin Microbiol 27:459, 1989.

386. Salimans MMM, Holsappel S, van de Rijke FM, et al. Rapid detection of human parvovirus B19 DNA by dot-hybridization and the polymerase chain reaction. J Virol Methods 23:19, 1989.

387. Clewley JP. Polymerase chain reaction assay of parvovirus B19 DNA in clinical specimens. J Clin Microbiol 27:2647, 1989.

388. Frickhofen N, Young NS. Polymerase chain reaction for detection of parvovirus B19 in immunodeficient patients with anemia. Behring Inst Mitt 85:46, 1990.

389. Koch WC, Adler SP. Detection of human parvovirus B19 DNA by using the polymerase chain reaction. J Clin Microbiol 28:65, 1990.

390. Frickhofen N, Young NS. A rapid method of sample preparation for detection of DNA viruses in human serum by polymerase chain reaction. J Virol Methods 35:65, 1991.

391. Sevall JS. Detection of parvovirus B19 by dot-blot and polymerase chain reaction. Mol Cell Probes 4:237, 1990.

392. Fridell E, Kékássy AN, Larsson B, Eriksson BM. Polymerase chain reaction with double primer pairs for detection of human parvovirus B19 induced aplastic crises in family outbreaks. Scand J Infect Dis 24:275, 1992.

393. Clewley JP. PCR detection of parvovirus B19. *In* Persing DH, Smith TF, Tenover FC, White TJ (eds). Diagnostic Molecular Microbiology: Principles and Applications. Washington DC, American Society for Microbiology. 1993, pp 367–373.

394. Sevall JS, Ritenhous J, Peter JB. Laboratory diagnosis of parvovirus B19 infection. J Clin Lab Anal 6:171, 1992.

395. Schwarz TF, Jäger G, Holzgreve W, Roggendorf M. Diagnosis of human parvovirus B19 infections by polymerase chain reaction. Scand J Infect Dis 24:691, 1992.

395a. *Wattre P, Dewilde A, Subtil D, et al. A clinical and epidemiological study of human parvovirus B19 infection in fetal hydrops using PCR Southern blot hybridization and chemiluminescence detection. J Med Virol 54:140–144, 1998.*

396. Nerlich A, Schwarz TF, Roggendorf M, et al. Molekularbiologischer nachweis einer parvovirusinfektion in fetalem gewebe. Verh Dtsch Ges Pathol 74:394, 1990.

397. Brown KE, Cohen BJ. Haemagglutination by parvovirus B19. J Gen Virol 73:2147, 1992.

398. Rogers BB. Case 5 histopathologic variability of finding erythroid inclusions with intrauterine parvovirus B19 infection. Pediatr Pathol 12:883, 1992.

399. Gentilomi G, Zerbini M, Musiani M, et al. In situ detection of B19 DNA in bone marrow of immunodeficient patients using a digoxigenin-labelled probe. Mol Cell Probes 7:19, 1993.

400. Nascimento JP, Hallam NF, Mori J, et al. Detection of B19 parvovirus in human fetal tissues by in situ hybridization. J Med Virol 33:77, 1991.

401. Mehraein Y, Rehder H, Draeger HG, et al. Die diagnostik fetaler virusinfektionen durch in-situ-hybirdisierung. Geburtshilfe Frauenheilkd 51:984, 1991.

402. Yun ZB, Hornsleth A. Production of digoxigenin-labelled parvovirus DNA probe by PCR. Res Virol 142:277, 1991.

403. Zakrzewska K, Ciappi S, Azzi A. Polymerase chain reaction for synthesis of digoxigenin-labelled DNA probe: application to parvovirus B19 and to polyomavirus BK. Mol Cell Probes 7:55, 1993.

404. Clewley JP, Cohen BJ, Field AM. Detection of parvovirus B19 DNA, antigen, and particles in the human fetus. J Med Virol 23:367, 1987.

405. Field AM, Cohen BJ, Brown KE, et al. Detection of B19 parvovirus in human fetal tissues by electron microscopy. J Med Virol 35:85, 1991.

406. Fritz B, Moore K, Naides SJ. A combined pseudoreplica-immunochemical technique for research and diagnostic virology. Microsc Res Tech 21:59, 1992.

407. Centers for Disease Control. Risks associated with human parvovirus B19 infection. Morb Mortal Wkly Rep 38:81, 93, 1989.

408. Gottlieb F, Deutsch J. Red cell aplasia responsive to immunoglobulin therapy as initial manifestation of human immunodeficiency virus infection. Am J Med 92:331, 1992.

409. Schwarz TF, Serke S, von Brunn A, et al. Heat stability of parvovirus B19: kinetics of inactivation. Int J Med Microbiol Virol Parasitol Infect Dis 277:219, 1992.

410. Fridell E. B19 human parvovirus in pregnancy. Scand J Infect Dis 71(Suppl):71, 1990.

411. American Academy of Pediatrics Committee on Infectious Diseases. Parvovirus, erythema infectiosum, and pregnancy. Pediatrics 85:131, 1990.

412. Cohen BJ, Brown KE. Laboratory infection with human parvovirus B19 (letter). J Infect 24:113, 1992.

413. Schwarz TF, Roggendorf M, Hottenträger B, et al. Immunoglobulins in the prophylaxis of parvovirus B19 infection (letter). J Infect Dis 162:1214, 1990.

414. Takahashi M, Koike T, Moriyama Y, Shibata A. Neutralizing activity of immunoglobulin preparation against erythropoietic suppression of human parvovirus (letter). Am J Hematol 37:68, 1991.

415. Bansal GP, Hatfield JA, Dunn FE, et al. Candidate recombinant vaccine for human B19 parvovirus. J Infect Dis 167:1034, 1993.

416. Bernstein IM, Capeless EL. Elevated maternal serum alpha-fetoprotein and hydrops fetalis in association with fetal parvovirus B-19 infection. Obstet Gynecol 74:456, 1989.

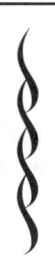

Fungal Infections

MICHAEL J. MILLER, M.D.

Fungal infections are rarely considered in newborns with signs of sepsis because bacterial, viral, and protozoan infections are more common causes of acute neonatal illness. Nevertheless, fungal infections do occur in infants and may be responsible for serious and occasionally fatal disease. Of even greater importance is the high incidence of mild mucocutaneous infections in newborns.

Mycotic infections, whether confined to epidermal structures or involving deep tissues, are caused by fungi free-living in soil, in bird or mammal excreta, or in decaying organic matter. In instances of fungal infections in newborns, organisms are most often acquired from the mother during birth of the infant or in utero from hematogenous or ascending vaginal infection. When inhaled, ingested, or inoculated directly into tissue, these saprophytic microorganisms may cause infection after birth in infants with undue susceptibility. Although much has been learned regarding pathogenesis, immune response, and treatment of fungal infections in humans, studies to determine the cause of increased susceptibility or resistances to infection with fungi, particularly in infants, are incomplete. However, advances have been made in both diagnosing and treating fungal infections in newborns. In this chapter, the acquisition, clinical manifestations, diagnosis, and data regarding fungal infections in adults are included and, to avoid confusion, are identified as such.

CANDIDIASIS

Species of *Candida*, particularly *Candida albicans*, account for the majority of fungal infections in infants and can be isolated from the mouth or oropharynx within days of birth[1] and with increasing frequency from those sites during the first few weeks of life.[2-4] In adults, *Candida* can be found as part of the normal flora in the mouth, feces, and vaginal secretions in the absence of clinical disease[5-8]; however, in infants, clinically apparent infection is frequent when the fungus is isolated from skin or mucous membranes.[9-11] Oral candidiasis, or thrush as it has been known for centuries,[12, 13] is the most common clinical disease in infants infected with *Candida* and has been reported in approximately 4% of newborns.[9] A high percentage of infants with oral candidiasis also have diaper dermatitis caused by *Candida*,[14, 15] but, in those instances of diaper rash in the absence of oral lesions, fungus is routinely found in feces.[1, 9, 16-19] In newborns whose defenses against infection may have been altered by disease or therapy, *Candida* may cause severe and even fatal disseminated infection, with involvement of almost all tissues of the body. Therapy with antibiotics or corticosteroids has been implicated as a factor predisposing infants to disseminated candidiasis.[20-26] Indwelling intravascular catheters for infusion of hyperalimentation fluids as well as other parenteral therapy may also contribute to infection with *Candida*.[25-34] In addition, contaminated monitoring equipment may be a source of disseminated *Candida* infection.[35, 36] Contaminated glycerin gel was suggested as the common source for an outbreak of infection due to *Candida parapsilosis*.[37]

The Organism

Candida exists in at least three morphologic forms. Blastospores, or yeast cells, measure 1.5 to 5 μm in diameter and bud asexually, which is the normal mode of reproduction. Chlamydospores measure 7 to 17 μm in diameter and are occasionally seen in human tissue in systemic infection.[38, 39] Pseudomycelia, or hyphae, are filamentous processes elongating from the yeast cell and have been considered to be the tissue phase of *Candida*, representing invasion rather than mere colonization.[40] However, blastospores have been shown to be more virulent than mycelia[41] and may invade tissue.[42]

C. albicans is the most frequent species of *Candida* encountered in humans, but *C. tropicalis*, *C. stellatoidea*, *C. krusei*, *C. pseudotropicalis*, *C. parapsilosis*, *C. guilliermondii*, and *C. lusitaniae* have also been shown to cause disease in humans.[43-57] Pathogenicity of *Candida* is thought to depend on toxin production and varies among species of *Candida* as well as among individual strains. The greater pathogenicity of *C. albicans* has been attributed to production of endotoxin from disrupted blastospores.[41] Hemolysins[58] and pyrogens[59] have also been demonstrated, as has a proteolytic enzyme.[60] Hasenclever and Mitchell described two antigenic groups of *C. albicans* and suggested that group A was more pathogenic than group B.[61] Confirmatory evidence of distinct antigenic groups of *C. albicans* with varying pathogenicity has not been presented, however.

Epidemiology and Transmission

EPIDEMIOLOGY

Species of *Candida* are distributed throughout the world in humans as commensals or pathogens. *Candida* has also been isolated from many other mammalian species[62-66] and birds, in which the fungus may be a cause of significant disease.[67-70] Direct transmission of the fungus from animals to humans has not, however, been demonstrated. Species of *Candida* have not been isolated from air[71] and have only rarely been isolated from soil,[65, 72, 73] where they are thought to result from contamination with infected animal feces.

TRANSMISSION

Candida may be acquired by the human fetus during gestation or at time of delivery. Intrauterine infection, which may result in either disseminated, pulmonary, or mucocutaneous infection,[46, 74-98] is usually caused by an ascending infection from the vagina of the mother.[46, 74, 97] Such vaginal infection is common during pregnancy, especially in the last trimester.[98-105] In the early 1980s, it was reported that intrauterine *Candida* infection may also result from diagnostic amniocentesis.[106-108] Although candidemia has been reported during pregnancy,[109] hematogenous transmission from mother to fetus has not been described. Flamm has suggested that the placenta may be an effective barrier to dissemination of *Candida* from maternal to fetal circulation.[110]

Perinatal infection with *Candida* may also be acquired from the infected vagina during birth of the infant and usually results in mucocutaneous candidiasis.[111, 112] In rare instances aspiration of infected vaginal secretions may result in severe and often fatal primary pulmonary candidiasis in the infant.[113–116] Infection in the first few months of life has also been considered to result from colonization at the time of birth.[111] However, intimate contact with the infected mother, particularly from breast-feeding, is another cause of high incidence of postnatal candidiasis.[117] Although cross-infection with Candida has been reported in an adult intensive care unit,[118] cross-contamination from infants with infection occurs rarely[119, 120] and precludes the necessity of isolation or segregation of infected infants.[121, 122] However, strict adherence to universal secretion precautions should be followed.

Pathogenesis

Saprophytic colonization in adults with pathogenic species of Candida has been demonstrated in the mouth (30%),[123] gastrointestinal tract (38%),[124] and vaginal secretions (39%).[125] Although Candida is rarely found on normal exposed skin, it is frequently isolated from moist intertriginous areas in the absence of clinical disease.[126] In infants, however, isolation of Candida from skin or mucous membranes is frequently associated with clinically apparent infection.

Mechanisms responsible for pathogenicity in infants have not been clearly defined. Although number of organisms, virulence of infecting strain, environmental conditions, and availability of nutrients (for optimal growth of the organism) appear likely to play a role, defense mechanisms in the host seem to be of greater importance in prevention of disease.[42, 127]

Susceptibility to infection with Candida is increased in patients receiving antimicrobial agents,[128, 129] but mechanisms responsible for enhanced susceptibility have been elusive. Antibiotic suppression of normal flora with proliferation of Candida has been proposed as the most likely mechanism,[130–132] but other explanations, such as direct stimulatory effect, removal of competition for nutrients, or removal of antifungal substances released by other organisms, also have been suggested.[133–138] Endotoxin-like substances released from proliferating Candida may cause tissue damage, enabling the fungus to more easily invade mucosa.[139]

There is considerable evidence that corticosteroids enhance tissue susceptibility to invasion and dissemination of fungi.[140, 141] Prolonged corticosteroid and other immunosuppressive therapy results in profound changes in host defenses,[142–144] and corticosteroids may also alter normal flora of the gastrointestinal tract[145, 146] or produce direct toxicity on the mucosa.[147–149]

In both adults and children with primary immunodeficiency and in those with immunodeficiency secondary to neoplastic disease or immunosuppressive therapy, mucocutaneous candidiasis and gastrointestinal candidiasis are common.[150–154] Despite widespread mucocutaneous infection in patients with primary cellular immunodeficiency, disseminated candidiasis is uncommon.[152] However, in older children and adults with acquired immunodeficiency syndrome (AIDS)[155] or immunodeficiency secondary to leukemia or lymphoma, or therapy received for these diseases, disseminated infection with Candida is frequent.[155–158] Severe or persistent mucocutaneous candidiasis may be an early manifestation of AIDS in the young infant and should alert the physician to perform appropriate diagnostic studies for human immunodeficiency virus (HIV) infection.

Although endocrinopathies are not common in infants, increased susceptibility to infection with Candida has been reported in patients with diabetes mellitus,[159, 160] hypoparathyroidism,[161, 162] Addison's disease,[163] and hypothyroidism.[164] Patients with extensive burns are susceptible to Candida infection,[165] which may be related to the loss of the usual barriers to infection, use of antimicrobial agents, or alteration in levels of immunoglobulins.[166] Candida infection may be a significant complication of indwelling intravascular catheters or infusion of contaminated intravenous solutions.[25–35, 167]

Infants have been considered to be especially susceptible to Candida infection during the first few months of life and subsequently become relatively resistant to such infection. This phenomenon has remained unexplained. In 1959, Roth and associates demonstrated a substance in normal human serum that would inhibit growth of Candida in vitro.[168] These authors showed a significant decrease in anti-Candida activity in serum of newborns compared with activity in the mother's serum. Adult levels of anti-Candida activity in serum were not achieved in infants until 6 to 8 months of age. Louria and Brayton demonstrated a candidicidal substance in alpha-and beta-globulin fractions of human serum but not in the gamma-globulin fraction.[169] This substance was present normally in cord blood[170] but was reduced in sera of patients with cirrhosis, hepatitis, diabetic acidosis, or mucocutaneous or disseminated candidiasis. Brody and Finch, using an immune adherence assay, also found normal levels of Candida antibodies in cord blood, but there was a significant decrease in antibody activity after birth and an increase after puberty.[171] In later studies, Candida antibodies were demonstrated in cord blood in titers comparable to those in the mother.[172] Such antibody is predominantly IgG and appears to be of maternal origin.[173] Candida antibody titers have been shown to be higher in the first few weeks of life, decreasing after 5 weeks of age, and subsequently increasing later in childhood.[173] Russell and Lay found no correlation between Candida antibody titers in newborns and isolation of the organism from their oral cavities.[4]

Other authors have demonstrated Candida antibodies in serum of healthy persons[40, 174, 175] and women with vaginal candidiasis,[176] but such antibodies were not protective. IgG and IgA antibodies to Candida have also been found in vaginal secretions, even in the absence of infection.[177] Candida antibodies as well as substances that inhibit the growth of Candida have been demonstrated in amniotic fluid, but it has not been determined if these substances alter susceptibility to infection with Candida in the newborn.[178–181] In studies by Xanthou and coworkers, phagocytosis of Candida by leukocytes in term and premature infants was similar to phagocytosis in adults, but ability to kill ingested organisms was reduced.[182] Hill and colleagues, however, described a premature infant with disseminated candidiasis whose neutrophils were capable of both phagocytosing and killing intracellular *Candida*.[183] Similar results were obtained by Oseas and co-workers in normal newborns.[184]

Although there are several reports of a higher incidence of *Candida* infection in premature infants,[24, 185–187] in those sustaining a prolonged or difficult delivery, and in those receiving resuscitation, Kozinn and associates found no difference in incidence of *Candida* infection between low- and normal-birth-weight infants, or between breast- and bottle-fed infants, or between those requiring extensive resuscitative measures and those needing none.[9] They did, however, find a higher incidence of mucocutaneous candidiasis in infants during warm weather.

There is considerable evidence that host factors play a major role in alteration of the yeast to mycelial forms. There are no confirmative studies that only hyphae are pathogenic, however. Blastospores have been found invading tissue,[42] and mycelia have been demonstrated in nonliving media.[188]

Pathology

The histologic study of lesions resulting from infection with *Candida* shows superficial ulceration with prominent polymorphonuclear leukocyte infiltration. There may be invasion of deeper tissues with mycelia or blastospores, and the presence in tissue of these forms indicates acute candidiasis. In disseminated infection, microabscesses may be found throughout the kidneys, liver, spleen, heart, and brain. Mycelia are frequently seen invading walls of vessels (Fig. 17–1).[189] In cases of intrauterine *Candida* infection, fetal membranes and the chorionic plate may show diffuse and extensive polymorphonuclear leukocyte infiltration.[83] Focal granulomatous lesions have been described in the umbilical cord,[91, 98]

and diffuse placentitis with karyorrhexis is prominent.[87] Studies by Hood and colleagues identified dense bands of fibrinoid exudate and inflammatory cells in the depth of the lesions. The lesions contained IgG, IgM, and IgA, with IgG being the most abundant.[106, 190] Blastospores and mycelia in tissue can best be demonstrated by Gridley or methenamine silver stains; they may be difficult to identify with hematoxylin-eosin.

Granuloma formation is occasionally found in the skin of patients with candidiasis at sites distant to the foci of infection and has been attributed to hypersensitivity to circulating *Candida* antigens.[191] This reaction is uncommon in infants with candidiasis.

Clinical Manifestations

Lesions on mucous membranes of the mouth and oropharynx usually appear on the seventh to tenth day of life as whitish-gray plaques that are easily scraped from the mucosa, exposing an inflamed base without bleeding. These plaquelike ulcerations may be found on buccal mucosa, soft palate, tongue, gums, or tonsils. Infection may extend from the oropharynx to the angles of the mouth. The dermatitis, consisting of vesicular or pustular lesions on an erythematous base, may be found on skin in the perineum, axillae, and intertriginous areas and around the umbilicus (Fig. 17–2). Lesions may be discrete, measuring a few millimeters in diameter, or they may coalesce, forming large patches of thickened, inflamed skin.

Disseminated candidiasis may involve most tissues of the body, but infection in one or two foci usually dominates the clinical picture. In newborns, meningitis and renal involvement are most common.[186, 192] Of interest is a report by Haruda and associates of two infants with *Candida* brain abscesses without evidence of meningeal involvement.[193] Goldsmith and colleagues reported an

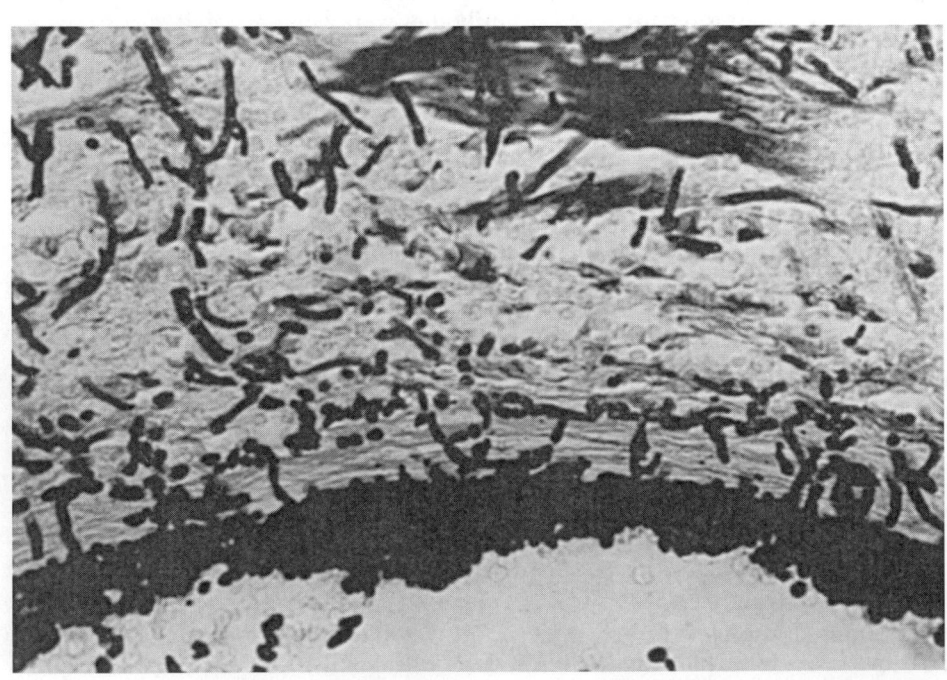

FIGURE 17–1 Gomori's methenamine silver stain demonstrating invasion of vessel wall by yeast forms and pseudohyphae. (From Dennis D, Miller MD, Peterson CG. *Candida* septicemia. Surg Gynecol Obstet 119:520, 1964. Used by permission of Surgery, Gynecology & Obstetrics.)

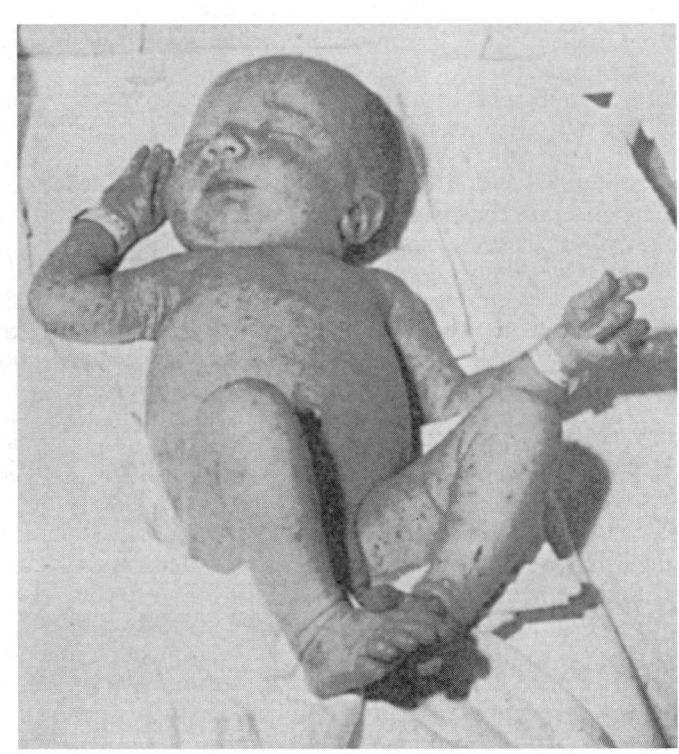

FIGURE 17–2 Cutaneous candidiasis at birth resulting from in utero infection. (From Jahn CL, Cherry JD. Congenital cutaneous candidiasis. Pediatrics 33:440, 1964. Reproduced by permission of Pediatrics, vol. 33, page 440. Copyright 1964.)

infant with candidemia who subsequently had multiple intracranial calcifications thought to be due to *Candida*.[194] Arthritis and osteomyelitis occur occasionally. Gastrointestinal candidiasis is not unusual in infants and may resemble enterocolitis resulting from other causes.

Although primary pulmonary infection with *Candida* has been reported in infants,[94, 96–100, 113–116] pulmonary infection more often occurs with disseminated infection.[115, 189] In some instances of intrauterine infection with *Candida*, the lungs may be the only site of infection.[96] Data regarding pulmonary candidiasis, however, may be difficult to evaluate because *Candida* is frequently isolated in the sputum of apparently healthy persons and in those hospitalized for reasons other than pulmonary disease.[123] This is due to the presence of *Candida* in the mouth in the normal host. These studies were performed with adults, and there are no comparable data on the incidence of *Candida* in the lower respiratory tract in infants. Blum and Elian have employed tracheal aspiration as a method of demonstrating intrauterine-acquired candidiasis in newborns and were able to isolate the organism in 6.5% of infants studied.[195] Pulmonary candidiasis has no characteristic features and cannot be distinguished on clinical grounds from most other causes of acute or chronic pulmonary infection.[96, 113–116]

Of particular interest are reports of endophthalmitis in some newborns with disseminated candidiasis.[48, 117, 183] Examination of the involved eye early in infection shows haziness of the vitreous surrounding fluffy white lesions. These exudates can be seen on the retina but may be floating free in the vitreous. The frequency with which such lesions occur in disseminated candidiasis is unknown, but Baley and co-workers reported eye involvement in four of eight infants with systemic infection.[196]

Diagnosis and Differential Diagnosis

Oral candidiasis may be confused with other infectious and noninfectious causes of oropharyngeal lesions. The most common are viral in origin. Oropharyngeal lesions caused by herpesvirus and coxsackievirus may appear similar to lesions caused by *Candida*. Most often, however, infants with herpetic stomatitis or herpangina caused by coxsackievirus have more discomfort and a moderate elevation in temperature. Vincent's infection, although uncommon in newborns, may result in oral lesions similar to those seen in thrush. There is usually a foul odor to the breath, and infection is frequently associated with fever, lethargy, and cervical lymphadenopathy. Occasionally, aphthous ulcers, which may appear similar to lesions caused by *Candida*, occur in infants.

Cutaneous infection with *Candida*, particularly when it occurs in the diaper area, may simulate dermatitis related to *Staphylococcus*, *Treponema pallidum*, herpesvirus, varicella-zoster virus, or primary irritants such as feces, ammonia, or detergent soaps.

Infants with disseminated infection may appear clinically identical to those with sepsis caused by other organisms. In infants who have sites of infection secondary to fungemia, signs and symptoms of infection in the secondary foci may prevail. Diagnosis of disseminated candidiasis may be made by isolation of the fungus from the blood of the sick infant. The use of buffy coat microscopy may allow for earlier diagnosis and initiation of therapy in patients with candidemia.[197] In adults, transient fungemia may occur in the absence of clinical disease, and the isolation of *Candida* from the blood of an asymptomatic person may not necessarily indicate systemic infection. But it is not known whether this ever occurs in newborns. If *Candida* is not isolated from the blood, a demonstration of the fungus in joint, cerebrospinal, pleural, or peritoneal fluid by direct microscopic examination or culture establishes the diagnosis.

In contrast, isolation of *Candida* from sputum, feces, or urine may be difficult to interpret because *Candida* may be found in these sites in the absence of invasion of tissue and clinical disease. The greatest difficulty occurs in the interpretation of isolation of *Candida* from urine. Transient candiduria may occur in patients receiving antibiotics, especially in the presence of urinary catheters, but *Candida* may also be a cause of significant disease in the urinary tract.[198–201] Persistent funguria after removal of catheters, especially if specimens are obtained by suprapubic aspiration, may indicate systemic or urinary tract candidiasis.[201–203] In infants with renal candidiasis, ureteropelvic obstruction may occur because of fungal masses.[204–207] Ultrasonography has been useful in such patients, as well as in infants with other foci of candidiasis.[207–211] Wise and colleagues have indicated that continuous irrigation of the bladder with amphotericin B for 5 days may distinguish between systemic candidiasis and lower urinary tract infection with *Candida*.[212]

Infective endocarditis in infants caused by *Candida* has become increasingly more common.[213–221] Both ultrasonography and echocardiography have been found to be useful in both diagnosis and determination of progression of intracardiac candidiasis in infants.

Because of difficulties in interpretation of isolation of *Candida* from sites normally inhabited by this fungus, numerous studies using immunologic or serologic techniques have been performed in an attempt to diagnose disease caused by *Candida*. Delayed hypersensitivity to oidiomycin and other skin test antigens of *Candida* has been unrewarding.[222–224] Systemic infection cannot be distinguished from saprophytic colonization in patients regardless of skin reactivity to *Candida* skin test antigens. In either situation, results may be positive or negative.[85, 225, 226] Although infants may show positive reactions to *Candida* skin test antigens, the results mentioned here were obtained with adults; comparable studies have not been performed with infants.

Several serologic tests have been described for demonstration of *Candida* antibodies, including complement fixation, indirect fluorescent antibody, precipitin, and agglutinin tests. Complement fixation and indirect fluorescent antibody techniques have been shown to be of little value in diagnosis of disseminated or local infection in adults,[227–229] and there are conflicting reports in the literature regarding the usefulness of agglutinin titers.[224, 230, 231] The demonstration of precipitating antibodies had been considered to be useful for diagnosis of systemic candidiasis in adults,[232–237] but data indicate a lack of sensitivity in many patients with disseminated infection.[238] Few data on *Candida*-precipitating antibodies in infants are available.[87, 239] Studies demonstrating *Candida* antigens in blood of patients with disseminated or invasive infection may enable earlier diagnosis of such infection in both adults and children,[240–244] and may be the best diagnostic test at this time. Schreiber and co-workers, using this technique, detected *Candida* antigen in

two premature infants with invasive candidiasis,[242] but further controlled studies in infants are needed to determine the sensitivity and specificity of this test.[245] Iwashita and co-workers found *Candida* antibodies in cerebrospinal fluid (CSF) in a child with *Candida* meningoencephalitis.[246] Although extensive studies employing this diagnostic test have not been performed, it may be helpful in certain cases of *Candida* meningitis.

Infection with *Candida* may be ascertained by direct microscopic examination of scrapings from lesions on the skin or mucous membranes, by culture, or by animal inoculation. Skin and nail scrapings should be mounted on a glass slide with a drop of 10 to 20 % potassium or sodium hydroxide, a coverslip added, and the specimen gently heated over a low flame. Gram stain may be employed for better definition of the fungus in dry mounts. Under the light microscope, species of *Candida* appear as homogeneous, small, oval, budding cells, measuring 2 to 4 μm in diameter. Hyphae may be present, with budding yeast cells attached along their length at points of constriction. Both yeast and hyphal forms are gram positive.

Prognosis

Oral candidiasis is a self-limited disease in normal infants and resolves without treatment within 1 to 2 months.[9, 10, 247] It has been assumed that cutaneous infection with *Candida* resolves in a similar period of time, but there are no reported studies of duration of cutaneous candidiasis in infants when either specific or symptomatic treatment was withheld. With treatment, lesions in the mouth and on the skin disappear in most instances in approximately 7 days. Relapses may occur from 1 week to 1 month after therapy in some cases, requiring additional treatment.[9, 248, 249] There is no apparent immunity to reinfection.

Mortality rates are high in infants with disseminated infection, especially if there is an associated debilitating disease.* There are reports, however, of spontaneous recovery from systemic infection with *Candida* without specific treatment.[189, 255] Transient fungemia may result from an infected intravascular catheter or a contaminated intravenous solution and may resolve when the catheter is removed or parenteral fluids are discontinued without specific antifungal therapy.

If a diagnosis of systemic candidiasis is suspected, specific therapy should be instituted promptly. In several studies that provide case reports of 13 infants, the diagnosis was not suspected, therapy was not given, and all 13 infants died.[89, 116, 251–254, 256, 257] Although there are no extensive studies of response to specific treatment in infants with systemic candidiasis, Faix[258] and Johnson and associates[259] reported favorable outcomes in most infants treated with amphotericin B and 5-fluorocytosine.[258, 259] Klein and co-workers reported an infant with *Candida* meningitis and arthritis who survived with treatment.[20] Dennis and colleagues reported five infants with disseminated candidiasis[189]; of the three who received

---

*See references, 21–24, 89, 116, 186, 187, 193, 198, and 250–254.

specific therapy, two died of causes other than *Candida* infection and the surviving infant was found to have severe mental retardation on follow-up. Of the two infants who were not treated, one died with *Candida* in almost all tissues of the body and the other survived, but with mental retardation. Lee and associates indicated that almost one third of premature infants with invasive candidiasis have neurodevelopmental disabilities.[260]

With better recognition of infection with *Candida* in infants and institution of specific therapy, mortality rates have decreased.* In a review of *Candida* meningitis in infants by Chesney and co-workers, the mortality rate was 29%,[263] although some infants did not receive antifungal therapy. In the infants who survived, mental retardation and hydrocephalus were common.

Prevention

Although it has been recommended that certain infants receive preventive therapy consisting of oral nystatin, there are no controlled studies that demonstrate the efficacy of prophylactic antifungal agents.[9]

CRYPTOCOCCOSIS

Although cryptococcosis is rare in the first month of life, seven infants have been reported with this infection.[271-275] All but one died, and in each, organisms with the morphologic appearance of *Cryptococcus* were identified by microscopic examination of tissue obtained at autopsy or by culture. The youngest patient reported with cryptococcal infection was 20 minutes of age[271] and had hydrocephalus and an enlarged liver and spleen. The infant died at 40 minutes of age, and encapsulated yeastlike organisms were identified in the brain, liver, and spleen. Neuhauser and Tucker, in their report of three infants with cryptococcosis, noted that one had disease at birth and died at 19 days of age.[272] At autopsy, organisms with the appearance of *Cryptococcus* were identified in the brain, liver, spleen, and bone. Similar organisms were recovered in culture from the infant and from the endocervix of the mother. Nassau and Weinberg-Heiruti reported one infant with cutaneous and disseminated cryptococcosis[273]; Heath described a newborn with endophthalmitis associated with widespread cryptococcal infection.[274] The only survivor reported by Gavai and associates had blood cultures that grew *C. neoformans* and received treatment.[275]

In adults, the respiratory tract has been considered to be the primary focus of infection with *Cryptococcus* in most instances[276-279] but the fungus appears to have a special predilection for the brain and meninges.[280, 281] Disseminated infection of the central nervous system (CNS) is common[281] and is more likely to occur in patients whose defenses against infection are compromised by disease or therapy.[127, 282-284]

---

*See references 27–30, 47, 48, 183, 196, 198, 239, 250, 251, and 261–270.

The Organism

The genus *Cryptococcus* is limited to spherical or oval encapsulated cells that reproduce by multilateral budding. Yeast cells vary in size but most often measure 5 to 10 μm in diameter exclusive of the mucinous capsule, which may be one half to five times the size of the cell proper. Although *Cryptococcus* usually appears on microscopic examination as an encapsulated yeast, some strains of *Cryptococcus neoformans* may produce true hyphae.[285] There are seven species of *Cryptococcus*, but only *C. neoformans* is pathogenic for humans. A saprophytic species, *C. neoformans* var. *innocuous*, is culturally and morphologically identical to *C. neoformans* and is frequently confused with it.

Three serologic types of *C. neoformans* have been identified by using type-specific capsular polysaccharide antisera.[286] However, cross-reactions have been noted with *C. albicans*, *Trichophyton* extract, and other antigens.[287]

Epidemiology and Transmission

EPIDEMIOLOGY

C. neoformans has been isolated from all areas of the world. The original isolate was made by San Felice from peaches,[288] and Klein recovered the fungus from cow's milk.[289] Emmons isolated *C. neoformans* from soil[290] and later related that finding to contamination of soil with excreta from pigeons.[291] Although natural cryptococcal infection in pigeons has not been demonstrated, many authors have thought that pigeons may be the primary source of pathogenic *Cryptococcus*.[292-294] Others, however, believe the soil to be the primary source, with pigeon excreta merely enhancing growth of *Cryptococcus*.[295, 296]

Some authors have reported recovery of *C. neoformans* from areas inhabited by birds other than pigeons,[297-299] but Fragner was able to isolate *C. neoformans* only from pigeon roosts and nonpathogenic species from roosts of other birds.[300] Nevertheless, it is generally accepted that avian habitats, particularly of feral pigeons, represent the major source of *C. neoformans* for humans and animals.

Sources of *C. neoformans* other than pigeon roosts have been reported. Clarke and colleagues isolated the fungus from apples,[301] and McDonough and associates recovered the organism from wood.[302] *Cryptococcus* has also been found occasionally in soil not contaminated with bird excreta.[303]

C. neoformans may cause disease in animals,[304] and epidemics of cryptococcal mastitis have occurred in dairy cows.[305, 306] None of the personnel caring for the cows acquired the infection.

Human cryptococcosis may occur at any age, but 60% of patients with cryptococcal infection are between the ages of 30 and 50 years.[307] Infection is three times more common in men than in women and is particularly frequent in white men. It has been suggested that this sex difference is related at least in part to the enhanced phagocytic activity of leukocytes for *Cryptococcus* in the presence of estrogens.[308]

TRANSMISSION

Infection with *C. neoformans* has been thought to result primarily from inhalation of the fungus from an exogenous source, and the respiratory tract is the primary focus of infection.[309] However, direct inoculation into the skin and ingestion of the fungus have been suggested as alternative routes of infection.[310–312] Tonsils have also been reported as a possible initial focus of infection.[313] Littman and Zimmerman[278] as well as others have suggested that *Cryptococcus* may be isolated from the oropharynx, normal skin, vagina, and intestinal tracts of humans with no apparent disease.[314] Whether isolates are actually *C. neoformans* has been questioned. Tynes and co-workers suggested that pathogenic *Cryptococcus* may be present in sputum as a saprophyte,[315] although, before their report, isolation of *C. neoformans* from humans had been considered indicative of disease.

None of the mothers giving birth to infected offspring[271–274] had any illness during pregnancy that could be attributed to infection with *Cryptococcus*,[271–274] and although inhalation of *Cryptococcus* cannot be excluded in newborns infected with it, the onset of disease at birth suggests that the transmission of the fungus occurred in utero. Isolation of encapsulated yeast from the endocervix of one of the mothers[272] suggests that transmission in this case may have occurred from an ascending vaginal infection in the mother. Kida and colleagues reported a woman with HIV infection and AIDS who died with disseminated cryptococcal infection 2 days after the birth of her infant, who was uninfected.[316] In no other instance reported of cryptococcal infection during pregnancy has transmission to the infant occurred.[317, 318]

Transmission from human to human, except for isolated cases of possible congenital transmission, has not been reported.

Pathogenesis

The presence of pathogenic *Cryptococcus* in humans has been considered to be an indication of disease related to that fungus. However, the possibility of saprophytic colonization of the skin, sputum, mucous membranes, and feces of healthy persons with *C. neoformans* has been suggested[288, 319, 320]; this would indicate an endogenous source of the fungus. The isolation of encapsulated yeast from the endocervix of an asymptomatic, apparently healthy mother lends support to this contention. Although clinically apparent infection with *C. neoformans* may occur in the normal host, there is a high incidence of infection in patients with Hodgkin's disease, lymphosarcoma, leukemia, and diabetes mellitus[127, 282–284, 320–322] as well as in those with HIV infection and AIDS.[155] The use of corticosteroids or other immunosuppressive therapy has been associated with a higher incidence of cryptococcosis.[323] Mechanisms of enhanced susceptibility in patients with these underlying disorders or methods of treatment are similar to those discussed earlier in connection with candidiasis. However, cryptococcal infections in these patients have not increased as strikingly as some of the other opportunistic fungal infections.[324]

There are no data specific to infants regarding increased susceptibility or resistances to infection with *Cryptococcus*. In the review by Siewers and Cramblett of cryptococcal infections in children, only one of four patients showed evidence of underlying disease.[325] Although gestational age was unknown in two of the seven infants with neonatal cryptococcosis, five of these were born prematurely. Only the surviving infant received antibiotics and none received corticosteroids. The surviving infant was also receiving hyperalimentation through a central venous catheter.

A factor in normal human serum that inhibits growth of *C. neoformans* has been demonstrated and may explain the low incidence of clinically apparent cryptococcal infections.[326–328] Alterations in this factor due to disease or therapy may account for the high incidence of cryptococcal infection in patients with diseases of the reticuloendothelial system and in those who are receiving treatment with immunosuppressive drugs. There are no data regarding inhibitory factors in the serum of newborns.

Pathology

In both infants and adults, the respiratory tract appears to be the primary focus of infection, which follows inhalation of the fungus. In some instances, the skin (by direct inoculation) or the gastrointestinal tract (by ingestion) may be the initial route of infection. In adults, respiratory infection is usually subacute or chronic and the lesion most commonly encountered is a solitary nodule measuring 2 to 7 cm in diameter and located at the periphery of the lung, at the hilar area or in the middle of a lobe.[278] There is usually minimal hilar lymphadenopathy. In infants and occasionally in adults, diffuse infiltration[329] or miliary disease similar to tuberculosis may be evident in the lung.[330] Fibrosis and calcification are rare, but cavitary disease may be found in 10% of adults with pulmonary cryptococcal infection.[307] Small subpleural nodules are frequently found at autopsy in these patients,[331] but pleuritic reaction is rare.

Microscopically, pulmonary lesions of cryptococcal infection may give the appearance of nonspecific granulomas. If tissue reaction is minimal, the mass has a mucoid appearance, a finding more commonly seen in infants. In most instances, there is an aggregate of encapsulated budding cells with intertwining loose connective tissue. Granulomatous reaction may occur with infiltration of lymphocytes and epithelioid cells but without caseation necrosis. Diffuse pneumonic infiltration seen in infants is characterized by accumulation of fungus in alveoli, and there is an outpouring of histiocytes and tissue macrophages with ingested organisms.

Cutaneous cryptococcal infection may occur in about 15% of adult cases[332] but has not been reported in infants.

Dissemination may occur via the bloodstream to any organ in the body, including the liver, spleen, kidneys, adrenal glands, bone, and eyes; but the CNS is the most common site of infection after dissemination. Lesions outside the CNS in both adults and infants may appear densely granulomatous, similar to tuberculous lesions.[277] In the CNS, there may be evidence of meningitis with a gray adherent exudate in the subarachnoid space. More extensive involvement may be present around the base of the brain in older patients. In some instances, there are small granulomas in the meninges and along the blood vessels. The underlying surface of the brain may show small cystlike lesions consisting of fungal or mucinous material. The cellular reaction may be minimal or extensive, with mononuclear inflammatory cells. The infection may extend along the vessels into varying depths of the brain substance, resulting in pinpoint cysts in gray matter. Parenchymatous lesions may result from embolization and are found in periventricular gray matter and basal ganglia and in white matter of the cerebral hemispheres. Such lesions are more often found in adults than in infants and appear as nonspecific granulomas or as cysts containing mucinous material from capsules of cryptococci. On occasion, discrete granulomas may be found in any part of the brain, spinal cord, or meninges and may act like space-occupying lesions.

Clinical Manifestations

ILLUSTRATIVE CASE[272]

A 19-day-old boy had been born 3 weeks prematurely. The mother was primigravid and had had no illnesses during pregnancy. The infant appeared normal at birth but was icteric. Jaundice became more pronounced during the first weeks of life. When he was 1 week of age, the infant's abdomen became distended, the urine became dark, and the feces were light in color. At the time of admission to the hospital, the infant appeared undernourished and icteric. The head was normal, but the sagittal suture was wide, the abdomen was protuberant, and the liver and spleen were markedly enlarged. Clinically, all other signs were normal.

Laboratory data included a white blood cell count of 12,800 per mm³—47% neutrophils, 40% lymphocytes and 2% eosinophils. The remaining cells were not identified. Total bilirubin concentration was 39.2 mg/dl, and the urine contained increased amounts of bile. Radiographs of the abdomen confirmed enlargement of liver and spleen; a chest radiograph was normal. Skull films showed extensive punctate calcifications overlying the cortex and within the brain substance.

During hospitalization, the infant had loose green stools and on two occasions a low-grade fever. Despite blood transfusions and intravenous fluid, his condition deteriorated. Respiration became shallow and rapid, and the heart rate slowed; the infant died 4 days after admission.

At autopsy, marked hydrocephalus with atrophy of the brain was found. Numerous small granulomas containing calcium were scattered over the entire surface of the brain. The liver and spleen were enlarged, and the kidneys contained miliary abscesses. The lungs showed only interstitial pneumonitis. Organisms with the morphologic appearance of *Cryptococcus* were seen in all organs except the lungs. ∎

Infants with cryptococcosis show evidence of multisystemic involvement characterized by enlargement of the liver or spleen or both, jaundice, hydrocephalus, and, in many instances, chorioretinitis. Roentgenologically, Neuhauser and Tucker found intracranial calcifications scattered over the cortex and within the brain substance in each of three newborns they reported.[272] It is noteworthy that these findings are compatible with those found in many congenital infections, including toxoplasmosis, rubella, syphilis, and cytomegalovirus infection. One infant was thought to have had toxoplasmosis as well as cryptococcal infection.[272]

Dissemination of *Cryptococcus* to other organs in infants usually produces signs of disease in one or more sites, most commonly the CNS. Signs vary with the location and extent of CNS involvement. Cryptococcal granuloma in the brain may produce signs similar to those of space-occupying lesions caused by other diseases. Meningitis most often manifests as headache, which may become progressively worse and is accompanied by nausea, vomiting, and lethargy. As infection continues, seizures may occur. On examination, there may be papilledema but nuchal rigidity is uncommon. When the brain is extensively involved, obtundation and coma often result. Cranial nerves may be involved, and amblyopia, diplopia, and optic atrophy are frequent findings. The infant who survived had no evidence of cryptococcosis beyond positive blood cultures. There was no meningitis or ophthalmic or pulmonary involvement.

Diagnosis and Differential Diagnosis

Neonatal cryptococcal infection may appear similar to congenital infection with *Toxoplasma gondii*, rubella virus, cytomegalovirus, and *T. pallidum*. Pulmonary cryptococcal infection may be confused with congenital or neonatal tuberculosis or infections with fungi other than *Cryptococcus*.

CNS infection in infants may be confused with tuberculous meningitis. In cases of localized granulomatous disease, the differential diagnosis must include brain abscess caused by bacteria, cerebrovascular thromboses, or hemorrhage.

Diagnosis of infection with *Cryptococcus* may be made by visualization of encapsulated yeast in sputum or in CSF, by culture, or by animal inoculation. Microscopic examinations of pus, sputum, exudates, and CSF are best performed by using India ink, which is displaced by the capsule. Thick specimens of sputum or pus may be mixed with an equal volume of 10% sodium or potassium hydroxide to dissolve tissue and cellular debris before addition of fresh India ink.

In cryptococcal meningitis, the CSF is usually under increased pressure, and pleocytosis may be present with a predominance of mononuclear cells. The CSF glucose level is decreased in only 55% of adult cases, and protein content is increased in 90%.[333] Direct microscopic examination of CSF using an equal volume of India ink may show encapsulated yeast in 50% of culturally proven cases. If yeast is found, the diagnosis is established because *Cryptococcus* is the only encapsulated yeast that infects the CNS in humans.

Specimens submitted for culture when diagnosis of

cryptococcal infection is suspected should include sputum, CSF, blood, urine, and bone marrow. If cutaneous lesions are present, pus should also be submitted.

Microscopic examination of tissue obtained by biopsy or at autopsy may strongly support the diagnosis of cryptococcal infection. Although Gridley and methenamine silver stains demonstrate the fungus very well, other fungi are also visualized with these stains. Specific stains for capsular mucin such as mucicarmine[334] and the Rhinehart-Abdul-Haj technique for acid mucopolysaccharide[335] are beneficial, especially for distinguishing *Cryptococcus* from *Histoplasma*.

Immunologic and serologic tests as aids in diagnosing infection with *Cryptococcus* have been proposed. Delayed hypersensitivity to cryptococcal antigens has been noted in adults, but dermal response has not been useful as a diagnostic test.[277, 336–341] No studies of response to cryptococcal skin test antigens in infants have been reported.

Agglutinins, complement-fixing hemagglutinating, and indirect fluorescent methods have been described.[342–346] Latex and complement fixation tests for detection of cryptococcal antigen in serum and body fluids have also been reported.[347–350] Circulating cryptococcal antigen has been demonstrated in serum and CSF in patients with meningeal and disseminated infections[348, 349, 351–353]; titers of antigen decrease with recovery. It has also been noted that cryptococcal antibody in serum may increase during recovery from infection with *Cryptococcus*. The latex particle agglutination test has proved to be valuable for detection of cryptococcal antigen in the CSF of patients in whom cultures and microscopic examination of CSF are negative.[354] There are no data on serologic studies in newborns with cryptococcal infection.

Prognosis

All of the newborns reported with cryptococcal infection who were given no treatment died within days to weeks of onset of the disease. One infant survived without apparent sequelae after receiving amphotericin B for 6 weeks.

Prevention

Preventive measures should be directed at elimination of exogenous sources of *Cryptococcus*. It is unlikely, however, that conservation laws will be changed to reduce the number of pigeons. A solution containing hydrated lime and sodium hydroxide has been shown to be effective in eradicating cryptococci from contaminated pigeon roosts when sprayed on soil containing the organism.[355]

Disseminated infection may be prevented by early recognition and adequate treatment of the primary focus of infection.

COCCIDIOIDOMYCOSIS

Clinically apparent infection with *Coccidioides immitis* in infants in the first month of life has been reported infrequently, despite the high incidence of infection in children living in areas where the fungus is endemic.[356] The first case of coccidioidomycosis in a neonate was reported by Cohen in 1949.[357] Although the diagnosis was not established until the infant was 15 weeks of age, signs of pulmonary disease were present at 1 week of age. Dactylitis was evident in the infant at 2 weeks of age; the infected finger was the site from which the fungus was finally isolated. Coccidioidomycosis has been reported in 11 other infants, in all of whom clinical disease began by 10 weeks of age.[358–366] Although pulmonary disease was prominent in each infant, disseminated infection was established at autopsy in all who died. Two of the infants had signs of meningitis,[358, 359] but the fungus was isolated from CSF obtained from only one of them.[359] Two additional infants have survived. In one the diagnosis was made by serologic studies,[365] and in the other the diagnosis was by identification of the fungus in tracheal secretions.[366]

The Organism

C. immitis is the only species of *Coccidioides* and is recognized in nature in two phases: saprophytic and parasitic. Saprophytic *Coccidioides* exists in a mycelial form in nonliving material, only rarely in tissue.[367]

Hyphae have regularly spaced septa with alternating infectious spores and sterile cells. Arthrospores are infectious components of hyphae and are barrel shaped, measuring 2 to 10 μm in width. Spores may be round or ovoid, in which case they are more typically chlamydospores. An annual rainfall of 5 to 20 inches in alkaline soil and a prolonged hot, dry season followed by precipitation favor the formation of spores.[368] Infectious spores become airborne with minimal disturbance during the hot, dry season and may remain infectious for several weeks. Arthrospores, which have been known to be transported on clothes or other inanimate objects containing contaminated dust, may cause infection great distances from endemic areas.[369]

The parasitic form of *C. immitis* is the spherule that forms in tissue from inhaled or inoculated arthrospores. It measures 10 to 80 μm in diameter and contains endospores, which form within the spherule by cleavage of cytoplasm. Mature spherules rupture, liberating a few hundred to several hundred endospores, which subsequently develop into new spherules.[367]

Epidemiology and Transmission

EPIDEMIOLOGY

C. immitis is found in soil 12 to 14 cm below the surface. Sunlight appears to destroy the fungus. *Coccidioides* is endemic in the Western Hemisphere in the San Joaquin Valley and southern counties of California, southern Arizona, New Mexico, and parts of Texas, as well as in Mexico, Guatemala, Honduras, Venezuela, Paraguay, Colombia, and Argentina. In endemic areas, naturally occurring infection has been reported in a variety of wild and domestic animals, including cattle[370] sheep,[371, 372] dogs,[373] horses and burros,[374] and rodents.[375]

Epidemiologic studies have estimated that approximately 10 million persons currently residing in endemic areas have been infected with *C. immitis*.[376] The rate of infection in susceptible persons arriving in an endemic area is 15 to 50% within the first year.[377] After residence in an endemic area for 5 years, 80% of susceptible persons will become infected. In more than 50% of these, infection is asymptomatic and can be demonstrated only by the presence of delayed hypersensitivity to coccidioidin skin test antigen. The incidence of infection is highest in the early summer and remains high until the first rains of winter. The rate of infection is also higher in dry seasons that follow a season of heavy rainfall.[378, 379]

There appears to be no racial or sex difference in incidence of primary coccidioidomycosis. However, primary infection is recognized more frequently in women because they are more likely to have cutaneous hypersensitivity reactions than men.[380, 381] In addition, there are considerable racial differences in the risk of disseminated disease. Mexican Indian men are three times more likely to disseminate the fungus than white men; black men are 14 times more prone to dissemination than white men; and Filipino men are reported to be 175 times more susceptible than white men.[376, 382, 383] In women dissemination is more common during pregnancy.[384–388] Before puberty, there appears to be no sex difference in clinical manifestations or extent of disease.

Studies to determine the mechanisms of increased susceptibility in men, nonwhite races, and pregnant women have not been reported. Patients with lymphomas, leukemia, and diabetes mellitus are reported to have no higher incidence of clinically significant or disseminated coccidioidal infection than other persons,[389] but disseminated infection may be more common in patients with AIDS[155, 390] and in those receiving corticosteroids or immunosuppressive therapy.[127, 391]

TRANSMISSION

Coccidioidomycosis in infants has been considered to result from inhalation of arthrospores. Transmission of fungus from mother to infant in utero has been reported by Shafai,[362] who reported twins born of a woman who died 24 hours later with disseminated coccidioidomycosis. Both infants died with widespread disease. Christian and associates described one case in which onset of disease was at 3 weeks of age in an infant living in a nonendemic area.[360] The infant's mother had inactive coccidioidal osteomyelitis but did not have pulmonary or cutaneous disease, suggesting that infection in the infant may have been acquired in utero or at the time of birth. An infant described by Cohen was born of a mother with active coccidioidomycosis during pregnancy; the infant had pulmonary disease at 1 week of age, again suggesting that the infection may have been acquired in utero.[357] Bernstein and co-workers reported an infant with onset of disease at 5 days of age, and although there was no evidence of disease in the mother, the onset of disease in the infant shortly after birth suggested in utero transmission of the fungus.[364] In contrast, there are several reports of disseminated coccidioidomycosis during pregnancy with only three instances of placental infection but no evidence of infection in any of the infants.[384, 387, 392–394]

Human-to-human transmission of *C. immitis* is rare. Even though infectious arthrospores may be found in residual pulmonary cavities and benign pulmonary granulomas in humans,[356] secondary cases within families are unusual. Eckmann and co-workers reported six cases of coccidioidomycosis acquired at the bedside of a patient with coccidioidal osteomyelitis whose cast was contaminated with spherule-containing exudate.[395]

Pathogenesis

The respiratory tract is the initial focus of infection by *C. immitis* in infants as well as in most adults, although direct inoculation of fungus into the skin has been reported rarely in adults and older children.[396] After arthrospores are inhaled, mature spherules develop in 4 to 7 days in bronchial mucosa.[397, 398] Granulomas form rapidly, involving lymphatics and tracheobronchial lymph nodes. In adults with mild disease, there may be a few scattered lesions; however, when pulmonary involvement is extensive, an outpouring of polymorphonuclear leukocytes filling alveoli and resembling bacterial pneumonia occurs. There may be ulceration of bronchi and bronchioles, with later development of bronchiectasis.

Pathology

The typical histologic appearance of lesions caused by *Coccidioides* is granulomatous formation with epithelioid cells and Langhans' giant cells. Granulomas occur in both infants and older patients. If resistant factors are deficient, suppuration may be prominent; but, with adequate host response hyalinization, fibrosis, and calcification occur.

Coccidioides may be disseminated by blood to any organ in the body. The most significant focus of infection after dissemination is the CNS, and the brain, meninges, or spinal cord may be involved. Dissemination to the CNS is most common in children and in white men and is the most common cause of death in patients with coccidioidomycosis.[367, 399] In cases of meningitis, there is a thick exudate encasing the brain and invariably resulting in noncommunicating hydrocephalus. Involvement around the base of the brain is usually more extensive than that above the cerebral cortex. On microscopic examination, the meninges are studded with small granulomas; similar lesions may be present in the underlying brain substance. In the spinal cord, infection may result in compression by the thick, tough inflammatory membrane, with subsequent loss of motor and sensory functions.

Other organs infected when the disease is disseminated include the skin, lungs and pleura, spleen, liver, kidneys, heart, genital tract, adrenal glands, and, occasionally, skeletal muscle. In infants, cutaneous infection most often makes its appearance as a papular rash in the diaper area. The gastrointestinal tract is almost always spared in infants, although the peritoneum and bowel serosa are frequently studded with granulomas. In each of three infants who died of disseminated coccidioidomycosis, there was infection in the lungs and spleen. One infant had infection in the liver, and one had documented meningitis. Skin infection was present in only one infant.[348] One of the surviving children had pulmonary infection and osteomyelitis,[357] and another had pulmonary infection and chorioretinitis.[365]

Clinical Manifestations

ILLUSTRATIVE CASE[359]

The patient was a 3-week-old white girl who was admitted to the hospital with a 2-day history of irritability, anorexia, and fever. The parents were well and had been living in the San Joaquin Valley for 12 years. On examination at time of admission to the hospital, the infant appeared acutely ill with a temperature of 104° F and a heart rate of 132 beats per minute. The throat was slightly erythematous, and there was questionable nuchal rigidity. The anterior fontanelle was full but not bulging. No other abnormalities were detected during examination.

Laboratory data included a CSF examination that showed 700 cells per mm³—80% neutrophils and 20% lymphocytes. The CSF glucose level was 15 mg/dl, and the protein level was 195 mg/dl. Culture of the CSF was negative for bacteria. The white blood cell count varied from 7100 to 19,800 cells per mm³ with a normal differential. Cultures of blood, bone marrow, and gastric washings were negative for *C. immitis*.

The child was treated with streptomycin, penicillin, and sulfonamides for suspected bacterial meningitis, and her temperature returned to normal 5 days after admission. Eight days after admission, the infant again became febrile but appeared in no distress. On the thirteenth hospital day, a chest radiograph showed patchy infiltration in both lungs; oxytetracycline was given, but no improvement occurred. Several days later, the spleen became enlarged. Repeat lumbar puncture was performed, this time showing 90 cells per mm³—72% neutrophils and 28% lymphocytes. CSF culture was positive for *C. immitis*. The condition of the infant began to deteriorate, scattered papules on the trunk developed, and the patient died 42 days after admission at 2 months of age.

At autopsy, a diagnosis of disseminated coccidioidomycosis was made. Granulomatous lesions were identified in the lungs, liver, spleen, kidneys, pancreas, and adrenals. Microscopic examination showed proliferative and destructive granulomatous reaction, and spherules of *C. immitis* were identified in most organs. Small nodules on the mitral and tricuspid valves proved on microscopic examination to be granulomas, but spherules could not be identified. Both brain and lymph nodes showed considerable disease, and, in some instances, caseous necrosis was seen in the centers of the granulomas. ■

Although primary pulmonary coccidioidal infection is asymptomatic in 60% of older children and adults,[400] and only 25% have an illness severe enough to seek medical attention, each of the reported infected newborns had symptoms of pulmonary disease. After an incubation period of 10 to 16 days, signs of a mild lower respiratory tract disease appear, characterized by a dry, nonproductive cough. There may be low-grade fever, anorexia, and malaise, as well as significant respiratory distress. Physical examination of the chest may demonstrate few abnormal findings, but roentgenograms may show bronchopneumonia or segmental or peribronchial disease in infants. Hilar nodes are often enlarged, and pleural fluid is common.

Cavitary lesions became apparent in one infant several months after birth and cleared by 30 months of age.[357] It is in such chronic lesions that the saprophytic form of *Coccidioides* has been demonstrated.[367]

In infants, dissemination of infection is frequent and, when dissemination to the CNS occurs, infection in brain and meninges may be overlooked.[401] Signs, which may be vague and nonspecific, include anorexia and lethargy. Nuchal rigidity is infrequent. As infection progresses, confusion, obtundation, coma, and seizures may occur. Papilledema is usually present at that time.

Diagnosis and Differential Diagnosis

Granulomatous pulmonary disease caused by *C. immitis* may mimic tuberculosis, Q fever, psittacosis, ornithosis, viral pneumonias, or other fungal infections, particularly histoplasmosis. In infants, pulmonary coccidioidomycosis may appear to be similar to bacterial infection. In patients with coccidioidal meningitis, the differential diagnosis includes tuberculous meningitis, cryptococcosis, histoplasmosis, blastomycosis, candidiasis, and partially treated bacterial meningitis.[364] In coccidioidal meningitis, CSF is usually under increased pressure. Pleocytosis with mononuclear cells is characteristic, but, in cases discovered early, a preponderance of polymorphonuclear cells may be found. Eosinophils are common in CSF in patients with coccidioidal meningitis. The CSF glucose level is decreased, and the protein level may be markedly elevated.

Diagnosis of coccidioidomycosis must be suspected in patients with unexplained pulmonary disease who reside in endemic areas. In addition, a history of travel to an endemic area or occupational hazards involving exposure to contaminated dust may be important clues leading to suspicion of coccidioidal infection.[402–404] Despite a history of exposure, a diagnosis of coccidioidomycosis may be difficult to establish. Identification of spherules in pus, sputum, or tissue is diagnostic of infection with *C. immitis*. Direct microscopic examination is best performed if the infected material is partially digested with 10% sodium or potassium hydroxide. Specimens treated by alkalinization are unsatisfactory for culture.

Spherules may be easier to identify if equal parts of iodine and Sudan IV are used. Iodine is absorbed into the wall of the spherule, and Sudan IV differentiates fat globules from spherules.[405] However, because spherulelike artifacts are commonly found in sputum and pus, direct examination may be misleading.

Direct microscopic examination of gastric juice and

CSF is usually unrewarding, and even cultures of CSF in cases of coccidioidal meningitis may be negative.[401]

Identification of spherules in tissue obtained by biopsy or at autopsy is best accomplished by using Gridley or Gomori methenamine silver stain. Hematoxylin-eosin may be used but often fails to give enough contrast between spherules and host tissue.

Coccidioides may be cultured on Sabouraud glucose agar; specimens submitted for culture should include sputum, pus from cutaneous lesions, cerebrospinal fluid, and urine. Because the morphology of mycelia is variable, the fungus can be injected into mice for demonstration of characteristic endosporulating spherules. Because culture and animal inoculation are time consuming and dangerous for laboratory personnel, most investigational studies employ immunologic and serologic tests for demonstration of infection with *Coccidioides*.

Studies of development of delayed hypersensitivity, with intradermal injections of 0.1 ml of coccidioidin, have demonstrated that positive reactions may occur 3 days to 2 weeks after the onset of symptoms and may persist for years.[367] In patients without erythema nodosum or erythema multiforme, a dilution of 1:100 of skin test antigen should be used. If no reaction occurs, a second test using a 1:10 dilution of coccidioidin should be applied. In patients with erythema nodosum or erythema multiforme, coccidioidin should be diluted to 1:10,000 before being applied. A positive reaction is manifested 24 to 48 hours after injection by induration of 5 mm or more. Cross-reactions may occur with coccidioidin in patients with histoplasmosis, and coccidioidin may evoke an antibody response to yeast-phase *Histoplasma* but not to *Coccidiodies*. False-negative reactions may occur in patients with disseminated infection or in those in whom skin testing is performed before development of cellular immune response to the fungus.

Cohen and Burnip performed coccidioidin skin tests in newborns in an endemic area.[393] Of 220 infants studied, 2 had positive reactions but neither had evidence of disease. Two infants born to women with coccidioidal meningitis during pregnancy had negative reactions to skin testing and no clinical or serologic evidence of infection.

Precipitin and complement fixation tests for antibodies to *Coccidioides* are important in the diagnosis of coccidioidomycosis.[406, 407] The complement fixation test is also useful in determining the extent of infection and the prognosis.[407] Precipitating antibodies appear to belong to the IgM class of immunoglobulins and are present in 90% of adults within 4 weeks of onset of symptoms.[408] In most instances, precipitins disappear in 4 to 6 weeks[409] Coccidioidal antibodies demonstrated by complement fixation tests appear more slowly and only in cases of severe infection. Antibody titers of greater than 1:16 may indicate disseminated infection. The presence of complement-fixing antibodies in CSF is diagnostic of coccidioidal meningitis; however, only 75% of patients with active meningeal infection have demonstrable antibody in CSF.[407]

An immunodiffusion technique is available for detection of coccidioidal antibody and appears to correlate with the complement fixation test.[410, 411] Huppert and associates have also described a latex particle agglutination test that measures antibody paralleling precipitin titers.[412] It is recommended that tests for precipitins and complement-fixing antibodies should both be employed for best results in diagnosing coccidioidomycosis.[412]

Other serologic tests for coccidioidal antibodies include counterimmunoelectrophoresis[413] and radioimmunoassay[414]; however, results of these techniques in neonates have not been reported.

Prognosis

The mortality rate in infants with coccidioidomycosis is high. With three exceptions, all of the infants in whom coccidioidal infection was identified died, with infection being recognized only at autopsy.

Prevention

Although dust control has been shown to reduce the incidence of infection in persons who are transients in endemic areas,[379, 415] there is little evidence that such control reduces infection in long-term residents in these areas. In persons at risk of developing severe or disseminated infection, attempting to control dust may be beneficial. Cohen suggested that the infant he reported acquired the infection from inhalation of dust blown into the nursery. Use of air conditioning, filters, and respirators in areas where individuals are at risk has been encouraged.[416] Masks have been recommended for persons working in heavily contaminated areas.[403] Others have suggested spraying soil with fungicides,[417] but such treatment reaches a depth of only 0.6 cm, which allows the fungus to survive below that level. Careful handling of heavily contaminated dressings by hospital personnel is recommended to prevent acquisition of infection. There appears to be no necessity for isolation or segregation of patients with coccidioidomycosis, however.

Levine and co-workers have employed a vaccine that has been effective in preventing disease in animals,[418] but results in humans as measured by serologic and skin tests have been erratic[377] and have not shown protection from infection.[419]

ASPERGILLOSIS

Aspergillosis has been reported in infants who ranged in age from 13 days to 7 weeks. In 1955, Zimmerman reported a 13-day-old neonate who became febrile and developed a subcutaneous abscess caused by *Staphylococcus*.[420] Despite antibiotic therapy, the infant subsequently developed pneumonia and hepatosplenomegaly and died at 1 month of age. *Aspergillus sydowi* was isolated from the lung, pericardial and pleural fluid, and brain. Allan and Andersen reported disseminated aspergillosis in an infant who showed the first signs of disease on the second day of life and who died at 18 days of age.[421] At autopsy, *Aspergillus* was identified in the lung, liver, spleen, heart, thyroid, bowel, and skin; *A. fumigatus* was cultured from the liver, spleen, and bowel. Luke and co-workers reported disseminated aspergillosis in a debilitated infant who died at 7 weeks of age.[422] At autopsy, *A. fumigatus* was isolated from the blood, heart, and kidneys, and the fungus was identified on microscopic examination in the endocardium, brain, and kidneys. Akkoyunlu and Yücell reported a case of aspergillosis in an infant in whom onset of respiratory and CNS disease occurred at 2 weeks of age.[423] The infant died at 20 days of age with pneumonia and meningitis. *Aspergillus* was identified and cultured from lung and brain tissue obtained at autopsy. The source of infection was thought to be infected grain on the farm where the infant lived. Infection in two of these four infants was considered secondary to prematurity or to antibiotic or corticosteroid therapy,[420, 422] but predisposing causes for disseminated aspergillosis were not found in the others.[421, 423]

Twenty-three additional cases of *Aspergillus* in infants have been reported.[424–442] Only 10 infants survived.[430, 432, 437–441] In only 2 who did not survive was the diagnosis made before death,[438] and none of the nonsurvivors received antifungal therapy. As in previously reported cases, *Aspergillus* infection was secondary to prematurity,[427] antibiotic therapy,[428] or serious underlying disease.[429, 430, 442]

The Organism

The genus *Aspergillus* contains about 70 distinct species,[443] but only 8 have been shown to be pathogenic for humans. Identification of species of *Aspergillus* is made by morphology and structural details of the conidia-producing structures on specialized media. A complete description may be found in the comprehensive study by Raper and Fennell.[443] The species groups that are pathogenic in humans and animals are *A. fumigatus* (which is the most common), *A. niger, A. flavus, A. glaucus, A. restrictus, A. nidulans, A. versicolor, A. terreus,* and *A. sydowi.*[444]

Pathogenic species of *Aspergillus* may produce both exotoxins and endotoxins in tissue or on food, and these may increase pathogenicity or produce disease in animals and humans. Endotoxin has been isolated from mycelia of *A. fumigatus,*[445–448] but it is not known what role it plays in disease in humans.[449] Toxins of *A. flavus* are important in disease in animals[450–452] and have been shown to be potent carcinogens.[453–455]

Epidemiology and Transmission

EPIDEMIOLOGY

Species of *Aspergillus* are found throughout the world in grains and decaying organic matter. Infection with *Aspergillus* is common in animals.[63, 456] Although it has been reported that infection is more common in individuals exposed to large numbers of conidia,[457–461] occupational predisposition has been questioned,[462–465] and a history of inordinate exposure is infrequent at present. There appears to be no racial or sexual predisposition in the infection rate, but clinical disease is more common in men than in women.[466]

TRANSMISSION

Species of *Aspergillus* are most often acquired by inhalation of spores into the respiratory tract, but saprophytic infection with *Aspergillus* may be found in the external auditory canal, skin, nails, nasal sinuses, and vagina.[466–470] Although infection in newborns may result from inhalation of conidia from the environment, the fungus may also be acquired during gestation or at the time of birth from an infection in the mother. None of the mothers in one study showed evidence of disseminated infection during pregnancy, and studies of vaginal flora were performed in only one.[421] In this case, onset of infection in the infant was at 2 days of age and studies were not performed in the mother until 1 month after birth of the infant. Cultures of vaginal secretions for *Aspergillus* were negative, and a chest roentgenogram was normal. Although interhuman transmission has not been reported, Allan and Andersen suggested that another source of infection in the infant described by them may have been another infant in the same nursery who had a similar clinical disease.[421] The child died, but, because an autopsy was not performed, the diagnosis of *Aspergillus* infection could not be confirmed.

Administration of parenteral fluids contaminated with *Aspergillus* has been reported as a source of infection.[158] Luke and colleagues suggested that an umbilical vein catheter in the case they reported may have been the route of *Aspergillus* infection.[422]

Granstein and associates[421] as well as others[471] have suggested that adhesive dressings and arm boards may be the source of *Aspergillus* infection. Outbreaks of *Aspergillus* have occurred among immunocompromised hospitalized patients exposed to nearby construction sites.[472, 473]

Pathogenesis

Four morphologic forms of the fungus representing stages of development from germination of conidia to fructification have been identified in humans infected with *Aspergillus.*[444] These progressive changes in morphology may reflect the host's susceptibility or resistance to the fungus. After inhalation, ingestion, or inoculation of the spore, primary hyphae form from the germinating conidia, evoking an intense polymorphonuclear leukocyte response. As infection continues, unbranched, straight, or spiraling hyphae may be seen. Later, characteristic branching occurs and vegetative forms of *Aspergillus* may be identified in devitalized tissue. In infants, the most common microscopic findings are acute inflammation, hemorrhagic infarction, and subsequent necrosis as well as invasion of tissue by characteristic hyphae. Vegetative forms are apparently not found in infants because the disease progresses so rapidly that death occurs first.

Pathology

The focus of primary *Aspergillus* infection in infants is most often the respiratory tract. In infants who have aspergillosis, prematurity or antibiotic or corticosteroid therapy may have contributed to infection. In two of the infants reported with aspergillosis,[420, 423] no predisposing causes were identified. Increased susceptibility to aspergillosis in premature and full-term infants has been previously suggested,[420, 474, 475] but the mechanisms of infection have not been defined. When species of *Aspergillus* infect infants, dissemination of the infection appears to be more common than locally invasive infection.[420–423, 475]

Aspergillus may invade tissue by direct extension, as in orbital or nasal sinus infection into the brain, or it may be widely disseminated by blood. In infants, dissemination appears to result from the primary focus of infection in the lung. The organs most often involved in invasive or disseminated infection are the lung, gastrointestinal tract, brain, liver, kidney, thyroid, and heart.[476] The skin and subcutaneous areas, genital tract, and adrenal glands are sometimes involved in disseminated aspergillosis. One of the infants who had aspergillosis had a skin infection also, and, at autopsy, *Aspergillus* was identified in the spleen.[422] Necrosis is the characteristic histologic finding in disseminated aspergillosis. Characteristic branching hyphae may be seen invading vessels. Although granulomatous lesions are occasionally seen throughout an infected organ, suppuration with polymorphonuclear leukocytes and abscess formation are more common. Because the fungus invades and occludes the vessels, hemorrhagic necrosis is frequently seen in the lung and gastrointestinal tract in both infants and adults.

Clinical Manifestations

ILLUSTRATIVE CASE[421]

The patient was an 18-day-old white boy born after a full-term gestation that had been complicated by pharyngitis and sinusitis in the mother at 4 months. At birth, the child was considered normal; on the second day of life, a nonspecific maculopapular rash over most of the body was seen. Episodes of cyanosis accompanied by crying were noted, but the infant did well and was discharged 7 days after birth. On the seventeenth day of life, he was seen by a physician because he was not nursing well. Examination at that time showed small crusted papules on the skin and an enlarged liver. The infant was somewhat listless but did not appear ill. Hospitalization was scheduled for the following day, and chloramphenicol and topical antibiotic ointment were prescribed. The following morning, the infant was found unresponsive, and, on arrival at the hospital, was pronounced dead.

Autopsy showed several circumscribed crusted papules on the scalp and body. There was a shallow grayish-yellow ulcer on the base of the tongue. Large granulomatous lesions were found throughout the abdominal viscera. Some had central necrosis. Both lungs contained large caseating granulomas, some extending through the diaphragm to involve the liver, which also contained some granulomas. There were small yellow nodules on the posterior aspect of the epicardium. Both kidneys and spleen contained numerous granulomas, and small hemorrhagic erosions

were noted on the mucosa of the jejunum. The brain was not examined.

On microscopic examination, the larger granulomas were found to have central caseation necrosis with massive infiltration by polymorphonuclear leukocytes. In adjacent tissue, there were numerous thrombosed arteries and veins. Branching septate hyphae were identified in the granulomas as well as in thrombosed vessels. Some of the hyphae appeared to be invading the vessel walls. Hyphae were identified in the skin and tongue lesions. *Aspergillus* was cultured from specimens of liver, spleen, and bowel obtained at autopsy. ∎

Most of the infants with aspergillosis had signs of pulmonary infection that were thought to be pneumonia, not pulmonary infarction. One infant had a cutaneous infection that appeared as a maculopapular rash on the second day of life.[421] Skin lesions became scaly and later pustular. In this infant, enlargement of the liver became apparent, and the infant failed to gain weight. The case reported by Luke and associates[422] was characterized by jaundice, hepatosplenomegaly, heart murmur, ascites, and melena. Cerebrospinal fluid in this infant contained white blood cells, but further details were not reported. Jaundice and enlargement of liver and spleen were prominent in the case reported by Zimmerman,[420] and the infant reported by Akkoyunlu and Yücell had pneumonia and meningitis.[423] Liver disease was also dominant in the cases reported by Mangurten and co-workers[427] and Gonzalez-Crussi and colleagues.[428] Widespread dissemination to the large and small bowel, liver, pancreas, peritoneum, and lung was demonstrated in the infant with aspergillosis and leukemia.[429]

There have been increasing reports of infection with *Aspergillus* in neonates limited to the skin.[433, 435, 437–441] Seven such infants have been reported, and all survived with medical or surgical treatment, or both. The cutaneous lesions may be pustules progressing to cellulitis with ulcerations and eschar formation. In only one infant was disseminated infection suspected; however, fungemia was not detected.

Diagnosis and Differential Diagnosis

Diagnoses that must be considered in patients with aspergillosis are infection with other fungi, particularly Phycomycetes and *Candida*. Granulomatous aspergillosis appears similar to infection with *Mycobacterium tuberculosis*, *Nocardia*, and *Actinomyces* as well as to infection with *Cryptococcus* and *Coccidioides*.

Although *Aspergillus* may be identified by direct microscopic examination or culture of secretions, its presence does not necessarily indicate infection even in the presence of clinical disease. Demonstration of *Aspergillus* by culture or by microscopic examination of tissue obtained by biopsy or from body fluids establishes the diagnosis.

Hematoxylin-eosin or methenamine silver stains may be used for tissue. Spores and branching septate hyphae measuring 4 μm in diameter may be seen. The presence of conidiospores in tissue is infrequent, but they may be seen in specimens of saprophytic infection. Mycelia of *Aspergillus* may be confused with pseudohyphae of *Candida*, which are usually smaller and have no branching; yeast forms are usually present. Phycomycetes may be distinguished from *Aspergillus* by its large size, irregularity, and absence of septa. The greatest difficulty is encountered in distinguishing *Aspergillus* in tissue from *Penicillium*, which may also cause infection in humans.[477] The hyphae of *Penicillium* are broader and contain fewer septa. Serologic studies, particularly detection of *Aspergillus* antigen, may be helpful in diagnosis, but no data on antigenemia are available for infants.[478, 479]

Prognosis

The prognosis of invasive or disseminated aspergillosis in infants is poor, and high mortality is reported.

PHYCOMYCOSIS

Infection with Phycomycetes occurs infrequently in newborns, but there are reports of 18 infants, ranging in age from 5 days to several weeks, who have been infected with these fungi.[480–495] All but 5 of the infants died, and in 8 the diagnosis was not suspected during life. One infant died 3 days after the diagnosis was made and therapy initiated. The gastrointestinal tract was the focus of infection in 8 of the 18 infants. Two neonates had infection only in the CNS, and a third infant had CNS involvement in addition to intestinal infection. In none of the 3 was there clinical evidence of nasopharyngeal or orbital infection. One infant, reported by Miller and co-workers,[487] had rhinocerebral infection and survived, and Lewis and colleagues reported an infant with methylmalonic aciduria and rhinocerebral mucormycosis who died[491] White and colleagues[488] reported an infant with cellulitis of the abdominal wall who also survived, and Ng and Dear reported an infant with multiple abscesses with *Rhizopus* who was also treated and survived.[490] There are three additional reports of infants with cutaneous infection.[493–495] Two of the 3 infants died despite medical and surgical therapy. One of the infants who died had progressive infection that involved the gastrointestinal and respiratory tracts.[494]

Although infection with Phycomycetes is common in adults receiving immunosuppressive therapy and in those with neoplastic diseases, particularly hematologic or reticuloendothelial malignancies,[127, 158, 496] none of the infants had received such drugs or had hematologic diseases. In adults, acidosis resulting from uncontrolled diabetes mellitus or from hepatic or renal failure appears to contribute significantly to infection with Phycomycetes.[496–502] Although none of the infants had diabetes mellitus or hepatic failure, diarrhea was a prominent finding in 6 to 10 infants; however, acidosis as a complication of diarrhea was not commented on in any of the reported cases of diarrhea. One patient had renal failure and acidosis,[489] and 4 others were acidotic, including the infant with methylmalonic aciduria.[489–491, 493] Twelve of 18 infants were born prematurely, and intensive antibiotic therapy was given to all but 1 infant. Two infants

were receiving nasogastric feedings,[484, 491] and 1 infant developed cellulitis beneath a jejunostomy dressing.[488] Another infant had a cutaneous infection that began under an abdominal adhesive tape to attach a radiant thermocensor.[495]

The Organism

There is some confusion regarding the taxonomy of Phycomycetes.[503] For purposes of simplicity here, Phycomycetes is considered a class and Mucorales the order of the three most common genera causing phycomycosis—*Mucor, Absidia,* and *Rhizopus.*[504] However, phycomycosis also includes infection with species of *Mortierella, Basidiobolus, Hyphomyces,* and *Entomophthora.*[503]

Hyphae are best stained by hematoxylin-eosin, for which they have an affinity; methenamine silver stains are inferior for this fungus. Characteristically, hyphae are randomly branched, are rarely septate, and appear empty. The diameter of hyphae is variable even within the length of the same mycelium.

Because these fungi are not sufficiently pathogenic for laboratory animals, attempts at isolation by inoculation are not useful as a diagnostic procedure.

Epidemiology and Transmission

EPIDEMIOLOGY

Phycomycetes is found throughout the world in soil, in animal manure, and on fruits. Fungi of this class are frequently found in refrigerators and are commonly known as bread molds.[505–507] *Basidiobolus* and *Entomophthora* may be isolated from decaying organic matter. Infection with Phycomycetes has been reported in both humans and animals.[508]

TRANSMISSION

In infants reported with phycomycosis, the infection may have been the result of either ingestion of the fungus and introduction into the gastrointestinal tract or inhalation into the nasopharynx or lung after birth, but saprophytic colonization in the vagina of the mothers and acquisition of the fungus at the time of delivery cannot be excluded. Little is known regarding the presence of Phycomycetes on the skin or in feces, or in pharyngeal or vaginal secretions in the absence of clinical disease. Emmons noted that, after exposure to this fungus, patients with bronchiectasis may cough up spores for several days in the absence of clinical infection.[508] Studies of isolation of these fungi from other sites without evidence of disease have not been reported, but data from newborns suggest that saprophytic colonization with Phycomycetes may be similar to the commensalism even with *Candida.* There is no indication that infection between humans occurs. In the case reported by Dennis and co-workers, *Rhizopus oryzale* was isolated from the Elastoplast that was used as an adhesive for the abdominal dressing.[485] Of interest is the infant with abdominal wall cellulitis reported by White and co-workers. Cellulitis developed beneath the adhesive dressing of a jejunostomy. In addition, Linder and colleagues isolated *Rhizopus* from the adhesive tape used to attach the thermocensor.[495] In both instances, cultures of similar dressings and tape in the same units failed to grow the fungus.[488, 495]

Pathogenesis

The bowel is a frequent site of infection in infants and appears to be associated with malnutrition or diarrhea.[482, 509]

Underlying disease seems to play a major role in most cases of phycomycosis. The high incidence of rhinocerebral infection in adults with diabetes mellitus has been noted, but the biochemical abnormality that increases susceptibility is considered to be acidosis rather than endocrine dysfunction.[484, 498] Straatsma and co-workers have suggested that acidosis from any cause, including hepatic and renal failure, may increase susceptibility to phycomycosis.[496] Of interest are infants and adults with gastrointestinal phycomycosis. Most had diarrhea, which may result in acidosis resulting from loss of bicarbonate, especially in infants. Whether diarrhea preceded or was the result of gastrointestinal phycomycosis in these cases cannot be determined. The mechanism of increased susceptibility to infection with Phycomycetes in an acidotic state is incompletely understood. Although optimum growth of Phycomycetes occurs at pH 4.0 in vitro but not at pH 2.7 or 7.3,[510] acidification is not suitable for the sexual cycle of Phycomycetes.[511] In the host, acidosis may delay polymorphonuclear response and limit fibroblastic reaction.[498, 502] Prematurity, antibiotics, and diarrhea may have been some of the predisposing causes of phycomycosis in the infants who died of this infection.

Pathology

The histopathology of infection with this class of fungi is characteristically vascular invasion with necrosis or hemorrhage. Necrotic and suppurative lesions containing massive infiltration by polymorphonuclear leukocytes are seen in invasive or disseminated phycomycosis. In patients with subcutaneous infection, lesions are usually granulomatous with epithelioid and Langhans' giant cells. Conspicuous infiltration with eosinophils occurs in subcutaneous infection, particularly with species of *Basidiobolus*. Vascular invasion in such cases is rare.

Clinical Manifestations

ILLUSTRATIVE CASE[481]

The patient was a white girl who was the product of a full-term uncomplicated pregnancy. During the first 4 days of life she did well; however, on the fifth day, she became febrile and irritable. Chloramphenicol was given; on the following day, otitis media was suspected and a myringotomy was performed. The abdomen was thought to be distended, and gastric suction was instituted. Roentgenograms of the chest and skull were normal, but abdominal radiographs were interpreted as showing adynamic ileus. On the seventh day of life, she began to vomit and had episodes of cyanosis. Diarrhea began on the ninth day. The infant's condition gradually worsened, and she died 16 days after birth.

At autopsy, fibrinous adhesions involving the serosa of the stomach were found, and the stomach was adherent to the colon, liver, spleen, and left hemidiaphragm. The base of the left lung was adherent to the diaphragm. Both lungs were red, but there was a hemorrhagic area in the base of the left lung. The wall of the stomach was thickened and indurated, and the mucosa was ragged and tan.

On microscopic examination, deposits of fibrin were identified on the pleural surface of the left lung. Adjacent alveoli and interstitial tissue contained large nonseptate hyphae, which were invading the vessel walls. Recent hemorrhage had occurred in that area. The gastric mucosa was necrotic, and nonseptate hyphae extended through the wall of the stomach, invading the liver, spleen, pancreas, and colon. There was extensive invasion of vessels by large nonseptate branching hyphae. Large numbers of mast cells and polymorphonuclear leukocytes were present in these areas. The brain was not examined. ■

The usual symptoms of gastrointestinal phycomycosis are bloody diarrhea and cramping abdominal pain. Because vascular invasion and necrosis occur, perforation and peritonitis with a rapidly fatal course are common. In seven of the eight infants with phycomycosis, diarrhea and abdominal distention or signs of peritoneal irritation or both were predominant findings. Two infants had free air in the peritoneal cavity from perforation. One infant without abdominal signs had CNS infection without other organ involvement.

Diagnosis and Differential Diagnosis

Infants with phycomycosis appear to be very similar to those with aspergillosis. Phycomycetes has the same affinity for vascular invasion, hemorrhage, necrosis, and suppuration. Bacterial infection in the lung may be indistinguishable from phycomycosis on clinical grounds. Hemorrhagic infarction of the lung or bowel from other causes has the same presenting signs as infection with Phycomycetes.

CSF in cases of CNS infection does not show a consistent pattern. Glucose and protein levels in CSF are frequently normal. Xanthochromia with small numbers of red blood cells is common, and a few mononuclear or polymorphonuclear cells may be present.[502]

Diagnosis of phycomycosis should be considered in debilitated patients, particularly those with acidosis related to diarrhea, diabetes mellitus, or hepatic or renal failure who do not respond to correction of the acidotic state. Sinus or orbital abnormalities in such patients should be investigated for the presence of Phycomycetes. Adults receiving immunosuppressive therapy or antimetabolites for hematologic diseases who develop pulmonary or gastrointestinal symptoms must be evaluated for possible Phycomycetes infection.

Diagnosis of infection with these fungi may be difficult because culture results are frequently negative.[512] Demonstration of the fungus is best accomplished by microscopic examination of tissue and visualization of the broad, branching, nonseptate hyphae. A 10% solution of potassium hydroxide may be used, although hematoxylin-eosin is preferred for specimens of tissue. Exudates from the nasopharynx or necrotic tissue obtained by debridement may be cultured on Sabouraud glucose agar. Because of the ubiquity of these fungi, demonstration of the organism in tissue is necessary to establish a diagnosis of phycomycosis. Media for culture may contain chloramphenicol to suppress growth of bacteria, but cyclohexamide should be eliminated because it prevents growth of Phycomycetes.

Although normal human serum contains substances that inhibit growth of *Rhizopus* in vitro,[513] serologic and immunologic tests have not been extensively studied as diagnostic aids for patients with phycomycosis. Bank and associates, using an extract of *Rhizopus* isolated from a patient, produced a cutaneous reaction with an intradermal injection in the patient but not in control subjects.[514] They also found complement-fixing antibodies in the serum of the patient but not in controls, although the same extract was used. Jones and Kaufman demonstrated antibodies to a homogenate of the fungus by immunodiffusion in 8 of 11 patients with mucormycosis.[515]

Prognosis

The diagnosis of phycomycosis in infants is most often made at autopsy. The diagnosis was not considered before death in nine of the reported patients. In seven patients, the organism was identified and therapy was given; four of the seven recovered.

BLASTOMYCOSIS

Infection with *Blastomyces* in the newborn has been reported only twice,[516, 517] although infection with this fungus has been reported in nine women during pregnancy.[517–523] Seven of the women had disseminated blastomycosis, and, in two, the infection was considered to be confined to the lungs. In all but three, the infection was diagnosed and treated before delivery. The untreated women had disseminated infection. Two of the infants were normal at birth, but one infant, born of an untreated mother, died at 3 weeks of age with *Blastomyces* identified in lung tissue. The other infant presented at 18 days of age with respiratory distress, and infection with *B. dermatitidis* was diagnosed by lung biopsy. He received amphotericin B but died 3 weeks after onset of therapy.[517] Infection with *Blastomyces* was not identified in any of the other infants.

The Organism

Blastomyces is a dimorphic fungus that has a mycelial form at room temperature and a yeast form at 37° C.[524]

The mycelial form is found in soil, where it may exist for long periods.[525, 526] Conidiophores arise at right angles to the hyphae and are believed to be infectious for humans when mycelia are disturbed. When inhaled, the fungus converts to the yeast form, which is multinucleated, containing 8 to 12 nuclei. It has a thick wall and reproduces by single budding with a broad connection to the parent.[527]

Epidemiology and Transmission

EPIDEMIOLOGY

Blastomycosis is endemic in the Mississippi and Ohio river valleys in the United States and in parts of Canada.[527–535] Sporadic cases have been reported in Central and South America and in Africa.[536] The infection is more common in middle-aged men,[528, 537, 538] particularly those who are employed outdoors in rural areas.[62, 539]

TRANSMISSION

Blastomyces is acquired by inhalation of contaminated soil, and the lung is the initial focus of infection.[540] Primary cutaneous blastomycosis by direct inoculation of the organism into skin has been reported.[540–542] It has been suggested that human-to-human transmission does not occur, but Craig and colleagues reported probable human-to-human transmission through sexual intercourse.[543] In addition, mother-to-fetus transmission has been suggested with blastomycosis reported by Watts and associates.[516]

Pathogenesis

Pulmonary infection has been identified as the initial site of infection due to *Blastomyces dermatitidis*.[540] In some instances, the pulmonary disease is self-limited and may resolve without therapy.[544] In some instances, however, both progressive pulmonary disease and dissemination may occur. Although there are no extensive studies of immunocompromised patients, both corticosteroid therapy and other immunosuppressive therapy may increase the risk of not only acquisition of the fungus but dissemination as well.[535, 545] Current published data also indicate that dissemination of the fungus may be more common during pregnancy.[516, 519–523] It has been suggested by some studies that a relative immunosuppressed state may occur during pregnancy, which may account for this increased risk of dissemination.[546–548] When dissemination occurs, the skin, bone, and genitourinary system are most commonly involved. The CNS, liver, spleen, and lymph nodes are not commonly affected. Cell-mediated immunity appears to decrease the risk of dissemination of *Blastomyces*.[549]

Pathology

The inflammatory response in the lung consists of polymorphonuclear leukocytes followed by noncaseating granulomatous formation with epithelioid and giant cells. Extrapulmonary sites of infection show a similar histologic pattern, with the exception of the skin, which shows pseudoepitheliomatous hyperplasia and microabscess formation.

Clinical Manifestations

Acute symptomatic pulmonary infection with *Blastomyces* is associated with abrupt onset of chills and fever, myalgias, and arthralgias. Pleuritic pain is common early, and cough is prominent and may become productive of purulent sputum late in the course of the disease. Resolution of symptoms without therapy is common. Pulmonary infection, however, may become chronic and slowly progressive, with chronic cough, hemoptysis, pleuritic chest pain, and weight loss.

When dissemination occurs, skin infections are reported in as many as 80% of cases.[528, 537, 550–553] These infections are most common on the exposed surfaces, and lesions have a verrucous appearance, particularly in the later stages. Abscesses may occur at the periphery of the lesions. In some patients, the skin lesions appear as shallow ulcerations with central granulation tissue that bleeds easily. Other sites of infection include subcutaneous tissue, bone, and joints and the genitourinary system, particularly the epididymis and prostate. CNS infection is uncommon; however, when it occurs, it usually involves the meninges with symptoms of headache and confusion.[554] Involvement of the liver and spleen does occur but is uncommon.

In nine women with blastomycosis during pregnancy, seven had disseminated infection; in four in whom studies were done, there was no evidence of placental infection in three.[465, 521, 522] One of these women had received amphotericin B for 35 days before the birth of her infant. *B. dermatitidis* was cultured from the placenta in the fourth woman, and the organism was visualized in both the fetal and the maternal placental tissue.[523] None of these infants were infected. In one woman in whom placental studies were not done, the fungus was isolated from urine, and her infant died at 3 weeks of age with pulmonary blastomycosis.[516] At autopsy, the infant had no evidence of extrapulmonary infection, suggesting that the fungus may have been acquired by aspiration of infected secretions during birth rather than by hematogenous spread in utero. In the other infant, although the original site of infection was the lung, the fungus was also found in the kidneys at autopsy.[517]

Diagnosis and Differential Diagnosis

Because of the rarity of neonatal blastomycosis, it is difficult to enumerate specific signs that may lead to its diagnosis. It is anticipated from both cases and extrapolated from data in infants with other nonopportunistic fungal infections that the diagnosis should be considered in an infant born in an endemic area and who has signs of indolent, progressive pulmonary disease. In older children and adults, acute pulmonary infection with *Blastomyces* appears similar to acute bacterial, mycoplasmal, and viral infections. Radiographic findings are also nonspecific. Chronic infection may simulate infection with *Mycobacterium* and other fungi, and mass lesions

may suggest carcinoma. There are few specific signs associated with extrapulmonary blastomycosis. However, the skin lesions may be mistaken for squamous cell carcinoma.

Diagnosis of blastomycosis is made by visualization of fungus in culture of secretions or tissue. Skin test antigens have been used, but studies indicate a lack of sensitivity and specificity.[528] Serologic studies to determine the presence of complement-fixing antibodies also lack sensitivity,[528] but immunodiffusion tests for precipitating antibody may be positive in as many as 80% of cases.[555, 556] No data regarding skin test reactivity or serology in infants with blastomycosis have been reported.

Prognosis

Both newborns with blastomycosis died. In one the diagnosis was not suspected, and in the other the infection progressed despite antifungal therapy.

DERMATOPHYTOSIS

The dermatophytes—*Epidermophyton*, *Microsporum*, and *Trichophyton*—are often responsible for infection of keratinized areas of the body, including skin, hair, and nails. Superficial infection with these "ringworm" fungi has been reported infrequently in newborns, although infants have been considered susceptible to infection with these specialized fungi.[557] In 1876, Lynch reported an infant with tinea faciei who was only 6 hours of age.[558] Unfortunately, in this report the diagnosis was made on clinical evidence, but there was no documentation of dermatophyte infection by microscopic examination or culture. More recently, Jacobs and colleagues reported an infant 8 days of age with tinea faciei related to *Microsporum canis*.[559] In the years between these two cases, dermatophyte infections in infants from a few weeks of age to several months of age have been described.[560–572]

Because of the infrequent reports of dermatophyte infections in infants, few investigative studies defining factors contributing to increased infantile susceptibility or resistance to infection by dermatophytes have been performed.[567, 568] Wyre and Johnson suggested that increased humidity in the incubator may have contributed to the infant reported with pityriasis versicolor,[568] and Lanska and associates indicated that prolonged exposure to humidified oxygen by hood may have contributed to cutaneous fungal infection in three infants.[570] *Malassezia furfur*, considered to be the cause of pityriasis versicolor, is a dimorphic, lipophilic yeast commonly found on the skin of infants in the absence of clinical disease.[573] However, 14 infants have been reported who had *Malassezia* isolated from blood. All had indwelling intravenous catheters and were receiving parenteral hyperalimentation containing fat emulsions.[573–576] Redline and Dahms reported an additional infant who had pneumonia considered to be caused by *M. furfur*.[577] That infant also had an indwelling intravenous catheter and was receiving Intralipid (Cutter Laboratories, Berkeley, Calif.). Nowak and co-workers[578] described intraluminal slime in a Hickman catheter containing mononuclear cells and *M. furfur*, and Marcon and colleagues[579] suggested that the fat emulsions contained the necessary fatty acids for proliferation of the organism in vivo. All of the infants survived; although some were given amphotericin B, removal of the intravenous catheter was curative in most instances.

The Organism

Dermatophytes have been placed in the class of imperfect fungi, Deuteromycetes, in the order Moniliales.[504] However, because of a sexual stage in some dermatophytes, other authors have preferred to classify some genera as belonging to the class Ascomycetes.[580, 581]

Hyphae of dermatophytes are long, undulant, and branching. Many septa are present along the length of hyphae. Hyphae break at the septa into barrel-shaped arthrospores. In culture, dermatophytes form conidiophores, with resulting microconidia and macroconidia. Genera and species identification is based on gross characteristics of colony and microscopic morphology of conidia. A complete review of distinguishing features may be found in standard mycology tests.[582, 583]

Epidemiology and Transmission

EPIDEMIOLOGY

Dermatophytes are distributed throughout the world in humans and animals; *Microsporum gypseum* is also found in soil.[583] The fungus may contaminate combs, hairbrushes, shoes, and shower floors and has been isolated from air.[584, 585] Contamination of soil with dermatophytes has been thought to occur in keratinous debris from infected animals and humans.[583] There is no evidence that these fungi are free-living saprophytes in soil.

TRANSMISSION

Dermatophyte infection is most often acquired from contact with infected persons or animals. Infections with *M. gypseum* may result from contact with soil contaminated with the fungus. Interhuman transmission may occur with *Epidermophyton floccosum*, *Microsporum audouinii*, *Trichophyton mentagrophytes*, *T. rubrum*, *T. schoenleinii*, *T. tonsurans* and *T. violaceum*.[586] Zoophilic dermatophytes include *M. canis*, *T. gallinae*, *T. mentagrophytes*, and *T. verrucosum*. Although *M. canis* is usually transmitted to humans from young animals, particularly kittens, transmission between persons is suggested in the case of an infant reported by Bereston and Robinson.[560] Pinetti and co-workers isolated *M. canis* and *M. gypseum* from flies, which suggests an additional mode of transmission.[587]

In newborns with dermatophyte infection, the fungus is most likely acquired after birth from contact with infected household members or animals. In the case reported by Lynch of clinically apparent infection at 6 hours of age, fungus may have been acquired in utero.[558] In this case, there was no evidence of infection in the mother, but the fungus has been demonstrated on skin in the absence of clinical disease.[588, 589]

Pathogenesis

Despite worldwide distribution of dermatophytes and frequency of exposure of humans to these fungi, the incidence of clinically apparent infection in both adults and infants is considerably lower than would be expected. Few studies defining host factors responsible for protection have been performed. Although Knight[590] has shown in experimental studies in humans that macerated moist skin is more susceptible to the infection than dry skin, the role of immunologic factors in the control of dermatophyte infection remains obscure. Repeated infection may occur at identical sites as long as 2 years after primary infection,[590, 591] despite reports that infection may offer partial immunity to reinfection.[592, 593]

Roth and colleagues[168] as well as others[594–598] have demonstrated antidermatophyte activity in normal human serum and have suggested that this substance may restrict dermatophyte infection to superficial layers of skin. No studies investigating the role of antifungal activity in sweat have been reported, although gamma globulins and antibodies have been demonstrated in sweat.[599] Although antidermatophyte activity has been reported in serum at birth,[585] there have been no specific studies in infants regarding other host factors or immunologic consequences of dermatophyte infection.

Pathology

Dermatophyte infection is generally confined to keratinized areas of the body and only rarely invades deeper tissues. There may be vesicles containing serous fluid. Inflammatory reaction with polymorphonuclear leukocyte infiltration is minimal and usually represents secondary bacterial infection. Occasionally, intense inflammatory reactions may occur in the absence of bacterial infection, especially in children with tinea capitis resulting from *T. mentagrophytes*. These pustular lesions, or kerions, surround infected hair follicles and appear to be reactions to virulent strains of fungus.[583]

Favus is a chronic infection usually caused by *T. schoenleinii* or *T. mentagrophytes*. Granulomatous formation occurs, with giant cells and masses of hyphae around the hair follicle. Overlying the infection is a crust of cellular debris and degenerating hyphae. This lesion is convex, and scarring and alopecia appear after healing.

Clinical Manifestations

Dermatophytosis is generally classified by focus of infection and less commonly by species of infecting fungus.

Tinea capitis is a fungus infection of the scalp and hair caused by species of *Microsporum* and *Trichophyton*. It occurs most often in infants and older children and adults. In infants, this infection has been reported more frequently than dermatophyte infection in other areas. Alteras reported that, in a group of 7000 patients, there were 70 infants between 2 and 12 months of age who had tinea capitis.[594] In this study, *M. audouinii* was the most common fungus in infants, as it is also in school children with tinea capitis. Other fungi reportedly caus-

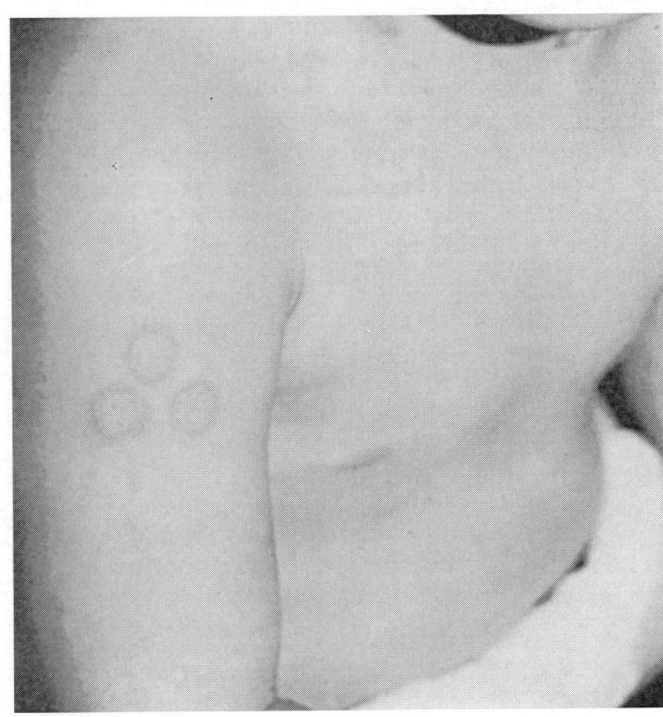

FIGURE 17–3 *Microsporum audouinii* infection in a 7-month-old infant.

ing tinea capitis include *M. canis*, *T. violaceum*, *T. tonsurans*, *T. mentagrophytes*, *T. schoenleinii*, *M. ferrugineum*, *E. floccosum*, and *T. rubrum*. Infection begins with small scaling papules that spread peripherally, forming circular pruritic patches (Fig. 17–3). Both kerion and favus formation may occur.

Tinea corporis, or ringworm of smooth skin, may result from infection with species of *Microsporum*, *Trichophyton*, or *Epidermophyton*, although infections with species of *Microsporum* are most common (Fig. 17–4). Infants and children appear to be more susceptible to tinea corporis than adults. King and co-workers reported five infants with tinea corporis who ranged in age from 3 weeks to 7 months[561] *Microsporum* species predominated in their study, but one infant, who was 8 weeks of age, was infected with *E. floccosum* (Fig. 17–5). In older children, *M. canis* and *T. mentagrophytes* are more common causes of tinea corporis. Lesions, which may be single or multiple, are round or oval scaling, erythematous patches. As infection spreads peripherally, the center of the lesion may show some clearing. In some instances, there may be an intense inflammatory reaction with vesiculation at the margins and severe pruritus. Patches of infected areas may coalesce, forming extensive plaques with serpiginous borders. Deep granulomas or nodules may form, especially when the infection is caused by *T. rubrum*.

Tinea cruris is a fungal infection of the groin, perineum, or perianal area and is most often caused by *E. floccosum*. *T. mentagrophytes* and *T. rubrum* are unusual causes of infection at these sites. Although *Candida* species account for the majority of fungal infections in the diaper area, King and co-workers reported one infant with *E. floccosum* infection in the perineum.[561] Infection with this fungus is characterized by brownish areas of scaly dermatitis with small, superficial pustules at the periphery of the lesion. Infection with *T. mentagrophytes*, which usually spreads from the feet, is associated with marked inflammation. Tinea cruris caused by *T. rubrum* may be unilateral and may be only one part of a generalized scaly, erythematous, plaquelike eruption (see Fig. 17–5).

Tinea pedis, or athlete's foot, is the most common dermatophyte infection in adults but is rare in infants and children. King and co-workers reported one 12-month-old infant with tinea pedis caused by *T. rubrum*.[561] Infection is usually accompanied by vesicles between the toes or on the soles. Skin may peel, forming fissures, and edema and lymphangitis may occur with secondary bacterial infection.

Diagnosis and Differential Diagnosis

Dermatophyte infection may be mistaken for seborrhea, impetigo or psoriasis. Tinea capitis may appear similar to alopecia areata, but there is usually an absence of scaling in the latter.

Definitive diagnosis of infection with dermatophytes may be made by direct microscopic examination of infected material. Areas to be examined should be cleansed with 70% alcohol, and scrapings should be made with a scalpel or scissors from the active periphery of the lesion. If vesicles are present, the tops should be removed for examination. Hairs infected with *M. audouinii* or *M. canis* may be identified by using Wood's light, which emits monochromatic ultraviolet rays. Infected hairs show a green-yellow fluorescence and may be removed for examination. Scrapings from nails, obtained from deep layers, should be thin. Specimens are placed on a glass slide, and a few drops of 10% sodium or potassium hydroxide are added. A coverslip is added, and the specimen is gently heated over a low flame. Examination

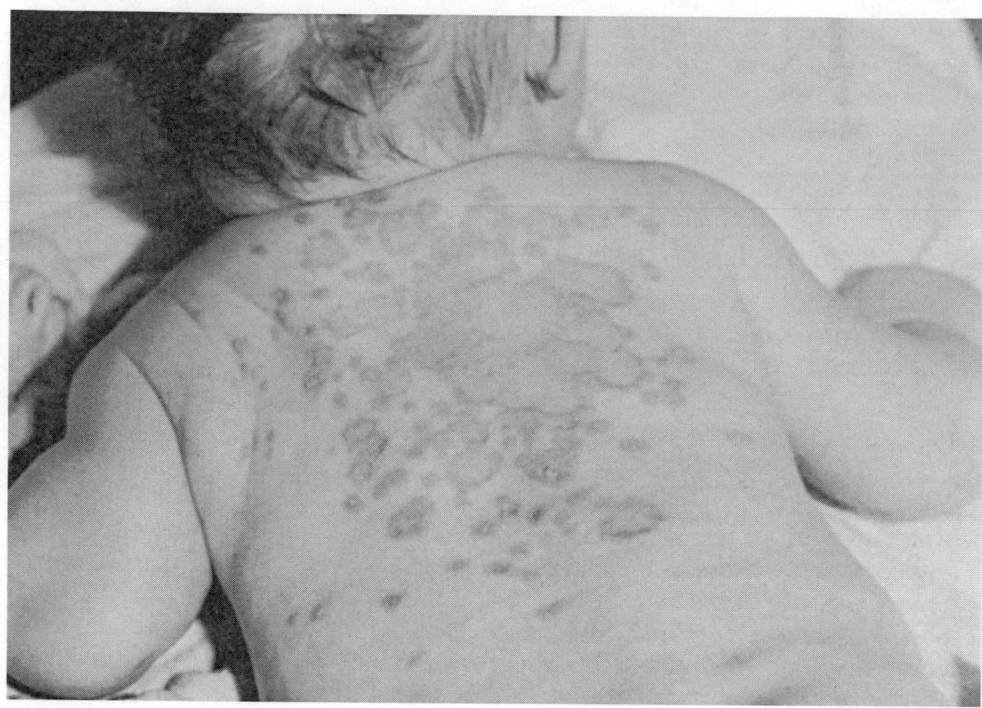

FIGURE 17–4 Tinea corporis caused by *Microsporum* sp. in a 4-month-old infant.

should take place immediately under low power of the microscope. The presence of hyphae on the specimen confirms the diagnosis of fungal infection. Young hyphae appear as long, thin threads, and older hyphae have many spores. Spores may be found either within the hair follicle or around its base. Shelley and Wood have described a technique of crushing the hair.[600] They found it to be superior to the use of potassium hydroxide for identifying the fungus in the hair.

Identification of the genus and species of dermatophyte may be made only by culture. Infected material should be cultured on a Sabouraud glucose agar slant, and microscopic examination of hyphae and conidia performed.

Skin test antigen that is group specific but not species specific is available. Delayed hypersensitivity reactions are common and do not correlate with active disease. Some patients may have an immediate reaction to intra-

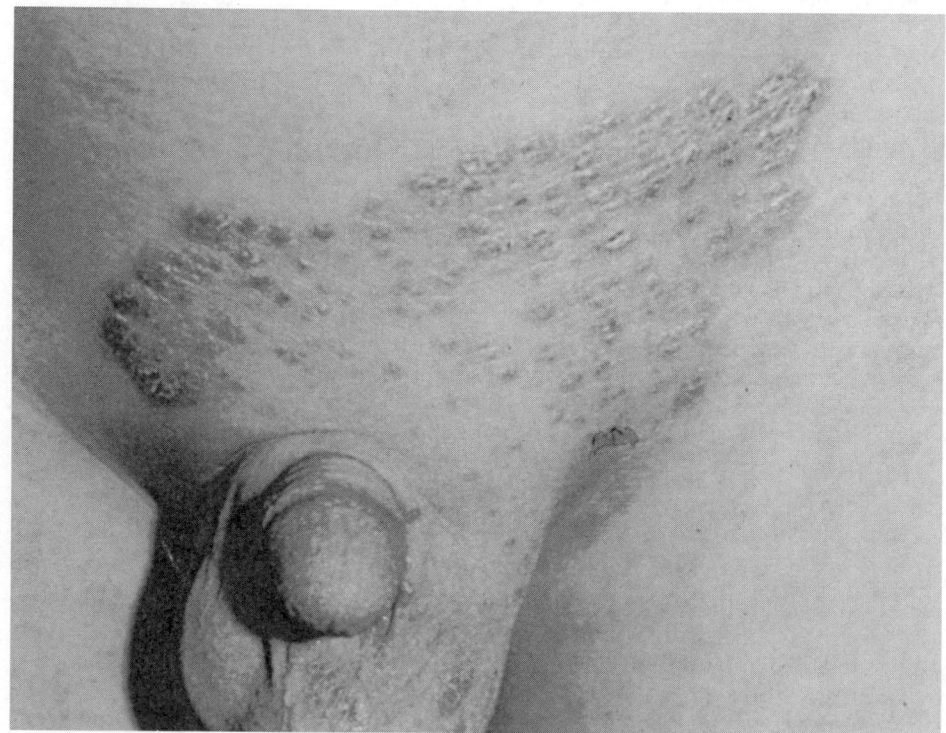

FIGURE 17–5 Tinea cruris infection with *Epidermophyton floccosum* in a young infant.

dermal injection of the skin test antigen, but this result does not appear to be correlated with increase or decrease in susceptibility. There are no studies of delayed hypersensitivity in infants.

Prognosis

Untreated dermatophyte infection is slowly progressive and may be disfiguring, especially in cases of kerion and favus reactions. Secondary bacterial infections are common, particularly in cases of tinea pedis. Unless severe underlying disease is present, deep tissue invasion does not occur.

Prevention

Separate combs, hairbrushes, and clippers should be available for the newborn and should not be shared with others in the household. Infected animals should be promptly treated.[601]

THERAPY

Amphotericin B

Amphotericin B is the most widely used antimicrobial agent for fungal infections, but alternative or adjunctive therapy has been employed successfully for specific fungi. Amphotericin B is a polyene antibiotic that reacts with sterols in cell membranes and results in cellular damage and lysis. The drug is effective topically for some cutaneous, mucocutaneous, and gastrointestinal fungal infections, but it is not absorbed from the gastrointestinal tract in quantities sufficient to give adequate serum levels in patients with disseminated or deep tissue fungal infections. In such instances, amphotericin B must be given intravenously. Serum levels in adults average 1.5 µg/ml 1 hour after intravenous injection of 0.6 to 1 mg/kg; the half-life is approximately 24 hours, but levels of 0.14 µg/ml have been detected in serum for at least 3 weeks.[602] Only one tenth to one twentieth of the serum level is distributed into CSF, and in some cases of fungal meningitis, it may be necessary to administer amphotericin B intrathecally.

There are few studies of the clinical pharmacology of amphotericin B in newborns or older infants from which an accurate recommendation for dosage can be made or that define toxicity in these age groups. For guidelines, the physician must turn to data that are available from studies of older children and adults. Cherry and associates reported levels of amphotericin B in serum and CSF of a child receiving 1.2 mg/kg intravenously on alternate days.[603] The serum level 44 hours after administration of the drug was 0.48 µg/ml, and the CSF level at the same time was 0.24 µg/ml. McCoy and co-workers, after infusion of 0.6 mg into a mother, found peak serum concentrations at 1 hour of 2.6 µg/ml in both the mother and arterial cord blood.[604] In that instance, the amphotericin B concentration in the amniotic fluid was 0.08 µg/ml. Ismail and Lerner found levels of amphotericin B in cord blood to be one third that of

the maternal serum.[519] Hager and associates obtained simultaneous amphotericin B levels in maternal blood, cord blood, and amniotic fluid 26 hours after an infusion of 20 mg.[522] The levels were 1.9, 1.3, and 0.3 µg/ml, respectively. Ward and co-workers reported a premature infant whose serum levels of amphotericin B were similar to those found in older children and adults, and those levels persisted for at least 17 days after amphotericin B had been discontinued.[605]

The toxicity of amphotericin B in humans is significant, and adults frequently experience nausea, vomiting, headache, chills, and fevor during infusion of the antibiotic.[606] Patients may become tolerant to these side effects, but pretreatment with salicylates and phenothiazines is helpful in reducing these symptoms, as is administration of hydrocortisone hemisuccinate before or with the infusion (in adults, the usual dose of hydrocortisone semisuccinate is 25 to 50 mg). Convulsions or cardiac arrhythmias may occur during infusion, especially if the drug is administered too rapidly or if the concentration of amphotericin B exceeds 0.1 mg/ml of diluent. In adults and older children, phlebitis at the site of infusion is common but may be reduced by careful technique and frequent changing of intravenous site. Anemia occurs frequently and may require blood transfusions. Hypokalemia can be corrected with potassium replacement and must be carefully watched for. Nephrotoxicity is the most important kind of toxicity associated with administration of amphotericin B. Renal damage appears to correlate with total dose of amphotericin B[607] and results from drug-induced renal vasoconstriction as well as from direct action of amphotericin B on renal tubules.[608] There may be a rise in serum creatinine and blood urea nitrogen levels and a decrease in creatinine clearance, as well as cylindruria, renal tubular acidosis, tubular necrosis, and nephrocalcinosis.

There are few data on toxicity of amphotericin B in children. Cherry and co-workers reviewed the use of amphotericin B in children and, despite the small numbers of patients in whom the dose of amphotericin B was recorded, suggested that toxicity in children was probably similar to that in adults.[603] These authors reviewed 13 children whose renal function was assessed 3 months after therapy was discontinued, and only 3 had slight to moderate loss of renal function. In one, renal abnormalities were thought to be caused by infection and not toxicity of amphotericin B. Of 19 children whose renal function was studied during treatment, only 7 had normal function. Seven of 12 children with abnormal function had only proteinuria, which cleared when the drug was discontinued. The remainder had either elevated blood urea nitrogen levels, proteinuria, or cylindruria. Faix reported that 11 of 12 children receiving amphotericin B and, in most instances, 5-fluorocytosine developed some toxicity, including hypokalemia, nephropathy, and hepatopathy.[258] In all but one infant, the toxicity was reversible when the drugs were discontinued. In addition, he found no difference in toxicity when the maximum daily dose of amphotericin B was 0.5 or 1 mg/kg. In contrast, Baley and co-workers found significant nephrotoxicity in very low birth weight infants when given amphotericin B at a dose of 1 mg/kg per day versus 0.5 mg/kg per day.[609]

The effect of amphotericin B on the fetus has not been extensively studied. There are now several reports of the use of amphotericin B in pregnant women.[518–522a, 604, 610–617] In no instance was there evidence of teratogenicity or fetal toxicity related to this antifungal agent.

Minimal inhibitory concentrations of amphotericin B for fungi causing disease in infants and recommended total dose of amphotericin B are presented in Table 17–1. Others have indicated that lower doses of amphotericin B may be effective.[618] Of importance are reports of resistance of some species of *Candida* to amphotericin B, necessitating species identification of *Candida* isolates as well as determination of minimal inhibitory concentrations to antifungal agents.[34, 50–52, 619]

The initial intravenous dose of amphotericin B in adults usually does not exceed 0.1 mg/kg and is given in 5% dextrose and water in a concentration no greater than 0.1 mg/ml. Amphotericin B should not be diluted in normal saline because a precipitate forms. After the initial dose, the amount of amphotericin B may be increased gradually until the maximum daily dose of 1 to 1.5 mg/kg is achieved.[621] The maximum daily dose and duration of therapy may depend on the focus and extent of fungal disease[622] as well as on the minimal inhibitory concentration of the organism with amphotericin B.[623] The speed at which maximum dosage can be reached is influenced by the side effects experienced by the infant. At that time, the antibiotic may be given daily or on alternate days. Many authors have suggested following serum levels of amphotericin B as a guide to therapy,[603, 624] although, because of the predictable pharmacokinetics of amphotericin B, obtaining levels may not be necessary.[625, 626] Rate of administration varies with tolerance to side effects, but the daily dose should be given slowly over at least 4 to 6 hours.

Intrathecal administration of amphotericin B may be necessary in patients with fungal meningitis, particularly if the fungus can be demonstrated in CSF after the maximum daily dose in intravenous therapy has been reached. The drug may be given into the lumbar sac, into the cisterna magna, or into the lateral ventricle either directly or by way of an indwelling intraventricular reservoir.[627] If the latter is to be employed alone, normal CSF circulation should be documented to ensure that amphotericin B will be distributed throughout the subarachnoid space. There are few data regarding the ideal intrathecal dose of amphotericin B in children with fungal meningitis. Klein and co-workers instilled 0.05 mg every third day for two administrations in an infant with *Candida* meningitis.[20] The initial intrathecal dose in infants should be 0.01 mg, gradually increased over a period of 5 to 7 days to 0.1 mg given every other day or every third day. Amphotericin B for intrathecal administration should be diluted in sterile distilled water containing no bacteriostatic agents. Concentration should not exceed 0.25 mg/ml diluent, and further dilution with CSF is recommended. Some infants with *Candida* meningitis have recovered with intravenous amphotericin B therapy alone.[189, 628] Complications of intrathecal amphotericin B administration include CSF pleocytosis (arachnoiditis), transient radiculitis, and sensory loss. Adults often complain of headache, and convulsions occur occasionally.

Administration of amphotericin B in other sites in infants has not been critically evaluated. Klein and co-workers employed intra-articular amphotericin B in the child they reported with septic arthritis caused by *Candida*.[20] The dose used was 0.5 mg on a single occasion. Hill and colleagues reported instillation of 0.4 ml of a 0.01% solution of amphotericin B into the anterior chamber of the eye in an infant with *Candida* endophthalmitis.[183]

Liposomal amphotericin B has been shown to be less nephrotoxic than amphotericin B,[629] and, although there is limited experience with this preparation in children, Lackner and co-workers reported its successful use in two premature infants with disseminated fungal infections using a dose of 5 mg/kg per day.[437] In addition, Weitkamp and associates reported use of this preparation in 21 lower-birth-weight infants with *Candida* infections using a dose of 1 to 5 mg/kg per day and demonstrated its efficacy without apparent nephrotoxicity.[630]

Scarcella and colleagues also reported using liposomal amphotericin B in 44 infants with severe fungal infections. Using a daily dose of 1 to 5 mg/kg per day, they reported successful outcomes in 32 infants. Twelve very low birth weight infants died. The researchers identified only transient hypokalemia during treatment.[631]

5-Fluorocytosine

5-Fluorocytosine, a fluoropyrimidine, has been shown to have in vitro activity against some fungi[606, 632–634] and has been effective in some patients with fungal infection.[269, 635] The drug is absorbed well from the gastrointestinal tract, and, with doses of 100 to 150 mg/kg daily, serum levels vary from 17 to 44 μg/ml.[636] In CSF, levels of 5-fluorocytosine may be as high as 88% of the serum concentration.[637] The drug is administered orally at a dose of 50 to 150 mg/kg per day in four divided doses for 2 to 6 weeks in adults. There is increasing experience with this agent in infants. Hill and co-workers treated a premature infant who had disseminated candidiasis with 5-fluorocytosine at a dose of 100 mg/kg per day.[183] After an initial oral dose of 25 mg/kg, serum levels of 5-fluorocytosine were 40 μg/ml at 2 hours and 27 μg/ml at 4 and 6 hours. The level in CSF at 6 hours was 40 μg/ml. Of interest was the rapid emergence of resistance

TABLE 17–1

Minimal Inhibitory Concentrations (MIC) of Amphotericin B and Recommended Total Dose

FUNGUS	MIC (μg/ml)	TOTAL DOSE (mg/kg)
Candida species[292–294]	0.09–3.12	25–30
Cryptococcus neoformans[294]	0.2–1.0	15–30
Coccidioides immitis[294]	0.78	70
Aspergillus species[294]	1.9–>4.0	15–45
Phycomycetes[620]	3.0–6.0	Unknown

of the *Candida* isolated from synovial fluid in their patient 12 days after initiation of 5-fluorocytosine therapy. This had previously been reported for *Candida* as well as for *C. neoformans*.[632–637] 5-Fluorocytosine has been used extensively in infants and children, usually with amphotericin B.[227, 258, 259, 638–641] Few untoward side effects have been noted, even with prolonged use. Schönebeck and Segerbrand reported a woman with *Candida* septicemia during pregnancy who was treated with 5-fluorocytosine with no apparent ill effects to her infant.[109]

Toxicity of 5-fluorocytosine includes transient neutropenia and hepatocellular damage.[642] Because the drug is cleared by the kidneys, the dose should be reduced and serum levels determined in patients with impaired renal function. Accumulation of 5-fluorocytosine in the blood can result in serious toxicity to the bone marrow, and monitoring levels in body fluids is recommended.[626]

There is experimental evidence that suggests that amphotericin B and 5-fluorocytosine act synergistically against some fungi, notably *Candida* and *Cryptococcus*.[642]

Miconazole

Miconazole is an imidazole derivative with activity against many species of fungi, including *Candida*,[261] *Coccidioides*[643] and *Cryptococcus*.[644] Sung and associates treated two infants with systemic candidiasis with miconazole, and both recovered.[261] One infant received 11.4 mg/kg per day, which was later increased to 15 mg/kg per day, also for 14 days. Serum levels in both were well above the minimal inhibitory concentration of the organism. Clarke and colleagues also reported a case of disseminated candidiasis in an infant treated with miconazole.[262] The drug was given initially intravenously at a dose of 10 mg/kg per day in two divided doses and then orally. This infant developed ventricular tachycardia while receiving the drug. It was discontinued, and the tachycardia did not recur when the drug was given for a second course. There is an additional report of cardiac toxicity in an infant who received an overdose of miconazole.[645] Casneuf and associates found miconazole to be effective for oral candidiasis and recommended a dosage schedule of 50 mg three times a day for infants weighing less than 10 kg and of 100 mg three times a day for children weighing more than 10 kg.[646] In a recent randomized trial, miconazole gel in a dose of 25 mg four times a day was far more effective than nystatin suspension in neonates with oral candidiasis.[647] There is a single report of resistance of *Candida* developing during therapy with miconazole.[648]

Although there are additional reports of successful results with miconazole alone or in combination with other antifungal agents,[649, 650] there are increasing reports of failure of miconazole therapy.[638–640] Data are insufficient and concerns are increasing regarding the routine use of miconazole in infants with infection caused by susceptible fungi.[651]

Clotrimazole

Clotrimazole is another imidazole derivative that has been used as a topical agent in infants with mucocutaneous candidiasis. Cohen and co-workers found clotrimazole to be as effective as nystatin in infants with thrush.[652] Montello and associates also reported an infant with thrush who was successfully treated with clotrimazole applied to the mouth and thumb.[653] Milne also found it to be effective in oral candidiasis, and although a longer course with it was necessary to cure the infection than with nystatin, there were fewer relapses.[654] Clotrimazole has been reported to increase myeloperoxidase activity within leukocytes, which may account for some of the drug's effectiveness.[655]

Ketoconazole

Ketoconazole, an oral, water-soluble imidazole derivative, has been demonstrated to have activity against *Candida*, *Coccidioides*, *Histoplasma*, *Blastomyces*, and dermatophytes as well as other fungi.[656] This antifungal agent has been effective in patients with a variety of cutaneous and systemic fungal infections.[657, 658] Of particular interest is the use of ketoconazole in patients with dermatophyte infections, especially when griseofulvin has failed.[659–661] In addition, it appears to be very effective in patients with chronic mucocutaneous candidiasis.[662–664] Heel[665] reviewed the use of ketoconazole in newborns and infants with candidasis, and Hensey and Cooke[666] successfully treated a premature infant who had systemic candidiasis with ketoconazole. Yinnon and colleagues reported the successful use of ketoconazole with 5-fluorocytosine in an infant infected with *C. lusitaniae* that was resistant to amphotericin B.[34]

Nystatin'

Nystatin has been used successfully in patients with mucocutaneous and dermal infections with *Candida*.[667, 668] The oral suspension contains 100,000 units of nystatin per ml; in infants with thrush, 1 ml should be slowly instilled into each side of the mouth every 6 hours and should be continued for several days after lesions have disappeared. Nystatin ointment, which contains 100,000 units per g, may be used liberally for cutaneous or oral candidiasis. In moist, intertriginous areas, nystatin powder is the preparation of choice; it may be used four times a day until skin infection has cleared. Occasional failures occur when *Candida* persists, resulting in a relapse 1 week to 1 month later. In such cases, therapy should be reinstituted and continued until smears or cultures are negative. In infants with gastrointestinal candidiasis, oral nystatin suspension, 400,000 to 1.6 million units per day in four to six divided doses, has been shown to be effective in eradicating *Candida* from feces within 3 days of initiation of therapy.[669] However, it is recommended that treatment be continued for 7 to 10 days. Diarrhea in the reported infants disappeared concomitant with eradication of the organism.

Nystatin may be used as an irrigating solution in patients with saprophytic or localized infection with *Aspergillus*[670, 671] at a concentration of 500 units per ml of sterile water.[672]

Griseofulvin

Griseofulvin has significantly altered morbidity of dermatophyte infection. This drug is deposited in epidermal structures before keratinization. As keratinized areas are exfoliated, they are replaced by noninfected tissue. In patients with tinea capitis, it may be necessary to clip the hair frequently because, as growth occurs, the ends of hairs may continue to harbor viable fungus. The oral dose of griseofulvin is 10 mg/kg per day for 7 to 10 days. Occasionally, a dose of 20 to 40 mg/kg per day is necessary for cure. In some instances, therapy must be continued for 3 weeks. There are few data on the use of griseofulvin in newborns. Ross reported use of griseofulvin in an infant 1 month of age at a dose of 10 mg/kg per day for 4 weeks without untoward effects.[673]

Griseofulvin is derived from a species of *Penicillium*, and cross-sensitivity may exist between penicillin and griseofulvin. The incidence of hypersensitivity reactions to griseofulvin in patients allergic to penicillin, however, has not been reported. The most common untoward reaction to griseofulvin is rash. Occasionally, urticaria and angioneurotic edema occur. In one report, griseofulvin was shown to cross the placenta in low concentrations, but fetal effects were not discussed.[674]

Fluconazole and Itraconazole

Fluconazole is an azole antifungal agent and is available in an intravenous as well as oral preparation. This agent has been shown to achieve good penetration into CSF, acular fluid, and skin.[675] It is effective against many fungi, including *Candida*, *Coccidioides*, and *dermatophytes*. Its use in neonates is limited. Wiest and associates used fluconazole in a premature infant with disseminated candidiasis unresponsive to amphotericin B and 5-fluorocytosine.[676] The infant received 6 mg/kg per day intravenously, achieving peak and trough serum levels of 10.3 and 6.98 mg/ml, respectively. Gürses and Kalayci reported successful use of fluconazole alone in a premature infant with candidal meningitis.[677] Dreissen and co-workers in two reports indicated fluconazole was effective and associated with fewer side effects than amphotericin B.[678, 679] Fluconazole has also been used in pregnancy without harmful effects on the fetus.[680]

Itraconazole, another azole antifungal agent, has not been used extensively in children. Bhandari and Narange reported its use in two premature infants with disseminated candidiasis.[681] Both received 10 mg/kg per day in two divided doses for 3 and 4 weeks, respectively. Both infants did well without any evidence of toxicity.

Suggested doses of antifungal agents are indicated in Table 17–2.

Adjunctive or Alternative Therapy

An important aspect of treatment of systemic or invasive fungal infection is attention to underlying disease or predisposing therapy. If feasible, indwelling intravenous catheters should be removed. Although use of antibiotics, corticosteroids, or cytotoxic drugs may be unavoidable, enhanced susceptibility to fungal infection in pa-

TABLE 17–2
Suggested Dosage of Antifungal Agents for Infants with Systemic or Severe Local Fungal Infection

AGENT	DOSAGE (mg/kg per day)
Amphotericin B	0.5–1
Liposomal amphotericin B	5
5-Fluorocytosine	100–150
Fluconazole	6
Ketoconazole	9
Itraconazole	10

tients receiving such therapy must be considered, and such agents should be discontinued or the dose reduced whenever possible.

CANDIDA

For many years, a 1% aqueous solution of gentian violet applied topically was the recommended treatment for oral candidiasis.[682–684] Although adequate treatment may be one or two applications, use of gentian violet has not been widely accepted by parents because of the temporary purple discoloration of the infant's mouth. Gentian violet may stain clothes and bed linen, but stains may be removed with a paste of sodium bicarbonate.

CRYPTOCOCCUS NEOFORMANS

There is substantial evidence in adults as well as in infants that administration of 5-fluorocytosine with amphotericin B appears to be optimal therapy for cryptococcal infection. A synergistic effect has been demonstrated with these two drugs against *Cryptococcus*, and their concomitant use may permit a lower total dose of amphotericin B in patients with infection with this fungus. Relapse of meningeal infection with *Cryptococcus* is common, necessitating additional courses of treatment.[354, 685–687] Despite intravenous or intrathecal amphotericin B, however, *Cryptococcus* may be visualized in cerebrospinal fluid, which is negative on culture. The presence of nonviable organisms in CSF does not warrant continued treatment. Determination of cryptococcal antigen in serum and CSF may be a useful guide to prognosis and to duration of treatment.[347]

COCCIDIOIDES IMMITIS

Coccidioidal infection appears to be less responsive to amphotericin B than other fungal infections and frequently requires prolonged treatment for control.[688, 689] In patients with coccidioidal meningitis, intrathecal therapy should always be employed. Duration of intrathecal amphotericin B may be monitored by coccidioidal complement fixation titer in CSF. In patients who never develop antibodies in CSF despite coccidioidal meningitis, the duration of therapy may be guided by the CSF findings.

In some patients who fail to respond to amphotericin

B therapy, use of transfer factor has been reported to be beneficial.[690]

ASPERGILLUS

In conjunction with antibiotic treatment, surgical resection of localized lesions may be indicated in some cases.[466, 606, 691] Although the experimental antifungal agent saramycetin has been used in several adults with aspergillosis,[692, 693] therapy with this agent has not been successful.

PHYCOMYCETES

Of paramount importance in the treatment of phycomycosis is correction of metabolic derangement, cessation of antibiotics, corticosteroids, or immunosuppressive agents whenever possible, and debridement or excision of necrotic tissue.[694] In conjunction with these measures, various antifungal agents in addition to amphotericin B have been employed. Iodides,[690–697] nystatin,[697, 698] and griseofulvin have been used with success in some cases.

DERMATOPHYTES

Topical therapy with keratolytic or fungicidal medications may be beneficial in some cases of dermatophyte infection, especially tinea pedis, in which results with griseofulvin are not encouraging. Whitfield's ointment, 1% solution of tolnaftate, or 3% each of sulfur and salicylic acid in an ointment may be used. Topical therapy should be continued until cultures and scrapings are negative for fungus.

References

1. Taschdjian CL, Kozinn PJ. Laboratory and clinical studies of candidiasis in the newborn. J Pediatr 50:426, 1957.
2. Lay KM, Russell C. Candida species and yeasts in mouths of infants from a special care unit of a maternity hospital. Arch Dis Child 52:794, 1977.
3. Blaschke-Hellmessen R, Hinkel GK, Kintzel HW. Zum problem des Candida-Hospitalismus bei Frühgeborenen. Dermatol Monatschr 159:403, 1973.
4. Russell C, Lay KM. Natural history of Candida species and yeasts in the oral cavities of infants. Arch Oral Biol 18:957, 1973.
5. Marples MJ, di Menna ME. The incidence of Candida albicans in Dunedin, NZ. J Path Bacteriol 64:497, 1952.
6. Benham RW, Hopkins AM. Yeast-like fungi found on skin and in the intestine of normal subjects. Arch Dermatol Syphilol 28:532, 1933.
7. Debré R, Mozziconacci P, Drouhet E, et al. Les infections à Candida chez le nourrisson. Ann Paediatr 184:129, 1955.
8. Sautter RL, Brown WJ. Sequential vaginal culture from normal young women. J Clin Microbiol 11:479, 1980.
9. Kozinn PJ, Taschdjian CL, Wiener H, et al. Neonatal candidiasis. Pediatr Clin North Am 5:803, 1958.
10. Anderson NA, Sage DN, Spaulding EH. Oral moniliasis in newborn infants. Am J Dis Child 67:450, 1944.
11. Ludlam GB, Henderson JL. Neonatal thrush in a maternity hospital. Lancet 1:64, 1943.
12. Pepys S. Pepys' Diary, June 17, 1665. Braybrooke's edition, 1825.
13. Hippocrates. Medical Works—Epidemics, Book 3. Translated by Chadwick J, Mann, WM. Oxford, Blackwell, 1950.
14. Bound JB. Thrush napkin rashes. BMJ 1:782, 1956.
15. Kozinn PJ, Taschdjian CL, Dragutsky D, et al. Cutaneous candidiasis in early infancy. Pediatrics 20:827, 1957.
16. Dobias B. Cutaneous moniliasis in pediatrics; diagnosis and therapy with nystatin. In Therapy of Fungus Diseases, an International Symposium. Boston, Little, Brown, 1955, p 205.
17. Ibrahim J. Ueber eine Soormykose der Haut in fruehen Saeuglingsalter. Arch Kinderheilkd 55:91, 1911.
18. Warin RP, Faulkner KE. Napkin psoriasis. Br J Dermatol 73:445, 1961.
19. Rebora A, Leyden JJ. Napkin (diaper) dermatitis and gastrointestinal carriage of Candida albicans. Br J Dermatol 105:551, 1981.
20. Klein JD, Yamauchi T, Horlick SP. Neonatal candidiasis, meningitis and arthritis: observations and a review of the literature. J Pediatr 81:31, 1972.
21. Schaberg A, Hildes JA, Wilt JC. Disseminated candidiasis. Arch Intern Med 94:112, 1954.
22. Gherardi GJ. Systemic moniliasis in infancy. JAMA 93:67, 1954.
23. Appleyard WJ, Lloyd JK. Candida septicemia. BMJ 1:577, 1969.
24. Larroche JC. Trois cas de moniliase pulmonaire chez dez prématurés. Etud Neo-Natales (Basel) 5:19, 1956.
25. Drouhet E. Some current aspects of deep visceral mycoses in children caused by opportunistic fungi. Ann Nestlé 34:5, 1975.
26. MacDonald L, Baker C, Chenoweth C. Risk factors for candidemia in a children's hospital. Clin Infect Dis 26:642, 1998.
27. Noble HB, Lyne ED. Candida osteomyelitis and arthritis from hyperalimentation therapy. J Bone Joint Surg Am 56:825, 1974.
28. Mazumdar PK, Marks MI. Candida albicans infections in hospitalized children: a survey of predisposing factors. Clin Pediatr 14:123, 1975.
29. Buscino L, Iannaccone G. Del Principe D, et al. Disseminated arthritis and osteitis by Candida albicans in a 2-month-old infant receiving parenteral nutrition. Acta Pediatr Scand 66:393, 1977.
30. Mercer HP, Gupta JM. Candida meningitis causing aqueductal stenosis following parenteral nutrition in an infant with meconium peritonitis. Aust Paediatr J 14:286, 1978.
31. Berant M, Kristal C, Wagner Y. Candida osteomyelitis as a complication of parenteral nutrition in an infant: successful treatment with 5-fluorocytosine. Helv Paediatr Acta 34:155, 1979.
32. Leibovitz E, Iuster-Reicher A, Amitai M, et al. Systemic candidal infections associated with use of peripheral venous catheters in neonates: 9-year experience. Clin Infect Dis 14:485, 1992.
33. Dato M, Dajani A. Candidemia in children with central venous catheters: role of catheter removal and amphotericin B therapy. Pediatr Infect Dis J 9:309, 1990.
34. Yinnon A, Woodin K, Powell K. Candida lusitaniae infection in the newborn: case report and review of the literature. Pediatr Infect Dis J 11:878, 1992.
35. Solomon SL, Alexander H, Eley JW, et al. Nosocomial fungemia in neonates associated with intravascular pressure-monitoring devices. Pediatr Infect Dis J 5:680, 1986.
36. Centers for Disease Control. Transducer-related

fungemia. National Nosocomial Infections Study Report. Annual summary 1974, issued April 1977, p 16.

37. Welbel SF, McNeil MM, Kuykendall RJ, et al. *Candida parapsilosis* bloodstream infections in neonatal intensive care unit patients: epidemiologic and laboratory confirmation of a common source outbreak. Pediatr Infect Dis J 15:998, 1996.

38. Heineman HS, Yunis EJ, Siemienski J, et al. Chlamydospores and dimorphism in *Candida albicans* endocarditis. Arch Intern Med 108:570, 1961.

39. Hurley R. The relationship between host and parasite in systemic moniliasis: a clinical and experimental study. M.D. thesis. University of London, England, 1962.

40. Winner HI, Hurley R. *Candida albicons.* Boston, Little, Brown, 1964, p 33.

41. Scherr GH. The effect of environmental temperature on cortisone toxicity for mice. Science 116:685, 1952.

42. Winner HI. The transition from commensalism to parasitism. Br J Dermatol 81(Suppl. 1):62, 1969.

43. Dobias B. Moniliasis in pediatrics. Am J Dis Child 94:234, 1957.

44. Richart R, Dammin GJ. *Candida tropicalis* as a pathogen for man. N Engl J Med 263:474, 1960.

45. Isacson M, Noah Z, Faber J, et al. Use of 5-fluorocytosine in systemic candidiasis in infancy. Arch Dis Child 47:954, 1972.

46. Bartizal FJ, Pacheco JC, Malkasian GD, et al. Microbial flora found in the products of conception in spontaneous abortions. Obstet Gynecol 43:109, 1979.

47. Svirsky-Fein S, Langer L, Milbauer B, et al. Neonatal osteomyelitis caused by *Candida tropicalis:* report of two cases and review of the literature. J Bone Joint Surg Am 61:455, 1979.

48. Palmer EA. Endogenous *Candida* endophthalmitis in infants. Am J Ophthalmol 89:388, 1980.

49. Kellogg SG, Davis C, Benirschke K. *Candida parapsilosis*: previously unknown cause of fetal infection: a report of two cases. J Reprod Med 12:159, 1974.

50. Guinet R, Chanas J, Goullier A, et al. Fatal septicemia due to amphotericin B–resistant *Candida lusitaniae.* J Clin Microbiol 18:443, 1983.

51. Sanchez P, Cooper B. *Candida lusitaniae:* sepsis and meningitis in a neonate. Pediatr Infect Dis J 6:758, 1987.

52. Christenson J, Guruswamy A, Mukwaya G, et al. *Candida lusitaniae:* an emerging human pathogen. Pediatr Infect Dis J 6:755, 1987.

53. Byers M, Chapman S, Feldman S, et al. Fluconazole pharmacokinetics in the cerebrospinal fluid of a child with *Candida tropicalis* meningitis. Pediatr Infect Dis J 11:895, 1992.

54. Yagupsky P, Dagan R, Chipman M, et al. Pseudooutbreak of *Candida guilliermondii* fungemia in a neonatal intensive care unit. Pediatr Infect Dis J 10:928, 1991.

55. Faix R. Invasive neonatal candidiasis: comparison of albicans and parapsilosis infection. Pediatr Infect Dis J 11:88, 1992.

56. Sherertz R, Gledhill K, Hampton K, et al. Outbreak of *Candida* bloodstream infections associated with retrograde medication administration in a neonatal intensive care unit. J Pediatr 120:455, 1992.

57. Zenker P, Rosenberg E, Van Dyke R, et al. Successful medical treatment of presumed *Candida* endocarditis in critically ill infants. J Pediatr 119:472, 1991.

58. Salvin SB. Haemolysin from the yeast-like phase of some pathogenic fungi. Proc Soc Exp Biol Med 76:852, 1951.

59. Braude AL, McConnell J, Douglas H. Fever from pathogenic fungi. J Clin Invest 39:1266, 1960.

60. Kim YP, Adachi K, Chow D. Leucine aminopeptidase in *Candida albicans.* J Invest Dermatol 38:115, 1962.

61. Hasenclever HF, Mitchell WO. Antigenic studies of *Candida*: I. Observations of two antigenic groups of *Candida albicans.* J Bacteriol 82:570, 1961.

62. Parle JN. Yeasts isolated from the mammalian alimentary tract. J Gen Microbiol 17:363, 1957.

63. Ainsworth GC, Austwick PKC. A survey of animal mycoses in Britain—general aspects. Vet Rec 67:88, 1955.

64. Coutelen F, Cochet G. Les rongeurs domestiques réservoirs de virus en mycopathologie humaine et vétérinaire. Ann Parasit Hum Comp 19:85, 1942.

65. Marples MJ. Some extrahuman reservoirs of pathogenic fungi in New Zealand. Trans R Soc Trop Med Hyg 55:216, 1961.

66. Quin AH. Newer problems in swine diseases—control and treatment. Can J Comp Med 16:265, 1952.

67. Gentry RF, Bubash GR, Chutes HL. *Candida albicans* in turkeys: I. Treatment of crop infection with mycostatin. Poult Sci 39:1252, 1960.

68. Hinshaw WR. Moniliasis (thrush) in turkeys and chickens. World's Poultry Congress, 5th Rome. Proceedings 3:190, 1934.

69. Keymer IF, Austwick PK. Moniliasis in partridges (*Perdix perdix*). Sabouraudia 1:22, 1961.

70. Kuprowski M. Zur Pathogenese und Morphologie der Moniliasis der Huhnervogel. Dtsch Tieraerztl Wochenschr 67:185, 1960.

71. Nilsby I, Norden A. Studies on the occurrence of *Candida albicans.* Acta Med Scand 133:340, 1949.

72. Ajello L. Soil as natural reservoir for human pathogenic fungi. Science 123:876, 1956.

73. di Menna ME. A search for pathogenic species of yeasts in New Zealand soil. J Gen Microbiol 12:54, 1955.

74. Blanc WA. Pathways of fetal and early neonatal infection. J Pediatr 59:473, 1961.

75. Sonnenschein H, Taschdjian CL, Clark DH. Congenital cutaneous candidiasis. Am J Dis Child 107:260, 1964.

76. Sonnenschein H, Clark HL, Taschdjian CL. Congenital cutaneous candidiasis in a premature infant. Am J Dis Child 99:97, 1959.

77. Ho CY, Aterman K. Infection of the fetus by *Candida* in a spontaneous abortion. Am J Obstet Gynecol 106:705, 1970.

78. Lopez E, Aterman K. Intra-uterine infection by *Candida.* Am J Dis Child 115:663, 1968.

79. Dvorak AM, Gavaller B. Congenital systemic candidiasis. N Engl J Med 274:540, 1966.

80. Jahn CL, Cherry JD. Congenital cutaneous candidiasis. Pediatrics 33:440, 1964.

81. Burry AF. Hydrocephalus after intra-uterine fungal infection. Arch Dis Child 32:161, 1957.

82. Sonnenschein H, Clark HL, Taschdjian CL. Congenital cutaneous candidiasis in a premature infant. Am J Dis Child 99:81, 1960.

83. Rhatigan RM. Congenital cutaneous candidiasis. Am J Dis Child 116:545, 1968.

84. van der Harten JJ. Proceedings: intrauterine *Candida albicans* infection. Arch Dis Child 50:662, 1975.

85. Kam LA, Giacocia GP. Congenital cutaneous candidiasis. Am J Dis Child 129:1215, 1975.

86. Gellis SS, Feingold M. Picture of the month: congenital cutaneous candidiasis. Am J Dis Child 130:291, 1976.

87. Rudolph N, Tariq AA, Reale MR, et al. Congenital cutaneous candidiasis. Arch Dermatol 113:1101, 1977.

88. Levin S, Zaidel L, Bernstein D. Intrauterine infection of fetal brain by *Candida.* Am J Obstet Gynecol 130:597, 1978.

89. Ehlers RE, Jarrett PB, Kaplan AM. Mixed bacterial and fungal meningitis in a neonate. Dev Med Child Neurol 21:643, 1979.

90. Buchanan R, Sworn MJ, Noble AD. Abortion associated with intrauterine infection by *Candida albicans*. Case report. Br J Obstet Gynaecol 86:741, 1979.

91. Schirar A, Rendu C, Vielh JP, et al. Congenital mycosis (*Candida albicans*). Biol Neonate 24:273, 1974.

92. Schweid AI, Hopkins GB. Monilial chorionitis associated with an intrauterine contraceptive device. Obstet Gynecol 31:719, 1968.

93. Cabaniss WH Jr, Manley WF Jr, Swan RE. Cutaneous moniliasis in a premature infant: report of a case with unusual clinical manifestations. J Pediatr 50:480, 1957.

94. Johnson EE, Thompson TR, Ferrieri P. Congenital candidiasis. Am J Dis Child 135:273, 1981.

95. Chapel TA, Gagliardi C, Nichols W. Congenital cutaneous candidiasis. J Am Acad Dermatol 6:926, 1982.

96. Mamlok RJ, Richarson CJ, Mamlok V, et al. A case of intrauterine pulmonary candidiasis. Pediatr Infect Dis 4:692, 1985.

97. Marelli G, Mariani A, Frigerio L, et al. Fetal *Candida* infection associated with an intrauterine contraceptive device. Eur J Obstet Gynecol Reprod Biol 68:209, 1996.

98. Schwartz D, Reef S. *Candida albicans* placentitis and funisitis: early diagnosis of congenital candidemia by histopathologic examination of umbilical cord vessels. Pediatr Infect Dis J 9:661, 1990.

99. Whyte RK, Hussain Z, deSa D. Antenatal infections with *Candida* species. Arch Dis Child 57:528, 1982.

100. Delprado WJ, Baird PJ, Russell P. Placental candidiasis: report of three cases with a review of the literature. Pathology 14:191, 1982.

101. Spaun E, Klinder K. *Candida* chorioamnionitis and intrauterine contraceptive device. Acta Obstet Gynecol Scand 65:183, 1986.

102. Honore LH. Placental candidiasis: report of two cases, one associated with an IUCD in situ. Contraception 30:555, 1984.

103. Candidiasis: colonization vs. infection. Editorial. JAMA 215:285, 1971.

104. Frerich W, Gad A. The frequency of *Candida* infections in pregnancy and their treatment with clotrimazole. Curr Med Res Opin 4:640, 1977.

105. Sparks RA, Williams GL, Boyce JMH, et al. Antenatal screening for candidiasis, trichomoniasis and gonorrhea. Br J Vener Dis 51:110, 1975.

106. Hood IC, deSa DJ, Whyte RK. The inflammatory response in candidal chorioamnionitis. Hum Pathol 14:984, 1983.

107. Bobitt JR, Hayslip CC, Damato JD. Amniotic fluid infections as determined by transabdominal amniocentesis in patients with intact membranes in premature labor. Am J Obstet Gynecol 140:947, 1981.

108. Delaplane D, Wiringa KS, Shulman ST, et al. Congenital mucocutaneous candidiasis following diagnostic amniocentesis. Am J Obstet Gynecol 147:342, 1983.

109. Schönebeck J, Segerbrand E. *Candida albicans* septicemia during first half of pregnancy successfully treated with 5-flurocytosine. BMJ 4:337, 1973.

110. Flamm H. Dic pránatalen Infektionen des Menschen. Stuttgart, Georg Thieme, 1959, p 70.

111. Kozinn PJ, Taschdjian CL, Wiener H. Incidence and pathogenesis of neonatal candidiasis. Pediatrics 21:421, 1958.

112. Montes LF, Pittillo RF, Hunt D, et al. Microbial flora of infant's skin. Arch Dermatol 103:400, 1971.

113. Linhartova A, Chung W. Bronchopulmonary moniliasis in the newborn. J Clin Pathol 16:56, 1963.

114. Pulmonary candidiasis in infants. BMJ 3:322, 1971.

115. Kassner EG, Kauffman SL, Yvon JJ, et al. Pulmonary candidiasis in infants: radiologic and pathologic features. AJR 135:863, 1980.

116. Dixon BL, Houston CS. Fatal neonatal pulmonary candidiasis. Radiology 129:132, 1978.

117. Gonzalez-Ochoa A, Dominguez L. Algunas observaciones epidemiologicas y patogenicas sobre la moniliasis oral del recien nacido. Rev Inst Salubr Enferm Trop Mexico City 17:1, 1957.

118. Burnie JP, Odds FC, Lee W, et al. Outbreak of systemica *Candida albicans* in intensive care unit caused by cross infection. [Clin Res] 290:746, 1985.

119. Vaudry W, Tierney A, Wenman W. Investigation of a cluster of systemic *Candida albicans* infections in a neonatal intensive care unit. J Infect Dis 158:1375, 1988.

120. Khateb R, Thirumoorthi MC, Reiderer KM, et al. Clustering of *Candida* infections in the neonatal intensive care unit: concurrent emergence of multiple strains simulating intermittent outbreaks. Pediatr Infect Dis J 17:130, 1998.

121. Kozinn PJ, Wiener H, Taschdjian CL, et al. Is isolation of infants with thrush necessary? JAMA 170:1172, 1959.

122. Harris LJ. Further observations on a simple procedure to eliminate thrush from hospital nurseries. Am J Obstet Gynecol 80:30, 1959.

123. Baum G. The significance of *Candida albicans* in human sputum. N Engl J Med 263:70, 1960.

124. Van Uden N. The occurrence of *Candida* and other yeasts in the intestinal tracts of animals. Ann N Y Acad Sci 89:59, 1960.

125. Carter B, Jones CP, Creadick RN, et al. The vaginal fungi. Ann NY Acad Sci 83:265, 1959.

126. Recio PM, De Leon A. Candidiasis of the rectoanal tract. J Philippine Med Assoc 33:293, 1957.

127. Hart PD, Russel E Jr, Remington JS. The compromised host and infection: II. Deep fungal infection. J Infect Dis 120:169, 1969.

128. Seelig MS, Mechanisms by which antibiotics increase the incidence and severity of candidiasis and alter the immunological defenses. Bacteriol Rev 30:442, 1966.

129. Seelig MS. The role of antibiotics in the pathogenesis of *Candida* infections. Am J Med 40:887, 1966.

130. Johnson SAM. *Candida (Monilia) albicans*. Arch Dermatol Syphilol 70:49, 1954.

131. Moore M. In vivo and in vitro effect of aureomycin hydrochloride on *Syringosporu (Monilia, Candida) albicans*. J Lab Clin Med 37:703, 1951.

132. Pappenfort RB Jr, Schnall ES. Moniliasis in patients treated with aureomycin. Arch Intern Med 88:729, 1951.

133. Isenberg HD, Pisano MA, Carito SL, et al. Factors leading to overt monilial disease: I. Preliminary studies of the ecological relationship between *Candida albicans* and intestinal bacteria. Antibiot Chemother 10:353, 1960.

134. Koser SA, Hodges E, Tribby I, et al. Growth of lactobacilli in association with *Candida albicans*. J Infect Dis 106:60, 1960.

135. Smith DT. The disturbance of the normal bacterial ecology by the administration of antibiotics with the development of new clinical syndromes. Ann Intern Med 37:1135, 1952.

136. Rosebury T, Gale D, Taylor DF. An approach to the study of interactive phenomena among microorganisms indigenous to man. J Bacteriol 67:135, 1954.

137. Paine TF Jr. In vitro experiments with *Monilia* and *Escherichia coli* in patients receiving antibiotics. Antibiot Chemother 2:653, 1952.

138. Gale D, Sandoval B. Response of mice to the inoculations of both *Candida albicans* and *Escherichia coli:* I. The enhancement phenomenon. J Bacteriol 73:616, 1957.

139. Maibach HI, Kligman AM. The biology of experimental human cutaneous moniliasis (*Candida albicans*). Arch Dermatol 85:233, 1962.

140. Sidransky H, Pearl MA. Pulmonary fungus infections associated with steroid and antibiotic therapy. Dis Chest 39:630, 1961.

141. Frenkel JK. Role of corticosteroids as predisposing factors in fungal diseases. Lab Invest 11:1192, 1962.

142. Thompson J, van Furth R. The effect of glucocorticosteroids on the kinetics of mononuclear phagocytes. J Exp Med 131:429, 1970.

143. Cohen JJ. The effects of hydrocortisone on the immune response. Ann Allergy 29:358, 1971.

144. Halland JF, Senn H, Baenenjel T. Quantitative studies of localized leukocyte mobilization in acute leukemia. Blood 37:499, 1971.

145. Mankowski ZT, Littleton BJ. Action of cortisone and ACTH on experimental fungus infections. Antibiot Chemother 4:253, 1954.

146. McCoy E. Changes in the host flora induced by chemotherapeutic agents. Annu Rev Microbiol 8:257, 1954.

147. Craig AM, Farber S. Development of disseminated visceral mycosis during therapy for acute leukemia. Am J Pathol 29:601, 1953.

148. Keye JD Jr, Magee WE. Fungal diseases in a general hospital: study of 88 cases. Am J Clin Pathol 26:1235, 1956.

149. St. Geme JW Jr, Beerbaugh JL, Pajari KL, et al. Enhanced viral infection with mouse treated with 6-mercaptopurine. J Lab Clin Med 76:213, 1970.

150. Chilgren RA, Meuwissen HJ, Quie PG, et al. Chronic mucocutaneous candidiasis, deficiency of delayed hypersensitivity and selective local antibody defect. Lancet 2:688, 1967.

151. Rocklin RE, Chilgren RA, Hong R, et al. Transfer of cellular hypersensitivity in chronic mucocutaneous candidiasis monitored in vivo and in vitro. Cell Immunol 1:290, 1970.

152. Quie PG, Chilgren RA. Acute disseminated and chronic mucocutaneous candidiasis. Semin Hematol 8:227, 1971.

153. Eras P, Goldstein MJ, Sherlock P. *Candidia* infection of the gastrointestinal tract. Medicine 51:367, 1972.

154. Schlegel RJ, Bernier GM, Bellanti JA, et al. Severe candidiasis associated with thymic dysplasia. IgA deficiency and plasma antilymphocyte effects. Pediatrics 45:926, 1970.

155. Diamond RD. The growing problem of mycoses in patients infected with the human immunodeficiency virus. Rev Infect Dis 13:480, 1991.

156. Silver RT. Infections, fever and host resistance in neoplastic diseases. J Chronic Dis 16:677, 1963.

157. Armstrong D, Young LS, Meyer RD, et al. Infectious complications of neoplastic disease. Med Clin North Am 55:729, 1971.

158. Hutter RVP, Collins HS. The occurrence of opportunistic fungus infections in a cancer hospital. Lab Invest 11:1035, 1962.

159. Akrawi YY. The biology of intestinal moniliasis. J Fac Med Baghdad 2:36, 1960.

160. Urbach E, Lentz W. Carbohydrate metabolism and the skin. Arch Dermatol Syphilol 52:106, 1945.

161. Louria DB, Shannon D, Johnson G, et al. The susceptibility to moniliasis in children with endocrine hypofunction. Trans Assoc Am Physicians 80:236, 1967.

162. O'Malley BW, Kohler PO. Hypoparathyroidism. Postgrad Med 44:77, 1968.

163. Hermans PE, Ulrich JA, Markowitz H. Chronic mucocutaneous candidiasis as a surface expression of deep seated abnormalities. Am J Med 47:503, 1969.

164. Montes LF, Pittman CS, Moore WJ, et al. Chronic mucocutaneous candidiasis: influence of thyroid status. JAMA 221:156, 1972.

165. Law EJ, Kim OJ, Stieritz DD, et al. Experience with systemic candidiasis in the burned patient. J Trauma 12:543, 1972.

166. Arturson G, Hogman CF, Johansson SGO, et al. Changes in immunoglobulin levels in severely burned patients. Lancet 1:546, 1969.

167. Salter W, Zinneman HH. Bacteremia and *Candida* septicemia: review of 185 cases during a four-year period. Minn Med. 50:1489, 1967.

168. Roth FJ Jr, Boyd CC, Sagami S, et al. An evaluation of the fungistatic activity of serum. J Invest Dermatol 32:549, 1959.

169. Louria DB, Brayton RG. A substance in blood lethal for *Candida albicans*. Nature 201:309, 1964.

170. Louria DB, Smith KJ, Brayton RG, et al. Anti-*Candida* factors in serum and their inhibitors: I. Clinical and laboratory observations. J Infect Dis 125:102, 1972.

171. Brody JI, Finch SC. *Candida* reacting antibody in the serum of patients with lymphomas and related disorders. Blood 15:830, 1960.

172. Mathur S, Mathur RS, Landgrebe SC, et al. Antibiotics to *Candida albicans* and steroid hormones during late pregnancy and in the umbilical circulation. Clin Immunol Immunopathol 12:335, 1979.

173. Seebacher C. Zum *Candida albicans*—agglutinationstiter bei jungen Säuglenzen. Mykosen 20:1, 1977.

174. Drake CH. Natural antibodies against yeast-like fungi as measured by slide agglutination. J Immunol 50:185, 1945.

175. Winner HI. A study of *Candida albicans* agglutinins in human sera. J Hyg 53:509, 1955.

176. Warnock DW, Milne JD, Fielding AM. Immunoglobulin classes of human serum antibodies in vaginal candidiasis. Mycopathologia 63:173, 1978.

177. Milne JD, Warnock DW. Antibodies to *Candida albicans* in human cervicovaginal secretions. Br J Vener Dis 53:375, 1977.

178. Auger P, Marquis G, Dallaire L, et al. Natural occurrence of a humoral response to *Candida* in amniotic fluid. Am J Obstet Gynecol 136:1075, 1980.

179. Bergman N, Bercovici B, Sacks T. Antibacterial activity of human amniotic fluid. Am J Obstet Gynecol 114:520, 1972.

180. Miller J, Michel J, Bercovici B, et al. Studies on the antimicrobial activity of amniotic fluid. Am J Obstet Gynecol 125:212, 1976.

181. Auger P, Marquis G, Dallaire L, et al. Stunted growth of *Candida albicans* in human amniotic fluid in vitro. J Lab Clin Med 95:272, 1980.

182. Xanthou M, Valassi-Adam E, Kintzonidom E, et al. Phagocytosis and killing ability of *Candida albicans* by blood leukocytes of healthy term and preterm babies. Arch Dis Child 50:72, 1975.

183. Hill HR, Mitchell TG, Matsen JM, et al. Recovery from disseminated candidiasis in a premature infant. Pediatrics 53:48, 1974.

184. Oseas R, Lehrer RI. A micromethod for measuring neutrophil candidicidal activity in neonates. Pediatr Res. 12:828, 1978.

185. Borderon JC, Drouhet E, Boulard P, et al. Environne-

ment fongique et infections c *Candida albicans* dans une collectivité de prématures. Bull Soc Fr Mycol Med 18:19, 1970.

186. Baley JE, Kliegman RM, Fanaroff AA. Disseminated fungal infections in very low birth weight infants: clinical manifestations and epidemiology. Pediatrics 73:144, 1984.

187. Faix RG, Kovarik SM, Shaw TR, et al. Mucocutaneous and invasive candidiasis among very low-birth-weight (<1,500 grams) infants in intensive care nurseries: a prospective study. Pediatrics 83:101, 1989.

188. McClary DO. Factors affecting the morphology of *Candida albicans*. Ann Mo Bot Gard 39:137, 1952.

189. Dennis D, Miller MJ, Peterson CG. *Candida* septicemia. Surg Gynecol Obstet 119:520, 1964.

190. Hood IC, Browning D, deSa DJ, et al. Fetal inflammatory response in second trimester candidal chorioamnionitis. Early Hum Dev 11:1, 1985.

191. Emmons CW, Binford CH, Utz JP. Medical Mycology. Philadelphia, Lea & Febiger, 1970.

192. Butler KM, Baker CJ. *Candida*: an increasingly important pathogen in the nursery. New Top Pediatr Infect Dis 35:543, 1988.

193. Haruda F, Bergman MA, Headings D. Unrecognized *Candida* brain abscess in infancy: two cases and a review of the literature. Johns Hopkins Med J 147:182, 1980.

194. Goldsmith LS, Rubenstein SD, Wolfson BJ, et al. Cerebral calcifications in a neonate with candidiasis. Pediatr Infect Dis J 9:451, 1990.

195. Blum M, Elian I. Tracheal aspirate screening for the detection of intrauterine or intrapartum candidiasis in the newborn. Mykosen 21:95, 1978.

196. Baley JE, Annable WL, Kliegman RM. *Candida* endophthalmitis in the premature infant. J Pediatr. 98:458, 1981.

197. Reddy TCS, Chakrabanti A, Singh M, Singh S. Role of buffy coat examination in the diagnosis of neonatal candidemia. Pediatr Infect Dis J 15:718, 1996.

198. Heckmatt JZ, Meadow SR, Anderson CK. Acute anuric renal failure in an infant with systemic candidiasis. Arch Dis Child 54:70, 1979.

199. Keller MA, Sellers BB Jr, Melish ME, et al. Systemic candidiasis in infants: a case presentation and literature review. Am J Dis Child 131:1260, 1977.

200. Patriquin H, Lebowitz R, Perreault G, et al. Neonatal *Candida*: renal and pulmonary manifestations. AJR 135:867, 1980.

201. Pappu LD, Purohit DM, Bradford BF, et al. Primary renal candidiasis in two preterm neonates. Am J Dis Child 138:923, 1984.

202. Haley LD. Yeast infections of the lower urinary tract: I. In vitro studies of the tissue phase of *Candida albicans*. Sabouraudia 4:98, 1965.

203. Kozinn PJ, Taschdjian CL. *Candida albicans*: saprophyte or pathogen? A diagnostic guideline. JAMA 198:170, 1966.

204. Eckstein CW, Kass EJ. Anuria in a newborn secondary to bilateral ureteropelvic fungus balls. J Urol 127:109, 1982.

205. Ekkelkamp S. Re: anuria in a newborn secondary to bilateral ureteropelvic fungus balls. J Urol 128:1131, 1982.

206. Laufer J, Reichman B, Graif M, et al. Anuria in a premature infant due to ureteropelvic fungal bezoars. Eur J Pediatr 145:125, 1986.

207. Cohen HL, Haller JQ, Schechter S, et al. Renal candidiasis of the infant: ultrasound evaluation. Urol Radiol 8:17, 1986.

208. Khoss AE, Ponhold W. Pollak A, et al. Abdominal aortic aneurysm in a premature neonate with disseminated candidiasis: ultrasound and angiography. Pediatr Radiol 15:420, 1985.

209. Kirpekar M, Abiri MM, Hilfer C, et al. Ultrasound in the diagnosis of systemic candidiasis (renal and cranial) in very low birth weight premature infants. Pediatr Radiol 16:17, 1986.

210. Bozynski ME, Naglil RA, Russell EJ. Real-time ultrasonographic surveillance in the detection of CNS involvement in systemic *Candida* infection. Pediatr Radiol 16:235, 1986.

211. Rehan VK, Davidson DC. Neonatal renal candidal bezoar. Arch Dis Child 67:63, 1992.

212. Wise GP, Wainstein S, Goldberg P, et al. *Candida* cystitis: management by continuous bladder irrigation with amphotericin B. JAMA 224:1636, 1973.

213. Schey WL, Brandt T. Pulmonary valve candidiasis in an infant. Am J Radiol 141:663, 1983.

214. Stopfkuchen H, Benzing F, Jungst BK, et al. Echocardiographic diagnosis of *Candida* endocarditis of the tricuspid valve and of the right atrium in a young infant. Pediatr Cardiol 4:49, 1983.

215. Johnson EE, Bass JL, Thompson TR, et al. *Candida* septicemia and right atrial mass secondary to umbilical vein catheterization. Am J Dis Child 135:275, 1981.

216. Foker JE, Bass JL, Thompson T, et al. Management of intracardiac fungal masses in premature infants. J Thorac Cardiovasc Surg 87:244, 1984.

217. Sanchez PJ, Siegel JD, Fishbein J. *Candida* endocarditis: successful medical management in three preterm infants and review of the literature. Pediatr Infect Dis J 10:239, 1991.

218. O'Callaghan C, McDougall P. Infective endocarditis in neonates. Arch Dis Child 63:53, 1988.

219. Heydarian M, Werthammer JW, Kelly PJ. Echocardiographic diagnosis of *Candida* mass of the right atrium in a premature infant. Am Heart J 113:402, 1984.

220. Gorlach G, Hagel KJ, Mulch J, et al. Surgical therapy of pulmonary thrombosis due to candidiasis in a premature infant. J Cardiovasc Surg 27:341, 1986.

221. Mayayo E, Moralejo J, Camps J, Gerarro J. Fungal endocarditis in premature infants: case report and review. Clin Infect Dis 22:366, 1996.

222. Comaish JS, Gibson B, Green CA. Candidiasis: serology and diagnosis. J Invest Dermatol 40:139, 1963.

223. Salvin SB. Immunologic aspects of the mycoses. Prog Allergy 7:213, 1963.

224. Louria DB. Deep-seated mycotic infections, allergy to fungi and mycotoxins. N Engl J Med 277:1065, 1967.

225. Lewis GM, Hopper ME, Montgomery RM. Infections of the skin due to *Monilia albicans*: I. Diagnostic value of intradermal testing with a commercial extract of *Monilia albicans*. NY State Med J 37:878, 1937.

226. Good RA, Kelly WD, Rotstein J, et al. Immunological deficiency diseases; agammaglobulinemia, hypogammaglobulinemia, Hodgkin's disease and sarcoidosis. Prog Allergy 6:187, 1962.

227. Peck SM, Bergamini R, Kelcec LC, et al. The serodiagnosis of moniliasis: its value and limitations. J Invest Dermatol 25:301, 1955.

228. Lehner T. Immunofluorescence study of *Candida albicans* in candidiasis carriers and controls. J Pathol Bacteriol 9:97, 1966.

229. Esterly NB. Serum antibody titers to *Candida albicans* utilizing an immunofluorescent technique. Am J Clin Pathol 50:291, 1968.

230. Salvin SB. Current concepts of diagnostic serology and skin hypersensitivity in the mycoses. Am J Med 27:97, 1959.

231. Preisler HD, Hasenclever HF, Levitan AA, et al. Serologic diagnosis of disseminated candidiasis in patients with acute leukemia. Ann Intern Med 70:19, 1969.

232. Stallybrass FC, *Candida* precipitins. J Pathol Bacteriol 87:89, 1964.

233. Taschdjian CL, Dobkin GB, Caroline L, et al. Immune studies relating to candidiasis: II. Experimental and preliminary clinical studies on antibody formation in systemic candidiasis. Sabouraudia 3:129, 1964.

234. Taschdjian CL, Kozinn PJ, Okas A, et al. Serodiagnosis of systemic candidiasis. J Infect Dis 117:180, 1967.

235. Remington JS, Gaines JD, Gilmer MA. Demonstration of *Candida* precipitins in human sera by counterimmunoelectrophoresis. Lancet 1:413, 1972.

236. Gaines JD, Remington JS. Diagnosis of deep infection with *Candida*: a study of *Candida* precipitins. Arch Intern Med 132:699, 1973.

237. Kozinn PJ, Hasenclever HF, Taschdjian CL, et al. Problems in the diagnosis and treatment of systemic candidiasis. J Infect Dis 126:548, 1972.

238. Edwards JE Jr, Lehrer RI, Stiehm ER, et al. Severe candidal infections: clinical perspective, immune defense mechanisms, and current concepts of therapy. Ann Intern Med 80:91, 1978.

239. Rao HKM Myers GJ. *Candida* meningitis in the newborn. South Med J 72:468, 1979.

240. Weiner MH, Coats-Stephen M. Immunodiagnosis of systemic candidiasis: mannan antigenemia detected by radioimmunoassay in experimental and human infections. J Infect Dis 140:989, 1979.

241. New approaches speed Dx of candidiasis and neonate strep. Hosp Pract 14:34, 1979.

242. Schreiber JR, Maynard E, Lew MA. *Candida* antigen detection in two premature neonates with disseminated candidiasis. Pediatrics 74:838, 1984.

243. de Repentigny L. Serodiagnosis of candidiasis, aspergillosis, and cryptococcosis. Clin Infect Dis 14(Suppl 1):S11, 1992.

244. McNeill MM, Gerber AR, McLaughlin DW, et al. Mannan antigenemia during invasive candidiasis caused by *Candida tropicalis*. Pediatr Infect Dis J 11:493, 1992.

245. Kerkering TM, Espinel-Ingroff A, Shadomy S. Detection of *Candida* antigenemia by counterimmunoelectrophoresis in patients with invasive candidiasis. J Infect Dis 140:659, 1979.

246. Iwashita H Araki K, Kuroiwa Y, et al. Occurrence of *Candida*-specific oligoclonal IgG antibodies in CSF with *Candida* meningoencephalitis. Ann Neurol 4:579, 1978.

247. Epstein B. Studien zur Saarkrankheit. Jahrb Kinderheilkd 104:29, 1924.

248. Strigl R, Lappy K. Treatment of oral candidiasis in the newborn. Mykosen 22:341, 1979.

249. Munz D, Powell KR, Pai CH. Treatment of candidal diaper dermatitis: a double-blind placebo-controlled comparison of topical nystatin with topical plus oral nystatin. J Pediatr 101:1022, 1982.

250. Michelson PE, Rupp R, Efthimiadis B. Endogenous *Candida* endophthalmitis leading to bilateral corneal perforation. Am J Ophthalmol 80:800, 1975.

251. Shapira Y, Drucker M, Russell A, et al. *Candida* endocarditis and encephalitis in an infant. Clin Pediatr 13:542, 1974.

252. Walsh TJ, Hutchins GM. Postoperative *Candida* infections of the heart in children: clinicopathologic study of a continuing problem of diagnosis and therapy. J Pediatr Surg 15:325 1980.

253. Bayer AS, Edwards JE, Seidel JS, et al. *Candida* meningi-

254. Ferry AP. Endogenous *Candida* endophthalmitis in childhood. J Pediatr Ophthalmol 11:189, 1974.

255. Roberts FB. Recovery from *Monilia* septicemia. Can Med Assoc J 83:857, 1960.

256. Hughes JM, Remington JS. Systemic candidiasis, a diagnostic challenge. Calif Med. 116:8, 1972.

257. Turner RB, Donowitz LG, Hendley JO. Consequences of candidemia for pediatrics patients. Am J Dis Child 139:178, 1985.

258. Faix RG. Systemic *Candida* infections in infants in intensive care nurseries: high incidence of central nervous system involvement. J Pediatr 105:616, 1984.

259. Johnson EE. Thompson TR, Green TP, et al. Systemic candidiasis in very low-birth-weight infants (1,500 grams). Pediatrics 73:138, 1984.

260. Lee BE, Cheung P, Robinson JL, et al. Comparative study of mortality and morbidity in premature infants (birth weight < 1250 g) with candidemia or candidal meningitis. Clin Infect Dis 27:559, 1998.

261. Sung JP, Rajani K, Chopra DR, et al. Miconazole therapy for systemic candidiasis in a conjoined (Siamese) twin and a premature newborn. Am J Surg 138:688, 1979.

262. Clarke M, Davies DP, Odds F, et al. Neonatal systemic candidiasis treated with miconazole. BMJ 281:354, 1980.

263. Chesney PJ, Justman RA, Bogdanowicz WM. *Candida* meningitis in newborn infants: a review and report of combined amphotericin B-fluorocytosine therapy. Johns Hopkins Med J 142:155, 1978.

264. Kühner U, Ströder J. Die *Candida albicans* meningitis im Sauglingsalter. Mykosen 18:81, 1975.

265. Salet J, Weissgerber G, Sarraf Chirazi MT, et al. Atrésic du grêle, muscoviscidose et septicémie à *Candida* chez un nouveau-né. Ann Pediatr 23:233, 1976.

266. Mahboubi S, Kaufmann HJ, Schut L. Two instances of inflammatory aqueductal occlusion in prematures after neonatal *Candida* septicemia. Clin Pediatr 15:651, 1976.

267. Adler S, Randall J, Plotkin SA. Candidal osteomyelitis and arthritis in a neonate. Am J Dis Child 123:595, 1972.

268. Pittard WB, III, Thullen JD, Fanaroff AA. Neonatal septic arthritis. J Pediatr 88:621, 1976.

269. Vandevelde AG, Mauceri AA, Johnson JE. 5-Fluorocytosine in the treatment of mycotic infections. Ann Intern Med 77:43, 1972.

270. Butler KM, Rench MA, Baker CA. Amphotericin B as a single agent in the treatment of systemic candidiasis in neonates. Pediatr Infect Dis J 9:51, 1990.

271. Oliverio Campos J. Congenital meningoencephalitis due to torulosis neoformans: preliminary report. Bol Clin Hopit Civis Lisbon 18:609, 1954.

272. Neuhauser EBD, Tucker A. The roentgen changes produced by diffuse torulosis in the newborn. AJR 59:805, 1948.

273. Nassau E, Weinberg-Heiruti C. Torulosis of the newborn. Harefuah 35:50, 1948.

274. Heath P. Massive separation of retina in full-term infants and juveniles. JAMA 144:1148, 1950.

275. Savai M, Gaur S, Frenkel LD. Successful treatment of cryptococcosis in a premature neonate. Pediatr Infect Dis J 14:1009, 1995.

276. Freeman W. Torula infection of central nervous system. J Psychol Neurol 43:236, 1931.

277. Cox LB, Tolhurst JC. Human Torulosis. Melbourne, Melbourne University Press, 1946.

278. Littman ML, Zimmerman LE. Cryptococcosis (Torulosis). New York, Grune & Stratton, 1956.

279. Khan MJ, Myers R, Koshy G. Pulmonary cryptococcosis:

a case report and experimental study. Dis Chest 36:656, 1959.

280. Carton CA. Treatment of central nervous system cryptococcosis: a review and report of four cases treated with Actidione. Ann Intern Med 37:123, 1952.

281. Carton CA, Mount LA. Neurosurgical aspects of cryptococcosis. J Neurosurg 8:143, 1951.

282. Zimmerman LE, Rappaport H. Occurrence of cryptococcosis in patients with malignant disease of the reticuloendothelial system. Am J Clin Pathol 24:1050, 1954.

283. Butler WT, Alling DW, Spickard A, et al. Diagnostic and prognostic value of clinical and laboratory findings in cryptococcal meningitis, a follow-up study of forty patients. N Engl J Med 270:59, 1964.

284. Gruhn JG, Sanson J. Mycotic infection in leukemic patients at autopsy. Cancer 16:61, 1963.

285. Shadomy JJ, Utz JP. Preliminary studies on a hyphae-forming mutant of *Cryptococcus neoformans*. Mycologia 58:383, 1966.

286. Evans EE. The antigenic composition of *Cryptococcus neoformans*: I. A serologic classification by means of the capsular and agglutination reactions. J Immunol 64:423, 1950.

287. Evans EE, Sorensen LJ, Walls KW. The antigenic composition of *Cryptococcus neoformans*: V. A survey of cross-reactions among strains of *Cryptococcus* and other antigens. J Bacteriol 66:287, 1953.

288. San Felice F. Contributo alla morfologia e biologia del blastomiceti che si sviluppano nei succhi di alcuni frutti. Annali dell'Instituto d'Igiene Sperimentale della R Universita di Roma 4:463, 1894.

289. Klein E. Pathogenic microbes in milk. J Hyg 1:78, 1901.

290. Emmons CW. The significance of saprophytism in the epidemiology of the mycoses. Trans N Y Acad Sci 17:157, 1954.

291. Emmons CW. Saprophytic source of *Cryptococcus neoformans* associated with the pigeon *(Columbia livia)*. Am J Hyg 62:227, 1955.

292. Kao CJ, Schwartz J. The isolation of *Cryptococcus neoformans* from pigeon nests, with remarks on the identification of virulent cryptococci. Am J Clin Pathol 27:652, 1957.

293. Littman ML, Borok R. Relation of the pigeon to cryptococcosis: natural carrier state, host resistance and survival of *Cryptococcus neoformans*. Mycopathol Mycol Appl 36:329, 1968.

294. Littman ML, Schneierson SS. *Cryptococcus neoformans* in pigeon excreta in New York City. Am J Hyg 69:49, 1959.

295. Ajello L. Comparative ecology of respiratory mycotic disease agents. Bacteriol Rev 31:6, 1967.

296. Schneidau JD Jr. Pigeons and cryptococcosis. Science 143:525, 1964.

297. Hajsig M, Curoija Z. Kriptokoki u fekalijama fazana golubova s osvrlom na nalaze *Cryptococcus neoformans*. Vet Arch 35:115, 1965.

298. Tsubura E. Experimental studies in cryptococcosis: I. Isolation of *Cryptococcus neoformans* from avian excreta and some considerations on the source of infection. Fungi Fungous Dis 3:50, 1962.

299. Staib F. Vorkommen von *Cryptococcus neoformans* in vogelmist. Zentralbl Bakteriol 182:562, 1961.

300. Fragner P. The findings of cryptococci in excrements of birds. Cesk Epidemiol Mikrobiol Immunol 11:135, 1962.

301. Clarke DS, Wallace RH, David JJ. Yeasts occurring on apples and in apple cider. Can J Microbiol 1:145, 1954.

302. McDonough ES, Auseherman RJ, Balows A, et al. Human pathogenic fungi recovered from soil in an area endemic for North American blastomycosis. Am J Hyg 73:75, 1961.

303. Ajello L. Occurrence of *Cryptococcus neoformans* in soils. Am J Hyg 67:72, 1968.

304. McGrath JT. Cryptococcosis of the central nervous system in domestic animals. Am J Pathol 30:651, 1954.

305. Simon J, Nichols RE, Morse EV. An outbreak of bovine cryptococcosis. J Am Vet Med Assoc 122:31, 1953.

306. Pounden WD, Amberson JM, Jaeger RF. A severe mastitis problem associated with *Cryptococcus neoformans* in a large dairy herd. Am J Vet Res 13:121, 1952.

307. Campbell GD. Primary pulmonary cryptococcosis. Am Rev Respir Dis 94:236, 1966.

308. Mohr JA, Tacker RJ, Devlin RF, et al. Estrogen-stimulated phagocytic activity in human cryptococcosis. Am Rev Respir Dis 99:979, 1969.

309. Littman ML, Walter JE. Cryptococcosis: current status. Am J Med 45:922, 1968.

310. Gandy WM. Primary cutaneous cryptococcosis. Arch Dermatol Syphilol 62:97, 1950.

311. Brier RL, Mopper C, Stone J. Cutaneous cryptococcosis. Arch Dermatol 75:262, 1957.

312. Takos MJ. Experimental cryptococcosis produced by the ingestion of virulent organisms. N Engl J Med 254:598, 1956.

313. Freeman W. Torula meningo-encephalitis: comparative histopathology in seventeen cases. Trans Am Neurol Assoc 56:203, 1930.

314. Randhawa HW, Palewal DK. Occurrence and significance of *Cryptococcus neoformans* in the oropharynx and on the skin of a healthy human population. J Clin Microbiol 6:325, 1977.

315. Tynes B, Mason KN, Jennings AE, et al. Variant forms of pulmonary cryptococcosis. Ann Intern Med 69:1117, 1968.

316. Kida A, Abramowsky CR, Santoscoy C. Cryptococcosis of the placenta in a woman with acquired immunodeficiency syndrome. Hum Pathol 20:920, 1989.

317. Silberfarb PM, Sarosi GA, Tosh FE. Cryptococcosis and pregnancy. Am J Obstet Gynecol 112:714, 1972.

318. Curole DN. Cryptococcal meningitis in pregnancy. J Reprod Med 26:317, 1981.

319. Reiss F, Szilagyi G. Ecology of yeast-like fungi in a hospital population: detailed investigation of *Cryptococcus neoformans*. Arch Dermatol 91:611, 1965.

320. Collins VP, Gellhorn A, Trimble JR. The coincidence of cryptococcosis and disease of the reticulo-endothelial and lymphatic systems. Cancer 4:883, 1951.

321. Burrows B, Barclay WR. Combined cryptococcal and tuberculous meningitis complicating reticulum cell sarcoma. Am Rev Tuberc Pulm Dis 78:760, 1958.

322. Annual report of the Division of Epidemiology. Bureau of Preventable Diseases, Department of Health, New York, N.Y. 1963–1964.

323. Goldstein E, Rambo ON. Cryptococcal infection following steroid therapy. Ann Intern Med 56:114, 1962.

324. Levine AS, Graw RG Jr, Young RC. Management of infections in patients with leukemia and lymphoma: current concepts and experimental approaches. Semin Hematol 9:141, 1972.

325. Siewers CMF, Cramblett HG. Cryptococcosis (torulosis) in children: a report of four cases. Pediatrics 34:393, 1964.

326. Baum GL, Artis D. Growth inhibition of *Cryptococcus neoformans* by cell-free human serum. Am J Med Sci 241:613, 1961.

327. Igel HJ, Bolande RP. Humoral defense mechanisms in cryptococcosis: substances in normal human serum, saliva

and cerebrospinal fluid affecting the growth of *Cryptococcus neoformans*. J Infect Dis 116:75, 1966.

328. Szilagyi G, Reiss F, Smith JC. The anticryptococcal factor of blood serum: a preliminary report. J Invest Dermatol 46:306, 1966.

329. Hamilton JB, Tyler GR. Pulmonary torulosis. Radiology 47:149, 1946.

330. Greening RR, Menville LJ. Roentgen findings in torulosis: report of four cases. Radiology 48:381, 1947.

331. Haugen RK, Baker RD. The pulmonary lesions in cryptococcosis with special reference to subpleural nodules. Am J Clin Pathol 24:1381, 1954.

332. Moore M. Cryptococcosis with cutaneous manifestations. J Invest Dermatol 28:159, 1957.

333. Spickard A. Diagnosis and treatment of cryptococcal disease. South Med J 66:26, 1973.

334. Lillie RD. Histopathologic Technique. Philadelphia, Blakiston, 1954.

335. Rhinehart JF, Abdul-Haj SK. An improved method for histologic demonstration of acid mucopolysaccharides in tissues. Arch Pathol 52:189, 1951.

336. Berghausen O. *Torula* infection in man. Ann Intern Med 1:235, 1927.

337. Kessel JF, Holtzwart F. Experimental studies with *Torula* from a knee infection in man. Am J Trop Med 15:467, 1935.

338. Dienst RB. *Cryptococcus histolyticus* isolated from subcutaneous tumor. Arch Dermatol Syphilol 37:461, 1938.

339. Salvin SB, Smith RF. An antigen for detection of hypersensitivity to *Cryptococcus neoformans*. Proc Soc Exp Biol Med 108:498, 1961.

340. Bennett JE, Hasenclever HF, Baum GL. Evaluation of a skin test for cryptococcosis. Am Rev Respir Dis 91:616, 1965.

341. Newberry WH, Walter JE, Chandler JW Jr, et al. Epidemiologic study of *Cryptococcus neoformans*. Ann Intern Med 67:724, 1967.

342. Rappaport BZ, Kaplan B. Generalized torula mycosis. Arch Pathol Lab Med 1:720, 1926.

343. Pollock AQ, Ward LM. A hemagglutination test for cryptococcosis. Am J Med 32:6, 1962.

344. Vogel R.A, Seelers TF, Woodward P. Fluorescent antibody techniques applied to the study of human cryptococcosis. JAMA 178:921, 1961.

345. Vogel RA. The indirect fluorescent antibody test for the detection of antibody in human cryptococcal disease. J Infect Dis 116:573, 1966.

346. Walter JE, Atchison RW. Epidemiological and immunological studies of *Cryptococcus neoformans*. J Bacteriol 92:82, 1966.

347. Bloomfield N, Gordon MA, Elmendorf DF Jr. Detection of *Cryptococcus neoformans* antigen in body fluid by latex particle agglutination. Proc Soc Exp Biol Med 114:64, 1963.

348. Gordon MA, Vedder DK. Serologic tests in diagnosis and prognosis of cryptococcosis. JAMA. 197:961, 1966.

349. Walter JE, Jones RD. Serodiagnosis of clinical cryptococcosis. Am Rev Respir Dis 97:275, 1968.

350. Young EJ, Hirsch DD, Fainstein V, et al. Pleural effusions due to *Cryptococcus neoformans*: a review of the literature and report of two cases with cryptococcal antigen determination. Am Rev Respir Dis 121:743, 1980.

351. Bennett JE, Hasenclever HF, Tynes BS. Detection of cryptococcal polysaccharide in serum and spinal fluid: value in diagnosis and prognosis. Trans Assoc Am Physicians 77:145, 1964.

352. Kaufman L, Blumer S. Value and interpretation of serological tests for the diagnosis of cryptococcosis. Appl Microbiol 16:1907, 1968.

353. Bindschadler DD, Bennett JE. Serology of human cryptococcosis. Ann Intern Med 69:45, 1968.

354. Goodman JS, Kaufman L, Koenig MG. Diagnosis of cryptococcal meningitis: value of immunologic detection of cryptococcal antigen. N Engl J Med 285:434, 1971.

355. Walter JE, Coffee EG. Control of *Cryptococcus neoformans* in pigeon coops by alkalinization. Am J Epidemiol 87:173, 1968.

356. Hughes WT. The deep mycoses. *In* Kelley VC (ed). Brennemann's Practice of Pediatrics. Hagerstown, Md, Harper & Row, 1970, p 1.

357. Cohen R. Coccidioidomycosis: case report in children. Arch Pediatr 66:241, 1949.

358. Hyatt HW. Coccidioidomycosis in a three week old infant. Am J Dis Child 105:127, 1963.

359. Townsend TE, McKey RW. Coccidioidomycosis in infants. Am J Dis Child 86:51, 1953.

360. Christian JR, Sarre SG, Peers JH, et al. Pulmonary coccidioidomycosis in a 21 day old infant. Am J Dis Child 92:66, 1956.

361. Westley CR, Haak W. Neonatal coccidioidomycosis in a Southwestern Pima Indian. South Med J 67:855, 1974.

362. Shafai T. Neonatal coccidioidomycosis in premature twins. Am J Dis Child 132:634, 1978.

363. Larwood TR. Transactions of the 7th Annual Meeting of the Veterans Administration and Armed Forces Coccidioidomycosis Study Group, San Francisco, 1962, pp 28–29.

364. Bernstein DI, Tipton JR, Schott SF, et al. Coccioidomycosis in a neonate; maternal-infant transmission. J Pediatr 99:752, 1981.

365. Golden SE, Morgan CM, Bartley DL, et al. Disseminated coccidioidomycosis with chorioretinitis in early infancy. Pediatr Infect Dis J 5:272, 1986.

366. Child DD, Newell JD, Bjelland JC, et al. Radiographic findings of pulmonary coccidioidomycosis in neonates and infants. AJR 145:261, 1985.

367. Fiese MJ Coccidioidomycosis. Springfield, Ill, Charles C Thomas, 1958.

368. Maddy KT. The geographic distribution of *Coccidioides immitis* and possible ecologic implications. Ariz Med 15:178, 1958.

369. Albert BL, Sellers TF. Coccidioidomycosis from fomites. Arch Intern Med 112:253, 1963.

370. Giltner LT. Occurrence of coccidioidal granuloma (oidiomycosis) in cattle. J Agric Res 14:533, 1918.

371. Beck MD. Occurrence of *Coccidioides immitis* in lesions of slaughtered animals. Proc Soc Exp Biol Med 26:534, 1929.

372. Davis CL, Stiles GW, Jr, McGregor AN. Pulmonary coccidioidal granuloma: a new site of infection in cattle. J Am Vet Med Assoc 91:209, 1937.

373. Reed RE. Diagnosis of disseminated canine coccidioidomycosis. J Am Vet Med Assoc 128:196, 1956.

374. Reed RE, Prchal CJ, Maddy KT. Veterinary aspects of coccidioidomycosis; panel discussion. Proceedings of a symposium on coccidioidomycosis. U.S. Public Health Service Publication No. 575, Washington, DC, U.S. Government Printing Office, 1957, p 101.

375. Emmons CW. Isolation of *Coccidioides* from soil and rodents. Public Health Rep 57:109, 1942.

376. Rhoads JP. Coccidioidomycosis. J Okla State Med Assoc 58:410, 1965.

377. Pappagianis D. Coccidioidomycosis. *In* Hoeprich PD (ed). Infectious Diseases. Hagerstown, Md, Harper & Row, 1972.

378. Smith CE. An epidemiological study of acute cocoidioi-domycosis with erythema nodosum. Proc Sixth Pacific Science Congress 5:797, 1939.

379. Smith CE, Beard RR, Rosenberger HG, et al. Effect of season and dust control on coccidioidomycosis. JAMA 132:833, 1946.

380. Overholt EL, Hornick RB. Primary cutaneous coccidioidomycosis. Arch Intern Med 114:14, 1964.

381. Winn WA. Coccidioidomycosis and amphotericin. Med Clin North Am 47:1131, 1963.

382. Gifford MA, Buss WC, Douds RJ. *Coccidioides* fungus infection. Kern County, 1900–1936. Kern County Health Dept. Annual Report 1936–1937, p 39.

383. Beck MD. Epidemiology, coccidioidal granuloma. Calif State Dept Public Health Special Bull 57:19, 1931.

384. Smale LE, Birsner JW. Maternal deaths from coccidioidomycosis. JAMA 140:1152, 1949.

385. Vaughan JE, Ramirez H. Coccidioidomycosis as a complication of pregnancy, Calif Med 74:121, 1951.

386. Wack EE, Ampel NM, Galgiani JN, et al. Coccidioidomycosis during pregnancy: an analysis of ten cases among 47,120 pregnancies. Chest 94:376, 1988.

387. Peterson CM, Johnson SL, Kelly JV, et al. Coccidioidal meningitis and pregnancy: a case report. Obstet Gynecol 73:835, 1989.

388. Barbee RA, Hicks MJ, Grosso D, et al. The maternal immune response in coccidioidomycosis. Chest 100:709, 1991.

389. Hildick-Smith G. International symposium on opportunistic fungous infections. Arch Dermatol 87:8, 1963.

390. Ampel NM, Wieden MA, Galgiani JN. Coccidioidomycosis clinical update. Rev Infect Dis 2:897, 1989.

391. Anderson FG, Guckian JC. Systemic lupus erythematosus associated with fatal pulmonary coccidioidomycosis. Tex Rep Biol Med 20:93, 1968.

392. Cohen R. Placental *Coccidioides*; proof that congenital coccidioides is non-existent. Arch Pediatr 68:59, 1951.

393. Cohen R, Burnip R. Coccidioidin skin testing during pregnancy and in infants and children. Calif Med 72:31, 1950.

394. McCaffree MA, Altshuler G, Benirschke K. Placental coccidioidomycosis without fetal disease. Arch Pathol Lab Med 102:512, 1978.

395. Eckmann BH, Schaefer GL, Huppert M. Bedside interhuman transmission of coccidioidomycosis via growth on fomites: epidemic involving 6 persons. Am Rev Respir Dis 89:175, 1964.

396. Wilson JM. Smith CE, Plunkett OA. Primary cutaneous coccidioidomycosis: the criteria for diagnosis. Calif Med 79:233, 1953.

397. Faber HK, Smith CE, Dickson EC. Acute coccidioidomycosis with erythema nodosum in children. J Pediatr 15:163, 1939.

398. Birsner JW. The roentgen aspects of five hundred cases of pulmonary coccidioidomycosis. AJR 72:556, 1954.

399. Riley HD. Systemic mycoses in children. Curr Probl Pediatr 2:3, 1972.

400. Smith CE, Beard RR, Rosenberger HG, et al. Varieties of coccidioidal infection in relation to epidemiology and control of the disease. Am J Public Health 36:1394, 1946.

401. Caudill RG, Smith CE, Reinarz JA. Coccidioidal meningitis: a diagnostic dilemma. Am J Med 49:360, 1970.

402. Plunkett OA. Ecology and spread of pathogenic fungi. *In* Sternberg TH, Newcomer VD (eds). Therapy of Fungus Diseases, an International Symposium. Boston, Little, Brown, 1955, p 18.

403. Werner SB, Pappagianis D, Heindle I, et al. An epidemic of coccidioidomycosis among archeology students in Northern California. N Engl J Med 286:507, 1972.

404. Gehlbach SH, Hamilton JD, Conant NF. Coccidioidomycosis: an occupational disease in cotton-mill workers. Arch Intern Med 131:254, 1973.

405. Creitz JR, Puckett JF. A method for cultural identification of *Coccidioides immitis*. Am J Clin Pathol 24:1318, 1954.

406. Smith CE, Saito MT, Beard RR, et al. Serological tests in the diagnosis and prognosis of coccidioidomycosis. Am J Hyg 52:1, 1950.

407. Smith CE, Saito MT, Simons SA. Pattern of 39,500 serologic tests in coccidioidomycosis. JAMA 160:546, 1956.

408. Swaki Y, Huppert M, Bailey JW, et al. Patterns of human antibody reactions in coccidioidomycosis. J Bacteriol 91:422, 1966.

409. Campbell CC. Use and interpretation of serologic and skin tests in the respiratory mycoses: current considerations. Dis Chest 54(Suppl 1):49, 1968.

410. Huppert M, Bailey JW. The use of immunodiffusion tests in coccidioidomycosis: I. The accuracy and reproducibility of the immunodiffusion test which correlates with complement fixation. Am J Pathol 44:364, 1965.

411. Huppert M, Bailey JW. The use of immunodiffusion tests in coccidioidomycosis: II. An immunodiffusion test as a substitute for the tube precipitin test. Am J Clin Pathol 44:369, 1965.

412. Huppert M, Peterson ET, Sun SH, et al. Evaluation of a latex particle agglutination test for coccidioidomycosis. Am J Clin Pathol 49:96, 1968.

413. Graham AR, Ryan KJ. Counter immunoelectrophoresis employing coccidioidin in serologic testing for coccidioidomycosis. Am J Clin Pathol 73:574, 1980.

414. Cotanzaro A, Flatauer F. Detection of serum antibodies in coccidioidomycosis by solid-phase radioimmunoassay. J Infect Dis 147:32, 1983.

415. Drips W, Smith CE. Epidemiology of coccidioidomycosis. JAMA 190:1010, 1964.

416. Schnelzer LL, Tabershaw IR. Exposure factors in occupational coccidioidomycosis. Am J Public Health 52:107, 1968.

417. Elconin AF, Egeberg MO, Bald JG, et al. A fungicide effective against *Coccidioides immitis* in the soil. *In* Ajello L (ed). Coccidioidomycosis. Tucson, University of Arizona Press, 1967, p 319.

418. Levine HB, Cobb JM, Smith CE. Immunogenicity of spherule-endospore vaccines of *Coccidioides immitis* for mice. J Immunol 85:218, 1961.

419. Pappagianis D. Evaluation of the protective efficacy of the killed *Coccidioides immitis* vaccine in man. *In* Proceedings of the 26th Interscience Conference on Antimicrobial Agents and Chemotherapy, Washington, DC, American Society for Microbiology, 1986 (abstract).

420. Zimmerman LE. Fatal fungus infections complicating other diseases. Am J Clin Pathol 25:46, 1955.

421. Allan GW, Andersen DH. Generalized aspergillosis in an infant 18 days of age. Pediatrics 26:432, 1960.

422. Luke JL. Bolande RP, Grass S. Generalized aspergillosis and *Aspergillus* endocarditis in infancy. Pediatrics 31:115, 1963.

423. Akkoyunlu A, Yücell FA. Aspergillose bronchopulmonaire et encéphalomeningel chez un nouvedau-né de 20 jours. Arch Fr Pediatr 14:615, 1957.

424. Matturi L, Fasolis S. L'aspergillosi generalizzata neonetale. Folia Hered Pathol 12:87, 1962.

425. Paradis AJ, Roberts L. Endogenous ocular aspergillosis:

report of a case in an infant with cytomegalic inclusion disease. Arch Ophthalmol 69:765, 1963.

426. Brass K. Infecciones hospitalarias asporgilosas broncopulmonares en lactantes y ninos menores. Mycopathologia 57:149, 1975.

427. Mangurien HH, Fernandez B, Neonatal aspergillosis accompanying fulminant necrotizing enterocolitis. Arch Dis Child 54:559, 1979.

428. Gonzalez-Crussi F, Mirkin LD, Wyllie RM, et al. Acute disseminated aspergillosis during the neonatal period: report of an instance of a 14-day-old infant. Clin Pediatr 18:137, 1979.

429. Raaf JH, Donahoe PK, Truman JT, et al. *Aspergillus*-induced small bowel obstruction in a leukemic newborn. Surgery 81:111, 1977.

430. Mouy R, Ropent JC, Donadieu J, et al. Granulomatose septique chronique revelée par une aspergillose pulmonaire neonatale. Arch Pediatr 2:861, 1995.

431. Bruyere A, Bourgeois J, Cochat P, et al. Entérocolite ulcéro-nécrotique néonatale et aspergillose. Pediatrie 38:185, 1983.

432. Rhine WD, Arvin AA, Stevenson DK. Neonatal aspergillosis: a case report and review of the literature. Clin Pediatr 25:400, 1986.

433. Granstein RD, First LR, Sober AJ. Primary cutaneous aspergillosis in a premature neonate. Br J Dermatol 103:681, 1980.

434. Shiota R, Agaewal HC, Grover AK, et al. *Aspergillus* endophthalmitis. Br J Ophthalmol 71:611, 1987.

435. Roth JG, Troy JL, Esterly NB. Multiple cutaneous ulcers in a premature neonate. Pediatr Dermatol 8:253, 1991.

436. Schwartz DA, Jacquette M, Chawla HS. Disseminated neonatal aspergillosis: report of a fatal case and analysis of risk factors. Pediatr Infect Dis J 7:349, 1988.

437. Lackner H, Schwinger W, Urban C, et al. Lipsomal amphotericin-B (AmBisome) for treatment of disseminated fungal infections in two infants of very low birth weight. Pediatrics 89:1259, 1992.

438. Rowen JL, Correa AG, Sokol DM, et al. Invasive aspergillosis in neonates: report of five cases and literature review. Pediatr Infect Dis J 11:576, 1992.

439. Perzigian RW, Faix RG. Primary cutaneous aspergillosis in a preterm infant. Am J Perinatol 10:269, 1993.

440. Gupta M, Weinberger B, Whitley-Williams PN. Cutaneous aspergillosis in a neonate. Pediatr Infect Dis J 15:464, 1996.

441. Papouli M, Roilides E, Bebashi E, Andreau A. Primary cutaneous aspergillosis in neonates: case report and review. Clin Infect Dis 22:1102, 1996.

442. Scroll AH, Jaeger G, Allendorf A, et al. Invasive pulmonary aspergillosis in a critically ill neonate: case report and review of invasive aspergillosis during the first 3 months of life. Clin Infect Dis 27:437, 1998.

443. Raper KB, Fennell DJ (eds). The Genus *Aspergillus*. Baltimore, Williams & Wilkins, 1965.

444. Austwick PKC. Pathogenicity. *In* Raper KB, Fennell DI (eds). The Genus *Aspergillus*. Baltimore, Williams & Wilkins, 1965, p. 82.

445. Salvin SB. Endotoxin in pathogenic fungi. J Immunol 69:89, 1952.

446. Rau EM. Koenig VL, Tilden EB. Partial purification and characterization of the endotoxin from *Aspergillus fumigatus*. Mycopathologica 14:347, 1961.

447. Tilden EB, Hatton EH, Freeman S, et al. Preparation and properties of the endotoxins of *Aspergillus fumigatus* and *Aspergillus flavus*. Mycopathologica 14:325, 1961.

448. Tilden EB, Freeman S, Lombard L. Further studies of the *Aspergillus* endotoxins. Mycopathologica 20:253, 1963.

449. Utz JP. Aspergillosis. *In* Hoeprich PD, (ed). Infectious Diseases. Hagerstown, Md, Harper & Row, 1972, p 425.

450. Asplin FD, Carnaghan RBA. The toxicity of certain groundnut meals for poultry with special references to their effects on ducklings and chickens. Vet Rec 73:1215, 1961.

451. Loosmore RM, Markson LM. Poisoning of cattle by Brazilian groundnut meal. Vet Rec 73:813, 1961.

452. Spensley PC. Aflatoxin, the active principle in turkey "X" disease. Endeavour 22:75, 1963.

453. Lancaster MC, Jenkins FP, Philip JM. Toxicity associated with certain samples of groundnuts. Nature 192:1095, 1961.

454. LeBreton E, Frayssinet G, Boy J. Sur l'apparition d'hépatomes "spontanés" chez le rat Wister: kôle de la toxine de l'*Aspergillus flavus*: intérêt en pathologie humaine et concérologie expérimentale. CR Acad Sci 255:784, 1962.

455. Carnaghan RBA. Fungi in human and animal disease: some biologic effects of aflatoxin. Proc R Soc Med 57:414, 1964.

456. Austwick PKC, Gitter M, Watkins CV. Pulmonary aspergillosis in lambs. Vet Rec 72:19, 1960.

457. Merchant RK, Louria DB, Geisler PH, et al. Fungal endocarditis: a review of the literature and report of three cases. Ann Intern Med 48:242, 1958.

458. Renon L. Recherches cliniques et expérimentales sur la pseudotuberculose aspergillaire. These No. 89. Paris, G. Steinheil, 1893.

459. Renon L l'Étude sur l'Aspergillose chez les Animaux et chez l'Homme, Paris, Masson, 1897.

460. Dieulafoy G, Chantemesse A, Widal GFI. Une pseudotuberculose myosique. Congres Int Berlin Gaz Hop (Paris) 63:821, 1890.

461. Wahl EF, Erickson MJ. Primary pulmonary aspergillosis. J Med Assoc Ga 17:341, 1928.

462. Hinson KPW, Moon AJ, Plummer NS. Bronchopulmonary aspergillosis: a review and a report of eight new cases. Thorax 7:317, 1952.

463. Macartney JM. Pulmonary aspergillosis: a review and description of three new cases. Thorax 19:287, 1964.

464. Hunter D, Perry KMA. Bronchiolitis resulting from the handling of bagasse. Br J Ind Med 3:64, 1946.

465. Stallybrass FC. A study of *Aspergillus* spores in the atmosphere of a modern mill. Br J Ind Med 18:41, 1961.

466. Conant NF, Smith DT, Baker RD, et al. Aspergillosis. *In* Manual of Clinical Mycology, 3rd ed. Philadelphia, WB Saunders, 1971.

467. Castellani A. Fungi and fungous diseases. Arch Dermatol Syphilol 17:61, 1928.

468. Finegold SM, Murray JF. Aspergillosis: a review and report of twelve cases. Am J Med 27:463, 1959.

469. Sartory A, Sartory R. Un cas d'onychomycose dû à l'*Aspergillus fumigatus* Fresenius. Bull Acad Med (Paris) 109:482, 1945.

470. Gregson AEW, La Touche CJ. Otomycosis: a neglected disease. J Laryngol Otol 75:45, 1961.

471. McCarty JM, Fram MS, Pullen G, et al. Outbreak of primary cutaneous aspergillosis related to intravenous arm boards. J Pediatr 108:721, 1986.

472. Dewhurst AG, Cooper MJ, Khan SM, et al. Invasive aspergillosis in immunocompromised patients: potential hazard of hosptial building work. BMJ 301:802, 1990.

473. Collins PW, Kelsey SM, DeLord C, et al. Invasive aspergillosis in immunosuppressed patients. Letter. BMJ 301:1046, 1990.

474. Tobler W, Minder W. Generalized chronic aspergillosis

in the child and its relation to antibiotic therapy. Helv Paediatr Acta 9:209, 1954.

475. Cawley EP. Aspergillosis and the aspergilli: report of a unique case of the disease. Arch Intern Med 80:423, 1947.

476. Young RC, Bennett JE, Vogel CL, et al. Aspergillosis: the spectrum of disease in 98 patients. Medicine 49:147, 1970.

477. Huang S, Harris LS. Acute disseminated penicilliosis. Am J Clin Pathol 39:167, 1963.

478. Weiner MH. Antigenemia detected by radioimmunoassay in systemic aspergillosis. Ann Intern Med 92:793, 1980.

479. Haynes KA, Latge JP, Rogers TR. Detection of *Aspergillus* antigens associated with invasive infection. J Clin Microbiol 28:2040, 1990.

480. Levin SE, Isaacson C. Spontaneous perforation of the colon in the newborn. Arch Dis Child 35:378, 1960.

481. Gatling RR. Gastric mucormycosis in a newborn infant. Arch Pathol 67:249, 1959.

482. Neame P, Raaner D. Mucormycosis. Arch Pathol 70:261, 1960.

483. Jackson JR, Karnauchow PN. Mucormycosis of the central nervous system. Can Med Assoc J 76:130, 1957.

484. Isaacson C, Levin SE. Gastrointestinal mucormycosis in infancy. S A fr Med J 35:582, 1961.

485. Dennis JE, Rhodes KH, Cooney DR, et al. Nosocomial *Rhizopus* infection (zygomycosis) in children. J Pediatr 96:824, 1980.

486. Michalak DM, Cooney DR, Rhodes RH, et al. Gastrointestinal mucormycosis in infants and children: a cause of gangrenous intestinal cellulitis and perforation. J Pediatr Surg 15:320, 1980.

487. Miller RD, Steinkuller PG, Naegele D. Nonfatal maxillocerebral mucormycosis with orbital involvement in a dehydrated infant. Ann Ophthalmol 12:1065, 1980.

488. White CB, Barcia PJ, Bass JW. Neonatal zygomycotic necrotizing cellulitis. Pediatrics 78:100, 1986.

489. Varricchio F, Wilks A. Undiagnosed mucormycosis in infants. Pediatr Infect Dis J 8:660, 1989.

490. Ng PC, Dear PRF. Phycomycotic abscesses in a preterm infant. Arch Dis Child 64:862, 1989.

491. Lewis LL, Hawkins HK, Edwards MS. Disseminated mucormycosis in an infant with methylmalonic aciduria. Pediatr Infect Dis J 9:851, 1990.

492. Crim PF III, Demello D, Keenan WJ. Disseminated zygomycosis in a newborn. Pediatr Infect Dis J 3:61, 1984.

493. Arisoy AE, Arisoy ES, Correa-Calderon A, Kaplan SL. Rhizopus necrotizing cellulitis in a preterm infant: a case report and review of the literature. Pediatr Infect Dis J 12:1029, 1993.

494. Craig NM, Leuden FL, Pensler JM, et al. Disseminated rhizopus infection in a premature infant. Pediatr Dermatol 11:346, 1994.

495. Linder N, Keller N, Huri C, et al. Primary cutaneous mucormycosis in a premature infant: case report and review of the literature. Am J Perinatol 15:35, 1998.

496. Straatsma BR, Zimmerman LE, Gass JDM. Phycomycosis: a clinicopathologic study of fifty-one cases. Lab Invest 11:963, 1962.

497. Sheldon WH, Bauer H. Activation of quiescent mucormycotic granulomas in rabbits by induction of acute alloxan diabetes. Am J Pathol 34:575, 1958.

498. Bauer H, Flanagan JF, Sheldon WH. Experimental cerebral mycormycosis in rabbits with alloxan diabetes. Yale J Biol Med 28:29, 1955.

499. Elder TD, Baker RD. Pulmonary mucormycosis in rab-

bits with alloxan diabetes: increased invasiveness of fungus during acute toxic phase of diabetes. Arch Pathol 61:159, 1956.

500. Schofield RA, Baker RD. Experimental mucormycosis (*Rhizopus* infection) in mice. Arch Pathol 61:407, 1956.

501. Johnson JE. Infection and diabetes. *In* Ellenberg M, Rifkin H (eds). Diabetes Mellitus: Theory and Practice. New York, McGraw-Hill, 1969.

502. Sheldon WH, Bauer H. The development of the acute inflammatory response to experimental cutaneous mucormycosis in normal and diabetic rabbits. J Exp Med 110:845, 1959.

503. Emmons CW, Binford CH, Utz JP. Medical Mycology, 2nd ed. Philadelphia, Lea & Febiger, 1970, p 230.

504. Alexopoulos CJ. Introductory Mycology, 2nd ed. New York, John Wiley, 1962.

505. Whittaker RH. New concepts of kingdoms of organisms. Science 163:150, 1969.

506. Dodge CW. Phycomycetes. *In* Medical Mycology. St. Louis, CV Mosby, 1935, p 97.

507. Conant NF, Smith DT, Baker RD, et al. Mucormycosis. *In* Manual of Clinical Mycology, 3rd ed. Philadelphia, WB Saunders, 1971.

508. Emmons CW. Phycomycosis in man and animals. Riv Patol Veg 4:329, 1964.

509. Hale LM. Orbital-cerebral phycomycosis: report of a case and a review of the disease in infants. Arch Ophthalmol 86:39, 1971.

510. Burkholder PR, McVeigh I. Growth of *Phycomyces blakesleeanus* in relation to varied environmental conditions. Am J Botany 27:634, 1940.

511. Bergman K, Burke PV, Cerda-Olmeda E, et al. Phycomyces. Bacteriol Rev 33:99, 1969.

512. Meyer RD, Rosen MD, Armstrong D. Phycomycosis complicating leukemia and lymphoma. Ann Intern Med 77:871, 1972.

513. Gale GR, Welch AM. Studies of opportunistic fungi: I. Inhibition of *Rhizopus oryzae* by human serum. Am J Med Sci 241:604, 1961.

514. Bank H, Shibolet S, Gilat T, et al. Mucormycosis of head and neck structures: a case with survival. BMJ 1:766, 1962.

515. Jones KW, Kaufman L. Development and evaluation of an immunodiffusion test for diagnosis of systemic zygomycosis (mucormycosis): preliminary report. J Clin Microbiol 7:97, 1978.

516. Watts EA, Gard PD Jr, Tuthill SW. First reported case of intrauterine transmission of blastomycosis. Pediatr Infect Dis 2:308, 1983.

517. Maxson S, Miller SF, Tayka F, Schutze G. Perinatal blastomycosis: a review. Pediatr Infect Dis J 11:760, 1992.

518. Neiberg AD, Mavromatis F, Dyke et al. *Blastomycos dermatitidis* treated during pregnancy: report of a case. Am J Obstet Gynecol 128:911, 1977.

519. Ismail MD, Lerner SA. Disseminated blastomycosis in a pregnant woman: review of amphotericin B usage during pregnancy. Am Rev Respir Dis 126:350, 1982.

520. Cohen I. Absence of congenital infection and teratogenesis in three children born to mothers with blastomycosis and treated with amphotericin B during pregnancy. Pediatr Infect Dis 6:76, 1987.

521. Daniel L, Salit IE. Blastomycosis during pregnancy. Can Med Assoc J 131:759, 1984.

522. Hager H, Welt SI, Cardasis JP, et al. Disseminated blastomycosis in a pregnant woman successfully treated with amphotericin-B: a case report. J Reprod Med 33:485, 1988.

522a. King CT, Rogers PD, Cleasy JD, Chapman SW. Antifungal therapy during pregnancy. Clin Infect Dis 27:1151, 1998.

523. MacDonald D, Alguire P. Adult respiratory distress syndrome due to blastomycosis during pregnancy. Chest 98:1527, 1990.

524. Rippon JW. Medical Mycology: The Pathogenic Fungi and the Pathogenic Actinomycetes, 2nd ed. Philadelphia, WB Saunders, 1982, p 428.

525. Denton JF, McDonough ES, Ajello L, et al. Isolation of *Blastomyces dermatitidis* from soil. Science 133:1126, 1961.

526. Denton JF, DiSalvo AF. Isolation of *Blastomyces dermatitidis* from natural sites at Augusta, Georgia. Am J Trop Med 13:716, 1964.

527. Tenenbaum MJ, Greenspan J, Kerkering TM. Blastomycosis. CRC Crit Rev Microbiol 3:139, 1982.

528. Blastomycosis Cooperative Study of the Veterans Administration. Blastomycosis: I. A review of 198 collected cases in Veterans Administration hospitals. Am Rev Respir Dis 89:659, 1964.

529. Furcolow ML, Chick EW, Busey JF, et al. Prevalence and incidence studies of human and canine blastomycosis: I. Cases in the United States, 1885–1968. Am Rev Respir Dis 102:60, 1970.

530. Furcolow ML, Busey JF, Mangis RW, et al. Prevalence and incidence studies of human and canine blastomycosis: II. Yearly incidence studies in three selected states, 1960–1967. Am J Epidemiol 92:121, 1970.

531. Kepron MD, Schoemperlen B, Hershfield ES, et al. North American blastomycosis in Central Canada. Can Med Assoc J 106:243, 1972.

532. Sekhon AS, Bogorus MS, Sems HV. Blastomycosis: report of three cases from Alberta with a review of Canadian cases. Mycopathologia 68:53, 1979.

533. Sekhon AS, Jackson FL, Jacobs HJ. Blastomycosis: report of the first case from Alberta, Canada. Mycopathologica 79:65, 1982.

534. Robertson SA, Kimball PL, Magtibay LZ. Pulmonary blastomycosis diagnosed by cytologic examination of sputum. Can Med Assoc J 126:387, 1982.

535. Kane J, Righter J, Krajden S, et al. Blastomycosis: a new endemic focus in Canada. Can Med Assoc J 129:728, 1983.

536. Chick EW. The epidemiology of blastomycosis. *In* Al-Doory Y: (ed). The Epidemiology of Human Mycotic Disease. Springfield, Ill, Charles C Thomas, 1975, p 103.

537. Witorsch P, Utz JP. North American blastomycosis: a study of 40 patients. Medicine 47:169, 1968.

538. Habte-Gabr E, Smith IM. North American blastomycosis in Iowa: review of 34 cases. J Chronic Dis 26:585, 1973.

539. Denton JF, DiSalvo AF. Additional isolations of *Blastomyces dermatitidis* from natural sites. Am J Trop Med Hyg 28:697, 1979.

540. Schwartz J, Baum GL. Blastomycosis. Am J Clin Pathol 11:999, 1951.

541. Larson DM, Eckman MR, Alber RL, et al. Primary cutaneous (inoculation) blastomycosis: an occupational hazard to pathologists. Am Soc Clin Pathol 79:253, 1983.

542. Gnann JW Jr, Bressler GS, Bodet CA III, et al. Human blastomycosis after a dog bite. Ann Intern Med 98:484, 1983.

543. Craig MW, Davey WN, Green RA. Conjugal blastomycosis. Am Rev Respir Dis 102:86, 1970.

544. Recht LD, Philips JR, Eckman MR. et al. Self-limited blastomycosis: a report of thirteen cases. Am Rev Respir Dis 120:1109, 1979.

545. Recht LD, Davies SF, Eckman MR, et al. Blastomycosis in immunocompromised patients. Am Rev Respir Dis 125:359, 1982.

546. Gall SA. Maternal adjustments in the immune system in normal pregnancy. Clin Obstet Gynecol 26:521, 1983.

547. Sridama V, Pacini F, Yang SL, et al. Decreased levels of helper T cells: a possible cause of immunodeficiency in pregnancy. N Engl J Med 307:352, 1982.

548. Weinberg ED. Pregnancy associated depression of cell-mediated immunity. Rev Infect Dis 6:814, 1984.

549. Cozad GC, Chang CT. Cell mediated immunoprotection in blastomycosis. Infect Immun 28:398, 1980.

550. Cherniss EI, Wisbren BA. North American blastomycosis: a clinical study of 40 cases. Ann Intern Med 44:105, 1956.

551. Abernathy RS. Clinical manifestation of pulmonary blastomycosis. Ann Intern Med 51:707, 1959.

552. Lockwood WR, Allison F, Batson BE, et al. The treatment of North American blastomycosis: ten years' experience. Am Rev Respir Dis 100:314, 1969.

553. Duttera MJ, Osterhout S. North American blastomycosis: a survey of 63 cases. South Med J 62:295, 1969.

554. Kravitz GR, Davies SF, Eckman MR, et al. Chronic blastomycotic meningitis. Am J Med 71:501, 1981.

555. Kaufman L, McLaughlin DW, Clar MJ, et al. Specific immunodiffusion test for blastomycosis. Appl Microbiol 26:244, 1973.

556. Williams JE, Murphy R, Standard PG, et al. Serologic response in blastomycosis: diagnostic value of double immunodiffusion assay. Am Rev Respir Dis 123:209, 1981.

557. Duhring LA. Diseases of the Skin, 3rd ed. Philadelphia, JB Lippincott, 1888.

558. Lynch JR. Case of ringworm occurring in an infant within 6 hours of birth. Med Press Circ 21:235, 1876.

559. Jacobs AH, Jacobs PH, Moore N. Tinea facei due to *Microsporum canis*. JAMA 219:1476, 1972.

560. Bereston EW, Robinson HM. Tinea capitis and corporis in an infant 4 weeks old. Arch Dermatol Syphilol 68:582, 1953.

561. King WC, Walter IK, Livingood CS. Superficial fungus infections in infants. Arch Dermatol 68:664, 1953.

562. Hubener LF. Tinea capitis (*Microsporum canis*) in a 30 day old infant. Arch Dermatol 76:242, 1957.

563. Alden ER, Chernila SA. Ringworm in an infant. Pediatrics 44:261, 1969.

564. Weston WL, Thorno, EG. Two cases of tinea in the neonate treated successfully with griseofulvin. Clin Pediatr 16:601, 1977.

565. Ross CM. Ringworm of the scalp at 4 weeks. Br J Dermatol 78:554, 1966.

566. Yesudian P, Kamalam A. *Epidermophyton floccosum* infection in a three week old infant. Trans St John's Hosp Dermatol Soc 59:66, 1973.

567. Kleibl K, Al-Ghareer HA, Sakr MF. Neonatal tinea circinata. Mykosen 26:152, 1982.

568. Wyre HW Jr, Johnson WT. Neonatal pityriasis versicolor. Arch Dermatol 117:752, 1981.

569. Gondim Goncalves HM, Mapurunga AC, Melo-Monteiro C, et al. Tinea capitis caused by *Microsporum canis* in a newborn. Int J Dermatol 31:367, 1992.

570. Lanska MJ, Silverman R, Lansaka DJ. Cutaneous fungal infections associated with prolonged treatment in humidified oxygen hoods. Pediatr Dermatol 4:346, 1987.

571. Kamalan A, Thambish AS. Tinea faciei caused by *Microsporum gypseum* in a two day old infant. Mykosen 24:40, 1981.

572. Smith EB, Gellerman GL. Tinea versicolor in infancy. Arch Dermatol 93:362, 1984.

573. Powell DA, Aungst J, Snedden S, et al. Broviac catheter-related *Malassezia furfur* sepsis in five infants receiving intravenous fat emulsions. J Pediatr 105:987, 1984.

574. Long JG, Keyserling HL. Catheter-related infection in infants due to an unusual lipophilic yeast—*Malassezia furfur*. Pediatrics 76:896, 1985.

575. Dankner WM, Spector SA. *Malassezia furfur* sepsis in neonates. Letter to the editor. J Pediatr 107:643, 1985.

576. Powell DA, Brady MT. Reply. J Pediatr 107:644, 1985.

577. Redline RW, Dahms BB. *Malassezia* pulmonary vasculitis in an infant on long-term intralipid therapy. N Engl J Med 305:1395, 1981.

578. Nowak JA, Ruppert VA, Menegus MA. *Pityrosporum ovale* colonization of a Hickman catheter. Abstract of the 85th Annual Meeting of the American Society for Microbiology, Las Vegas, March 1985. Washington, DC. American Society for Microbiology, 1985.

579. Marcon MJ. Powell DA, Durrell DE. Methods for optimal recovery of *Malassezia furfur* from blood culture. J Clin Microbiol 24:696, 1986.

580. Ajello L. A taxonomic review of the dermatophytes and related species. Sabouraudia 6:147, 1968.

581. Dawson CO, Gentles JC. Perfect stage of *Keritinomyces ajelloi*. Nature 183:1345, 1959.

582. Rebell G, Taplin D, Blank H. Dermatophytes. Their Recognition and Identification. Miami, Dermatology Foundation of Miami, 1964.

583. Emmons CW, Binford CH, Utz JP. Dermatophytoses. *In* Medical Mycology, 2nd ed. Philadelphia, Lea & Febiger, 1970.

584. English MP, Gibson MD. Studies in epidemiology of tinea pedis. BMJ 1:1442, 1959.

585. Rothman S, Knox G, Windhourst D. Tinea pedis as a source of infection in the family. Arch Dermatol 75:270, 1957.

586. Ajello L. Geographic distribution and prevalence of the dermatophytes. Ann N Y Acad Sci 89:30, 1960.

587. Pinetti P, Lostia A, Tarentino F. The role played by flies in the transmission of the human and animal dermatophytic infection. Mycopathologia 54:131, 1974.

588. Baer RL, Rosenthal SA, Furnari D. Survival of dermatophytes applied on the feet. J Invest Dermatol 24:619, 1955.

589. Baer RL, Rosenthal SA, Litt JZ, et al. Experimental investigations on mechanism producing acute dermatophytosis of feet. JAMA 160:184, 1956.

590. Knight AG. A review of experimental fungus infections. J Invest Dermatol 59:354, 1972.

591. Mackenzie DWR. The extra human occurrence of *Tricophyton tonsurans* var. *sulfureum* in a residential school. Sabouraudia 1:58, 1961.

592. Hildick-Smith G. Blank H, Sarkany I. Tinea capitis. *In* Fungus Diseases and Their Treatment. Boston, Little, Brown, 1964.

593. Roig MA, Rodriguez JMT. The immune response in childhood dermatophytoses. Mykosen 30:574, 1987.

594. Alteras I. Tinea capitis in suckling. Mykosen 13:567, 1970.

595. Weidman FD. Laboratory aspects of epidermophytosis. Arch Dermatol 15:415, 1929.

596. Goodman RS, Temple DE, Lorinez AL. A miniaturized system for extracorporeal hemodialysis with application to studies on serum anti-dermophyte activity. J Invest Dermatol 37:535, 1961.

597. Greenbaum SS. Immunity in ringworm infections. Arch Dermatol 10:279, 1924.

598. Lorincz AL, Priestly JO, Jacobs PH. Evidence for humoral mechanism which prevents growth of dermatophytes. J Invest Dermatol 31:15, 1958.

599. Page CO, Remington JS. Immunologic studies in normal human sweat. J Lab Clin Med 69:634, 1967.

600. Shelley WB, Wood MG. New technic for instant visualization of fungi in hair. J Am Acad Dermatol 2:69, 1980.

601. Burke RC. Tinea versicolor: susceptibility factors and experimental infection in human beings. J Invest Dermatol 36:389, 1961.

602. Fields BT Jr, Bates JH, Abernathy RS. Amphotericin B serum concentrations during therapy. Appl Microbiol 19:955, 1970.

603. Cherry JD, Lloyd CA, Quilty JF, et al. Amphotericin B therapy in children. J Pediatr 75:1063, 1969.

604. McCoy MJ, Ellenberg JF, Killum AP. Coccidioidomycosis complicating pregnancy. Am J Obstet Gynecol 137:739, 1980.

605. Ward RM, Sattler FR, Dotton AS Jr. Assessment of antifungul therapy in an 800-gram infant with candidal arthritis and osteomyelitis. Pediatrics 72:234, 1983.

606. Abernathy RS. Treatment of systemic mycoses. Medicine 52:385, 1973.

607. Miller RP, Bates JH. Amphotericin B toxicity. Ann Intern Med 71:1089, 1969.

608. McCurdy DK, Frederic M, Elkington JR. Renal tubular acidosis due to amphotericin B. N Engl J Med 278:124, 1968.

609. Baley JE, Kliegman RM, Fanaroff AA. Disseminated fungal infections in very low-birth-weight infants: therapeutic toxicity. Pediatrics 73:153, 1984.

610. Feldman R. Cryptococcosis (torulosis) of the central nervous system treated with amphotericin B during pregnancy. South Med J 52:1415, 1959.

611. Aitken GWE, Symonds EM. Cryptococcal meningitis in pregnancy treated with amphotericin B: a case report. J Obstet Gynaecol Br Commonw. 69:677, 1962.

612. Kuo D. A case of torulosis of the central nervous system during pregnancy. Med J Aust 49:558, 1962.

613. Sanford WG, Rosch JR, Stonehill RB. A therapeutic dilemma: the treatment of disseminated coccidioidomycosis with amphotericin B. Ann Intern Med 56:553, 1962.

614. Harris RE. Coccidioidomycosis complicating pregnancy: report of 3 cases and review of the literature. Obstet Gynecol 28:401, 1966.

615. Smale LE, Waechter KG. Dissemination of coccidioidomycosis in pregnancy. Am J Obstet Gynecol 107:356, 1970.

616. Hadsall FJ, Acquarelli JJ. Disseminated coccidioidomycosis presenting as facial granulomas in pregnancy: a report of two cases and a review of the literature. Laryngoscope 83:51, 1973.

617. Curole DN. Cryptococcal meningitis in pregnancy. J Reprod Med 26:317, 1981.

618. Glick C, Graves GR, Feldman S. Neonatal fungemia and amphotericin B. South Med J 86:1368, 1993.

619. Pappagianis HD, Collins MS, Hector R, et al. Development of resistance to amphotericin B in *Candida lusitaniae* infecting a human. Antimicrob Agents Chemother 16:123, 1979.

620. Meyers BR, Wormser G, Hirschman SZ, et al. Rhinocerebral mucormycosis postmortem diagnosis and therapy. Arch Intern Med 139:557, 1979.

621. Shirkey HC. Pediatric Therapy, 4th ed. St. Louis, CV Mosby, 1972, p 489.

622. Jacobs RF, Yasuda K, Smith AL, et al. Laryngeal candidiasis presenting as inspiratory stridor. Pediatrics 69:234, 1982.

623. Faix RG. *Candida parapsilosis* meningitis in a premature infant. Pediatr Infect Dis J 2:462, 1983.

624. Drutz DJ, Spickard A, Rogers DE, et al. Treatment of disseminated mycotic infections: new approach to therapy with amphotericin B. Am J Med 45:405, 1968.

625. Christiansen KJ, Bernard EM, Gold JWM, et al. Distribution and activity of amphotericin B in humans. J Infect Dis 152:1037, 1985.

626. Drutz DJ. In vitro antifungal susceptibility testing and measurement of levels of antifungal agents in body fluids. J Infect Dis 9:392, 1987.

627. Diamond RD, Bennett JE. A subcutaneous reservoir for intrathecal therapy of fungal meningitis. N Engl J Med 288:186, 1973.

628. Kozinn PJ, Taschdjian CL, Pishvazadeh P, et al. *Candida* meningitis successfully treated with amphotericin B. N Engl J Med 268:881, 1963.

629. Meunier F, Prentice H, Ringden O. Liposomal amphotericin B (AmBisome): safety data from a phase II/III clinical trial. J Antimicrob Chemother 28(Suppl B):83, 1991.

630. Weitkamp JH, Poets CF, Sievers R, et al. *Candida* infection in very low birth-weight infants: outcome and nephrotoxicity of treatment with liposomal amphotericin B (AmBisome). Infection 26:11, 1998.

631. Scarcella A, Pasquariello MB, Giugliano B, et al. Liposomal amphotericin B treatment for neonatal fungal infections. Pediatr Infect Dis J 17:146, 1998.

632. Shadomy S. In vitro studies with 5-fluorocytosine. Appl Microbiol 17:871, 1969.

633. Shadomy S. Further in vitro studies with 5-fluorocytosine. Infect Immun 2:484, 1970.

634. Shadomy S. What's new in antifungal chemotherapy. Clin Med 79:14, 1972.

635. Steer PL, Marks MI, Klite PD, et al. 5-Fluorocytosine: an oral antifungal compound: a report on clinical and laboratory experience. Ann Intern Med 76:15, 1972.

636. Harrison IIR, Galgiani JN, Reynolds AF Jr, et al. Amphotericin B and imidazole therapy for coccidioidal meningitis in children. Pediatr Infect Dis 2:216, 1983.

637. Sarosi GA, Parker JD, Doto IL, et al. Amphotericin B in cryptococcal meningitis. Ann Intern Med 70:1079, 1969.

638. McDougall PN, Fleming PJ, Speller DCE, et al. Neonatal systemic candidiasis: a failure to respond to intravenous miconazole in two neonates. Arch Dis Child 57:884, 1982.

639. Sutton A. Miconazole in systemic candidiasis. Arch Dis Child 58:319, 1983.

640. Duffty P, Lloyd DJ. Neonatal systemic candidiasis. Arch Dis Child 58:318, 1983.

641. Lilien LD, Ramamurthy RS, Pildes RS. *Candida albicans* with meningitis in a premature neonate successfully treated with 5-flucytosine and amphotericin B: a case report and review of the literature. Pediatrics 61:57, 1978.

642. Bennett JE. Therapy of cryptococcal meningitis with 5-fluorocytosine. Antimicrob Agents Chemother 10:28, 1970.

643. Stevens DA, Levine HB, Deresinski SC. Miconazole in coccidioidomycosis. II. Therapeutic and pharmacologic studies in men. Am J Med 60:191, 1976.

644. Graybill JR, Levine HB. Successful treatment of cryptococcal meningitis with intraventricular miconazole. Arch Intern Med 138:814, 1978.

645. Kanarek KS, Williams PR. Toxicity of intravenous miconazole overdosage in a preterm infant. Pediatr Infect Dis 5:486, 1986.

646. Casneuf J, de Loore F, Dhondt F, et al. Oral thrush in children treated with miconazole gel. Mykosen 23:75, 1980.

647. Hoppe JE and the Antifungals Study Group. Treatment of oropharyngeal candidiasis in immunocompetent infants: a randomized multicenter study of meconazole gel vs nystation suspension. Pediatr Infect Dis J 16:288, 1997.

648. Holt RJ, Azmi A. Miconazole-resistant *Candida*. Lancet 1:50, 1978.

649. Tuck S. Neonatal systemic candidiasis treated with miconazole. Arch Dis Child 55:903, 1980.

650. Tudehape DL, Rigby B. Neonatal systemic candidiasis treated with miconazole and hepaconazole. Med J Aust 1:480, 1983.

651. Bennett JE, Remington JS. Miconazole in cryptococcosis and systemic candidiasis: a word of caution. Ann Intern Med 94:708, 1981.

652. Cohen M, Harkness RA, Renz M, et al. Trials of the use of clotrimazole in the treatment of oral candidiasis in newborn babies. Postgrad Med J 50(Suppl 1):28, 1974.

653. Montello JM, Darby MH, Faubil K, et al. Clotrimazole by thumb. N Engl J Med 301:1005, 1975.

654. Milne LJR. Mycological studies in the use of clotrimazole in bronchopulmonary aspergillosis and neonatal and vaginal candidiasis. Postgrad Med J 50(Suppl 1):20, 1974.

655. Renz M, Farquhar JW, Cohen M, et al. Elevation of myeloperoxidase activity in infants with oral candidiasis treated with clotrimazole. Postgrad Med J 50(Suppl 1):30, 1974.

656. Dixon D, Shadomy S, Shadomy HJ, et al. Comparison of the in vitro antifungal activities of miconazole and a new imidazole, R 41,400. J Infect Dis 138:245, 1978.

657. Drouhet E, Dupont B. Chronic mucocutaneous candidiasis and other superficial and systemic mycoses successfully treated with ketoconazole. Rev Infect Dis 2:606, 1980.

658. Graybill JR, Lundberg D, Donovan W, et al. Treatment of coccidioidomycosis with ketoconazole: clinical and laboratory studies of 18 patients. Rev Infect Dis 2:661, 1980.

659. Robertson MH, Hanifin JM, Parker F. Oral therapy with ketoconazole for dermatophyte infections unresponsive to griseofulvin. Rev Infect Dis 2:578, 1980.

660. Welsh O, Rodriguez M. Treatment of dermatomycoses with ketoconazole. Rev Infect Dis 2:582, 1980.

661. Legendre R, Steltz M. A multi-center, double-blind comparison of ketoconazole and griseofulvin in the treatment of infections due to dermatophytes. Rev Infect Dis 2:586, 1980.

662. Kirkpatrick CH, Petersen EA, Alling DW. Treatment of chronic mucocutaneous candidosis with ketoconazole: preliminary results of a controlled, double-blind clinical trial. Rev Infect Dis 2:599, 1980.

663. Hay RJ, Wells RS, Clayton YM, et al. Treatment of chronic mucocutaneous candidiasis with ketoconazole: a study of 12 cases. Rev Infect Dis 2:600, 1980.

664. Graybill JB, Herndon JH Jr, Kniker WT, et al. Ketoconazole treatment of chronic mucocutaneous candidiasis. Arch Dermatol 116:1137, 1980.

665. Heel RC. Ketoconazole treatment of candidiasis in neonates and infants. *In* Levine HB (ed). Ketoconazole in the Management of Fungal Disease. Baltimore, Williams & Wilkins, 1982, p 147.

666. Hensey O, Cooke RW. Systemic candidiasis. Arch Dis Child 57:962, 1982.

667. Hazen EL, Brown R. Two antifungal agents produced by a soil Actinomycete. Science 112:423, 1950.

668. Petru A, Azimi PH. Esophagitis associated with *Candida* infection in a neonate. Clin Pediatr 23:179, 1984.

669. Kozinn PJ, Taschdjian CL. Enteric candidiasis. Pediatrics 30:71, 1962.

670. Walter JE, Jones RD. Serologic tests in diagnosis of aspergillosis. Dis Chest 53:729, 1968.

671. Young RC, Bennett JE. Invasive aspergillosis: absence of detectable antibody response. Am Rev Respir Dis 104:710, 1971.

672. Landau JW, Newcomer VD, Schulz J. Aspergillosis: report of two instances in children associated with acute leukemia and review of the pertinent literature. Mycopathologia 10:177, 1963.

673. Ross CM, Ringworm of the scalp at four weeks. Br J Dermatol 78:554, 1966.

674. Rubin, A, Dvornik D. Placental transfer of griseofulvin. Am J Obstet Gynecol 92:882, 1965.

675. Brammer KW, Farrow PR, Faulkner JK. Pharmacokinetics and tissue penetration of fluconazole in humans. Rev Infect Dis 12(Suppl):SB18, 1990.

676. Wiest DB, Fowler SL, Garner SS, et al. Fluconazole in neonatal disseminated candidiasis. Arch Dis Child 66:1002, 1991.

677. Gürses N, Kalayci AG: Fluconazole monotherapy for candidal meningitis in a premature infant. Clin Infect Dis 23:645, 1996.

678. Driessen M, Ellis JB, Cooper PA, et al. Fluconazole vs amphotericin B for the treatment of neonatal fungal septicemia: a prospective randomized trial. Pediatr Infect Dis J 15:1107, 1996.

679. Driessen M, Ellis JB, Muwazi F, DeVilliers FP: The treatment of systemic candidiasis in neonates with oral fluconazole. Ann Trop Paediatr 17:263, 1997.

680. Wiesinger EC, Mayerhofer S, Wenisch C, et al. Fluconazole in *Candida albicans* sepsis during pregnancy: case report and review of the literature. Infection 24:263, 1996.

681. Bhandari V, Narange A. Oral itraconazole therapy for disseminated candidiasis in low birth weight infants. J Pediatr 120:330, 1992.

682. Faber HK, Dickey LB. The treatment of thrush with gentian violet. JAMA 85:900, 1924.

683. Leung AKC. Gentian violet in the treatment of oral candidiasis. Pediatr Infect Dis J 7:304, 1988.

684. Grossman ER. Treatment of thrush. Pediatr Infect Dis J 7:303, 1988.

685. Beeson PB. Cryptococcic meningitis of nearly sixteen years' duration. Arch Intern Med 89:797, 1952.

686. Hildic-Smith G, Blank H, Sarkany I. Fungus Diseases and Their Treatment. Boston, Little, Brown, 1964.

687. Spickard A, Butler W, Utz JP. The improved prognosis of cryptococcal meningitis with amphotericin B therapy. Ann Intern Med 56:691, 1962.

688. Alznauer RL, Rolle C Jr, Pierce WF. Analysis of focalized pulmonary granulomas due to *Coccidioides immitis*. Arch Pathol 59:641, 1955.

689. Cotton BH, Paulsen GA, Birsner JW. Surgical considerations in pulmonary coccidioidomycosis: report of 100 cases. Am J Surg 90:101, 1955.

690. Graybill JR, Silva J, Whitsell W, et al. Immunologic deficits in coccidioidomycosis. Clin Res 21:57, 1973.

691. Longbottom JL, Pepys J. Pulmonary aspergillosis: diagnostic and immunologic significance of antigens and C-substance in *Aspergillus fumigatus*. J Pathol Bacteriol 88:141, 1964.

692. Weller WA, Joseph DJ, Hora JF. Deep mycotic involvement of the right maxillary and ethmoid sinuses, the orbit and adjacent structures. Laryngoscope 70:999, 1960.

693. Hildick-Smith G, Blank H, Sarkany I. Fungus Diseases and Their Treatment. Boston, Little, Brown, 1964, p 337.

694. Roberts HJ, Cutaneous mucormycosis: report of a case with survival. Arch Intern Med 110:108, 1962.

695. Dillon ML, Sealy WC, Fetter BL. Mucormycosis of the bronchus successfully treated by lobectomy. J Thorac Cardiovasc Surg 35:464, 1958.

696. Harris JS, Mucormycosis: report of a case. Pediatrics 16:857, 1955.

697. McCall W, Strobos RR. Survival of a patient with central nervous system mucormycosis. Neurology 7:290, 1957.

698. Oswald H, Seeliger HPR. Tierexperimentelle Untersuchungen mit antimycotischen Mitteln. Arzneim Forsch 8:370, 1958.

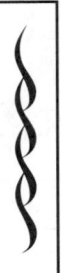

Other Viral Infections of the Fetus and Newborn

ANN M. ARVIN, M.D., and YVONNE A. MALDONADO, M.D.

HUMAN PAPILLOMAVIRUS (CONDYLOMA ACUMINATUM)

Human papillomavirus (HPV) is the cause of condyloma acuminatum (genital warts) and cervical condylomata.[1-3] The risk to the infant born to a mother with HPV infection is the development of juvenile laryngeal papillomatosis. Hajek associated the presence of condyloma acuminatum in a mother at the time of delivery with the subsequent development of laryngeal papilloma in her infant[4] (Table 18–1). Cook and colleagues described a similar association in five of nine children with laryngeal papilloma.[5] All five of the children who developed laryngeal papilloma when younger than 6 months of age were born to mothers who had condylomata acuminata at the time of delivery. The mothers of two of four other children with laryngeal papilloma had genital warts but did not have them at the time of delivery. Therefore, seven of the nine (78%) children with laryngeal papilloma had mothers with condylomata acuminata. The expected incidence of condylomata acuminata in women in the population studied by Cook and colleagues was 1.5%. Six of the nine children also had skin warts. Quick and co-workers also described a strong association between laryngeal papilloma in young children and maternal condylomata.[6] Twenty-one of the 31 (68%) patients with laryngeal papilloma they studied had been born to mothers who had had condylomata. The basis for this epidemiologic relationship is evident from the detection of HPV DNA sequences in both genital and laryngeal papilloma tissues.[3] Rare associations have been made between maternal genital HPV infections and neonatal giant cell hepatitis[7] and vulvar genital papillomas among stillborns.[8] Both of these associations were documented in small numbers of gestations but were confirmed by HPV-DNA polymerase chain reaction (PCR) or by electron microscopy.

HPV cannot be isolated by means of tissue culture, but HPV DNA sequences can be detected in cervical cells. Cervical infection is caused by several types of HPV, including types 6, 11, 16, 18, and 31, and is very common in the United States and Europe. HPV can be detected in epithelial cells that have a normal histologic appearance and from tissue samples of patients whose papillomatous lesions are in remission.[9] Clinically, most genital HPV infection is asymptomatic. The frequency of HPV detection has ranged from 5 to 15% in recent studies of women of childbearing age, with the highest incidence occurring among younger women.[10-13] Pregnancy was not associated with a higher rate of infection. Although the incidence of cervical infection was 20% in women with a past history of condyloma, most pregnant women with HPV infection do not have a history of genital warts. Infection of the infant probably occurs by exposure to the virus at delivery, although papillomatosis has been described in infants delivered by cesarean section. Tang and associates described an infant who was born with condylomata acuminata around the anal orifice.[14] The mother also had condylomata acuminata. Whether these cases reflect transplacental hematogenous spread or direct extension across intact membranes is not known.

Despite the prevalence of genital HPV infection, juvenile laryngeal papillomatosis remains a rare disease. The risk of subclinical transmission of HPV from mothers to infants is not known. HPV-6 and HPV-16 DNA sequences were detected in the cells from foreskin tissue of 3 of 70 infants.[15] These HPV types are also found in genital warts. Because of the prevalence of asymptomatic HPV infection, the feasibility of preventing the rare cases of laryngeal papillomatosis by considering maternal condyloma acuminatum as an indication for cesarean delivery is uncertain.

Treatment of anogenital warts is not optimal, but podophyllum resin or podofilox are often used in older children and adults. Neither has been tested for safety or efficacy in children, and both are contraindicated for use in pregnancy. Laryngeal papillomas recur even after repeated surgical removal. Interferon has been used with some success for treatment of laryngeal papillomas for more than 10 years as investigational treatment.[16] More recently, isotretinoin has also been used as investigational treatment.[17, 18]

EPSTEIN-BARR VIRUS

Epstein-Barr virus (EBV) is a human herpesvirus that is most familiar as the cause of infectious mononucleosis.

TABLE 18-1
Effects of Other Viral Infections of the Fetus and Newborn

INFECTIOUS AGENT	INCREASED INCIDENCE OF ABORTION	INCREASED RISK OF PREMATURITY	MAJOR CLINICAL MANIFESTATIONS IN INFANTS
Human papillomavirus	No	No	Laryngeal papilloma, condyloma acuminatum
Epstein-Barr virus	Possibly	Possibly	?
Human herpesvirus 6	No	No	Febrile illness in postnatal period
Influenza viruses	No	No	Probably none
Respiratory syncytial virus	No	No	Pneumonia, bronchiolitis, in postnatal period
Lymphocytic choriomeningitis virus	Yes	No	Hydrocephalus, chorioretinitis, viral meningitis, jaundice, ? thrombocytopenia
Molluscum contagiosum virus	No	No	Rash
Rabies	No	No	None known

However, most women of childbearing age have been infected asymptomatically in childhood. Because EBV cannot be isolated directly in tissue culture, serologic tests are used to detect recent primary or past infection.

Persons infected with EBV form both IgG and IgM antibodies to viral capsid antigens (VCA) soon after infection.[19] About 80% form antibodies to early antigens (EA), which usually fall to undetectable levels by 6 months after infection. The presence of antibodies to EA at later times after acute infection has been considered to indicate possible viral reactivation.[20] Antibodies to EBV-associated nuclear antigen (EBNA) develop 3 to 4 weeks after primary infection and probably persist for life, as do IgG antibodies to VCA.

Prospective studies using antibodies to EA as a marker of recent maternal EBV infection have yielded conflicting results. In a group of 719 women evaluated by Icart and Didier, pregnancies associated with early fetal death, birth of infants with a congenital abnormality, prematurity or intrauterine growth retardation, and deaths or illnesses during the first week of life were more common in women who were EA antibody positive during the first 3 months of pregnancy than in those who were not.[21] Whether these women had a recent primary EBV infection or reactivation of an infection cannot be determined because EBV EA antibodies persist in some otherwise healthy adults and are also associated with the reactivation of past EBV infection. In contrast, Fleisher and Bolognese noted that the frequency of antibodies to EA in pregnant women was 55%, compared with 22 to 32% among nonpregnant adults, but the incidence of low birth weight, neonatal jaundice, and congenital anomalies was not increased among infants of women with anti-EA antibodies.[22]

Primary EBV infection during pregnancy is unusual[23] because only 3.0 to 3.4% of pregnant women are susceptible.[24, 25] Recent primary EBV infection is diagnosed by the presence of VCA IgG and IgM antibodies in the absence of antibodies to EBV-associated nuclear antigen.[26] Six women were studied who had primary EBV infections during pregnancy as established by the presence of IgM antibody to VCA and the absence of antibody to EBNA in their sera.[24] Of these, only one had symptoms compatible with mononucleosis during pregnancy; she gave birth to a normal infant. Four of the

remaining five pregnancies terminated abnormally. One woman had a spontaneous abortion, and the other three were delivered of premature infants. All three of the premature infants were abnormal. One was stillborn, one had multiple congenital anomalies, and one was small for gestational age. The products of abortion and the premature infants were not studied for evidence of an EBV infection. The abnormal infants in this study did not have a characteristic syndrome but instead had a variety of abnormalities.

Fleisher and Bolognese identified three infants born to women who had had silent EBV seroconversion during the first trimester.[27] Two infants were normal; one infant had tricuspid atresia. EBV IgM was not detected in cord blood serum, and EBV was not recovered from the cord blood lymphocytes. Three infants of mothers with a primary EBV infection and infectious mononucleosis were normal at birth and had no serologic or virologic evidence of intrauterine infection.[28]

Early reports implicated EBV as a cause of congenital anomalies, particularly congenital heart disease; however, Tallqvist and colleagues were unable to show an increase in incidence of antibodies to EBV in 6- to 23-month-old children with congenital heart disease compared with normal age-matched controls.[29] EBV might cause congenital heart disease in an individual case, but this study suggests that it is not a common cause of cardiac defects. Brown and Stenchever described an infant with multiple congenital anomalies who was born to a mother who had a positive Monospot test 4 weeks before conception as well as at 16 and 36 weeks' gestation.[30] In addition to the anomalies, which involved many organs, the infant was small for gestational age. Normal chromosomal complements were found on standard and G-banded karyotypes. The total IgM level in the cord blood was not elevated. Studies were not performed for IgM VCA antibody or antibody to EA, and no attempts were made to isolate EBV. Therefore, although the evidence that the mother had mononucleosis near the time of conception is convincing, there is no virologic evidence that EBV was the cause of the anomalies. Goldberg and associates described an infant born with hypotonia, micrognathia, bilateral cataracts, metaphyseal lucencies, and thrombocytopenia.[31] Immunologic evidence suggesting possible EBV infection included elevated total IgM level, presence of IgM anti-VCA antibody at 22 days of age, and delay in development of anti-EBNA antibody until 42 days of age. Weaver and co-workers described an infant with extrahepatic bile duct atresia and evidence of intrauterine EBV infection; EBV IgM was noted in serum obtained from the infant at 3 and 6 weeks of age, and persistent EBV IgG was seen at 1 year.[32]

Although EBV cannot be recovered by standard tissue culture methods, the virus can be detected by its capacity to transform B lymphocytes into persistent lymphoblastoid cell lines. In studies to identify cases of intrauterine EPV infection, Visintine and colleagues[33] and Chang and Blankenship[34] observed spontaneous transformation of lymphocytes obtained from cord blood, but it was not associated with EBV. EBV-transformed cells were not found in any samples of cord blood from 2000 newborns studied by Chang and Seto[35] or from the 25 newborns tested by Joncas and associates.[36, 37] One study used nested PCR methods for amplifying EBV-DNA regions in circulating lymphocytes from 67 mother-infant pairs within 1 week of birth.[38] Approximately 50% of the women and 2 of the neonates were EBV PCR positive. Visintine and colleagues studied 82 normal term infants, 28 infants with congenital anomalies, and 29 infants suspected of having congenital infections; they were unable to isolate EBV from any of these infants.[33] Two infants have been described in whom there was evidence of infection with EBV at birth.[37, 39] A congenital cytomegalovirus (CMV) infection coexisted in both. Most of the clinical findings in the infants were compatible with those usually found in congenital CMV infections and included microcephaly, periventricular calcifications, hepatosplenomegaly, and inclusions characteristic of CMV in sections of tissues or cells in urinary sediments. One infant had deformities of the hands similar to those seen in arthrogryposis. Neither CMV nor EBV was isolated from the saliva or secretions of these infants. In the first infant, IgM antibody to EBV was present at birth and EBNA-positive permanent lymphoblastoid cell lines were established on five occasions between 3 and 30 months of age. In the second infant, permanent lymphoblastoid cell lines were established from the peripheral blood at birth and from heart blood at 3 days of age. EBNA and EBV RNA were identified in these cells, and CMV DNA was identified in the cells from the liver of the same infant.

Attempts to isolate EBV from secretions obtained from the maternal cervix have been unsuccessful,[33, 35] but the virus can be detected at this site by DNA hybridization.[40] There is little evidence suggesting that natal transmission of EBV occurs. However, EBV was recovered from genital ulcers in a young woman with infectious mononucleosis.[41] Fatal EBV infection was diagnosed by DNA hybridization of lymph node tissue from one infant who presented with failure to thrive, emesis, diarrhea, and a macular rash at 14 days of age, but this infection may have been acquired in utero.[42]

EBV can be transmitted to newborns in the perinatal period by blood transfusion.[33, 36] Permanent lymphoblastoid lines that contained EBV antigens were established by Joncas and co-workers[36] from the blood of two infants who had been transfused. One of these infants did not develop permanent antibodies to EBV.

There is no evidence at present that EBV causes congenital anomalies. Because both the early and the late serologic responses of young infants to a primary EBV infection differ from those found when a primary infection occurs at an older age,[20, 36, 43] it will be difficult to screen large numbers of newborns for serologic evidence of an EBV infection sustained in utero.

HUMAN HERPESVIRUS 6

Human herpesvirus 6 (HHV-6) is a newly recognized member of the herpesvirus family that has been identified as a cause of exanthema subitum (roseola).[44–46] The virus exhibits tropism for T lymphocytes and is most closely related to human CMV by genetic analysis.[47]

Seroepidemiologic studies have shown that HHV-6 is ubiquitous in the human population regardless of geographic area and that it infects more than 90% of infants during the first year of life. IgG antibodies to HHV-6 are detected in almost all infants at birth, with a subsequent decline in seropositivity rates by 4 to 6 months of age as transplacentally acquired antibody is lost. The highest rate of acquisition of HHV-6 infection appears to occur from 6 months to 1 year of age as maternal antibodies wane. The seroepidemiologic evidence and restriction enzyme analysis of paired virus isolates from mothers and their infants suggest that the usual route of transmission is perinatal or postnatal.[48] No cases of symptomatic intrauterine HHV-6 infection have been confirmed since the agent was identified in 1986. A case of intrauterine infection was documented by PCR in a fetus whose mother had human immunodeficiency virus infection and HHV-6 in peripheral blood mononuclear cells,[49] and 1 of 799 cord blood serum samples (0.28%) had IgM antibodies to HHV-6.[50] Another study utilizing HHV-6 DNA PCR applied to cord blood specimens from 305 infants demonstrated a 1.6% (5/305) PCR positivity rate, suggesting in utero transmission.[51] Evidence of reinfection after presumed congenital HHV-6 infection has also been demonstrated.[52] As diagnostic assays become more widely available, congenital infections may be recognized. However, primary HHV-6 infection, with its anticipated higher risk of transmission to the fetus, should be quite rare during pregnancy because almost all adult women have been infected in childhood. By analogy with human CMV, the reactivation of maternal HHV-6, although it may be common during pregnancy, would not be expected to cause symptomatic intrauterine infection.

In addition to the roseola syndrome, HHV-6 has been detected by PCR in peripheral blood lymphocytes obtained from infants younger than 3 months old with acute, nonspecific febrile illnesses.[53, 54] Two neonates who had fulminant hepatitis associated with HHV-6 infection have been described.[55, 56] Other associations among infants include a mononucleosis-like syndrome,[57] pneumonitis,[58] and one case report of possible immunodeficiency and pneumonitis associated with HHV-6 infection.[59] However, all clinical associations between disease in infants and HHV-6 infection must be evaluated with care because of the evidence that the majority of infants become infected with this virus within a few months after birth and that the virus persists after primary infection, as is characteristic of herpesviruses.[49] In clinical practice, it is also important to be aware of the potential for false-positive results in serologic assays and in attempts to detect the virus by PCR.[46]

INFLUENZA A AND B

Most investigations of the teratogenic potential of influenza virus have been epidemiologic studies in which the diagnosis of influenza was not confirmed serologically.[60] In 1959, Coffey and Jessup reported an incidence of 3.6% of congenital defects in 664 Irish women who had histories of having had influenza during pregnancy compared with 1.5% in 663 women who did not have symptoms compatible with influenza.[60] Central nervous system anomalies were the most common type of defect, and, of these, anencephaly was the most frequent. These investigators presented some evidence that women who had a history of having had influenza in the first trimester were more likely to give birth to children who had congenital anomalies than those who had influenza later in the pregnancy. This evidence lent credence to the report.

In a similar study conducted in Scotland, Doll and Hill were unable to confirm that congenital anomalies occurred with a higher frequency in infants of women who had histories of influenza during pregnancy than in infants of women who did not.[61] However, after reviewing the reported incidence of stillbirth related to anencephaly recorded by the Registrar-General for Scotland, they concluded that there was a small increase in risk of anencephaly if the mother had had influenza during the first 2 months of pregnancy. In performing this analysis, certain assumptions were made because of the lack of precise data. Record[62] and Leck[63] analyzed the same data and were unable to find an association between influenza and malformations of the central nervous system. An increase in congenital defects in infants of mothers who had influenza-like symptoms at 5 to 11 weeks of gestation was reported by Hakosalo and Saxen.[64] The majority of these anomalies involved the central nervous system, but there was no increase in incidence of anencephaly in infants of women who had symptoms compatible with influenza compared with those who remained asymptomatic.

All of these studies were undertaken during influenza epidemics. It was assumed that, under these circumstances, there would be a high correlation between a history of influenza as elicited from the patient and infection with influenza virus. However, during the 1957 outbreak, Wilson and Stein demonstrated that 60% of pregnant women who denied symptoms of influenza had serologic evidence of having been recently infected.[65] Conversely, 35% of those who stated that they had had influenza lacked serologic evidence of having been infected. Likewise, Hardy and co-workers found that 24% of those who stated that they had had influenza lacked serologic evidence of past infection with the epidemic strain and 39% of those with titers suggesting recent infection denied symptoms of influenza.[66] MacKenzie and Houghton have summarized the reports implicating influenza virus as a cause of maternal morbidity and congenital anomalies and have assessed the validity of the reports.[67]

Several studies have been performed in which infection by influenza virus has been serologically confirmed. Hardy and co-workers reported that the incidence of stillbirths was higher in 332 symptomatic pregnant women with serologically confirmed influenza infections than in 206 women with serologically confirmed infections who had remained asymptomatic or in 73 uninfected women.[66] The control group of uninfected women was smaller than expected because the attack rate during the period of the study was very high. Major congenital anomalies occurred in 5.3% of women whose infections occurred during the first trimester compared with 2.1% of 183 women infected during the second trimester and 1.1% of 275 women infected during the third trimester. Supernumerary digits, syndactyly, and skin anomalies were excluded from these figures. Among infants of mothers infected during the first trimester, cardiac anomalies were the most common type of anomaly; none of these infants had anencephaly. Griffiths and associates[68] noted a slight increase in congenital anomalies in infants born to women who had had serologically confirmed influenza during pregnancy compared with infants of women who had not; however, all of the infants with congenital anomalies were born to women who had had influenza in the second or third trimester. Monif and colleagues[69] did not document infection in any of eight infants born to mothers who had influenza A/Hong Kong infections in the second and third trimesters. Wilson and Stein noted no increase in congenital anomalies in women with serologic evidence of having been recently infected with influenza virus who had conceived during the 3-month period when influenza was epidemic.[65]

It can be said with certainty that intrauterine exposure to influenza virus does not cause a consistent syndrome. If there is a cause-and-effect association between influenza virus infections during pregnancy and congenital anomalies, the latter occur with low frequency. Hakosalo and Saxen have documented an increase in the use of nonprescription drugs during influenza outbreaks and have suggested that drugs rather than infection with influenza virus may exert an erratic teratogenic influence.[64]

Viremia is rare during influenza infections, but it does occur. Few attempts have been made to demonstrate transplacental passage of the virus to the fetus. Ruben and colleagues tested the cord sera of infants born to 22 mothers who had been pregnant during an influenza A/England/42/72 outbreak and who had had influenza hemagglutination inhibition titers to this virus of 1:16 or higher while pregnant.[70] In addition, 42 random cord serum samples were collected from infants who had been born on the same day as the selected infants. Of the 64 cord serum samples tested, in 4 a fall in titer of fourfold or more was noted after treatment with 2-

mercaptoethanol; this suggests that IgM antibody to influenza might have been present. Three of 16 cord blood samples tested gave positive lymphocyte transformation responses to influenza virus. All seven of the infants with evidence of antigenic recognition of influenza virus at birth had uncomplicated deliveries and remained healthy. Influenza A/Bangkok was isolated from the amniotic fluid of a mother with amnionitis and acute influenza infection at 36 weeks of gestation; the infant who was born at 39 weeks had serologic evidence of infection but was asymptomatic.[71]

Yawn and associates studied a woman who developed influenza in the third trimester and died of pulmonary edema.[72] A virus similar to the prototype strain A_2/Hong Kong/8/68 was isolated from the lung, hilar nodes, heart, spleen, liver, kidney, brain, and spinal cord of the mother and from the amniotic fluid and myocardium of the fetus. Ramphal and colleagues studied another woman who died of complications of an influenza infection at term.[73] A virus similar to strain A/Texas/77 was isolated from maternal tissues, but influenza virus was not isolated from any of the fetal tissues tested.

In contrast to intrauterine infections with influenza virus, which are rare, infections acquired by infants in the neonatal period are not uncommon. Passively transferred antibody to influenza virus may prevent symptomatic infections during the first few months of life if it is present in sufficient quantity.[74, 75] Two cases of influenza A/Hong Kong/68 infection in infants who were younger than 1 month of age were described by Bauer and associates.[76] The first infant developed high fever, irritability, and nasal discharge at 10 days of age; the second infant, who was premature, developed fever and nasal congestion at 14 days of age. Symptoms were restricted to the upper respiratory system, and both infants recovered within 4 days of onset of the illness. Influenza virus infection may, however, be fatal in the neonatal period.[77] Several outbreaks of influenza virus infection have occurred in neonatal intensive care units. In general, illness has been mild.[76, 78] Most of the eight infected neonates described by Meibalane and co-workers[78] had nonspecific symptoms, including apnea, lethargy, and poor feeding. Only two had cough or nasal congestion. None had tachypnea or respiratory distress, but three of five in whom chest roentgenograms were done had interstitial pneumonia.

Infants younger than 6 months of age cannot be protected by influenza vaccine. Therefore, it is important to encourage all health care professionals who care for high-risk newborns to receive the influenza A/influenza B vaccine annually in the fall. Pregnancy is not a contraindication for the administration of influenza vaccine.[79]

RESPIRATORY SYNCYTIAL VIRUS

Although respiratory syncytial virus (RSV) is a common cause of upper respiratory tract infection in adults, there is no evidence that the virus causes intrauterine infection. Maternal infection has no known adverse effect on the fetus.

RSV infections are frequently acquired by infants dur-

ing the first few weeks of life and are associated with a high mortality rate. Two thirds of all infants will be infected with RSV in the first year of life, one third of those will develop lower respiratory tract symptoms, 2.5% will be hospitalized, and 1 in 1000 infants will die as a result of RSV infection.[80] It was originally thought that passively transferred maternal antibody to RSV contributed to the severity of the infection in young infants by causing an immunopathologic reaction in the lung.[81] Later, studies of the age-corrected incidence of symptomatic RSV infections showed a relative sparing of infants who were younger than 3 weeks of age.[82, 83] This is the period during which maternal antibody is the highest. In subsequent studies, no evidence was found that the presence of maternal antibody adversely influenced the course of infection in the infant.[84] In fact, Lamprecht and colleagues found an inverse relationship between the level of maternal neutralizing antibody and the severity of the RSV infection in the infant.[85] Glezen and co-workers found that the quantity of neutralizing antibody to RSV in cord sera was lower in infants with proven RSV infections than in randomly selected infants.[86] None of the infected infants who had antibody titers of 1:16 or higher developed serious infections. Some have suggested that breast-feeding decreases the possibility that an infant will have a serious RSV infection early in life[87]; however, this has not been a consistent finding in every study. Because breast-feeding and crowded living conditions both affect the incidence of RSV infection in infants, studies have been difficult to perform.

Infection with RSV in infants who are younger than 4 weeks of age may be asymptomatic, consist of an afebrile upper respiratory syndrome, or be accompanied by fever, bronchiolitis or pneumonia, and apnea.[88] RSV accounted for 55% of cases of viral pneumonia in infants younger than 1 month of age in one study that evaluated hospitalized infants over a 5-year period.[89] Deaths occur most frequently in infants with underlying medical conditions that involve the heart or lungs.[90, 91] Premature infants who have recovered from hyaline membrane disease and who have bronchopulmonary dysplasia are especially likely to develop severe infections. The A subtype of RSV may have the potential to cause more severe disease than the B subtype.[92]

The nosocomial outbreaks that have occurred in nurseries caring for premature and ill term infants have varied in severity. Neligan and colleagues[93] described an outbreak in which eight infants were infected. The first symptom in all infants was the development of a clear nasal discharge at 10 to 52 days of age. Cough developed 2 to 7 days later. Three infants developed wheezing, and only one infant was seriously ill. In the outbreak described by Berkovich and Taranko,[94] 14 infants in a premature nursery became ill at 11 to 184 days of age. Of the 14 infants, 93% had coryza, 86% had dyspnea, 64% had pneumonia, and 36% had fever. Upper respiratory tract symptoms began 1 to 8 days before the first dyspnea in 11 infants. Changes compatible with pneumonia were demonstrable on chest roentgenograms 3 to 5 days before clinical evidence of lower respiratory tract involvement developed. The degree of illness in the nine infants studied by Mintz and associates was mild in four, moderate in two, and severe in two.[95] One infant was asymptomatic. The infants who were the most seriously ill had fever, cyanosis, pulmonary infiltrates, and respiratory deterioration. Infants with RSV infections have developed respiratory arrests as a result of apnea.[96, 97] Most infants infected during nosocomial outbreaks of RSV in nurseries were born prematurely but had attained 4 weeks or more in chronologic age at the time they developed the infections.[95, 96] Two nursery outbreaks were associated with dual infections caused by RSV and rhinovirus or parainfluenza virus 3.[98, 99] A diffuse viral pneumonia, which is indistinguishable from severe RSV pneumonia, can be caused in rare instances by parainfluenza viruses alone or, very rarely, by adenovirus.[100] Hall and co-workers have shown that infants who are younger than 3 weeks of age when they become infected with RSV have a higher incidence of nonspecific signs and a lower incidence of lower respiratory tract infection than infants who are more than 3 weeks of age at the time of infection.[101] RSV has been recovered from the oropharynx of infants who were younger than 48 hours old.[102] Thus, it may be difficult to recognize the index case when RSV is introduced into the nursery.[103]

Infants who are younger than 1 month of age have a higher mean maximal titer of virus in their secretions than those who are older.[104] Ninety-six percent of the infected infants studied by Hall and co-workers[104] shed virus for 9 days. Objects contaminated with secretions from infected infants may be important sources of infection in nursery personnel. It has been shown that RSV in infected secretions is viable for up to 6 hours on countertops, for up to 45 minutes on cloth gowns and paper tissues and for up to 20 minutes on skin.[105] Present evidence suggests that personnel are at least as important in spreading the infection to infants as are other infected infants housed in the same area and that infection control measures can reduce the risk of transmission.[106–108]

Any infant with rhinorrhea, nasal congestion, or unexplained apnea should be segregated and investigated for RSV infection. Personnel should be made aware that this agent, which causes only mild colds in adults, can cause fatal illnesses in infants. The specific diagnosis of RSV infection should be sought because aerosolized ribavirin treatment has some effectiveness in infants with lower respiratory infection caused by this virus.[109–112] Methods have been described for administering ribavirin safely to infants receiving mechanical ventilation.[113, 114] Questions concerning the benefits of ribavirin therapy for RSV pneumonia and the indications for its use remain.[115, 116] There is still a lack of consensus regarding appropriate management of the infant with RSV infection specifically with respect to the use of aerosolized ribavirin.[117, 118] To date, despite a number of studies in the United States and Canada regarding the use of aerosolized ribavirin, no clear improvement in clinical outcomes is consistent across all studies of both ventilated and nonventilated infants with RSV infection. However, infants who should be considered candidates for ribavirin therapy include those who are at increased risk for complications of RSV due to congenital heart disease, chronic lung disease, or immunodeficiency; infants with severe illness and signs of respiratory failure based on arterial oxygen concentrations of less than 65 mm Hg and rising $PaCO_2$ concentrations; and infants who might be compromised by a prolonged illness because of an underlying medical condition.[119] A number of studies have been published that have demonstrated the benefits of RSV intravenous immune globulin (RSV-IGIV) among selected infants at high risk for moderate to severe complications due to RSV infection.[120] In addition, palivizumab, an RSV monoclonal antibody preparation that is intramuscularly administered, has been demonstrated to reduce by 55% hospitalizations due to RSV infection in these high-risk infants.[120] Such high-risk infants include infants and children younger than 2 years of age with chronic lung disease who have required medical therapy for lung disease within 6 months of RSV season and premature infants who were 32 to 35 weeks' gestation at birth. Of importance, RSV-IGIV is contraindicated and palivizumab is not recommended for those with cyanotic congenital heart disease because of possible safety concerns.

Improved survival of infants with RSV infection and underlying cardiopulmonary disease has been reported with advances in intensive care management.[121, 122] Nevertheless, families of infants with medical conditions that predispose to severe RSV disease should be advised to avoid the higher risk of exposure associated with group day care.[123]

LYMPHOCYTIC CHORIOMENINGITIS VIRUS

Lymphocytic choriomeningitis virus (LCV) is spread from animals, primarily rodents, to humans. Person-to-person spread has not been described[124] (Table 18–2). Mice and hamsters have most often been implicated as the source of human infections. When mice acquire

TABLE 18–2
Sources of Maternal or Neonatal Infection

INFECTIOUS AGENT	OTHER PEOPLE WITH SAME INFECTION	ANIMAL
Human papillomavirus	Yes	No
Epstein-Barr virus	Yes	No
Human herpesvirus 6	Yes	No
Influenza viruses	Yes	No
Respiratory syncytial virus	Yes	No
Lymphocytic choriomeningitis virus	No	House mice, pet Syrian hamsters, laboratory rats, rabbits
Molluscum contagiosum virus	Yes	No
Rabies	—	Yes

LCV transplacentally or as newborns, they remain asymptomatic but shed the virus in their urine for months.[125, 126] This phenomenon of "tolerance" has been extensively studied in laboratory-bred strains of mice. Domestic household mice also have been implicated as a source of human cases of infection with LCV.[127] Several outbreaks in animal handlers and in families have been traced to pet Syrian (or golden) hamsters (Mesocricetus auratus).[128, 129] Adult and newborn hamsters remain asymptomatic after infection with LCV and shed the virus in feces and urine for months.[125] In outbreaks in which human cases have been associated with contact with infected hamsters, the location of the hamster's cage correlated with attack rate. When the hamster's cage was in a common living area, 52% of 42 family members in contact with the hamster became infected.[128] In contrast, no one became infected when the cage was located in a more remote area such as a basement or landing. LCV can be shed also by asymptomatic guinea pigs and rats.[125, 126, 129]

The illness caused by LCV is accompanied by fever, headache, nausea, and myalgia lasting 5 to 15 days.[124, 128, 130] In the outbreak of LCV described by Biggar and colleagues, fever occurred in 90% and headache in 85% of patients.[128] Myalgia occurred in 80% and was described as severe. The neck, shoulders, back, and legs were most often involved. Pain on eye movement occurred in 59%, nausea in 53%, and vomiting in 35%. About a fourth of the patients had a sore throat or photophobia. The illness was biphasic in 24% and was accompanied by swollen glands in 16%. Six percent of the patients had a mononucleosis-like illness characterized by intermittent fever, adenopathy, pharyngitis, extreme fatigue, and rash. Twelve percent of those with serologic evidence of having had an infection remained asymptomatic. Arthritis, encephalitis, and meningitis occurred in a minority of cases.

The diagnosis of infection with LCV can be made by isolation of the virus or by serology. The indirect fluorescent antibody titer may be positive as early as the first day of symptoms.[124, 130] The complement fixation titer generally does not rise until 10 days or longer after illness onset.[124, 129] The neutralization titer rises late, usually after the fourth week, but persists the longest.[124, 129] Therefore, a positive indirect fluorescent antibody titer, a falling indirect fluorescent antibody or complement fixation titer, or a rising neutralization titer suggests recent infection with LCV.

LCV infections during pregnancy appear to be associated with abortion, intrauterine infection, and perinatal infection. Ackermann and associates described a 23-year-old woman who developed a febrile illness beginning 4 weeks after she assumed the care of a Syrian hamster.[131] She was 7 months pregnant at the time of the illness and sustained a spontaneous abortion 4 weeks after onset of the fever. LCV was isolated from curettage material. Complement fixation antibodies to LCV were present initially, and neutralizing antibodies appeared later—a pattern compatible with recent infection. Diebel and co-workers[124] studied a pregnant woman who acquired LCV from a hamster and developed meningitis. One month after the onset of illness, a spontaneous abortion

occurred. Biggar and co-workers[128] described a woman who acquired LCV during the first trimester of pregnancy. She had a spontaneous abortion 1 month after onset of the illness. A review of U.S. cases of 26 serologically confirmed congenital LCV infections identified between 1955 and 1996 has been reported.[132] Eighty-five percent (22/26) were term infants with a median birth weight of 3520 g. The most common congenital anomalies identified were chorioretinopathy (88%), macrocephaly (43%), and microcephaly (3%). There was a 35% (n = 9) mortality rate with a 63% (10/16) rate of severe neurologic sequelae among reported survivors. One fourth of mothers had gestational exposure to rodents, and 50% of all women reported symptoms consistent with LCV infection.

Intrauterine infection of the fetus results in congenital hydrocephalus and chorioretinitis. In 1974, Ackermann and associates noted that two children who were born to mothers who had been in contact with hamsters during the second half of pregnancy had hydrocephalus and chorioretinitis.[133] Other problems included severe hyperbilirubinemia and myopia. The serologic pattern typical of recent infection was found in the mothers as well as in the infants and included a falling complement fixation titer and a rising neutralization titer to LCV. Sheinbergas found a statistically significant relationship between the presence of antibody to LCV and the occurrence of hydrocephalus in infants younger than 1 year of age.[130] Thirty percent of 40 infants with hydrocephalus had indirect fluorescent antibody to LCV, whereas only 2.7% of 110 infants with other nervous system diseases had antibody to LCV. Fourteen of 16 (87.5%) children who had serologically confirmed prenatal infection with LCV had hydrocephalus. Of these, 6 (37.5%) had been born with hydrocephalus and the remainder developed it at 1 to 9 weeks of age. Chorioretinal degeneration was found in 81%, and optic disk subatrophy was found in 56%.

Komrower and colleagues[127] described a mother who acquired LCV about a week before delivery. Despite segregation of the infant, LCV was acquired either transplacentally or natally and the infant subsequently became ill. The mother's initial symptoms included malaise, headache, fever, and cough. About 20 days after onset of symptoms and 12 days after delivery, an increase in cells and protein concentration in the cerebrospinal fluid was noted. The diagnosis of infection caused by LCV was confirmed by a rise in the mother's complement fixation titer from 1:2 to 1:64. The infant, who was probably premature, remained relatively stable until 11 days of age, at which time seizures, stiff neck, and mild pleocytosis were noted. The infant developed petechiae and died of a subarachnoid and intracerebral hemorrhage. LCV was isolated from the infant's cerebrospinal fluid and from mice caught in the home of the mother.

Because apparently healthy mice and hamsters may shed LCV chronically, pregnant women should avoid direct contact with these animals as well as with aerosolized excreta. Unless appropriate measures have been taken to ensure that laboratory animals are free of LCV, these precautions should apply to laboratory as well as domestic rodents. LCV causes spontaneous abortions. Hydrocephalus and chorioretinitis are common in infants who have survived intrauterine infection.[130, 133, 134] Women who acquire an LCV infection during the weeks immediately before delivery may transmit the virus to their infants. Although the total number of intrauterine and perinatal infections from LCV is not large, the incidence of serious sequelae in the infant appears to be high.

MOLLUSCUM CONTAGIOSUM

Molluscum contagiosum is a papular rash consisting of multiple discrete lesions that are acanthomas by histologic examination. The skin lesions are caused by a poxlike virus that has been difficult to study because it cannot be propagated in tissue culture. Epidemiologically, molluscum contagiosum is a disease of children and young adults. The virus may be transmitted by sexual conduct, given that the incidence increases among adolescents and young adults. Whether it is transmitted as a perinatal infection is not known.

Five women who delivered infants at a time when they had the lesions of molluscum contagiosum in the genital area have been described by Wilkin.[135] None of the infants developed molluscum contagiosum. Mandel and Lewis reported an infant who developed two papules on the thigh at 1 week of age.[136] These enlarged and were excised at 1 year of age. The results of histologic examination as well as the findings on electron microscopy were compatible with molluscum contagiosum. In 1926, Young reported an infant with molluscum contagiosum of the scalp. The lesions appeared at 1½ months of age.[137] No histologic studies were performed.

RABIES VIRUS

Transplacental transmission of rabies virus to the human fetus has not yet been described, although it is known that transplacental transmission occurs in experimental infections in many species.[138–143]

Spence and associates described an infant who was born 2 days before the onset of the mother's first symptom of encephalitis.[144] The mother died of rabies on the fourth postpartum day. Rabies virus antigens were demonstrated in the cornea, lacrimal gland, and various parts of the brain by fluorescent antibody stain. The child survived despite the fact that both mother and infant lacked neutralizing antibodies to rabies at the time of the birth.

Two reports describe the successful administration of horse antirabies hyperimmune serum and duck embryo vaccine to pregnant women.[138, 144] Unusual untoward effects were not noted, and the infants were delivered at term and were healthy. However, the mothers did not develop serum sickness, anaphylaxis, or neurologic complications. If they had, the viability of the fetus may have been threatened. Horse antiserum to rabies virus has been replaced by human rabies immune globulin. The chance of an adverse reaction to administration of human immune globulin is very small. The vaccine that was previously grown in duck embryos has been replaced with an inactivated vaccine derived from virus grown in human diploid fibroblast cells.[145] No serious reactions have been reported after administration of this vaccine, and it is possible to achieve titers that are about 10-fold higher than those found after administration of the duck embryo vaccine.

Because of the high likelihood of fatal disease after the bite of a rabid animal, postexposure prophylaxis should always be given. Pregnancy is not a contraindication. When it is necessary to administer this prophylaxis to a pregnant woman, human rabies immune globulin and human diploid cell vaccine should be used to minimize potential adverse effects on the pregnancy.

After reviewing the available data, the Advisory Committee on Immunization Practices of the Centers for Disease Control and Prevention has recommended human diploid cell vaccine to rabies virus as a pre-exposure immunization that is safe for use in pregnant women who will likely be exposed to wild rabies virus before completion of pregnancy.[146]

References

Human Papillomavirus (Condyloma Acuminatum)

1. Ono S, Saito H, Igarash M. The etiology of papilloma of the larynx. Ann Otol 66:1119, 1957.
2. Almeida JD, Oriel JD. Wart virus. Br J Dermatol 83:698, 1970.
3. Gissman L, Wolnik L, Ikenberg H, et al. Human papillomavirus types 6 and 11: DNA sequences in genital and laryngeal papillomas and in some cervical cancers. Proc Natl Acad Sci U S A 80:560, 1983.
4. Hajek EF. Contribution to the etiology of laryngeal papilloma in children. J Laryngol 70:166, 1956.
5. Cook TA, Brunschwig JP, Butel JS, et al. Laryngeal papilloma: etiologic and therapeutic considerations. Ann Otol 82:649, 1973.
6. Quick CA, Krzyzek RA, Watts SL, et al. Relationship between condylomata and laryngeal papillomata. Ann Otol 89:467, 1980.
7. Drut R, Gomez MA, Drut RM, et al. Human papillomavirus, neonatal giant cell hepatitis and biliary duct atresia. Acta Gastroenterol Latinoam 28:27–31, 1998.
8. Dias EP, Barcelos JM, Fonseca EF, Basso NG. Congenital papillomas and papillomatoses associated with the human papillomavirus (HPV)—report on 5 cases. Rev Paul Med 113:957–963, 1995.
9. Steinberg BM, Topp WC, Schneider PS, et al. Laryngeal papillomavirus infection during clinical remission. N Engl J Med 308:1261, 1983.
10. Hording U, Iversen AK, Sebbelov A, et al. Prevalence of human papillomavirus types 11, 16 and 18 in cervical swabs: a study of 1362 pregnant women. Eur J Obstet Gynecol Reprod Biol 35:191, 1990.
11. Peng T, Searle CP III, Shah KV, et al. Prevalence of human papillomavirus infections in term pregnancy. Am J Perinatol 7:189, 1990.
12. Kemp EA, Hakenewerth AM, Laurent SL, et al. Human papillomavirus prevalence in pregnancy. Obstet Gynecol 79:649, 1992.
13. Fife KH, Rogers RE, Zwickl BW. Symptomatic and asymptomatic cervical infections with human papillomavirus during pregnancy. J Infect Dis 156:904, 1987.

14. Tang CK, Shermeta DW, Wood C. Congenital condylomata acuminata. Am J Obstet Gynecol 131:912, 1978.
15. Roman A, Fife K. Human papillomavirus DNA associated with foreskins of normal newborns. J Infect Dis 153:855, 1986.
16. Avidano MA, Singleton GT. Adjuvant drug strategies in the treatment of recurrent respiratory papillomatosis. Otolaryngol Head Neck Surg 112:197–202, 1995.
17. Lippman SM, Donovan DT, Frankenthaler RA, et al. 13-*Cis*-retinoic acid plus interferon-alpha 2a in recurrent respiratory papillomatosis. J Natl Cancer Inst 86:859–861, 1994.
18. Eicher SA, Taylor-Cooley LD, Donovan DT. Isotretinoin therapy for recurrent respiratory papillomatosis. Arch Otolaryngol Head Neck Surg 120:405–409, 1994.

Epstein-Barr Virus

19. Henle W, Henle G, Horwitz CA. Epstein-Barr virus–specific diagnostic tests in infectious mononucleosis. Hum Pathol 5:551, 1974.
20. Fleisher G, Henle W, Henle G, et al. Primary Epstein-Barr virus infection in American infants: clinical and serological observations. J Infect Dis 139:553, 1979.
21. Icart J, Didier J. Infections due to Epstein-Barr virus during pregnancy. J Infect Dis 143:499, 1981.
22. Fleisher G, Bolognese R. Persistent Epstein-Barr virus infection and pregnancy. J Infect Dis 147:982, 1983.
23. Le CT, Chang S, Lipson MII. Epstein-Barr virus infections during pregnancy. Am J Dis Child 137:466, 1983.
24. Icart J, Didier J, Dalens M, et al. Etude prospective de l'infection à virus Epstein-Barr (EBV) au cours de la grossesse. Biomedicine 34:160, 1981.
25. Gervais F, Joncas JH. Seroepidemiology in various population groups of the greater Montreal area. Comp Immunol Microbiol Infect Dis 2:207, 1979.
26. Horowitz CA, Henle W, Henle G, et al. Long-term serologic follow-up of patients for Epstein-Barr virus after recovery from infectious mononucleosis. J Infect Dis 151:1150, 1985.
27. Fleisher G, Bolognese R. Epstein-Barr virus infections in pregnancy: a prospective study. J Pediatr 104:374, 1984.
28. Fleisher G, Bolognese R. Infectious mononucleosis during gestation: report of three women and their infants studied prospectively. Pediatr Infect Dis 3:308, 1984.
29. Tallqvist H, Henle W, Klemola E, et al. Antibodies to Epstein-Barr virus at the ages of 6 to 23 months in children with congenital heart disease. Scand J Infect Dis 5:159, 1973.
30. Brown ZA, Stenchever MA. Infectious mononucleosis and congenital anomalies. Am J Obstet Gynecol 131:108, 1978.
31. Goldberg GN, Fulginiti VA, Ray CG, et al. In utero Epstein-Barr virus (infectious mononucleosis) infection. JAMA 246:1579, 1981.
32. Weaver LT, Nelson R, Bell TM. The association of extrahepatic bile duct atresia and neonatal Epstein-Barr virus infection. Acta Paediatr Scand 73:155, 1984.
33. Visintine AJ, Gerber P, Nahmias AJ. Leukocyte transforming agent (Epstein-Barr virus) in newborn infants and older individuals. J Pediatr 89:571, 1976.
34. Chang RS, Blankenship W. Spontaneous in vitro transformation of leukocytes from a neonate. Proc Soc Exp Biol Med 144:337, 1973.
35. Chang RS, Seto DY. Perinatal infection by Epstein-Barr virus. Lancet 2:201, 1979.
36. Joncas J, Boucher J, Granger-Julien M, et al. Epstein-Barr virus in the neonatal period and in childhood. Can Med Assoc J 110:33, 1974.
37. Joncas JH, Wills A, McLaughlin B. Congenital infection with cytomegalovirus and Epstein-Barr virus. Can Med Assoc J 117:1417, 1977.
38. Meyohas MC, Marechal V, Sedire N, et al. Study of mother-to-child Epstein-Barr virus transmission by means of nested PCRs. J Virol 70:6816–6819, 1996.
39. Joncas J, Alfieri C, Leyritz M, et al. Dual congenital infection with the Epstein-Barr virus (EBV) and the cytomegalovirus (CMV). N Engl J Med 304:1399, 1981.
40. Sixbey JW, Lemon SM, Pagano JS. A second site for Epstein-Barr virus shedding: the uterine cervix. Lancet 2:1122, 1986.
41. Portnoy J, Ahronheim GA, Ghibu F, et al. Recovery of Epstein-Barr virus from genital ulcers. N Engl J Med 311:966, 1984.
42. Horwitz CA, McClain K, Henle W, et al. Fatal illness in a 2 week old infant: diagnosis by detection of Epstein-Barr virus genomes from a lymph node biopsy. J Pediatr 103:752, 1983.
43. Gervais F, Joncas JH. Correspondence—an unusual antibody response to Epstein-Barr virus during infancy. J Infect Dis 140:273, 1979.

Human Herpesvirus 6

44. Salahuddin SZ, Ablashi DV, Markham PD, et al. Isolation of a new virus, HBLV, in patients with lymphoproliferative disorders. Science 234:596, 1986.
45. Lopez C, Pellett P, Stewart J, et al. Characteristics of human herpesvirus-6. J Infect Dis 157:1271, 1988.
46. Leach CT, Sumaya CV, Brown NA. Human herpesvirus-6: clinical implications of a recently discovered, ubiquitous agent. J Pediatr 1231:173, 1992.
47. Lawrence GL, Chee M, Craxton MA, et al. Human herpes virus 6 is closely related to human cytomegalovirus. J Virol 64:287, 1989.
48. Yamaniski K, Okada K, Ueda K, et al. Exanthem subitum and human herpes virus 6. Pediatr Infect Dis J 12:204, 1993.
49. Aubi J-T, Poirel L, Agut H, et al. Intrauterine transmission of human herpes virus 6. Lancet 340:482, 1992.
50. Dunne WM, Demmler GJ. Serologic evidence for congenital transmission of human herpesvirus 6. Lancet 340:121, 1992.
51. Adams O, Krempe C, Kogler G, et al. Congenital infections with human herpesvirus 6. J Infect Dis 178:544–546, 1998.
52. van Loon NM, Gummuluru S, Sherwood DJ, et al. Direct sequence analysis of human herpesvirus 6 (HHV-6) sequences from infants and comparison of HHV-6 from mother/infant pairs. Clin Infect Dis 21:1017–1019, 1995.
53. Pruksananonda P, Hall CB, Insel RA, et al. Primary human herpes virus 6 infection in young children. N Engl J Med 22:1445, 1992.
54. Kawaguchi S, Suga S, Kozawa T, et al. Primary human herpesvirus 6 infection (exanthem subitum) in the newborn. Pediatrics 90:628, 1992.
55. Tajiri H, Nose O, Baba K, et al. Human herpesvirus-6 infection with liver injury in neonatal hepatitis. Lancet 335:863, 1990.
56. Asano Y, Yoshikawa T, Suga S, et al. Fatal fulminant hepatitis in an infant with human herpesvirus-6 infection. Lancet 335:862, 1990.
57. Kanegane C, Katayama K, Kyoutani S, et al. Mononucleosis-like illness in an infant associated with human herpesvirus 6 infection. Acta Paediatr Jpn 37:227–229, 1995.
58. Hammerling JA, Lambrecht RS, Kehl KS, Carrigan DR. Prevalence of human herpesvirus 6 in lung tissue from

children with pneumonitis. J Clin Pathol 49:802–804, 1996.

59. Knox KK, Pietryga D, Harrington DJ, et al. Progressive immunodeficiency and fatal pneumonitis associated with human herpesvirus 6 infection in an infant. Clin Infect Dis 20:406–413, 1995.

Influenza A and B

60. Coffey VP, Jessup WJE. Maternal influenza and congenital deformities. Lancet 2:935, 1959.
61. Doll R, Hill AB. Asian influenza in pregnancy and congenital defects. Br J Prev Soc Med 14:167, 1960.
62. Record RG. Anencephalus in Scotland. Br J Prev Soc Med 15:93, 1961.
63. Leck I. Incidence of malformations following influenza epidemics. Br J Prev Soc Med 17:70, 1963.
64. Hakosalo J, Saxen L. Influenza epidemic and congenital defects. Lancet 2:1346, 1971.
65. Wilson MG, Stein AM. Teratogenic effects of Asian influenza. JAMA 210:336, 1969.
66. Hardy JMB, Azarowicz EN, Mannini A, et al. The effect of Asian influenza on the outcome of pregnancy. Baltimore 1957–1958. Am J Public Health 51:1182, 1961.
67. MacKenzie JS, Houghton M. Influenza infections during pregnancy: association with congenital malformations and with subsequent neoplasms in children, and potential hazards of live virus vaccines. Bacteriol Rev 38:356, 1974.
68. Griffiths PD, Ronalds CJ, Heath RB. A prospective study of influenza infections during pregnancy. J Epidemiol Community Health 34:124, 1980.
69. Monif GRG, Soward DL, Eitzman DV. Serologic and immunologic evaluation of neonates following maternal influenza infection during the second and third trimesters. Am J Obstet Gynecol 114:239, 1972.
70. Ruben FL, Winkelstein A, Sabbagha RE. In utero sensitization with influenza virus in man (38918). Proc Soc Exp Biol Med 149:881, 1975.
71. McGregor JA, Burns JC, Levin MJ, et al. Transplacental passage of influenza A/Bangkok (H3N2) mimicking amniotic fluid infection syndrome. Am J Obstet Gynecol 149:856, 1984.
72. Yawn DH, Pyeatte JC, Joseph MM, et al. Transplacental transfer of influenza virus. JAMA 216:1022, 1971.
73. Ramphal R, Donnelly WH, Small PA. Fatal influenzal pneumonia in pregnancy: failure to demonstrate transplacental transmissions of influenza virus. Am J Obstet Gynecol 138:347, 1980.
74. Puck JM, Glezen WP, Frank AL, et al. Protection of infants from infection with influenza A virus by transplacentally acquired antibody. J Infect Dis 142:844, 1980.
75. Reuman PD, Ayoub EM, Small PA. Effect of passive maternal antibody on influenza illness in children: a prospective study of influenza A in mother-infant pairs. Pediatr Infect Dis J 6:398, 1987.
76. Bauer CR, Elie K, Spence L, et al. Hong Kong influenza in a neonatal unit. JAMA 223:1233, 1973.
77. Joshi VV, Escobar MR, Stewart L, et al. Fatal influenza A₂ viral pneumonia in a newborn infant. Am J Dis Child 126:839, 1973.
78. Meibalane R, Sedmak GV, Sasidharan P, et al. Outbreak of influenza in a neonatal intensive care unit. J Pediatr 91:974, 1977.
79. Sumaya CV, Gibbs RS. Immunization of pregnant women with influenza A/New Jersey/76 virus vaccine: reactogenicity and immunogenicity in mothers and infants. J Infect Dis 140:141, 1979.

Respiratory Syncytial Virus

80. Holberg CJ, Wright AL, Martinez FD, et al. Risk factors for respiratory syncytial virus–associated lower respiratory illnesses in the first year of life. Am J Epidemiol 133:1135–1151, 1991.
81. Chanock RM, Kapikian AZ, Mills J, et al. Influence of immunological factors in respiratory syncytial virus disease. Arch Environ Health 21:347, 1970.
82. Jacobs JW, Peacock DB, Corner BD, et al. Respiratory syncytial and other viruses associated with respiratory disease in infants. Lancet 1:871, 1971.
83. Parrott RH, Kim HW, Arrobio JO. Epidemiology of respiratory syncytial virus infection in Washington, D. C: II. Infection and disease with respect to age, immunologic status, race and sex. Am J Epidemiol 98:289, 1973.
84. Bruhn FW, Yeager AS. Respiratory syncytial virus in early infancy. Am J Dis Child 131:145, 1977.
85. Lamprecht CL, Krause HE, Mufson MA. Role of maternal antibody in pneumonia and bronchiolitis due to respiratory syncytial virus. J Infect Dis 134:211, 1976.
86. Glezen WP, Paredes A, Allison JE, et al. Risk of respiratory syncytial virus infection for infants from low-income families in relationship to age, sex, ethnic group, and maternal antibody level. J Pediatr 98:708, 1981.
87. Downham M, Scott R, Sims DG, et al. Breast-feeding protects against respiratory syncytial virus infections. BMJ 2:274, 1976.
88. Bruhn FW, Mokrohisky ST, McIntosh K. Apnea associated with respiratory syncytial virus infection in young infants. J Pediatr 90:382, 1977.
89. Abzug MJ, Beam AC, Gyorkos EA, et al. Viral pneumonia in the first month of life. Pediatr Infect Dis J 9:881, 1990.
90. MacDonald NE, Hall CB, Suffin SC, et al. Respiratory syncytial viral infection in infants with congenital heart disease. N Engl J Med 307:397, 1982.
91. Abman SH, Ogle JW, Butler-Simon N, et al. Role of respiratory syncytial virus in early hospitalizations for respiratory distress of young infants with cystic fibrosis. J Pediatr 113:826, 1988.
92. McConnochie KM, Hall CB, Walsh EE, et al. Variation in severity of respiratory syncytial virus infections with subtype. J Pediatr 117:52, 1990.
93. Neligan GA, Steiner H, Gardner PS, et al. Respiratory syncytial virus infection of the newborn. BMJ 3:146, 1970.
94. Berkovich S, Taranko L. Acute respiratory illness in the premature nursery associated with respiratory syncytial virus infection. Pediatrics 34:753, 1964.
95. Mintz L, Ballard RA, Sniderman SH, et al. Nosocomial respiratory syncytial virus infections in an intensive care nursery: rapid diagnosis by direct immunofluorescence. Pediatrics 64:149, 1979.
96. Goldson EJ, McCarthy JT, Welling MA, et al. A respiratory syncytial virus outbreak in a transitional care nursery. Am J Dis Child 133:1280, 1979.
97. Church NR, Anas NG, Hall CB. Respiratory syncytial virus–related apnea in infants: demographics and outcome. Am J Dis Child 138:247, 1984.
98. Valenti WM, Clarke TA, Hall CB, et al. Concurrent outbreaks of rhinovirus and respiratory syncytial virus in an intensive care nursery: epidemiology and associated risk factors. J Pediatr 100:722, 1982.
99. Meissner HC, Murray SA, Kiernan MA, et al. A simultaneous outbreak of respiratory syncytial virus and parainfluenza virus type 3 in a newborn nursery. J Pediatr 104:680, 1984.
100. Wensley DF, Baldwin VJ. Respiratory distress in the second week of life. J Pediatr 106:326, 1985.
101. Hall CB, Kopelman AE, Douglas RG, et al. Neonatal

respiratory syncytial virus infection. N Engl J Med 300:393, 1979.

102. Wilson CW, Stevenson DK, Arvin AM. A concurrent epidemic of respiratory syncytial virus and echovirus 7 infections in an intensive care nursery. Pediatr Infect Dis J 8:24, 1989.

103. Unger A, Tapia L, Minnich LL, et al. Atypical neonatal respiratory syncytial virus infection. J Pediatr 100:762, 1982.

104. Hall CB, Douglas RG Jr, Geiman JM. Respiratory syncytial virus infections in infants: quantitation and duration of shedding. J Pediatr 89:11, 1976.

105. Hall CB, Douglas RG Jr, Geiman JM. Possible transmission by fomites or respiratory syncytial virus. J Infect Dis 141:98, 1980.

106. Snydman DR, Greer C, Meissner HC, et al. Prevention of nosocomial transmission of respiratory syncytial virus in a newborn nursery. Infect Control Hosp Epidemiol 9:105, 1988.

107. Leclair JM, Freeman J, Sullivan BF, et al. Prevention of nosocomial respiratory syncytial virus infections through compliance with glove and gown isolation precautions. N Engl J Med 317:329, 1987.

108. Agah R, Cherry JD, Garakian AJ, et al. Respiratory syncytial virus (RSV) infection rate in personnel caring for children with RSV infections. Routine isolation procedure vs routine procedure supplemented by use of masks and goggles. Am J Dis Child 141:695, 1987.

109. Hall CB, McBride JT, Walsh EE, et al. Aerosolized ribavirin treatment of infants with respiratory syncytial viral infection: a randomized double-blind study. N Engl J Med 308:1443, 1983.

110. Hall CB, McBride JT, Gala CL, et al. Ribavirin treatment of respiratory syncytial viral infection in infants with underlying cardiopulmonary disease. JAMA 254:3047, 1985.

111. Rodriguez WJ, Kim HW, Brandt CD, et al. Aerosolized ribavirin in the treatment of patients with respiratory syncytial virus disease. Pediatr Infect Dis J 6:159, 1987.

112. Conrad DA, Christenson JC, Waner JL, et al. Aerosolized ribavirin treatment of respiratory syncytial virus infection in infants hospitalized during an epidemic. Pediatr Infect Dis J 6:152, 1987.

113. Outwater KM, Meissner HC, Peterson MB. Ribavirin administration to infants receiving mechanical ventilation. Am J Dis Child 142:512, 1988.

114. Frankel LR, Wilson CW, Demers RR, et al. A technique for the administration of ribavirin to mechanically ventilated infants with severe respiratory syncytial virus infection. Crit Care Med 15:1051, 1987.

115. American Academy of Pediatrics Committee on Infectious Diseases. Ribavirin therapy of respiratory syncytial virus. Pediatrics 79:475, 1987.

116. Wald ER, Dashefsky B, Green M. In re ribavirin: a case of premature adjudication? J Pediatr 112:154, 1988.

117. Prober CG, Wang EEL. Reducing the morbidity of lower respiratory tract infections caused by respiratory syncytial virus: still no answer. Pediatrics 99:472–475, 1997.

118. American Academy of Pediatrics. Committee on Infectious Diseases. Reassessment of the indications for ribavirin therapy in respiratory syncytial virus infections. Pediatrics 97:137–140, 1996.

119. Ribavirin therapy of respiratory syncytial virus. In Lepow PG, McCrachen ML, Phillips CF (eds). Report of the Committee on Infectious Diseases. Elk Grove Village, Ill, American Academy of Pediatrics, 1991, pp 581–586.

120. American Academy of Pediatrics. Committee on Infectious Diseases and Committee on Fetus and Newborn. Prevention of respiratory syncytial virus infections: indications for the use of palivizumab and update on the use of RSV-IGIV. Pediatrics 102:1211–1216, 1998.

121. Moler FW, Khan AS, Meliones JN, et al. Respiratory syncytial virus morbidity and mortality estimates in congenital heart disease patients: a recent experience. Crit Care Med 20:1406, 1992.

122. Navas L, Wang E, de Carvalho V, et al. Improved outcome of respiratory syncytial virus infection in a high-risk hospitalized population of Canadian children. J Pediatr 121:348, 1992.

123. Anderson LJ, Parker RA, Strikas RA, et al. Day-care center attendance and hospitalization for lower respiratory tract illness. Pediatrics 82:300, 1988.

Lymphocytic Choriomeningitis Virus

124. Diebel R, Woodall JP, Decher WJ, et al. Lymphocytic choriomeningitis virus in man: serologic evidence of association with pet hamster. JAMA 232:501, 1975.

125. Smadel JE, Wall MJ. Lymphocytic choriomeningitis in the Syrian hamster. J Exp Med 75:581, 1942.

126. Traub E. Persistence of lymphochoriomeningitis virus in immune animals and its relation to immunity. J Exp Med 63:847, 1936.

127. Komrower GM, Williams BL, Stones PB. Lymphocytic choriomeningitis in the newborn. Lancet 1:697, 1955.

128. Biggar RJ, Woodall JP, Walter PD, et al. Lymphocytic choriomeningitis outbreak associated with pet hamsters: fifty-seven cases from New York state. JAMA 232:494, 1975.

129. Hotchin J. The contamination of laboratory animals with lymphocytic choriomeningitis virus. Am J Pathol 64:747, 1971.

130. Sheinbergas MM. Hydrocephalus due to prenatal infection with the lymphocytic choriomeningitis virus. Infection 4:185, 1974.

131. Ackermann R, Stammler A, Armbruster B. Isolierung von Virus der lymphozytären Choriomeningitis aus Abrasionsmaterial nach Kontakt der Schwangeren mit einem Syrischen Goldhamster (Mesocricetus auratus). Infection 3:47, 1975.

132. Wright R, Johnson D, Neumann M, et al. Congenital lymphocytic choriomeningitis virus syndrome: a disease that mimics congenital toxoplasmosis or cytomegalovirus infection. Pediatrics 100:E9, 1997.

133. Ackermann R, Körver G, Turss R, et al. Pränatale Infektion mit dem Virus der lymphozytären Choriomeningitis. Dtsch Med Wochenschr 99:629, 1974.

134. Chastel C, Bosshard S, LeGoff F, et al. Infection transplacentaire par le virus de la choriomeningite lymphocytaire. Nouv Presse Med 7:1089, 1978.

Molluscum Contagiosum

135. Wilkin JK. Molluscum contagiosum venereum in a women's outpatient clinic: a venereally transmitted disease. Am J Obstet Gynecol 128:531, 1977.

136. Mandel MJ, Lewis RJ. Molluscum contagiosum of the newborn. Br J Dermatol 84:370, 1970.

137. Young WJ. Molluscum contagiosum with unusual distribution. Kentucky Med J 24:467, 1926.

Rabies Virus

138. Cates W Jr. Treatment of rabies exposure during pregnancy. Obstet Gynecol 44:893, 1974.

139. Martell MA, Montes FC, Alcocer RB. Transplacental transmission of bovine rabies after natural infection. J Infect Dis 127:291, 1973.

140. Geneverlay J, Dodero J. Note sur un enfant né d'une mere en etat du rage. Ann Inst Pasteur Paris 55:124, 1935.

141. Viazhevich VK. A case of birth of a healthy baby to a mother during the incubation period of rabies. Zh Mikrobiol Epidemiol Immunobiol 28:1022, 1957.

142. Machada CG, Zatz I, Saraiva PA, et al. Observations sur un enfant né de mere atteinte de rage et soumis du traitement prophylactique par le serum et le vaccome amtorabiques. Bull Soc Pathol Exp 59:764, 768, 1966.

143. Relova RN. The hydrophobia boy. J Philipp Med Assoc 39:765, 1963.

144. Spence MR, Davidson DE, Dill GS, et al. Rabies exposure during pregnancy. Am J Obstet Gynecol 123:655, 1975.

145. Meyer HM. FDA: rabies vaccine. J Infect Dis 142:287, 1980.

146. Public Health Service Advisory Committee on Immunization Practices. Rabies prevention. MMWR Morb Mortal Wkly Rep 29:265, 1980.

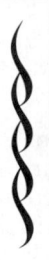

C H A P T E R 1 9

Protozoan and Helminth Infections (Including *Pneumocystis carinii*)

YVONNE A. MALDONADO, M.D.

Parasitic infections are highly prevalent in many developing areas of the world, and in developed countries may also be common among pregnant women. The placenta serves as an effective barrier, even in infections such as malaria and schistosomiasis in which systemic involvement and hematogenous spread are common. Although transplacental infections of the fetus are uncommon, in developing countries the prevalence of parasitic infections among infants younger than 1 month of age is high, primarily through transmission during or shortly after birth.

In a study conducted in Guatemala, Kotcher and colleagues found that 30% of newborns had acquired a protozoal infection by 2 weeks of age.[1] Although these infants were infected with *Entamoeba histolytica*, as well as with *Entamoeba coli*, *Endolimax nana*, and *Iodamoeba*

867

beutschlii, they remained asymptomatic. *Giardia lamblia* was found by the fifth week of life and *Trichuris trichiura* by the sixteenth week of life. A study conducted in a regional hospital in Togo revealed that 55% of infants and children from birth to 16 years of age demonstrated evidence of parasitic infections in stool or urine, with obvious neonatal infections occurring as well.[2]

Although *Pneumocystis* has been described as being a fungus by molecular biology criteria, its official taxonomic designation remains unsettled.

ASCARIS

Ascaris lumbricoides is the most prevalent parasitic infection worldwide, affecting up to 1 billion people. In humans, *Ascaris* eggs are ingested through fecal-oral contamination, hatch in the small intestine, and then penetrate the intestinal lumen to migrate extensively through blood and lymphatics. Larvae eventually reach the pulmonary circulation, where they migrate into the alveolar sacs, through the respiratory tree to the esophagus, and finally into the small intestine. Because *Ascaris* may migrate to many organs, worms are occasionally found in the uterus and the fallopian tubes.[3] Human fetuses are apparently able to mount an immune response to maternal *Ascaris* infection, but actual congenital infections are extremely rare. Sangeevi and associates studied the IgG and IgM reponses to *Ascaris* antigens from matched maternal and cord bloods in south India and found evidence of fetal IgM directed against *Ascaris* antigens in 12 of 28 samples.[4] Clinical status of the infants was not reported. Chu and co-workers, however, described an infant whose delivery was complicated by the simultaneous delivery of 12 adult *A. lumbricoides* worms.[5] During preparations for a cesarean section, which was being undertaken because of prolonged premature labor and fetal distress, one worm passed from the vagina and another was found in the vagina. When the placenta was removed, 10 worms were found on the maternal side of the placenta. The infant was delivered in good condition. The infant passed two female worms, which were 28 and 30 cm long, on the second and sixth days of life. He was treated with piperazine citrate, but no other worms were passed and no eggs were seen after the eleventh day of life. Fertilized ova of *A. lumbricoides* were found in the amniotic fluid and in the newborn's feces. It is known that an adhesion connected the mother's intestine and uterus, but it is uncertain whether the worms passed directly from the mother's intestine to the placenta and amniotic fluid and were swallowed by the fetus, whether larva passed hematogenously from the mother's lung to the placenta and thereby reached the fetal circulation, lung, and gastrointestinal tract, or whether female worms in the placenta produced fertile eggs that reached the amniotic fluid and were swallowed by the fetus. Other investigators have reported fetal evidence of *Ascaris* infection in infants as early as 1 to 2 weeks of age and in one infant with failure to thrive and bloody diarrhea at 3 weeks of age who responded to levamisole therapy.[6]

GIARDIASIS

G. lamblia causes a localized intestinal infection, with no systemic involvement. Hence, *G. lamblia* infection in pregnancy has not been associated with fetal infection. Severe maternal infection that compromises nutrition could affect fetal growth, but such a severe illness is rare.[7] Neonatal *G. lamblia* infection can result from fecal contamination at birth. Infected infants are usually asymptomatic.[8]

AMERICAN TRYPANOSOMIASIS (CHAGAS' DISEASE)

Millions of people in Central and South America are infected by *Trypanosoma cruzi* and related protozoa. Because of the chronicity of these infections, they have a significant impact on public health.

The Organism

The form of the organism that circulates in human blood is the trypomastigote. Cell division does not occur in the bloodstream. In tissue, the flagellum and undulating membrane are lost and the organism differentiates into a leishmanial form—the amastigote.[9, 10] Amastigotes multiply by binary fission, and masses of amastigotes are grouped into pseudocysts. The amastigotes in pseudocysts may evolve into trypanomastigotes and, on rupture of the pseudocyst, can gain access to the bloodstream or to new cells. Two strains of *T. cruzi* that cause human infections have been identified by biochemical differences among nine enzymes produced by the parasite.[11]

Epidemiology and Transmission

T. cruzi infects primates, marsupials, armadillos, bats, and many rodents, including guinea pigs, opossums, and raccoons; birds are not infected.[12] Infection of insects and mammals with *T. cruzi* is most common between the latitudes 39° N (northern California and Maryland) and 43° S (southern Argentina and Chile) and on the islands of Aruba and Trinidad.[1] The usual vectors are in the family Reduviidae, subfamily Triatominae. The main vector in Venezuela is *Rhodnius prolixus*; in Brazil, *Panstrongylus megistus*; and in Argentina, *Triatoma infectans*.[12] These species are well adapted to human dwellings. Triatominae are hematophagous insects. They both acquire and transmit the infection by biting infected vertebrates, including humans. The life span of the insect is not shortened by infection with *T. cruzi*; infected insects live up to a year after the onset of infection. In North America, the sylvatic habitat of the vector and the low virulence of the strains of *Trypanosoma* are responsible for the relative rarity of the disease. Colloquial terms used for the usual vector include the kissing or assassin bug in the southwestern United States; pito, hito, or vinchuca in Spanish America; and barbeiro in Portuguese America.[13]

The vector is most commonly found in huts of mud and sticks and in other housing containing cracks. In vectors infected with *T. cruzi*, metacyclic trypomastigotes congregate in the rectum. Bites become contaminated when defecation occurs. The infective form reaches the bloodstream through the site of the bite or by penetrating mucous membranes, conjunctivae, or abraded skin.[9] *Trypanosoma rangeli* is spread by a few species of the triatomid bug. These metacyclic trypanosomes develop, divide, and multiply in the salivary gland. They are injected directly into the site of the bite.

Infections can also be acquired by blood transfusion[14] and transplacentally. The isoenzyme patterns of *T. cruzi* recovered from congenitally infected infants and their mothers were identical, but transplacental transmission did not always follow maternal infection with enzymatically similar strains.[15]

Pathology

PLACENTA

The placenta is a relatively effective barrier to the spread of infection to the fetus.[10] The organism reaches the placenta by the hematogenous route and traverses the placental villi to the trophoblasts. After differentiation into amastigotes, the organism remains within Hofbauer's (phagocytic) cells of the placenta until it is liberated into the fetal circulation.[16-18]

Maternal parasitemia is greatest in the acute phase of infection; however, the period of intense parasitemia is short. Of the reported cases of congenital Chagas' disease, only four have originated during the acute phase of infection.[10] Most congenital infections occur in infants born to women with the chronic form of the disease.

Infected placentas are pale, yellow, and bulky. They have an appearance similar to the placentas of infants with erythroblastosis fetalis. Infection of the placenta is much more common than infection of the fetus.

BIOPSY AND AUTOPSY STUDIES

Two histologic types of lesions are recognized: those that contain parasites and those that do not.[10] In tissue sections, the parasite assumes the morphology of *Leishmania* bodies, which are round and contain an ovoid nucleus and a rodlike blepharoplast. Inflammation is not generally present unless there has been a rupture of a pseudocyst. Tissue reactions induced by antibody are believed to be responsible for lesions in which the parasite cannot be demonstrated. After infection, an antibody that cross reacts with the endocardium, the interstitium, and the blood vessels of the heart is formed and is referred to as endocardial-vascular-interstitial antibody.[19-21] This antibody has an affinity for the plasma membranes of the endocardium, endothelial cell, and striated muscle, as well as for *T. cruzi*. Endocardial-vascular-interstitial antibody is present in 95% of persons with Chagas' heart disease and in 45% of asymptomatic patients with serologic evidence of having had Chagas' disease.[21]

Tissue replication of the organism causes damage to the ganglia of the autonomic nervous system as well as to muscle.[12] Injury to Auerbach's plexus results in megaesophagus and megacolon as well as dilatation of other parts of the gastrointestinal tract and gallbladder. Similarly, the conducting system of the heart as well as the myocardium may be infected. Sudden death from arrhythmias can occur.

Clinical Manifestations

In the mother, urticaria is often present at the site of the bite regardless of whether the insect was infected or not.[9] The favored site for the bite is the face, presumably because this is the part of the body that is most often exposed during sleep. In acute infections, an inflammatory nodule, referred to as a chagoma, may develop at the site of the bite. If the bite is on the face, it is often associated with a unilateral, nonpurulent edema of the palpebral folds and an ipsilateral regional lymphadenopathy (Romaña's sign). Two or 3 weeks after the bite, parasitemia, fever, and a moderate local and general lymphadenopathy develop. The infection can extend and involve the myocardium, resulting in tachycardia, arrhythmia, hypotension, distant heart sounds, cardiomegaly, and congestive heart failure. The last is more severe in pregnant and postpartum women than in nonpregnant women. Hepatosplenomegaly and encephalitis also occur. The mortality rate during the acute phase is 10 to 20%. Death is usually cardiac in origin. Many survivors have abnormal electrocardiograms.

In the chronic phase, the placenta and fetus may be infected despite the fact that the mother is asymptomatic.[9] Chronic Chagas' disease often comes to medical attention because of the occurrence of an arrhythmia. These patients often do not have signs or symptoms of congestive heart failure.[12] Of 503 patients with myocardiopathy of chronic Chagas' disease studied by Vasquez, 19.8% died during an observation period of 6 years—37.5% suddenly and 55.2% with congestive heart failure.[22]

ABORTIONS AND STILLBIRTHS

Of 300 abortions in Argentina, 3 (1%) were due to Chagas' disease.[23] In Chile and Brazil, 10% of all abortions are attributed to Chagas' disease.[9] When the fetus is aborted, massive infection of the placenta is usually found.

CONGENITAL INFECTIONS

Bittencourt and co-workers found *T. cruzi* antibodies in 226 of 2651 pregnant women; 28.3% of seropositive mothers had parasitemia.[24] Nevertheless, the risk of transmission to the fetus is low, and live births of infants congenitally infected with *T. cruzi* are rare. Congenital infections occur in 1 to 4% of women with serologic evidence of having had Chagas' disease.[1, 9, 10, 18, 25] Among infants with a birth weight of 2500 g or more, congenital infections are very rare.[16, 26-29] Among low-birth-weight infants, congenitally infected infants can be either premature or small for gestational age or both. Congenital infections were found in 10 of 425 (2.3%) infants by Saleme and associates in Argentina,[23] in 10 of 500 (2%) infants weighing less than 2000 g by Bittencourt and co-workers in Brazil, and in 3 of 186 (1.6%) infants of more than 2000 g birth weight[24] and in 1 of 200 (0.5%) premature infants with birth weights of 2000 g or less by Howard in Chile.[30]

Congenitally infected infants may develop symptoms at birth or during the first few weeks of life. Early-onset jaundice, anemia, and petechiae are common. These symptoms are similar to those associated with erythroblastosis fetalis.[10] As may older patients, congenitally infected infants may have hepatosplenomegaly, cardiomegaly, and congestive heart failure, as well as involvement of the esophagus leading to dysphagia, regurgitation, and megaesophagus.[21, 31] Some infants have myxedematous edema. Pneumonitis has been associated with infection of the amnionic epithelium.[32] Congenitally infected infants can be born with encephalitis or can develop it postnatally. It is generally associated with hypotonia, a poor suck, and seizures.[9] The cerebrospinal fluid shows mild pleocytosis, which consists primarily of lymphocytes. Cataracts and opacification of the media of the eye have also been observed.[25] Twins may both be congenitally infected, or one may escape infection.[33]

Of 64 congenitally infected infants in whom the follow-up was known, Bittencourt reported that 7.8% died the first day, 35.9% died when younger than 4 months of age,[10] 9.3% died between the ages of 4 and 24 months, and 42.2% survived for more than 24 months. Of those who survived for 2 years or longer, 74% had no serious clinical symptoms despite continued parasitemia. However, subclinical abnormalities might have been found if electrocardiography or roentgenography had been performed.

As with other congenital infections, the immune system of the fetus is stimulated and both IgM antibody to *T. cruzi* and endocardial-vascular-interstitial antibody are formed.[10, 21]

Diagnosis

The diagnosis should be suspected at the time of abortions and stillbirths as well as in infants who develop symptoms compatible with congenital infection. An easy, but often omitted, means of making a diagnosis of congenital infection is to examine the placenta for the amastigote of *T. cruzi*. The gross appearance of the placenta is similar to that seen in erythroblastosis fetalis.

Motile trypomastigotes can also be demonstrated by examining blood under a coverslip.[10] The number of parasites is low initially but increases subsequently. Thin and thick smears can be examined after being stained with Giemsa stain. Microhematocrit concentration and examination of the buffy coat enhanced the detection of parasites in congenital Chagas' disease.[34] If more than 10 parasites per mm[3] are found, the infant generally dies.[23]

Xenodiagnosis is performed by allowing laboratory-bred uninfected insects to feed and ingest the patient's blood. The fecal contents of the insects are examined for trypomastigotes 30 to 60 days later. Blood may also

be injected into mice. In mothers with acute Chagas' disease, the parasites are present in blood smears beginning 3 weeks after onset of the infection and they persist for several months. Parasites can be demonstrated for years by xenodiagnosis.

In the chronic stages of the disease, the diagnosis can be made histologically by sampling skeletal muscle. The histologic appearance of the parasite in tissue sections is similar to that of toxoplasmosis. However, the amastigotes in Chagas' disease contain a blepharoplast that is lacking in toxoplasmosis.

Several tests for antibody are available. Complement-fixing antibody crosses the placenta from mother to infant. This test, referred to as the Machado-Guerreiro reaction, demonstrates antibodies that exhibit a cross-reaction with *Leishmania donovani* and with sera from patients with lepromatous leprosy. In uninfected infants, complement-fixing antibodies are no longer demonstrable after the fortieth day of life; in infected infants, these antibodies persist.[10]

Agglutinating antibodies may also be demonstrable. Uninfected infants with titers of agglutinating antibody of 1:512 or less at birth have negative titers by 2 months of age.[25] The titer of agglutinating antibody in uninfected infants with initial titers of 1:1024 or higher becomes negative by 6 months of age. IgM fluorescent antibodies can be demonstrated in some infants, but infected infants do not always have a positive test.[21, 33] Data suggest that fetal IgG to specific acute-phase antigens may be useful in the diagnosis of congenital Chagas' disease, but this is currently an experimental technique.[35]

Prognosis for Recurrence

Congenital infections can recur during subsequent pregnancies.[36] The same mother, however, often has healthy children both before and after the affected one.[21]

Therapy

In the past, various drugs, including nitrofurans, 8-aminoquinolines, and metronidazole, have been thought to have some effect on the blood-borne form of the parasite. They were ineffective in eliminating the tissue form—the amastigote. Nifurtimox (Lampit) is used to treat Chagas' disease,[23, 26] but its use in congenitally infected infants is still experimental. Current information regarding treatment can be obtained from the Parasitic Disease Drug Service, Centers for Disease Control and Prevention, Atlanta, Georgia.

Prevention

The main means of prevention is to improve housing so that the vector cannot reach the inhabitants, especially during sleep. In addition, in endemic areas potential blood donors should be tested, and only those who lack serologic evidence of having had Chagas' disease should be permitted to donate blood. The addition of gentian violet 1:4000 to blood has been found to be useful as a means of preventing transmission of the infection to the recipient of the blood.[12]

AFRICAN TRYPANOSOMIASIS (AFRICAN SLEEPING SICKNESS)

Whereas few cases of congenital disease have been reported, in adults infection with *Trypanosoma brucei gambiense* and *T. brucei rhodesiense* is severe and often fatal; and congenital infection is most likely under-reported. Humans are infected by the bite of an infected male or female tsetse fly, which injects trypomastigotes into the host. Humans are the primary reservoir for *T. gambiense* and large wild game the hosts for *T. rhodesiense*. Once injected, the organism disseminates throughout the bloodstream. Signs and symptoms of infection appear after 2 to 4 weeks, and a chronic infection develops 6 months to 1 to 2 years later. The chronic stage includes a progressive meningoencephalitis, which is often fatal if left untreated. Infection with *T. gambiense* is associated with lymphadenopathy and is slowly progressive, whereas infection with *T. rhodesiense* is rapidly progressive.

The parasite can be transmitted transplacentally, but few cases have been reported.[37, 38] Transplacental infection can cause prematurity, abortion, and stillbirth. Transplacental infection has been proved in infants who were born in nonendemic areas to infected mothers, or if the parasite was identified in the peripheral blood in the first 5 days of life. Central nervous system involvement is common in congenital infection and in some infants may be slowly progressive.

The diagnosis should be suspected in an infant with unexplained fever, anemia, hepatosplenomegaly, or progressive neurologic symptoms whose mother is from an endemic area. The parasite can be identified in thick smears from peripheral blood or in the cerebrospinal fluid. In infants, treatment with suramin or melarsoprol has been reported with good results; however, in a case report of congenital trypanosomiasis,[37] severe neurologic symptoms persisted after delayed diagnosis and treatment at 22 months of age.

ENTAMOEBA HISTOLYTICA

There is some evidence that amebiasis during pregnancy may be more severe and have a higher fatality rate than that expected in nonpregnant women of the same age.[39, 40] Abioye found that 68% of fatal cases of amebiasis in females 15 to 34 years of age occurred in pregnant women, whereas only 17.1 and 12.5% of fatal cases of typhoid or other causes of enterocolitis, respectively, in women in this age group occurred during pregnancy.[40] In addition, Czeizel and co-workers found a significantly higher incidence of positive stool cultures for *E. histolytica* among women who had spontaneous abortions than among those who gave birth to living infants at term.[41]

Amebiasis has been reported in infants as young as 3 to 6 weeks of age.[42–44] In most instances, person-to-person transmission was considered likely and the mother was the probable source of the infant's infection.[42] In one fatal case, the father had cysts of *E. histolytica* in his stool, whereas no evidence of infection with *E. histolytica* was found in the mother.[43] Perinatal infections have occurred in countries such as the United States in which the disease is rare.

Most infants reported with amebiasis in the perinatal period had illnesses with sudden, dramatic onset and were seriously ill. Bloody diarrhea was followed by development of hepatomegaly and hepatic abscess, rectal abscess, and gangrene of the appendix and colon with perforation and peritonitis. Persistent bloody diarrhea that is complicated by the development of a mass in or around the liver should lead to a thorough investigation as to whether infection with *E. histolytica* could be the cause.

Routine stool examinations for ova and parasites may be negative. Despite this, trophozoites of *E. histolytica* can usually be found in biopsy specimens of gastrointestinal ulcers and of the wall of the liver abscesses. The organisms cannot always be demonstrated in pus aspirated from the center of the abscess. An elevated indirect hemagglutination titer to *E. histolytica* can be helpful in diagnosing extraintestinal amebiasis. However, high titers are not usually seen until 2 weeks or more after onset of the infection in older patients and are not always present in neonates with severe extraintestinal infections.[42]

Infants have been successfully treated with oral metronidazole.[44] Critically ill children should receive intravenous therapy with dehydroemetine or metronidazole.

MALARIA

Although malaria is recognized as the major health problem of many countries, its impact on pregnancy and infant mortality has probably been underestimated.

The Organisms

Of the four species of malaria, *Plasmodium vivax* has the widest distribution, but *Plasmodium falciparum* tends to predominate in tropical areas. Malaria is spread to humans by the bite of anopheline mosquitoes. Of the many species of anopheline mosquito capable of becoming infected with malarial parasites, those that enter houses are more important than those preferring an outdoor habitat.[45] Mosquitoes that feed at night on human blood while the victim is asleep are the most important vectors.

After the bite of the mosquito, sporozoites are injected into the bloodstream but are cleared within half an hour. The parasites mature in the parenchymal cells of the liver and form a mature schizont, which contains 7500 to 40,000 merozoites depending on the species. The release of the merozoites results in the appearance of the ring stage in erythrocytes in the peripheral blood. Within hours, the parasite assumes an amoeboid form and is referred to as a trophozoite. The sexual form is called a gametocyte. In infections with *P. vivax*, *Plasmodium malariae*, and *Plasmodium ovale*, all forms are seen in the peripheral blood from early ring forms through mature schizonts and gametocytes. In infections with *P. falciparum*, usually only rings and gametocytes are found in the peripheral blood.

Epidemiology and Transmission

In addition to transmission by the bite of mosquitoes, malaria can be transmitted by transfusion of blood products. In infants, this has occurred after simple transfusion as well as after exchange transfusion.[46–49] The onset of symptoms in neonates infected by blood products has varied from 13 to 21 days.

Malaria parasites survive in blood for weeks. In addition, relapses can occur from *P. vivax* for up to 2 years and rarely for up to 4 years. Relapses from *P. malariae* have occasionally occurred 5 years or more after infection, but low-grade chronic parasitemia that is unassociated with symptoms is more common.

Malaria may be transmitted also by reuse of syringes and needles and has spread by this route among heroin addicts. Infection in heroin addicts who become pregnant can result in congenital infections.[50]

Pathology

EFFECT OF PREGNANCY ON MALARIA

Both the density and the prevalence of parasitemia are increased in pregnant women compared with women who are not pregnant but who reside in the same geographic area.[51–55] For *P. falciparum*, Campbell and colleagues found a parasite density of 6896 per mm³ in pregnant women and 3808 per mm³ in nonpregnant women; for *P. vivax*, the parasite density was 3564 per mm³ for pregnant women and 1949 per mm³ for nonpregnant women.[56] The prevalence as well as the density of the parasitemia decreases with increasing parity. Reinhardt and associates found that the placenta was infected in 45% of primiparous women compared with 19% of women with a parity of five.[52] This trend toward an increase in resistance to malaria with parity has been attributed by some to the increase in immunity that would be expected with an increase in age. However, both the prevalence and the density of parasitemia are increased in pregnant women of all parities compared with those in nonpregnant women of the same parity.[51–53] This suggests that pregnancy, as well as age, is an important factor in determining susceptibility to malaria.[51]

Infection of the Placenta

The intervillous spaces of infected placentas are packed with lymphoid macrophages, which contain phagocytosed pigment in large granules. Lymphocytes and immature polymorphonuclear leukocytes are also present in large numbers. Numerous young and mature schizonts are present. Trophozoites and gametocytes are uncommon.[57, 58] Jelliffe has suggested that the intensity of the infection in the placenta is related to the severity of the effect on the fetus.[59] In general, the inflammatory response in placentas infected with *P. falciparum* is more intense than that in those infected with *P. malariae*.

Effect of Malaria on Fetal Survival and Birth Weight

In 1941, Torpin reviewed 27 cases of malaria that had occurred in pregnant women during the preceding 20 years in a city in the United States.[60] The maternal mortality rate was 4%, and the fetal mortality rate was 60%. In 1951, in Vietnam, Hung found a fetal death rate of 14% among women who had infected placentas.[61] Many of these women had had severe attacks of malaria during the first trimester and had sustained spontaneous abortions at that time.

Low birth weight is more common when the placenta is infected by parasites than when the mother is infected but the placenta is not.[52, 53, 59, 62, 63] The mean birth weight is lower if the placenta is infected with *P. falciparum* than if it is infected with *P. malariae*. Maternal anemia as well as placental insufficiency probably affects the fetus. It has been postulated that heavy infiltrations of parasites, lymphocytes, and macrophages interfere with the circulation of maternal blood through the placenta and result in diminished transport of oxygen and nutrients to the fetus.[53] The transport through the placenta of antibody to malaria may also be decreased when placental inflammation is severe.[51]

Bruce-Chwatt found that when the placenta was infected, infant weight at birth was an average of 145 g less than the weight of infants born to women with uninfected placentas.[57] Similarly, Archibald[64] found infant weight at birth to be 170 g less, and Jelliffe[59, 63] found it to be 263 g less in infants of women with infected placentas than in infants of women with uninfected placentas. In the studies performed by Bruce-Chwatt and Jelliffe, 20% of the infants born to mothers with infected placentas weighed 2500 g or less, whereas 10 and 11%, respectively, of those born to mothers with uninfected placentas weighed 2500 g or less. Cannon found that 37% of women who had infected placentas gave birth to infants weighing 2500 g or less compared with 12% of those who had uninfected placentas.[53] For primiparous women, 44% of those with infected placentas and 27% of those with uninfected placentas gave birth to infants weighing 2500 g or less.[65] Infants who have parasites demonstrable in their cord blood appear to be more severely affected than those who do not have parasitemia at the time of delivery; the mean weight gain of the mothers of these infants and the head and chest circumferences of the infants at birth are lower than expected.[52] Larkin studied the prevalence of *P. falciparum* infection among 63 pregnant women and their newborns in southern Zambia and found peripheral parasitemia in 63% (40/63) of mothers and 29% (19/65) of newborns. Infected newborns had a mean average birth weight 469 g lower then uninfected newborns but did not have a higher incidence of preterm delivery.[66]

Using the method developed by Dubowitz and associates[67] for scoring gestational age, Reinhardt and colleagues[52] found no evidence that the incidence of infants who were small for gestational age was increased when the placenta was infected. This finding suggested that low birth weight was secondary to prematurity among infants born to women with malaria.

Jelliffe has pointed out that because malaria influences birth weight, it has an important effect on infant survival in countries in which it is endemic.[59] In 1925, Blacklock and Gordon noted that 35% of infants born to mothers with infected placentas died within the first 7 days of life, whereas only 5% of those born to mothers with uninfected placentas died during this period.[68] In 1958, Cannon found that the mortality among infants 7 days or younger in age was 6.9% for those whose mothers' placentas were infected compared with 3.4% for those whose mothers' placentas were uninfected.[53]

The data suggesting that malaria has an important influence on birth weight and therefore on infant survival have been given further credence by the demonstration by MacGregor and Avery that control of malaria in a region is followed by an increase in mean birth weight of infants born there.[65] After DDT spraying on the island of Malaita in the British Solomon Islands, the mean birth weight for infants of mothers of all parities increased by 165 g. For infants of primiparous women, the mean birth weight increased by 252 g.[65] There was a concomitant decrease in the number of infants with birth weights of 2500 g or less; the incidence of births in this weight range fell by 8% for all births and by 20% for infants of primiparous women.[65]

Malaria therefore contributes to fetal loss, stillbirth, prematurity, and neonatal death.[63, 69]

Influence of Maternal Antibody on Risk of Infection

Antimalarial antibodies are transferred from the mother to the infant. The prevalence of precipitating antibody to *P. falciparum* within 24 hours of birth in Gambia was 87% in newborns and 87.5% in their mothers.[70] The prevalence of antibody in these newborns reflected the extent to which malaria had been controlled in the area in which their mothers lived. In infants born in the provinces with more malaria, 97% had antibodies to malaria whereas 75.8% of infants born in an urban area had antibodies to malaria.

Antibodies to malaria can be detected by complement fixation, indirect hemagglutination, and indirect fluorescence. Agglutinating and precipitating antibodies are also formed.[71] Levels of both precipitating antibodies and antibodies detected by indirect hemagglutination decrease in the period from birth to 25 weeks of age.[72, 73] Subsequently, as a result of postnatal acquisition of infection, endogenous antibody synthesis begins and antibody levels rise.

Bray and Anderson have suggested that the amount of IgG transferred to the fetus is decreased when the placenta is heavily infested with parasites.[51] They found that women who were pregnant during the wet season in Gambia had higher mean antibody titers to *P. falciparum* than those who were pregnant during the dry season. This was due to the mothers' serologic responses to the increase in exposure to malaria during the wet season. The antibody titers of the infants born to women who were pregnant during the wet season were not higher than those of infants born to women who had been pregnant during the dry season. In fact, the infants

born to women who had been pregnant during the wet season had lower mean titers of antibody to malaria at birth than infants born during other seasons. In infants at 2 to 3 months of age, parasitemia was found in 32% born during the wet season but in only 3 to 15% born in other seasons.

Other Factors Influencing Risk of Infection

Infants younger than 3 months of age have a lower than expected incidence of clinical disease, death from malaria, and parasitemia.[70, 72] This has been attributed to a variety of factors, including the possibility that infants of this age are less exposed to and therefore less often bitten by mosquitoes. However, the two most important causes are probably the fact that the level of serologic immunity is high at this age and that fetal hemoglobin is present in the circulating red blood cells. Sehgal and associates studied the role of humoral immunity in acquired malaria infection among newborns in Papua New Guinea.[74] Among 104 newborns, there was a 3.8% incidence of congenital malaria and a cumulative incidence of acquired malaria of 3% at 12 weeks, 16% by 24 weeks, 24% by 36 weeks, and 38% by 48 weeks of age. Ninety-six percent of infants lost maternal antibody between 4 and 7 months, and the majority of asymptomatic malaria occurred among infants with detectable malaria antibody.

Gilles showed that, although there were seasonal fluctuations in overall incidence of parasitemia, the corrected rates were always lower for infants from birth to 2 months of age than for infants 3 to 4 or 5 to 6 months of age.[75] He did not find differences in sleeping habits or in the amount of exposure to mosquitoes among infants in these age groups. In June to October, parasitemia was found in 10% of those from birth to 2 months old, 42% of those 3 to 4 months old, and 53% of those 5 to 6 months old; in May, parasitemia was found in 0% of infants from birth to 2 months old, 11% of those 3 to 4 months old, and 16% of those 5 to 6 months old. The rise in prevalence of parasitemia corresponded with a fall in the amount of fetal hemoglobin in the red blood cells.[75] The fact that cells containing fetal hemoglobin are poor hosts for the malarial parasite had been previously suggested by Allison as one of the reasons for the selective advantage of sickle cell anemia and sickle cell trait in areas in which malaria is endemic.[76, 77] Although antibody is undoubtedly important in protecting newborns from malaria, Campbell and co-workers[56] and Reinhardt and associates[52] have pointed out that antibody levels in infants from birth to 2 months of age may be low or absent even when the mother has had parasitemia and placental infection.[56] The presence of fetal hemoglobin in the red cells may serve as a source of protection for infants who do not derive high levels of antibody from their mothers.

Placental infection as a risk for congenital malaria was studied in 197 infants in Cameroon. Infants born to placenta-infected mothers were more likely to develop malaria than infants born to women without placental infection.[78] Rates of infant infection and parasitemia were not related to maternally derived malaria antibodies.

Congenital Malaria

OCCURRENCE

There has been no consistently accepted definition of congenital malaria. Some have taken the position that parasites must be demonstrable in the peripheral blood of the infant during the first day of life; others have accepted cases that were confirmed within the first 7 days of life.[69] In areas in which malaria is endemic, infants are exposed to mosquitoes and may become infected by this route at a very young age. Thus, it may be difficult to distinguish congenital cases from acquired cases. However, a sufficient number of cases of congenital malaria have now been reported from countries that are free of malaria, thereby eliminating the possibility of postnatal transmission, to establish the fact that the clinical onset of disease in a congenitally infected infant can be delayed for weeks and rarely even for months.[49, 50, 79, 80] The prevalence of parasitemia in infants younger than 3 months of age was 0.7% among infants born during the dry season in the rural part of Gambia compared with 11.4% among those born during the wet season, which suggests that postnatal infection is a more common event than congenital malaria.[55] It is probable that IgG antibody transmitted from the mother to the infant is an important factor in determining whether parasites that reach the fetal circulation establish an infection. In addition, the presence of passively transferred antibody in the neonate may lengthen the incubation period over that which would be expected in the nonimmune host.

The frequency of placental infection varies according to the prevalence of malaria in the population, the vigor of measures of control, and the availability of nonprescription antimalarial drugs. However, among Nigerian women who did not receive antimalarial agents, three studies suggested that the frequency of infection of the placenta remained relatively stable over a 30-year period. In 1948 through 1950, Bruce-Chwatt found that 20% of the placentas from 228 pregnancies were infected.[57] One (0.4%) of the 235 neonates had the trophozoites of *P. falciparum* in a peripheral smear obtained on the fifth day of life. In 1958, Cannon[53] found that 26% of the placentas were infected; in 1970, Williams and McFarlane[81] found that 37% of the placentas were infected. None of the cord blood samples of the infants in these latter studies contained parasites. In 1964 through 1965 in Uganda, Jelliffe found that 16% of the 570 placentas were infected but only one (0.18%) infant was infected at birth.[59]

The studies of Kortmann,[82] Reinhardt and colleagues[52] and Schwetz and Peel[83] suggest that parasitemia in cord blood may be more common than had been previously believed and that the presence of parasites does not necessarily indicate that the infant will become infected. Reinhardt and colleagues found 33% of 198 placentas to be infected.[52] Thick smears of the cord blood were positive in 21.7% of the 198 infants and in 55% of the infants of mothers who had had parasitemia during the pregnancy. Thin smears were negative in all 198 infants. Kortmann was able to demonstrate parasites in 19.7% of the placentas of 1009 women but in only 3.8% of cord blood from their infants.[82] Eleven infants who had parasites in their cord blood also had peripheral smears performed; parasites were demonstrable in the peripheral blood of only two (18%). Lehner and associates found a 14.6% incidence of cord parasitemia and a 7.7% incidence of peripheral parasitemia among 48 newborns in Papua New Guinea.[84] Whereas all maternal and cord samples had malaria antibodies, low levels of cord malaria antibody were found to correlate with cord parasitemia. Schwetz and Peel demonstrated parasites in 6% of cord blood samples and 3.6% of peripheral blood samples of infants born to mothers in Central Africa.[83] Because the rate of infection of the placenta was 74%, this study demonstrates that the placenta, although frequently infected, serves as a relatively effective barrier and that parasites infrequently reach the fetus. The relative importance of transplacental infection or transmission by transfer from mother to infant during labor as mechanisms by which the infant acquires malaria remains uncertain.[85]

Despite massive involvement of the placenta, it is generally agreed that clinically apparent congenital infections are rare in areas in which malaria is endemic and levels of maternal immunity are high. Covell reviewed cases of congenital malaria that had been reported up to 1950 and estimated the incidence at 16 (0.3%) infections per 5324 live births.[70] This rate pertained to areas of the world in which malaria was endemic. For women having an overt attack of malaria during pregnancy, the rate of congenital infection was higher and was estimated to be 1 to 4%.[70] Congenital malaria is more common among infants of women who have clinical attacks of malaria during pregnancy than in those with chronic subclinical infections; however, congenital malaria may occur in infants of mothers who are asymptomatic throughout their pregnancy.[69, 80, 86] Often parasitemia is not demonstrable in the mother; splenomegaly is frequently present.[69] Congenital malaria is more common in infants of women who have immigrated to areas in which malaria is endemic than in women who have been raised to maturity in such areas because their levels of immunity are lower than those of the native population. Conversely, congenital malaria is also more common among women who immigrate from areas in which malaria is endemic to areas that are free of malaria. Loss of immunity results from lack of frequent exposure. Although rare, congenital malaria may also occur as a result of maternal infection by chloroquine-resistant *P. falciparum*. A number of reported cases of chloroquine-resistant congenital malaria in Africa and Indonesia responded to treatment with intravenous quinine.[87–89]

CLINICAL PRESENTATION

Cases of congenital malaria have been identified in countries in which malaria is endemic as well as in countries in which it is not, including Great Britain and the United States. The majority of infants with congenital malaria have had the onset of the first sign or symptom at 10 to 28 days of age.[49, 90–93] However, onsets as early as 14 hours of age and as late as 8 weeks of age have been reported.[69, 79, 80, 94–96]. Keitel and co-workers described a case of malaria in a 15-month-old child who had been separated from her mother at 6 weeks of age but who was breast-fed during this 6-week period.[50] The infection was due to *P. malariae*. The source of the mother's infection was probably contaminated needles and syringes used to inject heroin. The infant must have derived the infection from her mother because she had always lived in an area that was free of malaria. Hulbert reviewed the 49 cases of congenital malaria reported in the United States since 1950 and found that the mean age at onset of symptoms was 5.5 weeks (range 0 to 60 weeks) and that 96% of these children had signs or symptoms between 2 and 8 weeks of age.[93] There was no association found between age of symptom onset and *Plasmodium* species.

Most cases of congenital infection have occurred in infants of mothers who had overt attacks of malaria during pregnancy. However, Harvey and associates[80] and McQuay and colleagues[95] reported cases of congenital infection with *P. malariae* in which the mother had lived in an area that was free of malaria for 3 years or more. In these cases, it is likely that the mothers had had onset of their infection many years before their move from an endemic area.

The most common clinical findings in cases of congenital malaria are fever, anemia, and splenomegaly, which are present in more than 80% of cases.[49, 97] The anemia, which may be accompanied by pallor, is associated with a reticulocytosis in about half the cases. Jaundice and hyperbilirubinemia are found in about a third of the cases. Either the direct or the indirect bilirubin may be elevated, depending on whether liver dysfunction or hemolysis is the most important process in an individual case.[49] Hepatomegaly also may be present but is less common than splenomegaly. Nonspecific findings include failure to thrive, poor feeding, regurgitation, and loose stools. In developing countries, when malaria occurs during the first few months of life, it is frequently complicated by other illness, such as pneumonia, septicemia, and diarrhea.[96]

Of the 107 cases of congenital malaria summarized by Covell, 40% were due to *P. falciparum*, 32% to *P. vivax*, and 1.9% to *P. malariae*.[70] The clinical findings of congenital malaria are not distinguishable from the signs and symptoms of malaria that has been acquired by the bite of a mosquito. IgM antibody to *P. falciparum* was found in the cord blood of one infant.[94] The mother had probably had her first attack of malaria during that pregnancy and had high fever and parasitemia at delivery. Reinhardt and colleagues found that the total IgM levels in the cord blood of infants of infected mothers were similar to those of infants of uninfected mothers.[52] Although fever and parasitemia may occur within 24 hours of birth, hepatosplenomegaly and anemia at birth as a result of a chronic intrauterine infection have not been described. Normal red blood cells can cross from the maternal to the fetal circulation.[98] If parasitized cells cross, however, they must usually be destroyed by the immune defenses of the fetus and by the maternal antimalarial antibodies that have passed transplacentally.

TREATMENT

Chloroquine is the drug of choice for sensitive strains of *P. falciparum* and for *P. malariae*. For these infections, chloroquine phosphate should be administered orally in an initial dose of 10 mg/kg of chloroquine base (maximum 600 mg base) followed in 6 hours by a dose of 5 mg/kg of chloroquine base (maximum 300 mg base). Subsequent doses of 5 mg/kg of chloroquine base should be given 24 and 48 hours after the first dose (maximum 300 mg base). Parenteral therapy consists of quinidine gluconate at a dose of 10 mg/kg as a loading dose (maximum 600 mg) then 0.02 mg/kg/min until oral therapy can be given. Infections with *P. vivax* may also be treated with chloroquine alone because sporozoite forms are not transmitted and therefore there is no exoerythrocytic phase in congenital infections; administration of primaquine is not necessary.

The treatment of transfusion-acquired infections is the same as that for congenital infections because there is no exoerythrocytic phase in these infections.

In serious infections in infants of mothers who may have been exposed to chloroquine-resistant strains of *P. falciparum*, alternate therapy should be considered. In adults, combinations of quinine, pyrimethamine, and a sulfonamide or quinine and tetracycline have been used with success.[99] Intravenous quinidine in combination with exchange transfusion has been used in a severe case of maternal *P. falciparum* malaria.[100] Intravenous quinidine or the combination of quinine and trimethoprim-sulfamethoxazole has been suggested for treatment of infants with resistant *P. falciparum* infection.[87–89, 101] Intravenous quinine is no longer available in the United States, but in adults oral quinine may be useful in less severe cases of chloroquine-resistant *P. falciparum*. Mefloquine is an oral antimalarial effective against most *P. falciparum* strains. Recommended therapy for *P. falciparum* infection in areas with known chloroquine resistance is variable, depending on ability to appropriately diagnose resistant *P. falciparum*, the percentage of parasitemia, signs of organ involvement (especially of the central nervous system), and other systemic manifestations of malaria. Severe malaria may require intensive care, and exchange transfusion may be necessary if parasitemia is greater than 10%. Sequential smears should be monitored to ensure adequacy of therapy. The treatment regimen of choice is quinine sulfate in a dose of 25 mg/kg (maximum dose 2000 mg) in three doses for 3 to 7 days in addition to tetracycline in a dose of 5 mg/kg four times a day for 7 days (maximum individual dose 250 mg). The risk of dental staining in children younger than 8 years of age must be weighed against the risk of malaria morbidity and mortality. An alternative regimen is quinine sulfate alone in a dose of 30 mg/kg in three doses for 3 days or parenteral quinidine gluconate at the same dose recommended for non–chloroquine-resistant *P. falciparum* in addition to pyrimethamine-sulfadoxine or mefloquine hydrochloride in a dose of 15 to 25 mg/

kg in a single dose (maximum dose 1250 mg). Whereas the alternative regimen is not recommended for infants or pregnant women because pyrimethamine-sulfadoxine and mefloquine are not licensed for use in these populations by the Food and Drug Administration, data regarding use of mefloquine during pregnancy do not indicate a risk of adverse outcomes during pregnancy. Inadvertent use of mefloquine during the first trimester of pregnancy should be reported to the Centers for Disease Control and Prevention Malaria Center at 770-488-7760. Current recommendations regarding treatment can also be obtained from the Malaria Branch, Centers for Disease Control and Prevention, Atlanta, Georgia.

PREVENTION

Because malaria chemoprophylaxis may not be 100% effective, decreasing or eliminating exposure to mosquitoes is an important strategy for preventing malaria during pregnancy. Exposure to mosquitoes should be avoided by use of mosquito netting around beds, wire mesh screening on windows, insecticides, and mosquito repellants.

Although the possible toxicity of administering prophylactic antimalarial agents to women during pregnancy has been much discussed, controlled trials have shown that there is little risk and much to gain from such a practice. Treatment only for identified cases of maternal malaria rather than the administration of malaria prophylaxis failed to reduce the incidence of malaria-related low birth weight because only 12 of 65 women who had plasmodial pigmentation of the placenta had symptoms leading to an antenatal diagnosis of malaria.[102] Morley and associates showed that administration of a prophylactic monthly dose of 50 mg of pyrimethamine during pregnancy resulted in improved maternal weight gain and in an increase in the mean birth weight of 157 g compared with administration of antimalarial drugs only for febrile episodes.[103] Pyrimethamine prophylaxis is avoided in pregnant women because of concern that this dihydrofolate reductase inhibitor might cause abnormalities by interference with folic acid metabolism. Congenital defects have occurred in the offspring of animals ingesting pyrimethamine during pregnancy[104]; one possible case of pyrimethamine teratogenicity in a human fetus has been described,[105] and evidence of embryo resorption has been documented in pregnant Wistar rats given sulfadoxine-pyrimethamine.[106]

A recent retrospective review of 1627 reports of women exposed to mefloquine before or during pregnancy revealed a 4% prevalence of congenital malformations among infants of these women, reportedly similar to that observed in the general population.[107] A second report demonstrated a high rate of spontaneous abortions, but not congenital malformations, among 72 female U.S. soldiers who inadvertently received mefloquine during pregnancy.[108] Sufficient data do not exist to recommend the use of mefloquine in pregnant women, although its use in these women may be considered when exposure to chloroquine-resistant *P. falciparum* is unavoidable. The dose is 250 mg salt orally once a week

beginning 1 week before travel and ending 4 weeks after the last exposure. The combination of pyrimethamine and sulfadoxine for prophylaxis against chloroquine-resistant strains of *P. falciparum* is no longer recommended because the risk of Stevens-Johnson syndrome or neutropenia outweighs the potential benefit. Prophylaxis with chloroquine and proguanil is an alternative if a pregnant woman from a nonendemic area must risk exposure to resistant *P. falciparum*.[109]

Chloroquine alone also has been used as prophylaxis during pregnancy and has been shown to be of benefit.[54] Gilles found that parasitemia developed in more than 75% of pregnant women who received no prophylactic drug or who received folic acid but no antimalarial drugs. Sixty-three percent of these women developed anemia at 16 to 24 weeks' gestation. In contrast, only 2 (17%) of 12 pregnant women who received a dose of 600 mg of chloroquine base followed by a weekly dose of 25 mg of pyrimethamine developed parasitemia and only one developed anemia. Although anemia per se may be an important cause of low birth weight, as Harrison and Ibeziako maintained,[110] malaria appears to be an important cause of anemia in pregnant women.[110, 111]

Chloroquine and the other 4-aminoquinolines such as amodiaquine and hydroxychloroquine have similar activities and toxicities. The safety of administering chloroquine during pregnancy has been questioned. The usual recommendation for prophylaxis is 300 mg of chloroquine base once a week. Hart and Naunton attributed the abnormal outcome of four pregnancies in a single patient to the administration of chloroquine during the pregnancies.[112] This patient, who had systemic lupus erythematosus (SLE), took 150 to 300 mg chloroquine base daily. Two of the children who had had intrauterine exposures to chloroquine had severe cochleovestibular paresis and posterior column defects. Another had a Wilms tumor and hemihypertrophy. The fourth pregnancy ended in a spontaneous abortion at 12 weeks' gestation. As pointed out by Jelliffe[113] and Clyde,[114] the dose given to this pregnant patient was three to seven times higher than the dose recommended for prophylaxis against malaria. Two other studies reported pregnancy outcomes after exposure to antimalarials. Parke described 14 pregnancies among eight patients with SLE who took chloroquine or hydroxychloroquine during pregnancy.[115] Three pregnancies ended in spontaneous abortion or neonatal death during periods of increased SLE activity; of the remaining 11 pregnancies, 6 were normal full-term deliveries, 1 ended in stillbirth, and 4 ended in spontaneous abortion. No congenital deformities were noted. Levy and co-workers reviewed the cases of 24 women who took chloroquine or hydroxychloroquine during a total of 27 pregnancies.[116] Eleven women had SLE, 3 had rheumatoid arthritis, and 4 were taking malaria prophylaxis. There were 14 normal deliveries, six abortions secondary to severe underlying disease or social conditions, three stillbirths, and four spontaneous abortions. No congenital abnormalities were noted. The risk of poor outcome was higher among women with connective tissue disease, for which chloroquine and hydroxychloroquine doses are much higher than for malaria prophylaxis. Despite widespread use of weekly doses of chloroquine in pregnant women, teratogenic effects have not been confirmed in controlled trials.[117]

The consequences of an attack of malaria during pregnancy are serious. Hindi and Azimi described a woman who became pregnant while living in Nigeria but who stopped taking prophylactic doses of pyrimethamine at the onset of pregnancy.[79] At 6 months' gestation, she had a febrile illness and was treated with chloroquine for 2 weeks. At 8 months' gestation, she had a second attack of malaria and was delivered of an infant who was 4 weeks premature and small for gestational age. In addition to this, the infant developed malaria during the first few weeks of life and was treated with chloroquine. The total exposure of this infant to chloroquine would have been less if the mother had been taking it weekly in prophylactic doses.

Women living in or returning from areas in which malaria is endemic should continue to take prophylactic antimalarial agents. Although primaquine is not known to have teratogenic effects, experience with its use during pregnancy is limited; therefore, it is recommended that treatment with primaquine to eradicate the exoerythrocytic phase in *P. vivax* infections be deferred until after delivery.[104, 118]

Some have expressed the view that the widespread use of prophylaxis might lower the level of maternal immunity and increase the severity of cases of malaria seen in children who are younger than 1 year of age. To date, there is no evidence that administration of antimalarial drugs prophylactically to pregnant women has changed the expected incidence of infection during the first few months of life.

Because of the tremendous global burden of disease imposed by malaria infections, a key initiative in the prevention of malaria is the emphasis on development of malaria vaccines. The cloning of the *P. falciparum* receptor protein, which allows red blood cell attachment, should facilitate the development of a malarial vaccine.[119, 120] Vaccine candidates are in development, but no effective vaccine will likely be available in the near future.[121, 122] Other techniques for malaria prevention include use of improved chemoprophylactic regimens and development of animal models for malaria infection in which to test vaccines and antimalarial drugs. Recently, a rhesus monkey model mimicking human infection after exposure to *Plasmodium coatneyi* has been tested with potential for use in animal studies.[123] Current recommendations for malaria prophylaxis in pregnant women may be obtained from the Malaria Branch, Centers for Disease Control and Prevention, Atlanta, Georgia.

SCHISTOSOMIASIS (BILHARZIASIS)

Schistosomiasis contributes to infertility by causing sclerosis of the fallopian tubes or cervix.[124] The placenta usually does not become infected until the third month of pregnancy or thereafter.[125] Although the frequency of placental infection is as high as 25% in endemic areas,

the infestations are light and cause little histologic reaction.[125, 126] In their study of the impact of placental infection on the outcome of pregnancy, Renaud and co-workers concluded that there was little evidence that the size or weight of the infant was affected and that placental bilharziasis was not an important cause of intrauterine growth retardation or prematurity.[125]

TRICHOMONAS VAGINALIS

Infection of the vagina of the pregnant woman with *Trichomonas vaginalis* is not uncommon, but no adverse effect on the fetus has been documented.[127, 128] *T. vaginalis* was recovered from the tracheal secretions of three infants with respiratory illness whose viral and bacterial cultures revealed no other pathogens, but a causal relationship was not certain.[129, 130] During the first 2 weeks of life, female newborns may be particularly susceptible to infection because of the influence of maternal estrogens on the vaginal epithelium. By 3 to 6 weeks of age, the vaginal pH is no longer acid.[131] *T. vaginalis* has been found in 0 to 4.8% of sequentially studied female newborns.[131-133] Among infants younger than 3 weeks of age who had vaginal discharges, *T. vaginalis* was the probable cause of the discharge in 17.2%.[134] In addition to causing a vaginal discharge,[135] infection of the newborn with *T. vaginalis* may aggravate candidal infections and may be associated with urinary tract infections.[131] In most infants, the white blood cells found in the urine originate from the vagina rather than from the bladder.[136] However, several reports suggest that a bacterial urinary tract infection can be present concomitantly.[137, 138] In symptomatic cases, metronidazole has been used at a dosage of 50 mg every 8 hours for 5 to 7 days.[131, 136, 139]

TRICHINOSIS

Prenatal transmission of trichinosis from mother to infant is rare. Four larvae, however, were found in the diaphragm of a fetus by Kuitunen-Ekbaum.[140] No evidence of infection with trichinosis was found in 25 newborns studied by McNaught and Anderson.[141] Despite this, *Trichinella spiralis* has been found in the placenta and in the milk of nursing women as well as in the tissue from the mammary gland.[142] In 1939, Hood and Olson found *T. spiralis* in pressed muscle preparations from 4 to 48 (8.3%) infants from birth to 12 months of age.[143] Therefore, although transplacental transmission is rare, *T. spiralis* is present in the placenta of women with acute trichinosis and can be passed to the infant by means of breast milk.

BABESIOSIS

Babesia microti is a tick-borne protozoan that infects erythrocytes and causes a malaria-like illness. Most cases in the United States have occurred in the Northeast. Raucher and colleagues described a *B. microti* infection in a pregnant woman that began in the nineteenth week of gestation; the infant was born at term without evidence of infection.[144]

PNEUMOCYSTIS CARINII

Pneumocystis carinii, an organism of unsettled taxonomy, was discovered in the lungs of small mammals and humans in Brazil more than 80 years ago. It is today a widely known cause of often fatal pneumonic disease in patients with immunodeficiencies, hematologic malignancy, collagen-vascular disorders, or organ allografts who receive corticosteroids and immunosuppressive drug therapy. Although congenital or neonatal infection with *Pneumocystis* is unusual, the infection may occur in infants younger than 1 year of age in two well-defined epidemiologic settings: (1) in epidemics in nurseries located in impoverished areas of the world and (2) in isolated cases in which the infected child has an underlying primary immunodeficiency disease[145] or acquired immunodeficiency syndrome (AIDS) (see Chapter 9).

The intent of this chapter is to review the problem of *Pneumocystis* infection in the newborn. However, much of our knowledge of the epidemiologic, pathologic, and clinical features of pneumocystosis is drawn from observations of the infection in older children and adults. As a result, we have elected to include data derived from such observations to present a more complete picture of the infectious process caused by this unique organism.

History

In 1909, Chagas in Brazil first described the morphologic forms of *Pneumocystis* in the lungs of guinea pigs infected with *T. cruzi*.[146] However, he believed the forms to be a sexual state in the life cycle of the trypanosome and not a different organism. Carini, an Italian working in Brazil, later saw the same parasite-like cysts in the lungs of rats experimentally infected with *Trypanosoma lewisi*.[147] His slide material was subsequently reviewed by the Delanoes at the Pasteur Institute in Paris. They recognized that these alveolar cysts were present in the lungs of local Parisian sewer rats and thereby established that the "organisms" were independent of trypanosomes.[148] They proposed the name *P. carinii* for the new species.

At about this time, Chagas may have also unwittingly described the first human case of pneumocystosis when he reported the presence of similar organisms in the lungs of a patient with interstitial pneumonia who had died of American trypanosomiasis.[149] However, no definite etiologic connection was made between *P. carinii* and human pneumonic disease for another 30 years. The reason for this delay was the belief during this period that infantile syphilis was responsible for virtually all instances of interstitial plasmacellular pneumonia. In 1938, Benecke[150] and Ammich[151] identified a histologically similar pneumonic illness in nonsyphilitic children, which was characterized by a peculiar honeycombed exudate in alveoli. Subsequent scrutiny of photomicrographs in their reports revealed the presence of *P. carinii* organisms,[152] but it was not until 1942 that Van der Meer and Brug in the Netherlands unequivocally recognized the parasite in lungs from two infants and one adult.[153] The first epidemics of interstitial plasma cell pneumonia were reported shortly thereafter among premature debilitated babies in nurseries and foundling homes in central Europe, and in 1952, Vanek and Jirovec in Czechoslovakia provided the most convincing demonstration of the etiologic relationship of *P. carinii* to this disease entity in an autopsy study of 16 cases.[152]

Pneumocystosis was first brought to the attention of pediatricians in the United States in 1953 by Deamer and Zollinger, who reviewed the pathologic and epidemiologic features of the European disease.[154] Lunseth and associates are generally given credit for the initial case report of interstitial plasma cell pneumonia occurring in an infant born in the United States.[155] Curiously, the latter authors neither identified *Pneumocystis* organisms in their histologic sections nor even alluded to the parasite in their discussion of causation of the disease. During the next year, however, the presence of *Pneumocystis* pneumonia in the United States was documented in several published studies.[156-158]

In 1957, Gajdusek presented an in-depth perspective of the history of the infection that included an extensive bibliography.[159] This review was particularly timely because the next decade was to see the disturbing emergence of *P. carinii* pneumonia in the Western world—even while the epidemic disease in central Europe was waning—to the degree that it would become preeminent among the so-called opportunistic pulmonary infections of the compromised immunosuppressed host.

The Organism

The precise taxonomic status of *P. carinii* remains to be determined. Because the organism has only fairly recently been propagated in vitro, efforts to classify it and to elucidate its structure and life cycle have been based exclusively on morphologic observations of infected lungs from animals and humans. Because the earliest of these investigations was performed by parasitologists, the terminology applied to the forms of *Pneumocystis* seen in diseased tissue has been that reserved for protozoan parasites.

Three developmental forms of this presumably unicellular microbe[160] have been described: a thick-walled cyst, an intracystic sporozoite, and a thin-walled trophozoite.[153, 161, 162] The diagnostic form of *Pneumocystis* is the cyst, which may contain up to eight sporozoites. Each sporozoite is round to crescentic, measures 1 to 2 μm in diameter, and contains an eccentric nucleus. This cystic unit with its intracystic bodies is seen well in Giemsa-stained imprint smears of infected fresh lung.[159, 163] However, Giemsa stain results in staining of background alveoli and host cell fragments and does not stain empty cysts. Gomori methenamine silver nitrate stain, which highlights only the cyst wall of *Pneumocystis*, is preferable to Giemsa stain when tissues must be screened for the presence of organisms.[164-166]

The cysts stained with silver have a thin, often wrinkled, black capsule that may be round, crescentic, or disk-shaped. Each cyst measures 4 to 6 μm in diameter and must be distinguished from an erythrocyte. The cysts often occur in clusters within an alveolus (Fig. 19–1).

The typical honeycombed intra-alveolar exudate of *Pneumocystis* pneumonia is largely a collection of interlocking cysts whose walls flatten at points of contact, so that each cyst assumes a hexagonal shape. The internal structure of the silver-stained cyst is variable. In the lighter-stained round cysts, a pair of structures about 1 μm long resembling opposed commas or parentheses is often seen; these are occasionally connected end to end by thin, delicate strands.[164] Other cysts contain only a marginal nodule (Fig. 19–2). Whether these intracystic details correspond to the sporozoite-like bodies seen in Giemsa-stained preparations is not clear. However, there is evidence from both light and electron microscopy to suggest that they may not be located within cyst cytoplasm at all; instead, they may be thickened portions of the cyst wall.[167–169]

Staining procedures other than Giemsa and methenamine silver have been employed less frequently to delineate the cyst form of the organism. The cyst wall stains red with periodic acid–Schiff stain.[170] A modified Gram-Weigert method stains both the cyst wall and the intracystic sporozoites.[171] Gridley fungus stain may identify cyst outlines. More reliable stains for this purpose are the modified toluidine blue stain of Chalvardjian and Grawe[172] and the cresyl echt violet stain,[173] which color the cyst wall purple.

Electron microscopy has been an invaluable tool in morphologic studies of *P. carinii*.[161, 168, 174–182] It has helped to confirm that the structures regarded as *Pneumocystis* under light microscopy are, in fact, typical microorganisms and not just degradation products of host cells.[183]

Both trophozoite and cystlike stages have been delineated.[182] The trophozoite is thin walled and measures between 1.5 and 2.0 μm in diameter. It has numerous evaginations or pseudopodia-like projections, which appear to interdigitate with those of other parasites in the alveolar space.[177, 182] It has been postulated that the pseudopodia make up the reticular framework within which organisms reside in an alveolus and account for the fact that organisms remain clumped in lung imprints.[163, 172] It has also been suggested that the pseudopodia have also been shown to anchor *Pneumocystis* to the alveolar septal wall.[180] The prevailing opinion, however, is that there is no specialized organelle of attachment. Rather, the surfaces of *P. carinii* and alveolar cells (specifically, type I pneumonocytes) are closely opposed without fusion of cell membranes.[184] This adherence of *P. carinii* to alveolar lining cells may explain why organisms are not found commonly in expectorated mucus or tracheal secretions.[177]

The classic cystic unit of *P. carinii* is thick walled and measures 4 to 6 μm in diameter. The intracystic bodies measure 1.0 to 1.7 μm across and bear a marked similarity to small trophozoites[182] (Figs. 19–3 and 19–4). In addition, thick-walled cysts rich in glycogen particles but without intracystic bodies ("precysts"), partly empty cysts, and collapsed cystic structures have been identified. The collapsed cysts are crescentic and presumably are the same crescentic forms seen frequently in silver-stained specimens under light microscopy. They commonly have defects in their walls.

Life cycles for *P. carinii* have been proposed. They

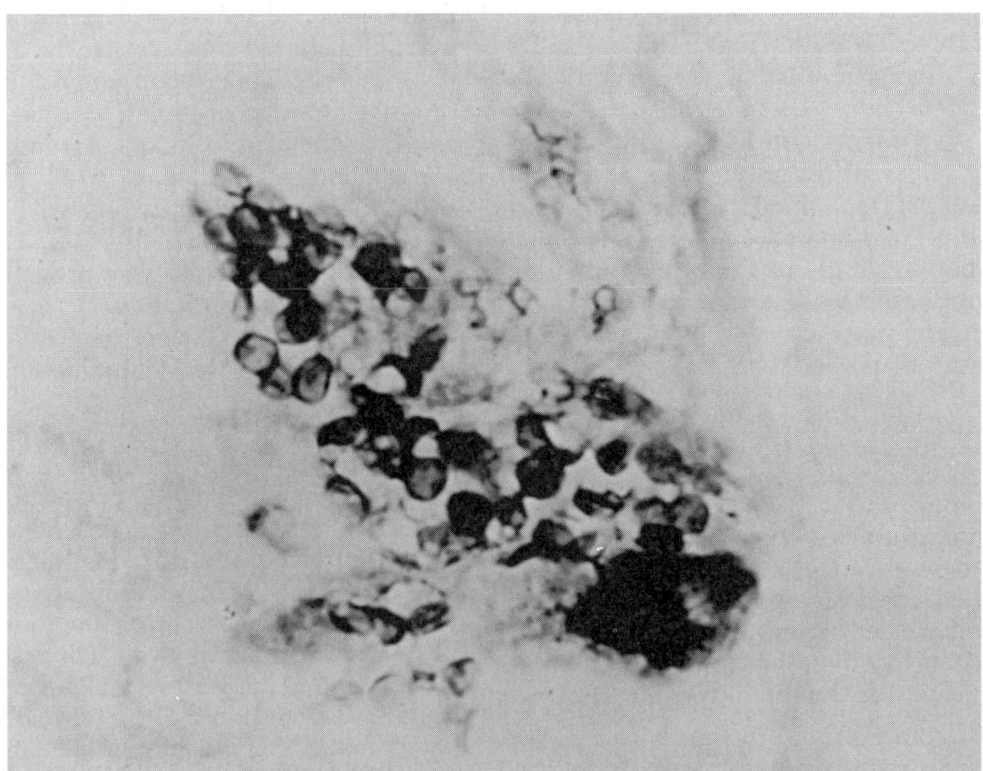

Figure 19–1 Section of lung tissue showing an alveolus filled with cystic forms of *Pneumocystis carinii*. Gomori methenamine silver stain, 400×. (From Remington JS. Hosp Pract 7:59, April 1972, with permission.)

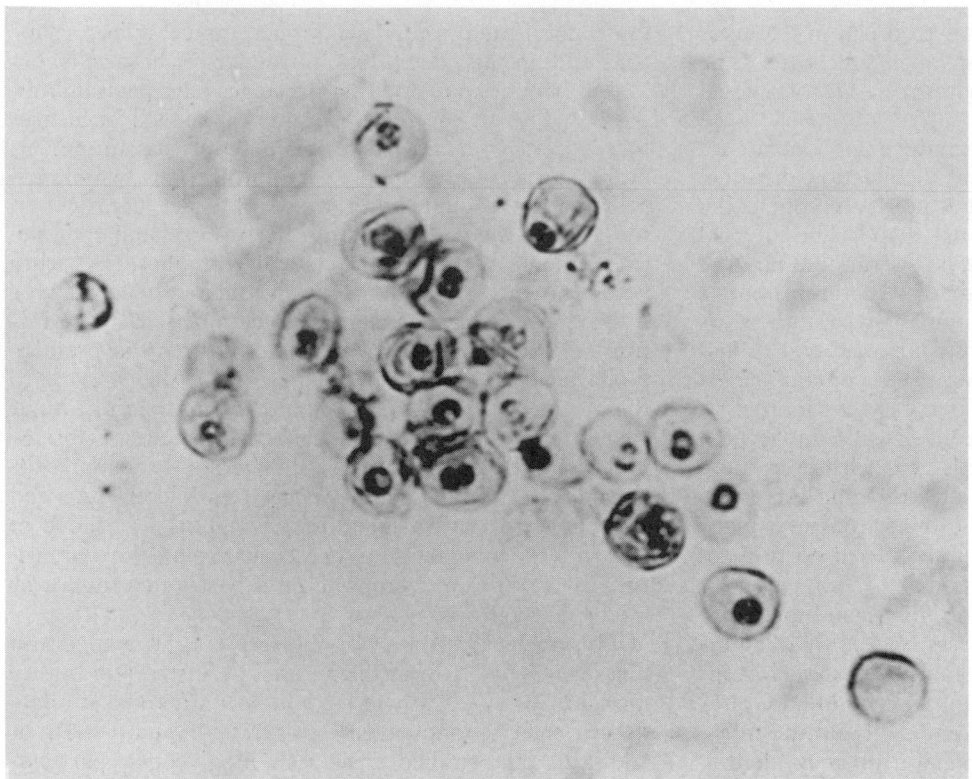

Figure 19–2 Imprint smear of fresh lung tissue stained with methenamine silver that shows a cluster of cysts of *Pneumocystis carinii*; typical comma-shaped bodies and marginal nodules are visible within cysts. 625×. (From Ruskin J, Remington JS. The compromised host and infection. JAMA 202:1070–1074, 1967. Copyright 1967, American Medical Association.)

have been based on the variant forms of the parasite detected by light[168, 169, 185–187] and electron[182, 188] microscopy. In one scheme[182] (Fig. 19–5), the thick-walled round cyst undergoes dissolution or "cracking" and the intracystic bodies pass through tears in the wall. It is not known whether the bodies escape from the cyst by active motility or whether they are extruded passively as a consequence of cyst collapse. At this stage, the intracystic bodies resemble free thin-walled trophozoites. It had been suggested that division of the intracystic body must occur soon after its expulsion from the mature thick-walled cyst to account for the large numbers of small (1 μm) trophozoites seen in infected lung.[168] However, electron microscopic observations indicate that another source for the smaller trophozoite is the immature thin-walled *Pneumocystis* cyst.[188] In any case, the small trophozoites evolve to larger forms, their walls thicken, and a precyst develops that is devoid of intracystic bodies. The cyclic process is completed when the mature cyst stage, containing eight daughter cysts, is achieved.

Despite these extensive morphologic studies of *P. carinii*, its taxonomic classification is unsettled.[189]

Controversy persists over whether the organism is a protozoan[190, 191] or a fungus.[192] Arguments in favor of a protozoan taxonomy are based mainly on the resemblance of its structural features to those of other protozoa. The organism has cystic and trophozoite stages, pseudopodia in cell walls, and pellicles around intracystic sporozoites.[180, 193] In addition, the disease caused by *Pneumocystis* responds to anti-protozoal—namely, antitrypanosomal or antitoxoplasmal—chemotherapy. On the other hand, proponents of a mycotic derivation of the organism note that, like fungi, *P. carinii* contains a paucity of cellular organelles, its nucleus is not visibly prominent, its cell membrane is layered throughout an entire life cycle, and its cell wall stains vividly with silver.[168]

The question of species specificity of *Pneumocystis* is similarly unanswered. Although most workers concur that human and rodent forms of the parasite are morphologically indistinguishable by light and electron microscopy,[161, 169, 182, 186] serologic studies designed to demonstrate identity between human and animal species[169, 190, 194–198] or even between human strains from diverse geographic locales[199, 200] yield conflicting results.

In Vitro Cultivation

Successful propagation of *P. carinii* in vitro was first reported in 1977 by Pifer and colleagues at the St. Jude Children's Research Hospital.[201, 202] These workers serially passed organisms in primary embryonic chick epithelial lung cells over 12 days and noted a 100-fold increase in numbers of cysts. Inoculation of trophozoites alone yielded modest numbers of cyst forms and typical cytopathogenic effects. However, continuing cultivation of *Pneumocystis* was not achieved. In addition, the organisms could not be grown in cell-free media employed commonly for the propagation of other parasites.[201]

Limited replication of *Pneumocystis* has since been accomplished in more widely available tissue culture cell lines (Vero, Chang liver, MRC 5, WI 38).[203–205] These tissue culture systems have not been used to isolate *P. carinii* from the lungs of animals or humans with suspected infection. However, examination of the organism in tissue culture has confirmed the existence of each of

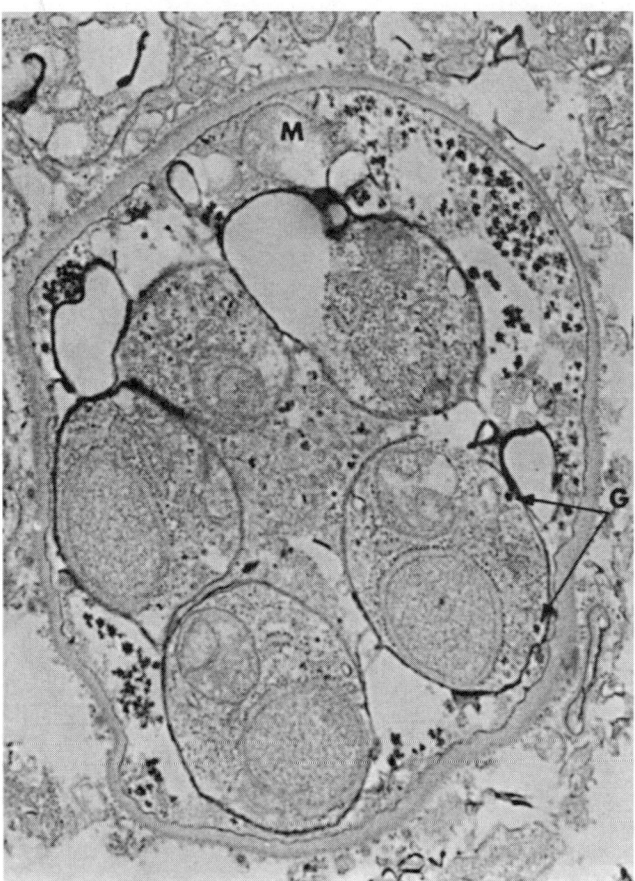

Figure 19–3 Formation of intracystic bodies in cyst of *Pneumocystis carinii*. Pellicle appears to be in the process of being formed from membranes within cytoplasm. Glycogen-like particles are almost entirely excluded from intracystic bodies. Arrows indicate two glycogen-like particles (G) within intracystic body. Mitochondrion (M) is also excluded from intracystic bodies. Lead citrate, original magnification 32,000×. (From Campbell WG Jr. Ultrastructure of *Pneumocystis* in human lung. Life cycle in human pneumocystosis. Arch Pathol 93:312–324, 1972. Copyright 1972, American Medical Association.)

its morphologic forms and has provided insight into the biologic interaction between the parasite and the host cells.[206]

Epidemiology

The natural habitat of *P. carinii* is unknown. However, it is clear that the distribution of human infection is worldwide[207-232] and that a variety of wild and domestic animal species harbor the organism without demonstrable pulmonary disease. Rarely, clinically evident *Pneumocystis* pneumonitis, not unlike the disease in humans, arises spontaneously in the animal host.[233-238]

The exact prevalence of infection with *Pneumocystis* remains to be determined because serologic methodology has not yet been employed on a sufficiently large scale to detect latent carriage of the parasite. However, serologic surveys indicate that infection is widespread and is acquired in early life. Meuwissen and colleagues

in the Netherlands noted that immunofluorescent antibodies to *P. carinii* are first detectable in normal children at the age of 6 months and by age 4 years nearly all children are seropositive.[239] Pifer and associates in the United States found significant titers of antibody to *Pneumocystis* in normal infants at age 7 months and in two thirds of normal children by age 4 years.[240] Gerrard and co-workers in England detected *P. carinii* antibodies in serum from 48% of 94 young healthy children.[241] Pifer and associates also found that normal rats possess serologic evidence of *Pneumocystis* infection before immunosuppressive therapy with corticosteroids causes them to develop overt *Pneumocystis* pneumonia.[242] Authors of a number of autopsy reviews have attempted to determine the incidence of *Pneumocystis* infection, but the results have been divergent, owing to the heterogeneity of the populations sampled.[229, 243-249] Those studies conducted in central Europe after World War II[244] or in cancer referral centers in the United States[249] have yielded higher rates of infection.

Few published reports have been devoted exclusively to the descriptive epidemiology of *Pneumocystis* pneumonia in the United States. In a literature review of the subject, Le Clair accumulated 107 accounts of the disease recorded from 1955 through 1967.[250] The male-to-female ratio of infected individuals was in excess of 2 to 1. The disease was reported from diverse geographic locales (21 of the 50 states). Climatic and ethnic factors were relatively unimportant in case distribution. The largest number of cases (33) occurred in infants younger than 1 year of age. Proved or presumptive congenital immunodeficiencies were identifiable in virtually all the children in this group. In patients 1 to 10 years of age, the next largest group (26), only 6 had a primary immune deficit, whereas most of the other children had an underlying hematologic malignancy. The remaining patients, ranging in age from 10 to 81 years, were individuals with assorted malignancies and renal allografts who almost always had prior exposure to corticosteroids or to radiation or cytotoxic drugs. The mortality rate for the entire group of patients was 95%.

The Centers for Disease Control and Prevention updated Le Clair's epidemiologic investigation in two separate communications, which related the epidemiologic as well as diagnostic and clinical aspects of all confirmed cases of pneumocystosis reported to its Parasitic Disease Drug Service between 1967 and 1970.[251, 252] The first of these reports has particular relevance here because it focused only on the infectious episodes in infants and young children.[251] A total of 194 documented cases of *P. carinii* pneumonia were analyzed, and the largest number of these (29) occurred, as in Le Clair's study, in infants younger than 1 year of age. The attack rate for this group (8.4 per million) was in fact calculated to be more than five times higher than that for other age groups. Eighty-three percent of these infants had an underlying primary immunodeficiency disease. Moreover, because the inheritance of the primary immunodeficiency state was often sex linked, the preponderance of infection (88%) occurred in males. The average age at the time of diagnosis of *Pneumocystis* pneumonia in the immunodeficient infants in this series was 7.5 months, whereas

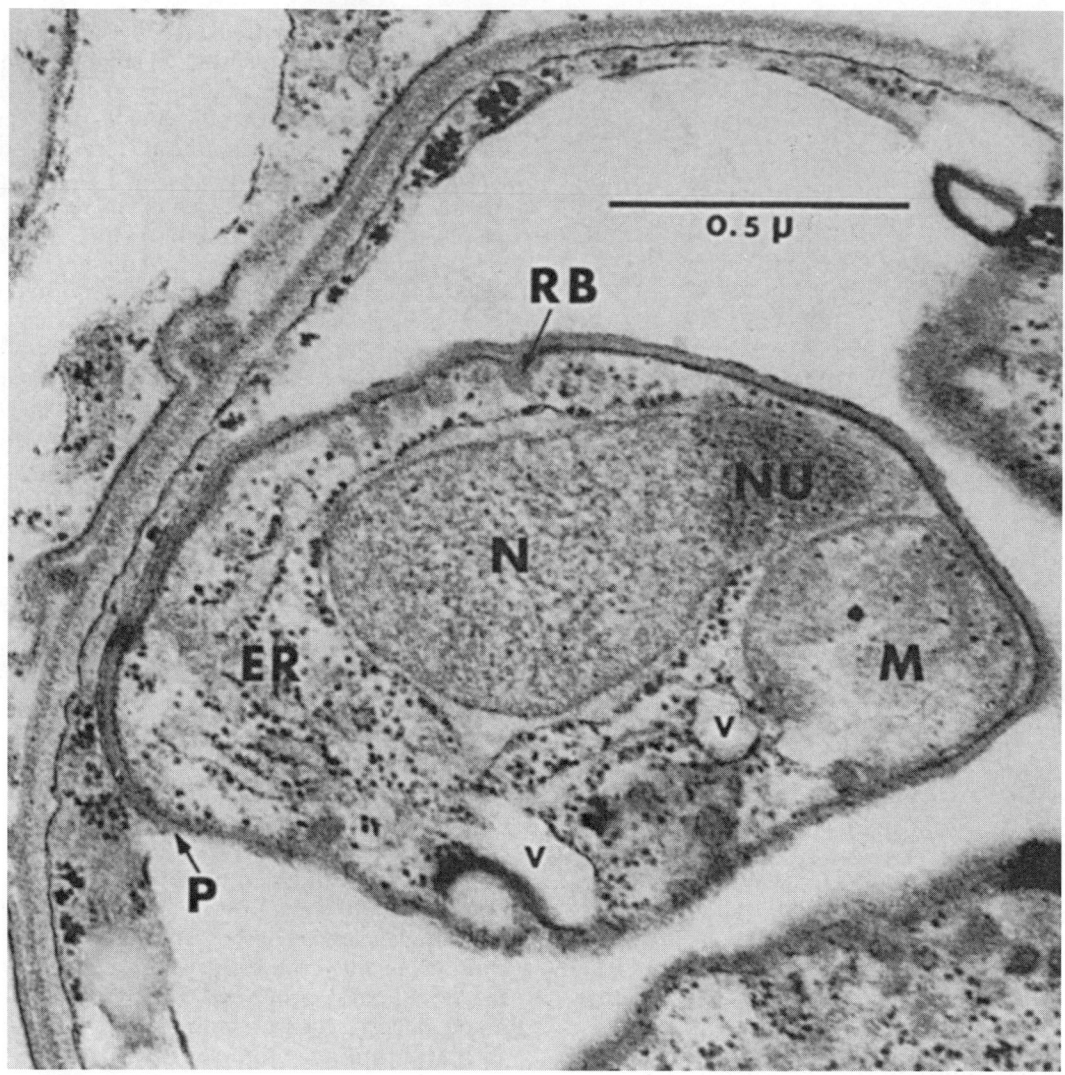

Figure 19–4 Intracystic body within mature cyst. Six-layer effect of cyst wall occurs only where there is contact with adjacent organisms. Note unit-membrane character of undulating membranes that form innermost layer of cyst wall and outer and inner membranes of pellicle (P). Round bodies (RB) appear to arise from pellicle (arrow). Rough endoplasmic reticulum (ER) is well developed. Ribosomes are attached to the external membrane of nucleus, and this membrane appears to communicate with membranes of rough endoplasmic reticulum. Cytoplasm also contains vacuoles (v). Nucleus (N) contains nucleolus (NU). Mitochondrion (M) is at the right. 80,000×. (From Campbell WG Jr. Ultrastructure of *Pneumocystis* in human lung. Life cycle in human pneumocystosis. Arch Pathol 93:312–324, 1972. Copyright 1972, American Medical Association.)

the epidemic form of the infection in European and Asian infants produced peak morbidity in the third and fourth months of life.[159, 163] Twenty-four percent of the infected children with immunodeficiencies had at least one sibling with an identifiable immune deficit who also developed *P. carinii* pneumonia.

After this analysis of cases indigenous to the United States was completed, it became evident that infantile pneumocystosis could be introduced into the United States from epidemics abroad. In reality, the first such case was reported as early as 1966, when a 3-month-old Korean infant suffered a fatal infection with *Pneumocystis* after being brought to the United States from an orphanage in Korea where the infection had been rampant.[253] The potential for imported pneumocystosis received renewed publicity with the cessation of hostilities

in Vietnam. Surveillance for *Pneumocystis* infection in American-adopted Vietnamese orphans was urged when it was recognized that large numbers of infants exposed to the hardships of war and malnutrition in Indochina had experienced fulminant *Pneumocystis* pneumonia.[254, 255] In quick succession, there appeared multiple reports of *Pneumocystis* infection in these refugee Vietnamese.[256–259] Of note is that most of the infants affected were about 3 months old; this was exactly the age at which pneumocystosis had emerged in the marasmic children infected during the earlier nursery epidemics in central Europe and Asia.

The epidemiology of *P. carinii* infection has changed in the United States and elsewhere as cases of human immunodeficiency virus (HIV) infection have occurred in infants[260] (see Chapter 9). Like adults with AIDS,

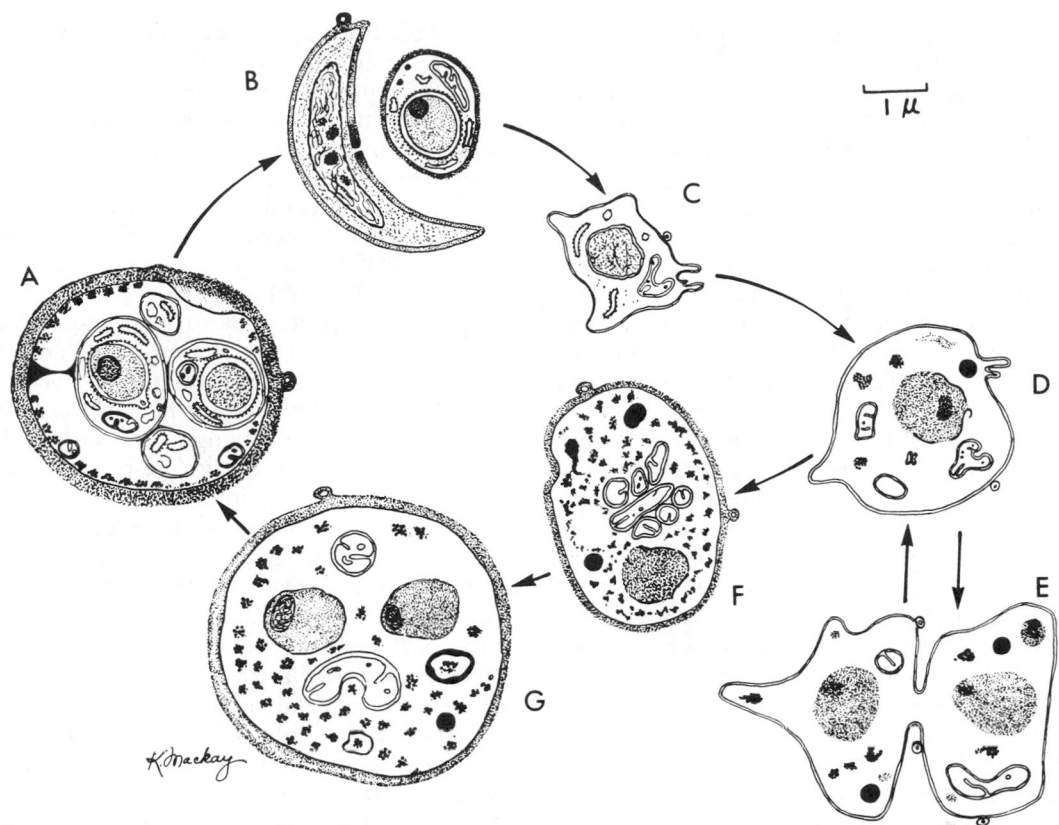

Figure 19–5 Probable life cycle of *Pneumocystis* within pulmonary alveoli. Mature cyst with intracystic bodies *(A)*; empty cyst and recently escaped intracystic body *(B)*; small trophozoite *(C)*; larger trophozoite *(D)*; possible budding or conjugating form *(E)*; large trophozoite undergoing thickening of pellicle *(F)*; precyst *(G)*. (From Campbell WG Jr. Ultrastructure of *Pneumocystis* in human lung. Life cycle in human pneumocystosis. Arch Pathol 93:312–324, 1972. Copyright 1972, American Medical Association.)

infants with AIDS are at high risk for this opportunistic infection. Among children with perinatally acquired HIV infection, *P. carinii* pneumonitis occurs most often among infants 3 to 6 months of age.[261]

The epidemiologic data presented thus far make it clear that congenital or acquired immunodeficiency disorders underlie most cases of *Pneumocystis* pneumonia. There have been only scattered reports of the infection in purportedly immunocompetent individuals.[175, 218, 243] However, it has been suggested[262–266] that *P. carinii* may be an important cause of pneumonitis in immunologically intact infants. In a prospective study of infant pneumonia, Stagno and co-workers detected *Pneumocystis* antigenemia in 10 (14%) of 67 infants.[267] None of these 10 subjects with serologic evidence of *Pneumocystis* infection had a primary immunodeficiency, nor had any received immunosuppressive medication. Antigenemia did not occur in control infants or in infants with pneumonitis caused by *Chlamydia trachomatis*, respiratory syncytial virus, cytomegalovirus, adenovirus, and influenza A and B viruses. Histopathologic confirmation of *Pneumocystis* pneumonia was possible in only the one child who underwent open lung biopsy. *P. carinii* also causes pneumonia in infants living in developing countries even when the child is not malnourished. Shann and associates found *P. carinii* antigen in serum from 23 of 94 children in Papua New Guinea who were hospitalized with pneu-

monia.[268] Nevertheless, more cases need to be confirmed histologically before it is accepted that *Pneumocystis* infection produces significant morbidity in infants who are not immunosuppressed.

Transmission

The mode of transmission of *P. carinii* remains unclear. Sporadic cases of pneumocystosis serve as poor models of infection transmission because they may not become clinically manifest until long after the host has acquired the organism. That person-to-person spread of *Pneumocystis* could occur was first suggested by the European nursery epidemics. However, even in these institutional outbreaks, it was readily appreciated that direct interpatient transfer of the organism happened rarely.[159] Rather, seroepidemiologic investigation indicated that healthy, subclinically infected nursery personnel transmitted the infection.[185, 199, 269]

The exact mode of spread of *Pneumocystis* from infected asymptomatic individuals to susceptible infants in the closed nursery environments was never settled. Airborne droplet transmission was suspected when "sterilization of air with ionizing radiation"[270] and isolation of uninfected infants from infected infants and their seropositive attendants[271] reduced the frequency of clinical disease. The thesis that *Pneumocystis* is transmissible through the air presupposes that the organism can be found in respiratory secretions. Although, as emphasized earlier, the intra-alveolar histopathology of pneumocystosis militates against this occurrence, *Pneumocystis* is occasionally detected in tracheal aspirates and sputum.[171, 187, 272–276]

Epidemiologic investigation of sporadic pneumocystosis indicates that person-to-person transmission of the infection is possible in specific situations. The sequential development of *Pneumocystis* pneumonia in immunosuppressed adults occupying adjoining hospital beds has been recorded.[277, 278] Jacobs and associates described a cluster of *P. carinii* pneumonia in adults without predisposing illnesses who were all inpatients between July and October 1989 at the same hospital.[279] Whereas all five patients were on different floors of the hospital on three different services, two of the patients were briefly in the intensive care unit at the same time. The mechanism of transmission was unknown. Immune evaluation of three of the five patients revealed essentially normal CD4, CD8, and CD4:CD8 ratios. However, all had depressed responses to T cell lectin phytohemagglutinin and T cell–dependent B-cell pokeweed mitogen. Although such episodes may have been coincidental, it seems reasonable to isolate patients with *Pneumocystis* pneumonia from other compromised hosts similarly prone to fulminant infection with the parasite. Occurrences of pneumocystosis in members of one family have also been reported.[264, 280–284] In a single instance, pneumonic disease developed in three family members in a strikingly related time sequence.[264] More commonly, however, cases within a family emerge over a period of several years and affected members are almost always infant siblings with either proven or suspected underlying immunodeficiencies. In at least three family studies, no fewer than three siblings succumbed to the infection.[280, 282, 283] However, it is unlikely that direct patient-to-patient transfer of the organism occurred in any of these settings because in the vast majority of them the siblings developed disease months or years apart, often long after the death of the initially infected child.[251]

Contagion could still be implicated in the family milieu if a reservoir of asymptomatic infection with *P. carinii* existed among healthy family members. In this regard, there are two published accounts of infants with primary immunodeficiencies and pneumocystosis whose parents were deemed to be possible sources of the infection because their sera contained specific anti-*Pneumocystis* antibody.[283, 285]

Maternal transfer of *Pneumocystis* to infants from colostrum or from the genital tract at parturition might also maintain *Pneumocystis* within a family, but screening of breast milk[281] or cervical secretions[282] with Giemsa and silver methenamine stains has failed to reveal the presence of the parasite. Alternatively, acquisition of *P. carinii* by infants in utero could occur. Unfortunately, it is difficult to test this hypothesis in the absence of reliable serologic tools to detect subclinical infection in the newborn. However, the paucity of documented cases of overt *Pneumocystis* pneumonia in stillborn infants or in the early neonatal period argues against frequent intrauterine passage of the organism.

In 1962, Pavlica, in Czechoslovakia, recorded the first instance of congenital infection.[286] The infant was stillborn. The parents and a female sibling were in good health. The mother's serum had complement-fixing antibodies against *Pneumocystis*. Subsequently, in a report detailing experience with *Pneumocystis* infection in southern Iran, a male child who had died at the age of 2 days was described; autopsy examination revealed scattered although definite alveolar foci of typical *Pneumocystis* infection.[287] The authors reasoned that this represented congenital infection rather than an acquired disease with an untenably short incubation period. Bazaz and colleagues, in the United States, described the striking development of *Pneumocystis* pneumonia in three otherwise normal female siblings who died at 3 months, 2 months, and 3 days of age, respectively; again, an in utero source of their infections was considered to be most likely.[282] In none of these cases of presumptive congenital pneumocystosis, however, was the placenta examined histologically for the presence of the parasite. One infant, born to a mother with AIDS and documented *P. carinii* pneumonia in the fourth month of gestation, did not have *P. carinii* infection in the newborn period.[288] Beach and co-workers reported an HIV-positive newborn with meconium aspiration and pneumonia, with *P. carinii* identified on open-lung biopsy at 19 days of age.[289] Of interest, despite the infant's positive HIV status, serum from the infant's mother was HIV-negative and the serum from the father HIV-positive. Because the parents disappeared shortly after the infant's birth, no follow-up was available; however, the parents had no previous history of *P. carinii* pneumonia and the mother had been noted to be markedly wasted.

The possibility that contagion is responsible for acquisition of the infection in older children was first explored in the United States at the University of Minnesota Hospitals[290] and at St. Jude Children's Research Hospital,[249] where in 1968 and 1969 an unusually high concentration of cases was recorded. At neither center was it possible to reconstruct the spread of pneumocystosis from one patient to another. In most cases, the onset of illness appeared to antedate admission to the hospital. No attempt was made in these studies, however, to incriminate asymptomatic carriers as point sources for seemingly isolated episodes of infection. At Memorial Hospital in New York, 11 patients, including 6 children, developed *Pneumocystis* pneumonia in a 3-month period.[291] Although no definite evidence of communicability could be discerned in this statistically significant cluster of cases, several of the *Pneumocystis*-infected children had had contact with each other and had shared rooms at various times; in addition, two physicians caring for these patients had had positive serologic tests for *Pneumocystis* infection. Similar outbreaks have since occurred in two pediatric hospitals in Indianapolis, Indiana,[292] and Milwaukee, Wisconsin.[293] At these centers, the increased rates of pneumocystosis were clearly related, as they were at St. Jude Children's Research Hospital,[249, 294] to the use of more intensive cancer chemotherapy protocols. However, in a seroepidemiologic investigation of the cases in the Indianapolis outbreak, it was found that transmission of *Pneumocystis* probably occurred within the hospital environment. A direct association was noted between length of hospitalization and subsequent *Pneumocystis* infection. Furthermore, a significantly higher prevalence of positive serologic tests for *Pneumocystis* was detected for staff members who had close contact with infected children than in personnel who had other duties. Precisely how *Pneumocystis* was originally introduced into the hospital was not determined.

Another intriguing possibility is that *Pneumocystis* pneumonia is a zoonotic disease and that infestation of rodents or even domesticated pets could provide a sizable reservoir for human infection. Indeed, abundant infection of rodents with *Pneumocystis* was discovered in the homes of many of the index cases in ward epidemics in Czechoslovakia.[295] In the United States at St. Jude Children's Research Hospital, a high rate of exposure to pets was noted among the *Pneumocystis*-infected children with malignancy.[296] Of course, these findings would have epidemiologic significance only if the species of *Pneumocystis* infecting both animals and humans was the same. This remains to be shown. On the contrary, experimental attempts to produce clinical pneumocystosis in multiple animal species by inoculation of infected human lung suspensions have not been successful,[166, 297 299] unless the animal was congenitally athymic[300] or immunosuppressed by treatment with corticosteroid (see later discussion).[301]

TRANSMISSION IN EXPERIMENTAL ANIMAL PNEUMOCYSTOSIS

Airborne transmission of *Pneumocystis* was first presumptively demonstrated by Hendley and Weller in 1971.[302] They observed that cesarean section–obtained, barrier-sustained (COBS) rats treated with corticosteroids developed patent infections with *Pneumocystis* when exposed to a common air supply from standard infected rats, whereas control corticosteroid-treated COBS animals remained free of infection. One potential flaw in this experimental design was that the corticosteroid therapy could have reactivated previously latent *Pneumocystis* infection in any of the challenged animals. To circumvent this problem, Walzer and co-workers challenged congenitally athymic (nude) mice.[300] These animals received no exogenous immunosuppressants and still contracted pneumocystosis after exposure to air from infected rats. Thus, these studies documented airborne transmission of *P. carinii* as well as spread of the organism between different animal species. Of note is that soon after these experiments were published, a natural epizootic of *Pneumocystis* pneumonia was uncovered in a colony of nude mice.[303]

Other studies with the murine model of pneumocystosis have suggested that subclinical transmission of the infection may also occur. Normal rats exposed to animals with *Pneumocystis* pneumonia remain well but develop titers of anti-*Pneumocystis* antibody consistent with acute acquisition of the infection.[304] In addition, rats with preexisting *Pneumocystis* antibody may become antigenemic on comparable exposure to overt infection; as such, they may be experiencing subclinical reinfection.[242]

Pathology

The gross and microscopic pathology of *P. carinii* pneumonia has been elucidated in a number of excellent reviews.[154, 159, 163, 166, 170, 270, 290, 305–307] At autopsy in typically advanced infection, both lungs are heavy and diffusely affected. The most extensive involvement is often located in posterior or dependent areas. At the lung margins anteriorly, a few remaining air-filled alveoli may constitute the only portion of functioning lung at the time of death.[154] Subpleural air blebs are not infrequently seen in these anterior marginal areas. Occasionally, there may even be prominent mediastinal emphysema or frank pneumothorax. The color of the lungs is variously described as dark bluish purple,[163, 287] yellow-pink,[164] or pale gray-brown.[154, 166] The pleural surfaces are smooth and glistening, with little inflammatory reaction. Hilar adenopathy is uncommon. Necrosis of tissue is not a feature of the disease.

Although these gross findings of widespread infection are strikingly characteristic, focal or subclinical pneumocystosis presents a less recognizable picture. In this condition, the lung has tiny 3- to 5-mm reddish brown retracted areas contained within peribronchial and subpleural lobules where hypostasis is greatest.[163, 170] However, even these features may be absent because of variable involvement of adjacent lung tissue by concomitant pathologic processes.

The microscopic appearance of both the contents and the septal walls of pulmonary alveoli in *Pneumocystis* pneumonia is virtually pathognomonic of the infection. The outstanding histologic finding with hematoxylin and eosin stain is an intensely eosinophilic, foamy, or honeycomb-like material uniformly filling the alveolar sacs (Fig. 19–6). This intra-alveolar material is composed largely of packets of *P. carinii*.[270, 308] Individually typical cysts or trophozoite forms of the parasite within alveoli are visible only after application of special stains such as silver methenamine.

The type and degree of cellular inflammatory response provoked by the intra-alveolar cluster of *Pneumocystis* organisms vary in different hosts.[270] The descriptive histologic term for pneumocystosis—interstitial plasma cell pneumonia—is derived from the pronounced plasmacellular infiltration of the interalveolar septa observed almost exclusively in newborns in European nursery epidemics. Distention of alveolar walls to 5 to 10 times normal thickness with resultant compression of alveolar spaces and capillary lumens is typically noted in this form of the disease. Hyaline membranes develop occasionally,[154] often when the foamy honeycomb pattern within alveoli is least prominent.[290] On the contrary, in sporadic pneumocystosis of older infants and children with primary or drug-induced impairment of immune reactivity, thickened septa and cellular infiltration are often less marked and plasma cells are either scant or lacking.[164, 309, 310] Although a variable degree of interstitial mononuclear infiltrate (i.e., lymphocyte or macrophage) and, less commonly, eosinophilic infiltrate is evident in

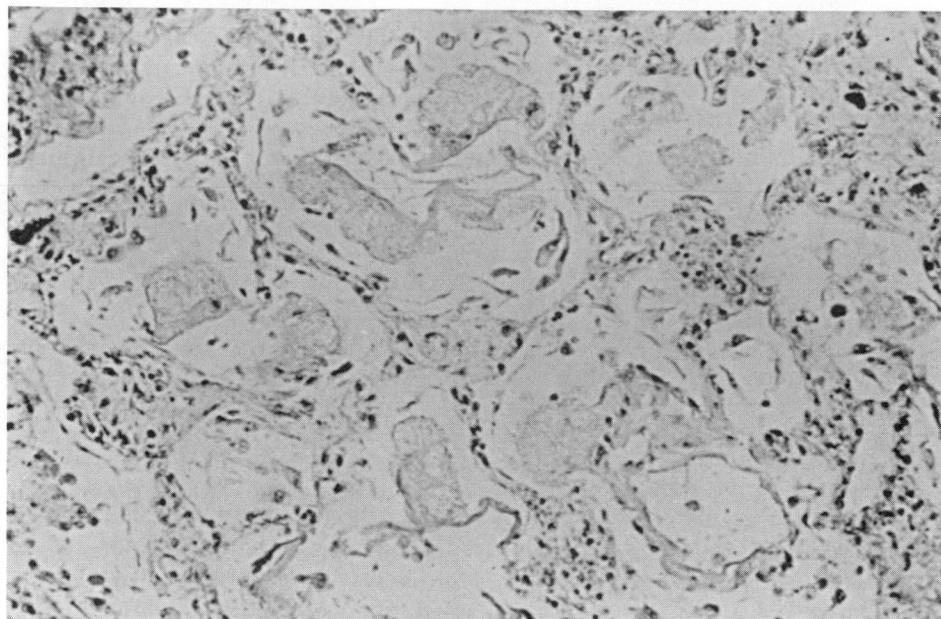

Figure 19–6 Section of lung tissue obtained at autopsy showing the amorphous, proteinaceous intra-alveolar infiltration characteristic of pneumonitis caused by *Pneumocystis carinii*. Hematoxylin and eosin stain. 160×. (From Remington JS. Hosp Pract 7:59, April 1972, with permission.)

infected immunodeficient patients, hyperplasia of alveolar lining cells rather than edema and inflammatory cell infiltration appears to be most responsible for septal thickening in the majority of cases.[247] Septal cell hyperplasia is apparently a nonspecific reaction of lung tissue to injury induced by infections of diverse etiology.[311]

Hughes and colleagues studied the histologic progression of typical *Pneumocystis* pneumonia based on the number and location of organisms and the cellular response in pulmonary tissue.[296] The lung samples were from children with underlying malignancy who had received intensive antitumor chemotherapy. The authors categorized three sequential stages in the course of the disease. In the first stage, there is no septal inflammatory or cellular response and only a few free cyst forms are present in the alveolar lumen; the remainder are isolated in the cytoplasm of cells on the alveolar septal wall. (In other histologic investigations[166, 170, 290, 312, 313] and in tissue culture systems,[201, 202, 206] an intracellular residence of *Pneumocystis* has not been confirmed.) The second stage is characterized by an increase in the number of organisms within macrophages fixed to the alveolar wall and desquamation of these cells into the alveolar space; again, only minimal septal inflammatory response is seen at this time. Finally, a third stage is identified in which there is extensive reactive and desquamative alveolitis. Such diffuse alveolar damage may be the major pathologic feature in certain cases.[314] Varying numbers of cysts of the organism, presumably undergoing dissolution, are present within the alveolar macrophages. These findings reinforce an earlier claim[315] that the so-called foamy exudate within alveoli is neither foamy edema fluid nor an exudative inflammatory reaction but largely a collection of coalesced alveolar cells and macrophages that contain sizable digestive vacuoles and remnant organisms.

The specific alveolar cell response in *Pneumocystis* pneumonia has not yet been studied in humans but

has been determined in an experimental rat model of pneumocystosis.[312, 313] Early in the infection, trophozoites line up along the alveolar wall and become attached closely to the type I pneumonocyte; the host cells are undamaged, and there is no inflammatory infiltrate. As the parasite burden increases, the type I pneumonocytes adjacent to organisms undergo focal necrosis, the type II cells become hyperplastic and alveolar macrophages become more numerous and phagocytose *Pneumocystis*. If comparable selective injury to the type I pneumonocyte occurs in human pneumocystosis, the consequent loss in integrity of the alveolar-capillary membrane could account in part for the acute onset and rapid evolution of respiratory failure that are seen so often in infected patients.

The mechanism of spread of *Pneumocystis* throughout pulmonary tissue is not completely understood. Direct invasion by the parasite through septal walls into the interstitium or the lymphatic or blood vascular spaces of the lung is considered unlikely,[170, 290, 296] except in rare instances when systemic dissemination of the organism occurs (see later discussion). Instead, it is probable that coughing expels cysts from alveoli into larger airways and that the organisms are then swept back into previously uninvolved alveolar areas.[270] This hypothesis of interairway transfer of *Pneumocystis* is supported by the fact that the heaviest concentration of parasites is usually found in dependent portions of the lung parenchyma.

UNUSUAL PATHOLOGIC CONSEQUENCES OF PNEUMOCYSTOSIS

Interstitial fibrosis is a distinctive but infrequently reported complication of *Pneumocystis* pneumonia in older children and adults but has been reported in infants only rarely.[155, 290, 297, 306, 307, 315–321] Nowak, in Europe, first emphasized that fibrosis was not unusual in the lungs of infants at autopsy who had especially protracted infection with *P. carinii*.[318] Similarly, mononuclear cell infiltration and fibrosis have been observed late in the course of experimental pneumocystosis in the rat treated with cortisone.[322, 323]

Pneumocystis-infected lungs sometimes demonstrate, in addition to fibrosis, other pathologic features compatible with a more chronic destructive inflammatory process. Multinucleate alveolar giant cells occasionally accompany alveolar cell proliferation.[163, 166, 170, 307] Whether this is more often a response to undetected concomitant viral infection is unknown. Typical granulomatous reactions with parasites visible in the granulomas have also been described.[307, 324, 325] Extensive calcification of *Pneumocystis* exudate and adjacent lung tissue may ultimately develop.[166, 290, 307] One child, with no apparent immunodeficiency, who had dual infection with *P. carinii* and cytomegalovirus in infancy developed fatal pulmonary hemosiderosis.[326] A composite histologic picture of giant cells, granuloma formation, calcification, and fibrosis has been seen in the few recorded cases of disseminated infection. Conceivably, these cases are caused by organisms possessing enhanced virulence.[327, 328]

Several instances of invasive or frankly generalized pneumocystosis have been reported in young children[327–329] (and in adults[212, 262, 297, 299]). Gajdusek[159] cited what was perhaps the first case in an infant in whom both parasitemia and widespread organ dissemination were demonstrable, but Dutz[163] rejected the validity of these findings. However, the latter investigator observed particles consistent with *Pneumocystis* merozoites in blood smears from infants with epidemic pneumocystosis.[163] That visceral spread of *Pneumocystis* can occur in congenitally immunodeficient infants is strikingly borne out by the case of a 13-month-old child with underlying thymic alymphoplasia and low serum IgG in whom organisms were found at autopsy in sections of heart, stomach, liver, spleen, kidney, bone marrow, and adrenal and thyroid glands.[329]

Common to many of these atypical cases of generalized pneumocystosis appears to be an unusually long duration (sometimes months) of objective illness, as well as extensive pulmonary parenchymal infection with calcification and granuloma formation. Alveolar walls are usually destroyed and parasitic invasion of pulmonary interstitium is apparent to such an extent that viable *Pneumocystis* organisms—perhaps within phagocytes— may have gained access to lymph and blood cells, thus permitting their eventual dissemination.[330]

Pathogenesis

The clinical conditions that predispose to the development of *Pneumocystis* pneumonia are given in Table 19–1. Because each of these conditions is associated with an impaired immune response, it may be assumed that *Pneumocystis* causes disease not because it is intrinsically virulent but because the host's antimicrobial immune mechanisms fail to contain it. The severity of *P. carinii* pneumonia in infants with AIDS illustrates this phenomenon dramatically. This would also explain in part why *Pneumocystis* pneumonia did not emerge as a serious health problem until the European epidemics, or more

---

TABLE 19–1

Conditions Associated with *Pneumocystis carinii* Pneumonia

1. Premature infants aged 2 to 4 months with marasmus and malnutrition, usually living in foundling homes in geographic locales endemic for pneumocystosis
2. Infants and children with congenital (primary) immunodeficiency disease
   a. Severe combined immunodeficiency
   b. X-linked agammaglobulinemia
   c. X-linked immunodeficiency
   d. Variable immunodeficiency
   e. Immunodeficiency with hyperimmunoglobulinemia
   f. Immunodeficiency associated with Wiskott-Aldrich syndrome
3. Children and adults with acquired immunodeficiency
   a. Disease-related: lymphoreticular malignancies; multiple myeloma; dysproteinemias
   b. Drug-related (corticosteroids, cyclophosphamide, busulfan, methotrexate, colloidal gold); organ transplantation; lymphoreticular malignancies; solid tumors; collagen vascular disorders; miscellaneous diseases treated with immunosuppressants
   c. Acquired immunodeficiency syndrome (human immunodeficiency virus infection)

Adapted from Burke BA, Good RA. *Pneumocystis carinii* infection. Medicine 52:23, 1972; and Walzer PD, et al. *Pneumocystis carinii* pneumonia in the United States; epidemiologic, diagnostic and clinical features. Ann Intern Med 80:83, 1974, with permission.

---

than 30 years after the disease was first recognized. The epidemics arose out of the devastation of World War II and widespread utilization of antibacterial drugs. Each of these two seemingly unrelated events served ultimately to disrupt the normal host-parasite immunologic interaction in favor of the parasite. The war created inordinate institutionalization of foundlings and orphans under conditions of overcrowding and malnutrition. At the same time, antibacterial therapy dramatically enhanced survival rates of these institutionalized infants, who would otherwise have succumbed to bacterial sepsis during the first days or weeks of life. Instead, they lived long enough to contract more chronic disease processes such as *Pneumocystis* pneumonia. In addition, it was realized that *Pneumocystis* infection appeared in these marasmic children at an age when their gamma globulin levels reached a physiologic nadir. By 1960, the orphanage epidemics had abated in Europe as environmental conditions became more normal, but they persisted in Asia, where poverty and overcrowding continued.[287, 331] Subsidence of the epidemic disease and more widespread antibacterial drug therapy, as well as sophisticated immunosuppressive drug treatment, contributed thereafter to awareness in Europe and North America of isolated instances of *Pneumocystis* infection among children suffering from a variety of identifiable immunodeficiencies.

The animal model of pneumocystosis, which has been alluded to several times in the preceding sections, has provided the experimental support for the hypothesis that clinical pneumocystosis emerges in states of impaired host defense mechanisms. Some of the more important aspects of these studies are described in the following discussion.

Weller, in Europe, was among the first to experimentally induce *Pneumocystis* pneumonia in animals.[332, 333] His crucial observation relative to pathogenesis of the infection was that rats pretreated with cortisone (and penicillin) and exposed to suspensions of *Pneumocystis*-containing lung tissue develop *Pneumocystis* pneumonia with the same frequency and severity as corticoid-treated animals that were not subsequently inoculated with parasites. The intensity of such artificially induced animal infection was also noted to be less marked than that in spontaneous human pneumocystosis of the epidemic variety. Comparable observations with the rabbit were made by Sheldon in the United States.[301] He showed that cortisone and antimicrobial agents were sufficient to induce *Pneumocystis* infection without direct exposure of animals to an exogenous source of organisms. The inescapable conclusion of these carefully designed studies was that *Pneumocystis* infection is latent in rats and rabbits and becomes clinically manifest only when host resistance is altered.

In 1966, Frenkel and colleagues published a hallmark study of rat pneumocystosis.[322] They showed that clinical and histopathologically significant involvement with *Pneumocystis* is regularly inducible in rats by "conditioning" them with parenteral cortisone over a period of 1 to 2 months. Premature death from complicating bacterial infection is warded off by simultaneous administration of antibacterial agents such as chlortetracycline. Of interest is their finding that regression of established interstitial pneumonitis occurs if cortisone conditioning is stopped early enough; on the other hand, rats continuing to receive cortisone die of coalescent alveolar *Pneumocystis* infiltration, which is almost devoid of inflammatory cells. These histologic changes are, in fact, an exact replica of those observed in sporadic cases of human *Pneumocystis* infection developing in congenitally immunodeficient and exogenously immunosuppressed patients. The authors attempted to precipitate clinical pneumocystosis with a variety of immunosuppressants other than cortisone. Of eight cytotoxic agents and antimetabolites tested, only cyclophosphamide was shown to activate latent infection. Total-body irradiation and lymphoid tissue ablation (splenectomy, thymectomy) by themselves were incapable of inducing overt *Pneumocystis* pneumonia.

The clinical association between pneumocystosis and protein-calorie deprivation has also been reproduced in a rat model.[334] Normal rats given either a regular or low-protein diet gain weight and exhibit little to no evidence of pneumocystosis post mortem. In contrast, rats fed a protein-free diet, which produces weight loss and hypoalbuminemia, regularly develop fatal infection; administration of corticosteroid only foreshortens their median survival time.[323, 334]

None of the experimental models described thus far permit a precise appraisal of the relative importance of the cellular and humoral components of host defense against *Pneumocystis*. Although corticosteroids, cytotoxic drugs, and starvation interfere primarily with cell-mediated immunity, they do not always induce purely functional cellular defects. For example, it is known from in vitro cell culture studies that corticosteroids do not inhibit the uptake of degradation of *Pneumocystis* by alveolar macrophages.[206, 335] Rather, the immunosuppressive effects of chemotherapeutic agents or of malnutrition are far more complex, and ultimately both cellular and humoral arms of the immune system may be impaired by them.

The production of pneumocystosis in the nude mouse without the mediation of exogenous immunosuppressants implies that susceptibility to the infection relates most to a defect in thymic-dependent lymphocytes.[300] Antibody deficiency must be less important because certain strains of nude mice are resistant to pneumocystosis, yet neither these animals nor their susceptible littermates produce measurable antibodies. This would not exclude a role for antibody in control of established infection with the organism; indeed, it has been shown in vitro that *P. carinii* adherent to rat alveolar macrophages become interiorized only after anti-*Pneumocystis* serum is added to the culture system.[206]

That primary immune deficits could predispose to sporadic pneumocystosis was first reported, unwittingly, by Hutchison in England in 1955.[227] He described male siblings with congenital agammaglobulinemai who died of a pneumonia of "similar and unusual" histology. *P. carinii* was implicated as the etiologic agent of these fatal infections only when the pathologic sections were reviewed by Baar,[336] who had himself reported the first case of *Pneumocystis* pneumonia in England earlier that year.[213] Numerous case studies of pneumocystosis occurring in single children or sibling pairs with hypogammaglobulinemia or agammaglobulinemia were subsequently recorded.[223, 281, 298, 310, 315, 317, 337–346] In one of the first such reports from the United States, Burke and her colleagues[310] stressed what was to become a typical histologic finding in *Pneumocystis*-infected agammaglobulinemic children—namely, the absence or gross deficiency of plasma cells in pulmonary lesions (and in hematopoietic tissues). This contrasted sharply to the extensive plasmacytosis seen in epidemic infections. In addition, sera from some of these hypogammaglobulinemic children did not contain antibody to a *Pneumocystis* antigen derived from lung tissue in "epidemic" European cases.[200]

In 1973, Walzer and co-workers summarized the reports of *Pneumocystis* pneumonia in infants and children with primary immunodeficiency diseases submitted to the Centers for Disease Control and Prevention.[251] Because all patients in this review had either decreased serum immunoglobulin levels or impaired antibody synthesis or both, the authors concluded that derangement in humoral immune function is important in the pathogenesis of pneumocystosis. There was no characteristic pattern of immunoglobulin abnormality. Depression of the serum IgG level was the most consistent finding. The serum IgA level was lowered more often than serum IgM level, but a selective decrease in either immunoglobulin was not observed.

None of these *Pneumocystis*-infected patients with a primary immunodeficiency disease had evidence of an isolated impairment of cellular immunity. (Indeed, only once has pneumocystosis been reported in association with a pure T cell deficiency—namely, in DiGeorge's syndrome.[347]) However, most of the *Pneumocystis* infections did occur in the infants with severe combined immunodeficiency, a state characterized by profound depression of both cellular and humoral immunity.

That the integrity of the cellular immune system is critical for resistance to *Pneumocystis* may be inferred from the hypercorticoid and congenitally athymic animal models of pneumocystosis described earlier and from clinical experience with the infection in older children with lymphoreticular malignancies, collagen-vascular disorders or organ allografts. These individuals receive broad immunosuppressive therapy designed to inhibit mainly the cellular arm of the immune system. Indeed, the incidence of *Pneumocystis* infection in these patients is related less to the nature of the underlying condition than to the intensity of immunosuppressive chemotherapy given for it.[270, 290, 294, 311, 348–350] Immunosuppression from adrenocorticotropic hormone given for the treatment of infantile spasms has been associated with *P. carinii* pneumonia in infancy.[351]

Until fairly recently, it had not been possible to study in vitro the cellular immune response to *P. carinii* because of the impurity of available antigens. Preliminary experiments with an antigen derived from a cell culture suggest that specific cell-mediated immunity may be depressed in children with active *Pneumocystis* pneumonia. Lymphocytes from two such children failed to transform in the presence of the antigen,[352] whereas lymphocytes from healthy, seropositive adults were in most cases stimulated specifically to undergo blastogenesis.[351, 353]

The humoral immune response to pneumocystosis has been measured in a variety of infected populations.[251, 290, 296, 306, 354, 355] The most detailed serosurveys have been conducted in Iran[163, 356] and central Europe[195, 357, 358] in infants with typical epidemic interstitial plasma cell pneumonia. The salient results of these studies are presented in the following discussion. However, it must be acknowledged that these results may not afford complete insight into the immunopathogenesis of present-day pneumocystosis in infants with congenital or acquired immunodeficiencies.

Infants in Iranian orphanages tended to show elevated levels of all immunoglobulins compared with values recorded in age-matched normal U.S. infants, presumably because of the abundance of infection in their institutional environments.[356] No statistical difference was detectable in immunoglobulin concentrations between *Pneumocystis* carriers ("focal pneumocystosis") and uninfected infants within an orphange. Prominent elevation in serum IgM levels correlated with the intensity of *Pneumocystis* disease as measured by clinical, radiographic and histologic (e.g., plasma cell infiltration) criteria. The peak values of IgM persisted for only a short "crisis" period and then rapidly decreased toward normal (Fig. 19–7). Serum IgG concentrations reached significantly depressed values of less than 200 mg/dl only in infants with massive interstitial pneumonia. A precipitous drop in serum IgA level was recorded in three *Pneumocystis*-infected children 2 to 3 days before marked respiratory impairment; the complete absence of alveolar IgA was also documented by fluorescent antibody techniques.

Iranian workers have proposed a provocative hypothesis relating these alterations in immunoglobulin levels to the pathogenesis of infant pneumocystosis (see Fig. 19–7). The infant's level of transplacentally transferred anti-*Pneumocystis* antibodies of the IgG class decreases by natural degradation. This reduction may be accentuated and occur earlier in premature infants, owing in part to malnutrition, diarrhea, and inordinate gastrointestinal protein loss.[163, 356, 359, 360] The low IgG concentration likely predisposes to intra-alveolar proliferation of *P. carinii*. Normally, IgA prevents surface spread of the parasite. If serum IgA levels then fall sharply, so that bronchoalveolar IgA secretion ceases (this remains to be proved in all cases), surface spread of the infection proceeds. This results in progression of focal pneumocystosis to clinically evident pneumonia. Increased IgM antibody formation reflects a humoral response to the highly antigenic cyst walls of the organism. If the child survives, active production of IgG antibodies with anti-*Pneumocystis* specificity occurs during the fifth to ninth months of life. Individuals with "hypoergic hypoimmune pneumocystosis," so named by Dutz,[163] with underlying congenital immunodeficiency (or acquired immune defects from immunosuppressive chemotherapy) would not exhibit such IgG responsiveness and thus would be subject to recurrence of clinically manifest pneumonic disease. An obstacle to complete acceptance of this attractive immunopathogenetic picture is that it assigns a major role to IgA antibody in host defense against *P. carinii* infection. Yet *Pneumocystis* pneumonia has not been reported in children who produce little or no IgA such as those with ataxia-telangiectasia.[290]

Brzosko and his colleagues in Poland have studied the immunopathogenesis of *Pneumocystis* pneumonia at a tissue level by elegant immunofluorescent methodology.[195, 357, 358, 361] These investigators first reported that gamma globulin is present in the intra-alveolar exudate of *Pneumocystis* infection.[361] Subsequently, they demonstrated that this collection of gamma globulin represents the specific antibody component of *Pneumocystis* antigen-antibody complexes.[357] Direct immunofluorescent staining of infected lung tissue with fluorescein-conjugated antihuman globulin or rheumatoid factor revealed a large amount of "immune" globulins bound to packets of *Pneumocystis*. Immunofluorescent complement fixation reactions performed on the same infected tissue blocks also resulted in marked fluorescence of *Pneumocystis*–gamma globulin complexes. The avidity of these conglomerates for rheumatoid factor and complement supports the assumption that the tissue-bound gamma globulin deposits are specific immune reactants to *P. carinii*.[357] The most intense fluorescence coincided with periodic acid–Schiff positive structures (presumably glycoproteins or mucoproteins) on the outer aspect of thick-walled cysts, suggesting that the major antigenicity of the parasite resides in its mucoid envelope.[195]

The Polish workers attempted to reconstruct the immunomorphologic events in typical epidemic pneumocystosis.[358] The intra-alveolar immunoglobulin masses bound to the surface of *Pneumocystis* were shown by light

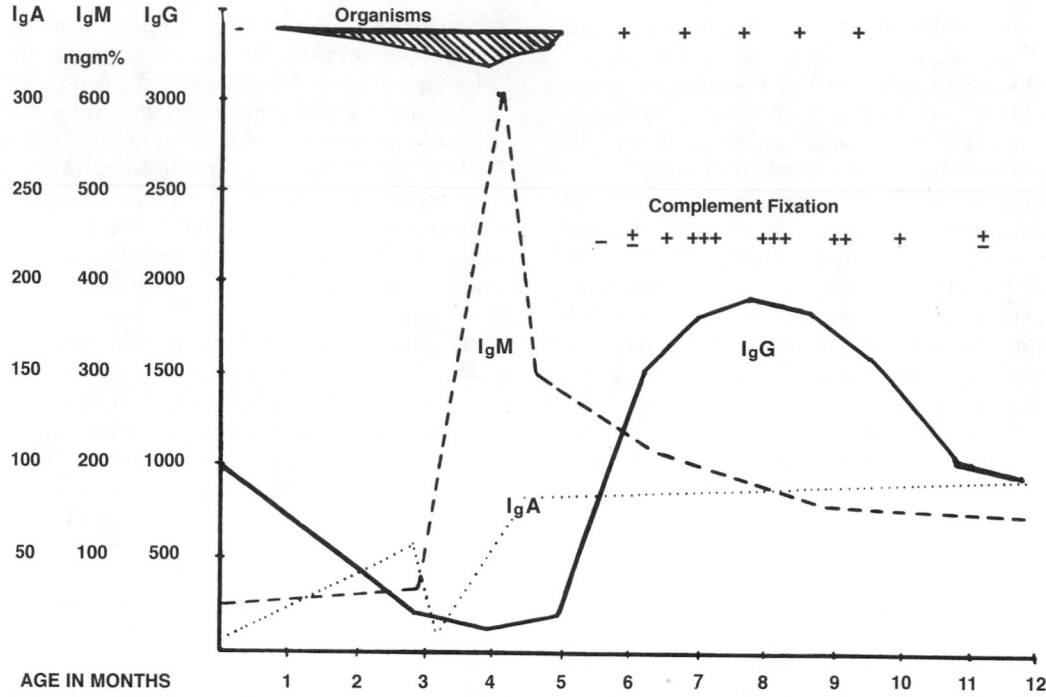

Figure 19–7 Summary of changes in interstitial plasmacellular pneumonia of infants. The IgG levels drop below their normal physiologic minimum. *Pneumocystis carinii* (as well as many other infectious agents) organisms proliferate during this period. Around the age of 4 months under certain circumstances—e.g., concomitant disease and advanced marasmus—the *Pneumocystis* growth starts to outstrip the phagocytic action. IgA levels drop, and massive proliferation with encystment of *Pneumocystis* occurs. The capsular antigens lead to a massive interstitial plasmacellular infiltration, widening the septa and, in severe cases, creating capillary block and respiratory death. The IgM produced at that time reaches high peaks, corresponding to the mass of cellular infiltrate.

If the child survives, massive collections of *Pneumocystis* in alveoli disappear; occasionally, however, later aspirates remain positive for organisms. The immunoglobulin production matures by the sixth month, and high levels of IgG antibodies are formed, reacting with the complement-fixing antigen produced from infantile and rat lungs.

The complement fixation test reaches its peak 6 to 8 weeks after the respiratory crisis and becomes borderline positive to negative with low titers by 6 to 8 months after the crisis.

Adults with cortisone-induced pneumocystosis and adults and children with congenital immunoglobulin deficiencies do not show the IgG response. Their complement fixation test remains negative.

The immunoglobulin patterns and quantitative immunoglobulin determinations were performed by Dr. E Kohout, Professor of Clinical Pathology, Pahlavi University, Shiraz, Iran. (From Dutz W. *Pneumocystis carinii* pneumonia. Pathol Annu 5:335, 1970, with permission.)

and immunoelectron microscopy to consist of a uniform mixture of IgG and IgM, with trace quantities of IgA and a small amount of beta-1-C globulin. As the pneumonitis progresses, immunoglobulins deposited on intra-alveolar organisms decrease, but increasing numbers of immunoglobulin-producing plasma cells (which initially release IgM, followed by IgG), accompanied by alveolar macrophages, surround the disintegrating *Pneumocystis* conglomerates. In summary, in the earliest stage of infection the antigenic constituents of *P. carinii* induce the formation of IgM and IgG anti-*Pneumocystis* antibodies, possibly in hilar and mediastinal lymph nodes. These antibodies bind to aggregates of alveolar *Pneumocystis* and form immune complexes. The latter then bind complement. This results in gradual disintegration of the masses of organisms and their eventual phagocytosis by alveolar macrophages. Immunoglobulin-forming plasma cells proliferate in the interstitium and, conceivably, contribute additional antibody to the *Pneumocystis* aggregates. Clearly, no impairment in immunoglobulin synthesis is recorded in this analysis of epidemic pneumocystosis, but retarded binding of complement components to the immune complexes is regularly observed. Because the ultimate destruction and removal of the *Pneumocystis*-antibody conglomerates are complement dependent and the complement system is, in general, physiologically deficient in the first few months of life, survival of a particular infant with epidemic *Pneumocystis* pneumonia may depend on the stage of development and relative functional competency of the complement system.

Clinical Manifestations

GENERAL CONSIDERATIONS

There are no pathognomonic clinical features of *P. carinii* infection. Organisms residing in scattered intra-alveolar foci may evoke no illness at all,[170, 362, 363] whereas histologically advanced infection may provoke variable symptoms and signs in different hosts. Features attributable to *Pneumocystis* infection per se may be obfuscated by concomitant infection with other opportunistic pathogens or by dramatic complications of an underlying condition.[166, 354] Furthermore, clinical syndromes ascribable to *Pneumocystis* may be simulated by other infections (cytomegalovirus[159]), or by inflammatory processes (drug-induced pulmonary toxicity,[364] radiation fibrosis[365]) and neoplasia (pulmonary leukemia[366]) capable of producing interstitial pulmonary infiltrates. Thus, recognition of pneumocystosis on clinical grounds alone requires above all a high index of suspicion whenever interstitial pneumonia occurs in settings known to predispose to infection with the parasite (see Table 19–1).

In spite of these caveats, *Pneumocystis* is distinguishable from other opportunistic microbes by the fact that infection with it commonly surfaces when underlying disorders are quiescent. For example, in the case of severe combined immunodeficiency disease, pneumocystosis may develop only after immunologic competence has been at least partially restored by bone marrow transplantation.[251, 290, 367] Apparently, reversal of immune paralysis elicits sufficient inflammation to convert subclinical infection to overt pneumonitis. Similarly, in children with lymphocytic leukemia, pneumocystosis most often occurs during periods of clinical and hematologic remission.[290, 296, 320, 368–371] It may be inferred from these observations that pneumocystosis is not merely an end-stage infection in a preterminal host; on the contrary, it often represents a potentially treatable cause of death in patients whose primary immunodeficiency or malignancy has been controlled or effectively cured.

SYMPTOMS AND SIGNS

Epidemic Infection in Infants

The onset of epidemic-type infection in infants is reported to be slow and insidious. Initially, nonspecific signs of restlessness or languor, poor feeding and diarrhea are common. Tachypnea and periorbital cyanosis gradually develop. Cough productive of sticky mucus, although not prominent, may appear later.[159, 170] Respiratory insufficiency progresses over 1 to 4 weeks, and patients exhibit increasingly severe tachypnea, dyspnea, intercostal retractions, and flaring of the nasal alae. Fever is absent or low grade.[372] Pulmonary physical findings are strikingly minimal and consist primarily of fine crepitant rales on deep breathing. In contrast, roentgenographic evidence of pulmonary infiltration regularly appears early. The total duration of untreated disease extends over a 4- to 6-week period, but this figure is necessarily inaccurate because of difficulty in establishing an exact date of onset of illness in an infected infant. Before the introduction of pentamidine therapy, the mortality rate of such epidemic infection is estimated to have been between 20 and 50%.[214, 355]

Sporadic Infection in Infants and Children

A typical clinical syndrome is less evident in sporadic cases of pneumocystosis occurring in acquired or congenitally immunodeficient infants and in older children with acquired immunodeficiency. In infants with primary immunodeficiency diseases, the onset of clinical infection may be insidious and illness may extend over weeks or possibly months,[290, 328] a course not unlike that seen in epidemic pneumocystosis. In contrast, in most infants with congenital immunodeficiency or AIDS and in older children with acquired immune deficits, *Pneumocystis* pneumonia presents abruptly and is a more asymptomatic short-lived disease.[181, 247, 252, 290, 296] Among infants with HIV infection, the median age at onset is 4 to 5 months of age and mortality is between 39 and 59%.[373] High fever and nonproductive cough appear initially, followed by tachypnea, coryza, and later cyanosis. Death may supervene within a week or so. If no treatment is given, essentially all patients with this form of pneumocystosis die.

RADIOLOGIC FINDINGS

Because the true extent of pulmonary involvement in *P. carinii* pneumonia is rarely detectable by physical examination, a chest roentgenogram showing diffuse infiltrative disease is the most useful indication of the presence of the infection in an appropriately susceptible host.[181, 277] Although certain characteristic patterns of radiographic involvement have been ascribed to *Pneumocystis* pneumonitis, it is worth re-emphasizing that the findings may vary depending on the presence of coincident pulmonary infection as well as on the nature of the underlying disease state.

Epidemic Infection in Infants

Ivady and colleagues in Hungary studied the radiographic progression of epidemic infantile *Pneumocystis* pneumonia and identified five developmental stages.[355] The first three stages are recognizable when the infant is virtually symptom-free and consist of perivascular and peribronchial peripheral shadows extending toward the pleura. The two later stages more closely coincide with clinical respiratory insufficiency and reveal changes resembling "butterfly" pulmonary edema and peripheral emphysematous blebs. The radiographic findings described by Vessal and associates in mild ("focal") cases of *Pneumocystis* pneumonia in infants from an Iranian orphanage include hilar interstitial infiltrate, thymic atrophy, pulmonary hyperaeration, and scattered lobular atelectasis.[374] Although in the authors' experience none of these signs is specific for *Pneumocystis* infection, they persist longer (3 weeks to 2 months) in serologically proven cases. Indeed, surviving infants may exhibit focal interstitial infiltrates after organisms are cleared from the lung[375] and for as long as 1 year.[376, 377]

Sporadic Infection in Infants and Children

The majority of radiologic characterizations of *Pneumocystis* pneumonia have emphasized the sporadic form of the infection. Minor differences in descriptive details usually reflect differences in the populations studied.[181, 290, 378–382] In infants, especially those with immunodeficiency syndromes, the initial roentgenogram often shows haziness spreading from the hilar regions to the periphery, which assumes a finely granular, interstitial pattern. An antecedent gross alveolar infiltrate is not usually seen.[290, 378] The peripheral granularity may progress to coalescent nodules. These changes resemble the "atelectatic" radiographic abnormalities of hyaline membrane disease. In both conditions, aeration is absent peripherally. Pneumothorax with subcutaneous and interstitial emphysema and pneumomediastinum are not uncommon and are associated with a poor prognosis.[372] Even in the face of effective anti-*Pneumocystis* therapy, radiographic clearing may lag far behind clinical improvement; indeed, the complications of residual interstitial fibrosis with calcification have already been discussed.

As experience with *Pneumocystis* has broadened, especially in older children and adults, a number of atypical roentgenographic abnormalities have been described.[181, 381–390] These include hilar and mediastinal adenopathy, pleural effusions, parenchymal cavitation, pneumatoceles, nodular densities, and unilateral or lobar distribution of infiltrates. In contrast, the chest roentgenogram may remain essentially normal well after the onset of fever, dyspnea, and hypoxemia.[391, 392] The presence of such roentgenographically silent lung disease may be suggested by abnormal pulmonary gallium scintigrams.[392–395]

LABORATORY STUDIES

Routine laboratory determinations yield little diagnostic information in *Pneumocystis* infection. Abnormalities in hemoglobin concentration or white blood cell count are more likely to result from the underlying disease of the hematopoietic system or cytotoxic drug effect. Neither laboratory value is consistently altered by secondary pneumocystosis. However, a subgroup of infants with primary immunodeficiency disease and infection caused by *P. carinii* may exhibit significant eosinophilia.[170, 214, 283, 290, 327, 328] Jose and associates first emphasized the association of peripheral blood eosinophilia and pneumocystosis in a report of three infected male siblings with infantile agammaglobulinemia.[283] In one of the infants in particular, eosinophilia developed very early in the course of the illness and ultimately attained a level of 42% as the respiratory disease worsened. Accordingly, it has been suggested that the combination of cough, tachypnea, diffuse haziness on chest roentgenograms, and eosinophilia in an infant with immunodeficiency may be indicative of *Pneumocystis* pneumonia.[283, 290]

Hypercalcemia with or without nephrocalcinosis has been reported in infants with epidemic pneumocystosis.[214] However, measurements of serum calcium levels in other patients with *Pneumocystis* infection have revealed normal values whether or not coincident foci of pulmonary or renal parenchymal calcification existed.[247, 290, 296] Elevated cold agglutinin titers have been noted in instances of epidemic infantile *Pneumocystis* disease,[395] as well as in *Pneumocystis*-infected recipients of renal allografts.[311, 348] Yet this finding has not been corroborated by subsequent studies of similarly infected immunosuppressed patients.[247, 306] It has been theorized that the development of cold agglutinins during the course of pneumocystosis results not from the latter infection but from coexistent infection with cytomegalovirus,[306] which is known to induce such nonspecific serologic abnormalities.[396]

A virtually constant pathophysiologic finding in pneumocystosis, as well as in other interstitial pulmonary diseases, is that of ventilation and perfusion defects most compatible with an "alveolar-capillary block" syndrome.[262, 268, 290, 348, 354, 397–400] Arterial blood gas determinations in infected patients may show severe hypoxemia and hypocapnia, often before profound subjective respiratory insufficiency or even radiologic abnormalities[391] supervene. Less commonly, modest hypercapnia with respiratory acidosis is recorded.[397]

This respiratory pathophysiology correlates well with the anatomic pulmonary lesion in *Pneumocystis* pneumonia. Concentration of parasites within alveoli and inflammation of the surrounding alveolar septa not unexpectedly lead to interference in gas transfer, whereas persistence of areas of normal lung parenchyma and lack of significant airway obstruction account for the usual absence of carbon dioxide retention.

CONCURRENT INFECTION

The clinical presentation of pneumocystosis may be altered by simultaneous infection with other organisms. Certainly, infection with a variety of opportunistic pathogens is not surprising in patients with broadly compromised immunologic defense mechanisms. Infection with one or more organisms was found in 56% of *Pneumocystis*-infected infants and children with primary immunodeficiency disease reported to the Centers for Disease Control and Prevention.[251] Comparable rates of multiple infection have also been noted in several large series of patients with acquired immune defects and pneumocystosis.[160, 290, 311, 401]

Infection with cytomegalovirus appears to be the most common "unusual" infection associated with pneumocystosis.* Indeed, in his 1957 review, Gajdusek was already able to cite numerous published studies referring to the "unexpectedly high frequency of association" of the two conditions.[159] He conceded that one infection most probably predisposes to the other. On the basis of electron micrographic observations of cytomegalovirus corelike particles within pneumocysts, Wang and coworkers hypothesized that *P. carinii* may even serve as an intermediate host or reservoir of the virus.[178] The possibility of viral parasitism of (or symbiosis with) *Pneumocystis* was also explored by Pliess and Seifert[405] and by Vawter and colleagues,[179] who were impressed by the resemblance of the outer membranes of *P. carinii* to an imperfect form of myxovirus. However, it is still unclear whether this inordinate concurrence of *Pneumocystis* and cytomegalovirus is caused by a specific and unique relationship between the two organisms or by coincidental infection of highly susceptible hosts with ubiquitous microbes.[193, 311] The pulmonary pathology of infants with

---

*See references 159, 178, 179, 220, 264, 311, 315, 326, and 402–404.

AIDS often demonstrates concomitant cytomegalovirus and *P. carinii* infections.[406, 407]

Diagnosis

Precise diagnosis of *Pneumocystis* pneumonia is still fraught with difficulty. The organism must be visualized in the respiratory tract of very ill individuals, and often this can be accomplished only by bronchoalveolar lavage and rarely by subjecting such patients to an invasive surgical procedure. Attempts to isolate *Pneumocystis* from clinical specimens on synthetic media or in tissue culture have not been successful, and serologic techniques to detect active infection have been too insensitive.

EXAMINATION OF PULMONARY SECRETIONS

Pneumocystis is not regularly detectable in expectorated sputum or hypopharyngeal and tracheal secretions.[177, 185, 408] However, during the European epidemics, parasitic forms were recognized in mucus from infected infants.[171, 187, 273] Specimens were usually obtained through a catheter or laryngobronchoscope passed into the hypopharynx, and smears of the aspirated secretions were fixed in ether-alcohol and stained by the Gram-Weigert technique. By this method, Le Tan-Vinh and associates in France reported antemortem diagnosis of *Pneumocystis* pneumonia in eight of nine infants.[171] Toth and co-workers in Hungary recovered *P. carinii* from tracheopharyngeal and gastric aspirates of 22 infants whose illness had just begun; in some cases, organisms were observed 7 to 10 days before the appearance of symptoms.[273] However, the mere presence of organisms in hypopharyngeal secretions did not always presage acute pneumonic disease in these environments where pneumocystosis was endemic. Rather, it often reflected chronic subclinical carriage of the parasite.[163]

Diagnosis of sporadic cases of pneumocystosis by examination of sputum or tracheal and gastric aspirates has never been as rewarding.[272, 276, 409] The rate of recovery of *Pneumocystis* from upper airway secretions in the cases compiled by the Centers for Disease Control and Prevention was estimated to be only about 6%.[252] Japanese investigators have described a method of concentrating sputum samples with acetyl-L-cysteine in 0.2 N sodium hydroxide solution, which permits filtration and centrifugation of a pellet of *Pneumocystis*.[410] Adoption of this technique may enhance the diagnostic sensitivity of sputum examination. Ognibene and associates reported the use of induced sputa in the diagnosis of pneumonia in 18 children with HIV infection or malignancies.[411] Nine sputum samples were positive for *P. carinii* by immunofluorescent antibody, and four of the patients with negative sputum samples subsequently underwent bronchoalveolar lavage and all were negative for *P. carinii*; the remaining five patients were treated for bacterial pneumonia and responded to therapy. This technique required ultrasonic nebulization of the children, and the youngest patient in this report was 2 years old.

PERCUTANEOUS LUNG ASPIRATION

The need to obtain lung tissue for a more accurate assessment of the presence of *Pneumocystis* pneumonia has been appreciated for some time. Percutaneous needle aspiration of the lung was already of proven value by the late 1950s in diagnosis of epidemic pneumocystosis in infants.[159] Subsequently, it was successfully employed in infected infants and children with underlying primary and acquired immunodeficiencies.[223, 296, 412, 413]

The procedure is performed without general anesthesia or sedation so that the child's respiratory function is not further compromised. The right side of the thorax is preferred as the site for aspiration to avoid cardiac trauma. Under fluoroscopy, a 20-gauge spinal needle with syringe in place is guided into the midportion of the lung. The resultant aspirate (usually <0.1 ml) may be transferred directly to slides as unsmeared drops or first cytocentrifuged to increase the concentration of organisms in the sample.[414] Slides are allowed to air dry and are then stained with Gram, Gomori methenamine silver nitrate, and toluidine blue O stains. The residual material in the syringe is diluted with 2 ml sterile saline and cultured for bacteria and fungi. Children with platelet counts of less than 60,000 per mm^3 receive fresh whole blood or platelet transfusions before the procedure. Pneumothorax appears to be the major complication encountered. In one series, it occurred in 37% of the patients and evacuation of air by thoracotomy tube was required in 14%.[413]

LUNG BIOPSY

It has been argued that aspiration is inferior to biopsy in that the former does not permit histologic examination of lung tissue. Open lung biopsy has therefore been proposed as the most reliable method for identifying and estimating the extent of *Pneumocystis* infection as well as for demonstrating the presence of complicating pathology such as coexistent infection, malignancy, or interstitial fibrosis.[290, 317, 342, 398, 401, 415–417] However, it may be hazardous to perform a thoracotomy under general anesthesia in patients with marginal pulmonary reserve.[252, 418] Although the procedure has had an acceptably low incidence of serious complications in critically ill children,[419–422] determination of its risk-to-benefit ratio based on the child's underlying disease, expected life span, and clinical condition is appropriate in individual cases.[423, 424] Unfortunately, these analyses have not yet been applied rigorously to infants and young children with suspected pneumocystosis. Technical modification in the performance of open biopsies that would avoid general anesthesia and endotracheal intubation (e.g., using thoracoscopy) may be particularly advantageous for diagnosis of *Pneumocystis* pneumonia in small children.[425]

A number of alternative diagnostic maneuvers, less invasive than surgical biopsy, have been used to recognize pneumocystosis. These include percutaneous needle biopsy,[404, 426–429] endobronchial brushing,[430] and transbronchial biopsy through rigid[431] and fiberoptic[432–434] bronchoscopes. Although extensive comparative studies of these methods have not been performed, closed biopsies carry inherent risks of pneumothorax and intrapulmonary hemorrhage,[401, 435] and the diagnostic yield of any of these modalities may fall short of open biopsy.[436]

Whichever invasive technique is employed for retrieval of tissue to test for the presence of *P. carinii*, there is general agreement that immediate examination and staining of frozen sections or imprints of fresh lung (or alveolar secretions) are critical.[159, 181, 342, 413, 415, 420, 437, 438] Processing of paraffin-embedded tissue incurs an unnecessary delay of one or more days in diagnosis, and the sections may actually reveal fewer organisms than the imprint smears. Although Giemsa stain is rapid and specific for the intracystic bodies of *P. carinii*, organisms are more readily located and identified against a background of tissue cells with a methenamine silver nitrate stain. It should be appreciated that other silver-positive organisms, such as *Torulopsis*[439] and zygomycete spores,[440] may mimic the cystic structure of *P. carinii* and that smears of *Pneumocystis* rather than fungi should be employed as controls for the stain.[441]

Unfortunately, the standard methenamine silver nitrate stain technique requires time (3 to 4 hours) and expertise usually found only in special histopathology laboratories. To circumvent these problems, several rapid (<30 minutes) and simpler modifications of the silver stain have been developed.[442–445] Because the results with these stains have not been as consistent as those achieved with the standard lengthier procedure, many laboratories have chosen not to use silver for rapid screening of specimens but prefer instead toluidine blue O[172, 446–449] and cresyl echt violet[173, 450] for this purpose.

BRONCHOALVEOLAR LAVAGE

Bronchoscopy with bronchoalveolar lavage has been a valuable alternative to lung biopsy for diagnosing *P. carinii* infection in adults.[451–453] New flexible fiberoptic instruments designed for pediatric use have made this diagnostic approach feasible for infants and children. *P. carinii* infection has been demonstrated from washings obtained by segmental bronchoalveolar lavage, thereby avoiding the morbidity of open lung biopsy in pediatric patients.[454, 455] Experience with flexible bronchoscopy and bronchoalveolar lavage in the diagnosis of pneumonia in children with HIV infection and malignancies has yielded positive results. Frankel and colleagues reported definitive diagnoses in six of seven children in one series; three of these children had *P. carinii* pneumonia.[456] Birriel and associates reported on 16 patients with AIDS who underwent fiberoptic bronchoscopy. For 10 patients, lavage revealed *P. carinii*; 2 others had lymphoid interstitial pneumonia, and 4 had prior trimethoprim-sulfamethoxazole or pentamidine therapy.[457] In contrast, Stokes and co-workers reviewed 60 flexible bronchoscopies in 48 children with malignancies and found a diagnostic yield in only 27%, with the most success from lavage compared with brushings. However, the majority of these patients were on broad-spectrum antimicrobial therapy before bronchoscopy. Of the 13 patients who underwent a second procedure after a negative bronchoscopy, only 1 had *P. carinii*.[458]

IMMUNOSEROLOGIC TESTS

It is clear that diagnostic maneuvers of any type that necessitate traumatic invasion of precariously ill patients leave much to be desired. Specific and reliable skin testing or serologic methods would be more suitable in such patients to detect active *Pneumocystis* infection. It is disappointing, therefore, that despite investigation of such tests, no method to be described in the following paragraphs has proved to be satisfactory for widespread use.

A reagent prepared from infected lung was employed in Europe for intradermal skin testing in a few cases, but little is known about its reproducibility or specificity.[185, 187] In epidemics of infantile pneumocystosis in both Europe and Asia, serologic tests received a more extensive evaluation. Complement-fixing antibodies to *P. carinii* were demonstrated in as many as 95% of infected infants.[199, 395, 459–461] In contrast, it was unusual to find positive complement-fixing tests in healthy children or in children with pneumonia not related to *Pneumocystis*. However, technical problems precluded universal application of the test; the antigenic material used was often impure, unstable, and not standardized. Moreover, a single positive test did not necessarily reflect acute infection. Although seropositivity occurred typically between 1 and 3 weeks after initial clinical symptoms, the test often did not become positive during the acute phase of the disease; instead, reactivity indicated only prior infection (i.e., infection acquired at least 1 month earlier).[163, 462]

The complement-fixing test has not been employed in diagnosis of sporadic pneumocystosis because sera from infected immunodeficient individuals appear to be generally devoid of complement-binding anti-*Pneumocystis* antibodies.[311, 398] This is perhaps not unexpected because these antibodies belong to the IgG class and their production may well be depressed in immunologically incompetent patients.[163, 286, 290] However, an alternative explanation for this difference in seroresponsiveness between children with epidemic pneumocystosis and those with sporadic infection rests on an as yet unproven premise that antigenic variation exists among parasites infecting these different hosts.[169, 200]

Serodiagnosis of *P. carinii* infection in infants by detection of immunofluorescent antibodies was first reported in 1964 in Europe.[463] It was found that IgM and IgG anti-*Pneumocystis* immunofluorescent antibodies appear sequentially in sera during the course of clinical infection. Both classes of antibodies are present in sera of diseased infants during the first weeks of pneumonia, but only IgG antibodies persist during convalescent periods or in cases of protracted infection.[464]

The worth of immunofluorescent antibody tests in diagnosis of sporadic pneumocystosis was examined subsequently in the United States by Norman and Kagan at the Centers for Disease Control and Prevention.[196] They observed generally low rates of serologic reactivity among patients with suspected and confirmed cases, positive tests in patients who seemed to have only cytomegalovirus and fungus infections and negative results in sera from six infants with primary immunodeficiency diseases and documented pneumocystosis.[251] Although it is possible to increase the specificity and sensitivity of these tests for *Pneumocystis*,[465, 466] such tests detect background levels of *Pneumocystis* antibody in clinically healthy subjects[239, 240, 466] and, as a result, fail to discriminate between patients with active disease and those who are latently infected with the parasite. This is analogous to the problem with the complement-fixing reaction in epidemic pneumocystosis in which a positive test is more an epidemiologic marker of previously acquired infection than a sign of acute pneumonia.[460, 461]

The performance of the immunofluorescent antibody test has been hampered for years by the crude *Pneumocystis* antigens employed. Impure antigen results in autofluorescence of uninfected lung tissue, and extensive absorption of sera risks undue reduction in intensity of staining of organisms. For this reason, several laboratories have attempted to prepare a *Pneumocystis* antigen that is isolated as nearly as possible from the lung parenchyma to which it characteristically clings. Techniques designed to extract free *P. carinii* from infected lung include bronchoalveolar saline lavage,[169, 401] enzymatic digestion of lung homogenates,[467] and differential centrifugation of lung homogenates on sucrose[468] or Ficoll-Hypaque[469] density gradients. These purified antigens have been used to generate immune sera that have been applied in immunofluorescent staining of *Pneumocystis* in lung tissue[470, 471] and in upper airway secretions.[450, 472, 473]

To avoid the problem posed by the insensitivity of antibody determinations per se in pneumocystosis, Pifer and colleagues developed a counterimmunoelectrophoretic assay for detecting circulating *Pneumocystis* antigen in suspected cases.[240] In an initial evaluation of the test, antigenemia was demonstrated in up to 95% of children with *Pneumocystis* pneumonia and was absent in normal control children. However, antigen was found in the sera of 15% of oncology patients who did not have pneumonia. Thus, although antigenemia appears to be superior to circulating antibody as a serologic correlate of *Pneumocystis* infection, antigenemia alone cannot be equated with a diagnosis of pneumocystosis without corroborating clinical data.

This was borne out by the findings in a subsequent study of older patients who were recipients of bone marrow transplants.[474] Although antigen was detected in the sera of 22 of 28 transplant patients with pneumocystosis, it was also identified in 35 of 52 of the transplant patients with viral or idiopathic pneumonia, in 11 of 25 without pneumonia, and in 22 of 28 nontransplant patients with pulmonary infiltrates. Whether all of the patients with positive tests and a variety of pulmonary insults were, in fact, experiencing subclinical infection with *Pneumocystis* is problematic. A more recent report by Pifer and colleagues studied the reliability of *P. carinii* antigen and IgG production in the diagnosis of *P. carinii* pneumonia and found 100% sensitivity and 90% specificity in 17 pediatric AIDS patients. IgG profiles were not useful in the diagnosis.[475]

Treatment

TRIMETHOPRIM AND SULFAMETHOXAZOLE

In 1974, Hughes and co-workers first demonstrated that the combination of trimethoprim and sulfamethoxazole (TMP/SMX) was active in treatment of cortisone-induced rat pneumocystosis.[476] The combination was then shown to be as efficacious as pentamidine in children infected with *Pneumocystis* who had underlying malignancy.[477] Several uncontrolled trials of TMP/SMX in congenitally immunodeficient infants[478, 479] and in older immunosuppressed children and adults[293, 478–481] confirmed the efficacy and low toxicity of the agent. The dosage employed is 20 mg of TMP and 100 mg of SMX per kilogram per day, given orally in four equally divided doses for 14 days. This daily dose is two to three times that used for conventional bacterial infection.

The equivalent efficacy of TMP/SMX and pentamidine has been confirmed in pediatric cancer patients with *P. carinii* pneumonia.[482]

TMP-SMX is the drug of choice for treatment of *P. carinii* pneumonia in infants and children. The oral route of administration can be used in mild cases at a dose of 20 mg TMP/100 mg SMX/kg per day in divided doses 6 to 8 hours apart. Infants with moderate or severe disease require treatment by the intravenous route with 15 to 20 mg TMP/75 to 100 mg SMX/kg per day in divided doses 6 to 8 hours apart. Generally, treatment is given for 2 to 3 weeks. Approximately 5% of children without HIV infection and 40% of children with HIV infection will develop adverse reactions to TMP/SMX, most commonly a maculopapular rash that clears after discontinuation of the drug. Other adverse reactions are uncommon and include neutropenia, anemia, renal dysfunction, and gastrointestinal symptoms.

Infants who do not respond to TMP/SMX or who develop adverse reactions may be treated with pentamidine isethionate at a single daily dose of 4 mg/kg per day intravenously. Other drugs have been tested in limited studies in children with HIV infection and *P. carinii* pneumonia, including atovaquone, trimetrexate-leucovorin, oral TMP-dapsone, pyrimethamine-sulfadoxine, clindamycin plus primaquine, and aerosolized pentamidine.

The ease with which TMP/SMX can be administered and the lack of adverse side effects make it an attractive combination for empirical therapy for suspected pneumocystosis. Such treatment is reasonable in infants who are gravely ill and whose outlook for recovery from underlying disease is bleak. However, there are several objections to the universal adoption of this approach. In at least half of the immunosuppressed children with typical clinical and roentgenographic features of *Pneumocystis* pneumonia, the illness is in fact not related to infection with *P. carinii*.[483] The correct etiology of the disorder and its proper management can be determined only by first performing a diagnostic procedure.

PENTAMIDINE

Until 1958, there was no known definitive chemotherapy specific for *P. carinii* infection. In that year Ivady and Paldy in Hungary recorded the first successful use of several aromatic diamidines, including pentamidine isethionate, in 16 of 19 infected infants.[484] By 1962, the Hungarian investigators had treated 212 patients with epidemic *Pneumocystis* pneumonia with pentamidine.[355]

During the next several years, favorable responses to the drug were observed in infants and children with both the epidemic and sporadic forms of the infection.[290, 296, 317, 342, 343, 485] Treatment effected a dramatic reduction in the mortality rate of the epidemic disease from 50% to less than 4%.[355] In the cases of sporadic infection reported to the Centers for Disease Control and Prevention,[252, 486, 487] recovery rates ranged from 42 to 63% for those patients who received the drug for 9 or more days. In cases confined largely to young children and managed at a single institution, cure rates were noted to be as high as 68 to 75%.[296, 477] Because spontaneous recovery from *Pneumocystis* pneumonia in immunodepressed individuals is rare,[488] it is clear that pentamidine therapy reduced mortality in such patients to nearly 25%. The recommended dose of the drug is 4 mg/kg intravenously once daily for 14 days. Clinical improvement becomes evident 4 to 6 days after initiation of therapy, but radiographic improvement may be delayed for several weeks.

Pentamidine toxicity from intravenous and intramuscular use has been reported. Although toxicity from pentamidine was apparently not a significant problem in the infected marasmic infants treated during the European epidemics,[489] the Centers for Disease Control and Prevention determined that 189 (47%) of 404 children and adults given the drug for confirmed or suspected *Pneumocystis* infection suffered one or more adverse effects.[252] Immediate systemic reactions, such as hypotension, tachycardia, nausea, vomiting, facial flushing, pruritus, and unpleasant taste, were noted particularly after intravenous administration of the drug. Herxheimer's reactions, although described well for patients given pentamidine for leishmaniasis,[490] occurred rarely.[491] Local reactions at injection sites—namely, pain, erythema, and frank abscess formation—developed in 10 to 20% of patients.[252, 487] Elevation in serum glutamic-oxalotransaminase levels was frequently recorded and may have resulted partly from this local trauma. Hypoglycemia ensued not uncommonly after the fifth day of pentamidine therapy but was often asymptomatic.[486] (Hypoglycemia was also observed in pediatric patients with AIDS who were treated with pentamidine for *P. carinii* pneumonia.[492]) Pentamidine-associated pancreatitis has also been reported in children and adults with HIV infection.[493, 494, 495] Although overt anemia was rare, megaloblastic bone marrow changes or depressed serum folate levels were noted.[486]

Renal tubular dysfunction, which was essentially unrecognized before 1969,[428, 496, 497] occurred in 23.5% of the 404 patients reported to the Parasitic Disease Drug Service.[252] It is arguable whether pentamidine alone was responsible for the renal dysfunction in all the reports.[252, 290, 296, 486, 498] In one unusual case, a 3-year-old child developed profound renal impairment in association with a severe toxic epidermal necrolysis.[499] The demonstration in humans and mice that pentamidine is concentrated in and highly bound to kidney tissue perhaps provides a pharmacodynamic basis for its apparent nephrotoxicity.[500, 501]

PYRIMETHAMINE AND SULFONAMIDE

In view of the toxicity of pentamidine, a number of other drugs were evaluated for their anti-*Pneumocystis* activity in the rodent model of the infection; only the combination of pyrimethamine and a sulfonamide was found to be as efficacious.[322] Subsequently, scattered reports appeared attesting to the efficacy of the combination in a few immunosuppressed adults[277, 311, 321, 502] and in one infant with a primary immunodeficiency who had not responded to pentamidine.[503] However, controlled trials of pyrimethamine plus sulfonamide in pneumocystosis were not carried out because it soon became apparent that the related fixed-drug combination of trimethoprim and sulfamethoxazole was a highly efficacious, less toxic therapeutic alternative.

TRIMETREXATE

Trimetrexate is an antifolate and potent inhibitor of dihydrofolate reductase and has been studied as an alternative treatment for *P. carinii* pneumonia in adults who are intolerant of or refractory to standard therapy.[504] Trimetrexate is being evaluated in pediatric HIV infection and is available only through clinical trials or on a compassionate basis.

SUPPORTIVE CARE

A critical component of the management of *Pneumocystis* pneumonia is carefully monitored oxygen therapy. Because hypoxemia may be profound, the fraction of inspired oxygen should be adjusted to maintain the arterial oxygen tension at 70 mm Hg or above. The inspired oxygen concentration should not exceed 50% so as to avoid oxygen toxicity. Assisted or controlled ventilation may be required. Three methods of ventilatory support have been used: the volume-regulated positive-pressure respirator,[505] membrane lung bypass,[506] and a continuous negative-pressure system.[507] The last method makes use of a modified tank respirator and has the advantage of not requiring intubation.

Other ancillary measures such as administration of gamma globulin[290, 478, 508] or granulocyte transfusions[509] to infected congenitally immunodeficient children have had limited application but warrant further study.

There is evidence that the use of early adjunctive corticosteroid therapy in the treatment of *P. carinii* pneumonia in adults with AIDS can increase survival and reduce the risk of respiratory failure.[510, 511] A national consensus panel has recommended the use of corticosteroids in adults and adolescents with HIV infection and documented or suspected *P. carinii* pneumonia.[512] Two recent studies have supported the use of corticosteroids in decreasing the morbidity and mortality of *P. carinii* pneumonia.[513, 514]

Prognosis

CHRONIC SEQUELAE

Little is known about the residual effects of successfully treated *Pneumocystis* pneumonia on pulmonary histopathology and function. This is understandable inasmuch as surviving patients may suffer additional "pulmonary" morbidity from other opportunistic infections or from noninfectious complications of underlying disease or its therapy. Robbins and associates were fortunate enough to be able to follow the course of an infected hypogammaglobulinemic child treated with pentamidine in 1964[317]; during the ensuing 5 years, despite intercurrent episodes of otitis media and bacterial pneumonia, she exhibited normal exercise tolerance and pulmonary function studies without evidence of reactivation of her *Pneumocystis* infection.[418] Hughes and co-workers furnished prognostic data in 18 surviving *Pneumocystis*-infected children with underlying malignancies.[296] The follow-up period after therapy ranged from 1 to 4 years. Although pulmonary function tests were not performed, none of the subjects demonstrated clinical or roentgenographic evidence of residual pulmonary disease. In a subsequent study from the same institution, pulmonary function was assessed serially in surviving children.[515] Significant improvement in function was noted within 1 month of the infection, and all abnormalities resolved by 6 months. This finding is in contrast to the observation of recurrent wheezing episodes and abnormal pulmonary function on follow-up of infants who had pneumonitis during the first 3 months of life.[326] Although later morbidity was independent of the original etiologic agent, 17% of these patients were thought to have *P. carinii* infection.

It seems inevitable that respiratory dysfunction may result from episodes of *Pneumocystis* pneumonia that are severe or protracted enough to provoke interstitial fibrosis or extensive calcification (see discussion under Pathology section). Cor pulmonale has been observed in infants with such protracted infection.[290] In one notably well-studied patient, an adult with biopsy-proven fibrosis 4 months after curative pentamidine therapy, serial tests of pulmonary function revealed persistent ventilatory defects of the restrictive type and impairment of carbon monoxide–diffusing capacity.[319] Although a possible link between pentamidine therapy per se and lung fibrosis was suggested by earlier observations in rat pneumocystosis,[322] healthy animals given the drug exhibit no histologic abnormalities.[516] Moreover, pulmonary fibrosis has been described after *Pneumocystis* pneumonia in patients treated with pyrimethamine and sulfonamide[321] and TMP/SMX.[517]

RECURRENT INFECTION

Recurrence of *Pneumocystis* pneumonia after apparently curative courses of therapy has been documented in infants and children with underlying congenital immunodeficiency or malignancy. As early as 1966, Patterson and colleagues reported the case of an infant with probable severe combined immunodeficiency who experienced one presumptive and two substantiated bouts of pneumocystosis at approximately 5-month intervals; treatment with pentamidine resulted in cessation of clinical illness on each occasion, although radiographic abnormalities persisted.[340, 518] A few years later, Richman and associates[519] and then Saulsbury[508] described recurrent pneumocystosis in two children with hypogammaglobulinemia; in the first case, three proven attacks responded to pentamidine; and in the second child, two separate

episodes of infection were treated successfully with TMP/SMX. At St. Jude Children's Research Hospital, a study of 28 children with malignancy whose pneumocystosis was treated with pentamidine revealed that 4 (14%) suffered a second infection.[300, 320] In each case, the clinical manifestations, roentgenographic findings, and response to therapy were similar in both infectious episodes. In addition, no differences in host factors were discernible in those patients who had recurrent infection and those who did not. Other examples of recurrent pneumocystosis emerging rather soon after clinical recovery have been observed in patients given either pentamidine or TMP/SMX.[520]

Whether recurrences of *Pneumocystis* pneumonia result from reinfection or from relapse of previously treated infection is not known. For relapse to occur, however, the anti-*Pneumocystis* therapy used to achieve clinical cure must allow viable organisms to persist in the host. To determine if pentamidine and TMP/SMX are in fact not pneumocysticidal would require in vitro systems that support unlimited replication of the organism, and these have not yet been developed. Although tests of drug activity in currently available tissue culture models indicate that pentamidine and TMP/SMX inhibit somewhat the growth of *Pneumocystis*[201, 521] and that organisms exposed to pentamidine (but not to TMP/SMX) fail to take up vital dyes,[522] such tests cannot be considered definitive assays of drug lethality to the organisms.

Clinical and morphologic studies have furnished conflicting views as to the completeness of parasitic killing by drugs. The Hungarian workers, who first utilized pentamidine in epidemic pneumocystosis of infants, witnessed progressive degeneration of *P. carinii* in tracheal mucus from the sixth day of therapy; by the tenth day, the organisms had almost entirely disintegrated.[355] In their review of sporadic pneumocystosis in the United States, Western and associates similarly concluded that pentamidine probably eliminates organisms from the lung.[486] In two patients, no microscopically visible *P. carinii* were present 5 and 14 days, respectively, after initiation of therapy. Also, none of 11 patients who died more than 20 days after starting pentamidine had demonstrable organisms in their lungs even though they survived an average of 189.5 days after administration of the drug. In ultrastructural studies, Campbell detected what he believed to be the destructive effects of pentamidine on the organisms.[182] In a lung biopsy obtained surgically 16 hours after onset of therapy, he was unable to find structurally normal trophozoites or mature cysts with intracystic bodies. Indeed, a few apparent "ghosts" of trophozoites were noted within phagosomes of intra-alveolar macrophages.

In contrast, there is documentation that pentamidine does not promptly eradicate potentially viable forms of the parasite. Hughes and co-workers identified intact *P. carinii* in lung aspirates (or autopsy material) 10 to 20 days after institution of drug treatment.[296] Richman and associates demonstrated normal-appearing *Pneumocystis* organisms in a lung aspirate from a clinically cured patient 3 days after completion of his 14-day course of pentamidine.[519] Similarly, Fortuny and colleagues[274] recovered organisms from induced sputa during each of 11 days of pentamidine injections, and Repsher and co-workers[430] detected rate but morphologically typical *Pneumocystis* in bronchial brushings obtained after a 10-day course of drug therapy that had otherwise resulted in clinical and radiologic improvement.

TMP/SMX appears to have only a limited and nonlethal effect on parasites. Experiments have shown that short-term treatment with the drug combination ultimately fails to prevent emergence of recrudescent *Pneumocystis* infection. In one study, a therapeutic dosage of TMP/SMX was given prophylactically to children with acute lymphocytic leukemia for a 2-week period beginning 28 days after initiation of antineoplastic treatment.[523] Although the incidence of *Pneumocystis* infection in these children after TMP/SMX was discontinued was not different from that observed in individuals who did not receive the drug, the time to development of patient infection was delayed. Reinfection rather than relapse may have accounted for the late infections, but relapse seems more likely in view of the following results in the experimental animal.[524] Immunocompetent rats were treated with TMP/SMX for as long as 6 weeks and then placed in individual isolator cages to exclude the possibility of acquisition of new organisms from the environmental air. After 12 weeks of immunosuppressive therapy with prednisone, *P. carinii* was still found in the lungs of at least 90% of both the animals treated with TMP/SMX and the untreated controls. These human and animal data are particularly relevant to the design of prophylactic programs to prevent *Pneumocystis* infection in humans (see later discussion). They provide a compelling argument for the need to continue a prophylactic regimen for as long as host defenses are considered to be too compromised to keep latent *Pneumocystis* infection in check.

Reactivation of pneumocystosis is not surprising in light of the pathogenesis and pathology of the infection in the immunodeficient subject. Frenkel and colleagues showed clearly in the earliest experimental animal models of *Pneumocystis* pneumonia that anti-*Pneumocystis* therapy alone was not completely curative and that relapse was to be anticipated unless factors provoking the infection (namely, corticosteroid administration) were minimized.[219] Long-term ultrastructural observations of *Pneumocystis* pneumonia in the rat confirmed that even with tapering of corticosteroid and apparent restoration of immune function, focal clusters of *P. carinii* are detectable in surviving animals for at least 21 weeks.[313] Furthermore, in humans, drugs might not reach organisms residing within the foci of fibrosis and calcification formed during especially severe infection.[328] Indeed, Dutz contended that drugs play no therapeutic role in epidemic pneumocystosis once the chronic plasmacellular infiltrate is established. Radiographic resolution is slow, and survival and permanent immunity to reinfection relate not to chemotherapy but to specific anti-*Pneumocystis* immunoglobulin production in the affected infants.[163] Unfortunately, the congenitally immunodeficient or exogenously immunosuppressed child does not possess such normal immune responsiveness and thus is subject to recurrent infection.

Prophylaxis

The first successful attempts to prevent pneumocystosis with drugs were reported in infants with the epidemic form of the infection. In a controlled trial conducted in an Iranian orphanage where the infection was endemic (attack rate of 28%), the biweekly administration of a pyrimethamine and sulfadoxine combination to marasmic infants before the second month of life entirely erased *Pneumocystis* pneumonia from the institution.[462] In a children's hospital in Budapest, Hungary, pentamidine given every other day for seven doses to premature infants from the second week of life provided equally effective prophylaxis. During the 6 years of the study, *Pneumocystis* infection did not develop among 536 premature babies so treated, whereas 62 fatal cases were recorded elsewhere in the city.[525]

Initial efforts to prevent pneumocystosis in the rat given cortisone produced less promising results. Disease in animals was not averted by pretreatment with pyrimethamine and sulfadoxine[526] or pentamidine[527] or by active vaccination with immunogenic suspensions of *Pneumocystis* organisms.[526] Later experiments employing the same rat model revealed, however, that TMP/SMX was a remarkably efficacious prophylactic agent.[476] Accordingly, the combination was evaluated in a randomized double-blind controlled trial in children with cancer at extremely high risk for *Pneumocystis* pneumonitis.[528] The dosages for prophylaxis were 5 mg of TMP and 20 mg of SMX per kilogram per day, administered orally in two divided doses. Seventeen (21%) of 80 children receiving placebo acquired pneumocystosis, whereas none of 80 patients given TMP/SMX developed the infection. No adverse effects of TMP/SMX administration were observed, although oral candidiasis was more prevalent in the drug-treated patients than in the controls. In a subsequent uncontrolled trial, the prophylactic efficacy of TMP/SMX was confirmed; cases of infection developed only in those children in whom the combination was discontinued while they were still receiving anticancer chemotherapy.[529] More recently, a regimen of TMP/SMX prophylaxis given 3 days a week was shown to be as effective as daily administration.[521]

The gratifying success of TMP/SMX in prevention of *Pneumocystis* infection has been duplicated in other medical centers caring for children with underlying malignancy.[293, 521, 530] It has become common practice to give the drug for as long as antineoplastic agents are being administered. It would seem prudent to reserve TMP/SMX prophylaxis for individuals at relatively high risk for *Pneumocystis* pneumonitis. Identification of such patients is best done by retrospective review of cases at one's own institution because attack rates of *Pneumocystis* among patients with the same risk factors vary from one medical center to another.[531] Congenitally immunodeficient children or infants with AIDS who have had a prior episode of *Pneumocystis* pneumonia would appear to be prime candidates for preventive therapy. The Centers for Disease Control and Prevention issued a set of guidelines for chemoprophylaxis against *P. carinii* pneumonia in children with HIV infection in 1991,[532] and updated these guidelines based on the most recent epidemiologic surveillance demonstrating that despite recommendations established for *P. carinii* prophylaxis, no substantial decrease in *P. carinii* pneumonitis has occurred.[533] Surveillance indicated that continued cases were the result of failure to identify HIV-infected infants and the poor sensitivity of CD4+ measurements to determine infants' risk for development of *P. carinii* pneumonitis, rather than because of treatment failures.[534] These updated guidelines recommend promptly identifying infants and children born to HIV-infected women, initiating prophylaxis at 4 to 6 weeks of age for all of these children, and continuing prophylaxis through 12 months of age for HIV-infected children and offer new algorithms based on clinical and immunologic status to continue prophylaxis beyond 12 months of age. Although no chemoprophylactic regimens for *P. carinii* pneumonia among HIV-infected children have been approved as labeling indications by the Food and Drug Administration, TMP-SMX is currently recommended as the drug of choice in children with HIV infection. This recommendation is based on the known safety profile of TMP-SMX and its efficacy in adults with HIV infection and in children with malignancies. Alternative regimens recommended for HIV-infected children who cannot tolerate TMP-SMX include aerosolized pentamidine in children more than 5 years of age, oral dapsanone, or intravenous pentamidine. One study suggests that TMP/SMX use is associated with a decreased incidence of *P. carinii* pneumonitis and an increased incidence of HIV encephalopathy as initial AIDS-defining conditions in infants and children.[535]

References

Introduction and *Ascaris*

1. Kotcher E, Mata LJ, Esquivel R, et al. Acquisition of intestinal parasites in newborn infants. Fed Proc 24:442, 1965 (abstract).
2. Agbere AD, Atakouma DY, Balaka B, et al. Gastrointestinal and urinary parasitic infection in children at a regional hospital center in Togo: some epidemiological aspects. Med Trop 55:65-67, 1995.
3. Sterling R, Guay AJL. Invasion of the female generative tract by *Ascaris lumbricoides*. JAMA 107:2046, 1936.
4. Sanjeevi CB, Vivekanandan S, Narayanan PR. Fetal response to maternal ascariasis as evidenced by anti–*Ascaris lumbricoides* IgM antibodies in the cord blood. Acta Paediatr Scand 80:1134, 1991.
5. Chu W, Chen P, Huang C, et al. Neonatal ascariasis. J Pediatr 81:783, 1972.
6. Costa-Macedo LM, Rey L. *Ascaris lumbricoides* in neonate: evidence of congenital transmission of intestinal nematodes. Rev Inst Med Trop São Paolo 32(5):351, 1991.

Giardiasis

7. Roberts NS, Copel JA, Bhutani V, et al. Intestinal parasites and other infections during pregnancy in Southeast Asian refugees. J Reprod Med 30:720, 1985.
8. Kreutner AK, Del Bene VE, Amstey MS. Giardiasis in pregnancy. Am J Obstet Gynecol 140:895, 1981.

American Trypanosomiasis (Chagas' Disease)

9. Edgcomb JH, Johnson CM. American trypanosomiasis (Chagas' disease). *In* Binford CH, Connor OH (eds).
10. Bittencourt AL. Congenital Chagas' disease. Am J Dis Child 130:97, 1976.
11. Miles MA. The epidemiology of South American trypanosomiasis—biochemical and immunological approaches and their relevance to control. Trans R Soc Trop Med Hyg 77:5, 1983.
12. Marsden PD. South American trypanosomiasis (Chagas' disease). Int Rev Trop Med 4:97, 1981.
13. Santos-Buch CA. American trypanosomiasis: Chagas' disease. Int Rev Exp Pathol 19:63, 1979.
14. Amato Neto V, Doles J, Russi A, et al. Rev Inst Med Trop São Paulo 10:46, 1968.
15. Bittencourt AL, Mota E. Isoenzyme characterization of *Trypanosoma cruzi* from congenital cases of Chagas' disease. Ann Trop Med Parasitol 4:393, 1985.
16. Bittencourt AL, Sadigursky M, Barbosa HA. Doenca de Chagas congenita: estudo de 29 cašos. Rev Inst Med Trop São Paulo 17:146, 1975.
17. Rassi A, Borges C, Koeberle F, et al. Sobre a transmissão congenita da doenca de Chagas. Rev Goiana Med 4:319, 1958.
18. Delgado MA, Santos Buch CA. Transplacental transmission and fetal parasitosis of *Trypanosoma cruzi* in outbred white Swiss mice. Am J Trop Med Hyg 27:1108, 1978.
19. Cossio PM, Dicz C, Szarfman A, et al. Chagasic cardiopathy: demonstration of a serum gamma globulin factor which reacts with endocardium and vascular structures. Circulation 49:13, 1974.
20. Cossio PM, Laguens RP, Diez C, et al. Antibodies reacting with plasma membrane of striated muscle and endothelial cells. Circulation 50:1252, 1974.
21. Szarfman A, Cossio PM, Arana RM, et al. Immunologic and immunopathologic studies in congenital Chagas' disease. Clin Immunol Immunopathol 4:489, 1975.
22. Vasquez AD. Doctoral thesis, Universidad del los Andes, Venezuela, 1959.
23. Saleme A, Yanicelli GL, Inigo LA, ct al. Enfermedad de Chagas-Mazza congenita en Tucuman. Arch Argent Pediatr 59:162, 1971.
24. Bittencourt AL, Mota E, Filho RR, et al. Incidence of congenital Chagas' disease in Bahaia, Brazil. J Trop Pediatr 31:242, 1985.
25. Barousse AP, Eposto MO, Mandel S, et al. Enfermedad de Chagas congenita en area no endemica. Medicina (Buenos Aires) 38:611, 1978.
26. Stagno S, Hurtado R. Enfermedad de Chagas congenita: studio immunologico y diagnostico mediante immunofluorescencia con anti IgM. Bol Chil Parasitol 26:20, 1971.
27. Bittencourt AL, Barbosa HS, Santos I, et al. Incidencia da transmissão congenita da doenca de Chagas em partos a termo. Rev Inst Med Trop São Paulo 16:197, 1974.
28. Rubio M, Howard BJ. Enfermedad de Chagas congenita: II. Halazgo anatomopatologico en 9 casos. Bol Chil Parasitol 23:113, 1968.
29. Azogue E, LaFuente C, Darras C. Congenital Chagas' disease in Bolivia: epidemiological aspects and pathological findings. Trans R Soc Trop Med Hyg 79:176, 1985.
30. Howard JE. La enfermedad de Chagas congenita. Thesis, Universidad de Chile, Santiago, 1962.
31. Bittencourt AL, Vieira GO, Tavares HC, et al. Esophageal involvement in congenital Chagas' disease. Am J Trop Med Hyg 33:30, 1984.
32. Bittencourt AL, Rodriguez de Freitas LA, De Araujo Galvao, MO, et al. Pneumonitis in congenital Chagas'

disease: a study of ten cases. Am J Trop Med Hyg 30:38, 1981.

33. Hoff R, Mott KE, Milanesi ML, et al. Congenital Chagas' disease in an urban population: investigation of infected twins. Trans R Soc Trop Med Hyg 72:247, 1978.

34. Feilij H, Muller L, Gonzalez Cappa SM. Direct micromethod for diagnosis of acute and congenital Chagas' disease. J Clin Microbiol 18:327, 1983.

35. Reyes MB, Lorca M, Munoz P, Frasch ACC. Fetal IgG specificities against *Trypanosoma cruzi* antigens in infected newborns. Proc Natl Acad Sci U S A 87:2846, 1990.

36. Bittencourt AL, Gomes MC. Gestacoes sucessivas de uma paciente chagasica com ocorrencia de casos de transmissao congenital da doenca. Gaz Med Bahia 67:166, 1967.

African Trypanosomiasis (African Sleeping Sickness)

37. Lingam S, Marshall WC, Wilson J, et al. Congenital trypanosomiasis in a child born in London. Dev Med Child Neurol 27:664–674, 1985.

38. Reinhardt MC, Macleod CL. Parasitic Infections in Pregnancy and the Newborn. Oxford University Press, 1988.

Entamoeba histolytica

39. Armon PJ. Amoebiasis in pregnancy and the puerperium. Br J Obstet Gynaecol 85:264, 1978.

40. Abioye AA. Fatal amoebic colitis in pregnancy and puerperium: a new clinico-pathological entity. J Trop Med Hyg 76:97, 1973.

41. Czeizel E, Hancsok M, Palkowich I, et al. Possible relation between fetal death and *E. histolytica* infection of the mother. Am J Obstet Gynecol 96:264, 1966.

42. Dykes AC, Ruebush TK II, Gorelkin L, et al. Extraintestinal amebiasis in infancy: report of three patients and epidemiologic investigations of their families. Pediatrics 65:799, 1980.

43. Botman T, Ruys PJ. Amoebic appendicitis in a newborn infant. Trop Geogr Med 15:221, 1963.

44. Axton JHM. Amoebic proctocolitis and liver abscess in a neonate. S Afr Med J 46:258, 1972.

Malaria

45. Young MD. Malaria. *In* Hunter GW III, Swartzwelder JC, Clyde DF (eds). Tropical Medicine. Philadelphia, WB Saunders, 1976, pp 353–396.

46. Shulman IA, Saxena S, Nelson JM, et al. Neonatal exchange transfusions complicated by transfusion-induced malaria. Pediatrics 73:330, 1984.

47. Piccoli DA, Perlman S, Ephros M. Transfusion-acquired *Plasmodium malariae* infection in two premature infants. Pediatrics 72:560, 1983.

48. Sinclair S, Mittal SK, Singh M. Neonatal transfusion malaria. Indian Pediatr 8:219, 1971.

49. Ghosh S, Patwari A, Mohan M, et al. Clinical and hematologic peculiarities of malaria in infancy. Clin Pediatr (Phila) 17:369, 1978.

50. Keitel HG, Goodman HC, Havel RJ, et al. Nephrotic syndrome in congenital quartan malaria. JAMA 161:521, 1956.

51. Bray RS, Anderson MJ. Falciparum malaria and pregnancy. Trans R Soc Trop Med Hyg 73:427, 1979.

52. Reinhardt MC, Ambroise-Thomas P, Cavallo-Serra R, et al. Malaria at delivery in Abidjan. Helv Paediatr Acta 33(Suppl 41):65, 1978.

53. Cannon DSH. Malaria and prematurity in the western region of Nigeria. BMJ 2:877, 1958.

54. Gilles HM, Lawson JB, Sibelas M, et al. Malaria, anae-

mia and pregnancy. Ann Trop Med Parasitol 63:245, 1969.

55. McGregor I. Epidemiology, malaria and pregnancy. Am J Trop Med Hyg 33:517, 1984.

56. Campbell CC, Martinez JM, Collins WE. Seroepidemiological studies of malaria in pregnant women and newborns from coastal El Salvador. Am J Trop Med Hyg 29:151, 1980.

57. Bruce-Chwatt LJ. Malaria in African infants and children in southern Nigeria. Ann Trop Med Parasitol 46:173, 1952.

58. Taufa T. Malaria and pregnancy. Papua New Guinea Med J 21:197, 1978.

59. Jelliffe EFP. Low birth-weight and malarial infection of the placenta. Bull World Health Organ 38:69, 1968.

60. Torpin R. Malaria complicating pregnancy with a report of 27 cases. Am J Obstet Gynecol 41:882, 1941.

61. Hung LV. Paludisive at grossesse a Saigon. Rev Palud Med Trop 83:75, 1951.

62. Spita AJ. Malaria infection of the placenta and its influence on the incidence of prematurity in eastern Nigeria. Bull World Health Organ 21:242, 1959.

63. Jelliffe EFP. Placental malaria and foetal growth. *In* Nutrition and Infection: CIBA Foundation Study Group No. 31. J & A Churchill, 1967, pp 18–40.

64. Archibald HM. The influence of malarial infection of the placenta on the incidence of prematurity. Bull World Health Organ 15:842, 1956.

65. MacGregor JD, Avery JG. Malaria transmission and fetal growth. BMJ 3:433, 1974.

66. Larkin GL, Thuma PE. Congenital malaria in a hyperendemic area. Am J Trop Med Hyg 45(5):587, 1991.

67. Dubowitz LMS, Dubowitz V, Goldberg G. Clinical assessment of gestational age in the newborn infant. J Pediatr 77:1, 1970.

68. Blacklock DB, Gordon RM. Malaria parasites in the placental blood. Ann Trop Med Parasitol 19:37, 1925.

69. Menon R. Pregnancy and malaria. Med J Malays 27:115, 1972.

70. Covell G. Congenital malaria. Trop Dis Bull 47:1147, 1950.

71. McGregor IA. Immunity to plasmodial infections; consideration of factors relevant to malaria in man. Int Rev Trop Med 4:1, 1971.

72. Molineaux L, Cornille-Brogger R, Mathews HM, et al. Longitudinal serological study of malaria in infants in the West African savanna. Bull World Health Organ 56:573, 1978.

73. Mathews HM, Lobel HO, Breman JG. Malarial antibodies measured by the indirect hemagglutination test in West African children. Am J Trop Med Hyg 25:217, 1976.

74. Sehgal VM, Siddiqui WA, Alpers MP. A seroepidemiological study to evaluate the role of passive maternal immunity to malaria in infants. Trans R Soc Trop Med Hyg 83(Suppl):105, 1989.

75. Gilles HM. The development of malarial infection in breast-fed Gambian infants. Ann Trop Med Parasitol 51:58, 1957.

76. Allison AC. Genetic factors in resistance to malaria. Ann Acad Sci 91:710, 1961.

77. Allison AC. Malaria in carriers of the sickle cell trait and in newborn children. Exp Parasitol 6:418, 1957.

78. Le Hesran JY, Cot M, Personne P, et al. Maternal placental infection with *Plasmodium falciparum* and malaria morbidity during the first two years of life. Am J Epidemiol 146:826–831, 1997.

79. Hindi RD, Azimi PH. Congenital malaria due to *Plasmodium falciparum*. Pediatrics 66:977, 1980.
80. Harvey B, Remington JS, Sulzer AJ. IgM malaria antibodies in a case of congenital malaria in the United States. Lancet 1:333, 1969.
81. Williams AIO, McFarlane H. Immunoglobulin levels, malarial antibody titres and placental parasitaemia in Nigerian mothers and neonates. Afr J Med Sci 1:369, 1970.
82. Kortmann HF. Malaria and pregnancy. Thesis, Manuel Drukkrig Elinkwijk, Utrecht, 1972.
83. Schwetz J, Peel M. Congenital malaria and placental infections amongst the Negroes of Central Africa. Trans R Soc Trop Med Hyg 28:167, 1934.
84. Lehner PJ, Andrews CJ. Congenital malaria in Papua New Guinea. Trans R Soc Trop Med Hyg 82:822, 1988.
85. Wyler DJ. Malaria resurgence, resistance and research. N Engl J Med 308:934, 1983.
86. Davies HD, Keystone J, Lester ML, Gold R. Congenital malaria in infants of asymptomatic women. Can Med Assoc J 146(10):1755, 1992.
87. Dianto, Rampengan TH. Congenital falciparum malaria with chloroquine resistance type II. Paediatr Indones 29:237, 1989.
88. Chabasse D, De Gentile L, Ligny C, et al. Chloroquine-resistant *Plasmodium falciparum* in Mali revealed by congenital malaria. Trans R Soc Trop Med Hyg 82:547, 1988.
89. Airede AI. Congenital malaria with chloroquine resistance. Ann Trop Paediatr 11:267, 1991.
90. Congenital malaria infection in an infant born to a Kampuchean refugee. MMWR Morb Mortal Wkly Rep 29:3, 1980.
91. Congenital malaria in children of refugees—Washington, Massachusetts, Kentucky. MMWR Morb Mortal Wkly Rep 30:53, 1981.
92. Woods WG, Mills E, Ferrieri P. Neonatal malaria due to *Plasmodium vivax*. J Pediatr 85:669, 1974.
93. Hulbert TV. Congenital malaria in the United States: report of a case and review. Clin Infect Dis 14:922, 1992.
94. Thomas V, Wing Chit C. A case of congenital malaria in Malaysia with IgM malaria antibodies. Trans R Soc Trop Med Hyg 74:73, 1980.
95. McQuay RM, Silberman S, Mudrik P, et al. Congenital malaria in Chicago: a case report and a review of published reports (U.S.A.). Am J Trop Med 16:258, 1967.
96. Dhatt PS, Singh H, Singhal SC, et al. A clinicopathological study of malaria in early infancy. Indian Pediatr 26:331, 1979.
97. Subramanian D, Moise KJ, White AC. Imported malaria in pregnancy: report of four cases and review of management. Clin Infect Dis 15:408, 1992.
98. Zarou DM, Lichtman HC, Hellman LM. The transmission of chromium 51 tagged maternal erythrocytes from mother to fetus. Am J Obstet Gynecol 88:565, 1964.
99. Miller LH. Malaria. *In* Hoeprich PD (ed). Infectious Diseases: A Modern Treatise of Infectious Processes, 2nd ed. Hagerstown, Md, Harper & Row, 1977, pp 1075–1087.
100. Wong RD, Murthy ARK, Mathiesen GE, et al. Treatment of severe falciparum malaria during pregnancy with quinidine and exchange transfusion. Am J Med 92:561, 1992.
101. Quinn TC, Jacobs RF, Mertz GJ, et al. Congenital malaria: a report of four cases and a review. J Pediatr 101:229, 1982.
102. Watkinson M, Rushton DI. Plasmodial pigmentation of placenta and outcome of pregnancy in West African mothers. BMJ 287:251, 1983.
103. Morley D, Woodland M, Cuthbertson WFJ. Controlled trial of pyrimethamine in pregnant women in an African village. BMJ 1:667, 1964.
104. Chemoprophylaxis of malaria. MMWR Morb Mortal Wkly Rep 27(Suppl):81, 1978.
105. Harpy JP, Darbois Y, Lefebvre G. Teratogenicity of pyrimethamine. Lancet 2:399, 1983.
106. Uche-Nwachi EO. Effect of intramuscular sulfadoxine-pyrimethamine on pregnant Wistar rats. Anat Rec 250:426–429, 1998.
107. Vanhauwere B, Maradi H, Kerr L. Post-marketing surveillance of prophylactic mefloquine (Lariam) use in pregnancy. Am J Trop Med Hyg 58:17–21, 1998.
108. Smoak BL, Writer JV, Keep LW, et al. The effects of inadvertent exposure of mefloquine chemoprophylaxis on pregnancy outcomes and infants of US Army servicewomen. J Infect Dis 176:831–833, 1997.
109. Ellis CJ. Antiparasitic agents in pregnancy. Clin Obstet Gynecol 13:269, 1986.
110. Harrison KA, Ibeziako PA. Maternal anaemia and fetal birthweight. J Obstet Gynaecol Br Commonw 80:798, 1973.
111. Schofield FD, Parkinson AD, Kelly A. Changes in hemoglobin values and hepatosplenomegaly produced by control of holoendemic malaria. BMJ 1:587, 1964.
112. Hart CW, Naunton RF. The ototoxicity of chloroquine phosphate. Arch Otolaryngol 80:407, 1964.
113. Jelliffe EFP. Letter to the editor. J Pediatr 88:362, 1976.
114. Clyde DF. Letter to the editor. J Pediatr 88:362, 1976.
115. Parke A. Antimalarial drugs and pregnancy. Am J Med 85(Suppl 4A):30, 1988.
116. Levy M, Buskila D, Gladman DD, et al. Pregnancy outcome following first trimester exposure to chloroquine. Am J Perinatol 8(3):174, 1991.
117. Wolfe MS, Cordero JF. Safety of chloroquine in chemosuppression of malaria during pregnancy. BMJ 290:1466, 1985.
118. Katz M. Treatment of protozoan infections: malaria. Pediatr Infect Dis 2:475, 1983.
119. Dame JB, Williams JL, McCutchan TF, et al. Structure of the gene and coding the immunodominant surface antigen of the sporozoite of the human malarial parasite. Science 225:593, 1984.
120. Enea V, Ellis J, Zavala F, et al. DNA cloning of *Plasmodium falciparum* circumsporozoite gene: amino acid sequence of repetitive epitope. Science 225:628, 1984.
121. Soares IS, Rodrigues MM. Malaria vaccine: roadblocks and possible solutions. Braz J Med Biol Res 31:317–332, 1998.
122. Graves PM. Comparison of the cost-effectiveness of vaccines and insecticide impregnation of mosquito nets for the prevention of malaria. Ann Trop Med Parasitol 92:399–410, 1996.
123. Davison BB, Cogswell FB, Baskin GB, et al. *Plasmodium coatneyi* in the rhesus monkey (*Macaca mulatta*) as a model of malaria in pregnancy. Am J Trop Med Hyg 59:189–201, 1998.

Schistosomiasis (Bilharziasis)

124. Bullough CHW. Infertility and bilharziasis of the female genital tract. Br J Obstet Gynaecol 83:819, 1976.
125. Renaud R, Brettes P, Castanier C, et al. Placental bilharziasis. Int J Gynaecol Obstet 10:25, 1972.
126. Bittencourt AL, de Almeida MAC, Iunes MAF, et al. Placental involvement in *Schistosomiasis mansoni*. Am J Trop Med Hyg 29:571, 1980.

Trichomonas vaginalis

127. Ross SM, Van Middelkoop A. *Trichomonas* infection in pregnancy—does it affect perinatal outcome? S Afr Med J 63:566, 1983.
128. Franjola RT, Anazco RR, Puente RP, et al. *Trichomonas vaginalis* en embarazadas y en recien nacidos. Rev Med Chile 117:142, 1989.
129. McLaren LC, Davis LE, Healy GR, et al. Isolation of *Trichomonas vaginalis* from the respiratory tract of infants with respiratory disease. Pediatrics 71:888, 1983.
130. Hiemstra I, Van Bel F, Berger HM. Can *Trichomonas vaginalis* cause pneumonia in newborn babies? BMJ 289:355, 1984.
131. Al-Salihi FL, Curran JP, Wang JS. Neonatal *Trichomonas vaginalis*: report of three cases and review of the literature. Pediatrics 53:196, 1974.
132. Feo LG. The incidence of *Trichomonas vaginalis* in the various age groups. Am J Trop Med 5:786, 1956.
133. Trussell RE, Wilson ME, Longwell FH, et al. Vaginal trichomoniasis: complement fixation, puerperal morbidity and early infection of newborn infants. Am J Obstet Gynecol 44:292, 1942.
134. Komorowska A, Kurnatowska A, Liniecka J. Occurrence of *Trichomonas vaginalis* (Donne) in girls in relation to hygiene conditions. Wiad Parazytol 8:247, 1962.
135. Danesh IS, Stephen JM, Gorbach J. Neonatal *Trichomonas vaginalis* infection. J Emerg Med 13:1–4, 1995.
136. Littlewood JM, Kohler HG. Urinary tract infection by *Trichomonas vaginalis* in a newborn baby. Arch Dis Child 41:693, 1966.
137. Postlethwaite RJ. *Trichomonas* vaginitis and *Escherichia coli* urinary infection in a newborn infant. Clin Pediatr (Phila) 14:866, 1975.
138. Dagenais-Perusse P, Baril E, Ouadahi S, et al. Vaginite á trichomonas du nourrison. Un Med Can 93:1228, 1964.
139. Crowther IA. *Trichomonas* vaginitis in infancy. Lancet 1:1074, 1962.

Trichinosis

140. Kuitunen-Ekbaum E. The incidence of trichinosis in humans in Toronto: findings in 420 autopsies. Can Public Health J 32:569, 1941.
141. McNaught JB, Anderson EV. The incidence of trichinosis in San Francisco. JAMA 107:1446, 1936.
142. Salzer BF. A study of an epidemic of 14 cases of trichinosis with cures by serum therapy. JAMA 67:579, 1916.
143. Hood M, Olson SW. Trichinosis in the Chicago area. Am J Hyg 29:51, 1939.

Babesiosis

144. Raucher HS, Jaffin H, Glass JL. Babesiosis in pregnancy. Obstet Gynecol 63:75, 1984.

Pneumocystis carinii

145. Fudenberg H, Good RA, Goodman HC, et al. Primary immunodeficiencies: report of a World Health Organization Committee. Pediatrics 47:927, 1971.
146. Chagas C. Nova trypanomiazaea humana. Mem Inst Oswaldo Cruz 1:159, 1909.
147. Carini A. Formas de eschizogonia do *Trypanosoma lewisii*. Soc. de Med. et Cir. de São Paulo. 16 Aŏut. Bull Inst Pasteur 9:937, 1911.
148. Delanoe P, Delanoe M. Sur les rapports des kystes de carini du poumon des rats avec le *Trypanosoma lewisii*. Presenté par M. Laveran. Note de Delanoe et Delanoe. C R Acad Sci 155:658, 1912.
149. Chagas C. Nova entidade morbida do homen; rezumo

geral de estudos etiologicos e clinicos. Mem Inst Oswaldo Cruz 3:219, 1911.
150. Benecke E. Eigenartige Bronchiolenerkrankung im ersten Lebensjahr. Verh Dtsch Pathol Ges 31:402, 1938.
151. Ammich O. Über die nichtsyphilitische interstitielle Pneumonie des ersten Kindesalters. Virchows Arch Pathol Anat 302:539, 1938.
152. Vanek J, Jirovec O. Parasitäre Pneumonie. "Interstitielle" plasmazellen Pneumonie der Frühgeborenen, verursacht durch *Pneumocystis carinii*. Zentralbl Bakteriol [Orig] 158:120, 1952.
153. Van der Meer G, Brug SL. Infection par *Pneumocystis* chez l'homme et chez les animaux. Ann Soc Belge Med Trop 22:301, 1942.
154. Deamer WC, Zollinger HU. Interstitial "plasma cell" pneumonia of premature and young infants. Pediatrics 12:11, 1953.
155. Lunseth JH, Kirmse TW, Prezyna AP, et al. Interstitial plasma cell pneumonia. J Pediatr 46:137, 1955.
156. Dauzier G, Willis T, Barnett RN. *Pneumocystis carinii* pneumonia in an infant. Am J Clin Pathol 26:787, 1956.
157. Hamperl H. *Pneumocystis* infection and cytomegaly of the lungs in the newborn and adult. Am J Pathol 32:1, 1956.
158. Russell HT, Nelson BM. *Pneumocystis* pneumonitis in American infants. Am J Clin Pathol 26:1334, 1956.
159. Gajdusek DC. *Pneumocystis carinii*—etiologic agent of interstitial plasma cell pneumonia of premature and young infants. Pediatrics 19:543, 1957.
160. LeClair RA. *Pneumocystis carinii* and interstitial plasma cell pneumonia: a review. Am Rev Respir Dis 96:1131, 1967.
161. Barton EG, Campbell WG. *Pneumocystis carinii* in lungs of rats treated with cortisone acetate. Am J Pathol 54:209, 1969.
162. Vavra J, Kucera K, Levine ND. An interpretation of the fine structure of *Pneumocystis carinii*. J Protozool 15:12, 1968.
163. Dutz W. *Pneumocystis carinii* pneumonia. Pathol Ann 5:309, 1970.
164. Esterly JA, Warner NE. *Pneumocystis carinii* pneumonia. Arch Pathol 80:433, 1965.
165. Sethi KK. *Pneumocystis carinii* pneumonia. Letter to the editor. Lancet 1:1387, 1967.
166. Minielly JA, Mills SD, Holley KE. *Pneumocystis carinii* pneumonia. Can Med Assoc J 100:846, 1969.
167. McNeal JE, Yaeger RG. Observations on a case of *Pneumocystis* pneumonia. Arch Pathol 70:397, 1960.
168. Vavra J, Kucera K. *Pneumocystis carinii* Delanoë, its ultrastructure and ultrastructural affinities. J Protozool 17:463, 1970.
169. Kim HK, Hughes WT, Feldman S. Studies of morphology and immunofluorescence of *Pneumocystis carinii*. Proc Soc Exp Biol Med 141:304, 1972.
170. Sheldon WH. Pulmonary *Pneumocystis carinii* infection. J Pediatr 61:780, 1962.
171. Le Tan-Vinh, Cochard AM, Vu Trieu-Dong, et al. Diagnostic "in vivo" de la pneumonie á "*Pneumocystis*." Arch Fr Pediatr 20:773, 1963.
172. Chalvardjian AM, Grawe LA. A new procedure for the identification of *Pneumocystis carinii* cysts in tissue sections and smears. J Clin Pathol 16:383, 1963.
173. Bowling MC, Smith IM, Wescott SL. A rapid staining procedure for *Pneumocystis carinii*. Am J Med Tech 39:267, 1973.
174. Bommer W. *Pneumocystis carinii* from human lungs under electron microscope. Am J Dis Child 104:657, 1962.
175. Huneycutt HC, Anderson WR, Hendry WS. *Pneumo-*

cystis carinii pneumonia: case studies with electron microscopy. Am J Clin Pathol 41:411, 1964.

176. Barton EG Jr, Campbell WG Jr. Further observations on the ultrastructure of *Pneumocystis*. Arch Pathol 83:527, 1967.

177. Huang SN, Marshall KG. *Pneumocystis carinii* infection: a cytologic, histologic and electron microscopic study of the organism. Am Rev Respir Dis 102:623, 1970.

178. Wang NS, Huang SN, Thurlbeck WM. Combined *Pneumocystis carinii* and cytomegalovirus infection. Arch Pathol 90:529, 1970.

179. Vawter GF, Uzman BG, Nowoslawski A. *Pneumocystis carinii*. Ann NY Acad Sci 174:1048, 1970.

180. Ham EK, Greenberg SD, Reynolds RC, et al. Ultrastructure of *Pneumocystis carinii*. Exp Mol Pathol 14:362, 1971.

181. Luna MA, Bodey GP, Goldman AM, et al. *Pneumocystis carinii* pneumonitis in cancer patients. Texas Rep Biol Med 30:1, 1972.

182. Campbell WG Jr. Ultrastructure of *Pneumocystis* in human lung: life cycle in human pneumocystosis. Arch Pathol 93:312, 1972.

183. Nietschke A. Zur Frage des histologischen Nachweises von Pneumocysten bei der interstitiellen Pneumonie. Monatsschr Kinderheilkd 108:142, 1960.

184. Yoneda K, Walzer PD. Attachment of *Pneumocystis carinii* to type I alveolar cells studied by freeze-fracture electron microscopy. Infect Immun 40:812, 1983.

185. Vanek J, Jirovec O, Lukes J. Interstitial plasma cell pneumonia in infants. Ann Paediatr 180:1, 1953.

186. Kucera K. On the morphology and developmental cycle of *Pneumocystis carinii* of human and rat origin. Progress in Protozoology, Proceedings of the First International Conference on Protozoology, Prague, August 22–31, 1961, p 482.

187. Kucera K, Valousek T. The direct proof of *Pneumocystis carinii* in alive nurslings and a new evolutive stage of *Pneumocystis*. Folia Parasitol 13:113, 1966.

188. Vossen M, Beckers P, Meuwissen J, et al. Developmental biology of *Pneumocystis carinii*, an alternative view on the life cycle of the parasite. Z Parasitenkd 55:101, 1978.

189. Mojon M. Critique de la place taxonomique de *Pneumocystis carinii*. Lyon Med 228:325, 1972.

190. Goetz O. Die Ätiologie der interstitiellen sogenannten plasmazellularen Pneumonie des jungen Säuglings. Arch Kinderheilkd 163:1, 1960.

191. Jirovec O. Das Problem der Pneumocystis Pneumonien vom parasitologischen Standpunkte. Monatsschr Kinderheilkd 108:136, 1960.

192. Giese W. Die Ätiologie der interstitielle plasmazellulären Säuglingspneumonie. Monatsschr Kinderheilkd 101:147, 1953.

193. Von Lichtenberg F. Enigmatic parasites of man and animal models: summation. Ann NY Acad Sci 174:1052, 1970.

194. Barta K, Lysek H. Experimental pneumocystosis: I. Studies on complement fixation antibodies. Cesk Epidemiol 11:196, 1962.

195. Brzosko WJ, Nowoslawski A. Identification of *Pneumocystis carinii* antigens in tissues. Bull Acad Pol Sci 13:49, 1965.

196. Norman L, Kagan IG. Some observations on the serology of *Pneumocystis carinii* infections in the United States. Infect Immun 8:317, 1973.

197. Walzer PD, Rutledge ME. Comparison of rat, mouse and human *Pneumocystis carinii* by immunofluorescence. J Infect Dis 142:449, 1980.

198. Walzer PD, Linke MJ. A comparison of the antigenic characteristics of rat and human *Pneumocystis carinii* by immunoblotting. J Immunol 138:2257, 1987.

199. Vivell O. Die Serologie der interstitiellen Pneumonie. Monatsschr Kinderheilkd 108:146, 1960.

200. Goetz O. Serologische Befunde interstitieller Pneumonien aus den vereinigten Staaten. Arch Kinderheilkd 170:60, 1964.

201. Pifer LL, Hughes WT, Murphy MJ. Cultivation of *Pneumocystis carinii* in vitro. Pediatr Res 11:305, 1977.

202. Murphy MJ, Pifer LL, Hughes WT. *Pneumocystis carinii* in vitro: a study by scanning electron microscopy. Am J Pathol 86:387, 1977.

203. Latorre CR, Sulzer AJ, Norman L. Serial propagation of *Pneumocystis carinii* in cell line cultures. Appl Environ Microbiol 33:1204, 1977.

204. Pifer LL, Woods D, Hughes WT. Propagation of *Pneumocystis carinii* in Vero cell culture. Infect Immun 20:66, 1978.

205. Bartlett MS, Verbanac PA, Smith JW. Cultivation of *Pneumocystis carinii* with WI-38 cells. J Clin Microbiol 10:796, 1979.

206. Masur H, Jones TC. The interaction in vitro of *Pneumocystis carinii* with macrophages and L-cells. J Exp Med 147:157, 1978.

207. Reye RDK, Ten Seldam REJ. *Pneumocystis* pneumonia. J Pathol Bacteriol 72:451, 1956.

208. da Silva GR, Gomes MC, Santos RF. *Pneumocystis* pneumonia in the adult: report of a case associated with corticosteroid therapy for rheumatoid arthritis. Rev Inst Med Trop São Paulo 7:31, 1965.

209. Gagne F, Hould F. Interstitial plasmacellular (parasitic) pneumonia in infants. Can Med Assoc J 74:620, 1956.

210. Pizzi T, Diaz M. Neumonia intersticial plasmocelular: II. Investigacion parasitologia del *Pneumocystis carinii*. Rev Chil Pediatr 27:294, 1956.

211. Thijs A, Janssens PG. Pneumocystosis in Congolese infant. Trop Geogr Med 15:158, 1963.

212. Jarnum S, Rasmussen EF, Ohlsen AS, et al. Generalized *Pneumocystis carinii* infection with severe idiopathic hypoproteinemia. Ann Intern Med 68:138, 1968.

213. Baar HS. Interstitial plasmacellular pneumonia due to *Pneumocystis carinii*. J Clin Pathol 8:19, 1955.

214. Ahvenainen EK. Interstitial plasma cell pneumonia. Pediatr Clin North Am 4:203, 1957.

215. Vlachos I. Necropsy findings in six cases of *Pneumocystis carinii* pneumonia in Pediatric Pathology Society. Arch Dis Child 45:146, 1970.

216. Desai AB, Shak RC, Schgal KN. *Pneumocystis carinii* pneumonia. Indian Pediatr 8:129, 1971.

217. Cahalane SF. *Pneumocystis carinii* pneumonia: report of a case and review of the literature. J Ir Med Assoc 50:133, 1962.

218. Kaftori JK, Bassan H, Gellei B, et al. *Pneumocystis carinii* pneumonia in the adult. Arch Intern Med 109:114, 1962.

219. Fontana G, Tamburello O. Epidemiologia della polmonite interstiziale plasmacellulare nell' I.P.A.I. di Roma. Minerva Nipiol 19:20, 1969.

220. Nakamura RM, Kimura K, Ichimaru M, et al. Coexistent cytomegalic inclusion disease and *Pneumocystis carinii* infection in adults. Acta Pathol Jpn 14:45, 1964.

221. Lim SK, Moon CS. Studies on *Pneumocystis carinii* pneumonia: epidemiological and clinical studies of 80 cases. Jonghap Med 6:69, 1960.

222. Ryan B. *Pneumocystis carinii* infection in Melanesian children. J Pediatr 60:914, 1962.

223. Becroft DMO, Costello JM. *Pneumocystis carinii* pneumonia in siblings: diagnosis by lung aspiration. N Z Med J 64:273, 1965.

224. Laerum OD, Flatmark AL, Enge I, et al. *Pneumocystis carinii* pneumonia in Norway. Scand J Respir Dis 53:247, 1972.

225. Byhosko Z. Pneumonia caused by *Pneumocystis carinii*. Pediatr Pol 31:493, 1956.

226. Mikhailov G. Pneumocystic pneumonia. Arch Patol (Moscow) 21:46, 1959.

227. Hutchison JH. Congenital agammaglobulinemia. Lancet 2:844, 1955.

228. Pepler WJ. *Pneumocystis* pneumonia. S Afr Med J 32:1003, 1958.

229. Moragas A, Vidal MT. *Pneumocystis carinii* pneumonia; first autopsy series in Spain. Helvet Paediatr Acta 26:71, 1971.

230. Nathorst-Windahl G, Hesselman BH, Sjostrom B, et al. Massive fatal *Pneumocystis* pneumonia in leukemia: Report of two cases. Acta Pathol Microbiol Scand 62:472, 1964.

231. Salfelder K, Schwarz J, Sethi KK, et al. Neumocistosis. Merida, Venezuela, Universidad de los Andes, Facultad de Medicina, 1966.

232. Abioye AA. Interstitial plasma cell pneumonia (*Pneumocystis carinii*) in Ibadan. W Afr Med J 16:130, 1967.

233. Farrow BRH, Watson ADJ, Hartley WJ, et al. *Pneumocystis* pneumonia in the dog. J Comp Pathol 82:447, 1972.

234. Shively JN, Dellers RW, Buergelt CD, et al. *Pneumocystis carinii* pneumonia in two foals. J Am Vet Med Assoc 162:648, 1973.

235. Van den Akker S, Goldbloed E. Pneumonia caused by *Pneumocystis carinii* in a dog. Trop Geogr Med 12:54, 1960.

236. Nikolskii CN, Shchetknin AN. *Pneumocystis* in swine. Veterinaria 44:65, 1967.

237. Chandler FW, McClure HM, Campbell WG, et al. Pulmonary pneumocystosis in nonhuman primates. Arch Pathol Lab Med 100:163, 1976.

238. Richter CV, Humason GL, Godbold JH Jr. Endemic *Pneumocystis carinii* in a marmoset colony. J Comp Pathol 88:171, 1978.

239. Meuwissen J, Tauber I, Leuwenberg A, et al. Parasitological and serologic observations of infection with *Pneumocystis* in humans. J Infect Dis 136:43, 1977.

240. Pifer LL, Hughes WT, Stagno S, et al. *Pneumocystis carinii* infection: evidence for high prevalence in normal and immunosuppressed children. Pediatrics 61:35, 1978.

241. Gerrard MP, Eden OB, Jameson B, et al. Serological study of *Pneumocystis carinii* infection in the absence of immunosuppression. Arch Dis Child 62:177, 1987.

242. Pifer L, Pifer D, Freeman-Shade L, et al. Subclinical *Pneumocystis carinii* infection: implications for the immunocompromised patient. Program and Abstracts of the 20th Interscience Conference on Antimicrobial Agents and Chemotherapy, New Orleans, September 22–24, 1980. Abstract 340.

243. Robinson JJ. Two cases of pneumocystosis: observation in 203 adult autopsies. Arch Pathol 71:156, 1961.

244. Weisse K, Wedler E. Über das Vorkommen der sogenannten "*Pneumocystis carinii*." Klin Wochenschr 32:270, 1954.

245. Hamlin WB. *Pneumocystis carinii*. JAMA 204:173, 1968.

246. Esterly JA. *Pneumocystis carinii* in lungs of adults at autopsy. Am Rev Respir Dis 97:935, 1968.

247. Vogel CL, Cohen MH, Powell RD Jr, et al. *Pneumocystis carinii* pneumonia. Ann Intern Med 68:97, 1968.

248. Sedaghatian MR, Singer DB. *Pneumocystis carinii* in children with malignant disease. Cancer 29:772, 1972.

249. Perera DR, Western KS, Johnson HD, et al. *Pneumocystis carinii* pneumonia in a hospital for children: epidemiologic aspects. JAMA 214:1074, 1970.

250. Le Clair RA. Descriptive epidemiology of interstitial pneumocystic pneumonia. Am Rev Respir Dis 99:542, 1969.

251. Walzer PD, Schultz MG, Western KA, et al. *Pneumocystis carinii* pneumonia and primary immune deficiency diseases of infancy and childhood. J Pediatr 82:416, 1973.

252. Walzer PD, Perl DP, Krogstad DJ, et al. *Pneumocystis carinii* pneumonia in the United States: epidemiologic, diagnostic and clinical features. Ann Intern Med 80:83, 1974.

253. Hyun BH, Varga CF, Thalheimer LJ. *Pneumocystis carinii* pneumonitis occurring in an adopted Korean infant. JAMA 195:784, 1966.

254. Danilevicius Z. A call to recognize *Pneumocystis carinii* pneumonia. Editorial. JAMA 231:1168, 1975.

255. Eidelman A, Nkongo A, Morecki R. *Pneumocystis carinii* pneumonitis in Vietnamese infant in U.S. Pediatr Res 8:424, 1974 (abstract).

256. Redman JC. *Pneumocystis carinii* pneumonia in an adopted Vietnamese infant: a case of diffuse fulminant disease, with recovery. JAMA 230:1561, 1974.

257. Gleason WA Jr, Roden VJ, DeCastro F. *Pneumocystis* pneumonia in Vietnamese infants. J Pediatr 87:1001, 1975.

258. Eidelman AI, Giebink GS, Stracener CE, et al. *Pneumocystis carinii* pneumonia in Vietnamese orphans. MMWR Morb Mortal Wkly Rep 25:15, 1976.

259. Giebink GS, Sholler L, Keenan TP, et al. *Pneumocystis carinii* pneumonia in two Vietnamese refugee infants. Pediatrics 58:115, 1976.

260. Update: acquired immunodeficiency syndrome—United States. MMWR Morb Mortal Wkly Rep 35:757, 1986.

261. Simonds RJ, Oxtoby MJ, Caldwell MB, et al. *Pneumocystis carinii* pneumonia among U.S. children with perinatally acquired HIV infection. JAMA 270:470–473, 1993.

262. Anderson CD, Barrie HJ. Fatal *Pneumocystis* pneumonia in an adult. Am J Clin Pathol 34:365, 1960.

263. Lyons HA, Vinijchaikul K, Hennigar GR. *Pneumocystis carinii* pneumonia unassociated with other disease. Arch Intern Med 108:929, 1961.

264. Watanabe JM, Chinchinian H, Weitz C, et al. *Pneumocystis carinii* pneumonia in a family. JAMA 193:685, 1965.

265. Weinberg AG, McCracken GH Jr, Lo-Spalluto J, et al. Monoclonal macroglobulinemia and cytomegalic inclusion disease. Pediatrics 51:518, 1973.

266. Rao M, Steiner P, Victoria MS, et al. *Pneumocystis carinii* pneumonia: occurrence in a healthy American infant. JAMA 238:2301, 1977.

267. Stagno S, Pifer LL, Hughes WT, et al. *Pneumocystis carinii* pneumonitis in young immunocompetent infants. Pediatrics 66:56, 1980.

268. Shann F, Walters S, Pifer LL, et al. Pneumonia associated with infection with pneumocystis, respiratory syncytial virus, *Chlamydia*, *Mycoplasma*, and cytomegalovirus in children in Papua New Guinea. BMJ 292:314, 1986.

269. Jirovec O. Dalsi poznatky o pneumonii kojencu zpusobene parasitem *Pneumocystis carinii*. Pediatr Listy 9:199, 1954.

270. Robbins JB. *Pneumocystis carinii* pneumonitis, a review. Pediatr Res 1:131, 1967.

271. Von Harnack GA. Organisatorische Probleme bei der Bekämpfung der interstitiellen Pneumonie. Monatsschr Kinderheilkd 108:159, 1960.

272. Erchul JW, Williams LP, Meighan PP. *Pneumocystis carinii* in hypopharyngeal material. N Engl J Med 267:926, 1962.

273. Toth G, Balogh E, Belay M. Demonstration in tracheal secretion of the causative agent of interstitial plasma cell pneumonia. Acta Paediatr Acad Sci Hung 7:25, 1966.

274. Fortuny IE, Tempero KF, Amsden TW. *Pneumocystis carinii* pneumonia diagnosed from sputum and successfully treated with pentamidine isethionate. Cancer 26:911, 1970.

275. Smith JA, Wiggins CM. Identification of *Pneumocystis carinii* in sputum. Letter to the editor. N Engl J Med 289:1254, 1973.

276. Lau WK, Young LS, Remington JS. *Pneumocystis carinii* pneumonia: diagnosis by examination of pulmonary secretions. JAMA 236:2399, 1976.

277. Ruskin J, Remington JS. The compromised host and infection: I. *Pneumocystis carinii* pneumonia. JAMA 202:1070, 1967.

278. Brazinsky JH, Phillips JE. *Pneumocystis* pneumonia transmission between patients with lymphoma. Letter to the editor. JAMA 209:1527, 1969.

279. Jacobs JL, Libby DM, Winters RA, et al. A cluster of *Pneumosystis carinii* pneumonia in adults without predisposing illnesses. N Eng J Med 324:246, 1991.

280. Robbins JD, Fodor T. *Pneumocystis carinii* pneumonia. MMWR Morb Mortal Wkly Rep 17:51, 1968.

281. Gentry LO, Remington JS. *Pneumocystis carinii* pneumonia in siblings. J Pediatr 76:769, 1970.

282. Bazaz GR, Manfredi OL, Howard RG, et al. *Pneumocystis carinii* pneumonia in three full-term siblings. J Pediatr 76:767, 1970.

283. Jose DG, Gatti RA, Good RA. Eosinophilia with *Pneumocystis carinii* pneumonia and immune deficiency syndromes. J Pediatr 79:748, 1971.

284. Yates JW, Ellison RR, Plager J. *Pneumocystis carinii* in a husband and wife. Letter to the editor. Lancet 2:610, 1975.

285. Meuwissen HJ, Brzosko WJ, Nowoslawski A, et al. Diagnosis of *Pneumocystis carinii* pneumonia in the presence of immunological deficiency. Letter to the editor. Lancet 1:1124, 1970.

286. Pavlica F. Erste Beobachtung von angeborener pneumozysten Pneumonie bei einem reifen, ausgetragenen Totgeborenen. Zentralbl Allg Pathol 103:236, 1962.

287. Post C, Dutz W, Nasarian I. Endemic *Pneumocystis carinii* pneumonia in South Iran. Arch Dis Child 39:35, 1964.

288. Brock P, Ninane J, Cornu G, et al. AIDS in two African infants born in Belgium. Acta Paediatr Scand 76:175, 1987.

289. Beach RS, Garcia ER, Sosa R, Good RA. *Pneumocystis carinii* pneumonia in a human immunodeficiency virus 1-infected neonate with meconium aspiration. Pediatr Infect Dis J 10:953–954, 1991.

290. Burke BA, Good RA. *Pneumocystis carinii* infection. Medicine 52:23, 1973.

291. Singer C, Armstrong D, Rosen PP, et al. *Pneumocystis carinii* pneumonia: a cluster of eleven cases. Ann Intern Med 82:772, 1975.

292. Ruebush TK, Weinstein RA, Baehner RL, et al. An outbreak of *Pneumocystis* pneumonia in children with acute lymphocytic leukemia. Am J Dis Child 132:143, 1978.

293. Chusid MJ, Heyrman KA. An outbreak of *Pneumocystis carinii* pneumonia at a pediatric hospital. Pediatrics 62:1031, 1978.

294. Hughes WT, Feldman S, Aur RJA, et al. Intensity of immunosuppressive therapy and the incidence of *Pneumocystis carinii* pneumonitis. Cancer 36:2004, 1975.

295. Kucera K. Some new views on the epidemiology of infections caused by *Pneumocystis carinii*. *In* Corradetti A (ed).

Proceedings of the First International Congress of Parasitology, Rome, Italy, September 26–28, 1964. Oxford, Pergamon Press, 1964, p 452.

296. Hughes WT, Price RA, Kim HK, et al. *Pneumocystis carinii* pneumonitis in children with malignancies. J Pediatr 82:404, 1973.

297. Hennigar GR, Vinijchaikul K, Roque AL, et al. *Pneumocystis carinii* pneumonia in an adult. Am J Clin Pathol 35:353, 1961.

298. Burke EC, Brown AL, Weed LA. *Pneumocystis carinii* pneumonia: report of case in infant with hypogammaglobulinemia. Staff Meet Mayo Clin 37:129, 1962.

299. Awen CF, Baltzan MA. Systemic dissemination of *Pneumocystis carinii* pneumonia. Can Med Assoc J 104:809, 1971.

300. Walzer PD, Schnelle V, Armstrong D, et al. Nude mouse: a new experimental model for *Pneumocystis carinii* infection. Science 197:177, 1977.

301. Sheldon WH. Experimental pulmonary *Pneumocystis carinii* infection in rabbits. J Exp Med 110:147, 1959.

302. Hendley JO, Weller TH. Activation and transmission in rats of infection with *Pneumocystis*. Proc Soc Exp Biol Med 137:1401, 1971.

303. Ueda K, Goto Y, Yamazaki S, et al. Chronic fatal pneumocystosis in nude mice. Jpn J Exp Med 47:475, 1977.

304. Walzer PD, Rutledge ME. Humoral immune responses in experimental *Pneumocystis carinii* pneumonia. Clin Res 28:381, 1980.

305. Price RA, Hughes WT. Histopathology of *Pneumocystis carinii* infestation and infection in malignant disease in childhood. Hum Pathol 5:737, 1974.

306. Rosen P, Armstrong D, Ramos C. *Pneumocystis carinii* pneumonia: a clinicopathologic study of 20 patients with neoplastic diseases. Am J Med 53:428, 1972.

307. Weber WR, Askin FB, Dehner LP. Lung biopsy in *Pneumocystis carinii* pneumonia: a histopathologic study of typical and atypical features. Am J Clin Pathol 67:11, 1977.

308. Hamperl H. Zur Frage des Parasitennachweises bei der interstitiellen plasmacellularen Pneumonie. Klin Wochenschr 30:820, 1952.

309. Robin E, Zak FG. *Pneumocystis carinii* pneumonia in the adult. N Engl J Med 262:1315, 1960.

310. Burke BA, Krovetz LJ, Good RA. Occurrence of *Pneumocystis carinii* pneumonia in children with agammaglobulinemia. Pediatrics 28:196, 1961.

311. Rifkind D, Faris TD, Hill RB. *Pneumocystis carinii* pneumonia: studies on the diagnosis and treatment. Ann Intern Med 65:943, 1966.

312. Lanken PN, Minda M, Pietra GG, et al. Alveolar response to experimental *Pneumocystis carinii* pneumonia in the rat. Am J Pathol 99:561, 1980.

313. Walzer PD, Yoneda K. Interaction of *Pneumocystis carinii* with host lungs: an ultrastructural study. Infect Immun 29:692, 1980.

314. Askin FB, Katzenstein AA. *Pneumocystis* infection masquerading as diffuse alveolar damage: a potential source of diagnostic error. Chest 79:420, 1981.

315. Kramer RI, Cirone VC, Moore H. Interstitial pneumonia due to *Pneumocystis carinii* and cytomegalic inclusion disease and hypogammaglobulinemia occurring simultaneously in an infant. Pediatrics 29:816, 1962.

316. Nicastri AD, Hutter RVP, Collins HS. *Pneumocystis carinii* pneumonia in an adult: emphasis on antemortem morphologic diagnosis. NY State J Med 65:2149, 1965.

317. Robbins JB, Miller RH, Arean VM, et al. Successful treatment of *Pneumocystis carinii* pneumonitis in a patient with congenital hypogammaglobulinemia. N Engl J Med 272:708, 1965.

318. Nowak J. Late pulmonary changes in the course of infection with *Pneumocystis carinii*. Acta Med Pol 7:23, 1966.

319. Whitcomb ME, Schwarz MI, Charles MA, et al. Interstitial fibrosis after *Pneumocystis carinii* pneumonia. Ann Intern Med 73:761, 1970.

320. Hughes WT, Johnson WW. Recurrent *Pneumocystis carinii* pneumonia following apparent recovery. J Pediatr 79:755, 1971.

321. Kirby HB, Kenamore B, Guckian JC. *Pneumocystis carinii* pneumonia treated with pyrimethamine and sulfadiazine. Ann Intern Med 75:505, 1971.

322. Frenkel JK, Good JT, Shultz JA. Latent *Pneumocystis* infection of rats, relapse and chemotherapy. Lab Invest 15:1559, 1966.

323. Walzer PD, Powell RD, Yoneda K, et al. Growth characteristics and pathogenesis of experimental *Pneumocystis carinii* pneumonia. Infect Immun 27:928, 1980.

324. Schmid KO. Studien zur *Pneumocystis*-erkrankung des Menschen: I. Mitteilung, das wechselnde Erscheinungsbild der *Pneumocystis* Pneumonie beim Säugling: konkordante und discordante Form, *Pneumocystosis* granulomatose. Frankfurt Z Pathol 74:121, 1964.

325. Cruickshank B. Pulmonary granulomatous pneumocystosis following renal transplantation: report of a case. Am J Clin Pathol 63:384, 1975.

326. Brasfield DM, Stagno S, Whitley RJ, et al. Infant pneumonitis associated with cytomegalovirus, *Chlamydia*, *Pneumocystis* and *Ureaplasma*: follow-up. Pediatrics 79:76, 1987.

327. Barnett RN, Hull JG, Vortel V, et al. *Pneumocystis carinii* in lymph nodes and spleen. Arch Pathol 88:175, 1969.

328. LeGolvan DP, Heidelberger KP. Disseminated, granulomatous *Pneumocystis carinii* pneumonia. Arch Pathol 95:344, 1973.

329. Rahimi SA. Disseminated *Pneumocystis carinii* in thymic alymphoplasia. Arch Pathol 97:162, 1974.

330. Salfelder K, Schwarz J. Pneumocystosis: current concepts and recent advances. Am J Dis Child 114:693, 1967.

331. Dutz W, Jennings-Khodadad E, Post C, et al. Marasmus and *Pneumocystis carinii* pneumonia in institutionalized infants: observations during an endemic. Z Kinderheilkd 117:241, 1974.

332. Weller R. Zur Erzeugung der Pneumocystosen im Tierver-such. Z Kinderheilkd 76:366, 1955.

333. Weller R. Weitere Untersuchungen über experimentele Rattenpneumocystose in Hinblick auf die interstitielle Pneumonie der Frühgeborenen. Z Kinderheilkd 78:166, 1956.

334. Hughes WT, Price RA, Sisko F, et al. Protein-calorie malnutrition: a host determinant for *Pneumocystis carinii* infection. Am J Dis Child 128:44, 1974.

335. Von Behren LA, Pesanti EL. Uptake and degradation of *Pneumocystis carinii* by macrophages in vitro. Am Rev Respir Dis 118:1051, 1978.

336. Baar, cited in Hutchison JH. Congenital agammaglobulinemia. Letter to the editor. Lancet 2:1196, 1955.

337. Bird T, Thompson J. *Pneumocystis carinii* pneumonia. Lancet 1:59, 1957.

338. Gerrard JW, Moore DF. Interstitial plasma cellular pneumonia due to *Pneumocystis carinii*. Can J Med Assoc J 76:299, 1957.

339. McKay E, Richardson J. *Pneumocystis carinii* pneumonia associated with hypogammaglobulinemia. Lancet 2:713, 1959.

340. Russell JGB. Pneumocystis pneumonia associated with agammaglobulinemia. Arch Dis Child 34:338, 1959.

341. Hendry WS, Patrick RL. Observations on thirteen cases of *Pneumocystis carinii* pneumonia. Am J Clin Pathol 38:401, 1962.

342. Marshall WC, Weston HJ, Bodian M. *Pneumocystis carinii* pneumonia and congenital hypogammaglobulinemia. Arch Dis Child 39:18, 1964.

343. Rodgers TS, Haggie MHK. *Pneumocystis carinii* pneumonia associated with hypogammaglobulinemia responding to pentamidine. Letter to the editor. Lancet 1:1042, 1964.

344. Allibone EC, Goldie W, Marmion BP. *Pneumocystis carinii* pneumonia and progressive vaccinia in siblings. Arch Dis Child 39:26, 1964.

345. Patterson JH, Lindsey IL, Edwards ES, et al. *Pneumocystis carinii* pneumonia and altered host resistance: treatment of one patient with pentamidine isethionate. Pediatrics 38:388, 1966.

346. Roberts FB, Nielsen HS. *Pneumocystis carinii* pneumonia: an unsuccessfully treated case. Can Med Assoc J 94:1235, 1966.

347. DiGeorge AM. Congenital absence of the thymus and its immunologic consequences: occurrence with congenital hypoparathyroidism. *In* Good RA, Bergsma D (eds). Immunologic Deficiency Diseases in Man. Birth Defects, Original Article Series. New York, National Foundation Press, 1968.

348. Rifkind D, Starzl TE, Marchioro TL, et al. Transplantation pneumonia. JAMA 189:808, 1964.

349. Fulginiti VA, Scribner R, Groth CG, et al. Infections in recipients of liver homografts. N Engl J Med 279:619, 1968.

350. LeClair RA. Transplantation pneumonia, associated with *Pneumocystis carinii*, among recipients of cardiac transplants. Am Rev Respir Dis 100:874, 1969.

351. Quittell LM, Fisher M, Foley CM. *Pneumocystis carinii* pneumonia in infants given adrenocorticotropic hormone for infantile spasms. J Pediatr 110:901, 1987.

352. Herrod HG, Valenski WR, Woods DR, et al. The in vitro response of human lymphocytes to *Pneumocystis carinii*. Clin Res 27:811, 1979.

353. Herrod HG, Valenski WR, Woods DR, et al. The in vitro response of human lymphocytes to *Pneumocystis carinii* antigen. J Immunol 126:59, 1981.

354. Ruskin J, Remington JS. *Pneumocystis carinii* infection in the immunosuppressed host. Antimicrob Agents Chemother 7:70, 1967.

355. Ivady G, Paldy L, Koltay M, et al. *Pneumocystis carinii* pneumonia. Letter to the editor. Lancet 1:616, 1967.

356. Kohout E, Post C, Azadeh B, et al. Immunoglobulin levels in infantile pneumocystosis. J Clin Pathol 25:135, 1972.

357. Brzosko WJ, Nowoslawski A, Madalinski K. Identification of immune complexes in lungs from *Pneumocystis carinii* pneumonia cases in infants. Bull Acad Pol Sci 12:137, 1964.

358. Brzosko WJ, Madalinski K, Krawczynski K, et al. Immunohistochemistry in studies on the pathogenesis of *Pneumocystis* pneumonia in infants. Ann NY Acad Sci 177:156, 1971.

359. Creamer B, Dutz W, Post C. The small intestinal lesion of chronic diarrhea and marasmus in Iran. Lancet 1:18, 1970.

360. Dutz W, Sadri S, Kohout E, et al. Bowel mucosal patterns and immunoglobulins in 100 infants from birth to one year of age. Pahlavi Med J 1:234, 1970.

361. Brzosko WJ, Nowoslawski A. Immunohistochemical studies on *Pneumocystis* pneumonia. Bull Acad Pol Sci 11:563, 1963.

362. Sheldon WH. Subclinical *Pneumocystis* pneumonitis. Am J Dis Child 97:287, 1959.

363. Charles MA, Schwarz MI. *Pneumocystis carinii* pneumonia. Postgrad Med 53:86, 1973.

364. Weiss RB, Muggia FM. Cytotoxic drug-induced pulmonary disease: update 1980. Am J Med 68:259, 1980.

365. Richards MJS, Wara WM. Radiation pneumonitis complicated by *Pneumocystis carinii*. Int J Radiat Oncol Biol Phys 4:287, 1978.

366. Wells RJ, Weetman RM, Ballantine TVN, et al. Pulmonary leukemia in children presenting as diffuse interstitial pneumonia. J Pediatr 96:262, 1980.

367. Solberg CO, Meuwissen HJ, Needham RN, et al. Infectious complications in bone marrow transplant patients. BMJ 1:18, 1971.

368. White WF, Saxton HM, Dawson IMP. Pneumocystis pneumonia: report of three cases in adults and one in a child with a discussion of the radiological appearances and predisposing factors. BMJ 2:1327, 1961.

369. Hughes WT. Infections during continuous complete remission of acute lymphocytic leukemia: during and after anticancer therapy. Int J Radiat Oncol Biol Phys 1:305, 1976.

370. Iacuone JJ, Wong KY, Bove KE, et al. Acute respiratory illness in children with acute lymphoblastic leukemia. J Pediatr 90:915, 1977.

371. Siegel SE, Nesbit ME, Baehner R, et al. Pneumonia during therapy for childhood acute lymphoblastic leukemia. Am J Dis Child 134:28, 1980.

372. Robillard G, Bertrand R, Gregoire H, et al. Plasma cell pneumonia in infants: review of 51 cases. J Can Assoc Radiol 16:161, 1965.

373. Hauger SB. Approach to the pediatric patient with HIV infection and pulmonary symptoms. J Pediatr 119(1):S25, 1991.

374. Vessal K, Post C, Dutz W, et al. Roentgenologic changes in infantile *Pneumocystis carinii* pneumonia. AJR Am J Roentgenol 120:254, 1974.

375. Vessal K, Dutz W, Kohout E, et al. Verlaufskontrolle der Pneumocystose im Röntgenbild. Radiologe 16:38, 1976.

376. Falkenbach KH, Bachmann KD, O'Laughlin BJ. *Pneumocystis carinii* pneumonia. AJR Am J Roentgenol 85:706, 1961.

377. Thomas SF, Dutz W, Khodadad EJ. *Pneumocystis carinii* pneumonia (plasma cell pneumonia): roentgenographic, pathologic and clinical correlations. AJR Am J Roentgenol 98:318, 1966.

378. Feinberg SB, Lester RG, Burke BA. The roentgen findings in *Pneumocystis carinii* pneumonia. Radiology 76:594, 1961.

379. Cohen WN, McAlister WH. *Pneumocystis carinii* pneumonia. AJR Am J Roentgenol 89:1032, 1963.

380. Capitanio MA, Kirkpatrick JA. *Pneumocystis carinii* pneumonia. AJR Am J Roentgenol 97:174, 1966.

381. Blank N, Castellino RA, Shah V. Radiographic aspects of pulmonary infection in patients with altered immunity. Radiol Clin North Am 11:175, 1973.

382. Bragg DG, Janis B. The roentgenographic manifestations of pulmonary opportunistic infections. AJR Am J Roentgenol 117:798, 1973.

383. Forrest JV. Radiographic findings in *Pneumocystis carinii* pneumonia. Radiology 103:539, 1972.

384. Doppman JL, Geelhoed GW, DeVita VT. Atypical radiographic features in *Pneumocystis carinii* pneumonia. Radiology 114:39, 1975.

385. Cross AS, Steigbigel RT. *Pneumocystis carinii* pneumonia presenting as localized nodular densities. N Engl J Med 291:831, 1974.

386. Rodriguez-Several RJ, Altieri PI, Castillo M. Unusual roentgenographic manifestation of *Pneumocystis carinii* pneumonia. Chest 69:422, 1976.

387. Byrd RB, Horn BR. Infection due to *Pneumocystis carinii* simulating lobar bacterial pneumonia. Chest 70:91, 1976.

388. Luddy RE, Champion LAA, Schwartz AD. *Pneumocystis carinii* pneumonia with pneumatocoele formation. Am J Dis Child 131:470, 1977.

389. Seigel R, Wolson AH. The radiographic manifestations of chronic *Pneumocystis carinii* pneumonia. AJR Am J Roentgenol 128:150, 1977.

390. Yamamoto A. A study of *Pneumocystis carinii* pneumonia. Jpn J Clin Radiol 24:259, 1979.

391. Friedman BA, Wenglin BD, Hyland RN, et al. Roentgenographically atypical *Pneumocystis carinii* pneumonia. Am Rev Respir Dis 111:89, 1975.

392. Sirotzky L, Memoli V, Roberts JL, et al. Recurrent *Pneumocystis* pneumonia with normal chest roentgenograms. JAMA 240:1513, 1978.

393. Levenson SM, Warren RD, Richman SD, et al. Abnormal pulmonary gallium accumulation in *P. carinii* pneumonia. Radiology 119:395, 1976.

394. Turbiner EH, Yeh SDJ, Rosen PP, et al. Abnormal gallium scintigraphy in *Pneumocystis carinii* pneumonia with a normal chest radiograph. Radiology 127:437, 1978.

395. Barta K, Dvoracek C, Kadlec A. Komplement-Bindungs-Reaktion bei Pneumocysten-pneumonien. Schweiz Z Allg Pathol Bakteriol 18:22, 1955.

396. Kantor GL, Goldberg LS, Johnson LB, et al. Immunologic abnormalities induced by postperfusion cytomegalovirus infection. Ann Intern Med 73:553, 1970.

397. Kerpel-Fronius E, Varga F, Bata G. Blood gas and metabolic studies in plasma cell pneumonia and in newborn prematures with respiratory distress. Arch Dis Child 39:473, 1964.

398. Smith E, Gaspar IA. Pentamidine treatment of *Pneumocystis carinii* pneumonitis in an adult with lymphatic leukemia. Am J Med 44:626, 1968.

399. Doak PB, Becroft DMO, Harris EA, et al. *Pneumocystis carinii* pneumonia—transplant lung. Q J Med 165:59, 1973.

400. Hughes WT, Sanyal SK, Price RA. Signs, symptoms, and pathophysiology of *Pneumocystis carinii* pneumonitis. Natl Cancer Inst Monogr 43:77, 1976.

401. Gentry LO, Ruskin J, Remington JS. *Pneumocystis carinii* pneumonia: problems in diagnosis and therapy in 24 cases. Calif Med 116:6, 1972.

402. Symmers WSC. Generalized cytomegalic inclusion-body disease associated with *Pneumocystis* pneumonia in adults. J Clin Pathol 13:1, 1960.

403. Theologides A, Lee JC. Concomitant opportunistic infection with *Toxoplasma*, *Pneumocystis* and cytomegalovirus. Minn Med 53:615, 1970.

404. Glaser JH, Schuval S, Burstein O, Bye MR. Cytomegalovirus and *Pneumocystis carinii* pneumonia in children with acquired immunodeficiency syndrome. J Pediatr 120(6):929, 1991.

405. Pliess G, Seifert K. Elektronenoptische Untersuchung bei experimenteller Pneumocystose. Beitr Pathol Anat 120:399, 1959.

406. Rubenstein A, Morecki R, Silverman B, et al. Pulmonary disease in children with acquired immunodeficiency syndrome and AIDS-related complex. J Pediatr 108:498, 1986.

407. Joshi VV, Oleske JM, Saad S, et al. Pathology of opportunistic infections in children with acquired immunodeficiency syndrome. Pediatr Pathol 6:145, 1986.

408. Case records of the Massachusetts General Hospital (case 15–1973). N Engl J Med 288:780, 1973.
409. Chan H, Pifer L, Hughes WT, et al. Comparison of gastric contents to pulmonary aspirates for the cytologic diagnosis of *Pneumocystis carinii* pneumonia. J Pediatr 90:243, 1977.
410. Yoshida Y, Ikai T, Ogino K, et al. Studies of *Pneumocystis carinii* and *Pneumocystis carinii* pneumonia: V. Diagnosis by cyst concentration from sputum. Jpn J Parasitol 27:473, 1978.
411. Ognibene FP, Gill VJ, Pizzo PA, et al. Induced sputum to diagnose *Pneumocystis carinii* pneumonia in immunosuppressed pediatric patients. J Pediatr 115(3):430, 1989.
412. Johnson HD, Johnson WW. *Pneumocystis carinii* pneumonia in children with cancer: diagnosis and treatment JAMA 214:1067, 1970.
413. Chaudhary S, Hughes WT, Feldman S, et al. Percutaneous transthoracic needle aspiration of the lung: diagnosing *Pneumocystis carinii* pneumonitis. Am J Dis Child 131:902, 1977.
414. Clink HM, Howard PF, Jameson B, et al. *Pneumocystis carinii* pneumonitis. Letter to the editor. Lancet 2:1265, 1975.
415. Rosen PP, Martini N, Armstrong D. *Pneumocystis carinii* pneumonia: diagnosis by lung biopsy. Am J Med 58:794, 1975.
416. Tyras DH, Campbell W, Corley C, et al. The role of early open lung biopsy in the diagnosis and treatment of *Pneumocystis carinii* pneumonia. Ann Thorac Surg 18:571, 1974.
417. Michaelis LL, Leight GS Jr, Powell RD, et al. *Pneumocystis* pneumonia: the importance of early open lung biopsy. Ann Surg 183:301, 1976.
418. Bradshaw M, Myerowitz RL, Schneerson R, et al. *Pneumocystis carinii* pneumonitis. Ann Intern Med 73:775, 1970.
419. Roback SA, Weintraub WH, Nesbit M, et al. Diagnostic open lung biopsy in the critically ill child. Pediatrics 52:605, 1973.
420. Wolff LJ, Bartlett MS, Baehner RL, et al. The causes of interstitial pneumonitis in immunocompromised children: an aggressive systematic approach to diagnosis. Pediatrics 60:41, 1977.
421. Ballantine TVN, Grosfeld JL, Knapek RM, et al. Interstitial pneumonitis in the immunologically suppressed child: an urgent surgical condition. J Pediatr Surg 12:501, 1977.
422. Mason WH, Siegel SE, Tucker BL. Diagnostic open lung biopsy in immunosuppressed pediatric patients. Clin Res 27:114, 1979.
423. Leight GS Jr, Michaelis LL. Open lung biopsy for the diagnosis of acute, diffuse pulmonary infiltrates in the immunosuppressed patient. Chest 73:477, 1978.
424. Rossiter SJ, Miller DC, Churg AM, et al. Open lung biopsy in the immunosuppressed patient: is it really beneficial? J Thorac Cardiovasc Surg 77:338, 1979.
425. Rodgers BM, Moazam F, Talbert JL. Thoracoscopy: early diagnosis of interstitial pneumonitis in the immunologically suppressed child. Chest 75:126, 1979.
426. Jacobs JB, Vogel C, Powell RD, et al. Needle biopsy in *Pneumocystis carinii* pneumonia. Radiology 93:525, 1969.
427. Lillehei JP, Funke JL, Drage CW, et al. *Pneumocystis carinii* pneumonia: needle-biopsy diagnosis and successful treatment. JAMA 206:596, 1968.
428. DeVita VT, Emmer M, Levine A, et al. *Pneumocystis carinii* pneumonia: successful diagnosis and treatment of two patients with associated malignant processes. N Engl J Med 280:287, 1969.
429. Cohen ML, Weiss EB. *Pneumocystis carinii* pneumonia: percutaneous lung biopsy and review of literature. Chest 60:195, 1971.
430. Repsher LH, Schroter G, Hammond WS. Diagnosis of *Pneumocystis carinii* pneumonitis by means of endobronchial brush biopsy. N Engl J Med 287:340, 1972.
431. Hodgkin JE, Andersen HA, Rosenow EC. Diagnosis of *Pneumocystis carinii* pneumonia by transbronchoscopic lung biopsy. Chest 64:551, 1973.
432. Scheinhorn DJ, Joyner LR, Whitcomb ME. Transbronchial forceps lung biopsy through the fiberoptic bronchoscope in *Pneumocystis carinii* pneumonia. Chest 66:294, 1974.
433. Feldman NT, Pennington JE, Ehrie MG. Transbronchial lung biopsy in the compromised host. JAMA 238:1377, 1977.
434. Chopra SK, Mohsenifar Z. Fiberoptic bronchoscopy in diagnosis of opportunistic lung infections: assessment of sputa, washings, brushings and biopsy specimens. West J Med 131:4, 1979.
435. Andersen HA. A safe procedure for diagnosis of *Pneumocystis carinii* pneumonia. Chest 66:222, 1974.
436. Toledo-Pereyra LH, DeMeester TR, Kinealey A, et al. The benefits of open lung biopsy in patients with previous nondiagnostic transbronchial lung biopsy: a guide to appropriate therapy. Chest 77:647, 1980.
437. Kim HK, Hughes WT. Comparison of methods for identification of *Pneumocystis carinii* in pulmonary aspirates. Am J Clin Pathol 60:462, 1973.
438. Rosen PP. Frozen section management of a lung biopsy for suspected *Pneumocystis carinii* pneumonia. Am J Surg Pathol 1:79, 1977.
439. Young RC, Bennett JE, Chu EW. Organisms mimicking *Pneumocystis carinii*. Letter to the editor. Lancet 2:1082, 1976.
440. Reinhardt DJ, Kaplan W, Chandler FW. Morphologic resemblance of zygomycete spores to *Pneumocystis carinii* cysts in tissue. Am Rev Respir Dis 115:170, 1977.
441. Demicco WA, Stein A, Urbanetti, JS, et al. False-negative biopsy in *Pneumocystis carinii* pneumonia. Chest 75:389, 1979.
442. Smith JW, Hughes WT. A rapid staining technique for *Pneumocystis carinii*. J Clin Pathol 25:269, 1972.
443. Churukian CJ, Schenk EA. Rapid Grocott's methenamine–silver nitrate method for fungi and *Pneumocystis carinii*. Am J Clin Pathol 68:427, 1977.
444. Mahan CT, Sale GE. Rapid methenamine-silver stain for *Pneumocystis* and fungi. Arch Pathol Lab Med 102:351, 1978.
445. Pintozzi RL. Modified Grocott's methenamine–silver nitrate method for quick staining of *Pneumocystis carinii*. J Clin Pathol 31:803, 1978.
446. Pifer LL, Woods DR. Efficacy of toluidine blue "O" stain for *Pneumocystis carinii*. Am J Clin Pathol 69:472, 1978.
447. Settnes OP, Larsen PE. Inhibition of toluidine blue O stain for *Pneumocystis carinii* by additives in the diethyl ether. Am J Clin Pathol 72:493, 1979.
448. Pintozzi RL, Blecka LJ, Nanos S. The morphologic identification of *Pneumocystis carinii*. Acta Cytol 23:35, 1979.
449. Cameron RB, Watts JC, Kasten BL. *Pneumocystis carinii* pneumonia: an approach to rapid laboratory diagnosis. Am J Clin Pathol 72:90, 1979.
450. Milder JE, Walzer PD, Coonrod JD, et al. Comparison of histological and immunological techniques for detection of *Pneumocystis carinii* in rat bronchial lavage fluid. J Clin Microbiol 11:409, 1980.
451. Drew WL, Finley TN, Mintz L, et al. Diagnosis of

Pneumocystis carinii pneumonia by bronchopulmonary lavage. JAMA 230:713, 1974.

452. Kelly J, Landis JN, Davis GS, et al. Diagnosis of pneumonia due to *Pneumocystis* by subsegmental pulmonary lavage via the fiberoptic bronchoscope. Chest 74:24, 1978.

453. Gosey LL, Howard RM, Witebsky FG, et al. Advantages of modified toluidine blue O stain and bronchoalveolar lavage for the diagnosis of *Pneumocystis carinii* pneumonia. J Clin Microbiol 22:803, 1985.

454. Leigh MW, Henshaw NG, Wood RE. Diagnosis of *Pneumocystis carinii* pneumonia in pediatric patients using bronchoscopic bronchoalveolar lavage. Pediatr Infect Dis 4:408, 1985.

455. Prober CG, Whyte H, Smith CR. Open lung biopsy in immunocompromised children with pulmonary infiltrates. Am J Dis Child 138:60, 1984.

456. Frankel LR, Smith DW, Lewiston NJ. Bronchoalveolar lavage for diagnosis of pneumonia in the immunocompromised child. Pediatrics 115(3):430, 1989.

457. Birriel JA, Adams JA, Saldana MA, et al. Role of flexible bronchoscopy and bronchoalveolar lavage in the diagnosis of pediatric acquired immunodeficiency syndrome–related pulmonary disease. Pediatrics 87:897, 1991.

458. Stokes DC, Shenep JL, Parham D, et al. Role of flexible bronchoscopy in the diagnosis of pulmonary infiltrates in pediatric patients with cancer. J Pediatr 115:561, 1989.

459. Vivell O. Ein neues stabiles Antigen für die Serodiagnose der interstitiellen plasmazellularen Pneumonie junger Säuglinge und Frühgeburten. Dtsch Med Wochenschr 80:1357, 1955.

460. Barta K. Complement fixation test for pneumocystosis (letter to the editor). Ann Intern Med 70:235, 1969.

461. Meuwissen JHET, Leeuwenberg ADEM. A microcomplement fixation test applied to infection with *Pneumocystis carinii*. Trop Geogr Med 24:282, 1972.

462. Post C, Fakoughi T, Dutz W, et al. Prophylaxis of epidemic infantile pneumocystosis with a 20:1 sulfadoxine and pyrimethamine combination. Curr Ther Res 13:273, 1971.

463. Nowoslawski A, Brzosko WJ. Indirect immunofluorescent test for serodiagnosis of *Pneumocystis carinii* infection. Bull Acad Pol Sci 12:143, 1964.

464. Brzosko W, Madalinski K, Nowoslawski A. Fluorescent antibody and immuno electrophoretic evaluation of the immune reaction in children with pneumonia induced by *Pneumocystis carinii*. Exp Med Microbiol 19:397, 1967.

465. Lau WK, Young LS. Immunofluorescent antibodies against *Pneumocystis carinii* in patients with and without pulmonary infiltrates. Clin Res 25:379, 1977.

466. Shepherd V, Jameson B, Knowles GK. *Pneumocystis carinii* pneumonitis: a serological study. J Clin Pathol 32:773, 1979.

467. Meuwissen JHET, Leeuwenberg ADEM, Heeren J, et al. New method for study of infections with *Pneumocystis carinii*. Letter to the editor. J Infect Dis 127:209, 1973.

468. Norman L, Kagan IG. A preliminary report of an indirect fluorescent antibody test for detecting antibodies to cysts of *Pneumocystis carinii* in human sera. Am J Clin Pathol 58:170, 1972.

469. Walzer PD, Rutledge ME, Yoneda K, et al. *Pneumocystis carinii*: new separation method from lung tissue. Exp Parasitol 47:356, 1979.

470. Minielly JA, McDuffie FC, Holley KE. Immunofluorescent identification of *Pneumocystis carinii*. Arch Pathol 90:561, 1970.

471. Lim SK, Jones RH, Eveland WC. Fluorescent antibody studies on experimental pneumocystosis. Proc Soc Exp Biol Med 136:675, 1971.

472. Lim SK, Eveland WC, Porter RJ. Development and evaluation of a direct fluorescent antibody method for the diagnosis of *Pneumocystis carinii* infections in experimental animals. Appl Microbiol 26:666, 1973.

473. Lim SK, Eveland WC, Porter RJ. Direct fluorescent antibody method for the diagnosis of *Pneumocystis carinii* pneumonitis from sputa or tracheal aspirates from humans. Appl Microbiol 27:144, 1974.

474. Meyers JD, Pifer LL, Sale GE, et al. The value of *Pneumocystis carinii* antibody and antigen detection for diagnosis of *Pneumocystis carinii* pneumonia after marrow transplantation. Am Rev Respir Dis 120:1283, 1979.

475. Williford Pifer LL, Wood DR, Edward CC, et al. *Pneumocystis carinii* serologic study in pediatric acquired immunodeficiency syndrome. Am J Dis Child 142:36, 1988.

476. Hughes WT, McNabb PC, Makres TD, et al. Efficacy of trimethoprim and sulfamethoxazole in the prevention and treatment of *Pneumocystis carinii* pneumonitis. Antimicrob Agents Chemother 5:289, 1974.

477. Hughes WT, Feldman S, Chaudhary SC, et al. Comparison of pentamidine isethionate and trimethoprim-sulfamethoxazole in the treatment of *Pneumocystis carinii* pneumonia. J Pediatr 92:285, 1978.

478. Lipson A, Marshall WC, Hayward AR. Treatment of *Pneumocystis carinii* pneumonia in children. Arch Dis Child 52:314, 1977.

479. Larter WE, John TJ, Sieber OF, et al. Trimethoprim-sulfamethoxazole treatment of *Pneumocystis carinii* pneumonitis. J Pediatr 92:826, 1978.

480. Lau WK, Young LS. Trimethoprim-sulfamethoxazole treatment of *Pneumocystis carinii* pneumonia in adults. N Engl J Med 295:716, 1976.

481. Yoshida Y, Ikai T, Takeuchi M, et al. Studies on *Pneumocystis carinii* and *Pneumocystis carinii* pneumonia: VII. Chemotherapy of 42 clnical cases. Jpn J Parasitol 6:455, 1979.

482. Seigel SE, Wolff LJ, Baehner RL, et al. Treatment of *Pneumocystis carinii* pneumonitis: a comparative trial of sulfamethoxazole-trimethoprim vs pentamidine in pediatric patients with cancer: report from the Children's Cancer Study Group. Am J Dis Child 138:1051, 1984.

483. Overturf GD. Use of trimethoprim-sulfamethoxazole in pediatric infections: relative merits of intravenous administration. Rev Infect Dis 9 (suppl 2):168, 1987.

484. Ivady G, Paldy L. Ein neues Behandlungsverfahren der interstitiellen plasmazelligen Pneumonie Frühgeborener mit fünfwertigen Stibium und aromatischen Diamidinen. Monatsschr Kinderheilkd 106:10, 1958.

485. Lörinczi K, Mérth J, Perényi K. Pentamidinnel szerzett tapasztalatink az interstitialis plasmasejtes pneumonia kezelésében. Gyermekgyogyaszat 15:207, 1964.

486. Western KA, Perera DR, Schultz MG. Pentamidine isethionate in the treatment of *Pneumocystis carinii* pneumonia. Ann Intern Med 73:695, 1970.

487. Parasitic Disease Drug Service—pentamidine releases for *Pneumocystis* pneumonia. MMWR Morb Mortal Wkly Rep 25:365, 1976.

488. Shultz JC, Ross SW, Abernathy RS. Diagnosis of *Pneumocystis carinii* pneumonia in an adult with survival. Am Rev Respir Dis 93:943, 1966.

489. Ivady G, Paldy L. Treatment of *Pneumocystis carinii* pneumonia in infancy. Natl Cancer Inst Monogr 43:201, 1976.

490. Schoenbach EB, Greenspan EM. The pharmacology, mode of action and therapeutic potentialities of stilbamidine, pentamidine, propamidine and other aromatic diamidines: a review. Medicine 27:327, 1948.

491. Stark FR, Crast F, Clemmer T, et al. Fatal Herxheimer

reaction after pentamidine in *Pneumocystis* pneumonia. Letter to the editor. Lancet 1:1193, 1976.

492. Stahl-Bayliss CM, Kalman CM, Laskin OL. Pentamidine-induced hypoglycemia in patients with the acquired immune deficiency syndrome. Clin Pharmacol Ther 39:271, 1986.

493. Pauwels A, Eliasewicz M, Larrey D, et al. Pentamidine-induced acute pancreatitis in a patient with AIDS. J Clin Gastroenterol 12(4):457, 1990.

494. Wood G, Wetzig N, Hogan P, Whitby M. Survival from pentamidine induced pancreatitis and diabetes mellitus. NZ J Med 21:341, 1991.

495. Miller TL, Winter HS, Luginbuhl LM, et al. Pancreatitis in pediatric human immunodeficiency virus infection. J Pediatr 120(2 pt. 1):223, 1992.

496. Emmer M, DeVita VT. *Pneumocystis carinii* pneumonia and pentamidine isethionate toxicity. Letter to the editor. Ann Intern Med 69:637, 1968.

497. DeVita VT, Emmer M. The successful treatment of *Pneumocystis carinii* pneumonitis in an adult with lymphosarcoma: a comment on pentamidine isethionate nephrotoxicity. Rev Fr Etud Clin Biol 14:55, 1969.

498. Western KA, Schultz MG. Pentamidine non-toxicity. Letter to the editor. Ann Intern Med 70:234, 1969.

499. Wang JJ, Freeman AI, Gaeta JF, et al. Unusual complications of pentamidine in the treatment of *Pneumocystis carinii* pneumonia. J Pediatr 77:311, 1970.

500. Waalkes TP, DeVita VT. The determination of pentamidine (4,4'-diamidinophenoxypentane) in plasma, urine and tissues. J Lab Clin Med 75:871, 1970.

501. Waalkes TP, Denham C, DeVita VT. Pentamidine: clinical pharmacologic correlations in man and mice. Clin Pharmacol Ther 11:505, 1970.

502. Young RC, DeVita VT. Treatment of *Pneumocystis carinii* pneumonia: current status of the regimens of pentamidine isethionate and pyrimethamine-sulfadiazine. Natl Cancer Inst Monogr 43:193, 1976.

503. Whisnant JK, Buckley RH. Successful pyrimethamine-sulfadiazine therapy of *Pneumocystis* pneumonia in infants with X-linked immunodeficiency with hyper-IgM. Natl Cancer Inst Monogr 43:211, 1976.

504. Amsden GW, Kowalsky ST, Morse GD. Trimetrexate for *Pneumocystis carinii* pneumonia in patients with AIDS. Ann Pharmacother 26:218, 1992.

505. Geelhoed GW, Levin BJ, Adkins PC, et al. The diagnosis and management of *Pneumocystis carinii* pneumonia. Ann Thorac Surg 14:335, 1972.

506. Geelhoed GW, Corso P, Joseph WL. The role of membrane lung support in transient acute respiratory insufficiency of *Pneumocystis carinii* pneumonia. J Thorac Cardiovasc Surg 68:802, 1974.

507. Sanyal SK, Avery TL, Hughes WT, et al. Management of severe respiratory insufficiency due to *Pneumocystis carinii* pneumonitis in immunosuppressed hosts: the role of continuous negative-pressure ventilation. Am Rev Respir Dis 116:223, 1977.

508. Saulsbury FT, Bernstein MT, Winkelstein JA. *Pneumocystis carinii* pneumonia as the presenting infection in congenital hypogammaglobulinemia. J Pediatr 95:559, 1979.

509. Pedersen FK, Johansen KS, Rosenkvist J, et al. Refractory *Pneumocystis carinii* infection in chronic granulomatous disease: successful treatment with granulocytes. Pediatrics 64:935, 1979.

510. Gagnon S, Boota AM, Fischi MA, et al. Corticosteroids as adjunctive therapy for severe *Pneumocystis carinii* pneumonia in the acquired immunodeficiency syndrome. N Engl J Med 323:1444, 1990.

511. Bozzette SA, Sattler FR, Chiu J, et al. A controlled trial of early adjunctive treatment with corticosteroids for *Pneumocystis carinii* pneumonia in the acquired immunodeficiency syndrome. N Engl J Med 323:1451, 1990.

512. NIH–University of California Expert Panel for Corticosteroids as Adjunctive Therapy for Pneumocystis Pneumonia. Special Report: Consensus statement on the use of corticosteroids as adjunctive therapy for pneumocystis pneumonia in the acquired immunodeficiency syndrome. N Engl J Med 323:1500, 1990.

513. McLaughlin GE, Virdcc SS, Schlcicn CL, et al. Effect of corticosteroids on survival of children with acquired immunodeficiency syndrome and *Pneumocystis carinii*–related respiratory failure. J Pediatr 126:821–824, 1995.

514. Bye MR, Cairns-Bazarian AM, Ewig JM. Markedly reduced mortality associated with corticosteroid therapy of *Pneumocystis carinii* pneumonia in children with acquired immunodeficiency syndrome. Arch Pediatr Adolesc Med 148:638–641, 1994.

515. Sanyal SK, Mariencheck WC, Hughes WT, et al. Course of pulmonary dysfunction in children surviving *Pneumocystis carinii* pneumonitis. Am Rev Respir Dis 124:161, 1981.

516. Kluge RM, Spaulding DM, Spain AJ. Combination of pentamidine and trimethoprim-sulfamethoxazole in the therapy of *Pneumocystis carinii* pneumonia in rats. Antimicrob Agents Chemother 13:975, 1978.

517. Ruskin J. Parasitic diseases in the immunocompromised host. *In* Rubin RH, Young LS (eds). Clinical Approach to Infection in the Compromised Host. New York, Plenum Publishing, 1981.

518. Patterson JH. *Pneumocystis carinii* pneumonia; pentamidine therapy. Letter to the editor. Pediatrics 38:926, 1966.

519. Richman DD, Zamvil L, Remington JS. Recurrent *Pneumocystis carinii* pneumonia in a child with hypogammaglobulinemia. Am J Dis Child 125:102, 1973.

520. Ross L, Ortega J, Fine R, et al. Recurrent *Pneumocystis carinii* pneumonia. Clin Res 25:183, 1977.

521. Hughes WT, Rivera GK, Schell MJ, et al. Successful intermittent chemoprophylaxis for *Pneumocystis carinii* pneumonitis. N Engl J Med 316:1627, 1987.

522. Pesanti EL. In vitro effects of antiprotozoan drugs and immune serum on *Pneumocystis carinii*. J Infect Dis 141:775, 1980.

523. Wolff LJ, Baehner RL. Delayed development of *Pneumocystis* pneumonia following administration of short-term high-dose trimethoprim-sulfamethoxazole. Am J Dis Child. 132:525, 1978.

524. Hughes WT. Limited effect of trimethoprim-sulfamethoxazole prophylaxis on *Pneumocystis carinii*. Antimicrob Agents Chemother 16:333, 1979.

525. Kemeny P, Adler T, Szokolai V, et al. Prevention of interstitial plasma-cell pneumonia in premature infants. Letter to the editor. Lancet 1:1322, 1973.

526. Hughes WT, Kim HK, Price RA, et al. Attempts at prophylaxis for murine *Pneumocystis carinii* pneumonitis. Curr Ther Res 15:581, 1973.

527. Western KA, Norman L, Kaufmann AF. Failure of pentamidine isethionate to provide chemoprophylaxis against *Pneumocystis carinii* infection in rats. J Infect Dis 131:273, 1975.

528. Hughes WT, Kuhn S, Chaudhary S, et al. Successful chemoprophylaxis for *Pneumocystis carinii* pneumonitis. N Engl J Med 297:1419, 1977.

529. Wilber RB, Feldman S, Malone WJ, et al. Chemoprophylaxis for *Pneumocystis carinii* pneumonitis: outcome of unstructured delivery. Am J Dis Child 134:643, 1980.

530. Harris RE, McCallister JA, Allen SA, et al. Prevention of *Pneumocystis* pneumonia: use of continuous sulfamethoxazole-trimethoprim therapy. Am J Dis Child 134:35, 1980.

531. Hughes WT. *Pneumocystis* pneumonia: a plague of the immunosuppressed. Johns Hopkins Med J 143:184, 1978.

532. U.S. Department of Health and Human Services. Guidelines for prophylaxis against *Pneumocystis carinii* pneumonia for children infected with human immunodeficiency virus. MMWR Morb Mortal Wkly Rep 40(RR-2):ii–13, 1991.

533. Centers for Disease Control and Prevention. 1995 Revised guidelines for prophylaxis against *Pneumocystis carinii* pneumonia for children infected with or perinatally exposed to human immunodeficiency virus. MMWR Morb Mortal Wkly Rep 44 (RR-4):1–11, 1995.

534. Simonds RJ, Lindegren ML, Thomas P, et al. Prophylaxis against *Pneumocystis carinii* pneumonia among children with perinatally acquired HIV infection in the United States. N Engl J Med 332:786–790, 1995.

535. Maldonado YA, Araneta RG, Hersh AL. *Pneumocystis carinii* pneumonia prophylaxis and early clinical manifestations of severe perinatal human immunodeficiency virus type 1 infection. Northern California Pediatric IIIV Consortium. Pediatr Infect Dise J 17:398–402, 1998.

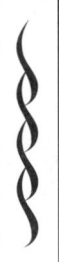

C H A P T E R   2 0

Hepatitis

CLYDE S. CRUMPACKER, M.D.

A remarkable explosion of knowledge about the viruses that cause hepatitis has occurred in the past 35 years. Five agents that cause clinical hepatitis have been identified: hepatitis A virus (HAV); hepatitis B virus (HBV); hepatitis D virus (HDV, or the "delta agent"); hepatitis C virus (HCV; post-transfusion and sporadic non-A, non-B hepatitis virus [NANB]); and hepatitis E virus (HEV; epidemic non-A, non-B virus [Et-NANB]). Since the discovery by Blumberg and co-workers in 1963 of the antigen ultimately associated with hepatitis B virus,[1, 2] HBV has been isolated, cloned, and sequenced and major inroads have been accomplished into the cell biology, immunology, and pathogenesis of the illness. Similarly, the epidemiology, serology, pathophysiology, and molecular structure of HAV and HDV have been determined. Both parenterally transmitted virus (HCV) and water-borne non-A, non-B hepatitis virus (HEV) have been isolated. An explosion of knowledge about the biology and clinical aspects of these agents is occurring. In this chapter, the initial focus is on the nature of the viruses that cause the clinical syndrome of viral hepatitis. It is virtually impossible to clinically distinguish an infection due to any one of these hepatitis agents from another. Diagnosis is, therefore, dependent on use of serologic tests and nucleic acid–based assays. Aspects related to the pathophysiology, transmission, clinical findings, diagnosis, prevention, and treatment are discussed.

THE VIRUSES

Hepatitis A

The virus was first identified in the stool of a patient with the acute phase of hepatitis A.[3] Subsequently, all sera from patients with hepatitis A were demonstrated to agglutinate the 27-nm particle observed in stools. These antibodies were found to develop in patients inoculated with the Krugman MS-1 strain.[4, 5]

HAV has properties of an enterovirus. Although the size (27 nm in diameter), density (1.32 to 1.4 g/ml in cesium chloride), and structure (genetic organization, no lipid membrane) are similar to other enteroviruses, HAV does not share any cross-reactive antigens, nucleic acid, or protein sequences with the other enteroviruses.[6–9] The RNA is 7478 nucleotides long and has been completely sequenced. Sequence variations have been observed between different isolates and attenuated strains of virus, but they have been much less diverse than those found in HBV.[8] The coat protein has only one antigenic class that is recognized by the anti-HAV antibody. Like other picornaviruses, the nucleic acid consists of a single-stranded RNA molecule that is polyadenylated and codes for a polyprotein that is subsequently cleaved into the component peptides that constitute the virus. HAV is also more stable than other picornaviruses.

The virus is stable to diethyl ether and to low pH,

indicating that it does not contain a lipid envelope. Complement-fixing antibody to the virus develops readily.[5] Heat (100°C for 5 minutes) completely destroys infectivity, but heating of the virus at 60°C for 1 hour reduces the infectivity only partially. Ultraviolet irradiation completely inactivates the virus, and treatment with formalin (1:400 dilution) for 3 days at 37°C inactivates the virus. The virus is infectious for marmosets, and the usual quantity of the virus found in patients is 10^4 to 10^6 50% infectious doses for marmosets per milliliter of stool from acutely infected patients. By electron microscopy, the virus has been seen in the cytoplasm of livers of infected marmosets. HAV has been cultured in a variety of human and nonhuman primate cells in vitro.[8] This has allowed the purification of viral antigens and the development of attenuated strains for vaccination. The virus can be neutralized by sera from patients recovering from HAV infection. Immune electron microscopy shows characteristic halos of antibody molecules around each virus particle; this pattern results in immune complexes of the virus and antibody (Fig. 20–1).

Hepatitis A is diagnosed in the laboratory by demonstration of hepatitis virus antigen (HA Ag) in the feces or by measurement of serum antibodies to HAV (anti-HAV). The presence of HA Ag in the feces establishes that an acute infection is in progress, but its absence does not exclude infection. The HAV can be detected in the liver, bile, blood, and stool earlier than 2 weeks after exposure. The average incubation period from ex-

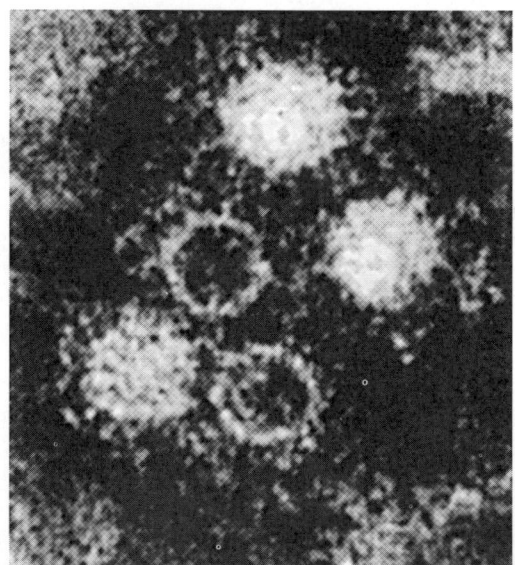

FIGURE 20–1 HAV particles. Electron micrograph of stool specimen of patient with hepatitis A. The stool specimen was incubated with convalescent serum from a patient with hepatitis A, and antibody produced clumping of the 27-nm particles. Two of the particles are empty, devoid of nucleic acid. This illustration demonstrates the technique of immune electron microscopy. (Reprinted with permission from Feinstone SM, Kapikian AZ, Purcell RH. Hepatitis A: detection by immune electron microscopy of a viruslike antigen associated with acute illness. Science 182:1026. Copyright 1973 by the American Association for the Advancement of Science.)

posure to onset of symptoms is 4 weeks. Once hepatitis develops, viremia, fecal shedding of the virus, and infectivity rapidly diminish. For example, HA Ag can be demonstrated in only 50% of patients in the first week of disease, in 25% in the second week, only rarely in the third week, and almost never in the fourth week of illness. Hepatitis A is spread by fecal-oral contamination. Even though HAV infection is self-limited, the prevalence of the disease is perpetuated by the physical stability of the virus and the reservoir of asymptomatic nonepidemic cases. Most infections are anicteric. Mild hepatitis is most often diagnosed. Despite the small percentage of icteric cases that result in fulminant hepatitis, the high prevalence of HAV infection worldwide results in hepatitis A being the most common cause of fulminant hepatitis in the world. Hepatitis A has been associated with both a prolonged "cholestatic" hepatitis and an immune complex disease.

Antibodies to HAV rise rapidly early in the acute phase and are always present at the onset of clinical disease. It may be difficult to detect a fourfold rise in antibody titer because the first serum often already shows a high titer of anti-HAV. A better diagnostic marker, therefore, is the determination of anti-HAV of the IgM class (anti-HAV IgM), an antibody that is always present at the first sign of disease and persists for several months to a year at most. Anti-HAV IgM can be measured by radioimmunoassay or enzyme-linked immunosorbent assay.[9]

A study of maternal-infant transmission of acute icteric hepatitis during pregnancy included six women with acute hepatitis A as diagnosed by the appearance of anti-HAV during convalescence. These six pregnant women were all icteric on admission to the hospital for delivery and had markedly increased serum alanine aminotransferase (ALT) levels. One had the onset of illness early in the second trimester, and five had hepatitis in the third trimester. Five patients had complete clinical and biochemical recovery. One patient, however, presented with acute hepatitis during the seventh month of pregnancy, was delivered of a premature infant, and died of fulminant hepatic failure 2 months later. None of the infants born to mothers with acute hepatitis A during pregnancy developed clinical or laboratory signs of hepatitis. The investigators concluded that transmission of HAV to infants does not occur, even when the mother has the onset of acute hepatitis at delivery.[10]

In two studies on the effects of hepatitis A and B in pregnancy in South Africa, the researchers concluded that hepatitis A during pregnancy offered no risk for the mother or the fetus.[11] In a study of 50 pregnancies complicated by acute viral hepatitis, Hieber and coworkers found acute hepatitis B in 20 (40%) and the rest were described as non-B hepatitis.[12] The course of the pregnancy was not affected by the hepatitis, and there was no difference between hepatitis B infection and non-hepatitis B infection on the incidence of congenital malformations, stillbirths, spontaneous abortion, or small-for-gestational-age neonates. The incidence of prematurity was increased in both groups, with 31.6% of infants born to mothers with hepatitis B during pregnancy being born prematurely and 25% of infants born to mothers with non–hepatitis B being premature. Similarly, in Shanghai, China, 34 anti-A HAV IgM-positive mothers did not transmit HAV to their neonates and no obvious birth defects were observed.[13] In one well-investigated outbreak of HAV infection in a newborn nursery, an acutely infected mother was implicated as the source of the infection.[14] She spread the infection to her neonate either during birth or while breast-feeding. In another outbreak of HAV in a neonatal intensive care unit due to blood transfusion, the premature infants were noted to have prolonged excretion of HAV.[15] This is not unexpected, since the competence of the immune system is essential for mediating viral clearance. In summary, the transmission of hepatitis A to infants from pregnant mothers with acute hepatitis does not appear to constitute a significant problem. Newborns may be at risk of infection, however, if acute hepatitis occurs less than 2 weeks before termination of pregnancy. Under these circumstances it has been suggested that a single intramuscular injection of immune serum globulin (ISG), 0.5 ml, be given shortly after birth. Measures designed to prevent fecal-oral contamination prevent the spread of HAV infection in nurseries. These include hand washing, use of disposable utensils and dishes, boiling and chlorine treatment of gowns and linens, and use of gowns and gloves when handling contaminated items. ISG contains a high enough titer of anti-HAV antibody to passively immunize an exposed individual.

Hepatitis B

The hepatitis associated with the HBV has been known by several terms. The terms *hepatitis-associated antigen* and *Australia antigen* refer to an antigen on the surface of the HBV that is now known as the hepatitis B surface antigen (HBsAg). The other terms are no longer used, and in this chapter HBsAg will be used to designate the surface antigen of the HBV. HBV is one of a family of viruses called hepadnavirus (*hepa*—liver, *dna*—DNA). Viruses with genetic organization and morphologic structure similar to those of HBV have been identified in the Eastern woodchuck (woodchuck hepatitis B virus, WHBV),[16] bushy ground squirrels[17] and flying squirrels (ground squirrel hepatitis virus, GSHV), ducks[18] and geese (duck hepatitis virus, DHBV), and herons (heron hepatitis virus). The WHBV can infect squirrels, and the GSHV can infect woodchucks, but other members of the hepadnavirus family cannot infect other species. The host range of HBV is limited to humans, gorillas, and chimpanzees.

The serum of patients with acute hepatitis B contains three morphologically distinct forms of virus or viral antigen (Fig. 20–2). These forms are distinct particles that can be readily aggregated by reaction with serum containing specific antibody against the HBsAg (anti-HBs). After aggregation, the particles are readily visualized by the technique of immune electron microscopy. The first particle to be described and the most common form in the serum is a spherical 22-nm particle composed of multiple subunits.[5] In addition, long microfilaments with the same 22-nm diameter as the spherical particles can be seen scattered throughout an electron

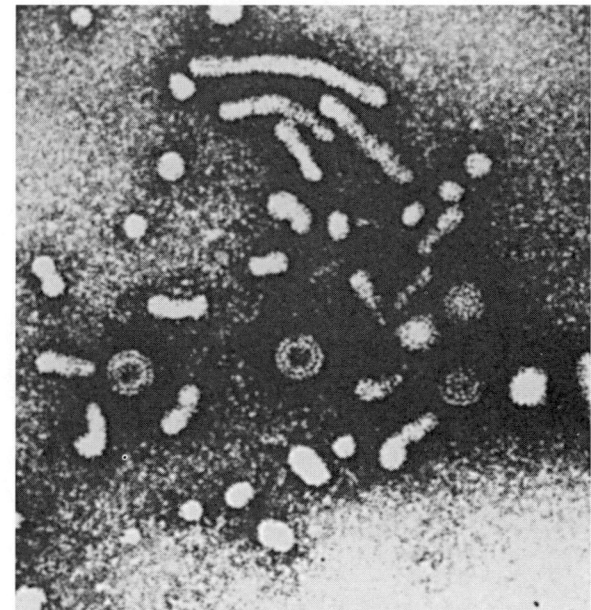

FIGURE 20–2 HBV particles. Electron micrograph of acute serum of patient with type B hepatitis. Three distinct particles are present. The long filamentous structures represent aggregates of HBsAg, the 20-nm spherical structures represent free HBsAg, and the 47-nm multilayered spheres with a dense core are the infectious Dane particles representing the complete virus. This electron micrograph was obtained after the reaction of serum containing anti-HBs, which produced clumping of viral particles. (Courtesy of Dr. June Almeida.)

microscopic field. The third particle to be described by Dane and co-workers is a large spherical particle, 42 nm in diameter, with an outer shell and a dense inner core.[19] The Dane particles have now been shown to be the complete infectious virus. The inner core of the virus contains a DNA polymerase enzyme[10] and an immunologically distinct antigen designated the hepatitis B core antigen (HBcAg).[12]

The virus particle contains a partially double-stranded DNA molecule. The long ("l") strand is approximately 3200 nucleotides long (molecular weight, 1.6 million), whereas the short ("s") strand is of variable length (Fig. 20–3).[20] The DNA genome codes for four families of polypeptides (open reading frames): the pre-S/S region, the pre-C/C/e antigen region, the P gene, and the X gene. The pre-S/S region codes for three polypeptides that exist as both glycosylated and nonglycosylated forms: the large S (pre-S1) protein, the middle S (pre-S2) protein, and the small or major S protein.[21, 22] The microfilamentous and 22-nm forms of HBsAg are mostly composed of the major S protein, with a minor component being the middle S protein. About 90% of the surface protein on the Dane particle is major S, whereas the remaining 10% is equally divided between the large and middle S molecules. The pre-S sequences on the middle and large S proteins are more hydrophilic than the major S sequences. Most likely, they are involved with receptor-mediated uptake of the virus.[23] The pre-S region binds glutaraldehyde-polymerized human serum

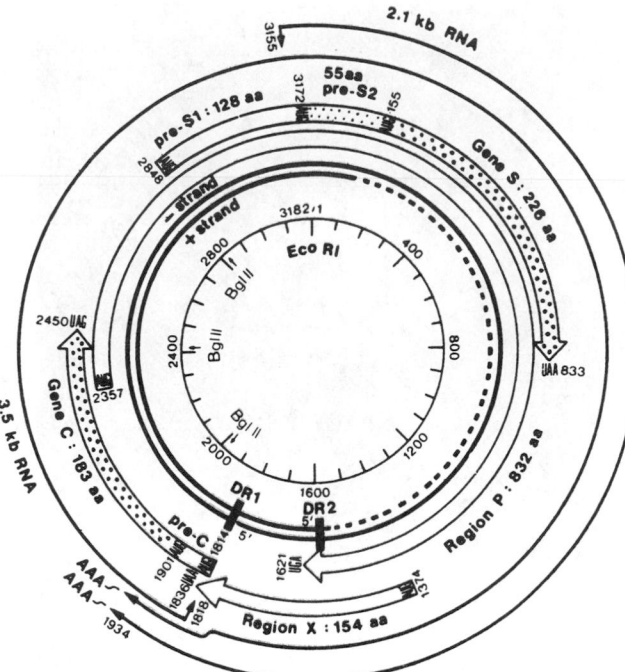

FIGURE 20–3 Structure, genomic organization, transcription, and translation products of HBV. The restriction map of HBV DNA is shown in the center, and outlying it is the partially double-stranded structure of HBV DNA. The 3182-nucleotide long (−) or "l" strand and the variable-length (+) or "s" strand are shown. Surrounding that are the four open-reading frames for the putative protein products and the two major RNA transcripts. (From Tiollais P, Pourcel C, Dejean A. The hepatitis B virus. Reprinted by permission from Nature, Vol. 317, pp. 489–495. Copyright © 1985 Macmillan Magazines Limited.)

albumin and denatured human albumin. Whether this affinity is fortuitous or may be related to receptor-mediated viral uptake has yet to be determined. The major S sequences are mostly hydrophobic and probably reside in the lipid bilayer that surrounds the core structure.

Possibly because of HBV's worldwide distribution, there is much diversity in its DNA sequences and the antigenicity of HBsAg. The nucleotide sequences of regions near the terminus of the l and s strands and the pre-S and pre-C regions are not as divergent as the rest of the DNA molecule.[24] Classically, three antigenic epitopes on HBsAg have been distinguished: the a, dy, and wr classifications.[25–27] The a antigen is common to HBsAg molecules derived from all strains of HBV and is the major neutralizing epitope. Because vaccination with HBsAg usually results in the development of antibodies to the a epitope, any form of HBsAg can be used to produce neutralizing antibodies. "Escape" mutants have been described that have an arginine for glycine substitution in amino acid 145 that results in the loss of the a epitope.[28] These mutants have been identified in children who were vaccinated with the HBsAg-containing HBV vaccine but who developed hepatitis B infection. Although other mutations have been identified, the most common is the amino acid 145 substitution. Currently, the prevalence of "escape" mutants is low, but the existence of these viral variants may necessitate a change in the composition of the current HBV vaccines. One vaccinated infant who was infected with an "escape" mutation during her first year was observed to be infected 5 years later. Usually HBsAg is exclusively w or r and d or y. Rarely, HBsAg can have the adyw serotype. With the development of monoclonal antibodies to HBsAg, more subtle differences in serotypes of HBsAg have become apparent.[29] Although the antigenic differences among viral isolates are of epidemiologic interest, the clinical outcome of HBV infection does not appear to be affected by any particular strain of virus except with one rare exception: papular acrodermatitis of children occurs more often with subtype ayw.[30, 31]

The inner core of the virus is composed of the core protein (HBcAg), the product of the c gene. The e antigen (HBeAg) is a polypeptide product of the c gene that is prematurely terminated.[24, 32] HBcAg exists in the serum free of the Dane particle. Both HBeAg and HBcAg share antigenic epitopes. Encapsulated in the core particle are a DNA polymerase,[1, 33] the partially double-stranded DNA, and a protein bound to the 5' end of the long strand of the viral DNA molecule.[24] The hepatitis B DNA polymerase also has reverse transcriptase activity, and hepatitis B can be inhibited by some reverse transcriptase inhibitors such as lamivudine. Both the DNA polymerase and the terminal protein on the 5' end of the l strand of HBV DNA are part of the viral-encoded DNA polymerase. The x gene is found in the cytoplasm of infected hepatocytes, and antibodies to the gene product can be detected in acute and chronically infected individuals.[24] The x gene protein may help to regulate c gene transcription. Because of the limited host range of the virus and the lack of in vitro infection models for HBV, not as much is known about how to inactivate the virus as with other viral agents. Although HBsAg antigenicity survives treatments of 10 hours' incubation at 60°C or 1 minute in boiling water,[34] infectivity is abolished. Similarly, viral infectivity is abolished by a combination of β-propiolactone and ultraviolet light treatments.[35]

In summary, the HBV contains four separate and distinct antigens: HBsAg, HBcAg, HBxAg, and HBeAg. The HBsAg is found on the surface of the hepatitis B virus. The HBcAg is detectable after removal of the lipid coat from the virus by detergents, is associated with the core of Dane particles, and is closely identified with the virus-associated DNA polymerase activity.

Serologic Testing for Hepatitis B Antigen and Antibody

The availability of reliable, reproducible methods for a variety of antigens and antibodies associated with HBV infection has played a major role in the rapid accumulation of knowledge on the epidemiology and clinical importance of HBV. Most of these tests are widely employed by community hospitals and blood banks. The clinical use of each test is briefly reviewed here.

HEPATITIS B SURFACE ANTIGEN (HBsAg)

The modern era in detecting viral-associated antigens was begun with Blumberg's detection of HBsAg.[1, 2] The concentration of this family of surface glycoproteins can be as high as 1 mg/ml, but usually it ranges from the picogram to microgram per milliliter concentration. HBsAg has been detected by the following assays: agar gel diffusion assay,[36, 37] counterimmunoelectrophoresis,[37] complement fixation assay, hemagglutination assay, hemagglutination-inhibition assay, reverse passive hemagglutination assay,[38] radioimmunoassay (RIA),[39–45] and enzyme-linked immunosorbent assay (EISA). Variations of the RIA and ELISA methods using polyclonal antisera and monoclonal antibodies are being employed. Most immunoassays have a limit of sensitivity in the tens of picogram per milliliter range. With the employment of ever more sensitive immunoassays for HBsAg, it may take a few months for sera to have undetectable concentrations of antigen even though viral protein synthesis has stopped. This is because the serum half-life of HBsAg is 1 to 2 weeks (longer in males than in females) and the concentration of HBsAg may be in the tens to hundreds of micrograms per milliliter range at the time viral protein synthesis ceases.

HBsAg is synthesized during viral replication and may also be synthesized from HBV DNA sequences integrated into the chromosomes of hepatocytes in the absence of viral production.[24] The small S and middle S (pre-S2, S) protein molecules are readily secreted from the liver cells, but large S (pre-S1, pre-S2, S) protein secretion is impaired (which may facilitate the incorporation of large S protein into the Dane particle).[46] Detection of serum HBsAg therefore correlates with HBV infection but does not elucidate the stage of the HBV-related disease or whether virus production is occurring. Approximately 90% of adults will be HBsAg positive using a conventional ELISA for HBsAg during the first 2 weeks of symptomatic acute viral hepatitis B; however, the prevalence of HBsAg-positive patients declines rapidly with time, and a positive reaction is much less even during the first 2 weeks in an asymptomatic infection.[47] Therefore, the absence of serum HBsAg does not exclude HBV infection because the antigen concentration may be below the sensitivity of the immunoassays.

Immunoassays for pre-S1 and pre-S2 epitopes are being clinically evaluated. Because the large and middle S proteins are mostly associated with the Dane particle, these assays may prove to be a direct measure of the potential infectivity of a given serum. Furthermore, the disappearance of pre-S sequences may be an early indication that the viral infection is resolving before the seroconversion from HBsAg positivity to negativity. This is especially relevant because of the long serum half-life of HBsAg and the rapid clearance of the virus. Until more studies are complete, these assays are available only in a research setting.

ANTIBODY TO HEPATITIS B CORE ANTIGEN (Anti-HBc)

Like HBsAg, anti-HBc is most commonly detected by RIA or ELISA. Furthermore, kits are now widely available that can determine whether the anti-HBc antibodies are predominantly of the IgM or IgG subtypes. As early as 4 weeks after exposure to HBV, infected persons may have circulating antibodies to the core antigen of the Dane particle. All symptomatic adults are anti-HBc positive 2 weeks after symptoms begin, and virtually all patients with asymptomatic HBV infections are anti-HBc positive at the time when other viral-associated antigens are detectable and the ALT rises. The anti-HBc response is initially of the IgM subclass, but with time the titer of IgM anti-HBc declines as the titer of IgG anti-A HBc rises. At 6 months the majority of patients' anti-HBc antibodies are IgG, although a minority may have detectable IgM anti-HBc for up to 2 years. The anti-HBc antibody titer slowly declines but remains detectable for many years after self-limited infection. The anti-HBc titer usually remains high during the course of chronic infection. This difference may be one way to distinguish a chronic carrier who is only anti-HBc positive from a patient who has resolved self-limited HBV infection and is no longer anti-HBs positive. The IgM anti-HBc may again become detectable during the reactivation of hepatitis that occurs during an HBeAg to anti-HBe seroconversion in chronic carriers.[47, 48]

The IgM anti-HBc assay is, therefore, helpful in diagnosing an HBV infection of recent origin or an HBeAg to anti-HBe seroconversion. The anti-HBc antibody may sometimes be the only marker that a patient had a previous HBV infection.

HEPATITIS B VIRUS e ANTIGEN (HBeAg) AND ANTIBODY (Anti-HBe)

Both HBeAg and anti-HBe are detectable by both RIA and ELISA. The HBeAg is usually detectable when a large quantity of viral replication is occurring. Later, a seroconversion from HBeAg to anti-HBe may presage the eventual clearance of virus during a self-limited infection or may be an isolated event during chronic HBV infection. The concentration of virus is usually higher in HBeAg-positive sera than HBeAg-negative, anti-HBe-negative sera, or anti-HBe-positive sera. The absence of HBeAg positivity, however, does not exclude the potential infectivity of HBsAg-positive sera.[49–62] For example, children born of HBsAg-positive, HBeAg-positive mothers have a 90% chance of acquiring an HBV infection by their first birthday if they are not vaccinated and have not received hepatitis B immune globulin (HBIG) at birth. Children born of HBsAg-positive, HBeAg-negative mothers have a lower incidence of HBV infection (approximately 20%). Similarly, health care providers who were stuck by needles contaminated with HBsAg-positive, HBeAg-positive blood have a 19% chance of contracting HBV infection. Those exposed to needles contaminated by HBsAg-positive, HBeAg-negative blood still have a 2.5% chance of infection.[63] The concentration of HBV DNA, a more direct measure of the presence of the virus, is usually higher in HBeAg-positive blood than HBeAg-negative and/or anti-HBe-positive blood.[57] Exceptions to this are mutant viral strains that contain nonsense mutations in the pre-C region.[49] These pre-core mutant HBV infections have been associated with both fulminant hepatitis B and very progressive HBeAg-negative chronic hepatitis.[52–62] In the

United States, most individuals who become HBeAg negative do not develop pre-core region nonsense mutations. At present, although the immunoassays for HBeAg and anti-HBe are readily available to the clinician, the clinical use of these assays is limited to helping to identify an HBeAg to anti-HBe seroconversion in a chronic HBV carrier. No other management decisions can be reliably based on these tests at this time. The decision of whether to perform immunoprophylaxis of a newborn of an HBsAg-positive mother with HBIG and HBV vaccine should not depend on her HBeAg/anti-HBe status.

ANTIBODY TO SURFACE ANTIGEN (Anti-HBs)

The widely available RIAs and ELISAs for anti-HBs most likely measure only the presence of antibodies directed against epitopes on the small S protein. Although immunoassays for antibodies to the pre-S epitopes are being used by research laboratories, currently their availability is limited and their use is unclear. In self-limited HBV infections, it is usually assumed that the patient is no longer infectious after the anti-HBs is detectable. With the development of more sensitive immunoassays for HBsAg and anti-HBs, patients with self-limited infection may be transiently HBsAg and anti-HBs positive.[64] Furthermore, in the woodchuck model of hepadnavirus infection, woodchucks who had a self-limited hepatitis who became anti-WHBs positive still had WHBV DNA detectable in their spleens.[65] Most patients with chronic HBV infections will never be anti-HBs positive. Conversely, less than 10% of chronic carriers have anti-HBs antibodies.[64] Whether the epitopes to which these antibodies are directed are identical to the anti-HBs antibodies in the patients with self-limited infection is still under study. Despite these reservations, anti-HBs positivity usually implies that the patient has had either an antibody response to the hepatitis B vaccine (see later) or has resolved an HBV infection. In the latter case, the person is usually also anti-HBc positive unless the infection was in the distant past.

OTHER TESTS FOR HEPATITIS B VIRUSES

HBV DNA Polymerase

The HBV DNA polymerase assay measures the ability of the core particle of the Dane particle to synthesize DNA using the partially double-stranded HBV DNA genome as a template.[66] The test is cumbersome, expensive, and less sensitive than the previously discussed immunoassays and the tests for HBV DNA to be described later. The test remains a direct measure of the presence of Dane particles and has use in assessing the responsiveness of HBV infections to antiviral agents.

HBV DNA

The HBV DNA test can be performed in three ways: (1) *hybridization assays* probe labeled nucleic acids to filters in which denatured serum has been spotted or to filters that were Southern-blotted after the nucleic acid

in the serum was electrophoretically separated.[67–69]; (2) *HBV DNA polymerase assays* use labeled deoxynucleotide triphosphates that are incorporated into the DNA, which is then electrophoresed and identified either by autoradiography or by enzymatic methods[70]; and (3) *HBV DNA polymerase chain reaction (PCR)* employs a segment of the viral genome that is amplified and identified by either its migration in agarose gels or by Southern blot hybridization to the amplified DNA-specific nucleic acid probe.

The hybridization assays are currently the most sensitive means to identify serum HBV DNA. When the HBV DNA concentration was determined in serum whose chimpanzee infectivity had been determined, the two results correlated very well; thus, HBV DNA is a direct measure of the presence of Dane particles. The currently available HBV DNA assays can detect a minimum of 2500 to 25,000 viruses per milliliter of serum. The minimum concentration of virus to infect a chimpanzee is about 100 viruses per milliliter; therefore, the sensitivity of the current HBV DNA assays is below that needed to determine that a biologic specimen is not potentially infectious. Although it is an adjunctive test in gauging the responsiveness of HBV infection to antiviral therapy, it is not clear whether the HBV DNA assay will be helpful in managing most HBV-infected patients. The absence of serum HBV DNA even by PCR in a chronic HBsAg-positive carrier may be only transient and should not be used to imply lack of infectivity.

Hepatitis X Antigen (HBxAg) and Antibody (Anti-HBx)

These immunoassays for hepatitis x antigen and antibody are available on a limited basis. The clinical utility of these assays is under investigation,[71] and their role is unclear.

Hepatitis C

After the development of definitive assays for both HAV and HBV in the mid 1970s, the realization occurred that other agents were also responsible for post-transfusion hepatitis, sporadic hepatitis, and occasional epidemics of maternally transmitted hepatitis.[72–83] HCV is the major agent for parenterally transmitted non-A, non-B virus and sporadic hepatitis. HCV is a positively stranded RNA virus that is related to flaviviruses, the agents that cause yellow fever, dengue fever, and other hemorrhagic fevers.[84] Although most flaviviruses are transmitted by insects (hence are called arboviruses), HCV is thought to be transmitted primarily by needle stick exposure (as in intravenous drug use), blood transfusion, or, rarely, sexually. Like the other flaviviruses, the 9300-nucleotide-long positively stranded RNA HCV genome is translated into a polyprotein that is cleaved by viral-encoded proteases to form at least three structural proteins (two envelope proteins and a core protein) and at least five nonstructural proteins with enzymatic activity, including RNA polymerase, helicase, and protease activity (Fig. 20–4). This lipid-containing RNA virus is 50 to 60 nm in diameter. Like other RNA viruses, HCV is

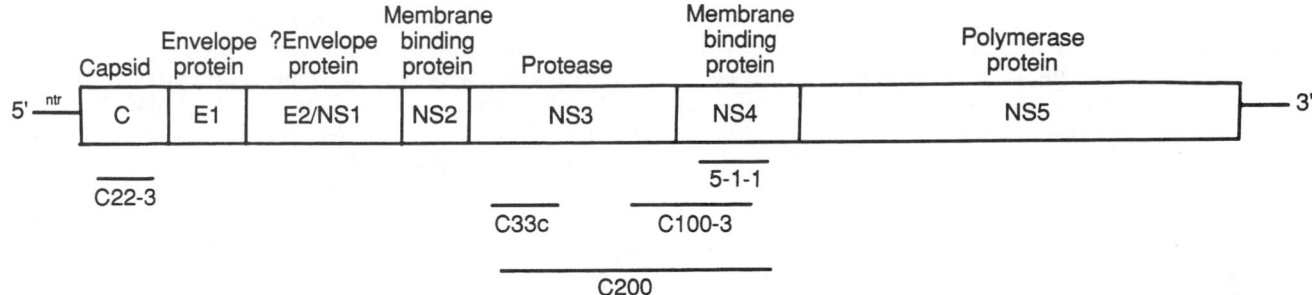

FIGURE 20–4 Putative genome organization of HCV based on similarities between the hydrophobicity/hydrophilicity of the HCV polyprotein; ntr is the 5′ nontranslated region. (From Zeldis JB. Molecular biology of viral hepatitis. *In* Kaplewitz, N [ed]. Liver and Biliary Diseases. Baltimore, Williams & Wilkins, 1992, p 78.)

genetically unstable and has areas that mutate at a high rate. These hypervariable regions may serve as a defensive mechanism by which the virus changes its antigenic epitopes, thus eluding immunologically mediated viral clearance.[85-92] At least six subtypes of HCV have now been identified. Although not definitive, evidence is emerging that the virulence of the infection and responsiveness to antiviral therapy may correlate with viral subtype.[92, 93]

The diagnosis of HCV infection mostly relies on the detection of antibodies to various viral antigens. Currently, the second-generation immunoassays detect antibodies to core (C22), protease (NS3, C33, C100), and membrane-binding protein (NS 4, C100) antigens.[85, 94] The currently available assays are either enzyme-linked immunoassays (EIAs) or recombinant immunoblot assays (RIBA) that are in a Western blot-type format. Nucleic acid detection assays using either PCR or direct hybridization to the HCV RNA genome are also being developed and are commercially available.[95-98] In a typical HCV infection, as early as 10 days after inoculation viral RNA can be detected in serum and liver.[98] Antibodies to HCV antigens develop as early as 1 month after infection; however, not all HCV-infected individuals seroconvert to anti-HCV antibody positivity. Currently, no serologic marker can distinguish acute from chronic infection.

Hepatitis D

Rizzetto and colleagues first noted that clinical deterioration of chronic HBV infection was associated with the appearance of a new (delta) antigen in the liver and antibody in the serum to this antigen.[99] This delta agent was subsequently isolated and analyzed and its nucleic acid cloned and sequenced.[100-102] The delta agent, or HDV, is a defective 37-nm double-shelled RNA agent that requires co-infection with HBV. Experimentally, HDV can infect WHBV-infected woodchucks and thus is not as species restricted as the hepadnaviruses for its host range.[103] HDV does not infect HBsAg-negative patients. The virus uses HBsAg as its surface coat, which covers a lipid bilayer surrounding the delta antigen that serves as a core protein. The circular RNA genome is 1700 nucleotides long and is completely unrelated to other known hepatitis viruses.[101, 102] The RNA genome

is capable of cleaving itself; therefore, it is classified as a ribozyme.[104, 105]

HDV infections occur in three clinical settings: acute HDV hepatitis with acute HBV hepatitis, acute HDV hepatitis with chronic HBV hepatitis, and chronic HDV hepatitis with chronic HBV hepatitis. Initially, the only means to diagnose HDV infection was by immunofluorescent staining of liver biopsy specimens. Although definitive, this test is usually impractical. Commercial anti-HD RIAs and ELISAs are now widely available. The IgM anti-HD test is still not widely commercially available. In acute self-limited HDV hepatitis, the IgM anti-HD antibody is only transiently positive; therefore, serial samples should be obtained to confirm the diagnosis. In any HBsAg-positive, IgM anti-HBc antibody-negative patient who has acute hepatitis, a screen for IgM anti-HD antibody may rule out HDV infection. In chronic HDV hepatitis, serum IgM or high-titer IgG anti-HD antibodies are detectable. Serial samples that are positive for anti-HD antibody confirm that the infection is chronic and not acute. Perhaps the best test for HDV will be an HDV RNA assay, which has yet to become commercially available.[106, 107]

As more experience is obtained with diagnostic assays, it is becoming clear that hepatitis D has a worldwide distribution and is not a new disease. Liver biopsies that were performed in the 1930s and 1940s in patients in South America have shown evidence of delta antigen.[108] Of the more than 37,000 chronic HDV carriers in the United States, most are drug addicts and hemophiliacs. HDV is present in 40 to 60% of all cases of fulminant HBV infection. The incidence, transmission, and clinical consequence of HDV infection in newborns and young children are currently being determined. The prevention of hepatitis D is the same as that for hepatitis B because there is no evidence that HDV can infect a person who is HBsAg negative.[107]

Hepatitis E

Hepatitis E virus (HEV), formerly called enterally transmitted non-A, non-B hepatitis (Et-NANB),[109, 110] is a calicivirus that has been isolated and cloned.[111] This virus is approximately 30 nm in diameter and is found in low concentrations in stool during the acute phase of the infection. The virus is quite labile and does not have a lipid membrane.[112] HEV contains a 7500-base polyadenylated positively stranded RNA whose sequence is unique from that of other known viruses. The virus is able to grow in marmosets and cynomolgus monkeys. An interesting aspect of the microbiology of hepatitis E is that it does not make a polyprotein like most other RNA viruses. Open reading frame 2 (ORF2) is thought to encode the major capsid protein and may be the major immunodominant antigen for this infection. Work is currently being performed to determine whether ORF2-related antigens may be used as a vaccine. Preliminary data have shown that antibodies to ORF2 epitopes neutralize HEV infection of cultured hepatocytes. Like other RNA viruses, the virus encodes proteases, helicases, and RNA replicases. HEV infection is found worldwide. Recently developed immunoassays have discovered antibodies to HEV-related epitopes in 1 to 2% of U.S. volunteer blood donors. Like hepatitis A, HEV infection becomes predominant during compromises in good public health, such as during flooding and other natural disasters. Most people infected with HEV infection are between the ages of 10 and 40. This agent differs from HAV in that mortality is exceedingly common in pregnant women.[110, 112] There is no evidence of perinatal transmission of this virus. This correlates with the enteral mode of HEV transmission.

PATHOGENESIS AND PATHOLOGY OF HEPATIC INFECTION

Knowledge of the pathogenesis of hepatocyte infection with HAV, HBV, HCV, HDV, and HEV remains incomplete, but some gains have been made both from advances in molecular and cellular biology and from the use of animal models. In both humans and marmosets, HAV replication is occurring before evidence of hepatocyte injury. In tissue culture, HAV is not cytotoxic. It is therefore believed that in clinical HAV infection, antibody-dependent or antibody-independent cytotoxic cells are involved in the etiology of the liver injury. The biochemical and histologic evidence of hepatitis occurs with the onset of the anti-HAV immune response. When the HAV-mediated hepatitis is occurring, the titer of virus in the blood, bile, and stool is markedly less than that a few weeks before. The cellular receptors involved in viral uptake and the cell biology of HAV-mediated liver injury have not yet been elucidated.[113] Like HBV, HAV also infects the bone marrow.[114] The physiologic significance of this is uncertain. By serially passaging the virus in tissue culture, attenuated strains of HAV have been isolated that do not cause as much liver injury as the wild-type HAV strains. The minor differences in nucleotide sequences among the attenuated and wild-type HAV strains vary with each attenuated isolate. In one viral isolate, base changes appear to produce a different secondary structure in the RNA genome that may affect the viral replicative cycle.[8]

The life cycle of HBV is largely understood because of extensive studies with DHBV, WHBV, and GSHV. The following description is based on work performed in these systems. Early after infection the virus is taken up by hepatocytes, Kupffer cells, bone marrow cells, and splenocytes. Although the mechanism of viral entrance is not yet known, it is believed that the relatively hydrophilic pre-S1 and pre-S2 sequences may be involved with cellular receptor-mediated viral uptake. Pre-S sequences bind glutaraldehyde-conjugated human serum albumin but not albumins of other species. Whether this observation is related to the mechanism of receptor-mediated viral uptake is yet to be determined. On entering the hepatocytes, the partially double-stranded DNA molecule becomes completely double-stranded through the action of the virion DNA polymerase, which has reverse transcriptase activity, and the protein bound to the l strand is cleaved. The genome becomes a covalently closed circular molecule with either a single copy of the virus or a head-to-tail dimer that resides in the nucleus. This supercoiled molecule elaborates a 3.5- to 3.6-kilobase pair (kbp) RNA that both serves as a replicative intermediate and as a messenger RNA for the pre-S/S, the pre-C/C, and the putative DNA polymerase (P gene). A 2.2- and a 0.7-kbp messenger RNAs are also transcribed that are translated into the major S and X proteins, respectively. The 3.6-kb RNA is terminally redundant at the DR1 and DR2 sequences and is reverse-transcribed into the l strand, a 3.2-kbp DNA molecule (see Fig. 20–3). The formation of the l strand occurs in core particles. On completion of the 3.2-kbp l strand, this single-stranded DNA molecule acts as a template for a DNA polymerase that starts synthesizing the s strand as the 3.5-kbp RNA template is degraded. The DNA polymerase is covalently bound to the l strand. This later is cleaved and results in the terminal protein being bound to the 5′ end of the l strand. The DNA polymerase also has RNAse H activity that destroys the RNA template as the l strand is synthesized.[115] As s strand synthesis is occurring, the core particle migrates to the surface of the hepatocyte, is coated with the different HBsAg molecules, and buds from the hepatocyte. Some Dane particles contain genomes that are DNA:RNA hybrid molecules; these represent intermediates in the reverse transcriptase reaction carried out by the virus DNA polymerase and are found in Dane particles released from the cell before synthesis of the s strand. The release of Dane particles may be partially regulated by the large and middle S molecules because hepatocytes do not readily secrete these proteins unless bound to Dane particles.[32, 47, 115–118]

The infected liver displays on its surface HBsAg, HBcAg, and HBeAg. In acute hepatitis, liver injury appears to coincide with the onset of circulating T cells with specificities for HBsAg, HBcAg, and HBeAg. Like HAV, HBV does not appear to directly injure the infected hepatocytes, but the immune response to the virally infected cells causes the liver cell inflammation and necrosis. The outcome of HBV infections is also immunologically mediated (Fig. 20–5). Although age, sex, and concomitant medical conditions affect the decision whether an acute infection becomes self-limited or chronic, the physiologic bases for this remain unresolved. As the chronic infection progresses, the viral DNA integrates into hepatocytes' chromosomes. There does not appear to be a preferential site of integration. Furthermore, the integrity of the viral genome structure appears to be affected by the integration event. Most

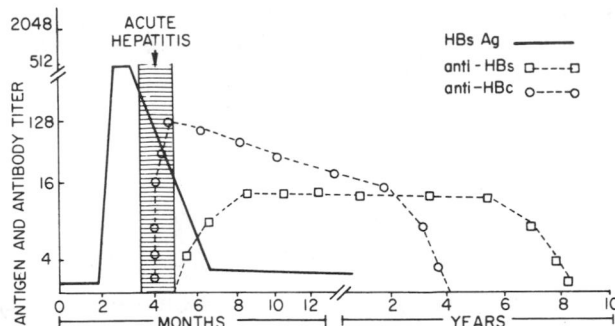

FIGURE 20–5 The time course of appearance of viral antigens and antibodies during a typical case of viral hepatitis, type B. The shaded area represents the period of clinical hepatitis with jaundice. Patient was inoculated at period 0 with HBV after being injected with HBsAg-positive blood.

integrated viral genomes are rearranged. The viral sequences near the junction between the host and viral DNA are usually the DR sequences that flank the 3.6 kbp RNA replicative intermediate. One hypothesis is that the RNA replicative intermediate is somehow involved in the mechanism of viral integration. Early in the chronic infection, the host develops a vigorous immune response to HBeAg and the liver is cleared of most cells that are actively replicating HBV. This is often accompanied by biochemical and histologic evidence of acute self-limited hepatitis, the so-called lobular hepatitis. The surviving cells mostly contain integrated HBV DNA sequences or no viral sequences at all. Because HBsAg and HBxAg can still be made from these integrated viral genomes, the patient may remain HBsAg positive and may still have continued inflammation of the liver related to immune responses to viral-associated antigens. The few hepatocytes that still harbor extra-chromosomal HBV DNA later will rarely replicate the virus and infect other hepatocytes. This may lead to an anti-HBe to HBeAg seroconversion. With the chronic inflammation of the liver, the host will elaborate antibodies and cells directed against hepatocyte-related antigens. Thus, a significant component of late chronic hepatitis B is autoimmune.[119–121]

Many chronic HBsAg-positive, anti-HBe–positive carriers harbor mutations in pre-core and core genes. There are "hot spots" for these mutations that may be areas of the core gene to which cytotoxic T cells are directed.[53–62] Whether these mutations change the natural history of the disease or the virulence of the infection or are needed for the HBeAg to anti-HBe seroconversion is yet to be determined.[126–129]

The serum concentration of HBV DNA, a reflection of the serum concentration of Dane particles, varies markedly from patient to patient with different states of chronic HBV disease. Asymptomatic HBeAg-positive chronic carriers with little or no hepatocellular injury usually have very high concentrations of serum HBV DNA. Anti-HBe–positive, HBsAg–positive patients with chronic active hepatitis and cirrhosis usually have much lower concentrations of virus.[73–75]

With the exception of the chimpanzee, all species

chronically infected with hepadnaviruses eventually develop primary hepatocellular carcinoma. One hundred percent of woodchucks that were neonatally infected with WHBV and that had chronic hepatitis developed primary hepatocellular carcinoma by their second year of life.[122] Viral DNA is integrated into chromosomes of most tumors. The viral DNA usually has been severely rearranged with deletions, duplications, inversions, and insertions.[123] To date, there is no evidence that tumors are associated with a particular site of integration.[124] Viral DNA has been found to be inserted in almost every chromosome. DNA was located near known oncogenes or was the site for an illegitimate recombination event between nonhomologous chromosomes.[124] The role of HBV in carcinogenesis may be that of an initiator that primes the liver for a subsequent event that leads to the development of cancer. Chronic inflammation results in expansion of a zone of replicating hepatocytes near the portal region that may be targets for oncogenic events.

HCV infection is associated with circulating and intrahepatic T cells with specificity for various structural and nonstructural proteins.[86, 92] At this juncture, it is not known whether a specific epitope or sets of epitopes are needed to cause chronic HCV-associated liver disease.[125] Evidence that the virus is not directly cytotoxic includes the observation that immune-suppressed individuals, such as liver and kidney transplant recipients, often normalize their aminotransferase level yet still have inflammation of their livers.[87] Furthermore, HCV-infected cancer patients who become immune competent after bone marrow transplantation often have reactivation (or exacerbation) of their liver disease. If the liver injury were due to direct cytotoxicity, immune suppression should not affect the level of the aminotransferase (an indirect measure of hepatocellular damage). However, if the injury were immunologic, immune suppression should decrease or modify the amount of liver injury. Furthermore, data are emerging that immune suppression is associated with at least a 10-fold rise in viral titer. HCV definitely infects peripheral blood mononuclear cells and bone marrow cells of chronic carriers.[87] Furthermore, replicative intermediates of hepatitis C (negative-stranded RNA) can be detected in these cells. Most likely, the cells are of the monocytic lineage. The role, if any, that HCV infection of nonhepatic cells has in the physiology of the infection is also currently being established.

Little is known about HDV infection. On entrance of the HDV into the hepatocyte, the replication of HBV all but ceases. Although HBsAg continues to be synthesized, most of the cellular machinery is involved in synthesizing the HDV-related proteins and HDV assembly. The virus may be directly cytotoxic to the hepatocyte because liver biopsies show less cell-mediated hepatocyte injury and necrosis than are found with either HAV or HBV infection. On clearing of the HDV infection, HBV replication and the synthesis of HBV-related proteins increase. Because the virus is coated with HBsAg, it is presumed that the virus is taken up by the same mechanism as HBV.[84]

Very little is known about the pathophysiology of HEV infection. The virus can be grown in primary cultures derived from cynomolgus macaque hepatocytes. Nothing is known about cellular immunology of hepatitis E or the possible modulatory role that hormones may have on viral replication.

Virtually nothing is known about the pathophysiology of non-A, non-B agents. Based on histology, it is believed that, like HBV, a good part of the liver injury is immune-mediated.[99, 125]

HISTOPATHOLOGY OF NEONATAL HEPATITIS

The most common response of neonatal exposure to HBV is a chronic hepatitis with the histologic features of unresolved hepatitis. Of 17 HBsAg-positive infants studied by Schweitzer and colleagues, 13 showed no signs of acute clinical hepatitis and remained consistently HBs-Ag positive.[130] The duration of documented antigenemia in these patients ranged from 4 to 39 months (mean, 18 months; total patient months tested, 242). Physical findings for 12 of the infants with persistent antigenemia remained normal; there was no evidence of liver disease. In one child, moderately firm hepatomegaly and splenomegaly were detected at 15 months of age. Liver biopsy specimens were obtained from 10 HBsAg-positive infants between 3 and 27 months of age. Liver biopsy results from 8 of the 10 infants were nearly identical. The lobular architecture was intact, and there was no suggestion of nodular regeneration or fibrosis. All the liver cells were hydropic and polyhedral, giving a cobblestone appearance to the liver lobule. No cytoplasmic condensations or displacement of cytoplasm to a peripheral position was seen. Liver cell nuclei were slightly enlarged, and small foci of hepatocytolysis were present. Foci of destroyed hepatocytes were filled in by Kupffer cells and macrophages. One liver biopsy specimen had increased amounts of fibrosis, but no bridging was apparent. On electron microscopy of the hepatic biopsy specimens, particles with the morphology of viruses were observed in the hepatocyte nuclei of six of nine HBsAg-positive infants. The virus-like particles were 24 nm in diameter and were randomly distributed in the nuclei; they were never seen in aggregates or in a crystalline array. Often fewer than 10 virus-like particles were visible in a single nucleus. These virus particles were probably the nucleocapsid HBV cores. Occasionally, hepatocytes with infected nuclei contained similar virus-like particles in the cytoplasm. Other pathologic changes consisted of cytoplasmic "ballooning," which caused the vesicles associated with the endoplasmic reticulum to be more conspicuous than normal and the mitochondria to appear aggregated throughout the cytoplasm. Very little glycogen remained in the hepatocytes, and many of the nuclei contained marginated chromatin. These histologic changes in the liver resemble the alterations seen in adults who have the sequelae of acute viral hepatitis known as unresolved hepatitis or persistent hepatitis.

The histology of neonatal hepatitis has not been definitively established. Hepatitis C is not associated with syncytial hepatitis of childhood or neonatal hepatitis. A paramyxovirus has been identified as an etiologic agent for syncytial hepatitis in a child as young as 5 months of age.

TRANSMISSION

Transmission from Mothers Who Are Chronic HBsAg Carriers

Such transmission of an infectious agent from mother to infant is termed *vertical transmission*. This mode of transmission may occur transplacentally in utero, at the time of delivery, or shortly after delivery. The term *horizontal transmission* refers to transmission between any two persons who may be close contacts or family members but in whom the special relationship defined by in utero life does not apply. Two distinct patterns of transmission emerged from studies reported by workers in Taiwan and Japan and from research done in Western Europe and America. In Taiwan, where the prevalence of HBsAg is 5 to 20% (one of the highest rates in the world), there is a high frequency of vertical transmission of HBsAg from asymptomatic carrier mothers.[131] When the HBsAg level was measured by radioimmunoassay and complement fixation, antigenemia was found in 63 infants born to 158 carrier mothers. Fifty-one of these infants became antigen positive within the first 6 months of life. This strikingly high frequency of transmission of the hepatitis virus from carrier mothers in Taiwan has also been observed in some Asian and African populations. The nearly linear relationship between the mother's HBsAg complement-fixation titer and the development of antigenemia in the infant suggests a direct relation between levels of HBsAg and those of infectious virus particles. When the mothers had a prenatal complement fixation titer (serum) of 1:64 or greater for HBsAg, more than 90% of the infants became positive. It seems unlikely that a source other than the mothers infected the infants because the presence of HBsAg in the father's serum or the presence of siblings who were HBsAg positive had no effect on the development of antigenemia in the infants. These findings make it tempting to speculate that the high prevalence of HBsAg in Taiwan may in part be explained by this high frequency of vertical transmission and the opportunity to develop immune tolerance to HBV.

A high incidence of maternal transmission of HBsAg from asymptomatic carrier mothers to infants was noted also in Japan.[132] In a study of 5993 mothers in five municipal hospitals in Tokyo, 139 (2.3%) were positive for HBsAg. These women were judged to be asymptomatic carriers by three criteria: (1) HBsAg was present in a high titer ($\geq$1:512) as determined by the immune adherence hemagglutination method; (2) the women were free of clinical liver disease; and (3) no laboratory-tested abnormalities of liver function were present. The incidence of HBsAg-positive carriers in a control population of Japanese adults living in Tokyo was 2.2%; therefore, the mothers studied were representative of the general population. Of the infants born to the 139 HBsAg-positive mothers, none had congenital malformations and none of 59 cord blood specimens tested by the technique of immune adherence hemagglutination were positive for HBsAg. Eleven infants of HBsAg-positive mothers were followed. In 8 of these 11, HBsAg appeared in the serum within 6 months and persisted for 8 to 26 months. Three remained HBsAg negative for 7 to 14 months. In 4 of the 8 HBsAg-positive infants, chronologic estimation of the appearance of HBsAg was possible. HBsAg was detected in serum on days 5 and 13 in 2 others. All of the infants were thriving and had no evidence of hepatic disease despite persistent antigenemia. The subtypes of HBsAg in the serum of mothers and infants in each pair were completely in accord; there were six adr and two adw pairs.

The high incidence of transmission of HBV from carrier mothers to infants found in both Taiwan and Japan suggests that the virus easily passes the placental barrier. This observation, however, differs distinctly from observations in other parts of the world. In a study of 1707 pregnant women at a hospital in Lahore, Pakistan, only 26 (1.5%) were found to be HBsAg-positive asymptomatic carriers.[133] Sixteen of these women and 1 other woman with clinical hepatitis were admitted for delivery; all 17 were positive for HBsAg. Eighteen specimens of cord blood from infants of these 17 positive mothers were negative for HBsAg and for antibody to HBsAg. When these HBsAg-positive mothers were followed for 6 months or longer after childbirth, all except 1 remained HBsAg positive. However, with the exception of one infant of a pair of twins who became positive between 22 and 36 weeks of age, all the children remained negative during a 4- to 12-month follow-up. In this study, HBsAg was detected by the methods of microimmunodiffusion and countercurrent immunoelectrophoresis, two methods that are relatively insensitive. However, the authors emphasized that it seemed unlikely that all positive cord specimens could have been missed by these techniques. The study concluded that under the conditions employed no evidence of transplacental transmission of the HBsAg was demonstrated. The one infant who became HBsAg positive probably did so at the time of birth by contamination

with the mother's blood or feces through the oral or conjunctival route. In contrast, the Taiwan study[131] showed that 21 of 103 infants born to carrier mothers had a positive cord blood sample and that 16 of them remained positive for HBsAg, thus confirming a high rate of transplacental transmission in Taiwan. The cord blood findings were thought to be especially significant because the authors claimed that special precautions were taken to avoid contamination with the mothers' blood.

In the United States, the rate of transmission of HBsAg from asymptomatic carrier mothers to their children also appears to be very low. Schweitzer and colleagues found that only 1 of 21 infants born to HBsAg-positive mothers became positive for HBsAg.[134] In this study, HBsAg was found in the cord blood in 9 of 18 specimens by the RIA method, but none of these infants became HBsAg positive. The authors concluded that the presence of HBsAg in the cord blood bore no relationship to the development of antigenemia in the infant of an asymptomatic carrier mother. In Denmark, Skinhoj and co-workers[135] found no infections among 28 infants studied for 3 to 5 months after birth to asymptomatic carrier mothers. None acquired antigenemia, and 16 of these infants had no HBsAg when retested at 1 year of age. In Greece, Papaevangelou[136] found only transient HBsAg in 2 of 11 infants born to carrier mothers, and Punyagupta and co-workers[137] reported from Thailand that none of 14 infants of carrier mothers became HBsAg positive in the first 6 months of life. Thus, in Taiwan and Japan, the risk of infants acquiring hepatitis B from asymptomatic carrier mothers appears to be high, whereas in Pakistan, the United States, Denmark, Greece, and Thailand, the risk of acquiring neonatal hepatitis from HBsAg carrier mothers is very low (Table 20–1).

A report from Japan[138] documented the presence of e antigen in the blood of 10 asymptomatic carrier mothers, all 10 of whose infants became HBsAg positive. The infants born to mothers whose sera contained antibodies to e antigen (anti-e) did not become HBsAg positive. The investigators concluded that the presence of e anti-

TABLE 20–1
Transmission of HBV from HBsAg Carrier Mothers to Neonates in Various Geographic Areas

| | | NO. INFANTS | | |
| | | Patients Studied | HBsAg-Positive | Vertical Transmission[a] (%) |
INVESTIGATORS	LOCATION			
Stevens et al.[131]	Taiwan	158	63	40
Okada et al.[132]	Japan	11[b]	8	73
Schweitzer et al.[134]	United States	21	1	4.8
Schweitzer et al.[152]	United States	36	3	8.3
Skinhoj et al.[137]	Denmark	36	0	0
Papaevangelou et al.[136]	Greece	12	1	8.3
Punyagupta et al.[137]	Thailand	14	0	0
Aziz et al.[133]	Pakistan	26	1	3.8
Derso et al.[153]	United Kingdom	122	17	14

[a]Vertical transmission means transmission from mother to infant and may occur in utero, at the time of delivery, or shortly after delivery.
[b]One hundred thirty-nine HBsAg-positive carrier mothers were studied, but only 11 infants participated in follow-up.

gen in the serum of an asymptomatic carrier mother was a good indicator that the infant would become HBsAg positive.

The importance of e antigen as a determinant in the transmission of HBV was confirmed in a prospective trial of 125 healthy mothers who were carriers of HBsAg. Seventy of these mothers delivered, and 38 of the mothers were HBeAg positive. Thirty-seven of 38 HBeAg-positive mother-infant pairs were followed for 5 months or more. By 5 months, 26 of the 37 infants (70.3%) born to HBeAg-positive mothers were HBsAg positive. There was a strong correlation between the presence of HBeAg in a carrier mother and the subsequent development of HBsAg in the infant ($p = 0.001$).[139] In a study from Taiwan, the sensitive RIA was employed to detect HBeAg.[140] A very strong correlation was found between the presence of HBeAg in the serum of HBsAg carrier mothers and the development of HBsAg in the newborns. All the infants who became chronic carriers for HBsAg were born to mothers who were positive for HBeAg. Nearly all infants born to HBeAg-positive women became infected with HBV during the first year of life, and 85% of those infants developed chronic antigenemia. The presence of maternal HBeAg was a better indicator for the development of chronic HBs antigenemia than the HBsAg titer in the mothers' serum. An earlier study from Taiwan that employed a less sensitive assay for the detection of HBeAg had concluded that a high complement fixation titer for HBsAg (>1:64) and the presence of maternal HBeAg were both good indicators for the vertical transmission of HBV.[141]

Hepatitis B can be transmitted more than once from an asymptomatic carrier mother to sequential infants, and this has been associated with fatal hepatitis.[142] Fawaz and co-workers described fatal hepatitis in two 3-month-old infants born successively to an asymptomatic carrier of HBsAg. Retrospective studies have implied that severe or fatal hepatitis B in the neonate may be more likely when the mother is an asymptomatic carrier of HBsAg, even though transmission of the infection itself is most likely when the mother has acute hepatitis late in pregnancy or in the postpartum period.[143, 144] In both of the fatal cases of hepatitis, the time of onset and the autopsy evidence of massive hepatic necrosis were identical. In one of the cases, immunotherapy with gamma globulin containing a large amount of anti-HBs was attempted. Within 9 hours of this treatment, the patient's HBsAg titer was undetectable by RIA and the serum anti-HBs was 1:256 by passive hemagglutination. However, the infant's condition, as defined by clinical and biochemical criteria, did not improve.

Another asymptomatic HBsAg carrier woman in Italy had six children from 1951 to 1973. Four of these children died between 38 and 75 days of age with clinical courses most compatible with neonatal hepatitis. A fifth child was a chronic healthy HBsAg carrier. The sixth child and last born was admitted to the hospital at age 3 months with clinical HBsAg-positive hepatitis.[145] This last child received infusions of hepatitis B immune plasma, and the authors suggested that this therapy may have contributed to a favorable outcome. This case illustrates that an asymptomatic HBsAg carrier mother may transmit the HBsAg and severe disease to successive children over a 22-year period.

In summary, it appears that the majority of infants become infected with HBV by transmission from mothers with acute hepatitis B either in the third trimester of pregnancy or near the time of delivery. Infection occurs at the time of delivery, although transplacental infection can occur in a minority of infants. Transmission of HBV from mothers who are carriers for HBsAg is rare in studies reported from Western industrialized countries but is common in studies from Taiwan and Japan. Although childhood infection with HBV is common in sub-Saharan Africa, only about 15% of children are infected in the neonatal period. Most acquire the disease before the 10th year of life, probably from their siblings.[146–148] The studies from Taiwan suggest that there is significant transplacental transmission and infection at time of birth from carrier mothers. Although infants may be infected through the fecal-oral route or from breast milk, this mode of transmission appears to be a problem in very few cases.

Transmission from Mothers with Acute Hepatitis B in Pregnancy

In the United States, Schweitzer and co-workers studied the presence of HBsAg in 56 mother-infant pairs; the mothers had acute viral hepatitis during pregnancy or within 6 months after delivery.[149] This study indicated that HBsAg was transmitted from mother to infant by 10 of 26 mothers who had HBsAg-positive hepatitis and by 8 of 17 mothers whose hepatitis developed within 2 months after delivery. All mothers of the 10 HBsAg-positive infants had acute HBsAg-positive hepatitis during the latter part of pregnancy or early in the postpartum period. Hepatitis was diagnosed in four mothers at the time of birth, and three of them became ill within 5 weeks after delivery. Seventeen women had HBsAg-positive hepatitis within 2 months after delivery, and eight of their infants were HBsAg positive. HBsAg was found in 2 of 19 cord blood samples tested. The authors concluded that HBsAg was transmitted transplacentally in three cases, but the high incidence of infected infants whose mothers had HBsAg-positive hepatitis near the time of delivery suggested that the majority were infected with HBV at birth. None of the HBsAg-positive infants were breast-fed, so transmission through mother's milk was excluded. In a subsequent report, Schweitzer and colleagues[130] demonstrated that the frequency of HBV transmission from mother to infant is high (76%) when acute hepatitis B occurs in the third trimester or early in the postpartum period and low (10%) when hepatitis occurs in the first two trimesters of pregnancy. Cossart also studied six mother-infant pairs and reviewed the literature on mother-to-infant transmission of HBV.[150] He concluded that neonatal hepatitis seldom occurred when the mother had hepatitis early in pregnancy or was a chronic carrier of HBsAg. The risk of neonatal hepatitis was about 50%, however, when the mother had hepatitis late in pregnancy. These results suggested strongly that the neonate became infected primarily during the process of birth itself, and this suggestion was further strengthened by the finding that three mothers who were seropositive at delivery had infants who were negative after birth and then became HBsAg positive between 34 and 94 days of age.[130] From observations on five mother-infant pairs, Merrill and co-workers[151] also concluded that the HBV was transmitted from HBsAg-positive mothers at the time of delivery or soon after and resulted in seropositivity in the infants at 6 to 12 weeks, thus fulfilling the criteria for asymptomatic carriers; that is, none had clinical evidence of liver disease, although all had concentrations of serum aminotransferase two to three times greater than the normal value, all maintained high serum levels of HBsAg for 8 to 22 months, and none had detectable HBsAg antibody (Table 20–2).

The difference between the low neonatal infection rate when the mother had hepatitis early in pregnancy or is an asymptomatic HBsAg carrier and the much higher rate when acute maternal hepatitis occurs near term may be explained. One possible suggestion is that there is a differential in the placental passage barrier for HBV and anti-HBs. Schweitzer has reported that antibody levels in maternal and cord blood are comparable, whereas the HBsAg cannot usually be detected in cord blood at all by counterimmunoelectrophoresis and is detectable only by the highly sensitive RIA. Thus, it appears that antibody crosses the placenta more readily than does HBsAg.[152]

Furthermore, these studies did not determine whether pre-S sequences or HBV DNA was present in the cord blood. Thus it is not known whether the Dane particle or just the major S protein complexes cross the placenta. Undoubtedly there is mixing of blood between the mother and fetus at the time of birth. It is likely, but still not yet proved, that this is when the infant receives a major inoculation of HBV. Because the infant has received transplacentally the anti-HBc IgG from its infected mother, the antibodies may bind to the surface of infected liver cells and "mask" the viral antigens from the infant's immune system. This may ultimately result in chronic infection. If the placenta is usually impervious to Dane particles, it is not surprising that women infected during the first two trimesters do not often transmit HBV to their offspring because they might not be viremic at the time of birth.[119]

Other Possible Methods of Transmission to Infants

A study from Japan, which failed to detect HBsAg in cord blood but showed that 8 of 11 infants had HBsAg in their serum within 6 months of birth, suggests that the virus is not frequently acquired in utero but most likely at delivery or in the early postnatal period.[132]

In addition to transplacental transmission of HBV and infection at the time of birth, two other methods of possible mother-infant transmission must be considered: (1) postpartum fecal-oral transmission and (2) transcolostral transmission. Postpartum fecal-oral spread from mother to infant undoubtedly does occur because HBV is highly contagious and HBsAg has been found in saliva, stool, urine, prostatic fluid, and seminal fluid.[153] The rate of transmission by this route between mother and child must be small, however, because when HBsAg-negative infants born to 17 mothers who were consistently positive were followed for 4 to 12 months, the infants remained negative throughout the period of observation.[133] An additional piece of indirect evidence can be obtained from the observations on four infants born to mothers who had HBsAg-positive hepatitis at the time of delivery or soon thereafter and whose umbilical cord serum samples were negative for both antigen and antibody. The infants were all initially negative and developed HBsAg only after 6 to 12 weeks of incubation. This incubation period corresponds closely to the incubation period after parenteral exposure reported by Krugman and colleagues.[154] The close similarity of the incubation periods in these cases suggests that the infection occurred at a common time around the moment of birth.

Additional evidence also supports the assertion that most infants are infected during labor, delivery, or the puerperium. In a study examining the gastric contents of newborns born to mothers who were HBsAg positive, 95.3% of the gastric contents of the infants contained HBsAg. The authors suggested that the universal presence of HBsAg in vaginal contents of the mother during labor and delivery and in the gastric fluid of the infant during resuscitation attempts indicates a probable mechanism of transmission. The direct demonstration of HBsAg in the gastric fluid of newborns born to mothers who are carriers of HBsAg provides evidence for the oral route of HBV infection at childbirth. It has been previously established that the oral route is effective in producing HBV infection, but 50 times more virus is required as there is in producing infection by the parenteral route.[155]

Transmission by breast-feeding is also possible because HBsAg is found in breast milk.[156, 157] Transmission by this route, however, is controversial. In the study of Merrill and co-workers,[151] who found that HBsAg was

TABLE 20–2
Transmission of HBV from Mothers with Acute Hepatitis B During or After Pregnancy

| INVESTIGATOR | ACUTE HEPATITIS B DURING FIRST AND SECOND TRIMESTERS | | | ACUTE HEPATITIS B DURING THIRD TRIMESTER TO WITHIN 2 MONTHS POST PARTUM | | |
	No. Mothers	No. Infants	% Transmission	No. Mothers	No. Infants	% Transmission
Schweitzer et al.[130]	10	1	10	21	16	76
Gossart et al.[150]	1	0	0	4	2	50
Merrill et al.[151]	1	0	0	4	4	100

present in the serum of mothers who had acute hepatitis at the time of delivery and whose infants became HBsAg positive, neither HBsAg nor antibody to HBsAg could be demonstrated in the colostrum. These mothers did not breast-feed their infants and still the infants became positive, a fact indicating that it was not necessary for HBsAg to be transmitted by way of the colostrum.

A study in Taiwan found no difference in the rate of antigenemia in 70 infants breast-fed by HBsAg carrier mothers and those fed on formula. This was cited as evidence against breast-feeding as a mechanism for vertical transmission of HBV. In a later study, however, in which RIA was employed to test for HBsAg, antigen was detected in the breast milk of 71% of the carrier mothers.[139] The authors concluded that breast-feeding could provide a mechanism for transmission of HBV and should be avoided in mothers who were carriers for HBsAg.

The discrepancy between the results from Taiwan and those from other studies may be explained by the observation that infants of carrier mothers in Taiwan are at such high risk of HBV infection that any additional exposure through breast milk is negligible. The high attack rate in Taiwan is attributed to the fact that most carrier mothers there are HBeAg positive and infants are born into an environment where the overall carrier rate is 10 to 20%. In the United States and Europe, most carrier mothers are HBeAg negative and probably have lower serum concentrations of virus. Their infants are at relatively low risk. Among 17 HBsAg-positive infants born to carrier mothers in the United Kingdom, only 4 were breast-fed and 11 were not breast-fed at any stage.[155] Of 64 antigen-negative infants born to carrier mothers on whom information is available, 28 (44%) were breast-fed for varying periods. The authors concluded that breast milk may contain small amounts of HBsAg but infection is much more likely to occur from exposure to antigen during birth either from ingestion of blood-contaminated fluid or from the presence of HBsAg in cord blood.

The decision to breast-feed or not to breast-feed needs to be individualized. It appears that breast-feeding should be recommended for infants who live in developing areas of the world where hepatitis B is endemic and artificial formulas are likely to be contaminated. The benefits of breast-feeding under these circumstances far outweigh the risks. In developed areas of the world, however, where artificial formulas are available and safe, the potential risks of breast-feeding may be greater than the benefits. Thus, even though no case of HBV transmission via breast-feeding has been documented, leading experts have recommended that HBsAg carrier mothers in developed countries avoid breast-feeding their infants if possible.[158, 159] The data in this report were reviewed by the Committee on Infectious Diseases of the American Academy of Pediatrics, who reached the following conclusion: "Studies in Taiwan and England failed to demonstrate that breast feeding by mothers with HBsAg increased HBV infection."[159] Thus the data suggest that breast-feeding of infants by HBsAg carrier mothers in developed countries does not increase the risk of HBV infection for the infants. If mothers strongly desire to breast-feed their infants, this can probably be carried out with minimal or no risk.

Another possible mechanism of transmission is scalp vein needles used for fetal monitoring.

Transmission Within the Family

Familial clustering of hepatitis B, including cases of asymptomatic carriage of HBsAg and of chronic hepatitis, has been described.[160, 161] A high degree of familial clustering of HBsAg carriers has been observed in some tropical areas.[162] In a survey of 449 family contacts of blood donors from 197 households containing carriers of HBsAg in the New York area, 6.7% were positive for HBsAg compared with 0.8% in control households.[163] The greatest prevalence of HBsAg occurred among siblings (19.7%) and among other related family contacts (8%). This study revealed that the frequency of antigen detection among offspring did not depend on whether the carrier was the father or the mother, and anti-HBs was detected more frequently in children of carrier fathers than in those of carrier mothers. The investigators concluded that whenever close and long-term contact exists, HBV may become widely disseminated, and that in the United States, vertical transmission was not of primary importance in the spread of HBV among the general population or in the formation of HBsAg-positive family clusters. They also concluded that sexual transmission was not a major means of spread of HBV because infection was 2.4 times more prevalent in parents of carriers than in spouses and 5.8 more prevalent in siblings than in spouses. The younger age of siblings at the time of primary infection might also favor the development of a chronic carrier state; studies among institutionalized patients revealed that the younger the subject at the time of primary infection, the greater the probability that chronic infection would ensue.[164] Horizontal transmission of HBV occurred in first-generation Asian children in a day-care facility in Atlanta. This evidence was used to argue that all first-generation children who could be in contact with HBV-infected children should be vaccinated against HBV. The presence of liver damage in family contacts was assessed, and 20% of family contacts with HBsAg-positive sera were found to have elevated levels of hepatic enzymes. In this study of nearly 200 families, the frequency of hepatitis B was exactly the same in households in which the carrier had elevated transaminase activity as in those in which the carrier had normal values. The authors concluded that intrafamilial spread was not determined by the presence of liver damage as much as by the common environment.

In another study of 54 household contacts of 29 carriers of HBsAg, the contacts of carriers with evidence of liver damage dysfunction were found to be at greater risk of becoming infected with HBV than were contacts of healthy HBsAg carriers.[165] Evidence of exposure was found to be more common in sexual partners than in blood relatives. Additional studies have also suggested the increased risk of hepatitis developing in sexual contacts of persons with acute type B hepatitis.[166–168] In conclusion, it appears that there is a definitely increased risk of HBV infection in family contacts of HBsAg carriers. This risk is increased for both blood relatives and sexual partners, although there is conflicting evidence about which of these is the more important route of transmission.

CLINICAL FINDINGS AND DIAGNOSIS

Neonatal Disease

The majority of infants who become positive for HBsAg after mother-to-infant transmission remain anicteric, show no signs of acute clinical hepatitis, and remain HBsAg positive for long periods. In the 56 mother-infant pairs studied by Schweitzer and colleagues,[149] the duration of documented antigenemia ranged from 4 to 39 months (mean, 18 months). During a total of 242 patient-months tested, no HBsAg-positive patient became antigen negative. In another series of 20 infants who became infected, two developed a significant anti-HBs titer 6 months after their hepatitis infection.[130] The mild hepatitis was an acute icteric hepatitis from which they rapidly recovered. The maximum ALT value was 570 Karmen units at age 2 months in one and 1000 units at age 4 months in the other. None of the remaining 18 patients developed overt hepatitis, and on follow-up (to 5 years of age), all remained HBsAg positive; seven of these children were older than 4 years of age.[152] These children all had variable ALT elevations, and biopsies taken from 10 of them between 3 and 27 months of age revealed persistent hepatitis, as described in the previous section. Among neonates who became HBsAg positive, there was a marked increase in frequency of low birth weight and early gestational age. In this study, 35% of the infants weighed less than 2500 g and had gestational ages of less than 37 weeks.[130] These findings were probably caused by the acute illness of the mother rather than by an incubating fetal infection. A similar high incidence of prematurity was also present in HBsAg-negative infants born to mothers with acute hepatitis B. Therefore, a high incidence of prematurity (35%) occurs in mothers who have hepatitis B during pregnancy, regardless of infection of the neonate. Physical findings in 12 of 13 infants with persistent antigenemia remained normal with no evidence of liver disease. In one child firm hepatomegaly and splenomegaly were detected at 15 months of age. Two infants were lost to follow-up after becoming HBsAg positive. In 12 of 13 infants who were seropositive for HBsAg, the ALT levels were consistently elevated. In two patients the elevation was pronounced (1500 Karmen units), in three patients it was moderate (200 to 800 Karmen units), and in seven patients it was only slight (≤100 Karmen units). The two patients with the markedly high aminotransferase levels showed early portal infiltration and fibrosis on liver biopsy. In the patients with persistent HBs antigenemia, results of other liver function tests (including serum albumin, total globulins, alkaline phosphatase, bilirubin, and prothrombin time) were within normal limits on all occasions. Antibody was never detected in four HBsAg-positive infants who remained persistently positive.[151]

In a study in which HBsAg-positive infants were observed for up to 10 years, all patients remained chronically HBsAg positive and some had periodic increase in serum ALT levels.[10] In a group of eight children with a long follow-up, three developed spider angiomas, three had hepatomegaly, and two had both spider angiomas and hepatomegaly. All eight of these children had previous liver biopsies that were consistent with persistent hepatitis. The authors concluded that the picture of chronic persistent hepatitis may not be clinically stable but may develop into a more serious type of liver disease.

In a study of 27 Greek infants who were all 4 months of age and who had hyperbilirubinemia and a neonatal hepatitis syndrome, Kattamis and co-workers found that 10 of the children were positive for HBsAg and 3 had suggestive evidence of HBV infection.[143] The clinical diagnoses for the other 14 who showed no evidence of hepatitis B were congenital malformation of the biliary tract (4); sepsis (3); cytomegalovirus infection (1); fructosemia (1); and hepatitis A (5). They found that the infants with neonatal hepatitis syndrome caused by HBV had a more prolonged course, more severe disease, and a graver prognosis when compared with those infants who were negative for HBsAg. Eight of the HBsAg-positive infants were born to healthy carrier mothers. Two of the mothers had had acute hepatitis B during pregnancy, one in the fourth month of pregnancy and one in the eighth month.

Among the conditions that may be associated with HBsAg-positive neonatal hepatitis is congenital α_1-antitrypsin deficiency.[167] A regional survey of neonatal hepatitis carried out in Great Britain showed that 5 of 28 infants with acute hepatitis had genetically determined deficiency of α_1-antitrypsin. HBsAg was found in the serum of three of these infants. The authors speculated that HBsAg may play a role in pathogenesis by serving as a trigger for the development of severe liver disease and cirrhosis in patients who are genetically predisposed. This association has been confirmed by additional studies.[168, 169] In one of these studies,[169] five patients with α_1-antitrypsin deficiency were described. All had neonatal hepatitis syndrome and two developed cirrhosis at ages 5 and 8 years. Three patients aged 1, 9, and 21 years were asymptomatic. The oldest of these patients had only mild histologic changes in the liver. The investigators concluded that the prognosis for patients with α_1-antitrypsin deficiency developing neonatal hepatitis is not necessarily grave.

In the Taiwan study, in which 158 women who were carriers of HBsAg gave birth to 63 antigen-positive infants (40%), all the infants remained healthy without signs or symptoms of hepatitis. Thus, it is evident that the majority of infants who became HBsAg positive by mother-to-infant transmission are clinically healthy, but they may have a persistently elevated level of ALT and signs of chronic hepatitis may be found on biopsy. The long-term effects of chronic neonatal HBV infection are not known. The subsequent development of serious liver disease and hepatic cancer and extrahepatic complications such as glomerulonephritis and systemic arteritis are possibilities that must be considered.

Neonatal hepatitis C in infants appears to be asymptomatic; however, no good clinical description of this has yet to be published. Most children who have been identified as being infected with HCV are asymptomatic but have serologic markers for HCV or are antibody negative but are viremic based on nucleic acid detection assays. All children born of anti-HCV reactive mothers will be anti-HCV reactive for the first 4 to 6 months of life until their maternal antibody is replaced by endogenous immunoglobulins. Perinatal HCV transmission occurs rarely, but more frequently in HIV-positive women or women with high viral titers.[170–177] In the United States co-infection of mothers with human immunodeficiency virus type 1 (HIV-1) and HCV is common. In a large study of 155 mothers who were dually infected with HCV and HIV-1, 8.4% of infants born to these mothers were infected with HCV.[178] This rate was similar to the 5.5% of 18 infants reported in Italy[179] and 5.2% infants reported in the United Kingdom.[180] In another study from Italy a very high rate of 36% infant infection in 22 infants born to mothers dually infected with HCV and HIV-1 was reported.[181] The study from the United States showed that HCV RNA concentration was higher in HIV-1–infected mothers who transmitted HCV. No HCV infection was detected in infants born to mothers with plasma HCV RNA concentration of less than 100,000 copies/ml.

The role of HCV viral load in transmission has also been suggested in smaller studies of HCV. This closely approximates the role of high plasma concentration of HBV DNA in perinatal transmission of HBV[182] and of high levels of maternal HIV-1 RNA in mother-to-infant transmission of HIV-1.[183] This information should reassure mothers who do not have detectable levels of HCV RNA and those with low levels of HCV RNA at the time of delivery that the risk of transmitting infection to their infants is very low. This study also provides support to reduce HCV RNA load in women with high levels of perinatal HCV RNA concentration to prevent transmission to the infant.

It has been shown that interferon alfa, the first effective therapy for HCV infection, will rapidly reduce plasma levels of HCV RNA and HCV core protein.[184] A decrease in serum HCV RNA level by 50% in 7.2 hours was observed on the first day of therapy in a pharmacokinetics study. This is followed by a slower decline in serum HCV RNA level after the first day. Therefore, interferon alfa therapy results in a biphasic reduction in HCV RNA. This pharmacokinetics of interferon alfa–induced reduction in HCV RNA has not been determined in pregnant women, but interferon alfa treatment would be expected to rapidly decrease HCV RNA in these patients as well. In some instances, serum HCV RNA is detected for only the first 9 months after birth. In one instance, a mother had a number of HCV variants, but only one viral species was found in the neonate.[172] HCV exists in plasma as either an immune complex or as a free circulating virus.[185] Work is currently being performed to determine whether the immune-complex virus or the free form can pass through the placenta.

Severe and Fulminant Hepatitis

As noted previously, neonatal hepatitis B is usually a benign disease; there are three reports in the literature of severe and fulminant hepatitis B in the neonate.[142–144] Dupuy and co-workers described 14 infants ranging in age from 2 to 5 months who were hospitalized with severe to fulminant hepatitis. Eleven of the 14 were positive for HBsAg or had a secondary rise in anti-HBs. Eight of these patients had received blood products during the neonatal period, and infection was believed to have been transmitted by the blood. However, the mothers of five of the remaining infants were found to be asymptomatic carriers of HBsAg, as judged by the presence of two serum samples collected 6 months apart. Three of these infants were positive for HBsAg, and two of the three infants died of massive hepatic failure. Two of the infants who died were members of the same family. At autopsy, examination of the liver revealed massive necrosis and collapse of liver cells, and this was associated with periportal fibrosis when the hepatitis was present for a long enough time. Eight of the patients who were positive for HBsAg died. The causes of death included sepsis, massive pulmonary hemorrhage, and overt hepatic coma. Most of the patients had moderate hepatomegaly and rises in bilirubin and serum ALT levels. All patients, however, had a prothrombin time that was less than 10% of normal. The most adequate evidence for liver regeneration was a spontaneous increase in clotting factor V. Despite intensive care, numerous exchange transfusions and passive immunotherapy with anti-HBs, the mortality rate was high (57%). The five HBsAg-positive patients who received anti-HBs globulin all developed seroconversion to anti-HBs positivity, but clinical improvement did not ensue. The severity of the disease appeared to be the same whether the infants received transfusions or developed hepatitis from a chronic carrier mother. The average incubation time, however, was 100 days after infection from an asymptomatic carrier mother and 77 days after transfusion. The authors concluded that those patients with a long incubation time and infection from a chronic carrier mother had sustained oral, massive, and repeated exposure to HBsAg rather than a transplacental contamination.

Kattamis and co-workers, as mentioned previously, described a severe hepatitis in 10 infants with neonatal hepatitis who were HBsAg positive.[143] The infants were all younger than 4 months of age, and two died in a short time in hepatic coma; four developed cirrhosis. All the patients showed marked elevation of serum ALT levels, high levels of alkaline phosphatase, and a severe prolongation of the prothrombin time. On liver biopsy, collapse of liver architecture, giant cell formation, bile duct proliferation and inspissated bile, and periportal fibrosis were noted. Treatment was generally unsuccessful, and, in particular, high doses of prednisone were of no use in decreasing serum bilirubin levels.

The cases of fatal hepatitis in two infants born successively to an asymptomatic carrier of HBsAg illustrate that particularly severe or fatal neonatal hepatitis appears to be more likely when the mother is an asymptomatic carrier of HBsAg, which is a reflection of the higher serum viral titer in these patients than the serum viral titer in other forms of HBV infection.[143] Fatal cases are rare; only five have been described. However, in the three reports of severe neonatal hepatitis, two fatal cases occurred in each of two families.[142, 144]

In the cases reported by Fawaz and co-workers, both children were the products of a normal gestation and full-term delivery and in both the onset of hepatitis occurred at 3 months of age.[142] The time of onset, clinical course, and autopsy evidence of massive hepatic necrosis were identical. The mother had another living child, the first born, who was 6 years old when the second fatal case occurred and whose serum contained neither HBsAg nor anti-HBs. The mother was persistently HBsAg positive, but she showed normal results from liver function tests and physical examination. The mother had no known source for acquisition of HBsAg, and her husband was negative for HBsAg. Both the mother and the infant with fatal hepatitis had large amounts of anti-HBc. The clinical course of the infant was one of rapid deterioration despite treatment with intravenous fluids, fresh frozen plasma, corticosteroids, and oral neomycin. Immunotherapy with 3 ml of gamma globulin containing anti-HBs (titer, 1:500,000 by passive hemagglutination) was unsuccessful, even though the HBsAg titer became undetectable within 9 hours and anti-HBs appeared. The total bilirubin level rose to 32 mg/dl, and the serum albumin value fell to 1.9 mg/dl. The liver shrank, severe ascites developed, and multiple-system hemorrhage appeared. Double-volume exchange transfusion failed to produce any clinical improvement, and the patient died on the 13th hospital day. Although the clinicians were concerned about possible harmful effects from the administration of anti-HBs, none appeared; in particular, no immune-complex manifestations could be documented.

There is little evidence that HCV is an agent for fulminant hepatic failure in adults or children. Although HEV has been associated with fulminant hepatic failure in pregnant women, it has not yet been implicated in fulminant hepatic failure in infants.[110]

Immune-Complex Manifestations

Although immune complexes containing HBsAg do form in hepatitis B and explain some of the clinical manifestations, they have not been described in neonatal hepatitis. The main purpose of describing them in this section is to point out that immune-complex formation may represent a special hazard in infants with hepatitis B who are passively immunized with serum containing anti-HBs. Theoretically, these patients could undergo immune-complex formation and show the clinical consequences of these immune complexes, such as glomerulonephritis, vasculitis, or arthritis. These immune-complex manifestations have not been observed in patients with fulminant hepatitis B who received transfusions with plasma containing high titers of anti-HBs.[186] Immune-complex complications were also not noted in an infant with fatal hepatitis B who received immunotherapy with high-titer anti-HBs and in whose serum HBsAg rapidly disappeared, presumably because HBsAg was bound to anti-HBs[142] Although the manifestations of immune-complex disease have not been observed in infants with

neonatal hepatitis, the clinician should keep in mind the possibility that they may occur.

HBV is the first virus pathogenic for humans whose antigens have been shown to play a role in circulatory immune complexes and in immune-complex disease. Although systemic lupus erythematosus is the prototype immune-complex disease, its etiology remains unclear and a viral association has not been definitely shown. In the immune-complex manifestations of hepatitis B, however, circulatory immune complexes containing HBsAg, antibody and complement have been documented, and deposition of these complexes in various tissues has been demonstrated. Presumably these complexes mediate tissue injury. The occurrence of allergic symptoms in hepatitis B was emphasized by Mirick and Shank in their analysis of an epidemic in a contained population. An estimated 70% of persons who received injections of human plasma while serving as controls in a study of the efficacy of an influenza vaccine developed hepatitis; the mean incubation period from inoculation to onset of liver disease was 79 days.[187] Of 272 cases studied, arthralgia occurred in 25%, urticaria in 21%, angioedema in 4%, and other types of rash in 14%. The overall incidence of allergic symptoms was 50% (Table 20–3).

When techniques for detection of HBsAg became available, it was possible to study the association of HBV with various immune-complex disorders. The occurrence of arthralgia, arthritis, and urticaria in 18 patients with acute HBsAg hepatitis was reported by Alpert and co-workers[188] in 1971; levels of complement, both CH_{50} and C4, were depressed in nine patients with acute joint and skin symptoms. These observations were confirmed and extended in a simultaneous report by data from three patients who presented during the prodrome of hepatitis B with rash and arthritis; they had HBsAg in association with low complement levels in both serum and synovial fluid. With the onset of jaundice, these signs resolved spontaneously and did not recur. The

TABLE 20–3
Immune-Complex Manifestations of Hepatitis B

Allergic symptoms[187]
   Arthralgia, 25%
   Urticaria, 21%
   Angioedema, 4%
   Rash, 14%
Arthritis
   Nine patients with joint symptoms and low level
      complement[188]
   Three patients with HBs and low complement level in
      synovial fluid[189]
Glomerulonephritis
   Membranous glomerulonephritis in an HBsAg carrier[190]
   Chronic membranous glomerulonephritis with chronic
      active hepatitis[191]
Periarteritis nodosa (PAN)
   Six patients with PAN and HBsAg[192]
   Thirty percent of 33 cases of PAN had HBsAg[193]
Circulating HBsAg—anti-HBs complexes have been found in
   cryoprecipitates[191]

level of complement in serum also returned to normal. The time course of these findings was remarkably similar to that in Dixon's "one-shot" serum-sickness model and suggested that a serum-sickness–like illness was present during the prodrome of hepatitis B.[189]

Combes and associates have obtained direct evidence for glomerulonephritis related to the HBsAg-anti-HBs immune complex.[190] They described a 53-year-old man who developed acute hepatitis B after a blood transfusion and remained positive for HBsAg for many months. One year after the hepatitis infection, the patient had severe proteinuria, his serum was positive for HBsAg, and renal biopsy showed membranous glomerulonephritis. Direct immunofluorescence revealed IgG, C'3, and HBsAg deposited in the glomeruli. Electron microscopy indicated that discontinuous electron-dense deposits were present in a thickened basement membrane and along the subepithelial surface of the glomerular capillary basement membrane. In addition to this patient, another case of chronic membranous glomerulonephritis with HBsAg–anti-HBs immune complexes in the glomeruli has also been described.[191]

Gocke and colleagues have reported widespread vasculitis in association with HBsAg in six patients with a clinicopathologic picture of periarteritis nodosa.[192] The clinical features included fever with polyarthralgia, myalgia, rash, urticaria, and abnormal results of hepatic tests. Fibrinoid necrosis and perivascular infiltration were present in the walls of small muscular arteries. In two patients, HBsAg and IgM deposits were present in arterial walls 3 and 6 months after the onset of symptoms. HBsAg was present in the serum of all six patients. Although high titers of HBsAg have been found in other patients, specific immune complexes in vessel walls or as circulating complexes have not been seen. In 33 cases of periarteritis nodosa described in three separate studies, 10 patients had HBsAg (incidence, 30%), and anti-HBs was found in 5 patients (15%). This association is greater than can be explained by chance alone and suggests that immune complexes containing HBsAg play a pathogenic role in periarteritis nodosa.[193]

In summary, these several manifestations of immune-complex disease in hepatitis B cover the spectrum of serum-sickness–like illness and should be looked for in infants with neonatal hepatitis, particularly those receiving immunotherapy with anti-HBs. In spite of this, immune-complex disease has not been observed in patients receiving both HBsAg as part of a vaccine and HBIG. Chronic HCV infection is associated with a mixed cryoglobulinemia. The mixed cryoglobulins have been demonstrated in coprecipitate with HCV RNA and to have anti-HCV specificity. This disease has so far been described only in adults.[92]

Hepatocellular Carcinoma

Neonatal infection with HBV has been suggested as playing a dominant role in the development of primary hepatocellular carcinoma in later life. A progression of events from vertical HBV transmission leading to chronic antigenemia, resulting in cirrhosis and hepatocellular carcinoma in adult life, has been implicated to explain findings in Senegal, West Africa, where primary hepatocellular carcinoma is a major cause of death in young adult men.[194] The finding that mothers of patients with hepatocellular carcinoma were positive for HBsAg four times more frequently than the fathers suggested that the virus was acquired from the mother by vertical transmission.

Neonatal HBV infection enhances the carrier state and progression to cirrhosis and hepatoma. In those areas of the world that possess a high incidence of hepatocellular carcinoma, vertical transmission of HBV from carrier mothers to infants occurs more frequently than in those areas possessing a low incidence of hepatocellular carcinoma. This may relate to an associated high incidence of HBeAg positivity in some HBsAg carriers. In the United States, only 3 to 5% of HBsAg carriers are also HBeAg positive and hepatocellular carcinoma is uncommon, whereas 30% of HBsAg carriers are also HBeAg positive in Taiwan, Japan, and Uganda; and these countries have a very high incidence of hepatocellular carcinoma. In several studies, between 37 and 90% of patients with hepatocellular carcinoma were HBsAg positive, a figure that is 10-fold greater than that for matched controls living in the same area.[195]

The Chinese-American population, for example, is at a very high risk for hepatitis B infection and hepatocellular carcinoma; this provides evidence supporting the indication that these conditions are causally related.[196] The HBsAg was present in 9.3% of 666 Chinese-Americans living in New York, and anti-HBs was detected in 57%. The anti-HBc antibody was found in 8.8%. Fifty percent of the mothers of HBs carriers and 66% of the siblings were also antigenemic. These rates are 10-to 40-fold higher than those in other ethnic groups. The death rate from hepatocellular carcinoma is also very high in Chinese-American males, being 4 times greater than that in black males and 10 times higher than that in white males. Among Chinese Americans in the United States who develop hepatocellular carcinoma, 70% have HBsAg antigen or anti-HBc alone in their sera.[197] This association with hepatocellular carcinoma seemed to be specific because even among patients with biliary duct carcinoma there was not an excess prevalence of HBV markers.

The two lines of evidence that support the association between HBV and hepatocellular carcinoma are the close correlation in the geographic distribution of hepatocellular carcinoma and chronic HBV infection and the high frequency of HBsAg positivity in hepatocellular carcinoma patients. Increasing evidence suggests that HBV is the single most important causative factor of hepatocellular carcinoma. If the vertical transmission of HBV is confirmed as a primary feature in the development of the chronic carrier of HBsAg progressing to the chronic active cirrhosis and hepatocellular carcinoma, prevention of mother-to-infant transmission might alter this progression and reduce the incidence of hepatocellular carcinoma.

Prevention programs combining passive immunization of infants with HBIG and active immunization with purified HBsAg have been effective in reducing hepatocellular carcinoma associated with HBV.[198, 205]

Chronic HCV infection is also a risk factor for the development of hepatocellular carcinoma.[87] In South Africa, the average age of a patient who develops hepatocellular carcinoma and who is HCV infected is approximately 12 years greater than those who are HBV infected.[88] This may reflect that the HBV-infected patients are infected at a younger age and that neonatal- and infant-acquired HCV is a rarer event than for HBV.

PREVENTION OF HEPATITIS B IN THE NEONATE

Hepatitis Vaccine

A safe, effective vaccine against hepatitis B composed of purified HBsAg from chronic carriers is available. This vaccine was administered to a large number of homosexual men in the United States known to be at high risk for hepatitis B. The vaccine was safe, and the incidence of side effects was very low. Within 2 months of vaccination, 77% of vaccinated persons had high levels of protective antibody against HBsAg.[199] These findings were confirmed and extended in a double-blind placebo-controlled trial of three 20-μg doses of hepatitis B vaccine (Merck) in 1330 high-risk health care personnel in six Boston teaching hospitals.[200] In the vaccine recipients, 58% responded within 1 month and 97% within 9 months, and there was no difference in immune response between men and women. This study established that vaccination with the 20-μg hepatitis B vaccine was highly immunogenic and safe in health care workers.[200] The efficacy of vaccination was evaluated after a mean follow-up of 13.2 months. Five HBV infections occurred in placebo recipients and only one in a vaccine recipient. The only HBV infection in a vaccine recipient occurred in an anesthesiologist within 1 month after vaccination and consisted of anti-HBc seroconversion. His serum ALT level remained within normal limits. A follow-up study was carried out on 28 health care workers who had a poor antibody response to the hepatitis B vaccine and received revaccination with three additional doses of vaccine.[201] Eight of 20 nonresponders and all eight of hyporesponders, who had anti-HBs levels of 8 RIA units, attained anti-HBs levels of 36 RIA units or more after revaccination. Tests for genetic markers suggested that genes present in the major histocompatibility complex may modulate the immune response because 45% of the poor responders had HLA-DR7 and 40% had HLA-DR3, compared with an expected rate of 23% in the general population.[201]

Workers in France have also prepared a similar inactivated hepatitis B vaccine from chronic carriers of HBsAg. This vaccine was administered to medical staff working in French hemodialysis units, where the annual incidence of hepatitis B in staff and patients was 40% in 1975. In this population, the vaccine was safe and effective, providing protection from hepatitis B within 63 days after vaccination.[202] More than 2500 persons in high-risk settings were immunized with three monthly injections. Anti-HBs responses were seen in 95% of staff and in 60% of hemodialysis patients. Of those patients with an anti-HBs response to immunization, none had clinical or biologic signs of hepatitis B. In an attempt to prevent early HBsAg carrier state in children, this vaccine was also evaluated in Senegal, an area of high endemicity.[203] Three doses of inactivated hepatitis B vaccine were given at 1-month intervals to Senegalese children younger than 2 years of age. A control group received diphtheria/tetanus/polio vaccine. Of those children who were HBsAg-negative before immunization, 94.5% had a specific anti-HBs response. Anti-HBs of maternal origin did not interfere with the active immunization. The hepatitis B vaccine was without ill effects, irrespective of hepatitis B marker status before immunization.

In 26 Senegalese infants who received their first injection of an alum hepatitis B vaccine at under 1 month of age and second and third doses at 1-month intervals, 94.7% of those neonates whose serum was negative for HBsAg and anti-HBs showed a specific anti-HBs response. The anti-HBs titers in neonates were similar to those previously obtained in Senegalese children aged 1 to 24 months. The hepatitis B vaccine was without side effects and was highly immunogenic in these neonates. The presence of anti-HBs of maternal origin did not interfere with the active immunization response of the neonates.[204] When vaccination was carried out in children older than 1 month of age, the mean titer of anti-HBs did not vary with age. Children younger than 6 months of age who received three injections of vaccine exhibited a 95% anti-HBs response. After 12 months of follow-up, the incidence of the HBsAg carrier state was reduced by 85% in susceptible children ($p<0.0001$). There were 238 HBsAg-, anti-HBs- and anti-HBc-negative children in the hepatitis B vaccine group and 195 in the control group. At the end of a 12-month follow-up, 4 children (1.7%) from the hepatitis B vaccine group were HBsAg carriers compared with 14 in the control group ($p=0.005$). Of the 4 children who became HBsAg carriers in the hepatitis B vaccine group, all were nonresponders to the vaccine. The vaccine must be given early in life because once HBsAg has been acquired, it does not lessen the chance of a chronic carrier state. Of children who were HBsAg positive at the time of immunization, 53.9% were still HBsAg carriers after 12 months of follow-up, a rate not statistically different from that seen in the HBsAg-positive control group in which 78.7% were still HBsAg carriers at 12 months.[203] In Senegal, hepatitis B occurs either perinatally or during childhood. To eliminate perinatal transmission from HBsAg-positive mothers to their infants, a program of passive-active immunization has been established. Infants born to HBsAg-positive mothers are immunized at birth with HBIG plus hepatitis B vaccine. Infants born to HBsAg-negative mothers are immunized with hepatitis B vaccine alone, beginning during the first 3 months of life. In this area of high prevalence for hepatitis B virus, it is hoped that this approach will eradicate the chronic carrier state and provide proof of a causal relationship between HBV infection and primary hepatocellular carcinoma.

The long-term efficiency of hepatitis B vaccinations among high risk infants was evaluated in 805 vaccine responders who were immunized at birth in Taiwan during 1981–1984 and followed to age 10 years[205] by life table and cox multivariate analyses. The study showed that there was a cumulative persistence of antibody at age 10 years of 85% and the cumulative incidence of HBV infection was only 15%. It also showed that in this population of high-risk infants, vaccination was enormously successful in preventing HBV infection. The most significant result was that it greatly reduced the rate of chronic carriage of HbsAg because only three children became chronic carriers. It is this outcome that has been associated with chronic liver disease. The 12-month anti-HBs titer was the strongest predictor of efficacy. The higher the initial titer, the lower the risk of anti-HBs loss. Of interest, it was also shown that maternal hepatitis B e antigen positivity but not hepatitis B immunoglobulin dose or gender predicted greater antibody persistence to age 10. The study also concluded that booster revaccination within 10 years was unnecessary because the level of antibody persistence remained high and so very few children became carriers. In another study from Taiwan between 1981 and 1994, the institution of a nationwide hepatitis B vaccination program in 1984 was shown to dramatically reduce the incidence of hepatocellular carcinoma in children.[198]

In adults who were given vaccine and HBIG simultaneously, the passively acquired antibody did not interfere with an active immune response to the vaccine. The timing of antibody appearance and the titer of antibody were similar at 8 months of follow-up in those who were given vaccine 1 month after HBIG, in those who were given vaccine and HBIG simultaneously, and in those who were given vaccine alone. This work showed that passive-active immunization against hepatitis B vaccine is both feasible and advantageous in humans.[204]

The Merck plasma-derived hepatitis B vaccine (Heptavax-B) contains the major S protein and lacks pre-S sequences.[206] Thus, immunity to the major S determinants are sufficient to protect against HBV infection. Despite the fact that the vaccine is derived from pooled infectious sera, the final products lack antigens for other known viruses, such as HIV-1.[207, 208] Vaccine recipients do not have a higher incidence of infection or antibodies to HIV antigens than matched patients who received placebo. The Pasteur Institute vaccine (Hevac B) contains pre-S sequences and elicits both anti-HBs and anti-pre-S responses.[209] Genetically engineered yeast-derived vaccines containing either just the major S protein or the pre-S and S polypeptides have been demonstrated to elicit anti-HBs responses and to protect neonates at high risk for contracting hepatitis.[210] The genetically engineered vaccines appear to be as safe and effective as the plasma-derived vaccines.

Hepatitis A vaccine is now available, and hepatitis C and E vaccines should be available in the next 2 years. In view of the fact that most people become infected with hepatitis A after weaning (between the age of 2 and 10 years) and that hepatitis E infection occurs mostly in people older than the age of 10, childhood immunizations against these viruses may become the norm. A single injection of hepatitis A virus prevented the acquisition of hepatitis A in Hasidic Jews in upstate New York. In this trial, no child obtained hepatitis A infection 5 weeks after vaccination. A chimpanzee immunized with *Escherichia coli*–derived complex of the first and second envelope protein of HCV and challenged with 100 CID_{50} of HCV developed a self-limited infection. Another chimpanzee developed chronic infection. In another trial, a HeLa cell–derived recombinant complex of the first and second envelope protein was used to vaccinate another set of chimpanzees. At least one chimpanzee was protected against 10 CID_{50} inoculation with hepatitis C. Antibodies against the open reading frame 2 (ORF2) of the hepatitis E virus prevented the in vitro HEV infection of cultured hepatocytes. This observation may become the basis for the development of a vaccine against HEV.

Hyperimmune Globulin

Because infants born to mothers with acute hepatitis B in the last trimester of pregnancy are at high risk of becoming HBsAg positive and developing chronic neonatal hepatitis, Kohler and colleagues sought to evaluate the efficacy of passive immunization of these infants with specific antibody to HBsAg (anti-HBs) in prevention of hepatitis B. They treated four infants from 1 to 6 days of age with antibody to HBsAg; the infants remained antigen-negative for 5 to 14 months.[211] In 6 of 11 similar infants who were untreated, chronic antigenemia developed within 5 to 12 weeks of birth and persisted up to the age of 36 months. The treated infants all had normal results of liver function tests. Seven umbilical cord serum samples were tested by RIA for HBsAg, and only two in the treated group were positive. This did not confirm in utero infection, however, because cord blood was negative for HBsAg when tested by electroimmunodiffusion and counterimmunoelectrophoresis and when tested by RIA at 1 and 6 days after delivery. The initial positive RIA for HBsAg probably represented contamination by maternal blood. This conclusion is further supported by the work of Schweitzer and colleagues, who used RIA to detect the presence of HBsAg in 11 of 22 cord blood and serum specimens, compared with only 1 of 22 detected by counterimmunoelectrophoresis.[149] The presence of HBsAg detected by RIA did not correlate with subsequent antigenemia because only 1 of 11 infants who were "cord positive" became a carrier of HBsAg. It is important to establish that the presence of HBsAg in cord blood does not indicate in utero HBV infection because antibody will not influence an existing infection. Although antibody has the potential for toxic immune-complex formation in the recipient through the interaction of autologous HBsAg and passively administered anti-HBs, this has not yet been observed. Several other studies have explored the use of high-titer HBIG in preventing hepatitis B. In Taiwan, administration of HBIG to infants born to chronic carrier mothers did not prevent hepatitis B but greatly delayed the onset for the development of HBsAg serum positivity to 9 months of age.[212] This treatment also decreased the frequency of antigenemia from 83 to 63% in the treated infants. Another study by Reesink and coworkers showed that HBIG was protective in four infants born to mothers with acute hepatitis B in the third trimester of pregnancy.[213] This report also described 21 infants who received HBIG within 48 hours of birth and every month thereafter for 6 months who did not become HBsAg-positive. Yano and co-workers have also reported that HBIG administered within 24 hours of birth and at 15-week intervals to infants born to HBcAg-, HBsAg-positive carrier mothers prevented the appearance of HBsAg in these infants.[214]

The use of immune serum globulin (ISG) for immunoprophylaxis in infants born to mothers with acute type B hepatitis has been controversial. In a study of seven infants born to mothers with acute hepatitis B during the third trimester, ISG containing a low titer of anti-HBs prevented HBV infection.[215] In this study, infants were given a 2-ml dose of ISG within 7 days of birth. Another study by Tong and colleagues, however, did not show that ISG was protective for infants born to mothers with acute hepatitis B at term.[216] This same group also demonstrated that ISG did not protect infants born to HBsAg carrier mothers even when administered as early as 12 hours after birth.

A study by Szmuness and associates revealed that there was no significant difference between the prophylactic efficacy of low-titer (1:16) compared with high-titer (1:262,144) anti-HBs human gamma globulin administered to children in institutions where HBV infection was endemic.[217] Serologic evidence for infection was reduced from 25% (13/52) in untreated children to 13.6% (6/44) in those receiving high-titer anti-HBs gamma globulin and to 8.1% (3/37) in those receiving low-titer gamma globulin. Antigenemia developed in one infant given standard gamma globulin (anti-HBs titer, 1:64) at 5 weeks of age.

Although the risk of neonatal hepatitis B is high in infants of mothers with acute hepatitis at the time of delivery, the risk of neonatal infection in infants of healthy HBsAg-carrier mothers is extremely variable. Schweitzer and co-workers[134] found that antigenemia occurred in only 1 of 21 infants born to chronic carriers, but Kohler and colleagues[211] observed antigenemia in 1 of 2 untreated infants born to HBsAg carriers. Mothers who are carriers can be highly infectious, however, and a family has been described in which the mother and three older siblings of an infant treated with anti-HBs were healthy carriers of HBsAg while the infant remained negative for HBsAg. Thus specific antibody prophylaxis of infants born to mothers with acute HBsAg-positive hepatitis at the time of delivery is effective in preventing neonatal hepatitis B. The role of specific antibody treatment of infants born to healthy carrier mothers is less clear, but one study[211] has suggested such treatment as a means of reducing the reservoir of chronic HBsAg carriers.

Fawaz and co-workers[142] reported that immunotherapy with anti-HBs globulin in an infant with a fatal hepatitis caused the patient's HBsAg to be undetectable within 9 hours of administration. The anti-HBs titer was 1:256 at 12 hours, peaked at 1:512 at 24 hours, and remained 1:256 for 5 days. No clinical improvement occurred, however, and the authors concluded that if immunotherapy with anti-HBs is to be useful in neonatal

hepatitis the infant of an HBsAg-positive mother should be treated soon after birth. Another method that has been suggested is immunization of the HBsAg-positive mother during pregnancy. When the mother develops acute hepatitis B late in pregnancy and the infant is at high risk for development of neonatal hepatitis, it is particularly important to explore the possibility that high-titer anti-HBs globulin may cross the placenta, neutralize the virus, and prevent neonatal hepatitis B.

The best hope for prevention of neonatal HBsAg-positive hepatitis appears to be prompt immunization of infants of HBsAg carrier mothers with purified HBsAg vaccine plus high-titer HBIG at birth.[145, 203]

A randomized double-blind placebo-controlled efficacy trial of HBIG for prevention of the vertically transmitted HBsAg carrier state was completed in Taiwan, where the carrier rate in the general population is 15 to 20%.[209] HBIG was given at birth to infants to HBeAg-positive HBsAg carrier mothers, and the infants were followed for 15 months. In 40 infants who received 0.5 ml of HBIG at birth and at age 3 and 6 months, a carrier rate of only 23% was present. In 42 infants who received only a single 1.0-ml dose of HBIG at birth, however, a 42% carrier rate was observed. In 35 infants who received only placebo, a carrier rate of 91% developed. These results strongly indicate that the three-dose series was 75% successful in preventing persistent HBs antigenemia.

The current recommendation to prevent HBV infection in infants born to mothers with acute hepatitis B in the last trimester of pregnancy or to infants born to chronic HBsAg carrier mothers is to immunize with HBIG, 0.5 ml at birth, at 3 months, and at 6 months.[209] If HBIG is not available, standard ISG should be administered at birth (2.0 ml) and at age 1 month. The first dose should be administered as soon as possible after delivery, preferably within 1 hour. It is not convincing, however, that ISG is effective. Other precautions to minimize vertical transmission of HBV include the following:

1. Elective cesarean section in the HBeAg-positive pregnant HBsAg carrier to minimize maternal-fetal transfusion during delivery or oral infection of the newborn from ingestion of vaginal contents during passage in the birth canal.
2. Gentle resuscitation of the infant to eliminate trauma to the pharyngeal mucosa that would create entry of HBV into the bloodstream.
3. Routine gastric aspiration to remove infected fluid that had been swallowed.
4. Avoidance of breast-feeding. In developed countries where artificial formula is available, the potential risks of breast-feeding may be greater than the benefits.[158]
5. Avoidance of use of scalp needles to administer intravenous fluids in these infants.
6. Screening for HBsAg of pregnant women who are suspected of parenteral drug abuse or possible HBsAg carriage.

HBV immune prophylaxis with HBIG and hepatitis

vaccine will also protect against HDV infection if the child is not yet infected with HBV.

At this juncture, it is not known whether ISG contains neutralizing antibodies for hepatitis C or E. Preparations of ISG in the past have transmitted antibodies to both viruses. In one study, post-transfusion NANB hepatitis was diminished by the use of ISG; however, the study did not evaluate the participants for HCV serology. In India, household contacts to HEV-infected individuals received ISG. Unfortunately, this did not prevent or ameliorate the illness. Thus, no recommendation about ISG can currently be given for exposures to these agents. Undoubtedly, once the neutralizing epitopes for these viruses are understood, hyperimmune globulins or monoclonal antibodies may be used for prophylaxis.

Little work has been performed on the use of antiviral agents for hepatitis A infection. This mainly reflects the self-limited nature of this infection and the low incidence of fulminant hepatic failure during acute infection (0.1% of fulminant hepatic failure of those who become jaundiced due to HAV). In adults, chronic HBV carriers who are HBeAg positive with elevated ALT and relatively low HBV DNA concentrations (<100 pg/ml) have an approximately 50% chance of seroconverting to anti-HBe positivity with interferon alfa therapy. Sixty-five percent of these responders will become HBsAg negative 4 years after interferon therapy and, for all intents and purposes, have suppressed their viral infection. The results of studies in HBV-infected children are pending. The nucleoside analogue lamivudine (3TC) is a reverse transcriptase inhibitor that inhibits HIV reverse transcriptase and has been effective in clinical trials of HIV-1–infected patients. Hepatitis B virus replication is also dependent on a viral reverse transcriptase that is very similar to the HIV-1 reverse transcriptase. In patients with chronic hepatitis B infection, lamivudine treatment has been associated with a rapid and profound decrease in serum HBV DNA levels[218] and histologic improvement of liver biopsies.[219] Adefovir dipivoxil is an experimental phosphonate drug that is also promising as a treatment for HIV-1 and hepatitis B infection.[220] There have been no studies of antiviral therapy for hepatitis B in neonates and infants, and these need to be carried out. Similarly, therapy with interferon alfa and interferon beta in adult chronic carriers for hepatitis C will normalize their ALT approximately 50% of the time after a 4- to 6-month course. Approximately half of these treated individuals will go into a long-term remission. The rest will experience relapse and have elevated ALT again. Evidence is now accumulating that 80 to 90% of patients in long-term remission are cured of their HCV infection (i.e., there is no evidence of continued viral replication in these individuals). The combination of ribavirin and interferon alfa has also been shown to be more effective than interferon alfa alone in inducing a response in patients with chronic hepatitis C. In a study of ribavirin and interferon alfa-2b as initial treatment for chronic hepatitis C, a substantial virologic response, defined as the absence of HCV RNA in patients' serum, was seen in 38% of recipients at 24 weeks after treatment was completed.[221] When the combination was used to treat a relapse of chronic hepatitis C,

49% of patients showed a sustained virologic response at 24 weeks after treatment was completed.[222] These are promising results. No infants or newborns have been treated with this combination. Studies in children are ongoing, and, to date, there are no data on treating infants with interferon alfa or beta. Although HEV infection does respond to ribavirin therapy, the self-limited nature of this infection also has precluded clinical trials. No studies in children or pregnant women have been reported.

RECOMMENDATIONS FOR NURSERY PERSONNEL

The HBV is highly contagious, and the presence of an HBsAg-positive infant in a newborn nursery presents definite risks to personnel and other infants. The children and spouses of women who are asymptomatic carriers of HBsAg have an increased risk of becoming HBsAg positive and of developing subclinical or clinical hepatitis.[163] HBsAg has been detected in saliva, urine, semen, vaginal secretions, and breast milk; the presence of this antigen indicates that all of these body fluids are capable of harboring infectious virus. Thus, nursery personnel coming in contact with an HBsAg-positive infant born to a mother with acute hepatitis in the last trimester must be aware that infection or transmission to susceptible infants is possible. In has been shown that the administration of HBIG may be effective in preventing hepatitis B in patients and staff at high risk for developing hepatitis after exposure in a renal dialysis unit[210] or in medical workers accidentally stuck with needles containing HBsAg blood.[223] If HBIG is not available, normal commercial globulin (ISG) may also provide protection against hepatitis B.[217] It is apparent that the conventional commercial immune globulin (ISG) prepared since 1970[224] has a significant titer of anti-HBs (≥1:1000 when tested by passive hemagglutination). Use of hepatitis B vaccine is recommended for selected personnel who are at significant risk for acquisition of infection. These facts should be kept in mind by all nursery personnel. The following recommendations are suggested for all personnel caring for HBsAg-positive infants:

1. Be scrupulous in hand-washing habits when working with HBsAg-positive infants or infants likely to be HBsAg positive.
2. Wear disposable gloves while working with HBs-positive infants, especially when drawing blood, removing excretions, feeding infants, and dismantling machinery used in caring for an infant. Disposable gloves should be kept at each patient's bedside, and staff personnel should remove gloves when moving from one infant's bedside to another.
3. Wear hospital gowns while working with HBsAg-positive infants; the gowns should be removed and discarded before working with another infant.
4. Cover all breaks in the skin when handling HBsAg-positive infants.
5. Avoid using needles whenever possible.

6. When needles are used, practice impeccable techniques.

7. Instead of recapping needles, deposit uncapped needle and syringe in a disposable plastic bottle. Bottles should be available at each bedside and, when filled, they should be capped, removed, and incinerated.

8. If a staff person is stuck by a needle, he or she should be tested for HBsAg and anti-HBs. Personnel who are already HBsAg-positive will receive no benefit from HBIG and it need not be given. A person who already has anti-HBs (28% of normal population) is not susceptible to type B hepatitis, and no immune globulin is necessary.

9. If a staff person is stuck with a needle containing HBsAg-positive blood and the criteria listed in No. 8 are fulfilled, the individual should be inoculated as soon as possible with HBIG, if this is available (3 ml of 16% solution). This should be repeated in 6 weeks. If HBIG is not available, standard commercial globulin (immune serum globulin, ISG) should be used (8 ml).[225]

10. Label all specimens from HBsAg-positive infants as infectious.

11. Instruct mothers recovering from HBsAg hepatitis and carrier mothers in proper hand-washing and precautionary techniques before contact with their infants. These mothers should be discouraged from breast-feeding their infants. No data suggesting that mother and infant should be separated in the hospital exist.

HAV is extraordinarily infectious because it is stable and transmitted by the fecal-oral route. Outbreaks of HAV infection have been reported among health care workers in nurseries.[226, 227] ISG has a high enough titer of protective anti-HAV antibody to protect against recent HAV exposure. If there is an outbreak of HAV in the nursery, injection with ISG is sufficient immune prophylaxis. Hand washing, using disposable dishes, boiling clothes and linens, using separate toilet facilities, and wearing gowns and gloves when handling virus-contaminated items are usually sufficient to contain the infection.

No recorded outbreaks of hepatitis C or E in a nursery setting have yet been documented. Whereas HEV is fecally-orally transmitted, HEV, unlike HAV, is quite labile. The prophylactic measures used to prevent hepatitis A, with the exception of ISG, probably apply to HEV infection.

References

1. Blumberg BS, Riddell NM. Inherited antigenic differences in human serum beta-lipoproteins: a second antiserum. J Clin Invest 42:867–875, 1963.
2. Blumberg BS. Polymorphisms of serum proteins and the development of isoprecipitins in transfused patients. Bull NY Acad Med 40:377–386, 1964.
3. Feinstone SM, Kapikian AZ, Purcell RH. Hepatitis A detection by immune electron microscopy of a virus-like antigen associated with acute illness. Science 182:1026–1028, 1973.
4. Provost PJ, Wolanski BS, Miller WJ. Physical, chemical and morphologic dimensions of human hepatitis A virus. Proc Soc Exp Biol Med 148:532–536, 1975.
5. Krugman S. Viral hepatitis A identified by CF and immune adherence. N Engl J Med 292:1141–1143, 1975.
6. Najarian R, Caput D, Gee W, et al. Primary structure and gene organization of human hepatitis A virus. Proc Natl Acad Sci U S A 82:2627–2631, 1985.
7. Baroudy BM, Ticehurst JR, Miele TA, et al. Sequence analysis of hepatitis A virus cDNA coding for capsid proteins and RNA polymerase. Proc Natl Acad Sci U S A 82:2143–2147, 1985.
8. Cohen JI, Rosenblum B, Ticehurst JR, et al. Complete nucleotide sequence of an attenuated hepatitis A virus: comparison with wild-type virus. Proc Natl Acad Sci U S A 84:2497–2501, 1987.
9. Denhardt F. Predictive value of markers of hepatitis virus infection. J Infect Dis 141:299–305, 1980.
10. Tong MJ, Thursby M, Rakela J, et al. Studies on the maternal-infant transmission of the viruses which cause acute hepatitis. Gastroenterology 80:999–1004, 1981.
11. Schwer M, Moosa A. Effects of hepatitis A and B in pregnancy on the mother and fetus. S Afr Med J, 54:1092–1095, 1978.
12. Heiber JP, Dalton D, Shorey J, et al. Hepatitis and pregnancy. J Pediatr 91:545–549, 1977.
13. Zhang RJ, Zeng JS, Zhang HZ. Survey of 34 pregnant women with hepatitis A and their neonates. Chin Med J 103:552–555, 1990.
14. Watson JC, Fleming DW, Borella AJ, et al. Vertical transmission of hepatitis A resulting in an outbreak in a neonatal intensive care unit. J Infect Dis 167:567–571, 1993.
15. Rosenblum LS, Villarino ME, Nainan OV, et al. Hepatitis A outbreak in a neonatal intensive care unit: risk factors for transmission and evidence of prolonged viral excretion among preterm infants. J Infect Dis 164:476–482, 1991.
16. Summers J, Smolec JM, Snyder R. A virus similar to human hepatitis B virus associated with hepatitis and hepatoma in woodchucks. Proc Natl Acad Sci U S A 75:4533–4537, 1978.
17. Siddiqui A, Marion PL, Robinson WS. Ground squirrel hepatitis virus DNA: molecular cloning and comparison with hepatitis B virus DNA. J Virol 38:393–397, 1981.
18. Mason WS, Seal G, Summers J. Virus of Pekin ducks with structural and biological relatedness to human hepatitis B virus. J Virol 36:829–836, 1980.
19. Dane DS, Cameron CH, Briggs M. Virus-like particles in serum of patients with Australia-antigen–associated hepatitis. Lancet 1:695, 1970.
20. Delius H, Gough NM, Cameron CH, et al. Structure of the hepatitis B virus genome. J Virol 47:337–343, 1983.
21. Stibbe W, Gerlich WH. Variable protein composition of hepatitis B surface antigen from different donors. Virology 123:436–442, 1982.
22. Heerman KH, Goldmann U, Schwartz W, et al. Large surface proteins of hepatitis B virus containing the pre-S sequence. J Virol 52:396–402, 1984.
23. Machida A, Kishimoto S, Ohnuma H, et al. A polypeptide containing 55 amino acid residues coded by the pre-S region of hepatitis B virus deoxyribonucleic acid bears the receptor for polymerized human as well as chimpanzee albumins. Gastroenterology 86:910–918, 1984.
24. Tiollais P, Dejean A, Brechot C, et al. Structure of hepatitis B virus DNA. In Vyas GN, Dienstag JL, Hoofnagle JH (eds). Viral Hepatitis and Liver Disease. New York, Grune & Stratton, 1984, pp 49–65.
25. Wands JR, Fujita YK, Isselbacher KJ, et al. Identification and transmission of hepatitis B virus-related variants. Proc Natl Acad Sci U S A 83:6608–6612, 1986.

26. Vitvitski L, Trepo C, Prince AM, et al. Detection of virus-associated antigen in serum and liver of patients with non-A, non-B hepatitis. Lancet 32:1263–1267, 1979.

27. Coursaget P, Bourdil C, Adamowicz P, et al. HB$_s$Ag positive reactivity in man not due to hepatitis B virus. Lancet 2:1354–1358, 1987.

28. Carman WF, Zanetti AR, Karayiannis P, et al. Vaccine-induced escape mutant of hepatitis B virus. Lancet 336:325–329, 1990.

29. Wands JR, Ben-Porath E, Wong MA. Monoclonal antibodies and hepatitis B: a new perspective using highly sensitive and specific radioimmunoassays. In Vyas GN, Dienstag JL, Hoofnagle JH (eds). Viral Hepatitis and Liver Disease. New York, Grune & Stratton, 1984, pp 543–559.

30. Ishimaru Y, Ishimaru H, Toda G, et al. An epidemic of infantile papular acrodermatitis (Gianotti's disease) in Japan associated with hepatitis B surface antigen subtype ayw. Lancet 1:707–709, 1976.

31. Gorden I, Berberian M, Stevenson D, et al. Distribution of hepatitis B antigenic determinants in different forms of viral hepatitis. J Infect Dis 126:569–574, 1972.

32. Magnius LO, Espmark JA. New specificities in Australia antigen positive sera distinct from the Le Bouvier determinants. J Immunol 109:1017–1021, 1972.

33. Kaplan PM, Greenman RL, Gerin JG, et al. DNA polymerase associated with human hepatitis B antigen. J Virol 12:995–1005, 1973.

34. Krugman S, Giles JP, Hammond J. Hepatitis virus: effect of heat on the infectivity and antigenicity of MS-1 and MS-2 strains. J Infect Dis 122:432–436, 1970.

35. Prince AM, Stephan W. Effect of combined beta propiolactone/ultraviolet treatment on hepatitis B virus. Letter to the editor. Lancet 2:917, 1980.

36. Prince AM. An antigen detected in the blood during incubation period of serum hepatitis. Proc Natl Acad Sci U S A 60:814–821, 1968.

37. Kissling RE, Barker LF. Evaluation of assay methods for hepatitis associated antigen. Appl Microbiol 23:1037–1046, 1972.

38. Juji T, Yokochi T. Hemagglutination technique with erythrocytes coated with specific antibody for detection of Australia antigen. Jpn J Exp Med 39:615–620, 1969.

39. Walsh JH, Yalow R, Berson SA. Detection of Australia antigen and antibody by means of radioimmunoassay technique. J Infect Dis 21:550–554, 1970.

40. Herbert V, Lan K, Gottlieb CW, et al. Coated charcoal immunoassay of insulin. J Clin Endocrinol 25:1376–1377, 1965.

41. Aach RO, Grisham JW, Parker CW. Detection of Australia antigen by radioimmunoassay. Proc Natl Acad Sci U S A 68:1056–1060, 1971.

42. Catt K, Niall HD, Tregear GW. Solid phase radio-immunoassay. Nature 312:825–827, 1967.

43. Hollinger FB, Aach RD, Gitnick GL, et al. Limitations of solid phase radioimmunoassay for HB Ag in reducing post-transfusion hepatitis. N Engl J Med 289:385–391, 1973.

44. Hollinger FB, Werch J, Melnick JL. A prospective study indicating that double antibody radioimmunoassay reduces the incidence of posttransfusion hepatitis B. N Engl J Med 290:1101–1109, 1974.

45. Londen WT, Alter H, Landers J, et al. Serial transmission in rhesus monkeys of an agent related to HAA. J Infect Dis 125:382–389, 1972.

46. Chisari FV, Filippi P, McLachlan A, et al. Expression of hepatitis B virus large envelope polypeptide inhibits hepatitis B surface antigen secretion in transgenic mice. J Virol 60:880–887, 1986.

47. Lindsay KL, Nizze JA, Koretz R, et al. Diagnostic usefulness of testing for anti-HBc IgM in acute hepatitis B. Hepatology 6:1325–1328, 1986.

48. Lemon, SM. What is the role of testing for IgM antibody to core antigen of hepatitis B virus? Mayo Clin. Proc. 63:201–204, 1988.

49. Matsuyama, Y., Omata, M., Yokosuka, O., et al. Discordance of hepatitis B e antigen/antibody and hepatitis B virus deoxyribonucleic acid in serum. Gastroenterology 89:1104–1108, 1985.

50. Brunetto MR, Stemler M, Bonino F, et al. A new hepatitis B virus strain in patients with severe anti-HBe positive chronic hepatitis B. J Hepatol 10:258–261, 1990.

51. Santantonio T, Jung MC, Miska S, et al. Prevalence and type of pre-C HBV mutants in anti-HBe positive carriers with chronic liver disease in a highly endemic area. Virology 183:840–844, 1991.

52. Brunetto MR, Giarin MM, Oliveri F, et al. Wild-type and e antigen-minus hepatitis B viruses and course of chronic hepatitis. Proc Natl Acad Sci U S A 88:4186–4190, 1991.

53. Raimondo G, Stemler M, Schneider R, et al. Latency and reactivation of a precore mutant hepatitis B virus in a chronically infected patient. J Hepatol 11:374–380, 1990.

54. Raimondo G, Schneider R, Stemler M, et al. A new hepatitis B virus variant in a chronic carrier with multiple episodes of viral reactivation and acute hepatitis. Virology 179:64–68, 1990.

55. Omata M, Ehata T, Yokosuka O, et al. Mutations in the precore region of hepatitis B virus DNA in patients with fulminant and severe hepatitis. N Engl J Med 324:1699–1704, 1991.

56. Liang TJ, Hasegawa K, Rimon N, et al. A hepatitis B virus mutant associated with an epidemic of fulminant hepatitis. N Engl J Med 324:1705–1709, 1991.

57. Okamoto H, Yotsumoto S, Akahane Y, et al. Hepatitis B viruses with precore region defects prevail in persistently infected hosts along with seroconversion to the antibody against e antigen. J Virol 64:1298–1303, 1990.

58. Kojima M, Shimizu M, Tsuchimochi T, et al. Posttransfusion fulminant hepatitis B associated with precore-defective HBV mutants. Vox Sang 60:34–39, 1991.

59. Kosaka Y, Takase K, Kojima M, et al. Fulminant hepatitis B: induction by hepatitis B virus mutants defective in the precore region and incapable of encoding e antigen. Gastroenterology 100:1087–1094, 1991.

60. Tong SP, Li JS, Trepo C. Active hepatitis B virus replication in the presence of anti-HBe is associated with viral variants containing an inactive pre-C region. Virology 176:596–603, 1990.

61. Akahane Y, Yamanaka T, Suzuki H, et al. Chronic active hepatitis with hepatitis B virus DNA and antibody against e antigen in the serum: disturbed synthesis and secretion of e antigen from hepatocytes due to a point mutation in the precore region. Gastroenterology 99:1113–1119, 1990.

62. Ulrich PP, Bhat RA, Kelly I, et al. A precore-defective mutant of hepatitis B virus associated with e antigen-negative chronic liver disease. J Med Virol 32:109–118, 1990.

63. Werner BG, Grady GF. Accidental hepatitis-B-surface-antigen-positive inoculations: use of 3 antigens to estimate infectivity. Ann Intern Med 97:367–369, 1982.

64. Shields MT, Taswell HF, Czaja AJ, et al. Frequency and significance of concurrent hepatitis B surface antigen and

antibody in acute and chronic hepatitis B. Gastroenterology 93:675–680, 1987.

65. Korba BE, Wells F, Tennant BC, et al. Lymphoid cells in the spleens of woodchuck hepatitis virus–infected woodchuck are a site of active viral replication. J Virol 61:1318–1324, 1987.

66. Kaplan PM, Greenman RL, Gerin JL, et al. DNA polymerase associated with human hepatitis B antigen. J Virol 12:995–1005, 1973.

67. Berninger MM, Hammer B, Hoyer BH, et al. An assay for the detection of the DNA genome of hepatitis B virus in serum. J Med Virol 9:57–68, 1982.

68. Scotto J, Hadchovel M, Hery C, et al. Detection of hepatitis B virus DNA in serum by simple spot hybridization technique: comparison with results for other viral markers. Hepatology 3:279–284, 1983.

69. Zeldis JB, Ben-Porath E, Enat R, et al. Correlation of HBV DNA and monoclonal reactivity to HBsAg in serum of patients with HBV infection. J Virol Methods 14:154–166, 1986.

70. Imazeki F, Omata M, Yokosuka O, et al. Analysis of DNA polymerase reaction products for detecting hepatitis B virus in serum—comparison with spot hybridization technique. Hepatology 5:783–788, 1985.

71. Moriarty AM, Alexander H, Lerner RA, et al. Antibodies to peptides detect new hepatitis B antigen: serological correlation with hepatocellular carcinoma. Science 227:429–433, 1985.

72. Tabor E, Geraty RJ, Dickes JA, et al. Transmission of non-A, non-B hepatitis from man to chimpanzee. Lancet 1:463–466, 1978.

73. Alter HJ, Holland PV, Morrow AG, et al. Clinical and serological analysis of transfusion-associated hepatitis. Lancet 2:838–841, 1975.

74. Balayan MS, Adnjaparidz AG, Savinskaya SS, et al. Evidence for a virus in non-A, non-B hepatitis transmitted via the fecal-oral route. Intervirology 20:23–31, 1983.

75. Khuroo MS. Study of an epidemic of non-A, non-B hepatitis: possibility of another human hepatitis virus distinct from post-transfusion non-A, non-B type. Am J Med 68:818–824, 1980.

76. Wong DC, Purcell RH, Screenivasan MA, et al. Epidemic and endemic hepatitis in India: evidence for a non-A, non-B hepatitis virus etiology. Lancet 2:876–879, 1980.

77. Chakraborty S, Datta M, Pasha ST, Kumar S. Non-A, non-B viral hepatitis: a common-source outbreak traced to sewage contamination of drinking water. J Commun Dis 14:41–46, 1982.

78. Kane MA, Bradley DW, Shrestha SM, et al. Epidemic non-A, non-B hepatitis in Nepal: recovery of a possible etiology agent and transmission studies in marmosets. JAMA 252:3140–3145, 1984.

79. Alter MJ, Gerety RJ, Smallwood LA, et al. Sporadic non-A, non-B hepatitis: frequency and epidemiology in an urban US population. J Infect Dis 145:886–893, 1982.

80. Bamber M, Thomas HC, Bannister B, et al. Acute type A, B, and non-A, non-B hepatitis in a hospital population in London: clinical and epidemiological features. Gut 24:561–564, 1983.

81. Caredda F, Antinori S, Re T, et al. Clinical features of sporadic non-A, non-B hepatitis possibly associated with fecal-oral spread. Lancet 2:444–445, 1985.

82. Khuroo MS, Teli MR, Skidmore S, et al. Incidence and severity of viral hepatitis in pregnancy. Am J Med 70:252–255, 1981.

83. Bradley DW, Maynard JE. Etiology and natural history of post-transfusion and enterically-transmitted non-A, non-B hepatitis. Semin Liver Dis 6:56–66, 1986.

84. Choo OL, Kuo G, Weiner AJ, et al. Isolation of a cDNA clone derived from a blood-borne non-A, non-B viral hepatitis genome. Science 244:359–362, 1989.

85. Kuo G, Choo OL, Alter HJ, et al. An assay for circulating antibodies to a major etiologic virus of human non-A, non-B hepatitis. Science 244:362–364, 1989.

86. McHutchinson JG, Kuo G, Houghton M, et al. Hepatitis C virus antibodies in acute icteric and chronic non-A, non-B hepatitis. Gastroenterology 101:1117–1119, 1991.

87. Houghton M, Weiner A, Han J, et al. Molecular biology of the hepatitis C viruses: implications for diagnosis, development and control of viral disease. Hepatology 14:381–388, 1991.

88. Bukh J, Miller, RH, Kew MC, Purcell RH. Hepatitis C virus RNA in Southern African blacks with hepatocellular carcinoma. Proc Nat Acad Sci U S A 90:1848–1851, 1993.

89. Okamoto H, Kurai K, Okada S, et al. Full-length sequence of a hepatitis C virus genome having poor homology to reported isolates: comparative study of four distinct genotypes. Virology 188:331–341, 1992.

90. Hijikata M, Kato N, Ootsuyama Y, et al. Hypervariable regions in the putative glycoprotein of hepatitis C virus. Biochem Biophys Res Commun 175:220–228, 1991.

91. Weiner AJ, Brauer MJ, Rosenblatt J, et al. Variable and hypervariable domains are found in the regions of HCV corresponding to the flavivirus envelope and NS1 proteins and the pestivirus envelope glycoproteins. Virology 180:842–848, 1991.

92. Weiner AJ, Geysen HM, Christopherson C, et al. Evidence for immune selection of hepatitis C virus (HCV) putative envelope glycoprotein variants: potential role in chronic HCV infections. Proc Natl Acad Sci U S A 89:3468–3472, 1992.

93. Inchauspe G, Zebedee S, Lee DH, et al. Genomic structure of the human prototype strain H of hepatitis virus: comparison with American and Japanese isolates: Proc Natl Acad Sci U S A 88:10292–10296, 1991.

94. Hosein B, Fang CT, Popovsky MA, et al. Improved serodiagnosis of hepatitis C virus infection with synthetic peptide antigen from capsid protein. Proc Natl Acad Sci U S A 88:3647–8651, 1991.

95. Busch MP, Wilber JC, Johnson P, et al. Impact of specimen handling and storage on detection of hepatitis C virus RNA. Transfusion 32:420–425, 1992.

96. Lau JY, Davis GL, Kniffen J, et al. Significance of serum hepatitis C virus RNA levels in chronic hepatitis C. Lancet 341:1501–1504, 1993.

97. Hu KO, Yu CH, Vierling JM. Direct detection of circulating hepatitis C virus RNA using probes from the 5' untranslated region. J Clin Invest 89:2040–2045, 1992.

98. Shimizu UK, Weiner AJ, Rosenblatt J, et al. Early events in hepatitis C virus infection of chimpanzees. Proc Natl Acad Sci U S A 87:6441–6444, 1990.

99. Rizzetto M, Canese MG, Gerin JL, et al. Transmission of the hepatitis B virus-associated delta antigen to chimpanzees J Infect Dis 141:590–602, 1980.

100. Denniston KJ, Hoyer BH, Smedile A, et al. Cloned fragment of the hepatitis delta virus RNA genome: sequence and diagnostic application. Science 232:873–875, 1986.

101. Wang KS, Choo QL, Weiner AJ, et al. Structure, sequence and expression of the hepatitis delta viral genome. Nature 323:508–514, 1986.

102. Kos A, Dijkema R, Arnberg AC, et al. The hepatitis

delta virus possesses a circular RNA. Nature 323:558–560, 1986.

103. Ponzetto A, Cote PJ, Popper H, et al. Transmission of the hepatitis virus associated delta agent to the eastern woodchuck. Proc Natl Acad Sci U S A 81:2208–2212, 1984.

104. Robertson HD, Branch AD. Comparative ribozyme structure and function of delta agent RNA and RNA of other circular subviral RNA pathogens. Prog Clin Biol Res 382:79–88, 1993.

105. Macnaughton TB, Wang YJ, Lai MM. Replication of hepatitis delta virus RNA: effect of mutations of the autocatalytic cleavage sites. J Virol 67:2228–2234, 1993.

106. Aragona M, Macagno S, Caredda F, et al. Serological response to the hepatitis delta virus in hepatitis D. Lancet 1:478–480, 1987.

107. Bonino F, Smedile A. Delta agent (type D) hepatitis. Semin Liver Dis 6:28–33, 1986.

108. Buitrago B, Hadler SC, Popper H, et al. Epidemiologic aspects of Santa Marta hepatitis over a 40 year period. Hepatology 6:1292–1296, 1986.

109. Balayan MS, Adnjaparidz AG, Savinskaya SS, et al. Evidence for a virus in non-A, non-B hepatitis transmitted via the fecal-oral route. Intervirology 20:23–31, 1983.

110. Balayan MS. HEV infection: historical perspectives, global epidemiology, and clinical features. In Hollinger FB, Lemon SM, Margolis HS (eds). Viral Hepatitis and Liver Disease. Baltimore, Williams & Wilkins, 1991, pp 498–501.

111. Reyes GR, Purdy MA, Kim JP, et al. Isolation of a cDNA from the virus responsible for enterically transmitted non-A, non-B hepatitis. Science 247:1335–1339, 1990.

112. Ticehurst J. Identification and characterization of hepatitis E virus. In Hollinger FB, Lemon SM, Margolis. HS (eds). Viral Hepatitis and Liver Disease. Baltimore, Williams & Wilkins, 1991, pp. 501–513.

113. Lemon SM. Type A viral hepatitis. N Engl J Med 313:1059–1067, 1985.

114. Busch FW, de Vos S, Flehmig B, et al. Inhibition of in vitro hematopoiesis by hepatitis A virus. Exp Hematol 15:978–982, 1987.

115. Seeger C, Ganem D, Varmus HE. Biochemical and genetic evidence for the hepatitis B virus replication strategy. Science 232:477–484, 1986.

116. Will H, Reiser W, Weimer T, et al. Replication strategy of human hepatitis B virus. J Virol 61:904–911, 1987.

117. Molnar-Kimber KL, Summers JW, Mason WS. Mapping of the cohesive overlap of duck hepatitis B virus DNA and of the site of initiation of reverse transcription. J Virol 51:181–191, 1984.

118. Blum HE, Haase AT, Harris JB, et al. Asymmetric replication of hepatitis B virus DNA in human liver: demonstration of cytoplasmic minus-strand DNA by blot analyses and in situ hybridization. Virology 139:87–96, 1984.

119. Thomas HC, Pignatelli M, Scully LJ. Viruses and immune reactions in the liver. Scand J Gastroenterol [Suppl] 114:105–117, 1985.

120. Shih C, Burke K, Chou MJ, et al. Tight clustering of human hepatitis B virus integration site in hepatomas near a "triple-stranded" region. J Virol 61:3491–3497, 1987.

121. Summers J. Replication of hepatitis B viruses. In Vyas GN, Dienstag JL, Hoofnagle JH (eds). Viral Hepatitis and Liver Disease. New York, Grune & Stratton, 1984, pp 87–96.

122. Popper H, Roth L, Purcell RH, et al. Hepatocarcinogenicity of the woodchuck hepatitis virus. Proc Natl Acad Sci U S A 84:866–870, 1987.

123. Moroy T, Marchio A, Etiemble J, et al. Rearrangement and enhanced expression of c-myc in hepatocellular carcinoma of hepatitis virus infected woodchucks. Nature 324:276–279, 1986.

124. Dejean A, Bougueleret L, Grzeschik KH, et al. Hepatitis B virus DNA integration in a sequence homologous to v-erb-A and steroid receptor genes in a hepatocellular carcinoma. Nature 322:70–72, 1986.

125. Dienstag JL, Alter HJ. Non-A, non-B hepatitis: evolving epidemiologic and clinical perspective. Semin Liver Dis 6:67–68, 1986.

126. Chen Y, Robinson WS, Marion PL. Naturally occurring point mutation in the C terminus of the polymerase gene prevents duck hepatitis B virus RNA packaging. J Virol 66:1282–1287, 1992.

127. Farugi AF, Roychoudhury S, Greenberg R, et al. Replication-defective missense mutations within the terminal protein and spacer/intron regions of the polymerase gene of human hepatitis B virus. Virology 183:764–768, 1991.

128. Wu TT, Condeay LD, Coates L, et al. Evidence that less-than-full length pol gene products are functional in hepadnavirus DNA synthesis. J Virol 65:2155–2163, 1991.

129. Kochel HG, Kann M, Thomssen R. Identification of a binding site in the hepatitis B virus RNA pregenome for the viral Pol gene product. Virology 182:94–101, 1991.

130. Schweitzer IL, Dunn AE, Peters RL, et al. Viral hepatitis B in neonates and infants. Am J Med 55:762–771, 1973.

131. Stevens CE, Beasley RP, Tsui J, et al. Vertical transmission of hepatitis B antigen in Taiwan. N Engl J Med 292:771–774, 1975.

132. Okada K, Yarnada T, Mijakawa Y, et al. Hepatitis B surface antigen in the serum of infants after delivery from asymptomatic carrier mothers. J Pediatr 87:360–363, 1975.

133. Aziz MA, Khan G, Khanum T, et al. Transplacental and postnatal transmission of the hepatitis associated antigen. J Infect Dis 127:110–112, 1973.

134. Schweitzer IL, Moseley JW, Ashcavai M, et al. Factors influencing neonatal infection by hepatitis B virus. Gastroenterology 65:227–283, 1973.

135. Skinhoj P, Sardemann H, Cohen J. Hepatitis associated antigen (HAA) in pregnant women and their newborn infants. Am J Dis Child 123:380–381, 1972.

136. Papaevangelou GJ. Hepatitis B infants. N Engl J Med 288:972–975, 1973.

137. Punyagupta S, Olson LC, Harsinatu U, et al. The epidemiology of hepatitis B antigen in a high prevalence area. Am J Epidemiol 97:349–354, 1973.

138. Okada K, Kamiyama I, Inomata M, et al. e antigen and anti-e in the serum of asymptomatic carrier mothers as indicators of positive and negative transmission of hepatitis B virus to their infants. N Engl J Med 294:746–749, 1976.

139. Lee AKY, Ip HMH, Wong VCW. Mechanisms of maternal-fetal transmission of hepatitis B virus. J Infect Dis 138:668–671, 1978.

140. Stevens CE, Neurath RA, Beasley P, et al. HBeAg and anti HBe detection by radioimmunoassay—correlation with vertical transmission of HBV in Taiwan. J Med Virol 3:237–241, 1979.

141. Beasley RP, Trapo C, Stevens CE, et al. The e antigen and vertical transmission of hepatitis B surface antigen. Am J Epidemiol 105:94–98, 1977.

142. Fawaz KA, Gray GF, Kaplan MM, et al. Repetitive maternal-fetal transmission of fatal hepatitis B. N Engl J Med 293:1357–1359, 1975.

143. Kattamis CA, Demetrios D, Matsaurotis NS. Australia

antigen and neonatal hepatitis syndrome. Pediatrics 54:157–164, 1974.

144. Dupuy JM, Frommel D, Alagille D. Severe viral hepatitis type B in infancy. Lancet 1:191–194, 1975.

145. Mollica F, Musumeci S, Fischer A. Neonatal hepatitis in five children of a hepatitis B surface antigen carrier woman. J Pediatr 90:949–951, 1977.

146. Bowry TR, Seroepidemiology of hepatitis B in an urban population in Nairobi, Kenya. J Infect Dis 148:1122–1126, 1983.

147. Darin F, Perrin J, Chotard J, et al. Cross-sectional and longitudinal epidemiology of hepatitis B in Senegal. Prog Med Virol 27:148–162, 1981.

148. Ben-Porath E, Hornstein L, Zeldis J, et al. Hepatitis B virus infection and liver disease in Ethiopian immigrants to Israel. Hepatology 6:662–666, 1986.

149. Schweitzer IL, Wing A, McPeak C, et al. Hepatitis and hepatitis-associated antigen in 56 mother-infant pairs. JAMA 220:1092–1095, 1972.

150. Cossart YE. Acquisition of hepatitis B antigen in the newborn period. Postgrad Med J 50:334–337, 1974.

151. Merrill DA, DuBois RS, Kohler PF. Neonatal onset of the hepatitis-associated antigen carrier state. N Engl J Med 287:1280–1282, 1972.

152. Schweitzer IL. Vertical transmission of the hepatitis B surface antigen. Am J Med Sci 270:287–291, 1975.

153. Villarejos VM, Visma KA, Gutierrez A, et al. Role of saliva, urine and feces in transmission of type B hepatitis. N Engl J Med 291:1375–1378, 1974.

154. Krugman S, Giles JP, Hammond J. Viral hepatitis, type B (MS-2 strain): prevention with specific hepatitis B immune serum globulin. JAMA 218:1665–1670, 1971.

155. Derso A, Boxall EH, Tarlow MJ, et al. Transmission of HB$_s$Ag from mother to infant in 4 ethnic groups. BMJ 1:949–952, 1978.

156. Linnemann CC, Goldberg S. HBAg in breast milk. Lancet 2:155, 1974.

157. Boxall EH, Flewett TH, Dane DS, et al. Hepatitis B surface antigen in breast milk. Lancet 2:1007–1008, 1974.

158. Stevens CE, Krugman S, Szmuness W, et al. Viral hepatitis in pregnancy: problems for the clinician dealing with the infant. Pediatr Rev 2:121–125, 1980.

159. Report of the Committee on Infectious Diseases, 19th ed. Edmonston, Ill, American Academy of Pediatrics, 1982, p 113.

160. Hadziyannis SJ, Merikas GE. Australia antigen in a family. Lancet 1:1057–1058, 1970.

161. Ohlayashi A, Okachi K, Mayumi M. Familial clustering of asymptomatic carriers of Australia antigen and patients with liver disease or primary liver cancer. Gastroenterology 62:618–624, 1972.

162. Blumberg BS, Friedlander JS, Woodside A, et al. Hepatitis and Australia antigen: autosomal recessive inheritance of susceptibilty to infection in humans. Proc Natl Acad Sci U S A 62:1108–1115, 1969.

163. Szmuness W, Prince AM, Hirsch RL, et al. Familial clustering of hepatitis B infection. N Engl J Med 289:1162–1166, 1973.

164. Hersh T, Melnick JL, Goyal RK, et al. Nonparenteral transmission of viral hepatitis type B. N Engl J Med 285:1363–1364, 1971.

165. Heathcote J, Gateau P, Sherlock S. Role of hepatitis B antigen carriers in nonparenteral transmission of hepatitis B virus. Lancet 2:370–371, 1974.

166. Jeffries DL, James WH, Jeffries FJG, et al. Australia (hepatitis associated) antigen in patients attending a venereal disease clinic. BMJ 2:455–456, 1973.

167. Szmuness W, Much ML, Prince AM. On the role of sexual behavior in the spread of hepatitis B infection. Ann Intern Med 83:489–496, 1975.

168. Bosch J, Bruquera M, Rodes J. Familial spread of type B hepatitis. Lancet 2:457, 1973.

169. Porter CA, Mowat AP, Cook PJL, et al. Alpha-1 antitrypsin deficiency and neonatal hepatitis. BMJ 3:435, 1972.

170. Ohto H, Terazawa S, Sasaki N, et al. Transmission of hepatitis C virus from mothers to infants. The Vertical Transmission of Hepatitis C Virus Collaborative Study Group. N Engl J Med 330:744–750, 1994.

171. Marcellin P, Bernuau J, Martinot-Peignoux M, et al. Prevalence of hepatitis C virus infection in asymptomatic anti-HIV1 negative pregnant women and their children. Dig Dis Sci 38:2151–2155, 1993.

172. Weiner AJ, Thaler MM, Crawford K, et al. A unique, predominant hepatitis C virus variant found in an infant born to a mother with multiple variants. J Virol 67:4365–4368, 1993.

173. Roudot-Thoraval F, Pawlotsky JM, Thiers V, et al. Lack of mother-to-infant transmission of hepatitis C virus in human immunodeficiency virus-seronegative women: a prospective study with hepatitis C virus RNA testing. Hepatology 17:772–777, 1993.

174. Lam JP, McOmish F, Burns SM, et al. Infrequent vertical transmission of hepatitis C virus. J Infect Dis 167:572–576, 1993.

175. Reinus JF, Leikin EL, Alter HJ, et al. Failure to detect vertical transmission of hepatitis C virus. Ann Intern Med 117:881–886, 1992.

176. Wejstal R, Widell A, Mansson AS, et al. Mother-to-infant transmission of hepatitis C virus. Ann Intern Med 117:887–890, 1992.

177. Inoue Y, Takeuchi K, Chou WH, et al. Silent mother-to-child transmission of hepatitis C virus through two generations determined by comparative nucleotide sequence analysis of the viral cDNA. J Infect Dis 166:1425–1428, 1992.

178. Thomas DL, Villano SA, Reister KA, et al. Perinatal transmission of hepatitis C virus from human immunodeficiency virus type 1-infected mothers. J Infect Dis 177:1480–1488, 1998.

179. Manzini P, Saracco G, Cerchier A, et al. Human immunodeficiency virus infection as a risk factor for mother to child hepatitis C virus transmission: persistence of anti-hepatitis C virus in children associated with the mother's anti-hepatitis C immunoblotting pattern. Hepatology 21:328–332, 1995.

180. Lam JPH, McOmish F, Burns SM, et al. Infrequent vertical transmission of hepatitis C virus. J Infect Dis 167:572–576, 1992.

181. Zanetti AR, Tanzi E, Paccagnini S. Mother to infant transmission of hepatitis C virus. Lombardy Study Group on Vertical HCV Transmission. Lancet 345:289–291, 1995.

182. Burk RD, Hwang LY, Ho GYF, et al. Outcome of perinatal hepatitis B virus exposure is dependent on maternal virus load. J Infect Dis 170:1418–1423, 1994.

183. Dickover RE, Garratty EM, Herman SA, et al. Identification of levels of maternal HIV-1 RNA associated with the risk of perinatal transmission: effect of maternal zidovudine treatment on viral load. JAMA 275:599–605, 1996.

184. Kohichiroh Y, Takeshi O, Yoshiki M, et al. Dynamics of hepatitis C viremia following interferon-α administration. J Infect Dis 177:1475–1479, 1998.

185. Shimuzu YK, Hijikata M, Iwamoto A, et al. Physical and biological properties of HCV inocula: useful markers

for prediction of in vivo infectivity (abstract). Tokyo, International Symposium on Viral Hepatitis and Liver Disease, 1993, p 57.

186. Mosley JW. Treatment of fulminant type B hepatitis with hepatitis B immune globulin: a cooperative study. Gastroenterology 66:698–752, 1974.

187. Mirick GS, Shank RE. An epidemic of serum hepatitis studied under controlled conditions. Am Clin Climat Assoc 71:176–178, 1959.

188. Alpert E, Isselbacher KJ, Shur PH. The pathogenesis of arthritis associated with viral hepatitis. N Engl J Med 285:185–189, 1971.

189. Onion D, Crumpacker C, Gilliland B. Arthritis of hepatitis associated with Australia antigen. Ann Intern Med 75:29–33, 1971.

190. Combes B, Stasny P, Shorey J, et al. Glomerulonephritis with deposition of Australia antigen-antibody complexes in glomerular basement membrane. Lancet 2:234–237, 1971.

191. Kohler PF, Cronin RE, Hammond WS, et al. Chronic membranous glomerulonephritis caused by hepatitis B antigen-antibody immune complexes. Ann Intern Med 31:448–451, 1974.

192. Gocke DS, Hsu K, Morgan C, et al. Association between polyarteritis and Australia antigen. Lancet 2:1149–1152, 1972.

193. Kohler PF. Clinical immune complex disease. Medicine 52:419–429, 1973.

194. Larouze B, et al. Host response to hepatitis-B infection in patients with primary hepatic carcinoma and families: a case/control study in Senegal, West Africa. Lancet 2:534–538, 1976.

195. Szmuness W. Hepatocellular carcinoma and the hepatitis B virus: evidence for a causal association. Prog Med Virol 24:40–69, 1978.

196. Szmuness W, Stevens CE, Ikram H, et al. Prevalence of hepatitis B virus infection and hepatocellular carcinoma in Chinese-Americans. J Infect Dis 137:822–829, 1978.

197. Tabor E, Geraty RJ, Vogel CL, et al. Hepatitis B virus infection and primary hepatocellular carcinoma. J Natl Cancer Inst 58:1197–1200, 1977.

198. Chang MH, Chen CJ, Lai MS, et al. Universal hepatitis B vaccination in Taiwan and the incidence of hepatocellular carcinoma in children: Taiwan Childhood Hepatoma Study Group. N Engl J Med 336:1855–1859, 1997.

199. Szmuness W, Stevens CE, Harley EJ, et al. Hepatitis B vaccine: demonstration of efficacy in a controlled clinical trial in a high risk population in the United States. N Engl J Med 303:833–841, 1980.

200. Dienstag JL, Werner BG, Polk BF, et al. Hepatitis B vaccine in health care personnel: safety, immunogenicity, and indicators of efficacy. Ann Intern Med 101:34–40, 1984.

201. Craven DE, Awdeh ZL, Kunches LM, et al. Nonresponsiveness to hepatitis B vaccine in healthcare workers: results of revaccination and genetic typings. Ann Intern Med 105:356–360, 1986.

202. Crosnier J, Jungers P, Courouce, AM, et al. Randomized placebo controlled trial of hepatitis B surface antigen vaccine in French hemodialysis units: I: Medical staff. Lancet 1:455–459, 1981.

203. Maynard P, Barin F, Chiron JP, et al. Efficacy of hepatitis B vaccine in prevention of early HBsAg carrier state in children. Lancet 1:289–292, 1981.

204. Szmuness W, Stevens CE, Oleszko WR, et al. Passive-active immunization against hepatitis B: immunogenicity studies in American adults. Lancet 1:575–577, 1981.

205. Wu JS, Hwang LY, Goodman KJ, Beasley RP. Hepatitis B vaccination in high-risk infants: 10-year follow-up. J Infect Dis 179:1319–1325, 1999.

206. Neurath AR, Stick N, Kent SB, et al. Enzyme-linked immunoassay of pre-S gene-coded sequences in hepatitis B vaccines. J Virol Methods 12:185–192, 1985.

207. Dienstag JL, Werner BG, McLane MF, et al. Absence of antibodies to HTLV-III in health workers after hepatitis B vaccination. JAMA 254:1064–1066, 1985.

208. Francis DP, Feorino PM, McDougal S, et al. The safety of the hepatitis B vaccine: inactivation of the AIDS virus during routine manufacture. JAMA 256:869–872, 1986.

209. Beasley RP, Hwang LY, Lin CC, et al. Hepatitis B immune globulin (HBIG) efficacy in the interruption of perinatal transmission of hepatitis B virus carrier state: initial report of randomized double-blind placebo controlled trial. Lancet 2:388–393, 1981.

210. Stevens CE, Taylor PE, Tong MJ, et al. Yeast-recombinant hepatitis B vaccine: efficacy with hepatitis B immune globulin in prevention of perinatal hepatitis B virus transmission. JAMA 257:2612–2616, 1987.

211. Kohler PF, Dubois RS, Merrill DA, et al. Prevention of chronic neonatal hepatitis B virus infection with antibody to hepatitis B surface antigen. N Engl J Med 291:1378–1380, 1974.

212. Beasley P, Stevens CE. Vertical transmission of HBV and interruption with globulin. In Vyas GN, Cohen SN, Schmiel R (eds). Viral Hepatitis. Philadelphia, Franklin Institute Press, 1978, pp 333–345.

213. Reesink HW, Reesink-Burger EE, Lafeber-Schut BJ. Prevention of chronic HBsAg carrier states in infants of HBsAg positive mothers by hepatitis B immunoglobulin. Lancet 1:436–438, 1979.

214. Yano M, Koga M, Sato A. Prevention of maternal transmission of hepatitis B virus (HBV) with high titer HB immunoglobin (HBIG). Gastroenterology 79:1131, 1980.

215. Varma RR. Hepatitis B surface antigen carrier state in neonates. JAMA 236:2303–2304, 1976.

216. Tong MJ, McPeak CM, Thursby MW. Failure of immune serum globulin to prevent hepatitis B virus infection in infants born to HBsAg positive mothers. Gastroenterology 76:535–539, 1979.

217. Szmuness W, Prince AM. Goodman M, et al. Hepatitis B immune serum globulin in prevention of nonparenterally transmitted hepatitis. N Engl J Med 290:701–706, 1974.

218. Dienstag JL, Perrillo RP, Schiff ER, et al. A preliminary trial of lamivudine for chronic hepatitis B virus infection. N Engl J Med 333:1657–1661, 1995.

219. Honkoop P, de Man RA, Zondervan PE, Schalm SW. Histological improvement in patients with chronic hepatitis B virus infection treated with lamivudine. Liver 17:103–106, 1997.

220. Deeks SG, Collier A, Lalezari J, et al. The safety and efficacy of adefovir dipivoxil, a novel antihuman immunodeficiency virus (HIV) therapy in infected adults: a randomized, double-blind placebo-controlled trial. J Infect Dis 176:1517–1523, 1997.

221. McHutchinson JG, Gordon SC, Schiff ER, et al. Interferon alfa-2b alone or in combination with ribavirin as initial treatment for chronic hepatitis C. N Engl J Med 339:1485–1492, 1998.

222. Davis GL, Esteban-Mur R, Rustgi V, et al. Interferon alfa-2b alone or in combination with ribavirin as initial treatment of relapse of chronic hepatitis C. N Engl J Med 339:1493–1499, 1998.

223. Grady GF, Lee VA. Prevention of hepatitis from accidental exposure among medical workers. N Engl J Med 293:1067–1070, 1975.

224. Grady GF, Rodman M, Larsen LH. Hepatitis B antibody in conventional globulin. J Infect Dis 132:474–476, 1975.

225. Barker LF, Smith KO, Gehle WD, et al. Some antigenic and physical properties of virus-like particles in sera of hepatitis patients. J Immunol 102:1529–1532, 1969.

226. Shaw FE Jr, Sudman JH, Smith SM, et al. A community-wide epidemic of hepatitis A in Ohio. Am J Epidemiol 123:1057–1065, 1986.

227. Klein BS, Michaels JA, Rytel MW, et al. Nosocomial hepatitis A: A multinursery outbreak in Wisconsin. JAMA 252:2716–2721, 1984.

Bacterial Sepsis and Meningitis

JEROME O. KLEIN, M.D.

SEPSIS IN THE NEWBORN RECENTLY
DISCHARGED FROM THE
HOSPITAL, 982
Congenital Infection

Late-Onset Disease
Infections in the Household
Fever in the First Month of Life

Bacterial sepsis in the neonate is a clinical syndrome characterized by systemic signs of infection and accompanied by bacteremia in the first month of life. Meningitis in the neonate is usually a sequela of bacteremia and is discussed in this chapter because meningitis and sepsis share a common etiology and pathogenesis. Infections of the bones, joints, and soft tissues and of the respiratory, genitourinary, and gastrointestinal tracts may be accompanied by bacteremia, but the features of these infections are sufficiently different to warrant separate discussions. Sepsis and meningitis caused by group B streptococci, *Staphylococcus aureus*, *Neisseria gonorrhoeae*, *Listeria monocytogenes*, *Salmonella* species, *Treponema pallidum*, *Mycoplasma* species, *Borrelia burgdorferi*, and *Mycobacterium tuberculosis* are described in other chapters.

Two patterns of disease, early-onset and late-onset, have been associated with systemic bacterial infections during the first month of life (Table 21–1). Early-onset disease presents as a fulminant, multisystemic illness during the first few days of life. Infants with early-onset disease may have a history of one or more significant obstetric complications, including premature rupture of maternal membranes, premature onset of labor, chorioamnionitis, and peripartum maternal fever, and many of the infants are premature or of low birth weight. Bacteria responsible for early-onset disease are acquired from the birth canal during delivery. The mortality rate is high, varying in some series between 5% and 50%. Late-onset disease may occur as early as 5 days of age but is more commonly recognized after the first week of life. Late, late onset infection due to group B *Streptococcus* (disease in infants older than 3 months of age) is discussed in Chapter 26. Infants may have a history of obstetric complications, but these are less characteristic than in early-onset disease. Bacteria responsible for late-onset sepsis and meningitis include those acquired from the maternal genital tract and organisms acquired after birth from human contacts or from contaminated equipment or materials. The mortality rate is lower than

that in early-onset sepsis—2 to 6%. Because different microorganisms are responsible for the two forms of disease, the choice of antimicrobial agents also differs. Some organisms, such as *Escherichia coli*, groups A and B streptococci, and *L. monocytogenes*, may be responsible for both early-onset and late-onset diseases, whereas others, such as *S. aureus*, coagulase-negative staphylococci, and *Pseudomonas aeruginosa*, are usually associated with late-onset disease only. The survival of very low birth weight (VLBW) infants with prolonged stays in the intensive care unit has been accompanied by increased risk for nosocomial infections (see Chapter 34).[1]

BACTERIOLOGY

The changing pattern of organisms responsible for neonatal sepsis is reflected in a series of reports by pediatricians at the Yale–New Haven Hospital covering the period 1928 to 1988 (Table 21–2).[2–6] Before development of the sulfonamides, gram-positive cocci caused most cases of neonatal sepsis. With the introduction of antimicrobial agents, gram-negative enteric bacilli, particularly *E. coli*, became the predominant cause of serious infection in the newborn. *S. aureus* was a major concern in the years 1950 to 1963 but subsequently diminished in importance (for reasons that are still unclear). The most recent reports for the periods 1966 to 1978 and 1979 to 1988 from Yale Medical Center indicate the current importance of group B streptococci, *E. coli*, and *Staphylococcus epidermidis* in neonatal sepsis. The latest reports also document the problem of sepsis in small infants who have survived with the aid of sophisticated life-support systems in neonatal intensive care units. The Yale neonatal intensive care unit was established in 1962.[4]

The pattern of microbial etiology observed at Yale has also been reported in studies of neonatal sepsis carried out at other centers during the same times (Table

TABLE 21–1
Characteristics of Early-Onset and Late-Onset Neonatal Sepsis

CHARACTERISTIC	EARLY-ONSET	LATE-ONSET
Time of onset (days)	4	5
Complications of pregnancy or delivery	+	±
Source of organism	Mother's genital tract	Mother's genital tract; postnatal environment
Usual clinical presentation	Fulminant	Slowly progressive
	Multisystem	Focal
	Pneumonia frequent	Meningitis frequent
Mortality rate (%)	5–50[a]	2–6

[a]Higher mortality rates in earlier studies.

TABLE 21–2
Bacteria Causing Neonatal Sepsis at Yale–New Haven Hospital, 1928–1988

ORGANISM	NO. OF CASES					
	1928–1932[a]	1933–1943[b]	1944–1957[b]	1958–1965[c]	1966–1978[d]	1979–1988[e]
Beta-hemolytic streptococci	15	18	11	8	86	83
Group A		16	5	0	0	0
Group B		2	4	1	76	64
Group D		0	1	7	9	19
Viridans streptococci						11
Staphylococcus aureus	11	4	8	2	12	14
Staphylococcus epidermidis						36
Streptococcus pneumoniae	2	5	3	2	2	2
Haemophilus species				1	9	9
Escherichia coli	10	11	23	33	76	46
Pseudomonas aeruginosa	1	0	13	11	5	6
Klebsiella and *Enterobacter* species	0	0	0	8	28	25
Others	0	6	4	9	21	38
Total no. of cases	39	44	62	73	239	270
Mortality rate for years	87%	90%	67%	45%	26%	16%

[a]Data from reference 2.
[b]Data from reference 3.
[c]Data from reference 4.
[d]Data from reference 5.
[e]Data from reference 6.

21–3). Studies indicate that group B streptococci and gram-negative enteric bacilli were the most important causes of sepsis, but other organisms were prominent in some centers: *S. aureus* was an important cause of sepsis in Finland[16] and East Africa[27] but not elsewhere; *Streptococcus viridans* was the most frequent isolate from cultures of blood in Philadelphia[13]; *S. epidermidis* was responsible for 53% of cases in Liverpool[18] and the most recent report from Yale[6]; and *Klebsiella-Enterobacter* species were the most common bacterial pathogens in Tel Aviv.[26] Neonatal sepsis and focal infections in developing countries is further discussed in Chapter 3.

The survey of five university hospitals in Finland[16] provided data about the association of the etiologic organism and mortality based on time of occurrence of signs (Table 21–4) and birth weight (Table 21–5). Infants with signs during the first 24 hours of life and weighing less than 1500 g had the highest mortality.

The mortality rates of neonatal sepsis over time are documented in the Yale reports. In the preantibiotic era, neonatal sepsis was usually fatal. Even with the introduction of penicillins and aminoglycosides in the reports from 1944 to 1965, death was the result in a majority of infants. Concurrent with the introduction of neonatal intensive care units and technologic support for cardiorespiratory and metabolic functions beginning in 1966, mortality was reduced to 16%.

The Yale data also provide information about the microorganisms responsible for early- and late-onset sepsis (Table 21–6). Group B streptococci were responsible for a majority of early-onset disease. *E. coli* and coagulase-negative staphylococci were the major pathogens of late-onset disease, and a wide variety of gram-positive cocci and gram-negative bacilli caused disease after 30 days.

Survival of VLBW infants (<1500 g) has been accompanied by an increased risk for invasive infection as a cause of morbidity and mortality. The danger of sepsis is documented in a multicenter trial that enrolled 2416 VLBW infants in a study of the efficacy of intravenous immunoglobulin in preventing nosocomial infections.[32] Sixteen percent of the VLBW infants developed septicemia at a median age of 17 days, with a mortality of 21% and a hospital stay that averaged 98 days; infants without sepsis had a mortality of 9% and average hospital stay of 58 days.

Organisms responsible for purulent meningitis in the newborn are listed in Table 21–7, which summarizes data collected during the period 1932 to 1992 at neonatal centers in the United States,[33–39] The Netherlands,[40] Great Britain,[22] and Panama.[41] Gram-negative enteric bacilli and group B streptococci are currently responsible for the majority of cases of purulent meningitis. Organisms that cause acute meningitis in older children and adults—*Streptococcus pneumoniae*, *Neisseria meningitidis*, and *Haemophilus influenzae* type b—are relatively infrequent causes of meningitis in the neonate. A nationwide survey of causative agents of neonatal meningitis in Sweden during the period 1976 to 1983 indicated a shift from bacterial to viral or unidentified microorganisms with lower mortality rates.[42]

Escherichia coli

Coliform organisms are prevalent in the maternal birth canal, and most infants are colonized during or just before delivery. The antigenic structure of *E. coli* is complex; members of this species account for more than 145 different somatic (O) antigens, approximately 50 flagellar (H) antigens, and 80 different capsular (K) anti-

TABLE 21–3
Surveys of Neonatal Bacteremia

	SITE	YEAR[a]	REFERENCE
United States	New Haven	1933	2
		1958	3
		1966	4
		1981	5
		1990	6
	New York	1949	7
	Minneapolis	1956	8
	Nashville	1961	9
	Baltimore	1965	10
	Los Angeles	1981	11
	Indianapolis	1982	12
	Philadelphia	1985	13
	Kansas City	1987	14
Canada	Montreal	1985	15
Europe	Finland	1985	16
		1989	17
	Liverpool	1985	18
	Göttingen	1985	19
	Götegorg	1990	20
	London	1981	21
		1991	22
	Mallorca	1993	23
	Denmark	1991	24
	Norway	1998	25
Middle East	Tel Aviv	1983	26
Africa	Nigeria	1984	27
	Ethiopia	1997	28
	South Africa	1998	29
Asia	Hyderabad	1985	30
Australia		1997	31

[a]Year of publication.

gens. Although there is a wide genetic diversity of human commensal isolates of *E. coli*, strains causing neonatal pathology are due to a limited number of clones.[43]

One of the capsular antigens of *E. coli*, K1, is uniquely associated with neonatal meningitis.[44-46] K1 antigen is an acidic polysaccharide that is immunochemically similar to the capsular antigen of group B *N. meningitidis*. McCracken and co-workers found K1 strains in the blood or cerebrospinal fluid (CSF) of most (65 of 77) infants with meningitis related to *E. coli*. These strains were also cultured from the blood of some infants (14 of 36) and adults (43 of 301) with sepsis but without meningitis.[43] The K1 capsular antigen was present in 88% of 132 cases of neonatal meningitis caused by *E. coli* in The Netherlands.[40] K1 antigen was related not only to invasive disease but also to a more severe outcome: those infants with meningitis caused by K1 strains had significantly higher mortality and morbidity rates

TABLE 21–4
Bacteremia in Finnish Neonates Related to Times of Onset of Signs and Mortality

	MORTALITY FOR ONSET OF SIGNS AT					
	<24 hr		24 hr–7 d		8–20 d	
ORGANISM	No. Died/Total	%	No. Died/Total	%	No. Died/Total	%
Group B streptococci	28/93	30	0/26	0	1/11	0
Escherichia coli	8/26	31	14/45	31	3/10	30
Staphylococcus aureus	3/14	21	7/64	11	1/12	8
Other	15/47	32	9/55	16	4/7	57
Total	54/180	30	30/190	16	9/40	23

Data from Vesikari R, Janas M, Gronroos P, et al. Neonatal septicemia. Arch Dis Child 60:542–546, 1985.

TABLE 21–5
Bacteremia in Finnish Neonates Related to Birth Weight and Mortality

| | MORTALITY FOR ONSET OF SIGNS AT | | | | | |
| | <1500 g | | 1500–2500 g | | >2500 g | |
ORGANISM	No. Died/Total	%	No. Died/Total	%	No. Died/Total	%
Group B streptococci	11/15	73	10/36	20	8/79	10
Escherichia coli	11/15	73	8/19	42	6/47	13
Staphylococcus aureus	4/9	44	4/26	15	3/55	5
Other	12/18	67	7/21	33	9/70	13
Total	38/57	67	29/102	28	26/251	10

Data from Vesikari R, Janas M, Gronroos P, et al. Neonatal septicemia. Arch Dis Child 60:542–546, 1985.

than did infants with meningitis caused by non-K1 strains.[45] The severity of the disease was directly related to the presence, amount, and persistence of K1 antigen in the CSF. Strains of *E. coli* with K1 antigens were isolated from cultures of stool of 7 to 38% (varying with time and location of the study) of normal newborns and from approximately 50% of nurses and mothers of the infants.[46, 47] The K1 strains were present in the birth canal of mothers and subsequently in cultures from their newborns, indicating that the infants acquired the organisms during birth.[47, 48] High rates of carriage of K1 strains by nursery personnel indicate that postnatal acquisition of the K1 strains may also occur in the nursery.[46, 47]

Pili or fimbriae are filamentous surface appendages that may play a role in the pathogenesis of disease caused by *E. coli*.[49] Pili assist adherence of *E. coli* to epithelial cell surfaces, an initial step in the development of invasive disease. Fimbriated strains of *E. coli* have been asso-

ciated with infections of the urinary tract in infants (see Chapter 24). The epidemiology of fimbriated *E. coli* and the relationship of these strains to fecal colonization of neonates and development of extraintestinal infections are discussed in a monograph by Tullus.[50]

Group B Streptococci

Group B beta-hemolytic streptococci were implicated in human disease shortly after the precipitin-grouping technique came into use.[51] Neonatal sepsis caused by this organism then became recognized as a clinical entity, but at first only a few sporadic cases were reported.[3, 52] However, in an 18-month period beginning in December 1961, group B streptococci were the most common organisms responsible for neonatal sepsis at the Boston City Hospital.[53] Since the report from the Boston City Hospital, group B streptococci have been identified throughout the United States and Western Europe as

TABLE 21–6
Microbiology of Neonatal Sepsis at Yale–New Haven Hospital, 1979–1988

| | NO. OF ISOLATES | | | | |
| | Age When Cultured (days) | | | Transported Infants | Total |
MICROORGANISM	0–4	5–30	>30		
Staphylococcus aureus	1	4	4	5	14
Coagulase-negative staphylococci	1	10	10	12	33
Group B streptococci	51	4	3	6	64
Enterococcus species	4	7	3	4	18
Viridans streptococci	2	3	2	4	11
Streptococcus pneumoniae	2	0	0	0	2
Listeria monocytogenes	2	0	0	0	2
Escherichia coli	13	17	6	10	46
Klebsiella pneumoniae	0	3	8	7	18
Enterobacter cloacae	1	1	3	2	7
Pseudomonas aeruginosa	0	1	3	2	6
Haemophilus influenzae	7	0	0	1	8
Candida species	0	2	5	4	11
Miscellaneous	9	2	6	10	27
Total	93	54	53	67	267

From Gladstone IM, Ehrenkranz RA, Edberg SC, Baltimore RS. A ten-year review of neonatal sepsis and comparison with the previous fifty-year experience. Pediatr Infect Dis J 9:819, 1990, with permission.

TABLE 21-7
Bacteria Associated with Neonatal Meningitis in Selected Studies

ORGANISM	NO. OF CASES OF ASSOCIATION								
	Boston (27)[a] 1932–1957 77 Cases	Cincinnati (28) 1948–1959 26 Cases	Los Angeles (29) 1963–1968 125 Cases	Dallas (30) 1966–1972 51 Cases	Houston (31) 1967–1972 51 Cases	Multihospital Survey[b] (32) 1971–1973 131 Cases	The Netherlands (33) 1976–1982 280 Cases	Great Britain (21) 1985–1987 329 Cases	Dallas (34) 1969–1989 257 Cases
Beta-hemolytic streptococci (group not stated)	9	5	12						
Beta-hemolytic streptococci									
Group A					1	2			
Group B				10	18	41	68	113	134
Group D				3		2	4		
Staphylococcus epidermidis	12	1	5			3		9	
Staphylococcus aureus	7	1	1		3	1	7	4	
Streptococcus pneumoniae			4		3	2	6	21	
Listeria monocytogenes	3	3	6	7	5	7	12	21	18
Escherichia coli	25	4	44	21	16[c]	50	132	2	42
Pseudomonas aeruginosa	4		1		2	2	4	3	
Klebsiella and Enterobacter species	3	3	13	4	[c]	3	19	8	10
Proteus species	2	1	5			4	5	8	3
Haemophilus influenzae	1	1	2		2	3	2	12	
Neisseria meningitidis						1	3	14	
Salmonella species	2		4	3		3	3	2	4
Miscellaneous	12	7	28	3	1	7	15	32	46

[a]Numbers in parentheses are reference numbers.

[b]Survey of 16 newborn nurseries participating in neonatal meningitis study of intrathecal gentamicin under the direction of Dr. George McCracken, Jr.

[c]Authors note 16 cases related to enteric bacteria including E. coli, Proteus species, and Klebsiella–Enterobacter group.

a major cause of invasive disease in the neonate (see Chapter 26).

Streptococcus agalactiae, the species designation of group B streptococci, has a characteristic colonial morphology on suitable solid media. The organism produces a mucoid colony with a narrow zone of beta-hemolysis on plates of fresh beef heart infusion agar containing 10% sheep's blood. A double hemolytic zone is characteristic of colonial growth on pour plates. The group B organisms can be differentiated immunochemically on the basis of their type-specific polysaccharides. Types Ia, Ib, Ic, II, and III have been distinguished, and most human strains can be classified into one of these types.

Group B streptococci have been isolated from various sites and body fluids including throat, skin, wounds, exudates, stool, urine, cervix, vagina, blood, joint fluid, and CSF. The organisms are commonly found in the genital tract of adult women and on the skin and in the upper respiratory tract of newborns.

Patterns of early-onset and late-onset disease have been associated with these organisms (see Table 21–1). The early-onset disease presents as a multisystemic illness with rapid onset during the first week of life and is frequently characterized by severe respiratory distress. The pathogenesis is presumed to be similar to that of other forms of early-onset sepsis of neonates. Isolates may belong to any of the five serotypes of group B streptococci. The mortality rate is 5% to 50% (higher mortality occurred in early studies).

Clinical manifestations of late-onset neonatal sepsis are more insidious than those of early-onset disease, and meningitis is usually a part of the clinical picture. Many of the infants are products of a normal pregnancy and delivery and have no problems in the nursery. The pathogenesis is obscure in most cases. It is also uncertain whether the group B *Streptococcus* was acquired at the time of birth and carried until disease developed or was acquired after delivery from the mother, other newborns, or nursery personnel. Almost all strains belong to serotype III. The mortality rate, 10 to 20%, is lower than that for early-onset disease.

In addition to sepsis and meningitis, other manifestations of neonatal disease caused by group B streptococci include pneumonia, empyema, facial cellulitis, ethmoiditis, orbital cellulitis, conjunctivitis, osteomyelitis, suppurative arthritis, and impetigo. Bacteremia without systemic or focal signs of sepsis may occur. Group B streptococcal infection in pregnant women may result in peripartum infections including chorioamnionitis, septic abortion, peripartum sepsis, and toxic shock syndrome.[54]

Group A Streptococci

Streptococcal puerperal sepsis has been recognized as a cause of morbidity and mortality among parturient women since the sixteenth century.[55–59] Group A streptococcal infection in the neonate is now reported infrequently[60–71] but may occur in epidemic form in nurseries.[60–64] The re-emergence of virulent group A streptococcal infections including invasive disease and toxic shock syndrome has been reflected in an increasing number of case reports of severe disease in the pregnant woman and her newborn.

Group A streptococcal disease in the mother can affect the fetus of newborn in three clinical patterns: first, maternal streptococcal bacteremia during pregnancy can lead to in utero infection resulting in fetal loss or stillbirth; second, acquisition of group A streptococci from the maternal genital tract can cause early-onset neonatal disease similar to early-onset group B streptococcal disease; and third, the fetus can be affected by transplacentally acquired group A streptococcal toxins resulting from maternal infection. In the first form of disease, previously healthy pregnant women presented with influenza-like signs and symptoms that rapidly progressed to disseminated intravascular coagulopathy and shock; four of five women died; stillbirth or fetal loss occurred in three cases; one neonate developed group A streptococcal sepsis and recovered; and a fifth infant was unaffected.[72–74] In the second form of disease, early-onset group A streptococcal infection in the neonate was acquired from maternal genital or pharyngeal infection and was frequently fatal. A review by Greenberg and colleagues[75] of 15 cases of neonatal sepsis due to group A streptococci reported between 1976 and 1999 identified nine cases of early-onset sepsis (three deaths) and six cases of late-onset sepsis (one death).

The third manifestation of fetal or neonatal group A streptococcal disease is due to production of toxins transferred across the placenta to the fetus. Babl and colleagues described the case of a woman who had bacteremia due to group A *Streptococcus* at term, extensive infection of the placenta, and a toxic shock syndrome leading to disseminated intravascular coagulopathy (personal communication, 1999). A severely depressed but uninfected infant was delivered by cesarean section with resulting hypoxic encephalopathy. Presumably, the infant was affected by transplacental passage of streptococcal toxins. The virulence factors produced by group A streptococci that are important in the systemic toxicity characteristic of streptococcal toxic shock syndromes are largely the extracellular toxins, such as pyrogenic exotoxin A, B, and C, mitogenic factor, and streptococcal superantigen. These toxins have the ability to induce cytokine production by monocytes and lymphocytes through superantigen mechanism. The result is T cell proliferation with production of interleukin-2, interferon-γ, and tumor necrosis factor-β.[76–79] It is not clear if the immune system of a fetus or neonate is sufficiently mature to respond to superantigens with subsequent cytokine production or whether the effect on the fetus was due to cytokines produced on the maternal side of the placenta and passed to the fetal circulation.

In addition to sepsis, meningitis, and toxin-mediated disease in the neonate, focal infections including cellulitis, omphalitis, Ludwig's angina,[80] pneumonia, and osteomyelitis have been reported. Because all group A streptococci are susceptible to β-lactam antibiotics, the current programs for prevention or treatment of infections due to group B streptococci are also applicable for infections due to group A streptococci.

Streptococci Other than Groups A and B

Group C streptococci have been associated with puerperal sepsis, but neonatal sepsis and meningitis related to these organism are rare.[81–83]

Group G streptococci are an infrequent cause of neonatal sepsis and pneumonia.[84-90] However, group G streptococci were isolated from the blood of seven neonates during a 5-year period beginning in 1974 at New York Hospital.[89] Maternal intrapartum transmission is the likely source for most cases, and concurrent endometritis and bacteremia in mother and sepsis in the neonate have been reported.[87] Dyson and Read[89] found very high rates of colonization in neonates born at New York Hospital in a 1-year survey of discharge cultures in 1979; the monthly incidence of cultures of group G streptococci from the nose and umbilicus varied between 41% and 70%. During this period, group B streptococcal colonization was only 1 to 11%.[89] Auckenthaler and colleagues[91] reviewed the literature about group G streptococcal bacteremia, including invasive disease in newborns.

Enterococci are now considered taxonomically separated from group D streptococci and a unique species. However, much of the earlier literature about neonatal sepsis combined enterococci (*Streptococcus faecalis* and *Streptococcus faecium*) and nonenterococci (*Streptococcus bovis* and *Streptococcus mitis*) and because of this historical context the two groups are considered together in this section. Enterococci are differentiated from nonenterococci by their ability to grow in 6.5% NaCl broth and to withstand heating at 60° C for 30 minutes. In general, enterococci are resistant to cephalosporins and relatively resistant to penicillin G and ampicillin and require the synergistic activity of a penicillin and aminoglycoside for maximal bactericidal action; nonenterococcal strains are susceptible to penicillin G, ampicillin, and most cephalosporins. Vancomycin-resistant enterococci have been reported from neonatal intensive care units and raise concerns about efficacy of antimicrobial agents currently approved for use in neonates.[92] Use of high doses of ampicillin is one option, but other drugs may be suggested by the susceptibility pattern (see Chapter 35). New agents, such as the streptogramin combination of quinupristin and dalfopristin and the oxazolidinone linezolid, are effective against vancomycin-resistant enterococci. However, no pharmacokinetic data are available to guide use in neonates. Most cases of group D streptococcal sepsis in the neonate are caused by *S. faecalis*, with a smaller number caused by *Enterococcus faecalis* and *S. bovis*[93-98]; rare cases are caused by *S. mitis*.[99, 100] In the 4 years beginning in 1974, 37 cases of group D streptococcal sepsis (including 30 related to enterococci and 7 to nonenterococcal strains) occurred in 30,059 deliveries at Parkland Memorial Hospital in Dallas. During this period, group D streptococci were second to group B streptococci (99 cases) as a cause of neonatal sepsis and were more common than *E. coli* (27 cases).[93] The clinical presentation in most cases was similar to that of early-onset sepsis.[95] In infants with respiratory distress, the chest radiographs were similar to those showing the hyaline membrane pattern of group B streptococcal infection. Enterococcal bacteremia occurred in 56 infants at Jefferson Davis Hospital in Houston, Texas, in the 10 years beginning January 1977 with the following features: early-onset presentation was a mild illness with respiratory distress or diarrhea; late-onset infection was often severe with apnea, bradycardia,

shock, and increased ventilatory requirements; and many cases were nosocomial.[101] Series of cases of neonatal sepsis or meningitis, or both, due to group D streptococci (including enterococci) have also been reported from Children's Hospital Medical Center of Cincinnati (13 cases from 1970 to 1976),[102] from the Hospital for Sick Children in Toronto (9 cases from 1985 to 1989),[103] and from New York Hospital/Cornell Medical Center (138 episodes of enterococcal bacteremia from 1974 to 1993).[92] Group D enterococci have also been recovered from CSF[93, 97] and from urine[93] in infants with sepsis. Outbreaks of bacteremia and meningitis related to *S. faecium* were reported from the neonatal intensive care units at the Medical College of Virginia[104] and Children's Hospital of Denver.[105]

Viridans streptococci are a heterogeneous group of alpha and nonhemolytic streptococci that are part of the normal mouth flora of infants and children. There are several classification schemata for these streptococci, and they may bear different designations in the literature. Viridans streptococci accounted for 23% of isolates from cultures of blood and CSF obtained from neonates in 1978 at the Jefferson Davis Hospital in Houston.[106] Only group B streptococci were more common (28%) as a cause of neonatal sepsis. Most infants had early-onset infection with signs similar to those of sepsis caused by other pathogens, but 22.6% had no signs of disease. One infant had meningitis. The case-fatality rate was 8.8%. Sepsis related to viridans streptococci has also been reported from Finland,[16] Liverpool,[17] Indianapolis,[13] and Montreal.[15]

Listeria monocytogenes

The prevalence of *Listeria monocytogenes* in packaged meat products and the danger to immunocompromised patients and pregnant women has been documented again in a 1998–1999 outbreak involving 72 cases in 14 states that occurred due to a rare strain of *L. monocytogenes* serotype 4b; the cases included 11 deaths in adults and miscarriages in five pregnant women.[107] *Listeria* can be found in unprocessed animal products, including milk, meat, poultry, cheese, ice cream, and processed meats, as well as on fresh fruits and vegetables. Most people exposed to *Listeria* do not develop illness, but the pregnant woman may suffer pregnancy loss and the neonate may develop sepsis and meningitis. Neonatal disease due to *Listeria* is discussed in Chapter 27.

Staphylococcus aureus and Staphylococcus epidermidis

S. aureus and *S. epidermidis* colonize skin and mucosa. Isolation of *S. aureus* from tissue, blood, or other body fluid is usually clearly associated with disease. Most episodes of sepsis due to *S. aureus* are hospital acquired, and mortality remains high (23% among 216 Swedish neonates with *S. aureus* bacteremia during the years 1967 to 1984), with low birth weight as the most important risk factor.[108] Disease in newborn infants caused by *S. aureus* and *S. epidermidis* is discussed in Chapter 30.

The apparent increased incidence of *S. epidermidis* sepsis[12, 109] has been associated with increased survival of very small premature infants with immature immune systems and with the introduction of invasive procedures for maintenance and monitoring of the infants, including long-term vascular access devices. Because *S. epidermidis* is present on the skin, isolation of the organism from cultures of blood may represent skin contamination but may also be an important episode of bloodstream invasion. A repeat culture of blood may assist in differentiating contamination from bloodstream invasion. The significance of a laboratory report of a positive blood culture of *S. epidermidis* is discussed later in the section Microbiologic Techniques.

Most hospital-acquired strains of *S. epidermidis* produce β-lactamase, and many are also resistant to β-lactamase–resistant penicillins. In nurseries with a significant incidence of invasive disease caused by *S. epidermidis*, initial antibiotic regimens must include a drug with uniform efficacy against these organisms, such as vancomycin.[110]

Many cases of sepsis caused by *S. epidermidis* are associated with the use of vascular catheters. *S. epidermidis* can adhere to and grow on surfaces of synthetic polymers used in the manufacture of catheters. Strains obtained from infected ventricular shunts or intravenous catheters produce a mucoid substance (a slime or glycocalyx) that stimulates adherence of microcolonies to various surfaces in the environment and on epithelium.[111] In addition to this adhesin function, the slime may protect staphylococci against antibiotics and host defense mechanisms such as opsonophagocytosis. Parenteral nutrition with a lipid emulsion administered through a venous catheter with organisms adherent to the polymer provides nutrients for growth of the bacteria leading to invasion of the bloodstream when the organisms reach an inoculum of sufficient size.[112]

Three cases of fatal sepsis caused by *S. epidermidis* occurred in VLBW infants with cytomegalovirus infection. At autopsy, the bacteria were cultured from the blood, spleen, and meninges. These cases suggest that concurrent cytomegalovirus infection may further suppress immune functions in the neonate and lead to increased virulence of the bacterial infection.[113]

Anaerobic Bacteria

Improvements in techniques for isolation and identification of the various genera and species of anaerobic bacteria have provided a better understanding of the anaerobic flora of humans and their role in disease.[114] With the exception of *Clostridium tetani* and *Clostridium botulinum*, all of the anaerobic bacteria belong to the normal flora of humans. Anaerobes are present on the skin, in the mouth, in the intestines, and in the genital tract. They account for the greatest proportion of the bacteria of the stool. All are present in the intestines, and all but *Actinomyces* species have been isolated from the external genitalia or vagina of pregnant and nonpregnant women.[115–117] Newborns are colonized with these organisms during or just before delivery. A review of the literature on neonatal bacteremia due to anaerobic bacteria by Brook in 1992 included 179 cases with a 26% mortality.[118] *Bacteroides* and *Clostridium* species were the most frequent isolates.

Anaerobic bacteria have been isolated from the blood of newborns with sepsis,[119–125] from various organs at autopsy,[119] from an infant with an adrenal abscess,[126] from an infant with an infected cephalhematoma,[127] and from infants with necrotizing fasciitis of the scalp caused by placement of a scalp electrode.[128] Feder reviewed meningitis caused by *Bacteroides fragilis*; seven of nine reported cases occurred in neonates.[129]

The incidence of neonatal sepsis caused by anaerobic bacteria remains uncertain, but data are available from some surveys: the proportion of bacterial sepsis related to anaerobes was 7.5% in Baltimore,[122] 8.7% in St. Louis,[121] 23% in San Francisco,[123] and 26% (including 8 of 23 isolates from cord blood) in Torrance, California.[125] Noel and colleagues identified 29 episodes of anaerobic bacteremia in neonates in the intensive care unit at New York Hospital during 18 years.[130] Chow and co-workers[119] analyzed 59 cases of systemic neonatal infection associated with anaerobic pathogens and classified them into four groups: transient bacteremia after premature rupture of membranes and maternal amnionitis; sepsis after postoperative complications; fulminant septicemia (in the case of clostridial infections); and intrauterine death associated with septic abortion. An additional 23 infants with anaerobic bacteremia were seen in a 3½-year period at Harbor General Hospital in Torrance, California. Of these 23 infants, organisms were isolated from peripheral blood in 15 and from cord blood in 8. The clinical presentation of anaerobic sepsis was similar to that of other types of sepsis in the newborn.

Infections caused by *Clostridium* species may be localized, as in the case of omphalitis,[131] cellulitis, and necrotizing fasciitis,[132] or may occur as sepsis or meningitis.[125] Disease in neonates has been related to *Clostridium perfringens*, *C. septicum*, *C. sordellii*, *C. butyricum*, *C. tertium*, and *C. paraputrificum*.[133] The presenting signs are usually similar to those of other forms of bacterial sepsis. Chaney reported a case of bacteremia caused by *C. perfringens* in mother and child in which the neonate had classic features of adult clostridial sepsis, including active hemolysis, hyperbilirubinemia, and hemoglobinuria.[125] Motz and colleagues reviewed five cases of clostridial meningitis due to *C. butyricum* and *C. perfringens*.[134]

The mortality rate of sepsis caused by anaerobic bacteria was low in Torrance (1 of 23 cases)[119] and in the small series from Baltimore (none of 4 cases),[122] but it was high in the series reported from St. Louis (three of eight infants died).[121] Also, two deaths occurred in three infants with *Bacteroides* sepsis in Santa Clara, California.[120] Clostridial sepsis is accompanied by a high mortality rate.[125]

Neonatal tetanus is caused by the gram-positive anaerobic spore-forming bacillus *C. tetani*. The organism is present in soil and may be present in human and animal feces. Infection usually occurs after contamination of the umbilical stump, which may result from unsanitary deliveries outside the hospital. In the United States, tetanus of the newborn is rare.[108] Five infants with neonatal tetanus were admitted to Baylor Affiliated Hospitals in Houston in the 30-month period beginning in October 1975.[135] Since 1984, only three cases of neonatal tetanus have been reported in the United

States.[136] The most recent case, reported from Montana in 1998, was an infant born to an unimmunized mother; the parents used a *C. tetani*–contaminated clay powder to accelerate drying of the umbilical cord. The use of this product had been promoted on an Internet site on "cord care" for use by midwives.[137]

In contrast to the United States, most cases of tetanus worldwide occur in neonates. In developing countries, the incidence and mortality of neonatal tetanus remain high.[138–141] In a rural area of Colombia, the rate of tetanus neonatorum was 11.6 per 100 births in the 1960s. In Juba, in southern Sudan, neonatal tetanus affects 1 of every 82 liveborn infants.[137] The mortality rate of neonatal tetanus in Djakarta in 1982 was 6.9 per 1000 live births; the mortality rate in island provinces of Indonesia was 10.7 per 1000 live births.[139] The mortality rate in areas of India and Iran is 72 and 64%, respectively. With early medical intervention, including use of intermittent positive pressure and muscle relaxants, the mortality has decreased to 10%.[142]

The mortality in neonates with tetanus in Lima, Peru, was 45% and was not improved with use of intrathecal tetanus antitoxin.[143] A meta-analysis of intrathecal therapy in tetanus suggested benefit for adults but not neonates.[144]

Application of contaminated materials to the umbilical cord is associated with deep-rooted customs and rituals in developing countries. A case-control study to identify risk factors for neonatal tetanus in rural Pakistan identified application of ghee (the clarified butter from the milk of water buffaloes or cows) to the umbilical wound as the single most important risk factor.[145] Although commercial ghee is available in Pakistan, the ghee used in rural areas is made at home from unpasteurized milk. Oudeslys-Murphy notes that application of some materials, including ghee and a stone wrapped in wet cloth, increased the risk of neonatal tetanus among Yoruba women but that other practices of cord care decreased the incidence, including searing of the cord with heat in China during the Ming dynasty and use of a candle flame to scar the cord in Guatemala.[146]

Neonatal tetanus is a preventable disease; use of sanitary techniques at delivery and a program of tetanus toxoid immunization of children and young adults, particularly of women in the childbearing years, are effective in eliminating the cause of the disease.[146–150]

Neisseria meningitidis, Haemophilus influenzae, and Streptococcus pneumoniae

Although *N. meningitidis*, *H. influenzae*, and *S. pneumoniae* are the most frequent causes of bacteremia and meningitis in infants and children, they are relatively uncommon in newborns. However, a survey of the age-specific incidence of bacterial meningitis in the United States for the years 1978 to 1981 indicated that meningitis caused by each of these three organisms is more common in the first month of life than any time after 2 years of age (Table 21–8). A survey of invasive disease reports from acute care hospitals in four states in 1995 identified the following incidence of cases in infants younger than 1 month per 100,000 for these pathogens: *H. influenzae* = 78.4, *S. pneumoniae* = 94.1, and *N. meningitidis* = 0. These data may be contrasted to the incidence of group B streptococci = 1984 and that of *L. monocytogenes* = 39.2.[151]

N. meningitidis may colonize the female genital tract[152, 153] and has been associated with pelvic inflammatory disease.[154] The infant may be infected at delivery by organisms present in the genital tract, or intrauterine infection may occur during maternal meningococcemia.[155] Meningococcal sepsis is rare in the neonate, but 45 cases (including 13 from the preantibiotic era) have been described.[156, 157] Both early-onset and late-onset forms[152, 153, 158] of meningococcal sepsis in neonates have been reported. Purpura similar to that of meningococcemia in older children was noted in a 15-day-old child.[158]

H. influenzae appears to be an increasing cause of maternal sepsis and neonatal sepsis and meningitis.[159–167] Most strains were nontypable; only 6% of 102 maternal, neonatal, and genital strains reviewed by Wallace and colleagues[163] were type b. The paucity of cases due to *H. influenzae* type b has been assumed to be due to protection provided to the fetus by the mother from passively transferred anticapsular antibody.[166, 167] *H. influenzae* type c is a rare cause of sepsis.[168] Four clinical syndromes have been associated with neonatal disease caused by *H. influenzae*: sepsis/respiratory distress syndrome; meningitis; soft tissue or joint infection; and otitis media/mastoiditis. The overall mortality rate was 5.5% among 45 cases reviewed by Friesen and Cho[167]; the mortality rate was 90% for 20 infants of gestational age younger than 30 weeks. Clinical and epidemiologic characteristics were similar to those of neonatal disease caused by group B streptococci, including early-onset (within 24 hours of birth) and late-onset presentations, signs simulating respiratory distress syndrome, and a high mortality rate. Autopsy of infants with bacteremia related to *H. influenzae* and signs of respiratory distress syndrome revealed hyaline membranes with gram-negative coccobacilli within the membranes similar to findings of hyaline membranes due to group B streptococci.[160] Examination of placentas from mothers of infants with sepsis caused by nontypable *H. influenzae* revealed acute chorioamnionitis and acute villitis in some.[161] *H. influenzae* has also been responsible for maternal disease, including bacteremia, chorioamnionitis,[169] acute or chronic salpingitis, and tubo-ovarian abscess.[163]

Neonatal sepsis caused by *Haemophilus parainfluenzae*[170, 171] and *Haemophilus aphrophilus*[172] has been reported.

Although pneumococci are isolated from cultures from the cervix or vagina of gynecologic patients or pregnant women, cases of early-onset pneumococcal sepsis in newborns have occurred that mimic neonatal disease caused by group B streptococci.[173–178] Bortolussi and colleagues[173] reported the cases of five infants with pneumococcal sepsis who had respiratory distress and clinical signs of infection in the first day of life. Three infants died, two within 12 hours of diagnosis. *S. pneumoniae* was isolated from the vagina of three of the mothers. Roentgenographic features were consistent

TABLE 21–8
Age-Specific Incidence of Bacterial Meningitis (United States, 1978–1981, per 10,000 Population)

| AGE | ORGANISM | | | | | TOTAL BACTERIAL MENINGITIS |
	Neisseria meningitidis	Haemophilus influenzae	Streptococcus pneumoniae	Group B streptococci	Listeria monocytogenes	
<1 mo	2.0	19	1.5	177	31	366
1–2 mo	18	48	19	26	1	141
3–5 mo	26	105	33	3	0.1	177
6–8 mo	13	135	18	3	0	176
9–11 mo	13	109	8		0.1	131
1–2 yr	5.8	3.9	3.2			49
3–4 yr	2.6	5.4	1.0			94
10–19 yr	1.0	0.1	0.3			1.2

Data were provided by J. Wenger, Centers for Disease Control, Atlanta. Modified from Wenger J, et al. Bacterial meningitis in the United States, 1986: report of a multistate surveillance study. J Infect Dis 162:1316, 1990, with permission.

with hyaline membrane disease or pneumonia, or both. The clinical features of these five patients had striking similarities to those of early-onset group B streptococcal infection, including the association of prolonged interval after rupture of membranes, early-onset respiratory distress, abnormal chest roentgenograms, hypotension, leukopenia, and rapid deterioration. Fatal pneumococcal bacteremia in a mother 4 weeks post partum and the same disease and outcome in her healthy term infant who died at 6 weeks of age suggested an absence of protective antibody in both mother and child.[174]

Citrobacter Species

Organisms of the genus Citrobacter are gram-negative bacilli that are occasional inhabitants of the intestinal tract and are responsible for disease in neonates and debilitated or immunocompromised patients. The genus has undergone frequent changes in nomenclature, making it difficult to relate the types identified in reports of newborn disease over the years. As an example, in 1990 Citerobacter koseri replaced Citerobacter diversus, which was eliminated as a valid species.[179] For the purposes of this section, C. koseri replaces C. diversus even though the original article may refer to the latter name.

Citrobacter species are responsible for sporadic and epidemic neonatal sepsis and meningitis, and C. koseri is uniquely associated with brain abscesses.[179–189] Neonatal disease may occur as early-onset or late-onset disease from infection acquired from the maternal birth canal. Outbreaks of C. koseri in neonatal intensive care units resulting in sepsis and meningitis, septic arthritis, and skin and soft tissue infections were reviewed by Doran.[179] Other focal infections in neonates due to Citrobacter species include bone, pulmonary, and urinary tract infections.[179]

During the period 1960 to 1980, 74 cases of meningitis caused by Citrobacter species were reported to the Centers for Disease Control of the U.S. Public Health Service.[184] In 1999, Doran reviewed an additional 56 cases of neonatal meningitis due to Citrobacter species.[179] Combining results from the two studies, brain abscess developed in 73 of 96 patients (76%) for whom informa-

tion was available. The pathogenesis of brain abscess caused by C. koseri is uncertain; cerebral vasculitis with infarction and bacterial invasion of necrotic tissues is the likely explanation.[188] Persistence of C. koseri in the central nervous system is suggested by a case report of recovery of the organism from the CSF during a surgical procedure 4 years after an episode of neonatal meningitis.[187] The case-fatality rate of meningitis due to Citrobacter species was about 30%; most of the infants who lived had some degree of mental retardation. A review of 110 survivors of Citrobacter meningitis revealed only 20 who were believed to be structurally intact and developmentally normal.[179]

Citrobacter species are usually resistant to ampicillin, variably susceptible to aminoglycosides, but usually susceptible to chloramphenicol. Most infants were treated with a combination of a penicillin or cephalosporin plus an aminoglycoside; chloramphenicol alone or in addition to the prior regimen was often administered once the microbiologic diagnosis was available. Surgical drainage has been used in some cases with variable success. Choosing antimicrobial agents with the most advantageous susceptibility pattern and selected surgical drainage appears to be the most promising approach to therapy, but no one regimen has been found to be more successful than another. Plasmid profiles, biotypes, serotypes, and chromosomal restriction endonuclease digests are useful as epidemiologic markers for the study of isolates of C. koseri. Morris and colleagues[189] used these markers to investigate an outbreak of six cases of neonatal meningitis caused by C. diversus (now C. koseri) in three Baltimore hospitals between 1983 and 1985. Identification of a specific outer membrane protein associated with strains isolated from CSF but uncommon elsewhere may provide a marker for virulent strains of C. koseri.[190]

Gardnerella vaginalis

Gardnerella vaginalis, previously known as Haemophilus vaginalis or Corynebacterium vaginalis, is a gram-negative coccobacillus that is present in the genital tract of up to one third of pregnant and nonpregnant women. The microbiology and clinical features of maternal and neonatal infections due to *G. vaginalis* are discussed in a review by Catlin.[191] The organism has been associated with nonspecific vaginitis and on rare occasion has been identified as a cause of septic abortion, endometritis, chorioamnionitis, peripartum or postpartum sepsis, and neonatal infection.[192, 193] A report from Johns Hopkins Hospital identified four infants with sepsis and congenital pneumonia who died and four infants who had mild or inapparent disease caused by *G. vaginalis*.[192] Meningitis has been reported in a 5-day-old neonate who survived without sequelae[194] and osteomyelitis as a complication of a cephalhematoma induced by a scalp electrode.[195] Pustules and cellulitis have been associated in neonates with injuries caused by the use of forceps (see Chapter 25).

Pseudomonas Species

P. aeruginosa is usually a cause of late-onset disease in infants who are presumably infected from their gut flora or from equipment, aqueous solutions, or, on occasion, the hands of health care personnel. Stevens and colleagues[12] reported nine cases of *Pseudomonas* sepsis, four of which presented in the first 72 hours of life. In three of these infants, the initial signs were those of respiratory distress, and chest radiographs were consistent with hyaline membrane disease. Noma (gangrenous lesions of the nose, lips, and mouth) has been associated with bacteremia caused by *P. aeruginosa*.[196]

P. aeruginosa conjunctivitis is of danger not only because it is rapidly destructive to the tissues of the eye but also because it may lead to sepsis and meningitis. Shah and Gallagher reviewed the course of 18 infants at Yale–New Haven Hospital newborn intensive care unit who had *P. aeruginosa* isolated from cultures of the conjunctiva during the 10 years beginning in 1986; five infants proceeded to bacteremia, including three with meningitis, and two infants died.[197]

Enterobacter Species

Among the *Enterobacter aerogenes* (synonym *Aerobacter aerogenes*) species, *E. cloacae*, *E. sakazakii*, and *E. hormaechei* have caused sepsis and a severe form of necrotizing meningitis in neonates.[198–203] *Enterobacter* septicemia was the most common nosocomial infection in neonates at the Ondokuz Mayis University Hospital in Samsun, Turkey, during the years 1988 to 1992.[204] Willis and Robinson[200] reviewed 17 cases of neonatal meningitis caused by *E. sakazakii*; cerebral abscess or cyst formation developed in 77% of the infants, and 50% of the infants died. Bonadio and colleagues reviewed 30 cases of *E. cloacae* bacteremia in children, including 10 cases in infants younger than 2 months of age.[198] Of importance is multiple drug resistance, reported in a strain of *E. cloacae* responsible for meningitis in a New Haven infant.[202]

Little is known about the source or mode of transmission of *Enterobacter* infections in the neonate. Contaminated infant formula has been identified as a source for infection.[205, 206] Parenteral nutrition and bladder catheterization were risk factors identified in 30 cases of

Enterobacter sepsis in the neonatal unit at Prince of Wales Hospital, Hong Kong.[207]

Salmonella Species

Salmonella is an uncommon cause of sepsis and meningitis in the first month of life, but a significant proportion of cases of salmonella meningitis occur in young infants. The Centers for Disease Control noted that approximately one third of 290 isolates from CSF reported during 1968 to 1979 were from patients younger than 3 months of age, and more than half were from infants younger than 1 year of age.[208] A 21-year review of gram-negative enteric meningitis in Dallas beginning in 1969 identified salmonella as being responsible for 4 of 72 cases.

Reed and Klugman[209] reviewed 10 cases of neonatal typhoid that occurred in a rural African hospital; 6 of the cases were early-onset sepsis with acquisition of the organism from the maternal genital tract, and 4 were late onset with acquisition from a carrier or an environmental source; two children developed meningitis, and three died.

Commensal Organisms

Species of bacteria and fungi that are normal flora of skin and mucous membranes may invade the bloodstream of selected infants. The bacteria include coagulase-negative *Staphylococcus* species, gram-positive rods other than *Listeria*, gram-negative cocci other than *N. meningitidis* and *N. gonorrhoeae*, and gram-positive anaerobes. The clinical significance of a blood culture positive for a commensal species is often obscure. Interpretation of culture results that identify commensal species and the management of infants with positive cultures are discussed later in the section on Diagnosis.

Mixed Infections

Multiple organisms are frequently present in brain, liver, or lung abscesses, aspiration pneumonia, or putrid empyema but are infrequently found in cultures of the blood or CSF. When several species are found, the significance of each is uncertain because it is possible that one or more of the organisms in a mixed culture is a contaminant.

Bacteremia due to more than one organism occurs in patients with immunodeficiency, major congenital abnormalities, or contamination of a body fluid with multiple organisms, as is present in peritonitis. Neonatal meningitis due to *S. pneumoniae* and *Acinetobacter calcoaceticus*[210] and sepsis due to *P. aeruginosa* and *Yersinia enterocolitica*[211] have been reported. Although included in a series of cases of neonatal sepsis by some investigators, mixed cultures are not identified by most. Mixed infections were noted by Tessin and co-workers in 5% of 231 Swedish neonates,[20] by Vesikari and associates in 4% of 377 Finnish infants,[17] and by Bruun and Paerregaard in 7% of 81 Danish neonates.[24] Faix and Kovarik reviewed the records of 385 specimens of blood or CSF submitted to the microbiology laboratories at the University of

Michigan Medical Center for the period September 1971 to June 1986: more than one organism was present in 38 specimens from 385 infants in the neonatal intensive care unit; 15 (3.9%) of the infants had multiple pathogens associated with clinical signs of sepsis or meningitis.[212] The mortality was high: 9 of the 15 infants died. Predisposing factors included prolonged rupture of membranes (> 24 hours); total parenteral nutrition; necrotizing enterocolitis; presence of vascular catheter or ventriculostomy; and disease associated with multiple pathogens, including peritonitis, pseudomembranous colitis, and hepatic necrosis. Chow and colleagues[119] reported polymicrobial bacteremia in eight newborns with anaerobic co-isolates or aerobic and anaerobic organisms in combination. An outbreak of polymicrobial bacteremia caused by *Klebsiella pneumoniae* and *E. cloacae* associated with use of a contaminated lipid emulsion was reported by Jarvis and colleagues.[213]

Mixed infections may also include bacteria and viruses. Sperra and Pacini reported mixed viral-bacterial meningitis in five patients, including neonates with CSF isolates of enterovirus and group B *Streptococcus* in a 10-day old and enterovirus and *Salmonella* in a 12-day old.[214]

Uncommon Bacterial Pathogens

Uncommon bacterial pathogens responsible for neonatal sepsis and meningitis are listed in Table 21–9, together with their references, and are reviewed by Giacoia.[215]

EPIDEMIOLOGY

Incidence of Sepsis and Meningitis

The incidence of neonatal sepsis varies from less than 1 to 8.1 cases per 1000 live births (Table 21–10).[11, 20, 23, 53, 279–283] A 2-year study beginning in January 1982 of 64,858 Atlanta infants (Table 21–11) revealed early-onset group B streptococcal disease in 1.09 of 1000 live births and late-onset group disease in 0.57 of 1000 live births.[283] The increased usage of antibiotic prophylaxis for women with suspected group B streptococcal infection or women with risk factors for infection has reduced the incidence of early-onset but not late-onset sepsis (see Chapter 26).

The incidence of meningitis is usually a fraction (approximately one fourth at the Boston City Hospital) of

---

TABLE 21–9
Unusual Pathogens Responsible for Neonatal Sepsis and Meningitis

ORGANISM	REFERENCE
Achromobacter species	Longe et al.[216]; Namnyaket et al.[217]
Acinetobacter species	Stone and Das[218]; McDonald[219]
Aerococcus viridans	Pack and Grossman[220]
Bacillus species	Doxiadis et al.[221]; Turnbullet et al.[222]; Wiedermann[223]; Patrick et al.[224], Feder et al.[225]
Borrelia species	Fuchs and Oyama[226]; Yagupsky and Moses[227]
Brucella melitensis	Singer et al.[228]; Al-Eissa and Al-Mofada[229]; Miller[230]
Burkholderia cepacia	Kahyaoglu[231]
Campylobacter species	Eden[232]; Simor et al.[233]; Goossens et al.[234]; Forbes and Scheifele[235]
Capnocytophaga species	Feldman et al.[236]; Mercer[237]; Iralu et al.[238]
Corynebacterium aquaticum	Beckwith et al.[239]
Edwardsiella tarda	Vohra et al.[240]
Escherichia hermanii	Ginsberg and Daum[241]
Flavobacterium species	Plotkin and McKitrick[242]; Linden et al.[243], Abrahamsen et al.[244]; Tizer[245]
Helicobacter cinaedi	Orlicek et al.[246]
Klebsiella species	Hill et al.[247]; John et al.[248]
Lactobacillus species	Boughton et al.[249]
Leptospira pomona	Goell et al.[250]
Leptospira icterohaemorrhagiae	Lindsay and Luke[251]
Leptospira canicola	Shaked et al.[252]
Leuconostoc species	Hardy et al.[253]; Handwerkeret et al.[254], Friedland et al.[255]; Carapetis[256]
Morganella morganii	Rowen and Lopez[257]
Pasteurella multocida	Frutos et al.[258]; Bhave and Guy[259]; Thompson et al.[260]; Clapp et al.[261]; Escande[262]
Plesiomonas (or Aeromonas) shigelloides	Pathak et al.[263]; Brenden et al.[264]; Applebaum et al.[265]
Proteus species	Burke et al.[266]
Pseudomonas pseudomallei	Osteraas et al.[267]
Pseudomonas testosteroni	Barbaro et al.[268]
Psychrobacter immobilis	Lloyd-Puryear et al.[269]
Serratia marcescens	Lewis et al.[270]; McCormack and Kunin[271]; Bollman et al.[272]
Shigella sonnei	Ruderman et al.[273]
Stomatococcus mucilaginosus	Langbaum and Eyal[274]
Staphylococcus haemolyticus	Xiao et al.[275]
Vibrio cholerae	Rubin et al.[276]
Yersinia enterocolitica	Pacifico et al.[211]; Challapalli and Cunningham[277]
Yersinia pestis	White et al.[278]

TABLE 21–10
Incidence of Bacterial Sepsis and Meningitis in Newborns

LOCATION[b]	PERIOD	NO. OF LIVE BIRTHS	NO. OF CASES	CASES PER 1000 BIRTHS		
				All	<2500 g	2500 g
Infants with Sepsis						
Leeds (284)	1947–1960	26,519	16	0.6	NS	NS
Boston (53)	1961–1963	5,421	28	5.2	NS	NS
Baltimore[c,d] (10)	1959–1963	2,906	116		40	
New York (280)	1953–1964	52,500	50	0.95	4.3	NS
New Haven (4)	1957–1965	39,283	72	1.8	NS	NS
Panorama City, Calif. (285)	1962–1987	58,256	126	2.2	18.6	1.2
Tel Aviv (26)	1978–1982	14,527	41	2.8	38[e]	0.8
Infants with Meningitis						
Chicago[c] (286)	1928–1947	7,129	12		1.6	
Cincinnati (34)	1948–1959	43,400	17	0.4	2.2	0.13
Leeds (284)	1947–1960	26,519	13	0.5	NS	NS
NIH Collaborative Study (286)	1959–1966	54,535	25	0.46	1.36	0.37
Panorama City, Calif. (285)	1962–1987	58,256	16	0.3	2.8	0.07

[a]Some infants had meningitis in addition to sepsis.
[b]Numbers in parentheses indicate reference numbers.
[c]Infants weighing less than 2500 g only.
[d]Excluding coagulase-negative staphylococci.
[e]Infants identified as premature or full term.
NS = not stated.

the number of infants with early onset sepsis. Meningitis is more frequent during the first month of life than in any subsequent period (see Table 21–6).

Characteristics of Infants Who Develop Sepsis

Host susceptibility, socioeconomic factors, obstetric and nursery practices, and the health and nutrition of mothers are all important in the pathogenesis of neonatal sepsis and meningitis. Infants who develop sepsis, particularly early-onset disease, usually have a history of one or more significant risk factors associated with the pregnancy and delivery; among these risk factors are premature delivery or low birth weight, premature rupture of membranes, prolonged time of rupture of membranes, maternal peripartum infection, septic or traumatic delivery, and fetal hypoxia.

BIRTH WEIGHT

The factor associated most significantly with bacterial sepsis and meningitis is low birth weight[32, 287–290] (see Tables 21–5, 21–10, and 21–11). Infection is the most common cause of death in VLBW infants.[291] In contrast, it is unusual for a full-term infant to develop early-onset sepsis after an uneventful pregnancy and delivery. In the Collaborative Perinatal Research Study sponsored by the National Institutes of Health,[287] low-birth-weight infants acquired meningitis three times more frequently than did term infants who weighed more than 2500 g. In a Cincinnati study,[34] meningitis was 17 times more frequent in the low-birth-weight group. The smaller the infant at birth, the higher the incidence of sepsis (see Table 21–5). In Israeli, Finnish, and American studies, the smallest infants (weighing 1000 to 1500 g) had a sepsis rate almost twice as high as that of larger infants (weighing 1500 to 2000 g) and almost eight times that of infants weighing 2000 g or more. Infants with a birth weight of less than 1000 g who lived more than 5 days and survived the physiologic problems associated with immaturity died of late-onset infection.[288] In the study of Atlanta infants (see Table 21–11), the importance of birth weight was identified for early-onset and late-onset sepsis. If VLBW infants survived the first days of life,

TABLE 21–11
Incidence and Mortality of Group B Streptococcal Disease by Birth Weight, Atlanta 1982–1983

BIRTH WEIGHT	TOTAL BIRTHS	EARLY ONSET		LATE ONSET	
		Cases (Deaths)	Cases/1000	Cases (Deaths)	Cases/1000
<1500 g	835	5 (1)	5.99	0	0
1500–2499 g	4,380	11 (2)	2.51	6 (0)	1.37
>2500 g	59,303	53 (5)	0.89	23 (0)	0.39

Modified from Schuchat A, Oxtoby M, Cochi S, et al. Population-based risk factors for neonatal group B streptococcal disease: Results of a cohort study in metropolitan Atlanta. J Infect Dis 162:672, 1990, with permission.

rates of sepsis decreased but remained a threat[283]; 16% of 2416 infants with birth weights of 501 to 1500 g who were enrolled in a study sponsored by the National Institute of Child Health developed sepsis at a median age of 17 days.[32]

RISK FACTORS IN INFANT AND MOTHER

The relative importance of other factors associated with systemic infection in the newborn is more difficult to define. Gluck and co-workers[4] noted that certain conditions were common in their series of 117 infants with sepsis: 23 (19.7%) had severely depressed respiratory function at birth and required intubation and resuscitation; 18 (15.4%) were associated with prolonged interval after rupture of maternal membranes (> 24 hours); and 17 (14.5%) were born to mothers who had peripartum infection or fever.

Attack rates of group B streptococcal sepsis in Chicago infants were affected by birth weight, duration of rupture of membranes, and occurrence of maternal fever. Infants with one of these perinatal risk factors had an attack rate of 8 per 1000 live births, compared with infants without such risk factors, who had a rate of 0.6 per 1000 live births; the mortality rate was 33% for infants with group B streptococcal sepsis plus a risk feature compared with 6% for infants with no risk features (Table 21–12).[292]

The evidence just cited notwithstanding, evaluation of the importance of the factors thought to predispose

TABLE 21–12
Relationship of Attack Rates and Fatalities of Neonatal Group B Streptococcal Early-Onset Disease to Perinatal Characteristics

CHARACTERISTIC	ATTACK RATE PER 1000 LIVE BIRTHS	% FATALITIES
Birth weight (g)		
<1000	26	90
1001–1500	8	25
1501–2000	9	29
2001–2500	4	33
>2500	1	3
Rupture of membranes (hr)		
<18	1	20
19–24	6	27
25–48	9	18
>48	11	33
Peak intrapartum temperature (°C)		
<37.5	2	29
>37.5	7	17
Perinatal risk factors		
Present	7.6	33
Absent	0.6	6
Total no. of infants = 32.384	2	26

Data from Boyer KM, Gadzala CA, Burd LI, et al. Selective intrapartum chemoprophylaxis of neonatal group B streptococcal early-onset disease: I. Epidemiologic rationale. J Infect Dis 148:795–801, 1983.

infants to neonatal sepsis requires knowledge of the frequency of these factors in all infants. A study of 483 infants at Boston City Hospital in 1970[293] showed the following incidence of factors related to sepsis:

Infants requiring resuscitation at birth: 7.7%
Mothers with temperature higher than 38.9° C (102° F) (oral) in the immediate postpartum period: 9.2%
Mothers with temperature higher than 37.8° C (100° F) (oral) in the immediate postpartum period: 38.2%

Maternal fever at or after delivery suggests a concurrent infectious event in mother and infant, but noninfectious events may be responsible for maternal fever. Use of epidural analgesia for pain relief during labor is associated with increases in maternal temperature. Intrapartum fever of more than 38° C (100.4° F) occurred an average of 6 hours after initiation of the epidural anesthesia in 14.5% of women receiving an epidural anesthetic contrasted to 1.0% of women not receiving an epidural agent; the rate of fever increased from 7% in women with labors of less than 6 hours to 36% for labors lasting longer than 18 hours. There was no difference in the incidence of neonatal sepsis in the infants born to 1045 women who received epidural analgesia (0.3%) contrasted to infants born to women who did not have epidural analgesia (0.2%).[294] Fetal core temperature may be elevated during maternal temperature elevation, and increased temperature may be present transiently in the neonate after delivery.

RACE

The Collaborative Perinatal Research Study provided information on 38,500 pregnancies[295]; selected data for white and black women are presented in Table 21–13. Black women had a higher rate of premature rupture of membranes lasting more than 24 hours (21.4%) compared with white women (10.8%); black women had a higher rate of puerperal infection (4.1%) compared with white women (3.6%); and more black infants weighed less than 2500 g at birth (13.4%) compared with white infants (7.1%).

In the study of group B streptococcal disease in Atlanta infants,[283] black infants had higher rates of disease than non-black infants; the risk of late-onset disease was 35 times the risk in non-black infants. Thirty percent of early-onset disease and 92% of late-onset disease could be attributed to black race after controlling for other significant risk factors of low birth weight and maternal age younger than 20 years. The increased incidence of group B streptococcal disease in blacks of all ages was corroborated in a survey by the Centers for Disease Control and Prevention in selected counties in California, Georgia, and Tennessee and the entire state of Oklahoma: the rate of disease was 13.5 cases per 100,000 population in blacks, significantly higher than the 4.5 cases per 100,000 population in whites; the differences were also significant for neonates—2.7 cases per 1000 live births for blacks and 1.3 cases per 1000 live births for whites.[296] Maternal factors such as socioeconomic status, nutrition, recently acquired sexually transmitted diseases, or racial differences in maternally acquired pro-

TABLE 21–13
Selected Characteristics of Women,[a] Their Pregnancies, and Newborns in the Collaborative Perinatal Study of the National Institute of Neurological Diseases and Stroke

CHARACTERISTIC	% WITH CHARACTERISTICS	
	White Women	Black Women
Premature rupture of membranes: time from rupture to onset of labor		
<8 hr	70.9	56.7
8–23 hr	18.3	21.9
24–48 hr	5.4	11.7
49+ hr	5.4	9.7
Puerperal infection	3.6	4.1
Type of delivery		
Vaginal vertex	91.7	92.4
Vaginal breech	3.3	2.6
Cesarean section	4.9	5.0
Birth weight <2500 g	7.1	13.4
Neutrophilic infiltration of:		
Amnion	9.0	7.9
Chorion	13.1	15.6
Umbilical vein	14.6	7.5

[a]Approximately 18,700 white women and 19,800 black women were evaluated. Data from reference 295.

tective antibodies may result in the increased risk of group B streptococcal disease among blacks.

SEX

A predominance of male infants is apparent in almost all studies of sepsis in the newborn but not among infants infected in utero (Table 21–14). Washburn and colleagues[298] studied infections in the fetus and newborn. The incidence of intrauterine infections (including tuberculosis, toxoplasmosis, syphilis, and listeriosis) was approximately equal in male and female infants. In contrast, bacterial sepsis and meningitis acquired during delivery or in the nursery were significantly more common in males. The greater susceptibility of the male infant is even more evident in cases of sepsis caused by gram-negative enteric bacilli than in sepsis caused by gram-positive cocci. The data for intrauterine and perinatal *Listeria* infections are of interest; intrauterine infection occurs with equal frequency in males and females, whereas perinatal infection is significantly more common in males than in females (ratio of 7:3).[298] Necrotizing enterocolitis, which is not primarily an infectious disease, occurs with equal frequency in both sexes.[299]

The usual male predominance in neonatal sepsis has suggested the possibility of a sex-linked factor in host susceptibility. A gene located on the X chromosome and involved with function of the thymus or with synthesis of immunoglobulins has been postulated.[298, 300] The female has double the number of genes affecting these factors and thus might possess a greater resistance to infection. The immunologic basis for the superior survival of female infants is reviewed by Purtillo and Sullivan.[301]

Female infants have lower rates of respiratory distress syndrome than do male infants. Torday and colleagues[302] studied fetal pulmonary maturity by determining lecithin:sphingomyelin ratios[302] and concentrations of saturated phosphatidylcholine and cortisol in amniotic fluid of fetuses between 28 and 40 weeks' gestation. Female infants had higher indices of pulmonary maturity than did male infants. These data provide a biochemical basis for the increased risk of respiratory distress syndrome in male infants, but the role of these factors of pulmonary maturation in the development of pulmonary infection remains uncertain.

GEOGRAPHIC FACTORS

The bacterial etiology of neonatal sepsis varies from hospital to hospital and from one community to another. These differences probably reflect characteristics of the

TABLE 21–14
Incidence of Fetal and Neonatal Infections by Sex

INFECTION	NO. OF INFANTS		RATIO OF MALE TO FEMALE
	Male	Female	
Intrauterine infections			
Syphilis	118	134	0.89
Tuberculosis	15	14	1.07
Toxoplasmosis	118	103	1.14
Listeriosis	26	37	0.70
Perinatal sepsis			
Gram-negative organisms	82	34	2.41
Gram-positive organisms	58	31	1.87
Perinatal meningitis			
Gram-negative organisms	126	44	2.87
Gram-positive organisms	45	39	1.15

Data based on a review of the literature and study of Johns Hopkins Hospital case records, 1930–1963.[297]

population served, including unique cultural features and sexual practices, local obstetric and nursery practices, and patterns of use of antimicrobial agents. The bacteriology of neonatal sepsis and meningitis in Western Europe[16-24, 303] (see Table 21-3) and Jamaica[304] is, in general, similar to that in the United States. In tropical areas, a different pattern is evident.[305-307] In Riyadh, Saudi Arabia, *E. coli* and *Klebsiella* and *Serratia* species were the dominant causes of neonatal sepsis; group B streptococci were infrequent causes.[308] At the University of Benin (Nigeria) Teaching Hospital between 1974 and 1982, 55 cases of neonatal meningitis were managed; a majority were due to gram-negative organisms, including *E. coli* and *Klebsiella* species.[216] In Ibadan, Nigeria, the agent most often responsible for neonatal meningitis was *Salmonella*, followed by other enterobacteria and *S. pneumoniae*.[305] In a later survey from the same hospital for 1976, *S. pneumoniae* was the most common cause of meningitis in neonates, but *Klebsiella* species and *S. aureus* were the most common causes of bacteremia.[306] *Klebsiella* was also the most frequent cause of sepsis (43 of 176 positive blood culture) in the neonatal unit at Chris Hani Baraqwanath Hospital in Johannesburg in the year beginning March 1996; group B *Streptococcus* was next in frequency (26 cases); of interest was group A streptococcal sepsis in 12 infants.[29]

Group B streptococcal disease is uncommon in Mexican infants, and Mexican women have a low rate of endocervical colonization.[309] Of interest is the report of lower rates of colonization with group B streptococci in Mexican-American women living in Los Angeles when compared with white and black women in the same community.[310] The genetic and sociocultural characteristics of the Mexican women living in Mexico City and Los Angeles are similar. The reasons for the low rate of group B streptococcal colonization and disease are uncertain but may reflect a genetic factor or differences in sexual practices, hygiene, or nutrition. In another country that is predominantly Roman Catholic—Spain—group B streptococcal infection is an important cause of neonatal sepsis[311]; this organism was the leading cause of neonatal sepsis at the Hospital Santa Creu i Sant Pau in Barcelona in 1980.[312]

SOCIOECONOMIC FACTORS

The lifestyle pattern of mothers, including cultural habits, housing, nutrition, and level of income, appears to be important in determining infants at risk of infection. The most significant factors in sepsis are low birth weight and prematurity, and the incidence of these is inversely related to socioeconomic position. Various criteria for determining socioeconomic status have been used, but no completely satisfactory and reproducible standard is available. Naeye and Blanc have analyzed income data derived from values developed by the U.S. Social Security Administration.[313] In their studies, neonates born to women from poor families had significantly more infection than infants born to women in higher income groups. Black infants had more infections than white or Puerto Rican children. Significantly fewer cases of pneumonia and splenitis were found at autopsy in children born to mothers who occupied private or semiprivate hospital suites or who had incomes significantly above the mean compared with children born to ward patients with low incomes.

PROCEDURES

Most VLBW infants have one or more procedures that place them at risk for infection. Any disruption of the protective capability of the intact skin or mucosa may be associated with infection. In a multicenter study of neonatal intensive care unit patients, increased risk of bacteremia was associated with hyperalimentation, mechanical ventilation, peripherally inserted central catheters, peripheral venous catheters, and umbilical artery catheters.[314]

Nursery Outbreaks

The nursery is a small community of highly susceptible patients cared for by many adults, including mothers, nurses, and physicians (see Chapter 34). Fathers and siblings are now encouraged to enter the nursery or mothers' hospital suites and represent an additional source of infection. Outbreaks of respiratory and gastrointestinal illness, most of which is caused by nonbacterial agents, are frequent. Spread of microorganisms to the infant occurs by droplets from the respiratory tracts of parents, nursery personnel, or other infants. Organisms may be transferred from infant to infant by the hands of nursery personnel. The greatest hazard, however, is the individual with an open or draining lesion.

Staphylococcal infection and disease are still a concern in many nurseries in the United States (see Chapter 34). In addition, epidemics associated with contamination of equipment and solutions and caused by *Proteus* species, *Klebsiella* species, *Serratia marcescens*, *Pseudomonas* species, and *Flavobacterium* have been reported. An unusual and unexplained outbreak of early-onset group B streptococcal sepsis with an attack rate of 14 per 1000 live births occurred in Kansas City during January through August 1990.[315]

The availability of markers to distinguish among bacterial strains provides an important epidemiologic tool in investigation of nursery outbreaks. In addition to antibiotic susceptibility patterns, recent technologic advances include use of biotypes, serotypes, plasmid profiles, outer membrane protein profiles, and chromosomal restriction endonuclease digests to identify strains as similar or different.[189, 232]

Antimicrobial agents play a major role in the ecology of the microbial flora in the nursery. Extensive use of these drugs helps to eliminate sensitive strains and allows proliferation of resistant strains. Thus, there is a selective pressure toward colonization by microorganisms that are resistant not only to the antimicrobial agents used in the hospital but, because of cross-resistance patterns, also to other similar drugs.

Examples of the selective pressure of systemic antimicrobial agents include the use by Gezon and co-workers of benzathine penicillin G to control an outbreak of group A streptococcal disease.[61] All infants entering the nursery during a 3-week period were treated with a single intramuscular dose. Before institution of this policy, the majority of strains of *S. aureus* in the nursery were sensitive to penicillin G. Within 1 week after initiation of the prophylactic regimen and for the next 2 years, almost all strains of *S. aureus* isolated from newborns in this nursery were resistant to penicillin G. Also, physicians in Gainesville, Florida,[316] substituted gentamicin for kanamycin to control a nursery outbreak of infections caused by gram-negative enteric bacteria with R factor–mediated resistance to kanamycin. Within a month, the number of kanamycin-resistant strains had decreased significantly, but resistance to gentamicin was noticed for the first time; within 15 months, 25% of the nursery strains were resistant to gentamicin. Development of resistance in gram-negative enteric bacilli has also been documented after use of aminoglycosides in Israel[317] and chloramphenicol in Canada.[318]

Data suggest that extensive use of third-generation cephalosporins in the nursery may lead to more rapid emergence of drug-resistant gram-negative enteric bacilli than has been identified with the standard regimen of a penicillin and an aminoglycoside. Use of cefotaxime in combination with ampicillin as usual therapy for presumed sepsis in a nursery in South Carolina led to the rapid emergence of cefotaxime-resistant *E. cloacae*.[319]

The effect of a topical agent is typified by the activity of hexachlorophene against bacterial flora of the neonate. Hexachlorophene bathing decreases staphylococcal colonization, but this chemical is ineffective against gram-negative enteric bacilli. Increased colonization by such organisms occurs in infants bathed with hexachlorophene. However, there is no evidence that the incidence of disease is increased because of gram-negative enteric bacilli in these infants.[320, 321] Nosocomial infections in the nursery and their epidemiology and management are further discussed in Chapter 34.

Unexplained Changes in the Pattern of Microorganisms in the Nursery

New strains of bacteria may appear in a nursery without changes in techniques, nursery practices, or antimicrobial use. Evans and co-workers noted marked annual variations in the prevalence of various bacteria colonizing newborns.[322] We are also still uncertain about the cause of the worldwide epidemic of *S. aureus* disease in the 1950s and equally uncertain about the reasons for its diminished importance in the 1960s. The incidence of serious infections caused by group B streptococci increased beginning in the 1960s, and there is no ready explanation for the appearance of this organism as a major cause of neonatal morbidity and mortality.

PATHOGENESIS

The developing fetus is relatively protected from the microbial flora of the mother. Procedures disturbing the integrity of the uterine contents, such as amniocentesis,[323] cervical cerclage,[324] transcervical chorionic villus sampling,[325] or percutaneous umbilical blood sampling,[323, 326] can, however, permit entry of skin or vaginal organisms, causing amnionitis and secondary fetal infection.

Initial colonization of the neonate usually takes place after rupture of the maternal membranes.[297, 327] In most cases, the infant is colonized with the microflora of the birth canal during delivery. If delivery is delayed, however, vaginal bacteria may ascend and in some cases produce inflammation of the fetal membranes, umbilical cord, and placenta.[328, 329] Fetal infection can then result from aspiration of infected amniotic fluid,[330] leading to stillbirth, premature delivery, or neonatal sepsis.[323, 329, 331, 332] The organisms most commonly isolated from infected amniotic fluid are anaerobic bacteria, group B streptococci, *E. coli*, and genital mycoplasmas.[323, 331]

Amniotic fluid is inhibitory to *E. coli* and other bacteria,[333] owing to the presence of lysozyme, transferrin, or immune globulins (IgA and IgG but not IgM) in the fluid.[332] If meconium or vernix is added to amniotic fluid in vitro, there is increased growth of *E. coli* and group B streptococci.[334–336] The implications of these findings are uncertain, but they suggest that amniotic fluid is bacteriostatic. The introduction of a small number of organisms (such as might occur during amniocentesis or placement of a fetal monitor) would be unlikely to lead to significant infection unless meconium or some other factor that promoted bacterial growth was present.[336, 337] For further information about bacterial inhibition by amniotic fluid, the reader is referred to Chapter 33.

Infection of the mother at the time of birth, particularly genital infection, can play a significant role in the development of infection in the neonate. Transplacental hematogenous infection during or shortly before delivery (including the period of separation of the placenta) is possible, although it seems more likely that the infant is infected during passage through the birth canal. Among reports of concurrent bacteremia in mother and child are cases caused by *H. influenzae* type b,[338] *H. parainfluenzae*,[171] *S. pneumoniae*,[339] group A beta-hemolytic streptococci,[340] and *N. meningitidis*[341]; and concurrent cases of meningitis have been reported as caused by *S. pneumoniae*,[342] *N. meningitidis*,[341] and group B streptococci.[343] Many infants are bacteremic at the time of delivery, which indicates that invasive infection occurred at some time ante partum.[344] Infants with signs of sepsis during the first 24 hours of life also have the highest mortality rate.[16] These data suggest the importance of beginning chemoprophylaxis for women with colonization related to group B streptococci and a risk factor for invasive disease in the neonate at the time of onset of labor rather than after delivery of the infant (see Chapter 26).[345]

Microorganisms acquired by the infant during birth colonize the skin and mucosa, including the nasopharynx and oropharynx, conjunctivae, and umbilical cord and, in the female infant, the external genitalia. The skin of infants delivered by cesarean section is sterile soon after birth, in contrast to that of infants born per vagina, who are colonized with organisms from the birth canal.[346] Normal skin flora of the newborn includes *S. epidermidis*, diphtheroids, and *E. coli*.[347] In most cases, the microorganisms proliferate at the initial site without resulting in illness. On occasion, contiguous areas may be infected by direct extension (e.g., sinusitis and otitis from upper respiratory tract colonization).

Bacteria can be inoculated through the skin by use of obstetric forceps, and organisms may infect the skin and soft tissues if abrasions or congenital defects are present. Scalp abscesses have been reported in infants who undergo scalp puncture for fetal blood sampling[348] or who have electrodes placed during labor for measurement of heart rate.[349–353] The incidence of this type of infection in the hands of experienced clinicians is, however, generally quite low (approximately 1 per 200 procedures).[349] A 10-year survey of neonatal enterococcal bacteremia discovered 6 of 44 infants with scalp abscesses as the probable source of their infection.[351] The investigators were unable, from the data available, to deduce whether these abscesses were associated with fetal scalp monitoring, intravenous infusion, or other skin trauma.

Transient bacteremia may accompany procedures that traumatize mucosal membranes. Bacteremia was identified in infants who received endotracheal suctioning; the bacteremia was present immediately after the procedure, but culture results were negative at 10 minutes.[353]

Invasion of the bloodstream may follow multiplication of organisms in the upper respiratory tract or other foci. The source for bacteremia is frequently inapparent, but careful inspection may reveal a focus, such as an infected circumcision site or infection of the umbilical stump. Metastatic foci of infection may follow bacteremia and may involve the lungs, kidney, spleen, bones, or central nervous system.

Most cases of meningitis result from bacteremia. Fetal meningitis followed by stillbirth[354] or hydrocephalus, presumably as a result of maternal bacteremia and transplacental infection, has been described but must be exceedingly rare. Although CSF leaks caused by spiral fetal scalp electrodes do occur, no cases of meningitis have been traced to this source.[355] After delivery, the meninges can be invaded directly from an infected skin lesion, with spread through the soft tissues and skull sutures and along thrombosed bridging veins,[327] but in most cases bacteria gain access to the brain through the bloodstream to the choroid plexus during the course of sepsis.[354] Infants with developmental defects such as a midline dermal sinus or myelomeningocele are particularly susceptible to invasion of underlying nervous tissue.[356]

Brain abscesses may result from hematogenous spread of microorganisms (septic emboli) and proliferation in tissue that is devitalized as a result of anoxia or vasculitis with hemorrhage or infarction. Certain organisms are more likely than others to invade nervous tissue and cause local or widespread necrosis.[356] A majority of cases of meningitis related to *C. diversus* (now *C. koseri*) and *E. sakazakii* are associated with cyst and abscess formation. Other gram-negative bacilli with potential to cause brain abscesses include *Proteus*, *Pseudomonas*, and *Serratia*.[190, 357–360] Volpe pointed out that bacteria associated with brain abscesses are those that cause meningitis and severe vasculitis.[361]

Host Factors

Infants with one or more predisposing factors (e.g., low birth weight, premature rupture of membranes, septic or traumatic delivery, fetal hypoxia, male gender, or maternal peripartum infection) are at increased risk for sepsis. Microbial factors, such as inoculum size[362] and virulence of the organism,[323] undoubtedly are significant. Immature function of phagocytes and decreased inflammatory and immune responses are characteristic of very small infants and may contribute to the unique susceptibility of the fetus and newborn (see Chapter 2).

Metabolic factors are likely to be important in increasing risk for sepsis and severity of the disease. Fetal hypoxia and acidosis may impede certain host defense mechanisms or allow localization of organisms in necrotic tissues. Infants with hyperbilirubinemia may suffer impairment of various immune functions, including neutrophil bactericidal activity, antibody response, lymphocyte proliferation, and complement functions (see Chapter 2). The indirect hyperbilirubinemia that commonly occurs with "breast-feeding jaundice" is rarely associated with neonatal sepsis.[363] Late-onset jaundice and direct hyperbilirubinemia, both of which have been observed in newborns with sepsis, are the result of the infectious process. Evidence of diffuse hepatocellular damage and bile stasis have been described in such infants.[364, 365]

Hypothermia in newborns, generally defined as a rectal temperature equal to or below 35° C (95° F), is associated with a significant increase in the incidence of sepsis, meningitis, pneumonia, and other serious bacterial disease.[366–369] In developing countries, it can represent a leading cause of death during the winter. Although frequently accompanied by abnormal leukocyte counts, acidosis, and uremia, all of which can interfere with resistance of infection, the exact cause of the increased morbidity remains poorly understood. In many cases, it is unclear whether hypothermia predisposes to, or results from, bacterial infection.

Infants with galactosemia are particularly susceptible to sepsis caused by gram-negative enteric bacilli.[370, 371] Among eight infants identified with "classic" galactosemia by routine newborn screening in Massachusetts, four had systemic infection caused by *E. coli*.[371] Three of these four infants died of bacteremia and meningitis; the fourth infant, who had an infection of the urinary tract, survived. A survey of state programs in which newborns are screened for galactosemia revealed that among 32 infants detected, 10 were known to have systemic infection and 9 died of bacteremia. *E. coli* was the infecting organism in 9 of the infants, and group D *Streptococcus* was the cause in the tenth. It appears that galactosemic neonates have an unusual predisposition to severe infection with *E. coli*. Bacterial sepsis is probably the primary cause of death among neonates with galactosemia. Depressed neutrophil function due to elevated serum galactose levels is the likely cause of the predisposition to sepsis.[372, 373]

Other inherited metabolic diseases have not been associated with a higher incidence of neonatal bacterial infection. A poorly documented increase in the "relative frequency" of sepsis has been stated to occur among infants with hereditary fructose intolerance.[374] Infants with methylmalonic acidemia and other inborn errors of branched-chain amino acid metabolism manifest neutropenia as a result of bone marrow suppression by accumulated metabolites; however, no increased incidence of infection has been described in this group of infants.[375] Shurin[372] noted that infants became ill while serum levels of galactose were high and blood levels of glucose were likely to be low and that susceptibility to infection diminished when dietary control was begun.

Iron may have an important role in the susceptibility of neonates to infection. Iron added to serum in vitro enhances the growth of many organisms, including *E. coli*, *Klebsiella* species, *Pseudomonas* species, *Salmonella* species, *L. monocytogenes*, and *S. aureus*. Iron-binding proteins, lactoferrin and transferrin, are present in serum, saliva, and breast milk. However, the newborn has low levels of these proteins.[376] Barry and Reeve demonstrated an increased incidence of sepsis in Polynesian infants who were administered intramuscular iron.[377] Prophylactic regimens of intramuscular iron dextran were administered to these infants soon after birth because of a high incidence of iron deficiency anemia. The regimen was shown to be effective in preventing anemia of infancy, but an extraordinary increase in bacterial sepsis occurred. The incidence of sepsis in newborns receiving iron was 17 per 1000 live births, whereas the incidence of sepsis in infants who did not receive iron was 3 per 1000 live births; during a comparable period, the rate of sepsis for European infants was 0.6 per 1000 live births. Special features of sepsis in the infants who received iron soon after birth were late onset of disease, paucity of adverse perinatal factors, and predominance of *E. coli* as the cause of sepsis. During the period studied, *E. coli* was responsible for 26 of 27 cases of sepsis in iron-treated Polynesian infants and for none of 3 cases of sepsis in the infants who did not receive iron. This study is similar to the experience reported by Farmer for New Zealand infants given intramuscular iron.[378] The incidence of meningitis caused by *E. coli* increased fivefold in infants who received iron and decreased when the use of iron was terminated.

Infection in Twins

The first born of twins is at higher risk of contracting ascending intrauterine infection than is the second born.[328] Pass and colleagues[379] showed that low-birth-weight twins were at higher risk for group B streptococcal infection than were low-birth-weight singletons; infection developed in 3 of 56 twin births, or 53.5 per 1000 live births, compared with 7 infections in 603 singleton births, or 11.6 per 1000. Edwards and colleagues studied group B streptococcal infection in 12 index cases of multiple pregnancies.[380] Early-onset disease occurred in both twins in one pair and in one of the pair of five others; late-onset infection occurred in both infants in two pairs and in only one twin in four others. The late-onset cases occurred closely in time: cases occurred at 19 and 20 days in one set and at 28 and 32 days in the other set.

The basis for the increased risk of infection in twins for infection acquired from the maternal genital tract includes the common features of presence of virulent organisms, absence of protective antibody, and similar genetic heritage. It seems logical that twins, particularly if monochorionic, should have high rates of simultane-

ous early-onset infection, but it is particularly intriguing that some cases of late-onset disease occur in twins almost simultaneously. Infections in twins, including disease related to *Toxoplasma gondii*, echoviruses 18 and 19, and *T. pallidum*, are discussed in other chapters (see Chapters 5, 10, and 12, respectively). Other examples of neonatal infections in twins are diseases caused by group A streptococci[381] (which includes a case report of streptococcal sepsis in a mother and infant twins) and *Salmonella* species,[382] malaria,[383] coccidioidomycosis,[384] cytomegalovirus infection,[385] and rubella.[386]

The Umbilical Cord as a Focus of Infection

The umbilical cord is a particularly common portal of entry for systemic infection in the newborn. The devitalized tissue is an excellent medium for bacterial growth, and the recently thrombosed umbilical vessels provide direct access to the bloodstream. Epidemics of erysipelas, staphylococcal disease, tetanus, and gas gangrene of the umbilicus were common in the nineteenth century. The introduction of simple hygienic measures in cord care resulted in a marked reduction of omphalitis.[387] In 1930, Cruickshank wrote, "in Prague, before antiseptic and aseptic dressing of the cord was introduced, sepsis neonatorum was as common as puerperal sepsis . . . after the introduction of cord dressing in the hospital the number of newborn children developing fever sank from 45% to 11.3%."[388, 389]

Closure of the umbilical vessels and the subsequent aseptic necrosis of the cord begin soon after the infant takes a first breath; the umbilical arteries contract, the blood flow stops, and the cord tissues, deprived of a blood supply, undergo aseptic necrosis.

The umbilical stump acquires a rich flora of microorganisms soon after birth. Within hours, it is colonized with large numbers of gram-positive cocci, particularly *Staphylococcus* species, and shortly thereafter with fecal organisms as well.[389, 390] These bacteria may invade the open umbilical wound, causing a localized infection with purulent discharge and, as a result of delayed obliteration of umbilical vessels, bleeding from the umbilical stump. From this site, infection can proceed into the umbilical vessels, along fascial planes of the abdominal wall, or into the peritoneum (Fig. 21–1).[387, 389, 391]

Although umbilical discharge or an "oozing" cord are the most common manifestations of omphalitis, periumbilical cellulitis and fasciitis are most often associated with hospitalization.[391] Infants presenting with fasciitis have a high incidence of bacteremia, coagulopathy, shock, and death.[391] Septic embolization arising from the infected umbilical vessels is uncommon but can produce metastatic foci in various organs, including the lungs, pancreas, kidneys, and skin.[387] Such emboli can arise not only from the umbilical arteries but also from the umbilical vein, because final closure of the ductus venosus and separation of the portal circulation from the inferior vena cava and the systemic circulation are generally delayed until the fifteenth to thirtieth days of life.[392]

Complications of omphalitis include a variety of infections such as septic umbilical arteritis,[387, 393] suppurative

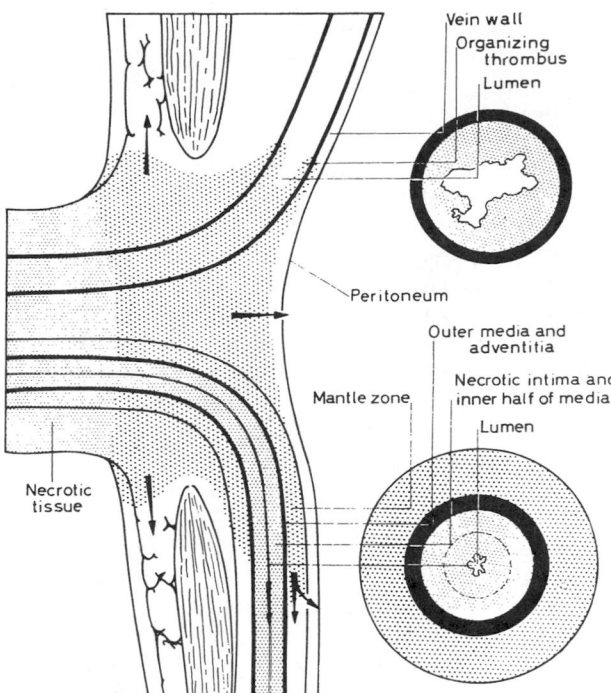

FIGURE 21–1 After birth, the necrotic tissue of the umbilical stump separates. This provokes some inflammation, which, however, is limited by fibroblastic reaction extending to the inner margin of the coarsely stippled area. The inner half of the media and the intima of the umbilical arteries become necrotic, but this does not stimulate an inflammatory reaction. Arrows indicate routes by which infection may spread beyond the granulation tissue barriers. Organisms invading the thrombus in the vein may disseminate by emboli. (From Morison JE. Foetal and Neonatal Pathology, 3rd ed. Washington, DC, Butterworths, 1970, with permission.)

thrombophlebitis of umbilical or portal veins or the ductus venosus,[393-395] peritonitis,[393, 394, 396] liver abscess, endocarditis, pylephlebitis,[397] and subacute necrotizing funisitis.[398] Some of these infections may occur in the absence of signs of omphalitis.[387, 393]

Administration of Drugs to the Mother Before Delivery

Almost all antimicrobial agents cross the placenta. Antimicrobial drugs administered to the mother at term may alter initial neonatal microflora and may impair the physician's ability to diagnose infection in the neonate. See Chapter 35 for a review of the clinical pharmacology of antimicrobial agents administered to the mother.

Several studies have shown that corticosteroids administered to mothers in anticipation of delivery to enhance pulmonary maturation in the fetus resulted in a significant decrease in incidence and severity of neonatal respiratory distress syndrome but an increase in maternal infection, particularly endometritis, when compared with a placebo.[399] A trend toward increased neonatal infection was also described among infants whose mothers received corticosteroid treatment.[399] Other investiga-

tors have found that corticosteroids administered to the mother at term had no effect on either maternal or neonatal infections.[399-402]

Substance abuse during pregnancy may affect certain immune functions in the neonate. Significant abnormalities in T cell function and an apparent increased incidence of infections have been found during the first year of life among infants born to alcohol-[403] and heroin-addicted[404, 405] mothers. The adverse effects of cocaine and opiates on placental function, fetal growth and development, and prematurity may also predispose to a greater likelihood of neonatal infection.[405, 406] Unfortunately, drug abuse is a multifactorial problem; it is virtually impossible to separate the consequences of direct pharmacologic effects on the fetus from those brought about by the inadequate nutrition, failure of prenatal care, and infectious medical complications encountered in addicted pregnant women.[405-407]

Administration of Drugs Other than Antibiotics to the Neonate

A survey of neonates who received indomethacin for closure of a patent ductus arteriosus indicates a higher incidence of sepsis in the indomethacin-treated groups compared with infants treated with surgery or other medications. The mechanism for the role of indomethacin in predisposing the low-birth-weight infant to sepsis is unknown.[408]

O'Shea described the outcomes of VLBW (500 to 1250 g) infants given dexamethasone at 15 to 25 days of age for prevention of chronic lung disease. Among 61 infants treated with tapering doses for 42 days, there was no increase in the incidence of sepsis or the number of sepsis workups when compared with a control population.[409]

A strong association between intravenous lipid administration to newborns and coagulase-negative staphylococcal bacteremia has been confirmed.[112] Although the infants studied were of low birth weight, ill, and utilizing nonumbilical central venous catheters for nutrition, administration of lipid emulsion could be isolated as an independent risk factor predisposing to bacteremia. The causes were thought to include the role of lipid as a growth medium for bacteria, mechanical blockage of the catheter by deposition of lipids in the lumen, and an effect of lipid emulsions on the function of neutrophils and macrophages.

The effects of prostaglandins and leukotrienes in the perinatal period were reviewed by Heyman.[410] Prostaglandin E_1 has been used in the management of congenital malformations in which it is critical to maintain the ductus arteriosus in a dilated position. Side effects of prostaglandin E_1 that might be confused with sepsis included temperature elevation, hypotension, and jitteriness.

PATHOLOGY

Infants with severe and rapidly fatal sepsis generally have minimal, if any, histologic indication of an infectious process.[327, 411] Findings typical of bacteremia such as multiple disseminated abscesses of similar size, purulent vasculitis, and intravascular identification of bacteria are evident in only a minority of infants.[411] Shock accompanying sepsis will sometimes cause superimposed findings, including periventricular leukomalacia and intraventricular hemorrhage, scattered areas of nonzonal hepatic necrosis, renal medullary hemorrhage, renal cortical or acute tubular necrosis, and adrenal hemorrhage and necrosis. Evidence of disseminated intravascular coagulopathy, manifested by strands of interlacing fibrin seen in the vessels or by the presence of a well-demarcated subarachnoid fibrinous hematoma, may also be present.[354, 411] The pathology of infections of the respiratory, genitourinary, and gastrointestinal tracts and focal suppurative diseases is discussed in subsequent chapters.

The pathology of neonatal meningitis[354, 412, 413] and brain abscess[414, 415] is similar to that in the older child and adult. The major features are ventriculitis (including inflammation of the choroid plexus), vasculitis, cerebral edema, infarction, cortical neuronal necrosis, and periventricular leukomalacia; chronic pathologic features include hydrocephalus, multicystic encephalomalacia and porencephaly, and cerebral cortical and white matter atrophy.[416] Significant collections of pus may be present in the sulci and subarachnoid space, particularly around the basal cisterns, of infants with meningitis. Because the fontanelles are open, exudate can collect around the base of the brain without a significant increase in intracranial pressure. Hydrocephalus may result from closure of the aqueduct or the foramina of the fourth ventricle by purulent exudate, or through inflammatory impairment of CSF resorption through the arachnoid channels.[354, 417] Ventriculitis has been described in 20 to 90% of cases[354, 356, 417] and is often the reason for persistence of bacteria in CSF and for slow clinical recovery.[418] Acute inflammatory cells infiltrate the ependymal and subependymal tissues, causing destruction of the epithelial lining of the ventricles. Hemorrhage, venous thrombosis, and subdural effusions are also often present.

Brain abscesses and cysts in the neonate are distinguished by the relatively large size of the lesions and relatively poor capsule formation. They occur most frequently in association with meningitis due to *C. diversus*, *E. sakazakii*, *Serratia marcescens*, and *Proteus* and are usually located in the cerebrum, involving several lobes.[190, 357, 360, 361] These organisms characteristically give rise to a hemorrhagic meningoencephalitis brought about by intense bacterial infiltration of cerebral vessels and surrounding tissues. The resulting vascular occlusion is followed by infarction and widespread necrosis of cerebral tissue with liquefaction and formation of multiple loculated cysts.[360, 361]

CLINICAL MANIFESTATIONS

Signs of fetal distress may be the earliest indication of infection among infants with sepsis beginning at or soon after delivery. Fetal tachycardia in the second stage of labor was evaluated as a sign of infection by Schiano and colleagues[419]: pneumonia or sepsis occurred in 3 of 8 infants with marked fetal tachycardia (> 180 beats per minute), in 7 of 32 infants with mild tachycardia (160 to 179 beats per minute), and in 1 of 167 infants with lower heart rates.

An Apgar score suggesting distress at or before delivery has also been correlated with sepsis in the newborn period. Infants delivered per vagina had a 56-fold risk of sepsis when the Apgar score was less than 7 at 5 minutes compared with infants with higher scores.[420] Among infants with rupture of the amniotic membranes for 24 hours or more, St. Geme and colleagues found a significant increase in the risk of perinatal bacterial infection among those with an Apgar score of less than 6 at 5 minutes but could find no association with fetal tachycardia (> 160 beats per minute).[329]

The Apgar score is well characterized in term infants but less so in premature infants who have the highest attack rates for sepsis. Because low Apgar scores (< 3 at 1 minute and < 6 at 5 minutes) were significantly associated with low birth weight and shorter gestational age, the use of the score is less valuable as an indicator of sepsis in premature than in term infants.[421]

The earliest signs of sepsis are often subtle and nonspecific. Poor feeding, diminished responsiveness, or just "not looking well" may provide the only evidence that infection is present. More prominent findings are respiratory distress, apnea, lethargy, fever or hypothermia, jaundice, vomiting, diarrhea, and skin manifestations, including petechiae, abscesses, and sclerema.[422]

The nonspecificity and subtle nature of signs of sepsis in newborns is even more a concern in identifying sepsis in the VLBW infant. The clinical signs of late-onset sepsis that presented in 325 infants weighing 501 to 1500 g included increasing apnea/bradycardia (55%), increasing oxygen requirement (48%), feeding intolerance, abdominal distention or guaiac-positive stools (46%), lethargy and hypotonia (37%), and temperature instability (10%). Unexplained metabolic acidosis (11%) and hypoglycemia (10%) were the most common laboratory indicators of metabolic derangement.[32]

Bonadio and co-workers attempted to determine the most reliable clinical signs of sepsis in more than 200 febrile infants aged birth to 8 weeks.[423] They found that changes in affect, peripheral perfusion, and respiratory status or effort best identified those infants with serious bacterial infection. Alterations in feeding pattern, level of alertness, level of activity, and muscle tone were often also present; however, these signs were less sensitive indicators.

Focal infection involving virtually any organ can occur in infants with sepsis. Evaluation of infants with suspected bacteremia must include a careful search for a primary or secondary focus such as meningitis, pneumonia, urinary tract infection, otitis media, septic arthritis, osteomyelitis, or peritonitis.

Serious bacterial infections are very uncommon in infants without any clinical evidence of illness,[423] even among those with risk factors for infection.[424] Occasionally, bacteremia occurs without signs.[425, 426] Albers and associates[425] described the case histories of three infants without signs of illness for whom blood cultures were performed as part of a nursery study involving 131

TABLE 21–15
Clinical Signs of Bacterial Sepsis in 455 Newborns Studied at Four Medical Centers

CLINICAL SIGN	% OF INFANTS WITH SIGN
Hyperthermia	51
Hypothermia	15
Respiratory distress	33
Apnea	22
Cyanosis	24
Jaundice	35
Hepatomegaly	33
Lethargy	25
Irritability	16
Anorexia	28
Vomiting	25
Abdominal distention	17
Diarrhea	11

Data from references 3, 4, 9 and 10.

infants. Blood was obtained from peripheral veins at different times during the first 10 days of life. The same pathogen was isolated repeatedly (three, three, and two times) from the blood of the three infants even though they remained well.[425] The infants were subsequently treated with appropriate antimicrobial agents. Bacteremia caused by group B streptococci may occur with minimal or no systemic or focal signs,[426–428] and it may be sustained over several days.[429] Almost all of these infants were born at term and had early-onset (< 7 days of age) infection. Similarly, among 44 neonates with enterococcal bacteremia, 3 of 18 (17%) with early-onset, but none with late-onset, infection appeared well.[101] The incidence of bacteremia without signs is uncertain because few cultures of blood are performed for infants who show no signs of sepsis.

Clinical signs of bacterial sepsis in 455 infants studied in four programs are presented in Table 21–15. Clinical signs of bacterial meningitis in 255 infants studied in six programs are given in Table 21–16. Noninfectious conditions that may present with clinical manifestations similar to those of sepsis are shown in Table 21–17.

TABLE 21–16
Clinical Signs of Bacterial Meningitis in 255 Newborns Studied at Six Medical Centers

CLINICAL SIGN	% OF INFANTS WITH SIGN
Hyperthermia	61
Lethargy	50
Anorexia or vomiting	49
Respiratory distress	47
Apnea	7
Convulsions	40
Irritability	32
Jaundice	28
Bulging or full fontanelle	28
Diarrhea	17
Nuchal rigidity	15

Data from references 33, 34, 287, 295, 412, 415, and 430.

Fever and Hypothermia

The temperature of the infant with sepsis may be elevated, depressed, or normal.[427–433] In a multicenter survey of almost 250 infants with early-onset group B streptococcal bacteremia, approximately 85% had a normal temperature (36° C to 37.2° C [96.8° F to 99° F]) at the time of their admission to the neonatal intensive care unit.[427] In comparing temperatures by gestational age, it was noted that term infants were more likely to have fever than preterm infants (12% versus 1%), whereas preterm infants more frequently had hypothermia (13% versus 3%). Phagocytes of the infant born after normal labor can produce adult concentrations of leukocytic pyrogen (interleukin-1). For reasons that remain unknown, the phagocytes of infants born after cesarean section have a markedly suppressed ability to make leukocytic pyrogen.[434] In the studies reviewed in Table 21–15, approximately half of the infants had fever. Hypothermia was specifically mentioned in only one study and was found in 15% of the infants.

Fever is variably defined for newborns. A temperature of 38.0° C (100.4° F) measured rectally is generally accepted as the lower limit of the definition of fever. Although some clinical studies indicate that umbilical,[435] axillary,[436, 437] skin-mattress,[436] and infrared tympanic membrane thermometry[437] are accurate and less dangerous alternatives to the rectal route for obtaining "core temperature," the reliability of these methods, particularly in febrile infants, has been questioned.[438–441] At present, the method of choice for determining the presence of fever in neonates is a rectal temperature taken at a depth of 2 to 3 cm past the anal margin for 3 minutes or until the temperature stabilizes. It has been shown that, in cases of suspected sepsis among infants without fever, a *difference* between core (rectal) and skin (sole of the foot) temperature of more than 3.5° C may be a more useful indicator of infection than measurement of core temperature alone.[433]

There is no study of temperatures in neonates that is prospective, assesses all infants (febrile and nonfebrile), includes rectal and axillary temperatures, includes premature and term infants, and uses data from cultures of blood or other body fluids to identify invasive bacterial disease. However, three studies provide useful information: Craig[442] reviewed the literature about temperature in newborns to 1962; Voora and colleagues[443] observed 100 full-term infants in Chicago with an axillary or rectal temperature of 37.8° C (100.1° F) or higher during the first 4 days of life; and Osborn and Bolus[443] did a retrospective review of 2656 full-term infants in Los Angeles. The pertinent features of the combined results may be summarized as follows:

1. Temperature elevation in full-term infants was uncommon. Approximately 1% of full-term infants had at least one episode of fever, measured as higher than 37.5° C (99.5° F) per axilla[447] or 37.8° C (100.1° F) or higher per axilla.[443]

2. Temperature elevation was infrequently associated with systemic infection when only a single elevated reading occurred. None of 32 Los Angeles infants and none of 32 Chicago infants who had only one episode of

TABLE 21–17

Differential Diagnosis of Clinical Signs Associated with Neonatal Sepsis and Some Noninfectious Conditions

Respiratory Distress (apnea, cyanosis, costal and sternal retraction, rales, grunting, diminished breath sounds, tachypnea)

Transient tachypnea of the newborn
Respiratory distress syndrome
Atelectasis
Aspiration pneumonia, including meconium aspiration
Pneumothorax
Pneumomediastinum
Central nervous system disease: hypoxia, hemorrhage
Congenital abnormalities, including tracheoesophageal fistula, choanal atresia, diaphragmatic hernia, hypoplastic lungs
Congenital heart disease
Cardiac arrhythmia
Hypothermia (neonatal cold injury)
Hypoglycemia
Neonatal drug withdrawal syndrome
Medication error with inhaled epinephrine[430]

Temperature Abnormality (hyperthermia or hypothermia)

Altered environmental temperature
Disturbance of central nervous system thermoregulatory mechanism, including anoxia, hemorrhage, kernicterus
Hyperthyroidism or hypothyroidism
Neonatal drug withdrawal syndrome
Dehydration
Congenital adrenal hyperplasia
Vaccine reaction

Jaundice

Breast milk jaundice
Blood group incompatibility
Red cell hemolysis, including blood group incompatibility, G6PD deficiency
Resorption of blood from closed space hemorrhage
Gastrointestinal obstruction, including pyloric stenosis
Extrahepatic or intrahepatic biliary tract obstruction
Inborn errors of metabolism, including galactosemia, glycogen storage disease type IV, tyrosinemia, disorders of lipid metabolism, peroxisomal disorders, defective bile acid synthesis (trihydroxycoprostanic acidemia)
Hereditary diseases, including cystic fibrosis, α_1-antitrypsin deficiency, bile excretory defects (Dubin-Johnson, Rotor, Byler, Aagenaes syndrome)
Hypothyroidism
Prolonged parenteral hyperalimentation

Hepatomegaly

Red cell hemolysis, including blood group incompatibility, G6PD deficiency
Infant of a diabetic mother
Inborn errors of metabolism, including galactosemia, glycogen storage disease, organic acidemias, urea cycle disorders, hereditary fructose intolerance, peroxisomal disorders
Biliary atresia
Congestive heart failure
Benign liver tumors, including hemangioma, hamartoma
Malignant liver tumors, including hepatoblastoma, metastatic neuroblastoma, congenital leukemia

Gastrointestinal Abnormalities (anorexia, regurgitation, vomiting, diarrhea, abdominal distention)

Gastrointestinal allergy
Overfeeding, aerophagia
Intestinal obstruction (intraluminal or extrinsic)
Necrotizing enterocolitis
Hypokalemia
Hypercalcemia or hypocalcemia
Hypoglycemia
Inborn errors of metabolism, including galactosemia, urea cycle disorders, organic acidemias
Ileus secondary to pneumonia
Congenital adrenal hyperplasia
Gastric perforation
Neonatal drug withdrawal syndrome

Lethargy

Central nervous system disease, including hemorrhage, hypoxia, or subdural effusion
Congenital heart disease
Neonatal drug withdrawal syndrome
Hypoglycemia
Hypercalcemia
Familial dysautonomia

Seizure Activity (tremors, hyperactivity, muscular twitching)

Hypoxia
Intracranial hemorrhage or kernicterus
Congenital central nervous system malformations
Neonatal drug withdrawal syndrome
Hypoglycemia
Hypocalcemia
Hyponatremia, hypernatremia
Hypomagnesemia
Inborn errors of metabolism, including urea cycle disorders, organic acidemias, galactosemia, glycogen storage disease, peroxisomal disorders
Pyridoxine deficiency

Petechiae and Purpura

Birth trauma
Blood group incompatibility
Neonatal isoimmune thrombocytopenia
Maternal idiopathic thrombocytopenic purpura
Maternal lupus erythematosus
Drugs administered to mother
Giant hemangioma (Kasabach-Merritt syndrome)
Thrombocytopenia with absent radii (TAR) syndrome
Disseminated intravascular coagulopathy
Coagulation factor deficiencies
Congenital leukemia
Child abuse

fever developed clinical evidence of systemic infection (cultures of blood or other body fluids were not obtained).

3. Temperature elevation that was sustained for more than 1 hour was frequently associated with infection. Of 7 Los Angeles infants with sustained fever, 5 had proven bacterial or viral infection. Of 65 Chicago infants, 10 had documented systemic bacterial disease.

4. Temperature elevation without other signs of infection is infrequent. Only 1 of the 5 Los Angeles infants, an infant with cytomegalovirus infection, had fever without other signs. Only 2 infants (with bacteremia caused by *E. coli* and group B streptococci) of the 10 Chicago infants with fever and proven bacterial disease had no other significant signs of infection.

In addition to infection, fever may be due to an elevation in ambient temperature, dehydration, retained blood or extensive hematoma, and damage to the temperature-regulating mechanisms of the central nervous system; the latter can result from hemorrhage, anoxia, or kernicterus. Less common noninfectious causes of fever are hyperthyroidism, cystic fibrosis, familial dysautonomia, and ectodermal dysplasia. When thermoregulatory devices that monitor and modify infant temperature are introduced, the use of fever or hypothermia as a diagnostic sign of sepsis is sometimes impeded.

Respiratory Distress

Signs of respiratory distress, including tachypnea, grunting, flaring of the alae nasi, retractions, rales, and decreased breath sounds, are common and important findings in the infant suspected of having sepsis. Respiratory distress syndrome and aspiration pneumonia must be considered in the differential diagnosis. Apnea is one of the most specific signs of sepsis but usually occurs late. Clinical signs of cardiovascular dysfunction, including tachycardia, arrhythmia, and poor peripheral perfusion, that occur in the absence of congenital heart disease are sensitive signs of sepsis.

Jaundice

Jaundice is present in approximately one third of infants with sepsis and is also a common sign in infants with urinary tract infection[445-447]; it may appear suddenly or develop slowly and steadily. Occasionally, it is the only sign of sepsis. Jaundice usually decreases in intensity after institution of appropriate chemotherapy. It occurs in septic infants irrespective of the type of bacterial pathogen.

Organomegaly

The liver edge is palpable in premature infants and may extend to 2 cm below the costal margin in normal term infants. Ashkenazi and colleagues measured the size of the liver and noted the liver edge in healthy term infants examined within 24 hours of birth and again between 72 and 96 hours.[448] Measurements ranged between 1.6 and 4.0 cm below the costal margin, and there was no

significant difference between early and late examinations. Reiff and Osborn suggested that determination of liver span by palpation and percussion is a more reliable technique for determination of liver size than identifying the liver projection below the costal margin.[449] Hepatomegaly is also a frequent sign of in utero infections, as well as of some noninfectious conditions, such as cardiac failure or metabolic diseases (including galactosemia and glycogen storage disease).

Splenomegaly is less common than hepatomegaly and is infrequently mentioned in reports dealing with bacterial sepsis of the newborn.

Lymph nodes are often palpable in newborns as young as 2 hours old. Bamji and colleagues examined 214 healthy neonates in New York and identified palpable nodes at one or more sites in one third of the infants.[450] The most common sites were inguinal (24%), cervical (17%), and axillary (6.5%). The size of the nodes ranged from 3 to 16 mm in vertical and horizontal axes. Embree and Muriithi examined 66 healthy term Kenyan neonates during the first 24 hours of life and found palpable axillary nodes (27.7%) but no palpable inguinal nodes.[451] Adenopathy may be a sign of congenital infection caused by rubella virus, *T. gondii*, *T. pallidum*, and enteroviruses. Adenitis may occur in drainage areas involved with cellulitis, but neither adenitis nor adenopathy has been identified as an important sign of systemic bacterial infection in neonates.

Gastrointestinal Signs

Gastrointestinal disturbances including anorexia, regurgitation or vomiting, diarrhea, and abdominal distention are common and significant early signs of sepsis. The first indications of illness are usually noticed by the nurse, who may observe a change in feeding pattern or inattention and lethargy during feedings.

Skin Lesions

A variety of skin lesions may accompany bacteremia, including cellulitis, abscesses, petechiae, purpuric lesions, sclerema, erythema multiforme, and ecthyma. These lesions are described in Chapter 25.

Neurologic Signs

The onset of meningitis in the neonate is accompanied by general signs similar to those of sepsis, including fever, lethargy, jaundice, respiratory distress, anorexia, vomiting, and diarrhea. Meningitis may be heralded by increasing irritability, an alteration in consciousness, poor tone, tremors, or twitching. Convulsions were present in 40% of the infants reviewed in Table 21–16, but Volpe[452] identified seizures, in many cases subtle, in 75% of cases; approximately half of the seizures were focal. Focal signs including hemiparesis, horizontal deviation of the eyes, and cranial nerve signs involving the seventh, third, and sixth nerves, in that order of frequency, may be identified.[452] Because sutures of the neonate are open, allowing for expansion of the intracranial contents and increasing head size, a full or bulging fontanelle is usually absent.[428, 453] The less mature the infant, the more likely it is that these signs will be absent. Groover and co-workers[34] reported that none of 16 premature infants with meningitis had a bulging fontanelle at any time during the illness, whereas 13 of 23 term infants with meningitis had bulging fontanelles. The presence of a bulging fontanelle is not related to gestational age; among 72 newborns with gram-negative enteric bacillary meningitis, a bulging fontanelle was noted in 18% and 17% of term and preterm infants, respectively.[356] Nuchal rigidity, an important sign in older children and adults, is very uncommon in neonates.[356]

In addition to the physical findings in infants with meningitis, several reports have noted the occurrence of fluid and electrolyte abnormalities associated with inappropriate antidiuretic hormone secretion, including hyponatremia, decreased urine output, and increased weight gain.[417, 420] On rare occasion, the onset of meningitis has been followed by a transient or persistent diabetes insipidus.[453]

Early clinical signs of brain abscess in the newborn may be subtle and are frequently unnoticed by the physician or parent. Presenting signs include signs of increased intracranial pressure (vomiting, bulging fontanelle, enlarging head size, and separated sutures), focal cerebral signs (hemiparesis, focal seizures), and acute signs of meningitis. Of six infants with brain abscesses described by Hoffman and colleagues,[414] only two were febrile and two had seizures, but five had increased head size.

Other foci of infection in the nervous system include pneumococcal endophthalmitis in a neonate with meningitis[454] and epidural abscess caused by *S. aureus* in 3-[455] and 4-week-old infants.[456, 457]

DIAGNOSIS

The diagnosis of systemic infection in the newborn is difficult to establish on the basis of clinical findings alone. A history of one or more significant risk factors associated with the pregnancy and delivery is usually present. The extensive list of conditions that must be considered in the differential diagnosis for the various signs that are associated with sepsis or meningitis and noninfectious conditions is given in Table 21–17. Laboratory tests to assist in the diagnosis of sepsis are discussed in Chapter 32.

Maternal History

Most infants who develop systemic infection at delivery are born to women who have one or more risk features. The following features are identified by the American College of Obstetricians and Gynecologists as the basis for identification of women who should receive intrapartum antibiotic chemoprophylaxis[458]:

1. Preterm labor, less than 37 weeks' gestation
2. Preterm premature rupture of membranes, less than 37 weeks' gestation

3. Fever during labor, defined by temperature of 38.1° C (100.5° F) or more, or fever subsequent to delivery
4. Multiple births
5. Rupture of membranes more than 18 hours

Microbiologic Techniques

Isolation of microorganisms from a significant source such as the blood, CSF, urine, other body fluids (peritoneal, pleural, joint, middle ear), or tissues (bone marrow, liver, spleen) remains the most valid method of diagnosing bacterial sepsis. Antigen detection techniques are available for group B streptococci (see Chapter 26). Infectious agents cultured from the nose, throat, skin, umbilicus, or stool indicate colonization and may include organisms that cause sepsis, but isolation of a microorganism from these materials does not establish the presence of active systemic infection. The limited sensitivity, specificity, and predictive value of body surface cultures in a neonatal intensive care unit was documented using a data base of 24,584 cultures from 3371 infants by Evans and colleagues.[459]

CULTURE OF BLOOD

Isolation of a pathogenic microorganism from the blood is the most specific method of diagnosis of neonatal sepsis.

Methods. Conventional broth culture remains the usual technique for detection of bacteremia, but DNA methods for rapid detection are now used in many laboratories. Campos has reviewed techniques for pediatric blood cultures including automated and semiautomated systems.[460–462]

Lysis direct plating consists of lysis of 0.5 to 1.5 ml of blood in a tube containing a cell membrane–active lysis reagent (Isolator 1.5 Microbial Tube, Dupont) followed by direct inoculation of 0.25-ml amounts to one or more agar plates. Positive cultures are recognized by growth of colonies on agar and provide a rapid means to obtain quantitative blood culture results from pediatric patients.[463] St. Geme and colleagues used this technique to investigate the distinction of sepsis from contamination in cultures of blood growing coagulase-negative staphylococci.[464]

Time to Detection of a Positive Blood Culture. Bacterial growth is evident in the vast majority of cultures of blood within 48 hours.[465] With use of conventional culture techniques and subculture at 4 and 14 hours, only 4 of 105 cultures that had positive results (one group B *Streptococcus* and three *S. aureus*) required more than 48 hours of incubation.[465] By use of a radiometric technique (BACTEC 460), 40 of 41 cultures showing group B *Streptococcus* and 15 of 16 cultures showing *E. coli* were identified within 24 hours.[466]

Optimal Number of Cultures. The optimal number of cultures to obtain for diagnosis of bacteremia in the newborn remains uncertain. It is possible that a single blood culture from an infant with sepsis will be negative. Sprunt[467] suggested the use of two blood cultures "not primarily to increase the yield of organisms. The purpose of two cultures is to minimize the insecurity and debates over the meaning of the findings." Two or more cultures of blood may yield more information than a single culture. At a minimum, one culture of blood should be obtained when sepsis is suspected and therapy is to be started as soon as possible. The debate about the value of one- or multiple-site blood cultures for diagnosing neonatal sepsis is discussed by Wiswell and Hachey.[468]

Optimal Volume of Blood. The optimal volume of blood needed to detect bacteremia in neonates has not been identified. Neal and colleagues[469] evaluated the volume of neonatal blood submitted for culture by physicians who were unaware of the study; the mean blood volume per patient was 1.05 ml. The data of Dietzman and co-workers[470] suggested that 0.2 ml of blood is sufficient to detect bacteremia caused by *E. coli* in neonates. The relationship between colony counts of *E. coli* for blood cultures from septic infants and meningitis and mortality rate in these infants is given in Table 21–18. Meningitis occurred only in infants with more than 1000 colonies per ml of blood. The mortality rate was 35% in infants with bacteremia whose colony counts were less than 1000 per ml, whereas it was 73% in infants with more than 1000 colonies per ml of blood. These data are corroborated by experimental results indicating that common pediatric pathogens can be reliably recovered from 0.5 ml of blood even when cultured at blood-to-broth ratios of 1:100.[471]

Capillary Blood Cultures. The use of capillary blood culture is of uncertain value.[472-475] Heel-stick cultures may be considered for infants with suspected sepsis who do not have available peripheral veins. However, contamination is frequent; and osteomyelitis, osteochondritis, and calcified nodules have been detected on the heels of neonates after multiple heel sticks were used to obtain blood samples (this problem is reviewed in Chapter 23).[476]

Cultures of Blood from Umbilical Vessels and Intravascular Catheters. Cultures of blood obtained from umbilical vessels have not come into general use because of the high incidence of positive results when results of cultures of peripheral venous blood are negative. However, it is possible that fastidious technique in obtaining the culture,[477-479] use of blood obtained from the umbilical artery, and use of the technique only in infants who are very young (< 9 hours of age) and therefore not extensively colonized[478] may provide reliable informa-

tion. Quantitative blood cultures using lysis direct plating techniques may also be useful in diagnosing intravenous catheter-associated infections.[480, 481]

Results of cultures of blood obtained from umbilical or Broviac indwelling catheters may present ambiguities in interpretation of results: does the positive culture represent colonization of the catheter or sepsis? Ruderman and colleagues used quantitative blood cultures to distinguish bacteremia associated with catheter colonization from catheter sepsis; infants with sepsis had higher colony counts.[480] Confusion may be avoided by obtaining blood for culture from a peripheral vein as well as through the catheter.

Distinguishing Clinically Important Bacteremia from Contamination. The increased use of intravascular catheters in neonates has resulted in an increase in positive cultures of blood, particularly as a result of coagulase-negative staphylococci, and uncertainty of the significance of the culture results. Investigators have considered criteria based on clinical signs and microbiologic factors.

Yale investigators[6] used the following criteria to define the role of commensal organisms for the purposes of their study of neonatal sepsis: one major clinical sign documented at the time the blood culture was obtained—apnea, bradycardia, core temperature greater than 38.0° C or less than 36.5° C, plus another blood culture positive for the same organism obtained within 24 hours of the first or an intravascular access device in place before signs.

Microbiologic features that may be used to distinguish sepsis from contamination include the following:

1. Time to grow in conventional media—the longer the time needed to detect growth (> 2 days), the more likely that skin or intravascular line contamination was present.
2. Number of cultures positive—if an intravascular catheter was used to obtain the blood specimen, ambiguity is avoided by obtaining a specimen from a peripheral site; if both or the peripheral specimen alone are positive, the presence of the organism in the blood is likely; if the catheter specimen alone is positive, intravascular line colonization is likely. Contamination is more likely when only one bottle of an aerobic-anaerobic set is positive.
3. Organism type—organisms that are part of normal

TABLE 21–18

Colony Counts for Blood Cultures and Prognosis of Newborns with *Escherichia coli* Bacteremia

COLONIES/ML	NO. OF CULTURES[a] (%)	NO OF INFANTS WITH MENINGITIS (%)	MORTALITY (%)
0–4[b]	5 (16)		
5–49	11 (34)	0/17 (0)	6/17 (35)
50–1000	5 (16)		
>1000	11 (34)	6/11 (55)	8/11 (73)

[a]Thirty-two cultures from 28 newborns.
[b]One culture positive in broth was negative on pour plates.
After Dietzman DE, Fischer GW, Schoenknecht FD. Neonatal *Escherichia coli* septicemia—bacterial counts in blood. J Pediatr 85:128, 1974.

skin flora (diphtheroids, *Bacillus* species, nonhemolytic streptococci, and coagulase-negative staphylococci) suggest contamination, whereas known bacterial pathogens must be considered to be associated with sepsis. Multiple species in one culture or different species in two bottles suggest contamination.

4. Clinical signs—if the child is well without use of antibiotics, a positive culture for a commensal organism is more likely to be a contaminant.

In an attempt to resolve issues of sepsis versus contamination, investigators have used multiple site blood cultures,[468] comparisons of results of cultures of blood and cultures of skin at the venipuncture site,[482] and quantitative blood cultures.[464] These techniques are of investigational interest, but the results do not suggest that any one is of sufficient value to be adopted for clinical practice. At present, management of the sick infant with a positive culture of blood for coagulase-negative staphylococci requires that the organism be considered a pathogen and managed with appropriate antimicrobial agents. If the infant is well, the microbiologic features noted earlier should be considered in the decision to use or continue use of an antimicrobial agent. Another culture of blood should be obtained when the initial culture result is ambiguous.

BUFFY-COAT EXAMINATION

The rapid diagnosis of bacteremia by identification of microorganisms in the "buffy" leukocyte layer of centrifuged blood has been used for many years and has been evaluated for the newborn period.[483–489]

By using Gram and methylene blue stains of the buffy-coat preparation, immediate and accurate information was obtained for 37 of 48 (77%) bacteremic clinically septic infants in the four studies reported to date.[484–486, 488] Positive results showed both gram-positive and gram-negative organisms. Gram stain was believed by one investigator to be most effective in identifying the former organisms, whereas methylene blue was more helpful for the latter. In contrast to studies reported for adult populations,[490] there were no false-positive smear results among almost 200 infants with negative blood culture results. Failure to identify organisms was attributed to extreme neutropenia in several patients.

The sensitivity of leukocyte smears in neonates may be explained by the large number of organisms in the blood of the neonate during bacteremia. Smears have shown positive results with as few as 50 colonies per milliliter of *S. aureus* in the peripheral blood; about half of newborns with *E. coli* bacteremia have higher concentrations.[470] *Candida* and *S. epidermidis* septicemia in young infants have also been diagnosed by use of this method.[491–493] Strom[494] reported that bacteria were identified in peripheral blood smears in 17 of 19 infants with septicemia. However, Rodwell and associates[495] were able to identify bacteria in direct blood smears in only 4 of 24 bacteremic neonates.

CULTURE OF URINE

Infants with sepsis may have a concomitant urinary tract infection. Urine should be considered for culture from infants before initiation of antimicrobial therapy for sepsis. The yield of culture of urine is relatively low in early-onset sepsis. Visser and Hall found positive cultures of urine in only 1.6% of infants with early-onset sepsis, whereas 7.4% of infants whose signs occurred late had positive urine cultures.[496] DiGeronimo performed a chart review of 146 septic infants who had cultures of blood and urine; 11 had positive cultures of blood with a pathogen; only one urine culture was positive, and this culture was obtained in an infant whose blood was also positive for group B *Streptococcus*.[497] These data suggest that cultures of urine yield limited information about the source of infection in infants with signs of sepsis in the first few days of life (early onset). Urine should be obtained for culture if possible, but therapy should not be withheld if there is any difficulty in obtaining the specimen.

Because of the difficulty of collecting satisfactory clean-voided specimens of urine from the newborn, needle aspiration of bladder urine is frequently performed. This method is simple and safe and avoids the ambiguities inherent in urine obtained by other methods.[498] If a suprapubic aspirate cannot be performed for technical reasons, catheterization is a satisfactory way to obtain urine.

CULTURES OF TRACHEAL ASPIRATES AND PHARYNX

Because of the association of pneumonia and bacteremia, investigators have sought to determine the risk of sepsis on the basis of colonization of the upper respiratory tract. Although infants who become septic are likely to have the organism present in the tracheal aspirate, cultures of the trachea for bacterial pathogens do not predict which infants proceed to sepsis. Similarly, cultures of the pharynx did not predict the causative organism in an episode of serious bacterial infection.[499] Among ventilated infants who became septic, the same organism was usually present in cultures of tracheal aspirate and blood.[500]

DIAGNOSTIC NEEDLE ASPIRATION AND TISSUE BIOPSY

Direct aspiration of tissues or body fluids through a needle into a syringe is used for the diagnosis of a wide variety of infectious and noninfectious diseases.[501] Needle aspiration of an infectious focus in lung, pleural space, middle ear, pericardium, bones, joints, and other sites provides immediate and specific information to guide therapy. Biopsy of the liver or bone marrow may assist in diagnosing occult infections.

AUTOPSY BACTERIOLOGY

Two factors must be considered in interpreting bacterial cultures obtained at autopsy: the frequent isolation of organisms usually considered to be nonpathogenic and the difficulty of culturing certain fastidious organisms such as anaerobic bacteria. To minimize these problems, it is important that specimens be collected with as nearly complete asepsis as possible and as early as possible after death.

It is a common belief that organisms in the intestinal and respiratory tracts gain access to tissues after death, but it is also possible that bacteremia occurs shortly before death and is not a postmortem phenomenon. Eisenfeld and colleagues identified similar organisms found in specimens obtained before and within 2 hours after death.[502] Confusion in interpretation of results of bacteriologic cultures is often obviated by review of slides prepared directly from tissues and fluids. If antibiotic treatment was administered before death, organisms may be seen on a smear, although they are not viable. Pathogens would be expected to occur in significant numbers in association with inflammatory cells, whereas contaminants or organisms that invade tissues after death would probably not be seen, and if they were seen, they would be present diffusely and in small numbers with no relation to the inflammatory process.[503, 504]

RAPID TECHNIQUES FOR DETECTION OF MICROORGANISMS IN BODY FLUIDS

The limulus lysate assay for endotoxin produced by gram-negative bacteria that is based on a gelation reaction between lysates of *Limulus* (horseshoe crab) amebocytes and bacterial endotoxin has been investigated for diagnosis of causes of neonatal meningitis with equivocal results.[505–509] McCracken and Sarff used the limulus assay to measure endotoxin in CSF from 84 neonates with meningitis caused by gram-negative bacteria. Endotoxin was detected by this method in 59% of samples of CSF that grew bacteria.[509]

Counterimmunoelectrophoresis has been used successfully for detecting the antigens of various pathogenic bacteria, including *S. pneumoniae*, *N. meningitidis*, *H. influenzae*, and group B streptococci (see Chapter 26), in body fluids such as CSF and urine.

The latex agglutination test, based on specific agglutination of antibody-coated latex particles by bacterial antigens, has been effective in early detection of bacterial antigens in the CSF of patients with acute meningitis. Although counterimmunoelectrophoresis was the first technique used extensively for antigen detection, latex agglutination is now preferred because of its speed, simplicity, and greater sensitivity for selected organisms. Commercially available kits are designed to detect cell wall or capsule carbohydrate antigen released into body fluids. Among the bacterial pathogens of importance to neonatal sepsis, only group B *Streptococcus* can be detected by latex agglutination. Kits are also available for *H. influenzae* type b, *N. meningitidis*, and *S. pneumoniae*. The sensitivity of latex agglutination for infants with group B streptococcal meningitis varies between 73% and 100% for CSF and 75% and 84% for urine.[510] Possible cross-reactions have occurred when concentrated urine was tested. Group B *Streptococcus* may cross react with *S. pneumoniae*, coagulase-negative staphylococci, enterococci, and gram-negative enteric bacteria, including *P. mirabilis* and *E. cloacae*. False-positive results in urine for a positive latex agglutination test for group B *Streptococcus* may be due to contamination of bag specimens of urine with the streptococci from rectal or vaginal colonization.[511]

Lumbar Puncture and Examination of Cerebrospinal Fluid

Because meningitis may accompany sepsis, a lumbar puncture should be considered for examination of the CSF in any neonate who is to be treated for sepsis. Approximately one fourth of infants with sepsis have accompanying meningitis; the overall incidence of bacterial meningitis (see Table 21–10) is less than 1 per 1000, but the number in low-birth-weight infants is approximately 10-fold that in larger infants. Examination of CSF may be of value for diagnosis of some noninfectious central nervous system diseases in the neonates, but computed tomography is now the diagnostic technique of choice for infants with suspected intracranial hemorrhage. For infants with hypoxic-ischemic encephalopathy, lumbar puncture should be considered only for those children in whom meningitis is a possible diagnosis.

Some investigators suggest that too many term and asymptomatic infants have septic workups including lumbar puncture based solely on maternal risk features and that the procedure is unlikely to yield information of importance. Other investigators have questioned the role of admission lumbar puncture in the premature infant with respiratory distress and note that the yield is also low.[512, 513] Of more than 1700 infants with respiratory distress syndrome evaluated for meningitis, bacterial pathogens were identified in the CSF of only 4. Three of the four infants with meningitis were bacteremic with the same pathogen.[513] Another retrospective study of a large number of neonates assessed the value of lumbar puncture in the evaluation of suspected sepsis in the first week of life and thereafter[514]; bacteria were isolated from 9 of 728 CSF specimens obtained during the first week of life, but only one infant was believed to have bacterial meningitis. Fielkow and colleagues found no cases of meningitis among 284 infants without clinical signs of sepsis who had lumbar punctures because of obstetric risk factors, whereas 2.5% of 799 neonates had meningitis when clinical signs were present whether or not obstetric risk factors were present.[515] In summary, the value of lumbar puncture is identified for infants with clinical signs of sepsis; lumbar puncture performed because of maternal risk features in a child without clinical signs is unlikely to be useful.

METHOD OF LUMBAR PUNCTURE

Lumbar puncture is more difficult to perform in the neonate than in the older child or adult, traumatic taps with resulting blood in the fluid are more frequent, and care must be observed for the infant who is in cardiac or respiratory distress. Gleason and colleagues suggest that the spinal tap be performed in the upright position or if performed in the flexed position be modified with neck extension.[516] Local anesthesia and preoxygenation have been suggested to reduce the risk to the neonate from hypoxia or from struggling during the procedure.

Pinheiro and associates evaluated the role of locally administered lidocaine before lumbar puncture and noted that the local anesthesia decreased the degree of struggling of the infant[517]; however, Porter and colleagues concluded that local anesthesia failed to influence physiologic changes during lumbar puncture in the neonate.[518] Fiser and colleagues suggest that preoxygenation before lumbar puncture prevents most hypoxemia resulting from the procedure in infants.[519]

Ventricular puncture should be considered in the infant with meningitis who does not respond appropriately to antimicrobial therapy because diagnosis of ventriculitis may necessitate revision of the plan of management. Ventriculitis is diagnosed on the basis of elevated white blood cell count (> 100 cells per mm³); identification of bacteria by culture, Gram stain, or antigen detection; increased intraventricular pressure; and dilated ventricles. Ventricular puncture is not without hazard; repeated punctures may be followed by development of intracerebral cysts.[520] The procedure should be performed only by a physician expert in the technique.

"Butterfly needle" sets that incorporate a thin-walled needle without stylet, a central plastic grip, and a clear plastic tube fitted at the distal end have been recommended to simplify the procedure.[521] However, the unoccluded needle has been criticized by some investigators, who believe that it may be associated with the development of epidermoid tumors.[522] Their hypothesis is that the cutting edge of the needle frees some epidermal tissue and deposits it in the subarachnoid space, where it may give rise to the tumor. A securely fitted stylet impedes introduction of epidermis into the subarachnoid space with decreased risk of epidermoid tumors.

RISKS OF LUMBAR PUNCTURE

The physician may choose to withhold or delay lumbar puncture in some infants who would be placed at risk of compromise of cardiac or respiratory function by the procedure. Transient hypoxemia occurred during lumbar puncture performed in the lateral position (left side with hips flexed to place knees to chest), but hypoxemia was less when the infant was in a sitting position or modified lateral position (left side with hips flexed to 90 degrees).[523] Other reasons for withholding lumbar puncture in older children are less likely to be a concern in a neonate: signs of increased intracranial pressure, signs of a bleeding disorder, and infection in the area that the needle will traverse to obtain CSF.

IF A LUMBAR PUNCTURE IS NOT PERFORMED

Is it sufficient to culture blood and urine for diagnosis of the neonate with bacterial meningitis? Visser and Hall demonstrated that the blood culture result was negative when the CSF result was positive in 6 of 39 infants (15%) with bacterial meningitis.[524] In contrast, Franco and colleagues identified positive cultures of blood in only 13 of 26 infants with meningitis.[525] Thus, there is a significant number of infants with meningitis whose condition will be undiagnosed if lumbar puncture is not performed.

Ideally, lumbar puncture should be performed before the initiation of therapy, but there are alternative strategies for the infant who may not tolerate the procedure. If the physician believes that lumbar puncture would endanger the infant with presumed sepsis and/or meningitis, therapy should be started after blood and urine are obtained for culture. When the infant is stabilized, lumbar puncture should be done. Even days after the start of antibiotic therapy, cytologic tests and CSF chemistry assays should identify the presence or absence of an inflammatory reaction. Culture of gram-negative bacilli from CSF on day 3 occurs in about half of infants who are appropriately treated. If the CSF culture result is negative, the limulus lysate test for endotoxin of gram-negative organisms or antigen detection of group B streptococci may yield information about the etiologic agent.

EXAMINATION OF CEREBROSPINAL FLUID

The cell content and chemistry of the CSF of "normal" newborns differ from those in older children and adults (Table 21–19). The values vary widely during the first weeks of life, and the normal range must be considered in evaluation of CSF in cases of suspected meningitis.[526-535] The cell content in the CSF of the neonate is higher than that in older children. Polymorphonuclear leukocytes are often present in the CSF of normal newborns, whereas more than a single polymorphonuclear neutrophil in the CSF of older children or adults should be considered abnormal. Total protein concentration is higher in preterm than in term infants and highest in VLBW infants (Table 21–20).[535] In term infants, the concentration decreases with age, reaching concentrations known for older infants (< 40 mg/dl) before the third month of life; in low birth weight or preterm infants, these concentrations may not occur for months. Blood glucose levels are lower in neonates than in older children, and these values may be related to the lower concentrations of glucose observed in CSF. Normal term infants may have blood glucose levels as low as 30 mg/dl, and preterm infants may have levels as low as 20 mg/dl.[536]

The physiologic basis for the higher concentration of protein and the increased numbers of white blood cells in CSF of normal preterm and term infants is unknown; the explanations that have been offered include possible mechanical irritation of meninges during delivery and an increased permeability of the blood-brain barrier.

In these studies of CSF in newborns, "normal" refers to the absence of clinical manifestations at the time of examination of CSF. Only the study by Ahmed and colleagues included in the definition of "normal" the absence of viral infection defined by lack of evidence of cytopathic effect in five cell lines and negative polymerase chain reaction for enteroviruses.[531] None of the studies included information about the health of the infant after the newborn period. It is now recognized that infants with congenital infections such as rubella, cytomegalovirus infection, toxoplasmosis, acquired immuno-

TABLE 21–19
Hematologic and Chemical Characteristics of Cerebrospinal Fluid in Normal Newborns: Results of Selected Studies

					WHITE BLOOD CELLS (MM³)				
	NEWBORNS			RED BLOOD CELLS (MM³)	No. of Cells	No. of Polymorphonuclear Cells	No. of Mononuclear Cells	PROTEIN (MG/DL)	GLUCOSE (MG/DL)
Group	Reference No.	Age (days)	No. of Infants	MEAN (RANGE)	Mean (Range)	Mean (Range)	Mean (Range)	MEAN (RANGE)	MEAN (RANGE)
Premature	470	1–3	22	Not given	2 (0–13)			105 (50–180)	
	471	0–7	21		9 (4–18)			100 (50–138)	
	472	1–7	21	(6–333)	27 (4–112)			150 (57–292)	
	475	<7–28a	28		9 (0–29)	5		115 (65–150)	50 (24–63)
	471	8–14	15		3 (4–44)		4	128 (50–269)	83b (66–106)
	472	8–19	28		20 (3–56)			110 (74–189)	
	471	15–28	30		9 (1–31)			75 (31–131)	79c (64–106)
	472	21–40	23		17 (2–70)			86 (55–166)	
Term	472	1	135	9 (0–1070)	5 (0–90)	3 (0–70)	2 (0–20)	63 (32–240)	51 (32–78)
	474	0–13	22		6 (0–15)			67 (52–120)	
	473	7	20	3 (0–48)	3 (0–9)	2 (0–5)		47 (27–65)	55 (48–62)
	475	<7–10	87		8 (0–32)	5	1 (0–4)	90 (20–170)	81 (44–248)
	474	14–27	14		5 (2–5)		3	52 (26–88)	
	474	28–55	16		2 (1–8)			48 (17–63)	

aTwenty-four of 28 infants younger than 7 days of age.
bThree cases, 0–14 days.
cNine cases, 0–28 days.

TABLE 21–20
Hematologic and Chemical Characteristics of Cerebrospinal Fluid in Normal Very Low Birth Weight Infants

BIRTH WEIGHT (g)	AGE (DAYS)	NO. OF SAMPLES	RED BLOOD CELLS (MM³) MEAN (RANGE)	WHITE BLOOD CELLS (MM³) MEAN (RANGE)	POLYMORPHONUCLEAR LEUKOCYTES (%) MEAN (RANGE)	GLUCOSE (MG/DL) MEAN (RANGE)	PROTEIN (MG/DL) MEAN (RANGE)
<1000	0–7	6	335 (0–1780)	3 (1–8)	11 (0–50)	70 (41–89)	162 (115–222)
	8–28	17	1465 (0–19,050)	4 (0–14)	8 (0–66)	68 (33–217)	159 (95–370)
	29–84	15	808 (0–6850)	4 (0–11)	2 (0–36)	49 (29–90)	137 (76–260)
1000–1500	0–7	8	407 (0–2450)	4 (1–10)	4 (0–28)	74 (50–96)	136 (85–176)
	8–28	14	1101 (0–9750)	7 (0–44)	10 (0–60)	59 (39–109)	137 (54–227)
	29–84	11	661 (0–3800)	8 (0–23)	11 (0–48)	47 (31–76)	122 (45–187)

Modified from Rodriguez AF, Kaplan SL, Mason EO. Cerebrospinal fluid values in the very low birth weight infant. J Pediatr 116:971, 1990, with permission.

deficiency syndrome, and syphilis may be asymptomatic during the newborn period. Observations of these infants over the course of months or years may reveal defects that were inapparent at birth. Until more data are available, it would appear prudent to observe carefully infants with many leukocytes (> 20 per mm³) or high CSF protein level (> 100 mg/dl) and, if clinical signs indicate, to obtain paired serum samples for assay of antibody and for isolation of the organism in body fluids and tissues for congenital central nervous system infections (*T. gondii*, rubella virus, cytomegalovirus, herpes simplex virus, human immunodeficiency virus, and *T. pallidum*).

In newborns with bacterial meningitis, cells may number in the thousands and polymorphonuclear leukocytes predominate early in the course of the disease.[33, 34, 286, 287, 532] The number of white blood cells in CSF is higher in infants with gram-negative meningitis than in infants with group B streptococcal meningitis; the median number of cells per cubic millimeter in CSF of 98 infants with gram-negative meningitis was more than 2000 (range 6 to 40,000), whereas the median number of cells per cubic millimeter in 21 infants with group B streptococcal meningitis was less than 100 (range 8 to > 10,000).[532] The concentration of glucose in CSF is usually less than two thirds of the concentration in blood. The concentration of protein may be low (< 30 mg/dl) or very high (> 1000 mg/dl). Thus, values found in the normal infant may overlap those of the infant with meningitis.

A Gram-stained smear of CSF should be prepared and examined for detection of bacteria, and appropriate media should be inoculated with the CSF. Sarff and colleagues detected organisms in Gram-stained smears of CSF in 83% of patients with group B streptococcal meningitis and in 78% of patients with gram-negative disease.[532] After initiation of appropriate antibiotic therapy, gram-positive bacteria usually clear rapidly from the CSF, whereas gram-negative enteric bacilli persist for many days.[534]

Microorganisms can be isolated from CSF that has no cells and normal chemistry test results. Visser and Hall reported "normal" CSF (cell count < 25; protein level < 200 mg/dl) in 6 of 39 (29%) infants with culture-proven meningitis.[524] Subsequent examination of CSF identified an increase in the number of cells and protein level. Presumably, the initial lumbar puncture was performed early in the course of meningitis when the CSF was seeded with bacteria but before an inflammatory response occurred. Other investigators reported isolation of enterovirus[537] and pneumococcus[536] from CSF of neonates in the absence of pleocytosis.

Identification of bacteremia without meningitis defined by absence of pleocytosis or positive culture of CSF may be followed by meningeal inflammation on subsequent examinations. Sarmen and colleagues identified six infants with gram-negative bacteremia and initial normal CSF who developed evidence of meningeal inflammation 18 to 59 hours after the first examination.[538] Although the authors suggest that identification of gram-negative bacteremia warrants repeat lumbar puncture to identify optimal duration of therapy, the recommendation should be broadened to include all infants with bacteremia and initial negative studies of CSF. Dissemination of the organisms from the blood to the meninges may occur subsequent to the first lumber puncture or before adequate sterilization of the blood and CSF.

Investigators have sought a sensitive and specific metabolic determinant of bacterial meningitis in CSF with little success. Among products that have been evaluated and found to be inadequate to distinguish bacterial meningitis from other neurologic disease (including cerebroventricular hemorrhage and asphyxia) are γ-aminobutyric acid,[539] lactate dehydrogenase,[540] and creatine kinase brain isoenzyme.[541] Cyclic-3',5'-adenosine monophosphate was elevated in the CSF of neonates with bacterial meningitis compared with CSF of infants who had nonbacterial meningitis or a control group.[542] Elevated CSF concentrations of C-reactive protein have been found in infants and children older than 4 weeks of age with bacterial meningitis[543, 544]; however, the test was found to be of no value in neonates.[544, 545] Current investigations of proinflammatory cytokines interleukin-6 and interleukin-8 indicate that there is a cytokine response in CSF after birth asphyxia and that these assays will not be useful in distinguishing the child with meningitis.[546, 547]

THE TRAUMATIC LUMBAR PUNCTURE

Blood in the CSF resulting from a traumatic lumbar puncture may obscure the significance of concentrations of cells and chemistries. The incidence of bloody specimens was determined by Schwersenski and colleagues[514]: 13.8% of 712 CSF specimens obtained during the first week of life had blood; an additional 14.5% were considered inadequate specimens.

If a lumbar puncture has been traumatic, a total cell count can be performed in a counting chamber. The red blood cells then can be lysed by acetic acid and a repeat cell count performed. If the total number of white blood cells compared with the number of red blood cells exceeds the value for whole blood, the presence of CSF pleocytosis is suggested. If the peripheral red blood cell and white blood cell counts are normal, 1 white blood cell per 700 red blood cells can be subtracted from the total white blood cell count in CSF before the use of acetic acid for lysis of the red cells.

Some investigators have noted that the observed white blood cell counts in bloody CSF are lower than would be predicted based on the ratio of white to red cells in peripheral blood; either white blood cells lyse more rapidly than red blood cells or there is a decrease of white cells for other reasons.[548–551] Several formulas have been used in an attempt to interpret cytologic findings in CSF contaminated by blood.[552–554] However, none of the corrections applied to bloody CSF can be used with confidence for ruling out possible meningitis.[555–557]

Protein in CSF is usually elevated after a traumatic lumbar puncture because of the presence of red blood cells. It has been estimated that an increase of 1 mg/dl in CSF protein occurs for every 1000 red blood cells per microliter. The concentration of glucose does not appear to be altered by blood from a traumatic lumbar puncture; a low CSF glucose concentration is an important result when associated with a traumatic tap.

Because of the difficulties in interpretation of the "bloody tap," it is often of value to repeat the lumbar puncture 12 to 72 hours later. Results of the second lumbar puncture, even if performed without trauma or apparent bleeding, may also be ambiguous because white blood cells may be induced by the inflammation created by the irritant effect of blood.

BRAIN ABSCESS

The CSF in the child with a brain abscess may include a pleocytosis of up to a few hundred cells with a predominance of mononuclear cells and with an elevated protein level. Bacteria may not be seen by Gram's stain of CSF if meningitis is not present. Sudden clinical deterioration and the appearance of many cells (> 1000 per mm³), most of which are polymorphonuclear cells, suggest rupture of the abscess into the CSF.

Laboratory Aids

Laboratory aids in the diagnosis of systemic and focal infection in the neonate include peripheral white blood cell and differential counts, platelet counts, acute-phase reactants, blood chemistries, histopathology of the placenta and umbilical cord, smears of gastric aspirate and fluid from the external ear canal, and radiologic examinations. New assays for diagnosis of early-onset sepsis including serum concentrations of neutrophil CD 11b,[558] granulocyte colony-stimulating factor,[559] interleukin receptor antagonist,[560] interleukin-6,[560–562] and procalcitonin[563] show promise for more sensitivity and specificity than current diagnostic tests. However, proinflammatory cytokines, including interleukin-1 and interleukin-6 and tumor necrosis factor-alpha, have been identified in serum and CSF in infants after perinatal asphyxia, raising doubts about the specificity of some of these markers.[546, 547, 564, 565] These tests and procedures are extensively discussed in Chapter 32.

MANAGEMENT

If the history and clinical signs lead the physician to consider an infant to be septic, culture of blood should be obtained, cultures of urine and CSF and a radiograph of the chest considered, and treatment with antimicrobial agents begun. Because of the subtlety of clinical manifestations of sepsis, the rapid progression of the disease, and the continuing high mortality rate, treatment must be started even when only minimal indications of sepsis are present. Many infants are treated for sepsis, but documentation of bacterial disease by positive blood, urine, or CSF culture results is accomplished in very few.

Choice of Antimicrobial Agents

INITIAL THERAPY FOR PRESUMED SEPSIS

The choice of antimicrobial agents for treatment of suspected sepsis is based on knowledge of the prevalent organisms responsible for neonatal sepsis and the patterns of their antimicrobial susceptibility. Initial therapy for the infant who becomes septic during the first days of life (early-onset disease) must include coverage for gram-positive cocci, particularly group B streptococci, and gram-negative enteric bacilli. Treatment of the infant who becomes septic after day 4 (late-onset disease) may need to include additional coverage for hospital-acquired organisms, such as *S. aureus* and *S. epidermidis*, and gram-negative enteric bacilli, such as *Pseudomonas* species.

Group B streptococci are uniformly sensitive to penicillins and cephalosporins. In a study in our laboratory of 231 isolates of group B streptococci, all strains were inhibited and killed by concentrations of penicillin G of less than 0.25 μg/ml[566]; ampicillin, the penicillinase-resistant penicillins, and third-generation cephalosporins are highly active and aminoglycosides are relatively ineffective. In vitro studies[567] and experimental infections in mice[568] indicate that antibacterial killing of group B streptococci was enhanced by addition of gentamicin to ampicillin. Some physicians prefer to continue the combination of ampicillin and gentamicin for 48 to 72 hours or the full course of treatment, especially when the minimal bactericidal concentration of ampicillin is many times greater than the minimal inhibitory concentration of the organism. However, there are no clinical data to suggest that the addition of aminoglycosides to a penicillin results in increased survival or more rapid recovery of infected neonates.

Most strains of *S. aureus* that cause disease in neonates produce β-lactamase and are thereby resistant to penicillin G, ampicillin, carbenicillin, and ticarcillin. These organisms are sensitive to the penicillinase-resistant penicillins and selected cephalosporins, and these drugs must be considered when staphylococcal disease is known or suspected. Methicillin-resistant staphylococci that are cross-resistant with other penicillinase-resistant penicillins and, in most cases, cephalosporins have been encountered in nurseries in the United States. Antibacterial susceptibility patterns must be monitored by surveillance of staphylococcal strains causing infection and disease in the nursery. Bacterial resistance must be considered as a possible cause of therapeutic failure whenever a patient with staphylococcal disease who is receiving an adequate dosage schedule of a penicillinase-resistant penicillin does not respond favorably. Most of these strains are sensitive to vancomycin. Vancomycin-resistant *S. aureus* has been reported from Japan and the United States, but no strains have as yet been identified in neonates.

S. epidermidis may be a cause of infection of prosthetic devices such as intravascular catheters for CSF. Most strains produce β-lactamase, and many are resistant to methicillin and other penicillinase-resistant penicillins and cephalosporins. Initial therapy for disease that may be caused by *S. epidermidis* must be considered carefully: vancomycin may be used and the initial choice reevaluated when results of susceptibility tests are available. Removal of the device is often necessary to effect a cure.

Group D streptococci vary in susceptibility to penicillins. Nonenterococcal strains, including *S. bovis*, are highly susceptible, but enterococci are moderately resistant to ampicillin and penicillin G and highly resistant to all cephalosporins. Optimal therapy for disease related to enterococci includes a penicillin and an aminoglycoside or vancomycin.

L. monocytogenes is susceptible to penicillin G and ampicillin and resistant to cephalosporins. Ampicillin is the preferred agent for *L. monocytogenes*, although the aminoglycoside, used for presumed sepsis or meningitis, can be continued with ampicillin until repeat cultures of CSF are sterile or for the entire course. Specific management is discussed in Chapter 27.

The choice of antibiotics for infections with gram-negative bacteria depends on the pattern of susceptibility in the hospital or nursery. These patterns vary in different hospitals or communities and from time to time within the same institution. Although information on strains from neonates should be monitored to determine the emergence of new strains with unique antimicrobial susceptibility, the general pattern of antibiotic susceptibility in the hospital is a good guide to initial therapy for neonates. The aminoglycosides kanamycin, tobramycin, gentamicin, netilmicin, and amikacin are highly effective against most isolates of *E. coli, Enterobacter, Klebsiella,* and *Proteus* species. All but kanamycin are also active against *P. aeruginosa.*

ROLE OF THIRD-GENERATION CEPHALOSPORINS

The third-generation cephalosporins cefotaxime, ceftriaxone, and ceftazidime possess attractive features for therapy for bacterial sepsis and meningitis in newborns. These features include excellent in vitro activity against group B streptococci and *E. coli* and other gram-negative enteric bacilli. Ceftazidime is highly effective in vitro against *P. aeruginosa.* None of the cephalosporins is active against *L. monocytogenes* and enterococci, and activity against *S. aureus* is variable. The cephalosporins provide high concentrations of drug in serum and adequate concentrations in CSF, and there is no dose-related toxicity. Clinical and microbiologic results of studies of sepsis and meningitis in neonates suggest that the third-generation cephalosporins are comparable but not superior to the traditional regimens of a penicillin and an aminoglycoside (see Chapter 35).[569–571] Because ceftriaxone can displace bilirubin from serum albumin, it is recommended for use in neonates only if it is uniquely effective against the bacterial pathogen.

The rapid development of resistance of gram-negative enteric bacilli when cefotaxime was used extensively for presumptive therapy for neonatal sepsis suggests that extensive use of newer cephalosporins may lead to emergence of drug-resistant bacteria more rapidly than has been identified with the standard regimen of a penicillin and an aminoglycoside.[319] Restriction of use of cefotaxime for infants with evidence of meningitis is warranted.

Current Practice

A combination of penicillin G or ampicillin plus an aminoglycoside such as gentamicin is considered to be most suitable for initial treatment of presumed early-onset neonatal sepsis.[572] If there is a concern for endemic or epidemic staphylococcal infection and disease, the initial treatment of late-onset neonatal sepsis should include a penicillinase-resistant penicillin or vancomycin (if resistance to penicillinase-resistant penicillin has been documented).

The increasing use of antibiotics, particularly in neonatal intensive care units, may result in alterations in the antibiotic susceptibility of bacteria; such shifts necessitate changes in consideration of initial therapy. The demonstrated alteration of the microbial flora in nurseries where use of different antimicrobial agents is widespread is persuasive argument for the judicious use of antibiotics. The hospital laboratory must regularly monitor isolates of pathogenic bacteria to assist the physician in the choice of the most appropriate initial therapy.

The clinical pharmacology and dosage schedules of the various antimicrobial agents considered for neonatal sepsis are provided in Chapter 35.

Continuation of Therapy When Results of Cultures Are Available

The choice of antibiotics should be reevaluated when results of cultures and susceptibility tests become available. The duration of therapy depends on the initial response to the appropriate antibiotics but should be 7 to 10 days in most infants with sepsis documented by positive culture of blood and minimal or absent focal infection; the minimal duration of therapy is 21 days for infants with meningitis caused by group B streptococci or gram-negative enteric bacilli.

The third-generation cephalosporins cefotaxime, ceftriaxone, and ceftazidime have important theoretical advantages for treatment of sepsis or meningitis when compared with therapeutic regimens that include an aminoglycoside or chloramphenicol. The cephalosporins are safe compared with aminoglycosides in terms of ototoxicity and nephrotoxicity and compared with chloramphenicol in terms of hematologic effects. Because there is no dose-related toxicity, measurements of serum concentrations, which are obligatory with the use of aminoglycosides and chloramphenicol, are unnecessary for the cephalosporins. A cephalosporin is advantageous in the infant with diminished renal function whose therapeutic alternative would be an aminoglycoside or in the infant with compromised hepatic function in whom chloramphenicol would be used. Routine use of the new cephalosporins for presumptive therapy for suggested sepsis may lead to problems with drug-resistant microorganisms. Extensive use of the third-generation cephalosporins in the nursery could result in emergence of resistance caused by derepression of chromosomally mediated β-lactamases.[573] Cefotaxime is preferred to other third-generation cephalosporins for use in neonates both because it has been used more extensively[570, 571] and because it is not excreted in bile, in which excretion could have an inhibitory effect on the bacterial flora of the intestinal tract.[573] Ceftazidime either alone or combined with an aminoglycoside should be considered for therapy for *P. aeruginosa* meningitis because of the excellent in vitro activity of the drug against these strains. Ceftriaxone use in the neonate is limited by its ability to displace bilirubin from serum albumin, but it may be of value in a once-daily dosage to complete outpatient therapy of uncomplicated group B streptococcal infection.[574]

Management of the Infant Whose Mother Received Intrapartum Antimicrobial Agents

Antimicrobial agents are now commonly used for women in labor who have risk factors associated with sepsis in the fetus, including premature delivery, prolonged rupture of membranes, and fever or other signs of endometritis. Antimicrobial agents cross the placenta and achieve concentrations in fetal tissues that are parallel to concentrations achieved in other well-vascularized organs. Placental transport of antibiotics is discussed in Chapter 35.

Protocols for prevention of group B streptococcal infection in the newborn by administration of a penicillin to the mother were published in 1992 by the American College of Obstetrics and Gynecology[574] and the American Academy of Pediatrics (AAP).[575] These guidelines were revised in 1996 by the Centers for Disease Control and Prevention[576] and in 1997 by the AAP,[577] and additional revisions have been suggested.[578] Concentrations of ampicillin are achieved in the fetus that are more than 30% of the concentrations in the blood of the mother.[579] Parenteral antibiotic therapy administered to the mother in labor is essentially treating the fetus earlier in the course of the intrapartum infection. Thus, if the fetus has been infected, the regimen is treatment not prophylaxis; for some infected fetuses the treatment administered in utero will be insufficient to prevent signs of early-onset group B streptococcal disease.[580] Although the prophylactic regimen has decreased the incidence of early-onset group B streptococcal disease (by more than 80% in a Pittsburgh survey),[581] the regimen has had no impact on the incidence of late-onset disease.

The various algorithms prepared to guide empirical management of the neonate born to a mother who had risk factors for group B streptococcal disease and received intrapartum antimicrobial prophylaxis for prevention of early-onset group B streptococcal disease focus on three clinical scenarios[577, 578]:

1. Infants who have signs of sepsis should receive a full diagnostic evaluation and should be treated with a combination of ampicillin and gentamicin.

2. Infants who are term, do not have clinical signs or suspicion of sepsis, and whose mothers received two or more doses of antibiotic before delivery do not have to be evaluated or treated but should be observed for 48 hours.

3. Infants who do not have signs of sepsis but who are less than 35 weeks' gestation and whose mothers received only one dose of antibiotic should be observed for 48 hours or more and should receive a limited evaluation (culture of blood and white blood cell count and differential).

The first two categories are readily identified, but the third category often leads to controversy because of the vague end points. Recent recommendations for prevention and treatment of early-onset group B streptococcal infection are more fully discussed in Chapter 26.

Management of the infant born to a mother who has received an antimicrobial agent within hours of delivery must include consideration of the effect of the drug on cultures obtained from the infant after birth. Intrapartum therapy is essentially initiating treatment of the infant in utero, and variable concentrations of drug will be present in the infant's body fluids and mucous membranes. If the infant is infected and the bacterial pathogen is susceptible to the drug administered to the mother, cultures of the infant may be falsely negative.

Treatment of the Infant Whose Bacterial Culture Results Are Negative

The physician must decide on the subsequent course of therapy for the infant who was treated for presumed sepsis and whose results of bacterial culture are negative whether or not the mother received antibiotics before delivery. If the child appears to be well and there is reason to believe that infection was an unlikely cause of early signs, treatment can be discontinued after an interval that would allow for growth of bacteria in cultures of blood. Three days should be sufficient to provide confidence in the absence of growth. If the clinical condition of the infant remains precarious and there is still suspicion of an infectious process, therapy should be continued as outlined for documented bacterial sepsis unless another diagnosis becomes apparent. Significant bacterial infection may be present without bacteremia, or bacteremia may be present before but not at the time blood for culture is obtained. Squire and colleagues noted that results of premortem blood cultures were negative in 7 of 39 infants (18%) with unequivocal infection at autopsy.[582] Thus, some infants with significant systemic bacterial infection may not be identified by the usual culture techniques. The physician must consider this limitation of current methods when results of bacterial cultures are negative.

Treatment of Neonatal Meningitis

Because the pathogens responsible for neonatal meningitis are the same as those that cause neonatal sepsis, initial therapy and subsequent therapy are the same. Meningitis caused by gram-negative enteric bacilli can pose special management problems. Eradication of the pathogen is often delayed, and brain abscess or other complications can occur.[583] The basis for persistence of gram-negative bacilli in CSF even when bactericidal titers of the antimicrobial agent were present led to evaluation of intrathecal gentamicin[584] and, subsequently, intraventricular gentamicin.[585] Mortality and morbidity were not significantly different in infants who received parenteral drug alone or parenteral plus intrathecal therapy.[584] The study of the intraventricular drug was stopped early because of the high mortality in the parenteral plus intraventricular therapy group.[585]

Treatment of neonatal meningitis was reviewed by Feigen and coworkers.[572] Ampicillin or penicillin G is preferred for infection caused by group B streptococci. Ampicillin and an aminoglycoside have been used for more than 20 years with satisfactory results, although bactericidal levels are often low. Cefotaxime has superior in vitro and CSF bactericidal activity.[570] Either cefotaxime alone or combined with an aminoglycoside or the conventional regimen of ampicillin and an aminoglycoside is satisfactory for treatment of enteric gram-negative bacillary meningitis.

If meningitis develops in a low birth weight infant who has been in the nursery for a prolonged period or in a neonate who has received previous courses of antimicrobial therapy for presumed sepsis, an alternative regimen should be considered. Enterococci and gentamicin-resistant gram-negative enteric bacilli are potential pathogens in these settings. A combination of ampicillin and another aminoglycoside (preferably amikacin) or ampicillin and cefotaxime could be used. In patients with long-term vascular catheters, an antistaphylococcal agent (a penicillinase-resistant penicillin or vancomycin) should be added to the regimen or substituted for penicillin because of possible sepsis due to *S. aureus* or coagulase-negative staphylococci. Ceftazidime alone or combined with an aminoglycoside should be considered for *P. aeruginosa* meningitis.

Other antibiotics may be necessary for treatment of highly resistant organisms. Chloramphenicol[586] or trimethoprim-sulfamethoxazole[587] may be uniquely effective against bacteria resistant to β-lactam drugs or aminoglycosides but would need to be carefully monitored because of toxicity unique to the newborn (see Chapter 25).

Continued treatment of meningitis caused by a gram-negative enteric bacillus is based on in vitro susceptibility tests. If facilities are not available for determining aminoglycoside concentrations or if the patient has abnormal renal function, one of the new cephalosporins would be advantageous.

If cultures of blood and CSF for bacterial pathogens by usual laboratory techniques are negative in the neonate with meningitis, the differential diagnosis of "aseptic meningitis" must be reviewed, particularly in view of diagnosing treatable infections (Table 21–21).

Treatment of the Infant with Meningitis Whose Bacterial Culture Results Are Negative

An aggressive diagnostic approach is necessary for the infant with meningitis (defined by increased number of white blood cells in the CSF and variable changes in concentration of protein and glucose) in the absence of a bacterial pathogen detectable in the CSF by usual laboratory techniques. The differential diagnosis of this event, frequently termed *aseptic meningitis*, is provided in Table 21–21 and the disease chapters should be consulted for diagnosis and management.

TABLE 21–21
Infectious and Noninfectious Causes of Aseptic Meningitis[a] in the Neonate

INFECTIOUS AGENT	DISEASE
Bacteria	Partially treated meningitis
	Parameningeal focus (brain or epidural abscess)
	Tuberculosis
Viruses	Herpes simplex meningoencephalitis
	Cytomegalovirus
	Enteroviruses
	Rubella
	Acquired immunodeficiency syndrome
	Lymphocytic choriomeningitis
	Varicella
Spirochetes	Syphilis
	Lyme disease
Parasites	Toxoplasmosis
	Chagas' disease
Mycoplasma	*M. hominis* infection
	Ureaplasma urealyticum infection
Fungi	Candidiasis
	Coccidioidomycosis
	Cryptococcosis
NONINFECTIOUS CAUSES	
Trauma	Subarachnoid hemorrhage
	Traumatic lumber puncture
Malignancy	Teratoma
	Medulloblastoma
	Choroid plexus papilloma and carcinoma

[a]*Aseptic meningitis* is defined as meningitis in the absence of evidence of bacterial pathogen detectable in cerebrospinal fluid by usual laboratory techniques.

The most frequent reason for "aseptic meningitis" in the neonate is likely to be prior antimicrobial therapy resulting in negative blood and CSF cultures. Congenital infections need to be ruled out. The most important diagnoses of aseptic meningitis in the newborn are those for treatable diseases, such as partially treated bacterial disease, meningoencephalitis due to herpes simplex virus, syphilis, Lyme disease, and toxoplasmosis. Rare causes of aseptic meningitis in the neonate such as tuberculosis and malignancy need to be considered in the differential diagnosis. With the list of possible diagnoses in mind, the physician must reconsider the history of illness and contacts in the mother and family and epidemiologic features (animal exposures, recent travel), reexamine the mother, reexamine the infant for focal signs of disease (including special techniques [slit-lamp examination]), and consider radiologic examination of the long bones, skull, and brain. Treatment of suggested bacterial or nonbacterial causes of aseptic meningitis may be necessary before the results of culture, antigen detection, polymerase chain reaction, or serology are available to indicate the diagnosis.

Treatment of Anaerobic Infections

The importance of anaerobic bacteria as a cause of serious neonatal infection is uncertain. *Clostridia, Pepto-*

coccus, and *Peptostreptococcus* are highly sensitive to penicillin G, but *B. fragilis* is usually resistant. If anaerobic organisms are known or suspected to be responsible for infection (as in peritonitis), chloramphenicol, clindamycin, or cefoxitin must be added to the penicillin-plus-aminoglycoside regimen.

Adjunctive Therapies for Treatment of Neonatal Sepsis

Despite appropriate antimicrobial and optimal supportive therapy, mortality resulting from neonatal sepsis remains distressingly high. With the hope of improving survival and decreasing the severity of sequelae in survivors, investigators have considered adjunctive modes of treatment, including granulocyte transfusion, exchange transfusion, and use of immune globulins for deficits in the host defenses of the neonate. These therapies are discussed in Chapter 2 by Lewis and Wilson and Chapter 26 by Edwards and Baker. Pentoxifylline was documented to reduce the plasma tumor necrosis factor-alpha concentrations in premature infants with sepsis, and survival improved, but the number of infants treated (five of five survived) and number of controls (one of four survived) was too small to provide more than a suggestion of efficacy.[588] The results of preliminary studies of granulocyte colony stimulating factor in neutropenic infants with sepsis were equivocal.[589, 590] Although the results of selected studies indicate that some of these techniques improved survival, the potential adverse effects (e.g., graft-versus-host reaction, pulmonary leukocyte sequestration) are of sufficient concern to warrant continued study only under experimental protocols.

Human immunoglobulin preparations for intravenous administration (IGIV) have been assessed for adjunctive therapy for early-onset sepsis based on the hypothesis that infected infants lack circulating antibody against the bacterial pathogen and that such materials could be provided by IGIV. The results of clinical trials suggest efficacy of IGIV for survival for infants with fulminant, early-onset neonatal infection. Hill reviewed four trials[591]: mortality was 15% (9 of 60) in the untreated and 3% (2 of 59) in the IGIV-treated infants. On the basis of these data, he suggested a single dose of 750 mg/kg in the infant with suspected sepsis. Other investigators are less sanguine; Noya concluded[592] that IGIV has not been demonstrated conclusively to be effective in the treatment of neonatal sepsis.

If purulent foci or abscesses are present, they should be drained. However, some brain abscesses resolve with medical therapy alone.[358, 593] Because brain abscesses may be polymicrobial or due to organisms that are uncommon causes of meningitis (including *Citrobacter*,[182, 184] *Enterobacter*,[200] *Proteus*,[594] and *Salmonella* species[595]), aspiration of the abscess provides identification of the pathogens to guide rational antimicrobial therapy.

Current Management of Infants with Sepsis

Criteria for therapy vary in different nurseries, but most physicians administer antibiotics to newborns at the least suspicion of sepsis because of the difficulty of clinical diagnosis and high mortality.

A survey of hospitalized patients in Pennsylvania indicated that 4.8% of children younger than 1 month of age were treated with antibiotics.[596] Because approximately 3.8 million infants are born in the United States each year, these data suggest that about 200,000 newborns may receive antibiotics annually, that most of them receive the antibiotics in the first few days of life, and that almost all receive two drugs—a penicillin and an aminoglycoside.

Many infants without infection should be treated to be certain of including those few with sepsis. The physician must evaluate the laboratory information and clinical signs during the course of therapy and must be ready to discontinue antimicrobial agents if the culture results are negative and the clinical course suggests that infection was unlikely.

PROGNOSIS

Before the advent of the antibiotic era, almost all infants with neonatal sepsis died.[5] Dunham[2] reported that physicians used various treatments, including "erysipelas serum" and transfusions, without altering the course of the disease. The introduction of the sulfonamides and penicillin and later of the broad-spectrum antibiotics such as chloramphenicol and streptomycin decreased the mortality rate to about 60%.[3, 5] During this period, some infants undoubtedly died because of the treatment rather than the disease, owing to the cardiovascular collapse (i.e., the gray baby syndrome) associated with high dosages of chloramphenicol.

The introduction of the aminoglycoside antibiotics—kanamycin in the early 1960s and gentamicin later in the decade—provided vastly improved therapy for bacteremia due to gram-negative organisms, the leading cause of sepsis at that time.[597] This factor, together with an improved understanding of neonatal physiology and an increased sophistication of life-support systems, combined to permit a steady decrease in neonatal mortality during the period 1960 to 1985, both in the United States[597] and in Europe.[17, 598–600] Mortality from sepsis, including infants of all weights and gestational ages, fell from 40 to 50% in the 1960s[4, 597, 598, 601] to 10 to 20% in the 1970s and 1980s.[16, 17, 427, 428, 597, 599, 600] During the 1990s in the United States fewer than 1070 of cases of neonatal sepsis due to group B *Streptococcus* were fatal.[602]

The postnatal age at which infection occurs, once thought to be of prognostic significance, has become less so within the past 10 years. Fulminant sepsis, with signs of illness present at birth or during the first day of life, still has a high mortality, varying from 20%[17, 592] or 30%[16] to as high as 70%.[603] However, when these early infections, most of which are caused by group B *Streptococcus*, are excluded from the analysis, the percentage of deaths due to early-onset sepsis (< 4 to 7 days of age) does not differ significantly from that associated with late-onset infection.[16, 17, 352, 428, 597–599]

Mortality from sepsis is higher for preterm than for

term infants in virtually all published studies[16, 17, 374, 427, 428, 599] but is approximately the same for all major bacterial pathogens (see Tables 21-4 and 21-5).[16, 599]

There are few data on morbidity after neonatal sepsis without meningitis. Alfven and colleagues[604] surveyed children 2½ to 6½ years old who had had sepsis as neonates; disabilities that could be regarded as related to sepsis were identified in 22% of these survivors. Sequelae due to osteomyelitis and bone destruction associated with sepsis were noted in 8% of more than 250 infants followed for up to 3 years after their hospitalization.[600] In one series of 92 infants with adequately treated early-onset group B streptococcal disease, recurrence of bacteremia during the second month of life was described in 3 children (3.8%).

In surveys conducted over the past decade, the case:fatality rate of neonatal meningitis has been remarkably consistent at 20 to 25%.[16, 356, 600, 605, 606] This represents a significant improvement from prior years, when most studies reported more than 30% deaths associated with meningitis.[34, 35, 415, 584, 585, 607] Mortality is greater among preterm than term infants.[356, 453, 584, 606, 608]

Significant sequelae develop in 20 to 50% of infants who survive neonatal meningitis caused by gram-negative enteric bacilli or group B streptococci.[356, 584, 585, 600, 601, 606, 609-611] These sequelae include mental and motor disabilities, convulsive disorders, hydrocephalus, hearing loss, and abnormal speech patterns.

The most extensive experience with long-term observation of infants who had group B streptococcal meningitis as neonates was reported by Edwards and colleagues.[612] Of 61 patients treated between 1974 and 1979, 21% died. Of the survivors, 38 were evaluated at 3 years of age or older: 29% had severe neurologic sequelae; 21% had minor deficits; and 50% were functioning normally. Factors associated with death or severe disability at presentation included comatose or semicomatose state, decreased perfusion, total peripheral white blood cell count less than 5000 per mm³, absolute neutrophil count less than 1000 per mm³, and CSF protein level greater than 300 mg/dl. A comparable study evaluating 35 newborns over a period of 3 to 18 years indicated even more favorable outcomes: 60% of survivors were considered normal at follow-up when compared with sibling controls, 15% had mild to moderate neurologic residua, and 25% had major sequelae.[607] The results of frequent and extensive neurologic, developmental, and psychometric assessments on a cohort of 10 group B streptococcal meningitis survivors followed for 1 to 14 years were reported by Franco and co-workers: one child had severe central nervous system damage; five children, including one with hydrocephalus, had mild academic or behavioral problems; and four were normal.[608]

The outcome described for infants with gram-negative bacillary meningitis is similar. Experience with this condition from 1969 to 1989 at two hospitals in Dallas, Texas, has been reviewed.[356] Among 72 patients, there were 60 survivors, 43 of whom were followed and evaluated for a period of at least 6 months. Neurologic residua caused by the meningitis, occurring alone or in combination, were described in 56% and included hydrocephalus, seizure disorder, and developmental delay each in about 30%; cerebral palsy in 25%; and hearing loss in 15%. Forty-four percent of the survivors were normal at follow-up. Data from the First Neonatal Meningitis Cooperative Study Group (1971 to 1975) indicate that among 78 infants whose conditions were evaluated for 9 to 13 years after their illness, 68% were considered normal, 23% had mild to moderate neurologic problems, and only 9% were severely damaged.[605] Factors at presentation of group B streptococcal meningitis associated with death or severe disability included comatose or semicomatose state, decreased perfusion, total peripheral white blood cell count less than 5000 per mm³, absolute neutrophil count less than 1000 per mm³, and CSF protein level greater than 300 mg/dl.[607] Among infants with gram-negative bacillary meningitis, thrombocytopenia, CSF white blood cell count greater than 2000 per mm³, CSF protein greater than 200 mg/dl, CSF/blood glucose ratio of less than 0.5, prolonged (> 48 hours) positive CSF cultures, and elevated endotoxin and interleukin-1 concentrations in CSF were indicators of a poor outcome.[356, 417, 613]

Computed tomography reveals a high incidence of central nervous system residua among newborns with meningitis. Among 44 infants with gram-negative bacillary meningitis, only 30% of computed tomographic scans were considered normal. Hydrocephalus was found in 20% of cases; areas of infarct, cerebritis, diffuse encephalomalacia, or cortical atrophy in 30%; brain abscess in about 20%; and subdural effusions in 7%. Two or more abnormalities were detected in about one third of infants.[605]

The prognosis of brain abscess in the neonate is guarded; about half of these children die, and sequelae such as hydrocephalus are frequent in survivors. Of 17 children who had brain abscess during the neonatal period and were observed for at least 2 years, only 4 had normal intellect and were free of seizures.[358] The poor outcome is likely due to destruction of brain because of hemorrhagic infarcts and necrosis in neonates with brain abscess.

PREVENTION

Obstetric Factors

It would seem reasonable to conclude that any improvements in the health of the pregnant woman and increased use of prenatal care facilities will lead to a lowering of the rate of prematurity and more appropriate management of prolonged interval after rupture of maternal membranes, maternal peripartum infections, and fetal distress. Because these factors are associated with sepsis in the newborn, improved care of the mother should decrease the opportunities for neonatal infection. Development of neonatal intensive care expertise and units with appropriate equipment has resulted in survival for VLBW infants. Increasingly, obstetric problems are anticipated and mothers are moved before delivery to medical centers with neonatal intensive care units; this procedure is safer than delivery in the local hospital followed by the hazardous step of transporting the newborn to the intensive care unit after birth.

Chemoprophylaxis

The use of antibiotics to prevent infection may be valuable when they are directed against specific microorganisms for a limited time. In the neonate, the use of silver nitrate eye drops to prevent gonococcal ophthalmia, vaccination with bacille Calmette-Guérin (BCG) or prophylactic use of isoniazid to reduce morbidity from tuberculosis in infants who must return to endemic areas, and use of hexachlorophene baths to prevent staphylococcal disease have been recognized as effective modes of chemoprophylaxis. The value of using antimicrobial agents against unknown pathogens in infants believed to be at high risk of infection or undergoing invasive procedures is uncertain. Studies of penicillin administered to the mother at term or the infant at delivery for prevention of neonatal disease caused by group B streptococci are reviewed earlier and in Chapter 26.

Daily administration of vancomycin has been investigated for prevention of coagulase-negative staphylococcal bacteremia in low-birth-weight infants. Vancomycin was effective in reducing colonization and bacteremia when added to parenteral nutrition fluids for infants weighing 500 to 1500 g. Baier and colleagues[614] randomized infants to receive vancomycin or no antibiotic for the duration of parenteral nutrition in a study blinded to the investigators: nine infants developed bacteremia or fungemia in the control group, and one infant developed candidemia in the vancomycin-treated group; all invasive episodes occurred in infants weighing less than 1000 g; there were no isolates of vancomycin-resistant strains of coagulase-negative staphylococci. Although the data are suggestive of a beneficial effect for the treated infants, the development of vancomycin-resistant strains of coagulase-negative staphylococci and other bacteria in the bowel of the treated infants and spread to other infants in the nursery would appear likely and restrain the use of this prophylactic regimen. The investigators suggest restriction of the prophylactic regimen to infants weighing less than 1000 g who would be most susceptible to invasive gram-positive infections, but even this limitation may be a concern in the neonatal intensive care unit.

Maternal Factors

The antiviral and antibacterial activity of human milk has been recognized for many years[615–617] and is extensively discussed in Chapter 4. Breast-fed infants have a lower incidence of gastroenteritis, respiratory illness, and otitis media than those who are formula fed. A protective effect of breast-feeding against infections of the urinary tract has also been suggested.[618]

Evidence that breast-feeding defends against neonatal sepsis and gram-negative meningitis was reported more than 20 years ago from Sweden.[619] More recent studies carried out in Pakistan have confirmed these findings and extended them, showing that even partial breast-feeding appears to be protective against clinical sepsis among neonates in a developing nation with a high mortality from this condition.[620] The degree to which this effect is based on anti-infective components in the milk, avoidance of contaminated foods and fluids, or both is the subject of ongoing investigation.

Observations that breast-feeding enhances lymphocyte responses to a purified protein derivative (PPD) of *M. tuberculosis* in infants given BCG vaccination at birth indicates that the effects of breast milk are not limited to those of an antibody-mediated mucosal protection.[621] The clinical significance of this increased specific cellular immune response during the first few weeks of life remains to be determined.

Immunoprophylaxis

The consequences of immaturity of the neonatal immune system include decreased levels of antibody against common pathogens; decreased complement activity; diminished polymorphonuclear leukocyte production, mobilization, and function; diminished T lymphocyte cytokine production; and reduced concentrations of plasma and cell surface fibronectin.[591] Recognition of these factors has engendered attempts at therapeutic intervention aimed specifically at each component of the deficient immune response.

Infants are protected from infection by passively transferred maternal antibody. To enhance the infants' ability to ward off potential severe infections, immunization of women in the child-bearing years or pregnant women has been selectively adopted.[622] Programs to immunize pregnant women in developing countries with tetanus toxoid have markedly decreased the incidence of neonatal tetanus. Investigational programs for immunization of pregnant women with polysaccharide pneumococcal, *H. influenzae* type b and group B streptococcal vaccines aim to provide infants with protection for the first months of life. Recent studies of safety and immunogenicity of polysaccharide conjugate vaccines for group B streptococci show promise of a reduction in incidence of late-onset as well as early-onset disease in newborns. Use of vaccines in pregnant women are discussed in Chapter 1.

Several clinical trials have explored the use of IGIV to overcome the antibody deficiency of neonates, particularly preterm newborns, and thereby reduce the incidence of sepsis. The results of these investigations were reviewed by Hill.[591] Two of six studies indicated that IGIV reduced the incidence of nosocomial infections, particularly those due to *Candida* and coagulase-negative staphylococci, but did not affect mortality. The remaining four studies failed to demonstrate any effect of IGIV on the rate of nosocomial infections, sepsis, mortality, or complications or on the length of hospital stay. The efficacy of IGIV in prevention of nosocomial infections among high-risk neonates thus remains unproven. The use of hyperimmune IGIV preparations and human monoclonal antibodies to prevent specific infections (e.g., group B streptococci, K1, *E. coli*) in high-risk neonates is being explored.[591]

Although IGIV appears to be of limited value in preventing neonatal infections, even when given within the first few days of life, it may be effective in special circumstances if administered *before* delivery. Sidiropoulos and co-workers studied the benefit of low-dose (12 gm in 12 hours) or high-dose (24 g daily for 5 days) IGIV given to pregnant women at risk for preterm delivery because of chorioamnionitis.[623] Maternal IgG serum concentrations were increased up to threefold following these regimens. Cord blood IgG levels were doubled in infants older than 32 weeks' gestational age whose mothers received the higher dosage schedule (compared with samples from control infants) but were unaffected in infants born earlier, suggesting little or no placental transfer of IGIV before the thirty-second week of gestation. Among the infants delivered after 32 weeks, 6 of 16 (37%) born to untreated mothers developed clinical, laboratory, or radiologic evidence of infection and required antimicrobial therapy; none of 7 infants born to treated mothers became infected. Although this study suggests that providing intrauterine fetal prophylaxis may be of benefit in select cases, the use of IGIV clearly cannot be recommended for all women having premature onset of labor.

The decreased number of circulating polymorphonuclear leukocytes and reduced myeloid reserves in the bone marrow of newborns have been ascribed to impaired production of cytokines interleukin-3, granulocyte colony-stimulating factor, granulocyte-macrophage colony-stimulating factor, tumor necrosis factor-alpha, and interferon-γ.[624, 625] Considerable experience with in vitro myeloid cell cultures and animal models[625, 626] as well as isolated human trials[627] suggest that cytokine therapy may prove to be an effective aid in preventing sepsis among newborns with hereditary or acquired congenital neutropenia. Treatment of small number of infants with early signs of sepsis with pentoxifylline to reduce the concentrations of tumor necrosis factor-alpha showed promise,[588] but there are no studies that have used pentoxifylline for prevention of sepsis. Similarly, preliminary studies of granulocyte colony-stimulating factor in neonates are inconsistent in demonstrating that absolute neutrophil counts are increased or that the incidence of sepsis is reduced.[589, 590, 628]

Fibronectins are high-molecular-weight glycoproteins, produced primarily by liver and endothelial cells, that serve to facilitate cell-to-cell and cell-to-substrate adhesion.[629, 630] They have been shown to be involved in numerous functions, including hemostasis; vascular integrity; tissue repair; T lymphocyte activation; leukocyte migration, adhesion, and phagocytosis; and reticuloendothelial clearance. Plasma fibronectin concentrations in newborns are about one third to one half those of adults; premature infants have levels significantly lower than those of term infants. These concentrations decrease even further in neonates with perinatal asphyxia, respiratory distress syndrome, and sepsis.[631] Studies in animal models and adults with sepsis suggest that fibronectin administration may be of value in improving host defenses and reducing the risk of nosocomial infection in neonates.

Decontamination of Fomites

Because contamination of equipment poses a significant infectious challenge for the newborn, disinfection of all materials that are involved in care of the newborn is an important responsibility of the physician in charge of the nursery. Use of disposable equipment and individual units, such as containers of sterile water for nebulization apparatus, is an important advance in prevention of infection. Intricate or large pieces of equipment may have disposable units, but the basic mechanisms must be cleaned appropriately, particularly because they have been implicated in nursery epidemics.

The frequency of catheter-associated coagulase-negative staphylococcal sepsis has led to attempts to prevent bacterial colonization of intravascular catheters through use of attachment-resistant polymeric materials, antibiotic impregnation, and immunotherapy directed against adherence factors.[632] These procedures are reviewed in Chapter 34.

Epidemiologic Surveillance

ENDEMIC INFECTION

Nursery-acquired infections may become apparent only several weeks to several months after discharge of the infant. Therefore, a surveillance system that not only provides information about infections within the nursery but also involves follow-up of infants after discharge should be established. Various techniques may be used; these are reviewed in Chapter 34.

EPIDEMIC INFECTION

The medical and nursing staff must be alert to the possibility of common-source outbreaks of infection in the nursery. Prevention of disease is based on the level of awareness of personnel. Infection in previously well infants who lack high-risk factors associated with sepsis must be viewed with suspicion. Several cases of infection occurring within a brief period or in physical proximity or caused by an unusual pathogen should be cause for concern. Techniques for management of outbreaks of infectious diseases in nurseries are considered in Chapter 34.

SEPSIS IN THE NEWBORN RECENTLY DISCHARGED FROM THE HOSPITAL

When fever or other signs of systemic infection occur in the first weeks after the newborn is discharged from the nursery, appropriate management requires consideration of the various sources of infection. Infection acquired from a household contact is the most likely etiology. Congenital infection may be present with signs of disease that are perceived first or occur first after discharge. Late-onset infection from microorganisms acquired at delivery or acquired in the nursery may occur weeks or even months after birth. Finally, signs of infection may occur after discharge as a result of underlying anatomic, physiologic, or metabolic abnormalities.

The newborn is susceptible to infectious agents that colonize or cause disease in other members of the household. If an infant who is well when discharged from the nursery and whose gestation and delivery were uneventful develops signs of an infectious disease in the first weeks of life, the infection was probably acquired from someone in the infant's environment. Respiratory and gastrointestinal infections are most common and may be accompanied by focal disease such as otitis media. The incidence of invasive disease caused by *H. influenzae* type b and *S. pneumoniae* is high by 2 months of age (see Table 21–6). A careful history of illness in household members may suggest the source of the infant's infection.

Congenital Infection

Signs of congenital infection may appear or may be identified after discharge from the nursery. Impairment of hearing related to congenital rubella, cytomegalovirus infection, or syphilis may be first noticed by the parent at home. Increasing head size indicative of hydrocephalus caused by congenital toxoplasmosis or rubella may be apparent only after serial examinations. Chorioretinitis, jaundice, or pneumonia may occur as late manifestations of congenital infection. If a lumbar puncture is performed in the course of a work-up for sepsis, CSF pleocytosis and increased concentration of protein may be caused by congenital infection and warrant appropriate diagnostic studies.

Late-onset disease acquired at the time of delivery may present weeks to months later as sepsis and meningitis. Infection from group B streptococci (see Chapter 26) is the most frequent cause of late-onset disease in the neonate. Neonatal disease related to *L. monocytogenes* resembles disease caused by group B streptococci, including early- and late-onset forms of sepsis and meningitis. The pathogenesis of late-onset disease is obscure in most cases. Mothers of infants with disease lack specific immunoglobulins for the infecting strain of group B streptococci; therefore, the infants receive no protective antibody through the placenta. However, the reason that an organism acquired at birth and carried for a prolonged period in the upper respiratory tract becomes invasive and causes sepsis or meningitis remains obscure. Other organisms acquired at delivery from the maternal genital tract that may cause disease in the neonate after discharge include herpes simplex virus, *Salmonella*, *Chlamydia trachomatis*, and cytomegalovirus.

Late-Onset Disease

Late-onset disease may also be caused by organisms acquired in the nursery. Lesions of the skin and soft tissues or other focal infections, including bone or lung from *S. aureus*, may not occur until the second to third week of life or later. Other nosocomially acquired organisms are discussed in Chapter 34.

Infections in the Household

Infection may be associated with an underlying anatomic defect, physiologic abnormality, or metabolic disease. The infant who fails to thrive or presents with fever may have infection of the urinary tract that is the first indication of a physiologic or anatomic abnormality. Infants with atresia of the lacrimal duct or choanae may develop focal infection. Sepsis caused by gram-negative enteric bacilli occurs frequently in infants with galactosemia (see Pathogenesis section).

The infected infant may be an important source of infection to family members. Staphylococcal disease has been found in family members after a newborn was brought into the home. In one study in New York,[633] 12.6% of household contacts developed suppurative lesions during the 10-month period after introduction into the home of an infant with a staphylococcal lesion. The incidence of suppurative infections in household contacts of infants without lesions was less than 2%. Damato and co-workers[634] demonstrated colonization of neonates with enteric organisms possessing R factor–mediated resistance to kanamycin and persistence of these strains for more than 12 months after birth. During the period of observation, one third of the household contacts of the infants became colonized with the same strain. Thus, organisms with R factor–mediated resistance to kanamycin spread within the household after the newborn was introduced.

Infections in infants have been associated with bites or licks of household pets. *Pasteurella multocida* is part of the normal flora of dogs, cats, and rodents. Meningitis caused by *P. multocida* was reported in seven infants younger than 2 months of age.[260] A 5-week-old infant with *P. multocida* meningitis was frequently licked by the family dog: the organism was identified in cultures of the mouth of the dog but not of the throats of the parents. *P. multocida* meningitis in a 3-week-old infant may have resulted from transmission of infection from the family cat to the mother and then to the infant.[259] The epidemiologic link between cats and dogs and infection in young infants suggests that parents should limit contact between pets and infants.

Fever in the First Month of Life

Reviews of fever in the first weeks of life indicate that elevation of temperature (> 38.8° C [101.8° F])[635–644] is relatively uncommon. However, when fever does occur in the young infant, the incidence of severe disease, including sepsis, meningitis, or pneumonia, is sufficiently high to warrant careful evaluation and conservative management. A careful history of the pregnancy, delivery, nursery experience, interval since discharge from the nursery, and infections in the household should be obtained. Physical examination should establish the presence or absence of signs associated with congenital infection and late-onset diseases. Culture of urine should be performed if no other focus is apparent, and cultures of blood and CSF and a chest radiograph should be considered if the infant is believed to have systemic infection.

Practice guidelines prepared by Baraff and colleagues[635] for management of infants and children with fever without source suggest that all febrile infants younger than 28 days should be hospitalized for parenteral antibiotic therapy. The group designated that 38.0°

C (100.4° F) should be used as the lower limit of the definition of fever. The sepsis evaluation in hospital includes a culture of blood, urine, and CSF; a complete blood cell and differential count; examination of CSF for cells, glucose, and protein; and a urinalysis.

ACKNOWLEDGMENT

Dr. S. Michael Marcy was a co-author of this chapter in the first four editions. The author is indebted to Dr. Marcy for his continued interest in the preparation of this chapter for the fifth edition.

References

1. Gaynes RP, Edwards JR, Jarvis WR, et al. Nosocomial infections among neonates in high-risk nurseries in the United States. Pediatrics 93:357–361, 1996.
2. Dunham EC. Septicemia in the newborn. Am J Dis Child 45:229, 1933.
3. Nyhan WL, Fousek MD. Septicemia of the newborn. Pediatrics 22:268, 1958.
4. Gluck L, Wood HF, Fousek MD. Septicemia of the newborn. Pediatr Clin North Am 13:1131, 1966.
5. Freedman RM, Ingram DL, Cross I, et al. A half century of neonatal sepsis at Yale. Am J Dis Child 35:140, 1981.
6. Gladstone IM, Ehrenkranz RA, Edberg SC, Baltimore RS. A ten-year review of neonatal sepsis and comparison with the previous fifty-year experience. Pediatr Infect Dis J 9:819, 1990.
7. Silverman WA, Homan WE. Sepsis of obscure origin in the newborn. Pediatrics 3:157, 1949.
8. Smith RT, Platou ES, Good RA. Septicemia of the newborn: current status of the problem. Pediatrics 17:549, 1956.
9. Moorman RS Jr, Sell SH. Neonatal septicemia. South Med J 54:137, 1961.
10. Buetow KC, Klein SW, Lane RB. Septicemia in premature infants. Am J Dis Child 110:29, 1965.
11. Hodgman JE. Sepsis in the neonate. Perinatol Neonatol 5:45, 1981.
12. Kumar SP, Delivoria-Papadopoulos M. Infections in newborn infants in a special care unit. Ann Clin Lab Sci 15:351, 1985.
13. Stevens DC, Kleiman MB, Schreiner RL. Early-onset *Pseudomonas* sepsis of the neonate. Perinatol Neonatol 6:75, 1982.
14. Hall RT, Kurth CG, Hall SL. Ten-year survey of positive blood cultures among admissions to a neonatal intensive care unit. J Perinatol 7:122, 1987.
15. Spigelblatt L, Saintonge J, Chicoine R, et al. Changing pattern of neonatal streptococcal septicemia. Pediatr Infect Dis J 4:56, 1985.
16. Vesikari R, Janas M, Gronroos P, et al. Neonatal septicemia. Arch Dis Child 60:542, 1985.
17. Vesikari T, Isolauri E, Tuppurainen N, et al. Neonatal septicaemia in Finland 1981–85. Acta Paediatr Scand 78:44, 1989.
18. Hensey OJ, Hart CA, Cooke RWI. Serious infection in a neonatal intensive care unit: a two-year survey. J Hyg (Camb) 95:289, 1985.
19. Speer C, Hauptmann D, Stubbe P, et al. Neonatal septicemia and meningitis in Gottingen, West Germany. Pediatr Infect Dis J 4:36, 1985.
20. Tessin I, Trollfors B, Thiringer K. Incidence and etiology of neonatal septicaemia and meningitis in Western Sweden 1975–1986. Acta Paediatr Scand 79:1023, 1990.
21. Battisi O, Mitchison R, Davies PA. Changing blood culture isolates in a referral neonatal intensive care unit. Arch Dis Child 56:775, 1981.
22. de Louvois J. Septicaemia and meningitis in the newborn. *In* de Louvois J, Harvey D (eds). Infection in the Newborn. New York, John Wiley & Sons, 1990.
23. Hervas JA, Alomar A, Salva F, et al. Neonatal sepsis and meningitis in Mallorca, Spain, 1977–1991. Clin Infect Dis 16:719, 1993.
24. Bruun B, Paerregaard A. Septicemia in a Danish neonatal intensive care unit, 1984 to 1988. Pediatr Infect Dis J 10:159, 1991.
25. Ronnestad A, Abrahamsen TG, Gaustad P, Finne PH. Blood culture isolates during 6 years in a tertiary neonatal intensive care unit. Scand J Infect Dis 30:245–251, 1998.
26. Karpuch J, Goldberg M, Kohelet D. Neonatal bacteremia: a 4-year prospective study. Isr J Med Sci 19:963, 1983.
27. Winfred I. The incidence of neonatal infections in the nursery unit at the Ahmadu Bello University Teaching Hospital, Zaria, Nigeria. East Afr Med J 61:197, 1984.
28. Ghiorghis B. Neonatal sepsis in Addis Ababa, Ethiopia: a review of 151 bacteremic neonates. Ethiop Med J 35(3):169–176, 1997.
29. Saloojee H, Liddle B, Gous H, Pooe M. Changing antibiotic resistance patterns in a neonatal unit and its implications for antibiotic usage. Presented at the International Congress of Paediatric Surgery and Paediatrics. Cape Town, South Africa. February 1–6, 1998 (abstract).
30. Karan S. Purulent meningitis in the newborn. Childs Nerv Syst 2:26, 1986.
31. Sanghvi KP, Tudehope DI. Neonatal bacterial sepsis in a neonatal intensive care unit: a 5-year analysis. J Paediatr Child Health 32:333–338, 1996.
32. Fanaroff AA, Korones SB, Wright LL, et al. Incidence, presenting features, risk factors and significance of late onset septicemia in very low birth weight infants. Pediatr Infect Dis 17:593–598, 1998.
33. Ziai M, Haggerty RJ. Neonatal meningitis. N Engl J Med 259:314, 1958.
34. Groover RV, Sutherland JM, Landing BH. Purulent meningitis of newborn infants. N Engl J Med 264:1115, 1961.
35. Mathies AW Jr, Wehrle PF. Management of bacterial meningitis. *In* Kagan BM (ed). Antimicrobial Therapy. Philadelphia, WB Saunders, 1974, pp 234–243.
36. Wilson HD, Eichenwald HF. Sepsis neonatorum. Pediatr Clin North Am 21:571, 1974.
37. Yow MD, Baker CJ, Barrett FF, et al. Initial antibiotic management of bacterial meningitis. Medicine 52:305, 1973.
38. McCracken GH Jr. Personal communication, 1976.
39. Unhanand M, Mustafa MM, McCracken GH Jr, Nelson JD. Gram-negative enteric bacillary meningitis: a twenty-one-year experience. J Pediatr 122:15, 1993.
40. Mulder CJJ, van Alphen L, Zanen HC. Neonatal meningitis caused by *Escherichia coli* in the Netherlands. J Infect Dis 150:935, 1984.
41. Moreno MT, Vargas S, Poveda R, Sáez-Llorens X. Neonatal sepsis and meningitis in a developing Latin American country. Pediatr Infect Dis J 13:516–520, 1994.
42. Bennhagen R, Svenningsen NW, Bekassy AN. Changing pattern of neonatal meningitis in Sweden: a comparative study 1976 vs. 1983. Scand. J Infect Dis 19:587, 1987.
43. Bingen E, Picard B, Brahimi N, et al. Phylogenetic analysis of *Escherichia coli* strains causing neonatal meningitis suggests horizontal gene transfer from a predominant

pool of highly virulent B2 group strains. J Infect Dis 177:642–650, 1998.

44. Robbins JB, McCracken GH Jr, Gotschuch EC, et al. *Escherichia coli* K₁ capsular polysaccharide associated with neonatal meningitis. N Engl J Med 290:1216, 1974.

45. McCracken GH Jr, Sarff LD, Glode MP, et al. Relation between *Escherichia coli* K₁ capsular polysaccharide antigen and clinical outcome in neonatal meningitis. Lancet 2:246, 1974.

46. McCracken GH Jr, Sarff LD. Current status and therapy of neonatal *E. coli* meningitis. Hosp Pract 9:57, 1974.

47. Sarff LD, McCracken GH Jr, Schiffer MS, et al. Epidemiology of *Escherichia coli* K₁ in healthy and diseased newborns. Lancet 1:1099, 1975.

48. Peter G, Nelson JS. Factors affecting neonatal *E. coli* K₁ rectal colonization. J Pediatr 93:866, 1978.

49. Guerina NG, Kessler TW, Guerina VJ, et al. The role of pili and capsule in the pathogenesis of neonatal infection with *Escherichia coli* K₁. J Infect Dis 148:395, 1983.

50. Tullus K. Epidemiological aspects of P-fimbriated *Escherichia coli* fecal colonization of newborn children and relation to development of extraintestinal *E. coli* infections. Kongl Carolinska Medico Chirurgiska Institut, Danderyl, 1986.

51. Lancefield RC. Serologic differentiation of human and other groups of hemolytic streptococci. J Exp Med 57:571, 1933.

52. Hood M, Janney A, Dameron G. Beta hemolytic *Streptococcus* group B associated with problems of the perinatal period. Am J Obstet Gynecol 82:809, 1961.

53. Eickhoff TC, Klein JO, Daly AK, et al. Neonatal sepsis and other infections due to group B beta-hemolytic streptococci. N Engl J Med 271:1221, 1964.

54. Schlievert PM, Gocke JE, Deringer JR. Group B streptococcal toxic shock-like syndrome: report of a case and purification of an associated pyrogenic toxin. Clin Infect Dis 17:26, 1993.

55. Charles D, Larsen B. Streptococcal puerperal sepsis and obstetric infections: a historical perspective. Rev Infect Dis 8:411, 1986.

56. Loudon I. Puerperal fever, the streptococcus, and the sulphonamides, 1911–1945. BMJ 295:485, 1987.

57. Watson BP. An outbreak of puerperal sepsis in New York City. Am J Obstet Gynecol 16:159–179, 1928.

58. Jewett JF, Reid DE, Safon LE, Easterday CL. Childbed fever: a continuing entity. JAMA 206:344–350, 1968.

59. McCabe WR, Abrams AA. An outbreak of streptococcal puerperal sepsis. N Engl J Med 272:615–618, 1965.

60. Geil CC, Castle WK, Mortimer EA. Group A streptococcal infections in newborn nurseries. Pediatrics 46:849–854, 1970.

61. Gezon HM, Schaberg MJ, Klein JO. Concurrent epidemics of *Staphylococcus aureus* and group A *Streptococcus* disease in a newborn nursery—control with penicillin G and hexachlorophene bathing. Pediatrics 51:383, 1973.

62. Peter G, Hazard J. Neonatal group A streptococcal disease. J Pediatr 87:454, 1975.

63. Nelson JD, Dillon HC Jr, Howard JB. A prolonged nursery epidemic associated with a newly recognized type of group A *Streptococcus*. J Pediatr 89:792, 1976.

64. Campbell JR, Arango CA, Garcia-Prats JA, Baker CJ. An outbreak of M serotype 1 group A *Streptococcus* in neonatal intensive care unit. J Pediatr 129:396–402, 1996.

65. Cartwright RY. Neonatal septicaemia due to group A beta-haemolytic *Streptococcus*. BMJ 1:146, 1977.

66. Wong VK, Wright HT Jr. Group A β-hemolytic streptococci as a cause of bacteremia in children. Am J Dis Child 142:831, 1988.

67. Murphy DJ Jr. Group A streptococcal meningitis. Pediatrics 71:1, 1983.

68. Rathore MH, Barton LL, Kaplan EL. Suppurative group A β-hemolytic streptococcal infections in children. Pediatrics 89:743, 1992.

69. Wilschanski M, Faber J, Abramov A, et al. Neonatal septicemia caused by group A beta-hemolytic *Streptococcus*. Pediatr Infect Dis J 8:536, 1989.

70. Panaro NR, Lutwick LI, Chapnick EK. Intrapartum transmission of group A *Streptococcus*. Clin Infect Dis 17:79, 1993.

71. Mahieu LM, Holm SE, Goossens HJ, Van Acker KJ. Congenital streptococcal toxic shock syndrome with absence of antibodies against streptococcal pyrogenic exotoxins. J Pediatr 127:987–989, 1995.

72. Acharya U, Lamont CAR, Cooper K. Group A beta-hemolytic *Streptococcus* causing disseminated intravascular coagulation and maternal death. Lancet 1:595, 1988.

73. Kavi J, Wise R. Group A beta-hemolytic *Streptococcus* causing disseminated intravascular coagulation and maternal death. Lancet 1:993–994, 1988.

74. Swingler GR, Bigrigg MA, Hewitt BG, McNulty CAM. Disseminated intravascular coagulation associated with group A streptococcal infection in pregnancy. Lancet 1:1456–1457, 1988.

75. Greenberg D, Leibovitz E, Shinnwell ES, et al. Neonatal sepsis caused by *Streptococcus pyogenes*—resurgence of an old etiology? Pediatr Infect Dis J 18:479–481, 1999.

76. Stevens DL, Tanner MH, Winship J, et al. Severe group A streptococcal infections associated with a toxic shock–like syndrome and scarlet fever toxin A. N Engl J Med 321:1–7, 1989.

77. Stevens DL. Invasive group A streptococcal infections. Clin Infect Dis 14:2–13, 1992.

78. Cleary PP, Kaplan EL, Handley JP, et al. Clonal basis for resurgence of serious *Streptococcus pyogenes* disease in the 1980s. Lancet 339:518–521, 1992.

79. Stevens DL, Bryant AS, Hackett SP, et al. Group A streptococcal bacteremia: the role of tumor necrosis factor in shock and organ failure. J Infect Dis 173:619–626, 1996.

80. Patamasucon P, Siegel JD, McCracken GH Jr. Streptococcal submandibular cellulitis in young infants. Pediatrics 67:378, 1981.

81. Stewardson-Krieger P, Gotoff SP. Neonatal meningitis due to group C beta hemolytic *Streptococcus*. J Pediatr 90:103, 1977.

82. Hervás JA, Labay MV, Rullán G, et al. Neonatal sepsis and meningitis due to *Streptococcus equisimilis*. Pediatr Infect Dis J 4:694, 1985.

83. Arditi M, Shulman ST, Davis AT, Yogev R. Group C β-hemolytic streptococcal infections in children: nine pediatric cases and review. Rev Infect Dis 11:34, 1989.

84. Baker CJ. Unusual occurrence of neonatal septicemia due to group G *Streptococcus*. Pediatrics 53:568, 1974.

85. Tsai TF, et al. Congenital yellow fever virus infection after immunization in pregnancy. Pediatr Infect Dis J 13:553–554, 1994.

86. Ancona RJ, Thompson TR, Ferrieri P. Group G streptococcal pneumonia and sepsis in a newborn infant. J Clin Microbiol 10:758, 1979.

87. Applebaum PC, Friedman Z, Fairbrother PF, et al. Neonatal sepsis due to group G streptococci. Acta Paediatr Scand 69:599, 1980.

88. Mohan VDKK, Tilton RC, Raye JR, et al. Fatal group G streptococcal sepsis in a preterm neonate. Am J Dis Child 134:894, 1980.

89. Dyson AE, Read SE. Group G streptococcal colonization and sepsis in neonates. J Pediatr 99:944, 1981.

90. Carstensen H, Pers C, Pryds O. Group G streptococcal neonatal septicemia: two case reports and a brief review of the literature. Scand. J Infect Dis 20:407, 1988.

91. Auckenthaler R, Hermans PE, Washington JA II. Group G streptococcal bacteremia: clinical study and review of the literature. Rev Infect Dis 5:196, 1983.

92. McNeeley DF, Brown AE, Noel GJ, et al. An investigation of vancomycin-resistant *Enterococcus faecium* within the pediatric service of a large urban medical center. Pediatr Infect Dis J 17:184–188, 1998.

93. Siegel JD, McCracken GH Jr. Group D streptococcal infections. J Pediatr 93:542, 1978.

94. McNeeley DF, Saint-Louis F, Noel GJ. Neonatal enterococcal bacteremia: an increasingly frequent event with potentially untreatable pathogens. Pediatr Infect Dis J 15:800–805, 1996.

95. Alexander JB, Giacoia GP. Early onset nonenterococcal group D streptococcal infection in the newborn infant. J Pediatr 93:489, 1978.

96. Headings DL, Herrera A, Mazzi E, et al. Fulminant neonatal septicemia caused by *Streptococcus bovis*. J Pediatr 92:282, 1978.

97. Fikar CR, Levy J. *Streptococcus bovis* meningitis in a neonate. Am J Dis Child 133:1149, 1979.

98. Bavikatte K, Schreiner RL, Lemons JA, et al. Group D streptococcal septicemia in the neonate. Am J Dis Child 133:493, 1979.

99. Hellwege HH, Ram W, Scherf H, et al. Neonatal meningitis caused by *Streptococcus mitis*. Lancet 1:743, 1984.

100. Bignardi GE, Isaacs D. Neonatal meningitis due to *Streptococcus mitis*. Rev Infect Dis 11:86, 1989.

101. Dobson SRM, Baker CJ. Enterococcal sepsis in neonates: features by age at onset and occurrence of focal infection. Pediatrics 85:165, 1990.

102. Buchino JJ, Ciambarella E, Light I. Systemic group D streptococcal infection in newborn infants. Am J Dis Child 133:270, 1979.

103. Boulanger JM, Ford-Jones EL, Matlow AG. Enterococcal bacteremia in a pediatric institution: a four-year review. Rev Infect Dis 13:847, 1991.

104. Coudron PE, Mayhall CG, Facklam RR, et al. *Streptococcus faecium* outbreak in a neonatal intensive care unit. J Clin Microbiol 20:1044, 1984.

105. Lugenbuhl LM, Rotbart HA, Facklan RR, et al. Neonatal enterococcal sepsis: case-control study and description of an outbreak. Pediatr Infect Dis J 6:1022, 1987.

106. Broughton RA, Krafka R, Baker CJ. Non-group D alpha-hemolytic streptococci: new neonatal pathogens. J Pediatr 99:450, 1981.

107. Centers for Disease Control and Prevention. Update: Multi-state outbreak of listeriosis—United States 1998–1999. MMWR Morb Mortal Wkly Rep 47:1117–1118, 1999.

108. Espersen F, Frimodt-Møller N, Rosdahl VT, Jessen O. *Staphylococcus aureus* bacteremia in children below the age of one year. Acta Paediatr Scand 78:56, 1989.

109. Sidebottom DG, Freeman J, Platt R, et al. Fifteen-year experience with bloodstream isolates of coagulase-negative staphylococci in neonatal intensive care. J Clin Microbiol 26:713, 1988.

110. Baumgart S, Hall SE, Campos JM, et al. Sepsis with coagulase-negative staphylococci in critically ill newborns. Am J Dis Child 137:461, 1983.

111. Hall RT, Hall SL, Barnes WG, et al. Characteristics of coagulase negative staphylococci from infants with bacteremia. Pediatr Infect Dis J 6:377, 1987.

112. Freeman J, Goldmann DA, Smith NE, et al. Association of intravenous lipid emulsion and coagulase-negative staphylococcal bacteremia in neonatal intensive care units. N Engl J Med 323:301, 1990.

113. Kumar ML, Jenson HB, Dahms BD. Experience and reason—briefly recorded. Pediatrics 76:110, 1985.

114. Gorbach SL, Bartlett JG. Anaerobic infections. N Engl J Med 290:1177, 1974.

115. Gorbach SL, Menda KB, Thadepalli H, et al. Anaerobic microflora of the cervix in healthy women. Am J Obstet Gynecol 117:1053, 1973.

116. Chow AW, Guze LB. Bacteroidaceae bacteremia: clinical experience with 112 patients. Medicine 53:93, 1974.

117. Finegold SM. Anaerobic infections. Surg Clin North Am 60:49, 1980.

118. Brook I. Bacteremia due to anaerobic bacteria in newborns. J Perinatol 10:351, 1990.

119. Chow AW, Leake RD, Yamauchi T, et al. The significance of anaerobes in neonatal bacteremia: analysis of 23 cases and review of the literature. Pediatrics 54:736, 1974.

120. Harrod JR, Stevens DA. Anaerobic infections in the newborn infant. J Pediatr 85:399, 1974.

121. Dunkle LM, Brotherton TJ, Feigen RD. Anaerobic infections in children: a prospective study. Pediatrics 57:311, 1976.

122. Crosson FJ Jr, Feder HM, Bocchini JA, et al. Neonatal sepsis at The Johns Hopkins Hospital, 1969–1975: bacterial isolates and clinical correlates. Johns Hopkins Med J 140:37, 1977.

123. Spector SA, Ticknor W, Grossman M. Study of the usefulness of clinical and hematologic findings in the diagnosis of neonatal bacterial infections. Clin Pediatr (Phila) 20:385, 1981.

124. Robinow M, Simonelli FA. *Fusobacterium* bacteremia in the newborn. Am J Dis Child 110:92, 1965.

125. Chaney NE. *Clostridium* infection in mother and infant. Am J Dis Child 134:1175, 1980.

126. Ohta S, Shimizu S, Fujisawa S, et al. Neonatal adrenal abscess due to *Bacteroides*. J Pediatr 93:1063, 1978.

127. Lee Y-H, Berg RB. Cephalhematoma infected with *Bacteroides*. Am J Dis Child 121:72, 1971.

128. Siddiqi SF, Taylor PM. Necrotizing fasciitis of the scalp: a complication of fetal monitoring. Am J Dis Child 136:226, 1982.

129. Feder HM Jr. *Bacteroides fragilis* meningitis. Rev Infect Dis 9:783, 1987.

130. Noel GJ, Laufer DA, Edelson PJ. Anaerobic bacteremia in a neonatal intensive care unit: an eighteen year experience. Pediatr Infect Dis J 7:858, 1988.

131. Gormley D. Neonatal anaerobic (clostridial) cellulitis and omphalitis. Arch Dermatol 113:683, 1977.

132. Kosloske A, Cushing AH, Borden TA, et al. Cellulitis and necrotizing fasciitis of the abdominal wall in pediatric patients. J Pediatr Surg 16:246, 1981.

133. Spark RP, Wike DA. Nontetanus clostridal neonatal fatality after home delivery. Arizona Med 40:697, 1983.

134. Motz RA, James AG, Dove B. *Clostridium perfringens* meningitis in a newborn infant. Pediatr Infect Dis J 15:708–709, 1996.

135. Adams JM, Kenny JD, Rudolph AJ. Modern management of tetanus neonatorum. Pediatrics 64:472, 1979.

136. Centers for Disease Control. Neonatal tetanus—Montana, 1998. MMWR Morb Mortal Wkly Rep 47:928–930, 1998.

137. U.S. Food and Drug Administration. Neonatal tetanus. FDA Med Bull, Summer 1998, p 4.

138. Woodruff AW, El Bashir EA, Yugusuk AZ, et al. Neona-

tal tetanus: mode of infection, prevalence, and prevention in southern Sudan. Lancet 1:378, 1984.

139. Arnold RB, Soewarso TI, Karyadi A. Mortality from neonatal tetanus in Indonesia: results of two surveys. Bull World Health Organ 64:259, 1986.

140. Athavale VB, Pai PN. Tetanus neonatorum—clinical manifestations. J Pediatr 67:649, 1965.

141. Salimpour R. Cause of death in tetanus neonatorum: study of 233 cases with 54 necropsies. Arch Dis Child 52:587, 1977.

142. Smythe PM, Bowie MD, Voss TJV. Treatment of tetanus neonatorum with muscle relaxants and intermittent positive-pressure ventilation. BMJ 1:223, 1974.

143. Herrero JIH, Beltran RR, Sanchanz AMM. Failure of intrathecal tetanus antitoxin in the treatment of tetanus neonatorum. J Infect Dis 164:619, 1991.

144. Abrutyn E, Berlin JA. Intrathecal therapy in tetanus. JAMA 266:2262, 1991.

145. Traverso HP, Kahn AJ, Rahim H, et al. Ghee application to the umbilical cord: a risk factor for neonatal tetanus. Lancet 1:486, 1989.

146. Oudesluys-Murphy AM. Umbilical cord care and neonatal tetanus. Lancet 1:843, 1989.

147. Newell KW, Lehmann AD, Leblanc CR, et al. The use of toxoid for the prevention of tetanus neonatorum: final report of a double-blind controlled field trial. Bull World Health Organ 35:863, 1966.

148. Black RE, Huber DH, Curlin GT. Reduction of neonatal tetanus by mass immunization of nonpregnant women: duration of protection provided by one or two doses of aluminum-adsorbed tetanus toxoid. Bull World Health Organ 58:927, 1980.

149. Schofield F. Selective primary health care: strategies for control of disease in the developing world: XXII. Tetanus: a preventable problem. Rev Infect Dis 8:144, 1986.

150. Stroh G, Kyu UA, Thaung U, et al. Measurement of mortality from neonatal tetanus in Burma. Bull World Health Organ 65:309, 1987.

151. Schuchat A, Robinson K, Wenger JD, et al. Bacterial meningitis in the United States in 1995. N Engl J Med 337:970–976, 1997.

152. Sunderland WA, Harris HH, Spence CA, et al. Meningococcemia in a newborn infant whose mother had meningococcal vaginitis. J Pediatr 81:856, 1972.

153. Jones RN, Stepack J, Eades A. Fatal neonatal meningococcal meningitis: Association with maternal cervical-vaginal colonization. JAMA 236:2652, 1976.

154. Cher DJ, Maxwell WJ, Frusztajer N, et al. A case of pelvic inflammatory disease associated with Neisseria meningitidis bacteremia. Clin Infect Dis 17:134, 1993.

155. Bhutta ZA, Khan IA, Agha Z. Fatal intrauterine meningococcal infection. Pediatr Infect Dis J 10:868, 1991.

156. Chugh K, Bhalla CK, Joshi KK. Meningococcal abscess and meningitis in a neonate. Pediatr Infect Dis J 7:136, 1988.

157. Arango CA, Rathore MH. Neonatal meningococcal meningitis: case reports and review of literature. Pediatr Infect Dis J 15:1134–1136, 1996.

158. Manginello FP, Pascale JA, Wolfsdorf J, et al. Neonatal meningococcal meningitis and meningococcemia. Am J Dis Child 133:651, 1979.

159. Khuri-Bulos J, McIntosh K. Neonatal Haemophilus influenzae infection: report of eight cases and review of the literature. Am J Dis Child 129:57, 1975.

160. Lilien LD, Yeh TF, Novak GM, et al. Early-onset Haemophilus sepsis in newborn infants: clinical, roentgenographic, and pathologic features. Pediatrics 62:299, 1978.

161. Campognone P, Singer DB. Neonatal sepsis due to nontypable Haemophilus influenzae. Am J Dis Child 140:117, 1986.

162. Lerman SJ. Systemic Hemophilus influenzae infection: a study of risk factors. Clin Pediatr (Phila) 21:360, 1982.

163. Wallace RJ Jr, Baker CJ, Quinones FJ, et al. Nontypable Haemophilus influenzae (biotype 4) as a neonatal, maternal and genital pathogen. Rev Infect Dis 5:123, 1983.

164. Meis JF, Bergman KA, Smedts F, Horrevorts AM. Fulminant neonatal sepsis due to Haemophilus influenzae. Scand J Infect Dis 23:649, 1991.

165. Falia TJ, Dobson SRM, Crook DWM, et al. Population-based study of non-typable Haemophilus influenzae invasive disease in children and neonates. Lancet 341:851, 1993.

166. Abdul-Rauf A, Schrieber JR. Neonatal Haemophilus influenzae type b sepsis. Pediatr Infect Dis J 9:918, 1990.

167. Friesen CA, Cho CT. Characteristic features of neonatal sepsis due to Haemophilus influenzae. Rev Infect Dis 8:777, 1986.

168. Barton LL, Cruz RD, Walentik C. Neonatal Haemophilus influenzae type C sepsis. Am J Dis Child 136:463, 1982.

169. Silverberg K, Boehm FH. Haemophilus influenzae amnionitis with intact membranes: a case report. Am J Perinatol 7:270, 1990.

170. Holt RN, Taylor CD, Schneider HJ, et al. Three cases of Hemophilus parainfluenzae meningitis. Clin Pediatr (Phila) 13:666, 1974.

171. Zinner SH, McCormack WM, Lee Y-H, et al. Puerperal bacteremia and neonatal sepsis due to Hemophilus parainfluenzae: report of a case with antibody titers. Pediatrics 49:612, 1972.

172. Miano A, Cipolloni AP, Casadei GP, et al. Neonatal Haemophilus aphrophilus meningitis. Helv Paediatr Acta 31:499, 1976.

173. Bortolussi R, Thompson TR, Ferrieri P. Early-onset pneumococcal sepsis in newborn infants. Pediatrics 60:352, 1977.

174. Shaw PJ, Robinson DL, Watson JG. Pneumococcal infection in a mother and infant. Lancet 2:47, 1984.

175. Westh H, Skibsted L, Korner B. Streptococcus pneumoniae infections of the female genital tract and in the newborn child. Rev Infect Dis 12:416, 1990.

176. Jacobs J, Garmyn D, Verhaegen J, et al. Neonatal sepsis due to Streptococcus pneumoniae. Scand J Infect Dis 22:493, 1990.

177. Robinson EN Jr. Pneumococcal endometritis and neonatal sepsis. Rev Infect Dis 12:799, 1990.

178. Kaplan M, Rudensky B, Beck A. Perinatal infections with Streptococcus pneumoniae. Am J Perinatol 10:1, 1993.

179. Doran TI. The role of Citrobacter in clinical disease of children: review. Clin Infect Dis 28:384–394, 1999.

180. Graham DR, Anderson RL, Ariel FE, et al. Epidemic nosocomial meningitis due to Citrobacter diversus in neonates. J Infect Dis 144:203, 1981.

181. Gwynn CM, George RH. Neonatal Citrobacter meningitis. Arch Dis Child 48:455, 1973.

182. Kaplan AM, Itabashi HH, Yoshimori R, et al. Cerebral abscesses complicating neonatal Citrobacter freundii meningitis. West J Med 127:418, 1977.

183. Ribeiro CC, Davis P, Jones DM. Citrobacter koseri meningitis in a special care baby unit. J Clin Pathol 29:1094, 1976.

184. Graham DR, Band JD. Citrobacter diversus brain abscess and meningitis in neonates. JAMA 245:1923, 1981.

185. Lin FYC, Devol WF, Morrison C, et al. Outbreak of neonatal Citrobacter diversus meningitis in a suburban hospital. Pediatr Infect Dis J 6:50, 1987.

186. Williams WW, Mariano J, Spurrier M, et al. Nosocomial meningitis due to *Citrobacter diversus* in neonates: new aspects of the epidemiology. J Infect Dis 150:229, 1984.

187. Eppes SC, Woods CR, Mayer AS, Klein JD. Recurring ventriculitis due to *Citrobacter diversus*: clinical and bacteriologic analysis. Clin Infect Dis 17:437, 1993.

188. Foreman SD, Smith EE, Ryan NJ, et al. Neonatal *Citrobacter* meningitis; pathogenesis of cerebral abscess formation. Ann Neurol 16:655, 1984.

189. Morris JG, Lin F-YC, Morrison CB, et al. Molecular epidemiology of neonatal meningitis due to *Citrobacter diversus*: a study of isolates from hospitals in Maryland. J Infect Dis 154:409, 1986.

190. Kline MW, Mason EO Jr, Kaplan SL. Characterization of *Citrobacter diversus* strains causing neonatal meningitis. J Infect Dis 157:101, 1988.

191. Catlin BW. *Gardnerella vaginalis*: characteristics, clinical considerations, and controversies. Clin Microbiol Rev 5:213, 1992.

192. Venkataramani TK, Rathbun HK. *Corynebacterium vaginale (Hemophilus vaginalis)* bacteremia: clinical study of 29 cases. Johns Hopkins Med J 139:93, 1976.

193. Platt MS. Neonatal *Hemophilus vaginalis (Corynebacterium vaginalis)* infection. Clin Pediatr (Phila) 10:513, 1971.

194. Berardi-Grassias L, Roy O, Berardi JC, et al. Neonatal meningitis due to *Gardnerella vaginalis*. Eur J Clin Microbiol Infect Dis 7:406, 1988.

195. Nightingale LM, Eaton CB, Fruehan AE, et al. Cephalhematoma complicated by osteomyelitis presumed due to *Gardnerella vaginalis*. JAMA 256:1936, 1986.

196. Ghosal SP, SenGupta PC, Mukherjee AK. Noma neonatorum: its aetiopathogenesis. Lancet 2:289, 1978.

197. Shah SS, Gallagher PG. Complications of conjunctivitis caused by *Pseudomonas aeruginosa* in a newborn intensive care unit. Pediatr Infect Dis J 17:97–102, 1998.

198. Kleiman MB, Allen SD, Neal P, et al. Meningoencephalitis and compartmentalization of the cerebral ventricles caused by *Enterobacter sakazakii*. J Clin Microbiol 14:352, 1981.

199. Muytjens HL, Zanen HC, Sonderkamp HJ, et al. Analysis of eight cases of neonatal meningitis and sepsis due to *Enterobacter sakazakii*. J Clin Microbiol 18:115, 1983.

200. Willis J, Robinson JE. *Enterobacter sakazakii* meningitis in neonates. Pediatr Infect Dis J 7:196, 1988.

201. Bonadio WA, Margolis D, Tovar M. *Enterobacter cloacae* bacteremia in children: a review of 30 cases in 12 years. Clin Pediatr 30:310, 1991.

202. Heusser MF, Patterson JE, Kuritza AP, et al. Emergence of resistance to multiple beta-lactams in *Enterobacter cloacae* during treatment for neonatal meningitis with cefotaxime. Pediatr Infect Dis 9:509, 1990.

203. Wenger PJ, Tokars JI, Brennan P, et al. An outbreak of *Enterobacter hormaechei* infection and colonization in an intensive care nursery. Clin Infect Dis 24:1243–1244, 1997.

204. Gürses N. *Enterobacter* septicemia in neonates. Pediatr Infect Dis J 14:638, 1995.

205. Muytjens HL, Kollee LAA. *Enterobacter sakazakii* meningitis in neonates: causative role of formula? Pediatr Infect Dis J 9:372, 1990.

206. Noriega FR, Kotloff KL, Martin MA, Schwalbe RS. Nosocomial bacteremia caused by *Enterobacter sakazakii* and *Leuconostoc mesenteroides* resulting from extrinsic contamination of infant formula. Pediatr Infect Dis J 9:447, 1990.

207. Fok TF, Lee CH, Wong EMC, et al. Risk factors for *Enterobacter* septicemia in a neonatal unit: case-control study. Clin Infect Dis 27:1204–1209, 1998.

208. Centers for Disease Control. Reported isolates of *Salmonella* from CSF in the United States, 1968–1979. J Infect Dis 143:504–506, 1981.

209. Reed RP, Klugman KP. Neonatal typhoid fever. Pediatr Infect Dis J 13:774–777. 1994.

210. Gromisch DS, Gordon SG, Bedrosian L, et al. Simultaneous mixed bacterial meningitis in an infant. Am J Dis Child 119:284, 1970.

211. Pacifico L, Chiesa C, Mirabella S, et al. Early-onset *Pseudomonas aeruginosa* sepsis and *Yersinia enterocolitica* neonatal infection: a unique combination in a preterm infant. Eur J Pediatr 146:192, 1987.

212. Faix RG, Kovarik SM. Polymicrobial sepsis among intensive care nursery infants. J Perinatol 9:131, 1989.

213. Jarvis WR, Hybsmith AK, Allen JR, et al. Polymicrobial bacteremia associated with lipid emulsion in a neonatal intensive care unit. Pediatr Infect Dis J 2:203, 1983.

214. Sferra TJ, Pacini DL. Simultaneous recovery of bacterial and viral pathogens from CSF. Pediatr Infect Dis J 7:552, 1988.

215. Giacoia GP. Uncommon pathogens in newborn infants. J Perinatol 14:134–144, 1994.

216. Longe AC, Omene JA, Okolo AA. Neonatal meningitis in Nigerian infants. Acta Paediatr Scand 73:477, 1984.

217. Namnyak SS, Holmes B, Fathalla SE. Neonatal meningitis caused by *Achromobacter xylosoxidans*. J Clin Microbiol 22:470, 1985.

218. Stone JW, Das BC. Investigation of an outbreak of infection with *Acinetobacter calcoaceticus* in a special care baby unit. J Hosp Infect 6:42, 1985.

219. McDonald LC, Walker M, Carson L, et al. Outbreak of *Acinetobacter* spp.: bloodstream infections in a nursery associated with contaminated aerosols and air conditioners. Pediatr Infect Dis J 17:716–722, 1998.

220. Park JW, Grossman O. *Aerococcus viridans* infection: case report and review. Clin Pediatr 29:525, 1990.

221. Doxiadis SA, Pavlaton M, Chryesostomidou O. *Bacillus faecalis alcaligenes* septicemia in the newborn. J Pediatr 56:648, 1960.

222. Turnbull PCB, Jorgensen K, Kramer JM, et al. Severe clinical conditions associated with *Bacillus cereus* and the apparent involvement of exotoxins. J Clin Pathol 32:289, 1979.

223. Wiedermann BL. Non-anthrax *Bacillus* infections in children. Pediatr Infect Dis J 6:218, 1987.

224. Patrick CC, Langston C, Baker CJ. *Bacillus* species infections in neonates. Rev Infect Dis 11:612, 1989.

225. Feder HM, Garibaldi RA, Nurse BA, Kurker R. *Bacillus* species isolates from CSF in patients without shunts. Pediatrics 82:909, 1988.

226. Fuchs PC, Oyama AA. Neonatal relapsing fever due to transplacental transmission of *Borrelia*. JAMA 209:690, 1969.

227. Yagupsky P, Moses S. Neonatal *Borrelia* species infection (relapsing fever). Am J Dis Child 139:74, 1985.

228. Singer R, Amitai Y, Geist M, et al. Neonatal brucellosis possibly transmitted during delivery. Lancet 338:127, 1991.

229. Al-Eissa YA, Al-Mofada SM. Congenital brucellosis. Pediatr Infect Dis J 11:667, 1992.

230. Miller MM. Persistent coccobacillary sepsis in a preterm newborn. Pediatr Infect Dis J 12:542, 1993.

231. Kahyaoglu O, Nolan B, Kumar A. *Burkholderia cepacia* sepsis in neonates. Pediatr Infect Dis J 14:815–816, 1995.

232. Eden AN. *Vibrio* fetus meningitis in a newborn infant. J Pediatr 61:33, 1962.

233. Simor AE, Karmali MA, Jadavji T, et al. Abortion and

perinatal sepsis associated with *Campylobacter* infection. Rev Infect Dis 8:397, 1986.

234. Goossens H, Kremp L, Boury R, et al. Nosocomial outbreak of *Campylobacter jejuni* meningitis in newborn infants. Lancet 2:146, 1986.

235. Forbes JC, Scheifele DS. Early onset *Campylobacter* sepsis in a neonate. Pediatr Infect Dis J 6:494, 1987.

236. Feldman JD, Kontaxis EN, Sherman MP. Congenital bacteremia due to *Capnocytophaga*. Pediatr Infect Dis J 4:415, 1985.

237. Mercer LJ. *Capnocytophaga* isolated from the endometrium as a cause of neonatal sepsis. J Reprod Med 30:67, 1985.

238. Iralu JV, Roberts D, Kazanjian PH. Chorioamnionitis caused by *Capnocytophaga*: case report and review. Clin Infect Dis 17:457, 1993.

239. Beckwith DG, Jahre JA, Haggerty S. Isolation of *Corynebacterium aquaticum* fron spinal fluid of an infant with meningitis. J Clin Microbiol 23:375, 1986.

240. Vohra K, Torrijos E, Jhaveri R, et al. Neonatal sepsis and meningitis caused by *Edwardsiella tarda*. Pediatr Infect Dis J 7:814, 1988.

241. Ginsberg HG, Daum RS. *Escherichia hermanii* sepsis with duodenal perforation in a neonate. Pediatr Infect Dis J 6:300, 1987.

242. Plotkin SA, McKitrick JC. Nosocomial meningitis of the newborn caused by a flavobacterium. JAMA 198:662, 1966.

243. Linden N, Karnan SH, Eyal F, et al. Trimethoprim-sulfamethoxazole in neonatal *Flavobacterium meningosepticum* infection. Arch Dis Child 59:582, 1984.

244. Abrahamsen TG, Finne PH, Lingass E. *Flavobacterium meningosepticum* infections in a neonatal intensive care unit. Acta Paediatr Scand 78:51, 1989.

245. Tizer KB, Cervia JS, Dunn A, et al. Successful combination vancomycin and rifampin therapy in a newborn with community-acquired *Flavobacterium meningosepticum* neonatal meningitis. Pediatr Infect Dis J 14:916–917, 1995.

246. Orlicek SI, Welch DF, Kuhls TL. Septicemia and meningitis caused by *Helicobacter cinaedi* in a neonate. J Clin Microbiol 31:569, 1993.

247. Hill HR, Hunt CE, Matsen JM. Nosocomial colonization with *Klebsiella*, type 26, in a neonatal intensive care unit associated with an outbreak of sepsis, meningitis, and necrotizing enterocolitis. J Pediatr 85:415, 1974.

248. John JF Jr, McKee KT, Twitty JA, et al. Molecular epidemiology of sequential nursery epidemics caused by multiresistant *Klebsiella pneumoniae*. J Pediatr 102:825, 1983.

249. Broughton RA, Gruter WC, Haffar AAM, et al. Neonatal meningitis due to *Lactobacillus*. Pediatr Infect Dis J 2:382, 1983.

250. Goell HO Jr, Olafsson A, Sonnabend W, et al. Intrauterine *Leptospirosis pomona*. Dtsch Med Wochenschr 31:1263, 1971.

251. Lindsay S, Luke IW. Fatal leptospirosis in a newborn infant. J Pediatr 7:90, 1947.

252. Shaked Y, Shpilberg O, Samra D, Samra Y. Leptospirosis in pregnancy and its effect on the fetus: case report and review. Clin Infect Dis 17:241, 1993.

253. Hardy S, Ruoff KL, Catlin E, et al. Catheter-associated infection with a vancomycin-resistant gram-positive coccus of the *Leuconostoc* species. Pediatr Infect Dis J 7:519, 1988.

254. Handwerger S, Horowitz H, Coburn K, et al. Infection due to *Leuconostoc* species: six cases and review. Rev Infect Dis 12:602, 1990.

255. Friedland IR, Snipelisky M, Khoosal M. Meningitis in a neonate caused by *Leuconostoc* sp. J Clin Microbiol 28:2125, 1990.

256. Carapetis J, Bishop S, Davis J, et al. *Leuconostoc* sepsis in association with continuous enteral feeding: two case reports and a review. Pediatr Infect Dis J 13:816–823, 1994.

257. Rowen JL, Lopez SM. *Morganella morganii* early onset sepsis. Pediatr Infect Dis J 17:1176–1177, 1998.

258. Frutos AA, Levitsky D, Scott EH, et al. A case of septicemia and meningitis in an infant due to *Pasteurella multocida*. J Pediatr 92:853, 1978.

259. Bhave SA, Guy LM. *Pasteurella multocida* meningitis in an infant with recovery. BMJ 2:741, 1977.

260. Thompson CM, Pappu L, Leukoff AH, et al. Neonatal septicemia and meningitis due to *Pasteurella multocida*. Pediatr Infect Dis J 3:559, 1984.

261. Clapp DW, Kleiman MB, Reynolds JK, et al. *Pasteurella multocida* meningitis in infancy: an avoidable infection. Am J Dis Child 140:444, 1986.

262. Escande F, Borde M, Pateyron F. Maternal and neonatal *Pasteurella multocida* infection. Arch Pediatr 4:1116–1118, 1997.

263. Pathak A, Custer JR, Levy J. Neonatal septicemia and meningitis due to *Plesiomonas shigelloides*. Pediatrics 71:389, 1983.

264. Brenden RA, Miller MA, Janda JM. Clinical disease spectrum and pathogenic factors associated with *Plesiomonas shigelloides* infections in humans. Rev Infect Dis 10:303, 1988.

265. Applebaum PC, Bowen AJ, Adhikari M, et al. Neonatal septicemia and meningitis due to *Aeromonas shigelloides*. J Pediatr 92:676, 1982.

266. Burke JP, Ingall D, Klein JO, et al. *Proteus mirabilis* infections in a hospital nursery traced to a human carrier. N Engl J Med 284:115, 1971.

267. Osteraas GR, Hardman JM, Bass JW, et al. Neonatal melioidosis. Am J Dis Child 122:446, 1971.

268. Barbaro DJ, Mackowiak PA, Barth SS, Southern PM. *Pseudomonas testosteroni* infections: eighteen recent cases and a review of the literature. Rev Infect Dis 9:124, 1987.

269. Lloyd-Puryear M, Wallace D, Baldwin T, Hollis DG. Meningitis caused by *Psychrobacter immobilis* in an infant. J Clin Microbiol 29:2041, 1991.

270. Lewis DA, Hawkey PM, Watts JA, et al. Infection with netilmicin resistant *Serratia marcescens* in a special care baby unit. BMJ 287:1701, 1983.

271. McCormack RC, Kunin CM. Control of a single source nursery epidemic due to *Serratia marcescens*. Pediatrics 37:750, 1966.

272. Bollmann R, Halle E, Sokolowska-Kohler W, et al. Nosocomial infections due to *Serratia marcescens*—clinical findings, antibiotic susceptibility patterns and fine typing. Infections 17:294.

273. Ruderman JW, Stoller KP, Pomerance JJ. Bloodstream invasion with *Shigella sonnei* in an asymptomatic newborn infant. Pediatr Infect Dis J 5:379, 1986.

274. Langbaum M, Eyal FG. *Stomatococcus mucilaginosus* septicemia and meningitis in a premature infant (letter). Pediatr Infect Dis J 11:334, 1992.

275. Ziao WS, Li S, Jun T. Neonatal septicemia caused by coagulase negative staphylococcus with plasmid analysis. Acta Paediatr Scand 77:308, 1988.

276. Rubin LG, Altman J, Epple LK, et al. *Vibrio cholera* meningitis in a neonate. J Pediatr 98:940, 1981.

277. Challapalli M, Cunningham DG. *Yersinia enterocolitica* septicemia in infants younger than three months of age. Pediatr Infect Dis J 12:168, 1993.

278. White ME, Rosenbaum RJ, Canfield TM, et al. Plague in a neonate. Am J Dis Child 135:418, 1981.

279. PHLS Report. Neonatal meningitis: a review of routine national data 1975–83. BMJ 290:778, 1985.

280. McCracken GH Jr, Shinefield HR. Changes in the pattern of neonatal septicemia and meningitis. Am J Dis Child 112:33, 1966.

281. Alden ER, Mandelkorn T, Woodrum DE, et al. Morbidity and mortality of infants weighing less than 1000 grams in an intensive care nursery. Pediatrics 50:40, 1972.

282. Baker CJ. Nosocomial septicemia and meningitis in neonates. Am J Med 70:698, 1981.

283. Schuchat A, Oxtoby M, Cochi S, et al. Population-based risk factors for neonatal group B streptococcal disease: results of a cohort study in metropolitan Atlanta. J Infect Dis 162:672, 1990.

284. Craig WS. Care of the Newly Born Infant, 2nd ed. Baltimore, Williams & Wilkins, 1962, p 324.

285. Miller A. Incidence of sepsis and meningitis in newborn infants at the Kaiser Foundation Hospitals, Panorama City, Calif. Unpublished data, 1988.

286. Kagan GM, Hess JH, Mirman B, et al. Meningitis in premature infants. Pediatrics 4:479, 1949.

287. Overall JC Jr. Neonatal bacterial meningitis. J Pediatr 76:499, 1970.

288. La Gamma EF, Drusin LM, Mackles AW, et al. Neonatal infections. Am J Dis Child 137:838, 1983.

289. Hemming VG, Britt MR, Overall JC Jr, et al. Infections in a newborn intensive care unit. Pediatr Res 9:297, 1975.

290. Simon C, Schröder H, Beyer C, Zerbst T. Neonatal sepsis in an intensive care unit and results of treatment. Infection 19:146–148, 1991.

291. Barton L, Hodgman JE, Pavlova Z. Causes of death in the extremely low birth weight infant. Pediatrics 103:446–451, 1999.

292. Boyer KM, Gadzala CA, Burd LI, et al. Selective intrapartum chemoprophylaxis of neonatal group B streptococcal early-onset disease: I. Epidemiologic rationale. J Infect Dis 148:795, 1983.

293. Braun P, Lee Y-H, Klein JO, et al. Epidemiology and clinical correlates of genital mycoplasmas in pregnancy and the newborn. Unpublished data, 1970.

294. Lieberman E, Lang JM, Frigoletto F Jr, et al. Epidural analgesia, intrapartum fever, and neonatal sepsis evaluation. Pediatrics 99:415–416, 1997.

295. Niswander KR, Gordon M. The women and their pregnancies. The Collaborative Perinatal Study of the National Institute of Neurological Diseases and Stroke. U.S. Department of Health, Education and Welfare Publication No. (NIH) 73–379. Washington, D.C., U.S. Government Printing Office, 1972.

296. Centers for Disease Control and Prevention. Group B streptococcal disease in the United States, 1990: report from a multistate active surveillance system. In CDC Surveillance Summaries, November 20, 1992. MMWR Morb Mortal Wkly Rep 41(No. SS–6):25, 1992.

297. Benirschke K, Driscoll S. The Pathology of the Human Placenta. New York, Springer-Verlag, 1967.

298. Washburn TC, Medearis DN Jr, Childs B. Sex differences in susceptibility to infections. Pediatrics 35:57, 1965.

299. Sweet AY. Epidemiology. In Brown EG, Sweet AY (eds). Neonatal Necrotizing Enterocolitis. New York, Grune & Stratton, 1980, p 11.

300. Schlegel RJ, Bellanti JA. Increased susceptibility of males to infection. Lancet 2:826, 1969.

301. Purtillo DT, Sullivan JL. Immunological bases for superior survival of females. Am J Dis Child 133:1251, 1979.

302. Torday JS, Nielsen HC, Fencl MD, et al. Sex differences in fetal lung maturation. Am Rev Respir Dis 123:205, 1981.

303. Bennet R, Eriksson M, Zetterström R. Increasing incidence of neonatal septicemia: causative organism and predisposing risk factors. Acta Paediatr Scand 70:207, 1981.

304. MacFarlane DE. Neonatal group B streptococcal septicaemia in a developing country. Acta Paediatr Scand 76:470, 1987.

305. Barclay N. High frequency of salmonella species as a cause of neonatal meningitis in Ibadan, Nigeria: a review of thirty-eight cases. Acta Paediatr Scand 60:540, 1971.

306. Montefiore D, Alausa KO, Sobayo E. Pyogenic meningitis in Ibadan, Nigeria: a 15-month prospective study. Scand J Infect Dis 10:113, 1978.

307. Alausa KO, Montefiore D, Sogbetun AO, et al. Septicaemia in the tropics: a prospective epidemiological study of 146 patients with a high case fatality rate. Scand J Infect Dis 9:181, 1977.

308. Ohlsson A, Bailey T, Takieddine F. Changing etiology and outcome of neonatal septicemia in Riyadh, Saudi Arabia. Acta Paediatr Scand 75:540, 1986.

309. Collado M de L, Kretschmer RR, Becker I, et al. Colonization of Mexican pregnant women with group B Streptococcus. J Infect Dis 143:134, 1981.

310. Anthony BF, Okada DM, Hobel CV. Epidemiology of group B Streptococcus: longitudinal observations during pregnancy. J Infect Dis 137:524, 1978.

311. Omenaca F, Quero J, Polo P, et al. Sepsis precoz por estreptococo des grupo B en el rec ién nacido: a propósito de 17 observaciones. An Esp Pediatr 12:607, 1979.

312. Ausina V, Coll P, Mirelis B. Letter to the editor. N Engl J Med 305:170, 1981.

313. Naeye RL, Blanc WA. Relation of poverty and race to antenatal infection. N Engl J Med 283:555, 1970.

314. Beck-Sague CM, Azimi P, Fonseca SN, Baltimore RS. Blood stream infections in neonatal intensive care unit patients: results of a multicenter study. Pediatr Infect Dis J 13:1110–1116, 1994.

315. Adams WG, Kinney JS, Schuchat A, et al. Outbreak of early onset group B streptococcal sepsis. Pediatr Infect Dis J 12:565, 1993.

316. Franco JA, Eitzman DV, Baer H. Antibiotic usage and microbial resistance in an intensive care nursery. Am J Dis Child 126:318, 1973.

317. Raz R, Sharir R, Shmilowitz L, et al. The elimination of gentamicin-resistant gram-negative bacteria in newborn intensive care unit. Infection 15:32, 1987.

318. Prober CG, Rajchgot P, Bannatyne RM, et al. Impact of chloramphenicol use on bacterial resistance in a neonatal intensive care unit. Lancet 2:158, 1983.

319. Bryan CS, John JF Jr, Pai MS, et al. Gentamicin vs. cefotaxime for therapy of neonatal sepsis. Am J Dis Child 139:1086, 1985.

320. Forfar JO, Gould JC, MacCabe AF. Effect of hexachlorophene on incidence of staphylococcal and gram-negative infection in the newborn. Lancet 2:177, 1968.

321. Light IJ, Sutherland SM, Cochran ML, et al. Ecologic relation between Staphylococcus aureus and a Pseudomonas in a nursery population. N Engl J Med 278:1243, 1968.

322. Evans HE, Akpata SO, Baki A, et al. Flora in newborn infants, annual variation in prevalence of Staphylococcus aureus, Escherichia coli, and streptococci. Arch Environ Health 26:275, 1973.

323. Gibbs RS, Duff P. Progress in pathogenesis and manage-

ment of clinical intraamniotic infection. Am J Obstet Gynecol 164:1317, 1991.

324. Charles D, Edwards WR. Infectious complications of cervical cerclage. Am J Obstet Gynecol 141:1065, 1981.

325. Fejgin M, Amiel A, Kaneti H, et al. Fulminant sepsis due to group B beta-hemolytic streptococci following transcervical chorionic villi sampling. Clin Infect Dis 17:142, 1993.

326. Wilkins I, Mezrow G, Lynch L, et al. Amnionitis and life-threatening respiratory distress after percutaneous umbilical blood sampling. Am J Obstet Gynecol 160:427, 1989.

327. Morison JE. Foetal and Neonatal Pathology, 3rd ed. Washington, D.C., Butterworth, 1970.

328. Benirschke K. Routes and types of infection in the fetus and newborn. Am J Dis Child 99:714, 1960.

329. St. Geme JW Jr, Murray DL, Carter J, et al. Perinatal bacterial infection after prolonged rupture of amniotic membranes: an analysis of risk and management. J Pediatr 104:608, 1984.

330. Blanc WA. Pathways of fetal and early neonatal infection: viral placentitis, bacterial and fungal chorioamnionitis. J Pediatr 59:473, 1961.

331. Hillier SL, Krohn MA, Kiviat NB, et al. Microbiologic causes and neonatal outcomes associated with chorioamnion infection. Am J Obstet Gynecol 165:955, 1991.

332. Yoder PR, Gibbs RS, Blanco JD, et al. A prospective, controlled study of maternal and perinatal outcome after intra-amniotic infection at term. Am J Obstet Gynecol 145:695, 1983.

333. Larsen B, Snyder IS, Galask RP. Bacterial growth inhibition by amniotic fluid: I. In vitro evidence for bacterial growth-inhibiting activity. Am J Obstet Gynecol 119:492, 1974.

334. Florman AL, Teubner D. Enhancement of bacterial growth in amniotic fluid by meconium. J Pediatr 74:111, 1969.

335. Kitzmiller JL, Highby S, Lucas WE. Retarded growth of E. coli in amniotic fluid. Obstet Gynecol 41:38, 1973.

336. Hoskins IA, Hemming VG, Johnson TRB, et al. Effects of alterations of zinc-to-phosphate ratios and meconium content on group B Streptococcus growth in human amniotic fluid in vitro. Am J Obstet Gynecol 157:770, 1988.

337. Larsen B, Galask RP. Host resistance to intraamniotic infection. Obstet Gynecol Surv 30:675, 1975.

338. Marston G, Wald ER. Hemophilus influenzae type b sepsis in infant and mother. Pediatrics 58:863, 1976.

339. Tarpay MM, Turbeville DV, Krous HF. Fatal Streptococcus pneumoniae type III sepsis in mother and infant. Am J Obstet Gynecol 136:257, 1980.

340. Panaro NR, Lutwick LI, Chapnick EK. Intrapartum transmission of group A Streptococcus. Clin Infect Dis 17:79, 1993.

341. Bhutta ZA, Khan IA, Agha A. Fatal intrauterine meningococcal infection. Pediatr Infect Dis J 11:868, 1991.

342. Tempest B. Pneumococcal meningitis in mother and neonate. Pediatrics 53:759, 1974.

343. Grossman J, Tompkins RL. Group B beta-hemolytic streptococcal meningitis in mother and infant. N Engl J Med 290:387, 1974.

344. Pyati SP, Pildes RS, Jacobs NM, et al. Penicillin in infants weighing two kilograms or less with early-onset group B streptococcal disease. N Engl J Med 308:1383, 1983.

345. Maberry MC, Gilstrap LC. Intrapartum antibiotic therapy for suspected intraamniotic infection: impact on the fetus and neonate. Clin Obstet Gynecol 34:345, 1991.

346. Sarkany I, Gaylarde CC. Skin flora of the newborn. Lancet 1:589, 1967.

347. Sacks LM, McKitrick JC, MacGregor RR. Surface cultures and isolation procedures in infants born under unsterile conditions. Am J Dis Child 137:351, 1983.

348. Balfour HH Jr, Bowe ET, James LS. Scalp abscesses following fetal blood sampling or monitoring. J Pediatr 79:344, 1971.

349. Cordero J Jr, Hon EH. Scalp abscess: A rare complication of fetal monitoring. J Pediatr 78:533, 1971.

350. Storm W. Transient bacteremia following endotracheal suctioning in ventilated newborns. Pediatrics 65:487, 1980.

351. Brook I, Frazier EH. Microbiology of scalp abscess in newborn. Pediatr Infect Dis J 11:766, 1992.

352. Dobson SRM, Baker CJ. Enterococcal sepsis in neonates: features by age at onset and occurrence of focal infection. Pediatrics 85:165, 1990.

353. Freedman RM, Baltimore R. Fatal Streptococcus viridans septicemia and meningitis: a relationship to fetal scalp electrode monitoring. J Perinatol 10:272, 1990.

354. Singer DB. Infections of fetuses and neonates. In Wigglesworth JS, Singer DB (eds). Textbook of Fetal and Perinatal Pathology. Boston, Blackwell Scientific Publications, 1991, pp 525–591.

355. Nieburg P, Gross SJ. Cerebrospinal fluid leak in a neonate with fetal scalp electrode monitoring. Am J Obstet Gynecol 147:839, 1983.

356. Unhanand M, Mustafa MM, McCracken GH Jr, et al. Gram-negative enteric bacillary meningitis: a twenty-one-year experience. J Pediatr 122:15, 1993.

357. Nagle RC, Taekman MS, Shallat RF, et al. Brain abscess aspiration in nursery with ultrasound guidance. J Neurosurg 65:557, 1986.

358. Renier D, Flandin C, Hirsch E, et al. Brain abscesses in neonates: a study of 30 cases. J Neurosurg 69:877, 1988.

359. Jadavji T, Humphreys RP, Prober CG. Brain abscesses in infants and children. Pediatr Infect Dis 4:394, 1985.

360. Campbell JR, Diacovo T, Baker CJ. Serratia marcescens meningitis in neonates. Pediatr Infect Dis J 11:881, 1992.

361. Volpe JJ. Neurology of the Newborn, 2nd ed. Philadelphia, WB Saunders, 1987, p 625.

362. Dillon HC, Khare S, Gray BM. Group B streptococcal carriage and disease: a 6-year prospective study. J Pediatr 110:31, 1987.

363. Maisels MJ, Kring E. Risk of sepsis in newborns with severe hyperbilirubinemia. Pediatrics 90:741, 1992.

364. Haber BA, Lake AM. Cholestatic jaundice in the newborn. Clin Perinatol 17:483, 1990.

365. Rooney JC, Hills DJ, Danks DM. Jaundice associated with bacterial infection in the newborn. Am J Dis Child 122:39, 1971.

366. Dagan R, Gorodischer R. Infections in hypothermic infants younger than 3 months old. Am J Dis Child 138:483, 1984.

367. Johanson RB, Spencer SA, Rolfe P, et al. Effect of post-delivery care on neonatal body temperature. Acta Paediatr 81:859, 1992.

368. Michael M, Barrett DJ, Mehta P. Infants with meningitis without CSF pleocytosis. Am J Dis Child 140:851, 1986.

369. El-Radhy AS, Jawad M, Mansor N, et al. Sepsis and hypothermia in the newborn infant: value of gastric aspirate examination. J Pediatr 104:300, 1983.

370. Kelly S. Septicemia in galactosemia. JAMA 216:330, 1971.

371. Levy HL, Sepe SJ, Shih VE, et al. Sepsis due to Escherichia coli in neonates with galactosemia. N Engl J Med 297:823, 1977.

372. Shurin SB. *Escherichia coli* septicemia in neonates with galactosemia. Letter to the editor. N Engl J Med 297:1403, 1977.

373. Kobayashi RH, Kettelhut BV, Kobayashi AL. Galactose inhibition of neonatal neutrophil function. Pediatr Infect Dis J 2:442, 1983.

374. Odievre M, Gentil C, Gautier M, et al. Hereditary fructose intolerance. Diagnosis management and course in 55 patients. Am J Dis Child 132:605, 1978.

375. Hutchinson RJ, Bunnell K, Thoene JG. Suppression of granulopoietic progenitor cell proliferation by metabolites of the branched-chain amino acids. J Pediatr 106:62, 1985.

376. Weinberg ED. Iron and susceptibility to infectious disease. Science 184:952, 1974.

377. Barry DMJ, Reeve AW. Increased incidence of gram-negative neonatal sepsis with intramuscular iron administration. Pediatrics 60:908, 1977.

378. Farmer K. The disadvantages of routine administration of intramuscular iron to neonates. N Z Med J 84:286, 1976.

379. Pass MA, Khare S, Dillon HC Jr. Twin pregnancies: incidence of group B streptococcal colonization and disease. J Pediatr 97:635, 1980.

380. Edwards MS, Jackson CV, Baker CJ. Increased risk of group B streptococcal disease in twins. JAMA 245:2044, 1981.

381. Nieburg PI, William ML. Group A beta-hemolytic streptococcal sepsis in a mother and infant twins. J Pediatr 87:453, 1975.

382. Larsen JG, Harra BA, Bottone EJ, et al. Multiple antibiotic resistant *Salmonella agora* infection in malnourished neonatal twins. Mt Sinai J Med 46:542, 1979.

383. Devlin HR, Bannatyne RM. Neonatal malaria. Can Med Assoc J 116:20, 1977.

384. Shafai T. Neonatal coccidioidomycosis in premature twins. Am J Dis Child 132:634, 1978.

385. Saigal S, Eisele WA, Chernesky MA. Congenital cytomegalovirus infection in a pair of dizygotic twins. Am J Dis Child 136:1094, 1982.

386. Montgomery RC, Stockdell K. Congenital rubella in twins. J Pediatr 76:772, 1970.

387. Forshall I. Septic umbilical arteritis. Arch Dis Child 32:25, 1957.

388. Cruickshank JN. Child Life Investigations: The Causes of Neo-natal Death. Medical Research Council Special Report Series No. 145. London, His Majesty's Stationery Office, 1930, p 26.

389. Cushing AH. Omphalitis: a review. Pediatr Infect Dis J 4:282, 1985.

390. Rotimi VO, Duerden BI. The development of the bacterial flora in normal neonates. J Med Microbiol 14:51, 1981.

391. Mason WH, Andrews R, Ross LA, et al. Omphalitis in the newborn infant. Pediatr Infect Dis J 8:521, 1989.

392. Meyer WW, Lind J. The ductus venosus and the mechanism of its closure. Arch Dis Child 41:597, 1966.

393. Morison JE. Umbilical sepsis and acute interstitial hepatitis. J Pathol Bacteriol 56:531, 1944.

394. Elliott RIK. The ductus venosus in neonatal infection. Proc R Soc Med 62:321, 1969.

395. Bedtke K, Richarz H. Nabelsepsis mit Pylephlebitis, multiplen Leberabscessen, Lungenabscessen und Osteomyelitis. Ausgang in Heilung. Monatsschr Kinderheilkd 105:70, 1957.

396. Beaven DW. Staphylococcal peritonitis in the newborn. Lancet 1:869, 1958.

397. Thompson EN, Sherlock S. The aetiology of portal vein thrombosis with particular reference to the role of infection and exchange transfusion. QJ Med 33:465, 1964.

398. Navarro C, Blanc WA. Subacute necrotizing funisitis: a variant of cord inflammation with a high rate of perinatal infection. J Pediatr 85:689, 1974.

399. Ohlsson A. Treatment of preterm premature rupture of the membranes: a meta-analysis. Am J Obstet Gynecol 160:890, 1989.

400. Taeusch WH Jr, Frigoletto F, Kitzmiller J, et al. Risk of respiratory distress syndrome after prenatal dexamethasone treatment. Pediatrics 63:64, 1979.

401. Fitzhardinge PM, Eisen A, Lejtenyi C, et al. Sequelae of early steroid administration to the newborn infant. Pediatrics 53:877, 1974.

402. Kitzmiller JL. Potential risks of maternal corticosteroid administration to prevent neonatal respiratory distress syndrome: infection, pulmonary edema, and fetal brain damage. *In* Gluck L (ed). Obstetrical Decisions and Neonatal Outcome. Report of the Seventy-Eighth Ross Conference on Pediatric Research. Columbus, Ohio, Ross Laboratories, 1979, p 118.

403. Johnson S, Knight R, Marmer DJ, et al. Immune deficiency in fetal alcohol syndrome. Pediatr Res 15:908, 1981.

404. Culver KW, Ammann AJ, Partridge JC, et al. Lymphocyte abnormalities in infants born to drug-abusing mothers. J Pediatr 111:230, 1987.

405. Chasnoff IJ (ed). Chemical dependency and pregnancy. Clin Perinatol 18:1, 1991.

406. Woods JR Jr (ed). Drug abuse in pregnancy. Clin Obstet Gynecol 36:221, 1993.

407. Chasnoff IJ (ed). Drug Use in Pregnancy: Mother and Child. Boston, MTP Press, 1986.

408. Herson VC, Krause PJ, Einsenfeld LI, et al. Indomethacin-associated sepsis in very-low-birth-weight infants. Am J Dis Child 142:555, 1988.

409. O'Shea TM, Kothadia JM, Klinepeter KL, et al. Follow-up of preterm infants treated with dexamethasone for chronic lung disease. Am J Dis Child 147:658, 1993.

410. Heymann MA Prostaglandins and leukotrienes in the perinatal period. Clin Perinatol 14:857, 1987.

411. Barson AJ. A postmortem study of infection in the newborn from 1976 to 1988. *In* de Louvois J, Harvey D (eds). Infection in the Newborn. New York, John Wiley & Sons, 1990, pp 13–34.

412. Berman PH, Banker BQ. Neonatal meningitis: a clinical and pathological study of 29 cases. Pediatrics 38:6, 1966.

413. Stocker JT, Dehner LP. Pediatric Pathology. Philadelphia, JB Lippincott, 1992.

414. Hoffman HJ, Hendrick EB, Hiscox JL. Cerebral abscesses in early infancy. J Neurosurg 33:172, 1970.

415. Watson DG. Purulent neonatal meningitis: A study of forty-five cases. J Pediatr 50:352, 1957.

416. Volpe JJ. Neurology of the Newborn, 3rd ed. Philadelphia, WB Saunders, 1995, pp 734–742.

417. Perlman JM, Rollins N, Sanchez PJ. Late-onset meningitis in sick, very-low-birth-weight infants: clinical and sonographic observations. Am J Dis Child 146:1297, 1992.

418. Gilles FH, Jammes JL, Berenberg W. Neonatal meningitis: the ventricle as a bacterial reservoir. Arch Neurol 34:560, 1977.

419. Schiano MA, Hauth JC, Gilstrap LC. Second-stage fetal tachycardia and neonatal infection. Am J Obstet Gynecol 148:779, 1984.

420. Soman M, Green B, Daling J. Risk factors for early neonatal sepsis. Am J Epidemiol 121:712, 1985.

421. Hegyi T, Carbone T, Anwar M, et al. The Apgar Score

and its components in the preterm infant. Pediatrics 101:77–81, 1998.

422. Powell KR. Evaluation and management of febrile infants younger than 60 days of age. Pediatr Infect Dis J 9:153, 1990.

423. Bonadio WA, Hennes H, Smith D, et al. Reliability of observation variables in distinguishing infectious outcome of febrile young infants. Pediatr Infect Dis J 12:111, 1993.

424. Fielkow S, Reuter S, Gotoff SP. Cerebrospinal fluid examination in symptom-free infants with risk factors for infection. J Pediatr 119:971, 1991.

425. Albers WH, Tyler CW, Boxerbaum B. Asymptomatic bacteremia in the newborn infant. J Pediatr 69:193, 1966.

426. Howard JB, McCracken GH. The spectrum of group B streptococcal infections in infancy. Am J Dis Child 128:815, 1974.

427. Weisman LE, Stoll BJ, Cruess DF, et al. Early-onset group B streptococcal sepsis: a current assessment. J Pediatr 121:428, 1992.

428. Yagupsky P, Menegus MA, Powell KR. The changing spectrum of group B streptococcal disease in infants: an eleven-year experience in a tertiary care hospital. Pediatr Infect Dis J 10:801, 1991.

429. Ramsey PG, Zwerdling R. Asymptomatic neonatal bacteremia. Letter to the editor. N Engl J Med 295:225, 1976.

430. Yu JS, Grauang A. Purulent meningitis in the neonatal period. Arch Dis Child 38:391, 1963.

431. Solomon SL, Wallace EM, Ford-Jones EL, et al. Medication errors with inhalant epinephrine mimicking an epidemic of neonatal sepsis. N Engl J Med 310:166, 1984.

432. Bonadio WA, Hegenbarth M, Zachariason M. Correlating reported fever in young infants with subsequent temperature patterns and rate of serious bacterial infections. Pediatr Infect Dis J 9:158, 1990.

433. Messaritakis J, Anagnostakis D, Laskari H, et al. Rectal-skin temperature difference in septicaemic newborn infants. Arch Dis Child 65:380, 1990.

434. Dinarello CA, Shparber M, Kent EF Jr, et al. Production of leukocytic pyrogen from phagocytes of neonates. J Infect Dis 144:337, 1981.

435. Kravitz H. Temperature of the umbilicus. J Pediatr 68:418, 1966.

436. Mayfield SR, Bhatia J, Nakamura K, et al. Temperature measurement in term and preterm neonates. J Pediatr 104:271, 1984.

437. Johnson KJ, Bhatia P, Bell EF. Infrared thermometry of newborn infants. Pediatrics 87:34, 1991.

438. Schuman AJ. The accuracy of infrared auditory canal thermometry in infants and children. Clin Pediatr 32:347, 1993.

439. Anagnostakis D, Matsaniotis N, Grafakos S, et al. Rectal-axillary difference in febrile and afebrile infants and children. Clin Pediatr 32:268, 1993.

440. Weisse ME, Reagen MS, Boule L, et al. Axillary vs. rectal temperatures in ambulatory and hospitalized children. Pediatr Infect Dis J 10:541, 1991.

441. Freed GL, Fraley JK. Lack of agreement of tympanic membrane temperature assessments with conventional methods in a private practice setting. Pediatrics 89:384, 1992.

442. Craig WS. The early detection of pyrexia in the newborn. Arch Dis Child 38:29, 1963.

443. Voora S, Srinivasan G, Lilien LD, et al. Fever in full-term newborns in the first four days of life. Pediatrics 69:40, 1982.

444. Osborn LM, Bolus R. Temperature and fever in the full-term newborn. J Fam Pract 20:261, 1985.

445. Seeler RA. Urosepsis with jaundice due to hemolytic *Escherichia coli*. Am J Dis Child 126:414, 1973.

446. Danks DM, Campbell PE, Connelly JF. An aetiological study of neonatal jaundice in a children's hospital. Aust Paediatr J 1:193, 1965.

447. Rooney JC, Hills DJ, Danks DM. Jaundice associated with bacterial infection in the newborn. Am J Dis Child 122:39, 1971.

448. Ashkenazi S, Mimouni F, Merlob P, et al. Size of liver edge in full-term, healthy infants. Am J Dis Child 138:377, 1984.

449. Reiff MI, Osborn LM. Clinical estimation of liver size in newborn infants. Pediatrics 71:46, 1983.

450. Bamji M, Stone RK, Kaul A, et al. Palpable lymph nodes in healthy newborns and infants. Pediatrics 78:573, 1986.

451. Embree J, Muriithi J. Palpable lymph nodes. Letter to the editor. Pediatrics 81:598, 1988.

452. Volpe JJ. Neurology of the Newborn, 2nd ed. Philadelphia, WB Saunders, 1987, p 608.

453. Bell AH, Brown D, Halliday HL, et al. Meningitis in the newborn: a 14 year review. Arch Dis Child 64:873, 1989.

454. Weintraub MI, Otto RN. Pneumococcal meningitis and endophthalmitis in a newborn. JAMA 219:1763, 1972.

455. Palmer JJ, Kelly WA. Epidural abscess in a 3-week old infant: case report. Pediatrics 50:817, 1972.

456. Aicardi J, Lepintre J. Spinal epidural abscess in a 1-month-old child. Am J Dis Child 114:665, 1967.

457. Walter RS, King JC, Manley J, et al. Spinal epidural abscess in infancy: successful percutaneous drainage in a nine-month-old and review of the literature. Pediatr Infect Dis J 19:860, 1991.

458. Hankins GV, Chalas E. Group B streptococcal infections in pregnancy: ACOG recommendations. ACOG Newletter, May 1993.

459. Evans ME, Schaffner W, Federspiel CF, et al. Sensitivity, specificity, and predictive value of body surface cultures in a neonatal intensive care unit. JAMA 259:248, 1988.

460. Campos JM. Pediatric blood cultures. Rep Pediatr Infect Dis 3:34, 1993.

461. Anderson JD, Trombley C, Cimolai N. Assessment of the BACTEC NR660 blood culture system for the detection of bacteremia in young children. J Clin Microbiol 27:721, 1989.

462. Kurlat I, Stoll BJ, McGowan JE Jr. Time to positivity for detection of bacteremia in neonates. J Clin Microbiol 27:1068, 1989.

463. Campos JM, Spainhour JR. Rapid detection of bacteremia in children with modified lysis direct plating method. J Clin Microbiol 22:674, 1985.

464. St. Geme JW III, Bell LM, Baumgart S, et al. Distinguishing sepsis from blood culture contamination in young infants with blood cultures growing coagulase-negative staphylococci. Pediatrics 86:157, 1990.

465. Pichichero MD, Todd JK. Detection of neonatal bacteremia. J Pediatr 94:958, 1979.

466. Rowley AH, Wald ER. Incubation period necessary to detect bacteremia in neonates. Pediatr Infect Dis J 5:590, 1986.

467. Sprunt K. Commentary. *In* Gellis SS (ed). The Year Book of Pediatrics 1973. Chicago, Year Book Medical Publishers, 1973, p 15.

468. Wiswell TE, Hachey WE. Multiple site blood cultures in the initial evaluation for neonatal sepsis during the first week of life. Pediatr. Infect Dis J 10:365, 1991.

469. Neal PR, Kleiman MB, Reynolds JK, et al. Volume of

blood submitted for culture from neonates. J Clin Microbiol 24:353, 1986.

470. Dietzman DE, Fischer GW, Schoenknecht FD. Neonatal *Escherichia coli* septicemia—bacterial counts in blood. J Pediatr 85:128, 1974.

471. Kennaugh JK, Gregory WW, Powell KR, Hendley JO. The effect of dilution during culture on detection of low concentrations of bacteria in blood. Pediatr Infect Dis J 3:317, 1984.

472. Holt RJ, Frankcombe CH, Newman RL. Capillary blood cultures. Arch Dis Child 49:318, 1974.

473. Mangurten HH, LeBeau LJ. Diagnosis of neonatal bacteremia by a microblood culture technique: a preliminary report. J Pediatr 90:990, 1977.

474. Knudson RP, Alden ER. Neonatal heel-stick blood culture. Pediatrics 65:505, 1980.

475. Paerregaard A, Bruun B, Andersen GE, Witt J. No advantage of capillary blood compared with venous blood for culture in neonates. Pediatr Infect Dis J 8:659, 1989.

476. Sell S, Hansen RC, Struck-Pierce S. Calcified nodules on the heels of neonates: a complication of neonatal intensive care. J Pediatr 96:473, 1980.

477. Polin JI, Knox I, Baumgart S, et al. Use of umbilical cord blood culture for detection of neonatal bacteremia. Obstet Gynecol 57:233, 1981.

478. Cowett RM, Peter G, Hakanson DO, et al. Reliability of bacterial culture of blood obtained from an umbilical artery catheter. J Pediatr 88:1035, 1976.

479. Pourcyrous M, et al. Indwelling umbilical arterial catheter: a preferred sampling site for blood cultures. Pediatrics 81:621, 1988.

480. Ruderman JW, Morgan MA, Klein AH. Quantitative blood cultures in the diagnosis of sepsis in infants with umbilical and Broviac catheters. J Pediatr 112:748, 1988.

481. Phillips SE, Bradley JS. Bacteremia detected by lysis direct plating in a neonatal intensive care unit. J Clin Microbiol 28:1, 1990.

482. Hammerberg O, Bialkowska-Hobrzanska H, Gregson D, et al. Comparison of blood cultures with corresponding venipuncture site cultures of specimens from hospitalized premature neonates. J Pediatr 120:120, 1992.

483. Humphrey AA. Use of the buffy layer in the rapid diagnosis of septicemia. Am J Clin Pathol 14:358, 1944.

484. Boyle RJ, Chandler BD, Stonestreet BS, et al. Early identification of sepsis in infants with respiratory distress. Pediatrics 62:744, 1978.

485. Faden HS. Early diagnosis of neonatal bacteremia by buffy-coat examination. J Pediatr 88:1032, 1976.

486. Storm W. Early detection of bacteremia by peripheral smears in critically ill newborns. Acta Paediatr Scand 70:415, 1981.

487. Kleiman MB, Reynolds JK, Schreiner RL, et al. Rapid diagnosis of neonatal bacteremia with acridine orange-stained buffy coat smears. J Pediatr 105:419, 1984.

488. Kite P, Millar MR, Gorham P, et al. Comparison of five tests used in diagnosis of neonatal bacteremia. Arch Dis Child 63:639, 1988.

489. Tak SK, Bhandari PC, Bhandari B. Value of buffy coat examination in early diagnosis of neonatal septicemia. Indian Pediatr 17:339, 1980.

490. Powers DL, Mandell GL. Intraleukocytic bacteria in endocarditis patients. JAMA 227:312, 1974.

491. Cattermole HEJ, Rivers RPA. Neonatal *Candida* septicaemia: diagnosis on buffy smear. Arch Dis Child 62:302, 1987.

492. Ascuitto RJ, Gerber MA, Cates KL, et al. Buffy coat smears of blood drawn through central venous catheters

as an aid to rapid diagnosis of systemic fungal infections. J Pediatr 106:445, 1985.

493. Selby DM, Gautier G, Luban NLC, Campos JM. Overwhelming neonatal septicemia diagnosed upon examination of peripheral blood smears. Clin Pediatr 29:706, 1990.

494. Strom W. Early detection of bacteremia by peripheral blood smears in critically ill newborns. Acta Paediatr Scand 70:415, 1981.

495. Rodwell RL, Leslie AL, Tudehope DI. Evaluation of direct and buffy coat films of peripheral blood for the early detection of bacteraemia. Aust Paediatr J 25:83, 1989.

496. Visser VE, Hall RT. Urine culture in the evaluation of suspected neonatal sepsis. J Pediatr 94:635, 1979.

497. DiGeronimo RJ. Lack of efficacy of the urine culture as part of the initial workup of suspected neonatal sepsis. Pediatr Infect Dis J 9:764, 1992.

498. Nelson JD, Peters PC. Suprapubic aspiration of urine in premature and term infants. Pediatrics 36:132, 1965.

499. Finelli L, Livengood JR, Saiman L. Surveillance of pharyngeal colonization: detection and control of serious bacterial illness in low birth weight infants. Pediatr Infect Dis J 13:854–859, 1994.

500. Lau YL, Hey E. Sensitivity and specificity of daily tracheal aspirate cultures in predicting organisms causing bacteremia in ventilated neonates. Pediatr Infect Dis J 10:290, 1991.

501. Klein JO, Gellis SS. Diagnostic needle aspiration in pediatric practice: with special reference to lungs, middle ear, urinary bladder, and amniotic cavity. Pediatr Clin North Am 18:219, 1971.

502. Eisenfeld L, Ermocilla R, Wirtschaffer D, et al. Systemic bacterial infections in neonatal deaths. Am J Dis Child 137:645, 1983.

503. Minckler TM, Newell GR, O'Toole WF, et al. Microbiology experience in human tissue collection. Am J Clin Pathol 45:85, 1966.

504. Pierce JR, Merenstein GB, Stocker JT. Immediate postmortem cultures in an intensive care nursery. Pediatr Infect Dis J 3:510, 1984.

505. Levin J, Poore TE, Zauber NP, et al. Detection of endotoxin in the blood of patients with sepsis due to gram-negative bacteria. N Engl J Med 283:1313, 1970.

506. Levin I, Poore TE, Young NS. Gram-negative sepsis. Detection of endotoxemia with the limulus test. Ann Intern Med 76:1, 1972.

507. Stumacher RI, Kovnat MJ, McCabe WR. Limitations of the usefulness of the limulus assay for endotoxin. N Engl J Med 288:1261, 1973.

508. Elin RJ, Robinson RA, Levine AS, et al. Lack of clinical usefulness of the limulus test in the diagnosis of endotoxemia. N Engl J Med 293:521, 1975.

509. McCracken GH Jr, Sarff LD. Endotoxin in CSF detection in neonates with bacterial meningitis. JAMA 235:617, 1976.

510. McGowan KL. Diagnostic value of latex agglutination tests for bacterial infections. Rep Pediatr Infect Dis 8:31, 1992.

511. Sanchez PJ, Siegel JD, Cushion NB, Threlkeld N. Significance of a positive urine group B streptococcal latex agglutination test in neonates. J Pediatr 116:601, 1990.

512. Eldadah M, Frenkel LD, Hiatt IM, Hegyi T. Evaluation of routine lumbar punctures in newborn infants with respiratory distress syndrome. Pediatr Infect Dis J 6:243, 1987.

513. Weiss MG, Ionides SP, Anderson CL. Meningitis in

premature infants with respiratory distress: role of admission lumbar puncture. J Pediatr 119:973, 1991.

514. Schwersendki J, McIntyre L, Bauer CR. Lumbar puncture frequency and CSF analysis in the neonate. Am J Dis Child 145:54, 1991.

515. Fielkow S, Reuter S, Gotoff SP. Clinical and laboratory observations: cerebrospinal fluid examination in symptom-free infants with risk factors for infection. J Pediatr 119:971, 1991.

516. Gleason CA, Martin FJ, Anderson JV, et al. Optimal position for a spinal tap in preterm infants. Pediatrics 71:31, 1983.

517. Pinheiro JMB, Furdon S, Ochoa LF. Role of local anesthesia during lumbar puncture in neonates. Pediatrics 91:379, 1993.

518. Porter FL, Miller JP, Cole S, Marshall RE. A controlled clinical trial of local anesthesia for lumbar punctures in newborns. Pediatrics 88:663, 1991.

519. Fiser DH, Gober GA, Smith CE, et al. Prevention of hypoxemia during lumbar puncture in infancy with preoxygenation. Pediatr Emerg Care 9:81, 1993.

520. Lorber J, Emery JL. Intracerebral cysts complicating ventricular needling in hydrocephalic infants: a clinicopathological study. Dev Med Child Neurol 6:125, 1964.

521. Greensher J, Mofenson HC, Borofsky LG, et al. Lumbar puncture in the neonate: a simplified technique. J Pediatr 78:1034, 1971.

522. Shaywitz BA. Spinal taps and epidermoid tumors. Hosp Pract 8:79, 1973.

523. Weisman LE, Merenstein GB, Steenbarger JR. The effect of lumbar puncture position in sick neonates. Am J Dis Child 137:1077, 1983.

524. Visser VE, Hall RT. Lumbar puncture in the evaluation of suspected neonatal sepsis. J Pediatr 96:1063, 1980.

525. Franco SM, Cornelius VE, Andrews BF. Should we perform lumbar punctures on the first day of life? Am J Dis Child 147:133, 1993.

526. Wolf H, Hoepffner L. The CSF in the newborn and premature infant. World Neurol 2:871, 1961.

527. Otila E. Studies on the CSF in premature infants. Acta Paediatr Scand 35(Suppl 8):9, 1948.

528. Gyllensward A, Malmstrom S. The CSF in immature infants. Acta Paediatr Scand 135(Suppl):54, 1962.

529. Naidoo BT. The CSF in the healthy newborn infant. S Afr Med J 42:933, 1968.

530. Widell S. On the CSF in normal children and in patients with acute abacterial meningoencephalitis. Acta Pediatr 47:711, 1958.

531. Ahmed A, Hickey SM, Ehrett S. Cerebrospinal fluid values in the term neonate. Pediatr Infect Dis J 15:298–303, 1996.

532. Sarff LD, Platt LH, McCracken GH Jr. Cerebrospinal fluid evaluation in neonates: comparison of high-risk infants with and without meningitis. J Pediatr 88:473, 1976.

533. Bonadio WA, Stanco L, Bruce R, et al. Reference values of normal CSF composition in infants ages 0 to 8 weeks. Pediatr Infect Dis J 11:589, 1992.

534. McCracken GH Jr. The rate of bacteriologic response to antimicrobial therapy in neonatal meningitis. Am J Dis Child 123:547, 1972.

535. Rodriguez AF, Kaplan SL, Mason EO Jr. Cerebrospinal fluid values in the very low birth weight infant. J Pediatr 116:971, 1990.

536. Moore CM, Ross M. Acute bacterial meningitis with absent or minimal CSF abnormalities: a report of three cases. Clin Pediatr (Phila) 12:117, 1973.

537. Yeager AS, Bruhn FW, Clark J. Cerebrospinal fluid: presence of virus unaccompanied by pleocytosis. J Pediatr 85:578, 1974.

538. Sarman G, Moise AA, Edwards MS. Meningeal inflammation in neonatal gram-negative bacteremia. Pediatr Infect Dis J 14:701–704, 1995.

539. Hedner T, Iversen K, Lundborg P. Aminobutyric acid concentrations in the CSF of newborn infants. Early Hum Dev 7:53, 1982.

540. Engelke S, Bridgers S, Saldanha RL, et al. Cerebrospinal fluid lactate dehydrogenase in neonatal intracranial hemorrhage. Am J Med Sci 29:391, 1986.

541. Worley G, Lipman B, Gewolb IH, et al. Creatine kinase brain isoenzyme: relationship of CSF concentration to the neurologic condition of newborns and cellular localization in the human brain. Pediatrics 76:15, 1985.

542. Lin C-Y, Ishida M. Elevation of cAMP levels in CSF of patients with neonatal meningitis. Pediatrics 71:932, 1983.

543. Corrall CJ, Pepple JM, Moxon ER, Hughes WT. C-reactive protein in spinal fluid of children with meningitis. J Pediatr 99:365, 1981.

544. BenGershom E, Briggeman-Mol GJJ, de Zegher F. Cerebrospinal fluid C-reactive protein in meningitis: diagnostic value and pathophysiology. Eur J Pediatr 145:246, 1986.

545. Philip AGS, Baker CJ. Cerebrospinal fluid C-reactive protein in neonatal meningitis. J Pediatr 102:715, 1983.

546. Martín-Ancel A, García-Alix A, Pascual-Salcedo D, et al. Interleukin-6 in the cerebrospinal fluid after perinatal asphyxia is related to early and late neurological manifestations. Pediatrics 100:789–794, 1997.

547. Sävman K, Blennow M, Gustafson K, et al. Cytokine response in cerebrospinal fluid after birth asphyxia. Pediatr Res 43:746–751, 1998.

548. Chow G, Schmidley JW. Lysis of erythrocytes and leukocytes in traumatic lumbar punctures. Arch Neurol 1984; 41:1084–1085.

549. Steele RW, Marmer DJ, O'Brien MD, et al. Leukocyte survival in CSF. J Clin Microbiol 23:965, 1986.

550. Osborne JP, Pizer B. Effect on the white cell count of contaminating CSF with blood. Arch Dis Child 56:400, 1981.

551. Novak RW. Lack of validity of standard corrections for white blood cell counts of blood-contaminated CSF in infants. Am J Clin Pathol 82:95, 1984.

552. Mayefsky JH, Roghmann KJ. Determination of leukocytosis in traumatic spinal tap specimens. Am J Med 82:1175, 1987.

553. Mehl AL. Interpretation of traumatic lumbar puncture: a prospective experimental model. Clin Pediatr 25:523, 1986.

554. Mehl AL. Interpretation of traumatic lumbar puncture: predictive value in the presence of meningitis. Clin Pediatr 25:575, 1986.

555. Bonadio WA, Smith DS, Goddard S, et al. Distinguishing CSF abnormalities in children with bacterial meningitis and traumatic lumbar puncture. J Infect Dis 162:251, 1990.

556. Naqvi SH, Dunkle LM, Naseer S, Barth C. Significance of neutrophils in CSF samples processed by cytocentrifugation. Clin Pediatr 22:608, 1983.

557. Bonadio WA. Bacterial meningitis in children whose CSF contains polymorphonuclear leukocytes without pleocytosis. Clin Pediatr 27:198, 1988.

558. Weirich E, Rabin RL, Maldonado Y, et al. Neutrophil CD11b expression as a diagnostic marker for early-onset neonatal infection. J Pediatr 132:445–451, 1998.

559. Kennon C, Overturf G, Bessman S, et al. Granulocyte

colony- stimulating factor as a marker for bacterial infection in neonates. J Pediatr 128:765–769, 1996.

560. Küster H, Weiss M, Willeitner AE, et al. Interleukin-1 receptor antagonist and interleukin-6 for early diagnosis of neonatal sepsis 2 days before clinical manifestation. Lancet 352:1271–1277, 1998.

561. Doellner H, Arntzen KJ, Haereid PE, et al. Interleukin-6 concentrations in neonates evaluated for sepsis. J Pediatr 132:295–296, 1998.

562. Panero A, Pacifico L, Rossi N, et al. Interleukin 6 in neonates with early and late onset infection. Pediatr Infect Dis J 16:370–375, 1997.

563. Chiesa C, Panero A, Rossi N, et al. Reliability of procalcitonin concentrations for the diagnosis of sepsis in critically ill neonates. Clin Infect Dis 26:664–672, 1998.

564. Yoon BH, Romero R, Yang SH, et al. Interleukin-6 concentrations in umbilical cord plasma are elevated in neonates with white matter lesions associated with periventricular leukomalacia. Am J Obstet Gynecol 174:1433–1440, 1996.

565. Dammann O, Leviton A. Maternal intrauterine infection, cytokines, and brain damage in the preterm newborn. Pediatr Res 42:1–8, 1997.

566. Fernandez M, Hickman ME, Baker CJ. Antimicrobial susceptibilities of group B streptococci isolated between 1992 and 1996 from patients with bacteremia or meningitis. Antimicrob Agents Chemother 42:1517–1519, 1998.

567. Schauf V, Deveikis A, Riff L, et al. Antibiotic-killing kinetics of group B streptococci. J Pediatr 89:194, 1976.

568. Deveikis A, Schauf V, Mizen M, et al. Antimicrobial therapy of experimental group B streptococcal infection in mice. Antimicrob Agents Chemother 11:817, 1977.

569. Odio CM, Umana MA, Saenz A, et al. Comparative efficacy of ceftazidime vs. carbenicillin and amikacin for treatment of neonatal septicemia. Pediatr Infect Dis J 6:371, 1987.

570. Begue P, Floret D, Mallet E, et al. Pharmacokinetics and clinical evaluation of cefotaxime in children suffering from purulent meningitis. J Antimicrob Chemother 14(Suppl):161, 1984.

571. Odio CM, Faingezicht I, Salas JL, et al. Cefotaxime vs. conventional therapy for treatment of bacterial meningitis of infants and children. Pediatr Infect Dis J 5:402, 1986.

572. Feigin RD, McCracken GH, Klein JO. Diagnosis and management of meningitis. Pediatr Infect Dis J 11:785–814, 1992.

573. Bradley JS, Ching DLK, Wilson TA, Compogiannis LS. Once-daily ceftriaxone to complete therapy of uncomplicated group B streptococcal infection in neonates: a preliminary report. Clin Pediatr 31:274–278, 1992.

574. Group B Streptococcal Infections in Pregnancy. ACOG Technical Bulletin, vol 170. Washington DC, American College of Gynecology, 1996.

575. American Academy of Pediatrics Committee on Infectious Diseases and Committee on Fetus and Newborn. Guidelines for prevention of group B streptococcal (GBS) infection by chemoprophylaxis. Pediatrics 90:775–778, 1992.

576. Centers for Disease Control and Prevention. Prevention of perinatal group B streptococcal: a public health perspective. MMWR Morb Mortal Wkly Rep 45:1–24, 1996.

577. American Academy of Pediatrics, Committee on Infectious Diseases/Committee on Fetus and Newborn. Revised guidelines for prevention of early-onset group B streptococcal infection. Pediatrics 99:489–496, 1997.

578. Gotoff SP, Boyer KM. Prevention of early-onset neonatal group B streptococcal disease. Pediatrics 99:866–869, 1997.

579. MacAulay MA, Abou-Sabe M, Charles D. Placental transfer of ampicillin. Am J Obstet Gynecol 96:943–950, 1966.

580. Yancey MK, et al. Risk factors for neonatal sepsis. Obstet Gynecol 87:188–194, 1966.

581. Brozanski BS, et al. Prevention of early-onset group B streptococcal sepsis (EOGBSS): implementation of the CDC guidelines. American Pediatric Society 108th Annual Meeting/Society for Pediatric Reserach 67th Annual Meeting, New Orleans, La, 1998.

582. Squire E, Favara B, Todd J. Diagnosis of neonatal bacterial infection: hematologic and pathologic findings in fatal and nonfatal cases. Pediatrics 64:60, 1979.

583. McCracken GH, Threlkeld N, Mize SB, et al. Moxalactam therapy for neonatal meningitis due to gram negative enteric bacilli: a prospective controlled evaluation. JAMA 252:1427, 1984.

584. McCracken GH Jr, Mize SG. A controlled study of intrathecal antibiotic therapy in gram-negative enteric meningitis of infancy. Report of the Neonatal Meningitis Cooperative Study Group. J Pediatr 89:66, 1976.

585. McCracken GH Jr, Mize SG, Threlkeld N. Intraventricular gentamicin therapy in gram-negative bacillary meningitis of infancy. Lancet 1:787, 1980.

586. Mulhall A, de Louvois J, Hurley R. Efficacy of chloramphenicol in the treatment of neonatal and infantile meningitis: a study of 70 cases. Lancet 1:284, 1983.

587. Levitz RE, Quintiliani R. Trimethoprim-sulfamethoxazole for bacterial meningitis. Ann Intern Med 100:881, 1984.

588. Lauterbach R, Zembala M. Pentoxifylline resues plasma tumour necrosis factor-alpha concentration in premature infants with sepsis. Eur J Pediatr 155:404–409, 1996.

589. Schibler KR, Osborn RA, Leung LY, et al. A randomized, placebo-controlled trial of granulocyte colony-stimulating factor administration to newborn infants with neutropenia and clinical signs of early-onset sepsis. Pediatrics 102:6–13, 1998.

590. Kocherlakota P, LaGamma EF. Preliminary Report: rhG-CSF may reduce the incidence of neonatal sepsis in prolonged preeclampsia-associated neutropenia. Pediatrics 102:1107–1111, 1998.

591. Hill HR. Intravenous immunoglobulin use in the neonate: role in prophylaxis and therapy of infection. Pediatr Infect Dis J 12:549, 1993.

592. Noya FDN. Use of intravenous immunoglobulin in neonates. Rep Pediatr Infect Dis 3:30, 1993.

593. Spirer Z, Jurgenson U, Lazewnick R, et al. Complete recovery from an apparent brain abscess treated without neurosurgery: the importance of early CT scanning. Clin Pediatr (Phila) 21:106, 1982.

594. Renier D, Flandin C, Hirsch E, Hirsch J-F. Brain abscesses in neonates: a study of 30 cases. J Neurosurg 69:877, 1988.

595. Wessalowski R, Thomas L, Kivit J, Voit T. Multiple brain abscesses caused by *Salmonella enteritidis* in a neonate: successful treatment with ciprofloxacin. Pediatr Infect Dis J 12:683, 1993.

596. Townsend T, Shapiro M, Rosner B, et al. The use of antimicrobial agents in general hospitals: IV. Infants and children. Pediatrics 64:573, 1979.

597. Gladstone IM, Ehrenkranz RA, Edberg SC, et al. A ten-year review of neonatal sepsis and comparison with the previous fifty-year experience. Pediatr Infect Dis J 9:819, 1990.

598. Speer CP, Hauptmann D, Stubbe P, et al. Neonatal septicemia and meningitis in Gottingen, West Germany. Pediatr Infect Dis J 4:36, 1985.

599. Tessin I, Trollfors B, Thiringer K. Incidence and etiology of neonatal septicaemia and meningitis in Western Sweden 1975–1986. Acta Paediatr Scand 79:1023, 1990.

600. Bennet R, Bergdahl S, Eriksson M, et al. The outcome of neonatal septicemia during fifteen years. Acta Paediatr Scand 78:40, 1989.

601. Zachman RD, Graven SN. A neonatal intensive care unit: a four-year summary. Am J Dis Child 128:165, 1974.

602. Zangwill KM, Schuchat A, Wenger JD. Group B streptococcal disease in the United States 1990: report from a multi-state active surveillance system. MMWR CDC Surveill Summ 41(SS-6):25–32, 1992.

603. Placzek MM, Whitelaw A. Early and late neonatal septicaemia. Arch Dis Child 58:728, 1983.

604. Alfven G, Bergqvist G, Bolme P, et al. Long-term follow-up of neonatal septicemia. Acta Paediatr Scand 67:769, 1978.

605. McCracken GH Jr, Threlkeld N, Mize S, et al. Moxalactam therapy for neonatal meningitis due to gram-negative enteric bacilli: a prospective controlled evaluation. JAMA 252:1427, 1984.

606. de Louvois J. Septicaemia and meningitis in the newborn. In de Louvois J, Harvey D (eds). Infection in the Newborn. New York, John Wiley & Sons, 1990, pp 107–115.

607. Wald E, Bergman I, Chiponis D, et al. Long-term outcome of group B streptococcal meningitis. Pediatrics 77:217, 1986.

608. Franco SM, Cornelius VE, Andrews BF. Long-term outcome of neonatal meningitis. Am J Dis Child 146:567, 1992.

609. Fitzhardinge PM, Kazemi M, Ramsay M, et al. Long-term sequelae of neonatal meningitis. Dev Med Child Neurol 16:3, 1974.

610. Schultz P, Leeds NE. Intraventricular septations complicating neonatal meningitis. J Neurosurg 38:620, 1973.

611. Horn KA, Zimmerman RA, Knostman JD, et al. Neurological sequelae of group B streptococcal neonatal infection. Pediatrics 53:501, 1974.

612. Edwards MS, Rench MA, Haffar AAM, et al. Long-term sequelae of group B streptococcal meningitis in infants. J Pediatr 106:717, 1985.

613. McCracken GH Jr, Mustafa M, Ramilo O, et al. Cerebrospinal fluid interleukin-1B and tumor necrosis factor concentrations and outcome from neonatal gram-negative enteric bacillary meningitis. Pediatr Infect Dis J 8:155, 1989.

614. Baier J, Bocchini JA Jr, Brown EG. Selective use of vancomycin to prevent coagulase-negative staphylococcal nosocomial bacteremia in high risk very low birth weight infants. Pediatr Infect Dis J 17:179–183, 1998.

615. Hanson LA, Karlsson B, Jalil F, et al. Antiviral and antibacterial factors in human milk. In Hanson LA (ed). Biology of Human Milk. New York, Raven Press, 1988, pp 141–157.

616. Mathus NB, Dwarkadas AM, Sharma VK, et al. Anti-infective factors in preterm human colostrum. Acta Paediatr Scand 79:1039, 1990.

617. Isaacs CF, Kashyap S, Heird WC, et al. Antiviral and antibacterial lipids in human milk and infant formula feeds. Arch Dis Child 65:861, 1990.

618. Coppa GV, Gabrielli OR, Giorgi P, et al. Preliminary study of breastfeeding and bacterial adhesion to uroepithelial cells. Lancet 1:569, 1990.

619. Winberg J, Wessner G. Does breast milk protect against septicaemia in the newborn? Lancet 1:1091, 1971.

620. Ashraf RN, Jalil F, Zaman S, et al. Breast feeding and protection against neonatal sepsis in a high risk population. Arch Dis Child 66:488, 1991.

621. Pabst HF, Godel J, Grace M, et al. Effect of breast-feeding on immune response to BCG vaccination. Lancet 1:295, 1989.

622. Englund JA, Glezen WP. Maternal immunization for the prevention of infection in early infancy. Semin Pediatr Infect Dis 2:225, 1991.

623. Sidiropoulos D, Herrman U Jr, Morell A, et al. Transplacental passage of intravenous immunoglobulin in the last trimester of pregnancy. J Pediatr 109:505, 1986.

624. Cairo MS, Dana R, Park L, et al. Reduced cytokine production (IL-3, G-CSF, GM-CSF) from stimulated cord monoculear cells compared to adult but normal cytokine receptor expression on newborn effector cells: possible mechanism in the dysregulation of neonatal granulopoiesis. Pediatr Res 29:273A, 1991.

625. Cairo MS. Cytokines: a new immunotherapy. Clin Perinatol 18:343, 1991.

626. Roilides E, Pizzo PA. Modulation of host defenses by cytokines: evolving adjuncts in prevention and treatment of serious infections in immunocompromised patients. Clin Infect Dis 15:508, 1992.

627. Roberts RL, Szelc CM, Scates SM, et al. Neutropenia in an extremely premature infant treated with recombinant human granulocyte colony-stimulating factor. Am J Dis Child 145:808, 1991.

628. Cairo MS, Agosti J, Ellis R, et al. A randomized, double-blind, placebo-controlled trial of prophylactic recombinant human granulocyte-macrophage colony-stimulating factor to reduce nosocomial infections in very low birth weight neonates. J Pediatr 134:64–70, 1999.

629. Yang KD, Bohnsack FJ, Hill HR. Fibronectin in host defense: implications in the diagnosis, prophylaxis and therapy of infectious diseases. Pediatr Infect Dis J 12:234, 1993.

630. Yoder MC. Therapeutic administration of fibronectin: current uses and potential applications. Clin Perinatol 18:325, 1991.

631. Dyke MP, Forsyth KD. Decreased plasma fibronectin concentrations in preterm infants with septicemia. Arch Dis Child 68:557, 1993.

632. Goldmann DA, Pier GB. Pathogenesis of infections related to intravascular catheterization. Clin Microbiol Rev 6:176, 1993.

633. Klein JO. Family spread of staphylococcal disease following a nursery outbreak. N Y State J Med 60:861, 1960.

634. Damato JJ, Eitzman DV, Baer H. Persistence and dissemination in the community of R-factors of nosocomial origin. J Infect Dis 129:205, 1974.

635. Baraff LJ, Bass JW, Fleisher GR, et al. Practice guidelines for the management of infants and children 0 to 36 months of age with fever without source. Pediatrics 91:1, 1993.

636. McCarthy PL, Dolan TF. The serious implications of high fever in infants during their first three months. Clin Pediatr (Phila) 15:794, 1976.

637. O'Shea JS. Assessing the significance of fever in young infants. Clin Pediatr (Phila) 17:854, 1978.

638. Roberts KB, Borzy MS. Fever in the first eight weeks of life. John Hopkins Med J 141:9, 1977.

639. Pantell RH, Naber M, Lamar R, et al. Fever in the first six months of life. Clin Pediatr (Phila) 19:77, 1980.

640. Greene JW, Hara C, O'Connor S, et al. Management of

febrile outpatient neonates. Clin Pediatr (Phila) 20:375, 1981.

641. Crain EF, Shelov SP. Febrile infants: predictors of bacteremia. J Pediatr 101:686, 1982.

642. Klein JO, Schlessinger PC, Karasic RB. Management of the febrile infant under three months of age. Pediatr Infect Dis J 3:75, 1984.

643. King JC Jr, Berman ED, Wright PF. Evaluation of fever in infants less than 8 weeks old. South Med J 80:948, 1987.

644. Dagan R, Sofer S, Phillip M, et al. Ambulatory care of febrile infants younger than 2 months of age classified as being at low risk for having serious bacterial infections. J Pediatr 112:355, 1988.

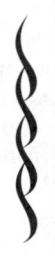

Bacterial Infections of the Respiratory Tract

ELIZABETH D. BARNETT, M.D., and JEROME O. KLEIN, M.D.

INFECTIONS OF THE ORAL CAVITY AND NASOPHARYNX

Pharyngitis, Retropharyngeal Cellulitis, and Retropharyngeal Abscess

Neonates with bacterial infection of the oropharynx may present with pharyngeal inflammation with or without exudate or with retropharyngeal cellulitis or abscess. Extension of infection to the surrounding structures may occur, leading to deep neck abscess formation. Microorganisms identified as the etiologic agents of these infections and their manifestations of disease include the following:

Staphylococcus aureus. Although many children are colonized in the throat and nasopharynx with *S. aureus*, this organism is rarely a primary agent in the etiology of pharyngitis in infants (or adults). There have, however, been reports of localized abscesses in the oral cavity related to *S. aureus*. Clark and Barysh, in 1936, reported a case of retropharyngeal abscess in a 6-week-old infant.[1] The child was critically ill but recovered after incision and drainage of the abscess. Steinhauer reported a case of cellulitis of the floor of the mouth (Ludwig's angina) in a 12-day-old infant.[2] The child was febrile and toxic; examination of the mouth revealed swelling under the tongue. Purulent material was subsequently drained from this lesion, and *S. aureus* was isolated from the pus. A laceration was noted in the floor of the mouth, and the author considered this wound to be the portal of entry of the infection.

Streptococcus pyogenes. Fever and pharyngeal inflammation may result from infection with this organism in the neonate.[3]

Streptococcus agalactiae. Retropharyngeal cellulitis has been associated with bacteremia caused by group B *Streptococcus*.[4, 5] These neonates presented with poor feeding, noisy breathing, and widening of the retropharyngeal space on radiographs of the lateral neck. A retropharyngeal abscess caused by group B *Streptococcus* occurred in one of three neonates reported in a series of 31 cases of retropharyngeal abscess seen in children in Camperdown, Australia, between 1954 and 1990.[6, 7] This infant was found to have a third branchial arch pouch that was subject to recurrent infection until age 5 years.

Listeria monocytogenes. Small focal granulomas on the mucous membrane of the posterior pharynx have been observed in neonates with *L. monocytogenes*. Necrosis of some of the granulomas results in ulcers on the pharynx and tonsils.

Treponema pallidum. Mucous patches occur on the lips, tongue, and palate of congenitally infected infants. Rhinitis may appear after the first week of life.

Neisseria gonorrhoeae. A yellow mucoid exudate of the pharynx may be present simultaneously with ophthalmia (A Yu, personal communication, 1981). A case report of in utero gonococcal infection with involvement of multiple tissues included pharyngeal abscess.[8]

Enterococcus faecalis. A case of retropharyngeal abscess in which culture of aspirated pus grew *E. faecalis* as well as two strains of coagulase-negative staphylococci occurred in a 2-week-old full-term infant from Australia.[7] The infant was severely ill and had atlantoaxial dislocation resulting in paraplegia. At autopsy he had bacterial endocarditis, diffuse bilateral pneumonia, and renal infarcts.

Escherichia coli. This organism can be a rare cause of infection of the pharyngeal cavity. Pus from a retropharyngeal abscess in a 1-week-old infant grew two strains of *E. coli*.[7] The infant was afebrile on presentation and had a large midline pharyngeal swelling.

Infants may have coryza and other signs of upper respiratory tract disease because of infection with respiratory viruses. Infections with respiratory viruses may damage the respiratory mucosa and increase susceptibility to bacterial infection of the respiratory tract. Eichenwald[9] described an apparent synergy of respiratory viruses and a staphylococcus that produced an upper respiratory tract infection called the "stuffy nose" syndrome. The syndrome occurred only when both organisms were present. He and his group also documented increased dissemination of bacteria by newborns carrying staphylococci and echovirus 20 or adenovirus type 2 in the nasopharynx and coined the term *cloud babies* for these infants.[10] These studies have not been repeated by other investigators, and the significance of synergy of two or more microorganisms in neonatal respiratory infections remains uncertain.

Noma

Noma (cancrum oris) is a destructive gangrenous process that may affect the nose, lips, and mouth. It occurs almost exclusively in malnourished children in developing countries; it has been postulated that nutrient deficiencies play a role in its pathogenesis.[11] Although it is usually a chronic, destructive process in older children, in neonates it may be rapidly fatal. Affected neonates are usually premature and have low birth weight. In older children and adults, noma is caused by fusospirochetes such as *Fusobacterium necrophorum*.[12] The disease in neonates is usually due to *Pseudomonas aeruginosa*. Ghosal and co-workers, from Calcutta, reported bacteriologic and histologic findings in 35 cases of noma in neonates.[13] *P. aeruginosa* was isolated from blood or the gangrenous area in more than 90% of the cases. An Israeli full-term infant with bilateral choanal atresia who required an airway developed gangrenous lesions of the cheek on day 11 and palatal lesions that progressed to ulceration and an oronasal fistula. Cultures from the lesions grew *P. aeruginosa*.[14]

Epiglottitis

Epiglottitis caused by *S. aureus* in an 8-day-old infant was reported by Baxter in a survey of experience with the disease at Montreal Children's Hospital between 1951 and 1965.[15] A second case of epiglottitis due to *S. aureus* in a 5-day-old infant was reported by Rosenfeld and associates.[16] The infant presented with bradycardia,

hoarseness, and inspiratory stridor and had diffuse inflammation of the arytenoids and epiglottis. *S. aureus* was cultured from pus on the epiglottic surface; blood culture was negative. Epiglottitis due to group B *Streptococcus* was reported in an 11-week old infant in 1996.[17]

Laryngitis

Laryngitis in the newborn is rare. The child with congenital syphilis may have laryngitis and an aphonic cry. Hazard and co-workers described a case of laryngitis caused by *Streptococcus pneumoniae*.[18] A term infant was noted at 12 hours to have a hoarse cry, which progressed to aphonia during the next 3 days. Direct examination of the larynx revealed swelling and redness of the vocal cords. The child was febrile (38.5° C), but the physical examination was unremarkable. *S. pneumoniae* was isolated from the amniotic fluid, the maternal cervix, and the larynx of the infant. The child responded rapidly to treatment with parenteral penicillin G.

Infection of the Paranasal Sinuses

The paranasal sinuses of the fetus begin to differentiate at about the fourth month of gestation. The sinuses develop by local evagination of nasal mucosa and concurrent resorption of overlying bone. The maxillary and ethmoid sinuses are developed at birth and may be sites for suppurative infection. The sphenoid and frontal sinuses are rudimentary at birth and are not well defined until about 6 years of age.[19, 20]

Inflammatory reaction may occur simultaneously in the paranasal sinuses, the middle ears, and the lungs. Autopsy may reveal that purulent exudate and leukocytic infiltration of the mucosa are present at one or more of these sites. Infection of the ethmoid and maxillary sinuses may be severe and life threatening in the newborn. Clinical manifestations include general signs of infection such as fever, lethargy, irritability, and poor feeding as well as focal signs indicative of sinus involvement (i.e., nasal congestion, purulent drainage from the nostrils, and periorbital redness and swelling). Proptosis may occur in severely affected children. Although any of the organisms responsible for neonatal sepsis may cause sinusitis, *S. aureus* and groups A and B streptococci are responsible for most infections.[21–23] Suppurative infection of the maxillary sinus may progress to osteomyelitis of the superior maxilla (see Chapter 23).[22]

Cultures of blood, nasopharynx, and purulent drainage (if present) should be obtained before treatment. Antibacterial therapy must include a penicillinase-resistant penicillin or cephalosporin for activity against *Staphylococcus* and groups A and B streptococci. If no material is available for examination of Gram-stained pus or if results of the preparation are ambiguous, initial therapy should include an aminoglycoside or a third-generation cephalosporin to ensure activity against gram-negative enteric bacilli (see discussion of management in Chapter 21). Surgical drainage of the infected site should be considered. Drainage of the suppurative maxillary sinus should be performed through the nose to avoid scars on the face and damage to the developing teeth.[22]

Diphtheria

Neonatal diphtheria, although now extremely rare in the United States, was common before the development and extensive use of immunization with diphtheria toxoid. Outbreaks occurred in hospital nurseries. One of the most striking reports describes three separate epidemics in a foundling hospital in Tipperary, Ireland, between 1937 and 1941; 36 infants younger than 1 month of age were afflicted, and 26 died.[24] Goebel and Stroder described 109 infants younger than 1 year of age with diphtheria in Germany during the period extending from the fall of 1945 to the summer of 1947: 59 infants were younger than 1 month of age, and 26 died.[25] In a report from the Communicable Disease Unit of the Los Angeles County Hospital covering the 10-year period ending June 1950, 1433 patients were admitted to the hospital with diphtheria; 19 patients were younger than 1 year of age, but just 2 patients were younger than 1 month of age.[26] Elsewhere, the disease also appears to be on the wane; only three cases of neonatal diphtheria were identified in India between 1974 and 1984 by Mathur and associates.[27]

Respiratory diphtheria has been well controlled in the United States since the introduction of diphtheria toxoid in the 1920s, although it remained endemic in some states through the 1970s.[28] The results of a survey of cases of diphtheria reported to the Centers for Disease Control (CDC) of the U.S. Public Health Service, Atlanta, Georgia, for the period 1971 to October 1975 showed that no cases involved children younger than 1 month of age and that only six cases occurred in children younger than 1 year of age (the youngest was 5 months old) (G Filice, personal communication, 1981). During the period 1980 through 1995, 41 cases of respiratory diphtheria were reported to the CDC; 4 (10%) were fatal, all of which occurred in unvaccinated children.[29] Importation of diphtheria from countries where diphtheria remains endemic, including areas of the world experiencing a resurgence of disease such as the independent states of the former Soviet Union, account for the majority of cases in industrialized nations.[30]

The newborn receives antibodies to *Corynebacterium diphtheriae* from the mother if she is immune, and the titers of mother and child at birth are approximately equivalent.[31] Protection of some degree results in the neonate from this passively transferred antibody. Serologic surveys performed in the United States in the 1970s and 1980s suggested that 20 to 60% of adults older than 20 years of age may be susceptible to diphtheria.[32, 33] Additional data from Europe confirmed that many adults remain susceptible to diphtheria.[33a, 33b] As is the case with other passively transferred immunity, protection depends on the level of maternal antibody at the time of the infant's birth, and protection decreases during the months after birth unless the infant is actively immunized.[34, 35]

Neonatal diphtheria is usually localized to the nares. Diphtheria of the fauces is less common. The skin and mucous membranes may be affected; the two infants in Los Angeles included an 8-day-old neonate with diphtheritic conjunctivitis.[26] Because isolation of *C. diphtheriae* requires inoculation of special culture media, notification of the laboratory of the possibility of diphtheria is important. Cultures of both nasal and pharyngeal secretions may improve yield of positive cultures.[36] Infants with suspected diphtheria should be isolated and treated with penicillin or erythromycin to eradicate the organism from the respiratory tract or other foci of infection to terminate toxin production and decrease likelihood of transmission. The mainstay of therapy, however, is diphtheria antitoxin, which should be administered as soon as the diagnosis of diphtheria is considered. This product is available in the United States from the CDC.[37]

Pertussis

Infants and young children in the United States are at the highest risk of pertussis and its complications.[38] Although the incidence of pertussis has declined markedly since 1934, when more than 250,000 cases were recorded, resurgence of disease since the early 1980s underscores the need for continued awareness of this disease.[39] Pertussis may occur in exposed and unprotected newborns.[40] Between 1959 and 1977 pertussis was diagnosed in 400 children in Dallas hospitals; 69 patients (17%) were younger than 12 weeks of age. An adult in the household with undiagnosed mild disease was the usual source of infection for these neonates and young infants.[41] A report of a nursery outbreak in Cincinnati highlights the persistent threat of pertussis in the young infant and in hospital personnel.[42] Between February and May 1974, six newborns, eight physicians, and five nurses developed pertussis (documented by isolation of *Bordetella pertussis* from the nasopharynx). Four additional infants had clinical illness, but the organism was not isolated from the upper respiratory tract. Two mothers of uninfected infants became ill. The initial case was a 1-month-old infant treated in a ward whose infection spread to the nursery when house officers became infected and transmitted the organism to newborns.

In the United States in the early 1990s, cases of pertussis were reported from every state, and large outbreaks occurred in Cincinnati and Chicago.[42a] In the Chicago outbreak, the highest attack rate was in infants younger than 6 months of age; factors associated with transmission of pertussis in this age group included young maternal age and cough lasting 7 days or more in their mothers.[43] Another risk factor for pertussis may be low birth weight. A study of cases of pertussis in Wisconsin infants and young children concluded that children of low birth weight were more likely than their normal birth weight counterparts to contract pertussis and to be hospitalized with the disease.[44]

Antibody to *B. pertussis* crosses the placenta, and titers in immune mothers and their newborns are approximately equal.[31, 45] If high titers of the passively transferred antibody are present, the antibody is protective for the newborn. This was demonstrated by Cohen and Scadron, who observed protection of 6 months' duration in the offspring of recently immunized women.[45] Three cases of clinical pertussis occurred among six infants who were exposed to infection and whose mothers had not been immunized, whereas no cases occurred among eight similarly exposed infants of immunized mothers. In the group of infants aged 7 to 12 months, there were two cases of clinical pertussis in offspring of immunized and unimmunized mothers, which suggests that passively transferred immunity was no longer present in the infant whose mother had been immunized during pregnancy. Many women who were vaccinated during infancy have low levels of antibody when they reach childbearing age, and this concentration of antibody may be insufficient to protect offspring if the infants are exposed to pertussis during the first few months of life (before they are actively immunized). Older children and adults are important sources of infection for infants.[46] The recent increase in pertussis cases in the United States despite the achievement of the highest levels of immunization ever is poorly understood.[38, 39]

Clinical presentation of pertussis in newborns is similar to that in older children. The incubation period may vary from 5 to 10 days. The initial sign is usually mild coughing that may progress, over a period of several days, to severe paroxysms with regurgitation and vomiting of food. The characteristic whoop may be absent. The most severely affected infants have marked respiratory distress, including cyanosis and apnea. Fever is usually absent. Lymphocyte counts are frequently in excess of 30,000 per mm³. Cockayne described a case of clinical pertussis in a neonate whose mother and brother were infectious at the time of birth.[47] The infant began to cough on the fifth day of life and had a high white blood cell count (36,000 per mm³), with a majority of lymphocytes. Phillips reported two cases of pertussis in newborns who were infected by an obstetric nurse.[48] The infants began to cough on the eighth and tenth days of life. Clinical signs of respiratory infection caused by *Chlamydia trachomatis* are similar to those of pertussis (see Chapter 15).

Complications of pertussis in young infants include convulsions, bronchopneumonia, and hemorrhage. In a study of 182 infants and children younger than age 2 hospitalized with pertussis from 1967 to 1986 in Dallas, apnea and convulsions occurred significantly more frequently in infants younger than 3 months of age; the three deaths were all in 1-month-old infants with secondary bacterial infection.[49] Mortality of infants aged younger than 3 months is high; in the earlier Dallas series, 5 of 69 infants (7%) with onset of signs at between 2 and 6 weeks died.[41] *B. pertussis* pneumonia may progress rapidly; pulmonary hypertension resulting from difficulty perfusing the congested lung may result in right-sided heart failure or fatal cardiac arrhythmias.[50] Long-term sequelae of whooping cough in infancy and early childhood were studied by Johnston and co-workers: there was a significant reduction in forced vital capacity in adulthood in those who had pertussis before age 7 compared with those who did not have pertussis.[51]

Diagnostic methods for pertussis depend on the age of the patient and the duration of cough. Children younger than 11 years of age and older patients with cough lasting less than 14 days should have nasopharyngeal specimens obtained using Dacron or calcium alginate swabs. Best results will be obtained if specimens are inoculated at the bedside or taken immediately to the laboratory in appropriate transport media. Specialized agar (Regan-Lowe or Bordet-Gengou) is required; thus, it is helpful to inform the laboratory of suspicion of pertussis. The organism is most easily isolated during the catarrhal or early paroxysmal stage of illness and rarely found after the fourth week of illness. Direct fluorescent antibody testing of nasopharyngeal secretions has low sensitivity and variable specificity and cannot be relied on to diagnose pertussis. Polymerase chain reaction shows promise as a diagnostic tool,[52] but it is not yet widely available or standardized between laboratories.

Serologic testing is the diagnostic method of choice for patients 11 years of age or older and has excellent sensitivity and specificity when done in an experienced laboratory on paired specimens, the first having been collected as early as possible during the course of illness. No single serologic marker has been identified as diagnostic for pertussis; efforts to standardize serologic studies are underway.

Antimicrobial therapy may ameliorate the disease if it is given in the catarrhal stage, but it has no clinical effect once paroxysms occur. The current antibiotic of choice for pertussis in infants and young infants is erythromycin, 40 to 50 mg/kg per day orally in four divided doses; maximum 2 g per day. Erythromycin eliminates carriage of the organisms from the upper respiratory tract and is of value in limiting communicability of infection even if given late in the course of disease. Resistance of *B. pertussis* to erythromycin has been reported[53] but does not appear to be widespread. Alternatives to erythromycin include trimethoprim-sulfamethoxazole (efficacy unproven) or clarithromycin or other macrolides. One study demonstrated clinical efficacy in treating pertussis with high-dose specific pertussis globulin from donors immunized with acellular pertussis vaccine,[54] although efficacy of this regimen on a larger scale has not been proven. One investigator has proposed a role for inhaled corticosteroids in the treatment of pertussis.[55]

Erythromycin is also of value in prevention of pertussis in exposed infants. Granstrom and colleagues described its use in 28 newborns of mothers with pertussis.[56] The women had serologic- or culture-confirmed pertussis at the time of labor. Mothers and their newborns received a 10-day course of erythromycin. The infected and treated mothers were allowed to nurse their infants. None of the infants developed signs or serologic evidence of pertussis. Erythromycin has also been shown to be effective in preventing secondary spread within households in which infants resided.[57]

Erythromycin (40–50 mg/kg per day, orally in four doses, maximum 2 g per day) for 14 days is recommended for household[57] and other close contacts, such as those in the hospital, including medical and surgical personnel.[58] Although their efficacies have not been established, clarithromycin, azithromycin, or trimethoprim-sulfamethoxazole may be alternatives for those who cannot tolerate erythromycin.

A recent report of a cluster of cases of pyloric stenosis among infants given erythromycin for prophylaxis after exposure to pertussis has raised concern about the use of erythromycin in this setting.[58a] Because erythromycin remains the only medication proven effective for this purpose, the drug remains the recommended agent until alternative regimens can be shown to be safe and effective. Health care professionals who prescribe erythromycin to newborns should inform parents of the risk of pyloric stenosis and counsel them about signs and symptoms of pyloric stenosis.

OTITIS MEDIA

Otitis media in the newborn may be an isolated infection, or it may be associated with sepsis, pneumonia, or meningitis. Acute otitis media is defined as the presence of fluid in the middle ear (middle ear effusion) accompanied by an acute sign of illness. Middle ear effusion may be present without other signs of acute illness. Autopsy studies indicated that inflammation in the lungs or paranasal sinuses is usually accompanied by inflammation in the middle ear.[59–62] Diagnostic criteria of otitis media in the newborn are the same as in the older child, but the microbiology of otitis media is different in the neonate and requires different considerations for antimicrobial therapy.

Pathogenesis and Pathology

During fetal life, amniotic fluid bathes the entire respiratory tree, including the lungs, paranasal sinuses, and middle ear cleft. Amniotic fluid and cellular debris are usually cleared from the middle ear in most infants within a few days after birth.[59] In term infants, the middle ear is usually well aerated and has normal middle ear pressure and normal tympanic membrane compliance within the first 24 hours.[63] A study of 68 full-term infants examined by otoscopy, tympanometry, and acoustic reflectometry within the first 3 hours of life revealed the presence of middle ear effusion in all neonates; fluid was absent at 72 hours of life in almost all infants.[64]

deSa's studies of the middle ear at autopsy provide important information about the development of otitis media in the neonate.[59] He examined 130 infants, including 36 stillborn infants, 74 neonates who died within 7 days of life, and 20 infants who died between 8 and 28 days. In 56 cases, the middle ear was aerated or contained a small amount of clear fluid. In 55 cases, amniotic debris was present; in 2 additional cases, cellular material was mixed with mucus. A purulent exudate was present in the middle ear of 17 infants; these exudates were cultured, and a bacterial pathogen was isolated from 13. Amniotic material was present in specimens obtained from most of the stillborn infants. Purulent exudate was not seen in the stillborns; the frequency of its presence increased with postnatal age at time of death. Of the 20 infants who lived for 7 or more days, 11 had purulent exudate in the middle ear. Each of the 17 infants with otitis media had one or more significant infections elsewhere; 12 had pneumonia, and 6 had meningitis. The author subsequently identified mucosal metaplasia and chronic inflammation in the middle ears of newborns receiving ventilatory support.[65]

Factors that may affect the development of otitis media in the neonate include the nature of the amniotic fluid, the presence of other infectious processes, the need for resuscitative efforts (especially positive-pressure ventilation), the presence of anatomic defects such as cleft palate, the immunologic status of the infant, and the general state of health of the infant. Aspiration of infected amniotic fluid through the eustachian tube may be one factor in the development of otitis media in the neonate; dysfunction of the eustachian tube, which is shorter, wider, and more horizontal than in the older child,[66] and failure to clear aspirated material from the middle ear probably have etiologic roles as well. Piza and associates[67] speculate that infants born through thick meconium fluid may be at greater risk for otitis media because of the inflammatory nature of this fluid. deSa noted that many infants who developed otitis media required assistance in respiration and speculated that the pressure of ventilation efforts was responsible for propelling infected material into the middle ear.[59] In infants, as in older children, middle ear effusion appears to be frequent in patients with nasotracheal tubes, and the effusion occurs first on the side of intubation.[68] Berman and colleagues[69] described an association between nasotracheal intubation for more than 7 days and the presence of middle ear effusion.

Infants with cleft palate are at high risk for recurrent otitis media and conductive hearing loss due to the persistence of middle ear effusion. Attempts to reduce the incidence of permanent hearing impairment have included intensive monitoring of children with cleft palate for middle ear effusion and repair of these defects earlier in infancy. A recent study, however, found that early cleft palate repair did not reduce significantly the subsequent need for ventilating tubes in these children.[70]

Breast-fed infants are at lower risk than bottle-fed infants for acute otitis media. Results of studies of Canadian Eskimo infants[71] and of infants in India,[72] Finland,[73] Denmark,[74] and the United States[75] indicate a significant decrease in the incidence of infection of the middle ear in breast-fed compared with bottle-fed infants. A study of infants in Cooperstown, New York, identified a significantly lower incidence of acute lower respiratory tract infection in infants who were breast fed compared with infants who were bottle fed; the incidence of otitis media was lower in the breast-fed infants, but this difference was not statistically significant.[76] Boston infants who were breast fed had a lower risk for either having had one or more episodes of acute otitis media or having had recurrent acute otitis media (three or more episodes) during the first year of life. Of interest was the fact that the protective association of breast-feeding did not increase with increased duration of breast-feeding; infants who were breast fed for 3 months had an incidence of otitis media in the first year of life that was as low as infants who were breast fed for 12 months.[77]

The beneficial effects of breast-feeding may be due to immunologic factors in breast milk or to development of musculature in the breast-fed infant that may affect eustachian tube function and assist in promoting drainage of middle ear fluid. Alternatively, the results may indicate harmful effects of bottle-feeding, including the reclining or horizontal position of the bottle-fed infant that allows fluid to move readily into the middle ear,[78, 79] allergy to one or more components in cow's or formula milk, or aspiration of fluids into the middle ear during feeding. The hypothesis that breast milk is protective is substantiated by the results of studies of a special feeding bottle for infants with cleft palate. Infants who were fed by this bottle containing breast milk had fewer days with middle ear effusion than did infants fed by this device containing formula, which suggests that protection was more likely to be a quality of the milk rather than of the mode of feeding.[80] Adherence of *S. pneumoniae* and *Haemophilus influenzae* to buccal epithelial cells was inhibited by human breast milk.[81]

Early onset of pneumococcal otitis media has been associated with low levels of cord blood pneumococcal antibodies.[82] Among a group of infants who had siblings with middle ear disease, low concentrations of cord blood antibody to pneumococcal serotypes 14 or 19F were associated with earlier onset of otitis media. These findings prompted study of immunization of pregnant women with pneumococcal vaccine. The role of antibodies to pneumococcus in human milk in prevention of nasopharyngeal colonization of infants with pneumococcus remains controversial. A study in Sweden involving 448 mother-infant pairs failed to demonstrate reduction in carriage of pneumococcus in neonates fed milk with anticapsular and antiphosphorylcholine activity and showed an increase in colonization when infants were fed milk with anti–cell-wall polysaccharide antibody activity.[83]

Other factors which may play a part in otitis media in the neonatal period include early colonization with pneumococcus or other bacteria[84] and heavy maternal smoking.[85]

Epidemiology

The incidence of acute otitis media or middle ear effusion in the newborn is uncertain because of the paucity of appropriate studies. Warren and Stool examined 127 consecutive infants whose birth weights were under 2300 g and found 3 with middle ear effusions (at 2, 7, and 26 days of life).[86] Jaffe and co-workers examined 101 Navajo infants within 48 hours of birth and identified 18 with impaired mobility of the tympanic membrane.[87] Berman and co-workers identified effusion in the middle ear of 30% of 125 consecutively examined infants who were admitted to a neonatal intensive care unit.[69] The clinical diagnosis was corroborated by aspiration of middle ear fluid. The basis for the differences in incidence in the various studies is uncertain but may be associated with procedures used in the nurseries.

Acute otitis media is common in early infancy. In the prospective study of Boston children, 9% of children had an episode of middle ear infection by 3 months of age.[77] Age at the time of first episode of acute otitis media appears to be an important predictor for recurrent otitis media.[77, 87, 88] Children who experience a first episode during the first months of life are more likely to experience repeated infection than children whose first episode occurs after the first birthday. Additional risk factors include parental smoking and low socioeconomic status.[89]

Some host factors that are also present in infants with neonatal sepsis have been identified in infants with middle ear infection. The incidence of infection is higher in premature infants than in those delivered at term in some studies,[90, 91] but not in the prospective study of Boston children.[77] Male infants are more frequently infected than female infants.[90] Otitis media is also associated with a prolonged interval after rupture of maternal membranes and with other obstetric difficulties.[59, 92] Middle ear infection is more severe in Native Americans and Canadian Eskimos than in the general population, and it is likely that this is true in neonates and older infants as well.[71, 87] Children with cleft palate have a high incidence of otitis media, which may begin soon after birth.[93]

Microbiology

The bacteriology of otitis media in infants is available from aspiration of middle ear fluid of 183 neonates with otitis media from studies in Honolulu,[90] Dallas,[91] Huntsville,[94] Boston,[94] Denver,[69] and Tampere Hospital in Finland[95] (Table 22–1). *S. pneumoniae* and *H. influenzae* are the bacteria isolated most frequently in the very young, as is the case in older infants and children. However, organisms associated with local and septic infection in the neonate, group B *Streptococcus*, *S. aureus*, and gram-negative enteric bacilli, are important pathogens in the newborn within 2 weeks after birth or in older infants who have remained in the nursery because

TABLE 22–1

Bacterial Pathogens Isolated from 183 Infants with Otitis Media in the First 6 Weeks of Life[a]

MICROORGANISM	% OF INFANTS WITH PATHOGEN
Respiratory bacteria	
Streptococcus pneumoniae	17.5
Haemophilus influenzae	12.6
S. pneumoniae and *H. influenzae*	2.7
Staphylococcus aureus	8.2
Streptococcus, groups A and B	2.7
Moraxella catarrhalis	6
Enteric bacteria	
Escherichia coli	5.5
Klebsiella-Enterobacter sp.	4.9
Pseudomonas aeruginosa	1.6
Miscellaneous	4.9
None or nonpathogens	34.4

[a]Reports from Honolulu,[90] Dallas,[91] Huntsville,[94] Boston,[94] Denver,[69] and Tampere Hospital in Finland.[95] The Denver report includes some infants 7 to 12 weeks of age.

of risk features (low birth weight or prematurity) or disease (respiratory distress syndrome). When term infants who have had no problems with delivery or in the nursery develop otitis media 2 or more weeks after hospital discharge, the bacterial pathogens are most likely *S. pneumoniae* and *H. influenzae.*

Gram-negative enteric bacilli have been the predominant organisms isolated at autopsy from purulent effusions of the middle ear. Of 17 infants studied by deSa, 7 had *E. coli* and 6 had *P. aeruginosa.*[59] Beta-hemolytic *Streptococcus* (not further identified) was isolated from one infant, and no organism was recovered from the remaining three. Because pneumonia and meningitis accompanied the otitis in all of these cases, the predominance of gram-negative pathogens in this series is not unexpected.

Congenital tuberculosis of the ear[96] and of the ear and parotid gland[97] have been reported recently in preterm infants from Hong Kong and Turkey. Both cases were notable for significant regional lymphadenopathy, lack of response to antibacterial therapy, and mothers with active pulmonary tuberculosis. Authors of both reports suggest that there is continued need to have a high index of suspicion of this disease in appropriate circumstances. Otitis media and bacteremia due to *P. aeruginosa* occurring at 19 days of life was thought to occur due to inoculation of the organism during a water birth.[98]

Diagnosis

During the first few weeks of life, examination of the ear requires patience and careful appraisal of all the structures of the external canal and the middle ear.[99] The diagnostic criteria for acute otitis media in the neonate are the same as those in the older child: presence of fluid in the middle ear accompanied by signs of acute illness. Middle ear effusion and its effect on tympanic membrane mobility are best measured with a pneumatic otoscope. The normal tympanic membrane moves inward with positive pressure and outward with negative pressure. The presence of fluid in the middle ear dampens tympanic membrane mobility.

In the first few days of life, the ear canal is filled with vernix caseosa; this material is readily removed with a small curette or suction tube. The canal walls of the young infant are pliable and tend to expand and collapse with insufflation during pneumatic otoscopy. Continuing pneumatic insufflation as the speculum is advanced is helpful because the positive pressure expands the pliable canal walls. The tympanic membrane often appears thickened and opaque, and mobility may be limited during the first few days of life.[100] In many infants, the membrane is in an extreme oblique position, with the superior aspect proximal to the observer (Fig. 22–1). The tympanic membrane and the superior canal wall may appear to lie almost in the same plane, so it is often difficult to distinguish the point where the canal ends and the pars flaccida of the membrane begins. The inferior canal wall may bulge loosely over the inferior position of the tympanic membrane and move with positive pressure, simulating movement of the tympanic membrane. The examiner must distinguish the movement of the canal walls and the movement of the membrane. The following should be considered to distinguish the movement of these structures: vessels are seen within the tympanic membrane but are less apparent in the skin of the ear canal; and the tympanic membrane moves during crying or respiration when the middle ear is aerated. The ear canals of most neonates permit entry of only a 2-mm-diameter speculum. Because the entire eardrum cannot be examined at one time, owing to the small diameter of the speculum, quadrants must be examined sequentially. By 1 month of age, the infant's tympanic membrane has assumed an oblique position that is less marked than in the first few weeks of life and one that is similar to the position in the older child.

Tympanometry is of limited value in diagnosis of middle ear effusion in the neonate. The flat tympanogram indicative of effusion in children 6 months of age or older is often not present in the younger infant even

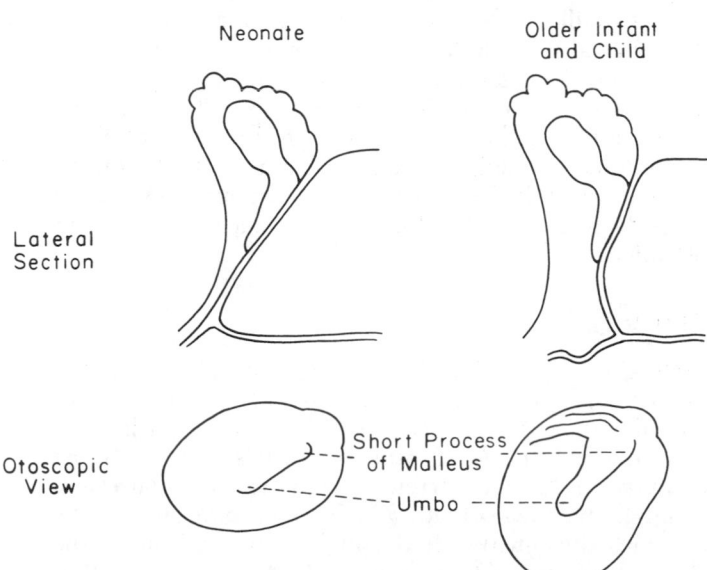

FIGURE 22–1 Lateral section of the middle ear and otoscopic view of the tympanic membrane in the neonate and older infant and child. (Courtesy of Charles D. Bluestone, M.D.)

when fluid is documented by aspiration.[101] Acoustic reflectometry may be of value in diagnosis of otitis media in the neonate because it does not require insertion into the ear canal or the achievement of a seal within the canal.[102]

Culture of the throat or nasopharynx is an imperfect method of identifying the bacterial pathogens responsible for otitis media. Many studies have demonstrated the diagnostic value of needle aspiration of middle ear effusions (tympanocentesis) in acute otitis media. The specific microbiologic diagnosis defines the appropriate antimicrobial therapy and is sufficiently important in the sick neonate to warrant consideration of aspiration of the middle ear fluid. Aspiration of middle ear fluid is more difficult in the neonate compared with the older child, and usually the assistance of an otolaryngologist (using an otoscope with a surgical head or an otomicroscope) is required.

When spontaneous perforation has occurred, the fluid exuding into the external canal from the middle ear is contaminated by the microflora from the canal. Appropriate cultures may be obtained by carefully cleaning the canal with 70% alcohol and obtaining cultures from the area of perforation as the fluid emerges or by needle aspiration through the intact membrane.

Treatment

Initial therapy for febrile infants with otitis media during the first 2 weeks of life is similar to that for neonatal sepsis. Both a penicillin and an aminoglycoside or third-generation cephalosporin should be used. Specific therapy can be provided if needle aspiration is performed and the pathogen is identified. Infants who remain in the nursery because of prematurity, low birth weight, or illness require similar management during the first 4 to 6 weeks of life. If the infant was born at term, had a normal delivery and course in the nursery, has been in good health since discharge from the nursery, and is 2 weeks of age or older, the middle ear infection is probably due to *S. pneumoniae* or *H. influenzae* and may be treated with an appropriate oral antimicrobial agent such as amoxicillin.[103] The infant may be managed outside the hospital if he or she does not appear to have a toxic condition. For infants born at term who have acute otitis media and are in a toxic condition, the physician must consider hospitalization, cultures of blood and cerebrospinal fluid, and use of parenterally administered antimicrobial agents because of possible systemic infection, a focus of infection elsewhere, or presence of a resistant organism.

Prognosis

Infants who have infections of the middle ear in the neonatal period appear to be susceptible to recurrent episodes of otitis media.[77, 87, 88] The earlier in life the child has an episode of otitis media, the more likely the child is to have recurrent infections. It is uncertain whether this means that an early episode of otitis media damages the mucosa of the middle ear and makes the child more prone to subsequent infection or whether early infection merely identifies children with dysfunction of the eustachian tube or subtle or undefined immune system abnormalities who have a propensity to infection of the middle ear because of these abnormalities.

MASTOIDITIS

The mastoid air cells are not developed at birth and usually consist of only a single space. Therefore, mastoiditis rarely occurs in the neonate. One report, however, cited a case of meningitis and mastoiditis caused by *H. influenzae* in a newborn.[104] Roentgenograms of the mastoid area demonstrated a cloudy right antrum. At operation, the middle ear was normal but the antrum was filled with infected mesenchymal tissue.

PNEUMONIA

Pneumonia, inflammation of the lungs, in the fetus and newborn can be classified into four categories according to the time and mode of acquisition of inflammation:

1. *Congenital pneumonia acquired by the transplacental route:* the pneumonia is one component of generalized congenital disease.

2. *Intrauterine pneumonia:* an inflammatory disease of the lungs found at autopsy in stillborn or live-born infants who die within the first few days of life, usually associated with fetal asphyxia or intrauterine infection and thus includes infectious and noninfectious causes.

3. *Pneumonia acquired during birth:* the signs of pneumonia occur within the first few days of life, and infection is due to microorganisms that colonize the maternal birth canal.

4. *Pneumonia acquired after birth:* the illness manifests itself during the first month of life, either in the nursery or at home; sources of infection include human contacts and contaminated equipment.

Although helpful as a general framework for understanding neonatal pneumonia, these four categories have clinical features and pathologic characteristics that overlap. Thus, management of pneumonia is essentially the same for all four categories, requiring aggressive supportive measures for the respiratory and circulatory systems along with treatment for the specific infectious etiology.

Pneumonia in the neonate may be caused by viruses, bacteria, and parasitic organisms. Detailed information about causative organisms mentioned in this chapter other than bacteria will be found in the appropriate chapters in this book; bacterial disease will be covered in detail here.

Pneumonia acquired by the transplacental route may be caused by rubella, cytomegalovirus, herpes simplex virus, adenoviruses,[105] mumps virus,[106] *Toxoplasma gondii*, *L. monocytogenes*, or *T. pallidum*. Some of these organisms and the enteroviruses, genital mycoplasmas, *C. trachomatis*, and *Mycobacterium tuberculosis* are also responsible for intrauterine pneumonia resulting from aspiration of infected amniotic fluid. Fatal pneumonitis due to echovirus has also been reported in newborns (see Chapter 10).[107] Isolation of *Trichomonas vaginalis* from the tracheal aspirates of infants with pneumonia suggests a possible association of this organism with respiratory tract disease in the neonate.[108, 109]

Group B *Streptococcus* is the most frequent cause of bacterial pneumonia acquired at delivery. Pneumonia due to Group B *Streptococcus*, and other bacteria such as *E. coli* or *L. monocytogenes*, may resemble hyaline membrane disease.

Pneumonias acquired after birth, either in the nursery or at home, include those caused by respiratory viruses such as respiratory syncytial virus, influenza, or adenoviruses; gram-positive bacteria such as pneumococcus and *S. aureus*; gram-negative enteric bacilli; *C. trachomatis*; *Mycoplasma*; and *Pneumocystis carinii*.[110] Pneumonia caused by nonbacterial microorganisms is discussed in the appropriate chapters. Bacterial pneumonia and neonatal sepsis acquired during or soon after birth share many features of pathogenesis, epidemiology, and management, and these aspects are discussed in Chapter 21. This section consists of a discussion of pneumonia in the fetus and newborn not presented elsewhere in the text.

Pathogenesis and Pathology

CONGENITAL OR INTRAUTERINE PNEUMONIA

Histologic features of congenital or intrauterine pneumonia have been described from autopsy findings in infants who are stillborn or who die shortly after birth (usually within 24 hours). An inflammatory reaction is found in histologic sections of lung. Polymorphonuclear leukocytes are present in the alveoli and are often mixed with vernix and squamous cells. Infiltrates of round cells may be present in interstitial tissue of small bronchioles and interalveolar septa.[111–116] Alveolar macrophages may be present and have been associated with both duration of postnatal life and inflammatory pulmonary lesions.[117] The inflammation is diffuse and usually uniform throughout the lung. Bacteria are seen infrequently, and cultures for bacteria are often negative. Davies and Aherne[114] noted that the usual characteristics of bacterial pneumonia are missing in congenital pneumonia; among these characteristics are pleural reaction, infiltration or destruction of bronchopulmonary tissue, and fibrinous exudate in the alveoli.

The pathogenesis of congenital pneumonia is not well understood.[118] Asphyxia and intrauterine infection, acting alone or together, appear to be the most important factors.[114] It is thought that microorganisms of the birth canal contaminate the amniotic fluid by ascending infection after early rupture of maternal membranes or through minimal and often unrecognized defects in the membranes. Evidence of aspiration of amniotic fluid is frequent.[114] Naeye and colleagues proposed that microbial invasion of the fetal membranes and aspiration of infected amniotic fluid is a frequent cause of chorioamnionitis and congenital pneumonia.[119–121] Bacteriologic studies, however, have given equivocal results. Many infants with congenital pneumonia do not have bacteria

in their lungs, yet cultures of the lung of some infants without pneumonia do yield bacteria.[122] Fetal asphyxia or hypoxia appears to be a factor in most cases of congenital pneumonia. The asphyxia may cause death directly or by eliciting a pulmonary response consisting of hemorrhage, edema, and inflammatory cells. From his studies of congenital pneumonia, Barter concluded that hypoxia or infection may produce similar inflammation in the lungs.[123] In addition, Bernstein and Wang found that evidence of fetal asphyxia was frequently present at autopsy in infants with congenital pneumonia who also had generalized petechial hemorrhage, subarachnoid and intracerebral hemorrhage, liver cell necrosis, or ulceration of the gastrointestinal mucosa.[124]

Although it is likely that either asphyxia or infection can produce similar inflammatory patterns in lungs of the fetus, available information is insufficient to determine which is more important or more frequent. In a review of fetal and perinatal pneumonia, Finland concluded that "pulmonary lesions certainly play a major role in the deaths of the stillborn and of infants in the early neonatal period. Infection, on the other hand, appears to play only a minor role in what has been called 'congenital pneumonia,' that is, the inflammatory lesion seen in the stillborn or in those dying within the first few hours, or possibly the first day or two; it assumes greater importance in pneumonias that cause death later in the neonatal period."[125] Davies noted that the histologic presentation of congenital pneumonia appears to represent aspiration of materials in amniotic fluid, including maternal leukocytes and amniotic debris, rather than infection originating in the pulmonary air spaces. Evidence of infiltration of alveoli or destruction of bronchopulmonary tissue is rarely present.[126]

PNEUMONIA ACQUIRED DURING THE BIRTH PROCESS AND IN THE FIRST MONTH OF LIFE

The pathology of pneumonia acquired during or after birth is similar to that of older children or adults. The lung contains areas of densely cellular exudate with vascular congestion, hemorrhage, and pulmonary necrosis.[114, 124, 127] Bacteria are often seen in sections of the lung. *S. aureus* (see Chapter 30) and *Klebsiella pneumoniae*[128, 129] may produce extensive tissue damage, microabscesses, and empyema. Pneumatoceles are a common manifestation of staphylococcal pneumonia but may also occur in infections with *K. pneumoniae*[128, 129] and *E. coli*.[130] Hyaline membranes similar to those seen in respiratory distress syndrome have been observed in the lungs of infants who died with pneumonia caused by group B streptococci. Cocci were present within the membranes, and, in some cases, exuberant growth that included masses of organisms was apparent. Although most thoroughly documented in cases of pneumonia caused by group B streptococci, similar membranes have been seen in histologic sections of the lungs of infants who died with pneumonia caused by *H. influenzae* and gram-negative enteric bacilli.[131]

The pathogenesis of pneumonia acquired at or immediately after birth is similar to that of neonatal sepsis and is discussed in Chapter 21. Presumably, aspiration of infected amniotic fluid or secretions of the birth canal are responsible for most cases of pneumonia acquired during delivery. After birth, the infant may become infected through human contact or contaminated equipment. Infants who receive assisted ventilation are at risk because of the disruption of the normal barriers to infection due to the presence of the endotracheal tube and possible irritation of tissues near the tube. Bacteria or other organisms may invade the damaged tissue, which may result in tracheitis or tracheobronchitis.[132] Ventilator-associated pneumonia may be prevented by reducing bacterial colonization of the aerodigestive tract and decreasing the incidence of aspiration. A recent review highlighted strategies for prevention of pneumonia in patients receiving mechanical ventilation, including nonpharmacologic strategies such as attention to hand washing and standard precautions, positioning of patients, avoiding abdominal distention, avoiding nasal intubation, and maintaining ventilator circuits and suction catheters and tubing, as well as pharmacologic strategies such as appropriate use of antimicrobial agents.[133] Newborns with congenital anomalies such as tracheoesophageal fistula, choanal atresia, and diaphragmatic hernia have an increased risk of developing pneumonia.

Lung abscess is uncommon in neonates. The abscess may occur as a result of infection of congenital cysts of the lung. Single or multiple abscesses are usually associated with staphylococcal pneumonia but may also be caused by group B *Streptococcus*, *E. coli*, and *K. pneumoniae*.[134, 135] Cavitary lesions may develop in pneumonia due to *Legionella pneumophila*.[136]

Empyema is often associated with extensive pneumonia and may occur with many different bacteria. During the 1950s and 1960s, outbreaks of staphylococcal pneumonia occurred; many times these infections were accompanied by empyemas and pneumatoceles. This is now seen infrequently. Although rare in newborns, *H. influenzae* was associated with pneumonia and empyema[137] until its virtual disappearance after initiation of universal immunization in the early 1990s. The decade of the 1990s has been characterized by emergence of increased incidence of invasive disease due to group A *Streptococcus*. Cases of pleural empyema due to group A *Streptococcus* have been reported[138, 139]; it remains to be seen whether these reports represent isolated cases or are part of a generalized increase in this disease.

Microbiology

Most information about the bacteriology of fetal and neonatal pneumonia has been derived from cultures taken at autopsy of stillborn infants and of infants who die during the first month of life. In addition, useful information has been obtained from cultures of blood, tracheal aspirates, pleural fluid, and needle aspiration of the lungs of living children with pneumonia.

The bacterial species responsible for fetal and neonatal pneumonia are those present in the maternal birth canal; included in this flora are gram-positive cocci such as groups A, B, and F[140] streptococci and gram-negative enteric bacilli, predominantly *E. coli* and, to a lesser extent, *Proteus*, *Klebsiella*, and *Enterobacter* species. Microorganisms acquired postnatally include *S. aureus*

(from human sources) and gram-negative bacilli such as *P. aeruginosa* and flavobacteria. The presence of pneumonia, empyema, and pneumatocele due to *Serratia marcescens* in a 15-day-old, 26-week gestation infant has been reported.[141] *S. pneumoniae*,[142–144] *H. influenzae*,[131, 145] and *Moraxella catarrhalis*[146] are infrequent causes of pneumonia in the newborn. Infants with pneumonia caused by these organisms are usually bacteremic, and some have meningitis.[114, 142, 144, 145] Nosocomial infection due to *L. pneumophila* has been reported, including cases of fatal necrotizing pneumonia and cavitary pneumonia.[147] Reports have identified *Citrobacter diversus* as a cause of lung abscess[148] and *Bacillus cereus* as a cause of a necrotizing pneumonia in premature infants.[149] Pneumonia and pleural empyema due to group A *Streptococcus* acquired during passage through the birth canal has been reported from the United Kingdom and Sweden.[138, 139] A fatal case of congenital pneumonia caused by *Pasteurella multocida* in a full-term neonate was associated with maternal infection and colonization of the family cat with the same organism.[150] A case of pneumonia and sepsis due to ampicillin-resistant *Morganella morganii* was reported from Texas[151]; the authors speculate about the role of increased use of intrapartum antibiotics in predisposing to colonization and infection with ampicillin-resistant organisms.

Bacteriologic studies at autopsy of infants with and without pneumonia were reported by Barter and Hudson.[122] The incidence of bacteria in the lungs increased with age in infants dying with and without pneumonia; of those infants with pneumonia, bacteria were cultured from the lungs of 55% of stillborn infants and infants who died during the first day of life, 70% of infants who died between 24 hours and 7 days of age, and 100% of infants who died between 7 and 28 days of age. However, of those infants without pneumonia, bacteria were cultured from the lungs of 36% of stillborn infants and infants who died within the first 24 hours, 53% of infants who died between 24 hours and 7 days of age, and 75% of infants who died between 7 and 28 days of age. The bacterial species were similar in the infants with and without pneumonia, with the exception of group B *Streptococcus*, which was found only in infants with pneumonia.

These results were corroborated by Penner and McInnis: bacteria were cultured from 92% of the lungs of fetuses and neonates with pneumonia and from 40% of the lungs of fetuses and neonates without pneumonia.[116] Davies did lung punctures in stillborn and liveborn infants immediately after death, and bacteria were cultured from the lungs of 74% of 93 infants, although pneumonia was diagnosed in only 9 cases.[152] Barson identified bacteria in lung cultures at autopsy of 252 infants dying with bronchopneumonia; positive cultures were obtained in 60% of infants dying on the first day of life and in 78% of infants dying between 8 and 28 days of age.[153] Thus, bacteria were cultured at autopsy from the lungs of many infants with and without pneumonia.

Epidemiology

Incidence. The incidence of pneumonia at autopsy of stillborn and live-born infants is given in Table 22–2.

TABLE 22–2

Incidence of Congenital and Neonatal Pneumonia Based on Findings at Autopsy

PLACE (REFERENCE NO.) AND YEAR(S) OF STUDY	NO. WITH PNEUMONIA/TOTAL NO. OF INFANTS (%)						AGE OR WEIGHT OF INFANTS AT DEATH
	Stillbirths			Live-Born Infants			
	Premature	Term	Total	Premature	Term	Total	
Helsinki (111) 1951	5/13 (38)	9/32 (28)	14/45 (31)				
Helsinki (127) 1946–1952				218/361 (60)	210/315 (67)	428/676 (63)	<29 days of age
Newcastle (112) 1955–1956			13/70 (19)			10/31 (32)	<7 days of age
Adelaide (113) 1950–1951	5/44 (11)	10/53 (19)	15/97 (15)	9/32 (28)	3/8 (38)	12/40 (30)	Lived <6 hours after birth
Detroit (124) 1956–1959						55/231 (24)	<7 days of age
Winnipeg (155) 1954–1960	15/46 (33)						<750 g
Winnipeg (156) 1954–1957						27/110 (25)	<7 days of age
Edinburgh (157) 1922						22/80 (26)	8 hours to 5 weeks of age
NIH Collaborative Study (158) 1959–1964				67/387 (17)	33/125 (26)	100/512 (20)	<48 hours of age
Manchester (115) 1950–1954		28/275 (10)				59/219 (27)	<7 days of age
Los Angeles (154) 1990–1993				25/111 (23)			<1000 g, <48 hr

Pneumonia remains a significant cause of death in the neonatal period,[154] and infection of amniotic fluid leading to pneumonia may be the most common cause of death in extremely premature infants.[155] The definition of pneumonia in the autopsy studies was usually based on the presence of polymorphonuclear leukocytes in the pulmonary alveoli or interstitium or both. The presence or absence of bacteria was not important in the definition of pneumonia. The incidences of congenital and neonatal pneumonia at autopsy are similar despite the different times of study (1922 to 1999) and different locations[111–113, 115, 124, 154–158] (with the single exception of a report from Helsinki[127]): 15 to 38% of stillborn infants and 20 to 32% of live-born infants had evidence of pneumonia. The incidence of pneumonia was similar in premature and term infants.

Race and Socioeconomic Status. In two studies, black infants had pneumonia at autopsy significantly more often than did white infants. The Collaborative Study of the National Institutes of Health[158] considered the incidence of pneumonia in live-born infants who died within the first 48 hours of life: 27.7% of black infants had evidence of pneumonia, whereas only 11.3% of white infants showed signs of this disease, and this difference was present in every weight group. In New York City, Naeye and co-workers studied 1044 consecutive autopsies of newborn and stillborn infants; black infants had significantly more pneumonia (38%) than Puerto Rican infants (22%) or white infants (20%).[119] The same study showed that the incidence of pneumonia

in the infant was inversely related to the level of household income. Infants from the families with the lowest income had significantly more pneumonia than infants from the families with the highest income. At comparable levels of household income, black infants had a higher incidence of neonatal pneumonia than did Puerto Rican or white infants. These racial and economic differences were not readily explained by the authors or by other investigators.

Epidemic Disease. Pneumonia may be epidemic in a nursery because of a single source of infection, such as a suppurative lesion caused by *S. aureus* in a nursery employee or contamination of a common solution or piece of equipment, usually caused by *Pseudomonas*, *Flavobacterium*, or *S. marcescens*. Infection may also spread by droplet nuclei among infants or between personnel and infants. Epidemics of respiratory infection related to viruses have also been reported (see Chapters 18 and 34).

Developing Countries. Pneumonia is a particular threat to neonates in developing countries. A survey of a rural area in central India revealed that mortality due to pneumonia in the first 29 days of life was 29 per 1000 live-born children (the rate during the first year was 49.6 per 1000 live-born children).[159] The aerobic bacteria grown from the vagina of rural women was used as a surrogate for likely pathogens of pneumonia in neonates.[160] Vaginal flora included *E. coli* and other gram-negative enteric bacilli and staphylococcal species in expected proportions but a relatively low rate of beta-hemolytic streptococci (3.2%). Management of pneumonia cases (those that did not demand immediate referral to a hospital) included continued breast-feeding and trimethoprim-sulfamethoxazole.

Singhi and Singhi studied the clinical signs of illness in Chandigarh infants younger than 1 month of age with radiologically confirmed pneumonia to determine how to increase accuracy of diagnosis of pneumonia by health care workers.[161] Rural health care workers (most were illiterate) used revised World Health Organization criteria of pneumonia in infants, including respiratory rate greater than 60 breaths per minute, presence of severe chest indrawing, or both.[162] Cough and respiratory rate greater than 50 breaths per minute missed 25% of cases; decreasing the threshold respiratory rate to 40 breaths per minute increased the sensitivity. In the absence of cough, chest retraction and/or respiratory rate greater than 50 breaths per minute had maximum accuracy.

Clinical Manifestations

Onset of respiratory distress at or soon after birth is characteristic of intrauterine or congenital pneumonia. Before delivery, fetal distress may be evident: the infant may be tachycardic, and the fetal tracing may be nonreassuring, with poor beat-to-beat variability or evidence of deep decelerations. Meconium aspiration may be present and may have occurred before delivery, suggesting fetal asphyxia and gasping. The infant may have episodes of apnea or may have difficulty establishing regular respiration. In some cases, severe respiratory distress is delayed, but it may be preceded by increasing tachypnea, apneic episodes, and requirement for increasing amounts of oxygen. The infant may have difficulty feeding, temperature instability, and other signs of generalized sepsis, including poor peripheral perfusion, disseminated intravascular coagulation, and lethargy.

Infants who acquire pneumonia during the birth process or postnatally may have signs of systemic illness such as lethargy, anorexia, and fever. Signs of respiratory distress may be present at the onset of the illness or may develop later; these signs include tachypnea, dyspnea, grunting, coughing, flaring of the alae nasi, irregular respirations, cyanosis, intercostal and supraclavicular retractions, rales, and decreased breath sounds. Infants with severe disease may have progression to apnea, shock, and respiratory failure. Signs of pleural effusion or empyema may be present in suppurative pneumonias associated with staphylococcal infections, groups A[163] and B streptococcal infections, and E. coli infections.[164]

An outpatient study demonstrated the rarity of pneumonia in infants younger than 60 days of age; infants with the following characteristics did not have pneumonia: illness in the summer; absence of cough, dyspnea, and respiratory distress (grunting, flaring, retracting); respiratory rate lower than 60 breaths per minute; absence of rales and decreased breath sounds; presence of normal color; and white blood cell count lower than 19,000 per mm³.[165]

Diagnosis

Clinical Diagnosis. A history of premature delivery, prolonged interval between rupture of maternal membranes and delivery, prolonged labor, excessive obstetric manipulation, and presence of foul-smelling amniotic fluid are frequently associated with neonatal infection, including sepsis and pneumonia. The clinical manifestations of pneumonia may be subtle and nonspecific at the onset, and specific signs of respiratory infection may not be evident until late in the course of illness. Most commonly, pneumonia is associated with evidence of respiratory distress, including tachypnea, retractions, flaring, and increasing requirement for oxygen.

Radiologic Diagnosis. A chest roentgenogram is the most helpful tool for making the diagnosis of pneumonia. The roentgenogram of the infant with intrauterine pneumonia, however, may contribute no information or show only the coarse mottling of aspiration. If done early in the course of meconium or other aspiration pneumonias, typical radiologic features may not yet have developed. The roentgenogram of the child with pneumonia acquired during or after birth may show streaky densities or confluent opacities. Peribronchial thickening, indicating bronchopneumonia, may be present. Pleural effusion, abscess cavities, and pneumatoceles are frequent in infants with staphylococcal infections but may also occur in pneumonia caused by group A Streptococcus, E. coli,[130] or K. pneumoniae.[129] Diffuse pulmonary granularity or air bronchograms similar to that seen in respiratory distress syndrome have been observed in infants with pneumonia related to group B Streptococcus.[166] Computed tomography with contrast medium enhancement is of benefit in localizing pulmonary lesions such as lung abscess and distinguishing abscess from empyema, pneumatoceles, or bronchopleural fistulas.[135] Ultrasound was used to diagnose hydrothorax in utero at 32 weeks of gestation.[167]

Although it is not possible to distinguish bacterial from viral pneumonia on the basis of a chest radiograph alone, there are several features that may help distinguish between the two. Findings that are more characteristic of viral pneumonias include hyperexpansion, atelectasis, parahilar peribronchial infiltrates, and hilar adenopathy, which is associated almost exclusively with adenovirus. Alveolar disease, consolidation, air bronchograms, pleural effusions, pneumatoceles, and necrotizing pneumonias are more characteristic of bacterial processes.[168]

Microbiologic Diagnosis. Because of the difficulty in accessing material from a suppurative focus in the lower respiratory tree, microbiologic diagnosis of pneumonia is problematic. Although cultures of material obtained from lung aspiration have been shown to yield bacterial pathogens in about one third of a group of seriously ill infants with lung lesions accessible to needle aspiration,[169] this rate of positive results is unlikely to be obtained in an unselected group of infants with pneumonia. Diagnosis may be based on isolating pathogens from other sites. When generalized systemic infection is present, cultures of blood, urine, or cerebrospinal fluid may yield a pathogen. Bacteremia may be identified in about 10% of febrile children with pneumonia.[170] If a pleural effusion is present and the bacterial diagnosis is not yet evident, pleural fluid biopsy and/or culture may be helpful. Bacterial cultures of the throat and nasopharynx are unrevealing or misleading because of the high numbers of respiratory pathogens present.

Tracheal aspiration through a catheter is frequently valuable when performed by direct laryngoscopy, but the aspirate may be contaminated when the catheter is passed through the nose or mouth. Sherman and colleagues performed a careful study of the use of tracheal aspiration in diagnosis of pneumonia in the first 8 hours of life.[171] Tracheal aspirates were obtained from 320 infants with signs of cardiorespiratory disease and an abnormal chest radiograph; 25 infants had bacteria present in the smear of the aspirate, and the same organisms were isolated from cultures of 14 of 25 aspirates. Thureen and colleagues found that tracheal aspirate cultures failed to define an infectious cause of deterioration in ventilated infants. Positive tracheal aspirates occurred with equal frequency among infants with a clinical suspicion of lower respiratory tract infection and in "well" controls.[172] Tracheal aspirate cultures may provide useful information about potential pathogens in pneumonia or bacteremia but rarely indicate the risk or timing of such complications.[173] Often, surveillance cultures of tracheal aspirate material are used to guide empirical therapy when an infant with a prolonged course on a ventilator develops a new illness.

Bronchoscopy can provide visual, cytologic, and microbiologic evidence of bacterial pneumonia.[174] Aspiration of pulmonary exudate (lung puncture or lung tap) can be used to provide direct, immediate, and unequivocal information about the causative agent of pneumonia.[175] This procedure is now performed rarely; most reports of its use in infants and young children precede the introduction of antimicrobial agents.[176, 177]

Open-lung biopsy has been used to identify the etiology of lung disease in critically ill infants and appears to have been most helpful at a time when corticosteroids for bronchopulmonary dysplasia were withheld if there was concern about pulmonary infection. Cheu and colleagues identified three infections in 17 infants who had open lung biopsies: respiratory syncytial virus in 1 infant and *Ureaplasma urealyticum* in 2 infants.[178] Although the optimal indications for use of corticosteroids in bronchopulmonary dysplasia remains a topic of controversy,[179] generally corticosteroids are not withheld because of low likelihood of an infectious process.

Histologic and Cytologic Diagnosis. The data of Naeye and co-workers indicate that congenital pneumonia or pneumonia acquired during birth is almost always accompanied by chorioamnionitis, although chorioamnionitis may be present in the absence of pneumonia or other neonatal infections.[119] These and other studies[180] suggest that the presence of leukocytes in sections of placental membranes and of umbilical vessels or in Wharton's jelly is valuable in pneumonia and sepsis. Other investigators are less certain and believe that the presence of inflammation in the placenta or umbilical cord does not distinguish changes caused by hypoxia from those caused by infection.[123, 124]

Culture of material obtained by aspiration of stomach contents is usually not helpful in diagnosing pneumonia because this material is contaminated by the flora of the upper respiratory tract. In addition, infants with pneumonia may have no evidence of the organism in the gastric aspirate.[166, 181] There is some evidence, however, that microscopic examination of gastric contents may be useful in defining the presence of an inflammatory process in the lung after the first day of life. Because infants so afflicted are unable to expectorate, they swallow bronchial secretions. During the first few hours of life, inflammatory cells present in the gastric aspirate are of maternal origin; however, after the first day, any polymorphonuclear leukocytes present are those of the infant. Tam and Yeung demonstrated that if more than 75% of the cells in the gastric aspirate obtained from infants after the first day of life were polymorphonuclear leukocytes, pneumonia was usually present.[181] However, a study by Pole and McAllister did not confirm the value of gastric aspirate cytology in the diagnosis of pneumonia.[182]

Primary ciliary dyskinesia is congenital and may be present in the newborn period as respiratory distress. Infants with situs inversus are at risk for this condition. Consultation with a geneticist may be warranted; a biopsy of nasal epithelium may be needed to identify the characteristic abnormal morphology of cilia of the immotile cilia syndrome.[183–185]

Immunologic Diagnosis. Immunologic response to various microorganisms responsible for pneumonia is used extensively as an aid to diagnosis, including infections related to group B *Streptococcus, S. aureus* (see Chapters 26 and 30) and the organisms that cause congenital infection (rubella virus, *T. gondii*, herpes simplex virus, cytomegalovirus, and *T. pallidum*). Giacoia and colleagues prepared antigens from microorganisms isolated from bronchial aspirates and correlated specific antibodies and nonspecific IgM antibody with clinical and radiologic evidence of pneumonia.[186] A significant immune response was identified in approximately one fourth of the patients studied. These data are of interest but remain of uncertain significance because of the difficulty of distinguishing immune response to organisms responsible for lower respiratory tract disease from the response to organisms colonizing the respiratory tree.[187]

In infants with generalized sepsis and pneumonia, testing of blood, urine, and cerebrospinal fluid for antigens to group B *Streptococcus*, pneumococcus, *H. influenzae*, and *Neisseria meningitidis* may provide helpful information. Interpretation of results must take into account possible contamination of results by organisms colonizing the area around the urethra (in the case of a bag specimen of urine) and possible interference to the test result caused by recent immunization against *H. influenzae* type b or pneumococcus or recent infection due to these organisms. Bedside cold agglutination testing may be helpful in the case of *Mycoplasma* infection, but the test has low sensitivity so a negative result remains undiagnostic. Though polymerase chain reaction testing has provided diagnostic information for many conditions, it does not at this time, offer any specific advantages in the diagnosis of pneumonia.

Differential Diagnosis

A variety of noninfectious diseases and conditions may simulate infectious pneumonia. Respiratory distress syndrome (hyaline membrane disease), atelectasis, aspiration pneumonia, pneumothorax or pneumomediastinum, pulmonary edema and hemorrhage, pleural effusions of the lung (e.g., chylothorax), cystic lung disease, hypoplasia or agenesis, pulmonary infarct, and cystic fibrosis all have some signs and symptoms similar to those of pneumonia. Meconium aspirated into the distal air passages may produce chemical pneumonitis or segmental atelectasis.[188] Multifocal pulmonary infiltrates have been associated with feeding supplements containing medium-chain triglycerides.[189] Infants with immotile cilia syndrome may present within the first 24 hours of life with tachypnea, chest retraction, and rales. Results of prospective epidemiologic studies of neonatal respiratory diseases from Sweden[190] for the period 1976 to 1977 and from Lebanon[191] for the period 1976 to 1984 indicate that infection was second in frequency to hyaline membrane disease in both surveys. Clues to the diagnosis of diseases and conditions producing respiratory distress based on information from the maternal history and signs in the infant were presented in a convenient table by Avery and co-workers (Table 22–3).[192]

Pneumonia may be superimposed on hyaline membrane disease. One survey showed that histologic evidence of pneumonia was present at autopsy in 16% of 1535 infants with hyaline membrane disease.[193] Foote and Stewart demonstrated, by chest roentgenograms, that pneumonia modifies the reticulogranular pattern of hyaline membrane disease by replacing the air in the alveoli with inflammatory exudate.[194] Therefore, any modification of the radiographic pattern typical of hyaline membrane disease should lead the physician to consider superinfection.

Ablow and colleagues reported that infants with pneumonia caused by group B *Streptococcus* who also had the clinical and radiologic appearance of respiratory distress syndrome were easier to ventilate than were infants who had hyaline membrane disease and the picture of respiratory distress syndrome unassociated with infection.[195] These findings are of limited value in identifying infection in individual infants and were not confirmed in a subsequent study by Menke and colleagues.[196]

Pleural fluid, usually limited to the lung fissures, occurs in many infants and may be related to slow resorption of fetal lung fluid, to transient tachypnea of the newborn, or to respiratory distress syndrome of noninfectious etiology. Large collections of fluid in the pleural space may represent bacterial empyema; noninfectious causes include chylothorax, hydrothorax (associated with hydrops fetalis, congestive heart failure, or transient tachypnea), meconium aspiration pneumonitis, or hemothorax related to hemorrhagic disease of the newborn.

The symptoms of cystic fibrosis may begin in early infancy. Thirty percent of patients with newly diagnosed cases seen in a 5-year period at Children's Hospital Medical Center in Boston were younger than 1 year of age.[197] The authors described the histories of four children whose respiratory symptoms began before the infants were 1 month of age. The clinical course of the disease in young infants is characterized by a bronchiolitis-like syndrome with secondary chronic obstructive pulmonary disease and respiratory distress, coughing,

TABLE 22–3
Clues to Diagnosis of Types of Respiratory Distress

INFORMATION FROM MATERNAL HISTORY	MOST PROBABLE CONDITION IN INFANT
Peripartum fever	Pneumonia
Foul-smelling amniotic fluid	Pneumonia
Excessive obstetric manipulation at delivery	Pneumonia
Infection	Pneumonia
Premature rupture of membranes	Pneumonia
Prolonged labor	Pneumonia
Prematurity	Hyaline membrane disease
Diabetes	Hyaline membrane disease
Hemorrhage in days before premature delivery	Hyaline membrane disease
Meconium-stained amniotic fluid	Meconium aspiration
Hydramnios	Tracheoesophageal fistula
Excessive medications	Central nervous system depression
Reserpine	Stuffy nose
Traumatic or breech delivery	Central nervous system hemorrhage; phrenic nerve paralysis
Fetal tachycardia or bradycardia	Asphyxia
Prolapsed cord or cord entanglements	Asphyxia
Postmaturity	Aspiration
Amniotic fluid loss	Hypoplastic lungs

SIGNS IN THE INFANT	MOST PROBABLE ASSOCIATED CONDITION
Single umbilical artery	Congenital anomalies
Other congenital anomalies	Associated cardiopulmonary anomalies
Situs inversus	Kartagener's syndrome
Scaphoid abdomen	Diaphragmatic hernia
Erb's palsy	Phrenic nerve palsy
Cannot breathe with mouth closed	Choanal atresia; stuffy nose
Gasping with little air exchange	Upper airway obstruction
Overdistention of lungs	Aspiration, lobar emphysema or pneumothorax
Shift of apical pulse	Pneumothorax, chylothorax, hypoplastic lung
Fever or rise in temperature in a constant-temperature environment	Pneumonia
Shrill cry, hypertonia or flaccidity	Central nervous system disorder
Atonia	Trauma, myasthenia, poliomyelitis, amyotonia
Frothy blood from larynx	Pulmonary hemorrhage
Head extended in the absence of neurologic findings	Laryngeal obstruction or vascular rings
Choking after feedings	Tracheoesophageal fistula or pharyngeal incoordination
Plethora	Transient tachypnea

From Avery ME, Fletcher BD, Williams RG. The Lung and Its Disorders in the Newborn Infant. Philadelphia, WB Saunders, 1981.

wheezing, poor exchange of gases, cyanosis, hypoxia, and failure to thrive.

Management

Infants with bacterial pneumonia must be treated promptly and with appropriate antimicrobial agents. Culture of blood and urine may identify a bacterial pathogen, especially in patients with generalized sepsis. Cerebrospinal fluid culture may be helpful if the infant is not too unstable for lumbar puncture. In intubated infants, tracheal aspirate smears may indicate presence of inflammatory cells and cultures may provide information about organisms colonizing the trachea.

Because the microbiology of pneumonia in the newborn is the same as that of sepsis, the guidelines for management discussed in Chapter 21 are applicable. Initial antimicrobial therapy should include a penicillin (penicillin G or ampicillin) or a penicillinase-resistant penicillin (if staphylococcal infection is a possibility) and an aminoglycoside or a third-generation cephalosporin. The initial therapy should be reevaluated when the results of the cultures are available. Duration of therapy depends on the causative agent: pneumonia caused by gram-negative enteric bacilli or group B *Streptococcus* is treated for 10 days; disease caused by *S. aureus* required 3 to 6 weeks of antimicrobial therapy according to the severity of the pneumonia and the initial response to therapy.

When clinical and radiologic signs of hyaline membrane disease are present, infection caused by group B *Streptococcus* or gram-negative organisms, including *H. influenzae*, is not readily distinguished from the respiratory distress syndrome of noninfectious etiology. Until techniques are developed that can distinguish infectious from noninfectious causes of respiratory distress syndrome, it is reasonable to treat all infants who present with clinical and radiologic signs of the syndrome. Therapy is instituted for sepsis, as outlined earlier, after appropriate cultures have been taken. If the results of cultures are negative and the clinical course subsequently indicates that the illness was not infectious, the antimicrobial regimen is stopped. Because of concern for respiratory signs as a part of the initial presentation of sepsis and the rapid progression and high mortality of bacterial pneumonia in the neonate, particularly that of group B *Streptococcus*, early and aggressive therapy is warranted in infants with respiratory distress syndrome.

Antibiotics are only part of the management of the newborn with pneumonia; supportive measures such as maintaining fluid and electrolyte balance, providing oxygen or support of respiration with continuous positive airway pressure, or intubation and ventilation are equally important. Drainage of pleural effusions may be necessary when the accumulation of fluid embarrasses respiration. Single or multiple thoracocenteses may be adequate when the volumes of fluid are small. If larger amounts are present, a closed drainage system with a chest tube may be needed. The tube should be removed as soon as its drainage function is completed because delay may result in injury to local tissues, secondary infection, and sinus formation. Empyema and abscess formation are uncommon but serious complications of pneumonia. They may occur in association with pneumonia due to *S. aureus* and are discussed in detail in Chapter 30.

Prognosis

Available data on the significance of pneumonia during early life have been obtained in large measure from autopsy studies. There is information about the natural course of pneumonia caused by *S. aureus* in infants (see Chapter 30), but few studies of the sequelae of pneumonia caused by other agents exist. Even autopsy studies are equivocal in determining the importance of pneumonia because respiratory disease may have been the cause of death, a contributing factor in death, or incidental to and apart from the main cause of death.[198, 199] Pneumonia was said to be the sole cause of death in about 15% of neonatal deaths studied by Ahvenainen.[127] In the British Perinatal Mortality Study,[200] pulmonary infections were considered to be the cause of death in 5.5% of stillbirths and neonatal deaths.

Ahvenainen[127] noted that pneumonia is often a fatal complicating factor in infants with certain underlying conditions; these children include those with central nervous system malformations or disease, congenital heart disease, and anomalies of the gastrointestinal tract such as intestinal atresia.

Presence of pneumonia in the neonatal period has been implicated as a cause of chronic pulmonary disease in infancy and childhood. Pacifico and associates found that isolation of *U. urealyticum* from the respiratory tract of premature low-birth-weight infants in the first 7 days of life was associated with early development of bronchopulmonary dysplasia and severe pulmonary outcome.[201] Brasfield and colleagues studied a group of 205 infants hospitalized with pneumonitis during the first 3 months of life and identified radiographic and pulmonary function abnormalities that persisted for more than a year.[202]

References

1. Clark RH, Barysh N. Retropharyngeal abscess in an infant of six weeks, complicated by pneumonia and osteomyelitis, with recovery: report of case. Arch Pediatr 53:417, 1936.
2. Steinhauer PF. Ludwig's angina: report of a case in a 12-day-old boy. J Oral Surg 25:251, 1967.
3. Langewisch WH. An epidemic of group A, type 1 streptococcal infections in newborn infants. Pediatrics 18:438, 1956.
4. Asmar BI. Neonatal retropharyngeal cellulitis due to group B streptococcus. Clin Pediatr (Phila) 26:183, 1987.
5. Smith WL, Yousefzadeh DK, Yiu-Chi VS, et al. Percutaneous aspiration of retropharyngeal space in neonates. AJR Am J Roentgenol 139:1005, 1982.
6. Coulthard M, Isaacs D. Retropharyngeal abscess. Arch Dis Child 66:1227, 1991.
7. Coulthard M, Isaacs D. Neonatal retropharyngeal abscess. Pediatr Infect Dis J 10:547, 1991.
8. Oppenheimer EH, Winn KJ. Fetal gonorrhea with deep tissue infection occurring in utero. Pediatrics 69:74, 1982.

9. Eichenwald HF. "Stuffy nose syndrome" of premature infants: an example of bacterial-viral synergism. Am J Dis Child 96:438, 1958.

10. Eichenwald HF, Kotsevalov O, Fasso LA. The "cloud baby": an example of bacterial-viral interaction. Am J Dis Child 100:161, 1960.

11. Enwonwu CO, Galkler WA, Idigbe EO, et al: Pathogenesis of cancrum oris (noma): confounding interactions of malnutrition with infection. Am J Trop Med Hyg 60:223–232, 1999.

12. Falkler WA, Enwonwu JCO, Idigbe EO. Isolation of *Fusobacterium necrophorum* from cancrum oris (noma). Am J Trop Med Hyg 60:150–156, 1999.

13. Ghosal SP, SenGupta PC, Mukherjee AK, et al. Noma neonatorum: its aetiopathogenesis. Lancet 2:289, 1978.

14. Alkalay A, Mogilner BM, Nissim F, et al. Noma in a full-term neonate. Clin Pediatr (Phila) 24:528, 1985.

15. Baxter JD. Acute epiglottitis in children. Laryngoscope 77:1358, 1967.

16. Rosenfeld RM, Fletcher MA, Marban SL. Acute epiglottitis in a newborn infant. Pediatr Infect Dis J 11:594–595, 1992.

17. Young N, Finn A, Powell C. Group B streptococcal epiglottitis. Pediatr Infect Dis J 15:95–96, 1996.

18. Hazard, GW, Porter PJ, Ingall D. Pneumococcal laryngitis in the newborn infant: report of a case. N Engl J Med 271:361, 1964.

19. Davis WB. Anatomy of the nasal accessory sinuses in infancy and childhood. Ann Otol Rhinol Laryngol 27:940, 1918.

20. Wasson WW. Changes in the nasal accessory sinuses after birth. Arch Otolaryngol 17:197, 1933.

21. Benner MC. Congenital infection of the lungs, middle ears and nasal accessory sinuses. Arch Pathol 29:455, 1940.

22. Cavanagh F. Osteomyelitis of the superior maxilla in infants: a report on 24 personally treated cases. BMJ 1:468, 1960.

23. Howard JB, McCracken GH Jr. The spectrum of group B streptococcal infections in infancy. Am J Dis Child 128:815, 1974.

24. O'Regan JB, Heenan M, Murray J. Diphtheria in infants. Ir J Med Sci 6:116, 1943.

25. Goebel F, Stroder J. Diphtheria in infants. Dtsch Med Wochenschr 73:389, 1948.

26. Naiditch MJ, Bower AG. Diphtheria: a study of 1433 cases observed during a ten-year period at the Los Angeles County Hospital. Am J Med 17:229, 1954.

27. Mathur NB, Narang P, Bhatia BD. Neonatal diphtheria. Indian J Pediatr 21:174, 1984.

28. Centers for Disease Control and Prevention. Toxigenic *Corynebacterium diphtheriae*—Northern Plains Indian Community, August–October 1996. MMWR Morb Mortal Wkly Rep 46:506–510, 1997.

29. Bisgard KM, Hardy IRB, Popovic T, et al. Virtual elimination of respiratory diphtheria in the United States (Abstract no. G12). *In* Abstracts of the 36th Interscience Conference on Antimicrobial Agents and Chemotherapy. Washington, DC, American Society for Microbiology, 1995, p 160.

30. Centers for Disease Control and Prevention. Diphtheria acquired by US citizens in the Russian Federation and Ukraine—1994. MMWR Morb Mortal Wkly Rep 44:237–244, 1995.

31. Vahlquist B. The transfer of antibodies from mother to offspring. Adv Pediatr 10:305, 1958.

32. Crossley K, Irvine P, Warren JB, et al. Tetanus and diphtheria immunity in urban Minnesota adults. JAMA 242:2298–3000, 1979.

33. Koblin BA, Townsend TR. Immunity to diphtheria and tetanus in inner-city women of child-bearing age. Am J Public Health 79:1297–1298, 1989.

33a. Maple PA, Efstratiou A, George RC, Andrews NJ, Sesardic D. Diphtheria immunity in UK blood donors. Lancet 345:963–965, 1995.

33b. Galazka A. The changing epidemiology of diphtheria in the vaccine era. J Infect Dis 181(Suppl 1):S2–9, 2000.

34. Barr M, Glenny AT, Randall KJ. Concentration of diphtheria antitoxin in cord blood and rate of loss in babies. Lancet 2:324, 1949.

35. Cohen P, Scadron SJ. The effects of active immunization of the mother upon the offspring. J Pediatr 29:609, 1946.

36. Farizo KM, Strebel PM, Chen RT, et al. Fatal respiratory disease due to *Corynebacterium diphtheriae*: case report and review of guidelines for management, investigation, and control. Clin Infect Dis 16:59–68, 1993.

37. Centers for Disease Control and Prevention. Availability of diphtheria antitoxin through an investigational new drug protocol. MMWR Morb Mortal Wkly Rep 46:380, 1997.

38. Centers for Disease Control and Prevention. Pertussis vaccination: use of acellular pertussis vaccines among infants and young children—recommendations of the Advisory Committee on Immunization Practices (ACIP). MMWR Morb Mortal Wkly Rep 46(No. RR-7):2–3, 1997.

39. Centers for Disease Control and Prevention. Pertussis—United States, January 1992–June 1995. MMWR Morb Mortal Wkly Rep 44:525–529, 1995.

40. Sutter RW, Cochi SL. Pertussis hospitalizations and mortality in the United States. JAMA 267:386, 1992.

41. Nelson JD. The changing epidemiology of pertussis in young infants. Am J Dis Child 132:371, 1978.

42. Linnemann CC Jr, Ramundo N, Perlstein PH, et al. Use of pertussis vaccine in an epidemic involving hospital staff. Lancet 2:540, 1975.

42a. Centers for Disease Control and Prevention. Resurgence of pertussis—United States, 1993. MMWR Morb Mortal Wkly Rep 42:952–960, 1993.

43. Izurieta HS, Kenyon TA, Strebel PM, et al. Risk factors for pertussis in young infants during an outbreak in Chicago in 1993. Clin Infect Dis 22:503–507, 1996.

44. Langkamp DL, Davis JP. Increased risk of reported pertussis and hospitalization associated with pertussis in low birth weight children. J Pediatr 128:654–659, 1996.

45. Cohen P, Scadron SJ. The placental transmission of protective antibodies against whooping cough by inoculation of the pregnant mother. JAMA 121:656, 1943.

46. Deen JL, Mink CM, Cherry JD, et al. Household contact study of *Bordetella pertussis* infections. Clin Infect Dis 21:1211–1219, 1995.

47. Cockayne EA. Whooping-cough in the first days of life. Br J Child Dis 10:534, 1913.

48. Phillips J. Whooping-cough contracted at the time of birth, with report of two cases. Am J Med Sci 161:163, 1921.

49. Gan VN, Murphy TV. Pertussis in hospitalized children. Am J Dis Child 144:1130–1134, 1990.

50. Lovell MA, Miller AM, Hendley O. Pathologic case of the month: pertussis pneumonia. Arch Pediatr Adolesc Med 152:925–926, 1998.

51. Johnston IDA, Strachan DP, Anderson HR. Effect of pneumonia and whooping cough in childhood on adult lung function. N Engl J Med 338:581–587, 1998.

52. Edelman K, Nikkari S, Ruuskanen O, et al. Detection of

Bordetella pertussis by polymerase chain reaction and culture in the nasopharynx of erythromycin-treated infants with pertussis. Pediatr Infect Dis J 15:54–57, 1996.

53. Centers for Disease Control and Prevention. Erythromycin-resistant *Bordetella pertussis*—Yuma County, Arizona, May–October 1994. MMWR Morb Mortal Wkly Rep 43:807–810, 1994.

54. Granstrom M, Olinder-Nielsen AM, Holmblad P, et al. Specific immunoglobulin for treatment of whooping cough. Lancet 33:1230, 1991.

55. Winrow AP. Inhaled steroids in the treatment of pertussis. Pediatr Infect Dis J 14:922, 1995.

56. Granstrom G, Sterner G, Nord CE, et al. Use of erythromycin to prevent pertussis in newborns of mothers with pertussis. J Infect Dis 155:1210, 1987.

57. Sprauer MA, Cochi JSL, Zell ER, et al. Prevention of secondary transmission of pertussis in households with early use of erythromycin. Am J Dis Child 146:177–181, 1992.

58. American Academy of Pediatrics. Report of the Committee on Infectious Diseases, 24th ed. Elk Grove Village, Ill, American Academy of Pediatrics, 1997, p 397.

58a. Centers for Disease Control and Prevention. Hypertrophic pyloric stenosis in infants following pertussis prophylaxis with erythromycin—Knoxville, Tennessee, 1999. MMWR Morb Mortal Wkly Rep 48:1117–1120, 1999.

59. deSa DJ. Infection and amniotic aspiration of middle ear in stillbirth and neonatal deaths. Arch Dis Child 48:872, 1973.

60. McLellan MS, Strong JP, Johnson QR, et al. Otitis media in premature infants: a histopathologic study. J Pediatr 61:53, 1962.

61. Johnson WW. A survey of middle ears: 101 autopsies of infants. Ann Otol Rhinol Laryngol 70:377, 1961.

62. Benner MC. Congenital infection of the lungs, middle ears and nasal accessory sinuses. Arch Pathol 29:455, 1940.

63. Keith RW. Middle ear function in neonates. Arch Otolaryngol 101:376, 1975.

64. Roberts DG, Johnson CE, Carlin SA, et al. Resolution of middle ear effusion in newborns. Arch Pediatr Adolesc Med 149:873–877, 1995.

65. deSa DJ. Mucosal metaplasia and chronic inflammation in the middle ear of infants receiving intensive care in the neonatal period. Arch Dis Child 158:24, 1983.

66. Bluestone CD. Pathogenesis of otitis media: role of eustachian tube. Pediatr Infect Dis J 15:281–291, 1996.

67. Piza J, Gonzalez M, Northrop CC, Eavey RD. Meconium contamination of the neonatal middle ear. J Pediatr 115:910–914, 1989.

68. Persico M, Barker GA, Mitchell DP. Purulent otitis media—a "silent" source of sepsis in the pediatric intensive care unit. Otolaryngol Head Neck Surg 93:330, 1985.

69. Berman SA, Balkany TJ, Simmons MA. Otitis media in neonatal intensive care unit. Pediatrics 62:198, 1978.

70. Nunn DR, Derkay CS, Darrow DH, et al. The effect of very early cleft palate closure on the need for ventilation tubes in the first years of life. Laryngoscope 105:905–908, 1995.

71. Schaefer O. Otitis media and bottle feeding: an epidemiological study of infant feeding habits and incidence of recurrent and chronic middle ear disease in Canadian Eskimos. Can J Public Health 62:478, 1971.

72. Chandra RK. Prospective studies of the effect of breast feeding on incidence of infection and allergy. Acta Paediatr Scand 68:691, 1979.

73. Pukander J. Acute otitis media among rural children in Finland. Int J Pediatr Otorhinolaryngol 4:325, 1982.

74. Saarinen UM. Prolonged breast feeding as prophylaxis for recurrent otitis media. Acta Paediatr Scand 71:567, 1982.

75. Dewey KG, Heinig J, Nommsen-Rivers LA. Differences in morbidity between breast-fed and formula-fed infants. J Pediatr 126:696–702, 1995.

76. Cunningham AS. Morbidity in breast fed and artificially fed infants. J Pediatr 90:726, 1977.

77. Teele DW, Klein JO, Rosner B, and the Greater Boston Otitis Media Study Group. Epidemiology of otitis media during the first seven years of life in children in Greater Boston: a prospective cohort study. J Infect Dis 160:83, 1989.

78. Duncan RB. Positional otitis media. Arch Otolaryngol 72:454, 1960.

79. Beauregard WG. Positional otitis media. J Pediatr 79:294, 1971.

80. Paradise JL, Elster BA. Breast milk protects against otitis media with effusion. Pediatr Res 18:283a, 1984.

81. Andersson B, Porras O, Hanson LA, et al. Inhibition of attachment of *Streptococcus pneumoniae* and *Haemophilus influenzae* by human milk and receptor oligosaccharides. J Infect Dis 153:232, 1986.

82. Salazar JC, Kaly KA, Giebink GS, et al. Low cord blood pneumococcal immunoglobulin G (IgG antibodies predict early onset acute otitis media in infancy). Am J Epidemiol 145:1048–1056, 1997.

83. Rosen IAV, Hakansson A, Aniansson G, et al. Antibodies to pneumococcal polysaccharides in human milk: lack of relationship to colonization and acute otitis media. Pediatr Infect Dis J 15:498–507, 1996.

84. Faden H, Duffy L, Wasielewski R, et al. Relationship between nasopharyngeal colonization and the development of otitis media in children. J Infect Dis 175:1440–1445, 1997.

85. Ey JL, Holberg CG, Aldous MB, et al. Passive smoke exposure and otitis media in the first year of life. Pediatrics 95:670–677, 1995.

86. Warren WS, Stool SJE. Otitis media in low-birth-weight infants. J Pediatr 79:740, 1971.

87. Jaffe BF, Hurtado F, Hurtado E. Tympanic membrane mobility in the newborn (with seven months' followup). Laryngoscope 80:36, 1970.

88. Howie VM, Ploussard JH, Sloyer J. The "otitis-prone" condition. Am J Dis Child 129:676, 1975.

89. Stahlberg M-R, Ruuskanen O, Virolainen E. Risk factors for recurrent otitis media. Pediatr Infect Dis J 5:30, 1986.

90. Bland, RD. Otitis media in the first six weeks of life: diagnosis, bacteriology and management. Pediatrics 49:187, 1972.

91. Tetzlaff TR, Ashworth C, Nelson JD. Otitis media in children less than 12 weeks of age. Pediatrics 59:827, 1977.

92. McLellan MS, Strong JP, Vautier T, et al. Otitis media in the newborn: relationship to duration of rupture of amniotic membrane. Arch Otolaryngol 85:380, 1967.

93. Paradise JL, Bluestone CD. Early treatment of universal otitis media of infants with cleft palate. Pediatrics 53:48, 1974.

94. Shurin PA, Howie VM, Pelton SI, et al. Bacterial etiology of otitis media during the first six weeks of life. J Pediatr 92:893, 1978.

95. Karma PH, Pukander, JS, Sipila, MM, et al. Middle ear fluid bacteriology of acute otitis media in neonates and very young infants. Int J Pediatr Otorhinolaryngol 14:141, 1987.

96. Ng PC, Hiu J, Fok TF, et al. Isolated congenital tuberculosis otitis in a pre-term infant. Acta Paediatr 84:955–956, 1995.

97. Senbil N, Sahin F, Caglar, et al. Congenital tuberculosis of the ear and parotid gland. Pediatr Infect Dis J 16:1090–1091, 1997.

98. Parker PC, Boles RG. *Pseudomonas* otitis media and bacteremia following a water birth. Pediatrics 99:653, 1997.

99. Eavey RD, Stool SE, Peckham GJ, et al. How to examine the ear of the neonate. Clin Pediatr 15:338, 1976.

100. Cavanaugh RM Jr. Pneumatic otoscopy in healthy full-term infants. Pediatrics 79:520, 1987.

101. Pestalozza G, Cusmano G. Evaluation of tympanometry in diagnosis and treatment of otitis media of the newborn and of the infant. Int J Pediatr Otorhinolaryngol 2:73, 1980.

102. Barnett ED, Klein JO, Hawkins KA, et al. Comparison of spectral gradient acoustic reflectometry and other diagnostic techniques for detection of middle ear effusion in children with middle ear disease. Pediatr Infect Dis J 17:556–559, 1998.

103. Dowell SF, Butler JC, Giebink S, et al. Acute otitis media: management and surveillance in an era of pneumococcal resistance—a report from the Drug-Resistant *Streptococcus pneumoniae* Therapeutic Working Group. Pediatr Infect Dis J 18:1–9, 1999.

104. Lee BT, Stingle WH, Ombres P, et al. Neonatal meningitis and mastoiditis caused by *Haemophilus influenzae*. JAMA 235:407, 1976.

105. Meyer K, Girgis N, McGravey V. Adenovirus associated with congenital pleural effusion. J Pediatr 107:433, 1985.

106. Reman O, Freymuth F, Laloum D, et al. Neonatal respiratory distress due to mumps. Arch Dis Child 61:80, 1986.

107. Boyd MT, Jordan SW, Davis LE. Fatal pneumonitis from congenital echovirus type 6 infection. Pediatr Infect Dis J 6:1138, 1987.

108. McLaren LC, Davis LE, Healy GR, et al. Isolation of *Trichomonas vaginalis* from the respiratory tract of infants with respiratory disease. Pediatrics 71:888, 1983.

109. Hiemstra I, Van Bel F, Berger HM. Can *Trichomonas vaginalis* cause pneumonia in newborn babies? BMJ 289:355, 1984.

110. Hostoffer RW, Litman A, Smith PG, et al. *Pneumocystis carinii* pneumonia in a term newborn infant with a transiently depressed T lymphocyte count, primarily of cells carrying the CD4 antigen. J Pediatr 122:792, 1993.

111. Ahvenainen EK. On congenital pneumonia. Acta Paediatr 40:1, 1951.

112. Anderson GS, Green CA, Neligan GA, et al. Congenital bacterial pneumonia. Lancet 2:585, 1962.

113. Barter R. The histopathology of congenital pneumonia: a clinical and experimental study. J Pathol Bacteriol 66:407, 1953.

114. Davies PA, Aherne W. Congenital pneumonia. Arch Dis Child 37:598, 1962.

115. Langley FA, McCredie Smith JA. Perinatal pneumonia: a retrospective study. J Obstet Gynaecol Br Commonw 66:12, 1959.

116. Penner DW, McInnis AC. Intrauterine and neonatal pneumonia. Am J Obstet Gynecol 69:147, 1955.

117. Alenghat E, Esterly JR. Alveolar macrophages in perinatal infants. Pediatrics 74:221, 1984.

118. Schaffer AJ. The pathogenesis of intrauterine pneumonia: I. A critical review of the evidence concerning intrauterine respiratory-like movements. Pediatrics 17:747, 1956.

119. Naeye RL, Dellinger WS, Blanc WA. Fetal and maternal features of antenatal bacterial infection. J Pediatr 79:733, 1971.

120. Naeye RL, Tafari N, Judge D, et al. Amniotic fluid infections in an African city. J Pediatr 90:965, 1977.

121. Naeye RL, Peters EC. Amniotic fluid infections with intact membranes leading to perinatal death: a prospective study. Pediatrics 61:171, 1978.

122. Barter RA, Hudson JA. Bacteriological findings in perinatal pneumonia. Pathology 6:223, 1974.

123. Barter RA. Congenital pneumonia. Lancet 1:165, 1962.

124. Bernstein J, Wang J. The pathology of neonatal pneumonia. Am J Dis Child 101:350, 1961.

125. Finland M. Fetal and perinatal pneumonia. *In* Charles D, Finland M (eds). Obstetric and Perinatal Infections. Philadelphia, Lea & Febiger, 1973, p 122.

126. Davies PA. Pathogen or commensal? Arch Dis Child 55:169, 1980.

127. Ahvenainen EK. Neonatal pneumonia: I. Incidence of pneumonia during first month of life. Ann Med Intern Fenn 42(Suppl 17):1, 1953.

128. Thaler MM. *Klebsiella-Aerobacter* pneumonia in infants: a review of the literature and report of a case. Pediatrics 30:206, 1962.

129. Papageovgiou A, Bauer CR, Fletcher BD, et al. *Klebsiella* pneumonia with pneumatocele formation in a newborn infant. Can Med Assoc J 109:1217, 1973.

130. Kunh JP, Lee SB. Pneumatoceles associated with *Escherichia coli* pneumonias in the newborn. Pediatrics 51:1008, 1973.

131. Jeffery H, Mitchison R, Wigglesworth JS, et al. Early neonatal bacteraemia: comparison of group B streptococcal, other gram-positive and gram-negative infections. Arch Dis Child 52:683, 1977.

132. Rojas J, Flanigan TH. Postintubation tracheitis in the newborn. Pediatr Infect Dis J 5:714, 1986.

133. Kollef MH. The prevention of ventilator-associated pneumonia. N Engl J Med 340:627–634, 1999.

134. Siegel JD, McCracken GH Jr. Neonatal lung abscess. Am J Dis Child 133:947, 1979.

135. Mayer T, Matlak ME, Condon V, et al. Computed tomographic findings of neonatal lung abscess. Am J Dis Child 139:39, 1982.

136. Famiglietti RF, Bakerman PR, Saubolle MA, Rudinsky M. Cavitary legionellosis in two immunocompetent infants. Pediatrics 99:899–903, 1997.

137. Brook I. Microbiology of empyema in children and adolescents. Pediatrics 85:722–726, 1990.

138. Thaarup J, Ellermann-Eriksen S, Sternholm J. Neonatal pleural empyema with group A *Streptococcus*. Acta Paediatr 86:769–771, 1997.

139. Nathavitharana KA, Watkinson M. Neonatal pleural empyema caused by Group A *Streptococcus*. Pediatr Infect Dis J 13:671–672, 1994.

140. Wells DW, Keeney GT. Group F *Streptococcus* associated with intrauterine pneumonia. Letter to the editor. Pediatrics 66:820, 1980.

141. Khan EA, Wafelman LS, Garcia-Prats, Taber LH. *Serratia marcescens* pneumonia, empyema and pneumatocele in a preterm neonate. Pediatr Infect Dis J 16:1003–1005, 1997.

142. Rhodes PG, Burry VF, Hall RT, et al. Pneumococcal septicemia and meningitis in the neonate. J Pediatr 86:593, 1975.

143. Moriartey RR, Finer NN. Pneumococcal sepsis and pneumonia in the neonate. Am J Dis Child 133:601, 1979.

144. Naylor JC, Wagner KR. Neonatal sepsis due to *Streptococcus pneumoniae*. Can Med Assoc J 133:1019, 1985.

145. Collier AM, Connor JD, Nyhan WL. Systemic infection with *Haemophilus influenzae* in very young infants. J Pediatr 70:539, 1967.

146. Ohlsson A, Bailey T. Neonatal pneumonia caused by *Branhamella catarrhalis*. Scand J Infect Dis 17:225, 1985.

147. Holmberg RE, Pavia AT, Montgomery D, et al. Nosocomial *Legionella* pneumonia in the neonate. Pediatrics 92:450, 1993.

148. Shamir R, Horev G, Merlob P, et al. *Citrobacter diversus* lung abscess in a preterm infant. Pediatr Infect Dis J 9:221, 1990.

149. Vevon GP, Dunne WM, Hicks MJ, et al. *Bacillus cereus* pneumonia in premature neonates: a report of two cases. Pediatr Infect Dis J 12:251, 1993.

150. Andersson S, Larinkari U, Vartia T. Fatal congenital pneumonia caused by cat-derived *Pasteurella multocida*. Pediatr Infect Dis J 13:74–75, 1994.

151. Rowen JL, Lopez SM. *Morganella morganii* early onset sepsis. Pediatr Infect Dis J 17:1176–1177, 1998.

152. Davies PA. Pneumonia in the fetus and newborn. Pediatr Digest 1996, p 93.

153. Barson AF. A postmortem study of infection in the newborn from 1976 to 1988. *In* de Louvois J, Harvey D (eds). Infection in the Newborn. New York, John Wiley, 1990, pp 13–34.

154. Barton L, Hodgman JE, Pavlova Z. Causes of death in the extremely low birth weight infant. Pediatrics 103:446–451, 1999.

155. Briggs EJN, Hogg G. Pneumonia found at autopsy in infants weighing less than 750 grams. Can Med Assoc J 85:6, 1961.

156. Briggs EJN, Hogg G. Perinatal pulmonary pathology. Pediatrics 22:41, 1958.

157. Browne FJ. Pneumonia neonatorum. BMJ 1:469, 1922.

158. Fujikura T, Froehlich LA. Intrauterine pneumonia in relation to birth weight and race. Am J Obstet Gynecol 97:81, 1967.

159. Bang AT, Bang RA, Morankar VJP, et al. Pneumonia in neonates: can it be managed in the community? Arch Dis Child 68:550, 1993.

160. Kishore K, Decorarai AK, Meharban S, et al. Early onset neonatal sepsis—vertical transmission from maternal genital tract. Indian Pediatr J 24:45, 1987.

161. Singhi S, Singhi PD. Clinical signs in neonatal pneumonia. Lancet 336:1072, 1990.

162. World Health Organization. Acute respiratory infections in children: case management in small hospitals in developing countries. Geneva, World Health Organization, 1990 (WHO/ARI/90.5).

163. Petersen S, Astvad K. Pleural empyema in a newborn infant. Acta Paediatr Scand 65:527, 1976.

164. Gustavson EE. *Escherichia coli* empyema in the newborn. Am J Dis Child 140:408, 1986.

165. Losek JD, Kishaba RG, Berens RF, et al. Indications for chest roentgenogram in the febrile young infant. Pediatr Emerg Care 5:149, 1989.

166. Ablow RC, Gross I, Effmann EL, et al. The radiographic features of early onset group B streptococcal neonatal sepsis. Radiology 124:771, 1977.

167. Thomas DB, Anderson JC. Antenatal detection of fetal pleural effusion and neonatal management. Med J Aust 2:435, 1979.

168. Steele RW, Thomas MP, Kolls JK. Current management of community-acquired pneumonia in children: an algorithmic guideline recommendation. Infect Med Jan 1999, pp 46–52.

169. Klein JO. Diagnostic lung puncture in the pneumonias of infants and children. Pediatrics 44:486–492, 1969.

170. Teele DW, Pelton SI, Grant MJA, et al. Bacteremia in febrile children under 2 years of age: results of cultures of blood of 600 consecutive febrile children seen in a "walk-in" clinic. J Pediatr 87:227–230, 1975.

171. Sherman MP, Goetzman BW, Ahlfor CE, et al. Tracheal aspiration and its clinical correlates in the diagnosis of congenital pneumonia. Pediatrics 65:258, 1980.

172. Thureen PJ, Moreland S, Rodden DJ, et al. Failure of tracheal aspirate cultures to define that cause of respiratory deteriorations in neonates. Pediatr Infect Dis J 12:560, 1993.

173. Lau YL, Hey E. Sensitivity and specificity of daily tracheal aspirate cultures in predicting organisms causing bacteremia in ventilated neonates. Pediatr Infect Dis J 10:290, 1991.

174. Fan LL, Sparks LM, Dulinski JP. Applications of an ultrathin flexible bronchoscope for neonatal and pediatric airway problems. Chest 89:673, 1986.

175. Klein JO. Diagnostic lung puncture in the pneumonias of infants and children. Pediatrics 44:486, 1969.

176. Alexander HE, Craig HR, Shirley RG, et al. Validity of etiology diagnosis of pneumonia in children by rapid typing from nasopharyngeal mucus. J Pediatr 18:31, 1941.

177. Bollowa JGM. Primary pneumonias of infants and children. Public Health Rep 51:1076, 1903.

178. Cheu MHW, Lally MKP, Clark MR, et al. Open lung biopsy in the critically ill newborn. Pediatrics 86:561, 1990.

179. Greenough A. Gains and losses from dexamethasone for neonatal chronic lung disease. Lancet 352:835–836, 1998.

180. Aherne W, Davies PA. Congenital pneumonia. Lancet 1:234, 1962.

181. Tam ASY, Yeung CY. Gastric aspirate findings in neonatal pneumonia. Arch Dis Child 47:735, 1972.

182. Pole VRG, McAllister TA. Gastric aspirate analysis in the newborn. Acta Paediatr Scand 64:109, 1975.

183. Whitelaw A, Evans A, Corrin B. Immotile cilia syndrome: a new cause of neonatal respiratory distress. Arch Dis Child 56:432, 1981.

184. Ramet J, Byloos J, Delree M, et al. Neonatal diagnosis of the immotile cilia syndrome. Chest 89:138, 1986.

185. Ciliary dyskinesia and ultrastructural abnormalities in respiratory disease. Annotation. Lancet 1:1370, 1988.

186. Giacoia GP, Neter E, Ogra P. Respiratory infections in infants on mechanical ventilation: the immune response as a diagnostic aid. J Pediatr 98:691, 1981.

187. Marks MI, Law B. Respiratory infections vs. colonization. J Pediatr 100:508, 1982.

188. Lung function in children after neonatal meconium aspiration. Annotation. Lancet 2:317, 1988.

189. Smith RM, Brumley GW, Stannard MW. Neonatal pneumonia associated with medium-chain triglyceride feeding supplement. J Pediatr 92:801, 1978.

190. Hjalmarson O. Epidemiology of classification of acute, neonatal respiratory disorders: a prospective study. Acta Paediatr Scand 70:773, 1981.

191. Mounla NA. Neonatal respiratory disorders. Acta Paediatr Scand 76:159, 1987.

192. Avery ME, Fletcher BD, Williams RE. The Lung and Its Disorders in the Newborn Infant. Philadelphia, WB Saunders, 1981.

193. Butler NR, Alberman ED. Clinicopathological associations of hyaline membranes, intraventricular haemorrhage, massive pulmonary haemorrhage and pulmonary

infection. *In* British Perinatal Mortality Survey, Second Report: Perinatal Problems. Edinburgh, E & S Livingstone 1969, pp 184–199.

194. Foote GA, Stewart JH. The coexistence of pneumonia and the idiopathic respiratory distress syndrome in neonates. Br J Radiol 46:504, 1973.

195. Ablow RC, Driscoll SG, Effman EL, et al. A comparison of early-onset group B streptococcal infection and the respiratory distress syndrome of the newborn. N Engl J Med 294:65, 1976.

196. Menke JA, Giacoia GP, Jockin H. Group B beta hemolytic streptococcal sepsis and the idiopathic respiratory distress syndrome: a comparison. J Pediatr 94:467, 1979.

197. Lloyd-Still JD, Khaw K-T, Schwachman H. Severe respiratory disease in infants with cystic fibrosis. Pediatrics 53:678, 1974.

198. Ahvenainen EK. A study of causes of neonatal deaths. J Pediatr 55:691, 1959.

199. Osborn GT. Discussion on neonatal deaths. Proc R Soc Med 51:840, 1958.

200. Butler NR, Bonham DG. Perinatal Mortality. London, E & S Livingstone, 1963.

201. Pacifico L, Panero A, Roggini M, et al. *Ureaplasma urealyticum* and pulmonary outcome in a neonatal intensive care population. Pediatr Infect Dis J 16:579–586, 1997.

202. Brasfield DM, Stagno S, Whitley RJ, et al. Infant pneumonitis associated with cytomegalovirus, *Chlamydia*, *Pneumocystis* and *Ureaplasma*: follow-up. Pediatrics 79:53–60, 1987.

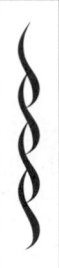

C H A P T E R   2 3

Bacterial Infections of the Bones and Joints

GARY D. OVERTURF, M.D., and S. MICHAEL MARCY, M.D.

OSTEOMYELITIS

Introduction

Osteomyelitis occurring in the first 4 weeks of life is uncommon. During the worldwide pandemic of staphylococcal disease of the 1950s and early 1960s, pediatric centers in Europe,[1–5] Australia,[6] and North America[7–11] reported the occurrence of neonatal osteomyelitis of one or two admissions per year at each institution.

With the advent of modern neonatal supportive care and the increased use of invasive diagnostic and therapeutic procedures, it appeared that osteomyelitis and septic arthritis secondary to bacteremia might occur more frequently in the newborn.[12] Yet subsequent experience in Europe,[13–15] Canada,[16, 17] and the United States[11, 18–20] during the decade 1970 to 1979 indicated little or no change in the incidence of this condition. Even in intensive care nurseries, despite an increasing problem with fungal (*Candida*) osteoarthritis,[21–25] the overall rate of nosocomial bone and joint infections remained low—2.6 or fewer per 1000 admissions.[23, 26, 27] It is clear, however, that infections associated with procedures such as placement of intravascular catheters may not appear or be recognized until after the perinatal period, sometimes several days or weeks after catheter removal.[12, 23]

Little has been published on the relative incidence of neonatal osteomyelitis during the 1980s and 1990s. An ongoing review of nursery infections at a Kaiser Permanente hospital in southern California revealed only three cases of osteomyelitis among 67,000 consecutive live births between 1963 and 1993; none occurred in the final years.[28] A similar survey performed at two pediatric referral centers in Texas showed no significant variation in the number of annual admissions for this condition from 1964 to 1986.[18, 29] Physicians working in intensive care nurseries in Great Britain,[30] France,[31] Spain,[32] and various parts of the United States[33, 34] observe, on the average, one to three cases of bone or joint infection per 1000 admissions, an incidence almost identical to that noted 15 years ago.[23, 26, 27] Thus, it appears that neonatal osteoarthritis continues to be an uncommon problem.

In a review of more than 300 cases of neonatal osteomyelitis, male infants predominated over females (1.6:1). Premature infants acquire osteomyelitis with relatively greater frequency than do term infants.[11, 13, 16, 35–44] In a series of osteomyelitis, 17 of 30 proven cases were in premature infants, 4 occurred in term infants receiving intensive care, and *Staphylococcus aureus* was responsible for 23 of the proven cases of osteomyelitis (16 methicillin sensitive and 7 methicillin resistant).[45] *Escherichia coli* and group B streptococci caused 3 and 2 cases, respectively. Risk factors for osteomyelitis and septic arthritis in premature infants have been mostly iatrogenic and include use of intravenous or intra-arterial catheters, ventilatory support, and bacteremia with nosocomial pathogens.

Microbiology

Because most cases of neonatal osteomyelitis arise as a consequence of an early bacteremia, it is not surprising that the bacteria responsible for osteomyelitis have reflected the changing trends in the etiology of neonatal sepsis. Before 1940, hemolytic streptococci were the predominant organisms responsible for sepsis in the newborn[46] and were also a frequent cause of osteomyelitis.[47, 48] In one large series, streptococci were implicated in the majority of cases of osteomyelitis in neonates and infants younger than 6 months of age.[49]

After 1950, the incidence of *S. aureus* osteomyelitis rose. A review of reports between 1952 and 1972 showed that 85% of the infections were caused by *S. aureus*, 6% were caused by hemolytic streptococci (no groups specified), and 2% were due to *Streptococcus pneumoniae*; either no organisms or miscellaneous organisms (particularly gram-negative bacilli) were isolated from 7% of the cases.[2–6, 11, 38, 41, 50–57]

Significant increases in the incidence of group B streptococcal sepsis in the 1970s were associated with a concomitant rise in the number of bone infections caused by this organism.[20, 58] This change in spectrum was reflected in U.S. reviews of osteomyelitis among infants hospitalized between 1965 and 1978 showing that group B *Streptococcus* had become the single most frequent agent.[11, 20, 59] However, this experience was not universal: newborn centers in Canada,[16] Sweden,[13] Spain,[32] Switzerland,[14] Nigeria,[60] and even sections of the United States[29] continued to find *S. aureus* as the predominant cause of osteomyelitis, with group B *Streptococcus* accounting for only a small number of cases. Although their relative importance may vary by region or institution, these two organisms have remained the most common cause of neonatal osteomyelitis.[34–36, 43] Recent cases of unusual sites of group B streptococcal osteomyelitis in the iliac wing[61] and the vertebrae[62] emphasize the renewed importance and frequency of this infection.

Osteomyelitis caused by gram-negative enteric bacilli is relatively uncommon despite the frequency of neonatal bacteremia.[35, 46, 63, 64] In Stockholm during 1969 to 1979, *E. coli* and *Klebsiella-Enterobacter* were responsible for about 30% of neonatal septicemia[15] but only 5% of bone infections.[13] *S. aureus*, on the other hand, although also causing about 30% of neonatal bacteremia, was responsible for 75% of osteomyelitis. The reasons for these discrepancies are unknown. Several other surveys performed within the past 20 years show about 10% of neonatal osteomyelitis to be due to gram-negative enteric bacilli.[11, 14, 16, 29, 34, 41] Although rates as high as 19%[60] and 45%[32, 42, 43] have been observed, they represent rare exceptions. A review of the literature has revealed isolated instances of hematogenous osteomyelitis in newborns caused by *E. coli*,* *Proteus* species,[13, 20, 30, 54, 71–75] *Klebsiella pneumoniae*,[13, 32, 43, 44, 70, 76–78] *Enterobacter*,[32, 72, 79, 80] *Serratia marcescens*,[20, 32] *Pseudomonas* species,[20, 32, 38, 41, 43, 48, 69, 82] and *Salmonella*.[16, 29, 42, 81–85]

Although suppurative arthritis is the most common manifestation of gonococcal sepsis involving the skeletal system,[86] osteomyelitis is often associated with this sepsis as well; it probably represents the site of primary infection in many cases.[41, 87, 88] Syphilitic osteitis and osteochondritis, so frequent in former years,[89] had been largely eliminated through serologic detection of disease during routine antenatal testing and institution of appropriate therapy for infected mothers. Unfortunately, a recent increase in the incidence of syphilis among women of childbearing age has been reflected in a parallel increase in the frequency of neonatal syphilis and attendant problems of treponemal bone infection.[90, 91]

Mycoplasma and *Ureaplasma* have now been reported as rare causes of osteomyelitis in infants. One infant experienced a sternotomy wound after cardiac surgery caused by *Mycoplasma hominis*,[65] whereas another 900-g infant had osteomyelitis of the hip and femur caused by *Ureaplasma urealyticum*.[66]

Tuberculous osteomyelitis is extremely rare in the neonate, even in the presence of disseminated congenital tuberculosis.[92, 93] Among a group of infants with widespread disease acquired in the perinatal or neonatal period, the youngest with skeletal involvement was 3 months of age.[88]

---

*See references 2, 8, 11, 13, 14, 20, 32, 37, 41–43, 48, 54, 65–70.

Pathogenesis

Complications of pregnancy, labor, or delivery precede the occurrence of neonatal osteomyelitis in one third to one half of patients.[11, 13, 16, 20, 32, 41–43] Although anoxia (placenta previa, breech extraction, fetal distress) or exposure to microorganisms (premature rupture of membranes) can explain this association in some cases, the means whereby maternal or obstetric problems influence the likelihood of acquiring bone infection is generally unknown.

Microorganisms may reach the skeletal tissues of the fetus and newborn in one of four ways: (1) by direct inoculation, (2) by extension from infection in surrounding soft tissues, (3) as a consequence of maternal bacteremia with transplacental infection and fetal sepsis, and (4) by blood-borne dissemination in the course of neonatal septicemia. Although hematogenous dissemination is responsible for most cases, examples of other routes of infection have appeared occasionally in the literature.

Direct inoculation of bacteria resulting in osteomyelitis has followed femoral venipuncture,[39, 60, 75, 94–96] radial artery puncture,[32] use of a fetal scalp monitor,[14, 97–100] great toe[86] or heel[14, 32, 34, 102–106] capillary blood sampling,[101] and serial lumbar punctures.[107] Infection after surgical invasion of bony structures (e.g., median sternotomy for cardiac surgery) is rare.[108] However, trauma has been associated with osteomyelitis of the neonate, similar to the concepts of osteomyelitis in older children; *S. aureus* osteomyelitis has occurred in a neonate at 3 weeks of age at the site of a perinatal fracture of the clavicle.[109]

Osteomyelitis caused by extension of infection from surrounding soft tissues is usually associated with organisms from an infected cephalhematoma involving the adjacent parietal bone.[110–113] A series of patients with *S. aureus* osteomyelitis of the skull associated with overlying scalp abscesses was reported more than 45 years ago and remains unexplained.[114] Predisposing factors in these patients were thought to be prolonged, excessive pressure on the fetal head when it lay against the sacral promontory or symphysis pubis, secondary ischemic necrosis, and localization of infection. Paronychia during the newborn period, although most frequently a source of sepsis and hematogenous dissemination of organisms, may extend into bony structures and cause phalangeal infection.[48]

Transplacental bacterial bone infection is almost exclusively syphilitic. A rare exception, published as a case report in 1933, described a premature infant who died at 19 hours of age with evidence of subacute parietal bone osteomyelitis, meningitis, and cerebritis. Rupture of the amniotic sac immediately before delivery, histopathologic evidence of the prolonged course (at least 2 weeks) of the infection, and the lack of involvement of the overlying scalp epidermis indicate that despite apparent absence of maternal illness this child was infected through the transplacental route. The authors postulated that the primary infection occurred in the parietal bone, with secondary extension to underlying meninges and brain. Although organisms were not isolated at autopsy, gram-positive diplococci were identified in infected tissues.[115]

Blood-borne dissemination of organisms, with metastatic seeding of the skeletal system through nutrient arteries, represents the major cause of neonatal osteomyelitis.[49, 116] Before the advent of antibiotics, the long bones reportedly became infected in as many as 10% of infants with bacteremia.[48, 117] Since that time, early recognition and effective empirical therapy for bacterial sepsis have caused a marked decrease in the incidence of this complication. In contrast, candidal invasion of the bloodstream, a condition difficult to diagnose and rarely treated expectantly because of toxicity of the drugs required, is being seen more frequently as a cause of bone and joint infections in small infants.[21, 23, 24, 36, 118, 119]

In recent years, the use of intravascular catheters—peripheral as well as central—has been associated with bacterial and fungal osteomyelitis in neonates.[11, 13, 16, 21, 23, 24, 43, 78–80, 118, 120–127] The reasons for this association are uncertain; however, it is believed that septic embolization from catheter-tip thrombi together with local hypoxia from partial occlusion of the vessels by the catheter are responsible for the bone infections.[121, 122] Whether the catheters become colonized initially as they are inserted or subsequently as the result of a transient bacteremia is also conjectural. The most common etiologic agent has been *S. aureus*, but other microorganisms, such as *Klebsiella*,[78, 80] *Proteus*,[64] *Enterobacter*,[79] and *Candida*,[21, 23, 72, 118] have also been implicated. Because the iliac arteries are the most likely pathway for an arterial embolus originating in an aortic catheter tip, the hips or knees or both are involved in more than three fourths of patients.[11, 78, 80, 121–123] There is a very close correlation between the site of the catheter and localization of osteomyelitis in the ipsilateral leg.[122] The distribution of infection originating in umbilical vein catheters is less predictable.[23, 79, 118, 124–126] Although the incidence of osteoarthritis varies greatly—from 1 in 30[121] to less than 1 in 600[122] infants with umbilical artery catheters—it can be reduced significantly by proper attention to aseptic technique and careful monitoring of catheter placement, combined with prompt catheter removal whenever possible.[122]

The disseminating focus of a bacteremia-producing metastatic abscess in bones is often unknown. Common primary sources include an omphalitis,* pustular dermatitis,[4, 11, 20, 32, 36, 42, 50, 54, 75] purulent rhinitis,[5, 56, 130] paronychia,[4, 5, 40, 51, 56, 75, 130] and mastitis.[4, 50] In a few infants, sepsis and subsequent osteomyelitis have arisen from infected circumcisions,[8, 39] operative sites,[8, 34, 75] intramuscular injections,[50, 75] or varicella lesions.[11] Although gonococcal osteoarthritis originates most commonly from a purulent conjunctivitis, virtually any orifice may provide a portal of entry.[86]

Hematogenous infection of long bones begins in the dilated capillary loops of the metaphysis, adjacent to the cartilaginous growth plate (physis), where the blood flow slows sufficiently to provide pathogenic bacteria with an ideal environment in which to multiply and form abscesses (Fig. 23–1).[116, 131, 132] Once the infectious process

*See references 4, 5, 11, 35, 42, 43, 50, 71, 75, 117, 128–130.

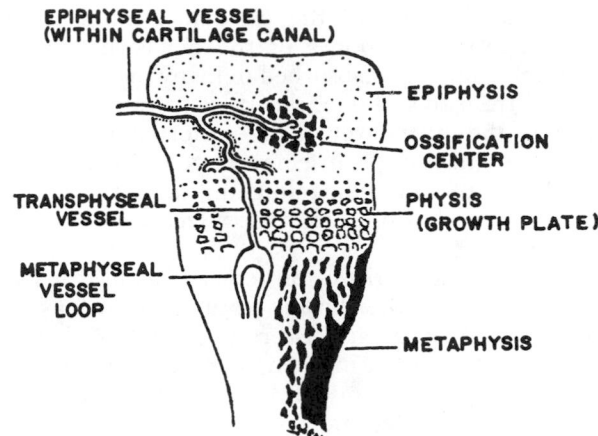

Figure 23–1 Schematic depiction of blood supply in the neonatal epiphysis. Normally in children there are two separate circulatory systems: (1) the metaphyseal loops, derived from the diaphyseal nutrient artery, and (2) the epiphyseal vessels, which course through the epiphyseal cartilage within structures termed cartilage canals. In the neonatal period, sinusoidal vessels, termed the transphyseal vessels, connect these two systems. With ensuing skeletal maturation, these vessels disappear and the epiphyseal and metaphyseal systems become totally separated. (From Ogden JA, Lister G. The pathology of neonatal osteomyelitis. Pediatrics 55:474, 1975, with permission.)

localizes at this site, there may occur (1) direct invasion and lysis of the cartilaginous growth plate; (2) spread from the metaphyseal vessel loops into the transphyseal vessel coursing through the growth plate and into the epiphyseal vessels; or (3) rupture laterally, out through the cortex into the joint, subperiosteal space, or surrounding soft tissues.[131, 132] Green and Shannon,[49] Blanche,[57] and others have pointed out that the large vascular spaces and thin spongy structure of the metaphyseal cortex in infants permit early decompression of this primary abscess into the subperiosteal space. For this reason, the bone marrow compartment is seldom involved in neonates, and the term *osteitis* is probably more accurate than *osteomyelitis*.

After rupture into the subperiosteal space, the abscess dissects rapidly beneath the loosely attached periosteum, often involving the entire length and circumference of the bone. As pressure increases from accumulating pus, there may be decompression through the thin, periosteal tissue into the surrounding soft tissues, and a subcutaneous abscess may form. In the absence of surgical intervention, this collection of pus will point and drain spontaneously through the skin, forming a sinus tract. Once adequate decompression and drainage have been established, general supportive care is often sufficient to permit complete healing and resolution of osseous and soft tissue foci of infection.[47, 49, 133, 134] Free communication between the original site of osteomyelitis and the subperiosteal space prevents the necrosis and extensive spread of infection through the bone structure of the shaft that occurs so frequently in older children and adults. Cortical sequestra are, therefore, less common in infants, and, because of the extreme richness of the blood supply to the bones of the newborn, they are rapidly and completely absorbed in many instances when they do form.[49] In addition, the efficient vasculature and fertility of the inner layer of the periosteum encourage early development of profuse new bone formation (involucrum) and permit remodeling of the shaft within a very short period of time after the infectious process has been controlled.[49, 116]

The same characteristics of neonatal bone that serve to prevent many of the chronic features of osteomyelitis seen in older children are also responsible for the complications that do occur in the neonate and young infant, namely, epiphysitis and pyarthrosis. It has been shown[116, 131, 132] that one manifestation of the excellent blood supply of the bones in newborns is persistent fetal vessels that penetrate the cartilaginous epiphyseal plate and end in large venous lakes within the epiphysis. Thus, organisms localizing at these sites early in the course of osteomyelitis lead to an epiphysitis and severe damage of the cartilage cells on the epiphyseal side of the growth plate. Once such damage occurs, it is generally irreparable[70, 116] and ultimately results in arrest or disorganization of growth at the ends of the bone. By the age of 8 to 18 months, the vascular connections between metaphysis and epiphysis are obliterated, and the cartilaginous growth plate provides a barrier against the spread of infection that persists throughout childhood and adult life.[116, 131, 132]

Rapid decompression of the primary metaphyseal abscess through the adjacent cortex also permits ready entrance of pus into the articular space of those bones whose metaphyses lie within the articular capsule of the joint. Therefore, suppurative arthritis of the hips, shoulders, elbows, and knees is frequently associated with osteomyelitis of the humerus or femur in infants.* When the infection originates in the epiphysis, pyarthrosis may also occur by direct extension of the primary abscess through the articular cartilage and into the joint space. Once pus enters the joint, it causes distention of the joint capsule and, owing to increasing pressure, may eventually produce a pathologic dislocation of the shoulder or hip joint. The lytic action of pyogenic (particularly staphylococcal) exudate within the joint[138, 139] and the ischemia produced by the high intra-articular tension are often sufficient to cause dissolution or separation of the entire head of the femur or humerus, both of which are composed almost completely of cartilage during the neonatal period.[3, 37, 38, 140–142] Although serious growth disturbances and deformities may result from septic arthritis at other sites, complete destruction of the joint is rare.

Clinical Manifestations

Drawing on their own observations and those of previous investigators, Greengard,[143] Thomson and Lewis,[40] and Dennison[3] described two distinct clinical syndromes that may be associated with suppurative bone involvement in the newborn period. In the first, a "benign form," there is little or no evidence of infection other than local swelling or disability related to an osteomyelitis involving one or more skeletal sites. In the second syndrome, a "severe form," systemic manifestations of sepsis predominate until multiple sites of bone and visceral involvement are noted as complications of the infant's underlying condition.

The most likely cause of the benign form of neonatal osteomyelitis is a mild, transient bacteremia that arises at a peripheral site and causes only minimal inflammation and suppuration. The experience of most investigators indicates that this form of illness represents the large majority of cases.* The few series in which high fever and evidence of sepsis were noted as common presenting signs probably represent instances in which delay in diagnosis resulted in more advanced disease being present at the time of admission.[2, 3, 42, 50]

Infants with mild illness are generally feeding well, gaining weight, and developing normally. Systemic manifestations are minimal, and the temperature is usually normal or only slightly elevated[4, 14, 34, 35, 57, 135, 140]; thus, parents sometimes fail to seek medical advice until 2 to 4 weeks have elapsed, by which time bone destruction may be severe and widespread.[48, 55, 57, 144] Even in hospital nurseries, where infants are under continuous professional observation, osteomyelitis may be missed. Usually discovered during a skeletal survey as additional unsuspected site or sites of infection in an infant with known bone involvement, osteomyelitis has also been diagnosed as an incidental finding on chest or abdominal radiographs.[16, 23, 145]

The signs first noted by the parents or physician are diffuse edema and swelling of an extremity or joint, usually without discoloration, accompanied by excessive irritability of the infant. Handling the infant causes increased discomfort, and prolonged episodes of crying during and after a diaper change constitute a common presenting complaint. Examination reveals diminished spontaneous and reflex movement of the affected extremity, either as a result of pain ("pseudoparalysis")[20, 34, 35, 43, 74, 77, 132] or because of weakness caused by a true neuropathy.[146–149] Pyarthrosis of the hip joint is characterized by a tendency of the hip to maintain a flexed, abducted, and externally rotated ("frog-leg") position.[146] Because the slightest degree of passive motion of an extremity may cause severe pain and prolonged crying, attempts to elicit a point of maximal bone tenderness often meet with little success.

As the suppurative process extends through the metaphyseal cortex into the surrounding subperiosteal and subcutaneous tissues, external signs of inflammation become more intense and points of maximal swelling, redness, and heat are more readily discernible. In most cases, the inflammatory mass is directly adjacent to the involved metaphysis or joint, although when deeper skeletal structures are involved, the abscess may point in distant sites. Thus, three infants have been described whose vertebral osteomyelitis was not discovered, or even suspected, until after a large retroperitoneal abscess

---

*See references 3, 4, 6, 11, 13, 16, 20, 21, 38, 59, 132, 135–139.

*See references 4, 6, 11, 13, 14, 16, 20, 34, 35, 41, 43, 52, 57, 133, 134.

had developed.[6] An abscess arising from the proximal femur, ilium, or hip joint usually appears in the upper thigh, buttocks, or groin, but occasionally also in the iliac fossa, where it can be palpated through the abdominal wall or by rectal examination.[52] Even when the infection is clearly localized in the distal extremities, it is difficult to determine solely on clinical grounds whether the bone or adjacent joint, or both, is involved. Radiologic examinations and diagnostic aspiration of suspected joints are generally necessary to establish a diagnosis.

The striking feature of the benign form of neonatal osteomyelitis is the satisfactory general condition of the infant, despite the intensity of the local process; feeding and weight gain are undisturbed, and there is no evidence of involvement of visceral structures. Although deformity and disability may follow such infections, the fatality rate is exceedingly low and healing is prompt.

In contrast, signs and symptoms of the severe form of neonatal osteomyelitis are predominantly those of a widespread septic process with prolonged and intense bacteremia. Infants with this condition usually fail to thrive; they manifest lethargy, refusal or regurgitation of feedings, abdominal distention, jaundice, and other signs characteristic of sepsis in the newborn. Infection of the bones and joints may be noted almost simultaneously with the onset of the septicemia, or it may appear later, despite administration of antibiotics. The appearance and evolution of the osteomyelitic process are identical with those in patients with the benign form of the disease. Despite this, early localizing signs and symptoms are frequently overshadowed by the more apparent constitutional manifestations and obtunded condition of the infant. Evidence of a suppurative process in the bone may be discovered accidentally in the course of routine radiographic examinations, or it may not be apparent until the formation of a local subcutaneous abscess directs the physician's attention to the underlying bone. The prognosis for these infants is guarded; death is generally caused by sepsis, with widespread and multiple foci of infection in the nervous system or viscera. The prognosis for the skeletal lesions among survivors is, however, not different from that described for the benign form.

As group B streptococcal infections have become increasingly prevalent, a distinctive clinical picture associated with osteomyelitis caused by this agent has emerged.[20, 34, 59, 150–154] Most cases are caused by type III streptococci and present as a late-onset illness during the third and fourth weeks of life (mean age at diagnosis, 25 days). Predisposing factors commonly seen with osteomyelitis caused by other agents, such as maternal obstetric complications, difficulties in the early neonatal period, use of vascular catheters, or other manipulative procedures, are unusual with group B streptococcal disease. The male preponderance usually identified with neonatal osteomyelitis is reversed, with a 1.5:1 excess of females. In almost 90% of the infants described with this condition, only a single bone has been involved, most commonly the humerus (50%) or femur (33%), affecting the shoulder or knee. In most cases, infants manifest the benign form of osteomyelitis without signs of systemic toxicity or involvement of other organ systems. Nevertheless, most are ill no more than 3 or 4 days before the diagnosis is established. Although the infected joints are typically neither warm nor erythematous, local swelling, tenderness, and diminished movement of the affected extremity are usually severe enough for the parents to seek early medical attention.

The distribution of bone involvement reported in the literature is represented in Table 23–1. There were 734 infected sites among 485 patients. A single bone was involved in 324 patients, and multiple foci were found in 161 patients.[155, 156] Because radiographic or radionuclide skeletal surveys, which often identify unsuspected foci of osteomyelitis,[13, 16, 23, 35, 127, 145] were generally not performed, the number of infants reported to have infection in multiple sites is probably falsely low. The high incidence of infections of the femur, humerus, and tibia in the neonate has also been noted in adults[157] and older infants and children.[8, 10, 135, 158] The relatively large number of cases of maxillary osteomyelitis is, however,

TABLE 23–1
Distribution of Bone Involvement in 485 Newborns with Osteomyelitis

BONE	NO. OF SITES[a]	% OF SITES
Femur	287	39
62 Proximal		
91 Distal		
81 Unspecified		
Humerus	133	18
66 Proximal		
16 Distal		
51 Unspecified		
Tibia	102	14
47 Proximal		
11 Distal		
44 Unspecified		
Radius	34	5
5 Proximal		
17 Distal		
12 Unspecified		
Maxilla	30	4
Ulna	22	3
Clavicle	18	2
Tarsal bones	15	2
2 "Tarsus"		
3 Talus		
10 Calcaneus		
Metacarpals	14	2
Phalanges	12	2
Ribs	12	2
Skull	9	1
Fibula	9	1
Ilium	8	1
Metatarsals	7	1
Mandible	7	1
Scapula	7	1
Sternum	6	1
Vertebrae	5	1
Ischium	3	0.4
Patella	1	0.1

[a]Thirty-three percent of infants had disease in more than one bone.
Data from references 2–6, 11, 14, 16, 32, 34–36, 40, 42, 43, 47, 48, 50–54, 56, 57, 74, 83, 127, 133, 134, 155, 156, and 174.

unique to the newborn period and is therefore discussed separately.

The exuberant new bone formation associated with osteomyelitis in the newborn period makes it difficult to determine the original foci of infection when radiographs are obtained late in the course of illness. For this reason, the site of the primary metaphyseal abscess was either unspecified or the infection was referred to as a "panosteitis" in many instances. In the femur, there was an equal distribution of proximal, distal, and uncertain sites of early infection, whereas localization in the tibia and humerus occurred most often at the proximal ends of the bones. In the radius, distal osteomyelitis predominated. The major consequence of these patterns of infection is the high incidence of secondary purulent arthritis of the hips, shoulders, knees, and wrists; this secondary arthritis has been noted in virtually every large series of newborns with bone infection.

Prognosis

Researchers who reported patients with neonatal osteomyelitis during the period between 1920 and 1940 recognized the existence of mortality rates of up to 40% in neonates and young infants[49] but stressed the overall benign nature of the disease and the good prognosis for life and function if sepsis was not present.[47, 49, 133, 134] The introduction of antimicrobial agents effective against the common infecting organisms was associated with a considerable reduction in mortality rates; only 24 deaths were reported among approximately 575 newborns with osteomyelitis acquired between 1945 and 1990.*

The improved survival rate served to direct greater attention to the high incidence of residual joint deformities that may follow neonatal osteomyelitis, particularly when the hip and knee joints are involved or when diagnosis is delayed for more than 3 or 4 days.[37–39, 41, 42, 57, 70, 75, 159–161] Destruction or separation of the capital femoral epiphysis may result in serious disturbances of growth, usually combined with a marked coxa vara, valga, or magna; an unstable hip joint; flexion contractures; and abnormalities of gait.† Damage to the cartilaginous growth plate in the knees is also often followed by disturbances in longitudinal growth and angulation at the site of infection, leading to genu varum or valgum, restricted motion, and instability of the joint.[11, 36, 57, 70, 130, 137] Although the consequences of shortening of bone and angular deformities are more serious in the lower extremities, analogous growth disturbances may follow osteomyelitis of the humerus, radius, or ulna.[3, 14, 40, 57, 70, 162] Most of these data have been collected from infants with staphylococcal bone or joint infection; in contrast, the prognosis for full recovery is excellent after group B streptococcal infection.[20, 33, 59]

Although vertebral osteomyelitis in the newborn is unusual, the consequences can be grave. Collapse or complete destruction of one or more vertebral bodies may occur,[13, 23, 162–166] with severe kyphosis or paralysis caused by spinal cord compression appearing as late complications.[13, 162, 163] In most cases, vertebral involvement is not recognized until after paraspinal abscesses appear.[6, 167–169]

The full clinical effect of osteomyelitis in the newborn period may not be fully appreciated for many years. Thus, despite a seemingly favorable outcome, even infants with minor bone or joint involvement should be followed to skeletal maturity to observe for the appearance of late deformity, dysfunction, or growth arrest.[70, 75] Early evidence of skeletal destruction, on the other hand, is almost always associated with the need for multiple orthopedic procedures to stabilize a joint or to straighten a limb or equalize its length with that of the opposite arm or leg. Descriptions of late regeneration of femoral epiphyses despite severe injury in the neonatal period emphasize, however, the remarkable healing potential and unpredictability of this illness.[170–176]

Chronic osteomyelitis and persistent sequestration of necrotic bone have been thought to be uncommon complications both before and after the availability of antibiotic therapy.[6, 40, 42, 49, 57, 133, 134] However, the apparent rarity of these complications in former years should be questioned because approximately 10% of infants with osteomyelitis who were studied by several groups formed sequestra and, in many cases, required sequestrectomy for complete cure.* A recently reported rare complication of neonatal osteomyelitis is osteochondroma (or exostosis) at the distal ulna, following *S. aureus* osteomyelitis.[176]

Diagnosis

Plain film radiographs are still the most useful means of establishing the diagnosis of neonatal osteomyelitis. Experience with computed tomography (CT) and magnetic resonance imaging (MRI) in the evaluation of neonatal disease, particularly bone infection, is limited and remains a final evaluation technique after plain radiographs, ultrasonography (of joints), and bone scans have been used.[177]

The earliest sign is swelling of soft tissue around the site of primary infection. Although this finding reflects the spreading edema and inflammation that occur as pus breaks through the metaphyseal cortex, it is nonspecific and serves only to define an area of inflammation. The first evidence of bone involvement appears as small foci of necrosis and rarefaction, most commonly located in the metaphysis adjoining the epiphyseal growth plate. This may be accompanied by capsular distention or widening of the joint space if inflammatory exudate or pus has entered the articular capsule. Unlike older children, in whom radiographic changes are commonly delayed for up to 3 weeks,[10, 158] neonates almost always show definite signs of bone destruction by the 7th to 10th day of illness.[5, 11, 20, 41, 54, 56, 122, 127, 175]

Extension of the suppurative process often produces widespread areas of cortical rarefaction, which, despite their appearance, infrequently result in significant bone sequestration. The presence of pus in the hip and shoul-

---

*See references 2, 4–6, 11, 13, 14, 16, 20, 32, 34, 41–43, 55, 57, 74, 127, 130.
†See references 38, 57, 75, 88, 95, 130, 141, 142, 162, and 163.

*See references 2, 5, 16, 51, 52, 74, 114, 137, 174, and 175.

der joints may cause progressive lateral and upward displacement of the head of the femur[35, 141, 142, 178] or humerus through stages of subluxation to pathologic dislocation. The absence during the newborn period of ossification centers, with the exception of those at the distal femur and proximal tibia, makes it very difficult to diagnose neonatal epiphysitis in any area but the knees.[137] Epiphyseal separation or destruction of the head of the femur or humerus is, for similar reasons, difficult to distinguish radiologically from simple dislocation.[141, 142]

In most infants, the reparative phase begins within 2 weeks after onset of infection. The first sign of healing is the formation of a thin layer of subperiosteal bone, which rapidly enlarges to form a thick involucrum between the raised periosteum and the cortex. Although bone destruction may continue at the same time, necrotic foci are rapidly absorbed and filled in as the new bone is deposited. The entire process from the first signs of rarefaction to restoration of the cortical structure may last no longer than 2 months; however, several months usually elapse before minimal deformities disappear and remodeling of the shaft is complete. In some cases, well-circumscribed defects involving the metaphysis and epiphysis may persist for years.[137]

The benefit of radiologic skeletal survey in newborns with osteomyelitis should be emphasized. Additional, clinically unsuspected sites of infection can be discovered in a significant proportion of infants, with delays of up to 3 weeks for radiographic appearance.[13, 16, 23, 36, 127, 179] Demonstration of such lesions may be more than academic: in one series,[16] 4 of 7 areas of occult infection required aspiration or drainage, whereas in another study,[13] 3 of 17 hip joint infections were discovered on routine radiographs taken because the infant had osteomyelitis elsewhere. A plain film skeletal survey for occult bone and joint infection should be performed on any infant with osteomyelitis.

As mentioned, experience with CT and MRI in the diagnosis of neonatal musculoskeletal infection is limited.[180, 181] Although both procedures can be helpful adjuncts to clinical diagnosis and conventional radiography, they are slow and require heavy sedation—usually undesirable in a febrile septic infant—to prevent movement artifact and loss of resolution.

CT provides good definition of cortical bone and is sensitive for the early detection of bone destruction, periosteal reaction, and formation of sequestra. It has been used to particular advantage in the diagnosis of osteomyelitis of the skull associated with infected cephalhematoma.[110, 111] Plain radiographs of uninfected cephalhematomas can show soft tissue swelling, periosteal elevation, calcification, and even underlying radiolucency caused by bone resorption[182]—findings also consistent with bone infection. In such cases, CT has been able to define foci of bone destruction more accurately, helping confirm the presence of osteomyelitis.

MRI, on the other hand, is of limited value in defining structural changes in cortical bone but provides excellent anatomic detail of muscle and soft tissue, superior to that of any other imaging technique.[181] It is therefore particularly useful in disclosing the early soft tissue edema seen adjacent to areas of bone involvement before the appearance of any osseous changes. It is also helpful in determining the presence of a periosteal abscess and assessing the need for surgical drainage. The major advantage of MRI over CT—the ability to detect inflammatory or destructive intramedullary disease—is of greater advantage in older children and adults than in neonates, in whom involvement of the marrow compartment is uncommon.

Both modalities provide excellent spatial resolution and anatomic detail; however, CT is best suited to cross-sectional views, whereas MRI can display anatomy with equal clarity in coronal and sagittal planes, permitting visualization in the plane most advantageous for accurate diagnosis. Absence of ionizing radiation is another distinct advantage of MRI over CT.

In recent years, there has been increasing interest in the use of ultrasonography for the detection of bone infection and joint effusions.[183–187] Diagnosis of osteomyelitis is based on the demonstration of periosteal thickening or the presence of abscess formation as indicated by periosteal elevation and separation from bone. Although the exact role of ultrasonography in the diagnosis of neonatal osteoarthritis has yet to be defined, it currently appears most useful as a tool for defining the presence of fluid collections in joints or adjacent to bone and as a guide for needle aspiration or surgical drainage of these collections. The occurrence of false-positive or false-negative examinations, although infrequent, requires that infants with conflicting clinical findings be evaluated further by other techniques. Recent reports of successful diagnosis of osteomyelitis in neonates with ultrasonography include the diagnosis of rib infection in a 650-g infant with staphylococcal osteomyelitis.[188] Other series have included 2- to 6-week-old infants with osteomyelitis of the costochondral junction and ribs as well.[189, 190]

Despite reports emphasizing the reliability of technetium-99m bone imaging in older infants and children,[191] experience with the use of this technique in neonates has been far less favorable.[16, 36, 43, 127, 192–196] In one study, among 10 newborns subsequently proved to have osteomyelitis involving 20 sites in all, only 8 of these sites were abnormal or equivocal by technetium scan.[192] Of the 12 sites that were normal by scan from 1 to 33 days (mean, 8 days) after the onset of symptoms, 9 showed destructive changes in the corresponding radiograph. The increased radioactivity in areas of inflammatory hyperemia surrounding an osteomyelitis, usually present in the early "blood-pool" images in children,[193] was also not seen, even in those infants with ultimately positive delayed bone scans. Although false-negative bone scans have also been described in older infants,[197, 198] the reason for the excessively high incidence among neonates is not known. It has been suggested that the discrepancy is due either to differences in the pathophysiology of neonatal disease or to the inability of earlier gamma cameras to separate the increased activity of the growth plate in the first weeks of life from that of infection.[145, 191] Clinical studies have indicated that the use of newer high-resolution cameras combined with electronic magnification can provide greater diagnostic accuracy.[145] In addition to more advanced technology, however, the authors also used significantly (four-fold to sixfold) larger doses of technetium, and almost all sites of involvement had radiographically detectable lesions at the time of diagnosis. At the present time, it appears reasonable to limit the use of technetium radionuclide scans to infants with normal or equivocal radiographs in whom there is a strong clinical suspicion of osteomyelitis.

Among older patients, gallium-67 bone imaging has been shown to be of value when the technetium scan and plain films are normal and osteomyelitis is strongly suspected.[198] Studies performed in small infants and neonates have shown similar results.[197, 199] Unfortunately, the radiation burden of this isotope is high and the probability that the results of a scan will, by themselves, influence therapy is low. Thus, the role of gallium bone imaging in the diagnosis of neonatal bone and joint infections is very limited.

Needle aspiration of an inflammatory area may provide a rapid means of establishing a diagnosis.[20, 34, 41, 43] Differentiation of subcutaneous from subperiosteal infection is often difficult; however, significant accumulations of pus aspirated from a periarticular abscess almost invariably originate in bone rather than in the soft tissues.[2, 132] Clinical or radiologic evidence of joint-space infection, particularly in the hip and shoulder, requires immediate confirmation through needle aspiration. If no effusion is found and clinical signs persist, aspiration should be repeated within 8 to 12 hours. If there is doubt about whether the joint was actually entered, limited arthrography with small amounts of dye can readily be performed with an aspirating needle.[141, 142] The usual iodinated contrast materials do not interfere with bacterial growth from subsequently aspirated specimens.[200] Inserting a needle into the metaphyseal region or joint up to 24 hours before scanning does not interfere with the scintigraphic detection of osteomyelitis.[194–196]

The total peripheral white blood cell count is of little value in diagnosing neonatal osteomyelitis. In more than 150 cases in which these values were recorded, the median peripheral leukocyte count was approximately 17,000 (mean, 20,000; range, 4,000 to 75,100). Polymorphonuclear leukocytes usually represented about 60% of the white blood cells counted; frequently, the number of immature forms was higher than normal. Neonates with osteomyelitis usually have a sedimentation rate higher than 20 mm per hour.[11, 34, 35, 59, 121, 152] Like the leukocyte count, the sedimentation rate is helpful for diagnosis and follow-up when elevated but cannot be used to rule out osteomyelitis when normal.[11, 13, 14, 201] Alternatively, the C-reactive protein may be as useful as the erythrocyte sedimentation rate as an acute phase reactant, and most methods for C-reactive protein determination require only 0.1 ml of blood, as opposed to the erythrocyte sedimentation rate, which may require 1 to 2 ml of blood.

Differential Diagnosis

The early descriptions of pyogenic neonatal osteomyelitis emphasized the difficulties of distinguishing the pseudoparalysis and irritability that are characteristic of this condition from the symptoms of congenital syphilis and from the true paralysis of congenital poliomyelitis.[202–204] The clinical course and radiologic examinations are generally sufficient to rule out polio; however, the periostitis and metaphyseal bone destruction that accompany congenital syphilis are frequently indistinguishable from bone alterations observed in infants with multicentric pyogenic osteomyelitis.[161–162] Similar osseous changes have been noted at birth in infants with congenital tumors or leukemia.[202, 205]

Serial radiologic examinations may be necessary to distinguish a superficial cellulitis, subcutaneous abscess, or bursitis[206, 207] from a primary bone infection, particularly when these conditions arise in a periarticular location. Similarly, a suppurative arthritis arising in the joint space rather than in the adjacent metaphysis can be defined as such only by determining that no destruction has occurred in bones contiguous to that joint.

The relative lack of any inflammatory sign other than edema is the only clinical feature that helps to differentiate between candidal and bacterial osteomyelitis.[21, 23] The former condition has been seen more frequently in recent years, particularly in premature infants, in whom antibiotic therapy, placement of umbilical catheters, and use of parenteral hyperalimentation, together with immature host defense mechanisms, predispose to candidal infection and dissemination.[21, 23–25, 37–40, 80, 118, 208, 209] The lesions of *Candida albicans* are typically seen radiologically as well-defined ("punched-out") metaphyseal lucencies, less aggressive in appearance than staphylococcal osteitis, and often surrounded by a slightly sclerotic margin.[21, 23, 37, 40, 41, 80, 209, 210] Even when the characteristic clinical circumstances and radiographic features are present, the diagnosis in almost all cases rests on identification of the organism by Gram stain or culture.

Several congenital viral lesions have also been associated with bone changes. Lesions caused by congenital rubella, although generally seen in the metaphyseal ends of the long bones, are distinct from those of bacterial osteomyelitis during the early stages of pathogenesis and show no evidence of periosteal reaction during the reparative phase.[211] There is little reason to confuse the radiographic features of bone pathology resulting from congenital cytomegalic inclusion disease[212, 213] or herpes simplex virus type 2 infections[214] with those of hematogenous osteomyelitis, particularly when roentgenograms are considered in context with the characteristic clinical signs and symptoms of these infections.

A number of noninfectious conditions causing bone destruction or periosteal reaction might be confused with osteomyelitis on clinical and radiographic grounds as well as by radionuclide scan. These include skeletal trauma caused by the birth process or parental abuse[145, 215–217] or associated with osteogenesis imperfecta; congenital infantile cortical hyperostosis (Caffey's disease)[145, 216, 218]; congenital bone tumors, metastases, and leukemia[145, 205]; extravasation of calcium gluconate at an infusion site[219]; and prostaglandin E₁ infusion.[220] The periosteal bone growth sometimes seen in normal infants, particularly the premature infant, may produce a "double-contour" effect in long bones that appears to be similar to the early involucrum of healing osteomyelitis but is unassociated with evidence of bone destruction and metaphyseal changes and is never progressive.[221]

Therapy

Successful treatment of osteomyelitis or septic arthritis depends on prompt clinical diagnosis and identification of the infectious agent. Every effort should be made to isolate the responsible organism(s) before therapy is initiated. Pus localized in skin, soft tissues, joint, or bone should be aspirated under strict aseptic conditions and sent to the laboratory for Gram stain, culture, and antibiotic susceptibility testing. Blood cultures, which may be the only source of the pathogen,[16, 18, 29, 38, 41, 56, 57, 222] should be obtained. Because osteomyelitis is generally the consequence of a systemic bacteremia, a lumbar puncture should also be performed. Any potential source of infection should be examined, including the tip of intravascular catheters.[223] Bacterial antigen testing of urine, blood, or cerebrospinal fluid can occasionally be helpful when direct examination of suppurative material fails to provide an etiologic diagnosis (see Chapter 21). Choice of therapy should be guided by results of Gram stain, culture, and antibiotic susceptibilities; in most cases, definitive data should be available within 48 hours.

When the cause of infection cannot be immediately determined, the initial choice of antimicrobial agents must be based on a presumptive bacteriologic diagnosis. The penicillinase-resistant penicillins are active against *S. aureus*, groups A and B streptococci, and *S. pneumoniae*, which together account for more than 90% of osteoarthritis in neonates. Osteomyelitis caused by enteric organisms is sufficiently common to justify additional therapy with an aminoglycoside such as gentamicin, tobramycin, or amikacin or an extended-spectrum agent (cefotaxime). Infants acquiring infection in nurseries where methicillin-resistant *S. aureus* is prevalent should be started on vancomycin rather than a penicillin.[127]

Once bacterial cultures and sensitivity data are available, treatment should be changed to the single safest and most effective drug. If group B streptococcal infection is confirmed, combination therapy with penicillin G and gentamicin should be given for 5 to 10 days, after which time penicillin G alone is adequate.[224] Standard disk susceptibility tests may falsely indicate sensitivity of methicillin-resistant *S. aureus* to cephalosporins.[225] Use of β-lactam antibiotics is inappropriate for infection with these agents, and vancomycin should be continued for the full course of therapy.

All antibiotics should be given by the parenteral route. There is no significant clinical advantage to intravenous rather than intramuscular administration, but the limited number of injection sites available in the newborn makes the intramuscular route impractical for use during prolonged periods. Intra-articular administration of antibiotics is unnecessary in the treatment of suppurative arthritis because adequate levels of activity have been demonstrated in joint fluid after parenteral doses of most drugs that would be used for therapy in this condition.[222] Antibiotic therapy for either osteomyelitis or suppurative arthritis should be continued for at least 3 or 4 weeks after defervescence. Monitoring serum acute phase proteins (particularly C-reactive protein) has been proposed as a useful way to determine resolution of infection and duration of therapy.[110, 226, 227]

There are insufficient data on the absorption and efficacy of orally administered antibiotics in the neonate to recommend their use in this age group for therapy for osteoarthritis. Nevertheless, after an initial course of intravenous therapy, newborns have been treated successfully with oral dicloxacillin,[201, 228, 229] flucloxacillin,[35] fusidic acid,[35, 36] and penicillin V[35, 179] for additional periods varying from 14 to 42 days. If sequential parenteral-oral therapy is used, adequacy of antibiotic absorption and efficacy must be closely monitored with regular clinical evaluation and serum bactericidal titers against the infecting organism.[179, 229, 230]

To overcome the uncertainties of oral absorption while still permitting discharge from the hospital, home intravenous antibiotic therapy has been advocated as an alternative form of treatment.[231] Although home management for older children and adults is now widely accepted, experience with newborns is still limited; however, with proper family and medical support, it can be a successful alternative to inpatient treatment.

Incision and drainage is indicated whenever there is a significant collection of pus in soft tissues. The need for drilling or windowing the cortex to drain intramedullary collections of pus is controversial.[11, 13, 14, 35] There is no evidence, based on controlled studies, that these procedures are of any value in either limiting systemic manifestations or decreasing the extent of bone destruction. Open surgical drainage for relief of intra-articular pressure is, however, a critical factor for preserving the viability of the head of the femur or humerus in infants with suppurative arthritis of the hip or shoulder joints.[6, 35, 38, 159] Intermittent needle aspiration with saline irrigation is usually adequate for drainage of other, more readily accessible joints. Lack of improvement after 3 days, rapid reaccumulation of fluid, or loculation of pus and necrotic debris in the joint may indicate the need for open drainage of these joints as well.[232]

The affected extremity should be immobilized until inflammation has subsided and there is radiologic evidence of healing. Prolonged splinting in a brace or cast is necessary when pathologic dislocation of the head of the femur accompanies pyarthrosis of the hip joint. Maintenance of adequate nutrition and fluid requirements is critical in determining the ultimate course of the illness. Before the advent of antibiotics, attention to these factors alone was often adequate to ensure prompt healing of osseous lesions in those infants who survived the initial septic process.[49]

PRIMARY SEPTIC ARTHRITIS

Although septic arthritis is often a complication of osteomyelitis in the newborn, it can also occur in the absence of demonstrable radiologic changes in the adjacent bone. Infection may be the result of synovial implantation of organisms in the course of a septicemia.

Infrequently, traumatic inoculation of organisms into the articular capsule may occur as a consequence of femoral venipuncture.[39, 60, 94–96] As is the case with osteomyelitis, there is also a strong association between septic arthritis and placement of an umbilical catheter.[233] Whatever the source of the infection, the presence of a concurrent osteomyelitis can never be completely ruled out because there always exists the possibility that the original suppurative focus lay in the radiolucent cartilaginous portion of the bone and that organisms entered the joint by direct extension from this site.

The spectrum of agents responsible for primary septic arthritis is similar to that causing arthritis secondary to a contiguous osteomyelitis. Bacteria that have been isolated from the blood or joints of newborns described in two representative series are given in Table 23–2.

Signs and symptoms of purulent arthritis are virtually identical to those seen in newborns with osteomyelitis.[234, 235] Limited use of an extremity progressing to pseudoparalysis is characteristic of both conditions and, although external signs of inflammation tend to be somewhat more localized in the periarticular area, recognition of this feature is of little diagnostic value in the individual case. Data are insufficient to provide any meaningful comparison between the skeletal distribution of septic arthritis and that of osteomyelitis; however, multiple joint involvement is common to both conditions. In one series of 16 consecutive newborns with pyarthrosis, 22 joints were involved; 4 infants had multifocal infections.[18, 29] A migratory polyarthritis, which may precede localization in a single joint by several days, is particularly characteristic of gonococcal arthritis, as is an extremely high frequency of knee and ankle involvement.[86] Recent series from Malaysia emphasize the frequency with which septic arthritis occurs within medical settings of newborn intensive care.[236] In this series the knee, hip, and ankle were involved in 10 cases of septic arthritis and 9 of 10 cases were caused by methicillin-resistant *S. aureus*, demonstrating the frequent occurrence of septic arthritis caused by nosocomial pathogens in premature infants in neonatal intensive care units.

The radiologic features, differential diagnosis, and therapy for septic arthritis have been discussed in the

TABLE 23–2

Organisms Isolated from Blood or Joints of Neonates with Primary Bacterial Arthritis (1972–1986)

BACTERIA	NO. OF INFANTS
Staphylococcus aureus	9
Group B *Streptococcus*	4
Streptococcus, unspecified	2
Staphylococcus epidermidis	1
Haemophilus influenzae, type b	1
Escherichia coli	1
Klebsiella pneumoniae	1
Pseudomonas aeruginosa	1
Neisseria gonorrhoeae	1

Data from references 18, 29, and 233.

section on osteomyelitis. Long-term evaluations are too scarce to permit an accurate overall assessment of the prognosis for this condition.

OSTEOMYELITIS OF THE MAXILLA

Although most large series dealing with neonatal osteomyelitis have emphasized the clinical features of infections of the tubular bones, there exists a significant literature dealing with neonatal osteomyelitis of the maxilla as a distinct clinical entity. Early reports of neonatal osteomyelitis were concerned almost exclusively with this problem; the specific aspects of infection in the extremities have received serious attention only within the past 50 years.

In terms of total numbers, maxillary osteomyelitis is a rare condition (there are fewer than 200 reported cases); yet in several surveys of neonatal bone infections, maxillary involvement was noted in approximately 25% of infants.[3, 6, 11, 49, 56, 237] The far lower incidence in children[8, 10] and adults[157] is probably explained by the earlier recognition and treatment of sinusitis in these age groups and by the lack of predisposing factors unique to the newborn period.

The causative organism is almost always *S. aureus*,[238–241] although hemolytic streptococci have been isolated on rare occasions from drainage sites.[240] More than 85% of all maxillary infections in infants occur in the first 3 months of life; the incidence is highest during the second to fourth weeks.[239–242]

In most cases, the predisposing cause remains obscure. Infants with sources of infection, such as skin abscesses or omphalitis, constitute a small minority.[240, 241] It has been postulated that there is a relationship between breast abscess in the nursing mother and maxillary osteomyelitis[240, 241, 243]; however, it is unclear whether the maternal infection is a source or a result of the infant's condition.[244] The pathogenesis of bone infection after colonization of the infant by staphylococci is equally uncertain. In some cases, osteomyelitis is believed to result from extension from a contiguous focus of infection in the maxillary antrum. Alternatively, the organisms may be blood-borne, establishing the infection in the rich vascular plexus surrounding the tooth buds.[242] Although the hematogenous route may be important in certain cases, particularly those involving the premaxilla,[238] this explanation is not compatible with the fact that mandibular osteomyelitis or the associated metastatic involvement of other structures is uncommon.[240] Another theory is that trauma or abrasion of the gum overlying the first molar is the primary route of introduction of organisms.[241]

The clinical course of maxillary osteomyelitis begins with acute onset of fever and nonspecific systemic symptoms. Shortly thereafter, redness and swelling of the eyelid appear and are frequently accompanied by conjunctivitis with a purulent discharge. Thrombosis of nutrient vessels and increasing edema may cause a proptosis or chemosis of the affected eye. In most infants, an early and diffuse swelling and inflammation of the cheek may localize to form an abscess or draining fistula below the inner or outer canthus of the eye. This is nearly always followed or accompanied by a purulent unilateral nasal discharge that is increased by pressure on the abscess. The alveolar border of the superior maxilla on the affected side is swollen and soft, as is the adjacent hard palate. Within a few days, abscesses and draining fistulas may form in these areas.[245] Sepsis and death frequently intervene in untreated cases. In most infants, the illness pursues a relatively chronic course characterized by discharge of premature teeth or numerous small sequestra of necrotic bone through multiple palatal and alveolar sinuses that have formed. The entire course may evolve over several days in severe cases, or it may extend for several weeks in mild or partially treated cases.

Neonatal maxillary osteomyelitis is frequently confused with either orbital cellulitis or dacryocystitis.[13, 241, 246] The early edema and redness of the cheeks that accompany acute osteomyelitis are an important differentiating feature, which is not observed in orbital cellulitis and occurs only as a late sign in infection of the lacrimal sac. Neither of the latter conditions is associated with a unilateral purulent nasal discharge. The early onset, limited area of involvement, and Gram stain characteristic of ophthalmia neonatorum should be sufficient, in most cases, to permit diagnosis of this condition. CT can be helpful in assessing the extent of infection as well as the presence of possible complications such as cerebral abscess.[245]

Therapy for maxillary osteomyelitis should be directed toward early adequate drainage of the maxillary empyema and contiguous abscess and should include appropriate antibiotics. Because most infections are due to *S. aureus* and the group A *Streptococcus*, systemic use of a penicillinase-resistant penicillin alone should be sufficient as initial therapy pending the results of bacterial cultures and sensitivity tests. The need or desirability for instillation of antibiotics into the maxillary antrum is uncertain.

Before the advent of penicillin therapy, the mortality rate for maxillary osteomyelitis was high, ranging from 15 to 75% in various series.[240, 241, 243, 247] Those who survived often had severe facial and dental deformities. Later studies[240, 241, 247] showed a mortality rate of closer to 5%, although sequelae such as stenosis of the lacrimal duct, ectropion, permanent loss of teeth, malocclusion, and facial hemiatrophy are still seen.[11, 239–241] In many instances, these complications could have been prevented through early recognition of the nature of the illness and prompt institution of appropriate therapy.

References

1. Craig WS. Care of the Newly Born Infant. Baltimore, Williams & Wilkins, 1962.
2. Boyes J, Bremner AD, Neligan GA. Haematogenous osteitis in the newborn. Lancet 1:544, 1957.
3. Dennison WM. Haematogenous osteitis in the newborn. Lancet 2:474, 1955.
4. Masse P. L'ostéomyelité du nouveau-né. Semaine Hôp Paris 34:2812, 1958.
5. Contzen H. Die sogennante Osteomyelitis des Neugeborenen. Dtsch Med Wochenschr 86:1221, 1961.
6. Clarke AM. Neonatal osteomyelitis: a disease different from osteomyelitis of older children. Med J Aust 1:237, 1958.
7. Hall JE, Silverstein EA. Acute hematogenous osteomyelitis. Pediatrics 31:1033, 1963.
8. Green M, Nyhan WL Jr, Fousek MD. Acute hematogenous osteomyelitis. Pediatrics 17:368, 1956.
9. Hung W, McGavisk DF. Acute hematogenous osteomyelitis: a report of 36 cases seen at Children's Hospital 1950 to 1958. Clin Proc Child Hosp 16:163, 1960.
10. Morse TS, Pryles CV. Infections of the bones and joints in children. N Engl J Med 262:846, 1960.
11. Fox L, Sprunt K. Neonatal osteomyelitis. Pediatrics 62:535, 1978.
12. Lim MO, Gresham EL, Franken EA Jr, et al. Osteomyelitis as a complication of umbilical artery catheterization. Am J Dis Child 131:142, 1977.
13. Bergdahl S, Ekengren K, Eriksson M. Neonatal hematogenous osteomyelitis: risk factors for long-term sequelae. J Pediatr Orthop 5:564, 1985.
14. Bamberger T, Gugler E. Die akute Osteomyelitis im Kindesalter. Schweiz Med Wochenschr 113:1219, 1983.
15. Bennet R, Eriksson M, Zetterström R. Increasing incidence of neonatal septicemia: causative organism and predisposing risk factors. Acta Paediatr Scand 70:207, 1981.
16. Mok PM, Reilly BJ, Ash JM. Osteomyelitis in the neonate with cerebral abscess. Radiology 145:677, 1982.
17. Dan M. Septic arthritis in young infants: Clinical and microbiologic correlations and therapeutic implications. Rev Infect Dis 6:147, 1984.
18. Nelson JD. Personal communication, 1987.
19. Barton LL, Dunkle LM, Habib FH. Septic arthritis in childhood: a 13-year review. Am J Dis Child 141:898, 1987.
20. Edwards MS, Baker CJ, Wagner ML, et al. An etiologic shift in infantile osteomyelitis: the emergence of the group B *Streptococcus*. J Pediatr 93:578, 1978.
21. Yousefzadeh DK, Jackson JH. Neonatal and infantile candidal arthritis with or without osteomyelitis: a clinical and radiographical review of 21 cases. Skeletal Radiol 5:77, 1980.
22. Pittard WB III, Thullen JD, Fanaroff AA. Neonatal septic arthritis. J Pediatr 88:621, 1976.
23. Brill PW, Winchester P, Krauss AN, et al. Osteomyelitis in a neonatal intensive care unit. Radiology 13:83, 1979.
24. Johnson DE, Thompson TR, Green TP, et al. Systemic candidiasis in very low-birth-weight infants (< 1,500 grams). Pediatrics 73:138, 1984.
25. Turner RB, Donowitz LG, Hendley JO. Consequences of candidemia for pediatric patients. Am J Dis Child 139:178, 1985.
26. Goldmann DA, Durbin WA Jr, Freeman J. Nosocomial infections in a neonatal intensive care unit. J Infect Dis 144:449, 1981.
27. Townsend TR, Wenzel RP. Nosocomial bloodstream infections in a newborn intensive care unit. Am J Epidemiol 114:73, 1981.
28. Miller A. Personal communication, 1993.
29. Jackson MA, Nelson JD. Etiology and medical management of acute suppurative bone and joint infections in pediatric patients. J Pediatr Orthop 2:313, 1982.
30. Hensey JO, Hart CA, Cooke RWI. Serious infections in a neonatal intensive care unit: a two year survey. J Hyg 95:289, 1985.
31. Lejeune C, Maudiev P, Robin M, et al. Fréquence des infections bactériennes néonatales dans les unites de réanimation et/ou néonatologie. Pediatrie 41:95, 1986.

32. Coto-Cotallo GD, Solis-Sanchez G, Crespo-Hernandez M, et al. Osteomielitis neonatal: estudio de una serie de 35 casos. Ann Esp Pediatr 33:429, 1990.

33. Pomerance J (Los Angeles, CA), Bradley JS (Portland, OR), Hall RT (Kansas City, MO), Cashore WJ (Providence, RI). Personal communications, 1987.

34. Asmar BI. Osteomyelitis in the neonate. Infect Dis Clin North Am 6:117, 1992.

35. Knudsen CJ, Hoffman EB. Neonatal osteomyelitis. J Bone Joint Surg Br 72:846, 1990.

36. Williamson JB, Galasko CSB, Robinson MJ. Outcome after acute osteomyelitis in preterm infants. Arch Dis Child 65:1060, 1990.

37. Baitch A. Recent observations of acute suppurative arthritis. Clin Orthop 22:157, 1962.

38. Obletz BE. Suppurative arthritis of the hip joint in premature infants. Clin Orthop 22:27, 1962.

39. Ross DW. Acute suppurative arthritis of the hip in premature infants. JAMA 156:303, 1954.

40. Thomson J, Lewis IC. Osteomyelitis in the newborn. Arch Dis Child 25:273, 1950.

41. Weissberg ED, Smith AL, Smith DH. Clinical features of neonatal osteomyelitis. Pediatrics 53:505, 1974.

42. Kumari S, Bhargava SK, Baijal VN, et al. Neonatal osteomyelitis: a clinical and follow-up study. Indian J Pediatr 15:393, 1978.

43. Deshpande PG, Wagle SU, Mehta SD, et al. Neonatal osteomyelitis and septic arthritis. Indian J Pediatr 27:453, 1990.

44. Brill PW, Winchester P, Krauss AN, et al. Osteomyelitis in a neonatal intensive care unit. Radiology 131:83, 1979.

45. Wong M, Isaacs D, Howman-Giles R, Uren R. Clinical and diagnostic features of osteomyelitis in the first three months of life. Pediatr Infect Dis 14:1047, 1995.

46. Freedman RM, Ingram DL, Gross I, et al. A half century of neonatal sepsis at Yale: 1928 to 1978. Am J Dis Child 135:140, 1981.

47. Dillehunt RB. Osteomyelitis in infants. Surg Gynecol Obstet 61:96, 1935.

48. Dunham EC. Septicemia in the newborn. Am J Dis Child 45:230, 1933.

49. Green WT, Shannon JG. Osteomyelitis of infants: a disease different from osteomyelitis of older children. Arch Surg 32:462, 1936.

50. Aractingi T-R. Etude de 32 cas d'ostéomyélite du nouveauné. Rev Chir Orthop 47:50, 1961.

51. Dennison WM, MacPherson DA. Haematogenous osteitis of infancy. Arch Dis Child 27:375, 1952.

52. DeWet IS. Acute osteomyelitis and suppurative arthritis of infants. S Afr Med J 28:81, 1954.

53. Hutter CG. New concepts of osteomyelitis in the newborn infant. J Pediatr 32:522, 1948.

54. Lindell L, Parkkulainen KV. Osteitis in infancy and early childhood: with special reference to neonatal osteitis. Ann Paediatr Fenn 6:34, 1960.

55. Kienitz M, Schulte M. Problematik bakterieller Infectionen des Früh- und Neuegeborenen. Munch Med Wochenschr 109:70, 1967.

56. Wolman G. Acute osteomyelitis in infancy. Acta Paediatr Scand 45:595, 1956.

57. Blanche DW. Osteomyelitis in infants. J Bone Joint Surg Am 34:71, 1952.

58. Howard JB, McCracken GH Jr. The spectrum of group B streptococcal infections in infancy. Am J Dis Child 128:815, 1974.

59. Memon IA, Jacobs NM, Yeh TF, et al. Group B streptococcal osteomyelitis and septic arthritis: its occurrence in infants less than 2 months old. Am J Dis Child 133:921, 1979.

60. Omene JA, Odita JC. Clinical and radiological features of neonatal septic arthritis. Trop Geogr Med 31:207, 1979.

61. Choma TJ, Davlin LB, Wagner JS. Iliac osteomyelitis in the newborn presenting as nonspecific musculoskeletal sepsis. Orthopedics 17:632, 1994.

62. Barton LL, Villar RG, Rice SA. Neonatal group B streptococcal vertebral osteomyelitis. Pediatrics 98:459, 1996.

63. Speer CP, Hauptmann D, Stubbe P, et al. Neonatal septicemia and meningitis in Göttingen, West Germany. Pediatr Infect Dis 4:36, 1985.

64. Karpuch J, Goldberg M, Kohelet D. Neonatal bacteremia: a 4-year prospective study. Isr J Med Sci 19:963, 1983.

65. Lequier L, Robinson J, Vaudry W. Sternotomy infection with Mycoplasma hominis in a neonate. Pediatr Infect Dis J 14:1010, 1995.

66. Gjuric G, Prislin-Muskic M, Nikolic E, Zurga B. Ureaplasma urealyticum osteomyelitis in a very low birth weight infant. Perinat Med 22:79, 1994.

67. Scott JES. Intestinal obstruction in the newborn associated with peritonitis. Arch Dis Child 38:120, 1963.

68. Seeler RA, Hahn K. Jaundice in urinary tract infections in infancy. Am J Dis Child 118:553, 1969.

69. Bayer AS, Chow AW, Louie JS, et al. Gram-negative bacillary septic arthritis: clinical, radiographic, therapeutic, and prognostic features. Semin Arthritis Rheum 7:123, 1977.

70. Peters W, Irving J, Letts M. Long-term effects of neonatal bone and joint infection on adjacent growth plates. J Pediatr Orthop 12:806, 1992.

71. Levy HL, O'Connor JF, Ingall D. Neonatal osteomyelitis due to Proteus mirabilis. JAMA 202:582, 1967.

72. Müller WD, Urban C, Haidvogel M, et al. Septische Arthritis und Osteomyelitis als Komplikation neonataler Intensivpflege. Paediatr Paedol 14:469, 1979.

73. Bogdanovich A. Neonatal arthritis due to Proteus vulgaris. Arch Dis Child 23:65, 1948.

74. Omene JA, Odita JC, Okolo AA. Neonatal osteomyelitis in Nigerian infants. Pediatr Radiol 14:318, 1984.

75. Choi IH, Pizzutillo PD, Bowen JR, et al. Sequelae and reconstruction after septic arthritis of the hip in infants. J Bone Joint Surg Am 72:1150, 1990.

76. Berant M, Kahana D. Klebsiella osteomyelitis in a newborn. Am J Dis Child 118:634, 1969.

77. White AA, Crelin ES, McIntosh S. Septic arthritis of the hip joint secondary to umbilical artery catheterization associated with transient femoral and sciatic neuropathy. Clin Orthop 100:190, 1974.

78. Nathanson I, Giacoia GP. Klebsiella osteoarthritis in prematurity: complication of umbilical artery catheterization. NY State J Med 79:2077, 1979.

79. Voss HV, Göbel U, Kemperdick H, et al. Enterobacter-Osteomyelitis bei zwei Säuglingen. Klin Paediatr 187:465, 1975.

80. Gordon SL, Maisels MJ, Robbins WJ. Multiple joint infections with Enterobacter cloacae. Clin Orthop 125:136, 1977.

81. Levinsky RJ. Two children with Pseudomonas osteomyelitis: the paucity of systemic symptoms may lead to delay in diagnosis. Clin Pediatr 14:288, 1975.

82. Gajzago D, Gottche O. Salmonella suipestifer infections in childhood. Am J Dis Child 63:15, 1942.

83. Konzert W. Über ein Salmonella-Osteomyelitis im Rahmen einer Salmonella-typhimurium Epidemia auf einer Neugeborenen Station. Wien Klin Wochenschr 81:713, 1969.

84. Tur AJ, Gartoch OO. Ein Fall von Erkrankung eines frühgeborenen Kindes im ersten Lebensmonate an multiplier Arthritis durch den Bacillus suipestifer. Z Kinderheilkd 56:696, 1934.

85. Adeyokunnu AA, Hendrickse RG. *Salmonella* osteomyelitis in childhood: a report of 63 cases seen in Nigerian children of whom 57 had sickle cell anemia. Arch Dis Child 55:175, 1980.

86. Kohen DP. Neonatal gonococcal arthritis: three cases and review of the literature. Pediatrics 53:436, 1974.

87. Gregory JE, Chison JL, Meadows AT. Short case report: gonococcal arthritis in an infant. Br J Vener Dis 48:306, 1972.

88. Cooperman MB. End results of gonorrheal arthritis: a review of seventy cases. Am J Surg 5:241, 1928.

89. Nabarro D. Congenital Syphilis. London, Edward Arnold, 1954.

90. Zenker PN, Berman SM. Congenital syphilis: trends and recommendations for evaluation and management. Pediatr Infect Dis J 10:516, 1991.

91. Brion LP, Manuli M, Rai B, et al. Long-bone radiographic abnormalities as a sign of active congenital syphilis in asymptomatic newborns. Pediatrics 88:1037, 1991.

92. Hughesdon MR. Congenital tuberculosis. Arch Dis Child 21:121, 1946.

93. Mallet R, Ribierre M, Labrune B, et al. Diffuse bony tuberculosis in the newborn (spina ventosa generalisata). Semaine Hôp Paris 44:36, 1968.

94. Nelson DL, Hable KA, Matsen JM. *Proteus mirabilis* osteomyelitis in two neonates following needle puncture. Am J Dis Child 125:109, 1973.

95. Asnes RS, Arendar GM. Septic arthritis of the hip: a complication of femoral venipuncture. Pediatrics 38:837, 1966.

96. Chacha PB. Suppurative arthritis of the hip joint in infancy: a persistent diagnostic problem and possible complication of femoral venipuncture. J Bone Joint Surg Am 53:538, 1971.

97. Overturf GD, Balfour G. Osteomyelitis and sepsis: severe complications of fetal monitoring. Pediatrics 55:244, 1975.

98. Plavidal FJ, Werch A. Fetal scalp abscess secondary to intrauterine monitoring. Am J Obstet Gynecol 125:65, 1976.

99. Brook I. Osteomyelitis and bacteremia caused by *Bacteroides fragilis*: a complication of fetal monitoring. Clin Pediatr 19:639, 1980.

100. McGregor JA, McFarren T. Neonatal cranial osteomyelitis: a complication of fetal monitoring. Obstet Gynecol 73:490, 1989.

101. Puczynski MS, Dvonch VM, Menendez CE, et al. Osteomyelitis of the great toe secondary to phlebotomy. Clin Orthop 190:239, 1984.

102. Lilien LD, Harris VJ, Ramamurthy RS, et al. Neonatal osteomyelitis of the calcaneus: complication of heel puncture. J Pediatr 88:478, 1976.

103. Myers MG, McMahon BJ, Koontz FP. Neonatal calcaneous osteomyelitis related to contaminated mineral oil. Clin Microbiol 6:543, 1977.

104. Blumenfeld TA, Turi GK, Blanc WA. Recommended site and depth of newborn heel skin punctures based on anatomical measurements and histopathology. Lancet 1:230, 1979.

105. Borris LC, Helleland H. Growth disturbance of the hind part of the foot following osteomyelitis of the calcaneus in the newborn: a report of two cases. J Bone Joint Surg Am 68:302, 1986.

106. Fernandez-Fanjul JL, Lopez-Sastre J, Coto-Cotallo D, et al. Osteomyelitis des Calcaneus beim Neugeborenen als Folge diagnostischer Fersenpunktionen. Monatsschr Kinderheilkd 127:515, 1979.

107. Bergman I, Wald ER, Meyer JD, et al. Epidural abscess and vertebral osteomyelitis following serial lumbar punctures. Pediatrics 72:476, 1983.

108. Edwards MS, Baker CJ. Median sternotomy wound infections in children. Pediatr Infect Dis 2:105, 1983.

109. Valerio PH. Osteomyelitis as a complication of perinatal fracture of the clavicle. Eur J Pediatr 154:497, 1995.

110. Mohon RT, Mehalic TF, Grimes CK, et al. Infected cephalohematoma and neonatal osteomyelitis of the skull. Pediatr Infect Dis 5:253, 1986.

111. Nightingale LM, Eaton CB, Fruehan AE, et al. Cephalohematoma complicated by osteomyelitis presumed due to *Gardnerella vaginalis*. JAMA 256:1936, 1986.

112. Plavidal FJ, Werch A. Fetal scalp abscess secondary to intrauterine monitoring. Am J Obstet Gynecol 125:65, 1976.

113. Lee PYC. Case report: infected cephalohematoma and neonatal osteomyelitis. J Infect 21:191, 1990.

114. McCarthy D, Walker AHC, Matthews S. Scalp abscesses in the newborn: a discussion of their causation. J Obstet Gynacol Br Emp 59:37, 1952.

115. Ladewig W. Über eine intrauterin entstandene umschriebene Osteomyelitis des Schädeldaches. Virchows Arch Pathol Anat 289:395, 1933.

116. Trueta J. Three types of acute haematogenous osteomyelitis. J Bone Joint Surg Br 41:671, 1959.

117. Todd RM. Septicaemia of the newborn: a clinical study of fifteen cases. Arch Dis Child 23:102, 1948.

118. Svirsky-Fein S, Langer L, Milbauer B, et al. Neonatal osteomyelitis caused by *Candida tropicalis*: report of two cases and review of the literature. J Bone Joint Surg Am 61:455, 1979.

119. Baley JE, Kliegman RM, Fanaroff AA. Disseminated fungal infections in very low-birth-weight infants: clinical manifestations and epidemiology. Pediatrics 73:144, 1984.

120. Randel SN, Tsang BHL, Wung J-T, et al. Experience with percutaneous indwelling peripheral arterial catheterization in neonates. Am J Dis Child 141:848, 1987.

121. Knudsen FU, Petersen S. Neonatal septic osteoarthritis due to umbilical artery catheterisation. Acta Paediatr Scand 66:225, 1977.

122. Lim MO, Gresham EL, Franken EA Jr, et al. Osteomyelitis as a complication of umbilical artery catheterization. Am J Dis Child 131:142, 1977.

123. Rhodes PG, Hall RT, Burry VF, et al. Sepsis and osteomyelitis due to *Staphylococcus aureus* phage type 94 in a neonatal intensive care unit. J Pediatr 88:1063, 1976.

124. deLorimier AA, Haskin D, Massie FS. Mediastinal mass caused by vertebral osteomyelitis. Am J Dis Child 111:639, 1966.

125. Qureshi ME. Osteomyelitis after exchange transfusion. BMJ 1:28, 1971.

126. Simmons PB, Harris LE, Bianco AJ. Complications of exchange transfusion: report of two cases of septic arthritis and osteomyelitis. Mayo Clin Proc 48:190, 1973.

127. Ish-Horowicz MR, McIntyre P, Nade S. Bone and joint infections caused by multiply resistant *Staphylococcus aureus* in a neonatal intensive care unit. Pediatr Infect Dis J 11:82, 1992.

128. Betke K, Richarz H. Nabelsepsis mit Pyelphlebitis, multiple Leberabscessen, Lungenabscessen, und Osteomyelitis. Ausgang in Heilung. Monatsschr Kinderheilkd 105:70, 1957.

129. Fraser J. Discussion on acute osteomyelitis. BMJ 2:605, 1924.

130. Lindblad B, Ekingren K, Aurelius G. The prognosis of acute hematogenous osteomyelitis and its complications during early infancy after the advent of antibiotics. Acta Paediatr Scand 54:24, 1965.

131. Chung SMK. The arterial supply of the developing proximal end of the human femur. J Bone Joint Surg Am 58:961, 1976.

132. Ogden JA. Pediatric osteomyelitis and septic arthritis: the pathology of neonatal disease. Yale J Biol Med 52:423, 1979.

133. Cass JM. *Staphylococcus aureus* infection of the long bones in the newly born. Arch Dis Child 15:55, 1940.

134. Stone S. Osteomyelitis of the long bones in the newborn. Am J Dis Child 64:680, 1942.

135. Ingelrans P, Fontaine G, Lacheretz M, et al. Les ostéoarthrites du nouveau-né et du nourrison: particularités étiologiques, diagnostiques et thérapeutiques: à propos de 35 observations. Lille Med 13:390, 1968.

136. Nicholson JT. Pyogenic arthritis with pathologic dislocation of the hip in infants. JAMA 141:862, 1949.

137. Roberts PH. Disturbed epiphyseal growth at the knee after osteomyelitis in infancy. J Bone Joint Surg Br 52:692, 1970.

138. Curtis PH, Klein L. Destruction of articular cartilage in septic arthritis: I. In vitro studies. J Bone Joint Surg Am 45:797, 1963.

139. Curtis PH, Klein L. Destruction of articular cartilage in septic arthritis: II. In vivo studies. J Bone Joint Surg Am 47:1595, 1965.

140. Obletz BE. Acute suppurative arthritis of the hip in the neonatal period. J Bone Joint Surg Am 42:23, 1960.

141. Glassberg GB, Ozonoff MB. Arthrographic findings in septic arthritis of the hip in infants. Radiology 128:151, 1978.

142. Kaye JJ, Winchester PH, Freiberger RH. Neonatal septic "dislocation" of the hip: true dislocation or pathological epiphyseal separation? Radiology 114:671, 1975.

143. Greengard J. Acute hematogenous osteomyelitis in infancy. Med Clin North Am 30:135, 1946.

144. Chung SMK, Pollis RE. Diagnostic pitfalls in septic arthritis of the hip in infants and children. Clin Pediatr 14:758, 1975.

145. Bressler EL, Conway JJ, Weiss SC. Neonatal osteomyelitis examined by bone scintigraphy. Radiology 152:685, 1984.

146. Clay SA. Osteomyelitis as a cause of brachial plexus neuropathy. Am J Dis Child 136:1054, 1982.

147. Young RSK, Hawkes DL. Pseudopseudoparalysis. Letter to the editor. Am J Dis Child 137:504, 1983.

148. Isaacs D, Bower BD, Moxon ER. Neonatal osteomyelitis presenting as nerve palsy. BMJ 1:1071, 1986.

149. Obando I, Martin E, Alvarez-Aldeau J, et al. Group B *Streptococcus* pelvic osteomyelitis presenting as footdrop in a newborn infant. Pediatr Infect Dis J 10:703, 1991.

150. Lai TK, Hingston J, Scheifele D. Streptococcal neonatal osteomyelitis. Am J Dis Child 134:711, 1980.

151. Ancona RJ, McAuliffe J, Thompson TR, et al. Group B streptococcal sepsis with osteomyelitis and arthritis: its occurrence with acute heart failure. Am J Dis Child 133:919, 1979.

152. McCook TA, Felman AH, Ayoub E. Streptococcal skeletal infections: observations in four infants. AJR 130:465, 1978.

153. Chilton SJ, Aftimos SF, White PW. Diffuse skeletal involvement of streptococcal osteomyelitis in a neonate. Radiology 134:390, 1980.

154. Broughton RA, Edwards MS, Haffar A, et al. Unusual manifestations of neonatal group B streptococcal osteomyelitis. Pediatr Infect Dis 1:410, 1982.

155. Einstein RAJ, Thomas CG Jr. Osteomyelitis in infants. AJR 55:299, 1946.

156. Stack JK, Newman W. Neonatal osteomyelitis. Q Bull Northwestern Univ Med Sch 27:69, 1953.

157. Waldvogel FA, Medoff G, Swartz MN. Osteomyelitis. Clinical Features, Therapeutic Considerations, and Unusual Aspects. Springfield, Ill, Charles C Thomas, 1971.

158. Dich VQ, Nelson JD, Haltalin KC. Osteomyelitis in infants and children: a review of 163 cases. Am J Dis Child 129:1273, 1975.

159. Samilson RL, Bersani FA, Watkins MB. Acute suppurative arthritis in infants and children. Pediatrics 21:798, 1958.

160. Hallel T, Salvati EA. Septic arthritis of the hip in infancy: end result study. Clin Orthop 132:115, 1978.

161. Bennett OM, Namyak SS. Acute septic arthritis of the hip joint in infancy and childhood. Clin Orthop 281:123, 1992.

162. Ekengren K, Bergdahl S, Eriksson M. Neonatal osteomyelitis: radiographic findings and prognosis in relation to site of involvement. Acta Radiol Diagn 23:305, 1982.

163. Mallet JF, Rigault P, Padovani JP, et al. Les cyphoses par spondylodiscite grave du nourrisson et du jeune enfant. Rev Chir Orthop 70:63, 1984.

164. Ammari LK, Offit PA, Campbell AB. Unusual presentation of group B *Streptococcus* osteomyelitis. Pediatr Infect Dis J 11:1066, 1992.

165. Altman N, Harwood-Nash DC, Fitz CR, et al. Evaluation of the infant spine by direct sagittal computed tomography. AJNR Am J Neuroradiol 6:65, 1985.

166. Bolivar R, Kohl S, Pickering LK. Vertebral osteomyelitis in children: report of 4 cases. Pediatrics 62:549, 1978.

167. Bode H, Kunzer W. Dornfortsatzosteomyelitis der Brustwirbel 10 und 11 bei einem Neugeborenen. Klin Paediatr 197:65, 1985.

168. McCook TA, Felman AH, Ayoub E. Streptococcal skeletal infections: Observations in four infections. AJR Am J Roentgenol 130:465, 1978.

169. Ein SH, Shandling B, Humphreys R, et al. Osteomyelitis of the cervical spine presenting as a neurenteric cyst. J Pediatr Surg 23:779, 1988.

170. Halbstein BM. Bone regeneration in infantile osteomyelitis: report of a case with 14-year follow-up. J Bone Joint Surg Am 49:149, 1967.

171. Miller B. Regeneration of the lateral femoral condyle after osteomyelitis in infancy. Clin Orthop 65:163, 1969.

172. Lloyd-Roberts GC. Suppurative arthritis of infancy: some observations upon prognosis and management. J Bone Joint Surg Br 42:706, 1960.

173. Singson RD, Berdon WE, Feldman F, et al. "Missing" femoral condyle: an unusual sequela to neonatal osteomyelitis and septic arthritis. Radiology 161:359, 1986.

174. Potter CMC. Osteomyelitis in the newborn. J Bone Joint Surg Br 36:578, 1954.

175. Troger J, Eissner D, Otte G, et al. Diagnose und Differentialdiagnose der akuten hämatogenen Osteomyelitis des Säuglings. Radiologe 19:99, 1979.

176. Vallcanera A, Moreno-Flores A, Gomez J, Cortina H. Osteochondroma post osteomyelitis. Pediatr Radiol 26:680, 1996.

177. Jaramillo D, Treves ST, Kasser JR, et al. Osteomyelitis and septic arthritis in children. Appropriate use of imaging to guide treatement. Am J Radiol 165:399, 1995.

178. Volberg FM, Sumner TE, Abramson JS, et al. Unreliabil-

ity of radiographic diagnosis of septic hip in children. Pediatrics 74:118, 1984.

179. Perkins MD, Edwards KM, Heller RM, et al. Neonatal group B streptococcal osteomyelitis and suppurative arthritis: outpatient therapy. Clin Pediatr 28:229, 1989.

180. Schauwecker DS, Braunstein EM, Wheat LJ. Diagnostic imaging of osteomyelitis. Infect Dis Clin North Am 4:441, 1990.

181. Moore SG, Bisset GS III, Siegel MJ, et al. Pediatric musculoskeletal MR imaging. Radiology 179:345, 1991.

182. Harris VJ, Meeks W. The frequency of radiolucencies underlying cephalohematomas. Pediatr Radiol 129:391, 1978.

183. Einhorn M, Howard DB, Dagan R. The use of ultrasound in the diagnosis and management of childhood acute hematogenous osteomyelitis. Presented at the 31st Interscience Conference on Antimicrobial Agents and Chemotherapy, Anaheim, Calif, October 1992 (abstract 77).

184. Williamson SL, Seibert JJ, Glasier CM, et al. Ultrasound in advanced pediatric osteomyelitis: a report of 5 cases. Pediatr Radiol 21:288, 1991.

185. Abiri MM, Kirpekar M, Ablow RC. Osteomyelitis: detection with US. Radiology 172:509, 1989.

186. Zeiger MM, Dorr U, Schulz RD. Ultrasonography of hip joint effusions. Skeletal Radiol 16:607, 1987.

187. Velkes S, Ganel A, Chechick A. Letter to the editor. Clin Orthop 260:309, 1990.

188. Rubin LP, Wallach MT, Wood BP. Radiological case of the month. Arch Pediatr Adolesc Med 150:217, 1996.

189. Riebel TW, Nasir R, Nazarenko O. The value of sonography in the detection of osteomyelitis. Pediatr Radiol 26:291, 1996.

190. Wright NB, Abbott GT, Carty HML. Ultrasound in children with osteomyelitis. Clin Radiol 50:623, 1995.

191. Harcke HT Jr. Bone imaging in infants and children: a review. J Nucl Med 19:324, 1978.

192. Ash JM, Gilday DL. The futility of bone scanning neonatal osteomyelitis: concise communication. J Nucl Med 21:417, 1980.

193. Gilday DL, Paul DJ. Diagnosis of osteomyelitis in children by combined blood pool and bone imaging. Radiology 117:331, 1975.

194. Canale ST, Harkness RM, Thomas PA, et al. Does aspiration of bones and joints affect results of later bone scanning? J Pediatr Orthop 5:23, 1985.

195. Traughber PD, Manaster BJ, Murphy K, et al. Negative bone scans of joints after aspiration or arthrography: experimental studies. AJR Am J Roentgenol 146:87, 1986.

196. Herndon WA, Alexieva BT, Schwindt ML, et al. Nuclear imaging for musculoskeletal infections in children. J Pediatr Orthop 5:343, 1985.

197. Lewin JS, Rosenfield NS, Hoffer PB, et al. Acute osteomyelitis in children: combined Tc-99m and Ga-67 imaging. Radiology 158:795, 1986.

198. Berkowitz ID, Wenzel W. "Normal" technetium bone scans in patients with acute osteomyelitis. Am J Dis Child 134:828, 1980.

199. Handmaker H, Giammona ST. Improved early diagnosis of acute inflammatory skeletal-articular diseases in children: a two-radiopharmaceutical approach. Pediatrics 73:661, 1984.

200. Melson GL, McDaniel RC, Southern PM, et al. In vitro effects of iodinated arthrographic contrast media on bacterial growth. Radiology 112:593, 1974.

201. Cole WG, Dalziel RE, Leitl S. Treatment of acute osteomyelitis in childhood. J Bone Joint Surg Br 64:218, 1982.

202. Rasool MN, Govender S. The skeletal manifestations of congenital syphilis: a review of 197 cases. J Bone Joint Surg Br 71:752, 1989.

203. Hiva SK, Ganapati JB, Patel JB. Early congenital syphilis: clinico-radiologic features in 202 patients. Sex Transm Dis 12:177, 1985.

204. McLean S. The roentgenographic and pathologic aspects of congenital osseous syphillis. Am J Dis Child 41:130, 363, 607, 887, 1128, 1411, 1931.

205. Ewerbeck V, Bolkenius M, Braun A, et al. Knochentumoren und tumorähnliche Veränderungen im Neugeborenen—und Säuglingsalter. Z Orthop 123:918, 1985.

206. Meyers S, Lonon W, Shannon, K. Suppurative bursitis in early childhood. Pediatr Infect Dis 3:156, 1984.

207. Brian MJ, O'Ryan M, Waagner D. Prepatellar bursitis in an infant caused by group B Streptococcus. Pediatr Infect Dis J 11:502, 1992.

208. Keller MA, Sellers BB Jr, Melish ME, et al. Systemic candidiasis in infants: a case presentation and literature review. Am J Dis Child 131:1260, 1977.

209. Reiser VM, Rupp N, Färber D. Röntgenologische Befunde bei der septischen Candida-Arthritis. Rofo 129:335, 1978.

210. Businco L, Iannaccone G, Del Principe D, et al. Disseminated arthritis and osteitis by Candida albicans in a two month old infant receiving parenteral nutrition. Acta Paediatr Scand 66:393, 1977.

211. Rudolph AJ, Singleton EB, Rosenberg HS, et al. Osseous manifestations of the congenital rubella syndrome. Am J Dis Child 110:428, 1965.

212. Merten DF, Gooding CA. Skeletal manifestations of congenital cytomegalic inclusion disease. Radiology 95:333, 1970.

213. Jenson HB, Robert MF. Congenital cytomegalovirus infection with osteolytic lesions: use of DNA hybridization in diagnosis. Clin Pediatr 26:448, 1987.

214. Chalhub EG, Baenziger J, Feigen RD, et al. Congenital herpes simplex type II infection with extensive hepatic calcification, bone lesions and cataracts: complete postmortem examination. Dev Med Child Neurol 19:527, 1977.

215. Madsen ET. Fractures of the extremities in the newborn. Acta Obstet Gynecol Scand 34:41, 1955.

216. Caffey J. Pediatric X-ray Diagnosis, 6th ed. Chicago, Year Book Medical Publishers, 1972.

217. Park H-M, Kernek CB, Robb JA. Early scintigraphic findings of occult femoral and tibial fractures in infants. Clin Nucl Med 13:271, 1988.

218. Marshall GS, Edwards KM, Wadlington WB. Sporadic congenital Caffey's disease. Clin Pediatr 26:177, 1987.

219. Ravenel SD. Cellulitis from extravasation of calcium gluconate simulating osteomyelitis. Am J Dis Child 137:402, 1983.

220. Ringel RE, Haney PJ, Brenner JI, et al. Periosteal changes secondary to prostaglandin administration. J Pediatr 103:251, 1983.

221. Ditkowsky SP, Goldman A, Barnett H, et al. Normal periosteal reactions and associated soft-tissue findings. Clin Pediatr 9:515, 1970.

222. Nelson JD. Follow up: the bacterial etiology and antibiotic management of septic arthritis in infants and children. Pediatrics 50:437, 1972.

223. Cooper GI, Hopkins CC. Rapid diagnosis of intravascular catheter-associated infection by direct Gram staining of catheter segments. N Engl J Med 312:1142, 1985.

224. Schauf V, Deveikis A, Riff L, et al. Antibiotic-killing kinetics of group B streptococci. J Pediatr 89:194, 1976.

225. Chambers HF, Hackbarth CJ, Drake TA, et al. Endocar-

ditis due to methicillin-resistant *Staphylococcus aureus* in rabbits: expression of resistance to β-lactam antibiotics in vivo and in vitro. J Infect Dis 149:894, 1984.

226. Sann L, Bienvenu F, Bienvenu J, et al. Evolution of serum prealbumin, C-reactive protein, and orosomucoid in neonates with bacterial infection. J Pediatr 105:977, 1984.

227. Philip AGS. Acute-phase proteins in neonatal infection. J Pediatr 105:940, 1984.

228. Fajardo JE, Bass JW, Lugo EJ, et al. Oral dicloxacillin for the treatment of neonatal osteomyelitis. Letter to the editor. Am J Dis Child 138:991, 1984.

229. Schwartz GJ, Hegyi T, Spitzer A. Subtherapeutic dicloxacillin levels in a neonate: possible mechanisms. J Pediatr 89:310, 1976.

230. Nelson JD. Options for outpatient management of serious infections. Pediatr Infect Dis J 11:175, 1992.

231. Sudela KD. Nursing aspects of pediatric home infusion therapy for the treatment of serious infections. Semin Pediatr Infect Dis 1:306, 1990.

232. Dunkle LM. Towards optimum management of serious focal infections: the model of suppurative arthritis. Pediatr Infect Dis J 8:195, 1989.

233. Pittard WB III, Thullen JD, Fanaroff AA. Neonatal septic arthritis. J Pediatr 88:621, 1976.

234. Howard PJ. Sepsis in normal and premature infants with localization in the hip joint. Pediatrics 20:279, 1957.

235. Borella L, Goobar JE, Summitt RL, et al. Septic arthritis in childhood. J Pediatr 62:742, 1963.

236. Halder D, Seng QB, Malik AS, Choo KE. Neonatal septic arthritis. Southeastern Asian J Tropical Med Public Health 27:600, 1996.

237. Gilmour WN. Acute hematogenous osteomyelitis. J Bone Joint Surg Br 44:841, 1962.

238. Allibone EC, Mills CP. Osteomyelitis of the premaxilla. Arch Dis Child 36:562, 1961.

239. Boete G. Zur Frage der Spätschäden nach Kieferosteomyelitis von Säuglingen und Kleinkindern. Arch Klin Exp Ohren Nasen Kehlkopfheilkd 187:674, 1966.

240. Cavanagh F. Osteomyelitis of the superior maxilla in infants: a report on 24 personally treated cases. BMJ 1:468, 1960.

241. McCash CR, Rowe NL. Acute osteomyelitis of the maxilla in infancy. J Bone Joint Surg Br 35:22, 1953.

242. Wilensky AO. The pathogenesis and treatment of acute osteomyelitis of the jaws in nurslings and infants. Am J Dis Child 43:431, 1932.

243. Bass MH. Acute osteomyelitis of the superior maxilla in young infants. Am J Dis Child 35:65, 1928.

244. Webb JF. Newborn infants and breast abscesses of staphylococcal origin. Can Med Assoc J 70:382, 1954.

245. Wong SK, Wilhelmus KR. Infantile maxillary osteomyelitis. J Pediatr Ophthalmol Strabismus 23:153, 1986.

246. Burnard ED. Proptosis as the first sign of orbital sepsis in the newborn. Br J Ophthalmol 43:9, 1959.

247. Hahlbrock KH. Über die Oberkieferosteomyelitis des Säuglings. Klin Monatsbl Augenheilkd 145:744, 1964.

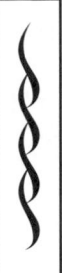

C H A P T E R   2 4

Bacterial Infections of the Urinary Tract

SARAH S. LONG, M.D., and JEROME O. KLEIN, M.D.

In 1918, Helmholz recognized the cryptogenic nature and underdiagnosis of urinary tract infection (UTI) in the newborn.[1] His observations are still true today. There are no specific signs of UTI in the newborn; the clinical presentation can vary from fever and other signs of septicemia to minimal changes such as alteration in feeding habits or poor gain in weight, or the infant may be without signs. The diagnosis of UTI in the neonate is made only by the examination and culture of a properly obtained specimen of urine.

The reported incidence, clinical manifestations, and prognosis of UTI in neonates have varied significantly. There are at least two reasons for discrepant results obtained in studies of UTI: different criteria have been used to define UTI, and infants with different characteristics have been studied. Before 1960, clean-voided specimens were used almost exclusively for examination and culture of urine. It is now clear that contamination is frequent when this method is used; Schlager and co-workers observed that 16 cultures of urine obtained by bag collection from 98 healthy newborns yielded greater than 10^4 colonies/ml of urine, with organisms that were found also on periurethral skin.[2] The only reliable method for obtaining urine for bacteriologic study is percutaneous aspiration or urethral catheterization of bladder urine.

In the neonate, bacterial infections of the kidney and urinary tract are usually acquired at or after delivery. Fungal infections develop as opportunistic infections, complicating a prolonged nursery course in infants with risk factors such as prematurity and use of intravascular catheters, parenteral alimentation, and broad-spectrum antibiotics, or after indwelling or intermittent catheterization of the urinary tract.[3] Viral infections, including rubella, herpes simplex, and cytomegalovirus, are responsible for in utero infection, although the organisms can be excreted in the urine for months after birth. Bacterial infections of the urinary tract (other than those related to *Neisseria gonorrhoeae*, *Staphylococcus aureus*, and group B *Streptococcus*) are reviewed here. For information

about infection and disease of the kidney and urinary tract caused by other microorganisms, the reader is referred to the chapters on toxoplasmosis, rubella, cytomegalovirus, herpes simplex, syphilis, the mycoplasmas, *Candida*, group B *Streptococcus*, gonorrhea, staphylococcal infection, and neonatal diarrhea (*Salmonella*).

EPIDEMIOLOGY

The incidence of UTI in infants in the first month of life varies from 0.1 to 1% in all infants[4–10] and may be as high as 10% in low-birth-weight infants[11] (Table 24–1). In contrast to the increased incidence of bacteriuria among females in other age groups, infection of the urinary tract in the first 3 months of life is more frequent in males.[2, 4–9, 12–14]

Infection of the urinary tract is usually sporadic, but clusters of cases, closely related in time, have been reported from nurseries in Cleveland[15] and Baltimore.[16] A nursery epidemic caused by *Serratia marcescens* was responsible for UTI and balanitis. The outbreak was caused by contamination of a solution applied to the umbilical cord.[17]

Surveys of infants born in U.S. Army medical centers and subsequently hospitalized for UTI indicate that uncircumcised males have more UTIs than do circumcised males in the first month and in months 2 to 12 of life (Table 24–2).[10, 18, 19] In 1982, Ginsburg and McCracken observed that 95% of 62 infant boys with UTI were uncircumcised.[20] A case-control study performed in 112 infant boys who had suprapubic aspiration or bladder catheterization performed for investigation of acute illness showed that all infants with UTI were uncircumcised, compared with 32% of controls.[21] Infection was associated with anatomic abnormalities in 26% of cases. The records of more than 136,000 boys born in U.S. Army hospitals from 1980 to 1985 were reviewed through the first month of life to compare courses of uncircumcised and circumcised boys.[22] Eighty-eight of

TABLE 24-1
Incidence of Urinary Tract Infections in Newborn Infants: Results of Seven Studies

STUDY[a]	METHODS USED TO OBTAIN URINE	NO. INFECTED/ NO. STUDIED (%)	SEX				BIRTH WEIGHT			
			Male		Female		<2500 g		>2500 g	
			No. Surveyed	No. Infected	No. Surveyed	No. Infected	No. Surveyed	No. Infected	No. Surveyed	No. Infected
Christchurch, N.Z. (4) 1968–1969	CVS, SPA	14/1460 (0.95)	757	11	703	3	N.S.	—	N.S.	—
Göteborg (5) 1960–1966	CVS	75[b]/57,000 (0.14)	N.S.	54	N.S.	21	N.S.	11	N.S.	64
New York (6) 1973[c]	CVS, SPA	12/1042 (1.2)	493	7	549	5	206	6	836	6
Leeds (7) 1967	CVS, SPA	8/600 (1.3)	309	7	291	1	N.S.	0	N.S.	8
Oklahoma City (11) 1974	SPA	10/102 (10)	N.S.	N.S.	N.S.	N.S.	102	10	—	—
Lausanne (8) 1978[c]	CVS, SPA	43/1762[d] (2.4)	1006	26	756	7	634[e]	10	1028[f]	33
Göteborg (9) 1977–1980[g]	CVS, SPA	26/3198 (0.81)	1502	23	1696	3	—	—	—	—
U.S. Army (10) 1975–1984[h]	SPA, Ca	320/422,328 (0.08)	217,116	162	205,212	158	—	—	—	—

[a]Location, reference number, years of study.
[b]Five male infants with infection and suspected or proven obstructive malformation of urinary tract not included.
[c]Date of published report; years of study not provided.
[d]Includes only infants younger than 28 days of age who were admitted to neonatal intensive care unit.
[e]Results reported for premature infants (<259 days' gestation).
[f]Results reported for term infants (≥259 days' gestation).
[g]Results reported for infants 1 wk to 2 mo of age.
[h]Results reported for infants 1 wk to 2 mo of age who were hospitalized.
CVS = clean-voided specimen; SPA = suprapubic aspiration of bladder urine; Ca = catheter; N.S. = not stated.

TABLE 24-2
Incidence of Urinary Tract Infections During the First Year of Life in Infants Born at U.S. Army Hospitals

STUDY LOCATION AND PARAMETERS	FEMALE INFANTS	MALE INFANTS Circumcised	Not Circumcised
Tripler Army Hospital[a]			
January 1982–June 1983			
No. infants	2759	1919	583
No. infants with UTI	13 (0.47%)	4 (0.21%)	24 (4.12%)
Mean age at diagnosis (mo)	2.5	1.4	1.7
Brooke Army Hospital[b]			
January 1980–December 1983			
No. infants	1905	1575	444
No. infants with UTI	8 (0.42%)	0	8 (1.8%)
Mean age at diagnosis (mo)	4.4	—	1.7
U.S. Army Hospital[b]			
January 1975–December 1984			
No. infants	205,212	175,317	41,799
No. infants with UTI	1164 (0.57%)	193 (0.11%)	468 (1.12%)
Mean age at diagnosis (mo)	3.9	2.7	2.5

[a]Data from Wiswell TE, Smith FR, Bass JW. Decreased incidence of urinary tract infection in circumcised males. Pediatrics 75:901–903, 1985.
[b]Data from Wiswell TE, Roscelli JD. Corroborative evidence for the decreased incidence of urinary tract infections in circumcised male infants. Pediatrics 78:96–99, 1986.

35,929 uncircumcised boys (0.24%) had UTI, 33 had concomitant bacteremia, 3 had meningitis, 2 had renal failure, and 2 died. Complications followed 0.19% of 100,157 circumcisions (including 20 UTIs) and were all minor except for three episodes of hemorrhage leading to transfusion. Meta-analysis of nine published studies through 1992 yielded an overall 12-fold increased risk of infection in uncircumcised boys.[23] In 1989, the American Academy of Pediatrics rescinded a 1971 position against circumcision, recognizing relative safety of the procedure and protection against UTI in the first year of life.[24] More recent studies using case-control and cohort design also support an association, although magnitude of risk for uncircumsized males is reduced to three- to seven-fold.[24a, 24b] In 1999, the American Academy of Pediatrics revised the recommendation, citing that although existing scientific evidence demonstrates potential medical benefits of newborn male circumcision, data are not sufficient to recommend its routine performance.[24c] Ritual Jewish circumcision performed on the eighth day of life, when periurethral bacterial colonization has been established, appears to have attendant risk for UTI. An epidemiologic study in Israel revealed excessive UTIs in males only from day 9 to 20 of life (the postcircumcision period).[25]

MICROBIOLOGY

Escherichia coli continues to be responsible for the vast majority of community-acquired infections of the urinary tract in infants younger than 3 months of age, accounting for 90 to 93% of approximately 400 cases in reports from 1990 to 1998.[26–28] Many O serotypes of *E. coli* have been associated with these infections. UTI in neonates was associated with a limited number of O:K:H

serotypes with P fimbria, adhesive capacity, hemolysin production, and serum resistance.[29–31] The serotypes of *E. coli* associated with diarrhea, however, rarely cause UTI. Cultures of urine can be positive in infants with septicemia caused by group B *Streptococcus*, but primary infection of the urinary tract without septicemia is rare (see Chapter 26).[14, 32] The incidence of neonatal UTIs as a complication of intensive care has risen sharply in recent years and occurs in patients with and without urinary catheters.[3] Microbiology of nosocomial UTI is dramatically different from that observed in the 1970s (Table 24–3), with *E. coli* supplanted by other Enterobacteriaceae, *Pseudomonas*, *Enterococcus*, *Candida*, and coagulase-negative staphylococci.[3, 33–35] Multiple pathogens can

TABLE 24-3
Pathogens Responsible for Urinary Tract Infections in Newborn Infants

ORGANISM	FREQUENCY (%) OF ISOLATION OF EACH PATHOGEN 1969–1978[a]	1989–1992[b]
Escherichia coli	75.3	10.5
Klebsiella sp.	13.4	10.5
Enterobacter sp.	1.4	12.3
Enterococcus sp.	2.1	14.0
Coagulase-negative staphylococci	1.4	31.6
Candida sp.	—	12.3
Other	6.4	8.8

[a]Data from 139 patients in nurseries and intensive care nurseries from references 4, 5, 7, and 8.
[b]Data from 50 patients in neonatal intensive care units from references 33 and 34.

occur; Maherzi and colleagues identified more than one bacterial pathogen in 4 of 43 infants with UTI documented by aspiration of bladder urine.[8]

S. aureus and E. coli have been responsible for localized suppurative disease of the urinary tract in the neonate, including prostatitis, orchitis, and epididymitis.[36–41] Other examples of focal disease in the urinary tract include orchitis caused by Pseudomonas aeruginosa[42] and testicular abscess caused by Salmonella enteritidis.[43] Blood cultures are frequently positive in these infants.

Bacteria responsible for infections of the circumcision site are discussed in the section Infections of the Skin and Subcutaneous Tissue in Chapter 25.

PATHOGENESIS

In older children and adults, most UTIs are thought to occur by the ascending route after introduction of bacteria through the urethral meatus. Less frequently, blood-borne infection of the kidney occurs. In the neonate, it is frequently difficult to know whether UTI was the cause or result of bacteremia. The predominance of males among infants younger than 3 months of age with UTI contrasts to the predominance of females in all other age groups. This may reflect increased risk of UTI in young uncircumcised males, increased prevalence of urinary and renal anomalies in males, transient urodynamic dysfunction, and vesicoureteral reflux (VUR) that predominantly affects male infants,[44] and the occasional UTI complicating circumcision. Additionally, bacteremia is more frequent in male infants, and it is likely that hematogenous invasion of the kidney can cause UTI in neonates.

Anatomic or physiologic abnormalities of the urinary tract play a role in the development and consequences of infection in some infants. Obstructive uropathy and vesicoureteral reflux are the most important. Infection is often the first indication of an abnormality. Infection was the presenting sign in half of 40 infants younger than 2 months of age with anomalies of the kidneys or ureters reported in 1980.[45] Congenital obstruction of the urinary tract was diagnosed in 5 of 80 children with UTI studied in Göteborg[5] and in 2 of 60 children studied in Leeds[46]; important radiologic abnormalities of the urinary tract were identified in 10 of 46 male infants and 3 of 13 female infants younger than 3 months of age from 1972 to 1982 in Christchurch, New Zealand.[47] Increasingly, antenatal ultrasonography identifies fetuses with significant anatomic abnormalities, and early neonatal intervention (with prophylactic use of antibiotics with or without surgery) decreases likelihood of infection.

VUR is identified in many infants with UTI who are examined by radiologic techniques. It is frequently the result of infection but also can be a primary defect predisposing to UTI. VUR is not a prerequisite for upper tract infection (i.e., pyelonephritis); fewer than half of children with pyelonephritis by scintigraphy had VUR in two studies.[48, 49] Majd and co-workers found that 23 of 29 (79%) children hospitalized for UTI who were found to have reflux had pyelonephritis by scintig-

raphy; so did 39 of 65 (60%) of children without reflux.[50] VUR can be a congenital abnormality. Fetal ultrasonography demonstrated that 30 of 107 infants with prenatally diagnosed urinary tract abnormalities had reflux, which was the only abnormality found postnatally in 10.[51] Gordon and colleagues observed that 16 of 25 infants with dilatation of the fetal urinary tract had reflux, 79% of whom had grade 3 to 5 severity.[52] Thirty-nine urinary tract abnormalities detected prenatally were compared with 46 urinary tract abnormalities found after first UTI in Austrian infants.[53] Obstructive lesions and multicystic dysplastic malformations of the kidneys accounted for 90% of all prenatally diagnosed malformations, and reflux accounted for only 10%. In contrast, reflux accounted for 59% of abnormalities detected after the first UTI. VUR detected prenatally has a male/female sex distribution of 6:1 (unlike VUR detected after UTI when females predominate[54]), may be determined developmentally by the site of the origin of the ureteral bud from the wolffian duct, and in severe cases can be associated with congenital renal damage consisting of global parenchymal loss (so-called reflux nephropathy).[55] Gunn and colleagues performed ultrasound examinations of 3228 fetuses: no renal tract abnormalities were detected before 28 weeks' gestation.[56] Subsequently, 3856 fetuses were examined by ultrasonography after 28 weeks of gestation. Urinary tract anomalies were identified in 313 fetuses: 15 had major structural abnormalities, all of which were confirmed postnatally; 298 (7.7% of fetuses) had dilated renal pelvis with normal bladder, the majority of which resolved spontaneously; however, 40 of these cases were confirmed postnatally to be due to serious abnormalities (usually obstruction or VUR).[57] Isolated mild renal pyelectasis (i.e., less than 10 mm) in fetuses and neonates is likely to be transient, unassociated with pathology or risk for UTI.[57a, 57b] VUR can be hereditary. Scott and co-workers performed cystography on 186 neonates born into families with known or probable VUR; 38 (20%) had VUR compared with an expected 1 to 2% of the general population.[58]

The relative contributions of reflux and infection in causing renal damage are debated, but there is growing consensus that postnatal damage correlates with episodes of infection. Follow-up of 108 cases of VUR diagnosed prenatally showed that when infections were prevented, 42% of those followed medically with VUR grade 4 or greater resolved and 16% improved within 18 months, and renal damage did not progress in any case.[55] In another study, patients identified with VUR in early childhood were followed prospectively for an average of 9.5 years.[58a] Either elimination of recurring UTIs or surgical correction of reflux prevented development of new renal scars. Four patients with unobstructed high-grade sterile reflux were followed for 6 to 10 years; none developed cortical scars.

Patrick suggested that infants born to mothers who were bacteriuric during pregnancy were more susceptible to UTI than infants born to mothers without bacteriuria.[59] Although the initial results were provocative, the group of infants used as controls was not studied at the same time as the patients, and a subsequent study[60] failed to corroborate the findings.

Bacterial virulence factors are likely to play an important role in the pathogenesis of UTIs. Strains of *E. coli* causing UTI are a selected sample of the fecal flora. Pyelonephritic isolates belong to a restricted number of serotypes, are resistant to the bactericidal effect of serum, attach to uroepithelial cells, and produce hemolysins.[61] Pili on the bacterial cell surface that adhere to specific receptors on epithelial cells may play a role in development of UTI.[29] Data from Stockholm,[29] Dallas,[30] and Copenhagen[31] suggest that some of these features of pyelonephritic strains of *E. coli* can be demonstrated in UTIs in newborns.

The increased rate of UTIs in the uncircumcised male is likely to be associated with periurethral bacterial flora. During the first 6 months of life, uncircumcised males have significantly higher total urethral bacterial colony counts and more frequent isolation and higher colony counts of uropathogenic organisms such as *E. coli*, *Klebsiella-Enterobacter* species, *Proteus*, and *Pseudomonas*.[62] With increasing age, the foreskin is more easily retracted and penile hygiene improves; by 12 months of age, both the excessive periuretheral flora and the frequency of UTI in uncircumcised males almost disappear.[19, 62]

Natural defenses in the urinary tract include antibacterial properties of urine, antiadherence mechanisms, mechanical effects of urinary flow and micturition, presence of phagocytic cells, antibacterial properties of the urinary tract mucosa, and immune mechanisms.[63] There is scant knowledge about these mechanisms in the newborn.

PATHOLOGY

The histologic appearance of acute pyelonephritis in newborns is similar to that in the adult.[64] Polymorphonuclear leukocytes are present in the glomeruli, the tubules, and the interstitial tissues. The renal pelvis can show signs of acute inflammation, with loss of the lining epithelium and necrosis. Focal suppuration can be present in the kidney, prostate, or testis. In disease of longer duration, the interstitial tissue is infiltrated with lymphocytes, plasma cells, and eosinophils. The number of glomeruli may be decreased, and some may be hyalinized. The epithelium of tubules is atrophic, and the lumen is filled with colloid casts. Pericapsular fibrosis is present in some infants. If the child dies within 6 months, there is little scarring or contraction of the kidney. Reversible hydronephrosis and hydroureter are observed manifestations of acute pyelonephritis in the neonate who has no anatomic abnormality or VUR. It is postulated that bacteria and endotoxins inhibit ureteral peristalsis.

Suppurative foci, such as otitis media, pneumonia, and meningitis, also can be seen in infants dying of acute infection of the urinary tract. Hepatocellular damage and bile stasis may be noted in liver sections from jaundiced infants.[65]

CLINICAL MANIFESTATIONS

The signs of UTI in neonates are varied and nonspecific. In general, five patterns are observed: (1) septicemia associated with early-onset (within the first 5 days of life) or late-onset (after 5 days of age) disease (see Chapter 21); (2) acute onset of fever without apparent source; (3) insidious illness marked by low-grade fever or failure to gain weight; (4) no apparent signs; and (5) localized signs of infection, including balanitis, prostatitis, urethritis, and orchitis.

The most frequent signs of acute UTI are fever or signs associated with septicemia or both (see Chapter 21 and Table 24–4).[4, 5, 7, 8] In infants with less acute infection, the presenting signs include poor weight gain or anorexia. Diarrhea and vomiting are common in these infants but do not appear to be the only factors responsible for failure to thrive. Fever is present in about half of such infants, although it may not be a presenting sign. Lethargy, irritability, seizures, and meningismus (in the absence of purulent meningitis) occur in some infants.[5] Enlargement of the liver and spleen and distention of the abdomen can be present. The kidneys may be enlarged or abnormal in shape or position, and anomalies of the urethra and penis also can occur. Signs associated with renal anomalies (e.g., a single umbilical artery, supernumerary nipples, spina bifida, and low-set ears) are seen in some infants. Jaundice is an important feature of UTI and may be the presenting sign[65–67]; it is frequently sudden in onset and clears rapidly after adequate antimicrobial therapy. Many infants with UTI and jaundice have positive blood cultures.[16, 67] Hyperbilirubinemia as the only manifestation of UTI in otherwise healthy neonates must be rare, however. Of 306 infants admitted to hospital within 21 days of birth solely because of indirect hyperbilirubinemia (mean peak serum bilirubin level 18.5 mg/dl), 90% were breast fed and none had a positive culture of urine or blood.[68] A reported case of severe methemoglobinemia observed in a 3-week-old infant with *E. coli* UTI was postulated to be caused by nitrite-forming bacteria, but concurrent diarrhea, dehydration, and acidosis may have been precipitating factors.[69] Hyperammonemic encephalopathy due to *Proteus* infection in children with urinary tract obstruction or atony also has been described.[70]

UTI without apparent signs of illness also can occur.

TABLE 24–4

Clinical Manifestations of Urinary Tract Infections in Newborn Infants as Described in Selected Reports[a]

CLINICAL MANIFESTATION	% OF INFANTS WITH MANIFESTATIONS[b]
Failure to thrive	50
Fever	39
Vomiting	37
Diarrhea	25
Cyanosis	23
Jaundice	18
Irritability or lethargy	17

[a]Data from references 4, 5, 7, and 8.
[b]When sign was not mentioned in report, the number of infants in the report was removed from the denominator used to determine percentage of infants with manifestation.

In some studies, infection detected during screening surveys was more frequent than infection identified after signs of illness[4, 6, 9, 71]; infection was detected in 9 of 14 infants in a screening program in Christchurch[4] and in 8 of 10 premature infants whose UTI was diagnosed in a program in Oklahoma City.[11]

Abscesses of the prostate, testis, or epididymis usually present as signs of septicemia, including fever, vomiting, and diarrhea.[36–43] Local signs of inflammation, including tenderness and swelling over the surface of the infected organ, may be present. Urinary retention occurs in infants with prostatitis.[38, 39] Renal abscess is rare in the neonate; one case report in a neonate (with congenital nephrosis) has been published.[72]

UTI should be considered in the differential diagnosis of unexplained fever in early infancy. UTI was frequent in infants younger than 3 months of age with nonspecific signs of illness brought to the walk-in clinic at the Boston City Hospital; 3 of 9 febrile children ($> 38.9°$ C) and 2 of 20 children with little or no temperature elevation ($< 38.9°$ C) had UTI.[73] Of 182 infants younger than 3 months of age presenting with fever at the Tripler Army Hospital in Hawaii, UTI was the most frequent bacterial infection; 20 of the infants (including 14 males) had UTI.[74] A 1-year study of children presenting to the emergency department of the Beilenson Hospital in Tel Aviv included 47 infants younger than 1 month of age; 8 of the infants had UTI, and 3 of these 8 also had bacteremia.[75] In Crain and Gershel's prospective study of 442 New York infants younger than 8 weeks of age with temperatures of 38.1° C (100.6° F) or more, 7.5% had UTI.[26] Of similarly aged infants studied by Hoberman and colleagues in Pittsburgh with temperatures of 38.3° C (101° F) or less, 14 of 306 (4.6%) infants had UTI.[76] Rate of circumcision in the population can effect the rate of UTI. In the New York study, prevalence of UTI in boys (82% of whom were not circumcised) was 12.4%. In the Pittsburgh study, prevalence of UTI in boys (2% of whom were not circumcised) was only 2.9%. In a study of 2411 febrile children younger than 24 months of age evaluated in an emergency department in Philadelphia, history of malodorous urine, prior history of UTI, and finding of abdominal tenderness were significantly associated with the diagnosis of UTI; findings, however, were present in less than 10% of infected infants and only 8 to 13% of infants with findings had UTI confirmed.[28] In a retrospective study of 354 Boston infants younger than 24 months of age with UTI confirmed, irritability and decreased appetite were each reported in half of children; diarrhea, vomiting, lethargy, and congestion in one fourth; and malodorous urine, apparent dysuria, frequency of urination, and abdominal pain in less than 10%.[14]

DIAGNOSIS

Infection of the urinary tract is defined as the presence of bacteria in urine that was obtained without contamination from the urethra or external genitalia. UTI should be considered in all infants older than 3 days of age who have fever or other signs of septicemia or who have subtle and nonspecific signs of "failure to thrive" during the first months of life. At present, no clinical finding or simple laboratory test adequately defines the location of infection in the urinary tract of the infant. It is assumed that bacteriuria in the neonate indicates infection throughout the urinary tract (including the kidney).

Culture of Urine

Suprapubic needle aspiration of bladder urine is the most reliable technique for identifying bacteriuria. Although a negative result from culture of bag-collected urine indicates that the urine is sterile, 12 to 21% of bag-collected specimens have results that are indeterminate or positive (10^4 or greater colonies/ml),[2, 26] and positive results must be verified by aspiration of bladder urine or by catheterization. There is infrequently time for this stepwise approach before instituting therapy. The technique of needle aspiration of the bladder has been used extensively, and the cumulative experience indicates that it is technically simple and safe and that it causes minimal discomfort to the infant.[77, 78] Although most infected urine specimens will have bacterial colony counts of 10^5/ml or greater, any bacterial growth in urine obtained by suprapubic aspiration is believed to be significant. Morbidity associated with suprapubic aspiration is minimal. Transient gross hematuria has been reported in 0.6% of 654 infants.[78] Gross bleeding that ceased only after cauterization was reported in one case.[79] Perforation of the bowel occurred in two cases, but this complication is avoided if the bladder is defined by palpation or percussion.[80] Hematoma of the anterior wall of the bladder,[81, 82] peritonitis,[83] and anaerobic bacteremia[84] also have been reported after suprapubic aspiration. These reports warranted publication because the cases are very uncommon. This should not deter the physician from using this technique for infants with suggested septicemia. However, suprapubic aspiration should not be performed if the infant has recently voided, has abdominal distention, has poorly defined anomalies of the urinary tract, or has a hematologic abnormality that might result in hemorrhage.

Suprapubic aspiration of bladder urine should be performed at least 1 hour after the patient has voided. The infant should lie supine, with the lower extremities held in a frog-leg position. The suprapubic area is cleansed with iodine and alcohol. A 20-gauge, 1½-inch needle attached to a syringe is used to pierce the abdominal wall and bladder approximately 1 inch above the symphysis pubis. The needle is directed caudally toward the fundus of the bladder, and urine is aspirated gently. Vigorous aspiration should be avoided because the mucosa can block the needle opening. The aspirated urine is sent to the laboratory immediately in a sterile tube. If the child urinates during the procedure or if it cannot be done properly for other reasons, aspiration should be repeated after 1 to 2 hours. Ultrasound may be useful in detecting the presence of urine in the bladder before suprapubic aspiration[85, 86]; with ultrasound, guided acquisition of urine improved from 60 to 96.4%.[86]

When it is important to obtain an immediate sample

of urine and suprapubic aspiration cannot be performed for technical reasons (lack of experience of the physician, dehydration, or recent voiding), catheterization of the bladder is appropriate. The incidence of infection related to catheterization in infants is unknown. Urine for culture should be transported to the laboratory as soon as possible, but if a delay is unavoidable, the specimen is refrigerated. Colony counts of 10^3/ml of urine obtained by catheter may represent significant bacteriuria in this age group.[87] In multiple studies of young children evaluated because of fever (relatively few of whom were neonates), approximately 80% of those with bacteriuria had colony counts of 10^5/ml or greater. Significant pyuria, elevated serum level of C-reactive protein, isolation of a single enteric organism, and abnormality on renal scintigraphy were each decreasingly associated with lower colony counts, with only rare positive tests in those children with colony counts of less than 10^4/ml.[13, 14, 27, 88]

Culture of Blood and Cerebrospinal Fluid

Because bacteremia and meningitis frequently accompany UTI, cultures of the blood and cerebrospinal fluid should be obtained before therapy for UTI is begun if the neonate has fever or any signs of illness. Blood (but not necessarily cerebrospinal fluid) should also be obtained for culture from the neonate with UTI but without specific or nonspecific signs of infection. In the Göteborg studies,[5] lumbar puncture was performed before therapy in 31 neonates with UTI: 6 infants had purulent meningitis, and in 9 infants the cerebrospinal fluid was sterile but pleocytosis (22 to 200 white blood cells [WBCs] per mm^3) was also present. Blood was obtained for culture in 32 infants and was positive in 12. Bacteremia was present in 11 of 35 (31%) Dallas infants younger than 30 days of age with UTI. The infants had been considered healthy when discharged from the nursery and were evaluated because of fever. Older infants with UTI were less likely to be bacteremic; positive cultures of blood occurred in 5 of 24 infants (21%) with UTI aged 1 to 2 months, 2 of 14 infants (14%) aged 2 to 3 months, and 1 of 18 infants (5.5%) aged 3 months or older.[20] Similarly, in Boston, bacteremia was present in 17 of 80 (21%) of febrile infants with UTI aged younger than 1 month, 8 of 59 (13%) aged 1 to 2 months, and 8 of 116 (7%) aged 2 to 6 months; 4 neonates had meningitis. No clinical finding or laboratory test discriminated between bacteremic and nonbacteremic infants.[14] In surveillance for UTI among 203,399 infants born in U.S. Army hospitals from 1985 to 1990, 23% of noncircumcised infant boys younger than 3 months of age with UTI had concomitant bacteremia; incidence of bacteremia associated with UTI was not different from that in circumcised boys, or girls with UTI.[23]

Examination of Urine Sediment

Many studies assessing presence of WBCs in the urine of newborn infants have been performed.[5, 20, 60, 89–94] Healthy infants can have up to 10 WBCs per mm^3 of clean-voided urine.[60, 93] Lincoln and Winberg obtained uninfected and clean-voided specimens of urine from infants younger than 1 week of age: male infants had up to 25 WBCs per mm^3 and female infants up to 50 WBCs per mm^3.[94]

Neither presence nor absence of pyuria is completely reliable evidence for or against UTI. Many studies have assessed urine specimens for predictive values for UTI of WBCs, organisms, or detection by dipstick of leukocyte esterase or reduction of nitrate. The following results are limited to studies of acutely ill, usually febrile infants whose urine was obtained by catheterization (or suprapubic aspiration where stated). Methods of assessing pyuria and definitions of UTI vary. In 27% of unspun urine samples collected by suprapubic aspiration from Dallas infants with UTI (bacterial colony counts of 10^5/ml or greater), fewer than 10 WBCs per high-power field were present.[20] Landau and co-workers reported that among infants younger than 4 months of age with positive urine cultures (colony counts of 10^4/ml or greater), 4 of 49 (8.2%) with renal scintigraphy diagnostic of acute pyelonephritis had fewer than 5 WBCs per high-power field (400×) in fresh centrifuged urine, compared with 27 of 79 (34.2%) of infants with UTI and negative scintigraphy.[13] Quantifying WBCs in uncentrifuged urine using a counting chamber is the most reproducible test for pyuria. Hoberman and colleagues found pyuria (at least 10 WBCs per mm^3 unspun urine) absent in 22 of 190 (20%) febrile infants younger than 24 months of age with positive urine cultures (colony counts of 5.0×10^4/ml or greater) and present in 6.7% with negative cultures; a single patient of 15 without pyuria who had renal scintigraphy performed under protocol had a positive study.[95] In Hansson and co-workers' study of 366 infants younger than 1 year of age with symptomatic UTI (colony counts of 10^3/ml or greater from suprapubic aspirate of urine), 80% had colony counts/ml of 10^5 or greater, 13% had 1 to 9 × 10^4, and 7% had 1 to 9 × 10^3. Pyuria was significantly associated with colony count. In children with UTI with less than 10^5 colonies/ml, sensitivity of pyuria (> 10 WBCs per mm^3) was 69% compared with 88% for those with at least 10^5 colonies/ml. Nitrate reduction test was highly insensitive; 44% had positive test when colony count was at least 10^5/ml and 11% had positive test with lower counts.[27] Renal scintigraphy was not performed in Hansson and co-workers' study to estimate significance of UTI, but VUR was present equally in infants with high (30%) and low (38%) colony counts.

Dipstick test for leukocyte esterase and nitrite is inadequate to exclude the diagnosis of UTI in infants. In Hoberman and colleagues' study, the test had sensitivity of 53% and positive predictive value of 82% for detecting 10 or more WBCs per mm^3; nitrite determination had sensitivity of 31% in identifying urine cultures with growth of at least 50,000 colonies/ml.[88] Shaw and co-workers reported dipstick results on 3873 febrile children younger than 2 years of age evaluated for UTI; sensitivity of positive test (trace or greater result for leukocyte esterase or positive nitrite) was 79% and positive predictive value was 46% for isolation of at least 10,000 colonies/ml from urine culture.[96]

Microscopic hematuria is present in some infants with UTI,[3, 37] but gross hematuria is usually associated with other diseases (e.g., renal vein thrombosis, polycystic disease of the kidney, obstructive uropathy, and Wilms' tumor).[97]

Usefulness of Gram stain of urine specimen in predicting bacteriuria has been studied prospectively in febrile infants younger than 24 months of age. Smears were prepared using 2 drops of uncentrifuged urine on a slide within a standardized marked area 1.5 cm in diameter, air dried, fixed, and stained. Presence of at least 1 organism per 10 fields examined using oil immersion lens was considered positive. Sensitivity and positive predictive value were 81% and 43%, respectively, for isolation of at least 1×10^4 colonies/ml in Shaw and colleagues' study[96] and 93% and 57%, respectively, for isolation of at least 5.0×10^4 colonies/ml in Hoberman and co-workers' study.[88] Presence of both pyuria and bacteriuria increased positive predictive value for positive cultures in both studies to 85 and 88%, respectively.

Studies of neonates with early-onset septicemia indicate that the yield of culture of urine is low.[98, 99] This study may be eliminated in evaluation of infants for presumed sepsis younger than 3 days of age. Examination of urine may occasionally assist in microbiologic diagnosis of early-onset septicemia, but initiation of antimicrobial therapy should not be delayed when there is difficulty in obtaining the specimen.

Examination of Blood

The peripheral blood leukocyte count varies among infants with UTI. Although significantly higher neutrophil and band counts and band/neutrophil ratios are documented in young children with UTI, these do not reliably discriminate presence, absence, or level of infection in the urinary tract or presence of bacteremia.[13, 14, 95] In studies from New Zealand,[4] half of the neonates had a peripheral blood leukocyte count of greater than 16,000 per mm[3], but no information was given about this measure in uninfected infants. Hemolytic anemia frequently accompanies jaundice when the latter is present in infants with UTI.[67] The direct Coombs test is usually negative. The reticulocyte count can be normal or elevated.[67]

Signs of inflammatory response such as elevated erythrocyte sedimentation rate (ESR) or C-reactive protein (CRP) have been shown to correlate significantly with abnormal renal scintigraphy suggestive of acute pyelonephritis in children with UTI. In 64 children studied, Majd and colleagues found abnormal scans in 78% of those with ESR of at least 25 mm/hr, compared with 33% of those with lower ESR.[50] Benador and co-workers found that ESR greater than 20 mm/hr or CRP level greater than 10 mg/ml had sensitivity of 89% and specificity of 25% for identifying renal lesions among 73 children with UTI.[49] Stokland and colleagues correlated CRP level greater than 20 μg/ml at the time of acute infection with resultant renal scar in 157 children reevaluated 1 year later; sensitivity of elevated CRP was 92%,

and positive and negative predictive values were 41% and 80%, respectively.[100] In 153 children with fever and positive urine culture (colony count 5.0×10^4/ml or greater), Hoberman and co-workers reported significant correlations between evidence of pyelonephritis versus cystitis versus asymptomatic bacteriuria with mean peripheral WBC count (22.4 vs. 14.6 vs. 11.7×10^3/μl, respectively); ESR (44.0 vs. 26.8 vs. 15.3 mm/hr, respectively); and CRP (10.1 vs. 2.7 vs. 1.3 μg/ml, respectively).[95]

Chemical Determinations

Hyperbilirubinemia is present in many infants with UTI; the percentage of conjugated bilirubin is often determined by the age of the infant at the onset of jaundice.[65] During the first week of life, almost all of the bilirubin is unconjugated, but in the second week and thereafter the fractionation is approximately equivalent. In 80 Boston infants younger than 1 month of age with UTI, 11 (14%) had jaundice and hyperbilirubinemia; only 4 had bacteremia.[14] With the exception of changes in serum bilirubin, the results of serum hepatic enzyme tests are normal generally or only slightly abnormal,[65, 67] although toxic hepatitis and cholestasis unassociated with hemolysis were documented by liver biopsy in an older child with jaundice associated with UTI.[101] Azotemia and hyperchloremic acidosis are not unusual; serum bicarbonate measured less than 20 mEq/liter in 34.1% of 354 young children with UTI in one study.[14]

Radiologic Examination of the Urinary Tract

The major goal of investigation of the urinary tract in infants with UTI (and those with abnormalities noted prenatally) is to identify important and correctable lesions (including urethral strictures, renal anomalies, severe VUR, obstructive uropathy, and urethral valves in males) and to provide the opportunity to begin antibiotic prophylaxis against recurring UTIs in those with reflux or hydronephrosis in whom surgery is not indicated. Multiple new imaging modalities are available and are safer than intravenous pyelography.[102] Each provides unique evaluations.[48, 54, 100, 103–107] Ultrasound is capable of showing the size, shape, and location of kidneys and contributes to diagnoses of hydronephrosis, hydroureter, ureterocele, bladder distention, and stones. It is the most noninvasive study, the accuracy of which is dependent on the experience of the interpreter. It is an insensitive test for pyelonephritis but sometimes shows enlarged kidney with abnormal echogenicity. Renal ultrasonography performed to follow up on fetal studies should be postponed for at least 48 hours after birth to avoid a false-negative result from dehydration or low glomerular filtration rate characteristic of newborns.[103]

Renal cortical scintigraphy using technetium-99m–labeled dimercaptosuccinic acid or gluceptate is the most sensitive test for identifying acute pyelonephritis (i.e., focally or diffusely decreased cortical uptake of tracer without evidence of cortical loss, sometimes in an enlarged kidney) or chronic scarring (i.e., decreased uptake with corresponding cortical volume loss); it also provides an estimate of renal function. Taken as the gold standard for acute pyelonephritis, 66% of 66 infants younger than 1 year of age with febrile UTI had positive renal scan in one study,[49] as did 75% of 153 children younger than 2 years of age in another study[95] and 66% of 94 children in another study.[50]

Voiding cystourethrography using radiographic or radionuclide methodology is the best study to visualize the bladder and urethra and to detect VUR; radionuclide scan is superior to the dye study to detect intermittent reflux but is inferior to detect urethral and bladder wall abnormalities and cannot be used to grade VUR. Both have invasiveness and discomfort attendant with catheterization. A 24-day-old male infant with ureterovesical junction obstruction had *E. coli* septicemia and UTI 6 days after elective vesicourethrography, which did not show VUR.[108] Toxic reaction to the cystourethrography dye can occur in infants but is very uncommon.

Ultrasonography and cystourethrography should be performed on all neonates with UTI judged to be other than that secondary to septicemia. Ultrasonography is performed at the time of infection to identify major renal and ureteral abnormalities. Cystourethrography sometimes can be delayed to permit resolution of inflammatory VUR; however, recent studies show that fewer than 50% of children with acute pyelonephritis have VUR.[27, 50, 104] Renal scintigraphy is useful in diagnosis and management of selective cases of UTI. Computed tomography is performed infrequently, for example, when a mass lesion or abscess is suspected.

MANAGEMENT

Management of UTI is aimed at halting infection rapidly, reconstituting normal fluid and acid-base status, and assessing medical or surgical interventions required to prevent subsequent episodes of UTI and kidney damage.

Antimicrobial Therapy

Antimicrobial agents should be administered as soon as cultures of the blood, cerebrospinal fluid (if indicated), and urine have been obtained. Because the physician must assume that bacteremia is present in the neonate who has UTI and signs of septicemia, the choice of antimicrobial agents for initial therapy and the dosage schedule is the same as that outlined in Chapter 21 for septicemia (a penicillin and an aminoglycoside). A penicillinase-resistant penicillin (methicillin or oxacillin) should be used if an abscess of the kidney, prostate, or testis is present, which suggests infection with *S. aureus*. Patients who have suspected hospital-acquired infection are frequently given vancomycin and an aminoglycoside as initial therapy because of the significant role of coagulase-negative staphylococci and *Enterococcus* species. Use of a third-generation cephalosporin is dependent on the patient's prior receipt of antibiotics, the patient's clinical state, and the knowledge of bacterial species indigenous in each neonatal intensive care unit. Gram stain of urine

sediment is helpful, especially when considering use of amphotericin for potential *Candida* infection. Treatment should be reconsidered when the results of cultures and antimicrobial susceptibility tests are available.

Effective antimicrobial agents sterilize the urine within 24 to 48 hours. A second specimen of urine often is obtained for examination and culture at about 48 hours. Persistence of bacteriuria implies that treatment is ineffective, a foreign body should be removed, or obstruction exists.

The duration of antimicrobial therapy for UTI in neonates is 10 to 14 days. Longer therapy (up to 3 weeks) is necessary if there is a poor response or if an anatomic or physiologic abnormality suggests that relapse may occur if administration of the drug is not continued. Timing of change from parenterally to orally administered agents depends on rapidity of clinical and microbiologic response and the presence of bacteremia or anatomic, functional, or physiologic abnormalities. Parenteral therapy is usually given for 5 to 7 days in uncomplicated cases. The urine should be examined and cultured frequently after conclusion of therapy so that relapse or recurrence of infection can be detected as soon as possible. Children with certain urinary tract anomalies, functional abnormalities, and higher grades of VUR are given prophylactic antibiotics continuously for extended periods of time until surgery is performed or the condition improves[56, 103]; amoxicillin, 20 mg/kg per day divided in doses administered every 12 hours, is the agent most frequently used in the neonate.

Ancillary Therapy

Severe dehydration, electrolyte imbalance, azotemia, and shock can accompany UTI in the newborn. Fluid replacement must be calculated carefully for correction of these abnormalities. Transfusion of blood may be necessary in infants with hemolytic anemia. Incision and drainage of abscesses of the prostate and testes should be considered.

PROGNOSIS

For patients with UTI and underlying genitourinary abnormalities, it is important to have long-term control of infection. After that, prognosis is dependent on severity of the lesion. The natural history of UTI in the newborn without underlying abnormality is incompletely described. Some infants with asymptomatic bacteriuria have infection that clears without use of antimicrobial agents.[4, 5, 71, 109] Some infants with symptomatic infection respond readily to therapy and have no subsequent infections, whereas others have recurrences, although the number appears to be smaller than that for older children and adults. In the series from Göteborg[5] and Leeds,[7] recurrences occurred in 26 and 19% of the infants, respectively; the second episode usually occurred during the first few months after the initial infection.

It is possible that inflammatory changes in the kidney early in life may lead to subsequent impairment of growth and development of the kidney and to epithelial damage, fibrosis, and vascular changes, but it is uncertain how frequently these events take place. In a study of 25 children with UTI who had acute pyelonephritis evident by renal scan and who had the scan repeated an average of 10.5 months later, 16 (64%) had corresponding scars.[49] In another study, 38% of 157 children (with median age 0.4 years at time of asymptomatic UTI) had renal scars documented 1 year later.[100] Infants do not appear to be at increased risk for scars; in 50 infants younger than 1 year of age with UTI and acute renal lesions, repeat scintigraphy after an average of 3 months showed scars in 40%.[110]

Obstructive lesions associated with reflux during the neonatal period may be associated with progressive renal damage, whereas children with unobstructive reflux regardless of severity appear not to have progressive renal damage if infection is assiduously prevented.[44, 51–53, 56, 103] Of 102 children with end-stage renal disease in Missouri from 1986 to 1995, damage from VUR and UTIs accounted for less than 1% of cases.[111]

References

1. Helmholz HF. Pyelitis in the newborn. Med Clin North Am 1:1451, 1918.
2. Schlager TA, Hendley JO, Dudley SM, et al. Explanation for false-positive urine cultures obtained by bay technique. Arch Pediatr Adolesc Med 149:170–173, 1995.
3. Lohr JA, Downs SM, Dudley S, et al. Hospital-acquired urinary tract infections in the pediatric patient: a prospective study. Pediatr Infect Dis J 13:8–12, 1994.
4. Abbott GD. Neonatal bacteriuria: a prospective study of 1460 infants. BMJ 1:267, 1972.
5. Bergström T, Larson H, Lincoln K, et al. Neonatal urinary tract infections. J Pediatr 80:859, 1972.
6. Edelman CM Jr, Ogwo JE, Fine BP, et al. The prevalence of bacteriuria in full-term and premature newborn infants. J Pediatr 82:125, 1973.
7. Littlewood JM, Kite P, Kite BA. Incidence of neonatal urinary tract infection. Arch Dis Child 44:617, 1969.
8. Maherzi M, Guignard JP, Torrado A. Urinary tract infection in high-risk newborn infants. Pediatrics 62:521, 1978.
9. Wettergren B, Jodal U, Jonasson G. Epidemiology of bacteriuria during the first year of life. Acta Paediatr Scand 74:925, 1985.
10. Wiswell TE, Roscelli JD. Corroborative evidence for the decreased incidence of urinary tract infections in circumcised male infants. Pediatrics 78:96, 1986.
11. Pendarvis BC Jr, Chitwood LA, Wenzl JE. Bacteriuria in the premature infant. Abstracts of papers presented at the Ninth Interscience Conference on Antimicrobial Agents and Chemotherapy, Washington, D.C., October 27–29, 1969. Washington, D.C., American Society for Microbiology, 1969.
12. Kunin CM. Detection, Prevention and Management of Urinary Tract Infections, 3rd ed. Philadelphia, Lea & Febiger, 1979.
13. Landau D, Turner M, Brennan J, et al. The value of urinalysis in differentiating acute pyelonephritis from lower urinary tract infection in febrile infants. Pediatr Infect Dis J 13:777–782, 1994.
14. Bachur R, Caputo GL. Bacteremia and meningitis among infants with urinary tract infections. Pediatr Emerg Care 11:280–284, 1995.

15. Sweet AY, Wolinsky E. An outbreak of urinary tract and other infections due to E. coli. Pediatrics 33:865, 1964.
16. Kenny JF, Medearis DN, Klein SW, et al. An outbreak of urinary tract infections and septicemia due to Escherichia coli in male infants. J Pediatr 68:530, 1966.
17. McCormack RC, Kunin CM. Control of a single source nursery epidemic due to Serratia marcescens. Pediatrics 37:750, 1966.
18. Wiswell TE, Smith FR, Bass JW. Decreased incidence of urinary tract infections in circumcised male infants. Pediatrics 75:901, 1985.
19. Wiswell TE, Enzenauer RW, Holton ME, et al. Declining frequency of circumcision: implications for changes in the absolute incidence and male to female sex ratio of urinary tract infections in early infancy. Pediatrics 79:338, 1987.
20. Ginsburg CM, McCracken GH Jr. Urinary tract infections in young infants. Pediatrics 69:409, 1982.
21. Herzog LW. Urinary tract infections and circumcision: a case-control study. Am J Dis Child 143:348, 1989.
22. Wiswell TE, Geschke DW. Risks from circumcision during the first month of life compared with those for uncircumcised boys. Pediatrics 83:1011, 1989.
23. Wiswell TE, Hachey WE. Urinary tract infections and the uncircumsized state: an update. Clin Pediatr 130–134, 1993.
24. Schoen EJ (chairman). American Academy of Pediatrics Task Force Report on Circumcision. Pediatrics 84:388, 1989.
24a. To T, Agha M, Dick PT, et al. Cohort study on circumcision of newborn boys and subsequent risk of urinary-tract infection. Lancet 352:1813, 1998.
24b. Craig JC, Knight JF, Sureshkumar P, et al. Effect of circumcision on incidence of urinary tract infection in preschool boys. J Pediatr 128:23, 1996.
24c. Lannon CM (chairman). American Academy of Pediatrics Task Force Report on Circumcision. Pediatrics 103:686, 1999.
25. Cohen HA, Drucker MM, Vainer S, et al. Post-circumcision urinary tract infection. Clin Pediatr 31:322, 1992.
26. Crain EF, Gershel JC. Urinary tract infections in febrile infants younger than 8 weeks of age. Pediatrics 86:363, 1990.
27. Hansson S, Brandström P, Jodal U, et al. Low bacterial counts in infants with urinary tract infection. J Pediatr 132:179–182, 1998.
28. Shaw KN, Gorelick M, McGowan KL, et al. Prevalence of urinary tract infection in febrile young children in the emergency department. Pediatrics 102:390, 1998.
29. Tullus K, Sjoberg P. Epidemiological aspects of P-fimbriated E. coli. Acta Paediatr Scand 75:205, 1986.
30. Israele V, Darabi A, McCracken GH Jr. The role of bacterial virulence factors and Tamm-Horsfall protein in the pathogenesis of Escherichia coli urinary tract infection in infants. Am J Dis Child 141:1230, 1987.
31. Marild S, Wettergren B, Hellstrom M, et al. Bacterial virulence and inflammatory response in infants with febrile urinary tract infection screening bacteriuria. J Pediatr 112:348, 1988.
32. Pena BM, Harper MB, Fleisher GR. Occult bacteremia with group B Streptococci in an outpatient setting. Pediatrics 102:67–72, 1998.
33. Lohr JA, Donowitz LG, Sadler JE III. Hospital-acquired urinary tract infection. Pediatrics 83:193, 1989.
34. Davies HD, Jones ELF, Sheng RY, et al. Nosocomial urinary tract infections at a pediatric hospital. Pediatr Infect Dis J 11:349, 1992.
35. Levy I, Leibovici L, Drucker M, et al. A prospective

study of Gram-negative bacteremia in children. Pediatr Infect Dis J 15:117–22, 1996.

36. Giannattasio RC. Acute suppurative prostatitis in the neonatal period. NY State J Med 60:3471, 1960.

37. Williams DI, Martins AG. Periprostatic haematoma and prostatic abscess in the neonatal period. Arch Dis Child 35:177, 1960.

38. Mann S. Prostatic abscess in the newborn. Arch Dis Child 35:396, 1960.

39. Heyman A, Lombardo LJ Jr. Metastatic prostatic abscess with report of a case in a newborn infant. J Urol 87:174, 1962.

40. Hendricks WM, Kellett GN. Scrotal mass in a neonate: testicular abscess. Am J Dis Child 129:1361, 1975.

41. Hemming VG. Bilateral neonatal group A streptococcal hydrocele infection associated with maternal puerperal sepsis. Pediatr Infect Dis 5:107, 1986.

42. McCartney ET, Stewart I. Suppurative orchitis due to *Pseudomonas aeruginosa*. J Pediatr 52:451, 1958.

43. Foster R, Weber TR, Kleiman M, et al. *Salmonella enteritidis*: testicular abscess in a newborn. J Urol 130:790, 1983.

44. Chandra M, Maddix H, McVicar M. Transient urodynamic dysfuncton of infancy: relationship to urinary tract infections and vesicoureteral reflux. J Urol 155:673–677, 1996.

45. Bensman A, Baudon JJ, Jablonski JP, et al. Uropathies diagnosed in the neonatal period: symptomatology and course. Acta Paediatr Scand 69:499, 1980.

46. Littlewood JM. 66 infants with urinary tract infection in first month of life. Arch Dis Child 57:218, 1972.

47. Bourcher D, Abbott ED, Maling TMJ. Radiological abnormalities in infants with urinary tract infection. Arch Dis Child 59:620, 1984.

48. Andrich MP, Majd M. Diagnostic imaging in the evaluation of the first urinary tract infection in infants and young children. Pediatrics 90:436–40, 1992.

49. Benador D, Benador N, Slosman DO, et al. Cortical scintigraphy in the evaluation of renal parenchymal changes in children with pyelonephritis. J Pediatr 124:17–20, 1994.

50. Majd M, Rushton HG, Jantausch B, et al. Relationships among vesicoureteral reflux, P-fimbriated *Escherichia coli*, and acute pyelonephritis in children with febrile urinary tract infection. J Pediatr 119:578, 1991.

51. Najmaldin A, Burge DM, Atwell JD. Pediatric urology: fetal vesicoureteric reflux. Br J Urol 65:403, 1990.

52. Gordon AC, Thomas DFM, Arthur RJ, et al. Prenatally diagnosed reflux: a follow-up study. Br J Urol 65:407, 1990.

53. Ring E, Zobel G. Urinary infection and malformations of urinary tract in infancy. Arch Dis Child 63:818, 1988.

54. Steele BT, De Maria J. A new perspective on the natural history of vesicoureteric reflux. Pediatrics 90:30–32, 1992.

55. Assael BM, Guez S, Marra G, et al. Congenital reflux nephropathy: a follow-up of 108 cases diagnosed perinatally. Br J Urol 82:252–257, 1998.

56. Gunn TR, Mora JD, Pease P. Outcome after antenatal diagnosis of upper urinary tract dilatation by ultrasonography. Arch Dis Child 63:1240, 1988.

57. Gunn TR, Mora JD, Pease P. Antenatal diagnosis of urinary tract abnormalities by ultrasonography after 28 weeks' gestation: incidence and outcome. Am J Obstet Gynecol 172:479–486, 1995.

57a. Dremsek PA, Gindl K, Void P, et al. Renal pyelectasis in fetuses and neonates: diagnostic value of renal pelvis diameter in pre- and postnatal sonographic screening. AJR 168:1017–1019, 1997.

57b. Thomas DFM, Madden NP, Irving HC, et al. Mild dilatation of the fetal kidney: a follow-up study. Br J Urol 74:236–239, 1993.

58. Scott J, Swallow V, Coulthard MG, et al. Screening of newborn babies for familial ureteric reflux. Lancet 350:396–399, 1997.

58a. Holland NH, Jackson EC, Kazee M, et al. Relation of urinary tract infection and vesicoureteral reflux to scars: follow-up of thirty-eight patients. J Pediatr 116:S65, 1990.

59. Patrick M. Influence of maternal renal infection on the foetus and infants. Arch Dis Child 42:208, 1967.

60. Gower PE, Husband P, Coleman JC. Urinary infection in two selected neonatal populations. Arch Dis Child 45:259, 1970.

61. Svanborg C, Hausson S, Jodal U, et al. Host-parasite interaction in the urinary tract. J Infect Dis 157:421, 1988.

62. Wiswell TE, Miller GM, Gelston HM Jr, et al. Effect of circumcision status on periurethral bacterial flora during the first year of life. J Pediatr 113:442, 1988.

63. Sobel JD. Pathogenesis of urinary tract infections. Infect Dis Clin North Am 1:751, 1987.

64. Porter KA, Giles HM. A pathological study of live cases of pyelonephritis in the newborn. Arch Dis Child 31:303, 1956.

65. Bernstein J, Brown AK. Sepsis and jaundice in early infancy. Pediatrics 29:873, 1962.

66. Ng SH, Rawstron JR. Urinary tract infections presenting with jaundice. Arch Dis Child 46:173, 1971.

67. Seeler RA, Hahn K. Jaundice in urinary tract infection in infancy. Am J Dis Child 118:553, 1969.

68. Maisels MJ, Kring E. Risk of sepsis in newborns with severe hyperbilirubinemia. Pediatrics 90:741–742, 1992.

69. Luk G, Riggs D, Luque M. Severe methemoglobinemia in a 3-week-old infant with a urinary tract infection. Crit Care Med 19:1325, 1992.

70. Das A, Henderson D. Your diagnosis, please. Pediatr Infect Dis J 15:922–923, 1996.

71. Abbott GD. Transient asymptomatic bacteriuria in infancy. BMJ 1:207, 1970.

72. Crawford DB, Rasoulpour M, Dhawan VM, et al. Renal carbuncle in a neonate with congenital nephrotic syndrome. J Pediatr 93:78, 1978.

73. Bauchner H, Philipp B, Dashefsky B, et al. Prevalence of bacteriuria in febrile children. Pediatr Infect Dis J 6:239, 1987.

74. Krober MS, Bass JW, Powell JM, et al. Bacterial and viral pathogens causing fever in infants less than 3 months old. Am J Dis Child 139:889, 1985.

75. Amir J, Alpert G, Reisner SH, et al. Fever in the first months of life. Isr J Med Sci 20:447, 1984.

76. Hoberman A, Chao H, Keller DM, et al. Prevalence of urinary tract infecton in febrile infants. J Pediatr 123:17–22, 1993.

77. Nelson JD, Peters PC. Suprapubic aspiration of urine in premature and term infants. Pediatrics 36:132, 1965.

78. Pryles CV, Saccharow, L. Further experience with the use of percutaneous suprapubic aspiration of the urinary bladder: bacteriologic studies in 654 infants and children. Pediatrics 43:1018, 1969.

79. Lanier B, Daeschner CW. Serious complication of suprabubic aspiration of the urinary bladder. J Pediatr 79:711, 1971.

80. Weathers WT, Wenzl JE. Suprapubic aspiration: perfora-

tion of a viscus other than the bladder. Am J Dis Child 117:590, 1969.

81. Morell RE, Duritz G, Oltorf C. Suprapubic aspiration associated with hematoma. Pediatrics 69:455, 1982.

82. Mandell J, Stevens PS. Supravesical hematoma following suprapubic urine aspiration. J Urol 119:286, 1978.

83. Schreiver RL, Skafish P. Complications of suprapubic bladder aspiration. Am J Dis Child 132:98, 1978.

84. Pass RF, Waldo FB. Anaerobic bacteremia following suprapubic bladder aspiration. J Pediatr 94:748, 1979.

85. Goldberg BB, Meyer H. Ultrasonically guided suprapubic urinary bladder aspiration. Pediatrics 51:70, 1973.

86. Kiernan SC, Pinckert TL, Kesler M. Ultrasound guidance of suprapubic bladder aspiration in neonates. J Pediatr 123:789–791, 1993.

87. Pryles CV, Lüders D, Alkan MK. A comparative study of bacterial cultures and colony counts in paired specimens of urine obtained by catheter versus voiding from normal infants and infants with urinary tract infection. Pediatrics 27:17, 1961.

88. Hoberman A, Wald ER, Reynolds EA, et al. Pyuria and bacteriuria in urine specimens obtained by catheter from young children with fever. J Pediatr 124:513–518, 1994.

89. Braude H, Forfar JO, Gould JC, et al. Cell and bacterial counts in the urine of normal infants and children. BMJ 4:697, 1967.

90. Houston IB. Urinary white cell excretion in childhood. Arch Dis Child 40:313, 1965.

91. Lam CN, Bremner AD, Maxwell JD, et al. Pyuria and bacteriuria. Arch Dis Child 42:275, 1967.

92. Hewstone AS, Lawson JS. Microscopic appearance of urine in the neonatal period. Arch Dis Child 39:287, 1964.

93. Littlewood JM. White cells and bacteria in voided urine of healthy newborns. Arch Dis Child 46:167, 1971.

94. Lincoln K, Winberg J. Studies of urinary tract infection in infancy and childhood: III. Quantitative estimation of cellular excretion in unselected neonates. Acta Paediatr Scand 53:447, 1964.

95. Hoberman A, Wald ER, Reynolds EA, et al. Is urine culture necessary to rule out urinary tract infection in young febrile children? Pediatr Infect Dis J 15:304–309, 1996.

96. Shaw KN, McGowan KL, Gorelick MH, et al. Screening for urinary tract infection in infants in the emergency department: which test is best? Pediatrics 101:1–5, 1998.

97. Emanuel B, Aronson N. Neonatal hematuria. Am J Dis Child 128:204, 1974.

98. Visser VE, Hall RT. Urine culture in the evaluation of suspected neonatal sepsis. J Pediatr 94:635, 1979.

99. DiGeronimo RJ. Lack of efficacy of the urine culture as part of the initial work up of suspected neonatal sepsis. Pediatr Infect Dis J 11:764–766, 1992.

100. Stokland E, Hellström M, Jacobsson B, et al. Renal damage one year after first urinary tract infection: role of dimercaptosuccinic acid scintigraphy. J Pediatr 129:815–820, 1996.

101. Hamdan JM, Rizk F. Jaundice complicating urinary tract infection in childhood. Pediatr Infect Dis 4:418, 1985.

102. Kassner EG, Elguezabal A, Pochaczevsky R. Death during intravenous urography: overdosage in young infants. NY State J Med 73:1958, 1973.

103. Fine RN. Diagnosis and treatment of fetal urinary tract abnormalities. J Pediatr 121:333, 1992.

104. Strife CF, Gelfand MJ. Renal cortical scintigraphy: effect on medical decision making in childhood urinary tract infection. J Pediatr 129:785–87, 1996.

105. Hellerstein S. Evolving concepts in the evaluation of the child with a urinary tract infection. J Pediatr 124:589–592, 1994.

106. Conway JJ, Cohn RA. Evolving role of nuclear medicine for the diagnosis and management of urinary tract infection. J Pediatr 124:87–90, 1994.

107. Dick PT, Feldman W. Routine diagnostic imaging for childhood urinary tract infections: a systematic overview. J Pediatr 128:15–22, 1996.

108. Slyper AH, Olson JC, Nair RB. Overwhelming Escherichia coli sepsis in ureterovesical junction obstruction without reflux. Arch Pediatr Adolesc Med 148:1102–1103, 1994.

109. Hoffpauir CW, Guidry DJ. Asymptomatic urinary tract infection in premature infants. Pediatrics 45:128, 1970.

110. Benador D, Benador N, Slosman D, et al. Are younger children at highest risk of renal sequelae after pyelonephritis? Lancet 349:17–19, 1997.

111. Sreenarasimhaiah S, Hellerstein S. Urinary tract infections per se do not cause end-stage kidney disease. Pediatr Nephrol 12:210–13, 1998.

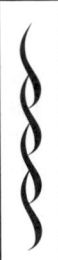

Focal Bacterial Infections

GARY D. OVERTURF, M.D., and S. MICHAEL MARCY, M.D.

INFECTIONS OF THE LIVER

Bacterial infection of the hepatic parenchyma is recognized most frequently in the form of multiple, small inflammatory foci (microabscesses) noted as an incidental finding in infants dying with sepsis. Diffuse hepatocellular damage—often in conjunction with infection of several organ systems—may be present after transplacental passage of microorganisms to the fetal circulation. On rare occasions, liver involvement may take the form of a solitary purulent abscess. Metastatic focal infections of the liver associated with bacteremia either resolve with antimicrobial therapy, are not recognized, or are found only at postmortem examination. Very rarely are they clinically apparent as solitary[1] or multiple[2] large abscesses and diagnosed during life.

Although metastatic infections are very uncommon, it is difficult to ascertain their true incidence. In a survey of more than 7500 autopsies of children performed between 1917 and 1967, Dehner and Kissane found only three neonates with multiple, small pyogenic hepatic abscesses,[3] whereas a review of approximately 4900 autopsies[4] performed at Los Angeles Children's Hospital between 1958 and 1978 revealed nine such infants.[5] Among 175,000 neonates admitted between 1957 and 1977 to the Milwaukee Children's Hospital, there were 2 who died with hepatic microabscesses[6]; 3 such patients were seen among 83,000 pediatric patients admitted to The New York Hospital between 1945 and 1983,[7] and 1 was reported at the University of Texas Medical Branch in Galveston between 1963 and 1984.[8] Most reviewers who have discussed postmortem observations of infants dying with neonatal sepsis either have not described the occurrence of such secondary sites of infection[9–16] or have presented them as an occasional ancillary finding.[17, 18]

Solitary hepatic abscesses in the newborn have also been reported rarely. About 30 such cases have been described in the literature.[1, 3, 4, 19–41] These infections have been associated frequently with prematurity and umbilical vein catheterization.[5, 6, 21, 22, 25, 28, 32, 34–41] Furthermore, solitary abscesses may occur as a result of bacteremia; Murphy and Baker describe a solitary abscess as a delayed consequence of sepsis caused by *Staphylococcus aureus.*[42]

Microbiology

Any bacteria that invade the bloodstream can cause multiple microabscesses in the liver. The etiologic agents in the infants described by Dehner and Kissane,[3] Moss and Pysher,[5] Chusid,[6] and Miedema and co-workers[7] were *Escherichia coli, S. aureus, Pseudomonas aeruginosa, Klebsiella* sp., *Enterobacter* sp., and *Listeria monocytogenes.*

The causative bacteria of solitary abscesses are generally those colonizing the umbilical stump,[43] including *S. aureus* (11 cases); *E. coli* alone (3 cases); *E. coli* with *S. aureus* (2 cases) or enterococcus (1 case); *Enterobacter* sp. (3 cases); *Klebsiella pneumoniae* alone (2 cases); *K. pneumoniae* with *Proteus* sp. (1 case); *P. aeruginosa* (1 case); *Staphylococcus epidermidis* with group F *Streptococcus* (1 case); and group A beta-hemolytic *Streptococcus* (1 case). In three infants, the abscesses were described as "sterile."[19, 28, 31] Although one of these infants had received penicillin for 9 days before surgical drainage, it is possible that in all three cases the abscesses were caused by anaerobic bacteria that failed to grow under the standard conditions of transport and culture. The presence of gas in seven abscesses[25, 28, 34, 35, 39] may indicate infection with anaerobes, a frequent cause of liver abscess in adults.[44]

The most common cause of intrauterine bacterial hepatitis—congenital listeriosis—characteristically involves the liver and adrenals (see Chapter 27). Typical lesions are seen histologically as sharply demarcated areas of necrosis (miliary granulomatosis) or as microabscesses containing numerous pleomorphic gram-positive bacilli.[15] Descriptions in the early 1900s of miliary necrosis of the liver related to "gram-positive argentophilic rodlike organisms" probably also represented infections with *L. monocytogenes*, which was not isolated and identified until 1926.[26]

Intrauterine tuberculosis results from maternal bacillemia with transplacental dissemination to the fetal bloodstream (see Chapter 28). Because the liver is perfused by blood with a high oxygen content[45] and is the first organ that encounters tubercle bacilli, it is often the most severely involved.[15, 44, 46] The presence of primary foci in the liver has, in fact, been considered prima facie evidence for the congenital nature of tuberculous lesions as a result of hematogenous spread along the umbilical vein.[47] However, it has been emphasized that hepatic granulomas may be less common than previously noted on closed (needle) biopsy or will require an open biopsy to confirm liver and regional node involvement.[48] Although generalized fetal infection may also arise through aspiration of contaminated amniotic fluid, the lesions acquired in this manner are usually most prominent in the lungs. In addition to hepatomegaly, a clinical picture of fever with elevated serum IgM and chorioretinitis (e.g., choroid tubercles) may simulate that caused by other congenital infectious agents.[49] In this review by Abughal and co-workers, positive sites of culture for tuberculosis include the liver (8/9), gastric aspirate (18/23), tracheal aspirate (7/7), ear (5/6), and cerebrospinal fluid (3/10).[49] Noncaseating granulomatous hepatitis, thought to be caused by a hypersensitivity reaction related to bacille Calmette-Guérin (BCG) vaccination, has also been described in a neonate.[50] Histologic and bacteriologic studies performed on liver biopsy specimens failed to identify the presence of acid-fast bacilli or BCG organisms.

On rare occasions, bacterial infection of the fetal liver has been reported in association with maternal tularemia,[51] anthrax,[52] typhoid fever,[53] and brucellosis.[54] It is uncertain whether the isolation of bacteria from the livers of stillborn fetuses is significant.[55, 56]

Treponema pallidum is the spirochete most commonly associated with transplacental hepatic infection (see Chapter 12). Pathologic changes in the liver, found in up to 95% of infants dying with congenital syphilis,[57] may include those of a diffuse hepatitis or focal areas of inflammation, both frequently accompanied by an increase of connective tissue with consequent enlargement of the liver.[15, 57-59] Involvement of the liver has also been documented, on the basis of isolation of organisms or their identification in histologic sections, in newborns with intrauterine infection caused by various *Leptospira* species (*L. icterohaemorrhagiae*,[60, 61] *L. pomona*,[62] *L. canicola*,[63] *L. kasman*[64]). Transplacental infection of the fetus with *Borrelia recurrentis* or *Borrelia burgdorferi* causes little or no inflammation of the liver parenchyma or biliary epithelium despite the presence of large numbers of spirochetes in the sinusoids.[65-68] Congenital infection has been described with *B. burgdorferi*[68a] (Lyme disease); and hepatic, central nervous system, and cardiac lesions are frequently observed as well as widely disseminated lesions in other tissues.

Pathogenesis

Infectious agents may reach the liver of the fetus or newborn by one of several pathways: (1) transplacental or transorificial intrauterine infection; (2) extension of thrombophlebitis of the umbilical vein; (3) via the hepatic artery during the course of a systemic bacteremia; (4) pylephlebitis secondary to a focus of infection in the areas of drainage of the portal vein (mesenteric or splenic veins); (5) direct invasion from contiguous structures or because of trauma or surgical inoculation; and (6) extension up the biliary passages in cases of suppurative cholangitis. Abscesses with no apparent focus of infection seem to be relatively more common in the newborn than in older children.[30] Three such cases, all in infants with solitary hepatic abscesses, have been described.[23, 24, 31] Descriptions of the findings at the time of surgery, together with the nature of the lesions, suggest, however, that an umbilical vein infection, obscured by the large collection of purulent material in the abscess, was the probable pathogenesis in all infants.

The mode of infection usually determines the pattern of hepatic involvement. Intense and prolonged seeding of the liver parenchyma, such as that which occurs in conjunction with intrauterine infection or neonatal sepsis, almost invariably results in diffuse hepatocellular damage or multiple small inflammatory lesions.[3, 5, 6] Umbilical vein thrombophlebitis, on the other hand, can cause an abscess of the falciform ligament[69] or extend into a single branch of the portal vein to produce a solitary pyogenic abscess,[6, 21, 22, 26, 29, 32, 33] or can lead to disseminated foci of infection through dislodgement of septic emboli.[6, 70–73]

The frequent use of umbilical catheters has been associated with an increase in the numbers of infants with solitary[5, 6, 20, 21, 22, 32, 34–40] or multiple[5, 74, 75] hepatic abscesses. In three large series, including almost 500 infants who died after placement of umbilical vein catheters, 29 infants were found to have purulent infections of the hepatic vessels or parenchyma.[37, 74, 76] Use of venous catheter for infusion of hypertonic or acidic solutions may provide a necrotic focus for abscess formation,[21, 32, 34–36, 75, 76] and prolonged[5, 22, 32, 76] or repeated[63] catheterization of a necrotic umbilical stump provides an ideal pathway for the introduction of pathogenic organisms. It has been postulated in some cases that hepatic abscesses were caused by the infusion of contaminated plasma[28] or by the use of nonsterile umbilical catheters.[74]

Although neonatal liver abscesses usually are caused by hematogenous dissemination of bacteria through the hepatic artery or umbilical vein, examples of infection arising from various other sources have been described. Solitary abscesses have followed a presumed portal vein bacteremia secondary to amebic colitis.[19, 20] Direct invasion of adjacent liver parenchyma from purulent cholecystitis[24] or postoperative perihepatic abscesses[5] also has been observed. Ascending cholangitis, the most frequent cause of hepatic pyemia in adults,[30] has not been implicated in the etiology of newborn infections.

Disease due to embryonic anatomic errors is unique to newborns. Shaw and Pierog[77] described a newborn with umbilical herniation of a pedunculated supernumerary lobe of the liver; histologic examination showed numerous small foci of early abscess formation. Although signs and symptoms of sepsis appeared at 18 days of age—possibly the result of bacterial spread from the liver to the umbilical vein—the infant improved and ultimately recovered after removal of the polypoid mass on the 19th day of life.

Descriptions of "umbilical sepsis" and "acute interstitial hepatitis" recorded by Morison seem to clearly indicate that his patients had acquired bacterial infections of the umbilical vessels with widespread extension into the portal tracts.[78] Although mild periportal parenchymal necrosis was observed in a few infants, hepatocellular damage was minimal or absent in most. Similar lesions have been found in infants dying with sepsis[79] and infantile diarrhea.[80]

Clinical Manifestations

Multiple hepatic abscesses and diffuse hepatitis related to neonatal sepsis or transplacental fetal infection are almost invariably diagnosed at autopsy; few clinical manifestations referable to hepatocellular damage are evident before death. The signs and symptoms associated with these conditions are those of the underlying sepsis or of secondary metastatic complications such as meningitis, pneumonitis, or peritonitis.[2, 3, 29, 33, 71, 74]

Solitary abscesses are indolent in terms of their development and clinical presentation. Although the suppurative umbilical focus or umbilical catheterization responsible for the introduction of microorganisms can usually be traced to the first week of life, evidence of hepatic involvement is usually not apparent before the second or third week. The abscess frequently becomes a source for the hematogenous dissemination of microorganisms, so that most infants have signs and symptoms referable to a bacteremia. Despite intense infection of the underlying vessels, inspection of the umbilical stump usually shows no evidence of inflammation or purulent discharge. The presence of hepatomegaly, a finding commonly associated with neonatal sepsis, also offers little aid in establishing a definitive diagnosis. In half of infants for whom physical findings are clearly described, a well-delineated, often fluctuant or tender mass could be palpated in the epigastrium or right upper quadrant. On a few occasions, this mass was noted by the infant's mother several days before the onset of systemic symptoms. Abscesses occur in the right or left lobe of the liver with almost equal frequency and are generally 3 cm or more in diameter at the time of surgical exploration.

Diagnosis

Hematologic studies are of little value in establishing a diagnosis. Leukocyte counts and sedimentation rates may be normal or elevated. The serum levels of liver enzymes may also be normal[25, 38] or elevated.[5, 23, 36]

Abdominal radiographs are usually normal or show nonspecific displacement of the lower edge of the liver. In five infants, the diagnosis was suspected from a plain x-ray film by the presence of gas within the hepatic shadow.[28, 32, 34, 39] Radiologic findings that commonly accompany hepatic abscess in older children, such as an altered contour of the diaphragm, right pleural effusion, and platelike atelectasis,[81] are rarely present in the neonate.

Ultrasonography should be the initial imaging study in newborns with clinical evidence of a hepatic abscess.[82–85] If negative, and the diagnosis is still strongly suspected, more sensitive techniques such as computed tomography (CT) or magnetic resonance imaging (MRI) should be performed.[82–87] Enhancement with contrast agents may increase the definition of smaller abscesses. Because congenital cysts, arteriovenous malformations, and tumors with central necrosis or hemorrhage can mimic hepatic abscess, the diagnosis should always be confirmed by aspiration of purulent material, either at laparotomy or by means of percutaneous drainage with ultrasound or CT guidance.[83, 88, 89]

Prognosis

The prognosis for infants with diffuse liver involvement related to fetal or neonatal sepsis is that of the underlying condition because hepatic function is rarely compromised sufficiently to determine the outcome. In most cases, pathologic changes in the liver are unsuspected before postmortem examination.

Eight of 24 infants with solitary hepatic abscesses

whose course was described died. Two infants died before antibiotics were available,[26] and the death of another could be ascribed directly to perforation of the cecum.[20] Four newborns died with sepsis caused by organisms that were identical to those isolated from the abscess.[21, 25, 33, 34] Prematurity was undoubtedly a major contributing factor in two of these deaths.[21, 25]

Treatment

Newborns with a solitary hepatic abscess have traditionally been treated with open surgical drainage in conjunction with antibiotic therapy. Developments in the therapy for pyogenic liver abscess during the past few years suggest that a reassessment of this approach may be in order.

Several investigators have described the use of percutaneous drainage of intrahepatic abscesses and cysts, guided by CT or ultrasonography, in neonates[41, 75, 89] and children.[7, 83, 88] When combined with antibiotic therapy and monitored by ultrasonography to ensure resolution, this treatment has been found highly effective. It is questionable whether the drainage contributed to recovery other than by aiding the selection of antibiotic coverage. Subsequently, patients were successfully treated with empirical antibiotic therapy alone.[90, 91] Conservative medical management in infants has been described in only two neonates and a 5-month-old infant.[33, 37, 77]

The risk of bacteremia and disseminated infection is high in neonates, and the need to identify infecting organisms to guide antibiotic coverage is of greater urgency in the first weeks of life. Therefore, it is appropriate for microbiologic diagnosis to attempt aspiration and drainage of any definable hepatic abscess in a newborn. When proper equipment (CT, ultrasonography) and experienced personnel are available, this can be attempted percutaneously.[88, 89] When they are not, open surgical drainage should be performed. Empirical antibiotic therapy should be reserved for the sickest infants for whom it is believed that the risk of open or closed drainage would exceed the potential benefits.

If purulent material is obtained, initial antibiotic therapy can be selected on the basis of the results of Gram staining. In addition to *S. aureus* and the aerobic enteric organisms commonly associated with hepatic abscesses, anaerobic bacteria have been suspected as the cause of infection in a substantial number of patients.[25, 28, 32, 33, 35, 39] Thus, if foul-smelling pus is aspirated or if Gram-stained smears show organisms with the characteristic morphology of anaerobes,[33] addition of metronidazole, beta-lactam/beta-lactamase inhibitor combinations (e.g., ampicillin/sulbactam), clindamycin, or imipenem should be included in the initial regimen. Cultures of blood, cerebrospinal fluid, and urine should also be obtained before initiation of therapy.

If empirical antibiotic therapy is required, it must be adequate for infections caused by *S. aureus*, enteric organisms, and anaerobic bacteria. Oxacillin, gentamicin, and clindamycin would be an appropriate combination. In nurseries where methicillin-resistant *S. aureus* or *S. epidermidis* infections have been a problem, substitution of vancomycin for oxacillin will provide coverage for these organisms. Gentamicin and vancomycin levels must be monitored and dosages adjusted as necessary.

Definitive therapy is based on the results of bacteriologic cultures that identify the pathogen and its antibiotic susceptibility. Adequate anaerobic transport and culture techniques must therefore be available if meaningful information is to be obtained. Duration of treatment is based on clinical response, cessation of drainage, and resolution of the abscess cavity as determined by serial ultrasonographic examinations. Parenteral therapy should be maintained for at least 2 weeks.

SPLENIC ABSCESS

Similar to hepatic abscesses, splenic abscesses have been rarely described in infants.[91a] Only 1 of 55 splenic abscesses occurred in an infant younger than 6 months of age. *S. aureus*, *Candida* sp., and streptococci were the most frequent causes. In 20 of 48 cases, hepatic abscesses co-existed with splenic abscess. In the single infant case, torsion of the splenic vessels was present, whereas in older children, other distant infections of hematologic conditions (e.g., hemoglobinopathy, hematogenous malignancy) were the associated comorbid conditions.

INFECTIONS OF THE BILIARY TRACT

The development of ultrasonography has provided a safe and rapid means for evaluating the neonatal gallbladder. Consequently, an increasing number of reports have appeared within the past 10 years describing ultrasonographic changes seen in the first month of life, with hydrops,[92, 93] cholelithiasis,[93–98] and transient distention of the gallbladder associated[92, 93, 97, 99–102] or unassociated[97, 100, 101, 103–106] with sepsis. Ultrasonographic criteria for separating normal from pathologically enlarged gallbladders and biliary tracts in neonates have also been described.[107, 108]

Despite advanced technology and increased surveillance, cholecystitis in the neonate is observed infrequently. The literature has documented about 25 cases, of which 9 were seen in association with an epidemic of neonatal enteritis caused by *Salmonella enteritidis*.[109] Of the remaining infants, 16 were the subjects of isolated case reports[24, 101, 110–121] and 3 died of other causes with inflammatory changes in the gallbladder described as an incidental finding at autopsy.[80, 93, 122] A tissue diagnosis of "chronic cholecystitis" was established in an infant whose biliary disease apparently began at 6 days of age.[123]

The pathogenesis of this condition is uncertain; all but three cases[97, 116, 120] of cholecystitis in the newborn period have been acalculous. It is postulated that sepsis, dehydration, prolonged fasting (e.g., total parenteral nutrition), congenital obstruction, or a stone impacted in the cystic duct leads to biliary stasis and acute distention of the gallbladder. In most cases, resolution of the primary process permits restoration of the flow of bile and relief of distention. In some cases, prolonged obstruction leads to hydrops.[92] On rare occasions, cholecystitis follows, perhaps because of a direct toxic effect of the retained bile or because of ischemia related to elevated intraluminal pressure. Bacterial invasion by fecal flora is probably a secondary phenomenon.[112, 113, 124] Organisms that have been isolated from gallbladder contents or tissue include *E. coli*,[112–114, 121] *Serratia marcescens*,[101, 115] *Pseudomonas* sp.,[113] *Streptococcus faecalis*,[121] "*Streptococcus viridans*,"[119] *S. aureus*,[121] and *Clostridium welchii*.[121] "Gram-positive cocci" were identified by Gram stain in one patient.[111]

The infant with cholecystitis may become ill at any time during the first weeks of life; most cases are diagnosed in the third or fourth week. The typical clinical picture is one of sepsis together with signs of peritoneal inflammation and a palpable tender right upper quadrant or epigastric mass. Diarrhea frequently accompanies these findings. Although ultrasonography and radionuclide scintigraphy are helpful in suggesting the presence of gallbladder enlargement or inflammation, the diagnosis can be confirmed only by surgical exploration.[92, 100, 101, 104, 106] Treatment consists of cholecystectomy or tube cholecystotomy, together with systemic antimicrobial therapy based on Gram stain, culture, and susceptibility studies. If a T tube is placed in the gallbladder, a cholangiogram should be done to confirm the patency of the biliary system before the tube is removed.

Changes compatible with a diagnosis of ascending cholangitis have been described in histologic sections of liver specimens from infants who died with diarrhea accompanied by hepatocellular injury with cholestasis.[90] Bacteria were also identified in the biliary tree of 2 of 178 premature infants who died after placement of an umbilical venous catheter for an exchange transfusion or for delivery of parenteral fluids.[74] The reasons for this association, if any, are unclear. An infant with spontaneous cholangitis caused by *Enterobacter agglomerans*, presenting as a fever of unknown origin at 3 weeks of age, has also been reported.[125]

Severe inflammation and fibrosis of the extrahepatic bile ducts and diffuse changes in the portal tracts, resembling those found in biliary atresia, were found in a premature infant who died at 3 hours of age with listeriosis.[126] The author postulated that occult prenatal infections with *L. monocytogenes* might be a rare cause of ascending cholangitis presenting as "idiopathic" biliary atresia at birth.

INFECTIONS OF THE ADRENAL GLANDS

Multiple adrenal microabscesses are occasionally found as metastatic lesions associated with neonatal sepsis. The presence of such abscesses is particularly characteristic of neonatal listeriosis (see Chapter 27). Solitary adrenal abscesses are, however, quite rare. About 25 such cases have been described in the literature.[17, 127–148]

The spectrum of organisms responsible for adrenal abscesses is the same as that seen in neonatal sepsis, including *E. coli* (7 cases),[17, 127, 128, 133–136] group B *Streptococcus* (4 cases),[136–139] *Proteus mirabilis* (3 cases),[129, 130, 142] *S.*

aureus,[140, 141] *Bacteroides* sp.,[131, 143] and 2 cases each with *Streptococcus pneumoniae*[132] and *Bacteroides* sp. and *Peptostreptococcus* sp.[144] recovered from 1 case. Drainage of foul-smelling pus at surgery suggests that anaerobic bacteria were also present in two infants from whom *E. coli* and *S. aureus* were isolated.[134, 140] Cultures were not obtained from four patients.[145–148]

Fourteen abscesses were located on the right side, seven were located on the left, and three[136, 137, 145] were bilateral. Three fourths of the infants were male. The same laterality and sex predominance are seen with adrenal hemorrhage in the newborn,[145, 148–150] and it has been postulated that formation of an adrenal abscess requires a preexisting hematoma as a nidus for bacterial seeding.[135, 136] This theory of pathogenesis is further supported by clinical observations,[132, 133, 137, 144, 145] as well as by objective evidence (e.g., curvilinear calcifications[128, 130]) documenting the presence of hemorrhage before development of an abscess.[132, 136, 140, 143, 148]

Most infants with adrenal abscess present in the third or fourth week of life with signs of sepsis and an abdominal or flank mass. A history of difficult delivery or intrapartum asphyxia is noted in about half of these infants; significant maternal fever or infection during labor is noted in about one fourth.[136, 138, 139, 148] Although a few infants are afebrile when first evaluated, a palpable mass is almost always present. Abscesses are usually 6 to 8 cm in diameter, with some containing as much as 200 ml of pus[131] and measuring up to 12 cm in diameter[132] or crossing the midline.[144]

Laboratory studies are helpful in the evaluation of a possible adrenal abscess. Most infants demonstrate a leukocytosis; about a third are anemic with a history of prolonged neonatal jaundice—features associated with adrenal hemorrhage. Urinary excretion of catecholamines and their metabolites (particularly vanillylmandelic acid and homovanillic acid), which is usually increased with neuroblastoma, is normal. Because most infants with adrenal abscess are seen for evaluation of possible sepsis, a blood culture, lumbar puncture, urine culture, and chest radiograph should be obtained.

Ultrasonography has become the most widely used modality for initial evaluation of abdominal masses. In an infant with adrenal abscess, not only can it help to define the extent and cystic nature of the lesion, but it also can often demonstrate movable necrotic debris in the abscess cavity.[130, 135, 136, 139, 140, 142–146] With serial examinations, abscesses can be distinguished from those masses associated with liquefying hematoma, adrenal cyst, hydronephrosis of an obstructed upper pole duplication, or necrotic neuroblastoma.[136, 138, 148, 151–152a] Intravenous pyelography demonstrates downward displacement of the kidney and compression of the upper calyces, which confirms the presence of a suprarenal mass.[128–130, 132, 134, 136, 139, 140, 142–144, 147] A round suprarenal radiopaque "halo" or "rim" with central lucency, which is characteristic of adrenal abscess, may also be seen on early films[135, 137, 141] but is not pathognomonic.[136] Intravenous pyelography adds little diagnostic information to that provided by ultrasound. Experience with radionuclide scanning,[138, 140, 141] CT,[136, 142] and MRI[124] in this condition is limited, but these modalities are likely to be as useful as ultrasonography.

Whichever diagnostic methods are used, concern about persisting signs of sepsis, more than the possible presence of an adrenal neoplasm, will generally encourage early efforts to establish a diagnosis. In the past, recommended management has been incision and drainage or resection of the abscess.[132, 136, 139, 142, 148] More recently, needle aspiration under ultrasonographic guidance, combined with placement of a catheter for drainage and irrigation, has proven to be a useful alternative method.[87, 128, 129, 141] Antibiotic therapy should be based on Gram stain, culture, and susceptibility studies of abscess fluid and should be continued for 10 to 14 days.

The adrenals are infected in about 15% of infants with congenital syphilis.[57, 58] In addition to the presence of spirochetes, the most frequent and characteristic change is an extraordinary amount of cellular connective tissue in the capsule.

APPENDICITIS

Acute appendicitis is extremely rare in infants younger than 4 weeks of age. Reviews of more than 25,000 cases of appendicitis in infants and children in Great Britain,[153] Ireland,[154] Norway,[155] Germany,[156] and the United States[157–162] revealed only eight infants who presented during the neonatal period. Pediatric surgery centers in Cologne in Germany,[163] Boston,[164] Cleveland,[165] Chicago,[166] and Detroit[167] found only four cases of neonatal appendicitis during the past 15 to 20 years. Since the condition was first described by Albrecht in 1905[168, 169] and Diess in 1908,[170] approximately 65 cases of neonatal suppurative appendicitis have been reported in the literature with sufficient details to permit tabulation of the clinical features of this condition.[153, 158, 159, 162, 171–207] The discussion that follows is based on a review of those cases. Only infants with acute intra-abdominal appendicitis were considered. Those with appendicitis secondary to other conditions, such as Hirschsprung's disease,[208, 209] necrotizing enterocolitis (NEC),[210] or incarceration in an inguinal hernia,[211, 212] have not been included. An additional 25 to 30 cases that have been reported with incomplete clinical observations, listed in series of patients with neonatal peritonitis (see Peritonitis section) or noted in other review articles but not available for analysis, are also not included.

Inflammation of the appendix is more common in male newborns than in female newborns. In those reports in which the sex was stated, 40 cases occurred in males and only 17 in females. Prematurity also appears to be a predisposing factor: 23 of the 49 infants whose birth weights were recorded weighed less than 2500 g at birth. The incidence of appendicitis in infants of multiple births—six twins and one triplet—appears to be higher than would be expected on the basis of their low birth weight alone.

Microbiology

Because obstruction of the appendiceal lumen is responsible for almost all cases of appendicitis,[164] it is not surprising that gram-negative enteric organisms resident in the bowel have been isolated from the peritoneal fluid or periappendiceal pus of about 75% of infants with this condition. Specific etiologic agents include *E. coli*, *Klebsiella*, *Enterobacter* sp., *Pseudomonas*, *Proteus* sp., untyped *Streptococcus*, *S. aureus*, and *Bacteroides* sp. These bacterial species have also been isolated from the peritoneal fluid of older children with appendicitis.[161, 164, 213] Attempts at isolation of anaerobic bacteria are rarely described.

A single case of perforated amebic appendicitis with secondary bacterial peritonitis and multiple hepatic abscesses in a premature infant born in Great Britain has been reported. The *Entamoeba histolytica* discovered in the wall of the necrotic appendix was presumably acquired from the patient's father, who was a carrier of the same organism.[20]

A patient with gangrenous appendicitis associated with *Rhizopus oryzae* has also been reported.[214] It was postulated that the fungus colonized the infant's gut by transfer from an adhesive bandage used to secure an endotracheal tube.

Pathogenesis

Obstruction of the appendiceal lumen has been generally accepted as the primary cause of appendicitis in all age groups. The relative rarity of this condition in the first month of life is therefore probably related to factors that serve to decrease the likelihood of obstruction. Such factors include a wide-based, funnel-shaped appendix; the predominantly liquid and soft-solid diet given to infants; the absence of prolonged periods in the upright position; and the infrequency of infections that cause hyperplasia of the appendiceal lymphoid tissue.[161, 215, 216]

The causes of luminal obstruction in the newborn period, when recognized, are often extrinsic to the appendix itself. Reports of appendicitis secondary to the presence of ectopic pancreatic tissue,[159] a fecalith,[172] or meconium plug[165] are unusual exceptions. It has been suggested since 1911 that sharp angulation of the appendix, bent on itself in the narrow retrocolic space, may be an important cause of obstruction.[217] The findings by this author of 11 neonates with inflammatory changes in the appendix, noted among 200 consecutive autopsies in infants younger than 3 months of age, have not been repeated in the past 80 years.

Inflammation of the appendix with perforation has been described as the presenting illness in several infants with neonatal Hirschsprung's disease.[209, 210] The association of these two conditions is attributed to the functional obstruction, increased intraluminal pressure, and fecal trapping that occur proximal to the aganglionic segments. Suppurative appendicitis related to incarceration and strangulation of the cecum within an inguinal or scrotal hernia has been found in a significant number of infants.[211, 212]

Clinical Manifestations

The onset of neonatal appendicitis generally occurs during the first 2 weeks of life. Only 3 of 54 infants with this condition presented between the twenty-first and thirtieth days. The reasons for this phenomenon are unclear, particularly in view of the relatively even distribution of cases during the remainder of the first year of life.[162] Five cases of "prenatal" appendicitis have been described.[218-222] Of the four available for analysis, only one showed definite evidence of a suppurative process in the appendix and signs of bowel obstruction clearly present at birth[218]; however, cultures and Gram stain of the pus found at surgery were free of bacteria. Poisoning by mercuric chloride was suspected in one[220] of the remaining three cases, and the other two, who were said to have prenatal rupture of the appendix, were asymptomatic until the second[219] and twelfth[222] days of life.

The signs of neonatal appendicitis are the same as those of any of the various forms of intestinal obstruction that occur during the newborn period[223] (Table 25-1). Prominent early findings include abdominal distention, progressive and frequently bilious vomiting, and evidence of pain, as manifested by persistent crying, irritability, or "colic." Clinical features such as diarrhea, constipation, lethargy, or refusal to feed may also be evident but are too nonspecific to be helpful in establishing a diagnosis. The presence or absence of fever is an unreliable sign in appendicitis as in other forms of neonatal infection; temperature has been recorded as normal or subnormal in more than 50% of newborns with this condition. Abdominal tenderness and guarding are inconstant findings and, when present, are rarely localized to the appendiceal area. Physical signs of sufficient specificity to indicate acute inflammation of the appendix are thus generally absent until late in the course of the illness, when gangrene and rupture may result in the formation of a localized intra-abdominal abscess or cellulitis of the anterior abdominal wall. Erythema or edema or both of the right lower quadrant have been observed in several patients. The presence of this finding, particularly when accompanied by a palpable mass in the right iliac fossa, indicates bowel perforation with peritonitis and should suggest a preoperative diagnosis of either NEC or appendicitis (see Necrotizing Enterocolitis section).

TABLE 25-1
Signs of Intra-abdominal Neonatal Appendicitis in 55 Infants

SIGN	% WITH FINDING
Abdominal distention	90
Vomiting	60
Refusal of feedings	40
Temperature ≥38° C	40
37° C to 38° C	30
≤37° C	30
Pain (crying, restlessness)	30
Lethargy	30
Erythema/edema of right lower quadrant	25
Mass in right lower quadrant	20
Diarrhea	20
Passage of bloody stools	20

Diagnosis

The diagnosis of appendicitis in the neonate is usually determined at surgery performed for evaluation of abdominal distention and suspected peritonitis. With the high incidence of prematurity associated with early appendicitis, bowel perforation from NEC has been a common preoperative consideration.[203] Indeed, the two conditions can coexist, and, in some cases, the appendix may participate in the process of ischemic necrosis and perforation.[202, 210]

Laboratory studies are of little value in establishing a diagnosis of appendicitis in the newborn. White blood cell counts of less than 10,000 per mm³ were found in 10 of 30 infants for whom this determination was performed. Urinalyses are usually normal, although ketonuria, which reflects diminished caloric intake, hematuria, and proteinuria may be seen. Because bacteremia may accompany appendiceal perforation and peritonitis, a blood culture and evaluation for metastatic infection with lumbar puncture and chest radiograph should be performed. The value of paracentesis for diagnosis of bowel perforation and peritoneal infection is discussed later (see Necrotizing Enterocolitis section).

Radiologic examinations are occasionally helpful, but in most cases they serve only to confirm the clinical impression of small bowel obstruction. The presence of an increased soft tissue density displacing loops of intestine from the right iliac fossa generally indicates appendiceal perforation with abscess formation and is perhaps the most reliable sign of acute appendicitis in the neonate. Extraluminal gas may be localized briefly to the right lower quadrant after rupture of the appendix.[209] The rapid development of an extensive pneumoperitoneum, however, obscures the site of origin of the escaping gas in most infants within a short time.[223] Ultrasonography may aid in the detection of a periappendiceal abscess[82] but lacks sensitivity and specificity to be of assistance in establishing an early diagnosis of appendicitis.

Prognosis

The overall mortality rate from appendicitis in the newborn is high but is improving. Eight of the newborns in the last 12 reported cases have lived, whereas of 60 infants with this condition for whom the outcome was recorded, 38 (64%) died. Survival was unrelated to birth weight. Among the many factors responsible for these discouraging figures, three appear to be of primary importance: (1) delay in diagnosis, (2) a high incidence of perforation, and (3) the rapid onset of diffuse peritonitis after appendiceal rupture.

Perforation has been noted at surgery or autopsy in 70% of newborns with acute appendicitis. The relative frequency of this complication has been attributed to delays in establishing a diagnosis as well as to certain anatomic features of the appendix in young infants that predispose it to early necrosis and rupture. These features include a meager blood supply that renders the organ more vulnerable to ischemia; a cecum that is relatively smaller and less distensible than that of adults, thereby forcing a greater intraluminal pressure on the appendix; and the presence of a thin muscularis and serosa that readily lose their structural integrity under the combined effects of ischemia and increased internal pressure.[161, 179, 180, 188]

Once the appendix has ruptured, infants are unable to contain the infection efficiently at the site of origin. Rapid dissemination of spilled intestinal contents produces a diffuse peritonitis within hours. The anatomic basis for this is the small size of the infant's omentum, which fails to provide an efficient envelope for escaping material; the relatively longer and more mobile mesenteries, which favor widespread contamination; and the small size of the peritoneal cavity, which permits easy access of infected material to areas removed from the site of spillage.[158, 164, 179, 180]

Peritonitis, accompanied not only by sepsis but also by the massive outpouring of fluids, electrolytes, and proteins from the inflamed serosal surfaces, is generally the terminal event in neonatal appendicitis. Deterioration of the patient's condition is often extremely rapid at this stage; failure to recognize the underlying illness and to institute appropriate therapy promptly is inevitably followed by a fatal outcome.

Treatment

Surgical intervention is essential for survival of young infants with appendicitis. Because vomiting, diarrhea, and anorexia frequently accompany this condition, restoration of fluid and electrolyte balance is a major factor in ensuring a favorable outcome. Loss of plasma into the bowel wall and lumen of the dilated intestine may require additional replacement with whole blood, plasma, or an albumin equivalent. Optimal preparation often necessitates a delay of several hours but remains, nonetheless, a major determining factor in the success of any surgical procedure done during the neonatal period.

The preoperative use of antibiotics has been recommended in infants with intestinal obstruction to achieve therapeutic blood levels of the drug before the time of incision and possible contamination.[165, 224, 225] Although there are few data to support such a recommendation in neonates, any controversy regarding the need for prophylactic antibiotics is generally moot: perforation, fecal spillage, and peritonitis occur so early in the course of neonatal appendicitis that almost all infants with this condition require treatment before the time of surgery. Once the diagnosis of gangrenous or perforated appendicitis has been established and surgery performed, parenteral antibiotic therapy should be continued for 10 days. The combination of clindamycin, gentamicin (or extended-spectrum cephalosporins), and ampicillin provides adequate coverage against most enteric pathogens and can be used for initial empirical therapy. Until the infant is able to tolerate alimentation, scrupulous attention to postoperative maintenance of body fluids, electrolyte balance, nutrition, and the correction of blood and plasma losses is vital to survival (see Peritonitis and Necrotizing Enterocolitis sections).

PERITONITIS

Peritonitis in the newborn is most commonly associated with perforation of the gastrointestinal tract, ruptured omphaloceles, or wound infections that follow abdominal surgery.[226, 227] For this reason, diagnosis and treatment of neonatal peritonitis are less frequently the responsibility of the pediatrician than of the surgeon. It has been estimated that as many as 20 to 40% of gastrointestinal surgical problems in the neonatal period are complicated by bacterial peritonitis (see also Necrotizing Enterocolitis section).[182, 228] Thus, between 1 and 10 cases per year have been reported in retrospective analyses of peritonitis diagnosed during the first month of life at pediatric surgical centers in the United States,[228–230] Great Britain,[227, 231] Hungary,[232] Germany,[233, 234] France,[235] and Zimbabwe.[236] Among almost 3000 infants admitted to a neonatal intensive care unit in Liverpool in 1981 to 1982, there were six cases of peritonitis, all secondary to NEC perforation of the gastrointestinal tract.[237] Peritonitis was present in 4 (all of low birth weight) of 501 infants on whom consecutive autopsies were performed from 1960 through 1966 at St. Christopher's Hospital for Children in Philadelphia. These cases represented approximately 3% of all patients with inflammatory lesions associated with death in this age group.[238] Potter considered the peritoneum "one of the most frequent points of localization" in infants dying with sepsis.[15] Among 121 such infants autopsied from 1976 to 1988 at St. Mary's Hospital in Manchester, England, generalized peritonitis was found in 9 (7.4%).[227]

A preponderance of males (2.5:1)[187, 236, 239] and a high incidence of prematurity (33%)[228, 231–233] have been found in unselected series of infants with this condition. These features are, however, probably less a characteristic of bacterial peritonitis in the newborn than of the primary surgical and septic conditions that are responsible for its occurrence (particularly NEC). Interestingly, among newborns with primary peritonitis, there appears to be a female preponderance.[232, 240] A high incidence of congenital anomalies not involving the intestinal tract has also been noted among neonates with peritonitis.[228, 233, 239, 241]

Microbiology

The condition that permits bacteria to colonize the peritoneal surface determines the nature of the infecting organisms. Most infants in whom rupture of a viscus and fecal spillage have caused peritonitis are infected by bacteria considered to be part of the normal enteric microflora; however, prior use of antimicrobial agents and colonization patterns within a nursery are important factors in determining which organisms predominate. Although a mixed flora of two to five species can often be recovered,[239] single isolates have been reported in as many as a third of infants with peritonitis.[242, 243] The predominant aerobic organisms usually include *E. coli*, *Klebsiella* sp., *Enterobacter* sp., *Pseudomonas* sp., *Proteus* sp., coagulase-negative and coagulase-positive staphylococci, ungrouped streptococci, *Enterococcus*, and *Candida*.[227, 228, 234, 236, 243–245]

Techniques adequate for the isolation of anaerobic organisms have been infrequently used. In a series of 43 consecutive infants with gastrointestinal perforation and bacterial growth from peritoneal fluid, about one fifth demonstrated a mixed aerobic-anaerobic flora with *Bacteroides* sp. the predominant anaerobes.[239] The remaining specimens grew aerobic or facultative organisms alone. No cultures yielded only anaerobes. In that series, as well as in others, the same organisms were frequently isolated from both the peritoneal cavity and blood.[229, 239, 241, 245]

In contrast to fecal flora isolated from infants with gastrointestinal perforation, gram-positive organisms predominated among neonates with "idiopathic primary peritonitis." This condition is presumably due to sepsis in most cases but also has often been associated with omphalitis. Specific organisms in one representative series included *S. pneumoniae* (three cases), ungrouped beta-hemolytic *Streptococcus* (three cases), and *S. aureus*, *Pseudomonas* sp., and *E. coli* (one case each).[228] Gram-positive cocci were also the major isolates in other series of peritonitis associated with hematogenous dissemination of organisms or extension from a peripheral suppurative focus.[10, 26, 33, 71, 240–250] Many of the cases caused by *S. aureus* occurred before the advent of antibiotics or during the worldwide pandemic of staphylococcal disease in the late 1950s, whereas streptococci, particularly group B, have been a prominent cause in recent years.[240, 246–250]

Rarely, peritonitis may be caused by *Candida albicans*, either in pure culture or mixed with the usual gram-negative enteric organisms.[227, 251] Because the clinical findings in this condition are no different from those seen with solely bacterial involvement, the diagnosis is usually established fortuitously by blood or peritoneal fluid culture. Severe hypothermia has been described as a possible predisposing cause of bowel perforation and peritonitis due to *Candida*.[252] In addition to well-recognized risk factors, such as prematurity, antibiotic therapy, and parenteral nutrition with deep venous catheters, NEC may also be a significant risk factor for systemic candidiasis, in which it was observed in 37% of 30 infants.[252a] However, only a single infant in this series had a positive culture of *Candida* species from the peritoneum. Peritoneal catheters or peritoneal dialysis may also be a risk for direct introduction of *Candida* organisms into the peritoneal space, which occurred in 1 of 26 children[252b] (see Chapter 17, Fungal Infections).

Pathogenesis

Acute bacterial peritonitis may occur whenever bacteria gain access to the peritoneal cavity, through fecal spillage, by extension from a suppurative focus, or by the hematogenous route. Intrauterine peritonitis due to *L. monocytogenes* has been reported[227]; however, cases of "fetal peritonitis" described in the early literature were actually examples of meconium peritonitis secondary to intrauterine intestinal perforation.[253, 254] Although bacterial colonization of the gastrointestinal tract in the first days of life often leads to infection in this condition, it is an aseptic peritonitis in its initial stages. A similar condition with focal perforation of the ileum or colon occurring postnatally has been described in very low birth weight infants. Blue-black discoloration of the abdomen, caused by meconium staining of the tissues of the underlying skin, was the first and most striking physical finding in these infants. Clinical, radiographic, and histopathologic evidence of infection or inflammation was notably absent in almost all cases.[225]

The various conditions that predispose to neonatal peritonitis are outlined in Table 25–2. The relative importance of each in the etiology of this condition can be estimated from data collected in several large series. Among almost 400 newborns with peritonitis studied between 1959 and 1978, perforation of the intestinal tract was responsible for 72% of cases, with ruptured omphaloceles or gastroschisis responsible for 12%, hematogenous dissemination or "primary" peritonitis for 12%, and omphalitis and postoperative complications for 2% each.[187, 226, 227, 234, 236, 257] A comprehensive review of neonatal peritonitis by Bell describes the common sites and causes of gastrointestinal perforation and their relative frequencies[226, 239] (Figs. 25–1 and 25–2).

TABLE 25–2
Etiology of Bacterial Peritonitis in the Neonatal Period

Gastrointestinal perforation[187, 227, 228, 231–236, 239, 241, 245, 256, 257]
  Necrotizing enterocolitis (see text)
  Ischemic necrosis
    Spontaneous focal gastrointestinal perforation[229, 242, 245, 255, 256, 258]
    Volvulus
    Hirschsprung's disease
    Meconium ileus (cystic fibrosis)[227, 260]
    Postoperative complications
    Congenital anomalies
    Internal hernia
    Catheter-associated vascular thrombosis[227]
    Indomethacin therapy (enteral or parenteral)[261, 262]
  Trauma
    Feeding tubes[263]
    Rectal thermometers, catheters, enema[264–269]
    Intrauterine exchange transfusion[227, 267]
    Paracentesis of ascites fluid
  Meconium peritonitis with postnatal bacterial contamination[239, 253, 254]
  Peptic ulcer: stomach, duodenum, ectopic gastric mucosa
  Acute suppurative appendicitis (see text)
  Infection
    Shigella or salmonella enterocolitis[268–270]
    Congenital luetic enteritis with necrosis[58]
Ruptured omphalocele or gastroschisis
Postoperative: anastomotic leaks, wound dehiscence, wound contamination
Primary peritonitis
  Prenatal sepsis: listeriosis, syphilis,[58] tuberculosis[46–49]
  Neonatal sepsis[10, 33, 227, 228, 236, 248–250, 257, 272]
  Suppurative omphalitis[26, 71, 236, 240, 246, 247, 257, 271]
Transmural migration (theory)[259, 273]

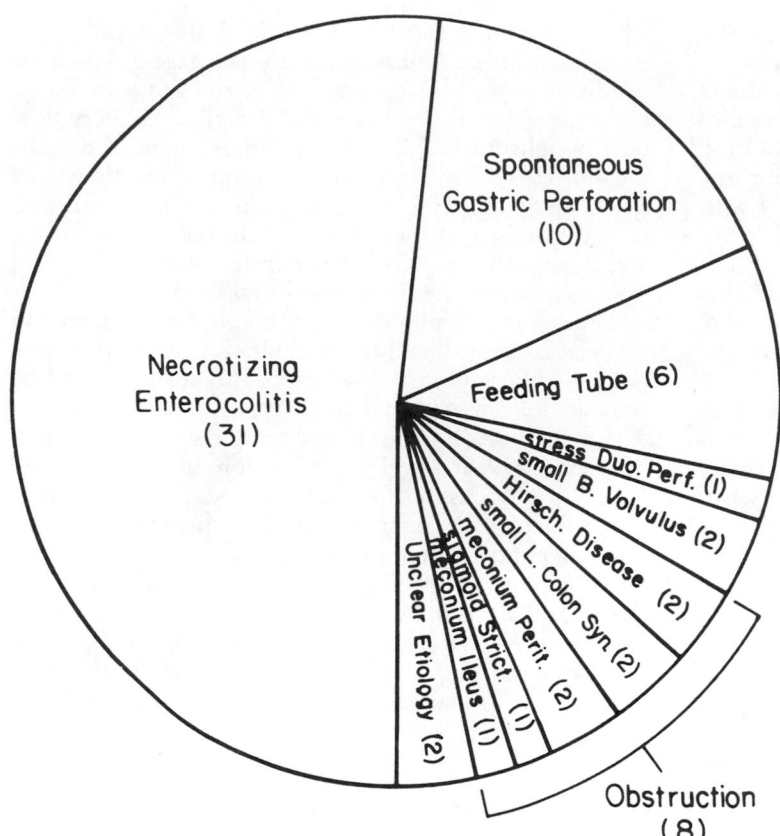

FIGURE 25–1 Etiology of perforation in 60 neonates. (From Bell MJ. Peritonitis in the newborn—current concepts. Pediatr Clin North Am 32:1181, 1985.)

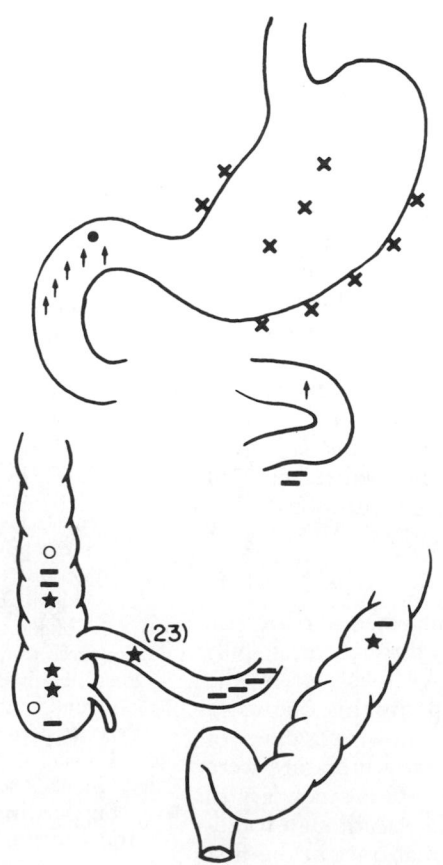

* Necrotizing enterocolitis (4 mult)
× Spontaneous gastric perforation
† Tube perforation
○ Hirschsprung's disease
● Stress ulcer
— Other

FIGURE 25–2 Site of perforation in 60 neonates. (From Bell MJ. Peritonitis in the newborn—current concepts. Pediatr Clin North Am 32:1181, 1985.)

No recent cases of neonatal peritonitis have been attributed to microorganisms entering the peritoneal cavity by traversing the bowel wall through the lymphatics or within macrophages, (i.e., transmural migration). Indeed, the evidence for the existence of this pathway is theoretical and is based primarily on retrospective analyses of data on pathology in humans together with supporting observations made on laboratory animals.[259, 273] Further confirmation will be necessary before the transmural pathway can be accepted as an established source of peritoneal colonization by bacteria.

Clinical Manifestations

Neonatal peritonitis is a disease primarily of the first 10 days of life; a significant number of infants have evidence of peritoneal infection within the first 24 hours.[228, 229, 236, 241] An analysis of the etiologic factors responsible for peritonitis in the newborn provides a ready explanation for this observation (see Table 25–2): most cases of NEC[239, 274] and "spontaneous" gastric perforation[229, 239, 245, 256] occur within the first week. Ruptured omphaloceles and gastroschisis, which are colonized not only by the maternal vaginal flora but also by the bacteria prevalent in the external environment, often manifest early infection. In the infant with congenital obstruction, the onset of alimentation during the first 12 to 24 hours accentuates distention and ischemic necrosis of the bowel wall, which leads to early intestinal perforation. Exchange transfusions are performed most frequently within the first 1 or 2 days of life and are followed by enterocolitis within 4 to 24 hours in most infants in whom perforation ultimately occurs.[275, 276] Finally, neonatal sepsis, with potential peritoneal seeding of microorganisms, is more frequent during the first 48 hours of life than during any subsequent period.[277]

The variety of signs and symptoms present in a young infant with peritonitis were summarized most succinctly by Thelander[245] in 1939:

> The little patient looks sick. He is cyanotic; the respirations are rapid and grunting; the abdomen is distended, and the abdominal wall, the flanks and the scrotum or vulva are usually edematous. Frequently brawny induration of the edematous area, which may resemble erysipelas, is also present. Food is taken poorly or not at all. Vomiting is frequent and persistent. The vomitus contains bile and may contain blood. The stools are either absent or scant; some mucus or blood may be passed. The temperature may be subnormal, but varying degrees of fever have been reported. The blood count is of little or no value. The hemoglobin content may be very high, which probably indicates only dehydration. The leukocytes may or may not respond with a rise.

Although her review was limited to neonates with perforation of the intestinal tract, subsequent reports have corroborated the presence of these findings in infants with peritonitis resulting from a wide variety of causes.[187, 228, 230–232, 236, 239, 244] All of the symptoms described may not be encountered in any one patient; however, some are always present (Table 25–3).

The large overlap between the signs of neonatal peritonitis and sepsis can make it difficult to differentiate the two conditions on the basis of clinical findings. Signs of intestinal obstruction such as abdominal distention

TABLE 25–3
Signs of Bacterial Peritonitis in the Neonate[a]

SIGN	INCIDENCE %
Abdominal distention	85
Shock	80
Vomiting	70
Constipation	60
Hypothermia	60
Respiratory distress	55
Fever	15
Diarrhea	15

[a]Data are based on patients described in references 228, 236 and 239. Redness, edema, and induration of the anterior abdominal wall, noted in only one series, are also recognized as characteristic signs.[239]

and vomiting, which are seen in 10 to 20% of newborns with sepsis,[9, 17, 241] may reflect a coexistent unrecognized peritonitis. Because the early use of antibiotics often cures hematogenous peritonitis in infants with septicemia, the diagnosis may be missed in infants who survive. It is noteworthy that peritonitis unassociated with perforation was found at postmortem examination in 4 of 20 infants with sepsis in 1933,[10] 9 of 73 premature infants dying with septicemia between 1959 and 1964,[9] and 9 of 121 such infants dying between 1976 and 1988.[226]

Diagnosis

Demonstration of free intraperitoneal fluid by ultrasonography[278] or abdominal radiographs taken in the erect and recumbent positions can be helpful in the diagnosis of peritonitis. This finding is sometimes the only evidence of perforation. Absence of definition of the right inferior hepatic margin, increased density of the soft tissue, and the presence of "floating" loops of bowel have been recorded as positive signs of ascites.[223, 279] Diagnostic paracentesis can be useful in determining whether the fluid is caused by bacterial peritonitis,[240, 248, 280, 281] hemoperitoneum, chylous ascites,[282] or bile peritonitis.[283]

The left lateral ("left-side down") decubitus film is of great value in showing small amounts of intraperitoneal gas.[239] Although pneumoperitoneum can be caused by mediastinal air dissecting down from the chest into the abdomen,[284, 285] free gas in the peritoneal cavity usually indicates intestinal perforation. An associated pneumatosis intestinalis should strongly suggest the diagnosis of NEC. Several patterns of intraperitoneal gas distribution have been described[275, 286, 287]: the air-dome sign, falciform ligament sign, football sign, lucent-liver sign, saddlebag sign, and gas in the scrotum. Absence of a gastric air–fluid level on an erect abdominal roentgenogram, together with a normal or decreased amount of gas in the small and large bowel, strongly favors a diagnosis of gastric perforation.[287] This finding is almost always accompanied by pneumoperitoneum.

In equivocal cases, metrizamide contrast studies of the bowel can be helpful in establishing a diagnosis of intestinal perforation.[242, 284] Serial abdominal transillumination with a bright fiberoptic light is a useful bedside method for the early detection of ascites or pneumoperitoneum in the newborn.[288]

Failure to demonstrate free air in the peritoneal cavity does not, however, rule out a diagnosis of perforation, particularly if air swallowing has been reduced or prevented through orotracheal intubation, nasogastric suction, or use of neuromuscular blocking agents.[280, 284, 289] In some cases, the amount of gas in the bowel lumen is so small that even if perforation occurs the gas could escape detection. Alternatively, small leaks may become walled off and the free air reabsorbed.[284, 290, 291] In three large series of infants with peritonitis in whom a patent site of perforation was found at surgery, pneumoperitoneum was absent in 35 to 75%.[228, 239, 241]

Radiographic evidence of intestinal obstruction, although a common cause or consequence of peritonitis, lacks sufficient specificity to be considered a reliable aid in making this diagnosis. A diffuse granular appearance of the abdomen, with one or more irregular calcific densities lying either within the bowel lumen or in the peritoneal cavity, should suggest a diagnosis of meconium peritonitis with possible bacterial superinfection.[254]

Prognosis

Prematurity, pulmonary infections, shock and hemorrhage related to perforation of the intestinal tract, sepsis, and disseminated intravascular coagulopathy are often the major factors responsible for the death of neonates, who may concurrently have peritonitis diagnosed at surgery or at postmortem examination. For this reason, case:fatality rates often represent the mortality rate among newborns dying with, rather than because of, infection of the peritoneal cavity.[227, 233, 239]

In the past, the incidence of fatalities was exceedingly high when peritonitis was associated with gastrointestinal perforation. Mortality rates of 70% were observed in large series of the 1960s and 1970s.[187, 228, 231, 232, 234–236, 241, 291] Heightened awareness of conditions associated with perforation, more rapid diagnosis, and improved surgical management have led to the percentage of survivors almost doubling in recent years.[233, 235] The cause of perforation appears to influence the likelihood of survival, with spontaneous gastric perforation having the lowest mortality rate (10%) and perforation of the duodenum caused by a feeding tube the highest (50%); NEC (40%) and all other causes (25%) occupy intermediate positions.[239]

As survival rates have improved, the number of nonlethal complications after perforation has risen proportionally. In one review, two thirds of surviving infants had significant postoperative complications pertaining to infection (bacteremia, wound infection, intra-abdominal abscess) or gastrointestinal tract dysfunction (esophageal reflux, obstruction, stomal stenosis).[239] Secondary surgical procedures to correct these problems were required in more than half of the infants. In addition, 60% required parenteral hyperalimentation for nutritional support during their recovery period.

The mortality rate among neonates with peritonitis from causes other than perforation of the bowel, such as sepsis,[187, 228, 232, 236] omphalitis,[236, 271] or a ruptured omphalocele,[228, 233, 236] although high in the past, has not been reassessed in the past few years.[239]

Early diagnosis and institution of appropriate surgical therapy are major factors in reducing the mortality rate.[239] It has been shown that infants operated on within 24 hours after the onset of symptoms had a survival rate that was almost double the rate for those who were operated on between 24 and 48 hours and two and one half times higher than the rate for those whose surgery was delayed more than 48 hours.[241] Factors with an apparent adverse influence on prognosis include low birth weight,[228, 233, 236, 239, 257] low birth weight for gestational age,[226] congenital malformations,[233] male sex,[227] and initial serum pH of less than 7.30.[227]

Treatment

The treatment of bacterial peritonitis is directed primarily toward correction of the causative condition.[227] Careful attention to preoperative preparation of the infant is essential to survival. As soon as bowel obstruction or perforation is diagnosed, continuous nasogastric suction should be instituted for decompression and prevention of aspiration pneumonitis. Diagnostic needle paracentesis is also useful for relief of pneumoperitoneum and may facilitate exchange of gas by reducing the intra-abdominal pressure. Shock, dehydration, and electrolyte disturbances should be corrected through parenteral administration of appropriate electrolyte solutions, plasma, or plasma substitutes. If blood is discovered in fluid recovered by gastric suction or abdominal paracentesis, use of whole blood may be necessary to correct depletion of blood volume. Persistent bleeding must be evaluated for disseminated intravascular coagulation or thrombocytopenia or both and treated accordingly. Hypothermia, which frequently accompanies neonatal peritonitis, should be corrected before induction of anesthesia. Infants who are unable to tolerate oral or tube feedings within 2 or 3 postoperative days should be started on parenteral hyperalimentation.

If a diagnosis of peritonitis is established at the time of paracentesis or surgery, both aerobic and anaerobic cultures of the peritoneal contents should be taken before initiation of antibiotic therapy. Parenteral administration of a combination of gentamicin or an extended-spectrum cephalosporin with clindamycin and ampicillin should be continued for 7 to 10 days.[212, 225] In the event of a poor clinical response, culture and susceptibility studies of the infecting organisms should be used as guides for modifying therapy.

Leakage of the intestinal contents sometimes results in formation of a localized abscess rather than contamination of the entire peritoneal cavity. Management of infants with such an abscess should include both antimicrobial therapy and surgical drainage of the abscess by the most convenient route.

NECROTIZING ENTEROCOLITIS

Necrotizing enterocolitis with necrosis of the bowel wall is a severe, often fatal, disease occurring with increasing frequency in recent years. The average annual NEC mortality rate is 13.1 per 100,000 live births; black infants (particularly males) are three times more likely to die of NEC than are white infants, and mortality rates are highest in the southern United States.[292-301] NEC occurs in about 5% of infants admitted to neonatal intensive care units; however, the incidence varies widely among centers and even from year to year at the same institution.[302-315] NEC predominantly affects infants with birth weights below 2000 g[292, 293, 308, 316-321]; in several series, the frequency in infants younger than 1500 g was as high as 10 to 15%.[292-294, 309, 310, 314, 320, 322-326] Only 5 to 10% of all cases of classic NEC occur in full-term infants.[301, 327-329] It has been stated that occasional cases of NEC may be the price to be paid for the benefits of modern neonatal intensive care.[330] Thus, although most reports of NEC emanate from the United States, Canada, and Great Britain, the condition occurs worldwide in countries maintaining neonatal intensive care units.

Pathology and Pathogenesis

Bowel wall necrosis of variable length and depth is the characteristic feature of NEC, with perforation in up to one third of affected infants generally in the terminal ileum or cecum, where microcirculation is poor.[239, 296, 300, 318, 327, 331-333] The pathogenesis of NEC is not yet established, but most investigators agree that the initiating event is some form of stress to the immature gastrointestinal tract, which leads to disruption of the mucosal barrier, bacterial invasion and proliferation, and gas formation within the bowel wall (Fig. 25–3).[308, 316, 317, 334] Surgical specimens from early stages of the disease show mucosal edema, hemorrhage, and superficial ulceration with very little inflammation or cellular response. By the second or third day, after progression to pneumatosis

and transmural necrosis of the bowel wall, bacterial proliferation and the acute inflammatory reaction become more prominent.[296, 318]

There has been a great deal of investigation and little agreement on the importance of various perinatal events in the causation of NEC.[308, 316, 317, 334] Except for immaturity and possibly polycythemia, other factors originally thought to predispose to NEC have, on further study, occurred with equal frequency in control populations of infants.[309, 314, 317, 319, 320, 329, 335, 336] Thus, maternal complications of pregnancy, labor, and delivery and neonatal respiratory distress syndrome are now thought to be unrelated to the development of NEC, whereas evidence linking NEC to birth asphyxia, hypotension, hypothermia, use of vascular catheters, exchange transfusion, feeding history, abnormalities of gut motility, neonatal achlorhydria, and the presence of patent ductus arteriosus is often contradictory. Each of these conditions, singly or together, may act as a stress leading to mucosal injury, but none has been consistently associated with NEC.[337, 338] NEC has occurred among apparently healthy infants with no known predisposing risk factors.[292, 301, 327, 334]

Several epidemiologic observations suggest that NEC is an infectious contagious disease of nosocomial origin. The temporal clustering of cases at institutions, the association of some outbreaks with single infectious agents or alterations in bowel flora, and the possible beneficial effects of breast-feeding, oral nonabsorbable antibiotics, or infection control measures in reducing the incidence of disease suggest a possible nosocomial etiology. Unfortunately, the evidence linking NEC to specific infectious agents is often circumstantial or open to alternative interpretation. Thus, current evidence suggests that NEC is the end response of the immature gastrointestinal tract to multiple factors acting alone or

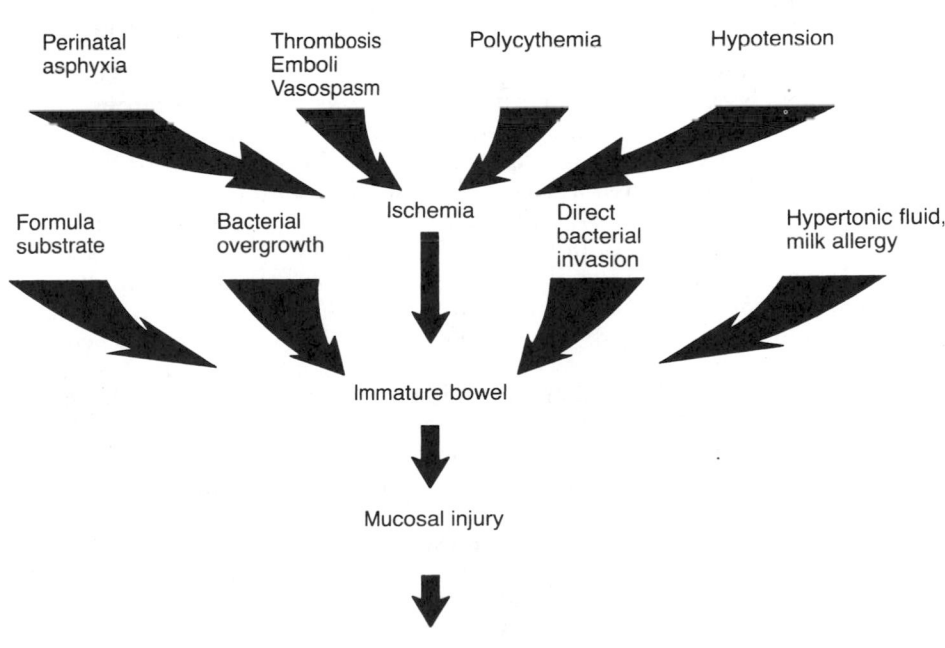

FIGURE 25–3 Pathogenesis of mucosal injury leading to necrotizing enterocolitis (NEC). (Adapted from Walsh MC, Kliegman RM. Necrotizing enterocolitis. Pediatric Basics 40:5, 1985, with permission.)

in concert to produce mucosal injury, with colonization or invasion by the microorganisms representing only one part of the continuum of that disease process.[276, 283, 284, 300]

Microbiology

Descriptions of sporadic outbreaks of NEC in neonatal intensive care units have led to a search for transmissible agents, including bacterial, viral, and fungal pathogens.[297, 308, 316, 317, 334, 339–344] Predominance of a single organism in the stool, blood, bowel wall, or peritoneal cavity of infants during epidemics of NEC has implicated *Klebsiella* species,[294, 305, 321, 333, 345–347] *Enterobacter* species,[348] *E. coli*,[349, 350] *Pseudomonas* species,[351, 352] *Salmonella* species,[353] *S. epidermidis* and other coagulase-negative staphylococci,[354] *S. aureus*,[355] rotavirus,[356, 357] coronavirus,[358] coxsackievirus B2,[359] and *Torulopsis glabrata*.[360]

The analogous pathology of necrotizing enteritis caused by *Clostridium septicum*[361] and *C. perfringens* in domestic animals,[307, 347, 362] older children, and adults[363] favored suggestions that *Clostridium* species might act as a primary pathogen in NEC.[308, 316, 317, 334, 344, 364] Several reports provided evidence that *C. perfringens*,[307, 365–368] *C. difficile*,[336, 369] or *C. butyricum*, acting alone[370, 371] or synergistically with *Klebsiella*,[372] was able to evoke NEC. Subsequent studies, however, indicated that these species were often acquired from the nursery environment[374, 375] and could frequently be recovered from healthy neonates.[363, 375–381] Furthermore, clostridial cytotoxin, which had been recovered from the stool of infants involved in an outbreak of NEC,[336, 369] has also been found in the stool of up to 90% of normal infants.[336, 368, 374, 380–382] The role of *Clostridium* spp. in NEC remains unclear.[344, 364]

Delta toxins, hemolysins of coagulase-negative staphylococci[383] and *S. aureus*, have also been proposed as possible primary toxins capable of producing NEC in infants. Frequent colonization by delta toxin staphylococci and higher levels of toxin production by associated strains causing NEC have both been noted,[384] as well as one outbreak with delta toxin–producing *S. aureus* strains.[355] Prospective studies have documented significant shifts in aerobic bacterial bowel flora within 72 hours before onset of clinical NEC[385]; therefore, the observed shift is secondary to preclinical changes in the intestinal environment. This would suggest that bacteria isolated at the time of onset were present as a result of possible intraluminal changes and are not directly involved in NEC.

Pending further experimental or epidemiologic observations, the weight of evidence at present indicates that although bacteria or bacterial toxins may play a primary or secondary role in the pathogenesis of NEC, the occasional association of this condition with a single organism probably reflects patterns of intestinal colonization prevalent in the nursery at the time of an outbreak.[308, 316, 317, 334] It is noteworthy that, despite intensive efforts to identify a specific infectious agent or toxin in the etiology of NEC, there have yet to be convincing reports implicating the same pathogen in more than one outbreak.[344]

Clinical Manifestations

Signs of NEC usually develop in the first 7 days of life.[301, 327, 386] More than half of the cases become apparent within 5 days of birth.[292, 318, 321, 387, 388] The most immature, smallest newborns usually develop illness later, in the second to the eighth week,[323, 325] whereas low-risk full-term infants may become ill shortly after delivery, sometimes within the first 24 hours.[328]

NEC is a disease with a wide spectrum of manifestations, ranging from a mild gastrointestinal disturbance to a fulminant course characterized by early bowel perforation, peritonitis, sepsis, and shock.[316, 389–391] A staging system (Table 25–4) taking these clinical variations into account has proved to be useful in guiding patient evaluation and therapy.[316, 392] A given patient's place in the spectrum of disease usually becomes apparent by the second day of illness. Thus, an infant who exhibits only mild systemic and intestinal signs 24 to 48 hours after onset is unlikely to develop a more serious condition.[316]

The classic presentation of NEC includes a triad of abdominal distention, retention of gastric contents, and gastrointestinal bleeding.* These findings are often preceded or accompanied by signs consistent with sepsis, such as lethargy, poor feeding, temperature instability, apnea, and bradycardia. Diarrhea is an inconstant feature, rarely seen in some series[316] but common in others.[325, 350] Progression of bowel wall necrosis leading to perforation, peritonitis, and sepsis is reflected in deteriorating vital signs accompanied by persistent acidosis,[393] clotting disorders, and circulatory collapse. Redness, induration, and edema of the anterior abdominal wall are commonly described in the advanced stages of NEC. In the absence of aggressive medical and surgical intervention, the course is rapidly downhill once late signs appear.

Diagnosis

Radiographic signs of NEC are largely nonspecific,[391] and interobserver variability in the interpretation of films is substantial.[395] However, roentgenographic examination of the abdomen is still the most reliable aid in establishing a diagnosis of NEC.[292, 312, 318, 393, 394] Ileus with generalized bowel dilatation and abdominal distention are the earliest radiologic findings. Increasing distention, separation of loops by peritoneal fluid or edema of the bowel wall, a gasless abdomen, pneumatosis intestinalis, and hepatic or portal air occur as the condition worsens. A persistent single dilated loop of bowel remaining relatively unchanged in shape and position in serial films is strongly suggestive[395–397] but not diagnostic[396, 398] of localized bowel ischemia with impending perforation.

If free air or ascites is absent on the initial abdominal examination, supine and left lateral decubitus films should be obtained every 6 to 8 hours until improvement or definitive surgery or invasive diagnostic measures have ruled out the presence of perforation. When perforation occurs, it is usually within the first day after

---

*See references 292, 303, 316, 318, 320, 325, 333, 338, 387, and 392.

☐ TABLE 25–4
Modified Bell's Staging Criteria and Recommendations for Therapy for Necrotizing Enterocolitis

| STAGE | SIGNS | | | TREATMENT |
	Systemic	Intestinal	Radiologic	
IA (suspected)	Temperature instability apnea, bradycardia, lethargy	Elevated residuals, mild abdominal distention, emesis guaiac-positive stools	Normal, mild ileus	NPO, antibiotics for 3 days
IB (suspected)	Same as IA	Frank rectal blood	Same as IA	Same as IA
IIA (definite), mild	Same as IB	Same as IB plus absent bowel sounds ± abdominal tenderness	Dilatation, ileus, pneumatosis intestinalis	NPO, antibiotics for 7–14 days if examination is normal in 24–48 hr
IIB (definite), moderate	Same as IIA with mild metabolic acidosis, mild thrombocytopenia	Same as IIA with definite abdominal tenderness ± abdominal cellulitis or right lower quadrant mass	Same as IIA plus portal gas ± ascites	NPO, antibiotics for 14 days
IIIA (advanced), bowel intact	Same as IIB plus hypotension, bradycardia, severe apnea, respiratory/ metabolic acidosis, disseminated intravascular coagulation, neutropenia	Same as IIB plus peritonitis, marked tenderness, abdominal distention	Same as IIB with ascites	Same as IIB plus 200 ml/kg fluid, inotropic agents, assisted ventilation, paracentesis
IIIB (advanced), bowel perforated	Same as IIIA	Same as IIIA	Same as IIIA plus pneumoperitoneum	Same as IIIA plus surgery

NPO = nothing by mouth.
Adapted from Walsh MC, Kliegman RM. Necrotizing enterocolitis: treatment based on staging criteria. Pediatr Clin North Am 33:179, 1986.

diagnosis[331] but may be delayed for as long as 5 or 6 days.[399] Although the presence of pneumoperitoneum[241, 275, 286] or intraperitoneal fluid generally indicates perforation, its absence does not exclude perforation.[218, 239, 241] In one study,[331] only 63% of infants with NEC and proven perforation had free air, 21% had ascites, and 16% had neither.

When plain films are normal or equivocal, other studies may be diagnostic. A metrizamide gastrointestinal series may demonstrate intestinal perforation or abnormalities of the bowel wall, mucosa, or lumen.[242, 284, 400] Real-time ultrasonography may reveal the presence of portal venous and hepatic parenchymal gas when plain films are normal.[331, 401, 402] Serial abdominal transillumination with a fiberoptic light is also a bedside method for early detection of ascites or pneumoperitoneum, although its sensitivity when compared with standard radiographic methods has not been determined.[288]

A rapid and direct means of establishing the presence of intestinal necrosis or perforation is by abdominal paracentesis.[403–405] Use of the procedure is unnecessary in infants to "rule out" NEC or in those improving on medical therapy. It is generally reserved for infants suspected, on the basis of clinical, radiographic, and laboratory findings, of having intestinal gangrene. When performed properly, paracentesis is both remarkably safe and accurate, as noted by Kosloske[405]:

The abdomen is palpated to locate any masses or enlarged viscera. After an antiseptic skin preparation, a small needle (22 or 25 gauge) is inserted carefully in the flank, at a 45 degree angle. It is advanced slowly and aspirated gently until free flow of 0.5 ml or more of peritoneal fluid is obtained. Any volume less than 0.5 ml is considered a "dry tap" and cannot be accurately interpreted. The color and appearance of the fluid are noted and it is transported immediately to the laboratory—preferably in the syringe with air expelled and the needle covered with a cork or rubber stopper—for Gram's stain and aerobic and anaerobic cultures. A positive paracentesis consists of brown fluid and/ or bacteria on the unspun fluid.

The accuracy of paracentesis in determining the need for an operation is between 90 and 95%.[404, 405] False-positive results are very rare; false-negative results are quite common. Thus, patients with a "dry tap" should be closely observed under medical therapy and serial paracenteses performed until indications for or against surgical intervention are clearly defined. Infants with a positive result should undergo exploratory surgery immediately.

Thrombocytopenia and disseminated intravascular coagulation are the most common hematologic complications,[292, 321, 343, 403, 406–408] particularly in the presence of bowel gangrene or perforation.[296, 408, 409] Leukopenia and absolute granulocytopenia, apparently caused by margination of white blood cells rather than bone marrow depletion,[410] have also been noted during the early stages of the illness.[406, 407] When persisting for more than 2 or 3 days, a low absolute granulocyte count is associated with a poor prognosis. Hemolytic anemia has been reported in association with NEC related to *C. perfringens*.[367] No consistent urinary abnormalities have been described for NEC, although increased D-lactate excretion, reflecting heightened enteric bacterial activity, may occur.[411] Increased amounts of fecal-reducing substances have been found in almost three fourths of formula-fed premature infants during the earliest stages of NEC, before the onset of abdominal distention, poor feeding, or emesis.[412] Although not readily available, urine growth factors have recently been found to be manyfold higher in children with stage II and III NEC[413]; such an analysis might identify children at higher risk of complications and the need for surgical intervention.

The evaluation of patients with NEC should include culture of the blood, cerebrospinal fluid, urine, and stool. The likelihood of bacteremia accompanying NEC depends on the severity of bowel involvement; the reported incidence has varied from 10 to 67% among symptomatic infants. Combined data from several large studies showed positive blood cultures in about one third of newborns with NEC.[296, 297, 342, 399] The usual organisms have been *E. coli*, *Klebsiella* sp., *S. aureus*, and *Pseudomonas* sp., whereas enterococci and anaerobic bacteria were isolated occasionally. A spectrum of organisms similar to those causing sepsis have been isolated from the peritoneal fluid.[296, 305, 325, 343, 399] Meningitis may accompany bacteremia, occurring in approximately 1% of NEC cases.[328, 414]

Treatment

Early and aggressive treatment must be initiated for any infant suspected of having NEC.[308, 316] The modified Bell staging system of NEC may guide diagnostic studies, management, antibiotics, and surgical intervention (see Table 25–4). Umbilical catheters should be removed whenever possible, oral feedings should be stopped, and nasogastric tube drainage should be instituted. Fluid and electrolyte deficits and maintenance require rigorous attention; blood, plasma, or colloid infusions are often necessary for volume expansion and maintenance of tissue perfusion.

After appropriate cultures (blood, cerebrospinal fluid, urine, and stool) are obtained, parenteral antibiotic therapy should be started with clindamycin and gentamicin, or an extended-spectrum cephalosporin, and ampicillin. In nurseries where coagulase-negative staphylococcal colonization or infection is prevalent, initial therapy with vancomycin may replace ampicillin.[415] Gentamicin and vancomycin dosages should be modified as necessary on the basis of serum levels. Despite anecdotal evidence that oral nonabsorbable aminoglycosides prevent gastrointestinal perforation in infants with NEC,[416] later controlled studies did not corroborate this finding[417]; thus, their use is not recommended. The need for inclusion of clindamycin to provide activity against anaerobic bacteria in the management of NEC has recently been questioned.[418]

After immediate treatment has been started, follow-up studies should be instituted. These include serial examinations with measurement of abdominal girth; testing of stools for blood; levels of serum electrolytes, blood glucose, and arterial blood gases; complete blood cell count and platelet count; urine-specific gravity; and supine and left lateral decubitus abdominal radiographs. These tests should be considered every 6 to 8 hours until the infant's clinical condition stabilizes. Attention to vital functions should be provided as necessary on the basis of clinical, laboratory, or radiographic studies. Parenteral nutritional support through a peripheral vein must be started as soon as possible.

Early recognition and prompt initiation of medical therapy may reduce the need for surgery. Generally accepted criteria for surgical exploration are a deteriorating clinical condition despite appropriate medical therapy, signs of peritonitis, presence of free air within the abdomen, or a positive paracentesis result. The principles of surgical preparation and management have been discussed by several authors.[298, 405, 419, 420] In addition to laparotomy with removal of necrotic bowel, closed peritoneal drainage has been proposed as an alternative in very small infants, with a resultant survival of more than 50%.[421]

Prevention

The first observations implicating bacterial proliferation as a factor in the pathogenesis of NEC prompted efforts at suppression of the gut flora with topical antibiotics in hopes of preventing the condition. Attempts to prevent NEC by giving oral kanamycin or gentamicin prophylactically in the first hours of life, before any signs of bowel involvement are recognized, have generated contradictory data. In controlled clinical trials, a significant reduction in the incidence of NEC in treated premature infants was shown in some,[322, 422–425] whereas in others the investigators were unable to demonstrate any protective effect.[425, 426] Studies of vancomycin[427] have shown a significant reduction in NEC in high-risk infants. Previous studies revealed selective growth of resistant organisms in the bowel flora[322, 426, 428] and evidence of significant systemic absorption of aminoglycoside antibiotics,[417, 429, 430] suggesting that the use of oral aminoglycoside prophylaxis is not free of potential risks. These potential risk factors, however, have not been examined in vancomycin trials. Thus, until additional evidence is presented indicating clear-cut benefits from the use of oral aminoglycosides or vancomycin, it does not appear that either should be used routinely for prevention of NEC in premature infants. Epidemiologic evidence that early use of parenteral ampicillin and aminoglycoside therapy may delay or decrease the risk of NEC has not been confirmed in controlled studies.[333]

Overly voluminous feedings or accelerated feeding advancements have been associated with increased frequency of endemic NEC[431]; therefore, some have recommended a schedule of slow (about 20 ml/kg/per day) advancement of daily feeding volumes. NEC infants are more likely to have been fed earlier, to have received full-strength formulas sooner, and to have received larger feeding volumes and increments; stress and associated respiratory problems may make such infants more vulnerable to NEC.[241, 302–307, 432] Use of a feeding regimen employing prolonged periods of bowel rest in high-risk infants has been extremely successful in preventing NEC in some nurseries[308] but totally without value in others.[310, 317] Carrion and Egan have suggested that relative hypochlorhydria of the neonate may contribute to NEC and found that hydrochloric acid supplements (0.01 to 0.02 1.0 N HCl/ml of formula) significantly reduced NEC rates and lowered gastric pH.[433]

Numerous NEC "epidemics" in neonatal intensive care units, lasting from 2 weeks to 7 months, have been reported from centers worldwide.[333, 343, 344, 434, 435] Although the microbiologic agents associated with these outbreaks have varied, institution of strict infection control measures was often useful in bringing about a significant decrease in the incidence of NEC; the reasons for success are less clear. However, results have been sufficiently impressive to recommend that enforcement of bedside enteric precautions together with cohorting of infants and staff be instituted whenever two or more cases of NEC occur in a nursery.[316, 344, 436]

The use of human breast milk has been claimed, largely on the basis of experimental evidence, to exert a protective effect against the development of NEC. Unfortunately, there are no prospective controlled studies demonstrating any benefit from the feeding of colostrum or breast milk to human neonates. A recent study demonstrating the protective effect of an orally administered IgA-IgG preparation suggests a possible way to provide benefits of high levels of functionally active antibodies in the gastrointestinal tract.[437]

Prognosis

The mortality rate of NEC is difficult to determine because mild cases with "suspected NEC" are probably more common than is recognized.[316, 389, 390] In studies in which analysis was limited to infants with "definite NEC," mortality figures vary from 20 to 40%.[301, 308, 317, 325-329, 386, 391, 393, 404] Several longitudinal studies have shown a significant improvement in outcome.[301, 312, 393, 438] A poor prognosis has been associated with very low birth weight, associated congenital defects, bacterial sepsis, disseminated intravascular coagulation, perforation, and persistent hemodynamic or respiratory instability.[320, 339, 386, 399] Surgical intervention, generally reserved for the sickest infants with more extensive bowel involvement, is also associated with higher mortality rates.[320, 386, 391, 393, 405]

Infants who survive the acute phase of the illness generally do well, although recurrences of NEC may occur in 5 to 10%.[301, 325, 438, 439] In addition to problems related to surgery (short-bowel syndrome, anastomotic leaks, fistula formation), enteric strictures are probably the most common delayed complication in surviving infants, occurring in 4 to 20%. Usually found at sites of ischemia and necrosis in the terminal ileum or colon,[292, 318, 440] these strictures often become apparent within a few weeks but may be delayed as long as 18 months. When multiple strictures occur, the intervening normal bowel may form an enterocyst.[394, 441] Clinically, strictures present as frequent episodes of abdominal distention, often with vomiting, obstipation, or hematochezia. Diagnosis is confirmed by gastrointestinal contrast studies.

Surgery with removal of the stenotic site is necessary to effect a cure.

Long-term follow-up of low-birth-weight infants with severe NEC (i.e., Bell's stages II and III) has documented higher rates of subnormal body weight (15 to 39%) and head circumference (30%) in addition to significant neurodevelopmental impairment (83%).[442] Recent clinical observations suggest that infants with bowel resection for NEC during the neonatal period are at increased risk of sepsis, occurring from 1 week to 3 years (mean, 4 months) later. Almost all had had a central venous catheter in place for parenteral nutrition at the time of infection. Enteric bacilli were responsible for more than 40% of the bacteremias; only 20% were caused by staphylococcal species usually associated with catheter sepsis. Several infants had two or more episodes of sepsis; 2 of 19 died as the direct result of infection.[443]

ENDOCARDITIS

Bacterial endocarditis in the neonate, although uncommon, has been recognized more frequently in recent years. About 60 cases that meet clinical and bacteriologic criteria sufficient to establish this diagnosis have been reported in the literature[444-472]; 35 have been reported in the past two decades. The prolonged survival of critically ill infants and the increased use of intravascular catheters, together with advances in the sensitivity and accessibility of echocardiography, are probably responsible for the rising incidence. In a recent 35-year review of 76 cases of endocarditis in children, 10% of patients were younger than 1 year of age; the youngest patient was 1 month of age.[473] Sixty-two (83%) had congenital heart disease, and 77% had had prior surgery. Central venous catheters were additional risk factors.

At the University of New Mexico in a level III nursery with 3200 to 3500 admissions annually, 12 cases of endocarditis occurred in children younger than 3 months of age.[474] Organisms isolated from these 10 cases included S. aureus (6 cases), Klebsiella pneumoniae (1 case), Enterobacter cloacae (2 cases), Candida sp. (1 case), alpha-streptococci (1 case), and coagulase-negative staphylococci (1 case). Three patients had congenital heart disease with early surgical intervention; all had surgically implanted catheters or intravenous access devices, one had NEC, and one had an associated osteomyelitis.

Etiologic agents of bacterial endocarditis in the newborn have been identified by either isolation from blood cultures or morphologic characteristics of organisms entrapped within valvular vegetations examined at autopsy. On this basis, the causative organisms were S. aureus in 36 infants*; streptococci in 6[447, 431, 476]; S. epidermidis[455, 456, 475] and group B Streptococcus[449, 459, 463] each in 5; S. pneumoniae,[447, 476] P. aeruginosa,[448, 454] and S. marcescens[452, 464] in 2 each; and Neisseria gonorrhoeae,[447] S. faecalis,[477] Streptococcus salivarius[470] and mixed alpha-hemolytic Streptococcus, K. pneumoniae, and P. mirabilis[455] in 1 each. Despite widespread cardiovascular involve-

---

*See references 445–447, 450, 453–455, 457, 458, 465–477, 479–500.

ment associated with congenital syphilis, there is no conclusive evidence that this disease produces valvular heart lesions in infected infants.[58]

Factors that predispose a newborn to endocarditis are not well understood, although intravascular catheters are commonly associated with endocarditis. Unlike the situation in older children, in whom congenital heart disease is often associated with endocarditis,[478] cardiac anomalies were found in only nine of the reported cases in neonates in series before 1994.[445, 450, 452, 455, 459, 460, 465, 480] Bacteremia arising from an infected umbilical stump,[446–448] conjunctivitis,[447] and skin lesions[447, 469] were the presumed sources of valvular involvement in six infants; indeed, the highly invasive organisms associated with these conditions and with neonatal endocarditis in general can infect normal heart valves.[481] Nevertheless, the greater frequency of bacterial and fungal[468, 479, 482–488] endocarditis in newborns in recent years, particularly in association with prematurity or placement of central vessel catheters or both, indicates that other, more complex mechanisms may also operate in some cases.[454–457, 471, 475, 479, 489]

Observations of laboratory animals and autopsy studies of adults have shown that damage to the intracardiac endothelium with formation of a sterile platelet-fibrin thrombus at the site of the injury is often the initiating event in a patient with endocarditis.[490] Endocardial trauma caused by placement of cardiac catheters, as well as disseminated intravascular coagulation and the various nonspecific stresses associated with prematurity such as hypotension and hypoxia, has been implicated in the genesis of thrombi.[455, 471, 475, 481, 491, 492] Nonbacterial thrombotic endocarditis or verrucous endocarditis usually remains uninfected and is described as an incidental finding at autopsy.[454, 471, 492, 493] With bacteremia, however, implantation of organisms may lead to valvular infection. Whether this mechanism or that of direct bacterial invasion is primarily responsible for the valvulitis is not known. A similar pathogenesis has been postulated for the formation of mycotic aortic aneurysms in newborns.[467, 496, 497]

Endocarditis should be suspected in any neonate, particularly a premature infant, with an indwelling vascular catheter, evidence of sepsis, and new or changing heart murmurs. When these findings are accompanied by persistent bacteremia or signs of congestive heart failure in the absence of underlying heart disease, the diagnosis must be considered seriously. Although Janeway's lesions,[471] a generalized petechial rash,[466, 479, 477] and splinter hemorrhages[477] have been noted, murmurs characteristic of semilunar valve insufficiency, Osler's nodes, Roth's spots, arthritis, and other findings typical of valvular infection in adults and older children have not been observed in neonates. However, multiple septic emboli with involvement of the skin, bones, viscera, and central nervous system are relatively common findings.*

Two-dimensional echocardiography has proved to be invaluable as a rapid, noninvasive method for diagnosing endocarditis.[456–459, 465, 490, 501] Although it cannot differen-

tiate between infected and sterile vegetations and other valvular lesions (see later discussion), imaging is quite specific, and false-positive readings are uncommon. Unfortunately, less certainty can be placed on a negative report. Despite the capability of echocardiography to detect vegetations as small as 2 mm, the number of false-negative examinations is significant[465, 471, 502]: in one series, two of three infants with thrombotic valvular lesions 3 to 7 mm in diameter had normal two-dimensional echocardiograms.[471] Thus, a diagnosis of bacterial endocarditis should be entertained in any infant with a compatible history and physical findings regardless of the results obtained by echocardiography.

More widespread use of new techniques such as transesophageal echocardiography, which provides detailed views of the mitral and tricuspid valves, and color flow Doppler imaging, which can identify areas of turbulence as blood passes over vegetations or through narrowed valve leaflets, should greatly improve diagnostic accuracy.[501]

When endocarditis is suspected, specimens of blood, cerebrospinal fluid, and urine obtained by catheterization or suprapubic aspiration should be sent for bacterial and fungal culture. Because blood drawn from a central catheter often contains organisms colonizing the line but not necessarily present in the systemic circulation, at least two *peripheral* venous blood cultures should be obtained before antimicrobial therapy is initiated. Volumes of 1 to 5 ml, depending on the infant's size, should be adequate.[490]

Routine laboratory studies are helpful in supporting a diagnosis of endocarditis in the newborn. The leukocyte count, differential, and platelet count are usually indicative of sepsis rather than cardiac valve infection in particular. Microhematuria has been reported, although rarely.[471, 477] A chest radiograph should be obtained to determine signs of cardiac failure or pulmonary or pleural space infection. CT or MRI of the brain can be helpful in an infant with neurologic signs, particularly if left-sided endocarditis or a right-to-left shunt is present.

Intravenous therapy with a penicillinase-resistant penicillin and an aminoglycoside should be started after appropriate cultures have been obtained. In nurseries where methicillin-resistant *S. aureus* or *S. epidermidis* infections have been a problem, vancomycin should be substituted initially for the penicillin.[490, 501, 502] Once the infecting organism is isolated and antibiotic susceptibilities are determined, specific antimicrobial therapy can be instituted. Four to 6 weeks of parenteral treatment is usually adequate. Dosage and efficacy should be monitored weekly with clinical and bacteriologic response with or without serum antibiotic and bactericidal levels.[501, 503] Determination of serum bactericidal titers (Schlichter's assay) is of uncertain value and has never been validated in neonatal endocarditis.[490, 501, 504] Efficacy of treatment can also be monitored with serial echocardiograms taken until vegetations remain stable in size or disappear.[465, 466, 468, 475, 479]

Intravascular catheters must be removed whenever possible and their tips cultured.[490, 505] Extremely large or mobile vegetations occluding an outflow tract or posing a high risk of embolism may have to be removed surgi-

---

*See references 445, 447, 449, 450, 454–456, 458–464, 468, 469, 471, 475, 477, 479, and 498–500.

cally.[463, 465, 468] In infants with right-sided endocarditis, demonstration of decreased pulmonary blood flow through the use of ventilation-perfusion scan can be of value in confirming the presence of emboli, particularly if there is clinical evidence of increasing respiratory effort and diminished peripheral oxygen saturation.[463]

With the availability of echocardiography, improved clinical awareness, and early diagnosis, prognosis has improved. Although there were infrequent survivors before 1973,[481] the first survivors with proven endocarditis were reported in 1983.[465, 466, 471] Approximately two thirds of subsequent cases have been cured. Death is usually the result of overwhelming sepsis, often in conjunction with cardiac failure. Early reconstructive surgery for infants who fail medical management may be helpful but has been reported in only a limited number of cases.[506, 507]

Inspection of the heart at autopsy has shown the mitral valve to be infected, alone or in combination with other valves, in about half the patients. The tricuspid valve was involved in 12 infants, pulmonary valve in 7, aortic valve in 6, infected mural thrombi in 12, and an unspecified site in 3. Microscopic examination of valve cusps has revealed the characteristic lesions of endocarditis, with multiple small, confluent, friable vegetations composed principally of bacteria and thrombi surrounded by inflammatory exudate.[445, 469, 471] On gross inspection, these vegetations are easily confused with noninflammatory lesions such as those of nonbacterial thrombotic endocarditis, blood cysts,[508] developmental valvular defects,[509] or hemangiomas or other vascular anomalies.[510] Cases of "fetal endocarditis" described in the literature are almost certainly examples of these types of lesions.[494, 509, 511]

PERICARDITIS

Purulent pericarditis is a very unusual complication of neonatal sepsis. Approximately 20 cases of proven bacterial etiology have been reported within the past 50 years.[498, 512–523] No single causative agent has predominated. S. aureus was responsible for seven cases,[498, 512–514] E. coli was isolated from three patients,[514, 519, 520] Haemophilus influenzae was found in two,[515, 522] and Salmonella wichita,[516] Klebsiella,[523] and P. aeruginosa[521] were isolated from single cases. One early review of Pseudomonas sepsis described suppurative pericarditis caused by that organism in four neonates.[517] Another report on the recovery of Pseudomonas from the pericardium of premature infants dying of septicemia and meningitis during a nursery outbreak is difficult to evaluate because details of clinical and autopsy findings were not given.[524] Cases caused by Candida sp. and Mycoplasma hominis have also been described.[479, 485, 525] The causes of a pericardial effusion in three fetuses with multiple congenital anomalies, myocardial hypertrophy, and pericarditis are uncertain. Although the inflammatory exudate found at autopsy contained polymorphonuclear leukocytes in addition to lymphocytes, no evidence of bacterial infection was found.[526]

Virtually every infant with pericarditis has associated septic foci; pneumonitis and multiple pulmonary abscesses are the most common. Involvement of the pericardium may occur in these patients either by direct extension from adjoining lung abscesses or by hematogenous spread of bacteria.[512] The presence of infectious processes elsewhere is sufficiently frequent to warrant the suggestion that pericarditis should be suspected in all infants who develop clinical signs of "heart failure" or a sudden increase in the size of the cardiac silhouette during the course of a purulent infection such as meningitis, pneumonia, or omphalitis.[515, 527]

Neonates with bacterial pericarditis generally present with signs and symptoms suggesting sepsis and respiratory distress. Thus, poor feeding, listlessness, emesis, or abdominal distention may be seen in the presence of tachypnea, tachycardia, and cyanosis of variable degree. More specific signs of cardiac involvement became apparent with the accumulation of increasing amounts of pericardial effusion. Unfortunately, the clinical findings of cardiac tamponade are extremely subtle and difficult to differentiate from those of myocardial disease with right-sided heart failure. A rapid pulse, quiet precordium, muffled heart sounds, neck vein distention, and hepatomegaly are findings common to both entities. More specific signs of tamponade, such as narrow pulse pressure or respiratory variations in pulse volume over 20 mm Hg (pulsus paradoxus), are technically difficult to obtain in neonates without an arterial catheter in place. A pericardial friction rub is absent in more than 50% of older infants and children and in most neonates with purulent pericarditis.

Rapid enlargement of the cardiac silhouette, a globular heart shape with widening of the base on tilting, and diminished cardiac pulsation on fluoroscopic examination are of little value in differentiating pericardial effusion from cardiac dilation.[528] The early ST segment elevation and subsequent T wave inversion seen on the electrocardiogram reflect subepicardial damage or inflammation and are similar to changes seen with primary myocarditis. Diminution in the amplitude of the QRS complex by fluid surrounding the heart is not a constant finding. Confirmation of the presence of a pericardial effusion is, therefore, almost always obtained by two-dimensional echocardiography.[498, 528] In some cases, CT scan can also be helpful in delineating the extent of a pericardial effusion.[529]

The causes of neonatal pericardial effusion include viral pericarditis,[530] intrapericardial teratoma,[531] maternal lupus,[532] immune and nonimmune[533] fetal hydrops, congenital diaphragmatic defects,[534] chylopericardium,[535] and central venous catheter perforation of the right atrium.[536]

A definitive diagnosis of purulent pericarditis can be made only by obtaining fluid at surgery or through needle aspiration. Care and experience are necessary to facilitate aspiration while avoiding the risks of cardiac puncture or laceration.[526] Accurate monitoring of needle position can usually be obtained through CT guidance, with echocardiographic or fluoroscopic imaging, or by attaching the exploring electrode (V lead) of an electrocardiograph to the needle and by looking for injury current if contact is made with the epicardial surface of the heart.

When fluid is obtained, it should be sent for analysis to the laboratory in the aspirating syringe with the air expelled and the needle covered with a cork or rubber stopper. In addition to cell count and protein and glucose levels, Gram and acid-fast stains should be performed together with cultures for bacteria, viruses, mycobacteria, and fungi. Rapid identification of bacterial antigens by latex agglutination or by counterimmunoelectrophoresis of pericardial fluid, urine, or serum may also help to establish an etiologic diagnosis.[537]

Purulent pericarditis is a medical and surgical emergency. Therapy must be directed both toward relief of the cardiac tamponade through adequate pericardial drainage and toward resolution of the infection. Both modes of treatment are essential for successful therapy for bacterial pericarditis in the newborn. Not a single infant with suppurative pericarditis has recovered when treated by antibiotics alone.[512] Although repeated needle aspirations or catheter drainage[538] may be sufficient, the frequent occurrence of loculations of pus, particularly with staphylococcal infection, suggests that open surgical pericardiostomy is the method of choice to achieve adequate drainage.

Cultures of blood, cerebrospinal fluid, and urine should be obtained before instituting antimicrobial therapy. Initial therapy should be based on results of Gram stain or antigen detection tests of the pericardial fluid. If no organisms can be identified, treatment can be started with a penicillinase-resistant penicillin and an aminoglycoside (or extended-spectrum cephalosporin) until definitive culture and susceptibility data are available. In nurseries where methicillin-resistant *S. aureus* infection has been a problem, vancomycin should be substituted for penicillin.[503]

The prognosis of neonatal purulent pericarditis is very poor; only three survivors have been reported[498, 514, 523] before the last decade of the twentieth century. Treatment in these patients consisted of needle aspiration(s), drainage, and systemic antibiotic therapy, and in one case it was combined with local instillation.

MEDIASTINITIS

Purulent mediastinitis has been reported in 11 infants younger than 6 weeks of age, although it is likely that a great many more cases occur than have been noted in the literature. Six of these patients acquired their mediastinal abscess either through blood-borne dissemination of organisms[539–541] or by extension from a focus of infection in an adjacent retropharyngeal abscess,[542] pleural or pulmonary abscess,[512, 540] or vertebral osteomyelitis.[543] One infant developed infection as a complication of surgery for esophageal atresia.[540] *S. aureus* was the causative organism in four infants, and *S. pneumoniae*, *Clostridium* sp., and mixed *S. aureus* and *E. coli* were causative in one infant each; organisms were not identified in four cases.

Traumatic perforation of the posterior pharynx or esophagus, usually the result of resuscitative efforts in premature infants involving either endotracheal or gastric intubation, produces a potential site for the entry of microorganisms.[544–551] Although retropharyngeal abscess,[552] an infected pseudodiverticulum, or pyopneumothorax may occur as a consequence, purulent mediastinitis has been reported only three times as a complication,[541, 545, 546] on one occasion as the result of overly vigorous passage of a nasogastric tube through an atretic esophageal pouch.[545] Low (intrathoracic) perforations are said to have a higher risk of mediastinitis and abscess formation than those in the cervical region.[547]

Early symptoms are nonspecific and are similar to those of any septic process in a neonate. As purulent fluid accumulates in the mediastinum, it places increasing pressure on the esophagus, trachea, and tributaries of the superior vena cava and thoracic duct, thus bringing about rapid development of dysphagia, dyspnea, neck vein distention, and facial cyanosis or edema. To maintain a patent tracheal airway, an afflicted infant will lie in an arched position with the head extended in a manner very similar to that seen in neonates with congenital vascular ring. A halting, inspiratory, staccato type of breathing, probably because of pain, is also characteristic. Ultimately, the abscess may come to a point on the anterior chest wall or in the suprasternal notch.

Usually the diagnosis is first suspected when widening of the mediastinum is noted on a chest film taken for evaluation of respiratory distress. Forward displacement of the trachea and larynx may accompany these findings when retropharyngeal abscess is associated with mediastinitis. Infection after traumatic perforation of the esophagus or pharynx is often accompanied by pneumomediastinum with or without a pneumothorax.[545, 547]

Contrast studies performed to define the cause of respiratory or feeding difficulties in infants with mediastinitis may result in flow of radiopaque fluid into an esophageal laceration, mimicking the findings of an atresia, duplication, or diverticulum of the esophagus.[547, 548] In such cases, endoscopy will often demonstrate a mucosal tear and confirm the true diagnosis.[548, 549]

Treatment should be directed toward immediate establishment of drainage and relief of pressure on vital structures through a mediastinostomy and placement of drainage tubes. The use of a tracheostomy or endotracheal tube may be necessary for maintenance of an adequate airway.

Initial empirical antimicrobial therapy with clindamycin, ampicillin, and an aminoglycoside should be started after cultures of the blood and cerebrospinal fluid have been obtained. Specific therapy can subsequently be determined by the results of bacteriologic studies of these sources or purulent fluid obtained at surgery.

ESOPHAGITIS

The esophagus is infrequently a focus for infection of the fetus or newborn.[553] Esophageal atresia is associated with congenital rubella (see Chapter 6). Severe esophagitis has also been reported in neonates with congenital cytomegaloviral infection.[553a] The esophagus may be involved in infants with congenital Chagas' disease identified by signs of dysphagia, regurgitation, and megaesophagus.[554] Esophageal disease may follow mediastinitis in the neonate (see earlier discussion). Only occasional cases of bacterial esophagitis in a neonate have been reported. A 940-g male infant developed signs of sepsis on the fifth day of life and died 5 hours later.[553] Premortem blood cultures were positive for *Bacillus* sp. Examination at autopsy revealed histologic evidence of esophagitis with pseudomembranous necrosis of squamous epithelium and many gram-positive bacilli. No other focus of infection was evident.

INFECTIONS OF ENDOCRINE ORGANS

Endocrine glands other than the adrenal are rarely involved in fetal or neonatal infection. Neonatal suppurative thyroiditis in a term Laotian infant was reported by Nelson.[555] The infant presented with a left anterior neck mass at 3 days of age. At surgery, a cystic mass within the left lobe of the thyroid was identified. Purulent material within the mass grew *S. viridans* and nonhemolytic streptococci.

Orchitis has been described in a 10-week-old neonate caused by *S. enteridis*.[555a] This infant presented with symptoms of sepsis and diarrhea, subsequently developing unilateral scrotal swelling and erythema on the fifth day after onset of illness. Ultrasound examination of the testis showed a patchy increased echo intensity; the diagnosis was confirmed at exploratory surgery to rule out testicular torsion. In addition, three other cases of infection of the testes caused by *Salmonella* sp. in infants younger than 3 months of age have been described.[555a]

INFECTIONS OF THE SALIVARY GLANDS

Infections of the salivary glands are uncommon in the neonate, but, when such infections occur, involvement of the parotid is the most frequent[556–561] and submandibular gland infection is infrequent.[557–562] Most infections are due to *S. aureus*,[556–559] but *E. coli*,[559] *P. aeruginosa*,[559] and group B *Streptococcus* (see Chapter 26) have also been implicated in suppurative parotitis. Not surprisingly, oral anaerobic bacteria, including *Bacteroides* sp. and *Peptostreptococcus* sp., may be found in mixed or isolated infections in more than half the cases.[560] Infections of the salivary glands occur more frequently in premature and male infants[559, 562] and most commonly present during the second week of life. The oral cavity is the probable portal of entry for the infecting organism. However, blood-borne bacteria may invade the salivary glands. In addition, dehydration with resultant decreased salivary flow may be a predisposing cause in some infants.

The clinical manifestations of salivary gland infection include fever, anorexia, irritability, and failure to gain weight. There may be swelling, tenderness, or erythema over the involved gland. Purulent material may be expressed from the ductal opening with or without gentle pressure over the gland.

The diagnosis is made by culture and/or Gram stain of the pus exuding from the duct or by percutaneous aspiration of a fluctuant area. If microscopic examination of the Gram stain does not suggest a responsible pathogen, initial antibiotic therapy should be directed against *S. aureus*, *E. coli*, and *P. aeruginosa* (e.g., penicillinase-resistant penicillin or vancomycin plus an aminoglycoside or ceftazidime). If there is a strong suspicion of involvement with anaerobic bacteria (i.e., negative aerobic cultures or failure to respond to therapy directed at aerobic pathogens), consideration should be given to adding or substituting antibiotics appropriate for anaerobic bacteria (e.g., clindamycin). The duration of therapy should extend throughout the period of inflammation, continuing 3 to 5 days after signs of local inflammation have disappeared. Incision and drainage may be helpful and at times essential; surgical drainage should be considered if there is not a prompt response to therapy within 72 hours or if fluctuance of the gland becomes apparent. Careful attention to preservation of the function of the seventh cranial nerve is important when considering incision and drainage.

INFECTIONS OF THE SKIN AND SUBCUTANEOUS TISSUE

Bacterial infections of the skin of the newborn may manifest as maculopapular rash, vesicles, pustules, bullae, abscesses, cellulitis, impetigo, erythema multiforme, and petechiae or purpura. Most infections of the skin are caused by *S. aureus;* such staphylococcal diseases include bullous impetigo, chronic furunculosis, the scalded skin syndrome, and breast abscesses (discussed in Chapter 30). Cellulitis frequently accompanied by adenitis and bacteremia may be caused by group B streptococci (see Chapter 26). Cutaneous infections caused by many other bacteria are discussed in this section; however, nearly all microorganisms that cause disease in the neonate may produce cutaneous infections, and, where relevant, those infections are discussed in other chapters. For additional information on bacterial infections of the skin, the reader is referred to the text by Solomon and Esterly[563] and the reviews by Swartz and Weinberg[564] and Frieden.[565] Excellent color photographs are included in Weinberg and co-workers' *Color Atlas of Pediatric Dermatology*.[566]

Pathogenesis

The skin of the newborn has unique characteristics, including absent microflora at birth; the presence of vernix caseosa; a less acid pH than that of older children; and, often, the presence of surgical wounds such as the severed umbilical cord, a circumcision site, and catheter wounds. In addition, the infant is immediately exposed to other infants, personnel, and the nosocomial environment. After the staphylococcal pandemic of the 1950s, information on the colonization of the skin, predisposing factors responsible for neonatal skin infection, bacterial transmission in the nursery, the inflammatory response of the skin to bacterial invasion, virulence factors of staphylococci, and methods of prevention of cross-infection became available. These studies are described in part in Chapters 30 and 34 and have been reviewed elsewhere.[567]

Cutaneous bacterial infection may be a primary event or the result of systemic infection. Thus, septicemic embolic infection may occur at widely separated sites, whereas local infections will often occur at a site with an identifiable predisposing cause. Procedures resulting in breaks in the cutaneous continuity, such as forceps abrasions or wounds at fetal electrodes or at venipuncture sites, may be readily identified. The necrotic umbilical cord is a site for proliferation of microorganisms that may invade local tissues.

Infection of the circumcision site remains a concern. It is the most common surgical procedure in children in the United States. Speert[568] noted that cleanliness was frequently disregarded by professional circumcisers as late as the nineteenth century. Operators were frequently uneducated, were dirty, and often spat on their instruments. Erysipelas, tetanus, and diphtheria have long been recognized as complications of unsterile surgical technique performed on newborns. In a now obsolete and prohibited part of the Orthodox Jewish circumcision ritual, the operator applied his lips to the fresh circumcision wound and sucked a few drops of blood. Such practices were responsible for syphilis and tuberculosis in neonates and may still occur in some parts of the world. In one report,[569] a 4-month-old infant presented with a penile ulcer, bilateral inguinal adenopathy, and a draining inguinal sinus caused by *Mycobacterium tuberculosis* after the "barber" spat on his razor before circumcision. Reports of 43 cases of tuberculosis associated with circumcision had been published by 1916.[568] Subsequent case reports of severe infection after circumcision include bacteremia related to group B streptococci,[570] local infection and fatal staphylococcal pneumonia,[571] staphylococcal scalded skin syndrome,[572, 573] necrotizing fasciitis,[574] and bullous impetigo.[575] Two recent reports of necrotizing fasciitis after Plastibell circumscision emphasize severe infection as a potential risk of this procedure.[576] One infection caused by *S. aureus* and *Klebsiella* sp. was associated with prolonged convalescent and multiple surgical repairs, whereas a second infant survived staphylococcal necrotizing fasciitis after 14 days of intravenous antibiotic treatment.

The incidence of infection after elective circumcision was investigated at the University of Washington Hospital[577] during the period 1963 to 1972. Infection, defined as the presence of pus or erythema, occurred in 0.41% of 5521 infants and was more frequently associated with the use of a disposable plastic bell (Plastibell; 0.72%) than with the use of a metal clamp (Gomco; 0.14%). Wound cultures were infrequently available, and thus microbiologic diagnosis was uncertain in most infants. It is clear that circumcision infection is uncommon, but local spread of infection may be devastating and lead to systemic infection.

Intrapartum fetal monitoring with scalp electrodes and intrauterine pressure catheters, as well as measurements of fetal blood gases via scalp punctures, has been associated with infections related to herpes (see Chapter 8), *Mycoplasma* (see Chapter 14), and a variety of aerobic and anaerobic bacteria. Bacterial infections have varied from pustules to abscesses or fasciitis.[578–581] Infection rates are relatively low, varying from 0.1 to 4.5%[580, 581]; however, severe infections, including fasciitis, meningitis, and osteomyelitis are severe complications. A review[582] of the causative organisms in fetal scalp monitor infections found that 61% of infections were polymicrobial, involving anaerobic bacteria, aerobic gram-positive cocci, and gram-negative bacilli.

A multitude of specific virulence factors may be important determinants of disease. Some phage types of *S. aureus* are responsible for local tissue damage and systemic disease; other staphylococci elaborate toxins that result in bullae and other cutaneous pathology. Groups A and B streptococci are responsible for cellulitis and impetigo in the infant. *P. aeruginosa* may invade and proliferate in small blood vessels, thereby causing local necrosis and eschar formation (ecthyma gangrenosum). Infections with *Clostridium* sp. cause disease in devitalized tissues such as the umbilical stump.[583] Similarly, organisms usually considered commensals, such as diphtheroids, may be responsible for infection of the cord and fetal membranes.[584]

Microbiology

The skin of the infant is colonized initially by microorganisms present in the maternal birth canal. The skin of infants delivered by cesarean section is usually sterile at birth. After birth, microorganisms may be transferred to the skin during handling by the parents and nursery personnel.

The prevalent organisms on the skin during the first few days of life include coagulase-negative staphylococci, diphtheroids, and gram-negative enteric bacilli (including *E. coli*).[585, 586] The umbilicus, genitalia, and adjacent skin areas (groin and abdomen) are colonized first; the organisms then spread to the nose, throat, conjunctivae, and other body sites. Organisms present in the nursery environment colonize the skin of the newborn after a few days in the nursery. *S. aureus*, group B streptococci, and various species of gram-negative bacilli may be present, but the microbiologic flora differs among nurseries and from time to time in the same nursery.

Use of soaps and antiseptic solutions modifies the flora on the skin of the newborn. Hexachlorophene decreases colonization with staphylococci and diphtheroids, but gram-negative organisms are unaffected or may increase after use of this agent.[587]

Epidemiology

Male infants are more susceptible to skin infections caused by *S. aureus* than are female infants. Thompson and co-workers[588] demonstrated that males were colonized more frequently in every body site cultured, including the nose, groin, rectum, and umbilicus. Their review of studies indicated that in England, the United

States, and Australia approximately 50% more males had skin lesions than did females. Although the incidence of breast abscesses is equal in males and females during the first 2 weeks of life, such abscesses are more frequent thereafter in females.[589] The reason for this pattern is unclear, but Rudoy and Nelson[589] hypothesized that physiologic breast enlargement may play a role. Hormone production in the female infant after the second week might account for the increase in abscesses of the breast.

Seasonal variation in the frequency of neonatal skin infections has been noted by Evans and co-workers, who conducted a series of studies at Harlem Hospital (New York).[590] The prevalence of *S. aureus, E. coli,* and streptococci in the nares and umbilicus of infants was lowest in the autumn and usually highest in the summer or spring. No seasonal variation was noted for *S. epidermidis* or *Enterobacter* sp. The authors concluded that seasonal differences must be considered in investigations of bacterial colonization of the newborn skin and that high humidity may favor gram-negative colonization.

The time of onset of skin lesions associated with sepsis may be early (during the first week of life) or late (up to several weeks or months after birth). Disease acquired in the nursery usually becomes apparent after 5 days of age. Therefore, many skin lesions do not appear until after the infant has left the nursery; thus, the observed incidence of skin disease caused by bacteria should include surveillance of infants in the home during the first month of life. Physicians responsible for neonatal care must be alert to the unusual occurrence of skin lesions. The introduction of a new and virulent bacterium, an alteration in technique, or the use of contaminated materials must be considered as possible causes of an increased incidence of such infections.

Clinical Manifestations

Infants who have skin infections that remain localized and are not invasive or part of a systemic infection have few general signs of disease, such as fever, alteration in feeding habits, vomiting, or diarrhea. These signs may be present when significant tissue invasion occurs, as in abscesses or extensive cellulitis. The various cutaneous manifestations that result from infectious diseases are listed in Table 25–5.

Among the most common and least specific lesions are the maculopapular rashes; these rashes may be due to viruses (measles, rubella, or enteroviruses), fungi (*Candida* sp.), or bacteria (streptococci or staphylococci), or they may be unassociated with any infectious process. Erythema multiforme lesions have been observed in cases of sepsis related to *S. aureus,*[591] streptococci,[563] and *P. aeruginosa.*[592] Virtually any rash may be associated with bacterial infection. In an outbreak of sepsis caused by *Achromobacter* in premature infants,[593] the illness was marked by respiratory distress, including apnea and cyanosis, but was characterized by a rash consisting of indurated, erythematous lesions with sharply defined borders that began on the cheeks or chest and spread rapidly to adjacent areas.

Cellulitis, erysipelas, and impetigo are usually associated with streptococcal infection (group A or B),[594] although impetigo caused by *S. aureus* or *E. coli* has also been reported in infants.

Vesicles, commonly associated with infections by herpesviruses, also are seen on occasion during the early stage of skin lesions caused by *S. aureus, H. influenzae,*[595] *L. monocytogenes,*[596] and *P. aeruginosa.* Group B *Streptococcus,*[597] *S. aureus, P. aeruginosa,* herpes simplex virus, and *T. pallidum* may also be responsible for bullous lesions. Pustules commonly occur in staphylococcal diseases but also occur in infections caused by *L. monocytogenes* and, rarely, in skin infections with *H. influenzae.*[598]

Ecthyma gangrenosum is a local manifestation of infection with *P. aeruginosa.*[599, 600] The lesion begins as a vesicular eruption on a wide erythematous base. The vesicles rupture and form an indurated black eschar. A larger but sharply demarcated, painless necrotic area follows. This ulcer results from a vasculitis of small vessels with necrosis of the adjacent tissue. The organism is present in purulent material underlying the necrotic membrane. These lesions are particularly more common adjacent to the nose, lip, ear, mouth, and perineum, resulting in avascular necrosis and loss of tissue. *P. aeruginosa* may be grown in pure culture from blood and lesions. Among 48 infants described in one outbreak, the lesions appeared within the first 2 weeks of life; most of the infants died within 3 days of onset.[601] Ecthyma is relatively specific for *Pseudomonas* infections, but similar or identical lesions have rarely been described in infections due to *S. aureus, Aeromonas hydrophila, S. marcescens, Aspergillus* sp., or *Mucor* sp.[602]

Many infants with *Candida* infections have cutaneous manifestations. In a report by Baley and Silverman,[603] 18 infants with systemic candidiasis were described; 8 had a burnlike truncal erythema, and 9 additional infants had typical candidal diaper rashes or maculopapular rashes of the axillae or neck.

Abscesses of the skin and subcutaneous tissue are usually due to *S. aureus* and, less frequently, to streptococci of groups A or B[604, 605] or to gram-negative enteric bacilli.[606–614] Organisms that colonize the skin over an area that has been disrupted by an abrasion or other wound may invade the subcutaneous tissue and produce an abscess. *Haemophilus* sp.,[615–617] *Gardnerella vaginalis,*[618] *Bacteroides* sp.[619] molluscum contagiosum,[620] *Drosophila myiasis,*[621] scabies,[622] and *Candida*[623] are examples of diverse pathogens that may produce cutaneous abscesses; thus, virtually any bacterial, fungal, or parasitic agent that is normally or transiently on the skin may become a pathogen. *E. coli, Klebsiella* sp., *P. aeruginosa,*[604, 609, 624] *N. gonorrhoeae,*[625] and *Bacteroides fragilis*[626] have caused wound infections in infants whose scalps were lacerated by forceps, fetal electrodes, or instruments used for obtaining blood from the scalp in utero. An extensive outbreak of systemic disease caused by *S. marcescens* in a neonatal intensive care nursery in Puerto Rico included wound infections at the site of intravenous infusions (see reference 686).

A cephalohematoma may become infected during sepsis or from manipulation of the cephalohematoma, such as through diagnostic or therapeutic needle puncture[627] or by puncture from a fetal monitor. Infections may be

TABLE 25–5
Manifestations and Etiologies of Some Infections of the Skin in Newborns

CLINICAL MANIFESTATION	ETIOLOGIC AGENT[a]	
	Bacterial	Nonbacterial
Maculopapular rash	*Treponema pallidum*[b, c]	Measles virus[b]
	Listeria monocytogenes	Rubella virus[b]
	Streptococcus[b]	Enteroviruses[b]
	Staphylococcus[b]	Molluscum contagiosum (620)
		Candida sp.[b]
Cellulitis (erysipelas)	Groups A and B streptococci	
	Achromobacter sp. (593)	
Impetigo	Groups A and B streptococci (594)[b]	
	Staphylococcus aureus[b]	
	Escherichia coli	
Erythema multiforme	Beta-hemolytic *Streptococcus* (591)	
	Staphylococcus aureus[b]	
	Pseudomonas aeruginosa (592)	
Vesicular or bullous lesions	*Staphylococcus aureus*	Herpes simplex virus[b, c]
	Pseudomonas aeruginosa	Cytomegalovirus[b]
	Treponema pallidum	Varicella virus[b, c]
	Haemophilus influenzae type b (595)	Variola virus[c]
	Listeria monocytogenes (596)	Coxsackieviruses[b]
		Candida sp.[b]
		Aspergillus sp.[b]
		Drosophila larvae (621)
		Sarcoptes scabei (622)
Pustular rashes	*Staphylococcus aureus*[b]	
	Listeria monocytogenes[b]	
	Haemophilus influenzae (598)	
Ecthyma gangrenosa	*Pseudomonas aeruginosa* (599–601)	
Abscesses and wound infections	*Staphylococcus aureus*[b]	*Mycoplasma hominis*[b]
	Staphylococcus epidermidis[b]	*Candida albicans* (623)
	Beta-hemolytic streptococci (604)	
	Group B streptococci (605)	
	Escherichia coli (606–608)	
	Klebsiella sp. (609)	
	Proteus mirabilis (610)	
	Pseudomonas aeruginosa (611)	
	Salmonella sp. (612)	
	Serratia marcescens (614)	
	Haemophilus influenzae (615)	
	Haemophilus parainfluenzae (616)	
	Corynebacterium vaginalis (617)	
	Neisseria gonorrhoeae (625)	
	Gardnerella vaginalis (618)	
	Bacteroides sp. (619)	
Petechiae, purpura, and ecchymoses	Gram-positive cocci[b] and gram-negative bacilli[b] associated with sepsis	Rubella virus[b, c]
	Listeria monocytogenes (596)	Cytomegalovirus[b, c]
	Streptococcus pneumoniae (596)	Herpes simplex virus[b, c]
	Treponema pallidum[b, c]	Coxsackievirus B[b, c]
		Toxoplasma gondii[b, c]

[a]Numbers in parentheses refer to references.
[b]See appropriate chapter for further discussion.
[c]Including infections acquired in utero.

due to *Bacteroides* sp.,[619] *E. coli*,[606, 607] and *P. aeruginosa*.[628] The infection may be associated with meningitis[628] or with osteomyelitis of the underlying skull.[606, 607]

S. aureus is the most frequent etiologic agent in breast abscess, but gram-negative enteric bacilli are becoming increasingly more common.[608, 612, 613] Of 36 cases with mastitis seen in Dallas during a 16-year period, 32 cases were due to *S. aureus*, 1 was due to *E. coli*, and 2 were

due to *Salmonella* sp.; and both *E. coli* and *S. aureus* were isolated from one abscess.[629] Forty-one cases of mastitis in neonates were managed at Children's Hospital (Boston) during the period 1947 to 1983.[630] *S. aureus* was responsible for 29 of 34 cases with an identifiable bacterial pathogen. All cases occurred in full-term infants during weeks 1 to 5 of life. Bilaterality and extramammary foci were rare. One third of the infants were febrile, and a majority had elevated white blood cell counts (>15,000 per mm³). Other reports identify group B streptococci[605] and *P. mirabilis*[610] as causes of breast abscesses. Brook[613] found that 5 of 14 breast abscesses contained anaerobic bacteria (i.e., *Bacteroides* sp. and *Peptostreptococcus*), but *S. aureus*, group B streptococci, or enteric bacteria predominated; anaerobic bacteria occurred alone in only 2 of 14 cases.

Paronychia may occur in neonates after injury to the cuticle. The lesion is usually caused by *S. aureus* or beta-hemolytic streptococci.[631] The authors of a report of an outbreak of paronychia in a Kuala Lumpur nursery suggest but do not prove that the lesions were due to an anaerobic *Veillonella* sp.[632]

Purpura may have many infectious and noninfectious causes but is of greatest concern because of its association with bacteremia in neonates.

Omphalitis is defined by the presence of erythema or serous or purulent discharge from the umbilical stump or the periumbilical tissues. A review by Cushing presents useful information about the pathophysiology, microbiology, diagnosis, and management of omphalitis.[633] The incidence of infection is more frequent in low-birth-weight infants and in those with complications of delivery. A survey of infants born at the Royal Woman's Hospital in Brisbane[634] identified an incidence of approximately 2% among term infants. The mean age of presentation of the disease was 3.2 days. Perhaps because hexachlorophene bathing was used, gram-negative bacilli were more frequently associated with infection than were gram-positive cocci. However, microbiologic results are difficult to interpret because swabs of the site of infection do not exclude surface contaminants unless cultures are taken with extreme care and precision.

A series from the United States[635] found that periumbilical fasciitis was more frequent in males but did not find that umbilical catheterization, low birth weight, or septic delivery was associated with a high risk; overall, the incidence of omphalitis was equal in males and females. In this series, omphalitis presented as discharge, cellulitis, or fasciitis; gram-positive organisms were found in 94% of cultures, and gram-negative bacteria were noted in 64%. *S. aureus* was the most frequent isolate, with *E. coli* and *Klebsiella* sp. the next most common. Group A streptococci have been responsible for nursery outbreaks that may include an indolent form of omphalitis characterized by erythema and oozing of the umbilical stump for days to weeks, accompanied by pustular lesions of the abdominal wall in some cases.[636] Neonatal tetanus usually occurs as a result of contamination of the umbilical wound by *Clostridium tetani* at delivery.

Acute necrotizing fasciitis is a bacterial infection of the subcutaneous tissue and fascial sheath.[611, 637, 638] The infection can arise in an operative wound or in a focal infection such as a breast abscess, or there may be no apparent predisposing cause. Necrotizing fasciitis has been reported after circumcision[574] and as a complication of a fetal monitor.[578] The trunk and extremities are the areas most commonly involved; the inflammation spreads rapidly along fascial planes, producing thrombosis and extensive necrosis, with infarcts developing in the

overlying skin. Vesicles and bullae appear, and the skin may become blue-gray or black. Myositis and bacteremia often accompany fasciitis. Staphylococci, group B streptococci,[639] *E. coli*, *P. aeruginosa*, anaerobic bacteria,[579] and mixtures of gram-positive and gram-negative bacteria have been associated with this disease. The bacteria are present in skin lesions, deep fascia, and, in some cases, blood. The mortality is high despite the use of fasciotomy, wide debridement, and antibiotics.

Perirectal abscesses may occur in newborns. Unlike older children, most newborns with perirectal abscess do not have underlying immunodeficiency, although infants with acquired or congenital immunodeficiency often present with this condition. The most common etiology for perirectal abscess is *S. aureus*, *E. coli*, or other enteric bacilli[640, 641]; however, anaerobic bacteria can also be involved. *S. aureus* and enteric bacilli may be more common in infants and newborns.[641] Recent rectal surgery for conditions such as Hirschsprung's disease or imperforate anus (myotomy or rectal dilatation) may be predisposing causes in infants; as in older children, neutropenia may also be associated with an increased risk for perirectal abscess.

Otitis externa is uncommon in the newborn. Victorin described an outbreak of neonatal infections in which *P. aeruginosa* was cultured from seven infants with suppuration of the auditory canal.[642] The author suggested that this outbreak was caused by contaminated bath water used in the nursery.

Diagnosis

The appearance of a skin lesion alone may be sufficiently typical to suspect certain etiologic agents (e.g., ecthyma gangrenosum), but more often the appearance is non-specific. A microbiologic diagnosis should be sought to provide specific therapy. The lesion and the surrounding tissue should be cleansed with 70% ethanol to prevent contamination from organisms that colonize the surface. If crusts are present, they should be lifted with a sterile swab to provide drainage, and cultures should be obtained from the base of the lesion. Vesicles and pustules can be aspirated with a needle (20 to 25 gauge) attached to a syringe, or they can be opened and exudate collected on a sterile swab. In general, swabs are not preferred for specimen collection because swab materials bind or inactivate bacterial organisms. Aspiration of abscesses is important; more than one aspiration may be required because the suppurative focus may not be easily distinguished from the surrounding inflammatory tissue. Aspiration of the leading edge or point of maximal inflammation of an area of cellulitis may be of value and should be performed if no other suppurative or purulent sites are available for culture. A small needle (e.g., 25 or 26 gauge) should be attached to a tuberculin or other small-volume syringe filled with 0.25 to 0.50 ml of sterile nonbacteriostatic saline; the needle should be inserted into the area of soft tissue to be sampled, with continuous, gentle aspiration applied to the syringe. If no fluid is returned to the syringe, a small amount of fluid should be injected and immediately aspirated back into the syringe. Collected material may be sent to the laboratory in the syringe for Gram stain and culture, or, alternatively, the contents may be washed into a tube of bacteriologic broth medium for transport and subsequent culture.

If swabs are used, care must be taken that the material does not dry before it is plated on bacteriologic media. Swabs preferentially should be directly inoculated and/or rinsed in bacteriologic media and immediately transported to the microbiology laboratory. Alternatively, they may be refrigerated or placed in appropriate transport media if more than a few hours will elapse before inoculation of media in the laboratory. Whenever sufficient material is available (on swabs or in liquid), several slides should be prepared for Gram staining.

It is often difficult to distinguish petechiae from vascular dilatation. Pressure with a glass slide on the border of the lesion is a simple and reliable method for detecting extravasation of red blood cells. If the lesion disappears on pressure, it is probably caused by dilatation of small vessels, whereas persistence of the lesion after application of pressure indicates extravasation of red blood cells. Bacteria may be present in petechial lesions that occur in infants with bacterial sepsis. Blood obtained by aspiration or gentle scraping with a scalpel at the center of the petechiae may reveal the causative organism on Gram stain or culture.

Differential Diagnosis

Sclerema neonatorum, milia, and erythema toxicum are noninfectious lesions that are often confused with infections of the skin.[643] Bullous and purpuric lesions may be due to noninfectious disorders, including mast cell diseases (e.g., urticaria pigmentosa), histiocytosis X, acrodermatitis enteropathica, dermatitis herpetiformis, epidermolysis bullosa, congenital porphyria,[563] and pemphigus vulgaris.[644] A syndrome of generalized erythroderma, failure to thrive, and diarrhea has been associated with various forms of immunodeficiency.[645]

Sclerema neonatorum is a diffuse, spreading, waxy hardness of the skin and subcutaneous tissue that occurs during the first weeks of life.[646, 647] The subcutaneous tissue seems to be bound to underlying muscle and bone. This condition is usually seen on the thighs, buttocks, and trunk. Although associated with sepsis in some infants, sclerema also afflicts infants with dehydration, acidosis, and shock. Most evidence supports the hypothesis that sclerema is a manifestation of shock and insufficiency of the peripheral circulation. Thus, when it occurs in infants with generalized infection, sclerema is associated with a poor prognosis. In a review of cases of sepsis at The New York Hospital, sclerema was detected in 6 of 71 infants, 5 of whom died.[648]

Milia are yellow or pearly white papules that are 1 mm in diameter and usually found scattered over the cheeks, forehead, and nose.[643, 649] The lesion is a small cyst formed from retention of sebum in sebaceous glands. Because the cyst is capped by a shiny surface of epidermis, it may be confused with a small pustule. Milia are common; Gordon estimated that 40% of healthy newborns have milia.[649] The lesions are frequent in the first few weeks of life. These cysts may be distinguished from staphylococcal pustules by aspiration and Gram stain of the material.

Erythema toxicum consists of several types of lesions, including 1- to 3-mm yellow-white papules or pustules on an erythematous base, erythematous macules, and/or diffuse erythema. These lesions are usually present on the trunk but may involve the head and neck and extremities as well. Most lesions appear within the first hours of life and are uncommon after 2 days of age. Erythema toxicum is uncommon in low-birth-weight or premature infants.[650] The affected infants have no signs of systemic illness or local irritation. A smear of the contents of pustules reveals the presence of eosinophils and an absence of bacteria. Other noninfectious pustular lesions of newborns include neonatal pustular melanosis, which is marked by a mixed infiltrate that has a predominance of neutrophils,[651] and infantile acropustulosis, which is characterized by an eosinophilic infiltration of the skin.[652, 653]

Bullae may occur on the skin of the wrist or forearm and usually are caused by trauma.[654] Sucking of the extremity by the infant is believed to cause the bullae, which contain sterile serous fluid.

Purpura may be due to noninfectious causes, including trauma, erythroblastosis fetalis, or, less frequently, coagulation disorders, maternal drug ingestion, congenital leukemia, and congenital Letterer-Siwe disease.

Diaper rash is primarily a contact dermatitis associated with soilage of the skin by urine and stool.[655-657] The rash may occur as a mild erythema or scaling, a sharply demarcated and confluent erythema, or discrete shallow ulcerations. A beefy red confluent rash with raised margins, satellite (e.g., folliculitis) oval-shaped lesions, or discrete vesicular-pustular lesions indicates secondary invasion by *C. albicans* or *S. aureus*. In addition, systemic infectious illnesses that manifest as disseminated rashes (e.g., herpes, varicella, syphilis) may be characterized by early typical lesions in the diaper area.

Treatment

The treatment of localized skin lesions consists of the use of local antiseptic materials, systemic antimicrobial agents, and appropriate incision and drainage or debridement.

Hexachlorophene (3% detergent emulsion) and chlorhexidene (4% solution) are of value in cleaning small abraded areas and discrete pustular lesions. Because of the concern over its neurotoxicity and cutaneous absorption, hexachlorophene should not be used on large open areas of skin (see Chapter 30).

Systemic antibiotics should be considered for therapy whenever there is significant soft tissue infection with abscess or cellulitis. The specific antibiotic choice should be made on the basis of the microbiology of the lesion; streptococci may be treated effectively with penicillin G, ampicillin, or extended-spectrum cephalosporins (i.e., cefotaxime or ceftriaxone), whereas staphylococci generally must be treated with penicillinase-resistant penicillins or vancomycin. Infections due to gram-negative enteric bacilli may be treated with aminoglycosides or extended-spectrum cephalosporins based on the results of susceptibility testing. Infections due to *Pseudomonas* organisms can be effectively treated with aminoglycosides or ceftazidime.

Local heat and moist dressings over areas of abscess formation may facilitate localization or spontaneous drainage. Indications for incision and drainage of abscesses in infants are the same as for those in older children and adults.

Prevention

Prevention of local skin infections is best provided by appropriate routine hygiene, maintenance of the integrity of skin (i.e., avoidance of drying, trauma, or chemical contact), frequent diaper changes, and hygienic care of the umbilicus or other wounds or noninfectious skin inflammation. The following measures of skin care are recommended by the Committee of the Fetus and Newborn of the American Academy of Pediatrics[657] to prevent infection:

1. The first bath should be postponed until the infant is thermally stable.
2. Nonmedicated soap and water should be used; sterile sponges (not gauze) soaked in warm water may be used.
3. The buttocks and perianal should be cleansed with fresh water and cotton, or with mild soap and water, at diaper changes.
4. Ideally, agents used on the newborn skin should be dispensed in single-use containers.
5. No single method of cord care has proved to be superior, and none is endorsed.[657]

Cord care may include application of alcohol, triple dye (brilliant green, proflavine hemisulfate, and crystal violet) or antimicrobial agents such as bacitracin. Alcohol hastens drying of the cord but is probably not effective in preventing cord colonization and omphalitis. A randomized study of triple dye, povidone-iodine, silver sulfadiazine, and bacitracin ointment showed comparability in antimicrobial control.[658]

During nursery outbreaks, the Centers for Disease Control and Prevention recommends the judicious use of hexachlorophene bathing.[659] Daily hexachlorophene bathing of the diaper area[660] and umbilical cord care with 4% chlorhexidene solution[661] have demonstrated efficacy for prevention of staphylococcal disease (see Chapter 30).

CONJUNCTIVITIS AND OTHER EYE INFECTIONS

Conjunctivitis in the newborn is usually due to one of four causes: (1) infection with *N. gonorrhoeae*, (2) infection with *S. aureus*, (3) inclusion conjunctivitis caused by *Chlamydia trachomatis*, or (4) chemical conjunctivitis induced by silver nitrate solution.[662, 663] Less commonly, other microorganisms have been implicated as a cause of conjunctivitis, including group A and B streptococci, *S. pneumoniae*, *H. influenzae* (nontypable[590] and group b[664]), *P. aeruginosa*, *Moraxella* (*Neisseria*) *catarrhalis*,[665]

Neisseria meningitidis,[666] *Corynebacterium diphtheriae*,[667] *Pasteurella multocida*,[668] *Clostridium* sp.,[669] herpes simplex virus, echoviruses, *M. hominis*, and *Candida* sp.. In addition to meningococcal infections, other neisserial species can be confused with gonococcal infections; *Neisseria cinerea* has been reported to cause conjunctivitis that was indistinguishable from gonococcal infection.[670] In addition, an epidemic of erythromycin-resistant *S. aureus* conjunctivitis affected 25 of 215 newborns during a 10-month period; control of the epidemic was achieved by identification of staff carriers and substitution of silver nitrate prophylaxis for erythromycin.[671] The major causes of conjunctivitis in the neonate are discussed in Chapter 29 (gonococcal infection) and Chapter 30 (staphylococcal infection). Cultures of the conjunctivae of neonates with purulent conjunctivitis and from the comparable eye(s) of a similar number of infants chosen as controls revealed significant differences, suggesting causality for *S. viridans*, *S. aureus*, *E. coli*, and *Haemophilus* sp.[672, 673]

In comparison to chemical (e.g., silver nitrate) conjunctivitis, other noninfectious causes for conjunctivitis occur only rarely. Eosinophilic pustular folliculitis has been described since 1970[674]; although this disease usually occurs after 3 months of age, occasional infants younger than 4 to 6 weeks of age have been described. These infants present with recurrent crops of pruritic papules primarily affecting the scalp and brow. Biopsy specimens reveal folliculitis with a predominant eosinophilic infiltrate; most infants also have a leukocytosis and eosinophilia. Other acute or chronic cutaneous conditions may also manifest as conjunctival or periorbital inflammation, such as seborrhea, atopic dermatitis, acropustulosis of infancy, and erythema toxicum (see discussion on skin infections).

In a review by Hammerschlag,[675] the incidence of the two major pathogens ranged from 17 to 32% for *C. trachomatis* and 0 to 14.2% for *N. gonorrhoeae* in four United States studies. In other developed countries such as England,[676] investigators found 8 cases of gonococcal infection and 44 cases of chlamydial infection among 86 newborns with ophthalmia neonatorum; in Denmark,[677] investigators found that 72% of infants with conjunctivitis at 4 to 6 days after birth had positive cultures but 70% were caused by staphylococci (both *S. aureus* and *S. epidermidis*) and that chlamydiae were isolated from only 2 of 300 newborns. Thus, the incidence and microbiology of neonatal conjunctivitis is dependent on the incidence of transmissible infections in the maternal genital tract or the nursery and the use and efficacy of chemoprophylaxis. In Nairobi, Kenya, in a hospital where ocular prophylaxis had been discontinued, the incidence of gonococcal and chlamydial ophthalmitis was 3.6 and 8.1 per 100 live births, respectively[678]; whereas in Harare, Zimbabwe, in a hospital where prophylaxis also was not used, the most common cause of conjunctivitis was *S. aureus*.[679] The introduction of tetracycline ointment for prophylaxis at Bellevue Hospital (New York City) led to an overall increase in conjunctivitis associated with an increase in the incidence of gonococcal infection[680] due to the emergence of tetracycline resistance among gonococci.

Infections related to *P. aeruginosa* deserve special attention. Although uncommon, pseudomonal conjunctivitis may be a devastating disease if not recognized and treated appropriately.[680] The infection is usually acquired in the nursery, and the first signs of conjunctivitis appear between the fifth and eighteenth days of life. At first, the clinical manifestations are localized to the eye and include edema and erythema of the lid and purulent discharge. In some children, the conjunctivitis progresses rapidly and there is a denuding of the corneal epithelium and infiltration with neutrophils. With extension of the corneal infiltration, perforation of the cornea may occur. The anterior chamber may fill with fibrinous exudate, and the iris can adhere to the cornea. Subsequent invasion of the cornea by small blood vessels (pannus) is characteristic of pseudomonal conjunctivitis. The late ophthalmic complications may be followed by bacteremia and septic foci in other organs.[681]

Pseudomonal eye infections in neonates can occur in epidemic form, with subsequent high rates of mortality and ophthalmic morbidity. Burns and Rhodes[681] reported a series of eye infections caused by *P. aeruginosa* in premature infants with purulent conjunctivitis rapidly progressing to septicemia, shock, and death in four infants. Five other children with conjunctivitis alone survived, but one child required enucleation. Drewett and co-workers[682] described a nursery outbreak of pseudomonal conjunctivitis believed to be due to contaminated resuscitation equipment; of 14 infected infants, 1 became blind and another had severe corneal opacities. Rapidity of the course of this infection is indicated in a case report of a 10-day-old infant who developed a corneal ulcer with perforation within 2 days after first observation of a purulent discharge.[683] An outbreak of four cases of *Pseudomonas* conjunctivitis in premature infants occurred within a period of 2 weeks at the American University of Beirut Medical Center[684]; no cause for the outbreak was found.

A review by Lohrer and Belohradsky of bacterial endophthalmitis in neonates underlines the importance of *P. aeruginosa* in invasive bacterial eye infections ranging from keratitis to panophthalmitis.[685] The literature review included 16 cases of invasive eye infections in neonates; 13 were due to *P. aeruginosa*, and the others were cases of endophthalmitis caused by group B streptococci and *S. pneumoniae*. Other opportunistic gram-negative pathogens associated with outbreaks of infections in nurseries may also include conjunctivitis as a part of the infection syndrome. In a report by Christensen and co-workers,[686] a multiply antibiotic-resistant *S. marcescens* was responsible for 15 cases of pneumonia, sepsis, and meningitis as well as 20 cases of conjunctivitis, cystitis, and wound infection over a 9-month period in a neonatal intensive care unit.

Dacryocystitis may complicate a congenital lacrimal sac distention (dacryocystocele). Harris and DiClementi described an infant who presented on day 4 of life with edema and erythema of the lower lid.[687] Purulent material emerged from the puncta after moderate pressure over the lacrimal sac; *S. marcescens* was grown from the material.

The physician responsible for management of the child with purulent conjunctivitis must consider the major causes of the disease and must be alert to the rare pathogen. In hospitals that practice Credé's method (i.e., silver nitrate application), purulent conjunctivitis during the first 48 hours of life is almost always due to chemical toxicity.[688] After the first 2 days, the pus of an exudative conjunctivitis must be carefully examined by Gram stain for the presence of gram-negative intracellular diplococci, gram-positive cocci in clusters, or gram-negative bacilli. Appropriate cultures should be used for isolation of the organisms concerned. If the smears are inconclusive and no pathogens are isolated on appropriate media and if the conjunctivitis persists, a diagnosis of inclusion or chlamydial infection is likely.[687, 689, 690]

The treatment of gonococcal and staphylococcal conjunctivitis is discussed in Chapters 29 and 30. Chlamydial conjunctivitis is reviewed in Chapter 15.

If infection with *Pseudomonas* species is suspected, treatment should be started at once with an effective parenteral antibiotic such as an aminoglycoside (e.g., tobramycin, amikacin, or gentamicin) with or without an antipseudomonal penicillin or ceftazidime (see Chapter 35) and with a locally applied ophthalmic ointment. The use of subconjunctival gentamicin or other antipseudomonal aminoglycoside is of uncertain value; however, if the cornea appears to be extensively involved, there is a risk of rapid development of endophthalmitis, and the subconjunctival injection of antibiotics should be considered in consultation with an ophthalmologist. If the diagnosis is confirmed, this regimen is continued until the local signs of *Pseudomonas* infection resolve.

Current recommendations for ocular chemoprophylaxis are discussed in the chapters on gonococcal and chlamydial infections. In addition, the reader is referred to the 2000 edition of the Report of the Committee on Infectious Diseases published by the American Academy of Pediatrics.[691]

References

Infections of the Liver

1. Murphy FM, Baker CJ. Solitary hepatic abscess: a delayed complication of neonatal bacteremia. Pediatr Infect Dis J 7:414, 1988.
2. Guillois B, Guillemin MG, Thoma M, et al. Staphylococcie pleuro-pulmonaire néonatale avec abcès hépatiques multiples. Ann Pediatr 36:681, 1989.
3. Dehner LP, Kissane JM. Pyogenic hepatic abscesses in infancy and childhood. J Pediatr 74:763, 1969.
4. Wright HT Jr. Personal communication, 1987.
5. Moss TJ, Pysher TJ. Hepatic abscess in neonates. Am J Dis Child 135:726, 1981.
6. Chusid MJ. Pyogenic hepatic abscess in infancy and childhood. Pediatrics 62:554, 1978.
7. Miedema BW, Dineen P, Yurt RW. Pyogenic liver abscesses in children. Infections in Surgery. April 1985, pp 295–305. (Personal communication, Peter Dineen, M.D., Cornell University Medical College, New York City, NY 10021.)
8. Bilfinger TV, Hayden CK, Oldham KT, et al. Pyogenic liver abscesses in nonimmunocompromised children. South Med J 79:37, 1986.
9. Beutow KC, Klein SW, Lane RB. Septicemia in premature infants: the characteristics, treatment, and preven-

tion of septicemia in premature infants. Am J Dis Child 110:29, 1965.

10. Dunham EC. Septicemia in the newborn. Am J Dis Child 45:229, 1933.

11. Nyhan W, Fousek MD. Septicemia of the newborn. Pediatrics 22:268, 1958.

12. Gotoff SP, Behrman RE. Neonatal septicemia. J Pediatr 76:142, 1970.

13. Hamilton JR, Sass-Kortsak A. Jaundice associated with severe bacterial infection in young infants. J Pediatr 63:121, 1963.

14. Hänninen P, Terhe P, Toivanen A. Septicemia in a pediatric unit: a 20-year study. Scand J Infect Dis 3:201, 1971.

15. Potter E. Pathology of the Fetus and Infant, 3rd ed. Chicago, Year Book Medical Publishers, 1975.

16. Silverman WA, Homan WE. Sepsis of obscure origin in the newborn. Pediatrics 3:157, 1949.

17. Smith RT, Platau ES, Good RA. Septicemia of the newborn: current status of the problem. Pediatrics 17:549, 1956.

18. Gersony WM, McCracken GH Jr. Purulent pericarditis in infancy. Pediatrics 40:224, 1967.

19. Axton JHM. Amoebic proctocolitis and liver abscess in a neonate. S Afr Med J 46:258, 1972.

20. Botman T, Ruys PJ. Amoebic appendicitis in newborn infant. Trop Geogr Med 15:221, 1963.

21. Brans YW, Ceballos R, Cassady G. Umbilical catheters and hepatic abscesses. Pediatrics 53:264, 1974.

22. Cohen HJ, Dresner S. Liver abscess following exchange transfusion for erythroblastosis fetalis. Q Rev Pediatr 16:148, 1961.

23. deBeaujeu J, Bethenod M, Mollard P, et al. Abcès hépatique à forme tumorale chez un nourrisson. Pediatrie 23:363, 1968.

24. Heck W, Rehbein F, Reismann B. Pyogene Leberabszesse im Säuglingsalter. Z Kinderchir Suppl 1:49, 1966.

25. Kandall SR, Johnson AB, Gartner LM. Solitary neonatal hepatic abscess. J Pediatr 85:567, 1974.

26. Kutsunai T. Abscess of the liver of umbilical origin in infants: report of two cases. Am J Dis Child 51:1385, 1936.

27. Madsen CM, Secouris N. Solitary liver abscess in a newborn. Surgery 47:1005, 1960.

28. Martin C, Saint-Supery G, Babin JP, et al. Abcès gazeux du foie avec coagulopathie chez le nouveau-né: guérison (à propos de 2 observations). Bordeaux Med 5:1181, 1972.

29. Pouyanne, Martin D. Abcès du foie à staphylocoques chez un nouveau-né, compliqué de suppuration sous-phrénique puis de péritonite à évolution subaiguë. Guérison J Med Bordeaux 130:929, 1953.

30. Pyrtek LJ, Bartus SA. Hepatic pyemia. N Engl J Med 272:551, 1965.

31. Sharma K, Kumar R. Solitary abscess of the liver in a newborn infant. Surgery 61:812, 1967.

32. Williams JW, Rittenberry A, Dillard R, et al. Liver abscess in newborn: complication of umbilical vein catheterization. Am J Dis Child 125:111, 1973.

33. Beaven DW. Staphylococcal peritonitis in the newborn. Lancet 1:869, 1958.

34. Fraga JR, Javate BA, Venkatessan S. Liver abscess and sepsis due to Klebsiella pneumoniae in a newborn. Clin Pediatr 13:1081, 1974.

35. Tariq AA, Rudolph NA, Levin EJ. Solitary hepatic abscess in a newborn infant: a sequel of umbilical vein catheterization and infusion of hypertonic glucose solutions. Clin Pediatr 16:577, 1977.

36. Cushman P, Ward OC. Solitary liver abscess in a neonate: complication of umbilical vein catheterization. Ir J Med Sci 147:374, 1978.

37. Wiedersberg H, Pawlowski P. Pyelophlebitis nach Nabelvenenkatheterismus. Monatsschr Kinderheilkd 128:128, 1980.

38. Gonzalez Rivera F, Montoro Burgos M, Cabrera Molina A. Absceso hepático en un recién nacido. An Esp Pediatr 23:59, 1985.

39. Nars PW, Klco L, Fliegel CP. Successful conservative management of a solitary liver abscess in a premature baby. Helv Paediatr Acta 38:489, 1983.

40. Larsen LR, Raffensperger J. Liver abscess. J Pediatr Surg 14:329, 1979.

41. Montoya F, Alam M-M, Couture A, et al. Abcès du foie chez un nouveau-né guerison après ponction percutanée sous controle échographique. Pediatrie 38:547, 1983.

42. Murphy SM, Baker CJ. Solitary hepatic abscess: a delayed complication of neonatal bacteremia. Pediatr Infect Dis J 7:414, 1988.

43. Anagnostakis D, Kamba A, Petrochilou V, et al. Risk of infection associated with umbilical vein catheterization: a prospective study in 75 newborn infants. J Pediatr 86:759, 1975.

44. Sabbaj J, Sutter V, Finegold SM. Anaerobic pyogenic liver abscess. Ann Intern Med 77:629, 1972.

45. Meyer WW, Lind J. Postnatal changes in the portal circulation. Arch Dis Child 41:606, 1966.

46. Hageman J, Shulman S, Schreiber M, et al. Congenital tuberculosis: critical reappraisal of clinical findings and diagnostic procedures. Pediatrics 66:980, 1980.

47. Hughesdon MR. Congenital tuberculosis. Arch Dis Child 21:121, 1946.

48. Cantwell MF, Shehab ZM, Costello AM, et al. Brief report: congenital tuberculosis. N Engl J Med 330:1051, 1994.

49. Abughali N, van der Kuyp F, Amable W, et al. Congenital tuberculosis. Pediatr Infect Dis J 13:738, 1994.

50. Simma B, Dietze O, Vogel W, et al. Bacille Calmette-Guérin–associated hepatitis. Eur J Pediatr 150:423, 1991.

51. Lide TN. Congenital tularemia. Arch Pathol 43:165, 1947.

52. Regan JC, Litvak A, Regan C. Intrauterine transmission of anthrax. JAMA 80:1769, 1923.

53. Hicks HT, French H. Typhoid fever and pregnancy with special reference to foetal infection. Lancet 1:1491, 1905.

54. Sarram M, Feiz J, Foruzandeh M, et al. Intrauterine fetal infection with Brucella melitensis as a possible cause of second-trimester abortion. Am J Obstet Gynecol 119:657, 1974.

55. Brim A. A bacteriologic study of 100 stillborn and dead newborn infants. J Pediatr 15:680, 1939.

56. Madan E, Meyer MP, Amortegui AJ. Isolation of genital mycoplasmas and Chlamydia trachomatis in stillborn and neonatal autopsy material. Arch Pathol Lab Med 112:749, 1988.

57. Oppenheimer EH, Hardy JB. Congenital syphilis in the newborn infant: clinical and pathological observations in recent cases. Johns Hopkins Med J 129:63, 1971.

58. Stokes JH, Beerman H, Ingraham NR Jr. Modern Clinical Syphilology: Diagnosis, Treatment, Case Study, 3rd ed. Philadelphia, WB Saunders, 1944.

59. Venter A, Pettifor JM, Duursma J, et al. Liver function in early congenital syphilis: does penicillin cause a deterioration? J Pediatr Gastroenterol Nutr 12:310, 1991.

60. Lindsay S, Luke JW. Fetal leptospirosis (Weil's disease) in a newborn infant: case of intrauterine fetal infection with report of an autopsy. J Pediatr 34:90, 1949.

61. Topciu V, Manu E, Strubert L, et al. Voie transplacen-

taire dans un cas de leptospirose humaine. Gynecol Obstet 65:617, 1966.

62. Gsell HO Jr, Olafsson A, Sonnabend W, et al. Intrauterine Leptospirosis pomona: Erster berichteter Fall einer intrauterin übertragenen und geheilten Leptospirose. Dtsch Med Wochenschr 96:1263, 1971.

63. Cramer HHW. Abortus bein Leptospirosis canicola. Arch Gynecol 177:167, 1950.

64. Chung H, Ts'ao W, Mo P, et al. Transplacental or congenital infection of leptospirosis: clinical and experimental observations. Chin Med J 82:777, 1963.

65. Fuchs PC, Oyama AA. Neonatal relapsing fever due to transplacental transmission of *Borrelia*. JAMA 208:690, 1969.

66. Yagupsky P, Moses S. Neonatal *Borrelia* species infection (relapsing fever). Am J Dis Child 139:74, 1985.

67. Fuchs PC. Personal communication, 1973.

68. Weber K, Bratzke H-J, Neubert U, et al. *Borrelia burgdorferi* in a newborn despite oral penicillin for Lyme borreliosis during pregnancy. Pediatr Infect Dis J 7:286, 1988.

68a. Steere AC. Lyme disease. N Engl J Med 321:586, 1989.

69. Lipinski JK, Vega JM, Cywes S, et al. Falciform ligament abscess in the infant. J Pediatr Surg 20:556, 1985.

70. Betke K, Richarz H. Nabelsepsis mit Pyelphlebitis, multiplen Leberabscessen, Lungenabscessen, und Osteomyelitis. Ausgang in Heilung. Monatschr Kinderheilkd 105:70, 1957.

71. Elliott RIK. The ductus venosus in neonatal infection. Proc R Soc Med 62:321, 1969.

72. McKenzie CG. Pyogenic infection of liver secondary to infection in the portal drainage area. BMJ 4:1558, 1964.

73. Menzel K, Buttenberg H. Pyelophlebitis mit multiplen Leberabszessen als Komplikation mehrfacher Sondierung der Nabelvene. Kinderaerztl Prax 40:14, 1972.

74. Sarrut S, Alain J, Alison F. Les complications précoces de la perfusion par la veine ombilicale chez le premature. Arch Fr Pediatr 26:651, 1969.

75. Santerne B, Morville P, Touche D, et al. Diagnostic et traitement d'une abcédation hépatique néo-natale multifocale par l'échographie. Presse Med 16:12, 1987.

76. Scott J. Iatrogenic lesions in babies following umbilical vein catheterization. Arch Dis Child 40:426, 1965.

77. Shaw A, Pierog S. "Ectopic" liver in the umbilicus: an unusual focus of infection in a newborn infant. Pediatrics 44:448, 1969.

78. Morison JE. Umbilical sepsis and acute interstitial hepatitis. J Pathol Bacteriol 56:531, 1944.

79. Bernstein J, Brown AK. Sepsis and jaundice in early infancy. Pediatrics 29:873, 1962.

80. Parker RGF. Jaundice and infantile diarrhea. Arch Dis Child 33:330, 1958.

81. Gwinn JL, Lee FA. Radiologic case of the month: pyogenic liver abscess. Am J Dis Child 123:50, 1972.

82. Martin DJ. Neonatal disorders diagnosed with ultrasound. Clin Perinatol 12:219, 1985.

83. Pineiro-Carrero VM, Andres JM. Morbidity and mortality in children with pyogenic liver abscess. Am J Dis Child 143:1424, 1989.

84. Caron KH. Magnetic resonance imaging of the pediatric abdomen. Semin Ultrasound CT MR 12:448, 1991.

85. Halvorsen RA Jr, Foster WL Jr, Wilkinson RH Jr, et al. Hepatic abscess: sensitivity of imaging tests and clinical findings. Gastrointest Radiol 13:135, 1988.

86. Weinreb JC, Cohen JM, Armstrong E, et al. Imaging the pediatric liver: MRI and CT. AJR Am J Roentgenol 147:785, 1986.

87. Cohen MD. Clinical utility of magnetic resonance imaging in pediatrics. Am J Dis Child 140:947, 1986.

88. Diament MJ, Stanley P, Kangarloo H, et al. Percutaneous aspiration and catheter drainage of abscesses. J Pediatr 108:204, 1986.

89. Rubinstein Z, Heyman Z, Morag B, et al. Ultrasound and computed tomography in the diagnosis and drainage of abscesses and other fluid collections. Isr J Med Sci 19:1050, 1983.

90. Reynolds TB. Medical treatment of pyogenic liver abscess. Ann Intern Med 96:373, 1982.

91. Loh R, Wallace G, Thong YH. Successful non-surgical management of pyogenic liver abscess. Scand J Infect Dis 19:137, 1987.

91a. Keidl CM, Chusid MJ. Splenic abscesses in childhood. Pediatr Infect Dis J 8:368, 1989.

Infections of the Biliary Tract

92. Bowen A. Acute gallbladder dilatation in a neonate: emphasis on ultrasonography. J Pediatr Gastroenterol Nutr 3:304, 1984.

93. Goldthorn JF, Thomas DW, Ramos AD. Hydrops of the gallbladder in stressed premature infants. Clin Res 28:122A, 1980.

94. Brill PW, Winchester P, Rosen MS. Neonatal cholelithiasis. Pediatr Radiol 12:285, 1982.

95. Callahan J, Haller JO, Cacciarelli AA, et al. Cholelithiasis in infants: association with total parenteral nutrition and furosemide. Radiology 143:437, 1982.

96. Keller MS, Markle BM, Laffey PA, et al. Spontaneous resolution of cholelithiasis in infants. Radiology 157:345, 1985.

97. Schirmer WJ, Grisoni ER, Gauderer MWL. The spectrum of cholelithiasis in the first year of life. J Pediatr Surg 24:1064, 1989.

98. Debray D, Pariente D, Gauthrer F, et al. Cholelithiasis in infancy: a study of 40 cases. J Pediatr 122:38, 1993.

99. Neu J, Arvin A, Ariagno RL. Hydrops of the gallbladder. Am J Dis Child 134:891, 1980.

100. Leichty EA, Cohen MD, Lemons JA, et al. Normal gallbladder appearing as abdominal mass in neonates. Am J Dis Child 136:468, 1982.

101. Peevy KJ, Wiseman HJ. Gallbladder distension in septic neonates. Arch Dis Child 57:75, 1982.

102. Dutta T, George V, Sharma GD, et al. Gallbladder disease in infancy and childhood. Progr Pediatr Surg 8:109, 1975.

103. Saldanha RL, Stein CA, Kopelman AE. Gallbladder distention in ill preterm infants. Am J Dis Child 137:1179, 1983.

104. El-Shafie M, Mah CL. Transient gallbladder distention in sick premature infants: the value of ultrasonography and radionuclide scintigraphy. Pediatr Radiol 16:468, 1986.

105. Modi N, Keay AJ. Neonatal gallbladder distention. Arch Dis Child 57:562, 1982.

106. Amodio JB, Fontanetta E, Cohen M, et al. Neonatal hydrops of the gallbladder: evaluation by cholescintigraphy and ultrasonography. NY State J Med 85:565, 1985.

107. McGahan JP, Phillips HE, Cox KL. Sonography of the normal pediatric gallbladder and biliary tract. Radiology 144:873, 1982.

108. Haller JO. Sonography of the biliary tract in infants and children. AJR 157:1051, 1991.

109. Guthrie KJ, Montgomery GL. Infections with *Bacterium enteritidis* in infancy with the triad of enteritis, cholecystitis, and meningitis. J Pathol Bacteriol 49:393, 1939.

110. Faller W, Berkelhamor JE, Esterly JR. Neonatal biliary

tract infection coincident with maternal methadone therapy. Pediatrics 48:997, 1971.

111. Jamieson PN, Shaw DG. Empyema of gallbladder in an infant. Arch Dis Child 50:482, 1975.

112. Arnspiger LA, Martin JG, Krempin HO. Acute noncalculous cholecystitis in children: report of a case in a 17-day-old infant. Am J Surg 100:103, 1960.

113. Ternberg JL, Keating JP. Acute acalculous cholecystitis: complication of other illnesses in childhood. Arch Surg 110:543, 1975.

114. Crystal RF, Fink RL. Acute acalculous cholecystitis in childhood: a report of two cases. Clin Pediatr 10:423, 1971.

115. Robinson AE, Erwin JH, Wiseman HJ, et al. Cholecystitis and hydrops of the gallbladder in the newborn. Radiology 122:749, 1977.

116. Snyder WH Jr, Chaffin L, Oettinger L. Cholelithiasis and perforation of the gallbladder in an infant, with recovery. JAMA 149:1645, 1952.

117. Washburn ME, Barcia PJ. Uncommon cause of a right upper quadrant abdominal mass in a newborn: acute cholecystitis. Am J Surg 140:704, 1980.

118. Thurston WA, Kelly EN, Silver MM. Acute acalculous cholecystitis in a premature infant treated with parenteral nutrition. Can Med Assoc J 135:332, 1986.

119. Pieretti R, Auldist AW, Stephens CA. Acute cholecystitis in children. Surg Obstet Gynecol 140:16, 1975.

120. Hanson BA, Mahour GH, Woolley MM. Discases of the gallbladder in infancy and childhood. J Pediatr Surg 6:277, 1971.

121. Dewan PA, Stokes KB, Solomon JR. Paediatric acalculous cholecystitis. Pediatr Surg Int 2:120, 1987.

122. Denes J, Gergely K, Mohacsi A, et al. Die Frühgeborenen-Appendicitis. Z Kinderchir 5:400, 1968.

123. Traynelis VC, Hrabovsky EE. Acalculous cholecystitis in the neonate. Am J Dis Child 139:893, 1985.

124. Aach RD. Cholecystitis in childhood. In Feigin RD, Cherry JD (eds). Textbook of Pediatric Infectious Diseases, 2nd ed. Philadelphia, WB Saunders, 1987, pp 742–743.

125. Wyllie R, Fitzgerald JF. Bacterial cholangitis in a 10-week-old infant with fever of undetermined origin. Pediatrics 65:164, 1980.

126. Becroft DMO. Biliary atresia associated with prenatal infection by *Listeria monocytogenes*. Arch Dis Child 47:656, 1972.

Infections of the Adrenal Glands

127. Favara BE, Akers DR, Franciosi RA. Adrenal abscess in a neonate. J Pediatr 77:682, 1970.

128. Mondor C, Gauthier M, Garel L, et al. Nonsurgical management of neonatal adrenal abscess. J Pediatr Surg 23:1048, 1988.

129. François A, Berterottiere D, Aigrain Y, et al. Abcès surrénalien neonatal à *Proteus mirabilis*. Arch Fr Pediatr 48:559, 1991.

130. Lizardo-Barahona JR, Nieto-Zermño J, Bracho-Blanchet E. Absceso adrenal en el recien nacido: informe de un caso y revision de la literatura. Bol Med Hosp Infant Mex 47:401, 1990.

131. Torres-Simon JM, Figueras-Aloy J, Vilanova-Juanola JM, et al. Absceso suprarenal en el recien nacido. An Esp Pediatr 31:601, 1989.

132. Zamir O, Udassion R, Aviad I, et al. Adrenal abscess: a rare complication of neonatal adrenal hemorrhage. Pediatr Surg Int 2:117, 1987.

133. Van de Water JM, Fonkalsrud EW. Adrenal cysts in infancy. Surgery 60:1267, 1966.

134. Blankenship WJ, Borgen H, Stadalnik R, et al. Suprarenal abscess in the neonate: a case report and review of diagnosis and management. Pediatrics 55:239, 1975.

135. Gibbons DM, Duckett JW Jr, Cromie WJ, et al. Abdominal flank mass in the neonate. J Urol 119:671, 1978.

136. Atkinson GO Jr, Kodroff MB, Gay BB Jr, et al. Adrenal abscess in the neonate. Radiology 155:101, 1985.

137. Carty A, Stanley P. Bilateral adrenal abscesses in a neonate. Pediatr Radiol 1:63, 1973.

138. Walker KM, Coyer WF. Suprarenal abscess due to group B *Streptococcus*. J Pediatr 94:970, 1979.

139. Camilleri R, Thibaud D, Gruner M, et al. Abcédation d'un hématome surrénal avec hypertension artérielle. Arch Fr Pediatr 41:705, 1984.

140. Rajani K, Shapiro SR, Goetsman BW. Adrenal abscess: complication of supportive therapy of adrenal hemorrhage in the newborn. J Pediatr Surg 15:676, 1980.

141. Wells RG, Sty JR, Hodgson NB. Suprarenal abscess in the neonate: technetium-99m glucoheptonate imaging. Clin Nucl Med 11:32, 1986.

142. Cadarso BA, Mialdea AMR. Absceso adrenal en la epoca neonatal. An Esp Pediatr 21:706, 1984.

143. Ohta S, Shimizu S, Fujisawa S, et al. Neonatal adrenal abscess due to *Bacteroides*. J Pediatr 93:1063, 1978.

144. Bekdash BA, Slim MS. Adrenal abscess in a neonate due to gas-forming organisms: a diagnostic dilemma. Z Kinderchir 32:184, 1981.

145. Gross M, Kottmeier PK, Waterhouse K. Diagnosis and treatment of neonatal adrenal hemorrhage. J Pediatr Surg 2:308, 1967.

146. Vigi V, Tamisari L, Osti L, et al. Suprarenal abscess in a newborn. Helv Paediatr Acta 36:263, 1981.

147. Suri S, Agarwalla ML, Mitra S, et al. Adrenal abscess in a neonate presenting as a renal neoplasm. Br J Urol 54:565, 1982.

148. Mittelstaedt CA, Volberg FM, Merten DF, et al. The sonographic diagnosis of neonatal adrenal hemorrhage. Radiology 131:453, 1979.

149. Rey A, Arena J, Nogues A, et al. Hemorragia suprarenal encapsulada en el recien nacido: estudio de ocho casos. An Esp Pediatr 21:238, 1984.

150. Black J, Williams DI. Natural history of adrenal hemorrhage in the newborn. Arch Dis Child 48:173, 1973.

151. Iklof O, Mortensson W, Sandstedt B. Suprarenal haematoma versus neuroblastoma complicated by haemorrhage: a diagnostic dilemma in the newborn. Acta Radiol Diagn 27:3, 1986.

152. White SJ, Stuck KJ, Blane CE, et al. Sonography of neuroblastoma. Am J Radiol 141:465, 1983.

152a. Shkolnik A. Applications of ultrasound in the neonatal abdomen. Radiol Clin North Am 23:141, 1985.

Appendicitis*

153. Etherington-Wilson WE. Appendicitis in newborn: report of a case 16 days old. Proc R Soc Med 38:186, 1945.

154. Puri P, O'Donnell B. Appendicitis in infancy. J Pediatr Surg 13:173, 1978.

155. Landaas B. Diagnosis of appendicitis in young children. Tidsskr Nor Laegeforen 68:335, 1948.

156. Reuter G, Krause I. Beitrag zur Problematik der Appendizitis des Neugeborenen. Kinderaerztl Prax 47:289, 1975.

157. Norris WJ. Appendicitis in children. West J Surg Obstet Gynecol 54:183, 1946.

---

*The list of references for intra-abdominal neonatal appendicitis is not exhaustive; additional cases can be found in the articles listed here.

158. Parsons JM, Miscall BG, McSherry CK. Appendicitis in the newborn infant. Surgery 67:841, 1970.

159. Schaupp W, Clausen EG, Ferrier PK. Appendicitis during the first month of life. Surgery 48:805, 1960. (Reviews 9 cases not included in this bibliography and adds 5 new cases of his own.)

160. Stanley-Brown EG. Acute appendicitis during the first five years of life. Am J Dis Child 108:134, 1964.

161. Snyder WH Jr, Chaffin L. Appendicitis during the first 2 years of life: report of 21 cases and review of 447 cases from the literature. Arch Surg 64:549, 1952.

162. Fields IA, Naiditch MJ, Rothman PE. Acute appendicitis in infants. Am J Dis Child 93:287, 1957.

163. Dick W, Hirt H-J, Vogel W. Die Appendizitis im Säglings-und Kleinkindesalter. Fortschr Med 94:125, 1976.

164. Gross RE. The Surgery of Infancy and Childhood: Its Principles and Techniques. Philadelphia, WB Saunders, 1953.

165. Grosfeld JL, Weinberger M, Clatworthy HW Jr. Acute appendicitis in the first two years of life. J Pediatr Surg 8:285, 1973.

166. Janik JS, Firor HV. Pediatric appendicitis: a 20-year study of 1,640 children at Cook County (Illinois) Hospital. Arch Surg 114:717, 1979.

167. Benson CD, Coury JJ Jr, Hagge DR. Acute appendicitis in infants: fifteen-year study. Arch Surg 64:561, 1952.

168. Massad M, Srouji M, Awdeh A, et al. Neonatal appendicitis: case report and a review of the English literature. Z Kinderchir 41:241, 1986.

169. Schorlemmer GR, Herbst CA Jr. Perforated neonatal appendicitis. South Med J 76:536, 1983.

170. Diess F. Die Appendizitis im Basler Kinderspital. Basle Dissertations, 1908, Case No. 36, p 63. Cited in reference 138 and in Abt. I A: Appendicitis in infants. Arch Pediatr 34:641, 1917.

171. Bartlett RH, Eraklis AJ, Wilkinson RH. Appendicitis in infancy. Surg Gynecol Obstet 130:99, 1970.

172. Broadbent NRG, Jardine JL. Acute appendicitis in a premature infant: a case report. Aust NZJ Surg 40:362, 1971.

173. Bryant LR, Trinkle JK, Noonan JA, et al. Appendicitis and appendiceal perforation in neonates. Am Surg 36:523, 1970.

174. Creery RDG. Acute appendicitis in the newborn. BMJ 1:871, 1953.

175. Hardman RP, Bowerman D. Appendicitis in the newborn. Am J Dis Child 105:99, 1963.

176. Klimt F, Hartmann G. Appendicitis perforata mit tiefsitzenden Dündarmverschluss beim Neugeborenen. Pädiatr Prax 1:271, 1962.

177. Kolb G, Schaeffer EL. Über Appendizitis mit Perforation in den ersten Lebenwochen. Kinderaerztl Prax 1:1, 1955.

178. Liechti RE, Snyder WH Jr. Acute appendicitis under age 2. Am Surg 29:92, 1963.

179. Meigher SC, Lucas AW. Appendicitis in the newborn: case report. Ann Surg 136:1044, 1952.

180. Meyer JF. Acute gangrenous appendicitis in a premature infant. J Pediatr 41:343, 1952.

181. Neve R, Quenville NF. Appendicitis with perforation in a 12-day-old infant. Can Med Assoc J 94:447, 1966.

181a. Nilforoushan MA. Fever and ascites in a newborn. Clin Pediatr 14:878, 1975.

182. Nuri M, Hecker WC, Duckert W. Beitrag zur Appendicitis im Neugeborenenalter. Z Kinderheilkd 91:1, 1964.

183. Parkhurst GF, Wagoner SC. Neonatal acute appendicitis. NY State J Med 69:1929, 1969.

184. Phillips SJ, Cohen B. Acute perforated appendicitis in newborn children. NY State J Med 71:985, 1971.

185. Smith AL, MacMahon RA. Perforated appendix complicating rhesus immunization in a newborn infant. Med J Aust 2:602, 1969.

186. Tabrisky J, Westerfeld R, Cavanaugh J. Appendicitis in the newborn. Am J Dis Child 111:557, 1966.

187. Vinz H, Erben U, Winkelvoss H. Neugeborenen peritonitis. Bruns Beitr Klin Chir 215:321, 1967.

188. Walker RH. Appendicitis in the newborn infant. J Pediatr 51:429, 1958.

189. Morehead CD, Houck PW. Epidemiology of Pseudomonas infections in a pediatric intensive care unit. Am J Dis Child 124:564, 1972.

190. Trojanowski JQ, Gang DL, Goldblatt A, et al. Fatal postoperative acute appendicitis in a neonate with congenital heart disease. J Pediatr Surg 16:85, 1981.

191. Ayalon A, Mogilner M, Cohen O, et al. Acute appendicitis in a premature baby. Acta Chir Scand 145:285, 1979.

192. Schellerer W, Schwemmle K, Decker R. Perforierte Appendizitis bei einem Frühgeborenen im Alter von 14 Tagen. Z Kinderchir 9:434, 1971.

193. Golladay ES, Roskes S, Donner L, et al. Intestinal obstruction from appendiceal abscess in a newborn infant. J Pediatr Surg 13:175, 1978.

194. Hemalatha V, Spitz L. Neonatal appendicitis. Clin Pediatr 18:621, 1979.

195. Tucci P, Holgersen L, Doctor D, et al. Congenital uretero-pelvic junction obstruction associated with unsuspected acute perforated appendicitis in a neonate. J Urol 120:247, 1978.

196. Fowkes GL. Neonatal appendicitis. BMJ 1:997, 1978.

197. Kwong MS, Dinner M. Neonatal appendicitis masquerading as necrotizing enterocolitis. J Pediatr 96:917, 1980.

198. Shaul WL. Clues to the early diagnosis of neonatal appendicitis. J Pediatr 98:473, 1981.

199. Grussner R, Pistor G, Engelskirchen R, et al. Appendicitis in childhood. Monatsschr Kinderheilkd 133:158, 1985.

200. Lassiter HA, Werner MH. Neonatal appendicitis. South Med J 76:1173, 1983.

201. Carol MJ, Creixell GS, Hernandez GJV, et al. Apendicitis neonatal: aportacion de un nuevo caso. An Esp Pediatr 20:807, 1984.

202. Bax NMA, Pearse RG, Dommering N, et al. Perforation of the appendix in the neonatal period. J Pediatr Surg 15:200, 1980.

203. Buntain WL. Neonatal appendicitis mistaken for necrotizing enterocolitis. South Med J 75:1155, 1982.

204. Heydenrych JJ, DuToit DF. Unusual presentations of acute appendicitis in the neonate: a report of 2 cases. S Afr Med J 62:1003, 1982.

205. Ruff ME, Southgate WM, Wood BP (eds). Radiological case of the month: neonatal appendicitis with perforation. Am J Dis Child 145:111, 1991.

206. Pathania OP, Jain SK, Kapila H, et al. Fatal neonatal perforation of appendix. Indian Pediatr J 26:1166, 1989.

207. Arora NK, Deorari AK, Bhatnagar V, et al. Neonatal appendicitis: a rare cause of surgical emergency in preterm babies. Indian Pediatr J 28:1330, 1991.

208. Srouji MN, Chatten J, David C. Pseudodiverticulitis of the appendix with neonatal Hirschsprung disease. J Pediatr 93:988, 1978.

209. Arliss J, Holgersen LO. Neonatal appendiceal perforation and Hirschsprung's disease. J Pediatr Surg 25:694, 1990.

210. Kliegman RM, Fanaroff AA. Necrotizing enterocolitis. N Engl J Med 310:1093, 1984.

211. Srouji MN, Buck BE. Neonatal appendicitis: ischemic infarction in incarcerated inguinal hernia. J Pediatr Surg 13:177, 1978.

212. Charif P. Perforated appendicitis in premature infants: a case report and review of the literature. Johns Hopkins Med J 125:92, 1969.

213. Stone HH, Sanders SL, Martin JD Jr. Perforated appendicitis in children. Surgery 69:673, 1971.

214. Dennis JE, Rhodes KH, Cooney DR, et al. Nosocomial *Rhizopus* infection (zycomycosis) in children. J Pediatr 96:824, 1980. (Same case as Michalak DM, Cooney DR, Rhodes KH, et al. Gastrointestinal mucormycoses in infants and children: a cause of gangrenous intestinal cellulitis and perforation. J Pediatr Surg 15:320, 1980.)

215. Buschard K, Kjaeldgaard A. Investigation and analysis of the position, fixation, length, embryology of the vermiform appendix. Acta Chir Scand 139:293, 1973.

216. Jones WR, Kaye MD, Ing RMY. The lymphoid development of the fetal and neonatal appendix. Biol Neonat 20:334, 1972.

217. Smith GM. Inflammatory changes in the appendix during early infancy. Am J Dis Child 1:299, 1911.

218. Hill WB, Mason CC. Prenatal appendicitis with rupture and death. Am J Dis Child 29:86, 1925.

219. Corcoran WJ. Prenatal rupture of the appendix. Am J Dis Child 39:277, 1930.

220. Jackson WF. A case of prenatal appendicitis. Am J Med Sci 127:710, 1904.

221. Kümmell EW. Cited in Etherington-Wilson WE. Appendicitis in newborn: report of a case 16 days old. Proc R Soc Med 38:186, 1945.

222. Martin LW, Glen PM. Prenatal appendiceal perforation: a case report. J Pediatr Surg 21:73, 1986.

223. Wilkinson RH, Bartlett RH, Eraklis AJ. Diagnosis of appendicitis in infancy: the value of abdominal radiographs. Am J Dis Child 118:687, 1969.

224. Holder TM, Leape LL. The acute surgical abdomen in the neonate. N Engl J Med 278:605, 1968.

225. Chang JHT. The use of antibiotics in pediatric abdominal surgery. Pediatr Infect Dis 3:195, 1984.

Peritonitis

226. Bell MJ. Peritonitis in the newborn—current concepts. Pediatr Clin North Am 32:1181, 1985.

227. Barson AJ. A postmortem study of infection in the newborn from 1976 to 1988. *In* deLouvois J, Harvey D (eds): Infection in the Newborn. New York, John Wiley & Sons, 1990, pp 13–34.

228. Fonkalsrud EW, Ellis DG, Clatworthy HW Jr. Neonatal peritonitis. J Pediatr Surg 1:227, 1966.

229. Lloyd JR. The etiology of gastrointestinal perforations in the newborn. J Pediatr Surg 4:77, 1969.

230. McDougal WS, Izant RJ, Zollinger RM Jr. Primary peritonitis in infancy and childhood. Ann Surg 181:310, 1975.

231. Rickham PP. Peritonitis in the neonatal period. Arch Dis Child 30:23, 1955.

232. Denes J, Leb J. Neonatal peritonitis. Acta Paediatr Acad Sci Hung 10:297, 1969.

233. Daum R, Schütze U, Hoffman H. Mortality of preoperative peritonitis in newborn infants without intestinal obstruction. Prog Pediatr Surg 13:267, 1979.

234. Schütze U, Fey KH, Hess G. Die Peritonitis im Neugeborenen-, Säglings-, und Kindesalter. Münch Med Wochenschr 116:1201, 1974.

235. Prevot J, Grosdidier G, Schmitt M. Fatal peritonitis. Prog Pediatr Surg 13:257, 1979.

236. Singer B, Hammar B. Neonatal peritonitis. S Afr Med J 46:987, 1972.

237. Hensey OJ, Hart CA, Cooke RWI. Serious infection in a neonatal intensive care unit: a two-year survey. J Hyg (Camb) 95:289, 1985.

238. Valdes-Dapeña MA, Arey JB. The causes of neonatal mortality: an analysis of 501 autopsies on newborn infants. J Pediatr 77:366, 1970.

239. Bell MJ. Perforation of the gastrointestinal tract and peritonitis in the neonate. Surg Gynecol Obstet 160:20, 1985.

240. Duggan MB, Khwaja MS. Neonatal primary peritonitis in Nigeria. Arch Dis Child 50:130, 1975.

241. Birtch AG, Coran AG, Gross RE. Neonatal peritonitis. Surgery 61:305, 1967.

242. Lacheretz M, Debeugny P, Krivosic-Horner R, et al. Péritonite néo-natale par pérforation gastrique: à propos de 21 observations. Chirurgie 109:887, 1983.

243. Mollitt DL, Tepas JJ, Talbert JL. The microbiology of neonatal peritonitis. Arch Surg 123:176, 1988.

244. Scott JES. Intestinal obstruction in the newborn associated with peritonitis. Arch Dis Child 38:120, 1963.

245. Thelander HE. Perforation of the gastrointestinal tract of the newborn infant. Am J Dis Child 58:371, 1939.

246. Dinari G, Haimov H, Geiffman M. Umbilical arteritis and phlebitis with scrotal abscess and peritonitis. J Pediatr Surg 6:176, 1971.

247. Forshall I. Septic umbilical arteritis. Arch Dis Child 32:25, 1957.

248. Chadwick EG, Shulman ST, Yogev R. Peritonitis as a late manifestation of group B streptococcal disease in newborns. Pediatr Infect Dis 2:142, 1983.

249. Reyna TM. Primary group B streptococcal peritonitis presenting as an incarcerated inguinal hernia in a neonate. Clin Pediatr 25:422, 1987.

250. Serlo W, Heikkinen E, Kouvalainen K. Group A streptococcal peritonitis in infancy. Ann Chir Gynaecol 74:183, 1985.

251. Johnson DE, Conroy MM, Foker JE, et al. *Candida* peritonitis in a newborn infant. J Pediatr 97:298, 1980.

252. Kaplan M, Eidelman AI, Dollberg L, et al. Necrotizing bowel disease with *Candida* peritonitis following severe neonatal hypothermia. Acta Paediatr Scand 79:876, 1990.

252a. Butler KM, Bench MA, Baker CJ. Amphotericin B as a single agent in the treatment of systemic candidiasis in neonates. Pediatr Infect Dis J 9:51, 1990.

252b. MacDonald L, Baker CJ, Chenoweth C. Risk factors for candidemia in a children's hospital. Clin Infect Dis 26:642, 1998.

253. Abt IA. Fetal peritonitis. Med Clin North Am 15:611, 1931.

254. Pan EY, Chen LY, Yang JZ, et al. Radiographic diagnosis of meconium peritonitis: a report of 200 cases including six fetal cases. Pediatr Radiol 13:199, 1983.

255. Aschner JL, Deluga KS, Metlay LA, et al. Spontaneous focal gastrointestinal perforation in very low birth weight infants. J Pediatr 113:364, 1988.

256. Holgersen LO. The etiology of spontaneous gastric perforation of the newborn: a reevaluation. J Pediatr Surg 16:608, 1981.

257. Rickham PP. Neugeborenen-peritonitis. Langenbeck's Arch Klin Chir 292:427, 1959.

258. Kadowaki H, Takeuchi S, Nakahira M, et al. Neonatal gastric perforations; a diagnostic clue in pre-perforative phase. Jpn J Surg 13:446, 1983.

259. Fowler R. Primary peritonitis: changing aspects 1956–1970. Aust Paediatr J 7:73, 1971.

260. Donnison AB, Schwachman H, Gross RE. A review of 164 children with meconium ileus seen at the Children's Hospital Medical Center, Boston. Pediatrics 37:833, 1966.

261. Alpan G, Eyal F, Vinograd I, et al. Localized intestinal perforations after enteral administration of indomethacin in premature infants. J Pediatr 106:277, 1985. (See also Letter to editor. J Pediatr 108:327, 1986.)

262. Wolf WM, Snover DC, Leonard AS. Localized intestinal perforation following intravenous indomethacin in premature infants. J Pediatr Surg 24:409, 1989.

263. Hayhurst EG, Wyman M. Morbidity associated with prolonged use of polyvinyl feeding tubes. Am J Dis Child 129:72, 1975.

264. Fonkalsrud EW, Clatworthy HW Jr. Accidental perforation of the colon and rectum in newborn infants. N Engl J Med 272:1097, 1956.

265. Frank JD, Brown S. Thermometers and rectal perforations in the neonate. Arch Dis Child 53:824, 1978.

266. Horwitz MA, Bennett JV. Nursery outbreak of peritonitis with pneumoperitoneum probably caused by thermometer-induced rectal perforation. Am J Epidemiol 104:632, 1976.

267. deVeber LL, Marshall DG, Robinson ML. Peritonitis, peritoneal adhesions and intestinal obstruction as a complication of intrauterine transfusion. Can Med Assoc J 99:76, 1968.

268. Haltalin KC. Neonatal shigellosis: report of 16 cases and review of the literature. Am J Dis Child 114:603, 1967.

269. Abramson H, Frant S, Oldenbusch C. *Salmonella* infection of the newborn: its differentiation from epidemic diarrhea and other primary enteric disorders of the newborn. Med Clin North Am 23:591, 1939.

270. Starke JR, Baker CJ. Neonatal shigellosis with bowel perforation. Pediatr Infect Dis 4:405, 1985.

271. Opitz K. Beitrag zur Klinik und Pathologie der Nabelschnurinfektionen. Arch Kinderheilkd 150:174, 1955.

272. Gluck L, Wood HF, Fousek MD. Septicemia of the newborn. Pediatr Clin North Am 13:1131, 1966.

273. Wells CL, Maddaus MA, Simmons RL. Proposed mechanisms for the translocation of intestinal bacteria. Rev Infect Dis 10:958, 1988.

274. Wilson R, Kanto WP Jr, McCarthy BJ, et al. Short communication: age at onset of necrotizing enterocolitis: an epidemiologic analysis. Pediatr Res 16:82, 1982.

275. Caralaps-Riera JM, Cohn BD. Bowel perforation after exchange transfusion in the neonate: review of the literature and report of a case. Surgery 68:895, 1970.

276. Touloukian RJ, Kadar A, Spencer RP. The gastrointestinal complications of neonatal umbilical venous exchange transfusion: a clinical and experimental study. Pediatrics 51:36, 1973.

277. Freedman RM, Ingram DL, Gross I, et al. A half century of neonatal sepsis at Yale: 1928 to 1978. Am J Dis Child 135:140, 1981.

278. Martin DJ. Neonatal disorders diagnosed with ultrasound. Clin Perinatol 12:219, 1985.

279. Griscom NT, Colodny AH, Rosenberg HK, et al. Diagnostic aspects of neonatal ascites: report of 27 cases. AJR Am J Roentgenol 128:961, 1977.

280. Kosloske AM, Lilly JR. Paracentesis and lavage for diagnosis of intestinal gangrene in neonatal necrotizing enterocolitis. J Pediatr Surg 13:315, 1978.

281. Töllner U, Pohlandt F. Aszitespunktion zur Differentialdiagnose beim akuten Abdomen des Neugeborenen. Klin Paediatr 196:319, 1984.

282. McKendry JBJ, Lindsay WK, Gerstein MC. Congenital defects of the lymphatics in infancy. Pediatrics 19:21, 1959.

283. Lees W, Mitchell JE. Bile peritonitis in infancy. Arch Dis Child 41:188, 1966.

284. Cohen MD, Weber TR, Grosfeld JL. Bowel perforation in the newborn: diagnosis with metrizamide. Radiology 150:65, 1984.

285. Rosenfeld DL, Cordell CE, Jadeja N. Retrocardiac pneumomediastinum: radiographic finding and clinical implications. Pediatrics 85:92, 1989.

286. Wind ED, Pillari GP, Lee WJ. Lucent liver in the newborn: a roentgenographic sign of pneumoperitoneum. JAMA 237:2218, 1977.

287. Pochaczevsky R, Bryk D. New roentgenographic signs of neonatal gastric perforation. Radiology 102:145, 1972.

288. Gellis SS, Finegold M. Picture of the month: pneumoperitoneum demonstrated by transillumination. Am J Dis Child 130:1237, 1976.

289. Thomas S, Sainsbury C, Murphy JF. Pancuronium belly. Lancet 2:870, 1984.

290. Ein SH, Stephens CA, Reilly BJ. The disappearance of free air after pediatric laparotomy. J Pediatr Surg 20:422, 1985.

291. Emanuel B, Zlotnik P, Raffensperger JG. Perforation of the gastrointestinal tract in infancy and childhood. Surg Gynecol Obstet 146:926, 1978.

Necrotizing Enterocolitis

292. Yu VYH, Tudehope DI, Gill GJ. Neonatal necrotizing enterocolitis: 1. Clinical aspects and 2. Perinatal risk factors. Med J Aust 1:685, 688, 1977.

292a. Holman RC, Stehr-Green JK, Zelasky MT. Necrotizing enterocolitis mortality in the United States, 1979–85. Am J Public Health 79:987, 1989.

293. Finer NN, Moriartey RR. Reply, letter to the editor. J Pediatr 96:170, 1980.

294. Book LS, Herbst JJ, Atherton SO, et al. Necrotizing enterocolitis in low-birth-weight infants fed an elemental formula. J Pediatr 87:602, 1975.

295. O'Neill JA Jr, Stahlman MT, Meng HC. Necrotizing enterocolitis in the newborn: operative indications. Ann Surg 182:274, 1975.

296. Moore TD (ed). Necrotizing Enterocolitis in the Newborn Infant: Report of the Sixty-Eighth Ross Conference on Pediatric Research. Columbus, Ohio, Ross Laboratories, 1975.

297. Virnig NL, Reynolds JW. Epidemiological aspects of neonatal necrotizing enterocolitis. Am J Dis Child 128:186, 1974.

298. Touloukian RJ. Neonatal necrotizing enterocolitis: an update on etiology, diagnosis, and treatment. Surg Clin North Am 56:281, 1976.

299. Bell MJ, Ternberg JL, Bower RJ. The microbial flora and antimicrobial therapy of neonatal peritonitis. J Pediatr Surg 15:569, 1980.

300. Emanuel B, Zlotnik P, Raffensperger JG. Perforation of the gastrointestinal tract in infancy and childhood. Surg Gynecol Obstet 146:926, 1978.

301. Kliegman RM, Fanaroff AA. Neonatal necrotizing enterocolitis: a nine-year experience: I. Epidemiology and uncommon observations. Am J Dis Child 135:603, 1981.

302. Goldman HI. Feeding and necrotizing enterocolitis. Am J Dis Child 134:553, 1980.

303. Brown EG, Sweet AY. Preventing necrotizing enterocolitis in neonates. JAMA 240:2452, 1978.

304. Book LS, Herbst JJ, Jung AL. Comparison of fast- and

slow-feeding rate schedules to the development of necrotizing enterocolitis. J Pediatr 89:463, 1976.

305. Bell MJ, Shackelford P, Feigin RD, et al. Epidemiologic and bacteriologic evaluation of neonatal necrotizing enterocolitis. J Pediatr Surg 14:1, 1979. (Same data as Bell MJ, Feigin RD, Ternberg JL, et al. Evaluation of gastrointestinal microflora in necrotizing enterocolitis. J Pediatr 92:589, 1978.)

306. Eidelman AI, Inwood RJ. Marginal comments: necrotizing enterocolitis and enteral feeding: is too much just too much? Am J Dis Child 134:545, 1980.

307. Kliegman RM, Fanaroff AA, Izant R, et al. Clostridia as pathogens in neonatal necrotizing enterocolitis. J Pediatr 95:287, 1979.

308. Brown EG, Sweet AY. Neonatal necrotizing enterocolitis. Pediatr Clin North Am 29:1149, 1982.

309. Kanto WP Jr, Wilson R, Breart GL, et al. Perinatal events and necrotizing enterocolitis in premature infants. Am J Dis Child 141:167, 1987.

310. Ostertag SG, LaGamma EF, Reisen CE, et al. Early enteral feeding does not affect the incidence of necrotizing enterocolitis. Pediatrics 77:275, 1986.

311. Merritt CRB, Goldsmith JP, Sharp MJ. Sonographic detection of portal venous gas in infants with necrotizing enterocolitis. AJR Am J Roentgenol 143:1059, 1984.

312. Cikrit D, Mastandrea J, Grosfeld JL, et al. Significance of portal venous air in necrotizing enterocolitis: analysis of 53 cases. J Pediatr Surg 20:425, 1985.

313. Maguire GC, Nordin J, Myers MG, et al. Infections acquired by young infants. Am J Dis Child 135:693, 1981.

314. Yu VYH, Joseph R, Bajuk B, et al. Perinatal risk factors for necrotizing enterocolitis. Arch Dis Child 59:430, 1984.

315. Uauy RD, Fanaroff AA, Korones SB, et al, for the National Institute of Child Health and Human Development Neonatal Research Network. Necrotizing enterocolitis in very low birth weight infants: biodemographic and clinical correlates. J Pediatr 119:630, 1991.

316. Walsh MC, Kliegman RM. Necrotizing enterocolitis: treatment based on staging criteria. Pediatr Clin North Am 33:179, 1986.

317. Kliegman RM, Fanaroff AA. Necrotizing enterocolitis. N Engl J Med 310:1093, 1984.

318. Santulli TV, Schullinger JN, Heird WC, et al. Acute necrotizing enterocolitis in infancy: a review of 64 cases. Pediatrics 55:376, 1975.

319. Kliegman RM, Hack M, Jones P, et al. Epidemiologic study of necrotizing enterocolitis among low-birth-weight infants: absence of identifiable risk factors. J Pediatr 100:440, 1982.

320. Stoll BJ, Kanto WP Jr, Glass RI, et al. Epidemiology of necrotizing enterocolitis: a case control study. J Pediatr 96:447, 1980.

321. Frantz ID III, L'Heureux P, Engel RR, et al. Necrotizing enterocolitis. J Pediatr 86:259, 1975.

322. Egan EA, Mantilla G, Nelson RM, et al. A prospective controlled trial of oral kanamycin in the prevention of neonatal necrotizing enterocolitis. J Pediatr 89:467, 1976. (See also reference 376.)

323. Wilson R, Kanto WP Jr, McCarthy BJ, et al. Age at onset of necrotizing enterocolitis: an epidemiologic analysis. Pediatr Res 16:82, 1982.

324. Gerard P, Bachy A, Battisti O, et al. Mortality in 504 infants weighing less than 1501 g at birth and treated in four neonatal intensive care units of South-Belgium between 1976 and 1980. Eur J Pediatr 144:219, 1985.

325. Yu VYH, Joseph R, Bajuk B, et al. Necrotizing enterocolitis in very low birthweight infants: a four-year experience. Aust Paediatr J 20:29, 1984.

326. Palmer SR, Biffin A, Gamsu HR. Outcome of neonatal necrotising enterocolitis: results of the BAPM/CDSC surveillance study, 1989–84. Arch Dis Child 64:388, 1989.

327. de Gamarra E, Helardot P, Moriette G, et al. Necrotizing enterocolitis in full-term neonates. Biol Neonate 44:185, 1983.

328. Thilo EH, Lazarte RA, Hernandez JA. Necrotizing enterocolitis in the first 24 hours of life. Pediatrics 73:476, 1984.

329. Wilson R, del Portillo M, Schmidt E, et al. Risk factors for necrotizing enterocolitis in infants weighing more than 2,000 grams at birth: a case-control study. Pediatrics 71:19, 1983.

330. Necrotizing enterocolitis. Editorial. Lancet 1:459, 1977.

331. Frey EE, Smith W, Franken EA Jr, et al. Analysis of bowel perforation in necrotizing enterocolitis. Pediatr Radiol 17:380, 1987.

332. Kliegman RM, Pittard WB, Fanaroff AA. Necrotizing enterocolitis in neonates fed human milk. J Pediatr 95:450, 1979.

333. Guinan M, Schaberg D, Bruhn FW, et al. Epidemic occurrence of neonatal necrotizing enterocolitis. Am J Dis Child 133:594, 1979.

334. Kosloske AM. Pathogenesis and prevention of necrotizing enterocolitis: a hypothesis based on personal observation and a review of the literature. Pediatrics 74:1086, 1984.

335. Gaynes RP, Palmer S, Martone WJ, et al. The role of host factors in an outbreak of necrotizing enterocolitis. Am J Dis Child 138:1118, 1984.

336. Han VKM, Sayed H, Chance GW, et al. An outbreak of *Clostridium difficile* necrotizing enterocolitis: a case for oral vancomycin therapy? Pediatrics 71:935, 1983.

337. McClead RE Jr (ed). Neonatal necrotizing enterocolitis: current concepts and controversies. J Pediatr 17 (Suppl):S1, 1990.

338. Jona JZ. Advances in neonatal surgery. Pediatr Clin North Am 45:605, 1998.

339. Milner ME, de la Monte SM, Moore GW, et al. Risk factors for developing and dying from necrotizing enterocolitis. J Pediatr Gastroenterol Nutr 5:359, 1986.

340. Wiswell TE, Hankins CT. Twins and triplets with necrotizing enterocolitis. Am J Dis Child 142:1004, 1988.

341. DeCurtis M, Paone C, Vetrano G, et al. A case control study of necrotizing enterocolitis occurring over 8 years in a neonatal intensive care unit. Eur J Pediatr 146:398, 1987.

342. Kliegman RM. Neonatal necrotizing enterocolitis: implications for an infectious disease. Pediatr Clin North Am 26:327, 1979.

343. Book LS, Overall JC Jr, Herbst JJ, et al. Clustering of necrotizing enterocolitis: interruption by infection-control measures. N Engl J Med 297:984, 1977.

344. Rotbart HA, Levin MJ. How contagious is necrotizing enterocolitis? Pediatr Infect Dis 2:406, 1983.

345. Roback SA, Foker J, Frantz IF, et al. Necrotizing enterocolitis. Arch Surg 109:314, 1974.

346. Stanley MD, Null DM Jr, deLemos RA. Relationship between intestinal colonization with specific bacteria and the development of necrotizing enterocolitis. Pediatr Res 11:543, 1977.

347. Hill HR, Hunt CE, Matsen JM. Nosocomial colonization with *Klebsiella*, type 26, in a neonatal intensive-care unit associated with an outbreak of sepsis, meningitis, and necrotizing enterocolitis. J Pediatr 85:415, 1974.

348. Powell J, Bureau MA, Paré C, et al. Necrotizing enterocolitis: epidemic following an outbreak of *Enterobacter cloacae* type 3305573 in a neonatal intensive care unit. Am J Dis Child 134:1152, 1980.

349. Speer ME, Taber LH, Yow MD, et al. Fulminant neonatal sepsis and necrotizing enterocolitis associated with a "nonenteropathogenic" strain of *Escherichia coli*. J Pediatr 89:91, 1976.

350. Cushing AH. Necrotizing enterocolitis with *Escherichia coli* heat-labile enterotoxin. Pediatrics 71:626, 1983.

351. Henderson A, Maclaurin J, Scott JM. *Pseudomonas* in a Glasgow baby unit. Lancet 2:316, 1969.

352. Waldhausen JA, Herendeen T, King H. Necrotizing colitis of the newborn: common cause of perforation of the colon. Surgery 54:365, 1963.

353. Stein H, Beck J, Solomon A, et al. Gastroenteritis with necrotizing enterocolitis in premature babies. BMJ 2:616, 1972.

354. Gruskay JA, Abbasi S, Anday E, et al. *Staphylococcus epidermidis*-associated enterocolitis. J Pediatr 109:520, 1986.

355. Overturf GD, Sherman MP, Wong L, et al. Neonatal necrotizing enterocolitis associated with delta toxin producing methicillin-resistant *S. aureus*. Pediatr Infect Dis J 9:88, 1990.

356. Rotbart HA, Nelson WL, Glode MP, et al. Neonatal rotavirus-associated necrotizing enterocolitis: case control study and prospective surveillance during an outbreak. J Pediatr 112:87, 1988.

357. Rotbart HA, Yolken RH, Nelson WL, et al. Confirmatory testing of Rotazyme results in neonates. J Pediatr 107:289, 1985.

358. Rousset S, Moscovici O, Lebon P, et al. Intestinal lesions containing coronavirus-like particles in neonatal necrotizing enterocolitis: an ultrastructural analysis. Pediatrics 73:218, 1984. (See also Letters to the editor. Pediatrics 74:560, 1984.)

359. Johnson FE, Crnic DM, Simmons MA, et al. Association of fatal coxsackie B2 viral infection and necrotizing enterocolitis. Arch Dis Child 52:802, 1977.

360. Baley JE, Kliegman RM, Annable WL, et al. *Torulopsis glabrata* sepsis appearing as necrotizing enterocolitis and endophthalmitis. Am J Dis Child 138:965, 1984.

361. *Clostridium septicum* and neutropenic enterocolitis. Editorial. Lancet 2:608, 1987.

362. Finegold SM. Anaerobic Bacteria in Human Diseases. New York, Academic Press, 1977.

363. Lawrence G, Walker PD. Pathogenesis of enteritis necroticans in Papua, New Guinea. Lancet 1:125, 1976.

364. Kliegman RM. The role of clostridia in the pathogenesis of neonatal necrotizing enterocolitis. *In* Borriello SP (eds). Clostridia in Gastrointestinal Disease. Boca Raton, Fla, CRC Press, 1985, pp 68–92.

365. Volsted-Pedersen P, Hansen FH, Halveg AB, et al. Necrotising enterocolitis of the newborn—is it gas gangrene of the bowels? Lancet 2:715, 1976.

366. Kosloske AM, Ulrich JA, Hoffman H. Fulminant necrotising enterocolitis associated with clostridia. Lancet 2:1014, 1978.

367. Warren S, Schreiber JR, Epstein MF. Necrotizing enterocolitis and hemolysis associated with *Clostridium perfringens*. Am J Dis Child 138:686, 1984.

368. Blakey JL, Lubitz L, Campbell NT, et al. Enteric colonization in sporadic neonatal necrotizing enterocolitis. J Pediatr Gastroenterol Nutr 4:591, 1985.

369. Cashore WJ, Peter G, Lauermann M, et al. Clostridia colonization and clostridial toxin in neonatal necrotizing enterocolitis. J Pediatr 98:308, 1981.

370. Sturm R, Staneck JL, Stauffer LR, et al. Neonatal necrotizing enterocolitis associated with penicillin-resistant, toxigenic *Clostridium butyricum*. Pediatrics 66:928, 1980.

371. Howard FM, Flynn DM, Bradley JM, et al. Outbreak of necrotising enterocolitis caused by *Clostridium butyricum*. Lancet 2:1099, 1977.

372. Riser E, Bradley J, Flynn D, et al. Synergy in necrotizing enterocolitis. Am J Dis Child 135:291, 1981.

373. Zedd AJ, Sell TL, Schaberg DR, et al. Nosocomial *Clostridium difficile* reservoir in a neonatal intensive care unit. Pediatr Infect Dis 3:429, 1984.

374. Al-Jumaili IJ, Shibley M, Lishman AH, et al. Incidence and origin of *Clostridium difficile* in neonates. J Clin Microbiol 19:77, 1984.

375. Smith MF, Borriello SP, Clayden GS, et al. Clinical and bacteriological findings in necrotizing enterocolitis: a controlled study. J Infect 2:23, 1980.

376. Gothefors L, Blenkharn I. *Clostridium butyricum* and necrotising enterocolitis. Lancet 1:52, 1978. (See reply in Bradley JM, Szawatkowski M, Noone P, et al. Clostridia in necrotising enterocolitis. Lancet 1:389, 1978.)

377. Laverdière M, Robert A, Chicoine R, et al. Clostridia in necrotising enterocolitis. Lancet 2:377, 1978.

378. Kelsey MC, Vince AJ. Clostridia in neonatal feces. Lancet 2:100, 1979.

379. Kindley AD, Roberts PJ, Tulloch WH. Neonatal necrotising enterocolitis. Lancet 1:649, 1977.

380. Lishman AH, Al-Jumaili IJ, Elshibly E, et al. *Clostridium difficile* isolation in neonates in a special care unit: lack of correlation with necrotizing enterocolitis. Scand J Gastroenterol 19:441, 1984.

381. Westra-Meijer CM, Degener JE, Dzoljic-Danilovic G, et al. Quantitative study of the aerobic and anaerobic faecal flora in neonatal necrotizing enterocolitis. Arch Dis Child 58:523, 1983.

382. Thomas DFM, Fernie DS, Bayston R, et al. Clostridial toxins in neonatal necrotizing enterocolitis. Arch Dis Child 59:270, 1984.

383. Scheifele DW, Bjornson GL. Delta toxin activity in coagulase-negative staphylococci from the bowel of neonates. J Clin Microbiol 26:279, 1988.

384. Scheifele DW, Bjornson GL, Dyer RA, et al. Delta-like toxin produced by coagulase-negative staphylococci is associated with neonatal necrotizing enterocolitis. Infect Immun 55:2268, 1988.

385. Hoy C, Millar MR, MacKay P, et al. Quantitative changes in faecal microflora preceding necrotizing enterocolitis in premature neonates. Arch Dis Child 65:1057, 1990.

386. Dykes EH, Gilmour WH, Azmy AF. Prediction of outcome following necrotizing enterocolitis in a neonatal surgical unit. J Pediatr Surg 20:3, 1985.

387. Wayne ER, Burrington JD, Hutter J. Neonatal necrotizing enterocolitis: evolution of new principles in management. Arch Surg 110:476, 1975.

388. Wilson R, Kanto WP Jr, McCarthy BJ, et al. Age at onset of necrotizing enterocolitis. Am J Dis Child 136:814, 1982.

389. Leonidas JC, Hall RT. Neonatal pneumatosis coli: a mild form of neonatal necrotizing enterocolitis. J Pediatr 89:456, 1976.

390. Richmond JA, Mikity V. Benign form of necrotizing enterocolitis. AJR Am J Roentgenol 123:301, 1975.

391. Barnard JA, Cotton RB, Lutin W. Necrotizing enterocolitis. Variables associated with the severity of the disease. Am J Dis Child 139:375, 1985.

392. Bell MJ, Ternberg JL, Feigin RD, et al. Neonatal necrotizing enterocolitis: therapeutic decisions based upon clinical staging. Ann Surg 187:1, 1978.

393. Buras R, Guzzetta P, Avery G, et al. Acidosis and hepatic portal venous gas: indications for surgery in necrotizing enterocolitis. Pediatrics 78:273, 1986.

394. Daneman A, Woodward S, de Silva M. The radiology of neonatal necrotizing enterocolitis (NEC): a review of 47 cases and the literature. Pediatr Radiol 7:70, 1978.

395. Mata AG, Rosengart RM. Interobserver variability in the radiographic diagnosis of necrotizing enterocolitis. Pediatrics 66:68, 1980. (See also Bowen A. Letter to the editor. Pediatrics 68:612, 1981.)

396. Johnson JF, Robinson LH. Localized bowel distension in the newborn: a review of the plain film analysis and differential diagnosis. Pediatrics 73:206, 1984.

397. Leonard T Jr, Johnson JF, Pettett PG. Critical evaluation of the persistent loop sign in necrotizing enterocolitis. Radiology 142:385, 1982.

398. Weinstein MM. The persistent loop sign in neonatal necrotizing enterocolitis: a new cause. Pediatr Radiol 16:71, 1986.

399. Kliegman RM, Fanaroff AA. Neonatal necrotizing enterocolitis: a nine-year experience: II. Outcome assessment. Am J Dis Child 135:608, 1981.

400. Keller MS, Chawla HS. Neonatal metrizamide gastrointestinal series in suspected necrotizing enterocolitis. Am J Dis Child 139:713, 1985.

401. Lindley S, Mollitt DL, Seiberty JJ, et al. Portal vein ultrasonography in the early diagnosis of necrotizing enterocolitis. J Pediatr Surg 21:530, 1986.

402. Malin SW, Bhutani VK, Ritchie WW, et al. Echogenic intravascular and hepatic microbubbles associated with necrotizing enterocolitis. J Pediatr 103:637, 1983. (See also Silverman NH. Letter to the editor. J Pediatr 104:639, 1984.)

403. Kosloske AM, Lilly JR. Paracentesis and lavage for diagnosis of intestinal gangrene in neonatal necrotizing enterocolitis. J Pediatr Surg 13:315, 1978.

404. Ricketts RR. The role of paracentesis in the management of infants with necrotizing enterocolitis. Am Surg 52:61, 1986.

405. Kosloske AM. Surgery of necrotizing enterocolitis. World J Surg 9:277, 1985.

406. Patel CC. Hematologic abnormalities in acute necrotizing enterocolitis. Pediatr Clin North Am 24:579, 1977.

407. Hutter JJ Jr, Hathaway WE, Wayne ER. Hematologic abnormalities in severe neonatal necrotizing enterocolitis. J Pediatr 88:1026, 1976.

408. Hyman PE, Abrams CE, Zipser RD. Enhanced urinary immunoreactive thromboxane in neonatal necrotizing enterocolitis: a diagnostic indicator of thrombotic activity. Am J Dis Child 141:688, 1987.

409. Scheifele DW, Olson EM, Pendray MR. Endotoxinemia and thrombocytopenia during neonatal necrotizing enterocolitis. Am J Clin Pathol 83:227, 1985.

410. Christensen RD, Rothstein G, Anstall HB, et al. Granulocyte transfusion in neonates with bacterial infection, neutropenia, and depletion of mature marrow neutrophils. Pediatrics 70:1, 1982.

411. Garcia J, Smith FR, Cucinell SA. Urinary D-lactate excretion in infants with necrotizing enterocolitis. J Pediatr 104:268, 1984.

412. Book LS, Herbst JJ, Jung AL. Carbohydrate malabsorption in necrotizing enterocolitis. Pediatrics 57:201, 1976.

413. Scott S, Rogers C, Angelus P, et al. Effect of necrotizing enterocolitis on urinary epidermal growth factor levels. Am J Dis Child 145:804, 1991.

414. Kliegman RM, Walsh MC. The incidence of meningitis in neonates with necrotizing enterocolitis. Am J Perinatol 4:245, 1987.

415. Scheifele DW, Olsen E, Ginter G, et al. Comparison of two antibiotic regimens in neonates with necrotizing enterocolitis. Clin Invest Med 8:A183, 1985 (abstract).

416. Bell MJ, Kosloske AM, Benton C, et al. Neonatal necrotizing enterocolitis: prevention of perforation. J Pediatr Surg 8:601, 1973.

417. Hansen TN, Ritter DA, Speer ME, et al. A randomized controlled study of oral gentamicin in the treatment of neonatal necrotizing enterocolitis. J Pediatr 97:836, 1980.

418. Faix RB, Polley TZ, Grasela TH. A randomized, controlled trial of parenteral clindamycin in neonatal necrotizing enterocolitis. J Pediatr 112:271, 1988.

419. Burrington JD. Necrotizing enterocolitis in the newborn infant. Clin Perinatol 5:29, 1978.

420. Ghory MJ, Sheldon CA. Newborn surgical emergencies of the gastrointestinal tract. Surg Clin North Am 65:1083, 1985.

421. Ein SH, Shandling B, Wesson D, et al. A 13-year experience with peritoneal drainage under local anesthesia for necrotizing enterocolitis perforation. J Pediatr Surg 25:1034, 1990.

422. Grylack LJ, Scanlon JW. Oral gentamicin therapy in the prevention of neonatal necrotizing enterocolitis: a controlled double-blind trial. Am J Dis Child 132:1192, 1978.

423. Egan EA, Nelson RM, Mantilla G, et al. Additional experience with routine use of oral kanamycin prophylaxis for necrotizing enterocolitis in infants under 1500 grams. J Pediatr 90:331, 1977.

424. Brantley VE, Hiatt IM, Hegyi T. The effectiveness of oral gentamicin in reducing the incidence of necrotizing enterocolitis (NEC) in treated and control infants. Pediatr Res 14:592, 1980.

425. Rowley MP, Dahlenburg GW. Gentamicin in prophylaxis of neonatal necrotizing enterocolitis. Lancet 2:532, 1978.

426. Boyle R, Nelson JS, Stonestreet B, et al. Alterations in stool flora resulting from oral kanamycin prophylaxis of necrotizing enterocolitis. J Pediatr 93:857, 1978.

427. Dear PRF, Thomas DEM. Oral vancomycin in preventing necrotizing enterocolitis. Arch Dis Child 63:1390, 1988.

428. Conroy MM, Anderson R, Cates KL. Complications associated with prophylactic oral kanamycin in preterm infants. Lancet 1:613, 1978.

429. Bhat AM, Meny RG. Alimentary absorption of gentamicin in preterm infants. Clin Pediatr 23:683, 1984.

430. Grylack LJ, Boehnert J, Scanlan JW. Serum concentration of gentamicin following oral administration to preterm newborns. Dev Pharmacol Ther 5:47, 1982.

431. Anderson DM, Kleigman RM. Relationship of neonatal alimentation practices to the occurrence of endemic neonatal necrotizing enterocolitis. Am J Perinatol 8:62, 1991.

432. McKeown RE, Marsh D, Amarnath U, et al. Role of delayed feeding and of feeding increments in necrotizing enterocolitis. J Pediatr 121:764, 1992.

433. Carrion V, Egan EA. Prevention of neonatal necrotizing enterocolitis. J Pediatr Gastroenterol Nutr 11:317, 1990.

434. Anderson CL, Collin MF, O'Keefe JP, et al. A widespread epidemic of mild necrotizing enterocolitis of unknown cause. Am J Dis Child 138:979, 1984.

435. Gerber AR, Hopkins SR, Lauer BA, et al. Increased risk of illness among nursery staff caring for neonates with necrotizing enterocolitis. Pediatr Infect Dis J 4:246, 1985.

436. Little GA (ed). American Academy of Pediatrics Committee on the Fetus and Newborn: Guidelines for Peri-

natal Care, 2nd ed. Elk Grove Village, Ill, American Academy of Pediatrics, 1988, pp 182–183.

437. Eibl MA, Wolf HM, Fürnkranz H, et al. Prevention of necrotizing enterocolitis in low-birth-weight infants by IgA-IgG feeding. N Engl J Med 319:1, 1988.

438. Schullinger JN, Mollitt DL, Vinocur CD, et al. Neonatal necrotizing enterocolitis: survival, management, and complications: a 25-year study. Am J Dis Child 136:612, 1981.

439. Abbasi S, Pereira GR, Johnson L, et al. Long-term assessment of growth, nutritional status and gastrointestinal function in survivors of necrotizing enterocolitis. J Pediatr 104:550, 1984.

440. Janik JS, Ein SH, Mancer K. Intestinal structure after necrotizing enterocolitis. J Pediatr Surg 16:438, 1981.

441. Ball TI, Wyly JB. Enterocyst formation: a late complication of neonatal necrotizing enterocolitis. AJR Am J Roentgenol 147:806, 1986.

442. Walsh MC, Simpser EF, Kliegman RM. Late onset of sepsis in infants with bowel resection in the neonatal period. J Pediatr 112:468, 1988.

443. Walsh MC, Kliegman RM, Hack M. Severity of necrotizing enterocolitis: influence on outcome at 2 years of age. Pediatrics 84:808, 1989.

Endocarditis

444. Scott J. Iatrogenic lesions in babies following umbilical vein catheterization. Arch Dis Child 40:426, 1965.

445. Blieden LC, Morehead RR, Burke B, et al. Bacterial endocarditis in the neonate. Am J Dis Child 124:747, 1972.

446. Lewis IC. Bacterial endocarditis complicating septicemia in an infant. Arch Dis Child 29:144, 1954.

447. Macaulay D. Acute endocarditis in infancy and early childhood. Am J Dis Child 88:715, 1954.

448. Shanklin DR. The pathology of prematurity. In Prematurity and the Obstetrician. New York, Appleton-Century-Crofts, 1969, p 471. (Personal communication, 1973.)

449. Steinitz H, Schuchmann L, Wegner G. Leberzirrhose, Meningitis, und Endocarditis ulceropolyposa bei einer Neugeborenensepsis durch B-Streptokokken (Streptokokkus agalactiae). Arch Kinderheilkd 183:382, 1971.

450. Johnson DH, Rosenthal A, Nadas AS. Bacterial endocarditis in children under 2 years of age. Am J Dis Child 129:183, 1975.

451. Mendelsohn G, Hutchins GM. Infective endocarditis during the first decade of life: an autopsy review of 33 cases. Am J Dis Child 133:619, 1979.

452. Liersch R, Nessler L, Bourgeois M, et al. Gegenwärtige Merkmale der bakteriellen Endokarditis im Kindesalter. Z Kardiol 66:501, 1977.

453. Colville J, Jeffries I. Bilateral acquired neonatal Erb's palsy. Ir Med J 68:399, 1975.

454. Symchych PS, Krauss AN, Winchester P. Endocarditis following intracardiac placement of umbilical venous catheters in neonates. J Pediatr 90:287, 1977.

455. Edwards K, Ingall D, Czapek E, et al. Bacterial endocarditis in 4 young infants: is this complication on the increase? Clin Pediatr 16:607, 1977.

456. McGuiness GA, Schieken RM, Maguire GF. Endocarditis in the newborn. Am J Dis Child 134:577, 1980.

457. Bender RL, Jaffe RB, McCarthy D, et al. Echocardiographic diagnosis of bacterial endocarditis of the mitral valve in a neonate. Am J Dis Child 131:746, 1977.

458. Lundström N-R, Björkhem G. Mitral and tricuspid valve vegetations in infancy diagnosed by echocardiography. Acta Paediatr Scand 68:345, 1979.

459. Weinberg AG, Laird WP. Group B streptococcal endo-

carditis detected by echocardiography. J Pediatr 92:335, 1978.

460. Barton CW, Crowley DC, Uzark K, et al. A neonatal survivor of group B beta-hemolytic streptococcal endocarditis. Am J Perinatol 1:214, 1984.

461. Agarwala BN. Group B streptococcal endocarditis in a neonate. Pediatr Cardiol 9:51, 1988. (Same case as Perelman MJ, et al. Aortic root replacement for complicated bacterial endocarditis in an infant. J Pediatr Surg 24:1121, 1989.)

462. Chattapadhyay B. Fatal neonatal meningitis due to group B streptococci. Postgrad Med J 51:240, 1975.

463. Cabacungan ET, Tetting G, Friedberg DZ. Tricuspid valve vegetation caused by group B streptococcal endocarditis: treatment by "vegetectomy." J Perinatol 13:398, 1993.

464. Kramer H-H, Bourgeois M, Liersch R, et al. Current clinical aspects of bacterial endocarditis in infancy, childhood, and adolescence. Eur J Pediatr 140:253, 1983.

465. Kavey R-EW, Frank DM, Byrum CJ, et al. Two-dimensional echocardiography assessment of infective endocarditis in children. Am J Dis Child 137:851, 1983.

466. Ward KE, Matson JR, Chartrand SR, et al. Successfully treated pulmonary valve endocarditis in a normal neonate. Am J Dis Child 137:913, 1983.

467. Nakayama DK, O'Neill JA Jr, Wagner H, et al. Management of vascular complications of bacterial endocarditis. J Pediatr Surg 21:636, 1986.

468. Morville P, Mauran P, Motte J, et al. Intérêt de l'échocardiographie dans le diagnostic des endocardites néonatales: à propos de trois observations. Ann Pediatr 32:389, 1985.

469. Eliaou J-F, Montoya F, Sibille G, et al. Endocardité infectieuse en période néo-natale. Pediatrie 38:561, 1983.

470. McCartney JE. A case of acute ulcerative endocarditis in a child aged three and a half weeks. J Pathol Bacteriol 25:277, 1922.

471. Oelberg DG, Fisher DJ, Gross DM, et al. Endocarditis in high-risk neonates. Pediatrics 71:392, 1983.

472. Gossius G, Gunnes P, Rasmussen K. Ten years of infective endocarditis: a clinicopathologic study. Acta Med Scand 217:171, 1985.

473. Noel GJ, O'Loughlin JE, Edelson PJ. Neonatal *Staphylococcus epidermidis* right-sided endocarditis: description of five catheterized infants. Pediatrics 82:234, 1988.

474. No reference provided.

475. Bannon MJ. Infective endocarditis in neonates. Letter to the Editor. Arch Dis Child 63:112, 1998.

476. Giddings ES. Two cases of endocarditis in infants. Can Med Assoc J 35:71, 1936.

477. Berkowitz FE, Dansky R. Infective endocarditis in Black South African children: report of 10 cases with some unusual features. Pediatr Infect Dis J 8:787, 1989.

477a. Soo SS, Boxman DL. *Streptococcus faecalis* in neonatal infective endocarditis. J Infect 23:209, 1991.

478. Zakrzewski T, Keith JD. Bacterial endocarditis in infants and children. J Pediatr 67:1179, 1965.

479. O'Callaghan C, McDougall P. Infective endocarditis in neonates. Arch Dis Child 63:53, 1988.

480. Prandstraller D, Marata AM, Picchio FM. *Staphylococcus aureus* endocarditis in a newborn with transposition of the great arteries: successful treatment. Int J Cardiol 14:355, 1987.

481. Weinstein L, Schlesinger JJ. Pathoanatomic, pathophysiologic and clinical correlations in endocarditis (1st of 2 parts). N Engl J Med 291:832, 1974.

482. Morand P, Laugier J, Lain J-L, et al. Endocardité triscup-

idienne calcifée du nourisson. Arch Mal Coeur 66:901, 1973.

483. Luke JL, Bolande RP, Gross S. Generalized aspergillosis and *Aspergillus* endocarditis in infancy: report of a case. Pediatrics 31:115, 1963.

484. Wiley EL, Hutchins GM. Superior vena cava syndrome secondary to *Candida* thrombophlebitis complicating parenteral alimentation. J Pediatr 91:977, 1977.

485. Walsh TJ, Hutchins GM. Postoperative *Candida* infections of the heart in children: clinicopathologic study of a continuing problem of diagnosis and therapy. J Pediatr Surg 15:325, 1980.

486. Faix R, Feick HJ, Frommelt P, et al. Successful medical treatment of *Candida parapsilosis* endocarditis in a premature infant. Am J Perinatol 7:272, 1990.

487. Zenker PN, Rosenberg EM, Van Dyke RB, et al. Successful medical treatment of presumed *Candida* endocarditis in critically ill infants. J Pediatr 119:472, 1991.

488. Sanchez PJ, Siegel JD, Fishbein J. *Candida* endocarditis: successful medical management in three preterm infants and review of the literature. Pediatr Infect Dis J 10:239, 1991.

489. Walsh TJ, Hutchins GM. Postoperative *Candida* infections of the heart in children: clinicopathologic study of a continuing problem of diagnosis and therapy. J Pediatr Surg 15:325, 1980.

490. Millard DD, Shulman ST. The changing spectrum of neonatal endocarditis. Clin Perinatol 15:587, 1988.

491. Morrow WR, Haas JE, Benjamin DR. Nonbacterial endocardial thrombosis in neonates: relationship to persistent fetal circulation. J Pediatr 100:117, 1982.

492. Kronsbein H. Pathogenesis of endocarditis verrucosa simplex in the newborn. Beitr Pathol 161:82, 1977.

493. Favara BE, Franciosi RA, Butterfield LJ. Disseminated intravascular and cardiac thrombosis of the neonate. Am J Dis Child 127:197, 1974.

494. Kunstadter RH, Kaltenekker F. Acute verrucous endocarditis in the newborn. J Pediatr 61:58, 1962.

495. Krous HF. Neonatal nonbacterial thrombotic endocarditis. Arch Pathol Lab Med 103:76, 1979.

496. Bergsland J, Kawaguchi A, Roland JM, et al. Mycotic aortic aneurysms in children. Ann Thorac Surg 37:314, 1984.

497. Thompson TR, Tilleli J, Johnson DE, et al. Umbilical artery catheterization complicated by mycotic aortic aneurysm in neonates. Adv Pediatr 27:275, 1980.

498. Bannon MJ. Infective endocarditis in neonates. Letter to the editor. Arch Dis Child 63:1112, 1988.

499. Hernandez I, Arcil G, Garru O, et al. Endocardités infecteuses néonatales: à propos de cinq observations. Arch Mal Coeur 83:627, 1990.

500. Bullaboy CA, Coulson JD, Jennings RB Jr, et al. Neonatal mitral valve endocarditis: diagnosis and successful management. Clin Pediatr 29:398, 1990.

501. Baltimore RS. Infective endocarditis in children. Pediatr Infect Dis J. 11:907, 1992.

502. Popp RL. Echocardiography and infectious endocarditis. Curr Clin Topics Infect Dis 4:98, 1983.

503. Watanakunakorn C. Treatment of infections due to methicillin-resistant *Staphylococcus aureus*. Ann Intern Med 97:376, 1982.

504. Wolfson JS, Swartz MN. Serum bactericidal activity as a monitor of antibiotic therapy. N Engl J Med 312:968, 1985.

505. Cooper GI, Hopkins CC. Rapid diagnosis of intravascular catheter-associated infection by direct Gram staining of catheter segments. N Engl J Med 312:1142, 1985.

506. Perelman MJ, Sugimoto J, Arcilla RA, et al. Aortic root replacement for complicated bacterial endocarditis in an infant. J Pediatr Surg 24:1121, 1989.

507. Tulloh RMR, Silove ED, Abrams LD. Replacement of an aortic valve cusp after neonatal endocarditis. Br Heart J 64:204, 1990.

508. Levinson SA, Learner A. Blood cysts on the heart valves of newborn infants. Arch Pathol 14:810, 1932.

509. Gross P. Concept of fetal endocarditis: a general review with report of an illustrative case. Arch Pathol 31:163, 1941.

510. Begg JG. Blood-filled cysts in the cardiac valve cusps in foetal life and infancy. J Pathol Bacteriol 87:177, 1964.

511. Menahem S, Robbie MJ, Rajadurai VS. Valvular vegetations in the neonate due to fetal endocarditis. Int J Cardiol 32:103, 1991.

511a. Charaf L, Lundell B, Abon P, et al. A case of neonatal endocarditis. Acta Pediatr Scand 79:704, 1990.

Pericarditis

512. Gersony WM, McCracken GH Jr. Purulent pericarditis in infancy. Pediatrics 40:224, 1967.

513. Schaffer AJ, Avery ME. Diseases of the Newborn, 3rd ed. Philadelphia, WB Saunders, 1971, p 252.

514. Neimann N, Pernot C, Gentin G, et al. Les péricardites purulentes néonatales: à propos du premier cas guéri. Arch Fr Pediatr 22:238, 1965.

515. Collier AM, Connor JD, Nyhan WL. Systemic infection with *Hemophilus influenzae* in very young infants. J Pediatr 70:539, 1967.

516. McKinlay B. Infectious diarrhea in the newborn caused by an unclassified species of *Salmonella*. Am J Dis Child 54:1252, 1937. (Later identified as *S. wichita* in Schiff F, Strauss L. A new *Salmonella* type [*Salmonella wichita*]. J Infect Dis 65:125, 1939.)

517. Chiari H. Zur Kenntnis der Pyozyaneus-infektion bei Säuglingen. Zentralb Allg Pathol 38:483, 1926.

518. Jaiyesimi F, Abioye AA, Anita AU. Infective pericarditis in Nigerian children. Arch Dis Child 54:384, 1979.

519. Wynn RJ. Neonatal *E. coli* pericarditis. J Perinatol Med 7:23, 1979.

520. Kachaner J, Nouaille J-M, Batisse A. Les cardiomegalies massives du nouveau-né. Arch Fr Pediatr 34:297, 1977.

521. Graham JPA, Martin A. *B. pyocyaneus* pericarditis occurring four days after birth. Cent Afr J Med 1:101, 1955.

522. Feldman WE. Bacterial etiology and mortality of purulent pericarditis in pediatric patients: review of 162 cases. Am J Dis Child 133:641, 1979.

523. Morgan RJ, Stephenson LW, Woolf PK, et al. Surgical treatment of purulent pericarditis in children. Thorac Cardiovasc Surg 85:527, 1983.

524. Jellard CH, Churcher GM. An outbreak of *Pseudomonas aeruginosa (pyocyanea)* infection in a premature baby unit, with observations on the intestinal carriage of *Pseudomonas aeruginosa* in the newborn. J Hyg 65:219, 1967.

525. Miller TC, Baman SI, Albers WW. Massive pericardial effusion due to *Mycoplasma hominis* in a newborn. Am J Dis Child 136:271, 1982.

526. Shenker L, Reed KL, Anderson CF, et al. Fetal pericardial effusion. Am J Obstet Gynecol 160:1505, 1989.

527. Cayler GG, Taybi H, Riley HD Jr. Pericarditis with effusion in infants and children. J Pediatr 63:264, 1963.

528. Noren GR, Kaplan EL, Staley NA. Nonrheumatic inflammatory diseases. *In* Adams FH, Emmanouilides GC (eds). Moss' Heart Disease in Infants, Children, and Adolescents, 3rd ed. Baltimore, Williams & Wilkins, 1983, pp 585–594.

529. Kanarek KS, Coleman J. Purulent pericarditis in a neonate. Pediatr Infect Dis J 10:549, 1991.

530. Cherry JD. Enteroviruses, polioviruses (poliomyelitis), coxsackieviruses, echoviruses, and enteroviruses. *In* Feigin RD, Cherry JD (eds). Textbook of Pediatric Infectious Diseases, 3rd ed. Philadelphia, WB Saunders, 1992, pp 1705–1752.

531. Zerella JT, Halpe DCE. Intrapericardial teratoma—neonatal cardiorespiratory distress amenable to surgery. J Pediatr Surg 15:961, 1980.

532. Doshi N, Smith B, Klionsky B. Congenital pericarditis due to maternal lupus erythematosus. J Pediatr 96:699, 1980.

533. Sasidharan P, Al-Mohsen I, Abdul-Karim A, et al. Nonimmune hydrops fetalis: case reports and brief review. J Perinatol 12:338, 1992.

534. deFonseca JMB, Davies MRQ, Bolton KD. Congenital hydropericardium associated with the herniation of part of the liver into the pericardial sac. J Pediatr Surg 22:851, 1987.

535. Jafa AJ, Barak S, Kaysar N, et al. Antenatal diagnosis of bilateral congenital chylothorax with pericardial effusion. Acta Obstet Gynaecol Scand 64:455, 1985.

536. Mupanemunda RH, Mackanjee HR. A life-threatening complication of percutaneous central venous catheters in neonates. Am J Dis Child 146:1414, 1992.

537. Dennehy PH. New tests for the rapid diagnosis of infection in children. *In* Aronoff S, Hughes W, Kohl S, et al (eds). Advances in Pediatric Infectious Disease, vol 8. St. Louis, Mosby–Year Book, 1993, pp 91–129.

538. Zeevi B, Perry S, Keane J, et al. Interventional cardiac procedures. Clin Perinatol 15:633, 1988.

Mediastinitis

539. Achenbach S. Mediastinalabszess bei einmen 3 Wochen alten Säugling. Arch Kinderheilkd 74:193, 1924.

540. Grewe HE, Martini Pape M. Die eitrige Mediastinitis im frühen Saüglingsalter. Kinderaerztl Prax 32:305, 1964.

541. Weichsel M. Mediastinitis in a newborn. Proc Rudolf Virchow Med Soc City NY 22:67, 1963. (Same infant as case 1 in Feldman R, and Gromisch DS. Acute suppurative mediastinitis. Am J Dis Child 121:79, 1971.)

542. Weber G. Retropharyngeal-und Mediastinalabszess bei einem 3 Wochen alten Säugling. Chirurg 21:308, 1950.

543. deLorimier AA, Haskin D, Massie FS. Mediastinal mass caused by vertebral osteomyelitis. Am J Dis Child 111:639, 1966.

544. Talbert JL, Rodgers BM, Felman AH, et al. Traumatic perforation of the hypopharynx in infants. J Thorac Cardiovasc Surg 74:152, 1977.

545. Grunebaum M, Horodniceanu C, Wilunsky E, et al. Iatrogenic transmural perforation of the oesophagus in the preterm infant. Clin Radiol 31:257, 1980.

546. Sands T, Glasson M, Berry A. Hazards of nasogastric tube insertion in the newborn infant. Lancet 2:680, 1989.

547. Krasna IH, Rosenfeld D, Benjamin BG, et al. Esophageal perforation in the neonate: an emerging problem in the newborn nursery. J Pediatr Surg 22:784, 1987.

548. Topsis J, Kinas HY, Kandall SR. Esophageal perforation—a complication of neonatal resuscitation. Anesth Analg 69:532, 1989.

549. Vandenplas Y, Delree M, Bougatef A, et al. Cervical esophageal perforation diagnosed by endoscopy in a premature infant. J Pediatr Gastroenterol Nutr 8:390, 1989.

550. Touloukian RJ, Beardsley GP, Ablow RC, et al. Traumatic perforation of the pharynx in the newborn. Pediatrics 59:1019, 1977.

551. Johnson DE, Foker J, Munson DP, et al. Management of esophageal and pharyngeal perforation in the newborn infant. Pediatrics 70:592, 1982.

552. Coulthard M, Isaacs D. Neonatal retropharyngeal abscess. Pediatr Infect Dis J 10:547, 1991.

Esophagitis

553. Bittencourt AL. Congenital Chagas disease. Am J Dis Child 130:97, 1976.

553a. Azimi PH, Willert J, Petru A. Severe esophagitis in a newborn. Pediatr Infect Dis J 15:385, 1966.

554. Walsh TJ, Belitsos NJ, Hamilton SR. Bacterial esophagitis in immunocompromised patients. Arch Intern Med 146:1345, 1986.

Endocrine Glands

555. Nelson AJ. Neonatal suppurative thyroiditis. Pediatr Infect Dis 2:243, 1983.

555a. Berner R, Schumacher RF, Zimmerhackl LB, et al. *Salmonella enteritidis* orchitis in a 10-week old boy. Acta Pediatr 83:922, 1994.

Salivary Glands

556. Sanford HN, Shmigelsky I. Purulent parotitis in the newborn. J Pediatr 26:149, 1945.

557. Shulman BH. Acute suppurative infections of the salivary glands in the newborn. Am J Dis Child 80:413, 1950.

558. Campbell WAB. Purulent parotitis in the newborn: report of a case. Lancet 2:386, 1951.

559. Leake D, Leake R. Neonatal suppurative parotitis. Pediatrics 46:203, 1970.

560. Brook I, Frazier EH, Thompson DH. Aerobic and anaerobic microbiology of acute suppurative parotitis. Laryngoscope 101:170, 1991.

561. David RB, O'Connell EJ. Suppurative parotitis in children. Am J Dis Child 119:332, 1970.

562. Banks WW, Handler SD, Glade GB, et al. Neonatal submandibular sialadentitis. Am J Otolaryngol 1:261, 1980.

Skin and Subcutaneous Tissue

563. Solomon LM, Esterly NB. Neonatal Dermatology. Philadelphia, WB Saunders, 1973.

564. Swartz MN, Weinberg AN. Bacterial diseases with cutaneous involvement. *In* Fitzpatrick TB, Arndt KA, Clark WH Jr, et al (eds). Dermatology in General Medicine. New York, McGraw-Hill, 1971.

565. Frieden IJ. Blisters and pustules in the newborn. Curr Probl Pediatr 19:553, 1989.

566. Weinberg S, Leider M, Shapiro L. Color Atlas of Pediatric Dermatology. New York, McGraw-Hill, 1975.

567. Maibach HI and Hildick-Smith G. (eds.). Skin Bacteria and Their Role in Infection. New York, McGraw-Hill, 1965.

568. Speert H. Circumcision of the newborn: an appraisal of its present status. Obstet Gynecol 2:164, 1953.

569. Annabil SH, Al-Hifi A, Kazi T. Primary tuberculosis of the penis in an infant. Tubercle 71:229, 1990.

570. Cleary TG, Kohl S. Overwhelming infection with group B beta-hemolytic *Streptococcus* associated with circumcision. Pediatrics 64:301, 1979.

571. Sauer L. Fatal staphylococcal bronchopneumonia following ritual circumcision. Am J Obstet Gynecol 46:583, 1943.

572. Annunziato D, Goldblum LM. Staphylococcal scalded skin syndrome. Am J Dis Child 132:1187, 1978.

573. Breuer GS, Walfisch S. Circumcision complications and indications for ritual recircumcision—clinical experience and review of the literature. Isr J Med Sci 23:252, 1987.

574. Woodside JR. Necrotizing fasciitis after neonatal circumcision. Am J Dis Child 134:301, 1980.

575. Stranko J, Ryan ME, Bowman AM. Impetigo in newborn infants associated with a plastic bell clamp circumcision. Pediatr Infect Dis 5:597, 1986.

576. Bliss DP, Healey PJ, Waldbraussen JHT. Necrotizing fasciitis after Plastibell circumscision. J Pediatr 131:459, 1997.

577. Gee WF, Ansell JS. Neonatal circumcision: a 10-year overview: with comparison of the Gomco clamp and the Plastibell device. Pediatrics 58:824, 1976.

578. Siddiqi SF, Taylor PM. Necrotizing fasciitis of the scalp. Am J Dis Child 136:226, 1982.

579. Okada DM, Chow AW, Bruce VT. Neonatal scalp abscess and fetal monitoring: factors associated with infection. Am J Obstet Gynecol 129:185, 1977.

580. Cordero L, Anderson CW, Hon EH. Scalp abscess: a benign and infrequent complication of fetal monitoring. Am J Obstet Gynecol 146:126, 1983.

581. Wagener MM, Rycheck RR, Yee RB, et al. Septic dermatitis of the neonatal scalp and maternal endomyometritis with intrapartum internal fetal monitoring. Pediatrics 74:81, 1984.

582. Brook I. Microbiology of scalp abscesses in newborns. Pediatr Infect Dis J 11:766, 1992.

583. Bogdan JC, Rapkin RH. Clostridia infection in the newborn. Pediatrics 58:120, 1976.

584. Fitter WF, DeSa DJ, Richardson H. Chorioamnionitis and funisitis due to *Corynebacterium kutscheri*. Arch Dis Child 55:710, 1979.

585. Sarkany I, Gaylarde CC. Skin flora of the newborn. Lancet 1:589, 1967.

586. Evans HE, Akpata SO, Baki A. Factors influencing the establishment of neonatal bacterial flora: I. The role of host factors. Arch Environ Health 21:514, 1970.

587. Sarkany I, Arnold L. The effect of single and repeated applications of hexachlorophene on the bacterial flora of the skin of the newborn. Br J Dermatol 82:261, 1970.

588. Thompson DJ, Gezon HM, Rogers KD, et al. Excess risk of staphylococcal infection and disease in newborn males. Am J Epidemiol 84:314, 1966.

589. Rudoy RC, Nelson JD. Breast abscess during the neonatal period: a review. Am J Dis Child 129:1031, 1975.

590. Evans HE, Akpata SO, Baki A, et al. Flora in newborn infants: annual variation in prevalence of *Staphylococcus aureus*, *Escherichia coli*, and streptococci. Arch Environ Health 26:275, 1973.

591. Starr HJ, Holliday PB Jr. Erythema multiforme as a manifestation of neonatal septicemia. J Pediatr 38:315, 1951.

592. Washington JL, Fowler REL, Guarino GJ. Erythema multiforme in a premature infant associated with sepsis due to *Pseudomonas*. Pediatrics 39:120, 1967.

593. Foley JF, Gravelle CR, Englehard WE, et al. *Achromobacter* septicemia—fatalities in prematures: I. Clinical and epidemiological study. Am J Dis Child 101:279, 1961.

594. Belgaumkar TK. Impetigo neonatorum congenita due to group B beta-hemolytic *Streptococcus* infection. Letter to the editor. J Pediatr 86:982, 1975.

595. Halal F, Delorme L, Brazeau M, et al. Congenital vesicular eruption caused by *Hemophilus influenzae* type b. Pediatrics 62:494, 1978.

596. Martin MO, Wallach D, Bordier C, et al. Les signes cutanés des infections bacteriennes néonatales. Arch Fr Pediatr 42:471, 1985.

597. Kline A, O'Connell E. Group B *Streptococcus* as a cause of neonatal bullous skin lesions. Pediatr Infect Dis J 12:165, 1993.

598. Khuri-Bulos N, McIntosh K. Neonatal *Haemophilus influenzae* infection: report of eight cases and review of the literature. Am J Dis Child 129:57, 1975.

599. Bray DA. Ecthyma gangrenosum: full thickness nasal slough. Arch Otolaryngol 98:210, 1973.

600. Heffner RW, Smith GF. Ecthyma gangrenosum in *Pseudomonas* septicemia. Am J Dis Child 99:524, 1960.

601. Ghosal SP, SenGupta PC, Mukherjee AK, et al. Noma neonatorum: its aetiopathogenesis. Lancet 1:289, 1978.

602. Bodey GP, Bolivar R, Fainstein V, et al. Infections caused by *Pseudomonas aeruginosa*. Rev Infect Dis 5:279, 1983.

603. Baley JE, Silverman RA. Systemic candidiasis: cutaneous manifestations in low birth weight infants. Pediatrics 82:211, 1988.

604. Cordero L Jr, Hon EH. Scalp abscess: a rare complication of fetal monitoring. J Pediatr 78:533, 1971.

605. Nelson JD. Bilateral breast abscess due to group B *Streptococcus*. Am J Dis Child 130:567, 1976.

606. Levy HL, O'Connor JF, Ingall D. Bacteremia, infected cephalhematoma, and osteomyelitis of the skull in a newborn. Am J Dis Child 114:649, 1967.

607. Ellis SS, Montgomery JR, Wagner M, et al. Osteomyelitis complicating neonatal cephalhematoma. Am J Dis Child 127:100, 1974.

608. Stetler H, Martin E, Plotkin S, et al. Neonatal mastitis due to *Echerichia coli*. J Pediatr 76:611, 1970.

609. Balfour HH Jr, Block SH, Bowe ET, et al. Complications of fetal blood sampling. Am J Obstet Gynecol 107:288, 1970.

610. McGuigan MA, Lipman RP. Neonatal mastitis due to *Proteus mirabilis*. Am J Dis Child 130:1296, 1976.

611. Wilson HD, Haltalin KC. Acute necrotizing fasciitis in childhood. Am J Dis Child 125:591, 1973.

612. Burry VF, Beezley M. Infant mastitis due to gram-negative organisms. Am J Dis Child 124:736, 1972.

613. Brook I. The aerobic and anaerobic microbiology of neonatal breast abscess. Pediatr Infect Dis J 10:785, 1991.

614. Centers for Disease Control. Nosocomial *Serratia marcescens* infections in neonates—Puerto Rico. MMWR Morbid Mortal Wkly Rep 23:183, 1974.

615. Todd JK, Bruhn FW. Severe *Haemophilus influenzae* infections: spectrum of disease. Am J Dis Child 129:607, 1975.

616. Zinner SH, McCormack WM, Lee Y-H, et al. Puerperal bacteremia and neonatal sepsis due to *Hemophilus parainfluenzae*: report of a case with antibody titers. Pediatrics 49:612, 1972.

617. Platt MS. Neonatal *Hemophilus vaginalis* (*Corynebacterium vaginalis*) infection. Clin Pediatr 10:513, 1971.

618. Leighton PM, Bulleid B, Taylor R. Neonatal cellulitis due to *Gardnerella vaginalis*. Pediatr Infect Dis 1:339, 1982.

619. Lee Y-H, Berg RB. Cephalhematoma infected with *Bacteroides*. Am J Dis Child 121:77, 1971.

620. Mandel MJ, Lewis RJ. Molluscum contagiosum of the newborn. Br J Dermatol 84:370, 1970.

621. Clark JM, Weeks WR, Tatton J. *Drosophila myiasis* mimicking sepsis in a newborn. West J Med 136:443, 1982.

622. Burns BR, Lampe RM, Hansen GH. Neonatal scabies. Am J Dis Child 133:1031, 1979.

623. Hensey OJ, Hart CA, Cooke RWI. *Candida albicans* skin abscesses. Arch Dis Child 59:479, 1984.

624. Turbeville DF, Heath RE Jr, Bowen FW Jr, et al. Complications of fetal scalp electrodes: a case report. Am J Obstet Gynecol 122:530, 1975.

625. Centers for Disease Control. Gonococcal scalp-wound infection—New Jersey. MMWR Morbid Mortal Wkly Rep 24:115, 1975.

626. Brook I. Osteomyelitis and bacteremia caused by *Bacteroides fragilis*. Clin Pediatr 19:639, 1980.

627. Mohon RT, Mehalic TF, Grimes CK, et al. Infected cephalhematoma and neonatal osteomyelitis of the skull. Pediatr Infect Dis 5:253, 1986.

628. Cohen SM, Miller BW, Orris HW. Meningitis complicating cephalhematoma. J Pediatr 30:327, 1947.

629. Rudoy RC, Nelson JD. Breast abscess during the neonatal period: a review. Am J Dis Child 129:1031, 1975.

630. Walsh M, McIntosh K. Neonatal mastitis. Clin Pediatr 25:395, 1986.

631. Langewisch WH. An epidemic of group A, type 1 streptococcal infections in newborn infants. Pediatrics 18:438, 1956.

632. Sinniah D, Sandiford BR, Dugdale AE. Subungual infection in the newborn: an institutional outbreak of unknown etiology, possibly due to *Veillonella*. Clin Pediatr 11:690, 1972.

633. Cushing AH. Omphalitis: a review. Pediatr Infect Dis 4:282, 1985.

634. McKenna H, Johnson D. Bacteria in neonatal omphalitis. Pathology 7:11, 1977.

635. Mason WH, Andrews R, Ross LA, et al. Omphalitis in the newborn infant. Pediatr Infect Dis J 8:521, 1989.

636. Geil CC, Castle WK, Mortimer EA Jr. Group A streptococcal infections in newborn nurseries. Pediatrics 46:849, 1970.

637. Kosloske AM, Cushing AH, Borden TA, et al. Cellulitis and necrotizing fasciitis of the abdominal wall in pediatric patients. J Pediatr Surg 16:246, 1981.

638. Goldberg GN, Hansen RC, Lynch PJ. Necrotizing fasciitis in infancy: report of three cases and review of the literature. Pediatr Dermatol 2:55, 1984.

639. Ramamurthy RS, Srinivasan G, Jacobs NM. Necrotizing fasciitis and necrotizing cellulitis due to group B *Streptococcus*. Am J Dis Child 131:1169, 1977.

640. Krieger RW, Chusid MJ. Perirectal abscess in childhood. Am J Dis Child 133:411, 1979.

641. Arditi M, Yogev R. Perirectal abscess in infants and children: report of 52 cases and review of the literature. Pediatr Infect Dis J 9:411, 1990.

642. Victorin L. An epidemic of otitis in newborns due to infection with *Pseudomonas aeruginosa*. Acta Paediatr Scand 56:344, 1967.

643. Laubo EJ, Paller AS. Common skin problems during the first year of life. Pediatr Clin North Am 41:1105, 1994.

644. Merlob P, Metzker A, Hazaz B, et al. Neonatal pemphigus vulgaris. Pediatrics 78:1102, 1986.

645. Glover MT, Atherton DJ, Levinsky RJ. Syndrome of erythroderma, failure to thrive, and diarrhea in infancy: a manifestation of immunodeficiency. Pediatrics 81:66, 1988.

646. Prod'hom LS, Choffat J-M, Frenck N, et al. Care of the seriously ill neonate with hyaline membrane disease and with sepsis (sclerema neonatorum). Pediatrics 53:170, 1974.

647. Hughes WE, Hammond ML. Sclerema neonatorum. J Pediatr 32:676, 1948.

648. McCracken GH Jr, Shinefield HR. Changes in the pattern of neonatal septicemia and meningitis. Am J Dis Child 112:33, 1966.

649. Gordon I. Miliary sebaceous cysts and blisters in the healthy newborn. Arch Dis Child 24:286, 1949.

650. Carr JA, Hodgman JE, Freedman RI, et al. Relationship between toxic erythema and infant maturity. Am J Dis Child 112:219, 1966.

651. Merlob P, Metzker A, Reisner SH. Transient neonatal pustular melanosis. Am J Dis Child 136:521, 1982.

652. Kahn G, Rywlin AM. Acropustulosis of infancy. Arch Dermatol 115:831, 1979.

653. Lucky AW, McGuire JS. Infantile acropustolosis with eosinophilic pustules. J Pediatr 100:428, 1982.

654. Murphy WF, Langley AL. Common bullous lesions—presumably self-inflicted occurring in utero in the newborn infant. Pediatrics 32:1099, 1963.

655. Weston WL, Lane AT, Weston JA. Diaper dermatitis: current concepts. Pediatrics 66:532, 1980.

656. Nappy rashes. Editorial. BMJ 282:420, 1981.

657. Hauth JC, Merenstein GB (eds). Guidelines for Perinatal Care, 4th ed. Elks Grove, Ill, American Academy of Pediatrics and American College of Obstetricians and Gynecologists, 1997.

658. Gladstone IM, Clapper L, Thorp JW, et al. Randomized study of six umbilical cord care regimens. Clin Pediatr 27:127, 1988.

659. Centers for Disease Control. National nosocomial infections study report: nosocomial infections in nurseries and their relationship to hospital infant bathing practices—a preliminary report. Atlanta, Ga, Centers for Disease Control, 1974, pp 9–23.

660. Gezon HM, Schaberg MJ, Klein JO. Concurrent epidemics of *Staphylococcus aureus* and group A *Streptococcus* disease in a newborn nursery—control with penicillin G and hexachlorophene bathing. Pediatrics 51:383, 1973.

661. Seeberg S, Brinkhoff B, John E, et al. Prevention and control of neonatal pyoderma with chlorhexidine. Acta Paediatr Scand 73:498, 1984.

Conjunctivitis and Other Eye Infections

662. de Toledo AR, Chandler JW. Conjunctivitis of the newborn. Infect Dis Clin North Am 6:807, 1992.

663. Whitcher JP. Neonatal ophthalmia: have we advanced in the last 20 years? Int Ophthalmol Clin 30:39, 1990.

664. Millard DD, Yogev R. *Haemophilus influenzae* type b: a rare case of congenital conjunctivitis. Pediatr Infect Dis 7:363, 1988.

665. McLeod DT, Ahmad F, Calder MA. *Branhamella catarrhalis* (beta lactamase positive) ophthalmia neonatorum. Lancet 2:647, 1984.

666. Ellis M, Weindling DC, Ho N, et al. Neonatal conjunctivitis associated with meningococcal meningitis. Arch Dis Child 67:1219, 1992.

667. Naiditch MJ, Bower AG. Diphtheria: a study of 1433 cases observed during a ten year period at Los Angeles County Hospital. Am J Med 17:229, 1954.

668. Khan MS, Stead SE. Neonatal *Pasteurella multocida* conjunctivitis following zoonotic infection of mother. J Infect Dis 1:289, 1979.

669. Brook I, Martin WJ, Finegold SM. Effect of silver nitrate application on the conjunctival flora of the newborn, and the occurrence of clostridial conjunctivitis. J Pediatr Ophthalmol Strabismus 15:179, 1978.

670. Bourbeau P, Holla V, Piemontese S. Ophthalmia neonatorum caused by *Neisseria cinerea*. J Clin Microbiol 28:1640, 1990.

671. Hedberg K, Ristinen TL, Soler JT, et al. Outbreak of erythromycin-resistant staphylococcal conjunctivitis in a newborn nursery. Pediatr Infect Dis J 9:268, 1990.

672. Paentice MJ, Hutchinson GR, Taylor-Robinson D. A microbiological study of neonatal conjunctivitis. Br J Ophthalmol 61:9, 1977.

673. Sandstrom KI, Bell TA, Chandler JW, et al. Microbial causes of neonatal conjunctivitis. J Pediatr 105:706, 1984.

674. Duarte AM, Kramer J, Yusk W, et al. Eosinophilic pustular folliculitis in infancy and childhood. Am J Dis Child 147:197, 1993.

675. Hammerschlag MR. Conjunctivitis in infancy and childhood. Pediatr Rev 5:285, 1984.

676. Wincelaus J, Goh BT, Dunlop EM, et al. Diagnosis of ophthalmia neonatorum. BMJ 295:1377, 1987.

677. Molgaard I-L, Nielsen PB, Kaern J. A study of the incidence of neonatal conjunctivitis and of its bacterial causes including *Chlamydia trachomatis.* Acta Ophthalmol 62:461, 1984.

678. Laga M, Nzanze H, Brunham RC, et al. Epidemiology of ophthalmia neonatorum in Kenya. Lancet 2:1145, 1986.

679. Nathoo KJ, Latif AS, Trijssenaar JES. Aetiology of neonatal conjunctivitis in Harare. Cent Afr J Med 30:123, 1984.

680. Stenson S, Newman R, Fedukowicz H. Conjunctivitis in the newborn: observations on incidence, cause, and prophylaxis. Ann Ophthalmol 13:329, 1981.

681. Burns RP, Rhodes DH Jr. *Pseudomonas* eye infection as a cause of death in premature infants. Arch Ophthalmol 65:517, 1961.

682. Drewett SE, Payne DJH, Tuke W, et al. Eradication of *Pseudomonas aeruginosa* infection from a special-care nursery. Lancet 1:946, 1972.

683. Cole GA, Davies DP, Austin DJ. *Pseudomonas* ophthalmia neonatorum: a cause of blindness. BMJ 281:440, 1980.

684. Traboulsi EI, Shammas IV, Ratl HE, et al. *Pseudomonas aeruginosa* ophthalmia neonatorum. Am J Ophthalmol 98:801, 1984.

685. Lohrer R, Belohradsky BH. Bacterial endophthalmitis in neonates. Eur J Pediatr 146:354, 1987.

686. Christensen GD, Korones SB, Reed L, et al. Epidemic *Serratia marcescens* in a neonatal intensive care unit: importance of the gastrointestinal tract as a reservoir. Infect Control 3:127, 1982.

687. Harris GJ, DiClementi D. Congenital dacryocystocele. Arch Ophthalmol 100:1763, 1982.

688. Nishida H, Risemberg HM. Silver nitrate ophthalmic solution and chemical conjunctivitis. Pediatrics 56:3368, 1975.

689. Kripke SS, Golden B. Neonatal inclusion conjunctivitis: a report of three cases and a discussion of differential diagnosis and treatment. Clin Pediatr 11:261, 1972.

690. Naib ZM. Cytology of TRIC agent infection of the eye of newborn infants and their mothers' genital tracts. Acta Cytol 14:390, 1970.

691. Peter G (ed). Prevention of neonatal opthalmia. *In* Report of the Committee on Infectious Diseases, 24th ed. Elk Grove Village, Ill, American Academy of Pediatrics, 1997, pp 601–603.

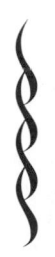
Group B Streptococcal Infections

MORVEN S. EDWARDS, M.D., and CAROL J. BAKER, M.D.

Lancefield group B beta-hemolytic streptococci were first recorded as a cause of human infection in 1938 when Fry described three patients with fatal puerperal sepsis.[1] Although sporadic cases were reported during the next three decades, this microorganism remained unknown to most clinicians until the 1970s when a dramatic increase in the incidence of septicemia and meningitis in neonates caused by group B streptococci was documented from geographically diverse regions.[2-11] The abrupt emergence of group B streptococcal infections in neonates also was accompanied by an increasing number of these infections in pregnant and nonpregnant adults.[12-15] In pregnant women, these were commonly manifested as localized uterine infections or chorioamnionitis, often with bacteremia, and had an almost uni-

formly good outcome with therapy.[16, 17] However, in nonpregnant adults who typically had underlying medical conditions, group B streptococcal infection often resulted in a fatal outcome.[18]

The reason for the appearance of group B streptococci as significant neonatal pathogens in the 1970s remains obscure. However, shifts in the prevalence of etiologic agents producing neonatal bacterial infections have been the rule in the past.[19] Reports in the early 1990s indicated that the incidence of perinatal infection associated with group B streptococci remained stable.[20-26] Case:fatality ratios have fallen but remain substantial compared with those reported for other invasive bacterial infections in infants. The severity and magnitude of infections attributed to group B streptococci have stimulated intense investigational effort in the past, with the hope that an understanding of the epidemiology and pathogenesis of these infections could result in the development of methods for their effective control and prevention.

Since the previous edition of this book was published in 1995, several notable events have occurred. Two additional capsular serotypes, VII and VIII, have been associated with human disease and immunochemically and structurally characterized. A shift in the distribution of serotypes causing invasive infection also has occurred. Serotype V group B streptococci now account for a substantial proportion of infections in the newborn, as well as among pregnant women and nonpregnant adults.[27–32] Infections caused by serotype Ia have increased, those due to type II have decreased, and type III remains a dominant cause of meningitis and of late-onset infection. The reason for this serotype shift is not known, but it has important implications for the development of vaccines to prevent group B streptococcal infections. The past 5 years also have provided insights that clarify the mechanism of invasion and the important role of inflammatory mediators in modulating host response to infection. The consensus guidelines developed in 1996 by the Centers for Disease Control and Prevention, the American College of Obstetricians and Gynecologists, and the American Academy of Pediatrics to prevent early-onset disease in neonates through intrapartum maternal chemoprophylaxis represent the greatest single achievement of the past 5 years.[33–35] The implementation of these guidelines has been associated with a substantial decline in the incidence of neonatal infection for the first time in two and a half decades.[35a] In addition, successful testing of group B streptococcal conjugate vaccines in healthy women during this same interval offers promise that immunoprophylaxis to prevent maternal and infant group B streptococcal disease may become a reality in the near future.

THE ORGANISM

Streptococcus agalactiae, the species designation for streptococci belonging to Lancefield group B, is a facultative gram-positive diplococcus with an ultrastructure similar to that of other gram-positive cocci.[36, 37] Before Lancefield's classification of hemolytic streptococci in 1933,[38] this microorganism was known to microbiologists by its characteristic colonial morphology, its narrow zone of beta hemolysis, and its double zone of hemolysis surrounding colonies on blood agar plates that appeared when plates were refrigerated an additional 18 hours beyond the initial incubation.[39, 40] Occasional strains (~1%) are alpha or nonhemolytic,[10, 41, 42] and these strains can cause human infection,[10, 43] although infrequently. Group B streptococci are readily cultivated in a variety of bacteriologic media. Isolation from certain body sites (respiratory, genital, gastrointestinal tracts) can be enhanced by use of broth medium containing antimicrobial agents that inhibit growth of other bacterial species indigenous to these sites.[6, 44–49]

Colonial Morphology and Identification

Colonies of group B streptococci on sheep blood agar medium are 3 to 4 mm in diameter, produce narrow zones of beta hemolysis, are gray-white, and are flat and mucoid. Beta hemolysis for some strains is apparent only when colonies are removed from the agar.

Although definitive identification of group B streptococci requires detection of the group B–specific antigen common to all strains through use of hyperimmune grouping antiserum, several laboratory tests have been employed for presumptive identification. These include bacitracin and sulfamethoxazole-trimethoprim disk susceptibility (92 to 98% of strains are resistant),[41, 42, 50, 51] hydrolysis of sodium hippurate broth (99% of strains are positive),[42, 50] hydrolysis of bile esculin agar (99 to 100% of strains fail to react),[42, 50] pigment production during anaerobic growth on certain media (96 to 98% of strains produce an orange pigment),[52–56] and CAMP (Christie, Atkins, and Munch-Petersen) testing (98 to 100% of strains are CAMP positive).[50, 57–59] This last test is based on the production of CAMP factor, a thermostable extracellular protein[60] that, in the presence of the beta toxin of *Staphylococcus aureus* (a sphingomyelinase), produces synergistic hemolysis on sheep blood agar. A spot CAMP test, employing a crude beta toxin–containing filtrate derived from a broth culture of *S. aureus*, allows rapid (30-minute) identification of group B streptococci from a single colony of the primary isolation plate with an accuracy equal to that of the standard CAMP test.[61, 62] Hippurate hydrolysis is an accurate method for presumptive identification of group B streptococci, but the requirement for 24 to 48 hours of incubation limits its usefulness. Group B strains can be differentiated from other streptococci by a combination of the CAMP test, the bile esculin reaction, and bacitracin sensitivity.[50] Biochemical micromethods identify group B streptococci with reasonable accuracy after a 4-hour incubation period.[63]

Definitive microbiologic identification of group B streptococci requires serologic methods to detect the group B carbohydrate antigen. Lancefield's original method[64] required acid treatment of large volumes of broth-grown cells to extract (solubilize) the group B antigen from the cell wall. Supernatants then were brought to neutral pH and mixed with hyperimmune rabbit antiserum prepared by immunization with the group B-variant strain (090R; devoid of type-specific antigen), and precipitins in capillary tubes were recorded. Less time-consuming techniques were subsequently developed. All employ hyperimmune group-specific antiserum to identify the group B antigen in intact cells, broth culture supernatants, or cell extracts. These methods include immunodiffusion, coagglutination, and latex agglutination.[65–68] Commercial availability and testing time make coagglutination and latex agglutination assays the most practical methods for use by hospital laboratories. Solubilization of the group-specific antigen with an enzyme contained in the culture supernatant of *Streptomyces globisporus* may facilitate effective serogrouping by latex agglutination.[69] The lectins of the tomato, *Lycopersicon esculentum*, and the potato, *Solanum tuberosum*, have been used for serogrouping in latex agglutination assays.[70]

Strains of Human and Bovine Origin

Before the dramatic increase in the incidence of human group B streptococcal infections in the 1970s, these microorganisms were principally associated with bovine mastitis.[10, 39, 71] Modern veterinary practices have largely controlled epidemics of bovine mastitis due to *S. agalactiae*, but sporadic cases still occur. The relationship between strains of human and bovine origin has been questioned for years. To date there is no evidence that cattle are a reservoir for transmission of group B streptococci to humans. In contrast, substantial data indicate several biochemical, biologic, and serologic differences between human and bovine isolates.[4, 53, 72–74] For example, Pattison and associates[72] were unable to serotype 75% of their bovine strains employing antisera that had enabled them to classify all of their human isolates. This nontypeability of bovine strains has been confirmed by others.[4, 71] Among typeable bovine strains, there are distinct patterns of serotype distribution when compared with those for human isolates. Using the concept of "herd type" for serologic typing, Jensen[75] demonstrated that the distribution of group B streptococci from newly infected herds was the same as that of human urogenital strains.[75] Other distinguishing characteristics for bovine strains include their unique fermentation reactions, their decreased frequency of pigment production,[53] and their usual susceptibility to bacitracin.[4] Protein X, rarely found in human strains, is commonly present in pathogenic bovine isolates.[76]

Serologic Classification

Lancefield defined two cell wall carbohydrate antigens for group B streptococci employing hydrochloric acid (HCl)-extracted cell supernatants and hyperimmune rabbit antisera: (1) the group B–specific or "C" substance common to all strains of this species and (2) the type-specific or "S" substance that allowed classification into four serotypes—Ia, Ib, II, and III.[77–83] Group B streptococcal strains were originally classified as serotypes I, II, and III. Strains designated as type I were later shown by Lancefield to have both cross-reactive and antigenically distinct polysaccharides.[79, 82, 83] When antisera raised to two different type I strains were made type specific by reciprocal cross absorption with streptococcal cells, the antigenically distinct type Ia and Ib polysaccharides were defined.[79] The serotype of group B *Streptococcus* historically designated as type Ic was characterized by Wilkinson and her co-workers.[84, 85] These strains possessed the type Ia capsular polysaccharide[86–88] and a protein antigen common to type Ib, up to 60% of type II,[89] and to rare type III strains.[10, 90] This protein antigen was historically called the type Ibc antigen and now is called C protein.

In an attempt to arrive at a uniform and more simple nomenclature, Jelínková and Motlová[91] introduced a revision adopted by the Workshop on Neonatal Group B Streptococcal Infections in Lund, Sweden, in 1983 in which it was proposed that the polysaccharide antigens of group B streptococci be designated as type antigens and the protein antigens as additional markers for supplementary characterization of serotypes.[92] The designation of the protein antigen Ibc was simplified to C protein. Thus, the former serotype Ic strains are now designated type Ia/c because they possess the Ia polysaccharide antigen and the C protein antigen. Type IV was introduced as an additional serotype by Perch and colleagues[93] in 1979. These investigators described 62 strains from 11 countries that possessed type IV polysaccharide alone or with one of the protein antigens. More recently, new antigenically distinct serotypes, V through VIII, have been recognized and characterized.[94–99] Strains of group B *Streptococcus* from patients with serious infections that cannot be serologically classified continue to account for less than 5% of isolates.[10, 99]

The serotyping scheme of Lancefield is based on microprecipitin reactions of acid extracts of whole cells with group B–specific and type-specific antisera.[64, 79] The biologic relevance of these serologically defined type-specific antigens has been investigated employing mouse protection experiments. Rabbit antibodies directed against the capsular polysaccharides provide passive protection to mice challenged with lethal doses of mouse virulent strains containing homologous but not heterologous antigens.[79, 80, 83, 96] Cross-protection also occurs when antibodies against the C protein and the type Ia and Ib strains that share this antigenic determinant are tested. Rabbit antibodies directed against the group B–specific antigen do not protect mice from lethal challenge,[83] nor do they mediate opsonophagocytosis of these organisms in vitro.

The C protein antigen was shown by Wilkinson and Eagon[85] to consist of two components, one sensitive to trypsin and pepsin and the other sensitive only to pepsin. Bevanger and Naess[100] designated these trypsin-resistant and trypsin-sensitive antigens alpha and beta, respectively, and found that antibodies to these proteins were partially mouse protective.[101] The beta C protein is present in about 10% of human group B streptococcal isolates. Alpha C proteins are present in approximately one half of isolates and in most of those strains bearing capsular polysaccharides other than III.[89] Strains expressing the alpha antigen are less readily opsonized, ingested, and killed by leukocytes in the absence of specific antibody than are alpha-negative strains.[102] Strains bearing both the alpha and beta C protein components have increased resistance to opsonization in vitro.

The alpha C protein consists of a series of tandem repeating units; and in naturally occurring strains, the repeat numbers may vary. The number of repeating units expressed alters antigenicity and influences the repertoires of antibodies elicited.[103] There are two distinct protective epitopes within the alpha C protein. The use of one or two repeat units of alpha C proteins elicits antibodies that bind all alpha C proteins with equal affinity, suggesting their potential usefulness as vaccine candidates.[104, 105] The beta antigen appears as a single protein of molecular mass between 124 and 134 kDa. The beta, but not the alpha antigen, binds the Fc region of human IgA.[106–108]

In addition to the group B, type-specific, and protein C antigens, some strains of group B streptococci contain surface proteins designated X and R antigens.[37, 109, 110] These were first described by Pattison and co-workers, who introduced reagents for their detection in an attempt to further classify nontypeable strains.[109] The X and R antigens are immunologically cross-reactive. The R antigen of type III group B streptococci is identical to that of type 28 group A streptococci.[110, 111] R antigens are found in the majority of type II and III strains but are rare in type Ia or Ib strains.[112] Four distinct immunologic species of R antigen have been described. Of these, R4 is the most prevalent in isolates recovered from humans, and it is expressed almost exclusively in type II and III strains.[113] A distinct surface protein, designated Rib, is expressed by most invasive strains, including almost all serotype III strains. It is immunologically unrelated, but like alpha C protein has an extremely repetitive structure.[114, 115] In contrast, a recently described laddering protein from type V group B *Streptococcus* does share sequence homology with alpha C protein.[116] Thus, there is a family of trypsin-resistant surface proteins with a repetitive structure that may have a role in immunity to infection. However, the role of the R proteins in human immunity, if any, remains to be defined.

Ultrastructure

Early concepts regarding the cellular structure of beta-hemolytic streptococci suggested a thick, rigid peptidoglycan layer external to the cytoplasmic membrane, which was surrounded by concentric layers of cell wall antigens. The group-specific carbohydrate was believed to be "covered" by the surface type-specific antigen, which for group A streptococci is M-protein and for group B is capsular polysaccharide. However, electron microscopic studies provided evidence for a mosaic structure of the group B streptococcal cell wall.[37] Other investigations employing both electron microscopic and immunologic techniques have suggested that, although a mosaic structure for the group B streptococcal cell wall is plausible, the group B antigenic determinant is not accessible for binding to group B-specific antibody when Lancefield prototype strains are studied.[36] The type-specific capsular polysaccharides appear to mask the group B–binding sites, suggesting that the group B antigen is a subcapsular cell wall structure. Only when these capsular polysaccharides are chemically modified or removed can group B carbohydrate-specific antibody attach to the cell surface.[36, 117, 118]

Standard techniques for demonstrating bacterial capsules (India ink or "quellung reaction") do not visualize capsules on group B streptococci,[10, 82] but these microorganisms are encapsulated.[36, 117] Immunoelectron techniques reveal abundant capsular polysaccharide on the surface of Lancefield prototype strains Ia (090), II (18RS21), and III (D136C), whereas less dense capsules are found on type Ib/c (H36b) and Ia/c (A909) strains[36] (Fig. 26–1). Similarly, incubation of the reference strains of serotypes IV, V, and VI with homologous type-specific antisera led to visualization of a thick capsular layer.[96, 119] The type-specific polysaccharides, therefore, are surface structures on group B streptococcal cells, although they may not be the exclusive surface component for some strains. Interestingly, study of serotype Ia strains has determined that invasive human isolates are much less encapsulated than in Lancefield's mouse-passed prototype Ia strain, 090.[120] The degree of encapsulation of group B streptococcal strains is a function of in vitro manipulation and of serotype. Expression of the capsular polysaccharide is not constitutive, but varies during growth in vitro and in primary cultures isolated from different sites of infection.[121, 122]

The ultrastructural location of the C protein antigen has been shown to have a surface location on both type Ia and Ib cells.[36] This surface location is consistent with the observation that antibodies to C protein as well as to capsular polysaccharides are protective against lethal challenge with organisms possessing these antigens.[82, 83]

Immunochemistry of Cell Wall Antigens

Lancefield's serologic definition of the cell wall antigens of group B streptococci was achieved by their extraction from whole cells by dilute HCl and heat treatment.[77, 79–82] Additional purification methods were necessary for isolation of the group B–specific from type-specific polysaccharide antigens.[80, 86, 123] The chemical composition of the group B polysaccharide initially was determined for B antigen extracted from whole cells of the laboratory-adapted variant strain 090R, devoid of capsular polysaccharide.[118, 123] In later studies, group B antigen was isolated from type III cells employing alcohol fractionation techniques with hot formamide extracts of whole cells.[124] With the use of rigorous biochemical methods for structural determination, the group B antigen was shown to contain L-rhamnose, D-galactose, 2-acetamido-2-deoxy-D-glucose and D-glucitol. It is composed of four different oligosaccharides, designated I, II, III, and IV, that are linked by one type of phosphodiester bond to form a complex, highly branched multiantennary structure.[124–126] The tetra-antennary structure proposed for arrangement of the component oligosaccharides is shown in Figure 26–2. Oligosaccharide IV has no glucitol and always is located at the reducing terminus of the antigen, where it probably functions as a linker molecule between the group B polysaccharide and the cell wall peptidoglycan of the organism. Inhibition studies have shown that antibodies to the group B polysaccharide are dominated by those specific for a trirhamnopyranoside epitope.

Extensive studies of the HCl-extracted type-specific polysaccharides have been reported in the past. The HCl antigens from type Ia, Ib, II, and III organisms are small-molecular-mass (1.5 to 5.0×10^4 daltons) neutral polysaccharides that contain identical constituents—galactose, glucose, and 2-acetamido-2-deoxyglucose—in repeating units of a core structure.[82, 86, 87, 118, 123] When more gentle techniques are employed for the extraction of these type-specific capsular polysaccharides from

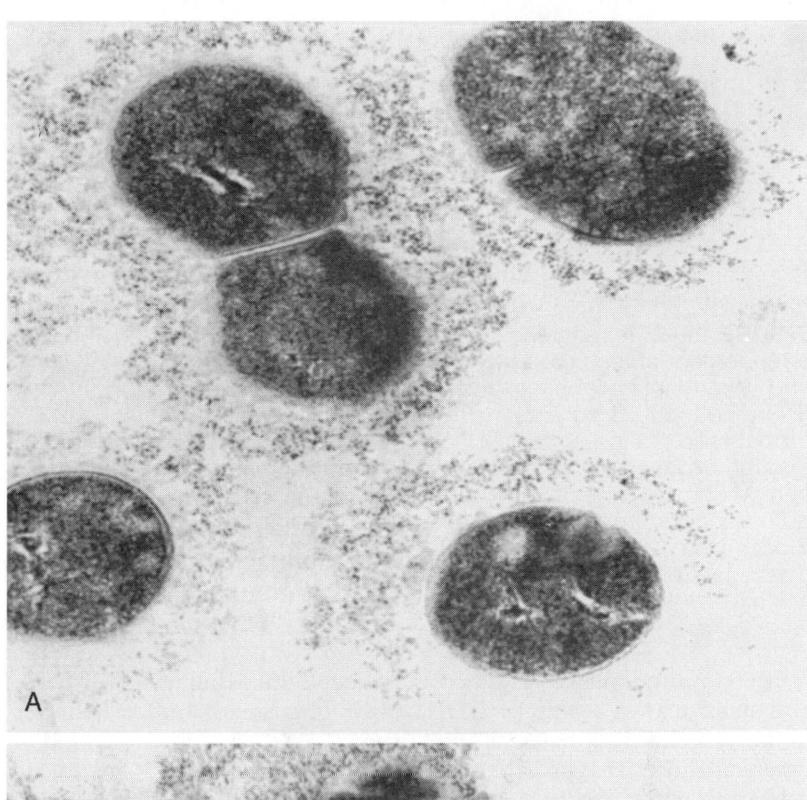

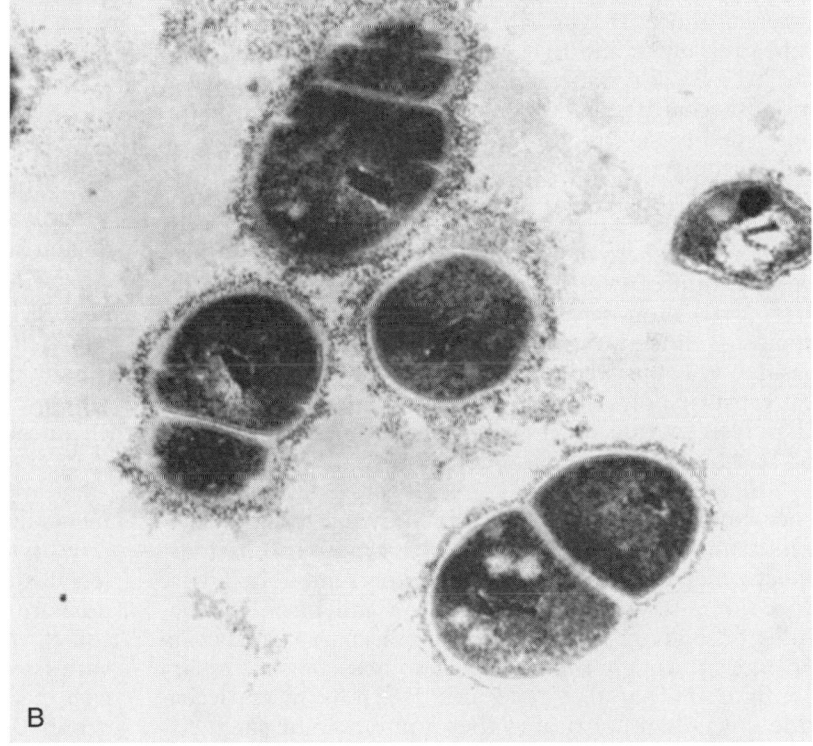

FIGURE 26–1 Electron micrographs of thin sections of group B streptococcal strains: *A*=type Ia (090) and *B*=type Ia/c (A909), stained with ferritin-conjugated type Ia-specific rabbit antibodies. The type Ia strain is representative of the large capsules found in Lancefield prototype II strain (18RS21) and type III isolates from infants with meningitis (M732), whereas the type Ia/c strain is representative of the much smaller capsules occurring in Lancefield prototype strains Ia/c (A909) and Ib/c (H36B). (Micrographs courtesy of Dennis L. Kasper, M.D.)

whole cells, large-molecular-mass (5×10^5 to 1×10^6 daltons) acidic polysaccharides with an additional antigenic determinant are isolated. These "native" antigens form a partial identity with the HCl antigens from homologous strains by immunodiffusion with type-specific antisera. The additional antigenic determinant on the more complete type-specific polysaccharides is the acid-labile sugar sialic acid.[81, 82, 86–88, 95, 118, 127–135] Acid hydrolysis of "native" polysaccharides results in degrada-

tion to core structures that are immunochemically identical to the homologous HCl-extracted antigens. Isolation of the immunologically more complete polysaccharides requires that growth of cells and extraction of antigens be performed under conditions that maintain neutral pH.[87, 127–135]

Analysis of the component monosaccharides of the capsular polysaccharides of type Ia, Ib, and III group B *Streptococcus* reveals that each has a five sugar repeating

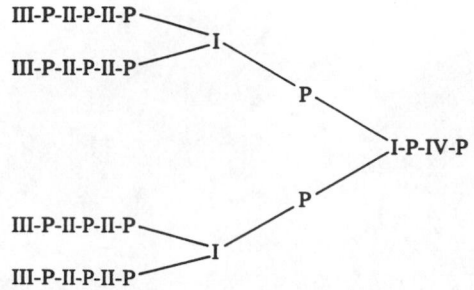

FIGURE 26–2 Tetraantennary structure proposed for arrangement of the component oligosaccharides (I, II, III, and IV) and interoligosaccharide phosphodiester linkages (P) in the group B polysaccharide. The group B antigen is probably linked to the cell surface of group B streptococci through oligosaccharide IV. (Reprinted with permission from Michon F, Brisson J-R, Dell A, et al. Multiantennary group-specific polysaccharide of group B *Streptococcus*. Biochemistry 27:5341–5351, 1988. © 1988, American Chemical Society.)

unit containing galactose, glucose, *N*-acetylglucosamine, and sialic acid in a ratio of 2:1:1:1.[127–129] The type II and V polysaccharides have a seven sugar repeating unit whereas those of types IV and VII consist of six sugar repeating units, and that of type VIII consists of four.[95–97, 130, 135, 136] The molar ratios vary, but the component monosaccharides are the same with only two exceptions described to date. First, no *N*-acetylglucosamine is present in the type VI polysaccharide. In addition, the recently described type VIII capsular polysaccharide is the only structure that contains rhamnose in the backbone structure.[98] Each of the antigens has a backbone repeating unit of two (Ia, Ib), four (II), or three (II, IV, V, VII, VIII) monosaccharides to which one or two side chains is linked. Sialic acid as a terminal side chain residue is a consistent feature of the group B streptococcal capsular polysaccharides. With the exception of type II polysaccharide, it is the exclusive sugar constituting or at the terminus of the side chain(s).

The repeating unit structures of the group B streptococcal polysaccharides, determined by methylation analysis combined with gas-liquid chromatography/mass spectrometry, are schematically represented in Figure 26–3. The structures of the type Ia and Ib polysaccharides differ only in a single monosaccharide side chain linkage, although there are differences in the tertiary configuration of the molecules.[131] These monosaccharide linkages are critical to their immunologic specificity and also explain their immunologic cross-reactivity.[79, 132]

Of interest, the type Ia, Ib, and III polysaccharides have a high degree of structural homology with two human serum glycoproteins. The terminal α-D sialic [2→3]-β-D-galactose of these native antigens is identical to the end group of human M and N blood group substances.[137] The type Ib polysaccharide has a repeating unit that is virtually identical to those of certain oligosaccharides present in human milk.[138] For the type III polysaccharide, a graded increase in relative affinity of antigen-antibody binding was observed as oligosaccharide size increased from 3 to 92 repeating units.[139] One

implication of this difference in antibody-binding affinity, estimated to exceed 300-fold, is that binding interaction with an oligosaccharide on a host glycoprotein would be of very low affinity, insufficient to result in activation of potentially damaging immune effector mechanisms. The type III polysaccharide also can form extended helices. The position of the conformational epitope along these helices is potentially important to binding site interactions.[140] Another structural homology is that between the HCl-extracted type III polysaccharide and the immunochemically identical type 14 pneumococcal polysaccharide.[141] This observation stimulated a number of investigations concerning the immunodeterminant specificity of human immunity to type III group B *Streptococcus* and of antibody recognition of conformational epitopes as a facet of the host immune response.[142, 143]

Because human immunity to type III strains correlates with antibody to the intact rather than to the desialylated capsular polysaccharide antigen, isolation of intact polysaccharides with sialic acid moieties has seemed a desirable goal for the study of human immunity. Growth of cells in highly buffered media[127] or by pH titration achieves the conditions of neutral pH necessary for isolation of immunologically complete antigens.[118] However, yield of polysaccharides extracted from whole cells by these gentle neutral buffer techniques is low.[127, 128] Improvements in preparative methods through use of chemically defined, pH-controlled growth medium, treatment of bacterial cells with enzymes[144] to release capsule into the medium, and serial chromatographic procedures to ensure purity[134] now allow for isolation of large quantities of "native" polysaccharides.

Growth Requirements and Bacterial Products

The nutritional requirements of several human and bovine strains of group B streptococci, examined in a chemically defined medium, reveal reasonable homogeneity in vitamin requirements.[145] Group B streptococci are also quite homogeneous in their amino acid requirements during aerobic or anaerobic growth.[146] Phenylalanine, tyrosine, tryptophan, glutamate, arginine, valine, leucine, lysine, methionine, isoleucine, cystine, and histidine are required by most strains. Serine is required by some type III strains, and the requirement for glycine varies from strain to strain.[146] Provision of a glucose-rich environment enhances both the number of viable group B streptococci during stationary phase and the amount of capsular polysaccharide on type III cells and elaborated into the growth medium.[147] In a modified chemically defined medium, the expression of capsule during continuous growth is regulated by the growth rate.[121]

Group B streptococci elaborate a number of bacterial products, including the soluble type-specific capsular polysaccharides,[127] hemolysin,[148, 149] pigment,[150] CAMP factor,[57] hippuricase,[42, 151] nucleases,[152] neuraminidase,[153] protease,[154] an oligopeptidase, and lipoteichoic acid.[155] The hemolysin or hemolysins of group B streptococci are an extracellular product of almost all strains and are

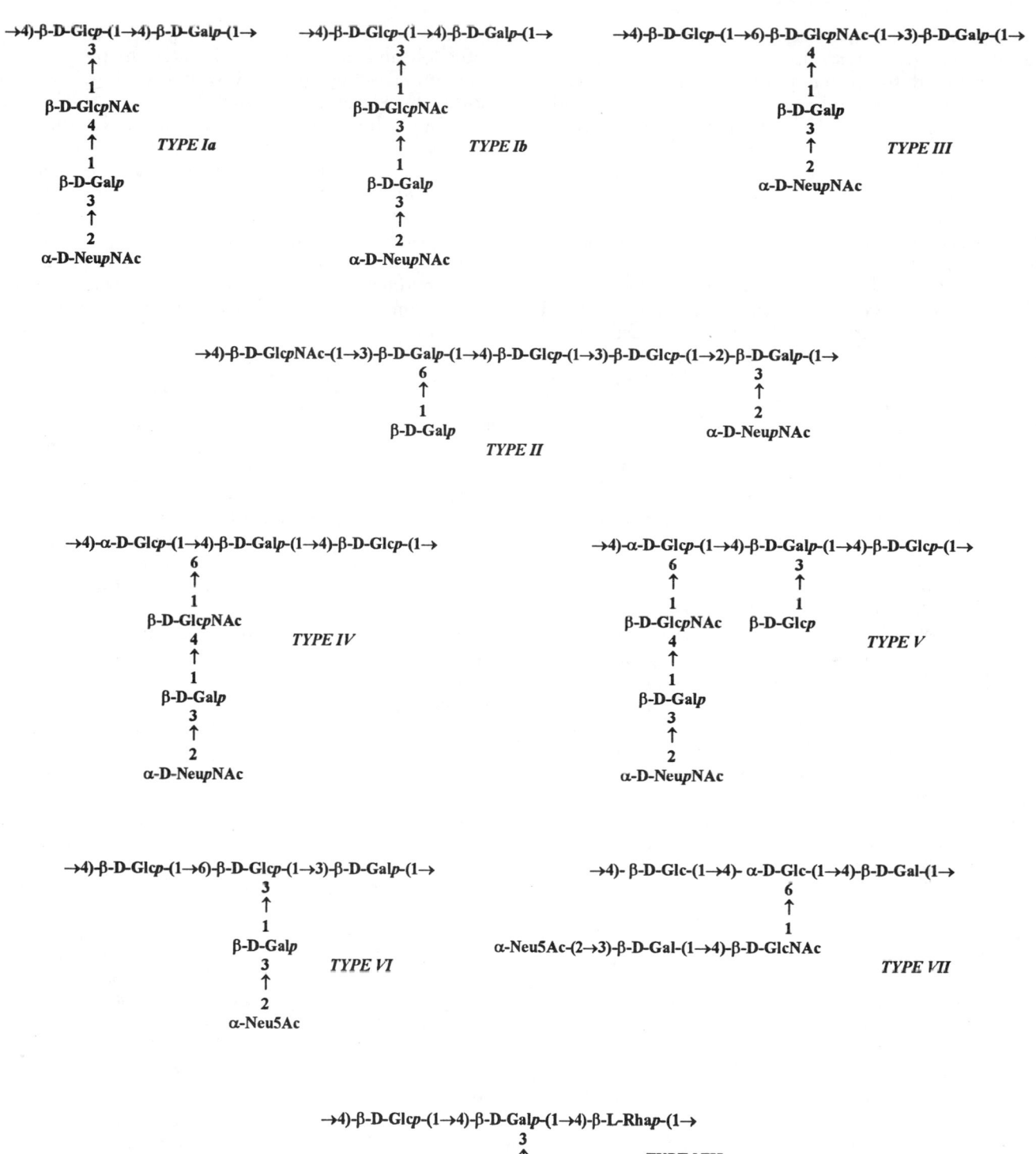

FIGURE 26–3 Repeating unit structures of group B streptococcal capsular polysaccharides type Ia,[131] type Ib,[131, 132] type II,[130, 136] type III,[129, 134] type IV,[135] type V,[95] type VI,[99] type VII,[97] and type VIII.[98]

active against the erythrocytes from several mammalian species. The hemolysin that produces the beta hemolysis surrounding group B colonies on blood agar plates has been isolated and characterized.[148] When it was tested with known inhibitors of other streptococcal hemolysins (phospholipids, trypan blue, proteases, cholesterol), it was inhibited only by phospholipids. The hemolysin was not detected in supernatants of broth cultures, suggesting either that it exists in a cell-bound form or that it is released by cells and rapidly inactivated. However, no measurable effect on virulence was observed when an isogenic mutant lacking hemolysin was compared with the parent group B streptococcal strain in a neonatal rat model of bacteremia.[149]

After growth to stationary phase, group B streptococci produce two types of pigment resembling a beta carotenoid.[150] Pigment, like hemolysin, may be formed and released by an active metabolic process, retaining its properties only in the presence of a carrier molecule. A potential role for pigment as a virulence factor is proposed but unproved. No relationship between the group B streptococcal hemolysin and CAMP factor has been determined.[148]

The CAMP phenomenon or the elaboration of CAMP factor by group B streptococci was described in 1944 by Christie, Atkins, and Munch-Petersen.[57] Skalka and Smola[156] reported that a partially purified CAMP factor was lethal in experimental infection. Subsequently, nonspecific binding of the CAMP factor to immunoglobulins in a protein A–like fashion led Jürgens and co-workers[157] to suggest the term *protein B* for CAMP factor. The cloning and expression of CAMP factor in *Escherichia coli* will aid investigations of its mode of action and role, if any, in the pathogenesis of human infections.

Group B streptococci can hydrolyze hippuric acid to benzoic acid and glycine, and this property has been useful in distinguishing group B streptococci from other beta-hemolytic groups.[42, 146] Ferrieri and co-workers isolated and characterized the hippuricase of group B streptococci.[151] This enzyme is cell associated and is sensitive to trypsin and heat. It is antigenic in rabbits, but its relationship to bacterial virulence has not been studied.

Most strains of group B streptococci have an enzyme that inactivates complement component C5a by cleaving a peptide at the carboxyl terminus.[158, 159] Group B streptococcal C5a-ase appears to be a serine esterase; it is distinct from the C5a-cleaving enzyme (termed *streptococcal C5a peptidase*) produced by group A streptococci,[160] although the genes that encode these enzymes are similar.[161] C5a-ase contributes to the pathogenesis of group B streptococcal disease by rapidly inactivating the neutrophil agonist C5a, thereby preventing the accumulation of neutrophils at the site of infection.[158] Naturally occurring IgG antibodies can neutralize the enzyme in serum or plasma, but C5a-ase associated with the bacterial surface of encapsulated type III group B *Streptococcus* is not inactivated by IgG, suggesting that the capsule provides protection from neutralization of the enzyme.[162]

Another group of enzymes elaborated by nearly all group B streptococci are the extracellular nucleases.[152] Three distinct nucleases—designated I, II, and III by Ferrieri and colleagues[151]—have been physically and immunologically characterized. All are maximally activated by divalent cations of calcium plus manganese. These group B nucleases are immunogenic in animals, and neutralizing antibodies to these antigens are detectable in sera from pregnant women known to be genital carriers of group B streptococci.[152] The relationship between this latter observation and the pathogenesis of human infection is unknown.

An extracellular product of group B streptococci that may relate to the virulence of group B streptococci in humans is neuraminidase (sialidase), considered by some to be a hyaluronate lyase.[163] Although the production of neuraminidase by group B streptococci was first reported by Hayano and Tanaka,[153] it was Milligan and associates who defined the conditions under which enzyme activity could be quantified.[154] Maximal levels were detected during late exponential growth in a chemically defined medium. Subsequently, proteases may degrade neuraminidase. The neuraminidases from some of the serotypes of group B streptococci have been purified and partially characterized. These have a molecular size of approximately 1×10^5 daltons and a limited range of activity on sialic acid substrates when compared with other bacterial neuraminidases. Type III polysaccharide (α-2,3 linkage) is resistant to type III group B streptococcal neuraminidase.[164, 165]

Elaboration of large quantities of neuraminidase may be a virulence factor for type III group B *Streptococcus*. Almost all type Ia, Ib, and II strains are low producers, whereas type III strains are either high producers or nonproducers.[166] When type III strains isolated from infants with invasive infection were compared with those isolated from asymptomatic infants, the former were significantly more often high neuraminidase producers. Musser and co-workers[167] identified a subset of type III strains that were high producers of extracellular neuraminidase that were responsible for the majority of serious group B streptococcal infections.

The role of type-specific polysaccharides as virulence factors acting independently has been evaluated in a murine model.[168] The amount of extracellular capsular polysaccharide produced by type III strains correlated with virulence in chick embryos[169] and mice[170] and with invasiveness in susceptible infants.[169] Mutants defective in capsular polysaccharide synthesis were cleared efficiently in a murine model.[171] The finding that group B streptococcal subpopulations with low buoyant density produce higher amounts of type-specific capsular polysaccharide and are more resistant to phagocytic killing than high-density variants also corroborates this concept as does the identification of a group of genetically related organisms with increased capsule production that causes the majority of invasive type III disease.[172]

Group B streptococci synthesize acylated (lipoteichoic) and deacylated glycerol teichoic acids that are cell associated and can be readily extracted and purified.[155] Strains from infants with early- or late-onset disease have higher levels of cell-associated and native deacylated lipoteichoic acid,[155] and this product may be the major cell-associated material responsible for attachment to human cells.[173, 174]

EPIDEMIOLOGY AND TRANSMISSION

Historically, *S. agalactiae* was known to cause bovine mastitis rather than human perinatal infection. When the organism became recognized as a human pathogen, epidemiologic studies examined whether bovine and human strains were biologically related and whether transmission from bovine sources to humans might occur.

Employing cultural, physiologic, and serologic properties as strain markers, investigators concluded that transmission from cows was exceedingly rare.[4, 71, 72, 74, 109, 175] In addition, during the past three decades when it has been a dominant human pathogen in the United States, the majority of our population has lacked exposure to the two possible modes of transmission: (1) proximity to dairy cattle (direct contact) and (2) ingestion of unpasteurized milk.

Asymptomatic Infection (Colonization) in Adults

Group B streptococcal infection limited to mucous membrane sites has been designated as *asymptomatic infection*, *colonization*, and *carriage*. Direct comparisons of the prevalence of colonization reported in the literature are virtually impossible because of differences in the ascertainment techniques employed for study.[10, 20, 176, 177] Several factors influence the accuracy of detecting colonization in a given population: the choice of bacteriologic media, the body sites sampled, the number of cultures obtained, and the time interval chosen for study. Isolation rates are significantly higher using broth rather than solid agar media, from media containing substances inhibitory for normal flora (usually antibiotics), and from selective broth rather than selective solid agar media.[178, 179] Among selective broth media chosen, Todd-Hewitt broth with gentamicin (4 to 8 μg/ml) or colistin (or polymyxin B) (10 μg/ml) *and* nalidixic acid (15 μg/ml) with or without sheep red blood cells has been the most useful for accurate detection of group B streptococci from genital and rectal cultures.[179, 180] These inhibit the growth of gram-negative enteric bacilli as well as other normal flora that make isolation of streptococci from these sites difficult. Broth media enable detection of low numbers of organisms that fail detection when inoculation of swabs is directly onto solid agar.[44, 45, 47, 49, 178–180]

Isolation rates are influenced by body sites selected for culture. Genital isolation rates from women double as one proceeds from the cervical os to the vulva.[181, 182] In addition, culture sampling of both lower genital tract *and* rectal sites increases group B streptococcal colonization rates 10 to 15% above that found if a single site is cultured.[20, 177, 183, 184] The urinary tract also is an important site of group B streptococcal infection, especially during pregnancy, when infection usually is manifested as asymptomatic bacteriuria.[178, 185, 186] Therefore, to accurately predict the likelihood of neonatal exposure to group B streptococci at delivery, maternal cultures of the lower vagina, vulva, or periurethral area *and* rectum should be collected (see Prevention).

In neonates, selection of optimal body sites for detection of colonization also influences prevalence rates. In the first 24 hours of life, external auditory canal cultures are more likely to yield group B streptococci than those from anterior nares, throat, umbilicus, or rectum[6, 9, 11, 183, 187]; and isolation of organisms from the ear canal is probably a measure of the degree of contamination from amniotic fluid and vaginal secretions sequestered during the birth process. After the first 48 hours of life, throat and rectal sites are the most common sources of group

B streptococci,[11, 187–189] and positive cultures indicate true colonization (multiplication of organisms at mucous membrane sites), not just maternal contamination. Beyond the neonatal period, throat and rectal sites continue to be the most common foci for group B streptococcal colonization, and this persists until the onset of sexual activity, when the genitourinary tract becomes a common site of colonization in both sexes.[10, 20, 190–196]

The prevalence of group B streptococcal colonization also is influenced by the number of cultures obtained from a single site and the interval during which these are collected in an individual patient. In a longitudinal study of 382 patients followed with sequential cultures of one body site (lower vagina) throughout pregnancy, 36% of 108 culture-positive women had chronic, 20% transient, 15% intermittent, and 29% indeterminant carriage of group B streptococci.[197] Other longitudinal studies found nearly one half of women vaginally colonized at delivery had negative antenatal cultures.[183, 198] In a longitudinal study of 5586 pregnant women, two thirds of whom were cultured initially during the second trimester, Boyer and associates found that the overall predictive value of a positive prenatal vaginal *or* rectal culture for colonization at delivery was 67%.[199] The predictive value of a positive prenatal culture was highest (73%) in women colonized at vaginal *and* rectal sites and lowest (60%) in those with rectal colonization only. Thus, if colonization is to be detected with maximal accuracy on a single occasion, lower vaginal and rectal cultures should be performed. Cultures performed from 1 to 5 weeks before delivery are accurate in predicting group B streptococcal colonization status at delivery in term parturients. Within this interval, the positive predictive value is 87% (95% confidence interval, 83–92%) and the negative predictive value is 96% (95% confidence interval, 95–98%). Cultures collected within this interval performed significantly better than those collected 6 or more weeks before delivery.[200]

The primary reservoir for group B streptococci is the lower gastrointestinal tract.[6, 46] Studies documenting the recovery of group B streptococci from the rectum alone three to five times more commonly than from the vagina alone,[184, 187] of a rectal-to-vaginal isolation ratio exceeding one,[184, 187, 199] and of the rectum as the site most accurately predicting persistence[184] or chronicity of carriage[186] support the importance of obtaining rectal cultures to define maternal carriage during pregnancy. Fecal carriage or rectal colonization with group B streptococci occurs in patients ranging in age from 1 day[201] to 70 to 80 years,[202] although rates are highest in adults.[201] Additional compelling evidence supporting the intestine as the primary reservoir of colonization by group B streptococci includes their isolation from the small intestine of adults[203] and their association with infections resulting from surgery of the upper or lower intestinal tract.[204] Rectal colonization also may contribute to the importance of group B streptococci as a urinary tract pathogen and for the resistance of genital tract colonization to eradication by antibiotics.[205, 206]

Group B streptococci are common constituents of the genital microflora at delivery, and the prevalence of colonization in a given population is similar for each trimester of gestation.[5, 9, 177, 178, 197, 198] Pregnancy does influence colonization rates, but few data are available for matched populations of pregnant and nonpregnant women.[20, 193] Several factors have been assessed for their possible influence on genital carriage in women. In one study of 499 college women, group B streptococci were isolated significantly more often from sexually experienced women, women studied during the first half of the menstrual cycle, those with an intrauterine device, and women 20 years of age or younger. The day of menstrual cycle and use of an intrauterine device probably increased rates of isolation by providing a local environment that increased the inoculum size, thus improving detection of organisms with a single culture. Both factors have been associated by others with higher colonization rates in nonpregnant women.[20, 207, 208]

A higher prevalence of colonization with group B streptococci has been found among pregnant diabetic patients than among controls.[209, 210] Prolonged carriage (over a 3-year interval) has been reported significantly more often in women who use tampons than in women who do not.[211] Colonization also appears to be more frequent among teenage women than those 20 years of age or older,[197, 198] and among women with three or fewer pregnancies than in those with more than three.[197, 198, 212] Ethnicity is related to colonization rates. In one large multicenter U.S. pregnancy study, colonization rates were highest in Hispanics of Caribbean origin, followed by African Americans, whites, and other Hispanics (predominantly Mexicans).[212] In another recent multicenter U.S. study, African Americans were significantly more likely to have group B streptococcal colonization at delivery than either whites or Hispanics.[213] Women of African-American ethnicity also are more likely to have a high inoculum of vaginal group B streptococcal colonization than are Hispanic women.[214]

Factors that do not influence the prevalence of genital colonization in nonpregnant women include use of oral contraceptives[193]; marital status; frequency of sexual intercourse or increasing number of sexual partners[192, 193, 212]; presence of vaginal discharge or other gynecologic symptoms[192, 193]; carriage of *Chlamydia trachomatis, Ureaplasma urealyticum, Trichomonas vaginalis,* or *Mycoplasma hominis*[212]; or infection with *Neisseria gonorrhoeae.*[181, 192]

Asymptomatic infection of the genital or lower gastrointestinal tract with group B streptococci occurs in men as well as in women (Table 26–1). Among sexual partners of genitally colonized women, urethral isolation of group B streptococci can be found in at least one half.[5, 20, 181, 194] This observation and those indicating that genital isolation rates are significantly greater in sexually active than in virgin women[193] and in patients attending venereal disease clinics than in those attending other outpatient facilities[181, 192, 216] led to the recognition that group B streptococci are sexually transmissible.[5, 10, 20, 177, 192, 194, 216] Phage-typing techniques have confirmed that several partners may carry identical strains. By contrast to agents such as *N. gonorrhoeae* or genital mycoplasmas, genital infection with group B streptococci is not related to number of sexual partners, promiscuity, or genital symptoms.[192, 193, 221]

Group B streptococci have been isolated from genital or lower gastrointestinal tract cultures or both of 15 to 40% of pregnant women (Table 26–2). These variations in colonization rates relate not only to intrinsic differences in populations (age, parity, socioeconomic status, geographic location) but also to lack of standardization in culture methods employed for study. True population differences also account for some of the disparity in these reported prevalence rates. When selective broth media is used and vagina and rectum are cultured, the overall prevalence of maternal colonization with group B streptococci by region is 12% in India and Pakistan, 19% in Asia and the Pacific, 19% in sub-Saharan Africa, 22% in the Middle East/North Africa, 14% in Central and South America, and 26% in the United

TABLE 26–1
Group B Streptococcal Colonization Rates in Diverse Populations of Women and Men

	SITE CULTURED	PREVALENCE RATES (%)	REPRESENTATIVE REFERENCE NO.
Pregnant women	Throat	2–5	5, 6, 9, 197, 198, 215
	Genital	2–29	2–6, 9, 11, 183, 197, 199, 215–219
	Rectal	16–22	46, 179, 199
Private care	Genital	7–18	183, 198, 216
Public care	Genital	11–27	6, 197, 215, 218
Nonpregnant women	Throat	3–12	6, 9, 47
	Genital	7–29	5, 6, 9, 181, 193
	Rectal	17–27	45, 46, 179
Venereal disease clinic enrollment	Genital	11–37	182, 192, 193, 216, 220, 221
	Rectal	24–40	220, 221
Heterosexual men	Throat	4–11	47, 218, 222
	Urethra	2–26	181, 192, 216
Homosexual men	Throat	19	223
	Urethra	23	223

TABLE 26–2
Group B Streptococcal Genital Colonization Rates in Geographically Diverse Populations of Women

COUNTRY	SITE(S) CULTURED	PREVALENCE RATES (%)[a]	REFERENCE NO.
Brazil	Vagina	18.6 [25.6]	224
Canada	Vagina	7.6–11.6	182
China	Endocervix, perineum, and rectum[b]	19.0	225
Colombia	Vagina, rectum, and throat	2	226
England	Vagina	10.5 [20]	227
Fiji	Cervix, vagina	2	228
India	Endocervix and vagina	5.8	229
Ireland	Vagina, perianal	25.6	230
Israel	Vagina or cervix	10.3	231
Italy	Cervix, vagina	6.0, 7.3 [7.5]	232
Japan	Vagina	2.9	233
Jordan	Vagina, rectum, and urine	30	234
Libya	Vagina	5	235
Mexico	Vagina, cervix	10	236, 237
Netherlands	Vagina, cervix	7.9, 6.3 [13.9]	187
Nigeria	Vagina	19.5	219
Peru	Cervix	6	238
Saudi Arabia	Vagina	5.1–9.2 [13.9]	239, 240
Scotland	Cervix and urethra	16	241
Spain	Vagina and/or rectum[b]	11.5	242
Thailand	Genital	6	243
The Gambia	Vagina and rectum	22	244
Trinidad	Vagina and rectum	31.4	245
United States	Vagina and rectum	25–28	212, 213, 246

[a]Overall carrier rate, multiple sites, given in brackets.
[b]Not specified by site positive.

States.[246, 247] The prevalence of pharyngeal colonization among pregnant and nonpregnant women and heterosexual men is similar[6, 47, 222]; however, it approaches nearly 20% in homosexual men.[223] No definite relationship between isolation of group B streptococci from throat cultures of adults or children with symptoms of pharyngitis has been proved,[248] but some have suggested that these organisms can produce acute pharyngitis.[222, 249]

Asymptomatic Infection in Infants and Children

The prevalence of group B streptococcal colonization in children appears to differ from that of adults. In a study of 100 girls between 2 months and 16 years of age, Hammerschlag and co-workers[190] isolated group B streptococci from cultures of lower vaginal, rectal, or pharyngeal sites or all three sites in 20%. Although the prevalence of positive pharyngeal cultures in girls 11 years of age or older (5%) was similar to that reported for women, that in younger girls (15%) resembled that reported for neonates.[6, 11, 188, 189] Rectal colonization was detected frequently in girls younger than 3 or older than 10 years of age (about 25%) but was uncommon in those between 3 and 10 years of age. In a similar study of prepubertal boys and girls, Mauer and colleagues[191] isolated group B streptococci from cultures of vaginal, anal, or pharyngeal areas or all three in 11% of patients. Pharyngeal (5% each) and rectal (10 and 7%) isolation rates were similar for boys and girls, respectively. Persson and co-workers[201] detected a lower (4%) rate of fecal carriage of group B streptococci among healthy boys and girls, and Cummings and Ross[250] found that only 2% of English schoolchildren had pharyngeal carriage of group B streptococci. Thus, the gastrointestinal tract is the most frequent site for carriage during infancy and childhood in both boys and girls, and genital colonization in girls is uncommon before puberty.[191, 192, 251, 252] Whether the latter finding is related to environmental influences in the prepubertal vagina or to lack of sexual experience before puberty or both awaits further study.

Transmission of Group B Streptococci to Neonates

The presence of group B streptococci in the maternal genital tract at delivery is a significant determinant of colonization and infection in the neonate. Exposure of the neonate to the organism occurs either by the ascending route in utero through ruptured membranes or by contamination during passage through the birth canal. Prospective studies have indicated vertical transmission rates of 29 to 85%, with a mean rate of approximately 50% (Table 26–3), among neonates born to women who at delivery have had group B streptococci isolated from cultures of vagina or rectum or both. Conversely, only about 5% of infants delivered of culture-negative women become asymptomatically infected at one or more sites during the first 48 hours of life.

TABLE 26–3
Transmission of Group B Streptococci to Neonates from Maternal or Nosocomial Sources

REFERENCE NO.	LOCATION	MATERNAL COLONIZATION AT DELIVERY (%)	COLONIZED NEONATES BORN TO MOTHERS COLONIZED AT DELIVERY[a] (%)	COLONIZED NEONATES BORN TO NONCOLONIZED MOTHERS (%)	NEONATES COLONIZED FROM NOSOCOMIAL SOURCE (%)
6	Houston	22.5	72	12	ND
218	Arkansas	16.0	57	0	~27[b]
183	Minneapolis	8.3	50	1	ND
9	Palm Beach	28.7	71	27	10
188	Houston	27.7	65	ND	~43[b]
11	Birmingham	19.0	47	3	ND
189	Los Angeles	28.8	63	9	ND
198	Houston	20.4	42	1.2	0
213	Houston	28.0	54	4.9	ND
217	Minneapolis	8.0	67	ND	ND
253	Atlanta	23.2	58	ND	13
254	Dallas	26.6	50	ND	ND
224	Brazil	25.6	55	ND	ND
229	India	5.8	56	0	ND
232	Italy	7.1	45	2.1	ND
219	Nigeria	19.5	29	4.4	ND
255	Pakistan	24.0	85	9	ND
241	Scotland	2.9	33	1.3	ND
256	Spain	ND	69	5.6	ND
257	Turkey	8.2	67	0	ND
258	London	15.0	35	4.7	22.2
259	London	15.0	43	4.2	17.8

[a]Time of newborn culture collection varied from <30 minutes after birth to 48–72 hours of age in these studies; therefore, rates of colonization depended on maternal inoculum when assessment was performed shortly after birth.
[b]Exact data are not listed.
ND = not determined.

The risk of a neonate acquiring colonization by the vertical route has been directly correlated to the intensity of maternal genital infection (inoculum size). Neonates born to heavily colonized women are more likely to acquire carriage at mucous membrane sites than those born to women with low colony counts of group B streptococci in vaginal cultures at delivery.[11, 217] Boyer and associates[199] found that rates of vertical transmission were substantially higher in women who had heavy compared with light colonization (65 vs. 17%) and that infants born to heavily colonized mothers were more likely to be colonized at multiple sites and to develop early-onset disease.

The likelihood of colonization in a neonate born to a woman culture-positive at delivery is unrelated to maternal age, race, parity, blood type, duration of labor, or method of delivery.[5, 6, 179, 188, 217, 225] Whether preterm or low-birth-weight neonates are at higher risk for colonization from maternal sources than term infants remains unclear.

Most neonates have group B streptococcal infection that is limited to surface or mucous membrane sites. This results from contamination of the oropharynx, gastric contents, or gastrointestinal tract by swallowing of infected amniotic fluid or maternal vaginal secretions. Infants asymptomatically colonized from a maternal source have persistence of infection at mucous membrane sites for weeks.[20, 188, 252] The distribution of serotypes of group B streptococcal isolates from mothers and neonates is comparable.

Besides exposure during birth, other sources for group B streptococcal colonization in the neonate have been established. Horizontal transmission from hospital[9, 188, 189, 253, 258–260] or community[188, 189] sources to neonates is an important, albeit less frequent, mode for transmission of infection. Cross-contamination from maternally infected to uninfected neonates can occur via hands of nursery personnel.[258] Unlike group A streptococci, which can produce epidemic disease in nurseries, group B streptococci rarely exhibit this potential, and isolation of neonates with positive skin, umbilical, throat, or gastric cultures is not indicated. An epidemic cluster of five infants with late-onset bacteremic infection related to type Ib group B *Streptococcus* has been observed among very low birth weight infants in a neonatal intensive care unit. Noya and associates[261] showed that none of the index cases was colonized at birth, establishing that nosocomial acquisition had occurred. Phage typing identified two overlapping patterns of susceptibility believed to represent a single epidemic strain. Epidemiologic analysis suggested infant-to-infant spread by means of the hands of personnel, although acquisition from two nurses colonized with the same phage type serotype Ib strain was not excluded. The control measures instituted prevented additional cases. This and other reports[218, 253, 258] indicate that, during an outbreak, cohorting of culture-positive infants and enforcing hand washing and gloving for infant contact significantly diminish nosocomial acquisition.

Another potential source for transmission of group B streptococci to the neonate is the community. Indirect evidence has suggested that this mode of infection occurs infrequently,[188, 198, 241, 258] and Gardner and co-workers[262] found that only 2 of 46 neonates culture-negative for group B streptococci when discharged from the newborn nursery had acquired mucous membrane infection at 2 months of age. Presumably, the mode of transmission is fecal-oral. Whether acquired by vertical or horizontal modes, infection of mucous membrane sites in neonates usually persists for weeks or months.[188, 251, 253, 263]

Serotype Distribution of Isolates

The differentiation of group B streptococcal strains into serotypes based on capsular polysaccharide or cell wall protein antigens has provided an invaluable tool in defining the epidemiology of human infection. In the 1970s and 1980s virtually all studies in which a large number of group B streptococcal strains were isolated from asymptomatic neonates, children, or adults revealed an even distribution into serotypes I, II, and III. This distribution also was reported for isolates from neonates with early-onset infection without meningitis.[25, 90, 177, 264–267] As late as 1990, serotypes other than I, II, or III accounted for less than 5% of isolates.

Since 1992, a number of reports from hospitals representing diverse regions throughout the United States have documented the emergence of serotype V as a frequent cause of colonization and invasive disease.[27–32, 268] The serotype distribution of group B streptococcal strains isolated from different patient groups from 1992 through 1998 is graphically summarized in Figure 26–4. In two reports, type V has been the predominant serotype among invasive isolates from nonpregnant adults.[28, 29] It also is responsible for a substantial proportion of early-onset disease and of infections among pregnant women. Serotype III strains, which account for approximately 90% of isolates from infants with meningitis, continue to be isolated from approximately two thirds of infants with late-onset disease. The emergence of type V is not due to a new pulsed-field gel electrophoresis clone. However, the majority of type V isolates do have one subtype pattern that has been present in the United States since 1975.[31] Serotypes VI, VII, and VIII rarely cause human disease in the United States, but one report indicates that types VI and VIII are the most common serotypes isolated from healthy Japanese women.[269]

Molecular Epidemiology

Epidemiologic investigation of group B streptococcal infections was hampered for many years by the lack of a discriminatory typing system.[270] Initial investigations employed phage-typing in combination with serologic classification to differentiate between infant acquisition of group B streptococci from maternal or nosocomial sources.[258, 271] This technique proved useful in determining the source of infection in the nursery environment.[253, 261, 272, 273] Although plasmids have been described in a few group B streptococci,[274] their usefulness as epidemiologic markers is limited.

More recently, multilocus enzyme electrophoresis,[275–277] restriction enzyme fragment length polymorphism analysis (RFLP), pulsed field gel electrophoresis (PFGE),[278] and a random-amplified polymorphic DNA (RAPD) assay[279] have been employed for molecular characterization of group B streptococcal isolates associated with human disease. RFLP analysis has indicated that some geographically and epidemiologically distinct isolates have identical patterns, suggesting dissemination of a limited number of clones.[280] These techniques have shown the molecular relatedness of mother-infant and twin-twin strains[270, 279] and have documented mother-to-infant transmission associated with ingestion of infected mother's milk.[280] Compared with conventional electrophoresis, PFGE generates more easily defined patterns with fewer and better separated bands.[278] Although additional study will be required to define their role for subspecies strain differentiation, it is clear that PFGE and RAPD have distinct advantages over some of the previously employed typing schemes.

Incidence of Infection in Neonates and Parturients

Two clinical syndromes occur among young infants with symptomatic group B streptococcal infection. These are epidemiologically distinct and relate to age at onset.[5, 281] The usual attack rates reported for the first, designated early-onset because it appears within the first 6 days of life (mean onset, 12–18 hours), have varied from 0.7 to 3.7 per 1000 live births (Table 26–4). The attack rates for late-onset infection (7 or more days of age) have ranged from 0.5 to 1.8 per 1000. A multistate active surveillance system with an aggregate population of 10.1 million persons in 1990 reported an incidence of 1.4 and 0.3 per 1000 live births for early- and late-onset disease, respectively.[285] The incidence of disease was significantly higher among African Americans than whites. The crude incidence was higher among white Hispanics than among the non-Hispanic white population. The multistate surveillance findings are in accord with a cohort study conducted in Atlanta indicating a higher risk for early- or late-onset disease among African-American infants than among those of other ethnic origins.[26] There was a statistically significant decline in the incidence of early-onset disease in some surveillance areas from 1993 to 1995.[288] The rates for late-onset and adult disease remained stable during the same interval. This decline occurred in association with the implementation of measures to prevent early-onset infection by interrupting mother-to-infant transmission. A more recent report from the same surveillance sites indicated that geographic areas in which a higher proportion of hospitals had prevention policies had significantly lower incidences of early-onset group B streptococcal disease.[289] The incidence of early-onset disease has decreased by

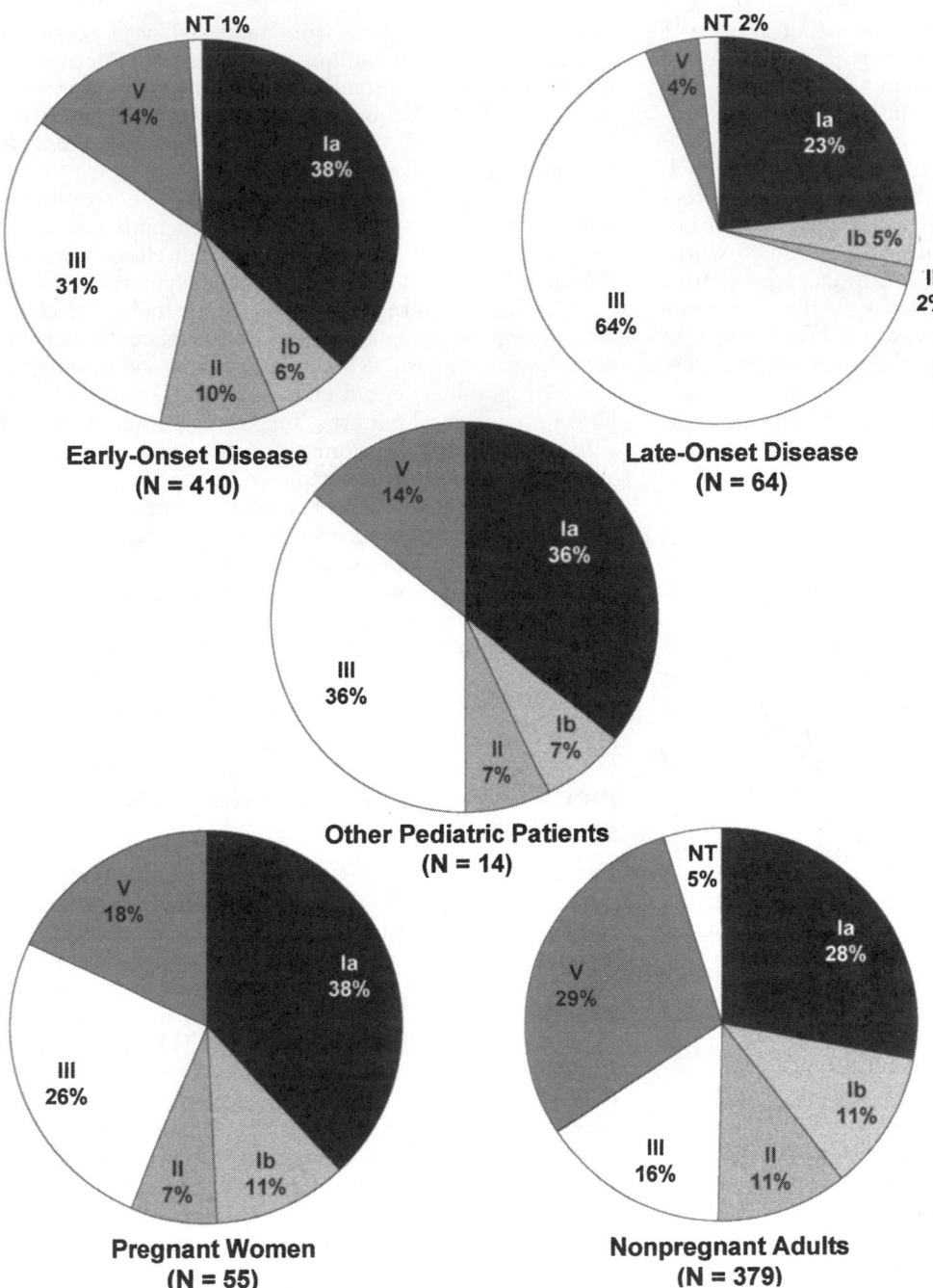

Early-Onset Disease
(N = 410)

NT 1%
V 14%
Ia 38%
III 31%
Ib 6%
II 10%

Late-Onset Disease
(N = 64)

NT 2%
V 4%
Ia 23%
Ib 5%
II 2%
III 64%

Other Pediatric Patients
(N = 14)

V 14%
Ia 36%
III 36%
Ib 7%
II 7%

Pregnant Women
(N = 55)

V 18%
Ia 38%
III 26%
Ib 11%
II 7%

Nonpregnant Adults
(N = 379)

NT 5%
Ia 28%
V 29%
Ib 11%
II 11%
III 16%

FIGURE 26–4 Schematic representation of group B streptococcal serotypes isolated from a variety of patient groups. NT = nontypable strains; ( ) = number of patient isolates studied. (Taken from data in refs. 27, 28, 29, and 246.)

65% from 1993 to 1998, from 1.7 to 0.6 per 1000 live births. It is estimated that 3900 early-onset infections and 200 neonatal deaths were prevented in 1998 by the use of intrapartum antibiotics.[35a]

The male:female ratio in both early- and late-onset group B streptococcal infection is nearly equal. Twenty to 25% of all infants with group B streptococcal disease have onset after 1 week of age. When attack rates for early-onset group B streptococcal disease are stratified by birth weight, the highest rates occur in lower birth weight categories.[25, 290–292] However, full-term infants still account for approximately three fourths of early-onset cases.

The importance of group B streptococci as a common

pathogen for the perinatal period includes the pregnant woman as well as her infant. Recent multistate surveillance data indicate that 10 to 15% of invasive group B streptococcal disease occurs in pregnant women.[26, 285] In addition to their role in infections such as chorioamnionitis and urinary tract infection, group B streptococci have been isolated from 20% of women with postpartum endometritis, and some authors estimate that 45,000 cases occur annually in the United States.[15, 17, 293, 294] Furthermore, group B streptococci are the second most common cause of bacteremia after cesarean section, accounting for 20 to 25% of cases, or in excess of 3000 cases annually.[15, 16, 20, 294] Pass and associates[295] estimated that the attack rate for puerperal sepsis related to group

TABLE 26–4
Attack Rates for Group B Streptococcal Disease in Infants

YEAR OF STUDY	LOCATION	ATTACK RATE PER 1000 FOR BACTEREMIC EARLY-ONSET INFECTION (LATE-ONSET RATE)	RATIO OF MATERNAL COLONIZATION AT DELIVERY TO NEONATAL INVASIVE DISEASE	REFERENCE NO.
1971	Denver	2.0	23:1[a]	5
1972	Houston	2.9	78:1	6
1972	Palm Beach	3.4	85:1	9
1976	Los Angeles	3.0 (1.6)[b]	100:1	10
1977	Birmingham	3.7 (1.7)	51:1	11
1978	Houston	2.3	102:1	20, 281
1977–1981	Dallas	1.2 (0.5)	225:1	254, 282
1978–1983	Birmingham	1.8 (1.8)	111:1	25
1982–1984	Madrid	0.7	164:1	242
1980–1989	Houston	2.1	175:1	283
1985–1994	Norway	0.4[b]	ND	284
1990	Multistate (USA)	1.4 (0.3)	ND	285
1991–1992	Multistate (USA)	1.8	ND	286
1992–1994	Australia	3.3 (0.1)	ND	287
1993–1995	Multistate (USA)	1.7 (0.5) (1993)	ND	288
		1.3 (0.5) (1995)	ND	288
1996	Multistate (USA)	0.6–1.8	ND	289

[a]Calculated from literature review.
[b]Based on surveys carried out during the first 25 months of 41-month study.
ND = not done.

B streptococci was 2 per 1000 deliveries. Cesarean section appears to enhance significantly the risk for bacteremia. Others have also shown that colonization with group B streptococci substantially increased the occurrence of post–cesarean section morbidity manifested as fever, endometritis, and bacteremia[296] as well as the overall frequency of pelvic infection in the puerperium.[297] Postpartum endometritis occurs with a frequency of 2.0%, and clinically diagnosed intra-amniotic infection occurs in 2.9% of women vaginally colonized with group B streptococci at the time of delivery. The risk of intra-amniotic infection was greater when associated with heavy colonization.[298]

IMMUNOLOGY AND PATHOGENESIS

Risk Factors for Early-Onset Infection

A number of factors increase infant risk for early-onset group B streptococcal infection. These are summarized in Table 26–5. The most obvious risk determinant is

TABLE 26–5
Risk Factors for Early-Onset Group B Streptococcal Disease

RISK FACTOR	REPRESENTATIVE REFERENCE NO.
Maternal colonization at delivery	6, 25, 193
High density of maternal colonization	11, 199, 217
Rupture of membranes before onset of labor	11, 286, 299
Preterm delivery	286
Prolonged rupture of membranes	11, 286, 299–301
Chorioamnionitis	302
Intrapartum fever	286
Intrauterine monitoring	286
Maternal postpartum bacteremia	17
Twin pregnancy	303, 304
Group B streptococcal bacteriuria or urinary tract infection	178, 286
Cesarean section	3, 10, 11, 177, 183
Low level of antibody to infecting serotype	305
African-American race	26, 285, 286
Young maternal age (<20 years)	286
Prior infant with group B streptococcal infection	303, 304

maternal colonization at delivery. Risk for penetration of infant mucous membrane barriers with resultant bacteremia directly correlates with maternal genital inoculum.[11, 25, 190, 217, 260, 306] Only 1 to 2% of neonates born to colonized women develop symptomatic early-onset septicemia. This rate is considerably increased if there is premature onset of labor (<37 weeks' gestation) (15%),[11] chorioamnionitis or interval between rupture of membranes and delivery longer than 18 hours (11%),[2, 3, 11, 272, 300, 301] twin pregnancy (35%),[303, 304] or maternal postpartum bacteremia (10%).[17] Given that the presence of group B streptococci in the mother is a prerequisite for fetal risk, the pathogenesis of early-onset infection is influenced by a number of factors that influence neonatal host-parasite interactions (Fig. 26–5).

The inverse relationship between duration of interval between membrane rupture and delivery and age at onset of symptoms of group B streptococcal bacteremia indicates that continuing exposure in utero by the ascending route increases risk for disseminated infection.[300] Amniotic fluid supports the proliferation of group B streptococci,[307] although some strains replicate more efficiently than others.[308] Fetal aspiration of infected amniotic fluid hours to a few days before delivery results in a continuum of intrapartum (still births) to early postpartum infant deaths.[2, 3, 11, 308–312] The attack rate of early-onset disease also has been related directly to interval between membrane rupture and delivery. In one study, when the duration was less than or equal to 18 hours, the attack rate was 0.7 per 1000 live births; when it was more than 30 hours, the attack rate increased to 18.3 per 1000.[301] Women who report a history of urinary tract infection are more likely to be delivered of infants with group B streptococcal infection. Group B streptococcal bacteriuria is a surrogate for high inoculum of colonization, which is a known risk

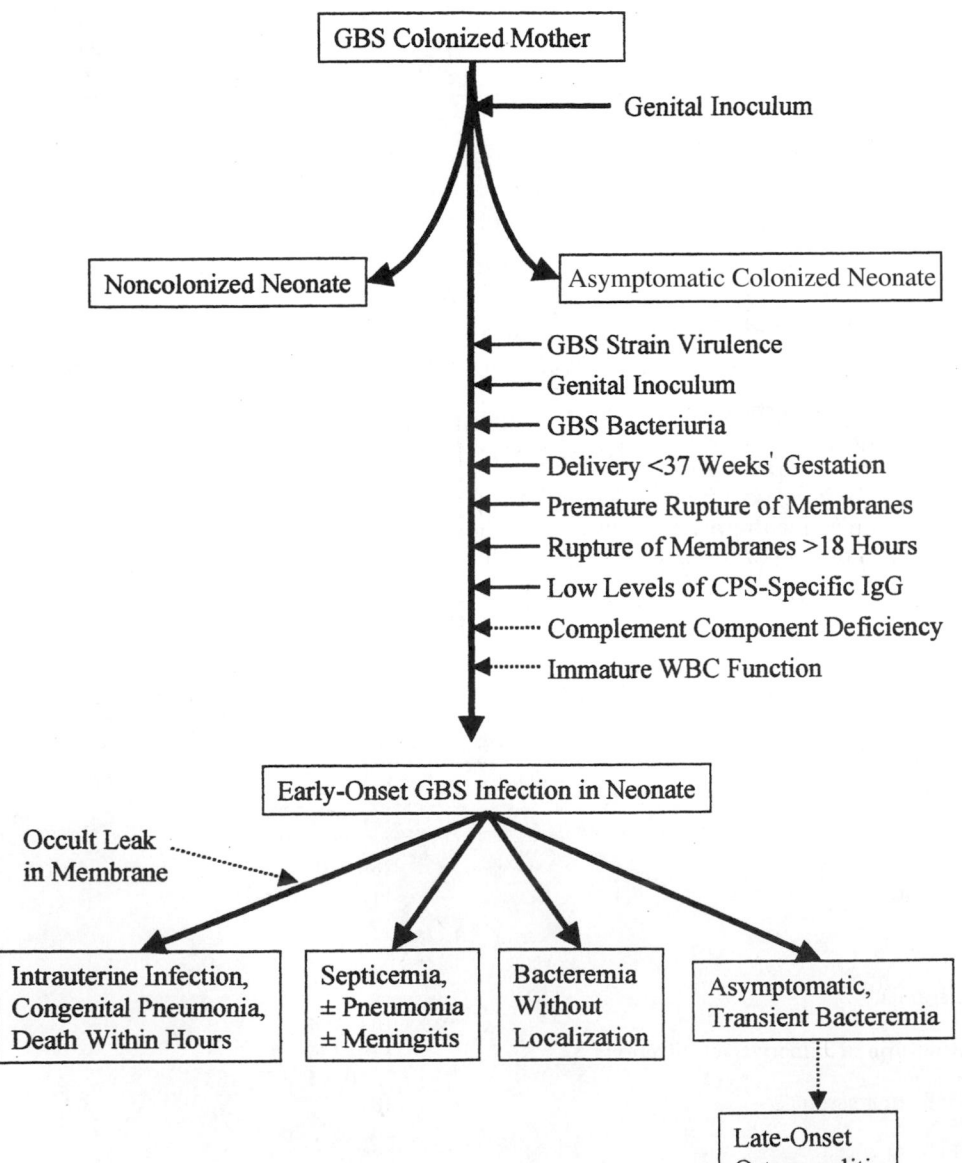

FIGURE 26–5 Hypothetical scheme of the pathogenesis of early-onset group B streptococcal (GBS) infection. → = strong evidence; ⚫⚫⚫→ = suggestive evidence.

factor.[286, 313] There is evidence supporting the hypothesis that ascending infection may be a primary pathogenetic event initiating membrane rupture and preterm labor.[314, 315] A significant correlation between the occurrence of group B streptococcal bacteriuria during pregnancy and rupture of membranes before the onset of labor supports the hypothesis that group B streptococci may cause disruption of the membranes, which leads to preterm delivery.[178] Regan and associates found that heavy group B streptococcal colonization in the second trimester of pregnancy was associated with increased risk of delivering a preterm, low-birth-weight infant.[316] Among infants born to mothers with premature rupture of membranes at term gestation, maternal chorioamnionitis and colonization with group B streptococci are predictors of neonatal infection.[317] Vaginal colonization with group B streptococci also is an independent risk factor for the development of chorioamnionitis.[318] Fulminant early-onset infection also can occur in infants delivered by cesarean section with ostensibly intact membranes[319] and in many with no known maternal factors predisposing to neonatal septicemia.[10, 20, 281] The presence of pulmonary symptoms and abnormal chest radiographs at birth, the maturity of the inflammatory changes in the lungs at autopsy, and the occurrence of death in the first few hours after birth all suggest ascending infection through intact membranes or membranes with microscopic tears. The suggestion that many infections may occur through intact membranes has been substantiated by clinical and pathologic evidence.[11, 301, 309–312, 319–321]

Group B streptococcal infection may begin in utero or during transit through the birth canal. In the prospective study of Pass and co-workers,[11] cases of sepsis resulting from intrauterine exposure and intrapartum acquisition of group B streptococci were clearly documented. One third to more than one half of infants with early-onset disease are symptomatic at birth or within 4 to 6 hours after delivery.[297, 301, 322] Clinical indicators of in utero acquisition include onset of symptoms within 6 hours of birth and 1-minute Apgar scores less than or equal to 5.[300, 301, 309] Among 19 neonates with histologic evidence of congenital pneumonia and isolation of group B streptococci from lung and premortem blood cultures, 95% were ill at or within 6 hours of birth and 84% had Apgar scores less than or equal to 5. By contrast, among 22 infants with early-onset septicemia without congenital pneumonia, only 36% had symptoms within 6 hours of birth and 23% had Apgar scores less than or equal to 5.[309]

Although prolonged interval after rupture of membranes (more than 18 hours) before delivery and preterm delivery (<37 weeks' gestation) are often concomitant risk factors in neonates with early-onset group B streptococcal infection, the latter is an independent contributor to neonatal risk, probably from immaturity of host defense mechanisms. It is estimated that the incidence of early-onset group B streptococcal infection is 10 to 15 times higher in premature than term neonates.[9–11, 20, 300, 301] Even when incidence is corrected for preterm gestation (<37 weeks) and low birth weight (<2500 g), Pass and co-workers[303] reported that twin pregnancy was an independent risk factor for invasive early-onset group B streptococcal septicemia. The explanation for this increased risk in twins[303, 304] is undefined but may be related to genetic factors regulating host susceptibility or to virulence of disease-producing strains.

PATHOPHYSIOLOGY OF INFECTION

In an attempt to understand the pathophysiology of early-onset group B streptococcal infection, experimental models of infection have been developed. These have addressed aspects of the pathophysiology of infection that otherwise could not be evaluated. A pregnant rabbit model has been used to document that upper vaginal inoculation with group B streptococci leads to ascending genital tract infection and fetal death.[323] An experimental model of pneumonia was used to show that surfactants used in clinical practice do not accelerate the growth of group B streptococci in the lungs.[324] Similarly, a surfactant protein A–deficient murine model showed the important role of this protein in enhancing clearance from the lung and preventing dissemination of the organism.[325] Live group B streptococci have been shown to injure and invade the lung microvascular endothelium and induce the release of vasoactive mediators.[326]

The hemodynamic consequences of infusion of whole group B streptococci into animals have been examined in detail. These include an early phase characterized by pulmonary hypertension, reduced cardiac output, and hypoxemia that is associated with increased thromboxane B_2 (a stable metabolite of the vasoconstrictor thromboxane A_2), followed by a late phase characterized by a progressive fall in cardiac output, systemic hypotension, granulocytopenia, granulocyte trapping in the lungs, and increased pulmonary vascular permeability.[327–330] This phase is associated with increased serum thromboxane B_2, 6-keto-prostaglandin $F_{1\alpha}$, and tumor necrosis factor-alpha (TNF-α).[331] The initial phase can be prevented by treatment with indomethacin, which inhibits the cyclooxygenase pathway of arachidonic acid metabolism.[332–334] Cyclooxygenase is the enzyme that produces prostaglandin intermediates that are subsequently converted to either pulmonary vasodilators or constrictors. Indomethacin inhibits the synthesis of thromboxane A_2, which is a potent vasoconstrictor, and prostacyclin, a mediator of hyperventilation-induced pulmonary vasodilation.[335] Inhibitors of the lipoxygenase products of arachidonic acid metabolism also can attenuate group B streptococcal–induced pulmonary hypertension.[336] Dazmegrel, a thromboxane synthesis inhibitor, as well as thromboxane receptor blockade also prevent the acute pulmonary hypertension and hypoxemia of the early phase.[337] Experiments with capsule-deficient mutants of types Ib and III group B streptococci indicate that capsular polysaccharide is not required for these serotypes to cause pulmonary hypertension and hypoxemia.[338, 339] Rather, nonencapsulated mutants cause a greater increase in pulmonary artery pressure and resistance than do encapsulated strains, suggesting that subcapsular structures promote the inflammatory response to infection.

The second hemodynamic phase can be attenuated by

the TNF-α inhibitor pentoxifylline,[331, 340] by the effect of combined pentoxifylline and indomethacin pretreatment,[341] and by leukotriene inhibition.[342] Antibodies to TNF-α as well as treatment with interleukin-1 receptor agonist also modify the response.[343, 344] Inhibitors of platelet-activating factor fail to reverse the pulmonary hypotensive response.[345] Dazmegrel elevates pulmonary vascular resistance but does not improve pulmonary gas exchange when administered after infection is established. Methylprednisolone also attenuates the late effects, suggesting that granulocytes may be involved in the production of the vascular injury.[327, 346] However, the findings that granulocytopenia and pulmonary leucostasis are not responses unique to group B streptococci[347] and that injury to vascular endothelium occurs despite granulocyte depletion[348] indicate that the role of granulocytes in the pulmonary response is not fully elucidated. The majority of organisms recovered after infusion of radiolabeled group B streptococci are localized in the lung, followed by the liver and spleen.[349] These organisms are cleared in part through an oxygen radical–dependent mechanism[350]; however, the oxygen radicals derived from cyclooxygenation of arachidonic acid do not contribute to microbicidal activity.[351] In addition, experimental group B streptococcal sepsis is accompanied by decreased mesenteric blood flow, myocardial dysfunction, and diminished diaphragmatic function, which may have a primary role in the pathogenesis of overwhelming infection.[352–356] A role for free oxygen radicals has been shown in the progressive pial arteriolar dilation caused by group B streptococci applied to the surface of the brain of adult rats.[357] Treatment with dimethylthiourea, a selective scavenger of hydroxyl radicals, protects against group B streptococci–induced pulmonary hypertension, edema, and hypoxemia, suggesting that hydroxyl radicals may have a role in the cardiopulmonary disturbances.[358]

Induction of nitric oxide synthase may play an important role in the hypotension and loss of systemic vascular responsiveness that occurs during group B streptococcal sepsis. Inhibition of nitric oxide synthase was shown to reverse hyporesponsiveness in group B streptococci–treated arteries isolated from the mesentery of neonatal piglets.[359] In experimental sepsis, the effect of nitric oxide synthase inhibitors alone worsened pulmonary hypertension and reduced cardiac output in neonatal piglets.[360]

In experimental models of group B streptococcal meningitis, cerebral blood flow changes consist of an early hyperemic phase and a later ischemic phase. There is an early and dramatic rise in TNF-α, suggesting that TNF-α has a role in initiating the inflammatory cascade.[361] Infusions of group B streptococci impair cerebrovascular reactivity and cause two distinct forms of neuronal injury: areas of necrosis in the cortex and apoptotic neuronal injury in the hippocampus.[362, 363] Production of nitric oxide by inducible nitric oxide synthase may ameliorate the extent of cortical neuronal injury by reducing cerebral ischemia.[364]

ANTIBODY TO CAPSULAR POLYSACCHARIDE

Lancefield's studies demonstrated that antibodies directed against the type-specific surface antigens of group B streptococci protected mice from lethal challenge with strains containing these antigens.[82, 83] Baker and Kasper,[305] in 1976, demonstrated that neonates at risk for early- or late-onset group B streptococcal infection with type III strains were those whose mothers had very low concentrations of antibodies to the type III capsular polysaccharide in their serum at delivery. A similar correlation was reported by Hemming and associates[365] for neonates with type II and III early-onset disease. Absent opsonic activity to the infecting strains was associated with a low concentration of these type-specific IgG antibodies in maternal serum or with failure to actively transport sufficient concentrations transplacentally before delivery of a premature infant.[365–371] Extremely premature infants have low total IgG concentrations in their sera because approximately 60% of maternally derived IgG is transported to the fetus during the last 10 weeks of pregnancy.[372]

Using a radioactive antigen-binding assay, Baker and colleagues[373] detected low levels (<1.7 μg/ml) of type III capsular polysaccharide-specific antibodies in sera from each of 32 infants with invasive diseases. Women with type III group B streptococcal genital colonization at delivery whose infants remained well had in excess of 2 μg/ml of type III-specific antibodies significantly more often than women whose infants developed type III early-onset disease. Quantitative determination of antibodies to type III group B streptococcal polysaccharide by enzyme-linked immunosorbent assay (ELISA) indicates that these are predominantly IgG class antibodies.[374, 375]

Capsular type-specific antibodies also are important in the pathogenesis of early-onset infection related to serotypes Ia, Ib, and II.[7, 365, 367, 376] Using ELISA standardized by quantitative precipitation,[377] 1.0, 0.2, and 1.3 μg/ml of IgG antibodies to serotypes Ia, Ib, and III, respectively, were protective in experimental models of infection.[370, 378–380] Among pregnant women at delivery, the prevalence of type-specific IgG antibodies in presumably protective concentrations range from 12 to 20%. However, "protective concentrations" of these antibodies are significantly more likely among women colonized with the homologous group B streptococcal serotype.[370, 380, 381] By contrast, women who deliver infants with invasive type III infection have very low concentrations of specific antibodies in delivery sera.[378, 380, 381] For serotype II infections, Gray and co-workers[382] noted a similar correlation between low concentrations of type II–specific antibodies in maternal delivery sera and susceptibility of some infants to invasive infection. Although human antibody to the group B polysaccharide is immunogenic as in experimental animals, it is *not* protective against invasive infant disease.[383, 384]

Antibodies to the capsular polysaccharides of group B streptococci correlate with in vitro opsonic activity (chemiluminescence[365, 385] and opsonophagocytic assays[120, 373, 385–389]) and with in vivo protection in experimental animal models of infection.[365, 367, 385, 390–393] Furthermore, in an uncontrolled study employing exchange transfusion as adjunctive therapy for early-onset group B streptococcal septicemia, infants receiving fresh donor blood containing type III opsonins in a volume more than or equal to 40% total blood volume were more likely to survive than those who received blood from donors without opsonic activity for type III organisms.[394] The factor or factors that explain the apparent relationship between asymptomatic mucosal infection and acquired specific humoral immunity in adults are unknown. However, whereas the majority of adults and children have very low, presumably nonprotective levels of serotype-specific antibodies in their sera,[190, 366, 370, 381] the pregnant woman most likely to infect her neonate with group B streptococci at birth is also the one who has the greatest probability of passively "immunizing" her infant.[367, 368, 370, 380, 381] These antibodies appear to persist at a given concentration throughout gestation in the overwhelming majority of women.[368]

Although neonates with early-onset type III group B streptococcal sepsis are uniformly deficient in type III–specific antibodies, most neonates born to women with type III genital colonization and low levels of type III antibody in their sera remain well.[366–368] Kim and co-workers[395] demonstrated opsonic and protective activity by cord sera that appeared to be independent of type-specific antibody or complement. Boyer and associates[396] reported that IgM-specific antibody, absent in serum from neonates, was detectable by 3 months of age and exceeded 0.5 µg/ml in all infants after 7 months. They proposed that the development of IgM-specific antibody in infancy may account for the marked decline in type III group B streptococcal infection after early infancy, but this finding has not been confirmed.

Pathogenesis of Late-Onset Infections

The epidemiology and pathogenesis of group B streptococcal infection occurring beyond the first week of life are less well defined than they are for early-onset disease. Although serotype III strains, which account for the majority of isolates from infants with late-onset infection,[7, 10, 11, 90, 264, 265, 397] must be uniquely virulent for the infant between 8 days and 3 months of age,[10, 20] virulence factors in these organisms (other than capsule) and specific host defense mechanisms other than type-specific IgG are incompletely elucidated.

It does not appear that type III strains of group B streptococci have an advantage over other serotypes with respect to acquisition or duration of asymptomatic mucous membrane infection.[5, 6, 9, 11, 183, 188, 189, 218] With the exception of epidemic clustering of cases,[261, 273, 334] acquisition of colonization by the neonate from maternal sources occurs at a frequency for each serotype expected for its prevalence. Duration of asymptomatic infection in colonized infants may be weeks or months irrespective of the serotype of the infecting strain.[188, 262, 263]

Because bacteremia is the presumed first event in the pathogenesis of most late-onset infections, factors that promote the entry of type III strains into the bloodstream are of interest. Baker and colleagues[281] suggested that viral upper respiratory tract infections, a common event just before late-onset meningitis, might alter epithelial cell surfaces in asymptomatically infected infants in a manner that allows type III but not other serotypes

of group B streptococci to enter the bloodstream. Upper respiratory tract infection frequently precedes late-onset meningitis,[3, 7, 281, 398, 399] but the relationship to pathogenesis, if any, has not been established. Of interest, concurrent influenza A virus infection significantly decreased the inoculum of a type Ia strain that produced lethal pulmonary infection in mice, but extrapulmonary dissemination and bacteremia were not observed in this model.[400]

Another possible virulence factor for type III strains is their ability to elaborate high levels of type-specific capsular polysaccharide antigen. Type III strains that produce high quantities of type III polysaccharide are more virulent in mice than are low producers,[168, 170] and mean values of capsule produced in supernatant fluid from infants with late-onset bacteremia or meningitis were significantly greater than those of type III strains from asymptomatically colonized infants or adults.[168] The finding of Rubens and colleagues[401] that a transposon mutant lacking surface expression of the type III capsule but not of the group B–specific polysaccharide lost virulence in a neonatal rat model substantiates the importance of the type III capsule as a virulence factor. The relationship between virulence and the relative amount of capsule when compared with other serotypes of group B streptococci or the potential effect of its extracellular elaboration has not been investigated in detail.

Early reports suggested that the presence of sialic acid in the type III capsular polysaccharide might account for the ability of strains of this serotype to penetrate the blood-brain barrier of the young infant.[127, 265] Among type III strains, those causing invasive infection and those more resistant to opsonization have greater amounts of cell-associated sialic acid than colonizing isolates or those strains easily opsonized by human sera.[402, 403] Wessels and associates[404] constructed a transposon mutant of type III group B *Streptococcus* that expresses a capsular polysaccharide differing from the wild type only in that the capsule of the mutant lacks sialic acid. Expression of an asialo capsular polysaccharide was associated with loss of virulence in a neonatal rat model of lethal infection. These observations demonstrated directly the role of capsular sialic acid as a critical determinant of virulence for type III group B *Streptococcus* and supports the hypothesis that surface sialylation aids in their evasion from host defense. For example, the asialo mutant adheres more avidly to epithelial cells and is phagocytosed more readily by neutrophils than the parent strain.[405] Molecular analysis of the region of the chromosome involved in type III capsule expression has been undertaken.[406, 407] Studies have identified a genetic locus essential for capsule sialylation.[408]

Some type III strains may possess additional, as yet not elucidated, characteristics potentiating their virulence. For example, a platelet-aggregating or "clumping factor" reaction influenced by type-specific antibody[409] has been identified in some type III strains that induced disseminated intravascular coagulation in mice.[410, 411] Protein antigens, such as R-protein, may contribute to the virulence of some type III strains.[412] Finally, the spectrum of disease severity produced by type III strains of group B streptococci in infants more than 7 days of age, from asymptomatic bacteremia to fatal meningitis within a few days' onset from first sign, suggests strain differences in virulence.

As in early-onset infection, low concentrations of antibodies to type III polysaccharide uniformly are found in the acute sera of infants with late-onset type III infection.[305, 365-367] In a study of 28 infants with late-onset bacteremia and 51 with meningitis, Baker and co-workers[373] detected less than 2 μg/ml of antibodies to type III polysaccharide in acute sera from all infants. These low levels of specific antibodies in term infants with late-onset type III group B streptococcal infection correlate with maternal levels at delivery.[366, 373]

It is important to employ antigens with "native" or intact type III polysaccharide specificity in evaluating human immunity to type III group B streptococci.[413, 414] Kasper and colleagues[414] used gently extracted (native) and HCl-treated (core) type III group B streptococcal and pneumococcal type 14 antigens to study sera from infants with invasive type III infection and their mothers. Concentrations of type III–specific antibodies in sera of sick infants and their mothers were uniformly low to "native," or fully sialylated, type III antigen. Concentrations of antibodies to "core," or desialylated, type III and type 14 pneumococcal antigens were similar in all patient sera. Opsonic immunity correlated with antibodies to "native" but not to "core" type III antigen or to type 14 pneumococcal antigen. Infants recovering from type III disease developing a significant increase in antibodies to the intact polysaccharide had no detectable rise to the acid-degraded or core antigen. Thus, human immunity to type III group B streptococci relates to antibodies to capsular type III polysaccharide with an intact protective epitope.[414] An extension of this concept comes from studies in which adults have been immunized with either type III polysaccharide or pneumococcal polysaccharide vaccine.[413-415] Adults with low concentrations of type III antibodies in their sera before immunization responded to type III polysaccharide vaccine with a significant increase in type III–specific antibodies.[415] This response was not observed when the structurally related type 14 pneumococcal polysaccharide was used as an immunizing agent. However, adults with moderate to high levels of antibodies to type III polysaccharide developed significant rises in level of this antibody after pneumococcal polysaccharide vaccine. This suggests that the structurally similar antigen could elicit secondary B cell proliferation in previously primed adults.[415]

Host-Bacterial Interactions Relating to Pathogenesis

The distinctive clinical and epidemiologic characteristics of the early- and late-onset group B streptococcal syndromes in infants serve to emphasize unique factors in their pathogenesis. There also are obvious similarities in the pathogenetic mechanisms of the two syndromes, such as the frequent occurrence of meningeal infection when bacteremia is caused by type III strains and the association of low concentrations of maternal type-spe-

cific antibodies in delivery serum with risk for invasive infant infection. Definition of immune mechanisms that restrict invasive infection to the first months of life are needed to fully understand the pathogenesis of neonatal infection.

ADHERENCE

Adherence of group B streptococci to mucosal surfaces presumably represents the initial event in colonization and invasion. Compared with other bacterial species, group B streptococci adhere efficiently to vaginal epithelial cells and to chorioamnionic membranes.[416-418] Type III strains also adhere to vaginal epithelial cells in vitro better than do other serotypes[419] and also to the buccal epithelial cells of neonates.[420] Strains causing neonatal sepsis adhere more avidly than colonizing strains.[421] Attachment occurs rapidly after organisms are exposed to epithelial cells,[422, 423] is pH dependent,[423, 424] and does not require bacterial viability.[423] The study of Jelínková and associates[425] provides evidence for strain-dependent differences in adherence and against specific tissue tropism. A number of strains adhere spontaneously to neonatal cord blood lymphocytes and promote lymphocyte proliferation.[426]

Several potential adhesins mediating attachment to epithelial surfaces have been proposed. Based on inhibition studies, Ofek and co-workers[427] and others[155, 173, 174, 428-430] have suggested that lipoteichoic acid may be a binding ligand. Group B streptococci isolated from infants with invasive disease have higher lipoteichoic acid content than do strains from asymptomatically colonized infants. Ayoub and Swingle[431] proposed that sialic acid masks a non–lipoteichoic acid cell wall–associated adhesin, a finding supported by the work of Jones and Menna.[432] Others suggest that the adhesin is a protein.[433-439] Wibawan and colleagues found an association between surface hydrophobicity and the adherence of group B streptococci to epithelial cells.[436] Removal of sialic acid enhanced and pronase treatment reduced surface hydrophobicity.

INVASION

Direct invasion of immortalized respiratory epithelial cell lines by type III group B streptococci has been demonstrated in vitro.[440] Bacterial protein, DNA, and RNA synthesis were required. Group B streptococcal beta-hemolysin expression correlates with lung epithelial cell injury and may be important in early events in the pathogenesis of early-onset disease.[441] Epithelial cell invasiveness correlates with the source of isolates, with strains causing disease invading more readily than strains obtained from vaginal carriers or colonized neonates.[442] Group B streptococci also invade chorion but not amnion cells at a high rate in vitro, suggesting that the amnion cell layer may be an effective barrier.[443] As to invasion of the meninges, the organism has been demonstrated to enter human brain microvascular endothelial cells, and serotype III strains invade these cells more efficiently than other common serotypes.[444]

MUCOSAL IMMUNE RESPONSE

Genital colonization with group B streptococci may elicit specific antibody responses in cervical secretions. Women with serotype Ia, II, or III rectal or cervical colonization have markedly elevated levels of both IgA and IgG antibodies to the colonizing serotype in their cervical secretions compared with women without group B streptococcal colonization. Elevated amounts of IgA and IgG antibodies to the protein antigen, R4, also have been found in women colonized with type III strains (most type III strains contain R4 antigen) compared with noncolonized women.[445, 446] These findings suggest that a mucosal immune response occurs in response to colonization with group B streptococci. Induction of mucosal antibodies to surface group B streptococcal polysaccharide or protein antigens may prevent genital colonization and thus diminish vertical transmission of infection from mothers to infants.

SERUM OPSONINS

The interactions between antibodies to group B streptococcal capsular polysaccharides and serum complement components have been explored in detail. Shigeoka and co-workers[447] demonstrated that type-specific antibody was required for opsonization of types Ia, II, and III group B streptococci by adult and neonatal sera and that classic complement pathway participation was necessary for maximal opsonization of type I, II, and several type III strains.[448] Capsular type–specific antibodies also facilitate alternative complement pathway–mediated opsonization and phagocytosis of type III group B streptococci.[143] A linear relationship between concentration of type III polysaccharide–specific antibodies and the rate constant of killing of type III strains has been reported.[449] Furthermore, Pincus and colleagues[450] showed that the efficacy of these specific antibodies is determined, at least in part, by the number of antibody molecules that bind to each bacterium.

Opsonic activity against type III group B streptococci has been shown in vitro for IgG subclass 1, 2, and 3 as well as for IgM antibodies.[451–454] Bohnsack and associates[455] demonstrated convincingly that an IgA monoclonal antibody to the type III capsular polysaccharide activated C3 and conferred protection against lethal infection. Type III–specific antibodies also facilitate C3 fragment deposition in the early phases of opsonization, although both encapsulated and genetically derived unencapsulated mutants can deposit C3 and support its degradation.[456] An inverse correlation between extent of encapsulation and C3 deposition by the alternative pathway has been verified.[457]

By contrast to these findings for type III strains, Baker and co-workers[120] demonstrated that clinical isolates of type Ia group B streptococci may be efficiently opsonized, phagocytosed, and killed by neutrophils from healthy adults by the classic complement pathway in the absence of immune globulin. Surface-bound capsular polysaccharide of type Ia strains mediates C1 binding and activation.[458–460] Thus, an intact classic complement pathway is necessary for opsonization of clinical isolates of type Ia group B streptococci.

For type Ib group B streptococci, a role for capsule size and density in modulating C3 deposition has been reported using a whole-bacterial-cell ELISA.[461] Variability among these strains in their capacity for C3 deposition by the alternative pathway also has been shown.[462]

The opsonic requirements of human sera for type II strains of group B streptococci have been delineated,[387–389, 463–465] and the strain-to-strain variability in opsonization of this serotype, originally identified by Shigeoka and associates,[447] has been confirmed. Type II strains possessing α and β components of the C protein antigen are more resistant to opsonization than strains lacking both components.[387] Strains lacking type II polysaccharide but having both components of protein antigen C are readily opsonized. However, neither the presence of the C antigen components nor the concentration of type II polysaccharide–specific antibodies in a serum fully explained all strain variation. Contribution by other opsonically active antigens (e.g., R-proteins) or an IgA-mediated blocking effect may modulate phagocytosis of some type II strains. The latter hypothesis is consistent with the report of Russell-Jones and co-workers,[466] who have shown that the beta antigen of C protein can bind IgA. In fact, nonimmune IgA binds to type II strains possessing the alpha component of the C protein and jacalin, an IgA1-binding lectin, and increases monocyte-mediated phagocytosis of C protein–bearing type II strains.[467, 468] The IgA receptor for group B streptococci is antigenically unrelated to that of group A streptococci, but it binds to the same region in IgA.[469, 470] Despite the complexity of type II opsonins, it is clear that the complement is essential for effective opsonophagocytosis and that integrity of the classic complement pathway is essential.

Evaluation of neutrophil-mediated killing of types IV and V group B streptococci also reveals that complement and capsule-specific antibodies are participants in opsonophagocytosis.[471, 472] When complement is limited, type-specific antibodies have an important role in facilitating killing. In sufficient concentration, however, the complement in agammaglobulinemic serum promotes opsonization, phagocytosis, and killing of type IV and V group B streptococci.

Quantitative deficiencies of complement components from both the classic and the alternative complement pathways have been defined in sera from normal newborns when compared with those of their mothers or with levels in healthy adults. Maturation occurs in an age-related fashion by 6 months of age.[473] Efficient function of the alternative pathway has been demonstrated in neonatal sera for a variety of bacteria, including group B streptococci.[474] Deficient classic pathway activity in newborn sera correlated significantly with low concentrations of C4 and C1q, and this could be corrected by addition of fresh-frozen plasma.[475] The results of the study of Baker and co-workers,[476] in which pregnant women were immunized with purified type III group B streptococcal polysaccharide, suggest that deficient function of the alternative pathway may be overcome in neonatal as in adult sera if the concentration of type III–specific antibodies is sufficient. Infants surviving type III group B streptococcal meningitis transiently develop type-specific antibodies, predominantly of the IgM isotype, and efficient opsonophagocytosis during convalescence.[477] However, once specific antibody concentrations decline and despite maturation of complement synthesis to adult capacity, opsonophagocytosis of type III organisms is poor to nil.

During the course of septic shock caused by group B streptococci, complement components are consumed. Cairo and co-workers[478] found a significant association between low levels of total hemolytic complement and fatal outcome from neonatal sepsis related to a variety of bacterial pathogens, including group B streptococci. It is unclear whether these findings are a consequence of severe infection or, less likely, important in pathogenesis.

INFLAMMATORY MEDIATORS

The production and effects of proinflammatory cytokines in the pathogenesis of group B streptococcal infections are being elucidated. Many of the associated findings in septic shock, including hypoxemia and pulmonary hypotension, are mediated by TNF-α (see Pathogenesis of Early-Onset Infection). High levels of TNF-α have been detected in cerebrospinal fluid (CSF) and serum of infants with group B streptococcal disease.[479] Capsule does not appear to be required for TNF-α production, because its release is similar in response to stimulation with encapsulated or unencapsulated group B streptococci.[480–482] The cell wall components, group B polysaccharide and peptidoglycan, are the major antigens evoking TNF-α release.[481] Other proinflammatory cytokines released in response to group B streptococci include interleukin-1α (IL-1α), IL-6, and interferon-γ (IFN-γ).[483–486] Pathologic concentrations of lactic acid enhance the secretion of these inflammatory mediators and are likely to contribute to septic shock caused by group B streptococci.[487] However, IFN-γ also can induce mediators, such as L-tryptophan, which have an inhibitory effect on group B streptococci in vitro, and recombinant IFN-γ can partially restore host defense.[488, 489] Group B streptococci also stimulate the release from human monocytes of the chemotactic cytokines IL-8 and leukotriene B$_4$. However, monocytes from newborn infants have a diminished response to bacterial stimulus.[490] The little information available regarding the cytokines involved in development of a T-helper response reveals a pattern characterized by interleukin-2, IFN-γ, and interleukin-12 in the absence of interleukin-4, interleukin-5, and interleukin-10.[484] By inducing a pattern that favors a T-helper 1 rather than a T-helper 2 response, group B streptococci may evade the specific antibody production important for host resistance. Of interest, exogenous IL-12, which regulates the production of some anti-inflammatory cytokines including IL-10, improves survival in experimental infection.[491, 492] Taken together, one may conclude that the inflammatory mediators have an important role in modulating the host response to infection and that these interactions are only partially elucidated.

PHAGOCYTIC FUNCTION

The role of neutrophil function in host defense to group B streptococci has been explored extensively. Dimin-ished chemotaxigenesis by type III group B streptococci in neonatal sera has been demonstrated and relates to low concentrations of capsular polysaccharide-specific antibodies and to abnormalities of complement component quantity and function.[493] Type-specific group B streptococcal antigens incubated in the absence of serum may enhance neutrophil adherence to endothelial cells and may impair the influx of neutrophils to sites of infection, such as the alveoli.[494] This enhanced adherence to endothelium could contribute to the pulmonary edema and hypertension observed in early-onset group B streptococcal infection.[494, 495] With granulocyte depletion, there is significant attenuation of the pulmonary hypertension and hypoxemia characterizing the early phase of experimental infection. Chemiluminescence responses elicited by a type III group B streptococcal strain were significantly depressed for neutrophils from infants with group B streptococcal infection compared with values for neutrophils from healthy infants or adults.[496] "Stressed" infants with infections caused by organisms other than group B streptococci or those with noninfectious illnesses had similarly depressed chemiluminescence responses.

Smith and associates[497] examined the role of complement receptors (CR) 1 and 3 in the opsonic recognition of types Ia and III group B streptococci by neutrophils from healthy neonates and adults. Selective blockade of CR3 or of both CR1 and CR3 inhibited killing for both serotypes by neutrophils from neonates. These experiments indicated the importance of CR function to opsonization, phagocytosis, and killing of group B streptococci by neutrophils. Whether deficient CR function contributes to susceptibility of neonates to invasive infection is not known. Of interest, a role for CR3 also has been shown in nonopsonic recognition of group B streptococci by macrophages.[498]

Yang and co-workers[499] carried out selective blockade of neutrophil receptors in experiments with type III group B streptococci opsonized with immune globulin. Antibodies to neutrophil Fc receptor III (FcR III) inhibited phagocytosis of opsonized bacteria to an extent exceeding that of CR3. Noya and colleagues[500] demonstrated a substantial role for neutrophil FcR II in mediating ingestion of type III group B streptococci opsonized in complement-inactivated serum. When CR function was allowed, FcR II participation no longer was requisite for phagocytosis to occur. Participation by FcR and CR in phagocytosis of group B streptococci by peritoneal macrophages also has been reported.[501]

Christensen and co-workers[502, 503] and others[504] have addressed the explanations for the profound neutropenia often observed in fulminant group B streptococcal infection in neonates. In experimental infection, neonatal but not adult rats developed neutropenia, exhaustion of neutrophil reserves, and decreased neutrophil production.[502] The finding that the proliferative rate of granulocytic stem cells is nearly maximal in noninfected neonatal animals and cannot respond to infection[503] led to the suggestion that neutrophil transfusion might improve the survival of human neonates with group B streptococcal infection in whom neutrophil storage pool depletion was documented.[478, 504] In experimental infection with type III group B streptococci, monoclonal IgM antibody to type III polysaccharide stimulated the release of neutrophil reserves into the bloodstream and improved neutrophil migration to the site of infection.[505] This facilitation of neutrophil function by type III–specific antibody improved survival in animals only when the antibody was administered when neutrophil reserves were intact (very early in infection).[506] Antibody recipients did not become neutropenic and did not experience depletion of their neutrophil reserve.[505] These and similar in vitro and in vivo studies using commercial preparations of immune globulin for intravenous administration[507–509] emphasize the importance of IgG in facilitating the neutrophil inflammatory response.

Reticuloendothelial clearance of opsonized group B streptococci also is less efficient in experimental infection of young animals,[510, 511] as are lung macrophage postphagocytic oxidative metabolic responses.[512, 513] An age-related impairment in clearance of group B streptococci from the lungs has been reported for infant compared with adult rats and for preterm compared with term animals.[514, 515] Animal age is a more important determinant of bacterial elimination from the lung than is amount of polysaccharide capsule, although encapsulated strains are ingested less efficiently and in fewer numbers in infant versus adult rats.[516]

OTHER FACTORS RELATING TO PATHOGENESIS

Fibronectin is a high-molecular-weight glycoprotein that participates in adherence and functions as a nonspecific opsonin. The observation that septic neonates have significantly lower fibronectin levels than those of healthy age-matched controls stimulated evaluation of its possible role in the pathogenesis of group B streptococcal infection.[517] Soluble fibronectin binds poorly to group B streptococci in the absence of other opsonins.[518] However, group B streptococci do adhere to immobilized fibronectin. Fibronectin also enhances ingestion by neutrophils, monocytes, or macrophages of group B streptococci opsonized with type-specific antibody,[519–521] and may promote TNF-α production by macrophages.[522]

It has been hypothesized that some individuals may have a genetically based predisposition to infection with group B streptococci. Grubb and co-workers[523] identified a surplus of individuals possessing G3m(5) and a deficit of those with G1m(1) among 34 Swedish mothers of infants with group B streptococcal disease. Thom and colleagues[524] found deficits of G1m(1) and Km(1) and an increased incidence of G2m(23) among mothers of infected infants. The distribution of allotypic markers may influence responses to protein and polysaccharide antigens. For example, G2m(23) is a marker of IgG₂, the subclass most commonly associated with response to polysaccharide antigens. Thus, there could be genetically determined explanations for the deficiency of IgG subclasses,[525] high IgM concentration with divergent ratio of IgG to IgM,[526, 527] and the chronic colonization state without immunologic response[528] described among Swedish mothers of infants with group B streptococcal

disease. However, in a study of U.S. women who delivered infants with invasive type III group B streptococcal disease, postpartum immunization with type III group B streptococcal polysaccharide elicited an immune response similar to control women.[436]

PATHOLOGY

The morphologic features of early-onset neonatal infection are dependent on the type and duration of exposure to group B streptococci before or during birth. Intrauterine death has been attributed to group B streptococcal infection,[2, 310, 528, 529] and it may be a relatively common cause of mid-gestational fetal loss in women who have experienced vaginal hemorrhage.[530, 531] There is increasing evidence that fetal membrane infection with group B streptococci may result in spontaneous abortion or premature rupture of membranes or both, as suggested by Hood and associates in 1961.[2, 178, 530, 532] Becroft and colleagues[533] noted histologic changes consistent with congenital pneumonia in live-born neonates whose autopsy lung cultures yielded group B streptococci. Six of 10 placentas available for study showed amnionitis, a finding in each of the infants with pneumonia who died within 36 hours of birth. The evidence was sufficient in four of six stillborn infants to suggest that death was a direct result of group B streptococcal amnionitis and intrauterine pneumonia. deSa and Trevenen[531] documented pneumonitis with pulmonary interstitial and intra-alveolar inflammatory exudates in each of 15 infants weighing less than 1000 g with intrauterine group B streptococcal infection. Six infants were stillborn and 9 died within 6 hours of birth. Placental examination revealed chorioamnionitis. In a nonhuman primate model of infection, intra-amniotic inoculation of group B streptococci elicited fulminant early-onset neonatal infection.[534] Transmission electron microscopy of lung tissue revealed group B streptococci within membrane-bound vacuoles of alveolar epithelial cells and interstitial fibroblasts. The presence of organisms within tissue macrophages of the liver, spleen, and brain document rapid dissemination to other viscera.

The finding of a high frequency of associated amnionitis and early death in the just described studies is somewhat less striking in others. However, it is clear that amnionitis in association with early-onset group B streptococcal sepsis (1) is more frequently detected when death occurs shortly after birth, (2) is a common finding when membranes have been ruptured 24 hours or more before delivery,[2, 312, 531] and (3) may be clinically silent in some women. It is obvious that group B *Streptococcus* can enter the amniotic cavity through ruptured or intact membranes,[535] thus allowing fetal aspiration of infected fluid and subsequent pulmonary lesions or bacteremia, *without* eliciting a local inflammatory response or maternal signs of amniotic fluid infection.

Among neonates with fatal early-onset group B streptococcal infection, pulmonary lesions represent the predominant pathology. The association between pulmonary inflammation and hyaline membrane formation was first noted by Franciosi and co-workers.[5] Subsequently, autopsy findings in 102 cases of early-onset disease indicated "atypical" pulmonary hyaline membranes in 59%,[5, 300, 309, 311, 312, 320, 536, 537] a figure that corresponds to radiographic findings consistent with hyaline membrane disease in about 50% of neonates with early-onset sepsis.[20] Morphologically, the distribution of these membranes may be typical of those found in hyaline membrane disease, but in neonates who survive more than 20 hours it may be more patchy and less uniform.[322] Group B streptococci are frequently found within these membranes,[311, 319, 320] and in some patients these are composed almost entirely of streptococci, rendering them basophilic rather than eosinophilic in hematoxylin and eosin preparations.[319] Katzenstein and colleagues[319] postulated that invasion of alveolar pneumatocytes and capillary endothelial cells by group B streptococci results in exudation of plasma proteins into the alveoli, deposition of fibrin, and hyaline membrane formation. Immune complex–mediated injury to the lung has been proposed by Pinnas and associates[320] as a mechanism for the hyaline membrane formation in early-onset group B streptococcal pneumonia. These investigators demonstrated C3, IgG, and fibrin deposition in the lungs of infants with fatal early-onset group B streptococcal sepsis.

Histologic evidence for pneumonia is found in approximately 80% of patients with fatal early-onset group B streptococcal pneumonia.[5, 300, 309, 311, 312, 319, 320, 536–538] The radiograph pattern may be focal or extensive, lobular, or bronchial, involving one or more lobes.[300, 312, 319] The typical histologic features of congenital pneumonia (i.e., alveolar exudates composed of neutrophils, erythrocytes and aspirated squamous cells, edema, and congestion) may be observed either independently or in association with hyaline membrane formation.[5, 20, 311, 536–538] In neonates with fulminant, rapidly fatal infection, the cellular inflammatory response is less pronounced.[536] A consistent feature is that of an interstitial inflammatory exudate.[311] Also noted is progressive atelectasis that is prominent in infants surviving more than 20 hours, a feature that distinguishes group B streptococcal pneumonia from fatal hyaline membrane disease. Some investigators have noted that the pattern of atelectasis is similar to that observed in hyaline membrane disease, except that the peripheral air spaces tend to be involved more extensively.[319] Group B streptococci have been detected in hyaline membranes, within the alveoli, or in the alveolar septa beneath the membranes in 86% of the neonates for whom the location has been specified.[309, 311, 312, 319, 320, 539] Pulmonary hemorrhage, varying from focal interstitial[311, 539] to extensive intra-alveolar,[300, 319, 538, 539] was a feature present at the time of autopsy in 77% of infants reported.

In central nervous system infection, age at onset predicts distinctive morphologic findings in the brain and meninges. In early-onset meningitis, little or no evidence of leptomeningeal inflammation has been detected in up to 77% of reported cases,[5, 11, 29, 539] although purulent meningitis may be observed occasionally.[300] This lack of inflammatory response may be the result of rapidly progressive infection with an interval of only a few hours from onset of symptoms until death[5] or of deficient host response to infection or of both. Bacteria generally are found in large numbers, and perivascular inflammation, thrombosis in small vessels, and parenchymal hemorrhage are frequently noted.[539] Some preterm infants surviving septic shock caused by early-onset group B streptococcal infection develop periventricular leukomalacia, a condition characterized by infarction of the white matter surrounding the lateral ventricles.[540] Those infants with late-onset meningitis almost always have diffuse purulent leptomeningitis, especially at the base of the brain, with or without perivascular inflammation and hemorrhage.[5, 21, 541, 542] In infants with severe meningitis who survive, multiple areas of necrosis and abscess formation may be found throughout the brain by neuroimaging or at later autopsy.

This age-related inflammatory response in infants with group B streptococcal infection has a parallel in the infant rat model of meningitis.[543] Infant rats 5 to 10 days of age have numerous bacteria distributed in a perivascular pattern, and, in some animals, organisms extend transmurally into vessel lumina. With a single exception, these animals had no evidence of acute inflammation or edema in the leptomeninges. By contrast, 11- to 15-day-old animals have leptomeningitis and cerebritis characterized by a pronounced infiltration of neutrophils and macrophages around meningeal vessels and in perivascular spaces within the cerebral cortex. Because host response to infection becomes more efficient within a few weeks after birth, the absence of inflammation in the brain and meninges of infant rats as well as of human neonates with early-onset group B streptococcal infection may relate to chemotactic defects,[493] exhaustion of neutrophil stores,[503, 544] immaturity of the reticuloendothelial system,[510] or other deficits in the host response to infection.[512, 513]

CLINICAL MANIFESTATIONS AND OUTCOME

Early-Onset Infection

When the incidence of neonatal infection caused by group B *Streptococcus* rose dramatically in the 1970s, a bimodal distribution of cases according to age at onset of signs became apparent. Thus, two syndromes related to age were described in 1973 by Franciosi and associates[5] (acute and delayed) and by Baker and colleagues[281] (early and late). Early-onset infection almost always manifests within 24 hours of birth (an estimated 85% of cases[10, 20]) (median age, 8 hours), but it may appear in the second 24 hours (an estimated 5% of cases[20]) or any time during the first 6 days of life.[5, 10, 20] Premature infants often have onset at or within 6 hours of birth, and those who have onset after the first 24 hours are term gestation.[300, 301, 303, 309] Late-onset infections occur at 7 to 90 days of age (median age, 27 days).[20] Although this classification of syndromes by age at onset has been useful to enhance our understanding of the pathogenesis of infection, there is a continuum in age at onset. A few patients with early-onset disease may present at 6 or 7 days of age, and late, late-onset infection occasionally affects 3- to 7-month-old infants, especially those with gestations of less than 28 weeks.[20, 281] Onset beyond 6 months of age may herald the presentation of human immunodeficiency virus (HIV) infection or other immune abnormality.[545]

Early-onset group B streptococcal infection often affects neonates whose mothers have had obstetric complications associated with risk for neonatal sepsis (onset of labor before 37 weeks' gestation, prolonged interval at any gestation between rupture of membranes and delivery, rupture of membranes 18 or more hours before delivery, intrapartum fever, chorioamnionitis, early postpartum febrile morbidity, and twin births) (Table 26–6). The incidence of infection correlates inversely with the degree of prematurity, and a contemporary report reveals group B streptococci to be the most frequent pathogen associated with early-onset sepsis in very low birth weight (<1500 g) neonates.[548] However, term neonates often develop early-onset group B streptococcal infection with no defined maternal risk factors other than colonization. In this situation, diagnosis and treatment often are delayed until the appearance of definite signs of sepsis (fever, tachypnea, apnea, hypotension), but more subtle signs usually precede these clinical manifestations.

The three most common manifestations of early-onset infection are septicemia (signs of sepsis in association with bacteremia *without* a defined focus of infection), pneumonia, and meningitis. Septicemia without a focus occurs in 25 to 40%, pneumonia in 35 to 55%, and meningitis in 5 to 10% of cases.[10, 20, 26, 546, 547] Bacteremia often is detected in neonates with the latter two presentations. Irrespective of site of involvement, respiratory signs (apnea, grunting respirations, tachypnea, or cyanosis) are the initial clinical findings in more than 80% of neonates. Hypotension is an initial finding in approximately 25%.[546] Infants with fetal asphyxia related to group B streptococcal infection in utero may have shock and respiratory failure at delivery.[510, 516] Other associated signs include lethargy, poor feeding, hypothermia or fever, abdominal distention, pallor, tachycardia,[541] and

jaundice. Five to 10% of neonates with early-onset infection have meningitis,[20, 26, 546, 547] indicating the propensity that group B streptococci have for meningeal invasion, especially when bacteremia is caused by serotype III strains.[177, 264] Neonates with meningitis frequently have a clinical presentation identical to those without meningeal involvement. Among 27 infants with early-onset meningitis, Chin and Fitzhardinge[549] described respiratory distress as the most common initial sign and noted that seizures were never a presenting feature of infection. Therefore, examination of CSF is the only means to exclude meningitis, a finding that would mandate modification of supportive and specific chemotherapy (see Treatment section). Seizures do occur during the first 24 hours in nearly 50% of infants with meningitis. The occurrence of persistent seizures, semicoma, or coma is associated with a poor prognosis.[281, 550–552]

Pulmonary involvement occurs in 35 to 55% of patients with early-onset infection, and virtually all of these infants have acute respiratory signs (grunting, tachypnea, apnea). Of 175 neonates with pulmonary involvement, 84% had respiratory signs in the first few hours of life (many at birth), and an additional 11% developed these within the first 24 hours of life.[300, 309, 311, 312, 319, 538] Among 19 infants with congenital pneumonia at autopsy, 89% had 1-minute Apgar scores of 4 or less, indicating in utero onset of infection.[309] Radiographically, features consistent with and indistinguishable from hyaline membrane disease are present in more than one half of these neonates with group B streptococcal bacteremia and pulmonary infection (Fig. 26–6). Infiltrates suggesting congenital pneumonia (Fig. 26–7) are present in one third. Increased vascular markings suggesting the diagnosis of transient tachypnea of the newborn or pulmonary edema may occur. Occasionally, respiratory distress may be present in the absence of radiographic abnormalities,[538, 553] appearing as persistent fetal circulation.[554, 555] Small pleural effusions[553, 556–558] and cardiomegaly[538, 558] have been described. The histologic finding of atypical hyaline membranes in the lungs of infants with fatal

TABLE 26–6
Features of Group B Streptococcal Disease in Neonates and Infants

	EARLY ONSET (<7 DAYS)	LATE ONSET (≥7 DAYS)	LATE, LATE ONSET
Median age at onset[26]	1 hour	27 days	>3 months
Incidence of prematurity	Increased	Not increased	Common
Maternal obstetric complications	Frequent (70%)	Uncommon	Varies
Common manifestations[10, 20, 26, 546]	Septicemia (25–40%)	Meningitis (30–40%)	Bacteremia without a focus (common)
	Meningitis (5–10%)	Bacteremia without focus (40–50%)	Bacteremia with a focus (occasional)
	Pneumonia (35–55%)	Osteoarthritis (5–10%)	
Serotypes isolated[10, 90, 265]	Ia, Ib, Ia/c (30%)	III (~75–80%)	Several
	II (30%)		
	III (40% nonmeningeal; 80% meningeal isolates)		
Mortality rate[20, 26, 546, 547]	5–10%	2–6%	Low

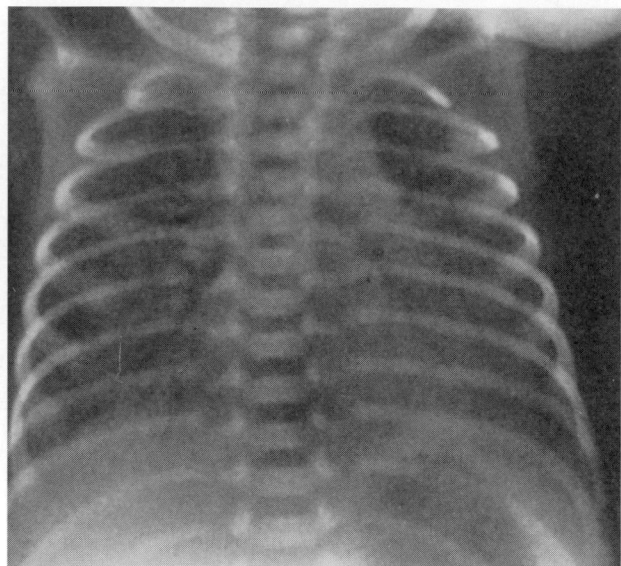

FIGURE 26–6 A chest radiograph from an infant with early-onset group B streptococcal septicemia showing features consistent with respiratory distress syndrome of the newborn.

infection provides an explanation for the clinical and radiographic mimicry of group B streptococcal pulmonary infection with noninfectious causes of respiratory distress syndrome.[311, 319]

The ratio of cases to fatalities for the nearly 300 neonates with early-onset infection summarized by Anthony and Okada[10] in 1977 was 55%. More recent reports[20, 546, 547] suggest lower rates ranging from 5 to 10%. Features associated with fatal outcome include a low 5-minute Apgar score, shock, neutropenia, pleural effu-

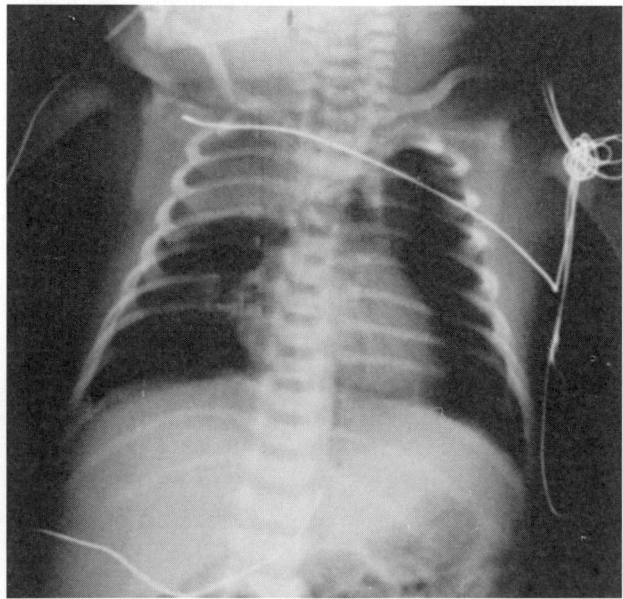

FIGURE 26–7 Chest radiograph of an infant with right upper and lower lobe infiltrates as manifestations of early-onset group B streptococcal pneumonia.

sion, apnea, and delay in treatment after the onset of symptoms.[26, 546, 558, 559] Fatal infection also occurs significantly more often among premature than term neonates (Table 26–7). Pyati and colleagues[561] reported a case: fatality ratio of 61% among 101 neonates who had early-onset group B streptococcal infection. However, infants with a birth weight in excess of 1500 g had a mortality rate of 14%. More recent data suggest a more than 20-fold increase when very low birth weight (<1500 g) neonates are compared with term infants.

Late-Onset Infection

Late-onset group B streptococcal infection typically affects the term infant from 7 days to 12 weeks of age. These infants frequently have an unremarkable early neonatal history, although late-onset disease does occur among premature infants.[25, 560] One report found that group B streptococci accounted for 2% of late-onset sepsis episodes in very low birth weight neonates. Late-onset disease has a lower case:fatality ratio (2 to 6%) than that reported for early-onset disease,[20, 26, 546, 547] and meningitis is a frequent clinical expression (an estimated 35 to 40% of reported cases). Serotype III strains are isolated from most patients (approximately 75 to 80%) irrespective of focus of infection.[28, 264, 281] An exception to the normal pattern for late-onset infection is the neonatal intensive care unit setting, where "clusters" of nosocomially acquired disease among low-birth-weight infants have been reported.[261, 273, 334, 547, 562] In these infants, the spectrum of clinical expression is similar to early-onset disease, and serotypes other than type III have been implicated.[261]

The initial signs in infants with late-onset meningitis almost always include fever, irritability or lethargy or both, poor feeding, and tachypnea. Preceding upper respiratory tract signs occur in 20 to 30% of infants.[5, 281, 300] In contrast to early-onset infection, grunting respirations and apnea are less frequent initial findings, and their presence suggests a more rapidly progressive, fulminant infection. Apnea or hypotension is observed in less than 15% of patients. However, for both early- and late-onset disease, there exists a spectrum in clinical severity of illness at presentation. For example, some neonates with late-onset meningitis are clinically well a few hours before their initial hospital evaluation, when they are noted to have seizures, poor perfusion, neutropenia, and large numbers of gram-positive cocci in their CSF Gram stain. Such patients often have a rapidly fatal course despite all attempts at specific and supportive therapy; or if they survive, they are left with devastating neurologic sequelae.[281, 563] The occurrence of leukopenia on admission (defined as fewer than 4000 cells per mm³ by Jacobs and associates[563]) or neutropenia (defined as fewer than 1500 polymorphonuclear leukocytes per mm³ by Payne and co-workers[558]) has been correlated with fatal outcome in such infants. Other admission findings associated with increased risk for fatal outcome or permanent neurologic sequelae include hypotension, coma or semicoma, status epilepticus, an absolute neutrophil count of fewer than 1000 per mm³, a CSF protein level exceeding 300 mg/dl, and a high concentration of type

TABLE 26–7
Birthweight-Specific Mortality Rates in Early-Onset Group B Streptococcal Infection

INVESTIGATOR	STUDY PERIOD	MORTALITY RATE (%) BY BIRTH WEIGHT (g)				
		500–1000	1001–1500	1501–2000	2001–2500	>2500
Boyer et al.[292]	1973–1981		71	29	33	3
Baker[560]	1982–1989	60	25	26	18	5
Weisman et al.[546]	1987–1989	75	40	20	15	6

III group B streptococcal antigen in CSF.[10, 281, 558] This last prognostic factor and the observation indicating prolonged antigenuria in meningitis survivors who are left with neurologic abnormalities probably reflect a higher bacterial inoculum in the CSF than is found in that of survivors with a normal outcome. Subdural effusions, which are usually small, unilateral, and asymptomatic, are found in up to 20% of patients with late-onset meningitis. These are not associated with any permanent sequelae.[10, 20, 281, 546] Subdural empyema as a complication is rare.[564–566]

The immediate and long-term outcomes from meningeal infection are based on reports of infants cared for nearly 20 years ago. Whether the prognosis has improved must await additional data. Among 292 neonates with early- or late-onset meningitis, 77 (26%) died in the hospital as the direct result of meningitis.[266, 281, 398, 549–552, 567] A substantial number of survivors (25 to 50%) had permanent neurologic sequelae of varying severity. In three series assessing a total of 112 survivors at mean intervals ranging from 2 to 8 years after diagnosis, major neurologic sequelae were observed in 21% of children. The most serious of these included global or profound mental retardation, spastic quadriplegia, cortical blindness, deafness, uncontrolled seizures, hydrocephalus, and hypothalamic dysfunction with poor thermal regulation and central diabetes insipidus.[549, 552, 564, 568] Mild or moderate sequelae persisted in 21% of survivors evaluated at a mean of 6 years after diagnosis.[552] These included profound unilateral sensorineural hearing loss, borderline mental retardation, spastic or flaccid monoparesis, and expressive or receptive speech and language delay. In a sibling-controlled follow-up study, Wald and coworkers[568] found that the psychometric performance did not differ significantly for children who had had group B streptococcal meningitis and their siblings. More postmeningitis children than control children had seizure disorders and hydrocephalus that required shunting procedures, but they were functioning in a manner comparable with that of their siblings. More subtle deficits such as delayed language development and mild hearing loss may not be detected by routine examination,[551] and all patients should have auditory brain stem–evoked response testing during convalescence as well as careful periodic neurologic and developmental assessments.

Bacteremia without a detectable focus of infection has been the second most common clinical expression of late-onset group B streptococcal disease until recently when it has been reported to exceed meningitis in frequency.[569] Osteomyelitis, septic arthritis, cellulitis, and adenitis are less frequent manifestations of late-onset disease. The infant with bacteremia without a focus has an uncomplicated perinatal course and presents with nonspecific signs (fever, poor feeding, irritability, rhinorrhea) in either an inpatient or an outpatient setting. Diagnosis results from the practice of obtaining blood cultures in febrile infants in the first few weeks of life to exclude serious bacterial infection as an etiology. These infants are mildly ill, but failure to initiate antimicrobial therapy *before* the availability of blood culture findings can result in extension of infection to distant sites, the most serious of which is the central nervous system. Both transient and persistent bacteremia have been described in symptomatic and asymptomatic patients.[7, 301, 570, 571] Fatal outcome has not been reported among patients with late-onset bacteremia without a focus, and survivors recover after treatment without sequelae.

Late, Late-Onset Infection

One report suggests that infants more than 3 months of age account for 20% of late-onset disease.[547] The terms *late, late-onset; very late onset;* and *beyond early infancy* have been applied to these infants. Most of these infants have gestations of less than 35 weeks. The need for prolonged hospitalization and its attendant monitoring as well as the immature host status of these infants probably contribute to infection beyond the usual interval. Bacteremia without a focus is a common presentation. Occasionally a focus for infection, including the central nervous system, intravascular catheter, or soft tissues, is identified (see Table 26–6). In the outpatient setting infants more than 3 months of age are likely to have a temperature of more than 39° C and a white blood cell count exceeding 15,000 per mm³.[569] When there are no other apparent risk factors, immune deficiency including infection should be considered in the setting of a late, late-onset of infection.[572, 573]

Septic Arthritis and Osteomyelitis

Group B streptococcal bone and joint infection has an indolent onset and a good prognosis. Less than 20% of these infants have had poor feeding,[574] respiratory distress,[575] meconium aspiration,[576] or mild elevation of serum bilirubin levels during the early neonatal period.[577] Manipulations known to predispose neonates to bone and joint infection caused by other pathogens (heel or needle puncture, umbilical vessel catheterization, exchange transfusion) have not been reported.

The clinical features of 20 infants with arthritis alone and 44 with osteomyelitis (with or without concomitant septic arthritis) related to group B streptococci are summarized in Table 26–8. The mean age at diagnosis of osteomyelitis (31 days) is greater than that of septic arthritis (20 days) or other manifestations of late-onset disease (27 days). In septic arthritis the onset is acute (mean duration of signs, 1.5 days), whereas in osteomyelitis the course is often protracted (mean, 9 days). In some infants with osteomyelitis, failure to move the involved extremity has been noted since hospital discharge after birth or shortly thereafter and has been associated with an interval as long as 4 weeks before correct diagnosis.[397]

Decreased motion of the involved extremity and pain with manipulation, such as lifting or diaper changing, are the most common signs of group B streptococcal bone or joint infection. Inflammatory signs (warmth or redness) occasionally are described[588, 589]; a history of fever has been reported in only 20% of infants. Lack of signs suggesting infection has led to an initial diagnosis of Erb's palsy.[397, 574] Several infants have had nerve conduction studies consistent with brachial plexus neuropathy associated with group B streptococcal osteomyelitis of the proximal humerus,[590, 593] and in one infant sciatic nerve injury at the level of the pelvis caused footdrop due to iliac osteomyelitis.[594]

Signs frequently observed include fixed flexion of the involved extremity, mild swelling, pain with passive motion, decreased spontaneous movement, and, in a minority of infants, erythema and warmth. Lack of associated systemic involvement is the rule, although osteomyelitis in association with meningitis,[574, 591] peritonitis,[589] and overwhelming sepsis with congestive heart failure[577, 595] have been reported.

When infants with septic arthritis alone are compared with those with osteomyelitis with respect to site involved, differences are evident. Infants with septic arthritis have had lower extremity involvement with the hip joint predominating.[4, 7, 577, 579, 581, 582] In contrast, 24 (56%) of the reported infants with osteomyelitis have had ex-clusive involvement of the humerus and, in those for whom the location was specified, the proximal humerus was affected in 94%.[7, 397, 574–577, 586, 591, 592] One infant with osteomyelitis involving both proximal humeri has been described.[591] The next most common site of involvement is the femur,[577, 583, 584, 591] and small, flat, and vertebral bone infections have been reported occasionally.[575, 578, 586, 589, 592, 596, 597] Single bone involvement predominates for group B streptococcal osteomyelitis, although infection involving two adjacent bones or multiple nonadjacent bones has been described.[575, 583, 591, 598] The rarity of multiple bone involvement contrasts to its common occurrence (estimated at 70%) in neonatal osteomyelitis caused by *S. aureus* or gram-negative enteric bacilli.[397] Although the majority of infants with humeral osteomyelitis have had concomitant infection in the shoulder joint, isolated septic arthritis of the shoulder joint has never been reported.

Impaired function after neonatal osteomyelitis caused by bacteria other than group B streptococci occurs in one fourth to one third of patients. In contrast, in 17 (90%) of the 19 infants with group B streptococcal osteomyelitis evaluated 6 months to 4 years after diagnosis, no functional impairment of the affected extremity was found.[7, 397, 576, 577, 579, 588, 590, 591] Residual shortening and limitation of motion of the humerus were noted in a patient who had the acute onset of overwhelming sepsis and congestive heart failure and osteomyelitis involving noncontiguous sites.[577] Growth disturbance as a consequence of subluxation of the hip joint has been described as a residual deficit from group B streptococcal arthritis.[598]

Although both group B streptococcal septic arthritis and osteomyelitis are considered manifestations of late-onset disease, osteomyelitis may represent early-onset asymptomatic bacteremia, secondary spread to a metaphysis, and late-onset expression of infection. An episode of asymptomatic bacteremia in the first few days of life in the neonate with a birth trauma–induced nidus in the proximal humerus could allow for localization of bacteria to the bone. Because lytic lesions take more

---

TABLE 26–8

Clinical Features of Group B Streptococcal Bone and Joint Infections[a]

FEATURE	SEPTIC ARTHRITIS WITHOUT OSTEOMYELITIS (20 PATIENTS)[4, 7, 366, 577–582]	OSTEOMYELITIS (44 PATIENTS)[7, 397, 574–577, 583–592]
Mean age at diagnosis (range)	20 days (5–37)	31 days (8–60)
Mean duration of symptoms (range)	1.5 days (<1–3)	9 days (1–28)
Male:female ratio	2:5	2:3
Site (%)	Hip (56)	Humerus (55)
	Knee (38)	Femur (24)
	Ankle (6)	Tibia, talus (5)
		Other[b] (16)
Group B streptococcal serotype (No. of patients)	III (12)	III (15), Ib/c (3), Ia/c (1)
Mean duration of parenteral therapy (range)	2 wk (2–3)	3 wk (1–6)

[a]Includes authors' unpublished data for seven patients.
[b]Ilium, acromion, clavicle, skull, digit, vertebrae; ribs—one patient each.

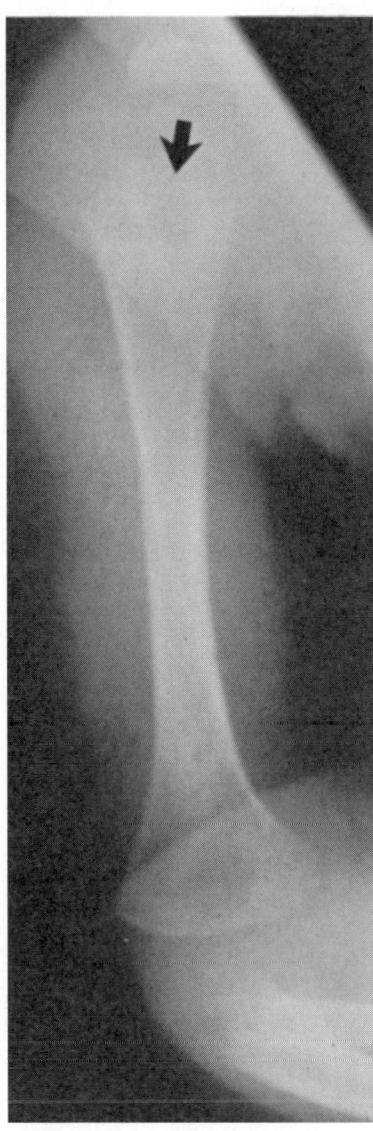

FIGURE 26–8 Radiograph showing a lytic lesion (arrow) of the proximal humerus in an infant whose bone biopsy proved osteomyelitis caused by type III group B *Streptococcus*.

than 10 days to become radiographically visible, the presence of lytic lesions on radiographs performed at hospital admission is suggestive of long-standing disease (Fig. 26–8). Also, whereas more than 90% of isolates from infants with other manifestations of late-onset group B streptococcal infection are serotype III,[90, 177] more than 20% of isolates from infants with osteomyelitis are other serotypes. These findings are consistent with the hypothesis that, in at least some patients, early-onset acquisition may have occurred.

Cellulitis or Adenitis

The manifestation of late-onset group B streptococcal infection designated facial cellulitis,[599] submandibular cellulitis,[600] or cellulitis/adenitis[601] has been reported in at least 24 infants.[602–605] Presenting signs include poor feeding, irritability, fever, and unilateral facial, preauric-

ular, or submandibular swelling usually accompanied by erythema. The mean age at onset is 5 weeks (range, 2 to 11 weeks) and, in contrast to all other patients with group B streptococcal infection, there is a striking male predominance (71%). The most common sites are the submandibular or parotid areas, and enlarged adjacent nodes become palpable within 2 days after onset of the soft tissue infection. Four of the 5 infants with facial or submandibular cellulitis reported by Baker[601] had ipsilateral otitis media at the time of diagnosis. Less common sites of involvement with cellulitis include the face, preauricular or inguinal areas, scrotum, anterior neck, and prepatellar spaces (Fig. 26–9).[601, 604, 605] In one patient, cellulitis of the neck occurred in association with an infected thyroglossal duct cyst.[601]

Bacteremia almost always is detected in these patients (92%), and cultures of soft tissue or lymph node aspirates have yielded group B streptococci in 83% of cases in whom aspiration was performed. These patients usually are not seriously ill, few have associated meningitis, and recovery within a few days of initiation of appropriate antimicrobial therapy is the rule. However, fulminant and fatal facial cellulitis has been described in a 7-hour-old neonate[7] and associated meningitis occurred in two infants.[606]

Unusual Manifestations of Infection

A number of uncommon clinical manifestations of early- and late-onset group B streptococcal infection have been recorded (Table 26–9). Peritonitis[607] and adrenal abscess[608, 610, 611] have been described as abdominal manifestations of early- and late-onset infection. The latter is thought to occur as the result of bacteremic seeding

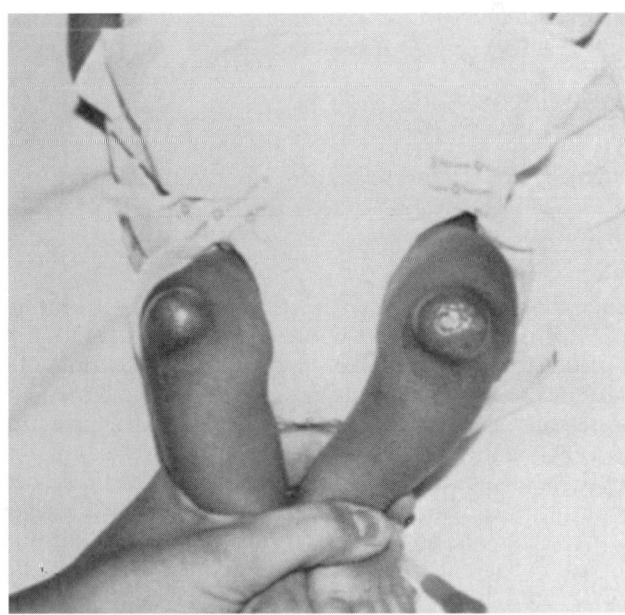

FIGURE 26–9 Prepatellar bursitis of both knees in an infant who had abraded his knees on the bedsheets. Aspiration of purulent material from the prepatellar space yielded type III group B streptococci. The knee joints were not affected.

TABLE 26–9
Unusual Clinical Manifestations of Group B Streptococcal Infections

SITE AND MANIFESTATION	ASSOCIATED WITH EARLY- OR LATE-ONSET INFECTION	REFERENCE NO.
Abdomen		
Peritonitis	Both	607
Adrenal abscess	Both	608–611
Gallbladder distention	Early	612
Brain		
Abscess	Late	613
Anterior fontanelle herniation	Both	614
Chronic meningitis	Late	615
Subdural empyema	Both	564–566
Cerebritis	Late	616
Myelopathy	Early	617
Ventriculitis complicating myelomeningocele	Both	618
Cardiovascular		
Asymptomatic bacteremia	Both	7, 301, 570, 571
Endocarditis	Both	261, 595, 619–621
Pericarditis	Not listed	622
Myocarditis	Late	576
Mycotic aneurysm	Late	623
Ear and Sinus		
Ethmoiditis	Late	7
Otitis media/mastoiditis	Both	565, 601, 624–626
Eye		
Conjunctivitis	Early	5, 627
Endophthalmitis	Late	628, 629
Respiratory Tract		
Supraglottitis	Late	630
Pleural empyema	Both	7, 631, 632
Tracheitis	Late	633
Skin and Soft Tissue		
Breast abscess	Late	634, 635
Bursitis	Late	636
Cellulitis/adenitis	Both	7, 560, 599–602, 637, 638
Fasciitis	Late	639, 640
Impetigo neonatorum	Early	641, 642
Purpura fulminans	Both	643, 644
Omphalitis	Both	541, 563
Rhabdomyolysis	Late	645
Scalp abscess	Both	646, 647
Abscess of cystic hygroma	Late	648
Dactylitis	Late	649
Urinary Tract Infection	Both	547, 650

associated with adrenal hemorrhage and subsequent abscess formation.[610] One neonate had the diagnosis of neuroblastoma and underwent en bloc resection of a large mass with nephrectomy before the diagnosis of adrenal abscess was established.[610] Gallbladder distention is a nonspecific manifestation of early-onset sepsis that usually resolves with medical management.[612] Late-onset bacteremia in association with jaundice, elevated levels of liver enzymes, and increased direct-reacting bilirubin fraction[644] has been reported. It was postulated that hemolysis and hepatocellular damage may have contributed to the development of jaundice. Underlying liver disease, a known predisposing feature to group B streptococcal bacteremia in adults, was suggested as an explanation for group B streptococcal bacteremia in a 22-month-old child.[651]

Siegel and co-workers[613] have described a patient with a brain abscess in association with recurrence of group B streptococcal meningitis. The infant recovered after craniotomy and excision of a well-encapsulated frontal mass but had neurologic sequelae. Sokol and colleagues[615] described a 5-week old with a cerebellar cyst believed to represent an astrocytoma. This infant proved to have obstructive hydrocephalus and chronic group B streptococcal ventriculitis. Rarely, anterior fontanelle herniation may complicate severe meningitis. The presence of a noncystic doughy mass over the fontanelle indicates that brain herniation may have occurred, and head ultrasonography or computed tomography may be used for confirmation. This finding is a poor prognostic sign.[614] One patient with cervical myelopathy initially had absence of extremity movement but made a good recovery and was able to walk at age 3 years.[617] Another unusual complication of group B streptococcal meningitis is subdural empyema, which has been described in patients with both early- and late-onset infections.[564-566] The diagnosis was established by needle aspiration of the subdural space at the time of admission[564] or within the first 5 days of treatment. Irritability, vomiting, seizures, increasing head circumference, focal neurologic signs, a tense anterior fontanelle, or a combination of these prompted evaluation.[565, 566, 652] Sterilization of the subdural space was accomplished by drainage, open or closed, in conjunction with antimicrobial therapy. Basal ganglia and massive cerebral infarction also have been described.[616]

Cardiovascular manifestations of group B streptococcal infection are rare. However, endocarditis,[261, 595, 620, 621] pericarditis,[622] myocarditis,[576] and mycotic aneurysm of the aorta[623] have been documented. Echocardiography has been useful in determining the nature of cardiac involvement, and this technique was employed successfully to delineate a 0.7-cm vegetation on the anterior leaflet of the mitral valve in a 4-week-old infant with endocarditis caused by a serotype III strain.[595] Paroxysmal atrial tachycardia may be a presenting feature of group B streptococcal bacteremia in the absence of focal infection of the heart.[20]

Group B streptococci are an uncommon cause of otitis media in the first few weeks of life (2 to 3% of cases).[591] However, otitis media is not infrequently found in infants with late-onset disease manifested as meningitis or submandibular cellulitis.[565, 625, 626] The finding of acute mastoiditis at autopsy in one infant with otitis media and meningitis suggests that the middle ear may serve as a portal of entry in some patients.[626]

Conjunctivitis related to group B streptococci occurs with such rarity that no cases were identified among 302 neonates with ophthalmia neonatorum reported by Armstrong and associates.[627] However, exudative conjunctivitis has been described in association with early-onset bacteremia.[7, 627] More severe ocular involvement is rare, but endophthalmitis has been noted in two patients in association with bacteremia and meningitis.[628, 629] As is the case for other agents producing endophthalmitis, high-grade bacteremia is a likely prelude to this unusual metastatic focus of group B streptococcal infection.

Supraglottitis was described in a 3-month-old infant with acute onset of stridor.[630] Swelling of the left aryepiglottic fold but not the epiglottis was noted at laryngoscopy. An infant with bacterial tracheitis had a similar presentation.[633] Although pulmonary infection caused by group B streptococci is common, pleural involvement is rare. However, it has been reported as a complication of both early-onset[7, 632] and late-onset[631] pneumonia. An interesting but as yet inexplicable association is that of delayed development of right-sided diaphragmatic hernia and early-onset group B streptococcal sepsis.[653-656] These infants invariably have the onset of respiratory distress at or within hours of birth, whereas the mean age at diagnosis of right-sided diaphragmatic hernia is 12 days (range, 3 to 35 days).[655] Ashcraft and associates[655] postulate that the insufficient diaphragmatic motion predisposes a neonate with peripartum exposure to group

B streptococci to the development of pneumonia and that subsequent respiratory effort accounts for the ultimate herniation of viscera into the pleural space. This phenomenon should be remembered and considered in the infant with group B streptococcal infection whose condition continues to deteriorate in spite of proper management. Radiographic features include increased density in the right lower lung or irregular aeration or both followed by progression to elevation of right bowel gas and liver shadow.

In addition to cellulitis and adenitis, a variety of unusual skin and soft tissue manifestations of group B streptococcal infection have been described. These include violaceous cellulitis,[657] perineal cellulitis and septicemia after circumcision,[658] scrotal ecchymosis as a sign of intraperitoneal hemorrhage,[638] purpura fulminans,[645] necrotizing fasciitis,[639, 640] impetigo neonatorum,[641, 642] omphalitis,[541, 631] scalp abscess secondary to fetal scalp electrode,[646, 647] abscess complicating cystic hygroma,[648] and breast abscess.[634] In patients with impetiginous lesions and abscess formation, bacteremia is unusual, but it is a frequent accompaniment to omphalitis and necrotizing fasciitis.

Although infants with early-onset bacteremia frequently have group B streptococci isolated from the urine when it is cultured,[281] primary urinary tract infection with these organisms is rare. A single infant with severe bilateral ureterohydronephrosis and group B streptococci in his urine has been reported.[650] The isolation of group B streptococci from a urine culture of a patient *without bacteremia* is an indication for evaluation of possible structural anomalies of the genitourinary tract.

Three infants ranging from 3 to 8 months of age have had sudden infant death attributed at the time of autopsy to group B streptococcal infection.[529]

Relapse or Recurrence of Infection

Relapse or recurrence of early- and late-onset type group B streptococcal infections has been reported in an estimated 0.5 to 3% of patients[603, 613, 637, 650, 658-665] who developed recrudescence of signs either during treatment or after an interval from 3 to 101 days after completion of antibiotic therapy. In one retrospective review, eight of nine infants were born at 25 to 36 weeks of gestation and one was born at term, and male infants predominated.[664] The first episode occurred at a mean age of 10 days (range 1 to 27) and recurrence occurred at a mean age of 42 days (range 23 to 68 days).[664] Two separate episodes of relapse have been documented in several infants.[662, 665-667] In some patients, circumstances that potentially could have predisposed to relapse or reinfection were reported (maternal mastitis, protracted focal seizures in an infant with a brain abscess,[613] endocarditis with underlying congenital heart disease[659]). Identical isolates were recovered from the maternal genital and breast milk cultures, suggesting that breastfeeding might have been the source of repeated exposure for one preterm infant with three episodes of bacteremia, even though the mother had no clinical findings of mastitis.[665] Although the initial episodes of infection were similar to those in patients with nonrecurrent disease, some infants have had new sites of involvement with the relapse or recurrence (meninges, ventricular or subdural fluid, or both,[659, 661, 662] brain parenchyma,[613] and soft tissue[603, 637]). Eradication of infection usually was achieved by treatment with a penicillin, either alone or in combination with an aminoglycoside. The penicillin dose was higher and the duration of therapy longer than was used for treatment of the first episode of infection.

One of the possible explanations for reported episodes of relapse or recurrence in the 1970s was failure to administer penicillin G or ampicillin at an optimal dosage or for a sufficient duration. In two patients, penicillin-tolerant organisms were isolated at the time of the second infection[613, 659]; isolates from the initial episode were not available for susceptibility testing. Because the finding of in vitro penicillin tolerance is not uncommon among group B streptococcal isolates (estimated at 4%[668]), the relationship between tolerance and relapse is unknown, but this in vitro phenomenon is unlikely to explain recurrent infections (see Treatment).

Because infants treated for invasive infection frequently remain colonized with group B streptococci at mucous membrane sites,[251] pharyngeal or gastrointestinal colonization may be the source for another episode of bacteremia. In addition, infants recovering from invasive infection with type III strains infrequently develop protective levels of antibody during convalescence. Denning and co-workers[667] used restriction endonuclease analysis to document that isolates from the second and third episodes of group B streptococcal disease in an infant were identical and were derived from a single clone. Green and colleagues[664] found that five of seven sets of isolates analyzed from first and second episodes were genotypically identical using pulsed field gel electrophoresis. Thus, recurrent infection in most infants results from reinvasion from persistently colonized mucous membrane sites. However, a minority of infants encounter a new strain and have a second episode based on exposure other than maternal.

Maternal Infections Caused by Group B Streptococci

In 1938, Fry[1] described three fatal cases of endocarditis in postpartum women. This was the first indication that group B *Streptococcus* was a human pathogen and could cause puerperal infection. For the next two decades, additional postpartum infections including septic abortion,[2, 3] bacteremia,[3, 4, 669] chorioamnionitis,[3] endometritis,[669, 670] pneumonia,[669] and septic arthritis[669] were recorded sporadically. However, before 1970, group B streptococcal infection in the postpartum woman, as in the neonate, was uncommon.[20, 671] The increase in neonatal infections during the past 30 years has been paralleled by an increasing number of infections in adults.[12-14, 17, 533] It is now obvious that these microorganisms are a common cause of significant febrile morbidity in pregnant women.

Reports by Ledger and co-workers[16] and Baker and Edwards[20] indicated that group B streptococci accounted for 10 to 20%, respectively, of blood culture isolates from febrile women on obstetric services. Most of these women have a clinical picture characterized by fever, malaise, moderate uterine tenderness with normal lochia, and occasionally chills. A more detailed study of group B streptococcal infection in postpartum patients was reported by Faro.[17] Forty women with endometritis and endoparametritis related to group B streptococci were observed among 3106 deliveries over a 12-month interval, an incidence of 1.3 per 1000 deliveries. The diagnosis was established by isolation of group B streptococci from the endometrium either alone (35%) or in addition to other organisms; one third had concomitant bacteremia. Many (94%) developed infection after cesarean section. These women characteristically developed fever in the early postpartum course (mean onset, 11.7 hours; range, 1 to 24 hours), a finding also reported by others.[295] Additional clinical features included chills, tachycardia, abdominal distention, and exquisite uterine, parametrial, or adnexal tenderness. Temperature more than or equal to 38.5° C correlated with an increased risk of concomitant bacteremia. Recovery was uniform after administration of one of a number of antimicrobial agents to which group B streptococci were susceptible. However, 6 of 45 (13.3%) infants delivered to these women developed group B streptococcal septicemia, and fatal infection occurred in 3. Febrile morbidity in a mother may be the single early clue of bacteremic infection in her neonate,[17, 20] and the infants of such women should be carefully evaluated.

Thirty-one cases of patients with postpartum group B streptococcal bacteremia were summarized by Gibbs and Blanco.[294] In their series, group B streptococci accounted for 15% of isolates from women with bacteremias. At initial evaluation (within 24 hours of delivery in 80%), approximately one half had no localizing signs of genital infection. Endometritis was subsequently diagnosed in 81% and chorioamnionitis in 19% of patients. Each recovered fully after antimicrobial therapy. Pass and associates[295] described similar features among 21 patients with puerperal sepsis caused by group B streptococci during a 36-month interval in which the attack rate was 2 per 1000 deliveries. Delivery by cesarean section was a significant risk factor. Although most obstetric patients with group B streptococcal infection, even in the presence of bacteremia, have a rapid response after initiation of appropriate therapy, several reports have documented the occasional occurrence of potentially fatal complications, including meningitis,[13, 672] abdominal abscess,[673] endocarditis,[13, 673-676] vertebral osteomyelitis,[677] epidural abscess,[678] and necrotizing fasciitis.[679]

The role of group B streptococcal bacteriuria during pregnancy as a potential risk factor for intrauterine or neonatal infection has been established. Asymptomatic bacteriuria and cystitis or pyelonephritis occur in 6 to 8% of women during pregnancy. In those with bacteriuria, 5 to 29% are caused by group B streptococci.[680-682] Pass and associates[295] observed three patterns of urinary tract infection among 20 patients: symptomatic lower urinary tract infection in the antenatal period (8); asymptomatic bacteriuria at delivery (7); and postpartum infection (5). Eleven infants born to these 20 women were colonized with group B streptococci, and 1 developed early-onset group B streptococcal sepsis. In the series of Moller and associates,[178] the 68 women with bacteriuria caused by group B streptococci had a significantly increased risk of delivery before 37 weeks' gestation compared with controls, but a causal relationship was not established. Among women with signs of spontaneous abortion, the occurrence of group B streptococci in the urine has been associated significantly with fetal loss.[683] More recent studies demonstrate that women with group B streptococcal bacteriuria are those with "heavy" ($>10^5$ colony-forming units per ml) colonization, and both conditions are associated with enhanced risk for maternal and neonatal infection.[199]

DIAGNOSIS

Isolation and Identification of the Organism

The diagnosis of invasive group B streptococcal infection is established by isolation of the organism from culture of blood, CSF, or site of suppurative focus (e.g., bone, joint fluid, empyema fluid). Isolation of group B streptococci from surfaces, such as the skin or umbilicus, or from mucous membranes is of no clinical significance.

Selective approaches to performing a lumbar puncture in the evaluation of neonates with possible sepsis has been advocated by some clinicians. However, exclusion of meningeal infection by lumbar puncture always is indicated when either early- or late-onset group B streptococcal infection is suspected because meningeal penetration occurs in 5 to 10% of cases[20, 26, 546, 547] and clinical features cannot distinguish between meningitis and bacteremia without meningitis. Further, whereas many neonates with meningitis have group B streptococci isolated from blood at initial evaluation, a substantial number (an estimated 10 to 15%) do not. Wiswell and colleagues found that if lumbar puncture was omitted as part of the early neonatal sepsis evaluation, the diagnosis of bacterial meningitis would have been missed or delayed in more than one third of infants.[684] Infants with late-onset infection can have meningitis even when another site of infection, such as cellulitis, is apparent.[606, 685] If lumbar puncture must be deferred initially because an infant is clinically unstable, penicillin G or ampicillin at the doses recommended for treatment of group B streptococcal meningitis (see Treatment) should be administered until meningeal involvement can be excluded.

ANTIGEN DETECTION METHODS

The difficulty of clinically differentiating neonates with group B streptococcal infection from those infected with other agents or with noninfectious disorders prompted the development of tests to provide a presumptive diagnosis. These included countercurrent immunoelectrophoresis (CIE),[92, 686–693] latex particle agglutination (LPA),[687, 689–691, 694–700] staphylococcal coagglutination (SCA),[688, 689, 701, 702] and enzyme immunoassay.[703] Each was based on the detection of group B or type-specific

polysaccharide antigens in body fluids using hyperimmune polyclonal antisera or monoclonal antibodies. The methods all have the attributes of simplicity, rapidity, and the ability to detect antigen after antimicrobial therapy has been initiated.

Antigen tests are an adjunct to diagnosis and are not a substitute for appropriately performed bacterial cultures in the diagnosis of group B streptococcal infection. A positive result indicates the presence of group B streptococcal antigen and not necessarily the presence of viable organisms. If antigen is detected, the finding should be confirmed by culture. The only specimens recommended for antigen detection testing are serum and CSF.[704] In neonates with meningitis, the reported sensitivity of CSF assays is 72 to 89%. Serum is less likely to have detectable antigen (estimated sensitivity, 30 to 40%). LPA is more sensitive than CIE.[689, 690, 694, 695, 700]

False-positive results have been encountered for antigen testing of serum[692] and CSF,[694, 699] and the estimated specificity of assays varies from 95 to 98%.

OTHER LABORATORY TESTS

Several laboratory tests for which positive results suggest the diagnosis of invasive group B streptococcal infection have been reported. These include the presence of gram-positive cocci in gastric[311, 692] or tracheal aspirates,[705] a positive gastric aspirate shake test in neonates with respiratory distress,[706] elevated C-reactive protein levels,[707, 708] depressed plasma fibronectin concentration,[517] and abnormalities of the neutrophil count.[312, 319, 538, 709, 710] The finding of gram-positive cocci in gastric or tracheal aspirates or in maternal amniotic fluid contents may indicate the presence of this or other organisms but does not give information regarding tissue invasion unless blood or lung tissue cultures or both grow group B streptococci.[20] The use of C-reactive protein for detecting bacteremia was documented by Sabel and Wadsworth,[708] who found initially elevated values in five of seven infants with group B streptococcal bacteremia. The findings of Philip[707] suggest that C-reactive protein may *not* be a good indicator of neonatal infection during the first 12 hours after birth. Depression of plasma fibronectin in neonatal sepsis may be caused by its behavior as an acute-phase reactant or by its increased consumption as a nonspecific opsonin.[517]

Abnormalities in the white blood cell count, including relative leukopenia,[709, 711] absolute neutropenia,[312, 319] leukocytosis,[319] and a tendency for a decline in the total white blood cell count in the first 24 hours of life,[706] are thought by some to be useful in identifying neonates with group B streptococcal pneumonia. In a study designed to determine the usefulness of the differential white blood cell count for distinguishing early-onset group B streptococcal infection from noninfectious forms of respiratory distress, Manroe and co-workers[709] found that each infected infant was identified by abnormalities in two or more of the following indices: (1) absolute neutrophil count indicating neutropenia or neutrophilia (87%), (2) elevation of the absolute immature neutrophil count (42%), and (3) abnormal ratio of immature neutrophils to the total number of neutrophils. The most useful index was the ratio of absolute immature neutrophils to absolute total neutrophils, which was elevated (>0.20) in 91% of infants with infection and in only 1 of 23 noninfected infants with respiratory disease.[709] Greenberg and Yoder[712] caution that repeat testing at 12 to 24 hours of age may enhance sensitivity when compared with testing between 1 and 7 hours of age. However, fatal early-onset group B streptococcal sepsis with a normal leukocyte count has been reported.[713] In general, measurements of peripheral blood leukocytes or inflammatory mediators are nonspecific and should never be employed for diagnosis except as adjuncts to blood and CSF cultures.

Differential Diagnosis

The clinical features in neonates with early-onset group B streptococcal infection mimic those in infants with sepsis caused by other etiologic agents and by some noninfectious illnesses. Radiographic findings characteristic of pneumonia are present in only one third of neonates with early-onset group B streptococcal sepsis. At least half of the neonates with proven bacteremia and pulmonary disease caused by group B streptococci have a radiographic pattern clinically indistinguishable from hyaline membrane disease or transient tachypnea of the newborn.[311, 312, 319] Neonates with early-onset group B streptococcal pulmonary disease are more likely to have an interval after rupture of membranes of more than 12 hours before delivery, apnea and shock within the first 24 hours of life, a 1-minute Apgar score of less than or equal to 5,[309] and an unusually rapid progression of pulmonary disease than are those with noninfectious causes for respiratory distress. Group B streptococcal infection also should be considered in a neonate with persistent fetal circulation associated with respiratory distress, neutropenia, and systemic hypotension.[554, 558]

The differential diagnosis for late-onset group B streptococcal infection depends on the clinical presentation. For infants with meningitis, the characteristic CSF Gram stain findings can provide a presumptive diagnosis. When this is inconclusive or if partial treatment may have altered the CSF culture, other organisms, including viruses, *Neisseria meningitidis*, *Streptococcus pneumoniae*, and nontypeable *Haemophilus influenzae*, must be considered in the differential diagnosis. Fever usually is a presenting feature for infants with late-onset bacteremia, and empirical therapy with broad-spectrum antibiotics customarily is employed until results of cultures permitting a specific diagnosis of bacteremia are available. The paucity of signs characteristic of group B streptococcal osteomyelitis and the occasional history that signs have been present since birth have caused this syndrome to be mistaken for Erb's palsy and neuromuscular disorders. However, the characteristic bony lesion in the affected metaphysis, the common finding of tenderness of the extremity when a careful examination is performed, and the isolation of the organism from bone or joint fluid usually provide a definitive diagnosis.[397] Finally, the lengthy list of uncommon manifestations of group B streptococcal infection between 1 week and 3 months of age and beyond indicates that group B streptococci should be suspected as etiologic agents, irrespective of site of infection, for infants in this age group.

TREATMENT

Group B streptococci have been the most frequent cause of infection in neonates for nearly three decades, resulting in increased awareness of associated risk factors and need for prompt and aggressive therapy. Despite striking declines, however, mortality and permanent sequelae from these infections remain all too frequent outcomes. In addition, relapses or reinfections, although rare, occur in the face of optimal therapy by conventional standards. These facts should prompt efforts to develop improved treatment modalities.

In Vitro Susceptibility

Uniform susceptibility of group B streptococci to penicillin G has continued for almost 50 years of usage.[3, 10, 581, 714–717] In vitro susceptibility of these organisms to ampicillin, vancomycin, teicoplanin, semisynthetic penicillins, and first-, second- (excluding cefoxitin) and third-generation cephalosporins also is the rule, although the degree of activity varies.[718–730] Ceftriaxone is the most active of the latter agents in vitro. Imipenem and meropenem are highly active.[716, 719, 731, 732] Ciprofloxacin has moderate in vitro activity.[722, 723] Resistance to erythromycin occurs in 7 to 21% and clindamycin resistance is found in 4 to 15% of isolates.[716, 733, 734] Tetracycline resistance has increased significantly from about 30% in 1957[725] to nearly 90%.[720, 735] Resistance of group B streptococci to bacitracin, nalidixic acid, trimethoprim-sulfamethoxazole, metronidazole, and aminoglycosides is uniform.

Despite the in vitro resistance of most group B streptococcal strains to aminoglycosides, when one of these drugs (especially gentamicin) is combined with a penicillin in vitro[736–740] and in vivo, synergy[737, 741–743] often is observed. The best combination to theoretically accelerate the killing of group B streptococci in vivo is ampicillin or penicillin and gentamicin. By contrast, the rapid and predictable bactericidal effect of penicillin or ampicillin on group B streptococci in vitro is ablated by the addition of either chloramphenicol or rifampin.[744–746] Although in vivo data are lacking, the in vitro antagonism of these two agents when combined with penicillins suggests that they not be employed in the treatment of proven or suspected group B streptococcal disease.

Of the new beta-lactam antibiotics reputed to attain high concentrations of drug in the CSF, only cefotaxime, ceftriaxone,[719, 727, 743] meropenem, and imipenem[716, 719, 731, 732] achieve minimal bactericidal concentrations (MBCs) comparable with those of penicillin G and ampicillin (0.008 to 0.4 μg/ml, respectively). Only a few infants have been treated with these agents,[747–749] and limited data suggest that their efficacy is equivalent to penicillin G. Thus, there is no compelling reason to consider these as alternative therapeutic agents.

Despite their uniform susceptibility to penicillin G,

group B streptococci require higher concentrations for growth inhibition in vitro than do strains belonging to group A. The minimal inhibitory concentration (MIC) of penicillin G to group B streptococci is 4- to 10-fold greater (range, 0.003 to 0.4 μg/ml) than that for group A strains.[3, 581, 714, 720, 736] This observation, combined with that indicating the significant influence of inoculum size on in vitro susceptibility to penicillin G,[714, 744, 750, 751] may have clinical relevance. If the inoculum of group B streptococci is reduced from 10^5 to 10^4 colony-forming units (CFU) per milliliter, a twofold decrease in the concentration of penicillin G is sufficient to inhibit in vitro growth.[714] Similarly, if the inoculum is increased from 10^4 to 10^7 CFU per ml, the MBC of ampicillin is increased from 0.06 to 3.9 μg/ml.[744, 750] Such in vitro findings may have in vivo correlates because some infants with group B streptococcal meningitis have been shown to have CSF bacterial concentrations of 10^7 to 10^8 CFU per ml.[750, 751] At the initiation of therapy for meningitis, achievable CSF levels of penicillin G or ampicillin may be only 10 to 20% of serum levels.[752] Therefore, the dose chosen to treat group B streptococcal meningitis may be crucial to the prompt sterilization of CSF. This in vitro inoculum effect also has been noted with cefotaxime and imipenem[720, 726, 731] and may portend failure of these new agents to demonstrate greater efficacy than penicillin G.

Although group B streptococci are susceptible to penicillin G, in vitro tolerance among 4 to 6% of strains has been noted.[613, 659, 668, 753] Defined as an MBC in excess of 16 to 32 times the MIC, tolerance in vitro corresponds with delayed bacterial killing, additive rather than synergistic effects when gentamicin is used in combination with penicillin G, and possibly an autolytic enzyme defect in such strains.[754, 755] Detection of tolerance among group B streptococcal isolates, however, is highly dependent on choice of growth medium, growth phase of bacterial inoculum, and quantitative definition of MBC employed for testing.[720] Although some infants with recurrence of group B streptococcal infection have had tolerant strains,[615, 659, 756] the clinical significance of this in vitro phenomenon is doubtful.

Antimicrobial Therapy

Although other penicillins are equally active against group B streptococci in vitro, penicillin G remains the drug of choice for the treatment of infant and adult infections caused by these microorganisms. This recommendation is undisputed, yet recommendations for dosage have varied considerably. Since 1973, the dosage for treatment of meningitis in neonates has increased from 100,000 to 250,000 to 500,000 units/kg per day.[757, 758] Several observations have prompted this upward adjustment in dosage: (1) the relatively high MIC of penicillin G to group B streptococci (median, 0.04 μg/ml) with respect to attainable levels of this drug in the CSF,[757] (2) the high initial inoculum in the CSF of some infants,[20, 750, 751] (3) the reports of relapse in infants with meningitis treated for 14 days with 200,000 units/kg per day of penicillin G, and (4) the known safety of higher doses of penicillin G in the newborn. To ensure rapid bactericidal effects, particularly in the CSF, we recommend relatively high doses of penicillin G (500,000 units/kg per day) or ampicillin (300 to 400 mg/kg per day) for the treatment of group B streptococcal meningitis (Table 26–10). There is no evidence to suggest increased risk for adverse reactions to these drugs at these higher doses in term or premature infants.

In the usual clinical setting, antimicrobial therapy will be initiated before definitive identification of the organism. Initial therapy should include ampicillin and an aminoglycoside appropriate for the treatment of early-onset neonatal pathogens including group B streptococci. Such a combination has been shown more effective than penicillin G or ampicillin alone in the in vitro and in vivo killing of group B streptococci.[724, 736, 737–739] It is our practice to continue combination therapy until the isolate has been identified as group B *Streptococcus* and, in patients with meningitis, until CSF obtained 24 to 48 hours into therapy is sterile. Kim[755] suggested that MIC and MBC determinations be considered in each of the following clinical circumstances: (1) a poor bacteriologic response to antimicrobial therapy, (2) relapse or recurrence of infection without a discernible cause, and

---

TABLE 26–10
Antimicrobial Regimens Recommended for Treatment of Group B Streptococcal Infections in Infants[a]

SITE OF INFECTION	DRUG	DOSE PER DAY (INTRAVENOUS)	DURATION
Bacteremia without meningitis	Ampicillin plus gentamicin	150–200 mg/kg plus 7.5 mg/kg	Initial treatment before culture results (48–72 hr)
	Penicillin G	200,000 units/kg	Complete a total treatment course of 10 days
Meningitis	Ampicillin plus gentamicin	300–400 mg/kg plus 7.5 mg/kg	Initial treatment (until cerebrospinal fluid is sterile)
	Penicillin G	500,000 units/kg	Complete a minimum total treatment course of 14 days[b]
Septic arthritis	Penicillin G	200,000 units/kg	2–3 wk
Osteomyelitis	Penicillin G	200,000 units/kg	3–4 wk
Endocarditis	Penicillin G	400,000 units/kg	4 wk[c]

[a]No modification of dose by postnatal age is recommended. Oral therapy is never indicated.
[b]Longer treatment (up to 4 wk) may be required for ventriculitis.
[c]In combination with gentamicin for the first 14 days.

(3) infections manifested as meningitis or endocarditis. If tolerance is demonstrated in one of these circumstances, the clinician has the choice of empirically continuing the combination of penicillin G or ampicillin and gentamicin, or of using penicillin G or ampicillin alone, or of employing cefotaxime. No data are available to indicate the best choice.[759]

For the infant with late-onset disease in whom the CSF Gram stain reveals gram-positive cocci in pairs or short chains, initial therapy should include ampicillin and gentamicin or cefotaxime rather than penicillin G alone. The rationale for this recommendation rests on several observations. First, group B streptococci are a frequent cause of meningitis in infants from 1 to 8 weeks of age. In this setting, combination therapy may provide for added efficacy early in the course of infection. Second, meningitis caused by *Listeria monocytogenes* may produce a CSF Gram stain difficult to distinguish from that of group B *Streptococcus*, especially to an inexperienced observer. Ampicillin and gentamicin are synergistic in vitro against most strains of *Listeria*. If pneumococcal meningitis is a consideration, cefotaxime in combination with vancomycin, should be included in the empirical regimen pending culture confirmation. Because group B streptococcal meningitis occurs uncommonly beyond 8 weeks of age, no change is suggested from the use of conventional agents as the initial treatment of meningitis beyond this period. For the premature infant remaining in the hospital since birth, empirical therapy can include vancomycin and an aminoglycoside. However, if meningitis is suspected, an additional agent should be added (i.e., either ampicillin or cefotaxime) because vancomycin achieves low CSF concentration and has a substantially higher MBC against group B streptococci than does ampicillin.

Once the bacteriologic diagnosis of group B streptococcal infection is known *and* the CSF of patients with meningeal infections 24 to 48 hours into therapy is shown to be sterile, treatment can be completed with penicillin G alone. Although the total duration of treatment is arbitrary, good outcomes have been noted when parenteral therapy is given 10 days for bacteremia without a focus or with soft tissue infection, 2 to 3 weeks for meningitis or pyarthrosis,[577] and 3 to 4 weeks for osteomyelitis[397] or endocarditis[12, 13, 760] (see Table 26–10). In the management of infants with meningitis, failure to achieve sterility suggests the presence of an unsuspected suppurative focus (subdural empyema, brain abscess, ventriculitis, septic thrombophlebitis) or failure to administer an appropriate drug in sufficient dosage. At the completion of therapy (minimum 14 days), another lumbar puncture should be considered to determine whether the CSF findings are compatible with adequacy of treatment or are of sufficient concern to warrant further treatment or further diagnostic evaluation. Examples of concerning results would include polymorphonuclear cells in excess of 20 to 30% of the total or a protein concentration in excess of 200 mg/dl. These findings also can be observed in patients with a fulminant course manifested by severe cerebritis, extensive parenchymal destruction with focal suppuration, severe vasculitis, or all three.

Infants with septic arthritis should receive at least 2 weeks of parenteral therapy; those with bone involvement require 3 to 4 weeks of therapy to ensure an uncomplicated outcome. Drainage of the suppurative focus is an adjunct to antibiotic therapy. In infants with septic arthritis excluding the hip or shoulder, needle aspiration of the involved joint on one or two occasions usually achieves adequate drainage.[7, 397, 577, 578] With hip or shoulder involvement, immediate open drainage is warranted. Approximately two thirds of infants with osteomyelitis have had open drainage procedures (arthrotomy and curettage of necrotic bone), and the remainder have had percutaneous needle aspiration of the metaphysis. For most patients, some type of drainage procedure, whether closed or open, is required for diagnosis because most patients have sterile blood cultures. Such procedures must be performed before or early in the course of antimicrobial therapy to ensure the successful isolation of the infecting strain.

In the circumstance of recurrent infection, three points should be considered. First, appropriate antimicrobial therapy fails to eliminate mucous membrane colonization with group B streptococci in up to 50% of infants.[251] Second, community exposure of the infant may result in colonization with a new strain that subsequently invades the bloodstream. Systemic infection in neonates does not result in protective levels of type-specific antibodies.[373] Therefore, even in the absence of an underlying immunologic abnormality or an unsuspected suppurative focus, recurrent systemic infections do occur. In this event, an evaluation to exclude underlying immune abnormality (e.g., HIV infection or hypogammaglobulinemia) should be considered. However, most infants will have no defined abnormalities. Therapy in those infants with recurrent infection need not be extended beyond that recommended by site of infection. Finally, while it is logical to suggest that colonization be eliminated, an efficacious regimen has not been identified. Rifampin has uniform in vitro activity against group B streptococci, but this agent is bacteriostatic. One small prospective study revealed that administration of oral rifampin (20 mg/kg per day for 4 days) to infants after completion of parenteral therapy eliminated mucous membrane colonization in some subjects.[761] Further study is needed.

Supportive Management

The importance of prompt, vigorous, and careful supportive therapy to the successful outcome of most group B streptococcal infections cannot be overemphasized. In neonates with early-onset disease accompanied by respiratory distress, the need for ventilatory assistance should be anticipated before apnea because its appearance can herald a poor outcome.[281, 300] The early treatment of shock, often not suspected during the initial phase when systolic pressure is maintained by peripheral vasoconstriction, is crucial. Persistent metabolic acidosis and reasonably normal color are characteristic of this early phase. Any indication of poor peripheral perfusion after initial attempts to achieve adequate volume expansion merits placement of a central venous pressure monitoring device and treatment with appropriate inotropic agents. This concept applies also to patients with late-onset meningitis. Fluid management should include packed red blood cell transfusions if anemia is significant. In patients with meningitis, effective seizure control is required to achieve proper oxygenation, to decrease metabolic demands, to prevent additional cerebral edema, and to optimize cerebral blood flow. Attention to the details of urine output and electrolyte balance and osmolality is necessary to detect and manage the early complications of meningitis, such as inappropriate secretion of antidiuretic hormone and increased intracranial pressure. Such intense and careful supportive management requires treatment in a tertiary care facility.

Extracorporeal membrane oxygenation (ECMO) has been used as rescue therapy for neonates with overwhelming early-onset group B streptococcal sepsis. Hocker and associates[762] reported a retrospective study that compared conventionally or ECMO-treated neonates with early-onset disease. A fatal outcome occurred in 3 of 28 (11%) of conventionally treated and 9 of 53 (17%) infants placed on ECMO. If only hypotensive neonates were considered, 13 of 15 ECMO patients survived compared with 11 of 18 of those treated conventionally ($p = .06$). These authors concluded that neonates with suspected early-onset sepsis who develop acidosis or hypotension should be considered for early referral to an ECMO center. Commenting on these results, LeBlanc[763] emphasizes the difficulty interpreting this study, citing the retrospective design and the fact that the most ill infants die before ECMO can be initiated. He also stressed that fatal complications of ECMO, such as brain hemorrhage, occur. Until a prospective, controlled trial is performed, this therapy should be considered controversial.

Adjunctive Therapies

Despite prompt initiation of antimicrobial therapy and aggressive supportive care, mortality and neurologic morbidity can result from group B streptococcal infection. Irreversible shock, often associated with persistent fetal circulation, is a frequent cause of death, and new methods for treatment of these complications have been sought. Nonsteroidal anti-inflammatory agents have improved survival in experimental models of endotoxin-mediated shock. The initial phase of shock with its associated pulmonary hypertension can be prevented in experimental infection by administration of indomethacin or dazmegrel, each of which inhibits synthesis of thromboxane A_2, a potent vasoconstrictor.[332–334, 764–766] The second hemodynamic phase appears to be independent of prostaglandin synthesis, but it can be inhibited by corticosteroids.[327, 346] The clinical significance of these and other experimental findings awaits controlled clinical trials.

Adjunctive therapy directed toward improvement of neonatal host defenses against group B streptococci has received considerable investigative effort. In an experimental rat model of group B streptococcal infection, both the neutrophil response and phagocytic efficiency in clearing bacteremia are deficient.[767] Rapid depletion of the neutrophil storage pool also occurs. Protection in this model can be achieved by injection of adult but not neonatal rat neutrophils.[768] These observations plus reports indicating the enhanced mortality in neutropenic neonates prompted clinical evaluation of granulocyte transfusions as adjunctive therapy for early-onset group B streptococcal sepsis.[478, 504, 769–771] In three trials, 13 infants with neutrophil storage pool depletion (documented by bone marrow aspiration) were assessed.[478, 504, 770] The results seemed promising, but the logistics of providing timely transfusion and the concern for adverse effects (graft-versus-host reaction, transmission of viral agents, pulmonary leukocyte sequestration) make this mode of therapy impractical.

Recombinant human cytokine molecules stimulatory for granulocyte progenitor cells, namely, granulocyte colony-stimulating factor (G-CSF) and granulocyte-macrophage colony-stimulating factor (GM-CSF), are widely available. G-CSF promotes proliferation of granulocyte progenitors in bone marrow, enhances chemotactic activities and superoxide anion production, and increases expression of neutrophil C3bi receptors. Because many of these attributes might improve the limited bone marrow neutrophil reserve and the defective neutrophil functions in human neonates, several investigators have evaluated their use as adjunctive therapy in experimental infection. Taken together, these studies suggest that G-CSF or GM-CSF might be useful as adjuncts in the treatment of group B streptococcal neonatal sepsis, possibly when they are used in combination with intravenous immune globulin (IGIV).[772–775] Any clinical recommendations must await evaluation of their safety and efficacy in controlled clinical trials.

Another proposed therapy is human immune globulin modified for intravenous use.[448] These preparations theoretically could provide type-specific antibodies for more efficient opsonization and phagocytosis of group B streptococci.[776–785] Also, IGIV has been shown in an animal model[786] and in septic neonates[787] to improve complement activation and chemotaxis by neonatal sera and to hasten resolution of neutropenia. Several investigators have demonstrated that administration with sufficient amounts of human type-specific antibodies against capsular polysaccharides to animals before lethal challenge with group B streptococci of the homologous serotype is protective.[380, 391, 777, 779–783]

Despite the sound theoretical basis on which use of IGIV as adjunctive therapy is based, several problems and questions have evolved. First, commercially available preparations contain relatively low concentrations of protective antibodies (directed at either protein or polysaccharide surface antigens),[782–785, 787–792] suggesting that large doses would be required and raising concern for reticuloendothelial system blockade.[780, 781, 784] Second, the in vitro functional activity of the currently licensed globulins varies by method of preparation and by lot.[503, 509, 779–781, 787–794] Third, the increase in type-specific antibodies after infusion may be only transient.[788, 795]

Development of hyperimmune group B streptococcal globulin or of human-human monoclonal antibodies would theoretically circumvent many of these potential problems. Raff and co-workers[796] developed a human

IgM monoclonal antibody specific for the group B cell wall polysaccharide. This antibody reacts with all group B streptococcal serotypes and was evaluated for safety and pharmacokinetics in two neonatal nonhuman primates.[797] Both it and a hyperimmune globulin[791] prepared by vaccination of healthy adults with polysaccharides from types Ia, Ib, II, and III group B streptococci were protective against experimental challenge with type I, II, and III strains in doses as low as 4 to 20 mg/kg.[798]

At the present time, the application, if any, of these intriguing experimental findings to the clinical setting remains unknown. However, clinical trials provide some insights. A prospective, multicenter, placebo-controlled trial was performed that entered 753 neonates with birth weights from 500 to 2000 g who were being empirically treated for possible sepsis; in 12 the causative agent was group B *Streptococcus*. Administration of IGIV at a dose of 500 mg/kg within 12 hours of birth was well tolerated and resulted in a survival rate among neonates with group B streptococcal sepsis that was similar to that of placebo recipients. The report by Christensen and colleagues[799] administered either IGIV (750 mg/kg) or albumin to 22 neonates with severe, early-onset sepsis. All infants survived. Eleven patients had neutropenia, but in all six IGIV recipients this resolved within 24 hours of infusion, whereas it persisted in each of the five albumin recipients. Furthermore, each of the IGIV recipients had a significant elevation of immature to total neutrophil ratios 1 hour after infusion when compared with controls. The IGIV was considered to stimulate release of neutrophils into the circulation from bone marrow storage pools. Based on limited data, it can be concluded that administration of IGIV in a single dose ranging from 500 to 750 mg/kg in neonates with clinical sepsis is safe and may provide hematologic and immunologic benefit.

PROGNOSIS

Considering the extensive investigation of group B streptococcal disease, there is a relative paucity of information concerning the prognosis for infants surviving invasive neonatal infection. Several reports have assessed sequelae among survivors of meningitis, but these do not reflect outcome for infants receiving intensive supportive care since the late 1980s. In 1977, Haslam and associates[551] reported major neurologic sequelae in 2 of 15 survivors of meningitis. No differences were evident between survivors and sibling controls in tests of hearing, speech, or adaptive skills. In a prospective assessment of 20 survivors of early-onset meningitis treated between 1974 and 1982, 14 (70%) were considered to be normal.[549] Major handicaps were found in 15%, and 3 had mild cognitive impairments. Similarly, 50% of children assessed at a mean age of 6 years after surviving meningitis during the 1970s were functioning normally.[552] Another 29% had severe sequelae, including global mental retardation, cortical blindness, and spasticity. Among the 21% with mild or moderate sequelae, deficits such as borderline mental retardation, spastic or flaccid monoparesis, or language delay still permitted

function at or near age-expected norms. In a study of 74 children who survived early- or late-onset group B streptococcal meningitis, 12% had major neurologic sequelae when evaluated at 3 to 18 years of age.[568] When these 9 children were excluded, there were no significant differences as rated by parents between the children with meningitis and their siblings for academic achievement, measures of intelligence quotient, fine motor dexterity, or behavior difficulties. These investigators concluded that "children not identified early, after appropriate examination, as having serious sequelae can be expected to perform intellectually, socially, and academically in a manner similar to other family members."[568]

Several clinical scoring systems for predicting a fatal outcome from neonatal group B streptococcal infection have been reported.[552, 558, 559] Payne and colleagues described a score derived from five variables, which, together with an initial blood pH less than 7.25, enabled prediction of outcome accurately in 93% of infants with early-onset group B streptococcal infection. These features were birth weight less than 2500 g, absolute neutrophil count less than 1500 cells per mm^3, hypotension, apnea, and a pleural effusion by initial chest radiograph.

Although a fatal outcome can be predicted with reasonable accuracy, little information is available concerning the long-term prognosis for survivors of neonatal group B streptococcal sepsis. One group at potential risk for sequelae is the preterm infant with septic shock who could develop periventricular leukomalacia. These survivors have had substantial neurodevelopmental sequelae at evaluation during the second year of life. However, the correlates of severity and duration of shock with periventricular leukomalacia and with long-term morbidity from group B streptococcal disease have not been evaluated. A poor prognosis also may be associated with very late-onset group B streptococcal disease, because a subset of these infants have HIV infection.[545]

PREVENTION

Theoretically, early- and late-onset group B streptococcal disease could be prevented if susceptible hosts were not exposed to the microorganism or if exposure occurred in the setting of protective immunity. Although several approaches to prevention have been advocated, the basic strategies are directed at either eliminating exposure or enhancing host resistance. These strategies are chemoprophylaxis and immunoprophylaxis. Both have limitations with respect to implementation, could be targeted for the prevention of maternal as well as neonatal infections, and are theoretically achievable.[15, 33, 176, 302, 800]

Chemoprophylaxis

HISTORICAL PRECEDENTS

Chemoprophylaxis as a method for preventing early-onset group B streptococcal infection was first suggested by Franciosi and colleagues in 1973.[5] Because vertical transmission was documented to be the prelude to early-onset disease, these and other investigators proposed oral penicillin treatment of colonized women late in pregnancy to interrupt maternal exposure of the neonate. This theoretically logical approach, however, has been demonstrated to be ineffective.

Early studies identified group B streptococcal carriers with third trimester vaginal cultures; culture-positive women were treated with oral antimicrobial agents for 1 to 2 weeks. Some 20 to 30% remained colonized at the end of therapy, and nearly 70% had group B streptococci isolated from vaginal cultures at delivery.[194, 801, 802] A suggested mechanism for these treatment failures was the possibility that pregnant women were being reinfected by colonized sexual partners.[5] In a study in which colonized pregnant women and their spouses were treated concurrently with oral penicillin for 14 days, Gardner and co-workers[194] found that 70% of women and 40% of their husbands remained infected after treatment. Somewhat better results were reported by Lewin and Amstey,[803] who administered 1.2 million units of benzathine penicillin G and 1.2 million units of procaine penicillin G intramuscularly to colonized, third-trimester women and their husbands. Only 18% of women remained colonized at delivery. One explanation for failure of antimicrobial therapy to eliminate group B streptococcal colonization is the inherent difficulty of eradicating a constituent of the bowel and genital flora even when high doses of intravenous penicillin G or ampicillin are employed.[194]

The next method evaluated in the attempt to prevent early-onset group B streptococcal neonatal infection by interrupting perinatal exposure was use of intravenously administered antibiotic to women during labor. This approach was first investigated by Yow and colleagues[804] in 1979. She treated 34 third-trimester women colonized with group B streptococci with intravenous ampicillin (500 mg) at hospital admission. Ampicillin uniformly interrupted vertical transmission to the neonates of treated women, contrasting with an expected rate of approximately 50%.[20] This observation was extended by others.[213, 805–807]

The first documentation that intrapartum chemoprophylaxis was effective in preventing early-onset neonatal disease as well as group B streptococcal–associated maternal morbidity was reported by Boyer and Gotoff in 1986.[807] In their prospective, randomized, and controlled trial, group B streptococcal colonization was detected at 26 to 28 weeks' gestation through use of lower vaginal and anorectal swabs incubated in selective broth medium.[44] Women who were carrying group B streptococci who had risk factors for early-onset infection were randomized to receive routine care or intrapartum intravenous ampicillin. Treated women did not vertically transmit group B streptococci to their infants, whereas the rate in neonates born to control women was 51%. Five of 79 neonates born to untreated women developed group B streptococcal sepsis (one death), whereas each of the 85 infants born to ampicillin-treated women remained well ($p = .024$). In a similarly designed study reported from Madrid, 1.8% of neonates born to ampicillin-treated and 13% born to untreated women developed early-onset group B streptococcal septicemia ($p =$

.04).[242] In a later report, these investigators also concluded that intrapartum ampicillin chemoprophylaxis for group B streptococcal carriers resulted in reduced maternal morbidity.[808] These and other studies[805, 809–811] established the efficacy of intrapartum chemoprophylaxis in group B streptococcal carriers identified antenatally in the prevention of early-onset neonatal disease and group B *Streptococcus*–associated maternal morbidity. Additional investigators have validated the cost effectiveness of this prevention method.[812–816]

RAPID ASSAYS FOR ANTENATAL DETECTION OF GROUP B STREPTOCOCCI

Controversy concerning the optimal gestation for antenatal group B streptococcal screening, the site or sites for maximal detection, and the predictive value of an antenatal culture result for carriage at delivery led to attempts at identifying candidates for selective intrapartum chemoprophylaxis at hospital admission. Morales and colleagues[805, 811] sought to detect vaginal colonization with a latex agglutination assay in 260 women admitted with premature rupture of membranes and a gestation of less than 34 weeks. A vaginal swab was placed into selective broth medium, which was incubated for 5 ("heavy" colonization) or 20 ("light" colonization) hours. The broth was then tested for group B antigen. Antigen-positive women received antimicrobial therapy. None of the neonates of women who received ampicillin had early-onset sepsis. Of women with a short latency period or in whom treatment delay occurred, 23% developed chorioamnionitis and 36% of their neonates had early-onset sepsis. In another study, the strategy of employing intrapartum screening followed by chemoprophylaxis of all group B antigen–positive women failed to prevent 13% of the cases of early-onset neonatal disease because the test result was delayed or the delivery was precipitous.[810]

These studies highlight the difficulties inherent in determining group B streptococcal colonization status at hospital admission, even when assays can be processed 24 hours a day. Several rapid methods using cervical or lower vaginal swab specimens have been evaluated in an attempt to more rapidly ascertain the colonization status at hospital admission. When vaginal swabs are immediately extracted (no incubation step) and tested for group B streptococcal antigen by LPA, the reported sensitivity ranges from 15 to 28% for all culture positives and from 57 to 67% for "heavily" colonized women; the specificity ranges from 95 to 99%.[810, 817–819] When swabs are tested by enzyme immunoassays, the reported sensitivity ranges from 12 to 44% for all colonized women and from 36 to 100% for "heavily" colonized women; the reported specificity is from 95 to 99%.[818, 820–823] Thus, these rapid antigen detection assays for vaginal swab specimens have limited sensitivity to detect group B streptococcal carriers, especially among women with a low inoculum of organisms. Although attack rates for early-onset disease are significantly higher in neonates born to "heavily" colonized women, risk also exists for those born to "lightly" colonized women (~0.5%).[25, 217, 810, 820] Alternatively, if commercially available latex assays are positive, the result is highly reliable. An optical immunoassay (Strep B OIA test, Biostar, Boulder, Colo) is more sensitive for detecting light (37–67%) and heavy (94–100%) colonization and outperforms enzyme immunoassays in direct comparisons.[823–825] Assays using a DNA hybridization methodology have shown variable sensitivity.[826, 827] None of these rapid tests is sufficiently accurate for routine use in the intrapartum detection of women colonized with group B streptococci. A bulletin from the Food and Drug Administration in 1995 provided guidelines stipulating that antigen tests "cannot be relied upon to exclude group B streptococcal colonization in a pregnant woman. Negative group B streptococcal antigen test results should be confirmed using selective broth culture which is more sensitive than antigen tests."[704]

INTRAPARTUM ANTIMICROBIAL PROPHYLAXIS

One approach to the prevention of early-onset group B streptococcal sepsis in neonates through intrapartum maternal chemoprophylaxis is to target all colonized women (nonselective). Garland and Fliegner[809] identified Australian vaginal carriers of group B streptococci at 32 weeks' gestation and treated all culture-positive women during labor with intravenous penicillin G (1 million units every 6 hours). From 1981 to 1988, no cases of early-onset disease occurred in neonates born to culture-positive women given intrapartum chemoprophylaxis.

In the United States, the rationale for offering intrapartum chemoprophylaxis to all women who have antenatal cultures positive for group B streptococci evolved from two concerns. First, selective intrapartum chemoprophylaxis fails to prevent an estimated 25 to 45% of cases and about 10% of deaths.[26, 299, 807] These cases represent term infants born to women with no identifiable risk factors for early-onset infant disease such as membrane rupture for more than 18 hours or fever during labor. However, the number of cases missed by selective chemoprophylaxis might be substantially diminished if the maternal risk factors were expanded to include premature rupture of membranes at any gestation,[219] asymptomatic bacteriuria caused by group B streptococci,[178, 286, 828] nongestational diabetes mellitus,[26, 828] women younger than 20 years, and black women.[26, 285, 302] Second, the pregnant woman informed that she carries a potential pathogen for her newborn often may desire prophylaxis in the absence of risk factors, especially when she is told that a risk factor–based prevention approach "misses" up to 50% of cases.[299]

For the prevention of early-onset disease, intrapartum maternal chemoprophylaxis ideally should be administered at least 4 hours before delivery. This allows sufficient time to achieve concentrations of ampicillin in the fetal blood (an estimated 30 minutes) and the amniotic fluid (~2 to 4 hours)[829, 830] that are bactericidal for group B streptococci. Also, when high doses of ampicillin (2 g) or penicillin G (5 million units) are given intravenously 4 or more hours before delivery, vertical transmission is interrupted[831] and infant disease prevented. Intrapartum chemoprophylaxis has no known efficacy in the prevention of late-onset infant infection.

In 1992, the American College of Obstetricians and Gynecologists[832] and the American Academy of Pediatrics[176] published separate documents regarding maternal intrapartum chemoprophylaxis for the prevention of early-onset group B streptococcal infection. Both documents concurred that selective intrapartum chemoprophylaxis has been demonstrated to prevent early-onset group B streptococcal disease and reduce maternal puerperal morbidity. Also, both documents indicated that the maternal factors enhancing risk for early-onset disease in the neonate were preterm labor at less than 37 weeks' gestation, preterm premature rupture of membranes at less than 37 weeks' gestation, rupture of membranes at any gestation beyond 18 hours, fever during labor, and previous delivery of a sibling with invasive group B streptococcal disease.[833, 834] Whereas the technical bulletin from the American College of Obstetricians and Gynecologists[832] was educational, the American Academy of Pediatrics guidelines[176] were more directive. The latter suggested that if culture screening were performed antenatally, cultures from both lower vaginal and anorectal sites should be obtained and that women with one or more risk factors and group B streptococcal colonization should be given intrapartum intravenous ampicillin or penicillin G. The American College of Obstetricians and Gynecologists proposed that culture screening could be avoided by treating all women with risk factors. Neither approach was widely implemented, and invasive disease rates remained high.

In 1996, consensus guidelines for the prevention of early-onset group B streptococcal disease were published by the Centers for Disease Control and Prevention (CDC), the American College of Obstetricians and Gynecologists, and the American Academy of Pediatrics.[33–35] These guidelines recommended that obstetric care providers and hospitals adopt a policy for group B Streptococcus prevention based on one of two strategies to identify women who require intrapartum chemoprophylaxis.[33–35] One strategy is culture based, and the other is risk factor based. When the culture-based approach is employed, the results of vaginal and rectal cultures obtained at 35 to 37 weeks' gestation and processed in selective broth media dictate prophylaxis. In this circumstance, it has been shown that most women prefer self-obtaining of cultures, and there is a high correlation with patient- and nurse-collected samples for accuracy.[835, 836] Furthermore, pregnant women place a high priority on knowing their group B streptococcal colonization status.[837] Thus, all women identified as carriers, and all unscreened women with a risk factor, would be offered intrapartum chemoprophylaxis. When the risk factor–based strategy is employed, women to be offered prophylaxis are identified by factors known to increase the likelihood of neonatal group B streptococcal disease; antenatal screening cultures are not performed. These risk factors include labor onset or membrane rupture before 37 weeks' gestation, intrapartum fever, or rupture of membranes more than 18 hours before delivery (Table 26–11). In both strategies, all women either with previous delivery of an infant with group B streptococcal disease or with group B streptococcal bacteriuria during the current pregnancy always receive prophylaxis. Each

TABLE 26–11

Strategies for Prevention of Early-Onset Group B Streptococcal Disease by Maternal Intrapartum Chemoprophylaxis

STRATEGY	TARGET POPULATION	ESTIMATED PROPORTION OF CASES PREVENTED	ESTIMATED PERCENT OF POPULATION TARGETED
Culture based	All GBS-positive women and women with ■ Previous GBS-infected infant or ■ GBS bacteriuria	85–90%	20–25%
Risk factor based	Women with any of the factors above or ■ Labor before 37 weeks' gestation ■ Rupture of membranes ≥18 hours or ■ Intrapartum fever (≥38° C)	50–65%	~15–25%

of these strategies results in the administration of antimicrobial agents intravenously to as many as 25% of pregnant women.[33] However, the proportion of disease theoretically prevented by the culture-based approach is higher (85–90%) than that using the risk factor–based approach (50–65%).[33, 320] Group B streptococcal carriers without risk factors can be delivered of infants with early-onset disease, and approximately 45% of infants with early-onset disease are born to such women.[299]

The recommended maternal intrapartum chemoprophylaxis regimen consists of penicillin G (5 million units initially and 2.5 million units every 4 hours thereafter until delivery).[33–35] Prophylaxis should be initiated as soon as possible because penicillin given 4 hours or more before delivery prevents vertical transmission and early-onset disease more reliably than doses given at shorter intervals. Ampicillin administered as a 2-g intravenous loading dose and then 1 g intravenously every 4 hours until delivery is the alternative antimicrobial regimen.[33–35] Regimens for the penicillin-allergic woman have not been evaluated for efficacy, and increasing in vitro resistance of group B streptococcal strains to the recommended alternative agents, clindamycin and erythromycin,[716, 733, 734] have led some experts to consider a first-generation cephalosporin, such as cefazolin, as the alternative drug.

The CDC has collected surveillance data to determine the impact of maternal intrapartum chemoprophylaxis on early-onset disease. For areas from which continuous data between 1993 and 1997 are available, representing approximately 190,000 annual births, a 53% decline in the incidence of early-onset disease has been documented (Fig. 26–10).[838] When data from 1998 are included, the incidence has decreased by 65%, to 0.6 per 1000 live births. There has not been a significant decline in the incidence of late-onset disease, although there is evidence to suggest a small downward trend.[35a]

MANAGEMENT OF NEONATES BORN TO MOTHERS RECEIVING INTRAPARTUM ANTIMICROBIAL PROPHYLAXIS

Management of the infant born to a mother given intrapartum chemoprophylaxis is based on the infant's clinical status at birth, the gestational age of the infant, and the duration of maternal chemoprophylaxis before delivery (Table 26–12).[34] If the infant has signs of infection, full diagnostic evaluation including a complete blood cell count and differential, blood culture, and chest radiograph (if the neonate has respiratory symptoms) should be performed. Lumbar puncture is performed at the discretion of the physician. The caveat that a minimum

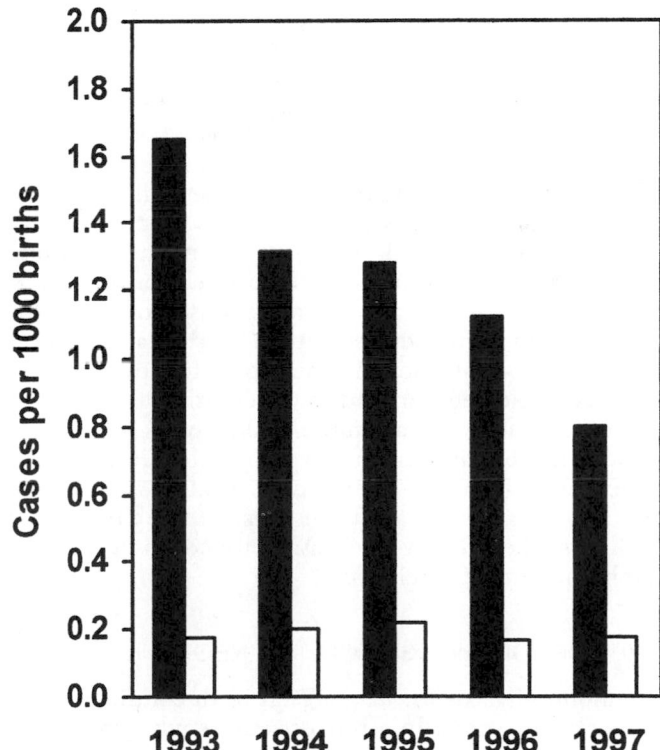

FIGURE 26–10 Incidence of early-onset (solid bars) and late-onset (open bars) group B streptococcal disease from 1993–1997. Data reflect aggregate disease rates from the state of Maryland as well as from three counties in California, eight in Georgia and five in Tennessee that represent approximately 190,000 births annually. (Adapted from Schuchat A. Group B *Streptococcus*. Lancet 353:51–56, 1999.)

TABLE 26–12
Management of Neonates Born to Women Receiving Intrapartum Chemoprophylaxis

CLINICAL STATUS/ GESTATION	DURATION OF MATERNAL CHEMOPROPHYLAXIS BEFORE DELIVERY	APPROACH	DURATION OF THERAPY
Symptomatic/Any	Any	Full diagnostic evaluation and initiation of empirical therapy for sepsis	As appropriate, based on results of cultures and clinical course of the infant
Asymptomatic/<35 Weeks	Any	Limited evaluation[a] Observe ≥48 hours[b]	None unless symptoms develop; then as dictated by results of cultures and clinical status of the infant
Asymptomatic/≥35 Weeks	≤4 hours	Limited evaluation[a] Observe ≥48 hours[b]	None unless symptoms develop; then as dictated by results of cultures and clinical status of the infant
Asymptomatic/≥35 Weeks	>4 hours	No evaluation Observe ≥48 hours[b]	None

[a]Consists of complete blood cell count and differential and a blood culture.
[b]If follow-up is assured and observation in home setting is reliable, this may be shortened to 24 hours.

of 10 to 15% of infants with meningitis will have a negative blood culture[684] should be kept in mind. Empirical therapy for neonatal sepsis then is initiated. The duration of therapy is based on results of cultures and the infant's clinical course (see Treatment section). If the infant is healthy in appearance but less than 35 weeks' gestation, a limited evaluation, including a blood culture, is performed without regard to the duration of maternal chemoprophylaxis. Empirical therapy need not be initiated unless the infant develops signs of sepsis or is very immature. Healthy-appearing infants of 35 weeks' gestation or more whose mothers had penicillin or ampicillin less than 4 hours before delivery also should be evaluated and observed closely. If the infant is asymptomatic, has a gestational age of 35 weeks or more, and has a mother given two or more doses of penicillin or ampicillin before delivery, then neither a diagnostic evaluation nor empirical antimicrobial therapy is recommended. The recommended observation interval for neonates undergoing a limited evaluation is 48 hours.[34] However, the management given in Table 26–12 is not an exclusive management pathway. It allows, for example, individual physicians to discharge these neonates at 24 hours when follow-up is assured and observation in the home setting is reliable.[839]

CHEMOPROPHYLAXIS FOR THE NEONATE

Chemoprophylaxis for neonates at birth continues to be advocated by some. In a retrospective study reported in 1978, Steigman and associates[840] indicated that among 130,000 newborns receiving a single intramuscular injection of penicillin G (50,000 units) at birth for gonococcal prophylaxis, no cases of early-onset group B streptococcal infection were recorded. The prevalence of maternal colonization was not determined, and a later report from the same hospital indicated that neonates with possible in utero acquisition of infection (those symptomatic at

birth) did not receive prophylaxis and were excluded from the analysis.[841] Investigators from the same institution using the same prophylactic regimen more recently reported an early-onset disease incidence of 0.34 per 1000 live births.[842] They continue to encourage consideration of this intervention to prevent early-onset disease, but as an adjunct to maternal chemoprophylaxis.

The lack of efficacy of chemoprophylaxis at birth in preventing early-onset infection was reported by Pyati and co-workers.[843] They evaluated 1187 neonates with birth weights less than 2000 g. Infants received penicillin within 90 minutes of birth or routine care. Infants had peripheral venous blood cultures obtained before treatment. Among 589 infants receiving prophylaxis, there were 10 with early-onset group B streptococcal bacteremia, 6 of whom died. Among the 598 control patients, there were 14 with group B streptococcal bacteremia during the first 72 hours of life; 8 died. Bacteremia within 90 minutes of birth was detected in 90% of treated and 86% of control infants. Thus, in these high-risk infants penicillin prophylaxis at birth was not effective in preventing bacteremia or in altering mortality rate.

Siegel and associates[21, 282] reported a prospective nonrandomized controlled study of a single intramuscular dose of penicillin G at birth that demonstrated that treated neonates had a significantly lower incidence of early-onset disease than did untreated controls. No cultures were obtained before penicillin prophylaxis. In an extension of these observations, the incidence of early-onset group B streptococcal disease from 1972 to 1994 in neonates receiving penicillin (0.25 to 0.63 per 1000) was significantly lower than that in untreated groups (1.19 to 1.95 per 1000) ($p = 0.03$).[844] These investigators propose that universal administration of single-dose penicillin at birth be considered in regions where a frequency of early-onset disease exceeds 1.5 per 1000 live births, either as an adjunct to maternal intrapartum chemoprophylaxis or as the sole means of prophylaxis in centers that lack universal culture screening or have not implemented protocols for intrapartum prophylaxis.

A special circumstance, however, merits consideration for infant chemoprophylaxis: the nonaffected sibling in a twin or multiple birth with early-onset[303, 304] or late-onset[304] group B streptococcal disease. In this situation, the infant sibling of a neonate with invasive infection has a 25-fold increased risk to develop group B streptococcal disease. At the time of diagnosis of group B streptococcal disease in one infant of a multiple birth, the other infant or infants should be clinically evaluated.[304] If any sign of infection is noted, cultures of blood *and* CSF are obtained, and empirical treatment is initiated and continued until cultures have been sterile for 48 hours. Obviously, if cultures are positive, a full course of treatment is recommended. If the initial clinical evaluation is unremarkable, management should be individualized. The high incidence of infection in both twins and the poor outcome noted when the second twin was not evaluated until the onset of symptoms[304, 845] merit caution in this circumstance. However, even when empirical therapy is given and invasive infection excluded, later onset may occur. This has been reported by Rubin and McDonald[846] in the noninfected sibling of a twin with early-onset infection. This nonaffected twin presented at 23 days of age with late-onset group B streptococcal bacteremia.

Immunoprophylaxis

The most promising and potentially lasting method for prevention of early- and late-onset infant infections as well as maternal infectious morbidity is immunoprophylaxis.[15, 177, 302, 800, 847] The underlying principle is that serum IgG directed against the type-specific capsular polysaccharide critical for protection against invasive group B streptococcal disease is provided by passive or active immunization. Human sera containing sufficient amounts of type III–specific antibody is protective against lethal challenge in animal models of infection.[848, 849] Studies of the other serotypes also indicate the importance of type-specific antibody in protection.[378–382, 850, 851] Provision of protective levels of type-specific immunity to the newborn theoretically may be achieved through passive or active immunization of the mother. Passive immune therapy for the mother would require development of hyperimmune preparations of human immune globulin for intravenous use, but animal studies indicate the potential usefulness of such an approach.[771, 852]

The capsular polysaccharides from the prevalent group B streptococcal serotypes including Ia, II, III, and V have been isolated, purified, and immunochemically characterized and tested as candidate immunogens in adults.[127, 130, 131, 415, 853, 854] Vaccination of adults with low serum levels of specific antibodies, the target population for the prevention of group B streptococcal maternal and infant infection, is safe, and an immune response occurs within 2 weeks of subcutaneous immunization in a mean of 40, 88, and 60% of adults given 50 μg of types Ia, II, or III polysaccharide vaccines, respectively.[853] Serum antibody levels among these vaccine re-

sponders have remained at presumably protective levels 5 to 7 years after immunization. Vaccine-induced antibodies are predominantly of the IgG class, the IgG_1 and IgG_2 subclasses, and are protective in vivo.[390, 449, 848]

In the only study of group B streptococcal vaccine in pregnant women, 40 were given type III polysaccharide at a mean of 30 weeks' gestation.[476] A significant antibody response was observed in 63% of these women. Cord serum concentrations of antibody to type III polysaccharide were significantly correlated with maternal delivery concentrations, with an estimated 70% transport via the placenta. Among infants born to the 25 vaccine responders, 83 and 75%, respectively, had protective levels of antibody in their sera at 1 and 2 months of age. Although this vaccine was not optimally immunogenic, the results of this clinical trial imply that maternal immunization with group B streptococcal vaccines can provide passive immunity against invasive infection in mothers and the majority of their infants during the critical period of susceptibility.[476]

The poor immunogenicity of most candidate group B streptococcal capsular polysaccharides in nonimmune adults suggested that protein-polysaccharide conjugates would be more suitable as vaccines.[800, 855] The first group B streptococcal conjugate vaccines were described in 1990.[854, 855] Such protein-polysaccharide vaccines are immunogenic and protective in experimental animals.[854, 856–859] Initial results using these candidate vaccines in which group B streptococcal polysaccharides are conjugated to tetanus toxoid by reductive amination, reveal their safety and excellent immunogenicity in nonpregnant adults.[860, 861] These candidate vaccines currently are undergoing additional clinical investigations that include administration as a multivalent preparation and testing of a monovalent vaccine in pregnant women.

An alternate method for the preparation of polysaccharide-protein conjugate vaccines is to employ the optimal oligosaccharide size by selective activation of the polysaccharide before conjugation.[855] Oligosaccharides may better elicit T cell help when conjugated to a protein antigen than polysaccharides. Paoletti and associates[862] reported the synthesis of a type III oligosaccharide and conjugation by reductive amination to tetanus toxoid. This conjugate was immunogenic in rabbits, producing antibodies that were functionally active and protective. Conjugate size, polysaccharide size, and the degree of polysaccharide-protein cross-linking all are important considerations in optimizing immunogenicity of candidate vaccines.[863]

Since the C protein of group B *Streptococcus* is common to several serotypes, and two of its four antigens—alpha and beta—have been characterized, cloned, and shown to be immunogenic and protective in experimental animals,[851, 859, 864] protein C may be a promising alternative to tetanus toxoid as the protein component of a conjugate vaccine. Based on the prevalence of group B streptococcal serotypes thought to cause perinatal disease, a type III polysaccharide–C protein conjugate vaccine composed of both the alpha and beta antigens theoretically could prevent 85% of systemic infections.[28] Once an optimal vaccine has been characterized and shown to be safe and immunogenic, its efficacy in women for prevention of neonatal and maternal disease can be assessed.

Because the majority of women have low concentrations of type-specific antibody in their sera, the most practical approach for future immunoprophylaxis is active immunization of all women of childbearing age, either before or later in pregnancy (i.e., early third trimester) or perhaps at the time of the adolescent vaccinations.[800] The strategy of targeting all women for active immunization as a means to prevent group B streptococcal disease also has difficulties. Even successfully vaccinated women may be delivered of infants so early in gestation that placental transfer of protective antibodies is inadequate. This group of infants, those born before 34 weeks' gestation, represents less than 2% of all early-onset cases.[313] More important, physicians *and* their patients must perceive this mode of prevention to be of high benefit and negligible risk, especially if pregnant women are to be the target population. Because as many as 65 to 85% of all infants with group B streptococcal disease (early- and late-onset) are born at term,[20, 21, 26, 547, 548] immunogenic group B streptococcal vaccines given to women early in the third trimester of pregnancy theoretically could prevent up to 95% of these infections. Finally, if active immunization is deemed unsuitable for pregnant women, effectively targeting nonpregnant women for vaccination will undoubtedly present the same difficulties noted for implementation of other vaccines among adults. The cost of developing suitable vaccines, although substantial, is considerably less than that of treating these infections and, for some infants, their lifelong sequelae.[15, 813, 816] However, if the prevention of group B streptococcal disease is to become a reality in the future, obstetricians, pediatricians, public health officials, parents, and legislators must join together as advocates for the pregnant woman and her neonate.

References

1. Fry RM. Fatal infections by haemolytic streptococcus group B. Lancet 1:199–201, 1938.
2. Hood M, Janney A, Dameron G. Beta-hemolytic *Streptococcus* group B associated with problems of perinatal period. Am J Obstet Gynecol 82:809–818, 1961.
3. Eickhoff TC, Klein JO, Daly AL, et al. Neonatal sepsis and other infections due to group B beta-hemolytic streptococci. N Engl J Med 271:1221–1228, 1964.
4. Butter MNW, de Moor CE. *Streptococcus agalactiae* as a cause of meningitis in the newborn, and of bacteremia in adults. Antonie van Leeuwenhoek 33:439–450, 1967.
5. Franciosi RA, Knostman JD, Zimmerman RA. Group B streptococcal neonatal and infant infections. J Pediatr 82:707–718, 1973.
6. Baker CJ, Barrett FF. Transmission of group B streptococci among parturient women and their neonates. J Pediatr 83:919–925, 1973.
7. Howard JB, McCracken GH Jr. The spectrum of group B streptococcal infections in infancy. Am J Dis Child 128:815–818, 1974.
8. Schauf V, Hlaing V. Group B streptococcal colonization in pregnancy. Obstet Gynecol 47:719, 1976.
9. Aber RC, Allen N, Howell JT, et al. Nosocomial trans-

10. mission of group B streptococci. Pediatrics 58:346–353, 1976.
10. Anthony BF, Okada DM. The emergence of group B streptococci in infections of the newborn infant. Ann Rev Med 28:355–369, 1977.
11. Pass MA, Gray BM, Khare S, et al. Prospective studies of group B streptococcal infections in infants. J Pediatr 95:437–443, 1979.
12. Bayer AS, Chow AW, Anthony BF, et al. Serious infections in adults due to group B streptococci. Am J Med 61:498–503, 1976.
13. Lerner PI, Gopalakrishna KV, Wolinsky E, et al. Group B *Streptococcus (S. agalactiae)* bacteremia in adults: analysis of 32 cases and review of the literature. Medicine 56:457–473, 1977.
14. Nicklas JM. Serious group B beta-hemolytic streptococcal infections in adults: report of two cases and review of the literature. Johns Hopkins Med J 142:39–45, 1978.
15. Institute of Medicine, National Academy of Sciences. Appendix P. New vaccine development: establishing priorities. *In* Diseases of Importance in the United States, vol 1. Washington, DC, National Academy Press, 1985, pp 242–439.
16. Ledger WJ, Norman M, Gee C, et al. Bacteremia on an obstetric-gynecologic service. Am J Obstet Gynecol 121:205–212, 1975.
17. Faro S. Group B beta-hemolytic streptococci and puerperal infections. Am J Obstet Gynecol 139:686–689, 1981.
18. Farley MM, Harvey RC, Stull T, et al. A population-based assessment of invasive disease due to group B *Streptococcus* in nonpregnant adults. N Engl J Med 328:1807-1811, 1993.
19. Freedman RM, Ingram DL, Gross I, et al. A half century of neonatal sepsis at Yale, 1928 to 1978. Am J Dis Child 135:140–144, 1981.
20. Baker CJ, Edwards MS. Group B streptococcal infections: perinatal impact and prevention methods. Ann N Y Acad Sci 549:193–202, 1988.
21. Siegel JD, McCracken GH Jr, Threlkeld N, et al. Single dose penicillin prophylaxis against neonatal group B streptococcal infections. N Engl J Med 303:769–775, 1980.
22. Broughton RA, Krafka R, Baker CJ. Non-group D alpha-hemolytic streptococci, new neonatal pathogens. Pediatrics 99:450–454, 1981.
23. Speer CP, Hauptmann D, Stubbe P, et al. Neonatal septicemia and meningitis in Göttingen, West Germany. Pediatr Infect Dis J 4:36–41, 1985.
24. Easmon CSF. Group B *Streptococcus*. Infect Control 7:S135–S137, 1986.
25. Dillon HC Jr, Khare S, Gray BM. Group B streptococcal carriage and disease: a 6-year prospective study. J Pediatr 110:31–36, 1987.
26. Schuchat A, Oxtoby M, Cochi S, et al. Population-based risk factors for neonatal group B streptococcal disease: results of a cohort study in metropolitan Atlanta. J Infect Dis 162:672–677, 1990.
27. Lin F-YC, Clemens JD, Azimi PH, et al. Capsular polysaccharide types of group B streptococcal isolates from neonates with early-onset systemic infection. J Infect Dis 177:790–792, 1998.
28. Harrison LH, Elliott JA, Dwyer DM, et al. Serotype distribution of invasive group B streptococcal isolates in Maryland: implications for vaccine formulation. J Infect Dis 177:998–1002, 1998.
29. Blumberg HM, Stephens DS, Modansky M, et al. Inva-

sive group B streptococcal disease: the emergence of serotype V. J Infect Dis 173:365–373, 1996.

30. Kvam AI, Efstratiou A, Bevanger L, et al. Distribution of serovariants of group B streptococci in isolates from England and Norway. J Med Microbiol 42:246–250, 1995.

31. Elliott JA, Farmer KD, Facklam RR. Sudden increase in isolation of group B streptococci, serotype V, is not due to emergence of a new pulsed-field gel electrophoresis type. J Clin Microbiol 36:2115–2116, 1998.

32. Lachenauer CS, Kasper DL, Shimada J, et al. Serotypes VI and VIII predominate among group B streptococci isolated from pregnant Japanese women. J Infect Dis 179:1030–1033, 1999.

33. Centers for Disease Control and Prevention. Prevention of perinatal group B streptococcal disease: a public health perspective. MMWR Morb Mortal Wkly Rep 45:1–24, 1996.

34. American Academy of Pediatrics Committee on Infectious Diseases and Committee on Fetus and Newborn. Revised guidelines for prevention of early-onset group B streptococcal (GBS) infection. Pediatrics 99:489–496, 1997.

35. American College of Obstetricians and Gynecologists Committee on Obstetric Practice: prevention of early-onset group B streptococcal disease in newborns. ACOG Committee Opinion. Washington, DC, American College of Obstetricians and Gynecologists (Bulletin No. 173), 1996.

35a. Schrag SJ, Zywicki S, Farley M, et al. Group B streptococcal disease in the era of intrapartum antibiotic prophylaxis. N Engl J Med 342:15–20, 2000.

36. Kasper DL, Baker CJ. Electron microscopic definition of surface antigens of group B Streptococcus. J Infect Dis 139:147–151, 1979.

37. Wagner B, Wagner M, Kubin V, et al. Immunoelectron microscopic study of the location of group-specific and protein type-specific antigens of group B streptococci. J Gen Microbiol 118:95–105, 1980.

38. Lancefield RC. A serological differentiation of human and other groups of hemolytic streptococci. J Exp Med 57:571–595, 1933.

39. Brown JH. Cultural differentiation of beta-hemolytic streptococci of human and bovine sources. J Exp Med 31:35–45, 1920.

40. Brown JH. Appearance of double-zone beta-hemolytic streptococci in blood agar. J Bacteriol 34:35–48, 1937.

41. Pollack HM, Dahlgren BJ. Distribution of streptococcal groups in clinical specimens with evaluation of bacitracin screening. Appl Microbiol 27:141–143, 1974.

42. Facklam RR, Padula JF, Thacker LG, et al. Presumptive identification of groups A, B and D streptococci. Appl Microbiol 27:107–113, 1974.

43. Roe MH, Todd JK, Favara BE. Non-hemolytic group B streptococcal infections. J Pediatr 89:75–77, 1976.

44. Baker CJ, Clark DJ, Barrett FF. Selective broth medium for isolation of group B streptococci. Appl Microbiol 26:884–885, 1973.

45. Baker CJ, Goroff DK, Alpert SL, et al. Comparison of bacteriological methods for the isolation of group B streptococcus from vaginal cultures. J Clin Microbiol 4:46–48, 1976.

46. Badri MS, Zawaneh S, Cruz AC, et al. Rectal colonization with group B Streptococcus: relation to vaginal colonization of pregnant women. J Infect Dis 135:308–312, 1977.

47. Ferrieri P, Blair LL. Pharyngeal carriage of group B streptococci: detection by three methods. J Clin Microbiol 6:136–139, 1977.

48. Lim DV, Morales WJ, Walsh AF. Lim group B strep broth and coagglutination for rapid identification of group B streptococci in preterm pregnant women. J Clin Microbiol 25:452–453, 1987.

49. Persson KM-S, Forsgren A. Evaluation of culture methods for isolation of group B streptococci. Diagn Microbiol Infect Dis 6:175–177, 1987.

50. Facklam RR, Padula JF, Wortham EC, et al. Presumptive identification of group A, B and D streptococci on agar plate medium. J Clin Microbiol 9:665–672, 1979.

51. Gunn BA. SXT and Taxo A disks for presumptive identification of group A and B streptococci in throat cultures. J Clin Microbiol 4:192–193, 1976.

52. Merritt K, Treadwell TL, Jacobs NJ. Rapid recognition of group B streptococci by pigment production and counterimmunoelectrophoresis. J Clin Microbiol 3:287–290, 1976.

53. Haug RH, Soderlund E. Pigment production in group B streptococci. Acta Pathol Microbiol Scand Sect B 85:286–288, 1977.

54. Merritt K, Jacobs NJ. Characterization and incidence of pigment production by human clinical group B streptococci. J Clin Microbiol 8:105–107, 1978.

55. Noble MA, Bent JM, West AB. Detection and identification of group B streptococci by use of pigment production. J Clin Pathol 36:350–352, 1983.

56. de la Rosa M, Perez M, Carazo C, et al. New Granada medium for detection and identification of group B streptococci. J Clin Microbiol 30:1019–1021, 1992.

57. Christie R, Atkins NE, Munch-Petersen E. A note on a lytic phenomenon shown by group B streptococci. Aust J Exp Biol Med Sci 22:197–200, 1944.

58. Tapsall JW, Phillips EA. Presumptive identification of group B streptococci by rapid detection of CAMP factor and pigment production. Diagn Microbiol Infect Dis 7:225–228, 1987.

59. Wilkinson HW. CAMP-disk for presumptive identification of group B streptococci. J Clin Microbiol 6:42–45, 1977.

60. Bernheimer AW, Linder R, Avigad LS. Nature and mechanism of action of the CAMP protein of group B streptococci. Infect Immun 23:838–844, 1979.

61. Di Persio JR, Barrett JE, Kaplan RL. Evaluation of the Spot-CAMP test for the rapid presumptive identification of group B streptococci. Am J Clin Pathol 84:216–219, 1985.

62. Ratner HB, Weeks LS, Stratton CW. Evaluation of Spot-CAMP test for identification of group B streptococci. J Clin Microbiol 24:296–297, 1986.

63. Facklam R, Bosley GS, Rhoden D, et al. Comparative evaluation of the API 20S and automicrobic gram-positive identification systems for non–beta-hemolytic streptococci and aerococci. J Clin Microbiol 21:535–541, 1985.

64. Lancefield RC. A microprecipitin-technic for classifying hemolytic streptococci, and improved methods for producing antisera. Proc Soc Exp Biol Med 38:473–478, 1938.

65. Hill HR, Riter ME, Menge SK, et al. Rapid identification of group B streptococci by counterimmunoelectrophoresis. J Clin Microbiol 1:188–191, 1975.

66. Edwards EA, Larson GL. New method for grouping beta-hemolytic streptococci directly on sheep blood agar plates by coagglutination of specifically sensitized protein A–containing staphylococci. Appl Microbiol 28:972–976, 1974.

67. Lue YA, Howit IP, Ellner PD. Rapid grouping of beta-hemolytic streptococci by latex agglutination. J Clin Microbiol 8:326–328, 1978.
68. Daly JA, Seskin KC. Evaluation of rapid, commercial latex techniques for serogrouping beta-hemolytic streptococci. J Clin Microbiol 26:2429–2431, 1988.
69. Lämmler C, Frede C, Blobel H. Effective murolytic solubilization of streptococcal group-specific antigen. J Clin Microbiol 24:903–904, 1986.
70. Slifkin M, Cumbie R. Identification of group B streptococcal antigen with lectin-bound polystyrene particles. J Clin Microbiol 25:1172–1175, 1987.
71. Stableforth AW. Incidence of various serological types of Streptococcus agalactiae in herds of cows in Great Britain. J Pathol Bacteriol 46:21–29, 1938.
72. Pattison IH, Matthews PRJ, Maxted WR. Type classification by Lancefield's precipitin method of human and bovine group B streptococci isolated in Britain. J Pathol Bacteriol 69:51–60, 1955.
73. Wilkinson HW, Thacker LG, Facklam RR. Nonhemolytic group B streptococci of human, bovine, and ichthyic origin. Infect Immun 7:496–498, 1973.
74. Finch LA, Martin DR. Human and bovine group B streptococci: two distinct populations. J Appl Bacteriol 57:273–278, 1984.
75. Jensen NE. Epidemiological aspects of human/animal interrelationships in GBS. Antibiot Chemother 35:40–48, 1985.
76. Wibawan IWT, Lämmler C. Properties of group B streptococci with protein surface antigens X and R. J Clin Microbiol 28:2834–2836, 1990.
77. Lancefield RC. A serological differentiation of specific types of bovine hemolytic streptococci (group B). J Exp Med 59:441–458, 1934.
78. Lancefield RC, Hare R. The serological differentiation of pathogenic and non-pathogenic strains of hemolytic streptococci from parturient women. J Exp Med 61:335–349, 1935.
79. Lancefield RC. Two serological types of group B hemolytic streptococci with related, but not identical, type-specific substances. J Exp Med 67:25–40, 1938.
80. Lancefield RC, Freimer EH. Type-specific polysaccharide antigens of group B streptococci. J Hyg 64:191–203, 1966.
81. Freimer EH. Type-specific polysaccharide antigens of group B streptococci: II. The chemical basis for serological specificity of the type II HCI antigen. J Exp Med 125:381–392, 1967.
82. Lancefield RC. Cellular antigens of group B streptococci. In Wannamaker LW, Matsen JM (eds). Streptococci and Streptococcal Diseases: Recognition, Understanding, and Management. New York, Academic Press, 1972, pp 57–64.
83. Lancefield RC, McCarty M, Everly WN. Multiple mouse-protective antibodies directed against group B streptococci. J Exp Med 142:165–179, 1975.
84. Wilkinson HW, Moody MD. Serological relationships of type I antigens of group B streptococci. J Bacteriol 97:629–634, 1969.
85. Wilkinson HW, Eagon RG. Type-specific antigens of group B type Ic streptococci. Infect Immun 4:596–604, 1971.
86. Wilkinson HW. Immunochemistry of purified polysaccharide type antigens of group B streptococcal types Ia, Ib, and Ic. Infect Immun 11:845–852, 1975.
87. Kane JA, Karakawa WW. Multiple polysaccharide antigens of group B Streptococcus, type Ia: emphasis on a sialic acid type-specific polysaccharide. J Immunol 118:2155–2160, 1977.
88. Kane JA, Karakawa WW. Existence of multiple immunodeterminants in the type-specific capsular substance of group B type Ia streptococci. Infect Immun 19:983–991, 1978.
89. Johnson DR, Ferrieri P. Group B streptococcal Ibc protein antigen: distribution of two determinants in wild-type strains of common serotypes. J Clin Microbiol 19:506–510, 1984.
90. Wilkinson HW. Analysis of group B streptococcal types associated with disease in human infants and adults. J Clin Microbiol 7:176–179, 1978.
91. Jelínková J, Motlová J. The nomenclature of GBS. Antibiot Chemother 35:49–52, 1985.
92. Henrichsen J, Ferrieri P, Jelínková J, et al. Nomenclature of antigens of group B streptococci. Int J Syst Bacteriol 34:500, 1984.
93. Perch B, Kjems E, Henrichsen J. New serotypes of group B streptococci isolated from human sources. J Clin Microbiol 10:109–110, 1979.
94. Jelínková J, Motlová J. Worldwide distribution of two new serotypes of group B streptococci: type IV and provisional type V. J Clin Microbiol 21:361–362, 1985.
95. Wessels MR, DiFabio JL, Benedí V-J, et al. Structural determination and immunochemical characterization of the type V group B Streptococcus capsular polysaccharide. J Biol Chem 266:6714–6719, 1991.
96. von Hunolstein C, D'Ascenzi S, Wagner B, et al. Immunochemistry of capsular type polysaccharide and virulence properties of type VI Streptococcus agalactiae (group B streptococci). Infect Immun 61:1272–1280, 1993.
97. Kogan G, Brisson J-R, Kasper DL, et al. Structural elucidation of the novel type VII group B Streptococcus capsular polysaccharide by high resolution NMR spectroscopy. Carbohydr Res 277:1–9, 1995.
98. Kogan G, Uhrín D, Brisson J-R, et al. Structural and immunochemical characterization of the type VIII group B Streptococcus capsular polysaccharide. J Biol Chem 271:8786–8790, 1996.
99. Kogan G, Uhrín D, Brisson J-R, et al. Structure of the type VI group B Streptococcus capsular polysaccharide determined by high resolution NMR spectroscopy. J Carbohydr Chem 13:1071–1078, 1994.
100. Bevanger L, Naess AI. Mouse-protective antibodies against the Ibc proteins of group B streptococci. Acta Pathol Microbiol Immunol Scand 93:121–124, 1985.
101. Bevanger L. Ibc proteins as serotype markers of group B streptococci. Acta Pathol Microbiol Immunol Scand 91:231–234, 1983.
102. Madoff LC, Hori S, Michel JL, et al. Phenotypic diversity in the alpha C protein of group B streptococci. Infect Immun 59:2638–2644, 1991.
103. Madoff LC, Michel JL, Gong EW, et al. Group B streptococci escape host immunity by deletion of tandem repeat elements of the alpha C protein. Proc Natl Acad Sci U S A 93:4131–4136, 1996.
104. Kling DE, Gravekamp C, Madoff LC, et al. Characterization of two distinct opsonic and protective epitopes within the alpha c protein of the group B Streptococcus. Infect Immun 65:1462–1467, 1997.
105. Gravekamp C, Horensky DS, Michel JL, et al. Variation in repeat number within the alpha c protein of group B streptococci alters antigenicity and protective epitopes. Infect Immun 64:3576–3583, 1996.
106. Jerlström PG, Chhatwal GS, Timmis KN. The IgA-binding β antigen of the c protein complex of group B streptococci: sequence determination of its gene and

detection of two binding regions. Mol Microbiol 54:843–849, 1991.

107. Brady LJ, Boyle MDP. Identification of non-immunoglobulin A–Fc-binding forms and low-molecular-weight secreted forms of the group B streptococcal β antigen. Infect Immun 57:1573–1581, 1989.

108. Jerlström PG, Talay SR, Valentin-Weigand P, et al. Identification of an immunoglobulin A binding motif located in the β-antigen of the c protein complex of group B streptococci. Infect Immun 64:2787–2793, 1996.

109. Pattison IH, Matthews PRJ, Howell DG. The type classification of group B streptococci with special reference to bovine strains apparently lacking in type polysaccharide. J Pathol Bacteriol 69:41–50, 1955.

110. Wilkinson HW. Comparison of streptococcal R antigens. Appl Microbiol 24:669–670, 1972.

111. Lancefield RC, Perlmann GE. Preparation and properties of a protein (R antigen) occurring in streptococci of group A, type 28 and in certain streptococci of other serological groups. J Exp Med 96:83–97, 1952.

112. Flores AE, Ferrieri P. Molecular species of R-protein antigens produced by clinical isolates of group B streptococci. J Clin Microbiol 27:1050–1054, 1989.

113. Fasola EL, Flores AE, Ferrieri P. Immune responses to the R4 protein antigen of group B streptococci and its relationship to other streptococcal R4 proteins. Clin Diagn Lab Immunol 3:321–325, 1996.

114. Stålhammar-Carlemalm M, Stenberg L, Lindahl G. Protein rib: a novel group B streptococcal cell surface protein that confers passive immunity and is expressed by most strains causing invasive infection. J Exp Med 177:1593–1603, 1993.

115. Wästfelt M, Stålhammar-Carlemalm M, Delisse A-M, et al. Identification of a family of streptococcal surface proteins with extremely repetitive structure. J Biol Chem 271:18892–18897, 1996.

116. Lachenauer CS, Madoff LC. A protective surface protein from type V group B streptococci shares N-terminal sequence homology with the alpha c protein. Infect Immun 64:4255–4260, 1996.

117. Mackie EB, Brown KN, Lam J, et al. Morphological stabilization of capsules of group B streptococci, types Ia, Ib, II and III, with specific antibody. J Bacteriol 138:609–617, 1979.

118. Kasper DL, Goroff DK, Baker CJ. Immunochemical characterization of native polysaccharides from group B Streptococcus: the relationship of the type III and group B determinants. J Immunol 121:1096–1105, 1978.

119. Rýc M, Jelínková J, Motlová J, et al. Immuno-electron-microscopic demonstration of capsules on group-B streptococci of new serotypes and type candidates. J Med Microbiol 25:147–149, 1988.

120. Baker CJ, Edwards MS, Webb BJ, et al. Antibody-independent classical pathway–mediated opsonophagocytosis of type Ia, group B Streptococcus. J Clin Invest 69:394–404, 1982.

121. Paoletti LC, Ross RA, Johnson KD. Cell growth rate regulates expression of group B Streptococcus type III capsular polysaccharide. Infect Immun 64:1220–1226, 1996.

122. Sellin M, Håkansson S, Norgren M. Phase-shift of polysaccharide capsule expression in group B streptococci, type III. Microb Pathog 18:401–415, 1995.

123. Russell H, Norcross NL. The isolation of some physiochemical and biologic properties of the type III antigen of group B Streptococcus. J Immunol 109:90–96, 1972.

124. Michon F, Katzenellenbogen E, Kasper DL, et al. Structure of the complex group-specific polysaccharide of group B Streptococcus. Biochemistry 26:476–486, 1987.

125. Michon F, Brisson J-R, Dell A, et al. Multiantennary group-specific polysaccharide of group B Streptococcus. Biochemistry 27:5341–5351, 1988.

126. Michon F, Chalifour R, Feldman R, et al. The α-L-(1→2)-trirhamnopyranoside epitope on the group-specific polysaccharide of group B streptococci. Infect Immun 59:1690–1696, 1991.

127. Baker CJ, Kasper DL, Davis CE. Immunochemical characterization of the native type III polysaccharide of group B Streptococcus. J Exp Med 143:258–270, 1976.

128. Tai JY, Gotschlich EC, Lancefield RC. Isolation of type-specific polysaccharide antigen from group B type Ib streptococci. J Exp Med 149:58–66, 1979.

129. Jennings HJ, Rosell K-G, Kasper DL. Structural determination and serology of the native polysaccharide antigen of the type III group B Streptococcus. Can J Biochem 58:112–120, 1980.

130. Kasper DL, Baker CJ, Galdes B, et al. Immunochemical analysis and immunogenicity of the type II group B streptococcal capsular polysaccharide. J Clin Invest 72:260–269, 1983.

131. Jennings HJ, Katzenellenbogen E, Lugowski C, et al. Structure of native polysaccharide antigens of type Ia and type Ib group B Streptococcus. Biochemistry 22:1258–1264, 1983.

132. Schifferle RE, Jennings HJ, Wessels MR, et al. Immunochemical analysis of the types Ia and Ib group B streptococcal polysaccharides. J Immunol 135:4164–4170, 1985.

133. De Cueninck BJ, Shockman GD, Swenson RM. Group B, type III streptococcal cell wall: composition and structural aspects revealed through endo-N-acetylmuramidase-catalyzed hydrolysis. Infect Immun 35:572–582, 1982.

134. Wessels MR, Pozsgay V, Kasper DL, et al. Structure and immunochemistry of an oligosaccharide repeating unit of the capsular polysaccharide of type III group B Streptococcus. J Biol Chem 262:8262–8267, 1987.

135. Wessels MR, Benedí V-J, Jennings HJ, et al. Isolation and characterization of type IV group B Streptococcus capsular polysaccharide. Infect Immun 57:1089–1094, 1989.

136. Jennings HJ, Rosell K-G, Katzenellenbogen E, et al. Structural determination of the capsular polysaccharide antigen of type II group B Streptococcus. J Biol Chem 258:1793–1798, 1983.

137. Sadler JE, Paulson JC, Hill RL. The role of sialic acid in the expression of human MN blood group antigens. J Biol Chem 254:2112–2119, 1979.

138. Pritchard DG, Gray BM, Egan ML. Murine monoclonal antibodies to type Ib polysaccharide of group B streptococci bind to human milk oligosaccharides. Infect Immun 60:1598–1602, 1992.

139. Wessels MR, Muñoz A, Kasper DL. A model of high-affinity antibody binding to type III group B Streptococcus capsular polysaccharide. Proc Natl Acad Sci U S A 84:9170–9174, 1987.

140. Brisson J-R, Uhrinova S, Woods RJ, et al. NMR and molecular dynamics studies of the conformational epitope of the type III group B Streptococcus capsular polysaccharide and derivatives. Biochemistry 36:3278–3292, 1997.

141. Lindberg B, Lönngren J, Powell DA. Structural studies of the specific type 14 pneumococcal polysaccharide. Carbohydr Res 58:117–186, 1977.

142. Wessels MR, Kasper DL. Antibody recognition of the type 14 pneumococcal capsule. Evidence for a conformational epitope in a neutral polysaccharide. J Exp Med 169:2121–2131, 1989.

143. Edwards MS, Kasper DL, Jennings HJ, et al. Capsular sialic acid prevents activation of the alternative complement pathway by type III group B streptococci. J Immunol 128:1278–1283, 1982.

144. Yeung MK, Mattingly SJ. Biosynthesis of cell wall peptidoglycan and polysaccharide antigens by protoplasts of type III group B *Streptococcus*. J Bacteriol 154:211–220, 1983.

145. Niven CF. The nutrition of group B streptococci. J Bacteriol 46:573–574, 1943.

146. Milligan TW, Doran TI, Straus DC, et al. Growth and amino acid requirements of various strains of group B streptococci. J Clin Microbiol 7:28–33, 1978.

147. Baker CJ, Kasper DL. Microcapsule of type III strains of group B *Streptococcus*: production and morphology. Infect Immun 13:189–194, 1976.

148. Marchlewicz BA, Duncan JL. Properties of a hemolysin produced by group B streptococci. Infect Immun 30:805–813, 1980.

149. Weiser JN, Rubens CE. Transposon mutagenesis of group B *Streptococcus* beta-hemolysin biosynthesis. Infect Immun 55:2314–2316, 1987.

150. Tapsall JW. Pigment production by Lancefield-group B streptococci (*Streptococcus agalactiae*). J Med Microbiol 21:75–81, 1986.

151. Ferrieri P, Wannamaker LW, Nelson J. Localization and characterization of the hippuricase activity of group B streptococci. Infect Immun 7:747–752, 1973.

152. Ferrieri P, Gray ED, Wannamaker LW. Biochemical and immunological characterization of the extracellular nucleases of group B streptococci. J Exp Med 151:56–68, 1980.

153. Hayano S, Tanaka A. Sialidase-like enzymes produced by group A, B, C, G, and L streptococci and by *Streptococcus sanguis*. J Bacteriol 97:1328–1333, 1969.

154. Milligan TW, Straus DC, Mattingly SJ. Extracellular neuraminidase production by group B streptococci. Infect Immun 18:189–195, 1977.

155. Nealon TJ, Mattingly SJ. Association of elevated levels of cellular lipoteichoic acids of group B streptococci with human neonatal disease. Infect Immun 39:1243–1251, 1983.

156. Skalka B, Smola J. Lethal effect of CAMP-factor and UBERIS-factor—a new finding about diffusible exosubstances of *Streptococcus agalactiae* and *Streptococcus uberis*. Zentralbl Bakteriol Mikrobiol Hyg 249:190–194, 1981.

157. Jürgens D, Sterzik B, Fehrenbach FJ. Unspecific binding of group B streptococcal cocytolysin (CAMP factor) to immunoglobulins and its possible role in pathogenicity. J Exp Med 165:720–732, 1987.

158. Hill HR, Bohnsack JF, Morris EZ, et al. Group B streptococci inhibit the chemotactic activity of the fifth component of complement. J Immunol 141:3551–3556, 1988.

159. Bohnsack JF, Mollison KW, Buko AM, et al. Group B streptococci inactivate complement component C5a by enzymic cleavage at the *C*-terminus. Biochem J 273:635–640, 1991.

160. Bohnsack JF, Zhou XN, Williams PA, et al. Purification of a protease from group B streptococci that inactivates human C5a. Biochim Biophys Acta 1079:222–228, 1991.

161. Cleary PP, Handley J, Suvorov AN, et al. Similarity between the group B and A streptococcal C5a peptidase genes. Infect Immun 60:4239–4244, 1992.

162. Bohnsack JF, Zhou X, Gustin JN, et al. Bacterial evasion of the antibody response: human IgG antibodies neutralize soluble but not bacteria-associated group B streptococcal C5a-ase. J Infect Dis 165:315–321, 1992.

163. Pritchard DG, Lin B, Willingham TR, et al. Characterization of the group B streptococcal hyaluronate lyase. Arch Biochem Biophys 315:431–437, 1994.

164. Milligan TW, Mattingly SJ, Straus DC. Purification and partial characterization of neuraminidase from type III group B streptococci. J Bacteriol 144:164–172, 1980.

165. Brown JG, Straus DC. Characterization of neuraminidases produced by various serotypes of group B streptococci. Infect Immun 55:1–6, 1987.

166. Milligan TW, Baker CJ, Straus DC, et al. Association of elevated levels of extracellular neuraminidase with clinical isolates of type III group B streptococci. Infect Immun 21:738–746, 1978.

167. Musser JM, Mattingly SJ, Quentin R, et al. Identification of a high-virulence clone of type III *Streptococcus agalactiae* (group B *Streptococcus*) causing invasive neonatal disease. Proc Natl Acad Sci U S A 86:4731–4735, 1989.

168. Durham DL, Straus DC. Extracellular products of type III *Streptococcus agalactiae* and their relationship to virulence. Curr Microbiol 8:89–94, 1983.

169. Klegerman ME, Boyer KM, Papierniak CK, et al. Type-specific capsular antigen is associated with virulence in late-onset group B streptococcal type III disease. Infect Immun 44:124–129, 1984.

170. Yeung MK, Mattingly SJ. Biosynthetic capacity for type-specific antigen synthesis determines the virulence of serotype III strains of group B streptococci. Infect Immun 44:217–221, 1984.

171. Yeung MK, Mattingly SJ. Isolation and characterization of type III group streptococcal mutants defective in biosynthesis of the type-specific antigen. Infect Immun 42:141–151, 1983.

172. Håkansson S, Granlund-Edstedt M, Sellin M, et al. Demonstration and characterization of buoyant-density subpopulations of group B *Streptococcus* type III. J Infect Dis 161:741–746, 1990.

173. Nealon TJ, Mattingly SJ. Role of cellular lipoteichoic acids in mediating adherence of serotype III strains of group B streptococci to human embryonic, fetal, and adult epithelial cells. Infect Immun 43:523–530, 1984.

174. Goldschmidt JC Jr, Panos C. Teichoic acids of *Streptococcus agalactiae*: chemistry, cytotoxicity, and effect on bacterial adherence to human cells in tissue culture. Infect Immun 43:670–677, 1984.

175. Wanger AR, Dunny GM. Identification of a *Streptococcus agalactiae* protein antigen associated with bovine mastitis isolates. Infect Immun 55:1170–1175, 1987.

176. Committee on Infectious Diseases and Committee on Fetus and Newborn. Guidelines for prevention of group B streptococcal (GBS) infection by chemoprophylaxis. Pediatrics 90:775–778, 1992.

177. Baker CJ. Summary of the workshop on perinatal infections due to group B *Streptococcus*. J Infect Dis 136:137–152, 1977.

178. Moller M, Thomsen AC, Borch K, et al. Rupture of fetal membranes and premature delivery associated with group B streptococci in urine of pregnant women. Lancet 2:69–70, 1984.

179. Anthony BF, Eisenstadt R, Carter J, et al. Genital and intestinal carriage of group B streptococci during pregnancy. J Infect Dis 143:761–766, 1981.

180. Skidmore AG, Henry DA, Smith A. Prevalence of type-specific group B streptococcal antibody in human sera: a study of 405 pregnant women. Am J Obstet Gynecol 152:857–860, 1985.

181. Christensen KK, Ripa T, Agrup G, et al. Group B streptococci in human urethral and cervical specimens. Scand J Infect Dis 8:74–78, 1976.

182. MacDonald SW, Manuel FR, Embil JA. Localization

of group B beta-hemolytic streptococci in the female urogenital tract. Am J Obstet Gynecol 133:57–59, 1979.

183. Ferrieri P, Cleary PP, Seeds AE. Epidemiology of group B streptococcal carriage in pregnant women and newborn infants. J Med Microbiol 10:103–114, 1976.

184. Dillon HC, Gray E, Pass MA, et al. Anorectal and vaginal carriage of group B streptococci during pregnancy. J Infect Dis 145:794–799, 1982.

185. Wood EG, Dillon HC Jr. A prospective study of group B streptococcal bacteriuria in pregnancy. Am J Obstet Gynecol 140:515–520, 1981.

186. Persson K, Bjerre B, Elfström L, et al. Longitudinal study of group B streptococcal carriage during late pregnancy. Scand J Infect Dis 19:325–329, 1987.

187. Hoogkamp-Korstanje JAA, Gerards LJ, Cats BP. Maternal carriage and neonatal acquisition of group B streptococci. J Infect Dis 145:800–803, 1982.

188. Paredes A, Wong P, Mason EO Jr, et al. Nosocomial transmission of group B streptococci in a newborn nursery. Pediatrics 59:679–682, 1976.

189. Anthony BF, Okada DM, Hobel CJ. Epidemiology of the group B Streptococcus: maternal and nosocomial sources for infant acquisitions. J Pediatr 95:431–436, 1979.

190. Hammerschlag MR, Baker CJ, Alpert S, et al. Colonization with group B streptococci in girls under 16 years of age. Pediatrics 60:473–477, 1977.

191. Mauer M, Thirumoorthi MC, Dajani AS. Group B streptococcal colonization in prepubertal children. Pediatrics 64:65–67, 1979.

192. Wallin J, Forsgren A. Group B streptococci in venereal disease clinic patients. Br J Vener Dis 51:401–404, 1975.

193. Baker CJ, Goroff DK, Alpert S, et al. Vaginal colonization with group B Streptococcus: a study in college women. J Infect Dis 135:392–397, 1977.

194. Gardner SE, Yow MD, Leeds LJ, et al. Failure of penicillin to eradicate group B streptococcal colonization in the pregnant woman. Am J Obstet Gynecol 135:1062–1065, 1979.

195. Manuel FR, MacDonald SW, Embil JA. Prevalence of group B beta-haemolytic streptococci in male urethra. Scand J Infect Dis 12:33–35, 1980.

196. Lewis RFM. Beta-haemolytic streptococci from the female genital tract: clinical correlates and outcome of treatment. Epidemiol Infect 102:391–400, 1989.

197. Anthony BF, Okada DM, Hobel CJ. Epidemiology of group B Streptococcus: longitudinal observations during pregnancy. J Infect Dis 137:524–530, 1978.

198. Yow MD, Leeds LJ, Thompson PK, et al. The natural history of group B streptococcal colonization in the pregnant woman and her offspring: I. Colonization studies. Am J Obstet Gynecol 137:34–38, 1980.

199. Boyer KM, Gadzala CA, Kelly PD, et al. Selective intrapartum chemoprophylaxis of neonatal group B streptococcal early-onset disease: II. Predictive value of prenatal cultures. J Infect Dis 148:802–809, 1983.

200. Yancey MK, Schuchat A, Brown LK, et al. The accuracy of late antenatal screening cultures in predicting genital group B streptococcal colonization at delivery. Obstet Gynecol 88:811–815, 1996.

201. Persson KM-S, Bjerre B, Elfström L, et al. Faecal carriage of group B streptococci. Eur J Clin Microbiol 5:156–159, 1986.

202. Kaplan EL, Johnson DR, Kuritsky JN. Rectal colonization by group B β-hemolytic streptococci in a geriatric population. J Infect Dis 148:1120, 1983.

203. Anthony BF, Carter JA, Eisenstadt R, et al. Isolation of group B streptococci from the proximal small intestine of adults. J Infect Dis 147:776, 1983.

204. Barnham M. The gut as a source of the haemolytic streptococci causing infection in surgery of the intestinal and biliary tracts. J Infect 6:129–139, 1983.

205. Easmon CSF. The carrier state: group B Streptococcus. J Antimicrob Chemother 18(Suppl A):59–65, 1986.

206. Anthony BF. Carriage of group B streptococci during pregnancy: a puzzler. J Infect Dis 145:789–793, 1982.

207. Farrag OA, Gawad AA, Antar S. Group B beta-haemolytic streptococcal colonization in women using intrauterine contraceptive devices. Contraception 31:595–602, 1985.

208. Chaudhary U, Sabharwal U, Gupta A, et al. Group B streptococci in IUCD users. Indian J Med Res 84:358–360, 1986.

209. Matorras R, Garcia-Perea A, Usandizaga JA, et al. Rectovaginal colonization and urinary tract infection by group B Streptococcus in the pregnant diabetic patient. Acta Obstet Gynecol Scand 67:617–620, 1988.

210. Ramos E, Gaudier FL, Hearing LR, et al. Group B Streptococcus colonization in pregnant diabetic women. Obstet Gynecol 89:257–260, 1997.

211. Christensen KK, Dykes A-K, Christensen, P. Relation between use of tampons and urogenital carriage of group B streptococci. BMJ 289:731–732, 1984.

212. Regan JA, Klebanoff MA, Nugent RP, et al. The epidemiology of group B streptococcal colonization in pregnancy. Obstet Gynecol 77:604–610, 1991.

213. Hickman ME, Rench MA, Ferrieri P, et al. Changing epidemiology of group B streptococcal (GBS) colonization. Pediatrics 104:203–209, 1999.

214. Newton ER, Butler MC, Shain RN. Sexual behavior and vaginal colonization by group B Streptococcus among minority women. Obstet Gynecol 88:577–582, 1996.

215. Beachler CW, Baker CJ, Kasper DL, et al. Group B streptococcal colonization and antibody status in lower socioeconomic parturient women. Am J Obstet Gynecol 133:171–173, 1979.

216. Embil JA, Martin TR, Hansen NH, et al. Group B beta haemolytic streptococci in the female genital tract: a study of four clinic populations. Br J Obstet Gynaecol 85:783–786, 1978.

217. Ancona RJ, Ferrieri P, Williams PP. Maternal factors that enhance the acquisition of group B streptococci by newborn infants. J Med Microbiol 13:273–280, 1980.

218. Steere AC, Aber RC, Warford LR, et al. Possible nosocomial transmission of group B streptococci in a newborn nursery. J Pediatr 87:784–787, 1975.

219. Dawodu AH, Damole IO, Onile BA. Epidemiology of group B streptococcal carriage among pregnant women and their neonates: an African experience. Trop Geogr Med 35:145–150, 1983.

220. Jackson DH, Hinder SM, Stringer J, et al. Carriage and transmission of group B streptococci among STD clinic patients. Br J Vener Dis 58:334–337, 1982.

221. Ross PW, Cumming CG. Group B streptococci in women attending a sexually transmitted diseases clinic. J Infect 4:161–166, 1982.

222. Chretien JH, McGinniss CG, Thompson, J, et al. Group B beta-hemolytic streptococci causing pharyngitis. J Clin Microbiol 10:263–266, 1979.

223. Sackel SG, Baker CJ, Kasper DL, et al. Isolation of group B Streptococcus from men [Abstract 467]. 18th Interscience Conference on Antimicrobial Agents and Chemotherapy, 1978.

224. Benchetrit LC, Fracalanzza SEL, Peregrino H, et al. Carriage of Streptococcus agalactiae in women and neonates

and distribution of serological types: a study in Brazil. J Clin Microbiol 15:787–790, 1982.

225. Liang ST, Lau SP, Chan SH, et al. Perinatal colonization of group B *Streptococcus:* an epidemiological study in a Chinese population. Aust N Z J Obstet Gynaecol 26:138–141, 1986.

226. Trujillo H. Group B streptococcal colonization in Medellín, Columbia. Pediatr Infect Dis J 9:224–225, 1990.

227. Needham JR. Neonatal group B *Streptococcus* infections: laboratory and animal studies. Med Lab Sci 39:261–270, 1982.

228. Gyaneshwar R, Nsanze H, Singh KP, et al. The prevalence of sexually transmitted disease agents in pregnant women in Suva. Aust N Z J Obstet Gynaecol 27:213–215, 1987.

229. Mani V, Jadhav M, Sivadasan K, et al. Maternal and neonatal colonization with group B *Streptococcus* and neonatal outcome. Indian Pediatr 21:357–363, 1984.

230. Kieran E, Matheson M, Mann AG, et al. Group B *Streptococcus* (GBS) colonisation among expectant Irish mothers. Ir Med J 91:21–22, 1998.

231. Schimmel MS, Eidelman AI, Rudensky B, et al. Epidemiology of group B streptococcal colonization and infection in Jerusalem, 1989–91. Isr J Med Sci 30:349–351, 1994.

232. Visconti A, Orefici G, Notarnicola AM. Colonization and infection of mothers and neonates with group B streptococci in three Italian hospitals. J Hosp Infect 6:265–276, 1985.

233. Yamane N, Yuki M, Kyono K. Isolation and characterization of group B streptococci from genitourinary tracts in Japan. Tohoku J Exp Med 141:327–335, 1983.

234. Sunna E, El-Daher N, Bustami K, et al. A study of group B streptococcal carrier state during late pregnancy. Trop Geogr Med 43:161–164, 1991.

235. Elzouki AY, Vesikari T. First international conference on infections in children in Arab countries. Pediatr Infect Dis J 4:527–531, 1985.

236. Solórzano-Santos F, Díaz-Ramos RD, Arredondo-García JL. Diseases caused by group B *Streptococcus* in Mexico. Pediatr Infect Dis J 9:66, 1990.

237. Solórzano-Santos F, Echaniz-Aviles G, Conde-Glez CJ, et al. Cervicovaginal infection with group B streptococci among pregnant Mexican women. J Infect Dis 159:1003–1004, 1989.

238. Collins TS, Calderon M, Gilman RH, et al. Group B streptococcal colonization in a developing country: its association with sexually transmitted disease and socioeconomic factors. Am J Trop Med Hyg 59:633–636, 1998.

239. Gosling PJ, Morgos FW. Group B streptococci: colonization of women in labour and neonatal acquisition in the western region of Saudi Arabia. J Hosp Infect 4:324, 1983.

240. Uduman SA, Chatterjee TK, Al-Mouzan MI, et al. Group B streptococci colonization among Saudi women in labor and neonatal acquisition. Int J Gynaecol Obstet 23:21–24, 1985.

241. Ross PW, Neilson JR. Group B streptococci in mothers and infants: Edinburgh studies. Health Bull 40:234–239, 1982.

242. Teres FO, Matorras R, Perea AG, et al. Prevention of neonatal group B streptococcal sepsis. Pediatr Infect Dis J 6:874, 1987.

243. Pengsa K, Puapermpoonsiri S, Taksaphan S, et al. Group B streptococcal colonization in mothers and their neonates. Ramathibodi Med J 7:83–90, 1984.

244. Suara RO, Adegbola RA, Baker CJ, et al. Carriage of group B streptococci in pregnant Gambian mothers and their infants. J Infect Dis 170:1316–1319, 1994.

245. Orrett FA, Olagundoye V. Prevalence of group B streptococcal colonization in pregnant third trimester women in Trinidad. J Hosp Infect 27:43–48, 1994.

246. Zaleznik DF, Krohn MA, Hillier SL, et al. Group B streptococcal colonization in parturient women differs among racial groups. Abstracts of the 35th Interscience Conference on Antimicrobial Agents and Chemotherapy, Abstract K188, 1995.

247. Stoll BJ, Schuchat A. Maternal carriage of group B streptococci in developing countries. Pediatr Infect Dis J 17:499–503, 1998.

248. Hayden GF, Murphy TF, Hendley JO. Non–group A streptococci in the pharynx. Pathogens or innocent bystanders? Am J Dis Child 143:794–797, 1989.

249. Hofkosh D, Wald ER, Chiponis DM. Prevalence of non–group A β-hemolytic streptococci in childhood pharyngitis. South Med J 81:329–331, 1988.

250. Cummings CG, Ross PW. Group B streptococci (GBS) in the upper respiratory tract of schoolchildren. Health Bull 40:81–86, 1982.

251. Paredes A, Wong P, Yow MD. Failure of penicillin to eradicate the carrier state of group B *Streptococcus* in infants. J Pediatr 89:191–193, 1976.

252. Shafer MA, Sweet RL, Ohm-Smith MJ, et al. Microbiology of the lower genital tract in postmenarchal adolescent girls: differences by sexual activity, contraception, and presence of nonspecific vaginitis. J Pediatr 107:974–981, 1985.

253. Band JD, Clegg HW, Hayes PS, et al. Transmission of group B streptococci. Am J Dis Child 135:355–358, 1981.

254. Siegel JD, McCracken GH Jr, Threlkeld N, et al. Single-dose penicillin prophylaxis against neonatal group B streptococcal infections: a controlled trial in 18,738 newborn infants. N Engl J Med 303:769–775, 1980.

255. Akhtar T, Zai S, Khatoon J, et al. A study of group B streptococcal colonization and infection in newborns in Pakistan. J Trop Pediatr 33:302–304, 1987.

256. Matorras R, Garcia-Perea A, Usandizaga JA, et al. Natural transmission of group B *Streptococcus* during delivery. Int J Gynecol Obstet 30:99–103, 1989.

257. Gökalp A, Oguz A, Bakici Z, et al. Neonatal group B streptococcal colonization and maternal urogenital or anorectal carriage. Turk J Pediatr 30:17–23, 1988.

258. Easmon CSF, Hastings MJG, Clare AJ, et al. Nosocomial transmission of group B streptococci. BMJ 283:459–461, 1981.

259. Easmon CSF, Hastings MJG, Blowers A, et al. Epidemiology of group B streptococci: one year's experience in an obstetric and special care baby unit. Br J Obstet Gynaecol 90:241–246, 1983.

260. Gerards LJ, Cats BP, Hoogkamp-Korstanje JAA. Early neonatal group B streptococcal disease: degree of colonization as an important determinant. J Infect 11:119–124, 1985.

261. Noya FJD, Rench MA, Metzger TG, et al. Unusual occurrence of an epidemic of type Ib/c group B streptococcal sepsis in a neonatal intensive care unit. J Infect Dis 155:1135–1144, 1987.

262. Gardner SE, Mason EO Jr, Yow MD. Community acquisition of group B *Streptococcus* by infants of colonized mothers. Pediatrics 66:873–875, 1980.

263. Wald ER, Snyder MJ, Gutberlet RL. Group B β-hemolytic streptococcal colonization. Am J Dis Child 131:178–180, 1975.

264. Wilkinson HW, Facklam RR, Wortham EC. Distribution

by serological type of group B streptococci isolated from a variety of clinical material over a five-year period (with special reference to neonatal sepsis and meningitis). Infect Immun 8:228–235, 1973.

265. Baker CJ, Barrett FF. Group B streptococcal infection in infants: the importance of the various serotypes. JAMA 230:1158–1160, 1974.

266. Christensen HO, Kamper J, Olsen H, et al. Treatment of meningitis in infants caused by group B-streptococci using benzylpenicillin and streptomycin. Dan Med Bull 30:416–418, 1983.

267. Mulder CJJ, Zanen HC. Neonatal group B streptococcal meningitis. Arch Dis Child 59:439–443, 1984.

268. Rench MA, Baker CJ. Neonatal sepsis caused by a new group B streptococcal serotype. J Pediatr 122:638–640, 1993.

269. Lachenauer CS, Kasper DL, Shimada J, et al. Serotypes VI and VIII predominate among group B streptococci isolated from pregnant Japanese women. J Infect Dis 179:1030–1033, 1999.

270. Blumberg HM, Stephens DS, Licitra C, et al. Molecular epidemiology of group B streptococcal infections: use of restriction endonuclease analysis of chromosomal DNA and DNA restriction fragment length polymorphisms of ribosomal RNA genes (ribotyping). J Infect Dis 166:574–579, 1992.

271. Stringer J. The development of a phage typing system for group-B streptococci. J Med Microbiol 13:133–144, 1980.

272. Boyer KM, Vogel LC, Gotoff SP, et al. Nosocomial transmission of bacteriophage type 7/11/12 group B streptococci on a special care nursery. Am J Dis Child 134:964–966, 1980.

273. Weems JJ Jr, Jarvis WR, Colman G. A cluster of late onset group B streptococcal infections in low birth weight premature infants: no evidence for horizontal transmission. Pediatr Infect Dis J 5:715–717, 1986.

274. Horodniceanu T, Bougueleret L, El-Solh N, et al. Conjugative R plasmids in *Streptococcus agalactiae* (group B). Plasmid 2:197–206, 1979.

275. Mattingly SJ, Maurer JJ, Eskew EK, et al. Identification of a high-virulence clone of serotype III *Streptococcus agalactiae* by growth characteristics at 40°C. J Clin Microbiol 28:1676–1677, 1990.

276. Musser JM, Mattingly SJ, Quentin R, et al. Identification of a high-virulence clone of type III *Streptococcus agalactiae* (group B *Streptococcus*) causing invasive neonatal disease. Proc Natl Acad Sci U S A 86:4731–4735, 1989.

277. Quentin R, Huet H, Wang F-S, et al. Characterization of *Streptococcus agalactiae* strains by multilocus enzyme genotype and serotype: identification of multiple virulent clone families that cause invasive neonatal disease. J Clin Microbiol 33:2576–2581, 1995.

278. Gordillo ME, Singh KV, Baker CJ, et al. Comparison of group B streptococci by pulsed field gel electrophoresis and by conventional electrophoresis. J Clin Microbiol 31:1430–1434, 1993.

279. Limansky AS, Sutich EG, Guardati MC, et al. Genomic diversity among *Streptococcus agalactiae* isolates detected by a degenerate oligonucleotide-primed amplification assay. J Infect Dis 177:1308–1313, 1998.

280. Bingen E, Denamur E, Lambert-Zechovsky N, et al. Analysis of DNA restriction fragment length polymorphism extends the evidence for breast milk transmission in *Streptococcus agalactiae* late-onset neonatal infection. J Infect Dis 165:569–573, 1992.

281. Baker CJ, Barrett FF, Gordon RC, et al. Suppurative meningitis due to streptococci of Lancefield group B: a study of 33 infants. J Pediatr 82:724–729, 1973.

282. Siegel JD, McCracken GH Jr, Threlkeld N, et al. Single-dose penicillin prophylaxis of neonatal group-B streptococcal disease. Lancet 2:1426–1430, 1982.

283. Baker CJ. Unpublished observations, 1993.

284. Aavitsland P, Høiby EA, Lystad A. Systemic group B streptococcal disease in neonates and young infants in Norway 1985–94. Acta Paediatr 85:104–105, 1996.

285. Zangwill KM, Schuchat A, Wenger JD. Group B streptococcal disease in the United States, 1990: report from a multistate active surveillance system. MMWR Morb Mortal Wkly Rep 41:25–32, 1992.

286. Schuchat A, Deaver-Robinson K, Plikaytis BD, et al. Multistate case-control study of maternal risk factors for neonatal group B streptococcal disease. Pediatr Infect Dis J 13:623–629, 1994.

287. Collignon PJ, Dreimanis DE, Vaughan TM, et al. Group B streptococcal infection in neonates. Med J Aust 164:125–126, 1996.

288. Centers for Disease Control and Prevention. Decreasing incidence of perinatal group B streptococcal disease—United States, 1993–1995. MMWR Morb Mortal Wkly Rep 46:473–477, 1997.

289. Centers for Disease Control and Prevention. Adoption of hospital policies for prevention of perinatal group B streptococcal disease—United States, 1997. MMWR Morb Mortal Wkly Rep 47:665–670, 1998.

290. Pyati SP, Pildes RS, Jacobs NM, et al. Penicillin in infants weighing two kilograms or less with early-onset group B streptococcal disease. N Engl J Med 308:1383–1389, 1983.

291. Cochi SL, Feldman RA. Estimating national incidence of group B streptococcal disease: the effect of adjusting for birth weight. Pediatr Infect Dis J 2:414–415, 1983.

292. Boyer KM, Gadzala CA, Burd LI, et al. Selective intrapartum chemoprophylaxis of neonatal group B streptococcal early-onset disease: I. Epidemiologic rationale. J Infect Dis 148:795–801, 1983.

293. Gibbs RS, Jones PM, Wilder CJ. Antibiotic therapy of endometritis following cesarean section. Obstet Gynecol 52:31–36, 1978.

294. Gibbs RS, Blanco JD. Streptococcal infections in pregnancy: a study of 48 bacteremias. Am J Obstet Gynecol 140:405–411, 1981.

295. Pass MA, Gray BM, Dillon HC Jr. Puerperal and perinatal infections with group B streptococci. Am J Obstet Gynecol 143:147–152, 1982.

296. Minkoff HL, Sierra MF, Pringle GF, et al. Vaginal colonization with group B beta-hemolytic *Streptococcus* as a risk factor for post-cesarean section febrile morbidity. Am J Obstet Gynecol 142:992–995, 1982.

297. Bobitt JR, Damato JD, Sakakini J. Perinatal complications in group B streptococcal carriers: a longitudinal study of prenatal patients. Am J Obstet Gynecol 151:711–717, 1985.

298. Krohn MA, Hillier SL, Baker CJ. Maternal peripartum complications associated with vaginal group B streptococcal colonization. J Infect Dis 179:1410–1415, 1999.

299. Rosenstein NE, Schuchat AE. Opportunities for prevention of perinatal group B streptococcal disease: a multistate surveillance analysis. Obstet Gynecol 90:901–906, 1997.

300. Tseng PI, Kandall SR. Group B streptococcal disease in neonates and infants. N Y State J Med 74:2169–2173, 1974.

301. Stewardson-Krieger PB, Gotoff SP. Risk factors in early-

onset neonatal group B streptococcal infections. Infection 6:50–53, 1978.

302. Schuchat A. Epidemiology of group B streptococcal disease in the United States: shifting paradigms. Clin Microbiol Rev 11:497–513, 1998.

303. Pass MA, Khare S, Dillon HC. Twin pregnancies: incidence of group B streptococcal colonization and disease. J Pediatr 97:635–637, 1980.

304. Edwards MS, Jackson CV, Baker CJ. Increased risk of group B streptococcal disease in twins. JAMA 245:2044–2046, 1981.

305. Baker CJ, Kasper DL. Correlation of maternal antibody deficiency with susceptibility to neonatal group B streptococcal infection. N Engl J Med 294:753–756, 1976.

306. Lim DV, Kanarek KS, Peterson ME. Magnitude of colonization and sepsis by group B streptococci in newborn infants. Curr Microbiol 7:99–101, 1982.

307. Hemming VG, Nagarajan K, Hess LW, et al. Rapid in vitro replication of group B *Streptococcus* in term human amniotic fluid. Gynecol Obstet Invest 19:124–129, 1985.

308. Abbasi IA, Hemming VG, Eglinton GS, et al. Proliferation of group B streptococci in human amniotic fluid in vitro. Am J Obstet Gynecol 156:95–99, 1987.

309. Baker CJ. Early onset group B streptococcal disease. J Pediatr 93:124–125, 1978.

310. Bergqvist G, Holmberg G, Rydner T, et al. Intrauterine death due to infection with group B streptococci. Acta Obstet Gynecol Scand 57:127–128, 1978.

311. Ablow RC, Driscoll SG, Effmann EL, et al. A comparison of early-onset group B streptococcal neonatal infection and the respiratory distress syndrome of the newborn. N Engl J Med 294:65–70, 1976.

312. Vollman JH, Smith WL, Ballard ET, et al. Early onset group B streptococcal disease: clinical, roentgenographic, and pathologic features. J Pediatr 89:199–203, 1976.

313. Schuchat A. Epidemiology of group B streptococcal disease in the United States: shifting paradigms. Clin Microbiol Rev 11:497–513, 1998.

314. Evaldson GR, Malmborg A-S, Nord CE. Premature rupture of the membranes and ascending infection. Br J Obstet Gynaecol 89:793–801, 1982.

315. Evaldson GR, Malmborg A-S, Nord CE, et al. *Bacteroides fragilis, Streptococcus intermedius* and group B streptococci in ascending infection of pregnancy. Gynecol Obstet Invest 15:230–241, 1983.

316. Regan JA, Klebanoff MA, Nugent RP, et al. Colonization with group B streptococci in pregnancy and adverse outcome. Am J Obstet Gynecol 174:1354–1360, 1996.

317. Seaward PG, Hannah ME, Myhr TL, et al. International multicenter term PROM study: evaluation of predictors of neonatal infection in infants born to patients with premature rupture of membranes at term. Am J Obstet Gynecol 179:635–639, 1998.

318. Yancey MK, Duff P, Clark P, et al. Peripartum infection associated with vaginal group B streptococcal colonization. Obstet Gynecol 84:816–819, 1994.

319. Katzenstein A, Davis C, Braude A. Pulmonary changes in neonatal sepsis due to group B β-hemolytic streptococcus: relation to hyaline membrane disease. J Infect Dis 133:430–435, 1976.

320. Pinnas JL, Strunk RC, Fenton LJ. Immunofluorescence in group B streptococcal infection and idiopathic respiratory distress syndrome. Pediatrics 63:557–561, 1979.

321. Naeye RL, Peters EC. Amniotic fluid infections with intact membranes leading to perinatal death: a prospective study. Pediatrics 61:171–176, 1978.

322. Hildebrand WL, Schreiner RL. Group B beta-hemolytic streptococcal sepsis in the neonate. Assoc Fam Pract 22:107–114, 1980.

323. McDuffie RS Jr, Gibbs RS. Ascending group B streptococcal genital infection in the rabbit model. Am J Obstet Gynecol 175:402–405, 1996.

324. Sherman MP, Campbell LA, Merritt TA, et al. Effect of different surfactants on pulmonary group B streptococcal infection in premature rabbits. J Pediatr 125:939–947, 1994.

325. LeVine AM, Bruno MD, Huelsman KM, et al. Surfactant protein A–deficient mice are susceptible to group B streptococcal infection. J Immunol 158:4336–4340, 1997.

326. Gibson RL, Soderland C, Henderson WR Jr. Group B streptococci (GBS) injure lung endothelium in vitro: GBS invasion and GBS-induced eicosanoid production is greater with microvascular than with pulmonary artery cells. Infect Immun 63:271–279, 1995.

327. Rojas J, Stahlman M. The effects of group B *Streptococcus* and other organisms on the pulmonary vasculature. Clin Perinatol 11:591–599, 1984.

328. Hemming VG, O'Brien WF, Fischer GW, et al. Studies of short-term pulmonary and peripheral vasculature responses induced in oophorectomized sheep by the infusion of a group B streptococcal extract. Pediatr Res 18:266–269, 1984.

329. O'Brien WF, Golden SM, Bibro MC, et al. Short-term responses in neonatal lambs after infusion of group B streptococcal extract. Obstet Gynecol 65:802–806, 1985.

330. Rojas J, Larsson LE, Hellerqvist CG, et al. Pulmonary hemodynamic and ultrastructural changes associated with group B streptococcal toxemia in adult sheep and newborn lambs. Pediatr Res 17:1002–1008, 1983.

331. Gibson RL, Redding GJ, Henderson WR, et al. Group B *Streptococcus* induces tumor necrosis factor in neonatal piglets. Am Rev Respir Dis 143:598–604, 1991.

332. Peevy KJ, Panus P, Longenecker GL, et al. Prostaglandin synthetase inhibition in group B streptococcal shock: hematologic and hemodynamic effects. Pediatr Res 20:864–866, 1986.

333. Rojas J, Larsson LE, Ogletree ML, et al. Effects of cyclooxygenase inhibition on the response to group B streptococcal toxin in sheep. Pediatr Res 17:107–110, 1983.

334. Runkle B, Goldberg RN, Streitfeld MM, et al. Cardiovascular changes in group B streptococcal sepsis in the piglet: response to indomethacin and relationship to prostacyclin and thromboxane A_2. Pediatr Res 18:874–878, 1984.

335. Hammerman C, Aramburo MJ. Effects of hyperventilation on prostacyclin formation and on pulmonary vasodilation after group B β-hemolytic streptococci–induced pulmonary hypertension. Pediatr Res 29:282–287, 1991.

336. Schreiber MD, Covert RF, Torgerson LJ. Hemodynamic effects of heat-killed group B β-hemolytic *Streptococcus* in newborn lambs: role of leukotriene D_4. Pediatr Res 31:121–126, 1992.

337. Tarpey MN, Graybar GB, Lyrene RK, et al. Thromboxane synthesis inhibition reverses group B *Streptococcus*–induced pulmonary hypertension. Crit Care Med 15:644–647, 1987.

338. Phillips JB III, Li J-X, Gray BM, et al. Role of capsule in pulmonary hypertension induced by group B *Streptococcus*. Pediatr Res 31:386–390, 1992.

339. Gibson RL, Redding GJ, Truog WE, et al. Isogenic group B streptococci devoid of capsular polysaccharide or β-hemolysin: pulmonary hemodynamic and gas exchange effects during bacteremia in piglets. Pediatr Res 26:241–245, 1989.

340. Del Moral T, Goldberg RN, Urbon J, et al. Effects of treatment with pentoxifylline on the cardiovascular manifestations of group B streptococcal sepsis in the piglet. Pediatr Res 40:469–474, 1996.

341. Gibson RL, Truog WE, Henderson WR Jr, et al. Group B streptococcal sepsis in piglets: effect of combined pentoxifylline and indomethacin pretreatment. Pediatr Res 31:222–227, 1992.

342. Goldberg RN, Suguihara C, Martinez O, et al. The role of leukotrienes in the late hemodynamic manifestations of group B streptococcal sepsis in piglets. Prostaglandins Leukot Essent Fatty Acids 33:191–198, 1988.

343. Givner LB, Gray L, O'Shea TM. Antibodies to tumor necrosis factor-α: use as adjunctive therapy in established group B streptococcal disease in newborn rats. Pediatr Res 38:551–554, 1995.

344. Vallette JD Jr, Goldberg RN, Suguihara C, et al. Effect of an interleukin-1 receptor antagonist on the hemodynamic manifestations of group B streptococcal sepsis. Pediatr Res 38:704–708, 1995.

345. Pinheiro JMB, Pitt BR, Gillis CN. Roles of platelet-activating factor and thromboxane in group B Streptococcus–induced pulmonary hypertension in piglets. Pediatr Res 26:420–424, 1989.

346. Rojas J, Palme C, Ogletree ML, et al. Effects of methylprednisolone on the response to group B streptococcal toxin in sheep. Pediatr Res 18:1141–1144, 1984.

347. Goldblum SE, Reed WP. Gram-positive bacteria-induced granulocytopenia and pulmonary leukostasis in rabbits. Infect Immun 37:336–343, 1982.

348. Engelhardt B, Sandberg K, Bratton D, et al. The role of granulocytes in the pulmonary response to group B streptococcal toxin in young lambs. Pediatr Res 21:159–165, 1987.

349. Bowdy BD, Aziz SM, Marple SL, et al. Organ-specific disposition of group B streptococci in piglets: evidence for a direct interaction with target cells in the pulmonary circulation. Pediatr Res 27:344–348, 1990.

350. Bowdy BD, Marple SL, Pauly TH, et al. Oxygen radical-dependent bacterial killing and pulmonary hypertension in piglets infected with group B streptococci. Am Rev Respir Dis 141:648–653, 1990.

351. Pauly TH, Aziz SM, Horstman SJ, et al. Impact of prostaglandin and thromboxane synthesis blockade on disposition of group B Streptococcus in lungs and liver of intact piglet. Pediatr Res 31:14–17, 1992.

352. Meadow WL, Meus PJ. Nonhomogeneous redistribution of mesenteric blood flow after tolazoline during group B streptococcal sepsis in piglets. Dev Pharmacol Ther 8:209–218, 1985.

353. Meadow WL, Meus PJ. Unsuspected mesenteric hypoperfusion despite apparent hemodynamic recovery in the early phase of septic shock in piglets. Circ Shock 15:123–129, 1985.

354. Peevy KJ, Chartrand SA, Wiseman HJ, et al. Myocardial dysfunction in group B streptococcal shock. Pediatr Res 19:511–513, 1985.

355. Sorensen GK, Redding GJ, Truog WE. Mechanisms of pulmonary gas exchange abnormalities during experimental group B streptococcal infusion. Pediatr Res 19:922–926, 1985.

356. Meadow WL, Meus PJ. Hemodynamic consequences of tolazoline in neonatal group B streptococcal bacteremia: an animal model. Pediatr Res 18:960–965, 1984.

357. McKnight AA, Keyes WG, Hudak ML, et al. Oxygen free radicals and the cerebral arteriolar response to group B streptococci. Pediatr Res 31:640–644, 1992.

358. Pauly TH, Bowdy BD, Haven CA, et al. Evidence for hydroxyl radical involvement in group B Streptococcus–induced pulmonary hypertension and arterial hypoxemia in young piglets. Pediatr Res 24:735–739, 1988.

359. Villamor E, Pérez-Vizcaíno F, Tamargo J, et al. Effects of group B Streptococcus on the responses to U46619, endothelin-1, and noradrenaline in isolated pulmonary and mesenteric arteries of piglets. Pediatr Res 40:827–833, 1996.

360. Gibson RL, Berger JI, Redding GJ, et al. Effect of nitric oxide synthase inhibition during group B streptococcal sepsis in neonatal piglets. Pediatr Res 36:776–783, 1994.

361. Ling EWY, Noya FJD, Ricard G, et al. Biochemical mediators of meningeal inflammatory response to group B Streptococcus in the newborn piglet model. Pediatr Res 38:981–987, 1995.

362. Rudinsky BF, Lozon M, Bell A, et al. Group B streptococcal sepsis impairs cerebral vascular reactivity to acute hypercarbia in piglets. Pediatr Res 39:55–63, 1996.

363. Leib SL, Kim YS, Chow LL, et al. Reactive oxygen intermediates contribute to necrotic and apoptotic neuronal injury in an infant rat model of bacterial meningitis due to group B streptococci. J Clin Invest 98:2632–2639, 1996.

364. Leib SL, Kim YS, Black SM, et al. Inducible nitric oxide synthase and the effect of aminoguanidine in experimental neonatal meningitis. J Infect Dis 177:692–700, 1998.

365. Hemming VG, Hall RT, Rhodes PG, et al. Assessment of group B streptococcal opsonins in human and rabbit serum by neutrophil chemiluminescence. J Clin Invest 58:1379–1387, 1976.

366. Baker CJ, Kasper DL, Tager IB, et al. Quantitative determination of antibody to capsular polysaccharide in infection with type III strains of group B Streptococcus. J Clin Invest 59:810–818, 1977.

367. Vogel LC, Kretschmer RR, Boyer KM, et al. Human immunity to group B streptococci measured by indirect immunofluorescence: correlation with protection in chick embryos. J Infect Dis 140:682–689, 1979.

368. Baker CJ, Webb BJ, Kasper DL, et al. The natural history of group B streptococcal colonization in the pregnant woman and her offspring: II. Determination of serum antibody to capsular polysaccharide from type III group B Streptococcus. Am J Obstet Gynecol 137:39–42, 1980.

369. Vogel LC, Boyer KM, Gadzala CA, et al. Prevalence of type-specific group B streptococcal antibody in pregnant women. J Pediatr 96:1047–1051, 1980.

370. Boyer KM, Papierniak CK, Gadzala CA, et al. Transplacental passage of IgG antibody to group B Streptococcus serotype Ia. J Pediatr 104:618–620, 1984.

371. Christensen KK, Christensen P, Duc G, et al. Correlation between serum antibody-levels against group B streptococci and gestational age in newborns. Eur J Pediatr 142:86–88, 1984.

372. Hyvarinen M, Zeltzer P, Oh W. Influence of gestational age on the newborn serum levels of alpha-1-fetoglobulin, IgG globulin, and albumin. J Pediatr 82:430–437, 1973.

373. Baker CJ, Edwards MS, Kasper DL. Role of antibody to native type III polysaccharide of group B Streptococcus in infant infection. Pediatrics 68:544–549, 1981.

374. Guttormsen H-K, Baker CJ, Edwards MS, et al. Quantitative determination of antibodies to type III group B streptococcal polysaccharide. J Infect Dis 173:142–150, 1996.

375. Berg S, Kasvi S, Trollfors B, et al. Antibodies to group B streptococci in neonates and infants. Eur J Pediatr 157:221–224, 1998.

376. Stewardson-Krieger PB, Albrandt K, Nevin T, et al.

Perinatal immunity to group B β-hemolytic *Streptococcus* type Ia. J Infect Dis 136:649–654, 1977.

377. Papierniak CK, Klegerman ME, Boyer KM, et al. An enzyme-linked immunosorbent assay (ELISA) for human IgG antibody to the type Ia polysaccharide of group B *Streptococcus*. J Lab Clin Med 100:385–398, 1982.

378. Klegerman ME, Boyer KM, Papierniak CK, et al. Estimation of the protective level of human IgG antibody to the type-specific polysaccharide of group B *Streptococcus* type Ia. J Infect Dis 148:648–655, 1983.

379. Boyer KM, Kendall LS, Papierniak CK, et al. Protective levels of human immunoglobulin G antibody to group B streptococcus type Ib. Infect Immun 45:618–624, 1984.

380. Gotoff SP, Odell C, Papierniak CK, et al. Human IgG antibody to group B *Streptococcus* type III: comparison of protective levels in a murine model with levels in infected human neonates. J Infect Dis 153:511–519, 1986.

381. Gotoff SP, Papierniak CK, Klegerman ME, et al. Quantitation of IgG antibody to the type-specific polysaccharide of group B *Streptococcus* type 1b in pregnant women and infected infants. J Pediatr 105:628–630, 1984.

382. Gray BM, Pritchard DG, Dillon HC Jr. Seroepidemiological studies of group B *Streptococcus* type II. J Infect Dis 151:1073–1080, 1985.

383. Anthony BF, Concepcion NF, Concepcion KF. Human antibody to the group-specific polysaccharide of group B *Streptococcus*. J Infect Dis 151:221–226, 1985.

384. Anthony BF, Concepcion NF, McGeary SA, et al. Immunospecificity and quantitation of an enzyme-linked immunosorbent assay for group B streptococcal antibody. J Clin Microbiol 16:350–354, 1982.

385. Anderson DC, Edwards MS, Baker CJ. Luminol-enhanced chemiluminescence for evaluation of type III group B streptococcal opsonins in human sera. J Infect Dis 141:370–381, 1980.

386. Edwards MS, Baker CJ, Kasper DL. Opsonic specificity of human antibody to the type III polysaccharide of group B *Streptococcus*. J Infect Dis 140:1004–1007, 1979.

387. Payne NR, Ferrieri P. The relation of the Ibc protein antigen to the opsonization differences between strains of type II group B streptococci. J Infect Dis 151:672–681, 1985.

388. Baker CJ, Webb BJ, Kasper DL, et al. The role of complement and antibody in opsonophagocytosis of type II group B streptococci. J Infect Dis 154:47–54, 1986.

389. Payne NR, Kim Y, Ferrieri P. Effect of differences in antibody and complement requirements on phagocytic uptake and intracellular killing of "c" protein-positive and -negative strains of type II group B streptococci. Infect Immun 55:1243–1251, 1987.

390. Vogel LC, Boyer KM, Gotoff SP, et al. Comparison of assays for antibody to group B *Streptococcus* type III. J Infect Dis 141:530, 1980.

391. Baltimore RS, Baker CJ, Kasper DL. Antibody to group B *Streptococcus* type III in human sera measured by a mouse protection test. Infect Immun 32:56–61, 1981.

392. Larsen JW Jr, Harper JS III, London WT, et al. Antibody to type III group B *Streptococcus* in the rhesus monkey. Am J Obstet Gynecol 146:958–962, 1983.

393. Itoh T, Yan X-J, Nakano H, et al. Protective efficacy against group B streptococcal infection in neonatal mice delivered from preimmunized pregnants. Microbiol Immunol 30:297–305, 1986.

394. Shigeoka AO, Hall RT, Hill HR. Blood transfusion in group B streptococcal sepsis. Lancet 1:636–638, 1978.

395. Kim KS, Wass CA, Hong JK, et al. Demonstration of opsonic and protective activity of human cord sera against type III group B *Streptococcus* that are independent of type-specific antibody. Pediatr Res 24:628–632, 1988.

396. Boyer KM, Klegerman ME, Gotoff SP. Development of IgM antibody to group B *Streptococcus* type III in human infants. J Infect Dis 165:1049–1055, 1992.

397. Edwards MS, Baker CJ, Wagner ML, et al. An etiologic shift in infantile osteomyelitis: the emergence of the group B *Streptococcus*. J Pediatr 93:578–583, 1978.

398. Barton LL, Feigin RD, Lins R. Group B beta hemolytic streptococcal meningitis in infants. J Pediatr 82:719–723, 1973.

399. Horn KA, Meyer WT, Wyrick BC, et al. Group B streptococcal neonatal infection. JAMA 230:1165–1167, 1974.

400. Jones WT, Menna JH, Wennerstrom DE. Lethal synergism induced in mice by influenza type A virus and type Ia group B streptococci. Infect Immun 41:618–623, 1983.

401. Rubens CE, Wessels MR, Heggen LM, et al. Transposon mutagenesis of group B streptococcal type III capsular polysaccharide: correlation of capsule expression with virulence. Proc Natl Acad Sci U S A 84:7208–7212, 1987.

402. Shigeoka AO, Rote NS, Santos JI, et al. Assessment of the virulence factors of group B streptococci: correlation with sialic acid content. J Infect Dis 147:857–863, 1983.

403. Håkansson S, Holm SE, Wagner M. Density profile of group B streptococci, type III, and its possible relation to enhanced virulence. J Clin Microbiol 25:714–718, 1987.

404. Wessels MR, Rubens CE, Benedí V-J, et al. Definition of a bacterial virulence factor: sialylation of the group B streptococcal capsule. Proc Natl Acad Sci U S A 86:8983–8987, 1989.

405. Wibawan IWT, Lämmler C. Influence of capsular neuraminic acid on properties of streptococci of serological group B. J Gen Microbiol 137:2721–2725, 1991.

406. Rubens CE, Heggen LM, Kuypers JM. IS*861*, a group B streptococcal insertion sequence related to IS*150* and IS*3* of *Escherichia coli*. J Bacteriol 171:5531–5535, 1989.

407. Kuypers JM, Heggen LM, Rubens CE. Molecular analysis of a region of the group B *Streptococcus* chromosome involved in type III capsule expression. Infect Immun 57:3058–3065, 1989.

408. Wessels MR, Haft RF, Heggen LM, et al. Identification of a genetic locus essential for capsule sialylation in type III group B streptococci. Infect Immun 60:392–400, 1992.

409. Wood EG, Gray BM. Type-specific antibody prevents platelet aggregation induced by group B streptococci type III. J Lab Clin Med 107:322–326, 1986.

410. Usui Y, Ohshima Y, Yoshida K. Platelet aggregation by group B streptococci. J Gen Microbiol 133:1593–1600, 1987.

411. Usui Y, Ichiman Y, Yoshida K, et al. Possible induction of disseminated intravascular coagulation in the mouse by group B streptococcal clumping factor. Br J Exp Pathol 67:629–635, 1986.

412. Linden V, Christensen KK, Christensen P. Correlation between low levels of maternal IgG antibodies to R protein and neonatal septicemia with group B streptococci carrying R protein. Int Arch Allergy Appl Immunol 71:168–172, 1983.

413. Baker CJ, Kasper DL, Edwards MS, et al. Influence of preimmunization antibody level on the specificity of the immune response to related polysaccharide antigens. N Engl J Med 303:173–178, 1980.

414. Kasper DL, Baker CJ, Baltimore RS, et al. Immunodeterminant specificity of human immunity to type III group B *Streptococcus*. J Exp Med 149:327–339, 1979.

415. Baker CJ, Edwards MS, Kasper DL. Immunogenicity of

polysaccharides from type III group B *Streptococcus*. J Clin Invest 61:1107–1110, 1978.

416. Mårdh P-A, Weström L. Adherence of bacteria to vaginal epithelial cells. Infect Immun 13:661–666, 1976.

417. Sobel JD, Myers P, Levison ME, et al. Comparison of bacterial and fungal adherence to vaginal exfoliated epithelial cells and human vaginal epithelial tissue culture cells. Infect Immun 35:697–701, 1982.

418. Galask RP, Varner MW, Petzold CR, et al. Bacterial attachment to the chorioamniotic membranes. Am J Obstet Gynecol 148:915–928, 1984.

419. Botta GA. Hormonal and type-dependent adhesion of group B streptococci to human vaginal cells. Infect Immun 25:1084–1086, 1979.

420. Broughton RA, Baker CJ. Role of adherence in the pathogenesis of neonatal group B streptococcal infection. Infect Immun 39:837–843, 1983.

421. Helmig R, Halaburt JT, Uldbjerg N, et al. Increased cell adherence of group B streptococci from preterm infants with neonatal sepsis. Obstet Gynecol 76:825–828, 1990.

422. Kubín V, Jirásková Z, Franék J. The effect of length of incubation on adherence of group B streptococci to epithelial cells. Folia Microbiol 28:241–243, 1983.

423. Zawaneh SM, Ayoub EM, Baer H, et al. Factors influencing adherence of group B streptococci to human vaginal epithelial cells. Infect Immun 26:441–447, 1979.

424. Kubín V, Jirásková Z, Franék J. The effect of pH on the adherence of group B streptococci to epithelial cells. Folia Microbiol 28:62–64, 1983.

425. Jelínková J, Grabovskaya KB, Rýc M, et al. Adherence of vaginal and pharyngeal strains of group B streptococci to human vaginal and pharyngeal epithelial cells. Zentralbl Bakteriol Mikrobiol Hyg 262:492–499, 1986.

426. Tietz H-J, Gantenberg R, Halle E, et al. Interactions between group B streptococci and human cord blood lymphocytes. Biomed Biochim Acta 49:1131–1137, 1990.

427. Ofek IE, Beachy EH, Eyal F, et al. Postnatal development of binding of streptococci and lipoteichoic acid by oral mucosal cells of humans. J Infect Dis 135:267–274, 1977.

428. Cox F. Prevention of group B streptococcal colonization with topically applied lipoteichoic acid in a maternal-newborn mouse model. Pediatr Res 16:816–819, 1982.

429. Nealon TJ, Mattingly SJ. Kinetic and chemical analyses of the biologic significance of lipoteichoic acids in mediating adherence of serotype III group B streptococci. Infect Immun 50:107–115, 1985.

430. Teti G, Tomasello F, Chiofalo MS, et al. Adherence of group B streptococci to adult and neonatal epithelial cells mediated by lipoteichoic acid. Infect Immun 55:3057–3064, 1987.

431. Ayoub EM, Swingle H. Pathogenic mechanisms in neonatal GBS infection. Antibiot Chemother 35:128–141, 1985.

432. Jones WT, Menna JH. Influenza type A virus–mediated adherence of type 1a group B streptococci to mouse tracheal tissue in vivo. Infect Immun 38:791–794, 1982.

433. Bagg J, Poxton IR, Weir DM, et al. Binding of type-III group-B streptococci to buccal epithelial cells. J Med Microbiol 15:363–372, 1982.

434. Bulgakova TN, Grabovskaya KB, Rýc M, et al. The adhesin structures involved in the adherence of group B streptococci to human vaginal cells. Folia Microbiol 31:394–401, 1986.

435. Miyazaki S, Leon O, Panos C. Adherence of *Streptococcus agalactiae* to synchronously growing human cell monolayers without lipoteichoic acid involvement. Infect Immun 56:505–512, 1988.

436. Wibawan IWT, Lämmler C, Pasaribu FH. Role of hydrophobic surface proteins in mediating adherence of group B streptococci to epithelial cells. J Gen Microbiol 138:1237–1242, 1992.

437. Smith LM, Laganas V, Pistole TG. Attachment of group B streptococci to macrophages is mediated by a 21-kDa protein. FEMS Immunol Med Microbiol 20:89–97, 1998.

438. Tamura GS, Kuypers JM, Smith S, et al. Adherence of group B streptococci to cultured epithelial cells: roles of environmental factors and bacterial surface components. Infect Immun 62:2450–2458, 1994.

439. Spellerberg B, Rozdzinski E, Martin S, et al. Lmb, a protein with similarities to the LraI adhesin family, mediates attachment of *Streptococcus agalactiae* to human laminin. Infect Immun 67:871–878, 1999.

440. Rubens CE, Smith S, Hulse M, et al. Respiratory epithelial cell invasion by group B streptococci. Infect Immun 60:5157–5163, 1992.

441. Nizet V, Gibson RL, Chi EY, et al. Group B streptococcal beta-hemolysin expression is associated with injury of lung epithelial cells. Infect Immun 64:3818–3826, 1996.

442. Valentin-Weigand P, Chhatwal GS. Correlation of epithelial cell invasiveness of group B streptococci with clinical source of isolation. Microb Pathog 19:83–91, 1995.

443. Winram SB, Jonas M, Chi E, et al. Characterization of group B streptococcal invasion of human chorion and amnion epithelial cells in vitro. Infect Immun 66:4932–4941, 1998.

444. Nizet V, Kim KS, Stins M, et al. Invasion of brain microvascular endothelial cells by group B streptococci. Infect Immun 65:5074–5081, 1997.

445. Hordnes K, Tynning T, Kvam AI, et al. Cervical secretions in pregnant women colonized rectally with group B streptococci have high levels of antibodies to serotype III polysaccharide capsular antigen and protein R. Scand J Immunol 47:179–188, 1998.

446. Hordnes K, Tynning T, Kvam AI, et al. Colonization in the rectum and uterine cervix with group B streptococci may induce specific antibody responses in cervical secretions of pregnant women. Infect Immun 64:1643–1652, 1996.

447. Shigeoka AO, Hall RT, Hemming VG, et al. Role of antibody and complement in opsonization of group B streptococci. Infect Immun 21:34–40, 1978.

448. Hill HR, Shigeoka AO, Hall RT, et al. Neonatal cellular and humoral immunity to group B streptococci. Pediatrics S64:787–794, 1979.

449. De Cueninck BJ, Eisenstein TK, McIntosh TS, et al. Quantitation of in vitro opsonic activity of human antibody induced by a vaccine consisting of the type III-specific polysaccharide of group B streptococcus. Infect Immun 39:1155–1160, 1983.

450. Pincus SH, Shigeoka AO, Moe AA, et al. Protective efficacy of IgM monoclonal antibodies in experimental group B streptococcal infection is a function of antibody avidity. J Immunol 140:2779–2785, 1988.

451. Givner LB, Baker CJ, Edwards MS. Type III group B *Streptococcus*: functional interaction with IgG subclass antibodies. J Infect Dis 155:532–539, 1987.

452. Kim JS, Kim KW, Wass CA, et al. A human IgG 3 is opsonic *in vitro* against type III group B streptococci. J Clin Immunol 10:154–159, 1990.

453. Anthony BF, Concepcion NF. Opsonic activity of human IgG and IgM antibody for type III group B streptococci. Pediatr Res 26:383–387, 1989.

454. Campbell JR, Baker CJ, Metzger TG, et al. Functional

activity of class-specific antibodies to type III, group B *Streptococcus*. Pediatr Res 23:31–34, 1988.

455. Bohnsack JF, Hawley MM, Pritchard DG, et al. An IgA monoclonal antibody directed against type III antigen on group B streptococci acts as an opsonin. J Immunol 143:3338–3342, 1989.

456. Campbell JR, Baker CJ, Edwards MS. Deposition and degradation of C3 on type III group B streptococci. Infect Immun 59:1978–1983, 1991.

457. Marques MB, Kasper DL, Pangburn MK, et al. Prevention of C3 deposition by capsular polysaccharide is a virulence mechanism of type III group B streptococci. Infect Immun 60:3986–3993, 1992.

458. Eads ME, Levy NJ, Kasper DL, et al. Antibody-independent activation of C1 by type Ia group B streptococci. J Infect Dis 146:665–672, 1982.

459. Levy NJ, Kasper DL. Surface-bound capsular polysaccharide of type Ia group B *Streptococcus* mediates C1 binding and activation of the classic complement pathway. J Immunol 136:4157–4162, 1986.

460. Levy NJ, Kasper DL. Antibody-independent and -dependent opsonization of group B *Streptococcus* requires the first component of complement C1. Infect Immun 49:19–24, 1985.

461. Smith CL, Pritchard DG, Gray BM. Role of polysaccharide capsule in C3 deposition by type Ib group B streptococci (GBS). Abstract 450. 31st Interscience Conference on Antimicrobial Agents and Chemotherapy, 1991.

462. Smith CL, Smith AH. Strain variability of type Ib group B streptococci: unique strains are resistant to C3 deposition by the alternate complement pathway. Clin Res 40:823A, 1992.

463. Gerards LJ, Fleer A, Westerdaal NAC, et al. Opsonic requirements of group B streptococci in human serum. *In* Gerards LJ (ed). Group B Streptococci in the Perinatal Period. Thesis, Utrecht, The Netherlands, 1985, pp 55–70.

464. Hindocha P, Hill R, Wood CBS, et al. Impaired opsonophagocytosis of serotypes Ib and II of group B streptococci as compared with serotypes Ia and III: role of the alternative pathway of complement in opsonization of serotype III of group B streptococci. J Clin Pathol 37:790–795, 1984.

465. Soderstrom C, Braconier JH, Christensen KK, et al. Opsonization of group B streptococci in properdin deficient serum. Acta Pathol Microbiol Immunol Scand 93:251–256, 1985.

466. Russell-Jones GJ, Gotschlich EC, Blake MS. A surface receptor specific for human IgA on group B streptococci possessing the Ibc protein antigen. J Exp Med 160:1467–1475, 1984.

467. Payne NR, Concepcion NF, Anthony BF. Opsonic effect of jacalin and human immunoglobulin A on type II group B streptococci. Infect Immun 58:3663–3670, 1990.

468. Anthony BF, Concepcion NF, Puentes SM, et al. Nonimmune binding of human immunoglobulin A to type II group B streptococci. Infect Immun 58:1789–1795, 1990.

469. Lindahl G, Åkerström B, Vaerman J-P, et al. Characterization of an IgA receptor from group B streptococci: specificity for serum IgA. Eur J Immunol 20:2241–2247, 1990.

470. Hedén L-O, Frithz E, Lindahl G. Molecular characterization of an IgA receptor from group B streptococci: sequence of the gene, identification of a proline-rich region with unique structure and isolation of N-terminal fragments with IgA-binding capacity. Eur J Immunol 21:1481–1490, 1991.

471. Hall MA, Edwards MS, Baker CJ. Complement and antibody participation in opsonophagocytosis of type IV and V group B streptococci. Infect Immun 60:5030–5035, 1992.

472. Hall MA, Hickman ME, Baker CJ, et al. Complement and antibody in neutrophil-mediated killing of type V group B *Streptococcus*. J Infect Dis 170:88–93, 1994.

473. Davis CA, Vallota EH, Forristal J. Serum complement levels in infancy: age-related changes. Pediatr Res 13:1043–1046, 1979.

474. Máródi L, Leijh PCJ, Braat A, et al. Opsonic activity of cord blood sera against various species of microorganism. Pediatr Res 19:433–436, 1985.

475. Edwards MS, Buffone GJ, Fuselier PA, et al. Deficient classical complement pathway activity in newborn sera. Pediatr Res 17:685–688, 1983.

476. Baker CJ, Rench MA, Edwards MS, et al. Immunization of pregnant women with a polysaccharide vaccine of group B *Streptococcus*. N Engl J Med 319:1180–1185, 1988.

477. Edwards MS, Hall MA, Rench MA, et al. Patterns of immune response among survivors of group B streptococcal meningitis. J Infect Dis 161:65–70, 1990.

478. Cairo MS, Worcester C, Rucker R, et al. Role of circulating complement and polymorphonuclear leukocyte transfusion in treatment and outcome in critically ill neonates with sepsis. J Pediatr 110:935–941, 1987.

479. Teti G, Mancuso G, Tomasello F. Cytokine appearance and effects of anti-tumor necrosis factor alpha antibodies in a neonatal rat model of group B streptococcal infection. Infect Immun 61:227–235, 1993.

480. Williams PA, Bohnsack JF, Augustine NH, et al. Production of tumor necrosis factor by human cells *in vitro* and *in vivo*, induced by group B streptococci. J Pediatr 123:292–300, 1993.

481. Vallejo JG, Baker CJ, Edwards MS. Roles of the bacterial cell wall and capsule in induction of tumor necrosis factor alpha by type III group B streptococci. Infect Immun 64:5042–5046, 1996.

482. Mancuso G, Tomasello F, von Hunolstein C, et al. Induction of tumor necrosis factor alpha by the group- and type-specific polysaccharides from type III group B streptococci. Infect Immun 62:2748–2753, 1994.

483. Mancuso G, Tomasello F, Migliardo M, et al. Beneficial effects of interleukin-6 in neonatal mouse models of group B streptococcal disease. Infect Immun 62:4997–5002, 1994.

484. Rosati E, Fettucciari K, Scaringi L, et al. Cytokine response to group B *Streptococcus* infection in mice. Scand J Immunol 47:314–323, 1998.

485. von Hunolstein C, Totolian A, Alfarone G, et al. Soluble antigens from group B streptococci induce cytokine production in human blood cultures. Infect Immun 65:4017–4021, 1997.

486. Vallejo JG, Baker CJ, Edwards MS. Interleukin-6 production by human neonatal monocytes stimulated by type III group B streptococci. J Infect Dis 174:332–337, 1996.

487. Steele PM, Augustine NH, Hill HR. The effect of lactic acid on mononuclear cell secretion of proinflammatory cytokines in response to group B streptococci. J Infect Dis 177:1418–1421, 1998.

488. MacKenzie CR, Hadding U, Däubener W. Interferon-γ–induced activation of idoleamine 2,3-dioxygenase in cord blood monocyte-derived macrophages inhibits the growth of group B streptococci. J Infect Dis 178:875–878, 1998.

489. Cusumano V, Mancuso G, Genovese F, et al. Role of

gamma interferon in a neonatal mouse model of group B streptococcal disease. Infect Immun 64:2941–2944, 1996.

490. Rowen JL, Smith CW, Edwards MS. Group B streptococci elicit leukotriene B₄ and interleukin-8 from human monocytes: neonates exhibit a diminished response. J Infect Dis 172:420–426, 1995.

491. Mancuso G, Cusumano V, Genovese F, et al. Role of interleukin 12 in experimental neonatal sepsis caused by group B streptococci. Infect Immun 65:3731–3735, 1997.

492. Cusumano V, Genovese F, Mancuso G, et al. Interleukin-10 protects neonatal mice from lethal group B streptococcal infection. Infect Immun 64:2850–2852, 1996.

493. Anderson DC, Hughes BJ, Edwards MS, et al. Impaired chemotaxigenesis by type III group B streptococci in neonatal sera: relationship to diminished concentration of specific anticapsular antibody and abnormalities of serum complement. Pediatr Res 17:496–502, 1983.

494. McFall TL, Zimmerman GA, Augustine NH, et al. Effect of group B streptococcal type-specific antigen on polymorphonuclear leukocyte function and polymorphonuclear leukocyte-endothelial cell interaction. Pediatr Res 21:517–523, 1987.

495. Olson TA, Fischer GW, Hemming VG, et al. A group B streptococcal extract reduces neutrophil counts and induces neutrophil aggregation. Pediatr Res 21:326–330, 1987.

496. Shigeoka AO, Chavette RP, Wyman ML, et al. Defective oxidative metabolic responses of neutrophils from stressed neonates. J Pediatr 98:392–398, 1981.

497. Smith CL, Baker CJ, Anderson DC, et al. Role of complement receptors in opsonophagocytosis of group B streptococci by adult and neonatal neutrophils. J Infect Dis 162:489–495, 1990.

498. Antal JM, Cunningham JV, Goodrum KJ. Opsonin-independent phagocytosis of group B streptococci: role of complement receptor type three. Infect Immun 60:1114–1121, 1992.

499. Yang KD, Bathras JM, Shigeoka AO, et al. Mechanisms of bacterial opsonization by immune globulin intravenous: correlation of complement consumption with opsonic activity and protective efficacy. J Infect Dis 159:701–707, 1989.

500. Noya FJD, Baker CJ, Edwards MS. Neutrophil Fc receptor participation in phagocytosis of type III group B streptococci. Infect Immun 61:1415–1420, 1993.

501. Noel GJ, Katz SL, Edelson PJ. The role of C3 in mediating binding and ingestion of group B Streptococcus serotype III by murine macrophages. Pediatr Res 30:118–123, 1991.

502. Christensen RD, Macfarlane JL, Taylor NL, et al. Blood and marrow neutrophils during experimental group B streptococcal infection: quantification of the stem cell, proliferative, storage and circulating pools. Pediatr Res 16:549–553, 1982.

503. Christensen RD, Hill HR, Rothstein G. Granulocytic stem cell (CFUc) proliferation in experimental group B streptococcal sepsis. Pediatr Res 17:278–280, 1983.

504. Wheeler JG, Chauvenet AR, Johnson CA, et al. Neutrophil storage pool depletion in septic neutropenic neonates. Pediatr Infect Dis J 3:407–409, 1984.

505. Christensen RD, Rothstein G, Hill HR, et al. The effect of hybridoma antibody administration upon neutrophil kinetics during experimental type III group B streptococcal sepsis. Pediatr Res 17:795–799, 1983.

506. Christensen RD, Rothstein G, Hill HR, et al. Treatment of experimental group B streptococcal infection with hybridoma antibody. Pediatr Res 18:1093–1096, 1984.

507. Harper TE, Christensen RD, Rothstein G, et al. Effect of intravenous immunoglobulin G on neutrophil kinetics during experimental group B streptococcal infection in neonatal rats. Rev Infect Dis 8:S401–S408, 1986.

508. Fischer GW, Hunter KW, Hemming VG, et al. Functional antibacterial activity of a human intravenous immunoglobulin preparation: in vitro and in vivo studies. Vox Sang 44:296–299, 1983.

509. Givner LB, Edwards MS, Anderson DC, et al. Immune globulin for intravenous use: enhancement of in vitro opsonophagocytic activity of neonatal serum. J Infect Dis 151:217–220, 1985.

510. Shigeoka AO, Bathras JM, Pincus SH, et al. Reticuloendothelial clearance of type III group B streptococci opsonized with type III specific monoclonal antibodies of IgM or IgG2a isotypes in an experimental rat model. Pediatr Res 21:334A, 1987.

511. Poutrel B, Dore J. Virulence of human and bovine isolates of group B streptococci (types Ia and III) in experimental pregnant mouse models. Infect Immunol 47:94–97, 1985.

512. Sherman M, Goldstein E, Lippert W, et al. Group B streptococcal lung infection in neonatal rabbits. Pediatr Res 16:209–212, 1982.

513. Sherman MP, Lehrer RI. Oxidative metabolism of neonatal and adult rabbit lung macrophages stimulated with opsonized group B streptococci. Infect Immunol 47:26–30, 1985.

514. Martin TR, Rubens CE, Wilson CB. Lung antibacterial defense mechanisms in infant and adult rats: implications for the pathogenesis of group B streptococcal infections in the neonatal lung. J Infect Dis 157:91–100, 1988.

515. Hall SL, Sherman MP. Intrapulmonary bacterial clearance of type III group B Streptococcus is reduced in preterm compared with term rabbits and occurs independent of antibody. Am Rev Respir Dis 145:1172–1177, 1992.

516. Martin TR, Ruzinski JT, Rubens CE, et al. The effect of type-specific polysaccharide capsule on the clearance of group B streptococci from the lungs of infant and adult rats. J Infect Dis 165:306–314, 1992.

517. Domula M, Bykowska K, Wegrzynowicz Z, et al. Plasma fibronectin concentrations in healthy and septic infants. Eur J Pediatr 144:49–52, 1985.

518. Butler KM, Baker CJ, Edwards MS. Interaction of soluble fibronectin with group B streptococci. Infect Immunol 55:2404–2408, 1987.

519. Hill HR, Shigeoka AO, Augustine NH, et al. Fibronectin enhances the opsonic and protective activity of monoclonal and polyclonal antibody against group B streptococci. J Exp Med 159:1618–1628, 1984.

520. Jacobs RF, Kiel DP, Sanders ML, et al. Phagocytosis of type III group B streptococci by neonatal monocytes: enhancement by fibronectin and gammaglobulin. J Infect Dis 152:695–700, 1985.

521. Yang KD, Bohnsack JF, Hawley MM, et al. Effect of fibronectin on IgA-mediated uptake of type III group B streptococci by phagocytes. J Infect Dis 161:236–241, 1990.

522. Peat EB, Augustine NH, Drummond WK, et al. Effects of fibronectin and group B streptococci on tumour necrosis factor-α production by human culture-derived macrophages. Immunology 84:440–445, 1995.

523. Grubb R, Christensen KK, Christensen P, et al. Association between maternal Gm allotype and neonatal septicaemia with group B streptococci. J Immunogenet 9:143–147, 1982.

524. Thom H, Lloyd DL, Reid TMS. Maternal immunoglobulin allotype (Gm and Km) and neonatal group B streptococcal infection. J Immunogenet 13:309–314, 1986.

525. Oxelius VA, Linden V, Christensen KK, et al. Deficiency of IgG subclasses in mothers of infants with group B streptococcal septicemia. Int Arch Allergy Appl Immunol 72:249–252, 1983.

526. Rundgren ÅK, Christensen KK, Christensen P. Increased frequency of high serum IgM among mothers of infants with neonatal group-B streptococcal septicemia. Int Arch Allergy Appl Immunol 77:372–373, 1985.

527. Christensen KK, Christensen P, Faxelius G, et al. Immune response to pneumococcal vaccine in mothers to infants with group B streptococcal septicemia: evidence for a divergent IgG/IgM ratio. Int Arch Allergy Appl Immunol 76:369–372, 1985.

528. Christensen KK, Christensen P, Hagerstrand I, et al. The clinical significance of group B streptococci. J Perinatol Med 10:133–146, 1982.

529. Christensen KK. Infection as a predominant cause of perinatal mortality. Obstet Gynecol 59:499–508, 1982.

530. Singer DB, Campognone P. Perinatal group B streptococcal infection in midgestation. Pediatr Pathol 5:271–276, 1986.

531. deSa DJ, Trevenen CL. Intrauterine infections with group B beta-haemolytic streptococci. Br J Obstet Gynaecol 91:237–239, 1984.

532. Novak RW, Platt MS. Significance of placental findings in early-onset group B streptococcal neonatal sepsis. Clin Pediatr 24:256–258, 1985.

533. Becroft DMO, Farmer K, Mason GH, et al. Perinatal infections by group B β-hemolytic streptococci. Br J Obstet Gynaecol 83:960–965, 1976.

534. Rubens CE, Raff HV, Jackson JC, et al. Pathophysiology and histopathology of group B streptococcal sepsis in *Macaca nemestrina* primates induced after intraamniotic inoculation: evidence for bacterial cellular invasion. J Infect Dis 164:320–330, 1991.

535. Varner MW, Turner JW, Petzold CR, et al. Ultrastructural alterations of term human amnionic epithelium following incubation with group B beta-hemolytic streptococci. Am J Reprod Immunol Microbiol 9:27–32, 1985.

536. Hemming VG, McCloskey DW, Hill HR. Pneumonia in the neonate associated with group B streptococcal septicemia. Am J Dis Child 130:1231–1233, 1976.

537. Robinson MJ, Eykyn SJ. Group B *Streptococcus*: the commonest pathogen in severe neonatal sepsis. J Infect 1:323–328, 1979.

538. Leonidas JC, Hall RT, Beatty EC, et al. Radiographic findings of early onset neonatal group B streptococcal septicemia. Pediatrics 59:S1006–S1011, 1977.

539. Quirante J, Ceballos R, Cassady G. Group B β-hemolytic streptococcal infections in the newborn. Am J Dis Child 128:659–665, 1973.

540. Faix RG, Donn SM. Association of septic shock caused by early-onset group B streptococcal sepsis and periventricular leukomalacia in the preterm infant. Pediatrics 76:415–419, 1985.

541. Van Peenen PF, Cannon RE, Seibert DJ. Group B beta-hemolytic streptococci causing fatal meningitis. Mil Med 130:65–67, 1965.

542. Jones HE, Howells CHL. Neonatal meningitis due to *Streptococcus agalactiae*. Postgrad Med J 44:549–562, 1968.

543. Ferrieri P, Burke B, Nelson J. Production of bacteremia and meningitis in infant rats with group B streptococcal serotypes. Infect Immunol 27:1023–1032, 1980.

544. Zeligs BJ, Armstrong CD, Walser JB, et al. Age-dependent susceptibility of neonatal rats to group B streptococcal type III infection: correlation of severity of infection and response of myeloid pools. Infect Immunol 37:255–263, 1982.

545. DiJohn D, Krasinski K, Lawrence R, et al. Very late onset of group B streptococcal disease in infants infected with the human immunodeficiency virus. Pediatr Infect Dis J 9:925–928, 1990.

546. Weisman LE, Stoll BJ, Cruess DF, et al. Early-onset group B streptococcal sepsis: a current assessment. J Pediatr 121:428–433, 1992.

547. Yagupsky P, Menegus MA, Powell KR. The changing spectrum of group B streptococcal disease in infants: an eleven-year experience in a tertiary care hospital. Pediatr Infect Dis J 10:801–808, 1991.

548. Stoll BJ, Gordon T, Korones SB, et al. Early-onset sepsis in very low birth weight neonates: a report from the National Institute of Child Health and Human Development Neonatal Research Network. J Pediatr 129:72–80, 1996.

549. Chin KC, Fitzhardinge PM. Sequelae of early-onset group B streptococcal neonatal meningitis. J Pediatr 106:819–822, 1985.

550. Horn KA, Zimmerman RA, Knostman JD, et al. Neurological sequelae of group B streptococcal neonatal infection. Pediatrics 53:501–504, 1974.

551. Haslam RHA, Allen JR, Dorsen MM, et al. The sequelae of group B β-hemolytic streptococcal meningitis in early infancy. Am J Dis Child 131:845–849, 1977.

552. Edwards MS, Rench MA, Haffar AAM, et al. Long-term sequelae of group B streptococcal meningitis in infants. J Pediatr 106:717–722, 1985.

553. Lilien LD, Harris VJ, Pildes RS. Significance of radiographic findings in early-onset group B streptococcal infection. Pediatrics 60:360–365, 1977.

554. Shankaran S, Farooki ZQ, Desai R. Beta-hemolytic streptococcal infection appearing as persistent fetal circulation. Am J Dis Child 136:725–727, 1982.

555. Hammerman C, Lass N, Strates E, et al. Prostanoids in neonates with persistent pulmonary hypertension. J Pediatr 110:470–472, 1987.

556. Weller MH, Katzenstein AA. Radiological findings in group B streptococcal sepsis. Radiology 118:385–387, 1976.

557. Long WA, Lawson EE, Harned HS Jr, et al. Pleural effusion in the first days of life: a prospective study. Am J Perinatol 1:190–194, 1984.

558. Payne NR, Burke BA, Day DL, et al. Correlation of clinical and pathologic findings in early onset neonatal group B streptococcal infection with disease severity and prediction of outcome. Pediatr Infect Dis J 7:836–847, 1988.

559. Lannering B, Larsson LE, Rojas J, et al. Early onset group B streptococcal disease. Seven year experience and clinical scoring system. Acta Paediatr Scand 72:597–602, 1983.

560. Baker CJ. Unpublished observations.

561. Pyati SP, Pildes RS, Ramamurthy RS, et al. Decreasing mortality in neonates with early-onset group B streptococcal infection: reality or artifact. J Pediatr 98:625–628, 1981.

562. Friis-Møller A, Busk HE, Korner B, et al. Infections and colonisations with haemolytic streptococci group B in a Danish neonatal intensive care unit. Dan Med Bull 31:494–499, 1984.

563. Jacobs MR, Koornhof HJ, Stein H. Group B streptococcal infections in neonates and infants. S Afr Med J 54:154–158, 1978.

564. McReynolds EW, Shane R. Diabetes insipidus secondary to group B beta streptococcal meningitis. J Tenn Med Assoc 67:117–120, 1974.

565. Sapir-Ellis S, Johnson A, Austin TL. Group B strepto-

coccal meningitis associated with otitis media. Am J Dis Child 130:1003–1004, 1976.

566. Ferguson L, Gotoff SP. Subdural empyema in an infant due to group B β-hemolytic *Streptococcus*. Am J Dis Child 131:97, 1977.

567. Carstensen H, Henrichsen J, Jepsen OB. A national survey of severe group B streptococcal infections in neonates and young infants in Denmark, 1978–1983. Acta Paediatr Scand 74:934–941, 1985.

568. Wald ER, Bergman I, Taylor HG, et al. Long-term outcome of group B streptococcal meningitis. Pediatrics 77:217–221, 1986.

569. Garcia Peña BM, Harper MB, Fleisher GR. Occult bacteremia with group B streptococci in an outpatient setting. Pediatrics 102:67–72, 1998.

570. Ramsey PG, Zwerdling R. Asymptomatic neonatal bacteremia. N Engl J Med 295:225, 1977.

571. Roberts KB. Persistent group B *Streptococcus* bacteremia without clinical "sepsis" in infants. J Pediatr 88:1059–1060, 1976.

572. Hussain SM, Luedtke GS, Baker CJ, et al. Invasive group B streptococcal disease in children beyond early infancy. Pediatr Infect Dis J 14:278–281, 1995.

573. De Witt CC, Ascher DP, Winkelstein J. Group B streptococcal disease in a child beyond early infancy with a deficiency of the second component of complement (C2). Pediatr Infect Dis J 18:77–78, 1999.

574. Ashdown LR, Hewson PH, Suleman SK. Neonatal osteomyelitis and meningitis caused by group B streptococci. Med J Aust 2:500–501, 1977.

575. McCook TA, Felman AH, Ayoub EM. Streptococcal skeletal infections: observations in four infants. Roentgenology 130:465–467, 1978.

576. Ancona RJ, McAuliffe J, Thompson TR, et al. Group B streptococcal sepsis with osteomyelitis and arthritis. Am J Dis Child 133:919–920, 1979.

577. Memon IA, Jacobs NM, Yeh TF, et al. Group B streptococcal osteomyelitis and septic arthritis. Am J Dis Child 133:921–923, 1979.

578. Pittard WB, Thullen JD, Fanaroff AA. Neonatal septic arthritis. J Pediatr 88:621–624, 1976.

579. McCracken GH Jr. Septic arthritis in a neonate. Hosp Pract 14:158–164, 1979.

580. Nelson JD. The bacterial etiology and antibiotic management of septic arthritis in infants and children. Pediatrics 50:437–440, 1972.

581. Anthony BF, Concepcion NF. Group B *Streptococcus* in a general hospital. J Infect Dis 132:561–567, 1975.

582. Dan M. Neonatal septic arthritis. Isr J Med Sci 19:967–971, 1983.

583. Siskind B, Galliguez P, Wald ER. Group B beta hemolytic streptococcal osteomyelitis/purulent arthritis in neonates: report of three cases. J Pediatr 87:659, 1975.

584. Fox L, Sprunt K. Neonatal osteomyelitis. Pediatrics 62:535–542, 1978.

585. Lai TK, Hingston J, Scheifele D. Streptococcal neonatal osteomyelitis. Am J Dis Child 134:711, 1980.

586. Hutto JH, Ayoub EM. Streptococcal osteomyelitis and arthritis in a neonate. Am J Dis Child 129:1449–1451, 1975.

587. Henderson KC, Roberts RS, Dorsey SB. Group B β-hemolytic streptococcal osteomyelitis in a neonate. Pediatrics 59:1053–1054, 1977.

588. Ragnhildstreit E, Ose L. Neonatal osteomyelitis caused by group B streptococci. Scand J Infect Dis 8:219–221, 1976.

589. Kexel G. Occurrence of B streptococci in humans. Z Hyg Infektionskr 151:336–348, 1965.

590. Clay SA. Osteomyelitis as a cause of brachial plexus neuropathy. Am J Dis Child 136:1054–1056, 1982.

591. Broughton RA, Edwards MS, Haffar A, et al. Unusual manifestations of neonatal group B streptococcal osteomyelitis. Pediatr Infect Dis J 1:410–412, 1982.

592. Mohon RT, Mehalic TF, Grimes CK, et al. Infected cephalhematoma and neonatal osteomyelitis of the skull. Pediatr Infect Dis J 5:253–256, 1986.

593. Sadleir LG, Connolly MB. Acquired brachial-plexus neuropathy in the neonate: a rare presentation of late-onset group-B streptococcal osteomyelitis. Dev Med Child Neurol 40:496–499, 1998.

594. Ammari LK, Offit PA, Campbell AB, et al. Unusual presentation of group B *Streptococcus* osteomyelitis. Pediatr Infect Dis J 11:1066–1067, 1992.

595. Weinberg AG, Laird WP. Group B streptococcal endocarditis detected by echocardiography. J Pediatr 92:335–336, 1978.

596. Obando I, Martin E, Alvarez-Aldean J, et al. Group B *Streptococcus* pelvic osteomyelitis presenting as footdrop in a newborn infant. Pediatr Infect Dis J 10:703–705, 1991.

597. Barton LL, Villar RG, Rice SA. Neonatal group B streptococcal vertebral osteomyelitis. Pediatrics 98:459–461, 1996.

598. Handrick W, Hörmann D, Kunze W, et al. Osteoarthritis durch B-streptokokken bei Neugeborenen und jungen Säuglingen. Dtsch Gesundheitswes 38:373–378, 1983.

599. Hauger SB. Facial cellulitis: an early indicator of group B streptococcal bacteremia. Pediatrics 67:376–377, 1981.

600. Patamasucon P, Siegel JD, McCracken GH Jr. Streptococcal submandibular cellulitis in young infants. Pediatrics 67:378–380, 1981.

601. Baker CJ. Group B streptococcal cellulitis/adenitis in infants. Am J Dis Child 136:631–633, 1982.

602. Pathak A, Hwu H-H. Group B streptococcal cellulitis. South Med J 78:67–68, 1985.

603. Haque KN, Bashir O, Kambal AMM. Delayed recurrence of group B streptococcal infection in a newborn infant: a case report. Ann Trop Paediatr 6:219–220, 1986.

604. Rand TH. Group B streptococcal cellulitis in infants: a disease modified by prior antibiotic therapy or hospitalization? Pediatrics 81:63–65, 1988.

605. Brady MT. Cellulitis of the penis and scrotum due to group B *Streptococcus*. J Urol 137:736–737, 1987.

606. Albanyan EA, Baker CJ. Is lumbar puncture necessary to exclude meningitis in neonates and young infants. lessons from group B *Streptococcus* cellulitis-adenitis syndrome. Pediatrics 102:985–986, 1998.

607. Chadwick EG, Shulman ST, Yogev R. Peritonitis as a late manifestation of group B streptococcal disease in newborns. Pediatr Infect Dis J 2:142–143, 1983.

608. Walker KM, Coyer WF. Suprarenal abscess due to group B streptococcus. J Pediatr 94:970–971, 1979.

609. Leitner M, Clarke TA, Feldman BH. Hyperbilirubinemia in association with late onset group B β-hemolytic streptococcal infection. Pediatrics 63:686, 1979.

610. Atkinson GO Jr, Kodroff MB, Gay BB, et al. Adrenal abscess in the neonate. Radiology 155:101–104, 1985.

611. Carty A, Stanley P. Bilateral adrenal abscesses in a neonate. Pediatr Radiol 1:63–64, 1973.

612. Peevy KJ, Wiseman HJ. Gallbladder distension in septic neonates. Arch Dis Child 57:75–76, 1982.

613. Siegel JD, Shannon KM, De Passe BM. Recurrent infection associated with penicillin-tolerant group B streptococci: a report of two cases. J Pediatr 99:920–924, 1981.

614. Cueva JP, Egel RT. Anterior fontanel herniation in group B *Streptococcus* meningitis in newborns. Pediatr Neurol 10:332–334, 1994.

615. Sokol DM, Demmler GJ, Baker CJ. Unusual presentation of group B streptococcal ventriculitis. Pediatr Infect Dis J 9:525–527, 1990.

616. Kim KS, Kaye KL, Itabashi HH, et al. Cerebritis due to group B *Streptococcus*. Scand J Infect Dis 14:305–308, 1982.

617. Coker SB, Muraskas JK, Thomas C. Myelopathy secondary to neonatal bacterial meningitis. Pediatr Neurol 10:259–261, 1994.

618. Ellenbogen RG, Goldmann DA, Winston KR. Group B streptococcal infections of the central nervous system in infants with myelomeningocele. Surg Neurol 29:237–242, 1988.

619. Chattopadhyay B. Fatal neonatal meningitis due to group B streptococci. Postgrad Med J 51:240–243, 1975.

620. Barton CW, Crowley DC, Uzark K, et al. A neonatal survivor of group B beta-hemolytic streptococcal endocarditis. Am J Perinatol 1:214–215, 1984.

621. Horigome H, Okada Y, Hirano T, et al. Group B streptococcal endocarditis in infancy with a giant vegetation on the pulmonary valve. Eur J Pediatr 153:140–142, 1994.

622. Harper IA. The importance of group B streptococci as human pathogens in the British Isles. J Clin Pathol 24:438–441, 1971.

623. Agarwala BN. Group B streptococcal endocarditis in a neonate. Pediatr Cardiol 9:51–53, 1988.

624. Shurin PA, Howie VM, Pelton SI, et al. Bacterial etiology of otitis media during the first six weeks of life. J Pediatr 92:893–896, 1978.

625. Tetzlaff TR, Ashworth C, Nelson JD. Otitis media in children less than 12 weeks of age. Pediatrics 59:827–832, 1977.

626. Ermocilla R, Cassady G, Ceballos R. Otitis media in the pathogenesis of neonatal meningitis with group B beta-hemolytic *Streptococcus*. Pediatrics 54:643–644, 1974.

627. Armstrong JH, Zacarias F, Rein MF. Ophthalmia neonatorum: a chart review. Pediatrics 57:884–892, 1976.

628. Greene GR, Carroll WL, Morozumi PA, et al. Endophthalmitis associated with group B streptococcal meningitis in an infant. Am J Dis Child 133:752, 1979.

629. Berger BB. Endophthalmitis complicating group B streptococcal septicemia. Am J Ophthalmol 92:681–684, 1981.

630. Lipson A, Kronick JB, Tewfik L, et al. Group B streptococcal supraglottitis in a 3-month-old infant. Am J Dis Child 140:411–412, 1986.

631. LeBovar Y, Trung PH, Mozziconacci P. Neonatal meningitis due to group B streptococci. Ann Pediatr 17:207–213, 1970.

632. Sokal MM, Nagaraj A, Fisher BJ, et al. Neonatal empyema caused by group B beta-hemolytic *Streptococcus*. Chest 81:390–391, 1982.

633. Park JW. Bacterial tracheitis caused by *Streptococcus agalactiae*. Pediatr Infect Dis J 9:450–451, 1990.

634. Nelson JD. Bilateral breast abscess due to group B *Streptococcus*. Am J Dis Child 130:567, 1976.

635. Rench MA, Baker CJ. Group B streptococcal breast abscess in a mother and mastitis in her infant. Obstet Gynecol 73:875–877, 1989.

636. Brian MJ, O'Ryan M, Waagner D. Prepatellar bursitis in an infant caused by group B *Streptococcus*. Pediatr Infect Dis J 11:502–503, 1992.

637. Ruiz-Gomez D, Tarpay MM, Riley HD. Recurrent group B streptococcal infections: report of three cases. Scand J Infect Dis 11:35–38, 1979.

638. Amoury RA, Barth GW, Hall RT, et al. Scrotal ecchymosis: sign of intraperitoneal hemorrhage in the newborn. South Med J 75:1471–1478, 1982.

639. Ramamurthy RS, Srinivasan G, Jacobs NM. Necrotizing fasciitis and necrotizing cellulitis due to group B *Streptococcus*. Am J Dis Child 131:1169–1170, 1977.

640. Goldberg GN, Hansen RC, Lynch PJ. Necrotizing fasciitis in infancy: report of three cases and review of the literature. Pediatr Dermatol 2:55–63, 1984.

641. Lopez JB, Gross P, Boggs TR. Skin lesions in association with β-hemolytic *Streptococcus* group B. Pediatrics 58:859–860, 1976.

642. Belgaumkar TK. Impetigo neonatorum congenita due to group B beta-hemolytic *Streptococcus* infection. J Pediatr 86:982–983, 1975.

643. Isaacman SH, Heroman WM, Lightsey AL. Purpura fulminans following late-onset group B beta-hemolytic streptococcal sepsis. Am J Dis Child 138:915–916, 1984.

644. Lynn NJ, Pauly TH, Desai NS. Purpura fulminans in three cases of early-onset neonatal group B streptococcal meningitis. J Perinatol 11:144–146, 1991.

645. Turner MC, Naumburg EG. Acute renal failure in the neonate: two fatal cases due to group B streptococci with rhabdomyolysis. Clin Pediatr 26:189–190, 1987.

646. Feder AM Jr, MacLean WC, Moxon R. Scalp abscess secondary to fetal scalp electrode. J Pediatr 89:808–809, 1976.

647. Handrick VW, Spencker F-B, Künzel R. Über eine Kopfschwarteninfektion durch B-streptokokken bei einem Neugeborenen nach interner Kardiotokographie. Zentralbl Gynaekol 106:1544–1546, 1984.

648. Wiswell TE, Miller JA. Infections of congenital cervical neck masses associated with bacteremia. J Pediatr Surg 21:173–174, 1986.

649. Frieden IJ. Blistering dactylitis caused by group B streptococci. Pediatr Dermatol 6:300–302, 1989.

650. St. Laurent-Gagnon T, Weber ML. Urinary tract *Streptococcus* group B infection in a 6-week-old infant. JAMA 240:1269, 1978.

651. Callanan DL, Harris GG. Group B streptococcal infection in children with liver disease. Clin Pediatr 21:99–100, 1982.

652. Dorand RD, Adams G. Relapse during penicillin treatment of group B streptococcal meningitis. J Pediatr 89:188–190, 1976.

653. Kenny JD. Right-sided diaphragmatic hernia of delayed onset in the newborn infant. South Med J 70:373–375, 1977.

654. Banagale RC, Watters JH. Delayed right-sided diaphragmatic hernia following group B streptococcal infection: a discussion of its pathogenesis, with a review of the literature. Hum Pathol 14:67–69, 1983.

655. Ashcraft KW, Holder TM, Amoury RA, et al. Diagnosis and treatment of right Bochdalek hernia associated with group B streptococcal pneumonia and sepsis in the neonate. J Pediatr Surg 18:480–485, 1983.

656. Suresh BR, Rios A, Brion LP, et al. Delayed onset right-sided diaphragmatic hernia secondary to group B streptococcal infection. Pediatr Infect Dis J 10:166–168, 1991.

657. Nudelman R, Bral M, Sakhai Y, et al. Violaceous cellulitis. Pediatrics 70:157–158, 1982.

658. Barton LL, Kapoor NK. Recurrent group B streptococcal infection. Clin Pediatr 21:100–101, 1982.

659. Broughton DD, Mitchell WG, Grossman M, et al. Recurrence of group B streptococcal infection. J Pediatr 89:183–185, 1976.

660. Walker SH, Santos AQ, Quintero BA. Recurrence of group B III streptococcal meningitis. J Pediatr 89:187–188, 1976.

661. Kenny JF, Zedd AJ. Recurrent group B streptococcal disease in an infant associated with the ingestion of infected mother's milk. J Pediatr 91:158–159, 1977.

662. McCrory JH, Au-Yeung YB, Sugg VM, et al. Recurrent group B streptococcal infection in an infant: ventriculitis complicating type Ib meningitis. J Pediatr 92:231–233, 1978.

663. Truog WE, Davis RF, Ray CG. Recurrence of group B streptococcal infection. J Pediatr 89:185–186, 1976.

664. Green PA, Singh KV, Murray BE, et al. Recurrent group B streptococcal infections in infants: clinical and microbiologic aspects. J Pediatr 125:931-938, 1994.

665. Atkins JT, Heresi GP, Coque TM, et al. Recurrent group B streptococcal disease in infants: who should receive rifampin? J Pediatr 132:537–539, 1998.

666. Simón JL, Bosch J, Puig A, et al. Two relapses of group B streptococcal sepsis and transient hypogammaglobulinemia. Pediatr Infect Dis J 8:729–730, 1989.

667. Denning DW, Bressack M, Troup NJ, et al. Infant with two relapses of group B streptococcal sepsis documented by DNA restriction enzyme analysis. Pediatr Infect Dis J 7:729–732, 1988.

668. Kim KS, Anthony BF. Penicillin tolerance in group B streptococci isolated from infected neonates. J Infect Dis 144:411–419, 1981.

669. Rantz LA, Keefer CS. The distribution of hemolytic streptococci groups A, B, and C in human infections. JAMA 111:128–132, 1928.

670. Ramsay AM, Gillespie M. Puerperal infection associated with haemolytic streptococci other than Lancefield's group A. J Obstet Gynaecol Br Emp 48:569–585, 1941.

671. Reinarz JA, Sanford JP. Human infections caused by non–group A or D streptococci. Medicine 44:81–96, 1965.

672. Aharoni A, Potasman I, Levitan Z, et al. Postpartum maternal group B streptococcal meningitis. Rev Infect Dis 12:273–276, 1990.

673. Sexton DJ, Rockson SG, Hempling RE, et al. Pregnancy-associated group B streptococcal endocarditis: a report of two fatal cases. Obstet Gynecol 66:44S–47S, 1985.

674. Backes RJ, Wilson WR, Geraci JE. Group B streptococcal infective endocarditis. Arch Intern Med 145:693–696, 1985.

675. Seaworth BJ, Durack DT. Infective endocarditis in obstetric and gynecologic practice. Am J Obstet Gynecol 154:180–188, 1986.

676. Vartian CV, Septimus EJ. Tricuspid valve group B streptococcal endocarditis following elective abortion. Rev Infect Dis 13:997–998, 1991.

677. Lischke JH, McCreight PHB. Maternal group B streptococcal vertebral osteomyelitis: an unusual complication of vaginal delivery. Obstet Gynecol 76:489–491, 1990.

678. Jenkin G, Woolley IJ, Brown GV, et al. Postpartum epidural abscess due to group B Streptococcus. Clin Infect Dis 25:1249, 1997.

679. Sutton GP, Smirz LR, Clark DH, et al. Group B streptococcal necrotizing fasciitis arising from an episiotomy. Obstet Gynecol 66:733–736, 1985.

680. Wood EG, Dillon HC. A prospective study of group B streptococcal bacteriuria in pregnancy. Am J Obstet Gynecol 140:515–520, 1981.

681. McFadyen IR, Eykyn SJ, Gardner NHN, et al. Bacteriuria in pregnancy. J Obstet Gynaecol Br Commonw 80:385–405, 1973.

682. Mead PJ, Harris RE. The incidence of group B beta hemolytic Streptococcus in antepartum urinary tract infections. Obstet Gynecol 51:412–414, 1978.

683. Daugaard HO, Thomsen AC, Henriques U, et al. Group B streptococci in the lower urogenital tract and late abortions. Am J Obstet Gynecol 158:28–31, 1988.

684. Wiswell TE, Baumgart S, Gannon CM, et al. No lumbar puncture in the evaluation for early neonatal sepsis: will meningitis be missed? Pediatrics 95:803–806, 1995.

685. Baker CJ. Unpublished observations.

686. Edwards MS, Baker CJ. Prospective diagnosis of early onset group B streptococcal infection by countercurrent immunoelectrophoresis. J Pediatr 94:286–288, 1979.

687. Bortolussi R, Wort AJ, Casey S. The latex agglutination test versus counterimmunoelectrophoresis for rapid diagnosis of bacterial meningitis. Can Med Assoc J 127:489–493, 1982.

688. Wasilauskas BL, Hampton KD. Determination of bacterial meningitis: a retrospective study of 80 cerebrospinal fluid specimens evaluated by four in vitro methods. J Clin Microbiol 16:531–535, 1982.

689. Hamoudi AC, Marcon MJ, Cannon HJ, et al. Comparison of three major antigen detection methods for the diagnosis of group B streptococcal sepsis in neonates. Pediatr Infect Dis J 2:432–435, 1983.

690. Rench MA, Metzger TG, Baker CJ. Detection of group B streptococcal antigen in body fluids by a latex-coupled monoclonal antibody assay. J Clin Microbiol 20:852–854, 1984.

691. Baker CJ, Rench MA. Commercial latex agglutination for detection of group B streptococcal antigen in body fluids. J Pediatr 102:393–395, 1983.

692. Jacobs RF, Yamauchi T, Eisenach KD. Detection of streptococcal antigen by counterimmunoelectrophoresis. Am J Clin Pathol 75:203–208, 1981.

693. Typlin BL, Koranyi K, Azimi P, et al. Counterimmunoelectrophoresis for the rapid diagnosis of group B streptococcal infections. Clin Pediatr 18:366–369, 1979.

694. Edwards MS, Kasper DL, Baker CJ. Rapid diagnosis of type III group B streptococcal meningitis by latex particle agglutination. J Pediatr 95:202–205, 1979.

695. Webb BJ, Baker CJ. Commercial latex agglutination test for rapid diagnosis of group B streptococcal infection in infants. J Clin Microbiol 12:442–444, 1980.

696. Bausch LC, Ecklund SS. Neonatal group B streptococcal septicemia. Nebr Med J 70:110–113, 1985.

697. Rabalais GP, Bronfin DR, Daum RS. Evaluation of a commercially available latex agglutination test for rapid diagnosis of group B streptococcal infection. Pediatr Infect Dis J 6:177–181, 1987.

698. Ingram DL, Suggs DM, Pearson AW. Detection of group B streptococcal antigen in early-onset and late-onset group B streptococcal disease with the Wellcogen Strep B Latex Agglutination Test. J Clin Microbiol 16:656–658, 1982.

699. Friedman CA, Wender DF, Rawson JE. Rapid diagnosis of group B streptococcal infection utilizing a commercially available latex agglutination assay. Pediatrics 73:27–30, 1984.

700. Kumar A, Nankervis GA. Latex agglutination test and countercurrent immunoelectrophoresis for detection of group B streptococcal antigen. J Pediatr 97:328–329, 1980.

701. Webb BJ, Edwards MS, Baker CJ. Comparison of slide coagglutination test and countercurrent immunoelectrophoresis for detection of group B streptococcal antigen in cerebrospinal fluid from infants with meningitis. J Clin Microbiol 11:263–265, 1980.

702. Drow DL, Welch DF, Hensel D, et al. Evaluation of the Phadebact CSF Test for detection of the four most common causes of bacterial meningitis. J Clin Microbiol 18:1358–1361, 1983.

703. Morrow DL, Kline JB, Douglas SD, et al. Rapid detection of group B streptococcal antigen by monoclonal

antibody sandwich enzyme assay. J Clin Microbiol 19:457–459, 1984.

704. FDA Alert. Safety alert re risk of misdiagnosis of group B streptococcal infection. JAMA 277:1343, 1997.

705. Rajani KB, Goetzman BW, Wennberg RP. Early diagnosis of group B streptococcal pneumonia using tracheal aspirates. Pediatrics 61:329, 1978.

706. Lewins MJ. The gastric aspirate shake test and group B streptococcal disease. N Engl J Med 298:1200, 1978.

707. Philip AGS. Response of C-reactive protein in neonatal group B streptococcal infection. Pediatr Infect Dis J 4:145–148, 1985.

708. Sabel K-G, Wadsworth C. C-reactive protein (CRP) in early diagnosis of neonatal septicemia. Acta Paediatr Scand 68:825–831, 1979.

709. Manroe BL, Rosenfeld CR, Weinberg AG, et al. The differential leukocyte count in the assessment and outcome of early-onset neonatal group B streptococcal disease. J Pediatr 91:632–637, 1977.

710. Menke JA, Giacoia GP, Jockin H. Group B beta hemolytic streptococcal sepsis and the idiopathic respiratory distress syndrome: a comparison. J Pediatr 94:467–471, 1979.

711. Manroe BL, Weinberg AG, Rosenfeld CR, et al. The neonatal blood count in health and disease: I. Reference values for neutrophilic cells. J Pediatr 95:89–98, 1979.

712. Greenberg DN, Yoder BA. Changes in the differential white blood cell count in screening for group B streptococcal sepsis. Pediatr Infect Dis J 9:886–889, 1990.

713. Christensen RD, Rothstein G, Hill HR, et al. Fatal early onset group B streptococcal sepsis with normal leukocyte counts. Pediatr Infect Dis J 4:242–245, 1985.

714. Baker CJ, Webb BJ, Barrett FF. Antimicrobial susceptibility of group B streptococci isolated from a variety of clinical sources. Antimicrob Agents Chemother 10:128–131, 1976.

715. Berkowitz K, Regan JA, Greenberg E. Antibiotic resistance patterns of group B streptococci in pregnant women. J Clin Microbiol 28:5–7, 1990.

716. Fernandez M, Hickman ME, Baker CJ. Antimicrobial susceptibilies of group B streptococci isolated between 1992 and 1996 from patients with bacteremia or meningitis. Antimicrob Agents Chemother 42:1517–1519, 1998.

717. Meyn LA, Hillier SL. Ampicillin susceptibilities of vaginal and placental isolates of group B Streptococcus and Escherichia coli obtained between 1992 and 1994. Antimicrob Agents Chemother 41:1173–1174, 1997.

718. Bayer AS, Morrison JO, Kim K-S. Comparative in vitro bactericidal activity of cefonicid, ceftizoxime, and penicillin against group B streptococci. Antimicrob Agents Chemother 21:344–346, 1982.

719. Jacobs MR, Kelly F, Speck WT. Susceptibility of group B streptococci to 16 β-lactam antibiotics, including new penicillin and cephalosporin derivatives. Antimicrob Agents Chemother 22:897–900, 1982.

720. Kim KS. Antimicrobial susceptibility of GBS. Antibiot Chemother 35:83–89, 1985.

721. Mulder C, Bol P, Nabbe A, et al. Susceptibility to six antibiotics of group B streptococci isolated from cerebrospinal fluid. Scand J Infect Dis 17:191–193, 1985.

722. Persson KM-S, Forsgren A. Antimicrobial susceptibility of group B streptococci. Eur J Clin Microbiol 5:165–167, 1986.

723. Rolston KVI. Susceptibility of group B and group G streptococci to newer antimicrobial agents. Eur J Clin Microbiol 5:534–536, 1986.

724. Baker CN, Thornsberry C, Facklam RR. Synergism kill-ing kinetics, and antimicrobial susceptibility of group A and B streptococci. Antimicrob Agents Chemother 19:716–725, 1981.

725. Jones WF, Feldman HA, Finland M. Susceptibility of hemolytic streptococci, other than those of group D, to eleven antibiotics in vitro. Am J Clin Pathol 27:159–169, 1957.

726. Landesman SH, Corrado ML, Cherubin CE, et al. Activity of moxalactam and cefotaxime alone and in combination with ampicillin or penicillin against group B streptococci. Antimicrob Agents Chemother 19:794–797, 1981.

727. Delaplane D, Yogev R, Shulman ST. Ceftriaxone therapy of group B streptococcal bacteraemia and meningitis in infant rats. J Antimicrob Chemother 11:69–73, 1983.

728. Liberto MC, Carbone M, Fera MT, et al. Cefixime shows good effects on group A and group B β-hemolytic streptococci. Drugs Exp Clin Res 17:305–308, 1991.

729. Sheppard M, King A, Phillips I. In vitro activity of cefpodoxime, a new oral cephalosporin, compared with that of nine other antimicrobial agents. Eur J Clin Microbiol Infect Dis 10:573–581, 1991.

730. Kim KS, Kang JH, Bayer AS. Efficacy of teicoplanin in experimental group B streptococcal bacteremia and meningitis. Chemotherapy 33:177–182, 1987.

731. Kropp H, Gerckens L, Sundelof JG. Antibacterial activity of imipenem: the first thienamycin antibiotic. Rev Infect Dis 7:S389–S410, 1985.

732. Kim KS. Efficacy of imipenem in experimental group B streptococcal bacteremia and meningitis. Chemotherapy 31:304–309, 1985.

733. Pearlman MD, Pierson CL, Faix RG. Frequent resistance of clinical group B streptococci isolates to clindamycin and erythromycin. Obstet Gynecol 92:258–261, 1998.

734. Rouse DJ, Andrews WW, Lin F-YC, et al. Antibiotic susceptibility profile of group B Streptococcus acquired vertically. Obstet Gynecol 92:931–934, 1998.

735. Borderon JC, Borderon E, Geslin P, et al. Sensibilité aux antibiotiques des streptocoques du groupe B. Pathol Biol 32:35–39, 1984.

736. Schauf V, Deveikis A, Riff L, et al. Antibiotic-killing kinetics of group B streptococci. J Pediatr 89:194–198, 1976.

737. Deveikis A, Schauf V, Mizen M, et al. Antimicrobial therapy of experimental group B streptococcal infection in mice. Antimicrob Agents Chemother 11:817–820, 1977.

738. Cooper MD, Keeney RE, Lyons SF, et al. Synergistic effects of ampicillin-aminoglycoside combinations on group B streptococci. Antimicrob Agents Chemother 15:484–486, 1979.

739. Overturf GD, Horowitz M, Wilkins J, et al. Bactericidal studies of penicillin-gentamicin combinations against group B streptococci. J Antibiot 30:513–518, 1977.

740. Swingle HM, Bucciarelli RL, Ayoub EM. Synergy between penicillins and low concentrations of gentamicin in the killing of group B streptococci. J Infect Dis 152:515–520, 1985.

741. Scheld WM, Alliegro GM, Field MR, et al. Synergy between ampicillin and gentamicin in experimental meningitis due to group B streptococci. J Infect Dis 146:100, 1982.

742. Backes RJ, Rouse MS, Henry NK, et al. Activity of penicillin combined with an aminoglycoside against group B streptococci in vitro and in experimental endocarditis. J Antimicrob Chemother 18:491–498, 1986.

743. Kim KS. Effect of antimicrobial therapy for experimental

infections due to group B *Streptococcus* on mortality and clearance of bacteria. J Infect Dis 155:1233–1241, 1987.

744. Weeks JL, Mason EO Jr, Baker CJ. Antagonism of ampicillin and chloramphenicol for meningeal isolates of group B streptococci. Antimicrob Agents Chemother 20:281–285, 1981.

745. Smith SM, Eng RHK, Landesman S. Effect of rifampin on ampicillin killing of group B streptococci. Antimicrob Agents Chemother 22:522–524, 1982.

746. Maduri-Traczewski M, Szymczak EG, Goldmann DA. In vitro activity of penicillin and rifampin against group B streptococci. Rev Infect Dis 5:S586–S592, 1983.

747. Hall MA, Ducker DA, Lowes JA, et al. A randomized prospective comparison of cefotaxime versus netilmicin/penicillin for treatment of suspected neonatal sepsis. Drugs 35(Suppl 2):169–188, 1988.

748. Bradley JS, Ching DLK, Wilson TA, et al. Once-daily ceftriaxone to complete therapy of uncomplicated group B streptococcal infection in neonates. Clin Pediatr 31:274–278, 1992.

749. Kim KS. Effect of antimicrobial therapy for experimental infections due to group B *Streptococcus* on mortality and clearance of bacteria. J Infect Dis 155:1233–1241, 1987.

750. Feldman WE. Concentrations of bacteria in cerebrospinal fluid of patients with bacterial meningitis. J Pediatr 88:549–552, 1976.

751. Fujita K, Yoshioka H. Relevance of concentration of pathogenic bacteria in cerebrospinal fluid to antibiotic therapy. J Pediatr 90:328–329, 1977.

752. Hieber JP, Nelson JD. A pharmacologic evaluation of penicillin in children with purulent meningitis. N Engl J Med 297:410–413, 1977.

753. Kim KS, Anthony BF. Penicillin tolerance in group B streptococci isolated from infected neonates. J Infect Dis 144:411–419, 1981.

754. Kim KS, Yoshimori RN, Imagawa DT, et al. Importance of medium in demonstrating penicillin tolerance by group B streptococci. Antimicrob Agents Chemother 16:214–216, 1979.

755. Kim KS. Clinical perspectives on penicillin tolerance. J Pediatr 112:509–514, 1988.

756. Steinbrecher UP. Serious infection in an adult due to penicillin-tolerant group B streptococcus. Arch Intern Med 141:1714–1715, 1981.

757. McCracken GH Jr, Feldman WE. Editorial comment. J Pediatr 89:203–204, 1976.

758. McCracken GH Jr. Group B streptococci: the new challenge in neonatal infections. J Pediatr 82:703–706, 1973.

759. Baker CJ. Antibiotic susceptibility testing in the management of an infant with group B streptococcal meningitis. Pediatr Infect Dis J 6:1073–1074, 1987.

760. Wilson WR. Antimicrobial therapy of streptococcal endocarditis. J Antimicrob Chemother 20(Suppl A):147–159, 1987.

761. Fernandez M, Albanyan EA, Rench MA, et al. Failure of rifampin to eradicate group B streptococcal (GBS) colonization in infants with invasive disease. Program and Abstracts of the 36th Annual Meeting of the Infectious Diseases Society of America, Abstract No. 41, 1998, p 82.

762. Hocker JR, Simpson PM, Rabalais GP, et al. Extracorporeal membrane oxygenation and early-onset group B streptococcal sepsis. Pediatrics 89:1–4, 1992.

763. LeBlanc MH. ECMO and sepsis. Pediatrics 90:127, 1992.

764. Truog WE, Gibson RL, Juul SE, et al. Neonatal group B streptococcal sepsis: effects of late treatment with dazmegrel. Pediatr Res 23:352–356, 1988.

765. Goldberg RN, Suguihara C, Streitfeld MM, et al. Effects of a leukotriene antagonist on the early hemodynamic manifestations of group B streptococcal sepsis in piglets. Pediatr Res 20:1004–1008, 1986.

766. Philips JB, Lyrene RK, Godoy G, et al. Hemodynamic responses of chronically instrumented piglets to bolus infections of group B streptococci. Pediatr Res 23:81–85, 1988.

767. Christensen RD, Shigeoka AO, Hill HR, et al. Circulating and storage neutrophil change in experimental type II group B streptococcal sepsis. Pediatr Res 14:806–808, 1980.

768. Santos JI, Shigeoka AO, Hill HR. Functional leukocyte administration in protection against experimental neonatal infection. Pediatr Res 14:1408–1410, 1980.

769. Hill HR. Phagocyte transfusion—ultimate therapy of neonatal disease? J Pediatr 98:59–61, 1981.

770. Christensen RD, Rothstein G, Anstall HB, et al. Granulocyte transfusions in neonates with bacterial infection, neutropenia, and depletion of mature marrow neutrophils. Pediatrics 70:1–6, 1982.

771. Givner LB, Baker CJ. The prevention and treatment of neonatal group B streptococcal infections. Adv Pediatr Infect Dis 3:65–90, 1988.

772. Cairo MS, Mauss D, Kommareddy S, et al. Prophylactic or simultaneous administration of recombinant human granulocyte colony stimulating factor in the treatment of group B streptococcal sepsis in neonatal rats. Pediatr Res 27:612–616, 1990.

773. Cairo MS, Plunkett JM, Nguyen A, et al. Effect of stem cell factor with and without granulocyte colony-stimulating factor on neonatal hematopoiesis: in vivo induction of newborn myelopoiesis and reduction of mortality during experimental group B streptococcal sepsis. Blood 80:96–101, 1992.

774. Iguchi K, Inoue S, Kumar A. Effect of recombinant human granulocyte colony-stimulating factor administration in normal and experimentally infected newborn rats. Exp Hematol 19:352–358, 1991.

775. Wheeler JG, Givner LB. Therapeutic use of recombinant human granulocyte-macrophage colony-stimulating factor in neonatal rats with type III group B streptococcal sepsis. J Infect Dis 165:938–941, 1992.

776. Yoder MC, Polin RB. Immunotherapy of neonatal septicemia. Pediatr Clin North Am 33:481–501, 1986.

777. Hill HR, Shigeoka AO, Pincus S, et al. Intravenous IgG in combination with other modalities in the treatment of neonatal infection. Pediatr Infect Dis J 5(Suppl):S180–S184, 1986.

778. Miller PS, Schauf V, Salo RJ. Enhanced killing of group B streptococci in vitro by penicillin and opsonophagocytosis with intravenous immunoglobulin. J Infect Dis 161:1225–1230, 1990.

779. Givner LB. Human immunoglobulins for intravenous use: comparison of available preparations for group B streptococcal antibody levels, opsonic activity, and efficacy in animal models. Pediatrics 86:955–962, 1990.

780. Weisman LE, Lorenzetti PM. High intravenous doses of human immune globulin suppress neonatal group B streptococcal immunity in rats. J Pediatr 115:445–450, 1989.

781. Kim KS. Efficacy of human immunoglobulin and penicillin G in treatment of experimental group B streptococcal infection. Pediatr Res 21:289–292, 1987.

782. Givner LB, Baker CJ. Pooled human IgG hyperimmune for type III group B streptococci: evaluation against multiple strains in vitro and in experimental disease. J Infect Dis 163:1141–1145, 1991.

783. Fischer GW, Hemming VG, Gloser HP, et al. Polyvalent group B streptococcal immune globulin for intravenous administration: overview. Rev Infect Dis 12(Suppl 4):S483–S491, 1990.

784. Kim KS. High-dose intravenous immune globulin impairs antibacterial activity of antibiotics. J Allergy Clin Immunol 84:579–588, 1989.

785. Baker CJ, Noya FJD. Potential use of intravenous immune globulin for group B streptococcal infection. Rev Infect Dis 12(Suppl 4):S476–S482, 1990.

786. Redd H, Christensen RD, Fischer GW. Circulating and storage neutrophils in septic neonatal rats treated with immune globulin. J Infect Dis 157:705–712, 1988.

787. Christensen KK, Christensen P. Intravenous gammaglobulin in the treatment of neonatal sepsis with special reference to group B streptococci and pharmacokinetics. Pediatr Infect Dis J 5(Suppl):S189–S192, 1986.

788. Christensen KK, Christensen P, Bucher HU, et al. Intravenous administration of human IgG to newborn infants: changes in serum antibody levels to group B streptococci. Eur J Pediatr 143:123–127, 1984.

789. van Furth R, Leijh PCJ, Klein F. Correlation between opsonic activity for various microorganisms and composition of gammaglobulin preparations for intravenous use. J Infect Dis 149:511–517, 1984.

790. Kim KS, Wass CA, Kang JH, et al. Functional activities of various preparations of human intravenous immunoglobulin against type III group B Streptococcus. J Infect Dis 153:1092–1097, 1986.

791. Gloser H, Bachmayer H, Helm A. Intravenous immunoglobulin with high activity against group B streptococci. Pediatr Infect Dis J 5(Suppl):S176–S179, 1986.

792. Linden V, Christensen KK, Christensen P. Low levels of antibodies to surface antigens of group B streptococci in commercial IgG preparation. Int Arch Allergy Appl Immunol 68:193–195, 1982.

793. Fischer GW, Hemming VG, Hunter KW, et al. Intravenous immunoglobulin in the treatment of neonatal sepsis: therapeutic strategies and laboratory studies. Pediatr Infect Dis J 5(Suppl):S171–S175, 1986.

794. Santos JI, Shigeoka AO, Rote NS, et al. Protective efficacy of a modified immune serum globulin in experimental group B streptococcal infection. J Pediatr 99:873–879, 1981.

795. Noya FJD, Rench MA, Garcia-Prats JA, et al. Disposition of an immunoglobulin intravenous preparation in very low birth weight neonates. J Pediatr 112:278–283, 1988.

796. Raff HV, Siscoe PJ, Wolff EA, et al. Human monoclonal antibodies to group B Streptococcus: reactivity and in vivo protection against multiple serotypes. J Exp Med 168:905–917, 1988.

797. Raff HV, Shuford W, Wolff E, et al. Pharmacokinetic and pharmacodynamic analysis of a human immunoglobulin M monoclonal antibody in neonatal Macaca fascicularis. Pediatr Res 29:310–314, 1991.

798. Hill HR, Gonzales LA, Knappe WA, et al. Comparative protective activity of human monoclonal and hyperimmune polyclonal antibody against group B streptococci. J Infect Dis 163:792–798, 1991.

799. Christensen RD, Brown MS, Hall DC, et al. Effect on neutrophil kinetics and serum opsonic capacity of intravenous administration of immune globulin to neonates with clinical signs of early-onset sepsis. J Pediatr 118:606–614, 1991.

800. Baker CJ. Immunization to prevent group B streptococcal disease: victories and vexations. J Infect Dis 161:917–921, 1990.

801. Gordon JS, Sbara AJ. Incidence, technique of isolation, and treatment of group B streptococci in obstetric patients. Am J Obstet Gynecol 126:1023–1026, 1976.

802. Hall RT, Barnes W, Krishnan L, et al. Antibiotic treatment of parturient women colonized with group B streptococci. Am J Obstet Gynecol 124:630–634, 1976.

803. Lewin EB, Amstey MS. Natural history of group B Streptococcus colonization and its therapy during pregnancy. Am J Obstet Gynecol 139:512–515, 1981.

804. Yow MD, Mason EO, Leeds LJ, et al. Ampicillin prevents intrapartum transmission of group B Streptococcus. JAMA 241:1245–1247, 1979.

805. Morales WJ, Lim DV, Walsh AF. Prevention of neonatal group B streptococcal sepsis by the use of a rapid screening test and selective intrapartum chemoprophylaxis. Am J Obstet Gynecol 155:979–983, 1986.

806. Boyer KM, Gadzala CA, Kelly PD, et al. Selective intrapartum chemoprophylaxis of neonatal group B streptococcal early-onset disease: III. Interruption of mother-to-infant transmission. J Infect Dis 148:810–816, 1983.

807. Boyer KM, Gotoff SP. Prevention of early-onset neonatal group B streptococcal disease with selective intrapartum chemoprophylaxis. N Engl J Med 314:1665–1669, 1986.

808. Matorras R, García-Perea A, Madero R, et al. Maternal colonization by group B streptococci and puerperal infection; analysis of intrapartum chemoprophylaxis. Eur J Obstet Gynecol Reprod Biol 38:203–207, 1990.

809. Garland SM, Fliegner JR. Group B Streptococcus (GBS) and neonatal infections: the case for intrapartum chemoprophylaxis. Aust NZ J Obstet Gynaecol 31:119–122, 1991.

810. Tuppurainen N, Hallman M. Prevention of neonatal group B streptococcal disease: intrapartum detection and chemoprophylaxis of heavily colonized parturients. Obstet Gynecol 73:583–587, 1989.

811. Morales WJ, Lim D. Reduction of group B streptococcal maternal and neonatal infections in preterm pregnancies with premature rupture of membranes through a rapid identification test. Am J Obstet Gynecol 157:13–16, 1987.

812. Strickland DM, Yeomans ER, Hankins GDV. Cost-effectiveness of intrapartum screening and treatment for maternal group B streptococci colonization. Am J Obstet Gynecol 163:4–8, 1990.

813. Mohle-Boetani JC, Schuchat A, Plikaytis BD, et al. Comparison of prevention strategies for neonatal group B streptococcal infection: an economic analysis. JAMA 270:1442–1448, 1993.

814. Rouse DJ, Goldenberg RL, Cliver SP, et al. Strategies for the prevention of early-onset neonatal group B streptococcal sepsis: a decision analysis. Obstet Gynecol 83:483–494, 1994.

815. Yancey MK, Duff P. An analysis of the cost-effectiveness of selected protocols for the prevention of neonatal group B streptococcal infection. Obstet Gynecol 83:367–371, 1994.

816. Committee to Study Priorities for Vaccine Development, Division of Health Promotion and Disease Prevention, Institute of Medicine. Stratton KR, Durch JS, Lawrence RS (eds). Vaccines for the 21st Century: A Tool for Decision Making. Washington, DC, National Academy of Sciences, 1999.

817. Kontnick CM, Edberg SC. Direct detection of group B streptococci from vaginal specimens compared with quantitative culture. J Clin Microbiol 28:336–339, 1990.

818. Skoll MA, Mercer BM, Baselski V, et al. Evaluation of two rapid group B streptococcal antigen tests in labor and delivery patients. Obstet Gynecol 77:322–326, 1991.

819. Green M, Dashefsky B, Wald ER, et al. Comparison of two antigen assays for rapid intrapartum detection of vaginal group B streptococcal colonization. J Clin Microbiol 31:78–82, 1993.

820. Towers CV, Garite TJ, Friedman WW, et al. Comparison of a rapid enzyme-linked immunosorbent assay test and the Gram stain for detection of group B *Streptococcus* in high-risk antepartum patients. Am J Obstet Gynecol 163:965–967, 1990.

821. Granato PA, Petosa MT. Evaluation of a rapid screening test for detecting group B streptococci in pregnant women. J Clin Microbiol 29:1536–1538, 1991.

822. Gentry YM, Hillier SL, Eschenbach DA. Evaluation of a rapid enzyme immunoassay test for detection of group B *Streptococcus*. Obstet Gynecol 78:397–401, 1991.

823. Baker CJ. Inadequacy of rapid immunoassays for intrapartum detection of group B streptococcal carriers. Obstet Gynecol 88:51–55, 1996.

824. Carroll KC, Ballou D, Varner M, et al. Rapid detection of group B streptococcal colonization of the genital tract by a commercial optical immunoassay. Eur J Clin Microbiol Infect Dis 15:206–210, 1996.

825. Park CH, Ruprai D, Vandel NM, et al. Rapid detection of group B streptococcal antigen from vaginal specimens using a new optical immunoassay technique. Diagn Microbiol Infect Dis 24:125–128, 1996.

826. Rosa C, Clark P, Duff P. Performance of a new DNA probe for the detection of group B streptococcal colonization of the genital tract. Obstet Gynecol 86:509–511, 1995.

827. Kircher SM, Meyer MP, Jordan JA. Comparison of a modified DNA hybridization assay with standard culture enrichment for detecting group B streptococci in obstetric patients. J Clin Microbiol 34:342–344, 1996.

828. Thomsen AC, Mørup L, Hansen KB. Antibiotic elimination of group-B streptococci in urine in prevention of preterm labour. Lancet 1:591–593, 1987.

829. Bray RE, Boe RW, Johnson WL. Transfer of ampicillin into fetus and amniotic fluid from maternal plasma in late pregnancy. Am J Obstet Gynecol 96:938–942, 1966.

830. Hirsch HA, Dreher E, Perrochet A, et al. Transfer of ampicillin to the fetus and amniotic fluid during continuous infusion (steady state) and by repeated single intravenous injections to the mother. Infection 2:207–212, 1974.

831. de Cueto M, Sanchez MJ, Sampedro A, et al. Timing of intrapartum ampicillin and prevention of vertical transmission of group B *Streptococcus*. Obstet Gynecol 91:112–114, 1998.

832. Group B streptococcal infections in pregnancy. ACOG Tech Bull 170:1–5, 1992.

833. Christensen KK, Dahlander K, Linden V, et al. Obstetrical care in future pregnancies after fetal loss in group B streptococcal septicemia: a prevention program based on bacteriological and immunological follow up. Eur J Obstet Gynecol Reprod Biol 12:143–147, 1981.

834. Dykes AK, Christensen KK, Christensen P. Chronic carrier state in mothers of infants with group B streptococcal infections. Obstet Gynecol 66:84–88, 1985.

835. Mercer BM, Taylor MC, Fricke JL, et al. The accuracy and patient preference for self-collected group B *Streptococcus* cultures. Am J Obstet Gynecol 173:1325–1328, 1995.

836. Taylor MC, Mercer BM, Engelhardt KF, et al. Patient preference for self-collected cultures for group B *Streptococcus* in pregnancy. J Nurse Midwifery 42:410–413, 1997.

837. Peralta-Carcelen M, Fargason CA Jr, Coston D, et al. Preferences of pregnant women and physicians for two strategies for prevention of early-onset group B strepto-

coccal sepsis in neonates. Arch Pediatr Adolesc Med 151:712–718, 1997.

838. Schuchat A. Group B *Streptococcus*. Lancet 353:51–56, 1999.

839. Mohle-Boetani JC, Lieu TA, Ray GT, et al. Preventing neonatal group B streptococcal disease: cost-effectiveness in a health maintenance organization and the impact of delayed hospital discharge for newborns who received intrapartum antibiotics. Pediatrics 103:703–710, 1999.

840. Steigman AJ, Bottone EJ, Hanna BA. Control of perinatal group B streptococcal sepsis: efficacy of single injection of aqueous penicillin at birth. Mt Sinai J Med 45:685–693, 1978.

841. Hodes HL. Penicillin prophylaxis and neonatal streptococcal disease. Hosp Pract 15:115–125, 1980.

842. Wedgwood JF, Carlin EB, Benjamin BL, et al. Penicillin at birth can help prevent early-onset group B streptococcal disease. Letter to the editor. Pediatrics 99:651, 1997.

843. Pyati SP, Pildes RS, Jacobs NM, et al. Early penicillin in infants ≤2,000 grams with early onset GBS: is it effective? Pediatr Res 16:1019, 1982.

844. Siegel JD, Cushion NB. Prevention of early-onset group B streptococcal disease: another look at single-dose penicillin at birth. Obstet Gynecol 87:692–698, 1996.

845. Moore DH, Schreiner RL. Fatal group B streptococcal septicemia in newborn twins. J Indiana State Med Assoc 69:630–631, 1976.

846. Rubin EE, McDonald JC. Group B streptococcal disease in twins: failure of empiric therapy to prevent late onset disease in the second twin. Pediatr Infect Dis J 10:921–923, 1991.

847. Coleman RT, Sherer DM, Maniscalco WM. Prevention of neonatal group B streptococcal infections: advances in maternal vaccine development. Obstet Gynecol 80:301–309, 1992.

848. Hemming VG, London WT, Fischer GW, et al. Immunoprophylaxis of postnatally acquired group B streptococcal sepsis in neonatal rhesus monkeys. J Infect Dis 156:655–658, 1987.

849. Rodewald AK, Onderdonk AB, Warren HB, et al. Neonatal mouse model of group B streptococcal infection. J Infect Dis 166:635–639, 1992.

850. Paoletti LC, Wessels MR, Michon F, et al. Group B *Streptococcus* type II polysaccharide-tetanus toxoid conjugate vaccine. Infect Immunol 60:4009–4014, 1992.

851. Madoff LC, Michel JL, Gong EW, et al. Protection of neonatal mice from group B streptococcal infection by maternal immunization with beta C protein. Infect Immun 60:4989–4994, 1992.

852. Paoletti LC, Pinel J, Rodewald AK, et al. Therapeutic potential of human antisera to group B streptococcal glycoconjugate vaccines in neonatal mice. J Infect Dis 175:1237–1239, 1997.

853. Baker CJ, Kasper DL. Group B streptococcal vaccines. Rev Infect Dis 7:458–467, 1985.

854. Wessels MR, Paoletti LC, Kasper DL, et al. Immunogenicity in animals of a polysaccharide-protein conjugate vaccine against type III group B *Streptococcus*. J Clin Invest 86:1428–1433, 1990.

855. Jennings H. Further approaches for optimizing polysaccharide-protein conjugate vaccines for prevention of invasive bacterial disease. J Infect Dis 165(Suppl 1):S156–S159, 1992.

856. Paoletti LC, Kennedy RC, Chanh TC, et al. Immunogenicity of group B *Streptococcus* type III polysaccharide-tetanus toxoid vaccine in baboons. Infect Immun 64:677–679, 1996.

857. Wessels MR, Paoletti LC, Pinel J, et al. Immunogenicity and protective activity in animals of a type V group B streptococcal polysaccharide-tetanus toxoid conjugate vaccine. J Infect Dis 171:879–884, 1995.

858. Paoletti LC, Wessels MR, Rodewald AK, et al. Neonatal mouse protection against infection with multiple group B streptococcal (GBS) serotypes by maternal immunization with a tetravalent GBS polysaccharide-tetanus toxoid conjugate vaccine. Infect Immun 62:3236–3243, 1994.

859. Madoff LC, Paoletti LC, Tai JY, et al. Maternal immunization of mice with group B streptococcal type III polysaccharide-beta C protein conjugate elicits protective antibody to multiple serotypes. J Clin Invest 94:286–292, 1994.

860. Kasper DL, Paoletti LC, Wessels MR, et al. Immune response to type III group B streptococcal polysaccharide-tetanus toxoid conjugate vaccine. J Clin Invest 98:2308–2314, 1996.

861. Baker CJ, Paoletti LC, Wessels MR, et al. Safety and immunogenicity of capsular polysaccharide-tetanus toxoid conjugate vaccines for group B streptococcal types Ia and Ib. J Infect Dis 179:142–150, 1999.

862. Paoletti LC, Kasper DL, Michon F, et al. An oligosaccharide-tetanus toxoid conjugate vaccine against type III group B *Streptococcus*. J Biol Chem 265:18278–18283, 1990.

863. Wessels MR, Paoletti LC, Guttormsen H-K, et al. Structural properties of group B streptococcal type III polysaccharide conjugate vaccines that influence immunogenicity and efficacy. Infect Immun 66:2186–2192, 1998.

864. Michel JL, Madoff LC, Kling DE, et al. Cloned alpha and beta C-protein antigens of group B streptococci elicit protective immunity. Infect Immun 59:2023–2028, 1991.

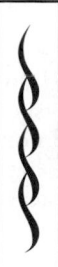

C H A P T E R 2 7

Listeriosis

ROBERT BORTOLUSSI, M.D., and WALTER F. SCHLECH III, M.D.

Listeria monocytogenes is a gram-positive, motile bacterium that is a frequent veterinary pathogen causing abortion and meningoencephalitis in sheep and cattle. Infection in a wide variety of other animals has been described. Infection in humans is uncommon but occurs most frequently in the neonatal period, during pregnancy, and in elderly or immunosuppressed patients. Nyfeldt described "*Listerella hominis*" as the cause of infectious mononucleosis in 1929,[1] but more recent descriptions suggest that human disease parallels that found in animals, with sepsis and meningoencephalitis occurring most commonly.

Murray and co-workers provided the first adequate description of the causative organism in 1926.[2] An epizootic among laboratory rabbits and guinea pigs provided an isolate, subsequently named *Bacterium monocytogenes*, that could produce infection in rabbits and other laboratory animals. The clinical characteristics were of dramatic wasting, lack of appetite, and lethargy leading to death. The greatest incidence and mortality occurred in animals that had recently been weaned. Pirie isolated the organism from South African gerbils and termed it *Listerella hepatolytica*, dedicating it in honor of Lord Lister.[3] Pirie subsequently revised the name to *Listeria monocytogenes*, the currently accepted species name.[4]

THE ORGANISM

Morphology

The morphologic characteristics of *L. monocytogenes* may vary with the age of the culture. In clinical specimens, Gram stain usually demonstrates short intracellular and extracellular gram-positive rods. Over-decolorized direct examinations may lead to a misdiagnosis of *Haemophilus influenzae* meningitis.[5] On primary culture, young cultures demonstrate a slightly pointed coccoid morphology and short chains are occasionally seen. Older cultures may be gram variable.

Motility

All strains of *L. monocytogenes* are motile, distinguishing the organism from *Erysipelothrix* and most species of *Corynebacterium*. Tumbling motility is seen in hanging drop preparations of primary cultures. Organisms show greater motility at room temperature than at 37°C.[6] Electron microscopic studies and protein electrophoresis have demonstrated that *L. monocytogenes* does not express flagellar protein at 37°C.[7]

Culture and Identification

L. monocytogenes grows well in broth cultures, including brain-heart infusion, trypticase soy, and thioglycollate broths. Primary isolation from normally sterile sites can be made on blood agar. Selected media, such as Oxford agar, modified Oxford agar, or other selection agar, should be used when isolation is attempted from contaminated specimens.[8]

Growth occurs between 20°C and 37°C, with fastest growth rates occurring between 30°C and 37°C. A cold enrichment technique may be useful in isolations from contaminated specimens but is unlikely to be useful in the clinical laboratory.[9]

After 48 hours at 37°C on 5% sheep blood, agar colonies reach the size of 0.2 to 1.5 mm in diameter. Narrow zones of beta hemolysis are present, and the colony may have to be moved to confirm hemolysis. *Listeria seeligeri* and *Listeria ivanovii* are also beta-hemolytic organisms but are not human pathogens. Speciation is aided by performance of the CAMP test using *Staphylococcus aureus* for *L. monocytogenes* and *L. seeligeri* and *Rhodococcus equi* for *L. ivanovii*.[10]

Discrimination between *Listeria* species is also aided by sugar fermentation patterns. *L. monocytogenes* produces acid from L-rhamnose and α-methyl-D-mannoside but not from xylose. *L. ivanovii* and *L. seeligeri* produce acid from D-xylose only. Nitrate reduction distinguishes *Listeria murrayi* from other *Listeria* species that cannot produce nitrate.[5]

Antigenic Structure and Typing Systems

Six serovars of *Listeria* have been described and are distinguished on the basis of O and H antigen difference.[11] Serovars 1/2a, 4a, and 4b are the most common isolates from animal and human disease. Other serovars are rarely seen and usually originate from soil and fecal specimens. Serotyping is not clinically useful and should be limited to epidemiologic investigations. *L. monocytogenes* shares common antigenic determinants with *Corynebacterium*,[10] *Escherichia coli* K8,[12] *Enterococcus faecalis*,[13] *S. aureus*,[14] and *Staphylococcus epidermidis*. Absorption studies with serovars of *L. monocytogenes* and with *S. aureus* and *Bacillus subtilis* may clarify cross-reactions.[15] Cross-reactions with *L. monocytogenes* do not involve the H antigen.

Bacteriophages are common in *L. monocytogenes* strains.[16] A phage-typing system has been developed for use in outbreak investigation based on lytic properties of 28 phages.[17] It has been useful in tracing sources of food-borne outbreaks of *Listeria*[17, 18] in which serotyping has not discriminated between epidemic and nonepidemic strains.

The development of multilocus enzyme electrophoresis has provided further insights into epidemic disease.[19] The limited availability of phage-typing makes this an attractive method for typing of outbreak-associated isolates.

Whereas plasmid profiling has not been useful in discriminating *L. monocytogenes* strains, newer techniques, including ribosomal RNA fingerprinting[20] and restriction fragment length polymorphism analysis,[21] may provide discrimination between epidemic and nonepidemic strains. Typing of *Listeria* strains on the basis of low-molecular-weight RNA profiles may not be feasible.[22]

Virulence Factors

Food-borne outbreaks of *L. monocytogenes* infections have precipitated an intense interest in organism-specific virulence factors to determine the pathogenesis of infection. *L. monocytogenes* has been used as a paradigm for intracellular parasitism, but organism-specific virulence has only recently been studied. A review of virulence factors has been published.[23]

Entry into host cells involves participation of several bacterial surface proteins. The internalin (Inl) family of bacterial surface proteins contributes to the attachment of the bacteria to mammalian cells.[24, 25] InlA is an 80-KDa protein needed for entry in human intestinal epithelial cells. Interaction between InlA and E-cadherin on mammalian cell surface promotes entry into the cell. E-cadherin is a glycoprotein expressed primarily in epithelial tissue including the digestive tract. InlB, a 67-KDa protein, mediates bacterial entry into cell lines derived from hepatocytes and fibroblasts. The receptor for InlB has not been identified. A third bacterial protein with a molecular mass of 60 KDa (p60) is secreted in large amounts by all strains of *Listeria* capable of invading host cells.[26]

All virulent strains of *L. monocytogenes* produce listeriolysin O (LLO), a sulfhydryl-activated cytolysin similar to streptolysin O. Nonhemolytic mutants are not virulent in animal models of *L. monocytogenes* infection.[27] Listeriolysin O (*hly* gene) lyses the bacteria-containing vacuole, allowing the organism access to the cytosol with subsequent intracellular growth.[28, 29] Once the organism has entered the cytosol it requires a second surface protein ActA, a product of the *actA* gene, to establish productive intracellular growth.[29] Environmental signals associated with the cytosolic environment modify expression of ActA, leading to a relative abundance of the protein.[29]

L. monocytogenes also produces phospholipase C (*plcA* gene) and a lecithinase (*plcB* gene), which may be involved in virulence. Mutations of the *plcA* and *plcB* gene cause diminished virulence, and these gene products may also be involved in cell-to-cell spread of *L. monocytogenes*.[25, 30, 31]

Another gene *(mpl)*, which encodes a metalloprotease, also appears to be permissive for lecithinase production, because isolates with an ineffective *mpl* gene have reduced virulence and lecithinase production.[33]

One regulatory promoter gene *(prfA)* has been described that appears to regulate the *hly*, *plc*, and *mpl* genes either directly or indirectly as well as regulating its own synthesis.[34] InlA or InlB and an internalin-related protein A gene (irpA) are transcribed by prfA-dependent and PrfA mechanisms.[35] Other, less well characterized virulence factors have been described; these include an extracellular hemorrhagic toxin,[36] a pyrogenic fraction,[37] a toxin causing cardiac abnormalities in animals,[38] and other toxins that enhance mortality caused by *Listeria* and other bacteria in mice.[39] A lipid-soluble extractable product having some characteristics of gram-negative endotoxin has also been studied.[40] *Listeria* cell wall fractions also have mitogenic and immunologic properties, which might be important in organism-specific virulence as well as in the host immune response.[41]

A monocytosis-producing agent (MPA) has also been isolated.[42] This produces monocytosis in rabbits and appears to be a phospholipid. Monocyte production is stimulated by an endogenous mediator induced by MPA.[43]

EPIDEMIOLOGY AND TRANSMISSION

Reservoir

L. monocytogenes is commonly present in soil, decayed matter, wood, and other material and is widespread in the natural environment.[44, 45] Spoiled silage appears to be a source of infection for animals.[46, 47] Fecal carriage of *L. monocytogenes* in animals allows recontamination of soil, and subsequent ingestion of contaminated silage completes the cycle in animals.

Transmission to Humans

Direct transmission of *L. monocytogenes* to humans and veterinarians delivering infected animals has been described.[48–50] Increased gastrointestinal carriage rates of *L. monocytogenes* and increased seropositivity rates have been noted in abattoir workers and farmers.[51, 52]

Evidence suggests that almost all human cases of *L. monocytogenes* are acquired through ingestion of contaminated food. In the early and mid 1980s, large outbreaks of *L. monocytogenes* infection occurred in both pregnant women and immunocompromised hosts. The first outbreak, reported from the Canadian Maritimes,[18] suggested indirect transmission from an animal reservoir. In this outbreak, *Listeria*-contaminated sheep manure was used to fertilize cabbage, which was placed in cold storage over the winter; clinical disease developed in pregnant women and immunocompromised patients who subsequently consumed the cabbage. Anecdotal cases of infection from unpasteurized dairy products in 1953[53] preceded large outbreaks caused by contaminated dairy products described more recently.[54–56] In the outbreak reported by Fleming and co-workers, with pasteurized milk as the vehicle, no evidence of improper pasteurization was noted.[54] Studies of thermal resistance of *L. monocytogenes* have failed to shed light on the source of this outbreak, although it may have been due to a very large inoculum. In recent years, outbreaks have been more commonly associated with meat products, including pork, paté, and hot dogs.[57–59]

Whether the development of these outbreaks is related to a high inoculum of *L. monocytogenes* or enhanced virulence of the epidemic strain is unknown. Host susceptibility appears to be constant in the population, although Schwartz and associates have proposed that other gastrointestinal pathogens may be a predisposing factor in translocation of *L. monocytogenes* from the intestine and development of disseminated disease.[60]

The improved ability to culture *L. monocytogenes* with selective media has offered the opportunity to examine food eaten by patients who have developed sporadic cases of listeriosis.[61] However, proof that the vast majority of cases of sporadic listeriosis are caused by ingestion of contaminated foodstuffs was not confirmed until studies in the United States by the Listeriosis Study Group at the Centers for Disease Control and Prevention (CDC) clearly demonstrated the role of food in sporadic listeriosis.[62, 63] These studies implicated undercooked chicken and soft cheeses as significant sources of disease and are supported by sampling surveys carried out by various regulatory agencies. A review of food-borne listeriosis has been published.[64]

Occurrence

Fecal carriage of listeriosis is uncommon but ranges from 1% in hospitalized patients to 26% in household contacts of patients with listeriosis.[65] In the Canadian Maritimes outbreak, fecal surveys demonstrated carriage rate in approximately 5% of family contacts.[18] During the California outbreak carriage rates in the community were approximately 8%.[66] *L. monocytogenes* may also cause a self-limited symptomatic gastrointestinal infection, but this is not a reportable condition. Surveillance systems for invasive listeriosis have focused on passive reporting of cases of meningitis and sepsis, and significant under-reporting probably occurs. Recent attempts at active surveillance suggest an annual incidence of 0.7 case per 100,000 population in the United States and 0.4 cases per 100,000 population in Canada.[67] An estimated 1700 cases of listeriosis occur annually in the United States, with a mortality rate of 40%. Slightly lower figures have been reported from Australia[68], England[69], and Denmark.[70] However, these studies depended on voluntary reporting of isolates to central public health laboratories.

Geographic differences in nonperinatal listeriosis have not been found, although rates for perinatal listeriosis may differ in geographic areas.[67]

In addition, the distribution of serovars does not appear uniform. In the United States, serovars 4b and 1/2 account for 95% of strains, with serotype 4b being the most common overall. In Canada, serovar 1/2b occurred in 42% of clinical isolates in 1988.[71] On the other hand, in what was formerly the Federal Republic of Germany, serovar 4b was clearly the predominant strain between 1969 and 1985.[72] The significance of these geographic differences is unknown.

Perinatal Listeriosis

In a pattern reminiscent of neonatal group B streptococcal infections, neonatal listeriosis is usually divided into "early-onset" and "late-onset" disease. The incidence in the United States for neonatal listeriosis is approximately 13 per 100,000 live births, approximately 30% of the total number of cases of listeriosis that occur,[67] with similar results reported in studies from Europe.[72, 73] Epidemics of food-borne listeriosis have disproportionately involved perinatal cases, and it is possible that higher infective doses are needed to infect pregnant women in comparison to immunocompromised hosts. No differences in carriage rates between pregnant women and nonpregnant individuals have been found in fecal and vaginal specimens.[74] Fecal carriage may lead to vaginal colonization and be responsible for the development of late-onset infection in infants born of healthy mothers.

Infection in the Compromised Host

Two thirds of cases of listeriosis occur in immunocompromised adults, and sepsis and meningitis are the most frequent presenting illnesses. Louria and co-workers initially described this infection in patients with malignancies,[75] but a wide variety of other conditions have been reported in association with invasive listeriosis.[76, 77] The human experience parallels studies of susceptibility in laboratory animals, which is increased by the administration of corticosteroids,[78] cyclosporin A,[79] and prostaglandins.[80] Renal transplantation appears to be a particularly significant risk factor, and a nosocomial outbreak of infection in this population has been reported.[81] Hemochromatosis with increased iron stores may also predispose to infection. Listeriosis is now reported in patients with acquired immunodeficiency syndrome who have a 1000-fold risk of acquiring invasive listeriosis.[82] Alcoholism, diabetes, and cirrhosis also contribute to infection, although community-acquired listeriosis may occur spontaneously in patients with no underlying predisposing conditions.[83] Animal studies[84] as well as one outbreak of human listeriosis[85] suggest that decreased gastric acidity may predispose to invasive infection in patients with immunosuppressive conditions.

Nosocomial Transmission

Although most large outbreaks of listeriosis have occurred in the community, case clusters of nosocomial listeriosis in both neonates and adults have been described.[86–91] Person-to-person transmission caused by poor infection-control techniques is likely to be responsible for most of these small clusters. Often the patient with the index case presents with early-onset infection, and subsequent cases have typical late-onset listeriosis. Cases with early-onset disease occurring within a day in the same unit may well have been caused by food-borne disease in the community. Nosocomial infection in adults in the Boston outbreak[85] was probably related to ingestion of contaminated food in a hospital environment or within 2 weeks of hospitalization. Clear-cut nosocomial infection has been demonstrated in an outbreak in Costa Rica.[92] In that outbreak, the index case had early-onset disease and was bathed with mineral oil that became contaminated with the epidemic isolate. Subsequent bathing of other infants with the same oil led to late-onset disease in those infants.

PATHOGENESIS

Host Response in Normal Adults

STAGES OF RESPONSE

At least three stages of host response to *Listeria* occur in normal adult animals.[93] Within hours after intravenous injection of the organism, macrophages of the liver and spleen capture and destroy 50% to 90% of the inoculum. Over the next 3 days, a nonspecific, T cell–independent phase of host resistance, termed natural resistance, appears to be operative. Since the 1960s, it was known that *L. monocytogenes* can survive within resident macrophages in the liver and spleen. In the late 1980s, it was also appreciated that *Listeria* can infect nonphagocytic cells (e.g., epithelial, hepatocellular, and fibroblast cell lines), thus providing the organism with an intracellular environment temporarily sheltered from more hostile host defense forces.[94–96]

Although proteins on the surface of *Listeria*, such as InlA, InlB, and p60 may identify important factors associated with entrance into the cell in vitro,[25, 26] they do not fully explain intracellular spread and multiplication of the organism in vivo.[97] During the early course of infection, *L. monocytogenes* resides within a vacuole (for nonphagocytic cells) or a phagosome (in monocyte/macrophage-derived cells) (Fig. 27–1). Lysis of the phagosome or vacuole is mediated by LLO and non–LLO-derived proteins.[29, 98–100] Bacterial-derived phospholipase C and a metalloprotease-mediated lysin may also contribute to escape of *L. monocytogenes* from vacuoles and phagosomes. Release of *L. monocytogenes* from intracellular vacuoles precipitates both intracellular growth and actin polymerization.[101] Actin polymerization is important in the cell-to-cell transfer of *L. monocytogenes* and is encoded by the *actA* gene.[32] Actin is the most abundant protein in the cytoplasm of mammalian cells. The single bacterial surface protein ActA causes host-cell actin to assemble into filaments around the bacterium. After 2 or 3 hours, the actin filaments polarize at one end of the organism. This "rocket tail" provides the propulsive force for the organism to move through the cytoplasm. When the bacterium reaches the cell membrane it forms a filipod that is ingested by adjacent cells. In the process, the organism avoids exposure to the extracellular environment. In addition to hepatocytes, enterocytes, and phagocytic cells, *Listeria* can grow and spread in fibroblasts, epithelial cells, vascular endothelial cells, and renal tubular epithelial cells.[101] The intracytoplasmic environment provides abundant growth conditions and a protected environment for this organism to survive.[94, 102]

Three or 4 days after infection begins there is normally a decrease in viable bacteria in the monocyte-macrophage phagocytic system. This heralds the onset of the immune T cell–dependent stage of antilisterial defense, termed *acquired resistance*.[103] Development of acquired anti-*Listeria* activity is seen by day 5 of infection and can be demonstrated by adoptive transfer of resistance using immune T cells. At this stage, the number of activated macrophages in infected tissue rapidly increases (Fig. 27–2).

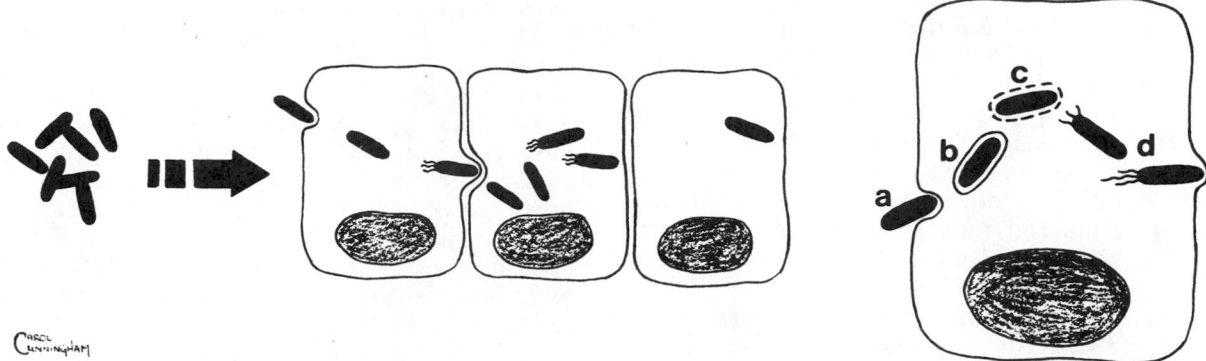

FIGURE 27–1 Cellular invasion by *Listeria monocytogenes*. Attachment of *L. monocytogenes* to the surface of cell membrane is determined by a family of bacterial surface proteins including internalins (IntA and IntB). Once internalized within a vacuole, listeriolysin O (LLO) can lyse the vacuole membrane, liberating the bacteria into the cytoplasm. Bacterial surface ActA induces polymerization of cellular actin which concentrates at one end of the bacterium. This "rocket tail" provides propulsion for the organism to move through the cytoplasm and into adjacent cells where the intracellular process will begin again.

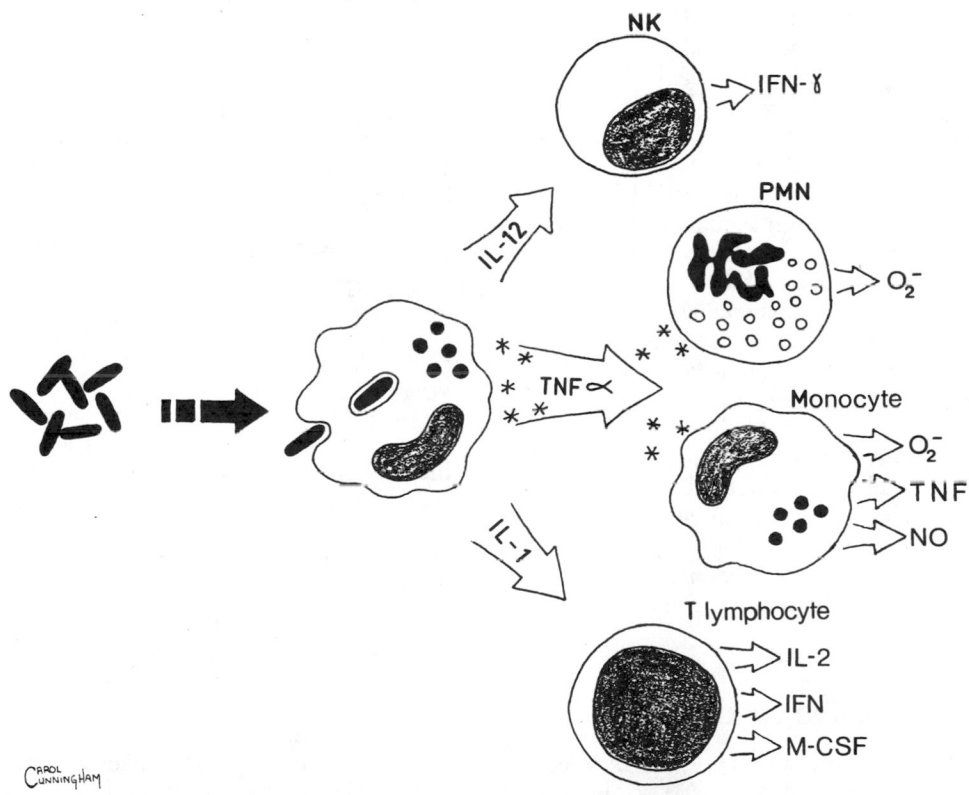

FIGURE 27–2 Interferon and cytokine production. Blood monocytes and tissue macrophages produce a variety of cytokines after ingestion of live *listeria*. Interleukin (IL)-12 causes activation of natural killer (NK) cells, which release high concentrations of interferon gamma (IFN-γ). Tumor necrosis factor-alpha (TNF-α) is produced in high concentrations by monocytes and macrophages after ingestion of *Listeria*. TNF-α leads to priming of polymorphonuclear leukocytes and activation of other macrophage cells, with increased production of superoxide (O_2^-), nitric oxide (NO), and TNF-α. Macrophage-produced IL-1 leads to proliferation of T cells, which, in turn, produce immunomodulating proteins such as IL-2, macrophage colony-stimulating factor (M-CSF), and IFN-γ.

CELLULAR RESPONSE

For adult animals, the process leading to acquired immunity to *Listeria* has been partially elucidated, and the sequence of cell-to-cell interaction resulting in cytolytic activity is now becoming clear. In adult immunocompetent animals, *Listeria* are phagocytosed by "professional" phagocytes (macrophages and monocytes) and by "nonprofessional" phagocytic cells (fibroblasts, hepatocytes, etc.) (see Fig. 27–1). Once ingested, partial degradation of *Listeria* occurs and transfer of the *Listeria* protein antigen fragments to the macrophage cell surface takes place.[104]

Peptides resulting from digestion of *Listeria* in the cytoplasm are actively processed by the endoplasmic reticulum where the peptides bind to major histocompatibility complex (MHC) class I molecules (Fig. 27–3).[104]

The *Listeria*-peptide-MHC complex is transported to the cell surface where it can be recognized by cytolytic T lymphocytes (CD8 phenotype). Bacterial peptides that are digested within a phagosome are transported to the plasma membrane where they attach to MHC class II molecules. CD4 T lymphocytes recognize specific antigens that are presented by MHC class II membrane receptors.[105] Development of T helper (T_H) subset during an immune response is important because *L. monocytogenes* infection is most effectively controlled by T_H1-type immune response.[105] *L. monocytogenes* induction of T_H1 development in vitro is stimulated by macrophage-produced interleukin-12 (IL-12). Cells with T_H1 phenotype secrete IL-2 and interferon gamma (IFN-γ) during primary infection.[106, 107] Although a small number of T_H2 cells may develop during listerial infection, they play little role in the clearance of *Listeria*.[108]

In the presence of listerial antigens and IL-2, T cells divide, producing *Listeria*-specific clones. In vitro evidence demonstrates that *L. monocytogenes*–immune CD8 T cells are cytolytic for *Listeria*-infected macrophages and hepatocytes[109, 110] (see Fig. 27–3). Neutrophils and monocytes that migrate to the site of primary infection may participate in the lysis of infected cells but, more importantly, play a role in the elimination of bacteria that are released to the surrounding tissue. By this stage of infection phagocytic cells have been primed or activated by IFN-γ or cytokines, making them more effective killers.[111–117]

ROLE OF INTERFERON AND CYTOKINES

In mature immunocompetent animals, *Listeria* infection induces circulating (IFN-γ) and (IFNα/β) on the second or third day in the acquired phase of immunity. Cytokines such as macrophage colony-stimulating factor (M-CSF)[118] and tumor necrosis factor-alpha (TNF-α) also appear during the first 5 days and have recently been implicated as mediators of listerial clearance.[116, 119–127] However, peak immunity to *Listeria* is expressed about the sixth day of infection, which coincides with maximal T_H1 cell synthesis of IFN-γ.[128–130] A role for endogenous IFN-γ for resolution for *L. monocytogenes* infection has been suggested.[131, 132] Adult animals treated with mono-

clonal antibody directed against IFN-γ do not develop activated macrophages, and clearance of *Listeria* from liver and spleen is decreased.[131]

There is growing evidence that TNF functions to enhance antibacterial or antiparasitic resistance mechanisms[133–139] (see Fig. 27–2). Many cell types produce TNF, including natural killer (NK) cells[140, 141]; however, monocytes and macrophages are probably the most abundant source.[142] Endotoxin (lipopolysaccharide) and other agents, including mitogens, viruses, protozoa, and cytokines such as M-CSF, IL-1, IL-2, and IFN-γ have been identified as inducers of TNF.[143–147] When administered before infection, TNF-inducing agents enhanced resistance of the host to bacterial infection.[148]

Endogenously produced TNF during sublethal *Listeria* infection in adult animals appears to function as an inducer of resistance.[119, 121–125] Injection of mice with anti-TNF immunoglobulin results in a striking increase in the number of bacteria during the first 2 or 3 days of infection; however, administration of anti-TNF immunoglobulin on day 5 of infection has virtually no effect on *Listeria* number in the spleen and liver.[116, 117, 123] These results suggest that TNF-dependent mechanisms limit intracellular infection early in the course of infection. Localized production of TNF is demonstrated in supernatants of organ homogenates from the liver or spleen.[149]

IL-12, originally called NK cell stimulatory factor, participates in the differentiation of T_H1 cells, IFN-γ production, and NK cell activation.[105, 127, 150] In the absence of T_H1 activation, animals are more susceptible to *L. monocytogenes* infection.[105, 150]

Host Response in the Neonate

CELL ACTIVATION

In newborn animals, susceptibility to *Listeria* appears to be associated with delayed activation of macrophages.[151, 152] The afferent and efferent arms of the immune system in newborn mice have been studied by Lu and others, who showed that macrophage/T lymphocyte interaction is impaired.[95, 149, 153–156] Macrophage activation does not occur. The relevance of animal studies to human infection remains to be determined; however, Issekutz and colleagues demonstrated a similar defect among infants surviving natural *Listeria* infection.[157]

Functional capacity of monocytic and macrophage cells is decreased in newborn animals. Chemotaxis, phagocytosis, and killing of *Candida albicans* were markedly impaired in neonatal rhesus monkey alveolar macrophages compared with those in juveniles and adults.[158] In newborn rabbits, lung macrophages have similar defects in oxygen radical generation.[159]

NK cells appear to be important in early response to *L. monocytogenes* infection. The proportion of mononuclear cells expressing NK cell phenotype and NK cell activity is decreased at birth, particularly in premature infants.[160, 161] Both NK cell phenotype and function increase rapidly in the weeks after birth.

INTERFERON AND CYTOKINE PRODUCTION

In adult animals, *Listeria* infection induces production of IL-12, which mediates several biologic activities such

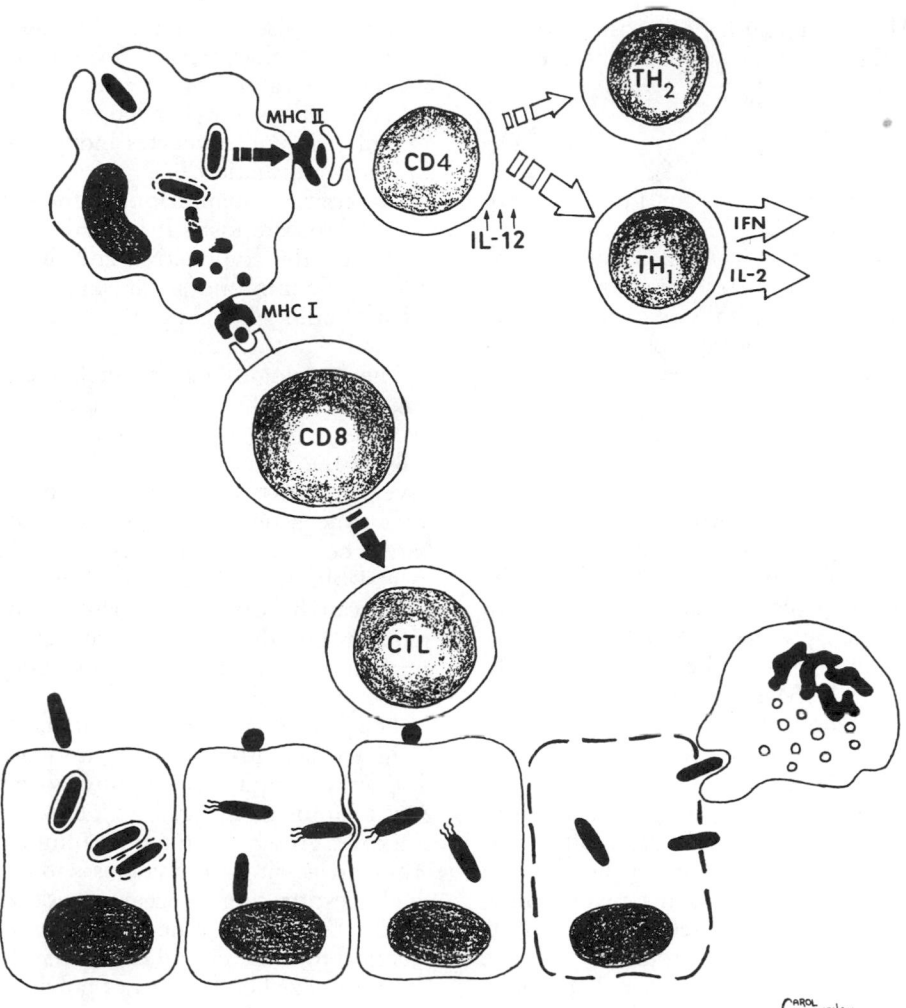

FIGURE 27–3 Activation of cytolytic cell mechanisms. Within an antigen presenting cell, organisms killed and digested within a phagosome release bacterial peptides that are transported to the plasma membrane where they attach to major histocompatibility complex (MHC) class II molecules. CD4 T lymphocytes recognize specific antigens that are presented by MHC class II receptors. CD4 T lymphocytes differentiate predominantly into T_H1 cells through stimulation by (IL)-interleukin 12. Such cells secrete high concentrations of IL-2 and interferon gamma during primary infection.

Bacterial peptides may also come from proteolytic digestion of intracytoplasmic organisms. Such peptides are processed by the endoplasmic reticulum where they bind to Major histocompatibility complex class I receptors. The bacterial-peptide-MHC I complex is transported to the cell membrane, where it is recognized by cytolytic T lymphocytes (CD8 phenotype). Such cells cause lysis of *Listeria*-infected cells, which are recognized by the presence of listerial peptides on their surface. Lysis of *Listeria*-infected cells leaves the organism exposed to phagocytosis and killing by activated phagocytic cells, polymorphonuclear leukocytes, and monocytes.

as T_H1 differentiation, NK cell activation, and IFN-γ production. The major cellular source of IL-12 are monocytes and macrophages. IL-12 messenger RNA (mRNA) expression and protein production in cord blood mononuclear cells is greatly decreased compared with adult cells stimulated with lipopolysaccharides.[162] In addition, the half-life of IL-12 p40 mRNA is shortened in activated cord blood cells compared with adult cells.[162] However, cord blood mononuclear cells from humans are capable of responding to exogenous IL-12 with production of IFN-γ and activation of NK cells.[163]

In adult animals, INF and agents that induce or augment INF production confer protection against lethal listeriosis.[120, 164, 165] Synthesis of interferon, IL-2 and IL-

4, all of which modulate the immune response and macrophage activation, is deficient in newborns.[156, 166–169] Although production of these factors may be defective, newborn animals do respond to exogenous INF; pretreatment with INF or its inducers[170] protects against subsequent infection.

The ontogeny of cytokine-related host defense mechanisms has not been studied in depth. TNF is decreased among newborn rats challenged with *L. monocytogenes*.[149] In one study on *L. monocytogenes*–infected newborn rats, TNF was detected only among animals older than 8 days of age. The age at which TNF is measurable corresponds to the approximate age at which increased resistance to *L. monocytogenes* is seen. In addition, the study showed that IFN-γ may enhance resistance to *L. monocytogenes* in newborn animals by permitting them to respond to exogenous TNF-α.

OPSONIC ACTIVITY

Opsonic activity of newborn serum for gram-negative organisms and *Listeria* is deficient.[171, 172] *Listeria* is opsonized primarily by IgM together with the classical complement pathway. Because newborn serum has negligible amounts of IgM and low concentrations of the classical complement pathway, its poor opsonic activity may contribute to the severity of infection in newborns.

PATHOLOGY

Human listeriosis is characterized by miliary granulomas and focal necroses or by suppuration in the affected tissues. The term *listerioma* has been coined for the granulomas associated with listeriosis. In the newborn, listeriosis is characterized by a disseminated involvement of numerous organs in which nodules of pinhead to millet-seed size are seen.[173] Massive involvement of the liver is almost always predominant. As in miliary tuberculosis, the liver is seeded with grayish yellow nodules. Analogous findings are observed in the spleen, adrenal glands, lungs, esophagus, posterior pharyngeal wall, and tonsils. Granulomas located subepithelially often undergo necrosis. Focal granulomas may also be detected in the lymph nodes, thymus, bone marrow, myocardium, testes, and skeletal muscles. The intestinal tract is affected to a variable degree, with a preference for the lymphatic structures of the small intestine and appendix. As was observed originally by Reiss,[174] listeriosis of the newborn is often accompanied by the development of cutaneous foci, commonly on the back and lumbar region (Fig. 27–4).

In listeriosis of the central nervous system, the tissue changes are also characterized by the formation of granulomas.[175] A characteristic histologic picture is seen in encephalitis caused by *Listeria*, consisting of necrosis of the cerebral tissue with a loosening of the reticulum and an infiltration of leukocytes and lymphocytes and, finally, an abscess formation.

Suppurative inflammation is the second form of tissue reaction to listeriosis. It is predominantly found in the meninges, the conjunctiva, and the epithelial linings of the middle ear and nasal sinuses. In meningitis, the subarachnoid space becomes filled with thick purulent exudate.

The histologic changes in human listeriosis are the same as those observed in animals. The organisms cause necrosis, which is followed by proliferative activity of cells of the reticuloendothelial system, resulting in the development of granulomas. The center of the granuloma is necrotic, and the periphery contains large numbers of chronic inflammatory cells. *Listeria* are detectable in variable numbers and positions in the necrotic foci. They can be easily demonstrated by means of Gram stain or Levaditi silver impregnation. Similar changes are found in all affected organs, independent of the age of the infected individual.

The gross and microscopic appearance of the placenta in listeriosis, although not pathognomic, is sufficiently distinct to permit a presumptive diagnosis by the experienced pathologist (Fig. 27–5). *Listeria* placentitis is characterized grossly by multiple minute white or gray necrotic areas within the villous parenchyma and decidua, the largest tending to occur in basal villi and the decidua basalis.[176–178] These necrotic foci are macroabscesses identical to those described in other fetal organs.[173] Typically, localized collections of polymorphonuclear leukocytes are found between the villous trophoblast and stroma, and inflamed or necrotic chorionic villi are enmeshed in intervillous inflammatory material and fibrin. Chorioamnionitis deciduitis, villitis, and fungisitis (in order of frequency) are seen. Cord lesions may be con-

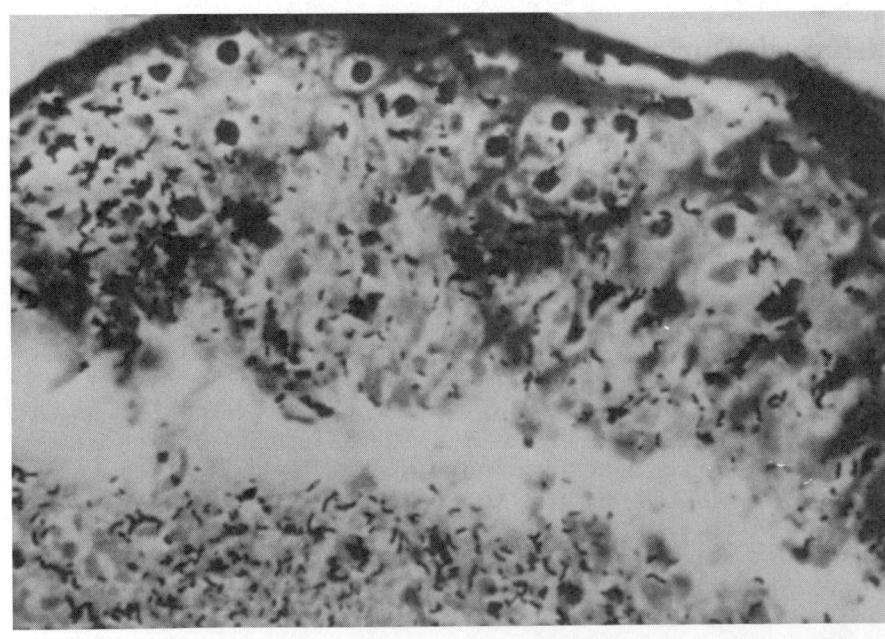

FIGURE 27–4 Cutaneous listeriosis. Note the numerous gram-positive rods that extend from the dermis below into the epidermis above.

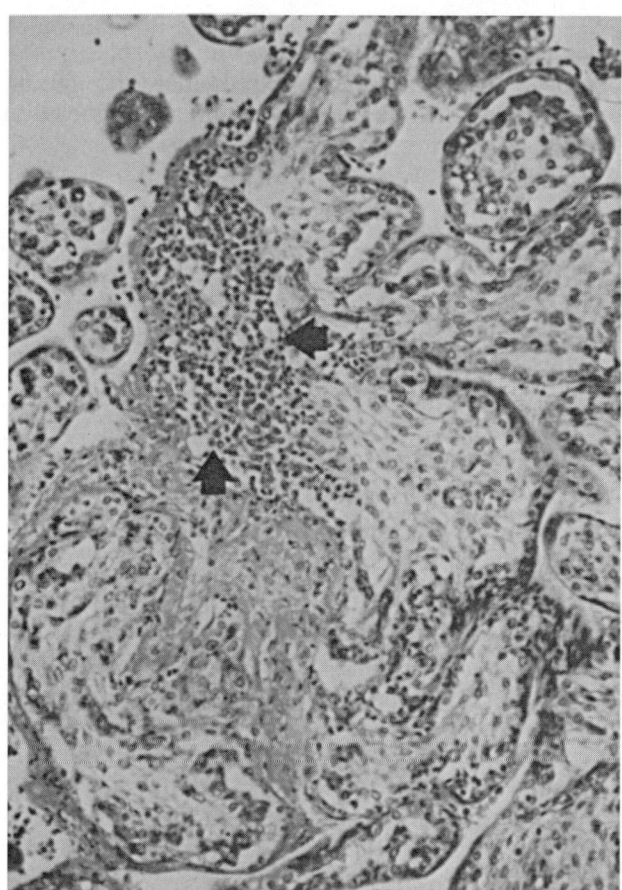

FIGURE 27–5 *Listeria* placentitis. Note the microabscess between the necrotic villous trophoblast and the stroma (arrows). Chorionic villi are enmeshed by intervillous and inflammatory material.

fined to superficial foci. Gram-positive rods are usually readily demonstrable within the necrotic centers of villous and decidual microabscesses as well as within the membranes and umbilical cord. An immunohistochemical stain using polyclonal antibody directed at LLO has also been used.[179]

CLINICAL MANIFESTATIONS

The clinical features of listeriosis have considerable variability and may mimic other infections or other disease states. Based on the most common clinical manifestations, four or more clinical groups may be distinguished.

Listeriosis During Pregnancy

The predilection of *Listeria* for the fetoplacental unit and intrauterine infection is well documented.[180–184] Maternal listeriosis can be transmitted to the fetus by an ascending or transplacental route. Early gestational listeriosis is associated with septic abortion; however, most cases of perinatal listeriosis are found after the fifth month of pregnancy, with premature delivery of a septic or stillborn infant the result.

Maternal influenza-like illness with fever and chills, fatigue, headache, and muscle pains often precedes delivery by 2 to 14 days. Although symptoms in the mother may subside before delivery, infection and fever precipitating delivery are common. Blood cultured from such women can yield *Listeria* at the time of initial symptoms or later. Premature labor in mothers with listeriosis is common; length of gestation is less than 35 weeks in approximately 70%. The mortality rate, including stillbirth and abortion, is 40% to 50%. Early treatment of *Listeria* sepsis in pregnancy, however, can prevent infection or sequelae.[185, 186] At the time of delivery, maternal symptoms of infection may be pronounced; however, these usually subside with or without antibiotic treatment soon after delivery.

The pathogenesis of fetal listeriosis is not clear. Because the heaviest foci for neonatal infection are lung and gut, the fetus is probably infected by swallowing contaminated amniotic fluid as well as through the transplacental hematogenous route. An ascending pathway from the lower genital tract may occur; however, infection through the transplacental route is favored by most authors. *L. monocytogenes* chorioamnionitis diagnosed by transabdominal amniocentesis (free from vaginal bacterial contamination), has been reported and thus favors a blood-borne route of infection.[173, 182, 186–188] Placental chorionic vascular thrombi can be associated with maternal coagulopathy. Emboli originating from *Listeria*-infected placental vessels has been described as a cause of congenital stroke in an infant.[179]

Susceptibility to *L. monocytogenes* is markedly increased in pregnant animals.[189, 190] Immunoregulation during pregnancy is poorly understood. The fetoplacental unit must survive in the potentially hostile maternal immunologic environment throughout gestation. Recent evidence is consistent with the hypothesis that the placenta and the immediately adjacent tissue constitute an immunologically privileged site, with local uterine immune response being suppressed.[184, 191] Such regulation may be necessary to protect the fetus from immunologic rejection by the mother. However, if infection in this area occurs, bacterial proliferation may be overwhelming because of slow cell-mediated immune response.

Listeriosis in the Newborn

The first descriptions of neonatal listeriosis were published in the 1930s by Burn.[192–194] Since then, it has become recognized that neonatal infection is the most common clinical form of human listeriosis. Infection in the neonatal period is usually divided into two clinical groups defined by age.

EARLY-ONSET INFECTION

Some clinical and laboratory manifestations of early-onset neonatal listeriosis are outlined in Table 27–1, which is compiled from clinical cases published since 1970 in which early and late forms of the disease could be differentiated.[77, 180, 188, 195–201] Classically, early-onset neonatal listeriosis develops within 1 or 2 days of life. However, in one outbreak involving 10 infants with

TABLE 27–1
Clinical and Laboratory Findings of Early-Onset and Late-Onset Neonatal Listeriosis

FEATURE	EARLY ONSET[a]	LATE ONSET[b]
Mortality (%)	25	15
Median age in days (range)	1 (0–6)	14 (7–35)
Male (%)	60	67
Preterm (%)	65	20
Respiratory involvement (%)	50	10
Meningitis (%)	25	95
Blood isolate (%)	75	20
Maternal perinatal illness (%)	50	0

[a] Data from references 77, 180, 188, 195–199.
[b] Data from references 195, 199–201, 264.

nosocomially acquired listeriosis, an atypical clinical picture was described.[92] Nine of these infants were bathed with *L. monocytogenes*–contaminated mineral oil shortly after birth. Clinical features of infection developed 4 to 8 days later and were similar to those seen in late-onset infection (insidious onset of illness with fever and meningitis was common).

Evidence of preceding maternal illness is often described in infants with early-onset disease. Although some symptoms in mothers are vague and nonspecific (malaise, myalgia), others are sufficiently distinctive (fever, chills) to alert physicians to the risk for prenatally acquired listeriosis. Blood cultures are often positive for *Listeria* from such mothers.

Although early-onset disease may occur up to 7 days of age, most cases are clinically apparent at delivery with meconium staining, cyanosis, apnea, respiratory distress and pneumonia. Meconium-stained amniotic liquor is a common feature in such infants and may occur at any gestational age, even less than 32 weeks. Pneumonia is also common, but radiographic features are not specific (peribronchial to widespread infiltration). In more long-standing infection, a coarse, mottled or nodular pattern has been described. Assisted ventilation is frequently necessary in such infants. Persistent hypoxia in spite of ventilatory assistance is seen in severely affected infants. One investigator has suggested that pulmonary vasospasms with right-to-left shunting of blood may aggravate this condition.

In severe infection, a granulomatous rash has been described (Fig. 27–6). Slightly elevated pale patches measuring 1 to 2 mm in diameter with a bright erythematous base are seen. If biopsies of such areas are performed, a leukocytic infiltrate with multiple bacteria is found (see Fig. 27–4).

Laboratory features are nonspecific; a leukocytosis with presence of immature cells may be seen, or, if infection is severe, neutropenia is noted. Similarly, thrombocytopenia may also occur.[180, 196] Many of the infants are anemic, perhaps attributable to hemolysin produced by the organism. These laboratory and clinical features do not help to distinguish listeriosis from early-onset group B streptococcal or other bacterial infection. The association of early-onset listeriosis with prematurity and maternal infection suggests the presence of intrauterine infection. The presence of chorioamnionitis in many of such cases[199] in the absence of ruptured membrane supports the hypothesis of *Listeria* infection occurring by a transplacental route, which differs from the common route of group B streptococcal infection.

LATE-ONSET INFECTION

Neonatal listerial infection that occurs after 7 days of life is termed *late-onset* infection. Although there is some overlap between early- and late-onset forms of listeriosis, the clinical pattern of the two is usually distinct. The common clinical and laboratory features of late-onset neonatal listeriosis are shown in Table 27–1. By far the most common form of *Listeria* infection over this period is meningitis, which is present in 94% of late-onset cases. In many centers, *Listeria* ranks second only to group B *Streptococcus* as a cause of bacterial meningitis in this age group, causing approximately 20% of such infections.[195]

Clinical features do not distinguish listerial meningitis in this age group from other causes. A striking predominance of males has been noted in most series. Fever and irritability are predominant clinical features. Often, infants do not appear excessively ill and may therefore elude diagnosis for several days.

Other clinical forms of disease at this age are less common but include *Listeria*-induced colitis with associated diarrhea and sepsis without meningitis.[202, 203]

Laboratory features of late-onset infection are not specific. Cell count in cerebrospinal fluid is usually high, with a predominance of polymorphonuclear neutrophil and band forms. Occasionally in long-standing disease, a relatively high number of monocytes may be seen. Gram stain of cerebrospinal fluid may not always suggest a diagnosis, both because the organism may be rare and because the morphology is atypical. Variable decolorization of the iodine stain may result in organisms appearing as gram-negative rods or gram-positive cocci. The appearance of organisms as illustrated in Figure 27–7 is characteristic of listeriosis in the early phase of severe meningitis.

Mortality of late-onset newborn infection is generally low unless diagnosis is delayed by more than 3 or 4 days after onset. Long-term sequelae and morbidity are uncommon.

Central Nervous System Infection

Acute or subacute bacterial meningitis accounts for two thirds of adult cases of listeriosis. Rhombencephalitis with ataxia, cranial nerve palsies, and multiple microabscesses on magnetic resonance imaging or computed tomography appears to be a distinct *Listeria* syndrome in humans, as it is in ruminants ("circling disease").[175] Both morbidity and mortality are high in this entity.[77]

Other Clinical Forms of Infection

Papular cutaneous lesions are often observed in newborns when listeriosis is disseminated. These are to be

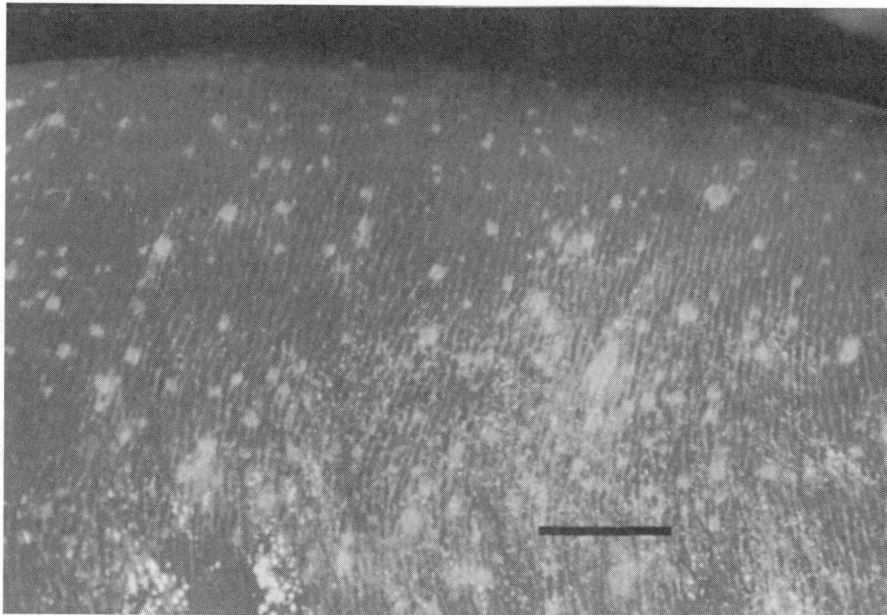

FIGURE 27–6 Rash of neonatal *Listeria monocytogenes* infection. Areas of small, elevated pale pustules surrounded by a deep-red erythematous base seen on the abdomen of a premature neonate. (Horizontal bar: ~1 cm in length.)

distinguished from the primary skin lesions caused by *Listeria* as observed in adults,[204, 205] which are the result of direct contact, such as the handling of a cow's placenta after abortion by a veterinarian or farmer.[50]

In the course of the septicemic form, an accompanying conjunctivitis is sometimes observed. Anton's eye test[206] actually resulted from a laboratory accident in which a technician accidentally contaminated his face. Other unusual forms of listeriosis, such as endocarditis,[207] liver abscess,[208] peritonitis,[209, 210] and osteomyelitis and septic arthritis[211] have been described in adults but appear to be rare in infants. Recently, a febrile gastroenteritis syndrome similar to salmonellosis has been described in adults and children in three outbreaks involving contaminated shrimp salad,[212] rice salad,[213] and chocolate milk.[203] Only a few patients developed invasive disease (sepsis) in these outbreaks, and the level of *Listeria* contamination appeared to be very high.[214]

DIAGNOSIS

The varied and often subtle symptoms and signs of listeriosis make an etiologic diagnosis difficult, if not impossible, based on clinical findings available when the patient is first seen.

Serology

The agglutination reaction (Widal's test) demonstrates antibodies against O and H antigens of the various *Listeria* serovars. Unfortunately, because of the antigen complexity of *L. monocytogenes*, no agreement has been reached as to the interpretation of agglutination reactions for diagnostic purposes.

Attempts to demonstrate complement-fixing *Listeria* antibodies date back to the 1930s.[215] In one study, serum samples collected from 32 mothers with perinatal *Liste-*

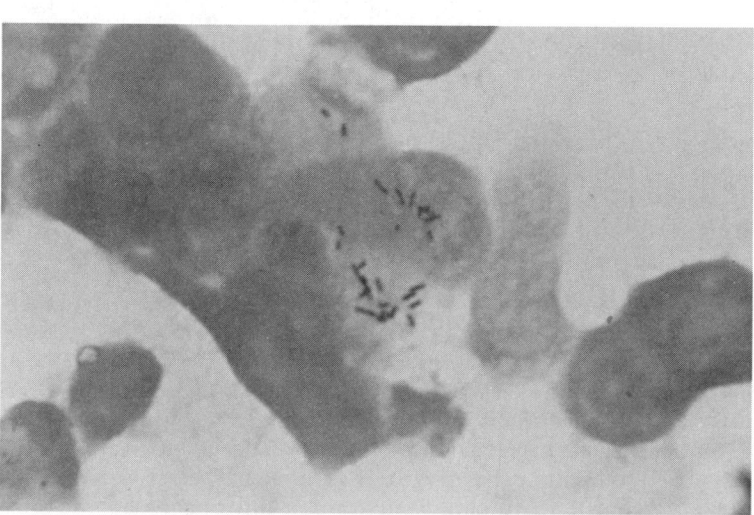

FIGURE 27–7 Short gram-positive intracellular organisms with variable length and rounded ends are arranged irregularly.

ria infection were compared with 128 samples from matched controls.[216] The sensitivity and specificity of the complement fixation test were found to be 78% and 91%, respectively; however, the positive predictive value was only 75%. A titer of 1:8 or more is accepted as significant.[216, 217] Thus, the complement fixation test can be regarded as reliable only in some patients with acute *Listeria* infection.

Detection of antibodies to LLO has been used to diagnose human listeriosis.[218] Purified LLO incorporated into nitrocellulose filters and then tested with serial dilutions of sera. Adsorbed anti-LLO was identified using enzyme-labeled anti-human IgG. Sensitivity and specificity of the test were over 90%. Although these results were impressive, the technique is not available commercially. It was recently used to identify patients in a febrile gastroenteritis outbreak with a good correlation with clinical illness.[203]

A precipitin test,[219] indirect hemagglutination reaction,[220] and antigen fixation test[221] have been described, showing apparent success.

Isolation of the Organism

Cultivation of *L. monocytogenes* is the only reliable means of proving that the cause of an infection is due to *Listeria*. Culture of venous blood, ascitic and other fluids, cervical material, urine, amniotic fluid, lochia and meconium, and tissues at biopsy or autopsy offers the best chances for identifying *Listeria* in persons with disease. Culture of the stool is not helpful. Feces are positive for *Listeria* in 1% to 5% of healthy women.[65, 222]

Microscopic diagnosis may be attempted by use of Gram stain only in specimens that normally do not contain bacteria: cerebrospinal fluid, meconium, and tissue smears. The finding of short, sometimes coccoid, gram-positive rods strongly supports a suspicion of listeriosis and is indicative of this infection in meconium smears. *L. monocytogenes* sometimes does not stain clearly as gram-positive. Particularly with long-standing disease or when the patient has received antibiotics, the organisms may appear gram-negative and be confused with *H. influenzae* when observed in the cerebrospinal fluid. In other instances, *Listeria* has been mistaken for pneumococci and corynebacteria.

The submission of clinical specimens for culture may be facilitated by the use of transport-enrichment fluid. It is, however, advisable to submit specimens such as blood, cerebrospinal fluid, and pus without any additives. For patients who have received antibiotics, the use of a commercial antibiotic-removing device is useful.

PROGNOSIS

Neonatal listeriosis accounts for the largest recognizable group of infections caused by *L. monocytogenes*. Fetal wastage with early gestational infection is a recognized complication of maternal infection. In late-gestational maternal infection, sparing of the fetus has been reported,[223] but it is probably uncommon unless antepartum antibiotic treatment has been given to the mother.[224, 225]

Although fetal or neonatal infection with *L. monocytogenes* is known to have a high fatality, the long-term morbidity is unclear. Rotheberg and associates[226] found an increased incidence of developmental delay assessed at a mean age of 29.5 months among small (<1250 g at birth) *Listeria*-infected infants who required assisted ventilation. Naege,[227] studying children 4 to 7 years after they recovered from early-onset listeriosis, also found increased neurodevelopmental handicaps. Others have reported hydrocephalus.[228]

In contrast, Evans and co-workers[229] found no evidence of neurodevelopmental sequelae in six of eight survivors studied at a mean age of 15 months and again at 32 months. The two infants with neurodevelopmental sequelae had severe acute perinatal sepsis with meningitis. Both had spastic diplegia. The authors concluded that long-term sequelae after neonatal early-onset listeriosis was uncommon. If meningitis is not present, the outcome may be generally good.

The prognosis for infants with late-onset neonatal sepsis and meningitis has not been studied extensively.

THERAPY

Listeria remains susceptible to antibiotics commonly used in its treatment.[230, 231] However, the high mortality rate and risk of relapse[232, 233] have prompted a search for newer therapeutic regimens, including quinolones,[234] trimethoprim-sulfamethoxazole,[235, 237] and rifampin.[238] Transferable plasmid-mediated antibiotic resistance has been reported[239] conferring resistance to chloramphenicol, tetracycline, and erythromycin.

In Vitro Studies

Conflicting reports of in vitro activity of antibiotics against clinical isolates of *L. monocytogenes* probably reflect a variable pattern of susceptibility for strains as well as differences in laboratory technique. Several large in vitro studies of antibiotic susceptibility of human clinical isolates of *L. monocytogenes* have been reported using broth dilution susceptibility methods.[240–242] Most studies found that the strains represented a homogeneous population susceptible to ampicillin, penicillin, erythromycin, and tetracycline. In vitro results, however, are greatly influenced by methodology: inoculum size, media, and definition of end points. Since 1988, several strains have been isolated showing various degrees of relative resistance to non–β-lactam antibiotics such as tetracycline and gentamicin.[241, 242] In addition, the minimal bactericidal concentration of antibiotics is often much higher than levels attainable clinically. Thus, most antibiotics tested are bacteriostatic but not bactericidal. Although bacteriostatic antibiotics have been used in the past, bactericidal antibiotics have a potential advantage for patients with impaired host defense mechanisms.[243]

Results of cephalosporin antibiotic in vitro and in vivo studies have been consistently disappointing.[244] The organism is uniformly highly resistant to all of the cephalosporin antibiotics tested. In fact, in one study, such antibiotics were incorporated into the medium to inhibit other bacteria while permitting growth of *Listeria*.[190]

In Vivo Studies

Several combinations of antibiotics,[228, 245–247] or altered methods of preparation such as liposome-entrapment,[248] have been compared for their bactericidal activity against *L. monocytogenes* in vivo. Animal models appear to provide the only practical way to assess therapeutic regimens, because large clinical studies in humans are not available. Murine models employing normal adults,[237, 248, 249] cortisone-treated adults,[250] immunodeficient adults,[251–253] or animals infected by inhalation of aerosolized *Listeria*[237] have been reported. A rabbit model using animals injected intracisternally with *Listeria* has also been described.[254] The model most analogous to neonatal disease was described by Hawkins and colleagues.[255] In their study, neonatal rats were injected intraperitoneally with bacteria and then randomized to begin antibiotic regimens 2 days later.

Interpretation of in vivo models is difficult because conflicting results have been reported. In addition to variability accounted for by technique (e.g., route of injection, bacterial strain, inoculum size), consideration should also be given to the pharmacokinetics for each antibiotic in the various animal species. For example, animal species differ widely in their metabolism of rifampin,[254–256] and the half-life of ampicillin is much longer in human neonates than in most of the adult animal models where it has been assessed. In one study involving adult mice infected with a virulent strain of *L. monocytogenes*, no synergy was demonstrated using a combination of ampicillin and gentamicin.[257] However, in the in vivo model of neonatal listeriosis described by Hawkins and associates, the combination of ampicillin with gentamicin gave significantly better eradication of organisms in spleen compared with ampicillin alone.[255] Similarly, the combination trimethoprim-sulfamethoxazole was found to be superior to either drug alone.[255] Reports of efficacy of other antibiotics in vivo are conflicting. Rifampin has been found by some authors to be highly effective in eradicating organisms,[237, 256] whereas others have found it to be ineffective.[258] Sensitivity of individual strains to rifampin may account for the widely discrepant results. Also, rifampin resistance may develop in vivo when it is used as a single drug. The use of ciprofloxacin in animal models has not suggested any therapeutic advantage over ampicillin.[250, 259]

Clinical Reports

There have been no prospective clinical trials reported for *L. monocytogenes* human infection. Anecdotal reports of single cases or reviews of outbreaks support the conclusions drawn from in vivo models. In one review of clinical management of 119 cases of listeriosis from three centers in the United States, excellent therapeutic results were seen for patients treated empirically with penicillin or ampicillin; all had a reduction of fever and clinical improvement. However, patients treated initially with cephalosporins had persistent fever and infection.[259] In the largest assessment of treatment regimens during a single outbreak,[260] a lower mortality was reported for children given ampicillin (16% of 57 children) compared with those treated with chloramphenicol, tetracycline, or streptomycin (33% of 82 children). As summarized by McLauchlin,[232] there have been several reports of treatment failure and recurrent human listeriosis. In some cases, weeks or months elapse between episodes. Patients have been treated with bacteriostatic (erythromycin) or β-lactam antibiotics during initial treatment. Nevertheless, in the absence of controlled clinical trials, a definitive recommendation for treatment cannot be made.

Suggested Management

LISTERIOSIS DURING PREGNANCY

If amnionitis is present, initial treatment should be given by the intravenous route to ensure adequate tissue levels (ampicillin, 4 to 6 g per day divided into four equal doses) plus an aminoglycoside. If amnionitis is not present or if acute symptoms of amnionitis have subsided, oral antibiotics are probably adequate (amoxicillin, 2 to 3 g per day divided into four equal doses). In both situations, treatment should continue for 14 days. If the patient has a significant allergy to ampicillin, therapeutic options are limited. Erythromycin may be given. The estolate form of this drug should be avoided because there is increased liver toxicity during pregnancy. Trimethoprim-sulfamethoxazole should not be used because premature delivery of the infant may occur as a consequence of infection, in which case the drug may be toxic to the infant.

EARLY-ONSET LISTERIOSIS

Ampicillin in combination with an aminoglycoside is the preferred management for early-onset infection. For infants with body weight less than 2000 g, 100 mg/kg per day (divided into two equal doses) should be administered for the first week of life. For infants with body weight of more than 2000 g, 150 mg/kg per day (divided into three equal doses) should be administered for the first week of life. For the second week of life, the appropriate dosages are 150 mg/kg per day and 200 mg/kg per day for infants weighing less than and more than 2000 g body weight, respectively. Aminoglycoside doses vary with the agent chosen. For gentamicin, the suggested dosages are 5 mg/kg per day (divided into two equal doses) for the first week of life and 7.5 mg/kg per day (divided into three equal doses) for the second week of life. Fourteen days of treatment is recommended for early-onset neonatal sepsis due to *L. monocytogenes*; however, a longer course of treatment should be given in the uncommon event of early-onset neonatal listeriosis with meningitis.

LATE-ONSET LISTERIOSIS

Meningitis is commonly present in late-onset listeriosis. Delayed eradication of the organism may be seen in such cases. Ampicillin (200 to 400 mg/kg kg per day divided into four to six equal doses) in combination with an aminoglycoside is recommended. Lumbar punctures should be repeated daily until the organism has been cleared. In the event of delayed clearance (more than 2 days), further investigations are indicated and should include computed tomography or cranial ultrasound evaluation to assess for the presence of cerebritis or intracranial hemorrhage. If the organism is present in the cerebrospinal fluid, the addition of rifampin or use of trimethoprim-sulfamethoxazole may be considered if the organism is sensitive in vitro. Experience with rifampin and trimethoprim-sulfamethoxazole in the neonatal period and with this organism is limited. Cephalosporin antibiotics have no role in treatment because the organism is uniformly resistant. Length of treatment is variable. If prompt clinical improvement and sterilization of cerebrospinal fluid occurs, 10 days of treatment is probably adequate. However, if response is slow, treatment for as long as 21 days may be considered.

PREVENTION AND OUTBREAK MANAGEMENT

Food-borne outbreaks of listeriosis are unpredictable and may occur in a wide geographic area. Therefore, reporting of sporadic cases of listeriosis to public health authorities may be the only method of distinguishing sporadic from epidemic disease. The epidemic threshold is unknown and may be determined only in retrospect. The recent studies suggesting that sporadic listeriosis is also food-borne have important public health implications.[261]

The sampling of foodstuffs associated with sporadic cases of listeriosis is not warranted. Case-control studies to determine potential vehicles of transmission in outbreaks may help define the source, and environmental sampling may be an important part of such outbreak investigations. Strains of *Listeria* from clinical and environmental isolates should be forwarded to a reference laboratory for appropriate epidemiologic typing. At a minimum, serotyping, phage-typing, and multifocus enzyme electrophoresis typing should be performed to characterize the epidemic strain.

During an outbreak of listeriosis, pregnant women presenting with sepsis syndrome or a flu-like illness should be empirically treated with ampicillin and an aminoglycoside after appropriate cultures of blood, rectum, and vagina have been obtained. Amniocentesis for diagnosis of chorioamnionitis may be appropriate.[187] If membranes have ruptured and contamination is suspected, use of selective media may enhance the isolation of *Listeria* from these patients.

Identification of early- or late-onset listeriosis in a newborn nursery should prompt appropriate epidemiologic and clinical history taking from the mother, as well as postpartum cultures of the rectum and vagina. Infection-control precautions with gowning, gloves, and careful hand washing will prevent nosocomial transmission between infected infants and is consistent with current procedures for all forms of neonatal sepsis.

TABLE 27–2
Dietary Recommendations for Preventing Foodborne Listeriosis

For All Persons

1. Thoroughly cook raw food from animal sources (e.g., beef, pork, and poultry).
2. Thoroughly wash raw vegetables before eating.
3. Keep uncooked meats separate from vegetables, cooked foods, and ready-to-eat foods.
4. Avoid consumption of raw (unpasteurized) milk or foods made from raw milk.
5. Wash hands, knives, and cutting boards after handling uncooked foods.

Additional Recommendations for Persons at High Risk[a]

1. Avoid soft cheeses (e.g., Mexican-style feta, Brie, Camembert, and blue veined cheeses). (There is no need to avoid hard cheeses, cream cheese, cottage cheese, or yogurt.)
2. Leftover foods or ready-to-eat foods (e.g., hot dogs) should be reheated until steaming hot before eating.
3. Although the risk for listeriosis associated with foods from delicatessen counters is relatively low, pregnant women and immunosuppressed persons may choose to avoid these foods or to thoroughly reheat cold cuts before eating them.

[a]Persons immunocompromised by illness or medications, pregnant women, and the elderly.
From Centers for Disease Control. Update: Foodborne Listeriosis—United States, 1988–1990. MMWR Morb Mortal Wkly Rep 41:251, 1992.

The recognition that sporadic cases of listeriosis are primarily food-borne has also prompted publication of preventive guidelines by the CDC[262] (Table 27–2). Following these guidelines may be difficult for all pregnant women, and their effectiveness in reducing sporadic cases of perinatal listeriosis will be difficult to ascertain. However, a decrease in the rates of listeriosis in some geographic areas in the United States has been temporally associated with the publication of these guidelines and industry efforts directed at removing foodborne pathogens from the food chain.[262, 263]

References

1. Nyfeldt A. Étiologie de la mononucléose infectieuse. Compt Rend Biol 101:590, 1929.
2. Murray EGD, Webb RA, Swann MBR. A disease of rabbits characterized by a large mononuclear leucocytosis, caused by a hitherto undescribed *Bacillus: Bacterium monocytogenes* (n. sp.). J Pathol Bacteriol 29:407, 1926.
3. Pirie JHH. A new disease of veld rodents, "Tiger River disease." Publ S Afr Inst Med Res 3:163, 1927.
4. Pirie JHH. Change of name for a genus of bacteria. Nature 145:264, 1940.
5. Bille J, Doyle MP. *Listeria* and *Erysipelothrix. In* Balows A, Hausler WJ Jr, Hermann, KL, et al (eds). Manual of Clinical Microbiology, 5th ed. Washington, D.C., American Society of Microbiology, 1991, pp 287–295.
6. Seeliger HPR. Listeriosis. Basel, S Karger, 1961.
7. Peel M, Donachie W, Shaw A. Temperature-dependent expression of flagella of *Listeria monocytogenes* studied by electron microscopy, SDS-PAGE, and Western blotting. J Gen Microbiol 134:2171, 1988.

8. van Netten P, Perales I, van de Moosdijk A, et al. Liquid and solid selected differential media for the detection and enumeration of *L. monocytogenes* on the *Listeria* species. Int J Food Microbiol 8:299, 1989.

9. Gray ML, Stafseth HJ, Thorp F Jr, et al. A new technique for isolating listerellae from the bovine brain. J Bacteriol 55:471, 1948.

10. Seeliger HPR, Jones D. Genus *Listeria*. *In* Sneath PHA, Mair HS, Sharp ME, et al (eds). Berge's Manual of Systematic Bacteriology, vol 2. Baltimore, Williams & Wilkins, 1986.

11. Seeliger HPR, Finger H. Analytical serology of *Listeria*. *In* Kwapinski JBG (ed). Analytical Serology of Microorganisms. New York, John Wiley, 1969, p 549.

12. Jaeger RF, Myers DM. *Listeria monocytogenes*—a study of two strains isolated from human listeriosis. Can J Microbiol 1:12, 1954.

13. Grönroos JA. Cross-reactivity of *Listeria monocytogenes* and *Streptococcus faecalis* types as revealed by agglutination and precipitin tests and immunofluorescent staining. Ann Med Exp Biol Fenn 45:131, 1967.

14. Seeliger HPR, Sulzbacher F. Antigenic relationship between *Listeria monocytogenes* and *Staphylococcus aureus*. Can J Microbiol 2:220, 1956.

15. Welshimer HJ. Staphylococcal antibody production in response to injections with *Listeria monocytogenes*. J Bacteriol 79:456, 1960.

16. Sword CP, Pickett MJ. Isolation and distribution of bacteriophages from *Listeria monocytogenes*. J Gen Microbiol 25:241, 1961.

17. McLauchlin J, Andurier A, Taylor AG. The evaluation of a phage typing system for *Listeria monocytogenes* for use in epidemiologic studies. J Med Microbiol 22:357, 1986.

18. Schlech WF III, Lavigne PM, Bortolussi R, et al. Epidemic listeriosis—evidence for transmission by food. N Engl J Med 308:203, 1983.

19. Piffaretti JC, Kressebuch H, Aeschbacher M, et al. Genetic characterization of clones of bacterium *Listeria monocytogenes* causing epidemic disease. Proc Natl Acad Sci U S A 86:3818, 1989.

20. Graves LM, Swaminathan B, Reeves MW, et al. Ribosomal DNA fingerprinting of *Listeria monocytogenes* using digoxin genum DNA probe. Eur J Epidemiol 7:77, 1991.

21. Carriere C, Allardet-Servent A, Bourg G, et al. DNA polymorphism in strains of *Listeria monocytogenes*. J Clin Microbiol 29:1351, 1991.

22. Slade PJ, Collins-Thompson DL. Differentiation of the genus *Listeria* from other gram-positive species based on low molecular weight (LMW) RNA profiles. J Appl Bacteriol 70:355, 1991.

23. Portnoy DA, Chakraborty T, Goebel W, et al. Molecular determinants of *Listeria monocytogenes* pathogenesis. Infect Immun 60:1263, 1992.

24. Gaillard JL, Berche P, Frehel C, et al. Entry of *L. monocytogenes* into cells is mediated by internallin, a repeat protein reminiscent of surface antigens from gram-positive cocci. Cell 65:1127, 1991.

25. Ireton K, Cossart P. Host-pathogen interactions during entry and actin-based movement of *Listeria monocytogenes*. Ann Rev Genet 31:113–138, 1997.

26. Hess J, Gentschev I, Szalay G, et al. *Listeria monocytogenes* p60 supports host cell invasion by and in vivo survival of attenuated *Salmonella typhimurium*. Infect Immun 63:2047–2053, 1995.

27. Cossart P, Vincente MF, Mengaud J, et al. Listeriolysin O is essential for virulence of *Listeria monocytogenes*: direct evidence by gene complementation. Infect Immun 57:3629, 1989.

28. Portnoy DA, Jacks PS, Hinrichs DJ. Role of hemolysin for the intracellular growth of *Listeria monocytogenes*. J Exp Med 167:1459, 1988.

29. Moors MM, Levitt B, Youngman P, Portnoy DA. Expression of listeriolysin O and ActA by intracellular and extracellular *Listeria monocytogenes*. Infect Immun 67:131–139, 1999.

30. Sun AN, Camilli A, Portnoy DA. Isolation of *Listeria monocytogenes* small plaque mutants defective for intracellular growth and cell-to-cell spread. Infect Immun 58:3770, 1990.

31. Vazquez-Boland J, Kocks C, Dramsi S, et al. Nucleotide sequence of lethicinase operon of *Listeria monocytogenes* and possible role of lethicinase in cell-to-cell spread. Infect Immun 60:219, 1992.

32. Kocks C, Gouin E, Tabouret M, et al. *Listeria monocytogenes* induced actin assembly requires the *actA* gene product, a surface protein. Cell 68:521, 1992.

33. Raveneau J, Jeoffroy C, Beretti JL, et al. Reduced virulence of a *Listeria monocytogenes* phospholipase-deficient mutant obtained by transposon insertion into the zinc metalloproteinase gene. Infect Immun 60:916, 1992.

34. Mengaud J, Dramsi S, Gouin E, et al. Pleotrophic control of *Listeria monocytogenes* virulence factors by a gene that is auto regulated. Mol Microbiol 5:2273, 1991.

35. Domann E, Zechel S, Lingnau A, et al. Identification and characterization of a novel PrfA-regulated gene in *Listeria monocytogenes* whose product, IrpA, is highly homologous to internalin proteins, which contain leucine-rich repeats. Infect Immun 65:101–109, 1997.

36. Liu PV, Bates JL. An extracellular haemorrhagic toxin produced by *Listeria monocytogenes* Can J Microbiol 7:107, 1961.

37. Zipplies G. Über bakterielle Reizstoffe aus *Listeria monocytogenes* und ihre Wirkung am Kaninchen (Intrakutantest). Arch Exp Vet Med 11:816, 1964.

38. McIlwain P, Eveleth DF, Doubly JA. Pharmacologic studies of a toxic cellular component of *Listeria monocytogenes*. Am J Vet Res 25:774, 1964.

39. Patočka F, Mara M, Schindler J. Studies on the pathogenicity of *Listeria monocytogenes*: II. Influence of substances isolated from cell of *Listeria monocytogenes* on experimental listeriosis in white mice. Zentralbl Bakteriol Hyg 174:586, 1959.

40. Wexler H, Oppenheim JD. Isolation, characterization, and biological properties of an endotoxin-like material from the gram-positive organism *Listeria monocytogenes*. Infect Immun 23:845, 1979.

41. Hether NW, Campbell PA, Baker LA, et al. Chemical composition and biologic function of *Listeria monocytogenes* cell wall preparation. Infect Immun 39:1114, 1983.

42. Stanley NF. Studies on *Listeria monocytogenes*: I. Isolation of a monocytosis-producing agent (MPA). Aust J Exp Biol 27:123, 1949.

43. Shum DT, Galsworthy SB. Stimulation of monocyte production by an endogenous mediator induced by a component of *Listeria monocytogenes*. Immunology 46:343, 1982.

44. Welshimer HJ, Donker-Voet, J. *Listeria monocytogenes* in nature. Appl Microbiol 21:516, 1971.

45. Welshimer HJ. Isolation of *Listeria monocytogenes* from vegetation. J Bacteriol 95:300, 1968.

46. Gray ML. Isolation of *Listeria monocytogenes* from silage. Science 132:1767, 1960.

47. Low JC, Renton CP. Septicemia, encephalitis, and abortions in a housed flock of sheep caused by *Listeria monocytogenes* type 1/2. Vet Rec 114:147, 1985.

48. Owen CR, Meis A, Jackson JW, et al. A case of primary cutaneous listeriosis. N Engl J Med 262:1026, 1960.

49. Dijkstra RG, DeVries J. Een bijzonder geval van listeriosis bij een schaap. Tijdschr Diergeneeskd 97:711, 1962.

50. McLauchlin J, Low JC. Primary cutaneous listeriosis in adults: an occupational disease in veterinarians and farmers. Vet Rec 135:615–617, 1994.

51. Elischerova K, Stupalova S. Listeriosis in professionally exposed persons. Acta Microbiol Acad Sci Hung 19:379, 1972.

52. Bojsen-Moller J. Human listeriosis: diagnostic, epidemiologic and clinical studies. Acta Pathol Microbiol Scand 229(Suppl):1, 1992.

53. Potel J. Atiologie der granulomatosis infantiseptica. Wissenschatt Z Martin Luther Univ 3:341, 1953.

54. Fleming DW, Cochi SL, MacDonald KL, et al. Pasteurized milk as a vehicle of infection in an outbreak of listeriosis. N Engl J Med 312:404, 1985.

55. Linnan JM, Mascola L, Lou XD, et al. Epidemic listeriosis associated with Mexican-style cheese. N Engl J Med 319:823, 1988.

56. Bille J, Rocourt J, Mean F, et al. Epidemic foodborne listeriosis in western Switzerland: II. Epidemiology. Presented at the 28th Interscience Conference on Antimicrobial Agents and Chemotherapy, October 23–26, 1988, Los Angeles, Calif (abstract 1107).

57. McLauchlin J, Hall SM, Velani SK, Gilbert RJ. Human listeriosis and pate: a possible association. BMJ 303:773–775, 1991.

58. Multistate outbreak of listeriosis—United States, 1998. MMWR Morbid Mortal Wkly Rep 47:1985–1986, 1998.

59. Lepoutre A, Moyse C, Roure C, et al. Epidemie de listerioses en France. Bull Epidemiol Hebdonv 25:115, 1992.

60. Schwartz B, Hexter D, Broome CV, et al. Investigation of an outbreak of listeriosis: new hypothesis for the etiology of epidemic Listeria monocytogenes infections. J Infect Dis 159:680, 1989.

61. McLaughlin J, Greenwood MH, Pini PM. The occurrence of Listeria monocytogenes in cheese from a manufacturer associated with a case of listeriosis. Int J Food Microbiol 10:255, 1990.

62. Schuchat A, Deaver K, Wenger JD, et al. Role of foods in sporadic listeriosis: I. Case-control study of dietary risk factors. JAMA 267:2041, 1992.

63. Pinner RW, Schuchat A, Swaminathan B, et al. Role of foods in sporadic listeriosis: II. Microbiologic and epidemiologic investigations. JAMA 267:2046, 1992.

64. Schlech WF III. Listeriosis: epidemiology, virulence and the significance of contaminated foodstuffs. J Hosp Infect 19:211, 1991.

65. Bojsen-Miller J. Human listeriosis: diagnostic, epidemiologic and clinical studies. Acta Pathol Microbiol Scand 229(Suppl):72, 1972.

66. Mascola L, Sorvillo F, Goulet V, et al. Fecal carriage of Listeria monocytogenes: observations during a community-wide, common-source outbreak. Clin Infect Dis 15:557–558, 1992.

67. Gellin BG, Broome CV, Bibb WF, et al. The epidemiology of listeriosis in the United States—1986. Am J Epidemiol 133:392, 1991.

68. Paul ML, Dwyer DE, Chow C, et al. Listeriosis—a review of eighty-four cases. Med J Aust 160:489–493, 1994.

69. Newton F, Hall SM, Pellerin N, et al. Listeriosis surveillance: 1990. CDR 1:R110, 1991.

70. Fredericksen B, Samuelsson S. Vito-maternalistic listeriosis in Denmark 1981–1988. J Infect 24:277, 1992.

71. Varughese PV, Carter AO. Human listeriosis in Canada—1988. Can Dis Wkly Rep 15:213, 1989.

72. Schmidt-Wolf G, Seeliger HPR, Schrettenbrunner A. Menschliche listeriosise-erkrankungen in der Bundesrepublik Deutschland, 1969–1985. Zentralbl Bakteriol Hyg 472, 1985.

73. McLaughlin J. Human listeriosis in Britain, 1967–1985, a summary of 722 cases: 1. Listeriosis during pregnancy and the newborn. Epidemiol Infect 104:181, 1990.

74. Lamont RJ, Postlethwaite R. Carriage of Listeria monocytogenes and related species in pregnant and non-pregnant women in Aberdeen, Scotland. J Infect 13:187, 1986.

75. Louria DB, Hentle T, Armstrong D, et al. Listeriosis complicating malignant disease: a new association. Ann Intern Med 67:261, 1967.

76. Schuchat A, Broome CV, Swaminathan B. Epidemiology of human listeriosis. Clin Microbiol Rev 4:169, 1991.

77. Lorber B. Listeriosis. Clin Infect Dis 24:1–9, 1997.

78. Miller JK, Hedberg M. Effects of cortisone on susceptibility of mice to Listeria monocytogenes. Am J Clin Pathol 43:248, 1965.

79. Hugin AW, Cerny A, Wrann M, et al. Effect of cyclosporin A on immunity to Listeria monocytogenes. Infect Immun 52:12, 1986.

80. Petit JC, Richard G, Burghoffer B, et al. Suppression of cellular immunity to Listeria monocytogenes by activated macrophages: mediation by prostaglandins. Infect Immun 49:383, 1985.

81. Stamm AM, Dismukes WE, Simmons BP, et al. Listeriosis in renal transplant recipients: report of an outbreak and review of 102 cases. Rev Infect Dis 4:665, 1982.

82. Gellin BG, Broome CV. Listeriosis. JAMA 261:1313, 1989.

83. Nieman RE, Lorber B. Listeriosis in adults: a changing pattern. Report of eight cases and review of the literature, 1968–1978. Rev Infect Dis 2:207, 1980.

84. Schlech WF III, Chase DP, Badley A. A model of foodborne Listeria monocytogenes infection in the Sprague-Dawley rats using gastric inoculation: development and effect of gastric acidity on infective dose. Int J Food Microbiol 18:15, 1993.

85. Ho JL, Shands KN, Friedland G, et al. An outbreak of type 4b Listeria monocytogenes infection involving patients from eight Boston hospitals. Arch Intern Med 145:520, 1986.

86. Florman AL, Sundararajan V. Listeriosis among nursery mates. Pediatrics 41:784, 1968.

87. Larson S. Listeria monocytogenes causing hospital-acquired enterocolitis and meningitis in newborn infants. BMJ 2:473, 1978.

88. Filice GA, Cantrell HF, Smith AB, et al. Listeria monocytogenes infection in neonates: investigation of an epidemic. J Infect Dis 138:17, 1978.

89. Campbell AN, Sill PR, Wardle JK. Listeria meningitis acquired by cross-infection in a delivery suite. Lancet 2:752, 1981.

90. Nelson KE, Warren D, Tomasi AM, et al. Transmission of neonatal listeriosis in a delivery room. Am J Dis Child 139:903, 1985.

91. Simmons MD, Cockcroft PM, Okubadejo OA. Neonatal listeriosis due to cross-infection in an obstetric theatre. J Infect 13:235, 1986.

92. Schuchat A, Lizano C, Broome CV, et al. Outbreak of neonatal listeriosis associated with mineral oil. Pediatr Infect Dis J 10:183, 1991.

93. Mitsuyama M, Takeya K, Nomoto K, et al. Three phases of phagocyte contribution to resistance against Listeria monocytogenes. J Gen Microbiol 106:165, 1978.

94. Cossart P, Mengaud J. Listeria monocytogenes: a model

system for the molecular study of intracellular parasitism. Mol Biol Med 6:463, 1989.

95. Lu CY. The delayed ontogenesis of Ia-positive macrophages: implications for host defense and self-tolerance in the neonate. Clin Invest Med 7:263, 1984.

96. Denis M. Growth of *Listeria monocytogenes* in murine macrophages and its modulation by cytokines; activation of bactericidal activity by interleukin-4 and interleukin-6. Can J Microbiol 37:253, 1991.

97. Gregory SH, Sagnimeni AJ, Wing EJ. Expression of the *inlAB* operon by *Listeria monocytogenes* is not required for entry into hepatic cells in vivo. Infect Immun 64:3983–3986, 1996.

98. Marquis H, Doshi V, Portnoy DA. The broad-range phospholipase C and a metalloprotease mediate listeriolysin O–independent escape of *Listeria monocytogenes* from a primary vacuole in human epithelial cells. Infect Immun 63:4531–4534, 1995.

99. Jones S, Portnoy DA. Characterization of *Listeria monocytogenes* pathogenesis in a strain expressing perfringolysin O in place of listeriolysin O. Infect Immun 62:5608–5613, 1994.

100. Bouwer HGA, Gibbins BL, Jones S, Hinrichs DJ. Antilisterial immunity includes specificity to listeriolysin O (LLO) and non–LLO-derived determinants. Infect Immun 62:1039–1045, 1994.

101. Southwick FS, Purich DL. Intracellular pathogenesis of listeriosis. N Engl J Med 334:770–776, 1996.

102. De Chastellier C, Berche P. Fate of *Listeria monocytogenes* in murine macrophages: evidence for simultaneous killing and survival of intracellular bacteria. Infect Immun 62:543–553, 1994.

103. McGregor DD, Chen-Woan M. The cell response to *Listeria monocytogenes* is mediated by a heterogeneous population of immunospecific T cells. Invest Med 7:243, 1984.

104. Shen H, Miller JF, Fan X, et al. Compartmentalization of bacterial antigens: differential effects on priming of CD8 T cells and protective immunity. Cell 92:535–545, 1998.

105. Kaufmann SHE, Ladel CH. Application of knockout mice to the experimental analysis of infections with bacteria and protozoa. Trends Microbiol 2:235–242, 1994.

106. Havell EA, Spitalny GL, Patel PJ. Enhanced production of murine interferon gamma by T-cells generated in response to bacterial infection. J Exp Med 156:112, 1982.

107. Hsieh C-S, Macatonia SE, Tripp CS, et al. Development of T_H^1 CD4$^+$ T cells through IL-12 produced by *Listeria*-induced macrophages. Science 206:547–549, 1993.

108. Serody JS, Poston RM, Weinstock D, et al. CD4$^+$ cytolytic effectors are inefficient in the clearance of *Listeria monocytogenes*. Immunology 88:544–550, 1996.

109. Harty JT, Bevan MJ. CD8 T-cell recognition of macrophages and hepatocytes results in immunity to *Listeria monocytogenes*. Infect Immun 64:3632–3640, 1996.

110. Conlan JW, North RJ. Early pathogenesis of infection in the liver with the facultative intracellular bacteria *Listeria monocytogenes*, *Francisella tularensis*, and *Salmonella typhimurium* involves lysis of infected hepatocytes by leukocytes. Infect Immun 60:5164–5171, 1992.

111. Chen-Woan M, McGregor DD, Noonan SK. Isolation and characterization of protective T cells induced by *Listeria monocytogenes*. Infect Immun 52:401, 1986.

112. Chen-Woan M, McGregor DD, Goldschneider I. Activation of *Listeria monocytogenes–induced* prekiller T cells by interleukin-2. Clin Invest Med 7:287, 1984.

113. Kaufmann SHE, Hug E, de Libero G. *Listeria monocytogenes*–reactive T lymphocyte clones with cytolytic activity against infected target cells. J Exp Med 164:363, 1986.

114. Guo Y, Neisel DW, Ziegler HK, et al. *Listeria monocytogenes* activation of human peripheral blood lymphocytes: induction of non–major histocompatibility complex–restricted cytotoxic activity and cytokine production. Infect Immun 60:1813, 1992.

115. Conlan W, North R. Neutrophil-mediated lysis of infected hepatocytes: selective lysis of permissive host cells is a strategy for controlling intracellular infection in the liver parenchyma. Am Soc Microbiol News 59:563–567, 1993.

116. Boockvar KS, Granger DL, Poston RM, et al. Nitric oxide produced during murine listeriosis is protective. Infect Immun 62:1089–1100, 1994.

117. Beckerman KP, Rogers HW, Corbett JA, et al. Release of nitric oxide during the T cell–independent pathway of macrophage activation: its role in resistance to *Listeria monocytogenes*. J Immunol 150:888–895, 1993.

118. Cheers C, Haigh AM, Kelso A, et al. Production of colony-stimulating factors (CSFs) during infection: separate determinations of macrophage-, granulocyte-, granulocyte-macrophage-, and multi-CSFs. Infect Immun 56:247, 1988.

119. Nakane A, Minagawa T, Kohanawa M, et al. Interactions between endogenous gamma interferon and tumor necrosis factor in host resistance against primary and secondary *Listeria monocytogenes* infections. Infect Immun 57:3331, 1989.

120. Nakane A, Numata A, Minagawa T. Suppression of host resistance against *Listeria monocytogenes* infection by 15-deoxyspergualin in mice. Immunology 71:560, 1990.

121. Havell EA. Production of tumor necrosis factor during murine listeriosis. J Immunol 139:4225, 1987.

122. Desiderio JV, Kiener PA, Lin P-F, et al. Protection of mice against *Listeria monocytogenes* infection by recombinant human tumor necrosis factor alpha. Infect Immun 57:1615, 1989.

123. Havell EA. Evidence that tumor necrosis factor has an important role in antibacterial resistance. J Immunol 143:2894, 1989.

124. Nakane A, Minagawa T, Kato K. Endogenous tumor necrosis factor (cachetin) is essential to host resistance against *Listeria monocytogenes* infection. Infect Immun 56:2563, 1988.

125. Roll JT, Young KM, Kurtz RS, et al. Human rTNFα augments anti-bacterial resistance in mice: potentiation of its effects by recombinant human rIL-1α. Immunology 69:316, 1990.

126. van Furth R, van Zwet TL, Buisman AM, van Dissel JT. Anti–tumor necrosis factor antibodies inhibit the influx of granulocytes and monocytes into an inflammatory exudate and enhance the growth of *Listeria monocytogenes* in various organs. J Infect Dis 170:234–237, 1994.

127. Wagner RD, Czuprynski CJ. Cytokine mRNA expression in livers of mice infected with *Listeria monocytogenes*. J Biol 53:525–531, 1993.

128. Buchmeier NA, Schreiber RD. Requirement of endogenous interferon-gamma production for resolution of *Listeria monocytogenes* infection. Proc Natl Acad Sci U S A 82:7404, 1985.

129. Murray HW. Interferon-gamma, the activated macrophage, and host defense against microbial challenge. Ann Intern Med 108:595, 1988.

130. Tsukada H, Kawamura I, Arakawa M, et al. Dissociated development of T cells mediating delayed-type hypersensitivity and protective T cells against *Listeria monocyto*-

genes and their functional difference in lymphokine production. Infect lmmun 59:3589, 1991.

131. Havell E. Augmented induction of interferons during *Listeria monocytogenes* infection. J Infect Dis 153:960, 1986.

132. Kiderlen AF, Kaufmann SHE, Lohmann-Matthes M-L. Protection of mice against the intracellular bacterium *Listeria monocytogenes* by recombinant immune interferon. Eur J Immunol 14:964, 1984.

133. Grau GE, Taylor TE, Molyneux ME, et al. Tumor necrosis factor and disease severity in children with falciparum malaria. N Engl J Med 320:1586, 1989.

134. Bermudez LEM, Young LS. Tumor necrosis factor, alone or in combination with IL-2, but not IFN-γ, is associated with macrophage killing of *Mycobacterium avium* complex. J Immunol 140:3006, 1988.

135. Black CM, Israelski DM, Suzuki Y, et al. Effect of recombinant tumor necrosis factor on acute infection in mice with *Toxoplasma gondii* or *Trypanosoma cruzi*. Immunology 68:570, 1989.

136. Djeu JY. Role of tumor necrosis factor and colony-stimulating factors in phagocyte function against *Candida albicans*. Diagn Microbiol Infect Dis 13:383, 1990.

137. Flesch IEA, Kaufmann SHE. Activation of tuberculostatic macrophage functions by gamma interferon, interleukin-4, and tumor necrosis factor. Infect Immun 58:2675, 1990.

138. Reiner NE, Ng W, Wilson CB, et al. Modulation of *in vitro* monocyte cytokine responses to *Leishmania donovani*. Interferon-γ prevents parasite-induced inhibition of interleukin-1 production and primes monocytes to respond to *Leishmania* by producing both tumor necrosis factor-α and TNF-α. J Clin Invest 85:1914, 1990.

139. Bazzoni F, Beutler B. The tumor necrosis factor ligand and receptor families. N Engl J Med 334:1717–1725, 1996.

140. Ostensen ME, Theile DL, Lipsky PE. Tumor necrosis factor-α enhances cytolytic activity of human natural killer cells. J Immunol 138:4185, 1987.

141. Sung SS, Jung LK, Walters JA, et al. Production of tumor necrosis factor cachectin by human B cell lines and tonsillar B cells. J Exp Med 168:1539, 1988.

142. Balkwill FR, Burke F. The cytokine network. Immunol Today 10:299, 1989.

143. Rosenblum MG, Donato NJ. Tumor necrosis factor-α multifaceted peptide hormone. Crit Rev Immunol 9:21, 1989.

144. Chouaib S, Branellec D, Buurman WA. More insights into the complex physiology of TNF. Immunol Today 12:141, 1991.

145. Stokes DC, Shenep JL, Fishman M, et al. Polymyxin B prevents lipopolysaccharide-induced release of tumor necrosis factor-α from alveolar macrophages. J Infect Dis 160:52, 1989.

146. Ferrante A, Staugas REM, Rowan-Kelly B, et al. Production of tumor necrosis factors alpha and beta by human mononuclear leukocytes stimulated with mitogens, bacteria, and malarial parasites. Infect Immun 58:3996, 1990.

147. Michie HR, Manogue KR, Spriggs DR, et al. Detection of circulating tumor necrosis factor after endotoxin administration. N Engl J Med 318:1481, 1988.

148. Galleli A, LeGarreo Y, Chadid L. Increased resistance and depressed delayed-type hypersensitivity to *Listeria monocytogenes* induced by pretreatment with lipopolysaccharide. Infect Immun 31:88, 1981.

149. Bortolussi R, Rajaraman K, Serushago B. Role of tumor necrosis factor-alpha and interferon gamma in newborn host defense against *Listeria monocytogenes* infection. Pediatr Res 32:460, 1992.

150. Brunda MJ. Interleukin-12. J Leukoc Biol 55:280–288, 1994.

151. McKay D, Lu C. Listeriolysin as a virulence factor in *Listeria monocytogenes* infection of neonatal mice and murine decidual tissue. Infect Immun 59:4286, 1991.

152. Bortolussi R. Neonatal listeriosis. Semin Perinatol 14:44, 1990.

153. Lu CY, Unanue ER. Ontogeny of murine macrophages: functions related to antigen presentation. Infect Immun 36:169, 1982.

154. Lu CY, Calamai EG, Unanue ER. A defect in the antigen-presenting function of macrophages from neonatal mice. Nature 282:327, 1979.

155. Kohl S. The neonatal human's immune response to herpes simplex virus infection: a critical review. Pediatr Infect Dis J 8:67, 1989.

156. Wilson CB. The ontogeny of T lymphocyte maturation and function. J Pediatr 118:S4, 1991.

157. Issekutz TB, Evans J, Bortolussi R. The immune response of human neonates to *Listeria monocytogenes* infection. Clin Invest Med 7:281, 1984.

158. Kurland G, Cheung ATW, Miller ME, et al. The ontogeny of pulmonary defenses: alveolar macrophage function in neonatal and juvenile rhesus monkeys. Pediatr Res 23:293, 1988.

159. Bellanti JA, Nerurkar LS, Zeligs BJ. Host defenses in the fetus and neonate: studies of the alveolar macrophage during maturation. Pediatrics 64:726, 1979.

160. McDonald T, Sneed J, Valenski WR, et al. Natural killer cell activity in very low birth weight infants. Pediatr Res 31:376, 1992.

161. Dominguez E, Madrigal JA, Layriss Z, Cohen SB. Fetal natural killer cell function is suppressed. Immunology 94:109–114, 1998.

162. Lee SM, Suen Y, Chang L, et al. Decreased interleukin-12 (IL-12) from activated cord versus adult peripheral blood mononuclear cells and upregulation of interferon-gamma, natural killer and lymphokine-activated killer activity by IL-12 in cord blood mononuclear cells. Blood 88:945–954, 1996.

163. Lau AS, Sigaroudinia M, Yeung MC, Kohl S. Interleukin-12 induces interferon-γ expression and natural killer cytotoxicity in cord blood mononuclear cells. Pediatr Res 39:150–155, 1996.

164. Bortolussi R, Issekutz T, Burbridge S, et al. Neonatal host defense mechanisms against *Listeria monocytogenes* infection: the role of lipopolysaccharides and interferons. Pediatr Res 25:311, 1989.

165. Murray HW. Gamma interferon, cytokine-induced macrophage activation, and antimicrobial host defense: in vitro, in animal models, and in humans. Diagn Microbiol Infect Dis 13:411, 1990.

166. Cederblad B, Riesenfeld T, Alm GV. Deficient herpes simplex virus–induced interferon-γ production by blood leukocytes of preterm and term newborn infants. Pediatr Res 27:7, 1990.

167. Frenkel L, Bryson YJ. Ontogeny of phytohemagglutinin-induced gamma interferon by leukocytes of healthy infants and children: evidence for decreased production in infants younger than 2 months of age. J Pediatr 111:97, 1987.

168. Lewis DB, Larsen A, Wilson CB. Reduced interferon-gamma mRNA levels in human neonates: evidence for an intrinsic T cell deficiency independent of other genes involved in T cell activation. J Exp Med 163:1018, 1986.

169. Lewis DB, Yu CC, Meyer J, et al. Cellular and molecular

mechanisms for reduced interleukin-4 and interferon-γ production by neonatal T cells. J Clin Invest 87:194, 1991.

170. Bortolussi R, Burbridge S, Durnford P, et al. Neonatal *Listeria monocytogenes* infection is refractory to interferon. Pediatr Res 29:400, 1991.

171. Bortolussi R. *Escherichia coli* infection in neonates: humoral defense mechanisms. Semin Perinatol 14:40, 1990.

172. Bortolussi R, Issekutz A, Faulkner A. Opsonization of *Listeria monocytogenes* type 4b by human adult and newborn sera. Infect Immun 52:493, 1986.

173. Klatt EC, Pavlova Z, Teberg AJ, et al. Epidemic perinatal listeriosis at autopsy. Hum Pathol 17:1278, 1986.

174. Reiss HJ. Zur pathologischen Anatomie der kindlichen Listeriosis. Kinderarztl Prax Separatum 92, 1953.

175. Armstrong RW, Fung PC. Brainstem encephalitis (rhombencephalitis) due to *Listeria monocytogenes*: case report and review. Clin Infect Dis 16:689–702, 1993.

176. Steele PE, Jacobs DS. *Listeria monocytogenes*: macroabscesses of placenta. Obstet Gynecol 53:124, 1979.

177. Topalovski M, Yang S, Boonpasat Y. Listeriosis of the placenta: clinicopathologic study of seven cases. Am J Obstet Gynecol 169:616–620, 1993.

178. Infections and inflammatory lesions of the placenta. *In* Fox H (ed). Pathology of the Placenta, 2nd ed. Toronto, WB Saunders, 1997, pp 309–311.

179. Presentation of case 15-1997. N Engl J Med 336:1439–1446, 1997.

180. Ahlfors CE, Goetzman BW, Halstad CC, et al. Neonatal listeriosis. Am J Dis Child 131:405, 1977.

181. Krause VW, Embree JE, MacDonald SW, et al. Congenital listeriosis causing early neonatal death. Can Med Assoc J 127:36, 1982.

182. Hood M. Listeriosis as an infection of pregnancy manifested in the newborn. Pediatrics 27:390, 1961.

183. Kelly CS, Gibson JL. Listeriosis as a cause of fetal wastage. Obstet Gynecol 40:91, 1972.

184. Redline RW, Lu CY. Specific defects in the anti-listerial immune response in discrete regions of the murine uterus and placenta account for susceptibility to infection. J Immunol 140:3947, 1988.

185. Kalstone C. Successful antepartum treatment of listeriosis. Am J Obstet Gynecol 164:57, 1991.

186. Liner RI. Intrauterine *Listeria* infection: prenatal diagnosis by biophysical assessment and amniocentesis. Am J Obstet Gynecol 163:1596, 1990.

187. Petrilli ES, d'Ablaing G, Ledger WJ. *Listeria monocytogenes* chorioamnionitis: diagnosis by transabdominal amniocentesis. Obstet Gynecol 55:5S, 1964.

188. Loeb MB, Ford-Jones EL, Styliadis S, et al. Perinatal listeriosis. J Soc Obstet Gynecol Can 18:164–170, 1996.

189. Luft BJ, Remington JS. Effect of pregnancy on resistance to *Listeria monocytogenes* and *Toxoplasma gondii* infections in mice. Infect Immun 38:1164, 1982.

190. Bortolussi R, Campbell N, Krause V. Dynamics of *Listeria monocytogenes* type 4b infection in pregnant and infant rats. Clin Invest Med 7:273, 1984.

191. Menu E, Kinsky R, Hoffman M, et al. Immunoactive products of human placenta: IV. Immunoregulatory factors obtained from cultures of human placenta inhibit in vivo local and systemic allogeneic and graft-versus-host reactions in mice. J Reprod Immunol 20:195, 1991.

192. Burn CG. Unidentified gram-positive bacillus associated with meningo-encephalitis. Proc Soc Exp Biol Med 31:1095, 1934.

193. Burn CG. Characteristics of a new species of the genus *Listerella* obtained from human sources. J Bacteriol 30:573, 1935.

194. Burn CG. Clinical and pathological features of an infection caused by a new pathogen of the genus *Listerella*. Am J Pathol 12:341, 1936.

195. Albritton WL, Wiggins GL, Feeley JC. Neonatal listeriosis: distribution of serotypes in relation to age at onset of disease. J Pediatr Infect Dis 4:237, 1976.

196. Evans JR, Allen AC, Stinson DA, et al. Perinatal listeriosis: report of an outbreak. Pediatr Infect Dis J 4:237, 1985.

197. Lennon D, Lewis B, Mantell C, et al. Epidemic perinatal listeriosis. Pediatr Infect Dis J 3:30, 1984.

198. Becroft DMO, Farmer K, Seddon RJ, et al. Epidemic listeriosis in the newborn. BMJ 3:747, 1971.

199. McLachlin J. Human listeriosis in Britain, 1967–85, a summary of 722 cases: I. Listeriosis during pregnancy and the newborn. Epidemiol Infect 104:181–189, 1990.

200. Filice GA, Cantrell HF, Smith AB, et al. *Listeria monocytogenes* infection in neonates: investigation of an epidemic. J Infect Dis 138:17, 1978.

201. Visintine AM, Oleske JM and Nahmias AJ. *Listeria monocytogenes* infection in infants and children. Am J Dis Child 131:339, 1977.

202. Pron B, Boumaila C, Jaubert F, et al. Comprehensive study of the intestinal stage of listeriosis in a rat ligated ileal loop system. Infect Immun 66:747–755, 1998.

203. Dalton CB, Austin CC, Sobel J, et al. An outbreak of febrile gastroenteritis and fever due to *Listeria monocytogenes* in milk. N Engl J Med 336:100–105, 1997.

204. Felsenfeld O. Diseases of poultry transmissible to man. Iowa State Coll Vet 13:89, 1951.

205. Owen RC, Meis A, Jackson JW, et al. A case of primary cutaneous listeriosis. N Engl J Med 262:1026, 1960.

206. Anton W. Kritisch-experimenteller Beitrag zur Biologie des Bacterium-monocytogenes mit besenderer Berücksichtigung seiner Beziehung zur infektiösen Mononukleose des Menschen. Zentralbl Bakteriol Hyg 131:89, 1934.

207. Spyrou N, Anderson M, Foale R. Listeria endocarditis: current management and patient outcome—world literature review. Heart 77:380–383, 1997.

208. Braun TI, Travis D, Dee RR, Nieman RE. Liver abscess due to *Listeria monocytogenes*: case report and review. Clin Infect Dis 17:267–269, 1993.

209. Sivalingam JJ, Martin P, Fraimow HS, et al. *Listeria monocytogenes* peritonitis: case report and literature review. Am J Gastroenterol 87:1839–1845, 1992.

210. Dylewski JS. Bacterial peritonitis caused by *Listeria monocytogenes*: case report and review of the literature. Can J Infect Dis 7:59–62, 1996.

211. Louthrenoo W, Schumacher HR. *Listeria monocytogenes* osteomyelitis complicating leukemia: report and literature review of *Listeria* osteoarticular infections. J Rheumatol 17:107–110, 1990.

212. Riedo FX, Pinner RW, Tosca ML, et al. A point-source foodborne listeriosis outbreak: documented incubation period and possible mild illness. J Infect Dis 170:693–696, 1994.

213. Salamina G, Niccolini A, Dalle Donne E, et al. A foodborne outbreak of gastroenteritis due to *Listeria monocytogenes*. Epidemiol Infect 117:429–436, 1996.

214. Schlech WF. *Listeria* gastroenteritis—old syndrome, new pathogen. N Engl J Med 336:130–132, 1997.

215. Kolmer JA. *Listerella monocytogenes* in relation to the Wasserman and flocculation reactions in normal rabbits. Proc Soc Exp Biol Med 42:183, 1939.

216. Hudak AP, Lee SH, Issekutz AC, et al. Comparison of three serological methods—enzyme-linked immunoabsorbent assay, complement fixation, and microagglu-

tination—in the diagnosis of human perinatal *Listeria monocytogenes* infection. Clin Invest Med 7:349, 1984.

217. Winblad S. Studies of antibodies in human listeriosis. Acta Pathol Microbiol Scand 58:123, 1963.

218. Berche P, Reiche KA, Bonnichon M, et al. Detection of anti-listeriolysin O for serodiagnosis of human listeriosis. Lancet 335:624, 1990.

219. Drew RM. Occurrence of two immunological groups within the genus *Listeria*: studies based upon precipitation reactions. Proc Soc Exp Biol Med 61:30, 1946.

220. Schierz G, Bürger A. The detection of *Listeria* antibodies by passive hemagglutination. Proceedings of the Third International Symposium on Listeriosis, Bilthoven, 1966, p 77.

221. Njoku-Obi AN. An antigen-fixation test for the serodiagnosis of *Listeria monocytogenes* infections. Cornell Vet 52:415, 1962.

222. Kampelmacher EH, Huysinga MT, van Noorle-Jansen ML. Het voorkomen van *Listeria monocytogenes* in faecesvan gravidae en pasgeborenen. Ned Tijdschr Geneeskd 116:1685, 1972.

223. Hune OS. Maternal *Listeria monocytogenes* septicemia with sparing of the fetus. Obstet Gynecol 48:335, 1976.

224. Katz VL, Weinstein L. Antepartum treatment of *Listeria monocytogenes* septicemia. South Med J 75:1353, 1982.

225. Fuchs S, Hochner-Celnikier D, Shalev O. First trimester listeriosis with normal fetal outcome. Eur J Clin Microbiol Infect Dis 13:656–658, 1994.

226. Rotheberg AD, Maisels MJ, Bagnato S, et al. Outcome for survivors of mechanical ventilation weighing less than 1200 gm at birth. J Pediatr 98:106, 1981.

227. Naege RL. Amnionic fluid infections, neonatal hyperbilirubinemia and psychomotor impairment. Pediatrics 62:497, 1978.

228. Line FG, Appleton FG. *Listeria* meningitis in a premature infant. J Pediatr 41:97, 1952.

229. Evans JR, Allen AC, Bortolussi R, et al. Follow-up study of survivors of fetal and early onset neonatal listeriosis. Clin Invest Med 7:329, 1984.

230. Espaze EP, Roubeix YG, LeBerre JY, et al. In vitro susceptibility of *Listeria monocytogenes* to some antibiotics and their combinations. Zentralbl Bakteriol Hyg 240:76, 1988.

231. Hof H. Therapeutic activities of antibiotics in listeriosis. Infection 19:S229, 1991.

232. McLauchlin J, Audurier A, Taylor AG. Treatment failure and recurrent human listeriosis. J Antimicrob Chemother 27:851, 1991.

233. Watson GW, Fuller TJ, Elms J, et al. *Listeria* cerebritis: relapse of infection in renal transplant patients. Arch Intern Med 138:83, 1978.

234. Hof H. Treatment of experimental listeriosis by CI 934, a new quinolone. J Antimicrob Chemother 25:121, 1990.

235. Spitzer PG, Hammer SM, Karchmer AW. Treatment of *Listeria monocytogenes* infection with trimethoprim-sulfamethoxazole: case report and review of the literature. Rev Infect Dis 8:427, 1986.

236. Winslow DL, Pankey GA. In vitro activities of trimethoprim and sulfamethoxazole against *Listeria monocytogenes*. Antimicrob Agents Chemother 22:51, 1982.

237. Armstrong RW, Slater B. *Listeria monocytogenes* meningitis treated with trimethoprim-sulfamethoxazole. Pediatr Infect Dis J 5:712, 1986.

238. Vischer WA, Rominger C. Rifampicin against experimental listeriosis in the mouse. Chemotherapy 24:104, 1978.

239. Poyart-Salmeran C, Carlier C, Trieu-Cuot P, et al.

Transferable plasmid-mediated antibiotic resistance in *Listeria monocytogenes*. Lancet 355:1422, 1990.

240. MacGowan AP, Holt HA, Bywater MJ, et al. In vitro antimicrobial isolated in the UK and other *Listeria* species. Eur J Clin Microbiol Infect Dis 9:767, 1990.

241. Soriano F, Zapardiel J, Nieto E. Antimicrobial susceptibilities of *Cornebacterium* species and other non–spore-forming gram-positive bacilli to 18 antimicrobial agents. Antimicrob Agents Chemother 39:208–214, 1995.

242. Charpentier E, Gerbaud G, Jacquet C, et al. Incidence of antibiotic resistance in *Listeria* species. J Infect Dis 172:277–281, 1995.

243. Hof H, Nichterlein L, Kretschmar M. Management of listeriosis. Clin Microbiol Rev 10:345–357, 1997.

244. Traub WH. Perinatal listeriosis: tolerance of a clinical isolate of *Listeria monocytogenes* for ampicillin and resistance against cefotaxime. Chemotherapy 27:423, 1981.

245. Gordon RC, Barrett FF, Clark DJ. Influence of several antibiotics, singly and in combination, on the growth of *Listeria monocytogenes*. J Pediatr 80:667, 1972.

246. Lavetter A, Leedom JM, Mathies AW Jr, et al. Meningitis due to *Listeria monocytogenes*: a review of 25 cases. N Engl J Med 285:598, 1971.

247. Eliopoulos GM, Moellering RC. Susceptibility of enterococci and *Listeria monocytogenes* to n-formimidoyl thienamycin alone and in combination with an aminoglycoside. Antimicrob Agents Chemother 19:789, 1981.

248. Fattal E, Rojas J, Youssef M, et al. Liposome-entrapped ampicillin in the treatment of experimental murine listeriosis and salmonellosis. Antimicrob Agents Chemother 35:770, 1991.

249. Edminsten CE, Gordon RC. Evaluation of gentamicin and penicillin as a synergistic combination in experimental murine listeriosis. Antimicrob Agents Chemother 16:862, 1979.

250. VanOgtrop ML, Mattie H, Razab SB, et al. Comparison of the antibacterial efficacies of ampicillin and ciprofloxacin against experimental infections with *Listeria monocytogenes* in hydrocortisone-treated mice. Antimicrob Agents Chemother 36:2375, 1992.

251. Hof P, Emmerling P, Seeliger HPR. Murine model for therapy of listeriosis in the compromised host. Chemotherapy 27:214, 1981.

252. Bakker-Woudenberg IAJM, de Bos P, van Leeuwen WB, et al. Efficacy of ampicillin therapy in experimental listeriosis in mice with impaired T-cell–mediated immune response. Antimicrob Agents Chemother 19:76, 1981.

253. Bakker-Woudenberg IAJM, Lokerse AF, Roerdink FH, et al. Free versus liposome-entrapped ampicillin in treatment of infection due to *Listeria monocytogenes* in normal and athymic (nude) mice. J Infect Dis 151:917, 1985.

254. Scheld WM, Fletcher DD, Fink FN, et al. Response to therapy in an experimental rabbit model of meningitis due to *Listeria monocytogenes*. J Infect Dis 140:287, 1979.

255. Hawkins AE, Bortolussi R, Issekutz AC. In vitro and in vivo activity of various antibiotics against *Listeria monocytogenes* type 4b. Clin Invest Med 7:335, 1984.

256. Dans PE, McGehee RF, Wilcox C, et al. Rifampin: antibacterial activity in vitro and absorption and excretion in normal young men. Am J Med Sci 259:120, 1970.

257. Hof H, Gukel H. Lack of synergism of ampicillin and gentamicin in experimental listeriosis. Infection 15:40, 1987.

258. Scheld WM. Evaluation of rifampin and other antibiotics against *Listeria monocytogenes* in vitro and in vivo. Rev Infect Dis 5:S593, 1983.

259. Cherubin CE, Appleman MD, Heseltine PNR, et al.

Epidemiologic spectrum and current treatment of listeriosis. Rev Infect Dis 13:1108, 1991.

260. Weingartner L, Ortel S. Zur Behandlung der Listeriose mit Ampicillin. Dtsch Med Wochenschr 92:1098, 1967.

261. Schlech WF. Expanding the horizons of foodborne listeriosis. JAMA 267:2081, 1992.

262. Centers for Disease Control. Update: foodborne listeriosis—United States, 1988–1990. MMWR Morbid Mortal Wkly Rep 41:251, 1992.

263. Tappero JW, Schuchat A, Deaver KA, et al. Reduction in the incidence of human listeriosis in the United States. JAMA 273:1118–1122, 1995.

264. Kessler SL, Dajani AS Listeria meningitis in infants and children. Pediatr Infect Dis J 9:61, 1990.

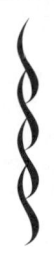

C H A P T E R   2 8

Tuberculosis

JEFFREY R. STARKE, M.D., and MARGARET H. D. SMITH, M.D.

Tuberculosis is a classic familial disease.[1] The household is the main setting throughout the world for the person-to-person spread of *Mycobacterium tuberculosis*. With the recent resurgence of tuberculosis in many industrialized nations, issues concerning pregnant women and their children have been reexamined by practitioners of tuberculosis control.

Before 1985, tuberculosis in the pregnant woman and newborn had become an infrequent event in the United States. Although specific statistics concerning tuberculosis in pregnancy are not reported, the increase in total tuberculosis cases in the late 1980s and 1990s and the shift in numbers to young adults and children imply that tuberculosis in pregnancy may be a more prevalent problem.[2, 3] This problem disproportionately affects minority urban populations because they have very high tuberculosis case rates, a greater relative shift in cases to adults of childbearing age, and, in general, less access to prenatal care and screening for tuberculosis disease and infection.

The influence of pregnancy on the occurrence and prognosis of tuberculosis has been discussed and debated for centuries. At various times, pregnancy has been thought to improve, worsen, or have no effect on the prognosis of tuberculosis. This controversy has lost much of its importance since the advent of effective antituberculosis chemotherapy. The greatest area of debate at present concerns the use of chemotherapy to prevent the progression of *M. tuberculosis* infection to tuberculosis during pregnancy and the postpartum period.

TERMINOLOGY

A practical approach to tuberculosis terminology is to follow the natural history of the disease, which can be divided into three stages: exposure, infection, and disease.[4] Exposure implies that the patient has had recent (less than 3 months) and significant contact with an adult with suspected or confirmed contagious pulmonary tuberculosis. For example, an infant born into a family in which an adult has active tuberculosis would be in the exposure stage. In this stage, the child's tuberculin skin test is negative, the chest radiograph result is normal, and the child is free of signs and symptoms of tuberculosis. Unfortunately, it is impossible to know whether a young child in the exposure stage is truly infected with *M. tuberculosis*, because the development of delayed-type hypersensitivity to a skin test for tuberculin may take up to 3 months after the organisms have been inhaled.

M. tuberculosis infection is present if an individual has a positive tuberculin skin test result but lacks signs or symptoms of tuberculosis. In this stage, findings on the chest radiograph either are normal or reveal only granuloma or calcification in the lung parenchyma or regional lymph nodes. The purpose of treating *M. tuberculosis* infection is to prevent future disease. In newborns, the progression from infection to disease can occur very rapidly, within several weeks to months.

Tuberculosis disease occurs if signs or symptoms or radiographic manifestations caused by *M. tuberculosis* become apparent. Because 25 to 35% of children with tuberculosis have extrapulmonary involvement, a thorough physical examination, in addition to a high-quality chest radiograph, is essential to rule out disease.[4] Genitourinary tuberculosis in women often causes only subtle symptoms until it is far advanced. Ten to 20% of immunocompetent adults and children with tuberculosis disease initially have a negative tuberculin skin test result, usually because of immunosuppression from tuberculosis itself. The rate of negative skin test results with tuberculosis disease, however, is much higher in newborns and small infants, especially if they have life-threatening forms of tuberculosis such as disseminated disease or meningitis.

MYCOBACTERIOLOGY

Mycobacteria are nonmotile, non–spore-forming pleomorphic, weakly gram-positive rods that are 1 to 5 μm long, usually slender, and slightly curved. *M. tuberculosis* may appear beaded or clumped. The cell wall constituents of mycobacteria determine their most striking biologic properties. The cell wall is composed of 20 to 60% lipids bound to proteins and carbohydrates. These and other properties make mycobacteria more resistant than most other bacteria to light, alkali, acid, and the bactericidal activity of antibodies. Growth of *M. tuberculosis* is slow, with a generation time of 12 to 24 hours.

Acid-fastness, the capacity to form stable mycolate complexes with certain aryl methane dyes that are not removed even by rinsing with 95% ethanol plus hydrochloric acid, is the hallmark of mycobacteria. The cells appear red when stained with carbol fuchsin (Ziehl-Neelsen or Kinyoun stains) or purple with crystal violet or exhibit yellow-green fluorescence under ultraviolet light when stained with auramine and rhodamine (Truant stain). Truant stain is considered the most sensitive stain, especially when small numbers of organisms are present. Approximately 10,000 cells per mm^3 must be present in a sample for them to be seen in an acid-fast stained smear.

Identification of mycobacteria depends on their staining properties and their biochemical and metabolic characteristics. Mycobacteria are obligate aerobes with simple growth requirements. *M. tuberculosis* can grow in classic media, whose essential ingredients are egg yolk and glycerin (Löwenstein-Jensen or Dorset media) or simple synthetic media (Middlebrook, Tween-albumin). Isolation on solid media takes 2 to 6 weeks, followed by another 2 to 4 weeks for drug-susceptibility testing. More rapid isolation (7 to 21 days) can be achieved using synthetic liquid medium in an automated radiometric system, the most common one being BACTEC (Becton-Dickinson, Towson, Md). A specimen is inoculated into a bottle of medium containing carbon-14–labeled palmitic acid as a substrate. As mycobacteria metabolize the palmitic acid, carbon dioxide-14 accumulates in the head space of the bottle, where radioactivity can be measured. Unfortunately, because bottles are often analyzed in series by repetitive needle aspiration in an automated, single-needle system, cross-contamination leading to a false-positive culture can occur. Drug susceptibility test-

ing can be performed on the same system using bottles with antimicrobial agents added to the medium. In this radiometric system, identification and drug-susceptibility testing often can be completed in 2 to 3 weeks, depending on the concentration of organisms in the patient sample.

Several types of nucleic acid amplification have been developed to detect *M. tuberculosis* in patient samples. The main form of nucleic acid amplification studied in children with tuberculosis is the polymerase chain reaction (PCR), which uses specific DNA sequences as markers for microorganisms. Various PCR techniques, most using the mycobacterial insertion element IS6110 as the DNA marker for *M. tuberculosis* complex organisms, have a sensitivity and specificity of more than 90% compared with sputum culture for detecting pulmonary tuberculosis in adults. However, test performance varies even among reference laboratories. The test is relatively expensive and requires fairly sophisticated equipment and scrupulous technique to avoid cross-contamination of specimens.

Use of PCR in childhood tuberculosis has been limited. Compared with a clinical diagnosis of pulmonary tuberculosis in children, sensitivity of PCR has varied from 25 to 83% and specificity has varied from 80 to 100%.[5] The PCR of gastric aspirates may be positive in a recently infected child even when the chest roentgenogram is normal, demonstrating the occasional arbitrariness of the distinction between *M. tuberculosis* infection and disease in children. The PCR may have a useful but limited role in evaluating children for tuberculosis. A negative PCR never eliminates tuberculosis as a diagnostic possibility, and a positive result does not confirm it. The major use of PCR will be in evaluating children with significant pulmonary disease when the diagnosis is not established readily on clinical or epidemiologic grounds. PCR particularly may be helpful in evaluating immunocompromised children with pulmonary disease, especially for children with human immunodeficiency virus (HIV) infection, although published reports of its performance in such children are lacking. PCR also may aid in confirming the diagnosis of extrapulmonary tuberculosis, although only a few case reports have been published. No information has been published concerning the accuracy of PCR or other techniques of nucleic acid amplification in samples from pregnant women or neonates with congenital or postnatally acquired tuberculosis.

Relatedness of strains of *M. tuberculosis* was determined in the past by analysis of bacteriophages, a cumbersome and difficult task. A newer technique, restriction fragment length polymorphism analysis of mycobacterial DNA, has become an accurate and powerful tool for determining strain relatedness. It is used frequently in some communities and may help determine if an infant with tuberculosis has true congenital infection or was infected by another source.

EPIDEMIOLOGY

Tuberculosis remains the leading infectious disease in the world.[6] The World Health Organization (WHO) estimates that during the 1990s 90 million individuals developed tuberculosis and 30 million people died of the disease worldwide. The WHO also estimates that, in the developing world, there are 1.3 million cases of tuberculosis and 400,000 tuberculosis-related deaths annually among children younger than 15 years of age. In most developing countries, the highest rates of tuberculosis occur among young adult men and women. Although much attention has been given recently to the growing number of children orphaned in developing countries by their parents' deaths from HIV-related illnesses, many orphans also are being created by tuberculosis.

In the United States from 1953 through 1984, the incidence of tuberculosis disease declined an average of 5% per year. From 1985 through 1992, there was a 20% increase in total cases of tuberculosis in the United States and a 40% increase in tuberculosis cases among children.[7] Most experts cite four major factors contributing to this increase: (1) the co-epidemic of HIV infection,[8] which is the strongest risk factor known for development of tuberculosis disease in an adult infected with *M. tuberculosis*; (2) the increase in immigration of people to the United States from countries with a high prevalence of tuberculosis, enlarging the pool of infected individuals[9, 10]; (3) the increased transmission of *M. tuberculosis* in congregate settings, such as jails, prisons, hospitals, nursing homes, and homeless shelters; and (4) the general decline in tuberculosis-related public health services and access to medical care for the indigent in many communities.[11]

In the early twentieth century, when tuberculosis was more prevalent, the risk of becoming infected with *M. tuberculosis* was high across the entire population. Currently, tuberculosis has retreated into fairly well-defined pockets of high-risk individuals, such as foreign-born persons from or persons who travel to high-prevalence countries; inmates of correctional institutions; illicit drug users; health care workers who care for high-risk patients; migrant families; homeless persons; and anyone likely to encounter people with contagious tuberculosis. One must distinguish the risk factors for becoming infected with *M. tuberculosis* from those that increase the likelihood that an infected individual will develop disease. Immune compromise and recent infection with *M. tuberculosis* are the major risk factors for progression of infection to disease. Although tuberculosis occurs throughout the United States, cases are disproportionately reported from large urban areas. Cities with populations exceeding 250,000 account for only 18% of the nation's population but almost 50% of its tuberculosis cases.

The number of tuberculosis cases in the United States is increasing among foreign-born persons from countries with a high prevalence of tuberculosis. The percentage of total cases of tuberculosis in the United States that occurs in foreign-born individuals has increased from 22% in 1986 to 42% in 1998.[10] In previous estimates, two thirds of foreign-born individuals with tuberculosis were younger than age 35 years when entering the United States and, in many cases, their disease could have been prevented if they had been identified as infected after immigration and given appropriate treatment for *M. tuberculosis* infection. Unfortunately, new immigrants to the United States older than 15 years of age are required to have a chest radiograph but no tuberculin skin test to detect asymptomatic infection; children younger than 15 years old receive no tuberculosis testing as part of immigration.[12] Studies have estimated that 30 to 50% of the almost 1 million annual new immigrants to the United States are infected with *M. tuberculosis*.[10] Clearly, foreign-born women and adolescents of childbearing age should be one group targeted for appropriate tuberculosis screening and prevention.[13]

Another factor that has had a great impact on tuberculosis case rates in the United States has been the epidemic of HIV infection.[8] The proportion of women with HIV infection is increasing, and because risk factors for HIV infection intersect with those for tuberculosis the number of co-infected women will increase.[14–16] In most locales experiencing recent increases in tuberculosis cases, the demographic groups with the greatest tuberculosis morbidity rates are the same as those with high morbidity rates from HIV infection. HIV-infected persons with a reactive tuberculin skin test develop tuberculosis at a rate of 5 to 10% per year compared with a historical average of 5 to 10% for the lifetime of an immunocompetent adult.

The current epidemiology of tuberculosis in pregnancy is unknown. From 1966 to 1972, the incidence of tuberculosis during pregnancy at New York Lying-In Hospital ranged from 0.6 to 1.0%.[17] During this time, 3.2% of the patients with culture-proven pulmonary tuberculosis were first diagnosed during pregnancy, a rate equal to that of nonpregnant women of comparable age. There have been only two series of pregnant women with tuberculosis reported from the United States in the past two decades.[18, 19] It is likely, however, that the number of women in the United States at risk for tuberculosis during or after pregnancy has increased over the past 10 years. The increased risk is most striking for foreign-born women, who have high rates of tuberculosis infection, and poor minority women. In the United States, almost 40% of tuberculosis cases in minority women occur before 35 years of age. Approximately 80% of tuberculosis cases among children in the United States occur in minority populations.[20] Most of these cases occur after exposure to an ill family member. In all populations, whether the disease incidence is high or low, tuberculosis infection and disease tend to occur in clusters, often centered on the close or extended family, meaning that minority newborns are at greatly increased risk of congenital and postnatally acquired tuberculosis infection and disease.

TUBERCULOSIS IN PREGNANCY

Pathogenesis

The pathogenesis of tuberculosis infection and disease during pregnancy is similar to that for nonpregnant individuals.[21, 22] The usual portal of entry for *M. tubercu-*

losis is the lung through inhalation of infected droplet nuclei discharged by an infectious individual. The inoculum of organisms necessary to establish infection is unknown but is probably less than 10.[23] Once tubercle bacilli are deposited in the lung, they multiply in the nonimmune host for several weeks. Usually, this uninhibited replication produces no symptoms, but a patient may experience low-grade fever, cough, or mild pleuritic pain. Shortly after infection, some organisms are carried from the initial pulmonary focus within macrophages to the regional lymph nodes.[24] From there, organisms enter lymphatic and blood vessels and disseminate throughout the body; the genitalia, endometrium, and, if the woman is pregnant, the placenta may be seeded. By 1 to 3 months after infection, the host usually develops cell-mediated immunity and hypersensitivity to the tubercle bacillus, reflected by the development of a reactive tuberculin skin test.[25] As immunity develops, the primary infection in the lung and foci in other organs begin to heal through a combination of resolution, fibrosis, and/or calcification.[26] Although walling-off of these foci occurs, viable tubercle bacilli persist. If the host later becomes immune suppressed, these dormant bacilli may become active, leading to "reactivation" tuberculosis.[27]

There are two major ways that tuberculosis infection in the mother can lead to infection of the fetus in utero. If dissemination of organisms through the blood and lymphatic channels occurs during pregnancy, the placenta may be infected directly. This can occur either during the asymptomatic dissemination that is part of the mother's initial infection or during pulmonary, miliary, or disseminated tuberculosis disease in the mother.[28-44] Miliary tuberculosis in women can arise from a long-standing dormant infection but more often complicates a recent infection (Fig. 28-1). Therefore, infection with *M. tuberculosis* that occurs during pregnancy, as opposed to dormant infection that occurred before the pregnancy, probably poses a greater risk to the fetus. This is a major reason why pregnant women with new onset of *M. tuberculosis* infection usually should be treated carefully during the pregnancy; delay could result in disease in the mother, the infant, or both.

The second mechanism by which a fetus can become infected with *M. tuberculosis* is directly from established genitourinary tuberculosis in the mother. Genital tuberculosis is most likely to start around the time of menarche and can have a very long and relatively asymptomatic course. The fallopian tubes most often are involved (in 90–100% of women), followed by the uterus (50–60%), ovaries (20–30%), and cervix (5–15%).[17] Sterility often is the presenting complaint of tuberculosis endometritis, which diminishes the likelihood of congenital tuberculosis occurring.[45, 46] If infection of the placenta occurs, it results more frequently from disseminated tuberculosis in the mother than from a local endometritis. Tuberculous endometritis, however, can lead to congenital infection of the newborn.[47-50] Tuberculosis in the mother as a complication of in vitro fertilization has been described.[51]

Effect of Pregnancy on Tuberculosis

Over the past two millennia, medical opinions regarding the interaction of pregnancy and tuberculosis have var-

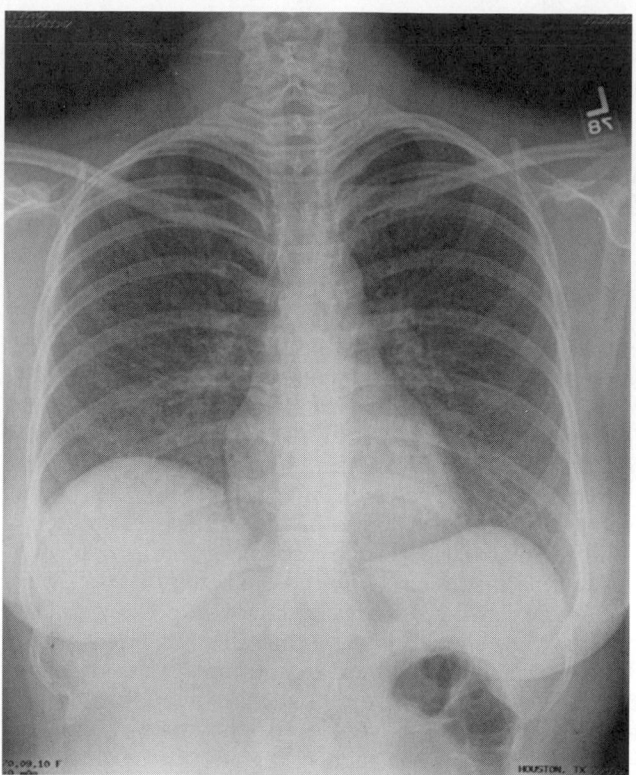

FIGURE 28–1 Chest radiograph from the mother of the child shown in Figure 28–2. This radiograph reveals early miliary tuberculosis.

ied considerably. Hippocrates believed that pregnancy had a beneficial effect on tuberculosis, a view that persisted virtually unchallenged well into the nineteenth century.[52] In 1850, Grisolle reported 24 cases of tuberculosis that developed during pregnancy.[53] In all patients the progression of tuberculosis during pregnancy was more severe than that usually seen in nonpregnant women of the same age. Shortly thereafter, several other papers were published that implied that pregnancy had a deleterious effect on tuberculosis. This view gained so much support that by the early twentieth century, the practice of induced abortion to deal with the consequences of tuberculosis during pregnancy became widely accepted.

The opinion that pregnancy had a deleterious effect on tuberculosis predominated until the late 1940s. In 1943, Cohen[54] detected no increased rate of progression of tuberculosis among 100 pregnant women with abnormal chest radiograph results. In 1953, Hedvall[53] presented a comprehensive review of published studies concerning tuberculosis in pregnancy. He cited studies totaling more than 1000 cases that reported deleterious effects of pregnancy on tuberculosis. He discovered a nearly equal number of reported cases, however, in which a neutral or favorable relationship between pregnancy and tuberculosis was observed. In his own study of 250 pregnant women with abnormal chest radiograph results thought to be due to tuberculosis, he noted that 9% improved, 7% worsened, and 84% remained unchanged during pregnancy. During the first postpartum year, 9% improved, 15% worsened, and 76% were stable. Cromie[55] noted that 31 of 101 pregnant women with quiescent tuberculosis experienced relapse after delivery. Twenty of the 31 relapses occurred in the first postpartum year. Several other investigators observed the higher risk of relapse during the puerperium. Several theories were proposed to explain this phenomenon, including postpartum descent of the diaphragm, nutritional stress of pregnancy and lactation, insufficient sleep for the new mother, rapid hormonal changes, and depression in immunity in late pregnancy and postpartum. A similar number of other studies, however, failed to support an increased risk of progression of tuberculosis in the postpartum priod.[56–60] Cohen's study failed to demonstrate an increase in activity of tuberculosis during pregnancy or any postpartum interval.[56] Rosenbach and Gangemi[58] and Cohen and colleagues[56] showed that only 9 to 13% of women with long-standing tuberculosis had progression of disease during the pregnancy or first postpartum year, a rate thought to be comparable to that in nonpregnant women. Few of these studies had adequate control populations. From all the studies reported, it became clear that the anatomic extent of disease, the radiographic pattern, and the susceptibility of the individual patient to tuberculosis were more important than pregnancy itself in determining the course and prognosis of the pregnant woman with tuberculosis.

The controversy concerning the effect of pregnancy or the postpartum period on tuberculosis has lost most of its importance with the advent of effective chemotherapy.[52, 61] With adequate treatment, pregnant women with tuberculosis have the same excellent prognosis as nonpregnant women. Several studies document no adverse effects of pregnancy, birth, the postpartum period, or lactation on the course of tuberculosis in women receiving chemotherapy.[62, 63]

Most studies have dealt with the risk of reactivation of tuberculosis among women with abnormal chest radiograph results but no evidence of active tuberculous lesions. It is not clear if women with asymptomatic *M. tuberculosis* infection but no radiographic findings are at increased risk of developing tuberculosis during pregnancy or the postpartum period. In 1959, Pridie and Stradling[64] found that the incidence of pulmonary tuberculosis among pregnant women was the same as in the nonpregnant female population of the area. From 1966 to 1972, Schaefer and associates[17] found that the annual pulmonary tuberculosis case rate among pregnant women in New York Lying-In Hospital was 18 to 29 per 100,000 population, comparable to the incidence of tuberculosis during the same period in women of childbearing age in of all New York City. Although no definitive study has been reported, it appears unlikely that progression from asymptomatic *M. tuberculosis* infection to tuberculosis disease is accelerated during pregnancy or the postpartum period.

Effect of Tuberculosis on Pregnancy

In the prechemotherapy era, active tuberculosis at an advanced stage carried a poor prognosis for both mother and child. Schaefer and associates[17] reported that the infant and maternal mortality rates from untreated tuberculosis were between 30% and 40%. In the chemotherapy era, the outcome of pregnancy rarely is altered by the presence of tuberculosis in the mother, except in the rare cases of congenital tuberculosis. One study from Norway revealed a higher incidence of toxemia, postpartum hemorrhage, and difficult labor in mothers with tuberculosis compared with control subjects.[65] The incidence of miscarriage was almost 10 times higher in the tuberculous mothers, but there was no significant difference in the rate of congenital malformations for children born to mothers with and without tuberculosis. Another study reported an incidence of prematurity for infants born to untreated mothers in a tuberculosis sanitarium ranging from 23% to 64%, depending on the severity of tuberculosis in the mother.[66] Most experts now believe, however, that with proper treatment of the pregnant woman with tuberculosis, the prognosis of the pregnancy should not be affected adversely by the presence of tuberculosis. Because of the excellent prognosis for the mother and child, the recommendation for therapeutic abortion has been abandoned.

Screening for Tuberculosis in Pregnancy

For all pregnant women, the history obtained in an early prenatal visit should include questions about a previously positive tuberculin skin test result, previous treatment for *M. tuberculosis* infection or disease, current symptoms compatible with tuberculosis, and known exposure to other adults with the disease.[67, 68] Membership in a high-risk group is a sufficient reason for a tuberculin skin test.[20] For many high-risk women prenatal or peripartum care represents their only contact with the health care system, and the opportunity to test them for tuberculosis infection or disease should not be lost. Some experts believe that all pregnant women should receive a tuberculin skin test.[69] Most experts believe, however, that only women with specific risk factors for *M. tuberculosis* infection or disease should be tested. It must be emphasized that women co-infected with HIV and *M. tuberculosis* may show no reaction to a tuberculin skin test. Pregnant women with high risk for or with known HIV infection should have a thorough investigation for tuberculosis.

Recent changes in the interpretation of the Mantoux tuberculin skin test have been promoted by the Centers for Disease Control and Prevention,[20] the American Thoracic Society, and the American Academy of Pediatrics.[70] The rationale for using different sizes of induration as representing a positive result in different populations has been discussed thoroughly in many publications. The current recommendation is that for those individuals at the highest risk of having *M. tuberculosis* infection progress to tuberculosis—contacts to adults with infectious tuberculosis, patients with an abnormal chest radiograph or clinical evidence of tuberculosis, or persons with HIV infection or other immunocompromise—a Mantoux tuberculin skin test reaction of at least 5 mm is classified as positive, indicating infection with *M. tuberculosis*. For other high-risk groups, a reaction of at least 10 mm is positive. For all other persons deemed at low risk for tuberculosis, a reaction of at least 15 mm is positive. Obviously, this classification scheme depends on the ability and willingness of the family and health care provider to develop a thorough epidemiologic history for tuberculosis exposures and risk. It also depends on accurate interpretation of the skin test. One recent study implied that pediatricians tend to underread induration in tuberculin skin tests.[71]

There have been no studies to verify whether the classification scheme for the Mantoux tuberculin skin test is valid in pregnant women, but there is no reason to suspect otherwise.[72, 73] The effect of pregnancy on tuberculin hypersensitivity as measured by the tuberculin skin test is controversial.[74] Some studies have shown a decrease in in vitro lymphocyte reactivity to purified protein derivative during pregnancy.[75] In vivo studies using patients as their own controls, however, have demonstrated no effect of pregnancy on cutaneous delayed hypersensitivity to tuberculin.[76, 77] Most experts believe the tuberculin skin test by the Mantoux technique is valid throughout pregnancy. There is no evidence that the tuberculin skin test has adverse effects on the pregnant mother or fetus or that skin testing reactivates quiescent foci of tuberculosis infection.[78]

One of the most difficult problems in the interaction of tuberculosis and pregnancy is deciding whether a pregnant woman with *M. tuberculosis* infection should receive immediate treatment or whether the treatment should be postponed until after the child is delivered.[79] Not all infected individuals have the same chance of developing tuberculosis during a short period of time. Individuals who were infected remotely (more than 2 years previously) have a low chance of developing tuberculosis during a given 9-month period. Individuals who have been infected more recently, however, particularly if their infection is discovered during a contact investigation of an adult with active tuberculosis, are at much higher risk; about half of the lifetime risk of progression of infection to disease occurs during the first 1 to 2 years after infection. Other vulnerable adults, particularly those co-infected with HIV, also are at greatly increased risk of having progression of infection to disease. In general, treatment for tuberculosis infection should be initiated during pregnancy if the woman likely has been infected recently (especially in the setting of a contact investigation of a recently diagnosed case) or she is at increased risk of rapid development of tuberculosis. Although isoniazid (INH) is not thought to be teratogenic, some experts recommend waiting until the second trimester of pregnancy to begin treatment. Unfortunately, patient adherence to INH treatment for tuberculosis infection appears to be very low if the initiation of treatment is delayed until after the child is delivered. The reason for this low adherence is not clear, but several problems include the perception of nonimportance because a treatment delay of many months is allowed, transfer of care from one segment of the health care system to another, and, perhaps, the lack of reinforcement by health care professionals concerning the importance of the treatment. Although screening and treatment of high-risk pregnant women may seem to be

an effective strategy to prevent future cases of tuberculosis, it has not yet been demonstrated that this strategy is successful in the U.S. health care system.[80]

Routine chest radiography is not advisable as a screening tool for pregnant women because the prevalence of tuberculosis remains fairly low.[81, 82] With appropriate shielding, however, pregnant women with positive tuberculin skin test results should have chest radiographs to rule out tuberculosis.[83] In addition, a thorough review of systems and physical examination should be carried out to exclude extrapulmonary tuberculosis.

CONGENITAL TUBERCULOSIS

Tuberculosis in the Mother

In general, the clinical manifestations of tuberculosis in the pregnant woman are the same as those in nonpregnant individuals. The most important determinants of the clinical presentation are the extent and anatomic location of disease. In one series of 27 pregnant and postpartum women with pulmonary tuberculosis, the most common clinical findings were cough (74%), weight loss (41%), fever (30%), malaise and fatigue (30%), and hemoptysis (19%).[19] Almost 20% of patients had no significant symptoms; other studies also have found less significant symptoms in pregnant women with tuberculosis.[18] The tuberculin skin test result was positive in 26 of 27 patients. The diagnosis was established in all cases by culture of sputum for *M. tuberculosis*. Sixteen of the patients in this series had drug-resistant tuberculosis; their clinical course was marked by more extensive pulmonary involvement, a higher incidence of pulmonary complications, longer sputum conversion times, and a higher incidence of death. In other series, 5 to 10% of pregnant women with tuberculosis have had extrapulmonary disease, a rate comparable with nonpregnant women of the same age.[18]

Although the female genital tract may be the portal of entry for a primary tuberculosis infection, more often infection at this site originates by continuity from an adjacent focus of disease or by blood-borne seeding of the fallopian tubes.[45] Progression of disease usually is by descent in the genital tract. Mucosal ulceration within the fallopian tube develops, and pelvic adhesions occur frequently. Many patients are asymptomatic. The most common complaints are sterility and menstrual irregularity with menorrhagia or amenorrhea. These findings greatly diminish the likelihood of congenital tuberculosis. Other less frequent signs and symptoms include lower abdominal pain and tenderness, weight loss, fever, and night sweats. Diagnosis in the nonpregnant woman is usually established by culture and histologic examination of tissue recovered after uterine curettage. The highest recovery rates of *M. tuberculosis* are obtained from scrapings obtained just before or during menstruation.

Tuberculosis mastitis is very rare in the United States but occurs almost exclusively in childbearing-aged women.[84–86] The most common finding is a single breast mass, with or without a draining sinus. Nipple retraction and peau d'orange skin changes suggestive of carcinoma also may be present. The ipsilateral axillary lymph nodes usually are enlarged. Diagnosis is confirmed by biopsy of the mass or axillary node and culture of the tissue for *M. tuberculosis*. Transmission of *M. tuberculosis* to the infant through breast milk is exceedingly rare, if it occurs at all.

In Utero Routes of Transmission

Tuberculosis in the neonate can be either truly congenital (i.e., acquired in utero) or truly neonatal (i.e., acquired early in life from the mother, contagious members of the family, friends, or caretakers). Each of these two kinds of perinatal tuberculosis may be subdivided. *Congenital tuberculosis* can be acquired in any one of three ways: (1) from the infected placenta via the umbilical vein, (2) by inhalation of infected amniotic fluid, and (3) by ingestion of infected amniotic fluid. *Neonatal tuberculosis* can be acquired in four different ways: (1) by inhalation of infected droplets, (2) by ingestion of infected droplets, (3) by ingestion of infected milk (theoretical), and (4) by contamination of traumatized skin or mucous membranes.

It is not always possible to be sure of the route of infection in a particular neonate, and, with effective chemotherapy at hand, it is not essential for the care of the infant. However, it is important to try to identify the source of infection so that the person infecting the infant can be treated and further transmission can be prevented.

The potential modes of inoculation of the fetus or newborn infant with *M. tuberculosis* from the mother are shown in Table 28–1. Infection of the fetus through the umbilical cord has been rare, with fewer than 300 cases reported in the English-language literature.[87] These infants' mothers frequently suffer from tuberculous pleural effusion, meningitis, or disseminated disease during pregnancy or soon after.[31, 34, 36, 37, 41, 88] In some series of congenital tuberculosis, however, fewer than 50% of the mothers were known to be suffering from tuberculosis at the time of delivery and beginning of symptoms in the newborn.[89, 90] In most of these cases, diagnosis of the child led to the discovery of the mother's tuberculosis. The intensity of lymphohematogenous spread during pregnancy is one of the factors that determines if congenital tuberculosis will occur. Hematogenous dissemination in the mother leads to infection of the placenta with subsequent transmission of organisms to the fetus. *M. tuberculosis* has been demonstrated in the decidua,

amnion, and chorionic villi of the placenta.[91] The organisms also have been shown to reach the placenta through direct extension from a tuberculous salpingeal tube. Even massive involvement of the placenta with tuberculosis, however, does not always give rise to congenital tuberculosis.[92] It is not clear if the fetus can be infected directly from the mother's bloodstream without a caseous lesion forming first in the placenta, although this phenomenon has been reported in experimental animal models.[93]

In hematogenous congenital tuberculosis, the organisms reach the fetus through the umbilical vein. If bacilli infect the liver, a primary focus develops with involvement of the periportal lymph nodes. The bacilli can pass through the liver, however, into the main circulation through the patent foramen ovale. Alternately, they can pass through the right ventricle into the pulmonary circulation, leading to a primary focus in the lung. The organisms in the lung often remain dormant until after birth when oxygenation and circulation increase significantly, leading to growth of organisms and pulmonary tuberculosis in the young infant. In many children with congenital tuberculosis, multiple lesions occur throughout the body; it is not possible to determine if they represent multiple primary foci or if some occur secondary to primary lesions in the lung or liver. The only lesion of the neonate that is unquestionably associated with congenital infection is a primary complex in the liver.

Congenital infection of the infant also can occur through aspiration or ingestion of infected amniotic fluid.[94] If the caseous lesion in the placenta ruptures directly into the amniotic cavity, the fetus can inhale or ingest the bacilli. Inhalation or ingestion of infected amniotic fluid is the most likely cause of congenital tuberculosis if the infant has multiple primary foci in the lung, gut, or middle ear.[95] In congenital tuberculosis caused by aspiration, the primary complex can be in the liver, the lung, or both organs.

The pathology of congenital tuberculosis in the fetus and newborn usually demonstrates the predisposition to dissemination ensured by the modes of transmission, particularly through the umbilical vein. The liver and lungs are the primary involved organs with bone marrow, bone, the gastrointestinal tract, adrenal glands, spleen, kidney, abdominal lymph nodes, and skin also involved frequently.[96, 97] The histologic patterns of involvement are similar to those in adults; tubercles and granulomas are common. Central nervous system involvement occurs in fewer than 50% of cases.[89, 97] In most recent series, the mortality rate of congenital tuberculosis has been close to 50%, primarily because of the failure to suspect the correct diagnosis. Most fatal cases are diagnosed at autopsy.[89, 90]

Postnatal acquisition of *M. tuberculosis* through airborne inoculation is the most common route of infection of the neonate.[98–100] It may be impossible to differentiate postnatal infection from prenatal acquisition on clinical grounds alone.[101] Any adult in the neonate's environment can be a source of airborne tuberculosis, including health care workers.[102, 103] Up to 40% of infants with untreated *M. tuberculosis* infection develop tuberculosis

TABLE 28–1
Modes of Inoculation of the Fetus or Newborn with *Mycobacterium tuberculosis*

MATERNAL FOCUS	MODE OF SPREAD
Placentitis	Hematogenous (umbilical vessel)
Amniotic fluid	Aspiration
Cervicitis	Direct contact
Pneumonitis	Airborne (postnatal)

disease within 1 to 2 years. There are few data concerning the time of onset of tuberculosis when the infection is acquired at or shortly after birth. In one series of 48 infants exposed postnatally to mothers with pulmonary tuberculosis in the pretreatment era, 21 became infected; of those who became ill, signs such as fever, tachypnea, weight loss, and hepatosplenomegaly developed in 4 to 8 weeks.[104] Because newborns infected with the organism are at extremely high risk of developing severe forms of disease, investigation of an adult with tuberculosis whose household contacts include a pregnant woman or newborn should be considered a public health emergency. In addition, all adults in contact with an infant suspected of having M. tuberculosis infection or disease should undergo a thorough investigation for disease.

The skin and mucous membranes are rare portals of entry for M. tuberculosis in neonates. Infection through the skin has been mentioned several times in association with lesions of the head and face, very likely related to minor traumatic lesions being infected by kissing. Primary lesions of the mucous membranes of the mouth also have been recognized, although usually in infants beyond the newborn period. In both of these situations, the primary lesion was insignificant but the enlarged regional lymph nodes called attention to the problem.

A previously well-known form of skin and mucous membrane infection was tuberculosis of the male genitalia after circumcision in the years when it was customary for the individual performing the circumcision to suck the blood around the incision. This procedure was obviously dangerous if that individual happened to have bacilli in the sputum. The primary focus of inoculation on the penis was often inconspicuous but, within 1 to 4 weeks, ulceration, suppuration, and bilateral inguinal lymphadenopathy would develop. At first firm and nontender, the nodes might later break down with sinus formation to the exterior. Holt,[105] in his review of circumcision tuberculosis, described a case with extensive ulceration of the penis and scrotum, greatly swollen lymph nodes, a generalized rash resembling varicella, hepatosplenomegaly, fever, cough, rales, and a positive tuberculin test, with recovery of tubercle bacilli from sputum and penile discharge. Of the 41 patients described by Holt, 16 died and 6 recovered, with the outcome of the others unknown.[105]

Criteria for Diagnosis of Congenital Tuberculosis

In 1935, Beitzke[91] suggested criteria for diagnosis of congenital tuberulosis in a thoughtful, detailed, and often-quoted review of the reported cases up to that time:

1. Tuberculosis in the child must be firmly established.
2. A primary complex in the liver is proof of congenital tuberculosis because this complex could arise only through perfusion of the liver with tubercle bacilli contained in umbilical cord blood.
3. If a primary complex is lacking in the liver, then tuberculosis can be considered to be congenital only if:

   a. Tuberculous lesions are present in a fetus or in a newborn only a few days old or,
   b. In an older infant, extrauterine infection can be excluded with certainty, that is, if the child was removed from the tuberculous mother at birth to a tuberculosis-free environment.

Cantwell and co-workers,[87] based on a review of cases of congenital tuberculosis published before and after 1980, proposed the following modification of Beitzke's criteria: the infant must have proven tuberculous lesions and at least one of the following: (1) lesions in the first week of life; (2) a primary hepatic complex or caseating hepatic granulomas; (3) tuberculosis infection of the placenta or maternal genital tract, or both; or (4) exclusion of postnatal transmission by a thorough contact investigation. Although Beitzke's criteria are in fact fully met by many of the 300 or so reported cases of congenital tuberculosis, in other cases it is impossible to be certain whether infection was transmitted in utero or was acquired during the early days or weeks of life. In many cases of true congenital tuberculosis, the mother was not known to be suffering from active tuberculosis. Two articles contain tables with detailed information on 26 cases and 15 cases.[89, 90] In only 10 of the 26 cases was tuberculosis diagnosed in the mother ante partum, although it became apparent in another 15 after diagnosis in the infant.[89] Five of the 26 mothers died of tuberculosis, an indirect confirmation of the fact that the diagnosis was made very late. In the series of 15 cases, 7 mothers were thought to be well at the time of delivery, but all 15 were subsequently found either to have had pleural effusion antepartum (four cases) or to have developed endometrial, miliary, or meningeal tuberculosis post partum.[90]

Clinical Features and Diagnosis of Congenital Tuberculosis

The clinical manifestations of tuberculosis in the fetus and newborn vary in relation to the site and size of the caseous lesions. Symptoms may be present at birth but more commonly begin by the second or third week of life. The most frequent signs or symptoms of true congenital tuberculosis are listed in Table 28–2.[87, 89, 106–129]

Most infants have an abnormal chest radiograph result, with about half having a miliary pattern.[130] Some infants with a normal chest radiograph early in the course develop profound radiographic abnormalities as the disease progresses (Fig. 28–2). The most common abnormalities are adenopathy and parenchymal infiltrates. Occasionally, the pulmonary involvement progresses very rapidly, leading to cavitation.[131, 132] Tuberculosis of the middle ear in children with congenital tuberculosis has been described fairly often.[37, 89, 95, 131, 133–136] The eustachian tube in newborns permits ready access to infected pharyngeal fluids or vomitus. Multiple perforation or total destruction of the tympanic membrane, otorrhea, enlarged cervical lymph nodes, and facial paralysis are all possible sequelae.

The clinical presentation of tuberculosis in the newborn is similar to that caused by bacterial sepsis and

TABLE 28–2
Most Frequent Signs and Symptoms of Congenital Tuberculosis

SYMPTOM OR SIGN	FREQUENCY (%)
Hepatosplenomegaly	76
Respiratory distress	72
Fever	48
Lymphadenopathy	38
Abdominal distention	24
Lethargy or irritability	21
Ear discharge	17
Papular skin lesions	14
Vomiting, apnea, cyanosis, jaundice, seizures, petechiae	<10 each

congenital infections with syphilis and cytomegalovirus.[137] The diagnosis of congenital tuberculosis should be suspected in any infant with signs and symptoms of sepsis or viral infection who does not respond to vigorous antibiotic therapy and whose evaluation for other congenital infections is unrevealing. Of course, suspicion also should be high if the mother has or has had tuberculosis or if she is in a high-risk group for tuberculosis. The importance of obtaining an adequate history for the presence of risk factors for tuberculosis in the mother cannot be overemphasized. Suspicion should increase if the mother has suffered from unexplained pneumonia, bronchitis, pleural effusion, meningeal disease, or endometritis during, shortly before, or even after pregnancy. Evaluation of both parents and other family members can yield important clues about the presence of tuberculosis within the family.

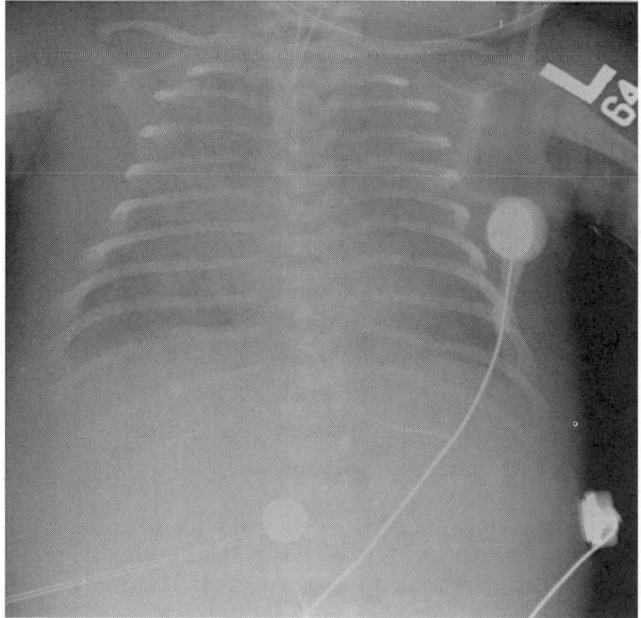

FIGURE 28–2 Chest radiograph from a 1-month-old infant with congenital tuberculosis.

The timely diagnosis of congenital or neonatal tuberculosis is often difficult.[138, 139] Whenever possible, the placenta should be examined and cultured for *M. tuberculosis*. The tuberculin skin test result essentially is always negative initially, although it may become positive after 1 to 3 months of treatment. The diagnosis must be established by finding acid-fast bacilli in body fluids or tissue or by culturing *M. tuberculosis*. A positive acid-fast bacilli smear of an early morning gastric aspirate obtained from a newborn should be considered indicative of tuberculosis, although false-positive results can occur.[140] Direct acid-fast bacilli smears from middle-ear fluid, bond marrow, tracheal aspirate, or biopsy tissue can be useful and should be obtained more often.[141] Hageman and colleagues[89] found positive cultures for *M. tuberculosis* in 10 of 12 gastric aspirates, three of three liver biopsies, three of three lymph node biopsies, and two of four bone marrow aspirations from children with congenital tuberculosis. Open-lung biopsy also has been used to establish the diagnosis.[142] The cerebrospinal fluid should be examined and cultured, although the yield for isolating *M. tuberculosis* is less than 20% and meningitis occurs in only one third of cases of congenital tuberculosis.

TREATMENT OF TUBERCULOSIS

The drugs used most commonly to treat *M. tuberculosis* infection and disease, their dosage forms, and doses are listed in Table 28–3. Detailed discussion of the pharmacokinetics of each drug is beyond the scope of this chapter. No published study has examined in detail the pharmacokinetics of drugs used as antituberculosis agents in premature or term neonates.[143]

INH is the mainstay of treatment for tuberculosis infection and disease in infants, children, and adults. It is inexpensive, highly effective in preventing the multiplication of tubercle bacilli, of low molecular weight and therefore readily diffusible to all tissues in the body, and relatively nontoxic to children. It can be administered orally or intramuscularly. When it is taken orally, high plasma, sputum, and cerebrospinal fluid levels are reached within a few hours and persist at least 6 to 8 hours. Because of the slow multiplication of *M. tuberculosis*, the total daily dose can be given at one time. The principal toxic effects of INH are peripheral neuritis and hepatitis. Peripheral neuritis, resulting from competitive inhibition of pyridoxine, is almost unknown in North American children because both cow's milk (or formula) and meat are the main dietary sources of pyridoxine. In some well-nourished children, serum pyridoxine concentrations are mildly depressed by INH but clinical signs are not apparent. For most children, therefore, it is not necessary to use supplementary pyridoxine. However, in pregnancy, for teenagers whose diets may be inadequate, in children from ethnic groups with a low milk and meat intake, and in breast-fed babies, pyridoxine supplementation (25 to 50 mg/day) is important. Hepatotoxicity from INH, rare in children, increases in frequency with age. Monitoring serum aspartate aminotransferase and serum alanine aminotransferase some-

☐ **TABLE 28–3**
☐ Antituberculosis Drugs in Children

DRUGS	DOSAGE FORMS	DAILY DOSE (mg/kg)	TWICE-WEEKLY DOSE (mg/kg/per dose)	MAXIMUM DOSE
Isoniazid	Scored tablets: 100 mg 300 mg Syrup: 10 mg/ml	10–15	20–40	Daily: 300 mg Twice weekly: 900 mg
Rifampin	Capsules: 150 mg 300 mg Syrup: formulated in syrup from capsules	10–20	10–20	600 mg
Pyrazinamide	Scored tablets: 500 mg	20–40	50–70	2 g
Streptomycin	Vials: 1 g, 4 g	20–40 (IM)	20–40 (IM)	1 g
Ethambutol	Scored tablets: 100 mg 400 mg	15–25	50	2.5 g

times reveals transient increases during treatment with INH, but the levels usually return spontaneously to normal without interruption of treatment. Liver enzyme abnormalities in adolescents receiving INH likewise are rather common and usually disappear spontaneously, but severe hepatitis can occur. Although neonates usually tolerate INH well, some experts recommend routine biochemical monitoring in the first several months of therapy. The usual dosage of INH in children is 10 to 20 mg/kg per day, to a maximum of 300 mg per day. INH is available in tablets of 100 and 300 mg. A syrup of INH in sorbitol (10 mg/ml) appears to be satisfactory; however, it is unstable at room temperature and should be kept cool. Many children develop significant gastrointestinal intolerance (nausea, vomiting) while taking the INH suspension, but neonates and infants tolerate the lower required volume of suspension well. If tablets are used, they are easily crushed in a dessert spoon and given with some soft food such as applesauce, mashed banana, thawed undiluted frozen orange juice, or another palatable medium. The crushed tablets should not be added to the nursing bottle or offered in milk or water because they will be ingested only partially.

Rifampin (RIF) is a semisynthetic drug derived from *Streptomyces mediterranei*. The drug is absorbed readily from the gastrointestinal tract in the fasting state. Excretion mainly is through the biliary tract; however, effective levels are achieved in the kidneys and urine. In many patients receiving RIF treatment, the tears, saliva, urine, and stool turn orange as a result of a harmless metabolite, and the patient and parents always must be warned of this in advance. RIF can be made into a suspension easily for use in children. RIF is very well tolerated by neonates and infants. The incidences of hepatitis, leukopenia, and thrombocytopenia are extremely low. RIF should be used alone only when treating *M. tuberculosis* infection due to an INH-resistant organism. If one uses INH, 20 mg/kg, and RIF, 15 to 20 mg/kg, there is an appreciable incidence of hepatox-

icity. Therefore, when using the two together, one would be wise to approximate INH, 10 mg/kg, and RIF, 15 to 20 mg/kg.

Pyrazinamide (PZA) contributes to the killing of *M. tuberculosis*, particularly at a low pH such as that within macrophages. The exact mechanism of action of PZA is a subject of controversy. PZA has no effect on extracellular tubercle bacilli in vitro but clearly contributes to the killing of intracellular bacilli. Primary resistance is very rare, except that *Mycobacterium bovis* is resistant. The drug diffuses readily into all areas, including the cerebrospinal fluid. The usual adult daily dose is 30 to 40 mg/kg. The optimal dose for infants and children has not been established firmly because no formal pharmacokinetic studies have been reported. The adult dose is tolerated well by infants and children, results in high cerebrospinal fluid concentrations, and clearly is effective in therapy trials for active tuberculosis in children. PZA appears to exert its maximum effect during the first 2 months of therapy. Hepatotoxicity can occur at high doses but is rare at the usual dose. PZA routinely causes an increase in the serum uric acid concentration by inhibiting its excretion through the kidneys. Toxic reactions in adults include flushing, cutaneous hypersensitivity, arthralgia, and overt gout; however, the considerable experience with this drug in children in Latin American countries, Hong Kong, and the United States has revealed few problems.

Ethambutol (EMB) has been used for many years as a companion drug for INH in adults. The usual oral dose is 15 mg/kg per day. At this dose, the drug primarily is bacteriostatic, its major role being to prevent emergence of resistance to other drugs. However, at doses of 25 mg/kg per day or 50 mg/kg given twice a week, EMB has some bactericidal action. Unfortunately, at these higher doses, optic neuritis or red-green color blindness has occurred in some adults. Although the incidence of ophthalmologic toxicity in children is extremely low, if it occurs at all, EMB is not recommended for routine use in young children in whom visual field and color discrimination tests are difficult and inaccurate. However, it is used frequently and safely in children with life-threatening forms of tuberculosis or with drug-resistant tuberculosis.

Streptomycin (STM) is a valuable drug to be used in conjunction with INH and RIF in life-threatening forms of tuberculosis. It is bactericidal and tolerated well by children in the usual dose of 20 to 40 mg/kg per day intramuscularly up to 1 g. Usually, STM can be discontinued within 1 to 3 months if clinical improvement is definite, whereas the other two or three drugs are continued with oral administration.

General Principles

The tubercle bacillus can be killed only during replication, which occurs among organisms that are active metabolically. In one model, bacilli in a host exist in different populations.[4] They are active metabolically and replicate freely where oxygen tension is high and the pH is neutral or alkaline. Environmental conditions for growth are best within cavities, leading to a large bacterial population. Older children with pulmonary tuberculosis and patients of all ages with only extrapulmonary tuberculosis are infected with a much smaller number of tubercle bacilli because the cavitary population is not present. However, neonates with congenital tuberculosis tend to have a large burden of organisms at diagnosis.

Naturally occurring drug-resistant mutant organisms occur within large populations of tubercle bacilli even before chemotherapy is started. All known genetic loci for drug resistance in *M. tuberculosis* are located on the chromosome; no plasmid-mediated resistance is known. The rate of resistance within populations of organisms is related to the rate of mutations at these loci. Although a large population of bacilli as a whole may be considered drug susceptible, a subpopulation of drug-resistant organisms occurs at a fairly predictable rate. The mean frequency of these drug-resistant mutations is about 10^{-6} but varies among drugs: STM, 10^{-5}; INH, 10^{-6}; and RIF, 10^{-7}. A cavity containing 10^9 tubercle bacilli has thousands of single drug-resistant mutant organisms, whereas a closed caseous lesion contains few, if any, resistant mutants.

The population size of tubercle bacilli within a patient determines the appropriate therapy. For patients with a large bacterial population (adults with cavities or extensive infiltrates), many single drug-resistant mutants are present and at least two antituberculosis drugs must be used. Conversely, for patients with *M. tuberculosis* infection but no disease, the bacterial population is very small (about 10^3 to 10^4 organisms), drug-resistant mutants are rare, and a single drug can be used. Older children with pulmonary tuberculosis and patients of all ages with extrapulmonary tuberculosis have medium-sized populations in which drug-resistant mutants may or may not be present. In general, these patients should be treated with at least two drugs. Neonates and infants with tuberculosis disease have large mycobacterial populations, and several drugs are required to effect a cure.

Pregnant Women

The only drug with well-documented efficacy against *M. tuberculosis* infection in pregnant women is INH. Infants and children tolerate INH very well, and adverse reactions are rare. However, adverse reactions are more common in adults. Between 5% and 10% of young adults taking INH have an asymptomatic increase in serum liver transaminase levels; 1 to 2% suffer from symptomatic hepatitis, which is reversible if the medication is stopped immediately. For most young adults, monitoring for hepatitis is done clinically. Routine or periodic evaluation of serum liver enzyme tests is reserved for adults with underlying liver disease or those taking other potentially hepatotoxic drugs. However, some experts think all pregnant women taking INH should have routine biochemical monitoring for hepatitis. Serum liver enzyme elevations of three to four times normal are common and do not necessitate discontinuation of the drug. There is no evidence that giving INH to a pregnant woman adversely affects the liver of the fetus. The other important adverse reaction of INH is peripheral neuritis caused by inhibition of pyridoxine metabolism. Pyridoxine should be given to pregnant adolescents or women and breast-feeding infants because breast milk has low concentrations of pyridoxine, even if the mother is receiving vitamin supplements.[144]

The current recommendation of the Centers for Disease Control and Prevention is to treat adults infected with *M. tuberculosis* with INH for 6 to 12 months.[20] Based on studies of cost-effectiveness of treatment, many health departments have opted to treat adults for 6 months. By contrast, the American Academy of Pediatrics recommends a 9-month course of treatment with INH for infants and children.[70] Usually, the medication is taken daily under self-supervision. If poor patient adherence is likely and resources are available, INH can be given twice weekly using directly observed therapy.[145] Directly observed therapy requires that a health care worker, often from the local health department, observe the patient take antituberculosis medications. In general, directly observed therapy should be used for all patients with tuberculosis disease because of the difficulty in predicting patient adherence and the consequences of poor adherence (relapse and development of drug resistance). Directly observed therapy is often used for high-risk newborns with tuberculosis exposure or infants with *M. tuberculosis* infection.

For patients who cannot take INH for treatment of *M. tuberculosis* infection either because of side effects of the medication or because they are infected with an INH-resistant but RIF-susceptible strain of *M. tuberculosis*, the treatment of choice for *M. tuberculosis* infection is RIF, which also can be given daily or twice a week under directly observed therapy.[146] If the mother is known to be infected with a strain of tuberculosis that is resistant to both INH and RIF (multidrug-resistant tuberculosis), an expert should be consulted for the management of the mother and the child after delivery.[147]

Although treatment of active tuberculosis during pregnancy is unquestioned, the treatment of a pregnant woman who has an asymptomatic *M. tuberculosis* infection is more controversial. Some clinicians prefer to delay therapy until after delivery, because pregnancy does not seem to increase the risk of developing active tuberculosis. Others believe that because recent infection can be accompanied by hematogenous spread to the placenta, it is preferable to treat without delay or to wait until the second trimester to start chemotherapy. A report by Franks and colleagues[148] suggests that the risk of INH-associated hepatitis and death is higher in women than in men and that women in the postpartum period are slightly more vulnerable to INH hepatotoxicity. These authors suggest that it might be prudent to avoid INH during the postpartum period or at least to monitor postpartum women taking INH with frequent examinations and laboratory studies. The possible increased risk of INH hepatotoxicity must be weighed against the risk of developing active tuberculosis as well as the consequences to both mother and infant should active tuberculosis develop.

The indications for treatment and the basic principles of management for the pregnant woman with tuberculosis disease are no different from those in the nonpregnant patient. The recommendations for which drugs to use and how long to give them are slightly different, however, mostly because of possible effects of several of the drugs on the developing fetus.

The currently recommended treatment for drug-susceptible pulmonary tuberculosis in the United States in nonpregnant individuals is 6 months of INH and RIF, supplemented during the first 2 months with PZA and either EMB or STM.[4, 149] With any of the regimens, the drugs usually are given every day for the first 2 weeks to 2 months; then they can be given daily or twice a week (under directly observed therapy) for the remainder of therapy with equal effectiveness and rates of adverse reactions.

There is no doubt that untreated tuberculosis represents a far greater risk to a woman and her fetus than does appropriate treatment of the disease.[150–155] Extensive experience with the use of INH in pregnancy has been reported. Even though it crosses the placenta, it is not teratogenic even when given during the first 4 months of gestation.[156] EMB also appears to be safe during pregnancy. In 650 cases in which pregnant women were treated with EMB, no evidence of fetal malformations, including eye abnormalities, was found.[78, 157–159] The action of RIF to inhibit DNA-dependent RNA polymerase combined with its ability to cross the placental barrier has created some concern about its use in pregnancy.[160] Only 3% of 446 fetuses exposed in utero to RIF had abnormalities, however, compared with 2% for EMB and 1% for INH.[78] The noted abnormalities included limb reductions, central nervous system abnormalities, and hypoprothrombinemia. Hemorrhagic disease of the newborn also has been described after the use of RIF in the mother. The incidence of abnormalities in fetuses not exposed to antituberculosis medications ranges from 1% to 6%. In general, the powerful antituberculosis effect of RIF outweighs concern about its effect on the fetus. Nonpregnant women receiving RIF should receive contraception counseling because receiving RIF can impair the efficacy of oral contraceptives, leading to unintended pregnancy in a tuberculous woman.[161]

Several antituberculosis drugs generally are not used in pregnant women because of possibly toxicity to the fetus.[162–164] STM has variable passage across the placental barrier. Its use in pregnancy is now limited by the availability of better drugs and its effect on the fetus.[165–167] In a review of 206 infants exposed in utero to STM, 34 (17%) had significant eighth nerve damage, the abnormalities ranging from mild vestibular damage to profound bilateral deafness.[78] The deleterious effects of STM are independent of the critical periods earlier in embryogenesis, and it is potentially hazardous throughout gestation. It is assumed that capreomycin, kanamycin, and amikacin, other aminoglycosides with antituberculosis activity, could have the same toxic potential as STM. Little is known about the specific effects of PZA on the fetus. Although there are no data, an increasing number of experts are using PZA during pregnancy with no reported adverse reactions. Nonspecific teratogenic effects have been attributed to ethionamide.[168] The central nervous system effects of cycloserine and the gastrointestinal effects of para-aminosalicylic acid in adults make their use in pregnancy undesirable.

The currently recommended initial treatment of drug-susceptible tuberculosis disease in pregnancy is INH and RIF daily, with the addition of EMB initially, under directly observed therapy.[169, 170] Pyridoxine (50 mg daily) always should be given with INH during pregnancy because of the increased requirements for this vitamin in pregnant women. After drug susceptibility testing of the isolate of *M. tuberculosis* reveals it to be susceptible to both INH and RIF, the EMB can be discontinued. If PZA is not used in the initial regimen, INH and RIF must be given for 9 months instead of 6 months. After the first 2 weeks to 2 months of daily treatment, the drugs can be given twice a week under directly observed therapy, which is the preferred method of treatment by most experts. The treatment of any form of drug-resistant tuberculosis during pregnancy is extraordinarily difficult and should be handled by an expert with great experience with the disease.[171, 172]

Because treatment of tuberculosis in pregnant women often continues after delivery, there is concern as to whether it is safe for the mother to breast-feed her infant. Snider and Powell[173] concluded that a breast-feeding infant would have serum levels of no more than 20% of the usual therapeutic levels of INH for infants and less than 11% of other antituberculosis drugs. Potential toxic effects of drugs delivered in breast milk have not been reported. Because pyridoxine deficiency in the neonate can cause seizures, however, and because breast milk has relatively low levels of pyridoxine, infants who are taking INH or whose breast-feeding mothers are taking INH should receive supplemental pyridoxine.[174]

Neonates and Infants

The optimal treatment of congenital tuberculosis has not been established, because the rarity of this condition precludes formal treatment trials. It would appear that the basic principles for treatment of other children and adults also apply to the treatment of congenital tuberculosis.[175] All children with suspected congenital tuberculosis should be started on four antituberculosis medications (INH, RIF, PZA, plus either EMB or STM) until the diagnostic evaluation and susceptibility testing of isolated organisms is concluded. Although the optimal duration of therapy has not been established, many experts treat infants with congenital or postnatally acquired tuberculosis for a total duration of 9 to 12 months because of the decreased immunologic capability of the young infant. INH given alone is known to be safe in the neonate, including premature infants. There are no comparable data for INH given in combination with other drugs or for other drugs alone. Several studies have shown that RIF can be given safely to premature infants for indications other than tuberculosis. In addition, anecdotal information supports the notion that PZA, STM, and kanamycin are safe in neonates. Young infants taking these drugs should have biochemical monitoring of serum liver enzymes and uric acid (for PZA) performed on a regular basis. Although the pharmacokinetics of antituberculosis drugs in the neonate are essentially unknown, extensive clinical experience suggests that the doses listed in Table 28–3 are effective and safe. Virtually all neonates and infants with tuberculosis should be treated by directly observed therapy.

Following the Infant on Therapy

Follow-up of children treated with antituberculosis drugs has become somewhat more streamlined in recent years. While receiving chemotherapy, the patients should be seen monthly, both to encourage regular taking of the prescribed drugs and to check, by a few simple questions (concerning appetite, well-being) and a few observations (weight gain; appearance of skin and sclerae; palpation of liver, spleen, and lymph nodes), that the disease is not spreading and that toxic effects of the drugs are not appearing. Repeat chest radiographs probably should be obtained 1 to 2 months after the onset of chemotherapy to ascertain the maximal extent of disease before chemotherapy takes effect; thereafter, radiographs rarely are necessary. Chemotherapy has been so successful that follow-up beyond its termination is not usually necessary, except for children with serious disease, such as congenital tuberculosis or meningitis, or those with extensive residual chest radiographic findings at the end of chemotherapy.

Every case of definite or suspected tuberculosis must, by law, be reported immediately by telephone to the health department to ensure (1) prompt contact investigation[176–182] and (2) free antituberculosis drugs, which are available for diagnosed cases and for intimate contacts in almost every state of the United States.

Prognosis

The prognosis for congenital tuberculosis was dismal in the prechemotherapy era.[183] In Hughesdon's report,[95] 3 infants died on the first day of life, 8 between 18 and 30 days, 15 between 31 and 60 days, and 3 between 65 and 112 days. Hageman and associates[89] reviewed 26 patients born since the introduction of INH in 1952: 12 died, and 9 of these were untreated, the diagnosis being established only at autopsy. The results in survivors were good, but the follow-up was usually short.[134, 184] The child reported by Nemir and O'Hare,[90] who was treated intensively with INH, STM, and aminosalicylic acid in the 1950s, recovered, was followed for 27 years, and is herself the mother of two tuberculin-negative children.

There is little question that today's multidrug, short-course chemotherapeutic regimens should be extremely effective in bringing the disease under rapid and permanent control, if due to drug-susceptible organisms. Experience with treatment of disease due to drug-resistant organisms is so limited as to preclude prognosis.

MANAGEMENT OF A NEONATE BORN TO A MOTHER WITH A POSITIVE TUBERCULIN SKIN TEST

If the mother is well and her chest radiograph result is normal, no separation of the mother and infant is required. Although the mother is a candidate for treatment of *M. tuberculosis* infection, the infant does not need special evaluation or therapy. Other family members should have a tuberculin skin test and further evaluation, if indicated. The local health department, however, often will not have the resources to do this testing, which should be performed by the treating physicians. It is not necessary to delay discharge of the infant from the newborn nursery pending the results of this family investigation. The need for further skin testing of the infant depends on whether disease is found in the family or cannot be excluded within the family's environment.

If the radiograph is abnormal, the mother and child should be separated until the mother has been evaluated thoroughly. If active tuberculosis is present in the mother, she should be started on effective antituberculosis medications right away. Examination of the mother's sputum for acid-fast organisms always is necessary even if obtaining a sample requires vigorous measures. All other household members and frequent visitors should be investigated for *M. tuberculosis* infection and disease.

If the mother's chest radiograph is abnormal but the history, physical examination, sputum smear, and evaluation of the radiograph reveal no evidence of active tuberculosis, it is reasonable to assume that the infant is at low risk for infection. The radiographic abnormality is due to another cause or a quiescent focus of previous infection with *M. tuberculosis*. If the mother remains untreated, however, she may develop reactivation tuberculosis and subsequently expose her infant. The mother, if not previously treated, should receive appropriate therapy, and she and her infant should receive frequent follow-up care. In this situation, the infant does not need chemotherapy. All household members should be evaluated for tuberculosis by a clinician.

If the mother has clinical and radiographic evidence of active, possibly contagious tuberculosis, the local health department should be informed immediately about the mother so that a contact investigation can be performed.

The infant should be evaluated for congenital tuberculosis with a physical examination and high-quality posteroanterior and lateral chest radiographs. If possible, serologic testing for HIV should be performed on the mother and/or her infant. The mother and infant should be separated until the infant is receiving chemotherapy or the mother is judged to be noncontagious.[185] Prophylactic INH (10 mg/kg per day) for newborns born to mothers with tuberculosis has been so efficacious that separation of the mother and infant is no longer considered mandatory once therapy is started.[186–188] Separation should occur only if the mother is ill enough to require hospitalization, if she has been or is expected to become nonadherent to her treatment, or if she is thought to be infected with a drug-resistant strain of *M. tuberculosis*. INH therapy should be continued in the infant at least until the mother has been shown to be culture negative for 3 months. At that time, a Mantoux tuberculin skin test is done on the child. If it is positive, the infant should be investigated for the presence of tuberculosis with a physical examination and chest radiograph and further appropriate workup if disease is suggested. If disease is absent, the infant should continue INH for a total of 9 months. If the follow-up skin test is negative and the mother or contact with tuberculosis has good adherence and response to treatment, INH many be discontinued in the infant. The infant needs close follow-up, and it is prudent to repeat a tuberculin skin test after 6 to 12 months.

If the mother or other family member with contagious tuberculosis has disease caused by a multidrug-resistant strain of *M. tuberculosis* or has poor adherence to treatment and better supervision of therapy for the adult and infant is not possible, the Centers for Disease Control and Prevention recommends that the infant should be separated from the contagious adult and vaccination with bacillus Calmette-Guérin (BCG) may be considered.[189–191] Vaccination with BCG appears to decrease the risk of tuberculosis in exposed infants, but the effect is variable.[192, 193] Kendig[194] reported 117 infants born to mothers with active tuberculosis around the time of delivery; none of the 30 BCG-vaccinated infants developed tuberculosis, and 38 cases of tuberculosis and three deaths occurred among the 75 infants who received neither BCG vaccine nor INH therapy. However, 24 of the 30 infants who received BCG vaccine also were separated from their mother for at least 6 weeks; it is impossible to determine what degree of protection was conferred by this separation. Similar studies in England and Canada also describe the apparent efficacy of BCG given to neonates.[195] BCG has some protective effect against the development of tuberculosis in newborns and appears to decrease the incidence of life-threatening forms of the disease.[196] Usually, the child must be kept out of the household, away from the contagious case, until the skin test result becomes reactive (marking protection from infection). However, many infants who receive a BCG vaccination do not develop a reactive tuberculin skin test. It is unknown if developing a reactive skin test correlates with protection. It is also unknown if a second BCG vaccination given to a child who maintains a negative tuberculin skin test reaction after the first BCG vaccination will cause an enhanced level of protection. Although BCG vaccines have some protective effect for the exposed newborn, most experts in the United States feel that appropriate separation and taking whatever steps are necessary to provide adequate chemotherapy for the child and the contagious adult is a superior approach to BCG vaccination. The use of directly observed therapy has made the need for BCG vaccination of infants in the United States almost nonexistent. The BCG vaccines are usually very safe, but fatal disseminated disease can occur in infants with underlying immune disorders.[197–204]

MANAGEMENT OF NEONATES AFTER POSTNATAL EXPOSURE

From time to time, workers in nurseries have been found to have infectious tuberculosis.[103, 205] These experiments of nature provide useful data on the risk to the infants. In general, risk of infection of neonates in a modern hospital nursery appears to be low. Most nurseries have large air volumes, flows, and adequate air exchanges to decrease risk of infection. Also, the minute volume of neonates is low, diminishing the risk of infection after a brief time of exposure. Light and co-workers[187] followed 437 infants exposed to a nurse with a cough and a sputum smear that was positive for tuberculosis. Of these infants, 160 were considered to be at greatest risk and received daily INH for 3 months; all infants remained tuberculin-negative. However, Steiner and colleagues[103] observed development of miliary tuberculosis in 2 of 1647 infants exposed in a nursery. Thus, infection is rare under nursery conditions, but it can and does occur. Strict control measures should prevent such episodes. Nursery personnel should undergo Mantoux testing before starting work and, if the result is negative, yearly thereafter. If the skin test is positive, a prospective employee should have a chest radiograph. If the radiograph is normal, appropriate therapy for *M. tuberculosis* infection should be given, accompanied by careful medical follow-up. Prospective employees with positive skin tests and abnormal chest radiographs must be carefully and thoroughly evaluated. Many require antituberculosis therapy.

Theoretically, these same guidelines apply to workers in licensed and unlicensed day-care facilities, but in many cases they have not yet been implemented.

Children with primary tuberculosis are rarely contagious because of the nature of their pulmonary disease, absence of forceful cough, and small number of organisms in the diseased tissue.[206] Infants with congenital tuberculosis often have extensive pulmonary involvement with positive acid-fast stains of tracheal aspirates and large numbers of tubercle bacilli in the lungs and airways.[207] In several cases, there has been evidence of transmission of *M. tuberculosis* from congenitally infected infants to health care workers; transmission to other infants has not been reported.[208, 209] Neonates with suspected congenital tuberculosis should be placed in appropriate isolation until it can be determined that they are not infectious, by acid-fast stain and culture of respiratory secretions.

If a member of the household other than the mother is found to have or to have had tuberculosis recently, the roles for chemotherapy and for BCG vaccine for the infant remain controversial. If the tuberculous family member has completed treatment in the past, that individual should undergo a checkup before the infant enters the home. If the family member is still being treated, he or she should have been sputum culture negative for at least 3 months before contact with the infant. If the infant must return to a home in which one of the family members has only recently started treatment, he or she should receive daily INH for at least 3 to 4 months, which Dormer and associates[186] showed to be very effective in preventing the development of tuberculosis in infants born to mothers in a sanatorium. If the family cannot be relied on to administer daily medication, if directly observed therapy is impossible, or if there are a number of household members suspected of having tuberculosis, BCG vaccination of the neonate should be considered.

CONCLUSION

Perinatal tuberculosis, although rare, will continue to occur, particularly among high-risk groups such as blacks, Hispanics, Asian/Pacific Islanders, and Native American/Alaskan natives, and particularly among recent immigrants to the United States. Intrauterine transmission to the unborn child occurs particularly in pregnant women experiencing initial *M. tuberculosis* infection and disease such as pleural effusion or miliary tuberculosis; less often it is a complication of endometrial tuberculosis. Postnatal tuberculosis, on the other hand, is usually acquired from a mother, other close family member, or caregiver with cavitary tuberculosis. Only by keeping the possibility of tuberculosis in mind and by carrying out appropriate history taking and tuberculin testing of pregnant patients, particularly those from high-risk groups, can tuberculosis be diagnosed and treated in time in the mother and newborn. If it does occur and is diagnosed in time, intensive treatment should result in an excellent outcome.

References

1. Dubos R, Dubos J. The White Plague: Tuberculosis, Man and Society. Boston, Little, Brown, 1952. Reissued as a paperback by Rutgers University Press, New Brunswick, N.J., 1987.
2. Adhikari M, Pillay T, Pillay DG. Tuberculosis in the newborn: an emerging disease. Pediatr Infect Dis J 16:1108–1121, 1997.
3. Margono E, Mroueh J, Garely A, et al. Resurgence of active tuberculosis among pregnant women. Obstet Gynecol 83:911–914, 1994.
4. Starke JR, Jacobs R, Jereb J. Resurgence of tuberculosis in children. J Pediatr 120:839–855, 1992.
5. Smith KC, Starke JR, Eisenach K, et al. Detection of *Mycobacterium tuberculosis* in clinical specimens from children using a polymerase chain reaction. Pediatrics 97:155–160, 1996.
6. Raviglione MC, Snider D Jr, Kochi A. Global epidemiology of tuberculosis: morbidity and mortality of a worldwide epidemic. JAMA 273:220–226 1995.
7. Ussery XT, Valway SE, Mckenna M, et al. Epidemiology of tuberculosis among children in the United States: 1985 to 1994. Pediatr Infect Dis J 15:697–704, 1996.
8. Barnes PF, Bloch AB, Davidson PT, et al. Tuberculosis in persons with human immunodeficiency virus infection. N Engl J Med 324:1644–1650, 1991.
9. Cantwell MF, McKenna M, McCray E, et al. Tuberculosis and race/ethnicity in the United States: impact of socioeconomic status. Am J Respir Crit Care Med 157:1016–1020, 1997.
10. McKenna MT, McCray E, Onorato IM. The epidemiology of tuberculosis among foreign-born persons in the United States, 1986 to 1993. N Engl J Med 332:1071–1076, 1995.
11. Asch S, Leake B, Anderson R, et al. Why do symptomatic patients delay obtaining care for tuberculosis? Am J Respir Crit Care Med 157:1244–1248, 1998.
12. Chin DP, DeReimer K, Small PM, et al. Differences in contributing factors to tuberculosis incidence in U.S.-born and foreign-born persons. Am J Respir Crit Care Med 158:1797–1803, 1998.
13. Lobato MN, Hopewell PC. *Mycobacterium tuberculosis* infection after travel to or contact with visitors from countries with a high prevalence of tuberculosis. Am J Respir Crit Care Med 158:1871–1875, 1998.
14. Coovadia HM, Wilkinson D. Childhood human immunodeficiency virus and tuberculosis co-infections: reconciling conflicting data. Int J Tuberc Lung Dis 2:844–851, 1998.
15. Jeena PM, Mitha T, Samber S, et al. Effects of the human immunodeficiency virus on tuberculosis in children. Tubercle Lung Dis 77:437–443, 1996.
16. Mofenson LM, Rodriguez EM, Hershow R, et al. *Mycobacterium tuberculosis* infection in pregnant and nonpregnant women infected with HIV in the women and infants transmission study. Arch Intern Med 155:1066–1072, 1995.
17. Schaefer G, Zervondakis IA, Fuchs FF, et al. Pregnancy and pulmonary tuberculosis. Obstet Gynecol 46:706–715, 1975.
18. Carter EJ, Mates S. Tuberculosis during pregnancy: the Rhode Island experience, 1987 to 1991. Chest 106:1466–1470, 1994.
19. Good JT Jr, Iseman MD, Davidson PT, et al. Tuberculosis in association with pregnancy. Am J Obstet Gynecol 140:492–498, 1981.
20. Centers for Disease Control and Prevention. Screening for tuberculosis and tuberculosis infection in high-risk populations. MMWR Morb Mortal Wkly Rep 44(RR-11):1–34, 1995.
21. Debré R, Lelong M, quoted by Rich AR. Pathogenesis of Tuberculosis, 2nd ed. Springfield, Ill, Charles C Thomas, 1951, p 72.
22. Weinberger SE, Weiss ST, Cohen WR, et al. Pregnancy and the lung. Am Rev Respir Dis 121:599–581, 1980.
23. Van Zwanenberg D. Influence of the number of bacilli on the development of tuberculous disease in children. Am Rev Respir Dis 83:31–44, 1960.
24. Rich AR. The Pathogenesis of Tuberculosis, 2nd ed. Springfield, Ill, Charles C Thomas, 1951.
25. Schluger NW, Rom WH. The host immune response to tuberculosis. Am J Respir Crit Care Med 157:679–691, 1998.
26. Wallgren A. The "time-table" of tuberculosis. Tubercle 29:245–251, 1948.

27. Smith S, Jacobs RF, Wilson CB. Immunobiology of childhood tuberculosis: a window on the ontogeny of cellular immunity. J Pediatr 131:16–26, 1997.

28. Abraham G, Teklu B. Miliary tuberculosis in pregnancy and puerperium: analysis of eight cases. Ethiop Med J 19:87–90, 1981.

29. Brar HS, Golde SH, Egan JE. Tuberculosis presenting as puerperal fever. Obstet Gynecol 70:488–491, 1987.

30. Brooks JH, Stirrat GM. Tuberculous peritonitis in pregnancy: case report. Br J Obstet Gynecol 93:1009–1010, 1986.

31. Centeno RS, Winter J, Bentson JR. Central nervous system tuberculosis related to pregnancy. J Comput Tomogr 6:141–145, 1982.

32. Freeman D. Abdominal tuberculosis in pregnancy. Tubercle 70:143–145, 1989.

33. Garrioch DB, Puerperal tuberculosis. Br J Clin Pract 29:280–281, 1975.

34. Golditch IM, Tuberculous meningitis and pregnancy. Am J Obstet Gynecol 110:1144–1146, 1971.

35. Govender S, Moodley SC, Grootboom MJ. Tuberculous paraplegia during pregnancy: a report of 4 cases. S Afr Med J 75:190–192, 1989.

36. Grenville-Mathers R, Harris WC, Trenchard HJ. Tuberculous primary infection in pregnancy and its relation to congenital tuberculosis. Tubercle 41:181–185, 1960.

37. Horley JF. Congenital tuberculosis. Arch Dis Child 17:167–172, 1952.

38. Kingdom JCP, Kennedy DH. Tuberculous meningitis in pregnancy. Br J Obstet Gynecol 96:233–235, 1989.

39. Maheswaran C, Neuwirth RS. An unusual cause of postpartum fever: acute hematogenous tuberculosis. Obstet Gynecol 41:765–769, 1973.

40. Manson N. Congenital tuberculosis after pleural effusion in the mother. BMJ 2:970, 1954.

41. Myers JP, Perlstein PH, Light IJ, et al. Tuberculosis in pregnancy with fatal congenital infection. Pediatrics 67:89–94, 1981.

42. Nsofor BI, Trivedi ON. Postpartum paraplegia due to spinal tuberculosis. Trop Doc 18:52–53, 1988.

43. Petrini B, Gente J, Winbladh B, et al. Perinatal transmission of tuberculosis: meningitis in mother, disseminated disease in child. Scand J Infect Dis 15:403–405, 1983.

44. Suvonnakote T, Obst D. Pulmonary tuberculosis with pregnancy. J Med Assoc Thor 64:26–30, 1981.

45. Bazaz-Malik G, Maheshwari B, Lal N. Tuberculosis endometritis: a clinicopathological study of 1000 cases. Br J Obstet Gynaecol 90:84–86, 1983.

46. Punnonen R, Kiilholma P, Meurman L. Female genital tuberculosis and consequent infertility. Int J Fertil 28:235–238, 1983.

47. Baumgartner W, Van Calker H, Eisenberger W. Congenital tuberculosis. Monatschr Kinderheilkd 128:563–566, 1980.

48. Cooper AR, Heneghan W, Mathew JD. Tuberculosis in a mother and her infant. Pediatr Infect Dis J 4:181–183, 1985.

49. Hallum JL, Thomas HE. Full term pregnancy after proved endometrial tuberculosis. J Obstet Gynaecol Br Emp 62:548–550, 1955.

50. Kaplan C, Benirschke K, Tarzy B. Placental tuberculosis in early and late pregnancy. Am J Obstet Gynecol 137:858–860, 1980.

51. Addis GM, Anthony GS, Semple P, et al. Miliary tuberculosis in an in-vitro fertilization pregnancy: a case report. Eur J Obstet Gynecol Reprod Biol 27:351–353, 1988.

52. Snider DE Jr. Pregnancy and tuberculosis. Chest 86 (Suppl):10S–13S, 1984.

53. Hedvall E. Pregnancy and tuberculosis. Acta Med Scand 147 (Suppl 286):1–101, 1953.

54. Cohen RC. Effect of pregnancy and parturition on pulmonary tuberculosis. BMJ 2:775–776, 1943.

55. Cromie JB. Pregnancy and pulmonary tuberculosis. Br J Tuberc 48:97–101, 1954.

56. Cohen JD, Patton EA, Badger TL. The tuberculous mother. Am Rev Tuberc 65:1–23, 1952.

57. Edge JR. Pulmonary tuberculosis and pregnancy. Br J Med 2:845–846, 1952.

58. Rosenbach LM, Gangemi CR. Tuberculosis and pregnancy. JAMA 161:1035–1037, 1956.

59. Stewart CJ, Simmonds FAH. Child-bearing and pulmonary tuberculosis. BMJ 2:726–729, 1947.

60. Stewart CJ, Simmonds FAH. Prognosis of pulmonary tuberculosis in married women. Tubercle 35:28–30, 1954.

61. Wilson EA, Thelin TJ, Dilts PV Jr. Tuberculosis complicated by pregnancy. Am J Obstet Gynecol 115:526–529, 1973.

62. de March AP. Tuberculosis and pregnancy: five to ten-year review of 215 patients in their fertile age. Chest 68:800–804, 1975.

63. Mehta BR. Pregnancy and tuberculosis. Dis Chest 39:505–511, 1961.

64. Pridie RB, Stradling P. Management of pulmonary tuberculosis during pregnancy. BMJ 2:78–79, 1961.

65. Bjerkedal T, Bahna SL, Lehmann EH. Course and outcome of pregnancy in women with pulmonary tuberculosis. Scand J Respir Dis 56:245–250, 1975.

66. Ratner B, Rostler AE, Salgado PS. Care, feeding and fate of premature and full term infants born of tuberculous mothers. Am J Dis Child 81:471–482, 1951.

67. Bernsee Rush JJ. Protocol for tuberculosis screening in pregnancy. J Obstet Gynecol Neonat Nurs 14:225–230, 1986.

68. Hamadeh MA, Glassroth J. Tuberculosis and pregancy. Chest 101:1114–1120, 1992.

69. McIntyre PB, McCormack JG, Vacca A. Tuberculosis in pregnancy—implications for antenatal screening in Australia. Med J Aust 146:42–44, 1987.

70. American Academy of Pediatrics Committee on Infectious Disease. Report of the Committee on Infectious Diseases. Elk Grove Village, Ill, American Academy of Pediatrics, 1997, pp 541–562.

71. Kendig EL, Kirkpatrick BV, Carter WH, et al. Underreading of the tuberculin skin test reaction. Chest 113:1175–1177, 1998.

72. Covelli HD, Wilson RT. Immunologic and medical consideration in tuberculin-sensitized pregnant patients. Am J Obstet Gynecol 132:256–259, 1978.

73. Keller MA, Rodriguez AL, Alvarez S, et al. Transfer of tuberculin immunity from mother to infant. Pediatr Res 22:277–281, 1987.

74. Gillum MD, Maki DG. Brief report: tuberculin testing, BCG in pregnancy. Infect Cont Hosp Epidemiol 9:119–121, 1988.

75. Smith JK, Caspary EA, Field EJ. Lymphocyte reactivity to antigen pregnancy. Am J Obstet Gynecol 113:602–606, 1972.

76. Montgomery WP, Young RC Jr, Allen MP, et al. The tuberculin test in pregnancy. Am J Obstet Gynecol 100:829–831, 1968.

77. Present PA, Comstock GW. Tuberculin sensitivity in pregnancy. Am Rev Respir Dis 112:413–416, 1975.

78. Snider DE Jr, Layde PM, Johnson MW, et al. Treatment

of tuberculosis during pregnancy. Am Rev Respir Dis 122:65–78, 1980.

79. Vallejo JG, Starke JR. Tuberculosis and pregnancy. Clin Chest Med 13:693–707, 1992.

80. Starke JR. Tuberculosis: an old disease but a new threat to the mother, fetus and neonate. Clin Perinatol 24:107–128, 1997.

81. Bonebrake CR, Noller KL, Loehnen PC, et al. Routine chest roentgenography in pregnancy. JAMA 240:2747–2748, 1978.

82. Maccato ML. Pneumonia and pulmonary tuberculosis in pregnancy. Obstet Gynecol Clin North Am 16:417–430, 1989.

83. Weinstein L, Murphy T. The management of tuberculosis during pregnancy. Clin Perinatol 1:395–405, 1974.

84. Hale JA, Peters GN, Cheek JH. Tuberculosis of the breast: rare but still extant. Am J Surg 150:620–624, 1985.

85. Jacobs RF, Abernathy RS. Management of tuberculosis in pregnancy and the newborn. Clin. Perinatol. 15:305–319, 1988.

86. Wapnir IL, Pallam TH, Gaudino J, et al. Latent mammary tuberculosis: a case report. Surgery 98:976–978, 1985.

87. Cantwell MF, Shehab ZM, Costello AM, et al. Brief report: congenital tuberculosis. N Engl J Med 330:1051–1054, 1994.

88. Micozzi MS. Skeletal tuberculosis, pelvic contraction and partuition. Am J Phys Anthropol 58:441–445, 1982.

89. Hageman J, Shulman S, Schreiber M, et al. Congenital tuberculosis: critical reappraisal of clinical findings and diagnostic procedures. Pediatrics 66:980–984, 1980.

90. Nemir RL, O'Hare D. Congenital tuberculosis: review and guidelines. Am J Dis Child 139:284–287, 1985.

91. Beitzke H. Ueber die angeborene tuberkuloese Infektion. Ergeb Gesamte Tuberkuloseforsch 7:1–30, 1935.

92. Rich AR, Follis RH Jr. Effect of low oxygen tension upon the development of experimental tuberculosis. Bull Johns Hopkins Hosp 71:345–357, 1942.

93. Vorwald AJ. Experimental tuberculous infection in the guinea-pig foetus compared with that in the adult. Am Rev Tuberc 35:260–295, 1937.

94. Hertzog AJ, Chapman S, Herring J. Congenital pulmonary aspiration tuberculosis. Am J Clin Pathol 19:1139–1142, 1949.

95. Hughesdon MR. Congenital tuberculosis. Arch Dis Child 21:121–139, 1946.

96. Corner BD, Brown NJ. Congenital tuberculosis: report of a case with necropsy findings in mother and child. Thorax 10:99–103, 1955.

97. Siegel M. Pathological findings and pathogenesis of congenital tuberculosis. Am Rev Tuberc 29:297–309, 1934.

98. Bate TWP, Sinclair RE, Robinson MJ. Neonatal tuberculosis. Arch. Dis. Child. 61:512–514, 1986.

99. Devi PK, Mujumdar SS, Modadam NG, et al. Pregnancy and pulmonary tuberculosis: observations on the domiciliary management of 238 patients in India. Tubercle 45:211–216, 1964.

100. Kendig EL Jr. Tuberculosis in the very young: report of three cases in infants less than one month of age. Am Rev Respir Dis 70:161–165, 1954.

101. Watchi R, Lu K, Kahlstrom E, et al. Tuberculous meningitis in a five-week-old child. Int J Tuberc Lung Dis 2:255–257, 1998.

102. Burk JR, Bahar D, Wold FS, et al. Nursery exposure of 528 newborns to a nurse with pulmonary tuberculosis. South Med J 71:7–10, 1978.

103. Steiner P, Rao M, Victoria MS, et al. Miliary tuberculosis in two infants after nursery exposure: epidemiologic, clinical and laboratory findings. Am Rev Respir Dis 113:267–271, 1976.

104. Kendig EL Jr, Rodgers WL. Tuberculosis in the neonatal period. Am Rev Tuberc Pulm Dis 77:418–422, 1958.

105. Holt LE. Tuberculosis acquired through ritual circumcision. JAMA 61:99–102, 1913.

106. Abughali N, Van der Kuyp F, Annable W, et al. Congenital tuberculosis. Pediatr Infect Dis J 13:738–741, 1994.

107. Amick FE, Alden MW, Sweet LK. Congenital tuberculosis. Pediatrics 6:384–390, 1950.

108. Arthur L. Congenital tuberculosis. Proc R Soc Med 60:19–20, 1967.

109. Asensi F, Otero MC, Perez-Tamarit D, et al. Congenital tuberculosis, still a problem. Pediatr Infect Dis J 9:223–224, 1990.

110. Blackall PB. Tuberculosis: maternal infection of the newborn. Med J Aust 42:1055–1058, 1969.

111. Davis SF, Finley SC, Hare WK. Congenital tuberculosis: case report. J Pediatr 57:221–224, 1960.

112. Foo AL, Tan KK, Chay DM. Congenital tuberculosis. Tubercle Lung Dis 74:59–61, 1993.

113. Hardy JB, Hartman JR. Tuberculous dactylitis in childhood. J Pediatr 30:146–156, 1947.

114. Hopkins R, Ermocilla R, Cassady G. Congenital tuberculosis. South Med J 69:1156, 1976.

115. Hudson FP. Clinical aspects of congenital tuberculosis. Arch Dis Child 31:136–138, 1956.

116. Koutsoulieris K, Kaslaris E. Congenital tuberculosis. Arch Dis Child 45:584–586, 1970.

117. Krishnan L, Vernekar AV, Diwakar KK, et al. Neonatal tuberculosis: a case report. Ann Trop Paediatr 14:333–335, 1994.

118. McCray MK, Esterly NB. Cutaneous eruptions in congenital tuberculosis. Arch Dermatol 117:460–464, 1981.

119. Morens DH, Baublis JV, Heidelberger KP. Congenital tuberculosis and associated hypoadrenocorticism. South Med J 72:160–165, 1979.

120. Niles RA. Puerperal tuberculosis with death of infant. Am J Obstet Gynecol 144:131–132, 1982.

121. Pai PM, Parikh PR. Congenital miliary tuberculosis: case report. Clin Pediatr 15:376–378, 1976.

122. Polansky SM, Frank A, Ablow RC, et al. Congenital tuberculosis. AJR 130:994–996, 1978.

123. Ramos AD, Hibbard LT, Graig JR. Congenital tuberculosis. Obstet Gynecol 43:61–64, 1974.

124. Reisinger KS, Evans P, Yost G, et al. Congenital tuberculosis: report of case. Pediatrics 54:74–76, 1974.

125. Sauer P, Kuss JJ, Lutz P, et al. La tuberculose congénital. Pédiatrie 36:217–224, 1981.

126. Soeiro A. Congenital tuberculosis in a small premature baby. S Afr Med J 45:1025–1026, 1971.

127. Todd RM. Congenital tuberculosis: report of a case with unusual features. Tubercle 41:71–73, 1960.

128. Voyce MA, Hunt AC. Congenital tuberculosis. Arch Dis Child 41:299–300, 1966.

129. Vucicevic Z, Suskovic T, Ferencic Z. A female patient with tuberculous polyserositis and congenital tuberculosis in her new-born child. Tubercle Lung Dis 76:460–462, 1995.

130. Dische MR, Krishnan C, Andreychuk R, et al. Congenital tuberculosis in a twin of immigrant parentage. Can Med Assoc J 119:1068–1070, 1978.

131. Cunningham DG, McGraw TT, Griffin AJ, et al. Neonatal tuberculosis with pulmonary cavitation. Tubercle 63:217–219, 1982.

132. Teeratkulpisarn J, Lumbigagmon P, Pairojkul S, et al.

Cavitary tuberculosis in a young infant. Pediatr Infect Dis J 13:545–546, 1994.

133. De Angelis P, Antonelli P, Esposito G, et al. Congenital tuberculosis in twins. Pediatrics 69:402–416, 1981.

134. Gordon-Nesbitt DC, Rajan G. Congenital tuberculosis successfully treated. Letter to the editor. BMJ 1:233–234, 1972.

135. Naranbai RC, Mathiassen W, Malan AF. Congenital tuberculosis localized to the ear. Arch Dis Child 63:738–740, 1989.

136. Senbil N, Sahin F, Coglar MK, et al. Congenital tuberculosis of the ear and parotid gland. Pediatr Infect Dis J 16:1090, 1997.

137. Vallejo J, Ong L, Starke J. Clinical features, diagnosis and treatment of tuberculosis in infants. Pediatrics 94:1–7, 1994.

138. Schaaf HS, Smith J, Donald PR, et al. Tuberculosis presenting in the neonatal period. Clin Pediatr 28:474–475, 1989.

139. Schaaf HS, Gie RP, Beyers N, et al. Tuberculosis in infants less than 3 months of age. Arch Dis Child 69:371–374, 1993.

140. Pomputius WF III, Rost J, Dennehy PH, et al. Standardization of gastric aspirate technique improves yield in the diagnosis of tuberculosis in children. Pediatr Infect Dis J 16:222–226, 1997.

141. Khan EA, Starke JR. Diagnosis of tuberculosis in children: increased need for better methods. Emerg Infect Dis 1:115–123, 1995.

142. Stallworth JR, Brasfield DM, Tiller RE. Congenital miliary tuberculosis proved by open lung biopsy specimen and successfully treated. Am J Dis Child 14:320–321, 1980.

143. Mieeli JN, Olson WA, Cohen SN. Elimination kinetics of isoniazid in the newborn infant. Dev Pharmacol Ther 2:235–239, 1981.

144. Atkins JN. Maternal plasma concentration of pyridoxal phosphate during pregnancy: adequacy of vitamin B_6 supplementation during isoniazid therapy. Am Rev Respir Dis 126:714–717, 1982.

145. Sumartojo E. When tuberculosis treatment fails: a social behavior account of patient adherence. Am Rev Respir Dis 147:1311–1320, 1993.

146. Villarino ME, Ridzon R, Weismuller PC, et al. Rifampin preventive therapy for tuberculosis infection: experience with 157 adolescents. Am J Respir Crit Care Med 155:1735–1738, 1997.

147. Centers for Disease Control. Management of persons exposed to multidrug-resistant tuberculosis. MMWR Morb Mortal Wkly Rep 41 (RR-11):1–8, 1992.

148. Franks AL, Binkin NJ, Snider DE Jr, et al. Isoniazid hepatitis among pregnancy and postpartum Hispanic patients. Public Health Rep 104:151–155, 1989.

149. Abernathy RS, Dutt AK, Stead WW, et al. Shortcourse chemotherapy for tuberculosis in children. Pediatrics 72:801–806, 1983.

150. Farqhuharson M, Turner B. Tuberculosis and the puerperium: a trial of chemotherapy and oestrogens. Br J Tuberc 50:320–325, 1956.

151. Flanagan P, Hensler NM. The course of active tuberculosis complicated by pregnancy. JAMA 170:783–787, 1959.

152. Schaefer G, Douglas RG, Silverman F. A re-evaluation of the management of pregnancy and tuberculosis. J Obstet Gynecol Br Emp 66:990–997, 1959.

153. Schaeffer G, Birnbaum SJ. Present-day treatment of tuberculosis and pregnancy. JAMA 165:2163–2167, 1957.

154. Varpela E. On the effect exerted by first-line tuberculosis medicines on the foetus. Acta Tuberc Scand 35:53–69, 1964.

155. Wall MA. Treatment of tuberculosis during pregnancy. Am Rev Respir Dis 122:989–993, 1980.

156. Scheinhorn DJ, Angelillo VA. Antituberculous therapy in pregnancy: risks to the fetus. West J Med 127:195–198, 1977.

157. Bobrowitz ID, Ethambutol in pregnancy. Chest 66:20–24, 1974.

158. Lewit T, Nebel L, Terracina S, et al. Ethambutol in pregnancy: observations on embryogenesis. Chest 68:25–27, 1974.

159. Place VA Ethambutol administration during pregnancy: a case report. J New Drugs 4:206–208, 1964.

160. Steen JSM, Stainton-Ellis DM. Rifampin in pregnancy. Lancet 2:604–605, 1977.

161. Skolnick JL, Stoler BS, Katz DB, et al. Rifampin, oral contraceptives, and pregnancy. JAMA 236:1382, 1976.

162. Brock PG, Rooch M. Antituberculosis drugs in pregnancy. Lancet 1:43–44, 1981.

163. Byrd, R.B. Treating the pregnant tuberculous patient: curing the mother without harming the fetus. J Respir Dis 3:27–32, 1982.

164. Lowe CR. Congenital defects among children born to women under supervision or treatment for pulmonary tuberculosis. Br J Prev Soc Med 18:14–16, 1964.

165. Donald PR, Sellars SL. Streptomycin ototoxicity in the unborn child. S Afr Med J 60:316–318, 1981.

166. Robinson GC, Cambon KG. Hearing loss in infants of tuberculous mothers treated with streptomycin during pregnancy. N Engl J Med 271:949–951, 1964.

167. Varpela E, Hietalahti J, Aro MJT. Streptomycin and dihydrostreptomycin medication during pregnancy and their effect on the child's inner ear. Scand J Respir Dis 50:101–109, 1969.

168. Potworowska M, Sianozecka E, Szufladowicz R. Ethionamide treatment and pregnancy. Polish Med J 5:1152–1158, 1966.

169. Davidson PT. Managing tuberculosis during pregnancy. Lancet 346:199–200, 1995.

170. Medchill MT, Gillum M. Diagnosis and management of tuberculosis during pregnancy. Obstet Gynecol Rev 44:81–91, 1989.

171. Bloch A, Cauthen G, Onorato I, et al. Nationwide survey of drug-resistant tuberculosis in the United States. JAMA 271:665–671, 1994.

172. Pablos-Mendez A, Raviglione MC, Laszlo A. Global surveillance for antituberculosis-drug resistance, 1994–1997. N Engl J Med 338:1641–1649, 1998.

173. Snider DE Jr, Powell KE. Should women taking antituberculosis drugs breast-feed? Arch Intern Med 144:589–590, 1984.

174. McKenzie SA, Macnab AJ, Katz G. Neonatal pyridoxine responsive convulsions due to isoniazid therapy. Arch Dis Child 51:567–569, 1976.

175. Steinhoff MC, Lionel J. Treatment of tuberculosis in newborn infants and their mothers. Indian J Pediatr, 55:240–245, 1988.

176. Doerr CA, Starke JR, Ong LT. Clinical and public health aspects of tuberculous meningitis in children. J Pediatr 127:27–33, 1995.

177. Gessner BD, Weiss NS, Nolan CM. Risk factors for pediatric tuberculosis infection and disease after household exposure to adult index cases in Alaska. J Pediatr 132:509–513, 1998.

178. MacIntyre CR, Plant AJ. Preventability of incident cases of tuberculosis in recently exposed contacts. Int J Tuberc Lung Dis 2:56–61, 1998.

179. Mehta JB, Bentley S. Prevention of tuberculosis in children: missed opportunities. Am J Prev Med 8:283–286, 1992.

180. Nolan R Jr. Childhood tuberculosis in North Carolina: a study of the opportunities for intervention in the transmission of tuberculosis in children. Am J Public Health 76:26–30, 1986.

181. Rodrigo T, Cayla JA, de Olalla PG, et al. Characteristics of tuberculosis patients who generate secondary cases. Int J Tuberc Lung Dis 1:352–357, 1997.

182. Spark RP, Pock NA, Pedron SL, et al. Perinatal tuberculosis and its public health impact: a case report. Texas Med 92:50–53, 1996.

183. Kendig EL. Prognosis of infants born of tuberculous mothers. Pediatrics 26:97–100, 1960.

184. Laurance BM. Congenital tuberculosis successfully treated. Letter to the editor. BMJ 2:55, 1973.

185. Avery ME, Wolfsdorf J. Diagnosis and treatment: approaches to newborn infants of tuberculous mothers. Pediatrics 42:519–521, 1968.

186. Dormer BA, Harrison I, Swart JA, et al. Prophylactic isoniazid protection of infants in a tuberculosis hospital. Lancet 2:902–903, 1959.

187. Light IJ, Saidleman M, Sutherland JM. Management of newborns after nursery exposure to tuberculosis. Am Rev Respir Dis 109:415–419, 1974.

188. Raucher HS, Grimbetz I. Care of the pregnant woman with tuberculosis and her newborn infant: a pediatrician's perspective. Mt Sinai J Med 53:70–75, 1986.

189. Centers for Disease Control and Prevention. The role of BCG vaccine in the prevention and control of tuberculosis in the United States: a joint statement by the Advisory Council for the Elimination of Tuberculosis and the Advisory Committee on Immunization Practices. MMWR Morb Mortal Wkly Rep 45 (RR-4):1–18, 1996.

190. Sedaghatian MR, Hashem F, Hossain MM. Bacille Calmette Guérin vaccination in pre-term infants. Int J Tuberc Lung Dis 2:679–682, 1998.

191. Sepulveda RL, Arredondo S, Rodriguez E, et al. Effect of human newborn BCG immunization on monocyte viability and function at 3 months of age. Int J Tuberc Lung Dis 1:122–127, 1997.

192. Lorber J, Menneer PC. Long-term effectiveness of B.C.G. vaccination of infants in close contact with infectious tuberculosis. BMJ 1:1430–1433, 1959.

193. Pabst HF, Godel J, Grace M, et al. Effect of breastfeeding on immune response to BCG vaccination. Lancet 1:295–297, 1989.

194. Kendig EL Jr. The place of BCG vaccine in the management of infants born to tuberculous mothers. N Engl J Med 281:520–523, 1969.

195. Curtis HM, Bamford FN, Leck I. Incidence of childhood tuberculosis after neonatal BCG vaccination. Lancet 1:145–148, 1984.

196. Colditz G, Berkey CS, Mosteller F, et al. The efficacy of bacillus Calmette-Guérin vaccination of newborns and infants in the prevention of tuberculosis: meta-analysis of the published literature. Pediatrics 96:29–35, 1995.

197. Besnard M, Sauvion S, Offredo C, et al. Bacillus Calmette-Guérin infection after vaccination of human immunodeficiency virus–infected children. Pediatr Infect Dis J 12:993–997, 1993.

198. Carlgren LE, Hansson CG, Henricsson L, et al. Fatal BCG infection in an infant with congenital lymphocytopenic agammaglobulinemia. Acta Pediatr Scand 55:636–644, 1966.

199. Esterly JR, Sturner WQ, Esterly NB, et al. Disseminated BCG in twin boys with presumed chronic granulomatous disease of childhood. Pediatrics 48:141–144, 1977.

200. Gonzalez B, Moreno S, Burdach R, et al. Clinical presentation of bacillus Calmette-Guérin infections in patients with immunodeficiency syndromes. Pediatr Infect Dis J 8:201–206, 1989.

201. Jovanguy E, Altare F, Lamhamedi S, et al. Interferon-γ-receptor deficiency in an infant with fatal bacille Calmette-Guérin infection. N Engl J Med 335:1956–1961, 1996.

202. Lallemant-le Couer S, Lallemant M, Cheynier D, et al. Bacillus Calmette-Guérin immunization in infants born to HIV-1-seropositive mothers. AIDS 5:195–199, 1991.

203. O'Brien K, Ruff A, Louis M, et al. Bacillus Calmette-Guérin complications in children born to HIV-1 infected women with a review of the literature. Pediatrics 95:414–418, 1995.

204. Peltola H, Salmi I, Vahuanen V, et al. BCG vaccination as a cause of osteomyelitis and subcutaneous abscess. Arch Dis Child 59:157–161, 1984.

205. Nivin B, Nicholas P, Gayer M, et al. A continuing outbreak of multidrug-resistant tuberculosis with transmission in a hospital nursery. Clin Infect Dis 26:303–307, 1998.

206. Centers for Disease Control and Prevention. Guidelines for preventing the transmission of Mycobacterium tuberculosis in health-care facilities. MMWR Morb Mortal Wkly Rep 43 (RR-13):1–133, 1994.

207. Lee HL, LeVea CM, Graman PS. Congenital tuberculosis in a neonatal intensive care unit: case report, epidemiological investigation, and management of exposures. Clin Infect Dis 27:474–477, 1998.

208. Machin GA, Honore LH, Fanning EA, et al. Perinatally acquired neonatal tuberculosis: report of two cases. Pediatr Pathol 12:707–716, 1992.

209. Rabalais G, Adams G, Stover B. PPD skin test conversion in healthcare workers after exposure to Mycobacterium tuberculosis infection in infants. Lancet 338:826, 1991.

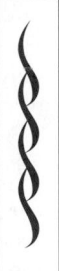

Gonococcal Infections

LAURA T. GUTMAN, M.D.

The word gonorrhea (from Greek, *gono*, meaning "seed," and German, *rhein*, meaning "to flow") refers to the purulent urethral discharge produced by *Neisseria gonorrhoeae* in males. The term has focused attention on urethritis alone and has obscured the other and varied manifestations of gonococcal infection. Recognition of the different anatomic sites that may become colonized or infected by the gonococcus in newborns has been particularly slow, and the only well-studied manifestation of gonococcal infection in the newborn is ophthalmia neonatorum. Recovery of *N. gonorrhoeae* from the newborn from an external site other than the eye was not well documented in the United States before 1971. However, a variety of syndromes and sites of infection in the newborn are now known to be caused by *N. gonorrhoeae* and are discussed in this chapter.[1–16]

BACTERIOLOGY AND PATHOGENESIS

Identification

N. gonorrhoeae was first observed in urethral exudate by Neisser in 1879 and was first isolated in 1882 by Liestikow and Loeffler. Gonococci are gram-negative diplococci having an ultrastructure similar to that of other gram-negative bacteria.

Sugar utilization tests are the primary means used to differentiate the gonococcus from the other *Neisseria* species indigenous to humans, which include *N. meningitidis*, *N. lactamica*, *N. cinerea*, *N. sicca*, *N. perflava*, *N. flava*, *N. subflava*, and *N. mucosa*.[17] *N. gonorrhoeae* utilizes glucose but not maltose, sucrose, or lactose. Other properties used to differentiate these species include colonial morphology, chromogenesis, growth on nutrient agar at 22° C, capacity to produce hemolysis, substrate growth requirements, DNA base content and DNA homologies, and serotype or serogroup.

Laboratory examination of specimens for *N. gonorrhea* also include direct specimen antigen detection methods, which may be used in addition to culture methods. Direct immunofluorescence methods are sometimes used to demonstrate organisms in tissue specimens. Solid-phase enzyme immunoassay may be used to confirm a positive pediatric specimen.

Two new tests for the diagnosis of *N. gonorrhoeae* are based on specific nucleic acid hybridization and have been approved by the Food and Drug Administration. These tests, when tested on adult specimens, show sensitivity and specificity that compare favorably with culture assays.[17, 18] However, as with all presentations of gonorrhea in children, it is recommended that a culture assay be used for diagnosis. Nonculture assays may be used as a secondary diagnostic method, or to confirm the culture result.[19] A complete review of gonococcal diagnostic methods is presented elsewhere.[20]

Strain Typing

N. gonorrhoeae forms four distinct types of colonies on agar medium. Only types 1 and 2 are seen on primary isolation, but, on repeated subculture at 37° C, these give rise to colonial types 3 and 4. Organisms obtained from type 1 or 2 colonies are more virulent than those from type 3 or 4 colonies. Types 1 and 2 cells have hairlike appendages called pili[21] that appear to be important in initial attachment of gonococci to a variety of mammalian cells and that interfere with phagocytosis of gonococci by polymorphonuclear leukocytes.

Gonococcal colonies are now also classified on the basis of colonial opacity, which is not related to pili. Opaque colonies (0⁻) have surface proteins (termed proteins II), which also influence the interactions of gonococci with host cells. Transparent (0^-) colonies lack proteins II and have increased serum resistance. Most gonococcal isolates from blood or fallopian tubes form 0^- colonies on primary culture. Gonococci from symptomatic genital sites are usually 0^-, and rapid shifts from 0^+ to 0^- commonly occur.[22]

Because all gonococci appear to be capable of producing all colony types, colonial morphology does not represent a useful means of differentiating between different types or strains of gonococci. However, other methods for typing gonococci have proved to be useful in epidemiologic studies. One method, called *auxotyping*, differentiates gonococci into several stable subtypes on the basis of their auxotrophic requirements for substrate amino acids, purines, pyrimidines, or vitamins. Marked antigenic heterogeneity exists among various strains of gonococci.[23]

The predominant protein in the gonococcal outer membrane is termed protein I. One typing system, using the enzyme-linked immunosorbent assay, identifies nine antigenic types of protein I. Types 1 and 2 predominate in strains from patients with disseminated disease. Serologic typing for protein I identifies three serogroups (WI to WIII).[24]

The typing method that offers greatest discrimination among strains is serologic and based on coagglutination and the use of monoclonal antibodies to outer membrane protein I.[25] Strains possessing this protein belong to one of two serogroups, 1A and 1B. These groups each contain serotypes, and at least 50 serotypes may be differentiated.

Outer membrane protein I is a stable characteristic of each gonococcal strain and does not exhibit rapid phase variation or antigenic shift. Epidemiologically related strains are almost always of similar serotype. Auxotyping and serotyping can be combined to facilitate epidemiologic studies of gonococcal infections.[26]

Bacteriology

Aspects of the microbiology of *N. gonorrhoeae* that pertain to virulence or to specific disease syndromes include the following:

1. Gonococcal lipopolysaccharide contains lipid A and core oligosaccharides. These cell wall components are produced and may be discharged as blebs from the outer membrane, and they appear to participate in toxic interactions with the fallopian tubes (see later).[27]

2. All virulent species of *Neisseria*, including *N. gonorrhoeae*, produce IgA1 protease, which cleaves human IgA1 at the hinge region, thereby rendering secretory IgA inactive.[28] This appears to facilitate mucosal colonization and invasion.

3. *N. gonorrhoeae* is particularly interesting in its interactions with atmospheric oxygen and with oxidative products of lysosomes of human polymorphonuclear leukocytes. *N. gonorrhoeae* is an obligate aerobe but appears to lack superoxide dismutase, the enzyme that is present in almost all other aerotolerant microorganisms and that moderates the toxic effects of oxygen radicals.[29] *N. gonorrhoeae* appears to compensate for exposure to

atmospheric oxygen through the production of a highly active terminal oxidase system and oxygen-stable catalase system.[30]

When grown in anaerobic conditions, virulent strains of *N. gonorrhoeae* produce an outer membrane protein, Pan 1. Pan 1 is a lipoprotein. Evidence that this lipoprotein is biologically significant comes from the demonstrations that it is the epitope for the majority of IgM antibody produced by patients with acute gonorrhea.[31]

The extent and mechanism of neutrophil killing of *N. gonorrhoeae* are an area of current uncertainty. However, data are accumulating to indicate that oxidative neutrophil systems may kill gonococci relatively inefficiently but that nonoxidative neutrophil systems may contribute to intraphagosomal lysis of gonococci. Cationic antimicrobial proteins, including cathepsin G, may participate in this process.[32]

The reader is referred to a recent review by Cohen and Sparling of the bacterial adaptations and interactions with host defenses that have made *N. gonorrhoeae* such a successful human pathogen.[33]

Several chromosomal loci have been identified in *N. gonorrhoeae* that influence the susceptibility of the organism to one or more antimicrobial agents.[34] Since the introduction of penicillin, strains of *N. gonorrhoeae* have shown the ability to acquire penicillin resistance, which is expressed as a wide spectrum of penicillin sensitivity. In 1983, an outbreak of gonorrhea occurred in North Carolina with a strain that was highly resistant to penicillin and in which the penicillin resistance was not conferred by plasmids. These strains exhibited chromosomally mediated alterations in penicillin-binding proteins, and the strains were termed CMRNG (chromosomally mediated resistant *N. gonorrhoeae*). These strains are now found across the United States and have occasioned several large outbreaks.[35]

Finally, as a measure of the rapidity with which *N. gonorrhoeae* may respond to altered patterns of antimicrobial use, strains with complex patterns of resistance are being reported that are resistant to tetracycline and produce penicillinase, are resistant to spectinomycin and produce penicillinase, or have chromosomally mediated resistance to multiple antibiotics. Infants and children have been infected with both penicillin-producing *N. gonorrhoeae* (PPNG) and CMRNG, although reports of newborn disease with either are still rare.[36–38]

In 1976, beta-lactamase–producing strains appeared nearly simultaneously in England (where they had been imported from Africa) and in the United States (where they had been imported from the Philippines). Infection with these strains is not cured by therapy with penicillin G, ampicillin, or amoxicillin. The beta-lactamases produced by these strains are coded on plasmids that show a high degree of homology with similar plasmids first found a few years earlier in strains of *Haemophilus parainfluenzae* and *Haemophilus influenzae*. Some strains of *N. gonorrhoeae* also contain a larger, conjugative plasmid capable of mobilizing the beta-lactamase plasmid into other bacterial cells. The early 1980s saw increasing numbers of these isolates in localized epidemics, and, in 1985, the rates of PPNG again increased sharply, primarily because of large outbreaks in Florida and New York. By 1991, 11% of all strains of *N. gonorrhoeae* in the United States were PPNG and 32% of all strains were resistant to one or more antimicrobial agents. Because of this, penicillin is no longer recommended for primary therapy for gonococcal disease and has been replaced by regimens using ceftriaxone and fluoroquinolones. Currently, most U.S. strains remain sensitive to the fluoroquinolones. However, resistant isolates have been reported and are increasing in other areas of the world.

Pathogenesis

Information concerning the pathogenesis of gonorrhea derives from histopathologic studies performed during the course of natural urethral infection,[39, 40] conjunctival infection[41] and perinatal infection[42] in humans; from studies of the interaction of *N. gonorrhoeae* with human sera, cells, or organ cultures[43, 44]; from limited observations on experimental urethral infection in the chimpanzee[45]; and from more extensive observations of gonococcal infection of nonmammalian experimental models, such as the chick embryo and small laboratory animal models,[46] which are quite dissimilar to human infection.

The first step in the pathogenesis of uncomplicated genital gonococcal infection is cell attachment to columnar or transitional epithelial cells. It seems likely that pili are important in the attachment of gonococci to epithelial cells in vivo and may confer target organ specificity. Pili are capable of phase variation, and pili-related genes are expressed in most isolates from urethral specimens but may be silent in isolates from other sites. Pili phase variation may be controlled by a mechanism in which specific DNA segments shift position nearer to or more distant from expression sites.[22] Outer membrane proteins II are also highly involved with attachment, replication, and successful colonization.[47]

The next step is penetration through or between epithelial cells. Penetration through cells occurs by a process resembling phagocytosis or endocytosis.[40, 43, 44] Several gonococci can be observed within individual epithelial cells of the urethra or fallopian tube because of entry of several organisms or multiplication within the epithelial cell.

A third step in the pathogenesis of gonococcal infection appears to be destruction of the infected epithelial cell, which is accomplished by gonococci but not by nonpathogenic *Neisseria*. This disrupts the continuity of the epithelial surface and presumably is one mechanism by which gonococci reach the subepithelial connective tissue, where they are demonstrable soon after acquisition of infection in uncomplicated human infections.[39, 41] One of the primary effects of *N. gonorrhoeae* on the human fallopian tube is the loss of the ciliary activity. The ciliated cells cease to function and then are sloughed off from the mucosa. Gonococci, however, adhere to nonciliated cells.[48] *N. gonorrhoeae* contains cytotoxic lipopolysaccharide and also produces proteases, phospholipases, and elastases that may play a role in pathogenesis. Although type 1 and 2 cells also appear to be more resistant than type 3 and 4 cells to phagocytosis

by neutrophils, gonococci within phagocytic vacuoles are in various stages of degeneration and appear to be fully susceptible to intracellular bactericidal mechanisms, regardless of colony type. The virulence of gonococcal strains may vary, depending on their ability to remove iron from lactoferrin on mucosal surfaces or from transferrin in blood.[49]

Humoral and local secretory antibodies to *N. gonorrhoeae* appear during uncomplicated gonorrhea, and a cellular immune response has been demonstrated in patients with recurrent gonococcal infection. The precise role of host defense mechanisms in affecting the course of gonococcal infection or in conferring immunity to infection or reinfection is unknown. Epidemiologic data suggest that only about one third of men become infected after exposure to infected women,[50] and a similar proportion of neonates exposed during vaginal delivery become infected. Components of the normal mucosal flora, such as *Candida albicans*, *Staphylococcus epidermidis* and lactobacilli, can inhibit *N. gonorrhoeae* in vitro and may provide natural resistance. Other nonspecific host immune factors in the neonate that are important in protecting against gonococcal infection have not been studied.

Before antibiotics became available for gonorrhea, the average duration of symptoms of gonococcal urethritis in men was only about 8 weeks, which suggests the development of at least some degree of strain-specific immunity. The duration of the subclinical gonococcal carrier state in men and women is unknown but is evidently finite. The human inoculation studies conducted in the 1940s by Mahoney and colleagues showed that men who had previously had gonorrhea had slightly but significantly increased resistance to experimental urethral infection.[57] Possible immune factors that protect against gonorrhea include local antibody to pili, which can block attachment of gonococci to epithelial cells. Pili also interfere with phagocytosis, and antibody to pili is opsonic.[52]

The pathogenesis of the complications of gonorrhea involves additional considerations. The temporal association of both gonococcemia[53] and gonococcal salpingitis[53] with menstruation, the increased incidence of salpingitis in women with an intrauterine contraceptive device,[54] the decreased risk of salpingitis in women using oral contraceptives,[54] the increased frequency of salpingitis in gonorrhea of adolescents[55] and the infrequent occurrence of salpingitis during pregnancy all suggest that local host defense mechanisms are decisive, especially in the pathogenesis of salpingitis.

There is evidence that one episode of gonococcal salpingitis protects against recurrent gonococcal salpingitis with the same protein I serotype.[56] Normal human serum contains IgM antibody directed against lipopolysaccharide antigens on the gonococcus and results in generation of the bactericidal C5 to C9 attack complex. Normal human serum also contains IgG antibody against a surface protein antigen present on serum-resistant gonococci; this antibody blocks the bactericidal action of the antilipopolysaccharide IgM antibody.[57, 58] These serum-resistant strains account for most cases of gonococcal bacteremia and gonococcal arthritis in adults.[59] Gonococcal strains that cause local or systemic complications are frequently resistant to normal serum-mediated killing mechanisms. Recent studies have shown that a mechanism by which gonococci express resistance to the bactericidal action of serum is through the expression of lipo-oligosaccharides, which are sialylated by human serum and red and white blood cells.[60]

Patients deficient in the terminal complement components C6, C7, or C8 are uniquely susceptible to bacteremia with serum-sensitive strains of *N. gonorrhoeae* as well as to meningococcemia.[61] It is of interest that infants in whom transplacental transfer of IgM antibody does not occur do not have serum bactericidal activity against gonococci, suggesting that infants may have increased susceptibility to gonococcemia.[62]

EPIDEMIOLOGY AND TRANSMISSION

Epidemiology

The incidence of gonorrhea in the United States fell rapidly after World War II as penicillin G came into use, but the annual incidence of reported cases began to rise slowly again in 1959, and, from 1963 to 1976, age-specific incidence rates tripled in the United States. After 1976, the incidence of gonorrhea leveled off and has fallen slowly. In 1996, 326,000 new cases of gonorrhea were reported to the Centers for Disease Control and Prevention (CDC), but it is estimated that only about one half of all new cases are actually reported. In 1996, there were approximately 120 cases per 100,000 population in the United States.

There is a seasonal variation in the incidence of gonorrhea, with the peak incidence in the United States occurring in the late summer.[63] The reported incidence is about 35 times as high in black as in other persons and is greater in urban than in nonurban populations. The reported incidence is highest in the 15- to 19-year-old age group. Among sexually active females, rates of gonorrhea are markedly higher in teenagers than in those 20 years of age or older; the rate of increase in incidence of gonorrhea during the 1960s and 1970s was greater in teenagers than in any other age group.[64, 65]

Studies of the prevalence of gonorrhea, as determined by routine culture, have helped to define the segments of the population that constitute the greatest reservoir of gonococcal infection in the community. Age, race, marital status, and socioeconomic status—risk factors influencing sexual behavior, illness behavior, and accessibility to health care—are each independently correlated with the prevalence of gonorrhea in asymptomatic women. The highest prevalence of infection has occurred in women who are younger than 30 years of age, nonwhite, and unmarried and who have low income; these are also risk factors for repeated gonococcal infections.[66] These data are useful in focusing efforts for gonorrhea case detection.

During the 1980s, an epidemic of use of crack cocaine coincided with a rise in the rate of drug-related sexually transmitted diseases, including human immunodeficiency virus, syphilis, and gonorrhea. Risk factors for gonococcal disease in large cities have included young age, minority status, poverty, exchange of sex for drugs, and history of other sexually transmitted disease.[67, 68] The progression of the acquired immunodeficiency syndrome epidemic is expected to continue to be associated with transmission of gonorrhea in susceptible populations, which include adolescents and young mothers.

Because of the risk of neonatal gonococcal infection and the possible adverse effect of gonorrhea on pregnancy, the performance of a test for gonorrhea is routine for pregnant women at the first prenatal visit to the physician. For populations who are at increased risk for acquiring disease, a second routine test should be made during the second trimester.[69]

Transmission

The usual site of gonococcal infection of the cervix of the adult female is the transitional zone and distal portion of the endocervix; intrapartum contamination of the newborn by *N. gonorrhoeae* usually occurs during passage through the birth canal. It is estimated that 30 to 35% of neonates acquire ophthalmic *N. gonorrhoeae* infection during vaginal delivery from infected mothers.[70] However, contamination may occur in utero after rupture of the membranes, and neonatal gonococcal infection of the eye[71, 72] and oropharynx[73] has been documented in infants delivered by cesarean section performed after membrane rupture. Contamination of the oropharynx and gastric contents probably results from swallowing of infected amniotic fluid or cervicovaginal secretions. *N. gonorrhoeae* has been isolated from conjunctival or orogastric aspirate samples from approximately 30% of neonates born to infected mothers. Table 29–1 shows estimated rates of gonococcal colonization or disease in infants born to mothers with untreated gonococcal disease; some of these infants received ocular prophylaxis. Data concerning the rate of septicemic dissemination of gonococcal disease in newborns are also included in Table 29–1.

POSTNATAL TRANSMISSION

Most gonococcal infections that become apparent during the first month of life are currently attributed to intrapartum infection. However, after the neonatal period, the method of acquisition of gonorrhea in young children is not always certain. An area of great concern to physicians who care for children with sexually transmitted diseases is the identification of the child who has been abused sexually. Throughout most of childhood, the diagnosis of gonorrhea is considered to be extremely strong evidence of sexual abuse, so strong that sexual abuse is considered to have occurred unless specifically disproved. Improved methods of examining children, of interviewing children and of interviewing the families indicate that almost all postneonatal gonorrhea is acquired during sexual contact and that the exceptions appear to be very rare. In one study, all children with gonorrhea who were older than 4 years of age had a defined episode of abuse, as did 6 of 17 (35%) children

TABLE 29–1

Incidence of Neonatal Gonococcal Disease in Exposed Infants

SITE OF NEONATAL INFECTION	INCIDENCE OF INFECTION	POPULATION	REFERENCE
Conjunctiva	5%; 0%; 2%	Exposed infants who had AgNO₃ ocular prophylaxis	Edwards et al.[74]; Allen and Barrere[75]; Armstrong et al.[76]
	2–30%	Exposed infants who had no ocular prophylaxis	Rothenberg[70]; Fransen et al.[1]
Orogastric fluid	40%; 26%	Infants of infected mothers	Handsfield et al.[77]; Edwards et al.[74]
Oropharynx	43/122 (35%)	Infants with gonococcal ophthalmia	Laga et al.[78]
Disseminated disease as a proportion of all neonatal gonorrhea	0–1% (rare)	Reported series of neonatal gonococcal disease	Folland et al.[79]; Tomeh and Wilfert[80]; Wald et al.[81]; Edwards et al.[74]; Fransen et al.[1]

younger than 4 years.[82] In view of the difficulties of obtaining information from children who are preverbal, these results support the contention that there is almost never any evidence of nonsexual transmission at any age other than the neonate.[83] Postnatal transmission of gonorrhea via sexual abuse has even occurred in children who are younger than 3 months of age after pharyngeal or rectal penetration and may be diagnosed when the physician recognizes the accompanying physical findings such as lax rectal tone or facial bruising.

Nonsexual transmission has been identified in case reports as unique events. One child acquired pharyngeal gonococcal disease after eating chocolate agar plates growing developed *N. gonorrhoeae* colonies.[84] A second child acquired gonococcal ophthalmia through intentional rinsing of the eye with human urine as a folk cure for viral conjunctivitis.[85]

In summary, in the first month of life, most cases of gonorrhea are probably acquired during passage through an infected birth canal. Thereafter, the physician must investigate the case for acquisition by abuse.

GONOCOCCAL OUTBREAKS

In the past, when gonorrhea occurred in the newborn nursery during the first month of life, it was attributed to transmission of infection via fomites. For example, a remarkable outbreak of gonorrhea involving 67 of 182 infants, including 53 who developed gonococcal arthritis, was reported by Cooperman in 1928[86] and was presumptively attributed to contamination of rectal thermometers, washbasins, or laundry. Gonococcal conjunctivitis, vaginitis, and arthritis apparently were endemic and epidemic in many babies' hospitals at the turn of the century, and it was said at that time that there was not an institution in New York City that was devoted to the care of infants and young children that had not had an outbreak of nosocomial gonococcal infections.[2] However, there were no investigations of any of these outbreaks that would have allowed for discovery of transmission by sexual abuse.

CLINICAL MANIFESTATIONS
Gonorrhea in Pregnancy

Gonococcal infections present several unique problems during pregnancy, some of which have important conse-

quences for the fetus or neonate. Although it has been proposed that pharyngeal infection may represent the sole site of gonococcal infection in pregnant women more often than in nonpregnant women, this has not been our experience. Similarly, pregnancy has been reported to be a risk factor for disseminated gonococcal infection.[53] Up to 40% of women in some series of disseminated gonococcal infection have been pregnant. However, in a series of consecutive patients with disseminated gonococcal infection (H. H. Handsfield, unpublished observation), no case occurred in pregnant women. Increased medical surveillance during pregnancy may have biased the identification of this syndrome in pregnant women in earlier studies of disseminated gonococcal infection.

The frequency with which ascending infection of the upper genital tract occurs with gonococcal infection is controversial. From 10 to 20% of nonpregnant women with gonorrhea have had clinical evidence of pelvic inflammatory disease in most studies, but up to 50% of women with recently acquired gonorrhea developed pelvic inflammatory disease in one study.[87] Pelvic inflammatory disease occurs much less often in pregnant women with gonorrhea, although surgically verified gonococcal salpingitis has been reported between 7 and 12 weeks' gestation, before obliteration of the endometrial cavity.[88] Local factors may decrease the risk for ascending gonococcal infection during pregnancy. Cervical mucus becomes impermeable to motile sperm and possibly to microorganisms under the influence of progesterone.[89] Most important, after the twelfth week of gestation, the chorion attaches to the endometrial decidua with obliteration of the intrauterine cavity, which obstructs the route for ascending intraluminal spread of gonococci.

The chorioamnion itself may become the site of ascending gonococcal infection after the twelfth week of gestation,[90] and the clinical spectrum of symptomatic gonococcal infection in pregnant patients has thus included septic abortion and premature rupture of membranes in 22% and 26% of cases in two studies.[91, 92] Several other retrospective studies have analyzed the relationship of antepartum gonococcal infection to the course of late pregnancy (Table 29–2). Charles and colleagues reported that premature rupture of membranes

TABLE 29–2

Outcome of Pregnancy in Mothers Who Were Infected with *Neisseria gonorrhoeae* at Delivery

OUTCOME	CHARLES ET AL.[93] (N = 14)[a]	SARREL AND PRUETT[91] (N = 37)	ISRAEL ET AL.[95] (N = 39)	AMSTEY AND STEADMAN[92] (N = 222)[a]	EDWARDS ET AL.[74] (N = 19)[a]	HANDSFIELD ET AL.[77] (N = 12)[a]
Normal or term infant	—	13 (35%)	30 (77%)	142 (64%)	7 (37%)	—
Aborted	—	13 (35%)	1 (2%)	24 (11%)	—	—
Perinatal death	—	3 (8%)	1 (2%)	15 (8%)	2 (11%)	—
Premature	—	6 (17%)	5 (13%)	49 (22%)	8 (42%)	8 (67%)
Perinatal distress	—	—	2 (5%)	—	2 (10%)	—
Premature rupture of membranes	6 (43%)	8 (21%)	—	52 (26%)	12 (63%)	9 (75%)

*Data were provided showing that the outcomes of pregnancies of mothers not infected with *N. gonorrhoeae* were significantly more favorable.

occurred in 43% of 14 women with untreated gonorrhea at the onset of labor as opposed to 4 (3%) of 144 women with gonococcal infection that was identified and treated during pregnancy.[93] Handsfield and associates reported that prematurity and delayed delivery after rupture of membranes were significantly correlated with intrapartum gonococcal infection.[77] Edwards and co-workers matched 19 pregnant women who had intrapartum gonococcal infection with 41 uninfected controls on the basis of age, race, parity, socioeconomic status, and date of delivery.[74] Patients with intrapartum gonococcal infection were significantly more likely than controls to have chorioamnionitis, premature rupture of membranes, delayed delivery after rupture of membranes, and prematurity. Finally, in a case-control study by Elliott of women delivering preterm and term infants, infection with *N. gonorrhoeae* was associated with preterm delivery and the attributable risk of gonococcal infection was 14%.[94] These studies all support the conclusion that gonococcal infection confers a substantial risk of preterm delivery and is an appropriate target for efforts to prevent preterm births.

The outcome for the fetus and infant when gonococcal disease of the mother is untreated has been reviewed by several authors (see Table 29–2). In these six studies, rates of premature delivery were 13 to 67%, of perinatal distress were 5 to 10%, and of perinatal deaths were 2 to 11%. The rates of apparently normal or term deliveries were only 35 to 77% of the reported pregnancies. The studies of Charles and colleagues,[93] Amstey and Steadman,[92] Edwards and co-workers,[74] and Handsfield and associates[77] included data concerning the outcomes of pregnancy of mothers who were not infected with *N. gonorrhoeae*, and those outcomes were significantly more favorable for the infant. In the study of Amstey and Steadman, the risk of adverse outcomes was the same in women who were treated for gonorrhea during pregnancy as in those who were not treated before delivery.

These studies provided scant information on other associated conditions or genital infections. However, there is increasing evidence that many or most infections of the lower genital tract of women, if they occur during pregnancy, carry a significant burden of adverse outcomes to the pregnancy, including premature rupture of membranes, abortions, perinatal mortality, and prematu-

rity. Included in this generalization are vaginal infections with *Mycoplasma hominis*,[96] *Ureaplasma urealyticum*,[97] bacterial vaginosis, and *Chlamydia trachomatis*.[98] The pathophysiology of such a general occurrence is uncertain but could be related to the reactivity of smooth muscle that accompanies inflammatory reactions and is well described in urinary tract infections of pregnancy.[99]

A final demonstration of ascending infection of the fetus before delivery is found in a report by Oppenheimer and Winn.[42] An infected stillborn infant was found at autopsy to have multiple areas of submucosal microabscesses containing gram-negative diplococci in the esophagus and upper respiratory tract. There was associated chorioamnionitis of the placenta, and the location of the lesions indicated that infection had been contracted during swallowing and respiration in utero.

Because of the possible adverse effects of gonococcal infection on pregnancy itself as well as because of the risk for neonatal infection, detection of *N. gonorrhoeae* by means of screening cultures during the initial antenatal visit is recommended in populations at risk for gonorrhea. Repeated cultures in the third trimester are also recommended for high-risk individuals (young, nonwhite, single, primigravida, low socioeconomic status, current or past history of sexually transmitted disease, particularly a past history of gonorrhea and especially gonorrhea earlier in pregnancy). In patients with premature rupture of membranes, intrapartum fever, or septic abortion, an endocervical culture for gonorrhea should be obtained.

Recommended treatment for gonorrhea in the pregnant patient is outlined in Table 29–3. Treatment of infants who are delivered to an infected mother or who develop perinatal disease is outlined in Table 29–4. Reinfection after treatment is common. If treatment of the sexual partner is not accomplished, monthly cultures are appropriate.

Gonococcal Ophthalmia Neonatorum

An association of conjunctivitis in the newborn with vaginal discharge in the mother was noted by Quellmaltz in 1750, but gonococcal ophthalmia neonatorum was not recognized as a distinct entity until 1881, 2 years after recognition of *N. gonorrhoeae* in genital exudate,

TABLE 29–3
Recommended Treatment of Gonococcal Infections in Pregnancy

Uncomplicated Urethral, Endocervical, and Rectal Disease

Pregnant women should have cultures for *Neisseria gonorrhoeae* (and be tested for *Chlamydia trachomatis* and syphilis) at the first prenatal care visit. For women at high risk of sexually transmitted diseases, a second culture for gonorrhea (and tests for chlamydial infection and syphilis) should be obtained late in the third trimester.

Recommended Regimen

Ceftriaxone, 125[a] IM mg once
                 or, if tolerant,
Spectromycin, 2 g IM once
                plus
Erythromycin base,[a] 500 mg PO qid for 7 days.
Amoxicillin, 500 mg PO tid for 7 days.

Pregnant women who are allergic to beta-lactams should be treated with spectinomycin, 2 g IM once (followed by erythromycin). Follow-up cervical and rectal cultures for *N. gonorrhoeae* should be obtained 4–7 days after treatment is completed.

Ideally, pregnant women with gonorrhea should be treated for chlamydial infection on the basis of diagnostic studies. If diagnostic testing for such infection is not available, treatment for chlamydia should be given. Tetracyclines (including doxycycline) and the quinolones are contraindicated in pregnancy because of possibly adverse effects on the fetus. Treatments for pregnant patients with chlamydial infection, acute salpingitis, and disseminated gonorrhea in pregnancy are described in respective sections of the CDC guidelines.

Pharyngeal Gonococcal Infection

Patients with uncomplicated pharyngeal gonococcal infection should be treated with ceftriaxone, 125 mg IM once.

Disseminated Gonococcal Infection (DGI)

Hospitalization is recommended for initial therapy, especially for patients who cannot reliably comply with treatment, have uncertain diagnoses, or have purulent synovial effusions or other complications. Patients should be examined for clinical evidence of endocarditis or meningitis.

Recommended Regimens: DGI Inpatient

Ceftriaxone, 1 g IM or IV every 24 hr
                or
Ceftizoxime, 1 g IV every 8 hr
                or
Cefotaxime, 1 g IV every 8 hr.

When the infecting organism is proven to be penicillin sensitive, parenteral treatment may be switched to ampicillin, 1 g every 6 hr (or equivalent). Patients treated for DGI should be tested for genital *C. trachomatis* infection.

Reliable patients with uncomplicated disease may be discharged 24–48 hr after all symptoms resolve and may complete the therapy (for a total of 1 wk of antibiotic therapy) with an oral regimen of amoxicillin, 500 mg with clavulanic acid in three times a day.

Special Considerations

All patients with gonorrhea should have a serologic test for syphilis and should be offered confidential counseling and testing for HIV infection. Most patients with incubating syphilis (those who are seronegative and have no clinical signs of syphilis) may be cured by any of the regimens containing beta-lactams (e.g., ceftriaxone).

Spectinomycin and the quinolones (ciprofloxacin, norfloxacin) have not been shown to be active against incubating syphilis. Patients treated with these drugs should have a serologic test for syphilis in 1 mo. These drugs are to be avoided in pregnancy.

Patients with gonorrhea and documented syphilis and patients with gonorrhea who are sex partners of syphilis patients should be treated for syphilis (see Syphilis section) as well as for gonorrhea.

Some practitioners report that mixing 1% lidocaine (without epinephrine) with ceftriaxone reduces the discomfort associated with the injection (see package insert). No adverse reactions have been associated with use of lidocaine diluent.

Management of Sex Partners

Persons who are exposed to gonorrhea within the 30 days should be examined, cultured, and treated presumptively.

Treatment Failures

Persistent symptoms after treatment should be evaluated by culture for *N. gonorrhoeae*, and any gonococcal isolate should be tested for antibiotic sensitivity. Symptoms of urethritis may also be caused by *C. trachomatis* and other organisms associated with nongonococcal urethritis (see Nongonococcal Urethritis section). Additional treatment for patients with gonorrhea should be ceftriaxone, plus other therapy as indicated by a thorough assessment. Infections occurring after treatment with one of the recommended regimens are commonly due to reinfection rather than to treatment failure and indicate a need for improved sex-partner referral and patient education.

[a]Erythromycin stearate, 500 mg, or erythromycin ethylsuccinate, 800 mg, or equivalent may be substituted for erythromycin base.
Adapted from Centers for Disease Control and Prevention. 1998 Sexually transmitted diseases treatment guidelines. MMWR Morb Mortal Wkly Rep 47(RR-1), 1998.

---

when Hirschberg and Krause[100] identified the gonococcus in conjunctival exudate from infants with purulent conjunctivitis. Inclusion conjunctivitis was subsequently differentiated from gonococcal ophthalmia by Lindner in 1909.[101]

Ophthalmia neonatorum occurred in 1 to 15% of infants born in European hospitals during the nineteenth century and in 9% of a large group of infants born in the United States before the introduction of prophylaxis.[102] In 1881, Credé reported the topical use of silver nitrate to prevent cases of ophthalmia neonatorum,[103] the great majority of which were presumably gonococcal. Credé reported a reduction in the rate of ophthalmia neonatorum from 10 to 0.3% with his method of prophylaxis, which consisted of cleansing the eyes with ordinary water, after which the eyelids were

☐ TABLE 29–4
Treatment of Gonorrhea in Infants and Children

Gonococcal Infections of Infants and Children

Child abuse should be carefully considered and evaluated for any child with documented gonorrhea.

Treatment of Infants Born to Mothers with Gonococcal Infection

Infants born to mothers with untreated gonorrhea are at high risk of infection (e.g., ophthalmia and disseminated gonococcal infection [DGI]) and should be treated with a single injection of ceftriaxone (50 mg/kg IV or IM, not to exceed 125 mg). Ceftriaxone should be given cautiously to hyperbilirubinemic infants, especially premature infants. Topical prophylaxis for neonatal ophthalmia is not adequate treatment for documented infections of the eye or other sites.

Treatment of Infants with Gonococcal Infection

Infants with documented gonococcal infections at any site (e.g., eye) should be evaluated for DGI. This evaluation should include a careful physical examination, especially of the joints, as well as blood and cerebrospinal fluid cultures. Infants with gonococcal ophthalmia or DGI should be treated for 7 days (10 to 14 days if meningitis is present) with one of the following regimens:

Recommended Regimen

Ceftriaxone, 25–50 mg/kg/day IV or IM in a single daily dose
or
Cefotaxime, 25 mg/kg IV or IM q12h.

Alternative Regimen

Limited data suggest that uncomplicated gonococcal ophthalmia among infants may be cured with a single injection of ceftriaxone (50 mg/kg up to 125 mg). A few experts use this regimen for children who have no clinical or laboratory evidence of disseminated disease.

Infants with gonococcal ophthalmia should receive eye irrigations with buffered saline solutions until discharge has cleared. Topical antibiotic therapy alone is inadequate. Simultaneous infection with *C. trachomatis* has been reported and should be considered for patients who do not respond satisfactorily. Therefore, the mother and infant should be tested for chlamydial infection.

Gonococcal Infections of Children

Children who weigh > 45 kg should be treated with adult regimens. Children who weigh < 45 kg who have uncomplicated vulvovaginitis, cervicitis, urethritis, pharyngitis, or proctitis should be treated as follows:

Recommended Regimen

Ceftriaxone, 125 mg IM once.

Patients who cannot tolerate ceftriaxone may be treated with spectinomycin, 40 mg/kg IM once.

Patients weighing < 45 kg with bacteremia or arthritis should be treated with ceftriaxone, 50 mg/kg (maximum 1 g) once daily for 7 days. For meningitis, treatment is for 10–14 days and the maximum dose is 2 g.

Children > 8 years of age should also be given doxycycline, 100 mg bid for 7 days. All patients should be evaluated for co-infection with syphilis and *C. trachomatis*. Follow-up cultures are unnecessary if ceftriaxone has been used.

Prevention of Ophthalmia Neonatorum

Instillation of a prophylactic agent into the eyes of all newborns is recommended to prevent gonococcal ophthalmia neonatorum and is required by law in most states. Although all regimens listed below effectively prevent gonococcal eye disease, their efficacy in preventing chlamydial eye disease is not clear. Furthermore, they do not eliminate nasopharyngeal colonization with *C. trachomatis*. Treatment of gonococcal and chlamydial infections in pregnant women is the best method for preventing neonatal gonococcal and chlamydial disease.

Recommended Regimen

Erythromycin (0.5%) ophthalmic ointment, once
or
Tetracycline (1%) ophthalmic ointment, once
or
Silver nitrate (1%) aqueous solution, once.

One of these agents should be instilled into the eyes of every neonate as soon as possible after delivery, and definitely within 1 hr after birth. Single-use tubes or ampules are preferable to multiple-use tubes. The efficacy of tetracycline and erythromycin in the prevention of TRNG and PPNG ophthalmia is unknown, although both are probably effective because of the high concentrations of drug in these preparations. Bacitracin is *not* recommended.

Adapted from Centers for Disease Control and Prevention. 1998 Sexually transmitted diseases treatment guidelines. MMWR Morb Mortal Wkly Rep 47 (RR-1), 1998.

---

held open and a single drop of 2% silver nitrate was instilled in each eye. This has since been modified by substituting 1% silver nitrate in individual dispensers for the stronger solution.

The success of prevention of ophthalmia neonatorum with use of Credé's method was reflected in a reduction in the importance of this syndrome as a cause of blindness. In the United States, the proportion of new entrants to schools for the blind with blindness attributable to ophthalmia neonatorum decreased from 28% in 1908 to 11% in 1933.[104] When sulfonamides and penicillin became available for antepartum care and for treatment

of gonococcal ophthalmia neonatorum, the acute morbidity attributable to this condition decreased still further,[105] and the proportion of new entrants to schools for the blind with blindness attributable to ophthalmia neonatorum further decreased to 1% by 1950[104] and to less than 0.1% by 1959.[105] *N. gonorrhoeae* was responsible for approximately half of the cases of ophthalmia neonatorum that occurred before 1940,[106] but the proportion of cases attributable to *N. gonorrhoeae* has decreased greatly since the availability of antibiotics.

In 1992, a study was made of reported cases of gonorrhea in children in Florida that had occurred between

1984 and 1988.[107] Eye infections represented 21% of cases in children younger than 1 year of age. Further review of records found a total of 68 cases of neonatal gonorrhea. Fifty-five (81%) of the 68 cases were gonococcal ophthalmia neonatorum, 4 were genital, 1 was nasal, 1 was skin, and 1 was scalp infection. Positive cultures at birth were obtained from three gastric samples and from two respiratory aspirate cultures.

A case-control study of mothers of infants with and without gonococcal disease showed that mothers of infected infants were more likely to be younger, black, and less well educated than were control mothers. Nineteen percent of mothers of infected infants were substance abusers.

The prevalence rate of clinical gonococcal ophthalmia neonatorum in hospitals from which any cases were reported was 1.7 per 100,000 live births, and the estimated prevalence of gonococcal infection in the mothers was 1.0 to 7.5%. The data suggested that prevalence rates of maternal and infant disease may be increasing.

ETIOLOGY AND DIFFERENTIAL DIAGNOSIS

The resurgence of gonorrhea during the 1960s and 1970s was associated with a reappearance of gonococcal ophthalmia neonatorum in the United States,[108–110] and, in a report from Glasgow,[111] N. gonorrhoeae was the most common cause of ophthalmia neonatorum in children who required hospitalization for this condition. In developing areas with high prevalence of gonococcal disease, this infection remains a common cause of serious visual deficiencies of children.[112] However, in most areas, gonococcal infection is now an infrequent, albeit the most serious, cause of bacterial conjunctivitis in the newborn. The main causes of ophthalmia neonatorum are given in Table 29–5 in decreasing order of frequency as seen in developed countries.

A mild chemical conjunctivitis can be expected after instillation of 1% silver nitrate drops. Evidence of epithelial desquamation and polymorphonuclear leukocytic exudate appears[112] usually within 6 to 8 hours and disappears usually within 24 to 48 hours.

In developing countries, where the prevalence of gonorrhea in prenatal patients may be high and antenatal

TABLE 29–5
Etiology of Ophthalmia Neonatorum, Listed in Decreasing Order of Frequency

ETIOLOGY	USUAL TIME OF ONSET AFTER BIRTH
Chemical conjunctivitis (silver nitrate)	6–24 hr
Chlamydia trachomatis	5 days–2 wk
Staphylococcus aureus	
Haemophilus sp.	
Streptococcus pneumoniae	5 days–3 wk
Enterococcus	
Herpes simplex virus, type 2 > type 1	2–3 days
Neisseria gonorrhoeae	2–5 days

screening for N. gonorrhoeae is not routine, the gonococcus remains a very common cause of neonatal conjunctivitis and of blindness.[112a] However, in developed countries, C. trachomatis is the most common cause of neonatal conjunctivitis, and N. gonorrhoeae is among the least common. The serotypes of C. trachomatis that are usually associated with inclusion conjunctivitis are those associated with genital infection and are sexually transmitted. Maternal chlamydial infection involves the transitional epithelium of the cervix, and contamination of the infant usually occurs during passage through the infected birth canal. The onset of inclusion conjunctivitis occurs from 5 to 14 days after delivery, although it may be as early as 2 days or as late as 4 weeks. Inflammation may be mild or severe but predominantly involves the tarsal conjunctivae. It produces a mixed polymorphonuclear and mononuclear leukocytic exudate. The preauricular lymph nodes are usually not enlarged. Conjunctival follicles usually do not develop in the neonate unless inflammation persists for 6 to 8 weeks or infection recurs. Acute inflammation subsides after 2 to 4 weeks without treatment and is followed by subacute or chronic inflammation that may rarely produce mild scarring of the cornea or conjunctiva.[113, 114]

Conjunctival infection caused by N. gonorrhoeae in the newborn usually produces an acute purulent conjunctivitis that appears from 2 to 5 days after birth. However, the initial course is occasionally indolent, and onset can occur later than 5 days after birth,[76, 110] perhaps because of partial suppression of infection by ophthalmic prophylaxis, because of small inoculum size or because of strain-to-strain variations in gonococcal virulence. Cases with incubation periods of up to 19 days have been reported after inoculation of the eye with contaminated urine,[115] and gonococcal infection without any signs of conjunctival inflammation has been detected by routine screening of neonates.[116] Chronic mild, intermittent gonococcal conjunctivitis of 3 months' duration has been reported in a 4-month-old child.[117] Prolonged incubation after perinatal acquisition is hard to distinguish from delayed onset caused by postnatal acquisition. Therefore, gonococcal infection must be ruled out in every case of conjunctivitis in infants, regardless of severity or time of onset. At the opposite extreme, gonococcal ophthalmia neonatorum has also been detected at birth or during the first few hours of life in infants born after a prolonged interval between rupture of membranes and delivery[71, 76]; and infection in utero may have also occurred in an infant who developed gonococcal ophthalmia after a cesarean section that was performed after membrane rupture.[71, 72]

As already noted, the risk of disease in the newborn caused by N. gonorrhoeae may be increased by premature rupture of membranes and by prematurity.[76, 118–120] Brown and associates[110] noted prematurity in 19 (83%) of 23 infants with gonococcal ophthalmia, perhaps because infants who are premature are also often delivered after premature rupture of membranes, and therefore the infection is established before delivery. Ocular silver nitrate is not efficacious for therapy for established gonococcal ophthalmia.[76] Gonococcal ophthalmia neonatorum has been more common in male than in female infants in some studies.[110] In contrast, in older children, gonococcal conjunctivitis is more common in girls, who usually have associated vulvovaginitis. Infants delivered of mothers with untreated gonococcal vaginitis have a significantly increased rate of ophthalmia, even if ocular prophylaxis was provided. Consequently, particular attention should be given to the postpartum follow-up of any child born under these circumstances.[120a]

Although gonococcal conjunctivitis is usually less severe and less rapidly progressive in the newborn than in the adult, permanent corneal damage after gonococcal ophthalmia neonatorum was usual in the preantibiotic era. The infant typically develops tense edema of both lids, followed by chemosis and a progressively purulent and profuse conjunctival exudate (Fig. 29–1), which may literally pour out of the lids when they are separated. If treatment is delayed, the infection extends beyond the superficial epithelial layers, reaching the subconjunctival connective tissue of the palpebral conjunctivae and, more significantly, the cornea. Corneal complications include ulcerations that may leave permanent nebulae or may cause perforation and lead to anterior synechiae, anterior staphyloma, panophthalmitis (rarely), and loss of the eye.[41] In the past, systemic spread occasionally caused peripheral manifestations of gonococcemia and death. Such local and systemic complications of gonococcal conjunctivitis are now rare in the newborn if treatment is begun promptly, while the cornea is still clear.

In addition to *N. gonorrhoeae* and *C. trachomatis*, herpes simplex virus is a third sexually transmittable agent that is a cause of severe neonatal ophthalmia. Herpes simplex virus infection can lead to keratitis and corneal scarring and may be the initial manifestation of disseminating herpes simplex virus infection in the neonate. Neonatal herpes simplex virus ophthalmia that is perinatally acquired occurs within a few days of birth, but, because of indolent progression, delayed recognition, or

postnatal acquisition, this condition may appear any time during the first month of life. Fluorescein staining should be routinely performed in neonatal conjunctivitis; corneal epithelial dendritic or ameboid (geographic) staining indicates presumptive herpes simplex virus keratitis. Management should include culture confirmation, careful examination for manifestations of disseminated or central nervous system infection, and initiation of local and systemic antiviral chemotherapy.

Although a variety of other bacteria are frequently recovered from the conjunctivae of infants with neonatal conjunctivitis, many bacteria are probably innocent bystanders because the conjunctivae normally become colonized by bacteria during the first few days of life. In a study of the bacteriology of normal and inflamed conjunctivae in the newborn, Kaivonen[106] found that only *Staphylococcus aureus* was recovered more often from purulent conjunctival exudates than from normal conjunctivae. *S. aureus* colonization occurred equally as often in children delivered by cesarean section as in those delivered vaginally, and it was thought that contamination of the newborn eye with *S. aureus* occurred in the nursery after delivery.

In addition to ocular complications from neonatal gonococcal ophthalmia, the disease may spread locally, cause primary disease of mucous membranes or other sites, or cause systemic disease. The ocular disease serves as a signal that the infant has been infected. Examples of extension of gonococcal disease beyond the eye include the observation that 35% of infants with gonococcal ophthalmia also yield *N. gonorrhoeae* from pharyngeal cultures[78] and the description of gonococcal meningitis[121] and arthritis[122] in infants with ophthalmia.

Systemic Gonococcal Disease in the Neonate

Other than septic arthritis, bacteremic spread of gonococcal disease in neonates is rare. No patient with proven gonococcal endocarditis during the first few months of life has been reported. Bradford and Kelley[121] reported one case of proven gonococcal meningitis in a 2-day-old infant with ophthalmia neonatorum and reviewed two other probable cases of gonococcal meningitis in infants with ophthalmia neonatorum. Septic arthritis has been the most commonly recognized manifestation of gonococcemia in the neonatal period. An association of arthritis in the newborn with ophthalmia neonatorum was noted by Lucas in 1885. Holt reported 26 cases of gonococcal arthritis in children, including two infants who developed arthritis within the first month of life.[2] One of these children also had ophthalmia neonatorum. However, it is remarkable that ophthalmia neonatorum has often been absent in subsequently reported cases of neonatal gonococcal arthritis. The primary focus of infection in most of the 53 infants with gonococcal arthritis reported by Cooperman[3] was uncertain. Only one had ophthalmia neonatorum. All of the female infants were said to have had vulvovaginitis, and several infants had proctitis. The source of bacteremia in other cases has been attributed to infection of the mouth,[123] nares,[124] and umbilicus.[14] It is of interest

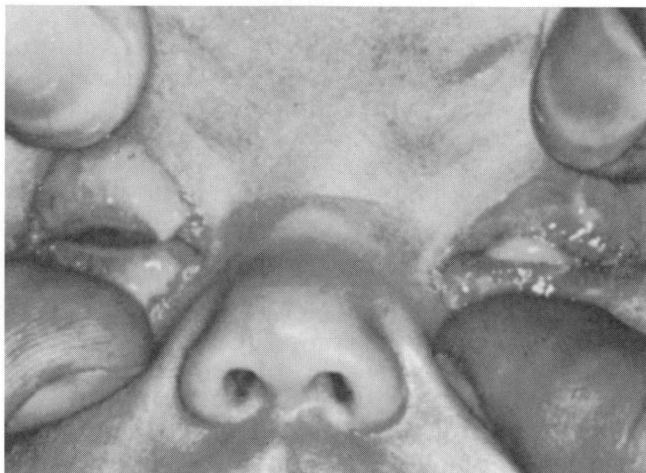

FIGURE 29–1 Bilateral acute gonococcal ophthalmia neonatorum. Appearance after inappropriate topical therapy for 2 weeks with neomycin–polymyxin B–bacitracin (Neosporin), sulfonamide, and chloramphenicol ophthalmic ointments.

that the mucosal source for bacteremic spread has been inapparent in many cases reported in the English language since the 1940s.[122, 123, 125–130]

The onset of clinical evidence of gonococcal arthritis in the newborn usually occurs from 1 to 4 weeks after delivery. One cannot distinguish between perinatal and postnatal acquisition of infection in most cases. The efficacy of ophthalmic prophylaxis, together with prompt recognition and treatment of gonococcal ophthalmia neonatorum when it occurs despite prophylaxis, may explain the absence of conjunctivitis in many cases of neonatal gonococcal arthritis reported since 1940. The pustular and necrotic skin lesions that characteristically appear during gonococcemia in the adult[53] have not yet been described in the newborn. The natural history of gonococcal arthritis in the infant is uncertain. Of the 53 cases described by Cooperman in newborns who were presumably infected by a single epidemic strain of *N. gonorrhoeae*, none had a fatal outcome, and permanent impairment of function was uncommon even without antibiotic therapy.[86] In contrast, 14 of 26 cases that occurred in a series of outbreaks described by Holt[2] in 1905 were fatal. No deaths have been reported among infants who received antibiotic therapy for gonococcal arthritis.

Infants with neonatal gonococcal arthritis share several important characteristics with neonates whose arthritis has other causes[127] (Table 29–6). In particular, polyarticular involvement is the norm.[122] The primary presentation is refusal to move the involved limb, which leads to the appearance of a paralytic process. Of special concern is the difficulty of providing an early diagnosis of bacterial infection of the hip in neonates and young children. Inflammatory disease of the hip does not present with visible external swelling, and because the hip joint capsule is relatively distensible, pain on movement may fail to provide a diagnosis. Nevertheless, infants with bacterial infections of the hips have a high incidence of subsequent development of aseptic necrosis of the head of the femur, and the physician must examine the child with particular care for this condition. If the infant with gonococcal disease fails to show normal spontaneous movement of a leg, a full workup, often including arthrocentesis, is indicated.[131]

TABLE 29–6
Signs of Disseminated Gonococcal Disease of the Newborn

SITE	CHARACTERISTICS
Associated mucosal sites	Conjunctivitis, ophthalmia
	Asymptomatic pyuria
	Urethritis, vaginitis, proctitis, pharyngitis
	Scalp abscess
	Contaminated orogastric contents
Systemic findings	Multiply involved joints
	Pseudoparesis of involved joints
	Sepsis of newborn
	Onset age 3–21 days

Localized Mucosal Disease

In infants as well as adults, most gonococcal disease represents an infection of mucosal membranes. Although ocular disease is the most widely recognized mucosal surface to be infected, infants may also present with gonococcal vaginitis,[6, 7] rhinitis,[132] anorectal infection,[1] funisitis, and urethritis.[5]

Primary mucosal infection by *N. gonorrhoeae* involves columnar and transitional epithelium. Anatomic sites that can be directly infected by the gonococcus include the anal canal, conjunctivae, and pharynx. Studies of gonococcal ophthalmia neonatorum have demonstrated concomitant pharyngeal colonization in 35% of cases, and coughing was a prominent finding in oropharyngeally infected infants.[1] Vulvovaginitis has been reported in the older literature to occur in the neonate,[2–4] as has neonatal gonococcal urethritis,[5] but clinically apparent gonococcal infections of the urethra or vagina occur rarely during the neonatal period, and inapparent colonization of these sites has not been systematically sought. In the more recent literature, the earliest reported onsets of gonococcal vaginitis in infants were at 25 and 34 days of age. These infections were attributed to perinatal infection, and signs of vaginitis presumably appeared only after the effects of maternal estrogen on the infant had disappeared.[6] One of these cases was associated with asymptomatic pyuria for 22 days before the onset of clinically apparent vaginitis.[7]

Neonatal Sepsis and Abscess

Case reports of gonococcal scalp abscesses attributed to intrauterine fetal monitoring have been cited.[9–13] *N. gonorrhoeae* may be an indirect or a direct cause of early neonatal sepsis and abscesses (see Table 29–2). Gonococcal gingival abscess has been reported in a 10-week-old infant,[8] and gonococcal infection of the umbilical stump has been reported in the past.[11] Gonococcemia commonly results in infection of the joints and skin and less commonly in infection of the meninges. Congenital ventriculoamniotic shunt placement has been complicated by gonococcal ventriculitis.[15] As noted, intrapartum gonococcal infection has been associated with premature delivery and premature rupture of membranes, which may lead to amniotic fluid infection with a variety of vaginal organisms capable of causing neonatal sepsis. Premature infants have increased susceptibility to sepsis. *N. gonorrhoeae* was the third most common pathogen (after *Escherichia coli* and group B streptococci) recovered from nasogastric aspirates in one study, usually in association with suspected neonatal sepsis.[77] *N. gonorrhoeae* has been isolated from blood of newborns with clinical sepsis without arthritis.[10, 124] The incidence of neonatal complications with *N. gonorrhoeae* reflects, of course, the incidence of disease in that community and the success or failure of maternal screening and treatment programs.

LABORATORY DIAGNOSIS

Diagnostic laboratory investigation of ophthalmia neonatorum is required if conjunctivitis appears to be more severe than the usual chemical conjunctivitis, persists longer than 2 or 3 days or progresses, or first appears after the first day of life. Initially, conjunctival exudate should be directly examined by Gram stain for the presence of gram-negative intracellular bean-shaped diplococci typical of *N. gonorrhoeae*; for gram-negative coccobacilli typical of *Haemophilus* species; or for gram-positive cocci suggestive of infection with gram-positive pathogens. The presence of one or more polymorphonuclear leukocytes per oil immersion field in a conjunctival smear supports the diagnosis of conjunctivitis. Detection of typical gram-negative diplococci by Gram stain warrants the presumptive diagnosis of gonococcal conjunctivitis, although other *Neisseria* species, such as *N. meningitidis*, have also been associated with purulent ophthalmia neonatorum.

Conjunctival exudate should also be inoculated directly onto blood agar, MacConkey's agar, and chocolate agar or chocolate inhibitory media. The inhibitory medium should be placed in a commercial carbon dioxide incubator or candle jar to provide an adequate concentration of carbon dioxide and should then be incubated at 36° C. If gonococcal conjunctivitis is suspected on the basis of examination of the Gram-stained smear of conjunctival exudate, cultures for *N. gonorrhoeae* should also be obtained from the oropharynx and anal canal because concomitant infection of these sites has been demonstrated in association with gonococcal ophthalmia neonatorum. Colonies resembling *N. gonorrhoeae* are further identified by Gram stain, by a positive oxidase test, and by utilization of glucose but not maltose, sucrose, or lactose.

Because other sexually transmitted diseases are commonly found in children and adults with a given sexually transmitted disease, infants with gonococcal ophthalmia should be evaluated for the other major neonatal ocular infection, *C. trachomatis*.[133] Epithelial cell scrapings may be obtained from the lower palpebral conjunctiva with a small platinum spatula or simply by swabbing the conjunctiva.[134] If infection by *C. trachomatis* is present, characteristic intracytoplasmic inclusions within epithelial cells are often but not always demonstrable by Giemsa stain, and chlamydial elementary bodies can be seen on conjunctival scrapings stained with fluorescein-conjugated *C. trachomatis*–specific monoclonal antibodies. Tissue cell culture techniques for recovery of *C. trachomatis* are more sensitive than Giemsa stain of conjunctival smears. Immunoassay methods and direct fluorescent antibody assays are available also.

Although the sensitivities and specificities of new and rapid methods for diagnosis of gonococcal disease have been studied in adult gonococcal syndromes, use of immunofluorescent methods or DNA hybridization for diagnosis of neonatal disease is unproved. Therefore, direct culture remains the method of choice for diagnosis of all forms of neonatal gonorrhea.

TREATMENT

Standard treatment regimens for gonococcal disease of the newborn and for infants born to mothers with gonococcal infection are outlined in Table 29–4.

Both parents of newborns with gonococcal diseases or colonization should be examined and treated because both parents of infants with ophthalmia neonatorum have a notably high incidence of infection with *N. gonorrhoeae* and *C. trachomatis*.[135]

By 1991, the CDC Gonococcal Isolate Surveillance Project showed that only 68% of strains had no resistance to antibiotics, 11% were penicillinase-producing, and an overall 32% were resistant to penicillin, tetracycline, or both. Because of the emergence of strains that are resistant to penicillin and tetracycline, recommendations for the treatment of gonococcal ophthalmia neonatorum now identify ceftriaxone as the first therapy of choice. This regimen has been highly successful in children.[136, 137] An alternative regimen with kanamycin has been studied and has demonstrated a failure rate of 5%.[138]

PREVENTION

The influence of Credé's method on reducing the incidence of blindness caused by gonococcal ophthalmia neonatorum represents one of the earliest achievements in preventive medicine, and the historical account of successful efforts to enact health legislation in the United States requiring use of Credé's method is both intriguing and instructive.[139] Opposition to the routine use of ophthalmic prophylaxis in the United States is still voiced, and debate continues as to which method of prophylaxis is optimal. Some physicians have urged discontinuation of silver nitrate prophylaxis, with or without substitution of systemic or topical prophylactic antibiotics, because of the occurrence of silver nitrate prophylaxis failures, the mild chemical conjunctivitis that is usually produced by instillation of the 1% solution, and the serious corneal damage that may be caused by mistaken use of stronger solutions.

Failure of properly administered silver nitrate prophylaxis to prevent ophthalmia neonatorum may, in some cases, be attributable to the following:

1. Occurrence of infection before delivery as a result of delayed delivery after rupture of membranes.
2. Irrigation with saline immediately after administration of silver nitrate rather than waiting a minimum of 15 seconds, although there are no data supporting this conjecture.
3. Acquisition of gonococcal infection subsequent to prophylaxis.
4. Occurrence of viral or inclusion conjunctivitis, which may not be preventable with silver nitrate.

Failures of gonococcal prophylaxis with other approved regimens also occur, including after erythromycin ophthalmic ointment.[140] Case reports of failures of antibiotic prophylaxis often include risk factors that are similar to those for silver nitrate failures, such as ophthalmia at delivery, prematurity, and prolonged time for rupture of membranes. From these experiences, it is becoming increasingly clear that no form of topical prophylaxis is adequate therapy for established infection. Therefore, children suspected of having established infection at birth should receive a systemic regimen for treatment.

The literature concerning comparative evaluations of various methods of prophylaxis has been reviewed well by Rothenberg and others.[70, 141, 142] Only recently have controlled evaluations of ophthalmic prophylaxis against gonococcal ophthalmia neonatorum been conducted in which (1) assignment to prophylaxis was randomized; (2) various methods of prophylaxis have been evaluated concurrently in sufficiently large numbers of infants in whom the incidence of gonococcal ophthalmia neonatorum is high enough that any existing differences in efficacy between methods would be detectable; or (3) the rate of exposure of the neonate to untreated maternal gonorrhea was known. Many of the earlier studies were performed at times or places at which gonococcal disease in the general population was relatively rare and identification of the efficacy of each regimen was correspondingly imprecise. Those uncontrolled studies that have compared the prophylactic use of 1% silver nitrate with no prophylaxis in large numbers of infants all have shown a lower incidence of gonococcal ophthalmia neonatorum among infants who were given the 1% silver nitrate. This is consistent with the observed reduction in blindness caused by ophthalmia neonatorum that accompanied the increased use of Credé's method and with the increased incidence of gonococcal ophthalmia noted in the past in areas where gonorrhea was prevalent and no prophylaxis or ineffective prophylaxis was substituted for Credé's method. For example, at Harlem Hospital in New York City, the rate of gonococcal ophthalmia increased sharply when no prophylaxis and bacitracin ointment treatments were intermittently substituted for the use of 1% silver nitrate[143, 144] (Table 29–7). Although assignment to prophylaxis or no prophylaxis was not randomized, the patients were drawn from the same population during a short period. A small outbreak of gonococcal ophthalmia neonatorum also occurred in a Seattle hospital when bacitracin ointment was used for a brief period in place of 1% silver nitrate (unpublished data). It is accepted that bacitracin ointment should not be employed for ophthalmic prophylaxis.

Because chlamydial conjunctivitis is now far more common than gonococcal conjunctivitis in the neonate (albeit this is partly because of antenatal screening for gonorrhea and the widespread use of 1% silver nitrate ophthalmic prophylaxis), there has been increasing interest in the use of ophthalmic prophylaxis to prevent both forms of neonatal conjunctivitis. A study of topical erythromycin and 1% silver nitrate in prevention of neonatal chlamydial conjunctivitis showed that neither regimen effectively prevented nasopharyngeal colonization of the neonate by *C. trachomatis*, and the efficacy of the erythromycin regimen has been challenged.[145] Experience in some centers where the prevalence of antenatal gonococcal infection is high suggests that topical erythromycin and tetracycline both provide effective prophylaxis against gonococcal neonatal conjunctivitis. Recent field studies of silver nitrate drops, erythromycin ophthalmic ointment, and tetracycline ophthalmic ointment have indicated that none of the regimens appears to be adequate in preventing chlamydial ophthalmia.[146, 147]

Topical antibiotics are slightly more expensive than silver nitrate for prophylaxis but are less irritating. Any form of ophthalmic prophylaxis is thought by some to interfere with parent–infant bonding, a matter of increasing public interest at the present time.[148] Some Western societies with a lower incidence of gonococcal and chlamydial infection currently do not routinely use any form of ophthalmic prophylaxis in the newborn, but this approach is not warranted in the United States. In choosing to use an antibiotic or silver nitrate as prophylaxis, it is important to recognize that ocular prophylaxis with a topical antibiotic (tetracycline or erythromycin) may lead to the emergence of strains of bacteria resistant to the prophylaxis in use at that institution. This has led to epidemics of clinically apparent disease.[149]

On the basis of these considerations, the American Academy of Pediatrics,[150] the National Society to Prevent Blindness,[151] and the CDC[19] recommend ophthalmic prophylaxis, which is required by law in nearly all states, by use of (1) 1% silver nitrate in single-dose ampules, (2) 0.5% erythromycin ophthalmic ointment in single-use tubes, or (3) 1% tetracycline ophthalmic ointment in single-use tubes. When silver nitrate is used, two drops can be instilled in each conjunctival sac. Whichever regimen is used, it should be administered as a single application immediately post partum, with no rinsing of the eyes. With prophylaxis, most infants born

TABLE 29–7
Efficacy of Prophylaxis of Gonococcal Neonatal Ophthalmia

AUTHOR, DATE, PLACE	STUDY DRUG	RATE OF MATERNAL GONORRHEA (%)	NO. OF INFANTS STUDIED	RATE OF OPHTHALMIA/ 1000 NEONATES	% REDUCTION
Greenberg, 1961,[144] New York (various hospitals not randomized)	1% AgNO$_3$	Unknown	7219	0.28	?
	Bacitracin	Unknown	1935	3.63	?
	No prophylaxis	Unknown	1996	4.0	—
Laga, 1986,[78] Kenya (randomized)	1% AgNO$_3$	100	52	96	80
	1% tetracycline	100	58	34	93
	No prophylaxis	100	—	480	—

to mothers with gonococcal infection do not develop gonococcal ophthalmia.

ACKNOWLEDGMENTS

The initial version of this chapter was authored by Dr. King K. Holmes. In 1988 and 1992, Dr. Gutman made extensive revisions of Dr. Holmes' work. The present chapter, the fourth version, was again revised by Dr. Gutman.

References

1. Fransen L, Nsanze H, Klaus V, et al. Ophthalmia neonatorum in Nairobi, Kenya: the roles of *Neisseria gonorrhoeae* and *Chlamydia trachomatis*. J Infect Dis 153:862–869, 1986.
2. Holt LE. Gonococcus infections in children with especial reference to their prevalence in institutions and means of prevention. NY Med J 81:521–527, 1905.
3. Cooperman MB. Gonococcus arthritis in infancy. Am J Dis Child 33:932–948, 1927.
4. Benson RA, Weinstock I. Gonorrheal vaginitis in children. Am J Dis Child 59:1083–1096, 1940.
5. Hunter GW, Fargo ND. Specific urethritis (gonorrhea) in a male newborn. Am J Obstet Gynecol 38:520–521, 1939.
6. Stark AR, Glode MP. Gonococcal vaginitis in a neonate. J Pediatr 94:298–299, 1979.
7. Barton LL, Shuja M. Neonatal gonococcal vaginitis. J Pediatr 98:171–172, 1981.
8. Urban MN, Heruada AR. Gonococcal gum abscess in a 10-week-old infant. Clin Pediatr 16:193–194, 1977.
9. D'Auria A, Tan L, Kreitzer M, et al. Gonococcal scalp wound infection. MMWR Morb Mortal Wkly Rep 24:115–116, 1975.
10. Thadepalli H, Rambhatla K, Maidman JE, et al. Gonococcal sepsis secondary to fetal monitoring. Am J Obstet Gynecol 126:510–512, 1976.
11. Plavidal FJ, Werch A. Gonococcal fetal scalp abscess: a case report. Am J Obstet Gynecol 127:437–438, 1977.
12. Reveri M, Krishnamurthy C. Gonococcal scalp abscess. J Pediatr 94:819–820, 1979.
13. Brook I, Rodriguez WJ, Controni G, et al. Gonococcal scalp abscess in a newborn. South Med J 73:396–397, 1980.
14. Butti IV, Cucullu AC. Arthritis gonococcia aguda del recien nacido. Arch Argent Pediatr 4:203–212, 1933.
15. Bland RS, Abramson JS, Nelson LH, et al. Gonococcal ventriculitis associated with ventriculoamniotic shunt placement. Pediatr Res 17:265A, 1983 (abstract).
16. Asnis DS, Brennessel DJ. Gonococcal scalp abscess: a risk of intrauterine monitoring. Clin Pediatr 31:316–317, 1992.
17. Stary A, Ching FF, Teodorowicz L, Lee H. Comparison of ligase chain reaction and culture for detection of *Neisseria gonorrhoeae* in genital and extragenital specimens. J Clin Microbiol 35:239–242, 1997.
18. Koumans EH, Johnson RE, Knapp JS, St. Louis ME. Laboratory testing for *Neisseria gonorrhoeae* by recently introduced nonculture tests: a performance review with clinical and public health considerations. Clin Infect Dis 27:1171–1180, 1998.
19. Centers for Disease Control and Prevention. 1998 Guidelines for treatment of sexually transmitted diseases. MMWR Morb Mortal Wkly Rep 47 (RR-1) 1–116, 1997.
20. Hook EW, Handsfield HH. Gonococcal infections in the adult. *In* Holmes KK, et al (eds). Sexually Transmitted Diseases, 3rd edition. New York, McGraw-Hill, 1998, pp 451–466.
21. Swanson J. Studies on gonococcus infection: IV. Pili: their role in attachment of gonococci to tissue culture cells. J Exp Med 137:571–589, 1973.
22. Sparling PF, Cannon JG, So M. Phase and antigenic variation of pili and outer membrane protein II of *Neisseria gonorrhoeae*. J Infect Dis 153:196–201, 1986.
23. Carifo K, Catlin BW. *Neisseria gonorrhoeae* auxotyping: differentiation of clinical isolates based on growth responses on chemically defined media. Appl Microbiol 26:223–230, 1973.
24. Sandstrom EG, Knapp JS, Buchanan TM. Serology of *Neisseria gonorrhoeae*: W-antigen serogrouping by coagglutination and protein I serotyping by enzyme-linked immunosorbent assay both detect protein I antigens. Infect Immun 35:229–239, 1982.
25. Knapp JS, Tam MR, Nowinski RC, et al. Serological classification of *Neisseria gonorrhoeae* with use of monoclonal antibodies to gonococcal outer membrane protein I. J Infect Dis 150:44–48, 1984.
26. Handsfield HH, Sandstrom EG, Knapp JS, et al. Epidemiology of penicillinase-producing *Neisseria gonorrhoeae* infections: analysis by auxotyping and serogrouping. N Engl J Med 306:950–954, 1982.
27. Gregg CR, Melly MA, Hellerqvist GG, et al. Toxic activity of purified lipopolysaccharide of *Neisseria gonorrhoeae* for human fallopian tube mucosa. J Infect Dis 143:432–439, 1981.
28. Mulks MA, Plaut AG. IgA protease production as a characteristic distinguishing pathogenic from harmless Neisseriaceae. N Engl J Med 299:973–976, 1978.
29. Archibald FS, Duong MN. Superoxide dismutase and oxygen toxicity defenses in the genus *Neisseria*. Infect Immun 51:631–641, 1986.
30. Sparling PF, Sax TE, Mohammed W, et al. Antibiotic resistance in the gonococcus: diverse mechanisms of coping with a hostile environment. *In* Brooks GF, et al. (eds). Immunobiology of *Neisseria gonorrhoeae*. Washington, DC, American Society for Microbiology, 1978, pp 44–52.
31. Clark VL, Knapp JS, Thompson S, et al. Presence of antibodies to the major anaerobically induced gonococcal outer membrane protein in sera from patients with gonococcal infections. Microb Pathog 5:381–390, 1988.
32. Shafer WM, Onunka VC, Marten LE. Antigonococcal activity of human neutrophil cathepsin G. Infect Immun 54:184–188, 1986.
33. Cohen MS, Sparling PF. Mucosal infection with *Neisseria gonorrhea*: bacterial adaptation and mucosal defenses. J Clin Invest 89:1699–1705, 1992.
34. Dougherty TJ. Genetic analysis and penicillin-binding protein alterations in *Neisseria gonorrhoeae* with chromosomally mediated resistance. Antimicrob Agents Chemother 30:649–652, 1986.
35. Rice RJ, Biddle JW, Jean Louis YA, et al. Chromosomally mediated resistance in *Neisseria gonorrhoeae* in the United States: results of surveillance and reporting, 1983–1984. J Infect Dis 153:340–345, 1986.
36. Thirumoorthy T, Rajan VS, Goh CL. Penicillinase-producing *Neisseria gonorrhoeae* ophthalmia neonatorum in Singapore. Br J Vener Dis 58:308–310, 1982.
37. Pang R, Teh LB, Rajan VS, et al. Gonococcal ophthalmia neonatorum caused by beta-lactamase-producing *Neisseria gonorrhoeae*. BMJ 1:380, 1979.
38. Doraiswamy B, Hammerschlag MR, Pringle GF, et al. Ophthalmia neonatorum caused by β-lactamase-producing *Neisseria gonorrhoeae*. JAMA 250:790–791, 1983.

39. Harkness AH. The pathology of gonorrhea. Br J Vener Dis 24:137–147, 1948.

40. Ward ME, Watt PJ. Adherence of *Neisseria gonorrhoeae* to urethral mucosal cells: an electron microscopic study of human gonorrhea. J Infect Dis 126:601–605, 1972.

41. Duke-Elder S. System of Ophthalmology: VIII. Diseases of the Outer Eye. St. Louis, CV Mosby, 1968, pp 115–127, 167–174.

42. Oppenheimer EH, Winn KJ. Fetal gonorrhea with deep tissue infection occurring in utero. Pediatrics 69:74–76, 1982.

43. McGee ZA, Jolinson AP, Taylor-Robinson D. Pathogenic mechanisms of *Neisseria gonorrhoeae*: observations on damage to human fallopian tubes in organ culture by gonococci of colony type 1 and type 4. J Infect Dis 143:413–422, 1981.

44. Ward ME, Glynn AA, Watt PJ. The fate of gonococci in polymorphonuclear leukocytes: an electron microscopic study of the natural disease. Br J Exp Pathol 53:289–294, 1972.

45. Lucas CT, Chandler F Jr, Martin JE Jr, et al. Transfer of gonococcal urethritis from man to chimpanzee: an animal model for gonorrhea. JAMA 216:1612–1614, 1971.

46. Arko RJ. *Neisseria gonorrhoeae*: experimental infection of laboratory animals. Science 177:1200–1201, 1972.

47. Bessen D, Gotschlich EC. Interactions of gonococci with HeLa cells: attachment, detachment, replication, penetration, and the role of protein II. Infect Immun 54:154–160, 1986.

48. Woods ML, McGee ZA. Molecular mechanisms of pathogenicity of gonococcal salpingitis. Drugs 31:1–6, 1986.

49. Mickelsen PA, Spariing PF. Ability of *N. gonorrhoeae*, *N. meningitidis* and commensal *Neisseria* species to obtain iron from transferrin and iron compounds. Infect Immun 33:554, 1981.

50. Hooper RR, Reynolds GH, Jones OG, et al. Cohort study of venereal disease: I. The risk of gonorrhea transmission from infected women to men. Am J Epidemiol 108:134–144, 1978.

51. Mahoney JF, Van Slyke CJ, Cutler JC, et al. Experimental gonococcic urethritis in human volunteers. Am J Syph Gonorrhea Vener Dis 30:1–39, 1946.

52. Siegal M, Olsen D, Critchlow C, et al. Gonococcal pili: safety and immunogenicity in humans and antibody function in vitro. J Infect Dis 145:300–310, 1982.

53. Holmes KK, Counts GW, Beaty HN. Disseminated gonococcal infection. Ann Intern Med 74:979–993, 1971.

54. Eschenbach DA, Harnisch JP, Holmes KK. Pathogenesis of acute pelvic inflammatory disease: role of contraception and other risk factors. Am J Obstet Gynecol 128:838–850, 1977.

55. Westrom L. Incidence, prevalence, and trends of acute pelvic inflammatory disease and its consequences in industrialized countries. Am J Obstet Gynecol 138:880–892, 1980.

56. Buchanan TM, Eschenbach DA, Knapp JS, et al. Gonococcal salpingitis is less likely to recur with *Neisseria gonorrhoeae* of the same principal outer membrane protein (POMP) antigenic type. Am J Obstet Gynecol 135:978–980, 1980.

57. Rice PA, Kasper DL. Characterization of serum resistance of gonococci that disseminate. J Clin Invest 70:157–167, 1982.

58. Joiner KA, Scales R, Warren KA, et al. Mechanism of action of blocking immunoglobulin G for *Neisseria gonorrhoeae*. J Clin Invest 76:1765–1772, 1985.

59. Schoolnik GK, Buchanan TM, Holmes KK. Gonococci causing disseminated gonococcal infection are resistant to the bactericidal action of normal human sera. J Clin Invest 58:1163–1173, 1976.

60. Schneider H, Griffiss JM, Boslego JW, et al. Expression of paragloboside like lipooligosaccharides may be a necessary component of gonococcal pathogenesis in men. J Exp Med 174:1601–1606, 1991.

61. Petersen BH, Lee TJ, Snyderman R, et al. *Neisseria meningitidis* and *Neisseria gonorrhoeae* bacteremia associated with C6, C7, or C8 deficiency. Ann Intern Med 90:917–920, 1979.

62. Schoolnik GK, Ochs HD, Buchanan TM. Immunoglobulin class responsible for bactericidal activity of normal human sera. J Immunol 122:1771–1779, 1979.

63. Cornelius CE III. Seasonality of gonorrhea in the United States. HSMHA Health Rep 86:157–160, 1971.

64. Mascola L, Albritton WL, Cates W, et al. Gonorrhea in American teenagers, 1960–1981. Pediatr Infect Dis 2:302–303, 1985.

65. Fox KK, Whittington WL, Levine WC, et al. Gonorrhea in the United States, 1981–1996. Demographic and geographic trends. Sex Transm Dis 7:386–393, 1998.

66. Klausner JD, Barrett DC, Dithmer D, et al. Risk factors for repeated gonococcal infections: San Francisco, 1990–1992. J Infect Dis 177:1766–1769, 1998.

67. Marx R, Aral SO, Rolfs RT, et al. Crack, sex, and STD. Sex Transm Dis 18:92–101, 1991.

68. Schwarcz SK, Bolan GA, Fullilove M, et al. Crack cocaine and the exchange of sex for money or drugs: risk factors for gonorrhea among black adolescents in San Francisco. Sex Transm Dis 19:7–13, 1992.

69. American College of Obstetricians and Gynecologists. Gonorrhea and chlamydial infections. Washington, DC, American College of Obstetricians and Gynecologists, March 1994 (ACOG Technical Bulletin No. 190).

70. Rothenberg R. Ophthalmic neonatorum due to *Neisseria gonorrhoeae*: prevention and treatment. Sex Transm Dis 6(Suppl. 2):187–191, 1979.

71. Thompson TR, Swanson RE, Wiesner PJ. Gonococcal ophthalmia neonatorum: relationship of time of infection to relevant control measures. JAMA 228:186–188, 1974.

72. Diener B. Cesarean section complicated by gonococcal ophthalmia neonatorum. J Fam Pract 13:739–744, 1981.

73. Nickerson CW. Gonorrhea amnionitis. Obstet Gynecol 48:815–817, 1973.

74. Edwards L, Barrada MI, Hamann AA, et al. Gonorrhea in pregnancy. Am J Obstet Gynecol 132:637–641, 1978.

75. Allen JH, Barrere LE. Prophylaxis of gonorrheal ophthalmia of the newborn. JAMA 141:522–525, 1949.

76. Armstrong JH, Zacarias F, Rein MF. Ophthalmia neonatorum: a chart review. Pediatrics 57:884–892, 1976.

77. Handsfield HH, Hodson WA, Holmes KK. Neonatal gonococcal infection: I. Orogastric contamination with *Neisseria gonorrhoeae*. JAMA 225:697–701, 1973.

78. Laga M, Naamara W, Brunham RC, et al. Single-dose therapy of gonococcal ophthalmia neonatorum with ceftriaxone. N Engl J Med 315:1382–1385, 1986.

79. Folland DS, Burke RE, Hinman AR, et al. Gonorrhea in preadolescent children: an inquiry into source of infection and mode of transmission. Pediatrics 60:153–156, 1977.

80. Tomeh MO, Wilfert CM. Venereal diseases of infants and children at Duke University Medical Center. NC Med J 34:109–113, 1973.

81. Wald ER, Woodward CL, Marston A, et al. Gonorrheal disease among children in a university hospital. Sex Transm Dis 7:41–43, 1980.

82. Ingram DL, White ST, Durfee MF, et al. Sexual contact

in children with gonorrhea. Am J Dis Child 136:994–996, 1982.

83. Matson N, Gutman LT. Child sexual abuse. *In* Holmes KK, et al. (eds). Sexually Transmitted Diseases, 3rd ed. New York, McGraw-Hill, 1998, pp 239–250.

84. Lipsitt HJ, Parmet AJ. Nonsexual transmission of gonorrhea to a child. Letter to the editor. N Engl J Med 311:470, 1984.

85. Alfonso E, Friedland B, Hupp S, et al. *Neisseria gonorrhoeae* conjunctivitis: an outbreak during an epidemic of acute hemorrhagic conjunctivitis. JAMA 250:794–795, 1983.

86. Cooperman MB. End results of gonorrheal arthritis review of 70 cases. Am J Surg 5:241–251, 1928.

87. Platt R, McCormack W. Pelvic inflammatory disease: a common early complication of gonococcal infection. New Orleans 20th Interscience Conference on Antimicrobial Agents and Chemotherapy 1980. Abstract 669.

88. Acosta AA, Mabray CR, Kaufman RH. Intrauterine pregnancy and coexistent pelvic inflammatory disease. Obstet Gynecol 37:282–285, 1971.

89. Moghissi KS. Composition and function of cervical secretion. *In* Greep FL (ed). Handbook of Physiology, Section 7, Endocrinology, vol. 2, Female Reproductive System, Part 2. Washington, DC, American Physiological Society, 1973, p. 25.

90. Rothbard MJ, Gregory T, Salerno LJ. Intrapartum gonococcal amnionitis. Am J Obstet Gynecol 121:565–566, 1975.

91. Sarrell PM, Pruett KA. Symptomatic gonorrhea during pregnancy. Obstet Gynecol 32:670–673, 1968.

92. Amstey MS, Steadman KT. Symptomatic gonorrhea and pregnancy. J Am Vener Dis Assoc 3:14–16, 1976.

93. Charles AG, Cohen S, Kass MB, et al. Asymptomatic gonorrhea in prenatal patients. Am J Obstet Gynecol 108:595–599, 1970.

94. Elliott B, Brunham RC, Laga M, et al. Maternal gonococcal infection as a preventable risk factor for low birth weight. J Infect Dis 161:531–536, 1990.

95. Israel KS, Rissing KB, Brooks GF. Neonatal and childhood gonococcal infections. Clin Obstet Gynecol 18:143–151, 1975.

96. Kass EH, McCormack WM, Lin J-S, et al. Genital mycoplasmas as a cause of excess premature delivery. Trans Assoc Am Physicians 94:261–266, 1981.

97. Kundsin RB, Driscoll SG, Monson RR, et al. Association of *Ureaplasma urealyticum* in the placenta with perinatal morbidity and mortality. N Engl J Med 310:941–945, 1984.

98. Gravett MG, Nelson HP, DeRouen T, et al. Independent associations of bacterial vaginosis and *Chlamydia trachomatis* infection with adverse pregnancy outcome. JAMA 256:1899–1903, 1986.

99. MacDonald PC, Porter JC, Schwartz BE, et al. Initiation of parturition in the human female. Semin Perinatol 2:273–286, 1978.

100. Hirschberg J, Krause F. Zentralbl Prakt Augen 5:39, 1881.

101. Lindner K. Wien Klin Wochenschr 22:1697, 1742, 1909.

102. Howe L. Credée's method for prevention of purulent ophthalmia in infancy in public institutions. Trans Am Ophthalmol Soc 8:52–57, 1897.

103. Forbes G, Forbes GM. Silver nitrate and the eyes of the newborn. Am J Dis Child 121:1–3, 1971.

104. Kerby CE. Blindness in preschool children. Sight Sav Rev 24:15–29, 1954.

105. Hatfield EM. Causes of blindness in school children. Sight Sav Rev 33:218–233, 1963.

106. Kaivonen M. Prophylaxis of ophthalmia neonatorum. Acta Ophthalmol Suppl 79:1–70, 1965.

107. Desenclos J-CA, Garrity D, Scraggs M, et al. Gonococcal disease of the newborn in Florida, 1984–1989. Sex Transm Dis 19:105–110, 1992.

108. Friendly DS. Gonococcal conjunctivitis in the newborn. Clin Proc Child Hosp DC 25:1–9, 1969.

109. Snowe RJ, Wilfert CM. Epidemic reappearance of gonococcal ophthalmia neonatorum. Pediatrics 51:110–114, 1973.

110. Brown WM, Cowper HH, Hodgman JE. Gonococcal ophthalmia among newborn infants at Los Angeles County General Hospital, 1957–1963. Public Health Rep 81:926–928, 1966.

111. Smith JA. Ophthalmia neonatorum in Glasgow. Scott Med J 14:272–276, 1969.

112. Norn MS. Cytology of the conjunctival fluid in newborn with references to Credé's prophylaxis. Acta Ophthalmol 38:491–495, 1960.

112a. Rahi JS, Sripathi S, Gilbert CE, Foster A. The importance of prenatal factors in childhood blindness in India. Dev Med Child Neurol 39:449–455, 1997.

113. Mordhorst CH, Dawson C. Sequelae of neonatal inclusion conjunctivitis and associated disease in parents. Am J Ophthalmol 71:861–867, 1971.

114. Goscienski PJ, Sexton RR. Follow-up studies in neonatal inclusion conjunctivitis. Am J Dis Child 124:180–182, 1972.

115. Valenton MJ, Abendanio R. Gonorrheal conjunctivitis. Can J Ophthalmol 8:421–427, 1973.

116. Podgore JK, Holmes KK. Ocular gonococcal infection with minimal or no inflammatory response. JAMA 246:242–243, 1981.

117. Fivush B, Woodward CL, Walt ER. Gonococcal conjunctivitis in a four-month-old infant. Sex Transm Dis 7:24–25, 1979.

118. Dundas GHG. Ophthalmia neonatorum before birth. Lancet 1:122, 1921.

119. Pearson HE. Failure of silver nitrate prophylaxis for gonococcal ophthalmia neonatorum. Am J Obstet Gynecol 73:805–807, 1957.

120. Wolffram E. Zentralbl Gynaekol 74:1729, 1952.

120a. Isenberg SJ, Apt L, Wood M. The influence of prenatal infective factors on ophthalmia neonatorum. J Pediatr Ophthalmol Strabismus 33:185–188, 1996.

121. Bradford WL, Kelley HW. Gonococcic meningitis in a newborn infant. Am J Dis Child 46:543–549, 1933.

122. Kohen DP. Neonatal gonococcal arthritis: three cases and review of the literature. Pediatrics 53:436–440, 1974.

123. Gaing E, Cossoy S, Giraldes DA. Arthritis gonococcica en un recien nacido prematuro: puerta de entrada gingival. An Soc Puericult Buenos Aires 7:83–91, 1941.

124. Canino R. Arthritis multiples post-rinitis gonococcia. Pediatria (Naples) 39:264–270, 1931.

125. Parrish PP, Console WA, Battaglia J. Gonococcic arthritis of a newborn treated with sulfonamide. JAMA 114:241–242, 1940.

126. Jones JB, Ramsey RC. Acute suppurative arthritis of hip in children. US Armed Forces Med J 7:1621–1628, 1956.

127. Soonzilli EE, Calabro JJ. Gonococcal arthritis in the newborn. JAMA 177:919–921, 1961.

128. Glaser S, Boxerbaum B, Kennell JH. Gonococcal arthritis in the newborn. Am J Dis Child 112:185–188, 1966.

129. Gregory JE, Chisom JL, Meadows AT. Gonococcal arthritis in an infant. Br J Vener Dis 48:306–307, 1972.

130. Kleiman MB, Lamb GA. Gonococcal arthritis in a newborn infant. Pediatrics 52:285–287, 1973.

131. Gutman LT. Acute, subacute and chronic osteomyelitis

and pyogenic arthritis in children. Curr Probl Pediatr 15:1–56, 1985.

132. Kirkland H, Storer RV. Gonococcal rhinitis in an infant. BMJ 1:263–267, 1931.

133. Herman-Giddens ME, Gutman LT, Berson NL, Duke Child Protection Team. Association of coexisting vaginal infections and multiple abusers in female children with genital warts. Sex Transm Dis 15:63–67, 1988.

134. Darougar S, Jones BR. Conjunctival swabbing for the isolation of TRIC agent (Chlamydia). Br J Ophthalmol 55:585–590, 1971.

135. Fransen L, Nsanze H, D'Costa LJ, et al. Parents of infants with ophthalmia neonatorum: a high-risk group for sexually transmitted diseases. Sex Transm Dis 12:150–154, 1985.

136. Haase DA, Nash RA, Nsanze H, et al. Single-dose ceftriaxone therapy for gonococcal ophthalmia neonatorum. Sex Transm Dis 13:53–55, 1986.

137. Rawston SA, Hammerschlag MR, Gullans C, et al. Ceftriaxone treatment of penicillinase-producing Neisseria gonorrhoeae infections in children. Pediatr Infect Dis J 8:445–448, 1989.

138. Fransen L, Nsanze H, D'Costa L, et al. Single dose kanamycin therapy of gonococcal ophthalmia neonatorum. Lancet 2:1234–1236, 1984.

139. Smith CA, Halse L. Ophthalmia neonatorum. Public Health Rep 70:462–470, 1955.

140. Neonatal gonococcal ophthalmia—California. MMWR Morb Mortal Wkly Rep 32:518–519, 1983.

141. Pearson HE. Failure of silver nitrate prophylaxis for gonococcal ophthalmia neonatorum. Am J Obstet Gynecol 73:805–807, 1957.

142. Oriel JD. Ophthalmia neonatorum: relative efficacy of current prophylactic practices and treatment. J Antimicrob Chemother 14:209–220, 1984.

143. Posner AA, Anderson GD, Prigot A. Observations on the prophylaxis of ophthalmia neonatorum in a municipal hospital. Antibiot Ann 1958–1959, pp. 134–137.

144. Greenberg M, Vandow JE. Ophthalmia neonatorum: evaluation of different methods of prophylaxis in New York City. Am J Public Health 51:836–844, 1961.

145. Bell TA, Sandstrom KI, Gravett MG, et al. Comparison of ophthalmic silver nitrate solution and erythromycin ointment for prevention of natally acquired Chlamydia trachomatis. Sex Transm Dis 14:195–200, 1987.

146. Hammerschlag MR, Cummings C, Roblin PM, et al. Efficacy of neonatal ocular prophylaxis for the prevention of chlamydial and gonococcal conjunctivitis. N Engl J Med 320:769–772, 1989.

147. Chen JY. Prophylaxis of ophthalmia neonatorum: comparison of silver nitrate, tetracycline, erythromycin and no prophylaxis. Pediatr Infect Dis J 11:1026–1030, 1992.

148. Butterfield PM, Emde RN, Sveijde MJ. Does the early application of silver nitrate impair maternal attachment? Pediatrics 67:737–738, 1981.

149. Hedberg K, Ristinan TL, Soler JT, et al. Outbreak of erythromycin-resistant staphylococcal conjunctivitis in a newborn nursery. Pediatr Infect Dis J 9:268–273, 1990.

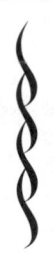

Staphylococcal Infections

HENRY R. SHINEFIELD, M.D., and JOSEPH W. ST. GEME III, M.D.

Staphylococcal disease as a recognized entity has troubled humans, including neonates, for hundreds of years. Pemphigus neonatorum was recognized in newborns probably as early as 1773, nearly 100 years before Tilbury Fox pointed out that this disease was contagious.[1] In 1880, both Louis Pasteur and Sir Alexander Ogston demonstrated a relationship between the *Staphylococcus* organism and the formation of abscesses.[2, 3] Nine years later, the first American nursery epidemic was described,[4] and in 1891 *Staphylococcus aureus* (coagulase-positive *Staphylococcus*) was identified as the cause.[5]

A description by Call in 1904 of a severe nursery outbreak of staphylococcal disease probably represents the first epidemiologic study of a nursery outbreak.[6] At that time, Call commented on the occurrence of associated breast abscess in mothers and stated, ". . . there is absolutely no means of stopping the spread of infection except by complete isolation of both mother and child." Such isolation was a control technique that again found favor in the 1950s, a time of worldwide nursery epidemics.[7] Outbreaks of staphylococcal disease in nurseries were first noted in the late 1920s[8] and peaked in the 1950s.[9] They continue to occur periodically but to a much lesser extent and severity than before. Nurseries are probably never completely free from sporadic or endemic infections, which fortunately are usually confined to the skin and are not serious.

Although *S. aureus* was the most common staphylo-coccal pathogen in the nursery from the 1950s to the 1970s,[10] in the past two decades, coagulase-negative staphylococci (CoNS) have assumed an equally important role as staphylococcal pathogens. These organisms are responsible for many serious infections in the newborn,[11–17] particularly in premature infants in neonatal intensive care units (NICUs). Indeed, in some NICUs CoNS account for almost half of all the cases of serious bacterial disease.[18–24] At present, the most troublesome isolates of *S. aureus* are methicillin-resistant strains, particularly when they are responsible for epidemics in NICUs.[25–34]

The severe hospital outbreaks throughout the world in the late 1950s stimulated intense interest in the problem of staphylococcal infection. Basic research on the biology of the organism and clinical investigations related to *S. aureus* disease led to considerable understanding of this complex organism and its interaction with the human host. Significant recent advances in the understanding of some of the molecular and genetic elements of this organism have been stimulated by the emergence of methicillin-resistant *S. aureus* (MRSA). This chapter summarizes current information about *S. aureus* and CoNS and their associated diseases, particularly as they relate to newborns. A detailed summary of the periodic advances made in the understanding of staphylococci has been published in four monographs.[35–38]

THE ORGANISMS

Taxonomists have decided that the genus *Staphylococcus* belongs to the *Bacillus-Lactobacillus-Streptococcus* cluster consisting of gram-positive bacteria with DNA of a low G + C content. Species of staphylococci are classified on the basis of DNA-DNA hybridization. They are further divided into two large groups on the basis of a variety of biologic and metabolic reactions, including the ability to ferment mannitol and produce the extracellular enzyme coagulase. Staphylococci with the ability to ferment mannitol and produce coagulase are known as coagulase-positive organisms or *S. aureus*.[39] Staphylococci that are negative for these products are refered to as CoNS. In general, the most important species of this group are *S. epidermidis*, *S. saprophyticus*, and *S. haemolyticus*. Among neonates, *S. epidermidis* predominates as a pathogen.

Staphylococci grow without difficulty on the usual laboratory media. A variety of available selective growth media incorporating 8% sodium chloride and 1% glucose facilitate the isolation of these organisms from clinical specimens. Gram staining shows gram-positive cocci, usually in irregular clusters. Growth in liquid culture often results in a predominance of single cocci, pairs, tetrads, and chains of three or four cells. Of note, bacteria in stationary phase or ingested by phagocytes may appear gram negative.

For clinical purposes many of the key characteristics of *S. aureus* can be determined by simple procedures performed with commercial rapid identification kits and automated systems.[39] *S. aureus* strains can be subdivided by their capacity to be lysed by certain bacteriophages.[40] Historically, phage typing has been among the most common systems for differentiating strains of *S. aureus* for epidemiologic purposes.[41] However, because of superior discriminating power and reproducibility, DNA finger printing using pulsed-field gel electophoresis (PFGE) has replaced phage, serologic typing, and other DNA and non-DNA technology as the most accurate method for distinguishing strains of *S. aureus*.[42-44]

Staphylococcus aureus

Studies of the subcellular structure of staphylococci have generated an increasing body of information. Of particular interest is knowledge about the chemical composition, biosynthesis, and antigenicity of the staphylococcal cell wall, which is made up of two major components, peptidoglycan and teichoic acid.[45] The cell wall also contains a small amount of group antigen known as protein A, small amounts of other proteins and carbohydrates that correspond to various type-specific precipitinogens, and agglutinogens. The peptidoglycan is composed of acetylglucosamine, acetylmuramic acid, alanine, glutamic acid, and lysine or diaminopimelic acid.[46] Studies on the inhibition of peptidoglycan biosynthesis have led to a recognition of the mode of action of several antibiotics and staphylolytic enzymes.[47] Important in the synthesis of peptidoglycan are four penicillin-binding proteins (PBP1, PBP2, PB23, and PBP4), which are inactivated by high concentrations of β-lactams.[48] MRSA contains the *mecA* gene, which encodes PBP2a, a low-affinity protein that permits continued integrity of the cell wall despite exposure to β-lactams.[49]

Teichoic acid is a polymer of ribitol phosphate that is held in the cell wall by covalent attachment to the insoluble peptidoglycan. Staphylococcal teichoic acid is antigenic, and antibodies to this substance cause agglutination of isolated staphylococcal cell walls.[50] Antibodies to teichoic acid enhance opsonophagocytic killing of nonencapsulated strains of *S. aureus*, but encapsulated strains are poorly killed even in the presence of a complement source.[51, 52] On the other hand, peptidoglycan antibody plays a key role in the opsonization of *S. aureus*.[53-56] Of note, antibodies to both teichoic acid and peptidoglycan are widespread in the population.[56] Teichoic acid mediates the binding of staphylococci to nasal mucosa cells,[57] interacting with fibronectin or the host cell surface.[58]

S. aureus produces a capsular layer external to the cell wall. Interest in the staphylococcal capsule has been aroused not only because of its disease-producing potential[59, 60] but also because of its ability to stimulate antibody production. The thick mucoid capsule produced by the Smith strain is uncommon. However, most *S. aureus* stains and some isolates of CoNS do produce a microcapsule.[61, 62]

One of the important advances in understanding *S. aureus* is related to characterization of the staphylococcal chromosome and other genetic elements including plasmids, bacteriophages, transposons, and insertion sequences.[63] Although the staphylococcal chromosome has not been completely sequenced, at least 100 genetic loci have been identified.[64] These loci encode proteins responsible for global control of staphylococcal activity, including regulated production of virulence factors involved in bacterial attachment, evasion of host defense, and tissue penetration and destruction. Also located on the chromosome are genes responsible for resistance to a variety of antimicrobial agents such as methicillin.[64] Resistance to inorganic ions and organic cations is encoded by plasmids and transposons.[65] These factors help explain the ability of *S. aureus* to preserve its pathogenicity and to survive in a noxious environment.

Coagulase-Negative Staphylococci

The composition of CoNS is similar to the makeup of *S. aureus*, except that ribitol takes the place of glycerol in the teichoic acid moiety and the cell wall does not contain protein A. CoNS are a heterogeneous group of organisms that have been divided into 31 species.[39] The following 13 species of *Staphylococcus* are found as members of the normal human flora: *S. epidermidis*, *S. haemolyticus*, *S. saprophyticus*, *S. capitis*, *S. warnerii*, *S. hominis*, *S. xylosus*, *S. cohnii*, *S. simulans*, *S. auricularis*, *S. saccharolyticus*, *S. lugdunensis*, and *S. schleiferi*.[39, 66]

Speciation of CoNS is accomplished on the basis of a series of biochemical characteristics. In recent years, species identification has been simplified by the introduction of commercially available miniaturized kits.[57] However, subspeciation, or distinction of two strains belonging to the same species, represents a more difficult problem. Biotyping combined with antibiotic susceptibility patterns has been used for this purpose with some success.[67] Phage-typing is another method that has been useful at times.[67–69] More powerful techniques for distinguishing strains of a given species include plasmid analysis, ribotyping, and chromosomal fingerprinting, especially PFGE.[39, 70–72]

CoNS have been recognized as pathogens in a number of clinical situations, including chronic skin infections,[73] bacterial endocarditis,[74] and otitis media.[75–77] In recent years these organisms have become major pathogens in additional settings, reflecting the more widespread use of invasive therapeutic modalities that require catheters, prosthetic devices, and immunosuppression.[11–24, 78–82] In most of these cases, the species responsible for disease is *S. epidermidis*. In the case of urinary tract infections, the etiologic agent is usually *S. saprophyticus*.[83–86] *S. haemolyticus*, *S. hominis*, *S. warnerii*, *S. simulans*, *S. lugdunensis*, and *S. schleiferi* are occasionally associated with human disease.[82, 87–94] The other species have been implicated in disease only rarely.

VIRULENCE AND PATHOGENESIS OF DISEASE

Role of the Organisms

STAPHYLOCOCCUS AUREUS

S. aureus has a diverse array of cellular and extracellular factors that contribute to the pathogenesis of disease.[95] The pathogenic process begins with bacterial attachment to host cells or extracellular matrices. To persist, the organism produces factors that impede phagocytosis and interfere with the function of specific antistaphylococcal antibodies or other specific host defense mechanisms. Ultimately, the organism expresses specific factors that attack host cells and others that degrade components of the extracellular matrix. Thus far, no single virulence factor has been shown to be either necessary or sufficient for the establishment of all cases of *S. aureus* disease, suggesting that the pathogenesis of disease involves the coordinate action of multiple factors. Furthermore, the importance of any given virulence factor often varies with the particular disease. However, there are three syndromes in which specific extracellular toxin(s) appears to be the prime virulence factors: staphylococcal scalded skin syndrome (SSSS), toxic shock syndrome (TSS), and staphylococcal food poisoning.

S. aureus produces a number of adhesive factors referred to as MSCRAMMS (microbial surface components recognizing adhesive matrix molecules), including clumping factor (ClfA), fibrinogen-binding protein (Fbp), fibronectin-binding protein A (FnbpA), fibronectin-binding protein B (FnbpB), and collagen-binding protein, among others.[96] In addition, *S. aureus* is capable of binding to laminin,[97] vitronectin,[98] elastin,[99] and thrombospondin,[100] although the specific genes and proteins responsible for these activities have not yet been identified. Studies suggest that the *S. aureus* MSCRAMMS and these additional adhesive activities play an important role in colonizing host tissues and binding to foreign objects such as prosthetic devices and catheters.[101–103]

Bacterial survival during infection is dependent on the ability of the organism to circumvent host defenses. Staphylococci have developed several strategies for this purpose. Protein A is a surface-associated protein that binds to the Fc portion of IgG antibodies, presumably blocking opsonization and providing the organism with a protective cover.[104, 105] *S. aureus* V8 protease is a serine protease that is capable of cleaving and inactivating IgG antibodies in vitro, leading to speculation that this protein functions to block the action of antibodies during natural infection. It is possible that V8 and other proteases also function to degrade antimicrobial peptides such as the neutrophil defensins or the platelet microbicidal proteins.[106, 107] Enterotoxins A through E, toxic shock syndrome toxin 1 (TSST-1), and exfoliative (epidermolytic) toxins A and B all have superantigen properties, binding to major histocompatibility complex class II proteins and activating specific subsets of T cells through the variable regions of T cell receptor beta chains.[108] These superantigens may serve to prevent the host from elaborating antibodies to other staphylococcal antigens. In response to an infection, the host can produce a variety of fatty acids and other lipid molecules that act as surfactants to disrupt the bacterial membrane, especially when an abscess is formed. Virtually all strains of *S. aureus* express lipases and are lipolytic,[35] potentially counteracting the effects of host lipids. Leukocidin and γ-hemolysin are two *S. aureus* extracellular proteins that have leukocytolytic activity.[109–113] and may enable the organism to circumvent neutrophil infiltration and phagocytosis. In addition, more than 90% of clinical isolates of *S. aureus* express a polysaccharide capsule, with 11 different known capsular types.[114] Although the role of capsule in pathogenesis is unclear, it is interesting that more than 75% of human isolates express either the type 5 or the type 8 polysaccharide.[115] One hypothesis is that the capsule prevents the interaction of antibodies with the bacterial surface.

A number of *S. aureus* factors have been postulated to promote tissue invasion. Perhaps best studied is α-toxin, also referred to as β-hemolysin, which forms a hexamer or heptamer on cell membranes, giving rise to a pore.[116] Pore formation is associated with release of nitric oxide from endothelial cells and appears to stimulate apoptosis in lymphocytes.[117, 118] Based on comparison of wild type and mutant strains, α-toxin has been implicated in virulence in models of keratitis and mastitis.[119, 120] β-Hemolysin is an enzyme with sphingomyelinase activity and acts on the membrane of red blood cells in vitro and potentially other cells during natural infection.[121] δ-Hemolysin is a 26 amino acid peptide that potentiates the activity of β-hemolysin in vitro, enhancing hemolysis.[122] Additional proteins that may facilitate tissue invasion include hyaluronidase and hyaluronate lyase,[123] enzymes that digest hyaluronic acid, which is a straight-chain polymer found in skin, bone, synovial fluid, umbilical cord, and vitreous humor.[124] Of note, individual isolates of *S. aureus* have been shown to produce multiple electrophoretic forms of these enzymes, suggesting that families exist.

Interestingly, many of the *S. aureus* cell wall–associated adhesive factors that facilitate the initial stages of infection are selectively produced during the exponential phase of in vitro growth.[125] It is noteworthy that these proteins can be anchored to the cell only while the cell wall is being assembled. In contrast, almost all *S. aureus* extracellular proteins presumed to participate in evasion of the immune system and to spread to adjacent tissues are synthesized predominantly during stationary phase.[125, 126] A notable exception is enterotoxin A, which is produced constitutively.[127] This differential expression of specific sets of virulence determinants is likely fundamental to the pathogenic process and is under control of the *agr* and *sar* regulatory loci.[128, 129]

COAGULASE-NEGATIVE STAPHYLOCOCCI

Until recently, the pathogenic potential of CoNS received little attention. With the emergence of these organisms as prominent pathogens, particularly in patients with central intravascular catheters, investigations have intensified in an effort to identify important virulence factors. Attention has centered on *S. epidermidis*, the species most frequently isolated in these cases.

In infections involving indwelling catheters and other prosthetic devices, bacterial adherence to the foreign body is an important step in the pathogenic process. Early evidence suggested that nonspecific factors, including long-range electromagnetic forces and surface hydrophobicity, promote initial attachment.[130] More recent studies have demonstrated that a polysaccharide capsular adhesin referred to as PS/A is also involved in adherence.[131] This material consists predominantly of galactose and glucosamine. It promotes adherence to plastic polymers and functions as an antiphagocytic capsule, preventing C3 deposition and phagocytosis. A second factor suggested to promote attachment to plastic surfaces is AtlE, which shows significant homology to the major autolysin of *S. aureus*.[132] AtlE contains two bacteriologically active domains, including a 60-kDa amidase and a 52-kDa glucosaminidase domain, generated by proteolytic processing.[132] The 60-kDa domain is located on the bacterial surface and is a prerequisite for AtlE-related adhesion. Of note, AtlE also has vitronectin-binding activity,[132] suggesting that this protein plays a role in bacterial attachment both to a naked plastic surface early in infection and to plasma protein-coated surfaces later in infection. SSP-1 is another protein that contributes to binding to plastic. This 280-kDa protein was identified in *S. epidermidis* strain 354 and forms fiber-like structures on the surface of the organism.[133, 134]

After initial attachment, organisms multiply and form multilayered aggregates, which involve intercellular adhesion and are referred to as biofilms. In recent work, Mack and colleagues found that an *S. epidermidis* transposon mutant lacking a polysaccharide antigen called PIA was unable to form multilayered cell clusters.[135] Purification and structural analysis revealed that PIA is a linear, β-1, 6-linked glucosaminoglycan composed primarily of at least 130 2-deoxy-2-amino-D-glucopyranosyl residues, 80 to 85% of which are *N*-acetylated.[136] A second factor important for *S. epidermidis*

intercellular adhesion and biofilm formation is a 140-kDa extracellular protein referred to as accumulation associated protein (AAP).[137] Elimination of expression of AAP has no effect on initial adhesion to glass and polystyrene surfaces but disrupts bacterial accumulation. Consistent with this result, antibody against AAP almost completely blocks accumulation.[138] Interestingly, expression of this protein is found only in bacteria grown under sessile conditions.[138]

After adherence and biofilm formation, most isolates of CoNS produce copious amounts of an extracellular material referred to as slime.[139] In a hospital-wide survey, Ishak and colleagues noted slime production in 13 of 14 clinically significant bloodstream isolates of *S. epidermidis*, compared with only 3 of 13 blood culture contaminants and 4 of 27 skin isolates.[140] Studies of infants have revealed similar results. For example, in independent studies, Hall and co-workers and Gruskay and associates detected slime production by 82% of isolates from infants with invasive disease.[141, 142] Slime presumably functions as a nonspecific physical barrier to cellular and humoral defense mechanisms. In addition, this material inhibits neutrophil chemotaxis and phagocytosis and suppresses lymphocyte blastogenesis.[143, 144] Furthermore, crude extracts of slime are capable of inhibiting the antimicrobial action of both vancomycin and teicoplanin.[145] Consistent with these in vitro results, in the murine model of catheter-related infection, slime-positive strains of CoNS produce disease in a significantly higher percentage of animals than do slime-negative isolates.[146] Relevant to the issue of treatment, the presence of slime makes eradication of CoNS infection more difficult.[147, 148]

Recent work indicates that CoNS produce a variety of exoproteins, including urease, lipase/esterase, fibrinolysin, DNase, and a number of proteases.[149] In addition, selected isolates produce delta-like toxin, an extracellular hemolysin that is similar in size, biologic properties, and antigenicity to the enteropathic δ-toxin of *S. aureus*. Studies by Scheifele and colleagues suggest that delta-like toxin may play a role in the pathogenesis of necrotizing enterocolitis.[150, 151] In particular, these investigators found a strong correlation between the presence of free toxin in the stool of premature infants and the development of necrotizing enterocolitis. Interestingly, under anaerobic conditions, toxin production is markedly reduced, raising the possibility that toxin-mediated bowel injury requires a favorable redox potential within the host bowel.

Selected strains of CoNS produce a polysaccharide capsule. By analogy with other encapsulated pathogens, it is possible that capsule plays a role in the pathogenesis of disease. However, among fresh clinical isolates, capsular material is present in fewer than 10%.[152, 153] Further studies are needed to establish the precise relationship between capsule production and disease.

Role of the Host

Even under the most ideal conditions, infants in the hospital are surrounded by staphylococci. As a result, physical barriers, including the skin and mucous membranes, represent a major defense against staphylococcal disease. Bacteremic disease most often develops when organisms colonizing the skin gain access to the bloodstream through the portal created by an intravascular catheter. Other routes for entry into the bloodstream include the intestinal tract after injury to the epithelial barrier and the respiratory tract, especially in patients being mechanically ventilated. Localized disease occurs when colonizing organisms are implanted into deeper tissues, often related to a break in skin or mucous membrane integrity and sometimes during placement of a foreign body. On occasion, a foreign body becomes contaminated after placement, either with organisms from the hands of medical personnel or from contaminated disinfectants.

Similar to the situation with other pathogenic bacteria, the presence of intact neutrophil phagocytic function is probably the single most important factor involved in controlling replication and spread of staphylococci.[154] Effective phagocytosis requires sufficient numbers of cells along with the ability to sense and migrate toward a site of infection and then ingest and kill microorganisms. At term, the peripheral neutrophil count is higher than that of adults, but there is little capacity to respond to infection with an outpouring of additional cells. As a result, the number of neutrophils at a site of infection is relatively low in infants compared with adults.[155] In addition, neutrophils from newborns show diminished motility toward chemoattractants compared with cells from older children and adults.[156] Potential mechanisms for this diminished chemotaxis include decreased circulating levels of fibronectin,[157] abnormal polymerization of actin,[158] and decreased production of chemotactic factors such as C5a and interleukin-8.[159, 160] Neutrophils from young infants also exhibit decreased migration across endothelium, possibly because of impaired capacity to upregulate endothelial cell expression of the CR3 receptor.[161, 162] Beyond decreases in neutrophil number, chemotaxis, and transepithelial migration, the capacity for neutrophil adherence and phagocytosis is reduced in neonates, largely due to deficiencies in opsonins, including complement, specific antibody, and fibronectin. Phagocytic killing appears to be intact in normal newborns but may be compromised in stressed infants, at least in part due to reduced production of hydroxyl radicals.[154, 163, 164]

Specific antibody is less important than complement in opsonization of S. aureus and plays a limited role in defense against neonatal staphylococcal disease, the possible exception being antibody directed against leukocidin.[165–167] For example, in general there is no correlation between antibody titers against S. aureus and the likelihood of asymptomatic carriage versus clinical disease.[168, 169] Consistent with this information, attempts to protect the newborn from staphylococcal disease by immunizing the mother near term have been unsuccessful.[170]

In most cases of neonatal staphylococcal disease, the role of T cells is unclear. However, T cells are centrally involved in the immune response to several S. aureus toxins, including TSST-1, the staphylococcal enterotoxins (SE A–E), and the staphylococcal exfoliative toxins (ETA, ETB). All of these toxins appear to function as superantigens, interacting with major histocompatibility complex class II proteins on the surface of T cells and activating specific subsets of cells through the variable regions of T cell receptor β chains. The consequence of this T cell activation is proliferation of a large proportion of T cells and release of a number of cytokines, including tumor necrosis factors alpha and beta, interleukin-1, interleukin-2, and interferon γ.[171] These molecules are thought to contribute to the systemic manifestations of SSSS, TSS, and food poisoning.

EPIDEMIOLOGY

Staphylococcus aureus

Many factors are involved in the transmission of staphylococci among newborns. The epidemiology of staphylococcal colonization and disease is influenced by nursery design, density of infant population, and obstetric and nursery practices. Other factors that likely affect transmission include biologic properties of the organism and undefined host factors. The difficulty of isolating and investigating each variable in the epidemiologic equation accounts for the disagreement among various workers about which factors predominate in transmission and prevention of staphylococcal disease. A particular event that is crucially important in one epidemic may not operate under different circumstances.

Quantitative studies demonstrate that very small numbers of S. aureus are capable of initiating colonization in the newborn. Fewer than 10 bacteria can initiate umbilical colonization in 50% of newborns, and approximately 250 organisms achieve a similar effect on the nasal mucosa.[172] These findings provide a plausible explanation for the difficulty encountered in isolating any factor in the environment (fomites, nurses' hands, and clothes or, indeed, any particular site) as a potential source of infection. In addition, it is likely that multiple sources of infection operate simultaneously.

Most evidence indicates that the initial and perhaps major source of infection is medical and nursing personnel.[172, 173] The S. aureus strain common among medical attendants is far more likely than the maternal strain to colonize a given infant.[9] Of note, the disseminating capacity of attendants varies.[174] In turn, there are marked differences in the ability of staphylococci to colonize infants.[175] Individuals with overt lesions or disease are often highly infectious, but asymptomatic carriers are sometimes equally so.[176] The suggestion that the infectiousness of a carrier is directly related to the number of staphylococci present in the anterior nares[177] has been disputed by Hare.[178] Staphylococci can be carried and disseminated from the perineal area without concomitant nasal carriage.[179]

Some reports emphasize the inability to incriminate personnel carriers as the source of infant infection and disease.[180] Infant-to-infant transmission has been postulated under these circumstances, and the major sources of spread that have been incriminated in the newborn are the nose,[181] skin,[175] and umbilical stump.[182]

The hands of hospital attendants are probably the most important source of infant contamination.[183] Data collected by Wolinsky and associates suggest that 85% of infant colonization with *S. aureus* results from an attendant's touch. Colonization of the other 15% takes place by way of air transfer. In one group of 37 infants handled by a study nurse for 10 minutes through the window of an isolette, 20 infants (54%) acquired the nurse's strain of *S. aureus*.[183, 184]

Colonization of the newborn umbilicus, nares, and skin takes place early in life. By the fifth day in the nursery, the colonization rate of nursery inhabitants may range from 40 to 90%.[185–187] The incidence of colonization is higher in males than in females,[188] suggesting that genetic factors may be important, although studies of twins argue against this hypothesis.[189] The umbilicus or rectum is usually colonized before the nares.[190, 191] During the next 4 to 8 weeks in the infant's life, colonization of the umbilicus falls off rapidly and approaches zero, and for the remainder of the first year of life averages about 20%.[186, 187] Despite the high rate of colonization during the newborn period, the incidence of disease in neonates is generally low, except when epidemic strains are involved. In one epidemic, the disease rate in infants and family members who were colonized with a virulent hospital strain of *S. aureus* approached 70%, but colonization with nonepidemic strains was associated with a disease rate of 3%.[192] Certain strains of *S. aureus* are more pathogenic for skin than are others. Epidemics of bullous impetigo and SSSS are caused mainly by strains of phage group II.[193–198] Exfolative toxins have been isolated from staphylococcal strains other than those in phage group II, and epidemics of SSSS have occurred with some of these strains.[199–201] Chesney and colleagues have suggested that the epidemics associated with phage group I may actually be TSS variants rather than staphylococcal strains causing SSSS.[202]

Although colonization of newborns with hospital strains may result in extensive disease, this outcome is not universal. We, as well as others, have noted epidemics of colonization with an 80/81 strain without any subsequent illness. It is not clear why on one occasion an 80/81 strain of *S. aureus* will colonize a large portion of the newborn population without causing disease, whereas on another, colonization by a seemingly identical type may lead to a subsequent incidence of disease as high as 50 to 70%.

Two other important epidemiologic factors related to nursery colonization merit comment. First, epidemics in full-term nurseries are usually not revealed by diseased infants in the nursery. It is more likely that skin disease in the infant appears from 1 to 3 weeks after discharge. Breast abscesses or pneumonia may not develop until 2 weeks to 2 months or more after delivery. Therefore, an accurate record of incidence of nursery-acquired infection requires surveillance outside the hospital.[203] Past experience has demonstrated that such surveillance can be performed by a telephone survey.[204] In NICUs, disease becomes apparent in the unit because of prolonged hospital stays.

Second, virulent strains of staphylococci that are good colonizers are often transmitted from infant to family.[205–207] The disease in the family, which can be maternal mastitis or furunculosis, can then "ping-pong" through the family members for periods as long as 6 to 7 years.[208] MRSA strains that have been the primary cause of epidemics as well as interepidemic *S. aureus* hospital strains do not have a tendency either to spread or to cause septic lesions in family members.[26, 30] However, there have been isolated reports of MRSA nursery epidemic strains with intrafamilial transmission.[209, 210]

There is no satisfactory explanation for the cyclic appearance and disappearance of virulent strains of *S. aureus*. The 80/81 strain that was so devastating in the 1950s is no longer a major problem, either in the United States or in Europe. Why has it disappeared? Two studies suggest that intensive control efforts, including hexachlorophene bathing, had little to do with its disappearance.[211–213] Studies in Denmark suggest that antibiotic sensitivity, together with infection of *S. aureus* strains with phage, have combined to alter strain predominance. It may well be that no strain can achieve a dominating epidemic position in an environment if it is sensitive to an antibiotic that is extensively used in that environment.[214] Therefore, the introduction of semisynthetic β-lactamase–resistant penicillins and the sensitivity of most staphylococcal strains to this group of antibiotics may have played a role in the disappearance of the 80/81 *S. aureus* strain. Against this theory is the fact that nursery epidemics caused by this organism were disappearing before the widespread use of methicillin in the United States.

Most full-term nursery outbreaks of staphylococcal disease in the United States are caused by staphylococcal strains that produce an exfoliative toxin.[193–200, 215, 216] Some cases have been reported in NICUs as well.[201, 217] A characteristic feature of these epidemics is the variety of skin lesions caused by a toxin elaborated by these strains. Similar epidemics first were reported in 1955 by Parker and co-workers in England[193] and later by Rycheck and associates in the United States.[195] Fortunately, these outbreaks have been easily controlled, and the incidence of serious disease has been small. In addition, these strains show little tendency toward transmission and are therefore responsible for little disease within households.

It is quite clear that the virulence of *Staphylococcus* is not enough to create a serious hospital problem; to be an epidemic strain, the organism must be a good colonizer as well. Perhaps another pandemic of serious staphylococcal disease awaits the development of virulent, easily transmissible MRSA. In this regard, since 1975 MRSA has emerged as an important nationwide nosocomial pathogen, usually involving adults but increasingly affecting children as well.[218, 219] In addition, community-acquired MRSA appears to be increasing as well.[220] Although epidemics of MRSA have been well documented since 1975, the extent of disease seen in adults has not been mirrored in infant nurseries.[25–34, 221–225]

It is clear that the severity and extent of disease seen in the 1950s with the *S. aureus* type 80/81 strain have not been replicated to date with MRSA organisms. Whether there is a specific biologic factor that confers on MRSA its ability to become an epidemic strain (EMRSA) remains to be determined.[226, 227] In any case, colonization and disease caused by MRSA may be a serious problem in infants who require invasive diagnostic or therapeutic procedures, or both.[225]

Temporal clustering of cases suggests that MRSA outbreaks generally are caused by a single strain. However, one report in which the MRSA organisms were characterized by genotypic as well as phenotypic analysis suggested that two separate strains of *S. aureus* were involved in an outbreak of disease among 10 infants.[31] Two different *S. aureus* (not MRSA) strains were isolated (from extremely low birth weight infants) in a second epidemic in an NICU, one producing disease and another in an asymptomatic infant.[217] It is clear that strain identity by phenotypic methods (i.e., phage types, antibiotograms, and even plasmid profiles) may not be precise enough to identify *S. aureus* strains for epidemiologic investigatory purposes. In these situations, strain identity requires characterization based on a molecular technique such as PFGE.

Coagulase-Negative Staphylococci

CoNS are common inhabitants of many human skin and mucous membrane sites.[228] *S. epidermidis* is the species found most commonly as a member of the normal flora of the nasal mucosa and the umbilicus of the newborn.[229] Colonization occurs early and at many sites. With sensitive culture techniques, the nose, umbilicus, and chest skin are colonized with CoNS in up to 83% of neonates by 4 days of age.[230] In one study, rates of colonization with *S. epidermidis* were as follows among 63 infants in an NICU: nose, 89%; throat, 84%; umbilicus, 90%; and stool, 86%. Comparable percentages for *S. aureus* were 17%, 17%, 21%, and 10%, respectively.[229]

In other studies in which isolates were characterized by species, biotype, antibiotic susceptibility pattern, and slime production, colonization rates were 50 to 80% by 4 to 7 days after admission to the NICU.[231–233] After 2 weeks in the unit, 75 to 100% of infants were colonized with CoNS at some mucosal site. In one study, slime-producing strains selectively colonized infants over a 4-week period, with nearly 90% of infants eventually harboring a single predominant *S. epidermidis* biotype.[232] Although most infants acquire CoNS from environmental sources, including hospital personnel, a small percentage are colonized by vertical transmission.[234, 235] The ubiquity of these organisms and their tolerance to both drying and temperature changes offer an explanation for the high prevalence of colonization among infants.

Ecologic relationships between the microbial flora of various body sites have been well studied, and factors that reduce colonization at one site with one organism tend to increase colonization at that site with others.[231] Current nursery practices that decrease colonization with *S. aureus* contribute to the increased presence of CoNS in neonates. These practices include the extensive use of antimicrobial agents and the use of skin and umbilical cleansing techniques. Furthermore, isolates of *S. epidermidis* and other CoNS resistant to multiple anti-

biotic agents are becoming increasingly common.[231] In a recent study, D'Angio and associates demonstrated that the incidence of strains resistant to multiple antibiotics rose from 32% to 82% by the end of the first week of life.[232]

The observation that CoNS are important nosocomial pathogens among newborns, especially low-birth-weight infants in NICUs, is explained by the prevalence of colonization with these organisms at multiple sites and the widespread use of invasive therapeutic modalities. Examples of invasive treatments include endotracheal intubation; mechanical ventilation; placement of umbilical catheters, central venous catheters, chest tubes, and ventriculoperitoneal shunts; and the use of feeding tubes.[16, 17, 19, 20, 23, 24] In many NICUs, disease due to *S. epidermidis* exceeds that caused by group B beta-hemolytic streptococci and *Escherichia coli*.[17, 19, 20]

Among newborns, an important risk factor for bacteremia due to CoNS is the administration of intralipids through a Teflon catheter. In a case-control study, infants with bacteremia were more likely than control infants to have received an intravenous lipid emulsion shortly before the onset of bacteremia.[236] The significant pathogenic factors included slime-producing CoNS, lipid infusion, and the Teflon catheter, all of which interfere with neutrophil and macrophage function. Whether lipids infused via catheters made of other materials are associated with a similar risk remains to be determined.

Thus, all the data, both clinical and experimental, suggest that CoNS have not become more virulent over time. Rather, these ubiquitous organisms have become more common pathogens because therapeutic approaches have become increasingly invasive and because premature infants, who already have compromised immunity, are surviving for longer periods of time.

CONTROL

Staphylococcus aureus

Control of nursery infection has been directed toward the three important links in the chain of events that leads to colonization of infants: the environment, nursery attendants, and the infants themselves.[237–239]

Attempts have been made to decrease colonization rates of infants by increasing the space allowance per child and by enforcing rigorous environmental controls that increase the level of asepsis.[240] *S. aureus* infection has not been controlled by such nursery policies, although such changes undoubtedly alter the level of environmental contamination. Other methods, such as ultraviolet light irradiation and marked increases of air flow, have likewise reduced the environmental contamination of nurseries but have not influenced infant colonization rates.[241]

Another approach to environmental control involves "rooming in," that is, placing the neonate in a room with his or her mother.[6, 7] However, because newborns may be colonized within the first few hours of life and the usual rooming-in technique involves at least a short time in a common nursery, this approach has often failed. A variation of rooming in is "cohort isolation," which involves clustering a small number of infants born within 1 or 2 days of each other in the same nursery so that they can be discharged as a "cohort." The intent is to prevent contact between newly born, uncolonized neonates and older, contaminated infants. Several reports describe the successful interruption of epidemics using this technique.[6, 215, 240]

The key to infant colonization is the nurse. Adequate staffing is important, particularly in an NICU. Maintaining an appropriate nurse-to-infant ratio is an important factor in reducing disease once a disease-associated *S. aureus* strain gains entrance to a nursery.[241, 242] In addition, there are a variety of preventive maneuvers directed at nurses, including frequent mask, gown, and glove changes before handling infants[243, 244]; nasal application of antimicrobial or antiseptic ointment and sprays[244–247]; and elimination of carriers from the nursery area.[180, 248] In special situations, when a strain of *Staphylococcus* does not easily spread from infant to infant but can colonize and produce disease when transferred directly by the nurse carrier, removal of the carrier from the nursery results in control of the epidemic.[249] Unfortunately, such situations are uncommon.

A fundamental means to reduce colonization rates is hand washing. Mortimer and associates reduced infant colonization rates from 92 to 53% by insisting that attendants wash their hands.[250] These observations led Williams and Oliver to abandon caps, masks, gowns, and hair nets for nurses.[251] Nurses who were *S. aureus* carriers were not removed from the nursery, and parents and medical students were permitted to enter the nursery. Colonization rates remained at about 5% during the time these traditional control measures were dropped.[251] The rule that was retained and reinforced was careful washing of hands before handling an infant. It must be emphasized that these observations were made at a time when the staphylococcal problem was at a low ebb. Although hand washing is an important prophylactic technique, it is doubtful that this procedure alone can interrupt a nursery epidemic of *S. aureus* disease caused by a virulent strain with good colonizing capacity. On the other hand, the importance of emphasizing hand washing by personnel in the nursery should not be minimized. In epidemic situations in which disease in infants was caused by multiple strains of *Staphylococcus* and was characterized in the main by pyoderma with little serious illness and no intrafamily spread of the organism, strict attention to hand washing was an important factor in curtailing the outbreak.[252, 253]

Because of the limited success in controlling colonization by these maneuvers, attempts have been made to protect the "target site"—the infant. Such protection consists of anointing or otherwise covering the skin or umbilicus of the newborn with some protective material. These measures have included the application of antimicrobial ointments[32, 254–256] or antiseptic dyes[182, 257–259] to the umbilicus or repeated washing of infants with hexachlorophene-containing powders or washes.[190, 258, 260–266] All of these approaches have had varying degrees of success. Because very few organisms are necessary for

colonization,[182] success or failure in particular instances probably was related to the strain involved and a variety of host and environmental factors.

Before the appearance of MRSA, some nursery epidemics were controlled with the use of systemic antibiotics.[267, 268] Because MRSA generally exhibits resistance to multiple antibiotics, it is doubtful that this approach would currently be successful if the epidemic strain is MRSA.

In the early 1960s attempts were made to stop virulent *S. aureus* epidemics in 10 NICUs throughout the United States using the technique of bacterial interference.[269–273] This technique involved deliberate implantation of an *S. aureus* strain of low virulence (502A) on the nasal mucosa and umbilicus of newborns to prevent colonization with the virulent *S. aureus* strain 80/81 and was successful in curtailing all 10 epidemics.[274] It is unlikely that 502A will be used in the future for such a purpose. However, recent information has accumulated regarding the local host factors and those related to the organism that are involved in colonization. Therefore, it may be possible to isolate a noninfectious fraction of *S. aureus*, successfully colonize particular sites, and thus prevent colonization with a virulent *S. aureus*.[57, 275]

It was also found in the early 1960s that meticulous hexachlorophene newborn infant body washes and cord care would reduce colonization with *S. aureus*.[261] This approach was used as an interepidemic technique in many nurseries in an attempt to prevent *S. aureus* epidemics.[260, 263, 264, 266] This was based on the hypothesis that control of infant colonization would prevent epidemics. Although epidemics of *S. aureus* have been associated with high colonization rates, they also occurred in some instances in NICUs with low colonization rates.[212, 276] On the other hand, there is a considerable body of evidence that high colonization rates are not always associated with *S. aureus* epidemic disease.[212, 252, 277] This has been true not only in infants colonized with β-lactam–sensitive *S. aureus* but also when nursery colonization rates are high with MRSA.[256]

If hexachlorophene is to be effective in reducing colonization rates, the application must be carried out in an almost ritualistic fashion and continued at home after hospital discharge.[255, 260, 263, 278] In addition, hexachlorophene washes have been shown to be neurotoxic, particularly to premature infants.[279–287] For these reasons, hexachlorophene is not recommended as a routine interepidemic newborn body cleansing preventative measure.

Other routine approaches to minimize interepidemic colonization of newborns have been investigated. These have included umbilical application of triple dye,[288] bacitracin,[289] silver sulfadiazine[290, 291] and mupirocin.[32, 256] All have shown some effect in reducing *S. aureus* colonization during the limited time of the study. Whether the long-term application of these materials results in the development of resistant organisms or some other undesirable bacterial or nonbacterial response remains to be seen.

To summarize, the following statements regarding control of epidemics and colonization seem to be warranted on the basis of available information:

1. All nurseries have a background of *S. aureus* coloni-

zation and disease with variation from nursery to nursery. Disease caused by these endemic strains is usually mild. The rate of illness varies from 3 to 6 infants per 1000 live births. Disease is usually not transmitted to family members.

2. Contact with the hands of nursery personnel is the usual manner by which infants are colonized with staphylococci. Although meticulous attention to hand washing does not eliminate colonization of infants with *S. aureus*, it can reduce the neonatal colonization rate. The importance of careful hand washing by any individual before handling infants should be emphasized at regular intervals.

3. An important element in preventing or controlling a nursery epidemic, particularly in an NICU, is maintaining an appropriate nurse-to-infant ratio.

4. Other techniques, such as gowns, masks, and caps, have little effect on colonization rates. Nurse and other personnel carriers need not be removed from the nursery routinely, but attendants with virulent strains should be removed during epidemics. No individual with a staphylococcal lesion should enter the nursery.

5. Because high colonization rates are not always associated with epidemics, the value of colonization surveillance is minimal. Cost outweighs benefit in carrying this out on a routine basis in most nurseries. Instead, close observation for disease, both in the nursery and at home, is a more reliable and less expensive method to identify a staphylococcal problem in the nursery.

6. Nowadays most epidemics in full-term nurseries are characterized by skin disease, little serious illness, and no intrafamily spread of infection. In the NICU, disease is often caused by MRSA and may result in more serious illness. In both situations, careful hand washing by nursery personnel and sequestration of infants may be effective in controlling the disease. Control in some circumstances may be achieved by local application of antimicrobial ointments, solutions, or dyes such as triple dye (brilliant green, proflavine hemisulfate, and crystal violet) to the umbilical cord. Hexachlorophene baths also may have limited effect. If hexachlorophene is used in these epidemic situations, the applications to infants should be carefully controlled. The bathing solution should not contain more than 3% hexachlorophene; it should be applied only to full-term infants, no more than two times to each infant, and then thoroughly washed off after the application.

7. Hexachlorophene bathing should not be used to reduce interepidemic colonization rates. There is some information on the use of modified chemoprophylactic techniques on a routine basis, which reduces colonization with *S. aureus*. Although some of these approaches seem safe and effective for short-term use, the potential problems of continual long-term application, particularly because of possible changes in infant biota, remain to be evaluated.

Coagulase-Negative Staphylococci

With the rise in prominence of CoNS as nosocomial pathogens, strategies for disease prevention have become increasingly important. Strict hand washing is of pri-

mary importance in minimizing staff-to-patient and patient-to-patient spread of CoNS. In addition, meticulous surgical technique to limit intraoperative bacterial contamination is critical in minimizing infection related to foreign bodies. Strict attention to protocols for the insertion and management of intravenous and intra-arterial catheters may decrease the risk of catheter-related infections. In patients who require intravenous access for prolonged periods of time, percutaneous placement of a small-diameter Silastic catheter is preferred when possible. In one study these catheters were maintained for as long as 80 days, with an infection rate of less than 10% in infants weighing less than 1500 g.[292]

Studies of CoNS using scanning and transmission electron microscopy suggest that attachment to catheters is a dynamic process, dependent on properties intrinsic to the catheter surface.[293-295] Peters and co-workers have suggested that catheter components may even serve as a nutrient source for these organisms.[293] With this information in mind, a number of investigators have explored the possibility of developing catheters that are inert and resistant to bacterial colonization. However, thus far these attempts have been disappointing.

Over the years, clinicians have employed prophylactic antibiotic therapy during implantation of a foreign body, intending to prevent infection due to CoNS and other nosocomial pathogens. Although this practice is now routine during neurosurgical, cardiac, and orthopedic surgery, efficacy remains unproven and selection for antibiotic resistance is a significant concern. More recent efforts have focused on the possibility of preventing infection by using catheters and other prosthetic materials that have been impregnated with antibiotics. Thus far, central catheters impregnated with cefazolin, minocycline-rifampin, or chlorhexidine–silver sulfadiazine have been studied in adults,[296-299] and these studies have generally shown a significant reduction in both catheter colonization and catheter-related bloodstream infection.[300] One study comparing catheters impregnated with either minocycline-rifampin or chlorhexidine–silver sulfadiazine demonstrated that the use of minocycline-rifampin is superior.[301]

In recent years, a number of investigators have examined the use of low-dose intravenous vancomycin to prevent nosocomial bacteremia due to CoNS in low-birth-weight infants. Spafford and associates performed a randomized, double-blind, controlled study involving 70 neonates weighing less than 1000 g, with central venous catheters in place.[302] Among these infants, 35 received the standard total parenteral nutrition (TPN) solution, and the remaining 35 received a constant infusion of vancomycin (25 µg/ml) mixed with their total TPN solution. In infants receiving vancomycin, the rate of colonization of catheters by CoNS was reduced from 40 to 18% and the rate of catheter-related sepsis was reduced from 15% to zero. Kacica and colleagues conducted a similar study in infants weighing less than 1500 g, and found that 1 of 71 infants receiving vancomycin compared with 24 of 70 control infants developed gram-positive bacteremia.[303] Cooke and co-workers employed a slightly different protocol, administering vancomycin in a dose of 5 mg/kg twice daily.[304] Among 72 neonates weighing less than 1500 g, 11 of 37 who received vancomycin compared with 17 of 35 who received standard TPN had one or more episodes of CoNS bacteremia. The results of these studies are certainly encouraging. On the other hand, the potential risks associated with prophylactic vancomycin, including ototoxicity, nephrotoxicity, and selection for resistant bacteria, remain poorly defined. At this point, the use of prophylactic vancomycin is not recommended routinely.

SPECIFIC STAPHYLOCOCCAL DISEASES

Skin Diseases

BULLOUS IMPETIGO

Bullous impetigo produces intraepidermal vesicles on a nonerythematous base with sharp margins. The vesicles contain clear yellow fluid and are easily ruptured. Lesions occur predominantly around the umbilicus, diaper area, and intertriginous areas of the axilla and neck; they are most commonly seen within the first 2 weeks of life and are usually not associated with fever or systemic illness. *S. aureus* of all phage groups has been isolated from these lesions, but *S. aureus* of phage group II is most frequently the causative agent. If there are only a few small lesions, local treatment consisting of artificial rupture of the vesicles followed by cleansing with soap and water or alcohol is usually sufficient to effect cure. Because metastatic dissemination can occur, the lack of immediate response to local therapy demands treatment with systemic antibiotics. (The dosage schedule for antibiotics useful in treatment of neonatal staphylococcal disease is given in Table 30–1.) The appearance of infants with such lesions should alert the physician to the existence of a staphylococcal problem in the nursery.

STAPHYLOCOCCAL SCALDED SKIN SYNDROME (TOXIC EPIDERMAL NECROLYSIS)

A much more extensive disease involving large surface areas of the skin, initially called Ritter's disease, is now referred to as the staphylococcal scalded skin syndrome (SSSS) or toxic epidermal necrolysis (TEN).[305] A similar exfoliative process described by Lyell in adults has multiple causes.[306] A scarlatiniform rash is noted initially, followed by wrinkling and desquamation of large areas of skin provoked by only light rubbing of skin surfaces (Nikolsky's sign). In some cases, the disease does not progress beyond the rash stage. Factors that are responsible for the expression of disease from the spectrum of rash to SSSS in a particular host remain to be determined.[307] If denudation occurs, drying and a secondary desquamation follow in about 48 hours and last for a few days (Fig. 30–1). Melish and Glasgow first described the toxin that was responsible for the disease.[308] It is now known that there are two toxins, each of which may be responsible for SSSS: ETA and ETB.[309] ETA was isolated from phage group II *S. aureus* cultured from the skin surface of some of these patients.[200–203] Subsequently, ETB was isolated from staphylococci of other phage groups that also have been associated with SSSS.[199–201] The skin manifestation is a result of the toxin[310]; the site of staphylococcal infection may be distant from the skin. Such primary areas of infection include the conjunctiva[311] and the circumcision site.[312] The patients are generally afebrile, and there may be difficulties with fluid balance and temperature regulation. Although initially noted in infants in full-term

TABLE 30–1
Drugs Useful in Treatment of Neonatal Staphylococcal Disease

AGENT	DOSAGE	
	Age Birth to 1 wk	Age 1–4 wk
Penicillin G	25,000–50,000 units/kg q12h	Same dose q8h
Methicillin ⎫		
Oxacillin ⎬	25–50 mg/kg q12h	25–40 mg/kg q6–8h
Nafcillin ⎭		
Cephalothin[a]	25–50 mg/kg q12h	25–40 mg/kg q6–8h
Cefazolin[a]	20 mg/kg q12h	Same dose

	DOSAGE BASED ON POSTCONCEPTIONAL AGE[b]		
	≤ 31 wk[c]	32–43 wk[c]	≥ 44 wk[c]
Vancomycin[d]	Loading dose 15 mg/kg 10 mg/kg q12h	Same dose q8h	Same dose q6h
Gentamicin[e]	2.5 mg/kg q12h	Same dose q12h	Same dose q8h

[a]To be used only in rare instances when neonate is sensitive to penicillin or related antibiotics; not to be used in treatment of methicillin-resistant organisms or staphylococcal meningitis.
[b]Postconceptional age = gestational age at birth + postnatal age.
[c]Dosing intervals are estimates only. Wide interpatient variability requires determination of peak and trough levels for appropriate intervals.
[d]Antibiotic of choice in treatment of methicillin-resistant staphylococci; should be given slowly over 30–60 min.
[e]If administered intravenously, should be given slowly over 30–60 min.

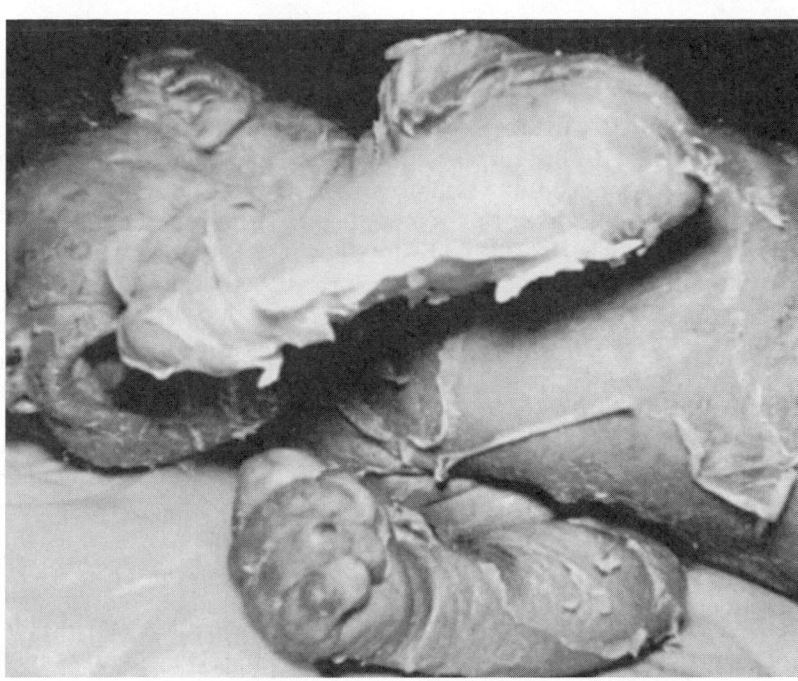

FIGURE 30–1 Ten-day-old infant with scalded skin syndrome caused by *Staphylococcus* phage group II. Good clinical response to β-lactamase–resistant penicillin was noted, and the child recovered in 1 week.

nurseries, epidemics of SSSS also have been reported in NICUs.[201, 217]

For clarity, it would be best to refer to exfoliation related to staphylococcal infection in either infant or adult as SSSS and to that caused by other causes in any age group as TEN. This is necessary because the diseases differ from each other in a number of important respects. Although they are clinically difficult to differentiate, rapid differentiation is accomplished by histologic examination of a frozen section of peeled skin or by cytodiagnosis of the denuded area obtained by a simple swab.[313–315] The cleavage plane of desquamation in SSSS is more superficial than that associated with TEN. A smear of the denuded area in individuals with SSSS reveals broad epithelial cells with relatively small nuclei and no inflammatory cells. The cytology in TEN, on the other hand, reveals cuboidal cells with a high nuclear cytoplasmic ratio plus inflammatory cells. In neither case should hexachlorophene be used to cleanse the denuded areas, because it may be absorbed and cause convulsions. Administration of a β-lactamase–resistant antistaphylococcal antimicrobial agent is indicated in SSSS but not in TEN. Although corticosteroids may be considered in TEN, they are contraindicated in SSSS.[316]

TOXIC SHOCK SYNDROME

Toxic shock syndrome (TSS) is caused by a toxin (TSST-1) or an enterotoxin produced by *S. aureus*.[317–320] Before the 1980s, disease occurred most commonly but not exclusively in menstruating women, particularly in those who used tampons.[321] The disease is characterized by sudden onset of fever, diarrhea, shock, hyperemia of the mucous membranes, and a diffuse macular erythematous rash, followed by desquamation of the hands and feet. Fluid loss and shock are a common cause of death in this disorder; therefore, primary attention should be paid to the replacement of fluid and electrolytes. Because most cases have been associated with penicillin-resistant *S. aureus*, a β-lactamase–resistant penicillin or cephalosporin should be used.

Beyond classic cases that involve menstrating women, TSS has also been reported in prepubertal girls, postmenopausal women, and men.[322, 323] The focus of infection in nonmenstrual cases is often inconspicuous but represents a site for *S. aureus* multiplication and elaboration of TSST-1, which then enters the bloodstream and is widely disseminated to distant organs.[318, 319]

Not surprisingly, TSS has been reported on occasion in newborns. Whitley and co-workers reported a fatal case in a 3-week-old infant who developed a staphylococcal abscess after a heel puncture.[324] Intravenous nafcillin was initiated, and the infant was improving but then developed profound shock and respiratory failure and died. Postmortem examination confirmed the clinical impression, with visceral and cutaneous histopathology characteristic of fatal TSS cases. Multiple blood cultures were negative, but cultures of the wound grew *S. aureus* that was penicillin resistant and nafcillin sensitive and produced exotoxin type C.

Chesney and associates described a 2-month-old premature infant with extensive exfoliative dermatitis with flaccid bullae.[202] Initially, the infant was thought to have SSSS. However, several points suggested a variant form of TSS: (1) Nikolsky's sign was negative; (2) mucosal involvement was present; (3) skin biopsy revealed subepidermal separation rather than intraepidermal separation; and (4) the organism belonged to phage type 29/52 (group I) and elaborated toxins associated with TSS rather than the exfoliation found with organisms responsible for SSSS.

It is possible that some of the nursery outbreaks described as SSSS that belong to phage group I are in reality TSS variants. Without isolation of specific toxins from the staphylococci, it is impossible to be sure of the disease entity.[199, 200]

CHRONIC RECURRENT FURUNCULOSIS

Furuncles and other skin afflictions are the most common lesions produced by staphylococci. They are commonly self-limited and either heal spontaneously or require only simple drainage. They may be particularly troublesome to the newborn. Complications occur when infection extends to areas more vulnerable than the skin.

Another problem is chronic recurrent furunculosis in individuals. Treatment of such individuals includes the elimination, when present, of the nasal carriage of the offending *S. aureus* strain. This often can be done with the use of systemic and/or local antibiotics. A variety of regimens have been suggested that include systemic trimethoprim-sulfamethoxazole with rifampin and topical nasal mupirocin.[325–328]

If this approach is unsuccessful, an effective treatment technique uses the concept of bacterial interference. Individuals and families with chronic recurrent furunculosis may be protected by artificial nasal colonization with a strain of *S. aureus* that has low virulence (strain 502A).[329, 330] This regimen includes the use of a topical nasal antibiotic and a systemic antibiotic before colonization. Patients with chronic recurrent furunculosis who are not likely to respond to this regimen include those with underlying diseases such as diabetes, eczema, and acne.[273] Success has been reported in 80% of treated patients. A controlled double-blind study has reconfirmed the value of recolonization in treating recurrent furunculosis.[331]

CERVICAL ADENITIS

In the newborn, *S. aureus* cervical adenitis can be another manifestation of nursery colonization. At least two outbreaks of cervical adenitis resulting from nursery infection have been described in England. One outbreak involving 25 infants had an attack rate of 1.9%, and another involving 9 infants had an attack rate of 5.6%.[332, 333] As with other manifestations of nursery-associated *S. aureus* disease, illness usually appears after discharge. The mean incubation period in the two epidemics in England was 86 and 72 days, respectively. Because of the delay in onset of disease, establishment of a nursery as the source of the infection may be difficult and necessitates careful epidemiologic investigation.

Although the disease may be mild, serious complications have occasionally been reported. Dissection of the infection along the fascial sheaths of the neck into the thorax can result in secondary pneumonia and pyothorax.[334]

To guide treatment of *S. aureus* cervical adenitis it is wise to obtain material for smear and culture by performing needle aspiration of the infected lymph node gland.[335, 336]

Eye, Ear, Nose, and Throat Infections

One of the common sites of staphylococcal infection is the conjunctiva. Purulent staphylococcal conjunctivitis cannot be distinguished clinically from conjunctivitis caused by other organisms. The disease responds to local, nonspecific treatment and, unlike gonococcal ophthalmitis, results in no residual damage.

Ethmoiditis with concomitant periorbital cellulitis is a serious infection that can evolve from *S. aureus* colonization of the nasopharynx. The periorbital tissues become red, edematous, and swollen. Disease progresses rapidly and leads to proptosis and limitation of eye movement. A variety of organisms other than staphylococci can cause this infection, which is dangerous because it is sometimes complicated by retrobulbar abscess and cavernous sinus infection and thrombosis. Intense parenteral treatment with antibiotics is required early.

Careful studies have suggested that staphylococci are occasionally true middle ear pathogens, with *S. epidermidis* being the species most frequently encountered. Staphylococci are recovered from middle ear fluid in about 3% of premature infants with otitis media and can result in recurrent purulent or serous otitis.[337]

Another infection seen primarily in premature infants is staphylococcal parotitis, usually due to *S. aureus*. Debilitated, dehydrated infants are particularly susceptible. The diagnosis can be made by collecting pus from Stensen's duct when the parotid gland is compressed.

Breast Abscesses

Infant and maternal breast abscesses occur frequently during nursery epidemics with virulent staphylococci. Maternal breast abscesses usually occur from 2 weeks to 2 months post partum. The causative organism is similar to the strain that colonizes the infant and probably gains access to the interstitial tissues of the breast through a crack in the skin or nipple. Alternatively, it may migrate through smaller ducts to the acini of the gland. Transmission of the organism is not always from infant to mother, because breast abscesses have been seen in women who were delivered of stillborn infants.[338]

During nursery epidemics, maternal breast abscesses are found almost exclusively in nursing mothers.[339, 340] In one epidemic, breast abscesses were noted in 5 of 15 nursing mothers but were absent from all 15 mothers who did not breast-feed their infants.[324] Both groups of infants were free of disease but were nasal carriers of *S. aureus* phage type 80/81. With this information in mind, during epidemics with virulent strains of staphylococci, it is debatable whether infants colonized with the epidemic organism should be breast-fed.

Clinically, the disease can range from a small area of mild erythema to extensive involvement with systemic signs of infection, including high fever. Care must be taken in making the diagnosis from a smear or culture expressed from the nipple, because staphylococci can be recovered from 25 to 50% of normal lactating women.[341–344] Many cases of maternal breast abscess respond simply to antibiotics and emptying the breast of milk. Other cases require surgery with incision and drainage, which usually leads to an uneventful recovery.

Sporadic puerperal mastitis without abscess differs from the maternal mastitis that occurs during epidemics caused by virulent organisms. In a large series of cases studied during a 2-year period in a nonindigent population, lactation continued during the course of therapy of the mother with no adverse effects on mother or infant.[345] In the great majority of cases, this proved to be a relatively mild disease and responded rapidly to therapy despite the continuation of breast-feeding. Complicating staphylococcal abscesses were seen in only 3 of 64 cases.

In neonates, breast disease usually occurs between the tenth and the fourteenth days of life. The disease can progress rapidly and involve not only the breast but also the entire subcutaneous tissue extending down to the abdomen and up around the shoulder to the back (Fig. 30–2). The extensive involvement is associated with a considerable amount of pus, toxicity, and systemic signs and symptoms of infection. Gram-negative organisms can also cause mastitis in the neonate,[346, 347] but the breast usually does not show the extensive involvement seen with staphylococcal infections. Generally, there are fewer toxic effects.[348] Diagnosis can be made by Gram stain and culture of milk expressed from the infant's breast. Collections of pus should be incised, drained, and examined by Gram stain and culture.

Neonatal breast abscess can affect subsequent breast development and result in a decrease in breast size in adult life.[349] The incidence of this complication is unknown. In one series of cases in which follow-up histories were obtained, a decrease in breast size was noted in two of six individuals who were examined at the ages of 8 and 15 years, respectively.[350]

Septicemia

CoNS and *S. aureus* are well-recognized causes of septicemia in the newborn period.[351, 352] Septicemia is the most common manifestation of neonatal infection with CoNS and usually occurs in the setting of a central intravascular catheter. With *S. aureus*, the incidence of septicemia increases when a virulent strain is present in the nursery and is more often associated with focal infection.

The signs and symptoms associated with staphylococcal septicemia are usually nonspecific and include disturbances of temperature regulation, respiration, circulation, gastrointestinal function, and central nervous system activity. Hypothermia is more common than fever and is often observed as the initial sign. Respiratory distress frequently manifests as episodes of apnea and bradycardia, particularly in infants who weigh less than 1500 g. Other abnormalities related to respiration include tachypnea, retractions, and cyanosis. From 20 to 30% of infants develop gastrointestinal findings, including poor feeding, regurgitation, abdominal distention, diarrhea, and bloody stools. Evidence of poor perfusion can include mottling, poor capillary refill, or metabolic acidosis. Some infants develop lethargy, irritability, or poor suck.

In infants who have septicemia associated with focal complications, these complications are often heralded by persistent bacteremia. Thus, when blood cultures remain positive for more than 72 hours on appropriate antibiotic therapy, a search for focal infection is advisable. The most common examples include skin or soft tissue infection, osteomyelitis, septic arthritis, endocarditis, and meningitis.

Interestingly, Patrick and co-workers recently described a group of 13 low-birth-weight infants with persistent CoNS bacteremia who had no indwelling central intravascular catheter and lacked evidence of focal infection.[353] These infants had positive blood cultures for 6 to 25 days despite appropriate antibiotic therapy. Abdominal distention and thrombocytopenia were especially common findings. Although the bacteremia eventually cleared without mortality, the explanation for the delayed response to therapy was elusive.

The diagnosis of staphylococcal septicemia is established by isolating organisms from the blood. To facilitate interpretation of positive cultures, especially those growing CoNS, multiple cultures should be obtained if at all possible. Recovery of the same strain (as defined by

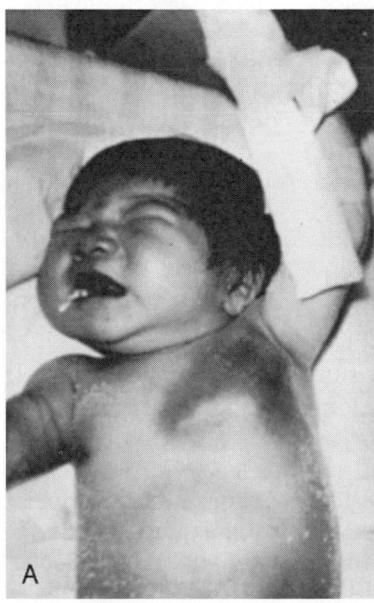
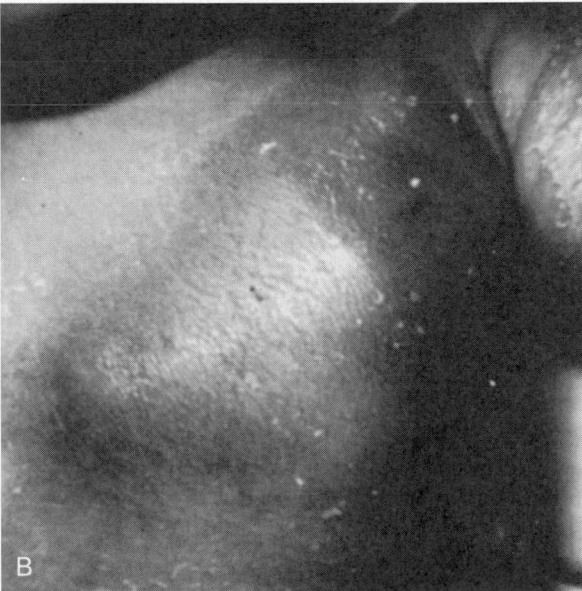

FIGURE 30–2 *A* and *B*, Left breast abscess in a 12-day-old infant. Abscess extends toward right side of chest and up over arm. Good response to incision and drainage and antimicrobial therapy was noted.

speciation, antibiotic susceptibility profile, and possibly molecular analysis) from two or more cultures provides strong evidence for true infection. On the other hand, when a single culture is collected and CoNS are recovered, assessment of the likelihood of true infection is often difficult. At least one study suggests that quantitative blood cultures may be useful in this situation.[354] In this study, peripheral blood cultures yielding more than 50 colony-forming units per milliliter (cfu/ml) occurred exclusively in infants with proven septicemia. In contrast, low colony counts were observed with both septicemia and culture contamination. Infants with septicemia, including those with colony counts of less than 50 cfu/ml, were significantly more likely to have a central catheter or an abnormal hematologic value (white blood cell count more than 20,000 per mm³ or less than 5000 per mm³, immature-to-total neutrophil ratio of more than 0.12, or platelet count of less than 150,000 per mm³). Infants who lacked these clinical features were more likely to have culture contamination. Several other studies have corroborated the usefulness of an elevated immature-to-total neutrophil ratio in identifying infants with CoNS septicemia.[353, 355, 356]

The elimination of staphylococcal septicemia in a patient with a central intravascular catheter in place can be difficult. However, it is not necessary to combine antimicrobial therapy with the removal of the catheter in all cases. Cure rates of up to 80% can be achieved with the use of an appropriate antibiotic without removal of the catheter.[357, 358] However, lack of bacteriologic response to antibiotics necessitates removal of the foreign body.

Pneumonia

The incidence of *S. aureus* pneumonia in infants younger than 6 months of age is directly related to outbreaks of severe *S. aureus* disease in nurseries. In the late 1950s and early 1960s, many nurseries throughout the United States harbored virulent staphylococci (phage type 80/81). A sharp rise in the incidence of *S. aureus* pneumonia was noted at that time.[359–361] Over the years, this disease has diminished in frequency, but the isolated cases that do occur are still serious and should be cause for grave concern.[362]

S. aureus pneumonia can be secondary to a primary distant site of staphylococcal infection that results in bacteremia and seeding of the lung.[363] Most cases of *S. aureus* pneumonia in infants, however, are preceded only by a mild respiratory infection. Bacteria descend from the upper respiratory tract to the alveoli and form microabscesses, which rupture and result in empyema. The occlusion of terminal bronchioles leads to formation of pneumatoceles. The course of *S. aureus* pneumonia in infants is usually fulminant. In older series, mortality as high as 12 to 15% has been reported.[359, 360] Because *S. aureus* pneumonia can be associated with either primary or secondary bacteremia, the possibility of distant metastatic staphylococcal lesions must be kept in mind.

The clinical course in infants is characterized by an antecedent viral infection followed by rapid onset of tachypnea, dyspnea, and tachycardia. Patients typically appear restless and acutely ill. Ileus and abdominal distention are not unusual. Temperature is sometimes normal, and it is not uncommon to find peripheral white blood cell counts of less than 10,000 per mm³. Early radiologic examination reveals extensive pulmonary infiltrates, pneumothorax, and pleural effusion (Fig. 30–3A).

S. aureus pneumonia in infants is almost always associated with empyema (see Fig. 30–3B), and needle aspiration of the pleural cavity is the most reliable way to establish a microbiologic diagnosis.[362] Ultimately the empyema must be drained by continuous closed underwater suction, which should be continued until the pleural space is evacuated and the lung is re-expanded (see Fig. 30–3C and D). A bactericidal drug, such as oxacillin or another semisynthetic penicillinase-resistant penicillin, is generally indicated in this disease. The duration of therapy is usually 3 weeks but depends on the clinical condition of the infant and the ancillary laboratory data. Supportive therapy includes blood transfusion if significant anemia is present, supplemental oxygen, and appropriate fluids.

After the patient recovers from the acute infection, residual pulmonary abnormalities such as pneumatoceles are relatively common (Fig. 30–4). They are not diagnostic of staphylococcal pneumonia because they are also occasionally seen with acute pyogenic lung infections caused by *Streptococcus pneumoniae*, *Streptococcus pyogenes*, or *Haemophilus influenzae*. They may persist for many months and usually require no therapy. The long-term prognosis for complete recovery is excellent, even after extensive bilateral lung disease.[364–366]

Pneumonia due to CoNS has also been described. In general, this diagnosis is assigned when an infant with respiratory distress and a pulmonary infiltrate has CoNS isolated from the blood. The largest series was described by Hall and colleagues, who identified 12 infants with hospital-acquired pneumonia among a total of 27 infants with CoNS bacteremia.[367] These authors noted an association between the presence of an endotracheal tube and development of pneumonia. Nine of their 12 patients were intubated at the time of the positive blood culture and pulmonary infiltrate, and the remaining 3 had been intubated previously.

Osteomyelitis

In interepidemic periods, *S. aureus* osteomyelitis is uncommon in neonates.[367] However, during nursery epidemics of *S. aureus* disease, osteomyelitis can occur secondary to skin infections and bacteremia.[368] Other factors that influence the pathogenesis of neonatal osteomyelitis include fetal monitoring[369] and manipulations related to the routine care of sick neonates, such as repeated heel punctures[370–372] and insertion of umbilical[373, 374] and peripheral[375] intravascular catheters. Neonatal osteomyelitis is a different disease from the bone infection that is seen in older children.[375–380] For example, in the neonate, membranous bones such as the scapula and maxilla are involved almost as frequently as are long bones.[377, 378, 381] As in older infants and children, infants develop bone infections at the metaphysis; how-

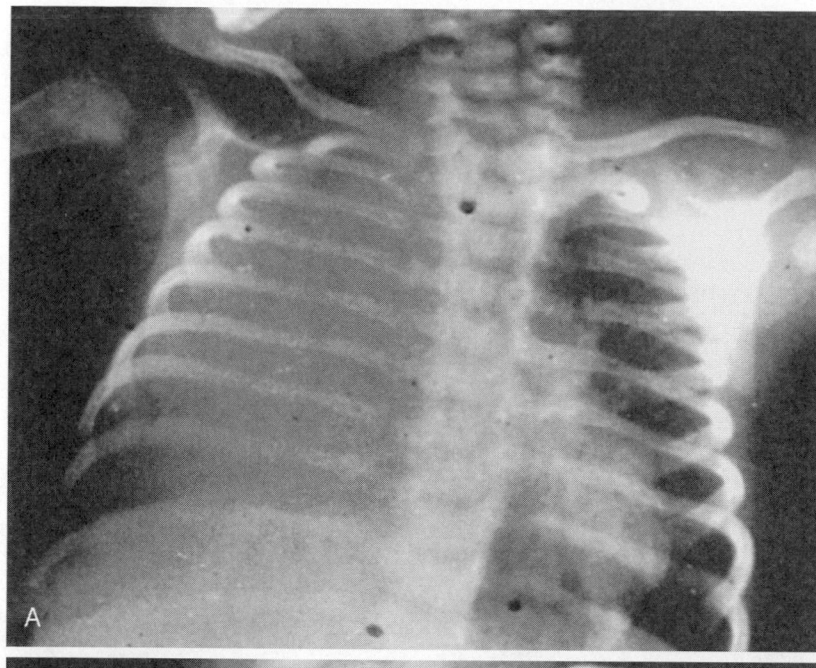

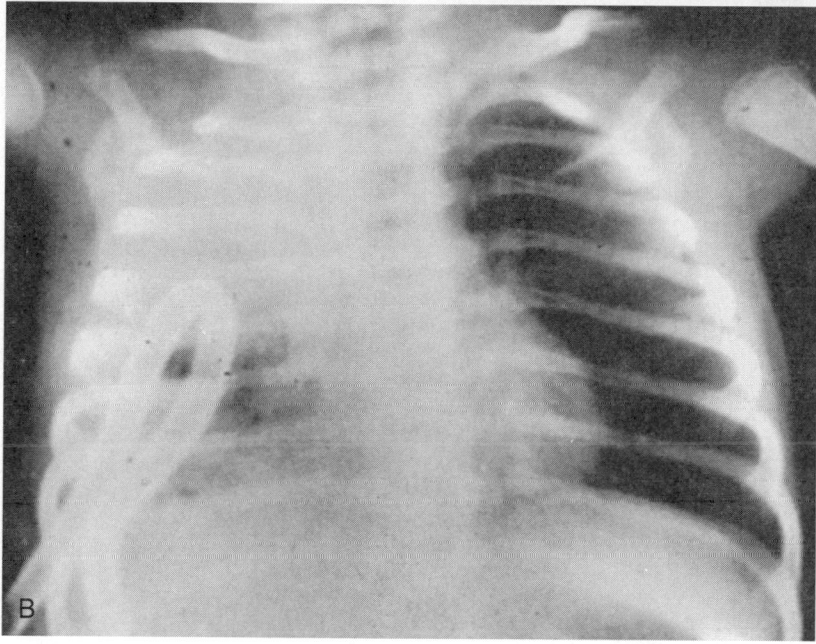

FIGURE 30–3 Serial chest roentgenograms of a 6-week-old infant with staphylococcal pneumonia taken over a 2-month period. *A,* Chest roentgenogram at admission of a 2-month-old infant with a history of fever, tachypnea, and dyspnea for 24 hours. Note complete opacity of right lung field. Empyema fluid grew *Staphylococcus aureus* 80/81. *B,* Film taken 5 days after initiation of therapy consisting of antibiotics and closed drainage with chest tube in the pleural space.

Illustration continued on following page

ever, because the infant cortex is thin and the periosteum strips easily, the sequestra that develop in older children are not usually seen.[382, 383] Greater diffusion of the infection is possible because the bones of neonates have larger intraosseous vascular spaces. Secondary joint involvement occurs occasionally, and the hip and shoulder are particularly vulnerable because in these joints the synovial capsule reaches beyond the metaphysis.

The classic signs and symptoms of an infection are not always present. In some cases the infant is afebrile, and the white blood cell count is normal.[384] In an infant who is inexplicably irritable, the loss of function as manifested by pseudoparalysis can be the only manifestation of disease. Osteomyelitis of the vertebrae can be particularly difficult to diagnose and should be suspected in an irritable infant who is uncomfortable on his or her back or has pain on palpation. The diagnostic problem is exaggerated with vertebral osteomyelitis, because roentgenographic evidence of disease may not become visible until 2 or 3 weeks after infection. Radioisotope studies may be helpful in these cases.[385] Rupture through the cortex of a vertebra can result in epidural abscess with attendant cord compression.[386]

In infants, roentgenographic evidence of bone destruction and new bone formation can be evident as early as 7 days after infection,[378] earlier than in older children. Roentgenograms sometimes reveal soft tissue changes around the site of a bone infection before changes in the bone itself are visible. The earliest changes are usually seen with radionuclide imaging. In some cases, evidence of bone infection is present as early as 16 hours after the appearance of clinical signs.[387, 388]

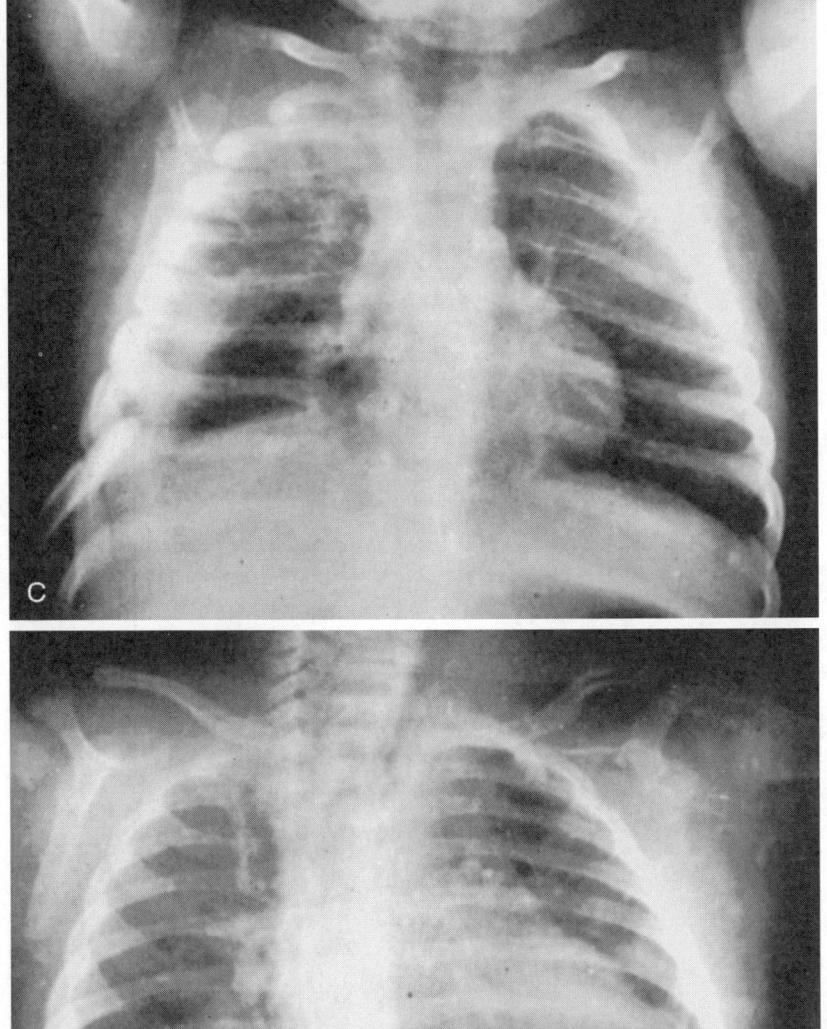

FIGURE 30–3 *Continued. C,* Eighteen days after admission, only the tip of the catheter remains in the pleural space. Signs of empyema and underlying pneumonia are resolving. *D,* Two months after admission, there is complete resolution of disease in the right lung. Minimal pleural thickening is the only sequela remaining.

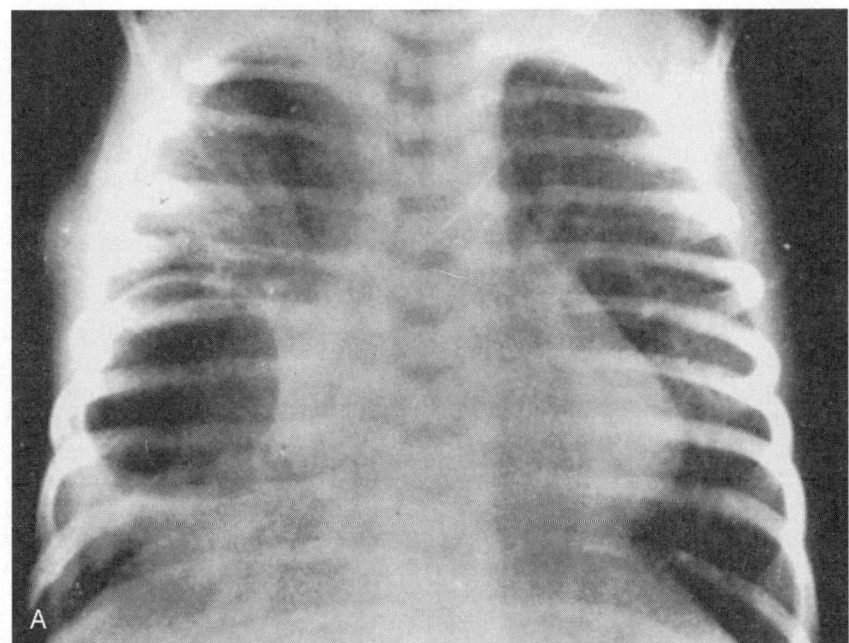

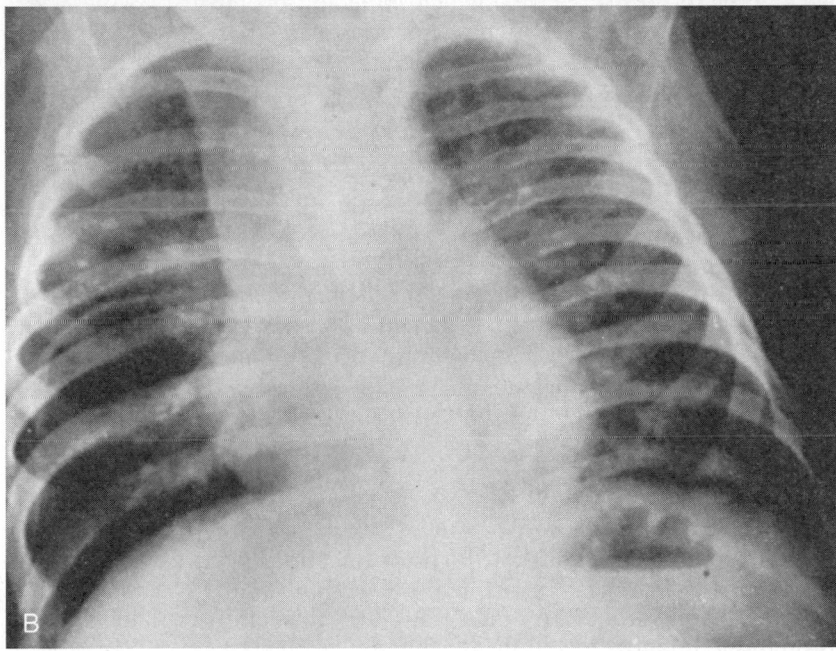

FIGURE 30–4 Roentgenogram of a 3-month-old infant who had been treated for 25 days for staphylococcal pneumonia at the time of the film shown in *A. A,* After intensive therapy, a large residual pneumatocele remains in the right lung. *B,* Five months later, the pneumatocele is markedly smaller without surgical intervention. Physiologic studies were within normal limits. (Roentgenograms courtesy of Dr. Heinz F. Eichenwald.)

Organisms can be obtained from the blood early in the course of disease in about 50% of cases.[378] Because optimal antibiotic therapy depends on isolation of the etiologic agent, a vigorous attempt should be made to recover the organism from the blood and from the lesion itself by needle aspiration or bone biopsy. Because sequestra seldom occur in the neonate and the infection is not localized, early operative intervention is not indicated. If there are signs of localized collections of pus, these must be evacuated.

In cases of osteomyelitis, antibiotic therapy should be parenteral and continued for 4 to 6 weeks. Regimens combining parenteral and oral antibiotics that are common for the management of osteomyelitis in older infants and children are not suitable for treating neonates.[389, 390] In the newborn, serum levels are unpredictable when antistaphylococcal antimicrobial agents are administered orally.[391] Following the sedimentation rate is a reasonable method for assessing the course of the disease. However, if there is concomitant joint involvement, the values may remain abnormal for a prolonged time.[392] Measurement of serum C-reactive protein is an alternative approach to monitor response to therapy.

Despite early intensive therapy, neonatal osteomyelitis can result in severe long-term sequelae. In a study of 40 neonates followed for 7 months to 11 years after infection, the prognosis of neonatal osteomyelitis was correlated with both appropriate surgical measures and perinatal risk factors.[393] Thirteen of 21 infants with sequelae had one or more risk factors, which included low birth weight, low gestational age, catheterization of a large vessel, and respiratory distress syndrome. However, in neonates without such risk factors, the prognosis for acute osteomyelitis after adequate therapy is excellent unless the epiphysis of the bone is completely destroyed. Partially destroyed epiphyses of neonates show a remarkable ability to regenerate.[394] Chronic disease that results in draining sinuses is rarely observed, although permanent sequelae may result if a joint is involved.

Neonatal osteomyelitis due to CoNS is unusual but has been reported at the site of a scalp clip.[369] In addition, osteomyelitis involving the sternum has been reported on occasion in neonates who have had sternotomy performed for intrathoracic surgery.[395]

Arthritis

Septic arthritis in the neonate can be secondary either to osteomyelitis or to a distant focus of infection. Some cases have been associated with femoral venipuncture.[396] S. aureus is the most common cause of this disease throughout infancy, including during the neonatal period. The disease is typically difficult to diagnose, because the only indication may be an irritable infant who cries when moved. Some edema or discoloration surrounding the affected joint is sometimes visible. Occasionally, localized findings are not detected when the infant is examined initially but are noted several days later. Roentgenograms can be normal or show soft tissue swelling or capsular distention.[397]

To facilitate appropriate treatment, it is important to establish an etiologic diagnosis. Joint fluid should be aspirated for Gram stain and culture. Blood cultures should also be collected because they will sometimes yield an organism even when the joint fluid culture is sterile. Analysis of joint fluid usually reveals a white blood cell count of over 50,000 per mm³, with a predominance of polymorphonuclear leukocytes and a depressed glucose concentration.

Although satisfactory treatment in many cases consists only of repeated needle aspirations of purulent material in combination with antibiotic therapy, open drainage is advisable in infants to prevent destructive debilitating disease, particularly if the hip joint is involved. The femoral head may disappear within 4 days after onset of symptoms because of the extreme susceptibility of the articular cartilage to the ravages of S. aureus.[397] After drainage, the hip should be immobilized until the infection subsides.

In most cases, patients should be treated with a parenteral antibiotic for 3 to 4 weeks, provided there is no evidence of osteomyelitis. If concomitant osteomyelitis is present, treatment should be continued for 4 to 6 weeks. In infants with delayed response to treatment, the possibility of a collection of pus should be explored, because even high concentrations of antibiotic may lack activity in the presence of pus. There is no evidence that instillation of antibiotics into the joint space itself hastens recovery.

Central Nervous System Infections

Staphylococci, including S. aureus and CoNS, have long been recognized as a cause of meningitis or ventriculitis, particularly in patients with intraventricular shunts or ventriculostomy catheters.[398–400] Before the extensive use of shunts and catheters to divert the flow of cerebrospinal fluid in patients with congenital or acquired obstructions, most staphylococcal infections of the central nervous system involved the dura and venous sinuses and were sequelae of infections near the face. In recent years, several authors have reported the development of neonatal meningitis in the absence of an intraventricular foreign body or a contiguous site of infection. These patients appear to develop meningitis as a sequela of bacteremia.[353, 401]

Neonatal staphylococcal meningitis is typically associated with nonspecific signs and symptoms and with minimal changes in the cerebrospinal fluid (CSF). Among patients with a shunt or catheter, examination of the CSF most often reveals a mild pleocytosis, typically with an elevated protein and sometimes with a slightly depressed glucose; however, sometimes the CSF is completely normal. Gruskay and associates described 10 infants with S. epidermidis bacteremia and meningitis who had unremarkable CSF cell counts and normal glucose and protein levels: the mean CSF white blood cell count was 6 per mm³ with a range of 0 to 14 per mm³, and the mean glucose and protein values were 2.8 mmol/L and 1.15 g/L, respectively.[401]

Traditionally, management of staphylococcal meningitis in an infant with a shunt or catheter involves removal of the contaminated foreign body and administration of appropriate antibiotic therapy. Recently, however, several investigators have advocated simply externalizing the distal end of the shunt, treating with both intravenous and intraventricular antibiotics (usually for 7 to 10 days after sterilization of the CSF), and then replacing the distal catheter.[402, 403] This approach can be effective in some patients but is less likely to succeed if the infecting organism is slime producing.[404, 405] For CoNS, vancomycin is usually the antibiotic of choice. In cases refractory to initial treatment, especially if the intraventricular shunt or catheter cannot be removed, combination therapy with rifampin may be useful.[406]

Diffuse glomerulonephritis can develop in patients with a ventriculoatrial shunt and CoNS bacteremia.[407] The renal disease results from an immunologic response to the staphylococcal infection rather than from direct bacterial embolization to the kidney. Improvement in renal function occurs after removal of the shunt.

Enteric Infections

On rare occasions, S. aureus is the cause of gastroenteritis or enterocolitis in the newborn. It may be difficult to assess the significance of S. aureus recovered from the stool, because this organism is recovered in 10 to 93% of asymptomatic normal infants.[408] When S. aureus is the predominant aerobic organism in the stool, symptoms of diarrhea are nearly always present, varying from mild to severe with dehydration. In 1947, Holst described an infant who died of S. aureus diarrhea.[409] Postmortem examination revealed pus in the intestinal lumen that yielded S. aureus on culture.

Some cases of S. aureus enteritis in neonates resemble the enterotoxin-mediated gastroenteritis that is commonly seen in older children and adults and is characterized by sudden onset of vomiting and diarrhea 3 to 8 hours after consumption of contaminated food.[410, 411] Abrupt cessation of symptoms is usually noted within 24 hours. Diagnosis is made by the appropriate epidemiology, clinical picture, and recovery of an enterotoxin-producing strain of S. aureus from the stool of patients or from contaminated food. The disease is self-limited, and usually no treatment is needed. Occasionally, parenteral fluid is required in severe cases. Death has been reported in neonates.

In the newborn, enterotoxin-mediated gastroenteritis has been associated with breast-feeding.[411] It is surprising that more breast-fed infants do not suffer from staphylococcal gastroenteritis or enterocolitis. Large numbers of S. aureus can be recovered from samples of breast milk expressed from normal breasts of lactating and nonlactating women.[343] The dose of enterotoxin ingested during feeding is probably too small to be of any consequence in a normal infant[344]; however, even small quantities of enterotoxin can be harmful in a debilitated, sensitive neonate.

Gutman and associates reported S. aureus enterocolitis in four infants fed with either indwelling nasoduodenal or gastric feeding catheters.[412] The disease was characterized by acute onset of nonbloody diarrhea or ileus. Gram stain of the stool revealed numerous gram-positive small cocci resembling staphylococci, and a stool culture yielded S. aureus as the sole or dominant isolate. No single phage type of S. aureus was implicated, and the organism isolated from the stool did not produce enterotoxin. The infants were treated with oral vancomycin (40 mg/kg per day) for 3 days with a good response.

Strains of S. aureus can be etiologic agents in cases of enterocolitis not only because of their ability to produce an enterotoxin but also because of their invasive capacity. In these cases, the pathogenic mechanisms are similar to those of Shigella. Enterocolitis in a 17-day-old malnourished infant infected with such a strain clearly demonstrates the ability of S. aureus to act as an enteric pathogen despite suggestions to the contrary.[413]

Thus far, the role of CoNS in neonatal enteric disease has been limited to necrotizing enterocolitis. Fabia and co-workers were the first to suggest a relationship between CoNS and this disease.[414] Just a few years later, Gruskay and colleagues described a series of 19 newborns with S. epidermidis bacteremia and associated acute enterocolitis.[415] By definition, all 19 infants in this series had bloody stools with mucus together with signs and symptoms of enterocolitis and an abnormal abdominal radiograph. Only one infant developed pneumatosis intestinalis, and none had portal venous or free intraperitoneal air. Furthermore, none of these patients developed prolonged feeding intolerance or evidence of an intestinal stricture as a complication of enterocolitis. Although the results of this report suggest that necrotizing enterocolitis associated with CoNS is relatively mild, other authors have described severe, even fatal cases of enterocolitis apparently due to S. epidermidis.[416–419]

Endocarditis

S. aureus endocarditis in the newborn is extremely rare. The peak incidence occurred between 1954 and 1959, during the height of nursery epidemics with virulent S. aureus. During this period, the fatality approached 100% and the disease was often associated with staphylococcal abscesses in other organs. In most cases, infection was acquired transplacentally in association with maternal sepsis or via infection of the umbilicus or skin.

In recent years, staphylococcal endocarditis in young infants has reemerged as a clinical problem concomitant with the frequent use of intravascular catheters and the predominance of CoNS in neonatal intensive care units. Most cases are right-sided and occur in association with an umbilical venous or Broviac catheter positioned in the right atrium.[420] The presence of a catheter in the right atrium for even a brief time can induce endocardial trauma, which enhances adherence of CoNS.[421–423] Although the mortality for S. aureus endocarditis in the neonate is quite high, the prognosis for infection due to CoNS is much more favorable. In the series reported by Noel and colleagues, four of five infants were cured of infection without subsequent sequelae.[420] The diagnosis should be suspected when bacteremia persists despite catheter removal and appropriate antibiotic therapy. The presence of persistent thrombocytopenia is often an important diagnostic clue. Diagnosis is confirmed by echocardiography, which typically reveals intracardiac lesions associated with a valve or the endocardial wall.

TREATMENT

Staphylococcus aureus

The therapeutic approach to *S. aureus* infection is conditioned by the special characteristics of this organism: its ability to persist under adverse conditions, its tendency to form deep-seated abscesses, and its capacity for resistance to chemotherapy. In general, therapy consists of a sound antimicrobial regimen coupled with surgery when indicated. Aside from superficial skin lesions, staphylococcal infection in the newborn is a serious disease, and thus infants should be hospitalized and treated early and intensively with parenteral antibiotics.

Approximately 95% of *S. aureus* isolates produce β-lactamase, a serine protease that hydrolyzes the β-lactam ring and confers resistance to penicillin. In addition, an increasing percentage of isolates contain the *mecA* gene, which encodes PBP2a and confers resistance to methicillin and all other penicillinase-resistant penicillins (oxacillin and nafcillin) and cephalosporins. Several laboratories have identified isolates with reduced (intermediate) susceptibility to vancomycin (minimal inhibitory concentration, 8 μg/ml). At this point, the mechanism of resistance in these isolates is still unclear.

For isolates susceptible to penicillin, this antibiotic remains the drug of choice. In cases caused by isolates that produce β-lactamase, a semisynthetic penicillin (usually either oxacillin or nafcillin) is preferred, although first-generation cephalosporins such as cephalothin and cefazolin are acceptable alternatives. Vancomycin has less activity and thus should be reserved for patients with infection due to β-lactamase–producing, methicillin-resistant strains. Other antibiotics that often have activity against *S. aureus* include trimethoprim-sulfamethoxazole, clindamycin, and fluoroquinolones (generally contraindicated in neonates). Studies of isolates with reduced susceptibility to vancomycin have reported sensitivity to gentamicin, rifampin, trimethoprim-sulfamethoxazole, chloramphenicol, and tetracycline.

The pharmacokinetics of aqueous penicillin G, the semisynthetic penicillins (oxacillin, nafcillin, and methicillin), and the first-generation cephalosporins (cephalothin and cefazolin) have been well characterized in newborns.[424–437] In general, clearance of these antibiotics increases as postnatal age advances from birth to 4 weeks, and dosing intervals should be adjusted accordingly. Recommended doses and dosing intervals are summarized in Table 30–1.

In treating *S. aureus* infection of the central nervous system, cephalothin and cefazolin should be avoided because of their poor penetration into the CSF. Compared with first-generation cephalosporins, third-generation cephalosporins such as cefotaxime and ceftriaxone penetrate the blood-brain barrier much better and have been used with some success to treat neonatal *S. aureus* meningitis. However, these agents possess relatively less activity against *S. aureus* and have been associated with occasional treatment failures.[424–427] Accordingly, their use in patients with meningitis should be limited.

Isolates of *S. aureus* that test resistant to methicillin are also resistant to oxacillin and nafcillin and should be considered resistant to penicillin and all cephalosporins as well, even if in vitro susceptibility testing suggests otherwise. With these isolates, vancomycin is the antibiotic of choice, in some cases in conjunction with gentamicin or rifampin. Doses for both vancomycin and gentamicin are best calculated on the basis of postconceptional age (gestational age at birth + postnatal age), as outlined in Table 30–1. Even with careful dosing, serum concentrations of these antibiotics exhibit significant interpatient variability. Furthermore, other medications such as indomethacin can impair glomerular filtration and delay excretion.[428] Accordingly, to maximize therapeutic effect and minimize renal toxicity and ototoxicity, serum levels of vancomycin and gentamicin should be determined. With vancomycin, peak levels should be between 20 and 40 μg/ml and predose trough levels should be less than 10 μg/ml. With gentamicin, peak levels of 4 to 8 μg/ml and trough levels less than 2 μg/ml are desirable.

Coagulase-Negative Staphylococci

Similar to the situation with *S. aureus*, antibiotic treatment is critical in the management of disease due to CoNS. Resistance to penicillin, the semisynthetic penicillins, and gentamicin is common among hospital-acquired isolates.[367, 416, 429] Resistance to vancomycin is rare but has been reported among isolates of *S. haemolyticus*.[430, 431] With this information in mind, most experts recommend vancomycin as empirical therapy when CoNS infection is suspected or proven. The treatment regimen is then modified based on antibiotic susceptibility testing.

In considering antibiotic susceptibility results, several caveats deserve mention. First, as with *S. aureus*, penicillin resistance in CoNS is frequently mediated by production of β-lactamase.[432] Because this resistance is often not detected by routine microdilution methods, all isolates that appear susceptible to penicillin or ampicillin should be tested for β-lactamase production. Such testing involves first exposing organisms to oxacillin, which induces expression of β-lactamase. Second, although each organism in a population may have the genetic information necessary for resistance to semisynthetic penicillins, only a small minority express resistance under in vitro testing conditions.[433] To avoid overlooking these organisms, the clinical microbiology laboratory should attempt to optimize expression of resistance by culturing on salt-containing media at 30 to 35° C.[434] Third, routine susceptibility testing frequently indicates that an isolate resistant to methicillin is susceptible to cephalosporins; however, as described with *S. aureus*, cross-resistance is extensive, and thus for clinical purposes, all isolates of CoNS found to be resistant to semisynthetic penicillins should also be considered resistant to cephalosporins.[435–437]

For the few isolates that are rigorously established

to be penicillin susceptible and β-lactamase negative, penicillin is a suitable antibiotic. For isolates that are resistant to penicillin but truly susceptible to the semisynthetic penicillins, therapy with oxacillin or nafcillin is appropriate. Vancomycin is the preferred antibiotic for CoNS that are resistant to semisynthetic penicillins and also for the rare neonate allergic to penicillin. One report indicates that the combination of rifampin and clindamycin is an alternative regimen for patients allergic to penicillin.[438] For multiresistant isolates, other glycopeptide antibiotics, including teicoplanin and daptomycin, and quinolone derivatives are considerations. However, resistance to these agents has also been reported.

In some cases, including endocarditis and CSF shunt infection, synergistic therapy may be indicated.[439, 440] In vitro synergy studies have been performed with vancomycin in combination with rifampin, gentamicin, or cephalothin (with isolates susceptible to each), and synergy has been demonstrated with all of these combinations.[441, 442] Given the high frequency of resistance to gentamicin and the β-lactams, vancomycin plus rifampin is probably the best regimen for most cases. Although rifampin alone also has good antistaphylococcal activity, resistance emerges rapidly unless this antibiotic is used together with other antimicrobial agents.[442]

CONCLUSION

Staphylococcus is an almost perfect parasite. Most of the time it enjoys a commensal status with the newborn host. On occasion, it can cause mild or even serious disease. Despite intensive study, the staphylococcal factors that cause disease or death in a majority of infections have not been elucidated. Perhaps of greater importance is our lack of understanding of the neonate's inability to deal with such a clever organism. This is particularly true of sick low-birth-weight infants compromised by a variety of invasive diagnostic and/or therapeutic procedures. With additional basic knowledge about the organism as well as a better understanding of the infant's defense mechanisms, it may be possible in the future to thwart a host-organism interaction that results in disease.

References

1. Fox T. Cited by Poole WH, Whittle CH. Epidemic pemphigus of newly born (impetigo contagiosa et bullosa neonatorum). Lancet 1:1323, 1935.
2. Pasteur L. De l'extension de la théorie des germes a l'étiologie de quelques maladies communes. Compt Rend 90:1033, 1880.
3. Ogston A. Über abscesse. Arch Klin Chir 25:588, 1880.
4. Kilham EB. An epidemic of pemphigus neonatorum. Am J Obstet 22:1039, 1889.
5. Almquist E. Pemphigus neonatorum. Z Hyg Infektionskr 10:253, 1891.
6. Call EL. An epidemic of pemphigus neonatorum. Am J Obstet 50:473, 1904.
7. Seidemann I, Andeisenoff H. Rooming-in service in a medium-sized community hospital. Report on four and one-half years observation. NY State J Med 56:2533, 1956.
8. Rulison ET. Control of impetigo neonatorum: advisability of a radical departure in obstetrical care. JAMA 93:903, 1929.
9. Schaffer TE, Sylvester RF Jr, Baldwin JN, et al. Staphylococcal infections in newborn infants: II. Report of 19 epidemics caused by an identical strain of *Staphylococcus pyogenes*. Am J Public Health 47:990, 1957.
10. Dixon RE, Kaslow RA, Mallinson GF, et al. Staphylococcal disease outbreaks in hospital nurseries in the United States—December 1971 through March 1972. Pediatrics 51:413, 1973.
11. Patrick CC. Coagulase-negative staphylococci: pathogens with increasing clinical significance. J Pediatr 116:497, 1990.
12. Hall SL. Coagulase-negative staphylococcal infections in neonates. Pediatr Infect Dis J 10:57, 1991.
13. Schmidt BK, Kirpalani HM, Corey M, et al. Coagulase negative staphylococci as true pathogens in newborn infants: a cohort study. Pediatr Infect Dis J 6:1026, 1987.
14. Ponce de Leon S, Wenzel EP. Hospital-acquired bloodstream infections with *Staphylococcus epidermidis*. Am J Med 77:639, 1984.
15. Kumar ML, Jenson HB, Dahms BB. Fatal staphylococcal epidermidis infections in very low-birth-weight infants with cytomegalovirus infection. Pediatrics 76:110, 1985.
16. Noel GJ, Edelson DJ. *Staphylococcus epidermidis* bacteremia in neonates: further observations and the occurrence of focal infection. Pediatrics 74:832, 1984.
17. Fleer A, Senders RC, Visser MR, et al. Septicemia due to coagulase-negative staphylococci in a neonatal intensive care unit: clinical and bacteriologic features and contaminated parenteral fluids as a source of sepsis. Pediatr Infect Dis J 2:426, 1983.
18. LaGamma EF, Drusin LM, Mackles AW, et al. Neonatal infections: an important determinant of late NICU mortality in infants less than 1,000 g at birth. Am J Dis Child 137:838, 1983.
19. Battisti O, Mitchison R, Davies DA. Changing blood culture isolates in a referral neonatal intensive care unit. Arch Dis Child 56:775, 1981.
20. Placzek MM, Whitelaw A. Early and late septicemia. Arch Dis Child 58:728, 1983.
21. Hall R, Kurth CG, Hall SL. Ten year survey of positive blood cultures among admissions to a neonatal intensive care unit. J Perinatol 7:122, 1987.
22. Donowitz LG, Haley CE, Gregory WW, et al. Neonatal intensive care unit bacteremia: emergence of gram-positive bacteria as major pathogens. Am J Infect Control 15:141, 1987.
23. Baumgart S, Hall SE, Campos JM, et al. Sepsis with coagulase-negative staphylococci in critically ill newborns. Am J Dis Child 137:461, 1983.
24. Munson DP, Thompson TR, Johnson DE, et al. Coagulase-negative staphylococcal septicemia: experience in a newborn intensive care unit. J Pediatr 101:602, 1982.
25. Dunkle LM, Naqvi SH, McCallum R, et al. Eradication of epidemic methicillin-gentamicin–resistant *Staphylococcus aureus* in an intensive care nursery. Am J Med 70:455, 1981.
26. Haley RW, Bregman DA. The role of understaffing and overcrowding in recurrent outbreaks of staphylococcal infection in a neonatal special-care unite. J Infect Dis 145:875, 1982.
27. Davies EA, Emmerson AM, Hogg GM, et al. An outbreak of infection with a methicillin-resistant *Staphylococcus aureus* in a special care baby unit: value of topical

mupirocin and of traditional methods of infection control. J Hosp Infect 10:120, 1987.

28. Millar MR, Keyworth N, Lincoln C, et al. Methicillin-resistant *Staphylococcus aureus* in regional neonatal unit. J Hosp Infect 7:187, 1987.

29. Reboli AC, John JF, Leukoff AH. Epidemic methicillin-gentamicin resistant *Staphylococcus aureus* in a neonatal intensive care unit. Am J Dis Child 143:34, 1989.

30. Rosenfeld CR, Laptook AR, Jeffery J. Limited effectiveness of triple dye in preventing colonization with methicillin-resistant *Staphylococcus aureus* in a special care nursery. Pediatr Infect Dis J 9:291, 1990.

31. Noel GJ, Kreiswirth BN, Edelson PJ, et al. Multiple methicillin-resistant *Staphylococcus aureus* strains as a cause for a single outbreak of severe disease in hospital neonates. Pediatr Infect Dis J 11:184, 1992.

32. Haddad Q, Sobayo EI, Basit OBA, Rotimi VO. Outbreak of methicillin-resistant *Staphylococcus aureus* in a neonatal-intensive care unit. J Hosp Infect 23:211, 1993.

33. Haley RW, Cushion NB, Tenover FC, et al. Eradication of endemic of methicillin-resistant *Staphylococcus aureus* infections from a neonatal intensive care unit. J Infect Dis 171:614, 1995.

34. Back NA, Linnemann CC, Staneck JL, Kotagal UR. Control of methicillin-resistant *Staphylococcus aureus* in a neonatal-intensive care unit: use of intensive microbiological surveillance and mupirocin. Infect Control Hosp Epidemiol 17:227, 1996.

35. Elek SD. *Staphylococcus pyogenes*. London, E & S Livingstone, 1959.

36. Cohen JO (ed). The Staphylococci. New York, John Wiley, 1972.

37. Easmon CFS, Adlam C (eds). Staphylococci and Staphylococcal Infections, vols. 1 and 2. London, Academic Press, 1983.

38. Crossley KB, Archer GL (eds). The Staphylococci in Human Disease. New York, Churchill Livingstone, 1997.

39. Kloos W. Taxony and Systemics of Staphylococci Indigenous to Humans. *In* Crossley KB, Archer GL (eds). The Staphylococci in Human Disease. New York, Churchill Livingstone, 1997, p 127.

40. Blair JE, Williams REO. Phage typing of staphylococci. Bull WHO 24:771, 1961.

41. Parker MT, Roundtree PM. Report (1966B1970) of the Subcommittee on Phage Typing of Staphylococci to the International Committee on Nomenclature of Bacteria. Int J Syst Bacteriol 21:167, 1971.

42. Mulligan ME, Arbeit RD. Epidemiologic and clinical utility of typing systems for differentiating among strains of methicillin-resistant *Staphylococcus aureus*. Infect Control Hosp Epidemiol 12:20, 1991.

43. Prevost G, Jaulhoc B, Piedmont Y. DNA fingerprinting of pulsed-field gel electrophoresis is more effective than ribotyping in distinguishing among methicillin-resistant *Staphylococcus aureus* isolates. J Clin Microbial 30:967, 1992.

44. Tenover FC, Arbeit R, Archer G, et al. Comparison of traditional and molecular methods of typing isolates of *Staphylococcus aureus*. J Clin Microbial 32:407, 1994.

45. Braddiley J, Brock JH, Davidson AL, et al. The wall composition of micrococci. J Gen Microbiol 54:393, 1968.

46. Strominger JL. The Bacteria. New York, Academic Press, 1962.

47. Strominger JL, Ghuysen JM. Mechanisms of enzymatic bacteriolysis: cell walls of bacteria are solubilised by action of either specific carbohydrases or specific peptidases. Science 156:213, 1967.

48. Labischinski H. Consequences of interaction of β-lactam antibiotics with penicillin binding proteins from sensitive and resistant *Staphylococcus aureus* stains. Med Microbiol Immunol 181:241, 1992.

49. de Lencastre H, de Jonge BLM, Mathews PR, Tomaz A. Molecular aspects of methicillin resistance in *Staphylococcus aureus*. J Antimicrob Chemother 33:7, 1994.

50. Juergens WG, Sanderson AR, Strominger JL. Chemical basis for the immunological specificity of a strain of *Staphylococcus aureus*. Bull Soc Chim Biol 42:110, 1960.

51. Mudd A, Yoshida A, Lenhart NA. Identification of a somatic antigen of *Staphylococcus aureus* critical for phagocytosis by human blood leucocytes. Nature 199:1200, 1963.

52. Lee JC, Pier GB. Vaccine-based strategies for prevention of staphylococcal diseases. *In* Crossley KB, Archer GL (eds). The Staphylococci in Human Disease. New York, Churchill Livingstone, 1997, 640.

53. Shayegani M. Failure of immune sera to enhance significantly phagocytosis-promoting factors. Infect Immun 2:742, 1970.

54. Shayegani M, Hisatsune K, Mudd S. Cell wall component which affects the ability of serum to promote phagocytosis and killing of *Staphylococcus aureus*. Infect Immun 2:750, 1970.

55. Peterson PK, Wilkinson BJ, Kim Y, et al. The key role of peptidoglycan in the opsonization of *Staphylococcus aureus*. J Clin Invest 61:597, 1978.

56. Verburgh HA, Peters R, Rozenberg-Arska M, et al. Antibodies to cell wall peptidoglycan of *Staphylococcus aureus* in patients with serious staphylococcal infections. J Infect Dis 144:1, 1981.

57. Aly R, Shinefield HR, Litz C, et al. Teichoic acid in the binding of *Staphylococcus aureus* to nasal epithelial cells. J Infect Dis 141:463, 1980.

58. Bibel JD, Aly R, Shinefield HR, et al. The *Staphylococcus aureus* receptor for fibronectin. J Invest Dermatol 80:494, 1983.

59. Wiley BB, Maverakis NH. Capsule production and virulence among strains of *Staphylococcus aureus*. Ann NY Acad Sci 236:221, 1974.

60. Morse SI. Isolation and properties of a surface antigen of *Staphylococcus aureus*. J Exp Med 115:295, 1962.

61. Wilkinson BJ, Staphylococcal capsules and slime. *In* Easmon CFS, Adlam C (eds). Staphylococci and Staphylococcal Infections. London, Academic Press, 1983, p 481.

62. Christensson B, Boutonnier A, Ryding U, et al. Diagnosing *Staphylococcus aureus* endocarditis by detecting antibodies against *S. aureus* capsular polysaccharide types 5 and 8. J Infect dis 163:530, 1991.

63. Novick PR. The *Staphylococcus* as a molecular genetic system. *In* Novick RP (ed). Molecular Biology of the Staphylococci. New York, VCH, 1990.

64. Iandolo JJ, Bannantine JP, Stewart GC. Genetic and Physical Map of the Chromosome of *Staphylococcus aureus*. *In* Crossley KB, Archer GL (eds). The Staphylococci in Human Disease. New York, Churchill Livingstone, 1997, p 46.

65. Paulsen IT, Firth N, Skurray RA. Resistance to Antimicrobial Agents Other Than β-Lactums. *In* Crossley KB, Archer GL (eds). The Staphylococci in Human Disease. New York, Churchill Livingstone, 1997, 175.

66. Pfaller MA, Herwaldt LA. Laboratory, clinical and epidemiological aspects of coagulase-negative staphylococci. Clin Microbiol Rev 1:281, 1988.

67. Christensen GD, Parisi JT, Bisno AL, et al. Characterization of clinically significant strains of coagulase-negative staphylococci. J Clin Microbiol 18:258, 1983.

68. Pulverer G, Pillich J, Klein A. New bacteriophages of *Staphylococcus epidermidis*. J Infect Dis 132:524, 1975.

69. Jefferson SH, Parisi JT. Bacteriophage typing of coagulase-negative staphylococci in critically ill newborns. Am J Dis Child 137:461, 1983.

70. Parisi JT, Hecht DW. Plasmid profiles in epidemiologic studies of infections by *Staphylococcus epidermidis* of ventriculoatrial shunts. J Infect Dis 141:637, 1980.

71. Archer GL, Vishniavsky N, Stiver HG. Plasmid pattern analysis of *Staphylococcus epidermidis* isolates from patients with prosthetic valve endocarditis. Infect Immun 35:627, 1982.

72. Parisi JT, Hecht DW. Plasmid profiles in epidemiologic studies of *Staphylococcus epidermidis*. J Infect Dis 141:637, 1980.

73. Castellani A. Note préliminaire sur un nouveau microcoque isolé d'une dermatite axillaire superficielle tropicale. Ann Inst Pasteur 89:475, 1955.

74. Quinn EL, Cox F, Drake EH. Staphylococcal endocarditis: disease of increasing importance. JAMA 196:815, 1966.

75. Feigin RD, Shackelford G, Campbell J, et al. Assessment of the role of *Staphylococcus epidermidis* as a cause of otitis media. Pediatrics 52:569, 1973.

76. Gibink GS, Mills EL, Huff JS, et al. The microbiology of serous and mucoid otitis media. Pediatrics 63:915, 1979.

77. Berman SA, Balkany TJ, Simmons MA. Otitis media in the neonatal intensive care unit. Pediatrics 62:198, 1978.

78. Holt R. The classification of staphylococci from colonized ventriculo-atrial shunts. J Clin Pathol 22:475, 1969.

79. Holt R. The early serological detection of colonization by *Staphylococcus epidermidis* of ventriculoatrial shunts. Infection 8:8, 1980.

80. Shurtleff DB, Foltz EL, Weeks RD, et al. Therapy of *Staphylococcus epidermidis*: infection associated with cerebrospinal fluid shunts. Pediatrics 53:55, 1974.

81. Christensen GD, Bisno AL, Parisi JT, et al. Nosocomial septicemia due to multiply antibiotic-resistant *Staphylococcus epidermidis*. Ann Intern Med 96:1, 1982.

82. Haslett TM, Isenberg HD, Hilton E, et al. Microbiology of indwelling central intravascular catheters. J Clin Microbiol 26:696, 1988.

83. Mabeck C. Significance of coagulase-negative staphylococcic bacteriuria. Lancet 2:1150, 1969.

84. Hermansson G, Bollgren J, Bergstrom T, et al. Coagulase-negative staphylococci as a cause of urinary tract infections in children. J Pediatr 84:807, 1974.

85. Gerber MA, Baldovi V. *Staphylococcus saprophyticus* urinary tract infection. Clin Pediatr 21:378, 1982.

86. Latham RH, Running K, Stamm WE. Urinary tract infections in young adult women cause by *Staphylococcus saprophyticus*. JAMA 250:3063, 1983.

87. Hall RT, Hall SL, Barnes WG, et al. Characteristics of coagulase-negative staphylococci from infants with bacteremia. Pediatr Infect Dis J 6:377, 1987.

88. Etienne J, Pangon B, Leport C. *Staphylococcus lugdunensis* endocarditis. Lancet 1:390, 1989.

89. Fleurette J, Bes M, Brun Y, et al. Clinical isolates of *Staphylococcus lugdunensis* and *S. schleiferi*: bacteriological characteristics and susceptibility to antimicrobial characteristics and susceptibility to antimicrobial agents. Res Microbial 140:107, 1989.

90. Martin MA, Pfaller MA, Wenzel RP. Coagulase-negative staphylococcal bacteremia. Ann Intern Med 110:9, 1989.

91. Freney J, Brun Y, Bes M, et al. *Staphylococcus lugdunensis* sp. nov., and *Staphylococcus schleiferi* sp. nov., two species

92. Fleurette Y, Brun Y, Bes M, et al. Infections caused by coagulase-negative staphylococci other than *S. epidermidis* and *S. saprophyticus*. In Pulverer G, Quie PG, Peters G (eds). Pathogenicity and Clinical Significance of Coagulase-Negative Staphylococci. Stuttgart, Gustav Fisher Verlag, 1987, p 195.

from human clinical specimens. Int J Syst Bacteriol 38:168, 1988.

93. Ponce de leon S, Guenther SH, Wenzel RP. Microbiologic studies of coagulase-negative staphylococci isolated from patients with nosocomial bacteremias. J Hosp Infect 7:121, 1986.

94. Gill VJ, Selepak ST, Williams EC. Species identification and antibiotic susceptibilities of coagulase-negative staphylococci isolated from clinical specimens. J Clin Microbial 18:1314, 1983.

95. Foster TJ, Höök M. Surface protein adhesions of *Staphylococcus aureus*. Trends Microbial 12:484, 1998.

96. Projan SJ, Novik RP. The medical basis for pathogenicity. *In* Crossley KB, Archer GL (eds). The Staphylococci in Human Disease. New York, Churchill Livingstone, 1997, p 61.

97. Vercellotti GM, McCarthy JB, Lindholm P, et al. Extracellular matrix proteins (fibronectin, laminin, and type IV collagen) bind and aggregate bacteria. Am J Pathol 120:13, 1985.

98. Chhatwal GS, Preissner KT, Muller-Berghaus G, Blobel H. Specific binding of the human S protein (vitronectin) to streptococci, *Staphylococcus aureus*, and *Escherichia coli*. Infect Immun 55:1878, 1987.

99. Park PW, Roberts DD, Grosso LE, et al. Binding of elastin to *Staphylococcus aureus*. J Biol Chem 266:23399, 1991.

100. Hermann M, Suchard SJ, Boxer LA, et al. Thrombospondin binds to *Staphylococcus aureus* and promotes staphylococcal adherence to surfaces. Infect Immun 59:279, 1991.

101. Cheung AL, Eberhardt KJ, Chung E, et al. Diminished virulence of a *sar-/agr*-mutant of *Staphylococcus aureus* in the rabbit model of endocarditis. J Clin Invest 94:1815, 1994.

102. Vaudaux P, Pittet D, Haeberli A, et al. Host factors selectively increase staphylococcal adherence on catheters: a role for fibronectin and fibrinogen or fibrin. J Infect Dis 160:865, 1989.

103. Pati JM, Allen BL, McGavin MJ, Hook M. MSCRAMM-mediated adherence of microorganisms to host tissues. Ann Rev Microbiol 48:585, 1994.

104. Forsgren A, Sjoquist J. "Protein A" from *S. aureus* pseudo-immune reaction with human gamma-globulin. J Immunol 97:822, 1966.

105. Verhoef J, Peterson PK, Verbrugh HA. Host-parasite relationship in staphylococcal infections: the role of the staphylococcal cell wall during the process of phagocytosis. Antonie Van Leeuwenhoek 45:49, 1979.

106. Selsted ME, Tang YQ, Morris WL, et al. Purification, primary structures, and antibacterial activities of beta-defensins, a new family of antimicrobial peptides from bovine neutrophils. J Biol Chem 268:6641, 1993.

107. Yeaman MR, Sullam PM, Dazin PF, Bayer AS. Platelet microbicidal protein alone and in combination with antibiotics reduces *Staphylococcus aureus* adherence to platelets in vitro. Infect Immun 62:3416, 1994.

108. Bohach GA, Dinges MH, Mitchell DT, et al. Exotoxins. *In* Crossley KB, Archer GL (eds). The Staphylococci in Human Disease. New York, Churchill Livingstone, 1997, p 83.

109. Supersac G, Prevost G, Piemont Y. Sequencing of leu-

cocidin R from *Staphylococcus aureus* P83 suggests that staphylococcal leucocidins and gamma-hemolysin are members of a single, two-component family of toxins. Infect Immun 61:580, 1993.

110. Rahman A, Izaki K, Kato I, Kamio Y. Nucleotide sequence of leukocidin S-component gene (*lukS*) from methicillin resistant *Staphylococcus aureus*. Biochem Biophys Res Commun 181:138, 1991.

111. Rahman A, Nariya H, Izaki K, et al. Molecular cloning an nucleotide sequence of leukocidin F-component gene (*lukF*) from methicillin-resistant *Staphylococcus aureus*. Biochem Biophys Res Commun 184:640, 1992.

112. Choorit W, Kaneko J, Muramoto K, Kamio Y. Existence of a new protein component with the same function as the LukF component of leukocidin or gamma-hemolysin and its gene in *Staphylococcus aureus* P83. FEBS Lett 357:260, 1995.

113. Cooney J, Kienle Z, Foster TJ, O'Toole PW. The gamma-hemolysin locus of *Staphylococcus aureus* comprises three linked genes, two of which are identical to genes for the F and S components of leukocidin. Infect Immun 61:768, 1993.

114. Sau S, Lee CY. Cloning of type 8 capsule genes and analysis of gene clusters for the production of different capsular polysaccharides in *Staphylococcus aureus*. J Bacteriol 178:2118, 1996.

115. Arbeit R, Karakawa WW, Van WF, Robbins JB. Predominance of two newly described capsular polysaccharide types among clinical isolates of *Staphylococcus aureus*. Diagn Microbiol Infect Dis 2:85, 1984.

116. Bhakdi S, Tranum-Jensen J. Alpha-toxin of *Staphylococcus aureus*. Microbiol Rev 55:733, 1991.

117. Suttorp N, Fuhrmann M, Tannert-Otto S, et al. Poreforming bacterial toxins potently induce release of nitric oxide in porcine endothelial cells. J Exp Med 178:337, 1993.

118. Jonas D, Walev I, Berger T, et al. Novel path to apoptosis: small transmembrane pores created by staphylococcal alpha-toxin in T lymphocytes evoke internucleosomal DNA degradation. Infect Immun 62:1304, 1994.

119. Callegan MC, Engels LS, Hill JM, O'Callaghan RJ. Corneal virulence of *Staphylococcus aureus*: roles of alpha-toxin and protein A in pathogenesis. Infect Immun 62:2478, 1994.

120. Bramley AJ, Patel AH, O'Reilly M, et al. Roles of alpha-toxin and beta-toxin in virulence of *Staphylococcus aureus* for the mouse mammary gland. Infect Immun 57:2489, 1989.

121. Wadstrom T, Mollby R. Studies on extracellular proteins from *Staphylococcus aureus*: VII. Studies on beta-hemolysin. Biochim Biophys Acta 242:308, 1972.

122. Ruzickova V. A rapid method for the differentiation of *Staphylococcus aureus* hemolysins. Fol Microbiol 39:112, 1994.

123. Farrell AM, Taylor D, Holland KT. Cloning, nucleotide sequence determination and expression of the *Staphylococcus aureus* hyaluronate lyase gene. FEMS Microb Lett 130:81, 1995.

124. Meyer K, Palmer JW. The polysaccharide of the vitreous humor. J Biol Chem 107:629, 1934.

125. Bjorklind A, Arvidson S. Mutants of *Staphylococcus aureus* affected in the regulation of exoprotein synthesis. FEMS Microbiol Lett 7:203, 1980.

126. Coleman G, Jakeman C, Martin N. Patterns of extracellular protein secretion by a number of clinically isolated strains of *Staphylococcus aureus*. J Gen Microbiol 107:189, 1978.

127. Tremaine M, Brockman DK, Betley MJ. Staphylococcal

128. enterotoxin A gene (*sea*) expression is not affected by the accessory gene regulator (*agr*). Infect Immun 61:356, 1993.

128. Peng HL, Novick RP, Kreiswirth B, et al. Cloning, characterization, and sequencing of an accessory gene regulator (*agr*) in *Staphylococcus aureus*. J Bacteriol 170:4365, 1988.

129. Cheung AL, Koomey JM, Butler CA, et al. Regulation of exoprotein expression in *Staphylococcus aureus* by a locus (*sar*) distinct from *agr*. Proc Natl Acad Sci U S A 89:6462, 1992.

130. Hogt AH, Dankert J, Hulstaert CE, et al. Cell surface characteristics of coagulase-negative staphylococci and their adherence to fluorinated poly (ethylenepropylene). Infect Immun 51,294, 1986.

131. Tojo M, Yamashita N, Goldmann DA, et al. Isolation and characterization of a capsular polysaccharide adhesin from *Staphylococcus epidermidis*. J Infect Dis 157:713, 1988.

132. Heilman C, Hussain M, Peters G, Götz F. Evidence for autolysin-mediated primary attachment of *Staphylococcus epidermidis* to a polystrene surface. Mol Microbiol 24:1013, 1997.

133. Timmerman CP, Fleer A, Besnier JM, et al. Characterization of a proteinaceous adhesion of *Staphylococcus epidermidis* which mediates attachment to polystrene. Infect Immun 59:4187, 1991.

134. Veenstra GJC, Cremers FFM, Van Dijk H, Fleer A. Ultrastructural organization and regulation of a biomaterial adhesion of *Staphylococcus epidermidis*. J Bacteriol 178:537, 1996.

135. Mack D, Nedelmann M, Krokotsch A, et al. Characterization of transposon mutants of biofilm-producing *Staphylococcus epidermidis* impaired in the accumulative phase of biofilm production: genetic identification of a hexosamine-containing polysaccharide intercellular adhesion. Infect Immun 62:3244, 1994.

136. Mack D, Fischer W, Krokotsch A, et al. The intercellular adhesin involved in biofilm accumulation of *Staphylococcus epidermidis* is a linear β-1-6-linked glucosaminoglycan: purification and structural analysis. J Bacteriol 178:175, 1996.

137. Schumacher-Perdreau F, Heilmann C, Peters G, et al. Comparative analysis of a biofilm forming *Staphylococcus epidermidis* strain and its adhesion-positive accumulation-negative isogenic mutant. FEMS Microbial Lett 117:71, 1994.

138. Hussain M, Herrmann M, von Eiff C, et al. A 140-kilodalton extracellular protein is essential for the accumulation of *Staphylococcus epidermidis* strains on surfaces. Infect Immun 65:519, 1997.

139. Christensen GD, Simpson WA, Bisno AL, et al. Adherence of slime producing strains to smooth surfaces. Infect Immun 37:318, 1982.

140. Ishak MA, Groschel DHM, Mandell GL, et al. Association of slime with pathogenicity of coagulase-negative staphylococci causing nosocomial septicemia. J Clin Microbial 22:1025, 1985.

141. Hall RT, Hall SL, Barnes WG, et al. Characteristics of coagulase-negative staphylococci from infants with bacteremia. Pediatr Infect Dis J 6:377, 1987.

142. Gruskay JA, Nachamkin I, Baumgart S, et al. Predicting the pathogenicity of coagulase-negative *Staphylococcus* in the neonate: slime production, antibiotic resistance, and predominance of *Staphylococcus epidermidis* species. Pediatrics 20:397A, 1986.

143. Gray ED, Peters G, Verstegen M, et al. Effect of extracellular slime substance from *Staphylococcus epidermidis* on

the human cellular immune response. Lancet 1:365, 1984.

144. Johnson GM, Lee DA, Regelmann WE, et al. Interference with granulocyte function by *Staphylococcus epidermidis* slime. Infect Immun 54:13, 1986.

145. Farber BF, Kaplan MH, Clogston AG. *Staphylococcus epidermidis* extracted slime inhibits the antimicrobial action of glycopeptide antibodies. J Infect Dis 161:37, 1990.

146. Christensen GD, Simpson WA, Bisno AL, et al. Experimental foreign body infections in mice challenged with slime producing *Staphylococcus epidermidis*. Infect Immun 40:407, 1983.

147. Kristinson KG, Spencer RC. Slime production as a marker for clinically significant infection with coagulase-negative staphylococci. J Infect Dis 154:728, 1986.

148. Younger JJ, Christensen GD, Bartley DL, et al. Coagulase-negative staphylococci isolated from cerebrospinal fluid shunts: importance of slime production, species identification, and shunt removal to clinical outcome. J Infect Dis 156:548, 1987.

149. Gemmel CG, Schumacher-Perdeau F. Extracellular toxins and enzymes elaborated by coagulase-negative staphylococci. *In* Easmon CSF, Adlam C (eds). Staphylococci and Staphylococcal Infections. New York, Academic Press, 1983, p 809.

150. Scheifele DW, Bjornson GL, Dyer RA, et al. Delta-like toxin produced by coagulase-negative staphylococci is associated with neonatal necrotizing enterocolitis. Infect Immun 55:2268, 1987.

151. Scheifele DW, Bjornson GL. Delta toxin activity in coagulase-negative staphylococci from the bowels of neonates. J Clin Microbiol 26:279, 1988.

152. Breckenridge JC, Bergdoll MS. Food borne gastroenteritis due to coagulase-negative *Staphylococcus*. N Engl J Med 284:541, 1971.

153. Males BM, Rogers WA, Parisi JT. Virulence factors of biotypes of *Staphylococcus epidermidis* from clinical sources. J Clin Microbiol 1:256, 1975.

154. Shigoeka AO, Santos JI, Hill HR. Functional analysis of neutrophil granulocytes from healthy, infected, and stressed neonates. J Pediatr 95:454, 1979.

155. Mease AD. Tissue neutropenia: the newborn neutrophil in perspective. J Perinatol 10:55, 1990.

156. Anderson DC, Hughes B, Smith CW, Abnormality motility of neonatal polymorphonuclear leukocytes. J Clin Invest 68:863, 1981.

157. Polin RA. Role of fibronectin in diseases of newborn infants and children. Rev Infect Dis 12(Suppl 4):S428, 1990.

158. Hilmo A, Howard TH. F-actin content of neonate and adult neutrophils. Blood 69:945, 1987.

159. Schibler KR, Trautman MS, Liechty KW, et al. Diminished transcription of interleukin-8 by monocytes from preterm neonates. J Leuk Biol 53:399, 1993.

160. Yoshimura TK, Matsuskima K, Tanaka S, et al. Purification of a human monocyte derived neutrophil chemotactic factor that shares sequence homology with other host defense cytokinese. Proc Natl Acad Sci U S A 84:9233, 1987.

161. Anderson DC, Rothlein R, Marlin SD, et al. Impaired transendothelial migration by neonatal neutrophils: abnormalities of Mac-1 (CD11b/CD18)–dependent adherence reactions. Blood 76:2613, 1990.

162. Zimmerman GA, Prescott SM, McIntyre TM. Endothelial cell, interactions with granulocytes: tethering and signaling molecules. Immunol. Today 13:93, 1992.

163. Shigeoka AO, Charette RP, Wyman ML, Hill HR. De-

164. Strauss RG, Snyder EL. Activation and activity of the superoxide-generating system of neutrophils from human infants. Pediatr Res 17:662, 1983.

165. Banffer JR. Anti-leucocidin and mastitis puerperalis. BMJ 2:1224, 1962.

166. Johanovsky J. Importance of antileucocidin and antitoxin in immunity against staphylococcal infections. Z Immunitaetsforsch 116:318, 1959.

167. Banffer JRJ, Franken JF. Immunization with leucocidin toxoid against staphylococcal infection. Pathol Microbiol 30:166, 1967.

168. Lack CH, Towers AG. Serological tests for staphylococcal infection. BMJ 2:1227, 1962.

169. Florman AL, Lamberston GH, Zepp H, et al. Relation of 7S and 19S staphylococcal hemagglutinating antibody to age of individual. Pediatrics 32:501, 1963.

170. Lavoipierre GJ, Newell KW, Smith MHD, et al. A vaccine trial for neonatal staphylococcal disease. Am J Dis Child 122:377, 1971.

171. Marrach P, Kappler J. The staphylococcal enterotoxin and their relatives. Science 248:705, 1990.

172. Shinefield HR, Ribble JC, Boris M, et al. Bacterial interference: its effect on nursery-acquired infection with *Staphylococcus aureus*: I. Preliminary observations. Am J Dis Child 105:646, 1963.

173. Allison VD, Hobbs BC. Inquiry into epidemiology of pemphigus neonatorum. BMJ 2:1, 1947.

174. Hare R, Thomas CGA. The transmission of *Staphylococcus aureus*. BMJ 2:840, 1956.

175. Shinefield HR, Boris M, Ribble JC, et al. Bacterial interference: its effect on nursery-acquired infection with *Staphylococcus aureus*: III. The Georgia epidemic. Am J Dis Child 105:663, 1963.

176. Shinefield HR, Ribble JC, Sutherland JM, et al. Bacterial interference: its effect on nursery-acquired infection with *Staphylococcus aureus*: II. The Ohio epidemic. Am J Dis Child 105:655, 1963.

177. White A. Quantitative studies of nasal carriers of staphylococci among hospitalized patients. J Clin Invest 40:23, 1961.

178. Hare R. Infection in hospitals, epidemiology, and control. *In* Williams REO, Shooter RA (eds). Infection in Hospitals. Philadelphia, FA Davis, 1963.

179. Ridely M. Perineal carriage of *Staphylococcus aureus*. BMJ 1:270, 1959.

180. Wysham DN, Mulhern ME, Navarre GC, et al. Staphylococcal infections in an obstetric unit: I. Epidemiologic studies of pyoderma neonatorum. N Engl J Med 257:295, 1957.

181. Eichenwald HF, Kotsevalov O, Fasso LA. Another example of bacterial-viral interaction: "cloud-baby," important factor in transmission of staphylococcal infection in nursery and home. Am J Dis Child 98:432, 1959.

182. Jellard J. Umbilical cord as reservoir of infection in a maternity hospital. BMJ 1:925, 1957.

183. Wolinsky E, Lipsitz PJ, Mortimer EA Jr, et al. Acquisition of staphylococci by newborns: direct versus indirect transmission. Lancet 2:620, 1960.

184. Rammelkamp CH Jr, Mortimer EA Jr, Wolinsky E. Transmission of streptococcal and staphylococcal infections. Ann Intern Med 60:753, 1964.

185. Fairchild JP, Graber CD, Vogel EH, et al. Flora of the umbilical stump: 2479 cultures. J Pediatr 53:538, 1958.

186. Torrey JC, Reese MK. Initial anaerobic flora of newborn infants; selective tolerance of upper respiratory tract bacteria. Am J Dis Child 69:208, 1945.

fective oxidative metabolic responses of neutrophils from stressed infants. J Pediatr 98:392, 1981.

187. Hurst V. *Staphylococcus aureus* in the infant upper respiratory tract: I. Observations on hospital-born babies. J Hyg 55:299, 1957.

188. Thompson DJ, Gezon HM, Hatch TF, et al. Sex distributions of *Staphylococcus aureus* colonization and disease in newborn infants. N Engl J Med 269:337, 1963.

189. Aly R, Shinefield HR. Staphylococcal colonization in identical and non-identical twins. Am J Dis Child 127:486, 1974.

190. Gillespie WA, Simpson K, Tozer RC. Staphylococcal infection in a maternity hospital: epidemiology and control. Lancet 2:1075, 1958.

191. Hurst V. Transmission of hospital staphylococci among newborn infants: II. Colonization of the skin and mucous membranes of the infants. Pediatrics 25:204, 1960.

192. Boris M, Shinefield HR, Ribble JC, et al. Bacterial interference: its effect on nursery-acquired infection with *Staphylococcus aureus*: IV. The Louisiana epidemic. Am J Dis Child 105:674, 1963.

193. Parker MT, Tomilinson AJH, Williams REO. Impetigo contagiosa: association of certain types of *Staphylococcus aureus* and of *Streptococcus pyogenes* with superficial skin infections. J Hyg 53:458, 1955.

194. Howells CHL, Everley-Jones H. Two outbreaks of neonatal skin sepsis caused by *Staphylococcus aureus* phage type 71. Arch Dis Child 36:214, 1961.

195. Rycheck RR, Taylor PM, Gezon HM. Epidemic staphylococcal pyoderma associated with Ritter's disease and the appearance of phage type 3B/71. N Engl J Med 269:332, 1963.

196. Albert S, Baldwin R, Czekajewski S, et al. Bullous impetigo due to group II *Staphylococcus aureus*. Am J Dis Child 120:10, 1970.

197. Kaplan MH, Chmel H, Hsieh HC, et al. Importance of exfoliatin Toxin A production by *Staphylococcus aureus* strains isolated from clustered epidemics of neonatal pustulosis. J Clin Microbiol 23:83, 1986.

198. Dancer SJ, Poston SM, East J, et al. An outbreak of pemphigus neonatorum. J Infect 20:73, 1990.

199. Faden HS, Burke JP, Glasgow LA, et al. Nursery outbreak of scalded-skin syndrome: scarlatiniform rash due to phage group I *Staphylococcus aureus*. Am J Dis Child 130:265, 1976.

200. Curran JP, Al-Salihi FL. Neonatal staphylococcal scalded skin syndrome: massive outbreak due to unusual phage type. Pediatrics 66:285, 1980.

201. Florman AL, Holzman RS. Nosocomial scalded skin syndrome: Ritter's disease caused by phage group 3 *Staphylococcus aureus*. Am J Dis Child 134:1043, 1980.

202. Chesney PJ, Jaucian R, McDonald RA, et al. Exfoliative dermatitis in an infant: association with enterotoxin F–producing staphylococci. Am J Dis Child 137:899, 1983.

203. Wentworth FH, Miller AL, Wentworth BB. Observations relative to the nature and control of epidemic staphylococcal disease. Am J Public Health 48:287, 1958.

204. Ravenholt RT, Ravenholt OH. Staphylococcal infections in the hospital and community: hospital environment and staphylococcal disease. Am J Public Health 48:277, 1958.

205. Hurst V. The hospital nursery as a source of staphylococcal disease among families of newborn infants. N Engl J Med 262:951, 1960.

206. Oliver VL, Sargent CA, Dammann GLA, et al. The spread of sepsis contracted in hospital to the family. Am J Hyg 79:302, 1964.

207. Blowers R, Hodgkin K, Sklaroff S. Spread of hospital staphylococci in healthy families—a study from general practice. BMJ 4:642, 1967.

208. Nahmias AJ, Lepper MH, Hurst V, et al. Epidemiology and treatment of chronic staphylococcal infections in the household. Am J Public Health 52:1828, 1962.

209. Lund GC, Green DW. Methicillin-resistant *Staphylococcus aureus* colonization in neonatal intensive care graduates. Arch Pediatr Adolesc Med 148:1106, 1994.

210. Hollis RJ, Barr JL, Doebbeling BN, et al. Familial carriage of methicillin-resistant *Staphylococcus aureus* and subsequent infection in a premature neonate. Clin Infect Dis 21:328, 1995.

211. Caswell HT, Groschel D, Roberg FB, et al. A ten-year study of staphylococcal disease: surveillance, control, and prevention of hospital infections, 1956 to 1965. Arch Environ Health 17:221, 1968.

212. Light IJ, Sutherland JM. What is the evidence that hexachlorophene is not effective? Pediatrics 51:345, 1973.

213. Light IJ, Atherton HD, Sutherland JM. Decreased colonization of newborn infants with *Staphylococcus aureus* 80/81: Cincinnati General Hospital, 1960B1972. J Infect Dis 131:281, 1975.

214. Jessen O, Rosendal K, Bulow P, et al. Changing staphylococci and staphylococcal infections—a ten-year study of bacteria and cases of bacteremia. N Engl J Med 281:627, 1969.

215. Anthong BF, Guiliano DM, Oh W. Nursery outbreak of staphylococcal scalded-skin syndrome: rapid identification of the epidemic bacterial strain. Am J Dis Child 124:41, 1972.

216. Light IJ, Brackvogel MS, Walton RL, et al. An epidemic of bullous impetigo arising from a central admission-observation nursery. Pediatrics 49:15, 1972.

217. Saiman L, Jakob K, Holmes KW, et al. Molecular epidemiology of staphylococcal scalded skin syndrome in premature infants. Pediatr Infect Dis J 17:329, 1998.

218. Maranan MC, Moreira B, Boyle-Vavra S, Daum RS. Antimicrobial resistance in staphylococci: epidemiology, molecular mechanism, and clinical relevance. Infect Dis Clin North Am 11:813, 1997.

219. Panlilio AL, Culver DH, Gaynes RP, et al. Methicillin-resistant *Staphylococcus aureus* in US hospitals, 1975–1991. Infect Control Hosp Epidemiol 13:582, 1992.

220. Herold BC, Immergluck LC, Maranan MC, et al. Community-acquired methicillin-resistant *Staphylococcus aureus* in children with no identified predisposing risk. JAMA 279:593, 1998.

221. Graham DR, Correa-Villasinor A, Anderson RJ, et al. Epidemic neonatal gentamicin-methicillin resistant *Staphylococcus aureus* infection associated with nonspecific topical use of gentamicin. J Pediatr 97:972, 1980.

222. Holzman RS, Florman AL, Lyman M. Gentamicin resistant and sensitive strains of *Staphylococcus aureus*: factors affecting colonization and virulence for infants in a special care nursery. Am J Epidemiol 112:352, 1980.

223. Dunkle LM, Naqvi SH, McCallum R, et al. Eradication of epidemic methicillin-gentamicin-resistant *Staphylococcus aureus* in an intensive care nursery. Am J Med 70:455, 1981.

224. Parks YA, Nuy MF, Aukett MA, et al. Methicillin-resistant *Staphylococcus aureus* in milk. Arch Dis Child 62:82, 1987.

225. Ribner BS. Endemic, multiply resistant *Staphylococcus aureus* in a pediatric population. Am J Dis Child 141:1183, 1987.

226. Jordens JZ, Duckworth GJ, Williams RJ. Production of "virulence factors": by "epidemic" methicillin-resistant *Staphylococcus aureus* in vitro. J Med Microbial 30:245, 1989.

227. Frenay HME, Theelen JPG, Schouls LM, et al. Discrimination of epidemic and nonepidemic methicillin-resis-

tant *Staphylococcus aureus* strains on the basis of protein A gene polymorphism. J Clin Microbial 32:846, 1994.

228. Noble WC, Somerville DA. Microbiology of Human Skin. London, WB Saunders, 1974.

229. Goldmann DA. Bacterial colonization and infection in the neonate. Am J Med 70:417, 1981.

230. Simpson RA, Spencer AF, Speller DCE, et al. Colonization by gentamicin-resistant *Staphylococcus epidermidis* in a special care baby unit. J Hosp Infect 7:108, 1986.

231. Speck WT, Driscoll JM, Polin RA, et al. Effect of bacterial flora on staphylococcal colonization of the newborn. J Clin Pathol 31:153, 1978.

232. D'Angio CT, McGowan KL, Baumgart S, et al. Surface colonization with coagulase-negative staphylococci in premature neonates. J Pediatr 114:1029, 1989.

233. Hall SL, Riddell SW, Barnes WG, et al. Evaluation of coagulase-negative staphylococcal isolates from serial nasopharyngeal cultures of premature infants. Diagn Microbiol Infect Dis 13:17, 1990.

234. Hall SL, Hall RT, Barnes WG, et al. Relationship of maternal to neonatal colonization with coagulase-negative staphylococci. Am J Perinatol 7:384, 1990.

235. Patrick CH, John JF, Levkoff A, et al. Relatedness of strains of methicillin-resistant coagulase-negative *Staphylococcus* colonizing hospital personnel and producing bacteremias in a neonatal intensive care unit. Pediatr Infect Dis J 11:935, 1992.

236. Freeman J, Goldmann DA, Smith NE, et al. Association of intravenous lipid emulsion and coagulase negative staphylococcal bacteremia in neonatal intensive care units. N Engl J Med 323:301, 1990.

237. Gezon HM, Roger KD, Thompson DJ, et al. Environmental aspects of staphylococcal infections acquired in hospitals: II. Some controversial aspects in the epidemiology of hospital nursery staphylococcal infections. Am J Public Health 50:473, 1960.

238. Shinefield HR, Ribble JC. Current aspects of infections and diseases related to *Staphylococcus aureus*. Annu Rev Med 16:263, 1965.

239. Daschner FD. Nosocomial infections in maternity wards and newborn nurseries: rooming-in or not? J Hosp Infect 7:1, 1986.

240. Frazer MJL. A study of neonatal infections in the nurseries of a maternity hospital. Arch Dis Child 23:107, 1948.

241. Haley RW, Bregman DA. The role of understaffing and overcrowding in recurrent outbreaks of staphylococcal infection in a neonatal special-care unit. J Infect Dis 145:875, 1982.

242. Haley RW, Cushion NB, Tenover FC, et al. Eradication of endemic methicillin-resistant *Staphylococcus aureus* infections from a neonatal intensive care unit. J Infect Dis 171:614, 1995.

243. Gillespie WA, Adler VG. Control of an outbreak of staphylococcal infection in a hospital. Lancet 1:632, 1957.

244. Rountree PM, Heseltine M, Rheuben J, et al. Control of staphylococcal infection of newborn by treatment of nasal carriers in staff. Med J Aust 1:528, 1956.

245. Monro JA, Markham NP. Staphylococcal infection in mothers and infants: maternal breast abscesses and antecedent neonatal sepsis. Lancet 2:186, 1958.

246. Martin WJ, Nichols DR, Henderson ED. The problem of management of nasal carriers of staphylococci. Proc Staff Meet Mayo Clin 35:282, 1960.

247. Williams JD, Waltho CA, Ayliffe GAJ, et al. Trials of five antibacterial creams in the control of nasal carriage of *Staphylococcus aureus*. Lancet 2:390, 1967.

248. Smith RT. The role of the chronic carrier in an epidemic of staphylococcal disease in a newborn nursery. Am J Dis Child 95:461, 1958.

249. Belani A, Sherertz RJ, Sullivan ML, et al. Outbreak of staphylococcal infection in two hospital nurseries traced to a single nasal carrier. Infect Control 7:487, 1986.

250. Mortimer EA Jr, Lipsitz PJ, Wolinksky E, et al. Transmission of staphylococci between newborns: importance of the hands of personnel. Am J Dis Child 104:289, 1962.

251. Williams CPS, Oliver TK Jr. Nursery routines and staphylococcal colonization of the newborn. Pediatrics 44:640, 1969.

252. Najem GR, Riley HD Jr, Ordway NK, et al. Clinical and microbiologic surveillance of neonatal staphylococcal disease: relationship to hexachlorophene whole-body bathing. Am J Dis Child 129:297, 1975.

253. Gehlbach SH, Gutman LT, Wilfert CM, et al. Recurrence of skin disease in a nursery: ineffectuality of hexachlorophene bathing. Pediatrics 55:422, 1975.

254. Klainer LM, Agrawal HS, Mortimer EA Jr, et al. Bacitracin ointment and neonatal staphylococci. Am J Dis Child 103:72, 1962.

255. Gezon HM, Thompson DJ, Rogers KD, et al. Control of staphylococcal infections and disease in the newborn through the use of hexachlorophene bathing. Pediatrics 51:331, 1973.

256. Davies EA, Emmerson AM, Hogg GM, et al. An outbreak of infection with a methicillin-resistant *Staphylococcus aureus* in a special care baby unit: value of topical mupirocin and of traditional methods of infection control. 10:120, 1987.

257. Rosenfield CR, Laptook AR, Jeffery J. Limited effectiveness of triple dye in preventing colonization with infection with methicillin-resistant *Staphylococcus aureus* in a special care baby unit. Pediatr Infect Dis J 9:290, 1990.

258. Pildes RS, Ramamurthy RS, Vidyasagar D. Effect of triple dye on staphylococcal colonization in the newborn infant. J Pediatr 82:987, 1973.

259. Ramamurthy RS, Pildes RS, Gorbach SL. Nursery epidemic caused by a nontypable gray colony variant of *Staphylococcus aureus*. Pediatrics 51:608, 1973.

260. Gluck L, Wood HF. Effect of an antiseptic skin-care regimen in reducing staphylococcal colonization in newborn infants. N Engl J Med 265:1177, 1961.

261. Simon HJ, Yaffe SJ, Gluck L. Effective control of staphylococci in a nursery. N Engl J Med 265:1171, 1961.

262. Plueckhahn VD, Banks J. Antisepsis and staphylococcal disease in the newborn child. Med J Aust 2:519, 1963.

263. Gezon HM, Thompson DJ, Rogers KD, et al. Hexachlorophene bathing in early infancy: effect on staphylococcal disease and infection. N Engl J Med 270:379, 1964.

264. Pleuckhahn VD. Hexachlorophene and the control of staphylococcal sepsis in a maternity unit in Geelong, Australia. Pediatrics 51:368, 1973.

265. Gezon HM, Schaberg MJ, Klein JO. Concurrent epidemics of *Staphylococcus aureus* and group A *Streptococcus* disease in a newborn nursery-control with penicillin G and hexachlorophene bathing. Pediatrics 51:383, 1973.

266. Hyams PJ, Counts WG, Monkus E, et al. Staphylococcal bacteremia and hexachlorophene bathing: epidemic in a newborn nursery. Am J Dis Child 129:595, 1975.

267. Shaffer TE, Baldwin JN, Rheins M, et al. Staphylococcal infections in newborn infants: study of epidemics among infants and nursing mothers. Pediatrics 18:750, 1956.

268. Mortimer EA. Personal communication, 1965.

269. Shinefield HR, Ribble JC, Boris M, et al. Bacterial interference: its effect on nursery-acquired infection with *Staphylococcus aureus*: V. An analysis and interpretation. Am J Dis Child 105:683, 1963.

270. Eichenwald HF, Shinefield HR, Boris M, et al. Bacterial interference and staphylococcal colonization in infants and adults. Ann NY Acad Sci 128:365, 1965.

271. Light IJ, Sutherland JM, Schott JE. Control of a staphylococcal outbreak in a nursery-use of bacterial interference. JAMA 193:699, 1965.

272. Light IJ, Walton RL, Sutherland JM, et al. Use of bacterial interference to control a staphylococcal nursery outbreak. Am J Dis Child 113:291, 1967.

273. Shinefield HR, Ribble JC, Boris M. Bacterial interference between strains of *Staphylococcus aureus*, 1960 to 1970. Am J Dis Child 121:148, 1971.

274. Shinefield HR. Bacterial interference. Ann NY Acad Sci 236:444, 1974.

275. Shuter J, Hatcher VB, Lowy FD. *Staphylococcus aureus* binding to human nasal mucin. Infect Immun 64:310, 1996.

276. Kwong MS, Loew AD, Anthony BF, et al. The effect of hexachlorophene on staphylococcal colonization rates in the newborn infant: a controlled study using a single-bath method. J Pediatr 82:982, 1973.

277. Gooch JJ, Britt EM. *Staphylococcus aureus* colonization and infection in newborn nursery patients. Am J Dis Child 132:893, 1978.

278. Neumann LL, Rager R, Brickman A, et al. Gram-positive umbilical flora in a nursery using alcohol cord care. Society for Pediatric Research, Atlantic City, April 28–May 1, 1971, p. 258 (abstract).

279. Kimbrough RD. Review of recent evidence of toxic effects of hexachlorophene. Pediatrics 51:391, 1973.

280. Mullick FG. Hexachlorophene toxicity. Pediatrics 51:395, 1973.

281. Kopelman AE. Cutaneous absorption of hexachlorophene in low birth-weight infants. J Pediatr 82:972, 1973.

282. Committee of the Fetus and Newborn, American Academy of Pediatrics. Skin care of newborns. Pediatrics 54:682, 1974.

283. Powell H, Swarner O, Gluck L, et al. Hexachlorophene myelinopathy in premature infants. J Pediatr 82:976, 1973.

284. Shuman RM, Leech RW, Alvord EC Jr. Neurotoxicity of hexachlorophene in the human: I. A clinical-pathologic study of 248 children. Pediatrics 54:90, 1974.

285. Shuman RM, Leech RW, Alvord EC Jr. Neurotoxicity of topically applied hexachlorophene in the young rat. Arch Neurol 32:315, 1975.

286. Shuman RM, Leech RW, Alvord EC Jr. Neurotoxicity of hexachlorophene in humans: II. A clinical-pathologic study of 46 premature infants. Arch Neurol 32:320, 1975.

287. Tyrala EE, Hillman CS, Hillman RE, et al. Clinical pharmacology of hexachlorophene in newborn infants. Pediatrics 91:481, 1977.

288. Pyati S, Ramamurthy RS, Krauss T, et al. Povidone-iodine (PI), ethyl alcohol (AL) and triple dye (TD): control of neonatal staphylococcal (*Staphylococcus aureus*) colonization. Pediatr Res 10:431, 1976.

289. Johnson JD, Malachowski NC, Vosti KL, et al. A sequential study of various modes of skin and umbilical care and the incidence of staphylococcal colonization and infection in the neonate. Pediatrics 58:354, 1976.

290. Speck WT, Driscoll JM, Polin RA, et al. Staphylococcal and streptococcal colonization of the newborn infant: effect of antiseptic cord care. Am J Dis Child 131:1005, 1977.

291. Barrett FF, Mason EO, Fleming D. The effect of three cord care regimens on bacterial colonization of normal neonates. Pediatr Res 11:497, 1977.

292. Durand M, Ramanathan R, Martinelli B, et al. Prospective evaluation of percutaneous central venous Silastic catheters in newborn infants with birth weights of 510 to 3,920 grams. Pediatrics 78:245, 1986.

293. Peters G, Locci R, Pulverer G. Adherence and growth of coagulase-negative staphylococci on surface of intravenous catheters. J Infect Dis 146:479, 1982.

294. Franson TR, Sheth NK, Rose HD, et al. Scanning electron microscopy of bacteria adherent to intavascular catheters. J Clin Microbiol 20:500, 1984.

295. Marrie TJ, Costerton JW. Scanning and transmission electron microscopy of in situ bacterial colonization of intervenous and intraarterial catheters. J Clin Microbiol 19:687, 1984.

296. Kamal GD, Pfaller MA, Rempe LE, Jebson PJ. Reduced intravascular catheter infection by antibiotic bonding: a prospective, randomized, controlled trial. JAMA 265:2364, 1991.

297. Bach A. Clinical studies on the use antibiotic- and antiseptic-bonded catheters to prevent catheter-related infection. Int J Med Microbiol Virol Parasitol 283:208, 1995.

298. Radd I, Darouiche R, Dupuis J, et al. Central venous catheters coated with minocycline and rifampin for the prevention of catheter-related colonization and blood-stream infections: a randomized, double-blind trial. Ann Intern Med 127:267, 1997.

299. Darouiche R, Raad I, Heard S, et al. A prospective randomized, multicenter clinical trial comparing central venous catheters impregnated with minocycline and rifampin vs. chlorhexidine gluconate and silver sulfadiazine. Crit Care Med 26 (Suppl):A128, 1998 (abstract).

300. Veenstra DL, Saint S, Saha S, et al. Efficacy of antiseptic-impregnated central venous catheters in preventing catheter-related bloodsteam infection. JAMA 281:261, 1999.

301. Darouiche R, Raad I, Heard S, et al. A comparison of two antimicrobial-impregnated central venous catheters. N Engl J Med 340:1, 1999.

302. Spafford PS, Sinkin RA, Cox C, et al. Prevention of central venous catheter-related coagulase-negative staphylococcal sepsis in neonates. J Pediatr 125:259, 1994.

303. Kacica MA, Horgan MJ, Ochoa L, et al. Prevention of Gram-positive sepsis in neonates weighing less than 1500 grams. J Pediatr 125:253, 1994.

304. Cooke RWI, Nycyk JA, Okuonghuae H, et al. Low-dose vancomycin prophylaxis reduces coagulase-negative *Staphylococcus* bacteraemia in very low birthweight infants. J Hosp Infect 37:297, 1997.

305. Melish ME, Glasgow LA. Staphylococcal scalded-skin syndrome: the expanded clinical syndrome. J Pediatr 78:958, 1971.

306. Lyell A. A review of toxic epidermal necrolysis in Britain. Dermatology 79:622, 1967.

307. Gemmell CG. Staphylococcal scalded skin syndrome. J Med Microbiol 43:318, 1995.

308. Melish ME, Glasgow LA. The staphylococcal scalded-skin syndrome: development of an experimental model. N Engl J Med 282:1114, 1970.

309. Kondo I, Sakurai S, Sarai Y, Futaki S. Two serotypes of exfoliation and their distribution in staphylococcal strains isolated from patients with scalded skin syndrome. J Clin Microbiol 1:397, 1975.

310. Dajani AS. The scalded-skin syndrome: relation to phage group II staphylococci. J Infect Dis 125:548, 1972.

311. Fox KR, Golomb HS. Staphylococcal ophthalmia neonatorum and the staphylococcal scalded skin syndrome. Am J Ophthalmol 88:1052, 1979.

312. Annunziato D, Goldblum LM. Staphylococcal scalded skin syndrome: a complication of circumcision. Am J Dis Child 132:1187, 1978.

313. Amon RB, Diamond RL. Toxic epidermal necrolysis: rapid differentiation between staphylococcal and drug-induced disease. Arch Dermatol 111:1433, 1975.

314. Elias PM, Fritsch P, Epstein EH. Staphylococcal scalded skin syndrome: clinical features, pathogenesis, and recent microbiological and biochemical development. Arch Dermatol 113:207, 1977.

315. Manzella JP, Hull CB, Green JL, et al. Toxic epidermal necrolysis in childhood: differentiation from staphylococcal scalded skin syndrome. Pediatrics 66:291, 1980.

316. Rudolph RI, Schwartz W, Leyden JJ. Treatment of staphylococcal toxic epidermal necrolysis. Arch Dermatol 110:559, 1974.

317. Todd J, Fishaut M, Kapral F, et al. Toxic shock syndrome associated with phage group I staphylococci. Lancet 2:1116, 1978.

318. Schlievert PM, Shands KN, Dan BB et al. Identification and characterization of an exotoxin from *Staphylococcus aureus* associated with toxic shock syndrome. J Infect Dis 143:509, 1981.

319. Bergdoll MS, Crass BA, Reiser RF, et al. An enterotoxin-like protein in *Staphylococcus aureus* strains from patients with toxic shock syndrome. Ann Intern Med 96:969, 1982.

320. Schlievert PM. Biological properties of toxic shock syndrome exotoxin. Surv Synth Pathol Res 3:54, 1984.

321. Shands KN, Schmid GP, Dan BB, et al. Toxic shock syndrome in menstruating women: association with tampon use and *Staphylococcus aureus* and clinical features in 52 cases. N Engl J Med 303:1436, 1980.

322. Broome CV. Epidemiology of TSS in the United States: overview. Rev Infect Dis 11 (Suppl 1):S14, 1989.

323. Gaventa S, Reingold AL, Hightower AW, et al. Active surveillance for TSS in the United States. Rev Infect Dis 11:S28, 1989.

324. Whitley CB, Thompson LR, Osterholm MT, et al. Toxic shock syndrome in a newborn infant. Pediatr Res 16:254A, 1982.

325. Reboli AC, John JF, Platt CG, Cantey JR. Methicillin-resistant *Staphylococcus aureus* outbreak at a Veterans Affairs medical center: importance of carriage of the organism by hospital personnel. Infect Control Hosp Epidemiol 11:291, 1990.

326. Darouiche R, Wright C, Hamill R, et al. Eradication of colonization by methicillin-resistant *Staphylococcus aureus* by using oral minocycline-rifampin and topical mupirocin. Antimicrob Agents Chemother 35:1612, 1991.

327. Strausbaugh LJ, Jacobson C, Sewell DL, et al. Antimicrobial therapy for methicillin-resistant *Staphylococcus aureus* colonization in residents and staff of a Veterans Affairs nursing home care unit. Infect Control Hosp Epidemiol 13:151, 1992.

328. Doebbeling BN, Breneman DL, Neu HC, et al. Elimination of *Staphylococcus aureus* nasal carriage in health care workers: analysis of six clinical trials with calcium mupirocin ointment. Clin Infect Dis 17:466, 1993.

329. Boris M, Shinefield HR, Romano P, et al. Bacterial interference. Am J Dis Child 115:521, 1968.

330. Boris M. Bacterial interference—protection against staphylococcal disease. Bull NY Acad Med 44:1212, 1968.

331. Steele RW. Recurrent staphylococcal infection in families. Arch Dermatol 116:189, 1980.

332. Ayliffe GA, Brightwell KM, Ball PM, et al. Staphylococcal infection in cervical glands of infants. Lancet 2:479, 1972.

333. Dewar J, Porter IA, Smylie HG. Staphylococcal infection in cervical glands of infants. Lancet 2:712, 1972.

334. Hieber HP, Davis AT. Staphylococcal cervical adenitis in young infants. Pediatrics 57:424, 1976.

335. Scobie WG. Acute suppurative adenitis in children. Scott Med J 14:352, 1969.

336. Barton LL, Feigin RD. Childhood cervical lymphadenitis: a reappraisal. J Pediatr 84:846, 1974.

337. Warren WS, Stool SE. Otitis in low birth-weight infants. J Pediatr 79:740, 1971.

338. Duncan J, Walker J. *Staphylococcus aureus* in the milk of nursing mothers and the alimentary canal of their infants. J Hyg 42:474, 1942.

339. Soltan DHK, Hatcher GW. Some observations on the aetiology of breast abscess in the puerperium. BMJ 1:1603, 1960.

340. Wysham DN, Mulhern ME, Navarre GC, et al. Staphylococcal infections in an obstetric unit: II. Epidemiologic studies of puerperal mastitis. N Engl J Med 257:304, 1957.

341. Foster D, Harris RE. The incidence of *Staphylococcus pyogenes* in normal human breast milk. J Obstet Gynaecol Br Emp 67:463, 1960.

342. Montgomery TL, Wise MDI, Land WR, et al. A study of staphylococci colonization of postpartum mothers and newborn infants. Am J Obstet Gynecol 66:1227, 1959.

343. Ottenheimer EJ, Minchew IBH, Cohen LS, et al. Studies of the epidemiology of staphylococcal infection. Bull Johns Hopkins Hosp 109:114, 1961.

344. Burbianka M, Dluzniewska A, Windyga B. Enterogenic staphylococci and enterotoxin in human milk. *In* Jeljaszewicz J, Hryniewicz W (eds). Staphylococci and Staphylococcal Infections: Recent Progress. Warsaw, Polish Medical Publishers, 1973, p 444.

345. Marshall BR, Hepper JK, Zirbel CC. Sporadic puerperal mastitis: an infection that need not interrupt lactation. JAMA 233:1377, 1975.

346. Stetler H, Martin E, Plotkin S, et al. Neonatal mastitis due to *Escherichia coli*. J Pediatr 76:611, 1970.

347. Burry BF, Beezley M. Infant mastitis due to gram-negative organisms. Am J Dis Child 124:736, 1972.

348. Nelson J. Suppurative mastitis in infants. Am J Dis Child 125:458, 1973.

349. Kalbow H. Über Mastitis neonatorum und ihre Folgen. Zentralbl Gynaekol 60:1821, 1936.

350. Rudoy RC, Nelson JD. Breast abscess during the neonatal period. Am J Dis Child 129:1031, 1975.

351. Buetow KC, Klein SW, Lane RB. Septicemia in premature infants. Am J Dis Child 110:29, 1965.

352. McCracken GH Jr., Shinefield HR. Changes in the pattern of neonatal septicemia and meningitis. Am J Dis Child 112:33, 1966.

353. Patrick CC, Kaplan SL, Baker CJ, et al. Persistent bacteremia due to coagulase-negative staphylococci in low birthweight neonates. Pediatrics 84:977, 1989.

354. St. Geme JW III, Bell LM, Baumgart S, et al. Distinguishing sepsis from blood culture contamination in young infants with blood cultures growing coagulase-negative staphylococci. Pediatrics 86:157, 1990.

355. Baumgart S, Hall SE, Campos JM, et al. Sepsis with coagulase-negative staphylococci I critically ill newborns. Am J Dis Child 137:461, 1983.

356. Schmidt BK, Kirpalani HM, Corey M, et al. Coagulase-negative staphylococci as true pathogens in newborn infants: a cohort study. Pediatr Infect Dis J 6:1026, 1987.

357. Scherer LR, West KW, Weber TR, et al. *Staphylococcus epidermidis* sepsis in pediatric patients: clinical and therapeutic considerations. J Pediatr Surg 19:358, 1984.

358. Prince A, Heller B, Levy J, et al. Management of fever

in patients with central venous catheters. Pediatr Infect Dis J 5:20, 1986.

359. Koch R, Carson MJ, Donnell G. Staphylococcal pneumonia in children: a review of 83 cases. J Pediatr 55:473, 1959.

360. Hendren WH III, Haggerty RJ. Staphylococcic pneumonia in infancy and childhood: analysis of 75 cases. JAMA 168:6, 1958.

361. Bevaen DW, Burry AF. Staphylococcal pneumonia in the newborn: an epidemic with eight fatal cases. Lancet 2:211, 1956.

362. Turner JAP. Staphylococcal pneumonia: a contemporary rarity. Clin Pediatr 2:69, 1972.

363. Kanof A, Kramer B, Carnes M. Staphylococcus pneumonia: a clinical, pathologic, and bacteriologic study. J Pediatr 14:712, 1939.

364. Huxtable KA, Tucker AS, Wedgwood RJ. Staphylococcal pneumonia in childhood. Am J Dis Child 108:262, 1964.

365. Wise MB, Beaudry PH, Bates DV. Long-term follow-up of staphylococcal pneumonia. Pediatrics 38:398, 1966.

366. Ceruti E, Contreras J, Neira M. Staphylococcal pneumonia in childhood: long-term follow-up including pulmonary function studies. Am J Dis Child 122:386, 1971.

367. Hall RT, Kurth CG, Hall SL. Ten-year survey of positive blood cultures among admissions to a neonatal intensive care unit. J Perinatol 7:122, 1987.

368. Rhodes PG, Hall RT, Burry VE, et al. Sepsis and osteomyelitis due to Staphylococcus aureus phage type 94 in a neonatal intensive care unit. Letter to the editor. J Pediatr 88:1063, 1976.

369. Overturf GD, Balfour G. Osteomyelitis and sepsis: severe complications of fetal monitoring. Pediatrics 55:244, 1975.

370. Lilien LD, Harris VJ, Ramamurthy RS, et al. Neonatal osteomyelitis of the calcaneus: complication of heel puncture. J Pediatr 88:478, 1976.

371. Lauer BA, Altenburger KM. Outbreak of Staphylococcus infections following heel puncture for blood sampling. Am J Dis Child 135:277, 1981.

372. Myers MG, McMahon BJ, Koontz FP. Neonatal calcaneous osteomyelitis related to contaminated mineral oil. J Clin Microbiol 6:543, 1977.

373. Lim MO, Gresham EL, Franken EA Jr, et al. Osteomyelitis as a complication of umbilical artery catheterization. Am J Dis Child 131:142, 1977.

374. Weeks JL, Garcia-Prat JA, Baker C. Methicillin-resistant Staphylococcus aureus osteomyelitis in a neonate. JAMA 245:1662, 1981.

375. Blanche DW. Osteomyelitis in infants. J Bone Joint Surg 34A:578, 1954.

376. Potter CMC. Osteomyelitis in the newborn. J Bone Joint Surg 36B:578, 1954.

377. Clarke AM. Neonatal osteomyelitis: a disease different from osteomyelitis of older children. Med J Aust 45:237, 1958.

378. Gilmour WN. Acute hematogenous osteomyelitis. J Bone Joint Surg 44B:841, 1962.

379. Ogden JA, Lister G. The pathology of neonatal osteomyelitis. Pediatrics 55:474, 1975.

380. Ogden JA. Pediatric osteomyelitis and septic arthritis: pathology of neonatal disease. Yale J Biol Med 52:423, 1979.

381. Fardon DF. Osteomyelitis of the scapula in an infant: case report. Miss Med 67:299, 1970.

382. Einstein RAJ, Thomas CG. Osteomyelitis in infants. AJR Am J Roentgenol 55:299, 1946.

383. Green WT. Osteomyelitis in infancy. JAMA 105:1835, 1935.

384. Weissberg ED, Smith AL, Smith DH. Clinical features of neonatal osteomyelitis. Pediatrics 53:505, 1974.

385. Ambrose GB, Alpert M, Neer CS. Vertebral osteomyelitis: a diagnostic problem. JAMA 197:101, 1966.

386. Miller WH, Hesch JA. Nontuberculous spinal epidural abscess: report of a case in a 5-week old infant. Am J Dis Child 104:269, 1962.

387. Treves S, Khettry J, Broher FH, et al. Osteomyelitis: early scintigraphic detection in children. Pediatrics 57:173, 1976.

388. Magd M. Radionuclide imaging in early detection of childhood osteomyelitis and its differentiation from cellulitis and bone infarction. Ann Radiol 20:9, 1977.

389. Tetzloff TR, McCracken GH, Nelson JD. Oral antibiotic therapy for skeletal infections of children: II. Therapy of osteomyelitis and suppurative arthritis. J Pediatr 92:485, 1978.

390. Prober CG, Yeager AS. Use of the serum bactericidal titer to assess the adequacy of oral antibiotic therapy in the treatment of acute hematogenous osteomyelitis. J Pediatr 95:131, 1979.

391. Schwartz GJ, Hegyi T, Spitzer A. Subtherapeutic dicloxacillin levels in a neonate: possible mechanisms. J Pediatr 89:310, 1976.

392. Dich VC, Nelson JD, Haltalin KC. Osteomyelitis in infants and children. Am J Dis Child 129:1273, 1975.

393. Bergdahl S, Ekengren K, Eriksson M. Neonatal hematogenous osteomyelitis: risk factors for long-term sequelae. J Pediatr Orthop 5:564, 1985.

394. Halbstein BM. Bone regeneration in infantile osteomyelitis. J Bone Joint Surg 49A:149, 1967.

395. Edwards MS, Baker CJ. Median sternotomy wound infections in children. Pediatr Infect Dis 2, 105, 1983.

396. Chacha PB. Suppurative arthritis of the hip in infancy: a persistent diagnostic problem and possible complication of femoral vein puncture. J Bone Joint Surg 53A:538, 1971.

397. Obletz BE. Acute suppurative arthritis of the hip in the neonatal period. J Bone Joint Surg 42A:23, 1960.

398. Wellman WE, Senft RA. Bacterial meningitis: III. Infections caused by Staphylococcus aureus. Proc Staff Meet Mayo Clin 39:263, 1964.

399. Mulcare RJ, Harter DH. Changing patterns of staphylococcal meningitis. Arch Neurol 7:114, 1962.

400. Shurtleff DB, Foltz EL, Weeks RD, et al. Therapy of Staphylococcus epidermidis: infection associated with cerebrospinal fluid shunts. Pediatrics 53:55, 1974.

401. Gruskay J, Harris MC, Costarino AT, et al. Neonatal Staphylococcus epidermidis meningitis with unremarkable CSF examination results. Am J Dis Child 143:580, 1989.

402. McLaurin RL, Frame PT. Treatment of infections of cerebrospinal fluid shunts. Rev Infect Dis 9:595, 1987.

403. Wald SL, McLaurin RL. Cerebrospinal fluid antibiotic levels during treatment of shunt infections. J Neurosurg 52:41, 1980.

404. Diaz-Mitoma F, Harding GKM, Hoban DJ, et al. Clinical significance of a test for slime production in ventriculoperitoneal shunt infections caused by coagulase-negative staphylococci. J Infect Dis 156:555, 1987.

405. Younger JJ, Christensen GD, Bartley DL, et al. Coagulase-negative staphylococci isolated from cerebrospinal fluid shunts: importance of slime production, species identification and shunt removal to clinical outcome. J Infect Dis 156:548, 1987.

406. Conners JM. Cure of Ommaya reservoir–associated Staphylococcus epidermidis ventriculitis with a simple regimen of vancomycin and rifampin without reservoir removal. Med Pediatr Oncol 10:549, 1982.

407. Stickler GB, Shin MH, Burke EC, et al. Diffuse glomerulonephritis associated with infected ventriculo-atrial shunt. N Engl J Med 279:1077, 1968.

408. Barrie D. Staphylococcal colonization of the rectum in the newborn. BMJ 1:1574, 1966.

409. Holst A. Cited by Selberg L. Fatal staphylococcal poisoning of breast-fed infant whose mother suffered from staphylococcal mastitis. Acta Obstet Gynaecol Scand 27:275, 1947.

410. Dolman CE. Bacterial food poisoning: II. *Staphylococcus* food poisoning. Can J Public Health 34:205, 1943.

411. Selberg L. Fatal staphylococcal poisoning of breast fed infant whose mother suffered from staphylococcal mastitis. Acta Obstet Gynaecol Scand 27:275, 1947.

412. Gutman LT, Idriss ZH, Gehlbach S, et al. Neonatal staphylococcal enterocolitis: association with indwelling feeding catheters and *S. aureus* colonization. J Pediatr 88:836, 1976.

413. Christie CDC, Lynch-Ballard E, Andiman WA. Staphylococcal enterocolitis revisited: cytotoxic properties of *Staphylococcus aureus* from a neonate with enterocolitis. Pediatr Infect Dis J 7:791, 1988.

414. Fabia C, Pearlman MA, Leon EF, et al. *Staphylococcus epidermidis*: a new pathogen in necrotizing enterocolitis (NEC). Pediatr Res 17:312A, 1983.

415. Gruskay JA, Abbasi S, Anday E, et al. *Staphylococcus epidermidis*–associated enterocolitis. J Pediatr 109:520, 1986.

416. Baumgart S, Hall SE, Campos JM, et al. Sepsis with coagulase-negative staphylococci in critically ill newborns. Am J Dis Child 137:461, 1983.

417. Noel GJ, Edelson PJ. *Staphylococcus epidermidis* bacteremia in neonates: further observations and the occurrence of focal infection. Pediatrics 74:832, 1984.

418. Curtis J, Stobie PE. Necrotizing enterocolitis and staphylococcal sepsis. J Pediatr 111:953, 1987.

419. Mollit DL, Tepas JJ, Talbert JL. The role of coagulase-negative staphylococci in neonatal necrotizing enterocolitis. J Pediatr Surg 23:60, 1988.

420. Noel JG, O'Loughlin JE, Edelson PJ. Neonatal *Staphylococcus epidermidis* right side endocarditis: description of five catheterized infants. Pediatrics 82:234, 1988.

421. Garrison PK, Freedman LR. Experimental endocarditis: I. Staphylococcal endocarditis in rabbits resulting from placement of polyethylene catheter in the right side of the heart. Yale J Biol Med 42:394, 1970.

422. Durack DT, Beeson PG. Experimental bacterial endocarditis: I. Colonization of a sterile vegetation. Br J Exp Pathol 53:44, 1972.

423. Durack DT, Beeson PG, Petersdorf RG. Experimental bacterial endocarditis: II. Production and progress of the disease in rabbits. Br J Exp Pathol 54:142, 1973.

424. Nu HC. Structure-activity relations of new beta-lactam compounds and in vitro activity against common bacteria. Rev Infect Dis 5(Suppl. 2):S319, 1983.

425. Nelson SJ, Boies EG, Shackelford PG. Ceftriaxone in the treatment of infections caused by *Staphylococcus aureus* in children. Pediatr Infect Dis J 4:27, 1985.

426. Odio CM, Umana MA, Saenz A, et al. Comparative efficacy of ceftazidime vs. carbenicillin and amikacin for treatment of neonatal septicemia. Pediatr Infect Dis J 6:371, 1987.

427. Beldhradsky BH, Bruch K, Geiss D, et al. Intravenous cefotaxime in children with bacterial meningitis. Lancet 1:61, 1980.

428. Spivey JM, Gal P. Vancomycin pharmacokinetics in neonates. Letter to the editor. Am J Dis Child 140:859, 1986.

429. Dunne WM, Nelson DB, Chusid MJ. Epidemiologic markers of pediatric infections caused by coagulase-negative staphylococci. Pediatr Infect Dis J 6:1031, 1987.

430. Schwalbe RS, Stapleton JT, Gilligan PH. Emergence of vancomycin resistance in coagulase-negative staphylococci. N Engl J Med 16:927, 1987.

431. Froggatt JW, Johnston JL, Galetto DW, et al. Antimicrobial resistance in nosocomial isolates of *Staphylococcus haemolyticus*. Antimicrob Agents Chemother 33:460, 1989.

432. Gill VJ, Manning CB, Ingalls CM. Correlation of penicillin minimum inhibitory concentrations and antibiotic susceptibilities of coagulase-negative staphylococcal isolated from clinical specimen. J Clin Microbiol 14:437, 1981.

433. Pfaller MA, Hewaldt LA. Laboratory, clinical and epidemiological aspects of coagulase-negative staphylococci. Clin Microbiol Rev 1:281, 1988.

434. Sabath LD. Chemical and physical factors influencing methicillin-resistance of *Staphylococcus aureus* and *Staphylococcus epidermidis*. J Antimicrob Chemother Suppl 3:47, 1977.

435. Archer GL. Antimicrobial susceptibility and selection of resistance among *Staphylococcus epidermidis* isolates recovered from patients with infections of indwelling foreign devices. Antimicrob Agents Chemother 14:353, 1978.

436. John JF Jr, McNeill WF. Activity of cephalosporins against methicillin-susceptible and methicillin-resistant coagulase-negative staphylococci: minimal effect of beta-lactamase. Antimicrob Agents Chemother 17:179, 1980.

437. Lowy FD, Hammer SM. *Staphylococcus epidermidis* infections. Ann Intern Med 99:834, 1983.

438. Arditi M, Yogev R. *In vitro* interactions between rifampin and clindamycin against pathogenic coagulase-negative staphylococci. Antimicrob Agents Chemother 33:245, 1989.

439. Massanari RM, Donta ST. The efficacy of rifampin as adjunctive therapy in selected cases of staphylococcal endocarditis. Chest 73:371, 1978.

440. Karchmer AW, Archer GL, Dismukes WE. *Staphylococcus* endocarditis prosthetic value endocarditis: microbiological and clinical observations as guide to therapy. Ann Intern Med 98:447, 1983.

441. Shurtleff DB, Foltz EL, Weeks RD, et al. Therapy of *Staphylococcus epidermidis*: infections associated with cerebrospinal fluid shunts. Pediatrics 53:55, 1974.

442. Lowy FD, Chang DS, Lash PR. Synergy of combinations of vancomycin, gentamicin, and rifampin against methicillin-resistant, coagulase-negative staphylococci. Antimicrob Agents Chemother 23:932, 1983.

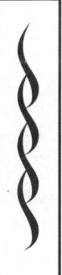

Microorganisms Responsible for Neonatal Diarrhea

THOMAS G. CLEARY, M.D., RICHARD L. GUERRANT, M.D., and LARRY K. PICKERING, M.D.

INTRODUCTION

Diarrheal diseases are second to respiratory tract infections as the most important cause of disability-adjusted years lost.[1–6] The U.S. Institute of Medicine estimated that the diarrheal case:fatality ratio in children younger

---

*In this chapter, references are numbered by section, starting with number one at the beginning of each major section. Headings in the list of references correspond to the major chapter sections.

than 5 years of age in developing countries was 0.2%.[7] The case:fatality ratio varies with age, being highest in youngest children. Estimates are that there are over 3 million deaths from diarrhea in children in developing countries each year with the rate being highest in the first year of life at 20 deaths per 1000 children.[2] Mortality rates decline with age and are lower after the first 5 years of life. These deaths account for 25% of all deaths in children younger than 5 years of age in developing countries.[4] In the United States, approximately 400 childhood deaths per year are reported,[8, 9] although the actual number may be higher.[9] Diarrheal diseases in children account for 2.1 to 3.7 million physician visits and 220,000 hospitalizations resulting in 924,000 hospital days and 10% of all hospitalizations for children younger than 5 years of age.[8] The morbidity rates in young children in the United States are two to three illnesses per child-year in children younger than 5 years of age or 21 to 36 million episodes per year among children younger than 5 years of age.[2, 10] Rates in children attending child care are higher.[11, 12] Overall rates of diarrhea in children in developing countries range from 3 to 15 illnesses per child-year among children younger than 5 years of age living in low socioeconomic conditions.[2, 13–15] In developing countries, diarrhea and malnutrition are closely related.[15, 16] The magnitude of the effect of diarrheal disease on growth in various studies has ranged from 10% to 80% of the growth retardation occurring in the first few years of life in comparison with an international reference population.[15] Perhaps because of breast-feeding in the neonatal period, deaths associated with this illness generally occur in infants older than 4 months of age, in whom the concept of weaning diarrhea is well-recognized.[17] The exception to this is the very low birth weight infant (<1500 g) in whom the death rate from diarrhea is 100-fold greater than in low- and normal-birth-weight (>1500 g) infants.[18]

This relative sparing of the newborn is probably the result of the interaction of several factors, including the almost universal practice of home delivery and breast-feeding in rural villages[19] and improved standards of education, sanitation, and medical care in many parts of the technologically more advanced nations. Worldwide, neonatal gastroenteritis occurs most commonly among the urban poor, who have rejected the protection afforded by older customs without acquiring the advantages available to the more affluent. Crowded together in large nurseries and later in tenements, where artificial feeding predominates, susceptible newborns are quickly thrust into an environment that provides ample opportunity for close and frequent exposure to enteric pathogens. As the incidence of neonatal gastroenteritis rises, there is a proportional increase in neonatal deaths because medical care for the poor is often unrecognized, unavailable, ignored, or inadequate.[4, 5]

The pathogenesis, diagnosis, treatment, and prevention of neonatal gastroenteritis are discussed in this chapter. Although emphasis is placed on currently recognized bacterial, fungal, parasitic, and viral enteropathogens, it has become increasingly necessary to recognize not just the organisms but also the virulence traits.[20, 21] Such traits as enterotoxin and cytotoxin production, invasiveness, and adherence are discussed in the section on *Escherichia coli*. This versatile species is capable of causing either prototypic inflammatory diarrhea, dysenteric colitis, or noninflammatory small bowel secretory diarrhea by totally different mechanisms, depending on the virulence traits, which are often encoded on transmissible plasmids.

Enteric Host Defense Mechanisms

Before specific causes of neonatal diarrhea are addressed, several general concepts about enteric host defense mechanisms are relevant to enteric infections, especially in the neonatal period. The neonate is a host that is uniquely susceptible to enteric infections. Not only have neonates not had the opportunity to develop local or systemic immune responses but, in the first few days of life, they have not yet acquired the highly important enteric flora that protects the normal adult gastrointestinal tract.[19, 22–24] Still less is known about the barrier effect of the neonate's gastric acidity,[25] intestinal mucus,[26] or motility,[27, 28] each of which provides protection against gastrointestinal tract infections. In many areas of the world the newborn infant is often fed formulas mixed with contaminated water, or, perhaps even worse, the critically ill newborn requires extensive antimicrobial and intensive care therapy, in which antibiotic-resistant nosocomial flora poses special risks.

The gastric acid barrier appears to be least effective during the first months of life. The average gastric pH of the newborn is high (pH 4 to 7; mean, 6).[29, 30] Although the pH falls to low levels by the end of the first day of life (pH 2 to 3),[29] it subsequently rises once again; by 7 to 10 days of life, the hydrochloric acid output of the neonatal stomach is far less than that of older infants and children.[30, 31] The buffering action of frequent milk feedings given to newborns and their short gastric emptying time[32–35] interpose additional factors that would be expected to permit most ingested organisms to reach the small intestine and thus would favor enteric infection.

Protective Factors in Human Milk

The importance of breast-feeding in prevention of diarrheal disease in infants has long been emphasized.[19, 36–49] Published studies reporting the association between breast-feeding and diarrhea are extensive and suggest that infants who are breast-fed suffer fewer episodes of diarrhea than those who are not. This protection is greatest during a child's first 3 months of life and declines with increasing age. During this period of weaning, partial breast-feeding confers protection that is intermediate between that gained by infants who are exclusively breast-fed and that by those who are exclusively bottle-fed.

A striking demonstration of the protection afforded by breast-feeding of newborns has been provided by Mata and Urrutia[19] in their studies of a population of infants born in a rural Guatemalan village. Despite extremely poor sanitation and the demonstration of fecal organisms in the colostrum and milk of almost a third of the mothers,[50] diarrheal disease did not occur in any newborns. The incidence of diarrhea rose significantly only after these infants reached 4 to 6 months of age, at which time solids and other fluids were used to supplement the human milk feedings. At this time *E. coli* and gram-negative anaerobes (*Bacteroides*) were noted to colonize the intestinal tract.[19] In contrast, urban infants of a similar ethnic background who were partly or totally artificially fed frequently acquired diarrheal disease caused by enteropathogenic *E. coli* (EPEC). An association between even limited supplementary bottle-feeding and the acquisition of infectious gastroenteritis has been noted frequently.

Several mechanisms by which breast-feeding protects

against diarrhea have been postulated. Methods of protection conferred by breast-feeding include the active components in human milk and the decreased exposure that a breast-fed infant has to organisms present on or in contaminated bottles, food, or water. Many protective components have been identified in human milk and generally are classified as belonging to the major categories of cells, antibody, anti-inflammatory factors, and glycoconjugates and other nonantibody factors.[51-54] Although many published studies of these potentially protective factors are descriptive in nature, others have shown by in vitro and in vivo experiments that various factors in milk interfere with or prevent many of the steps that occur in the pathogenesis of infection by bacteria, viruses, and parasites. In addition, the ability of human milk to initiate and maintain the growth of *Bifidobacterium* and low pH in the feces of newborn infants, thus creating an environment antagonistic to the growth of *E. coli*, has been shown.[19, 23, 24, 55]

Table 31–1 shows the association demonstrated between antibodies in human milk and protection against enteropathogens. The protective effect of human milk antibodies against enteropathogen-specific disease has been described for *Vibrio cholerae*,[56] *Campylobacter jejuni*,[57] EPEC,[58] enterotoxigenic *E. coli* (ETEC),[59, 60] *Shigella*,[61, 62] and *Giardia lamblia*[63, 64]; and for bovine milk concentrate, against ETEC,[65] rotavirus,[66] and *Shigella*.[67]

In 1933, the nonlactose carbohydrate fraction of human milk was found to consist mainly of oligosaccharides.[68] In 1960, Montreuil and Mullet[69] determined that up to 2.4% of colostrum and up to 1.3% of mature milk are oligosaccharides. Human milk contains a larger quantity of the oligosaccharides than does milk of other mammals, and its composition is singularly complex.[70] In 1970, Kobata and colleagues[71] described the synthesis of the milk oligosaccharides as being catalyzed by the same glycosyltransferases that function in the synthesis of the carbohydrate moieties of cellular glycolipids and glycoproteins. Enteropathogens use the oligosaccharide portion of glycolipids and glycoproteins as targets for attachment of whole bacteria and toxins. Evidence is emerging that these glycoconjugates could have an important role in protection of the breast-fed infant from disease.[52] Table 31–2 shows the association demonstrated

TABLE 31–2
Association Demonstrated Between Glycoconjugates in Human Milk and Protection Against Enteropathogens

ORGANISM	GLYCOCONJUGATES
Enterotoxigenic *Escherichia coli*	GM_1 ganglioside, glycoprotein
E. coli stable toxin, *Campylobacter jejuni*	Oligosaccharides
Enteropathogenic *E. coli*	Oligosaccharides
Shigella	Glycolipid Gb3
C. jejuni, *Vibrio cholerae*, *E. coli*	Glycolipids
Rotavirus	Lactadherin

between glycoconjugates in human milk and protection against enteropathogens.

The ganglioside fraction in human milk has been shown to inhibit the action of heat-labile toxin (LT) and cholera toxin on ileal loops more effectively than secretory IgA.[72, 73] Human milk protects suckling mice from the heat-stable enterotoxin (ST) of *E. coli*; on the basis of its chemical stability and physical properties, the protective factor was deduced to be a neutral fucosyloligosaccharide.[74, 75] Experiments have shown that EPEC attachment to HEp-2 cells can be inhibited by purified oligosaccharide fractions from human milk.[58] Globotriaosylceramide (Gb3), a glycolipid known to bind to both Shiga toxin and Shiga-like toxins, has been found in human milk and may contribute to the protective effect of human milk against infantile diarrhea associated with Shiga or Shiga-like toxin.[76] Lactadherin in human milk has been shown to bind to rotavirus and inhibit viral replication in vitro and in vivo.[77] A study of infants in Mexico showed that lactadherin in human milk protected infants from symptoms of rotavirus infection.[78]

The remainder of this chapter is devoted to several specific pathogens that cause inflammatory or noninflammatory diarrhea. The mainstay of management of all diarrheas is prompt and adequate fluid and electrolyte therapy followed by nutritional support.

ESCHERICHIA COLI

Nature of the Organism

E. coli promptly colonizes the lower intestinal tracts of healthy infants in their first few days of life[1-4] and constitutes the predominant aerobic coliform fecal flora throughout life in humans and in many animals. The concept that this species might cause enteric disease was first suggested in the late nineteenth and early twentieth centuries, when several veterinary workers described the association of diarrhea (scours) in newborn calves with certain strains of *E. coli*.[5-10]

In 1905, Moro[11] noted that *Bacterium coli* was found

TABLE 31–1
Association Demonstrated Between Antibodies in Human Milk and Protection Against Enteropathogens

ORGANISM	ANTIBODY
Vibrio cholerae	Lipopolysaccharide, enterotoxin
Campylobacter jejuni	Surface protein
Enteropathogenic *Escherichia coli*	Adherence protein
Enterotoxigenic *E. coli*	Enterotoxin, adherence proteins
Shigella	Lipopolysaccharide, virulence plasma-associated antigens
Giardia lamblia	Surface proteins

much more often in the small bowel of children with diarrhea than in children without diarrhea. Adam[12, 13] confirmed these findings and noted this similarity with Asiatic cholera and calf scours. He further extended these observations by suggesting that these *E. coli* strains could be separated from normal coliform flora by certain sugar fermentation patterns. Although he called these disease-producing organisms "dyspepsicoli" and thus initiated the important concept that *E. coli* could cause disease, their biochemical reactions have not proved to be a reliable means of distinguishing which *E. coli* are pathogenic. There are now evolving six or more pathogenic types of *E. coli* that cause diarrhea in infants and animals by apparently totally different mechanisms (Table 31–3).[14–20]

The first types of diarrheagenic *E. coli* are the two kinds of ETEC: those that produce an LT that acts like cholera toxin on intestinal adenylate cyclase,[21, 22] prostaglandin synthesis,[23, 24] and possibly platelet activating factor[25, 26] and those that produce a heat-stable enterotoxin (STa) that causes secretion by specifically activating intestinal mucosal guanylate cyclase.[27–29] Some types of *E. coli* produce both LT and STa. A third type of ETEC that causes noncyclic nucleotide-mediated bicarbonate secretion (STb) is important in neonatal animals, but its role in human disease remains unclear.[30–32] STa and STb are often grouped together and referred to as ST. The fourth type of *E. coli*, the enteroinvasive *E. coli* (EIEC), that causes diarrhea has the capacity to

invade the intestinal mucosa to cause an inflammatory enteritis much like shigellosis.[33, 34] The classically recognized EPEC types exhibit a characteristic localized pattern of adherence to HEp-2 cells with pedestal formation by mucosal epithelial cells or by HEp-2 cells in tissue culture. This localized EPEC adherence involves a complex array of plasmid-mediated adherence[14–18, 35, 36] followed by chromosomally mediated effacement, protein phosphorylation, and actin condensation in the host cell.[37] A second type of HEp-2 cell adherence is diffuse adherence, which is associated with diarrhea in older children in some areas[38, 39] but not in others.[40] A third type of adherence pattern is aggregative adherence or enteroaggregative adherence (EAggEC), in which bacteria adhere to cells alone or to cells plus glass or plastic. This type of adherence is associated with persistent diarrhea in several geographic areas and may cause intestinal inflammation, interleukin-8 (IL-8) release, and malnutrition.[19, 41–43] Some strains exhibiting each of these types of adherence can also be detected by one or more highly specific gene probes for specific adhesin or other traits.[44, 50] Another distinct group of *E. coli* is associated with enterohemorrhagic colitis (EHEC) and hemolytic-uremic syndrome and produces Shiga toxins.[51, 52] EHEC may also exhibit localized adherence to HEp-2 cells. Still other types of *E. coli* may cause diarrhea by a different mechanism of enteroadherence by colonization traits, hydrophobicity, or autoagglutination.[35, 53, 54]

A major problem in the recognition of ETEC, EIEC,

TABLE 31–3

Predominant Serogroups, Mechanisms, and Gene Codes Associated with Enterotoxigenic (ETEC), Enteroinvasive (EIEC), Enteropathogenic (EPEC), Enterohemorrhagic (EHEC), and Enteroaggregative (EAggEC) *Escherichia coli*

ETEC[a]	EIEC	EPEC	EHEC	EAggEC
LT	028ac	**"Class I"**	0157:H7	03:H2
06:K15	029, 0112	055:K59 (B5)	026:H11/H−	044
08:K40	0115, 0124	0111ab:K88 (B4)	0128, 0103:H2	078:H33
	0136, 0144	0119K6a (B14)	039	015:H11
LT and ST	0147, 0152	0125ac:K70 (B15)	0111:K58:H8/H−	077:H18
011:H27	0164	0126:K71 (B16)	0113:K75:H7/H21	051:H11
015, 020:K79		0127a:K63 (B8)	0121:H−, 0145:H−	and others
025:K7		0128abc:k67 (B12)	rough	
027, 063		0142, 0158	and others	
080, 085, 0139				
ST		**"Class II"**		
0 groups 78, 115		044:K74		
128, 148, 149, 153		086a:K61 (B7)		
159, 166, 167		0114:H2		
Mechanisms				
Adenylate or guanylate cyclase activation	Colonic invasiveness (like *Shigella*)	Localized attachment and effacement	Shigatoxins blocks protein synthesis	Aggregative adherence ?toxin (s)
Gene code(s)				
Plasmid	Plasmid	Chromosomal and plasmid	phage (? + chromosomal)	Plasmid (+ chromosomal)

[a]LT = heat-labile toxin; ST = heat-stable toxin.

EPEC, and EHEC strains of *E. coli* is that they are indistinguishable from normal coliform flora of the intestinal tract by the usual bacteriologic methods. Serotyping is of value in recognizing EPEC serotypes[55] and EIEC, because these organisms tend to fall into a limited number of specific serogroups[55, 56] (see Table 31–3). EIEC invasiveness is confirmed by inoculating fresh isolates into guinea pig conjunctivae, as described by Sereny.[57] The ability of organisms to produce enterotoxins (LT or ST) is encoded by a transmissible plasmid that can be lost by one strain of *E. coli* or transferred to a previously unrecognized strain.[58–60] Hence, although the enterotoxin plasmids do appear to prefer certain serogroups (that are different from EPEC or invasive serogroups, respectively),[61] one would not expect ETEC ever to be strictly limited to a particular set of serogroups. Instead, these strains can be recognized only by examining for the enterotoxin. This is done in ligated animal loops,[62] in tissue culture[63, 64] or by enzyme-linked immunosorbent assay (ELISA)[65] for LT or in suckling mice for ST.[66, 67] Specific DNA probes also are available for LT and ST.[47, 48] Whether there are yet other mechanisms involved in the ability of the versatile *E. coli* species to cause enteric disease, such as by producing other types of enterotoxins[68] or by fimbriate adherence traits alone,[35, 53, 69, 70] remains to be elucidated.

Enterotoxigenic *Escherichia coli*

Although early work on recognition of *E. coli* as a potential enteric pathogen focused on biochemical or serologic distinctions, there followed a shift in emphasis to the enterotoxins produced by previously recognized and entirely "new" strains of *E. coli*. Beginning in the mid-1950s with work by De and colleagues[71, 72] in Calcutta, *E. coli* strains from patients with diarrhea were found to cause a fluid secretory response in ligated rabbit ileal loops analogous to that seen with *V. cholerae*. Work by Taylor and associates[73, 74] showed that the viable *E. coli* strains were not required to produce this secretory response and that this enterotoxin production correlated poorly with classically recognized EPEC serotypes. In Sao Paulo, Trabulsi[75] made similar observations with *E. coli* isolated from children with diarrhea, and several veterinary workers demonstrated that ETEC was associated with diarrhea in piglets and calves.[76–79] A similar pattern was described in 1971 with acute undifferentiated diarrhea in adults in Bengal from whom *E. coli* could be isolated from the upper small bowel only during acute illness.[80, 81] These strains of *E. coli* produced a nondialyzable, heat-labile, ammonium sulfate–precipitable enterotoxin.[82]

Analogous to the usually short-lived diarrheal illnesses noted with *E. coli* by several workers, a short-lived time course of the secretory response to *E. coli* culture filtrates compared with the secretory response of cholera toxin was described.[22, 83] However, like responses to cholera toxin, secretory responses to *E. coli* were associated with activation of intestinal mucosal adenylate cyclase that paralleled the fluid secretory response.[21, 22, 84, 85]

The two types of enterotoxins produced by *E. coli*[86–88] have been found to be plasmid-encoded traits that are potentially separable from each other and from the equally important plasmid-encoded adherence traits for pathogenesis.[58–60, 89] It is now evident that ST causes an immediate and reversible secretory response,[62] whereas the effects of LT (like cholera toxin) follow a lag period and are relatively irreversible, perhaps depending on the renewal of gut epithelium.[21, 22, 63, 90, 91] It is also clear that only LT appears to cause fluid secretion by activating adenylate cyclase. The activation of adenylate cyclase by LT and by cholera toxin is highly promiscuous, occurring in many cell types, and resulting in development of nonintestinal tissue culture assay systems such as the Chinese hamster ovary (CHO) cell assay[63] and Y1 adrenal cell assay.[64] The antigenic similarity of LT and cholera toxin and their apparent binding to the monosialoganglioside GM_1 have enabled development of ELISAs for detection of LT and cholera toxin.[67, 92–94]

In contrast, ST fails to alter intracellular cyclic adenosine monophosphate (cAMP) concentration, is inactive in tissue culture assay systems used for LT or cholera toxin, and requires the suckling mouse bioassay for its detection.[66–67] ST is a much smaller molecule and is distinct antigenically from LT and cholera toxin. Although it fails to alter cAMP levels, ST has been shown to increase intracellular intestinal mucosal cyclic guanosine monophosphate (cGMP) concentrations and specifically activate intestinal guanylate cyclase.[27–29] Like cAMP analogues, cGMP analogues also cause intestinal secretion that mimics the response to ST.[27] Of considerable physiologic interest is the demonstration of ST effects in the kidney[95–98] and of ST-like compounds that activate guanylate cyclase isolated from mammalian intestine or kidney, demonstrating that ST has key counterparts in mammalian host cells.[99, 100]

Because the capacity to produce an enterotoxin may be transmissible between different organisms via a plasmid or even a bacteriophage,[58–60] one might expect that interstrain gene transfer may be responsible for occasional toxigenic non–*E. coli*. Indeed, enterotoxigenic *Klebsiella* and *Citrobacter* strains have been associated with diarrhea in a few reports, often in the same patients with ETEC.[100–102] Likewise, certain strains of *Salmonella* appear to produce a heat-labile, CHO cell–positive toxin that may play a similar role in the pathogenesis of watery, noninflammatory diarrhea sometimes seen with *Salmonella enteritidis* infection.[103, 104]

At least equally important as enterotoxigenicity for *E. coli* to cause disease is the ability of these organisms to colonize the upper small bowel, where the enterotoxin produced has its greatest effect. A separable, plasmid-encoded colonization trait was first recognized in the porcine *E. coli*. Veterinary workers demonstrated that the fimbriate K-88 surface antigen was necessary for ETEC to cause disease in piglets.[89] Furthermore, an autosomal dominant allele appears to be responsible for the specific intestinal receptor in piglets. In elegant studies by Gibbons and co-workers, the homozygous recessive piglets lacked the receptor for K-88 and were thus resistant to scours caused by ETEC.[105] At least five to seven analogous colonization factors have been described for human *E. coli* isolates[52, 69, 106–110] against which local IgA antibody may be produced. These antigens may potentially be useful in vaccine development.[111]

EPIDEMIOLOGY AND TRANSMISSION

Data on the epidemiology and transmission of ETEC remain scanty for the neonatal period. In the past two decades, these strains have been recognized among adults with endemic, cholera-like diarrhea in Calcutta and Dacca, Bangladesh[21, 80] and among travelers to areas such as Mexico and Central Africa.[112–114] Travelers to tropical areas have a 50% risk of acquiring a diarrheal illness, or *turista*, within 3 weeks of travel, most of which occurs during the second week after arrival and appears to be associated with ETEC.

The isolation of ETEC is uncommon in sporadic diarrheal illnesses in temperate climates where sanitation facilities are good and where winter viral patterns of diarrhea predominate. ETEC is commonly isolated from infants and children with acute watery summer diarrhea in areas where sanitary facilities are less than optimal.[101, 114–127] These include areas such as Africa,[101] Brazil,[114, 120, 125–127] Argentina,[116] Bengal,[117, 118] Mexico,[119] and Native American reservations in the southwestern United States.[121, 122] In a multicenter study of acute diarrhea among 3640 infants and children in China, India, Mexico, Myanmar, and Pakistan, 16% of cases (versus 5% of 3279 controls) had ETEC.[123] Furthermore, a case-control study from northwestern Spain showed a highly significant association of ETEC with 26.5% of neonatal diarrhea, often acquired in the hospital.[124] Although all types of ETEC (LT and ST, and LT or ST only) are associated with cholera-like noninflammatory watery diarrhea in adults in these areas, they probably constitute the major cause (along with rotaviruses) of dehydrating diarrhea in young children and infants in these areas as well. In this setting, peaks of illnesses tend to occur in the summer or rainy season and dehydrating illnesses may be life-threatening, especially in infants and small children.[120, 125, 126] Humans are probably the major reservoirs for the human strains of ETEC, and contaminated food and water probably constitute the principal vectors.[128–130] Although antitoxic immunity to LT and asymptomatic infection with LT-producing *E. coli* tend to increase with age, ST is poorly immunogenic and ST-producing *E. coli* continues to be associated with symptomatic illnesses into adulthood in endemic areas.[122, 127]

The association of ETEC with outbreaks of diarrhea in newborn nurseries is also well documented. Ryder and colleagues[131] isolated an ST-producing *E. coli* from 72% of infants with diarrhea as well as from the environment, and, in one instance, from an infant's formula, during a 7-month period in a prolonged outbreak in a special care nursery in Texas. Another ST-producing *E. coli* outbreak was reported in 1976 by Gross and associates[132] from a maternity hospital in Scotland. Furthermore, ETEC and EPEC were significantly associated with diarrhea among infants younger than 1 year of age in Bangladesh.[133]

An outbreak of diarrhea in a newborn special care nursery that was associated with enterotoxigenic organisms that were not limited to the same serotype or even the same species has also been reported.[100] The transiently ETEC, *Klebsiella*, and *Citrobacter* species in this outbreak raised the possibility that each infant's indigenous bowel flora might become transiently toxigenic, possibly by receiving the LT genome from a plasmid or even a bacteriophage.

CLINICAL MANIFESTATIONS

The clinical manifestations of ETEC diarrhea tend to be mild and self-limited, except in small or undernourished infants, in whom dehydration may constitute a major threat to life. Indeed, in many parts of the developing world, acute diarrheal illnesses are the leading recognized causes of death. There is some suggestion that the diarrheal illnesses associated with ETEC, especially ST-producing *E. coli*, may be more severe.[118]

Probably the best definition of the clinical manifestations of ETEC infection comes from volunteer studies with adults. Ingestion of 10^8 to 10^{10} human ETEC isolates that produce LT and ST or ST alone resulted in a 30 to 80% attack rate of mild to moderate diarrheal illnesses within 12 to 56 hours that lasted 1 to 3 days.[33, 134] These illnesses, typical for traveler's diarrhea, were manifested by malaise, anorexia, abdominal cramps, and sometimes explosive diarrhea. Nausea and vomiting occur relatively infrequently, and up to one third of patients may have a low-grade fever. Although illnesses usually resolve spontaneously within 1 to 5 days, they occasionally may persist for 1 week or longer. The diarrhea is noninflammatory, without fecal leukocytes or blood. In outbreaks in infants and neonates, the duration has been in the same range (1 to 11 days), with a mean of approximately 4 days.

PATHOLOGY

As in cholera, the pathologic changes associated with ETEC infection are minimal. From animal experiments in which Thiry-Vella loops were infected with these organisms and at a time when the secretory and adenylate cyclase responses were present, there was only a mild discharge of mucus from goblet cells and otherwise no significant pathologic change in the intestinal tract.[22] As previously noted, unless terminal complications of severe hypotension ensue, ETEC organisms rarely disseminate beyond the intestinal tract. Like cholera, ETEC diarrhea is typically limited to being an intraluminal infection.

DIAGNOSIS

The preliminary diagnosis of ETEC diarrhea can be suspected by the epidemiologic setting and the noninflammatory nature of stool specimens, which reveal few, if any, leukocytes. Although the ability of *E. coli* to produce enterotoxins may be lost or transmitted to other strains, there is a tendency for the enterotoxin plasmids to occur among certain predominant serotypes, as shown in Table 31–3.[135] These serotypes differ from either

EPEC or invasive serotypes, and their demonstration does not prove that they are enterotoxigenic.

The only definitive way to identify ETEC at present is to demonstrate the enterotoxin itself by a specific gene probe for the toxin codon or by a bioassay such as tissue culture or ileal loop assays for LT or the suckling mouse assay for ST or, in the case of LT, by immunoassay such as ELISA. However, it should be remembered that even these sensitive bioassays are limited by the unavailability of any selective media for culturing ETEC. Even though substantial improvements have been made in enterotoxin assay (particularly for LT), the necessary random selection of *E. coli* from a relatively nonselective stool culture plate resulted in a sensitivity of only 43% of epidemiologically incriminated cases in an outbreak when 5 to 10 isolates were randomly picked and tested for enterotoxigenicity.[129] By also examining paired serum samples for antitoxic antibody against LT, only 36% demonstrated significant serum antibody titer rises, for a total sensitivity of either ETEC isolation or serum antibody titer rises of only 64%. Some have suggested that isolates may be pooled for either LT or ST assay. The capacity to prove with radiolabeled or enzyme-tagged oligonucleotide gene sequences for the enterotoxins (LT or ST) now further facilitates the identification of enterotoxigenic organisms.[136, 137] A novel method of combining immunomagnetic separation (using antibody-coated magnetic beads) followed by DNA or even polymerase chain reaction (PCR) probing may enhance the sensitivity of screening fecal or food specimens for ETEC or other pathogens.[138, 139]

THERAPY AND PREVENTION

As discussed later under EPEC therapy, the mainstay of treatment of any diarrheal illness is rehydration.[140] This especially pertains to ETEC diarrhea, which is an intraluminal infection. The glucose absorptive mechanism remains intact in *E. coli* enterotoxin-induced secretion, much as it does in cholera, a concept that has resulted in the major advance of oral glucose-electrolyte therapy. This regimen can usually provide fully adequate rehydration in infants and children able to tolerate oral fluids, replacing the need for parenteral rehydration in most cases.[141, 142] Its use is particularly critical in rural areas and developing nations, where early application before dehydration becomes severe may be lifesaving.

The standard World Health Organization solution contains 3.5 g NaCl, 2.5 g $NaHCO_3$, 1.5 g KCl, and 20 g glucose per liter of clean or boiled drinking water.[140] This corresponds to (millimoles per liter): sodium, 90; potassium, 20; bicarbonate, 30; chloride, 80; and glucose, 110. A variety of recipes for homemade preparations have been described[143] but unless the cost is prohibitive, the premade standard solution is preferred. Each 4 ounces of this solution should be followed by 2 ounces of plain water. If there is concern about hypertonicity, especially in small infants in whom a high intake and constant direct supervision of feeding cannot be ensured, the concentration of salt can be reduced.[144] Indeed a reduced osmolality solution with 60 mmol sodium and 84 mmol glucose per liter and a total osmol-

ality of 224 (instead of 311) mOsm/kg has been found to reduce stool output by 28% and illness duration by 18% in a multicenter trial involving 447 children in four different countries.[145] Commercially available rehydration solutions are generally used in the United States.[140]

The role of antimicrobial agents in the treatment or prevention of ETEC is unclear at present. As noted, this illness usually does not require antimicrobial therapy. Furthermore, there is concern about the potential for coexistence of enterotoxigenicity and antibiotic resistance on the same plasmid, and, indeed, co-transfer of multiple antibiotic resistance and enterotoxigenicity has been well documented.[146] Therefore, widespread use of prophylactic antibiotics in areas where antimicrobial resistance is common has the potential for selecting for rather than against enterotoxigenic organisms. As discussed later for EPEC diarrhea, prolonged refractory illness may warrant empirical antimicrobial therapy.

The prevention and control of ETEC infections would be similar to those discussed under EPEC serotypes. In addition, the use of breast-feeding whenever possible should be encouraged.

Enteroinvasive *Escherichia coli*

There is a group of virulent *E. coli* that causes diarrhea by means of *Shigella*-like intestinal epithelial invasion.[33, 34] The somatic antigens of these invasive strains have been identified and seem to fall into 1 of 10 recognized O groups (see Table 31–3). Most, if not all, of these bacteria share cell wall antigens with one or another of the various *Shigella* serotypes and produce positive reactions with antisera against the cross-reacting antigen.[34] However, not all strains of *E. coli* belonging to the 10 serogroups associated with dysentery-like illness are pathogenic, because a large (140 MDa) invasive plasmid is also required.[147] Therefore, additional biologic tests, including the guinea pig conjunctivitis (Sereny) test, or a gene probe for the plasmid, are used to confirm the property of invasiveness.[33]

Although an outbreak of foodborne EIEC diarrhea has been well documented among adults who ate an imported cheese,[34] little is known about the epidemiology and transmission of this organism, especially in newborns and infants. Whether the infectious dose may be as low as it is for *Shigella* is not known; however, adult volunteer studies suggest that attack rates may be somewhat lower after ingestion of even large numbers of EIEC than one would expect with *Shigella*.

The outbreak of EIEC diarrhea resulted in a dysentery-like syndrome with an inflammatory exudate in stool and invasion and disruption of colonic mucosa.[34] Descriptions of extensive and severe ileocolitis in infants dying with *E. coli* diarrhea indicate that neonatal disease may also be caused by invasive strains capable of mimicking the pathologic features of shigellosis.[148] The immunofluorescent demonstration of *E. coli* together with an acute inflammatory infiltrate[149] in the intestinal tissue of infants tends to support this impression, although it has been suggested that the organisms may have invaded the bowel wall in the postmortem period.[33] There is still little direct evidence concerning the role of invasive strains of *E. coli* in the etiology of neonatal diarrhea.[114] The infrequency with which newborns manifest a dysentery-like syndrome makes it unlikely that this pathogen is responsible for a very large proportion of the diarrheal disease that occurs during the first month of life.

The diagnosis should be suspected in infants who have an inflammatory diarrhea as evidenced by fecal polymorphonuclear neutrophils or even bloody dysenteric syndromes from whom no other invasive pathogens, such as *Campylobacter, Shigella, Salmonella, Vibrio,* or *Yersinia,* can be isolated. In this instance, it may be appropriate to have the fecal *E. coli* isolated and serotyped or tested for invasiveness in the Sereny test. Plasmid pattern analysis and chromosomal restriction endonuclease digestion pattern analysis by pulsed-field gel electrophoresis have been used to evaluate strains involved in outbreaks.[150]

The management and prevention of EIEC diarrhea should be similar to those for acute *Shigella* or other *E. coli* enteric infections.

Enteropathogenic *Escherichia coli* (Classic Serotypes)

The serologic distinction of *E. coli* strains associated with epidemic and sporadic infantile diarrhea was first suggested by Goldschmidt in 1933[151] and confirmed by Dulaney and Michelson in 1935.[152] These researchers found that certain strains of *E. coli* that were associated with institutional outbreaks of diarrhea would agglutinate with antisera on slides. In 1943, Bray[153] isolated a serologically homogeneous strain of *E. coli* (subsequently identified as serogroup 0111) from 95% of infants with summer diarrhea in England. He subsequently summarized a larger experience with this organism isolated from only 4% of asymptomatic controls but from 88% of infants with diarrhea, half of which was hospital-acquired.[154] This strain (initially called *E. coli-gomez* by Varela in 1946) was also associated with infantile diarrhea in Mexico.[155] A second type of *E. coli* (called "beta" by Giles in 1948 and subsequently identified as 055) was associated with an outbreak of infantile diarrhea in Aberdeen, Scotland.[156, 157]

From this early work primarily on epidemic diarrhea in infants has developed an elaborate serotyping system for certain *E. coli* strains that were clearly associated with infantile diarrhea.[158–160] These strains were first termed enteropathogenic *E. coli* by Neter and colleagues[161] in 1955. The relationship of these EPEC serotypes to those that cause disease by invading the urinary tract, bloodstream, or cerebrospinal fluid remains unclear.[162–165] As noted in Table 31–1, these organisms are distinct from the enterotoxigenic or enteroinvasive organisms or those that inhabit the normal gastrointestinal tract. They exhibit localized HEp-2 cell adherence and the plasmid pMAR-2.[166] EHEC produces high levels of Shiga toxins and is discussed separately.[38, 39]

EPIDEMIOLOGY AND TRANSMISSION

Despite a large number of reports indicating that EPEC has been frequently shown to be a common identifiable cause of infantile gastroenteritis,[163, 167–172] illness caused by these organisms is rarely recognized as such by the practicing pediatrician. EPEC is, however, still an important cause of diarrhea in infants in developing or transitional countries.[16, 42, 172–176] Some have attributed the rarity of this recognition of illness in part to the declining severity of diarrheal disease caused by EPEC within the past 30 years, resulting in fewer cultures being obtained from infants with relatively mild symptoms.[177–180] There are, however, several other variables that influence the apparent incidence of this disease in the community.

A problem arises with "false-positive EPEC" on the basis of nonspecific cross-reactions noted with improper shortening of the serotyping procedure.[181, 182] Because of their complexity and relatively low yield, neither slide agglutination nor HEp-2 cell adherence nor DNA probe tests are provided as part of the routine identification of enteric pathogens by many clinical bacteriology laboratories. Failure to recognize the presence of EPEC in fecal specimens is the inevitable consequence.

The apparent incidence of EPEC gastroenteritis also varies with the epidemiologic circumstances under which stool cultures are obtained. The prevalence of enteropathogenic strains will obviously be higher among infants from whom cultures are obtained during a community epidemic compared with those obtained during sporadic diarrheal disease. Neither reflects the incidence of EPEC infection among infants involved in a nursery outbreak or hospital epidemic.

EPEC gastroenteritis is a worldwide problem, and socioeconomic conditions play a significant role in determining the incidence of this disease among different populations.[183] It is, for instance, unusual for newborn infants born in a rural environment to manifest diarrheal disease caused by EPEC; most infections of the gastrointestinal tract in these infants occur after the first 6 months of life.[184, 185] Conversely, among infants born in large cities, the attack rate of EPEC is high during the first 3 months of life. This age distribution reflects, in large part, the frequency with which EPEC causes cross-infection outbreaks among nursery populations[186–194]; however, a predominance of EPEC in infants in the first 3 months of life has also been described in community epidemics[195–197] and among sporadic cases of diarrhea acquired outside the hospital.[1, 198–204] The disparity in the incidence of neonatal EPEC infection between rural and urbanized societies has been ascribed to two factors[184, 185, 205]: (1) the trend away from breast-feeding among mothers in industrialized societies and (2) the crowding together of susceptible newborns in nurseries in those countries in which hospital deliveries predominate over home deliveries. Although the predominant serogroup may vary from year to year,[196, 199, 200, 203, 206, 207] the same strains have been prevalent during the past 40 years in Great Britain,[208] Puerto Rico,[209] Argentina,[167] Guatemala,[185] Panama,[210] Israel,[204] Newfoundland,[197] Indonesia,[201] Thailand,[211] Uganda,[212] and South Africa.[213]

When living conditions are poor and overcrowding of susceptible infants exists, there is a rise in the incidence of both neonatal diarrhea in general[214] and EPEC gastroenteritis in particular.[157, 195, 215] A higher incidence of asymptomatic family carriers also is found in such situations.[195, 196]

Newborn infants can acquire EPEC during the first days of life by one of several routes: (1) organisms from the mother ingested at the time of birth; (2) bacteria from other infants or toddlers with diarrheal disease, commonly transmitted on the hands of nursery personnel or parents; (3) bacteria from the contaminated hands of asymptomatic adults or older children who are secreting EPEC; (4) airborne or droplet infection; (5) fomites; or (6) organisms present in formulas or solid food supplements.[216] Only the first two routes have been shown conclusively to be of any real significance in the transmission of disease or the propagation of epidemics.

Most neonates acquire EPEC at the time of delivery through ingestion of organisms residing in the maternal birth canal or rectum. Stool cultures taken from women before, during, or shortly after delivery have shown that 10 to 15% carry EPEC at some time during this period.[1, 2, 4, 217, 218] Use of fluorescent antibody techniques[218] or cultures during a community outbreak of EPEC gastroenteritis[4] may reveal twice this number of persons excreting the organism. Virtually none of the women carrying pathogenic strains of E. coli had symptoms referable to the gastrointestinal tract.

Many of the mothers whose stools contain EPEC transmit these organisms to their infants,[1, 4] resulting in an asymptomatic infection rate of 2 to 5% among newborns cultured at random in nursery surveys.[1, 2, 195, 219] These results must be considered conservative and are probably an artifact of the sampling technique. One study using 150 O antisera to identify as many E. coli as possible in fecal cultures showed a correlation between the coliform flora in 66% of mother-infant pairs.[220] Of particular interest was the observation that the O groups of E. coli isolated from the infants' mucus immediately after delivery correlated with those subsequently recovered from their stools, supporting the contention that these organisms were acquired orally at the time of birth. In mothers whose stools contained the same O group as their offspring, the mean time from rupture of membranes to delivery was about 2 hours longer than in those whose infants did not acquire the same serogroups, suggesting that ascending colonization before birth also may play a role in determining the newborn's fecal flora.

The contours of the epidemiologic curves in both nursery[192, 221–226] and community[195–197] outbreaks are in keeping with a contact mode of spread. Transmission of organisms from one infant to another takes place by way of the fecal-oral route in almost all cases, most likely on the hands of persons attending to their care.[2, 224, 226, 227] Symptomatic infants represent the greatest risk to those around them because of the large numbers of organisms found in their stools[228–231] and vomitus.[232–234] Cross-infection also has been initiated by infants who were asymptomatic at the time of their admission to the nursery.[199–219, 221, 229, 235–237]

A newborn exposed to EPEC is likely to acquire enteric infection if contact with a person excreting the organism is intimate and prolonged, as in a hospital or family setting. Stool culture surveys taken during outbreaks have shown that between 20% and 50% of full-term neonates residing in the nursery carry EPEC in their intestinal tracts.[186, 187, 190, 222, 229] Despite descriptions of nursery outbreaks in which virtually every neonate or low-birth-weight infant became infected,[219, 221, 238] there is ample evidence that exposure to pathogenic strains of E. coli does not necessarily result in greater likelihood of illness for premature infants than for term infants.[218, 229, 236, 239] Any increased prevalence of cross-infections that may exist among premature infants can be explained more readily by the prolonged hospital stays, the increased handling, and the clustering of infants born in different institutions than by a particular susceptibility to EPEC based on immature defense mechanisms.

The most extensive studies on the epidemiology of gastroenteritis related to E. coli have dealt with events that took place during cross-infection outbreaks in newborn nurseries. Unfortunately, investigations of this sort frequently regard the nosocomial epidemic as an isolated phenomenon and ignore the strong interdependence that exists between community- and hospital-acquired illness.[177, 200, 237, 240, 241] Not surprisingly, the direction of spread is most often from the reservoir of disease within the community to the hospital. Thus, when the original source of a nursery outbreak can be established, it frequently turns out to be an infant born of a carrier mother who recently acquired her EPEC infection from a toddler living in the home. Cross-infection epidemics may also be initiated by infected newborns who have been admitted directly into a clean nursery unit from the surrounding district[227, 229, 242] or have been transferred from a nearby hospital.[204, 234, 235, 237, 243]

After a nursery epidemic has begun, it generally follows one of two major patterns. Some are explosive, with rapid involvement of all susceptible infants and a duration that seldom exceeds 2 or 3 months.[186, 221, 222, 233, 244] The fatality rate in these epidemics may be very high. Other nursery outbreaks start insidiously with a few mild, unrecognized cases; the patients may not even develop symptoms until after discharge from the hospital. During the next few days to weeks, neonates with an increased number of loose stools are reported by the nurses; shortly thereafter, the appearance of the first severely ill infants makes it apparent that a full-scale epidemic has been developing. Unless oral antimicrobial therapy is instituted (see Therapy section), nursery outbreaks like these may continue for months[189, 192, 223–227, 236, 241, 244] or years,[227] with cycles of illness followed by periods of relative quiescence. This pattern may be due to multiple strains (of different phage or antibiogram types) sequentially introduced into the nursery.[214, 235, 245, 246]

The nursery may be a source of infection for the community. The release of infants who either are in the incubation stages of their illness or are convalescent carriers about to relapse may lead to secondary cases of diarrheal disease among young siblings living in widely scattered areas.[1, 195, 196, 200] In turn, these children further disseminate infection to neighboring households, involving playmates of their own age, young infants, and mothers.[195, 196, 199] As the sickest of these contact cases are admitted to different hospitals, they contaminate new susceptible persons, thus completing the cycle and compounding the outbreak. This feedback mechanism has proved to be a means of spreading infantile gastroenteritis through entire cities,[157, 195, 196, 199] counties,[196, 242, 247] and even provinces.[197] One major epidemic of diarrhea related to EPEC 0111:B4 that occurred in the metropolitan Chicago–northwestern Indiana region during the winter of 1961 involved more than 1300 children and 29 community hospitals during a period of 9 months.[196, 248] Almost all of the patients were younger than 2 years of age, and 10% were younger than 1 month, producing an age-specific attack rate of close to 4% of neonates in the community. The importance of the hospital as a source of cross-infection in this epidemic was demonstrated through interviews with patients' families, indicating that a minimum of 40% of infants had either direct or indirect contact with a hospital shortly before the onset of their illness.

It has been suggested, but not proved, that asymptomatic carriers of EPEC in close contact with a newborn infant, such as nursery personnel or family members, might play an important role in its transmission.[177, 196, 200, 237, 241, 249] Stool culture surveys have shown that, at any one time, about 1% of adults[199, 250] and 1 to 5% of young children[2, 163, 169, 186, 195, 200, 201, 211, 212] who are free of illness harbor EPEC strains. Higher percentages have been recorded during community epidemics.[195, 196, 200] Because this intestinal carriage is transitory,[195, 237] the number of individuals who excrete EPEC at one time or another during the year is far higher than the 1% figure recorded for single specimens.[237, 250]

Nursery personnel feed, bathe, and diaper a constantly changing population of newborns, about 2 to 5% of whom excrete EPEC.[1, 2, 195, 237] Despite this constant exposure, intestinal carriage among nursery workers is surprisingly low. Even during outbreaks of diarrheal illness, when dissemination of organisms is most intense, less than 5% of the hospital staff in direct contact with infected neonates are themselves excreting pathogenic strains of E. coli.[187, 221, 224, 233, 239, 248, 251, 252]

Although adult asymptomatic carriers generally excrete fewer organisms than patients with acute illness,[229] large numbers of pathogenic bacteria may, nevertheless, be present in their stools.[199, 231] Yet no nursery outbreak and few family cases[197] have been traced to a symptomless carrier. Instead, passive transfer of bacteria from one infant to another on the hands of personnel appears to be of primary importance in these outbreaks.

EPEC can be recovered from the throat or nose of 5 to 80% of infants with diarrheal illness[163, 167, 188, 196, 224, 232, 251, 252] and from about 1% of asymptomatic infants.[188, 200] The throat and nasal mucosa may represent a portal of entry or a source of transmission for EPEC. Environmental studies have shown that EPEC is distributed readily and widely in the vicinity of an infant with active diarrheal disease, often within 1 day of admission to the ward.[188, 253] Massive numbers of organisms are shed in the diarrheal stool or vomitus of infected infants.[206, 253] Those E. coli organisms may survive 2 to 4 weeks in dust[200, 253] and can be found in the nursery air when the bedding or diapers of infected infants are disturbed during routine nursing procedures[188, 200, 253] or on floors, walls, and cupboards, as well as on nursery equipment such as scales, hand towels, bassinets, incubators, and oxygen tents of other infants.[4, 200, 224, 253] Documentation of the presence of EPEC in nursery air and dust does not, however, establish the importance of this route as a source of cross-infection. One study presented evidence of the respiratory transmission of EPEC; however, even in the cases described, the authors pointed out that fecal-oral transmission could not be completely ruled out.[195] More clinical and experimental data are required to clarify the significance of droplet and environmental infection.

Coliform organisms have also been isolated in significant numbers from human milk,[217, 254–256] prebottled infant formulas,[257] and formulas prepared in the home.[249] EPEC in particular has been found in stool cultures obtained from donors of human milk and workers in a nursery formula room.[217] In one instance, EPEC 0111:B4 was isolated from a donor, and subsequently the same serogroup was recovered in massive amounts in almost pure culture from her milk.[217] Pathogenic strains of E. coli have also been isolated from raw cow's milk[258] and from drinking water.[259] Likewise, EPEC has been isolated from flies during an epidemic, but this has not been shown to be of epidemiologic significance.[152, 163]

PATHOGENESIS

Infection of the newborn infant with EPEC takes place exclusively by the fecal-oral route. Attempts to induce disease in adult volunteers by rectal instillation of infected material have been unsuccessful.[259] There are no reports of disease occurring after transplacental invasion of the fetal bloodstream by either enteropathogenic or nonenteropathogenic strains of E. coli. Ascending intrauterine infection after prolonged rupture of the membranes has been reported only once; the neonate in this case suffered only from mild diarrhea.[2]

Bacterial cultures of the meconium and feces of newborns indicate that enteropathogenic strains of E. coli can colonize effectively the intestinal tract in the first days of life.[1–4] Although E. coli may disappear completely from stools of breast-fed children during the ensuing weeks, this disappearance is believed to be related to factors present in the human milk rather than the gastric secretions.[185, 260, 261] The use of breast-feeding or expressed human milk has even been effective in terminating nursery epidemics caused by EPEC 0111:B4, probably by reducing the incidence of cross-infections among infants.[262, 263] Although dose-effect studies have not been performed among newborns, severe diarrhea has occurred after ingestion of 10^8 EPEC organisms by very young infants.[264, 265] The high incidence of cross-infection outbreaks in newborn nurseries suggests that a far lower inoculum can often effect spread in this setting.

The role of circulating immunity in the prevention of gastrointestinal tract disease related to EPEC has not been clearly established. Virtually 100% of maternal sera have been found to contain hemagglutinating,[161, 266–270] bactericidal,[264, 269] or bacteriostatic[237, 271] antibodies against EPEC. The passive transfer of these antibodies across the placenta is extremely inefficient. Titers in blood of newborn infants are, on average, 4 to 100 times lower than those in the corresponding maternal sera. Group-specific hemagglutinating antibodies against the O antigen of EPEC are present in 10 to 20% of cord blood samples,[161, 266–271] whereas bactericidal[266, 270] or bacteriostatic[270] activity against these organisms can be found much more frequently. Tests for bacterial agglutination, which are relatively insensitive, are positive in only a small percentage of neonates.[161, 270]

The importance of circulating antibodies in the susceptibility of infants to EPEC infection is unknown. Experiments with suckling mice have failed to demonstrate any effect of humoral immunity on the establishment or course of duration of intestinal colonization with E. coli 0127 in mothers or their infants.[272] Similar observations have been made in epidemiologic studies among premature human infants using both enteropathogenic (0127:B8)[269] and nonenteropathogenic (04:H5)[226] strains of E. coli as the indicator organisms. It is of interest that in a cohort of 63 mothers and their infants followed from birth to 3 months of age, Cooper and associates[1] were able to show a far higher incidence of clinical EPEC disease in infants of EPEC-negative mothers than in infants born of mothers with positive EPEC stool cultures. This finding suggested to the authors the possibility that mothers harboring EPEC in their gastrointestinal tracts transfer specific antibodies to their infants that may confer some protection during the first weeks of life.

Protection against enteric infections in humans often correlates more closely with levels of local secretory antibodies than with serum antibody titers. Although it is known that colonization of newborns with E. coli leads to the production of coproantibodies against the ingested organisms,[273, 274] the clinical significance of this intestinal immunity is uncertain. The previously mentioned experiment with mice showed no effect of active intestinal immunity on enteric colonization.[272] In human infants, the frequency of bacteriologic and clinical relapse related to EPEC of the same serotype[157, 190, 221, 222, 236] and the capacity of one strain of EPEC to superinfect a patient already harboring a different strain[204, 215, 225] also cast some doubt on the ability of mucosal antibodies to inhibit or alter the course of intestinal infection. Studies on the protective effects of orally administered EPEC vaccines may help to resolve these questions.[177, 205]

The mechanism by which EPEC causes diarrhea involves a complex array of plasmid and chromosomally encoded traits. EPEC serotypes usually do not make one of the recognized enterotoxins (LT or ST) as usually measured in tissue culture or animal models,[275–279] nor do these serotypes cause a typical invasive colitis or positive Sereny test.[274, 275] Only relatively rarely do EPEC strains invade the bloodstream or disseminate.[245] Nevertheless, EPEC strains that are negative in the above tests are capable of causing diarrhea; inocula of 10^{10} E. coli 0142 or 0127 organisms caused diarrhea in 8 to 10 adult volunteers.[279] Researchers have been variably successful at demonstrating a cytotoxic or an enterotoxic effect of broth culture filtrates of EPEC on Vero cells[280] and in rat jejunum,[68] respectively. One report of an infant with protracted watery diarrhea with E. coli 0125 revealed the organism closely adherent to the small

bowel mucosal brush border with associated local destruction of the microvillous brush border, villus blunting, crypt hypertrophy, histiocytic infiltration in the lamina propria, and a reduction in the brush border enzymes,[15] analogous to that of the rabbit diarrhea E. coli described by Cantey and Blake.[281] Others have continued to show this close attachment of EPEC to the villous epithelium with effacement of the brush border epithelial surface in infants[282] and in experimental animals.[283, 284] Furthermore, this type of close attachment with host cell "pedicle" formation has been seen with the focal HEp-2 cell adherence by EPEC in tissue culture, the trait that has been associated with the 60-MDa plasmid pMAR-2, which seems to be critical to the capacity of most EPEC to cause diarrhea.[16, 35, 166] Furthermore, the 50- to 60-MDa plasmid in EPEC encodes inducible, bundle-forming pili that share amino-terminal sequence homology with toxin-coregulated pili in V. cholerae and are responsible for efficient adherence to HEp-2 cells in "localized" colonies.[285–287] Following colonization by plasmid-encoded, bundle-forming pili,[287] a 90-kDa bacterial protein cell Tir (translocated intimin receptor, formerly thought to be a host protein, Hp90) is transferred into the host cell where it is tyrosine-phosphorylated to be readied to act as the receptor for yet another bacterial product intimin (94 kDa) that triggers actin condensation, pedestal formation, and intimate adherence. The genes for the locus of enterocyte effacement traits are encoded with a type III secretion system on the chromosome and include many of these strains.[36, 37] The role of intracellular calcium-induced protein phosphorylation by a heat-labile product is unclear at present.[288, 289]

PATHOLOGY

The principal pathologic lesion with EPEC is the focal destructive adherence of the organism, effacing the microvillous brush border with villus blunting, crypt hypertrophy, histiocytic infiltration of the lamina propria, and reduced brush border enzymes as described earlier. Rothbaum and colleagues[282] described similar findings with dissolution of the glycocalyx and flattened microvilli with the nontoxigenic EPEC strain 0119:B14. There has been a wide range of pathologic findings reported in infants dying of EPEC gastroenteritis. Most newborns dying with diarrheal disease caused by EPEC show no morphologic changes of the gastrointestinal tract on either gross or microscopic examination of tissues.[151, 152, 157, 223] Bray described such "meager" changes in the intestinal tract that "the impression received was that the term gastroenteritis is incorrect."[153] At the other extreme, extensive and severe involvement of the intestinal tract, although distinctly unusual among neonates with EPEC diarrhea, has been noted in several reviews of the pathologic anatomy of this disease.[204, 278, 290] Changes virtually identical to those found in infants dying with necrotizing enterocolitis have been reported.[290] Drucker and co-workers noted that among 17 infants who were dying of EPEC diarrhea, "intestinal gangrene, and/or perforation, and/or peritonitis were present in five, and intestinal pneumatosis in five."[278]

The reasons for such wide discrepancies are not clear. The severity of intestinal lesions at the time of death does not correlate with the birth weight of the patient, the age of onset of illness, the serogroup of the infecting strain, or the prior administration of oral or systemic antimicrobial agents. The suggestion that the intensity of inflammatory changes might depend on the duration of the diarrhea[278] cannot be corroborated in either autopsy studies[157, 186, 219, 221, 291] or small intestinal biopsies.[292, 293] Furthermore, it is difficult to reconcile such a thesis with the observation that a wide range of intestinal findings may be seen at autopsy among newborns infected by a single serotype of EPEC during an epidemic. The nonspecific pathologic picture described by some researchers includes capillary congestion and edema of the bowel wall and an increase in the number of eosinophils, plasma cells, macrophages, and mononuclear cells in the mucosa and submucosa.[157, 186, 189, 196, 219, 278, 291] Villous patterns are generally well preserved, although some flattening and broadening of the villi are seen in the more severe cases. Almost complete absence of villi and failure of regeneration of small bowel mucosa have been reported in an extreme case.[294] Edema in and around the myenteric plexuses of Auerbach, a common associated finding, has been suggested as a cause of the gastrointestinal tract dilatation often seen at autopsy in infants with EPEC infections.[204, 291, 295] In general, the distal small intestine shows the most marked alterations; however, the reported pathologic findings may be found at all levels of the intestinal tract.

Several complications of EPEC infection have been reported. Candidal esophagitis, generally an uncommon autopsy finding, accounted for significant morbidity in two series collected before[152] and during[204] the antibiotic era. Oral thrush has been noted in 50% of EPEC-infected infants treated with oral or systemic antibiotics.[189, 202, 219, 221, 291] Fatty metamorphosis of the liver of varying degrees has been noted by several investigators[152, 157, 242, 291]; however, these changes are nonspecific and probably result from the poor caloric intake associated with persistent diarrhea or vomiting. Some degree of bronchopneumonia, probably a terminal event in most cases, is present in a large proportion of newborns dying of EPEC infection.[151, 152, 157, 251, 284, 295] In one reported series of infants, EPEC was demonstrated by immunofluorescent staining in the bronchi, alveoli, and interalveolar septa.

Mesenteric lymph nodes are often swollen and congested with reactive germinal centers in the lymphoid follicles.[157, 219, 250, 278, 291] Severe lymphoid depletion, unrelated to the duration or severity of the antecedent illness, also has been described.[242] The kidneys frequently show tubular epithelial toxic changes. Variable degrees of tubular degeneration and cloudy swelling of convoluted tubules are common findings.[157, 242, 291]

Renal vein thrombosis or cortical necrosis may be observed in infants with disseminated intravascular coagulation in the terminal phases of the illness. The heart is grossly normal in most instances but may show minimal vacuolar changes of nonspecific toxic myocarditis on microscopic examination.[291, 295] Candidal abscesses of the heart[295] and kidneys[242, 291, 295] have been described. With the exception of mild congestion of the pia arachnoid vessels and some edema of the meninges, examination of the central nervous system reveals few changes.[157, 219] Despite the observation of Bray[153] that "inflammation of the middle ear (is) exceptional," strains of EPEC have been isolated from a significant number of specimens of the middle ear in series in which dissection of the temporal bone has been performed.[151, 157, 204, 219]

CLINICAL MANIFESTATIONS

Exposure of newborns to EPEC may be followed by one of several possible consequences: (1) no infection; (2) asymptomatic infection; (3) illness with gastroenteritis of variable severity and duration; and, very rarely, (4) septicemia with or without metastatic foci of infection accompanying gastroenteritis.

When infants are exposed intimately to EPEC, a significant proportion become colonized as temporary stool[1, 4, 187, 191, 229, 237, 238] or pharyngeal[1, 195] carriers with no signs of clinical disease. Although Laurell[298] showed that the percentage of asymptomatic infections rises steadily as age increases, this observation has not been confirmed by other investigators.[156, 297] Similarly, the suggestion that prematurity per se is associated with a low incidence of inapparent EPEC infection has been documented in several clinical studies[219, 221, 222, 238] but refuted in others.[209, 236, 239, 262]

The majority of neonates who acquire infection with EPEC eventually show some clinical evidence of gastroenteritis. The incubation period is quite variable. Its duration has been calculated mostly from evidence in outbreaks in newborn nurseries, where the time of first exposure can be clearly defined in terms of birth or admission dates. Under these circumstances, almost all infants show signs or symptoms of infection between 2 and 12 days after exposure, and, in most cases, within the first 7 days.[157, 187, 221–223, 233, 236, 297, 298] In some naturally acquired[1, 2] and experimental[265] human infections with heavy exposure, the incubation period may be as short as 24 hours; the stated upper limit is 20 days.[188, 299] The first positive stool culture and the earliest recognizable clinical signs of disease occur simultaneously in most infants,[221, 223] although colonization may precede symptoms by 7 to 14 days.[219, 222, 223, 236, 299, 300]

The gastroenteritis associated with EPEC infection in the newborn is notable for its marked variation in clinical pattern. Symptoms range from those of a mild illness manifest only by transient anorexia and failure to gain weight to a sudden explosive fulminating diarrhea causing death within 12 hours of onset. Prematurity, underlying disease, and congenital anomalies are often associated with the more severe forms of illness.[156, 189, 200, 238, 240, 242, 278, 301, 302] Several experienced clinicians have observed that the severity of EPEC gastroenteritis has declined markedly during the past three decades.[169–180]

The onset of illness is usually slow, with vague signs of reluctance to feed, lethargy, spitting up of formula, mild abdominal distention, or even weight loss that may be present for 1 or 2 days before the first loose stool is passed. Diarrhea usually begins abruptly. It may be continuous and violent, or, in milder infections, it may run an intermittent course with 1 or more days of normal stools followed by 1 or more days of diarrhea. Vomiting is sometimes a prominent and persistent early symptom. Stools are loose and bright yellow initially, later becoming watery, mucoid, and green as they appear with increasing infrequency. Flecks or streaks of blood, which are commonly seen with enterocolitis caused by *Salmonella, Campylobacter,* or *Shigella,* are rarely present in EPEC diarrheal disease. A characteristic seminal smell may pervade the environment of infants infected with EPEC O111:B34,[188, 219, 303] and an odor variously described as "pungent," "musty," or "fetid" often surrounds patients excreting other strains in their stools.[187, 213, 242] Because the buttocks are repeatedly covered with liquid stools, excoriation of the perianal skin may be an early and persistent problem. Fever is an inconstant feature, and, when it is present, the patient's temperature rarely rises above 39° C. Convulsions are seen infrequently; their occurrence should alert the clinician to the possible presence of electrolyte disturbances, particularly hypernatremia. Prolonged hematochezia, distention, edema, and jaundice are ominous signs and suggest an unfavorable prognosis.[157, 197, 242, 290, 297]

Most infants receiving antimicrobial agents orally show a cessation of diarrhea, tolerate oral feedings, and resume weight gain within 3 to 7 days after therapy has been started.[199, 202, 221, 222] Those with mild illness who receive no treatment may continue to have intermittent loose stools for 1 to 3 weeks. In one outbreak related to EPEC O142:K86, more than one third of the untreated or inappropriately treated infants had diarrhea for more than 14 days in the absence of a recognized enteric pathogen on repeated culturing.[224]

Recurrence of diarrhea and vomiting after a period of initial improvement is characteristic of EPEC enteritis.[194, 196, 197] Although seen most frequently in newborns who have been treated either inadequately or not at all, clinical relapses also occur after appropriate therapy. Occasionally, the symptoms during a relapse may be more severe than those accompanying the initial attack of illness.[157, 188, 242]

Not all clinical relapses are the result of persisting infection. A significant number of relapses, particularly those that consistently follow attempts at reinstitution of formula feedings,[219, 222, 242, 247] turn out to be caused by disaccharide intolerance rather than bacterial proliferation. Intestinal superinfections, caused either by another serotype of EPEC[204, 304] or by completely different enteric pathogens, such as *Salmonella* or *Shigella,*[202] also may delay the resolution of symptoms. Rarely, infants may suffer a "relapse" caused by an organism from the same O group as the original strain but differing in its H antigen. Unless complete serotyping is performed on all EPEC isolates, such an event could easily be dismissed as being a recurrence rather than a superinfection with a new organism.[215, 225]

Antibiotics to which the infecting organisms are susceptible often may not eradicate the EPEC organism,[202, 222, 224] which may persist for weeks[221, 240, 300] or months[305] after the acute symptoms have subsided. Although reinfection cannot always be excluded, a significant number

of infants are discharged from the hospital with positive rectal cultures.[187, 189, 190, 199]

Dehydration is the most common and most serious complication of gastroenteritis caused by EPEC or a toxin-producing *E. coli.* Virtually all deaths directly attributable to the intestinal infection are caused by disturbances in the balance of body fluids and electrolytes. When stools are frequent in number, large in volume, and violent in release, as they often are in severe infections with abrupt onset, a neonate can lose up to 15% of body weight in a few hours.[188, 233] Rarely, fluid excretion into the lumen of the bowel proceeds so rapidly that reduction of circulating blood volume and shock may intervene before passage of even a single loose stool.[219] Before the discovery of the etiologic agent, epidemic diarrhea of the newborn was also known by the term *cholera infantum.*

Mild disease, particularly when aggravated by poor fluid intake, may lead to a subtle but serious deterioration of an infant's metabolic status. Sometimes a week or more of illness elapses before it becomes apparent that a patient with borderline acidosis and dehydration who seemed to be responding to oral fluids alone will require parenteral therapy for improvement.[229, 242] It is, therefore, incumbent on the clinician caring for small infants with gastroenteritis to follow them closely, with particular attention to serial weights, until full recovery can be confirmed.

There are few other complications, with the possible exception of aspiration pneumonia, directly related to EPEC gastroenteritis. Protracted diarrhea and nutritional failure may occur as a consequence of functional damage to the small intestinal mucosa, with secondary intolerance to dietary sugars.[222, 294, 306] Necrotizing enterocolitis, which occasionally results in perforation of the bowel and peritonitis, has not been causally related to infection with EPEC.[204, 221, 222, 278] Extraintestinal complications of EPEC enteritis are exceedingly uncommon. Several studies have shown that virtually no enteropathogenic strains have been isolated from nonenteric sources.[164, 165] A review of most of the large clinical series describing EPEC disease in infants who ranged in age from the newborn period to 2 years of age revealed only three proven instances of bacteremia,[222, 235] one possible urinary tract infection,[222] and one documented case of meningitis in an infant of unspecified age.[307] Focal infections among neonates were limited to several cases of otitis media[151, 157, 204, 219] and a subcutaneous abscess[251] from which EPEC could be isolated. Additional complications include interstitial pneumonia,[278] gastrointestinal bleeding with or without disseminated intravascular coagulation,[289, 290, 308] and methemoglobinemia caused by a mutant of EPEC O127:B8 that is capable of generating large quantities of nitrite from proteins present in the gastrointestinal tract.[309]

DIAGNOSIS

Classic EPEC has been recovered from the vomitus, stool, or bowel contents of infected newborns. Isolation from bile[189, 228] and the upper respiratory tract[1, 195, 196, 251, 265] has been accomplished in those instances in which a specific search has been made. Less commonly, EPEC is isolated from ascitic fluid[209] or purulent exudates[151, 157, 204, 219, 251]; occasionally it has been recovered from blood cultures,[222, 235] urine,[222] and cerebrospinal fluid.

Stool cultures are generally more reliable than rectal swabs in detecting the presence of enteric pathogens, although a properly obtained swab should be adequate to demonstrate EPEC in most cases.[159, 253, 310] Specimens should be obtained as early in the course of the illness as possible because organisms are present in virtually pure culture during the acute phase of the enteritis but diminish in numbers during the period of clinical improvement.* Because of the preponderance of EPEC in diarrheal stools, two cultures are adequate for isolation of these pathogens in almost all cases of active disease. Studies using fluorescent antibody methods for identification of EPEC in stool specimens have demonstrated, on the other hand, that during the incubation period of the illness, during convalescence, and among asymptomatic carriers of EPEC, organisms may be excreted in such small numbers that they would escape detection by standard bacteriologic methods in a significant proportion of infants.[195, 202, 229, 239, 311, 312] As many as 3 to 10 specimens may be required to detect EPEC with the relatively insensitive current techniques.[1, 187, 250, 302]

After a stool specimen is received, it should be either plated as quickly as possible onto noninhibiting media or placed in a preservative medium if it is to be held for longer periods. Deep freezing of specimens preserves viable EPEC when a prolonged delay in isolation is necessary.[160] No selective media, biochemical reactions, or colonial variations permit differentiation of pathogenic and nonpathogenic strains. Certain features may aid in the recognition of two important serogroups: cultures of serogroups O111:B4 and O55:B5, unlike many other coliforms, are sticky or stringy when picked with a wire loop and are rarely hemolytic on blood agar,[159, 163] whereas O111:B4 colonies emit a distinctive evanescent odor commonly described as "seminal."[152, 156, 221, 252] This unusual odor first led Bray to suspect that specific strains of E. coli might be responsible for infantile gastroenteritis.[303]

E. coli, like other Enterobacteriaceae, possesses cell wall somatic antigens (O), envelope or capsular antigens (K), and, if motile, flagellar antigens (H). Many of the O groups may be further divided into two or more subgroups (a, b, c), and the K antigens also are divisible into at least three varieties (B, L, A), based on their physical behavior. Organisms that do not possess flagellar antigens are nonmotile (designated NM). The EPEC B capsular surface antigen prevents agglutination by antibodies directed against the underlying O antigen. Heating at 100° C for 1 hour inactivates the agglutinability and antigenicity of the B antigen.

Slide agglutination tests with polyvalent O or OB antiserum may be performed on suspensions of colonies typical of E. coli that have been isolated from infants with diarrhea, especially in the nursery outbreak setting. However, because of numerous false-positive "cross-reactions," the O and K (or B) type must be confirmed by

titration with the specific antisera.[182] Finally, the presence of EPEC does not prove that EPEC is the cause of diarrhea in a particular case, nor does its absence exclude that other types of E. coli may cause the patient's diarrhea, which requires full identification of O, K, and H types, which usually requires a reference laboratory.[225, 245, 313] More recently, gene probes for one or more of the loci of enterocyte effacement traits as noted earlier under Pathogenesis and as detailed later are being used in diagnosis.

Isolation of a strain of EPEC from an infant with diarrhea does not necessarily exclude the presence of either another strain of EPEC or an entirely different enteric pathogen. Mixed cultures with two or three serotypes of EPEC have been demonstrated in 1 to 10% of patients.[163, 201, 202, 204, 242, 246, 308] This need not mean that two or three serotypes are causative agents. Superinfection with hospital-acquired strains may occur during convalescence,[189, 202, 204, 304] and some infants may have been asymptomatic carriers of one serotype at the time that another produced diarrheal disease. A similar explanation may pertain to mixed infections with EPEC and Salmonella or Shigella.[159, 163, 167, 171, 201, 240, 314] Nelson[202] noted the presence of these pathogens in combination with EPEC in 14% of infants who were cultured as part of an antibiotic therapy trial. Salmonella and Shigella that had not been identified on cultures obtained at admission were isolated only after institution of oral therapy with neomycin. The author postulated that the alteration in bowel flora brought about by the neomycin facilitated the growth of these organisms, which had previously been suppressed and obscured by coliform overgrowth. The importance of seeking all enteric pathogens in both primary and follow-up cultures of infantile diarrhea is apparent, particularly when the specimen originates from a patient in a newborn nursery or infants' ward.

Although EPEC gastroenteritis was once considered to be synonymous with "summer diarrhea," community outbreaks have occurred as frequently, if not more frequently, in the colder seasons.[156, 168, 196–198, 208, 215, 240] It has been suggested that the increased incidence at that time of year may be related to the heightened chance of contact between infants and toddlers that is bound to occur when children remain indoors in close contact.[215] Nursery epidemics, which depend on the chance introduction and dissemination of EPEC within a relatively homogeneous population and stable environment, demonstrate no seasonal prevalence. Average relative humidity, temperature, and hours of daylight have no significant effect in determining whether an outbreak will follow the introduction of enteropathogenic strains of E. coli into a ward of infants.[200]

There are no clinical studies of the variations in peripheral leukocyte count, urine, or cerebrospinal fluid in neonatal enteritis caused by EPEC. Microscopic examination of stools of infants with acute diarrheal illness caused by these organisms has usually shown an absence of fecal polymorphonuclear leukocytes,[156, 213, 251, 279, 315] although recent data with fecal lactoferrin in human volunteers suggest that an inflammatory process may be

---

*See references 157, 160, 178, 180, 221, 223, 224, 236, 238.

important in EPEC diarrhea.[316] Stool pH may be neutral, acid, or alkaline.[297, 318]

Serologic methods have not proved to be useful in attempting to establish a retrospective diagnosis of EPEC infection in neonates. Rising or significantly elevated agglutinin titers rarely could be demonstrated in early investigations[152, 157, 187, 297]; hemagglutinating antibodies showed a significant response in no more than 10 to 20% of cases.[202, 247, 319]

Fluorescent antibody techniques have become one of the most useful means available for preliminary identification of EPEC in acute infantile diarrhea. This method is both specific, with few false positives, and more sensitive than conventional plating and isolation techniques.[229, 239, 317, 320] The rapidity with which determinations can be performed makes them ideally suited for screening symptomatic infants, as well as possible carriers, in determining the extent and progression of a nursery[229, 239] or community[195, 248] outbreak. By avoiding the 24-hour and 48-hour delays necessitated by culture methods, it is possible to separate immediately the infected infants from the susceptible infants, thus breaking the cycle of transmission. Furthermore, because immunofluorescence is neither dependent on the viability of organisms nor affected by antibiotics that suppress growth on culture plates, it can be used to advantage in following bacteriologic response and relapses in patients receiving oral therapy.[152, 321] The use of fluorescent antibody techniques offers many advantages in the surveillance and epidemiologic control of EPEC gastroenteritis. Immunofluorescent methods should supplement but not replace standard bacteriologic and serologic methods for identification of enteric pathogens. Gene probes for specific virulence traits are becoming available and include the potential for probing directly for the focal enteroadherence plasmid.[16, 166] Alternatively, one can examine E. coli isolates for the characteristic localized HEp-2 cell adherence (LA)[35] or for a 94-MDa protein encoded by the focal enteroadherence plasmid.[322, 323] An ELISA for LA plus EPEC with this pMAR plasmid-encoded EAF (EPEC adherence factor) also has been described.[374] In addition, the capacity of LA plus EPEC to polymerize f-actin can be detected in tissue culture cells stained with rhodamine-labeled phalloidin.[325]

PROGNOSIS

The mortality rate recorded previously in epidemics of EPEC gastroenteritis is impressive for its variability. During the 1930s and 1940s, when organisms later recognized as classic enteropathogenic serotypes were infecting infants, the case:fatality ratio among neonates was about 50%.[151, 152, 157] During the 1950s and 1960s, many nursery epidemics still claimed about one of every four infected infants, but several outbreaks involving the same serotypes under similar epidemiologic circumstances had fatality rates of less than 3%.[190, 198, 208, 244, 262, 297] In the 1970s, reports appeared in the literature of a nursery epidemic with a 40% neonatal mortality rate[242] and of an extensive outbreak in a nursery for premature infants with 4% fatalities[222]; another report stated that among "243 consecutive infants admitted to the hospital

for enteropathogenic E. coli diarrheal disease . . . none died of diarrheal disease per se."[326]

A significant proportion of the infants who died during or shortly after an episode of gastroenteritis already were compromised either by preexisting disease[178, 189, 240, 292] or by congenital malformations[156, 187, 189, 197, 278, 301] at the time they acquired their illness. These underlying pathologic conditions appear to exert a strongly unfavorable influence, probably by reducing the infant's ability to respond to the added stresses imposed by the gastrointestinal tract infection. Although prematurity is often mentioned as a factor predisposing to a fatal outcome, the overall mortality rate among premature infants with EPEC gastroenteritis has not differed significantly over the years from that recorded for full-term infants.[189, 219, 221, 222, 236, 262]

THERAPY

The management of EPEC gastroenteritis should be directed primarily toward prevention or correction of problems caused by loss of fluids and electrolytes.[140] Most neonates have a relatively mild illness that can be treated with oral fluids and followed by means of regular visits on an outpatient basis. The reliability of the parents must be assured because clinical deterioration requiring medical attention can be rapid and subtle. Infants who appear to be in a toxic condition; those with voluminous diarrhea and persistent vomiting; and those with increasing weight loss should be hospitalized for observation and treatment with parenteral fluids and careful maintenance of fluid and electrolyte balance after initial fluid therapy, as well as possible antimicrobial therapy. Clinical studies suggest that slow nasogastric infusion of an elemental diet may be valuable in treating infants who have intractable diarrhea that is unresponsive to standard modes of therapy.[327]

There is no evidence that the use of proprietary formulas containing kaolin or pectin is effective in reducing the number of diarrheal stools in neonates with gastroenteritis. Attempts to suppress the growth of enteric pathogens by feeding lactobacillus to the infant in the form of yogurt, powder, or granules have not been shown to be of value.[328] A trial of cholestyramine in 15 newborns with EPEC gastroenteritis had no effect on the duration or severity of the diarrhea.[222] The use of atropine-like drugs, paregoric, or loperamide to reduce intestinal motility or cramping is to be avoided. Inhibition of peristalsis not only interferes with an efficient protective mechanism designed to rid the body of intestinal pathogens but may also lead to fluid retention in the lumen of the bowel that may be sufficient to mask depletion of extracellular fluid and electrolytes.

The value of antimicrobial therapy in management of neonatal EPEC gastroenteritis is still uncertain. There are no adequately controlled studies defining the benefits of any antibiotic in (1) eliminating EPEC from the gastrointestinal tract, (2) reducing the risk of cross-infection in community or nursery outbreaks, or (3) modifying the severity of the illness. Proponents of the use of antimicrobial agents have based their claims for efficacy on anecdotal observations or comparative studies.[202] Nonetheless, several clinical investigations have provided sufficient information to guide the physician faced with the dilemma of deciding whether to treat an individual infant or an entire nursery population suffering from EPEC diarrheal disease. It should be emphasized, however, that these guidelines must be considered to be tentative until rigidly controlled double-blind studies have established the efficacy of antibiotics on a more rational and scientific basis.

Oral therapy with neomycin,[190, 208, 221] colistin,[321] or chloramphenicol[300] appears to be effective in rapidly reducing the number of susceptible EPEC organisms in the stool of infected infants. Studies comparing the responses of infants treated orally with neomycin,[189] gentamicin,[222] polymyxin,[199] or kanamycin[329] with the responses of infants receiving supportive therapy alone have shown that complete eradication of EPEC occurs more rapidly in those receiving an antimicrobial agent. In most cases, stool cultures are free of EPEC 2 to 4 days after the start of therapy.[190, 202, 221, 321] Bacteriologic failure, that is, continued isolation of organisms during or after a course of antibiotics, can be expected to occur in 15 to 30% of patients.[189, 199, 202, 222] Such relapses are generally not associated with a recurrence of symptoms.[187, 190, 202, 221, 236]

This effectiveness of oral antimicrobial therapy in reducing the duration of EPEC excretion serves to diminish environmental contamination and the spread of pathogenic organisms from one infant to another. Breaking the chain of fecal-oral transmission by giving antimicrobial agents simultaneously to all carriers of EPEC and their immediate contacts in the nursery has appeared to be valuable in terminating outbreaks that have failed to respond to more conservative measures.[187, 190, 221, 222, 236, 330]

The apparent reduction in morbidity and mortality associated with oral administration of neomycin,[186, 189, 190, 203, 221, 236, 247] colistin[203, 224, 242] polymyxin,[199] or gentamicin[203] during nursery epidemics has led to the impression that these drugs also exert a beneficial clinical effect in severely or moderately ill infants. Reports describing clinical,[213] bacteriologic,[222] or histopathologic[278] evidence of tissue invasion by EPEC have persuaded some authors to suggest the use of systemic rather than oral drug therapy in debilitated or malnourished infants.

On the basis of these data, there appears to be sufficient evidence to recommend oral administration of nonabsorbable antibiotics in the treatment of severely or moderately ill newborns with EPEC gastroenteritis. The drug most frequently used for initial therapy is neomycin sulfate in a dosage of 100 mg/kg per day administered PO every 8 hours in three divided doses.[202] In communities in which neomycin-resistant EPEC has been prevalent, treatment should be started with colistin sulfate or polymyxin B in a dosage of 15 to 20 mg/kg PO daily, divided into three equal doses. However, it is rarely necessary to use this approach.

Treatment should be continued only until stool cultures become negative for EPEC.[202] Because of the unavoidable delay before cultures can be reported, most infants will receive therapy for 3 to 5 days. If fluorescent antibody testing of rectal swab specimens is available,

therapy can be discontinued as soon as EPEC is no longer identified in smears; this will take no more than 48 hours in more than 90% of cases.[202] Once diarrhea and vomiting have stopped and the infant tolerates formula feedings, shows a steady weight gain, and appears clinically well, discharge with outpatient follow-up is indicated. Bacteriologic relapses do not require therapy unless they are associated with symptoms or high epidemiologic risks to other young infants in the household. Because the infecting organisms in these recurrences generally continue to show in vitro susceptibility to the original drug, it should be reinstituted pending bacteriologic results.[202]

In circumstances in which clinical judgment suggests that a neonate may be suffering from bacterial sepsis as well as EPEC diarrheal disease, systemic antimicrobial therapy is indicated after appropriate cultures have been obtained. Supplemental oral drugs are not required in this situation. The routine use of systemic therapy in severe cases of EPEC enteritis is not appropriate on the basis of current clinical experience. Further information on the occurrence and significance of extraintestinal lesions produced by EPEC may require modification of this recommendation at some future time.

Antimicrobial susceptibility patterns of EPEC are an important determinant of the success of therapy in infections with these organisms.[189, 203, 204, 224] These patterns are unpredictable, depending not only on the ecologic pressures exerted by local antibiotic usage[203, 204] but also on the incidence of transmissible resistance factors (R-factors) in the enteric flora of the particular population served by an institution.[331–336] For these reasons, variations in susceptibility patterns are apparent in different nurseries[203, 334] and even from time to time within the same institution.[204, 205, 207] Sudden changes in clinical response may even occur during the course of a single epidemic as drug-susceptible strains of EPEC are replaced by strains with multiple-drug resistance.[189, 248, 304, 333] Because differences may exist in the susceptibilities of different EPEC serogroups to various antimicrobial agents, regional susceptibility patterns should be reported on the basis of OB group or serotype rather than for EPEC as a whole.[207] Knowledge of the resistance pattern in one's area may help in the initial choice of antimicrobial therapy.

PREVENTION

The prevention of hospital outbreaks of EPEC gastroenteritis is best accomplished by careful bacteriologic evaluation of all infants hospitalized with diarrhea. If the laboratory is equipped and staffed to perform fluorescent antibody testing, infants transferred from another institution to a newborn, premature, or intensive care nursery, as well as all infants with gastroenteritis on admission during an outbreak of EPEC diarrhea or in a highly endemic area, may be held in an observation area for 1 or 2 hours until the results of the fluorescent antibody tests are received. Those found to be excreting EPEC, even if asymptomatic, may then be separated from the others and given oral therapy until the tests are negative. Some experts have suggested that when the rapid results obtainable with fluorescent antibody procedures are not available, all infants admitted with diarrhea in a setting where EPEC is common may be treated as if they were excreting EPEC or some other enteric pathogen until contrary proof is obtained.[330] Stool cultures should be obtained on admission, and enteric precautions or isolation should be enforced among all who come into contact with the infant. Additional epidemiologic studies are needed to establish the advantages of careful isolation and nursing techniques, particularly in smaller community hospitals in which the number of infants in a "gastroenteritis ward" may be small. The use of prophylactic antibiotics has been shown to be of no value and may only select for increased resistance.[337]

Unfortunately, it is difficult to keep a nursery continuously free of EPEC. Specific procedures have been suggested for handling a suspected outbreak of bacterial enteritis in a newborn nursery or infant care unit.[191, 311, 338] Evidence indicating that a significant proportion of E. coli enteritis may be caused by nontypeable strains has required some modification of these earlier recommendations. The following infection control measures may be appropriate:

1. The unit is closed, when possible, to all new admissions.

2. Cultures for enteric pathogens are obtained from nursing personnel assigned to the unit at the time of the outbreak. Nurses are restricted from working in other areas of the hospital nursery until negative culture results are proved.

3. Stool specimens obtained from all infants in the nursery may be screened by the fluorescent antibody or another technique and cultured. Identification of a classic enteropathogenic serotype provides a useful epidemiologic marker; however, failure to isolate one of these strains does not eliminate the possibility of illness caused by a nontypeable EPEC.

4. Antibiotic therapy with oral neomycin or colistin may be considered for all infants with a positive fluorescent antibody test or culture. The initial drug of choice will depend on local patterns of susceptibility. Subsequent therapy may require modification depending on the results of susceptibility tests.

5. If an identifiable EPEC strain is isolated, second and third stool specimens from all infants in the unit are reexamined by the fluorescent antibody technique or culture at 48-hour intervals. If this is not practical, exposed infants should be carefully followed.

6. Early discharge for healthy, mature, uninfected infants is advocated.

7. An epidemiologic investigation should be performed to seek the factor or factors responsible for the outbreak. A surveillance system may be established for all those in contact with the nursery, including physicians, nursing personnel, housekeeping personnel, and postpartum mothers with evidence of enteric disease. A telephone, mail, or home survey may be conducted on all infants who were residing in the involved unit during the 2 weeks before the outbreak.

8. When all patients and contacts are discharged and control of the outbreak is obtained, a thorough terminal disinfection of the involved nursery is mandatory.

Above all, personnel and parents should pay scrupulous attention to hand washing when handling infants; physicians also must observe this rule and thus set the example.[224, 239]

Enterohemorrhagic *Escherichia coli*

Since a multistate outbreak of enterohemorrhagic colitis was associated with E. coli O157:H7,[38] numerous reports have arisen associating a limited number of serotypes of E. coli (some previously considered to be EPEC serotypes) with the production of Shiga toxin (also called Vero cytotoxin) and bloody diarrhea or the hemolytic-uremic syndrome.[16–18, 38, 39, 280, 340, 341] Enterohemorrhagic E. coli is also referred to in the literature as verotoxin-producing E. coli and Shiga toxin–producing E. coli. E. coli O157:H7 has a bovine reservoir and is transmitted by undercooked meat, unpasteurized milk, and contaminated vegetables such as lettuce, alfalfa sprouts, and radish sprouts (as occurred in over 9000 schoolchildren in Japan).[342, 343] It also spreads directly from person to person.[340, 342, 343] The clinical syndrome is that of bloody, noninflammatory (sometimes voluminous) diarrhea that is distinct from febrile dysentery with fecal leukocytes seen in shigellosis or EIEC infections. Most cases of EHEC infections have been recognized in outbreaks of bloody diarrhea or hemolytic-uremic syndrome in daycare centers, schools, nursing homes, and communities.[341–352] Although EHEC infections often involve infants and young children, the frequency of this infection in neonates remains unclear; indeed, animal studies suggest that receptors for the Shiga toxin may be developmentally regulated and thus susceptibility to disease may be age-related.[353]

As noted earlier, the capacity of EHEC to cause disease is related to the phage-encoded capacity of the organism to produce a Vero cell cytotoxin, subsequently shown to be one of the Shiga toxins.[16, 39, 341–345, 354–358] Shiga toxin 1 is neutralized by antiserum against Shiga toxin, whereas Shiga toxin 2, although biologically similar, is not neutralized by anti–Shiga toxin. Like Shiga toxin made by *Shigella dysenteriae*, both E. coli Shiga toxins act by inhibiting protein synthesis by cleaving an adenosine residue from position 4324 in the 28S ribosomal RNA (rRNA) to prevent elongation factor-1–dependent aminoacyl-tRNA (transfer RNA) from binding to the 60S rRNA.[359] The virulence of EHEC may also be determined in part by a 60-MDa plasmid that encodes for a fimbrial adhesin in O157 and O26.[360, 361] In addition, cytotoxigenic EHEC strains (from patients with hemorrhagic colitis or hemolytic-uremic syndrome) in O groups 157, 26, 111, 113, 121, and 145 (rough strains) exhibit close attaching and effacing adherence in the distal small bowel and colon in rabbits.[362] Clearly, we are just beginning to appreciate the mechanism, significance, and epidemiology of EHEC infections. The detection of sorbitol-negative E. coli O157 is further improved by use or rhamnose and cefixime containing sorbitol MacConkey's selective agar.[363] Alternatively, indirect hemagglutination assays or DNA toxin probes may prove useful.[364, 365] An ELISA for Shiga toxins is now available and helps to identify additional EHEC strains.[365] Supportive therapy with fluid and electrolytes is appropriate. The role of antimicrobial therapy is controversial at present, with little being known about the optimal treatment of EHEC infections.

Enteroaggregative and Other *Escherichia coli*

As noted earlier in the Nature of the Organism section, in addition to the locally adherent EPEC, there are *E. coli* serotypes that exhibit diffuse adherence or aggregative adherence to HEp-2 and other cells.[366] The diffusely adherent *E. coli* are variably seen in association with diarrhea in young infants and children[40–42, 367, 368] and represent several potential genotypes (as identified by different gene probes), including those for strain 1845[369] and for a 100-kb plasmid-encoded 100-kDa protein adhesin involved in diffuse adherence (AIDA-I) from strain 2787 (O126:H27).[370]

EAggEC exhibit a "stacked bricks" type of adherence to HEp-2, HeLa, or intestinal cells with or without adherence to glass slides via one or more bundle-forming fimbriate adhesins.[371–373] EAggEC, some of which are aggregative adherence probe–positive, are associated with persistent diarrhea in several areas, including India, Mexico, Brazil,[42–47] and Australia.[368] EAggEC 04 have been associated with an outbreak of diarrhea on a neonatal nursery ward.[374] Furthermore, the traditional EPEC serogroup 0125 can also be EAggEC.[375] It remains to be determined whether the diarrhea is related to a novel heat-stable toxin (EAST)[376] to yet another heat-labile "toxin" that is 120 kDa and antigenically related to the carboxy-terminal region of *E. coli* hemolysin that apparently induces host cell calcium-dependent protein phosphorylation from extracellular calcium (versus dantrolene-inhibitable intracellular calcium stores as with EPEC),[377] or to a product that triggers IL-8 release and intestinal inflammation.[19, 373] Detection of EAggEC depends on demonstration of their typical stacked bricks adherence to HEp-2 or other cells (with or without adherence to glass), hemagglutination by shaken L broth cultures of the organism with human erythrocytes, or by an aggregative adherence or other (ex AAF/I and AAF/II) DNA probe that detects some, but not all, of these strains.[51, 52, 371, 373, 378]

SALMONELLA

Nature of the Organism

Salmonella classification tends to be confusing. Although taxonomists classify *Salmonella* narrowly as a single species, with *S. typhi*, *S. choleraesuis*, and *S. enteritidis* technically being serovars or subspecies, conventionally for clinical purposes these subspecies are referred to as "species." For example clinical laboratories tend to use the shorthand *S. typhimurium* rather than the more formal designation *Salmonella enterica* serovar *typhimurium*. Biochemical traits are used routinely by hospital laboratories to differentiate *S. typhi*, *S. choleraesuis*, and *S. enteritidis* from each other. For example, *S. typhi* is unlike

other salmonellae in that it does not produce gas from glucose.[1] Because there are more than 1700 different serotypes included in the species *S. enteritidis*, serotyping of *S. enteritidis* is usually performed by state health departments rather than by hospital laboratories. The most common serogroups and representative serotypes are listed in Table 31–4. Infection of humans with the other serogroups (C_3, D_2, E_2, E_3, F, G, H, I, etc.) is uncommon.

There are differences in invasiveness of *Salmonella* strains related to serotype. *S. typhi*, *S. choleraesuis*, *S. heidelberg*[2, 3] and *S. dublin*[4] are particularly invasive, with bacteremia and extraintestinal focal infections occurring frequently. *Salmonella* species possess genes closely related to the *Shigella* invasion plasmid antigens; these genes are probably essential to intestinal infection.[5, 6] Virulence plasmids, which increase invasiveness in some serotypes, have been recognized, although the precise mechanisms of virulence remain to be elucidated; resistance to complement-mediated bacteriolysis by inhibition of insertion of the terminal C5b-9 membrane attack complex into the outer membrane may be important.[7, 8] Laboratory studies have demonstrated dramatic strain-related difference in the ability of *S. typhimurium* to evoke fluid secretion, to invade intestinal mucosa, and

TABLE 31–4

Common Serotypes and Serogroups of *Salmonella*

SEROGROUPS	SEROTYPES
A	*paratyphi A*
B	*agona*
	derby
	heidelberg
	paratyphi B (*schottmuelleri*)
	saint-paul
	typhimurium
C_1	*choleraesuis*
	eimsbuettel
	infantis
	montevideo
	oranienburg
	paratyphi C (*hirschfeldii*)
	thompson
C_2	*blockley*
	hadar
	muenchen
	newport
C_3	*kentucky*
D_1	*dublin*
	enteritidis
	javiana
	panama
	typhi
D_2	*maarssen*
E_1	*anatum*
E_2	*london*
	newington
E_3	*illinois*
E_4	*krefeld*
	senftenberg

to disseminate beyond the gut.[9] Production of an enterotoxin immunologically related to cholera toxin by about two thirds of *Salmonella* strains may be related to the watery diarrhea often seen.[10] The significance of protein synthesis–inhibiting cytotoxins[11] remains to be proved, although such toxins may damage gut epithelium, which could facilitate invasion. The cytotoxins produced by *Salmonella* are not immunologically related to Shiga toxin made by *Shigella dysenteriae* type 1[12] or *E. coli* O157:H7.

Salmonellae have the ability to penetrate epithelial cells and reach the submucosa, where they are ingested by phagocytes.[13] In phagocytes, salmonellae are resistant to killing, in part because of the properties of their lipopolysaccharides.[14, 15] Persistence of the organism within phagolysosomes of phagocytic cells may occur with any species of *Salmonella*. It is not completely clear how the organisms have adapted to survive in the harsh intracellular environment, but their survival has major clinical significance. It accounts for relapses after therapy. It explains the inadequacy of some antimicrobial agents that do not penetrate phagolysosomes. It perhaps is the reason for prolonged febrile courses that occur even with appropriate therapy. Although both humoral immunity and cell-mediated immunity are stimulated during *Salmonella* infections, it is believed that cell-mediated immunity plays a greater role in eradication of the bacteria.[16] T cell activation of macrophages appears to be important in killing intracellular *Salmonella*.[17] Defective interferon-γ production by monocytes of newborns in response to *S. typhimurium* lipopolysaccharide may explain in part the unusual susceptibility of infants to *Salmonella* infection.[18] Studies in mice suggest that helper T cell (Th1) responses in Peyer's patches and mesenteric lymph nodes may be central to protection of the intestinal mucosa.[19] Humans who lack IL-12 receptor and therefore have impaired Th1 responses and interferon-γ production are at increased risk for *Salmonella* infection.[20]

In typhoid fever, presence of an envelope antigen called Vi is known to enhance virulence. Patients who develop classic enteric fever have positive stool cultures in the first few days after ingestion of the organism and again late in the course after a period of bacteremia. This course reflects early colonization of the gut, penetration of gut epithelium with infection of mesenteric lymph nodes, and reseeding of the gut during a subsequent bacteremic phase.[21] Studies of *S. typhimurium* in monkeys suggest similar initial steps in pathogenesis (colonization of gut, penetration of gut epithelium, infection of mesenteric lymph nodes) but failure of the organism to cause a detectable level of bacteremia.[22]

Although *Salmonella* and *Shigella* both invade intestinal mucosa, the resultant pathologic changes are different. *Shigella* multiplies within and kills enterocytes with production of ulcerations and a brisk inflammatory response, whereas *Salmonella* passes through the mucosa and multiplies within the lamina propria, where the organisms are ingested by phagocytes; consequently, ulcer formation is less striking,[9] although villus tip cells are sometimes sloughed. Acute crypt abscesses may be seen in the stomach and small intestine, but the most dramatic changes occur in the colon, where acute diffuse inflammation with mucosal edema and crypt abscesses are the most consistent findings.[23, 24] With *S. typhi* there also is hyperplasia of Peyer's patches in the ileum, with ulceration of overlying tissues.

Epidemiology

Salmonella strains, with the exception of *S. typhi*, are well-adapted to a variety of animal hosts; human infection can often be traced to infected meat, contaminated milk, or contact with a specific animal. Half of commercial poultry samples are contaminated with *Salmonella*.[25] Definition of the serotype causing infection can sometimes suggest the likely source. For example, *S. dublin* is closely associated with cattle; human cases occur with a higher-than-predicted frequency in people who drink raw milk.[4] For *S. typhimurium*, which is the most common serotype and accounts for over a third of all reported human cases, a single source has not been established, although there is an association with cattle. Despite the 1975 ban by the U.S. Food and Drug Administration (FDA) on interstate commercial distribution of small turtles, these animals continue to be associated with infection, as illustrated by a series of cases in Puerto Rico.[26] Various pet reptiles are an important source of a variety of unusual *Salmonella* serotypes such as *S. marina*, *S. chameleon*, *S. arizonae*, *S. java*, *S. stanley*, *S. poona*, *S. jangwain*, *S. tilene*, *S. pomona*, *S. miami*, *S. manhattan*, *S. litchfield*, *S. rubislaw*, and *S. wassenaar*.[27–29] *Salmonella* organisms are hardy and capable of prolonged survival; organisms have been documented to survive in flour for nearly a year.[30] *S. tennessee* has been shown to remain viable for many hours on non-nutritive surfaces (glass, 48 hours; stainless steel, 68 hours; enameled surface, 114 hours; rubber mattress, 119 hours; linen, 192 hours; and rubber tabletop, 192 hours).[31]

Infection with *Salmonella* is, like most enteric infections, more common in young children than in adults. The frequency of infection is far greater in the first 4 years of life; roughly equal numbers of cases are reported during each decade beyond 4 years of age. Although the peak incidence occurs in the second through sixth months of life, infection in the neonate is relatively common. Researchers at the Centers for Disease Control and Prevention (CDC) have estimated the incidence of *Salmonella* infection in the first month of life at nearly 75 cases per 100,000 infants.[32]

Adult volunteer studies suggest that large numbers of *Salmonella* (10^5 to 10^9) need to be ingested to cause disease.[33] However, it is likely that lower doses cause illness in infants. The occurrence of nursery outbreaks[31, 34–59] and intrafamilial spread[60] suggests that organisms are easily spread from person to person; this pattern is typical of low-inoculum diseases transmitted by the fecal-oral route. The neonate with *Salmonella* infection infrequently acquires the organism from his or her mother during delivery. Although the index case in an outbreak can often be traced to a mother,[37–40, 58] subsequent cases are the result of contaminated objects in the nursery environment[61, 62] serving as a reservoir coming in contact with hands of attending personnel.[31, 46]

The mother of an index case may be symptomatic[42, 43, 63, 64] or asymptomatic with preclinical infection,[47] convalescent infection,[40, 44, 65] or chronic carriage.[66] The risk of the newborn becoming infected once *Salmonella* is introduced into a nursery has been reported to be as high as 20 to 27%,[50, 56] but the frequency of infection may be lower because isolated cases without a subsequent epidemic are unlikely to be reported.

Stomach acidity is an important barrier to *Salmonella* infection. Patients with anatomic or functional achlorhydria are at increased risk of developing salmonellosis.[67, 68] The hypochlorhydria[69] and rapid gastric emptying typical of early life[70] may in part explain the susceptibility of infants to *Salmonella*. Premature and low-birth-weight infants appear to be at higher risk of acquiring *Salmonella* infection than full-term infants.[46, 48] Whether this reflects increased exposure because of prolonged hospital stays or increased susceptibility on the basis of intestinal or immune function is unclear. Contaminated food or water is often the source of *Salmonella* infection in older patients; the limited diet of the infant makes contaminated food a less likely source of infection. Although human milk,[71–73] raw milk,[74] powdered milk,[75–77] formula,[56] and cereal[78] have been implicated in transmission to infants, more often fomites, such as delivery room resuscitators,[34] rectal thermometers,[49, 79] oropharyngeal suction devices,[80–82] water baths for heating formula,[82] soap dispensers,[83] scales,[31, 35, 84] "clean" medicine tables,[31] air-conditioning filters,[31] mattresses, radiant warmers,[61] and dust,[35] serve as reservoirs. One unusual outbreak involving 394 premature and 122 term infants was traced to faulty plumbing, which caused massive contamination of environment and personnel.[56] Once *Salmonella* enters a nursery, it is difficult to eradicate. Epidemics lasting 6 to 7 weeks,[49, 54] 17 weeks,[31] 6 months,[48, 53] 1 year,[43] and 27 to 30 months[50, 56] have been reported. Spread to nearby pediatric wards has occurred.[51, 57]

The incubation period in nursery outbreaks has varied widely in several studies where careful attention has been paid to this variable. In one outbreak of *Salmonella oranienburg* involving 35 newborns, 97% of cases occurred within 4 days of birth.[50] In an outbreak of *S. typhimurium*, all of the symptomatic infants presented within 6 days of birth.[40] These incubation periods are similar to those seen with *Salmonella newport* in older children and adults, 95% of whom have been reported to be ill within 8 days of exposure.[85, 86] Conversely, one outbreak of *Salmonella nienstedten* involving newborns was characterized by incubation periods of 7 to 18 days.[51]

The usual incubation period associated with fecal-oral nursery transmission is not found with congenital typhoid. During pregnancy, typhoid fever is associated with bacteremic infection of the fetus. The congenitally infected infants are symptomatic at birth. They are usually born during the second to fourth week of untreated maternal illness.[87] Usually the mother is a carrier; fecal-oral transmission of *S. typhi* can occur with delayed illness in the newborn.[88]

Clinical Manifestations

Several major clinical syndromes occur with nontyphoidal *Salmonella* infection in young infants. Asymp-

tomatic colonization may be the most common outcome of ingestion of *Salmonella* by the neonate. Such colonization is usually detected when an outbreak is under investigation. Most infected infants who become symptomatic have abrupt onset of loose, green, mucus-containing stools, or they have bloody diarrhea; an elevated temperature is also a common finding in *Salmonella* gastroenteritis in the first months of life.[3] Grossly bloody stools are found in the minority of patients although grossly bloody stools can occur in the first 24 hours of life. Hematochezia is more typically associated with noninfectious etiologies (swallowed maternal blood, intestinal ischemia, hemorrhagic diseases, anorectal fissures) at this early age.[89] There appear to be major differences in presentation related to the serotype of *S. enteritidis* causing infection. For example, in one epidemic of *S. oranienburg*[50] involving 46 newborns, 76% had grossly bloody stools, 11% were febrile, 26% had mucus in their stools, and only 11% were asymptomatic. In a series of *S. newport* infections involving 11 premature infants,[37] 90% of infants with gastroenteritis had blood in their stools, 10% had fever, 10% had mucus in their stools, and 9% were asymptomatic. In an outbreak of *S. typhimurium*[40] involving 11 symptomatic and 5 asymptomatic infants, none had bloody stools; all of the symptomatic infants were febrile and loose green stools were usually noted. Of 26 infants infected by *Salmonella virchow*, 42% were asymptomatic; the rest had mild diarrhea.[45] Seals and colleagues[51] described 12 infants with *S. nienstedten*, all of whom had watery diarrhea and low-grade fever; none had bloody stools. In a large outbreak in Zimbabwe of *S. heidelberg* infection reported by Bannerman,[48] 38% of 100 infants were asymptomatic, 42% had diarrhea, 16% had fever, 15% had pneumonia, and 2% developed meningitis. An outbreak of *Salmonella worthington* was characterized primarily by diarrhea, fever, and jaundice, although 3 of 18 infants developed meningitis and 17% died.[80] In dramatic contrast to these series, none of 27 infants with positive stool cultures for *S. tennessee* had symptoms in a nursery found to be contaminated with that organism.[32] A few infants with *Salmonella* gastroenteritis have developed necrotizing enterocolitis,[55, 90] but it is not clear whether *Salmonella* was the cause.

Although gastroenteritis is usually self-limited, chronic diarrhea has sometimes been attributed to *Salmonella*.[66, 91] Whether chronic diarrhea is caused by *Salmonella* is uncertain. Although some infants develop carbohydrate intolerance after a bout of *Salmonella* enteritis[92, 93] and *Salmonella* is typically listed as one of the causes of postinfectious protracted diarrhea,[94] it is difficult to be sure that the relationship is causal. The prolonged excretion of *Salmonella* after a bout of gastroenteritis may sometimes cause nonspecific chronic diarrhea to be erroneously attributed to *Salmonella*.

Major extraintestinal complications of *Salmonella* infection may develop in the neonate who becomes bacteremic. Extraintestinal spread may develop both in infants who initially present with diarrhea and in some who have no gastrointestinal tract symptoms. Bacteremia appears to be more common in the neonate than in the older child.[95] A study of over 800 children with *Salmonella* infection showed that extraintestinal infection occurred significantly more often (8.7% versus 3.6%) in the first 3 months of life.[96] Several retrospective studies suggest that infants in the first month of life may have a risk of bacteremia as high as 30 to 50%.[3] One retrospective study[2] suggests that the risk is not increased in infancy and estimates that the risk of bacteremia in childhood *Salmonella* gastroenteritis is between 8.5% and 15.6%. Prospective studies of infants in the first year of life suggest that the risk of bacteremia is 1.8 to 6.0%.[97, 98] Although selection biases in these studies limit the reliability of these estimates, the risk is substantial. The *Salmonella* species isolated from infants include some serotypes that appear to be more invasive in the first 2 months of life than in older children or healthy adults (*S. newport, S. agona, S. blockley, S. derby, S. enteritidis, S. heidelberg, S. infantis, S. javiana, S. saint-paul,* and *S. typhimurium*), as well as serotypes that are aggressive in every age group (*S. choleraesuis* and *S. dublin*). Other serotypes appear more likely to cause bacteremia in adults (*S. typhi, S. paratyphi* A and *S. paratyphi* B).[95]

Virtually any *Salmonella* serotype can cause bacteremic disease in neonates. A few infants with *Salmonella* gastroenteritis have died with *E. coli* or *Pseudomonas aeruginosa* sepsis,[57] but the role of *Salmonella* in these cases is unclear. Unlike the situation in older children in whom bacteremic salmonellosis is often associated with underlying disease, bacteremia may occur in young infants who have no immunocompromising conditions.[99] *Salmonella* bacteremia is often not suspected clinically because the syndrome is not usually distinctive.[2, 3] Even afebrile, well-appearing children with *Salmonella* gastroenteritis have been documented to have bacteremia that persists for several days.[100] Although infants with bacteremia may have spontaneous resolution without therapy,[101] a sufficient number develop complications to warrant empirical therapy when bacteremia is suspected. The frequency of complications is highest in the first month of life. Meningitis is the most feared complication of bacteremic *Salmonella* disease. Fifty to 75 percent of all cases of nontyphoidal *Salmonella* meningitis occur in the first 4 months of life.[102] The serotypes associated with neonatal meningitis (*S. typhimurium, S. heidelberg, S. enteritidis, S. saint-paul, S. newport,* and *S. panama*)[60] are serotypes frequently associated with bacteremia. Meningitis has a high mortality rate, in part due to the high relapse rates. Relapse has been reported in up to 64% of cases.[103] In some studies, more than 90% of patients with meningitis have died,[104] although more typically 30 to 60% of infants die.[105–107] The survivors suffer all the expected complications of gram-negative neonatal meningitis, including hydrocephalus, seizures, ventriculitis, abscess formation, subdural empyema, and permanent neurologic impairment. Neurologic sequelae have included retardation, hemiparesis, hydrocephalus, epilepsy, visual impairment, and athetosis.[102]

In large nursery outbreaks, it is common to find infants whose course is complicated by pneumonia,[48] osteomyelitis,[108, 109] or septic arthritis.[46, 48] Other rare complications of salmonellosis include pericarditis,[110] pyelitis,[111] peritonitis,[40] otitis media,[40] mastitis,[112] cholecystitis,[113] endophthalmitis,[114] cutaneous abscesses,[55] and infected cephalohematoma.[108] Other focal infections seen

in older children and adults, such as endocarditis and infected aortic aneurysms, have rarely or never been reported in neonates.[102, 115] Although mortality in two reviews of nursery outbreaks was 3.7 to 7.0%,[58, 59] in some series it has reached 18%.[48]

Enteric fever, most often related to *S. typhi* but also occurring with *S. paratyphi* A, *S. paratyphi* B, *S. paratyphi* C, and other *Salmonella* species, is reported much less commonly in infants than in older patients. Infected infants develop typical findings of neonatal sepsis and meningitis when infected in the first 3 weeks of life. Current data suggest that mortality is about 30%.[116] In utero infection with *S. typhi* has been well-described. Typhoid fever[83, 117] and nontyphoidal *Salmonella* infections[118] during pregnancy put women at risk of aborting the fetus. Premature labor usually occurs during the second to the fourth week of maternal typhoid if the woman is untreated.[87] In a survey of typhoid fever in pregnancy during the preantibiotic era, 24 of 60 women with well-documented cases delivered prematurely, with resultant fetal death; the rest delivered at term, although only 17 infants survived.[119] The outlook for carrying the pregnancy to term and delivering a healthy infant appears to have improved dramatically in the antibiotic era. However, one of seven women in a recent series was still delivered of a dead fetus with extensive liver necrosis caused by typhoid.[120] In the preantibiotic era, about 14% of pregnant women with typhoid fever died.[121] With appropriate antibiotic therapy, pregnancy does not appear to put the woman at increased risk of death from typhoid. Despite these well-described cases, typhoid fever is rare early in life.

Of 1500 cases of typhoid fever that Osler and McCrae[122] reported, only two were in the first year of life. In areas where typhoid fever is still endemic, systematic search for infants with enteric fever has failed to find many cases. The few infections with *S. typhi* documented in children in the first year of life often present as a brief nondescript "viral syndrome" or as pneumonitis.[123, 124] Fever, diarrhea, cough, vomiting, rash, and splenomegaly may occur; the fever may be high, and the duration of illness may be many weeks.[87]

Diagnosis

The current practice of early discharge of newborn infants, while potentially decreasing the risk of exposure, may make recognition of an outbreak difficult. Diagnosis of neonatal salmonellosis should trigger an investigation for other cases. Other than diarrhea, signs and symptoms of neonatal *Salmonella* infection are similar to the nonspecific findings seen in most neonatal infections. Lethargy, poor feeding, pallor, jaundice, apnea, respiratory distress, weight loss, and fever are common. Enlarged liver and spleen are common in those neonates with positive blood cultures.

Laboratory studies are required to establish the diagnosis because the clinical picture is not distinctive. The fecal leukocyte examination shows polymorphonuclear leukocytes in 36 to 82%[125, 126] of persons with *Salmonella* infection, but it has not been evaluated extensively in neonates. Obviously, the presence of fecal leukocytes is consistent with colitis of any cause and therefore is a nonspecific finding. Routine stool cultures usually detect *Salmonella* if two or three different enteric media (Mac-Conkey's, eosin–methylene blue, *Salmonella-Shigella*, Tergitol 7, xylose-lysine-deoxycholate, brilliant green, or bismuth sulfite agar) are used. Stool, rather than rectal swab material, is preferable for culture, particularly if the aim of culture is to detect carriers.[127] On the infrequent occasions when proctoscopy is performed, mucosal edema, hyperemia, friability, and hemorrhages may be seen.[24] Infants who are bacteremic often do not appear sufficiently toxic to raise the suspicion of bacteremia.[128] Therefore, blood cultures should be a routine part of evaluation of neonates with suspected or documented *Salmonella* infection. Symptomatic neonates with *Salmonella* infection should have a cerebrospinal fluid examination performed as part of their evaluation. Bone marrow cultures also may be indicated when enteric fever is suspected. There are no consistent abnormalities in the white blood cell count. Serologic studies are not helpful in making the diagnosis, although antibodies to somatic antigens[129, 130] and flagellar antigens[50] develop in many infected newborns. Currently, reagents are not commercially available for routine testing of infant sera against the vast number of O and H antigens.

If an outbreak of salmonellosis is suspected, further characterization of the organism is imperative.[131] Determination of somatic and flagellar antigens to characterize the specific serotype may be critical to investigation of an outbreak. When the serotype found during investigation of an outbreak is a common one (e.g., *S. typhimurium*), antimicrobial resistance testing[38, 132] and use of molecular techniques such as plasmid characterization[132] may be helpful in determining whether a single-strain, common-source outbreak is in progress.

Therapy and Prevention

As in all enteric infections, attention to fluid and electrolyte abnormalities is the first issue that must be addressed by the physician. Specific measures to eradicate *Salmonella* intestinal infection have met with little success. Multiple studies show that antibiotic treatment of *Salmonella* gastroenteritis prolongs the excretion of *Salmonella*.[133–140] Nearly half of the infected children in the first 5 years of life continue to excrete *Salmonella* 12 weeks after the onset of infection; more than 5% have positive cultures at 1 year.[141] No benefit of therapy has been shown in comparisons of ampicillin or neomycin versus placebo,[137] chloramphenicol versus no antibiotic treatment,[136] neomycin versus placebo,[138] ampicillin or trimethoprim-sulfamethoxazole versus no antibiotic,[135] and ampicillin or amoxicillin versus placebo.[139] In contrast to these studies, data suggest that in adults and children there may be a role for quinolone antibiotics[140, 142]; however, these drugs are not approved for use in persons younger than 18 years of age and resistance has been encountered.[143] Because these studies have few data on the risk:benefit ratio of therapy in the neonate, it is uncertain whether they should influence treatment decisions in neonates. Studies that have included a small number of neonates also suggest little

benefit from antibiotic therapy.[40, 50, 135, 144, 145] However, because bacteremia is common in neonates, antibiotic therapy for infants under 3 months of age who have *Salmonella* gastroenteritis is often recommended,[98, 128, 146] especially if the infant appears toxic. Premature infants and those who have other significant debilitating conditions also should probably be treated. The duration of therapy is debatable but should probably be no more than 3 to 5 days if the infant is not seriously ill and if blood cultures are sterile. If toxicity, clinical deterioration, or documented bacteremia complicates gastroenteritis, prolonged treatment is indicated. Even with antibiotic therapy, some infants develop complications. The relatively low risk of extraintestinal dissemination must be balanced against the well-documented risk of prolonging the carrier state. For infants who develop chronic diarrhea and malnutrition, hyperalimentation may be required; the role of antibiotics in this setting is unclear. The infant with typhoid fever should be treated with antibiotics; relapses sometimes occur after therapy.

Asymptomatically infected infants discovered by stool cultures during evaluation of an outbreak ought to be isolated but probably should not receive antibiotic therapy. Such infants should be discharged from the nursery as early as possible and followed carefully as outpatients.

Treatment of neonates who have documented extraintestinal dissemination must be prolonged. Bacteremia without localization is generally treated with at least a 10-day course of antibiotics. Therapy for *Salmonella* meningitis must be given for at least 4 weeks to lessen the risk of relapse. About three fourths of patients who have relapses have been treated for 3 weeks or less.[102] As in meningitis, treatment for osteomyelitis must be prolonged to be adequate. Although cures have been reported with 3 weeks of therapy, 4 to 6 weeks of therapy is recommended.

In vitro susceptibility data for *Salmonella* isolates must be interpreted with caution. The aminoglycosides show good in vitro activity but poor clinical efficacy, perhaps because of the low pH of the phagolysosome. They have poor activity in an acid environment. The stability of some drugs in this acid environment also may explain in vitro/in vivo disparities. The intracellular localization and survival of *Salmonella* within phagocytic cells also presumably explains the relapses encountered with virtually every regimen. Resistance to antibiotics has long been a problem with *Salmonella* infection.[133, 147, 148] There has been a steady increase in resistance to *Salmonella* in the United States over the last 20 years.[149] With the emergence of *S. enterica* serotype *typhimurium* type DT 104, resistance to ampicillin, chloramphenicol, streptomycin, sulfonamides, and tetracycline has increased from 0.6% in 1979–1980 to 34% in 1996.[150] Resistance plasmids have been selected and transmitted, partly because therapy has been given for mild illness that should not have been treated[133] and partly because of use of antibiotics in animal feeds. Resistance to chloramphenicol and ampicillin has made trimethoprim-sulfamethoxazole increasingly important for the treatment of *Salmonella* infection in those patients who require therapy. However, with increasing resistance to all three of these agents in Asia,[151] the Middle East,[152] Africa,[153]

Europe,[154, 155] Argentina,[148] and North America,[147, 156, 157] the third-generation cephalosporins and quinolones represent drugs of choice for invasive salmonellosis. The quinolones are not approved for persons younger than 18 years of age. Cefotaxime, ceftriaxone, and cefoperazone represent acceptable alternative drugs for both typhoidal and nontyphoidal salmonellosis when resistance is encountered.[158, 159] Because the second-generation cephalosporins, such as cefamandole and cefuroxime, are less active than the third-generation cephalosporins in vitro and are not consistently clinically effective, they should not be used.[158, 160] Data suggest that cefoperazone may sterilize blood and cause patients with typhoid fever to become afebrile more rapidly than chloramphenicol,[161] perhaps because cefoperazone is excreted into bile in high concentrations.[162] The third-generation cephalosporins may have higher cure and lower relapse rates than ampicillin or chloramphenicol in children with *Salmonella* meningitis.[163] The doses of ampicillin, chloramphenicol, or cefotaxime used in infants with gastroenteritis pending results of blood cultures are the same as those used in treatment of sepsis. Because of the risk of gray baby syndrome, chloramphenicol should not be used in neonates unless it is possible to monitor blood levels closely. Trimethoprim-sulfamethoxazole, although useful in older children and adults, is not used in neonates because of the risk of kernicterus. Nosocomial infection with strains of *Salmonella* resistant to multiple antibiotics, including third-generation cephalosporins, has emerged as a problem in South America.[148]

Non-antibiotic interventions are important in the control of *Salmonella* infections. Limited data suggest that intravenous immuneglobulin, 500 mg/kg on days 1, 2, 3, and 8 of therapy, along with antibiotic therapy may decrease the risk of bacteremia and death in preterm infants with *Salmonella* gastroenteritis.[164]

Early recognition and intervention in nursery outbreaks of *Salmonella* are the keys to control. When a neonate develops salmonellosis, a search for other infants who have been in the same nursery should be undertaken. When two or more cases are recognized, environmental cultures, cultures of all infants, cohorting and enteric isolation of infected infants, rigorous enforcement of hand-washing procedures, early discharge of infected infants, and thorough cleaning of all possible fomites in the nursery and delivery rooms are important elements of control. If cases continue to occur, the nursery should be closed to further admissions. Cultures of personnel are likely to be helpful in the unusual situation of an *S. typhi* outbreak in which a chronic carrier may be among the caretakers. Culture of health care personnel during outbreaks of salmonellosis caused by other *Salmonella* species is debatable, although often recommended. Data suggest that nurses infected with salmonellae rarely infect patients in the hospital setting.[165] The fact that nursing personnel are sometimes found to be colonized during nursery outbreaks[31, 37, 50, 52, 53] may be an effect rather than a cause of those epidemics.

The potential for a role of vaccines in control of neonatal disease is minimal. For the vast number of non–*S. typhi* serotypes, there is no prospect for an immunization strategy. A heat-phenol–inactivated, parenteral, whole-cell typhoid vaccine is available commercially in the United States but has limited use. The commercially available oral live attenuated vaccine (Vivotif Berna), manufactured from the Ty21a strain of *S. typhi*, has been shown in Chilean schoolchildren to reduce typhoid fever cases by more than 70%.[166, 167] However, the vaccine is not recommended for persons younger than 6 years of age, in part because immunogenicity of Ty21a is age-dependent; children younger than 24 months of age fail to respond with development of immunity.[168] Vi capsular polysaccharide vaccine is available for children older than 2 years of age. Whether some degree of protection of infants might occur due to reduced stool carriage or might be transferred to infants via milk of vaccinated mothers remains to be studied. There are data suggesting that breast-feeding may decrease the risk of other *Salmonella* infections.[169]

SHIGELLA

Nature of the Organism

On the basis of DNA relatedness, shigellae and *E. coli* belong to the same species.[1] However, for historical reasons and because of their medical significance, shigellae have been maintained as separate species. Shigellae are gram-negative bacilli that are unlike typical *E. coli* in that they do not metabolize lactose or do so slowly, are nonmotile, and in general produce no gas during carbohydrate utilization. They are classically divided into four species (serogroups) on the basis of both metabolic and antigenic characteristics (Table 31–5). The mannitol nonfermenters are in general classified as *S. dysenteriae*. Although the lipopolysaccharide antigens of the 13 currently recognized members of this group are not related to each other antigenically, these serotypes are grouped together as serogroup A. Serogroup D (*Shigella sonnei*) are ornithine decarboxylase–positive and slow lactose fermenters. All *S. sonnei* share the same lipopolysaccharide (O antigen). Those shigellae that ferment mannitol (unlike *S. dysenteriae*) but do not decarboxylate ornithine or ferment lactose (*S. sonnei*) belong to serogroups B and C. Of these, the strains that have lipopolysaccharide antigens immunologically related to each other are grouped together as serogroup B (*Shigella flexneri*), whereas those whose O antigens are not related to each other or to other shigellae are included in serogroup C (*Shigella boydii*). There are six major serotypes

TABLE 31–5
Shigella Serogroups Isolated from Humans

SEROGROUPS	SPECIES	NO. OF SEROTYPES
A	*S. dysenteriae*	13
B	*S. flexneri*	15 (including subtypes)
C	*S. boydii*	18
D	*S. sonnei*	1

of *S. flexneri* and 13 subserotypes (1a, 1b, 2a, 2b, 3a, 3b, 4a, 4b, 5a, 5b, 6, X and Y variant). There are 19 antigenically distinct serotypes of *S. boydii*. For *S. dysenteriae* and *S. boydii* serogroup confirmation, pools of polyvalent antisera are used.

The virulence of shigellae has been studied extensively since their recognition as major pathogens at the turn of the twentieth century. The major determinants of virulence are encoded by a 120- to 140-MDa plasmid.[2, 3] This plasmid, which is found in all virulent shigellae, encodes for the synthesis of several polypeptides, which are required for invasion of mammalian cells.[4, 5] Shigellae that have lost this plasmid, have deletions of genetic material from the region involved in synthesis of these proteins, or have the plasmid inserted into the chromosome lose the ability to invade eukaryotic cells and become avirulent.[6] The ability to invade cells is the basic pathogenic property shared by all shigellae[7, 8] and by the *Shigella*-like invasive *E. coli*, which also possesses the *Shigella* virulence plasmid.[4, 5, 9–11] In the laboratory, *Shigella* invasiveness is studied in tissue culture (HeLa cell invasion), in animal intestine, or in rabbit or guinea pig eye, where instillation of the organism causes keratoconjunctivitis (Sereny test).[12]

In addition to the virulence plasmid, several chromosomal loci produce materials that enhance virulence. This has been best studied in *S. flexneri* in which multiple virulence-enhancing regions of the chromosome have been defined.[3, 13–15] The specific gene products of some of the chromosomal loci are not known; one chromosomal virulence segment encodes for synthesis of the O repeat units of lipopolysaccharide. Intact lipopolysaccharide is necessary but not sufficient to cause virulence.[13, 16] At least two cell-damaging cytotoxins that also are chromosomally encoded are produced by shigellae. One of these toxins (Shiga toxin) is made in large quantities by *S. dysenteriae* serotype 1 (the Shiga bacillus) and is not made, or made only in small quantities, by other shigellae.[17] Shiga toxin is a major virulence factor. *E. coli* serotypes that make this toxin (EHEC) cause bloody diarrhea and hemolytic-uremic syndrome. This toxin kills cells by interfering with peptide elongation during protein synthesis.[18–20] A second toxin produced by shigellae and some *E. coli* strains is not firmly established as a virulence factor, although there is evidence suggesting that it may be important.[21]

Epidemiology

Although much of the epidemiology of shigellosis is predictable based on its infectious dose, certain elements are unexplained. Shigellae, like other organisms transmitted via the fecal-oral route, are commonly spread by food and water, but the low inoculum size required to cause infection allows person-to-person spread. Because of this low inoculum size, *Shigella* is one of the few enteric pathogens that can infect swimmers.[22] The dose required to cause illness in adult volunteers is as low as 10 organisms for *S. dysenteriae* serotype 1,[23] about 200 organisms for *S. flexneri*,[24] and 500 organisms for *S. sonnei*.[25] Person-to-person transmission of infection probably explains the continuing occurrence of *Shigella*

in the developed world. Enteropathogens that require large inocula and hence are best spread by food or drinking water are less common in industrialized societies because of sewage disposal facilities, water treatment, and food-handling practices. In the United States, day-care centers currently serve as a major focus for acquisition of shigellosis.[26] Numerous outbreaks of disease related to crowding, poor sanitation, and the low dose required for diseases have occurred in this setting.

Given the ease of transmission, it is not surprising that the peak incidence of disease is in the first 4 years of life. It is, however, paradoxical that symptomatic infection is uncommon in the first year of life.[27–30] The clearest data on the age-related incidence of shigellosis come from Mata's prospective studies of Guatemalan infants.[27] In these studies, stool cultures were performed weekly on a group of children followed from birth to 3 years of age. The rate of infection was more than 60-fold lower in the first 6 months of life than between 2 and 3 years of age (Fig. 31–1).[27] The same age-related incidence has been described in the United States[30] and in a rural Egyptian village.[29] This anomaly has been explained by the salutary effects of breast-feeding.[31–33] However, it is likely that breast-feeding alone does not

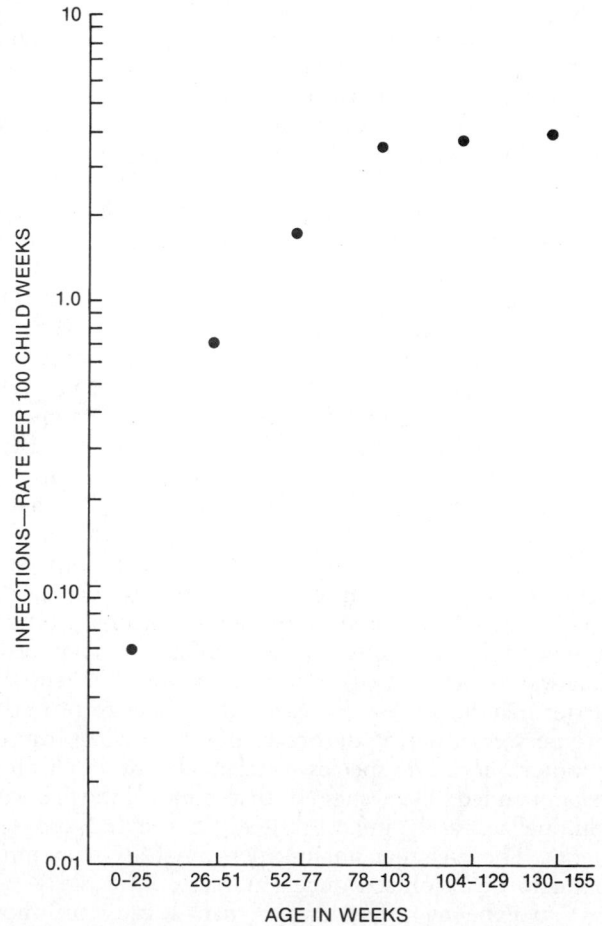

FIGURE 31–1 Age-related incidence of *Shigella* infection. (Adapted from the data of Mata LG. The Children of Santa Maria Cauque: a Prospective Field Study of Health and Growth. Cambridge, Mass, MIT Press, 1978.)

explain the resistance of infants to symptomatic shigellosis.

A review of three large series[34–36] suggests that about 1.6% (35 of 2225 cases) of shigellosis occurs in infants in the neonatal period. The largest series of neonatal shigellosis[33] suggests that the course, complications, and etiologic serogroups are different in neonates than in older children. Although newborns are routinely contaminated by maternal feces, neonatal shigellosis is rare.

Other aspects of the epidemiology of shigellosis elude simple explanation. The seasonality (summer-fall peak in the United States, rainy season peak in the tropics) is not well-explained. The geographic variation in species causing infection likewise is not well-understood. In the United States, most *Shigella* infections are due to *S. sonnei* or, less commonly, *S. flexneri*. In most of the developing world, the relative importance of these two species is reversed and other *Shigella* serotypes, especially *S. dysenteriae* serotype 1, are identified more frequently. As hygiene improves, the proportion of *S. sonnei* increases and that of *S. flexneri* decreases.[37] Data from Bangladesh suggest that *S. dysenteriae* is less common in neonates with *S. sonnei* and *S. boydii* is more common.[33]

Clinical Manifestations

There appear to be some important differences in the relative frequencies of various complications of *Shigella* infection related to age. Some of these differences and estimates are based on data that are undoubtedly contaminated by reporting biases.

S. dysenteriae serotype 1 characteristically causes a more severe illness than other shigellae with more complications, including pseudomembranous colitis, hemolysis, and hemolytic-uremic syndrome. However, in general, illnesses caused by various *Shigella* serotypes are indistinguishable from each other and therefore are conventionally discussed together.

The incubation period of shigellosis is related to the number of organisms ingested, but in general it is between 12 and 48 hours. Volunteer studies have shown that after ingestion, illness may be delayed for a week or more. Neonatal shigellosis seems to have a similar incubation period. More than half of the neonatal cases occur within 3 days of birth, consistent with fecal-oral transmission during parturition. Mothers of infected neonates are sometimes carriers, although more typically they are symptomatic during the perinatal period. Intrauterine infection is rare. In the older child, the initial symptoms are usually high fever, abdominal pain, vomiting, toxicity, and large-volume watery stools; diarrhea may be bloody or may become bloody. Painful defecation and severe crampy abdominal pain associated with frequent passage of small-volume stools with gross blood and mucus are characteristic findings in older children or adults who develop severe colitis. Many children, however, never develop bloody diarrhea. Adult volunteer studies have demonstrated that variations in presentation and course are not related to the dose ingested because some patients develop colitis with dysentery but others develop only watery diarrhea after ingestion of the same inoculum.[24] The neonate with shigellosis may have a mild diarrheal syndrome or a severe colitis.[34, 38–46] Fever in neonates is usually low-grade (<102° F) if the course is uncomplicated. The neonate has less bloody diarrhea, more dehydration, more bacteremia, and a greater likelihood of death than the older child.[33] Physical examination of the neonate may show signs of toxicity and dehydration, although fever, abdominal tenderness, and rectal findings are less striking than in the older child.[33]

Complications of shigellosis are common.[47] Although the illness is self-limited in the normal host, resolution may be delayed for a week or more. In neonates and malnourished children, chronic diarrhea may follow a bout of shigellosis.[38, 46] Ten to 35 percent of hospitalized children with *Shigella* have convulsions before or during the course of diarrhea.[47–49] Usually, the seizures are brief, generalized, and associated with high fever. Seizures are uncommon in the first 6 months of life, although neonates have been described with seizures.[40, 50] The cerebrospinal fluid is generally normal in these children, but a few have cerebrospinal fluid with a mild pleocytosis. The neurologic outcome is generally good even with focal or prolonged seizures, but fatalities do occasionally occur, often associated with toxic encephalopathy.[51] Although the seizures have been postulated to be due to the neurotoxicity of Shiga toxin, this explanation is now known to be incorrect because most shigellae make little or no Shiga toxin and the strains isolated from children with neurologic symptoms do not produce Shiga toxin.[17, 52] Hemolysis with or without development of uremia is a complication primarily of *S. dysenteriae* serotype 1 infection.[53]

Sepsis during the course of shigellosis may be caused either by the *Shigella* itself or by other gut flora that gain access to the bloodstream through damaged mucosa.[33, 54, 55] Sepsis occurs in up to 12% of neonates with shigellosis.[32, 47, 54, 56] The risk of sepsis is higher in the first year of life, particularly in neonates,[33, 38–40, 50, 57] in malnourished children, and in those with *S. dysenteriae* serotype 1 infection.[55] Given the infrequency of neonatal shigellosis, it is striking that 9% of reported cases of *Shigella* sepsis have involved infants in the first month of life.[58] One of the infants with bacteremia[59] was reportedly asymptomatic. Disseminated intravascular coagulation may develop in those patients whose course is complicated by sepsis. Meningitis has been described in a septic neonate. Colonic perforation has occurred in neonates,[31, 60] older children,[61] and adults.[62] Although this complication of toxic megacolon is rare, it appears to be more common in neonates than in older individuals. Bronchopneumonia may complicate the course of shigellosis, but shigellae are rarely isolated from lungs or tracheal secretions.[63] The syndrome of sudden death in the setting of extreme toxicity with hyperpyrexia and convulsions but without dehydration or sepsis (Ekiri syndrome)[64–66] is rare in neonates. In the nonbacteremic child, other extraintestinal foci of infection, including vagina[67, 68] and eye,[69] rarely occur. Reiter's syndrome, which rarely complicates the illness in children, has not been reported in neonates.

Although infection is less common in infants than in toddlers, mortality rates are highest in infants.[70, 71] The mortality rate in newborns appears to be about twice that of older children.[33] In industrialized societies, less than 1% of children with shigellosis die whereas in preindustrial cultures, up to 30% die. The relationship between age and mortality in a preindustrial society is shown in Figure 31–2. These differences in mortality rates are related to nutrition,[34] availability of medical care, antibiotic resistance of many shigellae, the frequency of sepsis, and the higher frequency of *S. dysenteriae* serotype 1 infection in the less-developed world.[55]

Diagnosis

Although the diagnosis of shigellosis may be suspected on clinical grounds, other enteropathogens can cause illnesses that are difficult or impossible to distinguish clinically. The neonate with watery diarrhea is more likely to be infected with *Salmonella* or rotavirus than *Shigella*. Infants presenting with bloody diarrhea may have necrotizing enterocolitis or infection with *Salmonella*, EIEC, EHEC, *Yersinia enterocolitica*, *Campylobacter jejuni*, *Clostridium difficile*, or *Entamoeba histolytica*. Shigellosis in the neonate is rare. Before cultures establish a diagnosis, clinical and laboratory data may aid in making a presumptive diagnosis. Abdominal radiographs that demonstrate pneumatosis intestinalis aid in establishing the diagnosis of necrotizing enterocolitis. Previous antibiotic use raises the possibility of antibiotic-associated diarrhea caused by *C. difficile*, although proof of this diagnosis in the first year of life is problematic. A history of several weeks of illness not associated with fever and with few fecal leukocytes suggests *E. histolytica* rather than *Shigella* infection.[72]

The definitive diagnosis of shigellosis depends on culture of the organism from stool. Unfortunately, culture is a relatively insensitive method of diagnosis.[73] In volunteer studies, daily stool cultures failed to detect shigellae in about 20% of symptomatic subjects.[24] Optimal recovery is achieved by immediate inoculation of stool (as opposed to rectal swabs) onto culture media. Use of transport media in general decreases the yield of cultures positive for *Shigella*[74] when compared with immediate inoculation.

Examination of stool for leukocytes as an indication of colitis is useful in support of the clinical suspicion of shigellosis. The white blood cell count and differential count also are used as supporting evidence for the diagnosis. Leukemoid reactions (white blood cells >50,000/mm^3) occur in almost 15% of children with *S. dysenteriae* serotype 1 but in less than 2% of other children with shigellosis.[52] Leukemoid reactions are more frequent in infants than in older children.[52] Even when the total white blood cell count is not dramatically elevated, there may be a striking left shift. Almost 30% of children with shigellosis have greater than 25% bands on the differential.[75-77] The few reports of the white blood cell count in newborns suggest that normal or low rather than elevated counts are more common. Although serum and fecal antibodies develop to lipopolysaccharides and the virulence plasmid-associated polypeptides,[78] serologic studies are not useful in the diagnosis of shigellosis. PCR can identify *Shigella* and EIEC in feces.[79]

Colonoscopy typically shows inflammatory changes that are most severe in the distal segments of colon.[80] Animal model studies have shown that bacteria penetrate and kill colonic mucosal cells and then elicit a brisk inflammatory response.[81, 82]

Therapy

Because dehydration is particularly common in neonatal shigellosis, attention to correction of fluid and electrolyte disturbances is always the first concern when the illness is suspected. Although debate continues over the indications for antibiotic therapy in the patient with shigellosis, in general the benefits of therapy outweigh the risks. The chief disadvantages of therapy include cost, drug toxicity, and emergence of antibiotic-resistant shigellae. Because of the self-limited nature of shigellosis, it has been argued that less severe illness should not be treated. However, children feel miserable during the typical bout of shigellosis, and appropriate antibiotic therapy shortens the duration of illness and eliminates shigellae from stool, decreasing secondary spread. Complications are probably decreased by antibiotics. Given the high mortality rates of neonatal shigellosis, therapy should not be withheld.

The empirical choice of an antibiotic is dictated by susceptibility data on the strains circulating locally at the time the patient's infection occurs. Multiply resistant shigellae complicate the choice of empirical therapy before availability of susceptibility data on the individual isolate. Plasmid-encoded resistance (R-factor) for multiple antibiotics has been a recurring theme in *S. dysenteriae* serotype 1 outbreaks[83] as well as with other shigel-

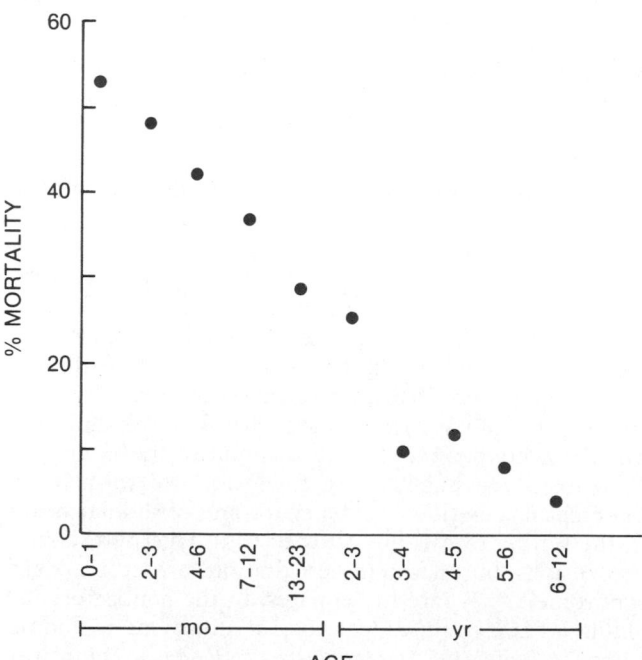

FIGURE 31–2 Age-related mortality of shigellosis based on 948 infants hospitalized in Durban, South Africa, between 1960 and 1975. (Adapted from the data of Scragg JN, Rubidge CJ, Appelbaum PCJ. Pediatrics 93:796, 1978.)

lae.[84–86] Antibiotic resistance patterns fluctuate from year to year in a given locale.[87] However, despite the guesswork involved, early presumptive therapy is indicated when an illness is strongly suggestive of shigellosis. In vitro susceptibility does not always adequately predict therapeutic responses. Cefaclor,[88] furazolidone,[89] cephalexin,[90] amoxicillin,[91] kanamycin,[92] and cefamandole[93] are all relatively ineffective therapies.

The optimal duration of therapy is debatable. Studies in children older than 2 years of age and in adults suggest that single-dose regimens may be as effective in relieving symptoms as courses given for 5 days. The single-dose regimens are generally not as effective in eliminating shigellae from the feces as are the longer courses. A third-generation cephalosporin such as ceftriaxone or cefixime may be the best empirical choice. Optimal doses for newborns with shigellosis have not been established. Trimethoprim at a dose of 10 mg/kg per day (maximum, 160 mg per day) and sulfamethoxazole at a dose of 50 mg/kg per day (maximum, 800 mg per day) in two divided doses for a total of 5 days is recommended for the older child if the organism is susceptible.[94–96] If the condition of the patient does not permit PO administration, the drug is usually divided into three doses given intravenously over 1 hour.[97] Ampicillin at a dose of 100 mg/kg per day in four divided doses PO for 5 days may be used if the strain is susceptible.[77]

For the rare newborn who acquires shigellosis, appropriate therapy is often delayed until susceptibility data are available. This occurs because shigellosis is so rare in newborns that it is almost never the presumptive diagnosis of the child with watery or bloody diarrhea before availability of culture data. Although sulfa is as efficacious as ampicillin when the infecting strain is susceptible,[76] sulfa is avoided in neonates because of concern about the potential risk of kernicterus. The risk of empirical ampicillin therapy is that shigellae are commonly resistant to the drug; 50% of shigellae currently circulating in the United States are resistant to ampicillin.[97, 98] For the neonate infected with ampicillin-resistant *Shigella*, there are few data on which to base a recommendation. Ceftriaxone is generally active against shigellae, and data in children and adults suggest that clinical improvement occurs with this drug.[99, 100] Quinolone antibiotics such as ciprofloxacin and ofloxacin have been shown to be effective agents for treating shigellae[101, 102] in adults, but they are not approved for use in persons younger than 18 years of age. Their potential usefulness in children may be limited by the potential risk of arthropathy. Other drugs sometimes used to treat diarrhea pose special risks to the infant with shigellosis. The antimotility agents, in addition to their intoxication risk, may pose a special danger in dysentery. In adults, diphenoxylate hydrochloride with atropine has been shown to prolong fever and excretion of the organism.[103]

The response to appropriate antibiotic therapy is generally gratifying. Improvement is often obvious in less than 24 hours. Complete resolution of diarrhea may not occur until a week or more after the start of treatment. In those who have severe colitis or those infected by *S. dysenteriae* serotype 1, the response to treatment is somewhat delayed.

Prevention

For most of the developing world, the best strategy for prevention of shigellosis is prolonged breast-feeding. Specific antibodies in milk prevent symptomatic shigellosis[104, 105]; nonspecific modification of gut flora and the lack of bacterial contamination of human milk also may be important. Breast-feeding, even when other foods are consumed, decreases the risk of shigellosis; children who continue to consume human milk into the third year of life are still partially protected from symptomatic illness.[106] In the United States, the best means of preventing infection in the infant may be good hygiene (e.g., increased hand washing) measures when an older sibling or parent develops diarrhea. Even in unsanitary environments, secondary spread of *Shigella* can be dramatically decreased by hand washing after defecation and before meals.[107] Spread of *Shigella* in the neonatal unit can presumably be prevented by the use of enteric isolation with attention to hand-washing technique. Although nursery personnel have acquired shigellosis from infected newborns,[86] further transmission to other infants in the nursery, although described,[108] is rare. In contrast to *Salmonella*, large outbreaks of neonatal nosocomial shigellosis are extremely rare.

Unfortunately, good hygiene is a particularly difficult problem in day-care centers. The gathering of susceptible children, breakdown in hand-washing technique, failure to use different personnel for food preparation and diaper changing, and difficulty controlling the behavior of toddlers all contribute to day care–focused outbreaks of shigellosis.

Immunization strategies have been studied since the turn of the twentieth century, but no satisfactory immunization has yet been developed. Even if immunizations are improved, it remains to be seen whether they will be useful in infants.

CAMPYLOBACTER

Campylobacter is a curved, gram-negative bacillus with a flagellum on one or both ends. *Campylobacter* was first recognized in an aborted sheep fetus in the early 1900s[1] and was named *Vibrio fetus* by Smith and Taylor in 1919.[2] This organism was subsequently identified as a major venereally transmitted cause of abortion and sterility as well as scours in cattle, sheep, and goats.[3, 4] It was not until 1947, when it was cultured from the blood of a pregnant woman who subsequently aborted at 6 months' gestation, that its significance as a relatively rare cause of bacteremia and perinatal infections in humans was appreciated.[5–7] It was recognized during the 1970s to be an opportunistic pathogen of debilitated patients.[8, 9] The possibility that *V. fetus* could be associated with enteric disease was first raised by King in 1957.[10] In 1963, *V. fetus* and related organisms were separated from the vibrios (such as *V. cholerae* and *Vibrio parahaemolyticus*) and placed in a new genus, *Campylo-*

bacter (Greek, meaning "curved rod").[11] Since 1973, several *Campylobacter* species have been recognized as a common cause of enteritis[12-28] and, in some cases, extraintestinal infections.

Nature of the Organism

The genus *Campylobacter* contains 18 species, the majority of which are recognized as animal and human pathogens. The most commonly considered causes of human disease are *C. fetus, C. jejuni, C. coli, C. lari,* and *C. upsaliensis* (Table 31–6),[26-28] although *C. mucosalis* has been isolated from stool of children with diarrhea.[29] DNA hybridization studies have shown that these species are distinct, sharing less than 35% DNA homology under stringent hybridization conditions.[30, 31] *Helicobacter pylori,* a cause of type B gastritis, was originally named *Campylobacter pylori,* but, owing to differences in DNA, it was reclassified and is no longer considered in the *Campylobacter* genus.

Strains of *C. fetus* are divided into two subspecies: *C. fetus* subsp. *fetus* and *C. fetus* subsp. *venerealis.* The first subspecies causes sporadic abortion in cattle and sheep[32, 33]; in the human fetus and newborn, it causes perinatal and neonatal infections that result in abortion, premature delivery, bacteremia, and meningitis.[5-7, 32-44] Outside the newborn period, it is a relatively infrequent cause of bacteremia, usually infecting those with impaired host defenses, including the elderly or the debilitated; less frequently it causes intravascular infection.[8-10, 45] Infection with *C. fetus* appears to be the most common type of *Campylobacter* infection in the first 3 weeks of life and is associated with a high incidence of fetal and neonatal mortality.

By far the most common syndrome produced by a *Campylobacter* species is enteritis caused by *C. jejuni* and *C. coli.* Both of these species cause gastroenteritis and are generally referred to collectively as *C. jejuni,* although DNA hybridization studies show them to be different. In the laboratory, *C. jejuni* can be differentiated from *C. coli* because it is capable of hydrolyzing hippurate, whereas *C. coli* is not. The majority of isolates that are associated with diarrhea (61 to 100%) are identified as *C. jejuni,*[46-49] and, in some cases, individuals have been shown to be simultaneously infected with both *C. jejuni* and *C. coli.*[47]

Because of the fastidious nature of *C. jejuni,* which is difficult to isolate from fecal flora, its widespread occurrence was not recognized until 1973.[12-28] Previously called "related vibrios" by King,[10] this organism had been associated with bloody diarrhea and colitis in infants and adults only when it had been associated with a recognized bacteremia.[50-52] In the late 1970s, development of selective fecal culture methods for *C. jejuni* enabled its recognition worldwide as one of the most common causes of enteritis in persons of all ages. It is an uncommon infection in neonates, who generally develop gastroenteritis when infected.[14, 53-66] Bacteremia with *C. jejuni* enteritis is uncommon.[14, 54, 59, 64, 67-73] Maternal symptoms considered to be related to *C. jejuni* infection are generally mild and include fever (75%) and diarrhea (30%). In contrast to serious disease in newborns caused by *C. fetus,* neonatal infections with *C. jejuni* usually result in a mild illness,[53, 55, 57, 58, 60-63, 66, 73] although meningitis occurs in rare instances.[56, 64] Perinatal infection related to either *C. fetus* or *C. jejuni* usually results in abortion or stillbirth.

Pathogenesis

C. fetus does not produce recognized enterotoxins or cytotoxins and does not appear to be locally invasive in the Sereny test.[9, 27] Instead, these infections tend to present more like enteric fever and may be associated with penetration of the organism through a relatively intact intestinal mucosa to the reticuloendothelial system and bloodstream.[9] Whether this reflects a capacity to resist normal serum factors or to multiply intracellularly remains to be determined.

C. jejuni is capable of producing illness by several mechanisms. These organisms have been shown to produce a heat-labile enterotoxin and a cytotoxin.[79-82] This enterotoxin is known to be a heat-labile protein with a molecular mass of 60 to 70 MDa.[79, 82] It shares functional and immunologic properties with cholera toxin and *E. coli* LT. *C. jejuni* and *C. coli* also elaborate a cytotoxin

---

TABLE 31–6

Campylobacter Species That Infect Humans

CURRENT NOMENCLATURE	PREVIOUS NOMENCLATURE	USUAL DISEASE PRODUCED
C. fetus	*Vibrio fetus*	Bacteremia, meningitis, perinatal infection, intravascular infection
	V. fetus var. *intestinalis*	
	C. fetus subsp. *intestinalis*	
C. jejuni	*Vibrio jejuni*	Diarrhea
C. coli	*C. fetus* subsp. *jejuni*	Diarrhea
C. lari	Grouped with *C. jejuni*	Diarrhea
	Nalidixic acid-resistant thermophilic, *Campylobacter, C. laridis*	Diarrhea
C. upsaliensis	None	Diarrhea, bacteremia
C. hyointestinalis	None	Diarrhea, bacteremia
C. concisus	None	
C. sputorum	None	Abscesses

that is toxic for a number of mammalian cells.[83, 84] The toxin is heat-labile, trypsin-sensitive, and not neutralized by immune sera to Shiga toxin or the cytotoxin of *Clostridium difficile*. The role of these toxins as virulence factors in diarrheal disease remains unproven.[79, 84]

Several animal models have been tested for use in the study of this pathogen.[85] Potential models for the study of *C. jejuni* enteritis include dogs, which may acquire symptomatic infection[86]; 3- to 8-day old chicks[87–89]; chicken embryo cells, which are readily invaded by *C. jejuni*,[21]; rhesus monkeys[90]; and rabbits via the removable intestinal tie adult rabbit technique. An established small mammal model that mimics human disease in the absence of previous treatment or surgical procedure has not been successful in adult mice.[91] An infant mouse model[92, 93] and a hamster model[94] of diarrhea appear promising. *C. jejuni* is negative in the Sereny test for invasiveness,[95] and most investigators report no fluid accumulation in ligated rabbit ileal loops.

Pathology

The pathologic findings of *C. fetus* infection in the perinatal period include placental necrosis[6] and, in the neonate, widespread endothelial proliferation, intravascular fibrin deposition, perivascular inflammation, and hemorrhagic necrosis in the brain.[96] The tendency for intravascular location and hepatosplenomegaly in adults infected with *C. fetus* has been shown.[9]

The pathologic findings in infants and children infected with *C. fetus* may include an acute inflammatory process in the colon or rectum, as evidenced by the tendency for patients to have bloody diarrhea with numerous fecal leukocytes.[97] There may also be crypt abscess formation and an ulcerative colitis or pseudomembranous colitis–like appearance[98, 99] or a hemorrhagic jejunitis or ileitis.[13, 23, 100, 101] Mesenteric lymphadenitis and acute appendicitis also have been described.

Epidemiology

Infection with *Campylobacter* species occurs after ingestion of contaminated food, including unpasteurized milk or poultry, and contaminated water.[22, 102–111] Many farm animals and pets, such as dogs and cats (especially young animals), are potential sources. The intrafamilial spread of infection in households,[13, 112] the occurrence of outbreaks in nurseries,[64, 65, 113] and the apparent laboratory acquisition of *C. jejuni*[114] all suggest that *C. jejuni* infection may occur following person-to-person transmission of the organism. Outbreaks of *C. jejuni* in the child daycare setting are not common. Volunteer studies[115] have shown a variable range in the infecting dose, with many volunteers developing no illness. The report of illness after ingestion of 10^6 organisms in a glass of milk[24] and production of illness in a single volunteer by 500 organisms[115] substantiate the variation in individual susceptibility. The potential for low-inoculum disease has significant implications for the importance of strict enteric precautions when infected persons are hospitalized, particularly in maternity and nursery areas. When diarrhea in neonates caused by *C. jejuni* has been re-

ported,[53–66] maternal-infant transmission during labor has generally been documented.[53–58, 60–63, 65, 66] One report used the Lior serotyping system to show that three culture-positive infants had the same serotype as their mothers.[61] The majority of mothers gave no history of diarrhea during pregnancy.[57, 58, 60, 61] Outbreaks have occurred in neonatal intensive care units because of person-to-person spread.

The frequency of asymptomatic carriage of *C. jejuni* ranges from 0 to 1.3%[12, 13] to as high as 13 to 85%.[12, 13, 28, 117–119] In a cohort study in Mexico, 66% of all infections related to *C. jejuni* were asymptomatic.[28] Infected children, if untreated, may be expected to excrete the organisms for 3 or 4 weeks; however, more than 80% are culture-negative after 5 weeks.[17, 18] Asymptomatic excretors pose a significant risk in the neonatal period, in which acquisition from an infected mother may be clinically important.[14, 55, 57, 61] *C. jejuni* has increasingly been recognized as a cause of both watery and inflammatory diarrhea in temperate and tropical climates throughout the world. It has been isolated from 2 to 11% of all fecal cultures from patients with diarrheal illnesses in various parts of the world.[12–18, 24, 28, 120–125] There is a tendency for *C. jejuni* enteritis to occur in the summer in countries with temperate climates.[121]

The reservoir of *Campylobacter* appears to be the gastrointestinal tract of domestic and wild birds and animals. It primarily infects sheep and cattle but has also been isolated from goats, antelope, swine, chickens, and domestic turkeys. *C. fetus* is often carried asymptomatically in the intestinal or biliary tracts of sheep and cattle. During the course of a bacteremic illness in pregnant animals, *C. fetus* organisms, which have a high affinity for placental tissue, invade the uterus and multiply in the immunologically immature fetus. The infected fetuses are generally aborted. Whether this organism is acquired by humans from animals or is carried asymptomatically for long periods in humans, who may then transmit the organism venereally, as appears to occur in animals, is unclear. It is believed that this subspecies is rarely found in the human intestine and that it is not a cause of human enteritis.[21] *C. fetus* infections predominantly occur in older men with a history of farm or animal exposure and in pregnant women in their third trimester.[5, 6, 12, 13] Either symptomatically or asymptomatically infected women may have recurrent abortions or premature deliveries and are the source of organisms associated with life-threatening perinatal infections of the fetus or newborn infant.[5, 35–44, 126] In several instances of neonatal sepsis and meningitis, *C. fetus* was cultured from the maternal cervix or vagina.[7, 43, 94] A nosocomial nursery outbreak has been associated with asymptomatic carriage in some infants.[127] Cervical cultures have remained positive in women who have had recurrent abortions and whose husbands have antibody titer elevations.[34]

The most commonly incriminated reservoir of *C. jejuni* is poultry.[107, 111, 128, 129] The majority of chickens cultured in several different geographic locations had a large number (mean, 4×10^6/g) of *C. jejuni* in the lower intestinal tract or feces. This occurred in some instances despite the use of tetracycline, to which the *Campylo-*

bacter was susceptible in vitro, in the chicken feed.[124] The internal cavities of chickens remain positive for *Campylobacter* even after they have been cleaned, packaged, and frozen.[128] However, unlike *Salmonella*, *C. jejuni* organisms that survive usually do not multiply to high concentrations.[21] Domestic puppies or kittens with *C. jejuni* diarrhea also may provide a source for spread, especially to infants or small children in the household.[13, 50, 111, 130–132]

C. jejuni enteritis has also been associated in a number of outbreaks with consumption of unpasteurized milk.[21, 108–110, 133–135] In retrospect, the first reported human cases of *C. jejuni* enteritis were probably in a milkborne outbreak reported in 1946.[136] Because *Campylobacter* infections of the udder are not seen, milk is probably contaminated from fecal shedding of the organism. These organisms are not spore formers and hence should be killed by adequate cooking.

Fecally contaminated water is a potential vehicle for *C. jejuni* infections. A large waterborne outbreak of *Campylobacter* enteritis involved an estimated 3000 people (19% of the population) in Bennington, Vermont.[137] Several phenotypic and genotypic methods have been used for distinguishing *C. jejuni* strains from animals and humans involved in epidemics.[138] There is also a tendency for *C. jejuni* to be associated with traveler's diarrhea among those traveling from England or the United States.[16]

Clinical Manifestations

Clinical manifestations of infection caused by *Campylobacter* depend on the species involved (see Table 31–6). Human infections with *C. fetus* are rare and are generally limited to bacteremia in patients with predisposing conditions,[10, 45] as well as to bacteremia or uterine infections with prolonged fever and pneumonitis lasting for several weeks in the third trimester of pregnancy. Unless appropriately treated, symptoms usually resolve only after abortion or delivery of an infected infant.[5, 7, 35–45] These infected neonates, who are often premature, develop signs suggesting sepsis, including fever, cough, respiratory distress, vomiting, diarrhea, cyanosis, convulsions, and jaundice. The condition typically progresses to meningitis, which may be rapidly fatal or may result in serious neurologic sequelae.[7] Other systemic manifes-

TABLE 31–7
Infections in Newborns with *Campylobacter fetus*

REFERENCE[a]	AGE AT ONSET	NO. OF PATIENTS	TYPE OF INFECTION	SOURCE OF ISOLATE	OUTCOME
Vinzent et al (1947)[5]	28 wk gestation	1	Stillbirth	Maternal blood	Stillbirth
Vinzent (1949)[34]	28 wk gestation	2	Not available; None	Maternal blood	Died, recovered
Hood and Todd (1960)[36]	28 wk gestation	1	Stillbirth	Brain	Stillbirth
van Wernig and Esseveld (1963)[37]	Premature	1	None	Placenta	No infection
Burgert and Hagstrom (1964)[38]	Premature	1	Meningitis	Cerebrospinal fluid	Died
Willis and Austin (1966)[39]	Premature	1	Bacteremia	Blood, cerebrospinal fluid	Died
Smith et al (1977)[40]	3 d	1	Bacteremia	Blood	Recovered
West et al (1982)[41]	19 wk gestation	1	Abortion	Cervix of mother	Abortion
Lee et al (1985)[42]	1 d	1	Meningitis, bacteremia	Cerebrospinal fluid, blood	Survived
Simor et al (1986)[43]	1 d	1	Bacteremia	Blood	Survived
Forbes and Scheifele (1987)[44]	1 d	1	Meningitis, bacteremia	Blood	Survived
Wong et al (1990)[35]	1 d	1	Bacteremia, meningitis	Blood	Survived
Morooka et al (1996)[127]		6	4 meningitis, 2 infants were asymptomatic	Nosocomial outbreak	Not stated

[a]See under *Campylobacter* in references.

TABLE 31–8
Infections in Newborns with *Campylobacter jejuni*

REFERENCE[a]	AGE AT ONSET	NO. OF PATIENTS	TYPE OF INFECTION	SOURCE OF ISOLATE	OUTCOME
Mawer and Smith (1979)[53]	1 d	1	Diarrhea	Stool	Recovered
CDR (1979)[54]	Not available	1	Diarrhea, bacteremia	Blood, stool	Recovered
Karmali and Tan (1980)[55]	3 d	1	Diarrhea	Stool	Recovered
Thomas et al (1980)[56]	12 d	1	Meningitis	Cerebrospinal fluid	Survived
Anders et al (1981)[57]	2–11 d	8	Diarrhea	Stool	Recovered
Vesikari et al (1981)[58]	2–11 d	8	Diarrhea	Stool	Recovered
Miller and Guard (1982)[59]	30 wk gestation	1	Bacteremia	Blood	Died
Buck et al (1982)[60]	2–3 d	2	Diarrhea	Stool	Recovered
Karmali et al (1984)[61]	2–3 d	4	Diarrhea	Stool	Recovered
Youngs et al (1985)[62]	1–3 d	3	Diarrhea	Stool	Recovered
Terrier et al (1985)[63]	3–6 d	25	Diarrhea	Stool	Recovered
Goossens et al (1986)[64]	5–16 d	11	Meningitis	Blood, cerebrospinal fluid	Recovered
DiNicola (1986)[65]	3 d	1	Diarrhea	Stool	Recovered
Hershkowici et al (1987)[66]	4–45 d	7	Diarrhea	Stool	Recovered
Others (1981, 1983, 1984)[67–72]	13–27 wk gestation	8	Abortion	Maternal blood and stool, spleen, lung	Abortion
Reina et al (1992)[73]	1 d	1	Diarrhea	Stool	Recovered

[a]See under *Campylobacter* in references.

tations include pericarditis, pneumonia, peritonitis, salpingitis, septic arthritis, and abscesses.[119] *C. upsaliensis*, like *C. fetus*, can cause abortion[139] (Table 31–7).

C. jejuni infection typically involves the gastrointestinal tract, producing watery diarrhea or a dysentery-like illness with fever and abdominal pain and stools that contain blood and mucus.[11, 28, 99] Older infants and children are generally affected, but neonates with diarrhea related to *C. jejuni* also have been reported (Table 31–8). Illness in neonates is generally mild or asymptomatic. Stools may contain blood, mucus, and pus[7, 17, 57, 58]; fever is often absent.[17, 57] The illness usually responds to appropriate antimicrobial therapy,[55, 57, 112] which shortens the period of fecal shedding.[140] Extraintestinal infections related to *C. jejuni* other than bacteremia are rare but include cholecystitis,[141] urinary tract infection,[142] and meningitis.[56] Bacteremia is a complication of gastrointestinal infection, particularly in malnourished children.[143] Meningitis that appears to occur secondarily to intestinal infection has also been reported in premature infants who have had intraventricular needle aspirations for neonatal hydrocephalus.[7] Complications in older children and adults that have been associated with *C. jejuni* enteritis include Reiter's syndrome,[144] Guillain-Barré syndrome,[145, 146] and reactive arthritis.[147, 148] Persistent *C. jejuni* infections have been described in patients infected with human immunodeficiency virus.[149] Extraintestinal manifestations generally occur in patients who are either immunosuppressed or at the extremes of age.[9] *Campylobacter lari* has caused chronic diarrhea and bacteremia in a neonate.[150]

Diagnosis

Most important in the diagnosis of *Campylobacter* infection is a high index of suspicion on clinical grounds. *C. fetus* and *C. jejuni* are both fastidious and may be overlooked on routine fecal cultures. The microbiology laboratory should be alerted to the possible diagnosis when specimens are obtained. Isolation of *Campylobacter* from blood and other sterile body sites does not represent the same problem as isolation from stool. Growth will occur on standard blood culture media, but it may be slow. In the case of *C. fetus* infecting the bloodstream or central nervous system, blood culture flasks should be blindly subcultured and held for at least 7 days or the organism may not be detected because of slow or inapparent growth.[38] The diagnosis of *C. fetus* infection should be considered when there is an unexplained febrile illness in the third trimester of pregnancy or in the event of recurrent abortion, prematurity, or neonatal sepsis and meningitis. A high index of suspicion and prompt, appropriate antimicrobial therapy may prevent the potentially serious neonatal complications that may follow maternal *C. fetus* infection. Although data are limited, a positive cervical culture for *Campylobacter* should be considered among potentially treatable causes of recurrent abortion.

Campylobacter is separated from the *Vibrio* organisms by its characteristics of carbohydrate nonfermentation as well as by its different nucleotide base composition.[11, 29-31, 34] *Campylobacter* measures 0.2 to 0.5 fm in width and 0.5 to 8.0 fm in length. It is a fastidious, microaerophilic, curved, motile gram-negative bacillus that has a single polar flagellum and is oxidase- and catalase-positive, except for *C. upsaliensis*, which is generally catalase-negative or weakly positive. *C. jejuni* and *C. fetus* are separated by growth temperature (*C. fetus* grows best at 25° C but can be cultured at 37° C; *C. jejuni* grows best at 42° C) and by nalidixic acid and cephalosporin susceptibilities because *C. jejuni* is susceptible to nalidixic acid and resistant to cephalosporins. *C. jejuni* grows best in a microaerobic environment of 5% oxygen and 10% carbon dioxide at 42° C. It will grow on a variety of media, including *Brucella* and Mueller-Hinton agars, but optimal isolation requires the addition of selective and nutritional supplements. Stool specimens or rectal swabs should be cultured.[137, 151] Growth at 42° C in the presence of cephalosporins is used to culture selectively for *C. jejuni* from fecal specimens. In a study of six media, charcoal-based selective media and a modified charcoal cefoperazone deoxycholate agar were the most selective for identification of *Campylobacter* species. Extending the incubation time from 48 to 72 hours led to an increase in the isolation rate regardless of the medium used.[152] Its typical darting motility may provide a clue to identification, even in fresh fecal specimens, when viewed by phase-contrast microscopy.[17, 153]

When the organism has been cultured, it is presumptively identified by motility and by its curved, sometimes "sea gull–like" appearance on carbolfuchsin stain. Polymorphonuclear leukocytes are usually found in stools when bloody diarrhea occurs and indicate the occurrence of colitis.[57, 97] To avoid potentially serious *C. jejuni* infection in the newborn infant, careful histories of any diarrheal illnesses in the family should be obtained, and pregnant women with any enteric illness should have cultures for this as well as other enteric pathogens. Detection of *C. jejuni* and *C. coli* by PCR has been reported[154] and in the future may be useful for the rapid and reliable identification of this organism.

The differential diagnostic considerations of *C. fetus* infections include the numerous agents that cause neonatal sepsis or meningitis, especially gram-negative bacilli. The other diagnostic considerations for an inflammatory or bloody enteritis include necrotizing enterocolitis, allergic proctitis, *Shigella*, *Salmonella*, and rarely *Shigella*, invasive *E. coli*, *E. coli* O157:H7, amebiasis, *Y. enterocolitica*, *Vibrio parahaemolyticus* infections, and pseudomembranous colitis associated with antibiotic use. Agglutination, complement fixation, bactericidal, immunofluorescence, and ELISA tests have been used for serologic diagnosis of *C. jejuni* infection and to study the immune response, but they are of limited value in establishing the diagnosis during an acute infection.[27]

Therapy

The prognosis is grave in newborn infants with sepsis or meningeal infection caused by *Campylobacter*. In infants with *C. jejuni* gastroenteritis, limited data suggest that appropriate, early antimicrobial therapy leads to improvement and rapid clearance of the organism from stool.[140] *Campylobacter* species are often resistant to penicillins, including ampicillin and cephalosporins.[155, 156] Most strains are susceptible to erythromycin, gentamicin, tetracycline, chloramphenicol, and the new quinolones, although sporadic resistance to these agents has been reported.[157, 158] It appears that a parenteral aminoglycoside is the drug of choice for *C. fetus* infections, pending in vitro susceptibility studies. In the case of central nervous system or meningeal involvement, cefotaxime and chloramphenicol are potential alternative drugs. Again, depending on in vitro susceptibilities, which vary somewhat with locale, erythromycin is the drug of choice for treating symptomatic *C. jejuni* enteritis.[13, 17, 18] If erythromycin therapy is initiated within the first 4 days of illness, a reduction in excretion of the organism and resolution of symptoms occur.[140] Although data regarding treatment of asymptomatic or convalescent carriers are not available, it would seem appropriate to treat colonized pregnant women in the third trimester of pregnancy, when there is a high risk of perinatal or neonatal infection. The failure of prophylactic parenteral gentamicin in a premature infant has been documented, followed by successful resolution of symptoms and fecal shedding with erythromycin stearate. Because there appears to be an increased risk of toxicity with erythromycin estolate during pregnancy and possibly in infants,[159] other forms of erythromycin should probably be used in these settings. Azithromycin appears to be effective if the organism is susceptible.[160] Strains that are erythromycin-resistant are often also resistant to azithromycin.[161] *Campylobacter* tends to have higher minimal inhibitory concentrations (MICs) for clarithromycin than for azithromycin.[162] Furazolidone has been used in children and ciprofloxacin in nonpregnant patients older than 17 years of age.

Prevention

Enteric precautions should be used during any acute diarrheal illness until *Campylobacter* can no longer be isolated from stools and diarrhea has subsided. Hand washing after handling raw poultry and washing cutting boards and utensils with soap and water after contact with raw poultry will prevent intrafamilial spread. Pasteurization of milk and chlorination of water are critical. Infected food handlers and hospital employees who are asymptomatic pose no known hazard for disease transmission if proper personal hygiene measures are maintained. Ingestion of human milk that contains anti–*C. jejuni* antibodies has been shown to protect infants from diarrhea due to *C. jejuni*.[163, 164]

CLOSTRIDIUM DIFFICILE

Nature of the Organism and Pathophysiology

Although pseudomembranous colitis was described before introduction of antibiotics into clinical practice,[1] it is now usually associated with antibiotic use. Before 1977, *Staphylococcus aureus* was assumed to be the cause,[2, 3] but the cause of essentially all cases of pseudomembranous colitis and a high percentage of antimicrobial-associated diarrhea is now established to be *Clostridium difficile*.[4–6] Rare cases of pseudomembranous colitis have been described in patients with dysentery related to *S. dysenteriae* serotype 1 and in the idiopathic hemolytic-uremic syndrome.[7, 8] It is now known that *S. dysenteriae* serotype 1 and the *E. coli* associated with hemolytic-uremic syndrome share the ability to make potent protein synthesis–inhibiting toxins, Shiga toxin, and the closely related Shiga-like toxins.[9]

C. *difficile* is a spore-forming, gram-positive anaerobic bacillus that produces two toxins. In the presence of antibiotic pressure, *C. difficile* colonic overgrowth and toxin production occur. The virulence properties of *C. difficile* are related to production of an enterotoxin that causes fluid secretion (toxin A) and a cytotoxin detectable by its cytopathic effects in tissue culture (toxin B).[10, 11] Both toxin genes have been cloned and sequenced, revealing that they encode proteins with estimated molecular masses of 308 kDa for toxin A and 270 kDa for toxin B.[12]

A wide variety of antibacterial, antifungal, antituberculosis, and antineoplastic agents have been associated with *C. difficile* colitis, although penicillin, clindamycin, and cephalosporins are associated most frequently. Rarely, no precipitating drug has been given.[13–17] *C. difficile* and its toxins can be demonstrated in up to one third of patients with antibiotic-associated diarrhea and in about 98% of patients with pseudomembranous colitis.[18]

Epidemiology

C. *difficile* may be isolated from soil and is frequently present in the hospital environment. Spores of *C. difficile* are acquired from the environment or by fecal-oral transmission from colonized individuals or from items in the environment such as thermometers and feeding tubes.[19–24] *C. difficile* has been demonstrated to persist on a contaminated floor for 5 months.[20] Nosocomial spread is related both to organisms on the hands of personnel[20, 21, 25] and to contaminated surfaces, which may serve as reservoirs.[6, 26] Although all groups are susceptible to infection, newborn infants represent a special problem. Less than 5% of healthy children older than 2 years of age[5] and healthy adults carry *C. difficile*,[18] but more than 50% of neonates can be demonstrated to have both *C. difficile* and its cytotoxin in their stools, usually in the absence of clinical findings.[6, 7, 21, 27, 28] Infants in neonatal intensive care units have high rates of colonization, in part because of frequent antibiotic use in these units.[27, 28] Clustering of infected infants suggests that much of the colonization of newborn infants represents nosocomial spread[6] rather than acquisition of maternal flora. The number of *C. difficile* organisms present in stools of well infants is similar to that found in older patients with pseudomembranous colitis.[28] The high frequency of colonization has led to justified skepticism about the pathogenic potential of this organism in the very young.[30] Although some episodes of diarrhea in early infancy may be due to *C. difficile*,[31] the diagnostic criteria used in older children and adults are inadequate to establish a definite diagnosis in this age group.

Clinical Manifestations

The usual manifestations of *C. difficile* disease in older children and adults include watery diarrhea, abdominal pain and tenderness, nausea, vomiting, and low-grade fever. Grossly bloody diarrhea is unusual, although occult fecal blood is common. Leukocytosis is present during severe illness. Diarrhea usually begins 4 to 9 days into a course of antimicrobial therapy but may be delayed until several weeks after completion of the therapeutic course. Usually, the illness is mild and self-limited if the offending drug is discontinued. Severe colitis with pseudomembranes is less common now than in previous years because the risk of diarrhea developing during antimicrobial therapy is recognized and the antimicrobial agent typically is stopped.

Complications of *C. difficile* infection include toxic megacolon, severe dehydration with electrolyte imbalance, and hypoalbuminemia. Several studies[6, 32, 33] suggest an association with necrotizing enterocolitis, but the relationship is debatable.[21] Chronic diarrhea without colitis after antibiotic therapy also has been described.[34]

Diagnosis

Endoscopic findings of pseudomembranes and hyperemic, friable rectal mucosa suggest the diagnosis of pseudomembranous colitis. Pseudomembranes are not always present in *C. difficile* colitis; mild cases are often described as nonspecific colitis. Several noninvasive techniques are used to establish the diagnosis and include culturing the organism using a selective agar medium, latex agglutination, cell culture assays, enzyme immunoassay (EIA) for toxin detection, and PCR.[35–38] Isolation of *C. difficile* from stool does not distinguish between toxigenic and nontoxigenic isolates. If *C. difficile* is isolated, testing for toxin by either cell culture or EIA should be performed to confirm the presence of a toxigenic strain. There are several commercially available EIAs that detect either toxin A or both toxins A and B.[35-37] These assays are sensitive and easy to use. Other assays are available for epidemiologic investigation of outbreaks of disease due to *C. difficile*.[38]

In older children and adults, the diagnosis is confirmed by culture of *C. difficile* and demonstration of toxin in feces. In neonates, these data are inadequate to prove that an illness is related to *C. difficile*. When the clinical picture is consistent, the stool studies are positive for *C. difficile* and no other cause for illness is found, a presumptive diagnosis of *C. difficile* is made. A favorable response to eradication of *C. difficile* is supportive evidence that the diagnosis is correct.[13] Because of the uncertainty implicit in the ambiguity of neonatal diagnostic criteria, other diagnoses must be considered.

Therapy and Prevention

When the decision is made that a neonate's symptoms are related to *C. difficile*, the initial approach should include both fluid and electrolyte therapy and discontinuation of the offending antibiotic. If this is done, symptoms usually resolve; however, if symptoms persist or worsen or if the patient has severe diarrhea, specific therapy with metronidazole,[6, 39] vancomycin,[40, 41] or bacitracin[40, 41] should be instituted. To decrease the emergence of vancomycin-resistant enterococci in hospitals, metronidazole is considered to be the first-line treatment of most patients with *C. difficile* colitis.[42] Oral vancomycin should be reserved for patients who do not respond to metronidazole. Resistance to metronidazole and bacitracin has been reported. The response rate to bacitracin is slower and less certain than that to vancomycin[40, 41] and potentially toxic if absorbed from an inflamed intestine. Patients who are unable to take oral therapy should be treated with both intravenous vancomycin and metronidazole as well as oral vancomycin delivered through a nasogastric tube, if possible, or an ostomy tube, if present.

After initiation of therapy, symptoms generally resolve within several days, and titer decreases and fecal toxins disappear eventually. Recurrence of colitis after discontinuation of metronidazole or vancomycin has been documented in 10 to 20% of patients.[43] Relapses are treated with a second course of either metronidazole or vancomycin. The combination of recommended antibiotics and *Saccharomyces boulardii* administered PO was effective and safe therapy for patients with recurrent disease due to *C. difficile*.[44] No benefit of *S. boulardii* was demonstrated for patients during their initial episodes. Drugs that decrease intestinal motility should not be given.

Neutralizing antibody against *C. difficile* cytotoxin has been demonstrated in human colostrum.[45] There are data showing that in addition to secretory IgA directed at toxin A, there are nonantibody factors present in milk that interfere with the action of toxin B.[46] Breast-feeding appears to decrease the frequency of colonization by *C. difficile*.[47]

In addition to standard precautions, contact precautions are recommended for the duration of illness. Meticulous hand-washing techniques, proper handling of contaminated waste and fomites, and limiting the use of antimicrobial agents are the best available methods for control of *C. difficile* infection.

VIBRIO CHOLERAE

V. cholerae is a gram-negative, curved bacillus with a polar flagellum. Of the many serotypes, only enterotoxin-producing organisms of serotype 01 and 0139 cause epidemics. *V. cholerae* 01 is divided into two serotypes, Inaba and Ogawa, and two biotypes, classic and E1 Tor; the latter is the predominant biotype. Nontoxigenic 01 strains and non-01 strains of *V. cholerae* can cause diarrhea and sepsis but do not cause outbreaks.[1-3]

V. cholerae 0 group 1 is the classic example of an enteropathogen whose virulence is due to enterotoxin production. Cholera toxin is an 84-MDa protein whose five B subunits cause toxin binding to the enterocyte membrane ganglioside GM_1, and whose A subunit causes adenosine diphosphate ribosylation of a guanosine triphosphate–binding regulatory subunit of adenylate cyclase.[4, 5] The elevated cAMP levels that result from stimulation of enterocytes by cholera toxin cause secretion of salt and water with concomitant inhibition of absorption. Two other toxins are also encoded within the virulence cassette that encodes choleratoxin. These toxins, zona occludens toxin (*zot*) and accessory choleratoxin (*ace*), are consistently found in illness-causing strains of both 01 and 0139 but not usually in *V. cholerae* organisms that are less virulent.

Since 1960, *V. cholerae* 01, biotype El Tor, has spread from India and Southeast Asia to Africa, the Middle East, southern Europe, and the southern, western, and central Pacific islands (Oceania). In late January of 1991, toxigenic *V. cholerae* 01, serotype Inaba, biotype El Tor, appeared in several coastal cities of Peru.[2, 3] It rapidly spread to most countries in South and North America. In reported cases, travel from the United States to Latin America or Asia and ingestion of contaminated food transported from Latin America or Asia have been incriminated. *V. cholerae* 0139 (Bengal) arose on the Indian subcontinent as a new cause of epidemic cholera in 1993.[6-11] In addition, in the United States, an endemic focus of a unique strain of toxigenic *V. cholerae* 01 exists on the Gulf Coast of Louisiana and Texas.[1, 12] This strain is different from the one associated with the epidemic in South America. Most cases of disease associated with the strain endemic to the U.S. Gulf Coast have been due to consumption of raw or undercooked shellfish. Humans are the only documented natural host, but free-living *V. cholerae* organisms can exist in the aquatic environment. The usual reported vehicles of transmission have included contaminated water or ice; contaminated food, particularly raw or undercooked shellfish; moist grains held at ambient temperature; and raw or partially dried fish. The usual mode of infection is ingestion of contaminated food or water. Boiling water or treating it with chlorine or iodine and adequate cooking of food kill the organism.[2] Direct person-to-person spread by contact has not been documented. Persons with low gastric acidity are at increased risk for cholera infection.

Cholera acquired during pregnancy, particularly in the third trimester, is associated with a high incidence of fetal death.[13] Miscarriage can be attributed to a fetal acidosis and hypoxemia resulting from the marked metabolic and circulatory changes that this disease induces in the mother. It is not surprising, therefore, that the likelihood of delivering a stillborn child is closely correlated with the severity of the maternal illness. The inability to culture *V. cholerae* from stillborn infants of infected mothers, together with the usual absence of bacteremia in cholera, suggests that transplacental fetal infection is not a cause of intrauterine death.

Neonatal cholera is a rare disease. This generalization applies to the new 0139 strains also, although both mild[14] and severe illness have rarely been described in newborns.[15] Among 327 children admitted to a cholera research hospital in Dacca, Bangladesh, there were no infants under 4 weeks of age.[16] Even infants born of mothers with active diarrheal disease may escape infection, despite evidence that rice-water stools, almost certain to be ingested during the birth process, may contain as many as 10^9 organisms per ml.[16] The reason for this apparently low attack rate among newborns is not known for certain; however, it is probably due in large part to the protection conferred by breast-feeding in those parts of the world in which cholera is most prevalent.[17] Human milk contains antibodies[18] as well as receptor-like glycoprotein that inhibit adherence of *V. cholerae*[19] and gangliosides that bind cholera toxin.[20] The role of transplacentally acquired vibriocidal maternal antibodies has not been determined.[21] Because *V. cholerae* causes neither bacteremia nor intestinal invasion, protection against illness is more likely to be a function of mucosal antibodies than of serologic titers.[22, 23] Additional factors that may reduce the incidence of neonatal cholera include the large inoculum required for infection[24] and the limited exposure of the newborn to the contaminated food and water by which infection is usually transmitted.[25]

Clinicians should request that appropriate cultures be performed for stool specimens from persons suspected of having cholera. The specimen is plated on thiosulfate citrate bile salts sucrose agar either directly or after optional enrichment in alkaline peptone water. Isolated specimens of *V. cholerae* should be confirmed at a state health department and then sent to the CDC for testing for production of cholera toxin. A fourfold rise in vibriocidal antibody titers between acute and convalescent serum samples or a fourfold decline in titers between early and late (> 2 months) convalescent serum specimens can confirm the diagnosis. Probes have been developed to test for cholera toxin.[26, 27]

The most important modality of therapy is administration of oral or parenteral rehydration therapy to correct dehydration and electrolyte imbalance and maintain hydration.[2] Antimicrobial therapy will eradicate vibrios, reduce the duration of diarrhea, and reduce requirements for fluid replacement. One cholera vaccine, which is administered parenterally, is currently licensed in the United States and is of very limited value. Several experimental oral vaccines are being tested.[28–30]

YERSINIA ENTEROCOLITICA

Y. enterocolitica is a major cause of enteritis in much of the industrialized world.[1, 2] Enteritis due to this organism primarily occurs in infants and young children, and infections in the United States are reported to be more common in the North than in the South.[3–8] *Y. enterocolitica* serogroup 0:3 is the most common serogroup in Europe, Japan, and Canada.[9] In the United States, serogroup 0:8 has been the most common, but outbreaks of diarrhea due to 0:3 have been reported.[3, 5] *Y. enterocolitica* can also cause extraintestinal disease[4, 8, 10] and has been associated with a variety of autoimmune manifestations, including arthritis and erythema nodosum. Animals, especially swine, have been shown to serve as the reservoir for *Y. enterocolitica* serogroup 0:3. Transmission has also occurred following ingestion of contaminated milk[11] and infusion of contaminated blood products.[12]

Virulence of *Y. enterocolitica* is related primarily to a virulence plasmid, which is closely related to the virulence plasmids of *Yersinia pseudotuberculosis* and *Yersinia pestis*.[13, 14] A heat-stable enterotoxin, which is closely related to the LT of ETEC,[15] may also be important. It is likely that additional virulence genes remain to be identified.[16]

Infection with *Y. enterocolitica* is recognized as one of the causes of bacterial gastroenteritis in young children, yet knowledge of neonatal infection with this organism is fragmentary. Even in large series, isolation of *Yersinia* from newborns is rare.[1, 2, 17]

The youngest infants whose clinical course has been described in detail were from 11 days to several months of age at the onset of their illness.[2, 17–25] There were no features of the gastroenteritis to distinguish it from that caused by other invasive enteric pathogens such as *Shigella* or *Salmonella*. Infants presented either with watery diarrhea or with stools containing mucus together with streaks of blood. Sepsis was common in these infants.[21, 22] Fever is not a consistent finding in children with bacteremia, and meningitis is rare. In older children, fever and right lower quadrant pain mimicking appendicitis are often found.[12]

Y. enterocolitica can be recovered from throat swabs, mesenteric lymph nodes, peritoneal fluid, blood, and stool. Because laboratory identification of organisms from stool requires special techniques, laboratory personnel should be notified when *Yersinia* is suspected. The yield of *Y. enterocolitica* stool cultures can be increased by cold enrichment.[26] Biotyping and serotyping are useful in assessing the clinical relevance of isolates. PCR has been used to detect pathogenic strains.[27, 28]

The effect of antimicrobial therapy on the outcome of gastrointestinal infection is uncertain. It has been recommended that antibiotics be reserved for sepsis or prolonged and severe gastroenteritis[1]; however, there are no prospective studies comparing the efficacy of various antibiotics with each other or with supportive therapy alone. Most strains of *Y. enterocolitica* are susceptible to trimethoprim-sulfamethoxazole, the aminoglycosides, piperacillin, imipenem, third-generation cepholosporins, amoxicillin–clavulanate potassium, and chloramphenicol, and resistant to amoxicillin, ampicillin, carbenicillin, ticarcillin, and macrolides.[29–31] Because there are serotype-related differences in susceptibility, therapy in individual cases should be guided by in vitro susceptibility testing.

OTHER BACTERIAL AGENTS AND FUNGI

Proving that an organism causes diarrhea is difficult, particularly when it may be present in large numbers in stools of healthy persons. Bacteria that have been associated with acute gastroenteritis may be considered to be causative when the following criteria are met:

1. A single specific strain of the organism should be found as the predominant organism in a majority of affected infants by different investigators in outbreaks of enteric disease in different localities.
2. This strain should be isolated in a much lower percentage and in smaller numbers from stool specimens of healthy infants.
3. Currently available methods must be used to exclude other recognized enteropathogens, including viruses and parasites, as well as enterotoxigenic agents and fastidious organisms such as *Campylobacter*.
4. Demonstration of effective specific antimicrobial therapy and specific antibody responses and, ultimately, production of experimental disease in volunteers are helpful in establishing the identity of a microorganism as a pathogen.

Optimally, the putative pathogen should have virulence traits that can be demonstrated in model systems. Most bacteria that have been suggested as occasional causes of gastroenteritis in neonates fail to fulfill one or more of these criteria. Their role in the etiology of diarrheal disease is questionable. This is particularly true of those microorganisms described in early reports in which the possibility of infection with more recently recognized agents cannot be excluded. Much of the clinical, bacteriologic, and epidemiologic data collected earlier linking unusual enteropathogens to infantile diarrhea should be reevaluated in light of current knowledge and methodology.

Diarrhea sometimes occurs as a manifestation of systemic infection. Patients with staphylococcal toxic shock syndrome, for example, often have diarrhea. Loose stools sometimes occur in sepsis, but it is unclear whether the diarrhea is a cause or an effect. The organisms isolated from blood cultures in a group of Bangladeshi infants and children with diarrhea included *Staphylococcus aureus*, *Haemophilus influenzae*, *Streptococcus pneumoniae*, *Pseudomonas aeruginosa*, and various gram-negative enteric bacilli.[1] It is unknown whether the bacteriology of sepsis associated with diarrhea is similar in the well-nourished infants seen in industrialized countries. Several potential causes of diarrhea are listed.

Aeromonas hydrophila

Of the potential enteric pathogens discussed in this section, *Aeromonas hydrophila* is the organism most likely to be a true enteropathogen. The organism is widely distributed in animals and the environment. Although wound infection, pneumonia, and sepsis (especially in compromised hosts) represent typical *Aeromonas* infections, gastroenteritis is being increasingly recognized. The organism is a gram-negative, oxidase-positive, facultatively anaerobic bacillus belonging to the family Vibrionaceae. Like other members of this family, it produces an enterotoxin[2] that causes fluid secretion in rabbit ileal loops.[3] Some strains cause fluid accumulation in the suckling mouse model,[4] whereas other strains are invasive[5] or cytotoxic.[6] The enterotoxin is not immunologically related to cholera toxin or the heat LT of *E. coli*.[7]

Although volunteer studies and studies with monkeys have failed to provide supportive evidence for enteropathogenicity,[8, 9] there is good reason to believe that *A. hydrophila* does cause diarrhea in children. The earliest description of *Aeromonas* causing diarrhea was an outbreak that occurred in a neonatal unit.[10] Although several studies have failed to show an association with diarrhea,[11–15] most studies have found more *Aeromonas* isolates among children with gastroenteritis than among controls.[16–18] Part of the controversy may be due to strain differences; some strains possess virulence traits related to production of gastroenteritis, whereas others do not.[12, 19]

The diarrhea described in children is a disease of summer, primarily affecting children in the first 2 years of life. In one study, 7 (13%) of 55 cases of *Aeromonas* detected during a 20-month period occurred in infants under 1 month of age. Typically, watery diarrhea with no fever has been described, although there are descriptions of watery diarrhea with fever.[20] However, in 22%, a dysentery-like illness occurred. Dysentery-like illness has been described in the neonate.[21] In one third of children, diarrhea has been reported to last for more than 2 weeks.[12] There may be species-related differences in clinical features of *Aeromonas*-associated gastroenteritis in children.[22] Organisms that were formerly classified as *A. hydrophila* are now sometimes labeled as *Aeromonas sobria* or *Aeromonas caviae*.[23, 24] Fever and abdominal pain appear to be particularly common with *A. sobria*. One series of *A. hydrophila* isolates from newborns in Dallas showed more blood cultures than stool cultures positive for *Aeromonas*.[25]

Diagnosis of enteric infection associated with *Aeromonas* is often not made because this organism is not routinely looked for in hospital laboratories. When the organism is suspected, the laboratory should be notified so that oxidase testing can be performed.

The organism is usually susceptible to aztreonam, imipenem, meropenem, third-generation cephalosporins, trimethoprim-sulfamethoxazole, and chloramphenicol.[26–28]

Plesiomonas shigelloides

Plesiomonas shigelloides is a gram-negative, facultative anaerobic bacillus that, like *Aeromonas*, is a member of the

Vibrionaceae family. It is widely disseminated in the environment; outbreaks of disease are usually related to ingestion of contaminated water or seafood.[29] Although it has been associated with outbreaks of diarrheal disease[30] and has been found more commonly in ill than well controls,[12] the role of *P. shigelloides* in diarrheal disease has remained controversial.[31] If it is a true enteropathogen, the mechanism by which it causes disease is unclear.[32, 33] The role of this organism in neonatal diarrhea has not been extensively investigated. Infections of neonates have been reported,[34–37] but most cases of enteric disease currently reported in the United States are in adults.[29] Typical illness consists of watery diarrhea and cramps; sometimes fever, bloody stools, and emesis occur and last for 3 to 42 days.

Diagnosis is not usually made by clinical microbiology laboratory testing because, as with *Aeromonas*, coliforms can be confused with *P. shigelloides* unless an oxidase test is performed.[38] Thus, the true frequency of infection is unknown. The organism has antibiotic susceptibilities similar to those of *Aeromonas*.[39, 40]

Miscellaneous Gram-Negative Rods

There are scant data suggesting that *P. aeruginosa* may cause neonatal gastroenteritis.[41–46] Enteric colonization with *Pseudomonas* in healthy newborns is usually detectable during the first few days of life.[49, 50] In most nurseries, the incidence of fecal carriage among neonates and young infants ranges from 0[51, 52] to 10%.[49, 53–55]

Neonates who carry *Pseudomonas* in the intestinal tract usually show no evidence of systemic or enteric disease,[42, 44, 46–49, 50, 56] even when the organisms are present in numbers sufficient to cause blue-green discoloration of the stools.[57] The symptoms of enteritis believed to be associated with *Pseudomonas* have varied from a few soft stools to a profuse watery diarrhea accompanied by vomiting.[42, 43, 45, 58] Descriptions of a green or blue-green color of diarrheal stools are difficult to evaluate because this finding may be seen with diarrhea from any cause.[47, 50, 59] The presence of cyanosis or a gray pallor of the skin has been specifically mentioned in several instances.[42, 43, 45, 59]

Klebsiella pneumoniae, considered alone or together with *Enterobacter* species, has been isolated from about one third of stool samples obtained from healthy infants.[53–55, 63] Several reports of acute gastroenteritis believed to have been caused by *Klebsiella* suggest that, rather than playing an etiologic role, these organisms had probably proliferated within an already inflamed bowel.[67, 71, 74] The recovery of *Klebsiella-Enterobacter* in pure culture from diarrheal stools has led several investigators to suggest that these bacteria may occasionally play a causative role in infantile gastroenteritis and enterocolitis.[63, 70, 75–78] Ingestion of infant formula contaminated with *Enterobacter sakazakii* has been associated with development of bloody diarrhea and sepsis.[79] However, *Klebsiella* species also may be isolated in pure culture from stools of newborns with no enteric symptoms.[56, 64, 66] In one study, certain capsular types of *Klebsiella* were more often isolated from infants with diarrheal disease than from normal infants.[63] More re-

cent work has shown that *K. pneumoniae*, *Enterobacter cloacae*, and *Citrobacter* species are capable of producing enterotoxins.[79–86] Reports of isolation of *Citrobacter* species, like those of *Klebsiella* species, note associations with enteric illnesses in up to 7% of cases.[89–91] At present, there is inadequate evidence to define the roles of *Klebsiella*, *Enterobacter*, and *Citrobacter* species as etiologic agents of enteric illnesses.

Proteus has been associated with infantile diarrhea since the early part of this century.[94, 95] Some investigators believe that there is sufficient evidence to implicate *Proteus* species as a definite, although uncommon, cause of outbreaks of infantile gastroenteritis.[94, 96–98] Others, noting that these organisms are generally recovered as frequently from healthy infants as from infants with diarrheal disease, ascribe little significance to their presence in stool cultures.[53–55, 72, 99, 100]

An association between *Providencia* and neonatal enteritis has been substantiated largely by anecdotal reports of nursery outbreaks.[91, 107–109] These bacteria are rarely isolated from infants with sporadic or community-acquired diarrheal disease.[53–55, 110–112]

Staphylococcus aureus

S. aureus was associated with pseudomembranous enterocolitis and the administration of antimicrobial agents before recognition of *C. difficile* as the usual cause of this syndrome. *S. aureus* is frequently recovered from stool specimens of healthy infants[101, 102] and infants with enteritis related to other causes.[103] The occurrence of primary staphylococcal infection of the gastrointestinal tract has rarely been described, even during the pandemic of the 1950s. A few outbreaks of gastroenteritis have suggested that this illness may, albeit infrequently, represent the principal manifestation of epidemic staphylococcal disease in the newborn infant.[104]

Group D Streptococci

There is insufficient evidence to confirm that group D streptococci, generally regarded as normal enteric flora, are capable of causing neonatal gastroenteritis.[106–108] It is more likely that their presence in increased numbers in the intestinal tract is the consequence rather than the cause of diarrheal disease.[48, 109]

Candida albicans

Candida albicans is generally acquired during passage through the birth canal and is considered a normal, although minor, component of the fecal flora of the neonate.[113] Intestinal overgrowth of these organisms frequently accompanies infantile gastroenteritis,[113–115] particularly after antimicrobial therapy.[114, 116] The upper small gut may become colonized with *Candida* in malnourished children with diarrhea[117]; whether the presence of the organism is cause or effect is unclear. Stool cultures obtained from infants with diarrheal disease are therefore inconclusive, and although *Candida* enteritis has been reported in adults,[118] the importance of this organism as a primary pathogen in the etiology of neonatal gastroenteritis has been difficult to prove. Clinical descriptions of nursery epidemics of candidal enteritis are poorly documented, generally preceding the recognition of EPEC and rotaviruses as a cause of neonatal diarrhea. Even well-studied cases of intestinal involvement add little in the way of substantive proof because secondary invasion of *Candida* has been shown to be a complication of coliform enteritis.[114–116]

Although diarrhea has sometimes been described as a finding in neonatal disseminated candidiasis,[119] more typically gastrointestinal tract involvement with disseminated *Candida* is associated with abdominal distention and bloody stools mimicking necrotizing enterocolitis.[116–122] Typically, affected infants are premature and have courses complicated by antibiotic administration, catheter use, and surgical procedures during the first several weeks of life. A trial of oral anticandidal therapy may be helpful in neonates suffering from diarrhea in the presence of oral or cutaneous candidiasis, particularly if mycelial elements of *Candida* can be demonstrated on a direct fecal smear. If the therapy is appropriate, a response should be forthcoming within 2 to 5 days.

PARASITES

The most important protozoa known to cause diarrhea in various parts of the United States are *Entamoeba histolytica*, *Giardia lamblia*, and four spore-forming protozoa: *Cryptosporidium parvum*, *Isospora belli*, *Microsporidium* species, and *Cyclospora cayetanensis*. Because of lack of data in the neonate, only *E. histolytica*, *G. lamblia*, and *Cryptosporidium* are discussed here.

Entamoeba histolytica

E. histolytica is an enteric pathogen that has been classified into two species that are morphologically identical but genetically distinct. *E. histolytica* is a noninvasive parasite that does not cause diarrhea. Asymptomatic colonization of neonates with various species of ameba is common in areas of high endemicity.[1] Infection probably results from ingestion of fecal material at birth, from unsterile oral fluids given as a supplement to breast-feeding, or from close contact with infected mothers.[2] Rates of acquisition and shedding of amebic infections, in contrast to giardial infections, appear to be independent of age.[3] On rare occasions, rapidly fatal colitis has been reported in infants.[4–7] Likewise, younger animals appear to be more susceptible than older animals to *E. histolytica* infection.[8, 9]

Diagnosis can be established by stool examination for cysts and trophozoites by serologic studies.[10] Through the use of PCR, isoenzyme analysis, and antigen detection assays, *E. histolytica* and *Entamoeba dupar* can be differentiated.[11, 12] Serum antibody assays may be helpful in establishing the diagnosis of amebic dysentery and extraintestinal amebiasis with liver involvement. The efficacy of treatment with metronidazole for colitis or liver abscess has not been established for the newborn period, although one investigator has used this therapy

with success.[4] Patients with colitis or liver abscess caused by *E. histolytica* are treated also with iodoquinol, as are asymptomatic carriers.

Giardia lamblia

G. lamblia is a binucleate flagellated protozoan parasite with trophozoite and cyst stages.[13] It is spread by the fecal-oral route after ingestion of cysts. Child-care center outbreaks reflecting person-to-person spread have demonstrated high infectivity.[14–17] Foodborne transmission and waterborne transmission also occur.[13, 18]

Infection is often asymptomatic. However, the younger the patient when infected, the more likely it is that symptomatic infection will occur.[19–26] Symptoms in giardiasis are related to the age of the patient, with diarrhea, vomiting, anorexia, and failure to thrive typical in the youngest infected children. Seroprevalence studies demonstrated evidence of past or present infection in 40% of Peruvian children by the age of 6 months.[24] In a study of lactating mothers and their infants, 82% of mothers and 42% of infants excreted *Giardia* once during the study, some infants as early as 3 months of age.[19] Of these infected infants, 86% had diarrhea, suggesting that the first exposure to the parasite results in disease.[19] In a prospective study of diarrhea conducted in Mexico,[26] infants frequently were infected with *Giardia* from birth to 2 months, with a crude incidence rate of first *Giardia* infection of 1.4 infections per child-year in infants from birth to 2 months of age.

Giardiasis is being increasingly recognized as a cause of chronic diarrhea or malabsorption, especially among children. The growing number of reports of giardiasis in infants, especially those who are not breast-fed, suggests that infants are at risk as soon as they eat or drink from a contaminated environment.[19, 24, 26, 27] Some cases have been recognized by stool or duodenal fluid examination in the first 4 weeks of life.[25, 26, 28] The diagnosis of giardiasis can be made on the basis of demonstration of antigen by EIA; of cysts or trophozoites in feces; or of trophozoites in duodenal fluid or, less frequently, on duodenal biopsy.[13, 18] Breast-feeding is believed to protect against symptomatic giardiasis.[26, 29, 30] This protection may be mediated by both cellular and humoral immunity[31–33] and nonspecifically by the antigiardial effects of unsaturated fatty acids.[34] Certainly, giardiasis should be considered among the treatable causes of chronic diarrhea, especially when associated with symptoms of malabsorption or malnutrition in infants. *Giardia* infections may result in severe diarrhea and may respond to metronidazole or furazolidone.[18]

Cryptosporidium

Cryptosporidium is a coccidian protozoon[35, 36] that is known to be an important cause of chronic diarrhea in patients with acquired immunodeficiency syndrome (AIDS)[37] and of acute diarrhea in immunocompetent patients, particularly young children.[38–44] The organism is related to *Toxoplasma gondii*, *I. belli*, and *Plasmodium* species. The species infecting humans and most other mammals is *Cryptosporidium parvum*.[35, 36] The life cycle involves ingestion of thick-walled oocysts; release of sporozoites, which penetrate intestinal epithelium; and development of merozoites. There is both asexual and sexual reproduction, with the latter resulting in formation of new oocysts that can be passed in stools.

Cryptosporidium species are ubiquitous. Infection often occurs in persons traveling to endemic areas.[45] Because *Cryptosporidium* infects a wide variety of animal species, there is often a history of animal contact among infected individuals.[46] Person-to-person spread, particularly in household contacts[42, 46-49] and day-care centers,[39-41] is well documented and suggests that the organism is highly infectious. Waterborne outbreaks also occur.[50] Asymptomatic carriage is rare. For reasons that are unclear, immunocompetent hosts appear to be infected more often in summer or fall.[42, 51, 52]

The clinical manifestations of illness in immunocompetent persons resemble those of *Giardia* infection but are somewhat shorter in duration.[53] Symptoms and signs include watery diarrhea, abdominal pain, myalgia, fever, and weight loss.[35, 40, 42, 45, 48, 53, 54] Although infection in the first month of life has been described,[43, 51] no reports have yet focused specifically on the neonate with cryptosporidiosis. The fact that symptoms resolve before excretion of oocysts suggests that a newborn whose mother has been ill with cryptosporidiosis in the month before delivery ought to be at risk even if the mother is asymptomatic at the time of the child's birth.[45] Furthermore, with the increasing frequency of AIDS, it is likely that women with symptomatic cryptosporidiosis occasionally will be delivered of infants who will become infected. Infants infected early in life may develop chronic diarrhea and malnutrition.[55]

The diagnosis of cryptosporidiosis is most typically made by examination of fecal smears using the Giemsa stain, Ziehl-Neelsen stain, auramine-rhodamine stain, Sheather's sugar flotation, an immunofluorescence procedure, a modified concentration-sugar flotation method, or an EIA.[56, 57] There is currently no consistently effective treatment for cryptosporidiosis. Because illness is usually self-limited in the normal host, attention to fluid, electrolyte, and nutritional status usually suffices. Enteric isolation of hospitalized infants with this illness is appropriate because of the high infectivity. Several studies suggest that the risk of infection early in life may be decreased by breast-feeding.[44, 51] Hyperimmune bovine colostrum raised against *Cryptosporidium* oocysts and sporozoites and monoclonal antibodies have reduced cryptosporidial infection in animals.[58-60]

VIRUSES

Acute viral gastroenteritis occurs in both endemic and epidemic forms worldwide. Most cases of acute gastroenteritis are caused by viruses, yet relatively few are confirmed in the laboratory. Several viruses are recognized to account for most cases of viral gastroenteritis in humans: (1) rotaviruses, (2) enteric adenoviruses, (3) caliciviruses, and (4) astroviruses (Table 31–9). These viruses differ in their epidemiology and pathogenesis in humans.[1-4] Other viruses have been identified from ani-

TABLE 31–9
Viruses Associated with Gastroenteritis in Humans

VIRUS	EXCRETION BY NEONATES DEMONSTRATED	SIZE (nm)
Rotavirus	+	70
Enteric adenovirus	+	70–80
Caliciviruses	+	28–40
Astrovirus	+	28

mals and humans with gastroenteritis, but their significance as a cause of diarrhea in humans is unknown.

The first human gastroenteritis virus discovered was the Norwalk agent, which was reported in 1972 from an outbreak of gastroenteritis that occurred in a primary school in Norwalk, Ohio, in 1968.[5] The agent they discovered has since been shown to be the prototype human calicivirus. A year later, a human rotavirus was observed in duodenal biopsies and stool specimens obtained from infants acutely ill with diarrhea and vomiting in Australia.[6] As epidemiologic studies confirmed the importance of rotavirus as a major cause of intestinal infection in childhood, a variety of other enteric agents, visualized by electron microscopy (EM) in stool preparations, were being reported as additional possible agents of diarrheal disease. By 1977, four more viruses had been detected in fecal specimens obtained from patients with acute enteritis: coronavirus, astrovirus, calicivirus, and "minireovirus." Although the first three, particularly the coronaviruses, were well-known in veterinary practice, they had not been associated before that time with human illness.

Enteric adenoviruses are another important viral agent of endemic diarrheal illness of infants and young children worldwide and cause outbreaks in child-care centers.[7-10] Caliciviruses and astroviruses cause sporadic cases and occasionally outbreaks of diarrheal illness in infants, young children, and adults.[11-17] Although agents other than rotavirus have been visualized in stool specimens of neonates, the incidence of infection and the severity of illness associated with these viruses in neonates are not defined adequately. The remainder of this section is limited to a discussion of rotaviruses and rotavirus gastroenteritis. Several reviews of the other viral agents responsible for gastroenteritis have been published.[1-4]

Nature of the Organism

Rotavirus derives its name from the distinctive wheel-like appearance of the virus when viewed under EM (Latin *rota*, meaning "wheel").[18, 19] Rotavirus particles contain a genome consisting of 11 segments of double-stranded RNA enclosed in a double-shelled capsid.[20] The inner capsid contains trimers of viral protein 6 (VP6), a potent immunogen that specifies group and subgroup antigens, encoded by gene 6. Six serologic groups (A through F) have been identified based on antigenic heterogeneity of VP6; groups A, B, and C occur in humans. Group A is the most common rotavirus that infects humans worldwide. The outer capsid contains a VP7 glycoprotein (G protein), encoded by gene 7, 8, or 9, and a VP4 protease-cleaved protein (P protein), encoded by gene 4. The latter (P protein) forms the viral spikes. Both G and P types independently are responsible for virus neutralization; therefore, a classification system has been proposed in which a strain would be identified by both its G-type and its P-type specificity.[21] Fourteen G types have been described from various animals, 10 of which have been isolated from humans. Each group A rotavirus has both subgroup and serotype designations, as well as a unique electropherotype identified by electrophoresis of its RNA genome segments. Rotavirus serotypes have been defined by plaque reduction neutralization in vitro, by tube neutralization, by fluorescent focus neutralization, by EIA using serotype-specific monoclonal antibodies, and by direct nucleotide sequence analysis of the VP7 gene.[22-24] The G types 2 to 4 account for over 95% of infections in humans, but other G types have been reported.[25] Although most human rotaviruses reported thus far have been group A, rotaviruses belonging to groups B and C have been associated with gastroenteritis in humans.[26, 27] These rotaviruses are morphologically identical to, but antigenically distinct from, group A rotaviruses.

The young of almost all mammalian species experience rotavirus infection. The virus has been detected in diarrheal stools from infant mice, calves, piglets, foals, lambs, kittens, rabbits, deer, antelope, gorillas, and chimpanzees, as well as humans. Rotaviruses have been identified in diarrheal stools, duodenal fluid, and small intestinal aspirates of infants and young children with acute gastroenteritis. The particle is structurally stable and ideally suited for intestinal infection since it resists degradation by trypsin, chymotrypsin, and pepsin and by a strongly acid (pH 3) environment.[28] Several studies with animal rotaviruses have indicated that pancreatic enzymes, primarily trypsin, enhance infectivity.[29] Rotavirus has been recognized by EM after storage for many years at $-20°$ C. The duration of infectivity of virus particles under various conditions of humidity and temperature has not been evaluated.

Pathogenesis

Infants with asymptomatic rotavirus infections in the nursery are less likely than uninfected nursery mates to experience severe rotavirus infection later in life.[30, 31] Several studies have indicated that serum and intestinal antirotavirus antibodies are associated with protection against infection,[32-37] although results have not been uniform.[38, 39] Studies performed in vitro, in animal models, and among naturally infected children and adult volunteers have shown an association between levels of antirotavirus antibodies to the neutralization epitopes, VP7 and VP4, and protection against homotypic virus infection and illness.[32, 33, 40-42] Protective isotopic-specific and G type–specific antibodies were achieved in a majority of children attending child-care centers after two seasons of exposure.[43] A high titer of fecal antirotavirus IgA antibody has been associated with protection against infection and illness.[44-51]

Presumably, antirotaviral antibodies acquired passively through breast-feeding should protect the neonate against infection. The high prevalence of such antibodies in colostrum and human milk has been demonstrated by numerous investigators in widely diverse geographic areas.[52] The presence of these antibodies correlates closely with that of serum antirotaviral antibodies.[53-57] Acquisition of circulating immunity in a susceptible woman during infection with rotavirus or following immunization with rotavirus is accompanied by the appearance of specific antibodies in her human milk, probably through stimulation of the enteromammary immune system.[55-58] Thus 90 to 100% of women examined in London, Bangladesh, Guatemala, Costa Rica, and the United States had antirotaviral IgA antibodies in their milk for periods of up to 2 years post partum.[52-59] Rotavirus-specific IgG antibodies have been found during the first few postpartum days in about one third of human milk samples assayed,[55, 57] whereas IgM antibodies were detectable in about one half[57] by EIA.

The actual demonstration of a beneficial effect of breast-feeding against rotavirus in neonates is poorly documented. Several studies have demonstrated no protective effect of breast-feeding against diarrhea caused by rotavirus.[54, 60, 61] In another study, there was no apparent difference in the infection rates of rotavirus diarrhea in breast-fed and formula-fed infants, but clinical manifestations of illness were milder in breast-fed infants.[62] Glycoproteins in human milk have been shown to prevent rotavirus infection in vitro and in an animal model,[63] and in humans lactadherin concentrations were significantly higher in human milk ingested by infants who developed asymptomatic rotavirus infection than by infants who developed symptomatic rotavirus infection.[64]

The essential pathologic feature of rotavirus infection is destruction of the absorptive cells lining the duodenum, jejunum, and possibly the ileum.[65] Lactase, which is present only in the brush border of the differentiated epithelial cells at these sites, may act as a combined receptor and uncoating enzyme for the virus, permitting transfer of the particles into the cell.[66] Perhaps for this reason, infection is limited to the mature columnar enterocytes on the distal half of the villi; crypt cells and crypt-derived cuboidal cells, which lack a brush border, appear to be resistant to rotaviral infection.[66, 67] This concept also may explain why rotavirus infection is less common in infants under 32 weeks of gestational age than in more mature infants[68]; between 26 and 34 weeks of gestational age, lactase activity is approximately 30% of that found in full-term infants.[69]

Fecal excretion of virus, probably a valid reflection of the intensity of mucosal infection, often begins a day or so before illness.[70-72] Maximal excretion usually occurs during the third and fourth days, as increasing numbers of virus-infected cells are shed into the bowel lumen,[73] and generally diminishes by the end of the first week, although low concentrations of virus have been detected in neonates for up to 2 weeks.[69]

Pathology

Limited autopsy studies in humans[74] and more extensive observations in experimental animals suggest that rotavirus infections generally remain localized in the gut and do not involve other organs, although hepatic and renal involvement has been reported in persons with T lymphocyte abnormalities.[75] In the intestine, the virus invades the villous epithelium of the proximal small bowel. Epithelial cells scraped from the intestinal mucosa show immunofluorescent virus antigen in cells from the duodenum and upper jejunum but not from the gastric mucosa, large bowel mucosa, or mesenteric lymph nodes. Although virtually all descriptions of intestinal morphology pertain to disease found in older infants and young children, there is little reason to believe that identical histopathologic features would not be found in the neonate.

Immunofluorescence,[74] electron microscopy,[6, 76, 77, 78] and immunocytochemical staining techniques[78] have shown that infection in the small intestine is limited to the mature columnar epithelial cells located on the distal half of the villi. The actively dividing enterocytes in the crypts, and the cuboidal epithelial cells that migrate up the villi to replace the columnar cells as they are destroyed and exfoliated prematurely, are resistant to infection by rotavirus and appear to be unaffected. The gross appearance of the bowel is usually normal; however, under the dissecting microscope, scattered focal lesions of the mucosal surface are apparent in most cases.[6] Light microscopy also shows patchy changes in villous morphology, compatible with a process of infection, inflammation, and accelerated mucosal renewal. The villi take on a shortened and blunt appearance as tall columnar cells are shed and replaced by less mature cuboidal enterocytes.[6, 77, 79] The infected cells may be vacuolated and are often scattered among apparently normal neighbors.[74, 76] Infiltration of the lamina propria with lymphocytes and plasma cells usually accompanies these findings. EM reveals distortion of microvilli, swelling of mitochondria, and distended cisternae of endoplasmic reticulum containing numerous rotavirus particles.[6, 76–78] In the experimental animal, even intense ultrastructural evidence of viral invasion may not be accompanied by changes in histology when examined by light microscopy.[78]

Not only morphologically but also functionally immature, the crypt-type epithelium shows diminished activity of several enzymes normally found in differentiated enterocytes, particularly Na$^+$, K$^+$-ATP are. It is postulated that diarrhea results from the disordered electrolyte and water transport secondary to this deficiency.[64, 80, 81] Clinical support for this concept comes from studies in infants showing markedly increased sodium and chloride concentrations in stools during the acute phase of the disease.[82] Abnormally low levels of maltase, sucrase, and lactase have been described in infants with rotaviral gastroenteritis,[6] and lactose malabsorption after rotavirus infection in infants has been described.[69] Xylose malabsorption also has been noted. Severity of the mucosal damage as seen by light microscopy does not correlate with the degree of enzyme depression.[6] Disaccharidase levels and xylose absorption both return to normal within a few days[79] to weeks following infection.[6]

Epidemiology

Rotaviral infection, like acute diarrheal disease in general, is uncommon in neonates.[30, 83–102] Starting in the third and fourth months of life, the number of infants with rotavirus gastroenteritis begins to increase, with a peak incidence, as indicated by virus shedding and serology, between 6 and 24 months of age.[84, 85, 103–105] In studies performed in Canada,[106] Argentina,[107] Kenya,[108] and Mexico,[103, 104] serious gastroenteritis was common in infants younger than 6 months of age. Data obtained among infants in Washington, D.C.,[109] and Australia[110] suggest that the socioeconomic status of families may be an important determining factor. Rotavirus has a mean incubation period of 2 days, with a range of 1 to 3 days in children as well as in experimentally infected adults.

One of the unexplained aspects of the epidemiology of rotavirus gastroenteritis is its marked seasonal variation.[111, 112] In countries with temperate climates, rotavirus rarely is associated with cases of diarrheal disease that occur during the warm season, whereas during the cooler months, 20% of clinic and 50% of hospitalized patients with acute gastroenteritis excrete the virus.[103–105, 109, 113, 114] In the tropics where high temperature and humidity are relatively constant, rotavirus is detected among infants with diarrhea, varying between 30% and 70%.[108, 115] Indications that the changes in prevalence that do occur may be related to other climatic factors, such as monthly rainfall,[116] have not been borne out in most studies.[115, 117–119]

Within newborn nurseries, where climate control usually maintains the temperature and relative humidity, attack rates are unpredictable and sometimes seem less dependent on outside environment than on other epidemiologic factors. In nurseries in which persisting endemic infection has permitted long-term surveillance of large numbers of neonates, rotavirus excretion is not always related to seasonal changes. Among 100 healthy infants examined during a 12-month study in a London maternity unit, the percentage of positive specimens varied from 10% in summer to almost 50% in winter.[62] In a premature nursery in Belgium, rotavirus was virtually absent from April through December after excretion rates of 10 to 20% during the colder months.[86] Conversely, there was no significant seasonal fluctuation in the attack rate among neonates in two nurseries studied continuously for almost a year in Sydney, Australia.[87] Rotaviruses were identified regularly in 40 to 50% of all stools examined. The controlling factors underlying cyclic variations that occur in one nursery but not in another remain unknown.

It also is not clear how units in which infection may remain endemic for months or years differ from those with a low incidence of rotavirus excretion in neonates. Several authors have reported their nurseries to be free of rotavirus infection[85, 87, 88] or minimally affected,[89, 120] whereas others have described diarrheal disease related to rotavirus throughout the year or during outbreaks involving 10 to 39% of resident neonates.[68, 94, 95, 121] The observation is not unique to rotavirus. Prolonged outbreaks of diarrhea caused by EPEC, usually associated with serious clinical disease, forced closure of many newborn nurseries in the 1950s and 1960s, whereas other nurseries were never involved.

Low birth weight does not seem to be an important factor in determining the attack rate among infants at risk but may be important in mortality.[122] Infants in premature or special-care nurseries, despite their prolonged stays and the increased handling necessary for their care, do not demonstrate a higher susceptibility to infection; none[88] or all[89] may shed the virus.

It is most likely, as suggested by analogy with rotavirus disease in animal colonies and child-care centers, that once infection is introduced into a nursery with a continuous flow of new arrivals, rotavirus will spread steadily and remain endemic until a change in admission policies or nursing practices permits interruption of the cycle.[123] Exactly how the virus is introduced and transmitted is uncertain, although limited observations and experience with other types of enteric disease in maternity units suggest several possibilities. The routes by which a newborn could acquire rotavirus infection include (1) ingestion of viral particles at or shortly before the time of delivery; (2) transfer from other infants or toddlers excreting the virus, via hands of nursery personnel or parents; (3) transmission by direct contact with adults or older children excreting the virus; (4) airborne or droplet infection; (5) fomites; or (6) contaminated foods or formula.

The early appearance of virus in stools of some neonates indicates that infection probably was acquired at delivery. Virus particles can be detected in the first[70, 89] or second[87] 24 hours of life in a significant number of infants. By day 3 or 4, most infants who will shed virus, with or without signs of illness, will have started to do so.[70, 87, 90] The large numbers of virus particles excreted[87, 90] suggest a fairly large, as well as early, oral inoculum. Studies with experimentally infected piglets have shown that ingestion of low doses, although not altering the clinical illness, causes a prolongation of the incubation period.[124] It is unlikely that contamination from any source other than maternal feces could provide an inoculum during the first few hours of life large enough to cause infection by the second day. Adults infrequently excrete rotavirus, at least at levels detectable by EM; attempts to demonstrate viral particles in the stools of mothers with infected newborns have been unsuccessful. Thus, although infants who excrete virus during the first 2 days of life probably acquired it during delivery, evidence is only circumstantial.

Transfer of particles from infant to infant on the hands of nursing and medical staff is probably the most important means of viral spread. With 10^8 to 10^{11} viral particles usually present in 1 g of stool, the hands of personnel easily could become contaminated once infection is introduced into a nursery. The numerous reports of nosocomial rotavirus gastroenteritis attest to the ease with which this agent spreads through a hospital or institutional setting.[91, 105, 112, 125-127] Admission of a symptomatic child usually is the initiating event, although transfer of a neonate with inapparent infection from one ward to another also has been incriminated. One group of investigators has shown that the most important factors influencing the incidence of rotavirus diarrhea in a nursery were the proximity to other newborns and the frequency of handling.[71] During the 4-month study, infants cared for by nursing staff and kept in communal nurseries experienced three epidemics of diarrhea with attack rates between 20% and 50%. During the same period, only 2% of infants rooming in with their mothers became ill, even though they had frequent contact with adult relatives and siblings during the visiting hours.

Family and child-care center outbreaks have shown how easily susceptible hosts can acquire rotavirus infection if they have prolonged and intimate contact with a person excreting the virus.[72, 111, 128, 129] In most homes, one third to one half of family members living with pediatric patients with diarrhea become infected.[31-35, 82, 129] Transmission usually originates with a toddler or young child and rapidly spreads to siblings (including newborns), parents, and other close contacts. The majority of adults will have some immunity from prior exposure in childhood and therefore experience only inapparent infection or mild clinical illness. That adults, particularly visitors to newborn nurseries, represent an important source of infection to their own or other infants has been postulated but not proved.[58, 89]

Epidemiologic observations indicate that infection among neonates is spread by the fecal-oral route. There is no evidence that airborne or droplet infection, originating in the upper respiratory tract or by aerosolization of diarrheal fluid while diapers are changed, is important. Under experimental conditions, rotavirus was transmitted in mice by aerosol droplets,[130] but the significance of this method of transmission in humans is unknown. There also is no evidence that transplacental or ascending intrauterine infection occurs. The respiratory isolation achieved by placing an infant in a closed incubator is not protective.[71] Transmission of virus through contaminated fomites, formula, or food has not been described. Rotavirus particles have not been found in human milk or colostrum.[57, 59]

Clinical Manifestations

Exposure of a newborn to rotavirus, presumably through ingestion of viral particles during delivery or shortly thereafter, may result in one of the following: (1) no infection, as determined by the absence of rotavirus in fecal samples and failure of seroconversion; (2) subclinical infection with excretion of virus or seroconversion without signs of illness; or (3) gastroenteritis. Reports of rotavirus infection in the newborn from different countries show an incidence rate of 23 to 56%,[62, 68, 86, 87, 97, 98, 131] whereas reports from the United States and Canada show a lower rate of 0 to 22%.[89, 101, 132, 133] In a study from Australia, rotavirus infection in neonates did not prevent reinfection but did confer significant resistance to disease severity during reinfection.[102]

It generally is believed that most neonates who excrete rotavirus will develop an asymptomatic infection,* but estimates of the incidence of clinically apparent disease differ considerably. This is due, at least in part, to varying definitions of diarrhea as well as to difficulties inherent in the clinical assessment of small infants, particularly breast-fed infants, who may have up to 10 loose or watery stools a day under normal conditions. When these inconsistencies are superimposed on differences in

---

*References 62, 86, 87, 89, 91, 95, 97–99, 120, 134, 135.

protocols used by various investigators to determine prevalence of viral excretion, meaningful comparisons are not possible. Thus, several reports described nurseries in which 10% or less of infected infants had minimal or no signs of illness,[62, 86, 89, 95, 99, 120, 134] and others noted some evidence of gastroenteritis in about half[70, 87, 91, 93, 121] or even three fourths[69] of those patients excreting the virus. Occasionally, neonatal rotavirus infection may cause severe gastrointestinal tract problems.[121]

RNA electrophoretic patterns of rotaviruses found in certain nurseries have shown uniform patterns,[96, 98, 100, 135] suggesting that the infective strains may have been attenuated and that this is why the infected neonates were asymptomatic. One study showed that infants in a tertiary care center can be infected with at least 10 different rotavirus strains within 2 months and that multiple strains can spread independently as part of a single outbreak.[136] Another study evaluated a cohort of infants hospitalized since birth who were exposed to other children with community-acquired rotavirus diarrhea. Rotavirus strains with identical electropherotype patterns produced asymptomatic infection in neonates and symptomatic infection in older infants,[99] suggesting that strains producing asymptomatic disease in neonates are not necessarily attenuated and that host factors may be important variables affecting the clinical course of rotavirus infection. Asymptomatic excretion of rotavirus in children beyond the neonatal period has been reported to range from 0 to 50%.[131] In studies of children in child-care centers in the United States, approximately 50% of infected children were found to asymptomatically excrete rotavirus during outbreaks of rotavirus diarrhea.[111]

No clinical features distinguish rotaviral gastroenteritis in the neonatal period. Early signs of illness, such as lethargy, irritability, and poor feeding, usually are followed in a few hours by the passage of watery yellow or green stools free of blood but sometimes containing mucus.[71, 82, 116, 137] The diarrhea is usually mild; severe dehydration and electrolyte imbalance are uncommon in neonates. A severe gastroenteritis known as "hakuri" (white stool diarrhea) or "pseudocholera infantum," characterized by a profuse milky diarrhea, has been reported from Japan.[138, 139] Once believed to be unique to that country, this type of gastroenteritis also has occurred in Kenya.[137] Fecal leukocytes have not been described in neonates with rotaviral diarrhea; they are no more prevalent in stools in older infants with this disease than among controls.[116, 140–142] Vomiting and a slight fever occasionally may precede or accompany the diarrhea. Upper respiratory tract illness, often prominent in older infants with rotaviral disease,[82, 104, 116] has not been observed in the neonate.[91]

Diarrhea usually remits by the second day of illness and is much improved by the third or fourth day. Occasionally, intestinal fluid loss and poor weight gain may continue for 1 or 2 weeks, particularly in infants of low birth weight.[91] Although excessive amounts of reducing substances frequently are present in early fecal samples from infants with rotaviral diarrhea,[68, 71, 91, 92] this finding is not necessarily abnormal in neonates, particularly those who are breast-fed.[143] Nevertheless, infants with prolonged diarrhea should be investigated for monosaccharide or disaccharide malabsorption or intolerance to cow's milk protein or both.[144]

Longitudinal studies in newborn nurseries and investigations of outbreaks among neonates rarely describe an adverse outcome. In a combined population of almost 400 nursery infants with diarrheal disease caused by rotavirus, not a single death could be attributed to gastroenteritis.[68, 71, 91] More than three fourths of the infants were housed in special-care nurseries for problems such as low birth weight, prematurity, or birth trauma.[68, 91] Because these infants were under constant observation, early detection of excessive fluid losses and the availability of immediate medical care were probably major factors in determining a favorable outcome. Rotavirus gastroenteritis may on occasion cause severe symptoms and even death. A series of 21 infant fatalities related to rotavirus gastroenteritis was recorded over a period of 5 years in Toronto.[75] Death was attributed to profound dehydration and electrolyte imbalance. Although the case: fatality ratio could not be calculated from the published data, a subgroup of 385 hospitalized patients in the same population included four deaths,[112] all occurring in infants over 4 months of age.[75] By contrast, in rural Bangladesh, only five deaths occurred among over 2100 patients with rotaviral diarrhea who were older than 2 years of age; this occurred despite moderate or severe dehydration in about one of six children younger than 2 years of age.[145, 146] Rotavirus has been associated with necrotizing enterocolitis,[147] but is not thought to be causal.

Diagnosis

There are many methods used for detection of rotavirus in stool specimens including EM, immune electron microscopy, EIA, latex agglutination, gel electrophoresis, culture of the virus, PCR, and reverse transcriptase–polymerase chain reaction. EM is the only method that can simultaneously detect and identify each of the enteroviruses, and EIA is most frequently used to identify rotavirus. In addition, there are many assays for serologic detection of a previous infection with rotavirus. Although cultivation of rotavirus is a cumbersome procedure and not a useful tool for diagnosis of rotavirus infection, the ability to grow rotaviruses in cell culture has been a critical step in understanding the virus genome as well as in producing rotavirus vaccine strains.[148, 149]

Fecal material for detection of rotavirus infection should be obtained during the acute phase of illness. Whole-stool samples are preferred, although suspensions of rectal swab specimens have been adequate for detection of rotavirus by immune electron microscopy[150] and EIA.[150, 151] Excretion of viral particles may precede signs of illness by several days.[70–72] Maximal excretion by older infants and children generally occurs 3 to 4 days after onset of symptoms[115]; excretion is usually no longer detectable by 10 days but can persist for up to 2 or 3 weeks when clinical illness is prolonged.[115, 125, 139] Virus excretion can be detected for weeks after recovery by the more sensitive PCR assay.[152] Neonates rarely excrete virus for more than 5 days when well[90] or ill.[70, 73]

Direct examination of fecal material by EM, although relatively insensitive, is the reference method against which others are compared. An experienced investigator can detect 10^5 viral particles per g of stool with diligent searching.[153] The distinctive morphologic appearance of rotaviruses and the large number of particles (between 10^7 and 10^{11} per g of stool) shed by most neonates[55, 62] and older infants make diagnosis by EM quite specific. The major disadvantages of direct examination of fecal material are the time and expertise required for each determination and the need for cumbersome and expensive equipment.[150] A major advantage of EM is the ability to detect non–group A rotavirus as well as other viral particles.

Several methods of identification of rotaviruses or their antigens in fecal material use antirotavirus antibodies. These methods include countercurrent immunoelectrophoresis, radioimmunoassay, immunofluorescence, latex agglutination, EIA, and PCR.[154] A number of EIA and latex agglutination polyclonal and monoclonal antibody–based assays have been developed commercially for detection of rotavirus in clinical specimens and have become the mainstay of diagnosis of rotavirus infection because of their ability to evaluate large numbers of specimens rapidly. Several comparisons of these assays with regard to sensitivity, specificity, and positive and negative predictive values have been reported.[155–158] In general, latex agglutination assays are more rapid than EIAs but are less sensitive. Use of all these assays is optimized by testing specimens obtained early in the course of illness when higher amounts of antigen are present.[158] These rapid detection assays also have contributed substantially to studies of rotavirus epidemiology. One drawback to these assays is their inability to detect non–group A rotaviruses. Rotazyme II has been reported to give a high percentage of false-positive reactions when tested with stools of neonates.[132, 133, 159–162] In addition, other laboratory practices have resulted in false-positive detections in stool specimens.[163]

All three methods of serodiagnosis, EIA, complement fixation, and fluorescent antibody testing, can distinguish between IgG and IgM subclasses of antirotavirus antibody. In the previously uninfected host with a primary immune response, IgM antibodies appear rapidly and usually are detected by 5 days after the start of the illness. IgG antibody rises usually occur by the second to third week in primary infections and earlier with secondary anamnestic responses. The presence of IgM antirotavirus antibodies in the absence of IgG antibodies is presumptive indication of recent infection with this agent. Their absence does not rule out infection.

Therapy

The primary goal of therapy is restoration and maintenance of fluid and electrolyte balance.[163] Despite the documented defect in carbohydrate digestion with rotavirus diarrhea, rehydration often can be accomplished with glucose-electrolyte or sucrose-electrolyte solutions given PO,[164–167] although intravenous fluids may be needed in neonates who are severely dehydrated, who

are vomiting, or who refuse to feed.[145, 146, 167] Persistent or recurrent diarrhea after introduction of milk-based formulas or human milk warrants investigation for secondary carbohydrate or cow's milk protein intolerance.[68, 144] Infants with intractable diarrhea related to severe morphologic and enzymatic changes of the bowel mucosa may require an elemental diet or parenteral nutrition. Data showing that a range of glycoproteins inhibit the in vivo and in vitro replication of rotaviruses suggest that the alteration in quantity or chemical composition of intestinal glycoproteins is a potential means for modulation of enteric infections.[63, 64, 168]

Hand washing before and after contact with each infant remains the single most important means of preventing the spread of infection. Because rotavirus is often excreted several days before illness is recognized,[70–72] isolation of an infant with diarrhea usually comes late in preventing cross-infection unless all nursing personnel and medical staff have adhered to this fundamental precaution. Infants who develop gastroenteritis should be moved out of the nursery area if adequate facilities are available and the infant's condition permits transfer. The use of an incubator is of value in reducing transmission of disease only by serving as a reminder that proper hand-washing and glove techniques are required when handling the infant, but is of little value as a physical barrier to the spread of virus.[71] Encouraging rooming-in of infants with their mothers has been shown to be helpful in preventing or containing nursery epidemics.[113]

Several live, orally administered rotavirus vaccines are being or have been evaluated, including use of attenuated animal (bovine and rhesus monkey) or human virus strains, use of generic reassortant rotaviruses, cloning of the rotavirus genome with expression of viral proteins in different vector systems, and production of synthetic peptide vaccines. In August 1998, the FDA licensed rhesus rotavirus tetravalent vaccine for oral administration of infants at 2, 4, and 6 months of age,[148, 149] including administration to premature infants if they are at least 6 months of age, discharged from the hospital, and clinically stable.

Provision of high-titer antirotavirus antisera orally to low-birth-weight infants was shown to delay rotavirus excretion and decrease the amount of excretion and the severity of the diarrhea.[169, 170] In studies of infants, provision of milk to hospitalized children had no effect on rotavirus excretion but reduced the severity of illness. Antirotavirus activity in the milk was not measured. Two immunodeficient children, one with severe combined immunodeficiency and one with agammaglobulinemia, responded to irradiated, lactose-free milk containing antibody to rotavirus.[171] Concentrates containing milk immunoglobulins prepared from rotavirus hyperimmunized cows, when fed to infants hospitalized for acute rotavirus gastroenteritis, significantly reduced excretion of virus[172] and prevented outbreaks of diarrhea caused by rotavirus.[173]

DIFFERENTIAL DIAGNOSIS

Diarrhea during the neonatal period is a clinical manifestation of a wide variety of disorders, all of which

TABLE 31–10
Differential Diagnosis of Neonatal Diarrhea

DIAGNOSIS	REFERENCE[a]	DIAGNOSIS	REFERENCE[a]
Anatomic Disorders		**Metabolic and Enzymatic Disorders** *(Continued)*	
Hirschsprung's disease	1, 2	Wolman's disease	31
Massive intestinal resection (short-bowel syndrome)	3	Transcobalamin II deficiency	32
Intestinal lymphangiectasis	4	Hereditary tyrosinemia (hepatorenal type)	31
Metabolic and Enzymatic Disorders		Methionine malabsorption (oasthouse urine disease)	31
Congenital disaccharidase deficiency (lactase, sucrase-isomaltose deficiency)	5, 6	Hartnup's disease	31
		Congenital Na$^+$ diarrhea	47
Congenital glucose-galactose malabsorption	7	**Inflammatory Disorders**	
Secondary disaccharide, monosaccharide malabsorption	8–16	Cow's milk protein intolerance	33, 55
After gastrointestinal surgery		Soy protein intolerance	34, 32
After infection		Regional enteritis	36
With milk-soy protein sensitivity		Ulcerative colitis	37, 38
Cystic fibrosis	17	**Primary Immunodeficiency Disorders**	
Syndrome of pancreatic insufficiency and bone marrow dysfunction (Shwachman's syndrome)	18	Wiskott-Aldrich syndrome	15, 39
		Thymic dysplasia	39
Physiologic deficiency of pancreatic amylase	19	Acquired immunodeficiency syndrome	48
Intestinal enterokinase deficiency	20	**Miscellaneous**	
Congenital bile-acid deficiency syndrome	21	Irritable colon of childhood (chronic nonspecific diarrhea)	40
Alpha/beta-lipoproteinemia	22	Phototherapy for hyperbilirubinemia	41
Acrodermatitis enteropathica	23, 24	Familial dysautonomia (Riley-Day syndrome)	42
Congenital chloride diarrhea	25, 26	Familial enteropathy	43, 46
Primary hypomagnesemia	27	High sulfates in water	44
Congenital adrenal hyperplasia	28	Phenolphthalein poisoning/child abuse	45
Intestinal hormone hypersecretion	29, 30		
Non-beta islet cell hyperplasia			
Neural crest tumors			

[a]See under Differential Diagnosis in references.

have in common a disturbance of intestinal motility and absorption. The initiating factor is usually a primary infection of the gastrointestinal tract, mild to moderate in severity, self-limited, and responsive to supportive measures. In addition to these acute enteritides, there are diseases leading to a chronic intractable diarrhea, which may in turn result in severe nutritional disturbances or even death unless the specific underlying condition is identified and treated appropriately. Because prolonged diarrhea of more than 2 weeks' duration is one of the features by which these syndromes are recognized, the diagnoses are most often established after the neonatal period. Nonetheless, the onset of symptoms occurs with sufficient frequency during the first few weeks of life to make their inclusion in the differential diagnosis of gastroenteritis of the newborn appropriate.

The differential diagnosis of diarrheal illnesses should first include an examination for fecal leukocytes to determine whether the process is inflammatory or noninflammatory. Causes of inflammatory diarrhea include *Shigella, Salmonella, Campylobacter, V. parahaemolyticus, Y. enterocolitica,* EIEC, *C. difficile,* necrotizing enterocolitis, antibiotic-associated colitis, and several noninfectious causes such as milk-soy intolerance, ulcerative colitis, and regional enteritis. Noninflammatory causes of diarrhea, by far the most common in most populations, include ETEC, EPEC, EAEC, rotaviruses, enteric adenoviruses, calicivirus, astrovirus, *G. lamblia* and *Cryptosporidium.* Although supportive fluid therapy is mandatory for all types of diarrhea, the brief examination for fecal leukocytes can direct the appropriate further diagnostic and therapeutic steps.

Some of the noninfectious diseases responsible for neonatal diarrhea are listed in Table 31–10 together with references to helpful investigative procedures.[1–48] More complete protocols for the evaluation of protracted infantile diarrhea are available in published reviews.[49–51]

References

Introduction

1. The World Bank. Health and developing countries: successess and challenges. *In* World Development Report 1993: Investing in Health. Oxford, Oxford University Press, 1993, pp 17–36.
2. Guerrant RL. Lessons from diarrheal diseases: demography to molecular pharmacology. J Infect Dis 169:1206, 1994.
3. Warren KS. Tropical medicine or tropical health: the Health Clark lectures, 1988. Rev Infect Dis 12:142, 1990.
4. Guerrant RL, Hughes JM, Lima NL, et al. Diarrhea in developed and developing countries: magnitude, special settings, and etiologies. Rev Infect Dis 12:S41, 1990.
5. World Health Organization. Forty-Fifth World Health Assembly. Implementation of the Global Strategy for Health for All by the Year 2000, Second Evaluation; and Eighth Report of the World Health Situation. Geneva, World Health Organization. 1992, A45/3.
6. Bern C, Martines J, deZoysa I, Glass RI. The magnitude of the global problem of diarrhoeal disease: a ten-year update. Bull World Health Organ 70:705, 1992.
7. Institute of Medicine. Committee on Issues and Priorities for New Vaccine Development. New Vaccine Development: Establishing Priorities. Diseases of Importance in Developing Countries, vol. 2. Washington DC, National Academy Press, 1986.
8. Ho MS, Glass RI, Pinsky PF, et al. Diarrheal deaths in American children: are they preventable? JAMA 260:3281, 1988.
9. Cohen ML. The epidemiology of diarrheal disease in the United States. Infect Dis Clin North Am 2:557, 1988.
10. Glass RI, Law JF, Gangarosa RE, et al. Estimates of morbidity and mortality rates for diarrheal disease in American children. J Pediatr 118:S27, 1991.
11. Holmes SJ, Morrow AL, Pickering LK. Child care practices: effects of social changes on epidemiology of infectious diseases and antibiotic resistance. Epidemiol Rev 18:10, 1996.
12. Pickering LK, Osterholm M. Infectious diseases associated with out-of-home child care. *In* Long SS, Pickering LK, Prober CG (eds). Principles and Practice of Pediatric Infectious Diseases. New York, Churchill-Livingstone, 1997, pp 31–39.
13. Schorling JB, Wanke CA, Schorling SK, et al. A prospective study of persistent diarrhea among children in an urban Brazilian slum: patterns of occurrence and etiologic agents. Am J Epidemiol 132:144, 1990.
14. Guerrant RL, Shorling JB, McAuliffe JF, de Souza MA. Diarrhea as a cause and effect of malnutrition: diarrhea prevents catch-up growth and malnutrition increases diarrhea frequency and duration. Am J Trop Med Hyg 47:28, 1992.
15. Black RE. Would control of childhood infectious diseases reduce malnutrition? Acta Paediatr Scand Suppl 374:133, 1991.
16. Rowland MGM, Rowland SGJG, Cole TJ. Impact of infection on the growth of children from 0 to 2 years in an urban West African community. Am J Clin Nutr 47:134, 1988.
17. Gordon JE. Diarrheal disease of early childhood—worldwide scope of the problem. Ann N Y Acad Sci 1976:9, 1971.
18. Parashar UD, Kilgore PE, Holman RC, et al. Diarrheal mortality in US infants. Arch Pediatr Adolesc Med 152:47, 1998.
19. Mata LJ, Urrutia JJ. Intestinal colonization of breastfed children in a rural area of low socioeconomic level. Ann N Y Acad Sci 176:93, 1971.
20. Guerrant RL, Steiner TS, Lima AAM, Bobak DA. How intestinal bacteria cause disease. J Infect Dis 179:S331, 1999.
21. Pickering LK, Cleary TG. Approach to patients with gastrointestinal tract infections and food poisoning. *In* Feigin RD, Cherry JC (eds). Textbook of Pediatric Infectious Diseases, 4th ed. Philadelphia, WB Saunders, 1997, p 567.
22. Bettelheim KA, Lennox-King SMJ. The acquisition of *Escherichia coli* by newborn babies. Infection 4:174, 1976.
23. Gorden J, Small PLC. Acid resistance in enteric bacteria. Infect Immun 61:364, 1993.
24. Pickering LK. Biotherapeutic agents and disease in infants. *In* Newburg DS (ed). Bioactive Substances in Human Milk. New York, Plenum Publishing. In press.
25. Giannella RA, Broitman SA, Zamcheck N. Influence of gastric acidity on bacterial and parasitic enteric infections: a perspective. Ann Intern Med 78:271, 1973.
26. Schrager J. The chemical composition and function of gastrointestinal mucus. Gut 11:450, 1970.
27. Challacombe DN, Richardson JM, Anderson CM. Bacterial microflora of the upper gastrointestinal tract in infants without diarrhea. Arch Dis Child 49:264, 1974.
28. Furuta GT, Walker WA. Nonimmune defense mechanisms of the gastrointestinal tract. *In* Blaser MJ, Smith PD, Ravdin JI, et al (eds). Infections of the Gastrointestinal Tract. New York, Raven Press, 1995, pp 89–97.
29. Avery G, Randolph JG, Weaver T. Gastric acidity in the first day of life. Pediatrics 37:1005, 1966.
30. Harries JT, Fraser AJ. The acidity of the gastric contents of premature babies during the first fourteen days of life. Biol Neonate 12:186, 1968.
31. Agunod M, Yamaguchi N, Lopez R, et al. Correlative study of hydrochloric acid, pepsin, and intrinsic factor secretion in newborns and infants. Am J Dig Dis 14:400, 1969.
32. Cavel B. Gastric emptying in infants. Acta Paediatr Scand 60:371, 1971.
33. Blumenthal I, Ebel A, Pildes RS. Effect of posture on the pattern of stomach emptying in the newborn. Pediatrics 66:482, 1980.
34. Silverio J. Gastric emptying time in the newborn and nursling. Am J Med Sci 247:732, 1964.
35. Cavell B. Gastric emptying in preterm infants. Acta Paediatr Scand 68:725, 1979.
36. Fallot ME, Boyd JL, Oski FA. Breast-feeding reduces incidence of hospital admissions for infection in infants. Pediatrics 65:1121, 1980.
37. Larsen SA, Homer DR. Relation of breast versus bottle feeding to hospitalization for gastroenteritis in a middle-class U.S. population. J Pediatr 92:417, 1978.
38. Cushing AH, Anderson L. Diarrhea in breast-fed and non–breast-fed infants. Pediatrics 70:921, 1982.
39. Guerrant RL, Kirchhoff LV, Shields DS, et al. Prospective study of diarrheal illnesses in northeastern Brazil: patterns of disease, nutritional impact, etiologies and risk factors. J Infect Dis 148:986, 1983.
40. Myers MG, Fomon SJ, Koontz FP, et al. Respiratory and gastrointestinal illnesses in breast- and formula-fed infants. Am J Dis Child 138:629, 1984.
41. Kovar MG, Serdula MK, Marks JS, et al. Review of the epidemiologic evidence for an association between infant feeding and infant health. Pediatrics 74:615, 1984.
42. Feachem RG, Koblinsky MA. Interventions for the control of diarrhoeal diseases among young children: promo-

tion of breast-feeding. Bull World Health Organ 62:271, 1984.

43. Forman MR, Graubard BI, Hoffman HJ, et al. The Pima infant feeding study: breastfeeding and gastroenteritis in the first year of life. Am J Epidemiol 119:335, 1984.

44. Leventhal JM, Shapiro ED, Aten CB, et al. Does breastfeeding protect against infections in infants less than 3 months of age? Pediatrics 78:8896, 1986.

45. Rubin DH, Leventhal JM, Krsilnikoff PA, et al. Relationship between infant feeding and infectious illness: a prospective study of infants during the first year of life. Pediatrics 85:464, 1989.

46. Victora CG, Smith PG, Vaughan JP, et al. Infant feeding and deaths due to diarrhea. Am J Epidemiol 129:1032, 1989.

47. Popkin BM, Adair L, Akin JS, et al. Breast-feeding and diarrheal morbidity. Pediatrics 86:874, 1990.

48. Morrow AL, Pickering LK. Human milk and infectious diseases. *In* Long SS, Pickering LK, Prober CG (eds). Principles and Practice of Pediatric Infectious Diseases. New York, Churchill-Livingstone, 1997, pp 87–95.

49. Newburg DS, Peterson JA, Ruiz-Palacios GM, et al. High levels of lactadherin in human milk are associated with protection against symptomatic rotavirus infection amongst breast fed infants. Lancet 351:1160, 1998.

50. Wyatt RG, Mata LJ. Bacteria in colostrum and milk in Guatemalan Indian women. J Trop Pediatr 15:159, 1969.

51. Grazioso CF, Werner AL, Alling DW, et al: Antiinflammatory effects of human milk on chemically induced colitis in rats. Pediatr Res 42:639, 1997.

52. Newburg DS. Oligosaccharides and glycoconjugates in human milk: their role in host defense. J Mammary Gland Biol Neoplasia 1:271, 1996.

53. Morrow AL, Pickering LK. Human milk protection against diarrheal disease. Semin Pediatr Infect Dis 5:236, 1994.

54. Pickering LK, Granoff DM, Erickson JE, et al. Modulation of the immune system by human milk and infant formula containing nucleotides. Pediatrics 101:242, 1998.

55. Ross CA, Dawes EA. Resistance of the breast fed infant to gastroenteritis. Lancet 1:994, 1954.

56. Glass RI, Svennerholm A, Stoll BJ, et al. Milk antibodies protect breastfed children against cholera. N Engl J Med 308:1389, 1983.

57. Ruiz-Palacios GM, Calva JJ, Pickering LK, et al. Protection of breastfed infants against *Campylobacter* diarrhea by antibodies in human milk. J Pediatr 116:707, 1990.

58. Cravioto A, Tello A, Villafan H, et al. Inhibition of localized adhesion of enteropathogenic *Escherichia coli* to HEp-2 cells by immunoglobulin and oligosaccharide fractions of human colostrum and breast milk. J Infect Dis 163:1247, 1991.

59. Holmgren J, Svennerholm AM, Lindblad M. Receptor-like glycocompounds in human milk that inhibit classical and El Tor *Vibrio cholerae* cell adherence (hemagglutination). Infect Immun 39:147, 1983.

60. Laegreid A, Otnaess ABK, Fuglesang J. Human and bovine milk: comparison of ganglioside composition and enterotoxin-inhibitory activity. Pediatr Res 20:416, 1986.

61. Hayani KC, Guerrero ML, Morrow AL, et al. Concentration of milk secretory immunoglobulin A against *Shigella* virulence plasmid-associated antigens as a predictor of symptom status in *Shigella*-infected breast-fed infants. J Pediatr 121:852, 1992.

62. Miotti PG, Gilman RH, Pickering LK, et al. Prevalence of serum and milk antibodies to *Giardia lamblia* in different populations of lactating women. J Infect Dis 152:1025, 1985.

63. Hayani KC, Guerrero ML, Ruiz-Palacios GM, et al. Evidence for long-term memory of the mucosal immune system: milk secretory immunoglobulin A against *Shigella* lipopolysaccharides. J Clin Microbiol 29:2599, 1991.

64. Walterspiel JN, Morrow AL, Guerrero ML, et al. Protective effect of secretory anti–*Giardia lamblia* antibodies in human milk against diarrhea. Pediatrics 93:28, 1994.

65. Tacket CO, Losonsky G, Link H, et al. Protection by milk immunoglobulin concentrate against oral challenge with enterotoxigenic *E. coli*. N Engl J Med 318:1240, 1988.

66. Davidson GP, Whyte PBD, Daniels E, et al. Passive immunization of children with bovine colostrum containing antibodies to human rotavirus. Lancet 2:709, 1989.

67. Tacket CO, Binion SB, Bostwick E, et al. Efficacy of bovine milk immunoglobulin concentrate in preventing illness after *Shigella flexneri* challenge. Am J Trop Med Hyg 47:276, 1992.

68. Polonovsky M, Lespagnol A. Nouvelles acquisitions sur les composés glucidiques du lait de femme. Bull Soc Chem Biol 15:320, 1933.

69. Montreuil J, Mullet S. Etude des variations des constituants glucidiques du lait de femme au cours de la lactation. Bull Soc Chem Biol 42:365, 1960.

70. Kobata A. Milk glycoproteins and oligosaccharides. *In* Horowitz MI, Pigman W (eds). The Glycoconjugates. I. New York, Academic Press, 1978, p 423.

71. Kobata A, Grollman EF, Torain BF, et al. Genes, glycosyltransferases and blood types. *In* Aminoff D (ed). Blood and Tissue Antigens. New York, Academic Press, 1970, p 497.

72. Otnaess AB, Svennerholm AM. Non-immunoglobulin fraction of human milk protects rabbits against enterotoxin-induced intestinal fluid secretion. Infect Immun 35:738, 1982.

73. Otnaess ABK, Laegreid A, Ertesvag K. Inhibition of enterotoxin from *Escherichia coli* and *Vibrio cholerae* by gangliosides from human milk. Infect Immun 40:563, 1983.

74. Cleary TG, Chambers JP, Pickering LK. Protection of suckling mice from heat-stable enterotoxin of *Escherichia coli* by human milk. J Infect Dis 148:1114, 1983.

75. Newburg DS, Pickering LK, McCluer RH, et al. Fucosylated oligosaccharides of human milk protect suckling mice from heat-stable enterotoxin of *Escherichia coli*. J Infect Dis 162:1075, 1990.

76. Newburg DS, Ashkenazi S, Cleary TG. Human milk contains the Shiga toxin and Shiga-like toxin receptor glycolipid Gb3. J Infect Dis 166:832, 1992.

77. Yolken RH, Peterson JA, Vonderfecht SL, et al. Human milk mucin inhibits rotavirus replication and prevents experimental gastroenteritis. J Clin Invest 90:1984, 1992.

Escherichia coli

1. Cooper ML, Keller HM, Walters EW, et al. Isolation of enteropathogenic *Escherichia coli* from mothers and newborn infants. Am J Dis Child 97:255, 1959.

2. Ocklitz HW, Schmidt EF. Enteropathogenic *Escherichia coli* serotypes: infection of the newborn through mother. BMJ 2:1036, 1957.

3. Gareau FE, Mackel DC, Boring JR III, et al. The acquisition of fecal flora by infants from their mothers during birth. J Pediatr 54:313, 1959.

4. Rosner R. Antepartum culture findings of mothers in relation to infantile diarrhea. Am J Clin Pathol 45:732, 1966.

5. Nocard E, Leclainche E. Les Maladies Microbiennes des Animaux, 2nd ed. Paris, Masson, 1898, p 106.
6. Joest E. Untersuchungen über Kalberruhr. Z Tiermed 7:377, 1903.
7. Titze C, Weichel A. Die Ätiologie der Kalberruhr. Berl Tierarztl. Wochenschr 26:457, 1908.
8. Jensen CO. Handbuch der pathogenen Microorganismen, vol. 6. Jena, G Fischer, 1913, p. 131.
9. Smith T, Orcutt ML. The bacteriology of the intestinal tract of young calves with special reference to the early diarrhea ("scours"). J Exp Med 41:89, 1925.
10. Tennant B (ed). Neonatal enteric infections caused by Escherichia coli. Ann N Y Acad Sci 176:1, 1971.
11. Moro E. Quoted in Adam A. Über die Biologie der Dyspepsiecoli und ihre Beziehungen zur Pathogenese der Dyspepsie und Intoxikation. Jahrb Kinderheilled 101:295, 1923.
12. Adam, A. Über die Biologie der Dyspepsiecoli und ihre Beziehungen zur Pathogenese der Dyspepsie und Intoxikation. Jahr Kinderheilkd 101:295, 1923.
13. Adam A. Zur Frage der bakteriellen Ätiologie der sogenannten alimentaren Intoxikation. Jahrb Kinderheilkd 116:8, 1927.
14. Guerrant RL. Yet another pathogenic mechanism for Escherichia coli diarrhea? N Engl J Med 302:113, 1980.
15. Donnenberg MS, Kaper JB. Enteropathogenic Escherichia coli. Infect Immun 60:3953, 1992.
16. Levine MM. Escherichia coli that cause diarrhea: enterotoxigenic, enteropathogenic, enteroinvasive, enterohemorrhagic, and enteroadherent. J Infect Dis 155:377, 1987.
17. Guerrant RL, Thielman NM. Types of Escherichia coli enteropathogens. In Blaser MJ, Smith PD, Ravdin JL, et al (eds). Infections of the Gastrointestinal Tract. New York, Raven Press, 1995, p 687.
18. Schlager TA, Guerrant RL. Seven possible mechanisms for Escherichia coli diarrhea. Infect Dis Clin North Am 2:607, 1988.
19. Steiner TS, Lima AM, Nataro JP, Guerrant R. Enteroaggregative Escherichia coli produce intestinal inflammation and growth impairment and cause interleukin-8 release from intestinal epithelial cells. J Infect Dis 177:88, 1998.
20. Guerrant R, Steiner T. Principles and syndromes of enteric infections. In Mandell GL, Bennett J, Dolin R (eds). Mandell, Douglas, and Bennett's Principles and Practice of Infectious Diseases, 5th ed. Philadelphia, WB Saunders, 1999.
21. Spanbler BD. Structure and function of cholera toxin and the related Escherichia coli heat-labile enterotoxin. Microbiol Rev 56:622, 1992.
22. Guerrant RL, Ganguly U, Casper AGT, et al. Effect of Escherichia coli on fluid transport across canine small bowel: mechanism and time-course with enterotoxin and whole bacterial cells. J Clin Invest 52:1707, 1973.
23. Peterson JW, Ochoa G. Role of prostaglandins and cAMP in the secretory effects of cholera toxin. Science 245:857, 1989.
24. Peterson JW, Reitmeyer JC, Jackson CA, et al. Protein synthesis is required for cholera toxin–induced stimulation or arachidonic acid metabolism. Biochim Biophys Acta 1092:79, 1991.
25. Thielman NM, Marcinkiewics M, Sarosiek J, et al. The role of platelet activating factor in Chinese hamster ovary cell responses to cholera toxin. J Clin Invest 99:1999, 1997.
26. Guerrant RL, Fang GD, Thielman NM, Fonteles MC. Role of platelet activating factor (PAF) in the intestinal epithelial secretory and Chinese hamster ovary (CHO) cell cytoskeletal responses to cholera toxin. Proc Natl Acad Sci U S A 91:9655, 1994.
27. Hughes JM, Murad F, Chang B, et al. Role of cyclic GMP in the action of heat-stable enterotoxin of Escherichia coli. Nature 271:755, 1978.
28. Field M, Graf LH Jr, Laird WJ, et al. Heat-stable enterotoxin of Escherichia coli: in vitro effects on guanylate cyclase activity, cyclic GMP concentration, and ion transport in small intestine. Proc Natl Acad Sci U S A 75:2800, 1978.
29. Guerrant RL, Hughes JM, Chang B, et al. Activation of intestinal guanylate cyclase by heat-stable enterotoxin of Escherichia coli: studies of tissue specificity, potential receptors and intermediates. J Infect Dis 142:220, 1980.
30. Kennedy DJ, Greenberg RN, Dunn JA, et al. Effects of E. coli heat stabile enterotoxin STb on intestines of mice, rats, rabbits, and piglets. Infect Immun 46:639, 1984.
31. Weikel CS, Nellans HN, Guerrant RL. In vivo and in vitro effects of a novel enterotoxin, STb, produced by E. coli. J Infect Dis 153:893, 1986.
32. Weikel CS, Tiemens KM, Moseley SL, et al. Species specificity and lack of production of STb enterotoxin by E. coli strains isolated from humans with diarrheal illness. Infect Immun 52:323, 1986.
33. DuPont HL, Formal SB, Hornick RB, et al. Pathogenesis of Escherichia coli diarrhea. N Engl J Med 285:1, 1971.
34. Tulloch EF, Ryan KJ, Formal SB, et al. Invasive enteropathic Escherichia coli dysentery. An outbreak in 28 adults. Ann Intern Med 79:13, 1973.
35. Nataro JP, Kaper JB, Robins-Browne R, et al. Patterns of adherence of diarrheagenic E. coli to HEp-2 cells. Pediatr Infect Dis J 6:829, 1987.
36. Rosenshine I, Donnenberg MS, Kaper JB, et al. Signal transduction between enteropathogenic Escherichia coli (EPEC) and epithelial cells. EPEC induces tyrosine phosphorylation of host cell proteins to initiate cytoskeletal rearrangement and bacterial uptake. EMBO J 11:3551, 1992.
37. Kenny B, DeVinney R, Stein M, et al. Enteropathogenic E. coli (EPEC) transfers its receptor for intimate adherence into mammalian cells. Cell 91:511, 1997.
38. Giron JA, Fry J, Frankel G, et al. Diffuse-adhering Escherichia coli (DAEC) as a putative cause of diarrhea in Mayan children in Mexico. J Infect Dis 163:507, 1991.
39. Baqui AH, Sack RB, Black RE, et al. Enteropathogens associated with acute and persistent diarrhea in Bangladeshi children <5 years of age. J Infect Dis 166:792, 1992.
40. Wanke CA, Schorling JB, Barrett LJ, et al. Adherence traits of Escherichia coli, alone and in association with other stool pathogens: potential role in pathogenesis of persistent diarrhea in an urban Brazilian slum. Pediatr J Infect Dis 10:746, 1991.
41. Bhan MK, Khoshoo V, Sommerfelt H, et al. Enteroaggregative Escherichia coli and Salmonella associated with non-dysenteric persistent diarrhea. Pediatr Infect Dis J 8:499, 1989.
42. Bhan MK, Raj P, Levine MM, et al. Enteroaggregative Escherichia coli associated with persistent diarrhea in a cohort of rural children in India. J Infect Dis 159:1061, 1989.
43. Cravioto A, Reyes RE, Trujillo F, et al. Risk of diarrhea during the first year of life associated with initial and subsequent colonization by specific enteropathogens. Am J Epidemiol 131:886, 1990.
44. Cravioto A, Tello A, Navarro A, et al. Association of Escherichia coli HEp-2 adherence patterns with type and duration of diarrhoea. Lancet 337:262, 1991.

45. Lima AAM, Fang G, Schorling JB, et al. Persistent diarrhea in Northeast Brazil: etiologies and interactions with malnutrition. Acta Paediatr Scand 381:39, 1992.

46. Fang G, Lima AAM, Martins CV, et al. Etiology and epidemiology of persistent diarrhea in Northeastern Brazil: A hospital-based prospective case control study. J Pediatr Gastroenterol Nutr 21:137, 1995.

47. Moseley SL, Echeverria P, Seriwatana J, et al. Identification of enterotoxigenic E. coli by colony hybridization using three enterotoxin gene probes. J Infect Dis 145:863, 1982.

48. Sommerfelt H, Svennerholm AM, Kallard KH, et al. Comparative study of colony hybridization with synthetic oligonucleotide probes and enzyme-linked immunosorbent assay for identification of enterotoxigenic E. coli. J Clin Microbiol 36:530, 1988.

49. Levine MM, Prado V, Robins-Browne R, et al. Use of DNA probes and HEp-2 cell adherence assay to detect diarrheagenic Escherichia coli. J Infect Dis 158:224, 1988.

50. Fang G. Intestinal E. coli infections. Curr Opin Infect Dis 6:48, 1993.

51. Riley LW, Remis RS, Helgerson SD, et al. Hemorrhagic colitis associated with a rare E. coli serotype. N Engl J Med 308:681, 1982.

52. Strockbine NA, Marques LRM, Newland JW, et al. Two toxin converting phages from E. coli 0157:H7 strain 933 encode antigenically distinct toxins with similar biologic properties. Infect Immun 53:135, 1986.

53. Wanke CA, Guerrant RL. Small bowel colonization alone is a cause of diarrhea. Infect Immun 55:1924, 1987.

54. Schlager TA, Wanke CA, Guerrant RL. Net fluid secretion and impaired villous function induced by colonization of the small intestine by non-toxigenic colonizing Escherichia coli. Infect Immun 58:1337, 1990.

55. Rowe B, Scotland SM, Gross RJ. Enterotoxigenic Escherichia coli causing infantile enteritis in Britain. Lancet 1:90, 1977.

56. Trabulsi LR, Fernandes MFR, Zuliani ME. Novas bacterias patogenicas para o intestino do homen. Rev Inst Med Trop Sao Paulo 9:31, 1967.

57. Sereny B. Experimental Shigella keratoconjunctivitis: a preliminary report. Acta Microbiol Acad Sci Hung 2:293, 1955.

58. Skerman FJ, Formal SB, Falkow S. Plasmid-associated enterotoxin production in a strain of Escherichia coli isolated from humans. Infect Immun 56:22, 1972.

59. Takeda Y, Murphy J. Bacteriophage conversion of heat-labile enterotoxin in Escherichia coli. J Bacteriol 133:172, 1978.

60. Lathe R, Hirth P. Cell-free synthesis of enterotoxin of E. coli from a cloned gene. Nature 284:473, 1980.

61. Merson MH, Rowe B, Black RE, et al. Use of antisera for identification of enterotoxigenic Escherichia coli. Lancet 2:222, 1980.

62. Evans DG, Evans DJ Jr, Pierce NF. Differences in the response of rabbit small intestine to heat-labile and heat-stable enterotoxins of Escherichia coli. Infect Immun 7:873, 1973.

63. Guerrant RL, Brunton LL, Schnaitman TC, et al. Cyclic adenosine monophosphate and alteration of Chinese hamster ovary cell morphology: a rapid, sensitive in vitro assay for the enterotoxins of Vibrio cholerae and Escherichia coli. Infect Immun 10:320, 1974.

64. Donta ST, Moon HW, Whipp SC. Detection of heat-labile Escherichia coli enterotoxin with the use of adrenal cells in tissue cultures. Science 183:334, 1974.

65. Yolken RH, Greenberg HB, Merson MH, et al. Enzyme-linked immunosorbent assay for detection of Escherichia coli heat-labile enterotoxin. J Clin Microbiol 6:439, 1977.

66. Dean AG, Ching YC, Williams RG, et al. Test for Escherichia coli enterotoxin using infant mice: application in a study of diarrhea in children in Honolulu. J Infect Dis 125:407, 1972.

67. Giannella RA. Suckling mouse model for detection of heat-stable Escherichia coli enterotoxin: characteristics of the model. Infect Immun 14:95, 1976.

68. Klipstein FA, Holdeman LV, Corcino JJ, et al. Enterotoxigenic intestinal bacteria in tropical sprue. Ann Intern Med 79:632, 1973.

69. Smith HW, Halls S. Observations by ligated intestinal segment and oral inoculation methods on Escherichia coli infections in pigs, calves, lambs and rabbits. J Pathol Bacteriol 93:499, 1967.

70. Evans DG, Silver RP, Evans DJ Jr, et al. Plasmid-controlled colonization factor associated with virulence in Escherichia coli enterotoxigenic for humans. Infect Immun 12:656, 1975.

71. De SN, Chatterjee DN. An experimental study of the mechanism of action of Vibrio cholerae on the intestinal mucous membrane. J Pathol Bacteriol 66:559, 1953.

72. De SN, Bhattachaya K, Sakar JK. A study of the pathogenicity of strains of Bacterium coli from acute and chronic enteritis. J Pathol Bacteriol 71:201, 1956.

73. Taylor J, Wilkins MP, Payne JM. Relation of rabbit gut reaction to enteropathogenic Escherichia coli. Br J Exp Pathol 42:43, 1961.

74. Taylor J, Bettelheim KA. The action of chloroform-killed suspensions of enteropathogenic Escherichia coli on ligated rabbit gut segments. J Gen Microbiol 42:309, 1966.

75. Trabulsi LR. Revelacao de colibacilos associados as diarreias infantis pelo metodo da infeccao experimental de alca ligade do intestino do coehlo. Rev Inst Med Trop Sao Paulo 6:197, 1964.

76. Moon HW, Sorensen DK, Sautter JH, et al. Association of Escherichia coli with diarrheal disease of the newborn pig. Am J Vet Res 27:1107, 1966.

77. Smith HW, Halls S. Studies on Escherichia coli enterotoxin. J Pathol Bacteriol 93:531, 1967.

78. Truszcynski M, Pilaszek J. Effects of injection of enterotoxin, endotoxin or live culture of Escherichia coli into the small intestine of pigs. Res Vet Sci 10:469, 1969.

79. Gyles CL, Barnum DA. A heat-labile enterotoxin from strains of Escherichia coli enteropathogenic for pigs. J Infect Dis 120:419, 1969.

80. Gorbach SL, Banwell JG, Chatterjee BD, et al. Acute undifferentiated human diarrhea in the tropics. I. Alterations in intestinal microflora. J Clin Invest 50:881, 1971.

81. Banwell JG, Gorbach SL, Pierce NF, et al. Acute undifferentiated human diarrhea in the tropics. II. Alterations in intestinal fluid and electrolyte movements. J Clin Invest 50:890, 1971.

82. Sack RB, Gorbach SL, Banwell JG, et al. Enterotoxigenic Escherichia coli isolated from patients with severe cholera-like disease. J Infect Dis 123:278, 1971.

83. Pierce NF, Wallace CK. Stimulation of jejunal secretion by a crude Escherichia coli enterotoxin. Gastroenterology 63:439, 1972.

84. Guerrant RL, Carpenter CCJ, Pierce NF. Experimental E. coli diarrhea: effects of viable bacteria and enterotoxin. Trans Assoc Am Physicians 86:111, 1973.

85. Kantor HS, Tao P, Gorbach SL. Stimulation of intestinal adenyl cyclase by Escherichia coli enterotoxin: comparison of strains from an infant and an adult with diarrhea. J Infect Dis 129:1, 1974.

86. Smith HW, Gyles CL. The relationship between two

apparently different enterotoxins produced by entero-pathogenic strains of *Escherichia coli* of porcine origin. J Med Microbiol 3:387, 1970.

87. Kohler EM. Observations on enterotoxins produced by enteropathogenic *Escherichia coli*. Ann N Y Acad Sci 176:212, 1971.

88. Moon HW, Whipp SC. Systems for testing the entero-pathogenicity of *Escherichia coli*. Ann N Y Acad Sci 176:197, 1971.

89. Smith HW, Linggood MA. Observations on the patho-genic properties of the K88, HLY and ENT plasmids of *Escherichia coli* with particular reference to porcine diar-rhea. J Med Microbiol 4:467, 1971.

90. Guerrant RL, Chen LC, Sharp GWG. Intestinal adenyl-cyclase activity in canine cholera: correlation with fluid accumulation. J Infect Dis 125:377, 1972.

91. Nalin DR, Bhattacharjee AK, Richardson SH. Cholera-like toxic effect of culture filtrates of *Escherichia coli*. J Infect Dis 130:595, 1974.

92. Holmgren J, Svennerholm AM. Enzyme-linked immuno-sorbent assays for cholera serology. Infect Immun 7:759, 1973.

93. Svennerholm AM, Holmgren J. Identification of *Esche-richia coli* heat-labile enterotoxin by means of a ganglio-side immunosorbent assay (G$_{m1}$ ELISA) procedure. Curr Microbiol 1:19, 1978.

94. Sack DA, Huda S, Neogi PKB, et al. Microtiter ganglio-side enzyme-linked immunosorbent assay for *Vibrio* and *Escherichia coli* heat-labile enterotoxins and antitoxin. J Clin Microbiol 11:35, 1980.

95. Lima AAM, Monteiro HSA, Fonteles MD. The effects of *E. coli* heat stable enterotoxin in renal sodium tubular transport. Pharmacol Toxicol 70:163, 1992.

96. Forte LR, Krause WJ, Freeman RH. *Escherichia coli* en-terotoxin receptors: localization in opossum kidney, in-testine, and testis. Am J Physiol 25770:F874, 1989.

97. White AA, Krause WJ, Turner JT, et al. Opossum kidney contains a functional receptor to the *Escherichia coli* heat-stable enterotoxin. Biochem Biophys Res Commun 159:363, 1989.

98. Fonteles MC, Lima AAM, Fang G, et al. Effect of STa and cholera toxin on renal electrolyte transport: possible roles of an endogenous ST-like compound in the isolated kidney. 27th U.S. Japan Cholera Meeting, Charlottes-ville, Va, 1991.

99. Currie MG, Fok KF, Kato J, et al. Guanylin: an endoge-nous activator of intestinal guanylate cyclase. Proc Natl Acad Sci USA 89:947, 1992.

100. Guerrant RL, Dickens MD, Wenzel RP, et al. Toxigenic bacterial diarrhea: nursery outbreak involving multiple bacterial strains. J Pediatr 89:885, 1976.

101. Wadstrom T, Aust-Kettis A, Habte D, et al. Enterotoxin-producing bacteria and parasites in stools of Ethiopian children with diarrhoeal disease. Arch Dis Child 51:865, 1976.

102. Wachsmuth K, Wells J, Shipley P, et al. Heat-labile enterotoxin production in isolates from a shipboard out-break of human diarrheal illness. Infect Immun 24:793, 1979.

103. Sandefur PD, Peterson JW. Isolation of skin permeability factors from culture filtrates of *Salmonella typhimurium*. Infect Immun 14:671, 1976.

104. Sandefur PD, Peterson JW. Neutralization of *Salmonella* toxin–induced elongation of Chinese hamster ovary cells by cholera antitoxin. Infect Immun 15:988, 1977.

105. Gibbons RA, Sellwood R, Burrows M, et al. Inheritance of resistance to neonatal *E. coli* diarrhoea in the pig:

examination of the genetic system. Theor Appl Genet 51:65, 1977.

106. Evans DG, Evans DJ Jr. New surface-associated heat-labile colonization factor antigen (CFA/II) produced by enterotoxigenic *Escherichia coli* of serogroup 06 and 08. Infect Immun 21:638, 1978.

107. Guerrant RL, Bergman MJ. Attachment factors among enterotoxigenic *Escherichia coli*. *In* Janowitz HD, Sachar DB (eds). International Colloquium in Gastroentero-logy—Frontiers of Knowledge in the Diarrheal Diseases. Upper Montclair, NJ, Projects in Health, 1979, p 137.

108. Deneke CF, Thorne GM, Gorbach SL. Attachment pili from enterotoxigenic *Escherichia coli* pathogenic for hu-mans. Infect Immun 26:362, 1979.

109. Bergman MJ, Updike WS, Wood SJ, et al. Attachment factors among enterotoxigenic *E. coli* from patients with acute diarrhea from diverse geographic areas. Infect Im-mun 32:881, 1981.

110. Honda T, Arita M, Miwatani T. Characterization of new hydrophobic pili of human enterotoxigenic *Escherichia coli*: a possible new colonization. Infect Immun 43:959, 1984.

111. McConnell MM, Thomas LV, Willshaw GA, et al. Ge-netic control and properties of coli surface antigens of colonization factor antigen IV (PCF8775) of enterotoxi-genic *Escherichia coli*. Infect Immun 56:1974, 1988.

112. Sack DA, Kaminsky DC, Sack RB, et al. Enterotoxigenic *Escherichia coli* diarrhea of travelers: a prospective study of American Peace Corps volunteers. Johns Hopkins Med J 141:63, 1977.

113. Guerrant RL, Rouse JD, Hughes JM, et al. Turista among members of the Yale Glee Club in Latin America. Am J Trop Med Hyg 29:895, 1980.

114. Guerrant RL, Moore RA, Kirschenfeld PM, et al. Role of toxigenic and invasive bacteria in acute diarrhea of childhood. N Engl J Med 293:567, 1975.

115. Echeverria P, Blacklow NR, Smith DH. Role of heat-labile toxigenic *Escherichia coli* and reovirus-like agent in diarrhoea in Boston children. Lancet 2:1113, 1975.

116. Viboud GI, Binsztein N, Svennerholm AM. Character-ization of monoclonal antibodies against putative coloni-zation factors of enterotoxigenic *Escherichia coli* and their use in an epidemiological study. J Clin Microbiol 31:558, 1993.

117. Ryder RW, Sack DA, Kapikian AZ, et al. Enterotoxigenic *Escherichia coli* and reovirus-like agent in rural Bangla-desh. Lancet 1:659, 1976.

118. Nalin DR, McLaughlin JC, Rahaman M, et al. Entero-toxigenic *Escherichia coli* and idiopathic diarrhea in Ban-gladesh. Lancet 2:1116, 1975.

119. Lopez-Vidal Y, Calva JJ, Trujillo A, et al. Enterotoxins and adhesins of enterotoxigenic *Escherichia coli*: are they risk factors for acute diarrhea in the community? J Infect Dis 162:442, 1990.

120. McLean M, Brennan R, Hughes JM, et al. Etiology and oral rehydration therapy of childhood diarrhea in northeastern Brazil. Bull Pan Am Health Organ 15:318, 1981.

121. Sack RB, Hirschhorn N, Brownlee I, et al. Enterotoxi-genic *Escherichia coli* associated diarrheal disease in Apache children. N Engl J Med 292:1041, 1975.

122. Hughes JM, Rouse JD, Barada AF, et al. Etiology of summer diarrhea among the Navajo. Am J Trop Med Hyg 29:613, 1980.

123. Huilan S, Zhen LG, Mathan MM, et al. Etiology of acute diarrhea among children in developing countries: a multicentre study in five countries. Bull World Health Organ 69:549, 1991.

124. Blanco J, Gonzalez EA, Blanco M, et al. Enterotoxigenic *Escherichia coli* associated with infant diarrhoea in Galicia, northwestern Spain. J Med Microbiol 35:162, 1991.

125. Nations MK, de Sousa MA, Correia LL, daSilva DM. Brazilian popular healers as effective promoters of oral rehydration therapy (ORT) and related child survival strategies. Bull Pan Am Health Organ 22:335, 1988.

126. Guerrant RL, Kirchhoff LV, Shields DS, et al. Prospective study of diarrheal illnesses in northeastern Brazil: patterns of disease, nutritional impact, etiologies and risk factors. J Infect Dis 148:986, 1983.

127. Korzeniowski OM, Dantas W, Trabulsi CR, et al. A controlled study of endemic sporadic diarrhea among adult residents of southern Brazil. Trans R Soc Trop Med Hyg 78:363, 1984.

128. Kudoh Y, Hiroshi ZY, Matsushita S, et al. Outbreaks of acute enteritis due to heat-stable enterotoxin-producing strains of *Escherichia coli*. Microbiol Immunol 21:175, 1977.

129. Rosenberg ML, Koplan JP, Wachsmuth IK, et al. Epidemic diarrhea at Crater Lake from enterotoxigenic *Escherichia coli*: a large waterborne outbreak. Ann Intern Med 86:714, 1977.

130. Sack RB, Sack DA, Mehlman IJ, et al. Enterotoxigenic *Escherichia coli* isolated from food. J Infect Dis 135:313, 1977.

131. Ryder RW, Wachsmuth IK, Buxton AE, et al. Infantile diarrhea produced by heat-stable enterotoxigenic *Escherichia coli*. N Engl J Med 295:849, 1976.

132. Gross RJ, Rowe B, Henderson A, et al. A new *Escherichia coli* O-group, 0159, associated with outbreaks of enteritis in infants. Scand J Infect Dis 8:195, 1976.

133. Albert MJ, Faruque SM, Faruque AS, et al. Controlled study of *Escherichia coli* diarrheal infections in Bangladeshi children. J Clin Microbiol 33:973, 1995.

134. Levine MM, Caplan ES, Waterman D, et al. Diarrhea caused by *Escherichia coli* that produce only heat-stable enterotoxin. Infect Immun 17:78, 1977.

135. Merson MH, Black RE, Gross RJ. Use of antisera for identification of enterotoxigenic *Escherichia coli*. Lancet 2:222, 1980.

136. Abe A, Komase K, Bangtrakulnonth A, et al. Trivalent heat-labile– and heat-stable–enterotoxin probe conjugated with horseradish peroxidase for detection of enterotoxigenic *Escherichia coli* by hybridization J Clin Microbiol 28:2616, 1990.

137. Sommerfelt H, Svennerholm AM, Kallard KH, et al. Comparative study of colony hybridization with synthetic oligonucleotide probes and enzyme-linked immunosorbent assay for identification of enterotoxigenic *E. coli*. J Clin Microbiol 26:530, 1988.

138. Lund A, Wasteson W, Olsvik O. Immunomagnetic separation and DNA hybridization for detection of enterotoxigenic *Escherichia coli* in a piglet model. J Clin Microbiol 29:2259, 1991.

139. Hornes E, Wasteson W, Olsvik O. Detection of *Escherichia coli* heat-stable enterotoxin genes in pig stool specimens by an immobilized, calorimetric, nested polymerase chain reaction. J Clin Microbiol 29:2375, 1991.

140. Duggan C, Santosham M, Glass RI. The management of acute diarrhea in children: oral rehydration, maintenance, and nutritional therapy. MMWR Morb Mortal Wkly Rep 41:1, 1992.

141. Pizarro D, Posada G, Mata L, et al. Oral rehydration of neonates with dehydrating diarrheas. Lancet 2:1209, 1979.

142. Santosham M, Daum RS, Dillman L, et al. Oral rehydration therapy for infantile diarrhea. A controlled study of well nourished children hospitalized in the United States and Panama. N Engl J Med 306:1070, 1982.

143. Molla AM, Molla A, Nath SK, et al. Food based oral rehydration salt solutions for acute childhood diarrhoea. Lancet 2:429, 1989.

144. Walker SH, Gahol VP, Quintero BA. Sodium and water content of feedings for use in infants with diarrhea. Clin Pediatr 20:199, 1981.

145. International Study Group on Reduced Osmolality ORS Solution. Multicentre evaluation of reduced-osmolality oral rehydration salts solution. Lancet 345:282, 1995.

146. Echeverria P, Ulyangco CV, Ho MT, et al. Antimicrobial resistance and enterotoxin production among isolates of *Escherichia coli* in the Far East. Lancet 2:589, 1978.

147. Harris JR, Wachsmuth IK, Davis BR, et al. High-molecular-weight plasmid correlates with *Escherichia coli* invasiveness. Infect Immun 37:1295, 1982.

148. De Assis A. *Shigella guanabara*, tipo serologico destacado do grupo B. ceylonensis-dispar. O Hospital 33:508, 1948.

149. Lapatsanis PD, Irving IM. A study of specific *E. coli* infections occurring in a unit for surgical neonates. Acta Paediatr 52:436, 1963.

150. Gordillo ME, Reeve GR, Pappas J, et al. Molecular characterization of strains of enteroinvasive *Escherichia coli* 0143, including isolates from a large outbreak in Houston, Texas. J Clin Microbiol 30:889, 1992.

151. Goldschmidt R. Untersuchungen zur Ätiologie der Durchfallserkrankungen des Säuglings. Jahr Kinderheilkd. 139:318, 1933.

152. Dulaney AD, Michelson ID. A study of *E. coli* mutable from an outbreak of diarrhea in the new-born. Am J Public Health 25:1241, 1935.

153. Bray J. Isolation of antigenically homogenous strains of *Bact. coli neopolitanum* from summer diarrhea of infants. J Pathol Bacteriol 57:239, 1945.

154. Bray J, Beaven TED. Slide agglutination of *Bacterium coli* var. *neopolitanum* in summer diarrhea. J Pathol Bacteriol 60:395, 1948.

155. Olarte J, Varela G. A complete somatic antigen common to *Salmonella adelaide*, *Escherichia coli-gomez* and *Escherichia coli* 0111:B4. J Lab Clin Med (London) 40:252, 1952.

156. Giles C, Sangster, G. An outbreak of infantile gastroenteritis in Aberdeen. J Hyg 46:1, 1948.

157. Giles C, Sangster G, Smith J. Epidemic gastroenteritis of infants in Aberdeen during 1947. Arch Dis Child 24:45, 1949.

158. Kaufman F, Dupont A. *Escherichia* strains from infantile epidemic gastroenteritis. Acta Pathol Microbiol Scand 27:552, 1950.

159. Edwards PR, Ewing WH. Identification of Enterobacteriaceae, 3rd ed. Minneapolis, Burgess Publishing, 1972.

160. Neter E, Korns RF, Trussell RF. Association of *Escherichia coli* serogroup 0111 with two hospital outbreaks of epidemic diarrhea of the newborn infant in New York State during 1947. Pediatrics 12:377, 1953.

161. Neter E, Westphal O, Luderitz O, et al. Demonstration of antibodies against enteropathogenic *Escherichia coli* in sera of children of various ages. Pediatrics 16:801, 1955.

162. Neter E. *Escherichia coli* as a pathogen. J Pediatr 89:166, 1976.

163. Gronroos JA. Investigations on certain *Escherichia coli* serotypes, with special reference to infantile diarrhoea. Ann Med 32:9, 1954.

164. Riley PD, Riley HD Jr. Serotypes and antibiotic susceptibility of *Escherichia coli* in nonenteric infections of children. Scand J Infect Dis 5:187, 1973.

165. Robbins JB, McCracken GH, Gotschlich EC, et al. *Esch-*

erichia coli K1 capsular polysaccharide associated with neonatal meningitis. N Engl J Med 290:1216, 1974.

166. Baldini MM, Kaper JB. Plasmid-mediated adhesion in enteropathogenic *E. coli*. J Pediatr Gastroenterol 2:534, 1983.

167. Lubin AH, Girola RA, Grinstein S. Prevalence of enteropathogenic bacteria isolated from infants with diarrhea in Buenos Aires. Am J Trop Med Hyg 12:771, 1963.

168. Goodwin MH Jr, Mackel DC, Ganelin RS, et al. Observation on etiology of diarrheal diseases in Arizona. Am J Trop Med Hyg 9:336, 1960.

169. Moffet HL, Shulenberger HK, Burkholder ER. Epidemiology and etiology of severe infantile diarrhea. J Pediatr 72:1, 1968.

170. Olarte J, Ramos-Alvarez M, Galindo E. Bol Med Hosp Infant Mex 14:263, 1957. Quoted in Ordway NK. Diarrhoeal disease and its control. Bull World Health Organ 23:73, 1960.

171. Ramos-Alvarez M, Olarte J. Diarrheal diseases of children. The occurrence of enteropathogenic viruses and bacteria. Am J Dis Child 107:218, 1964.

172. Moyenuddin M, Rahman KM. Enteropathogenic *Escherichia coli* diarrhea in hospitalized children in Bangladesh. J Clin Microbiol 22:838, 1985.

173. Toledo MRF, Alvariza MCB, Murahovschi J, et al. Enteropathogenic *Escherichia coli* serotypes and epidemic diarrhea in infants. Infect Immun 39:586, 1983.

174. Echeverria P, Orskov F, Orskov I, et al. Attaching and effacing enteropathogenic *Escherichia coli* as a cause of infantile diarrhea in Bangkok. J Infect Dis 164:550, 1991.

175. Ghosh AR, Nair GB, Naik TN, et al. Enteroadherent *Escherichia coli* is an important diarrhoeagenic agent in infants aged below 6 months in Calcutta, India. J Med Microbiol 36:264, 1992.

176. Echeverria P, Serichantalerg O, Changchawalit S, et al. Tissue culture adherent *Escherichia coli* in infantile diarrhea. J Infect Dis 165:141, 1992.

177. Braun OH. *E. coli* enteritis in Germany: epidemiology and recent research. Ann N Y Acad Sci 176:126, 1971.

178. Brown EH, Bailey EH. Infantile gastroenteritis: changing needs in treatment. Lancet 2:1218, 1957.

179. Neter E. Discussion. Ann N Y Acad Sci 176:136, 1971.

180. Taylor J. Host-parasite relations of *Escherichia coli* in man. J Appl Bacteriol 29:1, 1966.

181. Marker SC, Blazevic DJ. Enteropathogenic serotypes of *E. coli*. J Pediatr 90:1037, 1977.

182. Farmer JJ, Davis BR, Cherry WB, et al. "Enteropathogenic serotypes" of *Escherichia coli* which really are not. J Pediatr 90:1047, 1977.

183. Gordon JE. Diarrheal disease of early childhood—worldwide scope of the problem. Ann N Y Acad Sci 176:9, 1971.

184. Gordon JE, Chitkara ID, Wyon JB. Weanling diarrhea. Am J Med Sci 245:345, 1963.

185. Mata LJ, Urrutia JJ. Intestinal colonization of breastfed children in a rural area of low socioeconomic level. Ann N Y Acad Sci 176:93, 1971.

186. Bernet CP, Graber CD, Anthony CW. Association of *Escherichia coli* 0127:B8 with an outbreak of infantile gastroenteritis and its concurrent distribution in the pediatric population. J Pediatr 47:287, 1955.

187. Cooper ML, Walters EW, Keller HM, et al. Epidemic diarrhea among infants associated with the isolation of a new serotype of *Escherichia coli*: *E. coli* 0127:B8. Pediatrics 16:215, 1955.

188. Laurell G, Magnusson JH, Frisell E, et al. Epidemic infantile diarrhea and vomiting. Acta Paediatr 40:302, 1951.

189. Martineau B, Raymond R, Jeliu G. Bacteriological and clinical study of gastroenteritis and enteropathogenic *Escherichia coli* 0127:B8. Can Med Assoc J 79:351, 1958.

190. Wheeler WE, Wainerman B. The treatment and prevention of epidemic infantile diarrhea due to *E. coli* 0-111 by the use of chloramphenicol and neomycin. Pediatrics 14:357, 1954.

191. Kaslow RA, Taylor A Jr, Dweck HS, et al. Enteropathogenic *Escherichia coli* infection in a newborn nursery. Am J Dis Child 128:797, 1974.

192. Boyer KM, Peterson NJ, Farzaneh I, et al. An outbreak of gastroenteritis due to *E. coli* 0142 in a neonatal nursery. J Pediatr 86:919, 1975.

193. Masembe RN. The pattern of bacterial diarrhea of the newborn in Mulago Hospital (Kampala). J Trop Pediatr 23:61, 1977.

194. Gross RJ, Rowe B, Henderson A, et al. A new *Escherichia coli* O-group, 0159, associated with outbreaks of enteritis in infants. Scand J Infect Dis 8:195, 1976.

195. Boris M, Thomason BM, Hines VD, et al. A community epidemic of enteropathogenic *Escherichia coli* 0126:B16: NM gastroenteritis associated with asymptomatic respiratory infection. Pediatrics 33:18, 1964.

196. Kessner DM, Shaughnessy HJ, Googins J, et al. An extensive community outbreak of diarrhea due to enteropathogenic *Escherichia coli* 0111:B4. I. Epidemiologic studies. Am J Hyg 76:27, 1962.

197. Severs D, Fardy P, Acres S, et al. Epidemic gastroenteritis in Newfoundland during 1963 associated with *E. coli* 0111:B4. Can Med Assoc J 94:373, 1966.

198. Cooper ML, Keller HM, Walters EW. Comparative frequency of detection of enteropathogenic *E. coli*, *Salmonella* and *Shigella* in rectal swab cultures from infants and young children. Pediatrics 19:411, 1957.

199. Hinton NA, MacGregor RR. A study of infections due to pathogenic serogroups of *Escherichia coli*. Can Med Assoc J 79:359, 1958.

200. Hutchinson RI. *Escherichia coli* (O-types 111, 55, and 26) and their association with infantile diarrhea. A five-year study. J Hyg 55:27, 1957.

201. Joe LK, Sahab K, Yauw GS, et al. Diarrhea among infants and children in Djakarta, Indonesia, with special reference to pathogenic *Escherichia coli*. Am J Trop Med Hyg 9:626, 1960.

202. Nelson JD. Duration of neomycin therapy for enteropathogenic *Escherichia coli* diarrheal disease: a comparative study of 113 cases. Pediatrics 48:248, 1971.

203. Riley HD Jr. Antibiotic therapy in neonatal enteric disease. Ann N Y Acad Sci 176:360, 1971.

204. Rozansky R, Berant M, Rosenmann E, et al. Enteropathogenic *Escherichia coli* infections in infants during the period from 1957 to 1962. Pediatrics 64:521, 1964.

205. South MA. Enteropathogenic *Escherichia coli* disease: new developments and perspectives. J Pediatr 79:1, 1971.

206. Linzenmeier G. Wandel im Auftreten und Verhalten enteropathogene Colitypen. Zentralbl Bakteriol 184:74, 1962.

207. Nicolopoulos D, Arseni A. Susceptibility of enteropathogenic *E. coli* to various antibiotics. Letter to the editor. J Pediatr 81:426, 1972.

208. Ironside AG, Tuxford AF, Heyworth B. A survey of infantile gastroenteritis. BMJ 2:20, 1970.

209. Riley HD Jr. Clinical rounds. Enteropathogenic *E. coli* gastroenteritis. Clin Pediatr 3:93, 1964.

210. Kourany M, Vasquez MA. Enteropathogenic bacteria associated with diarrhea among infants in Panama. Am J Trop Med Hyg 18:930, 1969.

211. Gaines S, Achavasmith U, Thareesawat M, et al. Types

and distribution of enteropathogenic *Escherichia coli* in Bangkok, Thailand. Am J Hyg 80:388, 1964.

212. Buttner DW, Lado-Kenyi A. Prevalence of *Salmonella*, *Shigella*, and enteropathogenic *Escherichia coli* in young children in Kampala, Uganda. Tropenmed Parasitol 24:259, 1973.

213. Coetzee M, Leary PM. Gentamicin in *Esch. coli* gastroenteritis. Arch Dis Child 46:646, 1971.

214. Kahn E. The aetiology of summer diarrhoea. S Afr Med J 31:47, 1957.

215. Taylor J. The diarrhoeal diseases in England and Wales. With special reference to those caused by *Salmonella*, *Escherichia*, and *Shigella*. Bull World Health Organ 23:763, 1960.

216. Epidemiological Research Laboratory of the Public Health Laboratory Service, United Kingdom and Republic of Ireland. *E. coli* gastroenteritis from food. BMJ 1:911, 1976.

217. Ocklitz HW, Schmidt E. F. Über das Vorkommen von Dispepsie-Coli bei Erwachsenen. Helv Paediatr Acta 10:450, 1955.

218. Schaffer J, Lewis V, Nelson J, et al. Antepartum survey for enteropathogenic *Escherichia coli*. Detection by cultural and fluorescent antibody methods. Am J Dis Child 106:170, 1963.

219. Kirby AC, Hall EG, Coackley W. Neonatal diarrhoea and vomiting. Outbreaks in the same maternity unit. Lancet 2:201, 1950.

220. Bettelheim KA, Breaden A, Faiers MC, et al. The origin of O-serotypes of *Escherichia coli* in babies after normal delivery. J Hyg 72:67, 1974.

221. Stulberg CS, Zuelzer WW, Nolke AC. An epidemic of diarrhea of the newborn caused by *Escherichia coli* 0111:B$_4$. Pediatrics 14:133, 1954.

222. Farmer K, Hassall IB. An epidemic of *E. coli* type 055:k59(B5) in a neonatal unit. N Z Med J 77:372, 1973.

223. Hugh-Jones K, Ross GIM. Epidemics of gastroenteritis associated with *E. coli* 0119 infection. Arch Dis Child 33:543, 1958.

224. Senerwa D, Olsvik O, Mutanda LN, et al. Colonization of neonates in a nursery ward with enteropathogenic *Escherichia coli* and correlation to the clinical histories of the children. J Clin Microbiol 27:2539, 1989.

225. Wright J, Roden AT. *Escherichia coli* 055B5 infection in a gastroenteritis ward. Epidemiological applications of II antigen type determinations. Am J Hyg 58:133, 1953.

226. Balassanian N, Wolinsky E. Epidemiologic and serologic studies of *E. coli* 04:115 in a premature nursery. Pediatrics 41:463, 1968.

227. Jameson JE, Mann TP, Rothfield NJ. Hospital gastroenteritis. An epidemiological survey of infantile diarrhea and vomiting contracted in a children's hospital. Lancet 2:459, 1954.

228. Thomson S. The role of certain varieties of *Bacterium coli* in gastroenteritis in babies. J Hyg 53:357, 1955.

229. Page RH, Stulberg CS. Immunofluorescence in epidemiologic control of *E. coli* diarrhea. Incidence, cross-infections, and control in a children's hospital. Am J Dis Child 104:149, 1962.

230. Bertrams J, Pfortner M, Neusel H, et al. Colienteritis des Säuglings. Quantitative und fluoreszenzserologische Verlaufsuntersuchungen. Munch Med Wochenschr 112:38, 1970.

231. Thomson S. The numbers of pathogenic bacilli in faeces in intestinal diseases. J Hyg 53:217, 1955.

232. Herweg JC, Middlekamp JN, Thornton HK. *Escherichia coli* diarrhea. The relationship of certain serotypes of *Escherichia coli* to sporadic and epidemic cases of infantile diarrhea. J Pediatr 49:629, 1956.

233. Belnap WD, O'Donnell JJ. Epidemic gastroenteritis due to *Escherichia coli* 0-111. A review of the literature, with the epidemiology, bacteriology, and clinical findings of a large outbreak. J Pediatr 47:178, 1955.

234. Rogers KB, Koegler SJ. Inter-hospital cross-infection epidemic infantile gastroenteritis associated with type strains of *Bacterium coli*. J Hyg 49:152, 1951.

235. Stock AH, Shuman ME. Gastroenteritis in infants associated with specific serotypes of *Escherichia coli*. II. An epidemic of *Escherichia coli* 0111:B4 gastroenteritis involving multiple institutions. Pediatrics 17:196, 1956.

236. Stulberg CS, Zuelzer WW, Nolke AC, et al. *Escherichia coli* 0127:B$_8$, a pathogenic strain causing infantile diarrhea. Epidemiology and bacteriology of a prolonged outbreak in a premature nursery. Am J Dis Child 90:125, 1955.

237. Thomson S, Watkins AG, Grapy PO. *Escherichia coli* gastroenteritis. Arch Dis Child 31:340, 1956.

238. Olarte J, Ramos-Alvarez M. Epidemic diarrhea in premature infants. Etiological significance of a newly recognized type of *Escherichia coli* (0142:K86:H6). Am J Dis Child 109:436, 1965.

239. Nelson JD, Whitaker JA, Hempstead B, et al. Epidemiological application of the fluorescent antibody technique. Study of a diarrhea outbreak in a premature nursery. JAMA 176:26, 1961.

240. Buttiaux R, Nicolle P, LeMinor S, et al. Etude épidémiologique des gastroentérits à *Escherichia coli* dans un service hospitalier du nord de la France. Arch Mal Appar Dig 45:225, 1956.

241. Harris AH, Yankauer A, Green DC, et al. Control of epidemic diarrhea of the newborn in hospital nurseries and pediatric wards. Ann N Y Acad Sci 66:118, 1956.

242. Jacobs SI, Holzel A, Wolman B, et al. Outbreak of infantile gastroenteritis caused by *Escherichia coli* 0114. Arch Dis Child 46:656, 1970.

243. Curtin M, Clifford SH. Incidence of pathogenic serologic types of *Escherichia coli* among neonatal patients in the New England area. N Engl J Med 255:1090, 1956.

244. Greene DC, Albrecht RM. Recent developments in diarrhea of the newborn. N Y State J Med 55:2764, 1955.

245. Wheeler WE. Spread and control of *Escherichia coli* diarrheal disease. Ann N Y Acad Sci 66:112, 1956.

246. Buttiaux RR, Nicolle P, LeMinor L, et al. Etudes sur les *E. coli* de gastroentérite infantile. Ann Inst Pasteur 91:799, 1956.

247. Love WC, Gordon AM, Gross RJ, et al. Infantile gastroenteritis due to *Escherichia coli* 0142. Lancet 2:355, 1972.

248. Shaughnessy HJ, Lesko M, Dorigan F, et al. An extensive community outbreak of diarrhea due to enteropathogenic *Escherichia coli* 0111:B4. Am J Hyg 76:44, 1962.

249. Kendall N, Vaughan VC III, Kusakcioglu A. A study of preparation of infant formulas. A medical and sociocultural appraisal. Am J Dis Child 122:215, 1971.

250. Gamble DR, Rowson KEK. The incidence of pathogenic *Escherichia coli* in routine fecal specimens. Lancet 2:619, 1957.

251. Taylor J, Powell BW, Wright J. Infantile diarrhoea and vomiting. A clinical and bacteriological investigation. BMJ 2:117, 1949.

252. Modica RI, Ferguson WW, Ducey EF. Epidemic infantile diarrhea associated with *Escherichia coli* 0111, B$_4$. J Lab Clin Med 39:122, 1952.

253. Rogers KB. The spread of infantile gastroenteritis in a cubicled ward. J Hyg 49:140, 1951.

254. Wyatt RG, Matta LJ. Bacteria in colostrum and milk of Guatemalan Indian women. J Trop Pediatr 15:159, 1969.

255. Mossel DAA, Weijers HA. Uitkomsten, verkregen bij bacteriologisch onderzoek van vrouwenmelk van diverse herkomst en de betekenis daarvan de pediatrische praktijk. Maandschr Kindergeneeskd 25:37, 1957.

256. Rantasalo I, Kauppinen MA. The occurrence of Staphylococcus aureus in mother's milk. Ann Chir Gynaecol 48:246, 1959.

257. Edwards LD, Tan-Gatue LG, Levin S, et al. The problem of bacteriologically contaminated infant formulas in a newborn nursery. Clin Pediatr 13:63, 1974.

258. Thomson S. Is infantile gastroenteritis fundamentally a milk-borne infection? J Hyg 54:311, 1956.

259. Danielssen D, Laurell G. Fluorescent antibody technique in the diagnosis of enteropathogenic Escherichia coli, with special reference to sensitivity and specificity. Acta Pathol Microbiol Scand 76:601, 1969.

260. Bullen CL, Willis AT. Resistance of the breast-fed infant to gastroenteritis. BMJ 2:338, 1971.

261. Cravioto A, Tello A, Villafan H, et al. Inhibition of localized adhesion of enteropathogenic Escherichia coli to HEp-2 cells by immunoglobulin and oligosaccharide fractions of human colostrum and breast milk. J Infect Dis 163:1247, 1991.

262. Svirsky-Gross S. Pathogenic strains of coli (0,111) among prematures and the use of human milk in controlling the outbreak of diarrhea. Ann Paediatr 190:109, 1958.

263. Tassovatz B, Kotsitch A. Le lait de femme et son action de protection contre les infections intestinales chez le nouveau-né. Ann Paediatr 8:285, 1961.

264. Adam A. Fortschritte in der Pathogenese und Therapie der Ernährungsstörungen. Arztl Forschung 6:59, 1952.

265. Neter E, Shumway CN. E. coli serotype D433; occurrence in intestinal and respiratory tracts, cultural characteristics, pathogenicity, sensitivity to antibiotics. Proc Soc Exp Biol Med 75:504, 1950.

266. Arnon H, Salzberger M, Olitzki AL. The appearance of antibacterial and antitoxic antibodies in maternal sera, umbilical cord blood and milk: observations on the specificity of antibacterial antibodies in human sera. Pediatrics 23:86, 1959.

267. Kenny JF, Boesman MI, Michaels RH. Bacterial and viral coproantibodies in breast-fed infants. Pediatrics 39:202, 1967.

268. Sussman S. The passive transfer of antibodies to Escherichia coli 0111:B4 from mother to offspring. Pediatrics 27:308, 1961.

269. Stulberg CS, Zuelzer WW. Infantile diarrhea due to Escherichia coli. Ann N Y Acad Sci 66:90, 1956.

270. Yeivin R, Salzberger M, Olitzki AL. Development of antibodies to enteric pathogens: placental transfer of antibodies and development of immunity in childhood. Pediatrics 18:19, 1956.

271. Dancis J, Kunz HW. Studies of the immunology of the newborn infant. VI. Bacteriostatic and complement activity of the serum. Pediatrics 13:339, 1954.

272. Kenny JF, Weinert DW, Gray JA. Enteric infection with Escherichia coli 0127 in the mouse. II. Failure of specific immunity to alter intestinal colonization of infants and adults. J Infect Dis 129:10, 1974.

273. Lodinova R, Jouja V, Wagner V. Serum immunoglobulins and coproantibody formation in infants after artificial intestinal colonization with Escherichia coli 083 and oral lysozyme administration. Pediatr Res 7:659, 1973.

274. McNeish AS, Gaze H. The intestinal antibody response in infants with enteropathic E. coli gastroenteritis. Acta Paediatr Scand 63:663, 1974.

275. Goldschmidt MC, DuPont HL. Enteropathogenic Escherichia coli: lack of correlation of serotype with pathogenicity. J Infect Dis 133:153, 1976.

276. Echeverria PD, Chang CP, Smith D. Enterotoxigenicity and invasive capacity of "enteropathogenic" serotypes of Escherichia coli. J Pediatr 89:8, 1976.

277. Gross RJ, Scotland SM, Rowe B. Enterotoxin testing of Escherichia coli causing epidemic infantile enteritis in the U.K. Lancet 1:629, 1976.

278. Drucker MM, Pollack A, Yeivin R, et al. Immunofluorescent demonstration of enteropathogenic Escherichia coli in tissues of infants dying with enteritis. Pediatrics 46:855, 1970.

279. Levine MM, Bergquist EJ, Nalin DR, et al. Escherichia coli strains that cause diarrhea but do not produce heat-labile or heat-stable enterotoxins and are non-invasive. Lancet 1:1119, 1978.

280. Wade WG, Thom BT, Evans N. Cytotoxic enteropathogenic Escherichia coli. Lancet 2:1235, 1979.

281. Cantey JR, Blake RK. Diarrhea due to Escherichia coli in the rabbit: a novel mechanism. J Infect Dis 135:454, 1977.

282. Rothbaum RJ, Partin JC, McAdams AJ, et al. Enterocyte adherent E. coli 0119:B14: a novel mechanism of infant diarrhea. Gastroenterology 80:1265, 1981.

283. Polotsky Y, Dragunskaya EM, Seliverstova VG, et al. Pathogenic effect of enterotoxigenic Escherichia coli and Escherichia coli causing infantile diarrhea. Acta Microbiol Acad Sci Hung. 24:221, 1977.

284. Moon HW, Whipp SC, Argenzio RA, et al. Attaching and effacing activities of rabbit and human enteropathogenic Escherichia coli in pig and rabbit intestines. Infect Immun 41:1340, 1983.

285. Francis CL, Jerse AE, Kaper JB, et al. Characterization of interactions of enteropathogenic Escherichia coli 0127:H6 with mammalian cells in vitro. J Infect Dis 164:693, 1991.

286. Vuopio-Varkila J, Schoolnik GK. Localized adherence by enteropathogenic Escherichia coli is an inducible phenotype associated with the expression of new outer membrane proteins. J Exp Med 174:1167, 1991.

287. Giron JA, Ho ASY, Schoolnik GK. An inducible bundle-forming pilus of enteropathogenic Escherichia coli. Science 254:710, 1992.

288. Baldwin TJ, Brooks SF, Knutton S, et al. Protein phosphorylation by protein kinase C in HEp-2 cells infected with enteropathogenic Escherichia coli. Infect Immun 48:761, 1990.

289. Baldwin TJ, Ward W, Aitken A, et al. Elevation of intracellular free calcium levels in HEp-2 cells infected with enteropathogenic Escherichia coli. Infect Immun 59:1599, 1991.

290. Hopkins GB, Gould VE, Stevenson JK, et al. Necrotizing enterocolitis in premature infants. A clinical and pathologic evaluation of autopsy material. Am J Dis Child 120:229, 1970.

291. Rho Y, Josephson JE. Epidemic enteropathogenic Escherichia coli. Newfoundland, 1963: autopsy study of 16 cases. Can Med Assoc J 96:392, 1967.

292. Shwachman H, Lloyd-Still JD, Khaw KT, et al. Protracted diarrhea of infancy treated by intravenous alimentation. II. Studies of small intestinal biopsy results. Am J Dis Child 125:365, 1973.

293. Lucking T, Gruttner R. Chronic diarrhea and severe malabsorption in infancy following infections with pathogenic E. coli. Acta Paediatr Scand 63:167, 1974.

294. Handforth CP, Sorger K. Failure of regeneration of small

bowel mucosa following epidemic infantile gastroenteritis. Can Med Assoc J 84:425, 1961.

295. McKay DG, Wahle GH Jr. Epidemic gastroenteritis due to *Escherichia coli* 0111:B4. II. Pathologic anatomy (with special reference to the presence of the local and generalized Shwartzman phenomena). Arch Pathol 60:679, 1955.

296. Laurell G. Quoted in Ordway NK. Diarrhoeal disease and its control. Bull World Health Organ 23:93, 1960.

297. Braun OH, Henckel H. Über epidemische Säuglingsenteritis. Z Kinderheilkd 70:33, 1951.

298. Neter E. Enteritis due to enteropathogenic *Escherichia coli*. Present day status and unsolved problems. J Pediatr 55:223, 1959.

299. Rogers KB, Cracknell VM. Epidemic infantile gastroenteritis due to *Escherichia coli* type 0,114. J Pathol Bacteriol 72:27, 1956.

300. Todd RM, Hall EG. Chloramphenicol in prophylaxis of infantile gastroenteritis. BMJ 1:1359, 1953.

301. Gastroenteritis due to *Escherichia coli*. Editorial. Lancet 1:32, 1968.

302. Senerwa D, Olsvik O, Mutanda LN, et al. Enteropathogenic *Escherichia coli* serotype 0111:HNT isolated from preterm neonates in Nairobi, Kenya. J Clin Microbiol 27:1307, 1989.

303. Bray J. Bray's discovery of pathogenic *Esch. coli* as a cause of infantile gastroenteritis. Arch Dis Child 48:923, 1973.

304. Ironside AG, Brennand J, Mandal BK, et al. Cross-infection in infantile gastroenteritis. Arch Dis Child 46:815, 1971.

305. Linetskaya-Novgorodskaya EM. Acute intestinal infections of non-dysenteric etiology. Bull World Health Organ 21:299, 1959.

306. Lloyd-Still JD, Shwachman H, Filler RM. Protracted diarrhea of infancy treated by intravenous alimentation. 1. Clinical studies of 16 infants. Am J Dis Child 125:358, 1973.

307. Drimmer-Hernheiser H, Olitzki AL. The association of *Escherichia coli* (serotypes 0111:B4 and 055:B5) with cases of acute infantile gastroenteritis in Jerusalem. Acta Med Orient 10:219, 1951.

308. Linde K, Kodizt H, Funk G. Die Mehrfachinfektionen mit Dyspepsie-Coli, ihre Beurteilung in statistischer, bakteriologischer und klinischer Sicht. Z Hyg 147:94, 1960.

309. Fandre M, Coffin R, Dropsy G, et al. Epidemic of infantile gastroenteritis due to *Escherichia coli* 0127:B8 with methemoglobinemic cyanosis. Arch Fr Pediatr 19:1129, 1962.

310. Garcia de Olarte D, Trujillo H, Agudelo ON, et al. Treatment of diarrhea in malnourished infants and children. A double-blind study comparing ampicillin and placebo. Am J Dis Child 127:379, 1974.

311. Yow MD. Prophylactic antimicrobial agents—panel. Statement of panelist. *In* Centers for Disease Control Proceedings of the International Conference on Nosocomial Infections, August 3–6, 1970. Chicago, American Hospital Association, 1971, pp 315–316.

312. Bettelheim KA, Faiers M, Sheeter RA. Serotypes of *Escherichia coli* in normal stools. Lancet 2:1227, 1972.

313. Stock AH, Shuman ME. Gastroenteritis in infants associated with specific serotypes of *Escherichia coli*. I. Incidence of specific *Escherichia coli* serotypes 0111:B4 and 055:B5 in the Pittsburgh area. Pediatrics 17:192, 1956.

314. Mushin R. Multiple intestinal infection. Med J Aust 1:807, 1953.

315. Harris JC, DuPont HL, Hornick RB. Fecal leukocytes in diarrheal illness. Ann Intern Med 76:697, 1972.

316. Guerrant RL, Araujo V, Cooper WH, et al. Measurement of fecal lactoferrin as a marker of fecal leukocytes and inflammatory enteritis. J Clin Microbiol 30:1238, 1992.

317. Miller JR, Barrett LJ, Kotloff K, Guerrant RL. A rapid test for infectious and inflammatory enteritis. Arch Intern Med 154:2660, 1994.

318. Ross CA, Dawes EA. Resistance of the breast-fed infant to gastroenteritis. Lancet 1:994, 1954.

319. Cooper ML, Walters EW, Keller HM. *Escherichia coli* associated with infantile diarrhea. Ann N Y Acad Sci 66:78, 1956.

320. Cherry WB, Thomason BM. Fluorescent antibody techniques for *Salmonella* and other enteric pathogens. Public Health Rep 84:887, 1969.

321. Murray WA, Kheder J, Wheeler WE. Colistin suppression of *Escherichia coli* in stools. I. Control of a nosocomial outbreak of diarrhea caused by neomycin-resistant *Escherichia coli* 0111:B4. Am J Dis Child 108:274, 1964.

322. Jerse AE, Gicquelais KG, Kaper JB. Plasmid and chromosomal elements involved in the pathogenesis of attaching and effacing *Escherichia coli*. Infect Immun 59:3869, 1991.

323. Nataro JP, Scaletsky ICA. Plasmid-mediated factors conferring diffuse and localized adherence of enteropathogenic *E. coli*. Infect Immun 48:378, 1985.

324. Albert MJ, Ansaruzzaman M, Faruque SM, et al. An ELISA for the detection of localized adherent classic enteropathogenic *Escherichia coli* serogroups. J Infect Dis 164:986, 1991.

325. Knutton S, Baldwin T, Williams PH, et al. Actin accumulation at sites of bacterial adhesion to tissue culture cells: basis of a new diagnostic test for enteropathogenic and enterohemorrhagic *Escherichia coli*. Infect Immun 57:1290, 1989.

326. Nelson JD. Comment. *In* Gellis S (ed). Yearbook of Pediatrics, 1973. St Louis, Mosby–Year Book, 1973.

327. Sherman JO, Hamly CA, Khachadurian AK. Use of an oral elemental diet in infants with severe intractable diarrhea. J Pediatr 86:518, 1975.

328. Pearce JL, Hamilton JR. Controlled trial of orally administered lactobacilli in acute infantile diarrhea. J Pediatr 84:261, 1974.

329. Marie J, Hennequet A, Roux C. La kanamycin "per os" dans le traitement des gastroentérites à colibacilles du nourrison. Ann Paediatr 9:97, 1962.

330. Valman HB, Wilmers MJ. Use of antibiotics in acute gastroenteritis among infants in hospital. Lancet 1:1122, 1969.

331. Dailey KM, Sturtevant AB, Feary TW. Incidence of antibiotic resistance and R-factors among gram-negative bacteria isolated from the neonatal intestine. J Pediatr 80:198, 1972.

332. Neu HC, Cherubin C, Vogt M, et al. Antibiotic resistance of fecal *Escherichia coli*. A comparison of samples from children of low and high socioeconomic groups. Am J Dis Child 126:174, 1973.

333. Watanabe T. Transferable antibiotic resistance in Enterobacteriaceae: relationship to the problems of treatment and control of coliform enteritis. Ann N Y Acad Sci 176:371, 1971.

334. McCracken GH. Changing pattern of the antimicrobial susceptibilities of *Escherichia coli* in neonatal infections. J Pediatr 78:942, 1971.

335. Kunin CM. Resistance to antimicrobial drugs—a worldwide calamity. Ann Intern Med 118:559, 1993.

336. Silver LL, Bostian KA. Discovery and development of new antibiotics: the problem of antibiotic resistance. Antimicrob Agents Chemother 37:377, 1993.

337. Nelson JD. Commentary. J Pediatr 89:471, 1976.
338. Committee on Fetus and Newborn. Guidelines for Perinatal Care, 3rd ed. American Academy of Pediatrics and American College of Obstetricians and Gynecologists, 1992.
339. Sprunt K, Redman W, Leidy G. Antibacterial effectiveness of routine handwashing. Pediatrics 52:264, 1973.
340. Multistate outbreak of Escherichia coli 0157:H7 infections from hamburgers. MMWR Morb Mortal Wkly Rep 42:258, 1993.
341. MacDonald KL, Osterholm MT. The emergence of Escherichia coli 0157:H7 infection in the United States. JAMA 269:2264, 1993.
342. Watanabe H, Wadam A, Inagaki Y, et al. Outbreaks of enterohemorrhagic Escherichia coli 0157:H7 infection by two different genotype strains in Japan. Lancet 348:831, 1996.
343. Slutsker L, Ries AA, Maloney K, et al. A nationwide case-control study of Escherichia coli 0157:H7 infection in the United States. J Infect Dis 177:962, 1998.
344. Karmali MA. Infection by verocytotoxin-producing Escherichia coli. Clin Microbiol Rev 2:15, 1989.
345. Johnson WM, Lior H, Bezanson GS. Cytotoxic Escherichia coli 0157:H7 associated with haemorrhagic colitis in Canada. Lancet 1:76, 1983.
346. Pai CH, Gordon R, Sims HV, et al. Sporadic cases of hemorrhagic colitis associated with Escherichia coli 0157:H7. Clinical, epidemiologic and bacteriologic features. Ann Intern Med 101:738, 1984.
347. Remis RS, Macdonald KI, Riley LW, et al. Hemolytic-uremic syndrome and diarrhea associated with Escherichia coli 0157:H7. Ann Intern Med 101:264, 1984.
348. Spika JS, Parsons JE, Nordenberg D, et al. Hemolytic-uremic syndrome and diarrhea associated with Escherichia coli 0157:H7 in a day care center. J Pediatr 109:287, 1986.
349. Karmali MA, Petric M, Lim C, et al. The association between idiopathic hemolytic uremic syndrome and infection and verotoxin-producing Escherichia coli. J Infect Dis 151:775, 1985.
350. Hemolytic-uremic syndrome associated with Escherichia coli 0157:H7 enteric infections—United States. MMWR Morb Mortal Wkly Rep 34:20, 1985.
351. Belongia EA, Osterholm MT, Soler JT, et al. Transmission of Escherichia coli 0157:H7 infection in Minnesota child day-care facilities. JAMA 269:883, 1993.
352. Besser RE, Lett SM, Weber JT, et al. An outbreak of diarrhea and hemolytic uremic syndrome from Escherichia coli 0157:H7 in fresh-pressed apple cider. JAMA 269:2217, 1993.
353. Mobasellah M, Donohue-Rolfe A, Jacewicz M, et al. Pathogenesis of Shigella diarrhea: evidence for a developmentally regulated glycolipid receptor for Shigatoxin involved in the fluid secretory response of rabbit small intestine. J Infect Dis 157:1023, 1988.
354. O'Brien AD, Lively TA, Chang TW, et al. Purification of Shigella dysenteriae 1 (Shiga)-like toxin from Escherichia coli 0157:H7 strain associated with haemorrhagic colitis. Lancet 2:573, 1983.
355. O'Brien AD, Newland JW, Miller SF, et al. Shiga-like toxin-converting phages from Escherichia coli strains that cause hemorrhagic colitis or infantile diarrhea. Science 226:694, 1984.
356. Smith HR, Day NP, Scotland SM, et al. Phage-determined production of Vero cytotoxin in strains of Escherichia coli serogroup 0157. Lancet 2:1242, 1984.
357. Scotland SM, Smith HR, Rowe B. Two distinct toxins active on Vero cells from Escherichia coli 0157. Lancet 2:885, 1985.
358. Karmali MA, Petric M, Louie S, et al. Antigenic heterogeneity of Escherichia coli verotoxins. Lancet 1:164, 1986.
359. Cleary TG. Cytotoxin-producing Escherichia coli and the hemolytic uremic syndrome. Pediatr Clin North Am 35:485, 1988.
360. Karch H, Heeseman J, Laufs R, et al. A plasmid of enterohemorrhagic Escherichia coli 0157:H7 is required for expression of a new fimbrial antigen and for adhesion to epithelial cells. Infect Immun 55:455, 1987.
361. Levine MM, Jian-guo XU, Kaper JB. A DNA probe to identify enterohemorrhagic Escherichia coli of 0157:H7 and other serotypes that cause hemorrhagic colitis and hemolytic uremic syndrome. J Infect Dis 156:175, 1987.
362. Sherman P, Soni R, Karmali M. Attaching and effacing adherence of Vero cytotoxin–producing Escherichia coli to rabbit intestinal epithelium in vivo. Infect Immun 56:756, 1988.
363. Chapman PA, Siddons CA, Zadik PM, et al. An improved selective medium for the isolation of Escherichia coli 0157. J Med Microbiol 35:107, 1991.
364. Bitzan M, Karch H. Indirect hemagglutination assay for diagnosis of Escherichia coli 0157 infection in patients with hemolytic-uremic syndrome. J Clin Microbiol 30:1174, 1992.
365. Smith HR, Willshaw GA, Rowe TA. Applications of DNA probes for verocytotoxin-producing Escherichia coli. J Hosp Infect 18:438, 1991.
366. Yamamoto T, Koyama Y, Matsumoto M, et al. Localized, aggregative, and diffuse adherence to HeLa cells, plastic, and human small intestines by Escherichia coli isolated from patients with diarrhea. J Infect Dis 166:1295, 1992.
367. Echeverria P, Serichantalerg O, Changchawalit S, et al. Tissue culture–adherent Escherichia coli in infantile diarrhea. J Infect Dis 165:141, 1992.
368. Gunzburg ST, Chang BJ, Elliott SJ, et al. Diffuse and enteroaggregative patterns of adherence of enteric Escherichia coli isolated from aboriginal children from the Kimberley region of western Australia. J Infect Dis 167:755, 1993.
369. Bilge SS, Clausen CR, Lau W, et al. Molecular characterization of a fimbrial adhesin, F1845, mediating diffuse adherences of diarrhea-associated Escherichia coli to HEp-2 cells. J Bacteriol 171:4281, 1989.
370. Benz I, Schmidt MA. Isolation and serologic characterization of AIDA-I, the adhesin mediating the diffuse adherence phenotype of the diarrhea-associated Escherichia coli strain 2787 (0126:H27). Infect Immun 60:13, 1992.
371. Nataro JP, Deng Y, Maneval DR, et al. Aggregative adherence fimbriae 1 of enteroaggregative Escherichia coli mediate adherence to HEp-2 cells and hemagglutination of human erythrocytes. Infect Immun 60:2297, 1992.
372. Knutton S, Shaw RK, Bhan MK, et al. Ability of enteroaggregative Escherichia coli strains to adhere in vitro to human intestinal mucosa. Infect Immun 60:2083, 1992.
373. Nataro JP, Steiner T, Guerrant RL. Enteroaggregative Escherichia coli. Emerg Infect Dis 4:251, 1998.
374. Cobeljic M, Miljkovic-Selimovic B, Paunovic-Todosijevic D, et al. Enteroaggregative E. coli associated with an outbreak of diarrhea in a neonatal nursery ward. Epidemiol Infect 117:11, 1996.
375. doValle GR, Gomez TA, Irino K, Trabulsi LR. The traditional enteropathogenic E. coli (EPEC) serogroup 0125 comprises serotypes which are mainly associated with the category of enteroaggregative E. coli. FEMS Microbiol Lett 152:95, 1997.
376. Savarino SJ, Fasano A, Robertson DC, et al. Enteroaggregative Escherichia coli elaborate a heat-stable entero-

toxin demonstrable in an *in vitro* rabbit intestinal model. J Clin Invest 87:1450, 1991.

377. Baldwin TJ, Knutton S, Sellers L, et al. Enteroaggregative *Escherichia coli* strains secrete a heat-labile toxin antigenically related to *E. coli* hemolysin. Infect Immun 60:2092, 1992.

378. Jerse AE, Martin WC, Galen JE, et al. Oligonucleotide probe for detection of the enteropathogenic *Escherichia coli* (EPEC) adherence factor of localized adherent EPEC. J Clin Microbiol 28:2842, 1990.

Salmonella

1. Ewing WH. Edwards and Ewing's Identification of Enterobacteriaceae, 4th ed. New York, Elsevier, 1986.
2. Meadow WL, Schneider H, Beem MO. *Salmonella* enteritidis bacteremia in childhood. J Infect Dis. 152:185, 1985.
3. Hyams JS, Durbin WA, Grand RJ, et al. *Salmonella* bacteremia in the first year of life. J Pediatr 96:57, 1980.
4. Taylor DN, Bied JM, Munro JS, et al. *Salmonella dublin* infections in the United States, 1979–1980. J Infect Dis 146:322, 1982.
5. Kaniga K, Trollinger D, Galan JE. Identification of two targets of the type III protein secretion system encoded by the inv and spa loci of *Salmonella typhimurium* that have homology to the *Shigella* IpaD and IpaA proteins. J Bacteriol 177:7078, 1995.
6. Kaniga K, Tucker S, Trollinger D, Galan JE. Homologs of the *Shigella* IpaB and IpaC invasins are required for *Salmonella typhimurium* entry into cultured epithelial cells. J Bacteriol 177:3965, 1995.
7. Fierer J, Krause M, Tauxe R, et al. *Salmonella typhimurium* bacteremia: association with the virulence plasmid. J Infect Dis 166:639, 1992.
8. Heffernan EJ, Harwood J, Fierer J, et al. The *S. typhimurium* virulence plasmid complement resistance gene *rck* is homologous to a family of virulence related outer membrane protein genes, including *pagC* and *ail*. J Bacteriol 174:84, 1992.
9. Giannella RA, Formal SB, Dammin GJ, et al. Pathogenesis of salmonellosis: studies of fluid secretion, mucosal invasion, and morphologic reaction in the rabbit ileum. J Clin Invest 52:441, 1973.
10. Jiwa SF. Probing for enterotoxigenicity among the salmonellae: an evaluation of biological assays. J Clin Microbiol 14:463, 1981.
11. Koo FCW, Peterson JW, Houston CW, et al. Pathogenesis of experimental salmonellosis: inhibition of protein synthesis by cytotoxin. Infect Immun 43:93, 1984.
12. Ashkenazi S, Cleary T, Murray BE, et al. Cytotoxin production by *Salmonella* strains: quantitative analysis and partial characterization. Infect Immun 56:3089, 1988.
13. Takeuchi A. Electron microscope studies of experimental *Salmonella* infection. I. Penetration into the intestinal epithelium by *S. typhimurium*. Am J Pathol 50:109, 1967.
14. Modrazakowski MC, Spitznagel JK. Bactericidal activity of fractionated granule contents from human polymorphonuclear leukocytes: antagonism of granule cationic proteins by lipopolysaccharide. Infect Immun 25:597, 1979.
15. Weiss J, Victor M, Elsbach P. Role of charge and hydrophobic interaction in the action of the bactericidal/permeability increasing protein of neutrophils on gram-negative bacteria. J Clin Invest 71:540, 1983.
16. Mackaness GV. Resistance to intracellular infection. J Infect Dis 123:439, 1971.
17. Mackaness GV. Blander RV, Collins FM. Host parasite relations in mouse typhoid. J Exp Med 124:573, 1966.
18. McKenzie SE, Kline J, Douglas SD, Polin RA. Enhancement *in vitro* of the low interferon-gamma production of leukocytes from human newborn infants. J Leukoc Biol 53:691, 1993.
19. George A. Generation of gamma interferon responses in murine Peyer's patches following oral immunization. Infect Immun 64:4606, 1996.
20. de Jong R, Altare F, Haagen IA, et al. Severe mycobacterial and *Salmonella* infections in interleukin-12 receptor–deficient patients. Science 280:1435, 1998.
21. Hornick RB, Greisman SE, Woodward TE, et al. Typhoid fever: pathogenesis and immunologic control. N Engl J Med 283:686, 1970.
22. Kent TH, Formal SB, LaBrec EH. *Salmonella* gastroenteritis in rhesus monkeys. Arch Pathol 82:272, 1966.
23. Boyd JF. Pathology of the alimentary tract of *S. typhimurium* food poisoning. Gut 26:935, 1985.
24. Day DW, Mandel BK, Morson BC. The rectal biopsy appearances in *Salmonella* colitis. Histopathology 2:117, 1978.
25. Wilder AN, MacCready RA. Isolation of *Salmonella* from poultry, poultry products and poultry processing plants in Massachusetts. N Engl J Med 274:1453, 1966.
26. Pet turtle–associated salmonellosis—Puerto Rico. MMWR Morb Mortal Wkly Rep 33:141, 1984.
27. Sanyal D, Douglas T, Roberts R. *Salmonella* infection acquired from reptilian pets. Arch Dis Child 77:345, 1997.
28. Mermin J, Hoar B, Angulo FJ. Iguanas and *Salmonella marina* infection in children: a reflection of the increasing incidence of reptile-associated salmonellosis in the United States. Pediatrics 99:399, 1997.
29. Woodward DL, Khakhria R, Johnson WM. Human salmonellosis associated with exotic pets. J Clin Microbiol 35:2786, 1997.
30. Thomson S. Paratyphoid fever and Baker's confectionery: analysis of epidemic in South Wales 1952. Monthly Bull Ministry Health Public Health Serv 12:187, 1953.
31. Watt J, Wegman ME, Brown OW, et al. Salmonellosis in a premature nursery unaccompanied by diarrheal diseases. Pediatrics 22:689, 1958.
32. Hargrett-Bean NT, Pavia AT, Tauxe RV. *Salmonella* isolates from humans in the United States, 1984–1986. MMWR Morb Mortal Wkly Rep 37:25SS, 1988.
33. Blaser MJ, Newman LS. A review of human salmonellosis: I. Infective dose. Rev Infect Dis 4:1096, 1982.
34. Rubinstein AD, Fowler RN. Salmonellosis of the newborn with transmission by delivery room resuscitators. Am J Public Health 45:1109, 1955.
35. Bate JG, James U. *Salmonella typhimurium* infection dustborne in a children's ward. Lancet 2:713, 1958.
36. Rubbo SD. Cross-infection in hospital due to *Salmonella derby*. J Hyg 46:158, 1948.
37. Lamb VA, Mayhall CG, Spadora AC, et al. Outbreak of *S. typhimurium* gastroenteritis due to an imported strain resistant to ampicillin, chloramphenicol, and trimethoprim/sulfamethoxazole in a nursery. J Clin Microbiol 20:1076, 1984.
38. Abramas IF, Cochran WD, Holmes LB, et al. A *Salmonella newport* outbreak in a premature nursery with a one year follow up. Pediatrics 37:616, 1966.
39. Epstein HC, Hochwald A, Agha R. *Salmonella* infections of the newborn infant. J Pediatr 38:723, 1951.
40. Abramson H. Infections with *S. typhimurium* in the newborn. Am J Dis Child 74:576, 1947.
41. Leeder FS. An epidemic of *S. panama* infections in infants. Ann N Y Acad Sci 66:54, 1956.
42. Watt J, Carlton E. Studies of the acute diarrheal diseases.

XVI. An outbreak of *S. typhimurium* infection among newborn premature infants. Public Health Rep. 60(Pt 1):734, 1945.

43. Foley AR. An outbreak of paratyphoid B fever in a nursery of a small hospital. Can J Public Health 38:73, 1947.

44. Seligman E. Mass invasion of salmonellae in a babies' ward. Ann Paediatr 172:406, 1949.

45. Rowe B, Giles C, Brown GL. Outbreak of gastroenteritis due to *S. virchow* in a maternity hospital. BMJ 3:561, 1969.

46. Sasidharan CK, Rajagopal KC, Jayaram CK, et al. *S. typhimurium* epidemic in newborn nursery. Indian J Pediatr 50:599, 1983.

47. Borecka J, Hocmannova M, van Leeuwen WJ. Nosocomial infection of nurslings caused by multiple drug-resistant strain of *S. typhimurium*—utilization of a new typing method based on lysogeny of strains. Zentralbl Bakteriol 2336:262, 1976.

48. Bannerman CHS. *Heidelberg* enteritis—an outbreak in the neonatal unit of Harare Central Hospital. Cent Afr J Med 31:1, 1985.

49. McAllister TA, Roud JA, Marshall A, et al. Outbreak of *S. eimsbuettel* in newborn infants spread by rectal thermometers. Lancet 1:1262, 1986.

50. Szanton VL. Epidemic salmonellosis: a 30-month study of 80 cases of *S. oranienburg* infection. Pediatrics 20:794, 1957.

51. Seals JE, Parrott PL, McGowan JE, et al. Nursery salmonellosis: delayed recognition due to unusually long incubation period. Infect Control Hosp Epidemiol 4:205, 1983.

52. Hering E, Fuenzalida O, Lynch B, et al. Analises clinico-epidemiologica de un brote de infeccion por S. bredeney en recien nacidos. Rev Clin Pediatr 50:81, 1979.

53. Kumari S, Gupta R, Bhargava SK. A nursery outbreak with *S. newport*. Indian Pediatr 17:11, 1980.

54. Omland T, Gardborg O. *Salmonella enteritidis* infections in infancy with special reference to a small nosocomial epidemic. Acta Paediatr Belg 49:583, 1960.

55. Puri V, Thirupuram S, Khalil A, et al. Nosocomial *S. typhimurium* epidemic in a neonatal special care unit. Indian Pediatr 17:233, 1980.

56. Mendis NMP, de la Motte PU, Gunatillaka PDP, et al. Protracted infection with *S. bareilly* in a maternity hospital. J Trop Med Hyg 79:142, 1976.

57. Marzetti G, Laurenti F, deCaro M, et al. *Salmonella muenchen* infections in newborns and small infants. Clin Pediatr 12:93, 1973.

58. Baine WB, Gangarosa EJ, Bennett JV, et al. Institutional salmonellosis. J Infect Dis 128:357, 1973.

59. Schroeder SA, Aserkoff B, Brachman PS. Epidemic salmonellosis in hospitals and institutions. N Engl J Med 279:674, 1968.

60. Wilson R, Feldman RA, Davis J, et al. Salmonellosis in infants: the importance of intrafamilial transmission. Pediatrics 69:436, 1982.

61. Newman MJ. Multiple-resistant *Salmonella* group G outbreak in a neonatal intensive care unit. West Afr J Med 15:165, 1996.

62. Mahajan R, Mathur M, Kumar A, et al. Nosocomial outbreak of *Salmonella typhimurium* infection in a nursery intensive care unit (NICU) and paediatric ward. J Commun Dis 27:10, 1995.

63. Martyn-Jones DM, Pantin GC. Neonatal diarrhea due to *S. paratyphi* B. J Clin Pathol 9:128, 1956.

64. Rubinstein AD, Feemster RF, Smith HM. Salmonellosis as a public health problem in wartime. Am J Public Health 34:841, 1944.

65. Neter E. Observation on the transmission of salmonellosis in man. Am J Public Health 40:929, 1950.

66. Sanders DY, Sinal SH, Morrison L. Chronic salmonellosis in infancy. Clin Pediatr 13:640, 1974.

67. Waddell WR, Kunz LJ. Association of *Salmonella* enteritis with operations on the stomach. N Engl J Med 255:555, 1956.

68. Gray JA, Trueman AM. Severe *Salmonella* gastroenteritis associated with hypochlorhydria. Scott Med J 16:255, 1971.

69. Agunod M, Yamaguchi N, Lopez R, et al. Correlative study of hydrochloric acid, pepsin, and intrinsic factor secretion in newborns and infants. Am J Dig Dis 14:400, 1969.

70. Silverio B. Gastric emptying time in the newborn and the nursling. Am J Med Sci 247:732, 1964.

71. Fleischhacker G, Vutue C, Werner H-P. Infektion eines Neugeborenen durch *S. typhimurium*–haltige Muttermilch. Wien Klin Wochenschr 24:394, 1972.

72. Ryder RW, Crosby-Ritchie A, McDonough B, et al. Human milk contaminated with *S. kottbus*. A cause of nosocomial illness in infants. JAMA 238:1533, 1977.

73. Revathi G, Mahajan R, Faridi MM, et al. Transmission of lethal *Salmonella senftenberg* from mother's breast-milk to her baby. Ann Trop Paediatr 15:159, 1995.

74. Small RG, Sharp JCM. A milkborne outbreak of *S. dublin*. J Hyg 82:95, 1979.

75. Weissman JB, Deen RMAD, Williams M, et al. An island-wide epidemic of salmonellosis in Trinidad traced to contaminated powdered milk. West Indian Med J 26:135, 1977.

76. *Salmonella anatum* infection in infants linked to dried milk. Commun Dis Rep CDR Wkly 7:33, 1997.

77. Usera MA, Echeita A, Aladuena A, et al. Interregional foodborne salmonellosis outbreak due to powdered infant formula contaminated with lactose-fermenting *Salmonella virchow*. Eur J Epidemiol 12:377, 1996.

78. Silverstope L, Plazikowski U, Kjellander J, et al. An epidemic among infants caused by *S. muenchen*. J Appl Bacteriol 24:134, 1961.

79. Im SWK, Chow K, Chau PY. Rectal thermometer–mediated cross-infection with *S. wadsworth* in a pediatric ward. J Hosp Infect 2:171, 1981.

80. Khan MA, Abdur-Rab M, Israr N, et al. Transmission of *S. worthington* by oropharyngeal suction in hospital neonatal unit. Pediatr Infect Dis J 10:668, 1991.

81. Umasankar S, Mridha EU, Hannan MM, et al. An outbreak of *Salmonella enteritidis* in a maternity and neonatal intensive care unit. J Hosp Infect 34:117, 1996.

82. Riley LW, Cohen ML. Plasmid profiles and *Salmonella* epidemiology. Lancet 1:573, 1982.

83. Michel J, Malpeach G, Godeneche P, et al. Etude clinique et bactériologique d'une épidémie de salmonellose en milieu hospitalier (*S. oranienburg*). Pediatrie 25:13, 1970.

84. Adler JL, Anderson RL, Boring JR, et al. A protracted hospital-associated outbreak of salmonellosis due to a multiple antibiotic-resistant strain of *S. indiana*. J Pediatr 77:970, 1970.

85. Bilie BO, Mellbin T, Nordbring F. An extensive outbreak of gastroenteritis caused by *S. newport*. Acta Med Scand 175:557, 1964.

86. Horwitz M, Pollard R, Merson M, et al. A large outbreak of foodborne salmonellosis on the Navajo Nation Indian Reservation: epidemiology and secondary transmission. Am J Public Health 67:1071, 1977.

87. Griffith JPC, Ostheimer M. Typhoid fever in children. Am J Med Sci 124:868, 1902.

88. Freedman ML, Christopher P, Boughton CR, et al. Typhoid carriage in pregnancy with infection of neonate. Lancet 1:310, 1970.

89. Chhabra RS, Glaser JH. *Salmonella* infection presenting as hematochezia on the first day of life. Pediatrics 94:739, 1994.

90. Stein H, Beck J, Solomon A, et al. Gastroenteritis with necrotizing enterocolitis in premature babies. BMJ 1:616, 1972.

91. Guarino A, Spagnuolo MI, Russo S, et al. Etiology and risk factors of severe and protracted diarrhea. J Pediatr Gastroenterol Nutr 20:173, 1995.

92. Lifshitz F, Coello-Ramirez P, Gutirrez-Topete G, et al. Monosaccharide intolerance and hypoglycemia in infants with diarrhea. I. Clinical course of 23 infants. J Pediatr 77:595, 1970.

93. Iyngkaran N, Abdin Z, Davis K, et al. Acquired carbohydrate intolerance and cow milk protein–sensitive enteropathy in young infants. J Pediatr 95:373, 1979.

94. Lo CW, Walker WA. Chronic protracted diarrhea of infancy: a nutritional disease. Pediatrics 72:786, 1983.

95. Blaser MJ, Feldman RA. *Salmonella* bacteremia: reports to the Centers for Disease Control, 1968–1979. J Infect Dis 143:743, 1981.

96. Schutze GE, Schutze SE, Kirby RS. Extraintestinal salmonellosis in a children's hospital. Pediatr Infect Dis J 16:482, 1997.

97. Davis RC. *Salmonella* sepsis in infancy. Am J Dis Child 135:1096, 1981.

98. Torrey S, Fleisher G, Jaffe D. Incidence of *Salmonella* bacteremia in infants with *Salmonella* gastroenteritis. J Pediatr 108:718, 1986.

99. Sirinavin S, Jayanetra P, Lolekha S, et al. Predictors for extraintestinal infection of *Salmonella* enteritis in Thailand. Pediatr Infect Dis J 7:44, 1988.

100. Katz BZ, Shapiro ED. Predictors of persistently positive blood cultures in children with "occult" *Salmonella* bacteremia. Pediatr Infect Dis J 5:713, 1986.

101. Yamamoto LG, Ashton MJ. *Salmonella* infections in infants in Hawaii. Pediatr Infect Dis J 7:48, 1988.

102. Cohen JI, Bartlett JA, Corey GR. Extraintestinal manifestations of *Salmonella* infections. Medicine (Baltimore) 66:349, 1987.

103. West SE, Goodkin R, Kaplan AM. Neonatal *Salmonella* meningitis complicated by cerebral abscesses. West J Med 127:142, 1977.

104. Applebaum PC, Scragg J. *Salmonella* meningitis in infants. Lancet 1:1052, 1977.

105. Denis F, Badiane S, Chiron JP, et al. *Salmonella* meningitis in infants. Lancet 1:910, 1977.

106. Cherubin CE, Marr JS, Sierra MF, et al. *Listeria* and gram-negative bacillary meningitis in New York City 1973–1979. Am J Med 71:199, 1981.

107. Low LC, Lam BC, Wong WT, et al. *Salmonella* meningitis in infancy. Aust Paediatr J 20:225, 1984.

108. Diwan N, Sharma KB. Isolation of *S. typhimurium* from cephalohematoma and osteomyelitis. Indian J Med Res 67:27, 1978.

109. Konzert, W. Über eine *Salmonella*-Osteomyelitis in Rahmen einer *S. typhimurium* Epidemie auf einer Neugeborenen Station. Wien Klin Wochenschr 81:713, 1969.

110. McKinlay B. Infectious diarrhea of the newborn caused by an unclassified species of *Salmonella*. Am J Dis Child 54:1252, 1937.

111. Szumness W, Sikorska J, Szymanek E, et al. The microbiological and epidemiological properties of infections caused by *S. enteritidis*. J Hyg 64:9, 1966.

112. Nelson JD. Suppurative mastitis in infants. Am J Dis Child 125:458, 1973.

113. Guthrie KJ, Montgomery GI. Infections with *Bacterium enteritidis* in infancy with the triad of enteritis, cholecystitis and meningitis. J Pathol Bacteriol 49:393, 1939.

114. Corman LI, Poirier RH, Littlefield CA, et al. Endophthalmitis due to *S. enteritidis*. J Pediatr 95:1001, 1979.

115. Haggman DL, Rehm SJ, Moodie DS, et al. Nontyphoidal *Salmonella* pericarditis: a case report and review of the literature. Pediatr Infect Dis J 5:259, 1986.

116. Reed RP, Klugman KP. Neonatal typhoid fever. Pediatr Infect Dis J 13:774, 1994.

117. Stuart BM, Pullen RL. Typhoid: clinical analysis of 360 cases. Arch Intern Med 78:629, 1946.

118. Sengupta B, Ramachander N, Zamah N. *Salmonella* septic abortion. Int Surg 65:183, 1980.

119. Diddle AW, Stephens RL. Typhoid fever in pregnancy. Am J Obstet Gynecol 38:300, 1939.

120. Riggall F, Salkind G, Spellacy W. Typhoid fever complicating pregnancy. Obstet Gynecol 44:117, 1974.

121. Hicks HT, French H. Typhoid fever and pregnancy with special references to fetal infection. Lancet 1:1491, 1905.

122. Osler W, McCrae T. Typhoid fever. *In* Osler W. Principles and Practice of Medicine, 8th ed. New York, D Appleton, 1912, pp 1–46.

123. Ferreccio C, Levine MM, Manterola A, et al. Benign bacteremia caused by *S. typhi* and *S. paratyphi* in children younger than two years. J Pediatr 104:899, 1984.

124. Thisyakorn U, Mansuwan P, Taylor DN. Typhoid and paratyphoid fever in 192 hospitalized children in Thailand. Am J Dis Child 141:862, 1987.

125. Pickering LK, DuPont HL, Olarte J, et al. Fecal leukocytes in enteric infections. Am J Clin Pathol 68:562, 1977.

126. Harris JC, DuPont HL, Hornick RB. Fecal leukocytes in diarrheal illness. Ann Intern Med 76:697, 1972.

127. McCall CE, Martin WT, Boring JR. Efficiency of cultures of rectal swabs and fecal specimens in detecting *Salmonella* carriers: correlation with numbers of *Salmonella* excreted. J Hyg 64:261, 1966.

128. Raucher HS, Eichenfield AH, Hodes HL. Treatment of *Salmonella* gastroenteritis in infants. The significance of bacteremia. Clin Pediatr 22:601, 1983.

129. Gotoff SP, Cochran WD. Antibody response to the somatic antigen of *S. newport* in premature infants. Pediatrics 37:610, 1966.

130. Hodes HL, Zepp HD, Ainbender E. Production of O and H agglutinins by a newborn infant infected with *S. saint-paul*. J Pediatr 68:780, 1966.

131. Taylor DN, Bopp C, Birkness K, et al. An outbreak of salmonellosis associated with a fatality in a healthy child: a large dose and severe illness. Am J Epidemiol 119:907, 1984.

132. Rivera MJ, Rivera N, Castillo J, et al. Molecular and epidemiological study of *Salmonella* clinical isolates. J Clin Microbiol 29:927, 1991.

133. Aserkoff B, Bennett JV. Effect of antibiotic therapy in acute salmonellosis on the fecal excretion of salmonellae. N Engl J Med 281:636, 1969.

134. Dixon JMS. Effect of antibiotic treatment on duration of excretion of *S. typhimurium* by children. BMW 2:1343, 1965.

135. Kazemi M, Bumpert TG, Marks MI. A controlled trial comparing trimethoprim/sulfamethoxazole, ampicillin, and no therapy in the treatment of *Salmonella* gastroenteritis in children. J Pediatr 83:646, 1973.

136. Neill MA, Opal SM, Heelan J, et al. Failure of ciprofloxacin to eradicate convalescent fecal excretion after

acute salmonellosis: experience during an outbreak in health care workers. Ann Intern Med 114:195, 1991.

137. Pettersson T, Klemola E, Wager O. Treatment of acute cases of *Salmonella* infection and *Salmonella* carriers with ampicillin and neomycin. Acta Med Scand 175:185, 1964.

138. Association for Study of Infectious Diseases. Effect of neomycin in noninvasive *Salmonella* infections of the gastrointestinal tract. Lancet 2:1159, 1970.

139. Nelson JD, Kusmiesz H, Jackson LH, et al. Treatment of *Salmonella* gastroenteritis with ampicillin, amoxicillin, or placebo. Pediatrics 65:1125, 1980.

140. Asperilla MO, Smego RA, Scott LK. Quinolone antibiotics in the treatment of *Salmonella* infections. Rev Infect Dis 12:873, 1990.

141. Buchwald DS, Blaser MJ. A review of human salmonellosis: II. Duration of excretion following infection with nontyphi *Salmonella*. Rev Infect Dis 6:345, 1984.

142. Dutta P, Rasaily R, Saha MR, et al. Ciprofloxacin for treatment of severe typhoid fever in children. Antimicrob Agents Chemother 37:1197, 1993.

143. Piddock LJV, Griggs DJ, Hall MC, et al. Ciprofloxacin resistance in clinical isolates of *Salmonella typhimurium* obtained from two patients. Antimicrob Agents Chemother 37:662, 1993.

144. Edgar WM, Lacey BW. Infection with *S. heidelberg*. An outbreak presumably not foodborne. Lancet 1:161, 1963.

145. Rice PA, Craven PC, Wells JG. *S. heidelberg* enteritis and bacteremia. An epidemic on two pediatric wards. Am J Med 60:509, 1976.

146. Davis RC. *Salmonella* sepsis in infancy. Am J Dis Child 135:1096, 1981.

147. MacDonald KL, Cohen ML, Hargrett-Bean NT, et al. Changes in antimicrobial resistance of *Salmonella* isolated from humans in the United States. JAMA 258:1496, 1987.

148. Maiorini E, Lopez EL, Morrow AL, et al. Multiply resistant nontyphoidal *Salmonella* gastroenteritis in children. Pediatr Infect Dis J 12:139, 1993.

149. Lee LA, Puhr ND, Maloney EK, et al. Increase in antimicrobial-resistant *Salmonella* infections in the United States, 1989–1990. J Infect Dis 170:128, 1994.

150. Glynn MK, Bopp C, Dewitt W, et al. Emergence of multidrug-resistant *Salmonella enterica* serotype *typhimurium* DT104 infections in the United States. N Engl J Med 338:1333, 1998.

151. Koshi G. Alarming increases in multi-drug resistant *S. typhimurium* in Southern India. Indian J Med Res 74:635, 1981.

152. Anderson ES, Threlfall EJ, Carr JM, et al. Clonal distribution of resistance plasmid carrying *S. typhimurium*, mainly in the Middle East. J Hyg 79:425, 1977.

153. Wamola IA, Mirza NB. Problems of *Salmonella* infections in a hospital in Kenya. East Afr Med J 58:677, 1981.

154. Falbo V, Capriola A, Moncello F, et al. Antimicrobial resistance among *Salmonella* isolates from hospitals in Rome. J Hyg 88:275, 1982.

155. Threlfall EJ, Ward LR, Ashley AS, et al. Plasmid encoded trimethoprim resistance in multi-resistant epidemic *S. typhimurium* phagotypes 204 and 193 in Britain. BMJ 280:1210, 1980.

156. French GI, Lowry MF. Trimethoprim-resistant *Salmonella*. Lancet 2:375, 1978.

157. Smith SM, Palumbo PE, Edelson PJ. *Salmonella* strains resistant to multiple antibiotics: therapeutic implications. Pediatr Infect Dis J 3:455, 1984.

158. Soe GB, Overturf GD. Treatment of typhoid fever and other systemic salmonellosis with cefotaxime, ceftriazone,

159. Moosa A, Rubidge CJ. Once daily ceftriaxone vs. chloramphenicol for treatment of typhoid fever in children. Pediatr Infect Dis J 8:696, 1989.

160. deCarvalho EM, Martinelli R, de Oliveira MMG, et al. Cefamandole treatment of *Salmonella* bacteremia. Antimicrob Agents Chemother 21:334, 1982.

161. Pape JW, Gerdes H, Oriol L, et al. Typhoid fever: successful therapy with cefoperazone. J Infect Dis 153:272, 1986.

162. Demmerich B, Lode H, Boner K, et al. Biliary excretion and pharmacokinetics of cefoperazone in humans. J Antimicrob Chemother 12:27, 1983.

163. Kinsella TR, Yogev R, Shulman ST, et al. Treatment of *Salmonella* meningitis and brain abscess with the new cephalosporins: two case reports and a review of the literature. Pediatr Infect Dis J 6:476, 1987.

164. Gokalp AS, Toksoy HB, Turkay S, et al. Intravenous immunoglobulin in the treatment of *Salmonella typhimurium* infections in preterm neonates. Clin Pediatr (Phila) 33:349, 1994.

165. Tauxe RV, Hassan LF, Findeisen KO, et al. Salmonellosis in nurses: lack of transmission to patients. J Infect Dis 157:370, 1988.

166. Levine MM, Ferraccio C, Cryz S, et al. Comparison of enteric coated capsules and liquid formulation of Ty21a typhoid vaccine in randomised controlled field trial. Lancet 336:4, 1990.

167. Cryz SJ Jr, Vanprapar N, Thisyakorn U, et al. Safety and immunogenicity of *Salmonella typhi* Ty21a vaccine in young Thai children. Infect Immun 61:1149, 1993.

168. Murphy JR, Grez L, Schlesinger L, et al. Immunogenicity of *S. typhi* Ty21a vaccine for young children. Infect Immun 59:4291, 1991.

169. France GL, Marmer DJ, Steele RW. Breast-feeding and *Salmonella* infection. Am J Dis Child 134:147, 1980.

Shigella

1. Brenner DJ, Fannin GR, Skerman FJ, et al. Polynucleotide sequence divergence among strains of *E. coli* and closely related organisms. J Bacteriol 109:953, 1972.

2. Sansonetti PJ, Kopecko DJ, Formal SB. Involvement of a plasmid in the invasive ability of *Shigella flexneri*. Infect Immun 35:852, 1982.

3. Hale TL. Genetic basis of virulence in *Shigella* species. Microbiol Rev 55:206, 1991.

4. Hale TL, Sansonetti P, Schad PA, et al. Characterization of virulence plasmids and plasmid-mediated outer membrane proteins in *Shigella flexneri*, *Shigella sonnei* and *Escherichia coli*. Infect Immun 40:340, 1983.

5. Hale TL, Oaks EV, Formal SB. Identification and characterization of virulence associated, plasmid-coded proteins of *Shigella* spp. and enteroinvasive *E. coli*. Infect Immun 50:620, 1985.

6. Sasakawa C, Kamata K, Sakai T, et al. Molecular alteration of the 140-megadalton plasmid associated with the loss of virulence and Congo red binding activity in *Shigella flexneri*. Infect Immun 51:470, 1986.

7. LaBrec EH, Schneider H, Magnani TJ, et al. Epithelial cell penetration as an essential step in the pathogenesis of bacillary dysentery. J Bacteriol 88:1503, 1964.

8. Ogawa H. Experimental approach in studies on pathogenesis of bacillary dysentery—with special reference to the invasion of bacilli into intestinal mucosa. Acta Pathol Jpn 20:261, 1970.

9. Harris RJ, Wachsmuth IK, Davis BR, et al. High molecu-

lar weight plasmid correlates with *Escherichia coli* entero-invasiveness. Infect Immun 37:1295, 1982.

10. Sansonetti PJ, d'Hauteville H, Formal SB, et al. Plasmid-mediated invasiveness of "Shigella-like" *Escherichia coli*. Ann Microbiol 133A:351, 1982.

11. Sansonetti PJ, d'Hauteville H, Ecobiochon C, et al. Molecular comparison of virulence plasmids in *Shigella* and enteroinvasive *Escherichia coli*. Ann Microbiol 134A:295, 1983.

12. Sereny B. Experimental *Shigella* keratoconjunctivitis. Acta Microbiol Acad Sci Hung 2:293, 1955.

13. Sansonetti PJ, Hale TL, Dammin GI, et al. Alterations in the pathogenicity of *Escherichia coli* K-12 after transfer of plasmids and chromosomal genes from *Shigella flexneri*. Infect Immun 39:1392, 1983.

14. Tobe T, Sasakawa C, Okada N, et al. vacB, a novel chromosomal gene required for expression of virulence genes on the large plasmid of *S. flexneri*. J Bacteriol 174:6359, 1992.

15. Okada N, Sasakawa C, Tobe T, et al. Virulence associated chromosomal loci of *S. flexneri* identified by random Tn5 insertion mutagenesis. Mol Microbiol 5:187, 1991.

16. Okamura N, Nagai T, Nakaya R, et al. HeLa cell invasiveness and O antigen of *Shigella flexneri* as separate and prerequisite attributes of virulence to evoke keratoconjunctivitis in guinea pigs. Infect Immun 39:505, 1983.

17. Bartlett AV, Prado D, Cleary TG, et al. Production of Shiga toxin and other cytotoxins by serogroups of *Shigella*. J Infect Dis 154:996, 1986.

18. Olenick JG, Wolfe AD. *Shigella* toxin inhibition of binding and translation of polyuridylic acid by *Escherichia coli* ribosomes. J Bacteriol 141:1246, 1980.

19. Brown JE, Rothman SW, Doctor BP. Inhibition of protein synthesis in intact HeLa cells by *Shigella dysenteriae* 1 toxin. Infect Immun 29:98, 1980.

20. Obrig TG, Moran TP, Brown JE. The mode of action of Shiga toxin on peptide elongation of eukaryotic protein synthesis. Biochem J 244:287, 1987.

21. Prado D, Cleary TG, Pickering LK, et al. The relation between production of cytotoxin and clinical features in shigellosis. J Infect Dis 154:149, 1986.

22. Makintubee S, Mallonee J, Istre GR. Shigellosis outbreak associated with swimming. Am J Public Health 77:166, 1987.

23. Levine MM, DuPont HL, Formal SB, et al. Pathogenesis of *Shigella dysenteriae* 1 (Shiga) dysentery. J Infect Dis 127:261, 1973.

24. DuPont HL, Hornick RB, Dawkins AT, et al. The response of man to virulent *Shigella flexneri* 2a. J Infect Dis 119:296, 1969.

25. Levine MM. *Shigella* infections and vaccines: experiences from volunteer and controlled field studies. *In* Rahaman MM, Greenough WB, Novak NR, et al (eds). Shigellosis: A Continuing Global Problem. Dacca, Bangladesh, International Centre for Diarrhoeal Disease Research, 1983, p 208.

26. Pickering LK, Hadler SC. Management and prevention of infectious diseases in day care. *In* Feigin RD, Cherry JC (eds). Textbook of Pediatric Infectious Diseases. Philadelphia, WB Saunders, 1992, p 2308.

27. Mata LG. The Children of Santa Maria Cauque: A Prospective Field Study of Health and Growth. Cambridge, Mass, MIT Press, 1978.

28. Stoll BJ, Glass RI, Huq MI, et al. Surveillance of patients attending a diarrhoeal disease hospital in Bangladesh. BMJ 285:1185, 1982.

29. Floyd T, Higgins AR, Kader M. A. Studies in shigellosis. V. The relationship of age to the incidence of *Shigella* infections in Egyptian children, with special reference to shigellosis in the newborn and infant in the first six months of life. Am J Trop Med Hyg 5:119, 1956.

30. Summary of notifiable diseases, United States, 1981. MMWR Morb Mortal Wkly Rep 40:10, 1992.

31. Clemens JS, Stanton B, Stoll B, et al. Breast-feeding as a determinant of severity in shigellosis. Am J Epidemiol 123:710, 1986.

32. Mata LJ, Urrutia JM, Garcia B, et al. *Shigella* infections in breast fed Guatemalan Indian neonates. Am J Dis Child. 117:142, 1969.

33. Huskins WC, Griffiths JK, Faruque AS, Bennish ML. Shigellosis in neonates and young infants. J Pediatr 125:14, 1994.

34. Haltalin KC. Neonatal shigellosis. Am J Dis Child 114:603, 1967.

35. Scragg JN, Rubidge CJ, Appelbaum PC. *Shigella* infection in African and Indian children with special reference to *Shigella* septicemia. J Pediatr 93:796, 1978.

36. Burry VF, Thurn AN, Co TG. Shigellosis: an analysis of 239 cases in a pediatric population. Mo Med 65:671, 1968.

37. Enteric infection due to *Campylobacter, Yersinia, Salmonella* and *Shigella*. Bull World Health Organ 58:519, 1980.

38. Kraybill EN, Controni G. Septicemia and enterocolitis due to *S. sonnei* in a newborn infant. Pediatrics 42:529, 1968.

39. Moore EE. *Shigella sonnei* septicemia in a neonate. BMJ 1:22, 1974.

40. Aldrich JA, Flowers RP, Hall FK. *S. sonnei* septicemia in a neonate: a case report. J Am Osteopath Assoc 79:93, 1979.

41. Barton LL, Pickering LK. Shigellosis in the first week of life. Pediatrics 52:437, 1973.

42. Landsberger M. Bacillary dysentery in a newborn infant. Arch Pediatr 59:330, 1942.

43. Neter E. *S. sonnei* infection at term and its transfer to the newborn. Obstet Gynecol 17:517, 1961.

44. McIntire MS, Jahr HM. An isolated case of shigellosis in the newborn nursery. Nebr State Med J 39:425, 1954.

45. Greenberg M, Frant S, Shapiro R. Bacillary dysentery acquired at birth. J Pediatr 17:363, 1940.

46. Emanuel B, Sherman JO. Shigellosis in a neonate. Clin Pediatr 14:725, 1975.

47. Barret-Connor E, Connor JD. Extraintestinal manifestations of shigellosis. Am J Gastroenterol 53:234, 1970.

48. Fischler E. Convulsions as a complication of shigellosis in children. Helv Paediatr Acta 4:389, 1962.

49. Ashkenazi S, Dinari G, Zevalunov A, et al. Convulsions in childhood shigellosis. Am J Dis Child 141:208, 1987.

50. Whitfield C, Humphries JM. Meningitis and septicemia due to *Shigella* in a newborn infant. J Pediatr 70:805, 1967.

51. Goren A, Freier S, Passwell JH. Lethal toxic encephalopathy due to childhood shigellosis in a developed country. Pediatrics 89:1189, 1992.

52. Ashkenazi S, Cleary KR, Pickering LK, et al. The association of Shiga toxin and other cytotoxins with the neurologic manifestations of shigellosis. J Infect Dis 161:961, 1990.

53. Rahaman MM, Jamiul Alam AKM, Islam MR, et al. Shiga bacillus dysentery associated with marked leukocytosis and erythrocyte fragmentation. Johns Hopkins Med J 136:65, 1975.

54. Neglia TG, Marr TJ, Davis AT. *Shigella* dysentery with secondary *Klebsiella* sepsis. J Pediatr 63:253, 1976.

55. Struelens MJ, Patte D, Kabir I, et al. *Shigella* septicemia:

prevalence, presentation, risk factors, and outcome. J Infect Dis 152:784, 1985.

56. Haltalin KC, Nelson JD. Coliform septicemia complicating shigellosis in children. JAMA 192:441, 1965.

57. Levin SE. *Shigella* septicemia in the newborn infant. J Pediatr 71:917, 1967.

58. Martin T, Habbick BF, Nyssen J. Shigellosis with bacteremia: a report of two cases and a review of the literature. Pediatr Infect Dis J 2:21, 1983.

59. Raderman JW, Stoller KP, Pomerance JJ. Blood-stream invasion with *S. sonnei* in an asymptomatic newborn infant. Pediatr Infect Dis J 5:379, 1986.

60. Starke JR, Baker CJ. Neonatal shigellosis with bowel perforation. Pediatr Infect Dis J 4:405, 1985.

61. Azad MAK, Islam M. Colonic perforation in *Shigella dysenteriae* 1 infection. Pediatr Infect Dis J 5:103, 1986.

62. O'Connor JH, O'Callaghan U. Fatal *S. sonnei* septicemia in an adult complemented by marrow aplasia and intestinal perforation. J Infect 3:277, 1981.

63. Alam AN, Chowdhurg AAKM, Kabir IAKM, et al. Association of pneumonia with under-nutrition and shigellosis. Indian Pediatr 21:609, 1984.

64. Hoefnagel D. Fulminating, rapidly fatal shigellosis in children. N Engl J Med 258:1256, 1958.

65. Sakamoto A, Kamo S. Clinical, statistical observations on Ekiri and bacillary dysentery. A study of 785 cases. Ann Paediatr 186:1, 1956.

66. Dodd K, Buddingh GJ, Rapoport S. The etiology of Ekiri, a highly fatal disease of Japanese children. Pediatrics 3:9, 1949.

67. Davis TC. Chronic vulvovaginitis in children due to *S. flexneri*. Pediatrics 56:41, 1975.

68. Murphy TV, Nelson JD. *Shigella* vaginitis: report on 38 patients and review of the literature. Pediatrics 63:511, 1979.

69. Tobias JD, Starke JR, Tosi MF. *Shigella* keratitis: a report of two cases and a review of the literature. Pediatr Infect Dis J 6:79, 1987.

70. Butler T, Dunn D, Dahms B, et al. Causes of death and the histopathologic findings in fatal shigellosis. Pediatr Infect Dis J 8:767, 1989.

71. Bennish ML, Harris JR, Wojtyniak BJ, et al. Death in shigellosis: incidence and risk factors in hospitalized patients. J Infect Dis 161:500, 1990.

72. Speelman P, McGlaughlin R, Kabir I, et al. Differential clinical features and stool findings in shigellosis and amoebic dysentery. Trans R Soc Trop Med Hyg 81:549, 1987.

73. Taylor WI, Harris B. Isolation of shigellae. II. Comparison of plating media and enrichment broths. Am J Clin Pathol 44:476, 1965.

74. Stypulkowska-Misiurewics H. Problems in bacteriological diagnosis of shigellosis. *In* Rahaman MM, Greenough WB, Novak NR, et al. (eds). Shigellosis: A Continuing Global Problem. Dacca, Bangladesh, International Centre for Diarrhoeal Disease Research, 1983, p 87.

75. Haltalin KC, Nelson JD, Ring R, III, et al. Double-blind treatment study of shigellosis comparing ampicillin, sulfadiazine, and placebo. J Pediatr 70:970, 1967.

76. Haltalin KC, Nelson JD, Kusmiesz HT, et al. Optimal dosage of ampicillin in shigellosis. J Pediatr 74:626, 1969.

77. Haltalin KC, Nelson JD, Kusmiesz HT. Comparative efficacy of nalidixic acid and ampicillin for severe shigellosis. Arch Dis Child 48:305, 1973.

78. Oaks EV, Hale TL, Formal SB. Serum immune response to *Shigella* protein antigens in rhesus monkeys and humans infected with *Shigella* spp. Infect Immun 53:57, 1986.

79. Frankel G, Riley L, Giron JA, et al. Detection of *Shigella* in feces using DNA amplification. J Infect Dis 161:1252, 1990.

80. Speelman P, Kabir I, Islam M. Distribution and spread of colonic lesions in shigellosis: a colonoscopic study. J Infect Dis 150:899, 1984.

81. Formal SB, Kent TH, Austin S, et al. Fluorescent antibody and histological studies of vaccinated control monkeys challenged with *Shigella flexneri*. J Bacteriol 91:2368, 1966.

82. LaBrec EH, Formal SB. Experimental *Shigella* infections. IV. Fluorescent antibody studies of an infection in guinea pigs. J Immunol 87:562, 1961.

83. Frost JA, Rowe B, Vandepitte J, et al. Plasmid characterization in the investigation of an epidemic caused by multiply resistant *S. dysenteriae* type 1 in Central Africa. Lancet 2:1074, 1981.

84. Haider K, Hug MI, Samadi AR, et al. Plasmid characterization of *Shigella* spp. isolated from children with shigellosis and asymptomatic excretors. J Antimicrob Chemother 16:691, 1985.

85. Tauxe RV, Puhr ND, Wells JG, et al. Antimicrobial resistance of *Shigella* isolates in the USA: the importance of international travelers. J Infect Dis 162:1107, 1990.

86. Salzman TC, Scher CD, Moss R. Shigellae with transferable drug resistance: outbreak in a nursery for premature infants. J Pediatr 71:21, 1967.

87. Bennish ML, Salam MA, Hossain MA, et al. Antimicrobial resistance of *Shigella* isolates in Bangladesh, 1983–1990: increasing frequency of strains multiply resistant to ampicillin, trimethoprim/sulfamethoxazole, and nalidixic acid. Clin Infect Dis 14:1055, 1992.

88. Ostrower VG. Comparison of cefaclor and ampicillin in the treatment of shigellosis. Postgrad Med J 55:82, 1979.

89. Haltalin KC, Nelson JD. Failure of furazolidone therapy on shigellosis. Am J Dis Child 123:40, 1972.

90. Nelson JD, Haltalin KC. Comparative efficacy of cephalexin and ampicillin for shigellosis and other types of acute diarrhea in infants and children. Antimicrob Agents Chemother 7:415, 1975.

91. Nelson JD, Haltalin KC. Amoxicillin less effective than ampicillin against *Shigella* in vitro and in vivo: relationship of efficacy to activity in serum. J Infect Dis 129:S222, 1974.

92. Tong MJ, Martin DG, Cunningham JJ, et al. Clinical and bacteriological evaluation of antibiotic treatment in shigellosis. JAMA 214:1841, 1970.

93. Orenstein WA, Ross L, Overturf GD, et al. Antibiotic treatment of acute shigellosis: failure of cefamandole compared to trimethoprim/sulfamethoxazole and ampicillin. Am J Med Sci 282:27, 1981.

94. Yunus MD, Rahaman MM, Faruque ASG, et al. Comparative treatment of shigellosis with trimethoprim/sulfamethoxazole and ampicillin. *In* Rahaman MM, Greenough WB, Novak NR, et al (eds). Shigellosis: A Continuing Global Problem. Dacca, Bangladesh, International Centre for Diarrhoeal Disease Research, 1983, p 166.

95. Nelson JD, Kusmiesz H, Jackson LH, et al. Trimethoprim/sulfamethoxazole therapy for shigellosis. JAMA 235:1239, 1976.

96. Nelson JD, Kusmiesz H, Jackson LH. Comparison of trimethoprim/sulfamethoxazole and ampicillin for shigellosis in ambulatory patients. J Pediatr 89:491, 1976.

97. Nelson JD, Kusmiesz H, Shelton S. Oral or intravenous trimethoprim/sulfamethoxazole therapy for shigellosis. Rev Infect Dis J 4:546, 1982.

98. Gilman RH, Spira W, Rabbani H, et al. Single dose

ampicillin therapy for severe shigellosis in Bangladesh. J Infect Dis 143:164, 1981.

99. Varsano I, Elditz-Marcus T, Nussinovitch M, et al. Comparative efficacy of ceftriaxone and ampicillin for treatment of severe shigellosis in children. J Pediatr 118:627, 1991.

100. Kabir T, Butler T, Khanam A. Comparative efficacies of single intravenous doses of ceftriaxone and ampicillin for shigellosis in a placebo-controlled trial. Antimicrob Agents Chemother 29:645, 1986.

101. Bennish ML, Salam MA, Khan WA, et al. Treatment of shigellosis: III. Comparison of one- or two-dose ciprofloxacin with standard 5-day therapy. Ann Intern Med 117:727, 1992.

102. John JF Jr, Atkins LT, Maple PAH, et al. Activities of new fluoroquinolones against Shigella sonnei. Antimicrob Agents Chemother 36:2346, 1992.

103. DuPont HL, Hornick RB. Adverse effect of Lomotil therapy in shigellosis. JAMA 226:1525, 1973.

104. Hayani KC, Guerrero ML, Ruiz-Palacios GM, et al. Evidence for long-term memory of the mucosal immune system: milk secretory immunoglobulin A against Shigella lipopolysaccharides. J Clin Microbiol 29:2599, 1991.

105. Hayani KC, Guerrero ML, Morrow AL, et al. Concentration of milk secretory immunoglobulin A against Shigella virulence plasmid associated antigens as a predictor of symptom status in Shigella infected breast fed infants. J Pediatr 121:852, 1992.

106. Ahmed F, Clemens JD, Rao MR, et al. Community based evaluation of the effect of breast feeding on the risk of microbiologically confirmed or clinically presumptive shigellosis in Bangladeshi children. Pediatrics 90:406, 1992.

107. Khan MU. Interruption of shigellosis by handwashing. Trans R Soc Trop Med Hyg 76:164, 1982.

108. Farrar WE, Edison M, Guerry P, et al. Interbacterial transfer of R-factor in the human intestine: in vitro acquisition of R-factor mediated kanamycin resistance by a multi-resistant strain of S. sonnei J Infect Dis 126:27, 1972.

Campylobacter

1. McFadyean F, Stockman S. Report of the Departmental Committee Appointed by the Board of Agriculture and Fishcrics to Inquire into Epizootic Abortion, vol. 3, London, His Majesty's Stationery Office, 1909.

2. Smith T, Taylor MS. Some morphological and biochemical characters of the spirilla (Vibrio fetus, n. spp.) associated with disease of the fetal membranes in cattle. J Exp Med 30:200, 1919.

3. Jones FS, Orcutt M, Little RB. Vibrios (Vibrio jejuni, n. spp.) associated with intestinal disorders of cows and calves. J Exp Med 53:853, 1931.

4. Bryner JH, Estes PC, Foley JW, et al. Infectivity of three Vibrio fetus biotypes for gallbladder and intestines of cattle, sheep, rabbits, guinea pigs, and mice. Am J Vet Res 32:465, 1971.

5. Vinzent R, Dumas J, Picard, N. Septicémie grave au cours de la grossesse due à un vibrion. Avortement consécutif. Bull Acad Natl Med 131:90, 1947.

6. Eden AN. Perinatal mortality caused by Vibrio fetus: review and analysis. J Pediatr 68:297, 1966.

7. Torphy DE, Bond WW. Campylobacter fetus infections in children. Pediatrics 64:898, 1979.

8. Bokkenheuser V. Vibrio fetus infection in man. I. Ten new cases and some epidemiologic observations. Am J Epidemiol 91:400, 1970.

9. Guerrant RL, Lahita RG, Winn WC, et al. Campylo-

bacteriosis in man: pathogenic mechanisms and review of 91 bloodstream infections. Am J Med 65:584, 1978.

10. King EO. Human infections with Vibrio fetus and a closely related vibrio. J Infect Dis 101:119, 1957.

11. Sebald M, Veron M. Teneur en bases de l'ADN et classification des vibrions. Ann Inst Pasteur 105:897, 1963.

12. Butzler JP, Dekeyser P, Detrain M, et al. Related vibrio in stools. J Pediatr 82:493, 1973.

13. Skirrow MB. Campylobacter enteritis: a "new" disease. BMJ 2:9, 1977.

14. Communicable Disease Surveillance Centre and the Communicable Diseases (Scotland) Unit. Campylobacter infections in Britain 1977. BMJ 1:1357, 1978.

15. De Mol P, Bosmans E. Campylobacter enteritis in Central Africa. Lancet 1:604, 1978.

16. Lindquist B, Kjellander J, Kosunen T. Campylobacter enteritis in Sweden. BMJ 1:303, 1978.

17. Karmali MA, Fleming PC. Campylobacter enteritis in children. J Pediatr 94:527, 1979.

18. Pai CM, Sorger S, Lackman L, et al. Campylobacter gastroenteritis in children. J Pediatr 94:589, 1979.

19. Blaser MJ, Reller LB. Campylobacter enteritis. N Engl J Med 305:1444, 1981.

20. Dekeyser P, Gossuin-Detrain M, Butzler JP, et al. Acute enteritis due to related Vibrio: first positive stool cultures. J Infect Dis 125:390, 1972.

21. Butzler JP, Skirrow MB. Campylobacter enteritis. Clin Gastroenterol 8:737, 1979.

22. Blaser MJ, Berkowitz ID, LaForce FM, et al. Campylobacter enteritis: clinical and epidemiologic features. Ann Intern Med 91:179, 1979.

23. Karmali MA, Fleming PC. Campylobacter enteritis. Can Med Assoc J 120:1525, 1979.

24. Steele TW, McDermott S. Campylobacter enteritis in South Australia. Med J Aust 2:404, 1978.

25. Guandalini S, Cucchiara S, deRitis G, et al. Campylobacter colitis in infants. J Pediatr 102:72, 1983.

26. Walker RI, Caldwell MB, Lee EC, et al. Pathophysiology of Campylobacter enteritis. Microbiol Rev 50:81, 1986.

27. Penner JL. The genus Campylobacter: a decade of progress. Clin Microbiol Rev. 1:157, 1988.

28. Calva JJ, Ruiz-Palacios GM, Lopez-Vidal AB, et al. Cohort study of intestinal infection with Campylobacter in Mexican children. Lancet 1:503, 1988.

29. Figura N, Guglielmetti P, Zanchi A, et al. Two cases of Campylobacter mucosalis enteritis in children. J Clin Microbiol 31:727, 1993.

30. Harvey SM, Greenwood JR. Relationships among catalase-positive campylobacters determined by deoxyribonucleic acid–deoxyribonucleic acid hybridization. Int J Syst Bacteriol 33:275, 1983.

31. Owen RJ. Nucleic acids in the classification of campylobacters. Eur J Clin Microbiol 2:367, 1983.

32. Hoffer MA. Bovine campylobacteriosis: a review. Can Vet J 22:327, 1981.

33. Grant CA. Bovine vibriosis: a brief review. Can J Comp Med 19:156, 1955.

34. Vinzent R. Une affection méconnue de la grossesse: l'infection placentaire à "Vibrio fetus." Presse Med 57:1230, 1949.

35. Wong S-N, Tam Y-CA, Yeun K-Y. Campylobacter infection in the neonate: case report and review of the literature. Pediatr Infect Dis J 9:665, 1990.

36. Hood M, Todd JM. Vibrio fetus—a cause of human abortion. Am J Obstet Gynecol. 80:506, 1960.

37. van Wering RF, Esseveld H. Vibrio fetus. Ned Tijdschr Geneeskd 107:119, 1963.

38. Burgert W Jr, Hagstrom JWC. *Vibrio fetus* meningoencephalitis. Arch Neurol 10:196, 1964.

39. Willis MD, Austin WJ. Human *Vibrio fetus* infection: report of two dissimilar cases. Am J Dis Child 112:459, 1966.

40. Smith JP, Marymont JH Jr, Schweers J. Septicemia due to *Campylobacter fetus* in a newborn infant with gastroenteritis. Am J Med Technol 43:38, 1977.

41. West SE, Houghton DJ, Crock S, et al. *Campylobacter* spp. isolated from the cervix during septic abortion. Case report. Br J Obstet Gynaecol 89:771, 1982.

42. Lee MM, Welliver RC, LaScolea LJ. *Campylobacter* meningitis in childhood. Pediatr Infect Dis J 4:544, 1985.

43. Simor AE, Karmali MA, Jadavji T, et al. Abortion and perinatal sepsis associated with *Campylobacter* infection. Rev Infect Dis J 8:397, 1986.

44. Forbes JC, Scheifele DW. Early onset *Campylobacter* sepsis in a neonate. Pediatr Infect Dis J 6:494, 1987.

45. Francioli P, Herzstein J, Grobe JP, et al. *Campylobacter fetus* subspecies *fetus* bacteremia. Arch Intern Med 145:289, 1985.

46. Karmali MA, Penner JL, Fleming PC, et al. The biotype and biotype distribution of clinical isolates of *Campylobacter jejuni* and *Campylobacter coli* over a three-year period. J Infect Dis 147:243, 1983.

47. Albert MJ, Leach A, Asche V, et al. Serotype distribution of *Campylobacter jejuni* and *Campylobacter coli* isolated from hospitalized patients with diarrhea in Central Australia. J Clin Microbiol 30:207, 1992.

48. Riley LW, Finch MJ. Results of the first year of national surveillance of *Campylobacter* infections in the United States. J Infect Dis 151:956, 1985.

49. Georges-Courbot MC, Baya C, Beraud AM, et al. Distribution and serotypes of *Campylobacter jejuni* and *Campylobacter coli* in enteric *Campylobacter* strains isolated from children in the Central African Republic. J Clin Microbiol 23:592, 1986.

50. Wheeler WE, Borchers J. Vibrionic enteritis in infants. Am J Dis Child 101:60, 1961.

51. Middlekamp JN, Wolf HA. Infection due to a "related" *Vibrio*. J Pediatr 59:318, 1961.

52. Ruben FL, Wolinsky E. Human infection with *Vibrio fetus*. *In* Hobby GL (ed). Antimicrobial Agents and Chemotherapy. Bethesda, Md, American Society for Microbiology, 1967, p 143.

53. Mawer SL, Smith BAM. *Campylobacter* infection of premature baby. Lancet 1:1041, 1979.

54. *Campylobacter* in a mother and baby. Commun Dis Rep CDR 7917:4, 1979.

55. Karmali MA, Tan YC. Neonatal *Campylobacter* enteritis. Can Med Assoc J 122:192, 1980.

56. Thomas K, Chan KN, Riberiro CD. *Campylobacter jejuni/coli* meningitis in a neonate. BMJ 280:1301, 1980.

57. Anders BJ, Lauer BA, Paisley JW. *Campylobacter* gastroenteritis in neonates. Am J Dis Child 135:900, 1981.

58. Vesikari T, Huttunen L, Maki R. Perinatal *Campylobacter fetus* ss. *jejuni* enteritis. Acta Paediatr Scand 70:261, 1981.

59. Miller RC, Guard RW. A case of premature labour due to *Campylobacter jejuni* infection. Aust N Z Obstet Gynaecol 22:118, 1982.

60. Buck GE, Kelly MT, Pichanick AM, et al. *Campylobacter jejuni* in newborns: a cause of asymptomatic bloody diarrhea. Am J Dis Child 136:744, 1982.

61. Karmali MA, Norrish B, Lior H, et al. *Campylobacter* enterocolitis in a neonatal nursery. J Infect Dis 149:874, 1984.

62. Youngs ER, Roberts C, Davidson DC. *Campylobacter* enteritis and bloody stools in the neonate. Arch Dis Child 60:480, 1985.

63. Terrier A, Altwegg M, Bader P, et al. Hospital epidemic of neonatal *Campylobacter jejuni* infection. Lancet 2:1182, 1985.

64. Goossens H, Henocque G, Kremp L, et al. Nosocomial outbreak of *Campylobacter jejuni* meningitis in newborn infants. Lancet 2:146, 1986.

65. DiNicola AF. *Campylobacter jejuni* diarrhea in a 3-day old male neonate. Pediatr Forum 140:191, 1986.

66. Hershkowici S, Barak M, Cohen A, et al. An outbreak of *Campylobacter jejuni* infection in a neonatal intensive care unit. J Hosp Infect 9:54, 1987.

67. Gribble MJ, Salit IE, Isaac-Renton J, et al. *Campylobacter* infections in pregnancy: case report and literature review. Am J Obstet Gynecol 140:423, 1981.

68. Gilbert GL, Davoren RA, Cole ME, et al. Midtrimester abortion associated with septicaemia caused by *Campylobacter jejuni*. Med J Aust 1:585, 1981.

69. Jost PM, Galvin MC, Brewer JH, et al. *Campylobacter* septic abortion. South Med J 77:924, 1984.

70. Pearce CT. *Campylobacter jejuni* infection as a cause of septic abortion. Aust J Med Lab Sci 2:107, 1981.

71. Pines A, Goldhammer E, Bregman J, et al. *Campylobacter* enteritis associated with recurrent abortions in agammaglobulinemia. Acta Obstet Gynecol Scand 62:279, 1983.

72. Kist M, Keller KM, Niebling W, et al. *Campylobacter coli* septicaemia associated with septic abortion. Infection 12:88, 1984.

73. Reina J, Borrell N, Fiol M. Rectal bleeding caused by *Campylobacter jejuni* in a neonate. Pediatr Infect Dis J 6:500, 1992.

74. Benjamin J, Leaper S, Owen RJ, et al. Description of *Campylobacter laridis*, a new species comprising the nalidixic acid–resistant thermophilic *Campylobacter* (NARTC) group. Curr Microbiol 8:231, 1983.

75. Von Graevenitz A. Revised nomenclature of *Campylobacter laridis, Enterobacter intermedium,* and "*Flavobacterium branchiophila.*" Int J Syst Bacteriol 40:211, 1990.

76. Altwegg M, Burnens A, Zollinger-Iten J, et al. Problems in identification of *Campylobacter jejuni* associated with acquisition of resistance to nalidixic acid. J Clin Microbiol 25:1807, 1987.

77. Tauxe RV, Patton CM, Edmonds P, et al. Illness associated with *Campylobacter laridis*, a newly recognized *Campylobacter* species. J Clin Microbiol 21:222, 1985.

78. Nachamkin I, Stowell C, Skalina D, et al. *Campylobacter laridis* causing bacteremia in an immunocompromised host. Ann Intern Med 101:55, 1984.

79. Ruiz-Palacios GM, Torres J, Escamilla NI. Cholera-like enterotoxin produced by *Campylobacter jejuni*: characterization and clinical significance. Lancet 2:250, 1983.

80. Johnson WM, Lior H. Toxins produced by *Campylobacter jejuni* and *Campylobacter coli*. Lancet 1:229, 1984.

81. Guerrant RL, Wanke CA, Pennie RA. Production of a unique cytotoxin by *Campylobacter jejuni*. Infect Immun 55:2526, 1987.

82. McCardell BA, Madden JM, Lee EC. *Campylobacter jejuni* and *Campylobacter coli* production of a cytotonic toxin immunologically similar to cholera toxin. J Food Prot 47:943, 1984.

83. Klipstein FA, Engert RF. Purification of *Campylobacter jejuni* enterotoxin. Lancet 1:1123, 1984.

84. Klipstein FA, Engert RF, Short H, et al. Pathogenic properties of *Campylobacter jejuni*: assay and correlation with clinical manifestations. Infect Immun 50:43, 1985.

85. Newell DG. Experimental studies of *Campylobacter* enter-

itis. *In* Butzler JP (ed). *Campylobacter* Infection in Man and Animals. Boca Raton, Fla., CRC Press, 1984, p 113.

86. Prescott JF, Barker IK, Manninen KI, et al. *Campylobacter jejuni* colitis in gnotobiotic dogs. Can J Comp Med 45:377, 1981.

87. Ruiz-Palacios GM, Escamilla E, Torres N. Experimental *Campylobacter* diarrhea in chickens. Infect Immun 34:250, 1981.

88. Sanyal SC, Islam KM, Neogy PKB, et al. *Campylobacter jejuni* diarrhea model in infant chickens. Infect Immun 43:931, 1984.

89. Welkos SL. Experimental gastroenteritis in newly hatched chicks infected with *Campylobacter jejuni*. J Med Microbiol 18:233, 1984.

90. Fitzgeorge RB, Baskerville A, Lander KP. Experimental infection of rhesus monkeys with a human strain of *Campylobacter jejuni*. J Hyg 86:343, 1981.

91. Field LH, Underwood JL, Berry LJ. The role of gut flora and animal passage in the colonization of adult mice with *Campylobacter jejuni*. J Med Microbiol 17:59, 1984.

92. Jesudason MV, Hentges DJ, Pongpeeh P. Colonization of mice by *Campylobacter jejuni*. Infect Immun 57:2279, 1989.

93. Kazmi SU, Roberson BS, Stern NJ. Animal-passed, virulence-enhanced *Campylobacter jejuni* causes enteritis in neonatal mice. Curr Microbiol 11:159, 1984.

94. Humphrey CD, Montag DM, Pittman FE. Experimental infection of hamsters with *Campylobacter jejuni*. J Infect Dis 151:485, 1985.

95. Manninen KI, Prescott JF, Dohoo IR. Pathogenicity of *C. jejuni* isolates from animals and humans. Infect Immun 38:46, 1982.

96. Eden AN. *Vibrio fetus* meningitis in a newborn infant. J Pediatr 61:33, 1962.

97. Maki M, Maki R, Vesikari T. Fecal leucocytes in *Campylobacter*-associated diarrhoea in infants. Acta Paediatr Scand 68:271, 1979.

98. Lambert ME, Schofield PF, Ironside AG, et al. *Campylobacter* colitis. BMJ 1:857, 1979.

99. Blaser MJ, Parsons RB, Wang WL. Acute colitis caused by *Campylobacter fetus* spp. *jejuni*. Gastroenterology 78:448, 1980.

100. King EO. The laboratory recognition of *Vibrio fetus* and a closely related *Vibrio* isolated from cases of human vibriosis. Ann N Y Acad Sci 78:700, 1962.

101. Evans RG, Dadswell JV. Human vibriosis. BMJ 3:240, 1967.

102. Butzler JP, Oosterom J. *Campylobacter*: pathogenicity and significance in foods. Int J Food Microbiol 12:1, 1991.

103. Gill CO, Harris LM. Contamination of red meat carcasses by *Campylobacter fetus* subsp. *jejuni*. Appl Environ Microbiol 43:977, 1982.

104. Palmer SR, Gulley PR, White JM, et al. Water-borne outbreak of *Campylobacter* gastroenteritis. Lancet 1:287, 1983.

105. Rogol M, Sechter I, Falk H, et al. Water-borne outbreaks of *Campylobacter* enteritis. Eur J Clin Microbiol 2:588, 1983.

106. Shankers S, Rosenfield JA, Davey GR, et al. *Campylobacter jejuni*: incidence in processed broilers and biotype distribution in human and broiler isolates. Appl Environ Microbiol 43:1219, 1982.

107. Hood AM, Pearson AD, Shahamat M. The extent of surface contamination of retailed chickens with *Campylobacter jejuni* serogroups. Epidemiol Infect 100:17, 1988.

108. Harris NV, Kimball TJ, Bennett P, et al. *Campylobacter jejuni* enteritis associated with raw goat's milk. Am J Epidemiol 126:179, 1987.

109. Korlath JA, Osterholm MT, Judy LA, et al. A point-source outbreak of campylobacteriosis associated with consumption of raw milk. J Infect Dis 152:592, 1985.

110. Klein BS, Vergeront JM, Blaser MJ, et al. *Campylobacter* infection associated with raw milk. JAMA 255:361, 1986.

111. Deming MS, Tauxe RV, Blake PA, et al. *Campylobacter* enteritis at a university: transmission from eating chicken and from cats. Am J Epidemiol 126:526, 1987.

112. Blaser MJ, Waldman RJ, Barrett T, et al. Outbreaks of *Campylobacter* enteritis in two extended families: evidence for person-to-person transmission. J Pediatr 98:254, 1981.

113. Cadranel S, Rodesch P, Butzler JP, et al. Enteritis due to "related *Vibrio*" in children. Am J Dis Child. 126:152, 1973.

114. Prescott JF, Karmali MA. Attempts to transmit *Campylobacter* enteritis to dogs and cats. Can Med Assoc J 119:1001, 1978.

115. Black RE, Levine MM, Clements ML, et al. Experimental *Campylobacter jejuni* infection in humans. J Infect Dis 157:472, 1988.

116. Robinson DA. Infective dose of *Campylobacter jejuni* in milk. BMJ 282:1584, 1981.

117. Bokkenheuser VD, Richardson NJ, Bryner JH, et al. Detection of enteric campylobacteriosis in children. J Clin Microbiol 9:227, 1979.

118. Georges-Courbot MC, Beraud-Cassel AM, Gouandjika I, et al. Prospective study of enteric *Campylobacter* infections in children from birth to 6 months in the Central African Republic. J Clin Microbiol 25:836, 1987.

119. Rettig PJ. *Campylobacter* infections in human beings. J Pediatr 94:855, 1979.

120. Blaser MJ, Berkowitz ID, LaForce FM, et al. *Campylobacter* enteritis: clinical and epidemiological features. Ann Intern Med 91:179, 1979.

121. Butzler JP. Related vibrios in Africa. Lancet 2:858, 1973.

122. Lauwers S, DeBoeck M, Butzler JP. *Campylobacter* enteritis in Brussels. Lancet 1:604, 1978.

123. Severin WP. *Campylobacter* en enteritis. Ned Tijdschr Geneeskd 122:499, 1978.

124. Ribeiro CD. *Campylobacter* enteritis. Lancet 2:270, 1978.

125. Richardson NJ, Koornhof HJ. *Campylobacter* infections in Soweto. S Afr Med J 55:73, 1979.

126. Gribble MJ, Salit EI, Isaac-Renton J, et al. *Campylobacter* infections in pregnancy. Case report and literature review. Am J Obstet Gynecol 140:423, 1981.

127. Morooka T, Umeda A, Fujita M, et al. Epidemiologic application of pulsed-field gel electrophoresis to an outbreak of *Campylobacter fetus* meningitis in a neonatal intensive care unit. Scand J Infect Dis 28:269, 1996.

128. Smith MV, Muldoon AJ. *Campylobacter fetus* subspecies *jejuni* (*Vibrio fetus*) from commercially processed poultry. Appl Microbiol 27:995, 1974.

129. Grant IH, Richardson NJ, Bokkenheuser VD. Broiler chickens as potential source of *Campylobacter* infections in humans. J Clin Microbiol 2:508, 1980.

130. Blaser MJ, Weiss SH, Barrett TJ. *Campylobacter* enteritis associated with a healthy cat. JAMA 247:816, 1982.

131. Skirrow MB, Turnbull GL, Walker RE, et al. *Campylobacter jejuni* enteritis transmitted from cat to man. Lancet 1:1188, 1980.

132. Blaser MJ, Cravens J, Powers BW, et al. *Campylobacter* enteritis associated with canine infection. Lancet 2:979, 1978.

133. Taylor PR, Weinstein WM, Bryner JH. *Campylobacter fetus* infection in human subjects: association with raw milk. Am J Med 66:779, 1979.

134. *Campylobacter* enteritis in a household—Colorado. MMWR Morb Mortal Wkly Rep 27:273, 1979.

135. Robinson DA, Edgar WM, Gibson GL, et al. *Campylobacter* enteritis associated with the consumption of unpasteurized milk. BMJ 1:1171, 1979.

136. Levy AJ. A gastroenteritis outbreak probably due to bovine strain of *Vibrio*. Yale J Biol Med 18:243, 1946.

137. Vogt RL, Sours HE, Barrett T, et al. *Campylobacter* enteritis associated with contaminated water. Ann Intern Med 96:292, 1982.

138. Patton CM, Wachsmuth IK, Evins GM, et al. Evaluation of 10 methods to distinguish epidemic-associated *Campylobacter* strains. J Clin Microbiol 29:680, 1991.

139. Lathey JL, Fiscus SA, Rasheed S, et al. Optimization of quantitative culture assay for human immunodeficiency virus from plasma. J Clin Microbiol 31:3064, 1994.

140. Salazar-Lindo E, Sack B, Chea-Woo E, et al. Early treatment with erythromycin of *Campylobacter jejuni* associated dysentery in children. J Pediatr 109:355, 1986.

141. Darling WM, Peel RN, Skirrow MB. *Campylobacter* cholecystitis. Lancet 1:1302, 1979.

142. Davis JS, Penfold JB. *Campylobacter* urinary tract infection. Lancet 1:1091, 1979.

143. Reed RP, Friedland IR, Wegerhoff FO, Khoosal M. *Campylobacter* bacteremia in children. Pediatr Infect Dis J 15:345, 1996.

144. Johonsen K, Ostensen M, Christine A, et al. HLA-B27-negative arthritis related to *Campylobacter jejuni* enteritis in three children and two adults. Acta Med Scand 214:165, 1983.

145. Kaldor J, Speed BR. Guillain-Barré syndrome and *Campylobacter jejuni*: a serological study. BMJ 288:1867, 1984.

146. Kuroki S, Haruta T, Yoshioka M, et al. Guillain-Barré syndrome associated with *Campylobacter* infection. Pediatr Infect Dis J 10:149, 1991.

147. Ebright JR, Ryay LM. Acute erosive reactive arthritis associated with *Campylobacter jejuni*–induced colitis. Am J Med 76:321, 1984.

148. Schaad UB. Reactive arthritis associated with *Campylobacter* enteritis. Pediatr Infect Dis J 1:328, 1982.

149. Perlman DM, Ampel NM, Schifman RB, et al. Persistent *Campylobacter jejuni* infections in patients infected with human immunodeficiency virus (HIV). Ann Intern Med 108:540, 1988.

150. Chiu CH, Kuo CY, Ou JT. Chronic diarrhea and bacteremia caused by *Campylobacter lari* in a neonate. Clin Infect Dis 21:700, 1995.

151. Kaplan RL, Goodman LJ, Barrett JE, et al. Comparison of rectal swabs and stool cultures in detecting *Campylobacter fetus* spp. *jejuni*. J Clin Microbiol 15:959, 1982.

152. Endtz HP, Ruijs GJHM, Zwinderman AH, et al. Comparison of six media, including a semisolid agar for the isolation of various *Campylobacter* species from stool specimens. J Clin Microbiol 29:1007, 1991.

153. Paisley JW, Mirrett S, Lauer BA, et al. Darkfield microscopy of human feces for presumptive diagnosis of *Campylobacter fetus* subsp. *jejuni* enteritis. J Clin Microbiol 15:61, 1982.

154. Oyofo BA, Thornton SA, Burr DH, et al. Specific detection of *Campylobacter jejuni* and *Campylobacter coli* by using polymerase chain reaction. J Clin Microbiol 30:2613, 1992.

155. Kiehlbauch JA, Baker CN, Wachsmuth IK, et al. *In vitro* susceptibilities of aerotolerant *Campylobacter* isolates to 22 antimicrobial agents. Antimicrob Agents Chemother 36:717, 1992.

156. LaChance N, Gaudreau C, Lamothe F, et al. Susceptibilities of β-lactamase-positive and -negative strains of *Campylobacter coli* to β-lactam agents. Antimicrob Agents Chemother 37:1174, 1993.

157. Yan W, Taylor DE. Characterization of erythromycin resistance in *Campylobacter jejuni* and *Campylobacter coli*. Antimicrob Agents Chemother 35:1989, 1991.

158. Segretti J, Gootz TD, Goodman LJ, et al. High-level quinolone resistance in clinical isolates of *Campylobacter jejuni*. J Infect Dis 165:667, 1992.

159. Krowchuk D, Seashore JH. Complete biliary obstruction due to erythromycin estolate administration in an infant. Pediatrics 64:956, 1979.

160. Kuschner RA, Trofa AF, Thomas RJ, et al. Use of azithromycin for the treatment of *Campylobacter* enteritis in travelers to Thailand, an area where ciprofloxacin resistance is prevalent. Clin Infect Dis 21:536, 1995.

161. Rautelin H, Renkonen OV, Kosunen TU. Azithromycin resistance in *Campylobacter jejuni* and *Campylobacter coli*. Eur J Clin Microbiol Infect Dis 12:864, 1993.

162. Endtz HP, Broeren M, Mouton RP. *In vitro* susceptibility of quinolone-resistant *Campylobacter jejuni* to new macrolide antibiotics. Eur J Clin Microbiol Infect Dis 12:48, 1993.

163. Ruiz-Palacios GM, Calva JJ, Pickering LK, et al. Protection of breastfed infants against *Campylobacter* diarrhea by antibodies in human milk. J Pediatr 116:707, 1990.

164. Nachamkin I, Fischer SH, Yang XH, et al: Immunoglobulin A antibodies directed against *Campylobacter jejuni* flagellin present in breast-milk. Epidemiol Infect 112:359, 1994.

Clostridium difficile

1. Finney JMT. Gastroenterostomy for cicatrizing ulcer of the pylorus. Bull Johns Hopkins Hosp 4:53, 1893.

2. Altemeier WA, Hummel RP, Hill EO. Staphylococcal enterocolitis following antibiotic therapy. Ann Surg 157:847, 1963.

3. Tan TL, Drake CT, Jacobson MJ, et al. The experimental development of pseudomembranous colitis. Surg Gynecol Obstet 108:415, 1959.

4. Bartlett JG. Antibiotic-associated diarrhea. Clin Infect Dis 15:573, 1992.

5. Fekety R, Shah AB. Diagnosis and treatment of *Clostridium difficile* colitis. JAMA 269:71, 1993.

6. Johnson S, Gerding DN. *Clostridium difficile*–associated diarrhea. Clin Infect Dis 26:1027, 1998.

7. Kelber M, Ament ME. *Shigella dysenteriae* 1. A forgotten cause of pseudomembranous colitis. J Pediatr 89:595, 1976.

8. Tochen ML, and Campbell JR. Colitis in children with the hemolytic uremic syndrome. J Pediatr Surg 12:213, 1977.

9. Pickering LK, Obrig TG, Stapleton FB. Hemolytic-uremic syndrome and enterohemorrhagic *Escherichia coli*. Pediatr Infect Dis J 13:459, 1994.

10. Borriello SP, Davies HA, Kamiya S, et al. Virulence factors of *Clostridium difficile*. Rev Infect Dis 12:S185, 1990.

11. Sears CL, Kaper JB. Enteric bacterial toxins: mechanisms of action and linkage to intestinal secretion. Microbiol Rev 60:167, 1996.

12. Wren BW. Molecular characterisation of *Clostridium difficile* toxins A and B. Rev Med Microbiol 3:21, 1992.

13. Hyams JS, Berman MM, Helgason H. Nonantibiotic-associated enterocolitis caused by *Clostridium difficile* in an infant. J Pediatr 99:750, 1981.

14. Larson HE, Price AB. Pseudomembranous colitis: presence of clostridial toxin. Lancet 1:1312, 1977.

15. Peikin SR, Galdibin J, Bartlett JG. Role of *Clostridium difficile* in a case of nonantibiotic-associated pseudomembranous colitis. Gastroenterology 79:948, 1980.
16. Wald A, Mendelow H, Bartlett JG. Nonantibiotic-associated pseudomembranous colitis due to toxin producing clostridia. Ann Intern Med 92:798, 1980.
17. Adler SP, Chandrika T, Berman WF. *Clostridium difficile* associated with pseudomembranous colitis. Am J Dis Child 135:820, 1981.
18. Willey S, Bartlett JG. Cultures for *C. difficile* in stools containing a cytotoxin neutralized by *C. sordellii* antitoxin. J Clin Microbiol 10:880, 1979.
19. Tabaqchali S. Epidemiologic markers of *Clostridium difficile*. Rev Infect Dis 12:S192, 1990.
20. Kim KH, Fekety R, Batts D, et al. Isolation of *C. difficile* from the environment and contacts of patients with antibiotic-associated colitis. J Infect Dis 143:42, 1981.
21. Sheretz RJ, Sarubb FA. The prevalence of *C. difficile* and toxin in a nursery population: a comparison between patients with necrotizing enterocolitis and an asymptomatic group. J Pediatr 100:435, 1982.
22. Clabots CR, Johnson S, Olson MM, et al. Acquisition of *Clostridium difficile* by hospitalized patients: evidence for colonized new admissions as a source of infection. J Infect Dis 166:561, 1992.
23. Bliss DZ, Johnson S, Savik K, et al. Acquisition of *Clostridium difficile* and *Clostridium difficile*–associated diarrhea in hospitalized patients receiving tube feeding. Ann Intern Med 129:1012, 1998.
24. Jernigan JA, Siegman-Igra Y, Guerrant RC, Farr BM. A randomized crossover study of disposable thermometers for prevention of *Clostridium difficile* and other nosocomial infections. Infect Control Hosp Epidemiol 19:494, 1998.
25. Johnson S, Gerding DN, Olson NM, et al. Prospective controlled study of vinyl glove use to interrupt *Clostridium difficile* transmission. Am J Med 88:137, 1990.
26. Zedd AJ, Sell TL, Schabert DR, et al. Nosocomial *C. difficile* reservoir in a neonatal intensive care unit. Pediatr Infect Dis J 3:429, 1984.
27. Donta ST, Myers MG. *C. difficile* toxin in asymptomatic neonates. J Pediatr 100:431, 1982.
28. Al-Jumaili I, Shibley M, Lishman AH, et al. Incidence and origin of *C. difficile* in neonates. J Clin Microbiol 19:77, 1984.
29. Stark PL, Lee A, Parsonage BD. Colonization of the large bowel by *C. difficile* in healthy infants: quantitative study. Infect Immun 35:895, 1982.
30. Welch DF, Marks MT. Is *C. difficile* pathogenic in infants? J Pediatr 100:393, 1982.
31. Donta ST, Stuppy MS, Myers MG. Neonatal antibiotic-associated colitis. Am J Dis Child 135:181, 1981.
32. Cashmore WJ, Peter G, Lauermann M, et al. Clostridia colonization and clostridial toxin in neonatal necrotizing enterocolitis. J Pediatr 98:308, 1981.
33. Han VKM, Sayed H, Chance GW, et al. An outbreak of *C. difficile* necrotizing enterocolitis: a case for oral vancomycin therapy? Pediatrics 71:935, 1983.
34. Sutphen JL, Grand RJ, Flores A, et al. Chronic diarrhea associated with *C. difficile* in children. Am J Dis Child 137:275, 1983.
35. Barbut F, Kajzer C, Planas N, et al. Comparison of three enzyme immunoassays, a cytotoxicity assay, and toxigenic culture for diagnosis of *Clostridium difficile*–associated diarrhea. J Clin Microbiol 31:963, 1993.
36. Lyerly DM, Neville LM, Evans DT, et al. Multicenter evaluation of the *Clostridium difficile* TOX A/B TEST. J Clin Microbiol 36:184, 1998.
37. Kato H, Kato N, Watanabe K, et al. Identification of toxin A–negative, toxin B–positive *Clostridium difficile* by PCR. J Clin Microbiol 36:2178, 1998.
38. Rafferty ME, Baltch AL, Smith RP, et al. Comparison of restriction enzyme analysis, arbitrarily primed PCR, and protein profile analysis typing for epidemiologic investigation of an ongoing *Clostridium difficile* outbreak. J Clin Microbiol 36:2957, 1998.
39. Teasley DG, Gerding DN, Olson MM, et al. Prospective randomized trial of metronidazole vs. vancomycin for *C. difficile* associated diarrhoea and colitis. Lancet 2:1043, 1983.
40. Young GP, Ward PB, Bayley N, et al. Antibiotic-associated colitis due to *C. difficile*: double-blind comparison of vancomycin with bacitracin. Gastroenterology 89:1039, 1985.
41. Dudley MN, McLaughlin JC, Carrington G, et al. Oral bacitracin vs. vancomycin therapy for *C. difficile*–induced diarrhea. Arch Intern Med 146:1101, 1986.
42. Wenisch C, Parschalk B, Hasenhündl M, et al. Comparison of vancomycin, teicoplanin, metronidazole, and fusidic acid for the treatment of *Clostridum difficile*–associated diarrhea. Clin Infect Dis 22:813, 1996.
43. Bartlett JG, Tedesco FJ, Shull S, et al. Relapse following oral vancomycin therapy of antibiotic-associated pseudomembranous colitis. Gastroenterology 78:431, 1980.
44. McFarland LV, Surawicz CM, Greenberg RN, et al. A randomized placebo-controlled trial of *Saccharomyces boulardii* in combination with standard antibiotics for *Clostridium difficile* disease. JAMA 271:1913, 1994.
45. Wada N, Nishida N, Iwak S, et al. Neutralizing activity against *C. difficile* toxin in the supernatants of cultures of colostral cells. Infect Immun 29:545, 1980.
46. Kim K, Pickering LK, DuPont HL, et al. *In vitro* and in vivo neutralizing activity of *C. difficile* purified toxins A and B by human colostrum and milk. J Infect Dis 150:57, 1984.
47. Cooperstock MS, Steffen E, Yolken R, et al. *C. difficile* in normal infants and sudden death syndrome: an association with infant formula feeding. Pediatrics 70:91, 1982.

Vibrio cholerae

1. Levine WC, Griffin PM, and the Gulf Coast *Vibrio* Working Group. *Vibrio* infections on the Gulf Coast: results of first year of regional surveillance. J Infect Dis 167:479, 1993.
2. Swerdlow DL, Ries AA. Cholera in the Americas: guidelines for the clinician. JAMA 267:1495, 1992.
3. Glass RI, Libel M, Brandling-Bennett AD. Epidemic cholera in the Americas. Science 256:1524, 1992.
4. Spangler BD. Structure and function of cholera toxin and the related *Escherichia coli* heat-labile enterotoxin. Microbiol Rev 56:622, 1992.
5. Wachsmuth IK, Evins GM, Fields PI, et al. The molecular epidemiology of cholera in Latin America. J Infect Dis 167:621, 1993.
6. Siddique AK, Zaman K, Akram K, et al. Emergence of a new epidemic strain of *Vibro cholerae* in Bangladesh. An epidemiological study. Trop Geogr Med 46:147, 1994.
7. Fisher-Hoch SP, Khan A, Inam-ul-Haq, et al. *Vibrio cholerae* 0139 in Karachi, Pakistan. Lancet 342:1422, 1993.
8. Chongsa-Nguan M, Chaicumpa W, Moolasart P, et al. *Vibrio cholerae* 0139 Bengal in Bangkok. Lancet 342:430, 1993.
9. Cholera Working Group, International Centre for Diarrhoeal Diseases Research, Bangladesh. Large epidemic of cholera-like disease in Bangladesh caused by *Vibrio cholerae* 0139 synonym Bengal. Lancet 342:387, 1993.

10. Bhattacharya SK, Bhattacharya MK, Nair GB, et al. Clinical profile of acute diarrhoea cases infected with the new epidemic strain of *Vibrio cholerae* 0139: designation of the disease as cholera. J Infect 27:11, 1993.
11. Garg S, Saha PK, Ramamurthy T, et al. Nationwide prevalence of the new epidemic strain of *Vibrio cholerae* 0139 Bengal in India. J Infect 27:108, 1993.
12. Blake PA, Allegra DT, Snyder JD, et al. Cholera—a possible endemic focus in the United States. N Engl J Med 302:305, 1980.
13. Hirschhorn N, Chowdhury AAKM, and Lindenbaum J. Cholera in pregnant women. Lancet 1:1230, 1969.
14. Khan AM, Bhattacharyl MK, Albert MJ. Neonatal diarrhea caused by *Vibrio cholerae* 0139 Bengal. Diagn Microbiol Infect Dis 23:155, 1995.
15. Lumbiganon P, Kosalaraksa P, Kowsuwan P. *Vibrio cholerae* 0139 diarrhea and acute renal failure in a three day old infant. Pediatr Infect Dis J 14:1105, 1995.
16. Lindenbaum J, Akbar R, Gordon RS Jr, et al. Cholera in children. Lancet 1:1066, 1966.
17. Gunn RA, Kimball AM, Pollard RA, et al. Bottle feeding as a risk factor for cholera in infants. Lancet 2:730, 1979.
18. Glass RI, Svennerholm AM, Stoll BJ, et al. Protection against cholera in breast-fed children by antibodies in breast milk. N Engl J Med 308:1389, 1983.
19. Holmgren J, Svennerholm AM, Lindblad M. Receptor-like glycocompounds in human milk that inhibit classical and El Tor *V. cholerae* cell adherence (hemagglutination). Infect Immun 39:147, 1983.
20. Laegreid A, Otnaess AB, Fuglesang J. Human and bovine milk. Comparison of ganglioside composition and enterotoxin inhibitory activity. Pediatr Res 20:416, 1986.
21. Ahmed A, Bhattacharjee AK, Mosley WH. Characteristics of the serum vibriocidal and agglutinating antibodies in cholera cases and in normal residents of the endemic and non-endemic cholera areas. J Immunol 105:431, 1970.
22. Merson MH, Black RE, Sack DA, et al. Maternal cholera immunisation and secretory IgA in breast milk. Lancet 1:931, 1980.
23. Cash RA, Music SI, Libonati JP, et al. Response of man to infection with *Vibrio cholerae*. I. Clinical, serologic and bacteriologic responses to a known inoculum. J Infect Dis 129:45, 1974.
24. Nalin DR, Levine RJ, Levine MM. Cholera, non-*Vibrio* cholera, and stomach acid. Lancet 2:856, 1978.
25. Gordon JE, Chitkara ID, Wyon JB. Weanling diarrhea. Am J Med Sci 245:345, 1963.
26. Wright AC, Guo Y, Johnson JA, et al. Development and testing of a nonradioactive DNA oligonucleotide probe that is specific for *Vibrio cholerae* cholera toxin. J Clin Microbiol 30:2302, 1992.
27. Yoh M, Miyagi K, Matsumoto Y, et al. Development of an enzyme-labeled oligonucleotide probe for the cholera toxin gene. J Clin Microbiol 31:1312, 1993.
28. Kotloff KL, Wasserman SS, O'Donnell S, et al. Safety and immunogenicity in North Americans of a single dose of live oral cholera vaccine CVD 103-HgR: results of a randomized, placebo-controlled, double-blind crossover trial. Infect Immun 60:4430, 1992.
29. Clemens JD, Sack DA, Rao MR, et al. Evidence that inactivated oral cholera vaccines both prevent and mitigate *Vibrio cholerae* 01 infections in a cholera-endemic area. J Infect Dis 166:1029, 1992.
30. Levine MM, Noriega F. A review of the current status of enteric vaccines. P N G Med J 38:325, 1995.

Yersinia enterocolitica

1. Kohl S. *Yersinia enterocolitica* infections in children. Pediatr Clin North Am 26:433, 1979.

2. Marks MI, Pai CH, Lafleur L, et al. *Yersinia enterocolitica* gastroenteritis: a prospective study of clinical, bacteriologic, and epidemiologic features. J Pediatr 96:26, 1980.
3. Lee LA, Gerber AR, Lonsway DR, et al. *Yersinia enterocolitica* 0:3 infections in infants and children, associated with the household preparation of chitterlings. N Engl J Med 322:984, 1990.
4. Krogstad P, Mendelman PM, Miller VL, et al. Clinical and microbiologic characteristics of cutaneous infection with *Yersinia enterocolitica*. J Infect Dis 165:740, 1992.
5. Lee LA, Taylor J, Carter GP, et al. *Yersinia enterocolitica* 0:3: an emerging cause of pediatric gastroenteritis in the United States. J Infect Dis 163:660, 1991.
6. Morris JG Jr, Prado V, Ferreccio C, et al. *Yersinia enterocolitica* isolated from two cohorts of young children in Santiago, Chile: incidence of and lack of correlation between illness and proposed virulence factors. J Clin Microbiol 29:2784, 1991.
7. Metchock B, Lonsway DR, Carter GP, et al. *Yersinia enterocolitica*: a frequent seasonal stool isolate from children at an urban hospital in the southeast United States. J Clin Microbiol 29:2868, 1991.
8. Kane DR, Reuman PD. *Yersinia enterocolitica* causing pneumonia and empyema in a child and a review of the literature. Pediatr Infect Dis J 11:591, 1992.
9. Bissett ML, Powers C, Abbott SL, et al. Epidemiologic investigations of *Yersinia enterocolitica* and related species: sources, frequency, and serogroup distribution. J Clin Microbiol 28:910, 1990.
10. Milteer RM, Sarpong S, Poydras U. *Yersinia enterocolitica* septicemia after accidental oral iron overdose. Pediatr Infect Dis J. 8:537, 1989.
11. Black RE, Jackson RJ, Tsai T, et al. Epidemic *Yersinia enterocolitica* infection due to contaminated chocolate milk. N Engl J Med 298:76, 1978.
12. Pietersz RNI, Reesink HW, Pauw W, et al. Prevention of *Yersinia enterocolitica* growth in red blood cell concentrates. Lancet 340:755, 1992.
13. Kapperud G, Namork E, Skurnik M, et al. Plasmid-mediated surface fibrillae of *Y. pseudotuberculosis* and *Y. enterocolitica*. Relationship to the outer membrane protein YOP1 and possible importance for pathogenesis. Infect Immun 55:2247, 1987.
14. Brubaker RR. Factors promoting acute and chronic diseases caused by yersiniae. Clin Microbiol Rev 4:309, 1991.
15. Takao T, Tominaga N, Shimoniski Y, et al. Primary structure of heat-stable enterotoxin produced by *Y. enterocolitica*. Biochem Biophys Res Commun 125:845, 1984.
16. Grant T, Bennett-Wood V, Robins-Browne RM. Identification of virulence-associated characteristics in clinical isolates of *Yersinia enterocolitica* lacking classical virulence markers. Infect Immun 66:1113, 1998.
17. Paisley JW, Lauer BA. Neonatal *Yersinia enterocolitica* enteritis. Pediatr Infect Dis J 11:331, 1992.
18. Shapiro ED. *Yersinia enterocolitica* septicemia in normal infants. Am J Dis Child 135:477, 1981.
19. Chester B, Sanderson T, Zeller DJ, et al. Infections due to *Yersinia enterocolitica* serotypes 0:2, 3 and 0:4 acquired in South Florida. J Clin Microbiol 13:885, 1981.
20. Rodriguez WJ, Controni G, Cohen GJ, et al. *Y. enterocolitica* enteritis in children. JAMA 242:1978, 1979.
21. Challapalli M, Cunningham DG. *Yersinia enterocolitica* septicemia in infants younger than three months of age. Pediatr Infect Dis J 12:168, 1993.
22. Paisley JW, Lauer BA. Neonatal *Yersinia enterocolitica* enteritis. Pediatr Infect Dis J 11:332, 1992.
23. Antonio-Santiago MT, Kaul A, Lue Y, et al. *Yersinia*

enterocolitica septicemia in an infant presenting as fever of unknown origin. Clin Pediatr 25:213, 1986.

24. Sutton JM, Pasquariell PS. *Yersinia enterocolitica* septicemia in a normal child. Am J Dis Child 137:305, 1983.

25. Kohl S, Jacobson JA, Nahmias A. *Yersinia enterocolitica* infections in children. J Pediatr 89:77, 1976.

26. Kontianen S, Sivonen A, Renkonen OV. Increased yields of pathogenic *Yersinia enterocolitica* strains by cold enrichment. Scand J Infect Dis 26:685, 1994.

27. Ibrahim A, Liesack W, Stackebrandt E. Polymerase chain reaction–gene probe detection system specific for pathogenic strains of *Yersinia enterocolitica*. J Clin Microbiol 30:1942, 1992.

28. Kwaga J, Iversen JO, Misra V. Detection of pathogenic *Yersinia enterocolitica* by polymerase chain reaction and digoxigenin-labeled polynucleotide probes. J Clin Microbiol 30:2668, 1992.

29. Stolk-Engelaar VM, Meis JF, Mulder JA, et al. In-vitro antimicrobial susceptibility of *Yersinia enterocolitica* isolates from stools of patients in the Netherlands from 1982–1991. J Antimicrob Chemother 36:839, 1995.

30. Alzugaray R, Gonzalez Hevia MA, Landeras E, Mendoza MC. *Yersinia enterocolitica* 0:3. Antimicrobial resistance patterns, virulence profiles and plasmids. New Microbiol 18:215, 1995.

31. Preston MA, Brown S, Borczyk AA, et al. Antimicrobial susceptibility of pathogenic *Yersinia enterocolitica* isolated in Canada from 1972 to 1990. Antimicrob Agents Chemother 38:2121, 1994.

Other Bacterial Agents and Fungi

1. Struelens MJ, Bennish ML, Mondal G, et al. Bacteremia during diarrhea: incidence, etiology, risk factors, and outcome. Am J Epidemiol 133:451, 1991.

2. James C, Dibley M, Burke V, et al. Immunological crossreactivity of enterotoxins of *A. hydrophila* and cholera toxin. Clin Exp Immunol 47:34, 1982.

3. Sanyal SC, Singh SJ, Sen PC. Enteropathogenicity of *A. hydrophila* and *P. shigelloides*. J Med Microbiol 8:195, 1975.

4. Kirov SM, Rees B, Wellock RC, et al. Virulence characteristics of *Aeromonas* spp. in relation to source and biotype. J Clin Microbiol 24:827, 1986.

5. Watson IM, Robinson JO, Burke V, et al. Invasiveness of *Aeromonas* spp. in relation to biotype, virulence factors, and clinical features. J Clin Microbiol 22:48, 1985.

6. Kindshuh M, Pickering LK, Cleary TG, et al. Clinical and biochemical significance of toxin production by *A. hydrophila*. J Clin Microbiol 25:916, 1987.

7. Ljungh A, Eneroth P, Wadstrom T. Cytotonic enterotoxin from *Aeromonas hydrophila*. Toxicon 20:787, 1982.

8. Morgan D, Johnson PC, DuPont HL, et al. Lack of correlation between known virulence properties of *A. hydrophila* and enteropathogenicity for humans. Infect Immun 50:62, 1985.

9. Pitarangsi C, Echeverria P, Whitemire R, et al. Enteropathogenicity of *A. hydrophila* and *P. shigelloides*: prevalence among individuals with and without diarrhea in Thailand. Infect Immun 35:666, 1982.

10. Martinez-Silva R, Guzmann-Urrego M, Caselitz FH. Zur Frage der Bedeutung von Aeromonasstammen bei Saüglingsenteritis. Z Tropenmed Parasitol 12:445, 1961.

11. Figura N, Marri L, Verdiani S, et al. Prevalence, species differentiation, and toxigenicity of *Aeromonas* strains in cases of childhood gastroenteritis and in controls. J Clin Microbiol 23:595, 1986.

12. Gracey M, Burke V, Robinson J. *Aeromonas*-associated gastroenteritis. Lancet 2:1304, 1982.

13. Shread P, Donovan TJ, Lee JV. A survey of the incidence of *Aeromonas* in human feces. Soc Gen Microbiol 8:184, 1981.

14. Escheverria P, Blacklow NR, Sanford LB, et al. Travelers' diarrhea among American Peace Corps volunteers in rural Thailand. J Infect Dis 143:767, 1981.

15. Bhat P, Shanthakumari S, Rajan D. The characterization and significance of *P. shigelloides* and *A. hydrophila* isolated from an epidemic of diarrhea. Indian J Med Res 62:1051, 1974.

16. Agger WA, McCormick JD, Gurwith MJ. Clinical and microbiological features of *A. hydrophila*–associated diarrhea. J Clin Microbiol 21:909, 1985.

17. Agger WA. Diarrhea associated with *A. hydrophila*. Pediatr Infect Dis J 5:S106, 1986.

18. Deodhar LP, Saraswathi K, Varudkar A. *Aeromonas* spp. and their association with human diarrheal disease. J Clin Microbiol 29:853, 1991.

19. Santoso H, Agung IGN, Robinson J, et al. Faecal *Aeromonas* spp. in Balinese children. J Gastroenterol Hepatol 1:115, 1986.

20. Gomez CJ, Munozz P, Lopez F, et al. Gastroenteritis due to *Aeromonas* in pediatrics. An Esp Pediatr 44:548, 1996.

21. Diaz A, Velasco AC, Hawkins F, et al. *A. hydrophila*–associated diarrhea in a neonate. Pediatr Infect Dis J 5:704, 1986.

22. San Joaquin VH, Pickett DA. *Aeromonas*-associated gastroenteritis in children. Pediatr Infect Dis J 7:53, 1988.

23. George WL, Jones MJ, Nakata MM. Phenotypic characteristics of *Aeromonas* species isolated from adult humans. J Clin Microbiol 23:1026, 1986.

24. Janda JM. Recent advances in the study of the taxonomy, pathogenicity, and infectious syndromes associated with the genus *Aeromonas*. Clin Microbiol Rev. 4:397, 1991.

25. Freij BJ. *Aeromonas*: biology of the organism and diseases in children. Pediatr Infect Dis J 3:164, 1984.

26. Fainstein V, Weaver S, Bodey GP. *In vitro* susceptibilities of *A. hydrophila* against new antibiotics. Antimicrob Agents Chemother 22:513, 1982.

27. San Joaquin VH, Scribner RK, Pickett DA, et al. Antimicrobial susceptibility of *Aeromonas* species isolated from patients with diarrhea. Antimicrob Agents Chemother 30:794, 1986.

28. Jones BL, Wilcox MH. *Aeromonas* infections and their treatment. J Antimicrob Chemother 35:453, 1995.

29. Holmberg SD, Wachsmuth IK, Hickmann-Brenner FW, et al. *Plesiomonas* enteric infections in the United States. Ann Intern Med 105:690, 1986.

30. Tsukamoto T, Kinoshita Y, Shimada T, et al. Two epidemics of diarrhoeal disease possibly caused by *P. shigelloides*. J Hyg 80:275, 1978.

31. Holmberg SD, Farmer JJ. *A. hydrophila* and *P. shigelloides* as causes of intestinal infections. Rev Infect Dis 6:633, 1984.

32. Herrington DA, Tzipori S, Robins-Browne RM, et al. *In vitro* and *in vivo* pathogenicity of *P. shigelloides*. Infect Immun 55:979, 1987.

33. Brenden RA, Miller MA, Janda JM. Clinical disease spectrum and pathogenic factors associated with *P. shigelloides* infections in humans. Rev Infect Dis 10:303, 1988.

34. Pathak A, Custer JR, Levy J. Neonatal septicemia and meningitis due to *Plesiomonas shigelloides*. Pediatrics 71:389, 1983.

35. Fujita K, Shirai M, Ishioka T, Kakuya F. Neonatal *Plesiomonas shigelloides* septicemia and meningitis: a case review. Acta Paediatr Jpn 36:450, 1994.

36. Terpeluk C, Goldmann A, Bartmann P, Pohlandt F. *Plesi-*

omonas shigelloides sepsis and meningoencephalitis in a neonate. Eur J Pediatr 151:499, 1992.

37. Billiet J, Kuypers S, Van Lierde S, Verhaegen J. *Plesiomonas Shigelloides* meningitis and septicaemia in a neonate: report of a case and review of the literature. J Infect 19:267, 1989.

38. Alabi SA, Odugbemi T. Biochemical characteristics and a simple scheme for the identification of *Aeromonas* species and *Plesiomonas shigelloides*. J Trop Med Hyg 93:166, 1990.

39. Reinhardt JF, George WL. Comparative *in vitro* activities of selected antimicrobial agents against *Aeromonas* species and *P. shigelloides*. Antimicrob Agents Chemother 27:643, 1985.

40. Visitsunthorn N, Komolpis P. Antimicrobial therapy in *Plesiomonas shigelloides*–associated diarrhea in Thai children. Southeast Asian J Trop Med Public Health 26:86, 1995.

41. Kubota Y, Liu PV. An enterotoxin of *Pseudomonas aeruginosa*. J Infect Dis 123:97, 1971.

42. Bassett DCJ, Thompson SAS, and Page B. Neonatal infections with *Pseudomonas aeruginosa* associated with contaminated resuscitation equipment. Lancet 1:781, 1965.

43. Ensign PR, Hunter CA. An epidemic of diarrhea in the newborn nursery caused by a milk-borne epidemic in the community. J Pediatr 29:620, 1946.

44. Falcao DP, Mendonca CP, Scrassolo A, et al. Nursery outbreak of severe diarrhoea due to multiple strains of *Pseudomonas aeruginosa*. Lancet 2:38, 1972.

45. Henderson A, Maclaurin J, Scott JM. *Pseudomonas* in a Glasgow baby unit. Lancet 2:316, 1969.

46. Jellard CH, Churcher GM. An outbreak of *Pseudomonas aeruginosa (pyocyanea)* infection in a premature baby unit, with observations on the intestinal carriage of *Pseudomonas aeruginosa* in the newborn. J Hyg 65:219, 1967.

47. Linde K, Koditz H, Kittlick M. Untersuchungen zur Frage der Säuglingsenteritis durch *Pseudomonas aeruginosa* (Pyocyaneus-Bakterien). Monatschr Kinderheilkd 110:62, 1962.

48. Coello-Ramirez P, Lifshitz F, Zuniga V. Enteric microflora and carbohydrate intolerance in infants with diarrhea. Pediatrics 49:233, 1972.

49. Cole AP, Thom AR, Watrasiewicz K. Infant carriers of *Pseudomonas aeruginosa*. Lancet 2:1155, 1971.

50. Neter E, Weintraub DH. An epidemiological study of *Pseudomonas aeruginosa (Bacillus pyocyaneus)* in premature infants in the presence and absence of infection. J Pediatr 46:280, 1955.

51. Cooke EM, Shooter RA, O'Farrell SM, et al. Faecal carriage of *Pseudomonas aeruginosa* by newborn babies. Lancet 2:1045, 1970.

52. McFarlan AM, Crone PB, Tee GH. Variations in bacteriology of throat and rectum of infants in two maternity units. BMJ 2:1140, 1949.

53. Moffet HL, Shulenberger HK, Burkholder ER. Epidemiology and etiology of severe infantile diarrhea. J Pediatr 72:1, 1968.

54. Mohieldin MS, Gabr M, el-Hefny A, et al. Bacteriological and clinical studies in infantile diarrhoea. II. Doubtful pathogens: Enterobacteriaceae, *Pseudomonas*, *Alcaligenes* and *Aeromonas*. J Trop Pediatr 11:88, 1966.

55. Singer JM, Bar-Hay J, Hoenigsberg R. The intestinal flora in the etiology of infantile infectious diarrhea. Am J Dis Child 89:531, 1955.

56. Ayliffe GAJ, Collins BJ, Pettit F. Contamination of infant feeds in a Milton milk kitchen. Lancet 1:559, 1970.

57. Libit SA, Ulstrom RA, Doeden D. Fecal *Pseudomonas*

58. Thom AR, Cole AP, Watrasiewicz K. *Pseudomonas aeruginosa* as a cause of the blue diaper syndrome. J Pediatr 81:546, 1972.

58. Thom AR, Cole AP, Watrasiewicz K. *Pseudomonas aeruginosa* infection in a neonatal nursery, possibly transmitted by a breast-milk pump. Lancet 1:560, 1970.

59. Ujvary G, Angyal T, Lanyi B, et al. Beobachtungen über die Ätiologie der Gastroenterocolitiden des Säuglings- und Kindesalters. V. Untersuchung der Rolle der *Pseudomonas aeruginosa*- und *Staphylococcus aureus*-Stamme. Acta Microbiol Acad Sci Hung 10:337, 1964.

60. Schaffer AJ, Oppenheimer EH. *Pseudomonas* (Pyocyaneus) infection of the gastro-intestinal tract in infants and children. South Med J 41:460, 1948.

61. Waldhausen JA, Herendeen T, King H. Necrotizing colitis of the newborn: common cause of perforation of the colon. Surgery 54:365, 1963.

62. Verger P, Bentegeat J. Une épidémie d'entérite à bacille pyocyanique (*Pseudomonas aeruginosa*) observée dans un centre de prématurés. Nourisson 43:141, 1955.

63. Ujvary G, Angyal T, Voros S, et al. Beobachtungen Über die Ätiologie der Gastroenterocolitiden des Säuglings- und Kindesalters. II. Untersuchung der Rolle der *Klebsiella*-Stamme. Acta Microbiol Acad Sci Hung 10:241, 1964.

64. Adler JL, Shulman JA, Terry PM, et al. Nosocomial colonization with kanamycin-resistant *Klebsiella pneumoniae*, types 2 and 11, in a premature nursery. J Pediatr 77:376, 1970.

65. Hable KA, Matsen JM, Wheeler DJ, et al. *Klebsiella* type 33 septicemia in an infant intensive care unit. J Pediatr 80:920, 1972.

66. Hill HR, Hunt CE, Matsen JM. Nosocomial colonization with *Klebsiella*, type 16, in a neonatal intensive-care unit associated with an outbreak of sepsis, meningitis, and necrotizing enterocolitis. J Pediatr 85:415, 1974.

67. Jampolis M, Howell KM, Calvin JK, et al. *Bacillus mucosus* infection of the newborn. Am J Dis Child 43:70, 1932.

68. Wyatt RG, Mata LJ. Bacteria in colostrum and milk of Guatemalan Indian women. J Trop Pediatr 15:159, 1969.

69. Gareau FE, Mackel DC, Boring JR III, et al. The acquisition of fecal flora by infants from their mothers during birth. J Pediatr 54:313, 1959.

70. Gergely K. Über eine Enteritis-Epidemie bei Frühgeborenen, verursacht durch den Bacillus *Klebsiella*. Kinderaerztl Prax 9:385, 1964.

71. Olarte J, Ferguson WW, Henderson ND, et al. *Klebsiella* strains isolated from diarrheal infants. Human volunteer studies. Am J Dis Child 101:763, 1961.

72. Bertrams J, Pfortner M, Neussel H, et al. Colienteritis des Säglings. Quantitative und fluoreszenzserologische Verlaufsuntersuchungen. Munch Med Wochenschr 112:38, 1970.

73. Lifshitz F, Coello-Ramirez P, Gutierrez-Topete G, et al. Monosaccharide intolerance and hypoglycemia in infants with diarrhea. I. Clinical course of 23 infants. J Pediatr 77:595, 1970.

74. Murdoch MM, Janovski NA, Joseph S. *Klebsiella* pseudomembranous enterocolitis. Report of two cases. Med Ann DC 38:137, 1969.

75. Walcher DN. "Bacillus mucosus capsulatus" in infantile diarrhea. J Clin Invest 25:103, 1946.

76. Cass JM. *Bacillus lactis aerogenes* infection in the newborn. Lancet 1:346, 1941.

77. Sternberg SD, Hoffman C, Zweifler BM. Stomatitis and diarrhea in infants caused by *Bacillus mucosus capsulatus*. J Pediatr 38:509, 1951.

78. Worfel MT, Ferguson WW. A new *Klebsiella* type (capsu-

lar type 15) isolated from feces and urine. Am J Clin Pathol 21:1097, 1951.

79. Simmons BP, Gelfand MS, Haas M, et al. *Enterobacter sakazakii* infections in neonates associated with intrinsic contamination of a powdered infant formula. Infect Control Hosp Epidemiol 10:398, 1989.

80. Klipstein FA, Holdeman LW, Corcino JJ, et al. Enterotoxigenic intestinal bacteria in tropical sprue. Ann Intern Med 79:632, 1973.

81. Guerrant RL, Dickens MD, Wenzel RP, et al. Toxigenic bacterial diarrhea: nursery outbreak involving multiple bacterial strains. J Pediatr 89:885, 1976.

82. Guerrant RL, Moore RA, Kirschenfeld PM, et al. Role of toxigenic and invasive bacteria in acute diarrhea of childhood. N Engl J Med 293:567, 1975.

83. Wadstrom T, Aust-Kettis A, Habte D, et al. Enterotoxin-producing bacteria and parasites in stools of Ethiopian children with diarrhoeal disease. Arch Dis Child 51:865, 1976.

84. Wachsmuth K, Wells J, Shipley P, et al. Heat-labile enterotoxin production in isolates from a shipboard outbreak of human diarrheal illness. Infect Immun 24:793, 1979.

85. Panigrahi D, Roy P, Chakrabarti A. Enterotoxigenic *Klebsiella pneumoniae* in acute childhood diarrhea. Indian J Med Res 93:293, 1991.

86. Guarino A, Capano G, Malamisura B, et al. Production of *E. coli* STa-like heat stable enterotoxin by *Citrobacter freundii* isolated from humans. J Clin Microbiol 25:110, 1987.

87. Skerman FJ, Formal SB, Falkow, S. Plasmid-associated enterotoxin production in a strain of *Escherichia coli* isolated from humans. Infect Immun 5:622, 1972.

88. Takeda Y, Murphy J. Bacteriophage conversion of heat-labile enterotoxin in *Escherichia coli*. J Bacteriol 133:172, 1978.

89. Lipsky BA, Hook EW, Smith AA, et al. *Citrobacter* infections in humans: experience at the Seattle Veterans Administration Medical Center and a review of the literature. Rev Infect Dis 2:746, 1980.

90. Kahlich R, Webershinke J. A contribution to incidence and evaluation of *Citrobacter* findings in man. Cesk Epidemiol Mikrobiol Imunol 12:55, 1963.

91. Parida SN, Verma IC, Deb M, et al. An outbreak of diarrhea due to *Citrobacter freundii* in a neonatal special care nursery. Indian J Pediatr 47:81, 1980.

92. Rowe B, Gross RJ, Allen HA. *Citrobacter koseri* II. Serological and biochemical examination of *Citrobacter koseri* strains from clinical specimens. J Hyg 75:129, 1975.

93. Kalashnikova GK, Lokosova AK, Sorokina RS. Concerning the etiological role of bacteria belonging to *Citrobacter* and *Hafnia* genera in children suffering from diseases accompanied by diarrhea, and some of their epidemiological peculiarities. Zh Mikrobiol Epidemiol Immunobiol 6:78, 1974.

94. Graber CD, Dodd MC. The role of *Paracolobactrum* and *Proteus* in infantile diarrhea. Ann N Y Acad Sci 66:136, 1956.

95. Neter E, Goodale ML. Peritonitis due to the *Morgani bacillus*. With a brief review of literature on the pathogenicity of this organism. Am J Dis Child 56:1313, 1938.

96. Neter ER, Farrar RH. *Proteus vulgaris* and *Proteus morgani* in diarrheal disease of infants. Am J Dig Dis 10:344, 1943.

97. Neter E, Bender NC. *Bacillus morgani*, type I, in enterocolitis of infants. J Pediatr 19:53, 1941.

98. Ujvary G, Lanyi B, Gregacs M, et al. Beobachtungen über die Ätiologie der Gastroenterocolitiden des Säu-

glings- und Kindesalters. III. Untersuchung der Rolle der *Proteus vulgaris*- und der *Proteus mirabilis*-Stamme. Acta Microbiol Acad Sci Hung 10:315, 1964.

99. Williams S. The bacteriological considerations of infantile enteritis in Sydney. Med J Aust 2:137, 1951.

100. Ujvary G, Voros S, Angyal T, et al. Beobachtungen über die Ätiologie der Gastroenterocolitiden des Säuglings-und Kindesalters. IV. Untersuchung der Rolle der *Proteus morgani*-Stamme. Acta Microbiol Acad Sci Hung 10:327, 1964.

101. Braun OH. *E. coli* enteritis in Germany: epidemiology and recent research. Ann N Y Acad Sci 176:126, 1971.

102. Rosebury T. Microorganisms Indigenous to Man. New York, McGraw-Hill, 1962.

103. Hone R, Keane CT, Fitzpatrick S. Faecal carriage of *Staphylococcus aureus* in infantile enteritis due to enteropathic *Escherichia coli*. Scand J Infect Dis 6:329, 1974.

104. Smith RT. Epidemic staphylococcal gastroenteritis in a newborn nursery. Am J Dis Child 92:45, 1956.

105. Gutman LT, Idriss ZH, Gehlbach S, et al. Neonatal staphylococcal enterocolitis: association with indwelling feeding catheters and *S. aureus* colonization. J Pediatr 88:836, 1976.

106. Erwa HH. Enterococci in diarrhoea of neonates. Trans R Soc Trop Med Hyg 66:359, 1972.

107. Giles D, Sangster G, Smith J. Epidemic gastro-enteritis of infants in Aberdeen during 1947. Arch Dis Child 24:45, 1949.

108. Sharpe ME. Group D streptococci in the faeces of healthy infants and of infants with neonatal diarrhea. J Hyg 50:209, 1952.

109. Thomson S. The role of certain varieties of *Bacterium coli* in gastroenteritis of babies. J Hyg 53:357, 1955.

110. Kohler H, Kite P. Neonatal enteritis due to *Providencia* organisms. Arch Dis Child 45:709, 1970.

111. Ridge LEL, Thomas MEM. Infection with the Providence type of *Paracolon bacillus* in a residential nursery. J Pathol Bacteriol 69:335, 1955.

112. Bhat P, Myers RM, Feldman RA. Providence group of organisms in the aetiology of juvenile diarrhoea. Indian J Med Res 59:1010, 1971.

113. Bishop RF, Barnes GL, Townley RRW. Microbial flora of stomach and small intestine in infantile gastroenteritis. Acta Paediatr Scand 63:418, 1974.

114. Martineau B, Raymond R, Jeliu G. Bacteriological and clinical study of gastroenteritis with enteropathogenic *Escherichia coli* 0127:B8. Can Med Assoc J 79:351, 1958.

115. Bray J. Isolation of antigenically homogeneous strains of *Bact. coli neopolitanum* from summer diarrhea of infants. J Pathol Bacteriol 57:239, 1945.

116. Rozansky R, Berant M, Rosenmann E, et al. Enteropathogenic *Escherichia coli* infections in infants during the period from 1957 to 1962. Pediatrics 64:521, 1964.

117. Omoike IU, Abiodun PO. Upper small intestine microflora in diarrhea and malnutrition in Nigerian children. J Pediatr Gastroenterol Nutr 9:314, 1989.

118. Kane JG, Chretien JH, Garagusi VF. Diarrhea caused by *Candida*. Lancet 1:335, 1976.

119. VonGerloczy F, Schmidt K, Scholz M. Beiträge zur Frage der Moniliasis in Säuglingsalter. Ann Pediatr (Paris) 187:119, 1956.

120. Hill HR, Mitchell TG, Matsen JM, et al. Recovery from disseminated candidiasis in a premature neonate. Pediatrics 53:748, 1974.

121. Faix RG. Systemic *Candida* infections in infants in intensive care nurseries: high incidence of central nervous system involvement. J Pediatr 105:616, 1984.

122. Baley JE, Kliegman RM, Fanaroff AA. Disseminated fun-

gal infections in very low birth weight infants: clinical manifestations and epidemiology. Pediatrics 73:144, 1984.

Parasites

1. Kotcher E, Mata LJ, Esquivel R, et al. Acquisition of intestinal parasites in newborn human infants. Abstract. Fed Proc 24:442, 1965.
2. Nnochiri E. Observations on childhood amoebiasis in urban family units in Nigeria. Am J Trop Med Hyg 68:231, 1965.
3. Knight R. Surveys for amoebiasis. Interpretations of data and their implications. Ann Trop Med Parasitol 69:35, 1975.
4. Axton JHM. Amoebic proctocolitis and liver abscess in a neonate. S Afr Med J 46:258, 1972.
5. Botman T, Rusy PJ. Amoebic appendicitis in a newborn infant. Trop Geogr Med 15:221, 1963.
6. Hsiung CC. Amebiasis of the newborn: report of three cases. Chin J Pathol 4:14, 1958. Quoted in Paracher UD, Holman RC, Breese JS, et al. Epidemiology of diarrheal disease among children enrolled in four West Coast health maintenance organizations. Pediatr Infect Dis J 17:605, 1998.
7. Dykes AC, Ruebush TK, Gorelkin L, et al. Extraintestinal amebiasis in infancy: report of three patients and epidemiologic investigations of their families. Pediatrics 65:799, 1980.
8. Mattern CFT, Deister DB. Experimental amebiasis. II. Hepatic amebiasis in the newborn hamster. Am J Trop Med Hyg 26:402, 1977.
9. Diamond LS, Tanimoto WM, Martinez-Palomo A. Lesions in newborn guinea pigs with anexically cultivated *Entamoeba histolytica*. Arch Invest Med (Mex) 9:233, 1978.
10. Ravdin JI. Amebiasis. Clin Infect Dis 20:1453, 1995.
11. Mirelman D, Nuchamowitz Y, Stolarsky T. Comparison of use of enzyme-linked immunosorbent assay-based kits and PCR amplification of rRNA genes for simultaneous detection of *Entamoeba histolytica* and *E. dispar.* J Clin Microbiol 35:2405, 1997.
12. Haque R, Ali IKM, Petri WA Jr. Comparison of PCR, isoenzyme analysis, and antigen detection for diagnosis of *Entamoeba histolytica* infection. J Clin Microbiol 36:449, 1998.
13. Adam RD. The biology of *Giardia* spp. Microbiol Rev 55:706, 1991.
14. Black RE, Dykes AC, Sinclair SP, et al. Giardiasis in day care centers. Evidence of person-to-person transmission. Pediatrics 60:486, 1977.
15. Keystone JS, Krajden S, Warren MR. Person-to-person transmission of *G. lamblia* in day care nurseries. Can Med Assoc J 119:241, 1978.
16. Pickering LK, Evans DG, DuPont HL, et al. Diarrhea caused by *Shigella*, rotavirus, and *Giardia* in day care centers: prospective study. J Pediatr 99:51, 1981.
17. Pickering LK, Woodward WE, DuPont HL, et al. Occurrence of *G. lamblia* in children in day care centers. J Pediatr 104:522, 1984.
18. Pickering LK, Engelkirk PG. *Giardia lamblia.* Pediatr Clin North Am 35:565, 1988.
19. Islam A, Stoll BJ, Ljungstrom I, et al. *Giardia lamblia* infections in a cohort of Bangladeshi mothers and infants followed for one year. J Pediatr 103:996, 1983.
20. Mahmud MA, Chappell C, Hossain MH, et al. Risk factors for development of first symptomatic *Giardia* infection among infants of a birth cohort in rural Egypt. Am J Trop Med Hyg 53:84, 1995.
21. Court JM, Stanton C. The incidence of *G. lamblia* infection of children in Victoria. Med J Aust 2:438, 1959.
22. Fraser D, Dagan R, Naggan L, et al. Natural history of *Giardia lamblia* and *Cryptosporidium* infections in a cohort of Israeli Bedouin infants: a study of a population in transition. Am J Trop Med Hyg 57:544, 1997.
23. Meuwissen JHE, Tongeren JHM, Werkman HPT. Giardiasis. Lancet 2:32, 1977.
24. Miotti PG, Gilman RH, Santosham M, et al. Age-related rate of seropositivity and antibody to *Giardia lamblia* in four diverse populations. J Clin Microbiol 24:972, 1986.
25. Burke JA. Giardiasis in childhood. Am J Dis Child 129:1304, 1975.
26. Morrow AL, Reves RR, West MS, et al. Protection against infection with *Giardia lamblia* by breast-feeding in a cohort of Mexican infants. J Pediatr 121:363, 1992.
27. Rosenthal P, Liebman WM. Comparative study of stool examinations, duodenal aspiration, and pediatric enterotest for giardiasis in children. J Pediatr 96:278, 1980.
28. Monaghan H, Garvey RG, Egan-Mitchell B, et al. Giardiasis in infancy diarrhoea. Arch Dis Child 55:715, 1980.
29. Walterspiel JN, Morrow AL, Guerrero ML, et al. Protective effect of secretory anti–*Giardia lamblia* antibodies in human milk against diarrhea. Pediatrics 93:28, 1994.
30. Gendrel D, Richard-Lenoble D, Kombila M, et al. Giardiasis and breastfeeding in urban Africa. Pediatr Infect Dis J 8:58, 1989.
31. Stevens DP, Frank DM. Local immunity in murine giardiasis: is milk protective at the expense of maternal gut? Trans Assoc Am Physicians 91:268, 1978.
32. Andrews JS Jr, Hewlett EL. Protection against infection with *Giardia muris* by milk containing antibody to *Giardia.* J Infect Dis 143:242, 1981.
33. Miotti P, Gilman R, Pickering LK, et al. Prevalence of serum and milk antibodies to *G. lamblia* in different populations of lactating women. J Infect Dis 152:1025, 1985.
34. Rohrer L, Winterhalter KH, Eckert J, et al. Killing of *G. lamblia* by human milk mediated by unsaturated fatty acids. Antimicrob Agents Chemother 30:254, 1986.
35. Current WL, Garcia LS. Cryptosporidiosis. Clin Microbiol Rev 4:325, 1991.
36. Heyworth MF. Immunology of *Giardia* and *Cryptosporidium* infections. J Infect Dis 166:465, 1992.
37. Manabe YC, Clark DP, Moore RD, et al. Cryptosporidiosis in patients with AIDS: correlates of disease and survival Clin Infect Dis 27:536, 1998.
38. Weikel CS, Johnston LI, deSousa ME, et al. Cryptosporidiosis in northeastern Brazil: association with sporadic diarrhea. J Infect Dis 151:963, 1985.
39. Navin TR. Cryptosporidiosis in humans: review of recent epidemiologic studies. Eur J Epidemiol 1:77, 1985.
40. Alpert G, Bell LM, Kirkpatrick CE, et al. Outbreak of cryptosporidiosis in a day care center. Pediatrics 77:152, 1986.
41. Taylor JP, Perdue JN, Dingley D, et al. Cryptosporidiosis outbreak in a day care center. Am J Dis Child 139:1023, 1986.
42. Wolfson IS, Richter JM, Waldron MA, et al. Cryptosporidiosis in immunocompetent patients. N Engl J Med 312:1278, 1985.
43. Enriquez FJ, Avila CR, Santos JI, et al. *Cryptosporidium* infections in Mexican children: clinical, nutritional, enteropathogenic, and diagnostic evaluations. Am J Trop Med Hyg 56:254, 1997.
44. Agnew DG, Lima AAM, Newman RD, et al. Cryptosporidiosis in northeastern Brazilian children: association

with increased diarrhea morbidity. J Infect Dis 177:754, 1998.

45. Jokipii L, Jokipii AMM. Timing of symptoms and oocyst excretion in human cryptosporidiosis. N Engl J Med 313:1643, 1986.

46. Tzipori S. Cryptosporidiosis in animals and humans. Microbiol Rev 47:84, 1983.

47. Stehr-Green JK, McCaig L, Remsen HM, et al. Shedding of oocysts in immunocompetent individuals infected with *Cryptosporidium*. Am J Trop Med Hyg 36:338, 1987.

48. Soave R, Ma P. Cryptosporidiosis travelers' diarrhea in two families. Arch Intern Med 145:70, 1985.

49. Collier AC, Miller RA, Meyers JD. Cryptosporidiosis after marrow transplantation, person-to-person transmission and treatment with spiramycin. Ann Intern Med 101:205, 1984.

50. Hoxie NJ, Davis JP, Vergeront JM, et al. Cryptosporidiosis-associated mortality following a massive waterborne outbreak in Milwaukee, Wisconsin. Am J Public Health 87:2032, 1997.

51. Mata L, Bolanos H, Pizarro D, et al. Cryptosporidiosis in children from some highland Costa Rican rural and urban areas. Am J Trop Med Hyg 33:24, 1984.

52. Montessori GA, Bischoff L. Cryptosporidiosis: a cause of summer diarrhea in children. Can Med Assoc J 132:1285, 1985.

53. Jokipii L, Pohiola S, Jokipii AM. *Cryptosporidium*: a frequent finding in patients with gastrointestinal symptoms. Lancet 2:358, 1983.

54. Current WL, Reese NC, Ernst JV, et al. Human cryptosporidiosis in immunocompetent and immunodeficient persons: studies of an outbreak and experimental transmission. N Engl J Med 308:1252, 1983.

55. Sallon S, Deckelbaum RI, Schmid II, et al. *Cryptosporidium*, malnutrition and chronic diarrhea in children. Am J Dis Child 142:312, 1988.

56. MacPherson DW, McQueen R. Crytosporidiosis: multiattribute evaluation of six diagnostic methods. J Clin Microbiol 31:198, 1993.

57. Garcia LS, Shimizu RY. Evaluation of nine immunoassay kits (enzyme immunoassay and direct fluorescence) for detection of *Giardia lamblia* and *Cryptosporidium parvum* in human fecal specimens. J Clin Microbiol 35:1526, 1997.

58. Arrowood MJ, Mead JR, Mahrt JL, et al. Effects of immune colostrum and orally administered anti-sporozoite monoclonal antibodies on the outcome of *Cryptosporidium parvum* infections in neonatal mice. Infect Immun 57:2283, 1989.

59. Perryman LE, Riggs MW, Mason PH, et al. Kinetics of *Cryptosporidium parvum* sporozoite neutralization by monoclonal antibodies, immune bovine serum, and immune bovine colostrum. Infect Immun 58:257, 1990.

60. Peterson C, Gut J, Doyle PS, et al. Characterization of a >900,000-M$_r$ *Cryptosporidium parvum* sporozoite glycoprotein recognized by protective hyperimmune bovine colostral immunoglobulin. Infect Immun 60:5132, 1992.

Viruses

1. Kapikian AZ. Viral gastroenteritis. JAMA 269:627, 1993.
2. Christensen ML. Human viral gastroenteritis. Clin Microbiol Rev 2:51, 1989.
3. Blacklow NR, Greenberg HB. Viral gastroenteritis. N Engl J Med 325:252, 1991.
4. O'Ryan M, Matson DO, Pickering LK. Rotavirus, enteric adenoviruses, Norwalk virus and other gastroenteri-

tis viruses. *In* Spector S, Lancz G (eds). Clinical Virology Manual, 2nd ed. New York, Elsevier, 1992, pp 361–396.

5. Kapikian AZ, Wyatt RG, Dolin R, et al. Visualization by immune electron microscopy of a 27-nm particle associated with acute infectious nonbacterial gastroenteritis. J Virol 10:1075, 1972.

6. Bishop RF, Davidson GP, Holmes IH, et al. Virus particles in epithelial cells of duodenal mucosa from children with acute nonbacterial gastroenteritis. Lancet 2:1281, 1973.

7. Brandt CD, Kim HW, Rodriguez WJ, et al. Adenoviruses and pediatric gastroenteritis. J Infect Dis 151:437, 1985.

8. Grohmann G, Glass RI, Gold J, et al. Outbreak of human calicivirus gastroenteritis in a day-care center in Sydney, Australia. J Clin Microbiol 29:544, 1991.

9. Van R, Wun CC, O'Ryan ML, et al. Outbreaks of human enteric adenovirus types 40 and 41 in Houston day care centers. J Pediatr 120:516, 1992.

10. Jarecki-Khan K, Tzipori SR, Unicomb LE. Enteric adenovirus infection among infants with diarrhea in rural Bangladesh. J Clin Microbiol 31:484, 1993.

11. Matson DO, Estes MK, Glass RI, et al. Human calicivirus-associated diarrhea in children attending day care centers. J Infect Dis 159:71, 1989.

12. Fankhauser RL, Noel JS, Monroe SS, et al. Molecular epidemiology of "Norwalk-like viruses" in outbreaks of gastroenteritis in the United States. J Infect Dis 178:1571, 1998.

13. Herrmann JE, Taylor DN, Echeverria P, et al. Astroviruses as a cause of gastroenteritis in children. N Engl J Med 324:1757, 1991.

14. Kotloff KL, Herrmann JE, Blacklow NR, et al. The frequency of astrovirus as a cause of diarrhea in Baltimore children. Pediatr Infect Dis J 11:587, 1992.

15. Esahli H, Breback K, Bennet R, et al. Astroviruses as a cause of nosocomial outbreaks of infant diarrhea. Pediatr Infect Dis J 10:511, 1991.

16. Mitchell DK, Van R, Morrow AL, et al. Outbreaks of astrovirus gastroenteritis in day care centers. J Pediatr 123:725, 1993.

17. Jiang X, Graham DY, Wang K, et al. Norwalk virus genome cloning and characterization. Science 250:1580, 1990.

18. Flewett RH, Bryden AS, Davies H, et al. Relation between viruses from acute gastrocntcritis of children and newborn calves. Lancet 2:61, 1974.

19. Martin ML, Palmer EL, Middleton PJ. Ultrastructure of infantile gastroenteritis virus. J Virol 68:146, 1975.

20. Estes MK, Cohen J. Rotavirus gene structure and function. Microbiol Rev 53:410, 1989.

21. Taniguchi K, Urasawa T, Kobayashi N, et al. Nucleotide sequence of vp4 and vp7 genes of human rotaviruses with subgroup 1 specificity and long RNA pattern: implication for new G serotype specificity. J Virol 64:5640, 1990.

22. Gouvea V, Ramirez C, Li B, et al. Restriction endonuclease analysis of the vp7 genes of human and animal rotaviruses. J Clin Microbiol 31:917, 1993.

23. Gerna G, Sarasini A, Coulson BS, et al. Comparative sensitivities of solid-phase immune microscopy and enzyme-linked immunosorbent assay for serotyping of human rotavirus strains with neutralizing monoclonal antibodies. J Clin Microbiol 26:1383, 1988.

24. Green KY, Sears JF, Taniguchi K, et al. Prediction of human rotavirus serotype by nucleotide sequence analysis of the VP7 protein gene. J Virol 62:1819, 1988.

25. Ramachandran M, Gentsch JR, Parashar UD, et al. Detection and characterization of novel rotavirus strains in the United States. J Clin Microbiol 36:3223, 1998.

26. Gouvea V, Allen JR, Glass RI, et al. Detection of group B and C rotaviruses by polymerase chain reaction. J Clin Microbiol 29:519, 1991.

27. Kuzuya M, Fujii R, Hamano M, et al. Rapid detection of human group C rotaviruses by reverse passive hemagglutination and latex agglutination tests using monoclonal antibodies. J Clin Microbiol 31:1308, 1993.

28. Palmer EL, Martin ML, Murphy FA. Morphology and stability of infantile gastroenteritis virus: comparison with reovirus and bluetongue virus. J Gen Virol 35:403, 1977.

29. Graham DY, Estes MK. Proteolytic enhancement of rotavirus infectivity: biologic mechanisms. J Virol 101:432, 1980.

30. Bishop RF, Barnes GL, Cipriani E, et al. Clinical immunity after neonatal rotavirus infection. A prospective longitudinal study in young children. N Engl J Med 309:72, 1983.

31. Bhan MK, Lew JF, Sazawal S, et al. Protection conferred by neonatal rotavirus infection against subsequent rotavirus diarrhea. J Infect Dis 168:282, 1993.

32. Chiba S, Nakata S, Urasawa T, et al. Protective effect of naturally acquired homotypic and heterotypic rotavirus antibodies. Lancet 1:417, 1986.

33. Greene KY, Kapikian AZ. Identification of VP7 epitopes associated with protection against human rotavirus illness or shedding in volunteers. J Virol 66:548, 1992.

34. Hjelt K, Grauballe PC, Paerregaard A, et al. Protective effect of pre-existing rotavirus-specific immunoglobulin A against naturally acquired rotavirus infection in children. J Med Virol 21:39, 1987.

35. Matson DO, O'Ryan ML, Estes MK, et al. Characterization of serum antibody responses to natural rotavirus infections in children by VP7-specific epitope-blocking assays. J Clin Microbiol 30:1056, 1992.

36. Ward RL, Knowlton DR, Schiff GM, et al. Relative concentrations of serum neutralizing antibody to VP3 and VP7 protein in adults infected with human rotavirus. J Virol 62:1543, 1988.

37. Clemens JD, Ward RL, Rao MR, et al. Seroepidemiologic evaluation of antibodies to rotavirus as correlates of the risk of clinically significant rotavirus diarrhea in rural Bangladesh. J Infect Dis 165:161, 1992.

38. Zheng BJ, Lo SK, Tam Jr J, et al. Prospective study of community-acquired rotavirus infection. J Clin Microbiol 27:2083, 1989.

39. Ward RL, Clemens JD, Knowlton DR, et al. Evidence that protection against rotavirus diarrhea after natural infection is not dependent on serotype-specific neutralizing antibody. J Infect Dis 166:1251, 1992.

40. Dyall-Smith ML, Lazdins I, Tregear GW, et al. Location of the major antigenic sites involved in rotavirus serotype-specific neutralization. Proc Natl Acad Sci USA 83:3465, 1986.

41. Matsui SM, Offit PA, Vo PT, et al. Passive protection against rotavirus-induced diarrhea by monoclonal antibodies to the heterotypic neutralization domain of VP7 and the VP8 fragment of VP4. J Clin Microbiol 27:780, 1989.

42. O'Ryan ML, Matson DO, Estes MK, et al. Anti-rotavirus G type-specific and isotype-specific antibodies in children with natural rotavirus infection. J Infect Dis 169:504, 1994.

43. Matson DO, O'Ryan ML, Pickering LK, et al. Assessment of epitope-blocking assays to measure antibody to rotavirus. J Virol Methods 48:293, 1994.

44. Hjelt K, Grauballe PC, Schiotz PO, et al. Intestinal and serum immune response to a naturally acquired rotavirus gastroenteritis in children. J Pediatr Gastroenterol Nutr 4:60, 1985.

45. Grimwood K, Lund JCS, Coulson BS, et al. Comparison of serum and mucosal antibody responses following severe acute rotavirus gastroenteritis in young children. J Clin Microbiol 26:732, 1988.

46. Hjelt K, Grauballe PC, Andersen L, et al. Antibody response in serum and intestine in children up to six months after a naturally acquired rotavirus gastroenteritis. J Pediatr Gastroenterol Nutr 5:74, 1986.

47. Losonsky GA, Reymann M. The immune response in primary asymptomatic and symptomatic rotavirus infection in newborn infants. J Infect Dis 161:330, 1990.

48. Coulson BS, Grimwood K, Masendycz PJ, et al. Comparison of rotavirus immunoglobulin A coproconversion with other indices of rotavirus infection in a longitudinal study in childhood. J Clin Microbiol 28:1367, 1990.

49. Losonsky GA, Rennels MB, Lim Y, et al. Systemic and mucosal immune responses to rhesus rotavirus vaccine MMU18006. Pediatr Infect Dis J 7:388, 1988.

50. Coulson BS, Grimwood K, Hudson IL, et al. Role of coproantibody in clinical protection of children during reinfection with rotavirus. J Clin Microbiol 30:1678, 1992.

51. Matson DO, O'Ryan ML, Herrera I, et al. Fecal antibody responses to symptomatic and asymptomatic rotavirus infections. J Infect Dis 167:577, 1993.

52. Morrow AL, Pickering LK. Human milk protection against diarrheal disease. Semin Pediatr Infect Dis 5:236, 1994.

53. Brhssow H, Sidoti J, Lerner L, et al. Antibodies to seven rotavirus serotypes in cord sera, maternal sera, and colostrum of German women. J Clin Microbiol 29:2856, 1991.

54. Brhssow H, Benitez O, Uribe F, et al. Rotavirus-inhibitory activity in serial milk samples from Mexican women and rotavirus infections in their children during their first year of life. J Clin Microbiol 31:593, 1993.

55. Totterdell BM, Chrystie IL, Banatvala JE. Cord blood and breast milk antibodies in neonatal rotavirus infection. BMJ 1:828, 1980.

56. Yolken RH, Wyatt RG, Zissis G, et al. Epidemiology of human rotavirus types 1 and 2 as studied by enzyme-linked immunosorbent assay. N Engl J Med 299:1156, 1978.

57. McLean B, Holmes IH. Transfer of anti-rotaviral antibodies from mothers to their infants. J Clin Microbiol 12:320, 1980.

58. McLean BS, Holmes IH. Effects of antibodies, trypsin, and trypsin inhibitors on susceptibility of neonates to rotavirus infection. J Clin Microbiol 13:22, 1981.

59. Yolken RH, Wyatt RG, Mata L, et al. Secretory antibody directed against rotavirus in human milk—measurement by means of enzyme-linked immunosorbent assay. J Pediatr 93:916, 1978.

60. Weinberg RJ, Tipton G, Klish WJ, et al. Effect of breast-feeding on morbidity in rotavirus gastroenteritis. Pediatrics 74:250, 1984.

61. Glass RI, Stoll BJ, Wyatt RG, et al. Observations questioning a protective role for breast-feeding in severe rotavirus diarrhea. Acta Paediatr Scand 75:713, 1986.

62. Duffy LC, Riepenhoff-Talty M, Byers TE, et al. Modulation of rotavirus enteritis during breast-feeding. Am J Dis Child 140:1164, 1986.

63. Yolken RH, Peterson JA, Vonderfecht SL, et al. Human milk mucin inhibits rotavirus replication and prevents experimental gastroenteritis. J Clin Invest 90:1984, 1992.

64. Newburg DS, Peterson JA, Ruiz-Palacios GM, et al.

High levels of lactadherin in human milk are associated with protection against symptomatic rotavirus infection amongst breast-fed infants. Lancet 351:1160, 1998.

65. Shepherd RW, Gall DG, Butler DG, et al. Determinants of diarrhea in viral enteritis. The role of ion transport and epithelial changes in the ileum in transmissible gastroenteritis in piglets. Gastroenterology 76:20, 1979.

66. Holmes IH, Rodger SM, Schnagl RD, et al. Is lactase the receptor and uncoating enzyme for infantile enteritis (rota) viruses? Lancet 1:1387, 1976.

67. Shepherd RW, Butler DG, Cutz E, et al. The mucosal lesion in viral enteritis. Extent and dynamics of the epithelial response to virus invasion in transmissible gastroenteritis of piglets. Gastroenterology 76:770, 1979.

68. Cameron DJS, Bishop RF, Veenstra A, et al. Noncultivable viruses and neonatal diarrhea. Fifteen-month survey in a newborn special care nursery. J Clin Microbiol 8:93, 1978.

69. Lebenthal E. Lactose malabsorption and milk consumption in infants and children. Am J Dis Child 133:21, 1979.

70. Jesudoss ES, John TJ, Maiya PP, et al. Prevalence of rotavirus infection in neonates. Indian J Med Res 70:863, 1979.

71. Bishop RF, Cameron DJS, Veenstra AA, et al. Diarrhea and rotavirus infection associated with differing regimens for postnatal care of newborn babies. J Clin Microbiol 9:525, 1979.

72. Pickering LK, Bartlett AV, Reves RR, et al. Asymptomatic rotavirus before and after rotavirus diarrhea in children in day care centers. J Pediatr 112:361, 1988.

73. Vesikari T, Sarkkinen HK, Maki M. Quantitative aspects of rotavirus excretion in childhood diarrhoea. Acta Paediatr Scand 70:717, 1981.

74. Carlson JAK, Middleton PH, Szymanski MT, et al. Fatal rotavirus gastroenteritis. An analysis of 21 cases. Am J Dis Child 132:477, 1978.

75. Gilger MA, Matson DO, Conner ME, et al. Extraintestinal spread of rotavirus infections in children with immunodeficiency. J Pediatr 120:912, 1992.

76. Holmes IH, Ruck BJ, Bishop RF, et al. Infantile enteritis viruses: morphogenesis and morphology. J Virol 16:937, 1975.

77. Suzuki H, Konno T. Reovirus-like particles in jejunal mucosa of a Japanese infant with acute infectious nonbacterial gastroenteritis. Tohoku J Exp Med 115:199, 1975.

78. Graham DY, Estes MK. Comparison of methods for immunocytochemical detection of rotavirus infections. Infect Immun 26:686, 1979.

79. Saulsbury FT, Winklestein JA, Yolken RH. Chronic rotavirus infection in immunodeficiency. J Pediatr 97:61, 1980.

80. Kerzner B, Kelly MH, Gall DG, et al. Transmissible gastroenteritis: sodium transport and the intestinal epithelium during the course of viral gastroenteritis. Gastroenterology 72:457, 1977.

81. Gall DG, Chapman D, Kelly M, et al. Na$^+$ transport in jejunal crypt cells. Gastroenterology 72:452, 1977.

82. Tallet S, MacKenzie C, Middleton P, et al. Clinical, laboratory, and epidemiologic features of a viral gastroenteritis in infants and children. Pediatrics 60:217, 1977.

83. Pullan CR, Dellagrammatikas H, Steiner H. Survey of gastroenteritis in children admitted to hospital in Newcastle upon Tyne in 1971–1975. BMJ 1:619, 1977.

84. Madeley CR, Cosgrove BP, Bell EJ, et al. Stool viruses in babies in Glasgow. I. Hospital admissions with diarrhoea. J Hyg 78:261, 1977.

85. Soenarto Y, Sebodo T, Ridho R, et al. Acute diarrhea and rotavirus infection in newborn babies and children in Yogyakarta, Indonesia from June 1978 to June 1979. J Clin Microbiol 14:123, 1981.

86. van Renterghem L, Borre P, Tilleman J. Rotavirus and other viruses in the stool of premature babies. J Med Virol 5:137, 1980.

87. Murphy AM, Albrey MB, Crewe EB. Rotavirus infections in neonates. Lancet 2:1149, 1977.

88. Appleton H, Buckley M, Robertson MH, et al. A search for faecal viruses in newborn and other infants. J Hyg 81:279, 1978.

89. Santosham M, et al. Neonatal rotavirus infection. Lancet 1:1070, 1982.

90. Madeley CR, Cosgrove BP, Bell EJ. Stool viruses in babies in Glasgow. 2. Investigation of normal newborns in hospital. J Hyg 81:285, 1978.

91. Glasgow JFT, McClure BG, Connolly J, et al. Nosocomial rotavirus gastroenteritis in a neonatal nursery. Ulster Med J 47:50, 1978.

92. Cameron DJS, Bishop RF, Davidson G, et al. New virus associated with diarrhoea in neonates. Med J Aust 1:85, 1976.

93. Bryden AS, Thouless ME, Hall CJ, et al. Rotavirus infections in a special-care baby unit. J Infect 4:43, 1982.

94. Grillner L, Broberger U, Chrystie I, et al. Rotavirus infections in newborns: an epidemiological and clinical study. Scand J Infect Dis 17:349, 1985.

95. Tufvesson B, Polberger L, Svanberg L, et al. A prospective study of rotavirus infections in neonatal and maternity wards. Acta Paediatr Scand 75:211, 1986.

96. Hoshino Y, Wyatt RG, Flores J, et al. Serotypic characterization of rotaviruses derived from asymptomatic human neonatal infections. J Clin Microbiol 21:425, 1985.

97. Crewe E, Murphy AM. Further studies on neonatal rotavirus infection. Med J Aust 1:61, 1980.

98. Perez-Schael I, Daoud G, White L, et al. Rotavirus shedding by newborn children. J Med Virol 14:127, 1984.

99. Vial PA, Kotloff KL, Losonsky GA. Molecular epidemiology of rotavirus infection in a room for convalescing newborns. J Infect Dis 157:668, 1988.

100. Haffejee IE. Neonatal rotavirus infections. Rev Infect Dis 13:957, 1991.

101. Rodriguez WJ, Kim HW, Brandt CD, et al. Rotavirus: a cause of nosocomial infection in a nursery. J Pediatr 101:274, 1982.

102. Bishop RF, Barnes GL, Cipriani E, et al. Clinical immunity after neonatal rotavirus infection. N Engl J Med 309:72, 1983.

103. Velazquez FR, Calva JJ, Guerrero ML, et al. Cohort study of rotavirus serotype patterns in symptomatic and asymptomatic infections in Mexican children. Pediatr Infect Dis J 12:54, 1993.

104. Velazquez FR, Matson DO, Calva JJ, et al. Rotavirus infections in infants as protection against subsequent infections. N Engl J Med 335:1022, 1996.

105. Tufvesson B, Johnsson T. Occurrence of reo-like viruses in young children with acute gastroenteritis. Acta Pathol Microbiol Scand [B] 84:22, 1976.

106. Gurwith MJ, Williams TW. Gastroenteritis in children: a two year review in Manitoba. I. Etiology. J Infect Dis 136:239, 1977.

107. Muchinik GR, Grinstein S. Rotavirus in Buenos Aires, Argentina. Intervirology 13:253, 1980.

108. Mutanda LN, Epidemiology of acute gastroenteritis in early childhood in Kenya. III. Distribution of the etiological agents. East Afr Med J 57:317, 1980.

109. Brandt CD, Kim HW, Yolken RH, et al. Comparative epidemiology of two rotavirus serotypes and other viral

agents associated with pediatric gastroenteritis. Am J Epidemiol 110:243, 1979.

110. Schnagl RD, Holmes IH, MacKay-Scollay EM. A survey of rotavirus associated with gastroenteritis in aboriginal children in western Australia. Med J Aust 1:304, 1978.

111. Bartlett AV, Reves RR, Pickering LK. Rotavirus in infant-toddler day care centers: epidemiology relevant to disease control strategies. J Pediatr 113:435, 1988.

112. Middleton PJ, Szymanski MT, Petric M. Viruses associated with acute gastroenteritis in young children. Am J Dis Child 131:733, 1977.

113. Birch CJ, Lewis FA, Kennett ML, et al. A study of the prevalence of rotavirus infection in children with gastroenteritis admitted to an infectious disease hospital. J Med Virol 1:69, 1977.

114. Cruickshank JG, Zilberg B. Winter diarrhoea and rotaviruses in Rhodesia. S Afr Med J 50:1895, 1976.

115. Viera de Torres B, Mazzali de Ilja R, Esparza J. Epidemiological aspects of rotavirus infection in hospitalized Venezuelan children with gastroenteritis. Am J Trop Med Hyg 27:567, 1978.

116. Hieber JP, Shelton S, Nelson JD, et al. Comparison of human rotavirus disease in tropical and temperate settings. Am J Dis Child 132:853, 1978.

117. Dossetor JFB, Chrystie IL, Totterdell BM. Rotavirus gastroenteritis in northern Nigeria. Trans R Soc Trop Med Hyg 73:115, 1979.

118. Espeja RT, Calderon E, Gonzalez N, et al. Presence of two distinct types of rotavirus in infants and young children hospitalized with acute gastroenteritis in Mexico City, 1977. J Infect Dis 139:474, 1979.

119. Bantavala JE. The role of viruses in acute diarrhoeal disease. Clin Gastroenterol 8:569, 1979.

120. Schnagl RD, Morey F, Holmes IH. Rotavirus and coronavirus-like particles in aboriginal and non-aboriginal neonates in Kalgoorlie and Alice Springs. Med J Aust 2:178, 1979.

121. Dearlove J, Latham P, Dearlove B, et al. Clinical range of neonatal rotavirus gastroenteritis. BMJ 286:1473, 1983.

122. Parashar UD, Holman RC, Bresee JS, et al. Epidemiology of diarrheal disease among children enrolled in four West Coast health maintenance organizations. Pediatr Infect Dis J 17:605, 1998.

123. Leece JC, King MW, Dorsey WE. Rearing regimen producing piglet diarrhea (rotavirus) and its relevance to acute infantile diarrhea. Science 199:776, 1978.

124. Woode GN, Bridger J, Hall GA, et al. The isolation of reovirus-like agents (rotaviruses) from acute gastroenteritis in piglets. J Med Microbiol 9:203, 1976.

125. Flewett TH, Bryden AS, Davies H, et al. Epidemic viral enteritis in a longstay children's ward. Lancet 1:4, 1975.

126. Ryder RW, McGowan JE Jr, Hatch MH, et al. Reovirus-like agent as a cause of nosocomial diarrhea in infants. J Pediatr 90:698, 1977.

127. Chiba S, Akihara M, Kogasaka R, et al. An outbreak of acute gastroenteritis due to rotavirus in an infant home. Tohoku J Exp Med 127:265, 1979.

128. O'Ryan ML, Matson DO, Estes MK, et al. Molecular epidemiology of rotavirus in children attending day care centers (DCC) in Houston. J Infect Dis 162:810, 1990.

129. Pickering LK, Evans DG, DuPont HL, et al. Diarrhea due to *Shigella*, rotavirus, and *Giardia* in day-care centers: prospective study. J Pediatr 99:51, 1981.

130. Prince DS, Astry C, Vonderfecht S, et al. Aerosol transmission of experimental rotavirus infection. Pediatr Infect Dis J 5:218, 1986.

131. Champsaur H, Questiaux E, Prevot J, et al. Rotavirus carriage, asymptomatic infection, and disease in the first

132. Krause PJ, Hyams JS, Middleton PJ, et al. Unreliability of Rotazyme ELISA test in neonates. J Pediatr 103:259, 1983.

133. Rotbart HA, Yolken RH, Nelson WL, et al. Confirmatory testing of Rotazyme results in neonates. J Pediatr 107:289, 1985.

134. Albrey MB, Murphy AM. Rotaviruses and acute gastroenteritis of infants and children. Med J Aust 1:82, 1976.

135. Steele AD, Alexander JJ. Molecular epidemiology of rotavirus in black infants in South Africa. J Clin Microbiol 25:2384, 1987.

136. Rodriguez WJ, Kim HW, Brandt CD, et al. Use of electrophoresis of RNA from human rotavirus to establish the identity of stains involved in outbreaks in a tertiary care nursery. J Infect Dis 148:34, 1983.

137. Mutanda LN. Epidemiology of acute gastroenteritis in early childhood in Kenya. VI. Some clinical and laboratory characteristics relative to the aetiological agents. East Afr Med J 57:599, 1980.

138. Morishima T, Ichikawa T, Yamaguchi H, et al. Acute infantile gastroenteritis caused by rotavirus in Japan. Eur J Pediatr 129:259, 1978.

139. Nagayoshi S, Yamaguchi H, Ichikawa T, et al. Changes of the rotavirus concentration in faeces during the course of acute gastroenteritis as determined by the immune adherence hemagglutination test. Eur J Pediatr 134:99, 1980.

140. Rodriguez WJ, Kim HW, Brandt CD, et al. Sequential enteric illness associated with different rotavirus serotypes. Letter to the editor. Lancet 2:37, 1978.

141. Pickering LK, DuPont HL, Olarte J, et al. Fecal leukocytes in enteric infections. Am J Clin Pathol 68:562, 1977.

142. Goldwater PN. Gastroenteritis in Auckland: an aetiological and clinical study. J Infect Dis 1:399, 1979.

143. Whyte RK, Homes R, Pennock CA. Faecal excretion of oligosaccharides and other carbohydrates in normal neonates. Arch Dis Child 53:913, 1978.

144. Hyams JS, Krause PJ, Gleason PA. Lactose malabsorption following rotavirus infection in young children. J Pediatr 99:916, 1981.

145. Taylor PR, Merson MH, Black RE, et al. Oral rehydration therapy for treatment of rotavirus diarrhoea in a rural treatment centre in Bangladesh. Arch Dis Child 55:376, 1980.

146. Black RE, Merson MH, Rahman ASMM, et al. A two-year study of bacterial, viral, and parasitic agents associated with diarrhea in rural Bangladesh. J Infect Dis 142:660, 1980.

147. Rotbart HA, Levin MJ, Yolken RH, et al. An outbreak of rotavirus-associated neonatal necrotizing enterocolitis. J Pediatr 103:454, 1983.

148. American Academy of Pediatrics, Committee on Infectious Diseases. Prevention of rotavirus disease: guidelines for use of rotavirus vaccine. Pediatrics 102:1483, 1998.

149. Recommendations of the Advisory Committee on Immunization Practices (ACIP), Centers for Disease Control and Prevention. Rotavirus vaccine for the prevention of rotavirus gastroenteritis among children. MMWR Morb Mortal Wkly Rep 48:1, 1999.

150. Brandt CD, Kim HW, Rodriguez WJ, et al. Comparison of direct electron microscopy, immune electron microscopy, and rotavirus enzyme-linked immunosorbent assay for detection of gastroenteritis viruses in children. J Clin Microbiol 13:976, 1981.

151. Yolken RH, Kim HW, Clem T, et al. Enzyme-linked

two years of life. I. Virus shedding. J Infect Dis 149:667, 1984.

immunosorbent assay (ELISA) for detection of human reovirus-like agent of infantile gastroenteritis. Lancet 2:263, 1977.

152. Wilde J, Van R, Pickering LK, et al. Rotaviruses in the day care environment—detection by reverse transcriptase polymerase chain reaction. J Infect Dis 166:507, 1992.

153. Flewett TH. Electron microscopy in the diagnosis of infectious diarrheas. J Am Vet Med Assoc 173:538, 1978.

154. Kapikian AZ, Chanock RM. Rotaviruses. In Fields BN, Knipe DM, Howley PM, et al (eds). Fields Virology, 3rd ed. Philadelphia, Lippincott-Raven, 1996, p. 1657.

155. Gilchrist MJR, Bretl TS, Moultney K, et al. Comparison of seven kits for detection of rotavirus in fecal specimens with a sensitive, specific enzyme immunoassay. Diagn Microbiol Infect Dis 8:221, 1987.

156. Knisley CV, Bednarz-Prashad A, Pickering LK. Detection of rotavirus in stool specimens with monoclonal and polyclonal antibody–based assay systems. J Clin Microbiol 23:897, 1986.

157. Thomas EE, Puterman ML, Kawano E, et al. Evaluation of seven immunoassays for detection of rotavirus in pediatric stool samples. J Clin Microbiol 26:1189, 1988.

158. Miotti PG, Eiden J, Yolken RH. Comparative efficacy of commercial immunoassays for the diagnosis of rotavirus gastroenteritis during the course of infection. J Clin Microbiol 22:693, 1985.

159. Chrystie IL, Totterdell BM, Banatvala JE. False positive Rotazyme tests on fecal samples from babies. Lancet 2:1028, 1983.

160. Herrmann JE, Blacklow NR, Perron DM, et al. Enzyme immunoassay with monoclonal antibodies for the detection of rotavirus in stool specimens. J Infect Dis 152:830, 1985.

161. Prey MU, Lorelle CA, Taff TA. Evaluation of three commercially available rotavirus detection methods for neonatal specimens. Am J Clin Pathol 89:675, 1988.

162. Rand KH, Houck HJ, Swingle HM. Rotazyme assay in neonates without diarrhea. Am J Clin Pathol 84:748, 1985.

163. Lebaron CW, Allen JR, Hebert M, et al. Outbreaks of summer rotavirus linked to laboratory practices. Pediatr Infect Dis J 11:860, 1992.

164. Provisional Committee on Quality Improvement, Subcommittee on Acute Gastroenteritis. Practice parameter: the management of acute gastroenteritis in young children. Pediatrics 97:424, 1996.

165. Pizarro D, Posada G, Mata L, et al. Oral rehydration of neonates with dehydrating diarrhoeas. Lancet 2:1209, 1979.

166. Sack DA, Eusof A, Merson MH, et al. Oral hydration in rotavirus diarrhoea: a double-blind comparison of sucrose with glucose electrolyte solution. Lancet 2:280, 1978.

167. Black RE, Merson MH, Taylor PR, et al. Glucose vs. sucrose in oral rehydration solutions for infants and young children with rotavirus-associated diarrhea. Pediatrics 67:79, 1981.

168. Yolken RH, Willoughby R, Wee SB, et al. Sialic acid glycoproteins inhibit in vitro and in vivo replication of rotaviruses. J Clin Invest 79:148, 1987.

169. Barnes GL, Hewson PM, McLellan JA, et al. A randomized trial of oral gammaglobulin in low birth weight infants infected with rotavirus. Lancet 1:1371, 1983.

170. Guarino A, Guandalini S, Albano F, et al. Enteral immunoglobulins for treatment of protracted rotaviral diarrhea. Pediatr Infect Dis J 10:612, 1991.

171. Berger R, Hadziselimovic F, Just M, et al. Influence of breast milk on nosocomial rotavirus infections in infants. Infection 12:171, 1984.

172. Hilpert H, Brhssow H, Mietens C, et al. Use of bovine milk concentrate containing antibody to rotavirus to treat rotavirus gastroenteritis in infants. J Infect Dis 156:158, 1987.

173. Ebina T, Sato A, Umezu K, et al. Prevention of rotavirus infection by oral administration of cow colostrum containing antihuman rotavirus antibody. Med Microbiol Immunol 174:177, 1985.

Differential Diagnosis

1. Bill AH Jr, Chapman ND. The enterocolitis of Hirschsprung's disease. Its natural history and treatment. Am J Surg 103:70, 1962.

2. Stockdale EM, Miller CA. Persistent diarrhea as the predominant symptom of Hirschsprung's disease (congenital dilatation of colon). Pediatrics 19:91, 1957.

3. Wilmore DW. Factors correlating with a successful outcome following extensive intestinal resection in newborn infants. J Pediatr 80:88, 1972.

4. Fried D, Gotlieb A, Zaidel L. Intractable diarrhea of infancy due to lymphangiectasis. Am J Dis Child 127:416, 1974.

5. Lebenthal E. Small intestinal disaccharidase deficiency. Pediatr Clin North Am 22:757, 1975.

6. Ament ME, Perera DR, Esther LJ. Sucrase-isomaltose deficiency—a frequently misdiagnosed disease. J Pediatr 83:721, 1973.

7. Marks JF, Norton JB, Fordtran JS. Glucose-galactose malabsorption. J Pediatr 69:225, 1969.

8. Burke V, Anderson CM. Sugar intolerance as a cause of protracted diarrhea following surgery of the gastrointestinal tract in neonates. Aust Paediatr J 2:219, 1966.

9. Bishop RF, Davidson GP, Holmes IH, et al. Virus particles in epithelial cells of duodenal mucosa from children with acute non-bacterial gastroenteritis. Lancet 2:1281, 1973.

10. Coello-Ramirez P, Lifshitz F, Zuniga V. Enteric microflora and carbohydrate intolerance in infants with diarrhea. Pediatrics 49:233, 1972.

11. Akesode F, Lifshitz F, Hoffman KM. Transient monosaccharide intolerance in a newborn infant. Pediatrics 51:891, 1973.

12. Lucking T, Gruttner R. Chronic diarrhea and severe malabsorption in infancy following infections with pathogenic E. coli. Acta Paediatr Scand 63:167, 1974.

13. Iyngkaran N, Davis K, Robinson MJ, et al. Cow's milk protein–sensitive enteropathy. An important contributing cause of secondary sugar intolerance in young infants with acute infective enteritis. Arch Dis Child 54:39, 1979.

14. Iyngkaran N, Abdin Z, Davis K, et al. Acquired carbohydrate intolerance and cow milk protein–sensitive enteropathy in young infants. J Pediatr 95:373, 1979.

15. Ament ME. Malabsorption syndromes in infancy and childhood. I, II. J Pediatr 81:685, 867, 1972.

16. Whyte RK, Homer R, Pennock CA. Faecal excretion of oligosaccharides and other carbohydrates in normal neonates. Arch Dis Child 53:913, 1978.

17. Schwachman H, Redmond A, Khaw KT. Studies in cystic fibrosis. Report of 130 patients diagnosed under 3 months of age over a 20 year period. Pediatrics 46:335, 1970.

18. Aggett PJ, Cavanagh NPC, Matthew DJ, et al. Schwachman's syndrome. A review of 21 cases. Arch Dis Child 55:331, 1980.

19. Lilibridge CB, Townes PL. Physiologic deficiency of

pancreatic amylase in infancy: a factor in iatrogenic diarrhea. J Pediatr 82:279, 1973.

20. Lebenthal E, Antonowicz I, Schwachman H. Enterokinase and trypsin activities in pancreatic insufficiency and diseases of the small intestine. Gastroenterology 70:508, 1979.

21. Powell GK, Jones LA, Richardson J. A new syndrome of bile acid deficiency—a possible synthetic defect. J Pediatr 83:758, 1973.

22. Lloyd JK. Disorders of the serum lipoproteins. I. Lipoprotein deficiency states. Arch Dis Child 43:393, 1968.

23. Cash R, Berger CK. Acrodermatitis enteropathica: defective metabolism of unsaturated fatty acids. J Pediatr 74:717, 1969.

24. Garretts M, Molokhia M. Acrodermatitis enteropathica without hypozincemia. J Pediatr 91:492, 1977.

25. McReynolds EW, Roy S III, Etteldorf JN. Congenital chloride diarrhea. Am J Dis Child 127:566, 1974.

26. Minford AMB, Barr DGD. Prostaglandin synthetase inhibitor in an infant with congenital chloride diarrhea. Arch Dis Child 55:70, 1980.

27. Woodard JC, Webster PD, Carr AA. Primary hypomagnesemia with secondary hypocalcemia, diarrhea and insensitivity to parathyroid hormone. Am J Dig Dis 17:612, 1972.

28. Iversen T. Congenital adrenal hyperplasia with disturbed electrolyte regulation. Pediatrics 16:875, 1955.

29. Iida Y, Nose O, Kai H, et al. Watery diarrhoea with a vasoactive intestinal peptide–producing ganglioneuroblastoma. Arch Dis Child 55:929, 1980.

30. Ghishan FK, Soper RT, Nassif EG, et al. Chronic diarrhea of infancy: nonbeta islet cell hyperplasia. Pediatrics 64:46, 1979.

31. Stanbury JB, Wyngaarden JB, Fredrickson DS. (eds.). The Metabolic Basis of Inherited Disease, 6th ed. New York, McGraw-Hill, 1989.

32. Hakami N, Neiman PE, Canellos GP, et al. Neonatal megaloblastic anemia due to inherited transcobalamin II deficiency in 2 siblings. N Engl J Med 285:1163, 1971.

33. Bayna SL, Heiner DC. Cow's milk allergy: manifestations, diagnosis and management. Adv Pediatr 25:1, 1978.

34. Halpin TC, Byrne WJ, Ament ME. Colitis, persistent

35. Powell GK. Milk- and soy-induced enterocolitis of infancy. Clinical features and standardization of challenge. J Pediatr 93:553, 1978.

36. Miller RC, Larsen E. Regional enteritis in early infancy. Am J Dis Child 122:301, 1971.

37. Avery GB, Harkness M. Bloody diarrhea in the newborn infant of a mother with ulcerative colitis. Pediatrics 34:875, 1964.

38. Ein SH, Lynch MJ, Stephens CA. Ulcerative colitis in children under one year: a twenty-year review. J Pediatr Surg 6:264, 1971.

39. Sunshine P, Sinatra FR, Mitchell CH. Intractable diarrhoea of infancy. Clin Gastroenterol 6:445, 1977.

40. Davidson M, Wasserman R. The irritable colon of childhood (chronic nonspecific diarrhea syndrome). J Pediatr 69:1027, 1966.

41. Ebbesen F, Edelsten D, Hertel J. Gut transit time and lactose malabsorption during phototherapy. I, II. Acta Paediatr Scand 69:65, 69, 1980.

42. Perlman M, Benady S, Saggi E. Neonatal diagnosis of familial dysautonomia. Pediatrics 63:238, 1979.

43. Davidson GP, Cutz E, Hamilton JR, et al. Familial enteropathy: a syndrome of protracted diarrhea from birth, failure to thrive, and hypoplastic villous atrophy. Gastroenterology 75:783, 1978.

44. Chien L, Robertson H, Gerrard JW. Infantile gastroenteritis due to water with high sulfate content. Can Med Assoc J 99:102, 1968.

45. Fleisher D, Ament ME. Diarrhea, red diapers, and child abuse. Clin Pediatr (Phila) 17:820, 1978.

46. Candy DCA, Larcher VF, Cameron DJS, et al. Lethal familial protracted diarrhea. Arch Dis Child 56:15, 1981.

47. Holmberg C, Perheentipa J. Congenital Na$^+$ diarrhea: a new type of secretory diarrhea. J Pediatr 106:56, 1985.

48. Scott GB, Buck BE, Leterman JG, et al. Acquired immunodeficiency syndrome in infants. N Engl J Med 310:76, 1984.

49. Lo CW, Walker WA. Chronic protracted diarrhea of infancy: a nutritional disease. Pediatrics 72:786, 1983.

50. Levine JJ, Seidman E, Walker WA. Screening tests for enteropathy in children. Am J Dis Child 141:435, 1987.

51. Gleason W, Pickering LK. Chronic diarrhea in children. Curr Pediatr Ther 12:231, 1986.

diarrhea, and soy protein intolerance. J Pediatr 91:404, 1977.

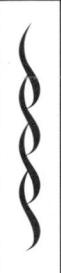

Laboratory Aids for Diagnosis of Neonatal Sepsis

GEOFFREY A. WEINBERG, M.D., and KEITH R. POWELL, M.D.

For years, investigators have sought a test or panel of tests able to identify septic neonates accurately and more rapidly than by the isolation of microorganisms from specimens of sterile body fluids or tissues. Although results of some studies have been encouraging, the isolation of microorganisms from sources such as the blood, cerebrospinal fluid (CSF), urine, other body fluids (peritoneal, pleural, joint, middle ear), or tissues (bone marrow, liver, spleen) remains the most valid method of diagnosing bacterial sepsis. Many advances in nonculture methods, which may nevertheless remain microorganism specific, such as tests employing polymerase chain reaction (PCR) amplification technology, hold the promise of more rapid diagnosis of infection. In this chapter, nonspecific laboratory aids for the diagnosis of invasive bacterial infections are discussed. Specific microbiologic techniques are discussed in Chapter 21 and in chapters dealing with specific pathogens.

DIAGNOSTIC UTILITY OF LABORATORY TESTS

In establishing the usefulness of any laboratory determination, a balance must be reached between sensitivity and specificity.[1] For the clinician faced with a decision to institute or withhold therapy on the basis of a test result, the predictive value (and perhaps likelihood ratios[2]) of that test is also of importance. In relation to neonatal infection, these terms can be defined as follows (Fig. 32–1):

Sensitivity: If infection is present, how often is the test result abnormal?
Specificity: If infection is absent, how often is the test result normal?

Positive predictive value: If the test result is abnormal, how often is infection present?
Negative predictive value: If the test result is normal, how often is infection absent?
Likelihood ratio, positive test result: If the result is abnormal, how much does that result raise the pretest probability of disease?
Likelihood ratio, negative test result: If the result is normal, how much does that result lower the pretest probability of disease?

In attempting to discover the presence of a serious illness such as neonatal bacteremia, which is life-threatening yet treatable, diagnostic tests with maximal (100%) sensitivity and negative predictive value are desirable. In other words, if infection is present, the result would always be abnormal; if the result is normal, infection would always be absent. The reduced specificity and positive predictive value that this may engender are usually acceptable because overtreatment with antibiotics on the basis of a false-positive result is likely to be of limited harm compared with withholding therapy on the basis of a false-negative result. Some authorities prefer the use of likelihood ratios.[3] Large likelihood ratios (>5–10) imply that a test result will conclusively raise the probability of disease being present, whereas small likelihood ratios (<0.1–0.2) minimize the probability of the disease being present.

Any analysis of the reliability of laboratory tests in the diagnosis of neonatal sepsis must consider that among infants who died with unequivocal evidence of infection at autopsy, bacteria were grown from 32 of 39 ante mortem blood or CSF cultures (sensitivity of 82%).[4] Among 50 infants without pathologic findings of infection at autopsy, 48 had negative blood culture results (specificity of 96%). When examined from the perspec-

		Bacterial Infection Present		
		Yes	**No**	
Laboratory Test	**Positive**	TRUE POSITIVES (a)	FALSE POSITIVES (b)	POSITIVE PREDICTIVE VALUE (a)/(a+b)
	Negative	FALSE NEGATIVES (c)	TRUE NEGATIVES (d)	NEGATIVE PREDICTIVE VALUE (d)/(c+d)
		SENSITIVITY (a)/(a+c)	SPECIFICITY (d)/(b+d)	PREVALENCE (a+c)/(a+b+c+d)
		LIKELIHOOD RATIO, POSITIVE sensitivity/1−specificity	LIKELIHOOD RATIO, NEGATIVE 1−sensitivity/specificity	

FIGURE 32–1 Diagnostic test characteristics. Sensitivity, specificity, postive predictive value, and negative predictive value are commonly expressed as percentages; likelihood ratios represent fold-increases or fold-decreases in probability.[1-3]

tive of the laboratory test, a positive blood or CSF culture result had a 94% chance of being associated with serious neonatal infection (positive predictive value of 94%), whereas a negative blood culture result indicated absence of serious infection only 87% of the time (negative predictive value of 87%). Thus, the lack of perfection of the generally used gold standard of bacterial culture complicates the analysis of new laboratory aids in the diagnosis of neonatal sepsis, because it may be unclear whether a new test is truly functioning better than culture.

Two further considerations confound the value of nonmicrobiologic laboratory tests in the diagnosis of neonatal sepsis. First, because the body's response to an infection necessarily begins after the invasion of a pathogen, it may never be possible to immediately diagnose an infection—there may always be a lag in the physiologic response on which the diagnostic test is based. On the other hand, it may not be clinically necessary to require detection of only bacterial sepsis. Tests that yield results considered "falsely positive" in the absence of bacterial disease may still be clinically useful in assigning normal versus abnormal status if the reults register positive because of serious viral disease that may require antiviral therapy (e.g., neonatal enterovirus or herpes simplex infections). Each report of a new test claiming superiority to bacterial culture must be critically evaluated in the field. Standardization both within clinical laboratories and between institutions is required.

WHITE BLOOD CELL COUNTS AND RATIOS

Total Leukocyte Count, Differential Leukocyte Count, and Morphology

It has been known for many years that total leukocyte counts are of limited value in the diagnosis of septicemia

of the newborn.[5-9] Normal at the time of initial evaluation in more than one third of infants with proven bacteremia,[4, 10-22] total leukocyte counts are particularly unreliable indicators of infection during the first several hours of early-onset (<48 hours) sepsis. Conversely, among neonates evaluated for suspected sepsis, less than half of those with reduced (<5000 per mm³) or elevated (>20,000 per mm³) cell counts are ultimately identified as being infected.[4, 13, 15]

Except for recent attention devoted to changes in the number of circulating neutrophils (see later discussion), differential leukocyte counts have not been extensively studied as markers for infectious disease in the newborn period. Increased percentages of lymphocytes have been described in association with pertussis and congenital syphilis, whereas minor changes of little diagnostic value have been noted in infants with ABO incompatibility, in sepsis, and in maternal hypertension.[23, 24] Monocyte counts, normally higher in neonates than in older children or adults,[25] may be further elevated in some cases of congenital syphilis,[26] perinatal listeriosis,[27] ABO incompatibility,[21] and recovery from sepsis.[24] Eosinophilia, a common finding in premature infants,[24, 28, 29] has been related to a number of factors, including low birth weight, immaturity, establishment of positive nitrogen balance, improved nutritional status, and use of total parenteral nutrition or blood transfusions.[29-33] A syndrome of maculopapular rash, eosinophilia, and thrombocytopenia after multiple exchange transfusions has been reported.[34] A dramatic fall in the absolute number of eosinophils, detectable only if serial counts have been performed, frequently accompanies sepsis or serious infection.[24, 31, 35] Basophil counts tend to follow the fluctuations in eosinophil numbers in ill or healthy newborns.[35]

An attempt to use the differential leukocyte count for identifying neonates with bacterial meningitis has been reported.[36] A "complete blood cell count differential ratio" (percent lymphocytes plus percent monocytes/percent polymorphonuclear leukocytes plus percent bands) of less than 1.5 was 100% sensitive for distinguishing infants with bacterial meningitis from those with meningitis due to other causes. However, subsequent evaluation failed to validate the reliability of this test.[37]

Several investigators have shown that, in association with serious bacterial infection, there are significant changes in neutrophil morphology with the appearance of toxic granules, Döhle bodies, and vacuolization.[18, 35-40] These features are of limited value in establishing a diagnosis; their presence has, at best, a positive predictive value for sepsis of only slightly more than 50%[4, 18, 38-40] and, at worst, 33 to 37%.[41, 42] Identical morphologic findings can occur as artifacts in citrate-anticoagulated blood samples stored for longer than 1 hour before smears are made.[43]

Total Neutrophil Count

Recognizing the low predictive value of total leukocyte counts in serious neonatal bacterial disease, several investigators initiated studies of the dynamics of neutrophil counts during the first month of life.[28, 35, 44-46] These researchers and others uncovered patterns of change sufficiently constant to establish limits of normal variation (Fig. 32-2) and defined noninfectious conditions involving the mother or infant that might have significant effects on neutrophil values (Tables 32-1 and 32-2). It was suggested, largely on the basis of these data, that calculation of the absolute number of circulating neutrophils (polymorphonuclear plus immature forms) might provide a useful index of neonatal infection. Clinical experience has only partly supported this premise.

Most series of consecutive cases of neonatal sepsis have shown abnormal neutrophil counts *at the time of onset of symptoms* in only about two thirds of infants.[4, 8, 10, 11, 20, 38, 39, 56-61] However, in some series, up to 80 to 90% of infected infants have had abnormal values,[16, 41, 44, 62] whereas in other series, initial neutrophil counts were reduced or elevated in only one fourth to one third of infants with bacteremia, particularly when counts were obtained early in the course of illness.[22, 48, 63] Thus, the neutrophil count, although slightly more sensitive than the total leukocyte count, is too often normal in the face of serious infection to be used as a guide for treatment.

Baley and associates investigated the causes of neutropenia among consecutive admissions to a neonatal intensive care unit.[45] Low neutrophil counts were found in 6% of these infants, most of whom were premature and of low birth weight. Less than one half of the episodes of neutropenia could be attributed to infection (bacterial, viral, necrotizing enterocolitis); the majority were of unknown cause or occurred in infants with perinatal complications. Similar findings have been described by Rodwell and co-workers among 1000 infants evaluated for sepsis in the first 24 hours of life.[50]

In specific clinical situations, however, the neutrophil count can be of value. Although the association between neutropenia, respiratory distress, and early-onset (<48 hours) sepsis caused by group B streptococci is well documented,[11, 16, 54, 64-68] the recognition that a similar association exists for early sepsis caused by other microorganisms has not been adequately emphasized. Several authors have described infants with septicemia related to *Haemophilus influenzae*,[69, 70] pneumococci,[71-73] *Escherichia coli*,[70] or nonenterococcal group D streptococci[74] whose clinical course was similar to that described for group B streptococcal infection. Because all were noted to be ill

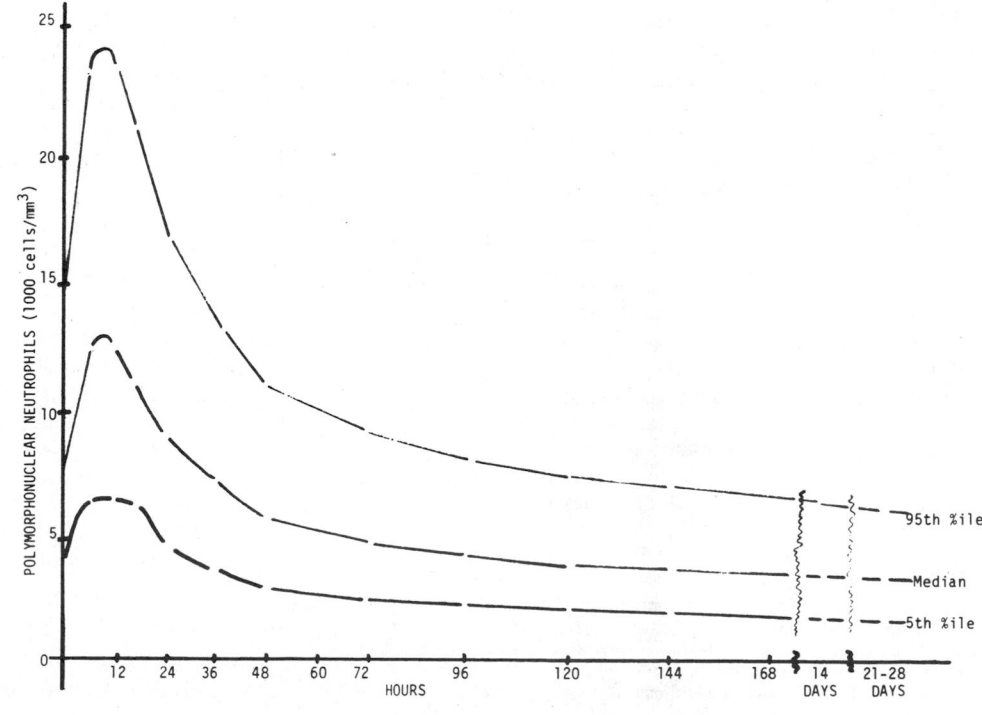

FIGURE 32-2 Total neutrophil counts in normal term infants. These limits are close to those defined by Xanthou[28] and Marks and co-workers[46] but are significantly higher during the first 18 hours of life than the reference values of Manroe and colleagues.[38] Premature infants have significantly fewer neutrophils at birth and during the first 5 days of life in most[28, 38, 44, 47] but not all[33] series. Median values for premature infants approximate the fifth percentile values for term infants. (Constructed based on data from reference 44.)

TABLE 32–1
Clinical Factors Affecting Neutrophil Counts

	NEONATES WITH ABNORMAL VALUES IN[a]				
	Total Neutrophils		Total Immature Increase	Increased I:T[b] Ratio	Approximate Duration (hr)
COMPLICATIONS	Decrease	Increase			
Maternal hypertension[48–50]	+ + + +	0	+	+	72
Maternal fever, neonate healthy	0	+ +	+ + +	+ + + +	24
≥6 hr intrapartum oxytocin	0	+ +	+ +	+ + + +	120
Asphyxia (5 min Apgar ≤5)[48, 51]	+	+ +	+ +	+ + +	24–60
Meconium aspiration syndrome[51]	0	+ + + +	+ + +	+ +	72
Pneumothorax with uncomplicated hyaline membrane disease	0	+ + + +	+ + + +	+ + + +	24
Seizures—no hypoglycemia, asphyxia, or central nervous system hemorrhage	0	+ + +	+ + +	+ + + +	24
Prolonged (≥4 min) crying[52]	0	+ + + +	+ + + +	+ + + +	1
Asymptomatic blood sugar ≤30	0	+ +	+ + +	+ + +	24
Hemolytic disease[35]	+ +	+ +	+ + +	+ +	7–28 days
Surgery[44]	0	+ + + +	+ + + +	+ + +	24
High altitude[53]	0	+ + + +	+ + + +	0	6[c]

[a]+ = 0 to 25% of neonates affected; + + = 25 to 50%; + + + = 50 to 75%; + + + + = 75 to 100%.
[b]Immature forms/total neutrophil count.
[c]Not tested after 6 hours.
Data from reference 38, with additional references as cited.

at birth or shortly thereafter, when neutrophil counts are normally rising, low counts (0 to 4000 per mm³) in this clinical setting are highly significant findings. In many cases, the low number of circulating neutrophils reflects a depletion of bone marrow granulocyte reserves[70, 75] and usually indicates a poor prognosis.[4, 11, 20, 44, 70, 76] The absolute neutrophil count may therefore be useful for screening infants with respiratory distress in the first few hours of life and for separating early-onset sepsis from other causes of pulmonary disease.

Total Nonsegmented Neutrophil Count

The blood smear and differential cell count during the newborn period are strikingly different from those seen

TABLE 32–2
Clinical Factors with No Effect on Neutrophil Counts

Race
Sex
Maternal diabetes
Fetal bradycardia
Route of delivery[a]
Premature rupture of membranes, mother afebrile
Meconium staining, no lung disease
Uncomplicated hyaline membrane disease[54]
Uncomplicated transient tachypnea of the newborn
Hyperbilirubinemia, physiologic, unexplained[11]
Phototherapy
Diurnal variation[28, 44]
Brief (≤3 min) crying[55]

[a]Total neutrophil counts in cord blood of infants delivered vaginally or by cesarean section after labor (2–14 hr) are twice those of infants delivered by cesarean section without labor.[55]
Data from reference 38, with additional references as cited.

at any other time of life. Immature forms are present in relatively large numbers, particularly among premature infants and during the first few days of life.[28, 38, 39, 77] The number of immature neutrophils, mostly nonsegmented (band, stab) forms, rises from a maximal normal value of 1100 cells per mm³ in cord blood to 1500 cells per mm³ at 12 hours of life and gradually falls to 600 cells per mm³ by 60 hours of life. Between 60 and 120 hours, the maximum count falls from 600 to 500 cells per mm³ and remains unchanged through the first month of life.[38] For unexplained reasons, possibly related to differences in the definition of a nonsegmented neutrophil,[56] higher counts have been recorded by other authors.[11, 62] Metamyelocytes and myelocytes also are often present in significant numbers during the first 72 hours after delivery but disappear almost entirely toward the end of the first week of life.[28] Even occasional promyelocytes and blast cells may be seen during the early days of life in healthy infants.[28]

As neutrophils are released from the bone marrow in response to infection, an increasing number of immature cells enter the bloodstream and produce a differential cell count with a "shift to the left" even greater than that normally present in the neonate.[62] This response is so inconstant, however, that, with few exceptions,[11, 56, 57] the absolute band or immature (bands, metamyelocytes) neutrophil count has been found to be of little diagnostic value.* In many infants, despite an increased proportion of immature cell types in the differential leukocyte count, exhaustion of the bone marrow reserves prevents a rise in the absolute number of band neutrophils in the circulation.[75, 79, 80] This is particularly common in the more seriously ill patients, in whom early diagnosis is most critical.[4, 62, 69, 70, 75]

*See references 4, 20, 41, 48, 54, 63, 65, 66, 69, and 78.

Despite its relative insensitivity, the immature neutrophil count has been found to have good positive predictive value in some,[4, 39, 42, 62, 66] although not all,[41] studies. Infants with clinical evidence of sepsis and high band counts in whom culture results remain negative should have follow-up cultures and should be investigated for a history of perinatal events that might explain the discrepancy (see Table 32–1), or should be evaluated for the possibility of infection related to other causes, such as enteroviruses.[81]

Neutrophil Ratios

The unreliability of absolute band counts led to the investigation of neutrophil ratios as an index of neonatal infection. These include the ratio of either bands or all immature neutrophils (e.g., bands, metamyelocytes, and myelocytes) to either segmented neutrophils (the immature to mature, or I:M, ratio) or all neutrophils (the immature to total, or I:T, ratio). Despite the early enthusiasm of researchers, the clinical studies that include these determinations have failed to show a consistent correlation with the presence of serious bacterial disease. As might be expected, low band counts caused by exhaustion of marrow can cause misleading low ratios in the presence of serious or overwhelming infection.[39, 66, 69, 74, 75]

There is not enough clinical experience with ratios of either band to segmented neutrophil[39, 62] or I:M ratios to verify their accuracy. However, initial studies in which the former ratio was used have been disappointing, with normal values recorded in more than one third of infected infants.

Band:total neutrophil ratios, although more extensively studied, have also proved to be too unpredictable to be of much diagnostic help. With 0.2 as the maximal normal ratio, the most favorable report would have missed 10% of neonates with sepsis while recording falsely abnormal values in almost 20% of uninfected infants.[13] The sensitivity of this determination in other series varies from 70% to as low as 30%, which precludes its use in a clinical setting.[17, 18, 20, 61, 62]

The proportion of immature to total neutrophils (I:T ratio) is perhaps the best studied of the ratios.[61, 82] Inclusion in the numerator of all immature forms, rather than just band cells, heightens accuracy by accounting for the increase in metamyelocytes that is sometimes seen with accelerated release from the neutrophil storage pool.[62] Use of total rather than segmented neutrophils in the denominator has the advantage of always yielding a value between 0 and 1 inclusive. The maximum ratio for the first 24 hours is 0.16.[38, 51] It falls gradually to around 0.12 by 60 hours of age and remains unchanged for the remainder of the first month.[38] A normal value up to 0.2, with age unspecified, has been found in some laboratories.[13] Immature:total neutrophil ratios during the first 5 days of life among healthy premature infants with a gestational age of 32 weeks or less are less than 0.2 in 96%.[77]

A large number of clinical studies have evaluated the I:T ratio. Results have been widely disparate, but, in most series, they indicate that this ratio is too unreliable to achieve more than limited usefulness. Sensitivities ranging from more than 90%[11, 14, 16, 38, 41, 66, 83] to as low as 70%,[15, 84] 60%,[48, 60, 63] or less[85, 86] have been reported. Furthermore, elevated ratios caused by a variety of perinatal conditions have been seen in 25 to 50% of uninfected ill infants (see Table 32–1).[14, 15] Perhaps the ratio's greatest value lies in its good negative predictive value: if the I:T ratio is normal, the likelihood that infection is absent is extremely high (99%).[3, 13–15, 41, 60, 66, 82]

In addition, serial determinations of the I:T ratio may lead to increased sensitivity.[42, 82, 87] However, some authors have found that inter-reader variability leads to enough bias to limit the usefulness of leukocyte ratios for general use.[88]

PLATELET COUNT

Several extensive studies have established that the normal platelet count in newborns, regardless of birth weight, is rarely less than 100,000 per mm^3 during the first 10 days of life or less than 150,000 per mm^3 during the next 3 weeks.[11, 19, 60, 89–93] Although it would behoove the clinician to perform a workup for sepsis in any infant with unexplained thrombocytopenia,[93–95] a reduction in the number of circulating platelets has been shown to be an insensitive, a nonspecific, and a relatively late indicator of serious bacterial infection during the neonatal period.

Only 10 to 60% of newborns with proven bacterial invasion of the bloodstream or meninges have platelet counts of less than 100,000 per mm^3.[10–12, 16, 18–20, 41, 63, 92] The average duration of thrombocytopenia is about 1 week but can last as long as 2 to 3 weeks. The nature of the organism involved (whether gram-positive or gram-negative) does not appear to be a determining factor,[11, 63, 92] with the possible exception of *Acinetobacter calcoacetius*, which was strongly associated with thrombocytopenia in one study.[96] Although platelet counts may begin to fall several days before the onset of clinical signs of infection, in most cases values remain elevated until 1 to 3 days after serious illness is already apparent.[12, 19, 20, 40, 56, 92] Thrombocytopenia accompanying bacterial infection is thought to be caused by a direct effect of bacteria or bacterial products on platelets and vascular endothelium leading to increased aggregation and adhesion or by increased platelet destruction caused by immune mechanisms.[39, 56, 92–94, 97]

In addition to the widely known association between thrombocytopenia and intrauterine infections related to toxoplasmosis, rubella, cytomegalovirus infection, herpes simplex virus infection, and syphilis, reduced platelet counts have also been described with postnatal viral infections with enteroviruses,[94, 97, 98] cytomegalovirus,[99] and herpes simplex virus, all of which can cause an illness clinically indistinguishable from bacterial sepsis. Conditions that predispose to sepsis, such as umbilical line placement, birth asphyxia, mechanical ventilation, meconium aspiration, multiple exchange transfusions, and necrotizing enterocolitis, have independently caused thrombocytopenia in the absence of positive blood culture results.[34, 95, 100–102] Neonatal thrombocytopenia has also been reported with various conditions causing maternal thrombocytopenia, including pregnancy-induced hypertension.[34] Infants with moderate to severe Rh hemolytic disease are also thrombocytopenic.[103] The use of platelet counts is clearly of limited value in establishing the diagnosis of bacterial infection during the newborn period.

Automated measurements of mean platelet volume (MPV) and platelet distribution width (PDW) are becoming more widely available as a noninvasive method to determine the etiology of thrombocytopenia. A preliminary study showed that MPV and PDW were significantly higher in infants infected after 3 days of age than in infants with perinatal sepsis.[104] Overall, the sensitivity of increased MPV and PDW was 48% with a specificity of 98%,[104] adding little to the platelet count as a diagnostic aid.

ACUTE-PHASE REACTANTS

In the presence of inflammation caused by infection, trauma, or other cellular destruction, the liver, under the influence of interleukin-1 and interleukin-6 (IL-1β, IL-6) and tumor necrosis factor-α (TNF-α), rapidly synthesizes large amounts of certain proteins collectively known as acute-phase reactants.[105–108] Serum levels of these proteins usually rise together, and, in general, the degree of change in one is proportional to the degree of change in the others (two important exceptions are albumin and transferrin, which decrease together) (Fig. 32–3). Acute-phase reactants are produced very early in fetal life, beginning in the fourth to fifth week of gestation,[109] and their exact role in the inflammatory process is unknown; most appear to be part of a primitive nonspecific defense mechanism. Several acute-phase reactants have been extensively evaluated in neonatal sepsis, including C-reactive protein (CRP), fibrinogen, and other proteins that influence the erythrocyte sedimentation rate; haptoglobin; and α₁-acid glycoprotein (orosomucoid). The most useful of these appears to be measurement of the CRP. Measurement of proinflammatory cytokines and their receptors holds promise to further increase diagnostic accuracy; these tests are discussed later in this chapter.

The development during the last decade of rapid and precise quantitative immunoassays that lend themselves readily to automation has encouraged re-evaluation of the acute-phase response, particularly in Europe. In general, these assays make use of specific and high-affinity antibodies that, in combining with the protein or glycoprotein antigen to be measured, produce a precipitate and turbidity in solution. Quantitative measurement of the light absorption or reflection produced by this immunoprecipitate is referred to as turbidimetry or nephelometry, respectively.[110] Studies comparing these methods with older assays (e.g., gel immunodiffusion) have shown comparable or superior precision with far greater speed, sensitivity, and reproducibility.[61, 107, 110]

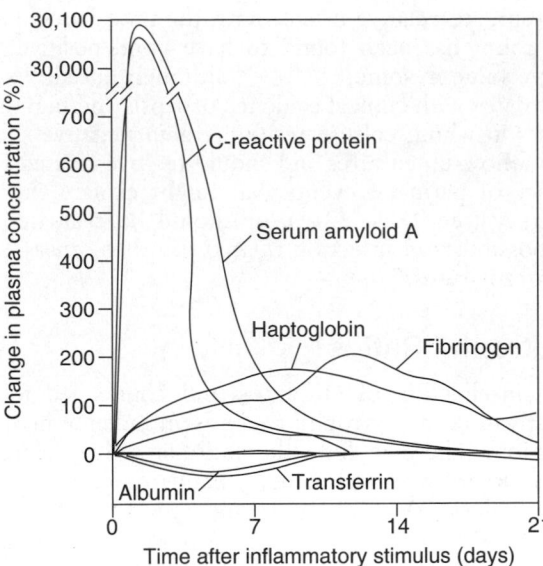

FIGURE 32–3 Acute-phase reactants in patients with inflammatory illnesses. The response of C-reactive protein (CRP) is greater than that of all other acute-phase proteins except serum amyloid A. Levels of certain plasma proteins decrease during the acute-phase response. (Reproduced with permission from Gabay C, Kushner I. Acute-phase proteins and other systemic responses to inflammation. N Engl J Med 340:448–454, 1999.)

C-Reactive Protein

CRP is a globulin that forms a precipitate when combined with the C-polysaccharide of *Streptococcus pneumoniae*.[107, 108] Because appearance of CRP in the blood has been closely associated with tissue injury, particularly when caused by an acute inflammatory process, it has been suggested that its primary function is to act as a carrier protein, to bind and facilitate clearance of potentially toxic foreign or altered materials released from invading microorganisms or damaged tissues. Its roles in activation of the classic complement pathway, promotion of phagocytosis, regulation of lymphocyte function, and platelet activation are under investigation.[61, 105–108]

Differences in laboratory techniques and in interpretation of what constitutes a positive value for CRP have been responsible for conflicting opinions about the reliability of this test during the neonatal period.[61, 107] Thus, early clinical reports must be interpreted in light of the knowledge that the capillary tube precipitation technique used for assay of CRP in those studies was less sensitive and less specific than more modern immunochemical methods.[61, 111] Furthermore, a comparison of reactions obtained by different investigators using the capillary tube method revealed widely disparate results, depending on the sensitivity of the commercial antiserum used in the assay.[112, 113]

Rapid and reliable quantitative methods have been developed in which monoclonal CRP-specific antibody is used.[114–117] These immunoassays can be divided into two groups: (1) those that permit direct visualization of a CRP-antibody complex through particle agglutination (e.g., latex agglutination) or through precipitation (e.g., radial immunodiffusion, immunoturbidimetry, nephelometry) and (2) those that enlist a marker for detection (e.g., radioimmunoassay, enzyme-multiplied immunoassay technique). Although the slide latex agglutination test is rapid (15 minutes) and convenient, it is only semiquantitative and subject to reagent variability.[114] Fully automated turbidimetric and nephelometric methods can provide quantitative results in 30 to 60 minutes, whereas enzyme immunoassays, such as the enzyme-multiplied immunoassay technique, can give results in less than 10 minutes.

Determination of CRP levels in serum by radial immunodiffusion, electroimmunodiffusion, spot immunoprecipitate assay, enzyme-multiplied immunoassay technique, and nephelometry has shown upper limits of about 1 mg/dl during the neonatal period.[42, 107, 108, 114, 118–123] Gestational age does not appear to influence the validity of results.[17, 107, 118–121, 124, 125]

CRP is detectable in the blood of healthy pregnant women; its level increases throughout pregnancy, labor, and the early postpartum period. Approximately one third of women have significantly elevated levels of CRP during labor,[117, 126, 127] and almost all women have CRP in the serum at some time during the first week after delivery.[127, 128] Analysis of paired serum specimens obtained from mothers and their infants (fetuses and premature infants as well as full-term neonates) has shown that CRP crosses the placenta either in very low concentrations or not at all.[107, 112, 117, 119, 126–130]

A strong correlation between elevated CRP levels and chorioamnionitis has been described in women with premature rupture of membranes.[131, 132] It has been shown, moreover, that increased CRP levels are also present significantly more often in the cord blood of infants born to mothers with these problems.[119, 120] Whether this response is caused by inflammation of fetal tissues exposed to the infected amniotic fluid or by transplacental passage of an inducer such as IL-1 is not known. Increases of CRP levels in neonates, up to 10 times normal, have also been associated with noninfectious conditions causing tissue injury or inflammation, such as fetal asphyxia, respiratory distress syndrome, intracerebral hemorrhage, and meconium aspiration pneumonitis.[119, 120, 123, 133, 134] Because these conditions are often confused, or associated, with newborn bacterial infection, such false-positive elevations greatly reduce the positive predictive value of CRP determinations and their usefulness in diagnosis. The mean incidence of falsely elevated CRP values in apparently healthy neonates is approximately 8%.[19, 83, 86, 118, 133–136]

Most surveys of CRP levels in sera of neonates with systemic bacterial infections have shown significant elevations *at the time of onset of signs* in 50 to 90% of cases.* A poor response is particularly frequent among infants whose infection occurs during the first 12 to 24 hours of life and among infants with infection caused by gram-positive bacteria including group B streptococci.[16, 83, 121, 133] Although the intensity of the response does not always reflect the severity of the infection, the relationship between formation of CRP and the degree of tissue injury indicates that positive reactors are usually those with systemic infections or involvement of deeper tissues.[16, 143] Thus, superficial bacterial infections of the skin cause little or no response in the host, whereas cellulitis or abscesses evoke increased levels of CRP.[112] Serum levels are occasionally elevated in infants with nonspecific acute diarrheal illness and urinary tract infections[120]; however, no effort has been made to correlate these rises with the site of infection (e.g., bladder as opposed to kidney) or with the pathogenesis of the illness (secretory diarrhea as opposed to inflammatory ileocolitis). The response of CRP to nonbacterial infections is variable; raised serum levels have been found in infants with viral infections.[144] Thus, the overall sensitivity of CRP at the onset of signs of sepsis ranges between 50 and 90%, and the specificity between 60 and 90%. The positive and negative predictive values, respectively, may be as low as 30% and as high as more than 95%.

It is clear from the foregoing discussion that despite new technology permitting more rapid and precise measurement, reliance on CRP levels alone as an early indicator of neonatal bacterial infection cannot be recommended. Although CRP levels are possibly helpful in combination with other tests as part of a "sepsis screen" (see later discussion), when used alone as an initial test for infection, even if the most favorable results are assumed, approximately 10% of cases will be missed and 5% of healthy infants will be overdiagnosed.

Nevertheless, determination of *serial* CRP levels does appear to be of some value in excluding serious infection.[61, 107, 108] Despite the large number of infants whose assays are normal at the onset of invasive bacterial disease, with a doubling time of about 8 hours,[107] rising CRP levels are usually apparent within a day, and levels peak at 2 to 3 days and remain elevated until infection is controlled and resolution of the inflammatory process begins.[14, 16, 83, 96, 118–121, 144a] Thereafter, by virtue of a relatively short serum half-life of about 19 hours,[108] CRP levels fall promptly and return to normal within 5 to 10 days in most infants with a favorable outcome.[16, 17, 118, 120, 143] Some studies conducted over the past 15 years reported that serial measurements of CRP levels may provide an index for determining the effectiveness of antibiotics, the duration of therapy, and the occurrence of relapse or of complications during or after treatment of known infection.[16, 119–121, 143, 145, 146]

Several more recent studies document that serial determination of CRP levels over 1 to 3 days after onset of possible neonatal bacterial infection yields diagnostic sensitivity of 75 to 98%, specificity of 90%, and perhaps, most notably, negative predictive value of 99%.[42, 133, 137–139] These studies suggest that although the relatively low sensitivity of initial CRP determination precludes the firm diagnosis of bacterial infection, the very high negative predictive value of several normal CRP determinations in combination allows the early discontinuance of empirical administration of intravenous antibiotics.[42, 133, 137–139] It is less certain whether there are enough distinctions between decay patterns of elevated CRP

---

*See references 13, 16, 19, 42, 61, 86, 107, 108, 121, 133, and 136–142.

levels to differentiate those newborns with positive bacterial cultures from those with negative cultures.[144a]

Erythrocyte Sedimentation Rate

The development over 50 years ago of an erythrocyte sedimentation rate by use of a microhematocrit tube and a few drops of capillary blood permitted the application of this test to very small infants.[147, 148] Attempts at standardization have shown the microerythrocyte sedimentation rate to increase slowly during the first weeks of life, perhaps as a result of rising fibrinogen and falling hematocrit levels. Maximal normal rates have varied so widely, however, that any laboratory attempting to use this test in neonates must establish its own normal values.[149–153] The upper (ninety-fifth percentile) limits established by Adler and Denton[149] lie almost on a mean between those of other investigators. An approximation of these limits for the first 2 weeks of life can be made by adding 2 or 3 to the age of the infant in days (i.e., 4 mm per hour at 2 days of age, 12 mm per hour at 9 days of age, and about 17 mm per hour at 14 days of age).

Rates do not vary significantly with gestational age, birth weight, or sex but are related inversely to the hematocrit level, particularly in infants with hematocrit readings of less than 0.40.[149, 150, 153] Comparisons between the microerythrocyte sedimentation rate and standard methods have shown good correlation in simultaneous analyses of samples obtained from cord blood, from infants with physiologic jaundice, and from healthy older children.[149, 153] Rapid alternative methods such as determination of the zeta sedimentation ratio[154] and plasma viscosity[155] compared well with standard erythrocyte sedimentation rate assays and were thought to reflect a change in the same plasma proteins; however, they have not been evaluated in newborns and their clinical use is dwindling.

The microerythrocyte sedimentation rate is generally normal or only mildly elevated in noninfectious conditions such as respiratory distress syndrome, aspiration pneumonia, and asphyxia, as well as in superficial infections.[149–153] Significant elevations are unusual in healthy infants but can occur in the presence of Coombs'-positive hemolytic disease[14, 149, 151, 152] and physiologic hyperbilirubinemia.[153]

Although extensive clinical experience has shown that sedimentation rates eventually become elevated in most infants with systemic bacterial infections,[141, 149, 150, 153, 156] this rise may be delayed at the time of the initial evaluation in 30 to 70% of infants with proven sepsis, particularly when disseminated intravascular coagulopathy is present.[13, 14, 76, 149–151, 153] Furthermore, once the rate is elevated, its return to normal can be exceedingly slow despite clinical recovery, sometimes taking several weeks from the time of onset of illness.[149, 152] Thus, use of the microerythrocyte sedimentation rate is of little value in either diagnosing or monitoring serious bacterial infection during the newborn period.

Other Acute-Phase Reactants

The rise in plasma *fibrinogen* level associated with infection has been recognized for many years through its effects on the erythrocyte sedimentation rate. Normal values during the first 48 hours of life are less than 340 mg/dl and rise to levels that plateau between 400 and 500 mg/dl during the third to twelfth days.[56, 157, 158] Concentrations may be affected by birth weight and test methodology.[159] Clinical experience with the use of fibrinogen levels is limited but generally disappointing. The median fibrinogen concentrations in infected infants overlapped greatly with levels obtained from normal infants.[56, 158, 160] Low values despite severe infection have been associated with disseminated intravascular coagulopathy,[56] respiratory distress syndrome,[158] and exchange transfusion. Furthermore, falsely high values were noted in almost 10% of newborns admitted to an intensive care nursery for a variety of conditions unrelated to intrauterine or postnatal infection.[158]

Haptoglobin is an α_2-glycoprotein that reacts with free hemoglobin to form a complex, which is removed by the reticuloendothelial system. Normal values of haptoglobin in cord blood are up to 10 mg/dl, increasing by 1 month of age to concentrations up to 50 mg/dl.[161, 162] Gestational age, neonatal asphyxia, sex, and hemolytic ABO/Rh disease have no significant influence on levels in cord blood or during the postnatal period; however, elevated levels usually persist for several days after exchange transfusion, probably as a result of passive transfer of blood with adult concentrations of haptoglobin. Inaccuracies related to phenotypic variants of haptoglobin, although seen when levels are measured by radial immunodiffusion, have not presented a problem when concentrations are determined by laser nephelometry. Because haptoglobin determinations, measured as plasma hemoglobin-binding capacity or by laser nephelometry, can be performed in 1 to 2 hours, they were thought to be potentially of great value in the early detection of bacterial infection in the newborn. Unfortunately, clinical studies have raised serious doubts about the reliability of this test. The earliest and most extensive investigation concluded that haptoglobin levels were a highly specific and sensitive index of neonatal septicemia, with abnormal determinations in 35 of 38 infants with positive blood culture results or clinical illness compatible with sepsis or both.[161] A second study, although it confirmed the positive predictive value, detected elevated plasma haptoglobin concentrations in only 9 of 30 infants with positive blood culture results.[13] The most recent investigations have found the test to be extremely unreliable, with normal levels in a considerable proportion of infected infants and with elevated levels in healthy infants.[17, 123, 136] Finally, in one study 60% of healthy term infants and 80% of healthy preterm infants had undetectable levels of haptoglobin by nephelometry, which might make it problematic to detect increased but low levels of haptoglobin in infection.[162] Until more favorable data become available, determination of haptoglobin levels cannot be considered a useful index for the early diagnosis of neonatal bacterial infection.

α_1–*Acid glycoprotein (orosomucoid)* is produced by lymphocytes, monocytes, and neutrophils as well as hepatocytes. It exists as an integral membrane protein of leukocytes and is liberated into the plasma as the cells disintegrate.[106] Its function is unknown, but it may have a role in forming collagen, binding steroid hormones, and modifying lymphocyte responsiveness.[145, 163] The maximal normal cord concentration of α_1-acid glycoprotein in infants of any gestational age is 40 mg/dl,[164] although very premature newborns have lower mean concentrations than those born closer to term.[160, 163, 165] In full-term infants, concentrations rise steadily to 75 mg/dl by the second week of life and to 90 mg/dl during the third and fourth weeks. Among premature infants, 75 mg/dl is achieved earlier (by 3 to 4 days), 90 mg/dl by 10 to 15 days, and a peak of 110 mg/dl at 3 to 4 weeks.[162, 164] Although early studies suggested that α_1-acid glycoprotein might be a specific and sensitive indicator of neonatal bacterial infection,[166, 167] subsequent surveys have not been able to confirm this favorable experience. Falsely low values have been recorded in 15 to 50% or more of newborns at the time of onset of serious bacterial infection,[13, 49, 121, 123, 143, 160, 164, 165, 168] and false-positive values have been recorded in 10 to 26% of infants who were ill but free of bacterial infection.[123, 164–166]

The failure of any of the acute-phase proteins discussed earlier to provide definitive guidelines for the early diagnosis of neonatal sepsis has led to a search for other, perhaps better, indicators. Among those evaluated have been α_1-proteinase inhibitor (α_1-antitrypsin)[17, 136]; the complex of elastase and α_1-proteinase inhibitor[169, 170]; α_1-antichymotrypsin[136]; lactoferrin[136]; prealbumin[86, 121, 123, 152]; human complement and complement split products[171]; and ceruloplasmin.[172] Further clinical studies will be required before any of these reactants can be considered to be helpful in managing the neonate suspected of having a bacterial infection.

ADDITIONAL LABORATORY STUDIES

Cytokine Concentrations

Cytokines, such as IL-1β, IL-6, TNF-α, and others, are thought to be endogenous mediators of the immune response to bacterial infections. Cytokine production and kinetics have not been well studied in newborns, but preliminary data suggest that cord plasma concentrations may vary with clinical complications during the perinatal period. IL-1β was elevated in cord plasma specimens from infants born after induced vaginal or urgent cesarean deliveries, whereas IL-6 was markedly elevated in infants with infectious complications.[173] Studies suggest that elevated IL-6 levels detected after birth may provide an early and sensitive parameter for the diagnosis of neonatal bacterial infection.[123, 125, 142, 174–177] Elevated concentrations have also been correlated with a fatal outcome in older children[178] and in newborns with sepsis. IL-8 was found to be elevated in cord blood from infants for whom there was histologic evidence of chorioamnionitis.[179] IL-8 concentrations were markedly suppressed in infants when corticosteroids were given to the mother to promote fetal lung maturation.[179] TNF-α and E-selectin have also been suggested as discriminators of bacterial sepsis.[137, 180]

Other substances associated with the inflammatory response, in some cases induced by cytokines, have also been evaluated as possible indicators of newborn infection. Studies have demonstrated an early and specific elevation in serum levels of procalcitonin[180–185] and intercellular adhesion molecule–1 (ICAM-1)[176, 186] in small numbers of infants with invasive bacterial disease. Procalcitonin has a natural fluctuation in the first 48 hours of life, however, mandating very careful (perhaps hourly) adjustments in the normal reference ranges and thus complicating its use as a diagnostic aid.[184] Cytokine receptors and receptor antagonists such as soluble IL-2 receptor and IL-1 receptor antagonist are among the most recently studied substances in the search to aid the laboratory diagnosis of neonatal sepsis.[187, 188] In one study, soluble IL-2 receptor was unique in showing 100% positive predictive value (as opposed to the high negative predictive value shown by most other laboratory aids discussed in this chapter).[188] If this observation is consistent in further studies, diagnosis of infection after an abnormal test result rather than diagnosis of the absence of infection after a normal result might lessen unnecessary use of antibiotics at onset of therapy. Further clinical data will be needed to determine whether measurement of these inflammatory products is truly useful for the diagnosis and follow-up of neonatal sepsis.

Lymphocyte and Neutrophil Marker Analysis

Two recent studies suggest that flow cytometric analysis of surface markers of white cell populations may help exclude early onset neonatal infection. Activation of T-lymphocytes after infection results in up-regulation of the CD45RO isoform and loss of the CD45RA isoform. Sequential analysis of the distribution of early CD45RA/CD45RO dual expression and later CD45RO expression alone discriminated bacterial (and viral) infection from respiratory distress or erythrocyte incompatibility in a small number of infants.[189] In a small retrospective pilot study, the surface expression of the neutrophil surface marker CD11b yielded sensitivity, specificity, and predictive values all greater than 95% in diagnosing neonatal bacterial infection.[190] The expression of CD11b may be affected by length of labor, however, so further studies will be required.[191]

Miscellaneous Analytes

Fibronectin is an adhesive, high-molecular-weight (450,000 kDa) glycoprotein that has been identified on cell surfaces and in extracellular fluids. It is thought, by virtue of its stickiness, to act as an intercellular cement and maintain microvascular integrity, and to act as an opsonin and aid in the phagocytic function of neutrophils and macrophages.[106, 192, 193] In general, the concentration of fibronectin in fetal plasma increases with gestational age to concentrations at term of approximately one half those found in healthy adults.[192–195] The value in normal adults measured by enzyme-linked immunosorbent assay (ELISA) ranges from 300 to 400 fg/ml, whereas that in term newborns is 216 ± 70 fg/ml and that in premature infants is 182 ± 45 fg/ml.[192, 193] Plasma concentrations usually fall significantly during the course of neonatal sepsis, probably as a result of clearance by the reticuloendothelial system of products of the inflammatory response. The rate of recovery of fibronectin concentrations as infection resolves is relatively rapid over 5 to 7 days.[192, 193, 195] However, attempts to characterize a fall in fibronectin concentrations as a marker for sepsis have been disappointing.[14, 193, 195] Concentrations not only remain elevated in a significant proportion of infants with sepsis[14, 193, 195] but also may decrease in a variety of conditions unrelated to bacterial infection, such as respiratory distress syndrome, perinatal asphyxia, and intrauterine growth retardation,[196] and may increase coincident with intravenous gamma-globulin therapy.[197] The role of fibronectin administration for the treatment of neonatal sepsis remains under investigation.[193, 198]

Demonstration of increased amounts of *total IgM* in umbilical cord sera was once thought to be helpful in detecting infants with intrauterine infections, particularly those caused by rubella virus, cytomegalovirus, *Treponema pallidum*, and *Toxoplasma gondii*.[199] On the basis of this experience, there were several attempts, mainly in the late 1960s and early 1970s, to use serially determined IgM concentrations in the evaluation of infants suspected of having acute postnatal bacterial infections. Most authors considered the upper limit of normal IgM concentrations in the cord blood of term infants to be 20 mg/dl for the first 2 weeks of life, slowly rising to 30 mg/dl during the remainder of the first month. Lower values are found in infants of shorter gestation or lower birth weight or both.[200, 201] The results of these and more recent[123] investigations were fairly consistent: a significant elevation in IgM concentrations in approximately three of five infants with bacterial sepsis, meningitis, pneumonia, or urinary tract infection was demonstrated.[128, 140, 202, 203] These studies were, however, disappointing in several crucial aspects. Not only did concentrations of IgM remain normal in up to half of all infants with sepsis,[123, 166, 202] but also, in patients in whom the concentration of IgM did rise, detectable elevations were often delayed for 2 to 9 days.[202, 203] In addition, viral infections,[123, 202] minor localized bacterial infections,[130, 200, 202–204] and meconium aspiration[123] were associated with a significant increase in IgM concentrations almost as frequently as were serious systemic illnesses. In one study of infants with suspected sepsis, elevated IgM concentrations of 30 mg/dl or higher determined by latex agglutination or immunodiffusion methods were present in 45 of 376 neonates, only 3 of whom proved to have bacterial sepsis.[13] Determination of IgM concentrations as an index of neonatal bacterial infection has largely been abandoned.

The discovery that neutrophils that have phagocytized bacteria reduce nitroblue tetrazolium dye to purple formazan led to development of several tests using this *leukocyte enzyme activity* for detection of bacterial infections involving the systemic circulation.[205] It was shown that in most cases the majority of peripheral neutrophils reduce nitroblue tetrazolium during the course of an untreated or ineffectively treated infection, whereas only a small proportion of neutrophils do so in healthy individuals. Unfortunately, attempts to incorporate this assay into the newborn period were hampered by difficulty in establishing standard techniques and normal values, and the predictive value of the test was found to be lower than expected.[199, 206–216] It is now rarely used in the diagnosis of neonatal infection.[85] Changes in leukocyte lactate dehydrogenase[217] and alkaline phosphatase[218–221] concentrations were thought a number of years ago to be potentially useful indices of neonatal infection. These determinations have received little further attention since that time and have apparently fallen into disuse.

Bacterial infections are known to alter *carbohydrate metabolism* in neonates. Although hypoglycemia[222] and hyperglycemia[223] have been described in infants with sepsis, the association between changes in blood glucose concentrations and neonatal infection is of only limited value as a diagnostic aid.

Microscopic Examination of Placenta, Umbilical Cord, Gastric Aspirates, and External Ear Canal Fluid

Microscopic examination of tissues or body fluids is a time-honored but rather insensitive and nonspecific aid to the diagnosis of neonatal sepsis. An association of neonatal sepsis with pathologic changes in the placenta and umbilical cord was suggested nearly 40 years ago.[224–226] Neonatal infection acquired at or about the time of birth is usually associated with chorioamnionitis or funisitis, but inflammation of these structures is not uncommon in the absence of sepsis.[227–229] The histologic sections show acute inflammatory changes with infiltration of the umbilical vein by polymorphonuclear leukocytes and gross or microscopic evidence of chorioamnionitis. The probability of finding inflammatory changes in these tissues is inversely related to birth weight[226] and directly related to the duration of rupture of membranes before delivery,[226, 230, 231] the presence of meconium in amniotic fluid,[230] and fetal distress and hypoxia.[232] As many as 30% of live-born infants show some inflammatory changes in the placenta and its membranes or the umbilical cord.[226, 227] Thus, the incidence of chorioamnionitis and placentitis exceeds the possible incidence of significant neonatal infection. It appears likely that signs of inflammation in the cord and placenta are frequently indicative of exposure to infection and perhaps other influences but are not specific signs of systemic infection in the newborn. A normal placenta and cord, however, usually exclude bacterial infection acquired during birth.[226]

The stomach of the newborn contains fluid swallowed before and during delivery. The presence of polymorphonuclear leukocytes and bacteria in a stained smear of the gastric aspirate indicates inflammation of the amniotic fluid, placenta, and other tissues of the birth canal.[233, 234] The polymorphonuclear leukocytes in the gastric aspirate obtained during the first day of life are from the mother and do not indicate a fetal inflammatory response.[235] Therefore, the presence of these maternal leukocytes indicates exposure to possible infection and does not necessarily identify an infectious disease in the newborn. However, after the first day, the gastric aspirate contains swallowed bronchial secretions, and examination of a stained preparation may suggest pneumonia in the neonate if inflammatory cells are present.[236]

As in examination of the gastric aspirate during the first day of life, the presence of polymorphonuclear leukocytes in the aspirated ear canal fluid indicates exposure to an infected environment. Data obtained by examination of gastric or external ear canal fluids appear to be of only limited value in identifying the infant at risk of sepsis.[237] The information obtained offers little more than that already available from a careful history of events occurring at the time of delivery[238] and does not seem to influence decision making regarding antimicrobial therapy.[239] Bacterial cultures of neonatal gastric aspirate or external ear canal fluid reflect the flora of the birth canal, and results parallel those of cultures obtained from the maternal vagina, endocervix, endometrium, and placenta.[240, 241] Thus, whereas the presence of organisms or inflammatory cells has low positive predictive value, the absence of organisms or polymorphonuclear neutrophils in preparations of gastric aspirates or ear canal fluid indicates that bacterial infection acquired during delivery is unlikely.[242] Similarly, pathogens are frequently isolated when daily tracheal aspirates for intubated infants are cultured.[243] However, because many (if not all) intubated newborns will eventually have pathogens isolated from their tracheal aspirate, the positive predictive value of this test is less than 30%.[243] Again, similar to gastric aspirates or external ear canal fluid, tracheal aspirates reflect environmental influences but do not necessarily imply sepsis.

To date, further tests on amniotic fluid, cord blood, or neonatal blood using more sophisticated techniques such as limulus assay for endotoxin or PCR amplification of bacterial DNA have not proved useful.[244, 245]

Screening Panels

The inability of any single laboratory test to provide rapid, reliable, and early identification of neonates with bacterial sepsis has led to efforts to devise a panel of screening tests, combining data from several different determinations, as a means of increasing predictive value. In general, the results have shown little increase in positive predictive value (if a test result is abnormal, disease is present) compared with most of the individual screening tests, although negative predictive value (if a result is normal, disease is absent) has been remarkably good, approaching 100% in some studies.

The most ambitious attempt to diagnose neonatal sepsis through multiple standard laboratory determinations involved more than 500 infants younger than 7 days old studied by Philip and Hewitt[13] and Philip.[60, 246] The authors devised a "sepsis screen" for use with infants believed to be at risk for, or demonstrating clinical evidence of, serious bacterial infection. In addition to the standard procedures (blood, CSF, and urine cultures; chest film), the evaluation included a screening panel consisting of total leukocyte count and ratio of bands to neutrophils, CRP and haptoglobin determinations, and microerythrocyte sedimentation rate. Results were available to the attending physician within an hour. An abnormality in any two or more of these items was considered to be a "positive sepsis screen," and in one or none, a "negative sepsis screen."

Analysis of the results[13, 60] showed a 39% probability that serious bacterial infection is present if two or more test results are positive (positive predictive value) and a 99% probability that it is not present if only one result is positive (negative predictive value). In actual numbers, as a result of the sepsis screen, 60 of 524 infants with clinically suspected sepsis were treated unnecessarily with antimicrobial agents, and 3 with subsequently proven bacterial infection were missed.[60] Comparable results have been reported by Gerdes and Polin,[14] who used a sepsis screen similar to that used by Philip, and by others[10, 19, 38, 41, 50, 87] who used only hematologic or clinical indices. It should be noted, however, that predictions of sepsis from a panel of screening tests have been little better than those obtained by relying solely on the I:T neutrophil ratio, particularly in the first week of life.[13–15, 41, 50, 60, 66]

By virtue of its high negative predictive value, a screening panel used in an intensive care nursery resulted in a significant decrease in the use of antimicrobial agents.[246] Not only did fewer neonates receive antimicrobial agents, but infants who were being administered these agents could more confidently be discontinued from treatment earlier. The author of the reported study was careful to emphasize, however, that screening tests are intended only to augment clinical evaluation. When the evidence obtained by history or physical examination conflicts with a negative screen, antimicrobial therapy should be started. Thus, clinical signs of sepsis remain the most important criteria for use of antimicrobial agents. Newer diagnostic tests are also being included in screening panels. Some examples are included in Table 32–3. These include using the combination of IL-6 and CRP[125, 137] and various cytokine panels.[137, 176]

PERSPECTIVES AND CONCLUSIONS

It is difficult to choose one cytokine, acute-phase reactant, or screening panel for current use as the "best" test when examining all of the data published to date (Table 32–3). Many of the studies discussed previously have analyzed only small numbers of infants. Different definitions of sepsis (e.g., culture-documented, probable, possible), inclusion or exclusion of microorganisms which may be commensal or pathogenic (e.g., coagulase-negative staphylococci), variable sampling routines, and different cutoffs for normal test values used by various investigators each will alter the diagnostic characteristics of a particular test and confound the comparison of published reports.

Faced with the diagnostic uncertainty of currently available laboratory aids for the diagnosis of neonatal sepsis, what is today's practitioner to do? First, it should be remembered that history, physical examination, and clinical impression still comprise a large part of clinical

TABLE 32–3
Selected Reports of Diagnostic Characteristics of Various Tests and Screening Panels for Neonatal Bacterial Infection

TEST	PREVALENCE OF CULTURE-DOCUMENTED BACTERIAL SEPSIS[a] (%)	SENSITIVITY (%)	SPECIFICITY (%)	POSITIVE PREDICTIVE VALUE (%)	NEGATIVE PREDICTIVE VALUE (%)
Individual Tests					
CRP[137]	45				
At initial evaluation		60	100	100	75
At 48 hr later		84	95	93	88
IL-6[137]	45				
At initial evaluation		89	96	95	91
At 48 hr later		58	84	75	71
Neutrophil CD11b expression[190]	5	100	81	22	100
Procalcitonin sampled twice over 48 hr[184]	12	93	88	75	97
sIL-2R, sampled thrice over 7 d[188]	30	71	100	100	88
Screening Panels					
IL-6 and/or CRP at 0 and 48 hr[137]	45	98	91	90	98
IL-6 and/or CRP[125]	4	96	74	49	99
Any two or more positive tests of:[13] I:T ratio, total WBC, CRP, ESR, haptoglobin	8	93	88	39	99
Any three or more positive tests of:[41] I:T ratio, total neutrophils, total WBC, I:M ratio, degenerative changes of neutrophils, thrombocytopenia	9	96	78	31	99

CRP = C-reactive protein; IL-6 = interleukin-6; sIL-2R = soluble interleukin-2 receptor; I:T ratio = immature to total neutrophil ratio; WBC = total leukocyte count; ESR = erythrocyte sedimentation rate; I:M ratio = immature to mature neutrophil ratio (see text).
[a]A higher prevalence of sepsis tends to inflate the predictive values of a test or panel.

medicine, even in the era of molecular diagnostics and therapeutics. A single normal laboratory test should not sway a clinician against empirical therapy for a newborn if it appears to be clinically indicated, nor should the presence of an isolated abnormal test result be enough to demand therapy. This concept may be restated in diagnostic terminology as follows: The negative predictive values of available tests are not yet high enough when results are normal to lead to withholding therapy for a possibly life-threatening disease (neonatal sepsis), nor are the positive predictive values of available tests high enough when results are abnormal to lead to institution of antimicrobial therapy. When laboratory testing is combined with clinical impression (and perhaps serial laboratory monitoring), predictive values may increase enough to help the clinician make decisions. However, when the risk of a poor outcome of disease is high and the risk of therapy is low (as is the case for neonatal sepsis and antimicrobial therapy), it may be difficult to find a test with predictive values high enough to "rule in" or "rule out" disease with complete confidence. In the final analysis, simple, rapid, standardized, and inexpensive (albeit imperfect) tests such as total neutrophil counts, total leukocyte counts, and I:T ratios, combined with clinical acumen, still appear to be as useful as the newer acute-phase reactant and cytokine tests. Clearly, future work is needed in the area of rapid diagnosis of neonatal sepsis.

References

1. Feinstein AR. Clinical biostatistics: XXXI. On the sensitivity, specificity, and discrimination of diagnostic tests. Clin Pharmacol Ther 17:104–116, 1975.
2. Jaeschke R, Guyatt GH, Sackett DL, et al. Users' guides to the medical literature: III. How to use an article about a diagnostic test. B. What are the results and will they help me in caring for my patients? JAMA 271:703–707, 1994.
3. Radetsky M. The laboratory evaluation of newborn sepsis. Curr Opin Infect Dis 8:191–199, 1995.
4. Squire E, Favara B, Todd J. Diagnosis of neonatal bacterial infection: hematologic and pathologic findings in fatal and nonfatal cases. Pediatrics 64:60–64, 1979.
5. Dunham EC. Septicemia in the newborn. Am J Dis Child 45:229–253, 1933.
6. Nyhan WL, Fousek MD. Septicemia of the newborn. Pediatrics 22:268–278, 1958.
7. Buetow KC, Klein SW, Lane RB. Septicemia in premature infants. Am J Dis Child 110:29–41, 1965.
8. Moorman RS Jr, Sell SH. Neonatal septicemia. South Med J 54:137–141, 1961.
9. Hänninen P, Terho P, Toivanen A. Septicemia in a pediatric unit: a 20-year study. Scand J Infect Dis 3:201–208, 1971.
10. Spector SA, Ticknor W, Grossman M. Study of the usefulness of clinical and hematologic findings in the diagnosis of neonatal bacterial infections. Clin Pediatr 20:385–392, 1981.
11. Kuchler H, Fricker H, Gugler E. La formule sanguine

dans le diagnostic précoce de la septicémie du nouveau-né. Helv Paediatr Acta 31:33–46, 1976.

12. Töllner U, Pohlandt F. Septicemia in the newborn due to gram-negative bacilli: risk factors, clinical symptoms, and hematologic changes. Eur J Pediatr 123:243–254, 1976.

13. Philip AGS, Hewitt JR. Early diagnosis of neonatal sepsis. Pediatrics 65:1036–1041, 1980.

14. Gerdes JS, Polin RA. Sepsis screen in neonates with evaluation of plasma fibronectin. Pediatr Infect Dis J 6:443–446, 1987.

15. King JC Jr, Berman ED, Wright PF. Evaluation of fever in infants less than 8 weeks old. South Med J 80:948–952, 1987.

16. Philip AGS. Response of C-reactive protein in neonatal group B streptococcal infection. Pediatr Infect Dis J 4:145–148, 1985.

17. Speer CH, Bruns A, Gahr M. Sequential determination of CRP, alpha-1 antitrypsin and haptoglobin in neonatal septicaemia. Acta Paediatr Scand 72:679–683, 1983.

18. Liu C-H, Lehan C, Speer ME, et al. Degenerative changes in neutrophils: an indicator of bacterial infection. Pediatrics 74:823–827, 1984.

19. Moodley GP. The micro-erythrocyte sedimentation rate in black neonates and children: II. A comparative study of the micro-erythrocyte sedimentation rate, C-reactive protein test and total white cell count. S Afr Med J 60:545–547, 1981.

20. Jahnke S, Bartiromo G, Maisels MJ. The peripheral white blood cell count in the diagnosis of neonatal infection. J Perinatol 5:50–56, 1985.

21. Rozycki HJ, Stahl GE, Baumgart S. Impaired sensitivity of a single early leukocyte count in screening for neonatal sepsis. Pediatr Infect Dis J 6:440–442, 1987.

22. Christensen RD, Rothstein G, Hill HR, et al. Fatal early onset group B streptococcal sepsis with normal leukocyte counts. Pediatr Infect Dis J 4:242–245, 1985.

23. Marks MI, Stacy T, Krous HF. Progressive cough associated with lymphocytic leukemoid reaction in an infant. J Pediatr 97:156–160, 1980.

24. Weinberg AG, Rosenfeld CR, Manroe BL, et al. Neonatal blood cell count in health and disease: II. Values for lymphocytes, monocytes, and eosinophils. J Pediatr 106:462–466, 1985.

25. Roth P. Colony stimulating factor 1 levels in the human newborn infant. J Pediatr 119:113–116, 1991.

26. Karayalcin G, Khanijou A, Kim KY, et al. Monocytosis in congenital syphilis. Am J Dis Child 131:782–783, 1977.

27. Visintine AM, Oleske JM, Nahmias AJ. *Listeria monocytogenes* infection in infants and children. Am J Dis Child 131:393–397, 1977.

28. Xanthou M. Leucocyte blood picture in healthy full-term and premature babies during neonatal period. Arch Dis Child 45:242–249, 1970.

29. Lawrence R Jr, Church JA, Richards, W, et al. Eosinophilia in the hospitalized neonate. Ann Allergy 44:349–352, 1980.

30. Burrell JM. A comparative study of the circulating eosinophil level in babies: II. In full term infants. Arch Dis Child 28:140–142, 1953.

31. Gibson EL, Vaucher Y, Corrigan JJ Jr. Eosinophilia in premature infants: relationship to weight gain. J Pediatr 95:99–101, 1979.

32. Gunn T, Reaman G, Outerbridge EW, et al. Peripheral total parenteral nutrition for premature infants with the respiratory distress syndrome: a controlled study. J Pediatr 92:608–613, 1978.

33. Bhat AM, Scanlon JW. The pattern of eosinophilia in premature infants: a prospective study in premature infants using the absolute eosinophil count. J Pediatr 98:612–616, 1981.

34. Chudwin DS, Ammann AJ, Wara DW, et al. Posttransfusion syndrome: rash, eosinophilia, and thrombocytopenia following intrauterine and exchange transfusions. Am J Dis Child 136:612–614, 1982.

35. Xanthou M. Leucocyte blood picture in ill newborn babies. Arch Dis Child 47:741–746, 1972.

36. Bonadio WA, Smith DS. CBC differential profile in distinguishing etiology of neonatal meningitis. Pediatr Emerg Care 5:94–96, 1989.

37. Metrov M, Crain EF. The complete blood count differential ratio in the assessment of febrile infants with meningitis. Pediatr Infect Dis J 10:334–335, 1991.

38. Manroe BL, Weinberg AG, Rosenfeld CR, et al. The neonatal blood count in health and disease: I. Reference values for neutrophilic cells. J Pediatr 95:89–98, 1979.

39. Zipursky A, Palko J, Milner R, et al. The hematology of bacterial infections in premature infants. Pediatrics 57:839–853, 1976.

40. Amato M, Howald H, von Muralt G. Qualitative changes of white blood cells and perinatal diagnosis of infection in high-risk preterm infants. Pädiatr Pädol 23:129–134, 1988.

41. Rodwell RL, Leslie AL, Tudehope DI. Early diagnosis of neonatal sepsis using a hematologic scoring system. J Pediatr 112:761–767, 1988.

42. Berger C, Uehlinger J, Ghelfi D, et al. Comparison of C-reactive protein and white blood cell count with differential in neonates at risk for septicemia. Eur J Pediatr 154:138–144, 1995.

43. Christensen RD. Morphology and concentration of circulating neutrophils in neonates with bacterial sepsis. Pediatr Infect Dis J 6:429–430, 1987.

44. Gregory J, Hey E. Blood neutrophil response to bacterial infection in the first month of life. Arch Dis Child 47:747–753, 1972.

45. Baley JE, Stork EK, Warkentin PI, et al. Neonatal neutropenia: clinical manifestations, cause, and outcome. Am J Dis Child 142:1161–1166, 1988.

46. Marks J, Gairdner D, Roscoe JD. Blood formation in infancy: III. Cord blood. Arch Dis Child 30:117–120, 1955.

47. Coulombel L, Dehan M, Tchernia G, et al. The number of polymorphonuclear leukocytes in relation to gestational age in the newborn. Acta Paediatr Scand 68:709–711, 1979.

48. Engle WD, Rosenfeld CR. Neutropenia in high-risk neonates. J Pediatr 105:982–986, 1984.

49. Brazy JE, Grimm JK, Little VA. Neonatal manifestations of severe maternal hypertension occurring before the thirty-sixth week of pregnancy. J Pediatr 100:265–271, 1982.

50. Rodwell RL, Tudehope DI, Gray PH. Hematologic scoring system in early diagnosis of sepsis in neutropenic newborns. Pediatr Infect Dis J 12:372–376, 1993.

51. Merlob P, Amir J, Zaizov R, et al. The differential leukocyte count in full-term newborn infants with meconium aspiration and neonatal asphyxia. Acta Paediatr Scand 69:779–780, 1980.

52. Christensen RD, Rothstein G. Pitfalls in the interpretation of leukocyte counts of newborn infants. Am J Clin Pathol 72:608–611, 1979.

53. Carballo C, Foucar K, Swanson P, et al. Effect of high altitude on neutrophil counts in newborn infants. J Pediatr 119:464–466, 1991.

54. Menke JA, Giacoia GP, Jockin H. Group B beta hemo-

lytic streptococcal sepsis and the idiopathic respiratory distress syndrome: a comparison. J Pediatr 94:467–471, 1979.

55. Frazier JP, Cleary TG, Pickering LK, et al. Leukocyte function in healthy neonates following vaginal and cesarean section deliveries. J Pediatr 101:269–272, 1982.

56. Zipursky A, Jaber HM. The haematology of bacterial infection in newborn infants. Clin Haematol 7:175–193, 1978.

57. Akenzua GI, Hui YT, Milner R, et al. Neutrophil and band counts in the diagnosis of neonatal infections. Pediatrics 54:38–42, 1974.

58. Rooney JC, Hill DJ, Danks DM. Jaundice associated with bacterial infection in the newborn. Am J Dis Child 122:39–41, 1971.

59. Benuck I, David RJ. Sensitivity of published neutrophil indexes in identifying newborn infants with sepsis. J Pediatr 103:961–963, 1983.

60. Philip AGS. Detection of neonatal sepsis of late onset. JAMA 247:489–492, 1982.

61. Da Silva O, Ohlsson A, Kenyon C. Accuracy of leukocyte indices and C-reactive protein for diagnosis of neonatal sepsis: a critical review. Pediatr Infect Dis J 14:363–366, 1995.

62. Christensen RD, Bradley PP, Rothstein G. The leukocyte left shift in clinical and experimental neonatal sepsis. J Pediatr 98:101–105, 1981.

63. Speer CP, Hauptmann D, Stubbe P, et al. Neonatal septicemia and meningitis in Göttingen, West Germany. Pediatr Infect Dis J 4:36–41, 1985.

64. Faden HS. Early diagnosis of neonatal bacteremia by buffy-coat examination. J Pediatr 88:1032–1034, 1976.

65. Leonidas JC, Hall RT, Beatty EC, et al. Radiographic findings in early onset neonatal group B streptococcal septicemia. Pediatrics 59:1006–1011, 1977.

66. Manroe BL, Rosenfeld CR, Weinberg AG, et al. The differential leukocyte count in the assessment and outcome of early-onset neonatal group B streptococcal disease. J Pediatr 91:632–637, 1977.

67. Payne NR, Burke BA, Day DL, et al. Correlation of clinical and pathologic findings in early onset neonatal group B streptococcal infection with disease severity and prediction of outcome. Pediatr Infect Dis J 7:836–847, 1988.

68. Neiburg PI. Prognostic/diagnostic factors in group B beta hemolytic streptococcal (GBBS) and other neonatal sepsis. Pediatr Res 10:402, 1976.

69. Courtney SE, Hall RT. *Haemophilus influenzae* sepsis in the premature infant. Am J Dis Child 132:1039–1040, 1978.

70. Christensen RD, Rothstein G, Anstall HB, et al. Granulocyte transfusions in neonates with bacterial infection, neutropenia, and depletion of mature marrow neutrophils. Pediatrics 70:1–6, 1982.

71. Bortolussi R, Thompson TR, Ferrieri P. Early-onset pneumococcal sepsis in newborn infants. Pediatrics 60:352–355, 1977.

72. Johnsson H, Bergström S, Ewald U, et al. Neonatal septicemia caused by pneumococci. Acta Obstet Gynecol Scand 71:6–11, 1992.

73. Jacobs J, Garmyn K, Verhaegen J, et al. Neonatal sepsis due to *Streptococcus pneumoniae*. Scand J Infect Dis 22:493–497, 1990.

74. Alexander JB, Giacoia GP. Early onset nonenterococcal group D streptococcal infection in the newborn infant. J Pediatr 93:489–490, 1978.

75. Christensen RD, Rothstein G. Exhaustion of mature marrow neutrophils in neonates with sepsis. J Pediatr 96:316–318, 1980.

76. Boyle RJ, Chandler BD, Stonestreet BS, et al. Early identification of sepsis in infants with respiratory distress. Pediatrics 62:744–750, 1978.

77. Lloyd BW, Oto A. Normal values for mature and immature neutrophils in very preterm babies. Arch Dis Child 57:233–235, 1982.

78. Sherman MP, Goetzman BW, Ahlfors CE, et al. Tracheal aspiration and its clinical correlates in the diagnosis of congenital pneumonia. Pediatrics 65:258–263, 1980.

79. Wheeler JG, Chauvenet AR, Johnson CA, et al. Neutrophil storage pool depletion in septic, neutropenic neonates. Pediatr Infect Dis 3:407–409, 1984.

80. Christensen RD, Harper TE, Rothstein G. Granulocyte-macrophage progenitor cells in term and preterm neonates. J Pediatr 109:1047–1051, 1986.

81. Lake AM, Lauer BA, Clark JC, et al. Enterovirus infections in neonates. J Pediatr 89:787–791, 1976.

82. Gerdes JS. Clinicopathologic approach to the diagnosis of neonatal sepsis. Clin Perinatol 18:361–381, 1991.

83. Mathers NJ, Pohlandt F. Diagnostic audit of C-reactive protein in neonatal infection. Eur J Pediatr 146:147–151, 1987.

84. Sherman, MP, Chance KH, Goetzman BW. Gram's stains of tracheal secretions predict neonatal bacteremia. Am J Dis Child 138:848–850, 1984.

85. Kite P, Millar MR, Gorham P, et al. Comparison of five tests used in diagnosis of neonatal bacteraemia. Arch Dis Child 63:639–643, 1988.

86. Schmidt BK, Kirpalani HM, Corey M, et al. Coagulase-negative staphylococci as true pathogens in newborn infants: a cohort study. Pediatr Infect Dis J 6:1026–1031, 1987.

87. Greenberg DN, Yoder BA. Changes in the differential white blood cell count in screening for group B streptococcal sepsis. Pediatr Infect Dis J 9:886–889, 1990.

88. Schelonka RL, Yoder BA, Hall RB, et al. Differentiation of segmented and band neutrophils during the early newborn period. J Pediatr 127:298–300, 1995.

89. Appleyard WJ, Brinton A. Venous platelet counts in low birth weight infants. Biol Neonate 17:30–34, 1971.

90. Wolff JA, Goodfellow AM. Hematopoiesis in premature infants with special consideration of the effect of iron and of animal-protein factor. Pediatrics 16:753–762, 1955.

91. Aballi AJ, Puapondh Y, Desposito F. Platelet counts in thriving premature infants. Pediatrics 42:685–689, 1968.

92. Modanlou HD, Ortiz OB. Thrombocytopenia in neonatal infection. Clin Pediatr 20:402–407, 1981.

93. Andrew M, Kelton J. Neonatal thrombocytopenia. Clin Perinatol 11:359–390, 1984.

94. Tate DY, Carlton GT, Johnson D, et al. Immune thrombocytopenia in severe neonatal infections. J Pediatr 98:449–453, 1981.

95. Mehta P, Vasa R, Neumann L, et al. Thrombocytopenia in the high-risk infant. J Pediatr 97:791–794, 1980.

96. Ng PC, Herrington RA, Beane CA, et al. An outbreak of *Acinetobacter* septicemia in a neonatal intensive care unit. J Hosp Infect 14:363–368, 1989.

97. Kekomäki R, Kekomäki M, Elfving J. Platelet-associated IgG in septicemia. N Engl J Med 301:271, 1979.

98. Modlin JF. Fatal echovirus 11 disease in premature neonates. Pediatrics 66:775–780, 1980.

99. Ballard RA, Drew L, Hufnagle KG, et al. Acquired cytomegalovirus infection in preterm infants. Am J Dis Child 133:482–485, 1979.

100. Ballin A, Koren G, Kohelet D, et al. Reduction of plate-

let counts induced by mechanical ventilation in newborn infants. J Pediatr 111:445–449, 1987.

101. Patel CC. Hematologic abnormalities in acute necrotizing enterocolitis. Pediatr Clin North Am 24:579–584, 1977.

102. Hutter JJ Jr, Hathaway WE, Wayne ER. Hematologic abnormalities in severe neonatal necrotizing enterocolitis. J Pediatr 88:1026–1031, 1976.

103. Koenig JM, Christensen RD. Neutropenia and thrombocytopenia in infants with Rh hemolytic disease. J Pediatr 114:625–631, 1989.

104. Patrick CH, Lazarchick J. The effect of bacteremia on automated platelet measurements in neonates. Am J Clin Pathol 93:391–394, 1990.

105. Gabay C, Kushner I. Acute-phase proteins and other systemic responses to inflammation. N Engl J Med 340:448–454, 1999.

106. Pepys MB, Baltz ML. Acute phase proteins with special reference to C-reactive protein and related proteins (pentaxins) and serum amyloid A protein. Adv Immunol 34:141–212, 1983.

107. Jaye DL, Waites KB. Clinical applications of C-reactive protein in pediatrics. Pediatr Infect Dis J 16:735–747, 1997.

108. Hanson L-O, Lindquist L. C-reactive protein: its role in the diagnosis and follow-up of infectious diseases. Curr Opin Infect Dis 10:196–201, 1997.

109. Gitlin D, Biasucci A. Development of IgG, IgA, IgM, β1C/β1A, C'1 esterase inhibitor, ceruloplasmin, transferrin, hemopexin, haptoglobin, fibrinogen, plasminogen, α₁-antitrypsin, orosomucoid, β-lipoprotein, α₂-macroglobulin, and prealbumin in the human conceptus. J Clin Invest 48:1433–1446, 1969.

110. Nakamura RM. Nephelometric immunoassays. In Boguslaski RC, Maggio ET, Nakamura RM (eds). Clinical Immunochemistry: Principles of Methods and Applications. Boston/Toronto, Little, Brown, 1984, pp 199–211.

111. Nilsson LA. Comparative testing of precipitation methods for quantitation of C-reactive protein in blood serum. Acta Pathol Microbiol Scand 73:129–144, 1968.

112. Felix NS, Nakajima H, Kagan BM. Serum C-reactive protein in infections during the first six months of life. Pediatrics 37:270–277, 1966.

113. Kagan BM, Stanincova V, Felix N. IgM determination in neonate and infants for diagnosis of infection. J Pediatr 77:916, 1970.

114. Hanson LA, Jodal U, Sabel K-G, et al. The diagnostic value of C-reactive protein. Pediatr Infect Dis J 2:87–90, 1983.

115. Wassunna A, Whitelaw A, Gallimore R, et al. C-reactive protein and bacterial infection in preterm infants. Eur J Pediatr 149:424–427, 1990.

116. Vallance H, Lockitch G. Rapid, semi-quantitative assay of C-reactive protein evaluated. Clin Chem 37:1981–1982, 1991.

117. O'Callaghan C, Franklin P, Elliott TSJ, et al. C reactive protein concentrations in neonates: determination by a latex enhanced immunoassay. J Clin Pathol 37:1027–1028, 1984.

118. Ewerbeck H, Khnzer W, Uhlig T. Serum C-reactive protein in early diagnosis of bacterial infections in premature infants. Acta Paediatr Hung 25:55–58, 1984.

119. Ainbender E, Cabatu EE, Guzman DM, et al. Serum C-reactive protein and problems of newborn infants. J Pediatr 101:438–440, 1982.

120. Forest J-C, Larivière F, Dolcé P, et al. C-reactive protein as biochemical indicator of bacterial infection in neonates. Clin Biochem 19:192–194, 1986.

121. Sann L, Bienvenu F, Bienvenu J, et al. Evolution of serum prealbumin, C-reactive protein, and orosomucoid in neonates with bacterial infection. J Pediatr 105:977–981, 1984.

122. Gill CW, Bush WS, Burleigh WM, et al. An evaluation of a C-reactive protein assay using a rate immunonephelometric procedure. Am J Clin Pathol 75:50–55, 1981.

123. Pourcyrous M, Bada HS, Korones SB, et al. Acute phase reactants in neonatal bacterial infection. J Perinatol 11:319–325, 1991.

124. Kisbán G, Bartalics L, Korányi G. Diagnostic value of C-reactive protein in premature babies weighing less than 1500 g. Acta Paediatr Hung 26:335–340, 1985.

125. Doellner H, Arntzen KJ, Haereid PE, et al. Interleukin-6 concentrations in neonates evaluated for sepsis. J Pediatr 132:295–299, 1998.

126. Kindmark C-O. The concentration of C-reactive protein in sera from healthy individuals. Scand J Clin Lab Invest 29:407–411, 1972.

127. Rozansky R, Bercovici B. C-reactive protein during pregnancy and in cord blood. Proc Soc Exp Biol Med 92:4–6, 1956.

128. Hanson LA, Nilsson L-A. Studies on C-reactive protein: II. The presence of C-reactive protein during the pre- and neonatal period. Acta Pathol Microbiol Scand 56:409–414, 1962.

129. Nesbitt REL Jr, Hays RC, Mauro J. The behavior of C-reactive protein in pregnant and puerperal women, fetal blood, and in the newborn infant under normal and abnormal conditions. Obstet Gynecol 16:659–666, 1960.

130. Khan WN, Ali RV, Werthmann M, et al. Immunoglobulin M determinations in neonates and infants as an adjunct to the diagnosis of infection. J Pediatr 75:1282–1286, 1969.

131. Hawrylyshyn P, Bernstein P, Milligan JE, et al. Premature rupture of membranes: the role of C-reactive protein in the prediction of chorioamnionitis. Am J Obstet Gynecol 147:240–246, 1983.

132. Salzer HR, Genger H, Muhar U, et al. C-reactive protein: an early marker for neonatal bacterial infection due to prolonged rupture of amniotic membranes and/or amnionitis. Acta Obstet Gynecol Scand 66:365–367, 1987.

133. Pourcyrous M, Bada HS, Korones SB, et al. Significance of serial C-reactive protein responses in neonatal infection and other disorders. Pediatrics 92:431–435, 1993.

134. Schouten-Van Meeteren NYN, Rietveld A, Moolenaar AJ, et al. Influence of perinatal conditions on C-reactive protein production. J Pediatr 120:621–624, 1992.

135. Lorber J, Emery JL. Intracerebral cysts complicating ventricular needling in hydrocephalic infants: a clinicopathological study. Dev Med Child Neurol 6:125–139, 1964.

136. Gutteberg TJ, Haneberg B, Jergensen, T. Lactoferrin in relation to acute phase proteins in sera from newborn infants with severe infections. Eur J Pediatr 142:37–39, 1984.

137. Ng PC, Cheng SH, Fok TF, et al. Diagnosis of late onset neonatal sepsis with cytokines, adhesion molecule, and C-reactive protein in preterm very low birthweight infants. Arch Dis Child 77:F221–F227, 1997.

138. Benitz WE, Han MY, Madan A, et al. Serial C-reactive protein levels in the diagnosis of neonatal infection. Pediatrics 102(4), 1998; electronic pages, available at URL: http://www.pediatrics.org/cgi/content/full/102/4/e41.

139. Ehl S, Gering B, Bartmann P, et al. C-reactive protein is a useful marker for guiding duration of antibiotic therapy

in suspected neonatal bacterial infection. Pediatrics 99:216–221, 1997.

140. Nakamura H, Uetani Y, Nagata T, et al. Serum C-reactive protein in the early diagnosis of neonatal septicemia and bacterial meningitis. Acta Pediatr Jpn 31:567–571, 1989.

141. Shortland DB, MacFadyen U, Elston A, et al. Evaluation of C-reactive protein values in neonatal sepsis. J Perinat Med 18:157–163, 1990.

142. Buck C, Bundschu J, Gallati H, et al. Interleukin-6: a sensitive parameter for the early diagnosis of neonatal bacterial infection. Pediatrics 93:54–58, 1994.

143. Isaacs D, North J, Lindsell D, et al. Serum acute phase reactants in necrotizing enterocolitis. Acta Paediatr Scand 76:923–927, 1987.

144. Saxstad, J Nilsson L-Å, Hanson L-Å. C-reactive protein in serum from infants as determined with immunodiffusion techniques: II. Infants with various infections. Acta Paediatr Scand 59:676–680, 1970.

144a. Ehl S, Gehring B, Pohlandt F. A detailed analysis of changes in serum C-reactive protein levels in neonates treated for bacterial infection. Eur J Pediatr 158:238–242, 1999.

145. Philip AGS. Acute-phase proteins in neonatal infection. J Pediatr 105:940–942, 1984.

146. Peltola H, Luhtala K, Valmari P. C-reactive protein as a detector of organic complications during recovery from childhood purulent meningitis. J Pediatr 104:869–872, 1984.

147. Barratt BA, Hill PI. A micromethod for the erythrocyte sedimentation rate suitable for use on venous or capillary blood. J Clin Pathol 33:1118, 1980.

148. Lascari AD. The erythrocyte sedimentation rate. Pediatr Clin North Am 19:1113–1121, 1972.

149. Adler SM, Denton RL. The erythrocyte sedimentation rate in the newborn period. J Pediatr 86:942–948, 1975.

150. Evans HE, Glass L, Mercado C. The micro-erythrocyte sedimentation rate in newborn infants. J Pediatr 76:448–451, 1970.

151. Ibsen KK, Nielsen M, Prag J, et al. The value of the micromethod erythrocyte sedimentation rate in the diagnosis of infections in newborns. Scand J Infect Dis 23(Suppl):143–145, 1980.

152. Prag J, Nielsen M, Horlyk H, et al. Micromethod erythrocyte sedimentation rate as a diagnostic tool in neonatal bacterial infections. Dan Med Bull 31:483–486, 1984.

153. Moodley GP. The micro-erythrocyte sedimentation rate in black neonates and children. S Afr Med J 59:943–945, 1981.

154. Bennish M, Vardiman J, Beem MC. The zeta sedimentation ratio in children. J Pediatr 104:249–251, 1984.

155. Stuart J, Whicher JT. Tests for detecting and monitoring the acute phase response. Arch Dis Child 63:115–117, 1988.

156. Silverman WA, Homan WE. Sepsis of obscure origin in the newborn. Pediatrics 3:157–176, 1949.

157. Sell EJ, Corrigan JJ Jr. Platelet counts, fibrinogen concentrations, and factor V and factor VIII levels in healthy infants according to gestational age. J Pediatr 82:1028–1032, 1973.

158. Jensen AH, Josso F, Zamet P, et al. Evolution of blood clotting factor levels in premature infants during the first 10 days of life: a study of 96 cases with comparison between clinical status and blood clotting factor levels. Pediatr Res 7:638–644, 1973.

159. Koçak Ü, Ezer Ü, Vidinlisan S. Serum fibronectin in neonatal sepsis: is it valuable in early diagnosis and outcome prediction? Acta Pediatr Jpn 39:428–432, 1997.

160. Boichot P, Schirrer J, Menget A, et al. L'orosomucoide à la période néonatale: étude chez le nouveau-né sain et le nouveau-né infecté. Pédiatrie 35:577–588, 1980.

161. Salmi TT. Haptoglobin levels in the plasma of newborn infants with special reference to infections. Acta Paediatr Scand 241:7–55, 1973.

162. Kanakoudi F, Drossou V, Tzimouli V, et al. Serum concentrations of 10 acute-phase proteins in healthy term and preterm infants from birth to age 6 months. Clin Chem 41:605–608, 1995.

163. Lee SK, Thibeault DW, Heiner DC. α_1-Antitrypsin and α_1-acid glycoprotein levels in the cord blood and amniotic fluid of infants with respiratory distress syndrome. Pediatr Res 12:775–777, 1978.

164. Bienvenu J, Sann L, Bienvenu F, et al. Laser nephelometry of orosomucoid in serum of newborns: reference intervals and relation to bacterial infections. Clin Chem 27:721–726, 1981.

165. Philip AGS, Hewitt JR. $\alpha_1\beta$-Acid glycoprotein in the neonate with and without infection. Biol Neonate 43:118–124, 1983.

166. Gotoh H, Ishikawa N, Shioiri R, et al. Diagnostic significance of serum orosomucoid level in bacterial infections during neonatal period. Acta Paediatr Scand 62:629–632, 1973.

167. Philip AGS. The protective effect of acute phase reactants in neonatal sepsis. Acta Paediatr Scand 68:481–483, 1979.

168. Treluyer JM, Bompard Y, Gantzer A, et al. Septicémies néonatales: diagnostic biologique et antibiothérapie: à propos d'une série de 46 cas. Arch Fr Pédiatr 48:317–321, 1991.

169. Rodwell RL, Taylor KM, Tudehope DI, et al. Capillary plasma elastase alpha-1-proteinase inhibitor in infected and non-infected neonates. Arch Dis Child 67:436–439, 1992.

170. Speer CP, Rethwilm M, Gahr M. Elastase-α_1-proteinase inhibitor: an early indicator of septicemia and bacterial meningitis in children. J Pediatr 111:667–671, 1987.

171. Adinolfi M. Human complement C9 and factor B in the diagnosis of infections in infants. Acta Paediatr Scand 71:845–846, 1982.

172. Suri M, Sharma VK, Thirupuram S. Evaluation of ceruloplasmin in neonatal septicemia. Indian Pediatr 28:489–493, 1991.

173. Miller LC, Isa S, Lo Preste G, et al. Neonatal interleukin-1β, interleukin-6, and tumor necrosis factor: cord blood levels and cellular production. J Pediatr 117:961–965, 1990.

174. Messer J, Eyer D, Donato L, et al. Evaluation of interleukin-6 and soluble receptors of tumor necrosis factor for early diagnosis of neonatal infection. J Pediatr 129:574–580, 1996.

175. Gomez R, Romero R, Ghezzi F, et al. The fetal inflammatory response syndrome. Am J Obstet Gynecol 179:194–202, 1998.

176. Lehrnbecher T, Schrod L, Rutsch P, et al. Immunologic parameters in cord blood indicating early-onset sepsis. Biol Neonate 70:206–212, 1996.

177. Panero A, Pacifico L, Rossi N, et al. Interleukin-6 in neonates with early and late onset infection. Pediatr Infect Dis J 16:370–375, 1997.

178. Shimoya K, Matsuzaki N, Taniguchi T, et al. Interleukin-8 in cord sera: a sensitive and specific marker for the detection of preterm chorioamnionitis. J Infect Dis 165:957–960, 1992.

179. Sullivan JS, Kilpatrick L, Costarino AT Jr, et al. Correla-

tion of plasma cytokine elevations with mortality rate in children with sepsis. J Pediatr 120:510–515, 1992.

180. Girardin EP, Berner ME, Grau GE, et al. Serum tumor necrosis factor in newborns at risk for infections. Eur J Pediatr 149:645–647, 1990.

181. Assicot M, Gendrel D, Carsin H, et al. High serum procalcitonin concentrations in patients with sepsis and infection. Lancet 1:515–518, 1993.

182. Gendrel D, Assicot M, Raymond J, et al. Procalcitonin as a marker for the early diagnosis of neonatal infection. J Pediatr 128:570–573, 1996.

183. Monneret G, Labaune JM, Isaac C, et al. Procalcitonin and C-reactive protein levels in neonatal infections. Acta Paediatr 86:209–212, 1997.

184. Chiesa C, Panero A, Rossi N, et al. Reliability of procalcitonin concentrations for the diagnosis of sepsis in critically ill neonates. Clin Infect Dis 26:664–672, 1998.

185. Lapillone A, Basson E, Monneret G, et al. Lack of specificity of procalcitonin for sepsis diagnosis in premature infants. Lancet 351:1211–1212, 1998.

186. Kuster H, Degitz K. Circulating ICAM-1 in neonatal sepsis. Lancet 1:506, 1993.

187. De Bont ESJM, De Leij LHFM, Okken A, et al. Increased plasma concentrations of interleukin-1 receptor antagonist in neonatal sepsis. Pediatr Res 37:626–629, 1995.

188. Spear ML, Stefano JL, Fawcett P, et al. Soluble interleukin-2 receptor as a predictor of neonatal sepsis. J Pediatr 126:982–985, 1995.

189. Hodge S, Hodge G, Flower R, et al. Surface activation markers of T lymphocytes: role in the detection of infection in neonates. Clin Exp Immunol 113:33–38, 1998.

190. Weirich E, Rabin RL, Maldonado Y, et al. Neutrophil CD11b expression as a diagnostic marker for early-onset neonatal infection. J Pediatr 132:445–451, 1998.

191. Weinschenk NP, Farina A, Bianchi DW. Neonatal neutrophil activation is a function of labor length in preterm infants. Pediatr Res 44:942–945, 1998.

192. Gerdes JS, Yoder MC, Douglas SD, et al. Decreased plasma fibronectin in neonatal sepsis. Pediatrics 72:877–881, 1983.

193. Yang KD, Bohnsack JF, Hill HR. Fibronectin in host defense: implications in the diagnosis, prophylaxis and therapy of infectious diseases. Pediatr Infect Dis 12:234–239, 1993.

194. McCafferty MH, Lepow M, Saba TM, et al. Normal fibronectin levels as a function of age in the pediatric population. Pediatr Res 17:482–485, 1982.

195. Koenig JM, Patterson LER, Rench MA, et al. Role of fibronectin in diagnosing bacterial infection in infancy. Am J Dis Child 142:884–887, 1988.

196. Yoder MC, Douglas SD, Gerdes J, et al. Plasma fibronectin in healthy newborn infants: respiratory distress syndrome and perinatal asphyxia. J Pediatr 102:777–780, 1983.

197. Caliouli C, Liossis G, Bakoleas B, et al. Fibronectin levels in septicemic neonates before and after the administration of immunoglobulin. Acta Paediatr Scand 80:1229–1230, 1991.

198. Yoder MC. Therapeutic administration of fibronectin: current uses and potential applications. Clin Perinatol 18:325–341, 1991.

199. Alford CA Jr. Immunoglobulin determinations in the diagnosis of fetal infection. Pediatr Clin North Am 18:99–113, 1971.

200. Haider SA. Serum IgM in diagnosis of infection in the newborn. Arch Dis Child 47:382–393, 1972.

201. Cederqvist LL, Ewool LC, Litwin SD. The effect of fetal age, birth weight, and sex on cord blood immunoglobulin values. Am J Obstet Gynecol 131:520–525, 1978.

202. Blankenship WJ, Cassady G, Schaefer J, et al. Serum gamma-M globulin responses in acute neonatal infections and their diagnostic significance. J Pediatr 75:1271–1281, 1969.

203. Korones SB, Roane JA, Gilkeson MR, et al. Neonatal IgM response to acute infection. J Pediatr 75:1261–1270, 1969.

204. Rothberg RM. Immunoglobulin and specific antibody synthesis during the first weeks of life of premature infants. J Pediatr 75:391–399, 1969.

205. Baehner RL. Use of the nitroblue tetrazolium test in clinical pediatrics. Am J Dis Child 128:449–451, 1974.

206. Cocchi P, Mori S, Becattini A. NBT tests in premature infants. 2:1426–1427, 1969.

207. Cocchi P, Mori S, Becattini A. Nitroblue-tetrazolium reduction by neutrophils of newborn infants in in vitro phagocytosis test. Acta Paediatr Scand 60:475–478, 1971.

208. Goel KM, Vowels MR. Leucocyte function in normal and pre-term infants. Acta Paediatr Scand 63:122–124, 1974.

209. Humbert JR, Kurtz ML, Hathaway WE. Increased reduction of nitroblue tetrazolium by neutrophils of newborn infants. Pediatrics 45:125–128, 1970.

210. Park BH, Holmes BM, Rodey GE, et al. Nitroblue-tetrazolium test in children with fatal granulomatous disease and newborn infants. Lancet 1:157, 1969.

211. Park BH, Holmes B, Good RA. Metabolic activities in leukocytes of newborn infants. J Pediatr 76:237–241, 1970.

212. Chandler BD, Kapoor N, Barker BE, et al. Nitroblue tetrazolium test in neonates. J Pediatr 92:638–640, 1978.

213. McCracken GH Jr, Eichenwald HF. Leukocyte function and the development of opsonic and complement activity in the neonate. Am J Dis Child 121:120–126, 1971.

214. Anderson DC, Pickering LK, Feigin RD. Leukocyte function in normal and infected neonates. J Pediatr 85:420–425, 1974.

215. Shigeoka AO, Santos JI, Hill HR. Functional analysis of neutrophil granulocytes from healthy, infected, and stressed neonates. J Pediatr 95:454–460, 1979.

216. Shigeoka AO, Charette RP, Wyman ML, et al. Defective oxidative metabolic responses of neutrophils from stressed neonates. J Pediatr 98:392–398, 1981.

217. Powers DW, Ayoub EM. Leukocyte lactate dehydrogenase in bacterial meningitis. Pediatrics 54:27–33, 1974.

218. Donato H, Gebara E, de Cosen RH, et al. Leukocyte alkaline phosphatase activity in the diagnosis of neonatal bacterial infections. J Pediatr 94:242–244, 1979.

219. Horner R, Elidan J, Sadovsky E, et al. Leukocyte alkaline phosphatase in newborn infants after delivery and and in the puerperium. J Perinat Med 3:68–72, 1975.

220. Sadovsky E, Matz D, Diamant YZ, et al. Leukocyte alkaline phosphatase in the newborn. Biol Neonate 27:96–101, 1975.

221. Nagy P, Szabó I, Csaba I. Changes in the alkaline phosphatase activity of granulocytes from the first to the sixth day of life in newborns. Biol Neonate 27:121–124, 1975.

222. Leake RD, Fiser RH Jr, Oh W. Rapid glucose disappearance in infants with infection. Clin Pediatr 20:397–401, 1981.

223. James T III, Blessa M, Boggs TR Jr. Recurrent hyperglycemia associated with sepsis in a neonate. Am J Dis Child 133:645–646, 1979.

224. Benirschke K. Routes and types of infection in the fetus and the newborn. Am J Dis Child 99:714–721, 1960.

225. Blanc WA. Pathways of fetal and early neonatal infection:

viral placentitis, bacterial and fungal chorioamnionitis. J Pediatr 59:473–496, 1961.

226. Driscoll SG. Pathology and the developing fetus. Pediatr Clin North Am 12:493–514, 1965.

227. Kelsall GRH, Barter RA, Manessis C. Prospective bacteriological studies in inflammation of the placenta, cord and membranes. J Obstet Gynecol Br Commonw 74:401–411, 1967.

228. Overbach AM, Daniel, SJ, Cassady G. The value of umbilical cord histology in the management of potential perinatal infection. J Pediatr 76:22–31, 1970.

229. Wilson MG, Armstrong DH, Nelson RC, et al. Prolonged rupture of fetal membranes: effect on the newborn infant. Am J Dis Child 107:138–146, 1964.

230. Morison JE. Foetal and Neonatal Pathology, 3rd ed. Washington, DC, Butterworth, 1970.

231. Fox H, Langley FA. Leukocytic infiltration of the placenta and umbilical cord: a clinico-pathologic study. Obstet Gynecol 37:451–458, 1971.

232. Dominguez R, Segal AJ, O'Sullivan JA. Leukocytic infiltration of the umbilical cord: manifestation of fetal hypoxia due to reduction of blood flow in the cord. JAMA 173:346–349, 1960.

233. Anderson GS, Green CA, Neligan GA, et al. Congenital bacterial pneumonia. Lancet 2:585–587, 1962.

234. Ramos A, Stern L. Relationship of premature rupture of the membranes to gastric fluid aspirate in the newborn. Am J Obstet Gynecol 105:1247–1251, 1969.

235. Vasan U, Lim DM, Greenstein RM, et al. Origin of gastric polymorphonuclear leukocytes in infants born after prolonged rupture of membranes. J Pediatr 91:69–72, 1977.

236. Yeung CY, Tam ASY. Gastric aspirate findings in neonatal pneumonia. Arch Dis Child 47:735–740, 1972.

237. Scanlon J. The early detection of neonatal sepsis by examination of liquid obtained from the external ear canal. J Pediatr 79:247–249, 1971.

238. Hosmer ME, Sprunt K. Screening method for identification of infected infant following premature rupture of maternal membranes. Pediatrics 49:283–285, 1972.

239. Zuerlein TJ, Butler JC, Yeager TD. Superficial cultures in neonatal sepsis evaluations: impact on antibiotic decision making. Clin Pediatr 29:445–447, 1990.

240. Handsfield HH, Hodson WA, Holmes KK. Neonatal gonococcal infection: I. Orogastric contamination with N. gonorrhoeae. JAMA 225:697–701, 1973.

241. MacGregor RR, Tunnessen WW Jr. The incidence of pathogenic organisms in the normal flora of the neonate's external ear and nasopharynx. Clin Pediatr 12:697–700, 1973.

242. Mims LC, Medawar MS, Perkins JR, et al. Predicting neonatal infections by evaluation of the gastric aspirate: a study in two hundred and seven patients. Am J Obstet Gynecol 114:232–238, 1972.

243. Lau YL, Hey E. Sensitivity and specificity of daily tracheal aspirate cultures in predicting organisms causing bacteremia in ventilated neonates. Pediatr Infect Dis J 10:290–294, 1991.

244. Laforgia N, Coppola B, Carbone R, et al. Rapid detection of neonatal sepsis using polymerase chain reaction. Acta Paediatr 86:1097–1099, 1997.

245. Hazan Y, Mazor M, Horowitz S, et al. The diagnostic value of amniotic Gram stain examination and limulus amebocyte lysate assay in patients with preterm birth. Acta Obstet Gynecol Scand 74:275–280, 1995.

246. Philip AGS. Decreased use of antibiotics using a neonatal sepsis screening technique. J Pediatr 98:795–799, 1981.

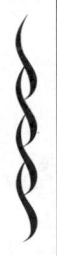

C H A P T E R   3 3

Obstetric Factors Associated with Infections of the Fetus and Newborn Infant

JILL K. DAVIES, M.D., and RONALD S. GIBBS, M.D.

Early-onset neonatal infection often has its origin in utero. Thus, risk factors for neonatal sepsis include prematurity, premature rupture of the membranes (PROM), and maternal fever during labor (which may be caused by clinical intra-amniotic infection). This chapter focuses on these major obstetric conditions. In addition to these three "classic" topics we have added a discussion of new information that indicates intrauterine exposure to bacteria is linked to major neonatal sequelae, including cerebral palsy, bronchopulmonary dysplasia, and respiratory distress syndrome.

INTRA-AMNIOTIC INFECTION

Clinically evident intrauterine infection during the latter half of pregnancy develops in 1 to 10% of pregnancies and leads to increased maternal morbidity as well as perinatal mortality and morbidity. In general, the diagnosis is clinically based on the presence of fever and other signs and symptoms, such as maternal or fetal tachycardia, uterine tenderness, foul odor of the amniotic fluid, and maternal leukocytosis. Although not invariably present, rupture of the membranes (ROM) or labor also occurs in most cases. Some prospective reports have noted higher rates (4.2 to 10.5%)[1–3] than in older retrospective studies (1 to 2%).[4] A number of terms have been applied to this infection, including chorioamnionitis, intrapartum infection, amniotic fluid infection, and intra-amniotic infection (IAI). We use the last designa-

tion to distinguish this clinical syndrome from bacterial colonization of amniotic fluid (also referred to as microbial invasion of the amniotic cavity) and from histologic inflammation of the placenta (histologic chorioamnionitis).

Pathogenesis

Before labor and ROM, amniotic fluid is nearly always sterile. With the onset of labor or with ROM, bacteria from the lower genital tract usually enters the amniotic cavity. This ascending route is the most common pathway for development of IAI.[4]

Occasional instances of documented IAI in the absence of ROM or of labor support a presumed hematogenous or transplacental route of infection. Fulminant IAI without labor and without ROM may be caused by Listeria monocytogenes.[5–9] Maternal sepsis with this organism often manifests as maternal flulike illness and may result in death of the fetus. In an outbreak caused by Mexican-style cheese contaminated with Listeria, several maternal deaths occurred.[10] Other virulent organisms, such as group A streptococci, have also been the cause of transplacental infection.[11] IAI may develop less commonly as a consequence of obstetric procedures such as cervical cerclage, diagnostic amniocentesis, cordocentesis (percutaneous umbilical cord sampling), or intrauterine transfusion. The absolute risk is small with all of these procedures: IAI develops in 2 to 8% of patients after cerclage,[12–15] 0 to 1% of patients after amniocentesis,[16] and 5% of patients after intrauterine transfusion.[17]

Higher risks are encountered, however, when cerclage is performed when the cervix is dilated and effaced.

In 1989, two large studies of risk factors for IAI identified characteristics of labor as the major risks by logistic regression analysis. These features were low parity, increased number of vaginal examinations in labor, as well as increased duration of labor, membrane rupture, and internal fetal monitoring.[3, 4] More recently, risk factors for IAI have been stratified for term versus preterm pregnancies.[18] For patients at term with IAI, these investigators observed, by logistic regression analysis, that the independent risk factors were ROM greater than 12 hours (odds ratio 5.81), internal fetal monitoring (odds ratio 2.01), and more than four vaginal examinations in labor (odds ratio 3.07). For preterm pregnancies, these three risk factors were again identified as being independently associated with IAI, but with differing odds ratios. Specifically, in the preterm pregnancies for ROM longer than 12 hours, the odds ratio was 2.49; for internal fetal monitoring, the odds ratio was 1.42; and for more than four examinations, the odds ratio was 1.59. One interpretation of these data regarding risk factors among preterm pregnancies is that there was some other risk factor not detected in this survey.

In 1996 a multivariate analysis demonstrated quantitatively the importance of chorioamnionitis in neonatal sepsis.[19] The odds ratio for neonatal sepsis accompanying clinical chorioamnionitis was 25, whereas for preterm delivery, ROM longer than 12 hours, endometritis, and group B streptococcal colonization, the odds ratios were all less than 5. Epidural anesthesia has been associated with fever in labor (independent of infection).[20] This knowledge must be considered in determining the etiology of fever in a patient who has an epidural anesthetic in place.

Although Naeye had reported an association between recent coitus and development of chorioamnionitis defined by histologic study,[21] further analysis of the same population refuted this association.[22] Other studies have not demonstrated any relationship between coitus and PROM, premature birth, or perinatal death.[23]

Microbiology

The cause of IAI is often polymicrobial. Gibbs and colleagues reported a microbiologic case-control study of amniotic fluid from 52 patients with clinical IAI.[24] Characteristics of these cultures are shown in Table 33–1. The following organisms were found in the amniotic fluid from patients with IAI: *Bacteroides* species, 25%; group B streptococci, 12%; other aerobic streptococci, 13%; *Escherichia coli*, 10%; other aerobic gram-negative rods, 10%; *Clostridium* species, 9%; *Peptococcus* species, 7%; and *Fusobacterium* species, 6%. For the 52 patients with clinical IAI, aerobes and anaerobes were isolated from 48%; aerobes only from 38%; anaerobes alone from 8%; and no aerobes or anaerobes from 6%. Cultures of amniotic fluid from patients with IAI were more likely to have more than 10^2 colony-forming units (cfu) of any isolate per milliliter, any number of high-virulence isolates, and more than 10^2 cfu/ml of high-virulence isolates. Only 8% of these cultures from control patients had 10^2 cfu/ml or more of high-virulence isolates. The isolation rate of low-virulence organisms, such as lactobacilli, diphtheroids, and *Staphylococcus epidermidis*, was similar in both the IAI and the control groups. In smaller studies, a similar spectrum of organisms was reported.[12, 25]

Neisseria gonorrhoeae was not isolated in any of these studies, but it appears to be an infrequent cause of amnionitis.[26, 27]

A role for genital mycoplasmas has been suggested by case reports describing their isolation from amniotic fluid of clinically infected patients and by epidemiologic studies showing an association between the isolation of *Mycoplasma hominis* or *Ureaplasma* and placental inflammation.[28, 29] Unfortunately, these latter studies did not demonstrate correlation of isolation of genital mycoplasmas with clinical infection in the mother or neonate. In a controlled study of IAI, Blanco and co-workers reported that 35% of cultures of amniotic fluid from patients with IAI yielded *M. hominis*, whereas only 8% of matched control cultures showed *M. hominis*

TABLE 33–1

Characteristics of Amniotic Fluid from Patients with Intra-amniotic Infection (IAI) and from Control Patients

CHARACTERISTICS	PATIENTS WITH IAI (N = 52)	p	MATCHED CONTROL PATIENTS (N = 52)
Mean no. of isolates	2.2		1.2
No. with > 10^2 cfu/ml (%)	42 (81)	<0.001	16 (31)
No. with > 10^5 cfu/ml (%)	23 (44)	<0.001	2 (4)
No. with no bacterial growth (%)	3 (6)	<0.01	13 (25)
No. with high-virulence isolates (%)	42 (81)	<0.001	12 (23)
No. with > 10^2 cfu/ml high-virulence isolates	36 (69)	<0.001	4 (8)

cfu = colony-forming units.
From Gibbs RS, Blanco JD, St. Clair PJ, et al. Quantitative bacteriology of amniotic fluid from patients with clinical intra-amniotic infection at term. J Infect Dis 145:1, 1982, with permission. University of Chicago, publisher.

($p < 0.001$).[30] *U. urealyticum* was isolated from amniotic fluid from 50% of the infected and uninfected patients. In a subsequent study, Gibbs and colleagues found *M. hominis* in the blood of 2% of women with IAI and reported a serologic response in 85% of women with IAI who also had *M. hominis* in the amniotic fluid.[31] This rate of serologic response was significantly higher than that in asymptomatic control women or in infected women without *M. hominis* in the amniotic fluid ($p < 0.001$).[31] Cultures of blood and serologic results did not clarify the role of *U. urealyticum*. Thus, the pathogenic potential of *M. hominis* is high in IAI, but the pathogenic status of *U. urealyticum* is unclear in this infection.

Data related to the role of *Chlamydia trachomatis* in infections of amniotic fluid are in conflict. Martin and co-workers prospectively studied perinatal mortality in women whose pregnancies were complicated by antepartum maternal chlamydial infections.[32] Two of the six fetal deaths in the *Chlamydia*-positive group were associated with chorioamnionitis compared with one of eight in the control group. Wager and colleagues showed that the rate of occurrence of intrapartum fever was higher in patients with antepartum *C. trachomatis* infection (9%) than in patients without *C. trachomatis* isolated from the cervix (1%).[33] The data are interesting but must be interpreted with caution because of the limited number of patients and because the control group may not have been sufficiently similar to the infected group. Furthermore, *C. trachomatis* has not been isolated from amniotic cells or placental membranes of patients with IAI.[34, 35] In a preliminary study, no difference was found in the rate of serologic response to *C. trachomatis* in women with IAI compared with that in asymptomatic women.[36]

In a large prospective study, Sperling and colleagues reported amniotic fluid culture results from 408 cases of IAI. The most commonly isolated organisms were *U. urealyticum* (47%), *M. hominis* (31%), *Bacteroides bivius* (29%), *Gardnerella vaginalis* (24%), group B streptococci (15%), anaerobic streptococci (9%), *E. coli* (8%), *Fusobacterium* species (6%), enterococci (5%), and other aerobic gram negative rods (5%).[37] A summary of representative data for five microbiologic studies is given in Table 33–2. Because of differences among these studies in microbiologic and collection techniques and in reporting format for isolates, Table 33–2 is meant to show broad, overall results.

Evidence has shown that maternal bacterial vaginosis is causally linked to IAI.[38] The evidence may be categorized as follows: (1) the microorganisms in bacterial vaginosis and in chorioamnionitis are similar; (2) bacterial vaginosis is associated with the isolation of organisms in the chorioamnion; and (3) bacterial vaginosis is associated with development of clinical chorioamnionitis in selected populations.[39–41] It has been demonstrated that treatment of bacterial vaginosis prenatally decreases the risk of chorioamnionitis.

Amniotic fluid cultures from cases of intra-amniotic fluid accompanying a low-birth-weight infant are more likely to contain the anaerobes *Fusobacterium* species (21.6 versus only 3.8% in non–low-birth-weight cases, $p < 0.001$) and *B. bivius* (46 versus 28%, $p = .035$). However, there were no significant differences in the

TABLE 33–2
Microbes Isolated in Amniotic Fluid from Cases of Intra-amniotic Infection: A Summary of Studies

MICROBE	REPRESENTATIVE % ISOLATED
Genital Mycoplasmas	
Ureaplasma urealyticum	47–50
Mycoplasma hominis	31–35
Anaerobes	
Bacteroides bivius	11–29
Peptostreptococcus	7–33
Fusobacterium sp.	6–7
Aerobes	
Group B streptococci	12–19
Enterococci	5–11
Escherichia coli	8–12, 55
Other aerobic gram-negative rods	5–10
Gardnerella vaginalis	24

Data from references 12, 24, 25, 30, and 37. See text.

isolation rates of group B streptococci, *E. coli*, other aerobes, or genital mycoplasmas between cases from low-birth-weight and non–low-birth-weight infants.[37]

Bloodstream isolates from newborns in 408 cases of IAI were reported as follows: *E. coli*, 5 cases; group B streptococci, 4 cases; *Staphylococcus aureus*, 2 cases; enterococci, 2 cases; other streptococci, 3 cases; and 1 case each for *Enterobacter* species, *Haemophilus influenzae*, *H. parainfluenzae*, and microaerophilic streptococci.[37] Thus, of 20 isolates, group B streptococci and *E. coli* accounted for 45% of isolates even though these organisms were present in the amniotic fluid of just 20% of cases.

Diagnosis

Diagnosis of IAI requires a high index of suspicion because the clinical signs and symptoms may be subtle. Moreover, usual laboratory indicators of infection, such as positive strains for organisms or leukocytes and positive culture results, are found more frequently than is clinically evident infection.

Diagnosis of IAI is usually based on maternal fever, maternal or fetal tachycardia, uterine tenderness, foul odor of amniotic fluid, and leukocytosis. Other causes of fever in the parturient patient include concurrent infection of the urinary tract or other organ systems and perhaps dehydration. The differential diagnosis of fetal tachycardia consists of prematurity, medications, arrhythmias, and hypoxia, whereas for maternal tachycardia other possible causes are drugs, hypotension, dehydration, and anxiety. In general, the most common clinical and laboratory criteria for diagnosis of IAI are fever, leukocytosis, and ruptured membranes; fetal tachycardia and maternal tachycardia are noted in variable percentages of cases.[1, 42, 43] Foul-smelling amniotic fluid and uterine tenderness, although more-specific signs, occur in a minority of cases. Bacteremia occurs in only 10% of cases or less. Because peripheral blood leukocytosis is common during normal labor, this result does not always indicate infection. As a predictor of IAI, leukocytosis (>12,000 per mm³) had a sensitivity of 67%, specificity of 86%, positive predictive value of 82%, and negative predictive value of 72%.[44]

Direct examination of the amniotic fluid may provide important diagnostic information. Samples can be collected by aspiration of an intrauterine pressure catheter, by needle aspiration of the forewaters, or by amniocentesis.

There is a significant association between detecting white blood cells or bacteria in a stain of uncentrifuged amniotic fluid and clinical infection.[24, 45] In a case-control study, white blood cells were seen on smear in 67% of cases of IAI and in only 12% of controls (p = 0.001). Bacteria were seen on smear in 81% of cases of IAI and in 29% of controls (p < 0.001).[24] With suspected IAI, detection of bacteria or white blood cells on a smear of uncentrifuged fluid supports the diagnosis, but there are frequent false-positive and false-negative results.

Several other recent tests of amniotic fluid have been evaluated as predictors of IAI. In a small case-control study, Hoskins and co-workers found that the leukocyte esterase test showed excellent performance (91% sensitivity, 95% specificity, 95% positive and 91% negative predictive values) when the clinical diagnosis of chorioamnionitis was used as the "gold standard."[44] Low concentrations of amniotic fluid glucose (variably reported as <10 to 20 mg/dl) are strongly associated with positive amniotic fluid culture and less strongly associated with clinical IAI.[46–48]

Interleukin (IL)-6 is an immunostimulatory cytokine and a key mediator of host response to infection. Several lines of investigation indicate that IL-6 may be the future diagnostic test of choice. For example, elevated levels of IL-6 in the amniotic fluid have been a more sensitive rapid test for the detection of microbial invasion of the amniotic cavity than amniotic fluid glucose, amniotic Gram stain, or amniotic fluid white blood cell count. Amniotic fluid IL-6 levels have also been shown to be increased with positive cultures of either the amniotic fluid or the amniochorion.[49] Elevated IL-6 levels are also a very sensitive test for acute histologic chorioamnionitis and the identification of neonates at risk for significant morbidity and mortality.[50] Maternal serum IL-6 levels also have been reported to be elevated when preterm labor is associated with intrauterine infection.[51] Finally, fetal production of IL-6 (as determined by cordocentesis) is an independent risk factor for the occurrence of severe neonatal morbidity, including sepsis and pneumonia.[52, 53]

Management and Short-Term Outcome

Traditionally, the effectiveness of management has been viewed in terms of short-term maternal and neonatal outcomes, including maternal sepsis and neonatal sepsis, pneumonia, meningitis, and perinatal death. In this section we discuss the management principles of these short-term outcomes.

In the past there was debate regarding timing of antibiotic administration, but it has now become the standard to begin treatment during labor, as soon as possible after the maternal diagnosis of IAI is made. Three studies, including a randomized clinical trial, have demonstrated benefits from intrapartum antibiotic therapy compared with immediate postpartum treatment (Table 33–3).[54–56] In a large, nonrandomized allocation of intrapartum versus immediate postpartum treatment, the former treatment was associated with a significant

TABLE 33–3
Comparative Studies of Intrapartum Versus Postpartum Maternal Antibiotic Therapy in the Treatment of Intra-amniotic Infection

AUTHOR, YEAR (REFERENCE)	DESIGN/SETTING	N	MATERNAL INTRAPARTUM ANTIBIOTIC REGIMEN	BENEFITS OF INTRAPARTUM TREATMENT
Sperling, 1987 (54)	Retrospective/public teaching hospital in San Antonio, Texas	257	Penicillin G plus gentamicin IV	NNS reduced from 19.6% in postpartum treatment group to 2.8% in intrapartum treatment group (p = 0.001).
Gilstrap, 1988 (56)	Retrospective/public teaching hospital in Dallas, Texas	273	Varied[a]	NNS reduced from 5.7% in postpartum treatment group to 1.5% in intrapartum treatment group (p = 0.06). Group B streptococcal bacteremia reduced from 5.7 to 0% (p = 0.004).
Gibbs, 1988 (55)	Randomized clinical trial/same as Sperling (1987)	45	Ampicillin plus gentamicin IV	NNS reduced from 21 to 0%. Maternal morbidity also decreased (p = 0.05).

[a]Antibiotic regimens noted as 47% received ampicillin or penicillin in combination with gentamicin and clindamycin; 22%, ampicillin or penicillin with gentamicin; 20%, cefoxitin; and 11%, other antibiotics.
NNS = neonatal sepsis confirmed by blood culture.

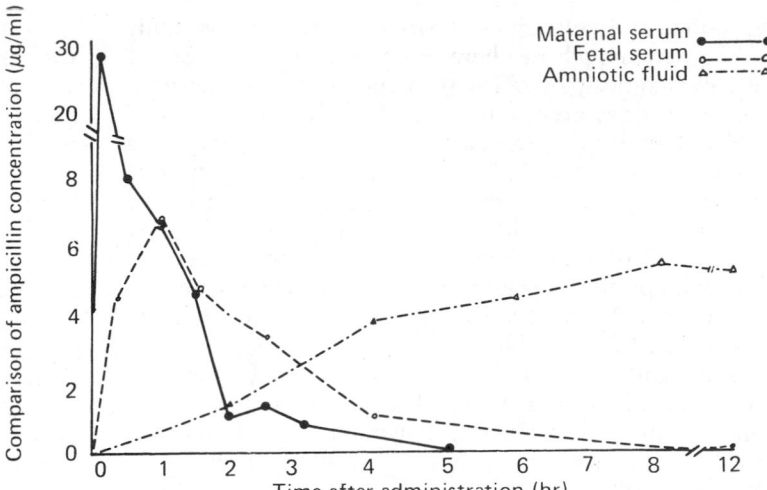

FIGURE 33–1 Ampicillin levels achieved with systemic administration to the mother. (From Bray RE, Boe RW, Johnson WL. Transfer of ampicillin into fetus and amniotic fluid from maternal plasma in late pregnancy. Am J Obstet Gynecol 96:938, 1966, with permission.)

decrease in neonatal bacteremia (2.8 versus 19.6%, $p < 0.001$) and a reduction in neonatal death from sepsis (0.9 versus 4.3%, $p = 0.07$).[54] Another large study showed an overall reduction in neonatal sepsis ($p = 0.06$), especially bacteremia due to group B streptococci (0 versus 4.7%, $p = 0.004$), by use of intrapartum treatment.[56] Then, in a randomized clinical trial, Gibbs and associates demonstrated that intrapartum treatment provided both maternal benefits (decreased hospital stay, lower mean temperature postpartum) and neonatal benefits (decreased sepsis, 0 versus 21%, $p = 0.03$ and decreased hospital stay). In this study, neonatal treatment was identical and consisted of intravenous ampicillin and gentamicin begun within 1 to 2 hours of birth and continued for at least 72 hours. If bacteremia or neonatal pneumonia was diagnosed, antibiotics were continued for 10 days.[55]

Pharmacokinetic studies[57] done during early pregnancy show that ampicillin concentrations in maternal and fetal sera are comparable 60 to 90 minutes after administration (Fig. 33–1). Penicillin G levels in fetal serum are one third of the maternal levels 120 minutes after administration.[58] In addition, ampicillin has some activity against *E. coli*. Accordingly, ampicillin is preferable to penicillin G for treatment of IAI. When used in combination with an aminoglycoside, ampicillin should be administered first, because it has the broader antimicrobial spectrum. In late pregnancy, gentamicin also crosses the placenta rapidly, but peak fetal levels may be low, especially if maternal levels are subtherapeutic.[59] An initial gentamicin dose of at least 1.5 to 2.0 mg/kg followed by 1.0 to 1.5 mg/kg every 8 hours is indicated because of the potential for unfavorable gentamicin kinetics. As an alternative, a newer penicillin or cephalosporin with excellent activity against aerobic gram-negative bacteria might be used. However, there is little published experience with these antibiotics in IAI. Levels of ampicillin and aminoglycosides in amniotic fluid are usually below fetal serum levels, and peak concentrations in amniotic fluid may be attained only after 2 to 6 hours.[57–59] The kinetics of newer penicillin and cephamycin antibiotics have not been studied extensively in pregnancy.

The duration of maternal treatment postpartum in cases of chorioamnionitis is debatable. One randomized trial compared single versus multidose postpartum treatment of mothers and reported that single-dose treatment was accompanied by a shorter time to discharge (33 hours in the single-dose group versus 57 hours in the multidose group, $p = 0.001$).[60] However, the single-dose group had a nearly threefold increase in failure of therapy, but this did not achieve statistical significance (11% in the single-dose treatment group versus 3.7% in the multidose group, $p = 0.27$). Our preference is to treat patients for 24 hours or more after resolution of fever.

With regard to timing of delivery, there is excellent short-term outcome without the use of arbitrary time limits.[1, 61, 62] Cesarean delivery is usually reserved for standard obstetric indications, not for IAI itself. In nearly all cases, delivery occurred within 8 hours after diagnosis of IAI (mean time was 3 to 5 hours). No critical interval from diagnosis of amnionitis to delivery could be identified. Yet nearly all of these cases were at or near term. Rates of cesarean section are two to three times higher among patients with IAI than in the general population, owing to patient selection (most cases occur in women with dystocia already diagnosed) and a poor response to oxytocin.[63, 64] There is no demonstrated advantage of the extraperitoneal technique over the transperitoneal technique in decreasing maternal complications of IAI.[65–68]

In the past, we used a combination of an intravenous penicillin and intravenous gentamicin as soon as the diagnosis was made and cultures had been obtained.[1, 43] Several studies have reported good results with similar regimens.[61] When a cesarean section is necessary, clindamycin should be added postpartum to these antibiotics because of the importance of anaerobes in post-cesarean section infection and the high (20%) failure rate of penicillin-gentamicin after cesarean section for IAI.[4] Other initial regimens with cefoxitin alone or ampicillin plus a newer cephalosporin may be equally effective, but no comparative trials have been performed.

Since 1979, retrospective studies have shown a vastly improved perinatal outcome compared with earlier studies. Gibbs and colleagues reported a retrospective study of 171 patients whose therapy was usually begun at the time of diagnosis of IAI with penicillin G and kanamycin.[4] The mean gestational age of the neonate was 37.7 weeks. There were no maternal deaths, and bacteremia was found in only 2.3% of mothers. Among women with IAI, the rate of cesarean delivery was increased approximately threefold to 35%, mainly because of dystocia. In all mothers the outcome was good. There was only one episode of septic shock and no pelvic abscesses or maternal deaths. Similar results were reported from Los Angeles County Hospital.[42]

Gibbs and colleagues found that when IAI is present, the perinatal mortality rate (140 per 1000 births) was approximately seven times the overall perinatal mortality rate for infants weighing more than 499 g (which was 18.2 per 1000 births).[4] Yet none of the perinatal deaths was clearly attributable to infection; among live-born infants weighing more than 1000 g, none died of infection. In the study of Koh and co-workers, the perinatal mortality rate was lower (28.1 per 1000 births), which probably reflected the higher mean gestational age (39.3 weeks).[42] There were no intrapartum fetal deaths and only four neonatal deaths. Again, no deaths were due to infection.

Neither perinatal nor maternal complications correlated with more prolonged diagnosis-to-delivery intervals. Because patients who had cesarean section had more complicated courses, it was concluded that cesarean section should be reserved for patients with standard obstetric indications for this procedure in addition to IAI.

Yoder and colleagues later provided a prospective, case-control study of 67 neonates with microbiologically confirmed IAI at term.[43] There was only one perinatal death, which was unrelated to infection. Cerebrospinal fluid culture results were negative for all 49 infants tested, and there was no clinical evidence of meningitis. Chest radiographs were interpreted as possible pneumonia in 20% of patients and as unequivocal pneumonia in only 4%. Neonatal bacteremia was documented in 8%. There was no significant difference in the frequency of low Apgar scores between the IAI and control groups.

Two other retrospective studies have been confirmatory. In 1984, Looff and Hager reported the outcome of 104 pregnancies with clinical chorioamnionitis.[61] The mean gestational age was 36 weeks. The perinatal mortality rate was 123 per 1000 births. Nearly all of the excess mortality was attributed to prematurity rather than to sepsis. These authors also reported an increase in the cesarean delivery rate (26%). In 1985, Hauth and co-workers reviewed 103 pregnancies with clinical chorioamnionitis at term.[62] There was a mean interval from diagnosis of amnionitis to delivery of 3.1 hours, which confirmed the absence of a critical interval for delivery. In this study, the overall perinatal mortality rate was 9.7 per 1000 births and the cesarean delivery rate was 42%.

Neonates born prematurely have a higher frequency of complications if their mothers have IAI. Garite and Freeman noted that the perinatal death rate was significantly higher in 47 preterm neonates with IAI than in 204 neonates with similar birth weights but without IAI.[69] The group with IAI also had a significantly higher percentage (13 versus 3%, $p < 0.05$) with respiratory distress syndrome (RDS) and total infection. A larger but similar comparative study of 92 patients with chorioamnionitis and 606 controls of similar gestational age also demonstrated significant increases in mortality, RDS, intraventricular hemorrhage (IVH), and clinically diagnosed sepsis in the group with chorioamnionitis[70] (see Table 33–4). When Sperling and associates stratified outcomes in cases of IAI by birth weight, cases leading to low-birth-weight infants had more frequent maternal bacteremia (13.5 versus 4.9%, $p = 0.06$), early-onset neonatal sepsis (16.2 versus 4.1%, $p = 0.005$), and neonatal death from sepsis (10.8 versus 0%, $p < 0.001$).[37]

In a retrospective, case-control study, Ferguson and co-workers reported neonatal outcome after chorioamnionitis.[71] Seventy percent of newborns weighed less than 2500 g. In 116 matched pairs, the authors found more deaths (20 versus 11%), more sepsis (6 versus 2%), and more asphyxia (27 versus 16%) in the group with chorioamnionitis. None of these differences, however, achieved statistical significance.

TABLE 33–4
Perinatal Outcome in Preterm Amnionitis (Intra-amniotic Infection)

| MEASURE (%) | AMNIONITIS[a] | | CONTROL[a] | |
	Reference 69 (N = 47)	Reference 70 (N = 92)	Reference 69 (N = 204)	Reference 70 (N = 606)
Perinatal death	13	25	3[b]	6[b]
Respiratory distress syndrome	34	62	16[b]	35[b]
Total infections	17	28	7[b]	11[b]
Intraventricular hemorrhage	NR	56	Nr[b]	22[b]

[a]At centers reporting these results, there were active referral services. In these series of consecutive patients with preterm premature rupture of membranes, those with amnionitis are compared with those without.
[b]Rates are significantly lower than for amnionitis group in corresponding study.
NR = not reported.

Long-Term Outcome

Hardt and colleagues followed preterm infants (weighing <2000 g) born after chorioamnionitis and found a significantly lower mental development index (Bayley's score) compared with preterm control infants (104 ± 18 versus 112 ± 14, p = 0.017).[72] Morales reported 1-year follow-up of preterm infants born after chorioamnionitis and of control infants. He did not observe differences in mental and physical development, but adjustments were made for IVH and RDS, both of which were more frequent in the amnionitis group.[70]

Exciting new information strongly suggests that intrauterine exposure to bacteria is associated with long-term serious neonatal complications, including cerebral palsy or its histologic precursor (periventricular leukomalacia) and major pulmonary problems of bronchopulmonary dysplasia (BPD) and RDS. The unifying hypothesis states that intrauterine exposure of the fetus to infection leads to overexuberant fetal production of cytokines. This, in turn, leads to fetal cellular damage in the brain, lung, and potentially other organs. This has been likened to the systemic inflammatory response syndrome (SIRS) in adults. The evidence linking infection to cerebral palsy may be summarized as follows:

1. Intrauterine exposure to maternal or placental infection is associated with an increased risk of cerebral palsy both in preterm and term infants.[73, 74]
2. Clinical chorioamnionitis in very low birth weight infants is significantly associated with an increase in periventricular leukomalacia (p = 0.001).[75]
3. The levels of inflammatory cytokines are increased in the amniotic fluid of infants with white matter lesions (periventricular leukomalacia [PVL]), and there is overexpression of these cytokines in neonatal brain with PVL.[76]
4. Experimental intrauterine infection in rabbits leads to brain white matter lesions.[77]

In addition to cellular and tissue damage in the fetal brain, an overexuberant cytokine response induced by bacteria may damage other fetal tissues, such as the lung, contributing to RDS and BPD.[78] In support of this hypothesis, a case-control study of infants with and without RDS was conducted. Those with RDS were significantly more likely to have elevated levels of amniotic fluid tumor necrosis factor (TNF)-α, a positive culture of the amniotic fluid, and severe histologic chorioamnionitis (p < 0.05 for each association). Elevated amniotic fluid IL-6 levels were also twice as common in the group with RDS, but this association did not achieve statistical significance. Furthermore, preterm fetuses with elevated cord blood IL-6 concentrations (>11 pg/mL) are more likely to develop RDS (64 versus 24%, p < 0.005) when compared with those without elevated cord IL-6 levels. BPD was also increased (11 versus 5%), but the p value was not statistically significant.[52]

In summary, IAI has a significant adverse effect on the mother and neonate, but vigorous antibiotic therapy and reasonably prompt delivery result in an excellent short-term prognosis, especially for the mother and the term neonate. If the combination of prematurity and amnionitis occurs, serious sequelae are more likely for the neonate. Newly developing information suggests that intrauterine infection is linked to major neonatal long-term complications.

Prevention

As categorized in Table 33–5, numerous approaches have recently been proposed for the prevention of IAI. Among these, prompt management of dystocia has been shown to decrease chorioamnionitis as well as to shorten labor and reduce the cesarean section rate.[79] Similarly, induction of PROM at term most likely results in fewer maternal infections than does expectant management.[80] Antibiotic prophylaxis for patients with preterm PROM decreases chorioamnionitis as well as other complications.[81, 82] Antibiotic prophylaxis for patients in preterm labor (but with intact membranes) does not appear to decrease chorioamnionitis.[83] Intrapartum prophylaxis for the prevention of neonatal group B streptococcal sepsis is now a national standard in known group B streptococcal colonized parturients or those in at risk categories. It is presumed that this also decreases chorioamnionitis, but there are no definitive data to support this. Prenatal treatment of bacterial vaginosis (by topical treatment), chlorhexidine vaginal washes in labor, and specific infection control measures have not been demonstrated to be effective.[84–86, 18]

SUBCLINICAL GENITAL INFECTION AS A CAUSE OF ADVERSE PREGNANCY OUTCOME

Preterm birth is the leading perinatal problem in the United States. Infants born before the thirty-seventh week of gestation account for approximately 6% of births but 80% of all perinatal deaths.[87] In most cases, the underlying cause of premature labor is not evident. Evidence from many sources points to a relationship between preterm birth and genitourinary tract infections.[88, 89]

In addition to the association between symptomatic urinary tract infection and preterm birth, infection of the genital tract—either clinical or subclinical—has been

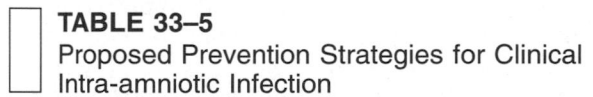

TABLE 33–5
Proposed Prevention Strategies for Clinical Intra-amniotic Infection

Prompt management of dystocia
Induction of labor with premature rupture of membranes at term
Antibiotic prophylaxis with preterm premature rupture of membranes
Antibiotic prophylaxis with preterm labor, but with intact membranes
Antibiotic prophylaxis for group B streptococcal infection
Prenatal treatment of bacterial vaginosis
Chlorhexidene vaginal irrigations in labor
Infection control measures

TABLE 33–6

Evidence Supporting a Relationship Between Preterm Births and Subclinical Genital Tract Infection

The incidence of histologic chorioamnionitis is increased after preterm birth.

The incidence of clinical infection is increased after preterm birth in both mother and neonate.

Some lower genital tract microbes or infections are associated with an increased risk of preterm birth.

There are biochemical mechanisms linking prematurity and infection.

Infection and inflammation cause cytokine release and prostaglandin production.

Bacteria and bacterial products induce preterm delivery in animal models.

Amniotic fluid culture results are positive in some patients in premature labor.

Some antibiotic trials have shown a decrease in numbers of preterm births.

implicated as a cause of premature birth or of low-birth-weight infants. Evidence supporting this relationship is categorized in Table 33–6.

Histologic Chorioamnionitis and Prematurity

One of the most consistent observations is that placentas in premature births are more likely to have evidence of inflammation (i.e., histologic chorioamnionitis) (Fig. 33–2). In a series of 3500 consecutive placentas, Driscoll found infiltrates of polymorphonuclear cells in 11%.[90] Few of the women developed clinically evident infection, but the likelihood of neonatal sepsis and death was increased.[91]

In recent studies, an association has been established between histologic chorioamnionitis and chorioamnion infection (defined as a positive culture).[91] Odds ratios have been reported from 2.8 to 14, this relationship being stronger among preterm deliveries than among term deliveries. Yet it is striking that 18 to 49% of placentas with histologic chorioamnionitis are culture negative and 15 to 45% of culture-positive membranes do not show inflammation. Overall, the organisms found in the chorioamnion are similar to those found in the amniotic fluid in cases of clinical IAI. This array of organisms supports an ascending route for chorioamnion infection in most cases.

Although it is not clear how histologic chorioamnionitis and membrane infection cause preterm delivery or preterm PROM, studies suggest that they lead to weakening of the membranes (as evidenced by lower bursting tension, less work to rupture, and less elasticity[92] in vitro) and to production of prostaglandins by the amnion.[93, 94]

Clinical Infection and Prematurity

Additional evidence linking prematurity and infection is the persistent observation that both premature infants

and women who were delivered of premature infants are more likely to develop clinically evident infection.[95] In a large study of more than 9500 deliveries, confirmatory evidence has shown that chorioamnionitis, endometritis, and neonatal infection were all significantly increased in preterm pregnancies, even after correcting for the presence of PROM.[96] These observations suggest that subclinical infection led to the delivery and that infection became clinically evident after delivery. Other physicians argue that there is no causal relationship but that premature infants develop infection more often because, for example, they are compromised hosts or because they have more invasive monitoring in the nursery.

Associations of Lower Genital Tract Organisms or Infections with Prematurity

Premature birth has been associated with isolation of several organisms from the maternal lower genital tract and with subclinical infections (Table 33–7). Some investigators have found a relationship between isolation of mycoplasmas from the genital tract and adverse pregnancy outcome. More than 20 years ago, Braun and colleagues showed that women with genital mycoplas-

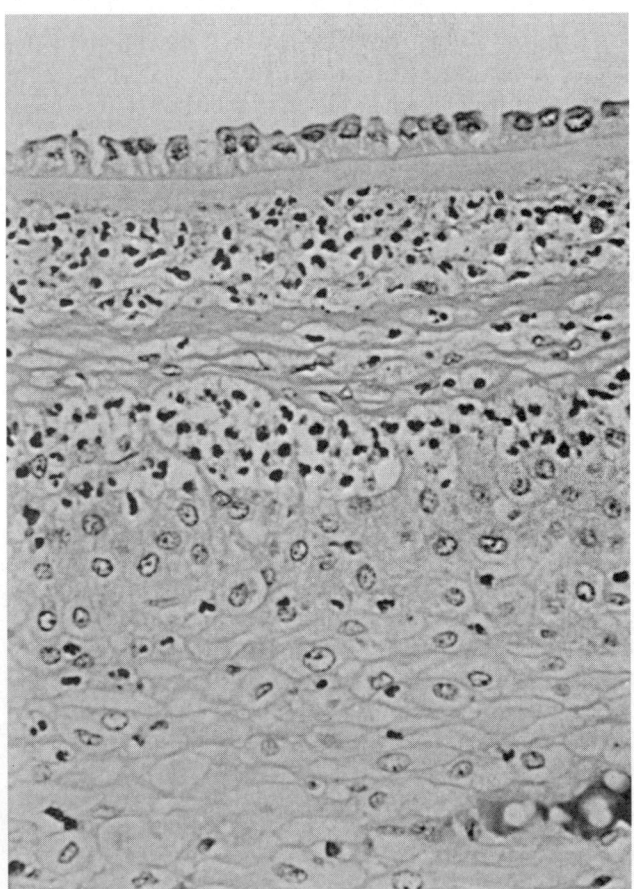

FIGURE 33–2 Infiltrates of polymorphonuclear cells are seen in the fetal membranes. Inflammation of the placenta and membranes has been consistently observed more often after preterm births than after term births.

TABLE 33–7
Organisms and Infections Associated with Premature Birth

Genital mycoplasmas
Chlamydia trachomatis
Group B streptococci
Bacteroides sp.
Trichomonas vaginalis
Bacterial vaginosis and anaerobes
Neisseria gonorrhoeae
Pyelonephritis
Bacteriuria

mas in the cervix or urine or both were delivered of neonates with a mean birth weight that was 202 g less than that of neonates delivered to women without genital mycoplasmas.[97] This difference in birth weight was statistically significant, but there was no significant difference in gestational age between the two groups. These investigators also reported associations between neonatal colonization with genital mycoplasmas and low birth weight and between significant rises in titer to *U. urealyticum* in pregnancy and low birth weight ($p < 0.02$). However, several recent studies have failed to confirm such associations. Of 11 cohort studies summarized recently, none supports an association between *U. urealyticum* and low-birth-weight or preterm birth.[89] Treatment of patients demonstrated to have *U. urealyticum* with up to 8 weeks of oral erythromycin had no effect on low birth weight, prematurity, or PROM. This treatment trial was large, well designed, and powerful.[98]

The effect of lower genital tract infection with *C. trachomatis* on the outcome of pregnancy has been the subject of several conflicting studies. In a longitudinal study, Martin and colleagues found *C. trachomatis* in the endocervix of 18 (6.7%) of 268 women at 19 weeks of pregnancy or earlier.[32] Pregnant women with endocervical *C. trachomatis* infection were significantly more likely to be delivered of stillborn infants or infants dying neonatally (6 of 18; 33%) than were women not infected in early pregnancy (8 of 238; 3.4%). In a matched cohort analysis of these data, the authors reported a perinatal mortality risk ratio for pregnancies with antepartum chlamydial infection versus pregnancies without infection of 10.18 ($p = 0.004$). Harrison and colleagues later found *C. trachomatis* cervical infection in 8% of pregnant women. *C. trachomatis*—infected women with IgM antibody had more low-birth-weight infants ($p < 0.02$) and more PROM ($p < 0.01$) than either *C. trachomatis*—infected women with no IgM antibody or women whose culture results were negative for *C. trachomatis*.[99]

Gravett and colleagues also reported that cervical *C. trachomatis* infection was an independent risk factor for preterm labor ($p < 0.01$), preterm PROM ($p < 0.05$), and low birth weight ($p = 0.01$).[100] However, larger studies in other institutions have failed to show any significant association between *C. trachomatis* infection and prematurity.[101-104]

N. gonorrhoeae, if untreated, is associated with clinical chorioamnionitis,[26] and its isolation from the neonate is associated with prematurity, prolonged ROM, and histologic chorioamnionitis.[27] However, this organism is probably not an important cause of prematurity in view of its relatively low prevalence as well as maternal screening and treatment of all patients with positive gonorrhoeae culture results.

Maternal genital tract colonization with group B streptococci may lead to neonatal sepsis, especially when birth occurs prematurely or when the membranes have been ruptured for prolonged intervals. In addition, an association between colonization of the cervix with these organisms and premature birth has been found by Regan and co-workers.[105] These investigators noted delivery at less than 32 weeks in 1.8% of the total population but in 5.4% of women colonized with group B streptococci ($p < 0.005$). PROM also occurred significantly more often in the colonized group (15.3 versus 8.1%, $p < 0.005$). Of the six studies evaluating the association between group B streptococci genital colonization and preterm labor or delivery, in five no association was found.[89] Yet in three of four studies, group B streptococci genital colonization was associated with preterm PROM. In contrast to the conflicting data regarding group B streptococci genital colonization, group B streptococci bacteriuria has been consistently associated with preterm delivery, and treatment of this bacteriuria resulted in a marked reduction in prematurity (37.5% in placebo versus 5.4% in treated group).[106-108] Current recommendations for treatment for group B streptococci in pregnancy from the Centers for Disease Control and Prevention (CDC) is intrapartum only, with the exception of group B streptococcal bacteriuria, which should be treated antepartum. Intrapartum the CDC recommends adoption of either a risk factors–based approach or universal screening. With the *risk factors–based approach*, intrapartum narrow spectrum antibiotics (intravenous penicillin G or ampicillin or clindamycin in the penicillin-allergic patient) should be given if the patient has any of the following: fever in labor at any gestational age, preterm labor or preterm rupture of membranes at less than 37 weeks' gestation, prolonged ROM (>18 hours), or a history of either group B streptococcal bacteriuria or a previously affected neonate. The *universal screening approach* involves screening women at 35 to 37 weeks' gestation with proper collection and culture techniques, followed by intrapartum treatment of all women with positive cultures.[109]

Infection of the maternal vagina with *Trichomonas vaginalis* has been associated with preterm labor in a teenage population in Baltimore and in the large Vaginal Infections and Prematurity Study. *T. vaginalis* was associated with low birth weight and PROM (Cotch MF, Interscience Conference on Antimicrobial Agents and Chemotherapy, 1990). However, *T. vaginalis* was not significantly associated with low birth weight or preterm labor in other women.[104, 110, 111]

Bacteroides species in the vagina have been implicated in preterm delivery and preterm PROM in several studies in Brooklyn, Seattle, and Australia.[104, 112, 113] Bacterial vaginosis, characterized by high concentrations of anaerobes, *G. vaginalis*, and *M. hominis*, with a corresponding decrease in the normal vaginal lactobacilli, has been linked to low birth weight and PROM.[100, 114] The largest study of bacterial vaginosis in pregnancy is the Vaginal Infections in Prematurity study involving 10,397 pregnant women. In this study, bacterial vaginosis was associated with preterm birth of low-birth-weight infants (odds ratio [OR] 1.4; 95% confidence interval [CI] 1.1–1.8). Primigravidity, black race, previous pregnancy loss, and previous preterm delivery were significantly associated with bacterial vaginosis.[115] Bacterial vaginosis has also been associated with an increased risk of IAI.[41] Currently, oral therapy rather than topical therapy is recommended for treatment of women at high risk of preterm birth with bacterial vaginosis. Treatment of bacterial vaginosis in low-risk women is not currently recommended.[116]

Gravett and colleagues found bacterial vaginosis (formerly called nonspecific vaginitis or *Gardnerella* vaginitis) in 14% of patients in labor. In a matched cohort study, bacterial vaginosis was associated with premature labor occurring at less than 34 weeks ($p < 0.05$).[117] Minkoff and colleagues found that isolation of *Bacteroides* species from the vagina carried a 1.4 relative risk ($p < 0.01$) for preterm delivery and a 1.6 relative risk ($p < 0.04$) for low birth weight.[104]

Untreated acute pyelonephritis has been found to be consistently associated with a 30% risk of preterm labor and delivery. More debatable, however, has been the relationship between asymptomatic bacteriuria and low birth weight. Although individual cohort studies often failed to show a significant association, a meta-analysis[118] showed that women with asymptomatic bacteriuria had a 60% higher rate of low birth weight (95% CI 1.4–1.9) and a 90% higher rate of preterm delivery (95% CI 1.3–1.9).

Amniotic Fluid Cultures in Preterm Labor

Within the past 15 years, several small studies of amniotic fluid bacteriology have supported the hypothesis that subclinical infection leads to premature birth. Amniocentesis was performed in patients in premature labor who had no overt signs of infection. Bobitt and colleagues found subclinical infections in 6 (24%) of 25 patients and noted that perinatal morbidity was greater among infants when the amniotic fluid culture result was positive.[119] Gravett and colleagues isolated microorganisms from 10 (26%) of 39 patients. Patients with such cultures were less responsive to tocolytic agents.[117] Others have found positive culture results in 3 to 21% of amniotic fluid samples from asymptomatic patients in labor.[120–122] In a large series of 264 women in preterm labor, 11% had positive cultures. Yet in the 111 women who had preterm delivery within 48 hours, fully 22% had positive culture.[123] The explanation for the difference in these percentages may be related to patient selection or to differences in microbiologic technique. Patients in preterm labor with a positive culture of the amniotic fluid are likely to have delivery within 24 to 48 hours, whereas culture-negative patients tend to have longer intervals (often up to 30 days) until delivery. Because amniotic fluid culture may be an insensitive

test for infection, other markers of infection have been assessed. Most women in preterm labor and with an elevated serum C-reactive protein do not respond to tocolytics (86 to 88%), whereas most with a normal value do respond (77 to 94%).[124–126]

Biochemical Links of Prematurity and Infection

To complement these clinical observations, Bejar and co-workers noted that a number of common genital tract bacteria elaborate phospholipase A_2, an enzyme involved in the synthesis of prostaglandins.[127] These authors postulated that premature labor may be initiated by high activity of phospholipase A_2 from these bacteria involved in endocervical or intrauterine contamination or infection. Other authors[128, 129] have demonstrated elevated concentrations of prostaglandins in the amniotic fluid of women with PROM and with positive amniotic fluid cultures. Metabolites of arachidonic acid (5-OH and 15-OH eicosatetraenoic acids and leukotriene B_4) are increased in the amniotic fluid of women in preterm labor and with positive amniotic fluid cultures. In addition, amnion from preterm placentas with histologic chorioamnionitis release more leukotriene B_4 in vitro than does amnion from preterm placentas without chorioamnionitis. Bacterial products such as endotoxin (lipopolysaccharide) have been detected in higher concentrations in the amniotic fluid of women with PROM and labor than in corresponding women not in labor.[89] Preterm labor triggered by infection may be signaled by cytokines such as IL-1 and IL-6 and TNF. Supporting evidence has been reported. IL-1 stimulates prostaglandin production by amnion and decidua in vitro, and amniotic fluid IL levels are increased in patients in preterm labor with positive amniotic fluid cultures. Similar observations have been made for TNF.[89]

The widely accepted working hypothesis is that bacteria ascending into the uterine cavity are able to directly stimulate cytokine activity. IL-1, IL-6, and TNF-α, the proinflammatory cytokines, have been shown to be produced by the fetal membranes, decidua, and myometrium. Those patients with elevated levels of these cytokines in the amniotic fluid have shorter amniocentesis to delivery intervals than those without elevated cytokine levels. Levels are also elevated when preterm labor is associated with IAI.[53] In addition, elevated amniotic fluid IL-6 levels have been found to prospectively identify those fetuses destined for significant neonatal morbidity and mortality.[50] Similarly, Romero and associates demonstrated that elevated fetal plasma levels of IL-6 in patients with preterm PROM, but not in labor, had a higher rate of delivery within 48 hours compared with those who delivered more than 48 hours after cordocentesis. These important finds suggest a fetal inflammatory cytokine response triggers spontaneous preterm delivery.[52]

Immunomodulatory cytokines such as IL-1 receptor antagonist (IL-1ra), IL-10, and growth factor (TGF)-β play a regulatory role in the cytokine response, allowing for a down-regulation of this response. IL-1ra has been shown in humans to increase in response to IAI.[130] Similarly, IL-10 inhibits IL-1β induced preterm labor in a rhesus model.[131]

Animal models have also evaluated cytokine-mediated initiation of preterm birth. Romero and colleagues demonstrated that systemic administration of IL-1 induced preterm birth in a murine model.[132] Similarly, Kaga and co-workers gave low-dose lipopolysaccharide (LPS) intraperitoneally to preterm mice causing preterm delivery.[133] Again in the murine model, Hirsch and colleagues demonstrated preterm birth after intrauterine inoculation of *E. coli*. Intrauterine inoculation is a more physiologic model of ascending infection and infection-mediated preterm birth in humans.

McDuffie and Gibbs recently reviewed animal models of ascending infection during pregnancy.[134]

Antibiotic Trials

In view of the data just discussed, studies of antibiotic treatment in pregnancy are especially interesting. These treatment trials have been of varying design but may be categorized into three general types as follows: (1) antibiotics given during prenatal care to patients at increased risk of preterm delivery; (2) antibiotics given adjunctively to tocolytics in women with preterm labor; and (3) antibiotics given to women with preterm PROM but not yet in labor (Table 33–8).

In the prototype of the first category of antibiotic trial, Kass and colleagues[135] and McCormack and associates[136] noted a reduction in the percentage of low-birth-weight infants delivered to women who were treated with oral erythromycin for 6 weeks in the third trimester compared with women who were given a placebo. The decrease was from 12% in the placebo-treated group to 3% in the erythromycin-treated group ($p = 0.047$). The infants in the placebo-treated group weighed significantly less (3187 versus 3331 g, $p = 0.042$). In a National Institutes of Health–sponsored, multi-institutional study, more than 900 women with genital *U. urealyticum* were randomized to placebo or erythromycin beginning at 26 to 28 weeks' gestation and continuing until 35 weeks. No improvement was detected in any outcome measure (Table 33–9).[98] In the third study, one involving 229 patients, subjects were randomized to a short course (7 days) of erythromycin or to placebo. There was no significant improvement in preterm birth, birth weight, or preterm PROM, but the authors observed a significant decrease in term PROM (16 versus 6%, $p =$

TABLE 33–8
Summary of Prospective Antibiotic Trials to Prevent Premature Birth

DESIGN	AUTHOR, YEAR (REFERENCE)	ANTIBIOTIC REGIMEN	PATIENT SELECTION
Administration during prenatal care	Kass, 1981 (135)	Erythromycin in third trimester	
	McCormack, 1987 (136)	Erythromycin or clindamycin for 6 wk	Vaginal mycoplasmas
	Eschenbach, 1991 (98)	Erythromycin from 28–35 wk	Vaginal *Ureaplasma urealyticum*
	McGregor, 1990 (137)	Erythromycin for 7 days	
Administration during premature labor, adjunctively with tocolytics	McGregor, 1986 (140)	Erythromycin	1 and <5 cm dilated
	Newton, 1986 (141)	Ampicillin *and* erythromycin	
	Morales, 1988 (142)	Ampicillin *or* erythromycin	
	Winkler, 1988 (143)	Erythromycin	
Administration after preterm premature rupture of membranes	Amon, 1988 (144)	Ampicillin	20–34 wk
	Morales, 1989 (145)	Ampicillin	26–34 wk
	Johnston, 1990 (146)	Mezlocillin/ampicillin	20–34 wk
	Christmas, 1990 (147)	Clindamycin/gentamicin/ampicillin	
	McGregor, 1991 (245)	Oral erythromycin 333 mg for 7 days	23–34 wk
	Owen, 1993 (246)	Intravenous ampicillin followed by oral ampicillin	24–33 wk
	Ernest, 1994 (247)	Intravenous penicillin then oral penicillin	21–37 wk

TABLE 33–9

A Randomized Trial of Erythromycin for Treatment of Vaginal *Ureaplasma urealyticum* in Pregnancy

OUTCOME	TREATMENT GROUP		P-VALUE
	Erythromycin (N = 605)	Placebo (N = 576)	
Birth weight (g, mean ± SD)	3302 ± 557	3326 ± 558	NS
Birth weight < 2500 g (%)	7	6	NS
Gestational age at delivery ≥ 36 wk (%)	8.6	8.2	NS
Premature rupture of membranes at ≥ 36 wk (%)	2.5	2.5	NS
Stillbirth (%)	0.5	0.5	NS
Neonatal death (%)	0.2	0	NS

NS = not significant.

0.01).[137] Two retrospective, nonrandomized studies have reported reductions in PROM, low birth weight, and preterm labor through antenatal treatment of *C. trachomatis*.[138, 139]

The prototype of the second category of antibiotic trial was reported by McGregor and colleagues. They randomized patients in premature labor to adjunctive oral erythromycin (in addition to clinically indicated tocolytics).[140] They found that among small groups of women with cervical dilatation (between 1 and 5 cm), the erythromycin-treated group (N = 8) had significantly prolonged pregnancy (32.5 versus 22.4 days, *p* = 0.02) and higher infant birth weight (2943 versus 2605 g, *p* = 0.07) when compared with the placebo group (N = 9). Additional studies of similar design have resulted in varying results regarding short-term delay in delivery and increase in term delivery.[141–143] None showed a decrease in perinatal mortality.

In 1988, Amon and colleagues reported the first antibiotic trial of the third type and noted a significant increase in pregnancies delivered more than 1 week after preterm PROM in the ampicillin group (47%) versus the no ampicillin group (26%, *p* = 0.05).[144] Three other trials of this type have uniformly reported significant short-term delays in delivery but varying effects in increases in birth weight, neonatal hospital stay, and term delivery. Here also, no study showed a significant decrease in perinatal mortality.[145–147]

More recently, Egarter and associates published a meta-analysis studying the effects of prophylactic antibiotics in seven randomized clinical trials and 795 patients. These authors concluded that prophylactic antibiotic administration in preterm labor with intact membranes without systemic signs or symptoms of IAI does not significantly reduce the rate of neonatal morbidity (chorioamnionitis, endometritis, maternal infection, neonatal death, neonatal sepsis, neonatal pneumonia, or necrotizing enterocolitis [NEC]).[83]

For reasons other than prevention of preterm birth, detection and treatment of *N. gonorrhoeae*, *C. trachomatis*, and bacteriuria are appropriate, but other antibiotic approaches, such as routine use of antibiotics for the prevention of premature birth, should be limited to investigational trials. In addition, bacterial vaginosis and trichomoniasis should be screened for and treated in the high-risk patient (Table 33–10).

PREMATURE RUPTURE OF THE MEMBRANES

PROM is a common but poorly understood problem. Because there is little understanding of its etiology, management has been largely empirical and obstetricians have been sharply divided about what constitutes the best approach to care. Indeed, the problem is complex. Gestational age and demographic factors influence the outcome of PROM. Therapeutic modalities added within the past 20 years include corticosteroids, tocolytics, and more potent antibiotics, but their place in therapy remains debatable in part. Of major importance is the marked improvement in survival of low-birth-weight infants. This chapter emphasizes developments since 1970. The literature has been reviewed periodically.[148–151]

Lack of standard, clear terminology has hindered our understanding of PROM. Most authors define PROM as rupture at any time before the onset of contractions, but "premature" also carries the connotation of preterm pregnancy. To avoid confusion, we use preterm to refer to gestational age less than 37 weeks. Others using the expression "prolonged rupture of the membranes" have used the same acronym, PROM.

The latent period is defined as the time from membrane rupture to onset of contractions. It is to be distinguished from the latent phase, which designates the phase of labor that precedes the active phase.

Terms used to describe maternal or perinatal infections during labor include *fever in labor*, *intrapartum fever*, *chorioamnionitis*, *amnionitis*, *intrauterine infection*, and *IAI*. In most reports, clinical criteria used for these diagnoses include fever, uterine irritability or tenderness, leukocytosis, and purulent cervical discharge. After delivery, maternal uterine infection is referred to as *endometritis*, *endomyometritis*, or *metritis*. These clinical diagnoses are usually based on fever and uterine tenderness. In few studies, however, were presumed maternal infections confirmed by blood or genital tract cultures.

For neonates, the most common term used to report

TABLE 33–10
Summary of Opinions for Use of Antibiotics to Prevent Preterm Birth

OPINION	COMMENT
During Prenatal Care	
1. Treat *Neisseria gonorrhoeae* and *Chlamydia trachomatis*	Screening and treatment of these two sexually transmitted organisms should follow standard recommendations to prevent spread to sexual partner(s) and the newborn. Published nonrandomized trials show improved pregnancy outcome with treatment.
2. Treat bacteriuria, including group B streptococcal bacteriuria	Screening and treatment for bacteriuria is a standard practice to prevent pyelonephritis. A meta-analysis had concluded that bacteriuria is directly associated with preterm birth.
3. Screen for and treat bacterial vaginosis in patients at high risk for preterm birth	Two double-blind randomized trials have shown a benefit in women with high-risk pregnancies. No published trials have assessed this approach in women at low risk.
4. Screen for and treat *Trichomonas vaginalis* in patients at high risk for preterm birth	This opinion is based on the association of this parasite with adverse pregnancy outcome in some studies, the degree of inflammation accompanying the infection, and the safety of treatment after the first trimester. There are no published trials to support its treatment to prevent preterm birth.
5. Do not treat *Ureaplasma urealyticum* genital colonization	One double-blind treatment trial that corrected for confounding infections showed no benefit.
6. Do not treat group B streptococcal genital colonization	One double-blind treatment trial showed no benefit.
With Preterm Labor and Intact Membranes	
1. Give group B streptococcal prophylaxis to prevent neonatal sepsis	As recommended by the Centers for Disease Control and Prevention and The American College of Obstetricians and Gynecologists.
2. Do not give antibiotics routinely to prolong pregnancy	Most trials and one meta-analysis concluded that antibiotics gave no benefit, to date.
3. In patients with bacterial vaginosis or *T. vaginalis*, treatment should be undertaken	This opinion is based on extrapolation of data from treatment during prenatal care.
With Preterm Premature Rupture of Membranes	
1. Give group B streptococcal prophylaxis to prevent neonatal sepsis	As recommended by the Centers for Disease Control and Prevention and The American College of Obstetricians and Gynecologists.
2. Give additional antibiotics in pregnancies at 24 to 32 weeks	One recent well-designed trial and two meta-analyses concluded there was substantial benefit to the neonate.
3. Give corticosteroids to enhance fetal organ maturation if 24 to 32 weeks	Not enough data to recommend weekly corticosteroids.

infection is *neonatal sepsis*, but some authors use a positive blood or cerebrospinal fluid culture result, whereas others use clinical signs of sepsis without bacteriologic confirmation.

Incidence

In several reports, the incidence of PROM has ranged from 4 to 7% of total deliveries,[95, 152, 153] whereas PROM related to preterm birth has occurred in approximately 1% of all pregnancies.[154–156] In some referral centers, however, preterm PROM accounted for 30% of all preterm births.[157]

Etiology

Several clinical variables have been associated with PROM,[155, 158] including cervical incompetence, cervical operations and lacerations, multiple pregnancies, polyhydramnios, antepartum hemorrhage, and heavy smoking. However, in most instances, none of these clinical variables is present. No association has been found between the frequency of PROM and maternal age, parity, maternal weight, fetal weight and position, maternal trauma, or type of work.[148, 159]

Physical properties of membranes that rupture prematurely have also been investigated. Studies of the collagen content of amnion in patients with PROM have led to conflicting results, perhaps because of important differences in methodology. Other reports have shown that membranes from women with PROM are thinner than membranes from women without PROM.[160] Using in vitro techniques to measure rupturing pressure, investigators have found that the membranes from patients with PROM withstand either the same or higher pressure before bursting than do membranes from women without PROM.[161-163] Such observations have suggested a local defect at the site of rupture, rather than a diffuse weakening, in membranes that rupture before labor. These studies of physical properties should be interpreted with caution because of differences in measuring techniques, possible deterioration of membrane preparations, and need for proper controls. In addition to being a possible cause of premature labor, subclinical infection may be a cause of PROM (see previous section). Acute inflammation of the placental membranes is twice as common when membranes rupture within 4 hours before labor than when they rupture after the onset of labor, which suggests that this "infection" may be the cause of PROM.[159]

Several reports have suggested a relationship between coitus, histologic inflammation, and PROM. In additional analyses, two successive singleton pregnancies in each of 5230 women (10,460 pregnancies) were considered.[164] Preterm PROM occurred in only 2% of 773 pregnancies when there was no recent coitus and histologic chorioamnionitis, but it occurred in 23% of 96 pregnancies when both of these features were present. However, a causal role of coitus or infection was not established because there may have been other factors that were not considered. Evaluation of successive pregnancies would not necessarily have eliminated these confounding variables. In the South African black population, the rates of histologic chorioamnionitis and PROM were increased when coitus had occurred within the last 7 days. Use of a condom during coitus resulted in less placental inflammation. In addition, PROM occurred more often ($p < 0.01$) when there had been male orgasm during coitus.[165] Because organisms may attach to sperm, it has been hypothesized that sperm carry organisms into the endocervix or uterus.

Further evidence is provided by bacteriologic studies. Patients with PROM before term or with prolonged ROM are more likely to have anaerobes in the endocervical cultures than are women without PROM at term.[166, 167] These observations may be interpreted as showing that subclinical anaerobic "infection" leads to PROM. However, the increased presence of anaerobes in cervical cultures may reflect hormonal or other influences at different stages of gestation.

Investigations of risk factors for preterm PROM are likely to provide insight into the etiology of this condition. In the largest case-control study, Harger and colleagues reported 341 cases and 253 controls.[168] Only three independent variables were associated with preterm PROM in a logistic regression analysis. These were previous preterm delivery (OR 2.5, 95% CI 1.4–2.5), uterine bleeding in pregnancy, and cigarette smoking. The OR accompanying bleeding increased with bleeding in late pregnancy and with the number of trimesters in which bleeding occurred (OR for first-trimester bleeding 2.4, 95% CI 1.5–3.9; OR for third-trimester bleeding 6.5, 95% CI 1.9–23; OR for bleeding in more than one trimester 7.4, 95% CI 2.2–26). For cigarette smoking, the OR was higher for those who continued smoking (2.1, 95% CI 1.4–3.1) than for those who stopped (1.6, 95% CI 0.8–3.3). Because previous preterm pregnancy is a historical feature and little can be done to

prevent bleeding in pregnancy, this study provides additional reason to encourage all patients, especially women of reproductive age, to stop smoking.

Diagnosis

In most cases, PROM is readily diagnosed by history, physical findings, and simple laboratory tests such as determination of pH (Nitrazene [phenaphthazine] test [Bristol-Myers Squibb, Princeton, NJ]) or detection of ferning. Although these tests are accurate in approximately 90% of cases, they yield false-positive and false-negative results, especially in women with small amounts of amniotic fluid in the vagina. Other biochemical and histochemical tests and intra-amniotic injection of various dyes have been suggested, but they have not gained wide acceptance. Ultrasound examination has also been used as a diagnostic technique because finding oligohydramnios suggests PROM. Oligohydramnios, however, has many additional causes.

Natural History

The onset of regular uterine contractions occurs within 24 hours after ROM in 80 to 90% of term patients.[148] The latent period exceeds 24 hours in 19% of patients at term and exceeds 48 hours in 12.5%.[169, 170] Only 3.6% of term patients do not begin labor within 7 days.[169]

Before term, latent periods are longer among patients with PROM. Confirming earlier studies, more recent investigations have shown latent periods of 24 hours in 57 to 83%,[170, 171] of 72 hours in 15 to 26%,[153, 172, 173] and of 7 days in 19 to 41% of patients.[154, 158, 170] There is an inverse relationship between gestational age and the proportion of patients with latent periods of 3 days.[172] There is also an inverse relationship between advancing gestation and a decreased risk of chorioamnionitis.[96] One third of women with pregnancies between 25 and 32 weeks' gestation had latent periods of 3 days, whereas for pregnancies between 33 and 34 and between 35 and 36 weeks, the values were 16 and 4.5%, respectively. In 53 cases of PROM at 16 to 25 weeks (mean, 22.6 weeks), the median length of time from PROM to delivery was 6 days (range, 1 to 87 days; mean, 17 days).[174] In a population-based study of 267 cases of PROM before 34 weeks, fully 76% of women were already in labor at the time of admission and an additional 5% had an indicated delivery. Only 19% were candidates for expectant management, and, of these women, 60% went into labor within 48 hours.[175] Thus, the natural history of PROM reveals that labor usually develops within a few days.

In a minority of cases of PROM, the membranes can "reseal," especially with rupture of membranes after amniocentesis. With expectant management, 2.8 to 13% may anticipate the cessation of leakage of amniotic fluid.[176, 177]

Complications

Analysis of complications described in recent studies is complex because of differences in study design. Table

TABLE 33-11
Complications in Newborns After Premature Rupture of Membranes[a]

COMPLICATION	RATE (%)
Perinatal mortality, overall	0–43
Term	0–2.5
All preterm	2–43
1000–1500 g	29
1501–2500 g	7
RDS, all preterm	10–42
1000–1500 g	42
1501–2500 g	7
Infection	
Amnionitis	4–33
Maternal (overall)	3–29
Endometritis	3–29
Neonatal sepsis	0–7
Neonatal overall (including clinically diagnosed sepsis)	3–281

[a]Studies with more than 100 infants.
RDS = respiratory distress syndrome.

33–11, however, attempts to summarize complications observed in studies with more than 100 infants. Direct comparisons of data from one study to another require extreme caution. The wide-ranging differences are attributable to major differences in populations at risk, gestational age, definitions, and management.

The most common complication among cases with PROM before 37 weeks is RDS, which is found in 10 to 40% of neonates. (A small number of studies have reported RDS in as many as 60 to 80% of newborns.) Neonatal sepsis was documented in less than 10%, whereas amnionitis (based on clinical criteria only) occurred in 4 to 60%.[178] Endometritis developed in 3 to 29% of patients in most reports, but it is not clear whether patients with amnionitis are included in the endometritis category. In selected groups, such as patients with cesarean section after PROM, endometritis occurs in up to 70% of patients.

When latent periods in preterm pregnancies are prolonged, pulmonary hypoplasia is an additional neonatal complication. In cases in which PROM occurred before 26 weeks and with long intervals (e.g., more than 5 weeks) between rupture and delivery, Nimrod and colleagues noted a 27% incidence of pulmonary hypoplasia.[179] Other studies demonstrate a lower incidence of pulmonary hypoplasia.[180] Pulmonary hypoplasia is rare if PROM occurs after 26 weeks' gestation.[181] In addition, pulmonary hypoplasia is poorly predicted antenatally by ultrasound.[182] An additional 20% of neonates had fetal skeletal deformities due to compression.

Asphyxia, defined as an Apgar score of less than 7 at 5 minutes of life, is noted in 15 to 64% of live-born infants.[153, 155, 183, 184] This complication is most common among very low birth weight infants. Other complications of PROM, especially in the preterm pregnancy, are malpresentation, cord prolapse, and congenital anomalies. In view of the long list of potential hazards, it is not surprising that premature infants surviving after PROM are often subject to prolonged hospitalization.

Perinatal mortality depends mainly on gestational age. The wide variation in results in Table 33–10 for preterm infants reflects different groupings of gestational ages. It is not certain whether infants with PROM have higher mortality than infants of the same gestational age without PROM.

Causes of perinatal death may be determined by examining data from four large series (Table 33–12).[152, 158, 185] Two of these studies included stillbirths; two studies excluded them. Overall, RDS was the leading cause of death. Deaths were presumed to be due to anoxia when there was an antepartum or intrapartum death of a very small infant. In both frequency and severity, RDS was a greater threat than infection to the preterm fetus.

Maternal mortality as a complication of PROM is rare. Studies document only one maternal death (related to chorioamnionitis, severe toxemia, and cardiorespiratory arrest) in more than 3000 women with PROM.[186] Case reports of maternal death from sepsis complicating PROM appear sporadically.[187]

Diagnosis of Infection

Because of the frequency and potential severity of maternal and fetal infections after PROM, various tests have been studied as predictors of infection. One review has critically appraised eight tests and found no test to be ideal[188] (Table 33–13). Several authors have evaluated the use of amniocentesis and microscopic examination of amniotic fluid for the presence of bacteria. This approach is limited, however, because amniotic fluid is available in only half the patients. Clinical infection is more common in women with positive smears or cultures, but 20 to 30% of these women or neonates had no clinical evidence of infection.[189–192] In addition, amniocentesis may potentially be accompanied by trauma, bleeding, initiation of labor, or introduction of infection, although Yeast and co-authors reported no increase in onset of labor and no trauma in their retrospective series.[193]

Because the value of amniocentesis in patients with preterm PROM has not been determined precisely, most practitioners do not employ this test routinely for several reasons. Most patients with PROM and positive amni-

TABLE 33-12
Primary Causes of Death Among Preterm Infants Born with Premature Rupture of Membranes

CAUSE	% OF PERINATAL DEATHS[a]
RDS	29–70
Infection	3–19
Congenital anomaly	9–27
Asphyxia-anoxia	5–46[b]
Others[c]	9–27

[a]Overall perinatal mortality was 13–24%.
[b]Includes stillbirths with birth weight between 500 and 1000 g.
[c]Includes atelectasis, erythroblastosis fetalis, intracranial hemorrhage, and necrotizing enterocolitis.
RDS = respiratory distress syndrome.
Data from references 129, 135, 161, and 162.

TABLE 33–13

Appraisal of Various Tests as Predictors of Clinical Chorioamnionitis in Preterm Premature Rupture of Membranes

TEST	NO. OF STUDIES	PPV (%)	NPV (%)
Maternal leukocytosis	3	40–50	89–90
C-reactive protein	4	10–45	80–97
Gram's stain or culture of amniotic fluid	2	67–45	85–95
Leukocyte esterase	1	4	92
Oligohydramnios	3	33–47	86–93
Low biophysical profile[a] within 24 hr of delivery	2	31–60	96–97

[a]Biophysical profile assigns 0 to 2 points for amniotic fluid volume, fetal tone, fetal breathing movements, fetal breathing, and fetal heart rate reactivity. A low score is 4 or less.

PPV = positive predictive value; NPV = negative predictive value.

After Ohlsson A, Wang E. An analysis of antenatal tests to detect infection in preterm premature rupture of membranes. Am J Obstet Gynecol 162:809, 1990.

otic fluid culture results are in labor within 48 hours, and culture results are often delayed and available after the fact. Because at least some patients have positive culture results with no clinical evidence of infection, there is concern regarding unnecessary delivery of preterm infants. Finally, it has not been demonstrated that clinical decisions based on data from amniocentesis lead to an improved perinatal outcome. Feinstein and colleagues evaluated 73 patients with preterm PROM who underwent amniocentesis.[192] When the Gram stain or culture result was positive, delivery was achieved. Results were compared with those of 73 matched patients from a historical group. Compared with controls, patients managed by amniocentesis had less clinically diagnosed amnionitis (7 versus 20%, $p < 0.05$) and fewer low Apgar scores at 5 minutes (3 versus 12%, $p < 0.05$). There were, however, no significant differences in rates of overall infection (22 versus 30%), "possible neonatal sepsis" (12 versus 14%), or perinatal deaths (1 versus 3%). Although there were apparent advantages to management by amniocentesis, there are serious limits to historically controlled studies, and there were no significant decreases in overall infection of perinatal mortality. In a small comparative study of expectancy versus the use of amniocentesis, Cotton and colleagues reported a significantly shorter neonatal hospital stay in the amniocentesis group ($p < 0.01$), but more than 25% of patients were excluded because no amniotic fluid pocket was seen.[194] Also, there were no significant differences in rates of maternal infection, neonatal sepsis, or neonatal death. Ohlsson and Wang found Gram stain and culture of amniotic fluid had a modest positive predictive value for clinical chorioamnionitis.[188] Thus, clear evidence for the widespread use of amniocentesis in PROM is not available. Given the more recent information regarding the association of cerebral palsy and infection, these issues should be reinvestigated in a controlled fashion.

Noninvasive procedures such as measuring the level of maternal serum C-reactive protein and amniotic fluid volume have also been suggested as predictors of infection. Several groups have evaluated C-reactive protein as such a predictor.[195–198] An elevated level of C-reactive protein in serum from patients with PROM has a modest positive predictive value for histologic amnionitis (40 to 96%), but its predictive value for clinically evident infection is poor (10 to 45%). The value of a normal level of C-reactive protein for predicting absence of clinical chorioamnionitis is better (80 to 97%). In view of the low predictive value of a positive test, it does not appear wise to attempt delivery solely on the basis of an elevated C-reactive protein level.

Women who have PROM with oligohydramnios appear to be at increased risk for clinically evident infection, but the positive predictive value is modest (33 to 47%). In 1985, Gonik and co-workers noted that "amnionitis" developed in 8 (47%) of 17 patients with no pocket of amniotic fluid larger than 1 by 1 cm on ultrasound examination, whereas amnionitis developed in 3 (14%) of 22 patients with adequate pockets (i.e., $>1 \times 1$ cm) ($p < 0.05$).[199] To improve the predictability of these tests, Vintzileos and colleagues used a biophysical profile that included amniotic fluid volume, fetal movement and tone, fetal respirations, and a nonstress test.[200] However, positive predictive value of the biophysical profile has been variable (31 to 60% for clinical chorioamnionitis and 31 to 47% for neonatal sepsis).[188]

Treatment of Preterm Premature Rupture of the Membranes in the Second Trimester

Because fetal viability is nil throughout nearly all of the second trimester, the traditionally recommended approach to PROM in this period of gestation has been to induce labor. However, retrospective reports have provided pertinent data on expectant management for PROM before fetal viability.[201–204] As expected, the latent period is relatively long (mean, 12 to 19 days; median, 6 to 7 days). Although maternal clinically evident infections were common (amnionitis in 39 to 59% and endometritis in 13 to 17%), none of these infections was serious. Of note, there was an appreciable neonatal survival rate of 13 to 50%, depending on gestational age at PROM and duration of the latent period. In cases with PROM at less than 23 weeks, the perinatal survival was 13%; whereas with PROM at 24 to 26 weeks, it was 50%.[204] Accordingly, with appropriate counseling, expectant management may be offered even in the second trimester for selected cases of PROM (Table 33–14). As

TABLE 33–14
Summary of Management Plans for Premature Rupture of Membranes

	STATUS
In Second Trimester (<26–28 wk)	
A. Induction	
B. Expectant management	Retrospective works show high maternal infection rate but 13–50% neonatal survival
In Early Third Trimester (26–34 wk)	
A. Tocolytics to delay delivery	Randomized trials show no important benefits
B. Corticosteroids to accelerate lung maturity	CDC consensus statement recommends use between 24–32 wk
C. Antibiotics for prophylaxis of neonatal group B streptococcal infection	Efficiency established in randomized trial
D. Antibiotics to prolong latent period	Risk:benefit ratio unresolved; limit to randomized trials; optimal duration of antibiotics unresolved
E. Expectant management	Approach followed most commonly; if premature rupture of membranes occurs > 32 weeks, randomized trials show no neonatal benefit to expectant management
At or Near Term (>35 wk)	
A. Early induction, within 12–24 hr	
B. Late induction, after approximately 24 hr	
C. Expectant management until labor or infection develop	Recent evidence supports both option A and option C
D. Prostaglandin E_1 and E_2 preparations to ripen cervix/induce labor	Randomized trials and historical data support safety and efficacy

neonatal survival in the periviable periods continue to improve, the numbers of infants afflicted by moderate to severe disabilities continues to be substantial.[205] These concerns should be clearly communicated to the mother before delivery. As discussed subsequently, a plan for group B streptococcal surveillance and treatment would also be indicated.

Treatment of Preterm Premature Rupture of the Membranes Early in the Third Trimester

It is at this gestational age interval (26 to 34 weeks) that management is most controversial. Yet new information has become available, and sophisticated meta-analyses have been performed. Controversial components of therapy are corticosteroids (after 32 weeks), tocolytics, and antibiotics to prolong pregnancy (see Table 33–14).

Corticosteroids. Many investigators have used corticosteroids in at least some patients with PROM.[206-218] In some studies, the investigators found evidence for an increased rate of maternal postpartum infection after administration of corticosteroids. The infections occurred mainly after vaginal delivery and were mild. Of still greater concern is the observation of some investigators that the rate of neonatal sepsis was increased when corticosteroids were used. However, most studies have not found this association.

Some studies reported significant (or nearly significant) decreases in the rate of RDS, but others found no significant decrease when corticosteroids were used in patients with PROM. There are major difficulties in interpreting these studies. In some of the more rigorously designed studies of corticosteroid use, the numbers

of patients with PROM were small. Thus, real differences may have been missed (a beta error). In most studies, there were at least small decreases in the incidence of RDS in the corticosteroid group. A relatively wide range of gestational ages was studied. The minimum number of weeks of gestation for entry into a study varied from 25 to 32, and the maximum varied from 32 to 37. Because an equal effect of corticosteroids on the rate of RDS is unlikely at all gestational age intervals, real differences may have been missed in some intervals because data for these intervals were combined with data for other gestational ages. Finally, experiments measuring the surfactant-inducing potency of corticosteroids suggest differences in the efficacy of various corticosteroid preparations and various dosages.

Several studies, including three meta-analyses, have attempted to resolve the confusion.[219-221] Unfortunately, the authors reached differing conclusions. Ohlsson concluded that in preterm PROM, corticosteroid treatment "cannot presently be recommended to prevent RDS . . . outside a randomized controlled trial.[219] The reasons for this are that the evidence that it decreases RDS is weak and its use increases the incidence of endometritis and may increase neonatal infections." On the other hand, Crowley and associates concluded that corticosteroids were effective in preventing RDS after preterm PROM (OR 0.44, 95% CI 0.32–0.60) and that they were not associated with a significant increase in perinatal infection (OR 0.84, 95% CI 0.57–1.23) or neonatal infection (OR 1.61, 95% CI 0.9–3.0).[220] Lovett and colleagues in a prospective, double-blind trial of preterm PROM did use corticosteroids in all patients. They also found significant decreases in mortality, sepsis, and RDS as well as increased birth weight when corticosteroids and antibiotics were given compared with use of corticosteroids alone. In addition, Lewis and co-workers investigated use of ampicillin-sulbactam in preterm PROM and then randomized patients to receive weekly corticosteroids versus placebo between 24 and 34 weeks. They found a decrease in RDS (44 versus 18%, $p = 0.03$ or 0.29, 95% CI 0.10–0.82) in the corticosteroid-treated group with no increase in maternal or neonatal infection complications.[221] Leitich and associates, however, concluded that corticosteroids appear to diminish the beneficial effects of antibiotics in the treatment of preterm PROM. This was based on the results of their meta-analysis of five randomized trials of antibiotics and preterm PROM in which corticosteroids were used, which they compared with those of their previous meta-analysis of preterm PROM without corticosteroids. They found nonsignificant differences in mortality, sepsis, RDS, IVH, and NEC when both antibiotics and corticosteroids were used. In contrast, when antibiotics but not corticosteroids were used, they found a significant decrease in chorioamnionitis (OR 0.37, $p = .0001$), postpartum endometritis (OR 0.47, $p = 0.03$), neonatal sepsis (OR 0.27, $p = 0.002$), and IVH (OR 0.48, $p = 0.02$).[222]

The NIH Consensus Development Panel in 1995 recommended that corticosteroids be given in the absence of IAI to women with preterm PROM at less than 30 to 32 weeks' gestation because the benefits of corticosteroids may outweigh the risk at this gestational age. Because the number of patients receiving corticosteroids with PROM at more than 32 weeks' gestation was small, the consensus panel chose to restrict their recommendation to less than 32 weeks' gestation. It is unclear if repeated courses of corticosteroids should be given if a woman remains pregnant longer than the expected period of benefit of 7 days.[223]

Antibiotics. Patients with preterm PROM are candidates for prophylaxis against group B streptococci.[109, 224, 225] In addition, one innovative report noted use of combination antibiotics in an asymptomatic patient in premature labor because of bacterial colonization of the amniotic fluid, which was detected by amniocentesis. A second amniocentesis 48 hours after therapy revealed a sterile culture.[226]

Some studies of preterm pregnancies have found an increased rate of amnionitis to be associated with an increasing length of the latent period,[152, 153, 227] whereas others[184] have not. In patients with preterm PROM, vaginal examination should be avoided until labor develops.[228] Some studies noted that prolonged ROM decreased the incidence of RDS[185, 186]; others noted no significant effect.[152, 154, 158, 184, 207, 210, 229] These discrepancies may be explained by differences in experimental design (such as grouping of various gestational ages and using different sample sizes) or in definitions of clinical complications. Antibiotics of several classes have been found to prolong pregnancy in the setting of preterm PROM. Mercer and Arheart[81] evaluated the subject of antibiotics in PROM with a meta-analysis. They evaluated such outcomes as length of latency, chorioamnionitis, postpartum infection, neonatal survival, neonatal sepsis, RDS, IVH, and NEC. Several classes of antibiotics were used, including penicillins and cephalosporins, although few studies used either tocolytics or corticosteroids. Benefits of antibiotics in this analysis included a significant reduction in chorioamnionitis, IVH, and confirmed neonatal sepsis. There was a significant decrease in the number of women delivering within 1 week of membrane rupture (OR 0.56, CI 0.41–0.76), but no significant differences were seen in NEC, RDS, or mortality. The evidence currently supports use of antibiotics in preterm PROM to prolong latency and to decrease maternal and neonatal infectious complications, but further studies to select the preferred agent have yet to be performed. The Maternal-Fetal Medicine Unit Network of the NICHD conducted a large, multicenter trial of antibiotics after PROM but also did not use tocolytics or corticosteroids. They demonstrated a significant decrease in perinatal morbidity, RDS, and NEC with use of ampicillin and erythromycin.[82] Egarter and associates found in a meta-analysis of seven published studies a 68% reduction of neonatal sepsis and a 50% decreased risk of IVH in infants born to mothers receiving antibiotics after preterm PROM. They did not, however, find any significant differences in either RDS or neonatal mortality.[230]

These trials, however, have not evaluated the efficacy of one antibiotic regimen versus another. Both of the above regimens will cover group B *Streptococcus*, but this was not the intent of use of the antibiotics. With the onset of labor, appropriate intrapartum antibiotics are recommended for both the preterm gestation or known group B *Streptococcus*–positive patient.

Tocolytics and Development of RDS. Older studies suggested a decrease in the rate of RDS with use of beta-adrenergic drugs, but in the National Collaborative Study use of tocolytics in patients with ruptured membranes increased the likelihood of RDS by about 350%.[231] In addition, two randomized controlled trials have assessed tocolytics in the presence of PROM.[232, 233] Neither found any significant increase in time to delivery or birth weight or any decrease in RDS or neonatal hospital stay. However, these studies did not use antibiotics or corticosteroids. Tocolytics have been shown to prolong pregnancy by about 48 hours in patients with intact membranes, but their efficacy with preterm PROM remains debatable. In the patient with preterm PROM and no contractions, tocolytics should not be given. In the patient with preterm PROM and contractions, IAI should be ruled out before consideration of tocolytics. Tocolytics could be considered in the early third trimester to maximize impact of antenatal corticosteroids (48-hour delay) on neonatal morbidity and mortality.

Determination of Fetal Lung Maturity. Some clinicians determine the status of fetal pulmonary maturity and proceed with delivery if the lungs are mature. Amniotic fluid may be collected by amniocentesis or by collection from the posterior vagina. Presence of either phosphatidylglycerol or a lecithin:sphingomyelin ratio higher than 2 in amniotic fluid has been reported to be a good predictor of pulmonary maturity. In a series of patients with PROM before 36 weeks, Brame and MacKenna determined whether phosphatidylglycerol was present in the vaginal pool and delivered patients when there was presence of phosphatidylglycerol, spontaneous labor, or evidence of sepsis.[234] Of 214 patients, 47 had phosphatidylglycerol present initially and were delivered. Of the remaining 167, 36 (21%) developed phosphatidylglycerol and were induced or delivered by cesarean section. Evidence of maternal infection developed in 8 (5%) and spontaneous labor developed in 123 (74%) of the 167 patients. Phosphatidylglycerol in amniotic fluid from the vagina reliably predicted fetal lung maturity. However, its absence did not necessarily mean that RDS would develop. Of 131 patients who did not show phosphatidylglycerol in the vaginal pool in any sample, 82 (62%) were delivered of infants who had no RDS.

Intentional Preterm Induction in the Mid-Third Trimester. Even with PROM, delivery of a premature infant simply because its lungs show biochemical maturity may be questioned in view of other potential hazards of prematurity and the potential difficulties of the induction.

Two recent papers have examined this controversial issue. With respect to the new information regarding the association between preterm PROM, chorioamnionitis, and subsequent development of cerebral palsy, the use of intentional mid–third-trimester induction is receiving increased attention.

Mercer and colleagues compared expectant management to immediate induction in 93 pregnancies complicated by PROM between 32 and 36 weeks, 6 days when mature fetal lung profiles were documented. They found significant prolongation of latent period, maternal hospitalization as well as increased neonatal length of stay, and increased antimicrobial use in the expectant management group despite no increase in documented neonatal sepsis. Thus, they concluded that in women with preterm PROM at 32 through 36 weeks with a mature fetal lung profile, immediate induction of labor reduces the duration of hospitalization in both mother and neonates.[235] Cox and Leveno similarly studied pregnancies complicated by preterm PROM at 30 to 34 weeks' gestation. Consenting patients were randomly assigned to expectant versus immediate induction. Corticosteroids, tocolytics, and antibiotics were not used in either group. Fetal lung profiles were not determined. They found a significant increase in the incidence of chorioamnionitis and antepartum hospitalization in the expectant management group. In addition, they found no clinically significant differences in birth weight, IVH, NEC, neonatal sepsis, RDS, or perinatal death. They concluded that there were no clinically significant neonatal advantages to expectant management of ruptured membranes and decreased antepartum hospitalization in those women managed with immediate induction.[236]

Fetal Surveillance. Due to concerns regarding cord compression and cord prolapse as well as the development of intrauterine and fetal infection, daily fetal monitoring in the setting of preterm PROM has been studied. Vintzileos and colleagues demonstrated that infection developed when the nonstress test became nonreactive 78% of the time compared with only 14% when the nonstress test remained reactive.[237] Similarly, the bio-physical profile score of six or less also predicted perinatal infection.[238] As a result, we recommend daily monitoring with nonstress tests. If the nonstress test is nonreactive, further workup with biophysical profiles should be performed. Because there are currently no large studies evaluating outpatient management of preterm PROM, we recommend hospitalization until delivery.

Conclusion. Despite availability of recent data and sophisticated meta-analyses, we believe the evidence supports the use of expectant management in the absence of IAI and in the absence of documented fetal lung maturity in the third trimester until 34 completed weeks. If expectant management is chosen, corticosteroids to enhance fetal organ maturation should be given until 32 weeks. In addition, broad-spectrum antibiotics consisting of ampicillin and erythromycin should be administered for 7 days. Bacterial vaginosis should also be treated if present. In general, tocolytics should be avoided. Daily fetal surveillance is also recommended. Appropriate group B streptococcal prophylaxis in this high risk group is strongly encouraged during labor.

Treatment of Term Premature Rupture of the Membranes

Approximately 8% of pregnant women at term experience PROM, although contractions commence spontaneously within 24 hours of membrane rupture in 80 to 90% of patients.[178] For many years, the practice in most institutions had been to induce labor in term patients within 12 hours of PROM primarily because of concerns about development of chorioamnionitis and neonatal infectious complications. However, three studies demonstrated that in most patients expectant management can be safely applied (see Table 33–14). The designs of these three reports were different. Kappy and associates reported a retrospective review in a private population.[169] Duff and colleagues performed a randomized study in indigent patients with unfavorable cervix characteristics (<2 cm dilated, <80% effaced) and with no complications of pregnancy (e.g., toxemia, diabetes, previous cesarean section, malpresentation, or meconium-stained fluid).[239] Patients assigned to the induction group generally had induction started 12 hours after rupture of membranes. The excess cesarean deliveries in the induction group were for failed induction. In the induction group, there was a higher probability of IAI. In the study by Conway and colleagues, all patients were observed until the morning after admission.[240] Induction of labor was then undertaken if the patient was not in labor. Wagner and co-workers provided yet another variant by comparing early induction (at 6 hours after PROM) to late induction (at 24 hours after PROM).[241] In their population at a Kaiser Permanente hospital, the results favored early induction by shortening maternal hospital stay and decreasing neonatal sepsis evaluations. Recent work has also evaluated use of oral and vaginal prostaglandin preparations (E_1, E_2) to ripen the cervix or induce labor after PROM at term. These preparations appear to be effective in shortening labor without increasing maternal or neonatal infection.[242–244] Hannah and colleagues evaluated four management schemes in women with PROM at term: (1) immediate induction with oxytocin, (2) immediate induction with vaginal prostaglandin E_2, (3) expectant management for up to 4 days followed by oxytocin induction, and (4) expectant management followed by prostaglandin E_2 induction. Although no differences in cesarean section rates or neonatal sepsis were found, an increase in chorioamnionitis was noted in the expectantly managed groups, and all deaths not caused by congenital anomalies occurred in the expectant management group. Of note, patient satisfaction was higher in the immediate induction group.

We endorse immediate induction with oxytocin in women with PROM at term if the cervix is favorable and the patient is agreeable. If the cervix is unfavorable, induction with appropriate doses of prostaglandins may be used before use of oxytocin. Intrapartum antibiotic prophylaxis against group B streptococci should be used according to the 1996 guidelines.[109]

References

1. Gibbs RS, Duff P. Progress in pathogenesis and management of clinical intra-amniotic infection. Am J Obstet Gynecol 164:1317, 1991.
2. Newton ER, Prihoda TJ, Gibbs RS. Logistic regression analysis of risk factors for intra-amniotic infection. Obstet Gynecol 73:571, 1989.
3. Soper DE, Mayhall CG, Dalton HP. Risk factors for intra-amniotic infection: a prospective epidemiologic study. Am J Obstet Gynecol 161:562, 1989.
4. Gibbs RS, Castillo MS, Rodgers PJ. Management of acute chorioamnionitis. Am J Obstet Gynecol 136:709, 1980.
5. Halliday HL, Hirata T. Perinatal listeriosis: a review of twelve patients. Am J Obstet Gynecol 133:405, 1979.
6. Shackleford PG. *Listeria* revisited. Am J Dis Child 131:391, 1977.
7. Fleming AD, Ehrlich DW, Miller NA, et al. Successful treatment of maternal septicemia due to *Listeria monocytogenes* at 26 weeks' gestation. Obstet Gynecol 66:52S, 1985.
8. Petrilli ES, D'Ablaing G, Ledger WJ. *Listeria monocytogenes* chorioamnionitis: diagnosis by transabdominal amniocentesis. Obstet Gynecol 55:5S, 1980.
9. Boucher M, Yonekura ML. Perinatal listeriosis (early-onset): correlation of antenatal manifestations and neonatal outcome. Obstet Gynecol 68:593, 1986.
10. Listeriosis outbreak associated with Mexican-style cheese—California. MMWR Morbid Mortal Wkly Rep 34:357, 1985.
11. Monif GRG. Antenatal group A streptococcal infection. Am J Obstet Gynecol 123:213, 1975.
12. Charles D, Edwards WR. Infectious complications of cervical cerclage. Am J Obstet Gynecol 141:1065, 1981.
13. Kuhn RJP, Pepperell RJ. Cervical ligation: a review of 242 pregnancies. Aust NZ J Obstet Gynaecol 17:79, 1977.
14. Aarnoudse JG, Huisjes HJ. Complications of cerclage. Acta Obstet Gynecol Scand 58:255, 1979.
15. Harger JH. Comparison of success and morbidity in cervical cerclage procedures. Obstet Gynecol 56:543, 1980.
16. Burnett RG, Anderson WR. The hazards of amniocentesis. J Iowa Med Soc 58:133, 1968.
17. Queenan JT. Modern Management of the Rh Problem, 2nd ed. Hagerstown, Md, Harper & Row, 1977, p 180.
18. Soper DJ, Mayhall CG, Froggatt JW. Characterization and control of intra-amniotic infection in an urban teaching hospital. Am J Obstet Gynecol 175:304–309, 1996.
19. Yancey MK, Duff P, Kubilis P, et al. Risk factors for neonatal sepsis. Obstet Gynecol 87:188–194, 1996.
20. Herbst A, Wolner-Hanssen P, Ingemarsson I. Risk factors for fever in labor. Obstet Gynecol 86:790–794, 1995.
21. Naeye RL. Coitus and associated amniotic-fluid infections. N Engl J Med 301:1198, 1979.
22. Klebanoff MA, Nugent RP, Rhoads GG. Coitus during pregnancy: is it safe? Lancet 2:914, 1984.
23. Mills JL, Harlap S, Harley EE. Should coitus late in pregnancy be discouraged? Lancet 2:136, 1981.
24. Gibbs RS, Blanco JD, St. Clair PJ, et al. Quantitative bacteriology of amniotic fluid from patients with clinical intra-amniotic infection at term. J Infect Dis 145:1, 1982.
25. Gravett MG, Eschenbach DA, Speigel-Brown CA, et al. Rapid diagnosis of amniotic fluid infection by gas-liquid chromatography. N Engl J Med 306:725, 1982.
26. Nickerson CW. Gonorrhea amnionitis. Obstet Gynecol 42:815, 1973.
27. Handsfield HH, Hodson WA, Holmes KK. Neonatal gonococcal infection: I. Orogastric contamination with *Neisseria gonorrhoeae*. JAMA 225:697, 1973.
28. Brunnel PA, Dische RM, Walker MB. Mycoplasma, amnionitis, and respiratory distress syndrome. JAMA 207:2097, 1969.
29. Shurin PA, Alpert S, Rosner B, et al. Chorioamnionitis and colonization of the newborn infant with genital mycoplasmas. N Engl J Med 293:5, 1975.
30. Blanco JD, Gibbs RS, Malherbe H, et al. A controlled study of genital mycoplasmas in amniotic fluid from patients with intra-amniotic infection. J Infect Dis 147:650, 1983.
31. Gibbs RS, Cassell GH, Davis JK, et al. Further studies on genital mycoplasmas in intra-amniotic infection: blood cultures and serologic response. Am J Obstet Gynecol 154:717, 1986.
32. Martin DH, Koustsky L, Eschenbach DA, et al. Prematurity and perinatal mortality in pregnancies complicated by maternal *Chlamydia trachomatis* infections. JAMA 247:1585, 1982.
33. Wager GP, Martin DH, Koustsky L, et al. Puerperal infectious morbidity: relationship to route of delivery and to antepartum *Chlamydia trachomatis* infection. Am J Obstet Gynecol 138:1028, 1980.
34. Pankuch GA, Applebaum PC, Lorenz RP, et al. Placental microbiology and histology and the pathogenesis of chorioamnionitis. Obstet Gynecol 64:803, 1984.
35. Dong Y, Ramzy I, Kagan-Hallet SK, et al. A microbiologic clinical study of placental inflammation at term. Obstet Gynecol 70:175, 1987.
36. Gibbs RS, Schachter JS. Chlamydial serology in patients with intra-amniotic infection and controls. Sex Transm Dis 14:213, 1987.
37. Sperling RS, Newton E, Gibbs RS. Intra-amniotic infection in low birth weight infants. J Infect Dis 157:113, 1988.
38. Gibbs RS. Chorioamnionitis and bacterial baginosis. Am J Obstet Gynecol 169:460–462, 1993.
39. Silver HM, Sperling RS, St. Clair PJ, et al. Evidence relating bacterial vaginosis to intra-amniotic infection. Am J Obstet Gynecol 161:808, 1989.
40. Gravett MG, Nelson HP, DeRouen T, et al. Independent associations of bacterial vaginosis and *Chlamydia tracho-*

matis infection with adverse pregnancy outcome. JAMA 256:1899–1903, 1986.

41. Newton ER, Piper J, Peairs W. Bacterial vaginosis and intra-amniotic infection. Am J Obstet Gynecol 176:672–677, 1997.

42. Koh KS, Chan FH, Monfared AH, et al. The changing perinatal and maternal outcome in chorioamnionitis. Obstet Gynecol 53:730, 1979.

43. Yoder RP, Gibbs RS, Blanco JD, et al. A prospective, controlled study of maternal and perinatal outcome after intra-amniotic infection at term. Am J Obstet Gynecol 145:695, 1983.

44. Hoskins IA, Johnson TRB, Winkel CA. Leukocyte esterase activity in human amniotic fluid for the rapid detection of chorioamnionitis. Am J Obstet Gynecol 157:730, 1987.

45. Miller JM, Pupkin MJ, Hill GB. Bacterial colonization of amniotic fluid from intact fetal membranes. Am J Obstet Gynecol 136:796, 1980.

46. Romero R, Jimenez C, Lohda A, et al. Amniotic fluid glucose concentration: a rapid and simple method for the detection of intra-amniotic infection in preterm labor. Am J Obstet Gynecol 163:968, 1990.

47. Kirshon B, Rosenfeld B, Mari G, et al. Amniotic fluid glucose and intra-amniotic infection. Am J Obstet Gynecol 164:818, 1991.

48. Kiltz R, Burke M, Porreco R. Amniotic fluid glucose concentration as a marker for intra-amniotic infection. Obstet Gynecol 78:619, 1991.

49. Andrews WW, Hauth JC, Goldenberg RL, et al. Amniotic fluid interleukin-6: Correlation with upper genital tract microbial colonization and gestational age in women delivered after spontaneous labor versus indicated delivery. Am J Obstet Gynecol 173:606–612, 1995.

50. Yoon BH, Romero R, Kim CH, et al. Amniotic fluid interleukin-6: A sensitive test for antenatal diagnosis of acute inflammatory lesions of preterm placenta and prediction of perinatal morbidity. Am J Obstet Gynecol 172:960–970, 1995.

51. Greig PC, Murtha AP, Jimmerson CJ, et al. Maternal serum interleukin 6 during pregnancy and during term and preterm labor. Obstet Gynecol 90:465–469, 1997.

52. Gomez R, Romero R, Ghezzi F, et al. The fetal inflammatory response syndrome. Am J Obstet Gynecol 179:194–202, 1998.

53. Gomez R, Ghezzi F, Romero R, et al. Premature labor and intra-amniotic infection. Clin Perinatol 22:281–342, 1995.

54. Sperling RS, Ramamurthy RS, Gibbs RS. A comparison of intrapartum versus immediate postpartum treatment of intra-amniotic infection. Obstet Gynecol 70:861, 1987.

55. Gibbs RS, Dinsmoor MJ, Newton ER, et al. A randomized trial of intrapartum vs immediate postpartum treatment of women with IAI. Obstet Gynecol 72:823, 1988.

56. Gilstrap LC, Laveno KJ, Cox SM, et al. Intrapartum treatment of acute chorioamnionitis: impact on neonatal sepsis. Am J Obstet Gynecol 159:579, 1988.

57. Bray RE, Boe RW, Johnson WL. Transfer of ampicillin into fetus and amniotic fluid from maternal plasma in late pregnancy. Am J Obstet Gynecol 96:938, 1966.

58. Charles D. Dynamics of antibiotic transfer from mother to fetus. Semin Perinatol 1:89, 1977.

59. Weinstein AJ, Gibbs RS, Gallagher M. Placental transfer of clindamycin and gentamicin. Am J Obstet Gynecol 124:688, 1976.

60. Chapman SJ, Owen J. Randomized trial of single-dose versus multiple-dose cefotetan for the postpartum treatment of intrapartum chorioamnionitis. Am J Obstet Gynecol 177:831–834, 1997.

61. Looff JD, Hager WD. Management of chorioamnionitis. Surg Gynecol Obstet 158:161, 1984.

62. Hauth JC, Gilstrap LC, Hankins GDV, et al. Term maternal and neonatal complications of acute chorioamnionitis. Obstet Gynecol 66:59, 1985.

63. Duff P, Sanders R, Gibbs RS. The course of labor in term patients with chorioamnionitis. Am J Obstet Gynecol 147:391, 1983.

64. Silver RK, Gibbs RS, Castillo M. Effect of amniotic fluid bacteria on the course of labor in nulliparous women at term. Obstet Gynecol 68:587, 1986.

65. Perkins RP. The merits of extraperitoneal cesarean section: a continuing experience. J Reprod Med 19:154, 1977.

66. Hanson H. Revival of the extraperitoneal cesarean section. Am J Obstet Gynecol 130:102, 1978.

67. Imig JR, Perkins RP. Extraperitoneal cesarean section: a new need for old skills: a preliminary report. Am J Obstet Gynecol 125:51, 1976.

68. Yonekura ML, Wallace R, Eglinton WR. Amnionitis—optimal operative management: extraperitoneal cesarean section vs low cervical transperitoneal cesarean section. Proceedings of the Third Annual Meeting of the Society of Perinatal Obstetricians, San Antonio, January 1983. Abstract 24A.

69. Garite TJ, Freeman RK. Chorioamnionitis in the preterm gestation. Obstet Gynecol 59:539, 1982.

70. Morales WJ. The effect of chorioamnionitis on the developmental outcome of preterm infants at one year. Obstet Gynecol 70:183, 1987.

71. Ferguson MG, Rhodes PG, Morrison JC, et al. Clinical amniotic fluid infection and its effect on the neonate. Am J Obstet Gynecol 151:1058, 1985.

72. Hardt NS, Kostenbauder M, Ogburn M, et al. Influence of chorioamnionitis on long-term prognosis in low birth weight infants. Obstet Gynecol 65:5, 1985.

73. Murphy DJ, Seller S, MacKenzie IZ, et al. Case-control study of antenatal and intrapartum risk factors for cerebral palsy in very preterm singleton babies. Lancet 346:1449–1454, 1995.

74. Grether JK, Nelson KB. Maternal infection and cerebral palsy in infants of normal birth weight. JAMA 278:207–211, 1997.

75. Alexander JM, Gilstrap LC, Cox SM, et al. Clinical chorioamnionitis and the prognosis for very low birth weight infants. Obstet Gynecol 91:725–729, 1998.

76. Yoon BH, Romero R, Kim CJ, et al. High expression of tumor necrosis factor-alpha and interleukin-6 in periventricular leukomalacia. Am J Obstet Gynecol 177:406–411, 1997.

77. Yoon BH, Kim CJ, Romer R, et al. Experimentally induced intrauterine infection causes fetal brain white matter lesions in rabbits. Am J Obstet Gynecol 177:797–802, 1997.

78. Hitti J, Krohn MA, Patton DL, et al. Amniotic fluid tumor necrosis factor-β and the risk of respiratory distress syndrome among preterm infants. Am J Obstet Gynecol 177:50–56, 1997.

79. Lopez-Zeno JA, Peaceman AM, Adashek JA, et al. A controlled trial of a program for the active management of labor. N Engl J Med 326:450–454, 1992.

80. Mozurkewich EL, Wolf FM. Premature rupture of membranes at term: a meta-analysis of three management schemes. Obstet Gynecol 89:1035–1043, 1997.

81. Mercer BM, Arheart KL. Antimicrobial therapy in ex-

pectant management of preterm premature rupture of the membranes. Lancet 346:1271–1279, 1995.

82. Mercer BM, Miodovnik M, Thurnau GR, et al. Antibiotic therapy for reduction of infant morbidity after preterm premature rupture of the membranes. JAMA 278:989–995, 1997.

83. Egarter C, Leitich H, Husslein P, et al. Adjunctive antibiotic treatment in preterm labor and neonatal morbidity: a meta-analysis. Obstet Gynecol 88:303–309, 1996.

84. Eschenbach DA, Duff P, McGregor JA, et al. 2% Clindamycin vaginal cream treatment of bacterial vaginosis in pregnancy. Infect Dis Soc Obstet Gynecol. Abstract. 1993.

85. Rouse DJ, Hauth JC, Andrews WW, et al. Chlorhexidine vaginal irrigation for the prevention of peripartal infection: a placebo-controlled randomized clinical trial. Am J Obstet Gynecol 176:617–622, 1997.

86. Sweeten KM, Erikse NL, Blanco JD. Chlorhexidine versus sterile water vaginal wash during labor to prevent peripartum infection. Am J Obstet Gynecol 176:426–430, 1997.

87. Brans YW, Escobedo MB, Hayashsi RH, et al. Perinatal mortality in a large perinatal center: five-year review of 31,000 births. Am J Obstet Gynecol 148:284, 1984.

88. Minkoff H. Prematurity: infection as an etiologic factor. Obstet Gynecol 62:137, 1983.

89. Gibbs RS, Romero R, Hillier SL, et al. A review of premature birth and subclinical infection. Am J Obstet Gynecol 166:1515, 1992.

90. Driscoll SG. The placenta and membranes. In Charles D, Finlands M (eds). Obstetrical and Perinatal Infections. Philadelphia, Lea & Febiger, 1973, p 532.

91. Russell P. Inflammatory lesions of the human placenta: I. Clinical significance of acute chorioamnionitis. Am J Diagn Gynecol Obstet 1:127, 1979.

92. Schoonmaker JN, Lawellin DW, Lunt B, et al. Bacteria and inflammatory cells reduce chorioamniotic membrane integrity and tensile strength. Obstet Gynecol 74:590, 1989.

93. Bernal A, Hansell DJ, Khong TY, et al. Prostaglandin E production by the fetal membranes in unexplained preterm labour and preterm labour associated with chorioamnionitis. Br J Obstet Gynaecol 96:1133, 1989.

94. Lamont RF, Anthony F, Myatt L, et al. Production of prostaglandin E_2 by human amnion in vitro in response to addition of media conditioned by microorganisms associated with chorioamnionitis and preterm labor. Am J Obstet Gynecol 162:819, 1990.

95. Daikoku NH, Kaltzeider F, Johnson TR, et al. Premature rupture of membranes and preterm labor: neonatal infection and perinatal mortality risks. Obstet Gynecol 58:417, 1981.

96. Seo K, McGregor JA, French JA. Preterm birth is associated with increased risk of maternal and neonatal infection. Obstet Gynecol 79:75, 1992.

97. Braun P, Lee Y, Klein JO, et al. Birth weight and genital mycoplasmas in pregnancy. N Engl J Med 284:167, 1971.

98. Eschenbach DA, Nugent RP, Rao AV, et al. A randomized placebo-controlled trial of erythromycin for the treatment of Ureaplasma urealyticum to prevent premature delivery. Am J Obstet Gynecol 164:734, 1991.

99. Harrison RM, Alexander R, Weinstein L, et al. Cervical Chlamydia trachomatis and mycoplasmal infections in pregnancy. JAMA 250:1721, 1983.

100. Gravett MG, Nelson HP, DeRouen T, et al. Independent associations of bacterial vaginosis and Chlamydia trachomatis infection with adverse pregnancy outcome. JAMA 256:1899, 1986.

101. Ismail MA, Chandler AE, Beem MO, et al. Chlamydial colonization of the cervix in pregnant adolescents. J Reprod Med 30:449, 1985.

102. Fitzsimmons J, Callahan C, Shanahan B, et al. Chlamydial infections in pregnancy. J Reprod Med 31:19, 1986.

103. Heggie AD, Lumicao GG, Stuart LA, et al. Chlamydia trachomatis infection in mothers and infants: a prospective study. Am J Dis Child 135:507, 1981.

104. Minkoff H, Grunebaum AN, Schwartz RH, et al. Risk factors for prematurity and premature rupture of membranes: a prospective study of the vaginal flora in pregnancy. Am J Obstet Gynecol 150:965, 1984.

105. Regan JA, Chao S, James LS. Premature rupture of membranes, preterm delivery, and group B streptococcal colonization of mothers. Am J Obstet Gynecol 141:184, 1981.

106. Moller M, Thomsen AC, Borch K, et al. Rupture of fetal membranes and premature delivery associated with group B streptococci in urine of pregnant women. Lancet 2:69, 1989.

107. White CP, Wilkins EGL, Roberts C, et al. Premature delivery and group B streptococcal bacteriuria. Lancet 2:586, 1984.

108. Thomsen AC, Morup L, Hansen KB. Antibiotic elimination of group-B streptococci in urine in prevention of preterm labour. Lancet 1:591, 1987.

109. U.S. Department of Health and Human Services. Prevention of perinatal group B streptococcal disease: a public health perspective. MMWR Morbid Mortal Wkly Rep 45(RR7):1–24, 1996.

110. Hardy PH, Nell EE, Spence MR, et al. Prevalence of six sexually transmitted disease agents among pregnant inner-city adolescents and pregnancy outcome. Lancet 2:333, 1984.

111. Mason PR, Brown IM. Trichomonas in pregnancy. Letter to the editor. Lancet 2:1025, 1980.

112. Krohn MA, Hillier SL, Lee ML, et al. Vaginal Bacteroides are associated with an increased rate of preterm delivery among women in preterm labor. J Infect Dis 164:88, 1991.

113. McDonald HM, O'Loughlin JA, Jolley P, et al. Vaginal infections and preterm labour. Br J Obstet Gynaecol 98:427, 1991.

114. Eschenbach DA, Gravett MG, Chen KCS, et al. Bacterial vaginosis during pregnancy: an association with prematurity and postpartum complications. In Mardh PA, Taylor Robinson D (eds). Bacterial Vaginosis. Stockholm, Almqvist & Wiksell, 1984, p 214.

115. Hillier SL, Nugent RP, Eschenbach DA, et al. Association between bacterial vaginosis and preterm delivery of low birth weight infant. N Engl J Med 333:1737–1742, 1995.

116. Gibbs RS, Eschenbach DA. Use of antibiotics to prevent preterm birth. Am J Obstet Gynecol 177:375–380, 1997.

117. Cotch MF, Pastorek JG, Nugent RP. Trichomonas vaginalis associated with low birth weight and preterm delivery. Sex Transm Dis 24:353–360, 1997.

118. Romero R, Mazor M. Infection and preterm labor. Clin Obstet Gynecol 31:553, 1988.

119. Bobitt JR, Hayslip CC, Damato JD. Amniotic fluid infection as determined by transabdominal amniocentesis in patients with intact membranes. Am J Obstet Gynecol 140:947, 1981.

120. Wallace RL, Herrick N. Amniocentesis in the evaluation of premature labor. Obstet Gynecol 57:483, 1981.

121. Leigh J, Garite TJ. Amniocentesis and the management of premature labor. Obstet Gynecol 67:500, 1986.

122. Wahbeh CJ, Hill GB, Eden RD, et al. Intra-amniotic

bacterial colonization in premature labor. Am J Obstet Gynecol 148:739, 1984.

123. Romero R, Sirtori M, Oyarzun E, et al. Infection and labor: V. Prevalence, microbiology, and clinical significance of intra-amniotic infection in women with preterm labor and intact membranes. Am J Obstet Gynecol 161:817, 1989.

124. Handwerker SM, Tejani NA, Erma US, et al. Correlation of maternal serum C-reactive protein with outcome of tocolysis. Obstet Gynecol 63:220, 1984.

125. Potkul RK, Moawad AH, Ponto KL. The association of subclinical infection with preterm labor: the role of C-reactive protein. Am J Obstet Gynecol 153:642, 1985.

126. Dodds WG, Iams JD. Maternal C-reactive protein and preterm labor. J Reprod Med 32:527, 1987.

127. Bejar R, Curbelo V, David C, et al. Premature labor: II. Bacterial sources of phospholipase. Obstet Gynecol 57:479, 1981.

128. Romero R, Emamion M, Quintero R, et al. Amniotic fluid prostaglandin levels and intra-amniotic infection. Lancet 1:1380, 1986.

129. Romero R, Kadar N, Hobbins JC. Infection and labor: detection of endotoxin in amniotic fluid. Am J Obstet Gynecol 157:815, 1987.

130. Fidel PL Jr, Romero R, Ramirez M, et al. Interleukin-1 receptor antagonist (IL-1ra) production by human amnion, chorion, and decidua. Am J Reprod Immun 32:1–7, 1994.

131. Gravett MG. Interleukin-10 (IL-10) inhibits interleukin-1β IL-1β induced preterm labor in Rhesus monkeys. IDSOG 1998 (abstract).

132. Romero R, Mazor M, Tartokovsky B. Systemic administration of interleukin-1 induces parturition in mice. Am J Obstet Gynecol 165:969–977, 1991.

133. Kaga N, Katsuki Y, Obsta M, et al. Repeated administration of low dose lipopolysaccharide induces preterm delivery in mice: a model for human preterm parturition and for assessment of the therapeutic ability of the drugs against preterm delivery. Am J Obstet Gynecol 174:754–759, 1996.

134. McDuffie RS, Gibbs RS. Animal models of ascending genital tract infection. Infect Dis Obstet Gynecol 2:60–70, 1994.

135. Kass EH, McCormack WM, Lin JS, et al. Genital mycoplasmas as a cause of excess premature delivery. Trans Assoc Am Physicians 94:261, 1981.

136. McCormack WM, Rosner B, Lee Y, et al. Effect on birth weight of erythromycin treatment of pregnant women. Obstet Gynecol 69:202, 1987.

137. McGregor JA, French JI, Richter R, et al. Cervicovaginal microflora and pregnancy outcomes: results of a double-blind, placebo-controlled trial of erythromycin treatment. Am J Obstet Gynecol 163:1580, 1990.

138. Cohen J, Valle JC, Calkins BM. Improved pregnancy outcome following successful treatment of chlamydial infection. JAMA 263:3160, 1990.

139. Ryan GM Jr, Abdella TN, McNeely SG, et al. *Chlamydia trachomatis* infection in pregnancy and effect of treatment on outcome. Am J Obstet Gynecol 162:34, 1990.

140. McGregor JA, French JI, Reller LB, et al. Adjunctive erythromycin treatment for idiopathic preterm labor: results of a randomized, double-blinded, placebo-controlled trial. Am J Obstet Gynecol 154:98, 1986.

141. Newton ER, Dinsmor MJ, Gibbs RS. A randomized, blinded, placebo-controlled trial of antibiotics in idiopathic preterm labor. Obstet Gynecol 74:562, 1989.

142. Morales WJ, Angel JL, O'Brien WF, et al. A randomized study of antibiotic therapy in idiopathic preterm labor. Obstet Gynecol 72:829, 1988.

143. Winkler M, Baumann L, Ruckhaberle KE, et al. Erthromycin therapy for subclinical intrauterine infections in threatened preterm delivery—a preliminary report. J Perinat Med 16:253, 1988.

144. Amon E, Lewis SV, Silbai BM, et al. Ampicillin prophylaxis in preterm premature rupture of membranes: a prospective randomized study. Am J Obstet Gynecol 159:539, 1988.

145. Morales WJ, Angel JL, O'Brien WF, et al. Use of ampicillin and corticosteroids in premature rupture of membranes: a randomized study. Obstet Gynecol 73:721, 1989.

146. Johnston MM, Sanchez-Ramos L, Vaughn AJ, et al. Antibiotic therapy in preterm premature rupture of membranes: a randomized, prospective, double-blind trial. Am J Obstet Gynecol 163:743, 1990.

147. Christmas JT, Cox SM, Gilstrap LC, et al. Expectant management of preterm ruptured membranes: effect of antimicrobial therapy on interval to delivery. *In* Proceedings of the 10th Annual Meeting of the Society of Perinatal Obstetricians, Houston, Texas, January 23–27, 1990. Houston, Society of Perinatal Obstetricians, 1990 (abstract).

148. Gunn GC, Mishell DR, Morton DG. Premature rupture of the fetal membranes: a review. Am J Obstet Gynecol 106:469, 1970.

149. Gibbs RS, Blanco JD. Premature rupture of the membranes. Obstet Gynecol 60:671, 1982.

150. Garite TJ. Premature rupture of the membranes: the enigma of the obstetrician. Am J Obstet Gynecol 151:1001, 1985.

151. ACOG Technical Bulletin No. 115. Washington, D.C., American College of Obstetricians and Gynecologists, 1988.

152. Bada HS, Alojipan LC, Andrews BF. Premature rupture of membranes and its effect on the newborn. Pediatr Clin North Am 24:491, 1977.

153. Fayez JA, Hasan AA, Jonas HS, et al. Management of premature rupture of the membranes. Obstet Gynecol 52:17, 1978.

154. Christensen KK, Christensen P, Ingemarsson L, et al. A study of complications in preterm deliveries after prolonged premature rupture of the membranes. Obstet Gynecol 48:670, 1976.

155. Evaldson G, Lagrelius A, Winiarski J. Premature rupture of the membranes. Acta Obstet Gynecol Scand 59:385, 1980.

156. Graham RJ, Gilstrap LC III, Lauth JC, et al. Conservative management of patients with premature rupture of fetal membranes. Obstet Gynecol 59:607, 1982.

157. Arias R, Tomich P. Etiology and outcome of low birth weight and preterm infants. Obstet Gynecol 60:277, 1982.

158. Eggers TR, Doyle LW, Pepperell RJ. Premature rupture of the membranes. Med J Aust 1:209, 1979.

159. Naeye RL, Peters EC. Causes and consequences of premature rupture of membranes. Lancet 1:192, 1980.

160. Artal R, Sokol RJ, Newman M, et al. The mechanical properties of prematurely and non-prematurely ruptured membranes, methods, and preliminary results. Am J Obstet Gynecol 125:655, 1976.

161. Parry-Jones E, Priya S. A study of the elasticity and tension of fetal membranes and of the relation of the area of the gestational sac to the area of the uterine cavity. Br J Obstet Gynecol 83:205, 1976.

162. Al-Zaid NS. Bursting pressure and collagen content of

fetal membranes and their relation to premature rupture of the membranes. Br J Obstet Gynecol 87:227, 1980.

163. Lavery JP, Miller CE. Deformation and creep in the human chorioamniotic sac. Am J Gynecol 134:366, 1979.

164. Naeye RI. Factors that predispose to premature rupture of the fetal membranes. Obstet Gynecol 60:93, 1982.

165. Naeye RL, Ross S. Coitus and chorioamnionitis: a prospective study. Early Hum Dev 6:91, 1982.

166. Creatsas G, Pavlatos M, Lolis D, et al. Bacterial contamination of the cervix and premature rupture of the membranes. Am J Obstet Gynecol 139:522, 1981.

167. DelBene VE, Moore E, Rogers M, et al. Bacterial flora of patients with prematurely ruptured membranes. South Med J 70:950, 1977.

168. Harger JH, Hsing AW, Tuomala RE, et al. Risk factors for preterm premature rupture of fetal membranes: a multicenter case-control study. Am J Obstet Gynecol 163:130, 1990.

169. Kappy KA, Cetrulo CL, Knuppel RA, et al. Premature rupture of the membranes at term: a comparison of induced and spontaneous labors. J Reprod Med 27:29, 1982.

170. Kappy KA, Cetrulo CL, Knuppel RA, et al. Premature rupture of the membranes: a conservative approach. Am J Obstet Gynecol 134:655, 1979.

171. Nochimson DJ, Petrie RH, Shah BL, et al. Comparisons of conservation and dynamic management of premature rupture of membranes/premature labor syndrome: new approaches to the delivery of infants which may minimize the need for intensive care. Clin Perinatol 7:17, 1979.

172. Johnson JW, Daikoku NH, Niebyl JR, et al. Premature rupture of the membranes and prolonged latency. Obstet Gynecol 57:574, 1981.

173. Miller JM Jr, Brazy JE, Gall SA, et al. Premature rupture of the membranes: maternal and neonatal infectious morbidity related to betamethasone and antibiotic therapy. J Reprod Med 25:173, 1980.

174. Taylor J, Garite TJ. Premature rupture of membranes before fetal viability. Obstet Gynecol 64:615, 1984.

175. Cox SM, Williams ML, Leveno KJ. The natural history of preterm ruptured membranes: what to expect of expectant management. Obstet Gynecol 71:558, 1988.

176. Johnson JWC, Egerman RS, Moorehead J. Cases with ruptured membranes that "reseal." Am J Obstet Gynecol 163:1024–1032, 1990.

177. Mercer BM. Management of premature preterm rupture of membranes before 26 weeks' gestation. Obstet Gynecol Clin North Am 19:339–351, 1992.

178. Mercer BM. Premature rupture of membranes. ACOG Pract Bulletin, 1998.

179. Nimrod C, Varela-Gittings F, Machin G, et al. The effect of very prolonged membrane rupture on fetal development. Am J Obstet Gynecol 148:540, 1984.

180. Vergani P, Ghidini A, Locatelli A, et al. Risk factors for pulmonary hypoplasia in second trimester PROM. Am J Obstet Gynecol 170:1359–1364, 1994.

181. Rotschild A, Lind EW, Puterman ML, et al. Neonatal outcome after prolonged preterm rupture of membranes. Am J Obstet Gynecol 162:46–52, 1990.

182. Lauria MR, Gonik B, Romero R. Pulmonary hypoplasia: pathogenesis, diagnosis, and antenatal prediction. Obstet Gynecol 86:466–475, 1995.

183. Perkins RP. The neonatal significance of selected perinatal events among infants of low birth weight: II. The influence of ruptured membranes. Am J Obstet Gynecol 142:7, 1982.

184. Schreiber J, Benedetti T. Conservative management of preterm premature rupture of the fetal membranes in a low socioeconomic population. Am J Obstet Gynecol 136:92, 1980.

185. Berkowitz RL, Kantor RD, Beck FJ, et al. The relationship between premature rupture of the membranes and the respiratory distress syndrome: an update and plan of management. Am J Obstet Gynecol 131:503, 1978.

186. Daikoku NH, Kaltreider F, Khouzami VA, et al. Premature rupture of membranes and spontaneous preterm labor: maternal endometritis risks. Obstet Gynecol 59:13, 1982.

187. Jewett JF. Committee on maternal welfare: prolonged rupture of the membranes. N Engl J Med 292:752, 1975.

188. Ohlsson A, Wang E. An analysis of antenatal tests to detect infection in preterm premature rupture of the membranes. Am J Obstet Gynecol 162:809, 1990.

189. Garite TJ, Freeman RK, Linzey EM, et al. The use of amniocentesis in patients with premature rupture of membranes. Obstet Gynecol 54:226, 1979.

190. Zlatnik FJ, Cruikshank DP, Petzold CR, et al. Amniocentesis in the identification of inapparent infection in preterm patients with premature rupture of the membranes. J Reprod Med 29:656, 1984.

191. Vintzileos AM, Campbell WA, Nochimson DJ, et al. Qualitative amniotic fluid volume versus amniocentesis in predicting infection in preterm premature rupture of the membranes. Obstet Gynecol 67:579, 1986.

192. Feinstein SJ, Vintzileos AM, Lodeiro JG, et al. Amniocentesis with premature rupture of membranes. Obstet Gynecol 68:147, 1986.

193. Yeast JD, Garite TJ, Dorchester W. The risks of amniocentesis in the management of premature rupture of the membranes. Am J Obstet Gynecol 149:505, 1984.

194. Cotton DB, Gonik B, Bottoms SF. Conservative versus aggressive management of prematerm rupture of membranes: a randomized trial of amniocentesis. Am J Perinatol 1:322, 1984.

195. Evans MI, Hajj SN, Devoe LD, et al. C-reactive protein as a predictor of infectious morbidity with premature rupture of membranes. Am J Obstet Gynecol 138:648, 1980.

196. Farb HF, Arnesen M, Geistler P, et al. C-reactive protein with premature rupture of membranes and premature labor. Obstet Gynecol 62:49, 1983.

197. Hawrylyshyn P, Bernstein P, Milligan JE, et al. Premature rupture of membranes: the role of C-reactive protein in the prediction of chorioamnionitis. Am J Obstet Gynecol 147:240, 1983.

198. Romem Y, Artal R. C-reactive protein as a predictor for chorioamnionitis in cases of premature rupture of the membranes. Am J Obstet Gynecol 150:546, 1984.

199. Gonik B, Bottoms SF, Cotton DB. Amniotic fluid volume as a risk factor in preterm premature rupture of the membranes. Obstet Gynecol 65:456, 1985.

200. Vintzileos AM, Campbell WA, Nochimson DJ, et al. The fetal biophysical profile in patients with premature rupture of the membranes—an early predictor of fetal infection. Am J Obstet Gynecol 152:510, 1985.

201. Beydoun SN, Yasin SY. Premature rupture of the membranes before 28 weeks: conservative management. Am J Obstet Gynecol 155:471, 1986.

202. Taylor J, Garite TJ. Premature rupture of membranes before fetal viability. Obstet Gynecol 64:615, 1984.

203. Major CA, Kitzmiller JL. Perinatal survival with expectant management of midtrimester rupture of membranes. Am J Obstet Gynecol 163:838, 1990.

204. Moretti M, Sibai BM. Maternal and perinatal outcome of expectant management of premature rupture of mem-

branes in the midtrimester. Am J Obstet Gynecol 159:390, 1988.

205. American Academy of Pediatrics. Perinatal care at the threshold of viability. Pediatrics 96:974–976, 1995.

206. Liggins GC. Prenatal glucocorticoid treatment: prevention of respiratory distress syndrome: lung maturation and prevention of hyaline membrane disease. Report of the 70th Ross Conference on Pediatric Research. Columbus, Ohio, Ross Laboratories, 1976, pp 97–105.

207. Block MF, Klin OR, Crosby WM. Antenatal glucocorticoid therapy for the prevention of respiratory distress syndrome in the premature infant. Obstet Gynecol 50:186, 1977.

208. Morrison JC, Whybrew WD, Bucovaz ET, et al. Injection of corticosteroids into mothers to prevent neonatal respiratory distress syndrome. Am J Obstet Gynecol 131:358, 1978.

209. Taeusch HW, Frigoletto F, Kitzmiller J, et al. Risk of respiratory distress syndrome after prenatal dexamethasone treatment. Pediatrics 63:64, 1979.

210. Papageorgiou AN, Desgranges MF, Masson M, et al. The antenatal use of betamethasone in the prevention of respiratory distress syndrome: a controlled double-blind study. Pediatrics 63:73, 1979.

211. Collaborative Group on Antenatal Steroid Therapy. Effect of antenatal dexamethasone administration on the prevention of respiratory distress syndrome. Am J Obstet Gynecol 141:276, 1981.

212. Garite TJ, Freeman RK, Linzey EM, et al. Prospective randomized study of corticosteroids in the management of premature rupture of the membranes and the premature gestation. Am J Obstet Gynecol 141:508, 1981.

213. Barrett JM, Boehm FH. Comparison of aggressive and conservative management of premature rupture of fetal membranes. Am J Obstet Gynecol 144:12, 1982.

214. Schmidt PL, Sims ME, Strassner HT, et al. Effect of antepartum glucocorticoid administration upon neonatal respiratory distress syndrome and perinatal infection. Am J Obstet Gynecol 148:178, 1984.

215. Iams JDE, Talbert ML, Barrows H, et al. Management of preterm prematurely ruptured membranes: a prospective randomized comparison of observation versus use of steroids and timed delivery. Am J Obstet Gynecol 151:32, 1985.

216. Simpson GF, Harbert GM Jr. Uses of β-methasone in management of preterm gestation with premature rupture of membranes. Obstet Gynecol 66:168, 1985.

217. Nelson LH, Meis PJ, Hatjis CG, et al. Premature rupture of membranes: a prospective, randomized evaluation of steroids, latent phase, and expectant management. Obstet Gynecol 66:55, 1985.

218. Morales WJ, Diebel ND, Lazar AJ, et al. The effect of antenatal dexamethasone administration on the prevention of respiratory distress syndrome in preterm gestations with premature rupture of membranes. Am J Obstet Gynecol 154:591, 1986.

219. Ohlsson A. Treatments of preterm premature rupture of the membranes: a meta-analysis. Am J Obstet Gynecol 160:890, 1989.

220. Crowley PA. Antenatal corticosteroid therapy: a meta-analysis of the randomized trials, 1972 to 1994. Am J Obstet Gynecol 173:322–335, 1995.

221. Lewis DF, Brody K, Edwards MS, et al. Preterm premature ruptured membranes: a randomized trial of steroids after treatment with antibiotics. Obstet Gynecol 88:801–805, 1996.

222. Leitich H, Egarter C, Reisenberger K, et al. Concomitant use of glucocorticoids: a comparison of two meta-analysis on antibiotic treatment in PROM. Am J Obstet Gynecol 178:899–908, 1998.

223. Liggins GC, Howie RN. A controlled trial of antepartum glucocorticoid treatment for prevention of the RDS in premature infants. Pediatrics 50:515–525, 1972.

224. Minkoff H, Mead P. An obstetric approach to the prevention of early-onset group B beta-hemolytic streptococcal sepsis. Am J Obstet Gynecol 154:973, 1986.

225. Boyer KM, Gotoff SP. Prevention of early-onset neonatal group B streptococcal disease with selective intrapartum chemoprophylaxis. N Engl J Med 314:1665, 1986.

226. Romero R, Scioscia AL, Edberg SC, et al. Use of parenteral antibiotic therapy to eradicate bacterial colonization of amniotic fluid in premature rupture of membranes. Obstet Gynecol 67:15S, 1986.

227. Thibeault DW, Emmanouilides GC. Prolonged rupture of fetal membranes and decreased frequency of respiratory distress syndrome and patent ductus arteriosus in preterm infants. Am J Obstet Gynecol 129:43, 1977.

228. Schutte MF, Treffess PE, Kloostrerman GJ, et al. Management of premature rupture of membranes: the risk of vaginal examination to the infant. Am J Obstet Gynecol 146:395, 1983.

229. Jones MD Jr, Burd LI, Bowes WA Jr, et al. Failure of association of premature rupture of membranes with respiratory-distress syndrome. N Engl J Med 292:1253, 1975.

230. Egarter C, Leitich H, Karas H, et al. Antibiotic treatment in PPROM and neonatal morbidity: a meta-analysis. Am J Obstet Gynecol 174:589–597, 1996.

231. Curet LB, Rao AV, Zachman RD, et al. Association between ruptured membranes, tocolytic therapy, and respiratory distress syndrome. Am J Obstet Gynecol 148:263, 1984.

232. Garite TJ, Keegan KA, Freeman RK, et al. A randomized trial of ritodrine tocolysis versus expectant management in patients with premature rupture of membranes at 25 to 30 weeks of gestation. Am J Obstet Gynecol 157:388, 1987.

233. Weiner CP, Renk K, Klugman M. The therapeutic efficacy and cost effectiveness of aggressive tocolysis for premature labor associated with premature rupture of the membranes. Am J Obstet Gynecol 159:216, 1988.

234. Brame RG, MacKenna J. Vaginal pool phospholipids in management of premature rupture of membranes. Am J Obstet Gynecol 145:992, 1983.

235. Mercer BM, Crocker LG, Boe NM, et al. Induction versus expectant management in premature rupture of the membranes with mature amniotic fluid at 32 to 36 weeks: a randomized trial. Am J Obstet Gynecol 169:775–782, 1993.

236. Cox SM, Leveno KJ. Intentional delivery versus expectant management with preterm ruptured membranes at 30 to 34 weeks' gestation. Obstet Gynecol 86:875–879, 1995.

237. Vintzileos AM, Campbell WA, Nochimson DJ, et al. The use of the nonstress test in patients with premature rupture of membranes. Am J Obstet Gynecol 155:149–153, 1986.

238. Hanley ML, Vintzileos AM. Biophysical testing in premature rupture of the membranes. Semin Perinatol 20:418–425, 1996.

239. Duff WP, Huff RW, Gibbs RS. Management of the term patient who has premature rupture of the membranes and a cervix unfavorable for induction. Obstet Gynecol 63:697, 1984.

240. Conway DI, Prendiville WJ, Morris A, et al. Management of spontaneous rupture of the membranes in the

absence of labor in primigravid women at term. Am J Obstet Gynecol 150:947, 1984.

241. Wagner MV, Chin VP, Peters CJ, et al. A comparison of early and delayed induction of labor with spontaneous rupture of membranes at term. Obstet Gynecol 74:93, 1989.

242. Meikle SF, Bissell ME, Freedman WL, et al. A retrospective review of the efficacy and safety of PGE_2 with premature rupture of the membranes at term. Obstet Gynecol 80:76, 1992.

243. Mahmood TA, Dick MJ, Smith NC, et al. Role of prostaglandin in the management of prelabour rupture of the membranes at term. Br J Obstet Gynaecol 99:112, 1992.

244. Ray DA, Garite TJ. Prostaglandin E_2 for induction in patients with premature rupture of membranes at term. Am J Obstet Gynecol 166:836–843, 1992.

245. McGregor JA, French JI, Seo K. Antimicrobial therapy in preterm premature rupture of membranes: results of a prospective, double-blind, placebo-controlled trial of erythromycin. Am J Obstet Gynecol 165:632–640, 1991.

246. Owen J, Groome LJ, Hauth JC. Randomized trial of prophylactic antibiotic therapy after preterm amnion rupture. Am J Obstet Gynecol 169:976–981, 1993.

247. Ernest JM, Givner LB. A prospective, randomized, placebo-controlled trial of penicillin in preterm premature rupture of membranes. Am J Obstet Gynecol 170:516–521, 1994.

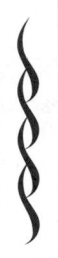

C H A P T E R   3 4

Infections Acquired in the Nursery: Epidemiology and Control

JO-ANN S. HARRIS, M.D., and DONALD A. GOLDMANN, M.D.

Nosocomial infections result in considerable morbidity and mortality among neonates.[1] Although most neonatal infections are maternal in origin, an increasing proportion is being acquired in the nursery.[1, 2] Nosocomial infections can occur in both the well-baby and special care nurseries, but the incidence is considerably higher in the latter. The incidence of hospital-acquired infections in the healthy term infant who is discharged within 48 hours from the well-baby nursery is very low as compared with that in preterm and sick infants in neonatal intensive care units (NICUs). Technologic advances and surfactant replacement therapy have improved the survival rate of infants with very low birth weights (<1.5 kg) and simultaneously created risks for nosocomial infection.[3] The frequency of these infections has increased in recent decades as a result of this increased survival of low-birth-weight infants, and rates for these infections are among the highest in hospitalized patient populations. NICU-acquired infections are associated with increased mortality rates, prolonged duration of hospitalization in survivors, and increased cost of neonatal health care. Prevention and control of hospital-acquired infections in infants who start life in an intensive care unit and whose immature defenses are compromised further by illness and invasive procedures are major challenges for nursery and infection control personnel.

UNIQUE ASPECTS OF THE NURSERY

Infections acquired in the nursery are unique in several respects. The population at risk has had no previous experience with microbes and has an immature immune system. Until birth, the newborn does not have an endogenous flora and can acquire almost any organism to which he or she is exposed. The resulting skin and mucosal flora reflects that of the maternal genital tract, the inanimate environment, and microorganisms transferred to the infant by nursery personnel. Newborns, especially premature infants, are at increased risk of infection from this newly acquired microbial flora. The skin is fragile and easily damaged, especially before 32 weeks of gestation, because the stratum corneum is poorly developed. The skin rapidly matures postnatally and is well developed by 2 weeks of age, even in premature neonates.[4]

The immune function of the newborn is incomplete. There is little antibody production in utero, and the newborn initially depends on passively transferred IgG antibodies from the mother. Transplacental transfer does not begin until approximately 34 weeks of gestation. The newborn also has a decreased granulocyte storage pool and defective neutrophil and monocyte chemotaxis. Although the newborn has a high total T cell count, the phenotypic surface markers are different from those in older children. Cytotoxic T cell and natural killer cell activity is decreased, and there is limited production of cytokines.[5] A more detailed discussion of host defenses of the neonate is presented in Chapter 2. The frequent exposure of critically ill neonates in NICUs to invasive devices and procedures further increases the risk of infection.

Determining the epidemiology of nosocomial infection in the nursery is complicated by the difficulties differentiating among intrapartum, peripartum, and postpartum acquisition of potential pathogens, as well as the short length of hospital stay of the normal newborn.[2] The Centers for Disease Control and Prevention (CDC) has arbitrarily defined all neonatal infections, whether acquired during delivery or during hospitalization (i.e., intrapartum or postpartum), as nosocomial unless known or proven to be transplacentally acquired, such as cytomegalovirus (CMV) disease or toxoplasmosis.[6, 7] Although all infections in newborns who are born in the hospital may be considered nosocomial, infections that manifest early in the first week of life usually are due to microorganisms transmitted from the mother to the infant and have a different epidemiology than nosocomial infections acquired later in the neonatal period.[8] Infection control measures designed to prevent acquisition of microorganisms within the nursery will not be effective with pathogens acquired perinatally.[2]

There is no time point that clearly distinguishes maternally transmitted infections from infections acquired in the nursery. Some investigators refer to infections developing within 24 to 72 hours of birth as "early onset infections," usually caused by organisms acquired from the mother, and infections developing 3 to 7 days or more after birth as "late onset infections," presumably caused by organisms acquired in the nursery.[8, 9] The problem of differentiating perinatal from nosocomial infections is exemplified by group B streptococcal infections, because late-onset group B streptococcal disease may result from colonization during delivery or post partum from the infant's mother, infant to infant spread from hands of personnel, or rarely, acquisition from colonized staff.[10, 11] With infants staying longer in the NICU, some have suggested that a third classification is needed—"late, late onset" infection, or infection after 30 days of age—because the microorganisms and risk factors for nosocomial infection differ from those in infants with shorter NICU stays.[12, 13]

Infections resulting from colonization in the nursery can occur either during or after hospitalization, particularly in full-term healthy newborns whose hospital stay is brief.[14, 15] Early discharge makes nosocomial infection surveillance more difficult, because infections acquired in the nursery are unlikely to become symptomatic in the hospital. Neonatal staphylococcal infections, for example, usually do not become apparent clinically until 5 to 7 days after birth, and substantial epidemics may be well established before they are recognized.[16] Accurate surveillance of infections requires routine postdischarge follow-up. Such programs have been developed but are cumbersome and may not be cost effective in the absence of an outbreak.[17] Case finding usually is obtained by voluntary reporting of community pediatricians, which is sporadic at best. Therefore, accurate nosocomial infection rates in well-baby nurseries are difficult to determine.

INCIDENCE

Nosocomial infections in the normal infant nursery are uncommon, whereas they are frequent in NICUs.[8] There are few data on infection rates in normal nurseries where the infant is healthy and the hospital stay is short. Reported rates are low, ranging from 0.3 to 1.7 per 100 newborns.[18, 19] In the National Nosocomial Infection Surveillance (NNIS) system, the infection rates ranged from 0.9% in nonteaching hospitals to 1.7% in large teaching hospitals in 1984. Similar rates for a small number of hospitals surveyed in Canada in 1984 were 1.4 to 3.1 per 100 discharges.[20, 21] Individual hospitals have reported similar rates of 0.6 to 1.7% in term infants.[19, 22] In a study at a large maternity hospital in Boston, questionnaires were mailed directly to mothers of infants 6 weeks after discharge. Infections were reported in 4% of infants.[17] More than 90% of the infants surveyed were from term nurseries. Postdischarge surveillance identified 12 times as many newborn infections as did concurrent prospective in-hospital surveillance. Because the questionnaires were returned in only 36% of cases, this rate is likely to be a minimal estimate. The most common infections were conjunctivitis, "diaper dermatitis," umbilical site infections, and pustules.

In contrast to the relatively low incidence of infections in term nurseries, the incidence of nosocomial infections in NICUs is often high, surpassing that reported for other hospital services and intensive care units.[19, 22–27] Reported infection rates in the NICU vary from 1.8 to 39.8 per 100 admissions or discharges.[19, 22, 24–31] There is some variability in the reported rates due to methodologic differences and the proportion of infants with severe underlying disease. The age range, methods for diagnosing infections, types of infections reported (e.g., whether viral infections are included), and referral patterns of infants to the study NICU may all have a significant impact on the reported incidence of nosocomial infections.[8]

A large review of nosocomial infections among neonates in high-risk nurseries was conducted by the CDC through the NNIS system from 1986 to 1994. There were 13,179 infections reported in 99 high-risk nurseries. The bloodstream was the most frequent site of infection, followed by nosocomial pneumonia, then gastrointestinal and eye, ear, nose, and throat sites.[1] The National Institutes of Child Health and Human Development (NICHD) Neonatal Research Network reported on a cohort of very low birth weight infants (401–1500 g) admitted to 12 participating centers from 1991 to 1993. Among 6911 infants who survived beyond 3 days, 25% developed a nosocomial bloodstream infection, with the rate of infection inversely proportional to birth weight and gestational age.[32]

Table 34–1, which shows the nosocomial infection rates in selected studies of high-risk nurseries, illustrates

TABLE 34–1
Nosocomial Infection Rates in the NICU

SOURCE	LOCATION	YEAR	INFECTION RATE[a]
Hemming, et al[25]	Salt Lake City	1970–1974	24.6
Wenzel, et al[27]	Charlottesville	1972–1975	24.0
Goldmann, et al[28]	Boston	1974–1978	7.7 (1.8)[b]
Maguire, et al[22]	Iowa City	1976–1977	16.9
Hoogkamp-Korstanje, et al[26]	Utrecht, The Netherlands	1977	39.8
Larson, et al[29]	Seattle	1977–1981	11.7 (9.6)[b]
Welliver, et al[19]	Buffalo	1980–1981	22.2
Brown, et al[30]	Springfield, Mass	1981–1983	5.9
Ford-Jones, et al[31]	Toronto	1984–1987	14.0
Moore[2]	Montreal	1986–1992	21.0
Josephson, et al[24]	Brooklyn	1988–1989	14.5
Beck-Sague, et al[34]	Oakland, Calif	1989–1991	11.2[c]
Stoll, et al[32]	U.S. Network	1991–1993	25[c]

[a]Rate per 100 admissions or discharges.
[b]Rates after move to new NICU in parentheses.
[c]Nosocomial bloodstream infections
Adapted from Moore D. Nosocomial infections in newborn nurseries and neonatal intensive care units. *In* Mayhall GC (ed). Hospital Epidemiology and Infection Control. Baltimore, Williams & Wilkins, 1996, pp 532–565; and Hauth JC, Merenstein GB. Infection control. *In* Hauth JC, Merenstein GB (eds). Guidelines for Perinatal Care, 4th ed. Elk Grove Village, Ill, American Academy of Pediatrics and American College of Obstetricians and Gynecologists, 1997, pp 251–277.

the wide variability among centers. In a frequently cited but somewhat dated study from the early 1970s, the nosocomial infection rate was 24.6 per 100 admissions in a regional NICU at the University of Utah Medical Center,[25, 33] with many infants having multiple infections. Among infants with a birth weight of less than 1.5 kg, the risk of infection was 33%, which was significantly higher than the 10% rate in infants whose birth weight was 1.5 kg or greater. By comparison, the nosocomial infection rate was 7.3% for the entire hospital, 5.4% for the general pediatric ward, and 0.6% for the well-baby nursery. This was a pioneering study because surveillance included viral as well as bacterial and fungal infections.

In a study of nosocomial infections in an NICU in Boston in the mid 1970s, the nosocomial infection rate was 5.8%. Possible explanations for this relatively low infection rate include strict case definitions, the unit's policy to transfer newborns who required surgery out of the nursery, and the lack of systematic testing for viral infections. It was hypothesized that proper staffing, adequate working space around incubators, control of traffic flow, and presence of convenient scrub areas would decrease the rate of nosocomial infections even further. This was confirmed in a retrospective cohort study, because the rate of major bacterial and fungal infections decreased from 5.8 to 1.8% when the NICU was moved to a new facility with improvement in all these areas.[28] Welliver and McLaughlin[19] reported a relatively high infection rate of 22.2%, perhaps because they made special efforts to diagnose viral infections. Maguire and associates[22] reported an infection rate of 16.9%, but they did not report any viral infections. Beck-Sague and colleagues focused on bloodstream infections. This multihospital NICU study demonstrated that most bloodstream infections in neonates were nosocomial and occurred at a rate approximately one half of that found in studies that measured the rate of all infections.[34] The

differences in methodology in each of these studies and the disparate time periods during which the studies were performed make meaningful comparison of nosocomial infection rates very difficult. For example, data from a study performed in 1976 are unlikely to be relevant to data gathered in a nursery in the year 2000 given the major advances in neonatal care in the interim.

SITES OF INFECTION

Infections occurring in the full-term nursery are commonly superficial, involving the skin, mouth, or eyes. Although oral and conjunctival infections are usually acquired during delivery, nursery-acquired infections are primarily cutaneous, including omphalitis, pustules, abscesses, and bullous impetigo. Outbreaks of infections with viral and gastrointestinal pathogens that commonly cause infections in the community may also occur.[16, 22] In the past, nursery epidemics of bacterial gastroenteritis were relatively common, but they have been reported infrequently in recent years except in countries with limited resources. However, the potential for rapid transmission of enteric bacterial and viral enteropathogens in full-term nurseries remains.

Although superficial infections are also a problem in the NICU, the leading categories of nosocomial infections are bloodstream infection, followed by pneumonia and eye, ear, nose, and throat infections (Table 34–2). The distribution of the most common pathogens identified in NICUs by site of infection is shown in Table 34–3.[1] The sites of nosocomial infections in the high-risk nursery differ from those in older children and adults.[1] Primary bloodstream infections account for 30 to 50% of episodes in NICUs depending on birth weight, but surgical site and urinary tract infections are rare. In contrast, more than 40% of nosocomial infections in adults are urinary tract infections and 20% are

TABLE 34–2
% Site Distribution of Nosocomial Infections in High-Risk Nurseries by Birth Weight (NNIS 1986–1994)

SITE	BIRTH WEIGHT			
	<1000 g	1001–1500 g	1501–2500 g	>2500 g
Bloodstream	49	45	32	36
Pneumonia	16	12	13	18
Eyes, ears, nose, throat	8	14	21	13
Skin and soft tissue	6	7	10	9
Gastrointestinal	7	10	11	5
Surgical site	1	1	3	7
Other	13	11	10	12

Adapted from Gaynes RP, Edwards JR, Jarvis WR, et al. Nosocomial infections among neonates in high-risk nurseries in the United States. Pediatrics 98:357–361, 1966.

surgical site infections. Many NICUs do not care for neonates after surgery, so the low reported rates of surgical site infections are not surprising. The relatively infrequent occurrence of urinary tract infections in newborns may reflect less reliance on urinary catheters in this population. Cutaneous sites are also more likely to be involved in neonates.[35]

ETIOLOGY

The diverse microorganisms that cause nursery-acquired infections include bacteria, fungi, and viruses and encompass virtually all human pathogens and commensal organisms. Given the appropriate circumstances, almost any microorganism can cause nosocomial infection in the neonate. Organisms causing infections in the normal nursery are usually pathogens acquired from the mother (group B *Streptococcus*) or acquired in the nursery (*Staphylococcus aureus*, group A *Streptococcus*, enteric pathogens,

enteroviruses, respiratory viruses). In the high-risk nursery, the spectrum of infections is broader to include organisms not usually pathogenic in the healthy newborn, such as coagulase-negative staphylococci (CONS) and *Candida*.[2]

There has been a shift in the etiology of nosocomial infections in high-risk nurseries over the past five decades, most likely related to increased use of technology, invasive procedures, and the prolonged survival of very low birth weight infants. Invasive strains of *S. aureus* were predominant in the 1950s, and gram-negative bacilli (*Pseudomonas aeruginosa*, *Klebsiella* species, and *Escherichia coli*) prevailed in the 1960s. There were numerous reports of group B streptococci in the 1970s, but these organisms were primarily maternally acquired and generally were not a major nosocomial problem. By the late 1970s, methicillin-resistant *S. aureus* (MRSA) and CONS became more prominent as pathogens of nosocomial infections in the high-risk nursery. Beginning in the 1990s, in addition to CONS, enterococci (including

TABLE 34–3
% Most Commonly Reported Pathogens from Neonates in NICUs by Site of Infection: NNIS 1986–1993 (N = 13,179)

PATHOGEN	BLOODSTREAM	EYE, EAR, NOSE, AND THROAT	GASTROINTESTINAL	PNEUMONIA	SSI
Coagulase-negative *Staphylococcus*	51	29.3	9.6	16.5	19.2
S. aureus	7.5	15.4		16.7	22.3
Group B streptococci	7.9			5.7	
Enterococci	6.2	3.4		4.6	8.9
Candida species	6.9				
Escherichia coli	4.3	6.1	13.9	5.8	12.0
Other *Streptococcus* species	2.7	7.4		3.3	
Enterobacter species	2.9	4.5	5.5	8.2	7.6
Klebsiella pneumoniae	2.5	2.8	9.8	5.8	6.3
Pseudomonas aeruginosa		6.6		11.7	
Haemophilus influenzae		2.7		1.4	
Viruses		5.1	30		
Gram-positive anaerobes			9.4		
Other enteric bacilli			0.8		
Others	8.1	16.7	21	21.7	23.7

Adapted from Gaynes RP, Edwards JR, Jarvis WR, et al. Nosocomial infections among neonates in high-risk nurseries in the United States. Pediatrics 98:357–361, 1996.

TABLE 34–4

Pathogens Causing Nosocomial Infection in Infants in NICUs

PATHOGEN	% OF INFECTIONS IN SELECTED STUDIES					
	Salt Lake City, Utah: 1970–1974	Utrecht, The Netherlands: 1977	Boston, Mass (Children's Hospital Medical Center): 1974–1978[a]	Selected U.S. Hospitals (NNIS): 1985–1986	Montreal, Canada: 1986–1992[b]	Selected U.S. Hospitals (NNIS): 1986–1993[c]
Staphylococcus aureus	47	27	10	12	8	11
Escherichia coli	27	16	9	9	13	6
Coagulase-negative staphylococci		27	11	31	23	36
Group B streptococci				6		5
Klebsiella species	8	7	26	6	10	4
Haemophilus species				1		1
Pseudomonas species	5	13	23	5	6	5
Group D streptococci, enterococci	5	4		1	8	5
Candida species	4	4	3	5	8	4
Other	20[d]	2	13	23	24	24

[a]Major infections only.
[b]Data from reference 2.
[c]Data from reference 1.
[d]Includes infections caused by multiple organisms.
Modified from Jarvis WR. Epidemiology of nosocomial infections in pediatric patients. Pediatr Infect Dis J 6:344–351, 1987.

vancomycin-resistant strains), multidrug-resistant gram-negative bacilli, and *Candida* became emerging problems.[2, 12] However, these temporal trends may not apply to individual nurseries, and it is important for infection control personnel to document the microbial ecology of the NICU in their institution.

Table 34–4 shows pathogens causing nosocomial infection in selected NICUs. A comparison of the etiology of early-onset infections (≤ 3 days) with late-onset infections (≥ 4 days) in an NICU from 1987 to 1995 is shown in Table 34–5. Early-onset infections were predominantly due to group B streptococci and late onset due to CONS.[12] These data are consistent with previously reported data from the NNIS system.[1]

Gram-Positive Bacteria

Although the major problem with *S. aureus* disease caused by a single phage type (often referred to as 80/81) that plagued nurseries in the 1950s has disappeared and life-threatening staphylococcal infection in young, otherwise healthy infants is much less frequent,[36] *S. aureus* continues to be a major cause of less serious infections (e.g., pustulosis, omphalitis, breast abscess) in well-baby nurseries.[37–42] The continuing occurrence of *S. aureus* infections has been associated with the discontinuation, two decades ago, of routine hexachlorophene bathing of newborns.[43, 44] Newborns seldom acquire staphylococci from their mothers at the time of birth, but in a matter of days colonization may reach 40 to 90% if these newborns are admitted to a nursery where many infants are already colonized.[45, 46] The umbilicus is usually the initial site of colonization,[47] but staphylococci quickly spread to the nose and other skin sites. Spread

from infant to infant occurs by means of the hands of personnel; airborne transmission rarely occurs, as shown by Rammelkamp and Mortimer in their classic studies.[48, 49] Droplet transmission from infants with coexisting viral respiratory tract infection ("cloud babies") is uncommon.[36] Staphylococci, including MRSA, survive well in the environment and on fomites, and indirect contact spread may occur by means of this route. Outbreaks due to heavy staphylococcal shedders on the

TABLE 34–5

Etiologies of Invasive Infections in Neonates at Parkland Memorial Hospital (January 1987–December 1995)

	EARLY ONSET (≤ 3 DAYS OF AGE) (N = 347) (%)	LATE ONSET (≥ 4 DAYS OF AGE) (N = 576) (%)
Coagulase-negative staphylococci	3	40
Gram-negative bacilli	15	16
Group B *Streptococcus*	68	10
Staphylococcus aureus	2	3
Methicillin-resistant *S. aureus*	—	13
Enterococcus	3	5
Fungal	—	3
Polymicrobial	1	9
Other	8	2

Adapted from Siegel JD. The newborn nursery. *In* Bennett JV, Brachman PS (eds). Hospital Infections, 4th ed. Boston, Little, Brown, 1998, pp 403–420.

nursery staff are quite rare. Colonization of the skin, nose, and umbilicus usually precedes infection, but rates of colonization correlate poorly with rates of infection.[14, 36, 50] The number of colonized infants may greatly exceed the number of infected infants, and, conversely, outbreaks of staphylococcal infection can occur in nurseries with low colonization rates.[36] Therefore, surveillance cultures to detect colonized infants are not recommended except under outbreak conditions.

Barrier precautions (e.g., gloves, gowns) and hand washing are effective means of preventing transmission of *S. aureus* from heavily colonized or infected infants. The use of hexachlorophene (3%) for bathing is effective in reducing colonization,[16] but this agent was found to cause cystic degenerative changes in the white matter of premature infants.[51–53] There was no evidence that this agent posed a hazard to full-term infants. A warning against use of hexachlorophene was issued by the U.S. Food and Drug Administration in 1972. The use of this agent for bathing of full-term infants remains an option during outbreaks of *S. aureus* infection (some recommend dilution of 1:4 to 1:5 in water), but hexachlorophene should not be used to bathe very low birth weight infants.[16] Chlorhexidine is a reasonable alternative because it has good antistaphylococcal activity, negligible absorption after bathing, and no documented toxicity.[54–56] Some MRSA strains appear to have reduced susceptibility to chlorhexidine, but the clinical significance is unclear.[57] A variety of antiseptic and antimicrobial agents have been used for umbilical cord care as a control measure with varying degrees of success.[58] (For more detailed discussion, see section on Skin and Cord Care.) In the past, when topical antiseptics and conventional infection control measures failed to halt epidemics of severe disease, artificial colonization with a relatively avirulent strain of *S. aureus* (502A) was used successfully to prevent colonization with virulent strains (bacterial interference), but this is not a practical or readily available intervention today.[59]

MRSA has become a problem in many nurseries throughout the world, causing a range of illness from minor skin disorders to scalded skin syndrome, sepsis, osteomyelitis, meningitis, and pneumonia.[57, 60–64] Although MRSA poses unique therapeutic challenges, studies to date have not demonstrated that the epidemiology of MRSA is fundamentally different from that of methicillin-susceptible *S. aureus*. MRSA may be introduced into the nursery by a colonized or infected infant or a health care worker.[65] High rates of colonization (30 to 70%), sometimes with more than one strain,[63] may occur before the problem is recognized.[61, 66] Molecular epidemiologic techniques are helpful in determining if a single strain or multiple strains of MRSA are causing a nursery outbreak.[67, 68] The major reservoir for MRSA colonization is infected newborns, and MRSA is most frequently transmitted by health care workers whose hands have become transiently contaminated during routine neonatal care. Environmental sources or chronic carriers[69, 70] do not commonly cause nosocomial infection.[35, 71] Once established in an institution, MRSA outbreaks have proved difficult to eradicate, despite intensive infection control measures. Epidemics can last

for months and frequently recur.[72] Cohorting and changes in hand-washing practices (such as switching to antiseptic soap) have been successful in some outbreaks.[63, 72, 73] Application of mupirocin to the cord and nares has also been shown to be effective in eradicating MRSA in some nurseries.[74] Haley and associates found that long-standing endemic MRSA in a nursery was not terminated even after institution of infection control measures such as hand-washing education, use of gowns and gloves, isolating colonized and infected infants, and treating colonized personnel, until the overcrowding and understaffing conditions in the nursery were corrected.[75, 76] Several sets of guidelines for the control and prevention of MRSA in hospitals have been published, some more rigid than others, and none specific to nurseries.[77–80]

Coagulase-negative staphylococci, especially *Staphylococcus epidermidis*, are the most frequent cause of nosocomial bacteremia in critically ill neonates[16, 26, 28, 81–85] and account for more than 50% of late-onset nosocomial infections in the NICU.[1, 32, 34, 86, 87] CONS are normal inhabitants of the newborn skin and nose and rarely cause disease in the healthy newborn.[88] However, it now is clear that the CONS strains that colonize and infect newborns are transmitted nosocomially from infant to infant on the hands of caregivers. In a study by Huebner and co-workers, two strains of CONS were shown to have persisted in an NICU for almost a decade.[81] The vast majority of CONS are resistant to methicillin, providing further confirmation of their nosocomial origin. The risk factors for CONS bacteremia include low birth weight, prolonged hospital stay, central venous catheterization, antibiotic use, and intravenous administration of lipids.[1–3, 89, 90] CONS has the ability to adhere to prosthetic materials such as intravascular catheters, because they produce capsular polysaccharide adhesin (poly-*N*-succinyl glucosamine).[91] Exopolysaccharide (slime) facilitates persistence of CONS on foreign bodies, providing a layer of protection against host defenses and antibiotic penetration.[92] CONS infections occasionally occur in full-term newborns in the absence of these predisposing factors.[93]

Molecular epidemiologic techniques such as pulse-field gel electrophoresis have helped distinguish strains of CONS and identified endemic and epidemic spread within the nursery.[81, 89, 94–97] Reservoirs of CONS include the feces, periauricular skin, and the axilla and nares of neonates, allowing for cross contamination among sites on the same infant as well as nosocomial spread among other infants in the nursery.[98] CONS, including clones of *Staphylococcus hemolyticus* and *S. epidermidis*, may become endemic in nurseries for prolonged periods and cause clusters of infections.[81, 89, 94, 99, 100]

The most common form of nosocomial infection due to CONS is bacteremia, which is generally less fulminant than bacteremia due to other organisms. CONS more rarely causes focal infections, such as neck and wound abscesses, omphalitis, mastitis, meningitis, and endocarditis.[88] Manifestations of disease are usually nonspecific, making diagnosis problematic. CONS infection in the neonate is associated with considerable morbidity (e.g., prolonged length of stay and increased costs), but not with excess mortality.[33, 88] Some investigators have suggested that CONS bacteremia may be associated with chronic lung disease in low-risk infants.[101] Infusion of vancomycin through central venous lines (i.e., added to parenteral nutrition fluids) has been found to be effective in reducing the incidence of nosocomial CONS infections in infants of less than 1500 g birth weight but has not been widely adopted because of concern over promoting vancomycin resistance in enterococci and CONS. Further studies are needed to evaluate the use of prophylactic vancomycin; and if this practice is adopted, it should be restricted to the highest risk group of infants (i.e., infants weighing less than 1000 g) in NICUs with high rates of CONS bacteremia.[8, 9, 102]

Enterococci are a well-established cause of nosocomial infection in the United States.[103] Enterococci have also been recognized as important pathogens in the high-risk nursery since the late 1970s, with reports of outbreaks of *Enterococcus faecium* and *Enterococcus faecalis* increasing over the past two decades.[104–111] In the past, it was thought that enterococci were acquired from the mother's flora. More recently, with the use of typing techniques such as pulse-field gel electrophoresis, nosocomial patient-to-patient transmission of identical strains has been documented. Enterococci can persist for long periods in the environment, and the environment is easily contaminated by incontinent infants. Caregivers can contaminate their hands either while caring for infants or by touching contaminated environmental objects or surfaces.[35, 112] Nosocomial enterococcal infections are more likely to occur in premature infants who have been in the nursery more than 30 to 60 days (late, late onset). Necrotizing enterocolitis or symptoms consistent with intra-abdominal disease occurred in more than one half of the patients in a study by McNeely and co-workers,[112] suggesting that the intestinal tract is the site of invasion in many cases. Moreover, most episodes are polymicrobial, including enteric organisms, providing further evidence of a gastrointestinal source. Other factors associated with enterococcal infections include prolonged use of central venous catheters and prior exposure to antibiotics. Although enterococcal infections can be severe (e.g., sepsis with associated focal infections such as soft tissue abscesses, pneumonia, meningitis, and endocarditis), the mortality rate generally is low.[35, 112]

The emergence of multiple antibiotic-resistant enterococci has raised serious concerns about the spread of resistance to other organisms and development of infections that may not be treatable by available antimicrobial agents. Vancomycin-resistant enterococci (VRE) are now endemic to many hospitals in the United States,[113] and VRE has been reported in NICUs.[109] The risk factors for VRE infections in NICUs, such as prolonged hospitalization, extensive use of broad-spectrum antibiotics, including vancomycin, and use of invasive medical devices, are particularly difficult to alter.[112] Standard infection control techniques, such as hand washing, patient isolation, barrier precautions, cohorting, and employee education, may be effective in containing the spread of these organisms.[112] Although guidelines for the control and prevention of VRE in the hospital setting have been published,[114] there are no guidelines specifically developed for the nursery.

Other less common nosocomial gram-positive pathogens have been reported in the nursery. These include *Listeria*,[115, 116] group B *Streptococcus*,[11] and group A beta-hemolytic *Streptococcus*.[117] *Clostridium difficile* has been associated with outbreak of necrotizing enterocolitis (NEC) in the nursery,[118] but its role as an etiologic agent for NEC is questionable.[35, 119] As many as 50% of healthy newborns may be colonized with toxin-producing strains of *C. difficile* (probably secondary to nosocomial transmission), and postnatal colonization has been detected in NICUs.[120–122] The lack of associated disease may be due to the immature intestinal mucosa of the neonate, which lacks receptors for the *C. difficile* toxin.[35]

Gram-Negative Bacteria

Nosocomial infections caused by gram-negative bacilli account for 18 to 19% of bloodstream infections[32, 34] and over 30% of nosocomial pneumonias in the NICU.[1] These infections are associated with high mortality rates ranging from 40 to 90%, although few studies have included appropriate controls required to demonstrate fatalities directly attributable to gram-negative infections.[32, 123] *E. coli*, *Klebsiella* species, and *Enterobacter* species cause the majority of gram-negative endemic nosocomial infections in the NICU.[1, 12, 32, 124–126] Other gram-negative bacilli associated with clusters or outbreaks of infection in the NICU include *P. aeruginosa*,[127–134] *Serratia* species,[135–138] *Proteus mirabilis*,[139] *Citrobacter diversus (koserii)*,[140–142] *Salmonella* species,[143–152] *Acinetobacter* species,[153–158] *Chryseobacterium (Flavobacterium) meningosepticum*,[159–162] and *Enterobacter* species. Nursery outbreaks of gram-negative infection have been associated with environmental contamination (i.e., contaminated water supply),[135, 163, 164] intravenous fluids,[165] respiratory therapy equipment,[134, 146, 166] suction machines,[146] and soap.[136, 137, 167–170] Outbreaks have also been associated with infant feeding (e.g., breast milk[171] and formula[172]). Other gram-negative bacilli identified less frequently as the etiology of nosocomial infection in the nursery include *Campylobacter* species,[173–176] nontypable strains of *Haemophilus influenzae*,[177, 178] *Bordetella* pertussis,[179] and *Legionella pneumophila*.[180–182]

Nosocomial gram-negative enteric pathogens in newborn nurseries, particularly those causing epidemics, often are resistant to multiple antibiotics.[183–188] Resistance to antibiotics commonly used to treat gram-negative infections in the NICU has been a progressive, persistent problem over the past several decades. Aminoglycoside resistance was observed early on, often due to plasmid-mediated production of aminoglycoside-inactivating enzymes.[123, 183–189] As cephalosporins were used more widely in NICUs, resistance to these agents developed rapidly. Third-generation cephalosporin resistance in *Enterobacter*, *Serratia*, and other enteric pathogens often is due to de-repression of chromosomal genes encoding cephalosporinases. In addition, resistance to third-generation cephalosporins may be mediated by so-called extended spectrum β-lactamases borne on conjugative plasmids.[190, 191] Recently, carbapenemases (both chromosomal and plasmid mediated) have been reported.[192] Other mechanisms of resistance may be relatively more important in some NICUs (e.g., aminoglycoside resistance in *P. aeruginosa* due to porin-mediated decreased permeability to this class of antibiotics). It is important to track resistance patterns in individual nurseries and limit unnecessary use of broad-spectrum antibiotics to ensure appropriate use of antimicrobial therapy.

Other Bacteria

Tuberculosis (TB) has recently been reported as a potential nosocomial pathogen in the NICU, and there has been at least one NICU outbreak of multidrug-resistant TB. Newborns are thought to be particularly susceptible to infection with *Mycobacterium tuberculosis*, even after brief periods of exposure, owing to paucity of alveolar macrophages in neonatal lungs and diminished rates of phagocytosis and killing of bacteria. In general, TB in infants is not very contagious. However, in the NICU setting, suctioning of newborns theoretically may generate infectious droplet nuclei. A recent case of congenital TB diagnosed at autopsy demonstrated that there is at least some risk of transmission to health care workers.[193] It might seem logical to assume that adults with smear-positive, cavitary TB would pose the greatest threat to neonates. However, several investigations involving hundreds of infants failed to demonstrate TB in exposed infants. Only one previous report identified active disease in two infants exposed to a nurse's aide with TB in the nursery.[193, 194] Nivin and co-workers[195] reported transmission of multidrug-resistant TB in a hospital nursery. Four infants born over a 2-week period developed disease between 4 and 15 months after birth. The exposure time was relatively short, because the average length of stay for these infants was 5 days. In addition, two health care workers in the nursery during the same period developed disease between 14 and 20 months after suspected exposure. A source case for the cluster of infections was not clearly identified. Information about the air ventilation patterns in the nursery at the time of exposure was not available, and the possibility of an unrecognized case of TB in a health care worker or visitor could not be excluded. The possibility of spread of TB within the nursery should be vigorously investigated. CDC guidelines for TB control should be followed.[196]

Fungi

Fungi have become increasingly important nosocomial pathogens in hospitalized patients over the past two decades, and investigators have noted the same trends in NICUs.[197] In an NNIS surveillance study done from 1986–1990, the highest rate of nosocomial fungal infections occurred in the burn/trauma, cardiac surgery, oncology, and general surgery units, and in the high-risk nursery.[197] During that period of time, the number of fungal nosocomial infections doubled in the nursery (4.7 to 9.6 fungal infections per 1000 discharges). Fungi have been reported to cause 7 to 13% of nosocomial bloodstream infections in high-risk nurseries.[1, 32, 197]

CANDIDA

Candida species account for the majority of fungal nosocomial infections in the nursery. Newborns acquire *Candida* from the mother at birth, with 4 to 19% being colonized, predominantly in the gastrointestinal tract, in the first week of life.[2] Many colonized full-term infants develop oral thrush or diaper dermatitis, which is not usually recognized until after discharge from the nursery. *Candida* can also be acquired postnatally in the NICU by infant-to-infant transmission through the hands of personnel[198–201] and occasionally from environmental sources such as contaminated solutions[202–204] and devices.[205] Molecular typing methods have allowed related strains of *Candida* to be identified, improving epidemiologic investigations of these organisms.[206] Invasion probably occurs most commonly from the colonized gastrointestinal tract. The rate of colonization in infants weighing less than 1500 g at birth has been reported to be 19 to 47%, with systemic disease occurring in 2.6 to 8% of colonized infants.[199, 207–210] Early colonization tends to be caused by *Candida albicans*, and later colonization is caused by species such as *Candida tropicalis* and *Candida parapsilosis*.[35] By using molecular typing methods, it has been shown that infants colonized or infected with *C. albicans* were colonized or infected with the same strain of *C. albicans* as their mothers. Infants colonized with *C. parapsilosis* had no maternal reservoir, and *C. parapsilosis* is the most common species of *Candida* found on the hands of health care providers, implicating horizontal transmission within the nursery.[211] The rate of candidemia increased by 11-fold over 15 years in one NICU, and the prevalent species has shifted from *C. albicans* to *C. parapsilosis*. The mortality rate from candidemia has been reported to be 25 to 54%,[212, 213] and the mortality rate for *C. albicans* was reported to be higher than for *C. parapsilosis* (26% vs. 4%, respectively).[213] C. parapsilosis has also been shown to be less virulent in animal models, although the relevance of this study to neonates is uncertain.[214] Other species of Candida that have been implicated in nosocomial infection in the NICU include *Candida lusitaniae*,[215, 216] Candida stellatoides,[217] and *Candida (Torulopsis) glabrata*.[218]

The development of candidemia in neonates has been associated with prolonged exposure to antibiotics, hyperalimentation, intravenous fat emulsion, and tracheal intubation.[219] Duration of antibiotic therapy was the most strongly and independently associated identified risk factor for invasive candidiasis in one study.[219] Central venous access has been reported as a risk factor,[220] but more recent studies could not document an association with use or duration of central catheterization. The contents of the infusate may be more relevant.[208, 217, 219] Detection of colonization in the first week of life, or the growth of *Candida* from an endotracheal aspirate at any given time during the NICU stay, may identify a group of very low birth weight infants with an increased risk of candidiasis. The relative risks of invasive candidiasis in very low birth weight infants colonized at any site during the first week of life or with colonization in the lungs while on a ventilator were 9.3 and 5.9, respectively.[208] Some investigators have suggested that selective antifungal prophylaxis targeted toward this high-risk group may be warranted, but further study is needed.

OTHER YEASTS

Other causes of nosocomial fungal infections in the nursery include yeasts, such as *Malassezia furfur*,[221–226] *Malassezia pachydermatis*,[227–229] *Trichosporin beigelii*,[230] and other dermatophytes.[231, 232] *M. furfur* is being recognized more frequently in the NICU as a cause of fungemia in infants receiving intravenous lipid emulsion through central venous catheters.[222, 225] *M. furfur* is a lipid-dependent fungus that causes tinea versicolor in older children and can frequently colonize the skin of neonates in intensive care.[223, 233] Skin colonization has been associated with younger gestational age, lower birth weight, and longer NICU stay.[223] The rate of skin colonization in high-risk neonates varies from 25 to 84%, in comparison to 5% of infants hospitalized in the non-NICU setting or attending a well-baby clinic.[224] Rectal colonization has been shown to increase in infants who receive antibiotics.[234] In addition to fungemia, *M. furfur* occasionally causes nosocomial pneumonia.[222, 223] *M. furfur* requires an exogenous source of lipid for its growth; isolation is enhanced by the use of lipid-supplemented media.[222] In an outbreak of *M. pachydermatis* fungemia in an intensive care nursery, Chang and co-workers[229] reported that the organism was introduced on a health care worker's hands after being colonized from pet dogs at home. The organism persisted in the nursery through patient-to-patient transmission and caused eight nosocomial bloodstream infections, two urinary tract infections, and one case of meningitis.

FILAMENTOUS FUNGI

Nosocomial infections with filamentous fungi,[235–240] such as *Aspergillus* and *Zygomycetes*, are unusual in the nursery, but sporadic cases have been reported. These infections occur as a result of environmental contamination. Dust that is generated by hospital construction or faulty cleaning practices can carry spores that settle in wounds or are inhaled. There have been reports of contaminated adhesive tape,[16, 235, 238] monitor leads,[241] and wooden tongue blades used for splints[242] causing nosocomial zygomatic (e.g., *Rhizopus*) infection in the NICU.

Aspergillus has become increasingly important as a nosocomial pathogen in the nursery. Aspergillosis presents as primary cutaneous disease and as pulmonary and/or disseminated disease. In a review of the literature over the past four decades, Groll and associates[243] found that prematurity, chronic granulomatous disease, and a complex of diarrhea, dehydration, malnutrition, and invasive bacterial infections accounted for the majority of underlying conditions predisposing to aspergillosis during the first 3 months of life. Exposure to antibiotics, corticosteroid use, and traumatized skin were risk factors for disease. Neutropenia did not appear to be a significant risk factor in neonates, but premature infants do not have normal chemotaxis or phagocytosis, which are major host defenses against the fungus. Aspergillosis was uniformly fatal in untreated infants, and the diagnosis often was made at autopsy. Careful attention to ventilation systems in the nursery, regular cleaning schedules to avoid buildup of dust contaminated with spores, and appropriate containment of dust during hospital renovation and construction work may prevent nosocomial aspergillosis in the high-risk neonate.[244]

Viral Infections

Viral nosocomial infections have been identified with increasing frequency in the NICU. The NNIS study[1] of nosocomial infections among high-risk neonates found that 5% of eye, ear, nose, and throat infections and 30% of gastrointestinal infections were caused by viruses. These NNIS data confirm earlier studies that emphasized the importance of performing appropriate viral studies.[19] Even so, it is likely that the NNIS data underestimate the true extent of the problem. High rates of infection in staff members characterize outbreaks of nursery viral infections.[245–247] Infected staff members usually have mild illness, continue to work, and therefore spread infection to the infants under their care.[35] Some viruses are well recognized to cause outbreaks in the nursery (i.e., respiratory viruses, enteroviruses, rotavirus, and hepatitis A virus [HAV]), whereas other viruses are not well transmitted horizontally in the nursery and are more likely due to vertical transmission from the mother (i.e., human immunodeficiency virus [HIV], hepatitis B [HBV] and C [HCV], and CMV). Transmission of herpes simplex virus (HSV) and varicella-zoster virus in the nursery is rare.

RESPIRATORY VIRUSES

Neonates are susceptible to the same respiratory viruses that infect older children and adults, including influenza, parainfluenza, adenovirus, respiratory syncytial virus (RSV), rhinovirus, and coronavirus. However, in the neonate, these pathogens are more likely to present as atypical features, such as apnea, lethargy, and poor feeding, in addition to signs of lower respiratory tract disease. Viral infections are rarely recognized in the full-term nursery owing to their incubation period, but it is well recognized that respiratory viruses, especially RSV, are important causes of infection in the NICU.[2] Two viruses may be epidemic in the nursery at the same time,[248–250] and the dual nature of the outbreak may be difficult to recognize without the availability of a diagnostic virology laboratory. An important clue to the etiologic agent or agents may be knowledge of the respiratory viruses circulating in the community at the time of the outbreak. Viral infections reflect community outbreaks and are often introduced into the nursery by parents, visitors, or members of the hospital staff.[245–247, 251, 252] Most respiratory viruses are spread by direct, indirect, and occasionally droplet contact, with the exception of influenza viruses, which may also be spread by droplet nuclei.[253, 254]

The best studied respiratory viral pathogen of importance in the NICU is RSV. RSV is spread primarily by means of the hands of caregivers.[255, 256] Personnel can contaminate their hands by direct contact with the secretions of infected infants, who excrete a high titer of viruses for prolonged periods,[257] or by touching soiled environmental surfaces, on which the virus can survive for minutes to hours.[258] If staff members rub their nose or eyes with contaminated hands, they may become ill, generally with symptoms of a cold, and serve as vectors for the transmission of RSV to infants under their care. Outbreaks are common, and attack rates among infants and personnel can reach high levels during the epidemic season.[248–250, 259–261] During one outbreak, 34% of the NICU staff developed RSV infection, as did 35% of infants remaining in the nursery for more than 6 days.[259] RSV was implicated in four deaths. Active surveillance, cohorting, strict visiting policies, gloving, gowning, and masking have been advocated to reduce the risk of transmission within the NICU,[261] but strict compliance with glove and gown precautions appears to be the most important control measure.[262]

Other respiratory viruses are associated with clusters of respiratory infections in the nursery, such as parainfluenza virus,[248, 263, 264] coronavirus,[265] and rhinovirus.[249] Risk factors for transmission include crowding, understaffing, nasogastric tubes, and endotracheal intubation.[248, 249, 263] Nosocomial infections due to influenza viruses are less frequent; symptoms may resemble bacterial sepsis.[247, 251, 266, 267] Nursery outbreaks of adenovirus respiratory infections have been reported.[247, 266–268] These infections may present as mild upper respiratory tract infections, conjunctivitis, or pneumonia or as severe sepsis syndrome with multiorgan involvement, cardiovascular collapse, and a case-fatality ratio of 84%.[247, 267, 268]

ENTEROVIRUSES

Enteroviruses have been reported to cause major outbreaks in the normal newborn nursery as well as in NICUs.[269–272] They are readily spread by the fecal-oral route once they have been introduced into the nursery. The index case may be an infant infected vertically by an ill mother or by an infected health care worker.[273, 274] During a community outbreak, 3.4% of mothers were found to have enterovirus in the stool at delivery, and transmission rates from mother to infant have been reported to be 29 to 57%.[274] Attack rates of 22 to 54% have been reported once the virus has been introduced into the nursery.[274] Risk factors for infection include procedures involving the mouths of newborns, such as nasogastric intubation or gavage feeding, and mouth care, as well as proximity to an infected infant and care by the same nurse.[271, 272] Newborns with severe underlying illness are more likely to be infected, presumably because prolonged intensive care with exposure provides more opportunities for transmission.[272, 274]

Echovirus and coxsackievirus B are the most frequent enteroviruses reported in the nursery setting.[273, 274] Coxsackievirus A infections are unusual in the newborn, but outbreaks of herpangina and aseptic meningitis have been reported.[269, 275] Nosocomial disease acquired in the nursery generally is less severe than infection acquired from the mother, the most frequent presentations being mild febrile illness and aseptic meningitis. However, nosocomial enteroviral disease can be severe (e.g., en-

cephalitis, myocarditis, hepatitis), and fatalities have been reported.[276, 277] Maternally derived antibody may play a role in limiting severity of disease in nursery-acquired enterovirus. Disease acquired from the mother is characterized by overwhelming viremia, meningitis, myocarditis, hepatic necrosis, and death.[16] Mothers who become ill near term do not have time to develop a type-specific antibody response before delivery. As a result, the infant is exposed to a large inoculum of virus without the presence of protective maternally derived antibody.[272, 274]

Control measures are similar to those used for other infections spread by the fecal-oral route. Emphasis on hand washing and barrier precautions, as well as cohorting of infected infants, is important for limiting transmission within the nursery.[278] However, control can be difficult because intestinal carriage may be widespread and long-lasting among infants and personnel, and rapid viral diagnostic tests are not generally available for enterovirus. Therefore, detection of carriers and definition of cohorts is not feasible. Immune serum globulin has been used in an attempt to interrupt outbreaks, with mixed success.[271, 277, 279, 280]

HEPATITIS A VIRUS

Nosocomial outbreaks of hepatitis A are uncommon because of the relatively brief duration and low titer of viral shedding in the stool.[281–283] However, the epidemiology of HAV infection in the nursery is unique because premature infants may excrete virus for as long as 4 to 5 months after acute infection.[282] HAV may be introduced into the nursery by an infant infected by blood transfusion[282–284] or by vertical transmission from a mother with acute infection.[281] Infection in the newborn usually is subclinical, and the first indication that there is a problem may be secondary symptomatic (e.g., jaundice) infection in a caregiver or parent.[281, 283–285] Therefore, major epidemics can occur before HAV infection is detected and contained. In one outbreak, two infants infected by the same blood transfusion were the source of transmission to 15 nurses and one parent.[283] In another outbreak, HAV spread among seven premature infants in a NICU, resulting in 15 secondary cases in adults.[285] Infections have spread to other nurseries when unrecognized infected infants have been transferred.[285]

HAV is transmitted to other infants, health care workers, and parents by fecal-oral spread. Direct contact is the route of transmission from infected infant to adult caregiver, and indirect contact is by the hands for transmission from one infant to another. Control of an outbreak can be difficult and often requires the assistance of the local health department when adult contacts or more than one institution are involved. Emphasis on hand washing, barrier precautions, and cohorting of infected infants, as well as administration of immune globulin to all exposed contacts, is usually necessary to limit transmission and halt an outbreak.[278, 286] The role of hepatitis A vaccine in the control of outbreaks has not yet been determined.

ROTAVIRUS

Rotavirus is a common cause of endemic and epidemic nosocomial gastrointestinal virus infection in the newborn nursery and NICU.[287–290] Rotavirus spreads rapidly among babies in the nursery by the fecal-oral route, and perhaps by respiratory secretions as well during the acute phase of the illness.[291] The principal mode of transmission is indirect contact from the hands of health care workers or contaminated equipment. The virus can survive on fomites for over an hour.[292] Introduction and transmission may be difficult to recognize and control because the majority of newborns remain asymptomatic, and symptomatic infants may shed virus intermittently for an extended period of time, creating an enduring reservoir of virus.

Unlike respiratory viruses, rotavirus infections in the nursery may be unrelated to concomitant community outbreaks and are usually acquired from nursery rather than maternal sources.[287] Studies have shown that neonatal rotavirus infection may occur with strains distinct from those circulating in the community.[287, 293]

Although infection in the newborn is primarily asymptomatic, mild, moderate, and severe cases of diarrhea have been reported. One study associated an outbreak of necrotizing enterocolitis in a nursery with concurrent rotavirus infection.[246] Another study showed that rotavirus infection was associated with a high incidence of bradycardia-apnea episodes in the neonate during the acute gastrointestinal phase of the disease; the authors speculated that the virus might involve the central nervous system.[294]

Control of rotavirus infections in the nursery depends on early and accurate identification of symptomatic and asymptomatic viral shedders. Rapid diagnostic techniques, such as enzyme immunoassays and latex agglutination assays, are commercially available. Use of gowns and gloves, hand washing, and appropriate disinfection of environmental surfaces are critical to prevent transmission. Chemical disinfection of rotavirus-contaminated inanimate surfaces is difficult because of high resistance to some chemical disinfectants and antiseptics commonly used in the nursery.[295] Disinfectants and antiseptics should contain a high proportion of alcohol to be effective against rotavirus. Lysol disinfectant spray (79% ethanol) successfully blocked transmission of rotavirus infection to humans when sprayed on inanimate surfaces experimentally contaminated with infectious rotavirus.[296] During peak months of rotavirus activity, or if infection is identified in the nursery, disinfection of environmental surfaces with Lysol or alcohol-containing disinfecting agents might decrease nosocomial spread.[297] Hand washing with plain soap is ineffective against rotavirus and may further spread virus over a larger area of the hands.[295] Hand antisepsis with waterless hand washing agents containing at least 70% alcohol may help limit rotavirus transmission.[297]

HERPES SIMPLEX VIRUS

Most neonates with HSV infection acquire it from their mother at the time of birth. Fetal scalp monitor electrodes may contribute to the pathogenesis of localized herpetic lesions in some cases.[298, 299] Transmission in the nursery is rare, but outbreaks have been reported.[300–304] Infants can also acquire the virus from health care workers in the postnatal period, although this also appears to be rare. Nurses with herpetic whitlow (HSV hand lesion) have been implicated in cross infections occurring in a pediatric intensive care unit.[305] Infection has been transmitted to an infant suctioned by a health care worker with herpes labialis (cold sores). Genotyping showed that strains from the health care worker and the infant were identical.[306] An estimate of 1% of nursery personnel per week have clinically apparent herpes labialis,[307] and as many as 24% of adults may shed virus asymptomatically into saliva.[308] Adults with herpes labialis often have virus on their hands.[309] In addition, the virus can survive for hours on environmental surfaces.[309] The magnitude of risk of adult to infant transmission is unknown and probably low.[303, 309] Asymptomatic persons are less infectious than persons with active lesions.[310, 311]

A practical infection control policy must be developed for personnel with orofacial lesions. They should be evaluated to determine their potential for transmitting HSV to high-risk patients such as neonates and should be excluded from care of such patients if possible.[312] On the other hand, such a policy may need to be tempered if exclusion of personnel with labial herpes would result in short-staffing and compromise the care of critically ill newborns. Personnel with oral lesions should be considered on an individual basis. The American Academy of Pediatrics (AAP) Committee on Infectious Diseases recommends that personnel with herpes labialis who have contact with infants should (1) cover and not touch their lesions; (2) carefully observe hand-washing policies; and (3) not kiss or nuzzle newborn infants.[313] Masks are of uncertain value in limiting viral shedding and would not necessarily reduce contamination of the hands of infected caregivers.[16] It is unknown whether the application of antiviral agents (e.g., acyclovir) to the lip would decrease the risk of transmission.[16] Personnel with HSV infection of the hands should be restricted from patient contact and contact with the patient's environment until the lesions have crusted. In addition, HSV lesions may be secondarily infected by *S. aureus* and group A *Streptococcus*, and personnel should be excluded from patient contact if secondary infection is documented.[312]

VARICELLA-ZOSTER VIRUS

Varicella (VZV) may be introduced into the nursery by mothers, health care workers, or visitors with unrecognized infection.[314, 315] However, outbreaks of VZV infection in nurseries are unusual, probably because most infants have transplacentally acquired antibody. Infants of less than 28 weeks' gestation may not have received a protective level of antibody from their mother before delivery, and infants born to seronegative mothers may be susceptible to infection and are at risk for more severe disease. Even infants who are more mature and have acquired detectable levels of serum antibody occasionally develop chickenpox after exposure, as can infants who have received varicella immune globulin to prevent infection.[316] Postnatal varicella exposure can result in serious disease[315, 317] in the infant, and exposed susceptible personnel can develop severe infection, including varicella pneumonia.

Prompt intervention, including administration of varicella immune globulin as quickly as possible after a varicella zoster exposure in the nursery and cohorting of potentially exposed or infected infants, is imperative. Some infection control professionals do not consider airborne or droplet transmission to be a risk if the neonate has been confined to a positive-pressure Isolette. Varicella is transmitted by contact with infected secretions or droplets and, rarely, by airborne transmission; therefore, strict adherence to airborne and contact precautions is necessary. Failure to control a potential outbreak can result in considerable expense, inconvenience, and potential closure of the nursery. Guidelines have been published regarding use of varicella immune globulin in newborns.[318] Guidelines have also been established for susceptible health care workers who are exposed to varicella, are potentially incubating infection, or have herpes zoster.[312] It is recommended that health care workers with herpes zoster be excluded from care of high-risk patients (including neonates) until all lesions dry and crust.[312] With more widespread use of the varicella vaccine, licensed in 1995, the number of susceptible mothers, visitors, or health care workers should decrease considerably.[35]

EPIDEMIOLOGY

Neonatal Colonization

The transition from the protective environment of the womb to an environment teeming with microbial life is abrupt. The newborn is a tabula rasa. Infants do not have a normal microbial flora to help them resist colonization by microorganisms they encounter in the birth canal, on the skin of their parents, on the hands of caregivers, or in the hospital and home environment. Healthy newborns begin to acquire their own unique normal flora within a few days after birth.[16] Alpha-streptococci colonize the throat and may play an important role in interfering with colonization by hospital bacteria, especially gram-negative bacilli.[319, 320] CONS predominate in the nose and umbilicus. Breast-fed infants have heavy gastrointestinal colonization with *Bifidobacterium*, and although they quickly acquire a diverse gastrointestinal flora, there is a paucity of pathogenic anaerobes such as *Clostridium* and facultative gram-negative bacilli.[321–324] Some investigators have postulated that lactose fermentation by *Bifidobacterium* lowers the stool pH to 4 in the presence of breast milk, which is a poor buffer, and that this acidic environment inhibits the multiplication of gram-negative bacilli such as *E. coli*.[325, 326] *E. coli* that do manage to colonize the gastrointestinal tract generally are identical to the strains in the maternal gastrointestinal flora. In contrast, formula-fed infants have a more complex gastrointestinal flora, which quickly comes to resemble that of adults. *Bifidobacterium* still is present in large numbers, but other anaerobes,

particularly *Bacteroides* and *Clostridium*, as well has gram-negative bacilli such as *E. coli* and *Klebsiella*, also can be recovered from careful stool cultures.

Full-term infants are now hospitalized for very brief periods, often less than 24 hours. Thus, the opportunity for colonization by nosocomial pathogens is limited. Moreover, the vast majority of infections occur post discharge, complicating nosocomial infection surveillance. Because most of the epidemiologic and microbiologic studies in the literature were written at a time when infants were hospitalized for at least several days, their relevance to the contemporary newborn population is unclear. Nonetheless, not all infants traverse the well-baby nursery without encountering nosocomial pathogens. The umbilicus is the initial colonization site for *S. aureus*, which then quickly populates the nose and skin.[327] Whereas colonization with *S. aureus* is a prerequisite for subsequent infection, recovery of this pathogen from the umbilicus or nose has a very low positive predictive value.[328] The majority of infants in an individual nursery may be colonized over a period of years, yet the nursery may escape a staphylococcal outbreak, whereas other nurseries experience an outbreak despite a long period of falsely reassuring low colonization rates. Other gram-positive bacteria that may colonize and infect infants during routine nursery care include group A streptococci[329] and group B streptococci.[11] *C. difficile* may spread among infants in the nursery,[121, 324, 330] but it ordinarily does not cause colitis in newborns, owing to the lack of the appropriate mucosal receptor.

Gastrointestinal pathogens, such as enteropathogenic *E. coli* and *Salmonella*, can also cause mischief in the well-baby nursery, and colonized infants may continue to harbor enteric pathogens in their gastrointestinal tracts for long periods. Fortunately, outbreaks caused by classic enteropathogenic strains are much less frequent today than they were in past decades.[331, 332] Similarly, nosocomial acquisition of *Salmonella* and other enteric pathogens, such as *Shigella* and *Campylobacter*, also is relative rare in nurseries in the United States.[333] Nevertheless, there always will be an explosive potential for fecal-oral spread of these microorganisms in a universally incontinent newborn population. Fecal-oral transmission is not confined to the usual pathogens that cause gastroenteritis. For example, *Citrobacter koserii (diversus)*, which may be acquired perinatally from maternal flora, also may be acquired in the nursery. Numerous nursery outbreaks of *Citrobacter* colonization and infection (including necrotizing meningitis) attest to the ease with which this microorganism can spread among hospitalized neonates.[142, 334, 335]

Critically ill babies who require care in NICUs have a different microbiological fate than infants who spend only a day or two in a routine nursery.[16] The NICU houses an extraordinarily vulnerable population of extremely premature infants, as well as infants with complex congenital anomalies and surgical problems. These infants often have very limited contact with their mothers and hence have little exposure to their mothers' normal flora and the resistance to nosocomial colonization that these bacterial strains might afford. Moreover, infants hospitalized in the NICU are almost commonly treated with broad-spectrum antibiotics, such as ampicillin and an aminoglycoside, or a third-generation cephalosporin, which wipe out whatever bacteria the infant might have transiently acquired during birth.[336] Not surprisingly, as many as one third of newborns hospitalized in the NICU have no detectable growth of microorganisms from surface sites during the first few days of life.[337] However, CONS begin to colonize the umbilicus, nose, and skin relatively quickly, and within the first week of life virtually all infants are colonized heavily with a multiplicity of staphylococcal strains.[321] Although some of these staphylococci are survivors from the infant's encounter with its mother, most are nosocomial strains derived from contact with caregivers. These strains tend to be resistant to multiple antibiotics, including methicillin.[321] In NICUs in which MRSA is prevalent, colonization of the umbilicus, nose, skin, and other sites with MRSA may also occur early in life, with far graver potential consequences for the colonized newborn.[63, 72, 74, 338, 339] Similarly, NICU infants are vulnerable to colonization and infection with antibiotic-resistant enterococci.[109, 340]

Gram-negative nosocomial pathogens may also colonize the throat, nose, and umbilicus. The respiratory tract often is an important site of colonization, because most newborns in the NICU require mechanical ventilation, and heavily contaminated respiratory secretions are an important reservoir for the transmission of nosocomial pathogens to other infants. However, the primary reservoir for these microorganisms generally is the gastrointestinal tract. Gastrointestinal colonization with the gram-negative, often antibiotic-resistant pathogens that are endemic or epidemic in the NICU progresses inexorably. A study performed at Children's Hospital, Boston, two decades ago remains relevant today.[337] Hospital strains of *Klebsiella*, *Enterobacter*, and *Citrobacter* were isolated from the stool of only 2% of infants on admission but from 60% and 91% of infants after 15 and 30 days, respectively. Under the selective pressure of broad-spectrum antibiotic therapy, the gram-negative pathogens that populate NICUs have only become more resistant over the ensuing years. Each NICU may have its own unique ecology. For example, 80% of infants hospitalized in one NICU for a month or more were colonized by *E. coli* K1, which ordinarily is a perinatally acquired pathogen but in this case appeared to have been spread from infant to infant.[341] It is important to recognize that pathogens colonizing the gastrointestinal tract reach prodigious concentrations, and it is not unusual to find 10^6 or even 10^8 bacteria per gram of stool. Thus, even a speck of stool contamination may inoculate a caregiver's hands with thousands of antibiotic-resistant bacteria. Moreover, colonization is enduring, and the majority of NICU graduates will have persistent antibiotic-resistant pathogens in their gastrointestinal tract up to a year after discharge from the hospital.[342] Because infants who require NICU care are frequently readmitted to the hospital subsequently, colonized infants can serve as a reservoir for the further spread of nosocomial pathogens to other areas of the hospital.

Recent years have witnessed a dramatic increase in fungal colonization and infection in NICUs, which is not surprising given the vulnerability of this patient population coupled with the intensive use of antibiotics and corticosteroids. *Candida* colonization of the gastrointestinal tract and other sites has been associated with prolonged antibiotic therapy, parenteral nutrition and lipid therapy, extreme prematurity, and mechanical ventilation.[3, 198, 199, 219] Candida may either be acquired from maternal sources or as the result of nosocomial transmission.[207] Although not as life threatening as *Candida*, *M. furfur* and *M. pachydermatis* have caused widespread colonization and bloodstream infection in the NICU.[224, 227] *M. furfur* colonization rates as high as 84% have been reported in the NICU, probably due in part to the extensive use of lipids (which favor the growth of *M. furfur*) in this population. Colonization and infection with invasive filamentous fungi, such as *Aspergillus* and *Rhizopus*, may also occur from environmental sources.[230, 242, 343, 344] Recovery of these serious pathogens from neonatal cultures is a cause for great concern.

Modes of Transmission

Epidemiologists usually categorize potential modes of transmission of nosocomial pathogens into the categories outlined in Table 34–6.[345] Microorganisms can spread in the nursery from any of these routes, although some clearly are much more important than others.

Contact is by far the dominant mode of transmission in most nurseries most of the time. *Direct contact* involves direct transfer of microorganisms from an infected or colonized person to a patient. The source may be a caregiver, family member, or other visitor or, under unusual circumstances, another patient. For example, a member of the nursery or NICU staff who has a staphylococcal or streptococcal infection might inoculate these pathogens onto a patient during the course of routine care. Although it might appear to be unseemly for a staff member with an obvious staphylococcal infection to care for highly vulnerable patients, providers with an infection sometimes do not report their condition for fear of uncompensated removal from work or because they are unaware that infection anywhere on the body greatly increases the chance that their entire skin surface will be heavily colonized. Moreover, personnel may be colonized with potential pathogens even in the absence of an apparent infection, and pathogens colonizing their hands can be easily transmitted to newborns, who are especially susceptible to colonization by microorganisms they encounter early in life. Classic studies by Rammelkamp demonstrated that 20% of infants in a well-baby nursery became colonized with their caregivers' staphylococcal strains during routine care.[48] Moreover, when three staphylococcal carriers handled 37 infants for 10 minutes each through the ports of an Isolette incubator, 54% of the infants were colonized. This study unequivocally demonstrated that so-called "Isolettes" do not effectively shield newborns from transmission of staphylococci from the hands. The emergence of MRSA has added a new dimension to the threat of direct-contact transmission of staphylococci.

Although *S. aureus* is the pathogen most frequently transmitted by direct contact in the nursery and NICU,

TABLE 34–6
Modes of Transmission of Selected Nosocomial Infections

MODE OF TRANSMISSION	NOSOCOMIAL INFECTION	RESERVOIR[b]	SOURCE[c]
Airborne	Measles, varicella,[a] pulmonary tuberculosis	Infected persons	Airborne droplet nuclei
Contact:			
Direct	Neonatal staphylococcal skin infection	Infected/colonized caregiver	Drainage from infected wound on the hand of a caregiver
Indirect	Respiratory syncytial virus (RSV) infection	Infected persons	Hands of caregivers, fomites
	Infection with antimicrobial-resistant bacteria	Infected/colonized persons	Hands of caregivers, fomites
Droplet	Pertussis, invasive meningococcal disease, group A streptococcal infection	Infected/colonized persons	Large respiratory droplets
Endogenous (Autoinfection)	Coagulase-negative staphylococcal bacteremia associated with a central venous line	Skin at the site of catheter insertion	Intravascular catheter
	Escherichia coli urinary tract infection associated with an indwelling urinary catheter	Periurethral skin and mucous membranes	Indwelling urinary catheter
Common vehicle	Gram-negative bacteremia associated with intravenous infusion	Liquid substances in the environment	Intrinsically or extrinsically contaminated IV fluids
	Post-transfusion infection with bloodborne, pathogen (HIV, HBV, HCV, CMV)	Infected persons	Blood products from infected donors
	Salmonellosis	Infected/colonized persons	Contaminated food
Vector	Enteric infection	Infected persons or infectious material	Flies, Pharaoh's ants

[a]Varicella-zoster virus may be transmitted by airborne, direct contact, and droplet contact transmission.
[b]Reservoir of infection.
[c]Sources involved in transmission of selected nosocomial infection.
Adapted from Huskins WC, Goldmann DA. Nosocomial infections. *In* Feigin RD, Cherry JD (eds). Textbook of Pediatric Infectious Disease, 4th ed. Philadelphia, WB Saunders, 1998, pp 2545–2585.

other microorganisms occasionally can be transmitted by this route. In one study, a caregiver who was colonized with *P. aeruginosa* apparently transmitted this pathogen to neonates in the NICU and was an important factor in initiating an epidemic of *Pseudomonas* infection in that unit. Investigation revealed that she was an avid swimmer and that both her ear and hands were heavily colonized with the epidemic strain.[346] In the same institution, independent risk factors for an outbreak of β-lactamase–producing, aminoglycoside-resistant enterococci included a nurse who was colonized with the epidemic strain in her gastrointestinal tract and on her hands, as well as hospitalization in a small surgical nursery.[340] In other nurseries, an outbreak of *Proteus mirabilis* infection was attributed to a nurse with vaginal and rectal colonization with this pathogen[139] and cases of *C. koserii (diversus)* meningitis were linked to the presence of personnel colonized with *Citrobacter*.[141, 142] Although gram-negative bacilli generally colonize the skin of the hands transiently, some caregivers develop chronic hand colonization and can directly transfer their microflora to newborns. Other investigators have noted this phenomenon as well.[347–349] *Candida* has been attributed to a colonized caregiver with onychomycosis.[201] Caregivers with infections due to respiratory viruses that are spread by contact, such as RSV, may also infect infants by direct contact. Although there is considerable concern about direct contact transmission of HSV to newborns, such transmission appears to occur relatively rarely. In one dramatic case, however, a caregiver with a cold sore transmitted herpes to an infant during resuscitation in the delivery room.[306]

Indirect contact transmission refers to spread of organisms through an intermediary person or inanimate object (fomite), although some epidemiologists prefer to reserve this term for spread from inanimate objects. Hardy microorganisms that can withstand the rigors of exposure to the environment, especially gram-positive pathogens such as staphylococci and enterococci and spore-forming microorganisms such as *C. difficile*, are particularly likely to be transmitted by fomites. However, even pathogens that persist for relatively short periods in the environment can be spread by indirect contact transmission.[16] For example, RSV survives for only an hour or so on environmental surfaces, yet this is sufficient for indirect contact spread to occur.[255] An outbreak of adenovirus was caused by contaminated ophthalmic equipment.[268] Commonly used objects, such as stethoscopes, may silently transmit nosocomial pathogens such as MRSA and vancomycin-resistant enterococci from patient to patient. Rectal thermometers are particularly dangerous and have been implicated in outbreaks of diverse pathogens, including VRE[350] and *Salmonella*.[351]

Indirect contact transmission from the hands of caregivers occurs far more frequently than transmission by contaminated fomites, and it could reasonably be argued that person-to-person transmission of microorganisms by contaminated hands is far and away the most important factor in endemic and epidemic nosocomial infections in nurseries and NICUs. As noted previously, the newborn gastrointestinal tract is the major reservoir for nosocomial pathogens, with concentrations of microorganisms exceeding billions per gram of feces. Because newborns are by definition incontinent and constantly contaminate themselves and their immediate environment, it is hardly surprising that the hands of caregivers can be contaminated even on casual contact with a colonized infant.[352-354] Gloves provide protection for the hands, but hands are easily contaminated when removing gloves and must be washed before moving on to the next newborn. Thus, fastidious attention to aseptic and barrier technique is critical if hand contamination and subsequent indirect contact spread are to be avoided. Innumerable studies have demonstrated that personnel frequently do not wash their hands when they should, even in the nursery.[355] Overcrowding and understaffing exacerbate the problem, as do inadequate hand-washing facilities and poor nursery design.[16, 76] Caregivers contaminate their hands with pathogens colonizing the infants under their care, fail to wash their hands, and inoculate new arrivals who require pharyngeal or gastrointestinal instrumentation, such as bag resuscitation, suctioning, or nasogastric feedings.[356] Endless opportunities exist for cross-contamination during care of vulnerable newborns, and if the infant has an invasive device, such as an intravenous catheter or endotracheal tube, that breaches normal host barriers, indirect contact transmission of nosocomial pathogens can produce infection in short order.

Indirect contact transmission from contaminated hands also plays a major role in the spread of viral pathogens among hospitalized neonates. RSV is transmitted primarily in this fashion, although caregivers who acquire an RSV upper respiratory tract infection also can inoculate neonates directly.[248-250, 259, 261] Adenovirus cross-infection probably occurs by the same route in many cases.[247, 266] Hands are the essential link in transmission of viruses that are spread by the fecal-oral route, such as hepatitis A.[283, 285] In one outbreak, the index case

was caused by a contaminated transfusion from a patient with hepatitis A, but subsequent transmission occurred by the fecal-oral route.[283] Fecal-oral spread from contaminated hands also plays a major role in the transmission of rotavirus.[246, 288, 289]

Endogenous infection (or autoinfection) originates from a patient's own flora. However, as outlined previously, newborns in the NICU do not have an opportunity to develop their own normal flora or even to acquire their mother's microorganisms. Rather, they are colonized by the nosocomial strains they encounter in the NICU, which are largely brought to them on the hands of their caregivers. Thus, endogenous infections in the NICU setting may be viewed as a special variation of direct and indirect contact transmission. These microorganisms populate their respiratory and gastrointestinal tracts, umbilicus, and skin, from where they can invade the bloodstream directly through the neonate's fragile cutaneous barriers, gain access to the bloodstream from intravascular devices, enter the lungs by means of ventilatory equipment or aspiration of pharyngeal secretions, or inoculate a surgical wound.

Even microorganisms that are widely assumed to be classic examples of endogenous infection, such as CONS and *Candida*, may be transmitted nosocomially from patient to patient from the hands of caregivers. Distinct strains of *S. haemolyticus*[94, 99] and *S. epidermidis*[81, 89, 94, 100] may become endemic or epidemic in the nursery and NICU. In one study, two strains of *S. epidermidis* were recovered from bloodstream infections over nearly a decade, and one of these strains was isolated from a nurse's hands at the end of this study period.[81] Similarly, outbreaks of *Candida* infection in newborns have been attributed to person-to-person transmission from the hands of nursery personnel.[198-201]

Droplet contact transmission involves transfer of microorganisms by large respiratory droplets, which may be generated by coughing, sneezing, or vigorously pronouncing the letters "t" or "p." Such droplets travel only a few feet, and transmission can be interrupted effectively by wearing a mask or staying 3 or 4 feet away from the patient. Important pathogens with the potential for nosocomial spread from droplet contact include *B. pertussis*, *Neisseria meningitidis*, and group A streptococci.[16, 44] Nosocomial spread of these pathogens in the nursery setting appears to be quite rare. Respiratory viral pathogens, such as adenovirus and parainfluenza viruses, are believed to be transmitted by large respiratory droplets, although rigorous data supporting this assumption are difficult to come by. RSV theoretically could be transmitted by droplets, but, as noted previously, both direct and indirect contact transmission appear to be much more important.

Airborne transmission may be subdivided into three distinct modes of spread: *droplet nucleus* transmission, *shedding*, and airborne dispersion of *fungal spores*. Droplet nuclei are the very small (several micron) particles aerosolized from the respiratory tract. Unlike the larger particles involved in droplet contact transmission, droplet nuclei can waft on air currents over long distances and can remain suspended in the air for minutes or even an hour or so. Because of their size, they are ideally suited to penetrating upper airway defenses and entering the lungs. Classic pathogens transmitted by droplet nuclei include measles, TB, *Legionella*, influenza, and varicella (under special circumstances, such as varicella pneumonia).[357, 358] However, data regarding droplet nucleus transmission in newborns are remarkably sparse. In general, nosocomial bacteria are not spread by droplet nuclei. Gram-negative bacilli may be detected in air samples using very sensitive techniques, but epidemiologists have been largely unsuccessful in attributing outbreaks due to these pathogens to airborne transmission. Group A streptococci may cause infections in operating rooms due to airborne inoculation of wounds, but airborne spread has not been documented in the nursery. As noted earlier, *S. aureus* is spread predominantly by contact in the nursery. In Rammelkamp's studies,[48] an infant known to be colonized with staphylococci was placed in a nursery and newborns were placed directly next to this infant or 4.5 or 11 feet away. Caregivers took extraordinary precautions not to transmit *S. aureus* person to person. Of the 91 newborns brought into the unit, only three became colonized with the index newborn's strain. It has been suggested that colonized newborns who have a concomitant upper respiratory viral infection might be more efficient disseminators of staphylococci—the so-called cloud baby phenomenon[359]—and a similar mechanism of spread has been reported in adults.[360]

Shedding refers to dissemination of microorganisms on colonized skin squames (or rafts) of caregivers. The vast majority of studies have been directed at shedding of *S. aureus*, although other microorganisms, such as group A streptococci and *Rhodococcus*, may be spread in this fashion as well.[44] Considering how frequently adults are colonized with *S. aureus* (up to 80% have staphylococci transiently in their nose at one time or another, and 20 to 40% are colonized for a longer period), it is remarkable how infrequently staphylococcal shedders have been implicated in nosocomial outbreaks. Nasal carriage often leads to skin colonization but rarely to significant shedding. Skin disease, such as eczema, or active infection may increase shedding greatly, but some shedders have no such risk factors. Shedding occurs predominantly from the perineum and is not blocked by standard scrub uniforms or surgical gowns. Colonized skin squames may be carried considerable distances on air currents but usually settle out in the general environment of the shedder. Because outbreaks of infection attributable to a shedder are the rare exception to the rule, care should be taken to avoid indiscriminate culturing of staff and sanctions against carriers unless careful epidemiology and characterization of staphylococcal strains have been performed.

Fungal spores from potential pathogens such as *Aspergillus* are ubiquitous in the environment, especially in soil and decaying organic material. It is not uncommon for such spores to be found in the environment of hospitals (e.g., on cultures of dust deposits). Fungal spores have a shape and size that are ideal for airborne dissemination over long distances, and they can easily enter the pulmonary tree or be deposited on the skin. Infections due to invasive filamentous fungi were not a significant problem before the advent of neonatal intensive care. Very premature or critically ill neonates clearly are vulnerable to such infections. Outbreaks of *Rhizopus*, *Aspergillus*, and other filamentous fungal infection have been reported in the literature.[227, 230, 242, 343, 344] The fragile skin of neonates appears to be a special risk factor, and the trauma (i.e., secondary to tape or adhesives) produced by trying to stabilize and secure intravenous catheters and endotracheal tubes may lead to inoculation of fungal spores and cutaneous infection. In one *Rhizopus* outbreak, contamination of wooden tongue depressors was linked to infection,[242] and latex finger stalls were linked to an *Aspergillus* outbreak in another NICU.[361] Careful housekeeping and good skin care are essential to prevent such infections, and strong consideration should be given to providing critically ill newborns with spore-free, HEPA-filtered air.

Common source (or common vehicle) infection is caused when a medication, solution, or piece of equipment becomes contaminated and subsequently colonizes infants who are exposed to the contaminated item. Common source outbreaks are a form of indirect contact spread by fomites run rampant. Such outbreaks should be rare in vigilant nurseries, but they remain surprisingly common, particularly when new devices or technologies are introduced. For example, blood pressure transducers caused numerous outbreaks before intensivists learned how to use them safely and refinements in design were made.[205, 362] A topical preparation designed to improve the integrity of neonatal skin and reduce the risk of infection[363] also has been responsible for a common source outbreak of infection.[364] Gram-negative bacilli can cause mischief if they are provided with even a modicum of moisture. For example, *Burkholderia cepacia* can survive in disinfectants, medications with preservatives, and antiseptics[365] and can even grow in distilled water for years with penicillin as its only carbon source.[365] Use of multidose medications and solutions and failure to properly disinfect medical devices open the door to contamination and common source outbreaks of infection. The list of published common source outbreaks is extensive and includes contaminated intravenous fluids,[165, 366] lipids,[367] multidose vials of glycerin,[203] breast milk,[368] enteral feeds (especially contamination with *Enterobacter*),[369, 370] blood products,[283, 284] a nonchlorinated water supply,[135] antiseptics,[136, 167, 168] hand lotions,[371, 372] suction machines,[146] delivery room resuscitators,[150] and laryngoscopes,[134] to mention just a few examples.

Vector transmission refers to spread by insects. Although this should occur rarely in a well-maintained hospital, it should be remembered that ants, roaches, and flies can carry nosocomial pathogens on their legs.[373-375] In tropical countries there is a danger of mosquito-borne dengue fever in hospitals. One of the authors has witnessed first hand the consequences of allowing insects into a newborn unit. In the course of investigating an outbreak of *S. aureus* in a nursery, maggots were observed crawling out of an infant's nose.

Risk Factors

Newborns, especially premature newborns, intrinsically have a higher risk of infection than older patients because of their immature immunologic system, fragile cutaneous barrier, and lack of endogenous microflora (see Chapter 2). Birth weight is an especially important risk factor for nosocomial infection in the neonate, and studies examining other potential risk factors must adjust assiduously for the neonate's degree of prematurity.[3, 8, 12, 25, 32, 376, 377] It is important to stratify neonates into narrow birthweight strata because Freeman and associates demonstrated that the risk of bloodstream infection with CONS increased precipitously only when birth weight fell below 1500 g.[376] Length of stay in the NICU is another extremely important risk factor for infection.[8,

[12, 32, 376] Thus, it is customary to present data on NICU infections stratified by birth weight and expressed as incidence density per 100 or 1000 patient-days of exposure to the unit.

However, it may be more useful to further adjust data regarding device-associated infections by the time of exposure to the device in question, as is routinely done by the NNIS study (Fig. 34–1). Even this may not adjust adequately for the risk of exposure to the device. For example, NNIS groups all umbilical and central venous catheters together when calculating days of exposure to these intravascular devices, even though each type of

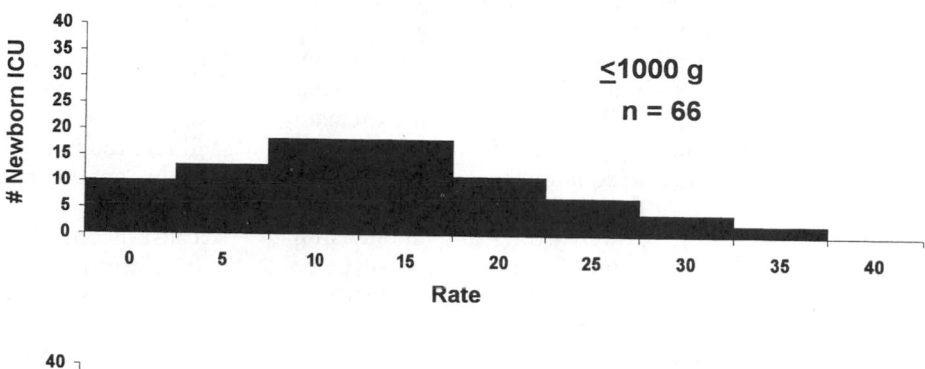

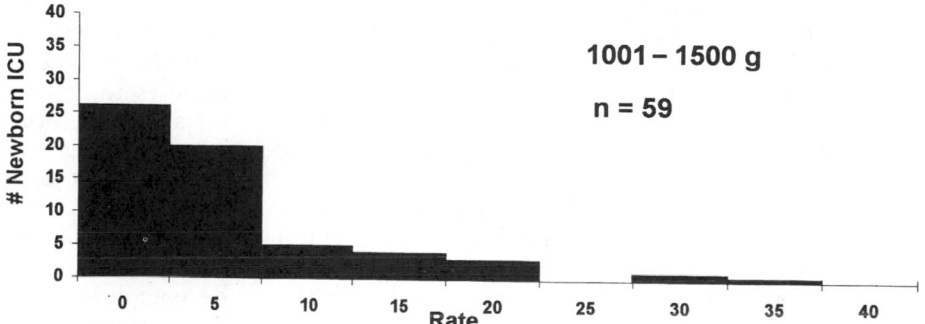

FIGURE 34–1 Central or umbilical intravascular catheter-associated bloodstream infection (BSI) rates by birth weight category for newborn intensive care units (NICU) in National Nosocomial Infections Surveillance System hospitals. Data for larger than 2500 g and 1501 to 2500 g birth weight categories are from October 1986 to September 1994; data for 1001 to 1500 g and 1000 g or less birth weight categories are from January 1992 to September 1994. Rate = the number of central or umbilical intravascular catheter–associated BSI per 1000 central or umbilical catheter-days. (Modified from Gaynes RP, Edwards JR, Jarvis WR, et al: Nosocomial infections among neonates in high-risk nurseries in the United States. Pediatrics 98:357–361, 1996, with permission.)

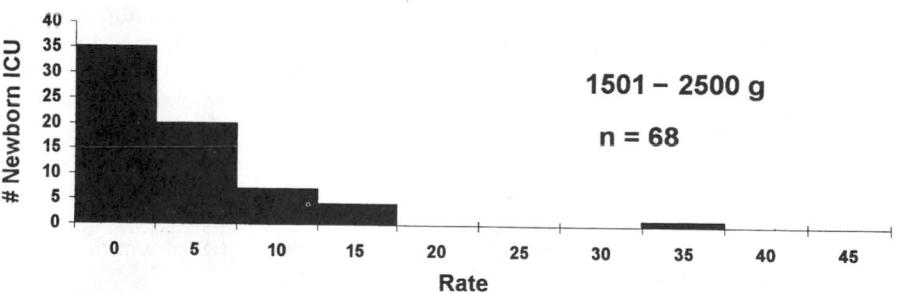

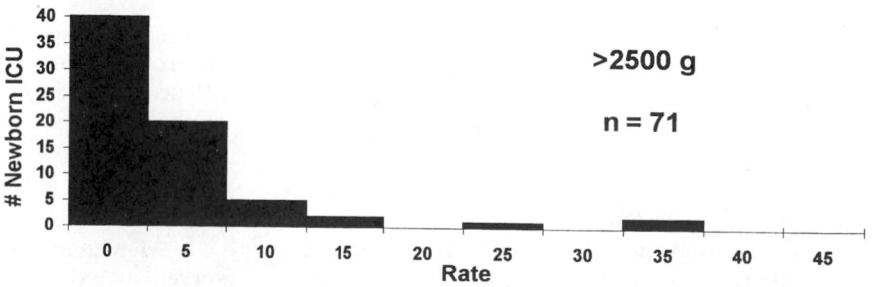

catheter confers a different degree of risk and some patients have more than one catheter type present at the same time. Despite the limitations of these data, it appears that patients in the NICU have a higher risk of intravascular catheter-related bacteremia and a lower risk of ventilator-associated pneumonia than their adult counterparts in the NNIS data base.[1]

Low birth weight may not accurately reflect the severity of illness of a newborn in the NICU. One infant with a birth weight of 1000 g may be much more critically ill as measured by physiologic parameters than another of the same weight. Scoring systems that reflect the physiologic severity of illness of newborns[378-380] and the intensity of therapeutic interventions[381] have been developed and validated. Although it may seem obvious that infants who have the greatest degree of physiologic instability at birth would have the greatest risk of infection, as suggested by a study using the Score for Neonatal Acute Physiology (SNAP),[382] it may be that including other risk factors, such as exposure to invasive devices, in the prediction model adequately accounts for most of the effect of underlying severity of illness.[383]

As noted previously, overcrowding and understaffing increase the risk of nosocomial transmission of pathogens and infection. It has been demonstrated that moving from an outdated NICU to a facility with 50% more nurses and far better design and sink placement reduced the rate of nosocomial infection from 5.8 to 1.8% after controlling for a variety of other potential risk factors.[28] Haley and colleagues showed that infant:nurse ratios exceeding 7:1 and high census increased the risk of colonization with MRSA in an intermediate-care nursery.[75, 76]

Exposure to invasive medical devices also exposes neonates to a substantially increased infection risk. Central venous catheters, especially percutaneous central venous and umbilical lines, appear to be associated with the greatest risk.[34, 384-386] Peripherally inserted soft catheters that are passed centrally ("spaghetti lines") may be safer, but studies in newborns are limited. In studies spanning a decade, risk of CONS infection was independently associated with central venous catheterization, especially when catheterization was prolonged.[90, 383] However, the independent contribution of central lines to infection risk appeared to be substantially less in the 1990s than in the previous decade, perhaps due to more reliance on peripherally inserted long lines and tunneled catheters. Interestingly, lipid therapy was at least as important a risk factor as central venous catheters in the earlier study, and in the later study the risk of lipid therapy far exceeded that of central venous catheters, independently accounting for the majority of infections. Lipids slow flow through catheters, provide fuel for proliferation of CONS in the presence of small amounts of protein, and may have an adverse impact on host defense.[90] Endemic risk does not appear to be related to contamination of lipids, although contamination can produce common source outbreaks, as noted previously. Lipid therapy also may predispose to *Candida* infections[217, 219, 387] as well as *Malassezia* infections.[203, 224]

Mechanical ventilation is the principal risk factor for nosocomial pneumonia in the NICU. Contamination of respiratory therapy equipment due to inadequate processing or in-use contamination used to be an important cause of gram-negative necrotizing pneumonia in neonatal intensive care. A number of outbreaks due to "water bugs," such as *Acinetobacter*, *Chryseobacterium* (*Flavobacterium*), and *Pseudomonas*, were reported in newborns, often linked to contamination of nebulizers that generated small particle aerosols.[163, 388, 389] Better processing practices, use of heated, rather than mechanical, humidification systems, and improved standards for the maintenance of small-volume mechanical nebulizers have drastically reduced the risk of pneumonia. However, nosocomial pneumonia remains a threat to ventilated neonates. Although few studies have been performed in newborns, it seems reasonable to extrapolate from studies in older patients, which have been summarized in a CDC guideline on prevention of nosocomial pneumonia.[390] Factors that increase colonization of the gastrointestinal tract, such as use of acid-reducing agents, and facilitate reflux of gastric contents into the pharynx, such as bolus enteral feedings, nasogastric tubes, and supine position, appear to be especially relevant in neonates. Because neonatal endotracheal tubes generally are uncuffed, aspiration of pathogens in oropharyngeal secretions occurs readily. Recent studies also have suggested that mechanical ventilation is a risk factor for CONS bacteremia, perhaps due to seeding of the bloodstream by CONS in the respiratory tract during suctioning.[3, 383]

Prolonged therapy with antibiotics undoubtedly predisposes to colonization and infection with antibiotic-resistant microorganisms, including *Candida*, posing substantial treatment challenges.[8, 391] A recent evaluation of the use of corticosteroids to reduce the impact of bronchopulmonary dysplasia found a significantly increased risk of nosocomial infection.[392] Surgical procedures, including placement of ventricular shunts, may be complicated by nosocomial surgical site infection. Patent ductus arteriosus was associated with a substantially increased risk of infection in an older study,[381] and complications such as bronchopulmonary dysplasia and necrotizing enterocolitis were associated with bacteremia in a more recent collaborative study,[32] although care must be taken in interpreting these data because adjustment for underlying severity of illness was incomplete. Fetal scalp electrodes are a clear risk factor for scalp abscesses, herpesvirus infection,[299, 348, 393, 394] and perhaps human immunodeficiency virus, but because these pathogens derive from the mother it may be debated whether they are truly nosocomial.

PREVENTION AND CONTROL

There are three principal goals for hospital infection control and prevention programs: (1) protect the patient; (2) protect the health care worker, visitors, and others in the health care environment; and (3) accomplish the previous two goals in a cost-effective manner if possible. The principal functions of infection control are listed below[395]:

1. Managing critical data and information, including surveillance of nosocomial infections

2. Setting and recommending policies and procedures

3. Intervening directly to interrupt the transmission of infectious diseases

4. Educating and training health care workers and providers

These basic principles of infection control are applicable to both the well-baby and the high-risk neonatal nurseries. Policies and procedures for infection control in nurseries should be established by the hospital infection control program based on valid scientific data and recommendations of national organizations, consensus groups, and regulatory agencies such as the AAP and the CDC. An infection control manual should be readily available to all health care workers in the nursery. The responsibilities of infection control program personnel include (1) coordination among relevant departments involved in the nursery (e.g., delivery room, central supply, microbiology, pharmacy, respiratory therapy, nursing, and physicians); (2) authority to institute appropriate precautions and isolation for individual patients, including closing the nursery to admission if necessary; (3) notification of nursery staff of specific diseases or potential infection control problems identified in the nursery; (4) assistance in implementing and evaluating infection control policies and procedures in the nursery; and (5) participation in continuing in-service education of nursery personnel.

Surveillance

Surveillance is an essential component of a hospital infection prevention and control program.[396] Surveillance data can help infection control programs focus their prevention and control efforts on the highest-risk patients and can provide a means of evaluating the effectiveness of these interventions. By establishing baseline endemic rates of nosocomial infections, surveillance also facilitates detection of outbreaks. Essential components of a neonatal surveillance program include (1) clear, objective definitions of infection; (2) reliable and valid data collection methods; (3) use of appropriate denominators when calculating and reporting rates (e.g., admissions, patient days, days of exposure to invasive devices); and (4) stratification of infection rates by birthweight category.[397]

The definitions of some neonatal nosocomial infections remain controversial and problematic. Valid criteria for distinguishing colonization of the respiratory tract from pneumonia in a ventilated newborn remain elusive. Contamination of blood cultures may be difficult to differentiate from true bloodstream infection, especially when relatively less pathogenic bacteria, such as CONS, are involved. Although most authorities recommend obtaining two independent cultures to work up an episode of suspected bloodstream infection, this is difficult to achieve in tiny newborns. Measuring the concentration of bacteria in the blood by quantitative culture is of questionable value because neonatal bacteremia can be very low grade. Criteria such as whether cultures turn positive in between 24 and 48 hours need to be studied further and may be of little practical utility.[398–400] Measurement of C-reactive protein or cytokine levels may be helpful but require further evaluation.[401, 402]

Routine cultures of body surfaces (skin, umbilicus, mucous membranes, tracheal aspirates, rectal swabs) of newborns or employees for colonization surveillance are generally not recommended. Colonization rates are not accurate predictors of infection, and correlation of isolates from surveillance cultures and invasive infections has been poor. Routine culturing is also very costly. During epidemics, surface cultures of skin, mucous membranes, and gastrointestinal sites may be helpful in identifying colonized infants and aid in cohorting infants colonized with the offending pathogen.[16, 189, 321] Such cultures may also serve as an indicator of compliance with outbreak control measures.[14, 38, 321, 397, 403–408] Stool surveillance for gentamicin and third-generation cephalosporin-resistant gram-negative rods and VRE, as well as surveillance of skin and mucosal sites for MRSA, may be useful in guiding empirical antibiotic therapy and in controlling the spread of these organisms.[16, 397] Also, in units with no clinical cases of VRE, it is now recommended that surveillance cultures be done at 6- to 12-month intervals to detect the presence of VRE before establishment of high colonization rates and clinical disease.[114] Recommendations for screening infants for MRSA and multiresistant gram-negative rods have not been published.

The intensity of surveillance will vary with the type of nursery and facilities available. In the NICU, all infections at all sites should be monitored. In the normal nursery, surveillance should concentrate on infections likely to be associated with outbreaks, such as staphylococcal or streptococcal skin infections, gastroenteritis, and respiratory viral infections. Various surveillance methods for nosocomial infection have been used. In the nursery, surveillance should include ward rounds, discussions with nursery staff, chart review, and concurrent review of culture reports. Data from culture reports should include bacterial isolates and the antimicrobial susceptibility patterns of pathogens.

Surveillance of nursery infections should also include identification of postdischarge infections. Although it is costly and difficult to capture a large proportion of nosocomial infections post discharge, review of readmission records and cultures, telephone reports from physicians and parents, and postcard surveillance (to parents or pediatricians or both) may be helpful. Computerized records of some managed-care organizations may facilitate identification of postdischarge infections, but very few hospitals have links to health care maintenance organization data bases. In hospitals with NICUs, surveillance of newborns transferred to other care units or other hospitals for at least 48 hours after transfer is also important.

Feedback of surveillance data (e.g., rates of infection, trends of antimicrobial resistance patterns) to clinicians should be performed regularly using an easy-to-understand graphic format. Surveillance data should be used to target areas for further investigation, additional staff education, and specific interventions.

Infection Rates

The numerator for reporting nosocomial infection rates is the number of verified cases of infection as defined by the infection control program. Selection of an appropriate denominator is more complex. It is important to calculate the cumulative incidence of nosocomial infections, for example, the number of infections per 100 patients admitted to the NICU. In addition, incidence density, or the number of infections occurring in a specified number of days in the NICU (e.g., per 1000 patient-days), should be calculated, because the risk of infection is related to an infant's total exposure to the unit. Because nosocomial infections generally are related to exposure to specific invasive devices, further information can be conveyed by presenting the incidence density in terms of device days (e.g., the number of nosocomial bacteremias per 1000 central venous catheter days, or the number of cases of nosocomial pneumonias per 1000 ventilator-days). Adjusting for exposure to specific devices may facilitate comparisons among NICUs.[377] Device utilization ratios have been shown to be useful for interhospital comparisons as long as the information has been obtained using the same surveillance definitions and techniques. The device utilization ratio is the measure of a neonatal unit's invasive device practices and, therefore, extrinsic risk of nosocomial infection. This ratio may also serve as a marker for severity of disease. If the device utilization ratio in a specific unit is above the 90th percentile, that is considered high for the particular device used and further investigation of that specific practice may be indicated.[35] Examples of how to calculate device-associated infection rates and device utilization rates are shown in Figure 34–2.

The association between birth weight and risk of nosocomial infection in the NICU patient is well recognized. For this reason, NNIS stratifies data regarding nosocomial infections in NICUs into the following birth weight categories: less than or equal to 1000 g; 1001 to 1500 g; 1501 to 2500 g; and greater than 2500 g (Table 34–7).[377] NICUs participating in the NNIS report wide variations in infection rates within birth categories, even after adjusting for duration of exposure to invasive devices. These disparities may be due to differences in exposure to other risk factors, such as use of total parenteral nutrition or lipids or surgical procedures that are not captured by the NNIS data. NICU programs with higher rates may also be tempted to claim that they care for a more critically ill neonatal population, because it is well known that birth weight alone is not a perfect proxy for severity of illness. The SNAP, a well-validated severity of illness scoring system, is a better predictor of mortality than birth weight alone.[378, 379, 381–383] A study by Gray and co-workers suggested that adjustment for SNAP plus birth weight predicted the risk of nosocomial infection better than birth weight alone.[381] However, a subsequent study in infants weighing less than 1500 gs suggested that SNAP adjustment was not required if exposure to risk factors such as lipids and central venous catheters was included in the analysis.[383] CRIB (clinical risk index for babies), a severity of illness scoring system popular in Europe, also has been used to adjust for

TABLE 34–7

Pooled Means of Device-Associated Infection Rates by Birth Weight Category in Newborn Intensive Care Units in National Nosocomial Infections Surveillance System Hospitals[a]

	POOLED MEANS	
BIRTH WEIGHT CATEGORY	Central or Umbilical Intravascular Catheter-Associated Bloodstream Infections/ 1000 Central or Umbilical Line Days	Ventilator-Associated Pneumonia/1000 Ventilator Days
≤ 1000 g	12.9	4.8
1001–1500 g	8.3	4.6
1501–2500 g	6.3	3.9
> 2500 g	4.9	3.0

[a]Data are from January 1992 to May 1995.
Modified from National Nosocomial Infections Surveillance System (NNIS). National Nosocomial Infections Surveillance System (NNIS) semi-annual report, May 1995. Am J Infect Control 23:377–385, 1995.

severity of illness in studies of NICU nosocomial infections.[380] Another study used the GRASP system workload quantification method to calculate a time and intensity-of-care adjusted nosocomial infection incidence density. Use of the sum of all infants' daily patient care hours (recorded by the nursing staff) as the denominator was found to effectively control for the difference in risk factors between units.[409] Incorporating adjustment for severity of illness into routine surveillance and use of composite risk indices appropriate for the NICU require further development and evaluation.[410] Until this happens, the validity of interhospital comparisons of nosocomial infection rates in NICUs will be uncertain.

Investigation of Outbreaks

An outbreak usually presents as a cluster of infections, but a single highly unusual infection may be sufficient to initiate an investigation.[411] Some outbreaks are difficult to recognize because they occur intermittently, involve multiple microorganisms, or involve infection at various anatomic sites.[412]

Recognition of a nursery outbreak is dependent on careful surveillance and appropriate criteria for differentiating endemic from epidemic rates of infection. Real-time trending of data is critical for outbreak recognition. Statistical process control, favored by quality improvement–oriented infection control programs, is a particularly powerful method for early outbreak detection. Common source outbreaks (e.g., due to contaminated solutions or equipment or to a carrier on the NICU staff) often present explosively with a fast up-tick in the infection rate. Person-to-person spread of an epidemic strain usually results in more sporadic cases rather than a sharp peak. However, common source

Device-associated infection rates:

$$\frac{\text{Number of device-associated infections for a specific site}}{\text{Number of device days}} \times 1000 = \text{Device-associated infection rate}$$

Device utilization ratio:

$$\frac{\text{Number of device days}}{\text{Number of patient days}} = \text{Device utilization ratio}$$

FIGURE 34–2 Calculation of device-associated infection: rate and device utilization ratio. (Adapted from NNIS Report, Data Summary from October 1996–April 1998, issued June 1998. Hospital Infections Program, National Center for Infectious Diseases, Centers for Diseases Control and Prevention, Public Health Service, US Department of Health and Human Service, Atlanta, Ga.)

outbreaks may be accompanied by person-to-person transmission from infected or colonized infants, so that the shape of the epidemic curve may be harder to interpret. Surveillance methods should be clearly specified and documented throughout the investigation, including case finding and laboratory techniques to identify pathogens.[413] Molecular genotyping techniques are a valuable adjunct to outbreak investigation and largely have replaced older phenotyping techniques such as phage typing and colicin typing. Genotyping is most useful when it is applied to test a epidemiologic hypothesis established during the course of an outbreak investigation. The most efficient epidemiologic method for investigating outbreaks is generally the case-control study.[414, 415]

Clusters of unusual or low-frequency events should be compared with past experience, including similar outbreaks in the literature and comparison with uniformly kept epidemiologic records for at least the preceding 6 to 12 months in the same hospital. An increase in infections involving a number of different organisms is likely to be related to breakdown in infection control techniques such as may occur with crowding, understaffing, or other major disruptions of nursery routine. An increase in infections due to a single organism should prompt a search for a point source, although person-to-person spread is more likely.[397] Once a cluster of nosocomial infections is identified, an epidemiologic investigation should be initiated. This includes identification of the responsible organism(s), reservoirs of infection, modes of transmission, and risk factors. Intensified surveillance for new cases should be initiated. Case finding during an outbreak investigation should include listing of admission and discharge dates for all cases, their location in the nurseries, and common caretakers, procedures, and equipment. A line listing of infected or colonized patients and key exposures and potential risk factors should be maintained during the investigation for later analysis.

It is essential to carefully consider which data elements are required for the investigation, and a paper or computerized data collection form should be developed and pilot tested. Failure to collect data in a standardized, rigorous fashion vastly complicates elucidation of the problem. In conducting a case-control study, care should be taken not to overmatch cases and controls early in the investigation because criteria used in matching cannot be studied as potential risk factors. A detailed record of all meetings and specific actions that were taken during the outbreak should be maintained. Approaches to the investigation of clusters of nosocomial infections have been published.[397, 412] Active surveillance should also be instituted for infants recently discharged from the hospital, especially when the nursery stay is short.

Infection control procedures such as hand washing, aseptic technique, cleaning, decontamination, disinfection, sterilization, and cohorting should be reviewed, and the importance of compliance with the policies should be emphasized. In many instances these general infection control procedures will end an outbreak before the source is identified.

Culturing of potential environmental sources or personnel should be performed only if epidemiologic information suggests an association with infection. Nursery epidemics have occasionally been traced to infected or chronically colonized personnel. Those implicated by epidemiologic data as sources during an outbreak investigation should be removed from patient care and when applicable receive treatment appropriate for the organism involved.[397, 411]

Infection Control Policies

Prevention of nosocomial infection requires establishment and rigorous adherence to well-defined policies and procedures necessary to optimize and standardize hospital routines and patient care practices. Written infection prevention and control policies and procedures must be established, implemented, maintained, and updated periodically. They should be scientifically valid, reviewed for practicality and cost, and lead to improved patient outcomes.[395] These policies may vary according to the level of care provided in the nursery (e.g., term infant vs. intensive care) and resources available in the hospital.[416] Numerous guidelines have been published that can help in the development of policies and procedures.[417]

Although many infection control policies have been evaluated and validated by epidemiologic studies, other nursery routines or rituals have evolved by custom or consensus. There is little evidence that such nursery rituals affect the incidence of nosocomial infection in either the well-baby or intensive care nurseries. For example, there is no evidence to support the routine use of gowns, masks, caps, or hair nets for personnel or sterile linens in bassinets or incubators.[16]

Numerous studies have shown poor compliance with policies and procedures such as hand washing and isolation precautions. To improve performance in such critical areas of infection control, nursery and hospital administrators need to make compliance with policies and procedures an organizational priority. They should support staff education, feed back nosocomial surveillance data to motivate staff members, and remove barriers to improve performance. For example, improved performance of isolation precautions cannot be expected if gloves are not readily available or inconveniently located. More studies need to be done to elucidate the reasons for noncompliance and to investigate ways to modify staff behavior.[412]

Ocular Prophylaxis

At delivery, the newborn's eyes should be cleaned with sterile cotton to remove secretions and debris.[397] Prevention of gonococcus neonatorum, although not a nursery-acquired infection, is an important infection control practice in the nursery and is mandatory for all neonates, including those born by cesarean delivery. A variety of topical agents appear to be equally effective, including application of two drops of 1% silver nitrate in single-dose containers or a 1- to 2-cm ribbon of sterile ophthalmic ointment containing 1% tetracycline or 0.5% erythromycin in single-use tubes. The eyes should not be irrigated after instillation of any of these agents.[416] A single dose of ceftriaxone, 125 mg (25–50 mg/kg for low-birth-weight infants, not to exceed 125 mg) administered intramuscularly or intravenously, is recommended for infants born to mothers with active gonorrhea at the time of delivery.[418] Topical erythromycin and tetracycline avoid the chemical conjunctivitis caused by silver nitrate, but neither agent is of proven benefit in the prevention of *Chlamydia trachomatis* ophthalmia. Recent studies have shown that none of the prophylactic agents significantly reduced the incidence of chlamydial conjunctivitis, and ocular prophylaxis cannot prevent chlamydial pneumonitis.[419, 420]

Eyes may become infected with water-borne organisms in humid incubators or from contaminated respiratory secretions. Nosocomial conjunctivitis has been reported frequently in NICUs. Care should be taken to avoid contaminating eyes with drips from suction catheters after suctioning the nasopharynx or endotracheal tube.[421]

Skin and Cord Care

Every effort should be made to promote colonization of the newborn with normal flora and to impede colonization with nosocomial pathogens. This is easier said than done, especially in the NICU. To do so, multiple methods of skin and cord care have been evaluated. These practices are divided into measures taken in the delivery room and daily routines in the nursery. Several approaches to skin and cord care have been used, but no optimal procedures have been recommended until recently. Lund and colleagues reviewed the literature addressing the care of neonatal skin and created a new and comprehensive practice guideline for clinicians, which is in the process of being evaluated in 58 sites in the United States.[422] Excessive drying, manipulation, exposure to irritating chemicals, or other trauma (e.g., adhesive tape) should be avoided to reduce the risk of damage to newborn skin. The skin of the premature infant is particularly fragile.[4] Bathing should be postponed until the neonate's thermal stability is ensured.[423]

After initial observation and stabilization of the newborn, meconium and blood may be wiped off with sterile cotton sponges soaked with warm water to remove potential blood-borne pathogens such as HBV or HIV and other contaminating microorganisms such as HSV. Personnel should wear gloves until cleaning is complete.[397] The skin should be carefully dried to minimize further heat loss. Except for cleansing and bathing as needed with water alone or a mild soap, the skin and cord may be kept dry for the rest of the hospital stay. The gelatinous skin of extremely immature neonates should be cleaned with sterile water and only when necessary.[423] The effectiveness of Aquafor ointment (Beiersdorf, Norwalk, Conn) in protecting neonatal skin and reducing nosocomial infections is being studied.[422]

Whole-body bathing and antiseptic soaps are not necessary for routine care, but they may be indicated in outbreaks or when the endemic rate of infection is high.[44] Various antiseptic compounds for skin care have been studied to determine their safety and efficacy in preventing colonization and infection in neonates. The most frequently used compounds capable of reducing bacterial colonization of the skin are iodophors, hexachlorophene, and chlorhexidine. Hexachlorophene, although relatively effective against gram-positive bacteria, is no longer recommended for routine daily bathing of newborns and is now seldom used in any circumstance in premature neonates because of its neurotoxicity when absorbed.[51, 52, 424] It may be useful as an alternative for term infants for control of *S. aureus* outbreaks. It should be used for a limited number of baths at a concentration of no more than 3% and should be carefully rinsed off after bathing.[423]

Preparations containing chlorhexidine, a compound that is poorly absorbed through intact skin, may be less toxic than hexachlorophene and have been found to be useful for bathing or for localized skin care. Chlorhexidine has also been used in outbreak control. It is less effective than hexachlorophene for *S. aureus* but more effective for gram-negative bacilli.[54–56, 423, 425–429] Iodophor detergents, widely used for surgical scrubs and nursery hand washing, are not recommended for routine bathing or cord care. Staining of the infant's skin with iodine is unattractive, and iodine-containing compounds may suppress neonatal thyroid function.[423, 430] The benefits of using an antiseptic agent for bathing should be weighed against the risk of toxicity.

No single method of cord care has proved to be superior in preventing colonization and disease.[423] The cord should be cut and tied using aseptic technique. Dry cord care is an acceptable regimen. A number of studies have evaluated the effectiveness of antimicrobial agents in cord care. Isopropyl alcohol, which is often applied daily or even more frequently during the hospitalization and after discharge, may accelerate drying and separation of the cord but does not affect colonization.[431] Triple dye (2.29 g of brilliant green, 1.14 g of proflavine hemisulfate, and 2.29 g of crystal violet per liter in an aqueous solution) delays drying and cord separation for 7 to 10 days and inhibits colonization, but colonization of the cord after discontinuation of its use can, of course, occur. In one NICU study, triple dye was shown to delay but not prevent colonization with MRSA, but in another report, application of triple dye after umbilical vessel catheterization in the first 12 hours after birth was instrumental in controlling a prolonged MRSA outbreak.[66, 75] Chlorhexidine cord care has been reported to be effective in reducing colonization and infection.[432-434] Topical mupirocin was shown to be effective in an outbreak of MRSA when applied to the cord and nares of infants in a special care unit.[74] Short-term use of mupirocin ointment for control of an outbreak associated with susceptible *S. aureus* or MRSA may be considered, but prolonged use has been associated with the emergence of resistant strains.[435] Other agents that have been studied include bacitracin ointment and silver sulfadiazine cream. The literature on cord care is confusing and inconsistent, as pointed out by a recent meta-analysis.[436]

Insertion and Maintenance of Invasive Devices

Advances in technology in the NICU have given rise to new nosocomial infection risks. Whenever a new invasive procedure or device is introduced into the nursery the potential risk for infection should be evaluated. Policies and procedures should be developed to minimize risk of infection and infection rates monitored. Infection control recommendations for the insertion and maintenance of endotracheal tubes, urinary catheters, and intravascular devices are similar to those recommended for adults.[437-439] There are limited data in the form of randomized controlled clinical trials from which to make specific recommendations for the NICU.

Nosocomial bloodstream infection is the most frequent device-related infection in the nursery. Of primary concern is the use of umbilical catheters and central venous catheters. Umbilical catheters are now used for initial management of the sick neonate and are no longer used for long-term vascular access. Umbilical lines should be inserted using aseptic technique. The nonsterile insertion site and devitalized cord tissue increase the risk of colonization. Several investigators have reported lower rates of umbilical catheter colonization among neonates receiving systemic antibiotics during umbilical catheterization.[440-442] However, a study of prophylactic antibiotic use in patients with chronic UACs found no clear benefit.[443]

There have been few prospective randomized trials evaluating the insertion and maintenance of central venous catheters in neonates. There are limited data examining the effect of dressing regimens, frequency of re-placement of catheters, or catheter material in reducing the incidence of catheter-related infection among neonates. Garland and colleagues found that 0.5% chlorhexidine gluconate in 70% isopropyl alcohol was more efficacious than 10% povidone-iodine for the prevention of peripheral intravenous catheter colonization in neonates.[444] The use of the biopatch dressing in neonates has been evaluated and found to reduce colonization of catheters, but it had unacceptable skin reactions in very low birth weight infants.[445] A study by Ford-Jones and associates demonstrated that infusion tubing in neonates receiving lipids should be changed at least every 24 hours, although less frequent changes are advocated if lipids are not being administered.[446] To prevent contamination of the catheter hub and internal lumen of the catheter, it is critical to minimize manipulation of the delivery system to prevent the introduction of contaminants. Some infection control authorities recommend disinfecting the hubs of disconnected systems with alcohol before reconnection. Complete recommendations, which in general are relevant to the NICU, have been published by the CDC.[439]

Nursery Staff

Because overcrowding and understaffing contribute to increased infection rates, adequate nursing staffing is important in the prevention of nursery-acquired infections.[16, 76, 322] There should be sufficient personnel to provide appropriate care of infants with adequate time for hand washing between patient contacts.[397] The AAP and American College of Obstetricians and Gynecologists, which have jointly developed guidelines for perinatal care, recommend one nurse per six to eight infants in the normal newborn nursery, one nurse per two to three infants in the intermediate care nursery, and one nurse per one to two infants in the intensive care nursery.[447] Nurseries with partial rooming-in require one nurse per shift for every three to four mother-infant pairs.[447] Nursing-to-infant ratios not meeting guidelines have been associated with increased rates of nosocomial infections[16] and invasive disease with susceptible *S. aureus* and MRSA in the nursery.[76]

Nursery Design and Environment

Nursery design should provide adequate space for appropriate care of the infant, room for necessary equipment, and sinks for hand washing.[447-449] The nursery should be located in a low traffic area with restricted access. Patient care areas should be separated from heavily used areas such as nursing stations and storage areas.

The AAP and the American College of Obstetricians and Gynecologists Perinatal Guidelines recommend an increasing amount of floor space per bassinet with increasing intensity of care. In the normal newborn nursery where fewer staff members are needed and there is no bulky equipment, 30 square feet of floor space per infant, with 3 feet between bassinets, is adequate. At least 100 square feet per infant, with 4 feet between incubators/warmers, is recommended in the intermediate care nursery, whereas 150 square feet per neonate, with incubators/warmers separated by at least 6 feet, is necessary in the intensive care unit owing to the large number of personnel and amount and complexity of equipment required.[447]

There should be sufficient numbers of strategically placed sinks for hand washing. The recommendation for the number of sinks in the normal nursery is one sink per six to eight infants; in intermediate care, one sink per three to four patients; and in intensive care, one sink for every two patients. In the NICU, sinks should be located so that personnel move no more than eight steps from any patient to reach a sink.[397, 447] All nursery entrances should have foot-operated, knee-operated, or photoelectric-operated sinks and soap dispensers. Paper towels, gowns and disposal facilities for laundry and contaminated waste should be readily available near each entrance.

The ventilation pattern should be designed to reduce the exposure of infants to particulate matter. A minimum of six air exchanges per hour is recommended, and at least two exchanges should be of outside air. Air delivered to the NICU should be filtered so as to remove particulate matter with at least 90% efficacy.[447] Some experts recommend 10 to 15 air exchanges per hour.[16, 448–450] Very high risk newborn care areas probably should receive HEPA-filtered air that is free of fungal spores. One or more isolation rooms with negative air pressure and discharge air to the outside should be provided to contain those few neonatal infections, such as varicella, that can be spread by the airborne route. Isolettes are at positive pressure with respect to the rest of the nursery and do not provide true isolation. Emphasis should be placed on keeping the environment free from dust buildup. Provision should be made for cleaning around delicate equipment and for periodic cleaning of each bed space. Phenolic disinfectants should be avoided because they have been associated with hyperbilirubinemia in neonates.[16] During dust-generating activities such as construction or renovation in the nursery, newborns and equipment should be protected from dust or debris that may contain fungal spores. Impermeable barriers must be set up to prevent dust or debris from construction areas entering the nursery. If this is impossible, the infants may have to be moved to a separate area of the hospital.[237, 449]

Patient placement techniques have been used to decrease the potential for transmission of infection in some normal newborn nurseries. Cohorting of infants may decrease risk of transmission in large nurseries by minimizing the number of other infants and personnel to whom each infant is exposed. All infants born or admitted within a 24- to 48-hour period are admitted to the same room and specific personnel are assigned to that cohort. The room is then closed and cleaned after the discharge of the last patient. However, cohorting requires additional personnel, is not practical for small nurseries or NICUs, and may not prevent contact spread of bacteria.[397, 451] Many hospitals promote rooming-in programs to encourage parental care of the infants. Limited studies indicate no increase in the incidence of nursery-acquired infection associated with rooming-in programs compared with that in nurseries without such programs.[452, 453] Rooming-in programs have the potential to reduce the risks from crowding and decrease the likelihood of cross-contamination in nurseries.

Hand Washing

Proper hand washing is of fundamental importance in decreasing the transmission of nosocomial pathogens from the contaminated hands of health care workers (Table 34–8). Hand washing is regarded as the single most important infection control and prevention measure in the nursery.[454, 455] Hand washing removes transient flora from caretakers' hands and controls the overgrowth of potentially pathogenic resident flora.[456] Vigorous scrubbing with plain soap and water for at least 10 to 15 seconds removes organic material and transient flora but does not necessarily reduce counts of microorganisms on the hands, especially counts of resident (colonizing) flora.[425] Recent data suggest that plain soap does not reliably eliminate transient carriage of antimicrobial-resistant organisms, such as vancomycin-resistant enterococci.[353] The quantity of soap or antibacterial agent also may enhance the effectiveness of hand washing.[457, 458] Various topical antimicrobial agents substantially reduce hand counts of transient and resident flora by 90% or more through their bactericidal and bacteriostatic effects. Certain agents used for hand washing (e.g., iodophors, triclosan, chlorhexidine gluconate) also have persistent residual antimicrobial activity.[425]

Indications and procedures for hand washing in the nursery are reviewed in several publications.[397, 416, 425, 455] In summary, hands should be washed before and after patient contact; after contact with body fluids, mucous membranes, nonintact skin, and objects that are likely to be contaminated; before performing invasive procedures; and after removing gloves. Gloves have been demonstrated to have macroscopic and microscopic holes that may lead to hand contamination, and hands may be contaminated in the process of removing soiled gloves.[459] Recommended procedures for hand washing by nursery personnel with patient contact are summarized in Table 34–8. Persons entering the nursery for patient contact should remove any jewelry, such as rings,

---

TABLE 34–8
Recommended Hand-Washing Procedures for Nursery Personnel

1. Roll sleeves above elbows and remove rings, watches, and other jewelry.
2. Wash hands thoroughly for 3 minutes with wet scrub brush and antiseptic hand washing agent over all areas; be certain to wash sides of all fingers.
3. Clean fingernails with orange stick or file.
4. Rinse thoroughly under running water.
5. Dry with paper towel.
6. Wash hands for 10 seconds or more between patients.

Adapted from American Academy of Pediatrics and American College of Obstetricians and Gynecologists. Infection control. *In* Guidelines for Perinatal Care, 4th ed. Elk Grove Village, Ill, American Academy of Pediatrics, 1997, pp 251–278, with permission.

watches, and bracelets, before washing their hands.[425] Finger nails should be trimmed short, and no false fingernails or nail polish should be permitted.[425] Authorities have recommended that hands, nails, and forearms should be washed with a suitable antibacterial detergent for 3 minutes,[416] but evidence supporting this recommendation is not well established.[458, 460] Because the greatest number of organisms are found around and under the fingernails, the nails should be cleaned meticulously. The hands should be rinsed thoroughly and dried with paper towels. After the hands are dried, only the patient and necessary equipment should be touched. Between handling of infants or after touching contaminated objects or surfaces, the hands should be washed again for at least 10 to 15 seconds with soap and water to remove transient flora. Hand contamination may be caused by touching one's self, another patient, another person, or a high-risk object after hand washing but before patient contact.[355]

Because plain (bland) soap does not reliably eliminate antibiotic-resistant microorganisms from contaminated hands, antimicrobial soap is recommended in NICUs.[352, 353] Available antiseptic agents include 4% chlorhexidine gluconate, 3% hexachorophene, 0.3% triclosan, and iodophors.

Hexachlorophene was widely used in the 1950s and 1960s, but its limited antibacterial spectrum (gram-positive organisms, principally S. aureus), irritant effects on the skin, and potential transcutaneous absorption have curtailed its use in nurseries.[424] It is best restricted to containment of S. aureus outbreaks.

Iodophor detergents have a broad spectrum of activity, including many gram-negative as well as gram-positive species, and they replaced hexachlorophene as a hand-washing agent in hospitals in the 1970s. However, many formulations of iodophors caused skin irritation and painful dermatitis, which resulted in employees limiting or avoiding hand washing in nurseries where iodophors were the only agents available. More recently, improved formulations have made iodophors more acceptable for routine use.

Chlorhexidine has replaced iodophors for routine hand washing and surgical scrubs in many nurseries. It is less irritating to the skin and also has a broad spectrum of antibacterial activity.[457] Chlorhexidine has the advantage of being tightly bound to the skin, leaving a residual antibacterial effect.[397, 425] Triclosan also has residual activity and has been shown to control MRSA outbreaks that persisted in the face of hand washing with chlorhexidine.[72, 425]

A variety of waterless hand-washing agents with antimicrobial activity are now available and appear useful when hand washing at a sink is inconvenient, such as on transport vehicles. For example, alcohol combined with emollients rapidly kills transient and colonizing flora and is inexpensive and well accepted by personnel.[425] These agents may not be as effective on soiled skin, and some caregivers may complain of irritation or drying of the hands.[416, 461]

Bar or liquid soap should also be available for employees whose skin does not tolerate the hospital's detergent of choice. Personnel with hand dermatitis usually have an increased number of bacteria with a potential for more pathogenic organisms on their hands. These workers should be treated, required to use gloves, and preferably removed from clinical patient care until their dermatitis has improved.[462] Moisturizing hand creams and lotions should not be used between hand washes for on-duty personnel because they may harbor bacteria, especially in open or multiple-use jars or vials, and may negate the residual antibacterial activity of antiseptics.[371, 372]

Compliance with hand-washing procedures has been shown to be poor in NICUs and other intensive care settings.[463, 464] Studies have shown that health care workers in critical care areas wash their hands only 20 to 30% of the time.[465, 466] Raju and Kobler assessed hand-washing compliance in a NICU and found that 37.5% of doctors and 53.9% of nurses demonstrated appropriate hand washing before handling an infant.[467] Brown and co-workers,[355] using video camera surveillance, reported that 24.7% of nurses, 31.8% of physicians, 20.5% of respiratory therapists, and 6.6% of parents complied with hand-washing procedures in a high-risk nursery. In addition, the rate of hand contamination after hand washing was 76.4% before the next patient contact. They concluded that infection control training in the intensive care setting should be directed not only to increasing hand-washing compliance but also to decreasing hand contamination before patient contact.[355]

Special Attire

There is no evidence that the traditional ritual of wearing a cover gown to enter the nursery is beneficial, and the routine use of cover gowns in nurseries for personnel with patient contact is no longer recommended. This practice has not been proved to decrease bacterial transmission or the incidence of infection in nurseries.[468–477] However, gowns should be worn when holding infants. A gown protects the infant from contact with the wearer's forearms and clothing and prevents contamination of the health care worker's exposed skin with infant flora. In practice, personnel rarely handle newborns outside of their bassinets or incubators, and most direct contact occurs from the hands.[397] It has also been shown that the routine use of gowns by visitors is not necessary. Ungowned, healthy visitors who are instructed on hand washing pose no hazard to newborns.[476] Although it is argued that gowns serve as reminders for hand washing, studies have shown that cover gowns may actually lead to a false sense of security and do not increase the frequency of hand washing.[35, 476, 478] The use of cover gowns does not decrease the traffic through the NICU.[472] Provision of short-sleeved scrub suits or other special attire with laundry services for personnel who spend most of the day in the nursery or NICU may have some benefits. This practice may prevent soiling of personal clothing and provide easy recognition of nursery personnel but is not considered an infection control measure.[397]

The current recommendations for the use of cover gowns include the following: (1) gowns are not required for staff or visitors on entrance to the nursery in nonoutbreak settings; (2) a long-sleeved gown should be worn if a newborn is to be handled outside the bassinet or incubator and either discarded after use or maintained for use exclusively with a single infant and changed every 8 to 12 hours; (3) gowns should be worn for anticipated soiling with blood or body fluids; (4) gowns should be worn in contact isolation or presence of clustered infections with epidemiologically important organisms that are considered to have been transmitted by contact; and (5) parents should wear gowns when they have concern for excessively soiled clothing.[35, 397] Other special attire such as caps, beard bags, and masks may be beneficial[397] during certain surgical procedures, including central line and umbilical vessel catheterization.[416] Masks also are used as part of droplet and airborne precautions.

Infection Control Precautions

The spread of infection within a nursery requires three elements: (1) a source of infecting microorganisms (e.g., patients, personnel, inanimate environment); (2) a susceptible host; and (3) a means of transmission for the microorganism (e.g., contact, droplet, or airborne). A variety of infection control measures are used for decreasing the risk of transmission of microorganisms in the nursery and make up the fundamentals of isolation precautions (Table 34–9). As previously discussed, hand washing is the single most important measure for preventing spread of infection. Gloves are worn for three different reasons: (1) to provide a protective barrier and prevent gross contamination when touching blood, body fluids, secretion, excretions, mucous membranes, and nonintact skin; (2) to reduce the likelihood that microorganisms on the hands of personnel will be transmitted to patients; and (3) to reduce the likelihood that hands of personnel contaminated with microorganisms from a patient or fomite can transmit these microorganisms to another patient (gloves must be changed between patient contacts and hands washed after glove removal).

Appropriate patient placement is an important component of isolation precautions. Published isolation guidelines recommend that patients with highly transmissible or epidemiologically important microorganisms

be placed in a private room.[278] These recommendations may not be appropriate for nurseries because the number of isolation rooms is limited and may be inadequate for the care of the critically ill newborn needing close observation. In addition, newborns are nonmobile and there is no direct contact between patients. Isolation requirements depend on (1) the overall condition of the neonate and type of care required; (2) the available space and facilities; (3) nurse:patient ratio; (4) the size and type of neonatal care service; (5) mode of transmission of the pathogen involved; and (6) the number of infected or colonized infants.[416]

Separate isolation rooms are seldom necessary to isolate infected neonates if certain criteria are met: (1) sufficient nursing and medical staff are on duty to provide comprehensive care; (2) sufficient space is provided for a 4- to 6-foot aisle between neonatal stations; (3) there is an adequate number of sinks available for hand washing in each area; (4) continuing instruction is provided about the mode of transmission of infections.[397, 416] One or more isolation rooms with the capacity for negative-pressure ventilation should be available to contain those few neonatal infections transmitted by the airborne route such as varicella, measles, TB, and possibly influenza.[397] Forced-air incubators do not provide adequate isolation for infected neonates. Although these incubators filter incoming air, they do not filter the air that is discharged into the nursery. Isolation areas in open nurseries for non-airborne infections can be defined by curtains, partitions, or other markers. A closed incubator may be helpful as a reminder for maintaining precautions, but outside surfaces and entry ports should be considered contaminated.[397] Cohorting of patients and personnel may be useful during outbreaks. In the normal nursery it may be more feasible to isolate the occasional newborn with gastroenteritis, respiratory tract infection, or skin infection in a single room or by rooming-in with the mother.[397]

Other components of isolation precautions include (1) limiting the movement and transport of newborns infected with virulent or epidemiologically important microorganisms; (2) utilizing appropriate barrier precautions in transit and notifying personnel in the areas to which colonized or infected patients will be arriving about necessary isolation precautions; (3) special attire such as masks, gowns, and other protective apparel (previously discussed); and (4) appropriate cleaning and disinfection of patient care equipment, articles, and bassinets/warmers/incubators. Autoclaving linen has not been shown to be effective in preventing infections in normal newborn or intensive care nurseries.[416, 462] Bacterial contamination of nonautoclaved linens is limited to skin flora in very low numbers. Linens and infant clothing have not been shown to be sources for nosocomial infections and do not warrant sterilization.[462]

After review and modification of existing isolation precautions, the CDC has developed the new "Guideline for Isolation Precautions in Hospitals." This system is designed to be as simple and user friendly as possible. There are two tiers of isolation precautions. The first and most important tier includes precautions designed for the care of all patients in hospitals regardless of

TABLE 34–9
Fundamentals of Isolation Precautions

Hand washing and gloving
Patient placement
Limiting transport of infected patients
Use of personal protective equipment:
   Masks
   Respiratory protection
   Eye protection
   Face shields
   Gowns and protective apparel
Handling and disposal of patient care equipment and articles
Cleaning of room, cubicle, or bedside equipment

Adapted from Garner JS, Hospital Infection Control Practices Advisory Committee (HICPAC). Guidelines for isolation precautions in hospitals. Infect Control Hosp Epidemiol 17:53–80, 1996, with permission.

their diagnosis or presumed infection status (standard precautions). The second tier of precautions is designed only for the care of patients known or suspected to be infected by epidemiologically important pathogens spread by airborne or droplet transmission or by contact with dry skin or contaminated surfaces (transmission-based precautions).[278]

Standard precautions represent a new system that combines the goals of protecting health care workers from blood-borne pathogens (universal precautions) and protecting health care workers and patients from transmission of microorganisms from moist body substances (body substance isolation).[278] Standard precautions apply to all patients at all times regardless of their diagnosis or presumed infection status and include any planned or potential contact with blood; all body fluids, secretions, and excretions, except sweat, regardless of whether they contain visible blood; nonintact skin; and mucous membranes. The components of standard precautions are outlined in Table 34–10. The prevention measures included in standard precautions comply with the OSHA standard for blood-borne pathogens (see Occupational Health and Bloodborne Pathogens in Table 34–10).

Transmission-based precautions are designed to provide necessary measures in addition to those already specified by standard precautions to prevent transmission of contagious diseases (e.g., varicella, measles, TB, pertussis) and other epidemiologically important microorganisms (e.g., multidrug-resistant microorganisms) from infected or colonized infants. There are three types of transmission-based precautions: airborne, droplet, and contact (Table 34–11). Airborne precautions are designed to prevent transmission of microorganisms spread by droplet nuclei (e.g., measles, varicella, TB), which can be carried on air currents over substantial distances. Special air handling and ventilation are required. Droplet precautions are designed to prevent transmission of microorganisms spread by large respiratory droplets that only travel short distances (less than 3 feet) before settling. Special air handling and ventilation are not required. Contact precautions are designed to prevent transmission of microorganisms spread by direct and indirect contact.

Some infections are spread by more than one route, so precaution systems may need to be combined for these infections (e.g., varicella requires both airborne and contact precautions). Patients infected or colonized with more than one microorganism also may need a combination of precaution systems (e.g., a patient with active pulmonary tuberculosis and *C. difficile* enterocoli-

---

TABLE 34–10
Standard Precautions[a]

Hand Washing
1. Necessary after touching blood, body fluids, secretions, excretions, and contaminated items.
2. Immediately after removing gloves, between patient contacts, and when otherwise indicated (e.g., touching patient care equipment or after hand contamination).

Gloves
1. Should be worn when touching blood, body fluids, secretions, excretions, and items contaminated by these fluids.
2. Clean gloves should be used before touching mucous membranes or nonintact skin.
3. Gloves should be removed promptly after use, before touching noncontaminated items and environmental surfaces, and before going to another patient.

Masks, Eye Protection, and Face Shields
1. Should be worn to protect mucous membranes of the eyes, nose, and mouth during procedures and patient care activities likely to generate splashes or sprays of blood, body fluids, secretions, or excretions.

Nonsterile Gowns
1. Worn to protect skin and prevent soiling of clothing during procedures or patient activities likely to generate splashes or sprays of blood, body fluids, secretions, or excretions.
2. Soiled gowns should be promptly removed.

Patient Placement
1. Place a patient who contaminates environment or who does not (or cannot) assist in maintaining appropriate hygiene or environmental control in a private room.
2. If private room not available, consult infection control professionals.

Patient Care Equipment
1. Used equipment should be handled in a manner that prevents skin and mucous membrane exposures and contamination of clothing.
2. Ensure reusable equipment has been cleaned and reprocessed before use for the care of another patient.

Linen
1. Handle, transport, and process used linen soiled with blood, body fluids, secretions, and excretions in a manner that prevents skin and mucous membrane exposure and contamination of clothing.

Occupational Health and Bloodborne Pathogens
1. Avoid exposure by taking all precautions to prevent injuries when using, cleaning, and disposing of needles, scalpels, and other sharp instruments and devices.
2. Mouthpieces, resuscitation bags, or other ventilation devices should be available in all patient care areas and used instead of mouth-to-mouth resuscitation.

---

[a]Used for all patients.
Adapted from Garner JS, Hospital Infection Control Practices Advisory Committee (HICPAC). Guidelines for isolation precautions in hospitals. Infect Control Hosp Epidemiol 17:53–80, 1996, with permission.

TABLE 34–11
Transmission-Based Precautions for Hospitalized Patients[a]

CATEGORY OF PRECAUTIONS	SINGLE ROOM	MASKS	GOWNS	GLOVES
Airborne	Yes	Yes	No	No
Droplet	Yes[b]	Yes, for close contact (< 3 ft)	No	No
Contact	Yes[b]	No	Yes	Yes

[a]These recommendations are in addition to those for standard precautions for all patients.
[b]Preferred but not required. Cohorting of infants infected with the same pathogen is acceptable.

tis requires airborne and contact precautions). Table 34–12 shows examples of infectious diseases requiring isolation precautions, and Table 34–13 shows examples of clinical syndromes and conditions warranting use of empirical transmission precautions.[278, 416, 479] Neonates on isolation precautions should have the designated type of isolation clearly stated on the incubator (Isolette), bassinet, or door to the room, with detailed instructions for gloving, gowning, and masking.

Visitors

The potential benefits of family and other visitors in the nursery must be weighed against the potential risks of transmission of pathogens to newborns. The AAP and American College of Obstetrics and Gynecology, in their "Guidelines for Perinatal Care," recommend that parents have access to their newborns 24 hours a day at all levels of care and should be encouraged to participate in the care of their newborns.[423] Whenever possible, parents of neonates in intermediate or intensive care areas should be allowed unrestricted visits. Flexible and liberal visiting policies for families should be encouraged. Sibling visitation is favorably received by parents[480] but is a concern because of possible transmission of infectious diseases.[423] Studies on the risks of transmission of infection from visitors are limited, but available data have demonstrated no effect on either bacterial colonization of normal neonates or infectious disease rates in NICUs resulting from sibling visitation.[481–483]

Each hospital should develop and enforce a clearly defined visiting policy for nurseries and NICUs. Physical contact with siblings (i.e., children younger than 12 years of age) is of particular concern because they are the most likely to be infected with easily transmitted pathogens, such as varicella, measles, pertussis, and respiratory and gastrointestinal viruses. The Committee on Fetus and Newborn of the AAP, as well as Association for Professionals in Inspection Control and Epidemiology (APIC) and others,[484] have developed basic guidelines for sibling visits that may serve as the basis for policy formulation in individual nursery and intensive care settings. These recommendations include the following:

1. Visitors should be restricted while infants are with their mothers. Normal newborns should be visited in the mother's private room or a special visiting area. The number of visitors at a time and the duration of visits should be limited to ensure adequate observation and monitoring of the visitor by the medical and nursing staff.

2. Before visitation, a nurse or physician should interview the parents at a site outside the unit to assess the current health of each sibling visitor.

3. Visitors should be screened for active infection and recent exposures and individually assessed for potential risk of transmission and ability to comply with instructions. No child with fever or symptoms of an acute illness, such as upper respiratory infection, gastroenteritis, or dermatitis, should be allowed to visit.

4. Persons with airborne infection (e.g., varicella, TB, measles) should not visit. Nonimmune visitors who have been recently exposed to known communicable disease (e.g., varicella, measles, rubella) and who may be in the infectious stage of the incubation period should not be allowed to visit.

5. Visiting in special care nurseries should be restricted to prevent the interruption of patient care activities.

6. Visiting siblings should be prepared in advance for the visit and parents should ensure adult supervision of visiting siblings at all times.

7. Visitors should be instructed in proper hand-washing technique, and the visiting child's hands should be washed carefully before contact with the newborn.

8. Visitors should not have contact with newborns other than the one being visited and should not handle patient care equipment.

To reduce inadvertent neonatal exposure to undetected infectious diseases among visitors, some obstetrical units have newborns returned to the nursery during general visiting hours and restrict visiting during community outbreaks of respiratory tract infections.[397] Many NICUs limit visitors to parents, grandparents, and other significant family members; some impose a limit of two visitors at a time; and others limit duration of visits. Scientific data supporting these recommendations are limited, and further studies of visitation and risks of acquiring infection from visitors need to be done.

Employee Health

People who work in health care settings are exposed more frequently to infectious diseases. They also may pose a risk to patients and other health care workers if they develop a communicable disease. Health care work-

TABLE 34–12

Type and Duration of Transmission-Based Precautions Needed for Selected Infections and Conditions

INFECTION/CONDITION	PRECAUTIONS	
	Type	Duration
Abscess, draining (no dressing or dressing does not contain drainage adequately)	C	DI
Adenovirus infection in infants and young children	D, C	DI
Bordetella pertussis (see Pertussis)		
Chickenpox (varicella)	A, C	F1
Chickenpox (varicella) exposure	A, F2	F2
Clostridium difficile	C	DI
Congenital rubella	C	F3
Conjunctivitis, acute viral (acute hemorrhagic)	C	DI
Enterococcus species (see Multidrug-resistant organisms, infection, or colonization if epidemiologically significant or vancomycin-resistant)		
Enterocolitis, *C. difficile*	C	DI
Enteroviral infections in infants and young children	C	DI
Furunculosis, staphylococcal, in infants and young children	C	DI
Gastroenteritis:		
C. difficile	C	DI
Escherichia coli	C, F4	DI
Rotavirus	C, F4	DI
Salmonella species (incl. *Salmonella typhi*)	C, F4	DI
Viral, other than rotavirus	C, F4	DI
German measles (rubella; also see Congenital rubella)	D	F5
Haemophilus influenzae	D	U$^{24 hr}$
Hepatitis A in diapered or incontinent patients	C	F6
Herpes simplex:		
Neonatal infection	C	DI
Neonatal exposure	C, F11	DI
Influenza	D, F7	DI
Multidrug resistant organisms, infection, or colonization:		
Gastrointestinal	C	CN
Respiratory	C	CN
Skin, wound, or burn	C	CN
Parainfluenza virus infection, respiratory, in infants and young children	C	DI
Parvovirus B19 infection	A or D, F12	F13
Pertussis (whooping cough)	D	F9
Pneumococcemia (pneumococcal sepsis), penicillin-resistant	D1, F8	U$^{24 hr}$
Pneumonia:		
Adenovirus	D, C	DI
H. influenzae in infants and children (any age)	D	D$^{24 hr}$
Neisseria meningitidis	D	U$^{24 hr}$
Streptococcus, group A, in infants and young children	D	U$^{24 hr}$
S. pneumoniae, penicillin-resistant	D, F8	U$^{24 hr}$
Respiratory infectious disease, acute	C	DI
Respiratory syncytial virus (RSV) in infants and young children	C	DI
Rotavirus infection (see Gastroenteritis, Rotavirus)		
Rubella (German measles; see also Congenital Rubella)	D	F5
Salmonellosis (see Gastroenteritis, *Salmonella* species)		
Staphylococcal disease (*Staphylococcus aureus*):		
Skin, wound, or burn, major (no dressing or dressing does not contain drainage adequately)	C	DI
Streptococcal disease (Group A *Streptococcus*):		
Skin, wound, or burn, major (no dressing or dressing does not contain drainage adequately)	C	U$^{24 hr}$
Pneumonia in infants and young children	D	U$^{24 hr}$
Streptococcus pneumoniae, penicillin-resistant	D, F8	U$^{24 hr}$
Tuberculosis, pulmonary or laryngeal, confirmed or suspected	A	F10
Varicella (chickenpox)	A, C	F1
Varicella (chickenpox) exposure	A, F2	F2
Whooping cough	D	F9
Wound infections, major (no dressing or dressing does not contain drainage adequately)	C	DI

1. Maintain precautions until all lesions are crusted.

2. Place exposed, susceptible patients on Airborne Precautions beginning 8 days after exposure and continuing until 21 days after the last exposure (up to 28 days if VZV immunoglobulin has been given).

3. Place infant on Contact Precautions during any admission until 1 year of age, unless nasopharyngeal and urine cultures are negative for virus after 3 months of age.

4. Use Contact Precautions for diapered or incontinent children and any child younger than 6 years of age for duration of illness.

5. Until 7 days after the onset of the rash.

6. Maintain precautions in infants and children younger than 3 years of age for the duration of the hospitalization; in children 3–14 years of age, until 2 weeks after onset of symptoms; and in others, until 1 week after onset of symptoms.

7. The "Guideline for Prevention of Nosocomial Pneumonia" recommends surveillance, vaccination, antiviral agents, and use of private rooms with negative air pressure as much as is feasible for patients in whom influenza is suspected or diagnosed. Many hospitals encounter logistic difficulties and physical plant limitations when admitting multiple patients with suspected influenza during community outbreaks. If sufficient private rooms are unavailable, consider cohorting patients or, at the very least, avoid room sharing with high-risk patients. See "Guideline for Prevention of Nosocomial Pneumonia" for additional prevention and control strategies.

8. The Centers for Disease Control and Prevention/Hospital Infection Control Practices Advisory Committee (CDC/HICPAC) guideline recommends only standard precautions for infections caused by penicillin-resistant *S. pneumoniae*. Based on reports of nosocomial transmission of penicillin-resistant *S. pneumoniae* in hospitals outside the United States and the possibility that these infections were spread by droplet transmission, we recommend the use of Droplet Precautions until 24 hours of effective antimicrobial therapy has been completed.

9. Maintain precautions until 5 days after patient is placed on effective therapy.

10. Discontinue precautions only when a patient with tuberculosis (TB) is on effective therapy, is improving clinically, and has three consecutive negative sputum smears collected on different days, or when TB is ruled out. Also see the CDC "Guideline for Preventing the Transmission of Tuberculosis in Health Care Facilities."

11. For infants delivered vaginally or by cesarean section and if the mother has active infection and membranes have been ruptured for more than 4–6 hours.

12. The CDC/HICPAC guideline recommends the use of Droplet Precautions.

13. Maintain precautions for duration of hospitalization when chronic disease occurs in an immunodeficient patient. For patients with transient aplastic crisis or red blood cell crisis, maintain precautions for 7 days.

A = airborne; C = contact; D = droplet; CN = until antimicrobial agents are discontinued and cultures are negative; DI = duration of illness (w/wound lesions, DI = until they stop draining); U = until time specified in hours after initiation of effective therapy; F = see footnote number.

Adapted from Huskins WC, Goldmann DA. Prevention and control of nosocomial infections in hospitalized children. *In* Feigin RD, Cherry JD (eds). Textbook of Pediatric Infections Diseases, 4th ed. Philadelphia, WB Saunders, 1998, pp 2585–2602.

TABLE 34–13

Clinical Syndromes or Conditions Warranting Empirical Use of Transmission-Based Precautions to Prevent Transmission of Epidemiologically Important Pathogens Until Infection with These Microorganisms Is Excluded[a]

CLINICAL SYNDROME OR CONDITION[b]	POTENTIAL PATHOGENS[c]	EMPIRICAL PRECAUTIONS
Diarrhea		
Acute diarrhea with a likely infectious cause	Enteric pathogens[d]	Contact
Diarrhea with a history of recent antibiotic use	*Clostridium difficile*	Contact
Meningitis	*Neisseria meningitidis*	Droplet
Rash or exanthems, generalized, etiology unknown		
Petechial/ecchymotic with fever	*Neisseria meningitidis*	Droplet
Vesicular	Varicella	Airborne and contact
Maculopapular with coryza and fever	Rubeola (measles)	Airborne
Respiratory infections		
Cough/fever/upper lobe pulmonary infiltrate in an HIV-negative patient or a patient at low risk for HIV infection	*Mycobacterium tuberculosis*	Airborne
Cough/fever/pulmonary infiltrate in any lung location in an HIV-infected patient or a patient at high risk for HIV infection	*Mycobacterium tuberculosis*	Airborne
Paroxysmal or severe persistent cough during periods of pertussis activity	*Bordetella pertussis*	Droplet
Respiratory infections, particularly bronchiolitis and croup, in infants and young children	Respiratory syncytial virus or parainfluenza virus	Contact
Risk of multidrug-resistant microorganisms[e]		
History of infection or colonization with multidrug-resistant organisms	Resistant bacteria	Contact
Skin, wound, or urinary tract infection in a patient in a facility where multidrug-resistant organisms are prevalent	Resistant bacteria	Contact
Skin or wound infection		
Abscess or draining would that cannot be covered	*Staphylococcus aureus*; group A *Streptococcus*	Contact

[a]Infection control professionals are encouraged to modify or adapt this table according to local conditions. To ensure that appropriate empirical precautions are always implemented, hospitals must have systems in place to evaluate patients routinely according to these criteria as a part of their preadmission and admission care.

[b]Patients with the syndromes or conditions listed may present with atypical signs or symptoms (e.g., pertussis in neonates and adults may not be associated with paroxysmal or severe cough). The clinician's index of suspicion should be guided by the prevalence of specific conditions in the community, as well as clinical judgment.

[c]The microorganisms listed are not intended to represent the complete, or even the most likely, diagnosis but rather possible etiologic agents that require precautions in addition to standard precautions until they can be ruled out.

[d]These pathogens include enterohemorrhagic *Escherichia coli* 0157:H7, *Shigella*, hepatitis A virus, and rotavirus.

[e]Resistant bacteria judged by the infection control program, based on current state, regional, or national recommendations, to be of special clinical or epidemiologic significance.

HIV = human immunodeficiency virus.

From Garner JS, Hospital Infection Control Practices Advisory Committee (HICPAC). Guidelines for isolation precautions in hospitals. Infect Control Hosp Epidemiol 17:53–80, 1996, with permission.

ers who work directly with, or in close proximity to, patients have the greatest risk of exposure. This may include medical and nursing staff, students, volunteers, and visitors. The infection control and employee health programs need to work collaboratively to develop policies and procedures for health care workers, such as placement evaluations; health and safety education; immunization programs; evaluation of potentially harmful infectious exposures; implementation of appropriate preventive measures; coordination of plans for managing outbreaks; provision of care to personnel with work-related illnesses or exposures; education regarding infection risks related to employment or special conditions; development of guidelines for work restrictions when an employee has (or is potentially incubating) an infectious disease; and maintenance of health records on all health care workers.[395]

Policies and procedures for assessing the health of nursery personnel should address screening for immunity to rubella, measles, mumps, VZV infection, and HBV infection. Immunizations should be provided for those nonpregnant personnel who are seronegative.[35, 278, 416] Annual immunization of nursery personnel against prevalent strains of influenza is highly recommended because young infants, especially those in the NICUs who have underlying chronic pulmonary disease, are vulnerable to complications of influenza and cannot be protected by either influenza immunization or chemoprophylaxis. Appropriate vaccine use protects both the health care worker and the patients, and immunization programs have been found to be highly cost effective.[395] Personnel should receive the Mantoux skin test with purified protein derivative for TB, and adequate treatment and noninfective status should be documented. Guidelines for immunization and TB screening of health care workers are available.[196, 278, 397]

Employees should understand the risks of transmission of contagious diseases to newborns and should report personal infections and skin conditions that might impair hand washing or facilitate dissemination of organisms colonizing the skin to their supervisors. If such conditions are present, the health care worker should be medically examined before working directly with neonates.[397, 416] Ideally, individuals with a respiratory, cutaneous, mucocutaneous, or gastrointestinal infection should not have direct contact with neonates, but removal of personnel may not be practical without compromising patient care due to understaffing. Decisions should be made on an individual basis, taking into consideration the mode of transmission of the particular infection and the ability of the employee to comply with preventive measures. Health care workers with airborne infections (e.g., TB, varicella, or measles), pertussis, exudative skin lesions, herpetic whitlow, or weeping dermatitis should be removed from direct patient care until they are no longer infectious.[397, 416] Personnel with oral herpetic lesions are unlikely to transmit HSV. Health care workers with herpes labialis are no longer routinely excluded from the nursery, provided that they are individually evaluated, cover their lesions and not touch them, carefully observe hand-washing policies, and avoid intimate contact with the infants (e.g., kissing or nuzzling).[313] Nonimmune personnel with significant exposure to varicella-zoster or measles should not work during the potentially contagious phase of the incubation period.[397] Specific detailed guidelines are available regarding work restrictions for health care workers in the nursery.[278, 397, 416, 479]

A structured approach to the assessment and management of exposures of health care workers to patients with infectious diseases, particularly blood-borne pathogens such as HIV, HBV, and HCV, is critical to provide employees with timely postexposure prophylaxis and to reduce anxiety and days lost from work. The federal Occupational Safety and Health Administration (OSHA) has issued regulations designed to minimize the transmission of HIV, HBV, and other potentially infectious agents in the workplace.[485] The OSHA regulations require the employer to implement an exposure control plan to minimize employees' exposure to blood-borne pathogens. The plan must contain the following components:

1. Personal protective equipment for employees exposed to blood or other body fluids
2. Adoption of certain workplace controls (hand-washing facilities, disposal of contaminated needles)
3. Housekeeping requirements
4. Provision of free HBV vaccination
5. Postexposure evaluation and follow-up procedures
6. Employee training
7. Record keeping

These requirements are enforced, and violations are punishable by fines. The first step is to develop criteria for assessing the nature of the exposure because many reported encounters are not significant. Some exposures may require an assessment of the susceptibility of the health care worker to infection (HBV, HIV, HCV), and procedures should describe the indications for laboratory tests and interpretation of results. Postexposure prophylaxis regimens should be developed. Counseling regarding the risks and consequences of the exposure is an important component of the plan.[416, 485]

The OSHA blood-borne pathogens standard requires testing the source patient for evidence of blood-borne infection, when consent can be obtained, and providing postexposure prophylaxis to the health care worker in accordance with CDC recommendations. Significant exposures are defined as percutaneous, mucous membrane, or nonintact skin exposure to blood and other potentially infectious body fluids (cerebrospinal fluid, pericardial fluid, pleural fluid, peritoneal fluid, synovial fluid, amniotic fluid, tissue or visibly bloody fluids, excretions, or secretions). A number of factors may affect the risk of infection in an individual case, including level of viremia in the source patient, amount of blood involved in the exposure, and the nature of the exposure. HBV is the most infectious blood-borne pathogen, and the risk of exposure is estimated to be 2 to 40%, with higher risk if the source patient is hepatitis B e-antigen positive. Transmission from mucous membrane or nonintact skin exposures have been well documented.[485, 486] The risk of HIV infection after percutaneous exposure is estimated to be 0.3%.[487] Infection after mucous membrane exposure has been reported, but it is considered much less likely. Independent risk factors for HIV infection include a deep injury, visible blood on the device causing injury, a procedure involving a needle placed directly in a vein or artery, and terminal illness in the source patient.[488] Studies have shown that antiviral chemoprophylaxis with zidovudine after occupational exposure to HIV has decreased the risk of transmission by 81%.[488] The efficacy and potential side effects of combination antiretroviral therapy for postexposure prophylaxis in uninfected health care workers exposed to HIV, as currently recommended by the CDC, are not as well studied. Updated recommendations will evolve as further data become available.[479, 489] The risk of hepatitis C after percutaneous exposure is less well defined (estimated at 3 to 10%). Recommendations for postexposure prophylaxis for HBV and HIV are outlined in Table 34–14 and Figure 34–3, respectively. There is no known effective prophylaxis for HCV.

There has been particular concern about the exposure of pregnant health care workers to infections they may acquire from direct care of neonates (e.g., CMV).[490] Pregnant health care workers, in general, do not have an increased risk for acquiring infections in the nursery, but certain infections cause a great deal of anxiety, especially CMV. Personnel in neonatal units are likely to be exposed to patients excreting CMV, because approxi-

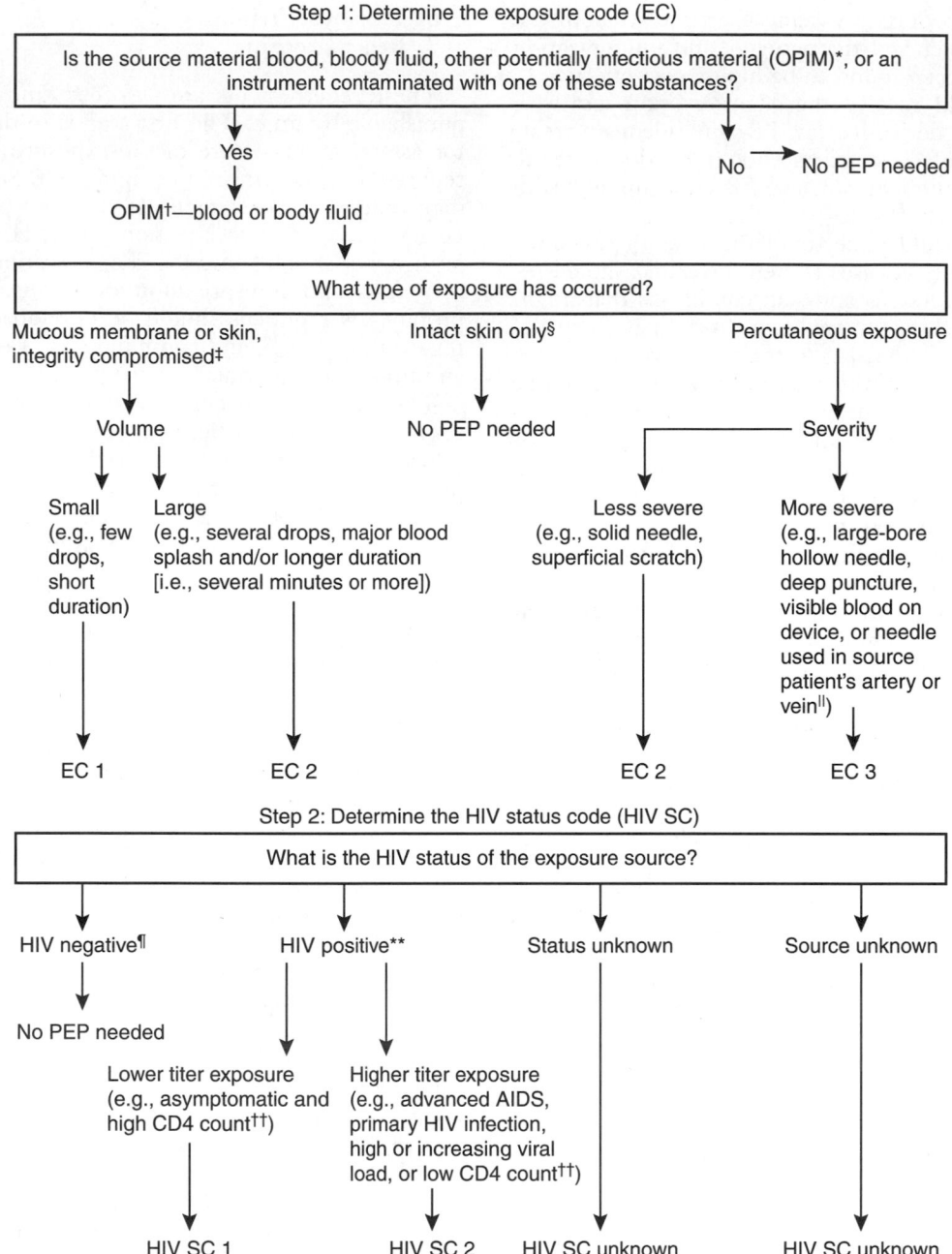

FIGURE 34–3 Determining the need for human immunodeficiency virus (HIV) postexposure prophylaxis (PEP) after an occupational exposure. (Adapted from Centers for Disease Control and Prevention. Public health service guidelines for the management of healthcare workers' exposure to HIV and recommendations for postexposure prophylaxis. MMWR Morb Mortal Wkly Rep 47[RR-7]:14, 1998.)

mately 1% of infants shed the virus. Although approximately 50% of American women are nonimmune to CMV, and the risk of severe fetal infection after primary CMV infection is estimated at 10 to 15%, studies have not shown nursery personnel to be at higher risk of CMV acquisition than the general population.[397, 491] No evidence exists that transfer to another area of the hospital or to a different group of patients decreases the risk, because many hospitalized patients asymptomatically shed CMV.[416] Acquisition of infection should be prevented by compliance with standard precautions.

Women of childbearing years should be counseled about the relatively low risk of exposure should they become pregnant and the importance of strict adherence to standard precautions. A routine program of serologic testing of health care workers is not recommended because seropositivity for CMV does not guarantee protection against reinfection or reactivation of the infection.[416, 490, 492] The only work restriction that is applied to pregnant health care workers is avoidance exposure to a child with RSV being treated with aerosolized ribiviran, because the medication has teratogenic potential.

Step 3: Determine the PEP recommendation

EC	HIV SC	PEP recommendation
1	1	**PEP may not be warranted.** Exposure type does not pose a known risk for HIV transmission. Whether the risk for drug toxicity outweighs the benefit of PEP should be decided by the exposed health care worker (HCW) and treating clinician.
1	2	**Consider basic regimen.**‡‡ Exposure type poses a negligible risk for HIV transmission. A high HIV titer in the source may justify consideration of PEP. Whether the risk for drug toxicity outweighs the benefit of PEP should be decided by the exposed HCW and treating clinician.
2	1	**Recommend basic regimen.** Most HIV exposures are in this category: no increased risk for HIV transmission has been observed, but use of PEP is appropriate.
2	2	**Recommend expanded regimen.**§§ Exposure type represents an increased HIV transmission risk.
3	1 or 2	**Recommend expanded regimen.** Exposure type represents an increased HIV transmission risk.
Unknown	Unknown	If the source or, in the case of an unknown source, the setting where exposure occurred suggests a possible risk for HIV exposure and the EC is 2 or 3, consider PEP basic regimen.

This algorithm is intended to guide initial decisions about PEP and should be used in conjunction with other guidance provided in MMWR reports.

* Semen or vaginal secretions; cerebrospinal, synovial, pleural, peritoneal, pericardial, or amniotic fluids; or tissue.

† Exposures to OPIM must by evaluated on a case-by-case basis. In general, these body substances are considered a low risk for transmission in health care settings. Any unprotected contact to concentrated HIV in a research laboratory or production facility is considered an occupational exposure that requires clinical evaluation to determine the need for PEP.

‡ Skin integrity is considered compromised if there is evidence of chapped skin, dermatitis, abrasion, or open wound.

§ Contact with intact skin is not normally considered a risk for HIV transmission. However, if the exposure was to blood, and the circumstance suggests a higher volume exposure (e.g., an extensive area of skin was exposed or there was prolonged contact with blood), the risk for HIV transmission should be considered.

‖ The combination of these severity factors (e.g., large-bore hollow needle and deep puncture) contributes to an elevated risk for transmission if the source person is HIV positive.

¶ A source is considered negative for HIV infection if there is a laboratory documentation of a negative HIV antibody, HIV polymerase chain reaction (PCR), or HIV p24 antigen test result from a specimen collected at or near the time of exposure and there is no clinical evidence of recent retroviral-like illness.

** A source is considered infected with HIV (HIV positive) if there has been a positive laboratory result for HIV antibody, HIV PCR, or HIV p24 antigen, or physician-diagnosed AIDS.

†† Examples are used as surrogates to estimate HIV titer in an exposure source for purposes of considering PEP regimens and do not reflect all clinical situations that may be observed. Although a high HIV titer (HIV SC2) in an exposure source has been associated with an increased risk for transmission, the possibility of transmission from a source with a lower HIV titer also must be considered.

‡‡ Basic regimen is 4 weeks of zidovudine, 600 mg per day in two or three divided doses, and lamivudine, 150 mg twice daily.

§§ Expanded regimen is the basic regimen plus either indinavir, 800 mg every 8 hours, or nelfinavir, 750 mg three times a day.

FIGURE 34–3 *Continued*

TABLE 34–14

Recommendations for Hepatitis B Prophylaxis After Percutaneous or Mucous Membrane Exposure

EXPOSED PERSON	TREATMENT WHEN SOURCE IS FOUND TO BE:		
	HBs-Ag Positive	HBs-Ag Negative	Not Tested or Unknown
Unimmunized	HBIG[a] × 1; initiate and complete HBV[b] series	Initiate and complete HBV[b] series	Initiate and complete HBV[b] series
Previously immunized:			
Known responder with adequate anti-HBs level[c]	No testing; no intervention	No testing; no intervention	No testing; no intervention
Known nonresponder	HBIG[a] × 2 or HBIG[a] × 1 plus 1 dose of HBV[b]	No treatment	If known high-risk source, treat as if source were HBsAg positive
Response unknown	Test exposed for anti-HBs; if adequate[c], no treatment; if inadequate, HBIG[a] × 1 plus HBV[b] booster dose	No treatment	Test exposed for anti-HBs; if adequate[c], no treatment; if inadequate, HBV[b] booster dose

[a]The HBIG dose is 0.06 mL/kg intramuscularly.
[b]HBV dosing requirements vary according to the manufacturer, the age of the recipient, and other factors (persons undergoing dialysis and immunocompromised persons require higher doses); follow the manufacturer's dosing recommendations.
[c]An adequate anti-HBs level is ≥10 mIU/mL.
HBsAg = hepatitis B surface antigen; HBIG = hepatitis B immunoglobulin; HBV = hepatitis B vaccine; anti-HBs = antibody to hepatitis B surface antigen.
Modified from Centers for Disease Control and Prevention. Protection against viral hepatitis: recommendations of the Immunization Practices Advisory Committee (ACIP). MMWR Morb Mortal Wkly Rep 46(No. RR-18):1–42, 1997, with permission.

TABLE 34–15
Management of Occupational Exposures to Infectious Agents in Pregnant Health Care Workers

AGENT	IN-HOSPITAL SOURCE	POTENTIAL EFFECT ON FETUS	RATE OF PERINATAL TRANSMISSION	MATERNAL SCREENING	PREVENTION
Cytomegalovirus (CMV)	Urine, blood; transplant pts; day-care toddlers	Hearing loss; congenital syndrome[a]	Total: 40% (symptomatic: <5–15%)	Antibody protects against most clinical disease; routine screening *not* recommended	Efficacy of CMV immune globulin not established; vaccine investigational; *standard precautions*
Hepatitis B	Blood, body fluids	Hepatitis; hepatocellular carcinoma as adult	$Hb_EAg +$:90%, $Hb_EAg -$:0.25%	HbsAg *is* recommended during pregnancy	Vaccine (safe during pregnancy); vaccine/ HBIG at birth; *standard precautions*
Hepatitis C (HCV)	Blood	Hepatitis	5% (0–25%)	Anti-HCV; HCV RNA in reference laboratories; routine screening *not* recommended	Immune globulin *not* recommended; *standard precautions*
Herpes simplex	Vesicular fluid, oropharyngeal secretions	Sepsis, encephalitis, mucocutaneous lesions; congenital malformations (rare)	Unlikely from nosocomial exposure; primary genital: 33–50%; recurrent genital: 4%	Antibody testing *not* useful; inspection for genital lesions during labor	*Standard precautions; contact precautions* when lesions present
Human immunodeficiency virus (HIV)	Blood, body fluids	AIDS by 2–3 yr of age; no congenital syndrome	20–30%	Antibody by immunoassay, Western blot	Avoid high-risk behaviors; antiretroviral chemoprophylaxis for high-risk needlesticks; intrapartum, postnatal chemoprophylaxis for HIV+ mothers and their babies; *standard precautions*
Influenza	Respiratory secretions	No congenital syndrome	Rare	None	Vaccine (safe during pregnancy); *contact precautions*
Measles (rubeola)	Respiratory secretions	Prematurity, abortion; no congenital syndrome	Rare	History, antibody	Vaccine,[b] immunoglobulin within 6 days of exposure if susceptible; *airborne precautions*

Disease	Source	Outcome	Rate	Screening	Prevention/Treatment
Parvovirus B19	Respiratory secretions, ?, blood; sicklers, immunocompromised patients	Fetal hydrops, stillbirth; no congenital syndrome	Total: 25%, but 1–9% maximum adverse outcome	Pre-pregnancy antibody selectively, *not* routinely	May choose to avoid care of sicklers w/ aplastic crises and immunocompromised patients with chronic anemia; *droplet precautions*
Rubella	Respiratory secretions	Congenital syndrome[a]	45–50% overall; 90% in first 12 wk of gestation	Antibody; pre-pregnancy screening recommended if immunization not well documented	Vaccine; *droplet precautions* for acute infections; *contact precautions* for congenital rubella ≤12 mo of age
Syphilis	Blood, vesicular fluid, amniotic fluid	Congenital syndrome[a]	10–90% determined by stage of maternal disease and trimester of infection	VDRL, RPR	Penicillin after percutaneous exposure from untreated patient; *standard precautions*; *contact precautions* when lesions present
Toxoplasmosis	*No* human-to-human spread; raw meat, cat feces, unwashed fruit and vegetables	Congenital syndrome[a]	30–50%; rate increases as pregnancy advances; severe disease after primary infection in first trimester	Antibody protects against disease; routine screening not recommended in United States	Freeze or cook meat; avoid or use glove for contact w/cat feces; wash fruits, vegetables
Tuberculosis	Sputum, skin lesions	Hepatic and/or pulmonary disease	Rare	Skin test (purified protein derivative)	Isoniazid and ethambutol ± rifampin for active maternal disease; *airborne precautions*
Varicella-zoster	Respiratory secretions, vesicular fluid	Malformations (skin, limb, central nervous system, eye); chickenpox, zoster	Total: 25%; congenital syndrome: 2% (0–4%)	History, antibody	Vaccine[b]; VZIG within 96 hr of exposure if susceptible; *airborne and contact precautions*

[a]Congenital syndrome: varying conditions of jaundice, hepatosplenomegaly; microcephaly, central nervous system abnormalities, thrombocytopenia, anemia, retinopathy, and skin and bone lesions.

[b]Live virus vaccines are given routinely before pregnancy.

AIDS = acquired immunodeficiency syndrome; RPR = rapid plasma reagin; VDRL = Veneral Disease Research Laboratory; VZIG = varicella-zoster immune globulin.

Adapted from Garner JS, Hospital Infection Control Practice Advisory Committee (HICPAC). Guidelines for infection control in healthcare personnel, 1998. Infect Contr Hosp Epidemiol 19:407–463, 1998, with permission. (Courtesy of Jane Siegel, M.D.)

Routine employee health screening of women of child-bearing age before pregnancy is critical so that they can be immunized against vaccine-preventable diseases. Certain vaccines are safe to give during pregnancy, including diphtheria and tetanus, hepatitis B, and annual influenza immunization. Immunity to these infections is highly desirable for pregnant health care workers. The CDC states that pregnancy is not a contraindication for the administration of influenza vaccine and specifically targets women who would be in the second or third trimester of pregnancy during influenza season, because there is an increased mortality in this group.[490, 493] Management of occupational exposures to infectious agents in a pregnant health care worker are summarized in Table 34–15. Other more detailed sources of information are available[397, 479, 492, 493] for the development of policy and procedures for pregnant employees.

References

1. Gaynes RP, Edwards JR, Jarvis WR, et al. Nosocomial infections among neonates in high-risk nurseries in the United States. Pediatrics 98:357–361, 1996.
2. Moore D. Nosocomial infections in newborn nurseries and neonatal intensive care units. In Mayhall GC (ed). Hospital Epidemiology and Infection Control. Baltimore, Williams & Wilkins, 1996, pp 532–565.
3. Mullett MD, Cook EF, Gallagher R. Nosocomial sepsis in the neonatal intensive care unit. J Perinatol 18:112–115, 1998.
4. Harpin VA, Rutter N. Barrier properties of the newborn infant's skin. J Pediatr 102:419–425, 1993.
5. Wilson CB, Lewis DB. Basis and implications of selectively diminished cytokine production in neonatal susceptibility to infection. Rev Infect Dis 12(Suppl 4):S410–S420, 1990.
6. Garner JS, Jarvis WR, Emori TG, et al. CDC definitions for nosocomial infections, 1988. J Infect Contr 16:128–140, 1988.
7. Gaynes RP, Horan JC. Surveillance of nosocomial infections: Appendix A: CDC definitions of nosocomial infections. In Mayhall GC (ed). Hospital Epidemiology and Infection Control. Baltimore, Williams & Wilkins, 1996, pp 1–14.
8. Baltimore RS. Neonatal nosocomial infections. Semin Perinatol 22:25–32, 1998.
9. Hauth JC, Merenstein GB. Infection control. In Hauth JC, Merenstein GB (eds). Guidelines for Perinatal Care, 4th edition. Elk Grove Village, Ill, American Academy of Pediatrics and American College of Obstetricians and Gynecologists, 1997, pp 251–277.
10. Dillon HC, Khare S, Gray BM. Group B streptococcal carriage and disease: a 6-year prospective study. J Pediatr 110:31–36, 1987.
11. Noya FJD, Rench MA, Metzger TG, et al. Unusual occurrence of an epidemic of type 1b/c group B streptococcal sepsis in a neonatal intensive care unit. J Infect Dis 155:1135–1144, 1987.
12. Gladstone IM, Ehrenkrantz RA, Edberg SC, Baltimore RS. A ten-year review of neonatal sepsis and comparison with the previous fifty-year experience. Pediatr Infec Dis J 9:819–825, 1990.
13. Baltimore RS. Late, late onset infections in the nursery. Yale J Biol Med 61:501–506, 1988.
14. Gooch JJ, Britt EM. Staphylococcus aureus colonization and infection in newborn nursery patients. Am J Dis Childhood 132:893–896, 1978.
15. Seals JE, Parrott PL, McGowan JE Jr, et al. Nursery salmonellosis: delayed recognition due to unusually long incubation period. Infect Control 4:205–208, 1983.
16. Goldmann DA. Prevention and management of neonatal infections. Infect Dis Clin North Am 3:779–813, 1989.
17. Holbrook KF, Nottebart VF, Hameed SR, Platt R. Automated post-discharge surveillance for postpartum and neonatal nosocomial infections. Am J Med 91(Suppl 3B):S125–S130, 1991.
18. Scheckler WE, Peterson PJ. Nosocomial infections in 15 rural Wisconsin hospitals—results and conclusions from 6 months of comprehensive surveillance. Infect Control 7:397–402, 1986.
19. Welliver RC, McLaughlin S. Unique epidemiology of nosocomial infection in a children's hospital. Am J Dis Child 138:131–135, 1984.
20. Horan TC, White JW, Jarvis WR, et al. Nosocomial infection surveillance, 1984. MMWR CDC Surveill Summ 35:17SS–29SS, 1986.
21. Bureau of Communicable Disease Epidemiology, Laboratory Centre for Disease Control, Health and Welfare, Canada. Canadian nosocomial infection surveillance program: Annual summary June 1984–May 1985. Can Dis Wkly Rep 12:S1, 1986.
22. Maguire GC, Nordin J, Myers MG, et al. Infections acquired by young infants. Am J Dis Child 135:693–698, 1981.
23. A Hospital Infection Program, Centers for Disease Control. Nosocomial infection rates for interhospital comparison: limitations and possible solutions. Infect Control Hosp Epidemiol 12:609–621, 1991.
24. Josephson A, Karanfil L, Alonso H, et al. Risk-specific nosocomial infection rates. Am J Med 91(Suppl 3B):131S–137S, 1991.
25. Hemming VG, Overall JC Jr, Britt MR. Nosocomial infections in a newborn intensive care unit: results of forty-one months of surveillance. N Engl J Med 294:1310–1316, 1976.
26. Hoogkamp-Korstanje JAA, Cats B, Senders RC, et al. Analysis of bacterial infections in a neonatal intensive care unit. J Hosp Infect 3:275–284, 1982.
27. Wenzel RP, Osterman CA, Hunting KJ. Hospital-acquired infections: II. Infection rates by site, service, and common procedures in a university hospital. Am J Epidemiol 104:645–651, 1976.
28. Goldmann DA, Durbin WA, Freeman J. Nosocomial infections in a neonatal intensive care unit. J Infect Dis 141:149–159, 1981.
29. Larson E, Hargiss CO, Dyk L. Effect of an expanded physical facility on nosocomial infections in a neonatal intensive care unit. Am J Infect Control 13:16–20, 1985.
30. Brown RB, Hosmer D, Chen C, et al. A comparison of infections in different ICUs within the same hospital. Crit Care Med 13:472–476, 1985.
31. Ford-Jones EL, Mindorff CM, Langley JM, et al. Epidemiologic study of 4684 hospital-acquired infections in pediatric patients. Pediatr Infect Dis J 8:668–675, 1989.
32. Stoll BJ, Gordon T, Korones SB, et al. Late-onset sepsis in very low birth weight neonates: a report from the National Institute of Child Health and Human Development Neonatal Research Network. J Pediatr 129:63–71, 1996.
33. Freeman J, Epstein MF, Smith NE, et al. Extra hospital stay and antibiotic usage with nosocomial coagulase-negative staphylococcal bacteremia in two neonatal intensive

care unit populations. Am J Dis Child 144:324–329, 1990.

34. Beck-Sague CM, Azimi P, Fonseca SN, et al. Bloodstream infections in neonatal intensive care unit patients: results of a multicenter study. Pediatr Infect Dis J 13:1110–1116, 1994.

35. Siegel JD. The newborn nursery. *In* Bennett JV, Brachman PS (eds). Hospital Infections, 4th ed. Boston, Little Brown, 1998, pp 403–420.

36. Sands KE, Goldmann DA. Epidemiology of *Staphylococcus aureus* and group A streptococci. *In* Bennett JV, Brachman PS (eds). Hospital Infections, 4th ed. Boston, Little Brown, 1998, pp 621–636.

37. Nakashima AK, Allen JR, Martone WJ, et al. Epidemic bullous impetigo in a nursery due to a nasal carrier of *Staphylococcus aureus*: role of epidemiology and control measures. Infect Control 5:326–331, 1984.

38. Belani A, Sheretz RJ, Sullivan ML, et al. Outbreak of staphylococcal infection in two hospital nurseries traced to a single nasal carrier. Infect Control 7:487–490, 1986.

39. Dancer SJ, Simmons NA, Poston SM, et al. Outbreak of staphylococcal scalded skin syndrome among neonates. J Infect 16:87–103, 1988.

40. Dave J, Reith S, Nash JQ, et al. A double outbreak of exfoliative toxin A–producing strains of *Staphylococcus aureus* in a maternity unit. Epidemiol Infect 112:103–114, 1994.

41. Mackenzie A, Johnson W, Heyes B, et al. A prolonged outbreak of exfoliative toxin A–producing *Staphylococcus aureus* in newborn nursery. Diagn Microbiol Infect Dis 21:69–75, 1995.

42. Saiman L, Jakob K, Holmes K, et al. Molecular epidemiology of staphylococcal scalded skin syndrome in premature infants. Pediatr Infect Dis J 17:329–334, 1998.

43. Kaslow RA, Dixon RE, Martin SM, et al. Staphylococcal disease related to hospital nursery bathing practices—a nationwide epidemiologic investigation. Pediatrics 51:418–429, 1973.

44. Johnson JD, Malachowski NC, Vosti KL, Sunshine P. A sequential study of various modes of skin and umbilical care and the incidence of staphylococcal colonization and infection in the neonate. Pediatrics 58:354–361, 1976.

45. Sands KE, Pursley D, Kalaidjian R, et al. Clinical and molecular epidemiology of *Staphylococcus aureus* in a neonatal intensive care unit. Infect Control Hosp Epidemiol 16(Suppl):P29, 1995 (abstract).

46. Fairchild JP, Gruber CD, Vogel EH. Flora of the umbilical stump: 2,479 cultures. J Pediatr 53:538, 1958.

47. Jellard J. Umbilical cord as a reservoir of infection in maternity hospital. Br J Med 1:925, 1957.

48. Rammelkamp CH, Mortimer EA, Wolinsky E. Transmission of streptococcal and staphylococcal infections. Ann Intern Med 60:753–758, 1964.

49. Mortimer EA, Lipsitz PJ, Wolinsky E, et al. Transmission of staphylococci between newborns: importance of the hands of personnel. Am J Dis Child 104:289–295, 1962.

50. Light IJ, Sutherland JM. What is the evidence that hexachlorophene is not effective? Pediatrics 51:345–359, 1973.

51. Powell H, Swarner O, Gluck L, et al. Hexachlorophene myelinopathy in premature infants. J Pediatr 82:976–981, 1973.

52. Shuman RM, Leech TW, Alvord EC Jr. Neurotoxicity of hexachlorophene in the human: I. A clinicopathologic study of 248 children. Pediatrics 54:689–695, 1974.

53. Shuman RM, Leech TW, Alvord EC Jr. Neurotoxicity of hexachlorophene in the human: II. A clinicopathologic

54. Aggett PJ, Cooper LV, Ellis SH, et al. Percutaneous absorption of chlorhexidine in neonatal cord care. Arch Dis Child 56:878–880, 1981.

55. Cowen J, Ellis SH, McAinsh J. Absorption of chlorhexidine from the intact skin of newborn infants. Arch Dis Child 54:379–383, 1979.

56. Johnsson J, Seeberg S, Kjellmer I. Blood concentrations of chlorhexidine in neonates undergoing routine cord care with 4% chlorhexidine gluconate solution. Acta Paediatr Scand 76:675–676, 1987.

57. Reboli AC, John JJ Jr, Levkoff AH. Epidemic methicillin-gentamicin–resistant *Staphylococcus aureus* in a neonatal intensive care unit. Am J Dis Child 143:34, 1989.

58. Shinefield HR. Staphylococcal infections. *In* Remington JS, Klein JO (eds). Infectious Diseases of the Fetus and Newborn Infant. Philadelphia, WB Saunders, 1990, pp 866–900.

59. Shinefield HR, Ribble JC, Boris M. Bacterial interference between strains of *Staphylococcus aureus* 1960 to 1970. Am J Dis Child 121:148–152, 1971.

60. Moore EP, Williams EW. A maternity hospital outbreak of methicillin-resistant *Staphylococcus aureus*. J Hosp Infect 19:5–16, 1991.

61. Webster J, Faoagali JL. Endemic methicillin-resistant *Staphylococcus aureus* in a special baby care unit: a 2 year review. J Paediatr Child Health 26:160–163, 1990.

62. Ish-Horowicz MR, McIntyre P, Nade S. Bone and joint infections caused by multiply resistant *Staphylococcus aureus* in a neonatal intensive care unit. Pediatr Infect Dis J 11:82–87, 1992.

63. Noel GJ, Kreiswirth BN, Edelson PJ, et al. Multiple methicillin-resistant *Staphylococcus aureus* strains as a cause for a single outbreak of severe disease in hospitalized neonates. Pediatr Infect Dis J 11:184–188, 1992.

64. Richardson JF, Quoraishi AH, Francis BJ, Marples RR. Beta-lactamase negative, methicillin-resistant *Staphylococcus aureus* in a newborn nursery: report of an outbreak and laboratory investigations. J Hosp Infect 16:109–121, 1990.

65. Hollis R, Barr J, Doebbeling B, et al. Familial carriage of methicillin-resistant *Staphylococcus aureus* and subsequent infection in a premature infant. Clin Infect Dis 21:328–332, 1995.

66. Rosenfeld CR, Laptook AR, Jeffery J. Limited effectiveness of triple dye in preventing colonization with methicillin-resistant *Staphylococcus aureus* in a special care nursery. Pediatr Infect Dis J 9:290–291, 1990.

67. Tenover FC, Arbeit R, Archer G, et al. Comparison of traditional and molecular methods of typing isolates of *Staphylococcus aureus*. J Clin Microbiol 32:407–415, 1994.

68. Fang F, McClelland M, Guiney D, et al. Value of molecular epidemiologic analysis in a nosocomial methicillin-resistant *Staphylococcus aureus* outbreak. JAMA 270:1323–1328, 1993.

69. Coovadia YM, Bhana RH, Johnson AP, et al. A laboratory-confirmed outbreak of rifampin-methicillin resistant *Staphylococcus aureus* (RMRSA) in a newborn nursery. J Hosp Infect 14:303–312, 1989.

70. Farrington M, Ling J, Ling T, French GL. Outbreaks of infection with methicillin-resistant *Staphylococcus aureus* on neonatal and burn units of a new hospital. Epidemiol Infect 105:215–228, 1990.

71. Boyce J. Methicillin-resistant *Staphylococcus aureus* infections. *In* Abrutyn E, Goldmann DA, Scheckler WE (eds). Saunders Infection Control Reference Service. Philadelphia, WB Saunders, 1998, p 641.

72. Zafar A, Butler R, Reese D, et al. Use of 0.3 triclosan (Bacti-Stat) to eradicate an outbreak of MRSA in a neonatal nursery. Am J Infect Control 23:200–208, 1995.

73. Millar MR, Keyworth N, Lincoln C, et al. Methicillin-resistant *Staphylococcus aureus* in a regional neonatal unit. J Hosp Infect 10:187–197, 1987.

74. Davies EA, Emmerson AM, Hogg GM, et al. An outbreak of infection with a methicillin-resistant *Staphylococcus aureus* in a special baby care unit: value of topical mupirocin and of traditional methods of infection control. J Hosp Infect 10:120–128, 1987.

75. Haley RE, Cushion NB, Tenover FC, et al. Eradication of endemic methicillin-resistant *Staphylococcus aureus* infections from a neonatal intensive care unit. J Infect Dis 171:614–624, 1995.

76. Haley RE, Bregman DA. The role of understaffing and overcrowding in recurrent outbreaks of staphylococcal infection in a neonatal special-care unit. J Infect Dis 145:875–885, 1982.

77. Combined Working Party. Revised guidelines for the control of epidemic MRSA. J Hosp Infect 16:351–377, 1990.

78. Working Group on Infection Prevention. Management policy for MRSA (abstract 35a). *In* Working Group on Infection Prevention. Leiden, The Netherlands, 1995, pp 1–8.

79. Boyce JM, Jackson MM, Pugliese G, et al. MRSA: a briefing for acute care hospitals and nursing facilities (the AHA technical panel on infections within hospitals). Infect Control Hosp Epidemiol 15:105–111, 1994.

80. Mulligan ME, Murray-Leisure KA, Ribner BS, et al. MRSA: a consensus review of the microbiology, pathogenesis and epidemiology with implications for prevention and management. Am J Med 94:313–328, 1993.

81. Huebner J, Pier G, Maslow J, et al. Endemic nosocomial transmission of *Staphylococcus* epidermidis bacteremia isolates in a neonatal intensive care unit over 10 years. J Infect Dis 169:526–531, 1994.

82. LaGamma EF, Drusin LM, Mackles AW, et al. Neonatal infections: an important determinant of late NICU mortality in infants less than 1000 gm at birth. Am J Dis Child 137:838–841, 1983.

83. Donowitz LG, Haley CE, Gregory WW, et al. Neonatal intensive care unit bacteremia: emergence of gram-positive bacteria as major pathogens. Am J Infect Control 15:141–147, 1987.

84. Hensey OJ, Hart CA, Cooke RWI. Serious infection in a neonatal intensive care unit: a two-year survey. J Hyg (Camb) 95:289–297, 1985.

85. Sidebottom DG, Freeman J, Platt R, et al. Fifteen-year experience with bloodstream isolates of coagulase-negative staphylococci in neonatal intensive care. J Clin Microbiol 26:713–718, 1988.

86. Baker CJ, Melish ME, Hall RT, et al. Intravenous immune globulin for the prevention of nosocomial infection in low birth weight neonates. N Engl J Med 327:213–219, 1992.

87. Fanaroff AA, Korones SB, Wright LL, et al. A controlled trial of intravenous immune globulin to reduce nosocomial infections in very low birth weight infants. N Engl J Med 330:1107–1113, 1994.

88. Hall SL. Coagulase-negative staphylococcal infections in neonates. Pediatr Infect Dis J 10:57–67, 1991.

89. Lyytikainen O, Saxen H, Ryhanen, et al. Persistence of a multiresistant clone of *Staphylococcus epidermidis* in a neonatal intensive care unit for a four-year period. Clin Infect Dis 20:24–29, 1995.

90. Freeman J, Goldmann DA, Smith NE, et al. Association

91. of intravenous lipid emulsion and coagulase-negative staphylococcal bacteremia in neonatal intensive care units. N Engl J Med 323:301–308, 1990.

91. McKenny D, Huebner J, Muller E, et al. The ICA locus of *Staphylococcus epidermidis* encodes production of the capsular polysaccharide/adhesin (PS/A). Infect Immun 66:4711–4720, 1998.

92. Kloos W, Bannerman T. Update on clinical significance of coagulase-negative staphylococci. Clin Microbiol Rev 7:117–140, 1994.

93. Noel GJ, Edelson PJ. *Staphylococcus epidermidis* bacteremia in neonates: further observations and the occurrence of focal infection. Pediatrics 74:832–837, 1984.

94. Patrick CJ, John LF, Levkoff AH, et al. Relatedness of strains of methicillin-resistant coagulase-negative *Staphylococcus* colonizing hospital personnel and producing bacteremias in a neonatal intensive care unit. Pediatr Infect Dis J 11:935–940, 1992.

95. Kacia MA, Horgan MJ, Preston KE, et al. Relatedness of coagulase-negative staphylococci causing bacteremia in low-birthweight infants. Infect Contr Hosp Epidemiol 15:658–662, 1994.

96. Camargo LFA, Strabelli TMV, Ribeiro FG, et al. Epidemiologic investigation of an outbreak of coagulase-negative staphylococcus primary bacteremia in a newborn intensive care unit. Infect Control Hosp Epidemiol 16:595–596, 1995.

97. Nesin M, Projan SJ, Kreisiverth B, et al. Molecular epidemiology of *Staphylococcus epidermidis* blood isolates from neonatal intensive care unit patients. J Hosp Infect 31:111–121, 1995.

98. Eastick K, Leening JP, Bennet D, et al. Reservoirs of coagulase-negative staphylococci in preterm infants. Arch Dis Child 74:F99–F104, 1996.

99. Low DE, Schmidt BK, Kirplani HM, et al. An endemic strain of *Staphylococcus haemolyticus* colonizing and causing bacteremia in neonatal intensive care unit patients. Pediatrics 89:696–700, 1992.

100. Neumeister B, Kastner C, Conrad S, et al. Characterization of coagulase-negative staphylococci causing nosocomial infections in preterm infants. Eur J Clin Microbiol Infect Dis 14:856–863, 1995.

101. Rojas MA, Gonzalez A, Bancalari E, et al. Changing trends in the epidemiology and pathogenesis of neonatal chronic lung disease. J Pediatr 126:605–610, 1995.

102. Baier JR, Bocchini JA, Brown EG. Selective use of vancomycin to prevent coagulase-negative staphylococcal nosocomial bacteremia in high risk very low birth weight infants. Pediatr Infect Dis J 17:179–183, 1998.

103. Schaberg DR, Culver DH, Gaynes RP. Major trends in the microbial etiology of nosocomial infection. Am J Med 91:72S–75S, 1991.

104. Buchino JJ, Ciamberella E, Light I. Systemic group D streptococcal infection in newborn infants. Am J Dis Child 133:270–273, 1979.

105. Bavikatte K, Schreiner RL, Lemons JA, et al. Group D streptococcal septicemia in the neonate. Am J Dis Child 133:493–496, 1979.

106. Dobson SRM, Baker CJ. Enterococcal sepsis in neonates: features by age at onset and occurrence of focal infection. Pediatrics 85:165–171, 1990.

107. Christie C, Hammond J, Reising S, et al. Clinical and molecular epidemiology of enterococcal bacteremia in a pediatric teaching hospital. J Pediatr 125:392–399, 1994.

108. Rice LB, Shlaes DM. Vancomycin resistance in the enterococcus: relevance in pediatrics. Pediatr Clin North Am 1995; 42:601–618, 1995.

109. McNeeley DF, Saint-Louis F, Noel GF. Neonatal entero-

coccal bacteremia: an increasingly frequent event with potentially untreatable pathogens. Pediatr Infect Dis J 15:800–805, 1996.

110. Coudron PE, Mayhall CG, Facklam RR, et al. *Streptococcus faecium* outbreak in a neonatal intensive care unit. J Clin Microbiol 20:1044–1048, 1984.

111. Luginbuhl LM, Rotbart HA, Facklan RR, et al. Neonatal enterococcal sepsis: case-control study and description of an outbreak. Pediatr Infect Dis J 6:1022–1030, 1987.

112. McNeeley DF, Brown AE, Noel GJ, et al. An investigation of vancomycin-resistant *Enterococcus faecium* within the pediatric service of a large urban medical center. Pediatr Infect Dis J 17:184–188, 1998.

113. Morris JG, Shay DK, Hebden JN, et al. Enterococci resistant to multiple antimicrobial agents, including vancomycin: establishment of endemicity in a university medical center. Ann Intern Med 123:250–259, 1995.

114. Centers for Disease Control and Prevention. Recommendations for preventing the spread of vancomycin resistance: recommendations of the Hospital Infection Control Practices Advisory Committee (HICPAC). MMWR Morb Mortal Wkly Rep 44(No. RR-12):1–13, 1995.

115. Nelson KE, Warren D, Tomasi AM, et al. Transmission of neonatal listeriosis in a delivery room. Am J Dis Child 139:903–905, 1985.

116. Schuchat A, Lizano C, Broome CV, et al. Outbreak of neonatal listeriosis associated with mineral oil. Pediatr Infect Dis J 10:183–189, 1991.

117. Campbell JR, Arango CA, Garcia-Prats JA, et al. An outbreak of M serotype 1 group A *Streptococcus* in a neonatal intensive care unit. J Pediatr 129:396–402, 1996.

118. Han VKM, Sayed H, Chance DW, et al. An outbreak of *Clostridium difficile* necrotizing enterocolitis: a case for oral vancomycin therapy? Pediatrics 71:935–941, 1983.

119. Enad D, Meislich D, Brodsky NL, Hurt H. Is *Clostridium difficile* a pathogen in the newborn intensive care unit? A prospective evaluation. J Perinatol 17:355–359, 1997.

120. Bacon AE, Fekety R, Schaberg DR, Faix RG. Epidemiology of *Clostridium difficile* colonization in newborns: results using a bacteriophage and bacteriocin typing system. J Infect Dis 158:349–354, 1988.

121. Zedd AJ, Sell TL, Schaberg DR, et al. Nosocomial *Clostridium difficile* reservoir in a neonatal intensive care unit. Pediatr Infect Dis J 3:429–432, 1984.

122. Delmee M, Verellen G, Avesani V, Francois G. *Clostridium difficile* in neonates: serogrouping and epidemiology. Eur J Pediatr 147:36–40, 1988.

123. Toltzis P, Blumer JL. Antibiotic-resistant gram-negative bacteria in the critical care setting. Pediatr Clin North Am 42:687–702, 1995.

124. Flibel-Rimon O, Leibovitz E, Juster-Reicher A, et al. An outbreak of antibiotic multiresistant *Klebsiella* at the neonatal intensive care unit, Kaplan Hospital, Rehovot, Israel, November 1991–April 1992. Am J Perinatol 13:99–102, 1996.

125. Al-Rabea AA, Burwen DR, Eldeen MAF, et al. *Klebsiella pneumoniae* bloodstream infections in neonates in a hospital in the kingdom of Saudi Arabia. Infect Contr Hosp Epidemiol 19:674–679, 1998.

126. Fok TF, Lee CH, Wong EMC, et al. Risk factors for *Enterobacter* septicemia in a neonatal unit: case control study. Clin Infect Dis 27:1204–1209, 1998.

127. Fierer J, Taylor PM, Gezon HM. *Pseudomonas aeruginosa* epidemic traced to delivery room resuscitators. N Engl J Med 276:991–996, 1967.

128. Bobo RA, Newton EJ, Jones LF, et al. Nursery outbreak of *Pseudomonas aeruginosa*: epidemiologic conclusions

from five different typing methods. Appl Microbiol 25:414–420, 1973.

129. Bassett DCJ, Thompson SAS, Page B. Neonatal infections with *Pseudomonas aeruginosa* associated with contaminated resuscitation equipment. Lancet 1:781–784, 1965.

130. Drewett SE, Payne DJH, Tuke W, Verdon PE. Eradication of *Pseudomonas aeruginosa* infection from a special-care nursery. Lancet 1:946–948, 1972.

131. Leigh L, Stoll BJ, Rohman M, et al. *Pseudomonas aeruginosa* infection in very low birth weight infants: a case control study. Pediatr Infect Dis J 14:367–371, 1995.

132. Grundmann H, Kropsec A, Harting D, et al. *Pseudomonas aeruginosa* in a neonatal intensive care unit: reservoirs and etiology of the nosocomial pathogen. J Infect Dis 168:943–947, 1993.

133. Verweij PE, Geven WB, van Belkum A, et al. Cross-infection with *Pseudomonas aeruginosa* in a neonatal intensive care unit characterized by polymerase chain reaction fingerprinting. Pediatr Infect Dis J 12:1027–1029, 1993.

134. Neal TJ, Hughes CR, Rothburn MM, et al. The neonatal laryngoscope as a potential source of cross-infection. J Hosp Infect 30:315–321, 1995.

135. Pegues DA, Arathoon EG, Samayoa B, et al. Epidemic gram-negative bacteremia in a neonatal intensive care unit in Guatemala. Am J Infect Control 22:163–171, 1994.

136. McNaughton M, Mazinke N, Thomas E. Newborn conjunctivitis associated with triclosan 0.5% antiseptic intrinsically contaminated with *Serratia marcescens*. Can J Infect Control 10:7–8, 1995.

137. Archibald LK, Corl A, Shah B, et al. *Serratia marcescens* outbreak associated with extrinsic contamination of 1% chlorxylenol soap. Infect Control Hosp Epidemiol 18:704–709, 1997.

138. van Ogtrop ML, van Zoern-Grobben D, Verbakel-Salomons E, et al. *Serratia marcescens* infections in neonatal departments: description of an outbreak and review of the literature. J Hosp Infect 36:95–103, 1997.

139. Burke JP, Ingall D, Klein JO, et al. *Proteus mirabilis* infections in a hospital nursery traced to a human carrier. N Engl J Med 284:115–121, 1971.

140. Goering RV, Ehrenkrantz J, Sanders CC, et al. Long-term epidemiological analysis of *Citrobacter diversus* in a neonatal intensive care unit. Pediatr Infect Dis J 11:99–104, 1992.

141. Kline MW. *Citrobacter* meningitis and brain abscess in infancy: epidemiology, pathogenesis, and treatment. J Pediatr 113:430–434, 1988.

142. Lin FC, Devor WF, Morrison C, et al. Outbreak of neonatal *Citrobacter diversus* meningitis in a suburban hospital. Pediatr Infect Dis J 6:50–55, 1987.

143. Khan MA, Abdur-Rab M, Isar N, et al. Transmission of *Salmonella worthington* by oropharyngeal suction in a hospital neonatal unit. Pediatr Infect Dis J 10:668–672, 1991.

144. Schroeder SA, Aserkoff B, Brachman PS. Epidemic salmonellosis in hospitals and institutions: a five-year review. N Engl J Med 279:674–678, 1968.

145. Kumar A, Nath G, Bhatia BD, et al. An outbreak of multidrug resistant *Salmonella typhimurium* in a nursery. Indian Pediatr 1995; 32:881–885, 1995.

146. Mahajan R, Mathur R, Kumar A, et al. Nosocomial outbreak of *Salmonella typhimurium* infection in a nursery intensive care unit (NICU) and pediatric ward. J Commun Dis 27:10–14, 1995.

147. Abroms IF, Cochran WD, Holmes LB, et al. A *Salmonella newport* outbreak in a premature nursery with a 1-year

follow-up: Effect of ampicillin following bacteriologic failure of response to kanamycin. Pediatrics 37:616–623, 1966.

148. Epstein HC, Hochwald A, Ashe R. *Salmonella* infection of the newborn infant. J Pediatr 38:723–731, 1951.

149. Leeder FS. An epidemic of *Salmonella panama* infections in infants. Ann NY Acad Sci 66:54–60, 1956.

150. Rubenstein AD, Fowler RN. Salmonellosis of the newborn with transmission by delivery room resuscitators. Am J Public Health 45:1109–1114, 1955.

151. Silverstolpe L, Plazikowski U, Kjellander J, et al. An epidemic among infants caused by *Salmonella muenchen*. J Appl Bacteriol 24:134–142, 1961.

152. Watt J, Wegman ME, Brown OW, et al. Salmonellosis in a premature nursery unaccompanied by diarrheal disease. Pediatrics 22:689–705, 1958.

153. Regev R, Dolfin T, Zelig S, et al. *Acinetobacter* septicemia: a threat to neonates? Special aspects in a neonatal intensive care unit. Infection 21:394–396, 1993.

154. Sakata H, Fujita K, Maruyama S, et al. *Acinetobacter calcoaceticus* biovar *anitratus* septicemia in a neonatal intensive care unit: epidemiology and control. J Hosp Infect 14:15–22, 1989.

155. Morgan MEI, Hart CA. *Acinetobacter* meningitis: acquired infection in a neonatal intensive care unit. Arch Dis Child 57:557–559, 1982.

156. Stone JW, Das BC. Investigation of an outbreak of infection with *Acinetobacter calcoaceticus* in a special baby care unit. J Hosp Infect 6:42–48, 1985.

157. Hartstein AI, Rashad AL, Lieber JM, et al. Multiple intensive care unit outbreak of *Acinetobacter calcoaceticus* subspecies *anitratus* respiratory tract infection and colonization associated with contaminated reusable ventilator circuits and resuscitation bags. Am J Med 85:624–631, 1988.

158. McDonald LC, Walker IM, Carson L, et al. Outbreak of *Acinetobacter* bloodstream infections in a nursery associated with contaminated aerosols and air conditioners. Pediatr Infect Dis J 17:716–722, 1998.

159. Pokrywka M, Vizanko K, Mednick J, et al. *Flavobacterium meningosepticum* outbreak among intensive care patients. Am J Infect Contr 21:394–396, 1993.

160. Abrahamsen TG, Finne PH, Lingaas E. *Flavobacterium meningosepticum* infections in a neonatal intensive care unit. Acta Paediatr Scand 78:51–55, 1989.

161. Plotkin SA, McKitrick JC. Nosocomial meningitis of the newborn caused by a flavobacterium. JAMA 198:194–196, 1966.

162. Cabrera HA, Davis GH. Epidemic meningitis of the newborn caused by flavobacterium. Am J Dis Child 101:289–295, 1961.

163. Wheeler WE. Water bugs in the bassinet [editorial]. Am J Dis Child 101:273–277, 1961.

164. Moffat HL, Allan D, Williams T. Survival and dissemination of bacteria in nebulizers and incubators. Am J Dis Child 114:13–20, 1967.

165. Matsaniotis NS, Syriopoulou VP, Theodoridou MC, et al. *Enterobacter* sepsis in infants and children due to contaminated intravenous fluids. Infect Control 1984; 5:471–477, 1984.

166. Lemaitre D, Elaichouni A, Hundhausen M, et al. Tracheal colonization with *Shigomonas paucimobilis* in mechanically ventilated neonates due to contaminated ventilator temperature probes. J Hosp Infect 32:199–206, 1996.

167. Simmons NA. Contamination of disinfectants. BMJ 1:842, 1969.

168. Ayliffe GA, Barrowcliff DF, Lowbury EJ. Contamination of disinfectants. BMJ 1:505, 1969.

169. Simmons NA, Gardner DA. Bacterial contamination of a phenolic disinfectant. BMJ 2:668–669, 1969.

170. Sanford JP. Disinfectants that don't. Editorial. Ann Intern Med 72:282, 1970.

171. Botsford KB, Weinstein RA, Boyer KB, et al. Gram-negative bacilli in human milk feedings: quantitation and clinical consequences for premature infants. J Pediatr 109:707–710, 1986.

172. Schreiner RL, Eitzen H, Gfell MA, et al. Environmental contamination of continuous drip feedings. Pediatrics 63:232–237, 1979.

173. Morooka T, Takeo H, Yasumoto S, et al. Nosocomial meningitis due to *Campylobacter fetus* subspecies *fetus* in a neonatal intensive care unit. Acta Paediatr Jpn 34:530–533, 1992.

174. Terrier A, Altwegg M, Bader P, von Graevenitz A. Hospital epidemic of neonatal *Campylobacter jejuni* infection. Lancet 2:1182, 1985.

175. Hershkowici S, Barak M, Cohen A, Montag J. An outbreak of *Campylobacter jejuni* infection in a neonatal intensive care unit. J Hosp Infect 9:54–59, 1987.

176. Goossens H, Henocque G, Kremp L, et al. Nosocomial outbreak of *Campylobacter jejuni* meningitis in newborn infants. Lancet 2:146–149, 1986.

177. Freisen CA, Cho CT. Characteristic features of neonatal sepsis due to *Haemophilus influenzae*. Rev Infect Dis 8:777–780, 1986.

178. Falla TJ, Dobson SRM, Crook DWM, et al. Population based study of nontypable *Haemophilus influenzae* invasive disease in children and neonates. Lancet 341:851–854, 1993.

179. Linnemann CC, Ramundo N, Perlstein PH, et al. Use of pertussis vaccine in an epidemic involving hospital staff. Lancet 2:540–543, 1975.

180. Holmberg RE, Pavia AT, Montgomery D, et al. Nosocomial *Legionella* pneumonia in the neonate. Pediatrics 92:450–453, 1993.

181. Aubert G, Bornstein N, Rayet I, et al. Nosocomial infection with *Legionella pneumophila* serogroup 1 and 9 in a neonate. Scand J Infect Dis 22:367–370, 1990.

182. Lowry PW, Blankenship RJ, Gridley W, et al. A cluster of *Legionella* sternal wound infections due to postoperative topical exposure to contaminated tap water. N Engl J Med 324:109–113, 1991.

183. Cook LN, Davis RS, Stover BH. Outbreak of amikacin-resistant Enterobacteriaceae in an intensive care nursery. Pediatrics 65:264–268, 1980.

184. McKee RT Jr, Cotton RB, Stratton CW, et al. Nursery epidemic due to multiply resistant *Klebsiella pneumoniae*: epidemiologic setting and impact on perinatal health care delivery. Infect Contr 3:150–156, 1982.

185. John JF, McKee KT, Twitty JA, et al. Molecular epidemiology of sequential nursery epidemics caused by multiresistant *Klebsiella pneumoniae*. J Pediatr 102:825–830, 1983.

186. Saravolatz LD, Arking L, Pohlod D, et al. An outbreak of gentamicin-resistant *Klebsiella pneumoniae*: analysis of control measures. Infect Control 5:79–84, 1984.

187. Gaynes RP, Simpson DS, Reeves SA, et al. A nursery outbreak of multiple-aminoglycoside–resistant *Escherichia coli*. Infect Control 5:519–524, 1984.

188. Eisenach KD, Reber R, Eitzman DV, et al. Nosocomial infections due to kanamycin-resistant, [R]-factor carrying enteric organisms in an intensive care nursery. Pediatr 50:395–402, 1972.

189. Morris JG, Lin FYC, Morrison CB, et al. Molecular epidemiology of neonatal meningitis due to *Citrobacter*

diversus: a study of isolates from hospitals in Maryland. J Infect Dis 154:409–414, 1986.

190. Modi N, Damjanovic V, Cooke RWI. Outbreak of cephalosporin-resistant *Enterobacter cloacae* infection in a neonatal intensive care unit. Arch Dis Child 62:148–151, 1987.

191. Bryan CS, John JF, Pai S, Austin TL. Gentamicin vs. ceftriaxone for therapy of neonatal sepsis. Am J Dis Child 139:1086–1089, 1985.

192. Cornaglia G, Riccio ML, Mazzariol A, et al. Appearance of IMP-1 metallo-beta-lactamase in Europe. Letter. Lancet 353:899–900, 1999.

193. Lee HL, LeVea CM, Graman PS. Congenital tuberculosis in a neonatal intensive care unit: case report, epidemiologic investigation, and management of exposures. Clin Infect Dis 27:474–477, 1998.

194. Steiner P, Rao M, Victoria MS, et al. Miliary tuberculosis in two infants after nursery exposure: epidemiologic, clinical, and laboratory findings. Am Rev Respir Dis 113:267–271, 1976.

195. Nivin B, Nicholas P, Gayer M, et al. A continuing outbreak of multidrug-resistant tuberculosis, with transmission in a hospital nursery. Clin Infect Dis 26:303–307, 1998.

196. Centers for Disease Control and Prevention. Guidelines for preventing the transmission of *Mycobacterium tuberculosis* in health care facilities, 1994. MMWR Morb Mortal Wkly Rep 43(No. RR-13); i–v, 1–132, 1994.

197. Beck-Sague CM, Jarvis WR. Secular trends in the epidemiology of nosocomial fungal infections in the United States, 1980–1990. J Infect Dis 167:1247–1251, 1993.

198. Saxen H, Virtanen M, Carlson P, et al. Neonatal *Candida parapsilosis* outbreak with a high case fatality rate. Pediatr Infect Dis J 14:776–781, 1995.

199. El-Mohandes AE, Johnson-Robbins L, Keiser JF, et al. Incidence of *Candida parapsilosis* colonization in an intensive care nursery population and its association with invasive fungal disease. Pediatr Infect Dis J 13:520–524, 1994.

200. Betremieux P, Chevrier S, Quindos G, et al. Use of DNA fingerprinting and biotyping methods to study a *Candida albicans* outbreak in a neonatal intensive care unit. Pediatr Infect Dis J 13:899–905, 1994.

201. Finkelstein R, Reinhartz G, Hashman N, et al. Outbreak of *Candida tropicalis* fungemia in a neonatal intensive care unit. Infect Control Hosp Epidemiol 14:587–590, 1993.

202. McNeil MM. *Candida. In* Mayhall GC (ed). Hospital Epidemiology and Infection Control. Baltimore, Williams & Wilkins, 1996, pp 408–419.

203. Welbel SF, McNeil MM, Kuykendall RJ, et al. *Candida parapsilosis* bloodstream infections in neonatal intensive care unit patients: epidemiologic and laboratory confirmation of a common source outbreak. Pediatr Infect Dis J 15:998–1002, 1996.

204. Sheretz RJ, Gledhill KS, Hampton KD, et al. Outbreak of *Candida* bloodstream infections associated with retrograde medication administration in a neonatal intensive care unit. J Pediatr 120:455–461, 1992.

205. Solomon SL, Alexander H, Eley JW, et al. Nosocomial fungemia in neonates associated with intravascular pressure-monitoring devices. Pediatr Infect Dis J 5:680–685, 1986.

206. Vazquez JA, Boikov D, Boikov SG, Dajani AS. Use of electrophoretic karyotyping in the evaluation of *Candida* infections in a neonatal intensive-care unit. Infect Control Hosp Epidemiol 18:32–37, 1997.

207. Baley JE, Kliegman RM, Boxerbaum B, et al. Fungal

208. Rowen JL, Rench MA, Kozinetz CA, et al. Endotracheal colonization with *Candida* enhances risk of systemic candidiasis in very low birth weight neonates. J Pediatr 124:789–794, 1994.

209. Huang YC, Li CC, Lin TY, et al. Association of fungal colonization and invasive disease in very low birth weight infants. Pediatr Infect Dis J 17:819–822, 1998.

210. Hageman JR, Stenske J, Keuler H, et al. *Candida* colonization and infection in very low birth weight infants. J Perinatol 6:251–254, 1985.

211. Waggoner-Fountain LA, Walker MW, Hollis RJ, et al. Vertical and horizontal transmission of unique *Candida* species to premature newborns. Clin Infect Dis 22:803–808, 1996.

212. Johnson DE, Thompson TR, Green TP, et al. Systemic candidiasis in very-low-birth-weight infants (<1500 grams). Pediatrics 73:138–143, 1984.

213. Weese-Mayer DE, Fondriest DW, Brouillette RT, et al. Risk factors associated with candidemia in the neonatal intensive care unit: a case-control study. Pediatr Infect Dis J 6:190–196, 1987.

214. Kossoff EH, Buescher ES, Karlowicz MG. Candidemia in a neonatal intensive care unit: trends during fifteen years and clinical features of 111 cases. Pediatr Infect Dis J 17:504–508, 1998.

215. Yinnon AM, Woodkin KA, Powell KR. *Candida lusitaniae* infection in the newborn: case report and review of the literature. Pediatr Infect Dis J 11:878–880, 1992.

216. Fowler SL, Rhoton B, Springer SC, et al. Evidence for person-to-person transmission of *Candida lusitaniae* in a neonatal intensive-care unit. Infect Control Hosp Epidemiol 19:343–345, 1998.

217. Leibovitz E, Iuster-Reicher A, Amitai M, Mogilner B. Systemic candidal infections associated with use of peripheral venous catheters in neonates: a 9-year experience. Clin Infect Dis 14:485–491, 1992.

218. Glick C, Graves GR, Feldman S. *Torulopsis glabrata* in the neonate: an emerging fungal pathogen. South Med J 86:969–970, 1993.

219. Weese-Mayer, Faix RG, Kovarik SM, et al. Mucocutaneous and invasive candidiasis among very low birth weight (<1500 grams) infants in intensive care nurseries: a prospective study. Pediatrics 83:101–107, 1989.

220. Baley JE, Kliegman RM, Fanaroff AA. Disseminated fungal infections in very low birth weight infants: clinical manifestation and epidemiology. Pediatrics 73:144–152, 1984.

221. Richet HM, McNeil MM, Edwards MC, et al. Cluster of *Malassezia furfur* pulmonary infections in infants in a neonatal intensive-care unit. J Clin Microbiol 27:1197–1200, 1989.

222. Dankner WM, Spector SA, Fierer J, et al. *Malassezia* fungemia in neonates and adults: complication of hyperalimentation. Rev Infect Dis 9:743–753, 1987.

223. Powell DA, Hayes J, Durrell DE, et al. *Malassezia furfur* skin colonization of infants hospitalized in intensive care units. J Pediatr 111:217–220, 1987.

224. Stuart SM, Lane AT. *Candida* and *Malassezia* as nursery pathogens. Semin Dermatol 11:19–23, 1992.

225. Powell DA, Aungst J, Snedden S, et al. Broviac catheter-related *Malassezia furfur* sepsis in five infants receiving intravenous fat emulsions. J Pediatr 105:987–990, 1984.

226. Long JG, Keyserling HL. Catheter-related infection in infants due to an unusual lipophilic yeast—*Malassezia furfur*. Pediatrics 76:896–900, 1985.

227. Welbel SF, McNeil MM, Pramanik A, et al. Nosocomial

Malassezia pachydermatis bloodstream infections in a neonatal intensive care unit. Pediatr Infect Dis J 13:104–108, 1994.

228. Larocco M, Dorenbaum A, Robinson A, Pickering LK. Recovery of *Malassezia pachydermatis* from eight infants in a neonatal intensive care nursery: clinical and laboratory features. Pediatr Infect Dis J 7:398–401, 1988.

229. Chang HJ, Miller HL, Watkins N, et al. An epidemic of *Malassezia pachydermatis* in an intensive care nursery associated with colonization of health care workers' pet dogs. N Engl J Med 338:706–711, 1998.

230. Fisher DJ, Christy C, Spafford P, et al. Neonatal *Trichosporin beigelii* infection: report of a cluster of cases in a neonatal intensive care unit. Pediatr Infect Dis J 12:149–155, 1993.

231. Snider R, Landers S, Levy ML. The ringworm riddle: an outbreak of *Microsporum canis* in the nursery. Pediatr Infect Dis J 12:145–148, 1993.

232. Mossovitch M, Mossovitch B, Alkan M. Nosocomial dermatophytosis caused by *Microsporum canis* in a newborn department. Infect Control 7:593–595, 1986.

233. Leeming JP, Sutton TM, Fleming PJ, et al. Neonatal skin as a reservoir of *Malassezia* species. Pediatr Infect Dis J 14:719–721, 1995.

234. Gross GJ, MacDonald NE, Mackenzie AMR. Neonatal rectal colonization with *Malassezia furfur*. Can Infect Dis J 3:9–13, 1992.

235. Dennis JE, Rhodes KH, Cooney DR, Roberts GD. Nosocomial *Rhizopus* infection (zygomycosis) in children. J Pediatr 96:824–828, 1980.

236. Grim PF, Demello D, Keenan WJ. Disseminated zygomycosis in a newborn. Pediatr Infect Dis J 3:61–63, 1984.

237. Krasinski K, Holzman RS, Hanna B, et al. Nosocomial fungal infection during hospital renovation. Infect Control 6:278–282, 1985.

238. White CB, Barcia PJ, Bass JW. Neonatal zygomycotic necrotizing cellulitis. Pediatrics 78:100–102, 1986.

239. Schwartz DA, Jacquette M, Chawla HS. Disseminated neonatal aspergillosis: report of a fatal case and analysis of risk factors. Pediatr Infect Dis J 7:349–353, 1988.

240. Varrichio F, Reyers MG, Wilks A. Undiagnosed mucormycosis in infants. Pediatr Infect Dis J 8:660, 1989.

241. Robertson AF, Vijay VJ, Ellison DA, Cedars JC. Zygomycosis in neonates. Pediatr Infect Dis J 16:812–815, 1997.

242. Mitchell SJ, Gray J, Hocking MD, Durbin GM. Nosocomial infection with *Rhizopus microsporus* in preterm infants: association with wooden tongue depressors. Lancet 348:441–443, 1996.

243. Groll AH, Jaeger G, Allendorf A, et al. Invasive pulmonary aspergillosis in a critically ill neonate: case report and review of invasive aspergillosis during the first 3 months of life. Clin Infect Dis 1998; 27:437–452, 1998.

244. Walmsley S, Devi S, King S, et al. Invasive *Aspergillus* infections in a pediatric hospital: a ten-year review. Pediatr Infect Dis J 12:673–682, 1993.

245. Agah R, Cherry JD, Garakian AJ, et al. Respiratory syncytial virus (RSV) infection rate in personnel caring for children with RSV infections. Am J Dis Child 141:695–697, 1987.

246. Rotbart HA, Levin MJ, Yolken RH, et al. An outbreak of rotavirus-associated neonatal necrotizing enterocolitis. J Pediatr 103:454–459, 1983.

247. Finn A, Anday E, Talbot GH. An epidemic of adenovirus 7a infection in a neonatal nursery: course morbidity and management. Infect Control Hosp Epidemiol 9:398–404, 1988.

248. Meissner HC, Murray SA, Kiernan MA, et al. A simulta-

neous outbreak of respiratory syncytial virus and parainfluenza virus type 3 in a newborn nursery. J Pediatr 104:680–684, 1984.

249. Valenti WM, Clarke TA, Hall CB, et al. Concurrent outbreaks of rhinovirus and respiratory syncytial virus in an intensive care nursery: epidemiology and associated risk factors. J Pediatr 100:722–726, 1982.

250. Wilson CW, Stevenson DK, Arvin AM. A concurrent epidemic of respiratory syncytial virus and echovirus 7 infection in an intensive care nursery. Pediatr Infect Dis J 8:24–29, 1989.

251. Bauer CR, Elie K, Spence L, et al. Hong Kong influenza in a neonatal unit. JAMA 223:1233–1235, 1973.

252. Chirico G, Rondini G, Piebani A, et al. Intravenous gammaglobulin therapy for prophylaxis of infection in high-risk neonates. J Pediatr 110:437–442, 1987.

253. Graman PS, Hall CB. Epidemiology and control of nosocomial viral infections. Infect Dis Clin North Am 3:815–841, 1989.

254. Moser MR, Bender TR, Margolis HS, et al. An outbreak of influenza aboard a commercial airliner. Am J Epidemiol 110:1–6, 1979.

255. Hall CB, Douglas RG Jr. Modes of transmission of respiratory syncytial virus. J Pediatr 99:100–103, 1981.

256. Hall CB, Douglas RG Jr, Schnabel KC, et al. Infectivity of respiratory syncytial virus by various routes of inoculation. Infect Immun 33:779–783, 1981.

257. Hall CB, Douglas RG Jr., Geiman JM. Possible transmission by fomites of respiratory syncytial virus. J Infect Dis 141:98–102, 1980.

258. Hall CB, Douglas RG Jr, Geiman JM. Respiratory syncytial virus infections in infants: quantitation and duration of shedding. J Pediatr 80:11–15, 1976.

259. Hall CB, Kopelman AE, Douglas RG Jr, et al. Neonatal respiratory syncytial virus infection. N Engl J Med 300:393–396, 1979.

260. Berkovich S, Taranko L. Acute respiratory illness in the premature nursery associated with respiratory syncytial virus infections. Pediatrics 34:753–760, 1964.

261. Snydman DR, Greer C, Meissner HC, McIntosh K. Prevention of nosocomial transmission of respiratory syncytial virus in a newborn nursery. Infect Control Hosp Epidemiol 9:105–108, 1988.

262. Leclair JM, Freeman J, Sullivan BF, et al. Prevention of nosocomial respiratory syncytial virus infections through compliance with glove and gown isolation precautions. N Engl J Med 317:329–334, 1987.

263. Singh-Naz N, Willy M, Riggs N. Outbreak of parainfluenza virus type 3 in a neonatal nursery. Pediatr Infect Dis J 9:31–33, 1990.

264. Moisiuk SE, Robson D, Klass L, et al. Outbreak of parainfluenza virus type 3 in an intermediate care nursery. Pediatr Infect Dis J 17:49–53, 1998.

265. Sizun J, Soupre D, Legrand MC, et al. Neonatal nosocomial respiratory infection with coronavirus: a prospective study in a neonatal intensive care unit. Acta Paediatr 84:617–620, 1995.

266. Abzug MJ, Levin MJ. Neonatal adenovirus infection: four patients and review of the literature. Pediatrics 87:890–896, 1991.

267. Piedra PA, Kasel JA, Norton IU, et al. Description of an adenovirus type 8 outbreak in hospitalized neonates born prematurely. Pediatr Infect Dis J 11:460–465, 1992.

268. Birenbaum E, Linder N, Varsano N, et al. Adenovirus type 8 conjunctivitis in a neonatal intensive care unit. Arch Dis Child 68:610–611, 1993.

269. Helin I, Widell A, Borulf S, et al. Outbreak of coxsackie-

virus A-14 meningitis among newborns in a maternity hospital ward. Acta Paediatr Scand 76:234–238, 1987.

270. Johnson I, Hammond GW, Verma MR. Nosocomial coxsackie B4 virus infections in two chronic-care pediatric neurological wards. J Infect Dis 151:1153–1156, 1985.

271. Kinney JS, McCray E, Kaplan JE, et al. Risk factors associated with echovirus 11 infection in a hospital nursery. Pediatr Infect Dis J 5:192–197, 1986.

272. Rabkin CS, Telzak EE, Ho MS, et al. Outbreak of echovirus 11 infection in hospitalized neonates. Pediatr Infect Dis J 7:186–190, 1988.

273. Modlin JF. Echovirus infections of newborn infants. Pediatr Infect Dis J 7:311–312, 1988.

274. Modlin JF. Perinatal echovirus and group B coxsackievirus infections. Clin Perinatol 15:233–246, 1988.

275. Chawareewong S, Kiangsiri S, Lokaphadhana K, et al. Neonatal herpangina caused by coxsackie A-5 virus. J Pediatr 93:492–494, 1978.

276. Nagington J. Echovirus 11 infection and prophylactic antiserum. Lancet 2:446, 1982.

277. Nagington J, Wreghitt TG, Gandy G, et al. Fatal echovirus 11 infections in outbreak in special-care baby unit. Lancet 1:725–728, 1978.

278. Garner JS, Hospital Infection Control Practices Advisory Committee (HICPAC). Guidelines for isolation precautions in hospitals. Infect Control Hosp Epidemiol 17:53–80, 1996.

279. Avoiding the danger of enteroviruses to newborn infants. Lancet 1:194–195, 1986.

280. Nagington J, Gandy G, Walker J. Use of normal immunoglobulin in an echovirus 11 outbreak in a special-care baby unit. Lancet 2:443–446, 1983.

281. Watson JC, Fleming DW, Borella AJ, et al. Vertical transmission of hepatitis A resulting in an outbreak in a neonatal intensive care unit. J Infect Dis 167:567–571, 1993.

282. Rosenblum LS, Villarino ME, Nainan OV, et al. Hepatitis A outbreak in a neonatal intensive care unit: risk factors for transmission and evidence of prolonged viral excretion among preterm infants. J Infect Dis 164:476–482, 1991.

283. Azimi PH, Roberto RR, Guralnik J, et al. Transfusion-acquired hepatitis A in a premature infant with secondary nosocomial spread in an intensive care nursery. Am J Dis Child 140:23–27, 1986.

284. Noble RC, Kane MA, Reeves SA, et al. Posttransfusion hepatitis A in a neonatal intensive care unit. JAMA 252:2711–2715, 1984.

285. Klein BS, Michaels JA, Rytel MW, et al. Nosocomial hepatitis A: a multinursery outbreak in Wisconsin. JAMA 252:2716–2721, 1984.

286. American Academy of Pediatrics. Hepatitis A infections. In Peter G (ed). 1997 Red Book: Report of the Committee on Infectious Diseases 24th ed. Elk Grove Village, Ill, American Academy of Pediatrics, 1997, pp 237–246.

287. Haffejee IE. Neonatal rotavirus infections. Rev Infect Dis 13:957–962, 1991.

288. Rodriguez WJ, Kim HW, Brandt CD, et al. Rotavirus: a cause of nosocomial infection in the nursery. J Pediatr 101:274–277, 1982.

289. Walther FJ, Bruggeman C, Daniels-Bosman MS. Rotavirus infections in high-risk neonates. J Hosp Infect 5:438–443, 1984.

290. Vial PA, Kotloff KL, Losonsky GA. Molecular epidemiology of rotavirus infection in a room for convalescing newborns. J Infect Dis 157:668–673, 1988.

291. Prince DS, Astry C, Vonderfecht S, et al. Aerosol transmission of experimental rotavirus infection. Pediatr Infect Dis 5:218–222, 1986.

292. Keswick BH, Pickering LK, Dupont HL, Woodward WE. Survival and detection of rotaviruses on environmental surfaces in day care centers. Appl Environ Microbiol 46:813–816, 1983.

293. Kilgore PE, Unicomb LE, Gentsch JR, et al. Neonatal rotavirus infections in Bangladesh: strain characterization and risk factors for nosocomial infection. Pediatr Infect Dis J 15:672–677, 1996.

294. Riedel F, Kroener T, Stein K, et al. Rotavirus infection and bradycardia-apnea episodes in the neonate. Eur J of Pediatr 155:36–40, 1996.

295. Ansari SA, Springthorpe S, Sattar SA. Survival and vehicular spread of human rotaviruses: possible relation to seasonality of outbreaks. Rev Infect Dis 13:448–461, 1991.

296. Ward RL, Bernstein DI, Knowlton DR, et al. Prevention of surface to human transmission of rotavirus by treatment with disinfectant spray. J Clin Microbiol 29:1991–1996, 1991.

297. Dennehy PH. Rotavirus infections. In Abrutyn E, Scheckler WE, Goldmann DA (eds). Saunders Infection Control Reference Service. Philadelphia, WB Saunders, 1998, pp 679–681.

298. Goldkrand JW. Intrapartum inoculation of herpes simplex virus by fetal scalp electrode. Obstet Gynecol 59:263–265, 1982.

299. Parvey LS, Chien LT. Neonatal herpes simplex virus infection introduced by fetal-monitor scalp electrodes. Pediatrics 65:1150–1153, 1980.

300. Light IJ. Postnatal acquisition of herpes simplex virus by the newborn infant: a review of the literature. Pediatrics 63:480–482, 1979.

301. Hammerberg O, Watts J, Chernesky M, et al. An outbreak of herpes simplex virus type 1 in an intensive care nursery. Pediatr Infect Dis J 2:290–294, 1983.

302. Sakoaka H, Saheki Y, Uzuki K, et al. Two outbreaks of herpes simplex virus type 1 nosocomial infections among newborns. J Clin Microbiol 24:36–40, 1986.

303. Kleiman MB, Schreiner RL, Eitzen H, et al. Oral herpesvirus infection in nursery personnel: infection control policy. Pediatrics 70:609–612, 1982.

304. Linnemann CC, Bushman TG, Light IJ, et al. Transmission of herpesvirus type 1 in a nursery for the newborn: identification of isolates by DNA fingerprinting. Lancet 1:964–966, 1978.

305. Adams G, Stover BH, Keenlyside RA, et al. Nosocomial herpetic infections in a pediatric intensive care unit. Am J Epidemiol 113:126–132, 1981.

306. Van Dyke RB, Spector SA. Transmission of herpes simplex virus type 1 to a newborn infant during endotracheal suctioning for meconium aspiration. Pediatr Infect Dis 3:153–156, 1984.

307. Francis DP, Herrmann KL, MacMahon JR, et al. Nosocomial and maternally acquired Herpesvirus hominis infections. Am J Dis Child 129:889–893, 1975.

308. Buddingh GJ, Schrum DI, Lanier JC, et al. Studies of the natural history of herpes simplex infections. Pediatrics 11:595–708, 1953.

309. Turner R, Shehab Z, Osborne K, et al. Shedding and survival of herpes simplex virus from fever blisters. Pediatrics 70:547–549, 1982.

310. Pereira FA. Herpes simplex: evolving concepts. J Am Acad Dermatol 35:503–520, 1996.

311. Spruance SL, Overall JC Jr, Kern ER, et al. The natural history of recurrent herpes simplex labialis: implications for antiviral therapy. N Engl J Med 297:69–75, 1977.

312. Bolyard EA, Tablan OC, Williams WW, et al. Guideline for infection control in health care personnel, 1998. Infect Control Hosp Epidemiol 19:410–463, 1998.

313. American Academy of Pediatrics. Herpes simplex. *In* Peter G (ed). 1997 Red Book: Report of the Committee on Infectious Diseases, 23rd ed. Elk Grove Village, Ill, American Academy of Pediatrics, 1994, pp 275–276.

314. Gershon AA, Raker R, Steinberg S, et al. Antibody to varicella-zoster virus in parturient women and their offspring during the first year of life. Pediatrics 58:692–696, 1976.

315. Gustafson TL, Shehab Z, Brunell PA. Outbreak of varicella in a newborn intensive care nursery. Am J Dis Child 138:548–550, 1984.

316. Bakshi SS, Miller TC, Kaplan M, et al. Failure of varicella-zoster immunoglobulin in modification of severe congenital varicella. Pediatr Infect Dis 5:699–702, 1986.

317. Rubin L, Leggiadro R, Elie MT, et al. Disseminated varicella in a neonate: implications for immunoprophylaxis of neonates postnatally exposed to varicella. Pediatr Infect Dis 5:100–102, 1986.

318. American Academy of Pediatrics. Varicella-zoster infections. *In* Peter G (ed). 1997 Red Book: Report of the Committee on Infectious Diseases, 24th ed. Elk Grove Village, Ill, American Academy of Pediatrics, 1997, pp 573–585.

319. Sprunt K, Leidy G, Redman W. Abnormal colonization of neonates in an ICU: conversion to normal colonization by pharyngeal implantation of alpha hemolytic streptococcus strain 215. Pediatr Res 14:303–313, 1980.

320. Sprunt K, Leidy G, Redman W. Abnormal colonization of neonates in an ICU: means of identifying neonates at risk of infection. Pediatr Res 12:998–1002, 1978.

321. Goldmann DA. Bacterial colonization and infection in the neonate. Am J Med 70:417–422, 1981.

322. Goldmann DA. The bacterial flora of neonates in intensive care—monitoring and manipulation. J Hosp Infect 11:340–351, 1988.

323. Blakey JL, Lubitz L, Barnes GL, et al. Development of gut colonization in pre-term neonates. J Med Microbiol 15:519–529, 1992.

324. Benno Y, Sawada K, Mitsuoka T. The intestinal microflora of infants: composition of fecal flora in breast-fed and bottle-fed infants. Microbiol Immunol 28:975–986, 1984.

325. Bullen CL, Tearle PV, Steward MG. The effect of "humanised" milks and supplemented breast feeding on the faecal flora of infants. J Med Microbiol 10:403–413, 1977.

326. Bullen CL, Tearle PV, Steward MG. Bifidobacteria in the intestinal tracts of infants: an in-vivo study. J Med Microbiol 9:325–333, 1976.

327. Gillespie WA, Simpson K, Tozer RC. Staphylococcal infection in maternity hospital: epidemiology and control. Lancet 2:1075, 1958.

328. Light IJ, Atherton HD, Sutherland JM. Decreased colonization of newborn infants with *Staphylococcus aureus* 80/81: Cincinnati General Hospital, 1960–72. J Infect Dis 131:281–285, 1975.

329. Nelson JD, Dillon HC, Howard JB. A prolonged nursery epidemic associated with a newly recognized type of group A *Streptococcus*. J Pediatr 89:792–796, 1976.

330. Al-Jumaili IJ, Shibley M, Lishman AH, Record CO. Incidence and origin of *Clostridum difficile* in neonates. J Clin Microbiol 19:77–78, 1984.

331. Boyer KM, Petersen NJ, Farzaneh I, et al. An outbreak of gastroenteritis due to *E. coli* 0142 in a neonatal nursery. J Pediatr 86:919–927, 1975.

332. Kaslow RA, Taylor A Jr, Dweck HS. Enteropathogenic *Escherichia coli* infection in a newborn nursery. Am J Dis Child 128:797–801, 1974.

333. DuPont HL, Ribner BS. Infectious gastroenteritis. *In* Bennett JV, Brachman PS (eds). Hospital Infections, 4th ed. Philadelphia, Lippincott–Raven, 1998, pp 537–550.

334. Parry MF, Hutchinson JH, Brown NA, et al. Gram-negative sepsis in neonates: a nursery outbreak due to hand carriage of *Citrobacter diversus*. Pediatrics 65:1105–1109, 1980.

335. Williams WW, Mariano J, Spurrier M, et al. Nosocomial meningitis due to *Citrobacter diversus* in neonates: new aspects of the epidemiology. J Infect Dis 150:229–235, 1984.

336. Fonseca SNS, Ehrenkrantz RA, Baltimore RS. Epidemiology of antibiotic use in a neonatal intensive care unit. Infect Control Hosp Epidemiol 15:156–162, 1994.

337. Goldmann DA, Leclair J, Macone A. Bacterial colonization of neonates admitted to an intensive care environment. J Pediatr 93:288–293, 1978.

338. Hare R, Thomas CGA. The transmission of *Staphylococcus aureus*. N Engl J Med 1:69–73, 1958.

339. Back NA, Linnemann CC Jr, Staneck JL, Kotugal UR. Control of methicillin-resistant *Staphylococcus aureus* in a neonatal intensive care unit: use of intensive microbiologic surveillance and mupirocin. Infect Control Hosp Epidemiol 17:227–231, 1996.

340. Rhinehart E, Smith NE, Wennerstein C, et al. Rapid dissemination of beta-lactamase-producing, aminoglycoside-resistant *Enterococcus faecalis* among patients and staff on an infant-toddler surgical ward. N Engl J Med 323:1814–1818, 1990.

341. Peter G, Nelson JS. Factors affecting neonatal *E. coli* K1 rectal colonization. J Pediatr 93:866–870, 1978.

342. Damato JJ, Eitzman DV, Baer H. Persistence and dissemination in the community of R-factors of nosocomial origin. J Infect Dis 129:205–209, 1974.

343. Rowen JL, Correa AG, Sokol DM, et al. Invasive aspergillosis in neonates: reports of five cases and literature review. Pediatr Infect Dis J 11:576–582, 1992.

344. Papouli M, Roilides E, Bibashi E, et al. Primary cutaneous aspergillosis in neonates: case report and review. Clin Infect Dis 22:1102–1104, 1996.

345. Goldmann DA. Transmission of infectious diseases in children. Pediatr Rev 13:283–292, 1992.

346. Potter-Bynoe G, Zawacki A, Psota C, et al. An unusual source of *Pseudomonas aeruginosa* infection in a neonatal ICU [abstract 131]. Presented at Eighth Annual Scientific Meeting of the Society for Healthcare Epidemiology of America (SHEA), Orlando, Fla, April 1998.

347. Guenther SH, Handley JO, Wenzel RP. Gram-negative bacilli as nontransient flora on the hands of hospital personnel. J Clin Microbiol 25:488–490, 1987.

348. Adams BG, Marrie TJ. Hand carriage of aerobic gram-negative rods may not be transient. J Hyg (Lond) 89:33–46, 1982.

349. Knittle MA, Eitzman DV, Baer H. Role of hand contamination of personnel in the epidemiology of gram-negative nosocomial infections. J Pediatr 86:433–437, 1975.

350. Brooks S, Khan A, Stoica D, et al. Reduction in vancomycin-resistant *Enterococcus* and *Clostridium difficile* infections following change to tympanic thermometers. Infect Control Hosp Epidemiol 19:333–336, 1998.

351. McAllister TA, Round JA, Marshall A, et al. Outbreak of *Salmonella eimsbuttel* in newborn infants spread by rectal thermometers. Lancet 1:1262–1264, 1986.

352. Ehrenkrantz NJ. Bland soap handwash or hand antisep-

sis? The pressing need for clarity. Infect Control Hosp Epidemiol 13:299–301, 1992.

353. Wade JJ, Desai N, Casewell MW. Hygienic hand disinfection for the removal of epidemic vancomycin-resistant *Enterococcus faecium* and gentamicin-resistant *Enterobacter cloacae*. J Hosp Infect 19:211–218, 1991.

354. Casewell M, Phillips I. Hands as route of transmission for *Klebsiella* species. BMJ 2:1315–1317, 1977.

355. Brown J, Froese-Fretz A, Luckey D, et al. High rate of hand contamination and low rate of hand washing before infant contact in a neonatal intensive care unit. Pediatr Infect Dis J 15:908–910, 1996.

356. Mayhall CG, Lamb VA, Bitar CM, et al. Nosocomial *Klebsiella* infection in a neonatal unit: identification of risk factors for gastrointestinal colonization. Infect Control 1:239–246, 1980.

357. Leclair JM, Zaia JA, Levin MJ, et al. Airborne transmission of chickenpox in a hospital. N Engl J Med 302:450–453, 1980.

358. Gustafson TL, Lavely GB, Brawner ER, et al. An outbreak of airborne nosocomial varicella. Pediatrics 70:550–556, 1982.

359. Eichenwald HF, Kotsevalor O, Fasco LA. The "cloud baby": an example of bacterial viral interactions. Am J Dis Child 100:161–173, 1960.

360. Sheretz RJ, et al. A cloud adult: the *Staphylococcus aureus*-virus interaction revisited. Ann Intern Med 124:539–547, 1996.

361. Singer S, Singer D, Ruchel R, et al. Outbreak of systemic aspergillosis in a neonatal intensive care unit. Mycoses 41:223–227, 1998.

362. Beck-Sague CM, Jarvis WR. Epidemic bloodstream infections associated with pressure transducers: a persistent problem. Infect Control Hosp Epidemiol 10:54–59, 1989.

363. Nopper AJ, Horii KA, Sookdeo-Drost S, et al. Topical ointment therapy benefits premature infants. J Pediatr 128:660–669, 1996.

364. Ramsey KM, Macone SG, Sey PD, et al. Aquaphor as a source of colonization and subsequent bloodstream infections among very low birth weight neonates [abstract 156]. Presented at Eighth Annual Scientific Meeting of the Society for Healthcare Epidemiology of America (SHEA), Orlando, Fla, April 1998.

365. Goldmann DA, Klinger JD. *Pseudomonas cepacia*—biology, mechanisms of virulence, epidemiology. J Pediatr 108:806–812, 1986.

366. Ross BS, Peter G, Dempsey JM, et al. *Klebsiella pneumoniae* nosocomial epidemic in an intensive care nursery due to contaminated intravenous fluid. Am J Dis Child 131:712, 1977.

367. Jarvis WR, Hingsmith AK, Allen JR, et al. Polymicrobial bacteremia associated with lipid emulsion in a neonatal intensive care unit. Pediatr Infect Dis J 1983; 2:203–208, 1983.

368. Donowitz LG, Marsik FJ, Fisher KA, et al. Contaminated breast milk: a source of *Klebsiella* bacteremia in a newborn intensive care unit. Rev Infect Dis 3:716–720, 1981.

369. Simmons BP, Gelfand MS, Haas M, et al. *Enterobacter sakasakii* infections in neonates associated with intrinsic contamination of a powdered infant formula. Infect Control Hosp Epidemiol 10:398–401, 1989.

370. Casewell MW, Cooper JE, Webster M. Enteral feeds contaminated with *Enterobacter cloacae* as a cause of septicemia. J Clin Res Ed 282:973, 1981.

371. Morse LJ, Williams HL, Grenn FP Jr, et al. Hand

372. Morse LJ, Williams HL, Grenn FP Jr, et al. Septicemia due to *Klebsiella pneumoniae* originating from a hand-cream dispenser. N Engl J Med 277:472–473, 1967.

373. Beatson SH. Pharaoh's ants as pathogen vectors in hospitals. Lancet 1:425–427, 1972.

374. Chadee DD, LeMaitre A. Ants: potential mechanical vectors of hospital infections in Trinidad. Trans R Soc Trop Med Hyg 84:297, 1990.

375. Fotedar R, Banerjee U, Singh S, et al. The housefly (*Musca domestica*) as a carrier of pathogenic microorganisms in a hospital environment. J Hosp Infect 20:209–215, 1992.

376. Freeman J, Platt R, Epstein MF, et al. Birth weight and length of stay as determinants of nosocomial coagulase-negative staphylococcal bacteremia in neonatal intensive care unit populations: potential for confounding. Am J Epidemiol 132:1130–1140, 1990.

377. National Nosocomial Infections Surveillance System (NNIS). National Nosocomial Infections Surveillance System (NNIS) semi-annual report, May 1995. Am J Infect Control 23:377–385, 1995.

378. Richardson DK, Gray JE, McCormick MC, et al. Score for Neonatal Acute Physiology: A physiologic severity index for neonatal intensive care. Pediatrics 91:617–623, 1993.

379. Richardson DK, Phibbs CS, Gray JE, et al. Birth weight and illness severity: independent predictors of neonatal mortality. Pediatrics 91:969–975, 1993.

380. The International Neonatal Network. The CRIB (clinical risk index for babies) score: a tool for assessing initial neonatal risk and comparing performance of neonatal intensive care units. Lancet 342:193–198, 1993.

381. Gray JE, Richardson DK, McCormick MC, et al. Neonatal therapeutic intervention scoring system: a therapy-based severity-of-illness index. Pediatrics 90:561–567, 1992.

382. Gray JE, Richardson DK, McCormick MC, et al. Coagulase-negative staphylococcal bacteremia among very low birth weight infants: relation to admission illness severity, resource use, and outcome. Pediatrics 95:225–230, 1995.

383. Avilla-Figueroa C, Goldmann DA, Richardson DK, et al. Intravenous lipid emulsions are the major determinant of coagulase-negative staphylococcal bacteremia in very low birth weight newborns. Pediatr Infect Dis J 17:10–17, 1998.

384. Landers S, Moise AA, Fraley JK, et al. Factors associated with umbilical catheter–related sepsis in neonates. Am J Dis Child 145:675–680, 1991.

385. Hruszkewycz V, Holtrop PC, Batton DG, et al. Complications associated with central venous catheters inserted in critically ill neonates. Infect Control Hosp Epidemiol 12:544–548, 1991.

386. Ramachandran P, Cohen RS, Kim EH, et al. Experience with double-lumen umbilical venous catheters in the low-birth-weight neonate. J Perinatol 14:280–284, 1994.

387. Davies HD, Jones EL, Sheng RY, et al. Nosocomial urinary tract infections at a pediatric hospital. Pediatr Infect Dis J 11:349–354, 1992.

388. Moffet MR, Bender TR, Margolis HS, et al. Colonization of infants exposed to bacterially contaminated mists. Am J Dis Child 114:21–25, 1967.

389. Barson AJ. Fatal *Pseudomonas aeruginosa* bronchopneumonia in a children's hospital. Arch Dis Child 46:55–60, 1971.

390. Tablan OC, Anderson LJ, Arden NH, et al. Guideline

lotions—a potential nosocomial hazard. N Engl J Med 278:376–378, 1968.

for prevention of nosocomial pneumonia. Infect Control Hosp Epidemiol 15:587–627, 1994.

391. Franco JA, Eitzman DV, Baer H. Antibiotic usage and microbial resistance in an intensive care nursery. Am J Dis Child 126:318–321, 1973.

392. Papile LA, et al. A multicenter trial of two dexamethasone regimens in ventilator-dependent premature infants. N Engl J Med 338:1112–1118, 1998.

393. Reveri M, Krishnamurthy C. Gonococcal scalp abscesses. J Pediatr 94:819–820, 1979.

394. Feder HM, MacLean WC, Moxon R. Scalp abscess secondary to fetal scalp electrode. J Pediatr 89:808–809, 1976.

395. Scheckler WE, Brimhall D, Buck AS, et al. Requirements for infrastructure and essential activities of infection control and epidemiology in hospitals: a consensus panel report. Infect Control Hosp Epidemiol 19:114–124, 1998.

396. Haley RW, Culver DH, White JW, et al. The efficacy of infection surveillance and control programs in preventing nosocomial infections in US hospitals. Am J Epidemiol 121:182–205, 1985.

397. Moore DL. Newborn nursery and neonatal intensive care unit. In Olmstead RN (ed). Association of Professionals in Infection Control (APIC): Infection Control and Applied Epidemiology. St. Louis, CV Mosby, 1996, pp 94-1–94-11.

398. St. Geme JW III, Bell LM, Baumgart S, et al. Distinguishing sepsis from blood culture contamination in young infants with blood cultures growing coagulase-negative staphylococci. Pediatrics 86:157–162, 1990.

399. Schelonka RL, Chai MK, Yonder BA, et al. Volume of blood required to detect common neonatal pathogens. J Pediatr 129:275–278, 1996.

400. Manroe BL, Weinberg AG, Rosenfeld CR, et al. The neonatal blood count in health and disease: I. Reference values for neutrophilic cells. J Pediatr 95:89–98, 1979.

401. Berner R, Niemeyer CM, Leititis JU, et al. Plasma levels and gene expression of granulocyte colony-stimulating factor, tumor necrosis factor-alpha, interleukin (IL)-1 beta, IL-6, IL-8, and soluble intercellular adhesion molecule-1 in neonatal early onset sepsis. Pediatr Res 44:469–470, 1998.

402. Franz AR, Steinbach G, Kron M, Pohlandt F. Reduction of unnecessary antibiotic therapy in newborn infants using interleukin-8 and C-reactive protein as markers of bacterial infections. Pediatr 104 (3 Part 1):447–453, 1999.

403. Hargiss C, Larson E. The epidemiology of *Staphylococcus aureus* in a newborn nursery from 1970 through 1976. Pediatrics 61:348–353, 1978.

404. White RD, Townsend TR, Stephens MA, et al. Are surveillance of resistant enteric bacilli and antimicrobial usage among neonates in a newborn intensive care unit useful? Pediatrics 68:1–4, 1981.

405. Evans ME, Schaffner W, Federspiel CF, et al. Sensitivity, specificity, and predictive value of body surface culture in a neonatal intensive care unit. JAMA 259:248–252, 1988.

406. Slagle TA, Bifano EM, Wolf JW, et al. Routine endotracheal cultures for the prediction of sepsis in ventilated babies. Arch Dis Child 64:34–38, 1989.

407. Lau YL, Hey E. Sensitivity and specificity of daily tracheal aspirate cultures in predicting organisms causing bacteremia in ventilated neonates. Pediatr Infect Dis J 10:290–294, 1991.

408. Lee PYC, Holliman RE, Davis EG. Surveillance cultures on neonatal intensive care units. J Hosp Infect 29:233–237, 1995.

409. Trofino J. JCAHO nursing standards, nursing care hours and LOS per DRG: part I. Nurse Manag 17:19–24, 1986.

410. Huskins WC, Goldmann DA. Nosocomial infections. In Feigin RD, Cherry JD (eds). Textbook of Pediatric Infectious Diseases, 4th ed. Philadelphia, WB Saunders, 1998, pp 2545–2585.

411. Harris JS. Infection control for neonatal gram-negative bacterial infections. Pediatr Infect Dis J 17:532–533, 1998.

412. Huskins WC, Goldmann DA. Prevention and control of nosocomial infections in hospitalized children. In Feigin RD, Cherry JD (eds). Textbook of Pediatric Infectious Diseases, 4th ed. Philadelphia, WB Saunders, 1998, pp 2585–2602.

413. Wendt C, Herwaldt LA. Epidemics: identification and management. In Wenzl RP (ed). Prevention and Control of Nosocomial Infections, 3rd ed. Baltimore, Williams & Wilkins, 1997, pp 175–213.

414. Bingen E. Applications of molecular methods to epidemiologic investigations of nosocomial infections in a pediatric hospital. Infect Control Hosp Epidemiol 15:488–493, 1994.

415. Jarvis WR. Usefulness of molecular epidemiology for outbreak investigations. Infect Control Hosp Epidemiol 15:500–503, 1994.

416. American Academy of Pediatrics and American College of Obstetricians and Gynecologists. Infection control. In Guidelines for Perinatal Care, 4th ed. Elk Grove Village, Ill, American Academy of Pediatrics, 1997, pp 251–278.

417. Abrutyn E, Goldmann DA, Scheckler WE (eds). Saunders Infection Control Reference Service. Philadelphia, WB Saunders, 1998.

418. American Academy of Pediatrics. Antimicrobial prophylaxis: prevention of neonatal ophthalmia. In Peter G (ed). 1997 Red Book: Report of the Committee on Infectious Diseases, 24th ed. Elk Grove Village, Ill, American Academy of Pediatrics, 1997, pp 601–603.

419. Hammerschlag MR, Cummings C, Roblin PM, et al. Efficacy of neonatal ocular prophylaxis for the prevention of chlamydial and gonococcal conjunctivitis. N Engl J Med 320:769–772, 1989.

420. Chen J-Y. Prophylaxis of ophthalmia neonatorum: comparison of silver nitrate, tetracycline, erythromycin and no prophylaxis. Pediatr Infect Dis J 11:1026–1030, 1992.

421. King S, Devi SP, Mindorff CC, et al. Nosocomial *Pseudomonas aeruginosa* conjunctivitis in a pediatric hospital. Infect Control Hosp Epidemiol 9:77–80, 1988.

422. Lund C, Kuller J, Lane A, et al. Neonatal skin care: the scientific basis for practice. Neonat Network 18(4):15–24, 1999.

423. American Academy of Pediatrics and American College of Obstetricians and Gynecologists. Postpartum and follow-up care. In Guidelines for Perinatal Care, 4th ed. Elk Grove Village, Ill, American Academy of Pediatrics, 1997, pp 147–182.

424. Lockhart JD. How toxic is hexachlorophene? Pediatrics 50:229–235, 1972.

425. Larson EL. APIC Guideline Committee. Guideline for hand washing and hand antisepsis in health care settings. Am J Infect Control 23:251–266, 1995.

426. Oneil J, Hosmer M, Challop R, et al. Percutaneous absorption potential of chlorhexidine in neonates. Curr Ther Res 31:485–489, 1982.

427. Larson E. Guideline for use of topical antimicrobial agents. Am J Infect Control 16:253–266, 1988.

428. Husak M, Wiltshire J, Carr H, et al. Effect of Hibiclens bathing on neonatal bactericidal colonization [abstract

714]. 21st Interscience Conference on Antimicrobial Agents and Chemotherapy, Chicago, Ill, 1981.

429. Maloney MH. Chlorhexidine: hexachlorophene substitute in the nursery. Nursing Times 71:21, 1975.

430. Chabrolle JP, Rossier A. Goitre and hypothyroidism in the newborn after cutaneous absorption of iodine. Arch Dis Child 53:495–498, 1978.

431. Barrett FF, Mason EO, Fleming D. The effect of three cord-care regimens on bacterial colonization of normal newborn infants. J Pediatr 94:796–800, 1978.

432. Bydgeman S, Hambraeus A, Henningsson A, et al. Influence of ethanol with and without chlorhexidine on the bacterial colonization of the umbilicus of newborn infants. Infect Control 5:275–278, 1984.

433. Seeberg S, Brinkhoff B, John E, et al. Prevention and control of neonatal pyoderma with chlorhexidine. Acta Paediatr Scand 73:498–504, 1984.

434. Smales O. A comparison of umbilical cord treatment in the control of superficial infections. NZ J Med 101:453–455, 1998.

435. Bradley SF. Effectiveness of mupiricin in the control of methicillin-resistant *Staphylococcus aureus*. Infect Med 10:23–31, 1993.

436. Zupan J, Garner P. Topical umbilical cord care at birth. The Cochrane Library 1:1–11, 1999.

437. Guidelines for the prevention of nosocomial pneumonia. MMWR Morb Mortal Wkly Rep 46(RR-1):1–79, 1997.

438. Wong ES, Hooton TM. Guidelines for the prevention of catheter-associated urinary tract infections. Infect Control 2:125, 1982.

439. Pearson ML, Hospital Infection Control Practices Advisory Committee (HICPAC). Guidelines for prevention of intravascular device-related infections. Infect Control Hosp Epidemiol 17:435–473, 1996.

440. Adam RD, Edwards LD, Becker CC, Schrom HM. Semiquantitive cultures and routine tip cultures on umbilical catheters. J Pediatr 100:123–126, 1982.

441. Krauss A, Albert RF, Kannan MM. Contamination of umbilical catheters in the newborn infant. J Pediatr 77:965–969, 1970.

442. Balagtas RC, Bell CE, Edwards LD, Levin S. Risk of local and systemic infections associated with umbilical vein catheterization: a prospective study in 86 newborn patients. Pediatrics 48:359, 1971.

443. Bard H, Albert G, Teasdale F, et al. Prophylactic antibiotics in chronic umbilical artery catheterization in respiratory distress syndrome. Arch Dis Child 48:630–635, 1973.

444. Garland JS, Buck RK, Maloney P, et al. A comparison of 10% povidone iodine and 0.5% chlorhexidine gluconate for the prevention of intravenous catheter colonization in neonates: a prospective trial. Pediatr Infect Dis J 14:510–516, 1995.

445. Personal communication with Donald A. Goldmann, M.D., Children's Hospital, Boston, 1999.

446. Matlow A, Kitai I, Kirplani H, et al. A randomized trial of 72- versus 24-hour intravenous tubing set changes in newborns receiving lipid therapy. Infect Control Hosp Epidemiol 20:487–493, 1999.

447. American Academy of Pediatrics and American College of Obstetricians and Gynecologists. Inpatient perinatal care services. *In* Guidelines for Perinatal Care, 4th ed. Elk Grove Village, Ill, American Academy of Pediatrics, 1997, pp 13–50.

448. Ross Planning Associates. Perspectives in Perinatal and Pediatric Design. Columbus, Ohio, Ross Laboratories, 1988.

449. Bureau of Communicable Disease Epidemiology, Health Protection Branch and Health Services Directorate, Health Services and Promotion Branch. Infection Control Guidelines for Perinatal Care. Ottawa, Health and Welfare Canada, 1988.

450. American Institute of Architects Committee on Architecture for Health. Mechanical standards. *In* Guidelines for Construction and Equipment of Hospital and Medical Facilities. Washington, DC, The American Institute of Architects Press, 1987, pp 46–54.

451. Ehrenkrantz NJ, Sanders CC, Eckert-Schollenberger D, et al. Lack of evidence of efficacy of cohorting nursery personnel in a neonatal intensive care unit to prevent contact spread of bacteria: an experimental study. Pediatr Infect Dis J 11:105–113, 1992.

452. Bishop RF, Cameron DJS, Veenstra AA, Barnes GL. Diarrhea and rotavirus infection associated with differing regimens for postnatal care of newborn babies. J Clin Microbiol 9:525–529, 1979.

453. Daschner F. Infectious hazards in rooming-in systems. J Perinat Med 12:3–6, 1984.

454. American Academy of Pediatrics Committee on Fetus and Newborn, American College of Obstetricians and Gynecologists Committee on Obstetrics. Maternal and Fetal Medicine: Guidelines for Perinatal Care, 3rd ed. Elk Grove Village, Ill, American Academy of Pediatrics, 1992, pp 23–29.

455. Garner JS, Favero MS. CDC guideline for hand washing and hospital environmental control, 1985. Infect Control Hosp Epidemiol 7:231–235, 1986.

456. Sprunt K, Redman W, Leidy G. Antibacterial effectiveness of routine hand washing. Pediatrics 52:264–271, 1973.

457. Doebbling BN, Stanley GL, Sheetz CT, et al. Comparative efficacy of alternative hand washing agents in reducing nosocomial infections in intensive care units. N Engl J Med 327:88–93, 1992.

458. Larson E. A casual link between hand washing and risk of infection? Examination of the evidence. Infect Control 9:28–36, 1988.

459. Korniewicz DM, Kirwin M, Cresci K, et al. Leakage of latex and vinyl exam gloves in high and low risk clinical settings. Am Ind Hyg Assoc J 54:22–26, 1993.

460. Steere AC, Mallison GF. Hand washing practices for the prevention of nosocomial infections. Ann Intern Med 83:683–690, 1975.

461. Larson EL, Eke PI, Laughon BE. Efficacy of alcohol-based hand rinses under frequent use conditions. Antimicrob Agents Chemother 30:542–544, 1986.

462. Waggoner-Fountain LA, Donowitz LG. Infection in the newborn. *In* Wengl RP (ed). Prevention and Control of Nosocomial Infections, 3rd ed. Baltimore, Williams & Wilkins, 1997, pp 1019–1038.

463. Conley JM, Hill S, Ross J, et al. Hand washing practices in an intensive care unit: the effects of an educational program and its relationship to infection rates. Am J Infect Control 17:330–339, 1989.

464. Larson E, Kretzer EK. Compliance with hand washing and barrier precautions. J Hosp Infect 30:88–106, 1995.

465. Albert RK, Condie F. Hand washing patterns in medical intensive care units. N Engl J Med 304:1465–1469, 1981.

466. Donowitz LG. Hand washing technique in a pediatric intensive care unit. Am J Dis Child 141:683–685, 1987.

467. Raju TNK, Kobler C. Improving hand washing habits in the newborn nursery. Am J Med Sci 302:355–358, 1991.

468. Forfar JO, MacCabe AF. Masking and gowning in nurseries for the newborn infant: effect on staphylococcal carriage and infection. Br J Med 1:76–79, 1958.

469. Silverman WA, Sinclair JC. Evaluation of precautions

before entering a neonatal unit. Pediatrics 40:900–901, 1967.

470. Evans HE, Akpata SO, Baki A. Bacteriologic and clinical evaluation of gowning in a premature nursery. J Pediatr 78:883–886, 1971.

471. Cloney DL, Donowitz LG. Overgown use for infection control in nurseries and neonatal intensive care units. Am J Dis Child 140:680–683, 1986.

472. Haque KN, Chagla AH. Do gowns prevent infection in neonatal intensive care units? J Hosp Infect 159–162, 1989.

473. Birenbaum HJ, Glorioso L, Rosenberger C, et al. Gowning on a postpartum ward fails to decrease colonization in the newborn infant. Am J Dis Child 144:1031–1033, 1990.

474. Rush J, Fiorino-Chiovitti R, Kaufman K, et al. A randomized controlled trial of a nursery ritual: wearing cover gowns to care for healthy newborns. Birth 17:25–30, 1990.

475. Pelke S, Ching D, Easa D, et al. Gowning does not affect colonization or infection rates in a neonatal intensive care unit. Arch Pediatr Adolesc Med 148:1016–1020, 1994.

476. Eason S. Are cover gowns necessary in the NICU for parents and visitors? Neonat Network 14:50, 1995.

477. Agbayani M, Rosenfeld W, Evans H, et al. Evaluation of modified gowning procedures in a neonatal intensive care unit. Am J Dis Child 135:650–652, 1981.

478. Donowitz LG. Failure of the overgown to prevent nosocomial infection in a pediatric intensive care unit. Pediatrics 77:35–38, 1986.

479. American Academy of Pediatrics. Infection control for hospitalized children. In Peter G (ed). 1997 Red Book: Report of the Committee on Infectious Diseases, 24th ed. Elk Grove Village, Ill, American Academy of Pediatrics, 1997, pp 100–107.

480. Renaud MT. Parental response to family centered maternity care and the implementation of sibling visit. Milit Med 146:850–852, 1981.

481. Wranesh BL. The effect of sibling visitation on bacterial colonization rates in neonates. JOGN Nursing 11:211–213, 1982.

482. Umphenour JH. Bacterial colonization in neonates with sibling visitation. J Obstet Gynecol Neonat Nursing 9:73–75, 1980.

483. Schwab F. Sibling visiting in a neonatal intensive care unit. Pediatrics 71:835–838, 1983.

484. Yamauchi T. Roles of the infection control professional. In Donowitz LG (ed). Hospital Acquired Infection in the Pediatric Patient. Baltimore, Williams & Wilkins, 1988, pp 351–368.

485. Occupational Safety and Health Administration (OSHA), Department of Labor. Occupational exposure to bloodborne pathogens: Final rule. Fed Reg 56:64175–64182, 1991.

486. Centers for Disease Control and Prevention. Protection against viral hepatitis: recommendations of the Immunization Practices Advisory Committee (ACIP). MMWR Morb Mortal Wkly Rep 39(No. RR-2):17–22, 1990.

487. Centers for Disease Control and Prevention. Public Health Service statement on management of occupational exposure to human immunodeficiency virus, including considerations regarding zidovudine postexposure use. MMWR Morbid Mortal Wkly Rep 39(No. RR-2):1–14, 1990.

488. Centers for Disease Control and Prevention. Case-control study of HIV seroconversion in health care workers after percutaneous exposure to HIV-infected blood: France, the United Kingdom, and the United States. MMWR Morbid Mortal Wkly Rep 44:929–933, 1995.

489. Centers for Disease Control and Prevention. Guidelines for the management of health care exposure to HIV and recommendations for post-exposure prophylaxis. MMWR Morb Mortal Wkly Rep 47(No. RR-7):1–33, 1998.

490. Mirza A, Wyatt M, Begue R. Infection control practices and the pregnant health care worker. Pediatr Infect Dis J 18:18–22, 1999.

491. Adler SP. Nosocomial transmission of cytomegalovirus. Pediatr Infect Dis J 5:239–246, 1986.

492. Hospital Infection Control Practices Advisory Committee. Guidelines for infection control in health care personnel, 1998. Am J Infect Control 26:289–327, 1998.

493. Centers for Disease Control and Prevention. Prevention and control of influenza: recommendations of the Advisory Committee on Immunization Practices (ACIP). MMWR Morb Mortal Wkly Rep 47(RR-6):1–26, 1998.

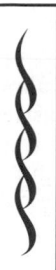

Clinical Pharmacology of Antibacterial Agents

XAVIER SÁEZ-LLORENS, M.D., and GEORGE H. McCRACKEN, JR., M.D.

Because of the susceptibility of newborns, particularly low-birth-weight premature neonates, to vertically and nosocomially acquired bacterial infections, pediatricians managing these infants often prescribe antibiotics for presumptive sepsis. Pharmacology of drugs is unique to the neonate and cannot be extrapolated from data derived from older infants and adults. For these reasons, safety and efficacy of antimicrobial products in the neonatal period must be established in term and premature infants.

The rapidly changing physiologic processes characteristic of the neonatal age profoundly affect the pharmacokinetic properties of antibiotics. These changes can result either in subtherapeutic drug concentrations, thereby delaying bacterial eradication, or in toxic drug concentrations that can cause morbidity and prolonged hospitalization. Therapeutic disasters such as kernicterus following use of sulfonamides, the chloramphenicol gray baby syndrome, tetracycline tooth staining, and kanamycin ototoxicity underscore the importance of pediatric pharmacology as an essential subspecialty. Clinical trials evaluating antimicrobial agents should include newborns, especially low-birth-weight premature neonates, who receive many courses of antimicrobial therapy during their nursery stays.

Since the previous edition of this book was published, a few new antibacterial agents have become available for use in newborns with suspected or proven bacterial infections. In this chapter, we update the data on β-lactamic agents and aminoglycosides and discuss the limited information available on antibiotics potentially useful for treatment of multiresistant microorganisms (ampicillin-sulbactam, carbapenems, ciprofloxacin, cefepime). Finally, it must be underscored that in the current era of alarming increase in widespread resistance of bacteria to multiple antimicrobial drugs, there is a need to develop stringent antibiotic-restriction policies to preserve the usefulness of selected antibiotics.

NEONATAL CLINICAL PHARMACOLOGY

Absorption, distribution, metabolism, and excretion are constantly changing during the neonatal period. The physiologic immaturity of enzymatic processes, the large extracellular fluid volume, the protein-binding affinities of antibiotic-competing substances, the fluctuations in renal clearance, and certain situations that provoke blood volume disturbances (e.g., exchange transfusions, patency of ductus arteriosus, extracorporeal membrane oxygenation [ECMO]) are among the numerous neonatal factors affecting the pharmacokinetic behavior of antimicrobial agents in newborns.

Absorption of drugs administered at extravascular sites occurs by passive diffusion across biologic membranes. This process is affected by chemical properties of the drug, such as its molecular weight, ionization, and lipid solubility, as well as by physiologic factors, such as local pH and blood flow, which undergo developmental changes as the newborn matures.

Oral absorption of antimicrobial agents can be affected by unique neonatal features, such as the alkaline gastric pH during the first hours of life, slow gastric emptying, high gastrointestinal:whole body surface area ratio, increased permeability of bowel mucosa, irregular peristalsis, prolonged intestinal transit time, and the deconjugational activity of the intestinal enzyme β-glucuronidase.[1] The net effect of these features on the oral absorption of specific antibiotics, however, is difficult to predict. For example, penicillin G, administered orally, achieves higher serum concentration in newborns than in older infants and children,[2] whereas the opposite occurs after oral administration of chloramphenicol palmitate.[3–5]

Although serum antibiotic concentrations are generally comparable after either intramuscular or intravenous administration, significant differences in peak values, half-lives, and plasma clearances can be observed for some antibiotics.[6, 7] Because the regional blood flow is the primary determinant of the extent and rate of antibiotic absorption after intramuscular administration, hypoxic and/or hypotensive infants with poor peripheral muscle perfusion can have profound reduction in absorption of some drugs.

Immaturity of enzymatic systems in the neonate can result from deficiency or absence of specific enzymes required for drug biotransformation. Deficiency of hepatic glucuronyl transferase leads to diminished conjugation of chloramphenicol to the inactive acid glucuronide, thus increasing the half-life with the consequent risk of free drug accumulation in serum. This event is probably the cause of cardiovascular collapse and death (gray baby syndrome) in some infants treated with chloramphenicol. In contrast, phenobarbital stimulates the activity of the hepatic enzymatic system, resulting in increased clearance of chloramphenicol and in reduced serum concentrations.[8] Newborns may lack the enzymes required to de-esterify antibiotic esters, notably pancreatic lipase, which is needed to convert oral chloramphenicol palmitate to the active agent. Another example is hemolysis produced by sulfonamides or nitrofurantoin given to infants who have erythrocyte glucose-6-phosphate dehydrogenase (G6PD) deficiency.[9]

The extracellular fluid volume of newborns is considerably greater than that of children and adults. It decreases from 7.3 to 5.8 liters per m² in the first 3 months of life and remains constant throughout infancy and childhood.[10] Several drugs distribute primarily in the extracellular space, which, because of the larger volume in newborns, can affect the pharmacokinetic profiles of these agents. For example, the peak serum concentrations of aminoglycosides in premature infants are lower than those in term infants after similar dosages, and it takes longer for these drugs to be excreted because of the expanded extracellular volume. This latter phenomenon may explain, in part, the longer half-lives of aminoglycosides in neonates than in older infants and children.[11]

There are quantitative and qualitative differences between the serum proteins of newborns and those of older infants; these differences affect the degree to which antimicrobial agents are protein bound and thus their kinetics.[12] The clinical significance of antibiotic protein binding, however, is unclear. Many variables, including the concentrations of both free albumin and antibiotic, drug affinity for protein-binding sites, presence of competing substances for these binding sites (furosemide, bilirubin), and plasma pH reversibly affect this process. Protein-bound drug has negligible antibacterial activity and remains in the intravascular space with limited distribution into tissues. Binding of some antibiotics, such as chloramphenicol, nafcillin, and ceftriaxone, to plasma proteins is lower in neonates compared with that in adults.[13, 14] Despite the different protein-binding capacities of individual antibiotics, there are inadequate clinical data in newborns to confirm the assumption that drugs with low protein binding are more efficacious than those with high protein binding.

Some antibacterial agents are capable of displacing bilirubin from albumin-binding sites. Theoretically, jaundiced neonates receiving these antibiotics are at increased risk of developing kernicterus. This complication, however, has been documented only for sulfonamides.[15] Most antimicrobial products have a much lower binding affinity for albumin than does bilirubin, thus explaining why these agents are unable to remove bilirubin once it is bound to this protein.[16] Antibiotics that have been shown to significantly displace bilirubin from albumin-binding sites include the sulfonamides, moxalactam, cefoperazone, and ceftriaxone.[17–19] Ampicillin has a weak displacing effect that can be minimized by slow infusion of the drug in jaundiced neonates.[20] In relatively normal physiologic conditions, the remaining commonly used antibacterial agents are generally not associated with bilirubin displacing.[21–23] Finally, the extent of protein binding by an antibiotic does not necessarily correlate with this potentially adverse event.[18]

Renal function in the newborn is different from that in older children. The glomerular filtration rate is 30 to 60% of adult levels. During the first 2 weeks of life, there is a remarkable increase in renal function. These changes and the rate at which they occur have a profound effect on antibiotic pharmacokinetics. As a result, sustained serum concentrations and prolonged half-life values of many drugs are observed in the first days of life, especially in premature infants. At 2 weeks of age, the half-life of β-lactam antibiotics is approximately twice that of adults. Drug elimination may be further reduced in the sick infant by conditions that decrease renal blood flow (e.g., severe respiratory distress syndrome, dehydration, hypotensive states).[24] For example, a prolonged serum half-life of aminoglycosides has been detected in hypoxemic infants.[25] Because renal function is constantly changing in the first month of life, a pharmacokinetic profile must be determined at various times during this period to define the proper dosage and frequency of administration of an antibiotic. Ototoxicity in newborns from aminoglycosides may develop if serum accumulation of these agents, because of reduced glomerular and renal tubular functions, goes unrecognized.

PHARMACOLOGIC EVALUATION OF ANTIBACTERIAL AGENTS IN NEONATES

The evaluation of antimicrobial agents in the treatment of neonatal infection is difficult. As a general rule, antibiotics must first be studied in adults and older children to obtain data concerning absorption, metabolism, excretion, efficacy, and safety before pharmacokinetic and clinical trials in newborns can be conducted. The data obtained in adults and children serve as guidelines for initial dosage and safety precautions in neonates.

There are relatively few comparative randomized controlled trials between an established antibiotic regimen and new compounds in newborns. If the standard regimen is highly effective, very large numbers of infants would be needed to determine the therapeutic superiority of a new regimen, especially when the prevalence of infection is relatively low (i.e., 1 to 5 cases per 1000 live births), as it is in developed countries. If the standard regimen has ceased to be effective, a randomized trial would be unethical. A less satisfactory alternative is to use open studies to establish that the new therapeutic modality is comparable with that used previously for that condition and then to determine whether a diminished risk of toxicity, more desirable pharmacokinetics, more convenient dosage schedules, and so on give the new agent significant advantage over the old one.

For the initial evaluation of any antibiotic, determination of the in vitro susceptibilities of commonly encountered bacterial pathogens in the neonatal period to that drug is imperative. Ideally, both the minimal inhibitory concentration (MIC) and the minimal bactericidal concentration (MBC) should be determined to avoid the potential occurrence of tolerant strains (i.e., organisms inhibited but not killed by up to 32 times the inhibiting concentration for that drug).[26] Because of the great variation in bacterial pathogens among different nurseries and geographic areas, antimicrobial agents to be evaluated should be tailored to those microorganisms prevalent in each unit. In general, potential therapeutic candidates should be effective against some or most of the following common neonatal pathogens: group B streptococci, coagulase-positive and coagulase-negative staphylococci, gram-negative enteric bacilli, enterococci, *Listeria monocytogenes*, and *Pseudomonas aeruginosa*.

The efficacy of combinations of antibiotics is often studied in vitro and in experimental animal models of infections. Demonstration of a synergistic or additive bacterial killing or of an antagonistic interaction is potentially important for the proper management of neonatal infections.[27–29] For instance, synergism has been demonstrated for ampicillin and aminoglycosides against group B streptococci,[30–32] enterococci,[33] *Listeria*,[34] and some gram-negative enteric rods[35]; for nafcillin and aminoglycosides against *Staphylococcus aureus*[36]; and for carbenicillin and gentamicin against enterococci, *Listeria*, and *P. aeruginosa*.[28, 37] The clinical significance of this in vitro synergism as it relates to therapy of infected neonates, however, remains to be established.

The next step in evaluating an antimicrobial agent is to obtain pharmacokinetic data by substitution of a single dose of the new drug for one dose of a standard antibiotic. Alternatively, the investigational drug can be given in addition to standard therapy, but drug concentrations in plasma would need to be determined by an assay that could discriminate between the drugs administered (e.g., high-pressure liquid chromatography). Substitution of only one dose does not expose the infant to the jeopardy of a prolonged period of possibly ineffective therapy that would occur if an untested new drug were given in repeated dosage. Subsequently, multiple serum and urine samples are obtained to determine concentrations of the drug at a given time after the dose. The serum half-life and volume of distribution are calculated by plotting the serum concentration-time curves and calculating the disappearance of drug from serum.[38]

These basic pharmacologic data are then analyzed with respect to age and birth weight, and predictions of dosage and intervals of administration are made by mathematical calculations. The distribution of many antibiotics in the body follows a biphasic pattern (i.e., initial distribution phase after the first dose and final tissue washout phase after the last dose) and most accurately fits a two-compartment pharmacokinetic model.[39–42] Accordingly, we can more precisely predict the serum concentrations of a specific drug and anticipate the persistence of subinhibitory concentrations of antibiotics in the urine several days after the drug is discontinued. This latter event may cause a selective pressure for development of resistant strains of nosocomial pathogens residing in the environment of neonatal intensive care units.

For an antimicrobial agent to be considered useful in the neonatal period, the drug should achieve good concentrations in the cerebrospinal fluid (CSF) compartment. This premise is based on the fact that approximately one fourth of septic newborns simultaneously have bacterial meningitis. In the 1980s, new antibiotics were tested in a rabbit model of meningitis before use in infants to determine the CSF penetration and bactericidal activity of the drug against commonly encountered meningeal pathogens.[43–45]

Only when all these preliminary steps are completed can a new antimicrobial agent be available for use with a reasonable assurance of effectiveness and safety.[46] Once the drug becomes approved by the U.S. Food and Drug Administration (FDA), usually after many years of basic and clinical research, additional measurements of serum drug concentrations and half-life determinations in different birth-weight groups are conducted. These determinations are especially useful when antibiotics with a narrow therapeutic index, such as aminoglycosides, chloramphenicol, and vancomycin, are administered to low-birth-weight premature infants. Drug concentrations are measured during the steady state, which is usually achieved after approximately four serum half-lives. Serum samples obtained just before and 15 minutes after the intravenous administration of a dose yield the trough and peak values, respectively. Peak values after the intramuscular and oral routes are achieved at approximately 30 minutes and 1 to 2 hours, respectively. Peak and trough serum concentrations for toxicity-prone antimicrobial agents (e.g., aminoglycosides, vancomycin) should be monitored if significant changes in renal or hepatic function occur and if prolonged therapy is required.

PLACENTAL TRANSPORT OF ANTIBIOTICS

Antimicrobial agents are prescribed for as many as 15 to 40% of pregnant women to treat a variety of conditions, ranging from mild upper respiratory tract infections to serious bacterial infections of the genitourinary system.[47–49] Many of these drugs are given at the end of pregnancy in an attempt to prevent or treat amnionitis or intrauterine bacterial infections. The selection of a specific agent is based on likely bacterial pathogens causing these infections and on transplacental passage of antimicrobial drugs from the pregnant woman to the fetus.

Drugs may be transported across the placenta either passively by simple diffusion or actively by energy-dependent processes. Factors influencing transplacental passage include lipid solubility, degree of ionization, molecular weight, protein-binding affinity, surface area of the fetal-maternal interface, placental blood flow, stage of pregnancy, and placental metabolism.[50] Placental drug biotransformation ensues by oxidation, reduction, hydrolysis, or conjugation with endogenous chemicals.[51] In addition, antibiotics concentrate in fetal tissues, depending on lipid solubility, specific binding to biologic constituents, changes in fetal circulation, and gestational age.

Ratios of infant to maternal serum concentrations of commonly used antimicrobial agents are shown in Table 35–1.[52–113] Maternal serum concentrations are generally lower than those reported in nonpregnant women owing to a larger plasma volume and an increased renal plasma clearance observed during pregnancy.[114, 115] The infant serum concentrations vary considerably because of differences in maternal dosage, route of administration, gestational age, timing of sample collection, and methods of measuring antimicrobial activity. As a result, a wide range of serum values for pregnant women and infants and of percentages of transplacental penetration is obtained for most drugs.

From Table 35–1 it can be seen that infant serum concentrations of some antibiotics, such as ampicillin,[57] carbenicillin,[59] cefotaxime,[65] chloramphenicol,[76, 77] and sulfonamides[100–102, 106, 107] approach or even exceed those in maternal serum. These high and rapidly attainable fetal ampicillin serum concentrations can explain, at least in part, the significant benefit of intrapartum administration of ampicillin to pregnant women colonized with group B *Streptococcus* in reducing colonization and early-onset neonatal sepsis caused by this pathogen. The ratio of infant to maternal serum values for methicillin[83, 92] is considerably higher than that for dicloxacillin[82, 83]; this may be a result of differences in serum protein binding (37 and 98%, respectively). Antibiotics with low transplacental penetration include cephalotin,[59, 75] dicloxacillin,[82, 83] erythromycin,[52, 84] nafcillin,[59] and tobramycin.[54, 59]

Complete evaluation of the possible adverse effects of drugs on the developing fetus must be performed before the drug is used during pregnancy. Some adverse events reported[116, 117] include fetal death and abortion (aminopterin), teratogenicity (thalidomide), neonatal death (heroin), kernicterus (sulfonamides), ototoxicity (streptomycin), inhibition of infant bone growth (tetracyclines), and discoloration of teeth (tetracyclines). Anecdotal clinical experience is not sufficient to assess properly the safety of antibiotic administration during pregnancy. Rather, carefully planned prospective toxicity

TABLE 35–1
Transplacental Passage of Antimicrobial Agents

ANTIMICROBIAL AGENT	TRIMESTER	SERUM INFANT TO MATERNAL RATIOS (%)	ADVERSE EFFECTS TO FETUS OR INFANT	REFERENCE NO.
Amikacin	1, 2	8–16	Potential ototoxicity	53
	3	30–50		55
Amoxicillin	3	30	None	56
Ampicillin	1, 2	50–250	None	57
	3	20–200		57
Azlocillin	3	50	Unknown	58
Carbenicillin	2, 3	60–100	None	59
Cefazolin	1, 2	2–27	None	59–61
	3	36–69		62
Cefoperazone	3	33–48	None	63–64
Cefotaxime	2	80–150	None	65
Cefoxitin	3	11–133	None	66–68
Ceftizoxime	3	13–130	None	69
Ceftriaxone	3	9–120	None	70
Cefuroxime	3	18–108	None	71–73
Cephalexin	3	33	None	74
Cephalothin	3	10–40	None	59, 75
Chloramphenicol	3	30–106	Potential circulatory collapse	76–78
Clindamycin	2	10–25	None	52, 59
	3	30–50		79
Cloxacillin	3	20–97	None	59, 80
Dicloxacillin	3	7–12	None	59, 82, 83
Erythromycin	2, 3	1–20	None	52, 84
Gentamicin	2, 3	21–44	Potential ototoxicity; potentiation of $MgSO_4$-induced neuromuscular weakness	78, 85, 86
Imipenem	3	14–52	Potential seizure activity	87
Kanamycin	3	26–48	Ototoxicity	59, 88, 89
Lincomycin	3	25–43	None	90, 91
Methicillin	3	30–140	None	83, 92
Nafcillin	3	16	None	59
Nitrofurantoin	3	38–92	Hemolysis in G-6-PD deficiency	93
Penicillin G	1, 2	26–70		59, 94
	3	15–100	None	59, 94–96
Streptomycin	3	13–100	Ototoxicity	97–99
Sulfonamides	3	13–275	Hemolysis in G-6-PD deficiency; jaundice and potential kernicterus	100–107
Tetracyclines	3	10–90	Depressed bone growth; abnormal teeth; possible inguinal hernia	59–64, 108–111
Tobramycin	1, 2	20	Potential ototoxicity	54, 59
Trimethoprim	1, 2	27–131	Teratogenic in animals	112, 113

studies in the fetus and neonate, first in animals and then in humans, are mandatory.

Because of the ease of transplacental passage of sulfonamides and their significant bilirubin-displacing capabilities with the theoretical risk for infants to develop kernicterus, these drugs should not be given to pregnant women near term.[104] The same cautionary statement might apply to other antibiotics with a high protein-binding affinity, such as ceftriaxone and cefoperazone. There are no clinical reports, however, confirming this potential association with these cephalosporins, and at present it is unknown whether this in vitro phenomenon will have clinical significance. In addition, jaundice and hemolytic anemia in newborns with G6PD deficiency have been noted after maternal sulfonamide administration near term.

The tetracyclines readily cross the placental barrier and concentrate in many tissues of the developing fetus.[111] Of particular interest is the deposition of tetracycline in fetal bones and deciduous teeth.[109, 118] The growth inhibition observed after tetracycline administration to premature infants, however, is reversible when short-term therapy is employed.[108] Calcification of deciduous teeth begins during the fourth month of gestation, and crown formation of the anterior teeth is almost complete at term. Tetracycline administered during this gestational period produces yellow discoloration, enamel hypoplasia, and abnormal development of those teeth. These effects have been documented for tetracycline, oxytetracycline, and demethylchlortetracycline.[109] One report found a possible association between ciprofloxacin therapy given to young infants and teeth discoloration,[119] but this association has not been confirmed by other investigators.

Chloramphenicol has been associated with circulatory collapse (gray baby syndrome) and death in premature infants who received the drug during the first weeks of life.[78] Chloramphenicol should not be administered to pregnant women near term because of the absence of glucuronyl transferase activity in the fetal liver and the potential danger of serum drug accumulation and shock in the newborn.[120]

Intrapartum administration of antimicrobial agents to women in labor creates a potential problem for the pediatrician by potentially suppressing fetal infection and delaying diagnosis and treatment of the neonate. Although there is evidence to support this contention for group B streptococcal early-onset neonatal infections,[121–123] it is less clear for other bacterial pathogens. With the advent of newer, more active β-lactam antibiotics, such as new-generation cephalosporins, it is possible that treatment of women in labor could prevent or even cure some bacterial infections in premature infants.

EXCRETION OF ANTIBIOTICS IN HUMAN MILK

As a general rule, the concentration of antimicrobial agents in breast milk is so low that neither therapeutic nor harmful effects are likely to occur. Sometimes, however, the amount of drug could be significant, depending on the volume of milk ingested by the newborn and the pharmacokinetic properties of that drug once it is absorbed through the infant's gastrointestinal mucosa.[124, 125] The safety of antibiotics in milk has primarily been determined by anecdotal clinical experience rather than by carefully controlled long-term studies.

Most drugs are transferred into breast milk by passive diffusion, and only a few are actively secreted. Factors influencing the transfer of antibiotics from plasma to milk include maternal serum concentration of unbound drug, water and lipid solubility, degree of ionization, serum and milk protein-binding capability, and molecular weight of the antibiotic.[125] Although drugs with a high lipid solubility tend to accumulate in milk, the extent varies with the fat content of the milk. Ionization power of drugs depends on the pH of the milk and the drug dissociation constant (pK_a). Human milk has a pH of 7.37; therefore, drugs that are weak bases ($pK_a > pH$), such as trimethoprim and tetracyclines, ionize and concentrate in milk,[126] whereas weak acids, such as ampicillin, do not.[125, 126] Drugs that are highly serum protein bound tend to remain in the intravascular space.

The maternal serum and breast milk concentrations of commonly used antimicrobial agents are given in Table 35–2.[64, 65, 70, 106, 125–144] Because the data for each drug are based on small numbers of women, the values vary considerably. In general, the concentrations of metronidazole, sulfonamides, and trimethoprim in breast milk are similar to those in maternal serum (milk:serum ratio of 1.0), whereas those of chloramphenicol, erythromycin, and tetracycline are 50 to 75%.[64, 135] Available data suggest that the concentrations of penicillins, oxacillin, various cephalosporins, and aminoglycosides in milk are low.[129, 140]

There are no data pertaining to antibiotic concentrations in the colostrum. Because blood flow and permeability are increased during the colostral phase,[145] it is possible that these drugs are present in concentrations equal to or greater than those found in mature milk.

There are very few reports of adverse effects to infants who were breast-fed by mothers receiving antimicrobial agents. Hemolytic anemia has been described in breast-fed newborns whose mothers were being treated with sulfonamides, nalidixic acid, or nitrofurantoin.[146] One report incriminated the administration of clindamycin to a mother with the development of antibiotic-induced colitis in her breast-fed infant.[147] A causal effect, however, could not be convincingly demonstrated. There are undoubtedly other examples of potential infant toxicity from antibiotics in milk that have not been recognized or reported.

The decision to allow or stop breast-feeding must be based on the likelihood that high milk concentrations are attained for a particular drug and that significant adverse events are commonly associated with this drug. For the vast majority of antibiotics, however, this does not appear to be an important issue. The American Academy of Pediatrics Committee on Drugs recommends that breast-feeding be transiently discontinued 12 to 24 hours before and during the course of treatment with metronidazole (in vitro mutagen) or chloramphenicol (theoretical risk of idiosyncratic bone marrow suppression) and warns about the use of nalidixic acid, nitrofurantoin, and sulfa drugs, which can cause hemolysis in G6PD-deficient infants.[146] In general, the severity of the woman's infection rather than the drug that she is receiving is most often the more important contraindication to breast-feeding.

PENICILLIN

Penicillin has been used for treatment of neonatal bacterial infections for more than three decades. It is safe and

TABLE 35–2
Excretion of Antimicrobial Agents in Human Breast Milk

ANTIBIOTIC	MATERNAL DOSAGE (ROUTE)	NO. OF PATIENTS	CONCENTRATION IN MILK (TIME)[a, b]	MILK/MATERNAL SERUM RATIO (%)	REFERENCE NO.
Amoxicillin	1 g (PO)	6	0.1 (1 hr)	1.4	127
			0.17 (2 hr)	1.2	
			0.37 (3 hr)	4	
Aztreonam	1 g (IM)	6	0.14 (2 hr)	0.4	128
	1 g (IV)	6	0.18 (2 hr)	0.6	
Cefadroxil	1 g (PO)	6	1.64 (6 hr)	8	130
Cefamandole	1 g (IV)	4	0.46 (1 hr)	2	130
Cefazolin	2 g (IV)	20	1.25 (2 hr)	2.3	130
Cefoperazone	1 g (IV)	4	0.41 (2 hr)	1	64
Cefotaxime	1 g (IV)	12	0.26 (1 hr)	2.8	65
			0.32 (2 hr)	8.6	
Cefoxitin	1 g (IV)	4	0.58 (1 hr)	3	132
Ceftazidime	2 g (IV)	11	5.2 (1 hr)	7	133
Ceftizoxime	1 g (IV)	6	0.25 (1 hr)	1	134
Ceftriaxone	1 g (IV)	10	0.47 (4 hr)	1.6	70
	1 g (IM)	10	0.63 (4 hr)	2.1	
Cephalexin	1 g (PO)	6	0.2 (1 hr)	1	127
			0.28 (2 hr)	2	
			0.39 (3 hr)	14	
Cephalotin	1 g (IV)	6	0.41 (1 hr)	7	127
			0.47 (2 hr)	25	
			0.36 (3 hr)	51	
Clindamycin	0.15 g (PO)	5	<1.4 (6 hr)	38	130
Doxycycline	0.1 g (PO)	15	0.77 (3 hr)	32	130
Erythromycin	0.4 g (PO)	—	0.4–1.6	50	64
Kanamycin	1 g (IM)	4	18.4 (1 hr)	33	137
Lincomycin	0.5 g (PO)	9	1.3 (6 hr)	93	64
Metronidazole	0.2 g (PO)	10	3.4 (4 hr)	87	130
Nitrofurantoin	0.2 g (PO)	4	0.2 (2 hr)	24	139
Penicillin G	10^5 units (IM)	10	<0.04 (2 hr)	<13	140
Sulfapyridine	0.5 g (PO)	3	10.3	54	106
	0.75 g (PO)	—	30–130	100	135
Tetracycline	0.5 g (PO)	5	0.5–2.6	62	135
Ticarcillin	5 g (IV)	10	2–2.5	—	142
Tobramycin	0.08 g (IM)	5	<0.5	—	143
Trimethoprim	—	50	2	125	64

[a]Concentrations are in micrograms per milliliter.
[b]Time refers to period from drug administration to mother until sample collection.
IM = intramuscular; IV = intravenous; PO = oral.

still effective for therapy against streptococci, susceptible staphylococci (currently most strains are resistant), the majority of pneumococci (though worldwide resistance is reaching alarming levels), and *L. monocytogenes*. In addition, most meningococcal strains and *Treponema pallidum* remain exquisitely susceptible to penicillin. Currently, many gonococcal isolates are resistant to this drug. Although penicillin (usually combined with an aminoglycoside) is used in some institutions as initial empirical therapy for neonatal septicemia and meningitis, ampicillin is preferred because it provides broader antimicrobial activity without sacrificing safety.

Mode of Action

Penicillin interferes with bacterial cell wall synthesis by reacting with one or more penicillin-binding proteins (PBPs) to inhibit transpeptidation.[148] The transpeptidase activity of PBPs is essential for cross-linking adjacent peptides and for incorporating newly formed peptidoglycan into an already existing strand. Subsequently, this event promotes bacterial cell lysis.

Several mechanisms of bacterial resistance to penicillin and some of the other β lactams have been identified. The most important is by inactivation through enzymatic hydrolysis of the β-lactam ring by β lactamases.[149] These enzymes are produced by most staphylococci and enteric gram-negative bacilli and by many *Neisseria gonorrhoeae* strains. Another mechanism of resistance is related to decreased permeability of the outer membrane of gram-negative bacteria, which can prevent this drug from reaching its target site.[150] In addition, by poorly defined mechanisms, some group B streptococcal organisms are inhibited but not killed by penicillin, a phenomenon termed *tolerance*.[151]

Usual MICs of penicillin against streptococci are between 0.005 and 0.1 μg/ml. For *T. pallidum*, the corresponding concentration ranges are between 0.02 and 0.2 μg/ml. Group B streptococcal-tolerant organisms (MBC 32 times MIC) are found in less than 5% of isolates.[152] Currently, 15 to 40% of pneumococcal strains isolated in many parts of the world are considered to be relatively (MICs of 0.1 to 1 μg/ml) or highly (≥2 μg/ml) resistant to penicillin.[153, 154] Many of these isolates are also resistant to multiple antibiotics, including third-generation cephalosporins. The mechanism of resistance is alteration of one or more penicillin-binding protein.

Pharmacokinetic Data

Aqueous Penicillin G. A mean peak serum concentration of 24 μg/ml (range, 8 to 41 μg/ml) is observed after a 25,000-units/kg dose of penicillin G given intramuscularly to infants with weights less than 2000 g at birth (Table 35–3).[155] The peak values do not change appreciably with birth weight or postnatal age up to 14 days. After a 50,000-units/kg dose, peak serum values of 35 to 40 μg/ml were detected in neonates of different ages. The concentrations at 4 and 8 hours after the dose were not substantially different from those after a dose of 25,000 units/kg.

The half-life of penicillin in serum is inversely correlated with birth weight and postnatal age. Half-life values of 1.5 to 10 hours are observed in the first week of life; the larger values are usually seen in infants with birth weights less than 1500 g. The half-life values for infants more than 7 days of age range from 1.5 to 4 hours. The half-life of penicillin in newborns is inversely correlated with clearance of creatinine. Plasma clearance of penicillin increases with the age of the newborn.

The concentrations of penicillin in urine after different dosages of penicillin G vary considerably. The highest values occur in the first 4 hours after a dose of 25,000 units/kg and range from 31 to 2000 μg/ml.[155] The urinary excretion of penicillin in infants is independent of age and dosage and is approximately 30% of the dose for a 12-hour period.

Procaine Penicillin G. Procaine penicillin G in a single daily intramuscular dose of 50,000 units/kg produces mean serum values of 7 to 9 μg/ml for up to 12

hours and 1.5 μg/ml at 24 hours after the dose in infants younger than 1 week of age (see Table 35–3).[155] Because the concentrations decrease more rapidly in older neonates, only 0.4 μg/ml is detected at 24 hours. These serum values are approximately twice those obtained when 22,000 units/kg is given to premature and term infants.[2] There is no accumulation of penicillin in serum after 7 to 10 days of daily doses of procaine penicillin G, and the drug is well tolerated without evidence of local reaction at the site of injection. The concentrations of penicillin in urine and the urinary excretion after equivalent doses are similar for both procaine penicillin G and aqueous penicillin G.

Benzathine Penicillin G. Penicillin can be detected in serum and urine for up to 12 days after a single 50,000-units/kg dose of benzathine penicillin G given intramuscularly to newborns. Peak serum concentrations of from 0.4 to 2.5 μg/ml (mean, 1.2 μg/ml) are observed from 12 to 24 hours after administration, and levels of from 0.07 to 0.09 μg/ml are present at 12 days.[156, 157] Urinary concentrations range from 4 to 170 μg/ml for 7 days and from 0.3 to 25 μg/ml for 8 to 12 days after a 50,000-units/kg dose of benzathine penicillin. This preparation is well tolerated by infants. Muscle damage from intramuscular injection as judged from creatinine kinase values does not appear to be appreciably different from that after intramuscular administration of the other penicillins.

Cerebrospinal Fluid Penetration

Penicillin does not penetrate CSF well, even when meninges are inflamed. Peak concentrations of 1 to 2 μg/ml are measured 30 minutes to 1 hour after a 40,000-units/kg intravenous dose of penicillin G is given to infants and children with bacterial meningitis.[158] These values are 2 to 5% of concomitant serum concentrations and exceed the MIC values of streptococci and susceptible pneumococci by 50- to 100-fold. CSF concentrations of penicillin are, however, not optimal to treat neonatal meningitis caused by penicillin-resistant pneumococci. When meningeal inflammation is decreased, however, the concentrations of penicillin are reduced substantially. Concentrations of penicillin in CSF during the first

TABLE 35–3
Pharmacokinetics of Penicillin G in Neonates

DRUG (DOSAGE)	BIRTH WEIGHT/ AGE GROUP	MEAN PEAK SERUM CONCENTRATION (μg/ml)	MEAN SERUM HALF-LIFE (hr)	PLASMA CLEARANCE (ml/min per 1.73 m²)
Crystalline penicillin G (25,000 units/kg)	2000 g			
	7 days	24	4.9	30
	8–14 days	23.6	2.6	48
	>2000 g			
	7 days	22.3	2.6	52
	8–14 days	21	2.1	75
Procaine penicillin G	7 days[a]	8.9	6.1	50
(50,000 units/kg)	8–14 days	6.2	5.4	93

[a]Average weight at time of study, 3100 g.

several days of therapy are maintained in the 0.5 to 1 μg/ml range; thereafter, the values are 0.1 μg/ml or less by 4 hours after the dose.

Most newborns with uninflamed meninges have undetectable concentrations of penicillin in the CSF after a 50,000-units/kg dose of intramuscular benzathine penicillin G.[156] With a 100,000-units/kg dose, the mean peak concentration obtained 12 to 24 hours later is 0.06 μg/ml but falls to very low values by 48 to 72 hours.[159] For this reason, we do not recommend this long-acting penicillin for therapy for infants with congenital neurosyphilis. By contrast, mean CSF concentrations range from 0.12 to 0.7 μg/ml between 4 and 24 hours after a 50,000-units/kg dose of intramuscular procaine penicillin G is administered to a newborn.[160, 161] These CSF values are at least severalfold greater than the required minimum spirocheticidal concentration.[161]

Oral Administration

Potassium penicillin G has been administered orally to premature and term infants.[2, 162] Mean peak serum concentrations at 2 and 6 hours after a 22,000-units/kg dose were 1.4 and 0.7 μg/ml, respectively, in premature infants. The corresponding values in term neonates were 1.7 and 0.2 μg/ml, respectively.

Elimination

Most of the penicillin dose is excreted in the urine in unchanged form. Tubular secretion accounts for approximately 90% of urinary penicillin, whereas glomerular filtration contributes the remaining 10%. Biliary excretion also occurs, and this may be an important route of elimination in newborns with renal failure.

Clinical Implications

Penicillin remains effective for therapy for infections caused by group B streptococci, susceptible pneumococci and staphylococci, meningococci, susceptible gonococci, and *T. pallidum*. The dosage recommended for neonatal sepsis or pneumonia is 50,000 to 100,000 units/kg per day administered in two to four divided doses, whereas that for meningitis is 150,000 to 200,000 units/kg per day in two to four divided doses depending on birth weight and postnatal age.[163] Neonatal meningitis caused by penicillin-resistant pneumococci must be treated with cefotaxime with or without vancomycin depending on the MIC values. There is no place for oral penicillin therapy in neonates with acute systemic infections.

Because central nervous system involvement in congenital syphilis is difficult to exclude with certainty, benzathine penicillin G should not be used for therapy for this disease unless new diagnostic modalities to rule out neurosyphilis are developed.[164] Its use for asymptomatic infants with normal CSF examinations and roentgenologic studies but who have positive treponemal serologies, presumably from maternal origin, is acceptable if follow-up can be ensured. For symptomatic infants and for asymptomatic infants with laboratory or radiologic evidence suggestive of congenital syphilis, the recommended regimens are either aqueous penicillin G, 50,000 units/kg daily for 10 to 14 days administered intramuscularly or intravenously in two divided doses, or procaine penicillin G, 50,000 units/kg daily for 10 to 14 days administered once daily intramuscularly.

All forms of penicillin are well tolerated in newborns. Cutaneous allergic manifestations to penicillin are rare in the newborn and young infant, and there is no evidence that infants receiving penicillin in the neonatal period are sensitized to the drug, thus increasing the risk of an allergic response on reexposure.

AMPICILLIN

Antimicrobial Activity

Ampicillin is commonly used alone or in combination with aminoglycosides for treatment of suspected or proven neonatal bacterial infections. Compared with penicillin G, ampicillin has increased in vitro efficacy against most strains of enterococci and *L. monocytogenes* as well as against some gram-negative pathogens, such as typable and nontypable *Haemophilus, Escherichia coli, Proteus mirabilis*, and *Salmonella* species. It is not as active, however, against groups A and B streptococci and susceptible strains of staphylococci and pneumococci. Approximately 90% of group B streptococci and *Listeria* are inhibited by 0.06 μg/ml or less of ampicillin. Almost two thirds of the gram-negative enteric bacilli isolated from CSF cultures of infants enrolled in the Second Neonatal Meningitis Cooperative Study (1976 to 1978) were inhibited by 10 μg/ml or less of ampicillin.[165] Recently, however, an increased rate of ampicillin-resistant gram-negative bacilli has been reported and possibly linked to the frequent use of intrapartum prophylaxis with ampicillin to prevent early-onset group B streptococcal neonatal infection.[166]

Pharmacokinetic Data

Serum ampicillin concentration-time curves after intramuscular doses of 5 to 25 mg/kg have been determined in newborns.[167–169] The mean peak serum concentrations 30 minutes to 1 hour after 5, 10, 20, and 25 mg/kg doses were 16, 25, 54, and 57 μg/ml, respectively, whereas the values at 12 hours were from 1 to 15 μg/ml (mean, 5 μg/ml). After 50-mg/kg doses, the mean peak values were from 100 to 130 μg/ml in low-birth-weight infants and from 80 to 85 μg/ml in larger term infants (Table 35–4). Peak serum concentrations as high as 300 μg/ml (mean values, 180 to 216 μg/ml) are observed 1 to 2 hours after the 100-mg/kg dose.[35] These latter values exceed the MIC_{90} values of group B streptococci by at least 3000-fold.

The elimination half-life of ampicillin is inversely correlated with birth weight and postnatal age. Half-life times of from 3 to 6 hours are noted in the first week of life and are 2 to 3.5 hours thereafter. Similar correlations with birth weight and chronologic age are observed with the plasma clearances of ampicillin.

TABLE 35–4
Pharmacokinetics of Ampicillin in Newborns

DOSAGE (ROUTE)	BIRTH WEIGHT/ AGE GROUP	MEAN PEAK SERUM CONCENTRATION (μg/ml)	MEAN SERUM HALF-LIFE (hr)	MEAN PLASMA CLEARANCE (ml/min per 1.73 m²)
50 mg/kg (IM)	2500 g			
	7 days	104	6.2	21
	8–14 days	130	2	30
	>2500 g			
	7 days	81	4.7	42
	8–14 days	84	2.3	63
100 mg/kg (IM)	2500 g			
	7 days	213	4.7	NA
	8–14 days	216	3.5	NA
	>2500 g			
	7 days	180	3.1	NA
	8–14 days	187	1.8	NA

IM = intramuscular; NA = not available.

Mean peak serum concentrations of 135 μg/ml for premature infants with gestational ages of 26 to 33 weeks were found after an intravenous 100-mg/kg dose of ampicillin, whereas for those infants with gestational ages of 34 to 40 weeks, they were 153 μg/ml.[170] When the loading dose was followed by maintenance ampicillin doses of 50 mg/kg intravenously at 12- to 18-hour intervals, the mean peak and trough serum concentrations in steady-state conditions were 113 and 30 μg/ml for premature neonates and 140 and 37 μg/ml for full-term neonates, respectively. The steady-state serum half-lives for ampicillin were about 9.5 and 7 hours for premature and full-term newborns, respectively.

Cerebrospinal Fluid Penetration

Concentrations of ampicillin in CSF vary greatly. The largest concentrations (3 to 18 μg/ml) occur approximately 2 hours after a 50-mg/kg intravenous dose and exceed the MIC values of group B streptococci and *Listeria* by 50- to 300-fold.[35] In contrast, against many *E. coli* strains, these peak concentrations equal or exceed the MIC values by only severalfold. The values in CSF are lower later than in the course of meningitis when meningeal inflammation subsides.

Oral Administration

Oral administration of 20- to 30-mg/kg doses of ampicillin trihydrate to normal, fasting full-term infants during the first 4 days of life produced peak values of 20 to 30 μg/ml 4 hours after the doses.[167] Higher peak serum concentrations are achieved by oral administration of the anhydrous form of ampicillin rather than the trihydrate preparation.[171] In our experience,[172] mean peak serum concentrations of 6.4 and 6.1 μg/ml occurred at 1 and 2 hours, respectively, after a 25-mg/kg dose of ampicillin trihydrate, and the drug was absorbed equally well in both fasting and concomitantly milk-fed infants. Because of better absorption, amoxicillin would be expected to achieve higher serum concentrations than ampicillin after equivalent doses.

Safety

Ampicillin is a safe drug when administered parenterally to newborns. Nonspecific rashes and urticaria are rarely observed, and diarrhea is uncommon. Elevations of serum glutamic-oxaloacetic transaminase and creatinine kinase values are frequently detected in neonates and most likely represent local tissue destruction at the site of intramuscular injection. Mild eosinophilia may be noted in newborns and young infants. Alteration of the microbial flora of the bowel may occur after parenteral administration of ampicillin, but overgrowth of resistant gram-negative organisms and *Candida albicans* occurs more frequently after oral administration.[173] Diarrhea usually subsides on discontinuation of therapy. Amoxicillin is better-tolerated, with fewer gastrointestinal side effects, than is orally administered ampicillin.

Clinical Implications

Vast clinical experience has demonstrated that ampicillin is a safe and effective drug for therapy for neonatal bacterial infections caused by susceptible organisms. Combined ampicillin and aminoglycoside therapy is appropriate initial empirical management of suspected bacterial infections of neonates because it provides broad antimicrobial activity and potential synergism against many strains of group B streptococci, *Listeria*, and enterococci.[31–34, 37]

For systemic bacterial infections other than meningitis, a dosage of 50 to 75 mg/kg per day in two to three divided doses in the first week of life and of 75 to 100 mg/kg per day in three to four divided doses thereafter is recommended. For therapy for bacterial meningitis, we recommend a dosage of 150 to 200 mg/kg per day given in three to four divided doses, although some consultants use dosages as high as 300 mg/kg per day.

We are not in favor of oral administration of ampicillin to newborns. As a general rule, infants with suspected or proven bacterial infections caused by susceptible organisms should be treated parenterally in the hospital. Otitis media in infants younger than 6 weeks of age may be better treated with other antimicrobial agents, such as amoxicillin-clavulanate or a cephalosporin, because *S. aureus* and resistant gram-negative organisms are possible etiologic agents.[174]

ANTISTAPHYLOCOCCAL PENICILLINS

S. aureus infections occur in nurseries either as sporadic cases or in the form of disease outbreaks. In recent years, multiply-resistant strains, especially coagulase-negative staphylococcal species, have been responsible for an increasing number of nosocomially acquired staphylococcal infections in many neonatal units. Familiarity with the antistaphylococcal penicillins is essential for physicians involved in the care of newborns with infections caused by susceptible staphylococci.

Antimicrobial Activity

The antistaphylococcal penicillins are resistant to hydrolysis by most staphylococcal β lactamases by virtue of a substituted side chain that acts by steric hindrance at the site of enzyme attachment. Most penicillinase-producing staphylococci are inhibited by 2.5 to 5 μg/ml or less of methicillin and by 0.5 μg/ml or less of nafcillin and oxacillin.[175] Currently, methicillin-resistant *S. aureus* (MRSA) strains are a relatively common cause of infection outbreaks in some nurseries, and methicillin-resistant *S. epidermidis* (MRSE) strains are an important cause of catheter-associated disease, particularly among low-birth-weight premature infants. These challenging isolates possess altered penicillin-binding proteins with low affinity to antistaphylococcal penicillins and cephalosporins.[176] Vancomycin is the drug of choice for infections caused by these resistant strains. The topical antimicrobial agent, mupirocin, has successfully been used to eradicate MRSA strains from sites of the newborn body

colonized with these strains and to prevent their spread to other infants.[177] In addition, tolerant staphylococci (MBC greater than five times MIC) have been described.[178] Infections caused by these uncommon staphylococcal isolates may require combined therapy with aminoglycosides or rifampin or the use of vancomycin alone.

Pharmacokinetic Data

Methicillin. Peak serum concentrations of methicillin are higher in the first week of life than during the remainder of the newborn period.[168, 169] For example, after 25-mg/kg intramuscular doses, mean peak values of 58 and 49 μg/ml are observed in 0- to 7-day-old infants who weigh 2000 g or less and more than 2000 g at birth, respectively; whereas for these same birth weights, values of 39 and 41 μg/ml, respectively, are achieved in infants 15 days old or more (Table 35–5).[179] A 50-mg/kg intramuscular dose produces a mean peak serum concentration of 80 μg/ml 30 minutes to 1 hour later. The half-life values become smaller with increasing birth weight and postnatal age. This correlates with the substantial increase in the plasma clearance of methicillin that occurs during the neonatal period. Urine concentrations of methicillin are from 275 to 880 μg/ml in the first 2 hours after a 20-mg/kg intramuscular dose and usually greater than 120 μg/ml for up to 12 hours after the dose. Approximately 30% of the dose is excreted in urine in the first 6 hours after administration.[168]

Nafcillin. The administration of 5-, 10-, 15-, and 20-mg/kg intramuscular doses of nafcillin to full-term newborns in the first 4 days of life produces mean peak serum concentrations 1 hour later of 10, 25, 30, and 37 μg/ml, respectively.[167, 180] These concentrations are significantly higher than those obtained in older children receiving comparable amounts of this drug.[180] Hepatic clearance is the principal route of nafcillin elimination because only 8 to 25% of this drug is excreted in the urine in a 24-hour period.[180]

Peak concentrations of nafcillin of from 100 to 160 μg/ml were obtained during steady-state conditions after 33- to 50-mg/kg intravenous doses were adminis-

TABLE 35–5
Pharmacokinetics of Methicillin and Nafcillin in Newborns

DRUG (DOSAGE)	BIRTH WEIGHT/ AGE GROUP	MEAN PEAK SERUM CONCENTRATION (μg/ml)	PEAK SERUM HALF-LIFE (hr)	MEAN PLASMA CLEARANCE (ml/min per 1.73 m²)
Methicillin	2000 g			
(25 mg/kg per dose)	0–7 days	58	2.8	32
	15 days	39	1.8	79
	>2000 g			
	0–7 days	49	2.2	62
	15 days	41	1.1	128
Nafcillin	2000 g			
(50 mg/kg per dose)[a]	0–7 days	±160	4	0.91[b]
	8–28 days		3.2	1.2[b]

[a]Data from reference 181.
[b]Total body clearance (ml/min per kg).

tered to premature infants weighing less than 2000 g at birth (see Table 35–5).[181] The half-life values ranged from 2.2 to 5.5 hours in these low-birth-weight neonates.

When nafcillin is given orally to newborns, mean peak serum concentrations are from 20 to 60% of those obtained after an identical dose is administered intramuscularly.[167, 182] Oral doses of 5 to 20 mg/kg of nafcillin result in mean peak serum concentrations of 3 to 21 μg/ml 2 to 4 hours after ingestion.

Oxacillin. The pharmacokinetics of oxacillin in neonates are similar to those of methicillin. Mean peak serum concentrations of approximately 50 and 100 μg/ml are produced by 20 and 50 mg/kg intramuscular doses, respectively.[168, 183] The serum half-life of oxacillin in premature infants is about 3 hours in the first week of life and 1.5 hours thereafter. Urinary concentrations are from 174 to 510 μg/ml in the first 2 hours after a 20-mg/kg dose, and 17 and 34% of the dose is excreted during 6 hours after administration in infants 8 to 14 days and 20 to 21 days of age, respectively.[168]

Cloxacillin. Oral administration of 5-, 10-, 20-, and 50-mg/kg single doses to full-term neonates during the first 4 days of life results in mean peak serum concentrations of 15, 24, 32, and 92 μg/ml, respectively, 1 to 2 hours after ingestion of this drug.[167] The mean concentrations 12 hours after the above doses are given fall to 0, 3, 8, and 19 μg/ml, respectively.

Safety

The antistaphylococcal penicillins are well tolerated and safe in newborn and young infants. Repeated intramuscular injections of methicillin frequently result in muscle damage and elevation of creatinine kinase concentrations. Sterile muscle abscesses occasionally follow intramuscular administration. Nephrotoxicity (interstitial nephritis or cystitis) is rare in newborns and occurs in 3 to 5% of children who receive large dosages of methicillin and possibly the other antistaphylococcal penicillins, with the exception of nafcillin.[184, 185] Reversible hematologic abnormalities such as neutropenia or eosinophilia are commonly observed in children treated with these drugs, but their incidence in newborns is unknown.[185–188] Because nafcillin has a predominant biliary excretion, accumulation of this drug in serum can occur in jaundiced neonates, and potential adverse effects can develop. Extravasation of nafcillin at the injection site can result in necrosis of local tissue.

Clinical Implications

Any of these antistaphylococcal drugs can be used for therapy for staphylococcal infections in neonates. The dosage of methicillin and oxacillin (preferred) is 25 to 50 mg/kg given every 8 to 12 hours (50 to 150 mg/kg per day) in the first week of life and every 6 to 8 hours (75 to 200 mg/kg per day) thereafter. The larger dosage is indicated for infants with disseminated disease or meningitis. For nafcillin, we recommend 25 mg/kg per dose given every 12 hours in the first week of life and every 6 to 8 hours thereafter.

In the unlikely circumstance that the *Staphylococcus* species is susceptible to penicillin, this agent is preferred for therapy. If an infant does not respond to antimicrobial therapy as anticipated, the physician should suspect occult sites of staphylococcal disease (e.g., abscesses, osteomyelitis, endocarditis), resistance of the pathogen to the drug given, or tolerance of the organism to the antibiotic. Appropriate drainage of purulent foci, addition of an aminoglycoside or rifampin to the regimen, and use of vancomycin are among several options to consider when dealing with unresponsive infections.

CARBENICILLIN

Carbenicillin is an α-carboxybenzyl penicillin that possesses activity against *P. aeruginosa* and some indole-positive *Proteus* strains. In addition, essentially all bacteria susceptible to ampicillin are also susceptible to carbenicillin. Although the combination of carbenicillin and an aminoglycoside provides a broader antimicrobial activity, ampicillin plus an aminoglycoside is the combination preferred in most nurseries. Carbenicillin is no longer available in the United States, having been replaced by newer, more active agents.

Antimicrobial Activity

Like ampicillin, carbenicillin is effective in vitro against the two most common pathogens of neonatal septicemia and meningitis, *E. coli* and group B *Streptococcus*. *L. monocytogenes* and enterococci are less susceptible in vitro to carbenicillin than to ampicillin. *Klebsiella* and many *Pseudomonas* species, other than *P. aeruginosa*, are resistant to carbenicillin.[37] Most hospital-acquired staphylococci are also resistant to this agent.[189] Combinations of carbenicillin and gentamicin are synergistic in vitro against *P. aeruginosa*, enterococci, and many *Listeria* isolates.[37]

Pharmacokinetic Data

The pharmacokinetic data of carbenicillin are similar to those of ampicillin in newborns. Peak serum concentrations of 180 to 190 μg/ml are observed after 100-mg/kg doses in all neonates except term infants more than 1 week of age, in whom peak values are from 140 to 150 μg/ml (Table 35–6).[190] Although peak serum concentrations after intravenous doses are about twice those obtained after identical intramuscular doses are given, the dose-response curves for both routes of administration are similar after the peak concentrations are achieved.[191] Serum half-life values are inversely correlated with birth weight, chronologic age, and rate of creatinine clearance.[190–192] During the first week of life, mean half-life values are from 3 to 6 hours; whereas for neonates aged 1 to 4 weeks, values of 2 to 3 hours are observed.[190] Plasma clearances of carbenicillin increase appreciably during the first 30 days of life.

Because carbenicillin is eliminated by renal mechanisms, extremely large concentrations are present in urine. Concentrations of from 800 to 5500 μg/ml (mean,

TABLE 35–6
Pharmacokinetics of Carbenicillin, Ticarcillin, and Piperacillin in Neonates

DRUG (DOSAGE, ROUTE)	BIRTH WEIGHT/ AGE GROUP	MEAN PEAK SERUM CONCENTRATION (μg/ml)	MEAN SERUM HALF-LIFE (hr)	MEAN PLASMA CLEARANCE (ml/min per 1.73 m²)
Carbenicillin (100 mg/kg; IM)	2000 g			
	7 days	180	5.7	25
	8–14 days	186	3.6	35
	>2000 g			
	7 days	185	4.2	45
	8–14 days	143	2.1	77
Ticarcillin (75 mg/kg; IM)	2000 g			
	Mean, 2.5 days	189	5.6	31
	>2000 g			
	Mean, 3 days	159	4.9	54
	Mean, 34 days[a]	125	2.2	118
Piperacillin (75 mg/kg; IV)	1000–1520 g (mean, 1300 g)			
	7 days	137	4.3	1.7[b]
	1500–3580 g (mean, 1930 g)			
	7 days	149	3.4	1.8[b]
	2265–3900 g (mean, 3108 g)			
	7 days	129	2.5	2.5[b]
	850–1400 g (mean, 1200 g)			
	8–14 days	110	3.2	3.2[b]
	1500–2170 g (mean, 1725 g)			
	8–14 days	100	2.5	3.4[b]
	2265–3900 g (mean, 3108 g)			
	8–14 days	97	1.7	4.4[b]

[a]Ticarcillin dosage of 100 mg/kg.
[b]Total body clearance (ml/min per kg).
IM = intramuscularly; IV = intravenously.

2689 μg/ml) are noted during the first 6 hours after 100-mg/kg doses.[191]

Clinical Implications

Carbenicillin alone or preferably in combination with an aminoglycoside was used for therapy for neonatal infections caused by *P. aeruginosa* or indole-positive *Proteus* species. New antimicrobial agents are now preferred for these infections. Although synergism between carbenicillin and gentamicin has been observed in vitro against enterococci, *L. monocytogenes*, and *P. aeruginosa*,[37] the clinical significance of this phenomenon is uncertain. The dosage schedule for carbenicillin is the following: 100 mg/kg given every 12 hours for all infants younger than 1 week of age, every 8 hours for infants older than 7 days weighing less than 2000 g at birth, and every 6 hours for neonates older than 7 days weighing more than 2000 g at birth. The drug should be administered intravenously in a 20- to 30-minute period.

The drug is well tolerated and safe in newborns. Platelet dysfunction, hypokalemia, and allergic manifestations observed in older patients have not been reported in neonates. Carbenicillin is a disodium salt that contains 4.7 mEq of sodium per gram of drug and should be used carefully in some newborns, such as those with heart failure.

TICARCILLIN

Ticarcillin is a semisynthetic penicillin with pharmacologic and toxic properties virtually identical to those of carbenicillin. Its in vitro activity is similar to that of carbenicillin, with the exception that ticarcillin is more active against *P. aeruginosa*.[189]

Mean peak serum concentrations of 189 μg/ml are seen 1 hour after 75-mg/kg intramuscular doses to low-birth-weight infants younger than 7 days of age and of 125 to 160 μg/ml to older neonates (see Table 35–6).[193] The half-life values and plasma clearances during the neonatal period are similar to those of carbenicillin.[193, 194]

There have never been comparative clinical studies of carbenicillin and ticarcillin to indicate an advantage of one drug over the other. In the United States, carbenicillin is no longer available. Ticarcillin alone or combined with clavulanate (Timetin) is preferred in patients with *P. aeruginosa* infections because of its greater in vitro activity against this organism. Although the quantity of sodium per gram is larger for ticarcillin than was the case for carbenicillin, the lower dosage schedule of ticarcillin recommended for neonates and young infants provides a smaller amount of sodium per dose of drug, which conceivably could be advantageous in infants with cardiac or renal disease. The dosage is 75 mg/kg administered every 12 hours to infants younger than 1 week of age, and every 8 and 6 hours to older infants weighing 2000 g or less and more than 2000 g at birth, respectively.

The co-administration of clavulanic acid with ticarcillin significantly enhances the antibacterial activity of the latter drug against several organisms, including some ticarcillin-resistant strains of *E. coli, Klebsiella pneumoniae, P. mirabilis*, and staphylococci.[195, 196] Clavulanic acid is a β-lactam with weak antibacterial activity, but it has the property of being a potent irreversible inhibitor of several β-lactamases produced by gram-positive and gram-negative bacteria.[197] Information regarding the use of this new compound in newborns is limited. Pharmacokinetic data obtained in three newborns with gram-negative infections treated with a ticarcillin:clavulanic acid weight ratio of 25:1 showed peak serum concentrations and half-life values similar to those observed after administration of ticarcillin alone.[198] This drug combination is potentially very useful in the treatment of neonatal infections. We have prescribed ticarcillin-clavulanate either alone or, more commonly, with an aminoglycoside for infants with nosocomial gram-negative enteric infections with satisfactory safety and effectiveness.

ACYLAMPICILLINS

The acylampicillins, a group of semisynthetic penicillins, include the ureidopenicillins (mezlocillin and azlocillin)
and a piperazine derivative of ampicillin called piperacillin.[199, 200] These drugs have not been approved by the FDA for use in newborns. Many pathogens incriminated in neonatal infections are susceptible in vitro to these antibiotics, but their most important feature is activity against *P. aeruginosa*.

Antimicrobial Activity

Mezlocillin, azlocillin, and piperacillin are active against a broad range of gram-positive and gram-negative bacteria (Table 35–7). In contrast to carbenicillin and ticarcillin, which show poor activity against *K. pneumoniae*, piperacillin is active against most isolates of this organism, whereas mezlocillin and azlocillin inhibit about 50%. They are also active against *P. mirabilis* and many strains of *Enterobacter* and *Serratia marcescens*. Because these antibiotics are susceptible to hydrolysis by β lactamases, they have very limited activity against β-lactamase–producing Enterobacteriaceae.[199, 200]

Piperacillin is the most active of these agents against *P. aeruginosa*. Mezlocillin, the least active of the three, is at least as effective as ticarcillin against this organism. Ninety percent of *P. aeruginosa* isolates are inhibited by approximately 16, 32, and 128 μg/ml of piperacillin, azlocillin, and mezlocillin, respectively.[201]

These drugs have good activity against penicillin-susceptible strains of *S. aureus*, streptococci, *H. influenzae*, *Neisseria meningitidis*, and *L. monocytogenes*. Penicillin- or ampicillin-resistant strains of these bacteria, however, are also resistant to these agents. In contrast to carbenicillin and ticarcillin, acylampicillins are active against enterococci. Activity against many anaerobes, such as *Bacteroides fragilis, Bacteroides melaninogenicus*, and *Clostridium perfringens*, is good.

When aminoglycosides are combined with any of

TABLE 35–7
Important Characteristics of Extended-Spectrum Penicillins

CHARACTERISTIC	EXTENDED-SPECTRUM PENICILLIN				
	Carbenicillin	Ticarcillin	Azlocillin	Mezlocillin	Piperacillin
Antibacterial Activity					
Gram-positive cocci					
Streptococci	+ +	+ +	+ +	+ +	+ +
Enterococci	–	–	+ +	+ +	+ +
Staphylococcus aureus[a]	–	–	–	–	–
Gram-negative bacilli					
Coliforms	+ +	+ +	+ +	+ +	+ +
Klebsiella sp.	–	–	+	+ +	+ +
Pseudomonas aeruginosa	+	+	+ +	+	+ +
Anaerobes					
Bacteroides fragilis	+	+	+	+ +	+ +
Body Clearance					
Renal	+ +	+ +	+	+	+
Hepatic	–	–	+	+	+
Sodium Content (mEq/g)	4.7	5.1	2.2	1.9	1.9

[a]Penicillin-resistant strains.
+ + = good; + = moderate; – = poor.

these three agents, in vitro synergistic activity against *P. aeruginosa*, coliforms, and susceptible *S. aureus* strains can be demonstrated.[199, 200] Both synergistic and antagonistic interactions have been observed when these penicillins were combined with various cephalosporins.[200–202] Antagonism may be related to the ability of certain cephalosporins to induce β-lactamase production, which, in turn, inactivates the penicillins.[200]

Pharmacokinetic Data

Mezlocillin. The pharmacokinetic behavior of mezlocillin has been studied in more than 150 premature and full-term infants.[203–206] Peak serum concentrations after 75 mg/kg intravenous doses occur at the end of drug infusion and range from a mean of about 260 μg/ml for newborns in the first week of life to 139 μg/ml for older neonates.[206] After intramuscular administration of an identical dose, peak concentrations were observed 30 minutes after the injection and ranged from a mean of 155 μg/ml for infants 1 week of age or younger to 121 μg/ml for those older than 7 days. No drug accumulation is observed after multiple doses of mezlocillin are administered.[205, 206] Plasma clearance of this drug increases with advancing gestational and postnatal ages. The half-life of mezlocillin is inversely related to gestational and postnatal ages. It decreases from about 4.5 hours in premature infants aged 1 week or younger to about 1.6 hours in full-term neonates older than 7 days.[206]

Available information on the CSF penetration of mezlocillin in newborns is limited. In one study, concentrations of from 20 to 90 μg/ml were measured at varying intervals after 75-mg/kg intravenous doses.[207] In another study, however, values of from 0 to 13.7 μg/ml (mean, 5.5 μg/ml) were found in nine neonates 1 to 3 hours after 100-mg/kg mezlocillin doses were intravenously injected.[208]

The mechanisms of mezlocillin elimination have not been studied in newborns. Renal excretion is the principal route of elimination in adults. Up to 30% of a mezlocillin dose, however, may be excreted in bile.[209]

Azlocillin. After a 50-mg/kg intravenous dose of azlocillin, concentrations of about 200 μg/ml are obtained at the end of drug infusion. Concentrations 1 and 5 hours after the dose are approximately 100 and 50 μg/ml, respectively.[203, 210, 211] The elimination half-life is about 2.5 hours. Most of the azlocillin dose is excreted unchanged in the urine. Biliary excretion accounts for only 5% of the dose.

Piperacillin. The mean peak serum concentration of piperacillin after an intravenous dose of 100 mg/kg is about 180 μg/ml, and it may be as high as 250 μg/ml in newborns with impaired renal function.[212] The half-life is prolonged and varies from 3.5 to 14 hours (median, 6.5 hours). In contrast, the reported half-life of piperacillin for infants 1 to 6 months of age is about 47 minutes.[213] Repeated administration of this drug does not result in its accumulation in serum. In one study,[214] a 75-mg/kg intravenous dose of piperacillin given to 28 neonates with gestational ages of 29 to 40 weeks and birth weights of 860 to 3900 g resulted in peak and trough serum concentrations ranging from 70 to 360 μg/ml and 5 to 34 μg/ml, respectively (see Table 35–6). The mean half-life values ranged from 1.7 to 4.3 hours and were inversely related to gestational and postnatal ages and birth weights.[214]

CSF piperacillin concentrations of from 2.6 to 6 μg/ml were measured in three neonates without meningitis within 7 hours of the intravenous administration of a 100-mg/kg dose.[212] In one infant with *Pseudomonas* meningitis, piperacillin achieved a concentration of 19 μg/ml in the CSF 2.5 hours after a 200-mg/kg intravenous dose was given.[212]

The major route of piperacillin excretion is the kidney. Up to 30 to 40% of the dose, however, may be eliminated by nonrenal mechanisms in children.[213, 215]

Safety

Adverse reactions from parenteral administration of mezlocillin, azlocillin, or piperacillin are rare in newborns. Hypersensitivity reactions, diarrhea, neutropenia, eosinophilia, and elevated serum concentrations of hepatic enzymes are infrequent compared with transient complications encountered in older children and adults treated with these drugs.[199] Impaired hemostasis secondary to platelet dysfunction occurs less frequently with these antibiotics than with carbenicillin and ticarcillin.[216] The sodium content of these drugs is less than half of that in carbenicillin or ticarcillin (see Table 35–7), which may be important in some newborns with cardiac or renal disease.

Clinical Implications

Mezlocillin and piperacillin, either alone or combined with aminoglycosides, have successfully been used for the treatment of bacteriologically proven neonatal infections. There is limited experience, however, using these agents routinely for the initial therapy of newborns with suspected sepsis. Accordingly, these agents should be reserved for situations in which a clear benefit can be derived from their use. Potential recipients include newborns with *P. aeruginosa* sepsis or meningitis, infants in whom sodium restriction is necessary, and neonates with bleeding problems in whom it would be desirable to minimize antibiotic-associated hemostatic impairment.

The dosage schedule for mezlocillin is 75 mg/kg given every 12 hours during the first week of life and every 8 hours thereafter. The proper dosage schedule for piperacillin for newborns has not been established. One study suggested that piperacillin doses of 100 mg/kg every 12 hours may be appropriate and that a dose of 200 mg/kg every 12 hours should be used for meningitis.[212] In a more complete pharmacokinetic study,[214] a dosage schedule of 75 mg/kg given every 12 and 8 hours for infants with gestational ages of less than 36 weeks and postnatal ages of 0 to 7 days and older than 1 week of age, respectively, was recommended. For full-term infants (>36 weeks' gestation), a 75-mg/kg dose given every 8 hours during the first week of life and every 6 hours thereafter was recommended. Additional data are required before a dosage schedule can be suggested for azlocillin.

CEPHALOSPORINS

All cephalosporins are semisynthetic derivatives of a 7-aminocephalosporanic acid nucleus. The individual derivatives differ chemically by the addition of various side chains. Cefoxitin and moxalactam are technically not cephalosporins[217] but are generally included in discussions of these antibiotics because of their close similarities to members of this group of drugs. Moxalactam is no longer available because of the potential for bleeding resulting from interference in prothrombin synthesis. It was ineffective against group B streptococci, limiting its usefulness in neonates. The cephalosporins exert their antibacterial action in a manner similar to that described earlier for penicillin.

It has become customary, albeit confusing at times, to group cephalosporins into generations of agents on the basis of their antibacterial spectrum of activity (see subsequent discussion) rather than their time of introduction for clinical use.[218] First-generation cephalosporins include cefazolin, cephalothin, cephalexin, and cefadroxil. Among the second-generation agents are cefaclor, cefprozil, cefamandole, cefuroxime, loracarbef, and cefoxitin. The most useful agents for the treatment of neonatal infections belong to the third-generation cephalosporins, which include cefoperazone, cefotaxime, ceftizoxime, ceftriaxone, and ceftazidime. Oral third-generation compounds include cefixime, cefpodoxime, ceftibuten, cefdinir, and cefetamet. A fourth-generation cephalosporin cefepime is still undergoing clinical evaluation in infants and children, and very limited information is available in the neonatal age. Cefepime has been shown to be effective for therapy for meningitis in children and should be useful for treatment of multiresistant gram-negative bacillary infections in pediatric patients. Cefpirome has not been studied in infants. The characteristics of many of the just-mentioned cephalosporins, particularly the oral agents, are not discussed because of the lack of neonatal studies evaluating these agents.

Antimicrobial Activity

The first-generation cephalosporins have good activity against gram-positive organisms but limited activity against gram-negative bacteria. Susceptible pathogens include streptococci, penicillin-susceptible and penicillin-resistant staphylococci, and penicillin-susceptible pneumococci. Enterococci, methicillin-resistant staphylococci, and *L. monocytogenes* are resistant to these agents. Although the activity against coliforms is usually good, other antibiotics are usually preferred for treatment of infections caused by these organisms. *Pseudomonas* species, *S. marcescens*, *Enterobacter* species, indole-positive *Proteus* species, and *B. fragilis* are all resistant to these antibacterial agents.[217]

Because of their improved stability to hydrolysis by β lactamases, the second-generation cephalosporins have increased activity against many gram-negative bacteria compared with that of first-generation antibiotics. Cefamandole has in vitro activity against gram-positive cocci comparable with that of cephalothin and is also active against *H. influenzae, Enterobacter cloacae, Klebsiella, E. coli,* and *Citrobacter.* Cefuroxime is more active than cephalothin against group B streptococci, pneumococci, and gram-negative enteric bacilli and is also active against *H. influenzae,* meningococci, gonococci, and staphylococci.[219] Cefoxitin has considerably less activity against gram-positive cocci compared with the first-generation cephalosporins, but its spectrum of activity against gram-negative enteric bacilli is at least as good as that of cefamandole. In addition, cefoxitin has excellent in vitro activity against *B. fragilis* and other anaerobes.[218] Cefaclor, an oral cephalosporin, has a spectrum of activity similar to that of cefamandole.[217] The second-generation agents have very poor activity against *P. aeruginosa,* enterococci, and *L. monocytogenes.*

The third-generation cephalosporins have excellent in vitro activity against *H. influenzae,* gonococci, meningococci, and many gram-negative enteric bacilli.[218] Ceftazidime and cefoperazone, however, are the only ones with adequate anti-*Pseudomonas* activity. Susceptibility of gram-positive organisms to these agents is variable but is generally lower than that to either first- or second-generation antibiotics. *L. monocytogenes* and enterococci are uniformly resistant to these agents.

The fourth-generation cephalosporins encompass activity against gram-positive and gram-negative bacterial pathogens and circumvent the development of resistance to other broad-spectrum cephalosporins that occurs with *Pseudomonas aeruginosa.* There is also evidence indicating that isolates of ceftazidime- and cefotaxime-resistant *Enterobacter* species are susceptible to cefepime.[220] Resistant organisms include enterococci, *L. monocytogenes,* methicillin-resistant *S. aureus* and *S. epidermidis,* and anaerobes.

There are several mechanisms of resistance to the cephalosporins. Cephalothin and cefazolin can be inactivated through enzymatic hydrolysis by β lactamases.[221] Exposure of some gram-negative bacteria, such as *P. aeruginosa* or *E. cloacae,* to second- or third-generation agents can induce the production of chromosomally mediated potent β lactamases by these bacteria that can hydrolyze even the β-lactamase–stable cephalosporins.[221] Several plasmid-mediated β lactamases have been shown to play a role in the resistance of certain gram-negative enteric bacilli to third-generation cephalosporins.[222] Other mechanisms of resistance include alterations in the permeability of the outer membranes of gram-negative bacteria to these drugs that limit their ability to reach the PBP target sites. Mutations leading to functional or quantitative changes in PBPs are an additional method by which bacteria can resist the antimicrobial action of these drugs.[221, 222]

Pharmacokinetic Data

Cephalothin. The intramuscular administration of a 10-mg/kg dose of cephalothin to full-term newborns in the first 4 days of life results in a 1-hour mean serum concentration of 12.4 μg/ml.[167] A 20-mg/kg dose given to a similar group of neonates produced mean concentrations of 47, 39, 10, and 2 µg/ml at 0.5, 1, 4, and 8 hours, respectively, after the injection.[167] In another study, premature newborns given 12.5-mg/kg intramuscular doses achieved concentrations of 22, 12, 2.4, and 0.5 µg/ml at 0.5, 2, 6, and 12 hours, respectively, after the injection, and these values were noted to be slightly lower than those for full-term newborns receiving an identical dose.[223]

After the intravenous infusion of 20 mg/kg of cephalothin to six newborns 3 to 21 days of age, serum concentrations of 61, 35, 7, and 2 µg/ml were detected 0.25, 1, 4, and 8 hours, respectively, after the end of the infusion.[224] The mean half-life was about 1.5 hours. The continuous intravenous infusion of 40 mg/kg per day of cephalothin produces serum values of from 24 to 35 µg/ml in premature infants and lower concentrations of from 7 to 22 µg/ml in full-term neonates. Increasing the dose to 80 mg/kg per day resulted in serum concentrations of from 50 to 120 µg/ml in the premature infants and from 32 to 50 µg/ml for those born at term.[225]

Cephalothin does not penetrate into the CSF to any appreciable extent even in the presence of meningeal inflammation. The drug is metabolized in the body to deacetylcephalothin, which is only 20% as active as cephalothin.[226] Both cephalothin and its metabolite are excreted in the urine primarily by tubular secretion. Approximately 60% of the cephalothin dose can be recovered in the urine within 8 hours of drug administration.[224]

Cefazolin. The intramuscular administration of 20 and 25 mg/kg doses of cefazolin produce serum concentrations of from 30 to 35 µg/ml and from 55 to 65 µg/ml, respectively, 1 hour after the dose. The concentrations at 12 hours drop to 2 to 3 µg/ml and to 13 to 18 µg/ml, respectively.[227] Intravenous doses of 25 mg/kg administered to six premature infants 2 to 12 days of age resulted in mean serum concentrations of 92, 79, 48, and 12 µg/ml 0.5, 1, 4, and 12 hours, respectively, after the end of the infusion.[224] The serum half-life of cefazolin decreases from 4.5 to 5 hours in the first week of life to approximately 3 hours by 3 to 4 weeks of age.

CSF penetration of cefazolin is poor. The drug is excreted in the urine in unchanged form.[226] About 45% of the dose can be recovered in the urine within 12 hours,[224] and 80 to 100% is recovered within 24 hours of administration.[226, 227]

Cephalexin. A 15-mg/kg oral dose of cephalexin given to newborns on their first day of life produces a mean peak serum concentration of about 10 µg/ml 4 hours after drug ingestion.[228] Increasing the dose to 50 mg/kg provides a mean peak serum value of about 29 µg/ml (range, 23 to 44 µg/ml) 2 hours after the dose. From 18 to 66% (mean, 39%) of the total dose is excreted in the urine over a 24-hour period.[228]

Cefaclor. Data on the pharmacokinetics of cefaclor in newborns are limited. After a single oral dose of 7.5 mg/kg given to 10 full-term neonates, peak serum concentrations of from 0.7 to 19 µg/ml (mean, 7.7 µg/ml) were observed 1 hour after drug ingestion.[229] The mean serum concentrations at 6 hours dropped to 3.5 µg/ml. A study

performed in infants and children revealed that peak serum value of from 3 to 22 µg/ml (means, 11 and 13 µg/ml, respectively) are observed 30 minutes after 15-mg/kg doses and that bioavailability is not affected by co-administration of drug and milk.[230]

Cefuroxime. After the administration of 10-mg/kg intramuscular doses, peak serum concentrations ranged between 15 and 25 µg/ml 30 minutes to 1 hour after the injection.[231] Serum values were inversely related to birth weight. Half-life times were from 3.6 to 5.6 hours. Repeated administration of the drug did not result in serum accumulation. About 70% of the daily cefuroxime dose could be recovered in the urine in a 24-hour period. Intramuscular doses of 25 mg/kg given to neonates weighing less than 2.5 kg during their first week of life produced mean serum concentrations of 49, 30, and 15 µg/ml 2, 4, and 8 hours after the injection, respectively.[232] For newborns weighing more than 2.5 kg, the corresponding values were lower (34, 21, and 9 µg/ml, respectively). Median serum concentrations of cefuroxime measured on the third or fourth day of therapy with 25-mg/kg intramuscular injections given every 12 hours to a group of premature and full-term infants were 45, 42, 26, and 11 µg/ml 0.5, 1, 5, and 12 hours, respectively.[233] The half-life values were from 2 to 11 hours (mean, 6 hours).

CSF cefuroxime concentrations of from 2.3 to 5.3 µg/ml were measured in three newborns with meningitis.[231] These values represented 12 to 25% of the corresponding serum concentrations. In three other neonates without meningeal inflammation, concentrations were lower and ranged from 0.4 to 1.5 µg/ml. In a brief publication, CSF cefuroxime concentration of 20 µg/ml was found after the third dose of the drug in one patient and concentrations of 50 and 47 µg/ml were detected 2.5 and 3 hours, respectively, after an intravenous dose in a second infant with hydrocephalus.[234]

Cefotaxime. Several investigators have evaluated the pharmacokinetic properties of cefotaxime in newborns.[235–240] A 25-mg/kg intravenous dose produces concentrations of from 60 to 80 µg/ml immediately after the end of drug infusion, which decreases to 35 to 50 µg/ml 30 minutes later.[236, 239] Serum cefotaxime concentrations are higher in premature newborns and in those younger than 1 week of age. The administration of a 50-mg/kg intravenous dose during the first week of life results in peak serum concentrations of 116 µg/ml (range, 46 to 186 µg/ml) in low-birth-weight infants compared with 133 µg/ml (range, 76 to 208 µg/ml) in term neonates (Table 35–8).[237] Values decline thereafter to about 34 to 38 µg/ml 6 hours after the dose. The mean half-life is 4.6 hours for low-birth-weight neonates and 3.4 hours for larger newborns.[237] When cefotaxime was administered intramuscularly at a dose of 50 mg/kg, a mean peak value of 93 µg/ml was measured 30 minutes after the injection.[238] The apparent discrepancy between the peak concentrations obtained after intravenous and intramuscular identical doses of cefotaxime is related to differences in the antibiotic assays employed. The former study[237] used a bioassay technique that measures the total concentration of both cefotaxime and its biologically active metabolite desacetyl cefotaxime, whereas the

TABLE 35–8
Pharmacokinetics of Selected Third-Generation Cephalosporins in Neonates

ANTIBIOTIC[a]	BIRTH WEIGHT OR GESTATIONAL AGE/AGE GROUP	MEAN PEAK SERUM CONCENTRATION (μg/ml)	MEAN SERUM HALF-LIFE (hr)	MEAN PLASMA CLEARANCE (ml/min per 1.73 m²)
Cefotaxime	<2000 g/0–7 days	116	4.6	23
	2000 g/0–7 days	133	3.4	44
Ceftriaxone	<1500 g/1–4 days	145	7.7[b]	17
	<1500 g/6–8 days	136	8.4	14
	1500 g/2–4 days	158	7.4	17
	1500 g/5–45 days	173	5.2	20
Cefoperazone	<33 wk/1–2 days	159	8.9	—
	33–36 wk/1–2 days	110	7.6	—
	>36 wk/1–2 days	109	7.2	—
Ceftazidime	32 wk	111	6.7	52
	33–37 wk	118	4.9	66
	38 wk	102	4.2	74

[a]Dosage of 50 mg/kg given intravenously.
[b]Longer serum half-life values (mean, 19 hr) have been reported by others.[14]

latter study[238] used a high-pressure liquid chromatography method that provides separate measurements of both compounds.

Cefotaxime is rapidly metabolized in the body to desacetyl cefotaxime through the action of esterases found in the liver, erythrocytes, and other tissues.[241] This metabolite is biologically active, but its antibacterial activity is generally lower than that of cefotaxime. Synergistic interactions against many organisms can be demonstrated when these two compounds are combined in vitro.[242] Desacetyl cefotaxime accounts for 15 to 45% of the peak and for 45 to 70% of the trough concentrations of total cefotaxime.[237–239]

Both cefotaxime and its metabolite penetrate well into the CSF of infants with meningitis.[236, 243, 244] Concentrations of from 7.1 to 30 μg/ml were detected 1 to 2 hours after a 50-mg/kg intravenous dose and represented 27 to 63% of simultaneously measured serum values. CSF concentrations as high as 20 μg/ml in neonates with or without meningitis have been reported.[243] Some investigators[244, 245] have noted that desacetyl cefotaxime achieves higher CSF concentrations and greater penetration than does cefotaxime. This suggests that the metabolite is either more capable of crossing the meninges than the parent compound or is cleared more slowly once it reaches the CSF.

About 80% of the cefotaxime dose is excreted in the urine. Only a third of the drug is eliminated in unchanged form.[241] Urine cefotaxime concentrations of from 300 to 1575 μg/ml have been measured in randomly collected urine specimens from neonates treated with this drug.[237]

Ceftriaxone. The administration of a 50-mg/kg intravenous dose of ceftriaxone to newborns of various birth weights and postnatal ages resulted in mean peak serum concentrations of from 136 to 173 μg/ml (see Table 35–8).[246] Concentrations 6 hours later were from 66 to 74 μg/ml. The mean plasma half-life values were longer in those weighing less than 1500 g. Repeated drug administration at 12-hour intervals resulted in drug accumulation in the serum.

Subsequent pharmacokinetic studies of ceftriaxone during the neonatal period have suggested that the drug's plasma half-life is actually longer than initially estimated.[14, 247–250] Elimination half-life ranged from 8 to 34 hours (mean, 19 hours) in 20 sick neonates receiving single 50-mg/kg intravenous doses of ceftriaxone.[14] In another study, neonates treated with single daily intravenous or intramuscular 50-mg/kg doses had mean peak serum concentrations after the first dose of about 149 μg/ml and the mean elimination half-life was 15.5 hours.[247, 248] After 3 or 4 days of treatment, however, both the mean peak serum concentration and elimination half-life decreased to 141 μg/ml and 9.4 hours, respectively. The observed decrease was believed to be a result of increasing postnatal age, which was associated with increased plasma clearance of ceftriaxone.

Intravenous administration of 50- to 144-mg/kg doses to neonates and infants with bacterial meningitis resulted in mean CSF concentrations of 18.3, 8.5, and 2.8 μg/ml 4, 12, and 24 hours after drug injection, respectively.[249] Penetration of ceftriaxone into the CSF was higher for patients with bacterial meningitis (17%) compared with that observed for infants with aseptic meningitis (4.1%). Smaller CSF penetration of ceftriaxone (2 to 7%) has been reported for older infants and children with bacterial meningitis.[251, 252]

About 70% of a ceftriaxone dose is excreted in unchanged form in the urine.[14] The remainder is cleared from the body by hepatic mechanisms.

Cefoperazone. Serum cefoperazone concentrations ranged from 109 to 159 μg/ml 30 minutes after an intravenous infusion of a 50-mg/kg dose given to 28 newborns of various gestational ages (see Table 35–8).[253] Values declined thereafter and were from 34 to 48 μg/ml and from 13 to 17 μg/ml by 12 and 24 hours after the dose, respectively.[254, 255] The serum half-life decreases with increasing birth weight, gestational age, or postnatal age.[163, 240, 253–255]

CSF concentrations of from 2.8 to 9 μg/ml were measured 1 to 4 hours after a 50-mg/kg intravenous dose given to three neonates with group B streptococcal meningitis. These values represented from 4.2 to 9% of the simultaneously obtained serum concentration. A fourth infant, with *E. coli* meningitis, had a CSF concentration of 9.5 μg/ml after 18 hours of drug administration.[253] Concentrations of from less than 1 to 7 μg/ml were detected at 2 to 4 hours in three neonates without meningitis. Other investigators have estimated the CSF penetration to be 3 to 5% in infants with meningitis.[163]

Hepatic clearance mechanisms play a major role in the elimination of cefoperazone from the body. At least 70% of the administered dose undergoes biliary excretion in adults.[63] Newborns excrete a greater proportion of the drug in their urine because of reduced hepatic function in this age group. About a third of a cefoperazone dose (range, 24 to 55%) can be recovered in the urine of neonates with a gestational age of 33 weeks or greater during their first 2 days of life. In contrast, more premature infants excrete about 55% (range, 28 to 93%) of the dose in their urine. By 5 to 7 days of age, the former group of infants will eliminate only a fourth of the dose (range, 7 to 35%) in the urine, whereas urinary recovery of the drug will not change appreciably in the latter group.[253]

Ceftazidime. Numerous reports on the pharmacokinetics of ceftazidime in neonates have been published in the last decade.[6, 240, 256–265] Peak serum concentrations of from 35 to 269 μg/ml (mean, 77 μg/ml) have been observed after intravenous administration of 25- to 30-mg/kg doses of ceftazidime to newborns of various gestational ages during their first week of life.[258, 261] Mean trough values measured 9 to 12 hours after the dose are from 15 to 19 μg/ml.[260–264] These concentrations are higher than those detected in older infants receiving identical ceftazidime dosages. When the dose is increased to 50 mg/kg intravenously, mean peak serum concentrations of from 102 to 118 μg/ml are obtained (see Table 35–8).[6, 259] Mean trough values 8 hours after the dose are from 29 to 41 μg/ml. The mean elimination half-life is inversely related to gestational age and varies from 4.2 to 6.7 hours. The peak serum concentrations after the intramuscular administration of 50 mg/kg of ceftazidime are lower (mean, 67 μg/ml) than those observed with intravenous infusion of the drug and are achieved 1 to 2 hours after the injection.[6, 263] Neonatal exposure to indomethacin or to asphyxia decreases glomerular filtration rate and clearance of ceftazidime.

Ceftazidime penetrates well into the CSF, especially when meningitis is present.[262, 266] Concentrations of from 1.8 to 7.9 μg/ml, corresponding to 6 to 46% of a simultaneous serum concentration, are obtained 2 to 7 hours after a 50-mg/kg dose of ceftazidime is given to infants with bacterial meningitis.[266] The extent of penetration is lower in patients with aseptic meningitis and relatively poor in those with uninflamed meninges.[262, 267]

Seventy to 90% of a ceftazidime dose is eliminated in unchanged form via the kidneys. Urinary ceftazidime concentrations of from 192 to 6028 μg/ml have been measured in specimens collected during a 12-hour period after drug administration.[261]

Safety

In general, cephalosporins are well tolerated by neonates. Adverse reactions that have been observed, mostly in older patients, include hypersensitivity reactions, diarrhea, thrombophlebitis, pain on intramuscular injection, eosinophilia, leukopenia, granulocytopenia, and seizures related to the administration of massive doses of these drugs.[268, 269] Falsely elevated serum creatinine concentrations have been observed in patients receiving cefoxitin or cephalothin. Alterations of the bowel bacterial flora are most pronounced with the third-generation agents, especially ceftriaxone and cefoperazone, and can lead to intestinal colonization by resistant organisms such as *Candida*, *Pseudomonas*, *Enterobacter*, or *Enterococcus* species. Subsequent superinfections by these drug-resistant pathogens have been described in neonates.[269, 270] Another potential adverse effect related to disruption of bacterial intestinal flora by potent cephalosporins is the induction of antibiotic-associated colitis, presumably caused by overgrowth of toxin-producing *Clostridium difficile* strains.

Bleeding disorders occurring with the use of cephalosporins have been well documented, mostly in adults. Immune-mediated platelet destruction with resultant thrombocytopenia is very rare but has been associated with the administration of cephalothin, cefazolin, cefamandole, cefaclor, and cefoxitin to older patients.[271] A second rare mechanism involves the development of antibodies, usually IgG, against certain clotting factors such as factor V or VIII. Hemostatic abnormalities associated with the use of cephalosporins can be mediated by several mechanisms. Platelet dysfunction can be observed after several days of therapy with any of the cephalosporins. These drugs may inhibit adenosine diphosphate–induced platelet aggregation with resultant prolongation of the bleeding time. The effect is slowly reversible after discontinuation of the drug.[216] A second mechanism is defective fibrinogen to fibrin conversion, which has been observed with drugs such as cefazolin and cefamandole. This phenomenon has been observed mostly in patients with renal failure who have very high serum antibiotic concentrations.[216, 271] The third and most important mechanism is interference with the production of vitamin K–dependent clotting factors (II, VII, IX, and X) with resultant hypoprothrombinemia.[216] This is most commonly observed with moxalactam and cefamandole therapy and is rare with cefotaxime and ceftriaxone. This effect is believed to be related to, but not necessarily caused by, the presence of the *N*-methylthiotetrazole side chain in cephalosporins such as moxalactam, cefamandole, and cefoperazone. This side chain appears to be capable of interfering with hepatic vitamin K metabolism. In patients with inadequate dietary intake, inhibition of colonic bacteria such as *E. coli* or *Bacteroides*, which are capable of vitamin K production, may lead to hypoprothrombinemia secondary to vitamin

K deficiency. This side effect is usually avoidable or reversible by the administration of supplemental vitamin K. An immune-mediated severe hemolytic reaction to ceftriaxone has been described in children and adults. Because ceftriaxone has a high avidity for protein binding, there is a theoretical concern that its use in the neonatal period can be associated with a significant displacement of bilirubin from albumin-binding sites, thereby inducing a hyperbilirubinemia. Ceftriaxone, when given to neonates in the first days of life, has been associated with an immediate and prolonged decrease in the reserve-albumin concentration, which could potentially predispose a vulnerable infant to bilirubin encephalopathy.

Clinical Implications

The usefulness of first-generation cephalosporins for therapy for neonatal bacterial infections is limited. Their activity against gram-negative bacteria is narrow and unpredictable, and their penetration into the CSF is relatively poor. These drugs are not indicated as initial therapy for suggested neonatal bacterial infections. If used in patients whose bacterial isolates are susceptible in vitro and in whom meningitis has been conclusively ruled out, the recommended dosage schedule for cephalothin is 20 mg/kg intravenously every 12 hours for newborns weighing less than 2000 g in the first week of life and every 8 hours for older infants. For infants weighing more than 2000 g, the dose is given every 8 hours in the first week of life and every 6 hours thereafter. Cefazolin can be given in a similar dosage schedule to that of cephalothin, except that a 6-hour schedule is not recommended. These first-generation agents can also be used for therapy for methicillin-susceptible *S. aureus* infections that do not involve the central nervous system.

Although second-generation cephalosporins have been successfully used to treat neonatal infections caused by susceptible bacteria, these antibiotics are not recommended for routine use because of limited experience in newborns and because of their inferior activity to that of third-generation agents against gram-negative bacteria. Cefaclor has been successfully used, however, for oral therapy for acute suppurative otitis media in infants younger than 6 weeks of age because middle ear disease in the first weeks of life is caused by a broad array of pathogens, including *S. pneumoniae* and *H. influenzae* and occasionally coliform organisms and staphylococci.[174] The drug is well tolerated in a dosage of 15 mg/kg given three times daily for 10 days. With the advent of multidrug resistant pneumococci, other antibiotics, such as amoxicillin-clavulanate, are preferred for treatment of neonatal otitis media.

As a group, third-generation cephalosporins are the most useful agents for the treatment of suspected or proven bacterial infections in newborns. Their advantages include excellent in vitro activity against the major pathogens for newborns, including aminoglycoside-resistant gram-negative bacilli, adequate CSF penetration with resultant high bactericidal activity in CSF of infants with meningitis and a proven record of safety and tolera-

bility.[272] Indications for use of individual agents vary in accordance with their pharmacologic properties.

The clinical efficacy and safety of cefotaxime in the treatment of neonatal infections have been well documented in several studies.[236, 270, 273, 274] Cefotaxime should not be used alone as initial therapy for suspected sepsis because of its poor activity against *L. monocytogenes* and enterococci. The addition of ampicillin provides antibacterial coverage against these organisms. One potential problem associated with the routine use of this drug is the possible emergence of cefotaxime-resistant gram-negative bacteria in the nursery.[270] Some nurseries, however, have not documented this problem even after 2 years of continuous use of this antibiotic.[273] Cefotaxime achieves CSF concentrations that are 50- to several-hundred-fold greater than the MIC_{90} of susceptible gram-negative enteric bacilli or group B streptococci isolated from newborns with meningitis and has been shown to be effective for the treatment of neonatal meningitis caused by susceptible bacteria.[275] The dosage of cefotaxime in newborns is 50 mg/kg given every 12 hours during the first week of life and every 8 hours thereafter. In full-term infants older than 3 weeks, a 6-hour regimen can be used for treatment of meningitis.

Although ceftriaxone has been used successfully for the treatment of severe neonatal infections,[247, 249] the limited experience with this antibiotic in newborns and concerns about its in vitro displacing ability of albumin-binding sites for bilirubin have limited the use of this antibiotic in the neonatal period. The most attractive features of ceftriaxone are its long serum half-life, which allows for a single daily administration, and its excellent bactericidal activity in the CSF against susceptible bacteria. The ceftriaxone dosage is 50 mg/kg once daily for all newborns except those older than 1 week of age who weigh more than 2000 g, in whom the dose is increased to 75 mg/kg once daily. In a Mexican study,[276] ceftriaxone (dosage, 100 mg/kg once daily) was administered to 27 premature and term newborns with bacteriologically proven sepsis and was found to be effective and safe, even when given to jaundiced infants. More studies are needed, however, before ceftriaxone can be recommended for routine therapy of neonatal sepsis.

Ceftazidime has been used alone as initial therapy for newborns with suspected sepsis.[262, 264, 265, 277] One study[278] compared the use of ceftazidime alone with a combination of carbenicillin and amikacin for the treatment of newborns with proven bacterial infections. It was found that all gram-negative enteric isolates were susceptible to ceftazidime, whereas 10 and 56% of these strains were resistant to amikacin and carbenicillin, respectively. Accordingly, failure rates were lower for the ceftazidime-treated group. Increased colonization and superinfection by resistant organisms such as enterococci and *C. albicans* have been encountered in ceftazidime-treated patients.[265, 278] We do not recommend using ceftazidime alone as initial therapy for suspected neonatal sepsis because this antibiotic is not active against enterococci and *L. monocytogenes* and because of the possibility for emergence of cephalosporin-resistant gram-negative organisms. In addition, several treatment failures have occurred when the offending organism proved to be a gram-positive bacteria.[262] We believe that it is preferable to reserve the use of ceftazidime for situations in which gram-negative bacteria, notably *P. aeruginosa*, have been isolated or strongly suspected of being the causative microorganisms in neonates with sepsis, meningitis, or other invasive infections. The dosage schedule is 100 mg/kg per day in two (birth weight <2000 g) or three (birth weight 2000 g) divided doses during the first week of life and 150 mg/kg per day in three divided doses for older neonates.

Experience with cefoperazone and the fourth-generation cephalosporin cefepime in neonatal infections is too limited to allow us to recommend their use in this age group or to suggest an appropriate dosage schedule.

AZTREONAM

Aztreonam is the first synthetic monocyclic β-lactam (monobactam) antibiotic approved for use in clinical medicine. Its aminoglycoside-like activity, good CSF penetration, and absence of nephrotoxic or ototoxic side effects make aztreonam potentially useful when combined with ampicillin for the initial empirical therapy for newborns with suspected sepsis.

Antimicrobial Activity

Aztreonam has good activity against a broad spectrum of aerobic gram-negative bacteria, but its activity against gram-positive or anaerobic organisms is poor.[279] The majority of Enterobacteriaceae, notably *E. coli, K. pneumoniae*, and *Citrobacter* species, are inhibited by less than 1 μg/ml of aztreonam.[279, 280] *Serratia* and *Enterobacter* are less susceptible (MIC_{90}, 1 to 4 μg/ml), whereas *H. influenzae* and *N. gonorrhoeae* are more susceptible (MIC_{90}, ≤0.2 μg/ml). *P. aeruginosa* requires MICs in the range of 8 to 12 μg/ml of aztreonam to be inhibited.[279–282]

Like other β lactams, aztreonam exerts its antimicrobial activity by interfering with bacterial cell wall synthesis by binding to PBPs, especially PBP-3 of aerobic gram-negative bacteria. This drug is stable to hydrolysis by chromosomal or plasmid-mediated β lactamases of Enterobacteriaceae and does not induce chromosomal β-lactamase production.

Pharmacokinetic Data

Mean peak serum concentrations of 83 and 98 μg/ml were found when a 30-mg/kg dose of aztreonam was given intravenously to 6 low-birth-weight infants younger than 1 week of age and to 11 larger and older neonates, respectively.[281] The serum half-lives were from 2.4 to 5.7 hours and were longest for premature infants during the first week of life. In contrast, the mean half-life was 1.7 hours for patients older than 1 month but younger than 12 years of age.

In another study, a 30-mg/kg intravenous dose of aztreonam administered to 26 infants weighing less than 2000 g during their first week of life resulted in mean peak serum concentrations of from 65 to 79 μg/ml after the first dose and from 77 to 83 μg/ml after 3 to 6 days of therapy.[282] Trough values ranged between 8.2 and 70.7 μg/ml. The mean serum half-life values on the first day of treatment were about 7, 10, and 6.4 hours for infants weighing 500 to 1001 g, 1001 to 1500 g, and 1501 to 2000 g, respectively, but decreased from 5.5 to 7.6 hours 3 to 6 days later. The mean plasma clearance increased from a range of 0.61 to 0.84 ml/minute per kg after the initial dose to a range of 0.96 to 1.13 ml/minute per kg after multiple doses of aztreonam.

Aztreonam has good penetration into the CSF of newborns with bacterial meningitis.[283] Concentrations of 13.3 μg/ml were obtained after 1.3 hours of an aztreonam dose 1 day after the diagnosis of bacterial meningitis was made in a 7-day-old newborn. This represented 18.8% of a simultaneously measured serum concentration. In a second neonate with meningitis, a CSF concentration of 2.4 μg/ml was detected 45 minutes after the dose (3.1% of a concomitant serum value), but this was measured after 14 days of treatment, when meningeal inflammation was substantially reduced.[281]

Aztreonam is excreted primarily in unchanged form in the urine. Urinary concentrations of from 24 to 461 μg/ml (mean, 254 μg/ml) have been obtained in the first spontaneously voided urine specimens collected after the end of drug infusion.[282] About 80% of the total aztreonam dose can be recovered in the urine during a 24-hour period.[281]

Safety

Aztreonam is well tolerated with no apparent side effects when given intravenously to newborns. Adverse reactions described in adults include rashes, nausea, diarrhea, and eosinophilia, but their incidence is low.[279] The effects on bowel flora are limited to a reduction in coliforms without significant changes in anaerobic bacteria. Colonization by resistant bacteria as a result of aztreonam therapy does not appear to be as much of a problem as that encountered with the use of the third-generation cephalosporins. Because aztreonam contains 780 mg of arginine per gram of antibiotic, concern has been raised regarding possible adverse effects such as an arginine-induced hypoglycemia.[284] Arginine is rapidly metabolized via urea and ornithine, the latter being transformed to glucose, which can provoke a significant rise in blood glucose concentration. As a result of this transient hyperglycemia, insulin concentrations immediately rise with the subsequent induction of hypoglycemia. These fluctuation in blood glucose can be potentially important in premature infants exposed to a metabolic stress. A study addressing this safety issue indicated that aztreonam was well tolerated and safe in premature infants when a glucose solution (>5 mg/kg per minute) was concomitantly infused.[285]

Clinical Implications

Aztreonam is still considered an investigational drug for neonates and infants younger than 3 months of age. Data from a prospective, randomized study of 58 neonates with infections caused by gram-negative bacilli, including *P. aeruginosa*, suggest that the use of aztreonam in combination with ampicillin is equally efficacious as the standard ampicillin and amikacin regimen.[284] Individual aztreonam doses of 30 mg/kg given two to four times daily can achieve median peak serum bactericidal titers of about 1:16 and can maintain trough serum concentrations that exceed the MIC_{90} of most gram-negative bacteria.

CARBAPENEMS

Imipenem is the first of a new class of β-lactam antibiotics, the carbapenems, to be used clinically. Its spectrum of activity includes most aerobic and anaerobic gram-positive and gram-negative bacteria. Cilastatin has no intrinsic antimicrobial activity but is a potent inhibitor of dehydropeptidase-I, the renal tubular brush border enzyme that metabolizes imipenem. The co-administration of both drugs increases the urinary concentration of imipenem, prolongs the imipenem serum half-life, and appears to prevent the nephrotoxicity induced by high doses of imipenem. In clinical practice, these drugs are co-administered to patients in a 1:1 ratio.

Meropenem is a newer carbapenem with similar clinical indications to those of imipenem. It has been recently approved by the FDA for use in children older than 3 months of age based on extensive pediatric investigations across a wide range of infections, including meningitis.[286] Compared with imipenem, the carbapenem ring structure of meropenem includes an additional β-methyl group in the C-1 position, providing stability against the human renal tubular enzyme dehydropeptidase, which is active against imipenem. A second major difference between these two compounds is the long, substituted pyrrolidine side chain present in the C-2 position in meropenem, which allows greater activity against intracellular target sites in organisms such as *Pseudomonas aeruginosa*. Antimicrobial activity against the vast majority of bacterial agents is similar for both antibiotics.[287]

Antimicrobial Activity

Imipenem and meropenem have an exceptionally broad spectrum of activity. The only three bacterial species considered resistant to these drugs are *Stenotrophomonas maltophilia*, *Burkholderia cepacia*, and *Enterococcus faecium*, none of which are significant neonatal pathogens.[288] It has been estimated that approximately 98% of unselected bacterial pathogens isolated from humans are susceptible to carbapenems at concentrations of 8 μg/ml or less.[288, 289]

Most streptococci and staphylococci are susceptible to imipenem and meropenem. The range of MIC_{90} values reported in different studies is 0.016 to 0.12 μg/ml for group B streptococci, 0.015 to 0.13 μg/ml for penicillin-susceptible *S. pneumoniae*, 0.12 to 1.0 μg/ml for penicillin-resistant *S. pneumoniae*, 0.01 to 4 μg/ml for *S. epidermidis*, 0.008 to 0.25 μg/ml for methicillin-sensitive *S. aureus*, 0.1 to 50 μg/ml for methicillin-resistant *S. aureus*, and 2 to 12.5 μg/ml for enterococci.[288] Imipenem and meropenem are also very active against *L. monocyto-*

genes and gram-positive anaerobes such as *Clostridium*, *Peptococcus*, and *Peptostreptococcus* species.

The range of MIC_{90} values against gram-negative bacteria has varied from 0.125 to 2 μg/ml for *E. coli*, 0.04 to 1.6 μg/ml for *K. pneumoniae*, 0.5 to 32 μg/ml for *P. mirabilis*, 2 to 4 μg/ml for indole-positive *Proteus* species, 0.7 to 1 μg/ml for *Citrobacter* species, 0.5 to 8 μg/ml for *Enterobacter* species, and 0.6 to 4 μg/ml for *Serratia* species.[288] Against *P. aeruginosa*, including multiresistant strains, values of from 0.5 to 16 μg/ml have been reported by different investigators, with meropenem being consistently more active than imipenem. These inhibitory concentrations against *P. aeruginosa* are comparable to those of ceftazidime. Imipenem and meropenem are also extremely active against gram-negative anaerobes such as *Bacteroides* species.

Synergistic interactions between carbapenems and aminoglycosides can be demonstrated in vitro against *P. aeruginosa* and *S. aureus* isolates. Antagonistic interactions are usually observed when imipenem is combined with other β lactams, probably as a result of chromosomal β-lactamase induction by imipenem.[288]

Carbapenem's unusually broad antibacterial spectrum is related to its ability to penetrate efficiently the outer membrane of gram-negative bacteria, its high binding affinity to PBP-2, and its resistance to hydrolysis by both plasmid- and chromosomally mediated β lactamases.[289, 290] Some β lactamases produced by *S. maltophilia*, *Aeromonas hydrophila*, and *B. fragilis*, however, are capable of hydrolyzing imipenem and meropenem. Emergence of carbapenem-resistant strains during therapy with this drug is rare except for *P. aeruginosa*, where resistance occurs in as many as 17% of isolates.[285] The mechanism for this resistance is unclear.

Pharmacokinetic Data

Serum concentrations of both imipenem and cilastatin are directly proportional to the administered dose.[291, 292] Cilastatin achieves higher serum concentrations than those observed with identical doses of imipenem. The intravenous administration during 30 to 60 minutes of 10-, 15-, and 20-mg/kg doses of both drugs to neonates results in mean peak imipenem concentrations of 11, 21, and 32 μg/ml, respectively, compared with mean cilastatin values of 28, 37, and 57 μg/ml, respectively.[291] In another study,[292] peak serum concentrations of 27 and 55 μg/ml for imipenem and 37 to 69 μg/ml for cilastatin were detected after intravenous doses of 15 and 25 mg/kg, respectively. After 3 to 4 days of treatment with 20 mg/kg intravenous doses of imipenem-cilastatin every 12 hours, peak serum concentrations were 35 and 86 μg/ml for imipenem and cilastatin, respectively.

The mean serum half-life of imipenem is about 2 hours, whereas that of cilastatin is 5.1 to 6.4 hours.[291] The half-lives for both drugs are inversely related to birth weight and gestational age and are considerably longer than the 1-hour half-life reported for both drugs in older infants and in healthy adult volunteers.[291–294] The plasma clearance of cilastatin is only 20 to 30% of that of imipenem during the neonatal period.[291]

Although both imipenem and cilastatin penetrate well

into the CSF in the presence of meningeal inflammation,[295, 296] data derived from neonatal studies are scant. One newborn receiving a 15-mg/kg intravenous dose had concentrations of 1.1 and 0.8 μg/ml for imipenem and cilastatin, respectively, and a second neonate receiving a 25 mg/kg dose had CSF values of 5.6 and 1.8 μg/ml for the same drugs 1.5 hours after injection.[292] It was not stated whether either of these infants had meningitis at the time of drug administration.

Imipenem is normally hydrolyzed by dehydropeptidase-I, a renal tubular enzyme, but cilastatin inhibits its enzymatic degradation. As a result, 70 to 80% of an imipenem dose can be recovered in the urine in unchanged form.[288] Urinary concentrations of imipenem were from 49 to 894 μg/ml in the first spontaneously voided urine specimen after the end of drug infusion in newborns.[291] Cilastatin is primarily excreted in unchanged form in the urine, but about 12% of the drug appears as the metabolite N-acetylcilastatin.[288] The urinary concentrations of cilastatin in newborns were from 72 to 2570 μg/ml in the first urine specimen collected after drug administration was completed.[291]

Limited pharmacokinetic data of meropenem in neonates are available for analysis. Studies has been performed in 25 premature infants (mean gestational age, 32.5 weeks; mean weight, 1.87 kg) and 15 full-term infants (mean gestational age, 39 weeks, mean weight, 3.17 kg).[297] The administration of increasing dosages of meropenem from 10 to 40 mg/kg resulted in approximately proportionate increases in area under the curve (AUC) and maximal concentration (C_{max}) values in each of the two patient groups. Therefore, meropenem, like imipenem, exhibits linear kinetics. A 20-mg/kg dose of meropenem resulted in a C_{max} similar to that produced by 25 mg/kg of imipenem. Half-life, volume of distribution, and total drug clearance of meropenem were 2.92 hours, 0.46 liter/kg, and 2.17 ml/min/kg, respectively for premature infants and 2.04 hours, 0.48 liter/kg, and 3.15 ml/min/kg, respectively for full-term neonates.[297] These values are similar to those observed for imipenem.

Safety

Both imipenem-cilastatin and meropenem appear to be well tolerated when administered intravenously to newborns. In a review of thousands of patients, most of whom were adults, treated with both drugs worldwide, it was observed that the nature and frequency of side effects were similar to those of other β-lactam antibiotics and consisted mainly of nausea, vomiting, diarrhea, thrombophlebitis, thrombocytosis, eosinophilia, and elevation of hepatic enzyme concentrations.[298] Colonization by *Candida* or imipenem-resistant bacteria occurred in about 16%, and secondary superinfection was noted in about 6%.[298] Alterations of bowel flora in children treated with imipenem-cilastatin have been minimal in the few patients studied in detail.[288, 299]

A worrisome report suggests that imipenem treatment of infants with bacterial meningitis was possibly associated with a drug-related seizure activity.[300] Seven (33%) of 21 infants, aged 3 to 48 months, with bacterial meningitis developed seizures after imipenem therapy was given. In this study,[300] CSF imipenem and cilastatin peak concentrations ranged from 1.4 to 10 μg/ml and 0.8 to 7.2 μg/ml, respectively. It is believed that interference of β-lactam antibiotics with the inhibitory effects of the neurotransmitter γ-aminobutyric acid results in epileptiform bursts.[301, 302] Of interest is that imipenem has been shown to induce seizure activity in mice at serum concentrations twofold to threefold lower than those of penicillin and cefotaxime.[303] Meropenem has less affinity than imipenem for the γ-aminobutyric acid receptor and consequently has demonstrated a lower propensity to cause seizures in animal models.[304] In infants and children with meningitis, treatment with meropenem was well tolerated and no drug-related seizure activity was observed.[286]

Clinical Implications

At present, imipenem-cilastatin and meropenem should be considered investigational drugs for newborns and young infants and cannot be recommended for routine use in the treatment of suspected or proved neonatal infections. Presently, use of the carbapenems in neonates should be limited to treat infections caused by multiresistant microorganisms. Preliminary data in 25 neonates with proven bacterial infections suggest that single-drug therapy with imipenem-cilastatin using a 25-mg/kg dose given two to four times daily is both efficacious and safe.[305] Because newborns have lower renal clearance capability and somewhat greater blood-brain permeability than older infants and children, high concentrations of imipenem-cilastatin could be achieved in the CSF of neonates, especially those with bacterial meningitis, and potentially result in drug-related seizure activity. Anecdotal evidence suggests that meropenem is also safe and effective for treatment of neonatal infections. Because meropenem therapy has not been linked to the potential induction of seizures, we believe that if a carbapenem is selected for therapy in a newborn, meropenem should be the agent of choice. Further studies are required, however, before these drugs can be recommended for routine use in newborns and before an appropriate dosage schedule can be formulated.

VANCOMYCIN

With the advent of staphylococcal strains that were resistant to the antistaphylococcal penicillins and the cephalosporins, it became necessary in 1978 to return to the use of vancomycin. This glycopeptidic agent had been used in the mid 1950s for treatment of penicillin-resistant staphylococcal disease, but its use was curtailed with the introduction of methicillin in the early 1960s.

Antimicrobial Activity

Vancomycin is bactericidal against most aerobic and anaerobic gram-positive cocci and bacilli but is ineffective against most gram-negative bacteria. The drug interferes with the phospholipid cycle of cell wall synthesis, alters plasma membrane function, and inhibits RNA synthesis.[306] It is not metabolized by the body and is excreted unchanged in the urine.

Pharmacokinetic Data

Peak concentrations of 17 to 30 μg/ml are produced at the end of a 30-minute infusion of a 15-mg/kg dose given to neonates weighing less than 2000 g at birth and 0 to 7 days of age (Table 35–9). Slightly higher values are observed in larger-birth-weight infants. In infants up to 12 months of age, doses of 10 mg/kg produce similar peak serum concentrations. The half-life decreases from 6 to 7 hours in the first week of life to 4 hours in early infancy to 2 to 2.5 hours in children. A corresponding increase in the plasma clearance values is seen during these periods.

Serum half-life of vancomycin was about 10 hours in three premature infants aged 27 to 32 days and weighing less than 1000 g at birth.[307] The half-life was shorter (mean, 5.4 hours) in a second group of six infants aged 26 to 62 days and weighing between 1120 and 1780 g. In a second study[308] of premature infants aged 2 months or younger, shorter mean half-life values of from 3 to 5 hours were found. There is a significant correlation between vancomycin serum half-life and clearance and a patient's body weight or postnatal age.[309, 310] Neonates undergoing ECMO have a larger volume of distribution, lower clearance, and longer half-life of vancomycin than other infants.[311]

The CSF concentrations of vancomycin are 10 to 15% of the concomitant serum concentrations in infants with minimal meningeal inflammation as seen in ventriculoperitoneal shunt infections.[41] The degree of penetration is similar to that of nafcillin. In premature infants, 26 to 31 weeks of gestational age, dosages of 20 mg/kg every 18 to 24 hours were associated with CSF vancomycin concentrations of 2.2 to 5.6 μg/ml, which were 26 to 68% of their correspondent serum values.[312]

In low-birth-weight, premature infants blood should be obtained to determine peak concentrations of vancomycin 15 to 30 minutes after a 60-minute infusion. This is usually measured after the third dose of vancomycin is given. Once a therapeutic peak serum concentration is achieved, concentrations should be monitored weekly if there is a change in renal function or if potentially nephrotoxic drugs are concomitantly given. The peak serum concentration that is considered to be therapeutic is 20 to 30 μg/ml, although concentrations of 30 to 40 μg/ml are preferred when treating meningitis. The upper limit of activity that must not be exceeded is unknown, but it is prudent to maintain serum concentrations below 50 μg/ml. Trough (predose) vancomycin values should be approximately 10 μg/ml or lower.

Safety

Initial experience with vancomycin in the 1950s suggested a moderate incidence of ototoxicity and nephrotoxicity. These adverse effects were presumably related to the impurities found in early preparations of the drug.[313] Further studies have indicated that vancomycin is well tolerated and safe when administered intravenously, particularly in newborns and young infants.[41] If it is administered in less than 30-minute infusions, some patients develop a histamine reaction characterized by an erythematous, pruritic rash on the upper part of the body and arms and on the neck and face. This reaction persists for several hours and tends to improve with antihistamine medications. Readministration of vancomycin with a slower infusion (i.e., 45 to 60 minutes) usually averts this adverse event.

Clinical Implications

The primary indication for vancomycin therapy in newborns is for infections caused by methicillin-resistant staphylococci and by ampicillin-resistant enterococci. Vancomycin is effective for therapy of MRSA strains, an increasing problem in many American nurseries. We believe that vancomycin is the initial drug of choice for documented infections caused by *S. epidermidis* because most strains are resistant to penicillin, methicillin, cephalosporins, and aminoglycosides. Vancomycin is not usually absorbed from the gastrointestinal tract, and oral preparations of this drug should be used only for the treatment of pseudomembranous colitis caused by *C. difficile*. However, because of the increasing isolation of vancomycin-resistant enterococci, vancomycin is not recommended for treatment of antibiotic-associated colitis.[314] Metronidazole is the drug of choice for this condition.

The dosage schedule for vancomycin in neonates is 10 to 15 mg/kg given every 12 hours (20 to 30 mg/kg per day) in the first week of life and every 8 hours (30 to 45 mg/kg per day) thereafter. For premature infants,

TABLE 35–9
Pharmacokinetics of Vancomycin in Newborns

AGE GROUP/WEIGHT	MEAN PEAK SERUM CONCENTRATION (μg/ml)	MEAN SERUM HALF-LIFE (hr)	MEAN PLASMA CLEARANCE (ml/min per 1.73²)
0–7 days (15 mg/kg per dose)			
2000 g	25	5.9	27
>2000 g	30	6.7	30
1–12 mo (average, 3 mo) (10 mg/kg per dose)	26	4.1	50

a different dosage schedule has been proposed that takes into account body weight and postnatal age to modify both the total daily dose and the dosing intervals for vancomycin.[309] Although this dosage schedule resulted in more consistent peak and trough serum concentrations within the desired therapeutic range, about 25% of trough and 33% of peak concentrations fell outside the recommended therapeutic values.[310] Accordingly, there is a need for monitoring serum vancomycin concentrations in low-birth-weight, premature infants treated with this drug and other infants with altered renal function. Beyond the newborn period, daily administration of 40 to 60 mg/kg (divided into three or four doses) is recommended. The larger dosage is used for treatment of central nervous system infection.

The dramatic increase in worldwide prevalence of vancomycin-resistant enterococci and the serious threat posed by the spread of vancomycin resistant to other gram-positive organisms such as staphylococci should discourage the use of this antibiotic for antimicrobial prophylaxis of very low birth weight infants and for empirical therapy for neonatal sepsis of unknown etiology. Thus, each nursery needs to implement a policy to restrict the liberal use of vancomycin for these situations.

AMINOGLYCOSIDES

For the past three decades, the aminoglycosides have been relied on for therapy for neonatal sepsis and meningitis because of their broad-spectrum antibacterial activity against gram-negative bacilli. Many neonatal units, however, have limited their use because of a low therapeutic index and the emergence of resistant strains among gram-negative enteric bacilli. For example, serum aminoglycoside concentrations are only one to five times the MBC_{90} of many gram-negative enteric organisms, and CSF concentrations are, at most, only one to two times greater. Streptomycin is no longer used, owing to the prevalence of resistant strains and to ototoxicity. Similarly, kanamycin is currently used infrequently in nurseries because of its lack of activity against *P. aeruginosa* and development of resistant coliform strains in many neonatal units during the 1970s.[315] Currently, gentamicin, tobramycin, or amikacin are the aminoglycosides of choice in most nurseries worldwide. Because amikacin is resistant to degradation by most of the plasmid-mediated bacterial enzymes that inactivate kanamycin, gentamicin, and tobramycin, some U.S. nurseries have held amikacin in reserve for treatment of nosocomially acquired, multiresistant gram-negative organisms. Gentamicin resistance occurs frequently in some European, Latin American, and U.S. centers to warrant use of amikacin as a first-line drug for therapy of life-threatening gram-negative infections, and its routine use has not resulted in emergence of resistant strains.

The history of aminoglycoside usage in the late 1950s and 1960s is an excellent example of the inherent problems of adapting dosages derived from studies in adults to newborns. Irreversible ototoxicity in neonates was caused by excessive dosages of streptomycin or kanamycin. By contrast, the pharmacokinetics of gentamicin, tobramycin, amikacin, and netilmicin were carefully defined in the neonate before routine use of these drugs; this provided a scientific basis for safe and effective dosage regimens. The risk of aminoglycoside toxicity has been proven to be minimal when these agents are administered to infants in the proper dosage and when serum concentrations are closely monitored and kept within the recommended therapeutic range.

Antimicrobial Activity

Aminoglycosides act on microbial ribosomes to irreversibly inhibit protein synthesis. Possible mechanisms of bacterial resistance to these drugs include alteration of the ribosomal binding site, changes in the cell surface proteins to prevent entrance of drug into the cell and induction of aminoglycoside-inactivating enzymes. Antibiotic resistance in clinical situations is most often a result of extrachromosomally controlled (R-factor) enzymes.[316, 317] Phosphorylation, adenylation, and acetylation are the three most common enzymatic mechanisms encountered.

In general, gentamicin, tobramycin, amikacin, and netilmicin have good antibacterial activity against most gram-negative strains isolated in many hospitals worldwide. On a weight-for-weight basis, tobramycin has the greatest anti-*Pseudomonas* activity[318] and amikacin is the only drug of this class that reliably provides activity against *Serratia* species and nosocomially acquired resistant coliforms. Although staphylococci are the only gram-positive organisms susceptible in vitro to aminoglycosides, infections caused by these pathogens usually do not respond satisfactorily to aminoglycoside therapy alone. Synergistic bactericidal activity between aminoglycosides and the penicillins has been demonstrated in vitro and in animals against *S. aureus*,[36] group B streptococci,[32, 33] *L. monocytogenes*,[34] and enterococci[37] in spite of low-level resistance of the microorganism to the aminoglycoside alone.

General Pharmacologic Considerations

Traditionally, the intramuscular route has been preferred for the administration of aminoglycosides to avoid potentially toxic peak serum concentrations. Pharmacokinetic studies of kanamycin,[319] gentamicin,[319, 320] and netilmicin[40] have, however, demonstrated that the serum concentration-time curves after an intramuscular injection and a 20-minute intravenous infusion are nearly superimposable. Although peak serum concentrations immediately after the intravenous dose may at times be considerably higher than the desired peak value, this elevation is transient and not clinically significant. The 6-hour serum concentrations, half-lives, and AUC values are also equivalent.

These drugs cannot be administered orally for treatment of systemic infection because they are not absorbed from the intact gastrointestinal tract.[321] Absorption through an inflamed gastrointestinal mucosa has, however, been suggested by studies of infants with gastroenteritis or necrotizing enterocolitis who were treated orally with neomycin[322, 323] and of infants with shigellosis[324] and necrotizing enterocolitis[325] receiving oral gentamicin. More than 10% of the administered dose of gentamicin was excreted in the urine during the acute phase of *Shigella* dysentery compared with only 2% after the acute inflammation had subsided. Peak serum gentamicin values of more than 10 μg/ml were detected in four children with necrotizing enterocolitis who received 2.5 mg/kg every 4 hours per nasogastric tube in addition to 7.5 mg/kg per day by the intramuscular route.[325] The mean peak gentamicin concentration was slightly higher than that detected in a control group of infants receiving the drug only intramuscularly. The mean trough gentamicin values, however, were similar. In contrast, the prophylactic use of oral gentamicin in neonates at high risk for developing necrotizing enterocolitis results in mean serum gentamicin concentrations below 2 μg/ml and only rarely achieves therapeutic serum values.[326, 327]

Pharmacokinetic studies have demonstrated a prolonged washout phase in neonates for netilmicin[40] and gentamicin.[42] Mean terminal half-lives of 62 to 110 hours and detectable serum and urine drug activity for as long as 11 and 14 days, respectively, after discontinuation of these drugs have been recorded. Presumably, this represents release of the drug that was bound to tissue, most likely renal, during the steady state. The practical significance of these findings is unknown. Persistent small serum concentrations could conceivably place the infant who requires a second course of therapy at increased risk of developing aminoglycoside-associated toxicity. It is also possible that the subinhibitory concentrations of aminoglycosides that persist in the urine could exert selective pressure for the emergence of resistant gram-negative organisms in neonatal intensive care units.

Finally, several studies have indicated that aminoglycoside pharmacokinetics in the very low birth weight premature infant are highly variable because of renal immaturity and unpredictable extracellular fluid volumes.[40, 328–334] Therefore, these infants may require frequent measurements of serum drug concentrations and individualization of dosage regimens. The pharmacokinetic properties of several aminoglycosides are compared in Table 35–10. Peak serum concentrations of gentamicin, tobramycin, and netilmicin should be maintained at 5 to 8 μg/ml and for kanamycin and amikacin at 15 to 25 μg/ml. Trough values should be kept below 2 μg/ml for the former drugs and below 10 μg/ml for the latter agents. To obtain peak serum concentrations a blood sample should be drawn 15 to 30 minutes after completion of the intravenous infusion (from another IV site) and 45 to 60 minutes after the intramuscular administration. Trough serum concentrations are measured just before the next dose of the aminoglycoside. In general, these peak and trough values should be determined every 72 to 92 hours while the patient is receiving aminoglycoside therapy.

Pharmacokinetic Data

Neomycin. Because neomycin is no longer used parenterally in newborns, pharmacokinetic data pertaining only to its oral administration are discussed. Poor absorption after oral administration has made this antibiotic useful for the control of nursery outbreaks of diarrhea caused by enteropathogenic *E. coli*. Although efficacy of this regimen has been questioned, a more

TABLE 35–10
Comparative Pharmacokinetics of Aminoglycosides in Neonates

DRUG (Dosage)	BIRTH WEIGHT/ AGE GROUP	PEAK SERUM CONCENTRATION (μg/ml)	SERUM HALF- LIFE (hr)	PLASMA CLEARANCE (ml/min per 1.73 m²)
Amikacin	2000 g			
(7.5 mg/kg)	7 days	17	6.5	22
	>7 days	18.9	5.5	24.6
	>2000 g			
	7 days	18–20	5–6.5	27–30
	>7 days	17.4	4.9	36.4
Gentamicin	2000 g/7 days	1.5–2.2	10.5–14	12–16.5
(1.5 mg/kg)[a]	>2000 g/7 days	2.5–2.7	4.5–5.5	30–34
	All infants >7 days	3	3.2	56.2
Tobramycin	2500 g			
(2 mg/kg)	<7 days	4.9–5.6	8.6	11
	7 days	5–5.4	6–9.8	8.6–14.3
	>2500 g			
	<7 days	4.9	5.1	25.3
	7 days	4.5	4	35.9
Netilmicin	2000 g			
(3 mg/kg)	<7 days	6	4.7	30.8
	7 days	5.6	4.1	34.1
	>2000 g			
	<7 days	6.9	3.4	38.8

[a]Recommended dosage, 2.5 mg/kg for all neonates.

rapid bacteriologic and clinical response was demonstrated in infants treated for 3 to 5 days compared with those given placebo.[335] Occasionally, neomycin may be absorbed from an inflamed gastrointestinal tract and cause ototoxicity or renal toxicity, particularly in patients with preexisting renal diseases.[322] Transient elevations of the blood urea nitrogen occurred in one infant who received 10 times the recommended dosage for several days in our institution.

Gentamicin. Gentamicin has been the most methodically studied aminoglycosidic antibiotic in newborns.[42, 320, 329, 336–349] Mean peak serum concentrations of 3.5 to 7 μg/ml occur within 1 hour after a 2.5-mg/kg dose. Mean serum values 12 hours after this dose were 0.5 to 1 μg/ml. Although most studies have not demonstrated drug accumulation during a 5- to 7-day course of therapy, one group of investigators showed accumulation in very low birth weight premature infants.[328] Serum aminoglycoside concentrations are reduced by 19 to 62% after a two-volume exchange transfusion; therefore, whenever possible, such procedures are best timed to precede the next scheduled dose of gentamicin.[350, 351] On the other hand, gentamicin, and probably other aminoglycosides, exhibits a higher volume of distribution, a lower clearance, and a longer half-life in neonates undergoing ECMO for severe respiratory failure.[352]

Urinary concentrations of gentamicin vary from 2 to 135 μg/ml, and values correlate directly with postnatal age and rates of creatinine clearance but are independent of birth weight and dosage. Approximately 10% of the dose administered to infants 0 to 3 days old was excreted within 12 hours compared with 40% excreted during the same period by infants 5 to 40 days of age.[336] After the final dose of gentamicin, urinary concentrations decrease in a biphasic pattern and remain detectable for 11 days (Fig. 35–1).

The serum half-life of gentamicin correlates inversely with the rate of creatinine clearance, gestational age, birth weight, and postnatal age.[320, 337, 343, 347–349] During the first week of life, half-life values as long as 14 hours have been observed in infants with birth weights of 800 to 1500 g compared with 4.5 hours in term infants. After the first 2 weeks of life, the half-life of gentamicin is approximately 3 hours, regardless of body weight (see Table 35–10). Both perinatal asphyxia and a patent ductus arteriosus are associated with prolonged serum gentamicin half-life values.[342, 353] One group of investigators recommended dosing intervals of 18 hours for infants of less than 35 weeks' gestation because of the occurrence of predose gentamicin serum concentrations greater than 2 μg/ml in 31 of 34 infants compared with 13 of 40 infants of more than 34 weeks gestational age.[329] Several other groups have made similar observations, and some have suggested prolonging the dosing interval to 24 hours in newborns weighing 1000 g or less or, alternatively, reducing individual gentamicin doses.[330, 343, 354–357]

CSF concentrations of gentamicin in infants with meningitis are from 0.3 to 3.7 μg/ml (mean, 1.6 μg/ml) 1 to 6 hours after a 2.5-mg/kg dose.[165] Peak values are observed 4 to 6 hours after the dose and are directly

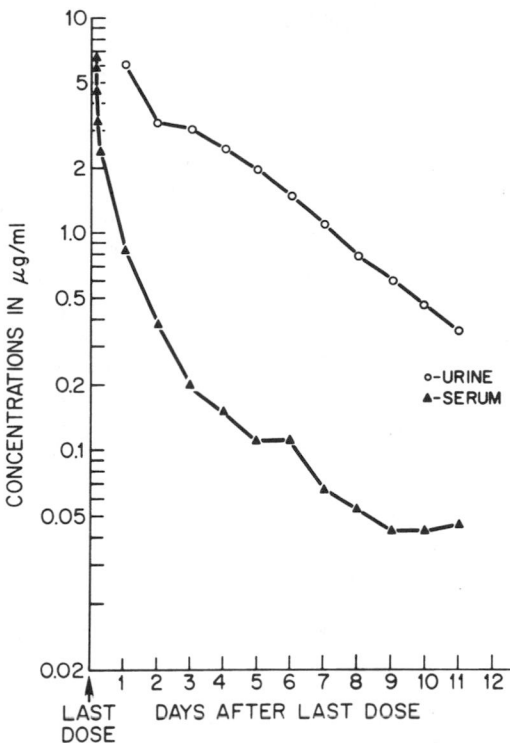

FIGURE 35–1 Washout concentrations after 2.5 mg/kg gentamicin in infants of 1500 g birth weight.

correlated with the degree of meningeal inflammation and dosage.

During the 1970s, the Neonatal Meningitis Cooperative Study Group evaluated lumbar intrathecal and intraventricular gentamicin administration in comparative studies with systemic antibiotic therapy alone (see Table 35–10).[165] The mean drug concentration in lumbar CSF obtained 2 to 4 hours after a 1-mg dose into the lumbar space was 30 μg/ml. By 18 to 24 hours, the mean concentration decreased to 1.6 μg/ml, a value similar to that seen after systemic therapy alone. Daily instillation of 2.5 mg gentamicin directly into the ventricles resulted in a mean ventricular fluid concentration of 48 μg/ml (range, 10 to 130 μg/ml) 1 to 6 hours after the dose compared with 1.1 μg/ml (range, 0.1 to 3 μg/ml) after systemic therapy only. An average concentration of 8.1 μg/ml (range, 1 to 24 μg/ml) was detected 16 to 24 hours after the intraventricular dose. Despite these higher CSF and intraventricular fluid concentrations, neither route of administration therapy was associated with a better outcome of infants with meningitis caused by gram-negative enteric organisms. Indeed, case:fatality rates were significantly greater in intraventricular gentamicin recipients. Subsequently, it was demonstrated that the rapid lysis of gram-negative bacteria by high ventricular fluid gentamicin concentrations resulted in significantly larger amounts of endotoxin released into the ventricular fluid and in a greater meningeal inflammation secondary to cytokine overproduction.[358] Poorer outcome of these infants can be explained, at least in part, by these findings.

Tobramycin. Tobramycin offers two theoretical advantages over gentamicin for therapy for neonatal infections: increased in vitro activity against *P. aeruginosa* and decreased nephrotoxicity.[359] The lower incidence of nephrotoxicity for tobramycin has been documented in laboratory animals and human adults but not in human neonates.[360] Because of the relative resistance of neonates to aminoglycoside nephrotoxicity, the applicability of such studies to young infants is uncertain. In addition, the overall clinical experience with tobramycin in this age group is small compared with that of gentamicin.

After a 2-mg/kg dose of tobramycin, mean peak serum concentrations of 4 to 6 μg/ml are observed at 30 minutes to 1 hour.[361] When an identical dose is given to low-birth-weight neonates, mean peak serum values are 8 μg/ml. Predose concentrations are inversely related to birth weight and gestational age and have been reported to be consistently greater than 2 μg/ml in premature neonates who receive 2.5 mg/kg doses every 12 hours.[331-333] There is no evidence for drug accumulation, but minimal serum values are detectable for at least 3 days after therapy is discontinued. The serum tobramycin half-life is inversely related to birth weight, gestational age, chronologic age, and creatinine clearance.[331, 361-363] In infants who weigh less than 1500 g at birth and are younger than 1 week of age, half-life values may be as long as 9 to 17 hours compared with half-lives of 3 to 4.5 hours for infants larger than 2500 g at birth and 1 to 4 weeks of age (see Table 35–10). Because of the markedly prolonged serum half-life values in infants of 30 weeks' gestational age or less, dosage intervals of 18 to 24 hours have been recommended.[331, 332, 364] Measurement of serum tobramycin concentrations and individualization of the dosage schedule provide the optimal therapy for these very low birth weight infants.

Concentrations of tobramycin in urine vary from 2 to 132 μg/ml after a 2-mg/kg dose.[361] Excretion in urine, expressed as percentage of the dose, correlates directly with postnatal age. Average excretion values are 15 to 25% of the administered dose during the first week of life and 25 to 40% in older infants.

Amikacin. Pharmacokinetic data of amikacin in neonates is limited because its use has been reserved for therapy for infections caused by multiresistant strains of Enterobacteriaceae. In general, the pharmacokinetic properties are similar to those of kanamycin, from which it is derived. Mean peak serum concentrations of 15 to 20 μg/ml occur 30 minutes to 1 hour after 7.5 mg/kg doses of amikacin (see Table 35–10). Mean trough concentrations of 3 to 6 μg/ml are detected 12 hours after the dose.[365] One study reported subtherapeutic peak serum values when a 7.5-mg/kg dose was administered to infants weighing less than 1500 g at birth. Doses of 10 mg/kg at 12-hour intervals were required to achieve a mean peak value of 21.5 μg/ml and an average trough concentration of 3.3 μg/ml. In contrast, other investigators[366] noted that subtherapeutic serum concentrations of amikacin given to premature infants in 7.5-mg/kg intravenous doses every 12 hours were present in only 10% of those younger than 2 weeks of age. However, as many as 38% of infants 29 days of age or older had peak serum concentrations below 15 μg/ml. Serum half-life values of amikacin in newborns are inversely correlated to gestational and chronologic ages.[365] Values of 7 to 8 hours occur in low-birth-weight infants 1 to 3 days old and of 4 to 5 hours in term infants who are older than 1 week of age. The serum half-life is prolonged in hypoxemic newborns.[25] Urinary amikacin concentrations range from 50 to 650 μg/ml, and the average urinary excretion of drug in 12 hours is 30 to 50% of the administered dose. Low concentrations of amikacin have been detected in serum and urine for as long as 10 to 14 days, respectively, after the final dose of a 5- to 7-day course of therapy.

There are few reports of CSF concentrations of amikacin.[365, 367-369] In the presence of uninflamed meninges in 1-day-old infants, CSF values ranged from 0.2 to 2.7 μg/ml when measured at 1 to 4 hours after a single 10-mg/kg dose administered by slow intravenous infusion.[368] Simultaneous concentrations in serum ranged from 15 to 29 μg/ml. The highest concentration reported has been 9.2 μg/ml after a 7.5-mg/kg dose was administered intramuscularly to an infant with meningitis.[365] Amikacin concentrations in ventricular fluid 12 hours after 1- or 2-mg intraventricular doses and 2 to 8 hours after intramuscular doses varies from 4.5 to 11.6 μg/ml (mean, 7.3 μg/ml).

The dosage schedule for neonates has not been established. The 10-mg/kg "loading" dose that was initially recommended by the manufacturer has been abandoned. Because of the similarity of amikacin and kanamycin pharmacokinetics, we recommend the following schedule: a 7.5-mg/kg dose to be used for infants weighing less than 2000 g and a 10-mg/kg dose for all other infants. A 12-hour dosing interval should be used for all neonates in the first week of life and an 8-hour interval used thereafter. Dosage schedules may require individualization for infants weighing less than 1500 g at birth or less than 30 weeks' gestational age or both because of the highly variable serum concentrations that may occur.[369] The appropriate regimen in these infants is best determined by monitoring serum concentrations.

Netilmicin. Numerous reports on the pharmacokinetics of netilmicin in newborns have been published.[40, 370-378] Mean peak serum concentrations vary from 5.6 to 7.7 μg/ml in infants tested 30 minutes to 1 hour after intramuscular administration of 2.5- to 3-mg/kg doses compared with mean peak values of 7 to 9 μg/ml after intravenous injection of similar doses.[40, 375-377] Average serum values of 1 to 2.8 μg/ml are observed 12 hours after the dose.[40, 376-378] The serum half-life of netilmicin is inversely related to birth weight, gestational age, and chronologic age. The mean half-life varies from 4.7 hours in infants weighing less than 2000 g at birth in the first week of life to 3.4 hours in infants larger than 2000 g at birth and older than 7 days of age (see Table 35–10). In another study,[377] half-life values of from 4.6 to 11.5 hours were found in 12 premature infants (mean weight, 1335 g) during their neonatal period. After the administration and rapid tissue distribution of the last dose of netilmicin, the drug is eliminated from the body in two phases. The first reflects the renal clearance of netilmicin by glomerular filtration, whereas the second is related to the slow release of the drug from tissues. The average terminal half-life for netilmicin is 52 to 62 hours and is within the range determined for gentamicin in adults.[40, 376] Despite this long terminal half-life[376] and tissue accumulation,[379] however, dosing intervals of two to three times per day appear to be appropriate for most neonates.

The steady-state serum concentration-time curves after 3-mg/kg doses of netilmicin or gentamicin are similar, with mean peak serum concentrations of 6.9 and 6.3 µg/ml and serum half-lives of 4 and 3.5 hours, respectively. Greater variability in serum concentrations was observed with gentamicin than with netilmicin.

The average concentrations of netilmicin in urine were 46 and 29 µg/ml for the first and second 3-hour study periods, respectively, after a 3-mg/kg dose. Netilmicin remains detectable in the urine for 14 days after the last dose of antibiotic is given. Information about penetration of netilmicin into the CSF of newborns is lacking.

Drug accumulation has been documented in premature infants of very low birth weight.[40] After 4-mg/kg doses of netilmicin given every 12 hours for an average of 6.4 days, the mean trough value in these infants increased from 2.2 µg/ml on the second day of therapy to 5.6 µg/ml on the final day. This same group of infants did not show the expected decrease in serum creatinine observed in term infants during the first 2 weeks of life, and they all required mechanical ventilation. Thus, hypoxemia superimposed on immature renal function is a possible explanation of drug accumulation in this special group of newborns.

On the basis of these pharmacokinetic studies, a dose schedule of 2.5 mg/kg administered every 12 hours to infants younger than 1 week of age should produce serum values that are within the therapeutic range. An 8-hour schedule should be given to infants older than 1 week of age. Trough serum concentrations greater than the 3 µg/ml recommended upper limit for netilmicin may be encountered in 25 to 50% of low-birth-weight (<2000 g) neonates,[375-378] thus necessitating monitoring of drug serum concentrations in these infants.

Safety

The major adverse effects of aminoglycosidic antibiotics are renal toxicity, ototoxicity, and, rarely, neuromuscular blockade. Hepatic and hematologic effects are not associated with this group of drugs. Acute toxic reactions and drug-induced fever are rare in the neonate.

It has been suggested that the immature kidney of the neonate may be protected from major toxic effects of aminoglycosides. Transient cylindruria and proteinuria may occur after prolonged administration of any of these drugs, but significant elevations in blood urea nitrogen and creatinine values are rarely observed and usually represent late manifestations of aminoglycoside nephrotoxicity.[380-386] One potential marker of early aminoglycoside nephrotoxicity that has been studied in newborns is the β2-microglobulin, a low-molecular-weight protein reabsorbed by proximal tubular cells after its glomerular filtration. Urinary excretion of this protein in aminoglycoside-treated infants has, however, been reported to increase (impaired tubular reabsorption),[385] decrease (de-

creased glomerular filtration rates),[384] or remain unchanged.[382] Other toxicity markers include increases in the urinary activity of enzymes of renal tubular origin such as N-acetyl-D-glucosaminidase and alanine aminopeptidase;[383] their increased urinary activity is believed to reflect damage to proximal renal tubular cells. The clinical significance of enzymuria and of the alleged tubular damage in terms of long-term renal damage after aminoglycoside therapy has not, however, been determined. Enzymuria is reversible on discontinuation of these drugs.

The criteria of maintaining peak and trough serum aminoglycoside concentrations within recommended values for older children and adults to prevent nephrotoxicity[387] have not been systematically assessed in newborns and should be considered as a guide rather than an established rule for formulating dosages of aminoglycosides in this age group. Factors that may be associated with increased risk for aminoglycoside nephrotoxicity include acidosis, hypovolemia, hypoalbuminemia, sodium depletion, duration of therapy, increased total aminoglycoside dose, and frequency of administration and co-administration of furosemide, vancomycin, or prostaglandin synthesis inhibitors such as indomethacin.[383, 384, 388, 389]

Because renal excretion accounts for the elimination of approximately 80% of an aminoglycoside dose, the greatest risk of toxicity occurs when drug elimination is impaired by reduction in renal function for any reason. After several doses of an aminoglycoside, measurements of serum drug concentrations are helpful to determine the intervals of administration to maintain therapeutic and potentially safe values.[390-392]

Neomycin,[322, 393] streptomycin,[394] kanamycin,[315] and gentamicin[165] have been implicated as a cause of sensorineural hearing loss in infants and children. Gentamicin and streptomycin have also been associated with vestibular impairment. It is, however, difficult to incriminate the aminoglycosides as the single causative agent of hearing loss in most studies because of the high-risk conditions present in these patients. For instance, asphyxia, hyperbilirubinemia, and incubator exposure have also been independently associated with ototoxicity.[395] Although animal studies have demonstrated a synergistic effect of noise combined with neomycin or kanamycin on development of ototoxicity, this has not been substantiated in the human neonate exposed to both incubator noise and kanamycin.[395, 396] A familial predisposition toward cochlear damage has been observed after therapy with streptomycin[394, 397] but not with the other aminoglycosides.

Kanamycin rarely causes toxicity when given in a dosage of 15 mg/kg per day for 10 or 12 days.[398] Ototoxicity is related primarily to total dosages: high-frequency sensorineural hearing loss in infants with normal renal function is more likely if the total dosage exceeds 500 mg/kg. In a prospective evaluation of long-term toxicity of kanamycin and gentamicin,[398] 86 infants who received one of these drugs during the neonatal period underwent yearly audiometric, vestibular, and psychometric examinations for 4 years. Neither gentamicin nor kanamycin could be incriminated as the sole agent responsible for hearing impairment. In another study,[399] long-term follow-up evaluations of 98 infants treated with short courses of streptomycin (mean dosage, 37 mg/kg per day) failed to ascribe any hearing loss to the use of this drug. Data from the first Neonatal Meningitis Cooperative Study[165] indicated that only 1 (1.3%) of 79 infants who received a minimum of 5 to 7.5 mg/kg per day of gentamicin for 3 weeks or longer developed profound deafness that may have been drug related. It is difficult, however, to establish a direct causal relationship in many of the published studies in which patients were treated with aminoglycosides because of their complicated clinical histories.

In recent years, the introduction of brain-stem response audiometry has facilitated assessment of hearing during the neonate's hospital stay.[400] A blinded, prospective controlled study of auditory brain-stem responses in neonates who were treated with amikacin or netilmicin was performed at our institution.[401] A high incidence of transient abnormalities was demonstrated, but permanent bilateral sensorineural hearing loss related to aminoglycoside therapy was documented in 2% of both amikacin- and netilmicin-treated infants as well as in the control group of untreated neonates. In another study,[402] significant delayed auditory brain-stem responses were detected in 15 neonates treated with 5 to 7.5 mg/kg per day for 6 to 10 days of either gentamicin or tobramycin compared with findings in 14 untreated controls. Long-term follow-up of these infants, however, was not performed to document whether the abnormalities were transient or permanent. Other investigators[403] failed to demonstrate permanent vestibular damage in 37 children aged 2 to 4 years treated with netilmicin during the neonatal period.

There are few reports of aminoglycoside-associated neuromuscular blockade.[404–406] The very young infant after undergoing surgery and having a highly variable fluid volume and renal function is at highest risk. The underlying mechanism appears to be inhibition of acetylcholine release at the neuromuscular junction by these drugs.[407] The aminoglycoside may act alone or synergistically with other neuromuscular blocking agents. Magnesium given to pregnant mothers with preeclampsia for prevention of seizures can be detected in the blood of their infants and potentiate the neuromuscular blocking effects of aminoglycosides. Diagnosis is made by nerve conduction studies, which reveal a progressive fatigue and post-tetanic facilitation characteristic of a nondepolarizing, curare-like neuromuscular block. Reversal is achieved by neostigmine or calcium or both. Potentiation of neuromuscular blockade can be observed in infant botulism when aminoglycosides are mistakenly administered because of suspicion of sepsis.[408] Prophylactic treatment with calcium is not indicated because this cation may interfere with the antimicrobial activity of aminoglycosides against certain organisms.

Clinical Implications

At present, the aminoglycosides still remain the first-line drugs in the newborn nursery for the initial empirical therapy of suspected gram-negative sepsis. The choice of aminoglycoside to be routinely used is mainly dependent on the patterns of microbial resistance within a nursery. Although the risk of toxicity may be smaller with tobramycin, netilmicin, or amikacin than with gentamicin, the comparative incidence rates of toxicity in neonates related to these drugs is unknown. Accordingly, selection of one agent over another should be based on other factors. Amikacin remains the drug of choice for empirical treatment when multiply-resistant coliforms are frequently isolated within an individual neonatal unit and when the infant has received one or more courses of aminoglycoside therapy previously. The aminoglycosides are usually safe in the newborn when administered according to the recommended dosage schedules and monitored carefully, particularly in very low birth weight, premature infants who have hypoxemia, renal dysfunction, or anesthetic effects. In addition, some investigators recommend that gentamicin and other aminoglycosides should be given in dosages that are about 25% lower than usual and at longer dosing intervals in ECMO-treated neonates.[352]

A systemic aminoglycoside remains the initial empirical treatment of choice when meningitis is present because, in combination with ampicillin, it offers potential synergistic activity against group B streptococci and *L. monocytogenes*.[409] In addition, aminoglycosides have been demonstrated to be effective for therapy for meningitis caused by susceptible gram-negative bacteria. We believe, however, that if gram-negative bacilli are seen on CSF smears or later isolated as the causative agents of meningitis, third-generation cephalosporins (i.e., cefotaxime or ceftazidime for *P. aeruginosa* infections) should be used. Although some comparative clinical trials between aminoglycosides and new-generation cephalosporins in newborns with gram-negative meningitis have failed to show any significant benefit of one therapy over the other, these studies have not evaluated a substantial number of infants to accurately make definitive conclusions. The high CSF bactericidal activity achieved with the use of these cephalosporins, with resultant rapid CSF sterilization, and the avoidance of monitoring serum concentrations are some of the attractive properties offered by these agents. Combined therapy with one of the new-generation cephalosporins and aminoglycosides is usually prescribed for the first 7 to 10 days of therapy to prevent emergence of bacterial resistance during the treatment of gram-negative meningitis, especially that caused by *Pseudomonas*, *Enterobacter*, and *Serratia* organisms, and for the possible synergistic activity on bacterial killing.

Oral administration of kanamycin or gentamicin has been recommended for the treatment[410] and prevention[411–413] of necrotizing enterocolitis in high-risk newborns. Although suppression of the gastrointestinal microflora has been suggested to prevent necrosis and perforation of the ischemic bowel,[410, 414, 415] this mode of therapy has been evaluated in a few studies in which conflicting results were observed.[325, 414, 416] In addition, serum gentamicin concentrations were substantially higher and potentially toxic in the infants who received systemic plus oral therapy.[325] Moreover, the potential increase in the prevalence of infants with aminoglycoside-resistant gram-negative enteric flora after the widespread use of these drugs is another factor to contraindicate their utilization for this purpose.[414]

Finally, considerable evidence generated in adults indicates that the daily dosage of an aminoglycoside given once daily is at least as safe and effective as given in two or three divided doses. The rationale for single daily dosing of these agents is based on the concentration-dependent bacterial killing and prolonged postantibiotic effect of the aminoglycosides.[417, 418] Some preliminary evidence with the use of gentamicin, tobramycin, and netilmicin suggests that this concept could also apply in the neonatal period.[419, 420] Recommendation of longer intervals of aminoglycoside administration in newborns must await, the results of carefully designed pharmacokinetic and clinical studies to determine safety and effectiveness in this age group.

CHLORAMPHENICOL

Although chloramphenicol has been used in newborns for more than 30 years, there are no reliable guidelines or methods, other than monitoring serum concentrations, on which to base dosage. Dosage regimens that have been recommended are as likely to produce subtherapeutic or toxic serum values as they are to produce concentrations that are within the desired range of 15 to 25 µg/ml. In the past, the major use of chloramphenicol was for therapy of meningitis because appreciable concentrations of drug diffuse into brain and CSF. Currently, however, new β-lactam antibiotics with excellent CSF penetration and greater safety have replaced chloramphenicol in this age group.

Antimicrobial Activity

Chloramphenicol competes with messenger RNA for binding sites on the ribosome, thus inhibiting bacterial ribosomal protein synthesis. The drug has broad antimicrobial activity, with bactericidal activity against *H. influenzae*, *S. pneumoniae*, and *N. meningitidis* but mainly static activity against group B streptococci and most coliform bacilli, the principal pathogens of the neonatal period.[8] Microbial resistance usually results from plasmid or R-factor–mediated acetyltransferase that catalyzes the acetylation of chloramphenicol. In addition, some gram-negative bacteria are probably resistant to chloramphenicol by altering the permeability of outer membrane proteins to the drug.[421, 422]

Pharmacokinetic Data

Chloramphenicol succinate is hydrolyzed in the body to the free, active drug, which in turn is conjugated in liver to the glucuronide salt. The free drug is excreted by glomerular filtration, whereas the conjugate is eliminated by tubular secretion. Unhydrolyzed chloramphenicol succinate is also excreted in the urine.[423] Approximately 65% of the total chloramphenicol in the serum of neonates is free drug, compared with 90% in adults. This is because excretion of the glucuronide by tubular

mechanisms is considerably reduced in the first weeks of life.

A large variability in serum concentrations and serum half-lives after recommended doses of chloramphenicol has been noted by many investigators.[424–430] This is particularly true for low-birth-weight infants, in whom peak serum concentrations ranged from 11 to 36 µg/ml after 14 to 25 mg/kg intravenous doses were administered during the first week of life. Half-life values were from 10 to more than 48 hours in these patients; the extremely long half-lives occurred in infants who tended to accumulate drug in serum between doses.[425] An inverse correlation between chloramphenicol half-life and postnatal age and weight has been demonstrated.[424]

Studies performed in the early 1960s[431, 432] reported serum concentrations of from 14 to 27 µg/ml (mean, 20 µg/ml) at 3 hours, 7 to 21 µg/ml (mean, 14 µg/ml) at 9 hours, and 2 to 18 µg/ml (mean, 6 µg/ml) at 21 hours after 25-mg/kg intramuscular doses to premature infants. The half-life values were estimated to be approximately 24 hours in the first week of life and 14 hours thereafter.

Oral administration of chloramphenicol in newborns results in significantly lower serum concentrations than those observed after intravenous infusion of similar doses.[5, 430] Peak serum concentrations of from 5.5 to 23.1 µg/ml were measured in seven premature and full-term neonates 4 hours or more after 12.5 mg/kg doses of chloramphenicol palmitate were given every 6 hours for several days. These erratic serum concentrations and the prolonged periods required to achieve peak values were ascribed to the immaturity of the newborn gastrointestinal tract.

Chloramphenicol concentrations in CSF are 35 to 90% of those in serum regardless of the extent of meningeal inflammation.[8, 424, 433] This highly diffusible drug attains concentrations of from 5 to more than 20 µg/ml after 10- to 20-mg/kg doses. These concentrations are usually bacteriostatic against gram-negative enteric bacilli.

Safety

The toxicity of chloramphenicol has been the major limiting factor for its routine use in newborns. A cardiovascular collapse reaction (gray baby syndrome) has been well documented in some chloramphenicol-treated neonates. The syndrome is characterized by vomiting, refusal to suck, respiratory distress, metabolic acidosis, abdominal distention, and passage of loose, green stools. The infant becomes gravely ill within 24 hours of the onset of symptoms. The reaction has been mostly documented in premature and full-term infants and occasionally in older infants and adults with very high (>70 µg/ml) serum chloramphenicol concentrations.[434]

The pathogenesis of the gray baby syndrome in newborns is related to excessive dosages, immaturity of the hepatic glucuronyl transferase system, and diminished glomerular and tubular function. As a result of these factors, elevated serum concentrations of free and conjugated drug are observed. Available evidence indicates that toxicity results from the free drug rather than its metabolic products and that multiple exchange transfusions or charcoal hemoperfusion may reverse the clinical syndrome by removing this free drug from the blood.[3, 435, 436] Chloramphenicol toxicity appears to be related to impaired mitochondrial protein synthesis as well as to direct inhibition of myocardial contractile activity.[437]

The most common untoward reaction is anemia caused by suppression of the marrow red blood cell precursors. Thrombocytopenia or leukopenia occurs less frequently. These three responses are dose related and are usually seen when serum concentrations consistently exceed 25 µg/ml.[438] The idiosyncratic reaction of bone marrow aplasia occurs in 1 in 30,000 to 1 in 50,000 treated patients and is not dose related, and it is not known whether it also applies to chloramphenicol-treated newborns. Other rare adverse effects of chloramphenicol therapy include sensorineural hearing loss, anaphylaxis, and retrobulbar neuritis, but these complications have been described only in older patients.[439, 440]

Clinical Implications

There is no rationale for the routine use of chloramphenicol in newborns. The agent can be considered an alternative to aminoglycosides for therapy for neonatal meningitis caused by gram-negative enteric bacilli in areas of the developing world, where third-generation cephalosporins are cost prohibitive. The main drawbacks of chloramphenicol therapy are the drug's toxicity and its bacteriostatic rather than bactericidal activity against gram-negative enteric pathogens.

There is considerable interpatient variation in serum chloramphenicol concentrations in the first weeks of life. Consequently, it is advisable to monitor serum values whenever possible to avoid either toxic or subtherapeutic concentrations. Peak serum concentrations should be within the 15 to 25 µg/ml range to be safe and effective. If the infant is also receiving phenobarbital, dosages may need to be increased because of induction of hepatic microsomal enzyme activity and accelerated conjugation of chloramphenicol. Simultaneous administration of phenytoin, rifampin, or acetaminophen can also affect chloramphenicol serum concentrations.[423]

SULFONAMIDES

The sulfonamides are structural analogues of p-aminobenzoic acid and differ from each other according to various substitutions on the sulfonamide group of the benzene ring. These drugs were commonly used in the prophylaxis and treatment of neonatal bacterial infections, but their usefulness in neonates has become greatly limited because of the availability of superior antimicrobial agents, the emergence of resistant bacteria, and the association of kernicterus with sulfonamide administration in some premature infants. Presently, there are no indications for their use in premature infants.

Antimicrobial Activity

The sulfonamides are bacteriostatic agents with a wide range of antimicrobial activity against both gram-posi-

tive and gram-negative organisms.[441] In addition, some sulfonamides are active against *Toxoplasma gondii*, the causative organism of congenital toxoplasmosis. Antimicrobial action is based on competition with the structurally similar p-aminobenzoic acid for the same enzyme, thus preventing normal utilization of p-aminobenzoic acid by microbes. Synthesis of folic acid is inhibited at the dihydropteroic acid step.

Acquired bacterial resistance to sulfonamides plays a significant role in therapeutic failures with this class of drugs. The origin of sulfonamide resistance is disputed, but the evidence indicates that mutations occurring randomly give rise to resistant variants, which are then favored by selection in the presence of the drug.[442] Resistance is more likely to develop if treatment is prolonged. Transfer of multiple drug resistance (R-factor mediated) among strains of coliform bacilli has been responsible for the emergence of sulfonamide-resistant *Shigella* strains worldwide.

Pharmacokinetic Data

There are a number of sulfonamide derivatives currently available. As a general rule, the short-acting sulfonamides, such as sulfadiazine, trisulfapyrimidine, and sulfisoxazole, are most commonly used for acute urinary tract infections. The first two agents are also employed, in combination with pyrimethamine, for the treatment of congenital toxoplasmosis (see Chapter 5). Sulfadiazine is slowly absorbed from the gastrointestinal tract, reaching peak values 8 hours after administration. Sulfisoxazole is more rapidly absorbed, attaining earlier peak values that are 50% higher than those of sulfadiazine.[443] The serum concentration-time curves for sulfisoxazole and triple sulfonamides are similar.

The pharmacokinetic properties for several of the sulfonamide derivatives have been studied in newborns. Sulfadiazine administered subcutaneously in an initial dose of 100 mg/kg, followed in 48 hours by 50 mg/kg given every 24 hours for 3 days, produces mean peak serum values of 170 µg/ml and trough values of 90 to 110 µg/ml. Although these concentrations are within the desired therapeutic range (50 to 150 µg/ml), the individual values vary considerably.[444] Serum concentrations of 110 to 180 µg/ml were found after an initial 100-mg/kg sulfadiazine dose given subcutaneously followed in 48 hours by a 50-mg/kg dose of triple sulfonamide given orally every 12 hours. Sulfisoxazole administered subcutaneously in a dose of 75 mg/kg every 12 hours results in serum concentrations of 60 to 120 µg/ml.[15]

The sulfonamides are excreted primarily by renal mechanisms.[445] Glomerular filtration is the major mechanism of excretion for both the free and the acetylated forms. Varying degrees of tubular reabsorption occur for most sulfonamides. Diminished renal function in neonates explains in part why they are able to maintain serum concentrations in the therapeutic range for longer periods than those observed in children or adults.

Safety

As a general rule, the sulfonamides are well tolerated by newborns; crystalluria and hematuria are uncommon in neonates. Use of these drugs in newborns has been greatly reduced by the demonstration that sulfonamides displaced bilirubin from albumin-binding sites and, as a result, were associated with the development of kernicterus in some prophylactically treated premature infants.[15] Sulfonamides may also cause hemolysis in neonates who have erythrocyte G6PD deficiency.[9] Cutaneous hypersensitivity reactions are rare in young infants.

Clinical Implications

Because of the availability of safer and more effective antimicrobial agents, the sulfonamides should not be used during the neonatal period for therapy for bacterial infections. Their principal usefulness is for dual treatment (pyrimethamine and sulfadiazine) of congenital toxoplasmosis. Neonates with acute urinary tract infections should be treated parenterally with ampicillin and an aminoglycoside until bloodstream invasion has been ruled out by blood culture. Bacteremia is found in approximately 20% of young infants with urinary tract infections.

TRIMETHOPRIM-SULFAMETHOXAZOLE

This combination of drugs provides sequential and synergistic inhibition of microbial folic acid synthesis.[446] Trimethoprim-sulfamethoxazole is currently used in the United States for therapy for urinary tract infections, otitis media and sinusitis, shigellosis, and *Pneumocystis carinii* infections. It is not approved for use in newborns because of insufficient pharmacokinetic, safety, and efficacy data in this age group. Nevertheless, this compound has been successfully used alone or in combination with an aminoglycoside for the treatment of neonatal meningitis caused by gram-negative enteric bacilli, particularly *Salmonella* organisms.[447–449] Treatment failures have also been observed.[448]

Mean peak and trough serum concentrations of trimethoprim were 3.4 µg/ml and 0.8 µg/ml, respectively, after administration of single daily intravenous doses of 5.25 mg/kg of trimethoprim and 26.25 mg/kg of sulfamethoxazole to 12 neonates.[450] On the third day of therapy, peak serum values were from 3 to 6.4 µg/ml. The mean serum half-life was 19 hours after one dose and about 25 hours after multiple doses. The peak serum concentrations for sulfamethoxazole were from 72 to 135 µg/ml after one dose but increased to values of 120 to 200 µg/ml after multiple doses. The mean trough serum value for sulfamethoxazole 24 hours after the first dose was 20 µg/ml. Mean serum half-live values for sulfamethoxazole were 16.5 hours after one dose and 23.3 hours after multiple doses. The half-life values for both drugs are longer in neonates than in older children and adults.

The paucity of information on trimethoprim-sulfamethoxazole in newborns precludes its use in this age group except under extraordinary circumstances, and even then it should be used with great caution. Physicians should be aware of the adverse effects of this compound before its use in neonates and in pregnant or nursing women; large concentrations are found in amniotic fluid, fetal serum, and breast milk after administration to the mother.[451]

The drug combination is available only at a fixed trimethoprim:sulfamethoxazole ratio of 1:5. One suggested dosage schedule is to give an initial loading dose consisting of 2 mg/kg of trimethoprim and 10 mg/kg of sulfamethoxazole.[450] This can then be followed by maintenance doses of 0.6 mg/kg of trimethoprim and 3 mg/kg of sulfamethoxazole given every 12 hours.

MACROLIDES

The macrolide antimicrobial agents that have been used in neonates include erythromycin and spiramycin. Although the lincomycins (e.g., clindamycin) are not macrolides, they are included in this section because of similarities in their antibacterial activities and clinical uses. These drugs were used to treat neonatal staphylococcal infections in the 1950s, when penicillin-resistant staphylococcal strains were prevalent and the penicillinase-resistant penicillins were not yet available. Erythromycin is useful in the young infant for therapy for infections caused by *Chlamydia trachomatis* and *Bordetella pertussis*, spiramycin for toxoplasmosis, and clindamycin for its activity against anaerobes, including *B. fragilis*. The role of the newer macrolides, such as clarithromycin and roxythromycin, and of the azalide azythromycin for treatment of neonatal infections has not yet been defined.

Erythromycin. Erythromycin is primarily a bacteriostatic agent that acts by interfering with protein synthesis through binding to ribosomes of susceptible bacteria and inhibiting the translocation steps.[452] Resistance to the macrolide antibiotics is due to demethylation of adenine in 23S ribosomal RNA, which results in reduced affinity between the antibiotic and the ribosome. Erythromycin is active against most gram-positive bacteria, including many penicillin-resistant strains of staphylococci. In some areas, penicillin-resistant pneumococci are also resistant to the macrolides; the higher the MIC of penicillin for pneumococci, the greater the MIC will be for the macrolides. In addition, most strains of *Neisseria* species, *T. pallidum*, *Mycoplasma pneumoniae*, *Ureaplasma urealyticum*, *B. pertussis*, and *C. trachomatis* are susceptible to this agent. Erythromycin is rarely administered parenterally, owing to the associated tissue damage.

Oral administration of erythromycin estolate to premature infants produced serum concentrations of 1 to 2 µg/ml 3 to 4 hours after a 10-mg/kg dose, and values of 0.5 µg/ml or greater were detected for a minimum of 6 hours.[453] Serum concentrations of erythromycin were independent of birth weight, postnatal age, and gastric acidity. Accumulation of drug in serum did not result from repeated doses every 6 hours for 8 days. Similar pharmacokinetic results have been observed in full-term newborns.[454]

In a comparative pharmacokinetic study of erythromycin estolate and ethylsuccinate, 28 infants younger than 4 months of age, 12 of whom were neonates, were evaluated.[455] The mean peak serum concentrations in infants taking the estolate were slightly greater than those taking the ethylsuccinate: 1.8 µg/ml as opposed to 1.3 µg/ml. During the steady state, the time of the peak serum concentration was achieved in 3.2 hours for the estolate preparation compared with 0.8 hour for the ethylsuccinate form of erythromycin (Fig. 35–2). When analyzed by the two-compartment model of pharmacokinetics, a similar difference was found in the mean absorption and elimination half-life values: 0.72-hour as opposed to 0.3-hour absorption half-life and 6.58 as opposed to 2.2 hours elimination half-life for the estolate and ethylsuccinate, respectively. Thus, 12-hour dosage intervals are appropriate for the estolate.

Erythromycin is excreted in the urine and bile, but only a fraction of the total dose can be accounted for by these two excretory routes. Although erythromycin is uniformly distributed throughout most of the body, concentrations in CSF are small, even in the presence of meningeal inflammation. Drug concentrations in tears 1 hour after the dose were greater than the highest serum concentration measured in 70% of infants, ranging from 2 to 5.4 µg/ml after the ethylsuccinate and from 0.6 to 5 µg/ml after the estolate.[455]

Erythromycin estolate is well tolerated by newborns. Cholestatic jaundice resulting from hypersensitivity to this preparation occurs primarily in teenagers and adults and has not been reported in infants younger than 6 weeks of age.[456] Loose stools as a side effect of erythromycin therapy were noted in about 2.5% of more than 10,000 children evaluated in one study, including 69 neonates.[457] The concomitant administration of erythromycin and theophylline can lead to reduced clearance of the latter drug, with resultant increased risk of theophylline toxicity.[458] Serum theophylline concentrations should, therefore, be monitored in these patients and the dosage reduced if necessary.*

Clindamycin. Clindamycin differs from its parent compound lincomycin in that it is more completely absorbed from the gut, has fewer adverse effects, and has greater antibacterial activity in vitro.[459] Indeed, lincomycin is only of historical interest in the United States. The drug is primarily a bacteriostatic agent that acts by inhibiting protein synthesis through binding to bacterial ribosomes.

Clindamycin is active against gram-positive cocci such as *S. aureus*, *S. pneumoniae* (including many multidrug resistant strains), and *S. pyogenes*. Aerobic gram-negative bacteria are usually not susceptible to this antibiotic. This drug's most notable feature is its activity against anaerobic bacteria, especially members of the *Bacteroides* group.[459] Resistance to clindamycin appears to be related to alterations of its target site and not to reduced uptake or to breakdown of the drug by resistant bacteria.[460]

---

*A recent report of a cluster of cases of pyloric stenosis among infants given erythromycin for prophylaxis after exposure to pertussis has raised concern about usage of erythromycin in neonates and young infants (Centers for Disease Control and Prevention. Hypertrophic pyloric stenosis in infants following pertussis prophylaxis with erythromycin, Knoxville, TN, 1999. Morb Mortal Wkly Rep 48:1117–1120, 1999.)

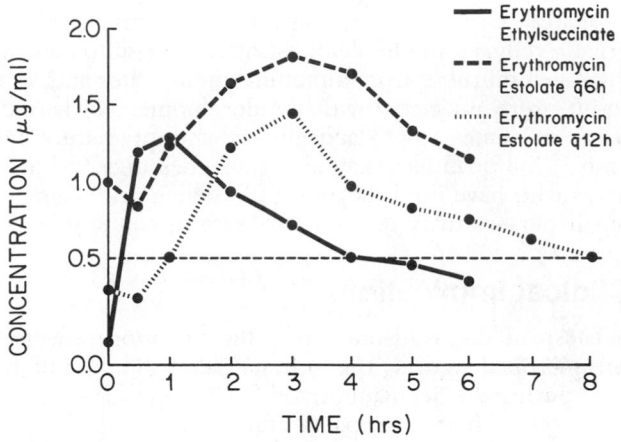

FIGURE 35–2 Serum concentration–time curves after administration of erythromycin ethylsuccinate and estolate to infants under 4 months of age.

Clindamycin administered intravenously at a dosage schedule of 20 mg/kg per day in three or four divided doses to premature and term infants results in mean peak serum concentrations of 11 µg/ml, whereas trough values are from 2.8 to 5.5 µg/ml.[461] The serum elimination half-life is inversely related to gestational age and birth weight. Premature neonates have a mean serum half-life of 8.7 hours compared with 3.6 hours for term newborns.[461] In another study,[462] 12 neonates receiving 3.2 to 11 mg/kg intravenous doses every 6 hours had serum elimination half-lives of from 3.5 to 9.8 hours (mean, 6.3 hours).

Clindamycin penetration into the CSF was once considered poor, but data in experimental meningitis models indicate excellent CSF concentrations after parenteral administration. The drug is primarily eliminated by the liver, with only about 10% excreted in unchanged form in the urine. Adverse effects of clindamycin include diarrhea, rashes, elevated values of hepatic enzymes, granulocytopenia, thrombocytopenia, and Stevens-Johnson syndrome. The most serious and potentially lethal complication is pseudomembranous colitis, but this condition is rare in newborns and young infants even though as many as 50 to 60% of such infants have gastrointestinal colonization with *C. difficile*. This adverse event is also observed with the use of β-lactam and other antimicrobials.

Clinical Implications

With the availability of newer penicillin analogues and vancomycin for treatment of staphylococcal infections, macrolides are no longer recommended for therapy for these infections in neonates. Erythromycin is currently the drug of choice for chlamydial conjunctivitis and pneumonitis as well as for pertussis. The dosage is 10 mg/kg given orally every 12 hours during the first week of life and every 8 hours thereafter. Peak serum concentrations of erythromycin are at least two to three times greater than the MICs reported for *C. trachomatis* (0.5 µg/ml)[463] and severalfold times greater than the MICs for *B. pertussis* (0.04 to 0.78 µg/ml).[452] A possible advantage of the estolate is the persistence for 8 hours or longer of serum drug concentrations that are greater than the MICs of these two organisms. Clindamycin use in newborns should be restricted because as many as 50% of asymptomatic neonates are colonized with *C. difficile*, the presumed etiologic agent of pseudomembranous colitis.[464] However, there is no evidence that *C. difficile* colonization is associated with colitis in newborns. For the rare *B. fragilis* infections in newborns, especially those involving the central nervous system, we prefer the use of either metronidazole or clindamycin, although the latter has been said to have poor penetration into the CSF,[465] and good penetration into brain tissue.[466] Accordingly, clindamycin has been used successfully for therapy for *Toxoplasma* encephalitis in adults with human immunodeficiency virus infections.[467] Whether neonates with congenital toxoplasmosis can be effectively treated with this agent remains undefined. Spiramycin is a macrolide antibiotic commonly used for the treatment of toxoplasmosis worldwide; its use and pharmacokinetic properties are discussed in Chapter 5.

OTHER ANTIBACTERIAL AGENTS

Mupirocin. Mupirocin, a topical antibiotic formerly called pseudomonic acid (derived from fermentation of *Pseudomonas fluorescens*), has been used extensively in recent years to eliminate MRSA carriers and prevent outbreaks of MRSA-infected newborns in several nurseries.[468, 469] Mupirocin interferes with bacterial RNA and protein synthesis by binding to bacterial isoleucyl-transfer RNA synthetase and preventing incorporation of isoleucine into protein chains.[470] Trace amounts absorbed into the systemic circulation are rapidly hydrolyzed, and the inactive metabolite has a plasma half-life of less than 30 minutes.[471] This antibiotic has little cross-resistance with other antimicrobial agents, probably because of its unique mechanism of action. Mupirocin inhibits the growth of staphylococci and streptococci (except enterococci) in low concentrations and is bactericidal in high concentrations readily achieved by topical application.[472] The drug is not active against Enterobacteriaceae, *P. aeruginosa*, or fungi. Emergence of resistant staphylococci has been reported with long-term topical therapy.[473] It is also possible that prolonged use of the drug may result in overgrowth of nonsusceptible organisms, such as fungi. Only local adverse effects such as itching or rash have been reported with mupirocin. Because mupirocin contains a polyethylene glycol vehicle, the possibility of absorption and serious renal toxicity should be kept in mind if the compound is applied to extensive open wounds or skin lesions.[474]

Rifampin. Because of the lack of pharmacokinetic studies in newborns, many potentially useful antimicrobial agents are not discussed in this chapter. For example, rifampin is usually used in other parts of the world for the treatment of congenital tuberculosis. It is possible that with the increasing number of tuberculosis cases seen worldwide amonge patients with acquired immunodeficiency syndrome, this antibiotic will be used more frequently in the future to treat newborns of tuberculosis-affected mothers. Rifampin might also provide a synergistic effect to antistaphylococcal drugs in the therapy

for selected neonates with systemic staphylococcal infections.[475] Italian investigators found mean peak serum rifampin concentrations of 5.8 µg/ml 12 hours after a 10-mg/kg dose was given orally to 18 male term newborns during their first 3 days of life.[476] By contrast, peak values were detected earlier (at 4 hours) and were substantially lower in older infants and children given a similar dosage of rifampin. These investigators proposed not to exceed a dosage of 10 mg/kg daily when rifampin is given orally to term newborn infants.

Metronidazole. Metronidazole is another example of a potentially useful antimicrobial agent that has been poorly evaluated in the neonatal period. This drug has been occasionally used for the treatment of newborns with anaerobic infections, such as necrotizing enterocolitis and *B. fragilis* meningitis. In one study, metronidazole pharmacokinetics were examined in 11 infants varying in gestational age from 28 to 40 weeks and in chronologic age from 0 to 3 days.[477] Elimination half-life was inversely related to gestational age, ranging from 22.5 to 109 hours. To achieve drug concentrations above the MIC required for treatment of anaerobic infections (i.e., 4 to 8 µg/ml), these investigators proposed an initial single intravenous dose of 15 mg/kg, followed 24 hours later in term infants and 48 hours later in preterm neonates by a dosage of 7.5 mg/kg every 12 hours.

Ciprofloxacin. Only case reports on the use of this quinolone in infected neonates have been published.[478–480] No pharmacokinetic studies on ciprofloxacin have been conducted in the neonatal period; therefore, neonatal dosages used have been extrapolated from data generated in older children and adults. Although quinolones have not been approved by the FDA for use in children younger than 18 years of age there are clinical pharmacologic data in many children but very few infants. The potential neonatal indications for parenteral administration of ciprofloxacin include treatment of multiresistant gram-negative infections (species of *Klebsiella*, *Enterobacter*, *Acinetobacter*, *Salmonella*, or *Pseudomonas* resistant to all other antibiotics) and meningitis caused by *Flavobacterium meningosepticum*. In these selected clinical situations dosages of 10 to 40 mg/kg per day, divided every 12 hours, have been used.[478–480]

Ampicillin-Sulbactam. Combination of a β-lactamase inhibitor (i.e., sulbactam or clavulanic acid) with ampicillin or amoxicillin offers the theoretical advantage of expanding the activity of the aminopenicillin against β-lactamase–producing bacteria, such as methicillin-susceptible *S. aureus*, coliform bacilli, and some anaerobes. There is very limited experience with the use of these agents in the neonatal period. Pharmacokinetic data are only available for ampicillin-sulbactam. This latter combination was administered to 16 newborns, 15 preterm infants, and 1 term infant.[481] A dosage of 50 mg/kg of each drug every 12 hours was associated with mean plasma concentrations of 110 µg/ml for sulbactam and 87µg/ml for ampicillin at 3 hours after dosing. Mean elimination half-lives were 7.9 hours for sulbactam and 9.4 hours for ampicillin. There was little evidence of accumulation of either drug, and both were well tolerated. Carefully designed pharmacokinetic studies are needed before this attractive combination can be used in the neonatal period.

TABLE 35–11
Suggested Dosage Schedules for Antibiotics Used in Newborns

		DOSAGE (mg/kg) AND INTERVAL OF ADMINISTRATION				
		Weight <1200 g[a]	Weight 1200–2000 g		Weight >2000 g	
ANTIBIOTICS	ROUTE	Age 0–4 Wk	Age 0–7 Days	Age >7 Days	Age 0–7 Days	Age >7 Days
Amikacin[b]	IV, IM	7.5 q12h	7.5 q12h	7.5 q8h	10 q12h	10 q8h
Ampicillin	IV, IM					
Meningitis		50 q12h	50 q12h	50 q8h	50 q8h	50 q6h
Other infections		25 q12h	25 q12h	25 q8h	25 q8h	25 q6h
Aztreonam	IV, IM	30 q12h	30 q12h	30 q8h	30 q8h	30 q6h
Cefazolin	IV, IM	20 q12h	20 q12h	20 q12h	20 q12h	20 q8h
Cefotaxime	IV, IM	50 q12h	50 q12h	50 q8h	50 q8h	50 q8h
Ceftazidime	IV, IM	50 q12h	50 q12h	50 q8h	50 q8h	50 q8h
Ceftriaxone	IV, IM	50 q24h	50 q24h	50 q24h	50 q24h	75 q24h
Cephalothin	IV	20 q12h	20 q12h	20 q8h	20 q8h	20 q6h
Chloramphenicol[b]	IV, PO	25 q24h	25 q24h	25 q24h	25 q24h	25 q12h
Ciprofloxacin[c]	IV	–	–	10–20 q24h	–	20–30 q12h
Clindamycin	IV, IM, PO	5 q12h	5 q12h	5 q8h	5 q8h	5 q6h
Erythromycin	PO	10 q12h	10 q12h	10 q8h	10 q12h	10 q8h
Gentamicin[b]	IV, IM	2.5 q18h	2.5 q12h	2.5 q8h	2.5 q12h	2.5 q8h
Imipenem	IV, IM	–	20 q12h	20 q12h	20 q12h	20 q8h
Methicillin	IV, IM					
Meningitis		50 q12h	50 q12h	50 q8h	50 q8h	50 q6h
Other infections		25 q12h	25 q12h	25 q8h	25 q8h	25 q6h
Metronidazole[d]	IV, PO	7.5 q48h	7.5 q24h	7.5 q12h	7.5 q12h	15 q12h
Mezlocillin	IV, IM	75 q12h	75 q12h	75 q8h	75 q12h	75 q8h
Meropenem[e]	IV, IM	–	20 q12h	20 q12h	20 q12h	20 q8h
Nafcillin	IV	25 q12h	25 q12h	25 q8h	25 q8h	37.5 q6h
Netilmicin[b]	IV, IM	2.5 q18h	2.5 q12h	2.5 q8h	2.5 q12h	2.5 q8h
Oxacillin	IV, IM	25 q12h	25 q12h	25 q8h	25 q8h	37.5 q6h
Penicillin G (units)	IV					
Meningitis		50,000 q12h	50,000 q12h	50,000 q8h	50,000 q8h	50,000 q6h
Other infections		25,000 q12h	25,000 q12h	25,000 q8h	25,000 q8h	25,000 q6h
Penicillin benzathine (units)	IM	–	50,000 (one dose)	50,000 (one dose)	50,000 (one dose)	50,000 (one dose)
Penicillin procaine (units)	IM		50,000 q24h	50,000 q24h	50,000 q24h	50,000 q24h
Piperacillin	IV, IM	–	50–75 q12h	50–75 q8h	50–75 q8h	50–75 q6h
Rifampin	PO, IV	–	10 q24h	10 q24h	10 q24h	10 q24h
Ticarcillin	IV, IM	75 q12h	75 q12h	75 q8h	75 q8h	75 q6h
Tobramycin[b]	IV, IM	2.5 q18h	2 q12h	2 q8h	2 q12h	2 q8h
Vancomycin[b]	IV	15 q24h	10 q12h	10 q12h	10 q8h	10 q8h

[a]Data from reference 482.
[b]Appropriate dosage schedule should be based on serum concentration measurements.
[c]Doses suggested based on anecdotic clinical experience.
[d]A loading intravenous dose of 15 mg/kg followed 24 hr later (term infants) and 48 hr later (preterm infants) by 7.5 mg/kg every 12 hr has been suggested by other investigators.[477]
[e]Dosages of meropenem suggested are the same as those of imipenem.
IM = intramuscular; IV = intravenous; PO = oral.

DOSAGE SCHEDULES FOR ANTIBIOTICS COMMONLY USED IN NEONATES

Dosage schedules for antibacterial agents commonly prescribed for the treatment of neonatal bacterial infections are presented in Table 35–11. For some drugs, the appropriate dosage schedules following initial doses should be based on measurement of serum concentrations.

References

1. Roberts RJ. Drug Therapy in Infants: Pharmacologic Principles and Clinical Experience. Philadelphia, WB Saunders, 1984, p 3.
2. Huang NN, High RH. Comparision of serum levels following the administration of oral and parenteral preparations of penicillin to infants and children of various age groups. J Pediatr 42:657, 1953.
3. Weiss CF, Glazko AJ, Weston JK. Chloramphenicol in the newborn infant: a physiologic explanation of its toxicity when given in doses. N Engl J Med 262:787, 1960.
4. Kauffman RE, Thirumoorthi MC, Buckley JA, et al. Relative bioavailability of intravenous chloramphenicol succinate and oral chloramphenicol palmitate in infants and children. J Pediatr 99:963, 1981.
5. Shankaran S, Kauffman RE. Use of chloramphenicol palmitate in neonates. J Pediatr 105:113, 1984.
6. Boccazzi A, Rizzo M, Caccamo ML, et al. Comparison of the concentrations of ceftazidime in the serum of newborn infants after intravenous and intramuscular administration. Antimicrob Agents Chemother 24:955, 1983.
7. Mulhall A. Antibiotic treatment of neonates—does route of administration matter? Dev Pharmacol Ther 8:1, 1985.
8. Ristuccia AM. Chloramphenicol: clinical pharmacology in pediatrics. Ther Drug Monit 7:159, 1985.
9. Beutler E. Drug-induced hemolytic anemia. Pharmacol Rev 21:73, 1969.
10. Friis-Hansen B. Body water compartments in children: changes during growth and related changes in body composition. Pediatrics 28:169, 1961.
11. McCracken GH Jr. Clinical pharmacology of gentamicin in infants 2 to 24 months of age. Am J Dis Child 124:884, 1972.
12. Wise R. The clinical relevances of protein binding and tissue concentrations in antimicrobial therapy. Clin Pharmacol 11:463, 1977.
13. Kurz H, Mauser-Ganshorn A, Stickel HH. Differences in the binding of drugs to plasma proteins from newborn and adult man: I. Eur J Clin Pharmacol 11:463, 1977.
14. Schaad UB, Hayton WL, Stoeckel K. Single-dose certriaxone kinetics in the newborn. Clin Pharmacol Ther 37:522, 1985.
15. Silverman WA, Andersen DH, Blanc WA, et al. A difference in mortality rate and incidence of kernicterus among premature infants allotted to two prophylactic antibacterial regimens. Pediatrics 18:614, 1956.
16. Brodersen R, Friis-Hansen B, Stern L. Drug-induced displacement of bilirubin from albumin in the newborn. Dev Pharmacol Ther 6:217, 1983.
17. Cashore WJ, Oh W, Brodersen R. Bilirubin-displacing effect of furosemide and sulfisoxazole: an in vitro and in vivo study in neonatal serum. Dev Pharmacol Ther 6:230, 1983.
18. Stutman HR, Parker KM, Marks MI. Potential of moxalactam and other new antimicrobial agents for bilirubin-albumin displacement in neonates. Pediatrics 75:294, 1985.
19. Gulian JM, Gonard V, Dalmasso C, et al. Bilirubin displacement by ceftriaxone in neonates: evaluation by determination of "free" bilirubin and erythrocyte-bound bilirubin. J Antimicrob Chemother 19:823, 1987.
20. Brodersen R, Ebbesen F. Bilirubin-displacing effect of ampicillin, indomethacin, chlorpromazine, gentamicin, and parabens in vitro and in newborn infants. J Pharm Sci 72:248, 1983.
21. Sakamoto H, Murakawa T, Hirose T, et al. Effect of ceftizoxime, a new cephalosporin antibiotic, on binding of bilirubin to human serum albumin. Chemotherapy 29:244, 1983.
22. Walker PC. Neonatal bilirubin toxicity: a review of kernicterus and the implications of drug-induced bilirubin displacement. Clin Pharmacokinet 13:26, 1987.
23. Robertson A, Fink S, Karp W. Effect of cephalosporins on bilirubin-albumin binding. J Pediatr 112:291, 1988.
24. Guignard JP. Drugs and the neonatal kidney. Dev Pharmacol Ther 4(Suppl 1):19, 1982.
25. Myers MG, Roberts RJ, Mirhij NJ. Effects of gestational age, birth weight, and hypoxemia on pharmacokinetics of amikacin in serum in infants. Antimicrob Agents Chemother 11:1027, 1977.
26. Handwerger S, Tomasz A. Antibiotic tolerance among clinical isolates of bacteria. Rev Infect Dis 7:368, 1985.
27. Moellering RC Jr. Rationale for use of antimicrobial combinations. Am J Med 75(Suppl 2A):4, 1983.
28. Giamarellou H. Aminoglycosides plus beta-lactams against gram negative organisms: evaluation of in vitro synergy and chemical interactions. Am J Med 80(Suppl. 6B):126, 1982.
29. Holm SE. Interactions between β-lactam and other antibiotics. Rev Infect Dis 8:S305, 1986.
30. Schauf V, Deveikis A, Riff L, et al. Antibiotic-killing kinetics of group B streptococci. J Pediatr 89:194, 1976.
31. Cooper MD, Keeney RE, Lyons SF, et al. Synergistic effects of ampicillin-aminoglycoside combinations on group B streptococci. Antimicrob Agents Chemother 15:484, 1979.
32. Scheld WM, Alliegro GM, Field MR, et al. Synergy between ampicillin and gentamicin in experimental meningitis due to group B streptococci. J Infect Dis 146:100, 1982.
33. Calderwood SA, Wennersten CBG, Moellering RC, et al. Resistance to six aminoglycosidic aminocyclitol antibiotics among enterococci: prevalence, evolution, and relationship to synergism with penicillin. Antimicrob Agents Chemother 12:401, 1977.
34. Scheld WM, Fletcher DD, Fink FN, et al. Response to therapy in an experimental rabbit model of meningitis due to Listeria monocytogenes. J Infect Dis 140:287, 1979.
35. Kaplan JM, McCracken GH Jr, Horton LJ, et al. Pharmacologic studies in neonates given large dosages of ampicillin. J Pediatr 84:571, 1974.
36. Watanakunakorn C, Glotzbecker C. Enhancement of the effects of antistaphylococcal antibiotics by aminoglycosides. Antimicrob Agents Chemother 6:802, 1974.
37. McCracken GH Jr, Nelson JD, Thomas ML. Discrepancy between carbenicillin and ampicillin activities against enterococci and Listeria. Antimicrob Agents Chemother 3:343, 1973.
38. Levy RH, Bauer LA. Basic pharmacokinetics. Ther Drug Monit 8:47, 1986.

39. Schentag JJ, Jusko WJ, Plaut ME, et al. Tissue persistence of gentamicin in man. JAMA 238:327, 1977.

40. Siegel JD, McCracken GH Jr, Nelson JD. Pharmacokinetic properties of netilmicin in newborn infants. Antimicrob Agents Chemother 15:246, 1979.

41. Schaad UB, McCracken GH Jr, Nelson JD. Clinical pharmacology and efficacy of vancomycin in pediatric patients. J Pediatr 96:119, 1980.

42. Haughey DB, Hilligoss DM, Grassi A, et al. Two-compartment gentamicin pharmacokinetics in premature neonates: a comparison to adults with decreased glomerular filtration rates. J Pediatr 96:325, 1980.

43. Schaad UB, McCracken GH Jr, Loock CA, et al. Pharmacokinetics and bacteriological efficacy of moxalactam (LY127935), netilmicin, and ampicillin in experimental gram-negative enteric bacillary meningitis. Antimicrob Agents Chemother 17:406, 1980.

44. Odio C, Thomas ML, McCracken GH Jr. Pharmacokinetics and bacteriological efficacy of mezlocillin in experimental Escherichia coli and Listeria monocytogenes meningitis. Antimicrob Agents Chemother 25:427, 1984.

45. McCracken GH Jr, Sakata Y, Olsen KD. Aztreonam therapy in experimental meningitis due to Haemophilus influenzae type b and Escherichia coli K1. Antimicrob Agents Chemother 27:655, 1985.

46. Jacobs MR, Myers C. Diagnostic microbiology and therapeutic drug monitoring in pediatric infectious diseases. Pediatr Clin North Am 30:135, 1983.

47. Doering PL, Stewart RB. The extent and character of drug consumption during pregnancy. JAMA 239:843, 1978.

48. Brocklebank JC, Ray WA, Federspiel CF, et al. Drug prescribing during pregnancy: a controlled study of Tennessee Medicaid recipients. Am J Obstet Gynecol 132:235, 1978.

49. Philipson A. The use of antibiotics in pregnancy. J Antimicrob Chemother 12:101, 1983.

50. Tropper PJ, Petrie RH. Placental exchange. In Lavery JP (ed). The Human Placenta: Clinical Perspectives. Rockville, Md., Aspen Publishers, 1987, p 199.

51. Juchau MR, Dyer DC. Pharmacology of the placenta. Pediatr Clin North Am 19:65, 1972.

52. Philipson A, Sabath LD, Charles D. Transplacental passage of erythromycin and clindamycin. N Engl J Med 288:1219, 1973.

53. Bernard B, Abate M, Thielen PF, et al. Maternal-fetal pharmacological activity of amikacin. J Infect Dis 135:925, 1977.

54. Bernard B, García-Cázares SJ, Ballard CA, et al. Tobramycin: maternal-fetal pharmacology. Antimicrob Agents Chemother 11:688, 1977.

55. Matsuda S, Mori S, Tanno M, et al. Evaluation of amikacin in obstetric and gynecological field. Jpn J Antibiot 27:633, 1974.

56. Buckingham M, Welply G, Miller JF, et al. Gastrointestinal absorption and transplacental transfer of amoxicillin during labour and the influence of metoclopramide. Curr Med Res Opin 3:392, 1975.

57. Nau H. Clinical pharmacokinetics in pregnancy and perinatology: II. Penicillins. Dev Pharmacol Ther 10:174, 1987.

58. Kafetzis DA, Brater DC, Fanourgakis JE. Materno-fetal transfer of azlocillin. J Antimicrob Chemother 12:157, 1983.

59. Charles D, Larsen B. Placental transfer of antibiotics. In Ristuccia AM, Cunha BA (eds). Antimicrobial Therapy. New York, Raven Press, 1984, p 519.

60. Bernard B, Barton L, Abate M, et al. Maternal-fetal transfer of cefazolin in the first twenty weeks trimester of pregnancy. J Infect Dis 136:377, 1977.

61. Dekel A, Elian I, Gibor Y, et al. Transplacental passage of cefazolin in the first trimester of pregnancy. Eur J Obstet Gynecol Reprod Biol 10:303, 1980.

62. Cho N, Ito T, Saito T, et al. Clinical studies on cefazolin in the field of obstetrics and gynecology. Chemotherapy 18:770, 1970.

63. Shimizu K. Cefoperazone: absorption, excretion, distribution, and metabolism. Clin Ther 3(Spec. Issue):60, 1980.

64. Briggs GG, Freeman RK, Yaffe SJ. Drugs in Pregnancy and Lactation: A Reference Guide to Fetal and Neonatal Risk, 2nd ed. Baltimore, Williams & Wilkins, 1986.

65. Kafetzis DA, Lazarides CV, Siafas CA, et al. Transfer of cefotaxime in human milk and from mother to foetus. J Antimicrob Chemother 6(Suppl. A):135, 1980.

66. Matsuda S, Tanno M, Kashiwakura T, et al. Laboratory and clinical studies on cefotaxin in the field of obstetric and gynecology. Chemotherapy (Tokyo) 26(Suppl 1):460, 1978.

67. Nankun C, Uerhara K, Sugizaki K, et al. Clinical studies of cefoxitin in the field of obstetrics and gynecology. Chemotherapy (Tokyo) 26(Suppl 1):468, 1978.

68. Bergongne-Berezin E, Morel C, Kafe H, et al. Étude pharmacocinètique chez l'homme de la cefoxitime: diffusion intrabronchique et transplacentaire. Therapie 34:345, 1979.

69. Motomura R, Kohno M, Mori H, et al. Basic and clinical studies of ceftizoxime in obstetrics and gynecology. Chemotherapy (Tokyo) 28(Suppl 5):888, 1980.

70. Kafetzis DA, Brater DC, Fanourgakis JE, et al. Ceftriaxone distribution between maternal blood and fetal blood and tissues at parturition and between blood and milk postpartum. Antimicrob Agents Chemother 23:870, 1983.

71. Craft I, Mullinger BM, Kennedy MRK. Placental transfer of cefuroxime. Br J Obstet Gynaecol 88:141, 1981.

72. Bousfield P, Browning AK, Mullinger BM, et al. Cefuroxime: potential use in pregnant women at term. Br J Obstet Gynaecol 88:146, 1981.

73. Coppi G, Berti MA, Chehade A, et al. A study of the transplacental transfer of cefuroxime in humans. Curr Ther Res 32:712, 1982.

74. Creatsas G, Pavlatos M, Lolis D, et al. A study of the kinetics of cephapirin and cephalexin in pregnancy. Curr Med Res Opin 7:43, 1980.

75. Morrow S, Palmisano P, Cassady G. The placental transfer of cephalothin. J Pediatr 73:262, 1968.

76. Scott WC, Warner RF. Placental transfer of chloramphenicol (Chloromycetin). JAMA 142:1331, 1950.

77. Ross S, Burke FG, Sites J, et al. Placental transmission of chloramphenicol (Chloromycetin). JAMA 142:1361, 1950.

78. Burns LE, Hodgman JE, Cass AB. Fatal circulatory collapse in premature infants receiving chloramphenicol. N Engl J Med 261:1318, 1959.

79. Weinstein AJ, Gibbs RS, Gallagher M. Placental transfer of clindamycin and gentamicin in term pregnancy. Am J Obstet Gynecol 124:688, 1976.

80. Herngren L, Ehrnebo M, Boréus LO. Drug binding to plasma proteins during human pregnancy and in the perinatal period: studies on cloxacillin and alprenolol. Dev Pharmacol Ther 6:110, 1983.

81. MacAulay MA, Charles D. Placental transmission of colistimethate. Clin Pharmacol Ther 8:578, 1967.

82. MacAylay MA, Berg SR, Charles D. Placental transfer of

dicloxacillin at term. Am J Obstet Gynecol 102:1162, 1968.

83. Depp R, Kind AC, Kirby WMM, et al. Transplacental passage of methicillin and dicloxacillin into the fetus and amniotic fluid. Am J Obstet Gynecol 107:1054, 1970.

84. Kiefer L, Rubin A, McCoy JB, et al. The placental transfer of erythromycin. Am J Obstet Gynecol 69:174, 1955.

85. Yoshioka H, Monma T, Matsuda S. Placental transfer of gentamicin. J Pediatr 80:121, 1972.

86. L'Hommedieu CS, Nicholas D, Armes DA, et al. Potentiation of magnesium sulfate–induced neuromuscular weakness by gentamicin, tobramycin, and amikacin. J Pediatr 102:629, 1983.

87. Heikkila A, Renkonen OV, Erkkola R. Pharmacokinetics and transplacental passage of imipenem during pregnancy. Antimicrob Agents Chemother 36:2652, 1992.

88. Good RG, Johnson GH. The placental transfer of kanamycin during late pregnancy. Obstet Gynecol 38:60, 1971.

89. Jones HC. Intrauterine ototoxicity: a case report and review of literature. J Natl Med Assoc 65:201, 1973.

90. Duignan NM, Andrews J, Williams JD. Pharmacological studies with lincomycin in late pregnancy. BMJ (Clin Res) 3:75, 1975.

91. Mickal A, Panzer JD. The safety of lincomycin in pregnancy. Am J Obstet Gynecol 121:1071, 1975.

92. MacAulay MA, Molloy WB, Charles D. Placental transfer of methicillin. Am J Obstet Gynecol 115:58, 1973.

93. Perry JE, LeBlanc AL. Transfer of nitrofurantoin across the human placenta. Tex Rep Biol Med 25:265, 1967.

94. Wasz-Höckert O, Nummi S, Vuopala S, et al. Transplacental passage of azidocillin, ampicillin and penicillin G during early and late pregnancy. Scand J Infect Dis 2:125, 1970.

95. Greene HJ, Hobby GL. Transmission of penicillin through human placenta. Proc Soc Exp Biol Med 57:282, 1944.

96. Woltz JHE, Zintel HA. The transmission of penicillin to amniotic fluid and fetal blood in the human. Am J Obstet Gynecol 50:330, 1945.

97. Woltz JHE, Wiley MM. Transmission of streptomycin from maternal blood to the fetal circulation and the amniotic fluid. Proc Soc Exp Biol Med 60:106, 1945.

98. Conway N, Birt BD. Streptomycin in pregnancy: effect on the foetal ear. BMJ (Clin Res) 2:260, 1965.

99. Donald PR, Sellars SL. Streptomycin ototoxicity in the unborn child. S Afr Med J 60:316, 1981.

100. Speert H. Placental transmission of sulfathiazole and sulfadiazine and its significance for fetal chemotherapy. Am J Obstet Gynecol 45:200, 1943.

101. Ziai M, Finland M. Placental transfer of sulfamethoxypyridazine. N Engl J Med 257:1180, 1957.

102. Sparr RA, Pritchard JA. Maternal and newborn distribution and excretion of sulfamethoxypyridazine (Kynex). Obstet Gynecol 12:131, 1958.

103. Kantor HI, Sutherland DA, Leonard JT, et al. Effect on bilirubin metabolism in the newborn of sulfisoxazole administered to the mother. Obstet Gynecol 17:494, 1961.

104. Brown AK, Cevik N. Hemolysis and jaundice in the newborn following maternal treatment with sulfamethoxypyridazine (Kynex). Pediatrics 36:742, 1965.

105. Perkins RP. Hydrops fetalis and stillbirth in a male glucose-6-phosphate dehydrogenase–deficient fetus possibly due to maternal ingestion of sulfisoxazole: a case report. Am J Obstet Gynecol 111:379, 1971.

106. Azad Khan AK, Truelove SC. Placental and mammary transfer of sulphasalazine. BMJ (Clin Res) 2:1553, 1979.

107. Esbjörner E, Järnerot G, Wranne, L. Sulphasalazine and sulphapyridine serum levels in children to mothers treated with sulphasalazine during pregnancy and lactation. Acta Paediatr Scand 76:137, 1963.

108. Cohlan SQ, Bevelander G, Tiamsic T. Growth inhibition of prematures receiving tetracycline: a clinical and laboratory investigation of tetracycline-induced bone fluorescence. Am J Dis Child 105:453, 1963.

109. Kline AH, Blattner RJ, Lunin M. Transplacental effect of tetracyclines on teeth. JAMA 188:178, 1964.

110. Kutscher AH, Zegarelli EV, Tovell HMM, et al. Discoloration of deciduous teeth induced by administration of tetracycline antepartum. Am J Obstet Gynecol 96:291, 1966.

111. LeBlanc AL, Perry JE. Transfer of tetracycline across the human placenta. Tex Rep Biol Med 25:541, 1967.

112. McEwen LM. Trimethoprim/sulphamethoxazole mixture in pregnancy. BMJ (Clin Res) 4:490, 1971.

113. Reid DWJ, Caillè G, Kauffman NR. Maternal and transplacental kinetics of trimethoprim and sulfamethoxazole separately and in combination. Can Med Assoc J 112:67S, 1975.

114. Philipson A. Pharmacokinetics of antibiotics in pregnancy and labour. Clin Pharmacokinet 4:297, 1979.

115. Mucklow JC. The fate of drugs in pregnancy. Clin Obstet Gynaecol 13:161, 1986.

116. Apgar V. Drugs in pregnancy. JAMA 190:840, 1964.

117. Sutherland JM, Light IJ. The effect of drugs upon the developing fetus. Pediatr Clin North Am 12:781, 1965.

118. Totterman LE, Saxen L. Incorporation of tetracycline into human fetal bones after maternal drug administration. Acta Obstet Gynecol Scand 48:542, 1969.

119. Lumbiganon P, Pengsaa K, Sookpranee T. Ciprofloxacin in neonates and its possible adverse effect on the teeth. Pediatr Infect Dis J 10:619, 1991.

120. Krasinski K, Perkin R, Rutledge J. Gray baby syndrome revisited. Clin Pediatr 21:571, 1982.

121. Boyer KM, Gottof SP. Prevention of early-onset neonatal group B streptococcal disease with selective intrapartum chemoprophylaxis. N Engl J Med 314:1665, 1986.

122. Teres FO, Matorras R, Perea AG, et al. Prevention of neonatal group B streptococcal sepsis. Pediatr Infect Dis J 6:874, 1987.

123. Yow MD, Mason EO, Leeds LJ, et al. Ampicillin prevents intrapartum transmission of group B *Streptococcus*. JAMA 241:1245, 1979.

124. Lewis PJ. Antibiotics and breast feeding. Clin Exp Obstet Gynecol 13:124, 1986.

125. Rivera-Calimlim L. The significance of drugs in breast milk: pharmacokinetic considerations. Clin Perinatol 14:51, 1987.

126. Wilson JT, Brown RD, Cherek DR, et al. Drug excretion in human breast milk: principles, pharmacokinetics and projected consequences. Clin Pharmacokinet 5:1, 1980.

127. Kafetzis DA, Siafas CA, Georgakopoulos PA, et al. Passage of cephalosporins and amoxicillin into the breast milk. Acta Paediatr Scand 70:285, 1981.

128. Fleiss PM, Richwald GA, Gordon J, et al. Aztreonam in human serum and breast milk. Br J Clin Pharmacol 19:509, 1985.

129. O'Brien TE. Excretion of drugs in human milk. Am J Hosp Pharm 31:844, 1974.

130. Gerding DN, Peterson LR, Hughes CE, et al. Extravascular antimicrobial distribution in man. *In* Lorian V (ed). Antibiotics in Laboratory Medicine, 2nd ed. Baltimore, Williams & Wilkins, 1986, p 960.

131. Dubois M, Delapierre D, Chanteux L, et al. A study of the transplacental transfer and the mammary excretion of cefoxitin in humans. J Clin Pharmacol 21:477, 1981.

132. Dresse A, Lambotte R, Dubois M, et al. Transmammary passage of cefoxitin: additional results. J Clin Pharmacol 23:438, 1983.

133. Blanco JD, Jorgensen JH, Castaneda YS, et al. Ceftazidime levels in human breast milk. Antimicrob Agents Chemother 23:479, 1983.

134. Gerding DN, Peterson LR. Comparative tissue and extravascular fluid concentrations of ceftizoxime. J Antimicrob Chemother 10(Suppl C):105, 1982.

135. Knowles JA. Excretion of drugs in milk—a review. J Pediatr 66:1068, 1965.

136. Steen B, Rane A. Clindamycin passage into human milk. Br J Clin Pharmacol 13:661, 1982.

137. Chyo N, Sunada H, Nohara S. Clinical studies of kanamycin applied in the field of obstetrics and gynecology. Asian Med J 5:265, 1962.

138. Singlas E. Tissue distribution of mezlocillin. Nouv Presse Med 11:373, 1982.

139. Varsano I, Fischl J, Shochet SB. The excretion of orally ingested nitrofurantoin in human milk. J Pediatr 82:886, 1973.

140. Greene HJ, Burkhart B, Hobby GL. Excretion of penicillin in human milk following parturition. Am J Obstet Gynecol 51:735, 1946.

141. Kauffman RE, O'Brien C, Gilford P. Sulfisoxazole secretion into human milk. J Pediatr 97:839, 1980.

142. von Kobyletzki D, Dalhoff A, Lindemeyer H, et al. Ticarcillin serum and tissue concentrations in gynecology and obstetrics. Infection 11:144, 1983.

143. Takase Z, Shirafuji H, Uchida M, et al. Laboratory and clinical studies on tobramycin in the field of obstetrics and gynecology. Chemotherapy (Tokyo) 23:1399, 1975.

144. Wilson JT, Brown RD, Hinson JL, et al. Pharmacokinetic pitfalls in the estimation of the breast milk/plasma ratio for drugs. Annu Rev Pharmacol Toxicol 25:667, 1985.

145. Catz CS, Giacoia GP. Drugs and breast milk. Pediatr Clin North Am 19:151, 1972.

146. American Academy of Pediatrics, Committee on Drugs. The transfer of drugs and other chemicals into human breast milk. Pediatrics 93:137, 1994.

147. Mann CF. Clindamycin and breast-feeding. Pediatrics 66:1030, 1980.

148. Neu HC. Penicillins. In Mandell GL, Douglas RG Jr, Bennett JE (eds). Principles and Practice of Infectious Diseases, 2nd ed. New York, John Wiley, 1985, p 166.

149. Neu HC. Contribution of beta-lactamases to bacterial resistance and mechanisms to inhibit beta-lactamases. Am J Med 79(Suppl 5B):2, 1985.

150. Nayler JHC. Resistance to β-lactams in gram-negative bacteria: relative contributions of β-lactamase and permeability limitations. J Antimicrob Chemother 19:713, 1987.

151. Tuomanen E, Durack DT, Tomasz A. Antibiotic tolerance among clinical isolates of bacteria. Antimicrob Agents Chemother 30:521, 1986.

152. Siegel JD, Shannon KM, DePasse BM. Recurrent infection associated with penicillin-tolerant group B streptococci: a report of two cases. J Pediatr 99:920, 1981.

153. Leggiadro RJ. Penicillin- and cephalosporin-resistant Streptococcus pneumoniae: an emerging microbial threat. Pediatrics 93:500, 1994.

154. Friedland IR, McCracken GH Jr. Management of infections caused by antibiotic-resistant Streptococcus pneumoniae. N Engl J Med 331:377, 1994.

155. McCracken GH Jr, Ginsberg C, Chrane DF, et al. Clinical pharmacology of penicillin in newborn infants. J Pediatr 82:692, 1973.

156. Kaplan JM, McCracken GH Jr. Clinical pharmacology of benzathine penicillin G in neonates with regard to its recommended use in congenital syphilis. J Pediatr 82:1069, 1973.

157. Klein JO, Scharberg MJ, Buntin M, et al. Levels of penicillin in serum of newborn infants after single intramuscular doses of benzathine penicillin G. J Pediatr 82:1065, 1973.

158. Hieber JP, Nelson JD. A pharmacologic evaluation of penicillin in children with purulent meningitis. N Engl J Med 297:410, 1977.

159. Speer ME, Taber LH, Clark DB, et al. Cerebrospinal fluid levels of benzathine penicillin G in the neonate. J Pediatr 91:996, 1977.

160. McCracken GH Jr, Kaplan JM. Penicillin treatment for congenital syphilis: a critical reappraisal. JAMA 228:855, 1974.

161. Speer ME, Mason EO, Scharnberg JT. Cerebrospinal fluid concentrations of aqueous procaine penicillin G in the neonate. Pediatrics 67:387, 1981.

162. Levin B, Neill CA. Oral penicillin in the newborn. Arch Dis Child 24:171, 1949.

163. McCracken GH Jr, Nelson JD. Antimicrobial Therapy for Newborns, 2nd ed. New York, Grune & Stratton, 1983.

164. Centers for Disease Control and Prevention. STD Treatment Guidelines. Atlanta, Centers for Disease Control, 1985.

165. McCracken GH, Mize SG, Threlkeld N. Intraventricular gentamicin therapy in gram-negative bacillary meningitis of infancy: report of the Second Neonatal Meningitis Cooperative Study Group. Lancet 1:787, 1980.

166. Joseph TA, Pyati SP, Jacobs N. Neonatal early-onset Escherichia coli disease: the effect of intrapartum ampicillin. Arch Pediatr Adolesc Med 152:35, 1998

167. Grossman M, Ticknor W. Serum levels of ampicillin, cephalothin, cloxacillin, and nafcillin in the newborn infant. In Hobby GL (ed). Antimicrobial Agents and Chemotherapy. Washington, DC, American Society for Microbiology, 1965, p 214.

168. Axline SG, Yaffe SJ, Simon HJ. Clinical pharmacology of antimicrobials in premature infants: II. Ampicillin, methicillin, oxacillin, neomycin, and colistin. Pediatrics 39:97, 1967.

169. Boe RW, Williams CPS, Bennett JV, et al. Serum levels of methicillin and ampicillin in newborn and premature infants in relation to postnatal age. Pediatrics 39:194, 1967.

170. Dahl LB, Melby K, Gutteberg TJ, et al. Serum levels of ampicillin and gentamycin in neonates of varying gestational age. Eur J Pediatr 145:218, 1986.

171. Silverio J, Poole JW. Serum concentrations of ampicillin in newborn infants after oral administration. Pediatrics 51:578, 1973.

172. McCracken GH Jr, Ginsburg CM, Clahsen JC, et al. Pharmacologic evaluation of orally administered antibiotics in infants and children: effect of feeding on bioavailability. Pediatrics 62:738, 1978.

173. Bass JW, Crowley DM, Steele RW, et al. Adverse effects of orally administered ampicillin. J Pediatr 83:106, 1973.

174. Tetzlaff TR, Ashwoth C, Nelson JD. Otitis media in children less than 12 weeks of age. Pediatrics 59:827, 1977.

175. Neu HC. Antistaphylococcal penicillins. Med Clin North Am 66:51, 1982.

176. Utsui Y, Yokota T. Role of an altered penicillin-binding protein in methicillin- and cephem-resistant *Staphylococcus aureus*. Antimicrob Agents Chemother 28:397, 1985.

177. Shanson DC, Johnstone D, Midgley J. Control of a hospital outbreak of methicillin-resistant *Staphylococcus aureus* infections: value of an isolation unit. J Hosp Infect 6:285, 1985.

178. Sabath LD, Wheeler N, Laverdiere M, et al. A new type of penicillin resistance of *Staphylococcus aureus*. Lancet 1:443, 1977.

179. Sarff LD, McCracken GH Jr, Thomas ML, et al. Clinical pharmacology of methicillin in neonates. J Pediatr 90:1005, 1977.

180. O'Connor WJ, Warren GH, Mandala PS, et al. Serum concentrations of nafcillin in newborn infants and children. *In* Sylvester JC (ed). Antimicrobial Agents and Chemotherapy. Washington, DC, American Society for Microbiology, 1964, p 188.

181. Banner W Jr, Gooch WM III, Burckart G, et al. Pharmacokinetics of nafcillin in infants with low birth weights. Antimicrob Agents Chemother 17:691, 1980.

182. O'Connor WJ, Warren GH, Edrada LS, et al. Serum concentrations of sodium nafcillin in infants during the perinatal period. *In* Hobby GL (ed). Antimicrobial Agents and Chemotherapy. Washington, DC, American Society for Microbiology, 1965, p 220.

183. Burns LE, Hodgman JE, Wehrle PF. Treatment of premature infants with oxacillin. *In* Sylvester JC (ed). Antimicrobial Agents and Chemotherapy. Washington DC, American Society for Microbiology, 1964, p 192.

184. Sarff LD, McCracken GH Jr. Methicillin-associated nephropathy or cystitis. J Pediatr 90:1031, 1977.

185. Kitzing W, Nelson JD, Mohs E. Comparative toxicities of methicillin and nafcillin. Am J Dis Child 135:52, 1981.

186. Greene GR, Cohen E. Nafcillin-induced neutropenia in children. Pediatrics 61:94, 1978.

187. Nahata MV, DeBolt SL, Powell DA. Adverse effects of methicillin, nafcillin and oxacillin in pediatric patients. Dev Pharmacol Ther 4:117, 1982.

188. Mallouh AA. Methicillin-induced neutropenia. Pediatr Infect Dis 4:262, 1985.

189. Neu HC. Carbenicillin and ticarcillin. Med Clin North Am 66:61, 1982.

190. Nelson JD, McCracken GH Jr. Clinical pharmacology of carbenicillin and gentamicin in the neonate and comparative efficacy with ampicillin and gentamicin. Pediatrics 52:801, 1973.

191. Morehead CD, Shelton S, Kusmiesz H, et al. Pharmacokinetics of carbenicillin in neonates of normal and low birth weight. Antimicrob Agents Chemother 2:267, 1972.

192. Yoshioka H, Takimoto M, Shimizu T, et al. Pharmacokinetics of intramuscular carbenicillin in the newborn. Infection 7:27, 1979.

193. Nelson JD, Kusmiesz H, Shelton S, et al. Clinical pharmacology and efficacy of ticarcillin in infants and children. Pediatrics 61:858, 1978.

194. Nelson JD, Shelton S, Kusmiesz H. Clinical pharmacology of ticarcillin in the newborn infant: relation to age, gestational age, and weight. J Pediatr 87:474, 1975.

195. Sutherland R, Beale AS, Boon RJ, et al. Antibacterial activity of ticarcillin in the presence of clavulanate potassium. Am J Med 79(Suppl 5B):13, 1985.

196. Pulverer G, Peters G, Kunstmann G. In-vitro activity of ticarcillin with and without clavulanic acid against clinical isolates of gram-positive and gram-negative bacteria. J Antimicrob Chemother 17(Suppl C):1, 1986.

197. Gould IM, Wise R. β-Lactamase inhibitors. *In* Peterson PK, Verhoef J (eds). The Antimicrobial Agents Annual 1. Amsterdam, Elsevier, 1986, p 51.

198. Bèguè P, Quiniou F, Quinet B. Efficacy and pharmacokinetics of Timentin in paediatric infections. J Antimicrob Chemother 17(Suppl):81, 1986.

199. Eliopoulos GM, Moellering RC Jr. Azlocillin, mezlocillin, and piperacillin: new broad-spectrum penicillins. Ann Intern Med 97:755, 1982.

200. Drusano GL, Schimpff SC, Hewitt WL. The acylampicillins: mezlocillin, piperacillin, and azlocillin. Rev Infect Dis 6:13, 1984.

201. Allan JD, Eliopoulos GM, Moellering RC Jr. The expanding spectrum of beta-lactam antibiotics. Adv Intern Med 31:119, 1986.

202. Moody JA, Peterson LR, Gerding DN. In vitro activities of ureidopenicillins alone and in combination with amikacin and three cephalosporin antibiotics. Antimicrob Agents Chemother 26:256, 1984.

203. Heimann G, Föster D. Pharmacokinetics of acylureidopenicillins (azlocillin, mezlocillin) in prematures and newborns. Drugs Exp Clin Res 7:287, 1981.

204. Rubio T, Wirth F, Karotkin E. Pharmacokinetic studies of mezlocillin in newborn infants. J Antimicrob Chemother 9(Suppl A):241, 1982.

205. Janicke DM, Rubio TT, Wirth FH Jr, et al. Developmental pharmacokinetics of mezlocillin in newborn infants. J Pediatr 104:773, 1984.

206. Odio C, Threlkeld N, Thomas ML, et al. Pharmacokinetics properties of mezlocillin in newborn infants. Antimicrob Agents Chemother 25:556, 1984.

207. Chiu T, Garrison RD, Fakhreddine F, et al. Mezlocillin in neonatal infections: evaluation of efficacy and toxicity. J Antimicrob Chemother 9(Suppl A):251, 1982.

208. Weingärtner L. Clinical aspects of mezlocillin therapy in childhood. J Antimicrob Chemother 9(Suppl A):257, 1982.

209. Bergan T. Review of the pharmacokinetics of mezlocillin. J Antimicrob Chemother 11(Suppl C):1, 1983.

210. Heimann G. Pharmacokinetics and clinical aspects of azlocillin in paediatrics. J Antimicrob Chemother 11(Suppl B):127, 1983.

211. Bergan T. Review of the pharmacokinetics and dose dependency of azlocillin in normal subjects and patients with renal insufficiency. J Antimicrob Chemother 11(Suppl B):101, 1983.

212. Placzek M, Whitelaw A, Want S, et al. Piperacillin in early neonatal infection. Arch Dis Child 58:1006, 1983.

213. Thirumoorthi MC, Asmar BI, Buckley JA, et al. Pharmacokinetics of intravenously administered piperacillin in preadolescent children. J Pediatr 102:941, 1983.

214. Kacet N, Roussel-DelVallez M, Gremillet C, et al. Pharmacokinetic study of piperacillin in newborns relating to gestational and postnatal age. Pediatr Infect Dis J 11:365, 1992.

215. Wilson CB, Koup JR, Opheim KE, et al. Piperacillin pharmacokinetics in pediatric patients. Antimicrob Agents Chemother 22:442, 1982.

216. Johnson GJ. Antibiotic-induced hemostatic abnormalities. *In* Peterson PK, Verhoef J (eds). The Antimicrobial Agents Annual 1. Amsterdam, Elsevier, 1986, p 408.

217. Bertino JS Jr, Speck WT. The cephalosporin antibiotics. Pediatr Clin North Am 30:17, 1983.

218. Eichenwald HF. Antimicrobial therapy in infants and children: update 1976–1985: I. J Pediatr 107:161, 1985.

219. Nelson JD. Cefuroxime: a cephalosporin with unique applicability to pediatric practice. Pediatr Infect Dis J 2:394, 1983.

220. Garau J. The clinical potential of fourth-generation cephalosporins. Diagn Microbiol Infect Dis 31:479, 1998.

221. Milatovic D, Braveny I. Development of resistance during antibiotic therapy. Eur J Clin Microbiol 6:234, 1987.

222. Sanders CC, Sanders WE Jr. The cephalosporins and cephamycins. *In* Peterson PK, Verhoef J (eds). The Antimicrobial Agents Annual 2. Amsterdam, Elsevier, 1987, p 70.

223. Sheng KT, Huang NN, Promadhattaveddi V. Serum concentrations of cephalothin in infants and children and placental transmission of the antibiotic. *In* Sylvester JC (ed). Antimicrobial Agents and Chemotherapy. Washington, DC, American Society for Microbiology, 1964, p 200.

224. Sakata Y. The pharmacokinetic studies of cephalothin, cefazolin and cefmetazole in the neonates and the premature babies. Kurume Med J 27:275, 1980.

225. Hallberg T, Svenningsen NW. Cephalothin in neonatal infections. Acta Paediatr Scand 206(Suppl):110, 1970.

226. Plaisance KI, Nightingale CH, Quintiliani R. Pharmacology of the cephalosporins. *In* Queener SF, Webber JA, Queener SW (eds). Beta-Lactam Antibiotics for Clinical Use. New York, Marcel Dekker, 1986, p 285.

227. Cho (Chang) N, Ito T, Saito H, et al. Studies on cefazolin in obstetrics and gynecology with special reference to its clinical pharmacology in the neonate. *In* Hejzlar M, Semonsky M, Masák S (eds). Advances in Antimicrobial and Antineoplastic Chemotherapy: Progress in Research and Clinical Application, vol 1. Baltimore, University Park Press, 1972, p 1187.

228. Boothman R, Kerr MM, Marshall MJ, et al. Absorption and excretion of cephalexin by the newborn infant. Arch Dis Child 48:147, 1973.

229. Chin KC, Kerr MM, Cockburn F, et al. A pharmacological study of cefaclor in the newborn infant. Curr Med Res Opin 7:168, 1981.

230. McCracken GH Jr, Ginsburg CM, Clahsen JC, et al. Pharmacokinetics of cefaclor in infants and children. J Antimicrob Chemother 4:515, 1978.

231. Renlund M, Pettay O. Pharmacokinetics and clinical efficacy of cefuroxime in the newborn period. Proc R Soc Med 70(Suppl 9):183, 1977.

232. Dash CH, Kennedy MRK, Ng SH. Cefuroxime in the first week of life. *In* Nelson JD, Grassi C (eds). Current Chemotherapy and Infectious Disease: Proceedings of the 11th International Congress of Chemotherapy and the 19th Interscience Conference on Antimicrobial Agents and Chemotherapy. Washington, DC, American Society for Microbiology, 1980, p 1161.

233. de Louvois J, Mulhall A, Hurley R. Cefuroxime in the treatment of neonates. Arch Dis Child 57:59, 1982.

234. Wilkinson PJ, Belohradsky BH, Marget WA. Clinical study of cefuroxime in neonates. Proc R Soc Med 70(Suppl 9):183, 1977.

235. von Hattingberg HM, Marget W, Belohradsky BH, et al. Pharmacokinetics of cefotaxime in neonates and children: clinical aspects. J Antimicrob Chemother 6(Suppl A):113, 1980.

236. Kafetzis DA, Brater DC, Kapiki AN, et al. Treatment of severe neonatal infections with cefotaxime: efficacy and pharmacokinetics. J Pediatr 100:483, 1982.

237. McCracken GH Jr, Threlkeld NE, Thomas ML. Pharmacokinetics of cefotaxime in newborn infants. Antimicrob Agents Chemother 21:683, 1982.

238. de Louvois J, Mulhall A, Hurley R. The safety and pharmacokinetics of cefotaxime in the treatment of neonates. Pediatr Pharmacol 2:275, 1982.

239. Crooks J, White LO, Burville LJ, et al. Pharmacokinetics

240. Bèguè P, Safran C, Quiniou F, et al. Comparative pharmacokinetics of four new cephalosporins: moxalactam, cefotaxime, cefoperazone and ceftazidime in neonates. Dev Pharmacol Ther 7(Suppl 1):105, 1984.

241. Chamberlain J, Coombes JD, Dell D, et al. Metabolism of cefotaxime in animals and man. J Antimicrob Chemother 6(Suppl A):69, 1980.

242. Jones RN, Barry AL, Thornsberry C. Antimicrobial activity of desacetyl-cefotaxime alone and in combination with cefotaxime: evidence of synergy. Rev Infect Dis 4:S366, 1982.

243. von Loewenich V, Miething R, Uihlein M, et al. Levels of cefotaxime and desacetyl-cefotaxime in the cerebrospinal fluid of newborn and premature infants. Padiatr Padol 18:361, 1983.

244. Wells TG, Trang JM, Brown AL, et al. Cefotaxime therapy of bacterial meningitis in children. J Antimicrob Chemother 14(Suppl B):181, 1984.

245. Cherubin CE, Corrado ML, Nair SR, et al. Treatment of gram-negative bacillary meningitis: role of the new cephalosporin antibiotics. Rev Infect Dis 4:S453, 1982.

246. McCracken GH Jr, Siegel JD, Threlkeld N, et al. Ceftriaxone pharmacokinetics in newborn infants. Antimicrob Chemother 23:341, 1983.

247. James J, Mulhall A, de Louvois J. Ceftriaxone—clinical experience in the treatment of neonates. J Infect 11:25, 1985.

248. Mulhall A, de Louvois J, James J. Pharmacokinetics and safety of ceftriaxone in the neonate. Eur J Pediatr 144:379, 1985.

249. Martin E, Koup JR, Paravicini U, et al. Pharmacokinetics of ceftriaxone in neonates and infants with meningitis. J Pediatr 105:475, 1984.

250. Guggenbichler JP, Parth J, Frisch H. Pharmacokinetic investigation of ceftriaxone in premature and newborn babies. Padiatr Padol 21:31, 1986.

251. del Rio M, McCracken GH Jr, Nelson JD, et al. Pharmacokinetics and cerebrospinal fluid bactericidal activity of ceftriaxone in the treatment of pediatric patients with bacterial meningitis. Antimicrob Agents Chemother 22:622, 1982.

252. Latif R, Dajani AS. Ceftriaxone diffusion into cerebrospinal fluid of children with meningitis. Antimicrob Agents Chemother 23:46, 1983.

253. Rosenfeld WN, Evans HE, Batheja R, et al. Pharmacokinetics of cefoperazone in full-term and premature neonates. Antimicrob Agents Chemother 23:866, 1983.

254. Philips JB III, Braune K, Ravis W, et al. Pharmacokinetics of cefoperazone in newborn infants. Pediatr Pharmacol 4:193, 1984.

255. Bosso JA, Chan GM, Matsen JM. Cefoperazone pharmacokinetics in preterm infants. Antimicrob Agents Chemother 23:413, 1983.

256. Assael BM, Boccazzi A, Caccamo ML, et al. Clinical pharmacology of ceftazidime in paediatrics. J Antimicrob Chemother 12(Suppl A):341, 1983.

257. Prinsloo JG, Delport SD, Moncrieff J, et al. A preliminary pharmacokinetic study of ceftazidime in premature, newborn and small infants. J Antimicrob Chemother 12(Suppl A):361, 1983.

258. Gooch WM III, Swenson E. Neonatal pharmacokinetic characteristics of ceftazidime. *In* Program and Abstracts of the 23rd Interscience Conference on Antimicrobial Agents and Chemotherapy. Washington, DC, American Society for Microbiology, 1983, p 237 (abstract).

259. McCracken GH Jr, Threlkeld N, Thomas ML. Pharma-

cokinetics of ceftazidime in newborn infants. Antimicrob Agents Chemother 26:583, 1984.

260. Prinsloo JG, Delport SD, Moncriegg J, et al. Pharmacokinetics of ceftazidime in premature, newborn and young infants. S Afr Med J 65:809, 1984.

261. Mulhall A, de Louvois J. The pharmacokinetics and safety of ceftazidime in the neonate. J Antimicrob Chemother 15:97, 1985.

262. Low DC, Bissenden JG, Wise R. Ceftazidime in neonatal infections. Arch Dis Child 60:360, 1985.

263. Padovani EM, Fanos V, Dal Moro A, et al. Ceftazidime pharmacokinetics in preterm newborns on the first day of life. Biol Res Pregnancy Perinatol 7:71, 1986.

264. Bègue P, Michel B, Chasalette JP, et al. Clinical efficacy and pharmacokinetics of ceftazidime in children and neonates. Pathol Biol 34:525, 1986.

265. de Louvois J, Mulhall A. Ceftazidime in the treatment of neonates. In Rubaltelli FF, Granati B (eds). Neonatal Therapy: Update. Amsterdam, Elsevier, 1986, p 249.

266. Blumer J, Reed M, Aronoff S, et al. CSF penetration and pharmacokinetics of ceftazidime in children with bacterial meningitis. In Program and Abstracts of the 23rd Interscience Conference on Antimicrobial Agents and Chemotherapy. Washington DC, American Society for Microbiology, 1983, p 237 (abstract).

267. Fong IW, Tomkins KB. Ceftazidime cerebrospinal fluid penetration in inflamed and non-inflamed meninges. In Program and Abstracts of the 23rd Interscience Conference on Antimicrobial Agents and Chemotherapy. Washington, DC, American Society for Microbiology, 1983, p 237 (abstract).

268. Schaad UB. The cephalosporin compounds in severe neonatal infection. Eur J Pediatr 141:143, 1984.

269. Roos R. New β-lactams. In Rubaltelli FF, Granati B (eds). Neonatal Therapy: An Update. Amsterdam, Elsevier, 1986, p 217.

270. Bryan CS, John JF Jr, Pai MS, et al. Gentamicin vs cefotaxime for therapy of neonatal sepsis: relationship to drug resistance. Am J Dis Child 139:1086, 1985.

271. Bang NU, Kammer RB. Hematologic complications associated with β-lactam antibiotics. Rev Infect Dis 5:S380, 1983.

272. McCracken GH Jr. Use of third-generation cephalosporins for treatment of neonatal infections. Am J Dis Child 139:1079, 1985.

273. Hall MA, Beech RC, Seal DV. The use of cefotaxime for treating suspected neonatal sepsis: 2 years experience. J Hosp Infect 8:57, 1986.

274. Parshina NV. Clinical efficacy and certain pharmacokinetics characteristics of cefotaxime in premature infants with pneumonia. Antibiot Med Biotekhnol 31:298, 1986.

275. Hoogkamp-Korstanje JAA. Activity of cefotaxime and ceftriaxone alone and in combination with penicillin, ampicillin and piperacillin against neonatal meningitis pathogens. J Antimicrob Chemother 16:327, 1985.

276. Macías-Parra M, González-Saldãna N, Saltigeral P, et al. Utilidad de la ceftriaxona en el tratamiento de la sepsis neonatal. Rev Enf Infect Pediatr 6:20, 1992.

277. Snelling S, Hart CA, Cooke RWI. Ceftazidime or gentamicin plus benzylpenicillin in neonates less than forty-eight hours old. J Antimicrob Chemother 12(Suppl A):353, 1983.

278. Odio CM, Umãna MA, Saenz A, et al. Comparative efficacy of ceftazidime vs. carbenicillin and amikacin for treatment of neonatal septicemia. Pediatr Infect Dis J 6:371, 1987.

279. Williams JD. Aztreonam. In Peterson PK, Verhoef J

280. Swabb EA, Cimarusti CM, Henry SA, et al. Aztreonam (SQ 26,776) and other monobactams. In Queener SF, Webber JA, Queener SW (eds). Beta-Lactam Antibiotics for Clinical Use. New York, Marcel Dekker, 1986, p 593.

281. Stutman HR, Marks MI, Swabb EA. Single-dose pharmacokinetics of aztreonam in pediatric patients. Antimicrob Agents Chemother 26:196, 1984.

282. Likitnukul S, McCracken GH Jr, Threlkeld N, et al. Pharmacokinetics and plasma bactericidal activity of aztreonam in low-birth-weight infants. Antimicrob Agents Chemother 31:81, 1987.

283. Greenman R, Arcey S, Dickinson G, et al. Penetration of aztreonam (SQ 26,776) into human cerebrospinal fluid in the presence of meningeal inflammation. In Program and Abstracts of the 23rd Interscience Conference on Antimicrobial Agents and Chemotherapy. Washington, DC, American Society for Microbiology, 1983, p 158 (abstract).

284. Umãna MA, Odio CM, Castro E, et al. Comparative evaluation of aztreonam/ampicillin versus amikacin/ampicillin in neonates with bacterial infections. Pediatr Infect Dis J 9:175, 1990.

285. Uauy R, Mize C, Argyle C, et al. Metabolic tolerance to arginine: implications for the safe use of arginine salt-aztreonam combination in the neonatal period. J Pediatr 118:965, 1991.

286. Bradley JS. Meropenem: a new, extremely broad spectrum beta-lactam antibiotic for serious infections in pediatrics. Pediatr Infect Dis J 16:263, 1997.

287. Blumer JL. Pharmacokinetic determinants of carbapenem therapy in neonates and children. Pediatr Infect Dis J 15:733, 1996.

288. Clissold SP, Todd PA, Campoli-Richards DM. Imipenem/cilastatin: a review of its antibacterial activity pharmacokinetic properties and therapeutic efficacy. Drugs 33:183, 1987.

289. Santos-Ferreira MO, Vital JO. In-vitro antibacterial activity of imipenem compared with four other β-lactam antibiotics (ceftazidime, cefotaxime, piperacillin and azlocillin) against 828 separate clinical isolates from a Portuguese hospital. J Antimicrob Chemother 18(Suppl E):23, 1986.

290. Williams RJ, Yang YJ, Livermore DM. Mechanisms by which imipenem may overcome resistance in gram-negative bacilli. J Antimicrob Chemother 18(Suppl E):9, 1986.

291. Freij BJ, McCracken GH Jr, Olsen KD, et al. Pharmacokinetics of imipenem-cilastin in neonates. Antimicrob Agents Chemother 27:431, 1985.

292. Gruber WC, Rench MA, Garcia-Prats JA, et al. Single-dose pharmacokinetics of imipenem-cilastin in neonates. Antimicrob Agents Chemother 27:511, 1985.

293. Jacobs RF, Kearns GL, Trang JM, et al. Single-dose pharmacokinetics of imipenem in children. J Pediatr 105:996, 1984.

294. Rogers JD, Meisinger MAP, Ferber F, et al. Pharmacokinetics of imipenem and cilastin in volunteers. Rev Infect Dis 7:S435, 1985.

295. Patamasucon P, McCracken GH Jr. Pharmacokinetics and bacteriological efficacy of N-formimidoyl thienamycin in experimental Escherichia coli meningitis. Antimicrob Agents Chemother 21:390, 1982.

296. Modai J, Vittecoq D, Decazes JM, et al. Penetration of imipenem and cilastin into cerebrospinal fluid of patients with bacterial meningitis. J Antimicrob Chemother 16:751, 1985.

297. Martinkova J, de Groot R, Chladek J, et al. Meropenem pharmacokinetics in pre-term and full-term neonates. *In* Programs and Abstracts of the 7th European Congress of Clinical Microbiology and Infectious Diseases, Vienna, March 26 to 30, 1995 (abstract 686).

298. Calandra GB, Brown KR, Grad LC, et al. Review of adverse experiences and tolerability in the first 2,516 patients treated with imipenem/cilastin. Am J Med 78(Suppl 6A):73, 1985.

299. Borderon JC, Rastegar A, Laugier J, et al. The effect of imipenem/cilastin on the aerobic faecal flora of children. J Antimicrob Chemother 18(Suppl E):121, 1986.

300. Wong VK, Wright HT, Ross LA, et al. Imipenem/cilastatin treatment of bacterial meningitis in children. Pediatr Infect Dis J 10:122, 1991.

301. Snavely SR, Hodges GR. The neurotoxicity of antibacterial agents. Ann Intern Med 101:92, 1984.

302. Hori S, Kurioka S, Matsuda M, et al. Inhibitory effect of cephalosporins on gamma-aminobutyric acid receptor binding in rat synapsis membranes. Antimicrob Agents Chemother 27:650, 1985.

303. Eng RH, Munsif AR, Yangco BG, et al. Seizure propensity with imipenem. Arch Intern Med 149:1881, 1989.

304. Day IP, Goudie J, Nishiki K, Williams PD. Correlation between in vitro and in vivo models of proconvulsive activity with the carbapenem antibiotics, biapenem, imipenem/cilastatin and meropenem. Toxicol Lett 76:239, 1995.

305. Collins MA, Tolpin M, and the Collaborative Imipenem-Cilastin Study Group. Clinical evaluation of imipenem-cilastin as a single agent therapy for sepsis neonatorum. *In* Program and Abstracts of the 27th Interscience Conference on Antimicrobial Agents and Chemotherapy. Washington, DC, American Society for Microbiology, 1987, p 188 (abstract).

306. Watanakunakorn C. Mode of action and in-vitro activity of vancomycin. J Antimicrob Chemother 14(Suppl 3):7, 1984.

307. Gross JR, Kaplan SL, Kramer WG, et al. Vancomycin pharmacokinetics in premature infants. Pediatr Pharmacol 5:17, 1985.

308. Naqvi SH, Keenam WJ, Reichley RM, et al. Vancomycin pharmacokinetics in small, seriously ill infants. Am J Dis Child 140:107, 1986.

309. James A, Koren G, Milliken J, et al. Vancomycin pharmacokinetics and dose recommendations for preterm infants. Antimicrob Agents Chemother 31:52, 1987.

310. Koren G, James A. Vancomycin dosing in preterm infants: prospective verification of new recommendations. J Pediatr 110:797, 1987.

311. Amaker PD, DiPiro JT, Bhatia J. Pharmacokinetics of vancomycin in critically ill infants undergoing extracorporeal membrane oxygenation. Antimicrob Agents Chemother 40:1139, 1996.

312. Reiter PD, Doron MW. Vancomycin cerebrospinal fluid concentrations after intravenous administration in premature infants. J Perinatol 16:331, 1996.

313. McHenry MC, Gavan TL. Vancomycin. Pediatr Clin North Am 30:31, 1983.

314. Spera RV, Farber BF. Multiply-resistant *Enterococcus faecium.* JAMA 268:2563, 1992.

315. McCracken GH Jr. Changing pattern of the antimicrobial suceptibilities of *Escherichia coli* in neonatal infections. J Pediatr 78:942, 1971.

316. Ristuccia AM, Cunha BA. The aminoglycosides. Med Clin North Am 66:303, 1982.

317. Davies JE. Resistance to aminoglycosides: mechanisms and frequency. Rev Infect Dis 5:S261, 1983.

318. Kluge RM, Standiford HC, Tatem B, et al. Comparative activity of tobramycin, amikacin, and gentamicin alone and with carbenicillin against *Pseudomonas aeuruginosa.* Antimicrob Agents Chemother 6:442, 1974.

319. McCracken GH Jr, Threlkeld N, Thomas ML. Intravenous administration of kanamycin and gentamicin in newborn infants. Pediatrics 60:463, 1977.

320. Paisley JW, Smith AL, Smith DH. Gentamicin in newborn infants: comparison of intramuscular and intravenous administration. Am J Dis Child 126:473, 1973.

321. Black J, Calesnick B, Williams D, et al. Pharmacology of gentamicin, a new broad-spectrum antibiotic. *In* Antimicrobial Agents and Chemotherapy. Washington, DC, American Society for Microbiology, 1963, p 138.

322. King JT. Severe deafness in an infant following oral administration of neomycin. J Med Assoc Ga 51:530, 1962.

323. Nation RL, Huang SM, Vidyasagar D, et al. Absorption of oral neomycin in premature infants with suspected necrotizing enterocolitis. Dev Pharmacol Ther 5:53, 1982.

324. Nunnery AW, Riley HD Jr. Gentamicin: pharmacologic observations in newborns and infants. J Infect Dis 119:402 1969.

325. Hansen TN, Ritter DA, Speer ME, et al. A randomized, controlled study of oral gentamicin in the treatment of neonatal necrotizing enterocolitis. J Pediatr 97:836, 1980.

326. Grylack L, Boehnert J, Scanlon J. Serum concentrations of gentamicin following oral administration to preterm newborns. Dev Pharmacol Ther 5:47, 1982.

327. Miranda JC, Schimmel MS, Mimms GM, et al. Gentamicin absorption during prophylactic use for necrotizing enterocolitis. Dev Pharmacol Ther 7:303, 1984.

328. Coyer WF, Wesbey GE, Cech KL, et al. Intravenous gentamicin pharmacokinetics in the small preterm infant. Pediatr Res 12:403, 1978 (abstract).

329. Szefler SJ, Wynn RJ, Clarke DF, et al. Relationship of gentamicin serum concentrations to gestational age in preterm and term neonates. J Pediatr 97:312, 1980.

330. Rameis H, Popow C, Graninger W. Gentamicin monitoring in low-birth-weight newborns. Biol Res Pregnancy Perinatol 4:123, 1983.

331. Arbeter AM, Saccar CL, Eisner S, et al. Tobramycin sulfate elimination in premature infants. J Pediatr 103:131, 1983.

332. Nahata MV, Powell DA, Durrell DE, et al. Effect of gestational age and birth weight on tobramycin kinetics in newborn infants. J Antimicrob Chemother 14:59, 1984.

333. Cordero L, Arwood L, Hann C, et al. Serum tobramycin levels in low and very low-birth-weight infants. Am J Perinatol 1:242, 1984.

334. Cookson B, Tripps J, Leung T, et al. Evaluation of amikacin dosage regimens in the low and very low-birth-weight newborn. Infection 8:S239, 1980.

335. Nelson JD. Duration of neomycin therapy for enteropathogenic *Escherichia coli* diarrheal disease: a comparative study of 113 cases. Pediatrics 48:248, 1971.

336. McCracken GH Jr, West NR, Horton LJ. Urinary excretion of gentamicin in the neonatal period. J Infect Dis 123:257, 1971.

337. McCracken GH Jr, Chrane DF, Thomas ML. Pharmacologic evaluation of gentamicin in newborn infants. J Infect Dis 124:S214, 1971.

338. Klein JO, Herschel M, Therakan RM, et al. Gentamicin in serious neonatal infections: absorption, excretion, and clinical results in 25 cases. J Infect Dis 124:S224, 1971.

339. Milner RDG, Ross J, Froud DJR, et al. Clinical pharmacology of gentamicin in the newborn infant. Arch Dis Child 47:927, 1972.

340. Zoumboulakis D, Anagnostakis D, Arseni A, et al. Gentamicin in the treatment of purulent meningitis in neonates and infants. Acta Paediatr Scand 62:55, 1973.

341. Chang MJ, Escobedo M, Anderson DC, et al. Kanamycin and gentamicin treatment of neonatal sepsis and meningitis. Pediatrics 56:695, 1975.

342. Friedman CA, Parks BR, Rawson JE. Gentamicin disposition in asphyxiated newborns: relationship to mean arterial blood pressure and urine output. Pediatr Pharmacol 2:189, 1982.

343. Hindmarsh KW, Nation RL, Williams GL, et al. Pharmacokinetics of gentamicin in very low birth weight preterm infants. Eur J Clin Pharmacol 24:649, 1983.

344. Edgren B, Karna P, Sciamanna D, et al. Gentamicin dosing in the newborn: use of a one-compartment open pharmacokinetic model to individualize dosing. Dev Pharmacol Ther 7:263, 1984.

345. Landers S, Berry PL, Kearns GL, et al. Gentamicin disposition and effect on development of renal function in very low birth weight infants. Dev Pharmacol Ther 7:285, 1984.

346. Kildoo C, Modanlou HD, Komatsu G, et al. Developmental pattern of gentamicin kinetics in very low birth weight (VLBW) sick infants. Dev Pharmacol Ther 7:345, 1984.

347. Husson C, Chevalier JY, Jezequel M, et al. Pharmacokinetics study of gentamicin in preterm and term neonates. Dev Pharmacol Ther 7(Suppl 1):125, 1984.

348. Miranda JC, Schimmel MM, James LS, et al. Gentamicin kinetics in the neonate. Pediatr Pharmacol 5:57, 1985.

349. Kasik JW, Jenkins S, Leuschen MP, et al. Postconceptional age and gentamicin elimination half-life. J Pediatr 106:502, 1985.

350. Kliegman RM, Bertino JS Jr, Fanaroff AA, et al. Pharmacokinetics of gentamicin during exchange transfusions in neonates. J Pediatr 96:927, 1980.

351. Bertino JS Jr, Kliegman RM, Myers CM, et al. Alterations in gentamicin pharmacokinetics during neonatal exchange transfusions. Dev Pharmacol Ther 4:205, 1982.

352. Cohen P, Collart L, Prober CG, et al. Gentamicin pharmacokinetics in neonates undergoing extracorporal membrane oxygenation. Pediatr Infect Dis J 9:562, 1990.

353. Watterberg KL, Kelly HW, Johnson JD, et al. Effect of patent ductus arteriosus on gentamicin pharmacokinetics in very low birth weight (<1,500 g) babies. Dev Pharmacol Ther 10:107, 1987.

354. Zarowitz BJM, Wynn RJ, Buckwald S, et al. High gentamicin trough concentrations in neonates of less than 28 weeks gestational age. Dev Pharmacol Ther 5:68, 1982.

355. Mulhall A, de Louvois J, Hurley R. Incidence of potentially toxic concentrations of gentamicin in the neonate. Arch Dis Child 58:897, 1983.

356. Koren G, Leeder S, Harding E, et al. Optimization of gentamicin therapy in very low birth weight infants. Pediatr Pharmacol 5:79, 1985.

357. Charlton CK, Needelman H, Thomas RW, et al. Gentamicin dosage recommendations for neonates based on half-life predictions from birthweight. Am J Perinatol 3:28, 1986.

358. Mustafa MM, Mertsola J, Ramilo O, et al. Increased endotoxin and interleukin-1 beta concentrations in cerebrospinal fluid of infants with coliform meningitis and ventriculitis associated with intraventricular gentamicin therapy. J Infect Dis 160:891, 1989.

359. Smith CR, Lipsky JJ, Laskin OL, et al. Double-blind comparison of the nephrotoxicity and auditory toxicity of gentamicin and tobramycin. N Engl J Med 302:1106, 1980.

360. Riff L, Schauf V. Use of aminoglycosides in the neonate. Semin Perinatol 6:155, 1982.

361. Kaplan JM, McCracken GH Jr, Thomas ML, et al. Clinical pharmacology of tobramycin in newborns. Am J Dis Child 125:656, 1973.

362. Williams G, Stroebel AB, Richardson H, et al. Pharmacokinetics of tobramycin in low-birth-weight newborn infants. In Nelson JD, Grassi C (eds). Current Chemotherapy and Infectious Disease: Proceedings of the 11th International Congress of Chemotherapy and the 19th Interscience Conference on Antimicrobial Agents and Chemotherapy. Washington, DC, American Society for Microbiology, 1980, p 1163.

363. Nahata MC, Powell DA, Gregoire RP, et al. Tobramycin kinetics in newborn infants. J Pediatr 103:136, 1983.

364. Nahata MC, Powell DA, Durrell DE, et al. Tobramycin pharmacokinetics in very low birth weight infants. Br J Clin Pharmacol 21:325, 1986.

365. Howard JB, McCracken GH Jr, Trujillo H, et al. Amikacin in newborn infants: comparative pharmacology with kanamycin and clinical efficacy in 45 neonates with bacterial diseases. Antimicrob Agents Chemother 10:205, 1976.

366. Prober CG, Yeager AS, Arvin AM. The effect of chronologic age on the serum concentrations of amikacin in sick term and premature infants. J Pediatr 98:636, 1981.

367. Trujillo H, Manotas R, Londono R, et al. Clinical and laboratory studies with amikacin in newborns, infants and children. J Infect Dis 134:S406, 1976.

368. Yow MD. An overview of pediatric experience with amikacin. Am J Med 62:954, 1977.

369. Philips JB, Cassady G. Amikacin: pharmacology, indications and cautions for use and dose recommendations. Semin Perinatol 6:166, 1982.

370. Henriksson P, Svenningsen N, Juhlin I, et al. Netilmicin in moderate to severe infections in neonates and infants: a study of efficacy, tolerance and pharmacokinetics. Curr Ther Res 24:108, 1978.

371. Peitersen B, Horlyk H, Nielsen M, et al. Netilmicin: efficacy and tolerance in the treatment of systemic infections in neonates. Scand J Infect Dis (Suppl) 23:151, 1980.

372. Henriksson P, Svenningsen N, Juhlin M, et al. Netilmicin in moderate to severe infections in newborns and infants: a study of efficacy, tolerance and pharmacokinetics. Scand J Infect Dis (Suppl) 23:155, 1980.

373. Chindasilpa V, Schauf V, Hamilton LR, et al. Netilmicin use in pediatric patients. Dev Pharmacol Ther 1:238, 1980.

374. Bergan T, Michalsen H. Pharmacokinetic assessment of netilmicin in newborns and older children. Infection 10:153, 1982.

375. Phillips AMR, Milner RDG. Clinical pharmacology of netilmicin in the newborn. Arch Dis Child 58:451, 1983.

376. Granati B, Assael BM, Chung M, et al. Clinical pharmacology of netilmicin in preterm and term newborn infants. J Pediatr 106:664, 1985.

377. Kuhn RJ, Nahata MC, Powell DA, et al. Pharmacokinetics of netilmicin in premature infants. Eur J Clin Pharmacol 29:635, 1986.

378. Cordero L, Arwood L, DeCenzo S, et al. Serum netilmicin levels in premature AGA infants. Am J Perinatol 4:36, 1987.

379. Phillips AMR, Milner RDG. Tissue concentrations of

netilmicin and gentamicin in neonates. J Infect Dis 149:474, 1984.

380. Parini R, Rusconi F, Cavanna G, et al. Evaluation of the renal and auditory function of neonates treated with amikacin. Dev Pharmacol Ther 5:33, 1982.

381. Heimann G. Renal toxicity of aminoglycosides in the neonatal period. Pediatr Pharmacol 3:251, 1983.

382. Rajchgot P, Prober CG, Soldin S, et al. Aminoglycoside related nephroxicity in the premature newborn. Clin Pharmacol Ther 35:394, 1984.

383. Aujard Y, Lambert-Zechovsky N, Laudignon N, et al. Gentamicin, nephrotoxic risk and treatment of neonatal infection. Dev Pharmacol Ther 7(Suppl 1):109, 1984.

384. Giacoia GP, Schentag JJ. Pharmacokinetics and nephrotoxicity of continuous intravenous infusion of gentamicin in low birth weight infants. J Pediatr 109:715, 1986.

385. Gouyon JB, Aujard Y, Abisror A, et al. Urinary excretion of N-acetyl-glucosaminidase and beta-2-microglobulin as early markers of gentamicin nephrotoxicity in neonates. Dev Pharmacol Ther 10:145, 1987.

386. Tessin I, Trollfors B, Bergmark J, et al. Enzymuria in neonates during treatment with gentamicin or tobramycin. Pediatr Infect Dis J 6:870, 1987.

387. Dahlgren JG, Anderson ET, Hewitt WL. Gentamicin blood levels: a guide to nephrotoxicity. Antimicrob Agents Chemother 8:58, 1975.

388. Zarfin Y, Koren G, Maresky D, et al. Possible indomethacin-aminoglycoside interaction in preterm infants. J Pediatr 106:511, 1985.

389. Gagliardi L. Possible indomethacin-aminoglycoside interaction in preterm infants. J Pediatr 107:991, 1985.

390. Sirinavin S, McCracken GH Jr, Nelson JD. Determining gentamicin dosage in infants and children with renal failure. J Pediatr 96:331, 1980.

391. Kalenga M, Devos D, Moulin D, et al. The need for pharmacokinetic monitoring of gentamicin therapy in critically ill neonates. Dev Pharmacol Ther 7(Suppl 1):130, 1980.

392. Herngren L, Broberger U, Wretlind B. A simplified model for adjustment of gentamicin dosage in newborn infants. Acta Paediatr Scand 75:198, 1986.

393. de Beukelaer MM, Travis LB, Dodge WF, et al. Deafness and acute tubular necrosis following parenteral administration of neomycin. Am J Dis Child 121:250, 1971.

394. Robinson GC, Cambon KG. Hearing loss in infants of tuberculous mothers treated with streptomycin during pregnancy. N Engl J Med 271:949, 1964.

395. Winkel S, Bonding P, Larsen PK, et al. Possible effects of kanamycin and incubation in newborn children with low birth weight. Acta Paediatr Scand 67:709, 1978.

396. Falk SA, Woods NF. Hospital noise-levels and potential health hazards. N Engl J Med 289:774, 1973.

397. Johnsonbaugh RE, Drexler HG, Light IJ, et al. Familial occurrence of drug-induced hearing loss. Am J Dis Child 127:245, 1974.

398. Finitzo-Hieber T, McCracken GH Jr, Roeser RJ, et al. Ototoxicity in neonates treated with gentamicin and kanamycin: results of a four-year controlled follow-up study. Pediatrics 63:443, 1979.

399. Johnsonbaugh RE, Drexler HG, Sutherland JM, et al. Audiometric study of streptomycin-treated infants. Am J Dis Child 112:43, 1966.

400. Starr A, Amile RN, Martin WH, et al. Development of auditory function in newborn infants revealed by auditory brainstem potentials. Pediatrics 60:831, 1977.

401. Finitzo-Hieber T, McCracken GH Jr, Brown KC. Prospective controlled evaluation of auditory function in neonates given netilmicin or amikacin. J Pediatr 106:129, 1985.

402. Bernard PA, Pecherè JC, Hèrbert R, et al. Detection of aminoglycoside antibiotic-induced ototoxicity in newborns by brain stem responses audiometry. In Nelson JD, Grassi C (eds). Current Chemotherapy and Infectious Disease: Proceedings of the 11th International Congress of Chemotherapy and the 19th Interscience Conference on Antimicrobial Agents and Chemotherapy. Washington, DC, American Society for Microbiology, 1980, p 602.

403. Hauch AM, Peitersen B, Peitersen E. Vestibular toxicity following netilmicin therapy in the neonatal period. Dan Med Bull 33:107, 1986.

404. Ream CR. Respiratory and cardiac arrest after intravenous administration of kanamycin with reversal of toxic effects by neostigmine. Ann Intern Med 59:384, 1963.

405. Pittinger CB, Eryasa Y, Adamson R. Antibiotic-induced paralysis. Anesth Analg 49:487, 1970.

406. Warner WA, Sanders E. Neuromuscular blockade associated with gentamicin therapy. JAMA 215:1153, 1971.

407. Yamada S, Kuno Y, Iwanaga H. Effects of aminoglycoside antibiotics on the neuromuscular junction: I. Int J Clin Pharmacol Ther Toxicol 24:130, 1986.

408. Santos JI, Swensen P, Glasgow LA. Potentiation of Clostridium botulinum toxin by aminoglycoside antibiotics: clinical and laboratory observations. Pediatrics 68:50, 1981.

409. McCracken GH Jr. New developments in the management of neonatal meningitis. In Sande MA, Smith AL, Root RK (eds). Bacterial Meningitis. New York, Churchill Livingstone, 1985, p 159.

410. Bell MJ, Kosloske AM, Benton C, et al. Neonatal necrotizing enterocolitis: prevention of perforation. J Pediatr Surg 8:601, 1973.

411. Egan EA, Mantilla G, Nelson RM, et al. A prospective controlled trial of oral kanamycin in the prevention of neonatal necrotizing enterocolitis. J Pediatr 89:467, 1976.

412. Grylack LJ, Scanlon JW. Oral gentamicin therapy in the prevention of neonatal necrotizing enterocolitis: a controlled double-blind trial. Am J Dis Child 132:1192, 1978.

413. Brantley VE, Hiatt IM, Hegyi T. The effectiveness of oral gentamicin in reducing the incidence of necrotizing enterocolitis in treated and control infants. Pediatr Res 14:592, 1980 (abstract).

414. Boyle R, Nelson JS, Stonestreet BS, et al. Alterations in stool flora resulting from oral kanamycin prophylaxis of necrotizing enterocolitis. J Pediatr 93:857, 1978.

415. Bell MJ, Shackelford PG, Feigin RD, et al. Alterations in gastrointestinal microflora during antimicrobial therapy for necrotizing enterocolitis. Pediatrics 63:425, 1979.

416. Rowley MP, Dahlenburg GW. Gentamicin in prophylaxis of neonatal necrotizing enterocolitis. Lancet 2:532, 1978.

417. Prins JM, Speelman P. Once-daily aminoglycosides. Practical guidelines. Neth J Med 52:1, 1998.

418. Mattie H, Craig WA, Pechere JC. Determinants of efficacy and toxicity of aminoglycosides. J Antimicrob Chemother 24:281, 1989.

419. Skopnik H, Heimann G. Once daily aminoglycoside dosing in full term neonates. Pediatr Infect Dis J 14:71, 1995.

420. Hayani KC, Hatzopoulos FK, Frank AL, et al. Pharmacokinetics of once-daily dosing of gentamicin in neonates. J Pediatr 131:76, 1997.

421. Burns JL, Mendelman PM, Levy J, et al. A permeability barrier as a mechanism of chloramphenicol resistance in

Haemophilus influenzae. Antimicrob Agents Chemother 27:46, 1985.

422. Gutmann L, Williamson R, Moreau N, et al. Cross-resistance to nalidixic acid, trimethoprim, and chloramphenicol associated with alterations in outer membrane proteins of *Klebsiella, Enterobacter*, and *Serratia*. J Infect Dis 151:501, 1985.

423. Ambrose PJ. Clinical pharmacokinetics of chloramphenicol and chloramphenicol succinate. Clin Pharmacokinet 9:222, 1984.

424. Friedman CA, Lovejoy FC, Smith AL. Chloramphenicol disposition in infants and children. J Pediatr 95:1071, 1979.

425. Glazer JP, Danish MA, Plotkin SA, et al. Disposition of chloramphenicol in low birth weight infants. Pediatrics 66:573, 1980.

426. Kauffman RE, Miceli JN, Strebel L, et al. Pharmacokinetics of chloramphenicol and chloramphenicol succinate in infants and children. J Pediatr 98:315, 1981.

427. Rajchgot P, Prober CG, Soldin S, et al. Initiation of chloramphenicol therapy in the newborn infant. J Pediatr 101:1018, 1982.

428. Nahata MC, Powell DA. Comparative bioavailability and pharmacokinetics of chloramphenicol after intravenous chloramphenicol succinate in premature infants and older patients. Dev Pharmacol Ther 6:23, 1983.

429. Rajchgot P, Prober C, Soldin S, et al. Chloramphenicol pharmacokinetics in the newborn. Dev Pharmacol Ther 6:305, 1983.

430. Mulhall A, de Louvois J, Hurley R. The pharmacokinetics of chloramphenicol in the neonate and young infant. J Antimicrob Chemother 12:629, 1983.

431. Hodgman JE, Burns LE. Safe and effective chloramphenicol dosages for premature infants. Am J Dis Child 101:140, 1961.

432. Ziegra SR, Storm RR. Dosage of chloramphenicol in premature infants. J Pediatr 58:852, 1961.

433. Dunkle LM. Central nervous system chloramphenicol concentration in premature infants. Antimicrob Agents Chemother 13:427, 1978.

434. Laferriere CI, Marks MI. Chloramphenicol properties and clinical use. Pediatr Infect Dis J 1:257, 1982.

435. Mauer SM, Chavers BM, Kjellstrand CM. Treatment of an infant with severe chloramphenicol intoxication using charcoal-column hemoperfusion. J Pediatr 96:136, 1980.

436. Kessler DL, Smith AL, Woodrum DE. Chloramphenicol toxicity in a neonate treated with exchange transfusion. J Pediatr 96:140, 1980.

437. Werner JC, Whitman V, Schuler HG, et al. Acute myocardial effects of chloramphenicol in newborn pigs: a possible insight into the gray baby syndrome. J Infect Dis 152:344, 1985.

438. Mulhall A, de Louvois J, Hurley R. Chloramphenicol toxicity in neonates: its incidence and prevention. BMJ 287:1424, 1983.

439. Iqbal SM, Srivatsav CBP. Chloramphenicol ototoxicity: a case-report. J Laryngol Otol 98:523, 1984.

440. Palchick BA, Funk EA, McEntire JE, et al. Anaphylaxis due to chloramphenicol. Am J Med Sci 288:43, 1984.

441. Hughes WT. Trimethoprim and sulfonamides. *In* Peterson PK, Verhoef J (eds). The Antimicrobial Agents Annual I. Amsterdam, Elsevier, 1986, p 197.

442. Pratt WB. Fundamentals of Chemotherapy. New York, Oxford University Press, 1973.

443. Daeschner CW, Clark JL, Yow EM. A comparative evaluation of sulfonamides. J Pediatr 50:531, 1957.

444. Fichter EG, Curtis JA. Sulfonamide administration in newborn and premature infants. Pediatrics 18:50, 1956.

445. Vree TB, Hekster YA, Lippens RJ. Clinical pharmacokinetics of sulfonamides in children: relationship between maturing kidney function and renal clearance of sulfonamides. Ther Drug Monit 7:130, 1985.

446. Smith LG, Sensakovic J. Trimethoprim-sulfamethoxazole. Med Clin North Am 66:143, 1982.

447. Sabel KG, Brandberg A. Treatment of meningitis and septicemia in infancy with a trimethoprim-sulfamethoxazole combination. Acta Pediatr Scand 54:25, 1975.

448. Ardati KO, Thirumoorthi MC, Dajani AS. Intravenous trimethoprim-sulfamethoxazole in the treatment of serious infections in children. J Pediatr 95:801, 1979.

449. Greene GR, Heitlinger L, Madden JD. *Citrobacter* ventriculitis in a neonate responsive to trimethoprim-sulfamethoxazole. Clin Pediatr 22:515, 1983.

450. Springer C, Eyal F, Michel J. Pharmacology of trimethoprim-sulfamethoxazole in newborn infants. J Pediatr 100:647, 1982.

451. Gleckman R, Alvarez S, Joubert DW. Drug therapy reviews: trimethoprim-sulfamethoxazole. Am J Hosp Pharm 36:893, 1979.

452. Washington JA, Wilson WR. Erythromycin: a microbial and clinical perspective after 30 years of clinical use. Mayo Clin Proc 60:189, 1985.

453. Burns L, Hodgman J. Studies of prematures given erythromycin estolate. Am J Dis Child 106:280, 1963.

454. Fujii R, Grossman M, Ticknor W. Micromethod for determination of concentration of antibiotics in serum for application in clinical pediatrics. Pediatrics 28:662, 1961.

455. Patamasucon P, Kaojarern S, Kusmiesz H, et al. Pharmacokinetics of erythromycin ethylsuccinate and estolate in infants under 4 months of age. Antimicrob Agents Chemother 19:736, 1981.

456. Krowchuk D, Seashore JH. Complete biliary obstruction due to erythromycin estolate administration in an infant. Pediatrics 64:956, 1979.

457. Kuder HV. Propionyl erythromycin: a review of 20,525 case reports for side effect data. Clin Pharmacol Ther 1:604, 1960.

458. Ludden TM. Pharmacokinetic interactions of the macrolide antibiotics. Clin Pharmacokinet 10:63, 1985.

459. LeFrock JL, Molavi A, Prince RA. Clindamycin. Med Clin North Am 66:103, 1982.

460. Hermans PE. Lincosamides. *In* Peterson PK, Verhoef J (eds). The Antimicrobial Agents Annual I. Amsterdam, Elsevier, 1986, p 103.

461. Bell MJ, Shackelford P, Smith R, et al. Pharmacokinetics of clindamycin phosphate in the first year of life. J Pediatr 105:482, 1984.

462. Koren G, Zarfin Y, Maresky D, et al. Pharmacokinetics of intravenous clindamycin in newborn infants. Pediatr Pharmacol 5:287, 1986.

463. Kuo CC, Wang SP, Grayston JT. Antimicrobial activity of several antibiotics and a sulfonamide against *Chlamydia trachomatis* organisms in cell culture. Antimicrob Agents Chemother 12:80, 1977.

464. Donta ST, Myers MG. *Clostridium difficile* toxin in asymptomatic neonates. J Pediatr 100:431, 1982.

465. Feldman WE. *Bacteroides fragilis* ventriculitis and meningitis: report of two cases. Am J Dis Child 130:880, 1976.

466. De Louvois J, Hurley R. Antibiotic concentrations in intracranial pus: a study from a collaborative project. Chemotherapy 4:61, 1975.

467. Danneman BR, Israelski DM, Remington JS. Treatment of toxoplasmic encephalitis with intravenous clindamycin. Arch Intern Med 148:2477, 1988.

468. Ayliffe GAJ, Duckworth GJ, Brumfitt W, et al. Guide-

lines for the control of epidemic methicillin-resistant *Staphylococcus aureus*. J Hosp Infect 7:193, 1986.

469. Dacre JE, Emmerson AM, Jenner EA. Nasal carriage of gentamicin and methicillin-resistant *Staphylococcus aureus* treated with topical pseudomonic acid. Lancet 2:1036, 1983.

470. Lamb YJ. Overview of the role of mupirocin. J Hosp Infect 19:S27, 1991.

471. Casewell MW, Hill RLR. Pharmacokinetics of mupirocin after its topical application. J Antimicrob Chemother 19:1, 1987.

472. Leyden JJ. Mupirocin: a new topical antibiotic. J Am Acad Dermatol 5:879, 1990.

473. Rahman M, Noble WC, Cookson BD. Mupirocin-resistant *Staphylococcus aureus*. Lancet 2:387, 1987.

474. Bruns DE. Renal toxicity caused by the topical application of polyethylene glycol to patients with extensive burns. Burns Incl Therm Inj 9:49, 1982.

475. Tuazon CA, Miller H. Comparative in vitro activities of teichomycin and vancomycin alone and in combination with rifampin and aminoglycosides against staphylococci and enterococci. Antimicrob Agents Chemother 25:411, 1984.

476. Acocella G, Buniva G, Flauto U, et al. Absorption and elimination of the antibiotic rifampin in newborns and children. *In* Progress in Antimicrobial and Anticancer Chemotherapy. Proceedings of the Sixth International Congress of Chemotherapists, Tokyo, 1969, p 755.

477. Jager-Roman E, Doyle PE, Baird-Lambert J, et al. Pharmacokinetics and tissue distribution of metronidazole in the newborn infant. J Pediatr 100:651, 1982.

478. Di Pentima MC, Mason EO, Kaplan SL. In vitro synergy against *Flavobacterium meningosepticum*: implications for therapeutic options. Clin Infect Dis 26:1169, 1998.

479. Green SD, Ilunga F, Cheesbrough JS, et al. The treatment of neonatal meningitis due to gram-negative bacilli with ciprofloxacin: evidence of satisfactory penetration into the cerebrospinal fluid. J Infect 26:253, 1993.

480. Wessalowski R, Thomas L, Kivit J, Voit T. Multiple brain abscesses caused by *Salmonella enteritidis* in a neonate: successful treatment with ciprofloxacin. Pediatr Infect Dis J 12:683, 1993.

481. Sutton AM, Turner TL, Cockburn F, McAllister TA. Pharmacokinetic study of sulbactam and ampicillin administered concomitantly by intraarterial or intravenous infusion in the newborn. Rev Infect Dis 5:S518, 1986.

482. Prober CG, Stevenson DK, Benitz WE. The use of antibiotics in neonates weighing less than 1200 grams. Pediatr Infect Dis J 9:111, 1990.

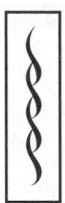

Index

Note: Page numbers in *italics* refer to illustrations; page numbers followed by t refer to tables.

ISBN 0-7216-7976-5

90038

9 780721 679761